PRINCIPLES AND PRACTICE OF GYNECOLOGIC ONCOLOGY

Fourth Edition

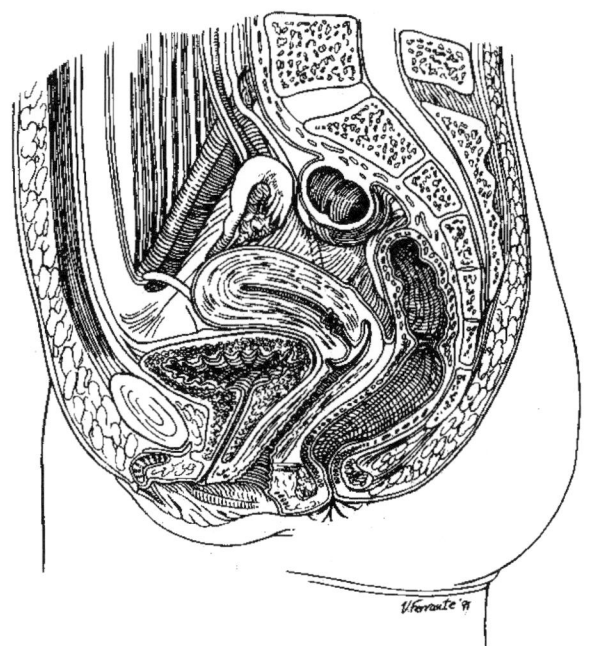

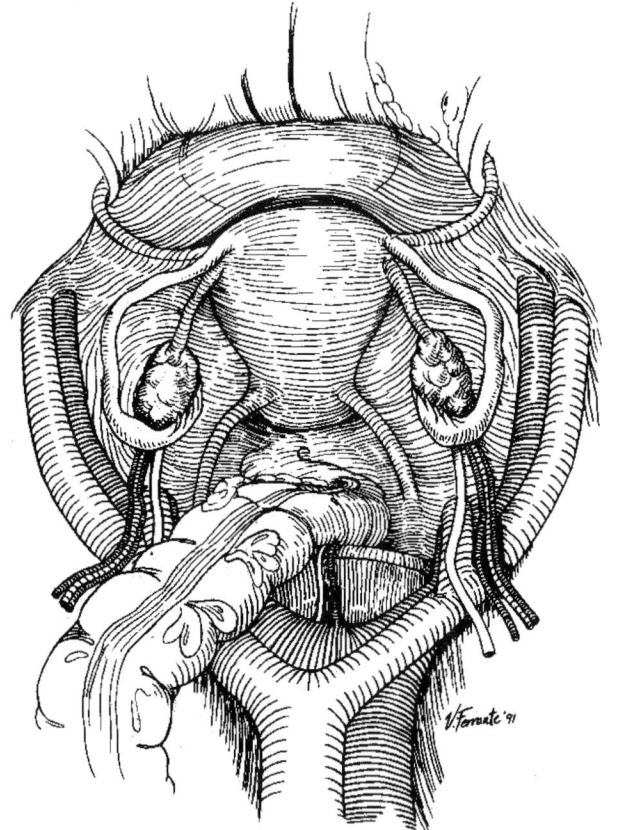

Sagittal view of the female pelvis. This view illustrates the relationship between the internal reproductive organs and the rectum, bladder, and pelvic vasculature.

Posteroanterior view of the female pelvis as viewed from a cephalad position. This view illustrates the relationship between the internal reproductive organs and the rectum and pelvic vasculature.

PRINCIPLES AND PRACTICE OF GYNECOLOGIC ONCOLOGY

Fourth Edition

William J. Hoskins, M.D.

Senior Vice President and Director, Curtis and Elizabeth Anderson Cancer Center
Memorial Health University Medical Center
Savannah, Georgia

Carlos A. Perez, M.D.

Chairman, Department of Radiation Oncology
Washington University School of Medicine
Radiation Oncologist-in-Chief
Barnes-Jewish Hospital
St. Louis, Missouri

Robert C. Young, M.D.

President, Fox Chase Cancer Center
Philadelphia, Pennsylvania

Richard R. Barakat, M.D.

Chief, Gynecology Service
Memorial Sloan–Kettering Cancer Center
New York, New York

Maurie Markman, M.D.

Vice President, Clinical Research
M. D. Anderson Cancer Center
Houston, Texas

Marcus E. Randall, M.D.

Chair and William A. Mitchell Professor of Radiation Oncology
Department of Radiation Oncology
Indiana University School of Medicine
Medical Director
Department of Radiation Oncology
Clarian–Indiana University Hospital
Indianapolis, Indiana

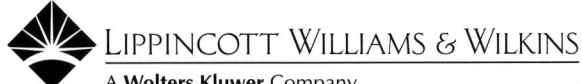

LIPPINCOTT WILLIAMS & WILKINS
A **Wolters Kluwer** Company

Philadelphia · Baltimore · New York · London
Buenos Aires · Hong Kong · Sydney · Tokyo

Acquisitions Editor: Jonathan W. Pine, Jr.
Developmental Editors: Raymond E. Reter and Lisa R. Kairis
Manufacturing Manager: Ben Rivera
Compositor: Maryland Composition
Printer: Courier-Westford

© **2005 by LIPPINCOTT WILLIAMS & WILKINS**
530 Walnut Street
Philadelphia, PA 19106 USA
LWW.com

Printed in the USA

Library of Congress Cataloging-in-Publication Data

Principles and practice of gynecologic oncology / [edited by] William J. Hoskins
... [et al.]. – 4th ed.
    p. ; cm.
Includes bibliographical references and index.
ISBN 0-7817-4689-2
1. Generative organs, Female—Cancer. I. Hoskins, William J., 1940-
[DNLM: 1. Genital Neoplasms, Female. WP 145 P957 2005]
RC280.G5P75 2005
616.99′465—dc22
                                                                    2004015835

10 9 8 7 6 5 4 3 2 1

This book is dedicated to our wives, Iffath Abbasi Hoskins, Susie Bradshaw Perez, Barbara Morris Young, Catherine Barakat, Brabham Morgan Randall, and Tomes Markman. Their patience, encouragement, guidance, and tolerance of our long hours at work have made the completion of this project possible.

Contents

Contributing Authors

Nadeem R. Abu-Rustum, M.D. Director, Minimally Invasive Surgery, Department of Surgery Memorial Sloan–Kettering Cancer Center, New York, New York

David S. Alberts, M.D. Regents Professor of Medicine, Pharmacology, and Public Health, Arizona Cancer Center, College of Medicine, University of Arizona, Tucson, Arizona

Kaled M. Alektiar, M.D. Associate Member, Department of Radiation Oncology, Memorial Sloan–Kettering Cancer Center, New York, New York

Donald Armstrong, M.D. Memorial Sloan–Kettering Cancer Center, Infectious Disease Service, New York, New York

Susan M. Ascher, M.D. Professor and Director of Abdominal Imaging, Department of Radiology, Georgetown University Medical Center, Washington, D.C.

Andrew Berchuck, M.D. F. Bayard Carter Professor, Division of Gynecologic Oncology, Duke University Medical Center, Durham, North Carolina

Ross S. Berkowitz, M.D. William H. Baker Professor of Gynecology, Harvard Medical School, Director of Gynecologic Oncology, Brigham and Women's Hospital and Dana Farber Cancer Institute, Boston, Massachusetts

Michael J. Birrer, M.D., Ph.D. Chief, Molecular Mechanisms Section, Cell and Cancer Biology Department, Center for Cancer Research, National Cancer Institute, Rockville, Maryland

Michael A. Bookman, M.D. Member, Division of Medical Science, Fox Chase Cancer Center, Philadelphia, Pennsylvania

Jeff Boyd, Ph.D. Attending Biologist, Departments of Surgery and Medicine, Memorial Sloan–Kettering Cancer Center, New York, New York

Mark Brady, Ph.D. Director of Statistics, Gynecology Oncology Group, Roswell Park Cancer Institute, Buffalo, New York

Otis W. Brawley, M.D. Associate Director for Cancer Control, Winship Cancer Institute, Emory University School of Medicine, Atlanta, Georgia

Louise A. Brinton, Ph.D. Chief, Hormonal and Reproductive Epidemiology Branch, National Cancer Institute, Rockville, Maryland

Brian Bundy, Ph.D. Research Associate Professor, Department of Biostatistics, State University of New York at Buffalo, Senior Biostatistician, Roswell Park Cancer Institute, Buffalo, New York

James J. Burke II, M.D. Assistant Professor, Department of Obstetrics and Gynecology, Mercer University School of Medicine, Associate Director, Division of Gynecologic Oncology, Memorial Health University Medical Center, Savannah, Georgia

Joanna M. Cain, M.D. Professor and Chair, Department of Obstetrics and Gynecology, Oregon Health Sciences University, Portland, Oregon

Higinia R. Cardenes, M.D., Ph.D. Clinical Associate Professor, Department of Radiation Oncology, Indiana University School of Medicine, Staff Physician, Clarian–Indiana University Hospital, Indianapolis, Indiana

David Cella, Ph.D. Professor, Psychiatry and Behavioral Science, Northwestern University Medical School, Director, CORE-Center on Outcomes, Research and Education, Evanston Northwestern Healthcare, Evanston, Illinois

David Z. Chang, M.D., Ph.D. Fellow, Department of Medicine, Memorial Sloan–Kettering Cancer Center, New York, New York

Dennis S. Chi, M.D. Assistant Surgeon, Gynecology Service, Department of Surgery, Memorial Sloan–Kettering Cancer Center, New York, New York

Cirrelda J. Cooper, M.D. Associate Professor, Department of Radiology, Georgetown MedStar Medical Center, Washington, D.C.

Daniel F. Dargent, M.D. Professor, Department of Gynecologic Surgery, Claude Bernard University, Lyon, France

D. David Dershaw, M.D. Professor of Radiology, Department of Radiology, Weill Medical College of Cornell University, Director, Breast Imaging Section, Memorial Sloan–Kettering Cancer Center, New York, New York

Chaitanya R. Divgi, M.D. Professor, Department of Radiology, Weill Medical College of Cornell University, Member, Departments of Radiology and Medicine, Memorial Sloan–Kettering Cancer Center, New York, New York

Robert T. Dorr, M.D. Department of Pharmacology, Arizona Cancer Center, College of Medicine, University of Arizona, Tucson, Arizona

James G. Douglas, M.D. Associate Professor, Department of Radiation Oncology, University of Washington Medical Center, Seattle, Washington

Paul F. Engstrom, M.D. Professor of Medicine, Department of Medical Oncology, Temple University Medical School, Senior Vice President, Population Science Division, Fox Chase Cancer Center, Philadelphia, Pennsylvania

Peter A. Fleming, M.D. Department of Radiation Oncology, The Cleveland Clinic Foundation, Cleveland, Ohio

Donald G. Gallup, M.D. Professor and Chair, Department of Obstetrics and Gynecology, Mercer University School of Medicine (Savannah), Director, Department of Gynecologic Oncology, Memorial Health University Hospital, Savannah, Georgia

Ginger J. Gardner, M.D. Department of Obstetrics, Gynecology and Reproductive Sciences, Division of Gynecologic Oncology, Mount Sinai School of Medicine, New York, New York

Mary L. Gemignani, M.D. Assistant Attending Physician, Department of Surgery, New York Hospital–Cornell Medical Center, Memorial Sloan–Kettering Cancer Center, New York, New York

David M. Gershenson, M.D. Ann Rife Cox Chair in Gynecology, Professor and Chairman, Department of Gynecologic Oncology, The University of Texas M. D. Anderson Cancer Center, Houston, Texas

Barbara A. Goff, M.D. Division of Gynecologic Oncology, University of Washington, School of Medicine, Seattle, Washington

Donald P. Goldstein, M.D. Professor, Department of Obstetrics, Gynecology, and Reproductive Biology, Harvard Medical School, Boston, Massachusetts

Benjamin E. Greer, M.D. Division of Gynecologic Oncology, University of Washington Medical Center, Seattle, Washington

Perry W. Grigsby, M.D. Mallinckrodt Institute of Radiology, Washington University School of Medicine, St. Louis, Missouri

Eric J. Hall, D.Phil, D.Sc. Higgins Professor of Radiation Biophysics, Professor of Radiology and Radiation Oncology, Center for Radiological Research, Columbia University Medical Center, New York, New York

Lynn C. Hartmann, M.D. Professor of Oncology, Department of Medical Oncology, Mayo Clinic College of Medicine, Rochester, Minnesota

Sabine Hawighorst-Knapstein, M.D. Hospital University, Mainz, Germany

Peter A. Heintz, M.D., Ph.D. Professor, Department of Gynecology, University of Utrecht, Head, Department of Gynecology University Medical Center of Utrecht, Utrecht, The Netherlands

David L. Hemsell, M.D. Professor, Department of Obstetrics and Gynecology, University of Texas Southwestern Medical Center, Dallas, Texas

Lisa M. Hess, M.A. Associate Scientific Investigator, College of Medicine, Arizona Cancer Center, University of Arizona, Tucson, Arizona

Carolyn J. Horowitz, M.D. Medical Director, The Radiation Oncology Center, Willow Ridge Complex, Marlton, New Jersey

Alan N. Houghton, M.D. Professor and Chairman of Immunology, Department of Medicine and Immunology, Weill Medical School of Cornell University; Chief, Department of Clinical Immunology, Memorial Sloan–Kettering Cancer Center, New York, New York

Hedvig Hricak, M.D. Professor of Radiology, Weill Medical College of Cornell University, Chairman, Department of Radiology, Memorial Sloan–Kettering Cancer Center, New York, New York

Clifford Hudis, M.D. Department of Medicine, Memorial Sloan–Kettering Cancer Center, New York, New York

Izumi Imaoka, M.D., Ph.D. Staff Radiologist, Department of Radiology, MR Division Tenri Hospital, Nara, Japan

Ian Jacobs, MD Professor of Gynaecological Oncology, Institute of Women's Health, London University, London, United Kingdom

Amir A. Jazaeri, M.D. Fellow, Department of Gynecologic Oncology, The University of Texas M. D. Anderson Cancer Center, Houston, Texas

John Kavanagh, M.D. Professor; Chairman ad interim, Department of Gynecologic Medical Oncology, The University of Texas M. D. Anderson Cancer Center, Houston, Texas

Paul-Georg Knapstein, M.D. Chief (retired), Department of Obstetrics and Gynecology, University Hospital, Mainz, Germany

Wui-Jin Koh, M.D. Professor, Department of Radiation Oncology, University of Washington Medical Center, Seattle, Washington

Elise C. Kohn, M.D. Head, Molecular Signaling Section, Laboratory of Pathology, Chair, Gynecologic Malignancies Faculty, Center for Cancer Research, National Cancer Institute, Bethesda, Maryland

Michael L. Krychman, M.D. Assistant Attending Surgeon, Department of Surgery, Memorial Sloan–Kettering Cancer Center, New York, New York

James V. Lacey Jr., M.P.H., Ph.D. Investigator, Hormonal and Reproductive Epidemiology Branch, Division of Cancer Epidemiology and Genetics, National Cancer Institute, Rockville, Maryland

Mary Jo Lechowicz, M.D. Assistant Professor, Department of Hematology and Oncology, Emory University School of Medicine, Atlanta, Georgia

Pauline Lesage, M.D., L.L.M. Attending Physician, Department of Pain Medicine/ Palliative Care, Beth Israel Medical Center, New York, New York

Douglas A. Levine, M.D. Assistant Member and Assistant Attending Surgeon, Gynecology Service/Department of Surgery, Memorial Sloan–Kettering Cancer Center, New York, New York

Zuofeng Li, D.Sc. Associate Professor, Department of Radiation Oncology, Washington University School of Medicine, St. Louis, Missouri

Philip O. Livingston, M.D. Professor of Medicine, Weill Graduate School of Medical Sciences of Cornell University, New York, New York

Katherine Y. Look, M.D. Professor of Obstetrics and Gynecology, Department of Obstetrics and Gynecology, Indiana University School of Medicine, Indianapolis, Indiana

Maurie Markman, M.D. Vice President, Clinical Research, M. D. Anderson Cancer Center, Houston, Texas

Daniela Matei, M.D. Assistant Professor, Department of Hematology Oncology, Indiana University, Indianapolis, Indiana

G. Larry Maxwell, M.D. Staff Gynecologic Oncologist, Division of Gynecologic Oncology, Walter Reed Army Medical Center, Washington, D.C.

Beryl McCormick, M.D. Attending and Clinical Director, Department of Radiation Oncology, Memorial Sloan–Kettering Cancer Center, New York, New York

William Patrick McGuire, M.D. Gynecologic Oncology Center, Mercy Medical Center, Baltimore, Maryland

Usha Menon, M.D. Senior Lecturer, Institute of Women's Health, University College of London, London, United Kingdom

Frank L. Meyskens, Jr., M.D. Professor of Medicine and Biological Chemistry, Director, Comprehensive Cancer Center, University of California, Irvine, Orange, California

Helen Michael, M.D. Professor of Pathology Indiana University School of Medicine, Chief, Pathology and Laboratory Medicine, Wishard Memorial Hospital, Indianapolis, Indiana

David H. Moore, M.D. Mary Fendrich Professor, Department of Obstetrics and Gynecology, Indiana University School of Medicine; Chief, Department of Gynecologic Oncology, Indiana University Hospital, Indianapolis, Indiana

Arno J. Mundt, M.D. Department of Radiation and Cellular Oncology, University of Chicago, Chicago, Illinois

David Gardner Mutch, M.D. Judith and Ira Gall Professor, Director, Division of Gynecologic Oncology, Washington University School of Medicine, St. Louis, Missouri

Steven A. Narod, M.D. Professor, Department of Public Health Sciences, University of Toronto, Chief, Breast Cancer Research on Women's Health, Sunnybrook and Women's Health Sciences Centre, Toronto, Ontario, Canada

Janet L. Osborne, M.D. Assistant Professor and Director, Division of Gynecologic Oncology, Department of Obstetrics and Gynecology, Medical College of Wisconsin, Director of Gynecologic Oncology, Department of Obstetrics and Gynecology, Medical College of Wisconsin, Milwaukee, Wisconsin

Robert F. Ozols, M.D., Ph.D. Senior Vice President, Department of Medical Science, Fox Chase Cancer Center, Philadelphia, Pennsylvania

Sergio Pecorelli, M.D. Department of Obstetrics and Gynecology, University of Brescia, Brescia, Italy

Carlos A. Perez, M.D. Chairman, Department of Radiation Oncology, Washington University School of Medicine, Radiation Oncologist-in-Chief, Barnes-Jewish Hospital, St. Louis, Missouri

Stephen Petersdorf, M.D. Associate Professor, Department of Medicine, University of Washington, Seattle, Washington

Marie Plante, M.D. Associate Professor, Department of Obstetrics and Gynecology, Laval University, Quebec City, Quebec, Canada

Russell K. Portenoy, M.D. Chairman, Department of Pain Medicine and Palliative Care, Beth Israel Medical Center, Professor of Neurology, Albert Einstein College of Medicine, New York, New York

Edwin M. Posadas, M.D. Medical Oncology Clinical Research Unit, National Cancer Institute, Bethesda, Maryland

James A. Purdy, Ph.D. Professor and Director, Department of Radiation Oncology, Washington University School of Medicine, St. Louis, Missouri

Marcus E. Randall, M.D. Department of Radiation Oncology, Indiana University School of Medicine, Medical Director, Department of Radiation Oncology, Clarian-Indiana University Hospital, Indianapolis, Indiana

Karina Reynolds, M.D. Senior Lecturer and Honorary Consultant in Gynecological Oncology, Gynecological Cancer Research Unit, St. Bartholomew's and The Royal London, Queen Mary School of Medicine, London, United Kingdom

Laurel W. Rice, M.D. Professor, Department of Obstetrics and Gynecology, University of Virginia, Vice Chairman, Gynecologic Oncology, Department of Obstetrics and Gynecology, University of Virginia Health Sciences Center, Charlottesville, Virginia

Stanley J. Robboy, M.D. Professor and Vice-Chairman of Pathology, Professor of Obstetrics and Gynecology, Duke University Medical Center, Durham, North Carolina

Lawrence M. Roth, M.D. Professor Emeritus Department of Pathology, Indiana University School of Medicine, Indianapolis, Indiana

Eric K. Rowinsky, M.D. Director, Institute for Drug Development, Cancer Therapy and Research Center, Clinical Professor of Medicine, University of Texas Health Sciences Center at San Antonio, San Antonio, Texas

Stephen C. Rubin, M.D. Franklin Payne Professor, Department of Obstetrics and Gynecology, University of Pennsylvania School of Medicine, Philadelphia, Pennsylvania

Anthony H. Russell, M.D. Associate Professor of Radiation Oncology, Department of Radiation Oncology, Massachusetts General Hospital, Boston, Massachusetts

Paul J. Sabbatini, M.D. Assistant Professor of Medicine, Weill Medical College of Cornell University, Assistant Attending Physician, Department of Medicine, Division of Solid Tumor Oncology, Memorial Hospital for Cancer and Allied Diseases, New York, New York

Mark Schattner, M.D. Instructor, Department of Medicine, Attending Physician, Department of Medicine, Memorial Sloan–Kettering Cancer Center, New York, New York

Leslie Scoutt, M.D. Professor, Diagnostic Radiology, Chief, Section of Ultrasound, Department of Radiology, Yale–New Haven Hospital, New Haven, Connecticut

Christopher K. Senkowski, M.D. Assistant Professor of Surgery, Mercer University School of Medicine: Attending Physician, Department of Surgery, Memorial Health University Medical Center, Savannah, Georgia

Kent A. Sepkowitz, M.D. Professor of Medicine, Weill Medical College of Cornell University, Director, Infection Control, Memorial Sloan–Kettering Cancer Center, New York, New York

Mark E. Sherman, M.D. Senior Research Fellow, Division of Cancer Epidemiology and Genetics, Hormonal and Reproductive Epidemiology Branch, National Cancer Institute, Rockville, Maryland

Moishe Shike, M.D. Cancer Prevention and Wellness Program, Memorial Sloan–Kettering Cancer Center, New York, New York

Elvio G. Silva, M.D. Department of Pathology, The University of Texas M.D. Anderson Cancer Center, Houston, Texas

Yukio Sonoda, M.D. Assistant Professor, Department of Obstetrics and Gynecology, Weill Medical College of Cornell University, Assistant Attending Surgeon, Department of Surgery, Gynecology Service, Memorial Sloan–Kettering Cancer Center, New York, New York

Fredrick B. Stehman, M.D. Clarence E. Ehrlich Professor and Chair, Department of Obstetrics and Gynecology, Indiana University School of Medicine, Indianapolis, Indiana

Christian A. Stief, M.D. Professor and Chair, Department of Urology, Ludwigs-Maximilians-University, Munich, Germany

Gregory P. Sutton, M.D. Chief, Department of Gynecologic Oncology, St. Vincent Hospitals and Health Services, Indianapolis, Indiana

Nikkie B. Swarte, M.D. Department of Gynecology, University Medical Center, Utrecht, The Netherlands

Ron E. Swensen, M.D. Assistant Professor, Department of Obstetrics and Gynecology, University of Washington School of Medicine, Seattle, Washington

Elizabeth M. Swisher, M.D. Assistant Professor, Department of Obstetrics and Gynecology, University of Washington School of Medicine, Seattle, Washington

Lee K. Tan, M.D. Department of Pathology, Memorial Sloan–Kettering Cancer Center, New York, New York

Marie E. Taylor, M.D. Assistant Professor, Department of Radiation Oncology, Washington University School of Medicine, Radiation Oncologist, Department of Radiation Oncology, Barnes-Jewish Hospital, St. Louis, Missouri

Gilliam M. Thomas, B.Sc., M.D. Professor of Radiation Oncology and Obstetrics and Gynecology, University of Toronto, Toronto, Ontario, Canada

Carmen Tornos, M.D. Attending Pathologist, Department of Pathology, Memorial Sloan–Kettering Cancer Center, New York, New York

Edward L. Trimble, M.D. Associate Chief, Surgery, Cancer Therapy Evaluation Program, National Cancer Institute, Bethesda, Maryland

Claes Tropi, M.D., Ph.D. Professor, Department of Gynecology, The Norwegian Radium Hospital, Oslo, Norway

Jan B. Vermorken, MD, Ph.D. Professor of Oncology, University of Antwerp, Head, Department of Medical Oncology, University Hospital of Antwerp, Antwerp, Belgium

Annette Vielhaber, M.D. Research Fellow, Department of Pain Medicine and Palliative Care, Beth Israel Medical Center, New York, New York

Daniel D. Von Hoff, M.D. Department of Medicine, Arizona Cancer Center, College of Medicine, University of Arizona, Tucson, Arizona

Lari B. Wenzel, Ph.D. Associate Adjunct Professor, College of Medicine, University of California, Irvine, Irvine, California

Stephen D. Williams, M.D. Indiana University Cancer Center, Indiana University School of Medicine, Indianapolis, Indiana

Edward J. Wilkinson, M.D. Professor and Vice Chairman, Department of Pathology, University of Florida College of Medicine, Medical Director, Anatomic Pathology, Department of Pathology, Shands Hospital at The University of Florida, Gainesville, Florida

Aaron Howard Wolfson, M.D. Professor, Department of Radiation Oncology, University of Miami School of Medicine, Attending Physician, Department of Radiation Oncology, University of Miami Affiliated Hospitals, Miami, Florida

Thomas C. Wright, Jr., M.D. College of Physicians and Surgeons, Columbia University, Department of Pathology, New York, New York

Robert H. Young, M.D. Department of Pathology, Massachusetts General Hospital, Boston, Massachusetts

Richard J. Zaino, M.D. Professor, Department of Pathology, Penn State Milton S. Hershey Medical Center, Hershey, Pennsylvania

Imran Zoberi, M.D. Instructor, Department of Radiation Oncology, Washington University School of Medicine, St. Louis, Missouri

Kristin K. Zorn, M.D. Molecular Mechanisms Section, Cell and Cancer Biology Department, Center for Cancer Research, National Cancer Institute, Rockville, Maryland

Preface

With the publication of the fourth edition of *Principles and Practice of Gynecologic Oncology*, the three Editors have worked together on this textbook for almost 15 years. It has been a rewarding experience, and all three of us are proud of the book and its place in the medical literature. Although we have not always agreed on all issues, we have always reached consensus, and our friendship has been one of the best parts of this experience. In this edition, we have added three Associate Editors: Richard Barakat, MD, Maurie Markman, MD, and Marcus Randall, MD. It is our intention for these Associate Editors to take over the position of Editors with the fifth edition of *Principles and Practice of Gynecologic Oncology*.

As Editors and as cancer specialists, we are committed to multidisciplinary cancer treatment, and as we pointed out in the preface to our last edition, multidisciplinary cancer therapies are ever increasing in their applicability to the management of malignant disease. (We remain committed to a text with disease-specific chapters written by a multidisciplinary team of authors, including a surgical oncologist, a medical oncologist, a radiation oncologist, and a pathologist.) As in previous editions, we have rotated approximately 30% of the chapter authors, and all chapters have either been completely rewritten or extensively updated. We are confident this edition contains the most up-to-date information available about gynecologic malignancies and the appropriate therapy for these diseases. As in previous editions, we have designed this text for the specialist in cancer care, whether that specialist is a surgeon, a medical oncologist, or a radiation oncologist. It is also designed to be of assistance to residents and fellows in training for a career in cancer care.

For the first three editions of this textbook, Stuart Freeman of Lippincott Williams & Wilkins was our guide through the process of creating *Principles and Practice of Gynecologic Oncology*. Stuart retired with the publication of the third edition. With this edition, Jonathan Pine has ably assumed the role of publisher, and we owe him our gratitude for his efforts on the behalf of Lippincott Williams & Wilkins.

Finally, the three editors of *Principles and Practice of Gynecologic Oncology* wish to thank all of their readers for their support and advice during these four editions and for all of the patients whose need for cancer care makes this text important. We are pleased with our contribution to the literature, and eagerly look forward to the new directions the text will take under the able leadership of Drs. Barakat, Markman, and Randall.

William J Hoskins, MD
Carlos A Perez, MD
Robert C Young, MD

Acknowledgments

The Editors acknowledge the contributions of the following individuals without whom this book would not have been possible: Jonathan Pine, Senior Executive Editor, Raymond Reter, Lisa Kairis, Eileen Muse, and Patrick Carr, of the Editorial Department of Lippincott Williams & Wilkins, provided invaluable encouragement, direction, and guidance during the development of the book. K. Alexandra MacDonald and George Monemvasitis, Editors of the Gynecology Service Academic Office, Department of Surgery, Memorial Sloan-Kettering Cancer Center (MSKCC), were major contributors in the coordination of editorial efforts. Al Beringer, Director of Maryland Publishing Services, efficiently and effectively oversaw the copyediting of the book. To all of them, our most sincere gratitude.

SECTION I

Epidemiology of Gynecologic Cancers

CHAPTER 1

Epidemiology of Gynecologic Cancers

Louise A. Brinton, James V. Lacey, Jr., and Mark E. Sherman

Disease-oriented texts often include a chapter on epidemiology or etiology, which is considered perfunctory if the book is used by therapists whose daily practice is rarely influenced by these considerations. This is not the case for physicians who treat patients with gynecologic cancers because these clinicians have frequent opportunities to interpret epidemiologic findings and make observations of etiologic importance. Moreover, public health measures based on epidemiologic findings influence gynecologic practice perhaps more than any other clinical discipline. In particular, epidemiologic data are critical for the prevention and treatment of cervical and endometrial cancers.

From the observation 150 years ago of the rarity of cervical cancer in nuns to the most recent follow-up studies of type-specific human papillomavirus infection, determining the cause, natural history, and prevention of this disease has focused on sexual practices and suspect infectious agents. Screening interventions based on natural history studies have fundamentally altered the usual presentation of this disease, and as more information about preceding infectious processes becomes available, even more radical changes in presentation and management are likely.

The probable estrogenic cause of endometrial cancer was proposed by etiologically oriented gynecologists decades before its demonstration by epidemiologists. Unfortunately, this did not prevent the largest epidemic of iatrogenic cancer in recorded history (i.e., endometrial cancer caused by estrogen replacement therapy). The resurgent interest in hormone replacement therapy, effects of progestins added to this regi-

men, and associated risk-benefit questions are certain to link the epidemiologist and the gynecologist for the foreseeable future. The iatrogenic chemoprevention of endometrial and ovarian cancer through oral contraception has similarly thrust the two disciplines together around issues ranging from basic biology to risk-benefit assessments.

The rich tradition of the mingling of epidemiology and gynecologic oncology has led to better opportunities for prevention, screening, and insights into basic mechanisms of disease than for any other subspecialty concerned with cancer. This chapter is written with the aim of clarifying how epidemiology is an integral part of the effort to reduce the morbidity and mortality from gynecologic cancer in women.

UTERINE CORPUS CANCER

Demographic Patterns

Cancer of the uterine corpus (hereafter referred to as uterine cancer) is the most common invasive gynecologic cancer and the fourth most frequently diagnosed cancer among American women today. One in 37 American women will develop uterine cancer before age 85 years (1), resulting in approximately 40,100 diagnoses during 2003 (2). The average annual age-adjusted (1970 U.S. standard) incidence from the Surveillance, Epidemiology and End Results (SEER) program, a cancer reporting system involving approximately 10% of U.S. residents, was 24.1 per 100,000 women for 1996–2000; the corresponding age-adjusted mortality rate was 2 per 100,000 women, reflecting the relatively good prognosis for this cancer (2). The 5-year survival rate is approximately 85%. It is estimated that approximately 6,800 women will die from uterine cancer during 2003.

Uterine cancer rates are highest in North America, intermediate in Europe and temperate South America, and low in Southern and Eastern Asia (including Japan) and in most of Africa (except southern Africa) (3). The disease is rare before the age of 45 years , but the risk rises sharply among women in their late forties to middle sixties. The age-adjusted incidence for whites is approximately twice the inci-

Louise A. Brinton: Hormonal and Reproductive Epidemiology Branch, Division of Cancer Epidemiology and Genetics, National Cancer Institute, Bethesda, Maryland 20892

James V. Lacey, Jr.: Hormonal and Reproductive Epidemiology Branch, Division of Cancer Epidemiology and Genetics, National Cancer Institute, Bethesda, Maryland 20892

Mark E. Sherman: Hormonal and Reproductive Epidemiology Branch, Division of Cancer Epidemiology and Genetics, National Cancer Institute, Bethesda, Maryland 20892

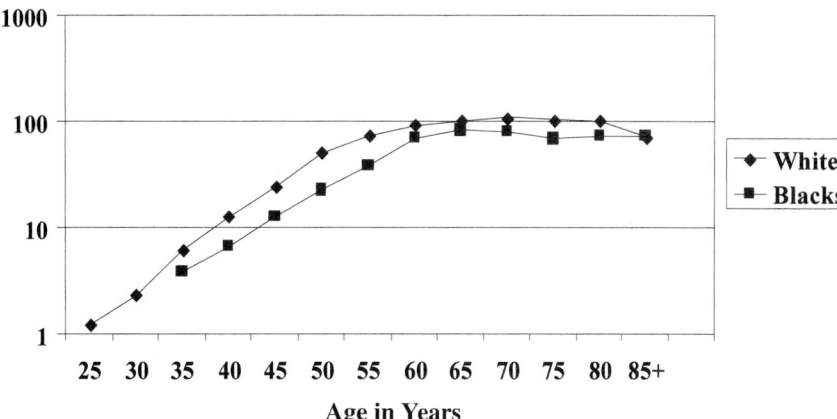

FIG. 1.1. Age-specific incidence of cancer of the corpus uteri by race. (Data from the Surveillance, Epidemiology and End Results Program, 1996–2000.)

dence for nonwhites. Reasons for the discrepancy remain largely undefined (Fig. 1.1). Within the last several decades in the United States, a dramatic change in the incidence pattern for uterine cancer has occurred, characterized by a marked increase that peaked about 1975 (Fig. 1.2) (4). Considerable evidence has linked this rise and fall with the widespread use of estrogen replacement therapy in the late 1960s and early 1970s. Mortality rates, albeit considerably lower, have generally mirrored incidence rates.

Risk Factors

Reproductive and Menstrual Risk Factors

Nulliparity is a recognized risk factor for uterine cancer. Most studies demonstrate a two- to threefold higher risk for nulliparous than parous women (5,6). The association of uterine cancer with nulliparity has been suggested to reflect prolonged periods of infertility. The hypothesis that infertility is a risk factor for uterine cancer is supported by studies showing higher risks for married nulliparous women than for unmarried women (7). Several studies have found that infertile women experience a three- to eightfold increase in risk (5,6,8). Mechanisms that may mediate the risk associated with infertility include anovulatory menstrual cycles (i.e., prolonged exposure to estrogens without sufficient pro-

gesterone); high serum levels of androstenedione (i.e., excess androstenedione is available for conversion to estrone); and the absence of monthly sloughing of the endometrial lining (i.e., residual tissue may become hyperplastic). In addition, nulliparity has been associated with lower levels of serum sex hormone– binding globulin (SHBG), leading to increased bioavailable estrogen (9).

In most studies, the risk of uterine cancer has been found to decrease with increasing parity, especially among premenopausal women (6,10). Although later ages at first live birth do not increase uterine cancer risk (unlike breast cancer) (5, 6), several recent studies have suggested that a last birth occurring late in reproductive life may reduce uterine cancer risk. Although this may reflect unique hormonal profiles of women who are able to conceive at older ages, mechanical clearing of neoplastic cells may account for the protective effect. The hypothesis is consistent with observations that the risk of uterine cancer increases with time since the most recent pregnancy (11,12). Further support for this hypothesis derives from several studies that have shown reductions in risk among users of intrauterine devices (13–15). However, it is also possible that these devices may affect risk by causing structural or biochemical changes that alter the sensitivity of the endometrium to circulating hormones.

The relationship of risk to breast-feeding remains contro-

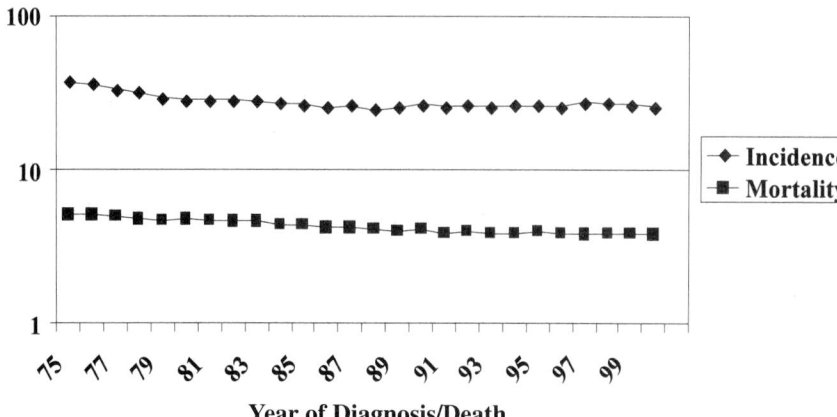

FIG. 1.2. Incidence and mortality trends among U.S. white females for cancer of the corpus uteri. (Data from the Surveillance, Epidemiology and End Results Program, 1975–2000.)

versial. Although a number of studies failed to show any relationship (5,16), more recent studies suggest that prolonged lactation may offer some protection (17,18); in one of these investigations, however, the reduced risk did not persist into the age range when uterine cancer becomes common (18).

Early ages at menarche were related to elevated risk for uterine cancer in several studies, although associations have generally been rather weak and trends inconsistent (5–7). Several studies found stronger effects of age at menarche among younger women, although this has not been consistently demonstrated (6,7). The extent to which these relationships reflect increased exposure to ovarian hormones or other correlates of early menarche (e.g., increased body weight) is unresolved.

Most studies have indicated that the age at menopause is directly related to the risk of developing uterine cancer (7). About 70% of all women diagnosed with uterine cancer are postmenopausal. Most studies support the estimate of Mac-Mahon (19) that there is about a twofold risk associated with natural menopause after the age of 52 years as compared to before age 49 years. It has been hypothesized that the effect of late age at menopause on risk may reflect prolonged exposure of the uterus to estrogen stimulation in the presence of anovulatory (progesterone-deficient) cycles. The interrelationships among menstrual factors, age, and weight are complex, and the biologic mechanisms of these variables operating in the pathogenesis of uterine cancer are subject to substantial speculation.

Exogenous Hormones

Oral Contraceptives

Studies have demonstrated significantly higher risks in users of sequential oral contraceptives (i.e., containing a high dose of estrogen and a weak progestin) as compared to users of estrogen-progestin combination pills. Studies have shown that women who used Oracon, a sequential preparation that employed dimethisterone (weak progestogen) with a large dose of a potent estrogen (ethinyl estradiol), had substantially elevated risks of uterine cancer (6,20). The risk associated with the use of other sequential oral contraceptives remains unclear, mainly because these drugs are no longer marketed.

In contrast, the use of combination oral contraceptives may reduce risk of uterine cancer by 50% compared to non-use, and long-term use may decrease risk further (20–23). Kaufman and others (22) showed that the reduced risk persisted for at least 5 years after discontinuation, but Weiss and Sayvetz (20) found that the protective effect waned within 3 years. In several studies, the greatest reduction in risk was associated with high–progestin-dose pills, although this finding was not replicated elsewhere (23,24). A number of studies indicate that the protective effect of the pill appears

greatest among nulliparous women (6,21). In other studies, the protection has been limited to nonobese women or those who have not been exposed to menopausal estrogens (6,25).

Postmenopausal Hormones

It is well established that the use of estrogen replacement therapy is associated with a 2- to 12-fold elevation in uterine cancer risk (26–29). In most investigations, the increased risk does not become apparent until the drugs have been used for at least 2 to 3 years, and longer use of estrogens is generally associated with higher risk (26,27,30). The highet relative risks (RRs) have been observed after 10 years of use (up to 20-fold), although it is unclear whether risk increases after 15 years. Most but not all studies have found that cessation of use is associated with a relatively rapid decrease in risk, although a number of studies have found significantly elevated risks to persist 10 or more years after last usage (26,27,29–31).

Higher doses of estrogen are associated with greatest elevations in risk. However, one study showed that even 0.3 mg of unopposed equine estrogen can result in a significant increase in risk (32). Fewer studies have focused on differences in risk according to cyclic versus continuous regimens or oral synthetic versus conjugated estrogen use. However, it appears that differences in modes of administration are less important predictors than duration of use and interval since last use (33). Unresolved is whether the use of estrogen patches, creams, or injections can affect risk; given relationships of risk with even low dose estrogens, it is plausible that these regimens may confer some increase in risk.

From a number of studies, it appears that estrogenic effects are strongest among women who are thin, nondiabetic, normotensive, and nonsmokers (26,30,34). These findings suggest either that estrogen metabolism differs among these women, or that risk is already high enough in women who are obese, diabetic, hypertensive, or smokers that exposure to exogenous estrogens has only a small additional effect. Tumors associated with estrogen use generally demonstrate favorable characteristics, including earlier stage at diagnosis, lower grade, and less frequent myometrial invasion (26,29). Estrogen users tend to be younger at diagnosis than nonusers, and the tumors are more frequently accompanied by hyperplasia or adenomyosis (35,36). The fact that estrogen remains linked to risk in studies limited to pathologically confirmed cases and that risk is increased for both early- and late-stage cancers (31,37) suggests that the increased risk is not related to pathologic overdiagnosis.

Progesterone has been shown to cause regression of endometrial hyperplasia, the presumed precursor of uterine cancers (38). This is consistent with the clinical recommendation that combined estrogen-progestin therapy be prescribed for all women with intact uteri. Recent studies indicate that the excess risk of uterine cancer can be significantly reduced if progestins are given for at least 10 days each month (28,

39–41). In several studies, however, subjects who used progestins for <10 days per month continued to experience some increased risk, with only a slight reduction compared to estrogen-only users (28,40–42). The sharp contrast between the effects of <10 and ≥10 days of progestin use has led to the suggestion that the extent of uterine sloughing or of ''terminal'' differentiation at the completion of the progestin phase may play a critical role in determining risk (28). It remains questionable whether 10 days of progestin administration per month is sufficient for complete protection, particularly for long-term users (43). Few studies have had large numbers of long-term sequential users, and in two studies there has been evidence that this pattern of usage may result in some persistence of risk (28,42).

Recently, there has been increased enthusiasm for prescribing estrogens continuously with progestins. Although Weiderpass and others in Sweden (40) observed a risk considerably below unity for this regimen, other studies in the United States have found either no alteration in risk (28) or an elevated risk (41). Discrepancies in findings may relate to the use of more potent progestins in Europe or to an imprecise risk estimate given the limited number of subjects in the Swedish study.

Tamoxifen

A number of clinical trials and one population-based case-control study have recently indicated an increased risk of uterine cancer among tamoxifen-treated breast cancer patients (44–46). This is consistent with tamoxifen's estrogenic effects on the endometrium. Elevated risks have been observed primarily among women receiving high cumulative doses of therapy, usually in the range of 15 g or greater. According to a recent investigation, the risk for malignant mixed mullerian tumors may be especially high (47). One recent study documented a poor prognosis among long-term tamoxifen users who developed uterine cancer, presumably reflecting less favorable histologies and higher stages of disease at diagnosis (48). Whether this finding is generalizable to other populations remains unclear.

Obesity

Obesity is a well-recognized risk factor for uterine cancer and may account for up to 25% of cases (49–53). Very heavy women appear to have exceptionally high risks (52). Although studies have demonstrated significant positive trends of uterine cancer with both weight and various measures of obesity, including Quetelet's index (weight/height^2), height has not been consistently associated with risk. Obesity appears to affect both premenopausal and postmenopausal uterine cancer (52).

Blitzer and others (54) found a positive association between uterine cancer and adolescent obesity, and hypothesized that long-standing obesity is a more important risk factor than adult weight. However, in several studies that have examined both weight during early adulthood and later in life, contemporary weight, and weight gain during adulthood appear to be most predictive of uterine cancer risk (50, 52).

Recent interest has focused on determining whether the distribution of body fat predicts uterine cancer risk. Upper-body fat has been found in several studies to have an effect on uterine cancer risk independent of body size (52,55,56). However, other studies suggest either no effect of body fat distribution or a more crucial role for central obesity (57–59).

Physical Activity

Several recent studies suggest a protective effect of physical activity on uterine cancer risk that appears independent of relationships with body weight (49,60–62). However, a number of these studies had internal inconsistencies. For instance, in a recent study (62), the absence of differences in risk by duration or intensity of physical activity levels suggested the need for caution before interpreting the association as causal. A potential relationship is biologically appealing given that physical activity can result in changes in the menstrual cycle, body fat distribution, and levels of endogenous hormones.

Dietary Factors

Despite the fact that obesity has been consistently related to uterine cancer, the role of dietary factors remains controversial. Geographic differences in disease rates (i.e., high rates in Western and low rates in Eastern societies) suggest that nutrition has a role, especially the high content of animal fat in Western diets . Armstrong and Doll (63) demonstrated a strong correlation between a country's total fat intake and uterine cancer incidence.

Although a number of studies have assessed uterine cancer risk in relation to consumption of dietary fat, the association remains unclear. A clear assessment of risk depends on careful control for effects of both body size and caloric intake (energy). One case-control study found a relationship with animal fat intake that was relatively independent of other dietary factors (64). Another case-control study (49) found that the risk associated with fat calories was partially explained by body size. Several other case-control studies did not confirm a relationship with fat intake (65,66). In addition, a recent cohort study found an opposite trend; namely, some decrease in risk with relatively high intakes of saturated or animal fat (53).

Reduced risks associated with consumption of certain micronutrients have been a more consistent finding. Barbone et al. (65) found no relationship with either animal or vegetable fat intake, but did find reduced risks related to high intake of certain micronutrients (including carotene and nitrate). A

European study found reduced risks among women reporting high intakes of fruits and vegetables, specifically those containing high levels of beta-carotene (67). Goodman and others (49) found inverse relationships of risk with consumption of cereals, legumes, vegetables, and fruits, particularly those high in lutein. McCann et al. (66) also found evidence for reduced risks among women in the highest quartiles of intake of protein, dietary fiber, phytoesterols, vitamin C, folate, alpha-carotene, beta-carotene, lycopene, lutein + zeaxanthin, and vegetables. However, not all studies support relationships with micronutrients, including recently reported results from a large Canadian prospective study (53).

Several studies have found that consumption of phytoestrogens and omega-3 fatty acids (found in fatty fish) may be protective (49,68,69), but confirmatory studies are needed. In addition, future studies are needed to assess whether risk reductions associated with certain dietary patterns reflect modified hormone metabolism, as suggested in both observational and intervention studies (70–73).

Alcohol Consumption

In several studies, regular consumption of alcoholic beverages has been linked to substantial reductions in uterine cancer risk (74–77). Several studies suggest more pronounced effects among premenopausal or overweight women, indicating that an attenuation in endogenous estrogen levels may be responsible for the reduced risk (75,77). However, other studies have failed to find a relationship between alcohol consumption and uterine cancer risk (78–80).

Cigarette Smoking

A reduced risk of uterine cancer among smokers has been reported, with current smokers having approximately half the risk of nonsmokers (81–83). Cigarette smoking has been linked to an earlier age at natural menopause in some populations and to reduced levels of endogenous estrogens. Reduced risk associated with long-term smoking is more pronounced in postmenopausal than premenopausal women (81, 84). In addition, reduced risk associated with smoking may be most apparent in parous or obese patients (5,82,83).

At present, biologic mechanisms underlying the inverse relationship of smoking to uterine cancer risk remain elusive. Alterations in endogenous hormones or metabolites are likely involved. In one report, the inverse association of smoking with uterine cancer risk appeared to be more strongly related to higher serum androstenedione levels than to lower serum estrogen levels except perhaps among overweight women (74).

Endogenous Hormones

Despite the recognition that uterine cancer is a hormonally responsive tumor, few studies have assessed relationships with endogenous hormones. To date, only three large epidemiologic studies have assessed associations with circulating estrogens (74,85,86). All three studies observed an increased risk of postmenopausal uterine cancer with increasing levels of estrone after adjustment for other factors, although in one study (85), the association was considerably attenuated after adjustment for body mass. In addition, two studies reported an increased risk with bioavailable (free and albumin-bound) fractions of estradiol and a reduced risk with increasing SHBG (85,86). In one investigation (85), estrogens appeared to be less predictive of premenopausal disease, suggesting that anovulation or progesterone deficiency might be more predictive of risk.

Less well investigated is whether other endogenous hormones are related to uterine cancer risk. Key and Pike (87) suggested that uterine carcinogenesis is dependent on uterine mitosis, which is increased by estrogens and reduced by progesterone, but risk associated with progesterone levels has not been well explored. Given that adrenal hormones play a central role in postmenopausal steroid biosynthesis, several studies have examined associations with cortisol, androstenedione, dehydroepiandrosterone (DHEA), and dihydroepiandrosterone sulfate (DHEA-S). Two large studies have shown positive associations of uterine cancer risk with serum androstenedione levels (74,85). In one of these investigations (85), this association remained after control for estrone levels, leading the investigators to speculate on the importance of aromatase and local conversion of estrone from androstenedione via abnormal endometrial cells.

Obesity, which is hypothesized to reflect elevated estrogen levels (87), seems to represent a key risk factor for both uterine carcinoma and endometrial hyperplasias, but the mechanisms mediating this are unclear. One case-control analysis of serum estrogen levels (85) reported that the risk associated with obesity was not entirely mediated by estrogen, especially among premenopausal women (88). This led to interest in a potential role for insulin levels (89); however, c-peptide levels were found to be unrelated to risk (90). In another cohort study of postmenopausal women, elevated serum estrogen levels appeared to account for the majority of the risk associated with obesity (86).

Medical Conditions

Numerous clinical reports link polycystic ovarian syndrome (PCOS) with an increase in the risk of uterine cancer, particularly among younger women (91–93); however, it is uncertain whether this risk is independent of obesity. In a follow-up study at the Mayo Clinic, women with chronic anovulation were found to be at a threefold increased risk of developing uterine cancer (94). Assessing histories of PCOS is challenging in case-control studies, but it is of interest that uterine cancer has been associated with histories of either hirsutism or acne (5,95), which are conditions often associated with hyperandrogenism.

A number of studies have noted a high risk of uterine cancer among diabetics, but again the issue is whether the association is independent of weight. Two cohort studies (96,97) and a number of case-control studies (5,98–100) suggest that the relationship persists when analyses are restricted to nonobese women or are adjusted for weight. However, in several other studies (51,101), the effect of diabetes on uterine cancer risk was apparent only among obese women, suggesting the possible involvement of selected metabolic abnormalities, including hyperinsulinemia. Further studies are needed to resolve the association, as well as to elaborate on how specific types of diabetes may be involved.

A variety of other diseases have been suggested as possibly predisposing to uterine cancer risk, including hypertension, arthritis, thyroid conditions, gallbladder disease, and cholesterolemia. In a number of studies, positive findings may be partially explained by the correlation of the diseases with other factors. Similar to breast cancer, patients with previous fractures have been found to have a reduced risk of uterine cancer (102,103), presumably reflecting the association of lowered bone density with altered endogenous hormone levels.

Genetic Factors

Several recent studies have suggested that a family history of uterine cancer is a risk factor for the disease (104–106). Data from a family-cancer database in Sweden (106) showed that risk was inversely related to age at diagnosis, with over a 10-fold excess risk among young (<50 years) daughters of mothers with early-onset diseases. In addition, subjects with a family history of colon cancer were at an increased risk, an association that is now recognized as reflective of hereditary nonpolyposis colorectal cancer, a dominantly inherited syndrome associated with mutations in the DNA mismatch repair genes MSH2, MLH1, and MSH6. Uterine cancer has not been linked to mutations in either the *BRCA1* or *BRCA2* genes (107). Several recent investigations have suggested possible disease associations with more common genetic polymorphisms, including the estrogen receptor methylenetetrahydrofolate reductase (MTHFR) and cytochrome P-450 1A1 (CYP1A1) genes (108–110), but confirmatory studies are needed.

Other Risk Factors

Women of upper socioeconomic status have been reported to be at a higher risk of uterine cancer (7). Findings related to socioeconomic status may be partially explained by other uterine cancer risk factors correlated with affluence (e.g., the use of estrogen replacement therapy or certain dietary consumption patterns).

Geographic variation in rates of uterine cancer, with high rates in certain industrial areas, has led to the suggestion that certain environmental agents may affect risk. Given the well-recognized influence of hormones on the disease, there has been particular concern about a potential role for certain endocrine disruptors, including dichlorodiphenyltrichloroethane (DDT). Several studies have addressed this issue by comparing dichlorodiphenyldichloroethylene (DDE) levels (the active metabolite of DDT) in the sera of cases and controls, finding no significant differences (111,112). Studies assessing the relationship of uterine cancer risk to exposure to electromagnetic radiation (electric blanket or mattress covers) have been negative (113). Data for occupational exposures are limited. One record linkage study in Finland found an association with exposure to animal dust and sedentary work (114).

Conclusions

A unified theory of how risk factors for uterine cancer might operate through one common hormonal pathway has been suggested. Estrogen promotes proliferation in the endometrium, which is opposed by progesterone. Therefore, exposure to estrogen, particularly bioavailable estrogen that is weakly bound or unbound to plasma protein, is viewed as a critical carcinogen. Functional ovarian tumors, the Stein-Leventhal syndrome, late menopause, and administration of exogenous estrogens and sequential oral contraceptives produce higher levels of estrogen exposure without the antiproliferative effects of progesterone. Obesity could also contribute in a variety of ways (115). Adipose tissue is the primary site for conversion of androstenedione to estrone, which is the primary source for estrogen after menopause. Obesity is associated with higher conversion rates and/or elevated plasma levels of estrogen. In addition, obesity is related to lower levels of SHBG and more frequent anovulatory menstrual cycles (i.e., less progesterone). Vegetarianism is associated with lower plasma estrogen levels, presumably on the basis of the relationship of diet composition to estrogen metabolism. The beneficial effects of combination oral contraceptives and cyclic progestins added to hormone replacement therapy presumably operate through the antiestrogenic effects of progesterone. The peculiar age incidence patterns for uterine cancer (i.e., extremely rare under age 45 years, followed by a rapid and progressive rise from ages 45 to 60 years) could also reflect the waning influence of progesterone. Nulliparity, hypertension, diabetes, the absence of smoking, and race may yet be added to the unifying scheme as knowledge of endocrinologic mechanisms in endometrial tissue increases.

Although there are several identified risk factors for uterine cancer (Table 1.1), important gaps in knowledge currently limit a full understanding of the proposed carcinogenic process. We need to understand when in a woman's life obesity matters most and how risk is influenced by weight loss; whether the number of adipocytes, their fat composition, or other factors determine peripheral conversion of an-

TABLE 1.1. *Risk factors for uterine cancer*

Factors Influencing Risk	Estimated Relative Risk*
Older ages	2–3
Residency in North America, Northern Europe	3–18
Higher levels of education or income	1.5–2.0
White race	2
Nulliparity	3
History of infertility	2–3
Menstrual irregularities	1.5
Late ages at natural menopause	2
Early ages at menarche	1.5–2.0
Late ages at natural menopause	2–3
Long-term use or high dosages of menopausal estrogens	10–20
Use of oral contraceptives	0.3–0.5
High cumulative doses of tamoxifen	3–7
Obesity	2–5
Stein-Leventhal disease or estrogen-producing tumors	>5
Histories of diabetes, hypertension, gallbladder disease, or or thyroid disease	1.3–3.0
Cigarette smoking	0.5

* Relative risks depend on the study and referent group employed.

drostenedione; and the precise hormonal mechanisms associated with vegetarianism. Perhaps the most important gap is in understanding the basic mechanism of estrogen carcinogenesis. Are estrogens complete carcinogens? Are they classic ''promoters'' that promote already initiated cells, or do they operate by stimulating growth and offering greater opportunity for abnormal cells to arise or for carcinogens to act on vulnerable genetic material? The epidemiologic data are consistent with estrogens acting at a relatively late stage of carcinogenesis. If this reflects their position as tumor promoters, then the need to identify initiators of the process becomes even more crucial.

OVARIAN CANCER

Demographic Patterns

Ovarian cancer accounts for 4% of all incident cancers in U.S. women (1). Approximately 1 in 70 American women develops ovarian cancer during her lifetime. The average annual age-adjusted incidence for all SEER areas between 1996 and 2000 was 16.9 per 100,000 women (2). An estimated 25,400 new cases will be diagnosed in the United States in 2003.

Diagnosis usually occurs at advanced stages; the overall 5-year survival between 1996 and 2000 was only 53%. The average annual age-adjusted mortality rate is 7.6 per 100,000

women (2). The estimated 14,300 deaths due to ovarian cancer in 2003 made it the fourth leading cause of cancer death among U.S. women (1).

After rising during the mid twentieth century, age-adjusted mortality rates have since remained relatively constant (1). Incidence rates show little variation over the past 30 years, but both incidence and mortality rates may be declining for U.S. women under age 40 years (116). U.S. blacks and whites have nearly identical mortality rates, but incidence rates remain higher for U.S. white women (117) (Fig. 1.3).

The highest incidence occurs in North American, Scandinavian, and Northern European countries, whereas the lowest rates occur in African nations and some eastern countries, such as China (3). Age-standardized rates vary 4.5-fold across countries. Mortality data show a similar but slightly less dramatic pattern. The estimated age-standardized mortality rates are 6.2 in developed countries and 2.8 in developing countries (118).

Risk Factors

Reproductive Variables

Gravidity is consistently associated with a decreased ovarian cancer risk (119–122). Compared with nulligravidous women, women with a single pregnancy have a RR of 0.6 to 0.8. Each additional pregnancy decreases risk another 10% to 15%. The number of full-term births seems most influential, but several studies have also found decreased risks associated with an increasing number of incomplete pregnancies (123,124). Most studies that adjusted for parity reported no residual association with age at first or last birth (125), but some investigators argue that both number and timing matter (126,127).

Whether these risk relationships reflect a hazardous role for infertility or merely the protective role of pregnancy is unclear. Comparing subfertile women with ovarian abnormalities to subfertile women with normal ovarian function has thus far shown no increased risk for the former, but the data are not definitive (128). Studies with higher risks among infertile women support some role for abnormal endocrine factors (129). In one study (119), sexually active women who were not using contraceptives and had not conceived for 10 or more years were at a sixfold excess risk compared with other women. Another large study similarly found a high risk associated with nulliparity despite unprotected intercourse, especially in women with long periods of ovulatory experience (129).

Infertility drugs, particularly ovulation-stimulating medications, have been linked to an increased ovarian cancer risk in some, but not in all, studies (122,130). Case-control studies have generally not found an association with fertility drug use, including specific medications (131–134). Some (8,130) but not all (135,136) cohort studies have reported

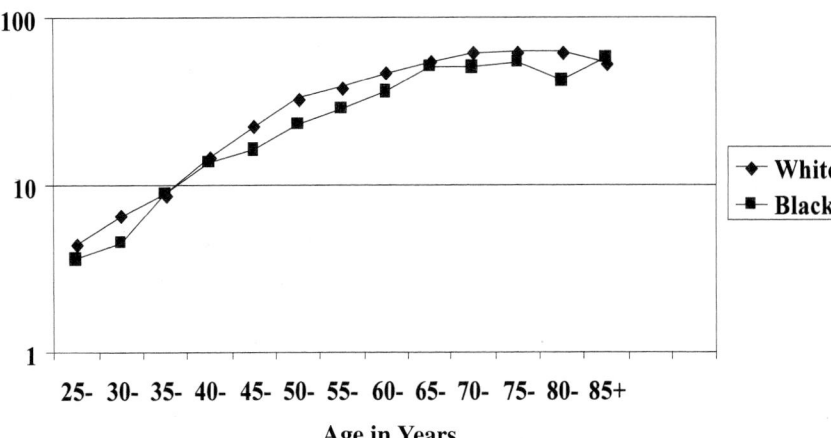

FIG. 1.3. Age-specific incidence of cancer of the ovary by race. (Data from the Surveillance, Epidemiology and End Results Program, 1996–2000.)

increased risks with particular medications. The reports of increased risk should be cautiously interpreted for a number of reasons, including small sample sizes. The prospect that the causes of subfertility and infertility, not the associated treatments, are the causative factors appears to be gaining support (128,137). Several ongoing studies will likely shed further light on this issue in the near future.

Some studies have not found an association between lactation and risk, whereas several others have shown reduced risks (119,121,138–140). However, those data lack clear trends of decreasing risk with increasing months of breast-feeding; most investigators conjectured that the weak correlation between duration of breast-feeding and suppression of ovulation may have contributed to the lack of significant trends.

Menstrual Factors and Gynecologic Surgery

Numerous studies have noted reduced risks among women who have had a simple hysterectomy or tubal ligation (119,141–144). These patients' risks were 30% to 40% lower than the risks among women who had not undergone surgery. Surgery offers an opportunity to remove abnormal-appearing ovaries, but this alone is unlikely to explain the protective effect (145). Partial devascularization and reduced ovarian function represent a possible alternative mechanism (146).

A 2001 publication (147) opposed earlier reports that linked late age at natural menopause to a slightly increased risk of ovarian cancer (119,148). The marked flattening in the age-specific incidence curves shortly after menopausal ages is consistent with the conclusion that early or late menopause has little effect on ovarian cancer risk. Most studies have not found earlier ages at menarche to increase risk, but some have reported weak positive associations (119,148).

Exogenous Hormones

Almost all epidemiologic studies show a reduced risk of ovarian cancer among women who use oral contraceptives.

Their use for only a few months introduces lasting protection, but long-term use generates the largest risk reduction (119,121,149). In one study, the protective effect of long-term use (≥10 years) reached 80% (150). The protection appears to persist for many years after their last use (119, 149–151). The lower-dose formulations now in use seem to reduce risk similarly to their higher dose predecessors (152–154).

In contrast, menopausal estrogen use seems to increase the risk of developing ovarian cancer. Early studies, which displayed null (122), inverse (155), and positive (156) associations, presented difficulties for deriving conclusions (157, 158). Questions still remain (159,160), but recent studies, including two large cohorts (161,162), have found that use of menopausal estrogens for ten or more years (163–165) increased risk. Very limited data have not shown that the use of estrogen plus progestin (161,163) increases risk. Additional data on associations with regimen, dose, and duration, especially for estrogen plus progestin, are desirable.

Endogenous Hormones

Two nested case-control studies have evaluated risks associated with endogenous hormone levels. One found higher levels of androgens and lower levels of gonadotropins among cases compared to controls (166). The second, a pooled analysis of three studies, reported null associations with estrogens, androgens, SHBG, insulin-like growth factor-1 (IGF-1), and the insulin-like growth factor–binding proteins (IGFBPs) (167,168). Despite these initial null results, the strong biologic rationale for these hormones in ovarian carcinogenesis warrants further investigation.

Medical Conditions

Several studies surveyed whether certain medical conditions predispose to ovarian cancer. Diabetes, hypertension, and thyroid diseases seem unrelated to risk (169,170). In line with a number of clinical studies showing simultaneous occurrences of endometriosis and ovarian cancer, several epidemiologic studies have found that women with a diagnosis of endometriosis have elevated risks for developing ovarian cancer (137,171). As discussed by Ness in a recent review article (172), the two conditions share a number of pathophysiologic processes, including estrogen excesses and progesterone deficits, immunologic responses, and inflammatory reactions. Pelvic inflammatory disease has also been found in several studies to be a possible risk factor for ovarian cancer (173,174). This finding supports a role for inflammation in ovarian carcinogenesis.

Obesity has recently received increased scrutiny as a possible risk factor. One study reported an increased risk among heavier women only for serous or endometrioid tumors (175). Attempts to replicate this finding, however, raised more uncertainty by reporting increased risks only among women who are clinically obese (176), whose body mass index (BMI; kg/m^2) is higher at age 18 years (177), who are diagnosed before menopause (178), who never used menopausal estrogens (179), or who are physically inactive (180). Other studies concluded obese women were at decreased ovarian cancer risk (169,181). These diverse results could reflect statistical chance or other systematic biases.

Although it appears from most investigations that obesity may be directly related to ovarian cancer risk, data for physical activity are inconclusive. Case-control studies in China (182) and the U.S. (183) have reported inverse associations with increasing activity, but the cohort analyses published to date (184,185) suggest that increasing activity might put women at increased, rather than decreased, risk.

Medications recently surfaced both as potential risk and protective factors. Several studies showed increased risks among users of psychotropic medications, particularly those operating through dopaminergic mechanisms (186). However, subsequent studies that employed cohort designs or improved exposure assessment reported null associations (187–190). Other data suggested a reduced risk among women who used antiinflammatory or other analgesic medications (191–193). As with the psychotropic medication data though, subsequent studies showed, at most, a weak and inconsistent association. Chemoprevention via the use of these medications remains a premature concept.

Dietary Factors

Correlations between ovarian cancer incidence and per capita fat availability and noted increased incidence rates among migrants who moved to areas with higher per capita fat availability have stimulated interest in dietary risk factors (63). Initial studies in unique populations, such as ovolacto-vegetarians (194) or meat abstainers (195), provided conflicting results. Since then, studies have targeted a few classes of foods: lactose and dairy foods, fats, vitamins, fiber, fruits, vegetables.

Higher consumption of yogurt, cottage cheese, and other lactose-rich dairy products was linked with increased risk in a case-control study (196). Galactose-related enzymes can influence gonadotropin levels, which are hypothesized to be crucial ovarian cancer risk determinants. The majority of subsequent studies showed no association with lactose consumption or galactose metabolism (197–200) despite an occasional positive (201) or inverse (202) report.

A survey of the literature on fat consumption finds case-control studies reporting more positive associations than prospective studies (203,204). The case-control data reported higher risks associated with particular fatty foods (e.g., butter and meats) as well as types of fat, but in two recent null studies that provided comprehensive pictures of different fat types, none stood out as a strong risk factor (205,206). Two cohort analyses (201,205) also reported null associations with increasing dietary fat consumption.

Vitamins, fiber, fruits, and vegetables might decrease ovarian cancer risk. Not all studies agree on what specifically reduces risk or by how much, but the pattern is surprisingly consistent. Total vegetable intake has been associated with reduced risk in several studies (200,201), as have different types of fiber (207,208). Some studies showed inverse associations with particular vitamins, such as beta-carotene (209) or vitamin A (210). Others found reduced risks with the full range of micronutrients (206), but one large cohort analysis reported null associations with any such exposures (211).

Host Factors

A family history of ovarian cancer is the strongest risk factor identified to date: Ovarian cancer in a first-degree relative approximately triples a woman's risk (212,213). Which family member was affected is less important than the total number of affected relatives or their age at diagnosis (214). Women with two or more affected relatives or whose relative was diagnosed before 50 years of age experience a higher increased risk (215). Approximately 5% to 10% of ovarian cancer patients have a first-degree relative with ovarian cancer (214).

Inherited mutations in two autosomal dominant genes—*BRCA1* and *BRCA2*—are strongly linked to familial ovarian cancer (and breast and other cancers) (216). Whereas the lifetime probability of developing ovarian cancer in most women is 2%, the probabilities in women with a family history or women with a *BRCA1/2* mutation are 9.4% (217) and 15% to 40% (218,219), respectively. Despite these increases, *BRCA1/2* mutations explain less than one-third of the elevated risk in women with familial ovarian cancer (215). Other candidate high-risk genes have not been identified but are almost certain to exist (214).

Other Risk Factors

Over-the-counter talc chemically resembles asbestos, a known cause of mesothelioma, and mesothelioma histologically resembles ovarian cancer. The published case-control studies generally report positive associations between ovarian cancer and perineal talc exposure. However, a lack of consistent statistical significance and inconsistent associations with different types of talc use raise questions about the validity of this association (220–222). One large cohort study reported no association with talc use (223).

In general, smoking is not considered a major risk factor for ovarian cancer. Some recent investigations suggest that smoking may increase the risk for mucinous tumors. A Canadian cohort of 89,835 women, followed for an average of 17 years (224); a large Australian case-control study (225); and two large U.S. case-control studies (226,227) observed increased risks for mucinous tumors after reporting null or weak positive associations based on all tumor histologies. Future studies that address this question would ideally possess adequate statistical power for a priori histology-specific analyses and employ standardized histologic review of the original pathology data. Passive smoking, addressed in a recent study (228), should also be pursued further.

Coffee consumption was linked to an elevated risk of ovarian cancer in several early studies (229,230), but a growing number of studies have not replicated that association (231–233).

The majority of studies do not support a relationship between alcohol consumption and ovarian cancer risk (231, 234,235). However, one case-control study reported an inverse association with two or more drinks per week (235), and a Swedish analysis of a cohort of women diagnosed with alcoholism over 30 years identified fewer than expected ovarian cancers (236). In the latter study, the investigators hypothesized that suppression of gonadotropin levels might account for the apparent reduced risk.

Certain occupations came under scrutiny when studies linked hair dyes and triazine herbicides to ovarian cancer (237,238). Record linkage studies in Finland (239), Sweden (240), and the United States (241) suggested a pattern of increased risks among certain professions (e.g., health care workers) or with particular occupational exposures (e.g., solvents). Until additional data address the potential for inconsistent or chance findings and the challenge of finding large populations with sufficient data on other potential confounding variables, occupation will likely not be considered a major risk factor for ovarian cancer (242).

Conclusions

Much of the clinical and epidemiologic evidence concerning risk factors for ovarian cancer implicates ovulatory activity (Table 1.2). Conditions associated with reduced ovulation, for example, pregnancy and oral contraceptives, consistently reduce risk. Combining these and other menstrual factors into single "ovulatory age" or "lifetime ovulatory cycles" indexes has generally produced the expected associations with ovarian cancer risk; that is, older ovulatory

TABLE 1.2. *Risk factors for ovarian cancer*

Factors Influencing Risk	Estimated Relative Risk*
Older ages	3
Residency in North America, Northern Europe	2–5
Higher levels of education or income	1.5–2.0
White race	1.5
Nulligravity	2–3
History of infertility	2–5
Early ages at menarche	1.5
Late ages at natural menopause	1.5–2.0
History of a hysterectomy	0.5–0.7
Use of oral contraceptives	0.3–0.5
Long-term use of menopausal estrogens	1 1.5–2.0
Perineal talc exposure	1.5–2.0
Female relative with ovarian cancer	3–4

* Relative risks depend on the study and referent group employed.

ages (243) or higher cycle counts (244) increase risk. However, the misclassification inherent in these indexes is sufficient to generate different risk estimates (245), and the magnitude of risk reduction for short-term oral contraceptive use or a single pregnancy exceeds the proportional decrease in ovulatory cycles that would be expected to be associated with these exposures.

The putative mechanisms behind ovulatory inhibition and the risk associated with "increased ovulation" (246) raise additional questions. An early report suggested, based on the associations with parity and infertility, that an unidentified endocrine abnormality predisposed women to relative or absolute infertility and ovarian cancer. The protection associated with oral contraceptives seems unlikely to fit this hypothesis unless, in some improbable manner, their use induces an endocrine milieu similar to that underlying fertility.

A second popular unifying hypothesis is that ovarian cancer is the result of accumulated exposure to circulating pituitary gonadotropins (247). Although this is consistent with the parity, menopause, and oral contraceptive associations, a study that directly measured gonadotropin levels failed to find a relationship with subsequent development of ovarian cancer (166). This theory also fails to account for the risks associated with clinical infertility, and it predicts that menopausal hormone therapy use would decrease risk, because both exposures are associated with reduced gonadotropin levels.

A third explanation points to a biologic effect of ovulation on ovarian surface epithelium. Ovulation prompts a cascade of epithelial events, including minor trauma, increased local concentrations of estrogen-rich follicular fluid, and increased epithelial proliferation. Such proliferation, particularly near the point of ovulation, can recruit inclusions into the ovarian parenchyma. Some or all of these "incessant

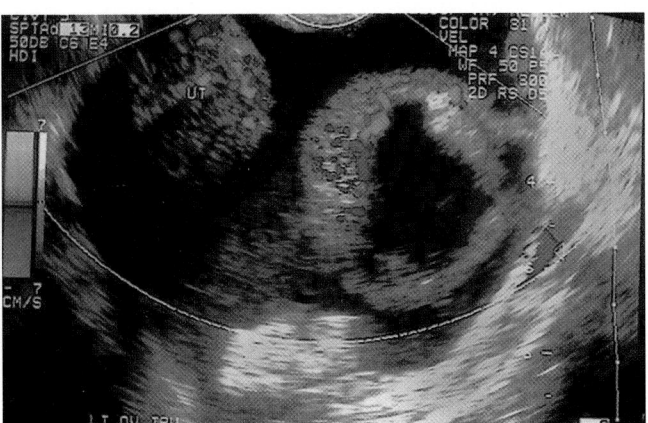

COLOR PLATE 10.35. Note irregular, thick walled left ovarian mass. The mass is highly vascular. Ascites is present.

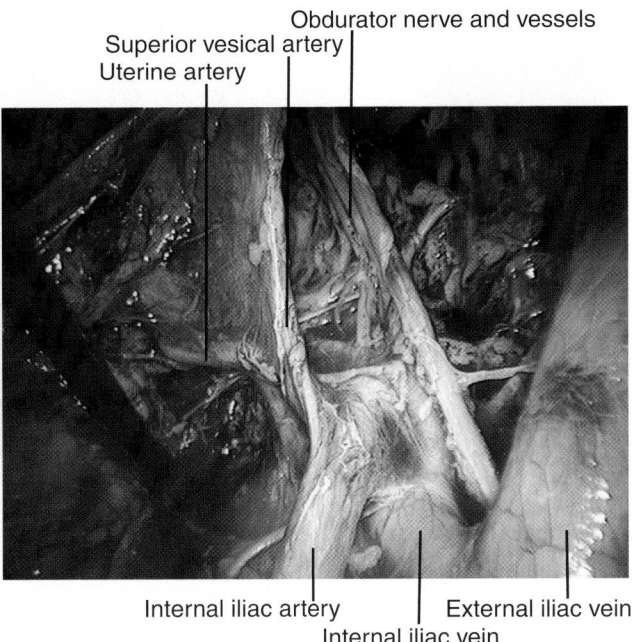

Uterine artery
Superior vesical artery
Obdurator nerve and vessels
Internal iliac artery
Internal iliac vein
External iliac vein

COLOR PLATE 13.3. Pelvic laparoscopic lymphadenectomy. The pelvic lymphadenectomy is complete. Picture of the dorsal part of the right pelvic sidewall.

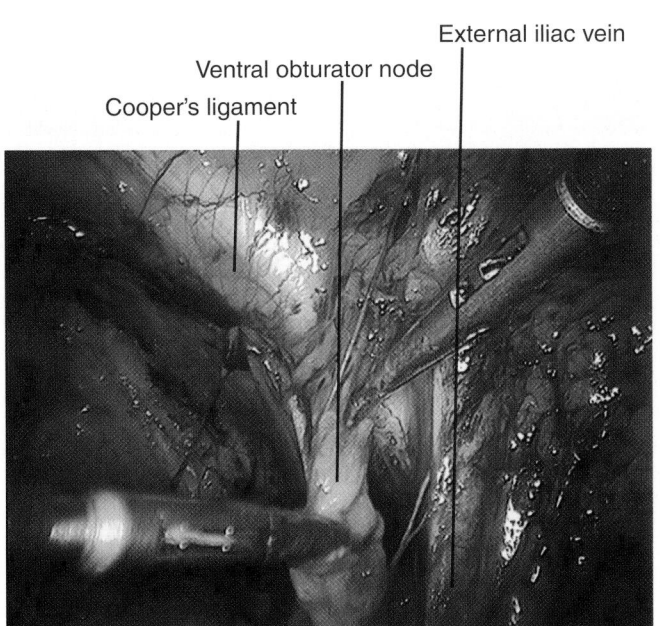

Cooper's ligament
Ventral obturator node
External iliac vein

COLOR PLATE 13.2. Pelvic laparoscopic lymphadenectomy. The pelvic lymphadenectomy is initiated. Picture of the ventral part of the right pelvic sidewall.

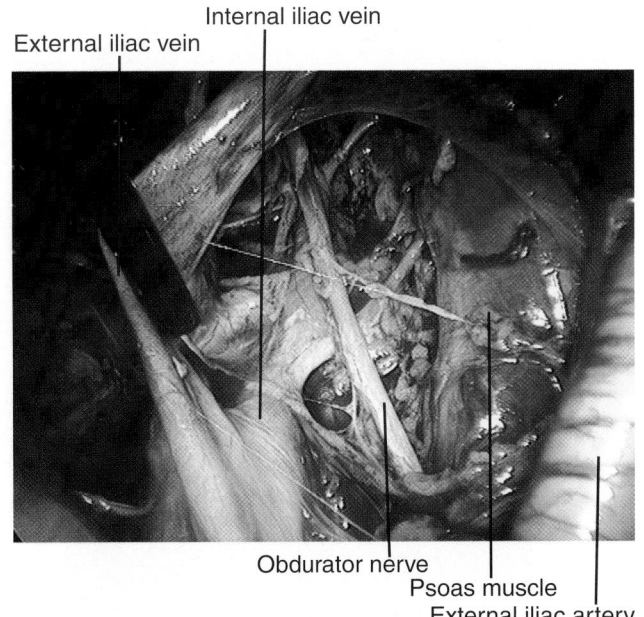

External iliac vein
Internal iliac vein
Obdurator nerve
Psoas muscle
External iliac artery

COLOR PLATE 13.4. Pelvic laparoscopic lymphadenectomy. The pelvic lymphadenectomy is complete. Same view as Figure 13.2, but the external iliac vein has been pushed medially.

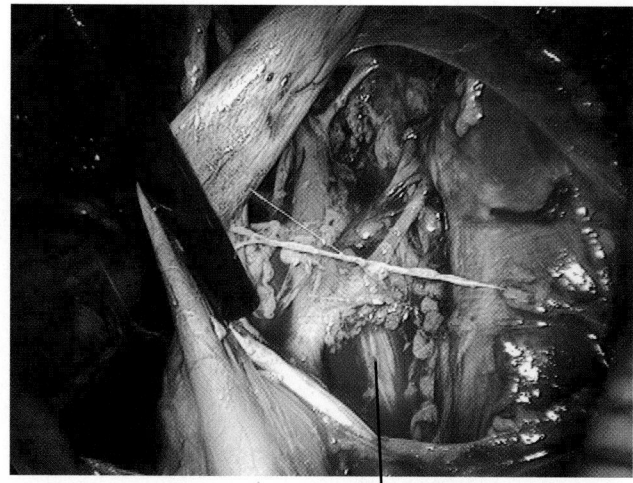

Lumbosacral nerve

COLOR PLATE 13.5. Pelvic laparoscopic lymphadenectomy. The pelvic lymphadenectomy is complete. Same view as Figure 13.3, but the external iliac vein and the obturator nerve have been pushed medially. The lumbosacral nerve is visible; this, more than the lymph node count, is proof that the pelvic lymphadenectomy has been done thoroughly.

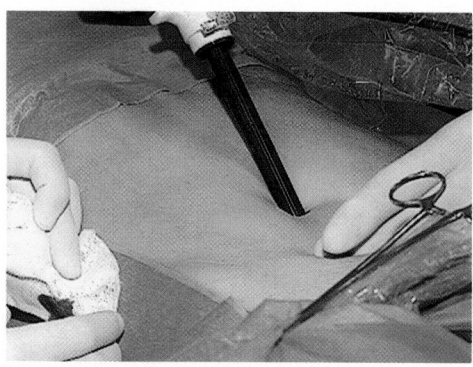

COLOR PLATE 13.6. Umbilical extraperitoneal laparoscopic approach. The instrument used is the Visiport (US Surgical Corporation, Norwalk, CT).

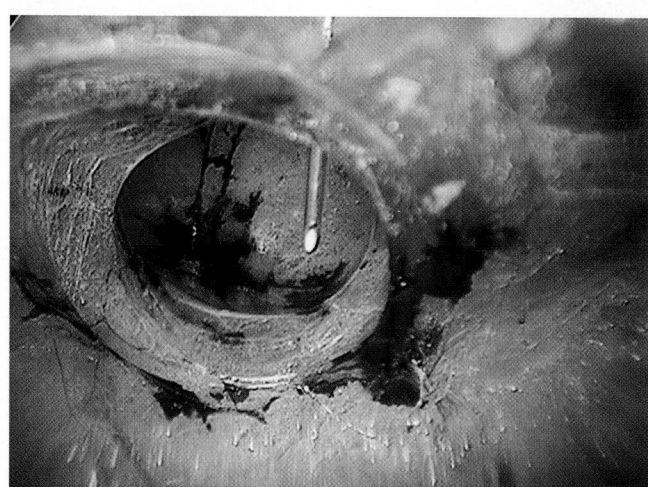

COLOR PLATE 13.7. Umbilical extraperitoneal laparoscopic approach. A spinal needle is introduced in the midline in the extraperitoneal space before the ancillary instruments are put in place.

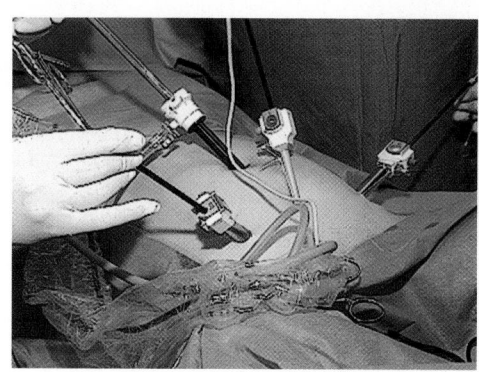

COLOR PLATE 13.8. Umbilical extraperitoneal laparoscopic approach. Position of laparoscopic trocar and ancillary trocars.

Cooper's ligament
Inferior epigastric vessels
Round ligament

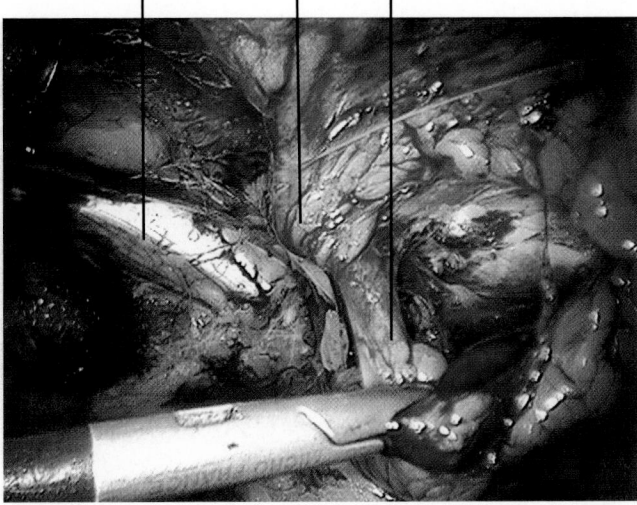

COLOR PLATE 13.9. Umbilical extraperitoneal laparoscopic approach. The round ligament on the right side is freed before being divided.

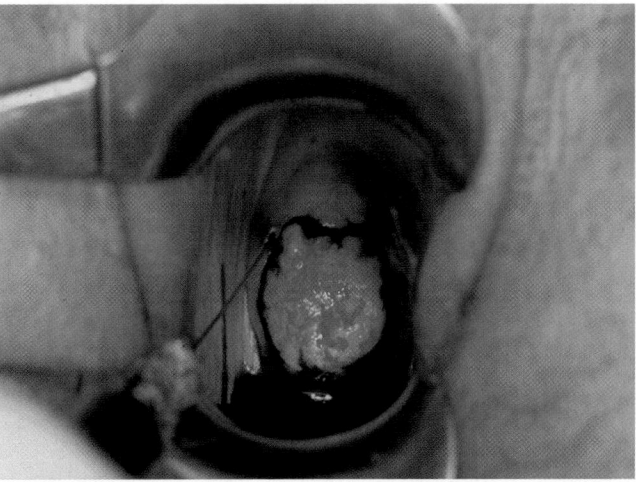

COLOR PLATE 13.10. Injection of the dye.[cf1] The dye is injected into the tissue surrounding the tumor. The sentinel lymph node procedure should only be used for early-stage cancers.

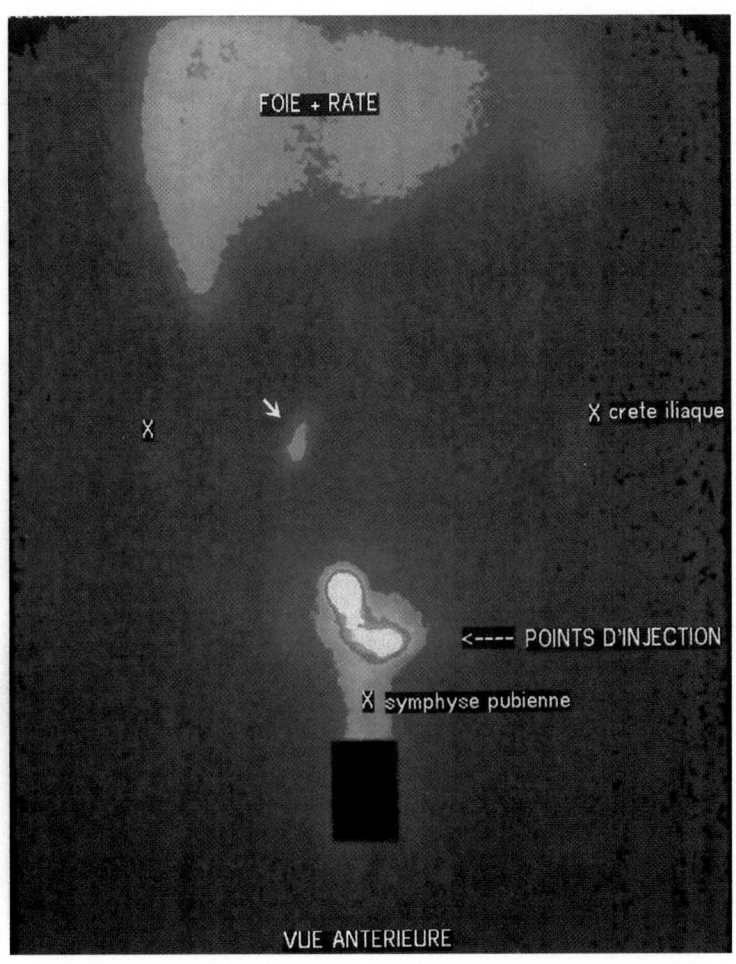

COLOR PLATE 13.11. Lymphoscintigraphy. One hot spot only is visible. No sentinel lymph node was detected on the left side. The sentinel lymph node on the right side was a common iliac node.

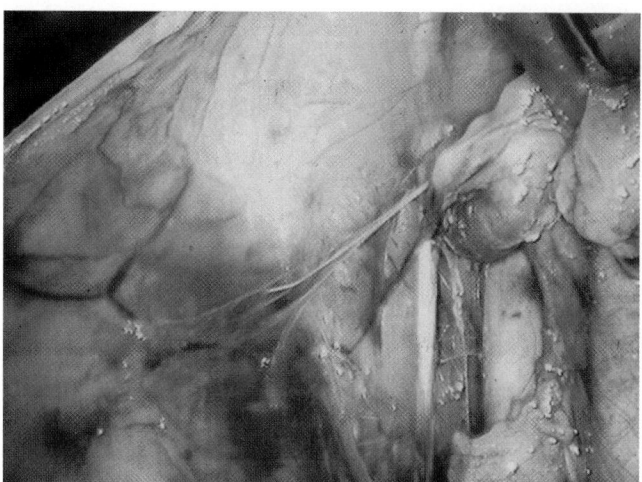

COLOR PLATE 13.12. Dissection of the sentinel node. The main lymphatic channel crosses the umbilical ligament and ends in a node situated between the external iliac vein and the obturator nerve.

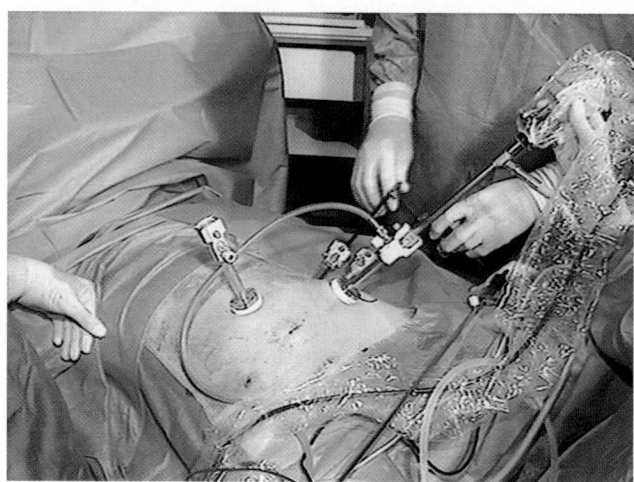

COLOR PLATE 13.15. Left-sided extraperitoneal laparoscopic approach. Position of laparoscopic trocar and ancillary trocars (the extraperitoneal approach is preceded by a transumbilical transperitoneal approach; the umbilical trocar is left in place after exsufflation).

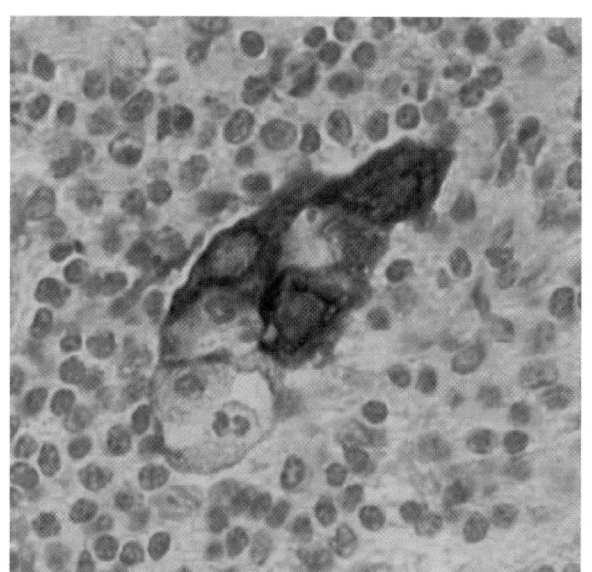

COLOR PLATE 13.14. Micrometastasis. Immunohistochemistry can be used to identify micrometastasis in the sentinel lymph node.

Left ureter

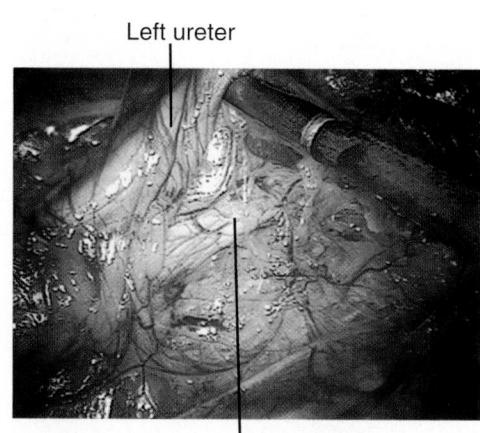

Left common iliac artery

COLOR PLATE 13.16. Left-sided extraperitoneal laparoscopic approach. The left ureter is pushed ventrally. The left common iliac artery is visible.

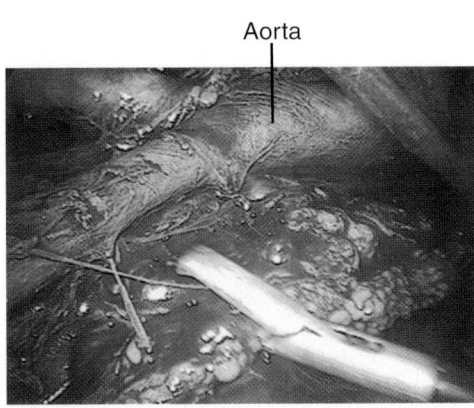

COLOR PLATE 13.17. Left-sided extraperitoneal laparoscopic approach. Picture taken at the end of the common iliac and lower aortic dissection.

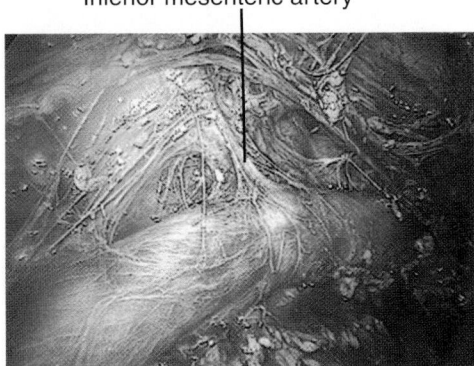

COLOR PLATE 13.18. Left-sided extraperitoneal laparoscopic approach. Picture taken at the end of the aortic dissection.

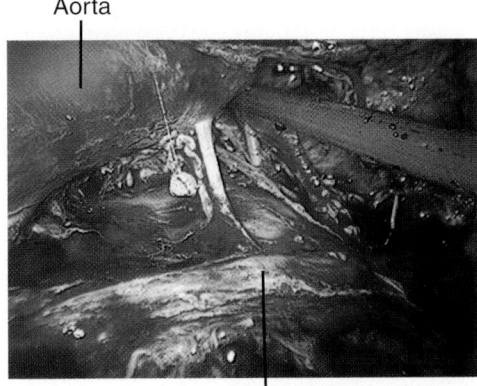

COLOR PLATE 13.19. Left-sided extraperitoneal laparoscopic approach. Picture taken at the beginning of the retroaortic dissection: the lumbar arteries and veins are visible.

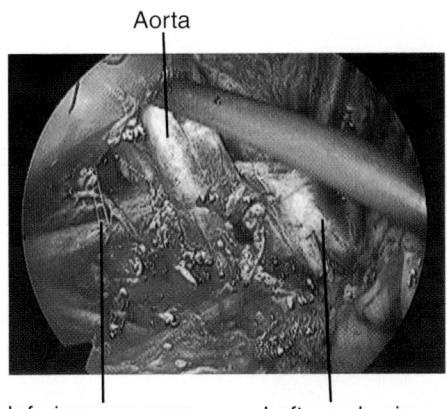

COLOR PLATE 13.20. Left-sided extraperitoneal laparoscopic approach. Picture taken after the lumbar arteries and veins have been divided and the interaorticocaval space appeared: the junction of the left renal vein and inferior vena cava is visible.

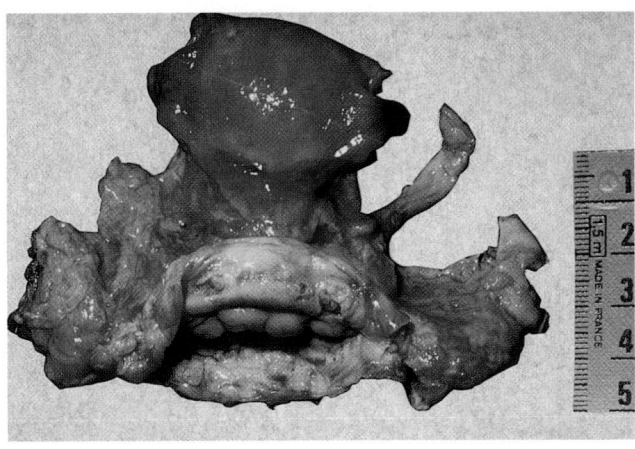

COLOR PLATE 13.21. Specimen of supraradical LAVRH (distal celio-Schauta).

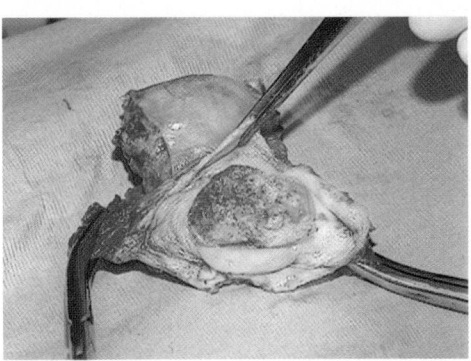

COLOR PLATE 13.22. Specimen of modified LAVRH (proximal celio-Schauta).

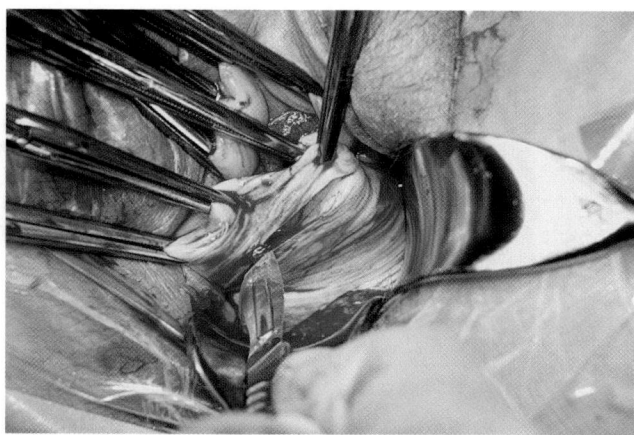

COLOR PLATE 13.23. Technique of modified LAVRH (proximal celio-Schauta). Incision of the vagina.

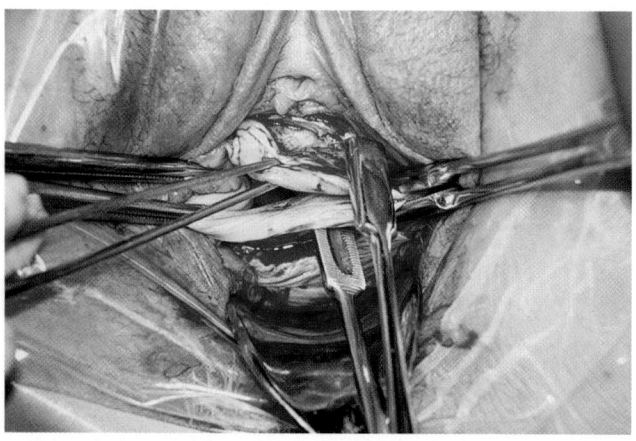

COLOR PLATE 13.24. Technique of modified LAVRH. Closing the vaginal cuff with Chroback forceps.

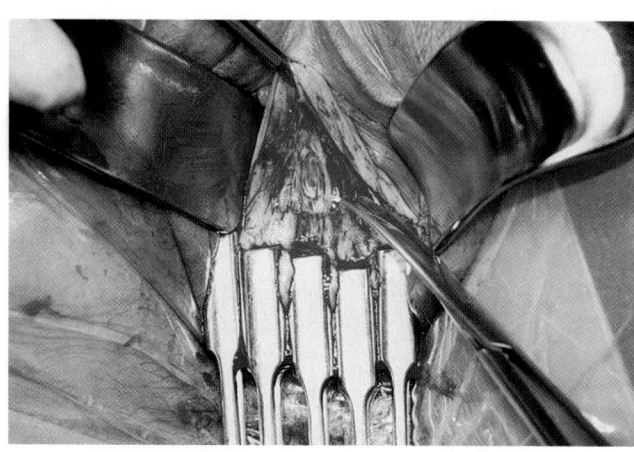

COLOR PLATE 13.25. Technique of modified LAVRH. Opening the vesicovaginal space.

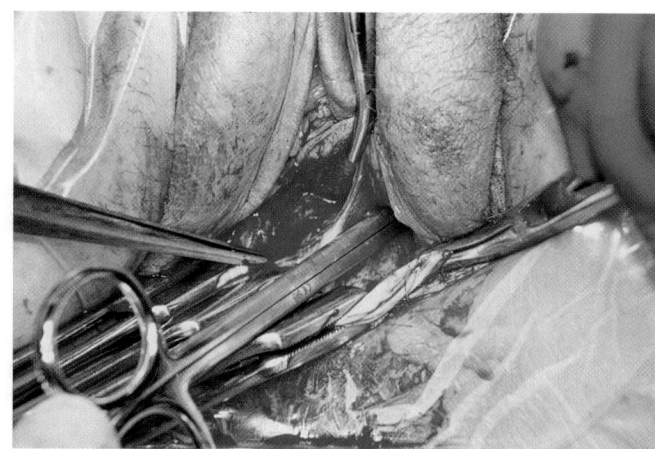

COLOR PLATE 13.26. Technique of modified LAVRH. Opening the paravesical space on the left side of the patient.

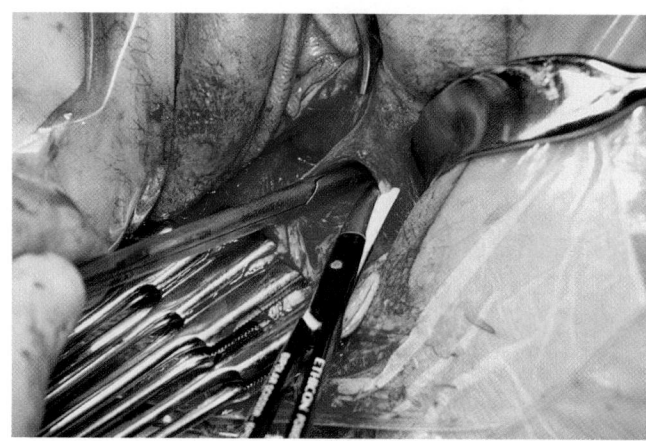

COLOR PLATE 13.27. Technique of modified LAVRH. Dividing the lateral fibers of the bladder pillar on the left side of the patient.

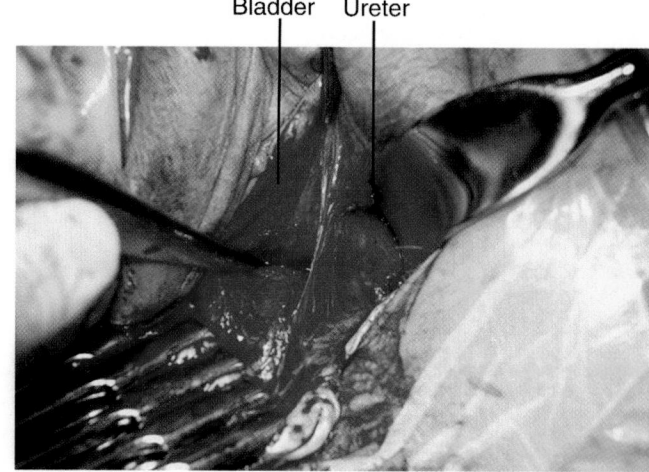

COLOR PLATE 13.28. Technique of modified LAVRH. The location where the ureter enters the bladder floor is visible. The medial fibers of the bladder pillar can be cut.

Ureter

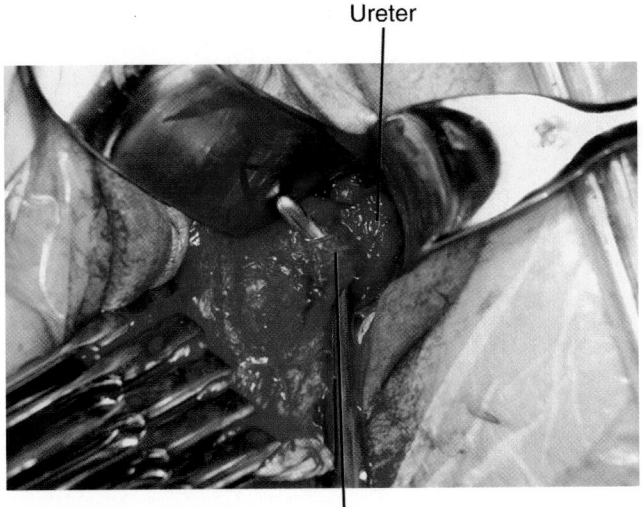

Uterine artery

COLOR PLATE 13.29. Technique of modified LAVRH. The medial fibers of the bladder pillar have been divided; the arch of the uterine artery is demonstrated.

Ureter

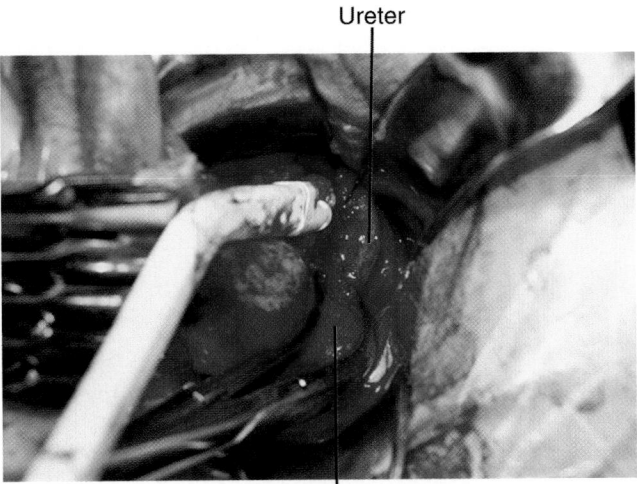

Paracervical ligament

COLOR PLATE 13.30. Technique of modified LAVRH. Two clamps are put on the paracervical ligament, the distal one being just underneath the tip of the knee of the ureter.

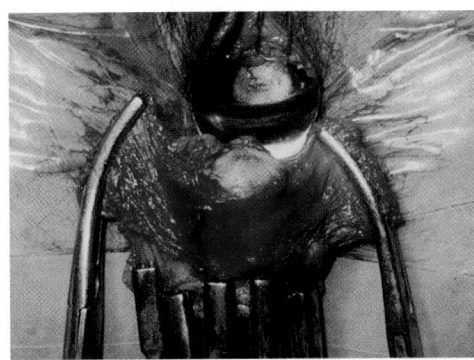

COLOR PLATE 13.31. Specimen of LVRT. The radicality is the same as in the modified LAVRH. The transected uterine isthmus is visible.

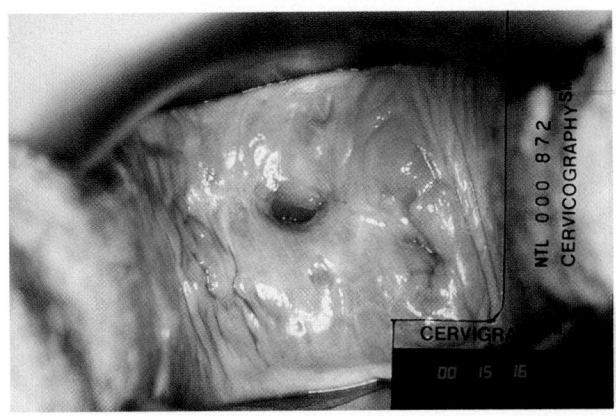

COLOR PLATE 13.32. Postoperative picture after LVRT. The contour of the cervix has disappeared but the uterine orifice remains patent.

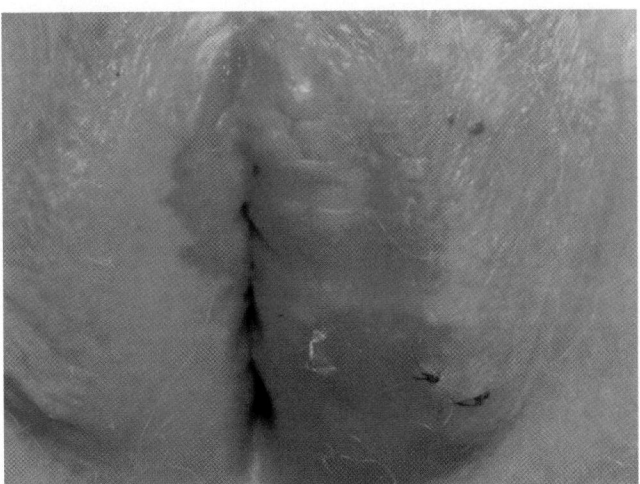

COLOR PLATE 20.4. This T1 lesion arose from a background of lichen sclerosus and demonstrates the typical irregular surface features and superficial ulceration of a squamous-cell carcinoma. The biopsy site is marked with a suture.

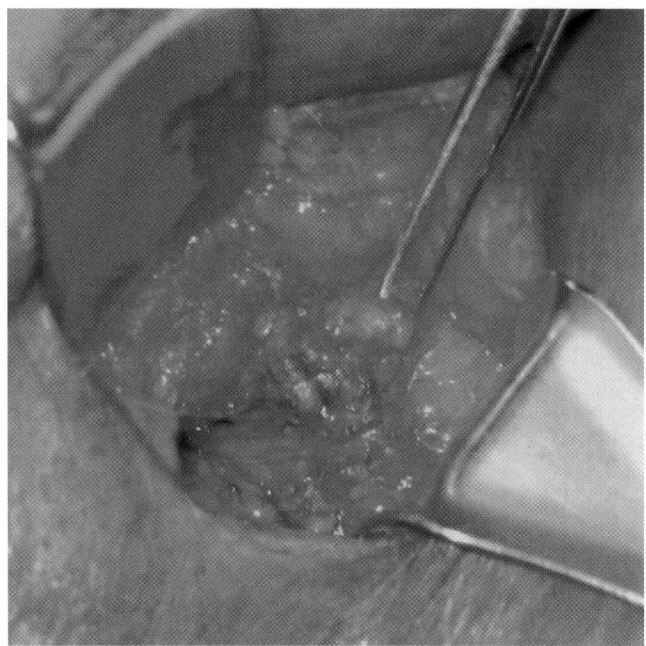

COLOR PLATE 20.17. Following isosulfan blue dye injection, sentinel lymph node biopsy is performed. In this case, the sentinel lymph node is easily identified by the visible presence of dye. (Photo courtesy of Charles Levenback, MD, Houston, TX).

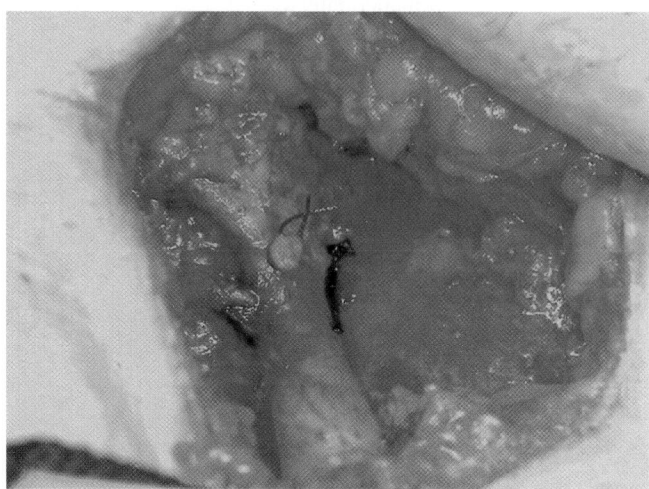

COLOR PLATE 20.21. The patient is undergoing superficial and deep dissection of the right groin nodes. At this point in the procedure, the saphenous vein, which is entering the surgical field from the right lower aspect, has been identified and preserved.

Supine: Transverse Plane

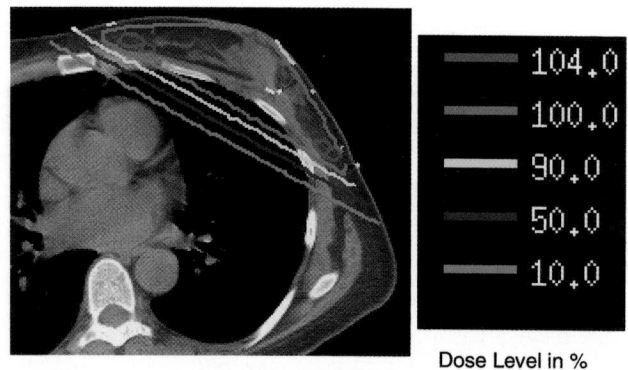

Dose Level in %

COLOR PLATE 30.28. Isodose curves for 6-MV x-rays, displayed in the transverse, sagittal and coronol planes, using IMRT planning. Prescription is to the 100% line. Prone position, compared with supine position, decreases lung dose.

ovulation'' events may lie on the causal path to ovarian cancer (248,249). This is consistent with most of the endocrine-related risk factors except for the risks associated with clinical infertility.

No single theory yet adequately incorporates the available data. A unifying hypothesis may lie in a combination of ovulation, hormones, and local effects. Additional factors, such as genetic alterations; androgens, progestagens, and other hormones (246,250–252); inflammation (173); and endometriosis (253), also appear to be important.

Each hypothesis identifies testable possibilities. Discriminating between the roles of voluntary versus involuntary infertility could identify the mechanisms underlying the role of parity. Characterizing the specific reproductive abnormalities associated with clinical infertility could reveal new biologic mechanisms involved in ovarian carcinogenesis. Determining why hysterectomy and tubal ligation reduce risk could generate insights into the role of gynecologic conditions and ovarian carcinogenesis. Exploring the interactive contributions of the hormones along the hypothalamic-pituitary-gonadal axis could explain how specific hormones seem to influence differentially risk at different time periods. In addition, verifying that inflammation or related conditions and pathways play an etiologic role in ovarian carcinogenesis could open new lines of inquiry.

Ovarian cancer epidemiology presents both simple and complex patterns. Rates have largely remain unchanged over the last 40 years, and virtually all studies show consistent associations with some exposures, such as oral contraceptives, parity, and family history. But where some uncertainty exists, it is substantial. Other reproductive or lifestyle factors that are consistently associated with other reproductive cancers—smoking, obesity, menopausal hormone therapy—have been published with such diversity that traditional attempts to summarize quantitatively the divergent data likely will not prove to be useful. Although it is tempting to attribute the differences to histology-specific associations, such hypotheses will require substantially more epidemiologic, clinical, genetic, and transitional data before their acceptance is certain. Careful a priori attempts to assess systematically the mechanisms of histologic differences may yet prove fruitful.

So where can epidemiology contribute to increasing the opportunities to reduce ovarian cancer's toll? The highly penetrant genes account for only a small proportion (10%) of women who develop ovarian cancer, but a better understanding of the mechanisms behind those risks could introduce immediate benefits for high-risk women. Continued close collaboration between geneticists and epidemiologist should pay dividends. By late 2003, a number of large, well-conducted ovarian cancer studies will be complete or ongoing. A clear picture has emerged for some protective factors, such as oral contraceptives and parity, but risk associated with other important public health issues, such as smoking, obesity, and physical activity, remains uncertain. Continued attempts to account for the differences between studies

should help delineate the spurious associations from the etiologically relevant risk factors. Doing so should help identify targets for improving detection, treatment, and prevention of this deadly tumor.

CERVICAL CANCER

Infection with one of approximately 15 different types of oncogenic human papillomaviruses (HPVs) is a necessary event for the development of cervical carcinoma and its precursors (254–256). Accordingly, the epidemiology of cervical cancer is best understood in terms of the effects that factors exert on the natural history of HPV infection including: (a) exposure/acquisition of infection; (b) persistence of HPV infection and progression to a cancer precursor [cervical intraepithelial neoplasia 3 (CIN3)]; and (c) development of invasion (Fig. 1.4) (257). The epidemiology of HPV infection has profoundly influenced clinical practice in that HPV testing has been used to clarify equivocal cytology (258) and augment primary screening (259,260). Additionally, knowledge regarding HPV has enabled refinement of the Bethesda System for reporting cervical cytology (261) and formulation of evidence-based management guidelines (262). In short, the last decade has witnessed the transformation of HPV epidemiology from a narrow field of research to essential knowledge for gynecologists.

Research on cervical carcinogenesis has focused on the pathogenesis of squamous carcinoma, the numerically predominant histologic tumor type. Accordingly, the bulk of this discussion is related to squamous carcinoma; essential findings for adenocarcinoma will be summarized separately.

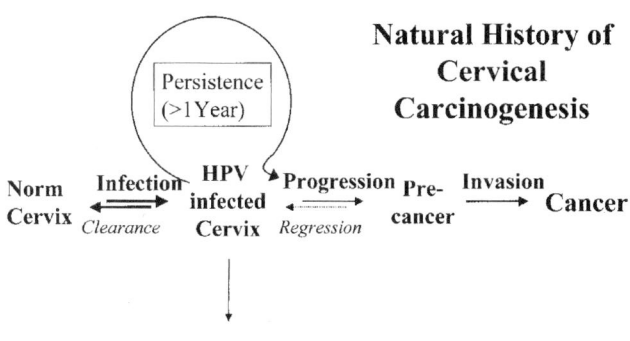

FIG. 1.4. An epidemiologic model of cervical carcinogenesis. The major steps in cervical carcinogenesis are human papillomavirus (HPV) infection (balanced by viral clearance), progression to precancer (partly offset by regression of precancer), and invasion. The persistence of oncogenic HPV types is necessary for progression and invasion. HPV infection is frequently, but not necessarily, associated with cytologic and histologic abnormalities. (From Schiffman M, Kjaer SK: Natural history of anogenital papillomavirus infection and neoplasia. *J Natl Cancer Inst Monogr Source* 2003; (31):14–19, with permission.)

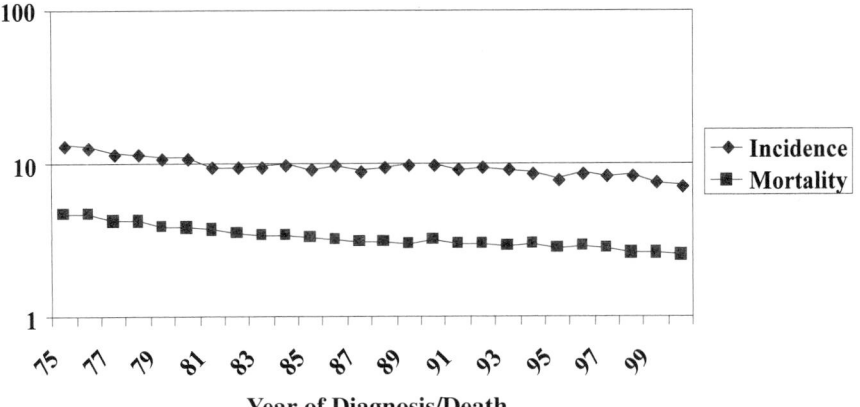

FIG. 1.5. Incidence and mortality trends among U.S. white women for cancer of the cervix uteri. (Data from the Surveillance, Epidemiology and End Results Program, 1975–2000.)

Demographic Patterns

It is estimated that approximately 470,000 women are diagnosed with cervical cancer and 233,000 die of the disease each year, making this tumor a leading cause of cancer death in developing nations throughout the world (263). Whereas rates of cervical cancer have remained stable over time in many poor nations without screening programs, rates have declined steadily in wealthier countries, including the United States (Fig. 1.5). The reason for the decline in rates during the early twentieth century is unknown, but reduced parity may have contributed (264), given that parity appears to be a co-factor for progression of HPV infection to cervical neoplasia. In the latter half of the last century, effective screening contributed to a further reduction in cancer incidence and mortality.

In the United States, approximately 1 in 117 women will develop invasive cervical cancer, resulting in an estimated 12,200 cases during 2003 (2). The average annual age-adjusted incidence for invasive cervical cancer in all SEER areas was 9.6 per 100,000 women for the period 1996 to 2000, with a corresponding age-adjusted mortality rate of 3.0 (2). The 5-year survival rate for cervical cancer is 72%. It is estimated that 4,100 women have died from cervical cancer in the United States in 2003.

Recent SEER data show that squamous carcinomas account for about 73% of cervical cancer, adenocarcinomas for about 14%, and other tumor types for the remainder (265). Age-specific rates for squamous carcinoma declined during this period for black women of all ages and white women 35 years of age and older. Among both blacks and whites, rates for squamous carcinoma *in situ* (CIS) peaked between ages 25 and 34 years, reflecting intensive screening in this age group in the United States. Rates for CIS among whites have increased steadily over this period in association with a reduction in invasive cancers, whereas among blacks, rates for CIS have risen only more recently. Although rates for invasive carcinoma remain higher for blacks than whites, the difference has narrowed over time, with major differences now being observed only among older women (Fig. 1.6). Data comparing clinical factors among blacks and whites suggest that health care disparities contribute to worse outcomes for blacks: Blacks are diagnosed more frequently with advanced stage tumors, they more often do not receive treatment, and when treated are more likely than whites to receive radiation as opposed to surgery (266). Although less data are available for U.S. Hispanics, a recent analysis found that rates for Hispanics are approximately twice that of non-Hispanics irrespective of stage (267).

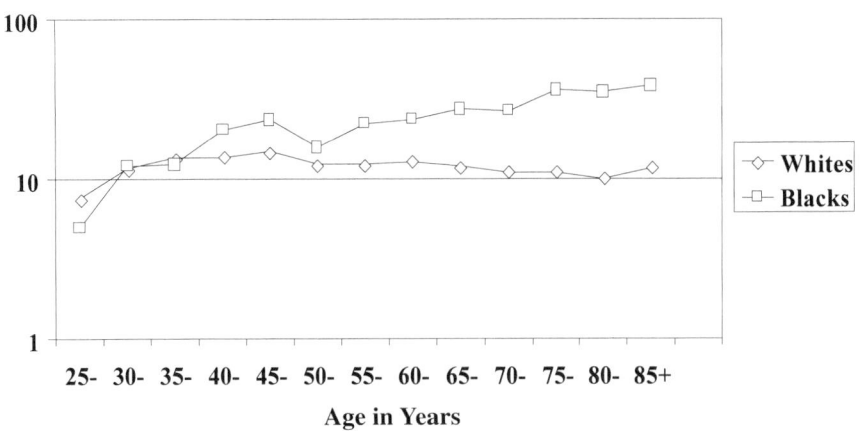

FIG. 1.6. Age-specific incidence of invasive cancer of the cervix uteri by race. (Data from the Surveillance, Epidemiology and End Results Program, 1996–2000.)

Risk Factors

HPV Infection

Proof that HPV is the cause of cervical cancer amassed quickly once accurate tests for detecting HPV DNA, optimized study designs, and improved study endpoints became routine (reviewed in ref. 254). In an international multicenter study involving 1,545 squamous carcinomas, HPV DNA detection was associated with a RR of 83.3 (95% confidence intervals, CI 54.9–105.3). HPVs 16, 18, 31, and 45 were the most common types detected both among cases and controls, with only slight variation in risk among commonly identified oncogenic types. Multiple infections were more frequent among cases than among HPV-positive controls, but did not confer increased risk. A strong association between HPV detection and squamous carcinoma, adenocarcinoma, and CIN3 has been found consistently in case-control studies. Data from prospective cohort studies in which the association between HPV detection at baseline and risk for future development of cervical neoplasia show similarly strong associations (268–271). In a study of 20,000 participants undergoing routine screening, the cumulative incidence ratio of cervical neoplasia among those who tested positive as compared to those who tested negative was 18.1 at 45 months and 8.0 after 120 months of passive follow-up. Cervical neoplasia was identified in 6.9% of women who tested positive at baseline (268).

HPV also shows specific relationships with different diseases, fulfilling another criterion for causality. For example, squamous carcinomas are more closely linked to HPV 16 and related viruses, whereas adenocarcinomas are more strongly associated with HPV 18 and related viruses. Viral infection has been shown to precede the development of disease and HPV type-specific persistence is a prerequisite for tumorigenesis (272,273). Furthermore, biopsy-proven disease has been associated with a higher viral load than subclinical infections (274), and high loads for HPV 16 have been associated with increased risk of neoplasia (275,276).

Sexual Acquisition of HPV

For centuries, anecdotal observations have suggested an association between sexual activity and cervical cancer, but proof that HPV is sexually transmitted was not achieved until sensitive methods for detecting HPV DNA were developed. Subsequently, it was demonstrated that virgins almost invariably test negative for HPV (277,278). A study of 100 virgins found that all but 1 was negative for both HPV DNA and antibodies to HPV 16; the single subject who tested positive demonstrated a weak signal for HPV 6 and had reported sexual contact without penetration (278). The cumulative detection of HPV over 2 years of follow-up among 78 monogamous women in this study was 7.7%.

Evidence linking HPV DNA detection to sexual behavior is compelling (256,279–281); however, the frequency of oc-currence and clinical relevance of vertical transmission have been debated. Rice et al. (282) have estimated that the frequency of perinatal transmission is 69% to 77% and that HPV is detected among at least 20% of children when determined using highly sensitive polymerase chain reaction (PCR)–based assays. They note that parturition leads to massive exposure of the newborn to HPV during passing through an infected birth canal, that ascending infection is possible with ruptured membranes, and that horizontal transmission may also occur. Based on a small longitudinal study, these investigators found HPV persistence in over 50% of subjects after 6 months and in some for 2 years. Failure to detect antibody against HPV in children was attributed to the insensitivity of the assays used or failure of the immature immune systems to mount a serologic response. Alternatively, it has been argued that contamination at the time of sample collection or in the laboratory may yield false-positive PCR results and perinatal immunoglobulin G (IgG) detection in infants may represent transplacental transport of maternal antibodies (283). In support of this, serologic responses have been noted as generally being absent until the age of 2 years, when children begin to develop cutaneous warts, which could provoke cross-reactive serologic responses against genital types. The absence of antibody detection in virgins has also been offered as evidence against the clinical relevance of vertical transmission apart from the rare instances of laryngeal papillomatosis, which mainly result from nononcogenic HPV types.

Numerous case-control and cohort studies have consistently shown that sexual behavior—variously determined as cumulative, new, or recent sexual partners—is the main determinant of incident HPV detection. Among girls and young women, the estimated cumulative incidence of HPV infection after 24 to 36 months of follow-up ranges from 39% to 55% (279–281,284). The vast majority of these infections are with specific oncogenic HPV types. In one report, new infections were identical among virgins and sexually experienced college-aged women (281). Nonpenetrative sexual contact was associated with risk among virgins but not sexually experienced women. In a study of teenagers, each new partner per month was associated with a tenfold increase in the risk of incident HPV detection (280). Risk for HPV detection may plateau among women with a history of many partners; for example, patients in sexually transmitted disease clinics and prostitutes (285).

In studies that have included women of widely varying ages, detection of oncogenic HPV infections declines sharply with increasing age (286,287), which is most likely as a function of acquired immunity (288). However, detection of nononcogenic types may not vary with age (279, 289).

A meta-analysis of studies examining the effect of condom use on HPV transmission and disease outcomes found that their use may afford modest protection against external warts and possibly other cervical lesions, but protection against HPV detection was found in only one of six studies. Given that users of condoms may not report sporadic unprotected contacts, and that the entire skin and mucosal genital area at risk for infection is not protected with this contraceptive method, only modest protection against transmission would be expected (290).

The Male Factor

Studies to increase an understanding of HPV transmission between sexual partners have proved challenging. Contact between women and multiple partners at different times, clearance of infection in one partner but not the other, and difficulties in collecting satisfactory specimens for HPV testing from men all complicate the demonstration of concordant infection among partners (291). Nonetheless, there is evidence that sexual behavior among men is an important determinant of risk, especially in regions with low cancer incidence (reviewed in refs. 292 and 293). Recognized factors supporting this view include the geographic clustering of cervical and penile cancer, the increased risk of cervical cancer among wives of men who have penile cancer, the increased risk among partners of men who have had a previous partner who died of cervical cancer, and the increased risk among women whose partners travel. In Spain, a country which has low cervical cancer rates, the disease was related to several risk factors among husbands including lifetime number of partners, number of contacts with prostitutes, early age at first intercourse, smoking, positive serology for *Chlamydia trachomatis*, and a history of oral or anal sex. Detection of oncogenic HPV DNA among men conferred a sevenfold risk of cervical cancer among their partners. Data for cervical cancer risk among monogamous women showed similar relationships for their partners. In contrast, data from Colombia, a country with an extremely high rate of cervical cancer in which men have many more sexual partners and contact with prostitutes than in Spain, risk was related only to lack of education and seropositivity for *C. trachomatis* among men. In combination, data from Spain and Colombia suggest that in some countries with high cervical cancer rates, sexually active women are at such a high risk for HPV exposure, acquisition of HPV is probably a weaker determinant of cancer risk than factors associated with progression. An international study reported that circumcision was associated with a reduced risk of HPV detection in penile samples, and that the wives of men with a history multiple partners were at lower risk of cervical cancer if the men had been circumcised (294).

Co-Factors for Persistence and Progression

Transient HPV infections are ubiquitous among sexually active young women, but progression to a cervical cancer precursor requires persistence of oncogenic types (271,284, 295–297). This has prompted epidemiologic studies to investigate "co-factors" that influence persistence. These studies pose many challenges: (a) identifying large stable cohorts that can be followed with repeated measurements for years; (b) performing repeated HPV testing and typing; (c) measuring exposures accurately; and (d) accommodating loss of progression due to censoring of lesions by treatment. To date, a widely accepted definition of persistence has not been developed; repeated detection of the same HPV type is common to all criteria, but minimum duration, assay sensitivity, and analytical considerations vary among researchers. Many women with persistent HPV infections have repeatedly abnormal cytology, leading to censoring for minor lesions. Persistence and progression to CIN3 occur concurrently, complicating the independent examination of these two processes. Based on a statistical model, Myers et al. concluded that the incidence of HPV infection and the rate of progression of HPV infections to high-grade lesions produce the greatest impact on age-specific cervical cancer incidence (298).

HPV Type and Viral Load. Oncogenic types, HPV 16 in particular, have a stronger tendency to persist than types not associated with cancer (284,295,299). Furthermore, intratypic sequence variants of HPV 16 and possibly HPVs 18 and 58 may confer different risks for cervical cancer. Non-European variants of HPV 16 in particular have been associated with a higher risk than European variants, although the latter do confer considerable cancer risk (reviewed in ref. 300). The role of elevated viral load (i.e., HPV content in samples obtained from infected women) in predicting persistence and progression of infection is debatable. Women with biopsy-proven lesions generally have higher HPV load than women with clinically occult infections (274). However, the high variable range of load (even within each grade of CIN) limits clinical utility (274,301). Several studies have associated higher loads of HPV 16 with high-grade CIN (301,302), and limited data suggest that high loads of HPV 16 increase the risk of subsequent high-grade CIN (276).

Although studies suggest that women with prevalent infections may be more likely to acquire additional infections, infection with one HPV type does not seem to influence the risk of persistence (303,304). In addition, the state of the virus (integrated into human host DNA vs episomal), methylation status, and transcript levels for the oncogenes E6 and E7 may also be associated with risk of persistence and subsequent neoplasia.

Host Factors. Human leukocyte antigens (HLAs) are important determinants of the efficiency of antigen presentation to immune effector cells and, therefore, may influence the outcome of HPV infections. A protective association with HLA DRB1*13 and/or DQB1*603 has been found consistently among studies, whereas specific HLA class II markers of increased risk have not been identified (reviewed in ref. 300). Data for risk associations with polymorphic variants of HLA class I antigens are sparse; a protective association with HLA C*0202 was reported in an analysis combining data from three diverse populations (305).

Whereas humoral immunity appears to play a central role in preventing HPV infection, elimination of HPV seems more closely related to mounting an effective cellular immune response (306–308). Variation in receptor variants on natural killer cells may represent an important source of genetically influenced risk; this topic, however, has not been adequately explored, in part because the required assays are technically challenging.

Impaired cellular immunity, attributable to human immunodeficiency virus (HIV) infection, transplantation, or immunosuppressive drugs, has been shown to increase HPV persistence, warts, CIN, and cancer (309–311). In contrast, deficiencies in humoral immunity appear unrelated to these conditions. The U.S. Centers for Disease Control and Prevention (CDC) has identified cervical cancer as an autoimmune deficiency syndrome (AIDS)–defining illness among women infected with HIV. Compared to the general population, women with AIDS have a fivefold excess risk of carcinoma *in situ* of the cervix, with risk increasing over time (312). Although risk was similarly elevated for invasive cancers, rates did not increase over time, suggesting that HIV infection probably has a limited impact on the transition from in situ to invasive disease. Although highly active antiretroviral therapy (HAART) improves CD4 levels, this has not been associated with regression of cervical cancer precursors (313).

In a cross-sectional study, HPV DNA was detected in cervical lavages among 63% of HIV-positive women as compared to 30% of high-risk HIV-negative women (313). Patients with peripheral CD4 counts below 200/mm^3 were at highest risk for HPV infection; above this level of CD4 detection, high levels of HIV viral load represented an additional risk factor for HPV DNA detection. Both HIV-negative and HIV-positive women were infected with a similarly broad range of HPV types, but multiple infections were found in 36% of HIV-infected patients as compared to 12% of HIV-uninfected women. HPV detection among HIV-positive women was associated with measures of lifetime HPV exposure but not recent exposures, suggesting that the high prevalence of HPV among HIV-positive women reflects increased HPV persistence rather than acquisition compared to HIV-negative women. Data from a cohort of high-risk women support this view; persistence was detected among 24% of HIV-positive women as compared to 4% of HIV-negative patients (311). In this cohort, the risk of new HPV infections was 11 per 100 examinations among HIV-positive women as compared to 9 per 100 visits among HIV-negative patients. Results of a meta-analysis suggested that HIV infection increases the risk of CIN among women who are HPV positive (314).

Parity. High parity has been associated with an increased risk of cervical neoplasia in multiple studies. In one multicenter study, seven or more full-term pregnancies were associated with nearly a fourfold increased risk for cervical cancer (315). Risks for cervical neoplasia generally persist when analyses are restricted to HPV-infected women. Some studies have failed to identify an association of cervical disease with parity (316,317), possibly reflecting overall low parity in these populations (318). Mechanisms underlying the association between parity and cervical neoplasia include trauma during parturition, hormonal changes associated with pregnancy, immunosuppression, and possibly altered anatomy of the transformation zone, specifically eversion. Other menstrual and reproductive factors, including miscarriages, abortions, stillbirths, ectopic pregnancies, cesarean sections, age at first pregnancy, age at menarche, and age at menopause, have not generally been associated with risk (315,319).

Cigarette Smoking. Geographic correlations of lung cancer in men and cervical cancer prompted the suggestion that smoking may relate to the risk of cervical neoplasia (320). Numerous studies have now confirmed an association, and in many the relationship has persisted after careful control for sexual behavior and HPV DNA detection. A review of over 50 studies concluded that smoking was a co-factor for HPV infection in the development of cervical cancer, and several recent reports have suggested that smoking approximately doubles the risk of cervical neoplasia among HPV-infected women, often with a demonstrable dose-response effect (321). Based on a multivariate analysis of a large cohort followed for up to 10 years, Castle et al. (317) found that HPV-positive women who smoked at least a pack of cigarettes per day experienced a fourfold increased risk for cervical neoplasia compared to nonsmokers. A similar strong dose-response relationship was found in another cohort study (322). Based on photographic assessment of lesion size among participants in a smoking-essation study, Szarewski et al. (323) found evidence of regression among 82% of women who stopped or markedly reduced their smoking for 6 months as compared to 28% of those who continued to smoke. Analysis of HPV DNA detection in a cohort of young women found that smokers maintained their infections longer than nonsmokers and had a reduced probability of clearing oncogenic HPV types (324).

A number of mechanisms could mediate the risk of cervical neoplasia associated with smoking (reviewed in ref. 321). These include the fact that cervical mucus contains both cotinine and nicotine, which can be converted to carcinogenic nitrosamines, with some studies showing concentrations exceeding those in serum. Smoking also increases the production of free radicals, which may be of magnified importance because smokers are relatively deficient in antioxidants. Data have also suggested that smoking may reduce both local and systemic immune functions.

Oral Contraceptives. The relationship of oral contraceptives to cervical neoplasia is difficult to study because sexually active women who are not using oral contraceptives and are not pregnant generally use alternative birth control measures, which may also modify risks for HPV infection, persistence, and /or progression. In addition, the ectropion associated with exogenous progesterone use may increase the vulnerability of the transformation zone to neoplastic influences, but also potentially increase the sensitivity of HPV DNA detection and cytologic screening. The use of oral contraceptives for at least 5 years has been shown to be related to over threefold significant increases in cervical neoplasia risk (325). Longer duration and recent use were most strongly related to risk, whereas risk declined to that of nonusers after cessation for 6 years. However, studies have not generally shown that ever or prolonged use of contraceptives is associated with HPV detection (326). These data have been interpreted as suggesting a promotional role for oral contraceptives. However, some studies have not found an association between cervical neoplasia and oral contraceptive use, including a recent analysis of data from a large cohort (317). Whereas case-control studies may suffer from detection biases (increased surveillance among birth control pill users compared to nonusers), cohort analyses also have acknowledged limitations. Some of the postulated mechanisms that could account for the possible risk of using birth control pills are similar to those related to the hormonal effects of pregnancy.

Other Co-Factors. Bosch et al. (254) concluded that HPV infection associated with one or more leading candidate cofactors (pregnancy, smoking, and oral contraceptive use) accounts for about 75% of cervical cancer, whereas in 25% of cases HPV has been implicated, but HPV co-factors have not been identified. Other factors that may influence the outcome of an HPV infection include diet, nutrition, unidentified genetic factors, and possibly other sexually transmitted diseases. One study found that inflammation in the cervix might represent a co-factor independent of the inciting cause, which might help clarify discrepancies in findings for different infectious agents (327).

Progression of HPV Infection

Although some data suggest slight differences between women who test HPV positive and have normal cytology as compared to those who have a low-grade squamous intraepithelial lesion (280), women with either of these conditions have a strong tendency to convert to HPV negative, especially if they are young. Results from the ASCUS Low-Grade Squamous Intraepithelial Lesion Triage Study (ALTS) found a similar risk of progression for women with histologic CIN1 and those with negative colposcopic examinations and/or biopsies (328). Data from a natural history study and inferred findings from ALTS suggest that whereas a substantial proportion of CIN2 lesions regress (329,330), CIN3 lesions tend to persist, at least in short follow-up. A meta-analysis found that HPV types associated with high-grade squamous intraepithelial lesions (HSILs) and carcinoma differ; in HSILs, types 31, 33, 52, and 58 (so-called ''intermediate-risk'' types) predominate, whereas in carci-

noma, types 16, 18, and 45 are more prevalent. Similarly, preliminary findings suggest that cytologic CIN2 is more strongly associated with intermediate-risk types than CIN3 and carcinoma, perhaps indicating that HPV typing may predict the risk of cancer in women with CIN2. Epidemiologic risk factors for women with CIN3 and carcinoma are similar. However, the wide difference in ages between women with CIN3 and those with carcinoma and the observation that microinvasion is uncommon in the absence of extensive CIN3 argue that progression from precursor to invasive tumor occurs slowly.

Cervical Adenocarcinoma

Interpreting rates for cervical adenocarcinomas over time poses challenges because of gradual improvements in clinical practices (including the use of devices to obtain better endocervical sampling), stricter criteria for adequate Pap tests, development of cytologic criteria for recognizing adenocarcinoma in situ (AIS), and recently, formal inclusion of the AIS category in the new Bethesda System (261). Incidence rates for invasive adenocarcinoma increased among whites in the interval 1988 to 2000 compared to 1976 to 1987, whereas rates for blacks have remained steady (265). Although rates for AIS rose among both blacks and whites from 1976 to 2000, rates for invasive adenocarcinomas have not declined in parallel. Proposed explanations for these upward trends include increased rates of HPV infection without improved cytologic detection of AIS, a specific increase in rates of HPV 18 infection (which accounts for a relatively higher percentage of adenocarcinomas as compared to squamous carcinomas), and increased exposure to HPV co-factors. Madeleine et al. (331) noted that the increased incidence of AIS in the United States was most notable among women born after 1945, which coincided with widespread use of oral contraceptives and increased numbers of reported sexual contacts.

Studies using refined assays have detected HPV DNA in over 90% of common invasive cervical adenocarcinomas; extremely rare types such as clear cell, serous, and mesonephric may be unrelated to HPV (254,332). HPV has also been identified in approximately 87% of population-based cases of AIS using fixed tissue, which may represent an underestimate of the true prevalence secondary to DNA degradation (331). In contrast to squamous carcinomas, the prevalence of HPV 18 in adenocarcinomas approximately equals that of HPV 16 (254,332). Whereas cytologic screening is highly protective for squamous carcinoma, a history of a negative cytologic examination provides limited risk reduction for adenocarcinoma. Mitchell et al. (333), reporting data from a large population-based registry, found that the protective effect of a history of a reportedly negative smear was entirely eliminated after 2 years, and never exceeded a modest relative protection of 1.6. Retrospective studies have found that the sensitivity of a single smear for

AIS was about 50% and only slightly higher for invasive adenocarcinoma (334,335). The cytologic recognition of AIS is notoriously difficult; incomplete sampling of lesions high in the endocervical canal or largely confined to deep endocervical invaginations, unfamiliarity with the morphology, and overlap with benign conditions pose serious problems (334–337). Hildesheim et al. (338) found that young white women with adenocarcinoma and adenosquamous carcinoma were overrepresented among patients who developed apparently rapid-onset diseases, defined mainly as a negative Pap smear within five years of diagnosis (confirmed on review) and the development of cancer within 10 years of initiation of sexual activity. Others, citing SEER data showing a difference of 13 years in the mean age of AIS and invasive adenocarcinoma, have argued that effective screening for preclinical glandular neoplasms should be possible (339).

Although our understanding of the etiology of cervical adenocarcinoma is incomplete, a picture is emerging in which adenocarcinoma seems to share some risk factors with cervical squamous carcinomas (acquisition of HPV through sexual contact) and others with uterine carcinoma (a tumor etiologically related to hormones). Two strongly linked factors for squamous carcinoma, parity and smoking, have not been shown to increase the risk for adenocarcinoma (340–342), in fact there is some evidence that both factors might be associated with decreases in risk. In contrast, increased weight (or related measures) appears to be related to increases in the risk of cervical adenocarcinomas (341, 343,344). Oral contraceptives have been linked to an increase risk for AIS or adenocarcinoma in a number of studies (267,331,341,345,346). In some studies, the association was strongest for long-term users (267,331,346) and in one study, young age at first usage, recent or current use, and high progesterone content were also related to risk. The increased risk of cervical adenocarcinoma associated with obesity and reduced risk with parity and smoking resemble the epidemiology of endometrial adenocarcinoma. However, the relationship between cervical adenocarcinoma and oral contraceptives is more similar to reported results for squamous carcinomas of the cervix. The association between estrogen replacement therapy and increased risk for adenocarcinoma has been inconsistent (347,348) and use of depo-medroxy-progesterone did not increase risk in one report (349).

As cancer control improves for squamous carcinoma in countries with screening programs, the proportion and relative importance of detecting AIS will increase. Additional studies that include pathologic review and HPV testing are needed. Recent findings suggest that endocervical adenocarcinomas infrequently express receptors for estrogen and progesterone even though normal endocervical epithelium does (350,351). Historical reports of receptor expression in the majority of these tumors may reflect misclassification of endometrial adenocarcinomas as endocervical tumors and problems with receptor assays. Expert review of cases, re-ceptor assays, and HPV testing using in situ hybridization or other molecular assays applied to microdissected samples may be needed to accurately classify some cases.

Conclusions

Knowledge of the epidemiology of HPV and its causal role in cervical carcinogenesis has been successfully translated into clinical practice (259). In many developed countries, women with equivocal cytology are tested for HPV DNA; a negative result provides strong reassurance that immediate follow-up is not required and can reduce patient anxiety and health costs (352). Comparison of HPV test results with cytologic interpretations provides important quality assurance for both tests (353,354). Repeated HPV testing is also finding application in following women without intervention and in determining the risk of recurrence among those treated for CIN. HPV testing as an adjunct to primary screening has been adopted in the United States, and screening studies are underway to develop new optimized approaches that focus resources on at-risk women (260). Finally, encouraging early results from vaccine trials suggest that primary prevention of HPV infection may be possible, potentially allowing eradication of cervical cancer in even the poorest nations of the world (355).

VULVAR CANCER

Demographic Patterns

Carcinoma of the vulva is a rare genital neoplasm with an average annual age-adjusted incidence in all SEER areas during 1996 to 2000 of 2.2 per 100,000 women (2). During 2003, an estimated 4,000 women will develop the disease and 800 will die as a consequence of it. Although vulvar cancer has been noted in clinical series to occur frequently among blacks, recent incidence data do not support any substantial differences in incidence by race. The disease occurs primarily in older women.

Cancer of the vulva occurs significantly more frequently among women with primary cancers of the cervix, and the two diseases often occur simultaneously (356,357). Approximately 15% to 20% of women with vulvar cancer have a second primary cancer occurring simultaneously or nonsimultaneously in the cervix, vagina, or anogenital area. As many as 10% to 15% of women with cancer of the vulva have a second primary lesion of the cervix. When multiple primaries are not diagnosed simultaneously, cancer of the cervix usually precedes cancer of the vulva. Many patients with vulvar cancer have multifocal genital lesions, commonly including a mixture of condyloma acuminatum planum and intraepithelial neoplasia. They may also have similar changes at other anogenital sites, including the vagina, cervix, and perianal region (358).

SEER incidence data indicate nearly a doubling in the rate

of vulvar cancer between 1973 and 1976 and 1985 and 1987 (359). This is in contrast to rates of invasive squamous cell carcinomas, which have remained relatively stable. Given that *in situ* cancers develop on average significantly earlier than invasive vulvar cancers, it may be that changes in certain risk factors (e.g., increased sexual activity) may have been too recent in order for effects to be seen for invasive cancers. Alternatively, successful treatment of *in situ* tumors may have prevented the occurrence of invasive disease. A third explanation for the patterns observed is that there may be etiologic differences, with HPV being more important for *in situ* cancers (360).

Risk Factors

HPV

Similar to cervical cancer, vulvar cancer has been strongly linked with HPV infections. Early case-control studies reported higher risks among women reporting multiple sexual partners (361,362). Subsequent studies postulated a role for HPV in the etiology of the tumors, finding high rates of detection of the virus in vulvar tumor tissue and high subsequent disease risks among patients with seropositive tests to HPV 16 (363–365). HPV type 16 appears to be the most predominant type detected among vulvar cancer patients (254).

Findings of elevated risks of vulvar cancer associated with cigarette smoking (361,365–367) have prompted several studies to examine interactions with HPV infection status. Two studies have found particularly high risks associated with HPV seropositivity among cigarette smokers, suggesting that the effect of HPV may depend on smoking as a cofactor (364,365).

Other Factors

Although the incidence of vulvar cancer has been discussed in relation to social class, results from one case-control study indicated that control for sexual factors eliminated this effect (361). Suggestions that the risk of vulvar cancer is elevated among nulliparous women and those with late ages at first birth were also not confirmed in this study.

Vulvar carcinomas often arise within genital warts, but more specific temporal associations between the two remain unclear. Several studies have suggested that a history of vulvar warts is associated with an elevated risk of vulvar cancer, with RRs ranging from 15 to 23 (361,368). In one study, a particularly high risk was associated with multiple episodes of genital warts, possibly reflecting poor immunologic response among these women (361).

Several clinical studies have suggested that vulvar cancer may be elevated among women with diabetes, obesity, or hypertension, but this has not been confirmed in the one epidemiologic study assessing these factors (361). An excess

risk of vulvar cancer among users of oral contraceptives was found in one study but not in another (361,367).

Recent attention has focused on the possible etiologic role of genetic factors. Although it has been hypothesized that some carcinogen-metabolizing genes might be involved, particularly those involved in the metabolism of cigarette smoke, studies have failed to find relationships of risk with either glutathione S-transferase (GST) or debrisoquine 4-hydroxylase (CYP2D6) genetic polymorphisms (369,370).

Most epidemiologic studies have focused on vulvar cancer as one disease entity, but tumors of different histologies may have distinctive etiologies. Basaloid and warty carcinomas have risk factor profiles similar to those of cervical cancer (including strong relationships with HPV), whereas keratinizing squamous carcinomas are less strongly linked to these factors (360). Vulvar intraepithelial neoplasias show risk factors that resemble basaloid and warty carcinomas.

Conclusions

The cervix and vulva are covered by squamous-cell epithelium with a common embryologic origin from the cloacogenic membrane. These similarities have led to the theory that the entire lower genital tract responds to various carcinogens as a single tissue field, resulting in a relatively high proportion of multicentric squamous carcinomas (371). The multicentric nature of the disease; its association with cervical, vaginal, and perianal malignancies; and several risk factors common to it and cervical cancer suggest that the etiologic mechanisms for vulvar and cervical cancer may be similar.

VAGINAL CANCER

Demographic Patterns

Cancer of the vagina is also rare, with an average annual age-adjusted incidence of 0.7 per 100,000 women in the SEER areas for the period from 1996 to 2000 (2). The incidence is higher for blacks than for whites, but the reasons for the discrepancy are unknown. During 2003, it is estimated that 2,000 women will develop the disease and 800 will die from it (2). The average 5-year survival rate is 46% for whites. Seventy-five percent of vaginal cancers are squamous-cell carcinomas, and they usually occur in the upper part of the vagina.

Vaginal cancer is primarily a disease of older women, with almost 60% occurring among women 60 years of age or older. In the past, carcinoma of the vagina was only rarely reported in infants and children but, beginning in the late 1960s, cases of clear-cell adenocarcinoma of the vagina, an uncommon cancer in any age group, began to be observed with much greater frequency than expected among women between 15 and 22 years of age. Most of these cases have been related to prenatal exposure to diethylstilbestrol (DES).

Risk Factors

The rarity of vaginal cancer has limited the conduct of definitive epidemiologic investigations. One case-control study of vaginal cancer, based on relatively few cases, found associations of risk with low socioeconomic status, histories of genital warts or other genital irritations, and previous abnormal Pap smears (372). A more recent and larger study linked risk with histories of multiple sexual partners, early ages at first intercourse, and current cigarette smoking (373). Epidemiologic studies have also shown high risks associated with prior hysterectomies, although this apparently is due to the predisposition of women with anogenital cancers (particularly those with cervical cancer) subsequently to develop vaginal cancers (373).

Findings that vaginal cancer is frequently found as a synchronous or a metachronous neoplasm with cervical cancer have led to the suggestion that there may be shared etiologic features between vaginal and cervical cancers. HPV has been related to disease risk through findings of HPV antigens or DNA in vaginal cancer tissue. In the largest study of this issue, HPV DNA was found in tumor blocks in over 80% of patients with *in situ* and over 60% of patients with invasive cancers (373). In addition, serologic antibodies to HPV have been linked to subsequent disease risk (363).

Diethylstilbestrol and Clear-Cell Adenocarcinomas

In 1971, seven clear-cell carcinomas of the vagina and one closely related endometrioid carcinoma developed in young women (ages 15 to 22 years) (374). An epidemiologic study found that the mothers of seven of the eight women had taken DES during the first trimester of pregnancy as opposed to none of the mothers of 32 matched controls. The relationship between DES exposure *in utero* and adenocarcinoma of the vagina was soon confirmed in New York State and at the Mayo Clinic (375,376). Since then, a registry of clear-cell cancer of the vagina and cervix has been established, and many more cases have been reported (377). Among these patients, about twice as many have clear-cell adenocarcinoma of the vagina as have clear-cell adenocarcinoma of the cervix.

Data from the Adenocarcinoma Registry revealed that most patients have been diagnosed between 14 and 23 years of age, with a peak at 19 years of age. This relatively narrow age range suggests that, in addition to DES exposure, some factors associated with the onset of puberty are necessary for the development of the cancer. Recent follow-up of three DES cohorts has found some cases developing at older ages, through age 29, but no cases after age 30 years (378). This latest follow-up has derived estimates that the risk of developing clear-cell adenocarcinoma of the vagina and cervix before 29 years of age is 1.5 per 1,000 DES-exposed daughters. Thus, DES exposure leads to a large relative increase in risk, but it affects only a small proportion of all exposed women. It remains to be seen what risk will be encountered by women when they reach their fifties and sixties, the peak ages of adenocarcinomas of the vagina in women unexposed to DES.

Conclusions

Even less is known about risk factors for vaginal cancer in the elderly than is known for vulvar cancer. However, it appears from limited data that further attention should focus on the role of sexually transmitted agents, specifically the HPVs. The rare occurrence of vaginal adenocarcinoma in young women is essentially an iatrogenic disease related to *in utero* exposure to DES and other estrogens. A proposed mechanism involves nests of abnormal cells of müllerian duct origin, which are stimulated by endogenous hormones during puberty and promoted into adenocarcinomas.

GESTATIONAL TROPHOBLASTIC DISEASES

Gestational trophoblastic diseases (GTDs) (which include hydatidiform moles, invasive moles, and choriocarcinoma) encompass a range of interrelated conditions characterized by abnormal growth of chorionic tissues with various propensities for local invasion and metastasis (379). Hydatidiform moles can be either complete or partial and have distinctive pathologies and etiologies. Complete moles have paternally derived nuclear DNA but maternally derived cytoplasmic DNA. In contrast, partial moles generally have a triploid karyotype, with the extra haploid set of chromosomes being of paternal origin.

Demographic Patterns

Choriocarcinoma is a rare malignancy in the United States, with a reported incidence in all SEER areas of 0.2 per 100,000 women, or approximately 1 per 22,623 live births (380). Hydatidiform mole occurs about once in every 1000 pregnancies, and approximately one of six occurrences results in invasive complications (either invasive mole or choriocarcinoma). Trophoblastic diseases have been reported to be more common in certain parts of the world, although some of the differences may be due to a variety of selection, detection, and reporting biases (381), including whether risk is expressed in relation to women at risk, conceptions, or live births.

The epidemiologic study of choriocarcinoma has been complicated by its relative infrequency. Most studies have, therefore, focused on defining risk factors for hydatidiform moles, but it is uncertain the extent to which these findings can be extrapolated to malignant trophoblastic disease.

Risk Factors

Host Factors

Trophoblastic disease rates are considerably higher in Asian and African countries, but the true extent of difference from Western rates is difficult to decipher because of variations in reporting practices. A recent survey in Britain showed that the incidence of gestational trophoblastic diseases in Asians was nearly twice as high as among non-Asians (382). One incidence survey in the United States showed that, even after adjustment for age and birth distribution effects, blacks had a 2.1-fold greater risk and other nonwhite races had a 1.8-fold greater risk than whites (380). American Indians have also recently been shown to have high rates of GTDs (383).

One clearly established risk factor for choriocarcinoma and hydatidiform mole is maternal age. A recent study showed women at extreme maternal ages (either very early or late) to have nearly twofold elevated rates, with even further age differences noted for the occurrence of complete moles (382).

Two studies have found an association between blood group A and choriocarcinoma (384,385). The combination of mother's group A and father's group O generated over a tenfold increased risk. Blood groups A and AB were associated with elevated risks of hydatidiform mole in one study but not in another (386,387). These findings may support a role for genetic factors or immunologic factors related to the histocompatibility of maternal and trophoblastic tissues.

Menstrual and Reproductive Factors

In several studies that have adjusted for the effects of late maternal age, parous women have remained at a substantially reduced risk of hydatidiform mole compared with nulliparous women, with some evidence of further reductions in risk with multiple births (386,388,389). Several studies found an increased risk associated with a prior spontaneous abortion, although this was not consistently observed (386, 388–390). An increased risk of hydatidiform mole was associated with induced abortions, although information was not available on reasons for the terminations (388). A history of infertility has also been suggested as a risk factor for gestational trophoblastic disease, although not confirmed in all studies (386,388,390). In one study, Chinese patients reporting the use of herbal medicines during the first trimester of a previous pregnancy were at elevated risk (388).

Low body mass, unrelated to dieting or exercise, has been reported as a risk factor for choriocarcinoma in one study (391). Patients also had later onset of menarche and lighter menstrual periods than controls, possibly reflecting lower estrogen levels.

Exogenous Hormones

Several studies have found an increased risk of trophoblastic diseases associated with long-term use of oral contraceptives (388,392–395). Two other case-control studies, however, found no influence of oral contraceptives on risk (386,390). In one study, the association was considerably stronger for partial than complete moles (394). Others have suggested that oral contraceptives may increase the risk of malignant sequelae after mole evacuation through a tumor-stimulating effect (396,397). In one study, this effect was restricted to users of high-dose estrogens, although in others, there were no effects of the pill on postmolar complications (392,398,399).

Other Risk Factors

Late paternal age was suggested in one study to increase the risk of trophoblastic diseases, but other investigations failed to confirm this (386,388,400). Cigarette smoking has also been linked with the occurrence of trophoblastic disease (390). One study suggested that low carotene intake affected the risk of hydatidiform mole, but no specific dietary associations were observed in another study (388,392).

Conclusions

Although a genetic role in the development of hydatidiform mole is now certain, little is known about genotypes that predispose to hydatidiform mole or environmental factors that may increase the risk of defective ova. Except for the possible role of oral contraceptives, few potential environmental promoters have been identified.

The trophoblast plays an active role in pregnancy, including metabolizing and detoxifying xenobiotic substances, regulating nutrient and waste product transfer, synthesizing steroid and protein hormones, and controlling the immune response of the maternofetal unit. Injury to the trophoblast can occur in pregnancy as a result of environmental exposure (e.g., heavy metals and polycyclic hydrocarbons), resulting in the breakdown of trophoblastic processes. When the trophoblast malfunctions, mutagenic, teratogenic, lethotoxic, and carcinogenic compounds gain access to the developing embryo, causing injury and death. The genotype of hydatidiform mole results in a trophoblast that malfunctions, and exposure to certain environmental agents during the molar pregnancy may promote choriocarcinoma. Before implantation, the trophoblast forms most of the embryonic tissue, which already metabolizes environmental agents. Even preimplanted moles, with their impaired metabolic capabilities, may increase the toxicity of environmental agents and promote carcinogenesis.

Recent advances in identifying genetic and molecular markers involved with partial versus complete moles (379) open a number of avenues for assessing the interaction of these markers with a variety of proposed environmental risk factors. This could include a focus on early stages in the disease process or on factors involved in the progression of molar pregnancies to more invasive complications.

SUMMARY

The goal of both medical practice and epidemiology is to reduce morbidity and mortality. For many diseases, the focus has turned to the ultimate aim of prevention. The link between identification of etiologic factors and possibilities for prevention is well illustrated for tobacco- and alcohol-related tumors and for those associated with specific pharmaceutical, radiogenic, and occupational exposures. Fortunately, for gynecologic cancers, there are a number of identified etiologic factors that are also amenable to preventive approaches.

Undoubtedly, the prospects for prevention are best for cervical cancer. For some time, secondary prevention in the form of screening for pathologic precursors of invasive disease has been the hallmark of the public health approach to this malignancy. The establishment of HPV as a central etiologic agent for the disease presents other avenues for prevention, including application of recently developed vaccines against the virus (355). Knowledge of when and how infection and other factors operate in the natural history of the disease has revolutionized screening strategies and shifted treatment from cell ablation to antiviral therapies. As always, combined laboratory, clinical, and epidemiologic research is needed to realize these propositions.

Many believe that more is known about the cause of endometrial carcinoma than for almost any other tumor. A unified theory of how all risk factors may operate through a final common estrogenic pathway is popular and well supported. A woman's hormonal milieu may prove to be favorable to modification at a practical level. There is substantial evidence that elimination of obesity and a reduction in fat in the diet—two interventions actively promoted for other reasons—should also reduce endometrial cancer risk. After the epidemic of endometrial cancer due to estrogen replacement therapy, changes in the management of menopause occurred, resulting in a marked decline in the rates of endometrial cancer. More care is devoted to identifying women who truly need estrogen therapy, treatment of menopausal symptoms is for a much shorter period of time, the use of cyclic progestin in combination with estrogen is advised if indicated, and regular endometrial sampling is frequently practiced for long-term estrogen users.

Although past alterations in patient management led to a decline in endometrial cancer, current events make future patterns less clear. Previous enthusiasm for long-term treatment of large segments of the population of menopausal women with hormones to control symptoms and prevent osteoporosis and heart disease may have implications for endometrial cancer in the future. On the other hand, current patterns of use of oral contraceptives could lead to reductions in endometrial cancer rates in the general population. The impact of widespread oral contraceptive use at young ages on endometrial cancer risk at older ages is not well studied. However, if it is anywhere near the reduced risk seen at young ages, the resulting reduction in endometrial cancer overall could be substantial.

With further research, it is also possible that pharmacologic interventions aimed specifically at groups at high risk

for endometrial cancer due to endogenous hormonal factors could be justified. More must be learned about the associations of risk for endometrial cancer and the quantitative levels of estrogens and other hormones and their relative proportions. Once these factors are known, women with polycystic ovarian disease, diabetes, morbid obesity, or other predisposing conditions could be evaluated for unfavorable hormone profiles and appropriately targeted for treatment.

Although a substantial amount has been learned about ovarian cancer risks, the prospects for meaningful preventive measures aimed at this tumor are probably worse than for the other gynecologic malignancies. Although several ovarian cancer risk factors seem to indict ovulatory activity as a common pathway to increased risk, the mechanism by which this occurs is unknown. Even if some of the hypothesized mechanisms prove to be correct (e.g., levels of circulating gonadotropins), it is unclear how reasonable any interventions may be. However, if the long-term effect of oral contraceptive use on ovarian cancer risk is similar to its short-term effect, a substantial decline in ovarian cancer rates should result from pill use patterns of the past 40 years. Another reason for the limited prospects for prevention is that for several risk factors (e.g., protection associated with hysterectomy), no credible mechanism has been suggested. The associations promising the greatest opportunities for preventive actions are several recently suggested dietary relationships; specifically, decreased risks with consumption of diets high in fruit and vegetable and certain micronutrients. However, these observations need to be replicated in additional studies. Because of the preventive implications, attempts at confirmation should have high priority.

For cervical cancer, endometrial cancer, and ovarian cancer, much is known about the risk factors. Less is known about the precise biologic mechanisms through which the known risk factors operate. There is substantial enthusiasm for current interdisciplinary studies that incorporate state of the art laboratory assays into robust epidemiologic research designs focused on answering these mechanistic questions. Even among some of the more conservative etiologists, there is a belief that the gynecologic oncologist may soon be able to intervene much earlier in the natural history of these diseases, and in some instances, engage in primary prevention.

REFERENCES

1. Jemal A, Murray T, Samuels A, et al. Cancer statistics, 2003. *CA Cancer J Clin* 2003;53(1):5–26.
2. Ries LAG, Eisner MP, Kosary CL, et al. *SEER Cancer Statistics Review 1975–2000*. http://seer.cancer.gov/csr/1975 2000. Bethesda, MD: National Cancer Institute, 2000.
3. Parkin DM, Pisani P, Ferlay J. Global cancer statistics. *CA Cancer J Clin* 1999;49(1):33–64, 1.
4. Weiss NS, Szekely DR, Austin DF. Increasing incidence of endometrial cancer in the United States. *N Engl J Med* 1976;294(23):1259–1262.
5. Brinton LA, Berman ML, Mortel R, et al. Reproductive, menstrual,

and medical risk factors for endometrial cancer: results from a case-control study. *Am J Obstet Gynecol* 1992;167(5):1317–1325.

6. Henderson BE, Casagrande JT, Pike MC, et al. The epidemiology of endometrial cancer in young women. *Br J Cancer* 1983;47(6): 749–756.

7. Kelsey JL, Li Volsi V, Holford TR. A case-control study of cancer of the endometrium. *Am J Epidemiol* 1982;116:333.

8. Modan B, Ron E, Lerner-Geva L, et al. Cancer incidence in a cohort of infertile women. *Am J Epidemiol* 1998;147(11):1038–1042.

9. Bernstein L, Pike MC, Ross RK, et al. Estrogen and sex hormone-binding globulin levels in nulliparous and parous women. *J Natl Cancer Inst* 1985;74(4):741–745.

10. La Vecchia C, Franceschi S, Decarli A, et al. Risk factors for endometrial cancer at different ages. *J Natl Cancer Inst* 1984;73(3):667–671.

11. Albrektsen G, Heuch I, Tretli S, et al. Is the risk of cancer of the corpus uteri reduced by a recent pregnancy? A prospective study of 765,756 Norwegian women. *Int J Cancer* 1995;61(4):485–490.

12. Lambe M, Wuu J, Weiderpass E, et al. Childbearing at older age and endometrial cancer risk (Sweden). *Cancer Causes Control* 1999; 10(1):43–49.

13. Castellsague X, Thompson WD, Dubrow R. Intra-uterine contraception and the risk of endometrial cancer. *Int J Cancer* 1993;54(6): 911–916.

14. Hill DA, Weiss NS, Voigt LF, Beresford SA. Endometrial cancer in relation to intra-uterine device use. *Int J Cancer* 1997;70(3):278–281.

15. Sturgeon SR, Brinton LA, Berman ML, et al. Intrauterine device use and endometrial cancer risk. *Int J Epidemiol* 1997;26(3):496–500.

16. Kelsey JL, Hildreth NG. *Breast and gynecologic cancer epidemiology.* Boca Raton, FL: CRC Press, 1983.

17. Newcomb PA, Trentham-Dietz A. Breast feeding practices in relation to endometrial cancer risk, USA. *Cancer Causes Control* 2000;11(7): 663–667.

18. Rosenblatt KA, Thomas DB. Prolonged lactation and endometrial cancer. WHO Collaborative Study of Neoplasia and Steroid Contraceptives. *Int J Epidemiol* 1995;24(3):499–503.

19. MacMahon B. Risk factors for endometrial cancer. *Gynecol Oncol* 1974;2(2–3):122–129.

20. Weiss NS, Sayvetz TA. Incidence of endometrial cancer in relation to the use of oral contraceptives. *N Engl J Med* 1980;302(10):551–554.

21. Combination oral contraceptive use and the risk of endometrial cancer. The Cancer and Steroid Hormone Study of the Centers for Disease Control and the National Institute of Child Health and Human Development. *JAMA* 1987;257(6):796–800.

22. Kaufman DW, Shapiro S, Slone D, et al. Decreased risk of endometrial cancer among oral-contraceptive users. *N Engl J Med* 1980;303(18): 1045–1047.

23. Voigt LF, Deng Q, Weiss NS. Recency, duration, and progestin content of oral contraceptives in relation to the incidence of endometrial cancer (Washington, USA). *Cancer Causes Control* 1994;5(3): 227–233.

24. Rosenblatt KA, Thomas DB. Hormonal content of combined oral contraceptives in relation to the reduced risk of endometrial carcinoma. The WHO Collaborative Study of Neoplasia and Steroid Contraceptives. *Int J Cancer* 1991;49(6):870–874.

25. Weiss NS, Lyon JL, Liff JM, et al. Incidence of ovarian cancer in relation to the use of oral contraceptives. *Int J Cancer* 1981;28(6): 669–671.

26. Brinton LA, Hoover RN. Estrogen replacement therapy and endometrial cancer risk: unresolved issues. The Endometrial Cancer Collaborative Group. *Obstet Gynecol* 1993;81(2):265–271.

27. Green PK, Weiss NS, McKnight B, et al. Risk of endometrial cancer following cessation of menopausal hormone use (Washington, United States). *Cancer Causes Control* 1996;7(6):575–580.

28. Pike MC, Peters RK, Cozen W, et al. Estrogen-progestin replacement therapy and endometrial cancer. *J Natl Cancer Inst* 1997;89(15): 1110–1116.

29. Shapiro S, Kelly JP, Rosenberg L, et al. Risk of localized and widespread endometrial cancer in relation to recent and discontinued use of conjugated estrogens. *N Engl J Med* 1985;313(16):969–972.

30. Levi F, La Vecchia C, Gulie C, Franceschi S, Negri E. Oestrogen replacement treatment and the risk of endometrial cancer: an assessment of the role of covariates. *Eur J Cancer* 1993;29A(10): 1445–1449.

31. Rubin GL, Peterson HB, Lee NC, et al. Estrogen replacement therapy and the risk of endometrial cancer: remaining controversies. *Am J Obstet Gynecol* 1990;162(1):148–154.

32. Cushing KL, Weiss NS, Voigt LF, et al. Risk of endometrial cancer in relation to use of low-dose, unopposed estrogens. *Obstet Gynecol* 1998;91(1):35–39.

33. Herrinton LJ, Weiss NS. Postmenopausal unopposed estrogens. Characteristics of use in relation to the risk of endometrial carcinoma. *Ann Epidemiol* 1993;3(3):308–318.

34. Newcomer LM, Newcomb PA, Trentham-Dietz A, Storer BE. Hormonal risk factors for endometrial cancer: modification by cigarette smoking (United States). *Cancer Causes Control* 2001;12(9): 829–835.

35. Elwood JM, Boyes DA. Clinical and pathological features and survival of endometrial cancer patients in relation to prior use of estrogens. *Gynecol Oncol* 1980;10(2):173–187.

36. Silverberg SG, Mullen D, Faraci JA, et al. Endometrial carcinoma: clinical-pathologic comparison of cases in postmenopausal women receiving and not receiving exogenous estrogens. *Cancer* 1980; 45(12):3018–3026.

37. Shapiro JA, Weiss NS, Beresford SA, Voigt LF. Menopausal hormone use and endometrial cancer, by tumor grade and invasion. *Epidemiology* 1998;9(1):99–101.

38. Randall TC, Kurman RJ. Progestin treatment of atypical hyperplasia and well-differentiated carcinoma of the endometrium in women under age 40. *Obstet Gynecol* 1997;90(3):434–440.

39. Persson I, Adami HO, Bergkvist L, et al. Risk of endometrial cancer after treatment with oestrogens alone or in conjunction with progestogens: results of a prospective study. *BMJ* 1989;298(6667):147–151.

40. Weiderpass E, Adami HO, Baron JA, et al. Risk of endometrial cancer following estrogen replacement with and without progestins. *J Natl Cancer Inst* 1999;91(13):1131–1137.

41. Newcomb PA, Trentham-Dietz A. Patterns of postmenopausal progestin use with estrogen in relation to endometrial cancer (United States). *Cancer Causes Control* 2003;14:195–201.

42. Beresford SA, Weiss NS, Voigt LF, et al. Risk of endometrial cancer following estrogen replacement with and without progestins: results of a prospective study. *Lancet* 1997;349(9050):458–461.

43. Archer DF. The effect of the duration of progestin use on the occurrence of endometrial cancer in postmenopausal women. *Menopause* 2001;8(4):245–251.

44. Andersson M, Storm HH, Mouridsen HT. Incidence of new primary cancers after adjuvant tamoxifen therapy and radiotherapy for early breast cancer. *J Natl Cancer Inst* 1991; 83(14):1013–1017.

45. Fisher B, Costantino JP, Wickerham DL, et al. Tamoxifen for prevention of breast cancer: report of the National Surgical Adjuvant Breast and Bowel Project P-1 Study. *J Natl Cancer Inst* 1998;90(18): 1371–1388.

46. van Leeuwen FE, Benraadt J, Coebergh JW, et al. Risk of endometrial cancer after tamoxifen treatment of breast cancer. *Lancet* 1994; 343(8895):448–452.

47. Curtis RE, Freedman M, Sherman ME, Fraumeni JF Jr. Elevated risk of malignant mixed mullerian tumors following tamoxifen therapy for breast cancer. *J Natl Cancer Inst* 2004 *(in press)*.

48. Bergman L, Beelen JLR, Gallee MPW, et al. Risk and prognosis of endometrial cancer after tamoxifen for breast cancer. *Lancet* 2000; 356(9233):881–887.

49. Goodman MT, Hankin JH, Wilkens LR, et al. Diet, body size, physical activity, and the risk of endometrial cancer. *Cancer Res* 1997;57(22): 5077–5085.

50. Olson SH, Trevisan M, Marshall JR, et al. Body mass index, weight gain, and risk of endometrial cancer. *Nutr Cancer* 1995;23(2): 141–149.

51. Shoff SM, Newcomb PA. Diabetes, body size, and risk of endometrial cancer. *Am J Epidemiol* 1998;148(3):234–240.

52. Swanson CA, Potischman N, Wilbanks GD, et al. Relation of endometrial cancer risk to past and contemporary body size and body fat distribution. *Cancer Epidemiol Biomarkers Prev* 1993;2(4):321–327.

53. Jain MG, Rohan TE, Howe GR, et al. A cohort study of nutritional factors and endometrial cancer. *Eur J Epidemiol* 2000;16(10): 899–905.

54. Blitzer PH, Blitzer EC, Rimm AA. Association between teen-age obe-

sity and cancer in 56,111 women: all cancers and endometrial carcinoma. *Prev Med* 1976;5(1):20–31.

55. Elliott EA, Matanoski GM, Rosenshein NB, et al. Body fat patterning in women with endometrial cancer. *Gynecol Oncol* 1990;39(3):253–258.

56. Schapira DV, Kumar NB, Lyman GH, et al. Upper-body fat distribution and endometrial cancer risk. *JAMA* 1991;266(13):1808–1811.

57. Austin H, Austin JM Jr, Partridge EE, et al. Endometrial cancer, obesity, and body fat distribution. *Cancer Res* 1991;51(2):568–572.

58. Folsom AR, Kaye SA, Potter JD, Prineas RJ. Association of incident carcinoma of the endometrium with body weight and fat distribution in older women: early findings of the Iowa Women's Health Study. *Cancer Res* 1989;49(23):6828–6831.

59. Shu XO, Brinton LA, Zheng W, et al. Relation of obesity and body fat distribution to endometrial cancer in Shanghai, China. *Cancer Res* 1992;52(14):3865–3870.

60. Colbert LH, Lacey JV Jr, Schairer C, et al. Physical activity and risk of endometrial cancer in a prospective cohort study (United States). *Cancer Causes Control* 2003;14(6):559–567.

61. Moradi T, Weiderpass E, Signorello LB, et al. Physical activity and postmenopausal endometrial cancer risk (Sweden). *Cancer Causes Control* 2000;11(9):829–837.

62. Littman AJ, Voigt LF, Beresford SA, et al. Recreational physical activity and endometrial cancer risk. *Am J Epidemiol* 2001;11(9):829–837.

63. Armstrong B, Doll R. Environmental factors and cancer incidence and mortality in different countries, with special reference to dietary practices. *Int J Cancer* 1975;15(4):617–631.

64. Potischman N, Swanson CA, Brinton LA, et al. Dietary associations in a case-control study of endometrial cancer. *Cancer Causes Control* 1993;4(3):239–250.

65. Barbone F, Austin H, Partridge EE. Diet and endometrial cancer: a case-control study. *Am J Epidemiol* 1993;137(4):393–403.

66. McCann SE, Freudenheim JL, Marshall JR, et al. Diet in the epidemiology of endometrial cancer in western New York (United States). *Cancer Causes Control* 2000;11(10):965–975.

67. Negri E, La Vecchia C, Franceschi S, et al. Intake of selected micronutrients and the risk of endometrial carcinoma. *Cancer* 1996;77(5):917–923.

68. Horn–Ross PL, John EM, Canchola AJ, et al. Phytoestrogen intake and endometrial cancer risk. *J Natl Cancer Inst* 2003;95(15):1158–1164.

69. Terry P, Wolk A, Vainio H, et al. Fatty fish consumption lowers the risk of endometrial cancer: a nationwide case-control study in Sweden. *Cancer Epidemiol Biomarkers Prev* 2003;11(1):143–145.

70. Armstrong BK, Brown JB, Clarke HT, et al. Diet and reproductive hormones: a study of vegetarian and nonvegetarian postmenopausal women. *J Natl Cancer Inst* 1981;67(4):761–767.

71. Barbosa JC, Shultz TD, Filley SJ, Nieman DC. The relationship among adiposity, diet, and hormone concentrations in vegetarian and nonvegetarian postmenopausal women. *Am J Clin Nutr* 1990;51(5):798–803.

72. Goldin BR, Adlercreutz H, Gorbach SL, et al. The relationship between estrogen levels and diets of Caucasian American and Oriental immigrant women. *Am J Clin Nutr* 1986;44(6):945–953.

73. Prentice R, Thompson D, Clifford C, et al. Dietary fat reduction and plasma estradiol concentration in healthy postmenopausal women. The Women's Health Trial Study Group. *J Natl Cancer Inst* 1990;82(2):129–134.

74. Austin H, Drews C, Partridge EE. A case-control study of endometrial cancer in relation to cigarette smoking, serum estrogen levels, and alcohol use. *Am J Obstet Gynecol* 1993;169(5):1086–1091.

75. Newcomb PA, Trentham-Dietz A, Storer BE. Alcohol consumption in relation to endometrial cancer risk. *Cancer Epidemiol Biomarkers Prev* 1997;6(10):775–778.

76. Swanson CA, Wilbanks GD, Twiggs LB, et al. Moderate alcohol consumption and the risk of endometrial cancer. *Epidemiology* 1993;4(6):530–536.

77. Webster LA, Weiss NS. Alcoholic beverage consumption and the risk of endometrial cancer. Cancer and Steroid Hormone Study Group. *Int J Epidemiol* 1989;18(4):786–791.

78. Gapstur SM, Potter JD, Sellers TA, et al. Alcohol consumption and postmenopausal endometrial cancer: results from the Iowa Women's Health Study. *Cancer Causes Control* 1993;4(4):323–329.

79. Weir HK, Sloan M, Kreiger N. The relationship between cigarette smoking and the risk of endometrial neoplasms. *Int J Epidemiol* 1994;23(2):261–266.

80. Weiderpass E, Baron JA. Cigarette smoking, alcohol consumption, and endometrial cancer risk: a population-based study in Sweden. *Cancer Causes Control* 2001;12(3):239–247.

81. Brinton LA, Barrett RJ, Berman ML, et al. Cigarette smoking and the risk of endometrial cancer. *Am J Epidemiol* 1993;137(3):281–291.

82. Parazzini F, La Vecchia C, Negri E, et al. Smoking and risk of endometrial cancer: results from an Italian case-control study. *Gynecol Oncol* 1995;56(2):195–199.

83. Terry PD, Miller AB, Rohan TE. A prospective cohort study of cigarette smoking and the risk of endometrial cancer. *Br J Cancer* 2002;86:1430–1435.

84. Lesko SM, Rosenberg L, Kaufman DW, et al. Cigarette smoking and the risk of endometrial cancer. *N Engl J Med* 1985;313(10):593–596.

85. Potischman N, Hoover RN, Brinton LA, et al. Case-control study of endogenous steroid hormones and endometrial cancer. *J Natl Cancer Inst* 1996;88(16):1127–1135.

86. Zeleniuch-Jacquotte A, Akhmedkhanov A, Kato I, et al. Postmenopausal endogenous oestrogens and risk of endometrial cancer: results of a prospective study. *Br J Cancer* 2001;84(7):975–981.

87. Key TJ, Pike MC. The dose–effect relationship between 'unopposed' oestrogens and endometrial mitotic rate: its central role in explaining and predicting endometrial cancer risk. *Br J Cancer* 1988;57(2):205–212.

88. Potischman N, Gail MH, Troisi R, et al. Measurement error does not explain the persistence of a body mass index association with endometrial cancer after adjustment for endogenous hormones. *Epidemiology* 1999;10(1):76–79.

89. Hale GE, Hughes CL, Cline JM. Endometrial cancer: hormonal factors, the perimenopausal "window of ris," and isoflavones. *J Clin Endocrinol Metab* 2002;87(1):3–15.

90. Troisi R, Potischman N, Hoover RN, et al. Insulin and endometrial cancer. *Am J Epidemiol* 1997;146(6):476–482.

91. Jafari K, Javaheri G, Ruiz G. Endometrial adenocarcinoma and the Stein-Leventhal syndrome. *Obstet Gynecol* 1978;51(1):97–100.

92. Wild S, Pierpoint T, Jacobs H, et al. Long-term consequences of polycystic ovary syndrome. *Hum Fertil (Camb)* 2000;3(2):101–105.

93. Wood GP, Boronow RC. Endometrial adenocarcinoma and the polycystic ovary syndrome. *Am J Obstet Gynecol* 1976;124(2):140–142.

94. Coulam CB, Annegers JF, Franz JS. Chronic anovulation syndrome and associated neoplasia. *Obstet Gynecol* 1983;61(4):403–407.

95. Dahlgren E, Friberg LG, Johansson S, et al. Endometrial carcinoma; ovarian dysfunction—a risk factor in young women. *Eur J Obstet Gynecol Reprod Biol* 1991;41(2):143–150.

96. Weiderpass E, Gridley G, Persson I, et al. Risk of endometrial and breast cancer in patients with diabetes mellitus. *Int J Cancer* 1997;71(3):360–363.

97. Wideroff L, Gridley G, Mellemkjaer L, et al. Cancer incidence in a population-based cohort of patients hospitalized with diabetes mellitus in Denmark. *J Natl Cancer Inst* 1997;89(18):1360–1365.

98. Weiderpass E, Persson I, Adami HO, et al. Body size in different periods of life, diabetes mellitus, hypertension, and risk of postmenopausal endometrial cancer (Sweden). *Cancer Causes Control* 2000;11(2):185–192.

99. Inoue M, Okayama A, Fujita M, et al. A case-control study on risk factors for uterine endometrial cancer in Japan. *Jpn J Cancer Res* 1994;85(4):346–350.

100. Parazzini F, La Vecchia C, Negri E, et al. Diabetes and endometrial cancer: an Italian case-control study. *Int J Cancer* 1999;81(4):539–542.

101. Anderson KE, Anderson E, Mink PJ, et al. Diabetes and endometrial cancer in the Iowa Women's Health Study. *Cancer Epidemiol Biomarkers Prev* 2001;10(6):611–616.

102. Newcomb PA, Trentham-Dietz A, Egan KM, et al. Fracture history and risk of breast and endometrial cancer. *Am J Epidemiol* 2001;153(11):1071–1078.

103. Persson I, Adami HO, McLaughlin JK, et al. Reduced risk of breast and endometrial cancer among women with hip fractures (Sweden). *Cancer Causes Control* 1994;5(6):523–528.

104. Gruber SB, Thompson WD. A population-based study of endometrial cancer and familial risk in younger women. Cancer and Steroid Hormone Study Group. *Cancer Epidemiol Biomarkers Prev* 1996;5(6): 411–417.

105. Parslov M, Lidegaard O, Klintorp S, et al. Risk factors among young women with endometrial cancer: a Danish case-control study. *Am J Obstet Gynecol* 2000;182(1 Pt 1):23–29.

106. Hemminki K, Vaittinen P, Dong C. Endometrial cancer in the family-cancer database. *Cancer Epidemiol Biomarkers Prev* 1999;8(11): 1005–1010.

107. Levine DA, Lin O, Barakat RR, et al. Risk of endometrial carcinoma association with BRCA mutation. *Gynecol Oncol* 2001;10(7): 793–798.

108. Esteller M, Garcia A, Martinez-Palones JM, et al. Germ line polymorphisms in cytochrome-P450 1A1 (C4887 CYP1A1) and methylenetetrahydrofolate reductase (MTHFR) genes and endometrial cancer susceptibility. *Carcinogenesis* 1997;18(12):2307–2311.

109. Esteller M, Garcia A, Martinez-Palones JM, et al. Susceptibility to endometrial cancer: influence of allelism at p53, glutathione S-transferase (GSTM1 and GSTT1) and cytochrome P-450 (CYP1A1) loci. *Br J Cancer* 1997;75(9):1385–1388.

110. Weiderpass E, Persson I, Melhus H, et al. Estrogen receptor alpha gene polymorphisms and endometrial cancer risk. *Carcinogenesis* 2002;21(4):623–627.

111. Sturgeon SR, Brock JW, Potischman N, et al. Serum concentrations of organochlorine compounds and endometrial cancer risk (United States). *Cancer Causes Control* 1998;9(4):417–424.

112. Weiderpass E, Adami HO, Baron JA, et al. Organochlorines and endometrial cancer risk. *Cancer Epidemiol Biomarkers Prev* 2000;9(5): 487–493.

113. McElroy JA, Newcomb PA, Trentham-Dietz A, et al. Endometrial cancer incidence in relation to electric blanket use. *Am J Epidemiol* 2002;156(3):262–267.

114. Weiderpass E, Pukkala E, Vasama-Neuvonen K, et al. Occupational exposures and cancers of the endometrium and cervix in Finland. *Am J Ind Med* 2001;39(6):572–580.

115. Siiteri PK. Steroid hormones and endometrial cancer. *Cancer Res* 1978;38(11 Pt 2):4360–4366.

116. Gnagy S, Ming EE, Devesa SS, et al. Declining ovarian cancer rates in U.S. women in relation to parity and oral contraceptive use. *Epidemiology* 2000;11(2):102–105.

117. Mink PJ, Sherman ME, Devesa SS. Incidence patterns of invasive and borderline ovarian tumors among white women and black women in the United States. Results from the SEER Program, 1978–1998. *Cancer* 2002;95(11):2380–2389.

118. Pisani P, Parkin DM, Bray F, Ferlay J. Estimates of the worldwide mortality from 25 cancers in 1990. *Int J Cancer* 1999;83(1):18–29.

119. Booth M, Beral V, Smith P. Risk factors for ovarian cancer: a case-control study. *Br J Cancer* 1989;60(4):592–598.

120. Hankinson SE, Colditz GA, Hunter DJ, et al. A prospective study of reproductive factors and risk of epithelial ovarian cancer. *Cancer* 1995;76(2):284–290.

121. Risch HA, Marrett LD, Howe GR. Parity, contraception, infertility, and the risk of epithelial ovarian cancer. *Am J Epidemiol* 1994;140(7): 585–597.

122. Whittemore AS, Harris R, Itnyre J. Characteristics relating to ovarian cancer risk: collaborative analysis of 12 US case-control studies. II. Invasive epithelial ovarian cancers in white women. Collaborative Ovarian Cancer Group. *Am J Epidemiol* 1992;136(10):1184–1203.

123. Chen MT, Cook LS, Daling JR, Weiss NS. Incomplete pregnancies and risk of ovarian cancer (Washington, United States). *Cancer Causes Control* 1996;7(4):415–420.

124. Greggi S, Parazzini F, Paratore MP, et al. Risk factors for ovarian cancer in central Italy. *Gynecol Oncol* 2000;79(1):50–54.

125. Voigt LF, Harlow BL, Weiss NS. The influence of age at first birth and parity on ovarian cancer risk. *Am J Epidemiol* 1986;124(3):490–491.

126. Negri E, Franceschi S, Tzonou A, et al. Pooled analysis of 3 European case-control studies: I. Reproductive factors and risk of epithelial ovarian cancer. *Int J Cancer* 1991;49(1):50–56.

127. Cooper GS, Schildkraut JM, Whittemore AS, Marchbanks PA. Pregnancy recency and risk of ovarian cancer. *Cancer Causes Control* 1999;10(5):397–402.

128. Klip H, Burger CW, Kenemans P, van Leeuwen FE. Cancer risk associated with subfertility and ovulation induction: a review. *Cancer Causes Control* 2000;11(4):319–344.

129. Whittemore AS, Wu ML, Paffenbarger RS Jr, et al. Epithelial ovarian cancer and the ability to conceive. *Cancer Res* 1989;49(14): 4047–4052.

130. Rossing MA, Daling JR, Weiss NS, et al. Ovarian tumors in a cohort of infertile women. *N Engl J Med* 1994;331(12):771–776.

131. Franceschi S, La Vecchia C, Negri E, et al. Fertility drugs and risk of epithelial ovarian cancer in Italy. *Hum Reprod* 1994;9(9):1673–1675.

132. Shushan A, Paltiel O, Iscovich J, et al. Human menopausal gonadotropin and the risk of epithelial ovarian cancer. *Fertil Steril* 1996;65(1): 13–18.

133. Parazzini F, Negri E, La Vecchia C, et al. Treatment for infertility and risk of invasive epithelial ovarian cancer. *Hum Reprod* 1997; 12(10):2159–2161.

134. Mosgaard BJ, Lidegaard O, Kjaer SK, et al. Infertility, fertility drugs, and invasive ovarian cancer: a case–control study. *Fertil Steril* 1997; 67(6):1005–1012.

135. Venn A, Watson L, Bruinsma F, et al. Risk of cancer after use of fertility drugs with in-vitro fertilisation. *Lancet* 1999;354(9190): 1586–1590.

136. Potashnik G, Lerner-Geva L, Genkin L, Chetrit A, Lunenfeld E, Porath A. Fertility drugs and the risk of breast and ovarian cancers: results of a long-term follow-up study. *Fertil Steril* 1999;71(5):853–859.

137. Ness RB, Cramer DW, Goodman MT, et al. Infertility, fertility drugs, and ovarian cancer: a pooled analysis of case-control studies. *Am J Epidemiol* 2002;155(3):217–224.

138. Rosenblatt KA, Thomas DB. Lactation and the risk of epithelial ovarian cancer. The WHO Collaborative Study of Neoplasia and Steroid Contraceptives. *Int J Epidemiol* 1993;22(2):192–197.

139. Siskind V, Green A, Bain C, Purdie D. Breastfeeding, menopause, and epithelial ovarian cancer. *Epidemiology* 1997;8(2):188–191.

140. Titus-Ernstoff L, Perez K, Cramer DW, et al. Menstrual and reproductive factors in relation to ovarian cancer risk. *Br J Cancer* 2001;84(5): 714–721.

141. Green A, Purdie D, Bain C, et al. Tubal sterilisation, hysterectomy and decreased risk of ovarian cancer. Survey of Women's Health Study Group. *Int J Cancer* 1997;71(6):948–951.

142. Hankinson SE, Hunter DJ, Colditz GA, et al. Tubal ligation, hysterectomy, and risk of ovarian cancer. A prospective study. *JAMA* 1993; 270(23):2813–2818.

143. Kreiger N, Sloan M, Cotterchio M, Parsons P. Surgical procedures associated with risk of ovarian cancer. *Int J Epidemiol* 1997;26(4): 710–715.

144. Rosenblatt KA, Thomas DB. Reduced risk of ovarian cancer in women with a tubal ligation or hysterectomy. The World Health Organization Collaborative Study of Neoplasia and Steroid Contraceptives. *Cancer Epidemiol Biomarkers Prev* 1996;5(11):933–935.

145. Weiss NS, Harlow BL. Why does hysterectomy without bilateral oophorectomy influence the subsequent incidence of ovarian cancer? *Am J Epidemiol* 1986;124(5):856–858.

146. Ellsworth LR, Allen HH, Nisker JA. Ovarian function after radical hysterectomy for stage IB carcinoma of cervix. *Am J Obstet Gynecol* 1983;145(2):185–188.

147. Schildkraut JM, Cooper GS, Halabi S, et al. Age at natural menopause and the risk of epithelial ovarian cancer. *Obstet Gynecol* 2001;98(1): 85–90.

148. Franceschi S, La Vecchia C, Booth M, et al. Pooled analysis of 3 European case-control studies of ovarian cancer: II. Age at menarche and at menopause. *Int J Cancer* 1991;49(1):57–60.

149. Rosenberg L, Palmer JR, Zauber AG, et al. A case-control study of oral contraceptive use and invasive epithelial ovarian cancer. *Am J Epidemiol* 1994;139(7):654–661.

150. The reduction in risk of ovarian cancer associated with oral-contraceptive use. The Cancer and Steroid Hormone Study of the Centers for Disease Control and the National Institute of Child Health and Human Development. *N Engl J Med* 1987;316(11):650–655.

151. Franceschi S, Parazzini F, Negri E, et al. Pooled analysis of 3 European case–control studies of epithelial ovarian cancer: III. Oral contraceptive use. *Int J Cancer* 1991;49(1):61–65.

152. Ness RB, Grisso JA, Klapper J, et al. Risk of ovarian cancer in relation to estrogen and progestin dose and use characteristics of oral contra-

ceptives. SHARE Study Group. Steroid Hormones and Reproductions. *Am J Epidemiol* 2000;152(3):233–241.

153. Royar J, Becher H, Chang-Claude J. Low-dose oral contraceptives: protective effect on ovarian cancer risk. *Int J Cancer* 2001;95(6): 370–374.

154. Schildkraut JM, Calingaert B, Marchbanks PA, et al. Impact of progestin and estrogen potency in oral contraceptives on ovarian cancer risk. *J Natl Cancer Inst* 2002;94(1):32–38.

155. Hartge P, Hoover R, McGowan L, et al. Menopause and ovarian cancer. *Am J Epidemiol* 1988;127(5):990–998.

156. Weiss NS, Lyon JL, Krishnamurthy S, et al. Noncontraceptive estrogen use and the occurrence of ovarian cancer. J Natl Cancer Inst 1982; 68(1):95–98.

157. Coughlin SS, Giustozzi A, Smith SJ, Lee NC. A meta-analysis of estrogen replacement therapy and risk of epithelial ovarian cancer. *J Clin Epidemiol* 2000;53(4):367–375.

158. Garg PP, Kerlikowske K, Subak L, Grady D. Hormone replacement therapy and the risk of epithelial ovarian carcinoma: a meta-analysis. *Obstet Gynecol* 1998;92(3):472–479.

159. Noller KL. Estrogen replacement therapy and risk of ovarian cancer. *JAMA* 2002;288(3):368–369.

160. Risch HA. Hormone replacement therapy and the risk of ovarian cancer. *Gynecol Oncol* 2002;86(2):115–117.

161. Lacey JV Jr, Mink PJ, Lubin JH, et al. Menopausal hormone replacement therapy and risk of ovarian cancer. *JAMA* 2002;288(3):334–341.

162. Rodriguez C, Patel AV, Calle EE, et al. Estrogen replacement therapy and ovarian cancer mortality in a large prospective study of US women. *JAMA* 2001;285(11):1460–1465.

163. Riman T, Dickman PW, Nilsson S, et al. Hormone replacement therapy and the risk of invasive epithelial ovarian cancer in Swedish women. *J Natl Cancer Inst* 2002;94(7):497–504.

164. Negri E, Tzonou A, Beral V, et al. Hormonal therapy for menopause and ovarian cancer in a collaborative re-analysis of European studies. *Int J Cancer* 1999;80(6):848–851.

165. Purdie DM, Bain CJ, Siskind V, et al. Hormone replacement therapy and risk of epithelial ovarian cancer. *Br J Cancer* 1999;81(3): 559–563.

166. Helzlsouer KJ, Alberg AJ, Gordon GB, et al. Serum gonadotropins and steroid hormones and the development of ovarian cancer. *JAMA* 1995;274(24):1926–1930.

167. Lukanova A, Lundin E, Micheli A, et al. Risk of ovarian cancer in relation to prediagnostic levels of C-peptide, insulin-like growth factor binding proteins-1 and -2 (USA, Sweden, Italy). *Cancer Causes Control* 2003;14(3):285–292.

168. Lukanova A, Lundin E, Akhmedkhanov A, et al. Circulating levels of sex steroid hormones and risk of ovarian cancer. *Int J Cancer* 2003; 104(5):636–642.

169. Parazzini F, Moroni S, La Vecchia C, et al. Ovarian cancer risk and history of selected medical conditions linked with female hormones. *Eur J Cancer* 1997;33(10):1634–1637.

170. Weiderpass E, Ye W, Vainio H, et al. Diabetes mellitus and ovarian cancer (Sweden). *Cancer Causes Control* 2002;13(8):759–764.

171. Brinton LA, Gridley G, Persson I, et al. Cancer risk after a hospital discharge diagnosis of endometriosis. *Am J Obstet Gynecol* 1997;176: 572–579.

172. Ness RB. Endometriosis and ovarian cancer: Thoughts on shared pathophysiology. *Am J Obstet Gynecol* 2003;189:289–294.

173. Ness RB, Cottreau C. Possible role of ovarian epithelial inflammation in ovarian cancer. *J Natl Cancer Inst* 1999;91(17):1459–1467.

174. Risch HA, Howe GR. Pelvic inflammatory disease and the risk of epithelial ovarian cancer. *Cancer Epidemiol Biomarkers Prev* 1995; 4(5):447–451.

175. Farrow DC, Weiss NS, Lyon JL, Daling JR. Association of obesity and ovarian cancer in a case-control study. *Am J Epidemiol* 1989; 129(6):1300–1304.

176. Schouten LJ, Goldbohm RA, van den Brandt PA. Height, weight, weight change, and ovarian cancer risk in the Netherlands cohort study on diet and cancer. *Am J Epidemiol* 2003;157(5):424–433.

177. Lubin F, Chetrit A, Freedman LS, et al. Body mass index at age 18 years and during adult life and ovarian cancer risk. *Am J Epidemiol* 2003;157(2):113–120.

178. Fairfield KM, Willett WC, Rosner BA, et al. Obesity, weight gain, and ovarian cancer. *Obstet Gynecol* 2002;100(2):288–296.

179. Rodriguez C, Calle EE, Fakhrabadi-Shokoohi D, et al. Body mass index, height, and the risk of ovarian cancer mortality in a prospective cohort of postmenopausal women. *Cancer Epidemiol Biomarkers Prev* 2002;11(9):822–828.

180. Purdie DM, Bain CJ, Webb PM, et al. Body size and ovarian cancer: case–control study and systematic review (Australia). *Cancer Causes Control* 2001;12(9):855–863.

181. Lukanova A, Toniolo P, Lundin E, et al. Body mass index in relation to ovarian cancer: a multi-centre nested case-control study. *Int J Cancer* 2002;99(4):603–608.

182. Zhang M, Lee AH, Binns CW. Physical activity and epithelial ovarian cancer risk: a case-control study in China. *Int J Cancer* 2003;105(6): 838–843.

183. Cottreau CM, Ness RB, Kriska AM. Physical activity and reduced risk of ovarian cancer. *Obstet Gynecol* 2000;96(4):609–614.

184. Bertone ER, Willett WC, Rosner BA, et al. Prospective study of recreational physical activity and ovarian cancer. *J Natl Cancer Inst* 2001; 93(12):942–948.

185. Mink PJ, Folsom AR, Sellers TA, Kushi LH. Physical activity, waist-to-hip ratio, and other risk factors for ovarian cancer: a follow-up study of older women. *Epidemiology* 1996;7(1):38–45.

186. Harlow BL, Cramer DW, Baron JA, et al. Psychotropic medication use and risk of epithelial ovarian cancer. *Cancer Epidemiol Biomarkers Prev* 1998;7(8):697–702.

187. Lacey JV Jr, Sherman ME, Hartge P, et al. Medication use and risk of ovarian carcinoma: a prospective study. *Int J Cancer* 2004;108(2): 281–286.

188. Dalton SO, Johansen C, Mellemkjaer L, et al. Antidepressant medications and risk for cancer. *Epidemiology* 1999;11:171–176.

189. Kato I, Zeleniuch-Jacquotte A, Toniolo PG, et al. Psychotropic medication use and risk of hormone-related cancers: the New York University Women's Health Study. *J Public Health Med* 2000;22(2): 155–160.

190. Dublin S, Rossing MA, Heckbert SR, et al. Risk of epithelial ovarian cancer in relation to use of antidepressants, benzodiazepines, and other centrally acting medications. *Cancer Causes Control* 2002;13(1): 35–45.

191. Cramer DW, Harlow BL, Titus-Ernstoff L, et al. Over-the-counter analgesics and risk of ovarian cancer. *Lancet* 1998;351(9096): 104–107.

192. Tzonou A, Polychronopoulou A, Hsieh CC, et al. Hair dyes, analgesics, tranquilizers and perineal talc application as risk factors for ovarian cancer. Int J Cancer 1993;55(3):408–410.

193. Rodriguez C, Henley SJ, Calle EE, Thun MJ. Paracetamol and risk of ovarian cancer mortality in a prospective study of women in the USA. *Lancet* 1998;352:1354–1355.

194. Phillips RL, Garfinkel L, Kuzma JW, et al. Mortality among California Seventh–Day Adventists for selected cancer sites. *J Natl Cancer Inst* 1980;65(5):1097–1107.

195. Kinlen LJ. Meat and fat consumption and cancer mortality: A study of strict religious orders in Britain. *Lancet* 1982;1(8278):946–949.

196. Cramer DW, Harlow BL, Willett WC, et al. Galactose consumption and metabolism in relation to the risk of ovarian cancer. *Lancet* 1989; 2(8654):66–71.

197. Herrinton LJ, Weiss NS, Beresford SA, et al. Lactose and galactose intake and metabolism in relation to the risk of epithelial ovarian cancer. *Am J Epidemiol* 1995;141(5):407–416.

198. Risch HA, Jain M, Marrett LD, Howe GR. Dietary lactose intake, lactose intolerance, and the risk of epithelial ovarian cancer in southern Ontario (Canada). *Cancer Causes Control* 1994;5(6):540–548.

199. Webb PM, Bain CJ, Purdie DM, et al. Milk consumption, galactose metabolism and ovarian cancer (Australia). *Cancer Causes Control* 1998;9(6):637–644.

200. Bosetti C, Negri E, Franceschi S, et al. Diet and ovarian cancer risk: a case-control study in Italy. *Int J Cancer* 2001;93(6):911–915.

201. Kushi LH, Mink PJ, Folsom AR, et al. Prospective study of diet and ovarian cancer. *Am J Epidemiol* 1999;149(1):21–31.

202. Goodman MT, Wu AH, Tung KH, et al. Association of dairy products, lactose, and calcium with the risk of ovarian cancer. *Am J Epidemiol* 2002;156(2):148–157.

203. Cramer DW, Welch WR, Hutchison GB, et al. Dietary animal fat in relation to ovarian cancer risk. *Obstet Gynecol* 1984;63(6):833–838.

204. Risch HA, Jain M, Marrett LD, Howe GR. Dietary fat intake and

risk of epithelial ovarian cancer. *J Natl Cancer Inst* 1994;86(18): 1409–1415.

205. Bertone ER, Rosner BA, Hunter DJ, et al. Dietary fat intake and ovarian cancer in a cohort of US women. *Am J Epidemiol* 2002; 156(1):22–31.

206. McCann SE, Moysich KB, Mettlin C. Intakes of selected nutrients and food groups and risk of ovarian cancer. *Nutr Cancer* 2001;39(1): 19–28.

207. Pelucchi C, La Vecchia C, Chatenoud L, et al. Dietary fibres and ovarian cancer risk. *Eur J Cancer* 2001;37(17):2235–2239.

208. McCann SE, Freudenheim JL, Marshall JR, Graham S. Risk of human ovarian cancer is related to dietary intake of selected nutrients, phytochemicals and food groups. *J Nutr* 2003; 133(6):1937–1942.

209. Slattery ML, Schuman KL, West DW, et al. Nutrient intake and ovarian cancer. *Am J Epidemiol* 1989;130(3):497–502.

210. Byers T, Marshall J, Graham S, et al. A case-control study of dietary and nondietary factors in ovarian cancer. *J Natl Cancer Inst* 1983; 71(4):681–686.

211. Fairfield KM, Hankinson SE, Rosner BA, et al. Risk of ovarian carcinoma and consumption of vitamins A, C, and E and specific carotenoids: a prospective analysis. *Cancer* 2001;92(9):2318–2326.

212. Stratton JF, Pharoah P, Smith SK, et al. A systematic review and meta-analysis of family history and risk of ovarian cancer. *Br J Obstet Gynaecol* 1998;105(5):493–499.

213. Koch M, Gaedke H, Jenkins H. Family history of ovarian cancer patients: a case-control study. *Int J Epidemiol* 1989;18(4):782–785.

214. Hemminki K, Granstrom C. Familial invasive and borderline ovarian tumors by proband status, age and histology. *Int J Cancer* 2003; 105(5):701–705.

215. Pharoah PD, Ponder BA. The genetics of ovarian cancer. *Best Pract Res Clin Obstet* Gynaecol 2002;16(4):449–468.

216. Venkitaraman AR. Cancer susceptibility and the functions of BRCA1 and BRCA2. *Cell* 2002;108(2):171–182.

217. Hartge P, Whittemore AS, Itnyre J, et al. Rates and risks of ovarian cancer in subgroups of white women in the United States. The Collaborative Ovarian Cancer Group. *Obstet Gynecol* 1994;84(5):760–764.

218. Wooster R, Weber BL. Breast and ovarian cancer. *N Engl J Med* 2003;348(23):2339–2347.

219. Struewing JP, Hartge P, Wacholder S, et al. The risk of cancer associated with specific mutations of BRCA1 and BRCA2 among Ashkenazi Jews. *N Engl J Med* 1997;336(20):1401–1408.

220. Cook LS, Kamb ML, Weiss NS. Perineal powder exposure and the risk of ovarian cancer. *Am J Epidemiol* 1997;146(5):459–465.

221. Cramer DW, Welch WR, Scully RE, Wojciechowski CA. Ovarian cancer and talc: a case-control study. *Cancer* 1982;50(2):372–376.

222. Harlow BL, Weiss NS. A case-control study of borderline ovarian tumors: the influence of perineal exposure to talc. *Am J Epidemiol* 1989;130(2):390–394.

223. Gertig DM, Hunter DJ, Cramer DW, et al. Prospective study of talc use and ovarian cancer. *J Natl Cancer Inst* 2000;92(3):249–252.

224. Terry PD, Miller AB, Jones JG, Rohan TE. Cigarette smoking and the risk of invasive epithelial ovarian cancer in a prospective cohort study. *Eur J Cancer* 2003;39(8):1157–1164.

225. Green A, Purdie D, Bain C, et al. Cigarette smoking and risk of epithelial ovarian cancer (Australia). *Cancer Causes Control* 2001; 12(8):713–719.

226. Marchbanks PA, Wilson H, Bastos E, et al. Cigarette smoking and epithelial ovarian cancer by histologic type. *Obstet Gynecol* 2000; 95(2):255–260.

227. Modugno F, Ness RB, Cottreau CM. Cigarette smoking and the risk of mucinous and nonmucinous epithelial ovarian cancer. *Epidemiology* 2002;13(4):467–471.

228. Goodman MT, Tung K-H. Active and passive smoking and the risk of borderline and invasive ovarian cancer (United States). *Cancer Causes Control* 2003;14:569–577.

229. La Vecchia C, Franceschi S, Decarli A, et al. Coffee drinking and the risk of epithelial ovarian cancer. *Int J Cancer* 1984;33(5):559–562.

230. Whittemore AS, Wu ML, Paffenbarger RS Jr, et al. Personal and environmental characteristics related to epithelial ovarian cancer. II. Exposures to talcum powder, tobacco, alcohol, and coffee. *Am J Epidemiol* 1988;128(6):1228–1240.

231. Kuper H, Titus-Ernstoff L, Harlow BL, et al. Population based study

232. of coffee, alcohol and tobacco use and risk of ovarian cancer. *Int J Cancer* 2000;88(2):313–318.

232. Polychronopoulou A, Tzonou A, Hsieh CC, et al. Reproductive variables, tobacco, ethanol, coffee and somatometry as risk factors for ovarian cancer. *Int J Cancer* 1993;55(3):402–407.

233. Snowdon DA, Phillips RL. Coffee consumption and risk of fatal cancers. *Am J Public Health* 1984;74(8):820–823.

234. Gwinn ML, Webster LA, Lee NC, et al. Alcohol consumption and ovarian cancer risk. *Am J Epidemiol* 1986;123(5):759–766.

235. Goodman MT, Tung KH. Alcohol consumption and the risk of borderline and invasive ovarian cancer. *Obstet Gynecol* 2003;101(6): 1221–1228.

236. Lagiou P, Ye W, Wedren S, et al. Incidence of ovarian cancer among alcoholic women: a cohort study in Sweden. *Int J Cancer* 2001;91(2): 264–266.

237. Boffetta P, Andersen A, Lynge E, et al. Employment as hairdresser and risk of ovarian cancer and non–Hodgkin's lymphomas among women. *J Occup Med* 1994;36(1):61–65.

238. Donna A, Crosignani P, Robutti F, et al. Triazine herbicides and ovarian epithelial neoplasms. *Scand J Work Environ Health* 1989;15(1): 47–53.

239. Vasama-Neuvonen K, Pukkala E, Paakkulainen H, et al. Ovarian cancer and occupational exposures in Finland. *Am J Ind Med* 1999;36(1): 83–89.

240. Shields T, Gridley G, Moradi T, et al. Occupational exposures and the risk of ovarian cancer in Sweden. *Am J Ind Med* 2002;42(3): 200–213.

241. Sala M, Dosemeci M, Zahm SH. A death certificate-based study of occupation and mortality from reproductive cancers among women in 24 US states. *J Occup Environ Med* 1998;40(7):632–639.

242. Shen N, Weiderpass E, Antilla A, et al. Epidemiology of occupational and environmental risk factors related to ovarian cancer. *Scand J Work Environ Health* 1998;24(3):175–182.

243. Franceschi S, La Vecchia C, Helmrich SP, et al. Risk factors for epithelial ovarian cancer in Italy. *Am J Epidemiol* 1982;115(5): 714–719.

244. Purdie DM, Bain CJ, Siskind V, et al. Ovulation and risk of epithelial ovarian cancer. *Int J Cancer* 2003;104(2):228–232.

245. Moorman PG, Schildkraut JM, Calingaert B, et al. Ovulation and ovarian cancer: a comparison of two methods for calculating lifetime ovulatory cycles (United States). *Cancer Causes Control* 2002;13(9): 807–811.

246. Risch HA. Hormonal etiology of epithelial ovarian cancer, with a hypothesis concerning the role of androgens and progesterone. *J Natl Cancer Inst* 1998;90(23):1774–1786.

247. Cramer DW, Welch WR. Determinants of ovarian cancer risk. II. Inferences regarding pathogenesis. *J Natl Cancer Inst* 1983;71(4): 717–721.

248. Fathalla MF. Incessant ovulation––a factor in ovarian neoplasia? *Lancet* 1971;2(7716):163.

249. Zajicek J. Ovarian cystomas and ovulation, a histogenetic concept. *Tumori* 1977;63(5):429–435.

250. Rodriguez GC, Nagarsheth NP, Lee KL, et al. Progestin-induced apoptosis in the Macaque ovarian epithelium: differential regulation of transforming growth factor-beta. *J Natl Cancer* Inst 2002;94(1): 50–60.

251. Schildkraut JM, Bastos E, Berchuck A. Relationship between lifetime ovulatory cycles and overexpression of mutant p53 in epithelial ovarian cancer. *J Natl Cancer Inst* 1997;89(13):932–938.

252. Webb PM, Green A, Cummings MC, et al. Relationship between number of ovulatory cycles and accumulation of mutant p53 in epithelial ovarian cancer. *J Natl Cancer Inst* 1998;90(22):1729–1734.

253. Ness RB. Endometriosis and ovarian cancer: thoughts on shared pathophysiology. *Am J Obstet Gynecol* 2003;189:280–294.

254. Bosch FX, Lorincz A, Munoz N, et al. The causal relation between human papillomavirus and cervical cancer. *J Clin Pathol* 2002;55(4): 244–265.

255. Munoz N, Bosch FX, de Sanjose S, et al. Epidemiologic classification of human papillomavirus types associated with cervical cancer. *N Engl J Med* 2003;348(6):518–527.

256. Schiffman MH, Bauer HM, Hoover RN, et al. Epidemiologic evidence

showing that human papillomavirus infection causes most cervical intraepithelial neoplasia. *J Natl Cancer Inst* 1993;85(12):958–964.

257. Schiffman M, Kjaer SK. Chapter 2: Natural history of anogenital human papillomavirus infection and neoplasia. *J Natl Cancer Inst Monogr* 2003;(31):14–19.

258. Solomon D. Chapter 14: Role of triage testing in cervical cancer screening. *J Natl Cancer Inst Monogr* 2003;(31):97–101.

259. Cuzick J. Role of HPV testing in clinical practice. *Virus Res* 2002; 89(2):263–269.

260. Franco EL. Chapter 13: Primary screening of cervical cancer with human papillomavirus tests. *J Natl Cancer Inst Monogr* 2003;(31): 89–96.

261. Solomon D, Davey D, Kurman R, et al. The 2001 Bethesda System: terminology for reporting results of cervical cytology. *JAMA* 2002; 287(16):2114–2119.

262. Wright TC Jr, Cox JT, Massad LS, et al. 2001 consensus guidelines for the management of women with cervical cytological abnormalities. *JAMA* 2002;287(16):2120–2129.

263. Bosch FX, de Sanjose S. Chapter 1: Human papillomavirus and cervical cancer—burden and assessment of causality. *J Natl Cancer Inst Monogr* 2003;(31):3–13.

264. Autier P, Coibion M, Huet F, Grivegnee AR. Transformation zone location and intraepithelial neoplasia of the cervix uteri. *Br J Cancer* 1996;74(3):488–490.

265. Wang SS, Sherman ME, Hildesheim A, et al. Incidence and trends for cervical adenocarcinoma and squamous cell carcinoma among white and black women in the United States from 1976–2000. *Cancer (in press).*

266. Howell EA, Chen YT, Concato J. Differences in cervical cancer mortality among black and white women. *Obstet Gynecol* 1999;94(4): 509–515.

267. Ursin G, Peters RK, Henderson BE, et al. Oral contraceptive use and adenocarcinoma of cervix. *Lancet* 1994;344(8934):1390–1394.

268. Sherman ME, Lorincz AT, Scott DR, et al. Baseline cytology, human papillomavirus testing, and risk for cervical neoplasia: a 10-year cohort analysis. *J Natl Cancer Inst* 2003;95(1):46–52.

269. Woodman CB, Collins S, Winter H, et al. Natural history of cervical human papillomavirus infection in young women: a longitudinal cohort study. *Lancet* 2001;357(9271):1831–1836.

270. Wallin KL, Wiklund F, Angstrom T, et al. Type-specific persistence of human papillomavirus DNA before the development of invasive cervical cancer. *N Engl J Med* 1999;341(22):1633–1638.

271. Ylitalo N, Josefsson A, Melbye M, et al. A prospective study showing long-term infection with human papillomavirus 16 before the development of cervical carcinoma in situ. *Cancer Res* 2000;60(21): 6027–6032.

272. Zur HH. Papillomaviruses causing cancer: evasion from host-cell control in early events in carcinogenesis. *J Natl Cancer Inst* 2000;92(9): 690–698.

273. Stanley MA. Human papillomavirus and cervical carcinogenesis. *Best Pract Res Clin Obstet Gynaecol* 2001;15(5):663–676.

274. Sherman ME, Schiffman M, Cox JT. Effects of age and human papilloma viral load on colposcopy triage: data from the randomized Atypical Squamous Cells of Undetermined Significance/Low-Grade Squamous Intraepithelial Lesion Triage Study (ALTS). *J Natl Cancer Inst* 2002;94(2):102–107.

275. Josefsson AM, Magnusson PK, Ylitalo N, et al. Viral load of human papilloma virus 16 as a determinant for development of cervical carcinoma in situ: a nested case-control study. *Lancet* 2000;355(9222): 2189–2193.

276. Ylitalo N, Sorensen P, Josefsson AM, et al. Consistent high viral load of human papillomavirus 16 and risk of cervical carcinoma in situ: a nested case-control study. *Lancet* 2000;355(9222):2194–2198.

277. Andersson-Ellstrom A, Hagmar BM, Johansson B, et al. Human papillomavirus deoxyribonucleic acid in cervix only detected in girls after coitus. *Int J STD AIDS* 1996;7(5):333–336.

278. Kjaer SK, Chackerian B, van den Brule AJ, et al. High-risk human papillomavirus is sexually transmitted: evidence from a follow-up study of virgins starting sexual activity (intercourse). *Cancer Epidemiol Biomarkers Prev* 2001;10(2):101–106.

279. Franco EL, Villa LL, Sobrinho JP, et al. Epidemiology of acquisition and clearance of cervical human papillomavirus infection in women from a high-risk area for cervical cancer. *J Infect Dis* 1999;180(5): 1415–1423.

280. Moscicki AB, Hills N, Shiboski S, et al. Risks for incident human papillomavirus infection and low-grade squamous intraepithelial lesion development in young females. *JAMA* 2001;285(23):2995–3002.

281. Winer RL, Lee SK, Hughes JP, et al. Genital human papillomavirus infection: incidence and risk factors in a cohort of female university students. *Am J Epidemiol* 2003;157(3):218–226.

282. Rice PS, Cason J, Best JM, Banatvala JE. High risk genital papillomavirus infections are spread vertically. *Rev Med Virol* 1999;9(1): 15–21.

283. Dillner J, Andersson-Ellstrom A, Hagmar B, Schiller J. High risk genital papillomavirus infections are not spread vertically. *Rev Med Virol* 1999;9(1):23–29.

284. Ho GY, Bierman R, Beardsley L, et al. Natural history of cervicovaginal papillomavirus infection in young women. *N Engl J Med* 1998; 338(7):423–428.

285. Bauer HM, Hildesheim A, Schiffman MH, et al. Determinants of genital human papillomavirus infection in low-risk women in Portland, Oregon. *Sex Transm Dis* 1993;20(5):274–278.

286. Jacobs MV, Walboomers JM, Daalmeijer N, et al. Distribution of 37 mucosotropic HPV types in women with cytologically normal cervical smears: the age-related patterns for high-risk and low-risk types. *Int J Cancer* 2000;87(2):221–227.

287. Melkert PW, Hopman E, van den Brule AJ, et al. Prevalence of HPV in cytomorphologically normal cervical smears, as determined by the polymerase chain reaction, is age-dependent. *Int J Cancer* 1993;53(6): 919–923.

288. Burk RD, Kelly P, Feldman J, et al. Declining prevalence of cervicovaginal human papillomavirus infection with age is independent of other risk factors. *Sex Transm Dis* 1996;23(4):333–341.

289. Kjaer SK, van den Brule AJ, Bock JE, et al. Determinants for genital human papillomavirus (HPV) infection in 1000 randomly chosen young Danish women with normal Pap smear: are there different risk profiles for oncogenic and nononcogenic HPV types? *Cancer Epidemiol Biomarkers Prev* 1997;6(10):799–805.

290. Manhart LE, Koutsky LA. Do condoms prevent genital HPV infection, external genital warts, or cervical neoplasia? A meta-analysis. *Sex Transm Dis* 2002;29(11):725–735.

291. Franceschi S, Castellsague X, Dal Maso L, et al. Prevalence and determinants of human papillomavirus genital infection in men. *Br J Cancer* 2002;86(5):705–711.

292. Munoz N, Castellsague X, Bosch FX, et al. Difficulty in elucidating the male role in cervical cancer in Colombia, a high-risk area for the disease. *J Natl Cancer Inst* 1996;88(15):1068–1075.

293. Bosch FX, Castellsague X, Munoz N, et al. Male sexual behavior and human papillomavirus DNA: key risk factors for cervical cancer in Spain. *J Natl Cancer Inst* 1996;88(15):1060–1067.

294. Castellsague X, Bosch FX, Munoz N, et al. Male circumcision, penile human papillomavirus infection, and cervical cancer in female partners. *N Engl J Med* 2002;346(15):1105–1112.

295. Kjaer SK, van den Brule AJ, Paull G, et al. Type specific persistence of high risk human papillomavirus (HPV) as indicator of high grade cervical squamous intraepithelial lesions in young women: population based prospective follow up study. *BMJ* 2002;325(7364):572.

296. Nobbenhuis MA, Walboomers JM, Helmerhorst TJ, et al. Relation of human papillomavirus status to cervical lesions and consequences for cervical-cancer screening: a prospective study. *Lancet* 1999; 354(9172):20–25.

297. Moscicki AB, Shiboski S, Broering J, et al. The natural history of human papillomavirus infection as measured by repeated DNA testing in adolescent and young women. *J Pediatr* 1998;132(2):277–284.

298. Myers ER, McCrory DC, Nanda K, et al. Mathematical model for the natural history of human papillomavirus infection and cervical carcinogenesis. *Am J Epidemiol* 2000; 151(12):1158–1171.

299. Hildesheim A, Schiffman MH, Gravitt PE, et al. Persistence of type-specific human papillomavirus infection among cytologically normal women. *J Infect Dis* 1994;169(2):235–240.

300. Hildesheim A, Wang SS. Host and viral genetics and risk of cervical cancer: a review. *Virus Res* 2002;89(2):229–240.

301. Swan DC, Tucker RA, Tortolero-Luna G, et al. Human papillomavirus (HPV) DNA copy number is dependent on grade of cervical disease and HPV type. *J Clin Microbiol* 1999;37(4):1030–1034.

302. Cuzick J, Terry G, Ho L, et al. Type-specific human papillomavirus DNA in abnormal smears as a predictor of high-grade cervical intraepithelial neoplasia. *Br J Cancer* 1994;69(1):167–171.

303. Rousseau MC, Pereira JS, Prado JC, et al. Cervical coinfection with human papillomavirus (HPV) types as a predictor of acquisition and persistence of HPV infection. *J Infect Dis* 2001;184(12):1508–1517.

304. Liaw KL, Hildesheim A, Burk RD, et al. A prospective study of human papillomavirus (HPV) type 16 DNA detection by polymerase chain reaction and its association with acquisition and persistence of other HPV types. *J Infect Dis* 2001;183(1):8–15.

305. Wang SS, Hildesheim A, Gao X, et al. Human leukocyte antigen class I alleles and cervical neoplasia: no heterozygote advantage. *Cancer Epidemiol Biomarkers Prev* 2002;11(4):419–420.

306. Konya J, Dillner J. Immunity to oncogenic human papillomaviruses. *Adv Cancer Res* 2001;82:205–238.

307. Man S, Fiander A. Immunology of human papillomavirus infection in lower genital tract neoplasia. *Best Pract Res Clin Obstet Gynaecol* 2001;15(5):701–714.

308. Woodworth CD. HPV innate immunity. *Front Biosci* 2002;7:d2058–d2071.

309. Birkeland SA, Storm HH, Lamm LU, et al. Cancer risk after renal transplantation in the Nordic countries, 1964–1986. *Int J Cancer* 1995;60(2):183–189.

310. Palefsky JM, Minkoff H, Kalish LA, et al. Cervicovaginal human papillomavirus infection in human immunodeficiency virus-1 (HIV)–positive and high-risk HIV-negative women. *J Natl Cancer Inst* 1999;91(3):226–236.

311. Sun XW, Kuhn L, Ellerbrock TV, et al. Human papillomavirus infection in women infected with the human immunodeficiency virus. *N Engl J Med* 1997;337(19):1343–1349.

312. Frisch M, Biggar RJ, Goedert JJ. Human papillomavirus–associated cancers in patients with human immunodeficiency virus infection and acquired immunodeficiency syndrome. *J Natl Cancer Inst* 2000;92(18):1500–1510.

313. Palefsky JM, Holly EA. Chapter 6: Immunosuppression and co-infection with HIV. *J Natl Cancer Inst Monogr* 2003;(31):41–46.

314. Mandelblatt JS, Kanetsky P, Eggert L, Gold K. Is HIV infection a cofactor for cervical squamous cell neoplasia? *Cancer Epidemiol Biomarkers Prev* 1999;8(1):97–106.

315. Munoz N, Franceschi S, Bosetti C, et al. Role of parity and human papillomavirus in cervical cancer: the IARC multicentric case-control study. *Lancet* 2002;359(9312):1093–1101.

316. Kruger-Kjaer S, van den Brule AJ, Svare EI, et al. Different risk factor patterns for high-grade and low-grade intraepithelial lesions on the cervix among HPV-positive and HPV-negative young women. *Int J Cancer* 1998;76(5):613–619.

317. Castle PE, Wacholder S, Lorincz AT, et al. A prospective study of high-grade cervical neoplasia risk among human papillomavirus-infected women. *J Natl Cancer Inst* 2002;94(18):1406–1414.

318. Castellsague X, Munoz N. Chapter 3: Cofactors in human papillomavirus carcinogenesis—role of parity, oral contraceptives, and tobacco smoking. *J Natl Cancer Inst Monogr* 2003;(31):20–28.

319. Hildesheim A, Herrero R, Castle PE, et al. HPV co-factors related to the development of cervical cancer: results from a population-based study in Costa Rica. *Br J Cancer* 2001;84(9):1219–1226.

320. Winkelstein W Jr. Smoking and cervical cancer—current status: a review. *Am J Epidemiol* 1990;131(6):945–957.

321. Szarewski A. Smoking and cervical neoplasia: a review of the evidence. *J Epidemiol Biostat* 1998;3:229–256.

322. Deacon JM, Evans CD, Yule R, et al. Sexual behaviour and smoking as determinants of cervical HPV infection and of CIN3 among those infected: a case-control study nested within the Manchester cohort. *Br J Cancer* 2000;83(11):1565–1572.

323. Szarewski A, Jarvis MJ, Sasieni P, et al. Effect of smoking cessation on cervical lesion size. *Lancet* 1996;347(9006):941–943.

324. Giulian AR, Sedjo RL, Roe DJ, et al. Clearance of oncogenic human papillomavirus (HPV) infection: effect of smoking (United States). *Cancer Causes Control* 2002;13(9):839–846.

325. Moreno V, Bosch FX, Munoz N, et al. Effect of oral contraceptives on risk of cervical cancer in women with human papillomavirus infection: the IARC multicentric case-control study. *Lancet* 2002;359(9312):1085–1092.

326. Green J, Berrington DG, Smith JS, et al. Human papillomavirus infection and use of oral contraceptives. *Br J Cancer* 2003;88(11):1713–1720.

327. Castle PE, Hillier SL, Rabe LK, et al. An association of cervical inflammation with high-grade cervical neoplasia in women infected with oncogenic human papillomavirus (HPV). *Cancer Epidemiol Biomarkers Prev* 2001;10(10):1021–1027.

328. Cox JT, Schiffman M, Solomon D. Prospective follow-up suggests similar risk of subsequent cervical intraepithelial neoplasia grade 2 or 3 among women with cervical intraepithelial neoplasia grade 1 or negative colposcopy and directed biopsy. *Am J Obstet Gynecol* 2003;188(6):1406–1412.

329. Nasiell K, Nasiell M, Vaclavinkova V. Behavior of moderate cervical dysplasia during long-term follow-up. *Obstet Gynecol* 1983;61(5):609–614.

330. ASCUS-LSIL Triage Study (ALTS) Group. Results of a randomized trial on the management of cytology interpretations of atypical squamous cells of undetermined significance. *Am J Obstet Gynecol* 2003;188(6):1383–1392.

331. Madeleine MM, Daling JR, Schwartz SM, et al. Human papillomavirus and long-term oral contraceptive use increase the risk of adenocarcinoma in situ of the cervix. *Cancer Epidemiol Biomarkers Prev* 2001;10(3):171–177.

332. Pirog EC, Kleter B, Olgac S, et al. Prevalence of human papillomavirus DNA in different histological subtypes of cervical adenocarcinoma. *Am J Pathol* 2000;157(4):1055–1062.

333. Mitchell H, Medley G, Gordon I, Giles G. Cervical cytology reported as negative and risk of adenocarcinoma of the cervix: no strong evidence of benefit. *Br J Cancer* 1995;71(4):894–897.

334. Schoolland M, Segal A, Allpress S, et al. Adenocarcinoma in situ of the cervix. *Cancer* 2002;96(6):330–337.

335. Schoolland M, Allpress S, Sterrett GF. Adenocarcinoma of the cervix. *Cancer* 2002;96(1):5–13.

336. Lee KR, Minter LJ, Granter SR. Papanicolaou smear sensitivity for adenocarcinoma in situ of the cervix. A study of 34 cases. *Am J Clin Pathol* 1997;107(1):30–35.

337. Krane JF, Granter SR, Trask CE, et al. Papanicolaou smear sensitivity for the detection of adenocarcinoma of the cervix: a study of 49 cases. *Cancer* 2001;93(1):8–15.

338. Hildesheim A, Hadjimichael O, Schwartz PE, et al. Risk factors for rapid-onset cervical cancer. *Am J Obstet Gynecol* 1999;180(3 Pt 1):571–577.

339. Plaxe SC, Saltzstein SL. Estimation of the duration of the preclinical phase of cervical adenocarcinoma suggests that there is ample opportunity for screening. *Gynecol Oncol* 1999;75(1):55–61.

340. Altekruse SF, Lacey JV Jr, Brinton LA, et al. Comparison of human papillomavirus genotypes, sexual, and reproductive risk factors of cervical adenocarcinoma and squamous cell carcinoma: Northeastern United States. *Am J Obstet Gynecol* 2003;188(3):657–663.

341. Ursin G, Pike MC, Preston-Martin S, et al. Sexual, reproductive, and other risk factors for adenocarcinoma of the cervix: results from a population-based case-control study (California, United States). *Cancer Causes Control* 1996;7(3):391–401.

342. Lacey JV Jr, Frisch M, Brinton LA, et al. Associations between smoking and adenocarcinomas and squamous cell carcinomas of the uterine cervix (United States). *Cancer Causes Control* 2001;12(2):153–161.

343. Parazzini F, La Vecchia C, Negri E, et al. Risk factors for adenocarcinoma of the cervix: a case-control study. *Br J Cancer* 1988;57(2):201–204.

344. Lacey JV Jr, Swanson CA, Brinton LA, Gravitt PE et al. Obesity as a potential risk factor for adenocarcinomas and squamous cell carcinomas of the uterine cervix. *Cancer* 2003;98(4):814–821.

345. Lacey JV Jr, Brinton LA, Abbas FM, et al. Oral contraceptives as risk

factors for cervical adenocarcinomas and squamous cell carcinomas. *Cancer Epidemiol Biomarkers Prev* 1999;8(12):1079–1085.

346. Thomas DB, Ray RM. Oral contraceptives and invasive adenocarcinomas and adenosquamous carcinomas of the uterine cervix. The World Health Organization Collaborative Study of Neoplasia and Steroid Contraceptives. *Am J Epidemiol* 1996;144(3):281–289.

347. Lacey JV Jr, Brinton LA, Barnes WA, et al. Use of hormone replacement therapy and adenocarcinomas and squamous cell carcinomas of the uterine cervix. *Gynecol Oncol* 2000;77(1):149–154.

348. Parazzini F, La Vecchia C, Negri E, et al. Case-control study of oestrogen replacement therapy and risk of cervical cancer. *BMJ* 1997;315(7100):85–88.

349. Thomas DB, Ray RM. Depot-medroxyprogesterone acetate (DMPA) and risk of invasive adenocarcinomas and adenosquamous carcinomas of the uterine cervix. WHO Collaborative Study of Neoplasia and Steroid Contraceptives. *Contraception* 1995;52(5):307–312.

350. Staebler A, Sherman ME, Zaino RJ, Ronnett BM. Hormone receptor immunohistochemistry and human papillomavirus in situ hybridization are useful for distinguishing endocervical and endometrial adenocarcinomas. *Am J Surg Pathol* 2002;26(8):998–1006.

351. Zaino RJ. The fruits of our labors: distinguishing endometrial from endocervical adenocarcinoma. *Int J Gynecol Pathol* 2002;21(1):1–3.

352. Kim JJ, Wright TC, Goldie SJ. Cost-effectiveness of alternative triage strategies for atypical squamous cells of undetermined significance. *JAMA* 2002;287(18):2382–2390.

353. Sherman ME, Schiffman MH, Lorincz AT, et al. Toward objective quality assurance in cervical cytopathology. Correlation of cytopathologic diagnoses with detection of high-risk human papillomavirus types. *Am J Clin Pathol* 1994;102(2):182–187.

354. Zuna RE, Moore W, Dunn ST. HPV DNA testing of the residual sample of liquid–based Pap test: utility as a quality assurance monitor. *Mod Pathol* 2001;14(3):147–151.

355. Koutsky LA, Ault KA, Wheeler CM, et al. A controlled trial of a human papillomavirus type 16 vaccine. *N Engl J Med* 2002;347(21):1645–1651.

356. Sherman KJ, Daling JR, Chu J, et al. Multiple primary tumors in women with vulvar neoplasms: a case-control study. *Br J Cancer* 1988;57(4):423–427.

357. Rose PG, Herterick EE, Boutselis JG, et al. Multiple primary gynecologic neoplasms. *Am J Obstet Gynecol* 1987;157(2):261–267.

358. Beckmann AM, Kiviat NB, Daling JR, et al. Human papillomavirus type 16 in multifocal neoplasia of the female genital tract. *Int J Gynecol Pathol* 1988;7(1):39–47.

359. Sturgeon SR, Brinton LA, Devesa SS, Kurman RJ. In situ and invasive vulvar cancer incidence trends (1973 to 1987). *Am J Obstet Gynecol* 1992;166(5):1482–1485.

360. Trimble CL, Hildesheim A, Brinton LA, et al. Heterogeneous etiology of squamous carcinoma of the vulva. *Obstet Gynecol* 1996;87(1):59–64.

361. Brinton LA, Nasca PC, Mallin K, et al. Case-control study of cancer of the vulva. *Obstet Gynecol* 1990;75(5):859–866.

362. Sherman KJ, Daling JR, Chu J, et al. Genital warts, other sexually transmitted diseases, and vulvar cancer. *Epidemiology* 1991;2(4):257–262.

363. Bjorge T, Dillner J, Anttila T, et al. Prospective seroepidemiological study of role of human papillomavirus in non-cervical anogenital cancers. *BMJ* 1997;315(7109):646–649.

364. Hildesheim A, Han CL, Brinton LA, et al. Human papillomavirus type 16 and risk of preinvasive and invasive vulvar cancer: results from a seroepidemiological case-control study. *Obstet Gynecol* 1997;90(5):748–754.

365. Madeleine MM, Daling JR, Carter JJ, et al. Cofactors with human papillomavirus in a population-based study of vulvar cancer. *J Natl Cancer Inst* 1997;89(20):1516–1523.

366. Daling JR, Sherman KJ, Hislop TG, et al. Cigarette smoking and the risk of anogenital cancer. *Am J Epidemiol* 1992;135(2):180–189.

367. Newcomb PA, Weiss NS, Daling JR. Incidence of vulvar carcinoma in relation to menstrual, reproductive, and medical factors. *J Natl Cancer Inst* 1984;73(2):391–396.

368. Daling JR, Chu J, Weiss NS, et al. The association of condylomata acuminata and squamous carcinoma of the vulva. *Br J Cancer* 1984;50(4):533–535.

369. Chen C, Madeleine MM, Weiss NS, Daling JR. Glutathione S-transferease M1 genotypes and the risk of vulvar cancer: a population-based case-control study. *Am J Epidemiol* 1999;150(5):437–442.

370. Chen C, Cook LS, Li XY, et al. CYP2D6 genotype and the incidence of anal and vulvar cancer. *Cancer Epidemiol Biomarkers Prev* 1999;8(4 pt 1):317–321.

371. Okagaki T. Female genital tumors associated with human papillomavirus infection, and the concept of genital neoplasm-papilloma syndrome (GENPS). *Pathol Annu* 1984;19(Pt 2):31–62.

372. Brinton LA, Nasca PC, Mallin K, et al. Case-control study of in situ and invasive carcinoma of the vagina. *Gynecol Oncol* 1990;38(1):49–54.

373. Daling JR, Madeleine MM, Schwartz SM, et al. A population-based study of squamous cell vaginal cancer: HPV and cofactors. *Gynecol Oncol* 2002;84(2):263–270.

374. Herbst AL, Ulfelder H, Poskanzer DC. Adenocarcinoma of the vagina. Association of maternal stilbestrol therapy with tumor appearance in young women. *N Engl J Med* 1971;284(15):878–881.

375. Greenwald P, Barlow JJ, Nasca PC, Burnett WS. Vaginal cancer after maternal treatment with synthetic estrogens. *N Engl J Med* 1971;285(7):390–392.

376. Noller KL, Decker DG, Lanier AP, Kurland LT. Clear-cell adenocarcinoma of the cervix after maternal treatment with synthetic estrogens. *Mayo Clin Proc* 1972;47(9):629–630.

377. Herbst AL, Anderson S, Hubby MM, et al. Risk factors for the development of diethylstilbestrol-associated clear cell adenocarcinoma: a case-control study. *Am J Obstet Gynecol* 1986;154(4):814–822.

378. Hatch EE, Palmer JR, Titus-Ernstoff L, et al. Cancer risk in women exposed to diethylstilbestrol in utero. *JAMA* 1998;280(7):630–634.

379. Fulop V, Mok SC, Gati I, Berkowitz RS. Recent advances in molecular biologic of gestational trophoblastic diseases. A review. *J Reprod Med* 2002;47(5):369–379.

380. Brinton LA, Bracken MB, Connelly RR. Choriocarcinoma incidence in the United States. *Am J Epidemiol* 1986;123(6):1094–1100.

381. Bracken MB, Brinton LA, Hayashi K. Epidemiology of hydatidiform mole and choriocarcinoma. *Epidemiol Rev* 1984;6:52–75.

382. Tham BW, Everard JE, Tidy JA, et al. Gestational trophoblastic disease in the Asian population of Northern England and North Wales. *BJOG* 2003;110(6):555–559.

383. Smith HO, Hilgers RD, Bedrick EJ, et al. Ethnic differences at risk for gestational trophoblastic disease in New Mexico: a 25-year population study. *Am J Obstet Gynecol* 2003;188(2):357–366.

384. Bagshawe KD, Rawlins G, Pike MC, Lawler SD. ABO blood-groups in trophoblastic neoplasia. *Lancet* 1971;1(7699):553–556.

385. Dawood MY, Teoh ES, Ratnam SS. ABO blood group in trophoblastic disease. *J Obstet Gynaecol Br Commonw* 1971;78(10):918–923.

386. Messerli ML, Lilienfeld AM, Parmley T, et al. Rosenshein NB. Risk factors for gestational trophoblastic neoplasia. *Am J Obstet Gynecol* 1985;153(3):294–300.

387. Parazzini F, La Vecchia C, Franceschi S, et al. ABO blood-groups and the risk of gestational trophoblastic disease. *Tumori* 1985;71(2):123–126.

388. Brinton LA, Wu BZ, Wang W, et al. Gestational trophoblastic disease: a case control study from the People's Republic of China. *Am J Obstet Gynecol* 1989;161(1):121–127.

389. Parazzini F, La Vecchia C, Pampallona S, Franceschi S. Reproductive patterns and the risk of gestational trophoblastic disease. *Am J Obstet Gynecol* 1985;152(7 Pt 1):866–870.

390. La Vecchia C, Franceschi S, Parazzini F, et al. Risk factors for gestational trophoblastic disease in Italy. *Am J Epidemiol* 1985;121(3):457–464.

391. Buckley JD, Henderson BE, Morrow CP, et al. Case-control study of gestational choriocarcinoma. *Cancer Res* 1988;48(4):1004–1010.

392. Berkowitz RS, Cramer DW, Bernstein MR, et al. Risk factors for complete molar pregnancy from a case-control study. *Am J Obstet Gynecol* 1985;152(8):1016–1020.

393. Palmer JR, Driscoll SG, Rosenberg L, et al. Oral contraceptive use

and risk of gestational trophoblastic tumors. *J Natl Cancer Inst* 1999;
91(7):635–640.

394. Parazzini F, Cipriani S, Mangili G, et al. Oral contraceptvies and
risk of gestational trophoblastic disease. *Contraception* 2002;65(6):
425–427.

395. Rosenberg L, Palmer JR, Shapiro S. Gestational trophoblastic disease
and use of oral contraceptives. *Am J Obstet Gynecol* 1989;161(4):
1087–1088.

396. Stone M, Dent J, Kardana A, Bagshawe KD. Relationship of oral
contraception to development of trophoblastic tumour after evacuation
of a hydatidiform mole. *Br J Obstet Gynaecol* 1976;83(12):913–916.

397. Yuen BH, Burch P. Relationship of oral contraceptives and the intrauterine contraceptive devices to the regressin of concentrations of the
beta subuit of human chorionic gonadotropin and invasive complications after molar pregnancy. *Am J Obstet Gynecol* 1983;145:214.

398. Curry SL, Schlaerth JB, Kohorn EI, et al. Hormonal contraception
and trophoblastic sequelae after hydatidiform mole (a Gynecologic
Oncology Group Study). *Am J Obstet Gynecol* 1989;160(4):805–809.

399. Morrow P, Nakamura R, Schlaerth J, et al. The influence of oral
contraceptives on the postmolar human chorionic gonadotropin
regression curve. *Am J Obstet Gynecol* 1985;151(7):906–914.

400. La Vecchia C, Parazzini F, Decarli A, et al. Age of parents and risk
of gestational trophoblastic disease. *J Natl Cancer Inst* 1984;73(3):
639–642.

CHAPTER 2

Clinical Genetics of Gynecologic Cancer

Steven A. Narod

GENETICS IN CLINICAL PRACTICE OF GYNECOLOGY ONCOLOGY

The identification of the *BRCA1* gene in 1994 and the *BRCA2* gene 1 year later has introduced a new component to gynecologic oncology. Genetic testing for ovarian cancer predisposition was generally available by 1996 and has been growing in volume steadily since. It now appears that the major genes for susceptibility to gynecologic cancer have been found (Table 2.1). The last important addition to the list of genes for cancer susceptibility, *HMSH6*, was added to the list in 1999. The ability to use laboratory testing to predict the later development of ovarian cancer requires clinicians to have a clear understanding of the role of genetic testing in patient care. This advance in preventive oncology has also had the effect of increasing the number of healthy women seeking advice from a gynecologic oncologist. Increasing numbers of prophylactic oophorectomies are performed on healthy women by surgeons who, for the large part, had previously treated patients with cancer. Information is now available that supports the use of genetic testing for *BRCA* mutations as a means to prevent ovarian cancer in high-risk women. The strategies for prevention include screening, prophylactic surgery, and chemoprevention with oral contraceptives.

OVARIAN CANCER

Genetic Epidemiology

Approximately 12% of all women with invasive ovarian cancer carry a *BRCA1* or *BRCA2* mutation (1), and it is reasonable therefore to offer genetic testing to a woman diag-

nosed with invasive, nonmucinous, epithelial ovarian cancer or to one of her first-degree female relatives. In general, if the patient is alive, testing is offered first to the affected woman. In the event of a positive test, testing is then extended to unaffected female relatives. However, if there is no living affected relative, then testing may be offered first to an unaffected woman. Of all the common forms of cancer in adults, only ovarian cancer has a hereditary proportion that exceeds 10%. The frequency of *BRCA* mutations among ovarian cancer patients is not the same in all ethnic groups. In some populations, there are recurrent (founder) mutations. In these populations, the overall frequency of *BRCA1* mutations tends to be higher and a large proportion of mutations will be accounted for by one, or a small number, of specific mutations. For example, approximately 30% to 40% of Jewish women with ovarian cancer will carry one of three founder mutations (two in *BRCA1* and one in *BRCA2*) (2,3). Moslehi et al. (2) found that 41% of Jewish women with ovarian cancer from North America carried a mutation, including the majority of those diagnosed with cancer between the ages of 40 and 60 years. Modan et al. (3) found one of the three mutations in 29% of 840 Jewish women with ovarian cancer in Israel. In Poland, 13.5% of unselected patients with ovarian cancer carried one of three common *BRCA1* mutations (4). One of these (*5382insC*) was also one of the three mutations found in these women . These three mutations account for 86% of all *BRCA* mutations found in Poland (5). The frequency of *BRCA* mutations has been esti-

TABLE 2.1. *Genes associated with common cancers*

Breast	Ovary	Colon	Endometrial
BRCA1	BRCA1		
BRCA2	BRCA2	APC	
ATM	HMSH2	HMSH2	HMSH2
CHEK2	HMLH1	HMLH1	HMLH1
NBS1	HMSH6	HMSH6	HMSH6
P53			PTEN

Steven A. Narod: The Centre for Research on Women's Health, Women's College Hospital, University of Toronto, Toronto, Ontario, Canada M5G 1N8

mated at 1 in 12.4 cases of ovarian cancer in the French-Canadian population (6) and 1 in 6.3 cases in Pakistan (7). In these populations, it may be possible to offer testing for only a limited number of mutations.

In the ethnically mixed populations of North America, approximately 10% to 13% of all patients with invasive ovarian cancer carry a mutation in *BRCA1* or *BRCA2* (1). However, the range of mutations is wide and genetic testing must be comprehensive (full genomic screening). In Ontario, a mutation was found in 59 of 515 (11.5%) unselected cases of ovarian cancer (1). Women with *BRCA1* mutations were diagnosed with ovarian cancer at an average age of 51.2 years compared to 57.5 years for carriers of *BRCA2* mutations. *BRCA1* mutations represented 83% of the mutations found in women diagnosed under age 50 years and *BRCA2* mutations represented 60% of those diagnosed after age 60 years. Among *BRCA1* carriers, the risk of ovarian cancer is substantial in women above the age of 35 years (approximately 1% per year), and preventive measures must therefore be initiated early. Women who carry a pathogenic mutation in the *BRCA1* gene carry a lifetime risk of approximately 40% of developing invasive ovarian cancer (8,9) (Table 2.2). Among *BRCA2* carriers, the risk is much lower [approximately 11% lifetime (9)] and ovarian cancer rarely occurs before age 50 years. Also, among *BRCA2* carriers, the risk of ovarian cancer varies with the position of the mutation. Thompson et al. (10) estimated that the risk of ovarian cancer to age 70 years was 20% for carriers of *BRCA2* mutations within the Ovarian Cancer Cluster Region (OCCR: nucleotides 4075–6503) and was 11% for mutations outside of this region.

Pathology and Surgical Presentation of Hereditary Ovarian Cancer

Ovarian cancers that occur in women with a *BRCA* mutation appear to be similar to their sporadic counterparts (1,2, 11,12) with the exception that mucinous tumors and tumors of low malignant potential (or ''borderline'' tumors) are rarely observed in women with a *BRCA* mutation. The great majority of *BRCA*-linked ovarian cancers show moderate to poor differentiation. Most hereditary tumors present at an advanced surgical stage (2,11), but stage I or II tumors are now being discovered in the context of high-risk screening programs, or as an incidental finding associated with a pro-

TABLE 2.2. *Lifetime risks of cancers associated with specific genes*

	BRCA1	BRCA2	MMR[a]
Breast	50%–85%	50%–85%	NI
Ovarian	30%–40%	15%–25%	5%–10%
Endometrial	NI	NI	40%–60%

NI, not increased.
[a] Mismatch repair genes *HMSH2, HMLH1,* and *HMSH6.*

phylactic oophorectomy in an asymptomatic woman. Several studies have reported the presence of early ovarian cancers among pathologic specimens obtained at the time of prophylactic surgery (13–15). In one study (13), 4 of 33 women (12%) at high risk were found to have clinically unsuspected ovarian cancer at the time of prophylactic oophorectomy. In a second study (14), two of eight women with germline *BRCA1* mutations had ovarian cancer at the time of prophylactic oophorectomy. Salazar et al. (15) reviewed the ovaries of 20 women who had a prophylactic oophorectomy and found two cases of microscopic cancer.

It is believed that most ovarian cancers originate in the epithelial component of the ovary, but it is not clear whether they originate in the single-cell layer of surface epithelium or in architectural aberrations of the surface epithelium. Examples of the latter include surface epithelium-lined clefts and cortical inclusion cysts. Among *BRCA1* carriers, a significant proportion of cancers arise originally in the fallopian tube and present clinically with multifocal disease (16). For stage III and IV ovarian cancer that presents clinically, it is often difficult to be certain about the exact site of origin of the malignancy.

Several study groups have asked whether morphologic alterations of the ovarian surface epithelium are prevalent in women with ovarian cancer (17,18) or who are at high genetic risk for ovarian cancer (19–22). Alterations of these types are common, and it has not yet been proven that they are present at a higher frequency than expected in cancer-prone ovaries. The existence of an identifiable premalignant lesion for ovarian carcinoma is controversial. Most ovarian carcinomas have reached an advanced stage at presentation and are associated with little or no residual preinvasive or normal epithelium. Benign and borderline (or low malignant potential) ovarian tumors are not believed to be precursors of invasive ovarian carcinoma (23).

Clinical Outcome and Treatment Effects

Several studies have reported that the survival of patients with *BRCA*-associated ovarian cancer is improved compared to women with sporadic ovarian cancer (11,24–26) but there have been negative studies as well (27). A recent study of consecutive cases of ovarian cancers, which compared *BRCA*-associated to sporadic ovarian cancer from the same institution, found that *BRCA* mutation status was a favorable and independent predictor of survival for women with advanced disease (11). It is not yet clear if the improved survival rates are the result of a difference in the natural history of ovarian cancer in the two subgroups or is the result of a better response of *BRCA*-associated tumors to current therapies. Laboratory data suggest that enhanced response to chemotherapy underlies the better survival. In support of this position, Cass et al. reported that *BRCA1* carriers with ovarian cancer had a higher response rate to primary therapy than did matched noncarriers, and carrier patients with advanced disease had improved survival (91 months for *BRCA1* carriers vs 54 months for noncarriers; $p = .05$) (28).

Prophylactic Oophorectomy

In 1995, a consensus panel of the National Institutes of Health (NIH) recommended prophylactic oophorectomy for high-risk women at age 35 years or after childbearing is complete (29). Fifty-four percent of 79 women with *BRCA* mutations counseled at Womens College Hospital in Toronto underwent a prophylactic oophorectomy within 3 years of receiving a positive result (30). It seems logical that prophylactic oophorectomy should eliminate the incidence of ovarian cancer, but there are two reasons for its failure to do so. First, it is possible that the removed ovaries contain foci of occult carcinoma and that cancer has spread locally to the peritoneum at the time of the resection. In this case, the peritoneal cancer is not a primary cancer but a metastatic ovarian cancer. Second, it is possible that de novo cancer of the peritoneum or of the fallopian tube arises in the peritoneum after oophorectomy. The peritoneum is derived from coelomic epithelium of the same embryologic origin as the surface epithelium of the ovary.

Liede et al. (31) followed a cohort of 33 Jewish women with *BRCA* mutations for a mean of 8 years. Five cases of primary peritoneal cancer were diagnosed. The 10-year risk of peritoneal cancer was 16%. However, the women in this study had both ovaries intact and the peritoneal origin of the tumors was not definite. It is difficult to measure the risk of peritoneal cancer in women with intact ovaries. Peritoneal, fallopian, and serous ovarian cancers are histologically indistinguishable, and symptomatic women often present with multiple foci of cancer involvement involving the peritoneum, tubes, omentum, and ovary. Tubal cancer is difficult to discriminate from ovarian cancer and is often misclassified as ovarian cancer (32).

It is easier to make the diagnosis of primary peritoneal cancer in women without ovaries. New serous cancers that arise in the abdominal peritoneum, following an oophorectomy, with pathologically normal ovaries are generally considered to be primary peritoneal cancers. The risk of peritoneal cancer after prophylactic oophorectomy in high-risk women has been addressed, but none of these studies is definitive. In many cases, the mutation status of the subject was not known. Piver et al. (33) reported that 6 of 324 women who underwent prophylactic oophrectomy experienced primary peritoneal cancer. The mutation status of these women was unknown and there was no standard period of follow-up. Struewing et al. (34) reported that the cancer risk in women after prophylactic oophorectomy was 13 times greater than that expected from population-based rates, but this was based on only two observed cases of peritoneal cancer. They estimated the risk reduction associated with prophylactic oophorectomy to be 50%. Kauff et al. (35) followed 170 *BRCA* carriers for an average of 2 years. They observed one peritoneal cancer among 98 women who chose salpingo-oophorectomy versus five ovarian/peritoneal cancers in 72 women with intact ovaries. In a historical cohort study of 551 *BRCA1* and *BRCA2* carriers, Rebbeck et al. (36) reported that the incidence of ovarian or peritoneal cancer was diminished by 96% (95% CI: 84% to 99%) in women who underwent prophylactic oophorectomy compared to those with intact ovaries. An additional benefit of prophylactic oophorectomy is a marked reduction in the risk of breast cancer (37,38). Oophorectomies performed at a relatively early age (<40 years) are associated with a greater degree of protection than those performed near the age of menopause.

Oral Contraceptives and Tubal Ligation

A protective effect of oral contraceptives against ovarian cancer has been reported in *BRCA* carriers (39–41). In a recent study of 232 ovarian cancer cases and 232 controls, oral contraceptive use was associated with a 56% reduction in the risk of ovarian cancer ($p = .002$) (46). Cases and controls were matched for year of birth, mutation (*BRCA1* or *BRCA2*), and country of residence. In a case-control study from Israel, oral contraceptives were not found to be protective against ovarian cancer in carriers of *BRCA* mutations (3). However, among the Israeli patients in the first study, a strong protective effect was seen (odds ratio 0.15; 95% CI 0.03 to 0.75) (41).

Tubal ligation has been found to be protective against ovarian cancer in the general population and among *BRCA1* carriers (40). Narod and colleagues reported an adjusted relative risk of 0.39 (95% CI 0.22 to 0.70) for tubal ligation and subsequent ovarian cancer (a risk reduction of 61%). The combination of tubal ligation and oral contraceptives provided 72% protection for *BRCA1* carriers. Surprisingly, no effect of tubal ligation was seen for *BRCA2* carriers. Piek et al. (42) suggest that the cells of origin of ovarian cancer in *BRCA1* carriers arise in the fallopian epithelium and are transported to the ovary, and that tubal ligation interrupts this passage.

Screening for Hereditary Ovarian Cancer

Screening for ovarian cancer using serial CA-125 levels and abdominal ultrasound has been proposed as a method of reducing mortality through early detection. There have been no randomized trials of screening in *BRCA1* carriers, but observational cohort studies have been disappointing. Liede et al. (31) identified seven ovarian/peritoneal cancers in a historical cohort of 33 *BRCA* carriers who underwent regular screening examinations. Six of the seven cases were stage III at the time of diagnosis. For the majority of cases, the ultrasound findings were normal prior to diagnosis and the women presented with pain or abdominal distension. In a randomized trial of CA-125 and ultrasound in women at average risk, Jacobs and colleagues (43) identified 16 ovarian cancers in the screened group. Eleven of the 16 tumors were diagnosed at stage III or IV. Neither CA-125 nor ultrasound has been proven to be a sensitive means of detecting stage I and stage II ovarian cancers. Mok et al. (44) reported that serum levels of prostasin are elevated in women with ovarian cancer, and proposed that this may qualify as a new tumor marker, possibly in combination with CA-125. New techniques for identifying patterns of serum proteins generated by mass spectroscopy are promising for the development of new sensitive and specific screening tests for ovarian cancer (45). Petricoin and colleagues were able to identify all 50 malignant ovarian cancers in a set of 116 serum samples, including 18 stage I cases (45). The specificity of the test was 95%. However, it is not yet known how long is the mean duration of an ovarian cancer in stage I, and therefore the optimal screening interval has not yet been defined.

CANCER OF THE FALLOPIAN TUBE

Carcinoma of the fallopian tube has been noted in several BRCA-linked breast and ovarian cancer kindreds.

In a population-based study of unselected cases of carcinoma of the fallopian tube, 7 of 44 (16%) tested patients were found to harbor a germline BRCA mutation, 5 in BRCA1 (11%) and 2 in BRCA2 (5%); implying that a substantial fraction of fallopian tube cancers may result from genetic predisposition (46). These prevalence figures are similar to those reported for unselected cases of ovarian cancer. There is also a high frequency of pathologic lesions found in the fallopian tubes of women with BRCA mutations. Colgan et al. (16) reviewed 60 tubal and ovarian specimens from women undergoing prophylactic oophorectomies. Among the 39 BRCA1-positive cases, there were five occult malignancies detected, and among the 21 women with no mutation identified, no malignancies were identified. The number of malignant foci ranged from one to seven. Paley et al. (47) discovered two occult cancers of the fallopian tube in women who carried germline BRCA1 mutations. In summary, cancer of the fallopian tube is rare but is an integral component of the breast–ovarian cancer syndrome and may be caused by mutations in either BRCA1 or BRCA2. It is necessary that the fallopian tube be completely removed when a prophylactic oophorectomy is performed.

ENDOMETRIAL CANCER

The most important factor in the etiology of endometrial cancer is prolonged estrogen exposure, but inherited factors are important for a proportion of cases as well. Susceptibility genes for endometrial cancer include BRCA1, PTEN, and the three mismatch repair genes HMSH2, HMLH1, and HMSH6. These genes are responsible for the hereditary breast–ovarian cancer syndrome, Cowden's syndrome, and hereditary nonpolyposis colon cancer (discussed below), respectively.

The Breast Cancer Linkage Consortium reported that some endometrial cancers were due to mutations in BRCA1 (48) but none was due to mutations in BRCA2 (49). Among BRCA1 carriers, the risk for endometrial cancer was reported to be 2.6 times higher than expected (95% CI 1.7 to 4.2). However, two smaller studies—one of patients with papillary serous endometrial tumors (50) and one of patients with endometrial carcinomas in general (51)—concluded that the risk of endometrial carcinoma in women with a germline BRCA1 mutation was not increased. These findings suggest that it is likely that some cases of endometrial carcinoma are likely to be due to an inherited BRCA1 mutation, but the penetrance of BRCA1 mutations for endometrial carcinoma is low and the hereditary fraction is small.

Somatic mutations in PTEN are common in endometrial cancers (52), and rarely are inherited constitutional mutations in PTEN present in women with endometrial cancer. In the latter case, endometrial cancer is seen in the context of Cowden's syndrome—a rare dominant disease of the skin that is associated with increased risks of cancer of the breast, thyroid, and endometrium (53).

Women in families with the syndrome of hereditary familial nonpolyposis colon cancer (HNPCC) are also at elevated risk for endometrial and ovarian cancers (54). This syndrome is characterized by an autosomal dominant inherited tendency to develop cancer of the colon and other cancers. The colon cancers tend to be of young onset, to be right-sided, and are often multicentric. Adenomatous polyps are seen, but florid polyposis is rare. Individuals in families with HNPCC are at risk for a range of cancer types, and among women, endometrial cancer is the second most frequent site of cancer (55). Genes that are responsible for repair of mismatched DNA (mismatch repair) are defective in families with this syndrome. HMSH2, HMLH1, and HMSH6 are the three major genes responsible. The risk of colon cancer is high in families with mutations in any of these genes, and the lifetime risk for endometrial cancer in women from these families is reported to be from 40% to 60% (54). The risk of endometrial cancer also depends on which gene carries the mutation in the particular family. Mutations in MSH2 and MSH6 have been implicated in most HNPCC families with endometrial cancer, but rare families with HMSH1 mutations have been reported as being well. Germline mutations in HMSH6 are relatively rare in HNPCC but are overrepresented in families with multiple cases of endometrial cancer (56). Goodfellow et al. reported that inactivating germline HMSH6 mutations were present in 7 of 441 women with unselected ovarian cancer (1.6%) (57). Cancers were diagnosed in women with mutations on average 10 years younger than in women without mutations.

The majority of tumors from individuals from HNPCC families demonstrate microsatellite instability. Microsatellite instability is a feature of tumors that are genetically unstable; that is, that are associated with error-prone DNA replication during cell division. Microsatellite instability is limited to tumor DNA, and the phenotype is visualized in the laboratory by comparison of tumor and lymphocyte DNA from the same individual. Microsatellite instability is highly predictive of colon and endometrial cancers that are attributable to mutations in one of three mismatch repair genes (*HMSH2, HMLH1,* and *HMSH6*). These mutations may be germline (inherited) but are more often somatic (restricted to tumor tissue only). Approximately one-quarter of women with nonhereditary endometrial cancer (sporadic cancer) have tumors that demonstrate microsatellite instability (58). If the mutation is present in the germline, it may be transmitted from the carrier parent to child. In this case, genetic counseling is warranted. This counseling should include a full pedigree review, and may involve predictive genetic testing for unaffected individuals. Other individuals found to carry the family mutation should be apprised of the risks and the range of tumor types involved. It is not necessary that genetic counseling be undertaken when the mutation is limited to the tumor tissue only, as this situation does not pose a risk to relatives. The gene may also be silenced by methylation of the gene regulatory regions. The *HMLH1* gene is usually found to be silenced through methylation in the tumor's tissues (59).

Individuals with inherited mutations in the mismatch repair genes are also at risk for additional cancers, including ovarian, gastric, urologic tract, and small bowel cancers, but the risk for these is much less than for the risk of colon or endometrial cancer. Members of the International Collaborative Group on HNPCC collected information on 80 women with ovarian cancer who were members of HNPCC families. The mean age of diagnosis was 43 years. The majority of cancers were highly, moderately, or well differentiated, and 85% were stage I or II. Synchronous endometrial cancer was reported in 21.5% of cases. The actual prevalence of mutations in the mismatch repair genes in unselected ovarian cancers has not yet been measured with accuracy but is likely to be low (1% to 2%).

There is currently no consensus on the screening and management of women with inherited mutations in the mismatch repair genes. Annual endometrial ultrasound surveillance has been recommended by the International Collaborative Group on HNPCC, but the effectiveness of this screening regimen has not been established. Although there are no data on the effectiveness of hysterectomy as a preventive measure for hereditary endometrial cancer, there have been no reports of failures of hysterectomy to prevent endometrial cancer. Because of the high lifetime risk of endometrial cancer in women with mutations in the mismatch repair genes, preventive hysterectomy may be warranted.

REFERENCES

1. Risch HA, McLaughlin JR, Cole DEC, et al. Prevalence and penetrance of germline *BRCA1* and *BRCA2* mutations in a population series of 649 women with ovarian cancer. *Am J Hum Genet* 2001;68:700–710.

2. Moslehi R, Chu W, Karlan B, et al. *BRCA1* and *BRCA2* mutation analysis of 208 Ashkenazi Jewish women with ovarian cancer. *Am J Hum Genet* 2000;66:1259–1272.

3. Modan B, Hartge P, Hirsh-Yechezkel G, et al. Parity, oral contraceptives, and the risk of ovarian cancer among carriers and non-carriers of a *BRCA1* or *BRCA2* mutation. *N Engl J Med* 2001;345:235–240.

4. Menkiszak J, Gronwald J, Gorski B, et al. Hereditary ovarian cancer in Poland. *Int J Cancer* 2003;106:942–945.

5. Gorski B, Jakubowska A, Huzarski T, et al. A high proportion of founder BRCA1 mutations in Polish breast cancer families. *Int J Cancer (in press).*

6. Tonin MP, Mes-Masson AM, Narod SA, et al. Founder *BRCA1* and *BRCA2* mutations in French-Canadian ovarian cancer cases unselected for family history. *Clin Genet* 1999;55:318–324.

7. Liede A, Malik IA, Aziz Z, et al. Contribution of *BRCA1* and *BRCA2* mutations to breast and ovarian cancer in Pakistan. *Am J Hum Genet* 2002;595–606.

8. Ford D, Easton DF, Stratton M, et al. Genetic heterogeneity and penetrance analysis of the *BRCA1* and *BRCA2* genes in breast cancer families. *Am J Hum Genet* 1998;62:676–689.

9. Antoniou A, Pharoah PD, Narod SA, et al. Average risks of breast and ovarian cancer associated with BRCA1 or *BRCA2* mutations detected in case series unselected for ovarian cancer: a combined analysis of 22 studies. *Am J Hum Genet* 2003;72:1117–1130.

10. Thompson D, Easton D (on behalf of the Breast Cancer Linkage Consortium). Variation in cancer risks, by mutation position, in *BRCA2* mutation carriers. *Am J Hum Genet* 2001;68:410–419.

11. Boyd J, Sonoda Y, Federici MG, et al. Clinicopathologic features of *BRCA*-linked and sporadic ovarian cancer. *JAMA* 2000;283:2260–2265.

12. Werness BA, Ramus SJ, Whittemore AS, et al. Histopathology of familial ovarian tumors in women from families with and without germline BRCA1 mutations. *Hum Pathol* 2000;31:1420–1424.

13. Lu KH, Garber JE, Cramer DE, et al. Occult ovarian tumours in women with *BRCA1* or *BRCA2* mutations undergoing prophylactic oophorectomy. *J Clin Oncol* 2000;18:2728–2732.

14. Johannsson OT, Ranstam J, Borg A, et al. Survival of BRCA1 breast and ovarian cancer patients: a population-based study from southern Sweden. *J Clin Oncol* 1998;16:397–404.

15. Salazar H, Godwin AK, Daly MB, et al. Microsoopic benign and invasive malignant neoplasms and a cancer-prone phenotype in prophylactic oophorectomies. *J Natl Cancer Inst* 1996;88:1810–1820.

16. Colgan TJ, Murphy J, Cole DEC, et al. Occult carcinoma in prophylactic oophorectomy specimens. Prevalence and association with BRCA germline mutation status. *Am J Surg Pathol* 2001;25:1283–1289.

17. Westhoff C, Murphy P, Heller D, Halim A. Is ovarian cancer associated with an increased frequency of germinal inclusion cysts? *Am J Epidemiol* 1993;138:90–93.

18. Tresserra F, Grases PJ, Labastida R, Ubeda A. Histological features of the contralateral ovary in patients with unilateral cancer: a case control study. *Gynecol Oncol* 1998;71:437–441.

19. Stratton JF, Buckley CH, Lowe D, et al. Comparison of prophylactic oophorectomy specimens from carriers and noncarriers of a *BRCA1* or *BRCA2* gene mutation. *J Natl Cancer Inst* 1999;91:626–628.

20. Deligdisch L, Gil J, Kerner H, et al. Ovarian dysplasia in prophylactic oophorectomy specimens. *Cancer* 1999;86:544–1550.

21. Barakat RR, Federici MG, Saigo PE, et al. Absence of premalignant histologic, molecular, or cell biological alterations in prophylactic oophorectomy specimens from BRCA1 heterozygotes. *Cancer* 2000;89:383–390.

22. Casey MJ, Bewtra C, Hoehne LL, et al. Histology of prophylactically removed ovaries from *BRCA1* and *BRCA2* mutation carriers compared with noncarriers in hereditary breast ovarian cancer syndrome kindreds. *Gynecol Oncol* 2000;78:278–287.

23. Chapman WB. Developments in the pathology of ovarian tumours. *Curr Opin Obstet Gynecol* 2001;13:53–59.

24. Rubin SC, Benjamin I, Behbakht K, et al. Clinical and pathologic features of ovarian cancer in women with germ-line mutations of *BRCA1*. *N Engl J Med* 1996;335:1413–1416.

25. Aida H, Takakuwa K, Nagata H, et al. Clinical features of ovarian cancer in Japanese women with germ-line mutations of *BRCA1*. *Clin Cancer Res* 1998;4:235–240.

26. Pharoah PDP, Easton DF, Stockton DL, et al. Survival in familial,

BRCA1-associated, and BRCA2-associated epithelial ovarian cancer. *Cancer Res* 1999;59:868–871.

27. McGuire V, Whittemore AS, Norris R, Oakley-Girvan I: Survival in epithelial ovarian cancer patients with prior breast cancer. *Am J Epidemiol* 2000;152:528–532.

28. Cass I, Baldwin RL, Varkey T, et al. Improved survival in women with BRCA-associated ovarian carcinoma. *Cancer* 2003;97:2127–2129.

29. NIH Consensus Development Panel on Ovarian Cancer. Ovarian cancer: screening, treatment and follow-up. *JAMA* 1995;273:491–497.

30. Metcalfe KA, Liede A, Hoodfar E, et al. An evaluation of the needs of female BRCA1 and BRCA2 carriers undergoing genetic counselling. *J Med Genet* 2000;37:866–874.

31. Liede A, Karlan BY, Baldwin RL, et al. Cancer incidence in a population of Jewish women at risk of ovarian cancer. *J Clin Oncol* 2002; 20:1570–1577.

32. Woolas R, Smith J, Paterson JM, Sharp F. Fallopian tube carcinoma: an under-reported primary neoplasm. *Int J Gynecol Oncol* 1997;7: 284–288.

33. Piver MS, Jishi MF, Tsukada Y, et al. Primary peritoneal carcinoma after prophylactic oophorectomy in women with a family history of ovarian cancer. A report from the Gilda Radner Family Ovarian Cancer Registry. *Cancer* 1993;71:2751–2755.

34. Struewing JP, Watson P, Easton DF, et al. Prophylactic oophorectomy in inherited breast/ovarian cancer families. *J Natl Cancer Inst Monogr* 1995;17:33–35.

35. Kauff ND, Satagopan JM, Robson ME, et al. Risk-reducing salpingo-oophorectomy in women with a BRCA1 mutation. *N Engl J Med* 2002; 346:1609–1615.

36. Rebbeck TR, Lynch HT, Neuhausen SL, et al. Prophylactic oophorectomy in carriers of BRCA1 and BRCA2 mutations. *N Engl J Med* 2002; 346:1616–1622.

37. Rebbeck TR, Levin AM, Eisen A, et al. Breast cancer risk after bilateral prophylactic oophorectomy in BRCA1 mutation carriers. *J Natl Cancer Inst* 1999;91:1475–1479.

38. Eisen A, Rebbeck TR, Lynch HT, et al. Reduction in breast cancer risk following bilateral prophylactic oophorectomy in BRCA1 and BRCA2 mutation carriers. *Am J Hum Genet* 2000;67:250.

39. Narod SA, Risch H, Mosleh R, et al. Oral contraceptives and the risk of hereditary ovarian cancer. *N Engl J Med* 1998;339:424–428.

40. Narod SA, Sun P, Ghadirian P, et al. Tubal ligation and the risk of ovarian cancer in carriers of BRCA1 or BRCA2 mutations. *Lancet* 2001; 357:1467–1470.

41. Narod SA, Sun P, Risch H. Effects of parity and use of oral contraceptives on the risk of ovarian cancer among carriers and non-carriers of BRCA1/2. *N Engl J Med (in press)*.

42. Piek JM, van Diest PJ, Zweemer RP, et al. Tubal ligation and risk of ovarian cancer. *Lancet* 2001;358:844.

43. Jacobs I, Skates SJ, MacDonald N, et al. Screening for ovarian cancer: a pilot randomized control trial. *Lancet* 1999;353:1207–1210.

44. Mok SC, Chao J, Skates S, et al. Prostasin: a potential serum marker for ovarian cancer: identification through microarray technology. *J Natl Cancer Inst* 2001;93:1458–1464.

45. Petricoin EF, Ardenaki AM, Hitt BA, et al. Use of proteomic patterns in serum to identify ovarian cancer. *Lancet* 2002;359:572–577.

46. Aziz S, Kuperstein G, Rosen B, et al. A genetic epidemiological study of carcinoma of the fallopian tube. *Gynecol Oncol* 2001;80:341–345.

47. Paley PJ, Swisher EM, Garcia RL, et al. Occult cancer of the fallopian tube in BRCA1 germline mutation carriers at prophylactic oophorectomy: a case for recommending hysterectomy at surgical prophylaxis. *Gynecol Oncol* 2001;80:176–180.

48. Thompson D, Easton DF, and the Breast Cancer Linkage Consortium. Cancer incidence in BRCA1 mutation carriers. *J Natl Cancer Inst* 2002; 94:1358–1365.

49. Breast Cancer Linkage Consortium Cancer risks in BRCA2 mutations carriers. *J Natl Cancer Inst* 1999;91:1310–1316.

50. Goshen R, Chu W, Elit L, et al. Is uterine papillary serous adenocarcinoma a manifestation of the hereditary breast-ovarian cancer syndrome? *Gynecol Oncol* 2000; 79:477–481.

51. Levine DA, Lin O, Barakat RR, et al. Risk of endometrial carcinoma associated with BRCA mutation. *Gynecol Oncol* 2001;80:395–398.

52. Zhou XP, Kusismanen S, Nystrom-Lahti M, et al. Distinct PTEn mutational spectrum in hereditary non-polyposis cancer syndrome—related endometrial carcinomas compared to sporadic microsatellite unstable tumors. *Hum Mol Genet* 2002;11:445–450.

53. Eng C. PTEN: one gene, many syndromes. *Hum Mutat* 2003;22: 183–198.

54. Watson P, Lynch HT. Cancer risk in mismatch repair gene carriers. *Fam Cancer* 2001; 1:57–60.

55. Watson P, Butzow R, Lynch HT, et al. The clinical features of ovarian cancer in hereditary non-polyposis colorectal cancer. *Gynecol Oncol* 2001;82:223–228.

56. Wijnen J, de Leeuw W, Vasen H, et al. Familial endometrial cancer in female carriers of MSH6 germline mutations. *Nat Genet* 1999;23: 142–144.

57. Goodfellow PJ, Buttin BM, Herzog TJ, et al. Prevalence of defective DNA mismatch repair and MSH6 mutation in an unselected series of endometrial cancers. *Proc Natl Acad Sci U S A* 2003;100:5908–5913.

58. Gurin CC, Federci MG, Kang L, Boyd J. Causes and consequences of microsatellite instability in endometrial carcinoma. *Cancer Res* 1999; 59:462–466.

59. Simpkins SB, Bocker T, Swisher EM, et al. MLH1 promoter methylation and gene silencing is the primary cause of microsatellite instability in sporadic endometrial cancers. *Hum Mol Genet* 1999;8:661–666.

CHAPTER 3

The Biology of Gynecologic Cancer

Kristin K. Zorn, Ginger J. Gardner, and Michael J. Birrer

INTRODUCTION TO THE BIOLOGY OF GYNECOLOGIC NEOPLASIA

Definitions and Spectrum of Histopathology

Nonneoplastic Versus Neoplastic

Nonneoplastic processes can alter the structure and/or function of a tissue, but are usually reversible. These conditions represent an adaptation to stress, such as an injury or infection, or a physiologic response to biochemical (e.g., hormonal) stimulation. *Hypertrophy* refers to an increase in cell size within a tissue, whereas hyperplasia is an increase in cell number. *Metaplasia* describes the process by which one differentiated cell type is replaced with another. *Dysplasia* is disordered cellular proliferation characterized by structural variability and disorganization of tissue architecture. When the full thickness of an epithelium is involved by this process, it is termed carcinoma *in situ*, and is considered to be a preinvasive process (1).

A neoplasm represents new growth and may be defined as an abnormal mass of tissue, the growth of which exceeds and is uncoordinated with that of the normal tissues and persists in the same excessive manner after cessation of the stimuli that evoked the change (2). Neoplasia has been traditionally classified as benign or malignant on the basis of structural and growth characteristics. Most benign tumors mimic their tissue of origin in both cellular form and function. Cancerous tumors exhibit a spectrum from well-differ-

entiated to anaplastic (undifferentiated, characterized by both cytologic pleomorphism and architectural disorganization). Benign masses are typically well demarcated, with a broad, expansive front, and do not invade local normal tissues. Although some malignancies may appear grossly to be encapsulated, they almost always infiltrate adjacent noncancerous tissue. In addition, malignancies tend to have a faster growth rate that is, in general, inversely related to the degree of differentiation. Finally, the ability to metastasize, a behavior that many malignant tumors exhibit, is a feature that benign tumors uniformly lack (1).

Biologic Properties of Transformed Cells and Tumors

Our understanding of the biologic behavior of malignant cells has been derived from *in vitro* comparisons of normal and transformed cells, the study of cell lines established by culturing human cancer cells, and the evaluation of tumors transplanted or induced in animals. Normal human cells display a finite ability to proliferate in cell culture, stopping after about 50 generations of cell division. These cells have specific requirements for growth, including the availability of nutrients and growth factors, attachment to a substratum, and lack of contact with other cells. In the event of temporary nutritional deprivation, they will arrest in a nonproliferative state but retain the capacity to resume replication with replenishment of growth-promoting substances.

Malignant cells, in contrast, demonstrate decreased reliance on exogenous growth factors, anchorage independence, and a lack of contact inhibition. As a result, transformed cells generally require less serum and supplements to grow, demonstrate nonadherent growth (such as growth in suspension or in a semisolid medium), and exhibit greater cell-population density. Cellular transformation produces disorganization of actin filaments, which results in more rounded, refractile cells.

Depending on location and accessibility to physical examination or imaging techniques, most tumors become clini-

Kristin K. Zorn: Molecular Mechanisms Section, Cell and Cancer Biology Department, Center for Cancer Research, National Cancer Institute, Rockville, Maryland 20850

Ginger J. Gardner: Department of Obstetrics, Gynecology and Reproductive Sciences, Division of Gynecologic Oncology, Mount Sinai School of Medicine, New York, New York 10029

Michael J. Birrer: Department of Obstetrics, Gynecology and Reproductive Sciences, Division of Gynecologic Oncology, Mount Sinai School of Medicine, New York, New York 10029

cally detectable at a mass of 1 to 10 g (10^9 to 10^{10} cells). A tumor mass of 1 kg (10^{12} cells) represents approximately 40 doublings and is generally lethal to the host in animal models. The time it takes for a given human malignancy to double in volume is usually constant, consistent with an exponential growth pattern (Fig. 3.1). Tumors frequently demonstrate a growth deceleration generally attributed to inadequate nutrition as they enlarge. Extrapolation into the preclinical phase reveals a slower rate of growth during this portion of the tumor's life span as well, which may be related to the early growth requirements of establishing a supporting vascular network and overcoming the host's immune surveillance (Fig. 3.1).

Doubling times for human malignancies range from a few days for certain lymphomas and leukemias to up to several months for epithelial tumors such as lung and colorectal carcinomas. The growth rates for tumors of identical origin and histology may also be quite variable. A formula that includes the growth fraction and duration of DNA synthesis may be used to estimate the theoretical doubling time for a given tumor. This potential tumor doubling time is often considerably shorter than the actual doubling time seen clinically (3). Reasons for this discrepancy include tumor cell death (apoptosis), or lowered growth fraction due to cellular senescence, due in part from the lack of an adequate vascular supply.

Cell Cycle, Senescence, and Cell Death (Apoptosis)

Cell Cycle

During the process of replication, a cell passes through a series of phases beginning with DNA synthesis (S phase) and culminating in mitosis (M phase), the process by which

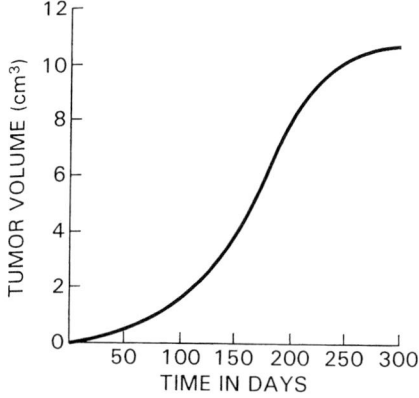

FIG. 3.1. An exponential growth curve with preclinical lag and terminal growth deceleration. The abscissa represents time of tumor growth in days. The ordinate displays tumor volume in square centimeters. A slower rate of tumor growth is shown during the tumor's preclinical phase as well as when it attains a large volume.

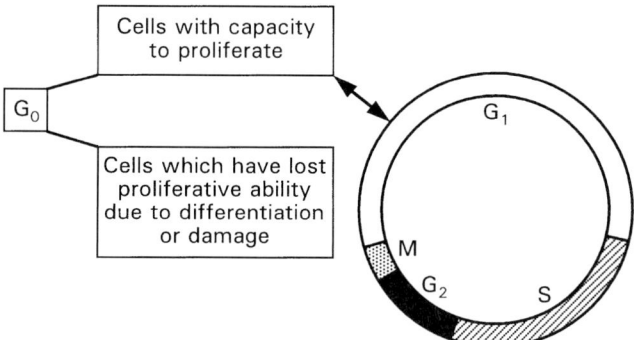

FIG. 3.2. The cell cycle. The normal cell cycle, with relative time spent in each phase, is illustrated. G_0 cells are "resting," with an ability to replicate given the appropriate conditions and stimulus, or they have lost the ability to proliferate secondary to damage, death, or differentiation. G_1 represents the presynthetic phase, DNA synthesis occurs during the S phase, G_2 is the premitotic phase, and M represents mitosis, the briefest portion of the cycle.

the cell actually divides (Fig. 3.2). These two periods are separated by the presynthetic (G_1) and premitotic (G_2) phases. Cells that are not actively proliferating are in the G_0 phase. Some of these nonproliferating cells retain the ability to progress through the cell cycle given the appropriate stimulus and environmental conditions. Others have lost the capacity for replication, which occurs secondary to terminal differentiation or damage sufficient to result in eventual cell death. The proportion of cells in a tumor that are actively proliferating is known as the tumor's growth fraction (3).

Entry into and transit through the cell cycle appear to be controlled by a number of regulatory proteins (3). Events necessary for G_0/G_1 cells to enter the S phase include the transduction of growth factor signals to the nucleus and the activation of "early response" genes whose products bind to DNA and regulate the expression of other genes necessary for progression through the cell cycle (Fig. 3.3). The proteins necessary for this progression include the cyclins, cyclin-dependent kinases (CDKs), and the CDK inhibitors (4,5). It is now abundantly clear that progression through the cell cycle requires the interaction of these proteins in a coordinated fashion.

The cyclins are a group of proteins that are synthesized and degraded during the cell cycle. They can be divided into two major classes depending on where in the cell cycle they are active: The G_1 cyclins include cyclins D, A, and E, whereas the mitotic cyclins include cyclins A and B. The cyclins bind to and activate the cyclin-dependent kinases (CDKs). The cyclin/CDK complex is critical for the phosphorylation and activation of proteins and enzymes involved in DNA replication. For instance, the cyclin D/CDK4, cyclin D/CDK6, cyclin E/CDK2, and cyclin A/CDK2 complexes phosphorylate the retinoblastoma gene product (pRb) (6). pRb is a protein with tumor-suppressor function. The Rb protein and a structurally related protein, p107, are modified

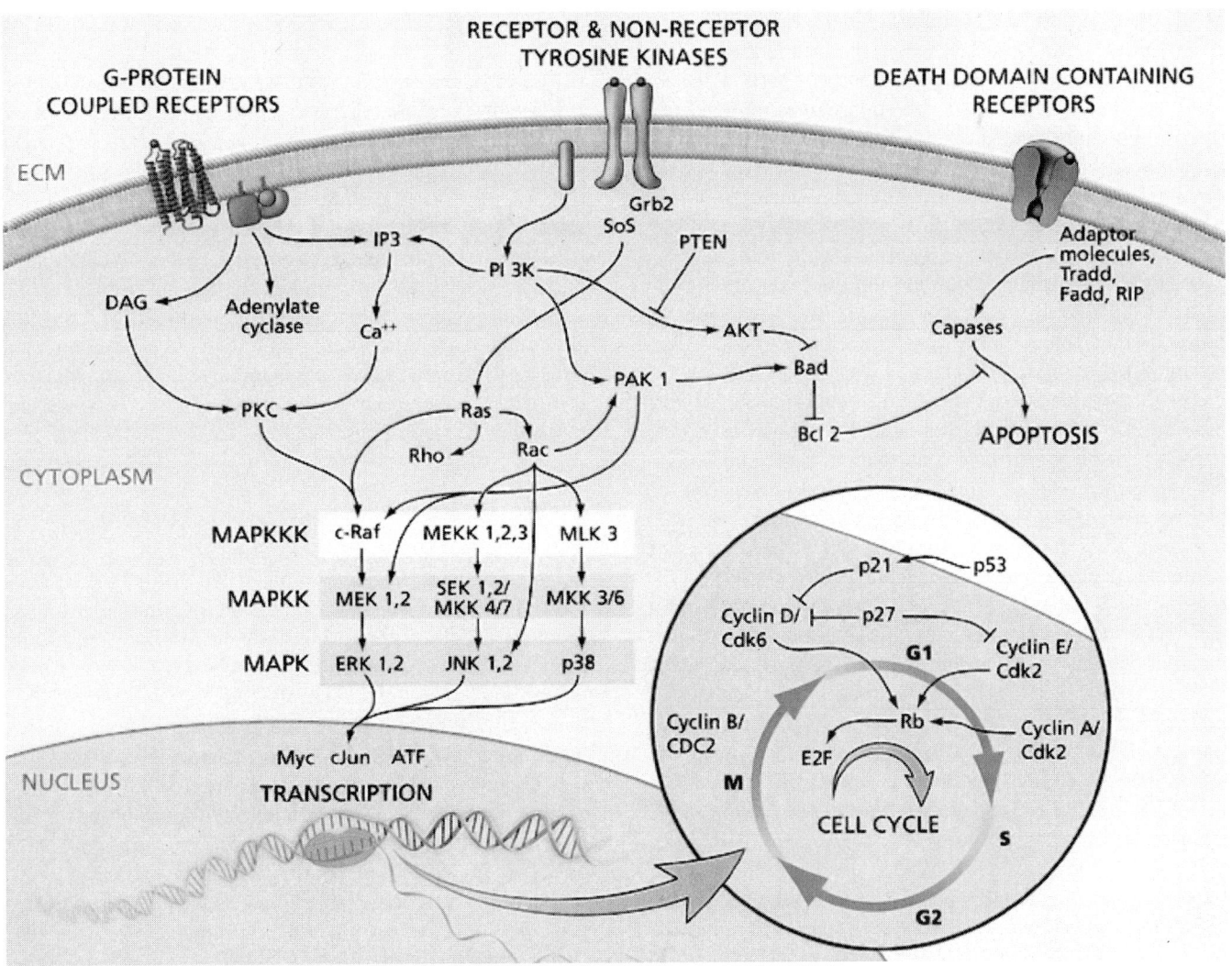

FIG. 3.3. Signal transduction, regulation of the cell cycle, and apoptotic pathways. The covalent modification of intracellular constituents is illustrated by receptor and nonreceptor protein tyrosine kinases. Input from the tyrosine kinases results in increased generation of activated ras bound to GTP, which in turn associates with raf (MAPKKK), raf propagates the signal to microtubule-associated protein kinase kinase (MAPKK), which activates MAPK. MAPK phosphorylates a host of substrates, including cytoplasmic phospholipase A_2, cytoskeletal components, protein synthesis machinery, and, most importantly, transcription factors such as myc, cJun, and ATF. Parallel pathways exist that use different MAPKKKs, MAPKKs, and MAPKs. Different MAPKs, such as ERK, JNK, and p38, phosphorylate and activate downstream targets that ultimately drive the cell cycle. The upstream activators of the MAPKKK are not as well characterized as other portions of the cascade and as such only ras, PAK 1, and rac have been listed for simplicity. Although the MAP kinase cascades are parallel in nature, there is extensive crosstalk between these pathways. The generation of "second messengers" that act upon intracellular receptor sites is exemplified by G-protein–coupled receptors. G-proteins interact with adenylate cyclase and certain phospholipases. Consequent hydrolysis of membrane phosphatidylinositol 4,5-bis-phosphate yields inositol 1,4,5-tris-phosphate (IP 3), which releases Ca^{2+} from internal stores, and diacylglycerol (DAG), which activates protein kinase C (PKC). Activation of PI 3′K by tyrosine kinases increases IP 3 levels, allowing cross-talk between growth factor and G-protein–coupled receptors. The ultimate effect of growth factors is to trigger the enzymatic cascade involving cyclins and cyclin-dependent kinases (CDKs) that play critical roles in stimulating cells to enter and transit through the cell cycle. Activation of a variety of receptors (Fas, TNF-R) containing death domains leads to the activation of caspases and programmed cell death (apoptosis). This pathway has extensive cross-talk with other cellular pathways, including the one depicted here. Elevated activity of PI 3′K leads to activation of AKT, which in turn phosphorylates Bad, leaving its protein partner Bcl-2 available to inhibit apoptosis.

by a variety of different cyclins and CDKs (7). Their phosphorylation results in the release of transcription factor E2F (8,9), which then drives the transcription of "growth genes" (10). Another example is the activation of the protein kinase p34^{cdc-2} by dephosphorylation and binding to a regulatory cofactor, which appears important for cell cycle transit. Kinase activity is maximal during mitosis, when p34^{cdc-2} is bound to the protein cyclin B.

The stimulatory activity of cyclin/CDK complexes is opposed by CDK inhibitors (4). The CDK inhibitors are a group of small proteins that are able to inhibit directly the activity of the cyclin/CDK complex. The G_1 cyclin/CDK complexes are inhibited by p15, p16, and p27.

The interaction of cyclins, CDKs, and CDK inhibitors provides for a regulated progression through the cell cycle (5). The cell passes through a number of checkpoints where assurance of proper completion of prior phases is required before proceeding further (11,12). If this has not been achieved, then the cell arrests. The p53 protein mediates two of these checkpoints (13). Overexpression of wild-type (nonmutated) p53 arrests cell cycle progression in G_1 at or near a restriction point regulating the G_1/S transition, in part by transcriptionally activating the expression of the CDK inhibitor p21 Waf1/Cip1 (13). Although routine cellular functions may not require the presence of p53, conditions such as DNA damage and cellular stress stimulate the expression of p53 and produce a G_1 arrest (5). If the DNA damage is minor, it is repaired during this arrest; extensive damage causes the cell to undergo apoptosis (discussed below) (14). Elevated levels of p53 can also produce a G_2/M arrest, providing another period of rest for the cell during which it can repair damaged chromosomes. Although the mechanism for G_2 arrest is less clear than that involved in the G_1 checkpoint, it appears to involve the inactivation of mitotic cyclins A and B (15–17) The formation of a functional mitotic spindle is critical for successful cell division. It is not surprising, therefore, that a checkpoint exists during mitotic spindle formation (18). The genes involved in this process have only recently been characterized, but some appear to be involved in human cancers (19).

Cellular Senescence

Cell growth slows as the finite number of cell doublings, known as the Hayflick limit, approaches (20). This process is governed by the loss of telomeres on chromosomal ends. Telomeres are protective DNA sequences rich in TTAGGG repeats that are shortened with successive replications. When the ends become critically shortened, the cell enters replicative senescence or mortality stage 1. Some cells escape senescence and continue to divide until they undergo crisis, which is also known as mortality stage 2. The rare cell that emerges from this stage still able to replicate is considered to be immortalized because it has acquired the ability to proliferate indefinitely. Immortalized cells are able to continue dividing because they are able to maintain telomere length, which is usually due to reactivation of telomerase (21,22) Telomerase is an RNA-dependent DNA polymerase that synthesizes the telomeric DNA sequences. It consists of an RNA template, which is universally expressed, and a catalytic component termed hTERT, whose expression is usually repressed after embryogenesis is complete. Approximately 90% of human tumors, however, express telomerase as a result of the upregulation of hTERT. Other tumors undergo a process independent of telomerase activation known as alternative lengthening of telomeres, which is less well understood. Although immortalized, these cell lines are generally not tumorigenic when implanted into animals. Further genetic alterations are required to convert these into tumor-forming cell lines.

Cellular Death (Apoptosis)

Apoptosis is an active and intricately regulated process in which cells undergo programmed cell death. It is a normal physiologic condition that is associated with involution and tissue remodeling during morphogenesis and a number of immunologic responses (23,24). Apoptosis consists of three phases known as the initiation, effector, and degradation phases. In the initiation phase, the cells receive a stimulus that triggers the apoptotic process. Hypoxia, ionizing radiation, chemotherapeutic agents, and viral infection can induce the process (25–28). Additionally, cytotoxic lymphocytes, mediated by the FAS ligand (29–31), and p53, mediated by *bax* (32,33), can induce apoptosis. The entire process is regulated by a myriad of oncogene and tumor-suppressor gene (*p53*, *Rb*, *ras*, *raf*, and c-*myc*) products (34). Apoptosis is still reversible in the effector phase; once degradation begins, though, the process is no longer reversible and cellular death ensues (24,28).

Histologically, apoptotic cells are characterized by cell shrinkage, chromatin condensation, and internucleosomal degradation of cellular DNA. This appearance differs from that of hypoxic necrosis, which is characterized by cellular swelling. The swelling is attributed to the loss of selective cell membrane permeability and to mitochondrial swelling, resulting in plasma membrane rupture with DNA, RNA, and protein degradation from the release of lysosomal hydrolases. The enzymatic degradation leads to an intense inflammatory response in the surrounding tissue, resulting in cellular necrosis (23,24,35). In contrast, this inflammatory response does not occur with apoptosis. During the final stages of apoptosis, the cell becomes convoluted and breaks into several membrane-bound vesicles containing intact organelles and nuclear fragments. Typically 180–200 bp in length, DNA fragments are the biochemical hallmark of apoptosis and can be used for morphologic analysis (24,35). Although apoptotic cells can be visualized and quantified with routine staining of tumor material, techniques using labeling of the "3' free ends" of the DNA fragments by radioactive or nonradioactive means allow for accurate identification of single apoptotic cells and quantification of the extent of apoptosis in tumor material via an "apoptotic index" (24,36,37). The index commonly measures either the number of apoptotic cells per 1,000 tumor cells or per ten high-power fields (24,38,39).

Apoptosis can be induced by cytotoxic lymphocytes (CD8$^+$ T lymphocytes) via the Fas ligand/receptor pathway (30,31). Fas (or Apo-1) is a glycosylated transmembrane receptor belonging to the tumor necrosis factor (TNF) receptor family. The binding of Fas receptor to Fas ligand (FAS-L), a transmembrane protein present on cytotoxic T lymphocytes, activates a pathway eventually leading to apoptotic cellular death (30, 31). Downstream of the Fas receptor is FADD (Fas-associated death domain), which binds to a conserved amino acid sequence known as the "death domain" of the cytoplasmic end of the Fas receptor. Together, these two proteins form an apoptotic signaling complex with FLICE, (FADD-like ICE, also known as caspase-8). Recently, caspases have been identified as the "common final pathway" in the execution of apoptosis in highly divergent systems (31). Caspase assays have been developed that, as with the DNA fragmentation index, provide a method of identifying cells undergoing apoptosis.

The bcl-2 family of proteins has been shown to play a major role in apoptosis. The bcl-2 protein was initially discovered as an overexpressed protein in B-cell lymphomas. For this reason, bcl-2 is considered to be an oncogene. Members of the bcl-2 protein family include both apoptosis-inhibiting (bcl-2, bcl-xl, bcl-w, bfl-1, brag-1, mcl-1, and A1) and apoptosis-promoting (bax, bak, bcl-xS, bad, bid, bik, and Hrk) members (24,40–45). Their actions can be independent of or in competition with one another. For instance, when bax is in excess, the bax homodimers predominate, favoring apoptosis. However, an excess of bcl-2 leads to bcl-2/bax heterodimers that inhibit apoptosis. In other examples, bcl-xl inhibits apoptosis by binding and sequestering bax, whereas bad promotes apoptosis by binding bcl-2 and bcl-xl, thereby releasing bax (24,43,44). The exact mechanism of action of each family member is currently under investigation. However, bcl-2, bcl-xl, and bax appear to exert their effects on the cell mitochondria either as ion channel or adapter/docking proteins. As these proteins form ion channel pores on the membrane surface of the mitochondria, disruption of the transmembrane potential releases caspase-activating substances, thereby activating the final common pathway in apoptosis (23,24,46).

Other oncogenes besides bcl-2 as well as tumor-suppressor genes are associated with the regulation and execution of apoptosis, including *p53*, *Rb*, *ras*, *raf*, and *c-my* (24,34). p53 Monitors the status of the DNA (Fig. 3.3). With DNA damage, p53 stalls the cell cycle through the induction of CIP/WAF/p21, a protein that prevents phosphorylation of CDKs (24,34,47,48). CDKs are positive regulators of the cell cycle. In the absence of this phosphorylated (active)

CDK, Rb will remain unphosphorylated, and the cell cycle will halt until the DNA is repaired. If the DNA is not repaired, p53 can promote apoptosis through the upregulation of bax and the downregulation of bcl-2 (24,34,49,50). Cells lacking p53 are resistant to some apoptotic induction events, such as ionizing radiation, chemotherapeutic agents, loss of Rb, and expression of c-myc. The effect of c-myc on the apoptotic process is growth-factor dependent. It induces proliferation in the presence of growth factors, but in their absence has apoptotic effects (24,51). Overexpression of ras may lead to increased or decreased apoptosis (24,52–54). Additionally, ras-induced apoptosis is inhibited by bcl-2. However, phosphorylation of bcl-2 negates its capacity to protect cells from ras-induced apoptosis (24,55).

Several investigators have examined differing aspects of apoptotic mechanisms in gynecologic malignancies (56–61). In general, overexpression of the oncogenes *bcl-2* and *bcl-xl* protect many cell types against inducers of apoptosis (hypoxia, ionizing radiation, chemotherapeutic agents, and viral infection), and therefore promotes tumorigenesis. Additionally, downregulation of the *p53* tumor-suppressor gene or of the proapoptotic *bax* gene also promotes tumorigenesis. In gynecologic malignancies, bcl-2 is strongly expressed in normal endometrial epithelium and is downregulated in atypical hyperplasia and endometrial adenocarcinoma. However, the use of bcl-2 expression as a prognostic factor is not well established (59). With respect to *p53*, immunohistochemical detection of p53 in tissue correlates closely with the presence of mutations in the gene, which is attributable to a much longer half-life of the mutated protein. Mutations of p53 are absent in normal endometrium but present in endometrial cancer, particularly the endometrioid subtype; p53 expression in endometrial cancer has been shown to correlate with tumor type, stage, and grade but not significantly with prognosis (57,60,62–66)

In Vivo Biology

Proliferation Indices

Various methods have been developed to measure the percentage of cells actively proliferating, the percentage of cells in specific phases of the cell cycle, the duration of different phases, and the total cell-cycle time. The labeling index (LI) is a crude estimate of the percentage of proliferating cells within a tumor. The LI identifies the proportion of cells that have completed S phase during the assay by using autoradiography to detect ^{3}H-thymidine that has been incorporated into cellular DNA. Another crude estimate of proliferation is given by the mitotic index (MI), which relies on enumeration of mitotic figures. This measure is limited by the relatively short duration of mitosis and the ability to identify correctly cells in mitosis. The percent labeled mitosis (PLM) method is used to estimate the duration of the cell cycle and its component phases. Serial biopsies are obtained after thymidine injection to follow the labeled cohort of cells as it passes through the cell cycle. Ideally, waves of labeled mitoses of width T_S (S-phase duration) are separated by T_C (cell-cycle duration). Phase duration variability, however, causes dampening of these waves, and computer models are required to generate approximations of the phase and cycle times. Drawbacks of the PLM method include the preferential collection of data from the cells with shorter cycle times and the inability to distinguish nonproliferating from slowly proliferating cells (3).

Flow cytometry has been used to analyze the cell cycle and growth fraction. The histogram generated by fluorescent emission allows estimation of the proportion of cells with DNA content that is diploid (G_1 and G_0 cells), tetraploid (G_2 and M cells), or intermediate (S-phase cells). The S-phase fraction (SPF) provides an approximation of the growth fraction. Phase determination may be complicated by background contamination due to cellular debris and by the imprecision involved in interpreting DNA distribution, especially in the presence of aneuploidy. A more specific method for estimating the SPF involves the administration of a nonradioactive DNA precursor, such as 5-bromodeoxyuridine or 5-iododeoxyuridine, followed by treatment with a DNA-intercalating fluorescent dye. The precursor may be recognized in denatured DNA by a fluorescent-labeled monoclonal antibody. Two-parameter flow cytometry is used to follow the labeled cohort of cells as it traverses the cell cycle. This method can generate estimates for T_S and LI from a single biopsy performed at a known interval after administration of the precursor. Similar to the PLM method, however, these flow cytometric measurements favor data collection from the most rapidly dividing cells. Another application of flow cytometry is the estimation of growth fraction via fluorescent-labeled antibody recognition of cellular antigens expressed only by actively proliferating cells (proliferation-dependent antigens) (3).

Estimates for the LI or SPF of solid human malignancies are generally in the range of 3% to 15%, a proliferation rate lower than that of normal bone marrow and intestinal epithelium but higher than that of other normal tissues such as liver and lung (31). Typical values for tumor T_S and T_C are 12 to 24 hours and 2 to 3 days, respectively. These values are somewhat longer than comparable estimates for nonmalignant, rapidly proliferating tissues. Many studies have addressed indices of proliferation for gynecologic malignancies. The PI (proliferation index, generally defined as %S + G_2 cells) or SPF are the measures that are commonly used. SPF and PI have been used as both discrete and continuous variables when establishing levels of significance.

Some retrospective investigations of epithelial ovarian cancer have found the SPF or PI to be prognostic indicators (67,68), whereas others have not (69,70). A prospective evaluation of 47 cases of ovarian carcinoma of all stages assessed SPF and expression of Ki-67, a proliferation-dependent nuclear antigen. Expression of Ki-67 and elevated SPF were both found to confer an adverse prognosis. When the cases were stratified by disease dissemination, stage I/II versus Stage III/IV, the SPF retained its significance within both groups (71).

Increasing SPF and PI have been noted to accompany increasing severity of endometrial hyperplasia (72), and several investigators have found a correlation between advanced grade and elevated indices in endometrial carcinoma (73–75). Two prospective studies, including 304 evaluable clinical stage I/II patients and 101 patients of all stages of endometrial cancer, reported SPF to be of independent prognostic significance in multivariate analyses (73,75). Another prospective study of 209 clinical stage I/II cases, however, found a high PI not to have adverse implications (76).

Increasing proliferative activity, as measured by mitotic index, has been reported to correlate with increasing degree of cervical dysplasia (77). One prospective evaluation of 242 squamous cell carcinoma patients of all stages found SPF to be significantly related to survival in both univariate and multivariate analyses, whereas another prospective study of 195 similar cases determined that SPF alone did not predict survival (78,79). A few investigators have noted the subset of diploid cases with high proliferative indices to have a significantly worsened prognosis (79–81).

Some studies of proliferation have assessed the less commonly occurring gynecologic malignancies. Retrospective analyses of uterine sarcomas have revealed the mitotic index or SPF to be useful for predicting clinical outcome (82–84) For discriminating molar versus nonmolar hydropic gestations, elevated SPF was found to be useful in one study, but not in another (85,86). In an evaluation of 51 complete mole patients with available follow-up, no significant difference was noted in the SPF for those with persistent disease versus those without (86). A retrospective evaluation of 42 cases with all stages of squamous-cell carcinoma of the vulva failed to show a significant association between SPF and recurrence or overall survival (87).

Precursor Lesions

A wide range of neoplasia is encountered in gynecology. Squamous-cell carcinoma of the cervix has the most well-defined precursor lesion among the gynecologic malignancies in the form of cervical dysplasia. High-grade cervical dysplasia has a known high propensity for eventual infiltration into the subepithelial tissue, whereas most low-grade dysplasia will spontaneously regress (88). Endometrial cancer has two forms of precursor lesions: Endometrioid endometrial cancer is associated with atypical hyperplasia arising in a setting of estrogen excess, whereas serous and some clear-cell endometrial cancer arises from endometrial intraepithelial neoplasia (EIN) in a setting of atrophy (89). A precursor lesion for epithelial ovarian cancer has not been identified consistently, although some researchers have found dysplasia of the ovarian surface epithelium, particularly in ovarian inclusion cysts, to be associated with ovarian cancer (90). Atypical endometriosis appears to be a preinvasive lesion for 28% of endometrioid and 49% of clear-cell ovarian cancer (90). Further evaluation of all of these precursor lesions is underway to define the critical events that cause a small fraction of them to progress to overt cancer while the rest remain premalignant or even regress.

Gynecologic neoplasms range from noninvasive benign tumors, such as uterine leiomyomata, to aggressive malignancies, such as high-grade epithelial ovarian carcinoma. Ovarian tumors of low malignant potential (LMP, also called borderline tumors) are relatively unique with respect to the criteria distinguishing benign from malignant neoplasia. Although originally thought to represent a preinvasive stage in ovarian malignancy, recent molecular evidence suggests a more complicated relationship between LMP and invasive tumors. Serous LMP tumors do not have p53 mutations and display LOH on the long arm of the inactivated X chromosome, whereas invasive serous ovarian cancer frequently displays p53 mutations and has a different pattern of loss of heterogeneity (LOH) involving multiple chromosomes (91). Mucinous LMP tumors, on the other hand, have similar patterns of K-ras mutation and LOH as invasive mucinous ovarian cancer (90). These results suggest that whereas mucinous LMP tumors may progress to invasive cancer, serous LMP tumors do not and, in fact, likely represent a distinct disease process. Other gynecologic neoplasms such as advanced endometriosis, with its ability to invade structures such as the bowel and ureter despite being a benign lesion, and pseudomyxoma peritonei, with an indolent but nevertheless potentially lethal course, also blur the boundaries between the behavior of benign and malignant tumors.

Genetic Alterations

Chromosomal Abnormalities

Karyotypic and molecular biologic analyses have provided evidence that most cancers arise in association with clonal genetic changes. Multiple genetic alterations appear necessary for conversion from the normal to the cancerous state, with primary events that are responsible for tumor initiation and secondary changes that account for tumor progression and heterogeneity. Gross chromosomal abnormalities include translocations, deletions, inversions, and amplifications affecting entire sections of a chromosome (92). Most forms of malignant neoplasia demonstrate both intertumoral and intratumoral heterogeneity with respect to chromosomal aberrations. Molecular chromosomal abnormalities in cancer consist of point mutations affecting a specific locus on the chromosome, frequently involving dominant (e.g., ras) or recessive (e.g., p53) oncogenes (93).

Classic examples of chromosomal abnormalities found in cancer are the reciprocal translocations that occur in chronic myelogenous leukemia (CML) [t(9;22)] and Burkitt's lym-

phoma [t(8;14)] and the inherited deletions of 13q14 in retinoblastoma (94). In CML, the protooncogene abl is translocated from chromosome 9 to 22. This results in the formation of a new protein that represents a fusion of the abl and bcr gene products. Experimental infection of mice with retroviruses carrying the gene encoding this fusion protein has produced a CML-like condition in these animals. In Burkitt's lymphoma, the myc protooncogene is repositioned near genes encoding the immunoglobulin heavy or light chains and is constitutively activated. Deregulated expression of the myc gene results in cellular proliferation. Characterization of chromosomal abnormalities at 13q14 in hereditary retinoblastoma resulted in the identification of the retinoblastoma gene (Rb). The identification of allelic loss in tumors from patients heterozygous at this locus (loss of heterozygosity or LOH analysis) has provided evidence that similar molecular mutations appear to be operating in the hereditary and sporadic forms of the disease. The Rb protein appears to have a major role in regulating cell division, and the consequences of alterations at the Rb locus have led to its characterization as a tumor-suppressor gene.

Gross chromosomal alterations have been described in both benign and malignant gynecologic neoplasia, but are more frequent and generally more extensive in the latter. In uterine leiomyomata, clonal chromosomal aberrations have been reported in 15% to 54% of tumors studied, with abnormalities involving chromosomes 12 and 14 being most frequently detected (95,96). In uterine sarcomas, up to 71% of tumors have demonstrable and often multiple abnormalities, with chromosomes 1, 7, and 11 most commonly involved, especially 11q22 (97,98). Cervical carcinoma is characterized by chromosome 1 alterations in greater than 90% of tumors, as well as by frequent deletions involving 3p, 11q, and 17p (99–102), and karyotypic analysis of epithelial ovarian cancers reveals frequent abnormalities of chromosomes 1, 3, 7, 11, and 12 (103–105).

In general, less aggressive malignancies are associated with less complex karyotypic changes. Simple chromosomal abnormalities have been reported for some granulosa-cell tumors (106), low–malignant-potential tumors (107), low-grade epithelial ovarian cancer (108), and early-stage endometrial and ovarian carcinomas (109,110), whereas advanced epithelial ovarian carcinoma frequently demonstrates complex chromosomal changes (103,108). In addition, specific changes for certain tumors may represent a later event in tumorigenesis or may confer a worse prognosis. The frequency of polysomy for chromosome 1 increases as the severity of cervical intraepithelial neoplasia increases (101). Gallion et al. detected LOH on 17p in benign, borderline, and invasive epithelial ovarian tumors, but found allelic loss on 11p in the invasive cancer cases only (111). LOH on 13q was noted in 58% of informative cases overall (18 of 31), including 80% (8 of 10) of stage I tumors. Worsham et al. analyzed six squamous cell carcinomas of the vulva, each containing multiple chromosomal rearrangements (112).

Two specific deletions, 10q23–25 and 18q22–23, were present in all four of the patients who died of disease but in neither of the long-term survivors.

Somatic Versus Germline Mutations

In addition to the above classification, genetic changes may be characterized as germline versus somatic. Whereas all of the cells in an individual with a germline mutation will manifest the genetic alteration, somatic mutations occur in a single cell and are detectable in tumors secondary to clonal proliferation. Germline genetic changes have been shown to be the basis of the hereditary cancers seen in syndromes such as BRCA1, BRCA2, and HNPCC. In general, these hereditary syndromes are thought to account for only a minority of gynecologic cancers (see Chapters 2 and 5 for full discussion). Somatic mutations, on the other hand, occur in the majority of cancers.

Clonality

Many human tumors exhibit extensive heterogeneity with respect to cellular properties such as morphology, surface markers, and chromosomal abnormalities. This diversity has raised the question of whether tumors originate from a monoclonal or polyclonal origin. One method of assessing clonality evaluates X-linked gene products such as the isozymic expression of glucose-6-phosphate dehydrogenase (G6PD) (113). Another technique utilizes restriction fragment length polymorphism (RFLP) analysis, exploiting the differential methylation patterns of X-linked genes such as hypoxanthine phosphoribosyl transferase (HPRT), phosphoglycerate kinase (PGK), and the human androgen receptor (HUMARA assay) (114). The use of proliferation-independent X chromosome–linked markers is based on lyonization, the phenomenon of random inactivation of one X chromosome in the embryonic cells of mammalian females. The somatic cells of heterozygous women will be mosaics, with approximately equal numbers of cells expressing either the maternal or paternal allele but no cells expressing both. A tumor arising in a woman heterozygous for an X-linked gene would be expected to express only one allele if it originated from a single antecedent cell, but to express both alleles if its origin were polyclonal (113). Although the studies utilizing these techniques have generally suggested a monoclonal origin for tumors, the interpretation of the results is complicated by technical issues with the assays, particularly the presence of monoclonal patches in many of the surrounding normal tissues, raising the possibility that the monoclonal tumor simply reflects the clonal composition of the normal tissue.

Genetic markers acquired secondary to somatic events have also been studied to assess clonality. Examples include the rearrangement of immunoglobulin and T-cell receptor genes in lymphoid malignancies (113), the allelic loss on autosomes described for a number of different cancers (115),

and point mutations. Immunohistochemistry or molecular probes are used to determine if the same gene product or gene arrangement is present in all of the cells within the tumor, suggesting their origin from a common precursor cell. LOH analysis is employed to discern whether or not the pattern of allelic loss is identical in all of the cells in a given tumor. Point mutations may be assessed by techniques such as RFLP analysis using restriction endonuclease digestion. Studies using these techniques have been performed on acute myelogenous leukemia, Burkitt's lymphoma, and many epithelial tumors. The results have provided overwhelming evidence for a monoclonal origin of most human malignancies.

Many studies have analyzed the clonal nature of gynecologic malignancies. Fialkow (116) reported the use of G6PD analysis for a variety of tumors, including cervical carcinoma, but this method was thought to be inconclusive, owing in part to its inability to reliably exclude the presence of contaminating normal tissue in the assay (113,117). Other problems noted with this method included the requirement for a relatively large amount of tissue and the low frequency of G6PD polymorphism in the female population. In contrast, Vogelstein et al. (114) demonstrated that RFLP analysis of the *HPRT* and *PGK* genes could be used to assess the clonality of tumors in greater than 50% of American women. Of 92 tumors tested with the *HPRT* and *PGK* probes, the X-inactivation patterns seen reflected clonality accurately in greater than 95%. Sawada et al. (117) evaluated the clonality of 25 gynecologic malignancies (4 cervical, 11 uterine, 7 ovarian, and 3 tubal) in women heterozygous for the BstXI polymorphism of the *PGK* gene. All 25 tumors were determined to be monoclonal, whereas adjacent normal tissue was polyclonal. DNA preparations from separate areas of the same primary tumor and from corresponding metastatic lesions again revealed identical allelic inactivation. The differential methylation patterns of the *PGK* gene on which this RFLP analysis is based could potentially limit the utility of this approach, however, since DNA methylation patterns are sometimes altered in malignancy.

Several investigators have employed a strategy of combined X-chromosome inactivation and autosomal LOH analysis to assess the clonality of metastatic epithelial ovarian cancer. Jacobs et al. (118) investigated the primary tumor and metastatic implants for LOH at five loci on chromosomes 5, 11, 13, and 17 and sequenced exons 5–8 of the *p53* gene in 17 cases. X-chromosome inactivation of the *PGK* gene could be assessed in five of these patients. Strong evidence for a single precursor cell was presented for 15 of 17 cases. In two cases, data were thought to be compatible with either a monoclonal origin or origin from two primary ovarian carcinomas. Tsao et al. (119) tested for LOH at 12 loci on chromosome 17 in 16 patients and were able to evaluate allelic inactivation of the *HPRT* gene in four of these 16. In all cases, the X-chromosome inactivations and LOH patterns were identical for all tumor deposits tested in each individual patient. Li et al. (120) examined eight cases of invasive and one case of borderline ovarian carcinoma. Analysis of LOH at 86 polymorphic autosomal loci and X-chromosome inactivation patterns of the RFLP DXS255 in five informative patients strongly suggested a monoclonal origin for all of the tumors tested.

In contrast, Muto et al. (121) has provided evidence for a polyclonal origin in four of six cases of papillary serous carcinoma of the peritoneum. Eight loci on chromosomes 1, 3, 4, and 17 were assessed for LOH at five or more different tumor sites within each patient. Screening for *p53* mutations was also performed. Four of the six patients demonstrated selective allelic loss at all sites tested. One of these four patients also had a *p53* mutation detected by single-strand conformational polymorphism (SSCP) analysis (and confirmed by DNA sequencing) at only half of the distinct anatomic sites tested. Recent analysis of borderline tumors, along with our own observations, has also determined that a small subset of these malignancies is multiclonal in origin (122). Additional studies of primary peritoneal serous carcinoma and borderline tumors are needed to clarify their clonal origin and their relationship to, or distinction from, primary ovarian serous carcinoma (123).

Ploidy

The cells in a tumor may be described in terms of their overall DNA content as compared to that of normal tissue. Normal tissue primarily contains cells that have a diploid (2n) complement of chromosomes, a subset of cells that have undergone DNA synthesis (4n) but have not yet divided, and a smaller number of cells with an intermediate amount of DNA. Deviation from this distribution is termed aneuploidy and occurs in approximately 70% of human tumors (124). Tumor ploidy status is frequently described by a ratio known as the DNA index. The numerator is the DNA content in tumor cells that are either not actively proliferating or are in the process of replicating but have not yet undergone DNA synthesis, whereas the denominator is the DNA content of normal diploid cells. Index values deviant from 1 are used to define aneuploidy (3).

Flow cytometry and, more recently, image cytometry are methods that have been used to assess the ploidy status of tumors. In flow cytometry, a DNA intercalating fluorescent dye, such as propidium iodide, is applied to a single-cell suspension. Laser excitation of the stained nuclei, which have been isolated from the cell, generates a fluorescent emission proportional to the amount of DNA in each cell. A histogram is generated, which is analyzed for evidence of tumor aneuploidy (Fig. 3.4) (3). Flow cytometry may be applied to paraffin-embedded as well as fresh-frozen tissue. In addition, because of the large number of cells evaluated, it may be used to describe other cellular parameters, such as the cell-cycle composition of the tumor cell population. Potential confounding factors associated with this method include cellular debris and normal cells contained in the suspension. In image cytometry, touch imprints of the tumor are stained with a stoichiometric nuclear dye, such as feulgen. To quantify DNA staining, a computer measures the optical density in intact cells that have been prescreened by light microscopy to exclude nontumorous cells. The number of cells analyzed is usually 100 to 200, which is in contrast to the 20,000 to 50,000 required by flow cytometry. Both paraffin-embedded and fresh-frozen tissue may be used for image cytometry. Other applications of image cytometry include the description of nuclear architecture and the quantification of hormone receptors (125–127). Although flow cytometry and image cytometry have provided comparable estimates of aneuploidy between series of cancer cases, the classification within series of cases evaluated by both methods may differ by as much as 15% (127).

Several important caveats regarding the use of ploidy status should be noted. Normal ploidy status should not be equated with a normal karyotype. Because ploidy determination provides an estimate of overall DNA content only, tumors with structural chromosomal abnormalities may still manifest a normal DNA content. Also, different areas of the same tumor may manifest heterogeneity with respect to ploidy status (69,128,129). Thus, differences in sampling technique (obtaining single versus multiple tissue specimens) may partially explain the discrepant results of various investigators examining the same tumor type.

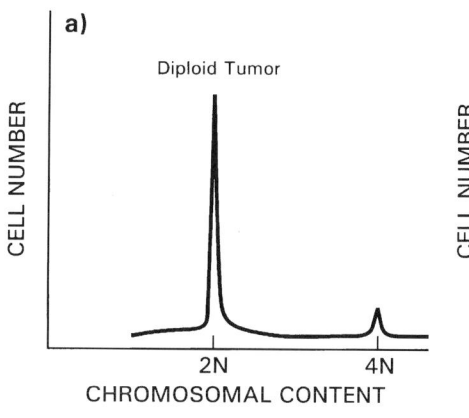

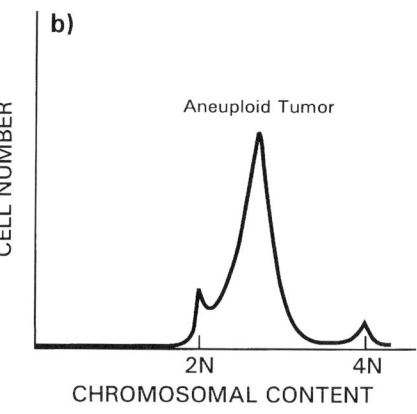

FIG. 3.4. DNA histograms for **(A)** diploid and **(B)** aneuploid tumors. **A:** The normal distribution of cells in somatic tissue is shown, with the majority possessing a 2N DNA content and a smaller fraction having a 4N or intermediate amount of DNA. **B:** In contrast, a tumor-cell population is shown that contains a prominent population of cells with an intermediate DNA content.

Ploidy studies of epithelial ovarian cancer have detected aneuploidy in 0% to 34% of LMP tumors (70,105,130–133) and in 50% to 80% of invasive carcinomas (68,69,71, 134–140). The three largest published series of LMP tumors are case-control studies involving 58 (132), 64 (141), and 92 (131) patients that reached conflicting conclusions regarding the significance of aneuploidy and prognosis. In invasive disease, studies have suggested that ploidy status may be of prognostic importance. Several studies have found ploidy status to be of independent prognostic significance in early-stage invasive disease (68,71,134,137,142). Many investigations that have included advanced-stage invasive disease have also reported a significant adverse association between aneuploidy and median time to recurrence or long-term survival (68–71,136–138). Subset analysis by stage in some of these studies, however, has shown the association to be significant only in patients with early-stage tumors (71, 137). Suboptimal tumor debulking at the primary surgery, a higher frequency of positive second-look laparotomies, and a greater likelihood of recurrence after a negative reassessment procedure have all been associated with aneuploidy (although the relationships have not always been statistically significant, as shown in Table 3.1) (67–71,75,76,78–81,125, 127,128,130–148). Overall, it appears that cytometric analysis of tumor DNA content is an important prognostic indicator in ovarian cancer and is associated with a shortened median time to recurrence and long-term survival. This association appears particularly true in early-stage tumors.

The clinical value of DNA ploidy status has also been analyzed in both endometrial hyperplasia and carcinoma (44, 72,76,142–145,149,150). Norris et al. (150) defined a set of combined morphometric and DNA content criteria to help distinguish between various forms of endometrial hyperplasia and carcinoma. Lindahl and Alm (72) prospectively evaluated 156 patients with endometrial hyperplasia (109 cystic glandular, 35 adenomatous, and 12 atypical). The frequency of aneuploidy was 21%, 20%, and 33%, respectively. Follow-up at 24 months for a subset of patients treated with dilatation and curettage only revealed nonhyperplastic endometria in 64% (21of 33) of those whose hyperplasias were initially diploid compared to 36% (5 of 14) of those whose lesions were nondiploid. The difference was not statistically significant, but they noted that this may have resulted from the small number of cases analyzed because a number of patients were lost to follow-up. Whereas earlier studies produced conflicting results with respect to the clinical value of DNA ploidy status on prognosis in endometrial carcinoma (76,142), more recent studies have shown DNA ploidy status to be an important prognostic indicator with respect to survival (143–145). In a subgroup of 293 women with early-stage disease from a Gynecologic Oncology Group protocol, Zaino et al. (143) found a significant increased risk of disease-related death for patients with aneuploid tumor type as compared to patients with diploid tumor type (144). Whereas this study examined early-stage disease, Nordstrom et al.

recently examined DNA ploidy status in 266 patients with advanced-stage or early-stage grade 3 tumors. In this study, World Health Organization (WHO), International Federation of Gynecology and Obstetrics (FIGO), and nuclear grading were evaluated for prognostic impact in relation to clinical variables and DNA ploidy. Patients with clinical stage I (grades 1–2) tumors were excluded. In univariate Cox analyses, WHO, FIGO, and especially nuclear grading ($p < .001$), as well as age, stage, and ploidy, were prognostic regarding survival. In the multivariate Cox analyses, WHO and FIGO grades yielded little further independent information beyond nuclear grade. When DNA ploidy was added to the analyses, nuclear grade lost most of its impact because aneuploidy was a powerful factor ($p < .001$) that covaried with nuclear grade. Thus, it appears that recent data would suggest aneuploidy as being an independent indicator of poor prognosis with respect to endometrial carcinomas.

Preinvasive and invasive cervical diseases have also been evaluated for the prognostic significance of aneuploidy. A good correlation has been demonstrated between normal and dysplastic Papanicolaou smears and normal and aneuploid DNA histograms, respectively (151,152). An increasing DNA index and a higher frequency of aneuploidy have been reported for increasing degrees of cervical intraepithelial neoplasia (CIN) (151,153–155). In a study of 292 dysplastic lesions of the cervix, Monsonego et al. (151) found a significant association between aneuploidy and the severity of lesions (94% for CIN 1, 55% for CIN 2, and 14% for CIN 3; $p < .0001$). They also noted that the severity of the lesions appeared to be independent of the human papillomavirus (HPV) type. Some investigators have suggested defining a subset of CIN at high risk for progression by quantitating the degree of aneuploidy (154,156). Bibbo et al. (157) found that polyploid CIN was more likely to revert to normal histology than aneuploid, nonpolyploid CIN. Additionally, in a prospective study examining the natural history of CIN, Kashyap et al. (155) noted that aneuploid lesions (CIN 1 and CIN 2) were more likely to progress to CIN 3 than nonaneuploid lesions. For invasive cancer, however, retrospective studies with fewer than 130 cases of varying stages, histology, and treatment modalities have failed to demonstrate a consistent relationship between aneuploidy and prognosis (80,146–148) One large retrospective study of invasive squamous cell carcinoma (344 stage IB/IIA patients treated with radical hysterectomy with or without postoperative irradiation) (81) and two sizable prospective studies of squamous-cell histology (307 patients of all stages who received irradiation and 195 patients of all stages who received either primary irradiation or radical hysterectomy) (79,127) found no significant association between aneuploidy and survival.

The less commonly occurring gynecologic malignancies have also been studied to assess the usefulness of ploidy status. Retrospective studies of 33 to 60 cases of uterine sarcoma have demonstrated a clear trend for nondiploid status to confer an adverse prognosis, but have not consistently

TABLE 3.1. *Selected studies of ploidy status in gynecologic tumors*

Tumor	Stages	No. eval pts	Endpoint eval	Results	Retro/prosp	Reference
Ov LMP	I–IV	53	Survival	NS	R	132
	I–III	64	Survival	S	R	141
	I–III	42	Recurrence	NS	R	130
	I–III	50	Survival	NS	R	133
	I–IV	92	Progression	S	R	131
Ov Inv	I/II	19	Survival	S	R	137
	I/II	21	Survival	S	P	71
	I/II	89	Survival	S	R	68
	I–IIA	48	Survival	S	R	142
	III/IV	68	Survival	NS	R	137
			2LL "+"	S		
			Recur post "−" 2LL	S		
	III/IV	23	Survival	NS	P	71
	III/IV	65	Survival	S	R	68
	III/IV	118	Survival	S	P	136
	I–IV	40	Survival	S	R	70
	I–IV	99	Survival	S	R	69
			2LL "+"	T		
			Recur post "−" 2LL	T		
	I–IV	42	Recurrence	NS	R	128
			Survival for subset			
			Diplold vs "mosaic"	S		
	I–IV	50	Survival	S	P	138
	I–IV	115	Survival	NS	R	67
			Time to recur	NS		
	I–IV	33	Progression	S	R	139
			Survival	S		
	I–IV	31	Survival	S	R	134
			Progression	S		
	I–IV	54	Survival	S	R	135
			Progression	S		
	III–IV	35	Survival	NS	R	140
Endomet	I/II[a]	245	Recurrence	S	P	76
	I/II[c]	37D	Survival	NS	P	75
		293	Survival	S	R	143
	I–IV	266	Survival	S	R	144
	I–IV	100	Survival	S	R	145
SCCA Cx	IB	53	Survival	NS	R	146
			Recurrence	NS		
	IB/IIA	65	Recurrence	S	R	80
	IB/IIA	344	Survival all pts	NS	R	81
			Survival for subset			
			HPP[b] diplold	S		
	IB–IV	121	Survival	NS	R	147
	IB–IV	307	Survival	NS	P	127
	IA–IV	195	Survival all pts	NS	P	79
			Survival for subset			
			HPP diplold	S		
	IB–IIIB	55	Survival	S	R	148

Tumor: Ov LMP, ovarian low–malignant potential tumors; Ov inv, invasive epithelial ovarian carcinoma; Endomet, endometrial adenocarcinoma; SCCA Cx, squamous-cell carcinoma of the cervix; No. eval pts, number of evaluable patients; Endpoint eval, endpoint evaluated; 2LL, second-look laparotomy; HPP, high proliferative phase; results, significant based on multivariate analysis, when available; NS, not significant; S. significant; T. trend: Retro/prosp: R. retrospective; P. prospective.

[a] Clinical staging.

[b] Method, image cytometry; all other studies peformed with flow cytometry.

[c] Included 13 adenocarcinoma pts.

shown aneuploidy to be a significant independent prognostic factor (82–84) Prospective evaluation of 56 cases (86,158) and retrospective examination of 51 cases (86) of complete hydatidiform mole found no association between ploidy status and risk of postmolar gestational trophoblastic neoplasia. A previously published retrospective complete mole study demonstrated that aneuploidy predicted persistence of disease (159). A retrospective series of 17 granulosa-cell tumors of all stages found ploidy to be prognostic, whereas a study of 29 stages IA and IC juvenile granulosa-cell tumors found no association (160,161) Dolan et al. (87) analyzed 42 patients with all stages of squamous-cell carcinoma of the vulva who had undergone surgical therapy with or without postoperative irradiation. The 5-year survival rate of the eight patients with aneuploidy was not significantly different from that of the 34 with diploid tumors. A retrospective evaluation of 61 cases of adenocarcinoma of the fallopian tube, which included all stages and grades of disease and a variety of postoperative therapies, found a 79% frequency of aneuploidy that was not significantly correlated with stage, grade, or median survival time (162).

Genomic and Proteomic Analysis Techniques

Recent advances in molecular techniques have provided new genomic and proteomic approaches that allow for a more precise analysis and definition of the genetic lesions within cancer cells (163). Loss of genetic material may reflect the presence of tumor-suppressor genes, whereas gain of chromosomal regions identifies the presence of dominant oncogenes.

Flourescent In Situ Hybridization

Gross chromosomal abnormalities are detected by the examination of cultured tumor cells arrested in mitosis by spindle poisons using standard cytogentic techniques. More recently developed techniques allow for more precise assessment of chromosomal abnormalities (101,233). Flourescent *in situ* hybridization (FISH) is an excellent technique for identifying the copy number and location of specific genes (or chromosomal regions) within a tumor. A nucleic acid probe that recognizes a specific gene (chromosomal region) is labeled with a flourescent dye and hybridized to chromosomal spreads. A control for chromosome number is accomplished by using a centromeric probe labeled with a different flourescent dye (Fig.3.5). Using these probes, total and relative (per chromosome) gene copy number can be derived.

A related technique know as comparative genomic hybridization (CGH) allows a much broader assessment of chromosomal imbalances (164). As described in a recent review, this technique utilizes total genomic DNA from control and test samples (164). After these samples are labeled with different fluorescent dye, they are then mixed and hybridized to normal metaphase spreads. A region that is deleted in the

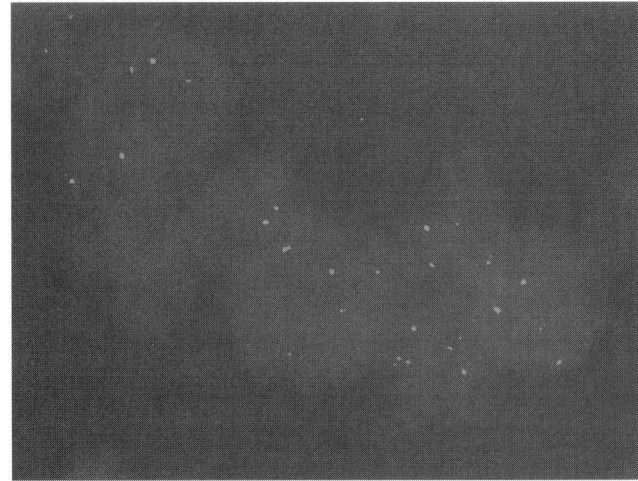
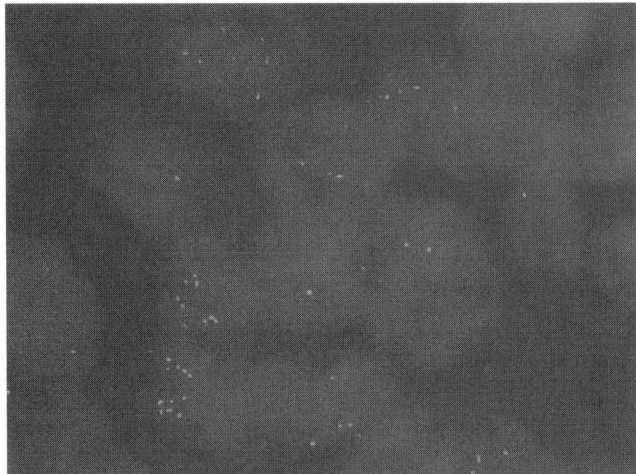

FIG. 3.5. FISH analysis. FISH analysis of advanced ovarian cancers for cyclin E. The BAC clone containing the CCNE1 (cyclin E) gene was labled with spectrum orange, whereas the BAC clone containing the INSR gene (to control for aneusomy) was labeled with spectrum green.

test sample will not hybridize to its chromosomal location, causing the control sample's dye to be in excess. Conversely, the test sample's dye will be in excess if a region is amplified. Thus, a global accessment of chromosomal imbalances can be determined. A more recently developed version of CGH utilizes microarrays (see below) that contain genomic DNA probes. Hybridization of the above-described labeled probes to microarrays containing genomic DNA from known chromosomal regions provides a quantitative assessment of chromosomal imbalances.

Microarrays

Microarray technology utilizes either cDNA or oligonucleotides spotted onto glass slides to evaluate the relative abundance of gene expression in a sample (Fig. 3.6) (165). RNA from tumor cells is converted to cDNA and is labeled

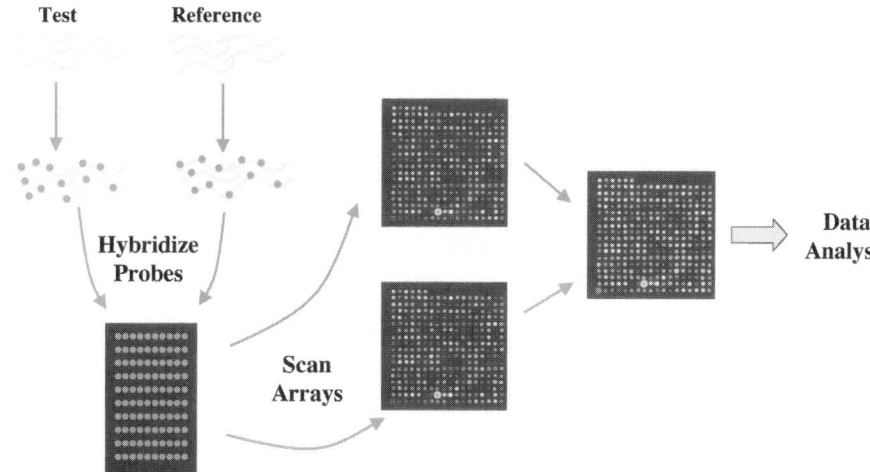

FIG. 3.6. Mircroarray technology RNA or DNA from tumor and reference sources are labeled with Cy-5 and Cy-3, respectively. Labeled probes are hybridized to glass microarray, washed, and scanned. A composite image is generated and analyzed.

with a fluorescent dye. The probe is hydrized to the glass array, washed, and scanned. Microarrays allow the simultaneous analysis of large numbers of genes (even the entire human genome of approximately 30,000 genes). These expression profiles can be established for tumors of different histology, stage, and grade and compared to those of normal tissues. These comparisons will yield those genes whose dysregulation are important for the development of the cancer.

Serial Analysis of Gene Expression

Serial analysis of gene expression (SAGE) is one of several new techniques that allow determination of the expression patterns of thousands of genes simultaneously (166). SAGE was developed based on the basic principles that a short sequence tag (10 bp) contains sufficient information to identify uniquely a transcript and that the concatenation of tags in a serial fashion allows for an increased efficiency in a sequence-based analysis. The procedure involves the synthesis of cDNA, which is then cleaved. The fragments eventually are amplified via polymerase chain reaction (PCR), concatenated, and sequenced. The identity and abundance for individual transcripts in a tissue can thus be determined (166). The advantage of SAGE is that it is an ''open'' technique that does not require prior knowledge of the sequences to be analyzed. Microarray technology requires the knowledge of the target sequences (cDNAs or oligonucleotides printed on the microarrays). However, microarrays tend to be easier to utilize.

BIOCHEMISTRY OF NEOPLASTIC CELLS

Morphology and Function of Cellular Constituents

Cell Structure

Malignant cells differ from normal cells by dramatic changes in their overall size and shape, as well as changes involving their intracellular components. The nuclei of malignant cells are often enlarged and irregular, containing coarse, clumped chromatin. The nucleus:cytoplasm ratio, normally in the range of 1:4 to 1:6, frequently approaches 1:1 (1). Nucleoli are often more prominent in cancerous cells than in normal cells. These differences can be quantitated and exploited as a measure of cellular transformation. For example, the technique of silver staining and counting nucleolar organizer regions (AgNORs) has been applied to cervical dysplasia and ovarian tumors. Wistuba et al. (167) demonstrated an increasing number of AgNORs with increasing severity of cervical dysplasia. In another study, involving 24 mucinous and 28 serous epithelial ovarian tumors, a higher number of AgNORs were found in the invasive carcinomas than in the borderline or benign tumors. The differences were not significant for the mucinous tumors, but a significant difference was demonstrated for the serous invasive versus other serous neoplasms (70).

Cellular fibrils appear to have important structural and functional roles in both normal and neoplastic cells. As presented in the description of the transformed cell, disorganization of actin microfilaments is thought to underlie some of the morphologic changes and random orientation manifested by these cells (168). Experimental evidence suggests that increased actin organization is associated with *in vitro* growth suppression (169). The distribution of intermediate filaments, such as desmin, vimentin, and the keratins, varies among different types of tumors. Monoclonal antibodies that recognize these filaments can aid in the diagnosis of poorly differentiated neoplasms (1). In addition to their traditionally ascribed functions, such as maintenance of cell structure and assistance with cell movement, intermediate filaments have been shown to play a role in cell division and nuclear function. They are demonstrated substrates for protein kinases involved with regulation of cellular proliferation, such as p34[cdc-2] and C-kinase. Phosphorylation of intermediate filaments is associated with their depolymerization during mitosis (170,171). Also, data suggest that lamin B, a component of the nuclear laminin complex, may be involved with the organization of chromatin during DNA replication (172).

Significant alterations in the structure and function of the cell membrane accompany malignant transformation. Modification of membrane glycoproteins, glycolipids, and cell surface adhesive properties are associated with the ability to invade and metastasize. An increased degree of branching in the glycan chains of glycoproteins has been noted as well as abnormal fucosylation and sialylation of membrane carbohydrate moieties (173,174). In some cases, new gangliosides or other novel structures are produced (61). These aberrantly glycosylated membrane components are recognized by monoclonal antibodies as tumor-associated carbohydrate antigens.

Tumor Metabolism

The process of malignant transformation produces profound changes in cellular metabolism. Tumor cells demonstrate a higher rate of both glycolysis and glutaminolysis, providing intermediary phosphometabolites for the biosynthesis of nucleotides, lipids, and complex carbohydrates. Alterations in the concentrations and activities of certain isoenzymes, such as the greatly increased activity of pyruvate kinase type M2, underlie these changes. Phosphometabolite levels are also higher secondary to lowered levels of their degradative enzymes (175–177). Other metabolic aberrations described in tumor cells include alterations in cholesterol biosynthesis and intramitochondrial aldehyde catabolism (177).

One consequence of altered tumor metabolism is the higher level of fucoproteins seen in the sera of cancer patients as compared to healthy individuals. Elevated serum levels of α-1,3 fucosyltransferase and fucosylated forms of α_1-antitrypsin and haptoglobin have been detected in patients with ovarian cancer, and these levels appeared to correlate with disease status (178). Another secondary effect of the abnormal metabolism of cancer cells is its effect on the host metabolism. When cancer strips its host of nutrients, the host metabolism adapts by processes such as increasing gluconeogenesis. Eventually, anorexia and depletion of energy stores are manifested in the clinical condition known as cachexia.

Tumor-associated Antigens, Oncofetal Proteins, Hormones, and Enzymes

Tumor cells may produce substances unique to the tissue cell of origin, such as prostate-specific antigen and human chorionic gonadotropin (1). Other substances that are secreted by tumors are infrequently or never elaborated by their normal cellular counterparts. These include ectopic hormones responsible for the paraneoplastic syndromes, tumor-associated antigens such as CA-125, and oncofetal antigens

such as α-fetoprotein (1). Oncofetal antigens, although absent from normal adult tissues, can be found in developmental precursor cells. Many of these tumor products are particularly useful as tumor markers that can assist with cancer diagnosis and surveillance. In addition, cancer cells frequently demonstrate an imbalance between the activities of proteolytic enzymes, such as plasminogen activator, metalloproteinases, and cathepsins, and their inhibitors. These deregulated enzyme activities are thought to play a role in the processes of tumor invasion and metastasis (179).

Protein Processing and Degradation

For proteins to serve their roles in cellular function, they require proper structure and carefully regulated levels that reflect a steady-state balance between synthesis, folding, and degradation. Recent discoveries have shown that protein folding, which is required for proper protein function, is mediated through a group of proteins called chaperones. Heat shock protein 90 (Hsp-90) is a typical chaperone that binds to a large number of client proteins and assists in their appropriate folding (180). Once appropriately folded, these proteins are fully functional till they become denatured and then targeted for degradation. Proteins are degraded in part by ubiquitination and targeting to the proteosome. Ubiquitination is accomplished by a family of ubiquitin ligases whose substrate specificity depends upon protein sequence and phosphorylation status. The proteosome is a complex of proteins including proteases that degrades a wide range of proteins. This complex process accounts for the tissue-specific and cell-cycle regulation of expression of many critical proteins.

The ubiquitination/proteosome process has received a great deal of attention in relation to its contribution to cancer development. Mutations and alterations in the phosphorylation state have been shown to change ubiquitination status and turnover of critical proteins including those involved in the cell cycle. Based in part upon these observations, the proteosome has been targeted for the development of novel small molecule inhibtors. It is hypothesized that these inhibtors would potentially be effective chemotherapeutic agents (180).

Signal Transduction Pathways

Neoplasia may be viewed fundamentally as a disorder of cell proliferation in both space and time. Central to the orderly occurrence of normal cell proliferation is the response to environmental cues. Growth factors, originally defined as peptides or proteins extractable from living tissues that promote cell proliferation in artificial (e.g., cell and organ cultures) systems, have come to be viewed as the means by which these signals are conveyed. In this way, neoplasia can also be viewed as a disorder of cellular communication.

''Signal transduction'' refers to the biochemical mechanisms by which small molecules alter the state or activities of the intracellular milieu. Two broad mechanisms for signal transduction have emerged. The first involves the generation consequent to the action of a growth factor of a covalent modification in intracellular constituents, with the "signal" lasting as long as the modification is present. The covalent modification par excellence is phosphorylation, which is accomplished by protein kinases, enzymes that transfer the gamma phosphate of ATP to substrate molecules whose function is altered owing to the attached phosphate. Two types of protein kinases of greatest importance in the regulation of cell growth are those that phosphorylate proteins on tyrosine residues and those that phosphorylate proteins on serine or threonine residues (14). The second general mechanism for signal transduction is found in the generation of "second-messenger" molecules, which are produced consequent to the action of a growth factor and which act upon intracellular receptor sites to effect functional changes, usually by allosteric mechanisms. The second messengers whose role in growth control are most clearly defined include, but are not limited to, Ca^{2+}, cyclic AMP (cAMP), and phospholipid metabolites. This section gives a broad overview of the growth-regulating pathways modified by growth factors employing these effector mechanisms.

Growth Factor Receptor–associated Tyrosine Kinases

The discovery of the importance of tyrosine kinases as mediators of carcinogenic stimuli came from the identification of their capture by acutely transforming RNA tumor viruses. Characterization of these captured genes revealed structures that identified them as kinases, and examination of the mass of phosphorylated amino acids in virally transformed cells demonstrated an increase in tyrosine phosphate, a normally minor phosphoamino acid constituent. Antisera specific for the transforming proteins immunoprecipitated proteins that have the ability to phosphorylate themselves and, in some cases, the precipitating antibody. Characterization of the phosphorylated proteins demonstrated the presence of phosphorylated tyrosine moieties. Subsequently, it was demonstrated that receptors for certain growth factors, truncated or mutated versions of which could also demonstrate oncogenic potential in certain instances, also possessed kinase activity for tyrosine. Conceptually, this links tyrosine kinase activity to the action of growth-regulatory substances.

As outlined in detail by Cadena and Gill (181), receptor–tyrosine kinases have at least four structural domains: (a) the extracellular domain binds ligand, and may be subgrouped into families of receptor-associated tyrosine kinases based on the presence of immunoglobulin-like domains or the number of cysteine-rich motifs; (b) a transmembrane domain links the external portion with the rest of the molecule; (c) an intracellular catalytic domain contains the core ATP binding and phosphoryl transfer elements (with reference again to pp60^{c-src}, this region is designated the SH1, or

Src homology region 1 domain); and (d) regulatory domains regulate the endogenous activity of the kinases by allosteric or intrachain "pseudosubstrate"-like mechanisms, or they mediate association of the receptor–tyrosine kinase with either substrates or regulatory molecules involved in the propagation of signals. Receptor-associated tyrosine kinases are divided into groups according to the structure of their extracellular domains, including the presence of a variable number of immunoglobulin-like domains, the number of cysteine-rich motifs, leucine-rich regions, cadherin domains, fibronectin type III repeats, discoid I–like domains, and epidermal growth factor (EGF)–like domains. These various structures result in at least 14 different families of receptor-associated tyrosine kinases.

In addition to causing autophosphorylation of the receptor, activation of growth-factor receptor–tyrosine kinases results in phosphorylation of key substrate molecules thought to be important in propagating the growth-promoting stimulus. Both of these reactions create tyrosine phosphates, which can then form complexes with SH2 (Src homology region 2) domains. SH2 domains are approximately 100 amino acid regulatory motifs originally defined by similarity to a portion of pp60^{c-src}. Importantly, SH2 domains are found in a number of signaling molecules, including phospholipase-C-gamma, phosphatidylinositol 3′-kinase (PI 3′K), the GTPase activator for ras proteins, protein phosphatase-1C, as well as a number of nonreceptor-tyrosine kinases, including pp60^{c-src}. An important family of "adapter" molecules, represented prototypically by grb2, are small molecules devoid of catalytic functions but simply consisting of two SH2 domains centered around another type of domain, the SH3 domain, capable of mediating protein-protein interactions. Through their SH2 domains, these adapter molecules function to associate physically proteins phosphorylated on tyrosine.

The important result of growth-factor receptor-kinase activation is, therefore, the assembly of multimeric complexes through SH2 domains of molecules with distinct signaling capabilities: (a) phospholipase-C-gamma (PLC-gamma) hydrolyzes membrane phosphatidylinositol bisphosphate (PIP_2), producing inositol triphosphate and increases in intracellular diacylglycerol (DAG). Inositol triphosphate interacts with the cell membrane and releases Ca^{2+}. Increased DAG and Ca^{2+} maximally activates PKC. (b) PI 3′K phosphorylates phosphatidylinositols at the 3′ position, creating new substrates for PLC-gamma. In addition, a substrate for PI 3′K is protein kinase B (AKT), which has been demonstrated to be important in suppressing apoptosis. (c) ras GTP hydrolysis is stimulated by ras GAP (GTPase-activating protein). It is also clear that in addition to the associations described above with receptor tyrosine-protein kinases, the adapter protein grb2 can form complexes with the mammalian homolog of the son of sevenless (Sos) protein originally described in the sevenless *Drosophila* mutant. The importance of this observation is that the Sos protein has

GDP-exchange activity for mammalian ras proteins. Thus, receptor–tyrosine kinase activation can both accelerate ras protein activation (through exchange of GDP for GTP) as well as lead to ras inactivation (through GAP). These findings provide a biochemical basis for the original observations that neoplastic transformation by receptor–tyrosine or nonreceptor–tyrosine kinases could be blocked by genetic maneuvers that inhibited ras function.

Non–Growth-Factor Receptor–associated Tyrosine Kinases

The prototype for oncogenic, non–growth-factor receptor–related tyrosine kinases is $pp60^{c-src}$, the cellular homolog of the transforming oncogene of Rous sarcoma virus, $pp60^{v-src}$. As the prototype of nonreceptor-associated tyrosine kinases, $pp60^{c-src}$ is representative of at least eight families of molecules with distinct domain structures. In addition to the Src family, these include the Abl, Fes/Fps, focal adhesion (FAK), c-Src kinase (CSK), Janus kinase (JAK), spleen tyrosine kinase (syk), and interleukin-2–inducible kinase (ITK) families. As reviewed by Bolen et al. (182), these kinases may have relatively ubiquitous expression (e.g., abl, src) or tissue-restricted distribution (e.g., fyn, lyn). Although they are anatomically distinct from the receptor–tyrosine kinases, they have certain functional similarities in that the kinase-specific activity of the nonreceptor-tyrosine kinases increases following ligand-stimulation of cell types in which they are found. Thus, as reviewed by Cantley et al. (183), thrombin activation of platelets and platelet-derived growth factor (PDGF) activation of fibroblasts results in increased $pp60^{c-src}$ activity, and activation of T lymphocytes through the CD4 or CD8 determinants activates $pp56^{c-lck}$, a $pp60^{c-src}$ family member (36).

The consequences of the activation of the nonreceptor–tyrosine kinases include the phosphorylation of many of the same substrates described above for the receptor-linked tyrosine kinases. In particular, the activation of ras through grb2/Sos underscores that ras activation can proceed through input from a number of different sources and points to the importance of the molecules "downstream" of ras as representing a "final common pathway" of cellular activation.

Ras Pathway

Nowhere in signal transduction research has more progress been achieved than in characterizing the downstream pathways from *ras*. Multiple protein kinases have been identified and their mode of interaction characterized (184). The view of growth factor–induced cellular activation that emerges from this train of recent investigation is represented in Figure 3.3, where input from either receptor-associated or non–receptor-associated tyrosine kinases is reflected in increased generation of activated *ras* bound to GTP. Activated *ras* in turn associates with *raf* and in some way in-

creases the catalytic activity of the latter protein, which propagates the signal to MAP kinase (185).

The c-*raf* protooncogene was originally defined as the cellular homolog of the transforming oncogene v-*raf*. However, accumulating evidence from genetic approaches, summarized by Van Aelst et al. (186), indicates that raf functions "downstream" of ras. Specifically, activated raf abrogated the need for ras to transform cells; mutations of *raf* could block ras transformation; growth-factor agonists that activated ras or constitutively activated ras-containing cells had hyperphosphorylated raf; and, most importantly, a family of serine threonine kinases, the microtubule-associated protein ("MAP," after a substrate used in their original purification) kinases, were themselves activated by "MAP kinase kinases" (MAPKK), which could be demonstrated to be substrates for raf. These genetic results led to a concerted effort to identify a biochemical association between ras or ras-associated molecules and raf. Indeed, several groups using recombinant-expressed protein or fusion proteins produced in yeast have clearly demonstrated a noncovalent association between ras and raf proteins (186,187). This association has been confirmed by precipitation of raf using ras affinity reagents (188). However, although it is clear that inactive raf is brought to the cell membrane by GTP-ras, the precise mechanism by which ras activates raf still remains unknown. Activated raf in turn phosphorylates MAPKK (MEK), which activates MAP kinases (185).

One dilemma in ras signaling was how a single protein could mediate such diverse biologic effects as apoptosis, proliferation, and differentiation. Recent work has identified two possible mechanisms: (a) a large family of *ras* effectors that could determine the specificity of ras signaling (189) and (b) a number of novel *ras*-like genes (190). Some of these ras effectors may play a role in the development of gynecologic cancer (189). Likewise, *ras*-like genes may also be important for the development of gynecologic cancers. For instance, Noey2 was originally described as a downregulated ras effector in ovarian cancer (191). This protein mediates growth inhibition and may function as a tumor suppressor gene. Several other ras effectors have recently been identified and characterized. The precise role for these effectors is not yet clear, but presumably they will serve important functions in a variety of biologic processes.

MAP Kinases

MAP kinase was originally defined as a distinctive protein whose phosphorylation on both tyrosine and threonine residues increased shortly after addition of growth factors to cells. It is now appreciated that there are multiple different MAP kinases and isoforms (192,193). Each family of MAP kinases has unique (although overlapping) downstream substrates and upstream activators (MAPKKs). MAP kinase families include the ERK, JNK, and the p38 families. The extracellular signal–regulated kinases (ERKs) are phosphorylated and activated by MEK 1,2, the JNKs are activated by JNKK1 (SAPKK1), and the p38s are activated by MKK 3 and 6. These MAPKKs are in turn activated by specific MAPKKKs. Thus, raf signals through MEK 1,2 to the ERK family members, whereas JNK and p38 receive their activation signals from other upstream kinases. These kinase cascades allow for rapid transduction and amplification of signals from the cell membrane. Recent work has demonstrated that activation of one MAPK pathway can suppress the activity of the others (194). Thus, although they are primarily vertical pathways, they supply ample lateral crosstalk between themselves, providing integration of multiple unique cell membrane signals.

As reviewed by Garrington and Johnson (195), MAP kinases in turn phosphorylate a diverse series of substrates, including cytoplasmic phospholipase A_2, cytoskeletal components, protein synthesis machinery, and, perhaps most importantly, transcription factors. The substrate specificity of different MAP kinase families, although overlapping, are unique (196). Thus, a unique combination of proteins is activated by each MAP kinase. It is proposed that activation of transcription of new genes in response to growth-factor action extends in part from these actions of MAP kinases. Included among the transcription factors affected are those that govern the synthesis of cyclins, which allow entry into the cell cycle (e.g., the E2F transcription factor controls the activity of promoters essential for transcription of genes necessary to complete the S phase) (197,198).

Phosphatidylinositol 3′-kinase

PI 3′K is a lipid kinase that appears to play an important role in mediating a wide variety of signals involved in diverse cellular processes including cellular proliferation, apoptosis, and vesicular trafficking (199). PI 3′K is a heterodimeric protein that is activated by a wide variety of receptor–tyrosine kinases such as the insulin, PDGF, and EGF receptors. It has been well established that phosphorylation of a tyrosine residue on the receptor will serve as a docking site a component of PI 3′K (p85) that in turn recruits the catalytic subunit of PI 3′K (p110). Alternatively, PI 3′K can be activated through a ras-dependent mechanism (demonstrating a connection between these two pathways). As mentioned above, PI 3′K has been widely recognized as being able to phosphorylate phosphatidylinositols at the 3′ position, which in turn activates protein kinase C (PKC). However, it is appreciated that there are other substrates of PI 3′K including p70 S6K and, most importantly, PKB/AKT. AKT is a protein kinase that has been demonstrated to mediate multiple biologic processes. Of particular importance, PI 3′K has been identified as amplified in breast and ovarian cancers. Increased PI 3′K activity has been detected in a large subset of ovarian cancers, and inhibiton of this pathway leads to inhibition of cellular proliferation (200).

AKT

AKT is a serine/threonine kinase and the primary mediator of the effects of PI 3′K (199). A broad spectrum of substrates is phosphorylated by AKT and includes transcription factors (Creb, Forkhead), proteins critical for apoptosis (caspase-9, BAD, IKK), and cell-cycle proteins (p21, p27) and other kinases (GSK-3). These substrates in turn activate multiple other pathways, including cross-talk to the MAPK pathway. The biologic downstream effects of activation of AKT includes suppression of apoptosis, induction of cell-cycle progression, and induced resistance to cytotoxic drugs. Given these effects, it is not suprising to note the evidence linking AKT to the development of cancer. AKT has been found to be activated and amplified in ovarian cancer (201). It has also been shown to play a major role in drug resistance in a variety of human malignancies.

Protein Kinase C

PKC was originally described as a Ca^{2+} (hence the C) and phospholipid-dependent kinase distinct from the c-AMP–dependent protein kinase A. It is now recognized that the term *protein kinase C* can refer to at least eight distinct molecular entities (isoforms) that, in some cases, may be actually independent of Ca^{2+}, but are related to other members of the family because of structural similarities.

The importance of PKC in tumorigenesis came from the finding that PKC isoforms were receptors for the tumor-promoting phorbol esters, one of the first demonstrations of a discrete molecular effector of a carcinogenetic stimulus (202). The relationship of this observation to growth-factor action came from the realization that the normal activators of PKC include diacylglycerols, which can be produced by phospholipase-C, an enzymatic activity that increases after the addition of growth factors of a variety of types. Thus, tyrosine kinase–linked growth factors could be shown to phosphorylate and activate the phospholipase-C-gamma isoform, whereas Ca^{2+}-linked growth factors (see discussion of G-protein and Ca^{2+}-related signals below) activate phospholipase-C-gamma. PKC, once activated, can directly influence the activity of the MAP kinase pathway by phosphorylating raf (203). Additional pathways leading to activation of transcription from PKC-sensitive promoter elements exist.

Cyclin-dependent Kinases

The ultimate consequence of growth-factor action is the entry of quiescent cells into the cell cycle. The molecular events responsible for this process are currently being elucidated. In particular, it was known as a result of classic biochemical experiments that at the onset of mitosis there was an increase in protein kinase activity directed at histones, and it was hypothesized that altered phosphorylation of nuclear proteins allows or promotes the morphologically apparent changes in chromosomal condensation. It was therefore of great interest when a protein with histone H1-kinase activity was found to complement a yeast mutation defective in cell-cycle progression. The responsible protein, p34^{cdc-2}, was found to be a serine/threonine kinase whose activity was cyclically regulated by the appearance during the normal yeast cell cycle of a family of molecules called cyclins, with the active H1-kinase enzyme consisting of a complex of cyclin and an appropriately phosphorylated p34^{cdc2} catalytic subunit (reviewed in a landmark series examining S and M phases) (204–208).

Subsequently, through the use of homology cloning and complementation of function in yeast, it became apparent that regulation of progression through G_1 is also regulated by a family of analogous molecules now collectively referred to as cyclin-dependent kinases (CDKs). This family is now known to include at least seven discrete molecular entities with at least eight cyclin-related putative regulators. Of great current interest is how growth factors regulate the enzymatic cascade that is directly responsible for entry into the cell cycle (Fig. 3.3). Of fundamental importance was the observation that the tumor-suppressor gene product of the retinoblastoma-related locus (pRb) was a substrate for CDK2, and that phosphorylation of Rb correlates with entry into the S phase (209, 210).

It is now well documented that cyclin D-CDK4/6 and cyclin E-CDK2 complexes phosphorylate Rb, causing it to release the transcription factor E2F. E2F in turn regulates the expression of S-phase genes, which are required for DNA replication. Thus, the G1–S-phase transition is critically dependent on sufficient CDK activity and, as expected, is a frequent target for alteration in cancer cells. For instance, recent analysis has demonstrated that cyclin E is frequently amplified and overexpressed in ovarian cancer (211). Genetic abnormalities such as these may provide important enzymatic targets for novel therapeutic agents.

G-Protein and Calcium-related Signals

Second-messenger control of intracellular events was first demonstrated convincingly in the case of cAMP control of glycolysis in liver treated with α-adrenergic agonists. Paramount to establishing the mechanism of this process was the observation that guanine nucleotides were necessary for the efficient generation of cAMP. This led to the purification of proteins that, in the GTP-bound state, stimulated adenylate cyclase, and thus were called ''G''-proteins (212). The class of receptor coupled to this effector system [G-protein-coupled receptors (GPCR)], the prototype of which is the adrenergic receptor, is structurally very distinct in comparison to receptor-linked tyrosine kinases. This receptor superfamily, with now over 200 members, has an external ligand-binding portion, seven transmembrane segments, and a carboxyl-terminal ''tail.'' These ''serpentine'' receptors (reviewed comprehensively in ref. 213) couple to G-proteins, which are now understood to interact not only with adenylate cyclase but also with certain phospholipases, including phospholipase-C-β. This entity hydrolyzes the membrane lipid phosphatidylinositol-4,5-bis-phosphate to yield the soluble metabolite inositol 1,4,5-tris-phosphate, which releases Ca^{2+} from internal stores as well as diacylglycerol, described above as the endogenous regulator of PKC (Fig. 3.3) (214).

Recent work has demonstrated that a subfamily of GPCRs that bind lysophospholipids appear to play a role in the development of ovarian cancer (215). These receptors include PSP24 and the EDG receptors. These receptors do not bind all lysophospholipids but are activated by lysophatidic acid (LPA) and sphingosine-1-phosphate (213,216,217). The combination of multiple receptor family members, different ligands, and the available intracellular G-proteins produces a wide range of biologic effects including proliferation, invasion, and cellular survival.

Protein Phosphatases

Protein phosphatases are a relatively newly described group of proteins that function in an opposing manner to protein kinases providing important regulatory mechanisms to the above-described signal cascades. In fact, it has been proposed that phosphatases play a critical role in cellular functions such as proliferation, differentiation, and apoptosis as protein kinases (218,219).

Protein phosphatases are divided into groups by different criteria, but the most commonly used is that of substrate specificity: protein tyrosine phosphatases (PTPs), serine/threonine phosphatases (PPs), and dual-specificity phosphatases (DSPs). Protein tyrosine phosphatases are further classified according to whether they contain a transmembrane domain or not. Transmembrane (TM) domain-containing PTPs [receptor PTPs (RPTPs)] have extracellular domains and possess a catalytic domain in their intracellular portion. Many RPTPs (such as CD45, LAR, and PTP beta, possess structural features that suggest a role in cellular adhesion (220). Indeed, studies have revealed that several RPTPs are important regulators of neuronal adhesion (36,41,221). Non-TM PTPs (membrane associated) are also important regulators of tyrosine phosphorylation, and some appear to associate with tyrosine kinases through the SH2 domains found within their structures (SHP-1, SHP-2). SHP-1 and SHP-2 appear to play critical roles in regulating tyrosine kinase signals within hematopoietic cells (206,222). PTEN is a tyrosine phosphatase that has been demonstrated to have an inhibitory effect on cellular proliferation (223). This inhibitory activity has been traced to a negative regulation of PI 3′K and AKT activity (224,225). Whether this is a direct effect of PTEN ability to dephosphorylate phosphotyrosine residues or its additional activity as a lipid phosphatase remains unclear. However, mutations in PTEN have been identified in a wide variety of tumors as well as in the germline of patients with Cowden's disease (226). Based upon these observations, it is widely concluded that *PTEN* is a tumor-suppressor gene. Recent work has identified mutations within this gene in endometrial cancers and endometrioid ovarian cancers (227,228). In a wider number of ovarian cancers, PTEN activity is suppressed, leading to an overactivity of the PI 3'K pathway.

Protein serine/threonine phosphatases (PSPs) comprise a group of protein phosphatases containing three subunits: regulatory, variable, and catalytic (229). Four major families have been identified (although a fifth family has recently been identifed): PP1, PP2A, PP2B, and PP2C. Multiple members exist within each family, and there is some evidence for substrate specificity differences between families. Type 2A PSPs have selective substrate specificity for PKC phosphorylated proteins and the ribosomal S6 protein. Type 2A PSPs are of particular interest because they have been found to associate with complexes formed by DNA tumor virus proteins and cellular proteins. The presence of PP2A in these complexes suggests it may play a role in the alteration of cellular proliferation mediated by DNA tumor viruses (230,231).

Dual-specificity phosphatases are frequently grouped with PTPs owing to their ability to dephosphorylate phosphotyrosine moieties. However, they are also able to use phosphoserine and phosphothreonine as substrates. DSPs such as MKP-1 and Cdi1 localize to the nucleus, where they have been shown to dephosphorylate MAP kinases (232). Thus, this represents an important family of proteins that may serve to regulate the incoming proliferative signals from various MAP kinase cascades. For instance, MKP-1/CL100 has been found to be differentially expressed between normal and malignant ovarian epithelium (233). Reexpression of this gene in ovarian cancer cells decreases the malignant phenotype.

Wnt/β-Catenin Pathway

The Wnt/β-catenin pathway is an important signal transduction pathway frequently disrupted in cancer cells (234). In the absense of Wnt signaling, β-catenin expression is controlled by the formation of a degradation complex that includes GSK3B, APC, and Axin (235). This complex produces ubiquitination of β-catenin and its degradation by the proteosome. When the Wnt ligand binds to its receptor Frizzled, the degradation complex is distablized, resulting in higher levels of nonphosphorylated β-catenin. High levels of β-catenin translocate to the nucleus, where it acts as a cofactor for TCF/LEF transcription factor.

This pathway has been extensivly studied in human cancers (234). Mutations in this pathway are very common in colorectal cancers. Germline mutations within the APC gene form the molecular basis for familial adenomatous polyposis (FAP). Somatic mutations of APC (and to a lesser extent β-catenin) are common in sporadic colorectal cancers. Activating mutations of the Wnt pathway are found in a wide variety of other cancers including gynecologic cancers. This is especially true for the endometriod phenotype of ovarian and endometrial cancers.

Growth Factors and Their Receptors

Epidermal Growth Factor

Epidermal growth factor (EGF) refers to a growth-promoting activity originally recognized by its ability to promote the normal formation of facial structures in neonatal mice. It is now recognized as the prototype for a family of growth factors widely distributed in a number of anatomic sites, including EGF, transforming growth factor-β (TGF-β), amphiregulin, "neu differentiation factor," and "neu/*erb*B2 ligand growth factor" (236,237). The growth factors have in common several structural motifs and combine with members of a receptor family that possesses intrinsic tyrosine kinase activity. These include the classic EGF receptor (EGF-R, also known as c-*erb*B1), which also binds to TGF-β, and the related receptor c-*erb*B2 (also known as p185*neu*), originally defined by its similar structure but distinct pattern of amplification and expression in tumors (149).

As outlined by Bast et al. (238), autocrine stimulation by TGF-β and overexpression of c-*erb*B2 appear to be of clear importance in ovarian carcinoma, where the level of c-*erb*B2 expression appears to correlate adversely with prognosis in some series (239,240). In addition, the expression and relation to tumor cell growth of c-*erb*B2 have been outlined in endometrial adenocarcinoma and cervical squamous cell and adenocarcinomas (65). Although receptors for EGF have been proposed as targets for the actions of antibodies that signal a negative growth regulatory signal (241), initial trials have been disappointing (242).

Insulin-like Growth Factors

Growth factors with metabolic effects analogous to insulin (in classic assays, such as the rat diaphragmatic muscle glycogen store assay) but with effects on other tissues that account for the activity of liver-derived, pituitary-growth-hormone–regulated "somatomedins" or "sulfation factors" (IGFs) also have, on amino acid sequence, a structure analogous to insulin. These "insulin-like growth factors" include IGF-I and IGF-II. The receptors for insulin and for IGF-I have been characterized as tyrosine kinase–linked receptors with a distinct repertoire of intracellular substrates in comparison to EGF. Recent studies have implicated these receptors and their cognate growth factors in the promotion of ovarian carcinoma (243).

Platelet-derived Growth Factor

The platelet-derived growth factor (PDGF) is of historic significance owing to its structural and functional homology to the v-*sis* viral oncogene. As reviewed in detail by Fantl et al. (244), the PDGF-R is a receptor-linked tyrosine kinase with distinctive features, including an extracellular domain with five regions with homology to immunoglobulins and an intracellular domain that interrupts the kinase region and is thought to serve as a "dock" for presentation of phosphotyrosines to molecules that can bind to phosphotyrosine through SH2 domains. Receptors with considerable homology to the PDGF-R include the macrophage colony-stimulating factor (M-CSF) and c-kit protein, which is the receptor for the "steel" ligand, which is important in normal melanocyte, germ-cell, and hematopoietic development.

Ovarian and choriocarcinoma cells have been reported to express PDGF and PDGF receptors (245,246). A number of ovarian and cervical carcinomas express either c-kit and/or steel ligand (247), and have receptors for M-CSF (248). Although the functional importance of these receptors has not been established, their presence raises the possibility that gynecologic neoplasms will depend at some point in their pathogenesis on the action of members of this growth-factor receptor family. In addition, the development of small molecule inhibitors that bind to the PDGF receptor (Gleevac) has raised the possiblity of inhibiting tumor progression *in vivo* by using this agent.

Fibroblast Growth Factor and Other Angiogenic Factors

The family of fibroblast growth factors (FGFs) comprises several members distinguished originally by binding to heparin and elution at a spectrum of pHs, thus allowing their characterization as basic or acidic FGFs (249). These entities have been proposed to mediate not only the direct promotion of tumor cell growth but also the stimulation of stroma formation and blood vessel growth to sustain tumors beyond the microscopic stage. Additional "angiogenic" factors include platelet-derived endothelial growth factor and vascular permeability factor. Basic FGF and its receptor is expressed in human ovarian carcinomas (250). Ovarian and endometrial neoplasms have recently been demonstrated to secrete both platelet-derived endothelial growth factor and vascular endothelial growth factor (251,252).

Transforming Growth Factor-β

TGF-β was originally recognized as a mediator of natural killer cell transformation distinct from TGF-β (4). It has a radically different receptor system than those described thus far, binding directly to a "receptor II," which is a constitutively active transmembrane serine/threonine kinase. After the binding of TGF-β, receptor II recruits another member (receptor I) into the complex, allowing propagation by receptor I of a serine/ threonine kinase signal to downstream substrates (253). The importance of TGF-β to gynecologic neoplasia extends in part from the recognition that the müllerian inhibitor substance (MIS), important in the embryogenesis of the normal genitourinary tract, is a member of the TGF-β family (254). TGF-β itself is recognized as a negative growth regulator of a variety of cell types, including ovarian tumor cells (174).

Tumor Necrosis Factor and Interleukin-1

It has recently been proposed that TNF and interleukin-1 (IL-1), cytokines originally defined as hematopoietic growth factors, operate via yet another distinct signaling mechanism. This involves the hydrolysis of membrane sphingomyelin, with the resulting ceramide acting as a second messenger to activate a ceramide-dependent protein kinase (255). Recent evidence has been accumulating that IL-1 can directly inhibit the growth of ovarian carcinoma cells (256) and is expressed by this cell type and endometrial carcinoma cells in culture (257). IL-1 has also been found to regulate the secretion of collagenase, which is important in mediating invasiveness in choriocarcinoma cells (258). TNF can act as an autocrine (213) and paracrine (259) growth factor for ovarian carcinoma cells.

Calcium-mobilizing Growth Factors

The importance of the G-protein–linked Ca^{2+}-mobilizing growth factors and their receptors to the growth of gynecologic neoplasms has been less completely characterized than the entities described above. However, it has recently been demonstrated that the peptide bombesin can modulate sensitivity of ovarian carcinoma cells to TNF and platinum, perhaps by modulating Ca^{2+} levels (260). In addition, pharmacologic treatments that seek to interfere with the increase in Ca^{2+} in response to growth factors of this class are under clinical evaluation in patients with gynecologic neoplasms (261).

CARCINOGENESIS

Chemical and Physical Carcinogenesis

Initiation and Promotion

The biologic processes of tumor initiation and promotion were first characterized from experiments that involved the induction of skin tumors in mice (262). Animals given high doses of an agent such as a polycyclic aromatic hydrocarbon (initiator or carcinogen) would eventually develop a low number of skin papillomas. If subtumorigenic doses of this agent were followed by multiple administrations of substances that by themselves could not produce tumors (promoters), such as croton seed oil, the animals developed papillomas at a high rate. Further treatment of these animals with a carcinogen converted some of the papillomas to carcinomas. From these classic studies, data from other animal models, and the direct study of human cancers, it has become clear that carcinogenesis is a multistep process.

Initiation is the first stage of carcinogenesis and is characterized by irreversible changes in the cellular DNA. Initiators can be chemical, physical, or viral agents. Chemical carcinogens are usually identified by their ability to cause malignancies when given as a single agent to animals or by epidemiologic studies of environmental/occupational exposures. Their mechanism of action stems in part from their ability to form reactive electrophilic species that can form covalent adducts with nucleophilic sites found in nucleic acids. These adducts can cause DNA structural distortions and, if not repaired prior to subsequent DNA synthesis, heritable mutations. The activity of a chemical carcinogen may vary depending on the dose received and host factors, such as age, sex, species, and target organ specificity. Examples of chemical carcinogens are aromatic amines, nitrosamines, hydrazines, chlorocarbons, reactive alkylating agents, and some natural products, including heavy metals such as cobalt, chromium, and nickel (262). Physical carcinogens include ionizing and ultraviolet radiation, which produce DNA mutations and chromosomal abnormalities through the formation of intermediates such as free radicals and pyrimidine dimers, respectively. Agents such as ultraviolet light, x-rays, certain viruses and chemicals, and tumor-cell DNA can be used to produce cell lines that are not only immortalized but capable of forming tumors in immunocompromised animals (168).

Promotion, the second stage of carcinogenesis, involves a series of generally reversible cellular and tissue changes that inevitably involve cellular proliferation. This proliferation results in the ''clonal'' expansion of ''initiated'' cells, which then accumulate more mutations, resulting eventually in a transformed cell. Most tumor promoters do not form electrophilic species. Activities associated with tumor promoters include changes in phospholipid, polyamine, and nucleic acid synthesis; enzyme induction; and release of prostaglandins, with concomitant alterations in cell morphology, differentiation, and mitotic rate. Some promoters bind to protein kinase C, a known second messenger in signal transduction pathways (262). Examples of substances classified as promoters include phorbol esters, phenobarbital, saccharin, and hormones such as estrogen (262,263).

The molecular mechanisms of tumor promotion involve proliferative stimuli from growth factors and hormones, the activation of second messenger cascades, stimulation of transcription factor activities, and ultimately changes in the expression of ''effector'' genes involved in the biologic processes of cellular growth and/or differentiation. The net effect is to alter cell division, produce clonal expansion of ''initiated'' cells, and allow for the continued accumulation of key mutations necessary for the development of the fully transformed phenotype (264).

Potential tumor promoters have been identified for gynecologic malignancies. For example, monocyte products IL-1, IL-6, and TNF-α have all been demonstrated to stimulate the growth of ovarian cancer cells (265). The role of these and other growth factors in the development of gynecologic cancer is more fully described above. In addition, another example is provided by the well-known growth stimulatory effect of estrogen on endometrial glands.

Occupational/environmental exposure to chemicals has not been identified as an important risk factor for the development of gynecologic malignancies, unlike other cancers such as those of the lung and bladder. The limited data that exist have been derived primarily from animal studies. Multiple chemicals have been shown to have the potential for causing ovarian granulosa-cell tumors, benign mixed neoplasms, or nonneoplastic toxic changes in some, but not all, rodent species tested (266,267). Examples of such agents include 1,3-butadiene, benzene, and tricresylphosphate. Chemical agents given in conjunction with an estrogen have also been used to generate endometrial carcinoma and uterine sarcoma in rodents (268,269).

Physical carcinogens may play a role in the development of some gynecologic tumors. History of prior pelvic irradiation is associated with the development of uterine sarcoma, particularly malignant mixed mesodermal tumor. Case series of patients developing endometrial adenocarcinoma following irradiation for cervical cancer have also been reported, with a disproportionate number of cases of papillary serous histology (270).

Agents that function as tumor promoters in the development of female genital cancers have been better characterized. Unopposed estrogen, whether exogenous or endogenous, is a well-known risk factor for endometrial carcinoma. More recently, concern has been raised over the partial agonist activity of the antiestrogenic agent tamoxifen, which is used most often in the treatment of breast cancer. Also, sequential oral contraceptives (OCPs) have been associated with an elevated risk of endometrial cancer, but have been replaced by combination preparations, which, in contrast, impart protection against both uterine and ovarian epithelial carcinoma.

Exposure to some hormonal agents has been associated with an increased risk for the development of other gynecologic malignancies as well, although their precise role (initiator versus promoter) in the pathogenesis remains unclear. For example, several studies have reported an increased rate of cervical cancer among long-time users of OCPs. Also, intrauterine exposure to diethylstilbestrol is associated with an increased risk of developing clear-cell adenocarcinoma of the vagina and cervix.

Viral Carcinogenesis

Experiments in the early 1900s in which inoculations of filtered, cell-free extracts from the cancer cells of one animal could induce a tumor in a healthy recipient provided evidence for the role of a transmissible agent in some forms of animal carcinogenesis (271). This phenomenon was initially demonstrated for chicken leukemia and sarcoma, with the responsible infectious agents isolated known as avian leukemia viruses (ALVs) and avian or Rous sarcoma viruses (ASV or RSV), respectively. Subsequently, the mouse mammary tumor viruses (MMTVs) were shown to transmit mammary carcinomas from nursing mothers to newborn mice via breast milk, and murine leukemia viruses (MuLV) were found to spread horizontally by means of cell-free extracts. These viruses are all examples of RNA-containing retroviruses.

The general structure and life cycle of a retrovirus are depicted in Figure 3.7. A retrovirus consists of an outer envelope and an inner core, within which resides the viral genome. The envelope is a lipid bilayer containing viral glycoproteins encoded by the *env* gene. The core contains capsid proteins specified by the *gag* gene, and two identical single viral RNA strands with bound reverse transcriptase enzyme encoded by the *pol* gene (271). A retrovirus enters a host cell by absorption and endocytosis via specific cell-surface receptors. For example, the human immunodeficiency virus (HIV) is a retrovirus with a known specificity for CD4$^+$ cells. Inside the host cell cytoplasm, the viral RNA is released from the envelope and capsid proteins are then reverse transcribed into DNA. An extension of a nucleotide repeat sequence on the ends of the viral RNA is also synthesized, forming a long terminal repeat (LTR) on the DNA that contains promoter, enhancer, and polyadenylation sequences required for viral RNA synthesis. Between the LTRs are located the *env*, *gag*, *pol*, and various other genes, depending on the type of retrovirus. This DNA localizes to the nucleus and is randomly integrated into the host genome by means of sequences at the ends of the LTR. The integrated DNA serves as a transcription template to replicate the viral genome or produce mRNA for structural and functional viral proteins. Virions are assembled from the viral RNA and processed proteins and are then released (271).

Transforming retroviruses may be classified into two basic types based on their mechanism of action (272). The first group consists of the acute transforming viruses, which can transform cells in culture within several days. These viruses contain viral oncogenes (v-*onc*) derived from normal host cell sequences called protooncogenes (c-*onc*) through the process of transduction, which involves recombination of viral and host genomes during viral integration. In the process of transduction, viral sequences necessary for reproduction are replaced by cellular DNA (c-*onc*), rendering the retrovirus replication defective and dependent on competent ''helper viruses'' to complete the replication process. In fact, oncogenes were first identified by the study of tumor-causing viruses. The v-*onc*s frequently differ from c-*onc*s by containing mutations and no intervening/noncoding sequences (introns). Protooncogene products include a wide range of proteins that are critical for the control of cell growth. They include growth factors and their receptors, nuclear transcription factors, and signal transduction proteins (see Chapter 5). Because retroviruses carrying these genes will express high levels of these products upon infection,

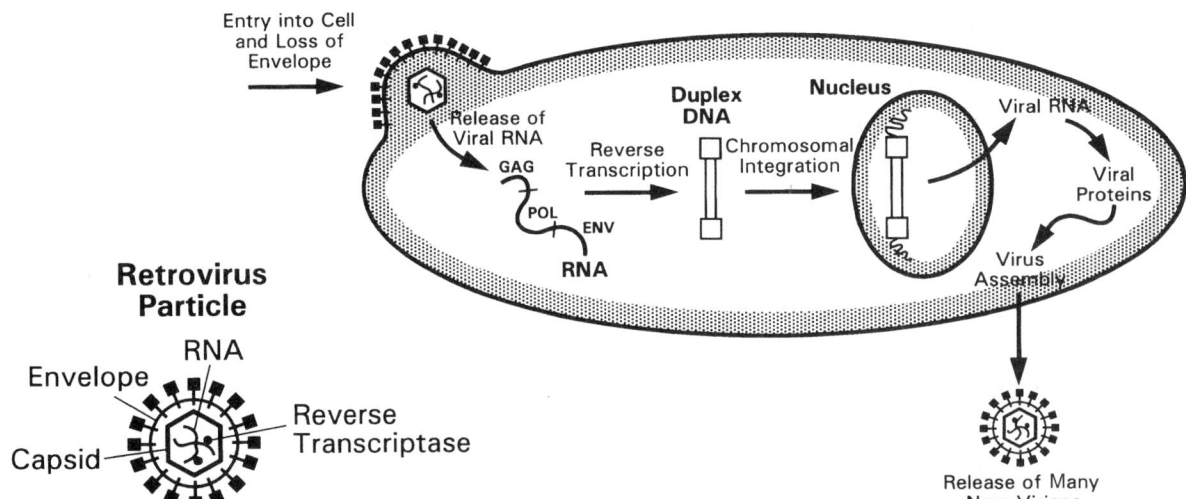

FIG. 3.7. The structure and life cycle of a retrovirus. The outer envelope of a retrovirus is a lipid bilayer containing viral glycoproteins encoded by the *env* gene. The inner core consists of capsid proteins, specified by the *gag* gene, and two identical single viral RNA strands with bound reverse transcriptase enzyme encoded by the *pol* gene. After entry into the host cell cytoplasm via absorption and endocytosis, the viral RNA is released from the viral particle and reverse transcribed into DNA. An extension of a nucleotide repeat sequence of the ends of the viral RNA is also synthesized, forming a long terminal repeat (LTR) on the DNA that contains sequences necessary for viral RNA synthesis. The DNA then localizes to the nucleus and is randomly integrated into the host genome. The viral genome is replicated and mRNA encoding viral proteins are produced and translated. New virions are assembled from their component parts and released from the cell.

the effects of these retroviruses on cell function are seen acutely.

Chronic or slow-acting retroviruses constitute the other major class of transforming retroviruses. They contain no oncogenes, are replication competent, and are associated with a long latency period. The mechanism of transformation by these viruses is via insertional mutagenesis (272). Random and rare viral genomic integration near a protooncogene or growth-effector gene (e.g., c-erbB, c-K-ras, or IL-2) results in abnormal transcriptional activation of the cellular gene. If the integration is upstream of the gene and in the same orientation for transcription as the gene, it is considered functionally a promoter insertion. When the integration occurs downstream from the target or upstream but in an opposite transcriptional orientation, the viral LTRs are thought to operate through enhancer insertion. An example of insertional mutagenesis is demonstrated by ALV, which can induce bursal lymphoma in chickens following integration of viral LTRs near the c-myc protooncogene by either promoter or enhancer insertion.

Viruses containing linear or circular double-stranded DNA have also been implicated in carcinogenesis. The Shope papillomaviruses, extracted from the warts of cottontail rabbits and transmitted horizontally to tumor-free animals, were the first such viruses isolated. Another early isolate was the polyoma virus, capable of causing murine salivary gland adenocarcinoma (271). The structures and activities of the DNA tumor viruses are more complex than those of the retroviruses. In general, the mechanisms of transformation may be direct or indirect (273). Direct methods include activation of cellular or viral oncogenes, alteration of host cell protein expression at the site of viral integration, and the interaction of viral oncoproteins with cellular proteins, such as the products of tumor-suppressor genes (273,274). Indirect actions include altering the host cell genome without persistence of the viral DNA or induction of host immunosuppression.

One example of a DNA tumor virus is simian virus 40 (SV40), a member of the papovavirus family (271). Although nonpathogenic in its natural adult monkey host, it can cause tumors when inoculated into newborn hamsters and certain strains of neonatal mice. Cell culture studies have shown that papovaviruses can cause either a lytic infection, in which the virus undergoes replication and subsequent release from the host cell via lysis and cell death, or an abortive infection, characterized by cell survival but with a subset undergoing transformation with viral DNA integrated in the host cell genome. Permissive cells that can support viral replication, like adult monkey cells, are subject to lytic infection. Nonpermissive or semipermissive cells, such as hamster cells, will typically be transformed.

Cells transformed by papovaviruses will often contain only a portion of the viral genome. The only consistent segment integrated in cells transformed by SV40 is the early viral region encoding proteins known as large-T and small-T antigens. The role of the small-T antigen is not well characterized, but several functions have been ascribed to the large-T antigen. By studying experimental mutants, functional domains of large-T have been identified. At least two domains appear to be involved in transformation. One of these includes amino acids 105–114, a segment necessary for binding to pRb (the product of the retinoblastoma tumor-suppressor gene) and p107 (a 107-kD cellular protein). Mutations within this domain will destroy the ability of SV40 to transform cells. Another domain includes that of amino acids 272–625, which contains binding sites for the p53 protein, DNA polymerase-α, and ATP, and is involved with helicase and self-oligomerization activities. Mutations within this portion of the SV40 genome will abolish its transforming ability in some, but not all, cell lines. Large-T antigen is also instrumental in the initiation and regulation of viral DNA replication and transcription.

The adenoviruses constitute another group of DNA tumor viruses studied in animal models and cell culture (271). In humans, they can cause acute infections of the eye and upper respiratory and intestinal tracts, whereas in rodents, they can cause tumors in neonates or transform cultured rodent cells. Similar to SV40, only a portion of the viral genome is consistently integrated. For the adenoviruses, this is represented by the E1A (early region 1A) and E1B gene sequences. Multiple gene products can be produced from both E1A and E1B as a result of differential splicing of transcripts. E1A products can immortalize cells but require the presence of E1B or an activated ras in cell culture to cause transformation. E1A can also regulate cellular and viral transcription. There are three conserved amino acid sequence domains for E1A. The first two are required for transformation and contain the binding sites for pRb. In addition, E1A can bind p107 and a 300-kD cellular protein, whereas E1B binds p53.

Despite our extensive investigations of the role of transforming viruses in animal models and in in vitro cell culture, their role in human cancer remains speculative. Human T-cell leukemia virus (HTLV-1) is a retrovirus that confers risk for human adult T-cell leukemia (ATL) (271). Infection is specific for CD4$^+$ lymphocytes, and can be transmitted vertically through breast milk or horizontally via sexual intercourse or blood transfusions. After random integration into the host genome, polyclonal expansion of T cells occurs during a latency period, which can last several years. Only a subgroup of infected patients actually develops leukemia, which is manifested by a clonal cell population that has the same viral site of insertion within all of the malignant cells of a given patient. In addition to the env, gag, and pol genes typical of retroviruses, the HTLV-1 genome encodes proteins known as Tax and Rex (275). The mechanism of transformation by HTLV-1 appears to be Tax protein transcriptional activation of cellular genes. Genes whose expression is altered include IL-2, c-sis, c-fos, granulocyte-macrophage colony-stimulating factor, and a subunit of the IL-2 receptor.

Acquired immune deficiency syndrome (AIDS) patients

are known to be at increased risk for developing certain malignancies, such as lymphoma and Kaposi's sarcoma (KS). HIV is a CD4$^+$ tropic retrovirus that causes AIDS, but its relationship to the above cancers remains unclear. For instance, although KS is commonly found in AIDS patients, its tumor cells lack evidence of viral genomic integration. However, supernatants from HIV-infected cells have been shown to be growth enhancing for the KS cells of AIDS patients secondary to the presence of the *tat* gene product encoded by the virus. In addition, germline insertion of the *tat* gene into mice precipitates skin tumors resembling KS (61). HIV, therefore, may act indirectly to induce and/or promote the development of KS. An increasing incidence of aggressive B-cell lymphomas has also been noted in HIV patients. Whether this is a result of reactivation of other viruses or an alteration in immune surveillance is unknown. Epstein-Barr virus (EBV) and c-myc overexpression appear to be involved in a large number of these cases (276).

EBV is a member of the DNA herpesvirus family. In addition to causing mononucleosis by acute infection, it has been associated with Burkitt's lymphoma (BL), lymphoma of the immunocompromised host, and nasopharyngeal carcinoma (277,278). The mechanisms of these associations remain to be defined. It is known that B cells and nasopharyngeal epithelium contain the cell-surface receptor CR2, which serves as a receptor for both C3d serum complement and EBV. In addition, B lymphocytes can be immortalized by EBV infection *in vitro*. Viral genes encoding EBV nuclear antigen 1 (*EBNA-1*), *EBNA-2*, and latent membrane protein (*LMP*) are the most likely candidates for effectors of immortalization (271). Although *EBNA-1* has been the only latent gene consistently expressed in BL, experiments with *LMP* mutants have suggested that *LMP* is required for the transformation of B lymphocytes, but which domain is necessary is currently unclear (279,280). BL characteristically contains chromosomal translocations, primarily t(8;14) but also t(2;8) and t(8;22), which reposition the protooncogene c-*myc* near immunoglobulin (Ig) genes. The resulting deregulation of c-*myc* favors cellular proliferation. Magrath et al. (280) have proposed a theory regarding the development of BL in African children. Infectious diseases such as malaria may alter the relative and absolute numbers of B-cell precursors in the bone marrow and perhaps mesentery, which are cells that are susceptible to the translocations found in BL. Ig enhancers may increase the frequency of translocations, and therefore play a role in c-*myc* deregulation. Magrath et al. believe that EBV probably increases Ig enhancer activity. BL is seen as a consequence of collaboration between EBV infection and these chromosoml aberrations. EBV may also cooperate with HIV in the development of some other B-cell lymphomas. When B lymphocytes from EBV-seropositive donors are infected with HIV, a subset of these cells is subsequently transformed. These transformed cells show marked elevations of c-*myc* transcripts and protein, as well as EBV DNA and RNA (276).

Another DNA virus associated with a human cancer is the hepatitis B virus (HBV). Chronic HBV infection is strongly associated with the development of hepatocellular carcinoma. HBV is hepatotropic secondary to the presence of HBV receptors on liver cells that recognize the viral coat protein. Acute infection is frequently hepatotoxic, resulting in destruction of liver cells. Chronic infection is associated with viral integration. The precise mechanism by which HBV increases the risk of developing hepatocellular carcinoma remains unknown. Although HBV is not an acutely transforming virus, two viral genes can be consistently demonstrated after integration. They are *ORF* (open reading frame) *X* and *preS2/S*, which encode proteins that can function as transcriptional activators (271). Insertional events may be important in the role of HBV in the pathogenesis of liver cancer. Modification of cyclin A has been reported secondary to HBV viral genomic integration into an intron of the cyclin A gene in cancerous liver cells. The resultant hybrid HBV-cyclin A transcript encodes a stabilized cyclin A resistant to degradation. This may play a role in the process of carcinogenesis, as cyclin A is intimately involved with cell-cycle control through its association with protein kinases such as p34^{cdc-2} and is a component of protein complexes involving E2F transcription factor and p107 (281, 282). Insertional mutagenesis involving the retinoic acid receptor-β gene and the mevalonate kinase gene owing to EBV integration have also been reported (283).

Herpes Simplex Virus 2

Historically, herpes simplex virus 2 (HSV-2) was the first viral agent suspected of playing a role in the pathogenesis of gynecologic malignancies. It is a member of the herpes family of DNA viruses. Epidemiologic studies showing a higher frequency of HSV-2 antibodies in women with cervical cancer than in healthy women suggested a possible link between HSV-2 infection and cervical cancer. Fragments of the HSV-2 genome have been identified in some cases of cervical and vulvar carcinoma, but are usually not integrated into the last genome (284,285). Genital keratinocytes previously immortalized by integration of human papillomavirus 16 have been transformed in cell culture by transfection with a subgenomic region of HSV-2 known as BglII N (286). However, with subsequent cell passages, the transformed phenotype was maintained despite loss of the HSV-2 genetic material. In addition, normal epithelial cells transfected with HSV-2/BglII N were not transformed. These data support the hypothesis that if HSV-2 plays a role in the development of cervical cancer, it most likely functions indirectly as a cofactor.

Human Papillomaviruses

The study of viral infections as possible contributors to the process of gynecologic carcinogenesis is now focused primarily on human papillomavirus (HPV). HPVs are epitheliotropic DNA viruses and members of the papovirus family (287). The HPV viral particle consists of an approximately 8,000-bp circular double-stranded DNA molecule surrounded by a 55-nm-diameter icosahedral capsid structure (288). The viral DNA contains seven early (E1–E7) and two late (L1 and L2) open reading frames (ORFs), plus a noncoding region (NCR) of about 1,000 bp involved in the control of replication and transcription (Fig. 3.8). E1 contains the DNA sequences for at least two proteins involved in DNA replication. Genes encoding activator and repressor proteins, which regulate viral mRNA synthesis, are located in E2. E4 may play a role in the maturation of viral particles. The E5 and E6/E7 ORFs were originally identified by their participation in the *in vitro* transformation of rodent cells by fragments of the bovine papillomavirus genome. L1 and L2 contain genes that encode the viral capsid proteins.

Over 60 HPV types have been identified by cross-hybridization procedures demonstrating less than 50% DNA sequence homology between any two types (287). Approximately 20 of these have been isolated from the anogenital tract. The lesions associated with HPV infections vary depending on the viral type involved. Lorincz et al. (289) analyzed the relationship between 15 common anogenital types of HPV and cervical dysplasia in 2,627 women. Evidence of HPV viral DNA was found in 84% of the 153 invasive carcinoma cases, predominantly HPV 16, 18, 45, or 56, with about 10% containing HPV 31, 33, 35, 51, 52, or 58. They referred to the former group of HPV types as "high risk" and to the latter group as "intermediate risk." Of the 261 cases of high-grade intraepithelial lesions (HGSILs), 54% contained high-risk HPV, 24% had intermediate-risk types, and 4% included viral DNA from their designated "low-risk" group, which included HPV 6, 11, 42, 43, and 44. The 377 low-grade intraepithelial lesions (LGSILs) contained high-risk types in 23%, intermediate-risk HPV in 17%, low-risk types in 20%, and no evidence of HPV in 30%. Nine percent of the LGSIL cases could not be classified. Multiple other investigators have also demonstrated the frequent association of HPV 16 and 18 with HGSILs and invasive carcinoma, whereas HPV 6 and 11 are more often found in condylomas and low-grade dysplasia. Squamous-cell histology has been studied more extensively than that of adeno and adenosquamous. The prevalence of HPV DNA in these less common types of cervical cancer has varied from 20% to 80%, depending on the method of detection used (260). The vast majority of vulvar condylomata acuminata are also associated with the low-risk HPV types, whereas high-risk types have been demonstrated in invasive vulvar carcinoma.

HPV DNA has been detected in host cells in both integrated and nonintegrated (episomal or extrachromosomal) states (288,290). Episomal viral DNA is characteristic of benign cervical precursor lesions, although integrated HPV is sometimes found in HGSILs. Invasive carcinoma almost always contains integrated viral DNA, but episomal forms of the viral genome have also been detected. Although integration has occurred near cellular protooncogenes, in general the site of viral integration appears to be random with respect to the host genome. However, there is a consistent pattern with respect to the site of disruption of the circular viral genome in the process of integration. The viral DNA is usually interrupted in the E1/E2 region, which is the viral transcriptional regulatory system. Upon integration into the host genome, two ORFs, E6 and E7, are consistently retained (287).

Human keratinocyte cell cultures and tumor cell lines have illustrated the participation of the HPV E6 and E7 proteins in the processes of immortalization and transformation. Transfection of human foreskin keratinocytes with high-risk HPV DNA, but not with low-risk HPV DNA, has been demonstrated to immortalize these cells (291). Integration and expression of both *E6* and *E7* are usually required for efficient immortalization, since *E7* alone has weak activity and *E6* alone has none (291). The role of HPV in the multistage process of cervical/vulvar carcinogenesis would appear to be early in the course of the disease since the effect of HPV has generally been limited to immortalization. Progression to the fully transformed phenotype has been described in an

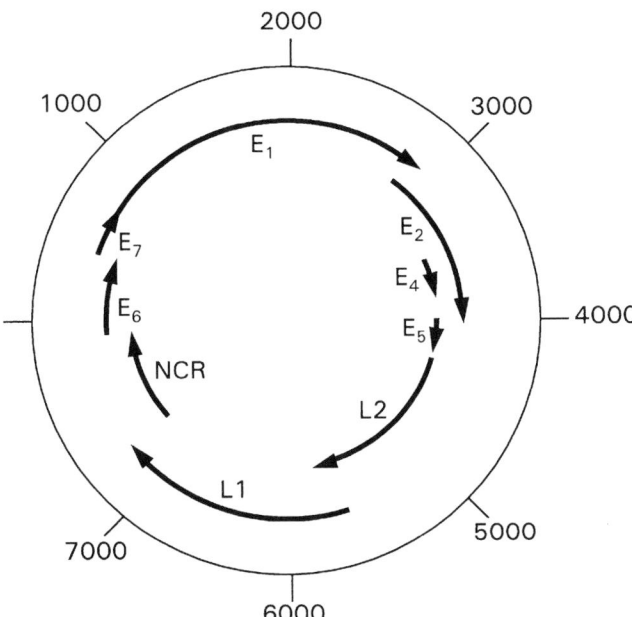

FIG. 3.8. The HPV genome. The HPV genome is an approximately 8,000-bp circular double-stranded DNA molecule containing seven early (E_1–E_7) and two late (L1 and L2) open reading frames (ORFs), plus a noncoding region (NCR) involved in the control of replication and transcription. E_1 contains sequences for proteins involved in DNA replication. E_2 encodes activator and repressor proteins that regulate viral mRNA synthesis. E_4 is thought to be involved in the maturation of viral particles. E_6 and E_7 can immortalize human keratinocytes and cooperate with oncogenes in the process of malignant transformation. L1 and L2 encode viral capsid proteins.

HPV 18–immortalized keratinocyte cell line after multiple passages, but in general, this phenomenon is quite rare (292). The transfection of an activated *Ha-ras* oncogene into HPV 16–immortalized cervical cells can render them tumorigenic, demonstrating the ability of HPV to cooperate with another cellular insult to effect carcinogenesis (293). Persistent expression of *E6* and *E7* appears to be necessary to maintain the transformed phenotype. The application of synthetic anti-*E6* and anti-*E7* oligonucleotides to cervical and oral cancer cell lines containing HPV 18 significantly inhibits cell growth (294). Treatment of the cells with both antisense oligonucleotides inhibits growth more effectively than either one applied alone.

An important property of the E6 and E7 oncoproteins is their biochemical interaction with tumor-suppressor gene products. Similar to adenovirus E1A and the SV40 large-T antigen, HPV E7 can bind pRb. The E7 proteins from HPV 16, 18, 6b, and 11 have all been demonstrated to bind pRb *in vitro*, although the binding affinities of the high-risk HPV types are higher (46). The E6 proteins of HPV 16 and 18 have been shown to bind p53 *in vitro*, which is analogous to adenovirus E1B and SV40 large-T (295). Inactivation of p53 and pRb, secondary to protein binding or mutation, may disrupt control of cellular proliferation. The small proportion of cervical cancer that is HPV negative frequently harbors a demonstrable p53 mutation. By use of p53-responsive reporter plasmids and a HeLa cervical cancer cell line, Hoppe-Seyler and Butz (296) have shown that HPV 16 E6, as well as mutant p53, can disrupt p53-mediated transactivation. Additional investigation is needed to define further the specific role of HPV in cellular transformation.

Molecular Basis of Carcinogenesis

Early epidemiologic studies suggested that the development of human epithelial cancers is a complex multistage process. The study of tumors that rise in frequency with age has revealed that cancer incidence is proportional to the *n*th power of age (297). This relationship may be interpreted to suggest that some *n* events, each time dependent but independent of each other, must occur before a tumor can develop. Two models have been proposed to explain how these events might take place. One proposal is that a single cell accumulates multiple genetic lesions (single target, multihit). The other suggests that multiple cells receive a single insult (multiple targets, single hit). Because of evidence suggesting that most human tumors have a monoclonal origin, the former theory has received the most support. Whether or not the *n* events need to occur in a certain order for a given malignancy to develop is unclear.

These epidemiologic data, combined with results from the aforementioned animal models of carcinogenesis, strongly suggested that human cancer results from a complex, multistage process. The application of modern molecular biologic techniques to the biologic mysteries of cancer has sup-

plied critical evidence for this multistage hypothesis. The identification and characterization of oncogenes as cancer-causing genes has provided the structural link between the carcinogen/promoter model of malignancy and the biochemical pathways known to be activated in the process of cellular transformation. A recent review proposed that despite the enormous variety of human cancers, five basic rules exist for making human tumor cells (298). According to these rules, malignant cells must have the ability to generate their own mitogenic signals, to resist exogenous growth-inhibitory controls, to evade apoptosis, to proliferate without limits, and to acquire vasculature. In addition, advanced tumors acquire the ability to invade and metastasize.

Oncogenes have been described by: (a) identification as transforming sequences found within retroviruses; (b) gene transfer experiments in which DNA sequences from tumor cells were shown to transform normal recipient cells; (c) characterization of fusion genes at chromosomal breakpoints; and (d) identification by nucleic acid sequence homology. Protooncogenes are cellular genes that play important roles in cellular proliferation. Activation of protooncogenes occurs secondary to point mutation, gene amplification, or loss of normal control mechanisms regulating gene expression. Overexpression and/or overactivity of the protein product results in and leads to the transformation of normal cells (299). Protooncogenes that have been well characterized include growth factors and their receptors, nuclear transcription factors, and components of signal transduction pathways (299).

Multiple activated oncogenes have been detected within gynecologic malignancies, some of which have been previously described in this chapter (300). For example, overexpression of c-*erb*B2, which encodes a transmembrane tyrosine kinase with 40% sequence homology to the EGF receptor, occurs in approximately 30% of epithelial ovarian carcinoma. The *ras* family of oncogenes encodes a protein with GTPase activity and is activated by point mutation. Activation of *ras* genes has been detected in endometrial carcinomas and ovarian LMP tumors. Overexpression of the nuclear transcription factor c-*myc* has been described in a large number of female genital cancers.

Another class of oncogenes known to be important in carcinogenesis are the tumor-suppressor genes. Historically, two independent lines of evidence supported their existence (299). Somatic cell hybrids, formed by the fusion of tumor cells with normal cells, frequently display a normal, rather than transformed, phenotype. This suggested that the normal cells harbored factors with tumor-suppressive activity. In addition, epidemiologic studies of the pediatric malignancy retinoblastoma strongly supported the existence of recessive oncogenes. Retinoblastoma occurs in two forms. The inherited form occurs early in life, with the tumors being frequently bilateral and multifocal. The sporadic form occurs later in life and is unilateral. Hethcote and Knudson (301) hypothesized that this tumor results from the loss of function of a key regulatory gene. In the hereditary form, a mutated allele is inherited and a tumor results when the second allele undergoes a somatic mutation. The sporadic form of the disease occurs as a result of two independent somatic events occurring in the same cell. Careful cytogenetic evaluation of retinoblastoma tumors revealed gross chromosomal abnormalities at 13q14. Molecular analysis of this area led to the identification and characterization of the retinoblastoma gene. Subsequently, other tumor-suppressor genes have been identified and shown to have dramatic effects on cellular proliferation. Mutational inactivation of these genes leads to deregulation of cell growth.

Mutation of the tumor-suppressor gene *p53* is the most common genetic alteration in human cancer. Mutation of this gene, which frequently leads to overexpression of the p53 protein, is associated with a large number of human malignancies, including tumors of the female genital tract. In advanced-stage ovarian carcinoma, for example, *p53* mutations occur in about 50% of cases. Multiple other tumor-suppressor genes have been proposed by the identification of other nonrandom allelic losses occurring within certain tumors.

Multistage Carcinogenesis Model and Human Cancers

Careful analysis of human epithelial cancers has provided substantial evidence for the general model of multistage carcinogenesis. For instance, the study of colorectal carcinoma has identified a series of histologic and molecular correlates in the progression from normal epithelium to hyperplasia, adenoma, and, ultimately, carcinoma. Some of the molecular events in this sequence are now known and include inactivation of the *APC* and *p53* tumor-suppressor genes and activation of the *ras* protooncogene (302). In other human cancers, such as lung cancer, activated *ras* genes, *p53* mutations, and 3p deletions are frequently found (303), whereas *p53* mutations, overexpression of EGF receptors, and gene amplifications of c-*myc* and *neu* are common genetic alterations in breast cancer (304).

Although our knowledge about the molecular biology of gynecologic malignancies has been steadily expanding, much remains unclear. Current research is directed at defining which molecular events are critical to tumor development and when these events occur. These efforts have allowed for the construction of hypothetical models of the development of gynecologic cancers, such as that for cervical carcinoma seen in Figure 3.9. The transition from normal to dysplastic to malignant cervical epithelium is shown in association with known risk factors for this process, such as HPV infection, tobacco use, and growth factor stimulation. Molecular mechanisms accompanying these histologic changes include the binding of tumor-suppressor gene products by HPV oncoproteins, activation of growth factor pathways, and genetic alterations such as c-myc amplification and LOH at 3p (300). Initiated cells are stimulated to divide

under the influence of tumor promoters–producing clonal expansion of partially transformed cells. As more oncogene/tumor-suppressor gene mutations occur, cells become fully transformed and invade the basement membrane.

The multistage model of carcinogenesis provides multiple opportunities for intervention that can have a positive clinical impact on this process for gynecologic cancers. Primary prevention involves risk factor modification. Smoking cessation, avoidance of unopposed estrogen, prophylactic oophorectomy, and dietary modification are activities aimed at preventing the initiation and/or promotion of gynecologic

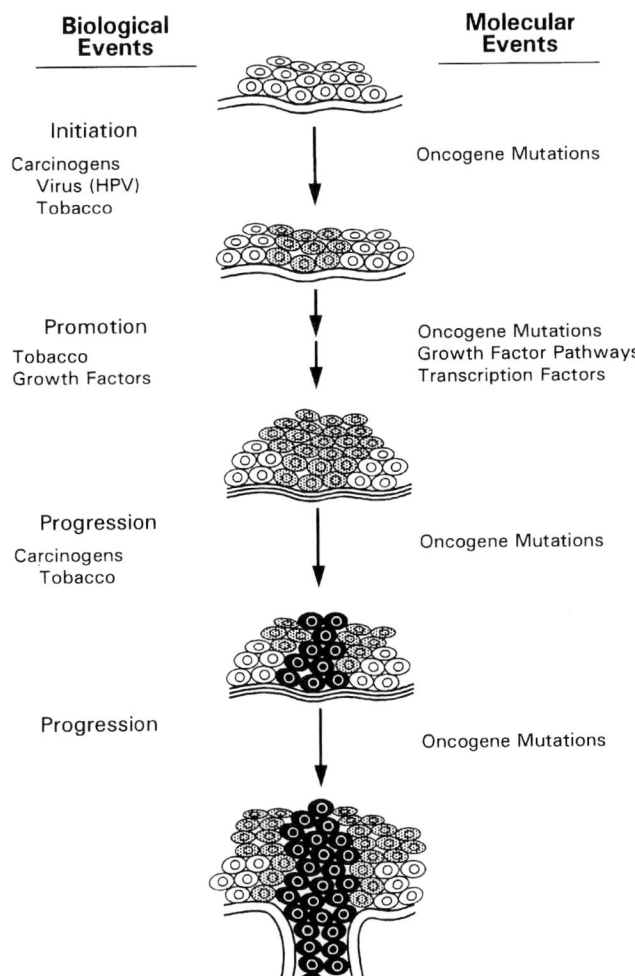

FIG. 3.9. Multistage model for the development of cervical carcinoma. The transition from normal to dysplastic to malignant cervical epithelium is shown in association with known risk factors, such as HPV infection, tobacco use, and growth-factor stimulation. Molecular mechanisms accompanying these changes include the binding of tumor-suppressor gene products by HPV oncoproteins, activation of growth-factor pathways, and genetic alterations such as c-*myc* amplification and LOH at 3p. Tumor promoters stimulate the division of initiated, partially transformed cells. Accumulation of additional oncogene/tumor-suppressor gene mutations effects full transformation and invasion of the basement membrane.

cancers. Secondary prevention implies intervening once the early events in tumor formation have occurred. This involves identification of the histologic stages of early carcinogenesis and treatment of the affected tissue. Traditionally, this has meant addressing preinvasive disease by surgery, topical applications, and hormonal manipulation. More recently, laser ablation and immunotherapy have been used. Identification of the molecular events occurring early in the development of gynecologic cancers may provide new, more sensitive, and specific markers for the early detection of these tumors.

Our new understanding of the molecular basis of the multistage process of human carcinogenesis has also provided novel approaches to cancer prevention and therapy. For initiation and progression events, we now have compounds that inhibit the activity of activated *ras* genes, antisense oligonucleotides that can reverse the transformed phenotype of HPV-associated cancer cells, and the potential ability to replace the lost functions of mutated tumor-suppressor genes by gene therapy (294). Our better understanding of the role of tumor promotion in the development of epithelial cancers has provided other excellent targets for intervention. The development of growth-factor antagonists might inhibit or reverse growth factor-induced cellular proliferation, which is critical for tumor promotion.

Another approach aimed at inhibiting tumor promoter–induced cellular proliferation has been suggested by the work of Brown et al. (305), who have created a dominant-negative mutant of the nuclear transcription factor c-jun. This mutant protein can block the activities of wild-type transcription factors in the c-jun and c-fos families and block cellular transformation by a wide range of oncogenes. Blocking transcriptional activity may be a potent method of inhibiting cellular proliferation associated with tumor promotion. A similar but more pharmacologic approach is the use of antioxidants for chemoprevention. Epidemiologic studies have found an association between decreased serum levels of the micronutrient beta-carotene and either a diagnosis of cervical dysplasia and carcinoma or a future risk of such disease (306,307). Research regarding the potential effect of beta-carotene therapy is ongoing.

Retinoids have been shown to retard the growth and differentiation of HPV 16–immortalized human cervical cells (308,309). These agents may trigger transcriptional factor pathways that either directly or indirectly interact with other proteins to redirect cellular programming. Meyskens et al. (310) have published the results of a randomized Phase III trial in which patients with moderate or severe cervical intraepithelial neoplasia (CIN) received either topical all-*trans* retinoic acid or a placebo. A significant increase in the complete regression rate of CIN 2 was achieved, but no significant treatment effect was seen for the CIN 3 group. More data regarding the clinical usefulness of retinoic acid are needed.

As our knowledge about tumor biology and the molecular mechanisms underlying the process of carcinogenesis continues to expand, so too will the potential for intervention. In this respect, basic science and clinical research will continue to complement each other in increasingly important ways.

REFERENCES

1. Cotran R, Robbins, SL., Kumar, V. *Pathologic basis of disease.* 5th ed. Philadelphia: Harcourt Brace Jovanovich; 1994.
2. Willis R. *The spread of tumors in the human body.* London: Butterworth; 1952.
3. Tannock I. *Cell proliferation.* Toronto: McGraw-Hill; 1992.
4. Roberts JM, Koff A, Polyak K, et al. Cyclins; CDKs; and cyclin kinase inhibitors. *Cold Spring Harb Symp Quant Biol* 1994;59:31–38.
5. Sherr CJ. Cancer cell cycles. *Science* 1996;274:1672–1677.
6. Knudsen ES, Buckmaster C, Chen TT, et al. Inhibition of DNA synthesis by RB: effects on G1/S transition and S-phase progression. *Genes Dev* 1998;12:2278–2292.
7. Ewen ME. The cell cycle and the retinoblastoma protein family. *Cancer Metastasis Rev* 1994;13:45–66.
8. Shirodkar S, Ewen M, DeCaprio JA, et al. The transcription factor E2F interacts with the retinoblastoma product and a p107–cyclin A complex in a cell cycle–regulated manner. *Cell* 1992;68:157–166.
9. Ludlow JW, Shon J, Pipas JM, et al. The retinoblastoma susceptibility gene product undergoes cell cycle–dependent dephosphorylation and binding to and release from SV40 large T. *Cell* 1990;60:387–396.
10. Weintraub SJ, Prater CA, Dean DC. Retinoblastoma protein switches the E2F site from positive to negative element. *Nature* 1992;358:259–261.
11. Elledge SJ. Cell cycle checkpoints: preventing an identity crisis. *Science* 1996;274:1664–1672.
12. Planas-Silva MD, Weinberg RA. The restriction point and control of cell proliferation. *Curr Opin Cell Biol* 1997;9:768–772.
13. el-Deiry WS, Tokino T, Velculescu VE, et al. WAF1; a potential mediator of p53 tumor suppression. *Cell* 1993;75:817–825.
14. Polyak K, Xia Y. Collins JL. A model for p53-induced apoptosis (see comments). *Nature* 1993;389:300.
15. Fiscella M, Ullrich SJ, Zambrano N, et al. Mutation of the serine 15 phosphorylation site of human p53 reduces the ability of p53 to inhibit cell cycle progression. *Oncogene* 1993;8:1519–1528.
16. Peng CY, Graves PR, Thoma RS, et al. Mitotic and G2 checkpoint control: regulation of 14–3–3 protein binding by phosphorylation of Cdc25C on serine–216. *Science* 1997;277:1501–1505.
17. Sanchez Y, Wong C, Thoma RS, et al. Conservation of the Chk1 checkpoint pathway in mammals: linkage of DNA damage to CDK regulation through Cdc25. *Science* 1997;277:1497–1501.
18. Hardwick KG. The spindle checkpoint. *Trends Genet* 1998;14:1–4.
19. Cahill DP, Lengauer C, Yu J, et al. Mutations of mitotic checkpoint genes in human cancers. *Nature* 1998;392:300–303.
20. Schmitt CA. Senescence; apoptosis and therapy––cutting the lifelines of cancer. *Nat Rev Cancer* 2003;3:286–295.
21. Stampfer MR, Yaswen P. Human epithelial cell immortalization as a step in carcinogenesis. *Cancer Lett* 2003;194:199–208.
22. Newbold RF. The significance of telomerase activation and cellular immortalization in human cancer. *Mutagenesis* 2002;17:539–550.
23. Granville DJ, Carthy CM, Hunt DW, McManus BM. Apoptosis: molecular aspects of cell death and disease. *Lab Invest* 1998;78:893–913.
24. Soini Y, Paakko P, Lehto VP. Histopathological evaluation of apoptosis in cancer. *Am J Pathol* 1998;153:1041–1053.
25. Kamesaki H. Mechanisms involved in chemotherapy-induced apoptosis and their implications in cancer chemotherapy. *Int J Hematol* 1998;68:29–43.
26. Mesner PW Jr., Budihardjo II, Kaufmann SH. Chemotherapy–induced apoptosis. *Adv Pharmacol* 1997;41:461–499.
27. Milas L, Gregoire V, Hunter N, et al. Radiation–induced apoptosis in tumors: effect of radiation modulating agents. *Adv Exp Med Biol* 1997;400B:559–564.
28. Susin SA, Zamzami N, Castedo M, et al. The central executioner

of apoptosis: multiple connections between protease activation and mitochondria in Fas/APO–1/CD95– and ceramide-induced apoptosis. *J Exp Med* 1997;186:25–37.

29. Berke G. The CTL's kiss of death. *Cell* 1995;81:9–12.

30. Nagata S. Fas–mediated apoptosis. *Adv Exp Med Biol* 1996;406:119–124.

31. Nagata S. Apoptosis by death factor. *Cell* 1997;88:355–365.

32. Miyashita T, Reed JC. Tumor suppressor p53 is a direct transcriptional activator of the human bax gene. *Cell* 1995;80:293–299.

33. Wu GS, Burns TF, McDonald ER 3rd, et al. KILLER/DR5 is a DNA damage–inducible p5-regulated death receptor gene. *Nat Genet* 1997;17:141–143.

34. Lane DP. Cancer. p53, guardian of the genome. *Nature* 1992;358:15–16.

35. Kerr JF, Winterford CM, Harmon BV. Apoptosis. Its significance in cancer and cancer therapy. *Cancer* 1994;73:2013–2026.

36. Gavrieli Y, Sherman Y, Ben-Sasson SA. Identification of programmed cell death in situ via specific labeling of nuclear DNA fragmentation. *J Cell Biol* 1992;119:493–501.

37. Wijsman JH, Jonker RR, Keijzer R, et al. A new method to detect apoptosis in paraffin sections: in situ end-labeling of fragmented DNA. *J Histochem Cytochem* 1993;41:7–12.

38. Lipponen P, Aaltomaa S, Kosma VM, Syrjanen K. Apoptosis in breast cancer as related to histopathological characteristics and prognosis. *Eur J Cancer* 1994;30A:2068–2073.

39. Shinohara T, Ohshima K, Murayama H, et al. Apoptosis and proliferation in gastric carcinoma: the association with histological type. *Histopathology* 1996;29:123–129.

40. Hockenbery DM. Bcl-2 in cancer; development and apoptosis. *J Cell Sci Suppl* 1994;18:51–55.

41. Krueger NX, Van Vactor D, Wan HI, et al. The transmembrane tyrosine phosphatase DLAR controls motor axon guidance in *Drosophila*. *Cell* 1996;84:611–622.

42. Reed JC. Bcl-2 and the regulation of programmed cell death. *J Cell Biol* 1994;124:1–6.

43. White E. Life, death, and the pursuit of apoptosis. *Genes Dev* 1996;10:1.

44. Yang E, Korsmeyer SJ. Molecular thanatopsis: a discourse on the BCL2 family and cell death. *Blood* 1996;88:386–401.

45. Yin XM, Oltvai ZN, Korsmeyer SJ. BH1 and BH2 domains of Bcl-2 are required for inhibition of apoptosis and heterodimerization with bax. *Nature* 1994;369:321–323.

46. Kroemer G. The proto-oncogene Bcl-2 and its role in regulating apoptosis. *Nat Med* 1997;3:614–620.

47. Martinez J, Georgoff I, Levine AJ. Cellular localization and cell cycle regulation by a temperature-sensitive p53 protein. *Genes Dev* 1991;5:151–159.

48. Michalovitz D, Halevy O, Oren M. Conditional inhibition of transformation and of cell proliferation by a temperature-sensitive mutant of p53. *Cell* 1990;62:671–680.

49. Miyashita T, Krajewski S, Krajewska M, et al. Tumor suppressor p53 is a regulator of bcl-2 and bax gene expression in vitro and in vivo. *Oncogene* 1994;9:1799–1805.

50. Yonish-Rouach E, Resnitzky D, Lotem J, et al. Wild-type p53 induces apoptosis of myeloid leukaemic cells that is inhibited by interleukin-6. *Nature* 1991;352:345–347.

51. Evan GI, Wyllie AH, Gilbert CS, et al. Induction of apoptosis in fibroblasts by c-myc protein. *Cell* 1992;69:119–128.

52. Kauffmann-Zeh A, Rodriguez-Viciana P, Ulrich E, et al. Suppression of c-Myc–induced apoptosis by Ras signalling through PI(3)K and PKB. *Nature* 1997;385:544–548.

53. Trent JC 2nd, McConkey DJ, Loughlin SM, et al. Ras signaling in tumor necrosis factor–induced apoptosis. *EMBO J* 1996;15:4497–4505.

54. Ward R, Todd, AV., Santiago, F., et al. Activation of the K-ras oncogene in colorectal neoplasms is associated with decreased apoptosis. *Cancer* 1997;79:1106.

55. Chen CY, Faller DV. Phosphorylation of Bcl-2 protein and association with p21Ras in ras-induced apoptosis. *J Biol Chem* 1996;271:2376–2379.

56. Chieng D, Ross JS, Ambros, RA. Bcl-2 expression and the development of endometrial carcinoma. *Mod Pathol* 1996;9:402.

57. Giatromanolaki A, Sivridis E, Koukourakis MI, et al. Bcl-2 and p53

58. Heatley MK. Association between the apoptotic index and established prognostic parameters in endometrial adenocarcinoma. *Histopathology* 1995;27:469–472.

59. Henderson GS, Brown KA, Perkins SL, et al. Bcl-2 is down-regulated in atypical endometrial hyperplasia and adenocarcinoma. *Mod Pathol* 1996;9:430–438.

60. Ioffe OB, Papadimitriou JC, Drachenberg CB. Correlation of proliferation indices, apoptosis, and related oncogene expression (bcl-2 and c-erbB-2) and p53 in proliferative, hyperplastic, and malignant endometrium. *Hum Pathol* 1998;29:1150–1159.

61. Saegusa M, Kamata Y, Isono M, Okayasu I. Bcl-2 expression is correlated with a low apoptotic index and associated with progesterone receptor immunoreactivity in endometrial carcinomas. *J Pathol* 1996;180:275–282.

62. Bur ME, Perlman C, Edelmann L, et al. p53 expression in neoplasms of the uterine corpus. *Am J Clin Pathol* 1992;98:81–87.

63. Kohler MF, Berchuck A, Davidoff AM, et al. Overexpression and mutation of p53 in endometrial carcinoma. *Cancer Res* 1992;52:1622–1627.

64. Koshiyama M, Konishi I, Wang DP, et al. Immunohistochemical analysis of p53 protein over-expression in endometrial carcinomas: inverse correlation with sex steroid receptor status. *Virchows Arch A Pathol Anat Histopathol* 1993;423:265–271.

65. Nielsen AL, Nyholm HC. p53 protein and c-erbB-2 protein (p185) expression in endometrial adenocarcinoma of endometrioid type. An immunohistochemical examination on paraffin sections. *Am J Clin Pathol* 1994;102:76–79.

66. Reinartz JJ, George E, Lindgren BR, Niehans GA. Expression of p53, transforming growth factor alpha, epidermal growth factor receptor, and c-erbB-2 in endometrial carcinoma and correlation with survival and known predictors of survival. *Hum Pathol* 1994;25:1075–1083.

67. Barnabei VM, Miller DS, Bauer KD, et al. Flow cytometric evaluation of epithelial ovarian cancer. *Am J Obstet Gynecol* 1990;162:1584–1590; discussion 1590–1592.

68. Kallioniemi OP, Punnonen R, Mattila J, et al. Prognostic significance of DNA index, multiploidy, and S-phase fraction in ovarian cancer. *Cancer* 1988;61:334–339.

69. Brescia RJ, Barakat RA, Beller U, et al. The prognostic significance of nuclear DNA content in malignant epithelial tumors of the ovary. *Cancer* 1990;65:141–147.

70. Griffiths AP, Cross D, Kingston RE, et al. Flow cytometry and Ag-NORs in benign, borderline, and malignant mucinous and serous tumours of the ovary. *Int J Gynecol Pathol* 1993;12:307–314.

71. Henriksen R, Strang P, Backstrom T, et al. Ki-67 immunostaining and DNA flow cytometry as prognostic factors in epithelial ovarian cancers. *Anticancer Res* 1994;14:603–608.

72. Lindahl B, Alm P. Flow cytometrical DNA measurements in endometrial hyperplasias. A prospective follow-up study after abrasio only or additional high-dose gestagen treatment. *Anticancer Res* 1991;11:391–395.

73. Strang P, Stendahl U, Tribukait B. Prognostic significance of S-phase fraction as measured by DNA flow cytometry in gynecologic malignancies. *Ann N Y Acad Sci* 1993;677:354–363.

74. Takahashi Y, Matsumoto H, Wakuda K, et al. Analysis of cell cycle kinetics using flow cytometry from paraffin-embedded tissues in endometrial adenocarcinoma. *Asia Oceania J Obstet Gynaecol* 1991;17:73–81.

75. Wagenius G, Bergstrom R, Strang P, et al. Prognostic significance of flow cytometric and clinical variables in endometrial adenocarcinoma stages I and II. *Anticancer Res* 1992;12:725–732.

76. Lindahl B, Gullberg B. Flow cytometrical DNA and clinical parameters in the prediction of prognosis in stage I-II endometrial carcinoma. *Anticancer Res* 1991;11:397–401.

77. Mariuzzi G, Sisti S, Santinelli A, et al. Evolutionary somatic cell changes in cervical tumour progression quantitatively evaluated with morphological, histochemical and kinetic parameters. *Pathol Res Pract* 1992;188:454–460.

78. Strang P, Stendahl U, Bergstrom R, et al. Prognostic flow cytometric information in cervical squamous cell carcinoma: a multivariate analysis of 307 patients. *Gynecol Oncol* 1991;43:3–8.

79. Willen R, Himmelmann A, Langstrom-Einarsson E, et al. Prospective

malignancy grading; flow cytometry DNA-measurements and adjuvant chemotherapy for invasive squamous cell carcinoma of the uterine cervix. *Anticancer Res* 1993;13:1187–1196.

80. Naus GJ, Zimmerman RL. Prognostic value of flow cytophotometric DNA content analysis in single treatment stage IB-IIA squamous cell carcinoma of the cervix. *Gynecol Oncol* 1991;43:149–153.

81. Zanetta GM, Katzmann JA, Keeney GL, et al. Flow-cytometric DNA analysis of stages IB and IIA cervical carcinoma. *Gynecol Oncol* 1992; 46:13–19.

82. Malmstrom H, Schmidt H, Persson PG, et al. Flow cytometric analysis of uterine sarcoma: ploidy and S-phase rate as prognostic indicators. *Gynecol Oncol* 1992;44:172–177.

83. Peters WA 3rd, Howard DR, Andersen WA, Figge DC. Deoxyribonucleic acid analysis by flow cytometry of uterine leiomyosarcomas and smooth muscle tumors of uncertain malignant potential. *Am J Obstet Gynecol* 1992;166:1646–1653; discussion 1653–1654.

84. Wolfson AH, Wolfson DJ, Sittler SY, et al. A multivariate analysis of clinicopathologic factors for predicting outcome in uterine sarcomas. *Gynecol Oncol* 1994;52:56–62.

85. Bocklage TJ, Smith HO, Bartow SA. Distinctive flow histogram pattern in molar pregnancies with elevated maternal serum human chorionic gonadotropin levels. *Cancer* 1994;73:2782–2790.

86. Fukunaga M, Ushigome S, Sugishita M. Application of flow cytometry in diagnosis of hydatidiform moles. *Mod Pathol* 1993;6:353–359.

87. Dolan JR, McCall AR, Gooneratne S, et al. DNA ploidy, proliferation index, grade, and stage as prognostic factors for vulvar squamous cell carcinomas. *Gynecol Oncol* 1993;48:232–235.

88. Hatch KD. Preinvasive cervical neoplasia. *Semin Oncol* 1994;21: 12–16.

89. Sherman ME. Theories of endometrial carcinogenesis: a multidisciplinary approach. *Mod Pathol* 2000;13:295–308.

90. Feeley KM, Wells M. Precursor lesions of ovarian epithelial malignancy. *Histopathology* 2001;38:87–95.

91. Teneriello MG, Ebina M, Linnoila RI, et al. p53 and Ki-ras gene mutations in epithelial ovarian neoplasms. *Cancer Res* 1993;53: 3103–3108.

92. Squire J, Phillips, RA. *Genetic basis of cancer*. 2nd ed. Toronto: McGraw-Hill; 1992.

93. Kurzrock R, Talpaz, M. *Molecular biology in cancer medicine*. London: Martin Dunitz, 1995.

94. Sandberg A, Chen, Z. *Cancer cytogenetics: nomenclature and clinical applications*. London: Martin Dunitz, 1995.

95. Hu J, Surti U. Subgroups of uterine leiomyomas based on cytogenetic analysis. *Hum Pathol* 1991;22:1009–1016.

96. Rein MS, Friedman AJ, Barbieri RL, et al. Cytogenetic abnormalities in uterine leiomyomata. *Obstet Gynecol* 1991;77:923–926.

97. Emoto M, Iwasaki H, Kikuchi M, Shirakawa K. Characteristics of cloned cells of mixed mullerian tumor of the human uterus. Carcinoma cells showing myogenic differentiation in vitro. *Cancer* 1993;71: 3065–3075.

98. Laxman R, Currie JL, Kurman RJ, et al. Cytogenetic profile of uterine sarcomas. *Cancer* 1993;71:1283–1288.

99. Hampton GM, Penny LA, Baergen RN, et al. Loss of heterozygosity in cervical carcinoma: subchromosomal localization of a putative tumor-suppressor gene to chromosome 11q22-q24. *Proc Natl Acad Sci U S A* 1994;91:6953–6957.

100. Kohno T, Takayama H, Hamaguchi M, et al. Deletion mapping of chromosome 3p in human uterine cervical cancer. *Oncogene* 1993;8: 1825–1832.

101. Segers P, Haesen S, Amy JJ, et al. Detection of premalignant stages in cervical smears with a biotinylated probe for chromosome 1. *Cancer Genet Cytogenet* 1994;75:120–129.

102. Sreekantaiah C, De Braekeleer M, Haas O. Cytogenetic findings in cervical carcinoma. A statistical approach. *Cancer Genet Cytogenet* 1991;53:75–81.

103. Gallion HH, Powell DE, Smith LW, et al. Chromosome abnormalities in human epithelial ovarian malignancies. *Gynecol Oncol* 1990;38: 473–477.

104. Kohlberger PD, Kieback DG, Mian C, et al. Numerical chromosomal aberrations in borderline, benign, and malignant epithelial tumors of the ovary: correlation with p53 protein overexpression and Ki-67. *J Soc Gynecol Investig* 1997;4:262–264.

105. Persons DL, Hartmann LC, Herath JF, et al. Fluorescence in situ hybridization analysis of trisomy 12 in ovarian tumors. *Am J Clin Pathol* 1994;102:775–779.

106. Gorski GK, McMorrow LE, Blumstein L, et al. Trisomy 14 in two cases of granulosa cell tumor of the ovary. *Cancer Genet Cytogenet* 1992;60:202–205.

107. Crickard K, Marinello MJ, Crickard U, et al. Borderline malignant serous tumors of the ovary maintained on extracellular matrix: evidence for clonal evolution and invasive potential. *Cancer Genet Cytogenet* 1986;23:135–143.

108. Pejovic T, Heim S, Mandahl N, et al. Chromosome aberrations in 35 primary ovarian carcinomas. *Genes Chromosomes Cancer* 1992;4: 58–68.

109. Milatovich A, Heerema NA, Palmer CG. Cytogenetic studies of endometrial malignancies. *Cancer Genet Cytogenet* 1990;46:41–53.

110. Tharapel SA, Qumsiyeh MB, Photopulos G. Numerical chromosome abnormalities associated with early clinical stages of gynecologic tumors. *Cancer Genet Cytogenet* 1991;55:89–96.

111. Gallion HH, Powell DE, Morrow JK, et al. Molecular genetic changes in human epithelial ovarian malignancies. *Gynecol Oncol* 1992;47: 137–142.

112. Worsham MJ, Van Dyke DL, Grenman SE, et al. Consistent chromosome abnormalities in squamous cell carcinoma of the vulva. *Genes Chromosomes Cancer* 1991;3:420–432.

113. Williams GT, Wynford-Thomas D. How may clonality be assessed in human tumours? *Histopathology* 1994;24:287–292.

114. Vogelstein B, Fearon ER, Hamilton SR, et al. Clonal analysis using recombinant DNA probes from the X-chromosome. *Cancer Res* 1987; 47:4806–4813.

115. Fearon ER, Hamilton SR, Vogelstein B. Clonal analysis of human colorectal tumors. *Science* 1987;238:193–197.

116. Fialkow PJ. Clonal origin of human tumors. *Biochim Biophys Acta* 1976;458:283–321.

117. Sawada M, Azuma C, Hashimoto K, et al. Clonal analysis of human gynecologic cancers by means of the polymerase chain reaction. *Int J Cancer* 1994;58:492–496.

118. Jacobs IJ, Kohler MF, Wiseman RW, et al. Clonal origin of epithelial ovarian carcinoma: analysis by loss of heterozygosity, p53 mutation, and X-chromosome inactivation. *J Natl Cancer Inst* 1992;84: 1793–1798.

119. Tsao SW, Mok CH, Knapp RC, et al. Molecular genetic evidence of a unifocal origin for human serous ovarian carcinomas. *Gynecol Oncol* 1993;48:5–10.

120. Li S, Han H, Resnik E, Carcangiu ML, et al. Advanced ovarian carcinoma: molecular evidence of unifocal origin. *Gynecol Oncol* 1993; 51:21–25.

121. Muto MG, Welch WR, Mok SC, et al. Evidence for a multifocal origin of papillary serous carcinoma of the peritoneum. *Cancer Res* 1995; 55:490–492.

122. Lu KH, Bell DA, Welch WR, et al. Evidence for the multifocal origin of bilateral and advanced human serous borderline ovarian tumors. *Cancer Res* 1998;58:2328–2330.

123. Gardner GJ, Birrer MJ. Ovarian tumors of low malignant potential: can molecular biology solve this enigma? *J Natl Cancer Inst* 2001; 93:1122–1123.

124. Barlogie B, Raber MN, Schumann J, et al. Flow cytometry in clinical cancer research. *Cancer Res* 1983;43:3982–3997.

125. Berchuck A, Boente MP, Kerns BJ, et al. Ploidy analysis of epithelial ovarian cancers using image cytometry. *Gynecol Oncol* 1992;44: 61–65.

126. Russack V. Image cytometry: current applications and future trends. *Crit Rev Clin Lab Sci* 1994;31:1–34.

127. Strang P, Stenkvist B, Bergstrom R, et al. Flow cytometry and interactive image cytometry in endometrial carcinoma. A comparative and prognostic study. *Anticancer Res* 1991;11:783–788.

128. Hamaguchi K, Nishimura H, Miyoshi T, et al. Flow cytometric analysis of cellular DNA content in ovarian cancer. *Gynecol Oncol* 1990; 37:219–223.

129. Kaern J, Trope CG, Kristensen GB, Pettersen EO. Flow cytometric DNA ploidy and S-phase heterogeneity in advanced ovarian carcinoma. *Cancer* 1994;73:1870–1877.

130. Demirel D, Laucirica R, Fishman A, et al. Ovarian tumors of low malignant potential. Correlation of DNA index and S-phase fraction

with histopathologic grade and clinical outcome. *Cancer* 1996;77: 1494–1500.

131. Guerrieri C, Hogberg T, Wingren S, et al. Mucinous borderline and malignant tumors of the ovary. A clinicopathologic and DNA ploidy study of 92 cases. *Cancer* 1994;74:2329–2340.

132. Harlow BL, Fuhr JE, McDonald TW, et al. Flow cytometry as a prognostic indicator in women with borderline epithelial ovarian tumors. *Gynecol Oncol* 1993;50:305–309.

133. Lai CH, Hsueh S, Chang TC, et al. The role of DNA flow cytometry in borderline malignant ovarian tumors. *Cancer* 1996;78:794–802.

134. Bakshi N, Rajwanshi A, Patel F, et al. Prognostic significance of DNA ploidy and S-phase fraction in malignant serous cystadenocarcinoma of the ovary. *Anal Quant Cytol Histol* 1998;20:215–220.

135. Eissa S, Khalifa A, Laban M, et al. Comparison of flow cytometric DNA content analysis in fresh and paraffin-embedded ovarian neoplasms: a prospective study. *Br J Cancer* 1998;77:421–425.

136. Friedlander ML, Hedley DW, Swanson C, Russell P. Prediction of long-term survival by flow cytometric analysis of cellular DNA content in patients with advanced ovarian cancer. *J Clin Oncol* 1988;6: 282–290.

137. Gajewski WH, Fuller AF Jr, Pastel-Ley C, et al. Prognostic significance of DNA content in epithelial ovarian cancer. *Gynecol Oncol* 1994;53:5–12.

138. Iversen OE. Prognostic value of the flow cytometric DNA index in human ovarian carcinoma. *Cancer* 1988;61:971–975.

139. Pietrzak K, Olszewski W. DNA ploidy as a prognostic factor in patients with ovarian carcinoma. *Pol J Pathol* 1998;49:141–144.

140. Resnik E, Trujillo YP, Taxy JB. Long-term survival and DNA ploidy in advanced epithelial ovarian cancer. *J Surg Oncol* 1997;64:299–303.

141. Kaern J, Trope C, Kjorstad KE, et al. Cellular DNA content as a new prognostic tool in patients with borderline tumors of the ovary. *Gynecol Oncol* 1990;38:452–457.

142. Wagner TM, Adler A, Sevelda P, et al. Prognostic significance of cell DNA content in early-stage ovarian cancer (FIGO stages I and II/A) by means of automatic image cytometry. *Int J Cancer* 1994;56: 167–172.

143. Zaino RJ, Davis AT, Ohlsson-Wilhelm BM, Brunetto VL. DNA content is an independent prognostic indicator in endometrial adenocarcinoma. A Gynecologic Oncology Group study. *Int J Gynecol Pathol* 1998;17:312–319.

144. Nordstrom B, Strang P, Lindgren A, et al. Carcinoma of the endometrium: do the nuclear grade and DNA ploidy provide more prognostic information than do the FIGO and WHO classifications? *Int J Gynecol Pathol* 1996;15:191–201.

145. Xue F, Jiao S, Zhao F. [A study on DNA content and cell cycle phase analysis in endometrial carcinoma]. *Zhonghua Fu Chan Ke Za Zhi* 1996;31:216–219.

146. Connor JP, Miller DS, Bauer KD, et al. Flow cytometric evaluation of early invasive cervical cancer. *Obstet Gynecol* 1993;81:367–371.

147. Jarrell MA, Heintz N, Howard P, et al. Squamous cell carcinoma of the cervix: HPV 16 and DNA ploidy as predictors of survival. *Gynecol Oncol* 1992;46:361–366.

148. Anton M, Nenutil R, Rejthar A, et al. DNA flow cytometry: a predictor of a high-risk group in cervical cancer. *Cancer Detect Prev* 1997;21: 242–246.

149. Yamamoto T, Ikawa S, Akiyama T, et al. Similarity of protein encoded by the human c-erb-B-2 gene to epidermal growth factor receptor. *Nature* 1986;319:230–234.

150. Norris HJ, Becker RL, Mikel UV. A comparative morphometric and cytophotometric study of endometrial hyperplasia, atypical hyperplasia, and endometrial carcinoma. *Hum Pathol* 1989;20:219–223.

151. Monsonego J, Valensi P, Zerat L, et al. Simultaneous effects of aneuploidy and oncogenic human papillomavirus on histological grade of cervical intraepithelial neoplasia. *Br J Obstet Gynaecol* 1997;104: 723–727.

152. Multhaupt H, Bruder E, Elit L, et al. Combined analysis of cervical smears. Cytopathology, image cytometry and in situ hybridization. *Acta Cytol* 1993;37:373–378.

153. Clavel C, Zerat L, Binninger I, et al. DNA content measurement and in situ hybridization in condylomatous cervical lesions. *Diagn Mol Pathol* 1992;1:180–184.

154. Hanselaar AG, Vooijs GP, Mayall BH, et al. DNA changes in progressive cervical intraepithelial neoplasia. *Anal Cell Pathol* 1992;4: 315–324.

155. Kashyap V, Das BC. DNA aneuploidy and infection of human papillomavirus type 16 in preneoplastic lesions of the uterine cervix: correlation with progression to malignancy. *Cancer Lett* 1998;123:47–52.

156. Bocking A, Hilgarth M, Auffermann W, et al. DNA-cytometric diagnosis of prospective malignancy in borderline lesions of the uterine cervix. *Acta Cytol* 1986;30:608–615.

157. Bibbo M, Dytch HE, Alenghat E, et al. DNA ploidy profiles as prognostic indicators in CIN lesions. *Am J Clin Pathol* 1989;92:261–265.

158. Lage JM, Mark SD, Roberts DJ, et al. A flow cytometric study of 137 fresh hydropic placentas: correlation between types of hydatidiform moles and nuclear DNA ploidy. *Obstet Gynecol* 1992;79:403–410.

159. Martin DA, Sutton GP, Ulbright TM, et al. DNA content as a prognostic index in gestational trophoblastic neoplasia. *Gynecol Oncol* 1989; 34:383–388.

160. Haba R, Miki H, Kobayashi S, Ohmori M. Combined analysis of flow cytometry and morphometry of ovarian granulosa cell tumor. *Cancer* 1993;72:3258.

161. Jacoby AF, Young RH, Colvin RB, et al. DNA content in juvenile granulosa cell tumors of the ovary: a study of early- and advanced-stage disease. *Gynecol Oncol* 1992;46:97–103.

162. Rosen AC, Graf AH, Klein M, et al. DNA ploidy in primary fallopian-tube carcinoma using image cytometry. *Int J Cancer* 1994;58: 362–365.

163. Baak JP, Path FR, Hermsen MA, et al. Genomics and proteomics in cancer. *Eur J Cancer* 2003;39:1199–1215.

164. Lichter P, Joos S, Bentz M, Lampel S. Comparative genomic hybridization: uses and limitations. *Semin Hematol* 2000;37:348–357.

165. Mohr S, Leikauf GD, Keith G, Rihn BH. Microarrays as cancer keys: an array of possibilities. *J Clin Oncol* 2002;20:3165–3175.

166. Velculescu VE, Zhang L, Vogelstein B, Kinzler KW. Serial analysis of gene expression. *Science* 1995;270:484–487.

167. Wistuba I, Roa I, Araya JC, et al. [Nucleolar organizer regions in uterine cervical cancer and its precursor epithelial lesions.] *Rev Med Chil* 1993;121:1110–1117.

168. Buick R, Tannock, I. Properties of malignant cells. In: Tannock IHR, ed. *The Basic Science of Oncology*. Toronto: McGraw-Hill, 1992:139.

169. Miyamoto S, Nishida M, Miwa K, et al. Increased actin cable organization after single chromosome introduction: association with suppression of in vitro cell growth rather than tumorigenic suppression. *Mol Carcinog* 1994;10:88–96.

170. Ando S, Tsujimura K, Matsuoka Y, et al. Phosphorylation of synthetic vimentin peptides by cdc2 kinase. *Biochem Biophys Res Commun* 1993;195:837–843.

171. Kusubata M, Matsuoka Y, Tsujimura K, et al. cdc2 kinase phosphorylation of desmin at three serine/threonine residues in the amino-terminal head domain. *Biochem Biophys Res Commun* 1993;190:927–934.

172. Moir RD, Montag-Lowy M, Goldman RD. Dynamic properties of nuclear lamins: lamin B is associated with sites of DNA replication. *J Cell Biol* 1994;125:1201–1212.

173. Dohi T, Nemoto T, Ohta S, et al. Different binding properties of three monoclonal antibodies to sialyl Le(x) glycolipids in a gastric cancer cell line and normal stomach tissue. *Anticancer Res* 1993;13: 1277–1282.

174. Hakomori S, Nudelman E, Levery SB, Kannagi R. Novel fucolipids accumulating in human adenocarcinoma. I. Glycolipids with di- or trifucosylated type 2 chain. *J Biol Chem* 1984;259:4672–4680.

175. Eigenbrodt E, Reinacher M, Scheefers-Borchel U, et al. Double role for pyruvate kinase type M2 in the expansion of phosphometabolite pools found in tumor cells. *Crit Rev Oncog* 1992;3:91–115.

176. Newsholme EA, Board M. Application of metabolic-control logic to fuel utilization and its significance in tumor cells. *Adv Enzyme Regul* 1991;31:225–246.

177. Baggetto LG. Deviant energetic metabolism of glycolytic cancer cells. *Biochimie* 1992,74:959–974.

178. Thompson S, Cantwell BM, Matta KL, Turner GA. Parallel changes in the blood levels of abnormally-fucosylated haptoglobin and alpha 1,3 fucosyltransferase in relationship to tumour burden: more evidence for a disturbance of fucose metabolism in cancer. *Cancer Lett* 1992,65: 115–121.

179. Hill R. *Metastasis*. 2nd ed. Toronto: McGraw-Hill, 1992.

180. Maloney A, Workman P. HSP90 as a new therapeutic target for cancer therapy: the story unfolds. *Expert Opin Biol Ther* 2002;2:3–24.

181. Cadena DL, Gill GN. Receptor tyrosine kinases. *Faseb J* 1992;6: 2332–2337.

182. Bolen JB, Rowley RB, Spana C, Tsygankov AY. The Src family of tyrosine protein kinases in hemopoietic signal transduction. *FASEB J* 1992;6:3403–3409.

183. Cantley LC, Auger KR, Carpenter C, et al. Oncogenes and signal transduction. *Cell* 1991;64:281–302.

184. Widmann C, Gibson S, Jarpe MB, Johnson GL. Mitogen-activated protein kinase: conservation of a three-kinase module from yeast to human. *Physiol Rev* 1999;79:143–180.

185. Morrison DK, Cutler RE. The complexity of Raf-1 regulation. *Curr Opin Cell Biol* 1997;9:174–179.

186. Van Aelst L, Barr, M, Marcus S, et al. Complex formation between RAS and RAF and other protien kinases. *Proc Natl Acad Sci U S A* 1993;90:6213.

187. Warne PH, Viciana PR, Downward J. Direct interaction of Ras and the amino-terminal region of Raf-1 in vitro. *Nature* 1993,364:352–355.

188. Moodie SA, Willumsen BM, Weber MJ, et al. Complexes of Ras.GTP with Raf-1 and mitogen-activated protein kinase kinase. *Science* 1993; 260:1658–1661.

189. Vos MD, Ellis CA, Bell A, et al. Ras uses the novel tumor suppressor RASSF1 as an effector to mediate apoptosis. *J Biol Chem* 2000;275: 35669–35672.

190. Ellis CA, Vos MD, Howell H, et al. Rig is a novel ras-related protein and potential neural tumor suppressor. *Proc Natl Acad Sci U S A* 2002;99:9876–9881.

191. Yu Y, Xu F, Peng H, et al. NOEY2 (ARHI), an imprinted putative tumor suppressor gene in ovarian and breast carcinomas. *Proc Natl Acad Sci U S A* 1999;96:214–219.

192. Gutkind JS. The pathways connecting G protein–coupled receptors to the nucleus through divergent mitogen-activated protein kinase cascades. *J Biol Chem* 1998;273:1839–1842.

193. Su B, Karin, M. Mitogen-activated protein kinase cascades and regulation of gene expression. *Curr Opin Immunol* 1996;8:402.

194. Shen YH, Godlewski J, Zhu J, et al. Cross-talk between JNK/SAPK and ERK/MAPK pathways: sustained activation of JNK blocks ERK activation by mitogenic factors. *J Biol Chem* 2003;278:26715–26721.

195. Garrington TP, Johnson GL. Organization and regulation of mitogen-activated protein kinase signaling pathways. *Curr Opin Cell Biol* 1999;11:211–218.

196. Cobb MH. MAP kinase pathways. *Prog Biophys Mol Biol* 1999;71: 479–500.

197. Davis RJ. The mitogen-activated protein kinase signal transduction pathway. *J Biol Chem* 1993,268:14553–14556.

198. Nevins JR. E2F: a link between the Rb tumor suppressor protein and viral oncoproteins. *Science* 1992;258:424–429.

199. Chang F, Lee JT, Navolanic PM, et al. Involvement of PI3K/Akt pathway in cell cycle progression, apoptosis, and neoplastic transformation: a target for cancer chemotherapy. *Leukemia* 2003;17: 590–603.

200. Shayesteh L, Lu Y, Kuo WL, et al. PIK3CA is implicated as an oncogene in ovarian cancer. *Nat Genet* 1999;21:99–102.

201. Cheng JQ, Godwin AK, Bellacosa A, et al. AKT2, a putative oncogene encoding a member of a subfamily of protein-serine/threonine kinases, is amplified in human ovarian carcinomas. *Proc Natl Acad Sci U S A* 1992;89:9267–9271.

202. Azzi A, Boscoboinik D, Hensey C. The protein kinase C family. *Eur J Biochem* 1992;208:547–557.

203. Rossomando A, Wu J, Weber MJ, Sturgill TW. The phorbol ester–dependent activator of the mitogen-activated protein kinase p42mapk is a kinase with specificity for the threonine and tyrosine regulatory sites. *Proc Natl Acad Sci U S A* 1992;89:5221–5225.

204. Heichman KA, Roberts JM. Rules to replicate by. *Cell* 1994;79: 557–562.

205. Hunter T, Pines J. Cyclins and cancer. II: Cyclin D and CDK inhibitors come of age. *Cell* 1994;79:573–582.

206. Klingmuller U, Lorenz U, Cantley LC, et al. Specific recruitment of SH–PTP1 to the erythropoietin receptor causes inactivation of JAK2 and termination of proliferative signals. *Cell* 1995;80:729–738.

207. Nurse P. Ordering S phase and M phase in the cell cycle. *Cell* 1994; 79:547–550.

208. Sherr CJ. G1 phase progression: cycling on cue. *Cell* 1994;79: 551–555.

209. Akiyama T, Ohuchi T, Sumida S, et al. Phosphorylation of the retinoblastoma protein by CDK2. *Proc Natl Acad Sci U S A* 1992;89: 7900–7904.

210. DeCaprio JA, Furukawa Y, Ajchenbaum F, et al. The retinoblastoma-susceptibility gene product becomes phosphorylated in multiple stages during cell cycle entry and progression. *Proc Natl Acad Sci U S A* 1992;89:1795–1798.

211. Farley J, Smith LM, Darcy KM, et al. Cyclin E expression is a significant predictor of survival in advanced, suboptimally debulked ovarian epithelial cancers: a Gynecologic Oncology Group study. *Cancer Res* 2003;63:1235–1241.

212. Casey PJ, Gilman AG. G protein involvement in receptor-effector coupling. *J Biol Chem* 1988;263:2577–2580.

213. Savarese TM, Fraser CM. In vitro mutagenesis and the search for structure-function relationships among G protein–coupled receptors. *Biochem J* 1992;283 (Pt 1):1–19.

214. Cockcroft S, Thomas GM. Inositol-lipid–specific phospholipase C isoenzymes and their differential regulation by receptors. *Biochem J* 1992;288 (Pt 1):1–14.

215. Fang X, Gaudette D, Furui T, et al. Lysophospholipid growth factors in the initiation, progression, metastases, and management of ovarian cancer. *Ann N Y Acad Sci* 2000;905:188–208.

216. Guo Z, Liliom K, Fischer DJ, et al. Molecular cloning of a high-affinity receptor for the growth factor-like lipid mediator lysophosphatidic acid from *Xenopus* oocytes. *Proc Natl Acad Sci U S A* 1996;93: 14367–14372.

217. Kelvin DJ, Michiel DF, Johnston JA, et al. Chemokines and serpentines: the molecular biology of chemokine receptors. *J Leukoc Biol* 1993;54:604–612.

218. Neel BG, Tonks NK. Protein tyrosine phosphatases in signal transduction. *Curr Opin Cell Biol* 1997;9:193–204.

219. Tonks NK, Neel BG. From form to function: signaling by protein tyrosine phosphatases. *Cell* 1996;87:365–368.

220. Brady-Kalnay SM, Tonks NK. Protein tyrosine phosphatases as adhesion receptors. *Curr Opin Cell Biol* 1995;7:650–657.

221. Peles E, Nativ M, Campbell PL, et al. The carbonic anhydrase domain of receptor tyrosine phosphatase beta is a functional ligand for the axonal cell recognition molecule contactin. *Cell* 1995;82:251–260.

222. Lorenz U, Bergemann AD, Steinberg HN, et al. Genetic analysis reveals cell type–specific regulation of receptor tyrosine kinase c-Kit by the protein tyrosine phosphatase SHP1. *J Exp Med* 1996,184: 1111–1126.

223. Li DM, Sun H. PTEN/MMAC1/TEP1 suppresses the tumorigenicity and induces G1 cell cycle arrest in human glioblastoma cells. *Proc Natl Acad Sci U S A* 1998;95:15406–15411.

224. Haas-Kogan D, Shalev N, Wong M, et al. Protein kinase B (PKB/Akt) activity is elevated in glioblastoma cells due to mutation of the tumor suppressor PTEN/MMAC. *Curr Biol* 1998;8:1195–1198.

225. Ramaswamy S, Nakamura, N., Vazquez, F., et al. Regulation of G1 progression by the PTEN tumor suppressor protein is linked to inhibition of the phosphatidylinositol 3-kinase/Akt pathway. *Proc Natl Acad Sci U S A* 1999;96:2110.

226. Eng C. Genetics of Coden syndrome: through the looking glass of oncology. *Int J Oncol* 1998;12:701.

227. Obata K, Morland SJ, Watson RH, et al. Frequent PTEN/MMAC mutations in endometrioid but not serous or mucinous epithelial ovarian tumors. *Cancer Res* 1998;58:2095–2097.

228. Risinger JI, Hayes AK, Berchuck A, Barrett JC. PTEN/MMAC1 mutations in endometrial cancers. *Cancer Res* 1997;57:4736–4738.

229. Villafranca JE, Kissinger CR, Parge HE. Protein serine/threonine phosphatases. *Curr Opin Biotechnol* 1996;7:397–402.

230. Goldberg Y. Protein phosphatase 2A: who shall regulate the regulator? *Biochem Pharmacol* 1999;57:321–328.

231. Schonthal AH. Role of PP2A in intracellular signal transduction pathways. *Front Biosci* 1998;3:D1262–D1273.

232. Tonks NK. Protein tyrosine phosphatases and the control of cellular signaling responses. *Adv Pharmacol* 1996;36:91–119.

233. Manzano RG, Montuenga LM, Dayton M, et al. CL100 expression is down-regulated in advanced epithelial ovarian cancer and its re-expression decreases its malignant potential. *Oncogene* 2002;21: 4435–4447.

234. Giles RH, van Es JH, Clevers H. Caught up in a Wnt storm: Wnt signaling in cancer. *Biochim Biophys Acta* 2003;1653:1–24.

235. Orford K, Crockett C, Jensen JP, et al. Serine phosphorylation-regulated ubiquitination and degradation of beta-catenin. *J Biol Chem* 1997;272:24735–24738.

236. Derynck R. The physiology of transforming growth factor-alpha. *Adv Cancer Res* 1992,58:27–52.

237. Wen D, Peles E, Cupples R, et al. Neu differentiation factor: a transmembrane glycoprotein containing an EGF domain and an immunoglobulin homology unit. *Cell* 1992;69:559–572.

238. Bast RC, Jr., Boyer CM, Jacobs I, et al. Cell growth regulation in epithelial ovarian cancer. *Cancer* 1993;71:1597–1601.

239. Meden H, Marx D, Rath W, et al. Overexpression of the oncogene c-erb B2 in primary ovarian cancer: evaluation of the prognostic value in a Cox proportional hazards multiple regression. *Int J Gynecol Pathol* 1994;13:45–53.

240. Slamon DJ, Godolphin W, Jones LA, et al. Studies of the HER-2/neu proto-oncogene in human breast and ovarian cancer. *Science* 1989;244:707–712.

241. Harwerth IM, Wels W, Schlegel J, et al. Monoclonal antibodies directed to the erbB-2 receptor inhibit in vivo tumour cell growth. *Br J Cancer* 1993;68:1140–1145.

242. Bookman MA, Darcy KM, Clarke-Pearson D, et al. Evaluation of monoclonal humanized anti–HER2 antibody, trastuzumab, in patients with recurrent or refractory ovarian or primary peritoneal carcinoma with overexpression of HER2: a phase II trial of the Gynecologic Oncology Group. *J Clin Oncol* 2003;21:283–290.

243. Resnicoff M, Ambrose D, Coppola D, Rubin R. Insulin-like growth factor-1 and its receptor mediate the autocrine proliferation of human ovarian carcinoma cell lines. *Lab Invest* 1993;69:756–760.

244. Fantl WJ, Johnson DE, Williams LT. Signalling by receptor tyrosine kinases. *Annu Rev Biochem* 1993;62:453–481.

245. Henriksen R, Funa K, Wilander E, et al. Expression and prognostic significance of platelet-derived growth factor and its receptors in epithelial ovarian neoplasms. *Cancer Res* 1993;53:4550–4554.

246. Versnel MA, Haarbrink M, Langerak AW, et al. Human ovarian tumors of epithelial origin express PDGF in vitro and in vivo. *Cancer Genet Cytogenet* 1994;73:60–64.

247. Inoue M, Kyo S, Fujita M, et al. Coexpression of the c-kit receptor and the stem cell factor in gynecological tumors. *Cancer Res* 1994; 54:3049–3053.

248. Baiocchi G, Kavanagh JJ, Talpaz M, et al. Expression of the macrophage colony–stimulating factor and its receptor in gynecologic malignancies. *Cancer* 1991;67:990–996.

249. Baird A, Bohlen, P. Peptide growth factors and their receptors I. In: Sporn MRA, ed. *Handbook of experimental pharmacology.* Berlin: Springer-Verlag, 1990:369.

250. Di Blasio AM, Cremonesi L, Vigano P, et al. Basic fibroblast growth factor and its receptor messenger ribonucleic acids are expressed in human ovarian epithelial neoplasms. *Am J Obstet Gynecol* 1993;169: 1517–1523.

251. Olson TA, Mohanraj D, Carson LF, et al. Vascular permeability factor gene expression in normal and neoplastic human ovaries. *Cancer Res* 1994;54:276–280.

252. Reynolds K, Farzaneh F, Collins WP, et al. Association of ovarian malignancy with expression of platelet-derived endothelial cell growth factor. *J Natl Cancer Inst* 1994;86:1234–1238.

253. Wrana JL, Attisano L, Wieser R, et al. Mechanism of activation of the TGF-beta receptor. *Nature* 1994;370:341–347.

254. Cate R, Donohoe P, MacLaughlin D. Mullerian inhibiting substance. In: Sporn MRA, ed. *Peptide growth factors and their receptors I. Handbook of experimental pharmacology.* Berlin: Springer-Verlag, 1990:179.

255. Kolesnick R, Golde DW. The sphingomyelin pathway in tumor necrosis factor and interleukin-1 signaling. *Cell* 1994;77:325–328.

256. Kilian PL, Kaffka KL, Biondi DA, et al. Antiproliferative effect of interleukin-1 on human ovarian carcinoma cell line (NIH: OVCAR–3). *Cancer Res* 1991;51:1823–1828.

257. Li BY, Mohanraj D, Olson MC, et al. Human ovarian epithelial cancer cells cultures in vitro express both interleukin 1 alpha and beta genes. *Cancer Res* 1992;52:2248–2252.

258. Lewis MP, Sullivan MH, Elder MG. Regulation by interleukin-1 beta

259. Wu S, Meeker WA, Wiener JR, et al. Transfection of ovarian cancer cells with tumor necrosis factor-alpha (TNF-alpha) antisense mRNA abolishes the proliferative response to interleukin-1 (IL-1) but not TNF-alpha. *Gynecol Oncol* 1994;53:59–63.

260. Isonishi S, Jekunen AP, Hom DK, et al. Modulation of cisplatin sensitivity and growth rate of an ovarian carcinoma cell line by bombesin and tumor necrosis factor-alpha. *J Clin Invest* 1992;90:1436–1442.

261. Kohn EC, Sandeen MA, Liotta LA. In vivo efficacy of a novel inhibitor of selected signal transduction pathways including calcium, arachidonate, and inositol phosphates. *Cancer Res* 1992;52:3208–3212.

262. Archer M. The basic science of oncology. In: Tannock IHR, ed. *Chemical carcinogenesis.* 2nd ed. Toronto: McGraw-Hill, 1992:102.

263. Sutherland D. *Hormones and cancer.* Toronto: McGraw-Hill, 1992.

264. Ames BN, Shigenaga MK, Gold LS. DNA lesions, inducible DNA repair, and cell division: three key factors in mutagenesis and carcinogenesis. *Environ Health Perspect* 1993,101[Suppl]:5:35–44.

265. Wu S, Rodabaugh K, Martinez-Maza O, et al. Stimulation of ovarian tumor cell proliferation with monocyte products including interleukin-1, interleukin-6, and tumor necrosis factor-alpha. *Am J Obstet Gynecol* 1992;166:997–1007.

266. Maronpot RR. Ovarian toxicity and carcinogenicity in eight recent National Toxicology Program studies. *Environ Health Perspect* 1987; 73:125–130.

267. Smith BJ, Mattison DR, Sipes IG. The role of epoxidation in 4-vinylcyclohexene–induced ovarian toxicity. *Toxicol Appl Pharmacol* 1990; 105:372–381.

268. Nagaoka T, Takeuchi M, Onodera H, et al. Experimental induction of uterine adenocarcinoma in rats by estrogen and N-methyl-N-nitrosourea. *In Vivo* 1993;7:525–530.

269. Turusov VS, Raikhlin NT, Smirnova EA, Trukhanova LS. Uterine sarcomas in CBA mice induced by combined treatment with 1,2-dimethylhydrazine and estradiol dipropionate. Light and electron microscopy. *Exp Toxicol Pathol* 1993;45:161–166.

270. Parkash V, Carcangiu ML. Uterine papillary serous carcinoma after radiation therapy for carcinoma of the cervix. *Cancer* 1992;69: 496–501.

271. Benchimol S. Viruses and cancer. In: Tannock IHR, ed. *The basic science of oncology.* Toronto: McGraw-Hill, 1992:88.

272. Varmus H. Retroviruses. *Science* 1988;240:1427–1435.

273. zur Hausen H. Viruses in human cancer. *Science* 1991;254:1167.

274. Van Dyke T. Analysis of viral–host protein interactions and tumorigenesis in transgenic mice. *Semin Cancer Biol* 1994;5:47.

275. Green PL, Chen IS. Regulation of human T cell leukemia virus expression. *FASEB J* 1990;4:169–175.

276. Laurence J, Astrin, SM. Human immunodeficiency virus induction of malignanat transformation in human B lymphocytes. *Proc Natl Acad Sci U S A* 1991;88:7635.

277. Stewart JP, Arrand JR. Expression of the Epstein-Barr virus latent membrane protein in nasopharyngeal carcinoma biopsy specimens. *Hum Pathol* 1993;24:239–242.

278. Young LS, Rowe M. Epstein-Barr virus, lymphomas and Hodgkin's disease. *Semin Cancer Biol* 1992;3:273–284.

279. Izumi KM, Kaye KM, Kieff ED. Epstein-Barr virus recombinant molecular genetic analysis of the LMP1 amino-terminal cytoplasmic domain reveals a probable structural role, with no component essential for primary B-lymphocyte growth transformation. *J Virol* 1994;68: 4369–4376.

280. Magrath I, Jain V, Bhatia K. Epstein-Barr virus and Burkitt's lymphoma. *Semin Cancer Biol* 1992;3:285–295.

281. Brechot C. Oncogenic activation of cyclin A. *Curr Opin Genet Dev* 1993;3:11–18.

282. Wang J, Zindy F, Chenivesse X, et al. Modification of cyclin A expression by hepatitis B virus DNA integration in a hepatocellular carcinoma. *Oncogene* 1992;7:1653–1656.

283. Graef E, Caselmann WH, Wells J, Koshy R. Insertional activation of mevalonate kinase by hepatitis B virus DNA in a human hepatoma cell line. *Oncogene* 1994;9:81–87.

284. Di Luca D, Costa S, Monini P, et al. Search for human papillomavirus, herpes simplex virus and c-myc oncogene in human genital tumors. *Int J Cancer* 1989;43:570–577.

285. Manservigi R, Cassai E, Deiss LP, et al. Sequences homologous to

two separate transforming regions of herpes simplex virus DNA are linked in two human genital tumors. *Virology* 1986;155:192–201.

286. DiPaolo JA, Woodworth CD, Popescu NC, Koval DL, Lopez JV, Doniger J. HSV-2–induced tumorigenicity in HPV16-immortalized human genital keratinocytes. *Virology* 1990;177:777–779.

287. Lancaster WD. Viral role in cervical and liver cancer. *Cancer* 1992; 70:1794–1798.

288. Gissmann L. Human papillomaviruses and genital cancer. *Semin Cancer Biol* 1992;3:253–261.

289. Lorincz AT, Reid R, Jenson AB, et al. Human papillomavirus infection of the cervix: relative risk associations of 15 common anogenital types. *Obstet Gynecol* 1992;79:328–337.

290. Howley PM, Munger K, Romanczuk H, et al. Cellular targets of the oncoproteins encoded by the cancer associated human papillomaviruses. *Princess Takamatsu Symp* 1991;22:239–248.

291. Woodworth CD, Doniger J, DiPaolo JA. Immortalization of human foreskin keratinocytes by various human papillomavirus DNAs corresponds to their association with cervical carcinoma. *J Virol* 1989;63: 159–164.

292. Hurlin PJ, Kaur P, Smith PP, et al. Progression of human papillomavirus type 18-immortalized human keratinocytes to a malignant phenotype. *Proc Natl Acad Sci U S A* 1991;88:570–574.

293. DiPaolo JA, Woodworth CD, Popescu NC, et al. J. Induction of human cervical squamous cell carcinoma by sequential transfection with human papillomavirus 16 DNA and viral Harvey ras. *Oncogene* 1989; 4:395–399.

294. Steele C, Cowsert LM, Shillitoe EJ. Effects of human papillomavirus type 18–specific antisense oligonucleotides on the transformed phenotype of human carcinoma cell lines. *Cancer Res* 1993;53: 2330–2337.

295. Werness BA, Levine AJ, Howley PM. Association of human papillomavirus types 16 and 18 E6 proteins with p53. *Science* 1990;248: 76–79.

296. Hoppe-Seyler F, Butz K. Repression of endogenous p53 transactivation function in HeLa cervical carcinoma cells by human papillomavirus type 16 E6, human mdm-2, and mutant p53. *J Virol* 1993;67: 3111–3117.

297. Stein WD. Analysis of cancer incidence data on the basis of multistage and clonal growth models. *Adv Cancer Res* 1991;56:161–213.

298. Hahn WC, Weinberg RA. Rules for making human tumor cells. *N Engl J Med* 2002;347:1593–1603.

299. Stancel GM, Baker VV, Hyder SM, et al. Oncogenes and uterine function. *Oxf Rev Reprod Biol* 1993;15:1–42.

300. Taylor RR, Teneriello MG, Nash JD, et al. The molecular genetics of gyn malignancies. *Oncology (Huntingt)* 1994;8:63–70, 73, discussion 73, 78–82.

301. Hethcote HW, Knudson AG Jr. Model for the incidence of embryonal cancers: application to retinoblastoma. *Proc Natl Acad Sci U S A* 1978;75:2453–2457.

302. Fearon ER, Vogelstein B. A genetic model for colorectal tumorigenesis. *Cell* 1990;61:759–767.

303. Perera F, Santella, R., Brandt-Rauf, P. *Molecular epidemiology of lung cancer.* New York: Cold Spring Harbor Laboratory Press, 1991.

304. Harris A. *Breast cancer, molecular oncology and cancer therapy.* New York: Cold Spring Harbor Laboratory Press, 1991.

305. Brown PH, Alani R, Preis LH, et al. Suppression of oncogene-induced transformation by a deletion mutant of c-jun. *Oncogene* 1993;8: 877–886.

306. Batieha AM, Armenian HK, Norkus EP, et al. Serum micronutrients and the subsequent risk of cervical cancer in a population-based nested case-control study. *Cancer Epidemiol Biomarkers Prev* 1993;2: 335–339.

307. Palan PR, Mikhail MS, Basu J, Romney SL. Beta-carotene levels in exfoliated cervicovaginal epithelial cells in cervical intraepithelial neoplasia and cervical cancer. *Am J Obstet Gynecol* 1992;167: 1899–1903.

308. Agarwal C, Hembree JR, Rorke EA, Eckert RL. Interferon and retinoic acid suppress the growth of human papillomavirus type 16 immortalized cervical epithelial cells, but only interferon suppresses the level of the human papillomavirus transforming oncogenes. *Cancer Res* 1994;54:2108–2112.

309. Agarwal C, Rorke EA, Irwin JC, Eckert RL. Immortalization by human papillomavirus type 16 alters retinoid regulation of human ectocervical epithelial cell differentiation. *Cancer Res* 1991;51: 3982–3989.

310. Meyskens FL Jr, Surwit E, Moon TE, et al. Enhancement of regression of cervical intraepithelial neoplasia II (moderate dysplasia) with topically applied all-trans-retinoic acid: a randomized trial. *J Natl Cancer Inst* 1994;86:539–543.

CHAPTER 4

Tumor Angiogenesis and Metastasis: Biology and Clinical Experience

Edwin M. Posadas and Elise C. Kohn

Genetic instability, sending aberrant signals down information cascades, is at the heart of malignant transformation. This is manifest in part by the activation of genetic and signaling messages stimulating malignant cells to activate their local microenvironment, invade locally, and then metastasize to distant sites (see Fig. 4.1). Invasive and metastatic disease is responsible for much of the morbidity and mortality associated with cancer. The search for factors affecting this process began as far back as 1889. Sir James Paget noted that women who died of breast cancer tended to have a higher frequency of metastases to bone and ovaries. He further commented that the process was not random and, even more importantly, represented a relationship between the ''seed,'' tumor cells of a given type, and ''soil,'' the microenvironment providing the growth advantage to the seeds (1). Scientists have turned much attention toward dissecting the sequence of events that comprise these key steps in the disease process and translating that understanding to development of targeted therapeutics. Signals in the cancers that stimulate and maintain the invasive and angiogenic phenotype can also drive survival. Recognition of the regulation and roles of angiogenesis, invasion, and tumor survival in the dissemination of gynecologic cancers has and will continue to lead to improved patient care and outcome.

CLINICAL IMPACT OF INVASION, ANGIOGENESIS, AND METASTASIS

Invasion

Patients die from metastasis. Survival, recurrence, and response to treatment, both local and systemic, strongly correlate with tumor invasion measured as nodal and distant me-

tastases (2). The importance of depth of invasion alone can be seen in cervical and endometrial cancer as recognized in their respective International Federation of Gynecology and Obstetrics (FIGO) staging systems (3). Invasion has been used as a discriminating clinical feature in the application of therapeutic modalities, especially local therapies such as radiation and intraperitoneal therapies. Further, invasion has prognostic importance, as shown in cancer of the uterine cervix where the risks of lymphovascular space involvement and risk of metastasis increase as the depth of invasion exceeds 5 mm (4,5). Finally, extent of invasion is a critical and significant predictor of disease-free survival in multivariate analyses of early cervical cancer and other cancers (6,7). Clinical outcome in endometrial cancer is also affected by depth of invasion. As myometrial invasion proceeds beyond the depth of 50%, the risks of development of nodal metastases and failure to respond to treatment escalate (8,9). In addition to FIGO stage and tumor type, depth of invasion in endometrial cancer was related to overall survival (10). Epithelial tumors of the ovary of low malignant potential (LMP/borderline) are characterized by their lack of penetration into the ovarian stroma (11). These tumors rarely metastasize, recur late, and have an overall survival at 5 years in excess of 95% (11). The presence of nodal metastases is a poor prognostic sign for gynecologic malignancies, a manifestation of invasion that results in upstaging, poor prognosis, and high risk of relapse. A study of fallopian tube cancer revealed a 76-month median survival in patients without lymph node metastases. This is in contrast to a 33-month median survival in patients with documented nodal disease (12). Invasion is thus an important event regulating the behavior and clinical outcome of gynecologic malignancies.

Angiogenesis

Angiogenesis is the process of formation of new blood vessels from a preexisting vascular network. Its role in can-

Edwin M. Posadas: Medical Oncology Clinical Research Unit, National Cancer Institute, Bethesda, Maryland 20892

Elise C. Kohn: Laboratory of Pathology, National Cancer Institute, Bethesda, Maryland 20892

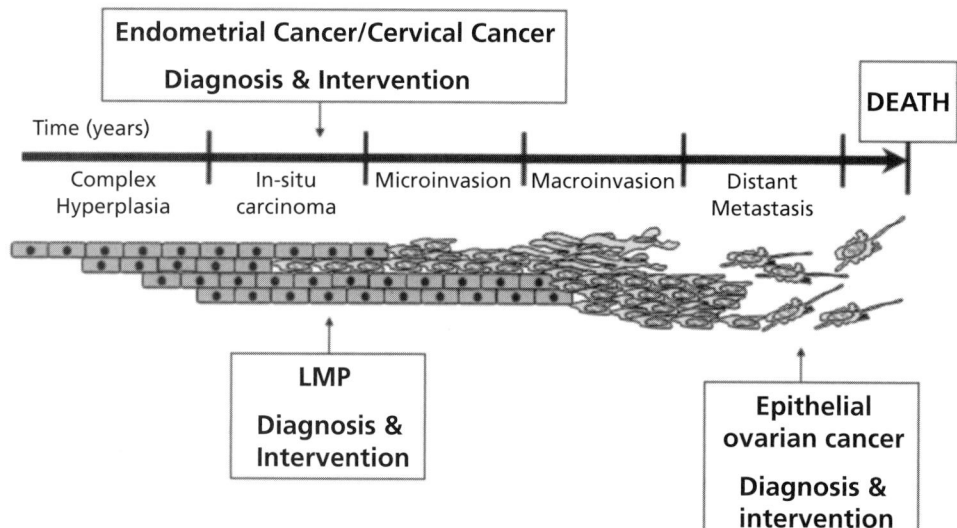

FIG. 4-1. Paradigm of cancer progression. The average age at diagnosis of cervical intraepithelial neoplasia III and/or carcinoma *in situ* (CIS) is approximately 42 years. Progression from CIS to invasive carcinoma occurs over 8 to 10 years. The majority of patients with invasive cervical cancer die within 10 to 15 years of their diagnosis. In comparison, a precursor or early detectable lesion for invasive ovarian cancer has not yet been found. Low malignant potential tumors, a less aggressive counterpart, are diagnosed between the fourth and fifth decade. Invasive ovarian cancer is diagnosed approximately 15 years later, with the majority of patients diagnosed dying of the disease within 5 years.

cer was first detailed by Folkman (13–15) and Liotta (16) in the 1970s. It is now known to be an invasive process itself. Initiated early in the process of malignant transformation, angiogenesis is prognostically important in tumor survival and progression, and has been shown to be a viable therapeutic target (14,17–19).

Several techniques have been applied to assess the extent of angiogenesis in clinical samples. Simple measurement of microvessel number and/or density has been done using immunohistochemical methods (20–23). Endothelial cells can be identified by antibodies to von Willebrand's factor, factor VIII, CD31, and CD34. High microvessel counts have been correlated with relapse of disease in all stages of cervical cancer (24–26), ovarian cancer (27), and endometrial cancer (21). High microvessel counts were found in a series of early-stage cervical cancer patients who developed disease recurrence within 14 months of diagnosis (28). Schlenger and colleagues (26) confirmed these results in cervical cancer patients of all stages. High microvessel counts in endometrial carcinomas have been also shown to correlate with depth of myometrial invasion, recurrent disease, progression-free survival, and overall survival (29–32). The extent of angiogenesis has been shown to correlate with progression-free survival and overall survival in ovarian cancers. Hollingsworth and colleagues (27) studied advanced-stage ovarian cancers and identified CD34 as the most useful discriminant of microvessels; counts and stage of disease were associated with overall survival and disease-free survival, respectively. The expression of vascular endo-

thelial growth factor (VEGF), a potent angiogenesis stimulator, has been used to complement microvessel density in the clinical assessment of angiogenesis. Paley and colleagues (33) first demonstrated that higher expression of VEGF correlated with poor outcome in early-stage and LMP ovarian tumors. A statistically significantly worse median disease-free survival was found in patients with VEGF-positive tumors. Although variability in methods exists, neoangiogenesis is a consistent clinical predictor of poor progression-free survival in gynecologic malignancies in univariate analysis and multivariate analysis. However, measures of angiogenesis have not been proven consistently as an independent variable for overall survival.

Metastasis

Activation of autocrine and paracrine signaling and growth factor or cytokine production programs for invasion and angiogenesis precede the development of invasive malignancy and may precede actual malignant transformation. Once activated, these events set the stage for local and distant dissemination. Activation and co-optation of the local microenvironment induces further permissive events supporting tumor metastasis. The specific and selective patterns of spread are variable between tumors and follow the biology and location of the primary tumor. Consider the distinct pattern of spread of gynecologic cancers. Cervical and endometrial cancers tend to follow the general adenocarcinoma pattern of early local extension with nodal involvement predicted by locally invasive behavior followed by later distant dissemination (34–36). Unlike other invasive adenocarcinomas, epithelial ovarian tumors disseminate broadly within the abdominal cavity prior to nodal and hematogenous dissemination (37,38). This occurs from tumor-cell shedding, followed by adhesion to the serosal and peritoneal surfaces and migration of the malignant epithelium. Common sites of early extension are bowel and bladder serosal surfaces and the abdominal and pelvic peritoneum. Disease can be found on the abdominal peritoneum of the diaphragm in patients before microscopic nodal involvement (FIGO stage IIIA vs IIIC). This was supported by a study of careful surgical assessment of early-stage disease that resulted in upstaging of over one-third patients, most commonly because of microscopic serosal surface disease in the upper abdomen (39). This is in sharp contrast to other gynecologic malignancies in which lymphatic invasion is an earlier event. Matsumoto and colleagues compared the process of lymphatic invasion of ovarian, cervical, and endometrial cancers (40) and showed that cervical and endometrial cancers tended to involve pelvic nodes earlier in the metastatic process than ovarian malignancies. Metastatic activity and pattern of spread is important in the presentation, extirpation, and treatment of all malignancies. The degree of surgical cytoreduction achieved strongly affects survival in ovarian cancer (41–44). The microscopic and insidious nature of the surface extension of ovarian cancer limits the success of complete surgical resection. Further, although metastasis is characterized as an inefficient process, the extent of surface shedding, development of a nurturing ascitic milieu in ascites, and the supportive local microenvironment of the serosa and peritoneum can result in a large microscopic tumor burden. Several studies of advanced-stage ovarian cancer patients indicated that only one-third of patients with distant metastasis are cytoreduced optimally (45). This alone has a significant impact on survival of advanced stage patients. Once a malignancy escapes the confines of a surgically manageable area, managing the case with favorable outcome becomes dramatically more difficult.

MECHANISMS AND REGULATION OF METASTASIS

Biology of Invasion

Invasion is the active translocation of a cell across tissue boundaries and through host cellular and extracellular matrix barriers. This process is tightly regulated in a variety of physiologic conditions, such as embryogenesis, wound healing, and trophoblast implantation. These regulatory mechanisms are disrupted or altered in the setting of malignancy. Invasion utilizes the triad of cellular adhesion, proteolysis, and migration coupled with activation of survival pathways (46). The components and events in physiological invasion and malignant invasion are the same. Quantity, activation, and regulatory status are what set the two forms of invasion apart. Intravasation occurs first. The tumor cell must migrate toward and adhere to the stromal side of the vascular basement membrane, degrade the matrix at that local site, and then migrate through the damaged basement membrane interpolating between endothelial cells in order to enter the vasculature (Fig. 4.2). Circulating tumor cells cannot complete the process of metastatic dissemination without reversing the process, extravasating at a favorable secondary site. That, coupled with stimulation of local angiogenesis and proliferation, leads to a metastatic focus. All these events are programmed into the cell. However, the metastatic cascade is a very inefficient process. Although millions of tumor cells are shed in to the circulation daily, less than 0.01% of the shed cells successfully lead to metastases (47). Such heterogeneity in metastatic competence implies that not all patients with circulating tumor cells will develop detectable metastatic disease. Thus, insight into these biological mechanisms may lead to new and better therapeutic targets and interventions.

Many stimulatory or inhibitory factors are involved, including tumor and stromal-derived cytokines and chemokines, growth factors, and matrix molecules (48–50). Cytokines and chemokines are small secreted peptides that control adhesion and transendothelial migration of tumor and inflammatory cells (51). Accumulating evidence shows that they play a role in solid tumor malignancies. This may be through interactions between tumor-infiltrating leukocytes and tumor cells or tumor cells and local stromal events (52,53). Like growth factors and matrix molecules, cytokines can stimulate production of other tumor-promoting factors, angiogenic factors, and survival factors. Emerging therapeutics targeted against these molecules have been developed to retard or prevent invasion of malignancies.

Biology of Adhesion

Both cell-cell and cell-stroma interactions play an important role in the cascade of events in physiologic and malignant invasion. Connections through cell adhesion molecules, integrins, and cadherins stabilize tissue integrity and provide survival and activation signals (54). Loss of these the same connections is associated with increased metastatic potential (55,56). Cell polarity and organization during spreading and migration are regulated by cell interaction with extracellular matrix (ECM) proteins through the integrin family, and with other cells through the transmembrane glycoproteins, cadherins. Activation of these cell surface receptors passes signals from the microenvironment to the intracellular environment thereby affecting cellular behavior. Differential expression and activation of adhesion molecules has been

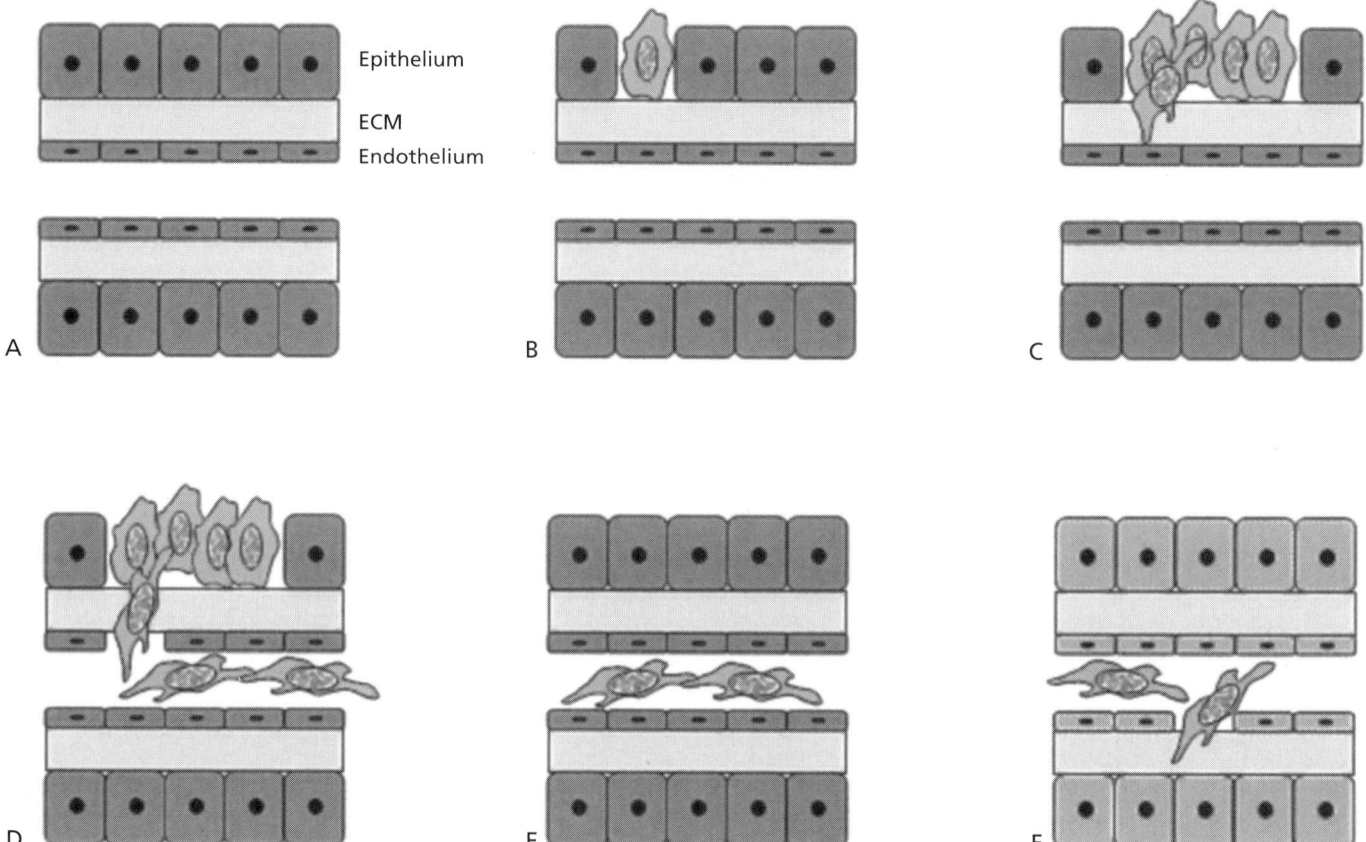

FIG. 4-2. Schema of invasion and metastasis. **(A)** Normal epithelium, extracellular matrix (ECM), and endothelium. **(B)** Early transformation and carcinoma *in situ*. **(C)** Stromal invasion requiring proteolysis and ECM degradation. **(D)** Intravasation requiring further proteolysis. **(E)** Migration. **(F)** Extravasation into distant sites.

described as differentiating normal from malignant cells and can play critical roles in regulation of the metastatic process.

Cadherins

Cadherins are transmembrane glycoproteins that mediate cell-cell interactions in a fashion dependent upon extracellular calcium. E-cadherin is the most extensively studied of the family. Cadherins are found in complex with the catenin family of cytoplasmic proteins (57,58). Cadherin-catenin complexes are linked to the cytoskeleton through direct interactions between α-catenin and α-actinin (59,60). E-cadherin has been demonstrated to function as a metastasis-suppressor molecule in several cell lines (61–64). Decreased E-cadherin expression in endometrial carcinoma has been associated with deep myometrial invasion and high tumor grade. E-cadherin-negative endometriotic cells had an invasive phenotype similar to metastatic carcinoma cells in a collagen invasion assay in vitro. In another study, human MCF-7 breast adenocarcinoma cells, but not normal mam-

mary epithelial cells, induced endothelial-cell dissociation that correlated with the loss of E-cadherin expression at the site of tumor-cell–endothelial-cell contact. Normal ovarian surface epithelium (OSE) rarely expresses E-cadherin (65–67) in contrast to other normal epithelial cells. In contrast, activated metaplastic OSE cells often express E-cadherin. It is almost always present in primary ovarian cancers, although scant or absent in metastases, which is consistent with its description as a metastastic suppressor (68–74). Forced expression of E-cadherin induced epithelial-differentiation markers associated with weakly preneoplastic, metaplastic ovarian surface epithelial and OSE-derived primary carcinomas, suggesting a role of E-cadherin in neoplastic progression in ovarian cancer (66,74). However, as tumors become more poorly differentiated or upregulate their metastasis gene cassette, E-cadherin expression is lost (67). Gain of E-cadherin expression early in the metaplastic process may affect gene transcription that may alter its expressed phenotype (74). This in turn may explain this paradoxical observation. Thus, intracellular adhesion mediated by cadherins/catenin complexes plays a role in both structural morphology and functional differentiation. Alterations associated with this control facilitate invasion in malignancy.

Integrins

The integrins are heterodimers composed of noncovalently linked α- and β-subunit transmembrane glycoproteins. Although originally identified as cell adhesion molecules, integrins are now recognized as signaling molecules for regulation of apoptosis, gene expression, cell proliferation, invasion, metastasis, angiogenesis, and survival. A variety of extracellular matrix proteins serve as ligands, including collagens, laminin, tenascin, fibronectin, vitronectin, von Willebrand's factor, and thombospondin. Matrix engagement is an important stimulant of invasive behavior through the integrin-linked kinase, focal adhesion kinase, and phosphatidylinositol 3' kinase (PI 3'K) to the AKT/protein kinase B pathway. There is interdependence between these proteins as shown experimentally by overexpression of AKT2 in ovarian cancer causing upregulation of β1 integrins, which results in increased invasion and metastasis (75). The signals and their regulation simultaneously advance adhesion and survival. Anoikis, or homelessness, first proposed by Frisch (76), is defined as apoptosis that occurs from loss of adhesion. Further investigation showed that anoikis apoptosis is due to loss of the adhesion-linked survival signals. It can be overcome by constitutive activation of the signaling events through genomic, transcriptional, and protein activation events. For example, in ovarian cancer, the PI 3'K p110 catalytic subunit is amplified genomically and that signal is conserved through overactivation of the PI 3'K protein. This in turn activates AKT and provides protection from anoikis in the absence of integrin engagement (77–81). Furthermore, expression of FAK protects cells from anoikis. Integrins also exhibit the capability of serving as mechanoreceptors allowing for the translation of mechanical external signals into biochemical messages such as during collagen matrix contraction (78). The αvβ3 integrin plays a fundamental role in angiogenesis, invasion, and survival. It mediates cellular adhesion to vitronectin, von Willebrand's factor, fibrinogen, fibronectin, and laminin. This integrin is expressed on epithelial, endothelial, and uterine smooth muscle cells, as well as leukocytes. Its activation initiates a calcium-dependent signaling pathway leading to an increase in cell motility and to survival signals. αvβ3 integrin is expressed minimally in normal or resting blood vessels and is upregulated both on activated vascular endothelium and tumor epithelium. It thus has a role in tumor activity as well as angiogenesis (82–86). There is increased expression of αvβ3 in cervical cancers (87) and ovarian cancers (88,89) with a gradient of expression of αvβ3 being reported in the progression from LMP tumors to invasive epithelial cancers (90). This integrin has been shown to be important in transducing survival signals in a paracrine and collateral fashion from angiogenic growth factors secreted by tumor cells in cross-talk from their tyrosine kinase receptors through the integrin and to survival proteins such as AKT/protein kinase B. Agents directed against integrins have been tested in a variety of models, but clinical results are still forthcoming. Examples of these agents can be found in Table 4.1.

Biology of Angiogenesis

Angiogenesis is a rate-limiting step in the growth of tumors and in the development of metastases (15,91,92). Tumor invasion is limited by nutrient requirements and waste removal from the tumor as well as by the ability of tumor cells to have access to the vasculature for hematogenous dissemination. Thus, vascularization is a crucial step in tumor progression (91,93–95). Net tumor volume represents a balance between cellular proliferation and apoptosis. Tumors enter dormancy when the proliferative rate and the apoptotic rate are equal, as modeled by Holmgren (93). In this model, lack of angiogenesis limits growth, creating a balance between proliferation and death rates (Fig. 4.3). A tumor mass larger than $0.125 \ mm^2$ has outgrown the capacity to acquire nutrients by simple diffusion. Further expansion of the tumor mass requires host vessels to initiate capillary sprouts in the direction of the tumor (14).

The formation of tumor neovasculature consists of multiple, interdependent steps similar to the process of invasion (96). Activation of endothelial cells by stimuli such as injury,

TABLE 4.1 *Examples of biological targets and novel therapies*

Target	Agent
Integrins	Cilengitide (EMD121974)
	Vitaxin
	Medi522
MMP	ABT-518
	Marimastat (BB-2516)
	COL-3
	BAY12-9566
	MMI270 (GCS27023A)
ras	RI157777
	SCH66336
	L-778,123
raf-kinase	ISIS 5132
	ISIS 2503
Angiogenesis	Thalidomide
	CAI
	Endostatin
	Angiostatin
	IL-12
	Ad-p53
	PI-88
Protein kinase C-α (PKC-α)	ISIS 3521 (LY900003)
	Bryostatin-1
mTOR/FRAP	CCI-779
	rapamycin

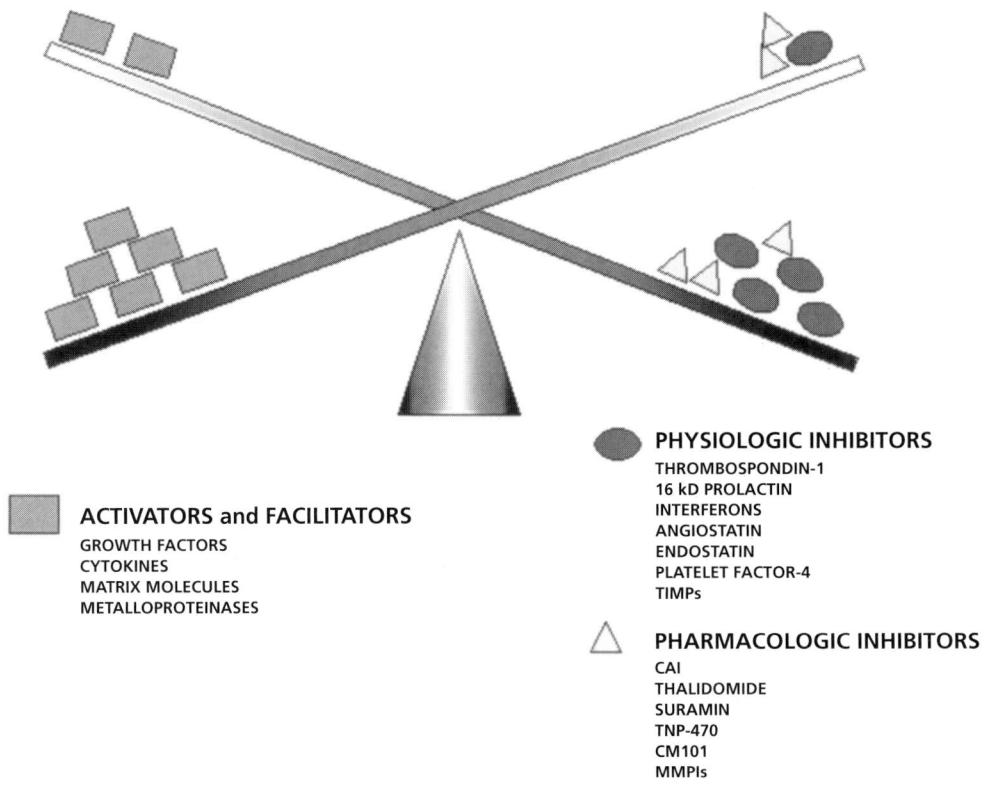

ACTIVATORS and FACILITATORS
GROWTH FACTORS
CYTOKINES
MATRIX MOLECULES
METALLOPROTEINASES

PHYSIOLOGIC INHIBITORS
THROMBOSPONDIN-1
16 kD PROLACTIN
INTERFERONS
ANGIOSTATIN
ENDOSTATIN
PLATELET FACTOR-4
TIMPs

PHARMACOLOGIC INHIBITORS
CAI
THALIDOMIDE
SURAMIN
TNP-470
CM101
MMPIs

FIG. 4-3. Schematic representation of angiogenesis. Vascular homeostasis represents a balance between physiologic activators and inhibitors of vessel formation. This balance is disrupted in cancer. Pharmacologic agents have been targeted at various elements of the angiogenic cascade in attempts to shift the balance away from an environment favorable to cancer.

inflammation, and tumor secretion of proangiogenic cytokines, growth factors, and matrix remodeling causes expression of a pro-invasive phenotype in the endothelial cells. This is manifest by local degradation of the capillary basement membrane, followed by endothelial-cell invasion into the surrounding stroma and migration of endothelial cells in the direction of the angiogenic stimulus. Proliferation of endothelial cells occurs at the leading edge of the migrating column, and the endothelial cells begin to organize into three-dimensional structures to form new capillary tubes (2, 97). The switch of endothelial cells from quiescent to invasive and proliferative is regulated by angiostimulatory and angiostatic signals (92). These include cytokines, fibrin, ECM molecules and fragments, and integrins, among others (98–101). Important factors in this process are listed in Table 4.2 (99,102–104). These different angioregulatory processes have been targeted for therapeutic inhibition in cancer and inflammation and stimulation in vascular deficiency diseases and chronic wounds. The results of these efforts are promising, as some cancers are highly responsive to antiangiogenic therapy. Investigators are characterizing a number of new molecular pathways that may be involved in the process of

angiogenesis. Examples of these pathways include the ephrin (105, 106), notch (107), hedgehog (108), sprouty (109), roundabouts and slits pathways (110). These may prove to be novel sites for molecular targeting. Table 4.3 lists a variety of biologic agents, and Figure 4.3 illustrates the balance between activators and inhibitors of angiogenesis in both physiologic and pathophysiologic states. Also shown are pharmacologic agents employed in the restoration of balance between the activating and inhibiting factors.

Vascular Endothelial Growth Factor

VEGF, also described initially as vascular permeability factor, was purified from ovarian cancer xenograft ascites (104,111). It is a mitogen for vascular endothelial cells, induces capillary tube formation, causes increased vascular permeability and protein extravasation, stimulates endothelial-cell migration, and stimulates a strong endothelial-cell survival signal (112). It has critical roles in normal gynecologic function, including endometrial cycling, ovarian follicle maturation and corpus luteum formation and regression (113), and in gynecologic pathologies, including endometri-

TABLE 4.2. *Overview of angiogenic growth factors and signals*

Factor	Function
Basic fibroblast growth factor (bFGF)	Induces tumor and endothelial cellular proliferation Stimulates endothelial cell migration Induces protease secretion Induces morphogenesis
Vascular endothelial growth factor (VEGF)	Induces proliferation of endothelial cells Increases vascular permeability Induces production of urokinase plasminogen activator by endothelial cells Induces lymphangiogenesis Induces Bcl-2 and A1 in endothelial cells (survival pathway)
Interleukin-8 (IL-8)	Cytokine stimulating growth, motility Pro-inflammatory cytokine
Platelet-derived growth factor (PDGF)	Stimulates endothelial cell proliferation Induces production of bFGF Promotes cellular motility Increases production of proteases
Hepatocyte growth factor/scatter factor (HGF/SF)	Increases endothelial cell migration Increases invasion Increases production of proteases Increases PDGF levels Survival pathway
Epidermal growth factor (EGF)	Increases endothelial cell migration Increases invasion Increase production of proteases Increases PDGF, VEGF, levels of others Survival pathway
Transforming growth factor-α (TGF-α)	Increases endothelial cell migration Increases invasion Increases production of proteases Increases PDGF levels Survival pathways
Transforming growth factor-β (TGF-β)	Increases endothelial cell migration Increases invasion Increases production of proteases

ovarian carcinoma where VEGF is expressed by tumor cells in primary and metastatic ovarian carcinoma (119). Additionally, the VEGF receptors Flt and KDR are also present and functional in ovarian cancer cells that co-express VEGF. This was the first example of localization of VEGFR-2/KDR expression in nonendothelial cells.

Circulating VEGF concentrations may be influenced by numerous factors including hormones, cytokines, and hypoxia, leading to increased levels of VEGF and a prolonged half-life of VEGF mRNA (120). A strong correlation exists between the degree of vascularization of a tumor and VEGF expression (121,122). The plasma and urine concentrations of VEGF increase during tumor progression. Similar data have also been published in ovarian cancer. In a study of advanced epithelial ovarian carcinomas, patients with tumors expressing higher levels of VEGF had shorter survival compared to those who did not express high levels of VEGF (123). Concordant results have also been found with serum levels of VEGF (124). VEGF is a product of known tumor growth-factor–signaling cascades, such as the lysophosphatidic acid (LPA) pathway in ovarian cancer (125,126). There it has been shown to be produced in and secreted into ascites, increasing the ascites burden through its vascular permeability activity (127,128). The role of VEGF in this has been confirmed by Hu and colleagues (128), who treated mice with A4.6.1, a monoclonal antibody to VEGF in combination with paclitaxel. When used in concert, both tumor burden and ascitic volume decreased. This diminution was larger than an additive effect between the two agents. Thus, VEGF is a prognostic factor and molecular target for gynecologic malignancies.

Bevacizumab is a recombinant humanized version of the murine antihuman VEGF monoclonal antibody. It has been shown that VEGF-neutralizing antibody inhibited VEGF-

TABLE 4.3. *Molecular targets of angiogenesis and corresponding agents*

Target	Drug
Vascular endothelial growth factor (VEGF)	Bevicizuamab HuMV833
Vascular endothelial growth factor receptor-1/2 (VEGFR-1/2)	Su5416 Su6668 Su101
Fibroblast growth factor receptor-1 (FGFR-1)	Su6668
Epidermal growth factor receptor (EGFR)	Gefitnib BiBx 1382 BS OSI-774 IMC-C225 Imatinib mesylate (Gleevec)
Platelet-derived growth factor receptor (PDGFR)	Su6668
Calcium influx	CAI
Tumor necrosis factor-α (TNF-αR)	Etanercept

osis (114,115) and polycystic ovarian disease (116). VEGF is expressed in the proliferative-phase endometrium and plays a role in fallopian tube function during ovulation (117). Expression is upregulated in a variety of tumors, including all gynecologic malignancies (33,118). It has been shown that VEGF is expressed in tumor cells and stromal support cells as well as in endothelial cells, which is an indication that VEGF is a paracrine mediator of angiogenesis in cancer. Autocrine stimulation with VEGF has been demonstrated in

induced signaling, resulting in reduced angiogenesis and tumor growth. Phase I and II studies have indicated that it is generally well tolerated as a single agent and in chemotherapeutic combination. It has been reported to reduce vascularity and tumor burden in a renal-cell cancer trial (129) and in colon cancer (130). A Phase II study of bevacizumab is ongoing in ovarian cancer at this writing, and preliminary discussion suggests that it may be an active agent. Preclinical studies have shown this agent to be at least additive when combined with chemotherapy for multiple cancers, including ovarian cancer. In addition to direct targeting of VEGF with bevacizumab, a number of small-molecule inhibitors of the VEGF receptors have been developed and have reached clinical trials. KDR is the most commonly targeted. Preclinical data have shown this approach to be active in reducing endothelial-cell proliferation, migration, and vascular development, and xenograft models have confirmed activity in a number of solid tumors (104,131–134). Several compounds have reached Phase II–III trials, although none has been reported as having single-agent efficacy.

Epidermal Growth Factor (EGF)

Epidermal growth factor (EGF) is a potent mitogen and motogen for many tumor-cell types and endothelial cells (135). It is presented as a prototype for growth-factor pathways that have successfully been subjects of molecularly targeted therapeutics. EGF expression has been correlated with malignant invasion and angiogenesis in a variety of tumors (136–142). This is a pathway that is both selective and/or inducible. It was shown that tumors that produce and secrete EGF can upregulate expression of EGFR in the local vasculature. This was associated with an antivascular and anti-tumor response to EGFR inhibition (143). This is important, as it also suggests a mechanism for escape from single molecular targeted therapies, as seen by tumor production of basic fibroblast growth factor (bFGF) when VEGF is downregulated (144–146).

The EGFR pathway has been shown to be important in gynecologic cancers. Patients with epithelial ovarian carcinoma with circulating EGF concentrations less than 1 ng/mL had significantly better survival than those with higher EGF concentrations (147). Increased expression of EGF receptor (ErbB1/HER-1) and HER-2/neu has been associated with risk of metastasis and reduced survival in ovarian carcinoma in some series (147–150). Nikura and colleagues (151) showed that the expression of EGF-related proteins correlated with the stage in ovarian cancers. Investigation of the putative anti-angiogenic activity of EGFR antagonists should be included in the translational investigation of this class of agents. Application of this approach is complicated by the EGFR (Her) family of receptors, as they have the ability to heterodimerize and activate downstream pathways regulating malignant proliferation and invasive behavior. Her-2/neu is not as overexpressed in gynecologic malignan-

cies as in breast cancer, but nonetheless is a poor prognostic factor (152). Overexpression of Her-2/neu has been shown to overcome therapeutic inhibition of EGFR kinase intervention owing to shifting the balance from EGFR homodimers to neu/EGFR heterodimers that overcome inhibition of the EGFR (153). Thus, it may be important to evaluate the expression of the family of receptors and/or to identify expression of the family of ligands to optimize therapeutic intervention of this pathway. Optimal intervention may require combinations of inhibitors that target multiple family members or multiple approaches to inhibition such as ligand competition and kinase inhibition concomitantly.

Platelet-derived Growth Factor

Platelet-derived growth factor (PDGF) expression has been demonstrated in epithelial ovarian carcinomas in contrast to borderline ovarian tumors (154). It may function as a paracrine stimulation of migration of endothelial cells. PDGF, a dimeric protein composed of two closely related A- and B-chain polypeptides encoded by independent genes (28), is a multifunctional cytokine that functions in an autocrine and paracrine fashion in ovarian cancer and angiogenesis. Three isoforms of PDGF (AA, AB, and BB) bind to two distinct receptors, PDGFRβ and α (155). The role of PDGF and PDGFR in promoting tumor angiogenesis is supported by various studies (156–159). Wang and colleagues showed that PDGF increased transcription and secretion of VEGF by PDGFRβ-expressing endothelial cells and demonstrated that activation of PI3K was important for this response, suggesting multiple levels of angiogenesis regulation (156). A similar study showed that PDGF-BB induced VEGF expression in pericytes and human vascular smooth muscle cells. This occurred through activation of the PI 3'K-AKT pathway in both human umbilical vein endothelial cells and human colon carcinoma cell lines, SW620 and HT29 (160). In addition, PDGF-mediated secretion of VEGF protected HUVECs from apoptosis caused by serum starvation, indicating an indirect role of PDGF in supporting tumor angiogenesis through activation of survival pathways (160). There is a greater expression of PDGF and PDGFRβ and α genes in ovarian cancer than in normal epithelial ovarian cells and borderline tumors (155,161). Henriksen and colleagues detected PDGF and PDGFRβ using immunohistochemistry in 73% and 36% of malignant tumor samples, respectively, with no staining in normal ovarian surface epithelial (OSE) cells or benign tumors (155). On the other hand, PDGFRβ was not detected in normal OSE or tumor cells but in the stroma of normal, benign, and malignant cells. Despite a short follow-up, cumulative survival probability at 40 months was 76% for those without detectable PDGFRα versus 28% for those expressing PDGFRβ, respectively. Those patients without detectable PDGFRβ had a survival equivalent to that of patients with early stage ovarian cancer. Stromal expression of PDGFRβ supports its role in angiogenesis and stromal reaction involved in tumor growth and invasion (54,155). The PDGFR is one of the molecular targets of imatinib mesylate (Gleevec). Preclinical studies have demonstrated that the use of imatinib will inhibit the PDGFR kinase, leading to the clinical hypothesis that it will have antiangiogenic activity and potentially direct anti-cancer activity. These hypotheses are the subjects of several phase II trials underway at this writing.

Non-growth-factor–related Angiogenic Molecular Targets

Several other molecular targets in invasion and angiogenesis have been tested in gynecologic malignancies. In addition to its cytoxic effect via stabilization of microtubules, paclitaxel had an antiangiogenic effect in xenografts apart from its cytoxic effect (162,163). As a control, cisplatin was shown to have little effect on angiogenesis. Several chemotherapeutic agents have been shown to have anti-angiogenic activity when administered in small doses in a more continuous exposures approach termed metronomic therapy (164). This approach has been studied in several model systems and is now in clinical trials.

Carboxyamido-triazole (CAI) is a synthetic compound that inhibits nonvoltage-gated calcium entry (96,165,166). Its inhibition of calcium influx-dependent signaling has resulted in blocking proliferation, adhesion, motility to extracellular matrix components, and proteolytic activity of tumor and endothelial cells (165,167). Disease stabilization in excess of 1 year was observed with limited toxicity (168,169). A Phase I trial of CAI with paclitaxel has resulted in a high proportion of objective responses in patients with gynecologic malignancies (170). A Phase II trial of CAI in ovarian cancer patients resulted in disease stabilization or objective response in 33% of patients (Kohn and colleagues, manuscript submitted).

Endostatin, a naturally occurring, 20-kD C-terminal fragment of collagen XVIII, was described as a naturally occurring antiangiogenic compound. With in vitro models, it has been shown to downregulate the expression of VEGF (171) and multiple genes involved in the process of angiogenesis including c-*myc*, c-*fos*, *max*, *cdc25B*, *MAPK-1*, *MAPK-2*, *preproendothelin-1*, *ET*$_B$ *receptor*, *AT*$_1$ *receptor* (172). At this time, a series of Phase I trials using endostatin have been completed (173–176). In all trials, the medication was very well tolerated. As a single agent, endostatin did not produce significant clinical benefits. No significant effects were seen in circulating levels of growth factors including bFGF and VEGF. However, noninvasive imaging suggested alterations in vascularization (173,175). Further data with endostatin in combination with other agents are forthcoming. Angiostatin, another anti-angiogenic peptide derived from collaged XV, has come under investigation (177). Although related by origin, the two molecules appear to differ slightly in their effects on the signaling cascade of angiogenesis.

Biology of Proteolysis

Local proteolysis occurs in both the tumor and stromal compartments. The process of intravasation and extravasation depends upon the ability to secrete proteolytic enzymes that are needed to degrade the barriers within the extracellular matrix. Overexpression of these enzymes occurs in almost all cells within the tumor-host microenvironment. Degradation of the basement membrane is affected by net proteolytic activity that is determined by the balance of activated proteolytic enzymes and their inhibitors. A positive correlation with tumor aggressiveness has been shown for a variety of degradative enzymes, including heparanases, and seryl-, thiol-, and metal-dependent enzymes. Comparisons were made between characterized cell lines such as Hep-3 and MDA-231, both highly malignant breast carcinomas and MCF-7, a less aggressive, hormone receptor–positive breast cancer cell line. The Hep-3 and MDA-231 cells demonstrated vascular intravasation, wherease the MCF-7 cells did not. Parallel results were seen comparing cells from characterized prostatic carcinomas including PC-3, a highly malignant, hormone-insensitive tumor, and LNCaP, a weakly malignant, hormone-sensitive cell line. This indicates that proteolytic behavior is a logical molecular target to interrupt the invasive and metastatic process in malignancy.

Matrix Metalloproteases

Matrix metalloproteases (MMPs) are a family of neutral metalloenzymes secreted as latent proenzymes. They require cleavage of the amino-terminal domain, and their activity depends on the presence of Zn^{2+} and Ca^{2+} (178,179). There are five subclasses grouped according to substrate specificity: interstitial collagenases, gelatinases, stromelysis, membrane-type MMPs, and elastases. Increased MMP activity has been detected and shown to correlate with invasion and metastatic potential in a wide rage of cancers, including gynecologic, lung, prostatic, breast, and pancreatic cancers (46,180,181). Fishman and colleagues (182) showed that epithelial ovarian carcinoma cells derived from primary ovarian tumors, metastatic lesions, or ascites overexpressed MMP-2 (gelatinase A) and MMP-9 (gelatinase B). Increased MT1-MMP (membrane type I metalloprotease) expression has been observed in invasive cervical carcinoma and lymph node metastases compared with its detection in noninvasive lesions (183). Expression of MMP-13 (collagenase-3) is abundant in vulvar carcinomas metastatic to lymph nodes. It was associated with tumor-cell expression of MTI-MMP and MMP-2 by stromal cells (184). Therefore, MMPs may serve as useful markers for detection of disease and/or as a target for therapeutic intervention in downregulation of tumor progression.

The activity of MMPs is regulated by a family of five proteins known as the tissue inhibitors of metalloproteases (TIMPs). In concert with MT1-MMP, TIMP-2 can regulate activation of MMP-2, whereas it can also directly inhibit MMP-2 function (185,186). The balance between levels of activated MT-MMPs, MMPs, and free TIMPs determines the balance between matrix degradation and matrix formation. Altering this equilibrium affects the progression of the invasive phenotype. MMPs and their inhibitors have been demonstrated to be present in most cervical adenocarcinomas independent of tumor grade or subtype, but with the exception of TIMP-1, they are not expressed in non-neoplastic endocervical epithelium (187). This has been used immunohistochemically to distinguish normal and malignant epithelia in cervical adenocarcinomas. Correlation with clinical outcomes did not suggest that the degree of positivity for MMP-1 correlated with prognosis (188). Similar data for MMPs and their inhibitors were found also for endometrial cancers and ovarian cancers (188). TIMPs have independent activities as well. TIMP-1 and TIMP-2 have been shown to inhibit tumor-induced angiogenesis in experimental systems (189) and to have antiapoptotic activity in lymphomas (190). It has been shown that TIMP-2 inhibits bFGF-induced stimulation of endothelial-cell proliferation independent of its ability to inhibit MMP activity (191). Such information has led to investigation of novel agents possessing the ability to affect the expression or activity of MMPs and TIMPs. Multiple synthetic inhibitors of MMPs have been studied in preclinical and clinical trials (192,193) demonstrating a variety of antineoplastic effects that have not translated successfully to the clinic. Clinical response to the MMP inhibitor class has been disappointing either from lack of activity and/or unexpected toxicity. A new generation of inhibitors has been developed and is reaching clinical testing (see Table 4.1 for examples) (194).

Seryl Proteases

Plasminogen activators (PAs) are serine-specific proteases that convert inactive plasminogen to active plasmin, a trypsin-like enzyme that degrades, a variety of proteins, including fibrin, fibronectin, type IV collagen, vitronectin, and laminin. Plasminogen activator exists in two forms: tissue-type plasminogen activator (tPA), the primary plasminogen activator in plasma, and urokinase plasminogen activator (uPA). uPA is involved primarily in cell-mediated proteolysis during macrophage invasion, wound healing, embryogenesis, and metastasis (195). Production of uPA in normal ovarian epithelial cells is reported as 17- to 38-fold lower than that found in ovarian carcinoma cells (196,197). The role of uPA in ovarian cancer has been shown in preclinical models. Its production is stimulated by multiple ovarian cancer-derived growth factors, such as lysophosphatidic acid (198). Approaches to molecular targeting of uPA and its related family of regulatory molecules have been limited to date; however, new agents are now reaching preclinical testing. These include a new drug, bikunin, a protease inhibitor found in amniotic fluid (199,200)

Biology of Migration

Neoplastic cells migrate from the primary tumor mass and successfully traverse tissue barriers to induce metastasis to a distant from the primary tumor (Fig. 4.1). This may involve simple cell locomotion from the primary into the interstitial stroma and subsequent shedding as seen in early ovarian cancer spread. Alternatively, it may require penetration and proteolysis of tissue obstacles as occurs in active invasion. Furthermore, tumor cells have to survive the stage of vascular transport and arrest in the capillary bed of distant organs to engage in a second round of invasion, called extravasation, whereby neoplastic cells exit from the vessel lumen into the surrounding stromal tissue (201). It is thus logical that most migration stimulation signals also activate cell survival signals. This key step in the cascade of events composing the invasive process of angiogenesis and metastasis is endothelial-cell and tumor-cell migration.

Tumor-cell motility responds to a number of stimuli including host-derived motility and growth factors, extracellular matrix components, and tumor-secreted autocrine factors. In order to achieve locomotion, cancer cells must initiate and maintain a complicated dynamic consisting of coordinated pseudopodal extension and attachment coupled with cell translocation and detachment. Examples of these include the insulin-like growth factors (IGF-I, IGF-II), hepatocyte growth factor (HGF, also known as scatter factor), FGFs, and PDGFs. IGF-I has been shown to induce a chemotactic response in human ovarian cancer (202).

HGF is a paracrine motility factor that acts at picomolar concentrations to stimulate motility of normal and malignant epithelial cells and normal and activated endothelial cells (203). The Ras mitogen-activated protein (MAP) kinase pathway has been implicated in most forms of growth-factor–induced motility (204,205), as has the PI 3′K pathway (204). In addition to growth factors, extracellular matrix proteins or fragment proteins have been shown to stimulate chemotaxis. This is an example of how the active process of invasion generates stimulants to further guide and sustain the process. Some of these ECM fragments, endostatin and angiostatin, have now been shown to have inhibitory activity (172,177,206). Thus, the dynamic process of migration in invasion and angiogenesis is the result of active positive and negative regulatory balance and the local environment. This process stops in physiologic invasion, such as in angiogenesis, when sufficient events have occurred. Regulation of migration is aberrant in malignancy, allowing for progression of the metastatic phenotype. Advancements in our understanding of autocrine and paracrine stimulation of migration have uncovered new molecular targets for therapeutic interruption.

Autotaxin and Lysophosphatidic Acid

The concept and role of autocrine growth factors is a long-standing and well-accepted biologic event. Many growth factors also stimulate motility. Autocrine motility factors that selectively regulate migration of normal and tumor cells have also now been identified. The defining member in this family is the cell surface-associated ectoenzyme, autotaxin (ATX), a potent motility-stimulating glycoprotein initially characterized and purified from the conditioned medium of a human melanoma cell line (207). ATX [or ATX/lyso-phospholipaseD (PLD)] expression in tissue has been shown to correlate with invasiveness of tumors such as breast cancer (208). ATX/lysoPLD has been shown to stimulate tumor-cell migration as well as endothelial-cell migration and tube formation (209). It has also been shown to stimulate angiogenesis in tumors in xenograft models. Dissection of the biochemistry of ATX is ongoing. Recent data indicate that ATX is involved in the production of lysophosphatidic acid (LPA) in the cellular microenvironment, cleaving lysophosatidylcholine (LPC) to release LPA. It is thus an important component of the LPA regulatory pathway and a novel extracellular molecular target.

LPA is known to induce tumor- and endothelial-cell proliferation, migration, and survival and is a driving growth and survival factor through its stimulation of the PI $3'$K pathway in ovarian cancer (127,210,211). ATX, by producing LPA, further amplifies the LPA signal by stimulating the generation of other growth and angiogenesis factors, such as VEGF (127). Significant levels of LPA can be found in body fluids, especially ascitic fluid from patients with ovarian cancer, the site from which it was first characterized. Our understanding of the metabolic pathways of LPA and characterization of its cloned and expressed G-protein-coupled LPA receptors have identified multiple therapeutic targets including its primary downstream PI $3'$K signaling pathway. G-protein-coupled receptors are the most successfully "druggable" targets; agents inhibiting the LPA receptor are awaited.

A myriad of forms of LPA exist, varying by the acyl groups at the SN1 and SN2 positions. These different isoforms convey overlapping and independent signals. More recently, the mechanisms through which biologically active forms of LPA are produced have been elucidated. ATX cleaves LPC to LPA by removal of the choline group (127, 212–214). Alternatively, LPA can be synthesized by hydrolysis of phosphatidic acid (PA) at the sn-2 position by soluble phospholipase A2 (sPLA2) or at the sn-1 position by phospholipase A1 (PLA1) (127). It is now logical that the pattern of expression and relationship to angiogenesis, invasion, and metastasis and aberrant expression is similar for both ATX and LPA. ATX/lysoPLD can promote angiogenesis both in vitro and in vivo (215). It is not clear whether this is due to generation of LPA or that ATX may have these properties directly. Interestingly, one study with ovarian cancer cells in vitro showed that LPA-induced migration could be inhibited by alendronate, a commercially available bisphosphonate (216) that is an agent used for osteoporosis treatment.

GENETICS OF INVASION, ANGIOGENESIS, AND METASTASIS

Malignant tumors consist of phenotypically heterogeneous populations that differ in their capacity to invade surrounding tissue, induce angiogenesis, and travel to distant sites, as only a few tumor cells that enter the circulation create metastatic foci (91,96,217–219). There are multiple levels of genetic and somatic factors that may be involved in regulating invasive and metastatic potential. As with cellular transformation, loss of function and gain of function events have been demonstrated in the regulation of metastatic suppression and promotion. Technologic advances and high-throughput systems are now being applied to the identification of new metastasis- and angiogenesis-associated genes. Table 3.3 provides examples of such agents and their associated targets.

NM23

NM23 is one of the earliest metastasis-suppressor genes described (220). NM23 is localized to chromosome 17q21 and encodes a nucleoside diphosphate (NDP) kinase. NM23-H1 and NM23-H2 expression has been associated inversely with lymph node metastases in several solid tumors including metastatic melanoma and ovarian, cervical, breast, gastrointestinal, and liver cancers. Consistent with these reports, Qian and colleagues (221) reported low levels of NM23 expression in ovarian tumors metastatic to lymph nodes. This finding has been described most markedly in ovarian tumors of the mucinous subtype. Marone and colleagues (222) have shown an inverse relationship between NM23 expression and lymph node involvement and myometrial invasion in cervical cancer and endometrial cancer. The mechanisms through which NM23 prevents metastasis remain unclear and under investigation. Current investigation suggests that there may be an effect on cytoskeletal organization and protein trafficking. Furthermore, NDP kinase may affect adhesion to the ECM. At this time, the role of NM23 in epithelial ovarian cancer remains unclear.

p53

p53, a tumor-suppressor gene localized to chromosome 17p13.1, regulates multiple cellular functions including gene transcription, DNA synthesis and repair, apoptosis, angiogenesis, invasion, and metastasis (223,224). p53 mutations have been described in many human cancers (225) including ovarian (226,227), endometrial (228), and cervical cancers (229). Studies have linked p53 to angiogenesis through several intermediates. Loss of wild-type p53 has been shown to downregulate thrombospondin-1, an ECM protein and potent inhibitor of angiogenesis. Higher levels of thrombospondin-1 expression were demonstrated in fibroblasts with wild-type p53, whereas loss of p53 was associated with a decrease in thrombospondin-1 (230). An inverse relationship between thombospondin-1 expression and angiogenic activity was also found. The migration of endothelial cells and cancer cell lines grown in media from wild-type *p53* fibroblasts was abrogated by antibody against thrombospondin-1. Thus, one mechanism of *p53*-mediated angiogenesis is its regulation of thrombospondin-1.

VEGF is expressed by numerous tumors under hypoxic stress and as a by-product of autocrine growth-factor loops. It is downstream of *p53* regulation through at least two mechanisms. Hypoxia-induced VEGF expression involves multiple intermediates, such as hypoxia-inducible factor-1? and *src* (231–234). Mukhopadhyay and colleagues (233) showed that hypoxia-induced *src*-mediated overexpression of VEGF may be augmented by mutant *p53*. VEGF expression was repressed 80% and VEGF promoter activity inhibited 70% in wild-type *p53* compared with *p53* mutant cell lines. They further demonstrated that *v-src* transfection increased VEGF promoter activity over empty vector transfectants. Wild-type *p53* had a dominant effect over *v-src*, causing a net decrease in VEGF expression. Mutant *p53* permitted the *v-src*–mediated VEGF induction (233). *p53* regulation of VEGF has been shown to correlate with mouse double minute-2 (MDM-2, the mouse analog of *p53*) oncoprotein expression. Zietz and colleagues (235) examined angiosarcomas for *p53* mutations, MDM-2 expression, and VEGF expression. Eighty percent of the angiosarcomas examined showed a correlation between elevated expression of MDM-2 and *p53* and increased VEGF expression. Mutant *p53* also has been shown to act through the protein kinase C pathway to increase VEGF expression (236,237). Thus, several mechanisms for *p53*-regulated VEGF expression exist, suggesting a key role for *p53* in the modulation of angiogenesis and multiple putative regulatory approaches that may be targeted for therapeutic gain.

PIK3CA

PIK3CA encodes the p110α catalytic subunit of PI 3'K. It sits in an amplicon on chromosome 3p26 identified by array-comparative genomic hybridization (77). Also within that amplicon is the p110β subunit of PI 3'K. It has been implicated in ovarian carcinogenesis and may act synergistically with RAS-mediated pathways to increase cell motility and metastasis (77). An increase in gene copy number, resulting in increased transcription and translation of *PIK3CA*, has been shown in ovarian cancer cell lines and patient samples (77). Increased protein was associated with phosphorylation of the PI 3'K p85 regulatory subunit, resulting in PI 3'K stimulation of the AKT/PKB survival pathway proteins and other downstream pathways (237,238). Further, PI 3'K has lipid kinase activity wherein it phosphorylates phosphatidylinositol 4,5-phosphate (PIP2) on the 3 position. PIP3 is a regulatory molecule for several other pathways involved in adhesion and motility, such as phospholipase C-δ (PLC-δ).

PLC-γ is involved in the detachment process required for motility (239). Like Her2-neu, this is an example of an amplification of a protein that in turn stimulates further augmentation of a signal that further promotes premetastatic function.

PTEN/MMAC-1

PTEN (phosphate and tensin homolog), also known as *MMAC-1*, has been identified as a tumor- and metastasis-suppressor gene. It is located at chromosome 10q23 and encodes a tyrosine and lipid phosphatase (240). *PTEN* mutations that result in the loss of the catalytic domain have been found in multiple human tumors, including glioblastoma, endometroid, endometrial and ovarian cancers, breast and prostatic cancers (241,242). *PTEN* inhibition of cell migration, spreading, and focal adhesion development has been shown to be mediated in part through focal adhesion kinase (FAK). Tamura and colleagues (243) demonstrated a 47% decrease in cell migration using stable wild-type PTEN transfections of NIH-3T3 cells. A significant decrease in integrin-mediated cell spreading and focal adhesion formation was associated with a 60% decrease in tyrosine phosphorylation of FAK in PTEN-overexpressing NIH-3T3 cells (243). Cell invasion, migration, and growth were downregulated by expressing *PTEN* and *FAK* in an ovarian cancer cell line, confirming the metastatic suppressor phenotype (244). Reversal of the metastatic phenotype was achieved also by inactivating phosphatase activity (244). *PTEN* is also important as a regulator of survival pathways. *PTEN* mutation functions similarly to genomic amplification and upregulation of the PI 3'K pathway and resultant upregulation of *AKt/PKB*. Loss of *PTEN* function removes inhibitory phosphatase activity and leaves AKT in its activated state, driving the proinvasive, proangiogenic, and prosurvival pathways. Thus, *PTEN* phosphatase activity and/or the regulatory status of the AKT pathway, immediately downstream of the PI 3'K oncogenic pathway in serous ovarian cancer and the *PTEN* suppressor pathway in endometroid endometrial and endometroid ovarian cancers, may be a critical signal for metastasis regulation.

ras Family

The ras family of oncoproteins function as integral modulators of signal transduction pathways and its members are potent inducers of mitogenesis and promoters of invasion when mutated or overexpressed (245). K-ras mutations have been found in 50% of mucinous ovarian cancers and 40% of LMP tumors but are generally uncommon in serous ovarian cancers (246). Approximately 10% to 30% of endometrial cancers show K-ras mutations (247,248). Harvey (H)-ras mutations have now been shown to be associated with the progression of papillomavirus-induced lesions in the uterine cervix (249). Although not always mutated or overexpressed, normal ras functions in invasion and angiogenesis in multiple ways. Several ras family members have been shown to regulate angiogenesis. Colorectal carcinoma cell lines constitutively expressing K-ras and H-ras-mutant cell lines have been shown to have increased VEGF expression (250). H-ras induction of VEGF expression was demonstrated to be mediated by TGF-β and bFGF expression, both of which are potent proangiogenic growth factors and are also produced in tumor autocrine and paracrine loops (251). Therapeutics directed at farnesylated proteins such as RAS have been shown to cause a decrease in VEGF expression in vitro and in vivo (252). This suggests that farnesyltransferase inhibitors may have a multifunctional role in cancer treatment (Table 4.1).

NOVEL TECHNOLOGIES TO STUDY THE MOLECULAR MECHANISM OF METASTASIS

Advances in technology are yielding new genes and new directions for studying the molecular mechanism of invasion, angiogenesis, and metastasis. To date, this information has been gained through examination of cultured cells and through animal models. Analysis from metastatic cell populations as they exist in their native environment may provide new insight into additional genes, proteins, and signal transduction pathways critical to metastastic events. Several technologies have been developed that may aid in the direct evaluation of metastatic cells.

Laser capture microdissection has provided more control in microdissection and markedly advanced our ability to evaluate events ongoing in human gynecologic and other tumors (253). Captured cells isolated from the appropriately fixed tissues can be used for genomic, expression, and protein studies. In one instance of the use of microdissected ovarian cancer cells from fixed tissues, a 50% loss of heterozygosity at chromosomal locus 8p21 was identified. This high rate of allelic loss, suggesting the presence of a tumor-suppressor gene at that locus, was missed by prior studies in which hand microdissection or no cell selection was performed and has led to further studies to identify the putative suppressor gene (254).

The use of frozen or ethanol-fixed tissues is necessary for gene and protein expression studies, and these products have been applied to investigative and high-throughput screening techniques. cDNA libraries from microdissected tissues have the advantage of representing the genes expressed from a specific cell population and can be compared to local stroma to discern differential gene regulation in the microenvironment. A relatively unknown growth factor, granulin-epithelin precursor (GEP), was identified as a possible ovarian cancer invasion gene from differential analysis of cDNA libraries from microdissected ovarian tumor epithelium (255,256). This finding would have been missed using non-

crodissected cells since this gene is expressed ubiquitously in stromal cells. GEP has been shown recently to be involved in angiogenesis and wound healing (257).

New proteomic technologies have been applied to gynecologic cancer tumors and serum samples through which to identify proteins and protein pathways involved in the development and progression of these cancers. Rho-guanine nucleotide dissociation inhibitor, Rho-GDI, is a protein that regulates the activation status of Rho, which is necessary for reorganization of the actin cytoskeleton and thus adhesion and migration. Rho-GDI was found to be upregulated in invasive epithelial ovarian cancers in the relatively crude approach of two-dimensional polyacrylamide gel electrophoresis. The finding has been validated using other proteomic approaches and immunohistochemical staining (258). This is another example of how the invasive and metastatic process can be investigated one gene or one protein at a time.

High-throughput approaches for global unbiased searches can also yield gene or protein family associations or signatures (259). Application of surface-enhanced or matrix-associated mass spectrometry with higher order artificial intelligence bioinformatics and mass sequencing is now being used to generate large volumes of information related to the malignant process. This will advance development of databases of proteomic information from which target validation and therapeutic application can proceed in a directed fashion.

CONCLUSIONS

Continued scientific, epidemiologic, and clinical advances are critically needed and will remain so until successful, reproducible and accurate early detection of gynecologic and other malignancies at the preinvasive or pretransformed stage becomes routine. Understanding the biology, regulation, and implications of the process of invasion and angiogenesis has and will continue to drive new biomarker and therapeutic target identification and intervention. The similarity in software and hardware between the dysregulated physiologic invasion of angiogenesis and the unregulated invasion of metastasis allows for a slightly more efficient scientific process and for duality of intervention. In fact, it could be described as stromal therapy, targeting the critical site of local microenvironmental interaction that is the important locale for scientific dissection and therapeutic application (54). Here, the process of autocrine and paracrine regulation, signal pathway activation, and cell-cell conversation are the most active, and the processes are similar between different histologic subtypes of gynecologic and other malignancies. The use of the newer and high-throughput technologies to identify collections of biologic targets rather than one gene or protein at a time can make the process more streamlined and provide a broader view of the interaction of events. Together, improved understanding, study of events in the patient populations, and cooperative and collaborative progress will allow us to overcome invasion and metastasis, the major causes of morbidity and mortality associated with gynecologic cancers.

REFERENCES

1. Paget S. The distribution of secondary growths in cancer of the breast. *Lancet* 1889;1:571–573.
2. Fidler IJ. Critical determinants of metastasis. *Semin Cancer Biol* 2002; 12:89–96.
3. Benedet JL, Bender H, Jones H 3rd, et al. FIGO staging classifications and clinical practice guidelines in the management of gynecologic cancers. FIGO Committee on Gynecologic Oncology. *Int J Gynaecol Obstet* 2000;70:209–262.
4. Creasman WT, Zaino RJ, Major FJ, et al. Early invasive carcinoma of the cervix (3 to 5 mm invasion): risk factors and prognosis. A Gynecologic Oncology Group study. *Am J Obstet Gynecol* 1998;178: 62–65.
5. Hirai Y, Takeshima N, Tate S, et al. Early invasive cervical adenocarcinoma: its potential for nodal metastasis or recurrence. *BJOG* 2003; 110:241–246.
6. Grisaru DA, Covens A, Franssen E, et al. Histopathologic score predicts recurrence free survival after radical surgery in patients with stage IA2-IB1–2 cervical carcinoma. *Cancer* 2003;97:1904–1908.
7. Sevin BU, Lu Y, Bloch DA, et al. Surgically defined prognostic parameters in patients with early cervical carcinoma. A multivariate survival tree analysis. *Cancer* 1996;78:1438–1446.
8. Bucy GS, Mendenhall WM, Morgan LS, et al. Clinical stage I and II endometrial carcinoma treated with surgery and/or radiation therapy: analysis of prognostic and treatment-related factors. *Gynecol Oncol* 1989;33:290–295.
9. Hicks ML, Piver MS, Puretz JL, et al. Survival in patients with para-aortic lymph node metastases from endometrial adenocarcinoma clinically limited to the uterus. *Int J Radiat Oncol Biol Phys* 1993;26: 607–611.
10. Steiner E, Eicher O, Sagemuller J, et al. Multivariate independent prognostic factors in endometrial carcinoma: a clinicopathologic study in 181 patients: 10 years experience at the Department of Obstetrics and Gynecology of the Mainz University. *Int J Gynecol Cancer* 2003; 13:197–203.
11. Taylor HC. Malignant and semimalignant tumors of the ovary. *Surg Gynecol Obstet* 1929;48:204.
12. di Re E, Grosso G, Raspagliesi F, et al. Fallopian tube cancer: incidence and role of lymphatic spread. *Gynecol Oncol* 1996;62:199–202.
13. Folkman J, Merler E, Abernathy C, et al. Isolation of a tumor factor responsible for angiogenesis. *J Exp Med* 1971;133:275–288.
14. Folkman J. Tumor angiogenesis: therapeutic implications. *N Engl J Med* 1971;285:1182–1186.
15. Folkman J, Hochberg M, Knighton D. Self-regulation of growth in three dimensions: the role of surface area limitations. In: Clarkson B, Baserga R, eds. *Control of proliferation in animal cells*. Cold Spring Harbor Conferences on Cell Proliferation 1. New York: Cold Spring Harbor Laboratory Press, 1974:833.
16. Liotta LA, Saidel GM, Kleinerman J. Diffusion model of tumor vascularization and growth. *Bull Math Biol* 1977;39:117–128.
17. Folkman J. What is the evidence that tumors are angiogenesis dependent? *J Natl Cancer Inst* 1990;82:4–6.
18. Folkman J. Angiogenesis in cancer, vascular, rheumatoid and other disease. *Nat Med* 1995;1:27–31.
19. Folkman J. The role of angiogenesis in tumor growth. *Semin Cancer Biol* 1992;3:65–71.
20. Weidner N, Semple JP, Welch WR, et al. Tumor angiogenesis and metastasis—correlation in invasive breast carcinoma. *N Engl J Med* 1991;324:1–8.
21. Abulafia O, Triest WE, Sherer DM, et al. Angiogenesis in endometrial hyperplasia and stage I endometrial carcinoma. *Obstet Gynecol* 1995; 86:479–485.
22. Ozuysal S, Bilgin T, Ozan H, et al. Angiogenesis in endometrial carcinoma: correlation with survival and clinicopathologic risk factors. *Gynecol Obstet Invest* 2003;55:173–177.
23. Ozalp S, Yalcin OT, Acikalin M, et al. Microvessel density (MVD) as a prognosticator in endometrial carcinoma. *Eur J Gynaecol Oncol* 2003;24:305–308.
24. Obermair A, Wanner C, Bilgi S, et al. Tumor angiogenesis in stage IB cervical cancer: correlation of microvessel density with survival. *Am J Obstet Gynecol* 1998;178:314–319.
25. Dellas A, Moch H, Schultheiss E, et al. Angiogenesis in cervical neoplasia: microvessel quantitation in precancerous lesions and invasive carcinomas with clinicopathological correlations. *Gynecol Oncol* 1997;67:27–33.
26. Schlenger K, Hockel M, Mitze M, et al. Tumor vascularity—a novel prognostic factor in advanced cervical carcinoma. *Gynecol Oncol* 1995;59:57–66.
27. Hollingsworth HC, Kohn EC, Steinberg SM, et al. Tumor angiogenesis in advanced stage ovarian carcinoma. *Am J Pathol* 1995;147: 33–41.
28. Wiggins DL, Granai CO, Steinhoff MM, et al. Tumor angiogenesis as a prognostic factor in cervical carcinoma. *Gynecol Oncol* 1995;56: 353–356.
29. Kaku T, Kamura T, Kinukawa N, et al. Angiogenesis in endometrial carcinoma. *Cancer* 1997;80:741–747.
30. Kirschner CV, Alanis-Amezcua JM, Martin VG, et al. Angiogenesis factor in endometrial carcinoma: a new prognostic indicator? *Am J Obstet Gynecol* 1996;174:1879–1882; discussion 1882–1874.
31. Behbakht K, Yordan EL, Casey C, et al. Prognostic indicators of survival in advanced endometrial cancer. *Gynecol Oncol* 1994;55: 363–367.
32. Obermair A, Tempfer C, Wasicky R, et al. Prognostic significance of tumor angiogenesis in endometrial cancer. *Obstet Gynecol* 1999; 93:367–371.
33. Paley PJ, Staskus KA, Gebhard K, et al. Vascular endothelial growth factor expression in early stage ovarian carcinoma. *Cancer* 1997;80: 98–106.
34. Beyer F. Patters of spread of invasive cancer of the human cervix. *Cancer* 1965;18:34.
35. Creasman WT, Morrow CP, Bundy BN, et al. Surgical pathologic spread patterns of endometrial cancer. A Gynecologic Oncology Group Study. *Cancer* 1987;60:2035–2041.
36. Guzick DS. Efficacy of screening for cervical cancer: a review. Am J Public Health 1978;68:125–134.
37. Jacobs A. Ovarian cancer. *Clin Symp* 1996;48:2–32.
38. Knapp RC, Friedman EA. Aortic lymph node metastases in early ovarian cancer. *Am J Obstet Gynecol* 1974;119:1013–1017.
39. Young RC, Decker DG, Wharton JT, et al. Staging laparotomy in early ovarian cancer. *JAMA* 1983;250:3072–3076.
40. Matsumoto K, Yoshikawa H, Yasugi T, et al. Distinct lymphatic spread of endometrial carcinoma in comparison with cervical and ovarian carcinomas. *Cancer Lett* 2002;180:83–89.
41. Chi DS, Liao JB, Leon LF, et al. Identification of prognostic factors in advanced epithelial ovarian carcinoma. *Gynecol Oncol* 2001;82: 532–537.
42. Hoskins WJ. Epithelial ovarian carcinoma: principles of primary surgery. *Gynecol Oncol* 1994;55:S91–S96.
43. Hoskins WJ, McGuire WP, Brady MF, et al. The effect of diameter of largest residual disease on survival after primary cytoreductive surgery in patients with suboptimal residual epithelial ovarian carcinoma. *Am J Obstet Gynecol* 1994;170:974–979; discussion 979–980.
44. Boente MP, Chi DS, Hoskins WJ. The role of surgery in the management of ovarian cancer: primary and interval cytoreductive surgery. *Semin Oncol* 1998;25:326–334.
45. Akahira JI, Yoshikawa H, Shimizu Y, et al. Prognostic factors of stage IV epithelial ovarian cancer: a multicenter retrospective study. *Gynecol Oncol* 2001;81:398–403.
46. Liotta LA, Stetler-Stevenson WG. Tumor invasion and metastasis: an imbalance of positive and negative regulation. *Cancer Res* 1991;51: 5054s–5059s.
47. Price JT, Bonovich MT, Kohn EC. The biochemistry of cancer dissemination. *Crit Rev Biochem Mol Biol* 1997;32:175–253.
48. Scotton CJ, Wilson JL, Scott K, et al. Multiple actions of the chemokine CXCL12 on epithelial tumor cells in human ovarian cancer. *Cancer Res* 2002;62:5930–5938.

49. Scotton CJ, Wilson JL, Milliken D, et al. Epithelial cancer cell migration: a role for chemokine receptors? *Cancer Res* 2001;61:4961–4965.

50. Scotton C, Milliken D, Wilson J, et al. Analysis of CC chemokine and chemokine receptor expression in solid ovarian tumours. *Br J Cancer* 2001;85:891–897.

51. Rossi D, Zlotnik A. The biology of chemokines and their receptors. *Annu Rev Immunol* 2000;18:217–242.

52. Balkwill F, Mantovani A. Inflammation and cancer: back to Virchow? *Lancet* 2001;357:539–545.

53. Vicari AP, Caux C. Chemokines in cancer. Cytokine Growth Factor Rev 2002;13:143–154.

54. Liotta LA, Kohn EC. The microenvironment of the tumour-host interface. *Nature* 2001;411:375–379.

55. Boyer B, Valles AM, Edme N. Induction and regulation of epithelial-mesenchymal transitions. Biochem Pharmacol 2000;60:1091–1099.

56. Stupack DG, Cho SY, Klemke RL. Molecular signaling mechanisms of cell migration and invasion. *Immunol Res* 2000;21:83–88.

57. Chen YT, Stewart DB, Nelson WJ. Coupling assembly of the E–cadherin/beta-catenin complex to efficient endoplasmic reticulum exit and basal-lateral membrane targeting of E-cadherin in polarized MDCK cells. *J Cell Biol* 1999;144:687–699.

58. Jou TS, Stewart DB, Stappert J, et al. Genetic and biochemical dissection of protein linkages in the cadherin-catenin complex. *Proc Natl Acad Sci U S A* 1995;92:5067–5071.

59. Pignatelli M. Integrins, cadherins, and catenins: molecular cross-talk in cancer cells. *J Pathol* 1998;186:1–2.

60. Klingelhofer J, Troyanovsky RB, Laur OY, et al. Exchange of catenins in cadherin–catenin complex. *Oncogene* 2003;22:1181–1188.

61. Christofori G, Semb H. The role of the cell–adhesion molecule E-cadherin as a tumour-suppressor gene. *Trends Biochem Sci* 1999;24:73–76.

62. Semb H, Christofori G. The tumor-suppressor function of E-cadherin. *Am J Hum Genet* 1998;63:1588–1593.

63. Mareel M, Vleminckx K, Vermeulen S, et al. Downregulation in vivo of the invasion-suppressor molecule E-cadherin in experimental and clinical cancer. *Princess Takamatsu Symp* 1994;24:63–80.

64. Mareel M, Vleminckx K, Vermeulen S, et al. E-cadherin expression: a counterbalance for cancer cell invasion. *Bull Cancer* 1992;79:347–355.

65. Kruk PA, Uitto VJ, Firth JD, et al. Reciprocal interactions between human ovarian surface epithelial cells and adjacent extracellular matrix. *Exp Cell Res* 1994;215:97–108.

66. Maines-Bandiera SL, Auersperg N. Increased E-cadherin expression in ovarian surface epithelium: an early step in metaplasia and dysplasia? Int J Gynecol Pathol 1997;16:250–255.

67. Davies BR, Worsley SD, Ponder BA. Expression of E-cadherin, alpha-catenin and beta-catenin in normal ovarian surface epithelium and epithelial ovarian cancers. *Histopathology* 1998;32:69–80.

68. Hashimoto M, Niwa O, Nitta Y, et al. Unstable expression of E-cadherin adhesion molecules in metastatic ovarian tumor cells. *Jpn J Cancer Res* 1989;80:459–463.

69. Inoue M, Ogawa H, Miyata M, et al. Expression of E–cadherin in normal, benign, and malignant tissues of female genital organs. *Am J Clin Pathol* 1992;98:76–80.

70. Veatch AL, Carson LF, Ramakrishnan S. Differential expression of the cell–cell adhesion molecule E-cadherin in ascites and solid human ovarian tumor cells. *Int J Cancer* 1994;58:393–399.

71. Peralta Soler A, Knudsen KA, Tecson–Miguel A, et al. Expression of E-cadherin and N-cadherin in surface epithelial-stromal tumors of the ovary distinguishes mucinous from serous and endometrioid tumors. *Hum Pathol* 1997;28:734–739.

72. Fujimoto J, Ichigo S, Hirose R, et al. Suppression of E-cadherin and alpha- and beta-catenin mRNA expression in the metastatic lesions of gynecological cancers. *Eur J Gynaecol Oncol* 1997;18:484–487.

73. Fujimoto J, Ichigo S, Hirose R, et al. Expression of E-cadherin and alpha- and beta-catenin mRNAs in ovarian cancers. *Cancer Lett* 1997;115:207–212.

74. Auersperg N, Pan J, Grove BD, et al. E-cadherin induces mesenchyma-to-epithelial transition in human ovarian surface epithelium. *Proc Natl Acad Sci U S A* 1999;96:6249–6254.

75. Arboleda MJ, Lyons JF, Kabbinavar FF, et al. Overexpression of AKT2/protein kinase Bbeta leads to up-regulation of beta1 integrins,

76. Frisch SM, Francis H. Disruption of epithelial cell-matrix interactions induces apoptosis. *J Cell Biol* 1994;124:619–626.

77. Shayesteh L, Lu Y, Kuo WL, et al. PIK3CA is implicated as an oncogene in ovarian cancer. *Nat Genet* 1999;21:99–102.

78. Tian B, Lessan K, Kahm J, et al. Beta 1 integrin regulates fibroblast viability during collagen matrix contraction through a phosphatidyl-inositol 3-kinase/Akt/protein kinase B signaling pathway. *J Biol Chem* 2002;277:24667–24675.

79. Bretland AJ, Lawry J, Sharrard RM. A study of death by anoikis in cultured epithelial cells. *Cell Prolif* 2001;34:199–210.

80. McFall A, Ulku A, Lambert QT, et al. Oncogenic Ras blocks anoikis by activation of a novel effector pathway independent of phosphatidyl-inositol 3-kinase. *Mol Cell Biol* 2001;21:5488–5499.

81. Lu Y, Lin YZ, LaPushin R, et al. The PTEN/MMAC1/TEP tumor suppressor gene decreases cell growth and induces apoptosis and an-oikis in breast cancer cells. *Oncogene* 1999;18:7034–7045.

82. Eliceiri BP, Cheresh DA. Role of alpha v integrins during angiogenesis. *Cancer J* 2000[6 Suppl 3]:S245–S249.

83. Naik MU, Mousa SA, Parkos CA, et al. Signaling through JAM-1 and alphavbeta3 is required for the angiogenic action of bFGF: dissociation of the JAM-1 and alphavbeta3 complex. *Blood* 2003;15:15.

84. Nam JO, Kim JE, Jeong HW, et al. Identification of the alphavbeta3 integrin-interacting motif of betaig-h3 and its anti-angiogenic effect. *J Biol Chem* 2003;278:25902–25909.

85. Sudhakar A, Sugimoto H, Yang C, et al. Human tumstatin and human endostatin exhibit distinct antiangiogenic activities mediated by alpha v beta 3 and alpha 5 beta 1 integrins. Proc Natl Acad Sci U S A 2003; 100:4766–4771.

86. Kerr JS, Slee AM, Mousa SA. The alpha v integrin antagonists as novel anticancer agents: an update. *Expert Opin Investig Drugs* 2002; 11:1765–1774.

87. Chattopadhyay N, Chatterjee A. Studies on the expression of al-pha(v)beta3 integrin receptors in non-malignant and malignant human cervical tumor tissues. *J Exp Clin Cancer Res* 2001;20:269–275.

88. Ahmed N, Riley C, Rice GE, et al. Alpha(v)beta(6) integrin—a marker for the malignant potential of epithelial ovarian cancer. *J Histochem Cytochem* 2002;50:1371–1380.

89. Ahmed N, Pansino F, Clyde R, et al. Overexpression of alpha(v)beta6 integrin in serous epithelial ovarian cancer regulates extracellular matrix degradation via the plasminogen activation cascade. *Carcinogenesis* 2002;23:237–244.

90. Liapis H, Adler LM, Wick MR, et al. Expression of alpha(v)beta3 integrin is less frequent in ovarian epithelial tumors of low malignant potential in contrast to ovarian carcinomas. *Hum Pathol* 1997;28:443–449.

91. Liotta LA, Kleinerman J, Saidel GM. Quantitative relationships of intravascular tumor cells, tumor vessels, and pulmonary metastases following tumor implantation. *Cancer Res* 1974;34:997–1004.

92. Hanahan D, Folkman J. Patterns and emerging mechanisms of the angiogenic switch during tumorigenesis. *Cell* 1996;86:353–364.

93. Holmgren L, O'Reilly MS, Folkman J. Dormancy of micrometastases: balanced proliferation and apoptosis in the presence of angiogenesis suppression. *Nat Med* 1995;1:149–153.

94. Klauber N, Parangi S, Flynn E, et al. Inhibition of angiogenesis and breast cancer in mice by the microtubule inhibitors 2-methoxyestra-diol and taxol. *Cancer Res* 1997;57:81–86.

95. Parangi S, O'Reilly M, Christofori G, et al. Antiangiogenic therapy of transgenic mice impairs de novo tumor growth. *Proc Natl Acad Sci U S A* 1996;93:2002–2007.

96. Kohn EC, Liotta LA. Molecular insights into cancer invasion: strategies for prevention and intervention. *Cancer Res* 1995;55:1856–1862.

97. Auerbach W, Auerbach R. Angiogenesis inhibition: a review. *Pharmacol Ther* 1994;63:265–311.

98. Dvorak HF. Tumors: wounds that do not heal. Similarities between tumor stroma generation and wound healing. *N Engl J Med* 1986; 315:1650–1659.

99. Folkman J, Klagsbrun M. Angiogenic factors. *Science* 1987;235:442–447.

100. Ingber DE, Folkman J. Mechanochemical switching between growth and differentiation during fibroblast growth factor–stimulated angio-

genesis in vitro: role of extracellular matrix. *J Cell Biol* 1989;109: 317–330.

101. O'Reilly MS. Angiostatin: an endogenous inhibitor of angiogenesis and of tumor growth. *EXS* 1997;79:273–294.

102. Joseph-Silverstein J, Silverstein RL. Cell adhesion molecules: an overview. *Cancer Invest* 1998;16:176–182.

103. Yancopoulos GD, Davis S, Gale NW, et al. Vascular-specific growth factors and blood vessel formation. *Nature* 2000;407:242–248.

104. Ferrara N, Gerber HP, LeCouter J. The biology of VEGF and its receptors. *Nat Med* 2003;9:669–676.

105. Pandey A, Shao H, Marks RM, et al. Role of B61, the ligand for the Eck receptor tyrosine kinase, in TNF-alpha–induced angiogenesis. *Science* 1995;268:567–569.

106. Ogawa K, Pasqualini R, Lindberg RA, et al. The ephrin-A1 ligand and its receptor, EphA2, are expressed during tumor neovascularization. *Oncogene* 2000;19:6043–6052.

107. Liu ZJ, Shirakawa T, Li Y, et al. Regulation of Notch1 and Dll4 by vascular endothelial growth factor in arterial endothelial cells: implications for modulating arteriogenesis and angiogenesis. *Mol Cell Biol* 2003;23:14–25.

108. Pola R, Ling LE, Silver M, et al. The morphogen Sonic hedgehog is an indirect angiogenic agent upregulating two families of angiogenic growth factors. *Nat Med* 2001;7:706–711.

109. Lee SH, Schloss DJ, Jarvis L, et al. Inhibition of angiogenesis by a mouse sprouty protein. *J Biol Chem* 2001;276:4128–4133.

110. Huminiecki L, Gorn M, Suchting S, et al. Magic roundabout is a new member of the roundabout receptor family that is endothelial specific and expressed at sites of active angiogenesis. *Genomics* 2002;79: 547–552.

111. Senger DR, Galli SJ, Dvorak AM, et al. Tumor cells secrete a vascular permeability factor that promotes accumulation of ascites fluid. *Science* 1983;219:983–985.

112. Ferrara N, Houck K, Jakeman L, et al. Molecular and biological properties of the vascular endothelial growth factor family of proteins. *Endocr Rev* 1992;13:18–32.

113. Ferrara N, Chen H, Davis–Smyth T, et al. Vascular endothelial growth factor is essential for corpus luteum angiogenesis. *Nat Med* 1998;4: 336–340.

114. McLaren J, Prentice A, Charnock–Jones DS, et al. Vascular endothelial growth factor (VEGF) concentrations are elevated in peritoneal fluid of women with endometriosis. *Hum Reprod* 1996;11:220–223.

115. Hull ML, Charnock-Jones DS, Chan CL, et al. Antiangiogenic agents are effective inhibitors of endometriosis. *J Clin Endocrinol Metab* 2003;88:2889–2899.

116. Ferrara N, Frantz G, LeCouter J, et al. Differential expression of the angiogenic factor genes vascular endothelial growth factor (VEGF) and endocrine gland–derived VEGF in normal and polycystic human ovaries. *Am J Pathol* 2003;162:1881–1893.

117. Gordon JD, Mesiano S, Zaloudek CJ, et al. Vascular endothelial growth factor localization in human ovary and fallopian tubes: possible role in reproductive function and ovarian cyst formation. *J Clin Endocrinol Metab* 1996;81:353–359.

118. Olson TA, Mohanraj D, Carson LF, et al. Vascular permeability factor gene expression in normal and neoplastic human ovaries. *Cancer Res* 1994;54:276–280.

119. Boocock CA, Charnock-Jones DS, Sharkey AM, et al. Expression of vascular endothelial growth factor and its receptors flt and KDR in ovarian carcinoma. *J Natl Cancer Inst* 1995;87:506–516.

120. Klagsbrun M, D'Amore PA. Vascular endothelial growth factor and its receptors. *Cytokine Growth Factor Rev* 1996;7:259–270.

121. Guidi AJ, Abu-Jawdeh G, Berse B, et al. Vascular permeability factor (vascular endothelial growth factor) expression and angiogenesis in cervical neoplasia. *J Natl Cancer Inst* 1995;87:1237–1245.

122. Guidi AJ, Abu-Jawdeh G, Tognazzi K, et al. Expression of vascular permeability factor (vascular endothelial growth factor) and its receptors in endometrial carcinoma. *Cancer* 1996;78:454–460.

123. Hartenbach EM, Olson TA, Goswitz JJ, et al. Vascular endothelial growth factor (VEGF) expression and survival in human epithelial ovarian carcinomas. *Cancer Lett* 1997;121:169–175.

124. Tempfer C, Obermair A, Hefler L, et al. Vascular endothelial growth factor serum concentrations in ovarian cancer. *Obstet Gynecol* 1998; 92:360–363.

125. Hu YL, Albanese C, Pestell RG, et al. Dual mechanisms for lysophos-

126. Hu YL, Tee MK, Goetzl EJ, et al. Lysophosphatidic acid induction of vascular endothelial growth factor expression in human ovarian cancer cells. *J Natl Cancer Inst* 2001;93:762–768.

127. Mills GB, Moolenaar WH. The emerging role of lysophosphatidic acid in cancer. *Nat Rev: Cancer* 2003;3:582–591.

128. Hu L, Hofmann J, Zaloudek C, et al. Vascular endothelial growth factor immunoneutralization plus paclitaxel markedly reduces tumor burden and ascites in athymic mouse model of ovarian cancer. *Am J Pathol* 2002;161:1917–1924.

129. Yang JC, Haworth L, Sherry RM, et al. A randomized trial of bevacizumab, an anti-vascular endothelial growth factor antibody, for metastatic renal cancer. *N Engl J Med* 2003;349:427–434.

130. Giantonio BJ, Levy D, O'Dwyer PJ, et al. Bevacizumab (anti-VEGF) plus IFL (irinotecan, fluorouracil, leucovorin) as front-line therapy for advanced colorectal cancer (advCRC): Results from the Eastern Cooperative Oncology Group (ECOG) Study E2200., American Society of Clinical Oncology 2003 Annual Meeting, Chicago, IL, 2003.

131. Giles FJ, Cooper MA, Silverman L, et al. Phase II study of SU5416—a small-molecule, vascular endothelial growth factor tyrosine–kinase receptor inhibitor—in patients with refractory myeloproliferative diseases. *Cancer* 2003;97:1920–1928.

132. Hunt S. Technology evaluation: IMC–1C11, ImClone Systems. *Curr Opin Mol Ther* 2001;3:418–424.

133. Hasselbalch HC. SU6668 in idiopathic myelofibrosis—a rational therapeutic approach targeting several tyrosine kinases of importance for the myeloproliferation and the development of bone marrow fibrosis and angiogenesis. *Med Hypotheses* 2003;61:244–247.

134. Baselga J, Rischin D, Ranson M, et al. Phase I safety, pharmacokinetic, and pharmacodynamic trial of ZD1839, a selective oral epidermal growth factor receptor tyrosine kinase inhibitor, in patients with five selected solid tumor types. *J Clin Oncol* 2002;20:4292–4302.

135. Boonstra J, Rijken P, Humbel B, et al. The epidermal growth factor. *Cell Biol Int* 1995; 19:413–430.

136. Takahashi Y, Kitadai Y, Ellis LM, et al. Multiparametric in situ mRNA hybridization analysis of gastric biopsies predicts lymph node metastasis in patients with gastric carcinoma. *Jpn J Cancer Res* 2002; 93:1258–1265.

137. Weber KL, Doucet M, Price JE, et al. Blockade of epidermal growth factor receptor signaling leads to inhibition of renal cell carcinoma growth in the bone of nude mice. *Cancer Res* 2003;63:2940–2947.

138. Kim SJ, Uehara H, Karashima T, et al. Blockade of epidermal growth factor receptor signaling in tumor cells and tumor-associated endothelial cells for therapy of androgen-independent human prostate cancer growing in the bone of nude mice. *Clin Cancer Res* 2003;9: 1200–1210.

139. Kedar D, Baker CH, Killion JJ, et al. Blockade of the epidermal growth factor receptor signaling inhibits angiogenesis leading to regression of human renal cell carcinoma growing orthotopically in nude mice. *Clin Cancer Res* 2002;8:3592–3600.

140. Baker CH, Solorzano CC, Fidler IJ. Blockade of vascular endothelial growth factor receptor and epidermal growth factor receptor signaling for therapy of metastatic human pancreatic cancer. *Cancer Res* 2002; 62:1996–2003.

141. Bruns CJ, Solorzano CC, Harbison MT, et al. Blockade of the epidermal growth factor receptor signaling by a novel tyrosine kinase inhibitor leads to apoptosis of endothelial cells and therapy of human pancreatic carcinoma. *Cancer Res* 2000;60:2926–2935.

142. Radinsky R, Risin, Fan, et al. Level and function of epidermal growth factor receptor predict the metastatic potential of human colon carcinoma cells. *Clin Cancer Res* 1995;1:19–31.

143. Mathur RS, Mathur SP, Young RC. Up-regulation of epidermal growth factor-receptors (EGF-R) by nicotine in cervical cancer cell lines: this effect may be mediated by EGF. *Am J Reprod Immunol* 2000;44:114–120.

144. Izumi Y, Xu L, di Tomaso E, et al. Tumour biology: herceptin acts as an anti-angiogenic cocktail. *Nature* 2002;416:279–280.

145. Jain RK, Carmeliet PF. Vessels of death or life. *Sci Am* 2001;285: 38–45.

146. Fidler IJ. Angiogenic heterogeneity: regulation of neoplastic angiogenesis by the organ microenvironment. *J Natl Cancer Inst* 2001;93: 1040–1041.

147. Shah NG, Bhatavdekar JM, Doctor SS, et al. Circulating epidermal growth factor (EGF) and insulin-like growth factor-I (IGF-I) in patients with epithelial ovarian carcinoma. *Neoplasma* 1994;41: 241–243.

148. Hogdall EV, Christensen L, Kjaer SK, et al. Distribution of HER-2 overexpression in ovarian carcinoma tissue and its prognostic value in patients with ovarian carcinoma: from the Danish MALOVA Ovarian Cancer Study. *Cancer* 2003;98:66–73.

149. Khalifa MA, Mannel RS, Haraway SD, et al. Expression of EGFR, HER-2/neu, P53, and PCNA in endometrioid, serous papillary, and clear cell endometrial adenocarcinomas. *Gynecol Oncol* 1994;53: 84–92.

150. Baron AT, Lafky JM, Boardman CH, et al. Serum sErbB1 and epidermal growth factor levels as tumor biomarkers in women with stage III or IV epithelial ovarian cancer. *Cancer Epidemiol Biomarkers Prev* 1999;8:129–137.

151. Niikura H, Sasano H, Sato S, et al. Expression of epidermal growth factor–related proteins and epidermal growth factor receptor in common epithelial ovarian tumors. *Int J Gynecol Pathol* 1997;16:60–68.

152. Cirisano FD, Karlan BY. The role of the HER–2/neu oncogene in gynecologic cancers. *J Soc Gynecol Invest* 1996;3:99–105.

153. Hellstrom I, Goodman G, Pullman J, et al. Overexpression of HER-2 in ovarian carcinomas. *Cancer* 2001;61:2420–2423.

154. Link CJ, Jr., Kohn E, Reed E. The relationship between borderline ovarian tumors and epithelial ovarian carcinoma: epidemiologic, pathologic, and molecular aspects. *Gynecol Oncol* 1996;60:347–354.

155. Henriksen R, Funa K, Wilander E, et al. Expression and prognostic significance of platelet-derived growth factor and its receptors in epithelial ovarian neoplasms. *Cancer* 1993;53:4550–4554.

156. Wang D, Huang HJ, Kazlauskas A, et al. Induction of vascular endothelial growth factor expression in endothelial cells by platelet–derived growth factor through the activation of phosphatidylinositol 3-kinase. *Cancer* 1999;59:1464–1472.

157. Sundberg C, Ljungstrom M, Lindmark G, et al. Microvascular pericytes express platelet-derived growth factor-beta receptors in human healing wounds and colorectal adenocarcinoma. *Am J Pathol* 1993; 143:1377–1388.

158. Plate KH, Breier G, Farrell CL, et al. Platelet–derived growth factor receptor-beta is induced during tumor development and upregulated during tumor progression in endothelial cells in human gliomas. *Lab Invest* 1992;67:529–534.

159. Westphal JR, Van't Hullenaar R, Peek R, et al. Angiogenic balance in human melanoma: expression of VEGF, bFGF, IL-8, PDGF and angiostatin in relation to vascular density of xenografts in vivo. *Int J Cancer* 2000;86:768–776.

160. Reinmuth N, Liu W, Jung YD, et al. Induction of VEGF in perivascular cells defines a potential paracrine mechanism for endothelial cell survival. *FASEB J* 2001;15:1239–1241.

161. Versnel MA, Haarbrink M, Langerak AW, et al. Human ovarian tumors of epithelial origin express PDGF in vitro and in vivo. *Cancer Genet Cytogenet* 1994;73:60–64.

162. Belotti D, Rieppi M, Nicoletti MI, et al. Paclitaxel (Taxol®) inhibits motility of paclitaxel-resistant human ovarian carcinoma cells. *Clin Cancer* 1996;2:1725–1730.

163. Belotti D, Vergani V, Drudis T, et al. The microtubule-affecting drug paclitaxel has antiangiogenic activity. *Clin Cancer* 1996;2: 1843–1849.

164. Bocci G, Nicolaou KC, Kerbel RS. Protracted low-dose effects on human endothelial cell proliferation and survival in vitro reveal a selective antiangiogenic window for various chemotherapeutic drugs. *Cancer* 2002;62:6938–6943.

165. Kohn EC, Alessandro R, Spoonster J, et al. Angiogenesis: role of calcium-mediated signal transduction. *Proc Natl Acad Sci U S A* 1995; 92:1307–1311.

166. Kohn EC, Sandeen MA, Liotta LA. In vivo efficacy of a novel inhibitor of selected signal transduction pathways including calcium, arachidonate, and inositol phosphates. *Cancer* 1992;52:3208–3212.

167. Alessandro R, Masiero L, Lapidos K, et al. Endothelial cell spreading on type IV collagen and spreading-induced FAK phosphorylation is regulated by Ca2 + influx. *Biochem Biophys Res Commun* 1998;248: 635–640.

168. Kohn EC, Figg WD, Sarosy GA, et al. Phase I trial of micronized formulation carboxyamidotriazole in patients with refractory solid tumors: pharmacokinetics, clinical outcome, and comparison of formulations. *J Clin Oncol* 1997;15:1985–1993.

169. Kohn EC, Reed E, Sarosy G, et al. Clinical investigation of a cytostatic calcium influx inhibitor in patients with refractory cancers. *Cancer* 1996;56:569–573.

170. Kohn EC, Reed E, Sarosy GA, et al. A phase I trial of carboxyamido-triazole and paclitaxel for relapsed solid tumors: potential efficacy of the combination and demonstration of pharmacokinetic interaction. *Clin Cancer* 2001;7:1600–1609.

171. Hajitou A, Grignet C, Devy L, et al. The antitumoral effect of endostatin and angiostatin is associated with a down-regulation of vascular endothelial growth factor expression in tumor cells. *FASEB J* 2002; 16:1802–1804.

172. Shichiri M, Hirata Y. Antiangiogenesis signals by endostatin. *FASEB J* 2001;15:1044–1053.

173. Thomas JP, Arzoomanian RZ, Alberti D, et al. Phase I pharmacokinetic and pharmacodynamic study of recombinant human endostatin in patients with advanced solid tumors. *J Clin Oncol* 2003;21: 223–231.

174. Herbst RS, Hess KR, Tran HT, et al. Phase I study of recombinant human endostatin in patients with advanced solid tumors. *J Clin Oncol* 2002;20:3792–3803.

175. Eder JP, Jr., Supko JG, Clark JW, et al. Phase I clinical trial of recombinant human endostatin administered as a short intravenous infusion repeated daily. *J Clin Oncol* 2002;20:3772–3784.

176. Mundhenke C, Thomas JP, Wilding G, et al. Tissue examination to monitor antiangiogenic therapy: a phase I clinical trial with endostatin. *Clin Cancer Res* 2001;7:3366–3374.

177. Dell'Eva R, Pfeffer U, Indraccolo S, et al. Inhibition of tumor angiogenesis by angiostatin: from recombinant protein to gene therapy. *Endothelium* 2002;9:3–10.

178. Coussens LM, Werb Z. Matrix metalloproteinases and the development of cancer. *Chem Biol* 1996;3:895–904.

179. Kelly T, Yan Y, Osborne RL, et al. Proteolysis of extracellular matrix by invadopodia facilitates human breast cancer cell invasion and is mediated by matrix metalloproteinases. *Clin Exp Metastasis* 1998;16: 501–512.

180. Liotta LA, Saidel MG, Kleinerman J. The significance of hematogenous tumor cell clumps in the metastatic process. *Cancer* 1976;36: 889–894.

181. Liotta LA, Tryggvason K, Garbisa S, et al. Metastatic potential correlates with enzymatic degradation of basement membrane collagen. *Nature* 1980;284:67–68.

182. Fishman DA, Bafetti LM, Banionis S, et al. Production of extracellular matrix–degrading proteinases by primary cultures of human epithelial ovarian carcinoma cells. *Cancer* 1997;80:1457–1463.

183. Gilles C, Polette M, Piette J, et al. High level of MT-*MMP* expression is associated with invasiveness of cervical cancer cells. *Int J Cancer* 1996;65:209–213.

184. Johansson N, Vaalamo M, Grenman S, et al. Collagenase-3 (MMP-13) is expressed by tumor cells in invasive vulvar squamous cell carcinomas. *Am J Pathol* 1999;154:469–480.

185. Toth M, Chvyrkova I, Bernardo MM, et al. Pro-MMP–9 activation by the MT1-MMP/MMP-2 axis and MMP-3: role of TIMP-2 and plasma membranes. *Biochem Biophys Res Commun* 2003;308: 386–395.

186. Bernardo MM, Fridman R. TIMP-2 (tissue inhibitor of metalloproteinase-2) regulates MMP-2 (matrix metalloproteinase-2) activity in the extracellular environment after pro-MMP-2 activation by MT1 (membrane type 1)-MMP. *Biochem J* 2003(Pt 3):739–745.

187. Davidson B, Goldberg I, Liokumovich P, et al. Expression of metalloproteinases and their inhibitors in adenocarcinoma of the uterine cervix. *Int J Gynecol Pathol* 1998;17:295–301.

188. Moser PL, Kieback DG, Hefler L, et al. Immunohistochemical detection of matrix metalloproteinases (MMP) 1 and 2, and tissue inhibitor of metalloproteinase 2 (TIMP 2) in stage IB cervical cancer. *Anticancer Res* 1999;19:4391–4393.

189. Ikenaka Y, Yoshiji H, Kuriyama S, et al. Tissue inhibitor of metalloproteinases-1 (TIMP-1) inhibits tumor growth and angiogenesis in the TIMP-1 transgenic mouse model. *Int J Cancer* 2003;105:340–346.

190. Guedez L, Stetler-Stevenson WG, Wolff L, et al. In vitro suppression of programmed cell death of B cells by tissue inhibitor of metalloproteinases-1. *J Clin Invest* 1998;102:2002–2010.

191. Murphy AN, Unsworth EJ, Stetler-Stevenson WG. Tissue inhibitor of metalloproteinases-2 inhibits bFGF-induced human microvascular endothelial cell proliferation. *J Cell Physiol* 1993;157:351–358.

192. Crul M, Beerepoot LV, Stokvis E, et al. Clinical pharmacokinetics, pharmacodynamics and metabolism of the novel matrix metalloproteinase inhibitor ABT–518. *Cancer Chemother Pharmacol* 2002;50: 473–478.

193. Nyormoi O, Mills L, Bar-Eli M. An MMP-2/MMP-9 inhibitor, 5a, enhances apoptosis induced by ligands of the TNF receptor superfamily in cancer cells. *Cell Death Differ* 2003;10:558–569.

194. Coussens LM, Fingleton B, Matrisian LM. Matrix metalloproteinase inhibitors and cancer: trials and tribulations. *Science* 2002;295: 2387–2392.

195. Conese M, Blasi F. The urokinase/urokinase–receptor system and cancer invasion. *Baillieres Clin Haematol* 1995;8:365–389.

196. Kiziridou AD, Toliou T, Stefanou D, et al. u-PA expression in benign, borderline and malignant ovarian tumors. *Anticancer Res* 2002;22: 985–990.

197. Moser TL, Young TN, Rodriguez GC, et al. Secretion of extracellular matrix–degrading proteinases is increased in epithelial ovarian carcinoma. *Int J Cancer* 1994;56:552–559.

198. Pustilnik TB, Estrella V, Wiener JR, et al. Lysophosphatidic acid induces urokinase secretion by ovarian cancer cells. *Clin Cancer* 1999;5:3704–3710.

199. Suzuki M, Kobayashi H, Tanaka Y, et al. Bikunin target genes in ovarian cancer cells identified by microarray analysis. *J Biol Chem* 2003;278:14640–14646.

200. Kobayashi H, Suzuki M, Tanaka Y, et al. A Kunitz-type protease inhibitor, bikunin, inhibits ovarian cancer cell invasion by blocking the calcium-dependent transforming growth factor-beta 1 signaling cascade. *J Biol Chem* 2003;278:7790–7799.

201. Quigley JP, Armstrong PB. Tumor cell intravasation alu-cidated: the chick embryo opens the window. *Cell* 1998;94:281–284.

202. Kohn EC, Francis EA, Liotta LA, et al. Heterogeneity of the motility responses in malignant tumor cells: a biological basis for the diversity and homing of metastatic cells. *Int J Cancer* 1990;46:287–292.

203. Stoker M, Gherardi E, Perryman M, et al. Scatter factor is a fibroblast–derived modulator of epithelial cell mobility. *Nature* 1987; 327:239–242.

204. Ueoka Y, Kato K, Wake N. Hepatocyte growth factor modulates motility and invasiveness of ovarian carcinomas via ras mediated pathway. *Mol Cell Endocrinol* 2003;202:81–88.

205. Ueoka Y, Kato K, Kuriaki Y, et al. Hepatocyte growth factor modulates motility and invasiveness of ovarian carcinomas via Ras-mediated pathway. *Br J Cancer* 2000;82:891–899.

206. Folkman J. Role of angiogenesis in tumor growth and metastasis. *Semin Oncol* 2002;29:15–18.

207. Stracke ML, Krutzsch HC, Unsworth EJ, et al. Identification, purification, and partial sequence analysis of autotaxin, a novel motility-stimulating protein. *J Biol Chem* 1992;267:2524–2529.

208. Yang SY, Lee J, Park CG, et al. Expression of autotaxin (NPP-2) is closely linked to invasiveness of breast cancer cells. *Clin Exp Metastasis* 2002;19:603–608.

209. Nam SW, Clair T, Campo CK, et al. Autotaxin (ATX), a potent tumor motogen, augments invasive and metastatic potential of ras-transformed cells. *Oncogene* 2000;19:241–247.

210. Tanyi JL, Morris AJ, Wolf JK, et al. The human lipid phosphate phosphatase-3 decreases the growth, survival, and tumorigenesis of ovarian cancer cells: validation of the lysophosphatidic acid signaling cascade as a target for therapy in ovarian cancer. *Cancer* 2003;63: 1073–1082.

211. Fang X, Schummer M, Mao M, et al. Lysophosphatidic acid is a bioactive mediator in ovarian cancer. *Biochim Biophys Acta* 2002; 1582:257–264.

212. Koh E, Clair T, Woodhouse EC, et al. Site-directed mutations in the tumor–associated cytokine, autotaxin, eliminate nucleotide phosphodiesterase, lysophospholipase D, and motogenic activities. *Cancer* 2003;63:2042–2045.

213. Ferry G, Tellier E, Try A, et al. Autotaxin is released from adipocytes, catalyzes lysophosphatidic acid synthesis, and activates preadipocyte proliferation. Up-regulated expression with adipocyte differentiation and obesity. *J Biol Chem* 2003;278:18162–18169.

214. Umezu-Goto M, Kishi Y, Taira A, et al. Autotaxin has lysophospholipase D activity leading to tumor cell growth and motility by lysophosphatidic acid production. *J Cell Biol* 2002;158:227–233.

215. Nam SW, Clair T, Kim YS, et al. Autotaxin (NPP-2), a metastasis-enhancing is an angiogenic factor. *Cancer* 2001;61:6938–6944.

216. Sawada K, Morishige K, Tahara M, et al. Alendronate inhibits lysophosphatidic acid–induced migration of human ovarian cancer cells by attenuating the activation of rho. *Cancer* 2002;62:6015–6020.

217. Woodhouse EC, Chuaqui RF, Liotta LA. General mechanisms of metastasis. *Cancer* 1997;80:1529–1537.

218. Kang Y, Siegel PM, Shu W, et al. A multigenic program mediating breast cancer metastasis to bone. *Cancer Cell* 2003;3:537–549.

219. Siegel PM, Shu W, Cardiff RD, et al. Transforming growth factor beta signaling impairs Neu-induced mammary tumorigenesis while promoting pulmonary metastasis. *Proc Natl Acad Sci U S A* 2003; 100:8430–8435.

220. Steeg PS, Bevilacqua G, Kopper L, et al. Evidence for a novel gene associated with low tumor metastatic potential. *J Natl Cancer Inst* 1988;80:200–204.

221. Qian M, Feng Y, Xu L, et al. Expression of antimetastatic gene nm23-H1 in epithelial ovarian cancer. *Chin Med J (Engl)* 1997;110: 142–144.

222. Marone M, Scambia G, Ferrandina G, et al. Nm23 expression in endometrial and cervical cancer: inverse correlation with lymph node involvement and myometrial invasion. *Br J Cancer* 1996;74: 1063–1068.

223. Greenblatt MS, Bennett WP, Hollstein M, et al. Mutations in the p53 tumor suppressor gene: clues to cancer etiology and molecular pathogenesis. *Cancer* 1994;54:4855–4878.

224. Levine AJ, Momand J, Finlay CA. The p53 tumour suppressor gene. *Nature* 1991;351:453–456.

225. Hollstein M, Sidransky D, Vogelstein B, et al. p53 mutations in human cancers. *Science* 1991;253:49–53.

226. Kohler MF, Marks JR, Wiseman RW, et al. Spectrum of mutation and frequency of allelic deletion of the p53 gene in ovarian cancer. *J Natl Cancer Inst* 1993;85:1513–1519.

227. Skilling JS, Sood A, Niemann T, et al. An abundance of p53 null mutations in ovarian carcinoma. *Oncogene* 1996;13:117–123.

228. Tsuda H, Hirohashi S. Frequent occurrence of p53 gene mutations in uterine cancers at advanced clinical stage and with aggressive histological phenotypes. *Jpn J Cancer* 1992;83:1184–1191.

229. Borresen AL, Helland A, Nesland J, et al. Papillomaviruses, p53, and cervical cancer. *Lancet* 1992;339:1350–1351.

230. Dameron KM, Volpert OV, Tainsky MA, et al. Control of angiogenesis in fibroblasts by p53 regulation of thrombospondin-1. *Science* 1994;265:1582–1584.

231. Carmeliet P, Dor Y, Herbert JM, et al. Role of HIF-1alpha in hypoxia-mediated apoptosis, cell proliferation and tumour angiogenesis. *Nature* 1998;394:485–490.

232. Mazure NM, Chen EY, Laderoute KR, et al. Induction of vascular endothelial growth factor by hypoxia is modulated by a phosphatidylinositol 3-kinase/Akt signaling pathway in Ha-ras-transformed cells through a hypoxia inducible factor-1 transcriptional element. *Blood* 1997;90:3322–3331.

233. Mukhopadhyay D, Tsiokas L, Sukhatme VP. Wild–type p53 and v-Src exert opposing influences on human vascular endothelial growth factor gene expression. *Cancer* 1995;5:6161–6165.

234. Mukhopadhyay D, Tsiokas L, Zhou XM, et al. Hypoxic induction of human vascular endothelial growth factor expression through c-Src activation. *Nature* 1995;375:577–581.

235. Zietz C, Rossle M, Haas C, et al. MDM-2 oncoprotein overexpression, p53 gene mutation, and VEGF up-regulation in angiosarcomas. *Am J Pathol* 1998;153:1425–1433.

236. Kieser A, Weich HA, Brandner G, et al. Mutant p53 potentiates protein kinase C induction of vascular endothelial growth factor expression. *Oncogene* 1994;9:963–969.

237. Khwaja A, Rodriguez-Viciana P, Wennstrom S, et al. Matrix adhesion and Ras transformation both activate a phosphoinositide 3-OH kinase and protein kinase B/Akt cellular survival pathway. *EMBO J* 1997; 16:2783–2793.

238. Bondeva T, Pirola L, Bulgarelli-Leva G, et al. Bifurcation of lipid and protein kinase signals of PI3Kgamma to the protein kinases PKB and MAPK. *Science* 1998;282:293–296.

239. Wells AR, Grandis JR. Phospholipase C-gamma1 in tumor progression. *Clin Exp Metastasis* 2003;20:285–290.
240. Steck PA, Pershouse MA, Jasser SA, et al. Identification of a candidate tumour suppressor gene, MMAC1, at chromosome 10q23.3 that is mutated in multiple advanced cancers. *Nat Genet* 1997;15:356–362.
241. Risinger JI, Hayes AK, Berchuck A, et al. PTEN/MMAC1 mutations in endometrial cancers. *Cancer* 1997;57:4736–4738.
242. Tashiro H, Blazes MS, Wu R, et al. Mutations in PTEN are frequent in endometrial carcinoma but rare in other common gynecological malignancies. *Cancer* 1997;57:3935–3940.
243. Tamura M, Gu J, Matsumoto K, et al. Inhibition of cell migration, spreading, and focal adhesions by tumor suppressor PTEN. *Science* 1998;280:1614–1617.
244. Tamura M, Gu J, Takino T, et al. Tumor suppressor PTEN inhibition of cell invasion, migration, and growth: differential involvement of focal adhesion kinase and p130Cas. *Cancer* 1999;59:442–449.
245. Bourne HR, Sanders DA, McCormick F. The GTPase superfamily: conserved structure and molecular mechanism. *Nature* 1991;349:117–127.
246. Teneriello MG, Ebina M, Linnoila RI, et al. p53 and Ki-ras gene mutations in epithelial ovarian neoplasms. *Cancer* 1993;53:3103–3108.
247. Matias-Guiu X, Catasus L, Bussaglia E, et al. Molecular pathology of endometrial hyperplasia and carcinoma. *Hum Pathol* 2001;32:569–577.
248. Enomoto T, Inoue M, Perantoni AO, et al. K-ras activation in neoplasms of the human female reproductive tract. *Cancer* 1990;50:6139–6145.
249. Alonio LV, Picconi MA, Dalbert D, et al. Ha-ras oncogene mutation associated to progression of papillomavirus induced lesions of uterine cervix. *J Clin Virol* 2003;27:263–269.
250. Okada F, Rak JW, Croix BS, et al. Impact of oncogenes in tumor angiogenesis: mutant K-ras up-regulation of vascular endothelial growth factor/vascular permeability factor is necessary, but not sufficient for tumorigenicity of human colorectal carcinoma cells. *Proc Natl Acad Sci U S A* 1998;95:3609–3614.
251. Breier G, Blum S, Peli J, et al. Transforming growth factor-beta and Ras regulate the VEGF/VEGF-receptor system during tumor angiogenesis. *Int J Cancer* 2002;97:142–148.
252. Rak J, Mitsuhashi Y, Bayko L, et al. Mutant ras oncogenes upregulate VEGF/VPF expression: implications for induction and inhibition of tumor angiogenesis. *Cancer* 1995;55:4575–4580.
253. Emmert-Buck MR, Bonner RF, Smith PD, et al. Laser capture microdissection. *Science* 1996;274:998–1001.
254. Brown MR, Chuaqui R, Vocke CD, et al. Allelic loss on chromosome arm 8p: analysis of sporadic epithelial ovarian tumors. *Gynecol Oncol* 1999;74:98–102.
255. Jones MB, Spooner M, Kohn EC. The granulin-epithelin precursor: a putative new growth factor for ovarian cancer. *Gynecol Oncol* 2003;88:S136–139.
256. Jones MB, Michener CM, Blanchette JO, et al. The granulin-epithelin precursor/PC-cell–derived growth factor is a growth factor for epithelial ovarian cancer. *Clin Cancer* 2003;9:44–51.
257. He Z, Ong CH, Halper J, et al. Progranulin is a mdiator of he wound response. *Nat Med* 2003;9:225–229.
258. Jones MB, Krutzsch H, Shu H, et al. Proteomic analysis and identification of new biomarkers and therapeutic targets for invasive ovarian cancer. *Proteomics* 2002;2:76–84.
259. Petricoin EF, Zoon KC, Kohn EC, et al. Clinical proteomics: translating benchside promise into bedside reality. *Nat Rev Drug Discov* 2002;1:683–695.

CHAPTER 5

Oncogenes and Tumor-Suppressor Genes

Jeff Boyd and Andrew Berchuck

HISTORICAL PERSPECTIVE

Discoveries over the past three decades have brought us to a new frontier in cancer research that is founded upon the identification and understanding of the basic cellular processes that become disrupted during cancer development. Historically, numerous empirical models have been proposed to explain the etiology of cancers. Attention has focused on viruses, environmental agents, chemical carcinogens, and congenital predisposition. We now know that all of these factors may contribute to carcinogenesis by disrupting genes whose products are involved in regulating cell proliferation, senescence, death, and the ability to invade and survive in ectopic locations. Most cancers are believed to arise from a single progenitor cell that has sustained mutations in several of these critical genes (1).

The genetic basis of human cancer development was implied by the work of some of the earliest cell biologists and is now considered among the most robust of biologic paradigms. In the mid nineteenth century, the great German pathologist Rudolph Virchow recognized that metastatic cancer cells resemble those of the corresponding primary tumor, and in the course of developing his cell theory, postulated that all cells of a cancer may arise from a single progenitor (2). Thus, the neoplastic phenotype is heritable from one tumor cell generation to the next, prompting the famous aphorism widely attributed to him, *"onmis cellulae cellula"* (every cell from a cell). In the early 1900s, Theodor Boveri extended this concept to the cytogenetic level, suggesting that gains and losses of specific chromosomes might lead to abnormal cell division and other aspects of the cancer phenotype. In his remarkable, landmark treatise, *Zur Frage*

der Entstehung maligner Tumoren ("On the Origin of Malignant Tumors"), Boveri initiated the age of cancer genetics, presaging the existence of tumor-suppressor genes, oncogenes, cell cycle checkpoints, multistep tumor progression, cancer predisposition through tumor-suppressor genes, the clonal origin of tumors, and other aspects of the neoplastic phenotype (3).

It required another half century, however, for Boveri's predictions to begin to be realized, with the discovery by Nowell and Hungerford in 1960 of a specific chromosomal translocation (the Philadelphia chromosome), which is characteristic of chronic myeloid leukemia (4). Nowell later provided a detailed and modernized version of the earlier notion of Virchow and Boveri that tumors are monoclonal with his theory on the clonal evolution of tumor cell populations (5). At this time in the mid 1970s, the stage was now set for the discovery by Bishop and Varmus that genetic sequences homologous to the transforming gene (v-*src*) of an avian cancer retrovirus exist in the host chicken genome (6), and indeed in the genomes of vertebrates including humans (7). This was the first direct evidence for the existence of cellular "oncogenes," which laid the groundwork for the field of cancer molecular genetics and was a discovery of sufficient magnitude to warrant awarding of the Nobel Prize to Bishop and Varmus in 1989.

This brief history of cancer genetics comes full circle with discoveries in 1973 that the Philadelphia chromosome represents a reciprocal translocation involving chromosomes 9 and 22 (8), in 1983 that this translocation results in the constitutive activation of the cellular oncogene c-*abl* (9), and in 2001 that a specific inhibitor of the ABL tyrosine kinase (Gleevec) is associated with extraordinary efficacy in the treatment of a subset of patients with leukemias harboring the Philadelphia chromosome (10). Although this "bench to bedside" success story is so far the exception rather than the rule, the molecular genetic basis of cancer has been defined in sufficient detail to allow an unprecedented optimism that we will eventually attain a thorough understanding of

Jeff Boyd: Departments of Surgery and Medicine, Memorial Sloan–Kettering Cancer Center, New York, New York 10021
Andrew Berchuck: Department of Obstetrics and Gynecology, Division of Gynecologic Oncology, Duke University Medical Center, Durham, North Carolina 27710

the molecular etiology of cancer. Although the number of genes that may be mutated and contribute to the development of the various cancer types is large, perhaps in the hundreds, the problem is clearly not intractable. Recent successes in elucidating the sequence of the human genome and in using comprehensive gene expression profiles to classify human malignancies in clinically relevant contexts contributes to this optimism. As our understanding of the molecular pathogenesis of cancer evolves, it is reasonable to assume that this knowledge will facilitate the development of new approaches to prevention, early diagnosis, and treatment.

GENETIC PARADIGM OF TUMORIGENESIS

All cancers are genetic in origin in the sense that the driving force of tumor development is genetic mutation. A given tumor may arise through the accumulation of acquired (somatic) mutations or through the inheritance of a mutation(s) through the germline followed by the acquisition of additional somatic mutations. These two genetic scenarios distinguish what are colloquially referred to as ''sporadic'' and ''hereditary'' cancers, respectively (Fig. 5.1).

Although alterations in gene expression also contribute to the malignant phenotype, the sequential mutation of cancer-related genes leading to outgrowth of a clonal population of cells is the major determinant of whether a cancer develops as well as the time required for its development and progression. The data supporting this multistep genetic paradigm are extensive (11,12), but perhaps the most compelling evidence is that the age-specific incidence rates for most epithelial tumors increase at roughly the fourth to eighth power of elapsed time, suggesting that a series of four to eight genetic alterations are rate limiting for cancer development (13). Additionally, it would seem rather self-evident that the well-characterized histopathologic progression of several common tumor types, for example, through hyperplasia, dysplasia, carcinoma *in situ*, and invasive carcinoma, reflects this multistep, multigenic model at the morphologic level.

Genetic alterations in cancer cells occur in two major families of genes: oncogenes and tumor-suppressor genes. Proteins encoded by oncogenes may generally be viewed as stimulatory and those encoded by tumor-suppressor genes as inhibitory to the neoplastic phenotype. Gain-of-function mutations resulting in the activation of ''proto-oncogenes'' to oncogenes and loss-of-function mutations resulting in the inactivation of tumor-suppressor genes both are requisite for cancer development. Proto-oncogene mutations are nearly always somatic, presumably because such cellular dominant mutations in the germline are incompatible with normal development. Two known exceptions involve the *RET* and *MET* proto-oncogenes, mutations of which may be inherited through the germline, predisposing to multiple endocrine neoplasia type II (14) and papillary renal carcinoma (15), respectively. Tumor-suppressor gene mutations may be inherited or acquired somatically, and nearly all hereditary cancer syndromes for which predisposing genes have been identified are linked to mutant tumor-suppressor genes. Genes encoding proteins involved in various pathways of DNA repair have been proposed to represent a third class of genes involved in cancer development (16), but as will be discussed below, these genes possess many of the features of tumor-suppressor genes and will be considered as such in this chapter.

A human cancer represents the endpoint of a long and complex process involving multiple cellular changes in genotype and phenotype. Human solid tumors generally are monoclonal, with every cell in a given cancer having arisen from a single progenitor cell. This does imply that all cells of a tumor are genetically identical, as the genetic instability characteristic of most malignancies results in substantial genetic heterogeneity as clonal evolution occurs (17). Clonal evolution, or clonal expansion (Fig. 5.2), is the process through which a cell and its offspring sustain and accumulate multiple mutations with the stepwise selection of variant sublines (5,18). A long-term goal of studying the molecular

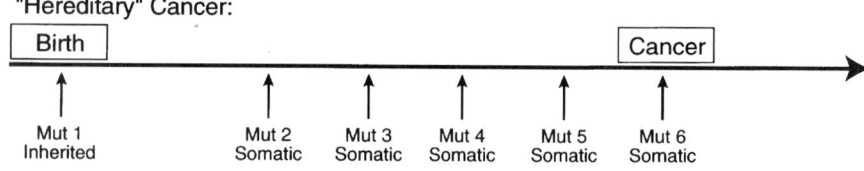

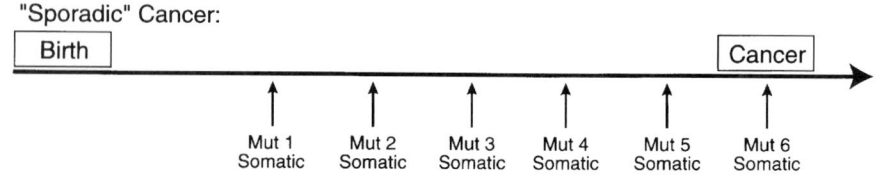

FIG. 5.1. All cancers are genetic. "Hereditary" cancers differ from "sporadic" cancers by virtue of association with a predisposing mutation inherited through the germline. In contrast, all of the mutations associated with sporadic tumorigenesis are acquired somatically.

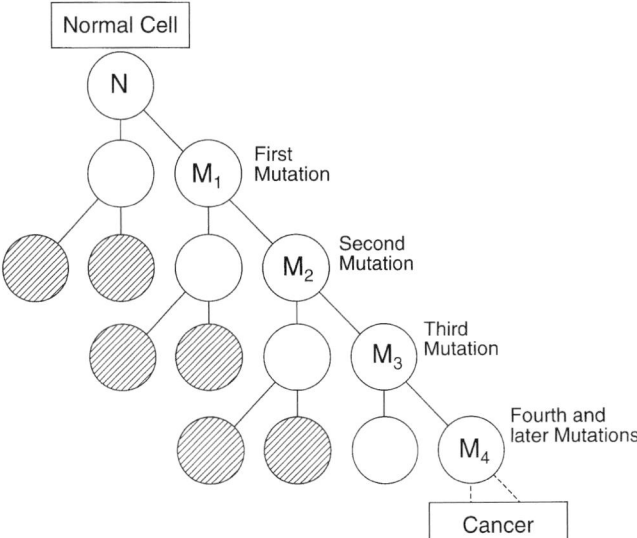

FIG. 5.2. Model of clonal evolution in neoplasia. Following the initiating mutation in a normal cell, stepwise genetic mutations and selective pressures result in a cancer consisting of a clonal population of cells all derived from the original progenitor cell. Each critical mutation in the evolving tumor may be viewed as having provided a selective advantage leading to clonal expansion.

genetics of a particular tumor type is to catalogue the specific genes that are affected by mutations and the relative order in which they are affected and, ultimately, to use this molecular genetic blueprint to improve methods of diagnosis, prognostication, and treatment. This task will undoubtedly prove to be difficult, however, because of the aforementioned genetic instability characteristic of cancers. There are multiple types of such instability that are operative at both the chromosomal and molecular levels (19). Distinguishing the genetic mutations that are simply the by-product of genetic instability from those that are critical to the neoplastic phenotype or, indeed, responsible for increasing genetic instability of one form or another is among the most formidable challenges to be faced in human cancer research.

The greatest progress in this context perhaps has been achieved for colorectal carcinoma, and a rudimentary model has been proposed that applies molecular detail to the general paradigm of multistep tumorigenesis and clonal evolution. In addition, most colon cancers are affected by one of two distinct types of genetic instability (19), and specific molecular genetic alterations have been shown to occur at discrete histologic stages of neoplastic progression in the colon; for example, mutation of the *APC* tumor-suppressor gene at a very early stage of hyperproliferation, mutation of the *KRAS* oncogene in the transition of early to intermediate adenoma, and mutation of the *TP53* gene tumor-suppressor gene in the transition of late adenoma to carcinoma (20). Several features of colorectal cancers facilitate this type of characterization, including the well-defined histopathologic progres-

sion of normal colonic epithelium to cancer and the accessibility of the various premalignant lesions for molecular analyses, as well as the occurrence of some of these genetic mutations in large fractions of colorectal tumors. This type of model is more difficult to apply to other cancer types, however, as premalignant precursor lesions for many solid tumor types (e.g., ovarian carcinoma) are not readily detectable, and few genetic alterations have been described that occur in major fractions of other cancer types.

TUMOR-SUPPRESSOR GENES

The protein products of tumor-suppressor genes normally function to inhibit various aspects of the neoplastic phenotype, such as cell proliferation, and are inactivated through loss-of-function mutations. Tumor-suppressor genes (having formerly been referred to variously as "recessive oncogenes" or "antioncogenes") are, by definition, recessive at the cellular level insofar as inactivation of both alleles (the copies present on both chromosomes) must occur for a phenotypic effect on tumorigenesis to be manifest. This is in contrast to the concept of mendelian recessivity, which refers to the necessity of germline transmission of two mutant alleles for a phenotype to be manifest. Most tumor-suppressor genes responsible for hereditary cancer syndromes are dominant at the mendelian level, which means that inheritance of a single mutant allele is sufficient to confer a high probability of developing the phenotype (cancer in this case); cellular recessivity must then occur through somatic inactivation of the second allele, and mechanisms through which this may occur are discussed below.

Several lines of evidence led to the discovery of tumor-suppressor genes. In addition to Boveri's predictions, a statistical analysis of carcinogen-induced mouse papillomas in 1942 led to the conclusion that a cellular recessive gene must be involved in carcinogenesis (21). Nearly 30 years later, Harris and colleagues demonstrated that somatic cell hybrids created from tumor cells and normal cells invariably expressed a nonmalignant phenotype, again implicating a cellular recessive class of cancer genes (22). Application of this notion of a recessive cancer gene was first applied to cancer predisposition by Knudson, who in 1971 published a statistical analysis of pediatric retinoblastoma and concluded that inactivation of both alleles of a single gene, one through the germline and one somatically, was necessary for tumor development (23). This concept became widely known as the "two-hit hypothesis" (a term not coined by Knudson), and is now inextricably linked to the more general concept of cellular recessivity of tumor-suppressor genes, the first of which to be discovered was the gene responsible for retinoblastoma, *RB1* (24).

This two-hit model for pediatric retinoblastoma is frequently misunderstood and misapplied, especially in the context of hereditary cancers generally, having become synonymous with the notion that inactivation of both alleles of a single gene is necessary *and* sufficient for tumorigenesis. It is important to recognize that this theory estimates only the number of events that are rate limiting for hereditary pediatric cancer development (25,26). As implied by Figure 5.1, most adult solid tumors, hereditary and sporadic, are likely to require mutations in multiple genes, most of which may occur at a relatively high frequency approaching zero-order kinetics, thus not appearing in the type of kinetic analysis performed by Knudson. This is especially true in cases where the inherited mutation affects a tumor-suppressor gene involved in DNA repair, with the result being increased genetic instability of one form or another.

The location and type of inactivating mutations in tumor-suppressor genes vary among genes and cancer types (Fig. 5.3). In some cases, most notably *TP53*, missense mutations occur that change a single amino acid in the encoded protein (27). More often, however, mutations in tumor-suppressor genes alter the base sequence such that the encoded protein product is truncated owing to generation of a premature stop codon. Truncated protein products may result from several types of mutational events. Included in this category are nonsense mutations in which a single base substitution changes the sequence from a specific amino acid to a stop codon (e.g., AAG to TAG). In addition, microdeletions or insertions of one or several nucleotides that disrupt the reading frame of the DNA (frameshifts) also lead to the generation of stop codons downstream in the gene. Less commonly, large genomic deletions are known sometimes to include

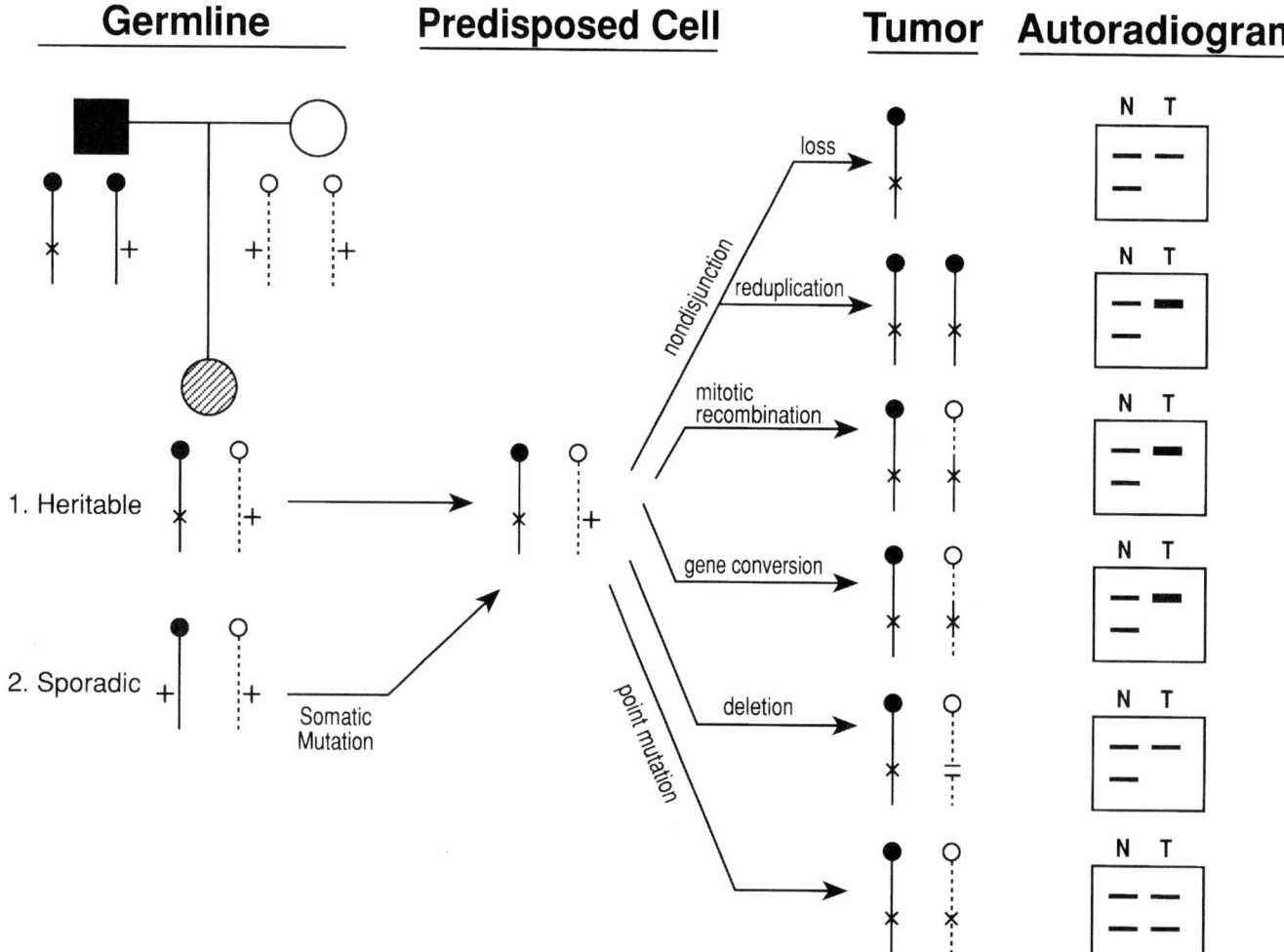

FIG. 5.3. Model for loss of tumor-suppressor gene function and recessivity at the cellular level. In hereditary tumorigenesis, one mutant allele is inherited from either parent, in which case the "predisposed cell" is, in effect, every cell in the body. In sporadic tumorigenesis, one allele is mutated somatically, in which case there is one predisposed cell in, for example, the ovarian surface epithelium. Loss of inactivation of the remaining wild-type allele may occur through any number of somatic chromosomal mechanisms, most commonly through nondisjunction or recombination. This so-called loss of heterozygosity is manifest through Southern blotting or polymerase chain reaction (PCR)–based procedures that allow visualization of loss of one or another polymorphic allele at or near the tumor-suppressor locus in tumor (T) DNA compared to nontumor (N) DNA from the same individual.

portions of tumor-suppressor genes. Any of these types of mutations in one allele, whether germline or somatic, is then "revealed" following somatic inactivation of the homologous wild-type allele, as discussed earlier. In theory, the same spectrum of mutational events could contribute to inactivation of the second allele, but what is typically observed in tumors is homozygosity or hemizygosity for the first mutation, indicating "loss" of the wild-type allele. As originally demonstrated for the retinoblastoma gene, loss of the second allele may occur through mitotic nondisjunction or recombination mechanisms or large deletions (Fig. 5.3) (28). This so-called "loss of heterozygosity" (LOH) has become recognized as the hallmark of tumor-suppressor gene inactivation. Table 5.1 lists some of the most well-characterized tumor-suppressor genes and the cancer syndromes and sporadic cancers with which they are associated.

Although some tumor-suppressor gene products reside outside the nucleus, many are nuclear proteins that prevent proliferation by arresting molecular pathways directly involved in cell cycle progression. The retinoblastoma gene (*RB1*) is a prototypical tumor-suppressor gene that encodes a nuclear protein involved in G_1 cell cycle arrest (29). Mutations in *RB1* have been noted primarily in retinoblastomas and sarcomas, but also occasionally in other types of cancers. In G_1, phosphorylated RB protein binds to the E2F transcription factor and prevents it from activating transcription of other genes involved in cell cycle progression (Fig. 5.4).

When RB is dephosphorylated, E2F is released and stimulates entry into the DNA synthetic (S) phase of the cell cycle. The phosphorylation of RB is regulated by a complex series of events that involves cyclins and cyclin-dependent kinases (CDKs). Cyclin-CDK complexes implicated in G_1 progression include cyclin D–CDK4/6, cyclin E–CDK2, and cyclin A–CDK2. Conversely, G_1 progression is restrained by CDK inhibitors such as p21, p16, and p27 (30,31). CDK inhibitors are classified as tumor-suppressor genes because of their ability to inhibit G_1 progression, and inactivation of CDK inhibitors, particularly the gene encoding p16 (*CDKN2A*), is a frequent event in human cancers (32). In contrast to the classic "two-hit" model of tumor-suppressor inactivation in which there is a mutation in one allele and deletion of the other, loss of p16 function usually involves deletion of both alleles or silencing of gene transcription due to promoter methylation. After DNA synthesis occurs in S phase, other classes of cyclins and genes such as *CHK1* and *CHK2* are involved in regulating progression from G_2 to mitosis (M phase). Germline mutations in the *CHK2* (*CHEK2*) gene have recently been implicated in Li-Fraumeni syndrome (33) and beast cancer predisposition (34).

Several tumor-suppressor genes involved in hereditary predisposition to cancer have been shown to function in the recognition and/or repair of various forms of DNA damage. The mutational inactivation of DNA repair genes contributes to tumorigenesis indirectly by promoting one or another type of genetic instability, which leads to the mutation of additional cancer-related genes. This unique mechanism of tumor suppression has led some to suggest that the DNA repair genes should represent a third cancer gene family. In all cases described to date, however, the genetic mechanism appears to involve a cellular recessive mechanism involving loss of function, which is consistent with the tumor-suppressor categorization. Perhaps more appropriate is the classifi-

TABLE 5.1. *Representative examples of tumor-suppressor genes mutated in human cancers*

Gene	Chromosomal location	Function	Hereditary cancers	Sporadic cancers
RB1	13q14	Cell cycle regulator	Retinoblastoma, osteosarcoma	Retinoblastoma, sarcomas, and others
WT1	11p13	Transcription factor	Wilms' tumor	Wilms' tumor
p53	17p13	Transcription factor; regulator of cell cycle, apoptosis	Li-Fraumeni syndrome	Many
APC	5q21-q22	Signal transduction	Familial adenomatous polyposis	Colorectal, gastric
VHL	3p26-p25	Transcriptional elongation	von Hippel-Lindau syndrome	Renal
MSH2, MLH1, MSH6	2p21, 3p21, 2p21	DNA mismatch repair	Hereditary nonpolyposis colorectal cancer	Colorectal, endometrial
BRCA1	17q12-21	DNA repair; transcription factor	Breast, ovary	Ovary (rare)
BRCA2	13q12	DNA repair, transcription factor	Breast, ovary	Ovary (rare)
NF1	17q11	Negative regulator of RAS	Neurofibromatosis	None
DPC4	18q21	TGF-beta signaling	None	Pancreatic
CDKN2A (p16)	9p21	Negative regulator of cyclin D	Melanoma	Many
PTEN (MMAC1)	10q24	Phosphatase	Cowden's disease	Many

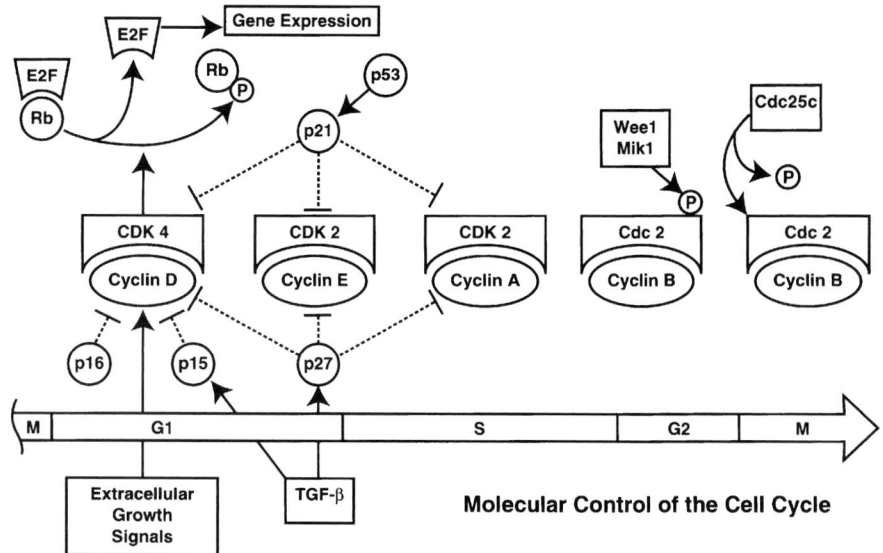

FIG. 5.4. Molecular control of cell cycle progression. A linear version of the various stages of the cell cycle is shown with the various cyclin/cyclin-dependent kinase complexes corresponding to the stages that they control.

cation scheme proposed by Kinzler and Vogelstein in which tumor-suppressor genes are subdivided into the categories of "gatekeepers" and "caretakers" (16). The former category includes those genes that function directly to inhibit cell proliferation or promote cell death (e.g., *RB1*, *TP53*, and *APC*), whereas the latter category consists of those genes that function to maintain genomic integrity (e.g., the mismatch repair genes involved in HNPCC, the nucleotide excision repair genes in involved in xeroderma pigmentosum, the *ATM* gene, and the *BRCA1* and *BRCA2* genes). It should be noted that some of these genes do not readily adhere to this distinction; *BRCA1* and *BRCA2*, for example, may function as both gatekeepers and caretakers.

Although numerous tumor-suppressor genes are mutated in various human cancers, only a limited number have been shown to play a significant role in gynecologic malignancies. Somatic mutations of *TP53* are observed at variable frequencies in gynecologic sarcomas and in ovarian and endometrial carcinomas, wherease viral inactivation of the p53 protein is a central mechanism in cervical tumorigenesis. Germline mutations in DNA mismatch repair genes, primarily *MSH2* or *MLH1*, lead to endometrial and ovarian carcinomas in association with the hereditary nonpolyposis colorectal cancer (HNPCC) syndrome, whereas epigenetic silencing of *MLH1* is associated with some cases of sporadic endometrial carcinoma. Most cases of hereditary ovarian carcinoma are associated with inherited mutation of *BRCA1* or *BRCA2*, whereas somatic mutations in these genes are occasionally observed in sporadic ovarian carcinomas. Finally, the *PTEN* gene is somatically mutated in many endometrial carcinomas. The role of these tumor suppressors in specific cancer types will be discussed in greater detail in a later section of this chapter following a discussion of the molecular function of these genes.

TP53

The *TP53* tumor-suppressor gene is the most frequently inactivated gene described thus far in both human cancers in general as well as specifically in gynecologic cancers. Originally identified through the physical interaction of its protein product with the SV40 large T antigen (35,36), *TP53* has been an intensely studied gene over the last 25 years. The gene was first classified as a cellular oncogene because of its apparent dominant transforming potential when transfected into rodent cells; subsequent studies confirmed, however, that the original cDNA clones used in the original studies all contained inactivating mutations, and that wild-type p53 is actually a tumor suppressor (37). Subsequently, several convergent lines of research provided unequivocal evidence that *p53* functions as a tumor-suppressor gene. Overexpression of exogenous wild-type p53 dramatically inhibits the growth of human colorectal carcinoma and osteosarcoma cell lines with endogenous *p53* mutations (38,39), and loss of heterozygosity at chromosome 17p, seen frequently in a variety of human tumors, correlates with mutational inactivation of *p53* in human colorectal carcinomas (40). Mutant p53 protein inactivates wild-type p53 protein by formation of inactive oligomeric complexes, reconciling the earlier observations of cellular transformation by the expression of exogenous mutant p53 constructs.

The most common class of mutation observed in *TP53* is the single nucleotide substitution that results in a missense alteration (change in one amino acid) (Fig. 5.5). Mutations that lead to truncated protein products are less common and include nonsense alterations, which directly encode premature stop codons, and frameshift mutations, which consist of small deletions or insertions. The vast majority (greater than 80%) of missense mutations occur within highly conserved regions in the middle third of p53 encoded by exons

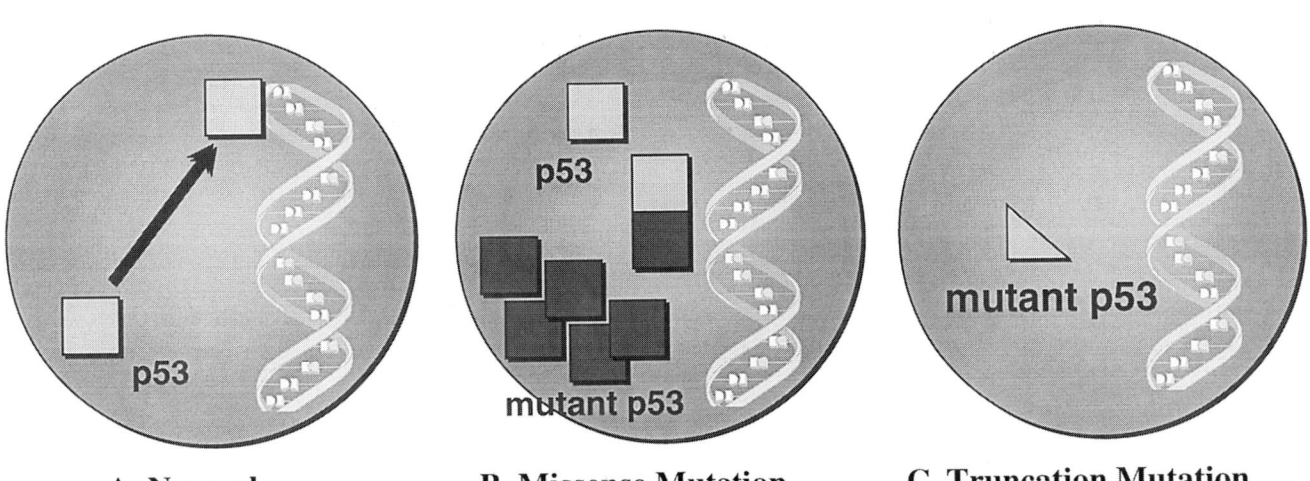

FIG. 5.5. Inactivation of the *p53* gene. **A:** Normal p53 protein binds to transcriptional regulatory elements in DNA. **B:** *p53* missense mutations encode proteins that no longer bind to DNA and the mutant protein complexes with and inactivates any remaining normal p53 in the nucleus. **C:** *p53* mutations that encode truncated protein products result in proteins that no longer bind to DNA, and these mutations usually are accompanied by deletion of the wild-type *p53* allele.

5 through 8 (41). Structural studies reveal that these regions are involved in a physical interaction between the p53 protein and DNA (42), consistent with the known role of p53 as a transcription factor. Disruption of the ability of p53 to interact with DNA appears to be a critical mechanism of p53 inactivation. Because p53 missense mutants are relatively resistant to degradation within the cell, mutant proteins accumulate within the nucleus leading to apparent "overexpression," which can be detected immunohistochemically. As a result, immunostaining of p53 has been used as a rapid method of screening cancers for *TP53* mutations. However, positive immunostaining usually is not observed in cancers with protein truncating (nonsense and frameshift) mutations; so immunohistochemical analysis is relatively imprecise when used as a surrogate for mutational analysis (43).

The mechanism through which the p53 protein functions as a central element in the suppression of tumorigenesis has now been revealed in great molecular detail (44–46). The *TP53* gene encodes a 53-kD nuclear phosphoprotein that exists at low levels in all normal cells. Functioning as a homotetrameric complex, p53 binds to DNA in a sequence-specific fashion to regulate gene transcription, and oncogenic forms of p53 inhibit this transcriptional activation. Expression of p53 can be downregulated when appropriate by the *MDM2* gene product, which targets it for degradation. Conversely, under other circumstances, p14^{ARF}, a negative regulator of MDM2, can increase expression of p53 leading to cell cycle arrest. It has become abundantly clear that the primary function of p53 is to activate the expression of genes involved in a DNA damage response pathway(s). Cell cycle arrest at the G_1-S checkpoint prior to DNA replication and at the G_2-M checkpoint prior to mitosis facilitates DNA damage repair and prevents mutations and aneuploidy, respec-

tively. Additionally, the induction of apoptosis (programmed cell death) may be considered to be a fail-safe mechanism in cases where irreparable DNA damage has occurred. The accumulation of p53 in response to DNA damage leads to an enhanced transcriptional activation of genes involved in apoptosis, such as *BAX*, *FAS*, and *BCL2*, as well as genes involved in cell cycle arrest, such as *CDKN1A* (encoding p21), which encodes a potent inhibitor of most CDKs. The molecular pathway linking DNA damage to p53 protein accumulation is still obscure. The carboxyl-terminal of p53 can bind nonspecifically to the ends of DNA molecules to catalyze renaturation and strand transfer, and can also bind to extrahelical regions of DNA affected by insertion or deletion mismatches. Double-strand breaks in DNA are especially efficient in causing p53 accumulation, probably through reduced ubiquitin-mediated proteolysis.

By activating transcription of these other genes, p53 induces cell cycle arrest in late G_1 phase or may induce apoptosis in response to DNA damage. Cells expressing mutant p53 do not pause in G_1 or undergo apoptosis, but continue directly into S phase before DNA repair is complete. *TP53* has therefore been referred to as the "guardian of the genome," as it prevents entry into S phase until the genome has been cleared of potentially carcinogenic mutations. As many chemotherapeutic drugs and radiation exert their cytotoxic effects through the induction of DNA damage and apoptosis, loss of p53 function may decrease sensitivity to these agents, enhancing the emergence of resistant populations of cancer cells. Indeed, p53 and p21 also are essential in maintaining the G_2-M checkpoint following γ irradiation (47). Although *TP53* mutation provides cells with a selective growth advantage, it also imposes a substantial cell cycle checkpoint deficit that permits cells to undergo DNA replication and mitosis in the presence of DNA damage. Theoretically, such checkpoint defects might be exploited to treat human cancers with abnormalities of p53 function (48).

DNA Mismatch Repair Genes

The hereditary nonpolyposis colorectal cancer syndrome (HNPCC) is an autosomal dominant cancer-predisposition syndrome described in detail in Chapter 2. In addition to colorectal cancers, HNPCC family members are at an increased risk for cancers of the endometrium, ovary, gastrointestinal sites, and upper urologic tract (49). This syndrome is believed to account for essentially all cases of hereditary endometrial carcinoma and up to 5% of cases of hereditary ovarian carcinoma. The estimated lifetime risk for endometrial cancer in female HNPCC gene carriers is 40% to 60%, corresponding to a relative risk of 13 to 20, whereas that of ovarian cancer is 6% to 20%, corresponding to a relative risk of 4 to 8 (50–55). Cloning and characterization of the genes responsible for HNPCC has provided substantial insight into the molecular etiology of HNPCC-associated malignancies as well as that of some sporadic gynecologic cancers.

Clues to the genetic basis of HNPCC first emerged in 1993 with several independent observations of somatic hypermutability of a class of DNA repetitive elements, known as "microsatellites," in sporadic and familial colorectal tumors (56–58). This observation was accompanied by reports of the genetic linkage of HNPCC kindreds to two loci: one on chromosome 2p (59) and another on chromosome 3p (60). Identification and cloning of the responsible genes at these loci, *MSH2* on chromosome 2 (61,62) and *MLH1* on chromosome 3 (63,64), quickly followed, together with the realization that these genes encoded human orthologs of yeast DNA mismatch repair proteins. Thus, the microsatellite instability phenotype previously observed in colorectal and other cancer types associated with the HNPCC syndrome could be explained by loss of function of these DNA mismatch repair (MMR) genes. In HNPCC, one of these genes is inherited in a mutant form through the germline followed by somatic loss of the wild-type allele, whereas in sporadic colorectal, endometrial, and gastric carcinomas affected by microsatellite instability, somatic silencing of *MLH1* through promoter hypermethylation appears to be the primary pathogenic mechanism (65).

Although most HNPCC kindreds appear to be linked to either *MSH2* or *MLH1*, a small fraction are linked to a third MMR gene, *MSH6*. There is some evidence that this gene may account for a substantial number of atypical or low-penetrance HNPCC kindreds, as well as those affected by a disproportionately high number of gynecologic cancers (66–69). Early evidence suggested that the MMR genes *PMS1* and *PMS2* may also play a role in HNPCC (70), but these observations were not widely confirmed, and a recent report involving investigators originally linking these genes

to HNPCC indicates that these genes are less likely to be involved in the syndrome (71).

The genetic instability phenotype associated with defective MMR genes is most readily observed through somatic length alterations in simple repeat sequences; for example, (CA)n, located throughout the genome and known as "microsatellites." Replication errors in these repeat sequences are probably common, and their inefficient repair results in the "microsatellite instability" phenotype. Since the discovery of mutant MMR genes and the corresponding microsatellite instability, a large number of studies have documented microsatellite instability in many sporadic tumor types, including those not associated with the HNPCC syndrome. Although mutations of the MMR genes have been readily identified in many HNPCC kindreds, somatic MMR gene mutations in sporadic tumors with the microsatellite instability phenotype are not commonly detected. It appears to be likely that hypermethylation of the *MLH1* promoter, resulting in downregulation of its expression, is the causative mechanism in most sporadic colorectal, gastric, and endometrial carcinomas with microsatellite instability (72–74).

It is not clear how microsatellite instability contributes to tumorigenesis in the endometrium, ovary, or other organs affected by the HNPCC syndrome. Microsatellites exist throughout the genome in predominantly noncoding regions of DNA. Simple repeat sequences are known to occur in the coding regions of genes, however, and their somatic mutation may result in loss of function for genes critical to the regulation of proliferation, invasion, or metastasis. Examples include genes encoding the transforming growth factor-β (TGF-β) receptor type II, the regulator of apoptosis BAX, and the insulin-like growth factor II receptor, all of which contain homopolymeric microsatellite repeats (e.g., A_8) that are mutated in some cancers with microsatellite instability (75). Frequently overlooked is the fact that the DNA mismatch repair system also functions in the repair of single nucleotide mismatches, so that defective mismatch repair would also lead to point mutations. Although the assay for this type of DNA damage is less straightforward than that for microsatellite instability, these single base-pair substitution mutations may play a more important role in tumorigenesis than microsatellite mutations.

BRCA1 and *BRACA2*

Approximately 10% of all epithelial ovarian carcinomas are associated with an autosomal dominant genetic predisposition. The great majority of these cases are attributable to the *BRCA1* or *BRCA2* tumor-suppressor genes and arise in the context of the hereditary breast and ovarian cancer syndrome, with a small fraction occurring in the HNPCC syndrome. (Clinical genetics aspects of this topic are discussed in Chapter 2.) Following the original reports of genetic linkage of early-onset breast cancer families (76) and some breast and ovarian cancer families (77) to the *BRCA1* locus on chromosome 17q, the *BRCA1* gene was cloned and characterized in 1994 (78). Shortly thereafter, the *BRCA2* locus on chromosome 13q was defined (79), and the gene was identified in 1995 (80). It is now clear that 60% to 90% of breast and ovarian cancer families are linked to *BRCA1*, with most of the remainder being linked to *BRCA2*, especially those with cases of male breast cancer.

The *BRCA1* and *BRCA2* genes share remarkable similarities in both structure and function, and will be discussed together. Both genes are unusually large, *BRCA1* consisting of 22 coding exons and a 7.8-kb mRNA transcript, and *BRCA2* consisting of 26 coding exons and a transcript exceeding 10 kb. Both genes contain a very large eleventh exon that encodes nearly half of the transcript, a start codon located in exon 2, and a high A/T to G/C content. Mutations occur throughout both genes, with no evidence of hotspots or clustering. Over 80% of detected mutations are nonsense or frameshift alterations that are predicted to lead to a truncated protein product, with the remainder representing missense and other miscellaneous "variants of uncertain significance" (81). Somatic LOH at the *BRCA* loci in breast and ovarian cancers invariably affects the wild-type allele, which is consistent with their function as classic tumor-suppressor genes (82–83). In the search for genotype/phenotype correlations in the *BRCA* genes, it has become clear that no strong association is likely to exist for *BRCA1*, but that *BRCA2* contains an "ovarian cancer cluster region" (OCCR) in exon 11; the ratio of ovarian to breast cancers is significantly higher in families segregating a *BRCA2* OCCR mutation (84) for reasons that remain obscure.

Prior to discovery of the *BRCA* genes, it was well documented that LOH affecting the relevant regions of chromosomes 17q and 13q was common in sporadic breast and ovarian cancers, and thus it came as a major surprise that somatic mutations in *BRCA1* and *BRCA2* are virtually nonexistent in sporadic breast cancers and rare in sporadic ovarian cancers. Gene silencing of *BRCA1* through promoter hypermethylation appears to play a role in the pathogenesis of a small fraction of sporadic ovarian cancers (85,86), whereas methylation of *BRCA2* has not been reported. Attempts to explain this paradox have centered on the argument that inactivation of *BRCA* genes early in development (i.e., through the germline) may be important for tumorigenesis, but not somatic inactivation in adult tissues. Recently, several lines of evidence suggest that inactivation of the *BRCA* pathway may play an important role in ovarian tumorigenesis through mechanisms other than inactivation of the *BRCA* genes themselves. Microarray-based gene expression profiling experiments indicate that rather than clustering as a third group, sporadic ovarian cancers all cluster as either *BRCA1*-like or *BRCA2*-like, implying the existence of a BRCA-deficient gene expression fingerprint in all ovarian cancers (87). Additionally, the novel EMSY protein was recently identified as a suppressor of BRCA2 activity, and the *EMSY* gene is amplified in 17% of ovarian cancers, providing a genetic

mechanism for inactivation of BRCA2 in some sporadic cancers (88).

Over the past 10 years, a large body of data has been generated with respect to BRCA function, which appears to be related for the two genes, but a coherent picture of precisely how these proteins function to suppress tumorigenicity remains elusive. Generally, there is substantial evidence for a role of BRCA1 and BRCA2 in cellular processes related to the prevention of genomic instability, including DNA damage recognition and repair, transcriptional regulation, and control of cell cycle checkpoints (89,90). A seminal research finding in this area was that BRCA1 colocalizes *in vivo* and physically associates *in vitro* with the RAD51 protein, known to function in the repair of double-strand DNA breaks, implying a role for BRCA1 in the control of recombination and genomic integrity (91). Other early work on the role of Brca2 in mouse development indicated that loss of the protein confers radiation hypersensitivity and also that Brca2 physically interacts with Rad51 in repair of double-strand DNA breaks (92). Remarkably, BRCA1 and BRCA2 proteins appear to be involved in the same biochemical pathway, mediated by RAD51, regulating genomic integrity.

Data derived from the study of embryonic cells and tissues from mice rendered nullizygous for *Brca1* or *Brca2* provide strong evidence for the role of these proteins in the response to DNA damage. An embryonic lethal phenotype is observed in mice with a homozygous null mutation in *Brca1* (93) or *Brca2* (92,94), suggesting their requirement for embryonic cellular proliferation prior to gastrulation. Partial rescue of this developmental lethality is achieved by simultaneous knockout of the *Tp53* gene (95,96), implying that the accumulation of DNA damage in *Brca* knockout mice leads to the arrest of cell division by p53, and that their concomitant knockout allows additional cell division to take place before eventual lethality. In cells from these Brca-deficient animals, gross chromosomal rearrangements are evident, and considerable data suggest that this chromosomal instability results from the inappropriate repair of DNA double-strand breaks during the S and G_2 phases of the cell cycle. Specifically, homology-directed repair of double-strand breaks, an error-free pathway, is defective in Brca1-deficient mouse cells (97–99) and in BRCA2-deficient human and mouse cells (100–102). The error-prone pathway of nonhomologous end joining remains intact in Brca-deficient cells, however, and the attempted repair of spontaneous and induced double-strand breaks because of inappropriate routing through this mechanism probably contributes to chromosomal instability observed in Brca-deficient cells. The precise roles of BRCA proteins in homology-directed repair remain to be determined, but evidence suggests that BRCA1 performs the general function of linking DNA damage sensing or signaling to effector components of the cellular response to DNA damage (90), whereas BRCA2 physically interacts with and controls the RAD51 recombinase (103), a catalytic activity essential for homologous recombination.

In contrast to BRCA2, there are considerable data linking the BRCA1 protein to other functions possibly involved in tumor suppression, especially the transcriptional regulation of gene expression. Fragments of BRCA1 are capable of transcriptional transactivation *in vitro* (104,105), and BRCA1 is a component of the RNA polymerase II holoenzyme (106) through its interaction with RNA helicase A (107). In response to DNA damage, BRCA1 functions as a p53-independent transactivator of the CDK inhibitor p21 (108,109). Ectopic expression of BRCA1 results in the p53-independent induction of GADD45 expression (110), as well as the selective coactivation of p53-dependent transcription (111), one target of which appears to be the gene encoding the G_2/M checkpoint control protein 14–3–3σ (112). Microarray-based expression profiling experiments indicate that the selective expression of BRCA1 in mouse and human cells leads to alterations in expression of numerous additional genes involved in cell cycle control and DNA repair (110,112,113).

Thus, the emerging model of BRCA function implies a dual role for the BRCA-deficient state in the initiation of tumorigenesis as well as targeted cancer therapy. In BRCA-deficient cells, the defective maintenance of genomic integrity may accelerate cancer initiation and progression, yet also render the resultant cancer more susceptible to therapeutic agents whose cytotoxic potential is mediated through the induction of the specific type of DNA damage that BRCA normally functions to repair. A number of commonly used cancer therapies are believed to cause DNA interstrand cross links, a lesion that appears to be repaired through creation of an intermediate double-strand break followed by homologous recombination. Prototypical agents from this mechanistic category include cisplatin, mitomycin C, and γ radiation (114). That BRCA-deficient cancers may respond favorably to this class of DNA damaging agents is suggested by studies in which modulation of BRCA1 expression in various isogenic cell clones is shown to affect sensitivity to cisplatin (115–117), mitomycin C (99), and γ radiation (118–121). This mechanism likely represents the underlying biologic basis for improved outcome in *BRCA*-linked hereditary ovarian cancer patients compared to matched sporadic cases (122–124). Further, this suggests a rational basis for trials investigating the efficacy of platinum-based chemotherapy in breast cancer patients with germline BRCA mutations.

PTEN

A novel tumor-suppressor gene responsible for the very rare, autosomal dominant hereditary cancer syndrome Cowden's disease was cloned and characterized in 1997 (125, 126). Cowden's disease, also known as multiple hamartoma syndrome, is characterized by benign hamartomas of multiple organs, including skin, intestine, breast, and thyroid. In addition to benign lesions, breast cancers develop in 30% to 50% of affected women and thyroid cancers occur in 10%

of affected individuals. Bannayan-Zonana syndrome, a closely related condition, was also subsequently found to be caused by the same gene (127). Named *PTEN*, this gene was originally noted to encode a likely tyrosine phosphatase with additional significant homologies to the cytoskeletal proteins tensin and auxilin. Early studies aimed at uncovering PTEN function indicated that its phosphatase activity may function to suppress tumorigenesis by negatively regulating cell interactions with the extracellular matrix, specifically the inhibition of integrin-mediated cell spreading and cell migration through dephosphorylation of focal adhesion kinase (FAK) (128). Additionally, expression of PTEN selectively inhibits activation of the extracellular signal-regulated kinase (ERK) mitogen-activated protein kinase (MAPK) pathway (129). Other cellular targets for the phosphatase activity of PTEN include elements of the phosphoinositide 3-kinase/AKT pathway (130). Because constitutive activation of either PI3-kinase or AKT is known to induce cellular transformation, an increase in the activity of this pathway caused by mutations in PTEN provided additional support for its complex role in tumor suppression. It is now well established that PTEN's lipid phosphatase activity, acting through the PI3K/AKT and MAPK pathways, plays a critical role in the regulation of growth arrest, apoptosis, and other important cellular functions (131).

Although endometrial carcinoma has been suggested to represent a component tumor of Cowden's syndrome according to revised diagnostic criteria (132), germline mutations in *PTEN* are not associated with a significant proportion of unselected endometrial carcinomas. Remarkably, however, sporadic endometrial carcinomas frequently exhibit loss of heterozygosity in a region of chromosome 10q that includes the *PTEN* gene (133,134). Mutation analyses of *PTEN* in endometrial carcinomas indicate that this gene is somatically inactivated in 30% to 50% of all such tumors (135–137), representing the most frequent molecular genetic alteration in endometrial cancers yet defined. Inactivation of *PTEN* may represent an early event in a subset of endometrial cancers, as mutations are detected at a significant frequency in premalignant endometrial hyperplasia specimens (138). Interestingly, *PTEN* mutations are also seen in a fraction of ovarian carcinomas of endometrioid histology (139), but not in those of serous or other histologic subtypes (137–140). More recent findings on the role of *PTEN* in specific gynecologic cancers will be discussed later in this chapter.

ONCOGENES

It has been convincingly demonstrated that alterations in genes whose products normally act to stimulate cell proliferation or other aspects of the neoplastic phenotype (oncogenes) can cause malignant transformation (Fig. 5.6) (141, 142). Oncogenes can be activated via several mechanisms. In solid tumors, the most common mechanism of oncogene

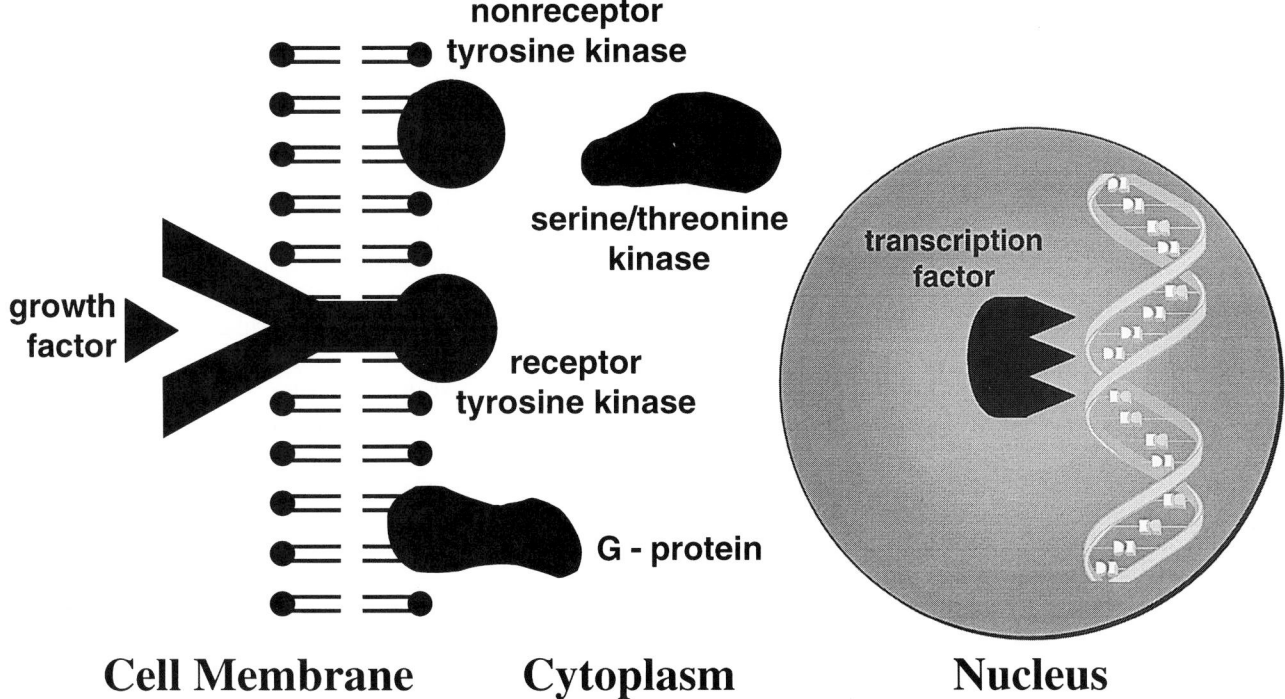

FIG. 5.6. Classes of oncogenes. Oncogene products generally are involved in stimulating proliferation from growth factors and their receptors on the outside of the cell to G-proteins and kinases inside the cell interior and ultimately nuclear transcription factors.

activation appears to be gene amplification with resultant overexpression of the corresponding protein. Instead of two copies of one of these genes, there may be as many as 40 copies. The *ERBB2* (HER-2/*neu*) oncogene is activated in this fashion. Some oncogenes may become resistant to inactivation when affected by specific point mutations in regulatory domains, resulting in constitutive signaling. The *RAS* family of oncogenes is prototypical in this regard. Finally, oncogenes may be translocated from one chromosomal location to another and then come under the influence of promoter sequences that cause overexpression of the gene. This mechanism frequently occurs in leukemias and lymphomas (e.g., the Philadelphia chromosome), but appears to be less common in solid tumors.

In various model systems and *in vitro*, many genes that are involved in normal pathways of cell proliferation, signal transduction, and transcriptional regulation can elicit neoplastic transformation when altered to overactive forms via amplification, mutation, translocation, or simple overexpression (Table 5.2). On this basis, a large number of genes have been classified as "oncogenic." However, the actual spectrum of such genes that have been shown to be altered mutationally in human cancers (the formal criterion for classification as an "oncogene") is much more limited. Presently, it appears that inactivation of tumor-suppressor genes is significantly more common than activation of oncogenes. This may reflect the fact that mutations are more apt to dis-

rupt the function of a gene than to create a product that is hyperactive. Alternatively, it is possible that the involvement of tumor-suppressor genes in malignant transformation has been more easily identifiable because of their association with hereditary cancer syndromes. In this section, the various

TABLE 5.2. *Classes of genes involved in growth stimulatory pathways*

Peptide growth factors	Corresponding receptors
Epidermal growth factor (EGF) and transforming growth factor (TGF-α)	EGF receptor (*ERBB1*)
Heregulln	*ERBB2* (HER-2/*NEU*), *ERBB3, ERBB4*
Insulin-like growth factors (IGF-I, IGF-II)	IGF-I and II receptors
Platelet-derived growth factor (PDGF)	PDGF receptor
Fibroblast growth factors (FGFs)	FGF receptors
Macrophage-colony stimulating factor (M-CSF)	M-CSF receptor (*FMS*)
Cytoplasmic factors	**Examples**
Nonreceptor tyrosine kinases	*ABL, SRC*
G proteins	*K-RAS, H-RAS*
Serine-threonine kinases	AKT2
Nuclear factors	**Examples**
Transcription factors	*MYC, JUN, FOS*
Cell-cycle progression factors	Cyclins, E2F

classes of oncogenes will be summarized with particular attention being paid to those that are altered in gynecologic cancers.

Peptide Growth Factors and Their Receptors

Peptide growth factors in the extracellular space can stimulate a cascade of molecular events that leads to proliferation by binding to cell membrane receptors. Unlike endocrine hormones, which are secreted into the blood stream to act in distant target organs, peptide growth factors usually act in the local environment. The concept that autocrine growth stimulation might be a key strategy by which cancer cell proliferation becomes autonomous has received considerable attention. In this model, it is postulated that cancers secrete stimulatory growth factors that then interact with receptors on the same cell. Although production of growth factors may play a role in enhancing proliferation associated with malignant transformation, they also are involved in development, stromal-epithelial communication, tissue regeneration, and wound healing. Thus, it remains unclear whether autocrine growth stimulation actually is a critical event in cancer development.

Cell membrane receptors that bind peptide growth factors are composed of an extracellular ligand-binding domain, a membrane-spanning region, and a cytoplasmic tyrosine kinase domain (143). More than a dozen receptor tyrosine kinases have been identified thus far that bind peptide growth factors. Binding of a growth factor to the extracellular domain results in aggregation and conformational shifts in the receptor and activation of the inner tyrosine kinase. This kinase phosphorylates tyrosine residues on both the growth factor receptor (autophosphorylation) and targets in the cell interior leading to activation of secondary signals. For example, phosphorylation of phospholipase C leads to breakdown of cell membrane phospholipids and generation of diacylglycerol and inositol-triphosphate (IP3), both of which play a role in propagation of the mitogenic signal.

Epidermal Growth Factor Receptor Family

The role of the epidermal growth factor (EGF) receptor family of transmembrane receptors and their ligands in growth regulation and transformation has been a prominent focus in cancer research over the past three decades (144). The salient findings will be summarized in this section. Initially, EGF and its receptor were found to be involved in growth and development in the mouse (145). EGF is a peptide growth factor of 53 amino acids that maintains its secondary structure by virtue of disulfide bonds between cysteine residues. At least five other peptide growth factors, including TGF-α, also interact with and activate the EGF receptor. TGF-α was so named because of its ability to act in concert with TGF-β to transform some types of cells in culture. EFG, TGF-α, and other EGF receptor ligands are produced as proforms that are inserted into the cell mem-

brane. The membrane anchored growth factor can interact with receptors on adjacent cells, a phenomenon known as juxtacrine growth regulation. Alternatively, the active peptide then can be cleaved and released into the extracellular space. The free peptide may interact with receptors on the same (autocrine) or nearby cells (paracrine) to stimulate growth.

The EGF family of receptors has been extensively characterized from both a genetic and biochemical standpoint. Similar to other growth factor receptors, the EGF family members are composed of an extracellular ligand-binding domain, a hydrophobic membrane-spanning region, and an intracellular tyrosine kinase domain (146,147). A truncated form of the EGF receptor that lacks the outer ligand-binding domain is the viral oncogene (v-erbB) responsible for avian erythroblastosis. The v-erbB gene encodes a receptor that is constantly activated and sending growth stimulatory signals to the nucleus. The EGF receptor is ubiquitously expressed in both epithelial and stromal cells and plays a role in growth stimulation of most cell types.

The EGF receptor has been shown to be massively amplified in the A431 human vulvar squamous cell carcinoma cell line, and these cells have been widely used as a model for studying the biochemical functions of the EGF receptor. In some head and neck and lung cancers, the EGF receptor also appears to be significantly amplified, and amplification may be associated with virulent behavior. In these cancers, the EGF receptor can be targeted therapeutically with monoclonal antibodies (148). In normal squamous epithelium, expression of EGF receptor is high in the basal proliferative layer and decreases as cells migrate toward the surface and differentiate. Although levels of EGF receptor vary between different primary squamous cancers of the lower genital tract in women, gene amplification rarely occurs, and EGF receptor levels do not appear to correlate closely with clinical behavior of these cancers (149). Similarly, EGF receptor is expressed in normal ovarian epithelium and endometrium, and although the level of expression varies between cancers, this is not a strong predictor of clinical behavior. In some human cancers, such a non–small-cell lung cancer, specific inhibitors of the EGF receptor, such as gefitinib (Iressa), have recently been proven to be effective in their treatment, and multiple clinical trials are now underway to test the efficacy of these agents alone or in combination with traditional chemotherapeutic agents (150).

The EGF receptor family of receptors also often is referred to as the ERBB family because the first member identified was the v-erbB oncogene. The second member of the family (ERBB2) initially was called neu because it was found to be the transforming gene responsible for the generation of neuroblastomas in rats treated with a chemical carcinogen. It subsequently was discovered that the neu gene encoded a 185-kD transmembrane receptor that is highly homologous with the EGF receptor (151). This human EGF receptor–like molecule was named both HER-2/neu and erbB2 by investigators working in the field. The transforming activity of *neu* in the animal model was due to the presence of a mutation in the transmembrane portion of the molecule that results in constitutive activation of the inner tyrosine kinase domain. Biochemical studies of HER-2/*neu* (formally designated ERBB2) have shown that activation of this receptor is not driven by ligand binding, but rather is dependent on activation of other members of the *ERBB* family (*ERBB3, ERBB4*) that heterodimerize with *ERBB2* and activate its tyrosine kinase domain (152).

In contrast to EGF receptor, which normally is expressed in both stromal and epithelial cells, ERBB2 is expressed primarily in epithelial cells. As originally shown for breast and ovarian cancers (153), the expression of ERBB2 is increased in several human cancer types as a result of gene amplification. In addition, artificial overexpression of this gene in some cell types in culture leads to acquisition of a malignant phenotype. In human cancers, *ERBB2* may also be overexpressed owing to alterations in regulation of transcription in the absence of gene amplification. Regardless of the underlying mechanism, it has been shown that overexpression correlates strongly with aggressive features in breast, ovarian, and endometrial cancers.

As noted above, activation of the ERBB3 and ERBB4 transmembrane receptors is requisite for ERBB2 kinase activity. At least four families of ligands, collectively called neuregulins (e.g., heregulin, *neu* differentiating factor), bind to ERBB3 and ERBB4 (152). Interestingly, there is considerable promiscuity between ERBB ligands and receptors. For example, amphiregulin can activate both the EGF receptor (ERBB1) and ERBB3. And one of the more recently described ligands (epiregulin) can activate heterodimers of any of the ERBB family members; these heterodimers are more potent growth stimulators than homodimers of any individual ERBB receptor. Finally, although their molecular signaling mechanisms have not yet been fully elucidated, the ERBB family of receptors also has been exploited as therapeutic targets. Success has been achieved with the anti-ERBB2 monoclonal antibody trastuzumab (Herceptin) that is approved for treatment of ERBB2-positive metastatic breast cancer. In combination with chemotherapy, trastuzumab provides significant clinical benefit in terms of increased response rate and extended survival compared with chemotherapy alone in patients with ERBB2-positive advanced breast cancer. Trastuzumab also has therapeutic activity as monotherapy in the front-line management of ERBB2-overexpressed or ERBB2-amplified metastatic breast cancer. Given its proven efficacy in the metastatic setting, the combination and sequential use of trastuzumab with adjuvant and neoadjuvant chemotherapy are the focus of several ongoing clinical studies (154). In ovarian cancers subject to *ERBB2* amplification and/or overexpression, however, trastuzumab has been proven to be disappointing in terms of efficacy compared to that observed in breast cancer (155). Nevertheless, the use of this agent in treatment of a select subset of breast cancer patients represents one of a very small number of success stories in translating knowledge of tumor-specific genetic defects into more effective targeted therapies, a major goal of translational research.

Extranuclear Signal Transduction

Following interaction of peptide growth factors and their receptors, secondary molecular signals are generated to transmit the mitogenic stimulus toward the nucleus. This function is served by a multitude of complex and overlapping signal transduction pathways that occur in the inner cell membrane and cytoplasm. Many of these signals involve phosphorylation of proteins by enzymes known as kinases. Cellular processes other than growth also are regulated by kinases, but one family of kinases appears to have evolved specifically for the purpose of transmitting growth stimulatory signals. These tyrosine kinases transfer a phosphate group from ATP to tyrosine residues of target proteins. Some kinases that phosphorylate proteins on serine and/or threonine residues (e.g., protein kinase C, AKT2) also are involved in stimulating proliferation. The activity of kinases is regulated by phosphatases, which act in opposition to the kinases by removing phosphates from the target proteins. Although several families of intracellular kinases have been identified that can elicit transformation when activated *in vitro* (e.g., SRC), structural alterations in these molecules appear to play a role in the development of human cancers only rarely.

RAS

G-proteins represent another class of molecules involved in transmission of growth stimulatory signals from the cell membrane to the nucleus (156). The RAS family of G-proteins functions as a relay switch that is positioned downstream of cell surface receptor tyrosine kinases and upstream of a cytoplasmic cascade of kinases that include the mitogen-activated protein (MAP) kinases (157,158). Activated MAP kinases in turn regulate the activities of nuclear transcription factors. RAS proteins are 21-kD molecules that localize to the inner aspect of the cell membrane. They have intrinsic GTPase activity that catalyzes the exchange of GTP for GDP. In their active GTP bound form, G-proteins interact with MAP kinases. Conversely, hydrolysis of GTP to GDP, which is stimulated by GTPase-activating proteins (GAPs), leads to inactivation of G-proteins.

It is estimated that point mutations in *RAS* genes are present in about one-third of cancers (11). Mutations in this family of G-proteins (*KRAS, HRAS*, and *NRAS*) are among the most frequently observed genetic alterations in human cancers (e.g., gastrointestinal and endometrial cancers). In human cancers and in a wide range of chemically induced rodent tumors, activating mutations in *RAS* are observed at codon 12, 13, or 61 (159). The encoded amino acids at these three locations appear to play a critical structural role in the active site of ras, such that missense mutations at one of these codons destroys the ability of RAS to convert GTP to GDP. The end result of such an activating mutation is accumulation of GTP-RAS protein that chronically transmits its growth stimulatory signal. In human epithelial malignancies, the most frequently observed mutation is that of *KRAS* codon 12; such is the case for gynecologic cancers, as will be discussed later in this chapter.

To be biologically active, RAS must move from the cytoplasm to the inner plasma membrane. A posttranslational modification, specifically addition of a farnesyl group to the C-terminal cysteine, is requisite for membrane localization. Farnesylation of RAS is catalyzed by the enzyme farnesyltransferase. Recently, several compounds have been developed that can inhibit farnesylation. Preclinical studies indicate that these molecules can suppress transformation and tumor growth *in vitro* and in animal models with little toxicity to normal cells (160).

Nuclear Factors

If proliferation is to occur in response to signals generated in the cytoplasm, these events must lead to activation of nuclear factors responsible for DNA replication and cell division. Expression of several genes that encode nuclear proteins increases dramatically within minutes of treatment of normal cells with peptide growth factors. Once induced, the products of these genes (e.g., FOS, JUN, MYC) bind to specific DNA regulatory elements and induce transcription of genes involved in DNA synthesis and cell division. When inappropriately amplified and/or overexpressed, however, these transcription factors can act as oncogenes.

Among the nuclear transcription factors involved in stimulating proliferation, amplification and/or overexpression of members of the *MYC* family has most often been implicated in the development of human cancers (161). MYC proteins are key regulators of mammalian cell proliferation, and treatment of cells with MYC antisense oligonucleotides inhibits proliferation. It has been shown that MYC acts as part of a heterodimeric complex with the protein MAX to initiate transcription of other genes involved in cell cycle progression (162). Ironically, in some instances in which myc expression is low, its inappropriate reexpression can elicit apoptosis (163).

GYNECOLOGIC MALIGNANCIES

Gynecologic cancers vary with respect to clinical features such as grade, histology, stage, response to treatment, and survival. It is now appreciated that this heterogeneity is attributable to differences in underlying molecular alterations. Some cancers arise in a setting of inherited mutations in cancer-susceptibility genes, but most occur sporadically in the absence of a strong predisposition. The spectrum of genes that are mutated varies both between cancer types and within a given type of cancer. In some instances, molecular features may be predictive of clinical phenotypes. As we gain a more complete understanding of the clinical implications of various genetic alterations in gynecologic cancers, the molecular profile may prove to be valuable in predicting clinical behavior and response to treatment. Insights into the molecular pathogenesis of gynecologic cancers also could provide opportunities for the development of new approaches to diagnosis, treatment, and prevention.

Endometrial Cancer

Epidemiologic and clinical studies of endometrial cancer have suggested that there are two distinct types of endometrial cancer (164). Type I cases are associated with unopposed estrogen stimulation and often develop in a background of endometrial hyperplasia. Type I lesions are characterized by well-differentiated, endometrioid histology, early-stage, and favorable outcome. In contrast, type II cancers are poorly differentiated and/or non-endometrioid and are more virulent. They often present at an advanced stage and survival is relatively poor. In practice, not all cases can be neatly characterized as either type I or II lesions, and endometrial cancers can also be viewed as a continuous spectrum with respect to etiology and clinical behavior. However, as the genetic events involved in the development of endometrial cancer have been elucidated, it has been found that specific alterations often, but not always, are seen primarily in either type I or II cases (Table 5.3).

About 5% of endometrial cancers occur in women with a strong hereditary predisposition due to germline mutations in DNA repair genes in the context of the HNPCC syndrome. An unresolved issue in the understanding of endometrial carcinogenesis is the role of unopposed estrogenic stimulation. It has long been thought that estrogens may contribute to the development of endometrial cancer by virtue of their mitogenic effect on the endometrium. A higher rate of proliferation in response to estrogens may lead to an increased frequency of spontaneous mutations. In addition, when genetic damage occurs, regardless of the cause, the presence of estrogens may facilitate clonal expansion. It also has been postulated that estrogens may act as ''complete carcinogens'' that both promote carcinogenesis by stimulating proliferation and act as initiating agents by virtue of their carcinogenic metabolites.

Cytogenetic studies have described gross chromosomal alterations in endometrial cancers including changes in the number of copies of specific chromosomes as well as deletions and translocations (165). More recently, comparative genomic hybridization (CGH) studies have demonstrated areas of chromosomal loss and gain in both endometrial cancers and atypical hyperplasias (166,167). The most common sites of chromosomal gain are 1q, 8q, 10p, and 10q (168–170). Chromosomal losses also are frequently ob-

TABLE 5.3. *Genetic alterations in sporadic endometrial carcinomas*

	Class	Mechanism	Approximate frequency (%)	Type I/II
Hereditary				
MSH2, MLH1, PMS1 PMS2, MSH6	DNA repair	Mutation	5%	I
Sporadic				
Oncogenes				
HER-2/neu	Tyrosine kinase	Amplification/overexpression	10	II
c-fms	Tyrosine kinase	Overexpression	?	II
K-ras	G-protein	Mutation	10–30	I/II
β-catenin	Transcription factor	Mutation	10	I
c-myc	Transcription factor	Amplification/overexpression	20–30	?
Tumor-suppressor genes				
p53	Transcription factor	Mutation/overexpression	20	II
PTEN	Phosphatase	Mutation/deletion	40	I
MLH1	Mismatch repair	Promoter methylation	10–20	I
CDC2	Cell cycle	Mutation/deletion	15	II

Type I, well differentiated, endometrioid, estrogen-associated cancers; type II, poorly differentiated, nonendometrioid cancers.

served both using CGH and in loss of heterozygosity studies (171). A correlation has been noted between higher numbers of chromosomal alterations on CGH and more virulent clinical features (172). The overall number of chromosomal alterations detected using CGH is lower in endometrial cancers relative to other cancer types.

Ploidy analysis simply measures total nuclear DNA content. About 80% of endometrial cancers have a normal diploid DNA content as measured by ploidy analysis. Aneuploidy occurs in 20% and is associated with advanced stage, poor grade, nonendometrioid histology, and poor survival (173). The frequency of aneuploidy is relatively low in endometrial cancers relative to ovarian cancers (80%). The differences in frequency of aneuploidy in between endometrial and ovarian cancers correlate well with the disparate outcome of these two diseases.

Finally, patterns of gene expression have been described using expression microarrays that distinguish between normal and malignant endometrium and between various histologic types of endometrial cancer (171,174). This approach has the potential to increase dramatically our understanding of the molecular pathogenesis of endometrial cancer and to enhance prediction of clinical phenotypes.

Tumor-suppressor Genes

Inactivation of the *p53* tumor-suppressor gene is among the most frequent genetic events in endometrial cancers (175). Overexpression of mutant p53 protein occurs in about 20% of endometrial adenocarcinomas and is associated with several known prognostic factors including advanced stage, poor grade, and nonendometrioid histology (Fig. 5.7) (173, 176).

Overexpression occurs in about 10% of stage I-II and 40% of stage III-IV cancers (176). Numerous studies have con-

firmed the strong association between p53 overexpression and poor prognostic factors and decreased survival (177–183). In some of these studies, p53 overexpression has been associated with worse survival even after controlling for stage (184,185). This suggests that loss of *p53* tumor-suppressor function confers a particularly virulent phenotype. Although little is known regarding molecular alterations in uterine sarcomas, overexpression of mutant *p53* occurs in a majority of mixed mesodermal sarcomas of the uterus (74%) and in some leiomyosarcomas (186,187).

Endometrial cancers that overexpress p53 protein usually harbor missense mutations in exons 5 through 8 of the gene that result in amino acid substitutions in the protein (Fig.

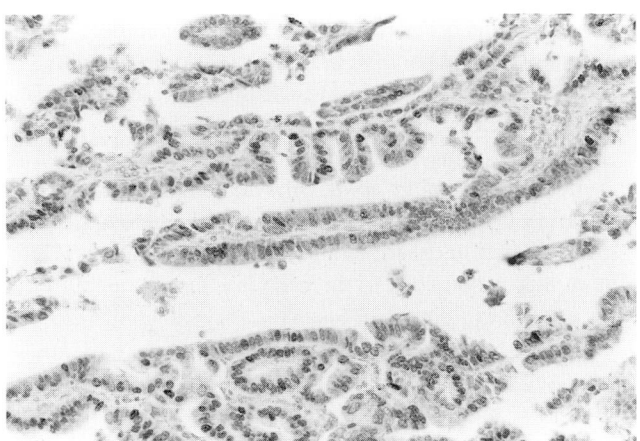

FIG. 5.7. Overexpression of p53. About 50% of ovarian cancers and 20% of endometrial cancers have missense mutations in the *p53* tumor-suppressor gene that result in protein products that are resistant to degradation. As is demonstrated in this endometrial cancer, these mutant p53 proteins overaccumulate in the nucleus of the cell and can be visualized using immunohistochemistry.

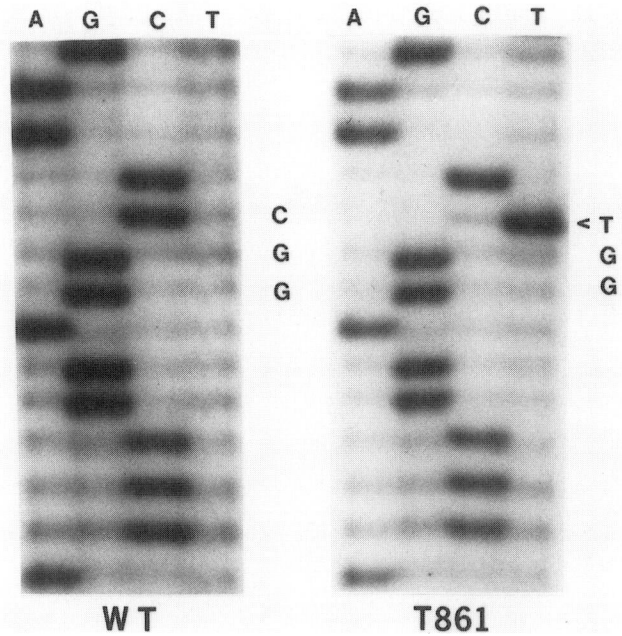

FIG. 5.8. Mutation of the *p53* gene. Endometrial cancer T861 has a missense mutation in codon 248 of the *p53* gene that changes the sequence from CGG to TGG and results in the substitution of tryptophan for arginine. On the left is the normal wild-type (WT) sequence.

5.8) (176,188–191). These mutations lead to loss of DNA-binding activity. Because *p53* mutations rarely, if ever, occur in endometrial hyplerplasias (188,192), this likely represents a late event in the development of endometrioid endometrial cancers. Alternatively, it is possible that acquisition of a *p53* mutation leads to development of a virulent poorly differentiated and/or serous type II endometrial cancer that does not transition through a phase of hyperplasia and is associated with rapid spread of disease. In a study of papillary serous carcinoma and its putative precursor (endometrial intraepithelial carcinoma), p53 overexpression was observed in 90% and 78% of cases, respectively (193).

Mutations in the *PTEN* tumor-suppressor gene on chromosome 10q occur in about 30% to 50% of endometrial cancers (135–137), and this represents the most frequent genetic alteration described thus far in these cancers. Deletion of the second copy of the gene is also a frequent event, which results in complete loss of *PTEN* function. Most of these mutations are deletions, insertions, and nonsense mutations that lead to truncated protein products, whereas only about 15% are missense mutations that change a single amino acid in the critical phosphatase domain. The *PTEN* gene encodes a phosphatase that opposes the activity of cellular kinases. For example, it has been shown that loss of *PTEN* in endometrial cancers is associated with increased activity of the PI 3 kinase with resultant phosphorylation of its downstream substrate Akt (194).

Mutations in the *PTEN* gene are associated with endome-

trioid histology, early stage, and favorable clinical behavior (195). Well-differentiated, noninvasive cases have the highest frequency of mutations. In addition, *PTEN* mutations have been observed in 20% of endometrial hyperplasias, suggesting that this is an early event in the development of some type I endometrial cancers (196). One group has reported that loss of PTEN may occur in normal-appearing endometrial glands even before the emergence of hyperplasia (197,198).

Synchronous endometrioid cancers are sometimes encountered in the endometrium and ovary that are indistinguishable microscopically. In some of these cases, identical *PTEN* mutations have been identified, suggesting that the ovarian tumor represents a metastasis from the endometrium (199). In other cases, the *PTEN* mutation seen in the endometrial cancer was not found in the ovarian tumor, suggesting that these represent two distinct primary cancers. *PTEN* mutations also have been observed in about 20% of endometrioid ovarian cancers that arise in the absence of endometrial cancers (139).

As noted in Chapter 2, inherited mutations in DNA mismatch repair genes are responsible for the HNPCC syndrome. Endometrial cancer is the second most common malignancy observed in women with HNPCC. Cancers that arise in these individuals are characterized by mutations in multiple microsatellite repeat sequences throughout the genome. This microsatellite instability also has been seen in about 20% of sporadic endometrial cancers (200,201). Endometrial cancers that exhibit microsatellite instability tend to be type I cancers. Because microsatellite instability has been noted in some sporadic endometrial cancers in women who do not carry germline DNA repair gene mutations that cause HNPCC syndrome (200), several groups have attempted to identify acquired somatic mutations in these genes. DNA repair gene mutations have been identified in only a minority of endometrial cancers with microsatellite instability (72, 202). Loss of mismatch repair in these cases appears to be most often due to silencing of the *MLH1* gene by way of promoter methylation (203,204). Methylation of the *MLH1* promoter also has been noted in endometrial hyperplasias (201,205) and normal endometrium adjacent to cancers, suggesting that this is an early event in the development of some of these cancers (206). It is thought that global changes in methylation that result in decreased expression of a number of tumor-suppressor and DNA repair genes may be a characteristic of some endometrial cancers, particularly type I cases (207,208). Loss of DNA mismatch repair may accelerate the process of malignant transformation by facilitating accumulation of mutations in microsatellite sequences present in genes involved in malignant transformation.

Finally, mutations in the *CDC4* gene, which is involved in regulating cyclin E expression during cell cycle progression, have been noted in 16% of endometrial cancers (209). Mutations were accompanied by loss of the wild-type allele and were more common in cancers with poor prognostic factors such as high grade and lymph node metastases. It is postulated that *CDC4* may act as a tumor suppressor by restraining the activity of cyclin E in promoting progression from G_1 to S phase.

Oncogenes

Alterations in some oncogenes have been demonstrated in endometrial cancers, but this occurs less frequently than inactivation of tumor-suppressor genes (Table 5.3). Increased expression of the HER-2/*neu* receptor tyrosine kinase has been noted in 10% to 15% of endometrial cancers (181,210–213) and is associated with advanced stage and poor outcome. In some studies, multivariate analysis revealed that high expression was an independent variable associated with poor survival (211). Papillary serous endometrial cancers most frequently overexpress HER-2/*neu*, and it has been suggested that this might represent an appealing therapeutic target (214). The levels of HER-2/*neu* overexpression in endometrial cancers are much less striking than in breast cancers, however, and thus far there is no evidence that Herceptin (anti–HER-2/*neu* antibody) is of therapeutic benefit in endometrial cancer.

The *fms* oncogene encodes a tyrosine kinase that serves as a receptor for macrophage-colony stimulating factor (M-CSF). Expression of fms in endometrial cancers was found to correlate with advanced stage, poor grade, and deep myometrial invasion (215, 216). Subsequently, it was shown that fms and its ligand (M-CSF) usually were coexpressed in endometrial cancers, and it was proposed that this receptor-ligand pair might mediate an autocrine growth stimulatory pathway (217). In support of this hypothesis, M-CSF serum levels are increased in patients with endometrial cancer. In addition, M-CSF increases the invasiveness of cancer cell lines that express significant levels of fms, but has no effect on cell lines with low levels of the receptor (218).

The *ras* oncogene undergoes point mutations in codon 12, 13, or 61 that result in constitutively activated molecules in many types of cancers. Initially, these codons of the K-*ras*, H-*ras*, and N-*ras* genes were examined in 11 immortalized endometrial cancer cell lines (219). Mutations in codon 12 of K-*ras* were seen in four cell lines, whereas three had mutations in codon 61 of H-*ras*. Subsequent studies of primary endometrial adenocarcinomas have confirmed that codon 12 of K-*ras* is mutated in about 10% of American cases and 20% of Japanese cases (188,220–226). These mutations occur more often, but not exclusively, in type I endometrial cancers. K-*ras* mutations also have been identified in some endometrial hyperplasias (221,226,227), which suggests that this may be a relatively early event in the development of some type I cancers

E-cadherin is a transmembrane glycoprotein involved in cell-cell adhesion, and its decreased expression in cancer cells is associated with increased invasiveness and metastatic potential. E-cadherin mutations occur only rarely in endometrial cancers (228), but cadherin expression may also be downregulated in the absence of mutations (229,230). The cytoplasmic tail of E-cadherin exists as a macromolecular complex with the β-catenin and *APC* gene products, which link it to the cytoskeleton. It appears that a critical function of the *APC* tumor-suppressor gene is to regulate phosphorylation of serine and threonine residues (codons 33, 37, 41, 45) in exon 3 of β-catenin, which results in degradation of β-catenin. Mutational inactivation of APC allows accumulation of β-catenin, which translocates to the nucleus and acts as a transcription factor to induce expression of cyclin D1 and perhaps other genes involved in cell cycle progression (230). Germline *APC* mutations are responsible for the adenomatous polyposis coli syndrome and somatic mutations are common in sporadic colon cancers; but *APC* mutations have not been described in endometrial cancers (231,232). The *APC* gene may be inactivated in some endometrial cancers owing to promoter methylation (233). In addition, it has been shown that missense mutations in exon 3 of *β-catenin* lead to the same end result—namely, abrogation of the ability of APC to induce β-catenin degradation—which results in abnormal transcriptional activity. In view of this, the *β-catenin* gene is considered an oncogene (234). *β-catenin* mutations have been observed in several types of cancers including hepatocellular, prostatic, and endometrial cancers. Mutation of *β-catenin* occurs in about 10% to 15% of endometrial cancers, but abnormal accumulation of β-catenin protein occurs in about one-third of cases, suggesting that mechanisms other than mutation might be involved in some cases (232,235).

Among nuclear transcription factors involved in stimulating proliferation, amplification of members of the *myc* family has most often been implicated in the development of human cancers. It has been shown that c-*myc* is expressed in normal endometrium (236) with higher expression in the proliferative phase. Several studies have suggested that *myc* may be amplified in a fraction of endometrial cancers (213, 237,238).

OVARIAN CANCER

About 10% of ovarian cancers arise in women who carry germline mutations in cancer-susceptibility genes—predominantly *BRCA1* or *BRCA2*. The vast majority of ovarian cancers are sporadic and arise because of accumulation of genetic damage. The causes of acquired genetic alterations in the ovarian epithelium remain uncertain, but exogenous carcinogens, with the possible exception of talc, have not been strongly implicated. Some mutations may arise spontaneously because of increased epithelial proliferation required to repair ovulatory defects. Oxidative stress and free radical formation due to inflammation and repair at the ovulatory site may also contribute to accumulation of DNA damage. Regardless of the mechanisms involved, reproductive events that decrease lifetime ovulatory cycles (e.g., pregnancy and birth control pills) are protective against ovarian cancer (239). However, the protective effect of these factors is greater in magnitude than one would predict based on the extent that ovulation is interrupted. Five years of oral contraceptive use provides a 50% risk reduction while only decreasing total years of ovulation by less than 20%. There is evidence to suggest that the progestagenic milieu of pregnancy and "the pill" might also protect against ovarian cancer by increasing apoptosis of ovarian epithelial cells, thereby cleansing the ovary of cells that have acquired genetic damage (240). The action of other reproductive hormones such as estrogens, androgens, and gonadotropins also may contribute to the development of ovarian cancers.

Epithelial ovarian cancers are heterogeneous with respect to behavior (borderline vs invasive) and histologic type (serous, mucinous, endometrioid, clear cell). Although most epidemiologic risk factors (e.g., parity) affect risk of all disease subsets, differences have been observed with respect to etiology and molecular alterations. For example, although it is thought that serous ovarian cancers arise from epithelial cells on the surface of the ovary or in underlying inclusion cysts, many endometrioid and clear cell cancers likely develop in deposits of endometriosis. Likewise, differences in the pattern of genetic alterations have been noted between serous and endometrioid/clear-cell ovarian cancers. As our understanding of the molecular pathogenesis of ovarian cancer continues to mature in the future, it is likely that the various disease subsets will increasingly be thought of as distinct entities that are defined by characteristic patterns of molecular signatures.

Global Genomic Changes

Invasive epithelial ovarian carcinoma generally is a monoclonal disease that develops as a clonal expansion of a single transformed cell in the ovary (241). However, there is evidence that some serous borderline tumors (212) as well as cancers that arise in the peritoneum of patients with *BRCA1* mutations may be polyclonal (242). Most ovarian cancers are characterized by a high degree of genetic damage that is manifest at the genomic and molecular levels. Gains and losses of various segments of the genome have been demonstrated using CGH (243). Likewise, LOH, indicative of deletion of specific genetic loci, also has been demonstrated to occur at a high frequency on many chromosomal arms (244). It is unclear whether the wide range of genetic alterations in ovarian cancers reflects the need to alter several genes in the process of malignant transformation or is the result of generalized genomic instability.

Both CGH and LOH studies have shown that advanced-stage, poorly differentiated cancers have a higher number of genetic changes than early-stage, low-grade cases (245–247). This finding could be interpreted as reflective of the fact that the number of genetic changes accumulates with progression from an early to an advanced cancer. Alter-natively, advanced-stage cancers may be intrinsically more virulent even at their early stages by virtue of their specific mutations and/or increased genomic instability. If this latter theory is correct, then early- and advanced-stage ovarian cancers could be thought of as different diseases rather than as steps in a progressive pathway. This could have significant implications for early diagnosis, treatment, and prevention of ovarian cancer.

It is estimated that the human genome contains about 30,000 genes. Recently, microarray chips that contain sequences complementary to thousands of genes have been created that allow global assessment of the level of expression of each gene. Expression arrays have been proven useful in predicting clinical phenotypes of various types of cancers. Several groups have applied expression array technology to the analysis of ovarian cancers. Many of these studies have compared gene expression between normal ovarian epithelial cells and ovarian cancers. Numerous genes have been identified that appear to be up or downregulated in the process of malignant transformation (248–250). In addition, microarrays have demonstrated patterns of gene expression that distinguish between histologic types (251) and between early- and advanced-stage cases (250,252).

Tumor-suppressor Genes

Alteration of the *p53* tumor-suppressor gene is the most frequent genetic event described thus far in ovarian cancers (Table 5.4) (43,253–259). The frequency of overexpression of mutant *p53* is significantly higher in advanced-stage (40% to 60%) relative to early stage cases (10% to 20%). The distribution of histologic types in early- and advanced-stage cases varies significantly, however, and this may account in part for the difference in *p53* mutation rate. The frequency of *p53* mutations is highest in serous and endometrioid ovarian cancers. Mutations in *p53* are a less prominent feature of clear-cell cases (260,261). The higher frequency of *p53* alterations in advanced-stage cases may indicate that this is a "late event" in ovarian carcinogenesis. Alternatively, it is possible that loss of *p53* confers an aggressive phenotype associated with more rapid progression. There is a suggestion that overexpression of mutant *p53* protein may be associated with slightly worse survival in advanced-stage ovarian cancers (253–259,262,263). Finally, although there is a high concordance between *p53* missense mutations in exons 5 through 8 and protein overexpression, about 20% of advanced ovarian cancers contain mutations that result in truncated protein products, which usually are not overexpressed (43,263). Some of these mutations may lie outside of exons 5 through 8. Overall, about 70% of advanced ovarian cancers have either missense or truncation mutations in the *p53* gene. Most *p53* missense mutations are transitions rather than transversions (264,265), which suggests that these mutations occur spontaneously rather than because of exogenous carcinogens.

TABLE 5.4. *Genetic alterations in epithelial ovarian cancers*

	Class	Mechanism	Approximate frequency (%)	Comments
Hereditary				
BRCA1	Double-stranded DNA repair	Mutation/deletion	6	Breast/ovarian syndrome
BRCA2	Double-stranded DNA repair	Mutation/deletion	3	Breast/ovarian syndrome
MSH2/MLH1	DNA mismatch repair	Mutation/deletion	1	HNPCC syndrome
Sporadic				
Oncogenes				
HER-2/neu	Tyrosine kinase	Amplification/overexpression	5–10	Gene amplification rare
K-ras	G-protein	Mutation	5	Common in serous borderline
AKT2	Serine/threonine	Amplification	5–10	
PIK3CA	Tyrosine kinase	Amplification	5–10	
c-myc	Transcription factor	Amplification	20–30	
EMSY	DNA repair	Amplification	17	
Tumor-suppressor genes				
p53	Transcription factor	Mutation/deletion	50–70	Most common in invasive
p16	CDK inhibitor	Deletion, promoter methylation	15	
p21, p27	CDK inhibitor	Promoter methylation	10–40	
BRCA1	Double-stranded DNA repair	Promoter methylation	10	

It has been postulated that loss of functional p53 might confer a chemoresistant phenotype because of its role in chemotherapy-induced apoptosis. In this regard, several studies have examined the correlation between chemosensitivity and *p53* mutation in ovarian cancers *in vitro* (266–271). Some have suggested a relationship between *p53* mutation and loss of chemosensitivity, but in other equally valid studies, such a relationship has not been observed. It is likely that the status of the *p53* gene is just one of a multitude of factors that determines chemosensitivity.

Overexpression of *p53* is rare in stage I serous borderline tumors, but occurs in as many as 20% of advanced-stage borderline cases (272,273). In a study of advanced serous borderline tumors, *p53* overexpression was associated with a sixfold higher risk of death (273). In some cases, invasive serous cancers may arise following an earlier diagnosis of borderline tumor. It has been shown that *p53* mutational status was not concordant between the original borderline tumor and the subsequent invasive cancer (274). This suggests that the invasive cancer either arises independently or as a clonal outgrowth within the original tumor.

Although mutations in the *Rb* tumor-suppressor gene are not a common feature of ovarian cancers, recent evidence suggests that inactivation of *Rb* greatly enhances tumor formation in ovarian cells with *p53* mutations (275). In a mouse model in which these genes were inactivated in the ovarian epithelium, few cancers developed in response to loss of either *p53* or *Rb* alone. When both genes were inactivated, epithelial ovarian cancers with serous features developed in almost all cases. Given that *Rb* mutations are rare in ovarian cancers, it is possible that inactivation of one of a number of genes in the *Rb* pathway can initiate transformation cooperatively with *p53*. Inactivation of *Rb* itself may not be requisite. This mouse model of ovarian cancer has the potential to add greatly to our understanding of epithelial ovarian carcinogenesis. A notable feature of this model is the development of dysplastic premalignant epithelium. Although ovarian dysplasia has long been thought to represent the precursor of serous ovarian cancers (276) and is an appealing target for early detection and prevention (277), the inaccessibility of the ovaries has presented a significant obstacle to studying its natural history. The ability to track the development of preinvasive and invasive lesions in this new mouse model presents the opportunity to develop chemoprevention approaches in a setting that appears to be similar to human ovarian carcinogenesis.

The CKK inhibitors act as tumor suppressors by virtue of their inhibition of cell cycle progression from G_1 to S phase. Expression of several CDK inhibitors appears to be decreased in some ovarian cancers. *p16* undergoes homozygous deletions in about 15% of ovarian cancers (278). There is evidence to suggest that *p16* (279) and some other tumor-suppressor genes, such as *BRCA1* (85,86,280), may be inactivated via transcriptional silencing owing to promoter methylation rather than mutation and/or deletion. Likewise, decreased expression of the p21 CDK inhibitor has been noted in a significant fraction of ovarian cancers despite the absence of inactivating mutations (281,282). Loss of the *p27*

CDK inhibitor also may occur and correlates with poor survival (283–286).

Normal ovarian epithelial cells are inhibited by the growth-inhibitory peptide TGF-β, whereas most immortalized ovarian cancer cell lines are unresponsive (287,288). The effect of TGF-β on primary ovarian cancer cells obtained directly from patients is less straightforward. In studies conducted using ovarian cancer cells grown in monolayer culture, most remain sensitive to the growth-inhibitory effect of TGF-β (288). In contrast, when ovarian cancer cells are grown in collagen matrix, they are unresponsive (289). There is some evidence that mutations may occur in cell surface TGF-β receptors or in the *Smad* family of genes that are involved in downstream signaling (290), but in other studies, these signaling pathways have been found to be intact (289). Thus far, it has not been convincingly demonstrated that derangement of the TGF-β pathway plays a role in the development of ovarian cancers.

Oncogenes

It has been shown that ovarian cancers produce and/or are capable of responding to various peptide growth factors. For example, EGF (291) and TGF-α (292) are produced by some ovarian cancers that also express the receptor that binds these peptides (EGF receptor) (293,294). Some cancers produce insulin-like growth factor-1 (IGF-1), IGF-1–binding protein, and express type 1 IGF receptor (295). Platelet-derived growth factor (PDGF) also is expressed by many types of epithelial cells including human ovarian cancer cell lines, but these cells usually are not responsive to PDGF (287,296, 297). In addition, ovarian cancers produce basic fibroblast growth factor (FGF) and its receptor, and basic FGF acts as a mitogen in some ovarian cancers (298). Ovarian cancers produce M-CSF, and serum levels of M-CSF are elevated in some patients (299). Since the M-CSF receptor (*fms*) is expressed by many ovarian cancers, this could comprise an autocrine growth-stimulatory pathway in some cancers (300). Ascites of patients with ovarian cancer also contains phospholipid factors such as lysophosphatidic acid (LPA) that stimulate proliferation and invasiveness of ovarian cancer cells (301). The edg-2 G-protein–coupled receptors act as functional receptors for LPA. The finding that neutralization of LPA activity decreases growth and increases apoptosis of ovarian cancers suggests that manipulation of this pathway may be therapeutically beneficial (302).

Several groups also have demonstrated that normal ovarian epithelial cells produce and are responsive to many of the same peptide growth factors as malignant ovarian epithelial cells (294,303–305). Thus, despite cell culture data demonstrating autocrine and paracrine growth regulation of ovarian cancer cells by peptide growth factors, it remains unclear whether alterations in expression of growth factors are critical early events involved in the development of ovarian cancers. Alternatively, it is possible that growth factors may primarily act as "necessary but not sufficient" cofactors that support growth and metastasis following malignant transformation.

The HER-2/*neu* tyrosine kinase is a member of a family of related transmembrane receptors that includes the EGF receptor (306). About 30% of breast cancers express increased levels of the HER-2/*neu* (153), often as a result of gene amplification. Overexpression of HER-2/*neu* in breast cancer has been associated with poor survival. Expression of HER-2/*neu* is increased in a fraction of ovarian cancers (Fig. 5.9), and overexpression has been associated with poor survival in some (153,307), but not all (308,309), studies. Unlike breast cancers, ovarian cancers that exhibit HER-2/*neu* overexpression rarely have high-level gene amplifica-

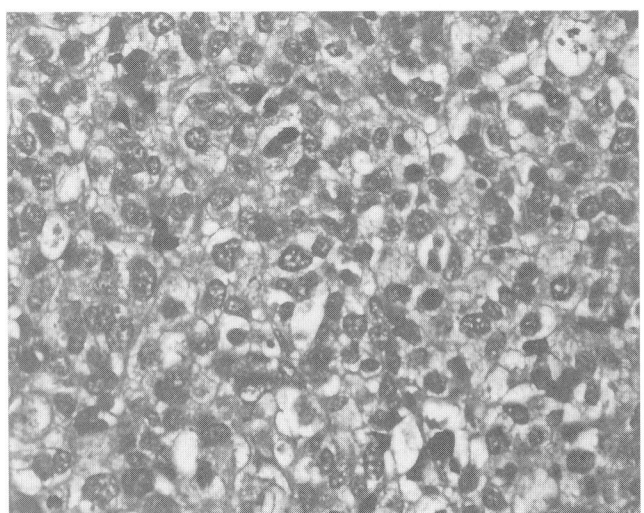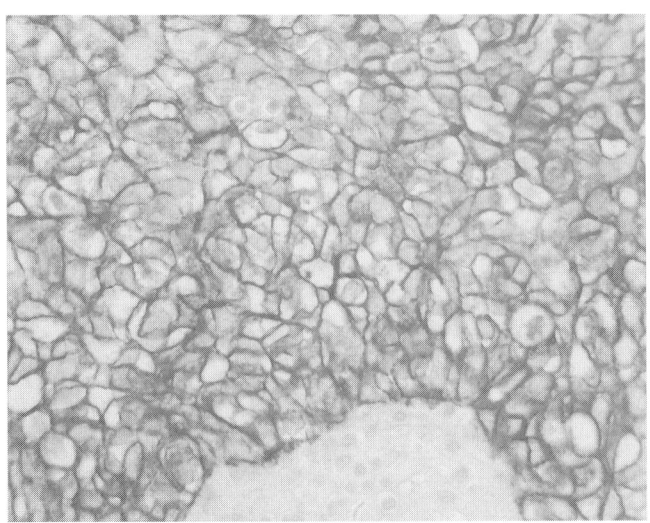

A   B

FIG. 5.9. Overexpression of HER-2/*neu* in ovarian cancer. **A:** Serous ovarian cancer. **B:** Immunostaining for HER-2/*neu* demonstrates intense cell membrane staining indicative of overexpression.

tion. Monoclonal antibodies that interact with HER-2/*neu* can decrease growth of breast and ovarian cancer cell lines that overexpress this receptor (310,311). Anti–HER-2/*neu* antibody therapy (Herceptin) has demonstrated efficacy in the treatment of breast cancer and often is administered in concert with paclitaxel (Taxol) (312). A study performed by the Gynecologic Oncology Group found only 11% of ovarian cancers exhibit significant HER-2/*neu* overexpression (155). The response rate to single-agent Herceptin therapy was disappointingly low (7.3%), but perhaps some benefit may be found in the future using combination regimens that also include taxanes or other cytotoxics.

Mutations in the *ras* genes are rare in invasive serous ovarian cancers (40,222,313–315). Although K-*ras* mutations have been noted in about 50% of mucinous ovarian cancers and some clear-cell cases, these tumors comprise only a small fraction of epithelial ovarian cancers. In contrast, K-*ras* mutations are common in borderline serous ovarian tumors, occurring in 20% to 50% of cases (316,317). This is supportive of the hypothesis that the molecular pathology of borderline tumors differs from that of invasive ovarian cancers.

Cytoplasmic kinases relay mitogenic signals from receptor tyrosine kinases and G-proteins on the cell membrane in toward the nucleus. The region of chromosome 3p26 that includes the phosphatidylinositol 3-kinase (*PIK3CA*) has been shown to be amplified in some ovarian cancer cell lines using comparative genomic hybridization (318). In addition, the *AKT2* serine/threonine kinase also has been shown to be amplified and overexpressed in some ovarian cancers (319). *PIK3CA* and *AKT2* kinase activity is opposed by the *PTEN* phosphatase. *PTEN* mutations may be uncommon in ovarian cancers because amplification of *PIK3CA* or *AKT2* in some cases abrogates the need for loss of this tumor suppressor.

As noted in the above section, mutations in the *β-catenin* gene are a feature of some endometrial cancers. Similarly, *β-catenin* mutations are present in about 30% of endometrioid ovarian cancers (320), but not other histologic types. This provides further evidence of the molecular heterogeneity of the various histologic types of ovarian cancer. In some endometrioid ovarian cancers with abnormal nuclear accumulation of β-catenin that lack mutations, the *APC, AXIN1,* or *AXIN2* genes that regulate β-catenin activity were found to be mutated (320). This suggests that alterations in the wnt signaling pathway are a feature of endometrioid ovarian cancers.

Increased activity of nuclear transcription factors also may enhance malignant transformation. In this regard, amplification of the c-*myc* oncogene has been reported to occur in some ovarian cancers. Several studies have suggested that the c-*myc* gene is amplified in about 30% of cases (321–326). In this study, c-myc overexpression was observed most often in advanced-stage serous cancers. Despite these reports of gene amplification, evidence of c-*myc* protein overexpression has been less convincing. Some ovarian

cancers have been reported to have increased expression of cyclin E, which is involved in cell cycle progression (327). In a study of advanced-stage suboptimally debulked ovarian cancers, high cyclin E expression was associated with a 6-month decrease in median survival (328). In some, but not all, cases amplification of the *cyclin E* gene was found to be the underlying cause of overexpression.

Finally, it has recently been discovered that the *EMSY* gene on chromosome 11q13.5 is amplified in 17% of high-grade ovarian cancers (88). It has been suggested that overexpression of EMSY is oncogenic by virtue of its ability to bind to the BRCA2 protein and to silence its DNA repair activity.

CERVICAL CANCER

Cervical cancer is the most common gynecologic malignancy worldwide and accounts for over 400,000 cases annually. Molecular and epidemiologic studies have demonstrated that sexually transmitted human papillomavirus (HPV) infections play a role in almost all cervical dysplasias and cancers (329–332). HPV infection also is involved in the development of dysplasias and cancers of the vagina and vulva. The peak incidence of HPV infection occurs in women in their 20s and 30s, and the incidence of cervical cancer increases from the 20s to a plateau between ages 40 and 50. Although HPV plays a major role in the development of most cervical cancers, only a small minority of women who are infected develop invasive cervical cancer. This suggests that other genetic and/or environmental factors also are involved in cervical carcinogenesis. For example, individuals who are immunosuppressed, either owing to human immunodeficiency virus (HIV) infection (333) or immunosuppressive drugs, are more likely to develop dysplasia and invasive cervical cancer following HPV infection.

Cervical screening programs in developed nations dramatically reduced both the incidence of invasive cervical cancer and disease-related mortality in the twentieth century. The recent report that an HPV 16 vaccine was highly effective in preventing HPV infection and dysplasia provides exciting evidence of the potential utility of this approach in the future (334). Although cervical cancer mortality is now low in the United States and Western Europe, it remains among the leading causes of cancer deaths in women in underdeveloped nations. Complete eradication of cervical cancer through screening and prevention strategies that are based on an understanding of HPV biology may be within reach in the twenty-first century.

Human Papillomavirus Infection

There are over 80 HPV subtypes, but not all infect the lower genital tract. HPVs 16 and 18 are the most common types associated with cervical cancer, and are found in over 80% of cases. Types 31, 33, 35, 39, 45, 51, 52, 56, 58, 59,

68, 73, and 82 should be considered high-risk types, and types 26, 53, and 66 should be considered probably carcinogenic (332). Low-risk types that may cause dysplasias or condylomata in the lower genital tract, but rarely cause cancers, include types 6, 11, 40, 42, 43, 44, 54, 61, 70, 72, and 81. The advent of HPV typing now allows assessment of whether patients carry high-risk or low-risk HPV types, and this has been proven to be clinically useful in the management of patients with low-grade Pap smear abnormalities.

The HPV DNA sequence consists of 7,800 nucleotides divided into ''early'' and ''late'' open reading frames (ORFs). ''Early'' ORFs are within the first 4,200 nucleotides of the genome and encode proteins (E1 to E8) and are important in viral replication and cellular transformation. ''Late'' ORFs (L1 and L2) are found within the latter half of the sequence and encode structural proteins of the virion. In oncogenic subtypes like HPV 16 and 18, transformation may be accompanied by integration of episomal HPV DNA into the host genome. Opening of the episomal viral genome usually occurs in the E1/E2 region, resulting in a linear fragment for insertion. The location of the opening may be significant since E2 acts as a repressor of the E6/E7 promoter and disruption of E2 can lead to unregulated expression of the E6/E7 transforming genes. HPV 16 DNA may be found in its episomal form in some cervical cancers, however, and unregulated E6/E7 transcription may occur independent of viral DNA integration into the cellular genome.

Examination of the biologic effects of HPV-encoded proteins has shed light on the mechanisms of HPV-associated transformation. Expression of the E4 transcript results in the production of intermediate filaments that colocalize with cytokeratins. E4 proteins of oncogenic subtypes disrupt the cytoplasmic cytokeratin matrix, whereas those of nononcogenic strains do not. It has been suggested that this may facilitate the release of HPV particles in oncogenic subtypes such as HPV 16. The E5 oncogene encodes a 44–amino acid protein that usually forms dimers within the cellular membrane. The transforming properties of E5 appear to involve potentiation of membrane-bound EGF receptors or PFG receptors. The E6 and E7 oncoproteins are the main transforming genes of oncogenic strains of HPV (Fig. 5.10) (335). Transfection of these genes in vitro results in immortalization and transformation of some cell lines. The HPV E7 protein acts primarily by binding to and inactivating the retinoblastoma (Rb) tumor-suppressor gene product. E7 contains two domains, one of which mediates binding to Rb, whereas the other serves as a substrate for casein kinase II (CKII) phosphorylation. Variations in oncogenic potential between HPV subtypes may be related to differences in the binding efficacy of E7 to Rb. High-risk HPV types contain E7 oncoproteins that bind Rb with more affinity than E7 from low-risk types. The transforming activity of E7 may be increased by CKII mutation, implying a role for this binding site in the development of HPV-mediated neoplasias. The E6 proteins of oncogenic HPV subtypes bind to and

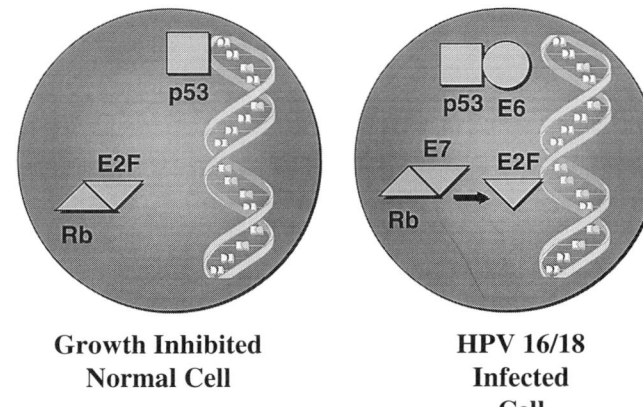

Growth Inhibited Normal Cell　　**HPV 16/18 Infected Cell**

FIG. 5.10. Role of *p53* and *Rb* genes in cervical carcinogenesis. The HPV 16/18 protein inactivates the p53 and Rb proteins, respectively.

inactivate the P53 tumor-suppressor gene product (336,337). There also is a correlation between oncogenicity of various HPV strains and the ability of their E6 oncoproteins to inactivate p53. Inactivation of Rb and p53 by E6/E7 circumvents the need for mutational inactivation of these key growth regulatory genes. HPV-negative cervical cancers are uncommon, but have been reported to exhibit overexpression of mutant p53 protein (338). This suggests that inactivation of the *p53* tumor-suppressor gene either by HPV E6 or by mutation is a requisite event in cervical carcinogenesis.

Genomic Changes

Comparative genomic hybridization techniques have been used to identify chromosomal loci that are either increased or decreased in copy number in cervical cancers. A strikingly consistent finding of various studies is the high frequency of gains on chromosome 3q in both squamous-cell cancers (339–344) and adenocarcinomas (345). Other chromosomes that exhibit frequent gains include 1q and 11q. The most common areas of chromosomal loss include chromosomes 3p and 2q. For the most part, with the exception of the *FHIT* gene on chromosome 3p, it has not been proven that these genomic gains and losses result in the recruitment of specific oncogenes and tumor-suppressor genes in the process of malignant transformation. It is conceivable that these chromosomal alterations may be frequent sequelae of infection with oncogenic HPVs, but play no significant role in the pathogenesis of cervical cancers. Abnormalities seen in invasive cancers using comparative genomic hybridization also have been identified in high-grade dysplasias, however, suggesting that these are early events in cervical carcinogenesis (340,343,346).

Oncogenes and Tumor-suppressor Genes

Only a small fraction of HPV-infected women develop cervical cancer. This suggests that additional genetic alterations are requisite for progression to high-grade dysplasia and cancer, but little is known regarding these events. Allelic loss suggestive of involvement of tumor-suppressor genes has been noted at loci on chromosomes 3p, 11p, and others, but alterations in specific genes have not yet been identified. In addition, alterations have not been found in a number of tumor-suppressor genes that are involved in other types of cancers.

The role of several oncogenes has been examined in cervical carcinomas including most prominently the *ras* and *myc* genes. Mutant *ras* genes are capable of cooperating with HPV in transforming cells *in vitro*. There is some evidence that mutations in either K-*ras* or H-*ras* may play a role in a subset of cervical cancers (338,347–350). Alterations in *ras* genes have not been seen in cervical intraepithelial neoplasia, suggesting that mutation of *ras* is a late event in the pathogenesis of some cervical cancers. In contrast, c-*myc* amplification and overexpression may be an early event in the development of some cervix cancers (351). Overexpression of c-*myc* has been demonstrated in one-third of early invasive carcinomas and some CIN 3 lesions, but not in normal cervical epithelium or lower grade dysplasia. It has been reported that overexpression of c-*myc*, gene may be due to amplification of the gene (4- to 20-fold) in some cases. In some studies, amplification correlated with poor prognosis in early-stage cases (352). However, other studies have not confirmed the finding of amplification of c-*myc* in cervical cancers. Integration of the HPV genome near c-*myc* on chromosome 8q may lead to increased expression due to enhanced transcription of the gene rather than amplification. Further studies are needed to clarify the role of *ras* genes, c-*myc*, and other oncogenes in cervical carcinogenesis.

The fragile histidine triad (*FHIT*) gene localized within human chromosomal band 3p14.2 is frequently deleted in many different cancers, including cervical cancer (353–355). Decreased expression of this putative tumor-suppressor gene is an early event in some cervical cancers (355, 356). In one study, FHIT protein expression was markedly reduced or absent in 71% of invasive cancers, 52% of HSILs associated with invasive cancer, and 21% of HSILs without associated invasive cancer (355). In addition, reduced expression is associated with poor prognosis in advanced cervical cancers (357).

As is the case in endometrial and ovarian cancers, it is thought that gene silencing due to promoter hypermethylation also may play a role in cervical carcinogenesis (358, 359). In this regard, the *RASSF1A* gene is located on chromosome 3p21.3 in an area that is frequently a site of deletions in cervical cancer. The function of this gene is not completely understood, but is thought to be involved in *ras*-mediated signal transduction pathways. Although mutations in *RASSF1A* do not occur in cervical cancers, inactivation of the gene due to promoter methylation occurs in a fraction of cases, particularly adenocarcinomas (360,361).

Molecular analyses can readily be performed using cell pellets obtained from liquid-based Pap smears. This promises to facilitate future investigation of the role of promoter methylation and other alterations in the molecular pathogenesis of cervical cancer (362).

GESTATIONAL TROPHOBLASTIC DISEASE

The genetic alterations that underlie gestational trophoblastic disease have been elucidated to a great extent. The most prominent feature of these tumors is an imbalance of parental chromosomes. In the case of partial moles, this involves an extra haploid copy of one set of paternal chromosomes, whereas complete moles generally are characterized by two complete haploid sets of paternal chromosomes and an absence of maternal chromosomes. Although the risk of repeat molar pregnancy is only about 1%, women who have had two molar pregnancies have about a 25% risk of developing another mole. Although this suggests a hereditary defect that affects gametogenesis, this remains speculative. Thus far there is no convincing evidence that damage to specific tumor-suppressor genes or oncogenes contributes to the development of gestational trophoblastic disease.

REFERENCES

1. Bishop, JM. Cancer: the rise of the genetic paradigm. *Genes Dev* 1995;9:1309–1315.
2. Virchow R. *Cellular pathology as based upon physiological and pathological histology*. London: John Churchill, 1860.
3. Boveri, T. *Zur Frage der Entstehung maligner Tumoren*. Jena: Verlag von Gustav Fischer, 1914.
4. Nowell PC, Hungerford DA. A minute chromosome in human chronic granulocytic leukemia. *Science* 1960;132:1497–1499.
5. Nowell P. The clonal evolution of tumor cell populations. *Science* 1976;194:23–28.
6. Stehelin D, Varmus HE, Bishop JM, et al. DNA related to the transforming gene(s) of avian sarcoma viruses is present in normal avian DNA. *Nature* 1976;260:170–173.
7. Spector D, Varmus HE, Bishop JM. Nucleotide sequences related to the transforming gene of avian sarcoma virus are present in DNA of uninfected vertebrates. *Proc Natl Acad Sci U S A* 1978;75:4102–4106.
8. Rowley JD. A new consistent chromosomal abnormality in chronic myelogenous leukaemia identified by quinacrine fluorescence and Giemsa staining. *Nature* 1973;243:290–293.
9. Heisterkamp N, Stephenson JR, Groffen J, et al. Localization of the c-abl oncogene adjacent to a translocation break point in chronic myelocytic leukaemia. *Nature* 1983;306:239–242.
10. Druker BJ, Talpaz M, Resta DJ, et al. Efficacy and safety of a specific inhibitor of the BCR-ABL tyrosine kinase in chronic myeloid leukemia. *N Engl J Med* 2001;344:1031–1037.
11. Vogelstein B, Kinzler KW. The multistep nature of cancer. *Trends Genet* 1993;9:138–141.
12. Hanahan D, Weinberg RA. The hallmarks of cancer. *Cell* 2000;100:57–70.
13. Renan MJ. How many mutations are required for tumorigenesis? Implications from human cancer data. *Mol Carcinog* 1993;7:139–146.
14. Hofstra RMW, Landsvater RM, Ceccherini I, et al. A mutation in the *RET* proto-oncogene associated with multiple endocrine neoplasia type 2B and sporadic medullary thyroid carcinoma. *Nature* 1994;367:375–378.
15. Schmidt L, Duh F-M, Chen F, et al. Germline and somatic mutations in the tyrosine kinase domain of the *MET* proto-oncogene in papillary renal carcinomas. *Nat Genet* 1997;16:68–73.

16. Kinzler KW, Vogelstein B: Gatekeepers and caretakers. *Nature* 1997; 386:761–763.

17. Loeb LA. A mutator phenotype in cancer. *Cancer Res* 2001;61: 3230–3239.

18. Foulds L. *Neoplastic development*. London: Academic Press, 1969.

19. Lengauer C, Kinzler KW, Vogelstein B. Genetic instability in colorectal cancers. *Nature* 1997;386:623–627.

20. Fearon ER, Vogelstein B. A genetic model for colorectal tumorigenesis. *Cell* 1990;61:759–767.

21. Charles DR, Luce-Clausen EM. The kinetics of papilloma formation in benzpyrene-treated mice. *Cancer Res* 1942;2:261–263.

22. Harris H, Miller OJ, Klein G, et al. Suppression of malignancy by cell fusion. *Nature* 1969;223:363–368.

23. Knudson AG. Mutation and cancer: statistical study of retinoblastoma. *Proc Natl Acad Sci U S A* 1971;68:820–823.

24. Friend SH, Bernards R, Rogelj S, et al. A human DNA segment with properties of the gene that predisposes to retinoblastoma and osteosarcoma. *Nature* 1986;323:643–646.

25. Haber DA, Housman DE. Rate limiting steps: the genetics of pediatric cancers. *Cell* 1991;64:5–8.

26. Knudson AG. Two genetic hits (more or less) to cancer. *Nat Rev Cancer* 2001;1:157–170.

27. Greenblatt MS, Bennett WP, Hollstein M, et al. Mutations in the *p53* tumor suppressor gene: clues to cancer etiology and molecular pathogenesis. *Cancer Res* 1994;54:4855–4878.

28. Cavenee WK, Dryja TP, Phillips RA, et al. Expression of recessive alleles by chromosomal mechanisms in retinoblastoma. *Nature* 1983; 305:779–784.

29. Bartek J, Bartkova J, Lukas J. The retinoblastoma protein pathway in cell cycle control and cancer. *Exp Cell Res* 1997;237:1–6.

30. Fischer PM, Endicott J, Meijer L. Cyclin-dependent kinase inhibitors. *Prog Cell Cycle Res* 2003;5:235–248.

31. Milde-Langosch K, Riethdorf S. Role of cell-cycle regulatory proteins in gynecological cancer. *J Cell Physiol* 2003;196:224–244.

32. Liggett WHJ Sidransky, D: Role of the p16 tumor suppressor gene in cancer. *J Clin Oncol* 1998;16:1197–1206.

33. Bell DW, Varley JM, Szydlo TE, et al. Heterozygous germ line hCHK2 mutations in Li-Fraumeni syndrome. *Science* 1999;286: 2528–2531.

34. Meijers-Heijboer H, van den Ouweland A, Klijn J, et al. Low-penetrance susceptibility to breast cancer due to CHEK2*1100delC in noncarriers of BRCA1 or BRCA2 mutations. *Nat Genet* 2002;31:55–59.

35. Lane DP, Crawford LV. T antigen is bound to a host protein in SV40-transformed cells. *Nature* 1979;278:261–263.

36. Linzer DIH, Levine AJ. Characterization of a 54K dalton cellular SV40 tumor antigen present in SV40-transformed cells and uninfected embryonal carcinoma cells. *Cell* 1979;17:43–52.

37. Finlay CA, Hinds PW, Levine AJ. The p53 proto-oncogene can act as a suppressor of transformation. *Cell* 1989;57:1083–1093.

38. Baker SJ, Markowitz S, Fearon ER, et al. Suppression of human colorectal carcinoma cell growth by wild-type p53. *Science* 1990;249: 912–915.

39. Chen PL, Chen YM, Bookstein R, et al. Genetic mechanisms of tumor suppression by the human p53 gene. *Science* 1990;250:1576–1580.

40. Baker SJ, Fearon ER, Nigro JM, et al. Chromosome 17 deletions and p53 gene mutations in colorectal carcinomas. *Science* 1989;244: 217–221.

41. Hollstein M, Sidransky D, Vogelstein B, et al. p53 mutations in human cancers. *Science* 1991;253:49–53.

42. Cho Y, Gorina S, Jeffrey PD, et al. Crystal structure of a p53 tumor suppressor-DNA complex: understanding tumorigenic mutations. *Science* 1994;265:346–355.

43. Casey G, Lopez ME, Ramos JC, et al. DNA sequence analysis of exons 2 through 11 and immunohistochemical staining are required to detect all known p53 alterations in human malignancies. *Oncogene* 1996;13:1971–1981.

44. Levine AJ. p53, the cellular gatekeeper for growth and division. *Cell* 1997;88:323–331.

45. Oren, M. Regulation of the p53 tumor suppressor protein. *J Biol Chem* 1999;274:36031–36034.

46. Vogelstein B, Lane D, Levine AJ. Surfing the p53 network. *Nature* 2000;408:307–310.

47. Bunz F, Dutriaux A, Lengauer C, et al. Requirement for p53 and p21 to sustain G_2 arrest after DNA damage. *Science* 1998;282:1497–1501.

48. Sherr CJ, McCormick F. The RB and p53 pathways in cancer. *Cancer Cell* 2002;2:103–112.

49. Lynch HT, Smyrk T. Hereditary nonpolyposis colorectal cancer: an updated review. *Cancer* 1996;78:1149–1167.

50. Watson P, Lynch HT. Extracolonic cancer in hereditary nonpolyposis colorectal cancer. *Cancer* 1993;71:677–685.

51. Watson P, Vasen HF, Mecklin JP, et al. The risk of endometrial cancer in hereditary nonpolyposis colorectal cancer. *Am J Med* 1994;96: 516–520.

52. Aarnio M, Mecklin JP, Aaltonen LA, et al. Life-time risk of different cancers in the hereditary non-polyposis colorectal cancer (HNPCC) syndrome. *Int J Cancer* 1995;64:430–433.

53. Vasen HF, Wijnen JT, Menko FH, et al. Cancer risk in families with hereditary nonpolyposis colorectal cancer diagnosed by mutation analysis. *Gastroenterology* 1996;110:1020–1027.

54. Dunlop MG, Farrington SM, Carothers AD, et al. Cancer risk associated with germline DNA mismatch repair gene mutations. *Hum Mol Genet* 1997;6:105–110.

55. Aarnio M, Sankila R, Pukkala E, et al. Cancer risk in mutation carriers of DNA-mismatch-repair genes. *Int J Cancer* 1999;81:214–218.

56. Ionov Y, Peinado MA, Malkhosyan S, et al. Ubiquitous somatic mutations in simple repeated sequences reveal a new mechanism for colonic carcinogenesis. *Nature* 1993;363:558–561.

57. Aaltonen LA, Peltomäki P, Leach FS, et al. Clues to the pathogenesis of familial colorectal cancer. *Science* 1993;260:812–816.

58. Thibodeau SN, Bren G, Schaid D. Microsatellite instability in cancer of the proximal colon. *Science* 1993;260:816–819.

59. Peltomäki P, Aaltonen LA, Sistonen P, et al. Genetic mapping of a locus predisposing to human colorectal cancer. *Science* 1993;260: 810–812.

60. Lindblom A, Tannergård P, Werelius B, et al. Genetic mapping of a second locus predisposing to hereditary non-polyposis colon cancer. *Nat Genet* 1993;5:279–282.

61. Fishel R, Lescoe MK, Rao MRS, et al. The human mutator gene homolog *MSH2* and its association with hereditary nonpolyposis colon cancer. *Cell* 1993;75:1027–1038.

62. Leach FS, Nicolaides NC, Papadopoulos N, et al. Mutations of a *mutS* homolog in hereditary nonpolyposis colorectal cancer. *Cell* 1993;75: 1215–1225.

63. Bronner CE, Baker SM, Morrison PT, et al. Mutation in the DNA mismatch repair gene homologue *hMLH1* is associated with hereditary non-polyposis colon cancer. *Nature* 1994;368:258–261.

64. Papadopoulos N, Nicolaides NC, Wei Y-F, et al. Mutation of a *mutL* homolog in hereditary colon cancer. *Science* 1994;263:1625–1629.

65. Peltomäki P. Deficient DNA mismatch repair: a common etiologic factor for colon cancer. *Hum Mol Genet* 2001;10:735–740.

66. Wijnen J, de Leeuw W, Vasen H, et al. Familial endometrial cancer in female carriers of *MSH6* germline mutations. *Nat Genet* 1999;23: 142–144.

67. Miyaki M, Konishi M, Tanaka K, et al. Germline mutation of *MSH6* as the cause of hereditary nonpolyposis colorectal cancer. *Nat Genet* 1997;17:271–272.

68. Akiyama Y, Sato H, Yamada T, et al. Germ-line mutation of the *hMSH6/GTBP* gene in an atypical hereditary nonpolyposis colorectal cancer kindred. *Cancer Res* 1997;57:3920–3928.

69. Kolodner RD, Tytell JD, Schmeits JL, et al. Germ-line *msh6* mutations in colorectal cancer families. *Cancer Res* 1999;59:5068–5074.

70. Nicolaides NC, Papadopoulos N, Liu B, et al. Mutations of two *PMS* homologues in hereditary nonpolyposis colon cancer. *Nature* 1994; 371:75–80.

71. Liu T, Yan H, Kuismanen S, et al. The role of hPMS1 and hPMS2 in predisposing to colorectal cancer. *Cancer Res* 2001;61:7798–7802.

72. Gurin CC, Federici MG, Kang L, et al. Causes and consequences of microsatellite instability in endometrial carcinoma. *Cancer Res* 1999; 59:462–466.

73. Herman JG, Umar A, Polyak K, et al. Incidence and functional consequences of *hMLH1* promoter hypermethylation in colorectal carcinoma. *Proc Natl Acad Sci U S A* 1998;95:6870–6875.

74. Leung SY, Yuen ST, Chung LP, et al. *hMLH1* promoter methylation and lack of *hMLH1* expression in sporadic gastric carcinomas with

high-frequency microsatellite instability. *Cancer Res* 1999;59: 159–164.

75. Duval A, Hamelin R. Mutations at coding repeat sequences in mismatch repair-deficient human cancers: toward a new concept of target genes for instability. *Cancer Res* 2002;62:2447–2454.

76. Hall JM, Lee MK, Newman B, et al. Linkage of early-onset familial breast cancer to chromosome 17q21. *Science* 1990;250:1684–1689.

77. Narod SA, Feunteun J, Lynch HT, et al. Familial breast-ovarian cancer locus on chromosome 17q12-q23. *Lancet* 1991;338:82–83.

78. Miki Y, Swensen J, Shattuck-Edens D, et al. A strong candidate for the breast and ovarian cancer susceptibility gene *BRCA1*. *Science* 1994;266:66–71.

79. Wooster R, Neuhausen SL, Mangion J, et al. Localization of a breast cancer susceptibility gene, *BRCA2*, to chromosome 13q12–13. *Science* 1994;265:2088–2090.

80. Wooster R, Bignell G, Lancaster J, et al. Identification of the breast cancer susceptibility gene *BRCA2*. *Nature* 1995;378:789–792.

81. Breast Cancer Information Core Database (http://research.nhgri.nih.gov/bic/).

82. Gudmundsson J, Johannesdottir G, Bergthorsson JT, et al. Different tumor types from BRCA2 mutation carriers show wild-type chromosome deletions on 13q12-q13. *Cancer Res* 1995;55:4830–4832.

83. Smith SA, Easton DF, Evans DG, et al. Allele losses in the region 17q12–21 in familial breast and ovarian cancer involve the wild-type chromosome. *Nat Genet* 1992;2:128–131.

84. Thompson D, Easton D, Breast Cancer Linkage Consortium. Variation in cancer risks, by mutation position, in BRCA2 mutation carriers. *Am J Hum Genet* 2001;68:410–419.

85. Esteller M, Silva JM, Dominguez G, et al. Promoter hypermethylation and BRCA1 inactivation in sporadic breast and ovarian tumors. *J Natl Cancer Inst* 2000;92:564–569.

86. Baldwin RL, Nemeth E, Tran H, et al. BRCA1 promoter region hypermethylation in ovarian carcinoma: a population-based study. *Cancer Res* 2000;60:5329–5333.

87. Jazaeri AA, Yee CJ, Sotiriou C, et al: Gene expression profiles of BRCA1-linked, BRCA2-linked, and sporadic ovarian cancers. *J Natl Cancer Inst* 2002;94:990–1000.

88. Hughes-Davies L, Huntsman D, Ruas M, et al. EMSY links the BRCA2 pathway to sporadic breast and ovarian cancer. *Cell* 2003;115:523–535.

89. Scully R, Livingston DM. In search of the tumour-suppressor functions of BRCA1 and BRCA2. *Nature* 2000;408:429–432.

90. Venkitaraman AR. Cancer susceptibility and the functions of BRCA1 and BRCA2. *Cell* 2002;108:171–182.

91. Scully R, Chen J, Plug A, et al. Association of BRCA1 with Rad51 in mitotic and meiotic cells. *Cell* 1997;88:265–275.

92. Sharan SK, Morimatsu M, Albrecht U, et al. Embryonic lethality and radiation hypersensitivity mediated by Rad51 in mice lacking *Brca2*. *Nature* 1997;386:804–810.

93. Hakem R, de la Pompa JL, Sirard C, et al. The tumor suppressor gene *Brca1* is required for embryonic cellular proliferation in the mouse. *Cell* 1996;85:1009–1023.

94. Suzuki A, de la Pompa JL, Hakem R, et al. *Brca2* is required for embryonic cellular proliferation in the mouse. *Genes Dev* 1997;11:1242–1252.

95. Hakem R, de la Pompa JL, Elia A, et al. Partial rescue of *Brca1*[5–6] early embryonic lethality by *p53* or *p21* null mutation. *Nat Genet* 1997;16:298–302.

96. Ludwig T, Chapman DL, Papaioannou VE, et al. Targeted mutations of breast cancer susceptibility gene homologs in mice: lethal phenotypes of *Brca1*, *Brca2*, *Brca1/Brca2*, *Brca1/p53*, and *Brca2/p53* nullizygous embryos. *Genes Dev* 1997;11:1226–1241.

97. Moynahan ME, Chiu JW, Koller BH, et al. Brca1 controls homology-directed DNA repair. Mol Cell 1999;4:511–518.

98. Snouwaert JN, Gowen LC, Latour AM, et al. BRCA1 deficient embryonic stem cells display a decreased homologous recombination frequency and an increased frequency of non-homologous recombination that is corrected by expression of a brca1 transgene. *Oncogene* 1999;18:7900–7907.

99. Moynahan ME, Cui TY, Jasin M. Homology-directed DNA repair, mitomycin-C resistance, and chromosome stability is restored with correction of a *Brca1* mutation. *Cancer Res* 2001;61:4842–4850.

100. Moynahan ME, Pierce AJ, Jasin M. BRCA2 is required for homology-directed repair of chromosomal breaks. *Mol Cell* 2001;7:263–272.

101. Tutt A, Bertwistle D, Valentine J, et al. Mutation in Brca2 stimulates error-prone homology-directed repair of DNA double-strand breaks occurring between repeated sequences. *EMBO J* 2001;20:4704–4716.

102. Xia F, Taghian DG, DeFrank JS, et al. Deficiency of human BRCA2 leads to impaired homologous recombination but maintains normal nonhomologous end joining. *Proc Natl Acad Sci U S A* 2001;98:8644–8649.

103. Yang H, Jeffrey PD, Miller J, et al. BRCA2 function in DNA binding and recombination from a BRCA2-DSS1-ssDNA structure. *Science* 2002;297:1837–1848.

104. Chapman, MS, Verma, IM. Transcriptional activation by BRCA1. *Nature* 1996;382:678–679.

105. Monteiro ANA, August A, Hanafusa H. Evidence for a transcriptional activation function for BRCA1 C-terminal region. *Proc Natl Acad Sci U S A* 1996;93:13595–13599.

106. Scully R, Anderson SF, Chao DM, et al. BRCA1 is a component of the RNA polymerase II holoenzyme. *Proc Natl Acad Sci U S A* 1997;94:5605–5610.

107. Anderson S, Schlegel B, Nakajima T, et al. BRCA1 protein is linked to the RNA polymerase II holoenzyme complex via helicase A. *Nat Genet* 1998;19:1–3.

108. Somasundaram K, Zhang H, Zeng Y-X, et al. Arrest of the cell cycle by the tumour-suppressor BRCA1 requires the CDK-inhibitor p21[WAF1/CIP1]. *Nature* 1997;389:187–190.

109. Li S, Chen P-L, Subramanian T, et al. Binding of CtIP to the BCRT repeats of BRCA1 involved in the transcription regulation of p21 is disrupted upon DNA damage. *J Biol Chem* 1999;274:11334–11338.

110. Harkin DP, Bean JM, Miklos D, et al. Induction of *GADD45* and JNK/SAPK–dependent apoptosis following inducible expression of *BRCA1*. *Cell* 1999;97:575–586.

111. Ouchi T, Monteiro ANA, August A, et al. BRCA1 regulates p53-dependent gene expression. *Proc Natl Acad Sci U S A* 1998;95:2302–2306.

112. Aprelikova O, Pace AJ, Fang B, et al. BRCA1 is a selective co-activator of 14-3-3σ gene transcription in mouse embryonic stem cells. *J Biol Chem* 2001;276:25647–25650.

113. MacLachlan TK, Somasundaram K, Sgagias M, et al. BRCA1 effects on the cell cycle and the DNA damage response are linked to altered gene expression. *J Biol Chem* 2000; 275:2777–2785.

114. Hoeijmakers JHJ. Genome maintenance mechanisms for preventing cancer. *Nature* 2001;411:366–374.

115. Husain A, He G, Venkatraman ES, et al. *BRCA1* up-regulation is associated with repair-mediated resistance to *cis*-diamminedichloroplatinum(II). *Cancer Res* 1998;58:1120–1126.

116. Bhattacharyya A, Ear US, Koller BH, et al. The breast cancer susceptibility gene BRCA1 is required for subnuclear assembly of Rad51 and survival following treatment with the DNA cross-linking agent cisplatin. *J Biol Chem* 2000;275:23899–23903.

117. Lafarge S, Sylvain V, Ferrara M, et al. Inhibition of BRCA1 leads to increased chemoresistance to microtubule-interfering agents, an effect that involves the JNK pathway. *Oncogene* 2001;20:6597–6606.

118. Abbott DW, Thompson ME, Robinson-Benion C, et al. BRCA1 expression restores radiation resistance in BRCA1-defective cancer cells through enhancement of transcription-coupled DNA repair. *J Biol Chem* 1999;274:18808–18812.

119. Scully R, Ganesan S, Vlasakova K, et al. Genetic analysis of BRCA1 function in a defined tumor cell line. *Mol Cell* 1999;4:1093–1099.

120. Cortez D, Wang Y, Qin J, et al. Requirement of ATM-dependent phosphorylation of Brca1 in the DNA damage response to double-strand breaks. *Science* 1999;286:1162–1166.

121. Lee J-S, Collins KM, Brown AL, et al. hCds1-mediated phosphorylation of BRCA1 regulates the DNA damage response. *Nature* 2000;404:201–204.

122. Rubin SC, Benjamin I, Behbakht K, et al. Clinical and pathologic features of ovarian cancer in women with germ-line mutations of *BRCA1*. *N Engl J Med* 1996;335:1413–1416.

123. Boyd J, Sonoda Y, Federici MG, et al. Clinicopathologic features of *BRCA*-linked and sporadic ovarian cancer. *JAMA* 2000;283:2260–2265.

124. Ben-David Y, Chetrit A, Hirsh-Yechezkel G, et al. Effect of BRCA

mutations on the length of survival in epithelial ovarian tumors. *J Clin Oncol* 2002;20:463–466.

125. Li J, Yen C, Liaw D, et al. *PTEN*, a putative protein tyrosine phosphatase gene mutated in human brain, breast, and prostate cancer. *Science* 1997;275:1943–1947.

126. Steck PA, Pershouse MA, Jasser SA, et al. Identification of a candidate tumour suppressor gene, *MMAC1*, at chromosome 10q23.3 that is mutated in multiple advanced cancers. *Nat Genet* 1997;15:356–362.

127. Marsh DJ, Dahia PLM, Liaw D, et al. Germline mutations in *PTEN* are present in Bannayan-Zonana syndrome. *Nat Genet* 1997;16:333–334.

128. Tamura M, Gu J, Matsumoto K, et al. Inhibition of cell migration, spreading, and focal adhesions by tumor suppressor PTEN. *Science* 1998;280:1614–1618.

129. Gu J, Tamura M, Yamada KM. Tumor suppressor PTEN inhibits integrin- and growth factor-mediated mitogen-activated protein (MAP) kinase signaling pathways. *J Cell Biol* 1998;143:1375–1383.

130. Wu X, Senechal K, Neshat MS, et al. The PTEN/MMAC1 tumor suppressor phosphatase functions as a negative regulator of the phosphoinositide 3-kinase/Akt pathway. *Proc Natl Acad Sci U S A* 1998; 95:15587–15591.

131. Waite KA, Eng C. Protean PTEN: form and function. *Am J Hum Genet* 2002;70:829–844.

132. Eng C. Will the real Cowden syndrome please stand up: revised diagnostic criteria. *J Med Genet* 2000;37:828–830.

133. Nagase S, Yamakawa H, Sato S, et al. Identification of a 790-kilobase region of common allelic loss in chromosome 10q25-q26 in human endometrial cancer. *Cancer Res* 1997;57:1630–1633.

134. Peiffer SL, Herzog TJ, Tribune DJ, et al. Allelic loss of sequences from the long arm of chromosome 10 and replication errors in endometrial cancers. *Cancer Res* 1995;55:1922–1926.

135. Kong D, Suzuki A, Zou T-T, et al. *PTEN* is frequently mutated in primary endometrial carcinomas. *Nat Genet* 1997;17:143–144.

136. Risinger JI, Hayes AK, Berchuck A, et al. *PTEN/MMAC1* mutations in endometrial cancers. *Cancer Res* 1997;57:4736–4738.

137. Tashiro H, Blazes MS, Wu R, et al. Mutations in *PTEN* are frequent in endometrial carcinoma but rare in other common gynecological malignancies. *Cancer Res* 1997;57:3935–3940.

138. Maxwell GL, Risinger JI, Gumbs C, et al. Mutation of the *PTEN* tumor suppressor gene in endometrial hyperplasias. *Cancer Res* 1998; 58:2500–2503.

139. Obat, K, Morland SJ, Watson RH, et al. Frequent PTEN/MMAC mutations in endometrioid but not serous or mucinous epithelial ovarian tumors. *Cancer Res* 1998;58:2095–2097.

140. Maxwell GL, Risinger JI, Tong B, et al. Mutation of the *PTEN* tumor suppressor gene is not a feature of ovarian cancers. *Gynecol Oncol* 1998;70:13–16.

141. Bishop JM. Molecular themes in oncogenesis. *Cell* 1991;64:235–248.

142. Weinberg RA. Oncogenes, antioncogenes, and the molecular basis of multistep carcinogenesis. *Cancer Res* 1989;49:3713–3721.

143. Madhani HD. Accounting for specificity in receptor tyrosine kinase signaling. *Cell* 2001;106:9–11.

144. Boerner JL, Danielsen A, Maihle NJ. Ligand-independent oncogenic signaling by the epidermal growth factor receptor: v-ErbB as a paradigm. *Exp Cell Res* 2003;284:111–121.

145. Carpenter G, Cohen S. Epidermal growth factor. *J Biol Chem* 1990; 265:7709–7712.

146. Cantley LC, Auger KR, Carpenter C, et al. Oncogenes and signal transduction. *Cell* 1991;64:281–302.

147. Pinkas-Kramarski R, Shelly M, Guarino BC, et al. ErbB tyrosine kinases and the two neuregulin families constitute a ligand-receptor network. *Mol Cell Biol* 1998;18:6090–6101.

148. Fan Z, Mendelsohn J. Therapeutic application of anti-growth factor receptor antibodies. *Curr Opin Oncol* 1998;10:67–73.

149. Berchuck A, Rodriguez G, Kamel A, et al. Expression of epidermal growth factor receptor and HER-2/neu in normal and neoplastic cervix, vulva, and vagina. *Obstet Gynecol* 1990;76:381–387.

150. Sridhar SS, Seymour L, Shepherd FA. Inhibitors of epidermal-growth-factor receptors: a review of clinical research with a focus on non–small-cell lung cancer. *Lancet Oncol* 2003;4:397–406.

151. Bargmann CI, Hung MC, Weinberg RA. The neu oncogene encodes an epidermal growth factor receptor–related protein. *Nature* 1986; 319:226–230.

152. Penuel E, Schaefer G, Akita RW, et al. Structural requirements for ErbB2 transactivation. *Semin Oncol* 2001;28[6 Suppl 18]:36–42.

153. Slamon DJ, Godolphin W, Jones LA, et al. Studies of the HER-2/*neu* proto-oncogene in human breast and ovarian cancer. *Science* 1989; 244:707–712.

154. Tan AR, Swain SM. Ongoing adjuvant trials with trastuzumab in breast cancer. *Semin Oncol* 2003;30[5 Suppl 16]:54–64.

155. Bookman MA, Darcy KM, Clarke-Pearson D, et al. Evaluation of monoclonal humanized anti-HER2 antibody, trastuzumab, in patients with recurrent or refractory ovarian or primary peritoneal carcinoma with overexpression of HER2: a phase II trial of the Gynecologic Oncology Group. *J Clin Oncol* 2003;21:283–290.

156. Neves SR, Ram PT, Iyengar R. G protein pathways. *Science* 2002; 296:1636–1639.

157. Campbell SL, Khosravi-Far R, Rossman KL, et al. Increasing complexity of Ras signalling. *Oncogene* 1998;17:1395–1413.

158. Gutkind JS. Cell growth control by G-protein–coupled receptors: from signal transduction to signal integration. *Oncogene* 1998;17: 1331–1342.

159. Bos JL. ras oncogenes in human cancer: a review. *Cancer Res* 1989; 49:4682–4689.

160. Baum C, Kirschmeier P. Preclinical and clinical evaluation of farnesyltransferase inhibitors. *Curr Oncol Rep* 2003;5:99–107.

161. Pelengaris S, Khan M. The many faces of c-MYC. *Arch Biochem Biophys* 2003;416:129–136.

162. Grandori C, Cowley SM, James LP, et al. The Myc/Max/Mad network and the transcriptional control of cell behavior. *Ann Rev Cell Dev Biol* 2000;16:653–699.

163. Nilsson JA, Cleveland JL. Myc pathways provoking cell suicide and cancer. *Oncogene* 2003;22:9007–9021.

164. Deligdisch L, Holinka CF. Endometrial carcinoma: two diseases? *Cancer Detect Prev* 1987;10:237–246.

165. Shah NK, Currie JL, Rosenshein N, et al. Cytogenetic and FISH analysis of endometrial carcinoma. *Cancer Genet Cytogenet* 1994;73: 142–146.

166. Baloglu H, Cannizzaro LA, Jones J, et al. Atypical endometrial hyperplasia shares genomic abnormalities with endometrioid carcinoma by comparative genomic hybridization. *Hum Pathol* 2001;32:615–622.

167. Kiechle M, Hinrichs M, Jacobsen A, et al. Genetic imbalances in precursor lesions of endometrial cancer detected by comparative genomic hybridization. *Am J Pathol* 2000;156:1827–1833.

168. Suzuki A, Fukushige S, Nagase S, et al. Frequent gains on chromosome arms 1q and/or 8q in human endometrial cancer. *Hum Genet* 1997;100:629–636.

169. Sonoda G, du Manoir S, Godwin AK, et al. Detection of DNA gains and losses in primary endometrial carcinomas by comparative genomic hybridization. *Genes Chromosomes Cancer* 1997;18:115–125.

170. Hirasawa A, Aoki D, Inoue J, et al. Unfavorable prognostic factors associated with high frequency of microsatellite instability and comparative genomic hybridization analysis in endometrial cancer. *Clin Cancer Res* 2003;9:5675–5682.

171. Risinger JI, Maxwell GL, Chandramouli GV, et al. Microarray analysis reveals distinct gene expression profiles among different histologic types of endometrial cancer. *Cancer Res* 2003;63:6–11.

172. Suehiro Y, Umayahara K, Ogata H, et al. Genetic aberrations detected by comparative genomic hybridization predict outcome in patients with endometrioid carcinoma. *Genes Chromosomes Cancer* 2000;29: 75–82.

173. Lukes AS, Kohler MF, Pieper CF, et al. Multivariable analysis of DNA ploidy, p53, and HER-2/neu as prognostic factors in endometrial cancer. *Cancer* 1994;73:2380–2385.

174. Moreno-Bueno G, Sanchez-Estevez C, Cassia R, et al. Differential gene expression profile in endometrioid and nonendometrioid endometrial carcinoma: STK15 is frequently overexpressed and amplified in nonendometrioid carcinomas. *Cancer Res* 2003;63:5697–5702.

175. Berchuck A, Kohler MF, Marks JR, et al. The p53 tumor suppressor gene frequently is altered in gynecologic cancers. *Am J Obstet Gynecol* 1994;170:246–252.

176. Kohler MF, Berchuck A, Davidoff AM, et al. Overexpression and mutation of p53 in endometrial carcinoma. *Cancer Res* 1992;52: 1622–1627.

177. Hachisuga T, Fukuda K, Uchiyama M, et al. Immunohistochemical study of p53 expression in endometrial carcinomas: correlation with

markers of proliferating cells and clinicopathologic features. *Int J Gynecol Cancer* 1993;3:363–368.

178. Hamel NW, Sebo TJ, Wilson TO, et al. Prognostic value of p53 and proliferating cell nuclear antigen expression in endometrial carcinoma. *Cancer Res* 1996;62:192–198.

179. Inoue M, Okayama A, Fujita M, et al. Clinicopathological characteristics of p53 overexpression in endometrial cancers. *Int J Cancer* 1994; 58:14–19.

180. Ito K, Watanabe K, Nasim S, et al. Prognostic significance of p53 overexpression in endometrial cancer. *Cancer Res* 1994;54: 4667–4670.

181. Khalifa MA, Mannel RS, Haraway SD, et al. Expression of EGFR, HER-2/*neu*, p53, and PCNA in endometrioid, serous papillary, and clear cell endometrial adenocarcinomas. *Cancer Res* 1994;53:84–92.

182. Kohlberger P, Gitsch G, Loesch A, et al. p53 protein overexpression in early stage endometrial cancer. *Cancer Res* 1996;62:213 –217.

183. Service RF. Research news: Stalking the start of colon cancer. *Science* 1994;263:1559–1560.

184. Clifford SL, Kaminetsky CP, Cirisano FD, et al. Racial disparity in overexpression of the p53 tumor suppressor gene in stage I endometrial cancer. *Am J Obstet Gynecol* 1997;176:S229–S232.

185. Kohler MF, Carney P, Dodge R, et al. p53 overexpression in advanced-stage endometrial adenocarcinoma. *Am J Obstet Gynecol* 1996;175:1246–1252.

186. Liu FS, Kohler MF, Marks JR, et al. Mutation and overexpression of the p53 tumor suppressor gene frequently occurs in uterine and ovarian sarcomas. *Obstet Gynecol* 1994;83:118–124.

187. Hall KL, Teneriello MG, Taylor RR, et al. Analysis of Ki-ras, p53, and MDM2 genes in uterine leiomyomas and leiomyosarcomas. *Cancer Res* 1997;65:330–335.

188. Enomoto T, Fujita M, Inoue M, et al. Alterations of the p53 tumor suppressor gene and its association with activation of the c-K-*ras*-2 protooncogene in premalignant and malignant lesions of the human uterine endometrium. *Cancer Res* 1993;53:1883–1888.

189. Okamoto A, Sameshima Y, Yamada Y, et al. Allelic loss on chromosome 17p and p53 mutations in human endometrial carcinoma of the uterus. *Cancer Res* 1991;51:5632–5636.

190. Risinger JI, Dent GA, Ignar-Trowbridge D, et al. Mutations of the p53 gene in human endometrial carcinoma. *Mol Carcinog* 1992;5: 250–253.

191. Yaginuma Y, Westphal H. Analysis of the p53 gene in human uterine carcinoma cell lines. *Cancer Res* 1991;51:6506–6509.

192. Kohler MF, Nishii H, Humphrey PA, et al. Mutation of the p53 tumor-suppressor gene is not a feature of endometrial hyperplasias. *Am J Obstet Gynecol* 1993;169:690–694.

193. Tashiro H, Isacson C, Levine R, et al. p53 gene mutations are common in uterine serous carcinoma and occur early in their pathogenesis. *Am J Pathol* 1997;150:177–185.

194. Kanamori Y, Kigawa J, Itamochi H, et al. Correlation between loss of PTEN expression and Akt phosphorylation in endometrial carcinoma. *Clin Cancer Res* 2001;7:892–895.

195. Risinger JI, Hayes K, Maxwell GL, et al. *PTEN* mutation in endometrial cancers is associated with favorable clinical and pathologic characteristics. *Clin Cancer Res* 1998;4:3005–3010.

196. Milner J, Ponder B, Hughes-Davies L, et al. Transcriptional activation functions in BRCA2. *Nature* 1997;386:772–773.

197. Mutter GL, Ince TA, Baak JP, et al. Molecular identification of latent precancers in histologically normal endometrium. *Cancer Res* 2001; 61:4311–4314.

198. Mutter GL, Lin MC, Fitzgerald JT, et al. Altered PTEN expression as a diagnostic marker for the earliest endometrial precancers. *J Natl Cancer Inst* 2000;92:924–930.

199. Lin WM, Forgacs E, Warshal DP, et al. Loss of heterozygosity and mutational analysis of the PTEN/MMAC1 gene in synchronous endometrial and ovarian carcinomas. *Clin Cancer Res* 1998;4:2577–2583.

200. Risinger JI, Berchuck A, Kohler MF, et al. Genetic instability of microsatellites in endometrial carcinoma. *Cancer Res* 1993;53: 5100–5103.

201. Faquin WC, Fitzgerald JT, Lin MC, et al. Sporadic microsatellite instability is specific to neoplastic and preneoplastic endometrial tissues. *Am J Clin Pathol* 2000;113:576–582.

202. Kowalski LD, Mutch DG, Herzog TJ, et al. Mutational analysis of MLH1 and MSH2 in 25 prospectively-acquired RER + endometrial cancers. *Genes Chromosomes Cancer* 1997;18:219–227.

203. Simpkins SB, Bocker T, Swisher EM, et al. MLH1 promoter methylation and gene silencing is the primary cause of microsatellite instability in sporadic endometrial cancers. *Hum Mol Genet* 1999;8:661–666.

204. Salvesen HB, MacDonald N, Ryan A, et al. Methylation of hMLH1 in a population-based series of endometrial carcinomas. *Clin Cancer Res* 2000;6:3607–3613.

205. Esteller M, Catasus L, Matias-Guiu X, et al. hMLH1 promoter hypermethylation is an early event in human endometrial tumorigenesis. *Am J Pathol* 1999;155:1767–1772.

206. Kanaya T, Kyo S, Maida Y, et al. Frequent hypermethylation of MLH1 promoter in normal endometrium of patients with endometrial cancers. *Oncogene* 2003;22:2352–2360.

207. Risinger JI, Maxwell GL, Berchuck A, et al. Promoter hypermethylation as an epigenetic component in Type I and Type II endometrial cancers. *Ann N Y Acad Sci* 2003;983:208–212.

208. Momparler RL. Cancer epigenetics. *Oncogene* 2003;22:6479–6483.

209. Spruck CH, Strohmaier H, Sangfelt O, et al. hCDC4 gene mutations in endometrial cancer. *Cancer Res* 2002;62:4535–4539.

210. Berchuck A, Rodriguez G, Kinney RB, et al. Overexpression of HER-2/neu in endometrial cancer is associated with advanced stage disease. *Am J Obstet Gynecol* 1991;164:t–21.

211. Hetzel DJ, Wilson TO, Keeney GL, et al. HER-2/*neu* expression: A major prognostic factor in endometrial cancer. *Cancer Res* 1992;47: 179–185.

212. Lu KH, Bell DA, Welch WR, et al. Evidence for the multifocal origin of bilateral and advanced human serous borderline ovarian tumors. *Cancer Res* 1998;58:2328–2330.

213. Monk BJ, Chapman JA, Johnson GA, et al. Correlation of c-*myc* and HER-2/*neu* amplification and expression with histopathologic variables in uterine corpus cancer. *Am J Obstet Gynecol* 1994;171: 1193–1198.

214. Santin AD, Bellone S, Gokden M, et al. Overexpression of HER-2/neu in uterine serous papillary cancer. *Clin Cancer Res* 2002;8: 1271–1279.

215. Kacinski BM, Carter D, Kohorn EI, et al. High level expression of *fms* proto-oncogene mRNA is observed in clinically aggressive endometrial adenocarcinomas. *Radiat Int J Oncol Biol Phys* 1988;15: 823–829.

216. Leiserowitz GS, Harris SA, Subramaniam M, et al. The proto-oncogene c-*fms* is overexpressed in endometrial cancer. *Cancer Res* 1993; 49:190–196.

217. Kacinski BM, Chambers SK, Stanley ER, et al. The cytokine CSF-1 (M-CSF), expressed by endometrial carcinomas *in vivo* and *in vitro*, may also be a circulating tumor marker of neoplastic disease activity in endometrial carcinoma patients. *Int J Radiat Oncol Biol Phys* 1990; 19:619–626.

218. Filderman AE, Bruckner A, Kacinski BMDN, et al. Macrophage colony-stimulating factor (CSF-1) enhances invasiveness in CSF-1 receptor-positive carcinoma cell lines. *Cancer Res* 1992;52:3661–3666.

219. Boyd J, Risinger JI Analysis of oncogene alterations in human endometrial carcinoma: prevalence of ras mutations. *Mol Carcinog* 1991; 4:189–195.

220. Ignar-Trowbridge D, Risinger JI, Dent GA, et al. Mutations of the Ki-*ras* oncogene in endometrial carcinoma. *Am J Obstet Gynecol* 1992;167:227–232.

221. Duggan BD, Felix JC, Muderspach LI, et al. Early mutational activation of the c-Ki-ras oncogene in endometrial carcinoma. *Cancer Res* 1994;54:1604–1607.

222. Enomoto T, Inoue M, Perantoni AO, et al. K-ras activation in neoplasms of the human female reproductive tract. *Cancer Res* 1990;50: 6139–6145.

223. Enomoto T, Inoue M, Perantoni AO, et al. K-*ras* activation in premalignant and malignant epithelial lesions of the human uterus. *Cancer Res* 1991;51:5308–5314.

224. Fujimoto I, Shimizu Y, Hirai Y, et al. Studies on *ras* oncogene activation in endometrial carcinoma. *Cancer Res* 1993;48:196–202.

225. Mizuuchi H, Nasim S, Kudo R, et al. Clinical implications of K-ras mutations in malignant epithelial tumors of the endometrium. *Cancer Res* 1992;52:2777–2781.

226. Sasaki H, Nishii H, Tada A, et al. Mutation of the Ki-*ras* protoonco-

gene in human endometrial hyperplasia and carcinoma. *Cancer Res* 1993;53:1906–1910.

227. Mutter GL, Wada H, Faquin WC, et al. K-ras mutations appear in the premalignant phase of both microsatellite stable and unstable endometrial carcinogenesis. *Mol Pathol* 1999;52:257–262.

228. Risinger JI, Berchuck A, Kohler MF, et al. Mutations of the E-cadherin gene in human gynecologic cancers. *Nat Genet* 1994;7:98–102.

229. Fujimoto J, Ichigo S, Hori M, et al. Expressions of E-cadherin and alpha- and beta-catenin mRNAs in uterine endometrial cancers. *Eur J Gynaecol Oncol* 1998;19:78–81.

230. Hirohashi S. Inactivation of the E-cadherin-mediated cell adhesion system in human cancers. *Am J Pathol* 1998;153:333–339.

231. O'Sullivan MJ, McCarthy TV, Doyle CT. Familial adenomatous polyposis: from bedside to benchside. *Am J Clin Pathol* 1998;109: 521–526.

232. Moreno-Bueno G, Hardisson D, Sanchez C, et al. Abnormalities of the APC/beta-catenin pathway in endometrial cancer. *Oncogene* 2002; 21:7981–7990.

233. Zysman M, Saka A, Millar A, et al. Methylation of adenomatous polyposis coli in endometrial cancer occurs more frequently in tumors with microsatellite instability phenotype. *Cancer Res* 2002;62: 3663–3666.

234. Mitra AB, Murty VV, Pratap M, et al. ERBB2 (HER2/neu) oncogene is frequently amplified in squamous cell carcinoma of the uterine cervix. *Cancer Res* 1994;54:637–639.

235. Fukuchi T, Sakamoto M, Tsuda H, et al. Beta-catenin mutation in carcinoma of the uterine endometrium. *Cancer Res* 1998;58: 3526–3528.

236. Odom LD, Barrett JM, Pantazis CG, et al. Immunocytochemical study of ras and myc proto-oncogene polypeptide expression in the human menstrual cycle. *Am J Obstet Gynecol* 1989;161:1663–1668.

237. Borst MP, Baker VV, Dixon D, et al. Oncogene alterations in endometrial carcinoma. *Cancer Res* 1990;38:364–366.

238. Williams JA, Jr., Wang ZR, Parrish RS, et al. Fluorescence in situ hybridization analysis of HER-2/neu, c-myc, and p53 in endometrial cancer. *Exp Mol Pathol* 1999;67:135–143.

239. Whittemore AS, Harris R, Itnyre J. Characteristics relating to ovarian cancer risk. Collaborative analysis of twelve US case-control studies: IV. The pathogenesis of epithelial ovarian cancer. *Am J Epidemiol* 1992;136:1212–1220.

240. Rodriguez GC, Walmer DK, Cline M, et al. Effect of progestin on the ovarian epithelium of macaques: cancer prevention through apoptosis? *J Soc Gynecol Invest* 1998;5:271–276.

241. Jacobs IJ, Kohler MF, Wiseman RW, et al. Clonal origin of epithelial ovarian carcinoma: analysis by loss of heterozygosity, p53 mutation, and X-chromosome inactivation. *J Natl Cancer Inst* 1992;84: 1793–1798.

242. Schorge JO, Muto MG, Welch WR, et al. Molecular evidence for multifocal papillary serous carcinoma of the peritoneum in patients with germline BRCA1 mutations. *J Natl Cancer Inst* 1998;90: 841–845.

243. Kallioniemi A, Kallioniemi OP, Sudar D, et al. Comparative genomic hybridization for molecular cytogenetic analysis of solid tumors. *Science* 1992;258:818–821.

244. Cliby W, Ritland S, Hartmann L, et al. Human epithelial ovarian cancer allelotype. *Cancer Res* 1993;53[Suppl]:8.

245. Dodson MK, Hartmann LC, Cliby WA, et al. Comparison of loss of heterozygosity patterns in invasive low-grade and high-grade epithelial ovarian carcinomas. *Cancer Res* 1993;53:4456–4460.

246. Iwabuchi H, Sakamoto M, Sakunaga H, et al. Genetic analysis of benign, low-grade, and high-grade ovarian tumors. *Cancer Res* 1995; 55:6172–6180.

247. Suzuki S, Moore DH, Ginzinger DG, et al. An approach to analysis of large-scale correlations between genome changes and clinical endpoints in ovarian cancer. *Cancer Res* 2000;60:5382–5385.

248. Welsh JB, Zarrinkar PP, Sapinoso LM, et al. Analysis of gene expression profiles in normal and neoplastic ovarian tissue samples identifies candidate molecular markers of epithelial ovarian cancer. *Proc Natl Acad Sci U S A* 2001;98:1176–1181.

249. Ono K, Tanaka T, Tsunoda T, et al. Identification by cDNA microarray of genes involved in ovarian carcinogenesis. *Cancer Res* 2000; 60:5007–5011.

250. Schummer M, Ng WV, Bumgarner RE, et al. Comparative hybridiza-

251. tion of an array of 21,500 ovarian cDNAs for the discovery of genes overexpressed in ovarian carcinomas. *Gene* 1999;238:375–385.

251. Schwartz DR, Kardia SL, Shedden KA, et al. Gene expression in ovarian cancer reflects both morphology and biological behavior, distinguishing clear cell from other poor-prognosis ovarian carcinomas. *Cancer Res* 2002;62:4722–4729.

252. Shridhar V, Lee J, Pandita A, et al. Genetic analysis of early- versus late-stage ovarian tumors. *Cancer Res* 2001;61:5895–5904.

253. Bennett M, Macdonald K, Chan SW, et al. Cell surface trafficking of Fas: a rapid mechanism of p53-mediated apoptosis. *Science* 1998; 282:290–293.

254. Eltabbakh GH, Belinson JL, Kennedy AW, et al. p53 overexpression is not an independent prognostic factor for patients with primary ovarian epithelial cancer. *Cancer* 1997;80:892–898.

255. Hartmann L, Podratz K, Keeney G, et al. Prognostic significance of p53 immunostaining in epithelial ovarian cancer. *J Clin Oncol* 1994; 12:64–69.

256. Henriksen R, Strang P, Backstrom T, et al. Ki-67 immunostaining and DNA flow cytometry as prognostic factors in epithelial ovarian cancers. *Anticancer Res* 1994;14:603–608.

257. Kohler MF, Kerns BJ, Humphrey PA, et al. Mutation and overexpression of p53 in early-stage epithelial ovarian cancer. *Obstet Gynecol* 1993;81:643–650.

258. Marks JR, Davidoff AM, Kerns B, et al. Overexpression and mutation of p53 in epithelial ovarian cancer. *Cancer Res* 1991;51:2979–2984.

259. van der Zee AG, Hollema H, Suurmeijer AJ, et al. Value of P-glycoprotein, glutathione S-transferase pi, c-erbB-2, and p53 as prognostic factors in ovarian carcinomas. *J Clin Oncol* 1995;13:70–78.

260. Okuda T, Otsuka J, Sekizawa A, et al. p53 mutations and overexpression affect prognosis of ovarian endometrioid cancer but not clear cell cancer. *Cancer Res* 2003;88:318–325.

261. Ho ES, Lai CR, Hsieh YT, et al. p53 mutation is infrequent in clear cell carcinoma of the ovary. *Cancer Res* 2001;80:189–193.

262. Berns EM, Klijn JG, van PWL, et al. p53 protein accumulation predicts poor response to tamoxifen therapy of patients with recurrent breast cancer. *J Clin Oncol* 1998;16:121–127.

263. Havrilesky L, Hamdan H, Darcy K, et al. Relationship between p53 mutation, p53 overexpression and survival in advanced ovarian cancers treated on Gynecologic Oncology Group studies #114 and #132. *J Clin Oncol* 2003;21:3814–3825.

264. Kohler MF, Marks JR, Wiseman RW, et al. Spectrum of mutation and frequency of allelic deletion of the p53 gene in ovarian cancer. *J Natl Cancer Inst* 1993;85:1513–1519.

265. Kupryjanczyk J, Thor AD, Beauchamp R, et al. p53 mutations and protein accumulation in human ovarian cancer. *Proc Natl Acad Sci U S A* 1993;90:4961–4965.

266. Brown R, Clugston C, Burns P, et al. Increased accumulation of p53 protein in cisplatin-resistant ovarian cell lines. *Int J Cancer* 1993;55: 678–684.

267. Eliopoulos AG, Kerr DJ, Herod J, et al. The control of apoptosis and drug resistance in ovarian cancer: influence of p53 and Bcl-2. *Oncogene* 1995;11:1217–1228.

268. Herod JJ, Eliopoulos AG, Warwick J, et al. The prognostic significance of Bcl-2 and p53 expression in ovarian carcinoma. *Cancer Res* 1996;56:2178–2184.

269. Perego P, Giarola M, Righetti SC, et al. Association between cisplatin resistance and mutation of p53 gene and reduced bax expression in ovarian carcinoma cell systems. *Cancer Res* 1996;56:556–562.

270. Righetti SC, Della TG, Pilotti S, et al. A comparative study of p53 gene mutations, protein accumulation, and response to cisplatin-based chemotherapy in advanced ovarian carcinoma. *Cancer Res* 1996;56: 689–693.

271. Havrilesky LJ, Elbendary A, Hurteau JA, et al. Chemotherapy-induced apoptosis in epithelial ovarian cancers. *Obstet Gynecol* 1995; 85:1007–1010.

272. Berchuck A, Kohler MF, Hopkins MP, et al. Overexpression of p53 is not a feature of benign and early-stage borderline epithelial ovarian tumors. *Cancer Res* 1994; 52:232–236.

273. Gershenson DM, Deavers M, Diaz S, et al. Prognostic significance of p53 expression in advanced-stage ovarian serous borderline tumors. *Clin Cancer Res* 1999;5:4053–4058.

274. Ortiz BH, Ailawadi M, Colitti C, et al. Second primary or recurrence? Comparative patterns of p53 and K-ras mutations suggest that serous

borderline ovarian tumors and subsequent serous carcinomas are unrelated tumors. *Cancer Res* 2001;61:7264–7267.

275. Flesken-Nikitin A, Choi KC, Eng JP, et al. Induction of carcinogenesis by concurrent inactivation of p53 and Rb1 in the mouse ovarian surface epithelium. *Cancer Res* 2003;63:3459–3463.

276. Plaxe SC, Deligdisch L, Dottino PR, et al. Ovarian intraepithelial neoplasia demonstrated in patients with stage I ovarian carcinoma. *Cancer Res* 1990;38:367–372.

277. Brewer MA, Johnson K, Follen M, et al. Prevention of ovarian cancer: intraepithelial neoplasia. *Clin Cancer Res* 2003;9:20–30.

278. Schultz DC, Vanderveer L, Buetow KH, et al. Characterization of chromosome 9 in human ovarian neoplasia identifies frequent genetic imbalance on 9q and rare alterations involving 9p, including CDKN2. *Cancer Res* 1995;55:2150–2157.

279. McCluskey LL, Chen C, Delgadillo E, et al. Differences in p16 gene methylation and expression in benign and malignant ovarian tumors. *Cancer Res* 1999;72:87–92.

280. Catteau A, Harris WH, Xu CF, et al. Methylation of the BRCA1 promoter region in sporadic breast and ovarian cancer: correlation with disease characteristics. *Oncogene* 1999;18:1957–1965.

281. Schmider A, Gee C, Friedmann W, et al. p21 (WAF1/CIP1) protein expression is associated with prolonged survival but not with p53 expression in epithelial ovarian carcinoma. *Cancer Res* 2000;77:237–242.

282. Levesque MA, Katsaros D, Massobrio M, et al. Evidence for a dose-response effect between p53 (but not p21WAF1/Cip1) protein concentrations, survival, and responsiveness in patients with epithelial ovarian cancer treated with platinum-based chemotherapy. *Clin Cancer Res* 2000;6:3260–3270.

283. Masciullo V, Ferrandina G, Pucci B, et al. p27Kip1 expression is associated with clinical outcome in advanced epithelial ovarian cancer: multivariate analysis. *Clin Cancer Res* 2000;6:4816–4822.

284. Sui L, Dong Y, Ohno M, et al. Implication of malignancy and prognosis of p27(kip1), cyclin E, and Cdk2 expression in epithelial ovarian tumors. *Cancer Res* 2001;83:56–63.

285. Hurteau JA, Allison BM, Brutkiewicz SA, et al. Expression and subcellular localization of the cyclin-dependent kinase inhibitor p27(Kip1) in epithelial ovarian cancer. *Cancer Res* 2001;83:292–298.

286. Korkolopoulou P, Vassilopoulos I, Konstantinidou AE, et al. The combined evaluation of p27Kip1 and Ki-67 expression provides independent information on overall survival of ovarian carcinoma patients. *Cancer Res* 2002;85:404–414.

287. Berchuck A, Olt GJ, Everitt L, et al. The role of peptide growth factors in epithelial ovarian cancer. *Obstet Gynecol* 1990;75:255–262.

288. Hurteau J, Whitaker RS, Rodriguez GC, et al. Effect of transforming growth factor-β on proliferation of human ovarian cancer cells obtained from ascites. *Soc Gynecol Invest* 1993;40:128–128.

289. Baldwin RL, Tran H, Karlan BY. Loss of c-myc repression coincides with ovarian cancer resistance to transforming growth factor beta growth arrest independent of transforming growth factor beta/Smad signaling. *Cancer Res* 2003;63:1413–1419.

290. Wang D, Kanuma T, Mizunuma H, et al. Analysis of specific gene mutations in the transforming growth factor-beta signal transduction pathway in human ovarian cancer. *Cancer Res* 2000;60:4507–4512.

291. Bauknecht T, Kiechle M, Bauer G, et al. Characterization of growth factors in human ovarian carcinomas. *Cancer Res* 1986;46:2614–2618.

292. Kommoss F, Wintzer HO, Von Kleist S, et al. In situ distribution of transforming growth factor-α in normal human tissues and in malignant tumours of the ovary. *J Pathol* 1990;162:223–230.

293. Morishige K, Kurachi H, Amemiya K, et al. Evidence for the involvement of transforming growth factor-α and epidermal growth factor receptor autocrine growth mechanism in primary human ovarian cancers in vitro. *Cancer Res* 1991;51:5322–5328.

294. Rodriguez GC, Berchuck A, Whitaker RS, et al. Epidermal growth factor receptor expression in normal ovarian epithelium and ovarian cancer. II. Relationship between receptor expression and response to epidermal growth factor. *Am J Obstet Gynecol* 1991;164:745–750.

295. Yee D, Morales FR, Hamilton TC, et al. Expression of insulin-like growth factor I, its binding proteins, and its receptor in ovarian cancer. *Cancer Res* 1991;51:5107–5112.

296. Henrikson R, Funa K, Wilander E, et al. Expression and prognostic significance of platelet-derived growth factor and its receptors in epithelial ovarian neoplasms. *Cancer Res* 1993;53:4550–4554.

297. Sariban E, Sitaras NM, Antoniades HN, et al. Expression of platelet-derived growth factor (PDGF)-related transcripts and synthesis of biologically active PDGF-like proteins by human malignant epithelial cell lines. *J Clin Invest* 1988;82:1157–1164.

298. Di Blasio AM, Cremonesi L, Vigano P, et al. Basic fibroblast growth factor and its receptor messenger ribonucleic acids are expressed in human ovarian epithelial neoplasms. *Am J Obstet Gynecol* 1993;169:1517–1523.

299. Kacinski BM, Stanley ER, Carter D, et al. Circulating levels of CSF-1 (M-CSF), a lymphohematopoietic cytokine, may be a useful marker of disease status in patients with malignant ovarian neoplasms. *Int J Radiat Oncol Biol Phys* 1989;17:159–164.

300. Toy EP, Chambers JT, Kacinski BM, et al. The activated macrophage colony-stimulating factor (CSF-1) receptor as a predictor of poor outcome in advanced epithelial ovarian carcinoma. *Cancer Res* 2001;80:194–200.

301. Furui T, LaPushin R, Mao M, et al. Overexpression of edg-2/vzg-1 induces apoptosis and anoikis in ovarian cancer cells in a lysophosphatidic acid-independent manner. *Clin Cancer Res* 1999;5:4308–4318.

302. Tanyi JL, Morris AJ, Wolf JK, et al. The human lipid phosphate phosphatase-3 decreases the growth, survival, and tumorigenesis of ovarian cancer cells: validation of the lysophosphatidic acid signaling cascade as a target for therapy in ovarian cancer. *Cancer Res* 2003;63:1073–1082.

303. Lidor YJ, Xu FJ, Martinez-Maza O, et al. Constitutive production of macrophage colony stimulating factor and interleukin-6 by human ovarian surface epithelial cells. *Exp Cell Res* 1993;207:332–339.

304. Siemans CH, Auersperg N. Serial propagation of human ovarian surface epithelium in culture. *J Cell Physiol* 1991;134:347–356.

305. Ziltener HJ, Maines-Bandiera S, Schrader JW, et al. Secretion of bioactive interleukin-1, interleukin-6 and colony-stimulating factors by human ovarian surface epithelium. *Biol Reprod* 1993;49:635–641.

306. Tzahar E, Yarden Y. The ErbB-2/HER2 oncogenic receptor of adenocarcinomas: from orphanhood to multiple stromal ligands. *Biochim Biophys Acta* 1998;1377:M25-M37.

307. Berchuck A, Kamel A, Whitaker R, et al. Overexpression of HER-2/*neu* is associated with poor survival in advanced epithelial ovarian cancer. *Cancer Res* 1990;50:4087–4091.

308. Kacinski BM, Mayer AG, King BL, et al. *Neu* protein overexpression in benign, borderline, and malignant ovarian neoplasms. *Cancer Res* 1992;44:245–253.

309. Rubin SC, Finstad CL, Wong GY, et al. Prognostic significance of HER-2/*neu* expression in advanced ovarian cancer. *Am J Obstet Gynecol* 1993;168:162–169.

310. Rodriguez GC, Boente MP, Berchuck A, et al. The effect of antibodies and immunotoxins reactive with HER-2/neu on growth of ovarian and breast cancer cell lines. *Am J Obstet Gynecol* 1993;168:228–232.

311. Pietras RJ, Pegram MD, Finn RS, et al. Remission of human breast cancer xenografts on therapy with humanized monoclonal antibody to HER-2 receptor and DNA-reactive drugs. *Oncogene* 1998;17:2235–2249.

312. Pegram MD, Lipton A, Hayes DF, et al. Phase II study of receptor-enhanced chemosensitivity using recombinant humanized anti-p185HER2/neu monoclonal antibody plus cisplatin in patients with HER2/neu-overexpressing metastatic breast cancer refractory to chemotherapy treatment. *J Clin Oncol* 1998;16:2659–2671.

313. Haas M, Isakov J, Howell SB. Evidence against *ras* activation in human ovarian carcinomas. *Mol Biol Med* 1987;4:265–275.

314. Feig LA, Bast RC, Jr., Knapp RC, et al. Somatic activation of *ras*K gene in a human ovarian carcinoma. *Science* 1984;223:698–701.

315. Gemignani ML, Schlaerth AC, Bogomolniy F, et al. Role of KRAS and BRAF gene mutations in mucinous ovarian carcinoma. *Cancer Res* 2003;90:378–381.

316. Teneriello MG, Ebina M, Linnoila RI, et al. p53 and ki-*ras* gene mutations in epithelial ovarian neoplasms. *Cancer Res* 1993;53:3103–3108.

317. Mok SCH, Bell DA, Knapp RC, et al. Mutation of K-*ras* protooncogene in human ovarian epithelial tumors of borderline malignancy. *Cancer Res* 1993;53:1489–1492.

318. Shayesteh L, Lu Y, Kuo WL, et al. PIK3CA is implicated as an oncogene in ovarian cancer. *Nat Genet* 1999;21:99–102.

319. Cheng JQ, Godwin AK, Bellacosa A, et al. AKT2, a putative oncogene encoding a member of a subfamily of protein-serine/threonine kinases, is amplified in human ovarian carcinomas. *Proc Natl Acad Sci U S A* 1992;89:9267–9271.

320. Wu R, Zhai Y, Fearon ER, et al. Diverse mechanisms of beta-catenin deregulation in ovarian endometrioid adenocarcinomas . *Cancer Res* 2001;61:8247–8255.

321. Baker VV, Borst MP, Dixon D, et al. c-myc amplification in ovarian cancer. *Cancer Res* 1990;38:340–342.

322. Berns EMJJ, Klijn JGM, Henzen-Logmans SC, et al. Receptors for hormones and growth factors (onco)-gene amplification in human ovarian cancer. *Int J Cancer* 1992;52:218–224.

323. Sasano H, Garrett C, Wilkinson D, et al. Protoocogene amplification and tumor ploidy in human ovarian neoplasms. *Hum Pathol* 1990; 21:4:382–391.

324. Serova DM. Amplification of c-*myc* proto-oncogene in primary tumors, metastases and blood leukocytes of patients with ovarian cancer. *Eksp Onkol* 1987;9:25–27.

325. Zhou DJ, Gonzalez-Cadavid N, Ahuja H, et al. A unique pattern of proto-oncogene abnormalities in ovarian adenocarcinomas. *Cancer* 1988;62:1573–1576.

326. Tashiro H, Niyazaki K, Okamura H, et al. c-*myc* overexpression in human primary ovarian tumors: its relevance to tumor progression. *Int J Cancer* 1992;50:828–833.

327. Marx J. Research news: how cells cycle towards cancer. *Science* 1994; 263:319–321.

328. Farley J, Smith LM, Darcy KM, et al. Cyclin E expression is a significant predictor of survival in advanced, suboptimally debulked ovarian epithelial cancers: a Gynecologic Oncology Group study. *Cancer Res* 2003;63:1235–1241.

329. Alani RM, Munger K. Human papillomaviruses and associated malignancies. *J Clin Oncol* 1998;16:330–337.

330. Arends MJ, Buckley CH, Wells M. Aetiology, pathogenesis, and pathology of cervical neoplasia. *J Clin Pathol* 1998;51:96–103.

331. Lowy DR, Schiller JT Papillomaviruses and cervical cancer: pathogenesis and vaccine development. *J Natl Cancer Inst Monogr* 1998; 27–30.

332. Munoz N, Bosch FX, de Sanjose S, et al. Epidemiologic classification of human papillomavirus types associated with cervical cancer. *N Engl J Med* 2003;348:518–527.

333. Sun XW, Kuhn L, Ellerbrock TV, et al. Human papillomavirus infection in women infected with the human immunodeficiency virus. *N Engl J Med* 1997;337:1343–1349.

334. Koutsky LA, Ault KA, Wheeler CM, et al. A controlled trial of a human papillomavirus type 16 vaccine. *N Engl J Med* 2002;347: 1645–1651.

335. Scheffner M, Werness BA, Huibregtse JM, et al. The E6 oncoprotein encoded by human papillomavirus types 16 and 18 promotes the degradation of p53. *Cell* 1990;63:1129–1136.

336. Scheffner M, Munger K, Byrne JC, et al. The state of the p53 and retinoblastoma gene in human cervical carcinoma cell lines. *Proc Natl Acad Sci U S A* 1991;88:5523–5527.

337. Werness BA, Levine AJ, Howley PM. Association of human papillomavirus types 16 and 18 E6 proteins with p53. *Science* 1990;248: 76–79.

338. Parker MF, Arroyo GF, Geradts J, et al. Molecular characterization of adenocarcinoma of the cervix. *Cancer Res* 1997;64:242–251.

339. Narayan G, Pulido HA, Koul S, et al. Genetic analysis identifies putative tumor suppressor sites at 2q35-q36.1 and 2q36.3-q37.1 involved in cervical cancer progression. *Oncogene* 2003;22:3489–3499.

340. Umayahara K, Numa F, Suehiro Y, et al. Comparative genomic hybridization detects genetic alterations during early stages of cervical cancer progression. *Genes Chromosomes Cancer* 2002;33:98–102.

341. Matthews CP, Shera KA, McDougall JK. Genomic changes and HPV type in cervical carcinoma. *Proc Soc Exp Biol Med* 2000;223: 316–321.

342. Hidalgo A, Schewe C, Petersen S, et al. Human papilloma virus status and chromosomal imbalances in primary cervical carcinomas and tumour cell lines. *Eur J Cancer* 2000;36:542–548.

343. Kirchhoff M, Rose H, Petersen BL, et al. Comparative genomic hybridization reveals a recurrent pattern of chromosomal aberrations in severe dysplasia/carcinoma in situ of the cervix and in advanced-stage cervical carcinoma. *Genes Chromosomes Cancer* 1999;24:144–150.

344. Heselmeyer K, Macville M, Schrock E, et al. Advanced-stage cervical carcinomas are defined by a recurrent pattern of chromosomal aberrations revealing high genetic instability and a consistent gain of chromosome arm 3q. *Genes Chromosomes Cancer* 1997;19:233–240.

345. Yang YC, Shyong WY, Chang MS, et al. Frequent gain of copy number on the long arm of chromosome 3 in human cervical adenocarcinoma. *Cancer Genet Cytogenet* 2001;131:48–53.

346. Lin WM, Michalopulos EA, Dhurander N, et al. Allelic loss and microsatellite alterations of chromosome 3p14.2 are more frequent in recurrent cervical dysplasias. *Clin Cancer Res* 2000;6:1410–1414.

347. Grendys ECJ, Barnes WA, Weitzel J, et al. Identification of H, K, and N-ras point mutations in stage IB cervical carcinoma. *Cancer Res* 1997;65:343–347.

348. Koulos JP, Wright TC, Mitchell MF, et al. Relationships between c-Ki-*ras* mutations, HPV types, and prognostic indicators in invasive endocervical adenocarcinoma. *Cancer Res* 1993;48:364–369.

349. Riou G, Barrois M, Sheng ZM, et al. Somatic deletions and mutations of c-Ha-*ras* gene in human cervical cancers. *Oncogene* 1988;3: 329–333.

350. Van Le L, Stoerker J, Rinehart CA, et al. H-*ras* codon 12 mutation in cervical dysplasia. *Cancer Res* 1993;49:181–184.

351. Riou G, Le MG, Favre M, et al. Human papillomavirus-negative status and c-*myc* gene overexpression: independent prognostic indicators of distant metastasis for early-stage invasive cervical cancers. *J Natl Cancer Inst* 1992;84:1525–1526.

352. Bourhis J, Le MG, Barrois M, et al. Prognostic value of c-myc proto-oncogene overexpression in early invasive carcinoma of the cervix. *J Clin Oncol* 1990;8:1789–1796.

353. Birrer MJ, Hendricks D, Farley J, et al. Abnormal Fhit expression in malignant and premalignant lesions of the cervix. *Cancer Res* 1999; 59:5270–5274.

354. Huang LW, Chao SL, Chen TJ. Reduced Fhit expression in cervical carcinoma: correlation with tumor progression and poor prognosis. *Cancer Res* 2003;90:331–337.

355. Connolly DC, Greenspan DL, Wu R, et al. Loss of fhit expression in invasive cervical carcinomas and intraepithelial lesions associated with invasive disease. *Clin Cancer Res* 2000;6:3505–3510.

356. Liu FS, Hsieh YT, Chen JT, et al. FHIT (fragile histidine triad) gene analysis in cervical intraepithelial neoplasia. *Cancer Res* 2001;82: 283–290.

357. Krivak TC, McBroom JW, Seidman J, et al. Abnormal fragile histidine triad (FHIT) expression in advanced cervical carcinoma: a poor prognostic factor. *Cancer Res* 2001;61:4382–4385.

358. Dong SM, Kim HS, Rha SH, et al. Promoter hypermethylation of multiple genes in carcinoma of the uterine cervix. *Clin Cancer Res* 2001;7:1982–1986.

359. Virmani AK, Muller C, Rathi A, et al. Aberrant methylation during cervical carcinogenesis. *Clin Cancer Res* 2001;7:584–589.

360. Wong YF, Selvanayagam ZE, Wei N, et al. Expression genomics of cervical cancer: molecular classification and prediction of radiotherapy response by DNA microarray. *Clin Cancer Res* 2003;9: 5486–5492.

361. Kuzmin I, Liu L, Dammann R, et al. Inactivation of RAS association domain family 1A gene in cervical carcinomas and the role of human papillomavirus infection. *Cancer Res* 2003;63:1888–1893.

362. Lin WM, Ashfaq R, Michalopulos EA, et al. Molecular Papanicolaou tests in the twenty-first century: molecular analyses with fluid-based Papanicolaou technology. *Am J Obstet Gynecol* 2000;183:39–45.

CHAPTER 6

Immunotherapy of Gynecologic Malignancies

David Z. Chang, Paul J. Sabatini, Chaitanya R. Divgi, Philip O. Livingston, and Alan N. Houghton

The natural clinical history of ovarian cancer makes it ideally suited for the evaluation of immune-based strategies. Although the majority of patients are diagnosed with advanced disease, 70% are in a complete clinical remission following initial cytoreductive surgery and platinum and taxane-based primary chemotherapy (1). However, data from second-look surgical assessments show that more than 60% of patients actually have persistent disease, which is supported by the fact that only 30% of optimally debulked stage III patients will remain disease free with a median progression-free interval of approximately 24 months (2). Despite the high relapse rate, many patients return to a complete or partial clinical remission following additional chemotherapy. With this chronic course of relapse and response, the median survival of optimally debulked patients exceeded 50 months in a study evaluating intraperitoneal therapy as part of primary treatment (3). Neither higher doses and protracted schedules nor non–cross-resistant consolidation chemotherapy has provided additional benefit. These ovarian cancer patients with minimal disease burdens are therefore appropriate candidates for the evaluation of immune-based strategies, which typically have excellent side effect profiles.

With regard to other gynecologic malignancies, the outcome of both early-stage and locally advanced cervix cancer has been improved with the addition of chemotherapy to radiation therapy, yet for those patients who relapse, survival in the metastatic setting is short (4,5). The bulk of immune strategies being evaluated in patients with cervical cancer target human papillomavirus, and this important subject is covered separately by Dr. Thomas Wright in Chapter 19 (6,7). The treatment of patients with metastatic recurrent endometrial cancer is also characterized by limited chemo-

therapy responses of short duration (8). There is a need in each of these gynecologic cancers for more effective therapy, especially in the adjuvant setting, when the target is circulating cancer cells and micrometastases or peritoneal implants. A variety of approaches utilizing the specificity and potency of the immune system are under evaluation including cytokines or other immunological modulators, monoclonal antibodies, and vaccines.

CANCER IMMUNOLOGY: OVERVIEW

The immune system evolved to fight foreign invaders such as bacteria, viruses, and parasites. However, recent evidence strongly suggests that the immune system also plays a crucial role in controlling or even rejecting incipient cancers. Mice that have major defects in immunity develop cancer more frequently, including carcinomas. This is called *immune surveillance* of cancer and has led to the idea that the immune system not only destroys incipient cancers, but that cancer cells in some circumstances are able to escape this early immunity leading to outgrowth of tumors with the capacity to escape recognition by the immune system. The process of tumor cells escaping from immunity is called *immune editing*.

The immune system is broadly divided into two arms. The innate arm of the immune system is present at birth and does not require adaptation to react against microorganisms or tumors. Examples of cells that are part of innate immunity include natural killer (NK) cells, macrophages, and dendritic cells. NK cells are lymphocytes that are programmed to recognize and destroy tissues that have been altered: for example, by viruses. Macrophages play many roles in immunity and inflammation, including production of soluble secreted proteins that are growth factors for other cells of the immune system. These growth factors are called *cytokines* and *chemokines*, and they support the growth and survival of immune and inflammatory cells. Macrophages play important roles

Memorial Sloan-Kettering Cancer Center, New York, New York 10021

in tissue remodeling during wound healing, orchestrating inflammatory responses, and presenting antigens to stimulate T cells. Macrophages may also play a counterproductive role, sometimes inhibiting immune responses.

Acquired immunity develops in response to infection (or potentially cancer progression). This arm of the immune system is not matured or activated at birth, but rather responds to infection. The two major cell types of acquired immunity are *T lymphocytes* (T cells) and *B lymphocytes* (B cells). T cells are set to recognize antigens sequestered inside cells; for instance, viral infections. T cells recognize antigens as short peptides, 8 to16 amino acids in length. Peptides must be presented by specialized antigen-presenting molecules called major histocompatibility complex (MHC) molecules. Examples are the HLA molecules present on almost every cell in the body of humans. On the other hand, B cells produce secreted *antibodies* that can recognize soluble and cell surface molecules. Both T cells and B cells initially develop with a very limited range for immune recognition, but in response to an antigen (e.g., from a virus or cancer cell), T cells or B cells with the best ''fit'' to the antigen are stimulated to proliferate, and this subpopulation can be quickly expanded.

Dendritic cells sit at the crossroads of innate immunity and acquired immunity. These are phagocytic cells that sit on epidermal surfaces, including skin and mucosa, looking for antigens or infectious organisms. Upon taking up antigens (including those expressed by microorganisms), dendritic cells are activated and move to draining lymph nodes. It is in draining lymph nodes that dendritic cells activate appropriate T cells recognizing that particular antigen. These T cells can then travel from a lymph node to a site of infection or tumor. Two types of T cells can be triggered by dendritic cells, depending on whether antigens are presented by MHC class I or MHC class II molecules on the dendritic cell. MHC class I molecules complexed with antigen stimulate CD8$^+$ T cells that are cytotoxic and kill target cells (infected cells or tumor cells). Class II MHC molecules stimulate CD4$^+$ helper T cells. Helper T cells produce chemokines and cytokines to help recruit and orchestrate other components of the immune system. There are two types of T cells. Th1 T cells produce interferon-α (INF-α) and interleukin-12 (IL-12) to recruit cytotoxic T cells and macrophages for *cellular immune responses*. On the other hand, Th2 T cells produce IL-4 and other cytokines that favor antibody responses, called *humoral immunity*. These are different types of immune responses with different characteristics. Cellular immunity may be particularly effective at attacking tumors in tissues, whereas humoral immunity may be better at controlling circulating metastatic tumor cells.

The notion that both the innate and acquired immune arm of the immune system can recognize and reject cancer had been controversial. Careful studies over the past three decades have shown that the immune system can recognize cancers. However, simple recognition by T cells, antibodies, or NK cells is not sufficient. Cytotoxic T cells and NK cells produce soluble and cell surface molecules that induce death of target tumor cells. Helper T cells can produce cytokines and chemokines that not only recruit cytotoxic T cells or B cells to make antibodies, but also inflammatory cells that create tissue destruction. Antibodies can recruit NK cells, macrophages, or other cells that have receptors for antibodies called Fc receptors, leading to activation of the recruited cells. Antibodies can also activate complement proteins in the blood that can directly kill tumor cells and recruit inflammatory cells to the tumor site.

Based on a solid set of evidence that the immune system can recognize antigens on tumor cells and that immunity is sufficient to destroy tumors, many strategies have been attempted at *immunotherapy*. These approaches can be generally divided into three groups. First, *immune modulation* uses nonspecific approaches to treat cancer. Examples include cytokines such as IL-2, INFs, BCG (bacille Calmette-Guérin, an attenuated *Mycobacterium* used successfully for treatment of early recurrent bladder cancer) and microbial products. This approach tends to rely on components from the innate immune arm. *Passive therapy* implies the transfer of specific components from the acquired immune system to the host with cancer. The first examples are monoclonal antibodies directed against antigens expressed on the surface of cancer cells. A second example is adopted cellular therapy, where cells from the patient or from a bone marrow donor in a transplant setting are grown or manipulated outside the body and reinfused. Cellular therapy has been particularly focused on T cells and to a lesser extent on NK cells. Finally, active immunization triggers the patient to make her or his own immune response. Vaccines fall into this category. Both passive and active immunotherapy must be directed against specific antigens on cancer cells. Simplistically, three classes of antigens have been defined on cancer cells that are recognized by the immune system. (a) Differentiation antigens are expressed by cancer cells and their normal cell counterparts. For instance, antigens expressed by ovarian carcinomas and normal ovarian epithelium are differentiation antigens. (b) Germ-cell antigens are expressed by germ cells, particularly in sperm, and are silenced in normal adult somatic tissues, but are reexpressed by certain tumors. (c) Genetic mutations and other alterations, such as translocations. Cancer vaccines take two approaches. First, there are vaccines that target differentiation antigens and germ-cell antigens. These vaccines can be composed of peptides, proteins, glycolipids, DNA, or RNA. Second are cellular vaccines, using the patient's own tumor cells or those from another patient. Autologous vaccines use the patient's own cells, and theoretically can trigger immunity against all three classes of antigens. However, cell-based vaccines are complex and have many regulatory hurdles.

In summary, cancer immunology has created a firm scientific footing over the last few decades. In particular, molecules on cancer cells that are recognized by the immune system provide new strategies for immunotherapy.

IMMUNOMODULATION AND CYTOKINE THERAPY

Cytokines play important roles in immune modulation. Many cytokines, including IL-2, IL-3, IL-4, IL-6, IL-10, and IL-12, tumor necrosis factor-α (TNF-α), macrophage colony-stimulating factor, and IFNs, have been studied for their roles in tumor cell killing. Some of these cytokines (IL-2 and IFN-α) have been approved by the U.S. Food and Drug Administration (FDA) for the treatment of melanoma and renal-cell carcinoma.

Gynecological cancers, particularly ovarian cancer, provide a unique environment for cytokine therapy in that the peritoneal cavity is a rich milieu for the elaboration of cytokines (9). The bulk of ovarian cancer occurs in the peritoneal cavity, making the regional administration of biologic therapy theoretically attractive. Distinct patterns of cytokine expression have been observed between the tumor and peritoneal compartments. Some of these cytokines may be counterregulatory components of T-lymphocyte networks that have the potential to either augment or inhibit host antitumor responses (10). The successful outcome of cytokine treatment in ovarian cancer may be the result of a number of mechanisms. Whereas some cytokines may inhibit tumor cell growth, downregulating the production of growth and survival factors, other cytokines may stimulate adaptive immunity or modulate angiogenesis. It is also possible that an individual cytokine has more than one role (11). The major cytokines that have been tested in gynecological cancers are IFN-α, IL-2, and IL-12.

Interferon

Cytokine therapy in gynecological cancers has been studied most extensively with IFN-α. There has been no head-to-head comparison between IFN-α and IFN-γ nonetheless, they appear to have similar antitumor efficacy in ovarian cancer (12–14), and most studies have focused on IFN-α. Although the exact mode of action of IFN in patients with ovarian cancer is unknown, several mechanisms have been proposed: (a) stimulation of NK cells and macrophages, both of which are known to have antitumor properties (15); (b) through antiangiogenic effects; and (c) inhibition of expression of dysregulated oncogenes (such as *HER-2/neu*) and thereby improving the responsiveness of cisplatin-resistant cells (16).

Initial trials with IFN evaluated administration of systemic IFN-α to patients with advanced ovarian cancer. The objective response rate was generally low at about 10% in a Gynecologic Oncology Group (GOG) study, where patients with measurable disease in whom higher priority treatment methods had failed were treated with IFN intramuscularly (17). The systemic IFN-α was also associated with frequent dose-limiting toxicity, including fatigue and flu-like symptoms, and moderate toxicity, such as leukopenia and thrombocytopenia. Because of the poor response rate and frequent toxic-

ity, further studies were focused on regional; that is, intraperitoneal (IP) administration of IFN-α. Multiple clinical trials with IP IFN therapy were carried out in women with persistent ovarian cancer (15,18–26). The surgically documented response rates from these studies ranged from 30% to 50%. An important finding was that the response rate was inversely correlated with tumor bulk and was not observed in patients with tumors >5 mm. For example, in a study where an overall response rate was 44%, patients with minimal residual disease (defined as < 5 mm) had a response rate of 71%, whereas none of the four patients whose tumors were ≥5 mm responded (18). Systemic IFN toxicity developed following peritoneal absorption, and the maximal tolerable dose (MTD) was defined as 50 MU IP once per week (9). A randomized, placebo-controlled GOG Phase III trial attempted to address the value of IP recombinant IFN-α as an adjuvant therapy in stage III ovarian patients with no evidence of disease at second-look surgery. Unfortunately, the study was prematurely terminated owing to slow accrual secondary to a decline of frequency of second-look surgery nationwide.

Some *in vitro* studies had suggested that IFN could increase the sensitivity of cytotoxic drugs, such as cisplatin and doxorubicin, in cancer cells (13,27). It was found that IFN produced no significant change in the uptake of cisplatin. Studies indicated that the mechanism of IFN-induced sensitization in human ovarian cancer cell lines is multifactorial. Several Phase I studies have been carried out to define the optimal dosing schedule of IP IFN-α in combination with cis-platinum–based chemotherapy (23,28,29). The MTD were generally 20 to 30 MU/m^2 of IFN-α with 60 to 75 mg/m^2 cis-platinum. The most common toxicities were myelosuppression, flu-like symptoms, abdominal pain and fatigue. In general, the combination of IP IFN-α with cis-platinum was less tolerated than IFN-α alone. Several Phase II studies have evaluated the efficacy of this combination with response rates in the range of 20% to 50% (21,23,30). IP carboplatin with or without IFN-α was also evaluated in a randomized trial in 111 patients with advanced ovarian cancer and minimal residual disease who had previously had platinum-based front-line chemotherapy (31). Median survival was 22 and 29 months in the carboplatin arm and in the carboplatin plus IFN-α arm, respectively. The IP IFN-α did not add any benefit to the results achievable with IP carboplatin alone, while the toxicity and the costs of the combination were consistently higher. Taking together all of these studies, there is no evidence that combinations of IP IFN with cytotoxic chemotherapy provide any benefit over single agents. A more recent study with IP IFN-α chemotherapy in ovarian cancer patients with minimal residual disease reported a total complete remission rate of 49% (32). This somewhat higher response rate remains to be confirmed by controlled trials.

In cervical cancer, IFN-α alone had minimal activity (33, 34). In a multiinstitutional, prospective Phase II clinical trial by the Eastern Cooperative Oncology Group (ECOG) evaluating the activity of IFN-α2b in women with metastatic or locally recurrent cervical cancer, only 10% achieved a clinical response. Further studies had been focused on the combination of IFN-α and retinoids because of observed synergistic antiproliferative, differentiating, and antiangiogenic activities in some human hematologic and solid-tumor systems. The proposed mechanisms include (a) the additive activation of transcription of a retinoic reporter gene (35); (b) the induction of higher levels of IFN-α–stimulated genes than the levels induced by either agent alone (36); (c) the upregulation of HLA class I and intracellular adhesion molecule-1 (ICAM-1) molecules, inducing an additive effect on the expression of immunologically important surface antigens on human cervical cancer cells (37). Several Phase II studies with this combination for locally advanced cervico-uterine cancer patients yielded response rates of 50%-58% (38,39). However, in heavily pretreated recurrent cervical cancers, this combination appears to be less active, with response rates of 0% to 31% (40–42). As a primary therapy for patients with locally advanced cervical cancer, this regimen had a response rate of 47% (33% complete remissions) with mild fever being the major toxicity, indicating that this combination is an active and tolerable therapy (43). In addition, the combination of IFN-α with cytotoxic agents, namely, cisplatin plus 5-fluorouracil (5-FU), has also been evaluated in the treatment of cervical cancer (44). It was relatively well tolerated, as toxicity was comparable to that of cisplatin plus 5-FU alone with a major response rate of 31%. Recent studies have shown that concurrent cisplatin-based radiotherapy and chemotherapy have significantly improved survival in both early- and locally advanced-stage cervical cancer (4,5,45), which have now become the standard of care. Future studies may test whether addition of IFN-α and/or retinoic acid will provide additional benefit.

Regional therapy with IFN-α gel for vulvar intraepithelial neoplasia was also evaluated in a prospective, randomized, double-armed crossover study comparing IFN-α with and without 1% nonoxynol-9. An overall response rate of 67% was achieved, and the toxicity was lower than previously reported for topical 5-FU. These data support the hypothesis that IFN-α is an active agent in the treatment of vulvar intraepithelial neoplasia III (46). Intralesional IFN-α was also evaluated for cervical intraepithelial neoplasia (47). However, with the good surgical success rate, this approach has received less enthusiasm.

In summary, IP IFN seems be well tolerated and may produce significant clinical responses in ovarian cancer patients with minimal residual disease. In advanced metastatic disease, combination of IFN with cytotoxic agents, for example, cisplatin or carboplatin, adds toxicity without significant antitumor activity. Combinations of IFN and retinoic acid or chemotherapy may have clinical benefit in cervical cancer not previously treated. The efficacy of IFN in combination with now standard chemoradiation regimens remains to be tested.

Interleukin-2

IL-2 is a T-cell growth factor that plays a central role in the immune system. Initial studies of IL-2 in the treatment of ovarian cancer involved continuous intravenous infusion therapy for patients with minimal residual disease at second-look surgery. The toxicity was significant and about 86% required dose reduction (48). Subsequent studies had been focused on IP administration of IL-2. A Phase I-II study (49) of IP IL-2 in patients with laparotomy-confirmed, persistent or recurrent ovarian cancer after ≥6 courses of prior platinum-based chemotherapy had shown an overall response rate of 25.7%, with an overall 5-year survival probability of 13.9%. For the patients who responded to therapy, the median survival time had not been reached (range 27 to 90+ months) at the time of the report, suggesting that this therapy may have long-term efficacy. This study also showed that IP IL-2 is better tolerated as a weekly infusion compared with a 7-day infusion. In their follow-up Phase II study of outpatient weekly infusion of IP IL-2 in patients with persistent ovarian cancer after primary paclitaxel (Taxol) and platinum therapy in patients with minimal residual disease (<2 cm), 17.6% had a surgically documented response and 41% of patients had stable disease. This study suggests that IP IL-2 has activity in persistent epithelial ovarian cancer and is well tolerated as an outpatient regimen (50). The combination of IL-2 and cytotoxic agents, for example, cisplatin, has been studied in mouse ovarian tumor models. In tumors that were hardly responsive to treatment with either of the drugs alone, combined local treatment with low doses of cisplatin and IL-2 resulted in an effective antitumor response with a complete response of 60%. Analysis of tumor-associated leukocytes showed that the combination of cisplatin and IL-2 resulted in enhanced nonspecific cytolytic activity of peritoneal leukocytes. Therefore, in the mouse model, combined local treatment with low doses of cis-platinum and IL-2 was more effective, suggesting that the same combination therapy may be more effective than cisplatin alone in human ovarian cancer (51).

A disadvantage of frequent administration of high-dose IL-2 is the occurrence of dose-limiting side effects. Therefore, delivery of IL-2-from an expression plasmid has been evaluated for the treatment of ovarian cancer. IP treatment of ovarian tumors with an IL-2–expressing plasmid resulted in an increase in local IL-2 levels, a change in the cytokine profile of the tumor ascites, and a significant antitumor effect in a mouse model (52). A Phase I trial with an IL-2 gene–modified tumor in refractory ovarian cancer patients was proposed and the result is not yet available (53). Other ongoing studies include a National Cancer Institute (NCI)–sponsored Phase I clinical trial of recombinant human IL-2 in patients with refractory, advanced-stage ovarian cancer and other abdominal carcinomatosis that is being conducted by University of Pittsburgh Cancer Institute and a CALGB pilot study of low-dose IL-2 plus recombinant human anti-HER-2 monoclonal antibody in patients with solid tumors, including ovarian cancers.

In summary, IL-2–based therapy may occasionally produce significant long-term remissions in ovarian cancer patients. The treatment, however, is hindered by significant toxicity. Approaches to minimize toxicity and optimize efficacy are being tested. The combination of low doses of cisplatinum with IL-2 seems to be a promising strategy in mouse models and warrants clinical trials to assess efficacy in humans.

Interleukin-12

IL-12 is a cytokine mainly produced by activated monocytes, tissue macrophages, and B cells. It can induce IFN-γ and together with IL-2 becomes a potent activator of cytotoxic T lymphocytes and NK cells (54,55). Whereas IL-4 and IL-10 mediate the development of Th2-type immunity, IL-12 initiates the differentiation of naive Th0 cells toward the Th1 phenotype. In addition, IL-12 production can be negatively or positively regulated by cytokines. For example, IL-10 and IL-4 have been shown to inhibit the production of IL-12 (10,56), whereas IL-2 and IFN-α enhance its production. In addition, IL-12 has potent antimetastatic and antitumor effects in several murine tumor models, as well as in human tumor cells *in vitro* and *in vivo* (55,57). IL-12 was better than IL-2 in enhancing the cytotoxicity against ovarian cancer cells of lymphocytes from ascites or peripheral blood from patients (58). IL-12 and IL-2 have a synergistic effect on the lymphokine-activated killer activity in peripheral blood mononuclear cells cultured in ovarian cancer ascitic fluid (59). It has been suggested that the antitumor effects of IL-12 involve enhanced IFN-γ production by antitumor T cells, their accumulation to tumor sites, and *in situ* IFN-γ production (60). In addition, IL-12 promotes IFN-γ–mediated upregulation of adhesion molecules [vascular cell adhesion molecule (VCAM-1) and ICAM-1] on tumor-associated blood vessels, providing access for circulating lymphocytes (58). However, ascitic IL-12 has also been shown to be an independent prognostic factor for adverse outcome in ovarian cancer (61).

A Phase II GOG clinical trial (62) evaluated intravenously administered recombinant human IL-12 in patients with recurrent or refractory ovarian cancer. The study showed that, as a single agent, IL-12 could be tolerated, and myelotoxicity and capillary leak syndrome were the major adverse events. However, the response rate was low: There were no complete responders—3.8% of the evaluable patients had a partial response and 50% had stable disease. Since antiangiogenesis might be one of the potential antitumor mechanisms of IL-12, the observed rate of stable disease may represent a significant response, and therefore patients with minimal residual disease may be a better model. IP administration of human recombinant IL-12 was also evaluated in patients with refractory ovarian and gastrointestinal

malignancies after primary standard therapy (63). Among the 29 patients, 2 patients (one with ovarian cancer and one with mesothelioma) had no remaining disease at laparoscopy, 8 patients had stable disease, and 19 had progressive disease. In this study, the dose-limiting toxicity was elevated transaminase. More frequent toxicities included fever, fatigue, abdominal pain, nausea, and catheter-related infections. Currently, a combination of IL-12 and trastuzumab in patients with HER-2/neu–overexpressing malignancies, including ovarian cancers, is being evaluated in a Phase I study at the Arthur C. James Cancer Hospital of the Ohio State University.

CANCER VACCINES DESIGNED TO AUGMENT T-LYMPHOCYTE RESPONSES

Options Available

There is a wide range of options for augmenting the immunogenicity of the antigenic targets for T-cell immunity (64–66). For these antigens, the options include (a) the full proteins or MHC-restricted peptides modified by amino acid substitutions to increase immunogenicity; (b) genes or minigenes for these proteins or peptides used as DNA vaccines; or (c) these genes expressed in viral or bacterial vectors. Co-stimulatory molecules, cytokines, or molecules targeting antigens to particular processing compartments can be incorporated into these vaccines. DNA vaccines are especially appealing in this regard because of ease of production, versatility, and adaptability to such combinations. Most of these approaches can also be applied to expressing these antigens in antigen-presenting cells, such as dendritic cells, that are then used to vaccinate the patient. Furthermore, since many tumor-rejection antigens detected by T cells in experimental animals are individually unique (mutated), a variety of individualized vaccines are being tested. Whole-cell vaccines can be prepared from each patient's cancer (if the tumor specimen is large enough) and immunogenicity may be increased by the use of an immunological adjuvant and transduction with genes for cytokines or co-stimulatory molecules, or treatment with haptens such as dinitrophenyl (DNP). Other approaches to increasing the immunogenicity of unique and shared antigens include the use of heat shock proteins that may carry the full range of cancer peptides, antiidiotype vaccines, and DNA or messenger RNA vaccines that may be obtained from smaller biopsy specimens. The range of options for augmenting T-cell immunity against cancer is daunting. Clinical trials with each of these approaches to augmenting T-cell immunity have been recently completed, are ongoing, or have been planned. There is no basis for selecting one over the other at this time.

Target Antigens for T Lymphocytes

Antigens shared by ovarian or endometrial cancers from different patients are KSA, MUC-16, WT1, carcinoembryonic antigen (CEA), MUC-1, HER-2/neu, and cancer-testis antigens (including the MAGE family) and NY-ESO-1. None of these cancer antigens defined as targets for T cells to date are perfect candidates for the majority of patients due to (a) overexpression on less than 50% of ovarian or endometrial cancers (HER-2/neu, CEA, and the cancer-testis antigens) and (b) wide expression (though at lower levels) on normal tissues (KSA, CEA, HER-2/neu, MUC-1). The highly polar extensive expression of KSA and some other antigens on cells apically at mucosal borders (lumens) in many normal epithelial tissues does not exclude them as a target for antibodies because IgG1, IgG3 and IgM antibodies are present in much lower concentrations in these lumens, or not at all, and there is little or no complement and no antibody-dependent cell-mediated cytotoxicity (ADCC) effector cells. Since antigen presentation to T cells in the context of HLA antigens is not known to have the same polar distribution, KSA would be a worrisome target for T cells. MUC-16 for ovarian cancers and human papillomavirus (HPV)–related antigens for cervical cancer are especially strong candidates at this time because of their widespread expression on the respective cancers and restricted expression on normal tissues.

Molecular analysis of endometrial carcinomas has identified a variety of proteins which may serve as target antigens for vaccine based therapy. For example, overexpression of Her-2/neu has correlated with advanced disease and poor outcome in both adenocarcinoma and uterine papillary serous carcinoma (67,68) More recent reports have implicated alterations in the hMLH1, p16(ink4a) (p16), and PTEN genes as promoters of carcinogenesis, as well as overexpression of the *SART-1* gene, which encodes the SART-1 (259) tumor antigen that is recognized by HLA-A26–restricted cytotoxic T lymphocytes (32% of tested specimens) (69,70).

CLINICAL TRIALS WITH SELECTED VACCINES DESIGNED PRIMARILY TO INDUCE T-CELL RESPONSES

NY-ESO-1 Vaccine

The NY-ESO-1 antigen belongs to the cancer-testis antigen family which includes the MAGE-1 protein (first human gene product recognized by CD8[+] T cells identified in a patient with cancer), and the GAGE and BAGE families (71, 72). NY-ESO-1 has shown consistent immunogenicity, and the existence of overlapping CD8[+] and CD4[+] T-cell epitopes within these antigens have provided the opportunity of using one short peptide, ESO 157–170, to generate both CD4[+] and CD 8[+] T cells (73). Immunoscreening studies have found NY-ESO—1 expression in ovarian cancers, and interestingly the cancer-testis family antigens are represented by the MAGE series (with the exception of MAGE-10), LAGE-1, and PRAME genes, but NY-ESO-1 expression is absent in patients with cervical cancer (74,75). The represented antigens would be appropriate targets for vaccines, and studies with a peptide vaccine targeted at NY-

ESO-1 have just been initiated in patients with ovarian cancer at the Memorial Sloan-Kettering and Roswell Park Cancer Centers. An existing Phase I clinical trial immunized 12 patients with metastatic NY-ESO-1–expressing tumors (7 were NY-ESO-1 serum antibody negative and five patients were NY-ESO-1 positive at the start of study) using intradermal administration of three HLA A2–restricted peptides. Primary peptide-specific CD8[+] T-cell reactions were generated in four of seven NY-ESO-1 antibody-negative patients. Although there were no complete or partial clinical responses, induction of a specific CD8[+] T-cell response to NY-ESO-1 in immunized antibody-negative patients was associated with disease stabilization and objective regression of single metastases. Stabilization of disease was observed overall in four of the seven seronegative patients who developed CD8[+] T-cell responses by ELISPOT and delayed-type hypersensitivity (DTH) reactions after vaccination (one of the two ovarian cancer patients had decreasing ascites and stable peritoneal carcinomatosis lasting 20 weeks) (76).

Granulocyte-Macrophage Colony-Stimulating Factor–Secreting Tumor-Cell Vaccines

Granulocyte-macrophage colony-stimulating factor (GM-CSF) has a variety of properties desirable for vaccine production including enhancing immune responses by inducing the proliferation, maturation, and migration of dendritic cells and the expansion of both T- and B-cell lymphocytes (77). A recent characterization of its adjuvant response has shown the early elevation of inflammatory molecules such as IL-6, TNF-α, and monocyte chemotactic protein-1 (MCP-1) followed later by IL-12 and IFN-δ production among others (78). *In vitro* characterization of a GM-CSF–secreting vaccine was performed by genetically engineering UCI-107 (ovarian cancer cell line) to secrete GM-CSF by retrovirus-mediated gene transduction with the LXSN retroviral vector containing the human GM-CSF gene and the neomycin resistance selection marker. A clone (UCI-107 GM-SF-MPS) was extensively characterized and shown to secrete high levels of GM-CSF over 6 months of study (79). In human trials, a variety of studies have shown that vaccination with irradiated tumor cells engineered to secrete GM-CSF stimulates long-lasting immunity in murine models and in patients with metastatic melanoma. A recent Phase I study evaluated patients with metastatic non–small-cell lung carcinoma. A metastatic site was resected, processed to single-cell suspension, infected with a replication-defective adenoviral vector encoding GM-CSF, irradiated, cryopreserved, and then given intradermally at weekly and biweekly intervals. Vaccines were made successfully for 34 of 35 patients. Dendritic cell, macrophage, granulocyte and lymphocyte infiltrates were elicited in 18 of 25 assessable patients. Two patients rendered disease free by metastasectomy for trial enrollment are disease free at 43 and 42 months, five patients had stable disease ranging from 3 to 33 months, and one patient had a mixed response (80). Additional trials in other solid tumor types, including gynecologic malignancies, are warranted.

Folate Receptor–Targeted Vaccines

Previous studies have identified the alpha isoform of the folate receptor (FR), which is a 38-kD GPI anchored protein constitutively expressed at high levels in 90% of nonmucinous ovarian cancer and at low levels in normal tissues (81). The reason for overexpression is unknown, but one hypothesis is that overexpression provides an alternate folate-processing pathway to compensate for deletion of the tetrahydrofolate reductase gene that is deleted frequently in cancer cells (82). FR expression has been shown in preclinical models to confer a growth advantage in FR-transfected cells, which suggests a role for the receptor in the control of cell proliferation (83). Growth regulation may be related to an inverse relationship between folate receptor expression and Cav-1, a 21- to 24-kD protein that may negatively regulate the activity of several cytoplasmic signaling proteins and tyrosine kinase inhibitors (84).

The preferential overexpression of the folate receptor in malignant tissue has prompted the investigation of this antigen in several preclinical immunization studies. Neglia et al. evaluated FR alpha cDNA after ligation into the VR1012 (Vical) expression vector under transcriptional control of the cytomegalovirus promoter. Purified plasma DNA was injected into BALB/c mice three times at 14-day intervals. At 10 days after the second injection, sera (100%) showed antibody titers against syngeneic C26 cells transduced with FR alpha, but not against unmodified C26 cells. Specific cytotoxic T-lymphocyte activity against FR alpha transduced C26 cells could be seen in splenocytes from all immunized animals. Challenge by subcutaneous injection with FR alpha–transduced C26 cells (administered 10 days after third injection) showed a statistically significant delay in tumor growth (85). Further studies by Peoples et al. showed that both immunodominant E39 (FBP, 191–199) and subdominant E41 (FBP, 245–53) epitopes of human high-affinity folate-binding protein (FBP) are presented by HLA-A2 in both ovarian and breast cancers (86). Tumor-associated lymphocytes stimulated with FBP peptides exhibit cytotoxicity not only against peptide loaded targets but also against FBP-expressing epithelial tumors of different histologies. Finally, FBP peptides induced E39-specific cytotoxic T lymphocytes (CTLs) and E39 and E41-specific IFN-δ and IP-10 secretion in a proportion of healthy donors. These studies provide motivation for proceeding to clinical trials with DNA and peptide FR vaccines in ovarian cancer patients.

Dendritic-Cell Approaches

Dendritic cells (DCs) are phenotypically distinct potent antigen-presenting cells well suited for vaccine strategies (87). They are found throughout the body, particularly at the portals of entry for infectious organisms, such as in the epidermis where they are called Langerhans cells. Multiple animal studies have demonstrated CTL-mediated protective immunity and even regression of established tumors with the administration of antigen pulsed DCs (88,89). A variety of approaches have been considered with regard to antigen type and loading techniques to include recombinant or fusion proteins (90), tumor-associated antigen-derived CTL epitopes (91), DC–tumor-cell hybrids (92), HLA-restricted antigens (93), and autologous antigens from tumor cell lysates (94,95). In a recent clinical study in metastatic colon cancer, pulsed DCs with CAP-1D, which is an HLA-A*0201–restricted epitope of CEA, and CTLs generated with this epitope retained their ability to lyse cells with native CEA (93). In a preliminary analysis of 10 HLA-A*0201–positive colon cancer patients receiving immunizations twice 28 days apart (required outpatient leukapheresis, *ex vivo* enrichment of DCs, co-incubation for 2 days with antigen, followed by vaccination), 7 developed CTL activity. The magnitude of tetramer + CD8 T-cell expansion correlated with clinical response (ANOVA, $p = 0.02$). Although not the trial endpoint, one patient had resolution of pulmonary metastasis and pleural effusion, and two patients had disease stabilization. Another patient had normalization of CEA, with no radiographically visible recurrence at 10 months. These observations support the plan for randomized efficacy trials for tumor-associated antigen pulsed DCs in colon cancer as well as a variety of solid tumors. The recent characterization of MUC-16 (CA-125) similarly will allow CA-125–directed DC therapy to be considered for patients with ovarian cancer (96).

Both the clinical relevance and presence of the target are obviously essential when using this tumor-associated antigen approach. For example, although several studies have demonstrated the marked effectiveness of using *in vitro*–generated DCs loaded with either a human leukocyte antigen A2-restricted peptide fragment of HER-2 (E75) or a HER-2 intracellular domain (ICD) in terms of immune response, recent data from a Gynecologic Oncology Group study showed that only 11.4% of 837 screened ovarian cancer tumor samples showed 2+ or 3+ fold overexpression of HER-2. Furthermore, using the monoclonal humanized anti-HER-2 antibody trastuzumab, an overall response rate of 7.3% was seen showing that even with appropriate overexpression, minimal single-agent activity is seen (97).

Using the autologous tumor antigen–pulsed DC approach in patients with ovarian cancer (n = 8) and uterine sarcoma (n = 2), Hernando et al. harvested DCs, and pulsed them with keyhole limpet hemocyanin (KLH) and autologous tumor cell lysate in the presence of GM-CSF (89). Significant tumor antigen specific lymphoproliferative responses were seen in two ovarian cancer patients. Progression free intervals of 25 to 45 weeks were seen in three patients (two with demonstrable immune responses), suggesting a disease-stabilization effect. These data combined with DC pulsed with lysates from other solid tumors such as melanoma, renal-cell carcinoma, and selected pediatric tumors showing specific T-cell immunity, and some objective responses further support evaluation of this approach in patients with gynecologic cancers (94,98,99).

DC approaches are potent at inducing T-cell responses. A variety of variables require further study to optimize the approach including choice of DC subtype, maturational status at immunization, adjuvant cytokines, antigen-loading method, and route and frequency of administration.

MECHANISMS FOR B-CELL RECOGNITION OF TUMOR ANTIGENS AND EFFECTOR ACTIONS

Whereas T lymphocytes recognize processed (partially digested) antigens, B cells recognize antigens in their natural configuration (100). For an individual to make antibodies against the full range of pathogens continually encountered, B lymphocytes expressing a diverse repertoire of immunoglobulins must be generated continually. Each B cell expresses immunoglobulin against a single antigenic epitope, with the immunoglobulin expressed at the cell surface where it acts as a specific receptor for that antigen. The diversity of specificities in different B cells is generated largely by gene rearrangements in new B cells, which continue to be generated throughout life. In their early development, B cells with immunoglobulins against ubiquitous self-antigens are eliminated. This elimination of B cells reactive with autoantigens is not absolute, however, as a broad array of monoclonal antibodies (mAbs) and serum antibodies against autoantigens have been derived from experimental animals and humans. Peripheral blood B cells consist of naive and relatively short-lived B cells, long-lived memory B cells resulting from maturation in response to antigenic stimulation, and a small population of B cells expressing germline specificities, also termed CD5 B cells (101).

B cells are not sessile; after maturation in the bone marrow they migrate through the peripheral blood to B cell rich areas such as follicles of lymph nodes, spleen and gastrointestinal tract and may continue re-circulating. If its antigen is encountered in these tissues, the B lymphocyte is detained in the T-cell–rich areas where if appropriate T cell help is provided, it may be activated to proliferate. This T-cell help does not have to be induced by the same antigen. Chemical conjugation of the original antigen to highly immunogenic bacterial or xenogeneic proteins, or expression of the antigen in bacterial or viral vectors, are widely used approaches to ensuring adequate T-cell help in vaccines. The result is antibody secreting plasma cells and germinal centers where hypermutation in variable genes and class and subclass switching occurs. The consequence is plasma cells secreting increasingly higher affinity IgG antibodies. In addition, some B cells which generally recognize nonprotein antigens can be stimulated to proliferate in the absence of T-cell help. Class switching, affinity maturation and memory B cells generally do not occur. Low-affinity IgM antibodies of shorter duration result.

The immunoglobulin variable region (Fv) determining antibody specificity is located in the Fab and is critical for effective recognition of tumor antigens (Fab and Fc are the immunoglobulin degradation products from papain digestion, in the hinge region). However, the constant region (Fc) where class and subclass are determined is equally critical. Binding of antibody to antigen results in a functional change in the Fc portion and activation of several effector mechanisms. IgM antibodies are synthesized early in the response against protein antigens but at all times in the response to most non-protein antigens and are found mainly in the blood. The IgM pentameric structure is specialized to increase avidity of binding to repeated antigens and to activate complement efficiently. Complement activation results in opsonization, activation of and uptake by macrophages, monocytes, neutrophils and dendritic cells, as well as membrane attack complex formation and complement dependent cytotoxicity (CDC). IgG antibodies are synthesized later in the response to protein antigens, are usually of higher affinity, and can be found in the extracellular fluid as well as in the blood. IgG1 and IgG3 antibodies in humans are especially effective at activating complement and also at sensitization of pathogens for killing by natural killer cells.

Opsonization for ingestion and destruction by phagocytes can occur through complement activation, but also occurs directly as a consequence of Fc receptors on phagocytic cells. Fc receptors on IgG1 and IgG3 bound at the cell surface are the primary targets for effector cells mediating ADCC of tumor cells. Fc receptors on a range of effector cells including especially NK cells, but also cells of myeloid lineage, react with these tumor-cell–bound antibodies, resulting in activation of inherent cytotoxic mechanisms in the effector cells. Although in some cases, antibody may have direct effects against tumor cells, for example, by inhibiting tumor-cell attachment or growth hormone receptors, in general, interaction of antibody and tumor cell antigen is without significance unless Fc-mediated secondary effector mechanisms are activated. Of these various effector mechanisms, activation of the complement system, opsonization, and ADCC are probably the most important.

BASIS FOR ANTIBODY-MEDIATED THERAPY OF CANCER

Antibodies are the primary mechanism for eliminating infectious pathogens from the blood stream. The effect of all commonly used vaccines against infectious agents is thought to be primarily a consequence of antibody induction. Antibodies are also ideally suited for elimination of circulating tumor cells and micrometastases. The importance of antibodies in mediating protection from tumor recurrence is well documented in experimental animals (102,103). Experiments involving administration of monoclonal antibody 3F8 against GD2 or induction of GD2 antibodies by vaccination after challenge with EL4 lymphoma (which expresses GD2) are two examples. Administration of 3F8 prior to intravenous tumor challenge or as late as 4 days after tumor challenge results in complete protection of a majority of mice (102). Comparable protection from EL4 challenge was induced by immunization with a GD2-KLH conjugate vaccine. This timing may be comparable to antibody induction, or administration, in patients in the adjuvant setting after surgical resection of the primary, or lymph node or peritoneal metastases, or after response to chemotherapy. In both cases, the targets may be circulating tumor cells and micrometastases.

There is also evidence in cancer patients that natural or passively administered antibodies in the adjuvant setting are associated with clinical benefit.

1. Natural antibodies (antibodies present in patient sera prior to vaccination) and vaccine-induced antibodies have been correlated with an improved prognosis. This is true for patients with paraneoplastic syndromes where high titers of antibodies against onconeural antigens expressed on particular cells in the nervous system and certain types of tumors have been associated both with debilitating autoimmune neurologic disorders and with delayed tumor progression and prolonged survival. Also patients with American Joint Commission for Cancer (AJCC) stage III melanoma and natural antibodies against GM2 ganglioside treated at two different medical centers have had an 80% to 100% 5-year survival compared to the expected 40% rate (104–106). Tumor vaccine induced antibodies in the adjuvant setting against GM2 and several other melanoma antigens at four different medical centers, and against sialyl Tn (sTn) antigen in adenocarcinoma patients, have correlated with prolonged disease-free interval and survival (reviewed in ref. 107).

2. A series of monoclonal antibodies have now been shown to have clinical efficacy in the advanced disease setting and have been approved by the FDA. These include Rituxan for B-cell lymphomas, Campath for chronic lymphocytic leukemias, and Herceptin for breast cancer.

Hence, passively administered and vaccine-induced antibodies have been shown to correlate with clinical responses or improved disease-free and overall survival in the mouse and human. Preclinical studies strongly suggest that the optimal setting for antibody therapy is the adjuvant setting. Since the great majority of gynecologic cancer patients are initially rendered free of detectable disease by surgery and or chemotherapy after initial diagnosis, administration of mAbs or vaccines inducing antibodies may have broad applicability. There are advantages to each approach. Titers of anticancer antibodies are generally higher acutely after administration of mAbs, and mAbs can be generated against virtually any antigen. On the other hand, human antimouse and antiidiotype antibodies may limit the usefulness of continued administration of mAbs, and maintenance of antibody titers with vaccines is more practical and less expensive than with mAbs.

BASIS FOR MONOCLONAL ANTIBODY THERAPY

Target Antigens for Antibodies

We have screened a variety of malignancies and normal tissues with a series of 40 mAbs against 25 antigens that were potential target antigens for immunotherapy of cancer (108–110). Since recognition of antigens on living cancer cells by antibodies is largely restricted to the cancer cell surface, the focus was on cell surface antigens. Antigen expression on ovarian and endometrial cancers and several other malignancies for the seven defined antigens expressed strongly in at least three of five biopsy specimens in our previous studies and CA-125 (MUC-16) are shown in Table 6.1 (108–112). The antigens expressed by ovarian and endometrial cancers are similar, and quite different from those expressed by melanomas, and similar to, although not the same as, those expressed by prostatic cancers. The 18 excluded antigens (including CEA and HER-2/neu) were expressed in one or zero of five specimens. With the possible exception of GM2 (for which there are no previous reports), our results are consistent with the separate studies describing the expression of these individual ovarian cancer antigens from other centers. Our studies identify ganglioside GM2 as an antigen present on many malignancies, which is a conclusion supported by an increasing number of recent reports (113,114).

The expression of these eight antigens on normal tissues is essentially restricted to apical epithelial cells at luminal borders, a site which appears not to be accessible to the immune system. Administered mAbs to several of these antigens have induced clinical responses but have not induced autoimmunity, indicating that antigen in these locations may not be accessible to antibodies. The exception is GM2, which is also expressed in the brain, although far less than the related ganglioside GD3, where the blood-brain barrier prevents autoimmune toxicity [infusions of monoclonal antibodies against GD3 have been associated with many clinical responses and no incidents of central nervous system (CNS) toxicity]. BR96 recognizes a broader specificity than Le^y (115,193), also including Le^x, which explains the reactivity with polymorphonucleocytes (which express Le^x but do not express Le^y). Hemorrhagic gastritis has been reported after high doses of BR96 (against Le^y), possibly related to a broader specificity of BR96, since treatment with another mAb, 3S193, against Le^y has not been associated with these toxicities. The extensive expression of CA-125 in over 80% of serous and endometrioid ovarian cancers has been well documented since the early 1980s (116). Following the successful cloning of CA-125 and identifying it as a complex mucin, it has been termed MUC-16 (96,117,118). Contribut-

TABLE 6.1. *Number of tumor biopsy specimens with 50% or more of tumor cells positive by immunohistology*

Tumor[a]	STn (CC49)	STn (B72.3)	TF (49H.8)	Le^y (3S193)	Le^y (BR96)	GM2 (696)	Globo H (Mbr1)	MUC-1 (HMFG2)	KSA (GA7333)	MUC-16 (CA-125)
Ovarian	4/5	3/5	5/5	4/5	99/133[b]	5/5	18/19	5/5	5/5	53/62[c]
Endometrial	4/5	2/5	4/5	3/5	2/5	5/5	4/5	3/5	5/5	–
Melanoma	0/5	0/5	0/5	0/5	0/5	10/10	0/10	0/5	0/5	0/4
Small-cell lung	0/5	0/5	0/5	2/5	1/5	6/6	4/6	2/5	4/5	0/2
Prostatic	4/5	3/5	1/5	3/5	3/5	5/5	2/5	1/5	5/5	0/5

[a]All the tumor tissues were stained by avidin-biotin complex immunoperoxidase methods (108–110).
[b]From ref. 111.
[c]From ref. 112.

ing to tumor mucin specificity is the less intense glycosylation of tumor mucins than normal mucins, involving shorter carbohydrate chains. The simplified structures of these antigens in relation to the cancer cell surface lipid bilayer are shown in Figure 6.1.

There is now sufficient experience from clinical trials with vaccine-induced antibody responses against GM2, TF, sTn, MUC-1, and KSA antigens, and passive administration of mAbs against sTn, MUC-16 (CA-125), and KSA to draw conclusions about the consequences of antigen distribution on various normal tissues. GM2 exposure on cells in the brain and GM2, sTn, TF, MUC-1, and KSA antigen expres-

sion in cells at the secretory borders of epithelial tissues induce neither immunological tolerance nor autoimmunity once antibodies are present, suggesting that they are sequestered from the immune system. Against this background, GM2, T, Tn, sTn, Globo H, MUC-1, MUC-16 (CA-125), and KSA all appear to be good cell surface targets for active immunotherapy with vaccines that induce antibodies.

Antibody Selection

Tumor cells have defined antigens and receptors on the cell surface that may differ from those present on normal

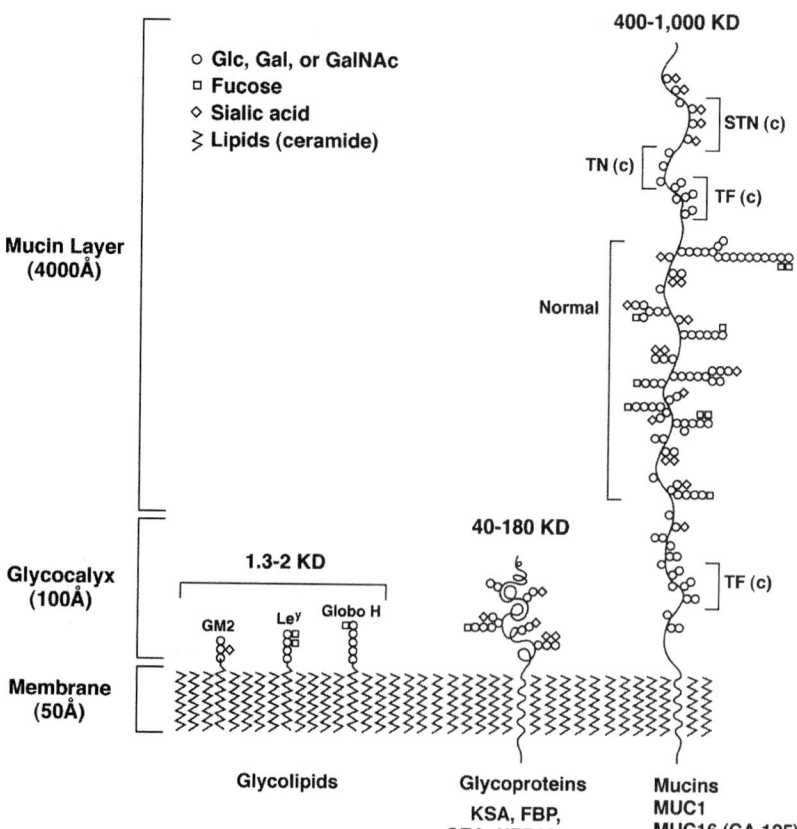

FIG. 6-1. Glycolipid and glycoprotein antigens expressed at the cell surface of gynecologic cancers. Symbols: ◇ = sialic acid; □ = fucose; ○ = glucose, galactose, N-acetylgalactosamine or N-acetylglucosamine.

TABLE 6.2. *Monoclonal antibodies targeting gynecologic malignancies*

Targeted antigens	Antibody examples	Therapeutic considerations
Mucins		
CA-125 (MUC-16)	OVAREX (B43.13), OC125 ACA-125 (anti-id OC-125)	Ovarian cancer
MUC-1	HMFGI, HMFG2	
Tumor-associated glycoprotein		
TAG-72 (sTn)	B72.3, CC49	Ovarian cancer
Human folate-binding protein (FBP)	MOv18, MOv 19	Ovarian cancer
Markers of epithelial differentiation		
CEA	MN-14	Ovarian cancer
Blood type substance		
Lewis-Y-related cell surface antigens	BR55, BR96, B3, 3S193	Ovarian cancer
Oncogene-associated growth factor receptor		
HER-2/neu receptor	Trastuzumab	Ovarian cancer
CAIX (MN antigen)	M75	Endometrial/cervical cancer

cells. mAbs directed against these targets have potential diagnostic and therapeutic applications. The selection of the optimal antigen-antibody system for clinical development depends on a number of biological and technical factors, including antigen density, pathways of catabolism, tumor specificity, heterogeneity of expression, effector mechanisms, and binding affinity. Antigens that have been used for immune targeting of gynecologic malignancies with mAbs for antibody development include (a) overexpressed tumor antigens [e.g., CA-125, TAG-72 (sTn), MUC-1, polymorphic epithelial mucin (PEM), folate binding protein (FBP), and Lewis-Y]; (b) overexpressed growth-factor receptors [e.g., HER-2/neu (erbB2), epidermal growth-factor receptor (EGFR), and vascular endothelial growth factor (VEGF)]; and (c) mutated tumor-suppressor genes (e.g., *p53* and *BRCA-1*). Binding of mAb to these antigens may have antitumor effect generated through these possible mechanisms: (a) antibody-mediated recruitment of human effector mechanisms in situ, ADCC against the tumor cells; (b) development of tumor specific CTLs; (c) activation of the complement system; (d) stimulation of granulocytes cytotoxic to the cancer cells; and (e) induction of an anti-idiotypic antibody that can elicit active immunity. The available antibodies and their targeting antigens that have been tested in gynecological malignancies are summarized in Table 6.2.

OBSTACLES IN ANTIBODY THERAPY AND ENGINEERING STRATEGIES

Despite decades of efforts, there are currently few nonimmunogenic antibodies against cell-surface antigens that are of therapeutic significance in gynecologic cancers. The major obstacles have been (a) development of human anti-murine antibodies (HAMA) that form immune complexes with subsequent antibody administration, which results in altered patterns of catabolism and host toxicity; (b) limited immunobiologic activity of nonconjugated antibody; (c) expression of antigens (e.g., growth-factor receptors on a wide range of normal host tissue); and (d) heterogeneity of antigen expression among different histologies and patients. Various engineering strategies have been tested to overcome these obstacles.

Overcoming HAMA

Because murine mAbs are xenotypic proteins, the immunocompetent human will recognize them as foreign and generate antibody responses (HAMA) against them. Although the resultant immune complexes may potentially boost the immune response to the antigen epitope, leading to enhanced recognition by the immune system and an increased processing by dendritic and antigen-presenting cells, the more likely outcome is increased blood clearance and less effective tumor targeting, precluding repeat administration. This has been one of the major obstacles in the application of murine mAbs to the treatment of human cancers. To minimize the effect of HAMA, various strategies have been explored, including: construction of smaller antibody fragments, design of recombinant antibodies with substitution of human for murine sequences, and direct cloning of human variable regions with the desired binding specificity. Chimeric or fully humanized antibodies have been developed to reduce HAMA responses associated with the administration of murine mAbs, with the concomitant possibility of manipulating the effector function (119). The reduced immunogenicity of humanized antibodies allows their repeated administration. Initial efforts involved development of a mouse-human chi-

TABLE 6.3. *Radionuclides, toxins, and cytotoxic agents used as mAb conjugates*

Reagents	Mechanistic considerations	Therapeutic considerations
Radionuclides		
^{125}I	Auger electron antitumor effects; $T_{1/2}$ 60 d	Standard iodination chemistry, subject to dehalogenation. Auger effects limited to 15 Å radius. β penetrates ~1 mm and can kill adjacent antigen-negative cells. γ Associated with wider penetration and dose-limiting marrow suppression.
^{131}I	364 KeVγ (imaging); 606 Kevβ (therapy); $T_{1/2}$8 d	
^{90}Y	2.27 Mev β; $T_{1/2}$2.7 d	Requires chelation. Almost pure β penetrates ~3 mm. Free ^{90}Y localizes to bone, associated with dose-limiting marrow suppression.
^{212}Bi	High LET 6.2 MeVα $T_{1/2}$ 1h	α Penetrates only several cell diameters (~20–100 μm). Toxicity not oxygen dependent, increased energy deposition compared to β. ^{212}Bi has very short $T_{1/2}$ (demanding rapid localization), requires chelation, and can be generated in laboratory. ^{211}At requires a cyclotron for generation, and can be directly conjugated.
^{211}At	High LET 6.0 ME11Vα $T_{1/2}$7.2 h	
^{186}Re	137 KeVγ (imaging) 1.1 Mevβ (therapy); $T_{1/2}$ 3.7 d	Techniques available for direct conjugation or chelation. Low abundance γ suitable for imaging.
^{177}Lu	208 KeVγ (imaging); 0.5 MeVβ (therapy); $T_{1/2}$ 6.7 d	Evaluated as chelate. Low-abundance γ suitable for imaging.
Toxins		
PE	Bacterial *Pseudomonas* exotoxin A. Enzymatic inactivation of protein synthesis by ADP ribosylation of elongation factor 2.	Both PE and RA require internalization and cytoplasmic translocation for protein synthesis inhibition. PE requires acid hydrolysis. No mechanisms for killing adjacent antigen-negative or nontargeted cells. Recombinant PE and RA fragments available for chemical conjugation or construction of single-chain chimeric proteins.
RA	Ricin A chain from castor beans. N-glycosidase–mediated inactivation of 28S ribosomal RNA.	
Cytotoxic agents		
DOX	Doxorubicin-associated free radical formation, DNA intercalation, inhibition of topoisomerase-II.	Toxicity requires internalization and acid hydrolysis to release free DOX.
Anti-CD	Effector activation via the T-cell receptor complex.	Requires simultaneous presence of activated effector cells, antibody, and antigen-positive tumor. Indirect cytokine effects, recruitment of inflammatory cells, and enhancement of immunity can occur.
Anti-FcR	Effector activation via NK/LGL FcγRIII complex.	
Biotin	Multistep amplification using biotin-streptavidin system.	Permits adding second- and third step reagents with high affinity for the primary antibody. Allows for systemic clearing with increased tumor localization and tumor to normal tissue ratios.

Source: Modified from Bookman MA, Boente MP, Bast R. Immunology and Immunotherapy of gynecologic cancer, *principles and practice of gynecologic oncology.* 3rd ed. Philadelphia: Lippincott Williams & Wilkins, 2000:129–163, with permission.

meric mAb by replacing the murine immunoglobin heavy- and light-chain constant regions with those of the human Ig (chimerization).

A widely used procedure for the humanization of xenogeneic antibodies is based on grafting the hypervariable or complementarity-determining regions (CDRs) of a xenogeneic antibody onto the human Ig framework. With this approach, a minimally immunogenic variant of humanized anti-CC49 mAb has been developed (120). Construction of smaller molecules has also been explored to decrease HAMA. Immunoglobulins have been engineered to retain only the domains that are required for antigen binding and/ or effector functions and have also been rebuilt into multivalent, high-affinity reagents to achieve the desired efficacy

(121). Studies with different forms of mAbs have shown that antibody fragments of lower molecular weight can penetrate tumor faster than whole IgG molecules (122,123). A humanized CC49 single-chain (scFv) construct (hu/muCC49 scFv) has been prepared, where the murine CC49 variable light chain was entirely replaced by a homologous human light chain. Pharmacokinetic studies in mice showed rapid blood and whole-body clearance with a half-life of 6 minutes, and biodistribution studies demonstrated equivalent tumor targeting to human colon carcinoma xenografts for muCC49 and hu/muCC49 scFv (124), indicating that it has potential diagnostic and therapeutic applications for TAG72-positive tumors. mAb constructs that have a deletion of the CH_2 portion of the constant region have been created: h-ΔCH_2CC49 is a humanized CC49 with its CH_2 region deleted, with identical affinity for TAG-72 (125). The clinical characteristics of these constructs and conjugates are being tested. Conjugates of these constructs with radionuclides, for example, ^{225}Ac, have also been made (126).

Antibody Conjugates

In view of limited efficacy of unconjugated antibody, efforts have been made to optimize the antitumor activity by conjugating with radionuclides, toxins, cytotoxic drugs, or second antibodies (Table 6.3) (9). Combinations of multiple antibodies to compensate for antigen heterogeneity in ovarian carcinomas have been evaluated. The choice of conjugates and specific antibodies are influenced by features such as antigen internalization, lysosomal degradation, shedding, and heterogeneity of expression. Although internalization is a prerequisite for cellular toxicity of some drug and toxin conjugates, it may result in reduced efficacy and increased host toxicity due to intracellular catabolism (9).

Radionuclides

A variety of radionuclides have been conjugated with antibodies for imaging and treatment. The optimal radionuclide for cancer therapy is not easy to define (9). Radioconjugates with β (i.e., ^{131}I and ^{90}Y) and α (i.e., ^{211}At and ^{212}Bi) emitters have been proposed for regional therapy of peritoneal implants. Estimates of dosimetry suggest that adequate therapy (i.e., 20 Gy) could be delivered to tumors with a depth <300 μg using ^{211}At, <0.1 cm using ^{131}I, and < 1 cm using ^{90}Y, when conjugated to antibodies. Delivery of effective radiation dose is greatly influenced by the extent of tumor binding, depth of tumor penetration, catabolism, and relative distribution between tumor and normal tissues. Although internalization is usually detrimental owing to enhanced catabolism, internalization is required for maximal Auger electron chromosomal toxicity from ^{131}I owing to an extremely limited sphere of penetration (15 Å). At the present time, β emitters are considered to be the optimal candidates for radiotherapy, as they avoid excessive systemic exposure as-

sociated with γ radiation. Conjugates with ^{131}I have been most extensively studied because of isotope availability, ease of chemical conjugation, and ability to perform γ imaging and β therapeutic studies with the same reagent. There has been an interest in finding alternatives to ^{131}I due to the nonspecific γ irradiation, bone marrow toxicity, and the tendency for rapid dehalogenation, which limits tumor retention. ^{90}Y provides 100% decay suitable for therapy over several millimeters (9), although it has no γ emission useful for imaging. Lutetium-177 (^{177}Lu) is a rare earth metal with a physical half-life of 6.7 days and β emissions that penetrate 0.2 to 0.3 mm in soft tissue. ^{177}Lu also emits two relatively low-abundance, low-energy rays (113–208 keV) that allow imaging with a gamma camera, but poses less radiation hazard to health care personnel compared with ^{131}I (127).

Immunotoxins, Drugs, and Cytokines

An important factor limiting the treatment of cancer is the low therapeutic index, which may be improved by targeted delivery of cytotoxic agents (Table 6.3) (9) to tumor sites. mAbs have been attractive carriers for tumor-directed therapy by increasing the intratumoral concentration of targeted agent, and to minimize toxicity by reducing systemic exposure (128). Drugs, toxins, and cytokines conjugated to mAb have been evaluated in gynecological cancers. Immunotoxins incorporate an antibody-binding domain and a toxin joined by a chemical cross-linker, peptide, or disulfide bond. The specific targeting afforded by mAbs and the relative potency of the toxin moiety present potential therapeutic advantages. The two most studied toxins have been *Pseudomonas* exotoxin A (PE), originally isolated from bacteria, and ricin, initially extracted from castor beans (9). In general, there has been less enthusiasm for antibodies conjugated with conventional cytotoxic drugs owing to concerns about quantitative drug delivery compared to treatment with maximally tolerated doses of the drug alone (9). The major drug conjugate that has been investigated in ovarian cancer is BR96-DOX, an immunoconjugate of doxorubicin (DOX) and an anti–Lewis-Y mAb. Studies utilizing these antibody conjugates are discussed in respective sections below and summarized in Table 6.4.

CLINICAL TRIALS WITH MONOCLONAL ANTIBODIES

Antibodies Targeting CA-125: OvaRex (mAb B43.13) and OC125 Conjugates

CA-125, a tumor-specific antigen that is found in 97% of patients with late-stage ovarian cancer, was first described by Bast et al. as an antigen that is elevated in the serum of patients with epithelial ovarian cancer (129). CA-125 has been cloned and identified as a mucin MUC-16 (117); its function is not clear. *In vitro* studies suggested that CA-125

(Text continues on page 140).

TABLE 6.4. *Clinical trials with mAbs in gynecologic malignancies*

Antibody	Phase	Disease	Antibody dose or combination	N	Responses	Toxicity	Remarks	Reference
B43.13	I	Recurrent ovarian cancer	2 mg, IV	13	HAMA:92%, Ab2: 66%, anti–CA-125: 33% 6 survived at least 50 wks 3 experienced a prolonged period of disease stability with survival approaching 2 years	Well tolerated	Administration of the antibody was well tolerated without infusion-related adverse events	136
B43.13	I	Recurrent ovarian cancer	IV B43.13/Chemo, sequential	—	HAMA:50%, Ab2: 75% Patients remained progression free for 50, 39, 18 and 36 weeks	Well tolerated	Subsequent chemotherapy did not abrogate the induced immune responses	137
							Patients with a T-cell response to CA-125 showed a highly significant benefit in time to progression and survival compared with non-responders ($p < 0.01$)	138
B43.13	I	Recurrent ovarian cancer	IV B43.13/Chemo, concurrent	19	HAMA/Ab2; 75% Functional T cells: 62.5%	Well tolerated		139
B43.13	II	Recurrent ovarian cancer	IV B43.13/Chemo, concurrent	16	2 CR TTP: 10.9 months	Side effects not additive between chemotherapy and B43.13	Chemotherapy did not abrogate the ability to generate an immune response	140
ACA-125	—	Recurrent ovarian cancer	IV ACA-125	42	Ab2: 66.7% Overall survival, 14.9± 12.9 months	Well tolerated	Patients with a positive immune response was 19.9 ± 13.1 months in contrast with 5.3 ± 4.3 months in those patients without detectable anti–CA-125 immunity	243
B43.13	III	Consolidation in CA-125 elevation patients	IV B43.13	55	DFS at 6 months: 75% (vs 35% in placebo group)	Well tolerated	Limited by early relapse	142
B43.13	III	Consolidation in CA-125 elevation patients	IV B43.13	345	55% generated Ab2 or HAMA responses Two-fold prolongation of survival compared with placebo control group	Well tolerated	Limited by early relapse	136

Agent	Phase	Indication	Route	No.	Results	Toxicity	Conclusion	Ref.
B43.13	III	Consolidation in CA-125 elevation patients	IV B43.13	345	HAMA: 51%; DFS: 24.0 months in the mAb B43.13 group and 10.8 months in the placebo group (Hazard ratio 0.53; $p = 0.06$)	Well tolerated	Limited by early relapse	144, 145
B43.13	III	Consolidation	IV B43.13	102	Awaits long term follow-up	Well tolerated		143
^{131}I-OC-125	I	Recurrent ovarian cancer	IV versus IP	10	IP ^{131}I-OC-125 resulted in a higher uptake of antibody in the tumor and a lower uptake of antibody in normal tissues	Well tolerated	IP is preferable route to IV	148
^{131}I-OC-125	I	Recurrent ovarian cancer	IP	20	12 of 20 patients were alive 3–17 months following therapy. Tumor progression was noted in the majority of patients, although 3 patients had documented decreases in tumor burden of short duration	Rare nausea and mild diarrhea. No dose-limiting toxicity has been observed for doses ≤120 mCi of ^{131}I	At doses ≤120 mCi, ^{131}I-OC-125 could be safely administered IP and may have antitumor effects	150
^{131}I-OC-125	II	Minimal residual disease ovarian cancer	IP ^{131}I-OC-125, 120 mCi	6	All 6 developed HAMA response. 2 patients without change, 3 with POD on biopsy at 3 months, 1 not biopsied	Grade III neutropenia and thrombocytopenia in 2 patients	Little therapeutic benefit from IP radioimmunotherapy in patients with residual ovarian carcinoma	151
^{131}I-HMFG1	I	Chemoresistant ovarian cancer	IP	24	9 of the 16 patients with small-volume disease at the time of treatment with radiolabeled antibody responded	Mild abdominal pain, pyrexia, diarrhea, and moderate reversible pancytopenia	IP of ≥140 mCi ^{131}I-HMFG1 is more effective than lower doses	154
^{90}Y-HMFG1	I–II	Adjuvant ovarian	IP	30 and 52	2 of 21 patients with minimal residual disease have died of their disease with a median follow-up of 35 months	The treatment was well tolerated and the only significant toxicity observed was reversible myelosuppression	With IV chelating agent, EDTA, allowed dose increased from 18 to 30 mCi without causing severe myelotoxicity. Suggests that patients with advanced ovarian cancer who achieve a CR following conventional therapy may benefit from further treatment with intraperitoneal radioactive mAb	155, 156

(Continued)

TABLE 6.4. *Continued*

Antibody	Phase	Disease	Antibody dose or combination	N	Responses	Toxicity	Remarks	Reference
^{90}Y-HMFG1	I	Adjuvant ovarian	IP 25 mg HMFG1 labeled with 18 mCi/m^2 ^{90}Y	52	All developed HAMA Survival at 5 years was 80%, vs 55% for controls ($p = 0.0035$)	Reversible myelosuppression	Shows a likely survival benefit for patients with ovarian cancer in the adjuvant setting Limited by historical control	157
^{90}Y-CITC-DTPA-HMFG1	I	Adjuvant ovarian	IP	19	11 of 12 evaluable patients developed anti-CITC-DTPA antibodies 5 patients developed hypersensitivity syndrome	Grade III platelet and granulocyte toxicity was observed at 19.3 mCi/m^2	Antichelate antibody responses developed against the macrocycle benzyl-DOTA, resulting in clinical side effects	157a
^{177}Lu-CC49	I	Chemoresistant ovarian cancer	IP ^{177}Lu-CC49	12	Localization of ^{177}Lu-CC49 in 11 of 12 patients 1 of 8 patients with gross disease had >50% tumor reduction, whereas 6 progressed and 1 went off study with stable disease Of the patients with microscopic or occult disease, 1 relapsed at 10 months and 3 remained free of disease after 18 months	Mild discomfort with administration, delayed transient arthralgia, and mild marrow suppression	The MTD had not been reached with levels ≤30 mCi/m^2	176
^{177}Lu-CC49	I–II	Chemoresistant ovarian cancer	IP ^{177}Lu-CC49	27	Antitumor effects were noted even at lower dose levels, and resulted in prolonged disease-free survival of most patients with microscopic disease	Dose-limiting toxicity was bone marrow suppression	MTD; 45 mCi/m^2	127
^{177}Lu-CC49	I	Chemoresistant ovarian cancer	IP ^{177}Lu-CC49 + IFN + Taxol	44	4 of the 17 patients with CT-measurable disease had a PR	Well tolerated with the expected reversible hematologic toxicity	MTD: 40 mCi/m^2 ^{177}Lu-CC49, when given with IFN-α in combination with 100 mg/m^2 Taxol did not have a significant effect on pharmacokinetic or dosimetry parameters	177
^{177}Lu-CC49	I	Chemoresistant ovarian cancer	SQ IFN-α2b, IP Taxol, and IP ^{90}Y- CC49	20	Of 9 patients with measurable disease, 2 had PR	Primarily hematological toxicity	MTD: 24.2mCi/m^2 of ^{90}Y-CC49	178

Agent	Phase	Disease	Treatment	No. of Patients	Results	Toxicity	Conclusion	Reference
^{131}I-MOv18	Pilot	Chemoresistant ovarian cancer	A single dose of IP ^{131}I-MOv18 (mean dose 14 mg) with 3700 GBq [131]I	16	Of the 11 patients with nonmeasurable disease, 7 patients had recurrence The majority of patients (15/16, 94%) produced HAMA responses CR: 5; SD: 6; POD: 5	The toxicity was negligible, with only mild and transient bone marrow suppression in 1 patient	^{90}Y-CC49-based radioimmunotherapy in combination with IFN-α2b and IP Taxol is feasible and well tolerated at a dose of ≤ 24.2 mCi/m^2	181
cMOv18	Pilot	Chemoresistant ovarian cancer	A single IV dose of cMOv18 (5 to 75 mg)	15	No HACA response was found up to 12 weeks post-injection	Only minor side effects at doses of ≥50 mg		183
cMOv18	Pilot	Recurrent ovarian cancer	IV injections of cMOv18 for 4 weeks	5	No HACA response was found Increased ADCC levels 3 patients had stable disease for up to 4 months, 9 months, and 14 months, respectively	Toxicity was mild and transient	Immunotherapy has minor effects in patients with ovarian cancer who have been heavily pretreated with chemotherapy Such strategies should be evaluated in patients who are more immunocompetent	184
[131]I-cMOv18	Pilot	Recurrent ovarian cancer	IV 3 GBq ^{131}I-cMOv18	3	No HACA responses All patients achieved an SD state	Only mild myelosuppression	Tumor-absorbed doses ranged from 600 to 3800 cGy	185
[111]In-mAb	I	Advanced ovarian cancer with Lewis-Y antigen	IV ^{90}Y-mAb B3 (5 to 25 mCi)	26	Definite tumor imaging was observed in 20 of 26 patients	DLT: myelosuppression	The MTD of ^{90}Y-mAb B3 was 20 mCi	198
LMB-1	I	Solid tumors that failed conventional therapy and whose tumors expressed the Lewis Y antigen	IV LMB-1	38	Objective antitumor activity was observed in 5 patients, 18 had SD, and 15 had POD	The major toxicity reported at this dose was vascular leak syndrome	The maximum tolerated dose of LMB-1 was 75 µg/kg given intravenously 3 times every other day	198a
MN-14	I	Ovarian cancer	Escalating IV doses of ^{131}I-MN-14 mAb	14	The mAb scan was positive in all 14 treated patients 1 CR	Myelosuppression was the only observed treatment-related toxicity	MTD: 50 mCi/m^2	207
[125]I- or ^{131}I-MX35	I	Ovarian cancer	Escalation doses, 2, 10, or 20 mg, administered by IV or IP injection	25	Specific localization of mAb in tumor was demonstrated by tumor:normal tissue ratios ranging from 2:3:1 to 34:1	Mild	mAb MX35 localizes well to tumor in selected patients with ovarian cancer	210

CR = complete response; DFS = disease-free survival; POD = progression of disease; PR = partial response; SD = stable disease; TTP = time to progression.

can produce a dose-dependent increase in invasiveness in a collagen gel invasion assay (130). It has also been shown that CA-125 can be induced by IL-1β, TNF-α, and TGF-α, whereas glucocorticoids and TGF-β can suppress the release of CA-125 from ovarian cancer cells (131). These findings may have a clinical implication on the measurement of CA-125 levels as an indicator of response to cytokine therapy (132). Two mAbs against CA-125 have been used in a series of clinical trials: OvaRex (mAb B43.13) and OC125 (Table 6.4).

OvaRex (mAb B43.13)

OvaRex (mAb B43.13), a murine anti–CA-125 mAb, was radiolabeled with ^{99m}Tc for detection of recurrent ovarian cancer. The therapeutic potential was serendipitously discovered when a retrospective study noted that patients who received radiolabeled mAb B43.13 for immunoscintigraphy exhibited unexpected prolonged survival times (119,133). It has been speculated that mAb B43.13 binds to circulating CA-125 antigens to form complexes that are recognized as foreign because they contain the foreign antibody. Several *in vitro* and *in vivo* studies have been carried out to explore the robustness of this finding. A series of prospective placebo-controlled and open-label studies in patients with ovarian cancer were carried out to assess therapeutic efficacy of naked mAb B43.13 or in combination with cytokines (e.g., IFN) or chemotherapy. Immunologic parameters in 100 patients with ovarian cancer who had been injected with mAb B43.13 were studied to explain the serendipitous observation of prolonged survival after such treatment (134). In addition to CA-125–specific humoral and cellular responses, IFN-γ was also found to be induced in those patients receiving the antibody. *In vitro* studies indicated that the expression of MHC I, MHC II, and ICAM-1 in ovarian tumor cells were upregulated in response to IFN-γ. Such tumor cells were also found to be more sensitive to CA-125–specific cytotoxic T cells compared with cells that were not incubated with IFN-γ. It was further noted that the clinical outcome was attributed to the induction of an antiidiotypic network by this antibody (133). In addition, these anti–CA-125 antibodies were able to conduct Fc-mediated tumor-cell killing (ADCC). In a multivariate analysis of clinical and immunologic profiles of 60 patients exposed to labeled mAb B43.13 compared to a contemporaneous historical cohort of 247 patients, the patients in the mAb B43.13 group were 2.7 times less likely to die from ovarian caner than were control patients managed with chemotherapy alone (*p* <0.001) (135). The mAb B43.13 group had a twofold higher median survival time compared with the control group. The 5-year survival rate was 40.7% in the mAb B43.13 group compared with 11.4% in the control group. Survival correlated with changes in three humoral immune parameters, including nonspecific HAMA responses, Ab2 and anti–CA-125 antibody development. This study suggested that mAb B43.13

exerts its therapeutic effects via stimulation of specific and nonspecific immune responses. Since then, anti–CA-125 antibodies have been tested in various settings of ovarian cancer.

OvaRex (mAb B43.13) in Recurrent Disease

Ehlen et al. reported a single-center, open-label trial to assess the induction of tumor protective immunity utilizing mAb B43.13 in a cohort of 13 patients with advanced chemorefractory recurrent ovarian cancer (136). It was noted that HAMA induction occurred in 12 of 13 patients, Ab2 was found in approximately two-thirds of the patients, and anti–CA-125–specific antibodies were elicited in one-third of the patients. These immunologic data demonstrate that the injection of a murine antibody to CA-125 can induce CA-125–specific antibody and T-cell responses even in late-stage cancer patients with substantial tumor burden. Administration of the antibody was well tolerated without infusion related adverse events. Notably, 6 patients survived at least 50 weeks and 3 patients experienced a prolonged period of disease stability with survival approaching 2 years. The use of mAb B43.13 in combination with second line chemotherapy in patients with recurrent ovarian cancer has been evaluated (137–140). The treatment has been well tolerated without significant added toxicities. Immune responses in this disease setting included HAMA and Ab2, as well as T-cell responses to CA-125 and autologous tumor cells. CA-125 measured prior to dosing of the antibody was noted to decline prior to additional chemotherapy. Patients remained progression free for prolonged periods of time. Subsequent or concurrent chemotherapy did not abrogate the induced immune responses, and T-cell responses to autologous tumor actually increased. Patients with a T-cell response to CA-125 on the autologous tumor showed a highly significant benefit in time to progression and survival compared with non-responders (*p* <0.01). Furthermore, the T-cell responses were MHC class I and II restricted, indicating the activation of CTLs and T helper cells. It was very encouraging to see that chemotherapy did not ablate the immune response as traditionally thought. A long-term follow-up study of 49 of the 218 patients who received injections of mAb B43.13 demonstrated notable periods of disease stabilization and showed that the magnitude of immunologic responses to mAb B43.13 assessed by serial evaluation of HAMA levels, anti–CA-125 antibody levels, and T-cell responses appeared to correlate with the treatment's clinical impact. A significant survival benefit post–antibody treatment was observed in patients with HAMA responses >2000 ng/mL (*p* = 0.001). Long-term survival was noted in 7 of these 49 patients who remained alive with disease 3 to 6 years after receiving mAb B43.13. These results suggest that treatment with mAb B43.13 can stimulate immune responses even in patients with relapsed ovarian cancer and can potentially slow the progression of their disease. In some cases, stabilization of the disease following immunotherapy may contribute to prolonged survival. Since mAb B43.13 has a benign safety profile, this treatment may be used as adjunctive therapy (141). Because the antiidiotypic response may have antitumor effects, antiidiotypic CA-125 antibodies have been evaluated in patients with ovarian cancer (described below).

OvaRex (mAb B43.13) in Consolidation

Standard surgery and chemotherapy for stage III-IV ovarian cancer give very good complete remission rates; however, the recurrence rate is high. Therefore, an effective consolidation regimen is desired after first-line therapy. While prolonged use of cytotoxic agents produces significant toxicities without proven survival benefits, the minimal disease state provides an ideal condition for immunotherapy-based consolidation. The goal is to stimulate the immune system to eradicate residual circulating microscopic cancer cells. mAb B43.13 has been studied as consolidation therapy following first-line surgery and chemotherapy.

One of the first randomized, double-blind, placebo-controlled studies of mAb B43.13 for adjuvant consolidation in epithelial ovarian cancer was reported by Bookman et al. (142). In this study, 55 patients who had no clinical or radiographic evidence of disease after surgery and first-line chemotherapy, but presented elevated CA-125 levels (>35 U/mL), were randomized to receive either mAb B43.13 or placebo. Immune responses were induced at a frequency similar to that reported by other studies. However, the limitation here was that the study population relapsed rapidly, and treatment was discontinued upon clinical relapse. Nevertheless, the subpopulation of patients who had time to mount an immune response had a trend of improved survival, with a 6-month progression-free survival of 75% for the mAb B43.13–treated group and 35% for the placebo cohort. In another study, 345 patients with stage III-IV epithelial ovarian cancer after surgery and chemotherapy were randomized to mAb B43.13 or placebo in a double-blind study to determine immune responses and clinical outcomes (136). Of the patients treated with mAb B43.13, 55% generated robust Ab2 or HAMA responses, associated with more than twofold prolonged median time to relapse compared with patients without immune responses (p <0.001). Adverse events were similarly distributed between the treatment and placebo groups. Repeat infusions were well tolerated throughout the treatment. These data demonstrate that mAb B43.13 also has clinical activity in the watchful waiting period following response to surgery and chemotherapy. The impact of different schedules on immune responses and clinical outcomes has been evaluated in a study of 102 patients with stage III-IV epithelial ovarian cancer treated with surgery and chemotherapy. Patients were randomized to adjuvant mAb B43.13 in three different schedules. Antibody responses specific for the constant (HAMA) and variable (Ab2) regions of mAb B43.13 were analyzed serially by enzyme-linked immunosorbent assay (ELISA) and T-cell responses by IFN-γ ELISPOT. It was noted that mAb B43.13 dosing can be increased without adversely affecting safety, and more than 2 doses were needed for optimal immune responses. Longer follow-up of time to relapse and survival will enable evaluation of the relationships between treatment schedule, immune responses, and clinical outcomes (143). A double-blind, placebo-controlled study of 345 patients following successful primary surgery and chemotherapy for stage III-IV ovarian cancer showed that immune responses were produced in patients treated with mAb B43.13 and correlated with an improved time to disease relapse (p <0.01) (144). A treatment effect was not detected in the absence of measurable antigen (CA-125 <5 U/mL). This finding supports the hypothesis that an immune complex forms between CA-125 and mAb B43.13 in the circulation, which leads to immune induction targeting CA-125 and its associated tumor source. The adverse event profiles were similar for the two treatments (145). To confirm the significant clinical benefit of mAb B43.13 for the consolidation treatment in advanced ovarian cancer, a 354-patient program with two confirmatory protocols [Immunotherapy Pivotal Ovarian Cancer Trial (IMPACT I & II)] has initiated patient recruitment at more than 50 centers throughout the United States. The study will assess disease-free survival, quality of life, and induction of immune responses by mAb B43.13 compared with placebo.

OvaRex (mAb B43.13) in First-Line Chemoimmunotherapy

The use of anti–CA-125 antibodies in chemoimmunotherapy as first-line therapy remains controversial. Traditionally, it has been thought that the combination of immunotherapy and chemotherapy was not desirable because of the immunosuppressive nature of cytotoxic agents. However, several reports have suggested that chemotherapy may selectively eliminate immunosuppressive lymphocyte populations and thereby may beneficially alter the characteristics of an immune response (146). The study with concurrent mAb B43.13 and chemotherapy in recurrent epithelial ovarian cancer reported above also supports the idea that favorable specific immune responses could be generated with this antibody despite concurrent chemotherapy (139). This observation, coupled with benign toxicity profiles and the proved survival prolongation in both recurrent ovarian cancer and during the watchful waiting stage, suggests that concurrent chemoimmunotherapy should be tested as a first-line therapy.

OvaRex (mAb B43.13) with Conjugates

A drug-antibody conjugate was tested in human ovarian serous adenocarcinomas after it showed selective toxicity *in vitro* against dividing cell populations of the human ovarian cancer cell lines expressing CA-125 (147). Daunorubicin (DNR)-OC125 was made from a new analog (PIPP-DNR) of daunorubicin that chemically links the drug to monoclonal antibodies. The immunofluorescence data show that the DNR-OC125 conjugate had high affinity and specificity for proliferating malignant cells from human ovarian tumors and indicated that the OC125 monoclonal antibody can indeed serve as a cancer-targeting carrier for daunorubicin and its analogs. The clinical efficacy has not yet been tested.

Immunoconjugated antibodies have been tested in the treatment of ovarian cancer. A distribution and pharmacokinetics study of ^{131}I-OC125 in patients with gynecologic tumors revealed that IP administration of the radiolabeled antibody resulted in a higher uptake of antibody in the tumor and a lower uptake of antibody in normal tissues (148). Therefore, this study suggested that for radioimmunotherapy of ovarian cancer, IP administration of radiolabeled antibodies is preferable to intravenous administration. This was also consistent with a study in nude mice with ovarian cancer xenografts (149). In a Phase I study, 20 patients with recurrent or persistent epithelial ovarian cancer failing conventional therapies were treated with a single IP injection of ^{131}I-OC125 mAb (150). Rare acute side effects were nausea and mild diarrhea, and no dose-limiting toxicity has been observed for doses ≤120 mCi of [131]I. Only three patients had partial responses of short duration. A Phase II study with IP radioimmunotherapy in patients with minimal residual ovarian adenocarcinoma after primary treatment with surgery and chemotherapy showed little therapeutic benefit (151). Toxicity was mainly hematologic, with grade III neutropenia and thrombocytopenia in two patients. In a retrospective study of patients with ovarian carcinoma who received 1 mg of ^{131}I-OC125 mAb one to five times after radical surgery and polychemotherapy, patients who developed high titers of Ab2 responses had a significantly higher survival rate than the ones with weak or no immunological response to ^{131}I-OC125 mAb treatment ($p < 0.05$) (152). The diagnostic value of ^{131}I-OC125 to localize ovarian tumors was tested prospectively. Scintigraphy revealed the presence of active disease, which was confirmed by laparotomy/laparoscopy in the majority of patients considered to be in clinical remission. Therefore, the sensitivity of scintigraphy with ^{131}I-OC125 was high enough and may have diagnostic value (153). Taken together, these studies showed that IP ^{131}I-OC125 may be well tolerated and patients with higher antiidiotypic responses may have a survival advantage. This may represent immunological competency required to the action of radioimmunotherapy, or simply represent the overall well being of the patients. Well controlled, randomized trials are needed to confirm these findings.

Antibodies Targeting MUC-1: HMFG1 and HMFG2

A murine immunoglobulin G1 mAb raised against human milkfat globules (HMFG1) reacts with an epitope in the pro-

tein core of polymorphic epithelial mucin (PEM) antigen (MUC-1) that is expressed by >90% of epithelial ovarian cancers and many other carcinomas. The therapeutic potential of HMFG1 has mainly been assessed in the form of conjugates with radionuclide. In one study, 24 patients with persistent epithelial ovarian cancer were treated with IP ^{131}I-labeled mAbs directed against tumor-associated antigens, including HMFG1 (154). Acute side effects were mild abdominal pain, pyrexia, diarrhea, and moderate reversible pancytopenia. Of the 16 patients with small-volume disease (<2 cm) at the time of treatment with radiolabeled antibody, 9 responded. Analysis of the data on relapse indicated that doses >140 mCi were more effective than lower doses. This study suggested that the IP administration of ≥140 mCi ^{131}I-labeled tumor-associated monoclonal antibodies represents a new and potentially effective form of therapy for patients with small-volume stage III ovarian cancer. In a Phase I-II trial of IP ^{90}Y-HMFG1 in patients with ovarian cancer, the dose was limited by myelotoxicity as described by bone deposition of free ^{90}Y carcinoma (155). The intravenous use of a chelating agent, Ledclair (ethylenediamine tetraacetic acid, EDTA), had allowed the dose to be increased from 18 to 30 mCi without causing severe myelotoxicity. An additional 52 patients with epithelial ovarian cancer were treated with IP ^{90}Y-HMFG1 following conventional surgery and chemotherapy and showed that patients with advanced ovarian cancer who receive conventional therapy and achieve a complete remission may benefit from further treatment with IP radioactive mAbs (156). Another adjuvant study with one dose of 25 mg of HMFG1 labeled with 18 mCi/m² ^{90}Y given intraperitoneally yielded a 5-year survival of 80% compared to 55% in control cases selected from the database ($p = 0.0035$). All patients developed serological evidence of HAMA. This study shows a likely survival benefit for patients with ovarian cancer who receive IP radioimmunotherapy in the adjuvant setting (157). To overcome the myelosuppression toxicity from bone deposition of ^{90}Y, stable chelating agents, such as the benzyl analog of DTPA, CITC-DTPA, was conjugated with ^{90}Y-HMFG1. However, antichelate antibody responses developed against the macrocycle benzyl-DOTA, resulting in clinical side effects with hypersensitivity syndrome (158). Whether ^{90}Y-HMFG1 antibody conjugate has a survival advantage over other forms of adjuvant IP therapy—for example, ^{32}P, IFN-γ, cisplatin, or paclitaxel, is unknown and remains to be tested.

Antibodies Targeting Tumor-Associated Glycoprotein-72 (TAG-72): CC49, B72.3

Human mammary and other carcinoma cells secrete and express on their cell surfaces complex, mucin-like glycoproteins that are recognized as tumor-associated antigens by a variety of mAbs. One such mAb, B72.3, was initially developed using a membrane-enriched fraction of human metastatic mammary carcinoma tissue as an immunogen (159).

This mAb has been extensively studied with respect to the range of reactivity for a variety of carcinomas versus normal tissues. TAG-72 is a tumor-associated glycoprotein recognized by mAb B72.3, which has more recently been shown to be specific for clusters of sTn (160). This high molecular weight mucin is expressed by the majority of common epithelial tumors. In an effort to improve the parental mAb B72.3, a series of second-generation mAbs have been developed that also recognize TAG-72 (161,162). Among the members of the initial library of antibodies produced, murine mAb CC49 was selected for further clinical studies because of its higher affinity and more rapid plasma clearance compared with mAb B72.3. mAb CC49 recognizes a different epitope than mAb B72.3 (although still sTn related) and exhibits higher reactivity to several carcinomas (163,164). The potential value of this mAb in immunotherapy has been tested for conjugates with various radionuclides in different cancers, including that of the breast (165,166), colon (167–171), and prostate (172–174). The studies in ovarian cancers are summarized below.

Animal model studies have shown considerable antitumor activity for ^{177}Lu-CC49 in TAG-72–positive human tumor xenograft models (127,175). Several Phase I trials (176) showed that treatment with ^{177}Lu-CC49 was well tolerated. Side effects included mild discomfort with administration, delayed transient arthralgia, and marrow suppression. The dose-limiting toxicity was bone marrow suppression with an MTD of 45 mCi/m^2. Antitumor effects were noted against chemotherapy-resistant ovarian cancer, even at lower dose levels, and resulted in prolonged disease-free survival of most patients with microscopic disease. The combination of IFN and Taxol with IP ^{177}Lu-CC49 was also evaluated in persistent ovarian cancer (177). Human recombinant IFN-α was administered to increase the expression of the tumor-associated antigen TAG-72. Taxol, which has radiosensitizing effects and antitumor activity against ovarian cancer, was given intraperitoneally 48 hours before radioimmunotherapy. The therapy was well tolerated with the expected reversible hematologic toxicity, and addition of IFN-α increased hematologic toxicity. The MTD was 40 mCi/m^2 ^{177}Lu-CC49 when given with IFN-α in combination with 100 mg/m^2 Taxol. A different radionuclide isotope, ^{90}Y, was also evaluated as an with mAb CC49. Treatment of patients with persistent ovarian cancer with a combination of subcutaneous IFN-α2b, IP paclitaxel, and of IP ^{90}Y-CC49 was associated with primarily hematologic toxicity (178). The MTD of IP ^{90}Y-CC49 was established at 24.2 mCi/m^2 in this combined regimen. Partial responses were observed in some of the patients with measurable disease.

The CC49 mAb was also evaluated as a drug conjugate with doxorubicin in mouse models. The immunoconjugate, designated CC49-BAMME-CH-DOX, was approximately a log less potent than unconjugated doxorubicin in an *in vitro* cytotoxicity assay (179). Immunoreactivity of the antibody was fully retained. When evaluated in a nude (*nu/nu*) mouse xenograft model with the antigen-positive human colorectal tumor target, CC49-BAMME-CH-DOX and free doxorubicin had similar tumor-suppressive activities. However, the immunoconjugate was clearly less toxic, as measured by weight loss and deaths. When evaluated in an NIH:OVCAR-3 human ovarian carcinoma xenograft model, CC49-BAMME-CH-DOX was superior at prolonging survival in comparison to free doxorubicin, unmodified CC49, and a non–tumor-binding doxorubicin immunoconjugate (179). These results indicate that targeting of doxorubicin with the CC49 antibody can improve the toxicity and/or the potency of the drug depending on the tumor target being evaluated.

In summary, these Phase I-II studies have shown that the IP treatment with radiolabeled antibodies is well tolerated. Although these studies were not designed to estimate response rate or survival, they do provide evidence of antitumor activities with this approach. The IP immunotherapy with radiolabeled antibodies for ovarian cancer has been investigated for over a decade. One advantage of administering isotopes conjugated to antibodies intraperitoneally is to ameliorate bowel complications associated with IP administration of unconjugated radioisotopes. Various forms of mAb CC49 have been engineered to improve delivery of radiation doses to tumors and minimize undesirable pharmacokinetics that lead to significant radiation exposure of normal tissues. The clinical efficacy of these different constructs will be tested.

Antibodies Targeting Folate-Binding Proteins: MOv18 and MOv19

The mAbs MOv18 and MOv19 were raised against a membrane preparation from an ovarian carcinoma surgical specimen. They reacted with a surface antigen present on the majority of nonmucinous ovarian malignant tumors tested but not with normal adult tissue (180). This antigen was subsequently identified to be folate-binding protein (FBP) (82), which is overexpressed in ovarian adenocarcinoma. The therapeutic potentials of these mAbs in ovarian cancer have been assessed in several pilot and Phase I studies. A pilot study in 16 patients with minimal residual ovarian cancer with a single dose of ^{131}I-MOv18 (mean dose 14 mg) with 3700 GBq ^{131}I showed complete response in 5 of 16 patients, and the majority of patients produced HAMA responses (181). The toxicity of radioimmunotherapy was negligible, with only mild and transient bone marrow suppression in one patient. A chimeric form of MOv18 (c-MOv18) was evaluated in several clinical trials with single or repeated injections of c-MOv18 (182–184). Toxicity was generally mild and transient. No human antichimeric antibody (HACA) response was found. Increased ADCC levels corresponding to a slight increase in CD4$^+$ and CD8$^+$ fractions were observed, whereas the CD4/CD8 ratio and the levels of CD25 remained unchanged. The radionuclide-labeled MOv18 (^{131}I-cMOv18) was also demonstrated to be safe with only mild myelosuppression; again without significant HACA response (185). These studies showed that immunotherapy aiming at boosting the patient's immunological capacity has minor effects in patients with ovarian cancer who have been heavily pretreated with chemotherapy and suggested such strategies should be evaluated in patients who are more immunocompetent; that is, before excessive chemotherapy and after achieving microscopic or small-volume disease.

A bispecific OC/TR mAb that cross links the CD3 molecule on T cells with human FBP was also generated and produced some complete and partial responses in clinical trials of patients with ovarian carcinoma (186). Most patients developed HAMA, which can inhibit OC/TR mAb-mediated lysis. An antibody-cytokine conjugate was constructed as a fusion protein between IL-2 and the scFv of MOv19 (187). This small molecule combines the specificity of MOv19 with the immunostimulatory activity of IL-2. The newly designed molecule may have improved tissue penetration and distribution within the tumor and reduced immunogenicity, and it may lack the toxicity related to the systemic administration of IL-2. In a syngeneic mouse model, IL-2/MOv19 scFv specifically targeted alpha-folate receptor gene–transduced metastatic tumor cells without accumulating in normal tissues owing to its fast clearance from the body. Treatment with IL-2/MOv19 scFv, but not with recombinant IL-2, significantly reduced the volume of subcutaneous venographic tumors. The pharmacokinetics and biological characteristics of IL-2/NMOV19 scFv may allow the combination of systemically administered IL-2/NMOV19 scFv and adoptive transfer of *in vitro* retargeted T lymphocytes for the treatment of ovarian cancer, thereby providing local delivery of IL-2 without toxicity.

It is worth noting that unlike other cancer-associated antigens, for example, CA-125, TAG-72, whose expression may be enhanced by IFN, expression of MOv18 and MOv19 was not modulated by IFN-α, INF-β, or IFN-γ (184,188). Addition of IL-2 *in vitro* also did not change any immunological parameters (184).

Antibodies Targeting The Lewis-Y (Le^y) Antigen: BR5, BR96, B3, 3S193

The Lewis-Y antigen is a type 2 blood group–related glycoprotein that is expressed by 60% to 90% of human carcinomas of epithelial cell origin, including breast, pancreas, ovary, colon, gastric, and lung cancer (109,189–193). A total of 75% of the analyzed ovarian cancer specimens expressed Lewis-Y (192). Because of its high frequency in tumors, high density and altered expression on the surface of tumor cells, and relatively homogeneous expression in primary and metastatic lesions, Lewis-Y has been an antigenic target for solid tumor immunotherapy (194). Several mAbs have been developed, including BR55 (195), BR64, and BR96 (193), B1 and B3 (196), and 3S193 (197). Some of these mAbs

have been evaluated for their potential therapeutic use in gynecological malignancies.

mAb B3 radiolabeled with ^{111}In demonstrated good tumor localization in patients with advanced epithelial tumors (198). The MTD of ^{90}Y-mAb B3 was 20 mCi, with myelosuppression as the dose-limiting toxicity. An immune toxin conjugate of B3 and *Pseudomonas* exotoxin, designated LMB-1, had excellent antitumor activity in nude mice bearing Lewis-Y–positive tumors (199). In a Phase I study in 38 patients with solid tumors who failed conventional therapy and whose tumors expressed the Lewis-Y antigen, LMB-1 produced objective antitumor activity. The MTD of LMB-1 was 75 μg/kg given intravenously three times every other day. The major toxicity reported at this dose was vascular leak syndrome.

A drug conjugate consisting of chimeric mAb BR96 and doxorubicin, BR96-Dox has been shown to cure 94% of athymic rats with subcutaneous human lung cancer (200). BR96-Dox conjugate was generally well tolerated with mild gastrointestinal toxicities, and did not show significant clinical antitumor activity in metastatic breast cancer (201–203). Another humanized anti–Lewis-Y mAb (hu3S193) was evaluated using a radionuclide conjugate of the ^{131}I isotope alone or in combination with Taxol in a MCF-7 xenografted BALB/c nude mouse, which is a breast cancer model (204). It has been noted that the combination of Taxol and ^{131}I-hu3S193 had a synergistic effect with significant tumor inhibition in 80% of the analyzed mice. Its value in the treatment of ovarian or other gynecological cancers has not been well studied and remains to be tested in the future.

Antibodies Targeting CEA: MN-14

CEA belongs to the class of tumor-associated antigens and has been most extensively studied in gastrointestinal cancers. The diagnostic and therapeutic value of CEA has been also evaluated in ovarian cancers. An anti-CEA mAb radiolabeled with ^{99}Tc was shown to be a promising radioimmunoimaging method for the detection of malignant ovarian tumors with excellent sensitivity and specificity (205). Complete clinical remission was observed in a patient with advanced ovarian cancer, refractory to paclitaxel therapy, treated with two cycles of ^{131}I-labeled murine MN-14 anti-CEA mAb (206). A follow-up Phase I therapy trial with intravenously administered ^{131}I-MN-14 anti-CEA mAb in patients with epithelial ovarian cancer showed that myelosuppression was the only observed treatment-related toxicity, and dose-limiting toxicity was seen at 50 mCi/m^2. It seems that MN-14 anti-CEA mAb is a suitable agent for tumor targeting, and it may have a therapeutic potential in patients with chemotherapy-refractive epithelial ovarian cancer, especially those with minimal disease (207).

Antibodies Targeting MX35 Antigen

mAb MX35 is a murine IgG1 that was initially developed at Memorial Sloan-Kettering Cancer Center (208,209). It detects an antigen expressed strongly and homogeneously on approximately 90% of human epithelial ovarian cancers (210), and was subsequently identified to be a 95-kD glycoprotein (211). The exact function of this antigen is yet to be defined; however, given its strong expression in ovarian cancers but not in normal peritoneum, mAb MX35 in the form of immune radionuclide conjugate has been tested for its therapeutic potential in ovarian cancer. In one study, 25 patients with advanced ovarian cancer were entered into a clinical trial using ^{125}I- or ^{131}I-labeled MX35 in escalation doses administered by intravenous or IP injection (210). Specific localization of mAb in tumor was demonstrated by tumor:normal tissue ratios ranging from 2.3:1 to 34:1 (mean 10.18:1), demonstrating that mAb MX35 localizes well to tumor in selected patients with ovarian cancer. Another study to quantify the targeting of the mAb MX35 to micrometastatic epithelial ovarian cancer demonstrated that mAb MX35 localizes to the micrometastatic ovarian carcinoma deposits within the peritoneal cavity (212). These two dosimetry results suggest a therapeutic potential for this antibody in patients with minimal residual disease (<5 mm).

Antibodies Targeting HER-2/neu and Vascular Endothelial Growth Factor

The rationale provided by preclinical studies, and the clinical data ultimately showing objective responses in 12% to 15% of metastatic breast cancer patients who overexpressed HER-2 and who received trastuzumab prompted evaluation in other malignancies (213). Original data had suggested that approximately 30% of ovarian cancer patients overexpress HER-2, providing a rationale for investigation (214). Furthermore, HER-2 overexpression appears inversely correlated with overall survival when considered in univariate and multivariate analysis among other usual prognostic factors (215). However, the most significant treatment experience in patients with recurrent or refractory ovarian or primary peritoneal cancer comes form the recently reported Gynecology Oncology Group study which screened 837 tumor samples for HER-2 expression, and showed the required 2+/3+ expression in only 95 (11.4%) of patients (216). Forty-five patients were entered into the study with an overall response rate of 7.3% with a median progression-free interval of 2 months. Based on infrequent HER-2 expression and the low rate of objective responses, the clinical value of single agent trastuzumab appears to be limited in these patients. It is unknown whether a clinical benefit could be seen by combining chemotherapy with trastuzumab in those patients with appropriate HER-2 expression, but this benefit would be limited by the frequency of expression. Recent intriguing results have been published from a small series evaluating HER-2 overexpression in the aggressive papillary serous variant of endometrial cancer. In ten consecutive specimens, 8 patients showed 2+/3+ expression, and this series is currently being expanded (217). The need for better

treatment for patients with uterine papillary serous cancer is apparent, and if this degree of overexpression is confirmed, clinical studies will be warranted.

Because the growth and metastasis of malignant neoplasms require the presence of an adequate blood supply, angiogenesis plays a central role in the development of neoplasms and their metastases. Therefore, pharmacologic inhibition of tumor-induced angiogenesis represents a promising target for antineoplastic therapy. The recent report at American Society of Clinical Oncology (ASCO) 2003 annual meeting that an anti–vascular endothelial growth factor (VEGF) mAb significantly improved survival in metastatic colon cancer when used in combination with chemotherapy represents a significant advancement in the field (218). The clinical efficacy of anti-VEGF mAb in patients with persistent or recurrent ovarian epithelial cancer and cervical cancer are being evaluated in two ongoing NCI-sponsored GOG trials.

Antibodies Targeting MN/CAIX Antigens: M75

The MN antigen was a tumor-associated antigen initially identified from a cervical carcinoma cell line HeLa (219), and was later identified to be CAIX, a carbonic anhydrase (220). It was found to be expressed in cervical intraepithelial neoplasia and 90% invasive cervical cancer but not in normal cervical tissue (219–221). Although the exact role of MN/CAIX antigen in carcinogenesis is not known, it has been suggested that it may facilitate acidification of the extracellular milieu surrounding cancer cells and in this way may promote tumor growth and spread (222). A retrospective study of 130 squamous cell cervical carcinomas demonstrated that a semiquantitative immunohistochemical analysis of CAIX expression in tumor biopsies is a significant and independent prognostic indicator of overall survival and metastasis-free survival after radiation therapy. Prospective studies have shown that MN/CAIX expression is upregulated in hypoxic human cervical tumors and is a significant and independent poor prognostic indicator (223). Therefore, CAIX may act as an intrinsic marker of tumor hypoxia and poor outcome after radiation therapy. The level of CAIX expression may be used to aid in the selection of patients who would benefit most from hypoxia-modification therapies or bio-reductive drugs. Mouse mAb M75 has been used in immunohistochemical staining in the above studies.

Summary of mAb Trials

Progress has been made in the application of mAb to the treatment of B-cell malignancies and breast cancer. However, currently, there are very few human or humanized antibodies against cell surface antigens that are of therapeutic significance in gynecologic cancers. Recently, a panel discussion of mAb in the treatment of ovarian cancers was held at the Helene Harris Memorial Trust 9th Biennial Forum on

Ovarian Cancer in Stratford, England (11). It was concluded that future trials should aim to develop humanized monoclonal antibodies to surface antigens that can be internalized. More effective radionuclide conjugates and chelates should be developed. Work should be encouraged with isotopes that are primarily α or possibly β emitters. The priorities in the development of effective mAb therapy, as nicely recommended by the panel, are (a) development of human/humanized mAbs to surface antigens that are internalized; (b) development of more effective radionuclides, chelates; (c) definition of suitable surrogate markers; (d) development of xenotypic antibodies that can induce immunity to autologous antigens; and (e) exploration of combinations with chemotherapy.

CANCER VACCINES DESIGNED TO AUGMENT ANTIBODY RESPONSES

Selection of KLH Conjugation Plus QS-21 for Vaccine Construction

We have explored a variety of approaches to increasing the antibody response against carbohydrate and peptide cancer antigens, including the use of autologous and allogeneic tumor cells modified in various ways, or not (reviewed in ref. 11), different immunological adjuvants (224–227), anti-idiotype vaccines (228,229), chemical modification of antigens to make them more immunogenic (230–232), and conjugation to various immunogenic carrier proteins (233). The conclusion from these studies is that the use of a carrier protein plus an immunological adjuvant is the optimal approach. The optimal immunological adjuvant in each case was one of two saponins (QS-21 or GPI-0100) obtained from the bark of *Quillaja saponaria* (234,235). The optimal carrier protein was in each case KLH (236–239). Each component of this approach is absolutely required; conjugate without adjuvant, antigen plus adjuvant, antigen plus KLH not conjugated plus adjuvant, all result in greatly diminished antibody responses. The rationale for this approach is reviewed above and in Table 6.5.

Conjugate Vaccines Against Cell Surface Antigens

Based on this background, GM2-KLH plus QS-21 (termed GMK) was tested in patients. It induced eight times higher titers of IgM antibody that lasted twice as long compared to our previous GM2/BCG vaccine, and for the first time GMK induced consistent IgG antibodies as well (240). Antibodies were induced in >95% of patients vaccinated with GMK instead of <85% as seen with the GM2/BCG vaccine. Consequently, a randomized multicenter intergroup trial comparing GMK to high-dose IFN-α was conducted by ECOG in stage III and high-risk stage II melanoma patients. Previous trials comparing high-dose IFN-α to no treatment (241) and GM2/BCG to BCG (106) resulted in comparable benefit for IFN and GM2/BCG, but the timing of the benefits was quite different. The beneficial effect of IFN was during the initial 6 to 8 months, whereas the effect of GMK vaccine was not clearly evident until after 2 years. An early look after 18 months median follow-up has demonstrated a significantly prolonged disease-free survival for the patients receiving IFN (242), and the trial has been stopped, although follow-up continues. If the late benefit of GMK is not seen with further follow-up, a possible explanation is the low or heterogeneous expression of GM2 in most melanomas. The solution may be a polyvalent vaccine.

A randomized adjuvant multicenter trial with a vaccine against sTn has recently been conducted by Biomira, Inc. (Edmonton, Alberta). The vaccine contains sTn disaccharide (also referred to as TAG-72) covalently linked to KLH and mixed with immunologic adjuvant Detox. Biomira is conducting the trial in patients with high-risk breast cancer at multiple centers in Canada, the United States, and Europe. This trial is based on the high-titer antibodies induced by this vaccine in this patient population, the correlation between expression of sTn on tumors and a more aggressive phenotype, and the correlation between antibody induction against sTn and longer disease-free and overall survival (107).

We have now applied the KLH conjugate plus QS21 vaccine approach to seven antigens expressed by gynecologic

TABLE 6.5. *Role of conjugate vaccine components in antibody induction againt cancer antigens*

Antigen	—Carrier (KLH) +	Adjuvant (QS-21)
1. Antigen configuration mimics expression on tumor cell. Conjugation site and tertiary structure are key.	1. Highly immunogenic carrier molecule is key for optimal cytokine release and overcoming tolerance.	The mechanism of action for most adjuvants includes:
2. High density of antigen per carrier molecule optimal.	2. Sequence of cytokine release may be important so an immunogenic carrier may be better than a cytokine, cytokine mixture or cytokine inducer.	1. Activation of APCs 2. B-cell activation 3. T-cell activation 4. Depot effect

malignancies. Antibody induction against GM2, MUC-1, and sTn occurred in 80% to 90% of vaccinated patients and against Globo H, LeY, TF, and Tn in 30% to 80% of patients. The antibody responses against these –KLH conjugate plus QS21 vaccines have reacted by flow cytometry with tumor cells expressing these antigens, and antibodies against the three glycolipids have effectively induced complement-mediated lysis. The IgG subclasses in all trials have been restricted to IgG1 and IgG3, which are the two subclasses known to mediate CDC and ADCC.

Clinical Impact of Conjugate Vaccines Against Ovarian Cancer

Markman et al. (242a) reviewed 179 patients primarily treated with platinum-based regimens as well as receiving platinum as second-line therapy. Of the 49% of responding patients to second-line therapy, only 3% of patients had a longer second remission than first remission. With the important objectives of (a) characterizing the second-remission population by evaluating a variety of prognostic factors to establish a benchmark for future consolidation trials and (b) evaluating our previously treated Phase I vaccine patients using methodology proposed by Markman et al., we have reviewed 81 patients treated on a series of Phase I monovalent vaccine studies at the Memorial Sloan-Kettering Cancer Center. The median duration of first and second remissions for our population was 15.6 (1.9 to 62.0) and 11 months (2.9 to 83.5), respectively, which fits with standard estimates. Interestingly, the number of patients with second remissions longer than first remissions in this second or greater complete clinical remission population treated with a variety of monovalent antigen vaccines (antigen-KLH + QS21 as adjuvant) was 22 of 81 (32%).

Based on this preliminary analysis, it is intriguing that such a large number of patients had second remission longer than the first when most were retreated with the same chemotherapeutic regimen with the vaccine as the most obvious variable. There are many reasons, however, why this population might differ from the population reviewed by Markman, including the fact that all of our patients were in complete clinical remission, most received IP consolidation therapy, and 40% had known negative second-look assessments, thus selecting a population with a "better" good prognosis. It is possible, however, that the improved outcomes are based on immunization with the selected antigens (the numbers are too small in each group to look at individual antigens) or on immune stimulation in general. This analysis is hypothesis generating and provides a rationale for moving forward with a definitive study to assess the effectiveness of these antibody-producing vaccines. Heterogeneity of antigen expression in different cancers of the same type, as well as different cells of the same cancer, and heterogeneity of immune response in different patients makes it likely that maximal benefit may not result from immunization against a single antigen.

ANTIIDIOTYPE VACCINES

Antiidiotype vaccines strive to augment both antibody and T-cell responses by using antibody facsimiles of the native antigens to overcome their poor immunogenicity and availability. Tumor-associated antigens are traditionally weakly immunogenic as the large majority of them in humans are nonmutated self-antigens. One approach has been to present the desired epitope to the now tolerant host in a different molecular environment, but the problem with many tumor antigens is that they are ill-defined chemically and difficult to purify and produce (243).

The "immune network hypothesis" attempts to transform epitope structures into idiotypic determinants expressed on the surface of antibodies, and was originally proposed in the 1970s (244,245). This approach assumes that immunization with a given antigen will generate the production of antibodies against this antigen (termed Ab1). Ab1 can generate antiidiotypic antibodies against Ab1, termed Ab2. Some of the antiidiotypic antibodies (Ab2β) express the internal image of the antigen recognized by the Ab1 antibody and can be used as surrogate antigens. Immunization with Ab2β can cause the production of anti–anti-Id antibodies (termed Ab3) that recognize the corresponding original antigen identified by Ab1 (246,247). (Since Ab3 can have Ab1-like reactivity, it is also called Ab1′ to distinguish it from the original Ab1.)

ACA-125

The generation and production of the murine anti-idiotypic antibody ACA-125 for clinical use has been described in detail (248). Briefly, BALB/c mice were immunized with murine monoclonal antibody OC125 (CIS; Bio International, Gif-Sur-Yvette, France) directed against the tumor-associated antigen CA-125. Splenic cells of immunized mice were fused with myeloma cells yielding an ACA-125–producing hybridoma that was adapted to serum-free medium. Large-scale production of mAb ACA-125 was performed in a hollow fiber system with yields of 10 to 15 mg antibody per day. mAb ACA-125 was purified from culture supernatant by affinity chromatography with protein G-sepharose and the preparation was checked by SDS-PAGE analysis (PHAST-System; Pharmacia Biotech, Uppsala, Sweden) to give >95% purity. The final product for vaccination in previous Phase I-II trials contained 2 mg of Ab2 IgG1 in sterile, pyrogen-free, polynucleotide-free, mycoplasma virus–free, and retrovirus-free phosphate-buffered saline (PBS) solution.

The antiidiotype approach has been used in a variety of clinical studies including patients with colon cancer, melanoma, small-cell lung cancer, and neuroblastoma. Immune responses have been demonstrated, and some have suggested a benefit in those patients in whom antibody develops (249–253). Problems with interpreting such Phase II studies have been appropriately recognized, and prospective Phase III studies are in development in several tumor types directed toward a variety of antigens.

A two-step study with ACA-125 has been conducted in Germany in patients with ovarian cancer and reported by Wagner et al. (254). Initially, 18 patients were enrolled in the Phase I portion, which was extended into a Phase II study with a total of 42 patients being treated. The objectives of the Phase I portion were to confirm safety. The objectives of the Phase II portion were to (a) further characterize the effect of ACA-125 vaccination on the Ab3 titer as a marker of a specific anti–ACA-125 immune response and (b) to evaluate overall survival comparing those patients in whom antibody was generated with those in whom it was not. Other immunologic parameters evaluated to characterize better the humoral response included assays of Ab1 and ADCC. The cytolytic activity of immunized patients' peripheral blood lymphocytes against human ovarian cancer cells (CA-125 expressing = OAW-42 and nonexpressing = SK-OV3) was also evaluated using a standard europium-release cytotoxicity assay.

Forty-two patients with advanced/recurrent epithelial ovarian carcinoma were enrolled with an average number of 2.1 prior regimens (range 1 to 5). All patients had tumors which strongly expressed CA-125 and received an intramuscular injection of 2 mg of alum-precipitated ACA-125 for four injections at 2-week intervals followed by monthly administration. A mean number of $16.6 + 10.8$ vaccinations was delivered (range 2 to 46). Minimal pain at the injection site was seen but no other systemic adverse effects. Hyperimmune sera of 27 of 42 patients (64.2%) showed an increase in HAMAs (>100 ng/mL). Ab3 responses were negative in all patients before ACA-125 administration; and 28 of 42 patients (66.7%) developed specific anti-antiidiotype antibodies (Ab3) during ACA-125 administration. The IgG subclass was evaluated in 10 patients: predominantly IgG1 and IgG2. No correlation could be shown between number of doses, serologic CA-125 concentration, and maximum Ab3 reactivity. The specificity of the immune responses induced after vaccination was demonstrated by a series of competition experiments showing that binding of patients Ab3 to the antiidiotype ACA-125 could be inhibited by the idiotypic mAb OC125 and the CA-125 antigen (254). Cell-mediated cytotoxicity from peripheral blood lymphocytes (PBLs) against CA-125–expressing and CA-125–nonexpressing human ovarian cancer cell lines in 18 patients were evaluated with measured cell kill increasing in 9 of 18 patients from $19.6 + 11.7\%$ to $52.7\% + 13.6\%$ at the effector:target cell ratio of 100:1 (254). Cell-mediated lysis was accompanied by the induction of Ab3 in eight of nine patients prompting only humoral response evaluation in the remaining patients. Overall survival of all patients vaccinated with ACA-125: 14.9 ± 12.9 months; of all patients with a positive response

to ACA-125: 19.9 ± 13.1 months; and of all patients with no detectable response to ACA-125: 5.3 ± 4.3 months; $p <.0001$.

Therefore, vaccination with a suitable antiidiotypic antibody may offer a way to induce immunity against undefined antigens or poorly immunogenic tumor antigen, such as CA-125. ACA-125 may also have had a positive impact on the survival of patients with recurrent ovarian cancer and was associated with few side effects. More recently, a study in mice has suggested that injection of the ACA-125 antibody fused to IL-6 may increase the specific humoral response against CA-125, although the clinical relevance has not been studied (255).

ADOPTIVE CELLULAR THERAPY

The goal of most immunotherapeutic approaches is to generate large numbers of highly reactive specific antitumor lymphocytes. Adoptive cellular therapy seeks to overcome tolerance hurdles by selecting and activating large numbers of lymphocytes in vitro, and manipulating the host environment to which they are introduced for maximum effect (146). Recent provocative data correlated progression-free and overall survival in patients with epithelial ovarian cancer to the presence or absence of tumor-infiltrating T cells. The 5-year overall survival rate was 38% among ovarian cancer patients whose tumor cells contained T cells and 4.5% among patients whose tumors did not contain T cells ($p <0.001$). This finding could represent a prognostic phenomenon, and the addition of T cells via the adoptive transfer approach or via vaccination may or may not be beneficial, but it warrants further exploration (256). The adoptive immunotherapeutic approach has resulted in striking clinical responses in melanoma patients after pretreatment with myeloablative chemotherapy (146), but no adoptive immunotherapy trials have been conducted in patients with gynecologic malignancies.

CONCLUSIONS

Most patients with cervical, endometrial, or ovarian cancer who will eventually die of their disease can be initially rendered free of detectable disease by surgery, radiation therapy, and/or chemotherapy. This adjuvant setting where the targets are circulating tumor cells or micrometastasis is ideal for treatment with immune interventions such as cytokines administered intraperitoneally, adoptive immunotherapy with monoclonal antibodies or cellular therapy, and vaccines that induce T cells or antibodies. This is especially true for cervical and ovarian cancers where HPV-related antigens and MUC-16 (CA-125) are uniquely specific target antigens. HPV-related interventions against cervical cancer are discussed in Chapter 19 by Dr. Thomas Wright. Initial studies in ovarian cancer patients using IFN or IL-2 administered IP have resulted in occasional partial or complete regressions of metastatic disease, especially of tumors less than 5 mm in diameter, but the impact on overall survival has yet to be demonstrated in randomized trials. Administration of mAbs MUC-16 and radiolabeled monoclonal antibodies against MUC-16, MUC-1 and sTn have resulted in occasional clinical responses and evidence of prolonged survival compared to historical controls, but results of randomized trials documenting the benefit of these approaches are not yet available. Vaccines have augmented T-cell or B-cell immunity, and these responses have been associated with stabilization of disease in some patients with advanced disease and prolongation of disease-free and overall survival compared to historical controls. Again, randomized trials confirming the benefit of vaccines remain to be accomplished. The suggestion of clinical efficacy in these trials with IP cytokines, monoclonal antibodies, and vaccines is encouraging but not definitive. As awareness of the unique features of the peritoneal cavity, radiolabeled mAb technologies, and vaccine design for augmentation of antibodies and T cells continue to evolve, there should be further progress. However, over the next several years, the focus will need to be on testing the clinical impact of these immunological interventions in appropriately controlled randomized trials in the adjuvant setting. Only in this way can a firm foundation be built on which to explore combinations of these treatments with each other and with surgery, radiation, and chemotherapy.

REFERENCES

1. McGuire WP, Hoskins WJ, Brady MF, et al. Cyclophosphamide and cisplatin compared with paclitaxel and cisplatin in patients with stage III and stage IV ovarian cancer. N Engl J Med 1996;334:1–6.
2. Muggia FM, Braly PS, Brady MF, et al. Phase III randomized study of cisplatin versus paclitaxel versus cisplatin and paclitaxel in patients with suboptimal stage III or IV ovarian cancer: a Gynecologic Oncology Group study. J Clin Oncol 2000;18:106–115.
3. Markman M, Bundy BN, Alberts DS, et al. Phase III trial of standard-dose intravenous cisplatin plus paclitaxel versus moderately high-dose carboplatin followed by intravenous paclitaxel and intraperitoneal cisplatin in small-volume stage III ovarian carcinoma: an intergroup study of the Gynecologic Oncology Group, Southwestern Oncology Group, and Eastern Cooperative Oncology Group. J Clin Oncol 2001;19:1001–1007.
4. Morris M, Eifel PJ, Lu J, et al. Pelvic radiation with concurrent chemotherapy compared with pelvic and para-aortic radiation for high-risk cervical cancer. N Engl J Med 1999;340:1137–1143.
5. Keys HM, Bundy BN, Stehman FB, et al. Cisplatin, radiation, and adjuvant hysterectomy compared with radiation and adjuvant hysterectomy for bulky stage IB cervical carcinoma. N Engl J Med 1999;340:1154–1161.
6. Koutsky LA, Ault KA, Wheeler CM, et al. A controlled trial of a human papillomavirus type 16 vaccine. N Engl J Med 2002;347:1645–1651.
7. Crum CP: The beginning of the end for cervical cancer? N Engl J Med 2002;347:1703–1705.
8. Lincoln S, Blessing JA, Lee RB, et al. Activity of paclitaxel as second-line chemotherapy in endometrial carcinoma: a Gynecologic Oncology Group study. Gynecol Oncol 2003;88:277–281.
9. Bookman MA, Boente MP, Bast R. Immunology and immunotherapy of gynecologic cancer, principles and practice of gynecologic oncology 3rd ed. Philadelphia: Lippincott Williams & Wilkins, 2000:129–163.
10. Nash MA, Lenzi R, Edwards CL, et al. Differential expression of cytokine transcripts in human epithelial ovarian carcinoma by solid tumour specimens, peritoneal exudate cells containing tumour, tumour-infiltrating lymphocyte (TIL)–derived T cell lines and established tumour cell lines. Clin Exp Immunol 1998;112:172–180.
11. Balkwill F, Schlom J, Berek J, et al. Discussion: immunological therapeutics in ovarian cancer. Gynecol Oncol 2003;88:S110–S113.
12. Allavena P, Peccatori F, Maggioni D, et al. Intraperitoneal recombinant gamma-interferon in patients with recurrent ascitic ovarian carcinoma: modulation of cytotoxicity and cytokine production in tumor-associated effectors and of major histocompatibility antigen expression on tumor cells. Cancer Res 1990;50:7318–7323.
13. Nehme A, Julia AM, Jozan S, et al. Modulation of cisplatin cytotoxicity by human recombinant interferon-gamma in human ovarian cancer cell lines. Eur J Cancer 1994;30A:520–525.
14. Saito T, Berens ME, Welander CE: Direct and indirect effects of human recombinant gamma-interferon on tumor cells in a clonogenic assay. Cancer Res 1986;46:1142–1147.
15. Berek JS: Intraperitoneal immunotherapy for ovarian cancer with alpha interferon. Eur J Cancer 1992;28A:719–721.
16. Windbichler GH, Hausmaninger H, Stummvoll W, et al. Interferon-gamma in the first-line therapy of ovarian cancer: a randomized phase III trial. Br J Cancer 2000;82:1138–1144.
17. Abdulhay G, DiSaia PJ, Blessing JA, et al. Human lymphoblastoid interferon in the treatment of advanced epithelial ovarian malignancies: a Gynecologic Oncology Group Study. Am J Obstet Gynecol 1985;152:418–423.
18. Berek JS, Hacker NF, Lichtenstein A, et al. Intraperitoneal recombinant alpha 2-interferon for 'salvage' immunotherapy in persistent epithelial ovarian cancer. Cancer Treat Rev 1985;12[Suppl B]:23–32.
19. Berek JS, Hacker NF, Lichtenstein A, et al. Intraperitoneal recombinant alpha-interferon for "salvage" immunotherapy in stage III epithelial ovarian cancer: a Gynecologic Oncology Group Study. Cancer Res 1985;45:4447–4453.
20. Berek JS: Intraperitoneal adoptive immunotherapy for peritoneal cancer. J Clin Oncol 1990;8:1610–1612.
21. Nardi M, Cognetti F, Pollera CF, et al. Intraperitoneal recombinant alpha-2-interferon alternating with cisplatin as salvage therapy for minimal residual-disease ovarian cancer: a phase II study. J Clin Oncol 1990;8:1036–1041.
22. Willemse PH, de Vries EG, Mulder NH, et al. Intraperitoneal human recombinant interferon alpha-2b in minimal residual ovarian cancer. Eur J Cancer 1990;26:353–358.
23. Berek JS, Welander C, Schink JC, et al. A phase I-II trial of intraperitoneal cisplatin and alpha-interferon in patients with persistent epithelial ovarian cancer. Gynecol Oncol 1991;40:237–243.
24. Pujade-Lauraine E, Guastella J, Colombo N, et al. Intraperitoneal administration of interferon gamma. An efficient adjuvant to the chemotherapy of ovarian cancers. Apropos of an European study of 108 patients. Bull Cancer 1993;163–170.
25. Pujade-Lauraine E, Guastalla JP, Colombo N, et al. Intraperitoneal recombinant interferon gamma in ovarian cancer patients with residual disease at second-look laparotomy. J Clin Oncol 1996;14:343–350.
26. Berek JS, Markman M, Stonebraker B, et al. Intraperitoneal interferon-alpha in residual ovarian carcinoma: a phase II gynecologic oncology group study. Gynecol Oncol 1999;75:10–14.
27. Welander CE, Morgan TM, Homesley HD, et al. Combined recombinant human interferon alpha 2 and cytotoxic agents studied in a clonogenic assay. Int J Cancer 1985;35:721–729.
28. Moore DH, Valea F, Walton LA, et al. A phase I study of intraperitoneal interferon-alpha 2b and intravenous cis-platinum plus cyclophosphamide chemotherapy in patients with untreated stage III epithelial ovarian cancer: a Gynecologic Oncology Group pilot study. Gynecol Oncol 1995;59:267–272.
29. Frasci G, Tortoriello A, Facchini G, et al. Intraperitoneal (ip) cisplatin-mitoxantrone-interferon-alpha 2b in ovarian cancer patients with minimal residual disease. Gynecol Oncol 1993;50:60–67.
30. Berek JS, Markman M, Blessing JA, et al. Intraperitoneal alpha-interferon alternating with cisplatin in residual ovarian carcinoma: a phase II Gynecologic Oncology Group study. Gynecol Oncol 1999;74:48–52.
31. Bruzzone M, Rubagotti A, Gadducci A, et al. Intraperitoneal carboplatin with or without interferon-alpha in advanced ovarian cancer

patients with minimal residual disease at second look: a prospective randomized trial of 111 patients. G.O.N.O. Gruppo Oncologic Nord Ovest. *Gynecol Oncol* 1997;65:499–505.

32. Ambrosio D, Piscopo L, Lauro C, et al. Trattamento del carcinoma ovarico con interferone alpha 2b somministrato per via intraperitoneale. *Minerva Ginecol* 2001;53:67–71.

33. Vasilyev RV, Bokhman Ja V, Smorodintsev AA, et al. An experience with application of human leucocyte interferon for cervical cancer treatment. *Eur J Gynaecol Oncol* 1990;11:313–317.

34. Wadler S, Burk RD, Neuberg D, et al. Lack of efficacy of interferon-alpha therapy in recurrent, advanced cervical cancer. *J Interferon Cytokine Res* 1995;15:1011–1016.

35. Lotan R, Dawson MI, Zou CC, et al. Enhanced efficacy of combinations of retinoic acid- and retinoid X receptor–selective retinoids and alpha-interferon in inhibition of cervical carcinoma cell proliferation. *Cancer Res* 1995;55:232–236.

36. Moore DM, Kalvakolanu DV, Lippman SM, et al. Retinoic acid and interferon in human cancer: mechanistic and clinical studies. *Semin Hematol* 1994;31:31–37.

37. Santin AD, Hermonat P, Ravaggi A, et al. Effects of retinoic acid combined with interferon-gamma on the expression of major-histocompatibility-complex molecules and intercellular adhesion molecule-1 in human cervical cancer. *Int J Cancer* 1998;75:254–258.

38. Lippman SM, Parkinson DR, Itri LM, et al. 13-Cis-retinoic acid and interferon alpha-2a: effective combination therapy for advanced squamous cell carcinoma of the skin [Comment]. *J Natl Cancer Inst* 1992; 84:235–241.

39. Paredes Espinoza M, Lippman SM, Kavanagh JJ, et al. Tratamiento de 32 pacientes con carcinoma cervico-uterino con acido 13-cis retinoico e interferon alfa. *Rev Invest Clin* 1994;46:105–111.

40. Hallum AV, 3rd, Alberts DS, Lippman SM, et al. Phase II study of 13-cis-retinoic acid plus interferon-alpha 2a in heavily pretreated squamous carcinoma of the cervix. *Gynecol Oncol* 1995;56:382–386.

41. Wadler S, Schwartz EL, Haynes H, et al. All-trans retinoic acid and interferon-alpha-2a in patients with metastatic or recurrent carcinoma of the uterine cervix: clinical and pharmacokinetic studies. New York Gynecologic Oncology Group. *Cancer* 1997;79:1574–1580.

42. Weiss GR, Liu PY, Alberts DS, et al. 13-cis-retinoic acid or all-trans-retinoic acid plus interferon-alpha in recurrent cervical cancer: a Southwest Oncology Group phase II randomized trial. *Gynecol Oncol* 1998;71:386–390.

43. Park TK, Lee JP, Kim SN, et al. Interferon-alpha 2a, 13-cis-retinoic acid and radiotherapy for locally advanced carcinoma of the cervix: a pilot study. *Eur J Gynaecol Oncol* 1998;19:35–38.

44. Gonzales-de Leon C, Lippman SM, Kudelka AP, et al. Phase II study of cisplatin, 5-fluorouracil and interferon-alpha in recurrent carcinoma of the cervix. *Invest New Drugs* 1995;13:73–76.

45. Rose PG, Bundy BN, Watkins EB, et al. Concurrent cisplatin-based radiotherapy and chemotherapy for locally advanced cervical cancer [Comment]. *N Engl J Med* 1999;340:1144–1153. [Erratum appears in *N Engl J Med* 1999;26;341(9):708.]

46. Spirtos NM, Smith LH, Teng NN: Prospective randomized trial of topical alpha-interferon (alpha-interferon gels) for the treatment of vulvar intraepithelial neoplasia III. *Gynecol Oncol* 1990;37:34–38.

47. Bornstein J, Ben-David Y, Atad J, et al. Treatment of cervical intraepithelial neoplasia and invasive squamous cell carcinoma by interferon. *Obstet Gynecol Surv* 1993;48:251–260.

48. Benedetti Panici P, Scambia G, Greggi S, et al. Recombinant interleukin-2 continuous infusion in ovarian cancer patients with minimal residual disease at second-look. *Cancer Treat Rev* 1989;16[Suppl A]:123–127.

49. Edwards RP, Gooding W, Lembersky BC, et al. Comparison of toxicity and survival following intraperitoneal recombinant interleukin-2 for persistent ovarian cancer after platinum: twenty-four-hour versus 7-day infusion. *J Clin Oncol* 1997;15:3399–3407.

50. Edwards RP, Gooding W, Lembersky BC, et al. Outpatient infusion of intraperitoneal interleukin-2 (ip IL-2) is safe and active for persistent ovarian cancer after Taxol and platinum. *Gynecol Oncol* 1998;68:111 (abst).

51. Bernsen MR, Van Der Velden AW, Everse LA, et al. Interleukin-2: hope in cases of cisplatin-resistant tumours. *Cancer Immunol Immunother* 1998;46:41–47.

52. Horton HM, Dorigo O, Hernandez P, et al. IL-2 plasmid therapy of murine ovarian carcinoma inhibits the growth of tumor ascites and alters its cytokine profile. *J Immunol* 1999;163:6378–6385.

53. Berchuck A, Lyerly H: A phase I study of autologous human interleukin-2 (IL-2) gene modified tumor cells in patients with refractory metastatic ovarian cancer. Human gene transfer protocols, Office of Recombinant DNA Activities. Bethesda, Maryland: National Institute of Health, 1995.

54. Gately MK: Interleukin-12: a recently discovered cytokine with potential for enhancing cell-mediated immune responses to tumors. *Cancer Invest* 1993;11:500–506.

55. Brunda MJ, Luistro L, Warrier RR, et al. Antitumor and antimetastatic activity of interleukin 12 against murine tumors. *J Exp Med* 1993; 178:1223–1230.

56. Coffman RL, Varkila K, Scott P, et al. Role of cytokines in the differentiation of CD4+ T-cell subsets in vivo. *Immunol Rev* 1991;123:189–207.

57. Nastala CL, Edington HD, McKinney TG, et al. Recombinant IL-12 administration induces tumor regression in association with IFN-gamma production. *J Immunol* 1994;153:1697–1706.

58. DeCesare SL, Michelini-Norris B, Blanchard DK, et al. Interleukin-12–mediated tumoricidal activity of patient lymphocytes in an autologous in vitro ovarian cancer assay system. *Gynecol Oncol* 1995;57:86–95.

59. Barton DP, Blanchard DK, Duan C, et al. Interleukin-12 synergizes with interleukin-2 to generate lymphokine-activated killer activity in peripheral blood mononuclear cells cultured in ovarian cancer ascitic fluid. *J Soc Gynecol Invest* 1995;2:762–771.

60. Fujiwara H, Hamaoka T. The anti-tumor effects of IL-12 involve enhanced IFN-gamma production by anti-tumor T cells, their accumulation to tumor sites and in situ IFN-gamma production. *Leukemia* 1997;11[Suppl 3]:570–571.

61. Zeimet AG, Widschwendter M, Knabbe C, et al. Ascitic interleukin-12 is an independent prognostic factor in ovarian cancer (comment). *J Clin Oncol* 1998;16:1861–1868.

62. Hurteau JA, Blessing JA, DeCesare SL, et al. Evaluation of recombinant human interleukin-12 in patients with recurrent or refractory ovarian cancer: a Gynecologic Oncology Group study. *Gynecol Oncol* 2001;82:7–10.

63. Lenzi R, Rosenblum M, Verschraegen C, et al. Phase I study of intraperitoneal recombinant human interleukin 12 in patients with mullerian carcinoma, gastrointestinal primary malignancies, and mesothelioma. *Clin Cancer Res* 2002;8:3686–3695.

64. Rosenberg, S.A. The identification of cancer antigens impact on the development of cancer vaccines. *Cancer J* 2000;S142–S149.

65. Moingeon, P. Review: Cancer vaccines. *Vaccine* 2001;19:1305–1326.

66. Guevara JA, Engelhorn M, Turk MJ, Houghton AN. Selectively altered self, an effective DNA vaccine for inducing anti-tumor immunity. In Preparation.

67. Santin AD, Bellone S, Gokden M, et al. Over expression of HER-2/neu in uterine serous papillary cancer. *Clin Cancer Res* 2002;8:1271–1279.

68. Khalifa MA, Mannel RS, Haraway SD, et al. Expression of EGFR, HER-2/neu, P53, and PCNA in endometrioid, serous papillary, and clear cell endometrial adenocarcinomas. *Gynecol Oncol* 1994;53:84–92.

69. Martini M, Ciccarone M, Garganese G, et al. Possible involvement of hMLH1, p16(INK4a) and PTEN in the malignant transformation of endometriosis. *Int J Cancer* 2002;102:398–406.

70. Matsumoto H, Shichijo S, Kawano K, et al. Expression of the SART-1 antigens in uterine cancers. *Jpn J Cancer Res* 1998;89:1292–1295.

71. van der Bruggen P, Traversari C, Chomez P, et al. A gene encoding an antigen recognized by cytolytic T lymphocytes on a human melanoma. *Science* 1991;254:1643–1647.

72. Chen YT, Scanlan MJ, Sahin U, et al. A testicular antigen aberrantly expressed in human cancers detected by autologous antibody screening. *Proc Natl Acad Sci U S A* 1997;94:1914–1918.

73. Zeng G, Li Y, El-Gamil M, et al. Generation of NY-ESO-1–specific CD4+ and CD8+ T cells by a single peptide with dual MHC class I and class II specificities: a new strategy for vaccine design. *Cancer Res* 2002;62:3630–3635.

74. Sarcevic B, Spagnoli GC, Terracciano L, et al. Expression of cancer/testis tumor associated antigens in cervical squamous cell carcinoma. *Oncology* 2003;64:443–449.

75. Stone B, Schummer M, Paley PJ, et al. Serologic analysis of ovarian tumor antigens reveals a bias toward antigens encoded on 17q. *Int J Cancer* 2003;104:73–84.

76. Jager E, Gnjatic S, Nagata Y, et al. Induction of primary NY-ESO-1 immunity: CD8 + T lymphocyte and antibody responses in peptide-vaccinated patients with NY-ESO-1 + cancers. *Proc Natl Acad Sci U S A* 2000;97:12198–12203.

77. Nasi ML, Lieberman P, Busam KJ, et al. Intradermal injection of granulocyte-macrophage colony-stimulating factor (GM-CSF) in patients with metastatic melanoma recruits dendritic cells. *Cytokines Cell Mol Ther* 1999;5:139–144.

78. Perales MA, Fantuzzi G, Goldberg SM, et al. GM-CSF DNA induces specific patterns of cytokines and chemokines in the skin: implications for DNA vaccines. *Cytokines Cell Mol Ther* 2003;7:125–133.

79. Santin AD, Ioli GR, Hiserodt JC, et al. Development and in vitro characterization of a GM-CSF secreting human ovarian carcinoma tumor vaccine. *Int J Gynecol Cancer* 1995;5:401–410.

80. Salgia R, Lynch T, Skarin A, et al. Vaccination with irradiated autologous tumor cells engineered to secrete granulocyte-macrophage colony-stimulating factor augments antitumor immunity in some patients with metastatic non–small-cell lung carcinoma. *J Clin Oncol* 2003;21:624–630.

81. Miotti S, Facheris P, Tomassetti A, et al. Growth of ovarian-carcinoma cell lines at physiological folate concentration: effect on folate-binding protein expression in vitro and in vivo. *Int J Cancer* 1995;63:395–401.

82. Coney LR, Tomassetti A, Carayannopoulos L, et al. Cloning of a tumor-associated antigen: MOv18 and MOv19 antibodies recognize a folate-binding protein. *Cancer Res* 1991;51:6125–6132.

83. Bottero F, Tomassetti A, Canevari S, et al. Gene transfection and expression of the ovarian carcinoma marker folate binding protein on NIH/3T3 cells increases cell growth in vitro and in vivo. *Cancer Res* 1993;53:5791–5796.

84. Bagnoli M, Canevari S, Figini M, et al. A step further in understanding the biology of the folate receptor in ovarian carcinoma. *Gynecol Oncol* 2003;88:S140–S144.

85. Neglia F, Orengo AM, Cilli M, et al. DNA vaccination against the ovarian carcinoma-associated antigen folate receptor alpha (FRalpha) induces cytotoxic T lymphocyte and antibody responses in mice. *Cancer Gene Ther* 1999;6:349–357.

86. Peoples GE, Anderson BW, Lee TV, et al. Vaccine implications of folate binding protein, a novel cytotoxic T lymphocyte-recognized antigen system in epithelial cancers. *Clin Cancer Res* 1999;5:4214–4223.

87. Santini SM, Belardelli F: Advances in the use of dendritic cells and new adjuvants for the development of therapeutic vaccines. *Stem Cells* 2003;21:495–505.

88. Mayordomo JI, Zorina T, Storkus WJ, et al. Bone marrow-derived dendritic cells serve as potent adjuvants for peptide-based antitumor vaccines. *Stem Cells* 1997;15:94–103.

89. Hernando JJ, Park TW, Kubler K, et al. Vaccination with autologous tumour antigen-pulsed dendritic cells in advanced gynecological malignancies: clinical and immunological evaluation of a phase I trial. *Cancer Immunol Immunother* 2002;51:45–52.

90. Hsu FJ, Benike C, Fagnoni F, et al. Vaccination of patients with B-cell lymphoma using autologous antigen-pulsed dendritic cells. *Nat Med* 1996;2:52–58.

91. Brossart P, Wirths S, Stuhler G, et al. Induction of cytotoxic T-lymphocyte responses in vivo after vaccinations with peptide-pulsed dendritic cells. *Blood* 2000;96:3102–3108.

92. Kugler A, Stuhler G, Walden P, et al. Regression of human metastatic renal cell carcinoma after vaccination with tumor cell-dendritic cell hybrids. *Nat Med* 2000;6:332–336.

93. Engleman EG, Fong L: Induction of immunity to tumor-associated antigens following dendritic cell vaccination of cancer patients. *Clin Immunol* 2003;106:10–15.

94. Geiger JD, Hutchinson RJ, Hohenkirk LF, et al. Vaccination of pediatric solid tumor patients with tumor lysate-pulsed dendritic cells can expand specific T cells and mediate tumor regression. *Cancer Res* 2001;61:8513–8519.

95. Nestle FO, Alijagic S, Gilliet M, et al. Vaccination of melanoma patients with peptide- or tumor lysate-pulsed dendritic cells. *Nat Med* 1998;4:328–332.

96. Yin, BWT, Dnistrian, A, and Lloyd, KO. Ovarian cancer antigen CA125 is encoded by the MUC16 mucin gene. *Int J Cancer* 2002;98:737–740.

97. Bookman MA, Darcy KM, Clarke-Pearson D, et al. Evaluation of monoclonal humanized anti-HER2 antibody, trastuzumab, in patients with recurrent or refractory ovarian or primary peritoneal carcinoma with overexpression of HER2: a phase II trial of the Gynecologic Oncology Group. *J Clin Oncol* 2003;21:283–290.

98. Lodge PA, Jones LA, Bader RA, et al. Dendritic cell-based immunotherapy of prostate cancer: immune monitoring of a phase II clinical trial. *Cancer Res* 2000;60:829–833.

99. Chakraborty NG, Sporn JR, Tortora AF, et al. Immunization with a tumor-cell-lysate-loaded autologous-antigen-presenting-cell-based vaccine in melanoma. *Cancer Immunol Immunother* 1998;47:58–64.

100. Parmiani G, Lotze MT, Livingston PO. In: *Tumor immunology: molecularly defined antigens and clinical applications.* Parmiani G, Lotze MT, eds. London: Taylor & Francis, 2002.

101. Fearon DT, Kelsoe G, Kinef JP, et al. The humoral immune response. In: Janeway CA Jr, Travers P, eds. *Immunobiology: the immune system in health and disease.* 3rd ed. New York: Garland, 1997:1–54.

102. Zhang H, Zhang S, Cheung NK, et al.. Antibodies can eradicate cancer micrometastases. *Cancer Res* 1998;58:2844–2849.

103. Livingston PO. The case for melanoma vaccines that induce antibodies. In: Kirkwood, JM, ed. *Molecular diagnosis and treatment of melanoma.* New York: Marcel Dekker, 1998.

104. Jones PC, Sze LL, Liu PY, et al. Prolonged survival for melanoma patients with elevated IgM antibody to oncofetal antigen. *J Natl Cancer Inst* 1981;66:249–254.

105. Livingston PO, Ritter G, Srivastava P, et al. Characterization of IgG and IgM antibodies induced in melanoma patients by immunization with purified GM2 gangliosic. *Cancer Res* 1989;49:7045–7050.

106. Livingston PO, Wong GYC, Adluri S, et al. Improved survival in AJCC stage III melanoma patients with GM2 antibodies: a randomized trial of adjuvant vaccination with GM2 ganglioside. *J Clin Oncol* 1994;12:1036–1044.

107. MacLean GD, Reddish MA, Koganty RR, Longenecker BM. Antibodies against mucin-associated sialyl-Tn epitopes correlate with survival of metastatic adenocarcinoma patients undergoing active specific immunotherapy with synthetic STn vaccine. *J Immunother* 1996;19:59–68.

108. Zhang S, Cordon-Cardo C, Zhang HS, et al. Selection of carbohydrate tumor antigens as targets for immune attack using immunohistochemistry. I. Focus on gangliosides. *Int J Cancer* 1997;73:42–49.

109. Zhang S, Zhang HS, Cordon-Cardo C, et al. Selection of tumor antigens as targets for immune attack using immunohistochemistry. II. Blood group–related antigens. *Int J Cancer* 1997;73:50–56.

110. Zhang S, Zhang HS, Cordon-Cardo C, et al. Selection of tumor antigens as targets for immune attack using immunohistochemistry: III. protein antigens. *Clin. Cancer Res.*1998;4:2669–2676.

111. Mark FF, Kudryashov V, Saigo PE, et al. Selection of carbohydrate antigens in human epithelial ovarian cancers as targets for immunotherapy: serous and mucinous tumors exhibit distinctive patterns of expression. *Int J Cancer* 1999;81:193–198.

112. Kabawat SE, Bast RC Jr, Welch WR, et al. Immunopathologic characterization of a monoclonal antibody that recognizes common surface antigens of human ovarian tumors of serous, endometrioid, and clear cell types. *Am J Clin Pathol* 1983;79(1):98–104.

113. Nakamura K, Koike M, Shitara K, et al. Chimeric anti-ganglioside GM2 antibody with antitumor activity. *Cancer Res* 1994;54:1511–1516.

114. Nishinaka Y, Ravindranath MNH, Ire RF. Development of a human monoclonal antibody to ganglioside GM2 with potential for cancer treatment. *Cancer Res* 1996;56:5666–5671.

115. Lloyd KO. Blood group antigens as markers for normal differentiation and malignant change in human tissues. *Am J Clin Pathol* 1987;87:129–139.

116. Bast RC, Feeney M, Lazarus H, et al. Reactivity of a monoclonal antibody with human ovarian carcinoma. *J Clin Invest* 1981;68:1331–1337.

117. Yin, BWT, and Lloyd, KO. Molecular cloning of the CA125 ovarian cancer antigen. *J Biol Chem* 2001;276:27371–27375.

118. O'Brien TJ, Beard JB, Underwood LJ, et al. The CA 125 gene: an

extracellular superstructure dominated by repeat sequences. *Tumor Biol* 2001;22:348–366.

119. Baum RP, Noujaim AA, Nanci A, et al. Clinical course of ovarian cancer patients under repeated stimulation of HAMA using MAb OC125 and B43.13. *Hybridoma* 1993;12:583–589.

120. Kashmiri SV, Iwahashi M, Tamura M, et al. Development of a minimally immunogenic variant of humanized anti-carcinoma monoclonal antibody CC49. *Crit Rev Oncol Hematol* 2001;38:3–16.

121. Goel A, Colcher D, Baranowska-Kortylewicz J, et al. Genetically engineered tetravalent single-chain Fv of the pancarcinoma monoclonal antibody CC49: improved biodistribution and potential for therapeutic application. *Cancer Res* 2000;60:6964–6971.

122. Kennel SJ, Chappell LL, Dadachova K, et al. Evaluation of 225Ac for vascular targeted radioimmunotherapy of lung tumors [Comment]. *Cancer Biother Radiopharmaceut* 2000;15:235–244.

123. Yokota T, Milenic DE, Whitlow M, et al. Rapid tumor penetration of a single-chain Fv and comparison with other immunoglobulin forms. *Cancer Res* 1992;52:3402–3408.

124. Pavlinkova G, Colcher D, Booth BJ, et al. Pharmacokinetics and biodistribution of a light-chain-shuffled CC49 single-chain Fv antibody construct. *Cancer Immunol Immunother* 2000;49:267–275.

125. Kashmiri SV, Shu L, Padlan EA, et al. Generation, characterization, and in vivo studies of humanized anticarcinoma antibody CC49. *Hybridoma* 1995;14:461–473.

126. Kennel SJ, Brechbiel MW, Milenic DE, et al. Actinium-225 conjugates of MAb CC49 and humanized delta CH2CC49. *Cancer Biother Radiopharmaceut* 2002;17:219–231.

127. Alvarez RD, Partridge EE, Khazaeli MB, et al. Intraperitoneal radioimmunotherapy of ovarian cancer with 177Lu-CC49: a phase I/II study. *Gynecol Oncol* 1997;65:94–101.

128. Trail PA, Bianchi AB. Monoclonal antibody drug conjugates in the treatment of cancer. *Curr Opin Immunol* 1999;11:584–588.

129. Bast RC Jr, Klug TL, St John E, et al. A radioimmunoassay using a monoclonal antibody to monitor the course of epithelial ovarian cancer. *N Engl J Med* 1983;309:883–887.

130. Gaetje R, Winnekendonk DW, Scharl A, et al. Ovarian cancer antigen CA 125 enhances the invasiveness of the endometriotic cell line EEC 145. *J Soc Gynecol Invest* 1999;6:278–281.

131. Marth C, Zeimet AG, Widschwendter M, et al. Regulation of CA 125 expression in cultured human carcinoma cells. *Int J Biol Markers* 1998;13:207–209.

132. Balkwill FR. Tumour necrosis factor and cancer. *Prog Growth Factor Res* 1992;4:121–137.

133. Schultes BC, Baum RP, Niesen A, et al. Anti-idiotype induction therapy: anti-CA125 antibodies (Ab3) mediated tumor killing in patients treated with Ovarex mAb B43.13 (Ab1). *Cancer Immunol Immunother* 1998;46:201–212.

134. Madiyalakan R, Yang R, Schultes BC, et al. OVAREX MAb-B43.13: IFN-gamma could improve the ovarian tumor cell sensitivity to CA125-specific allogenic cytotoxic T cells. *Hybridoma* 1997;16:41–45.

135. Berek JS, Dorigo O, Schultes B, et al. Specific keynote: immunological therapy for ovarian cancer. *Gynecol Oncol* 2003;88:S105–S109; Discussion S110–S113.

136. Ehlen TG, Gordon AG, Fingert HJ, et al. Adjuvant treatment with monoclonal antibody, OvaRex MAb-B43.13 (OV) targeting CA125, induces robust immune responses associated with prolonged time to relapse (TTR) in a randomized, placebo-controlled study in patients (pts) with advanced epithelial ovarian cancer (EOC). *Proc Am Soc Clin Oncol* 2002(abst 31).

137. Gordon A, Whiteside T, Nicodemus C, et al. An interim assessment of OvaRex® MAb-B43.13 in the management of recurrent ovarian cancer. *Proc Am Soc Clin Oncol* 2001;20:187b.

138. Schultes B, Gordon A, Ehlen T: Induction of tumor- and CA125-specific T cell responses in patients with epithelial ovarian cancer treated with OvaRex MAb B43.13. *Proc Am Assoc Cancer Res* 2002;43:144.

139. Gordon A, Stringer A, Edwards RP, et al. Clinical and immunologic outcomes of patients with recurrent epithelial ovarian cancer treated with OvaRex MAb and chemotherapy. *Gynecol Oncol* 2002;84:501(abst 74).

140. Schultes BC, Gordon AN, Whiteside TL, et al. Feasibility of combined

141. Bolle M, Niesen A, Korz W, et al. Possible role of anti-CA125 monoclonal antibody B43.13 (OvaRex) administration in long-term survival of relapsed ovarian cancer patients. *Proc Am Soc Clin Oncol* 2000; 19:476a.

142. Bookman MA, Rettenmaier M, Gordon A: Monoclonal antibody (Oregovomab) targeting of CA125 in patients (pts) with advanced epithelial ovarian cancer (EOC) and elevated CA125 after response to initial therapy. *Clin Cancer Res* 2001;7:3756s (abst 510).

143. Method MW, Gordon A, Finkler F, et al. Randomized evaluation of 3 treatment schedules to optimize clinical activity of OvaRex® MAb-B43.13 (OV) in patients (pts) with epithelial ovarian cancer (EOC). *Proc Am Soc Clin Oncol* 2002; (abst 80).

144. Berek J, Ehlen T, Gordon E, et al. Interim analysis of a double blind study of Ovarex® MAb B43.13 (OV) versus placebo (PBO) in patients with ovarian cancer. *Proc Am Soc Clin Oncol* 2001; (abst 837).

145. Berek JS, Taylor PT, Gordon AN, et al. Randomized pbo-controlled study of oregovomab (OV) for consolidation of clinical remission in pts with ovarian cancer (OC): Prolonged disease-free survival (DFS) in optimal chemosensitive pts. *Proc Am Soc Clin Oncol* 2003;

146. Dudley ME, Wunderlich JR, Robbins PF, et al. Cancer regression and autoimmunity in patients after clonal repopulation with antitumor lymphocytes. *Science* 2002;298:850–854.

147. Dezso B, Torok I, Rosik LO, et al. Human ovarian cancers specifically bind daunorubicin–OC-125 conjugate: an immunofluorescence study. *Gynecol Oncol* 1990;39:60–64.

148. Haisma HJ, Moseley KR, Battaile A, et al. Distribution and pharmacokinetics of radiolabeled monoclonal antibody OC 125 after intravenous and intraperitoneal administration in gynecologic tumors. *Am J Obstet Gynecol* 1988;159:843–848.

149. Thedrez P, Saccavini JC, Nolibe D, et al. Biodistribution of indium-111–labeled OC 125 monoclonal antibody after intraperitoneal injection in nude mice intraperitoneally grafted with ovarian carcinoma. *Cancer Res* 1989;49:3081–3086.

150. Finkler NJ, Muto MG, Kassis AI, et al. Intraperitoneal radiolabeled OC 125 in patients with advanced ovarian cancer. *Gynecol Oncol* 1989;34:339–344.

151. Mahe MA, Fumoleau P, Fabbro M, et al. A phase II study of intraperitoneal radioimmunotherapy with iodine-131–labeled monoclonal antibody OC-125 in patients with residual ovarian carcinoma. *Clin Cancer Res* 1999;5:3249s–3253s.

152. Schmolling J, Wagner U, Reinsberg J, et al. [Immune reactions and survival of patients with ovarian carcinomas after administration of 131I-F(Ab)2 fragments of the OC 125 monoclonal antibody.] *Geburtshilfe Frauenheilkd* 1995;55:200–203.

153. Kalofonos HP, Karamouzis MV, Epenetos AA. Radioimmunoscintigraphy in patients with ovarian cancer. *Acta Oncol* 2001;40:549–557.

154. Epenetos AA, Munro AJ, Stewart S, et al. Antibody-guided irradiation of advanced ovarian cancer with intraperitoneally administered radiolabeled monoclonal antibodies. *J Clin Oncol* 1987;5:1890–1899.

155. Hird V, Stewart JS, Snook D, et al. Intraperitoneally administered 90Y-labelled monoclonal antibodies as a third line of treatment in ovarian cancer. A phase 1–2 trial: problems encountered and possible solutions. *Br J Cancer* 1990;10[Suppl]:48–51.

156. Hird V, Maraveyas A, Snook D, et al. Adjuvant therapy of ovarian cancer with radioactive monoclonal antibody. *Br J Cancer* 1993;68:403–406.

157. Nicholson S, Gooden CS, Hird V, et al. Radioimmunotherapy after chemotherapy compared to chemotherapy alone in the treatment of advanced ovarian cancer: a matched analysis. *Oncol Rep* 5:223–226.

157a. Kosmas C, Maraveyas A, Gooden CS, et al. Anti-chelate antibodies after intraperitoneal yttrium-90-labeled monoclonal antibody immunoconjugates for ovarian cancer therapy. *J Nucl Med* 1995;36:746–753.

158. Maraveyas A, Snook D, Hird V, et al. Pharmacokinetics and toxicity of an yttrium-90-CITC-DTPA-HMFG1 radioimmunoconjugate for intraperitoneal radioimmunotherapy of ovarian cancer. *Cancer* 1994;73:1067–1075.

159. Colcher D, Hand PH, Nuti M, et al. A spectrum of monoclonal antibodies reactive with human mammary tumor cells. *Proc Natl Acad Sci U S A* 1981;78:3199–3203.

160. Zhang S, Walberg LA, Ogata S, et al. Immune sera and monoclonal

antibodies define two configurations for the sialyl Tn tumor antigen. *Cancer Res* 1995;55:3364–3368.

161. Colcher D, Minelli MF, Roselli M, et al. Radioimmunolocalization of human carcinoma xenografts with B72.3 second generation monoclonal antibodies. *Cancer Res* 1988;48:4597–4603.

162. Muraro R, Kuroki M, Wunderlich D, et al. Generation and characterization of B72.3 second generation monoclonal antibodies reactive with the tumor-associated glycoprotein 72 antigen. *Cancer Res* 1988; 48:4588–4596.

163. Sheer DG, Schlom J, Cooper HL. Purification and composition of the human tumor-associated glycoprotein (TAG-72) defined by monoclonal antibodies CC49 and B72.3. *Cancer Res* 1988;48:6811–6818.

164. Molinolo A, Simpson JF, Thor A, et al. Enhanced tumor binding using immunohistochemical analyses by second generation anti-tumor-associated glycoprotein 72 monoclonal antibodies versus monoclonal antibody B72.3 in human tissue. *Cancer Res* 1990;50:1291–1298.

165. Macey DJ, Grant EJ, Kasi L, et al. Effect of recombinant alpha-interferon on pharmacokinetics, biodistribution, toxicity, and efficacy of 131I-labeled monoclonal antibody CC49 in breast cancer: a phase II trial. *Clin Cancer Res* 1997;3:1547–1555.

166. Murray JL, Macey DJ, Grant EJ, et al. Enhanced TAG-72 expression and tumor uptake of radiolabeled monoclonal antibody CC49 in metastatic breast cancer patients following alpha-interferon treatment. *Cancer Res* 1995;55:5925s–5928s.

167. Rucker R, Bresler HS, Heffelfinger M, et al. Low-dose monoclonal antibody CC49 administered sequentially with granulocyte-macrophage colony-stimulating factor in patients with metastatic colorectal cancer. *J Immunol* 1999;22:80–84.

168. Triozzi PL, Kim JA, Martin EW, Jr., et al. Clinical and immunologic effects of monoclonal antibody CC49 and interleukin-2 in patients with metastatic colorectal cancer. *Hybridoma* 1997;16:147–151.

169. Divgi CR, Scott AM, Gulec S, et al. Pilot radioimmunotherapy trial with 131I-labeled murine monoclonal antibody CC49 and deoxyspergualin in metastatic colon carcinoma. *Clin Cancer Res* 1995;1: 1503–1510.

170. Divgi CR, Scott AM, Dantis L, et al. Phase I radioimmunotherapy trial with iodine-131-CC49 in metastatic colon carcinoma. *J Nucl Med* 1995;36:586–592.

171. Murray JL, Macey DJ, Kasi LP, et al. Phase II radioimmunotherapy trial with 131I-CC49 in colorectal cancer. *Cancer* 1994;73: 1057–1066.

172. Meredith RF, Khazaeli MB, Macey DJ, et al. Phase II study of interferon-enhanced 131I-labeled high affinity CC49 monoclonal antibody therapy in patients with metastatic prostate cancer. *Clin Cancer Res* 1999;5:3254s–3258s.

173. Meredith RF, Bueschen AJ, Khazaeli MB, et al. Treatment of metastatic prostate carcinoma with radiolabeled antibody CC49. *J Nucl Med* 1994;35:1017–1022.

174. Slovin SF, Scher HI, Divgi CR, et al. Interferon-gamma and monoclonal antibody 131I-labeled CC49: outcomes in patients with androgen-independent prostate cancer. *Clin Cancer Res* 1998;4:643–651.

175. Schlom J, Siler K, Milenic DE, et al. Monoclonal antibody-based therapy of a human tumor xenograft with a 177-lutetium-labeled immunoconjugate. *Cancer Res* 1991;51:2889–2896.

176. Meredith RF, Partridge EE, Alvarez RD, et al. Intraperitoneal radioimmunotherapy of ovarian cancer with lutetium-177-CC49. *J Nucl Med* 1996;37:1491–1496.

177. Meredith RF, Alvarez RD, Partridge EE, et al. Intraperitoneal radioimmunochemotherapy of ovarian cancer: a phase I study. *Cancer Biother Radiopharmaceut* 2001;16:305–315.

178. Alvarez RD, Huh WK, Khazaeli MB, et al. A phase I study of combined modality (90)yttrium-CC49 intraperitoneal radioimmunotherapy for ovarian cancer. *Clin Cancer Res* 2002;8:2806–2811.

179. Johnson DA, Briggs SL, Gutowski MC, et al. Anti-tumor activity of CC49-doxorubicin immunoconjugates. *Anticancer Res* 1995;15: 1387–1393.

180. Miotti S, Canevari S, Menard S, et al. Characterization of human ovarian carcinoma-associated antigens defined by novel monoclonal antibodies with tumor-restricted specificity. *Int J Cancer* 1987;39: 297–303.

181. Crippa F, Bolis G, Seregni E, et al. Single-dose intraperitoneal radioimmunotherapy with the murine monoclonal antibody I-131 MOv18:

clinical results in patients with minimal residual disease of ovarian cancer. *Eur J Cancer* 1995;31A:686–690.

182. Buist MR, Molthoff CF, Kenemans P, et al. Distribution of OV-TL 3 and MOv18 in normal and malignant ovarian tissue. *J Clin Pathol* 1995;48:631–636.

183. Molthoff CF, Prinssen HM, Kenemans P, et al. Escalating protein doses of chimeric monoclonal antibody MOv18 immunoglobulin G in ovarian carcinoma patients: a phase I study. *Cancer* 1997;80: 2712–2720.

184. van Zanten-Przybysz I, Molthoff C, Gebbinck JK, et al. Cellular and humoral responses after multiple injections of unconjugated chimeric monoclonal antibody MOv18 in ovarian cancer patients: a pilot study. *J Cancer Res Clin Oncol* 2002;128:484–492.

185. van Zanten-Przybysz I, Molthoff CF, Roos JC, et al. Radioimmunotherapy with intravenously administered 131I-labeled chimeric monoclonal antibody MOv18 in patients with ovarian cancer. *J Nucl Med* 2000;41:1168–1176.

186. Luiten RM, Warnaar SO, Sanborn D, et al. Chimeric bispecific OC/TR monoclonal antibody mediates lysis of tumor cells expressing the folate-binding protein (MOv18) and displays decreased immunogenicity in patients. *J Immunol* 1997;20:496–504.

187. Melani C, Figini M, Nicosia D, et al. Targeting of interleukin 2 to human ovarian carcinoma by fusion with a single-chain Fv of antifolate receptor antibody. *Cancer Res* 1998;58:4146–4154.

188. Greiner JW, Guadagni F, Goldstein D, et al. Intraperitoneal administration of interferon-gamma to carcinoma patients enhances expression of tumor-associated glycoprotein-72 and carcinoembryonic antigen on malignant ascites cells. *J Clin Oncol* 1992;10:735–746.

189. Sakamoto J, Furukawa K, Cordon-Cardo C, et al. Expression of Lewis-a, Lewis-b, X, and Y blood group antigens in human colonic tumors and normal tissue and in human tumor-derived cell lines. *Cancer Res* 1986;46:1553–1561.

190. Hakomori S: General concept of tumor-associated carbohydrate antigens: their chemical, physical and enzymatic basis. In: Oettgen HF, ed. *Gangliosides and cancer*. Weiheim, Germany: VHC Publishers, 1989:93–102.

191. Miyake M, Taki T, Hitomi S, et al. Correlation of expression of H/Le(y)/Le(b) antigens with survival in patients with carcinoma of the lung. (comment). *N Engl J Med* 1992;327:14–18.

192. Yin BW, Finstad CL, Kitamura K, et al. Serological and immunochemical analysis of Lewis y (Ley) blood group antigen expression in epithelial ovarian cancer. *Int J Cancer* 1996;65:406–412.

193. Hellström, I, Garrigues, HJ, Garrigues, U, and Hellström, KE. Highly tumor-reactive, internalizing, mouse monoclonal antibodies to Ley-related cell surface antigens. *Cancer Res* 1990;50:2183–2190.

194. Scott AM, Geleick D, Rubira M, et al. Construction, production, and characterization of humanized anti-Lewis Y monoclonal antibody 3S193 for targeted immunotherapy of solid tumors. *Cancer Res* 2000; 60:3254–3261.

195. Masucci G, Lindemalm C, Frodin JE, et al. Effect of human blood mononuclear cell populations in antibody dependent cellular cytotoxicity (ADCC) using two murine (CO17–1A and Br55–2) and one chimeric (17–1A) monoclonal antibodies against a human colorectal carcinoma cell line (SW948). *Hybridoma* 1988;7:429–440.

196. Pastan I, Lovelace E, Gallo M, et al. Characterization of monoclonal antibodies B1 and B3 that react with mucinous adenocarcinomas. *Cancer Res* 1991;51:3781–3787.

197. Kitamura K, Stockert E, Garin-Chesa P, et al. Specificity analysis of blood group Lewis-y (Le(y)) antibodies generated against synthetic and natural Le(y) determinants. *Proc Natl Acad Sci U S A* 1994;91: 12957–12961.

198. Pai-Scherf LH, Carrasquillo JA, Paik C, et al. Imaging and Phase I study of 111In- and 90Y-labeled anti-LewisY monoclonal antibody B3. *Clin Cancer Res* 2000;6:1720–1730.

198a. Pai LH, Wittes R, Setser A, et al. Treatment of advanced solid tumors with immunotoxin LMB-1: an antibody linked to *Pseudomonas* exotoxin. *Nature Med* 1996;2:350–353.

199. Pai LH, Batra JK, FitzGerald DJ, et al. Anti-tumor activities of immunotoxins made of monoclonal antibody B3 and various forms of Pseudomonas exotoxin. *Proc Natl Acad Sci U S A* 1991;88:3358–3362. [Erratum appears in *Proc Natl Acad Sci U S A* 1991;88:5066.].

200. Trail PA, Willner D, Lasch SJ, et al. Cure of xenografted human

carcinomas by BR96-doxorubicin immunoconjugates. *Science* 1993; 261:212–215. [Erratum appears in *Science* 1994;263:1076.]

201. Tolcher AW, Sugarman S, Gelmon KA, et al. Randomized phase II study of BR96-doxorubicin conjugate in patients with metastatic breast cancer [Comment]. *J Clin Oncol* 1999;17:478–484.

202. Tolcher AW: BR96-doxorubicin: been there, done that! [Comment]. *J Clin Oncol* 2000;18:4000.

203. Saleh MN, Sugarman S, Murray J, et al. Phase I trial of the anti–Lewis Y drug immunoconjugate BR96-doxorubicin in patients with Lewis Y–expressing epithelial tumors. [Comment]. *J Clin Oncol* 2000;18: 2282–2292.

204. Clarke K, Lee FT, Brechbiel MW, et al. Therapeutic efficacy of anti-Lewis(y) humanized 3S193 radioimmunotherapy in a breast cancer model: enhanced activity when combined with Taxol chemotherapy. *Clin Cancer Res* 2000;6:3621–3628.

205. Wu LY, Wu AR, Zhan J: Radioimmunoimaging assay of ovarian tumor with 99mTc labeled anti-carcinoembryonic antigen monoclonal antibody. *Chin J Obstet Gynecol* 1994;29:340–342, 381–382.

206. Juweid M, Sharkey RM, Alavi A, et al. Regression of advanced refractory ovarian cancer treated with iodine-131-labeled anti-CEA monoclonal antibody. *J Nucl Med* 1997;38:257–260.

207. Juweid M, Swayne LC, Sharkey RM, et al. Prospects of radioimmunotherapy in epithelial ovarian cancer: results with iodine-131-labeled murine and humanized MN-14 anti-carcinoembryonic antigen monoclonal antibodies. *Gynecol Oncol* 1997;67:259–271.

208. Mattes MJ, Lloyd KO, Lewis JL Jr. Binding parameters of monoclonal antibodies reacting with ovarian carcinoma ascites cells. *Cancer Immunol Immunother* 1989;28:199–207.

209. Mattes MJ, Look K, Furukawa K, et al. Mouse monoclonal antibodies to human epithelial differentiation antigens expressed on the surface of ovarian carcinoma ascites cells. *Cancer Res* 1987;47:6741–6750.

210. Rubin SC, Kostakoglu L, Divgi C, et al. Biodistribution and intraoperative evaluation of radiolabeled monoclonal antibody MX35 in patients with epithelial ovarian cancer. *Gynecol Oncol* 1993;51:61–66.

211. Welshinger M, Yin BW, Lloyd KO: Initial immunochemical characterization of MX35 ovarian cancer antigen. *Gynecol Oncol* 1997;67: 188–192.

212. Finstad CL, Lloyd KO, Federici MG, et al. Distribution of radiolabeled monoclonal antibody MX35 F(ab′)2 in tissue samples by storage phosphor screen image analysis: evaluation of antibody localization to micrometastatic disease in epithelial ovarian cancer. *Clin Cancer Res* 1997;3:1433–1442.

213. Cobleigh MS, Vogel CL, Tripathy D, et al. Multinational study of the efficacy and safety of humanized anti-HER-2 monoclonal antibody in women who have HER-2 over-expressing metastatic breast cancer that has progressed after chemotherapy for metastatic disease. *J Clin Oncol* 1999;17:2639–2648.

214. Slamon DJ, Godephin W, Jones LA, et al. Studies of the HER-2/neu proto-oncogene in human breast and ovarian cancer. *Science* 1989; 244:707–712.

215. Hogdall EV, Christensen L, Kjaer SK, et al. Distribution of HER-2 overexpression in ovarian carcinoma tissue and its prognostic value in patients with ovarian carcinoma: from the Danish MALOVA Ovarian Cancer Study. *Cancer* 2003;98:66–73.

216. Bookman M, Darcy K, Clarke-Pearson D, et al. Evaluation of monoclonal humanized anti–HER-2 antibody, trastuzumab, in patients with recurrent or refractory ovarian or primary peritoneal cancer with over expression of HER-2: a phase II trial of the Gynecologic Oncology Group. *J Clin Oncol* 2003;21:283–290.

217. Santin AD, Bellone S, Gokden M, et al. Overexpression of HER-2/neu in uterine serous papillary cancer. *Clin Cancer Res* 2002;8: 1271–1279.

218. Hurwitz H, Fehrenbacher L, Cartwright T, et al. Bevacizumab (a monoclonal antibody to vascular endothelial growth factor) prolongs survival in first-line colorectal cancer (CRC): results of a phase III trial of bevacizumab in combination with bolus IFL (irinotecan, 5-fluorouracil, leucovorin) as first-line therapy in subjects with metastatic CRC. Chicago: American Society of Clinical Oncology, 2003 (abst 3646).

219. Liao SY, Brewer C, Zavada J, et al. Identification of the MN antigen as a diagnostic biomarker of cervical intraepithelial squamous and glandular neoplasia and cervical carcinomas. *Am J Pathol* 1994;145: 598–609.

220. Pastorek J, Pastorekova S, Callebaut I, et al. Cloning and characterization of MN, a human tumor-associated protein with a domain homologous to carbonic anhydrase and a putative helix-loop-helix DNA binding segment. *Oncogene* 1994;9:2877–2888.

221. Zavada J, Zavadova Z, Pastorekova S, et al. Expression of MaTu-MN protein in human tumor cultures and in clinical specimens. *Int J Cancer* 1993;54:268–274.

222. Ivanov S, Liao SY, Ivanova A, et al. Expression of hypoxia-inducible cell-surface transmembrane carbonic anhydrases in human cancer. *Am J Pathol* 2001;158:905–919.

223. Loncaster JA, Harris AL, Davidson SE, et al. Carbonic anhydrase (CA IX) expression, a potential new intrinsic marker of hypoxia: correlations with tumor oxygen measurements and prognosis in locally advanced carcinoma of the cervix. *Cancer Res* 2001;61:6394–6399.

224. Kim S-K, Ragupathi G, Cappello S, et al. Effect of immunological adjuvant combinations on the antibody and T-cell response to vaccination with MUC-1-KLH and GD3-KLH conjugates. *Vaccine* 2000;19: 530–537.

225. Kim S-K, Ragupathi G, Musselli C, Livingston PO. Comparison of the effect of different immunological adjuvants on the antibody and T cell response to immunization with MUC1-KLH and GD3-KLH conjugate vaccines. *Vaccine* 1999;18:597–603.

226. Livingston PO, Adluri S, Raychaudhuri S, et al. A Phase I trial of the immunological adjuvant SAF-m in melanoma patients vaccinated with the anti-idiotype antibody MELIMMUNE-1. *Vaccine Res* 1994; 3:71–81.

227. Livingston PO, Adluri S, Helling F, et al. Phase I trial of immunological adjuvant QS-21 with a GM2 ganglioside-KLH conjugate vaccine in patients with malignant melanoma. *Vaccine* 1994;12:1275–1280.

228. Livingston PO, Adluri S, Zhang S, et al. Impact of immunological adjuvants and administration route on HAMA response after immunization with murine monoclonal antibody MELIMMUNE-1 in melanoma patients. *Vaccine Res* 1995;4:87–94.

229. Chapman PB, Livingston PO, Morrison ME, et al. Immunization of melanoma patients with anti-idiotypic monoclonal antibody BEC2 (which mimics GD3 ganglioside): pilot trials using no immunological adjuvant. *Vaccine Res* 1994;3:59.

230. Ritter G, Boosfeld E, Calves MJ, et al. Antibody response after immunization with gangliosides GD3, GD3 lactones, GD3 amide and GD3 gangliosidol in the mouse. GD3 lactone I induces antibodies reactive with human melanoma. *Immunobiology* 1990;182:32–43.

231. Ritter G, Boosfeld E, Adluri R, et al. Antibody response to immunization with ganglioside GD3 and GD3 congeners (lactones, amide and gangliosidol) in patients with malignant melanoma. *Int J. Cancer* 1991;48:379–385.

232. Ritter G, Ritter-Boosfeld E, Adluri R, et al. Analysis of the antibody response to immunization with purified O-acetyl GD3 gangliosides in patients with malignant melanoma. *Int J Cancer* 1995;62:1–5.

233. Helling F, Shang A, Calves M, et al. GD3 vaccines for melanoma: superior immunogenicity of keyhole limpet hemocyanin conjugate vaccines. *Cancer Res* 1994;54:197–203.

234. Kensil CR, Patel U, Lennick M, Marciani D. Separation and characterization of saponins with adjuvant activity from *Quillaja saponaria molina* cortex. *J Immunol* 1982;12:91–96.

235. Marciani DJ, Press JB, Reynolds RC, et al. Development of semisynthetic triterpenoid saponin derivatives with immune stimulating activity. *Vaccine* 2000;18:3141–3151.

236. Ragupathi G, Park TK, Zhang S, et al. Immunization of mice with the synthetic hexasaccharide Globo H results in antibodies against human cancer cells. *Angewandte Chem Int Engl* 1997;125–128.

237. Zhang S, Walberg LA, Helling F, et al. Augmenting the immunogenicity of synthetic MUC-1 vaccines in mice. *Cancer Res* 1996;55: 3364–3368.

238. Livingston PO: Approaches to augmenting the immunogenicity of melanoma gangliosides: from whole melanoma cells to ganglioside-KLH conjugate vaccines. *Immunol Rev* 1995;145:147–166.

239. Chapman PB, Morissey DM, Pangeas KS, et al. Induction of antibodies against GM2 ganglioside by immunizing melanoma patients using GM2-keyhole limpet hemocyanin + QS21 vaccine: a dose response study. *Clin Cancer Res* 2000;6:874–879.

240. Helling F, Zhang A, Shang A, et al. GM2-KLH conjugate vaccine: increased immunogenicity in melanoma patients after administration

with immunological adjuvant QS-21. *Cancer Res* 1995;55: 2783–2788.

241. Kirkwood JM, Strawderman MH, Ernstoff MS, et al. Interferon alfa-2b adjuvant therapy of high-risk resected cutaneous melanoma: the Eastern Co-operative Oncology Group trial EST 1684. *J Clin Oncol* 1996;14:7–17.

242. Kirkwood JM, Ibrahim JG, Sosman JA, et al. High-dose interferon alfa-2b significantly prolongs relapse-free and overall survival compared with the GM2-KLH/QS-21 vaccine in patients with resected stage IIB-III melanoma: Results of Intergroup Trial E1694/S9512/C509801. *J Clin Oncol* 2001;19:2370–2380.

242a. Markman M, Markman JR, Zanotti KM, et al. Duration of response to second-line platinum-based chemotherapy for ovarian cancer: implications for patient management and clinical trial design. *Proc Am Soc Clin Oncol* 2003;22:447 (abstract 1795).

243. Foon KA, Bhattacharya-Chatterjee M. Are solid tumor anti-idiotype vaccines ready for prime time? Commentary re: Wagner U, et al. Immunological consolidation of ovarian carcinoma recurrences with monoclonal anti-idiotype antibody ACA-125: immune responses and survival in palliative treatment. *Clin Cancer Res* 2001;7:1154–1162. *Clin Cancer Res* 2001;7:1112–1115.

244. Lindemann J. Speculations on idiotypes of homobodies. *Ann Immunol* 1973;124:171–184.

245. Jerne NK. Towards a network theory of the immune system. *Ann Immunol* 1974;125:373–389.

246. Birebent B, Somasundaram R, Purev E, et al. Anti-idiotypic antibody and recombinant antigen vaccines in colorectal cancer patients. *Crit Rev Oncol Hematol* 2001;9:107–113.

247. Herlyn D, Harris D, Zaloudik J, et al. Immunomodulatory activity of monoclonal anti-idiotypic antibody to anti-colorectal carcinoma antibody CO17-1A in animals and patients. *J Immunother Emphasis Tumor Immunol* 1994;15:303–311.

248. Saleh MN, Lalisan DY, Pride MW, et al. Immunologic response to the dual murine anti-Id vaccine Melimmune-1 and Melimmune-2 in patients with high risk melanoma without evidence of systemic disease. *J Immunother* 1998;21:379–388.

249. Wang X, Luo W, Foon KA, et al. Tumor associated antigen (TAA) mimicry and immunotherapy of malignant diseases from anti-idiotypic antibodies to peptide mimics. *Cancer Chemother Biol Response Modif* 2001;19:309–326.

250. Baral R, Sherrat A, Das R, et al. Murine monoclonal anti-idiotypic antibody as a surrogate antigen for human Her-2/neu. *Int J Cancer* 2001;92:88–95.

251. Safa MM, Foon KA. Adjuvant immunotherapy for melanoma and colorectal cancers. *Semin Oncol* 2001;28:68–92.

252. Foon KA, John WJ, Chakraborty M, et al. Clinical and immune responses in resected colon cancer patients treated with anti-idiotype monoclonal antibody vaccine that mimics the carcinoembryonic antigen. *J Clin Oncol* 1999;17:2889–2895.

253. Grant SC, Kris MG, Houghton AN, et al. Long survival of patients with small cell lung cancer after adjuvant treatment with the anti-idiotypic antibody BEC2 plus bacillus Calmette-Guerin. *Clin Cancer Res* 1999;5:1319–1323.

254. Wagner U, Kohler S, Reinartz S, et al. Immunological consolidation of ovarian carcinoma recurrences with monoclonal anti-idiotype antibody ACA-125: immune responses and survival in palliative treatment. See The biology behind: Foon KA, Bhattacharya-Chatterjee M. Are solid tumor anti-idiotype vaccines ready for prime time? *Clin Cancer Res* 2001;7:1112–1115. *Clin Cancer Res* 2001;7:1154–1162.

255. Reinartz S, Hombach A, Kohler S, et al. Interleukin-6 fused to an anti-idiotype Antibody in a vaccine increases the specific humoral immune response against CA125(+) (MUC-16) ovarian cancer. *Cancer Res* 2003;63:3234–3240.

256. Zhang L, Conejo-Garcia JR, Katsaros D, et al. Intratumoral T cells, recurrence, and survival in epithelial ovarian cancer. *N Engl J Med* 2003;348:203–213.

CHAPTER 7

Development and Identification of Tumor Markers

Karina Reynolds, Usha Menon, and Ian Jacobs

The term *tumor marker* is generally used to refer to biological substances that are produced by malignant tumors and enter the circulation in detectable amounts. The most useful biochemical markers in the management of cancer are the macromolecular tumor antigens, which include enzymes, hormones, receptors, growth factors, biological response modifiers, and glycoconjugates. As the human genome project has now reached the end of its first phase, functional and structural genomics projects have begun. The concept of one gene–one protein no longer holds and, consequently, the study of the human "proteome" is also gaining momentum (see section on proteomics below). Evidence is rapidly accumulating to show that global nondirected screening strategies at the DNA, RNA and protein levels can produce novel tumor markers to complement those previously identified by candidate gene or antibody-based approaches.

An ideal tumor marker would have 100% sensitivity, specificity, and positive predictive value. Table 7.1 gives an overview of the calculation of each of these attributes. *Sensitivity* refers to the percentage of patients with tumor who are correctly identified as a result of a positive test, whereas *specificity* refers to the percentage of the population without tumor who are correctly identified as a result of a negative test. *Positive predictive value* (PPV) refers to the percentage of patients with a positive test that have tumor (true positives). An ideal tumor marker for screening, diagnosis, monitoring therapeutic response and detecting recurrence would be tumor specific, and produced in sufficient amounts to allow detection of minimal disease and quantitatively reflect tumor burden. Few, if any, markers fulfill all of these criteria. The most frequent limitation is lack of spec-

ificity, as the vast majority of markers are tumor associated rather than tumor specific and are elevated in multiple cancers, in some benign and physiological conditions, and in the fetal circulation. This restricts their use, with a few exceptions, to monitoring therapeutic response and follow-up. The focus of this chapter is limited to markers that are clinically relevant to female genital tract malignancies.

OVARIAN AND FALLOPIAN TUBE CANCERS

Epithelial ovarian cancers represent the majority of ovarian malignancies, and numerous serum tumor markers have been investigated in the context of screening, prognosis, monitoring of response, and recurrence. The best known among them is CA-125.

CA-125

CA-125 is an antigenic determinant on a high molecular weight glycoprotein recognized by the murine monoclonal antibody OC-125 (1). It carries two major antigenic domains classified as A, the domain binding monoclonal antibody

TABLE 7.1. *Parameters of tumor marker assays*

Tumor marker result	True tumor status	
	Positive	Negative
Positive	a (True positives)	b (False positives)
Negative	c (False negatives)	d (True negatives)

Sensitivity = true positives/all with tumor = a/a + c
Specificity = true negatives/all tumor free = d/d +b
Positive predictive value (PPV) = true positives/all with positive tumor marker results = a /a + b

St. Bartholomew's and The Royal London Queen Mary School of Medicine, Gynaecological Cancer Research Unit, London, United Kingdom EC1M 6GR

OC-125, and B, the domain binding monoclonal antibody M11 (2). CA-125 is expressed by amniotic and coelomic epithelium during fetal development. In the adult, it is found in structures derived from coelomic epithelium (the mesothelial cells of the pleura, pericardium, and peritoneum) and in tubal, endometrial, and endocervical epithelium. Curiously, the surface epithelium of normal fetal and adult ovaries do not express the determinant except in inclusion cysts, areas of metaplasia, and papillary excrescences (3).

Serum CA-125 was originally quantified using a homologous assay based on the monoclonal antibody OC-125 alone. This has been replaced by a heterologous assay using OC-125 as the capture antibody and M11 as the detection antibody. There are a number of CA-125 assays now available, most of which correlate well with each other and are clinically reliable (4). A serum value of 35 U/mL, representing 1% of healthy female donors, is often accepted as the upper limit of normal in clinical practice (5). It should be noted that this is an arbitrary cut-off that may not be ideal for all applications of CA-125. For example, in postmenopausal women or in patients after hysterectomy, CA-125 levels tend to be lower than in the general population and lower cut-offs may be more appropriate; 20 and 26 U/mL have been suggested (6–8). Overall, approximately 85% of patients with epithelial ovarian cancer have CA-125 levels >35 U/mL (5,9). Elevated levels >35 U/mL are found in 50% of patients with stage I disease but raised levels are found in >90% of the women with more advanced stages (10). CA-125 is less often elevated in mucinous, clear-cell, and borderline tumors than in serous tumors (10–12). Elevation of serum CA-125 may also be associated with other malignancies (pancreatic, breast, colon, lung) and benign and physiological states, including pregnancy, endometriosis and menstruation (10). Many of these nonmalignant conditions are not found in postmenopausal women, thereby improving the diagnostic accuracy of an elevated level in this population.

Screening

The role of CA-125 in screening for early-stage ovarian cancer continues to be investigated. Like ultrasound, CA-125 lacks sufficient specificity to be a suitable screening test when used in isolation (13). However, there is good evidence that a multimodal strategy combining CA-125 with pelvic ultrasound in postmenopausal women can achieve high specificity (99.9%), positive predictive value (PPV 26.8%), and sensitivity (78.6%) (14). In addition, CA-125 elevation in apparently healthy postmenopausal women has been shown to be a powerful predictor of increased risk of ovarian cancer, especially when associated with abnormal ovarian morphology on ultrasound (15,16). Improvements to the sensitivity of CA-125 in screening have been achieved by the development of a statistical algorithm that incorporates the behavior of CA-125 with time in women with ovarian cancer and in normal controls (risk of ovarian cancer, ROC) (17,18). This together with refined interpretation of pelvic ultrasound in women with elevated CA-125 levels has also increased the specificity of the multimodal strategy (19). Skates et al. recently reported on a study conducted to assess the screening performance of the ROC calculation based on serial CA-125 levels from prospectively collected serum samples compared with a fixed CA-125 cutoff (20). The calculation was applied to data from a prospective trial of screening for ovarian cancer involving 22,000 postmenopausal women older than 45 years. They reported that the risk calculation significantly improved the area under the curve from 84% to 93% compared with a fixed cut-off for CA-125 ($p = .01$). For a target specificity of 98%, the risk achieved a sensitivity of 86% for preclinical detection of ovarian cancer, whereas CA-125 achieved a sensitivity of 62%. These results provide the first evidence that preclinical detection of ovarian cancer using serial CA-125 levels interpreted with the ROC calculation significantly improves screening performance compared with a fixed cut-off for CA-125.

With regard to specificity, it is of interest that Sjövall et al. (21), reporting on the cause of death among 5,550 women screened for ovarian cancer who did not have primary ovarian cancer but did have elevated CA-125 values, found that the difference between the incidence of malignant disease in women with elevated values and women with normal values was significant ($p = .02$). Furthermore, breast cancer and lung cancer were overrepresented among women with elevated CA-125 values ($p = .015$ and $<.001$, respectively). However, Jeyarajah et al. had reported in 1999 that elevated CA-125 in asymptomatic postmenopausal women is not a predictor of nongynecologic cancer or recurrence of cancer, and recommended that further investigation should be limited to the detection of gynecologic cancers (22). Their subjects consisted of a study group of 771 women with elevated CA-125 (> or =30 U/mL) and a control group of 771 women with CA-125 <30 U/mL that were selected from a prospective ovarian carcinoma screening trial of 22,000 postmenopausal women followed for a mean of 2,269 days. Nonetheless, this group did report that serum CA-125 elevation was associated with a significantly increased risk of death from all causes in the next 5 years (23). Although there is a discrepancy in findings from these two groups, they do agree that elevated CA-125 is a risk factor for death from malignant disease. These findings may have implications for asymptomatic postmenopausal women with CA-125 elevation.

Results of the first randomized trial to assess multimodal screening for ovarian cancer with sequential CA-125 antigen and ultrasonography were published in 1999 (24). In this pilot trial, postmenopausal women aged 45 years or older were randomized to a control group (n = 10,977) or screened group (n = 10,958). Women randomized to screening were offered three annual screens that involved measurement of serum CA-125, pelvic ultrasonography if CA-125 was 30 U/mL or more, and referral for gynecologic opinion if ovarian volume was 8.8 mL or more on ultrasonography. All women were followed up to see whether they developed invasive epithelial cancers of the ovary or fallopian tube (index cancers). Of 468 women in the screened group with a raised CA-125, 29 were referred for a gynecologic opinion; screening detected an index cancer in 6 and 23 had false-positive screening results. The positive predictive value was 20.7%. During 7-year follow-up, 10 further women with index cancers were identified in the screened group and 20 in the control group. Median survival of women with index cancers in the screened group was 72.9 months and in the control group was 41.8 months ($p = 0.0112$). The number of deaths from an index cancer did not differ significantly between the control and screened groups [18 of 10,977 vs 9 of 10,958; relative risk 2 (95% CI 0.78 to 5.13)]. These results show that a multimodal approach to ovarian cancer screening in a randomized trial is feasible and justify a larger randomized trial to see whether screening affects mortality.

There are currently two large randomized control trials of ovarian cancer screening in postmenopausal women in progress which incorporate CA-125 measurement. The study coordinated at St. Bartholomew's Hospital, London, aims to recruit 200,000 postmenopausal women (25), whereas the National Institutes of Health's (NIH) PLCO study in the United States will recruit 74,000 women (25a). These studies are designed to assess the impact of early intervention on ovarian cancer mortality in the general population.

Women with strong evidence of a hereditary predisposition to ovarian cancer are frequently offered screening using serum CA-125 and ultrasound. The benefit of screening is uncertain and it can be problematic among premenopausal women who have high false-positive rates for CA-125 and ultrasound. In two screening programs involving 983 women with a family history of ovarian cancer, CA-125 was elevated ($\geq$ 35 U/mL) in 11% of cases. No cases of invasive ovarian cancer were detected (26,27). Bourne et al. (28) retrospectively measured CA-125 levels in 1502 self-referred, asymptomatic women with a family history of ovarian cancer who had undergone ultrasound screening. The use of a threshold value for serum CA-125 $\geq$20 U/mL would have resulted in a 25% referral rate for ultrasonography and five of seven cancers (71%) would have been detected. In an initial report on a prospective screening study of 180 high-risk women (mean age 43.4 years) transvaginal ultrasound detected 7 of 9 ovarian cancers, whereas CA-125 was elevated ($\geq$ U/mL) in 4 of 9 cancers (29) . Women in the high-risk population who request screening should be counseled about the current lack of evidence for the efficacy of both CA-125 and ultrasound screening and the associated risk of false-positive results. Multifocal peritoneal serous papillary carcinoma may be a phenotypic variant of familial ovarian cancer, and screening strategies using ultrasonography and CA-125 testing are not reliable in detecting early disease

(30). Many will still opt for screening despite understanding the risks and limitations (31).

Differential Diagnosis of an Adnexal Mass

Serum CA-125 is of value in the differential diagnosis of benign and malignant adnexal masses, particularly in post-menopausal women (Table 7.2) . Einhorn et al. (32) measured CA-125 preoperatively in 100 women undergoing diagnostic laparotomy for palpable adnexal masses, 23 of whom were subsequently found to have a malignancy. Using an upper limit of 35 U/mL, serum CA-125 measurements had a sensitivity for malignant disease of 78%, a specificity of 95%, and a PPV of 82%. Numerous studies have since shown that in women with a pelvic mass, determination of CA-125 in addition to clinical examination and ultrasonography improves the sensitivity and specificity for ovarian cancer (33–35). Soper et al. (36) found that CA-125 >65 U/mL and elevations of either TAG-72 or CA-15-3 distinguished ovarian epithelial carcinomas from benign masses with a sensitivity of 73% and a specificity of 98%, which improved to 81% and 100%, respectively, among patients over 50 years of age. In the latter group of patients, Gadducci et al. (37), using multiple tumor markers [CA-125, CA-19-9, CA-15-3, CA-72-4, and tumor-associated trypsin inhibitor (TATI)], found the combination of serum CA-125 and CA-19-9 to have a significantly higher sensitivity (93.2% vs 81.1%) and a lower specificity (78.9% vs 86.0%) than CA-125 alone in the differential diagnosis of ovarian masses. More recently, the predictive value of the well-established tumor marker CA-125 with the newer tumor markers tetranectin (TN), OVX1, and cancer-associated serum antigen (CASA) in distinguishing benign and malignant pelvic masses in women was assessed: In comparison to the performance of CA-125, the additional discriminative value of TN and CASA was minor (38) . No significant correlations were found for OVX1; possibly because of the method used for collection and handling of serum samples. However, analyzing a panel of four selected tumor markers (CA-125 II, CA-72-4, CA-15-3, and lipid-associated sialic acid) collectively using an artificial neural network (ANN) approach to differentiate malignant from benign pelvic masses, the ANN classifier demonstrated a much improved specificity over

TABLE 7.2. *Sensitivity and specificity of CA-125 for detection of ovarian cancer in the presence of an adnexal mass*

Indicator	CA-125 reference value (U/mL)		
	>30	>35	>65
Sensitivity	81	78	56.5–72
Specificity	75	82–95	99–92.5
Positive predictive value	58	82	93

Source: Refs. 10, 32, and 34.

that of the assay CA-125 II alone (87.5% vs 68.4%) while maintaining a statistically comparable sensitivity (79.0% vs 82.4%) (39).

Jacobs et al. (40) combined serum CA-125 values with ultrasound scan results and menopausal status to calculate a risk of malignancy index (RMI). This approach achieved a sensitivity of 85% and specificity of 97%. Patients with an elevated RMI score had, on average, 42 times the background risk of cancer (40). The RMI was found to be superior to a panel of serum CA-125, CA-15-3, and TAG-72-3 for preoperative differential diagnosis of a pelvic mass (41). RMI has subsequently been validated prospectively and retrospectively in both specialized and nonspecialized gynecologic departments (42–48). Tingulstad et al. (42) performed a prospective validation in 173 women, 30 years of age or older, admitted for primary laparotomy of a pelvic mass. A sensitivity of 71%, specificity of 96%, and PPV of 89% was achieved. For stages II, III, and IV of ovarian cancer, the sensitivity increased to approximately 90% without any substantial loss in specificity. More recently, 447 patients with a pelvic mass were consecutively evaluated using RMI (43). The sensitivity was 70.6%, specificity 89.3%, PPV 66.1%, and NPV 91.1% for the study group as a whole. For patients undergoing surgery the sensitivity was 70.6%, specificity 87.7%, PPV 66.1%, and NPV 89.8%. The investigators concluded that although the method has significant limitations in borderline ovarian tumors, stage I invasive cancers, and nonepithelial tumors, RMI is a simple, easily applicable method in the primary evaluation of patients with adnexal masses. Using an RMI cut-off level of 200 to indicate malignancy, Ma et al. reported (45) that the RMI derived from a study group of 140 women with pelvic masses gave a sensitivity of 87.3%, a specificity of 84.4%, and a PPV of 82.1%. Artificial neural networks and alternative weightings in calculating the RMI have also been used to improve its performance of as a test for discriminating benign and malignant ovarian masses. These methods for differential diagnosis provide a rational basis for the selection of patients for referral to specialized gynecologic oncology centers (46–50).

Prognosis

In ovarian malignancy, preoperative serum CA-125 levels are related to tumor stage, tumor load, and histologic grade but initial studies did not find preoperative CA-125 to be an independent prognostic factor (51–54). Two more recent studies have questioned this view. Parker et al. (55), following a retrospective analysis of 114 consecutive patients with epithelial ovarian cancer, concluded that high serum CA-125 levels and low serum albumin levels at diagnosis can be used to identify poor prognostic subgroups independent of stage. In another retrospective multivariate analysis involving 201 patients with International Federation of Gynecology and Obstetrics (FIGO) stage I invasive epithelial ovarian cancer, Nagele et al. (56) identified preoperative

CA-125 ($\geq$65 U/mL) as the most powerful prognostic factor for survival, with the risk of dying of disease being sixfold higher in patients with CA-125 elevation.

Postoperative CA-125 levels and measurements taken during chemotherapy have been found to be significant prognostic indicators. It is, however, important to note that in the immediate postoperative period, CA-125 levels can be elevated as a result of abdominal surgery (57), and therefore measurements should be postponed for at least 4 weeks. Postoperative CA-125 levels >35 U/mL in women with no residual disease and >65 U/mL in those with residual disease were found to be independent prognostic factors in 687 patients with invasive epithelial ovarian cancer (52). A CA-125 prognostic score composed of two CA-125 values, one determined preoperatively and the other 1 month after surgery has been described by Rosen et al. (58). Patients with a lower score had significantly better prognosis in comparison to those with high scores.

During primary chemotherapy, serum CA-125 half-life is an independent prognostic factor both for the achievement of complete remission and for survival in patients with advanced epithelial ovarian cancer (59–61). The most commonly used cut-off is a CA-125 half-life of 20 days (61–63). Serum CA-125 levels, prior to the third course of chemotherapy (59,64,65), and the slope of the CA-125 exponential regression curve are other useful prognostic indicators of survival in patients with CA-125–positive tumors. Serum CA-125 continues to be of prognostic significance when disease recurs. Patients with normal serum CA-125 levels ($\leq$35 U/mL) at relapse have a better prognosis than those with elevated values (67).

Monitoring Response to Treatment

Serum CA-125 levels reflect progression or regression of disease in >90% of patients with ovarian cancer who have elevated preoperative levels (5,68) (Fig. 7.1). This has resulted in wide application of CA-125 measurements in monitoring clinical course and response to chemotherapy in women with epithelial ovarian cancer (69). Several studies have found an elevated CA-125 level prior to second-look laparotomy to be a good indicator of persistent disease. However, the overall accuracy is limited to 62% to 88% as values <35 U/mL do not exclude active disease (10,70). In patients with advanced-stage epithelial ovarian cancer, 92% of 13 patients with serum CA-125 of 20 to 35 U/mL and 49% of 82 patients with serum CA-125 values <20 U/mL had residual tumor at second-look laparotomy (71). The decrease in the use of second-look laparotomy over the past few years to determine response is largely due to the lack of the impact of this procedure on survival rather than the growing use of less invasive scanning techniques or CA-125 assay to determine disease status (72). Absolute values of CA-125 should not be used as the sole criterion to determine clinical response and evaluate chemotherapeutic efficacy (73).

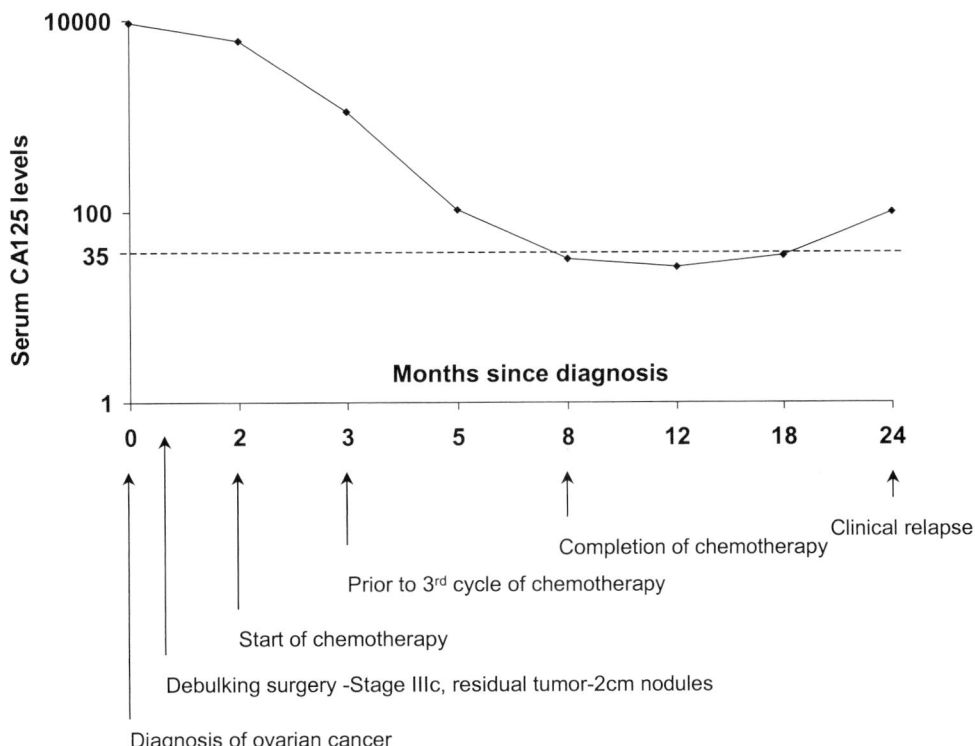

FIG. 7-1. Correlation between serum CA-125 and clinical course in ovarian cancer.

The pattern of CA-125 with time provides more useful information than an arbitrary cut-off level in the detection of residual tumor. Hawkins et al. (62) found that in patients with stage III or IV ovarian cancer, the odds of achieving complete remission during initial chemotherapy was 15% when serum CA-125 half-life was >20 days and 67% when it was <20 days. Buller et al. (74) accurately predicted therapeutic response by calculating the rate of CA-125 decline using an exponential regression model. Serum CA-125 levels prior to the third course of chemotherapy have also been used successfully to assess response (59,64). It has been suggested that women with CA-125 half-life of >20 days and an elevated level at the start of the third course of chemotherapy should be considered for a change of treatment regimen (75).

Rustin et al.(76) have described a more precise mathematical definition to evaluate response using strict CA-125 criteria based on an analysis of 277 patients in the North Thames Ovary Trial 3. Response to a specific treatment was defined as a 50% decrease in CA-125 after two samples, confirmed by a fourth sample (50% response), or a serial decrease over three samples of greater than 75% (75% response). The final sample had to be at least 28 days after the previous sample. This was subsequently validated in patients receiving first-line chemotherapy in 254 patients in the North Thames Ovary Trial 4 and the Gynaecologic Oncology Group protocol 97 (76). The definitions were also useful in

evaluating response in patients with relapsed ovarian cancer on second-line chemotherapy (77).

Detecting Recurrence

Among patients with elevated antigen levels at diagnosis, clinical detection of recurrence is often preceded by an elevation of serum CA-125. Rustin et al. (78) studied serial CA-125 levels in 255 patients undergoing first-line chemotherapy for ovarian cancer and found that a confirmed rise of serum CA-125 levels to more than twice the upper limit of normal predicted tumor relapse with a sensitivity of 84% and a false-positive rate of <2%. A median lead time prior to clinical progression of 63 to 99 days was demonstrated between marker detection of disease progression and clinically apparent progressive disease (78,79). The value of marker lead time depends ultimately on a patient's remaining therapeutic options. The influence on survival of therapeutic intervention at preclinical diagnosis of relapse remains to be tested in a randomized controlled trial. In a recent study on 78 patients with advanced ovarian cancer, CASA was reported to have similar characteristics to CA-125: In clinical situations with inconclusive or negative CA-125 serum values CASA may be useful in the identification and follow-up of such patients (80). A recent study has shown that CA-125 measurement together with thin-section CT and careful review of the clinical history is a valid alternative to exploratory laparotomy in the follow-up of ovarian carcinomas (80a).

Combination with Other Markers

TATI, CA-19-9, CA-72-4, and carcinoembryonic antigen (CEA) may be useful in addition to CA-125 in mucinous ovarian cancer (81). In patients with nonmucinous tumors, the addition of other serum markers to CA-125 sometimes improves the diagnostic sensitivity, but in general the effect is small (75,82–85). Human chorionic gonadotropin (hCG-β), macrophage colony-stimulating factor (M-CSF), and inhibin show promise of becoming useful supplements to CA-125 in ovarian cancer.

Carcinoembryonic Antigen

CEA was detected in 1965 using serum from rabbits immunized with a colon carcinoma (86). It is an oncofetal antigen found in small amounts in adult colon. Elevated levels are associated with colon and pancreatic carcinoma. Levels are also raised in benign diseases of the liver, gastrointestinal tract, and lung and in smokers. Immunohistochemistry of ovarian malignancies has revealed expression in most endometroid and Brenner tumors and in areas of intestinal differentiation in mucinous tumors. Unlike CA-125, it is not expressed in normal and inflammatory conditions of the adnexa. Serum CEA levels are elevated in 25% to 50% of women with ovarian cancer. Although there is some correlation with ovarian malignancy, this is less satisfactory than that obtained with the other described markers (87,88).

Alpha-Fetoprotein

Alpha-fetoprotein (AFP) is an oncofetal glycoprotein produced by the fetal yolk sac, liver, and upper gastrointestinal tract. Elevated levels occur in pregnancy and benign liver disease. Serum levels are raised in most patients with liver tumors and in some with gastric, pancreatic, colon and bronchogenic malignancies (87). In a study involving 135 women with germ-cell tumors, elevated levels were found in all with endodermal sinus tumors, 62% with immature teratomas and 12% with dysgerminomas (89). In women with endodermal sinus tumors and embryonal carcinomas, AFP is a reliable marker for monitoring therapeutic response and detecting recurrences (90,91). It accurately predicts the presence of yolk sac elements in mixed germ-cell tumors (92). On univariate analysis, serum AFP >1000 ng/mL together with age >22 years and histology were the major prognostic factors in a series of 43 patients with ovarian and extragonadal malignant germ-cell tumors. Although AFP production is extremely rare in ovarian epithelial cancers, a case has recently been described (93).

Human Chorionic Gonadotropin

hCG is synthesized in pregnancy by the syncytiotrophoblast. It is a glycoprotein hormone made up of two dissimilar noncovalently linked subunits termed α and β. Tumor production of hCG is accompanied by varying degrees of release of the free subunits into the circulation. Recent advances in our understanding of hCG/hCG-β beta synthesis by trophoblastic and nontrophoblastic tissues together with improved techniques for measuring hCG have helped define its role in clinical practice. In patients with gestational trophoblastic disease (hydatidiform mole, invasive mole, and choriocarcinoma), hCG is elevated in virtually all cases and serves as an ideal tumor marker. There is close correlation between hCG levels and tumor burden, and hCG levels are used in staging and clinical management. Serum hCG can also be detected in patients with nontrophoblastic cancers. Although gynecologic malignancies are prominent in this group, the sensitivity is below that of other markers in current use except in germ-cell tumors with a chorionic component (94).

A more promising approach is the measurement of hCG and its metabolic fragments in the urine. Urinary beta-core or urinary gonadotropin fragment (UGF) is a mixture of human chorionic gonadotropin, free beta-subunit, and its fragments. It has been found to be a general stage-dependent marker for gynecologic cancers. Levels were elevated in 56% to 84% of patients with ovarian cancer (95,96). In addition, Kinugasa et al. (96) found that using a combination of urinary beta-core and serum CA-125, elevated levels were present in all 45 patients with ovarian cancer in their series. Schwartz et al. (97) evaluated the marker for screening women at high risk for ovarian cancer and reported a false-positive rate of 1.5%.

Lysophosphatidic Acid

Lysophospahtidic acid (LPA) is a bioactive phospholipid with mitogenic and growth-factor–like activities that stimulates the proliferation of cancer cells. LPA has been implicated as a growth factor present in ascites of ovarian cancer patients (98): It increases cell proliferation, cell survival, resistance to cisplatin, and production of vascular endothelial growth factor in ovarian cancer cells but not in normal ovarian surface epithelial cells (99). In fact, LPA accounts for most of the ability of ascites to activate ovarian cancer cells (100). LPA levels were significantly higher in ascites from ovarian cancer patients than in malignant effusions from other cancer patients, suggesting a role for LPA-like lipids in the peritoneal spread of ovarian cancer (101). In a recent study of healthy control women, women with ovarian and other gynecologic cancers, benign gynecologic diseases, and breast cancer/leukemia, total plasma LPA levels were significantly higher in patients with ovarian cancer (mean 8.6 μmol/L; range 1.0 to 43.1 μmol/L) compared to healthy controls (mean 0.6 μmol/L; range <0.1 to 6.3 μmol/L). Elevated plasma LPA levels were detected in 9 of 10 patients with stage I ovarian cancer, all 24 patients with stage II, III, and IV ovarian cancer, and all 14 patients with recurrent ovarian cancer. In comparison, only 28 of 47 patients had elevated CA-125 levels, including 2 of 9 patients with stage I disease. LPA levels were also elevated in patients with other gynecologic cancers. Raised plasma LPA levels were detected in 5 of 48 controls and 4 of 17 patients with benign gynecologic diseases and in no women with breast cancer or leukemia (102). Using a new highly specific, sensitive, and reproducible assay, Bast and co-workers demonstrated elevated levels of LPA in more than 90% of ovarian cancer patients at stage I or II, less than 50% having elevated levels of CA-125 levels (103). Plasma LPA may represent a potential biomarker for ovarian and other gynecologic cancers (102).

Inhibin and Related Peptides

Inhibins and activins are structurally related dimeric proteins, which were first isolated from ovarian follicular fluid on the basis of their ability to modulate pituitary follicle-stimulating hormone secretion. They are members of a larger group of diverse proteins, the transforming growth factor-β superfamily, that are involved in cell growth and differentiation. Inhibin is a heterodimeric glycoprotein composed of a common α-subunit and one of two β-subunits, resulting in inhibin A ($\alpha\beta$A) and inhibin B ($\alpha\beta$B) for which specific immunoassays are now available. In addition, the serum also contains immunoreactive forms of the α-subunit that are not attached to the β-subunit, the most abundant of which is believed to be pro-αC and pro-αN-αC. These precursor forms of inhibin are measured using the pro-αC assay. The original Monash assay detected immunoreactive inhibin that included a range of inhibin-related peptides in addition to biologically active inhibin dimers.

In 1989, Lappohn et al. (104) reported serum immunoreactive inhibin concentration to be elevated in women with granulosa-cell tumors. Subsequently, numerous studies have confirmed serum inhibin elevation in ovarian sex cord/stromal tumors and established their role in the differential diagnosis and surveillance of these malignancies (105–107). Bioactive dimeric inhibins A and B are the major molecular forms detected (108,109). Antimüllerian hormone, or müllerian inhibitory factor, is another member of the transforming growth factor-β superfamily that is being investigated as a marker for granulosa-cell tumor (108,110,111).

In epithelial ovarian cancers, the role of the inhibin peptides remains to be defined. Using the initial nonspecific Monash assay, elevated serum inhibin levels were reported in 25% to 90% of women with epithelial ovarian cancers (112–114). More recently, using specific immunoassays that measure bioactive dimeric inhibin A, elevated serum levels have only been found in 5% to 31% of women with epithelial ovarian cancers (106,115,116). Mucinous ovarian cancers

are most likely to be associated with raised inhibin levels (106,115). Overall, the picture emerging is that dimeric inhibin A and B levels are not informative in epithelial ovarian cancer, and pro-αC immunoreactive forms are the most commonly elevated of the inhibin-related peptides (116,117). Furthermore, although there is preferential secretion of precursor forms of the α-subunit rather than dimeric inhibin A by epithelial ovarian cancer, pro-αC is unlikely to be a useful tumor marker when used alone (118). Combining proαC with CA-125 may increases the sensitivity for detection of epithelial ovarian cancer (116,119).

Activin is a dimer of the two β-subunits of inhibin and exists as activin A (βAβA), activin B (βBβB), and activin AB (βAβB). Serum activin A has been found to be significantly elevated in epithelial ovarian cancers (108,120,121), with highest levels being detected in undifferentiated tumors. Preliminary data suggest that there is poor correlation of activin with the clinical course of disease (108).

In conclusion, functional inhibin is secreted by most ovarian granulosa-cell tumors and may be superior to estradiol in determining therapeutic response and predicting recurrence. Dimeric inhibin A and B levels are probably not informative in epithelial ovarian cancer, but a more detailed analysis of pro-αC is needed before its exact role can be defined.

Estrogen/Androgen

Estrogen secretion is associated with granulosa cell tumors. Since the assessment of malignant potential of granulosa-cell tumors is difficult on histologic grounds, serial estradiol levels are of significant value in monitoring these patients after surgery. Androgen levels are elevated in women with Sertoli-Leydig cell tumors.

Cytokines

Cytokines are soluble mediator substances produced by cells that exercise a specific effect on other target cells. They have assumed increasing importance in tumor biology with the demonstration that many are produced by cancer cells and can influence the malignant process both positively and negatively (121). Cytokines do not fulfill the classic criteria for tumor markers. They are invariably produced by nonmalignant tissue, may be elevated in a number of pathologic conditions, are not specific for one cell type, and in the malignant scenario are often produced by the surrounding tissue in response to the tumor rather then by the tumor itself. Despite this, measurements of cytokines and their soluble receptors may provide valuable clinical information regarding prognosis and response to treatment.

Table 7.3 details some of the cytokines and their role as tumor markers in ovarian malignancy. Most are at an early stage of evaluation, and in some cases, studies have produced conflicting results. Serum M-CSF (or CSF-1) is the most important of the cytokines studied so far in the context of

TABLE 7.3. *Cytokines in ovarian cancer*

Cytokine	Description
Interleukin-6 (IL-6)	High levels of IL-6 in 50% of patients with primary ovarian cancer (202,203). Serum levels correlate with stage of disease (204). IL-6 sensitivity lower than that of CA-125, and the combination of both assays did not increase the sensitivity of CA-125 alone (203). Conflicting reports on the role of elevated IL-6 serum levels in predicting prognosis (203,205–207).
Soluble interleukin-2 receptor (SIL-2R)	Elevated in numerous malignancies and in liver, renal, and autoimmune diseases. Only patients with advanced epithelial ovarian cancer had elevated preoperative serum SIL-2Rα levels (208). Conflicting reports on the usefulness of SIL-2R as an adjunctive tool for the differential diagnosis of ovarian masses (209,210). Limited benefit for monitoring response to chemotherapy and follow-up of patients with epithelial ovarian cancer (211–213).
Tumor necrosis factor (TNF)	Raised levels documented in various malignancies and several benign conditions. Significantly higher levels in patients with epithelial ovarian cancer than in those with benign ovarian disease. No correlation of preoperative serum TNF values with common prognostic variables or the clinical outcome of patients (214).
Soluble receptors of TNF (sTNFR)	More sensitive than CA-125 in detecting primary as well as persistent or recurrent tumor and measuring response to therapy (215). Preoperative serum levels might have potential clinical relevance both for prognosis and for monitoring disease (214).
Macrophage colony-stimulating factor (M-CSF)	Levels significantly elevated in 61%–64% of patients with ovarian cancer compared to 6%–7% of patients with benign ovarian tumors. Elevation related to stage of disease and independent of histologic type (123,124). Serum M-CSF but not CA-125 significantly associated with outcome following adjustment for stage, grade, and degree of surgical clearance (53). May have a role in ovarian cancer screening (123,126).

ovarian cancer. It appears to be a marker with high specificity for ovarian malignancy with elevation being related to stage and independent of histologic type (122,123). Elevated serum levels were associated with poor outcome following adjustment for stage, grade, and degree of surgical clearance (53). In patients with advanced disease, low M-CSF levels in ascitic fluid were associated with longer overall survival and were better predictors of survival than any other prognostic factor except zero residual disease (124). Serum M-CSF was not useful in the follow up of women with advanced ovarian cancer (125), although it may have a role in ovarian cancer screening (122,126). Recent results have indicated that serum M-CSF may be highly sensitive and specific for malignant germ-cell tumors of the ovary, especially dysgerminoma (127).

Cytokeratins

Cytokeratins are intermediate filaments that are part of the cytoskeleton of all epithelial cells. They are specific markers of epithelial differentiation, and interestingly, they continue to be expressed by epithelial cells after malignant transformation. In contrast to cytokeratins themselves, fragments of cytokeratins are soluble in the serum and can therefore be detected and measured with the aid of monoclonal antibodies. They are currently being studied as tumor markers in various malignancies.

Tissue Polypeptide-Specific Antigen

Tissue polypeptide-specific antigen (TPS) is a proliferation marker closely related to the tumor marker TPA. It is recognized by a monoclonal antibody raised against the M3 epitope on cytokeratin 18. It is elevated in 50% to 77% of ovarian cancers studied with a specificity of 84% to 85% (128–131). Its measurement did not add to the diagnostic value of serum CA-125 (129). And there was no correlation between marker levels and survival. However serial measurement was useful in the follow-up of patients (128,129), with improved detection of recurrent disease when TPS was combined with CA-125 (130,131).

CYFRA 21-1

CYFRA 21-1 is a soluble serum fragment of cytokeratin 19. In a retrospective study, Hasholzner et al. (132) measured CYFRA 21-1 along with other tumor markers in stored serum from 72 women with primary ovarian cancer. The sensitivity of CYFRA 21-1 (44%) was similar to that of other markers (CA-25 II 47%, CA-72-4 47%, CASA 31%). Levels were elevated in 33% of serous and 36% of mucinous cancers (132). A similar sensitivity of 41% was reported by Tempfer et al. (133), leading to the conclusion that CYFRA 21-1 may not be suitable for screening. Reports of its role in the differential diagnosis of adnexal masses are conflicting.

Inaba et al. (134) found that CYFRA 21-1 was able to discriminate significantly better between ovarian cancer and benign adnexal tumors (PPV 94%) compared to CA-125 (PPV 69%), as CYFRA 21-1 levels were only elevated in 4% of women with benign ovarian masses, whereas CA-125 was elevated in 31%. However, this was not borne out on multivariate regression analysis by Tempfer et al. (133). They suggested that preoperative serum CYFRA 21-1 could be useful as an additional prognostic factor in ovarian cancer, as elevated levels were associated with poor overall and disease-free survival.

However, in a recent study, preoperative serum CYFRA 21-1 levels were retrospectively measured in 60 patients with ovarian cancer. The controls were 59 patients with benign ovarian disease (135). CYFRA 21-1 levels were also serially measured in 90 serum samples drawn from patients with advanced ovarian cancer in follow-up after surgery and chemotherapy. Preoperative serum CYFRA 21-1 levels were higher in patients with ovarian cancer compared with controls (median and range = 2.6 and 0.1 to 51.4 ng/mL vs 0.4 and 0.0–3.6 ng/mL; $p < .0001$). Among the former, antigen values were higher in the 39 patients with advanced-stage than in the 21 patients with early (FIGO stage I-II) disease ($p < .0001$), but Cox regression analysis failed to detect a significant association between preoperative CYFRA 21-1 assay and survival. With regard to patients in follow-up with a diagnosis of advanced ovarian cancer, CYFRA 21-1 levels were higher in the 42 samples drawn from patients with clinically detectable disease compared with the 48 specimens collected from patients with no clinical evidence of disease (median and range = 1.15 and 0.3 to 40.7 ng/mL vs 0.4 and 0.1 to 9.1 ng/mL; $p < .0001$). The investigators concluded that preoperative serum CYFRA 21-1 assay appears to be predictive of response to chemotherapy but is not prognostic of survival for patients with advanced ovarian cancer. Moreover, the serial measurement of CYFRA 21-1 levels might have a potential clinical relevance for the assessment of disease status in patients followed after surgery and chemotherapy (135). There is a need for further studies before the role of CYFRA 21-1 as a tumor marker for ovarian malignancy can be defined.

Tumor-Associated Trypsin Inhibitor

In ovarian cancer patients, a 6-kD polypeptide, TATI, can occur at elevated concentrations in both urine and serum. When used as a single marker in 180 patients with epithelial ovarian cancer and 214 women with benign pelvic pathology, serum TATI had lower sensitivity (63%) and specificity (72%) than CA-125 (80% and 82%, respectively). However, it was more sensitive than CA-125 in diagnosing mucinous adenocarcinomas (64% vs 50%), and unlike CA-125, TATI levels correlated with tumor grade (136). Although CA-125 remains the single tumor marker of choice in the diagnosis of epithelial ovarian cancer, TATI may prove to be a valuable complementary marker with a higher sensitivity in cases of poorly differentiated and mucinous carcinoma (137). The marker may also have a prognostic role in advanced ovarian cancer. Elevated preoperative serum TATI levels in patients with stage III or IV ovarian cancer were associated with a 5-year cumulative survival of 8% as opposed to 45% in patients with normal preoperative values. By contrast, the preoperative CA-125 levels in these women did not predict survival. In multivariate analysis that included age, stage, histologic grade, and preoperative TATI and CA-125 levels, patients with elevated TATI levels had a twofold increased risk of death compared with patients with normal levels (54). A further analysis based on preoperative serum TATI levels and residual tumor size after surgery has confirmed the possible prognostic role of TATI in advanced epithelial ovarian cancer (138).

Gene Expression (cDNA) Arrays

Cancer development is driven by the accumulation of changes in the 40,000 or so genes that make up the human genome and over the last two decades our understanding of the human gene and "genomics" have taken off. Although straightforward techniques for studying genes have been successful, the introduction of high-density oligonucleotide cDNA microarrays technology means that it is now possible to measure many thousands of gene-specific mRNAs in a single tissue sample (139). Using this approach, Schummer et al. used an array of 21,500 unknown ovarian cDNAs, which was hybridized with labeled first-strand cDNA from ten ovarian tumors and six normal tissues (140). They reported that 134 clones were overexpressed in at least five of the ten tumors. These cDNAs were sequenced and compared to public sequence databases. One of these, the gene *HE4*, was found to be expressed primarily in some ovarian cancers, and is thus a potential marker of ovarian carcinoma. Using gene-expression profiling, Hough et al. have identified a number of genes highly differentially expressed between nontransformed ovarian epithelia and ovarian carcinomas (141). Although some of the genes identified are already known to be overexpressed in ovarian cancer, several represent novel candidates.

Prostasin

Using microarray technology on RNA pooled from ovarian cancer and normal human ovarian surface epithelial cell lines, Mok et al. identified overexpressed genes for secretory proteins as potential serum biomarkers (142). From those identified, they selected prostasin, a serine protease normally secreted by the prostate gland, for further study.

They also demonstrated prostasin's potential as a biomarker through real-time polymerase chain reaction (PCR) in cancer and normal epithelial cell lines (significantly higher in cancer cell lines) and by differential staining in cancer tissue compared with normal tissue. They then demonstrated higher levels of serum prostasin in case patients with ovarian cancer than in control subjects (64 case patients with ovarian cancer and 137 control subjects; $p < .001$) and declining levels of prostasin after surgery for ovarian cancer: in 14 of 16 case patients with both preoperative and postoperative serum samples, postoperative prostasin levels were statistically significantly lower than preoperative levels ($p = .004$).

In 37 case patients with nonmucinous ovarian cancer and in 100 control subjects for whom levels of CA-125 and prostasin were available, the combination of markers gave a sensitivity of 92% (95% CI = 78.1% to 98.3%) and a specificity of 94% (95% CI = 87.4% to 97.7%) for detecting ovarian cancer (142). In contrast, the sensitivity of CA-125 alone at the same specificity was 24/37 = 64.9% (95% CI = 47.5% to 79.8%), and the sensitivity of prostasin alone at the same specificity was 19/37 = 51.4% (95% CI = 34.4% to 68.1%).

This study demonstrates that prostasin may be a biomarker with clinical potential. Moreover, it illustrates the immense potential of the powerful new technology of cDNA microarray in identifying overexpressed genes in ovarian cancer.

Osteopontin

Osteopontin is another biomarker that has been identified by exploiting gene-expression profiling techniques. In 2002, Kim et al. reported validation studies on this upregulated gene (143) previously identified using a cDNA microarray system (142). They showed that osteopontin expression was higher in ovarian cancer cell lines than in normal ovarian epithelial cell lines ($p = .03$), and in microdissected ovarian tumor tissue samples as compared to healthy ovarian epithelial tissue ($p = .06$). They also showed that tissue samples form 61 patients with invasive ovarian cancer and 29 patients with borderline ovarian tumors expressed higher levels of osteopontin than tissue samples from 6 patients with benign tumors and ovarian tissue samples from 3 healthy patients ($p = .03$). Finally, plasma levels of osteopontin were significantly higher ($p < .001$) in 51 patients with epithelial ovarian cancer compared with those of 107 healthy controls, 46 patients with benign ovarian disease, and 47 patients with other gynecologic cancers. Although future research to assess its clinical usefulness is required, these results provide evidence of an association between ovarian cancer and levels of this potential tumor marker.

Proteomics

The "proteome" is the expressed protein complement of a genome (144,145) or of a tissue or cell type. Proteomics is the study of the protein expression of a tissue or cell type, complements genomics-based approaches, and is increasingly being used to answer biomedical questions. Although proteins are the functional products of genes, it is not always clear from the genetic code which protein will be expressed, how much, and in which form. Futhermore, posttranslational modification and the effects of environmental factors or other processes such as disease and aging cannot be anticipated from the genetic code alone.

Proteomics is the study of the expression, structure, and function of all proteins as a function of state, time, age and environment (145–147]. Although methods to separate and define proteins on two-dimensional gels were developed in the 1970s, to date only a small proportion of the 100,000 to 1,000,000 proteins that make up the human proteome have been well described. This is at least in part due to the fact that, until recently, large-scale experiments were hampered by the technical difficulties of handling large numbers of samples. However, in the new era of proteomics, the study of plasma, urine, or other secretions from patients with the disease in question, with a high throughput but without prior knowledge of the disease process itself is now possible.

Two-dimensional gel electrophoresis continues to be the cornerstone of protein separation, with the two dimensions of separation being charge and molecular mass. Advances in this basic technique now allow 1,000 to 3,000 proteins to be visualized on a single gel (148). Multiple gels can be compared with the help of specialized software packages and differences between healthy and diseased samples found by using a process of subtraction. Those proteins of interest can then be identified and characterized by using a combination of methods. Methods exploiting mass spectrometry are being increasingly used, as they require ever-smaller sample sizes and have a high throughput.

There is now a wide range of techniques available for protein identification and characterization where high sensitivity and specificity are combined with high throughput. Surface-enhanced laser desorption ionization time-of-flight (SELDI-TOF) analysis and matrix-associated laser desorption ionization time-of-flight (MALDI-TOF) technology have the potential to identify patterns or changes in thousands of small proteins (<20 kD). When combined with matrices that selectively absorb certain serum proteins, these approaches can globally analyze almost all small proteins in complex solutions, such as serum or plasma (139,149). In a preliminary study, when linked to powerful computer algorithms, SELDI-TOF could identify a pattern of protein changes in serum with 100% sensitivity with 94% specificity for both early and late ovarian cancer in a limited set of samples (150). Protein bio-informatics packages are available to allow the identification and characterization of proteins studied in this way, and many proteome projects are currently underway to continue to provide ever-increasing information of this type.

In 2002, Petricoin et al. reported (151) that, by using SELDI-TOF to analyze the proteomic spectra patterns generated from 50 women with and 50 women without ovarian cancer, all ovarian cancers were correctly classified and distinguished from all non-malignant disorders, as were all stage I cancers confined to the ovary. Although the limitations of this study design and its analysis have been discussed in some detail in the literature (152–156), the implications of this type of proteomic spectrum analysis for the identification of novel tumor markers is huge. It is likely that in the future the early detection of ovarian cancer (and other cancers) will involve high throughput proteomic profiling either alone or in combination with markers already in use today.

Other Serum Markers

Multiple serum markers have been assessed in isolation and in various combinations in women with ovarian cancer, both in the context of screening and differential diagnosis, as well as in assessing prognosis, monitoring response and detecting recurrence. It is not possible in this chapter to describe the numerous studies in detail. A summary of some of the markers and their pertinent characteristics is detailed in Table 7.4, whereas Table 7.5 details their current role in ovarian cancer. The most significant finding is that in women with ovarian cancer no single marker or combination has emerged with a clear clinical advantage over CA-125 except in specific tumor subtypes such as germ-cell tumors with yolk sac or chorionic elements and granulosa cell tumors.

ENDOMETRIAL CANCERS

There are no serum markers with an established role in the clinical management of endometrial cancer. Serum CA-125 is elevated in 10% to 27% of patients (157–159) with elevated levels detected in 63% to 67% of patients with advanced-stage endometrial cancer as against 10% to 19% of those with early-stage disease (160,161). Preoperative assessment may therefore be useful in predicting the presence of extrauterine and metastatic disease and to a lesser extent myometrial invasion (162). Patsner et al. (158) suggested that serum CA-125 may be useful in the follow-up of patients with early-stage endometrial cancer, but levels can be falsely elevated in the presence of severe radiation injury. Isolated recurrences in the vagina do not cause elevation, whereas distant metastasis may. However, a more recent study has reported that CA-125 monitoring did not add to clinical findings and imaging in the follow up of women with endometrial cancer (162a).

Among the other tumor markers, CYFRA 21-1 has been found to be elevated in 52% of endometrial malignancies (134) and urinary beta-core or UGF levels in 38% to 48% (95,96). The more important of the other serum markers have been outlined in Table 7.6.

CERVICAL CANCERS

Screening for cervical cancer uses exfoliative cytology, and currently there are no serologic markers being explored in this context. However, in assessing prognosis, monitoring response to therapy, and detecting recurrence, a variety of serum markers is being investigated. The main among them are squamous-cell carcinoma antigen (SCC), tissue polypeptide antigen (TPA), CEA, and CYFRA 21-1.

Squamous-Cell Carcinoma Antigen

In 1977, Kato and Torigoe (163) isolated the tumor antigen TA-4 from a cervical squamous-cell carcinoma. SCC is one of 14 subfractions of tumor antigen TA-4. Elevated serum levels are found in 57% to 65% of women with primary squamous-cell carcinoma of the cervix (164,165). The release of SCC into the circulation is independent of local tissue content, as high antigen concentrations are found in the cytosol of normal cervical squamous epithelia, but in these cases, serum levels are always in the normal range (166). The antigen is, however, not specific for cervical squamous cell carcinoma. Elevated serum levels are also found in other squamous-cell cancers of the head and neck, esophagus, and lung and adenocarcinoma of the uterus, ovary, and lung. SCC levels can also be raised in skin diseases such as psoriasis and eczema (167).

SCC is probably a marker of cellular differentiation of squamous cells, as the incidence of elevated serum levels is higher in women with well-differentiated (78%) and moderately differentiated carcinomas (67%) than in those with poorly differentiated tumors (38%) (166). SCC pretreatment levels correlate with stage, tumor volume, lymph node status, and blood vessel invasion (168–172). However, there are conflicting reports on the prognostic significance of pretreatment SCC measurements (165,168,169,171,173,174). Duk et al. (169) found that even in node-negative patients, the risk of recurrence was three times higher if SCC levels were elevated prior to therapy.

In serum SCC-positive patients, serial determinations correlated with the clinical course in 72% of women (175), with levels decreasing with effective therapy (176,177). Normalization of elevated levels was associated with a complete response (178), whereas elevated posttreatment serum SCC levels were a predictor of treatment failure (174,179) and associated with poor survival rates (180). In patients affected by recurrent carcinoma, a raised SCC level was found in 50% to 71% of cases, with a lead time ranging from 0 to 12 months (164,178).

Tissue Polypeptide Antigen

TPA levels were raised in about 40% to 50% of women with squamous-cell carcinoma of the cervix (165,181). Serum levels were related to stage and grade. However, on multivariate analysis, pretreatment serum TPA levels were not predictive of survival (165,173,180,182).

(Text continues on page 170)

TABLE 7.4. *Other tumor markers for ovarian carcinoma that are not referred to in detail in the text*

Tumor marker	Description
CA-15-3	Tumor-associated antigen in human milkfat globule membrane. Most used in breast carcinoma. Elevated levels in 57%–71% of ovarian cancer patients and 2%–6% of patients with benign tumors (216,217). Not useful on its own (36), but in combination with CA-125 increases the specificity of the CA-125 assay in the differential diagnosis of adnexal masses (217).
CA-72-4 or TAG-72	Defines a glycoprotein surface antigen found in colon, gastric, and ovarian cancer. Levels elevated in 67% of ovarian cancers (218) with better sensitivity than CA-125 for mucinous tumors (219). In a retrospective study of 123 patients with ovarian carcinoma, CA-125 did not add to the sensitivity of CA-72-4 for mucinous ovarian carcinomas (220). The specificity of CA-72-4 for ovarian malignancy was >95%, and combination with CA-125 increased sensitivity without substantial change in specificity (221). The addition of serum CA-72-4 to the combination of pelvic examination, ultrasound, and serum CA-125 improved discrimination between malignant and benign pelvic masses (222)
CA-19-9	Defines an antigen that is part of the Lewis blood group antigens. Elevated in gastrointestinal, lung, ovarian, and endometrial carcinoma. Most useful in pancreatic carcinoma. Mucinous ovarian tumors express the antigen more frequently (76%) than serous tumors (27%). Unlike CA-125, not affected by pregnancy (223). Together with CA-125, was the most useful marker in patients with borderline ovarian tumors (11).
CA-130	A cancer-associated antigen recognized by two monoclonal antibodies, 130-22 and 145-9. Strong correlation with CA-125 levels as the epitopes recognized by monoclonal antibodies, 130-22 and 145-9, differ from the CA-125 epitope, but exist on the molecule bearing CA-125. Elevated in 91% of women with epithelial ovarian cancer, with levels correlating with regression or progression of ovarian cancer in >95% of cases. However, normalization of serum levels during treatment do not imply no microscopic residual disease (224).
OVX1	Antigenic determinant on a high molecular weight mucin-like glycoprotein present in ovarian and breast cancer cells. Recognized by a murine monoclonal antibody OVX1 (225). Elevated serum levels (>7.2 U/mL) found in 5% of 184 normal individuals and in 70% of 93 epithelial ovarian cancer patients (226). When combined with CA-125 and M-CSF, at least one marker was elevated in 98% of patients with stage I ovarian cancer, whereas CA-125 alone was elevated in only 67%. By the same criteria, 11% of healthy individuals and 51% of patients with benign pelvic masses had at least one elevated marker (126). The serial measurement of OVX1 in combination with CA-125 improved the sensitivity, specificity, and PPV of CA-125 alone in primary screening for epithelial ovarian cancer (227). OVX1 as part of a panel of eight different markers (CA-125, M-CSF, OVX1, LASA, CA-15-3, CA-72-4, CA-19-9, CA-54/61) improved the sensitivity for discriminating malignant from benign pelvic masses (228). However, the OVX1 radioimmunoassay is highly dependent on sample handling (85).
CASA/OSA	Tumor-associated antigens assayed by dual epitope ELISAs using the same capture monoclonal antibody (BC2) and different second antibodies (OM-1 AND BC3, respectively). Elevated levels in 58% of ovarian cancers. In addition, CASA elevated in patients with breast, lung, prostate, and bladder cancer (229). Initial results indicated that the OSA and CASA assays could be superior to CA-125 for detection of small-volume occult ovarian carcinoma (230). When used to predict the results of 41 second-look laparotomies, the PPV of CASA and CA-125 were 77% and 100%, respectively. The negative predictive values for CASA and CA-125 were 71% and 66%, respectively. CASA detected 50% of positive second-look laparotomies where microscopic disease only was found; the CA-125 test did not. Multivariate analysis of survival rates found that postoperative CASA levels ranked above all prognostic factors except age. CASA levels may be more accurate than surgical reporting of residual disease or they may define a subset of patients with biologically more aggressive ovarian carcinoma (231). Could supplement predictive and prognostic values of CA-125 measurements in monitoring disease (232,233).
TPA	Initially described as a tumor marker in ovarian malignancy in 1978 but does not have an established clinical role. Although it is detected in advanced stages of ovarian cancer, sensitivity is low in early-stage disease (234). In 1988, Panza et al. reported that in a series of 81 patients with ovarian cancer, combining TPA with CA-125 was useful in evaluating therapeutic response and in early detection of recurrence (235). However, this has not been substantiated (236).
Growth factors	Insulin-like growth factors (IGFs) and IGF-binding proteins (IGFBPs) have been shown to play a physiologic role in the female genital system, including the ovarian follicular system. A recent study has suggested that alterations in serum IGFBP-2 levels may serve as a potential additional marker for ovarian cancer. IGFBP-2 levels were high in serum of epithelial ovarian cancer patients, and the increment in serum IGFBP-2 correlated positively with CA-125 (237).

(Continued)

TABLE 7.4. *Continued*

Tumor marker	Description
Tetranectin	A tetrameric, plasminogen-binding plasma protein first discovered in 1986. Blood levels reduced in patients with a variety of cancers. At a false-positive rate of 1%, the sensitivity for ovarian cancer stages I and II was 33% for serum tetranectin against 76% for CA-125. Combining tetranectin with CA-125 increased sensitivity without causing a concomitant increase in the rate of false-positive results. However, neither markers rose to levels that would allow their use in the discrimination of localized cancer and benign tumors (238). Preoperative tetranectin levels correlated with survival (239). Chemotherapy induced significant increases in serum tetranectin levels with decrease in serum tetranectin during chemotherapy highly indicative of recurrence and a poor outcome (240). Høgdall et al. (241) measured serum tetranectin, CA-125, and CASA prior to 63 second-look and 5 third-look operations for ovarian cancer. Patients with residual tumor had significantly lower levels of tetranectin and higher levels of CASA and CA-125 compared with tumor-free patients. Using multivariate Cox analyses, it was found that all three markers were independent prognostic predictors for survival.
GAT (Galactosyltransferase associated with tumor)	Elevated in 4.5%–6.0% of women with endometriosis and 46%–48% of women with ovarian cancer. GAT may be useful in discriminating ovarian malignancy from endometriosis (242,243[a]).
LASA (lipid-associated sialic acid)	The assay predominantly determines glycoprotein-bound sialic acid and has high positivity rate in leukemia, Hodgkin's disease, melanoma, sarcoma, advanced ovarian carcinoma, and oropharyngeal tumors (244). The value of determination of LASA in addition to CA-125 was limited in a study of 152 patients with invasive epithelial ovarian cancer (245). This is due to lack of specificity. False-positive levels of LASA were found in 15.5% of 84 women at high risk for ovarian cancer who participated in an early ovarian cancer-detection program at Yale University (97). When used as part of a panel of serum markers, it may be useful in women with a pelvic mass (228).
Sialyl SSEA-1 antigen	Carbohydrate antigen detected using the monoclonal antibody FH-6. Rarely detected in normal tissues and is present in adenocarcinoma and fetal tissues. Elevated in 47%–64% of ovarian malignancies. Lower sensitivity than CA-125 in detection of ovarian cancer but associated with a lower false-positive rate. However, the combined determination of sialyl SSEA-1 and CA-125 did not markedly increase the detection rate (246,247). Diagnostic accuracy for ovarian cancer of the combination assay was increased (78.5%) by increasing the cut-off for sialyl SSEA-1 to >50 U/mL (CA-125 >35 U/mL). Twenty-seven of 37 patients who were only positive for CA-125 had endometriosis (248).
VEGF (vascular endothelial growth factor)	A promoter of angiogenesis, VEGF is believed to play a pivotal role in tumor growth and metastasis. In a preliminary study, serum VEGF had a sensitivity of 54% for ovarian cancer and was not useful in the differential diagnosis of adnexal masses (249).
IAP (immunosuppressive acid protein)	Increased levels detected in 70% of patients with ovarian cancer, 25% with benign tumors, and in 4.5% of normal women. The simultaneous determination of IAP and CA-125 allowed an overall sensitivity of 84% without any significant reduction of specificity (250). On multivariate analysis, there was significant association with survival (251).
Kallikrein	The human kallikrein gene family currently consists of 15 members. In addition to prostate-specific antigen (PSA, hK3)— an established tumor marker for prostate cancer diagnosis and follow-up—and human glandular kallikrein (hK2)—an emerging prostate cancer biomarker— accumulating evidence indicates that many other members of the human kallikrein gene family are also implicated in endocrine-related malignancies. Many kallikreins are differentially regulated in breast, prostate, ovarian, and testicular cancers. In addition, preliminary reports indicate that three newly identified kallikreins (hK6, hK10, and hK11) are serum biomarkers for diagnosis and monitoring of ovarian and prostate cancer (252,253).

[a] Abstract only.

TABLE 7.5. *Role of current tumor markers in ovarian cancer*

Ovarian cancer	Screening	Differential Diagnosis	Prognostic indicator	Monitoring response to treatment	Detection of recurrence
Epithelial cancers	CA-125 General population—research trials High-risk population—annual screening with CA-125 and ultrasound widely advocated but not yet validated.	CA-125 Significant contribution, especially in postmenopausal women. As part of the risk of malignancy index, a sensitivity of 71%–85% with a specificity of 96%–97% is achieved.	CA-125 Preoperative levels—conflicting evidence. Postsurgery levels—independent prognostic indicator. Criteria used include: 1. CA-125 >50 U/L 4 weeks after surgery 2. CA-125 score using pre- and post- operative values 3. CA-125 level prior to 3rd course of chemotherapy 4. Slope of CA-125 exponential regression curve	CA-125 Reflects clinical course in >90% of positive tumors. Serial values should be used. Criteria used include: 1. Half life—20 days most commonly used cut-off. 2. Level prior to 3rd course of chemotherapy 3. Slope of CA-125 exponential regression curve 4. Strict definitions using 50% and 75% reductions from pre-operative values	CA-125 Detects recurrence with a sensitivity of 84%–94% and a false-positive rate of <2%. Median lead time compared to clinical diagnosis of recurrence is 60–99 days
	OVX1[a] M-CSF[a]	CA-72–4[a] TATI[a]	TATI[a] M-CSF[a]	TPA + CA-125[a] Soluble receptors of TNF[a]	TPA[a] Soluble receptors of TNF[a]
	CA-72-4	CYFRA 21-1[a] Inhibin pro-αC[a] SIL-2R[a]—conflicting evidence GAT[a]	IL-6[a]—conflicting evidence Inhibin[a]—high levels associated with good response IAP[a] CASA + CA-125[a] CYFRA 21-1[a]	CASA[a]	TPS[a]
Germ-cell tumors		AFP—tumors with yolk sac elements hCG—tumors with chorionic elements	AFP	AFP—tumors with yolk sac elements hCG—tumors with chorionic elements	AFP—tumors with yolk sac elements hCG—tumors with chorionic elements
Sex cord stromal tumors		Inhibin[a], estradiol in granulosa-cell tumors		Inhibin in granulosa-cell tumors[a]	Inhibin, estradiol in granulosa-cell tumors[a]

Further discussion and references are to be found in the accompanying text.
[a] Potential role. Not yet used in routine clinical practice.

CYFRA 21-1

Following detection of elevated levels of CYFRA 21-1 in patients with squamous-cell carcinoma of the lung, various groups investigated their role in cervical carcinoma. Elevated levels were detected in 14% of controls, 35% of patients with stage Ib–IIa squamous-cell carcinoma of the cervix, and 64% of patients with stage IIb–IV squamous-cell carcinoma of the cervix (183). Although CYFRA 21-1 was related to tumor stage and size in patients with cervical cancer (184) and there was a positive correlation with SCC (185, 186), it was less sensitive and specific than SCC in detecting squamous-cell cancer of the cervix (181,183,187). In cervical adenocarcinoma, it was elevated in 63% of patients (187). CYFRA 21-1 may be useful in the follow-up of women with cervical cancer, but further investigation is needed (188).

TABLE 7.6. *Other potential tumor markers in endometrial cancer that are not referred to in detail in the text*

Tumor marker	Reference	Finding
CA-15-3	254	CA-15-3, CA-125, CA-19.9, CEA, and TPA were analyzed in 97 patients with endometrial cancer. The incidence of individual elevated tumor markers was 21%–31%. Elevations of CA-125 and CA-15.3 were significantly associated with poor prognostic clinical factors. In multivariate analysis, CA-15.3 was highly significant and had a larger hazard ratio than CA-125.
	255	CA-125, SCC, CA-19-9, and CA-15-3 were evaluated in the follow-up of 105 patients with endometrial carcinoma. The tumor markers were of limited value for the prediction of recurrences.
CA-19-9	159	CA-19-9 was elevated in 24% of 225 patients with primary endometrial carcinoma. Elevated CA-125 levels were found in 27% and the combined assay detected 39%. Serum levels of both CA-125 and CA-19-9 were significantly increased with surgical staging. The combined assay demonstrated a 72% positive rate at the time of detection of recurrence in 32 patients (66% for CA-125, 44% for CA-19-9). In 34% of the 32 recurrent cases, elevated levels of the tumor markers were the first sign of recurrence. The use of CA-19-9 in combination with CA-125 may be useful in the management of endometrial carcinoma.
Amino-terminal propeptide of type III procollagen (PIIINP)	256	PIIINP is an indicator of collagen metabolism. Serum levels were increased in 35% of 148 patients with endometrial carcinoma, and elevated levels were more often seen in advanced (63%) than early disease (31%). In monitoring advanced endometrial disease, the investigators found that it is of use when combined with CA-125.
Placental protein 4 (PP4)	257	Raised levels were detected in 48% of patients with endometrial carcinoma and 18% of patients with uterine myomata,
CYFRA 21-1	134	Elevated in 52% of endometrial malignancies.
CA-72-4	258	Increased levels in 32% of 72 patients with endometrial carcinoma. Levels correlated with depth of myometrial invasion, adnexal metastasis, lymphovascular space involvement, and pelvic and paraaortic lymph node metastasis. On multivariate analysis, significant correlation with adnexal metastasis.
OVX1 antigen	259	Levels elevated in 64% of 45 patients with endometrial cancer but only in 5% of 184 healthy persons and 9% of 58 patients with endometriosis. Elevation more frequent in patients with deep myometrial invasion and poorly differentiated tumors.
Soluble interleukin-2 receptor (SIL-2R)	260	Elevated serum levels of SIL-2R, CA-125, and SCC were detected in 52%, 11%, and 14% of 35 patients with endometrial cancer, respectively, rendering SIL-2R the most sensitive antigen for endometrial cancer among the three markers studied.
Macrophage colony-stimulating factor	157	Elevated in 73% of 183 patients with endometrial adenocarcinoma. Levels correlated with clinical course of disease, and measurement of CA-125 or the aminoterminal peptide of type III procollagen levels did not further enhance accuracy.

Further discussion and references are to be found in the accompanying text.

[a] Potential role. Not yet used in routine clinical practice.

CA-125/CEA

Serum CA-125 is elevated in only 13% to 21% of women with squamous cell carcinoma (161,175). However, in cervical adenocarcinoma, it is a better tumor marker than SCC (161,175,189). The combination of CA-19-9 and CA-125 was particularly useful with a sensitivity of 60% for cervical adenocarcinoma. The addition of CEA to the combination increased sensitivity to 70% (190). When levels are elevated, serum CA-125 has been found to be an important prognostic factor and an indicator of tumor virulence (191,192). Serial measurements of CA-125 can be used in the evaluation of chemotherapeutic response, with levels falling in 83% of women with previously untreated cervical carcinoma who responded to chemotherapy (193). In progressive disease, serum CA-125, SCC, and CEA levels were found to be elevated in patients with adenosquamous tumor, whereas only CA-125 was elevated in women with adenocarcinoma (189).

CEA is less useful in cervical cancers, with an overall sensitivity of 15% and a specificity of 90%. Levels are significantly higher among patients with cervical adenocarcinoma than squamous-cell cancers (194).

Multiple markers (TPA, SCC, CEA, CA-125, CYFRA 21-1) have been investigated for predicting prognosis and detecting recurrence in patients with cervical carcinoma. In the past, none was found to be an independent prognostic factor on multivariate analysis (165,173,180,195) except for CA-125 (190,197,198). More recently, however, there have been reports that SCC may be an independent predictor of response in women undergoing neoadjuvant chemotherapy (180,196,197), and one study (199) reports that, in patients with an elevated pretreatment SCC antigen, SCC antigen normalized more frequently with combined treatment and those patients had a better disease-free survival (DFS). Furthermore, in that study, elevated SCC antigen or CYFRA 21-1 levels after treatment completion indicated residual tumor in 92% and 70%, respectively. The investigators concluded that the presence of elevated posttreatment levels of SCC antigen or CYFRA 21-1 indicates the need for additional salvage surgery. SCC antigen proved to be superior to CYFRA 21-1 in predicting DFS and disease recurrence. Nonetheless, the evidence available so far does not justify the routine measurement of serum markers.

VULVAR AND VAGINAL CANCERS

Tumors of the vulva and vagina are rare, and there are relatively few studies of circulating markers in these conditions. TPS has been shown to be elevated in 80% of patients with vulvar or vaginal cancer (128), whereas SCC levels were elevated in 43% (200). Carter et al. (201) studied urinary core fragment of the β-subunit of hCG in these cancers. The sensitivity of beta-core was only 38%, but there was a highly significant difference in the survival curve between those with elevated beta-core levels and those with normal levels. Ninety percent of patients with elevated levels died within 24 months as opposed to 32% of those with normal levels. It might also be useful in detecting recurrence as rising UGF levels at an earlier clinic visit predicted recurrence in four of seven patients (200). Although the numbers are small, until larger studies become available, the data suggest that for lower genital tract cancer, the measurement of urinary beta-core may be valuable as a prognostic indicator, allowing a more informed approach to treatment and in follow-up.

CONCLUSIONS

The potential role of serologic tumor markers is hampered by the fact that the production of most of these markers is neither confined to the malignant tumor cell nor limited to the malignant phenotype. Of all those studied, hCG in gestational trophoblastic disease remains closest to the ideal tumor marker. Overall, serum CA-125 continues to the most useful marker in the context of gynecologic malignancies, especially ovarian epithelial cancers.

In summary, serum markers are of increasing diagnostic value in the differential diagnosis of adnexal masses. Numerous tumor markers have been recognized as promising prognostic factors, and this will aid the development of novel treatment strategies in the future. Recent technologic advances in genomics and proteomics have the potential to identify new tumor markers that may be used either alone or in combination with standard markers and strategies currently being used to screen for gynecologic malignancies. The role of markers in monitoring therapeutic response and detecting recurrence has yet to be fully exploited. In screening strategies, serial CA-125 in combination with ultrasonography is undergoing evaluation in randomized control trials of screening for ovarian cancer in the general population.

REFERENCES

1. Bast RC Jr, Feeney M, Lazarus H, et al. Reactivity of a monoclonal antibody with human ovarian carcinoma. *J Clin Invest* 1981;68(5): 133.
2. Nustad K, Bast RC Jr, Brien TJ, et al. Specificity and affinity of 26 monoclonal antibodies against the CA 125 antigen: first report from the ISOBM TD-1 workshop, International Society for Oncodevelopmental Biology and Medicine. *Tumour Biol* 1996;17(4):196.
3. Kabawat SE, Bast RC Jr, Bhan AK, et al. Tissue distribution of a coelomic-epithelium–related antigen recognized by the monoclonal antibody OC125. *Int J Gynecol Pathol* 1983;2(3):275.
4. Davelaar EM, van Kamp GJ, Verstraeten RA,, et al. Comparison of seven immunoassays for the quantification of CA 125 antigen in serum. *Clin Chem* 1998;44(7):1417.
5. Bast RC Jr, Klug TL, St John E, et al. A radioimmunoassay using a monoclonal antibody to monitor the course of epithelial ovarian cancer. *N Engl J Med* 1983;309(15):883.
6. Alagoz T, Buller RE, Berman M, et al. What is a normal CA125 level? *Gynecol Oncol* 1994;53(1):93.
7. Bon GG, Kenemans P, Verstraeten R, et al. Serum tumour marker immunoassays in gynecologic oncology: establishment of reference values. *Am J Obstet Gynecol* 1996;174:107.
8. Zurawski VR Jr, Orjaseter H, Andersen A, et al. Elevated serum CA 125 levels prior to diagnosis of ovarian neoplasia: relevance for early detection of ovarian cancer. *Int J Cancer* 1988;42(5):677–680.
9. Canney PA, Moore M, Wilkinson PM,, et al. Ovarian cancer antigen CA125: a prospective clinical assessment of its role as a tumour marker. *Br J Cancer* 1984;50(6):765.
10. Jacobs I, Bast RC Jr. The CA 125 tumour-associated antigen: a review of the literature. *Hum Reprod* 1989;4(1):1.
11. Tamakoshi K, Kikkawa F, Shibata K, et al. Clinical value of CA125, CA19-9, CEA, CA72-4, and TPA in borderline ovarian tumor. *Gynecol Oncol* 1996;62(1):67.
12. Vergote IB, Bormer OP, Abeler VM. Evaluation of serum CA 125 levels in the monitoring of ovarian cancer. *Am J Obstet Gynecol* 1987; 157(1):88.
13. Bell R, Petticrew M, Luengo S, et al. Screening for ovarian cancer: a systematic review. *Health Technol Assess.* 1998;2(2):i–iv, 1–84.
14. Jacobs I, Davies AP, Bridges J, et al. Prevalence screening for ovarian cancer in postmenopausal women by CA 125 measurement and ultrasonography. *BMJ* 1993;306(6884):1030.
15. Jacobs IJ, Skates S, Davies AP, et al. Risk of diagnosis of ovarian cancer after raised serum CA 125 concentration: a prospective cohort study. *BMJ* 1996;313:1355.
16. Menon U, Talaat A, Jeyerajah AR, et al. Ultrasound assessment of ovarian cancer risk in postmenopausal women with CA125 elevation. *Br J Cancer* 1999;80(10);1644.
17. Skates SJ, Xu FJ, Yu YH, et al. Toward an optimal algorithm for ovarian cancer screening with longitudinal tumor markers. *Cancer* 1995;76[10 Suppl]:2004.
18. Skates SJ, Chang Y, Xu FJ, et al. A new statistical approach to screening for ovarian cancer. *Tumor Biol* 1996;17:45.
19. Menon U, Talaat A, Rosenthal AN, et al. Performance of ultrasound as a second line test to serum CA125 in ovarian cancer screening. *BJOG* 1999 (in press).
20. Skates SJ, Menon U, MacDonald N, et al. Calculation of the risk of ovarian cancer from serial CA-125 values for preclinical detection in postmenopausal women. *J Clin Oncol* 2003;21[(10 Suppl]:206–210.
21. Sjövall K, Nilsson B, Einhorn N. The significance of serum CA 125 elevation in malignant and nonmalignant diseases. *Gynecol Oncol* 2002;85(1):175–178.
22. Jeyarajah AR, Ind TE, Skates S, et al. Serum CA125 elevation and risk of clinical detection of cancer in asymptomatic postmenopausal women. *Cancer* 1999;85(9):2068–2072.
23. Jeyarajah AR, Ind TE, MacDonald N, et al. Increased mortality in

postmenopausal women with serum CA125 elevation. *Gynecol Oncol* 1999;73(2):242–246.

24. Jacobs IJ, Skates SJ, MacDonald N, et al. Screening for ovarian cancer: a pilot randomised controlled trial. *Lancet* 1999;353(9160): 1207–1210.

25. Jacobs, I, UK Collaborative Trial of Ovarian Cancer Screening: full proposal for MRC grant, July 14, 1999.

25a. Kramer BS, Gohagan J, Prorok PC, et al. A National Cancer Institute sponsored screening trial for prostatic, lung, colorectal, and ovarian cancers. *Cancer* 1993;71[2 Suppl]:589.

26. Karlan BY, Raffel LJ, Crvenkovic G, et al. A multidisciplinary approach to the early detection of ovarian carcinoma: rationale, protocol design, and early results. *Am J Obstet Gynecol* 1993;169(3):494.

27. Muto MG, Cramer DW, Brown DL, et al. Screening for ovarian cancer: the preliminary experience of a familial ovarian cancer center, *Gynecol Oncol* 1993;51(1):12.

28. Bourne TH, Campbell S, Reynolds K, et al. The potential role of serum CA 125 in an ultrasound-based screening program for familial ovarian cancer. *Gynecol Oncol* 1994;52(3):379.

29. Dorum A, Kristensen GB, Abeler VM, et al. Early detection of familial ovarian cancer. *Eur J Cancer* 1996;32(10):1645.

30. Karlan BY, Baldwin RL, Lopez-Luevanos E, et al. Peritoneal serous papillary carcinoma, a phenotypic variant of familial ovarian cancer: implications for ovarian cancer screening. *Am J Obstet Gynecol* 1999; 180(4):917.

31. Bell R, Petticrew M. Screening people with a family history of cancer. Benefit of screening for ovarian cancer is unproved. *BMJ* 1997;15; 315(7118):1306.

32. Einhorn N, Bast RC Jr, Knapp RC, et al. Preoperative evaluation of serum CA 125 levels in patients with primary epithelial ovarian cancer. *Obstet Gynecol* 1986;67(3):414.

33. Curtin JP. Management of the adnexal mass. *Gynecol Oncol* 1994; 55(3):S42.

34. Maggino T, Gadducci A, D'Addario V, et al. Prospective multicenter study on CA 125 in postmenopausal pelvic masses. *Gynecol Oncol* 1994;54(2):117.

35. Parker WH, Levine RL, Howard FM, et al. A multicenter study of laparoscopic management of selected cystic adnexal masses in postmenopausal women. *J Am Coll Surg* 1994;179(6):733.

36. Soper JT, Hunter VJ, Daly L, et al. Preoperative serum tumor-associated antigen levels in women with pelvic masses. *Obstet Gynecol* 1990;75(2):249.

37. Gadducci A, Ferdeghini M, Prontera C, et al. The concomitant determination of different tumor markers in patients with epithelial ovarian cancer and benign ovarian masses: relevance for differential diagnosis. *Gynecol Oncol* 1992;44(2):147.

38. Høgdall EVS, Høgdall CK, Tingulstad S, et al. Predictive values of serum tumour markers tetranectin, OVX1, CASA and CA125 in patients with a pelvic mass. *International Journal of Cancer* 2000;89(6): 519–523.

39. Zhang Z, Barnhill SD, Zhang H, et al. Combination of multiple serum markers using an artificial neural network to improve specificity in discriminating malignant from benign pelvic masses. *Gynecol Oncol* 1999;73(1):56–61.

40. Jacobs I, Oram D, Fairbanks J, et al. A risk of malignancy index incorporating CA 125, ultrasound and menopausal status for the accurate preoperative diagnosis of ovarian cancer. *Br J Obstet Gynaecol* 1990;97(10):922.

41. Jacobs IJ, Rivera H, Oram DH, et al. Differential diagnosis of ovarian cancer with tumour markers CA 125, CA15-3 and TAG 72,3. *Br J Obstet Gynaecol* 1993;100(12):1120.

42. Tingulstad S, Hagen B, Skjeldestad FE, et al. Evaluation of a risk of malignancy index based on serum CA125, ultrasound findings and menopausal status in the pre-operative diagnosis of pelvic masses. *Br J Obstet Gynaecol* 1996;103(8):826.

43. Andersen ES, Knudsen A, Rix P, et al. Risk of malignancy index in the preoperative evaluation of patients with adnexal masses. *Gynecol Oncol* 2003;90(1):109–112.

44. Aslam N, Tailor A, Lawton F, et al. Prospective evaluation of three different models for the preoperative diagnosis of ovarian cancer. *Br J Obstet Gynaecol* 2000;107:1347–1353.

45. Ma S, Shen K, Lang J. A risk of malignancy index in preoperative diagnosis of ovarian cancer. *Chin Med J (Engl)* 2003;116(3):396–399.

46. Manjunath P, Pratapkumar, Sujatha K, et al. Comparison of three risk of malignancy indices in evaluation of pelvic masses. *Gynecol Oncol* 2001;81(2):225–229.

47. Morgante G, la Marca A, Ditto A, et al. Comparison of two malignancy indices based on serum CA 125, ultrasound score and menopausal status in the diagnosis of ovarian masses. *Br J Obstet Gynaecol* 1999;106(6):524–527.

48. Prys-Davies A, Iacobs I, Woolas R, et al. The adnexal mass: benign or malignant? Evaluation of a risk of malignancy index. *Br J Obstet Gynaecol* 1993;100:927–931.

49. Tingulstad, B, Hagen B, Skjeldestad FE, et al. Evaluation of a risk of malignancy index based on serum CA 125, ultrasound findings and menopausal status in the preoperative diagnosis of pelvic masses. *Br J Obstet Gynaecol* 1996;103:826–831.

50. Timmerman D, Verrelst H, Bourne TH, et al. Artificial neural network models for the preoperative discrimination between malignant and benign adnexal masses. *Ultrasound Obstet Gynecol* 1999;13 (1):17.

51. Tingulstad S, Hagen B, Skjeldestad FE, et al. The risk-of-malignancy index to evaluate potential ovarian cancers in local hospitals. *Obstet Gynecol* 1999;93(3):448–452.

52. Makar AP, Kristensen GB, Kaern J, et al. Prognostic value of pre- and postoperative serum CA125 levels in ovarian cancer: new aspects and multivariate analysis. *Obstet Gynecol* 1992;79(6):1002.

53. Scholl SM, Bascou CH, Mosseri V, et al. Circulating levels of colony-stimulating factor 1 as a prognostic indicator in 82 patients with epithelial ovarian cancer. *Br J Cancer* 1994;69(2):342.

54. Venesmaa P, Lehtovirta P, Stenman UH, Leminen A, Forss M, Ylikorkala O. Tumour-associated trypsin inhibitor (TATI): comparison with CA125 as a preoperative prognostic indicator in advanced ovarian cancer. *Br J Cancer* 1994;70(6):1188.

55. Parker D, Bradley C, Bogle SM, et al. Serum albumin and CA125 are powerful predictors of survival in epithelial ovarian cancer. *Br J Obstet Gynaecol* 1994;101(10):888.

56. Nagele F, Petru E, Medl M, et al. Preoperative CA 125: an independent prognostic factor in patients with stage I epithelial ovarian cancer. *Obstet Gynecol* 1995;86(2):259.

57. Yedema CA, Kenemans P, Thomas CM, et al. CA 125 serum levels in the early post-operative period do not reflect tumour reduction obtained by cytoreductive surgery. *Eur J Cancer* 1993;29A(7):966.

58. Rosen A, Sevelda P, Klein M, et al. A CA125 score as a prognostic index in patients with ovarian cancer. *Arch Gynecol Obstet* 1990; 247(3):125.

59. Gadducci A, Zola P, Landoni F, et al. Serum half-life of CA125 during early chemotherapy as an independent prognostic variable for patients with advanced epithelial ovarian cancer: results of a multicentric Italian study. *Gynecol Oncol* 1995;58(1):42.

60. Rosman M, Hayden CL, Thiel RP, et al. Prognostic indicators for poor risk epithelial ovarian carcinoma. *Cancer* 1994;74(4):1323.

61. Yedema CA, Kenemans P, Voorhorst F, et al. CA125 half-life in ovarian cancer: a multivariate survival analysis. *Br J Cancer* 1993; 67(6):1361.

62. Hawkins RE, Roberts K, Wiltshaw E, et al. The prognostic significance of the half-life of serum CA 125 in patients responding to chemotherapy for epithelial ovarian carcinoma. *Br J Obstet Gynaecol* 1989;96(12):1395.

63. Van der Burg ME, Lammes FB, et al. Ovarian cancer: the prognostic value of the serum half-life of CA125 during induction chemotherapy. *Gynecol Oncol* 1988;30(3):307.

64. Makar AP, Kristensen GB, Bormer OP, et al. Serum CA 125 level allows early identification of nonresponders during induction chemotherapy. *Gynecol Oncol* 1993;49(1):73.

65. Redman CW, Blackledge GR, Kelly K, et al. Early serum CA125 response and outcome in epithelial ovarian cancer. *Eur J Cancer* 1990; 26(5):593.

66. Buller RE, Vasilev S, DiSaia PJ. CA 125 kinetics: a cost-effective clinical tool to evaluate clinical trial outcomes in the 1990s. *Am J Obstet Gynecol* 1996;174(4):1241.

67. Makar AP, Kristensen GB, Bormer OP, et al. Is serum CA 125 at the time of relapse a prognostic indicator for further survival prognosis in patients with ovarian cancer? *Gynecol Oncol* 1993;49(1):3.

68. Hawkins RE, Roberts K, Wiltshaw E, et al. The clinical correlates of serum CA125 in 169 patients with epithelial ovarian carcinoma. *Br J Cancer* 1989;60(4):634.

69. Hempling RE, Piver MS, Natarajan N, et al. Predictive value of serum CA125 following optimal cytoreductive surgery during weekly cisplatin induction therapy for advanced ovarian cancer. *J Surg Oncol* 1993;54(1):38.

70. Fioretti P, Gadducci A, Ferdeghini M, et al. The concomitant determination of different serum tumor markers in epithelial ovarian cancer: relevance for monitoring the response to chemotherapy and follow-up of patients. *Gynecol Oncol* 1992;44(2):155.

71. Gallion HH, Hunter JE, van Nagell JR, et al. The prognostic implications of low serum CA 125 levels prior to the second-look operation for stage III and IV epithelial ovarian cancer. *Gynecol Oncol* 1992;46(1):29.

72. Fisken J, Leonard RC, Badley A, et al. Serological monitoring of epithelial ovarian cancer. *Dis Markers* 1991; 9(3–4):175.

73. Morgan RJ Jr, Speyer J, Doroshow JH, et al. Modulation of 5-fluorouracil with high-dose leucovorin calcium: activity in ovarian cancer and correlation with CA-125 levels. *Gynecol Oncol* 1995;58(1):79.

74. Buller RE, Berman ML, Bloss JD, et al. Serum CA125 regression in epithelial ovarian cancer: correlation with reassessment findings and survival. *Gynecol Oncol* 1992;47(1):87.

75. De Bruijn HW, van der Zee AG, Aalders JG. The value of cancer antigen 125 (CA 125) during treatment and follow-up of patients with ovarian cancer. *Curr Opin Obstet Gynecol* 1997;9(1):8.

76. Rustin GJ, Nelstrop AE, McClean P, et al. Defining response of ovarian carcinoma to initial chemotherapy according to serum CA 125. *J Clin Oncol* 1996b;14(5):1545.

77. Rustin GJ, Nelstrop AE, Crawford M, et al. Phase II trial of oral altretamine for relapsed ovarian carcinoma: evaluation of defining response by serum CA125. *J Clin Oncol* 1997;15(1):172.

78. Rustin GJ, Nelstrop AE, Tuxen MK, et al. Defining progression of ovarian carcinoma during follow-up according to CA125: a North Thames Ovary Group Study. *Ann Oncol* 1996a;7(4):361.

79. Cruickshank DJ, Terry PB, Fullerton WT. The potential value of CA125 as a tumour marker in small volume, non-evaluable epithelial ovarian cancer. *Int J Biol Markers* 1991;6(4):247.

80. Oehler MK, Sutterlin M, Caffier H. CASA and Ca 125 in diagnosis and follow-up of advanced ovarian cancer. *Anticancer Res* 1999;19(4A):2513–2518.

80a. Ferrozzi F, Bova D, De Chiara F, et al. Thin-section CT follow-up of metastatic ovarian carcinoma correlation with levels of CA-125 marker and clinical history. *Clin Imaging* 1998;22(5):364.

81. Stenman UH, Alfthan H, Vartiainen J, et al. Markers supplementing CA 125 in ovarian cancer. *Ann Med* 1995;27(1):115.

82. Padungsutt P, Thirapagawong C, Senapad S, et al. Accuracy of tissue polypeptide specific antigen (TPS) in the diagnosis of ovarian malignancy. *Anticancer Res* 2000;20(2B):1291–1295.

83. Sehouli J, Akdogan Z, Heinze T, et al. Preoperative determination of CASA (cancer associated serum antigen) and CA-125 for the discrimination between benign and malignant pelvic tumor mass: a prospective study. *Anticancer Res* 2003;23(2A):1115–1118.

84. Senapad S, Neungton S, Thirapakawong C, et al. Predictive value of the combined serum CA 125 and TPS during chemotherapy and before second-look laparotomy in epithelial ovarian cancer. *Anticancer Res* 2000;20(2B):1297–300.

85. Høgdall EVS, Høgdall CK, Kjaer SK, et al. OVX1 Radioimmunoassay results are dependent on the method of sample collection and storage. Clin Chem 1999;45:692–694.

86. Gold P, Freedman SO. Specific carcinoembryonic antigens of the human digestive system. *J Exp Med* 1965;122(3):467.

87. Onsrud M. Tumour markers in gynaecologic oncology. *Scand J Clin Lab Invest Suppl* 1991;206:60.

88. Roman LD, Muderspach LI, Burnett AF, et al. Carcinoembryonic antigen in women with isolated pelvic masses. Clinical utility? *J Reprod Med* 1998;43(5):403.

89. Kawai M, Kano T, Kikkawa F, et al. Seven tumor markers in benign and malignant germ cell tumors of the ovary. *Gynecol Oncol* 1992;45(3):248.

90. Chow SN, Yang JH, Lin YH, et al. Malignant ovarian germ cell tumors. *Int J Gynaecol Obstet* 1996;53(2):151.

91. Zalel Y, Piura B, Elchalal U, et al. Diagnosis and management of malignant germ cell ovarian tumors in young females. *Int J Gynaecol Obstet* 1996;55(1):1.

92. Olt G, Berchuck A, Bast RC Jr. The role of tumor markers in gynecologic oncology. *Obstet Gynecol Surv* 1990;45(9):570.

93. Mayordomo JI, Paz-Ares L, Rivera F, et al. Ovarian and extragonadal malignant germ-cell tumors in females: a single-institution experience with 43 patients. *Ann Oncol* 1994;5(3):225.

93a. Maida Y, Kyo S, Takakura M, et al. Ovarian endometrioid adenocarcinoma with ectopic production of alpha-fetoprotein. *Gynecol Oncol* 1998;71(1):133.

94. Mann K, Saller B, Hoermann R. Clinical use of HCG and hCG beta determinations. *Scand J Clin Lab Invest Suppl* 1993;216:97.

95. Cole LA, Tanaka A, Kim GS, et al. Beta-core fragment (beta-core/UGF/UGP), a tumour marker: a 7-year report. *Gynecol Oncol* 1996;60(2):264.

96. Kinugasa M, Nishimura R, Koizumi T, et al. Combination assay of urinary beta-core fragment of human chorionic gonadotropin with serum tumour markers in gonadotropin cancers. *Jpn J Cancer Res* 1995;86(8):783.

97. Schwartz PE, Chambers JT, Taylor KJ, et al. Early detection of ovarian cancer: preliminary results of the Yale Early Detection Program. *Yale J Biol Med* 1991;64(6):573.

98. Xu FJ, Yu YH, Daly L, et al. OVX1 as a marker for early stage endometrial carcinoma. *Cancer* 1994;73(7):1855.

99. Fang X, Gaudette D, Furui T, et al. Lysophospholipid growth factors in the initiation, progression, metastases, and management of ovarian cancer. *Ann NY Acad Sci* 2000;905:188–208.

100. Xu Y, Gaudette D, Boynton JD, et al. Characterization of an ovarian cancer activating factor (OCAF) in ascites from ovarian cancer patients. *Clin Cancer Res* 1995;1:1223–1232.

101. Westermann AM, Havik E, Postma FR, et al. Malignant effusions contain lysophosphatidic acid (LPA)–like activity. *Ann Oncol* 1998;9(4):437.

102. Xu Y, Shen Z, Wiper DW, et al. Lysophosphatidic acid as a potential biomarker for ovarian and other gynecologic cancers. *JAMA* 1998;280(8):719.

103. Bast, R.C., Xu F, Yu Y, et al. CA125: the past and the future. *Int J Biol Markers* 1998;13:179–187.

104. Lappohn RE, Burger HG, Bouma J, et al. Inhibin as a marker for granulosa-cell tumors. *N Engl J Med* 1989;321(12):790.

105. Boggess JF, Soules MR, Goff BA, et al. Serum inhibin and disease status in women with ovarian granulosa cell tumors. *Gynecol Oncol* 1997;64(1):64.

106. Cooke I, O'Brien M, Charnock FM, et al. Inhibin as a marker for ovarian cancer. *Br J Cancer* 1995;71(5):1046.

107. Jobling T, Mamers P, Healy DL, et al. A prospective study of inhibin in granulosa cell tumors of the ovary. *Gynecol Oncol* 1994;55(2):285.

108. Petraglia F, Luisi S, Pautier P, et al. Inhibin B is the major form of inhibin/activin family secreted by granulosa cell tumors. *J Clin Endocrinol Metab* 1998;83:1029.

109. Yamashita K, Yamoto M, Shikone T, et al. Production of inhibin A and inhibin B in human ovarian sex cord stromal tumors. *Am J Obstet Gynecol* 1997;177(6):1450.

110. Rey RA, Lhomme C, Marcillac I, et al. Antimullerian hormone as a serum marker of granulosa cell tumors of the ovary: comparative study with serum alpha-inhibin and estradiol. *Am J Obstet Gynecol* 1996;174(3):958.

111. Silverman LA, Gitelman SE. Immunoreactive inhibin, mullerian inhibitory substance, and activin as biochemical markers for juvenile granulosa cell tumors. *J Pediatr* 1996;129(6):918.

112. Blaakaer J, Micic S, Morris ID, et al. Immunoreactive inhibin-production in post-menopausal women with malignant epithelial ovarian tumors. *Eur J Obstet Gynecol Reprod Biol* 1993;52(2):105.

113. Healy DL, Burger HG, Mamers P, et al. Elevated serum inhibin concentrations in postmenopausal women with ovarian tumors. *N Engl J Med* 1993;329(21):1539.

114. Phocas I, Sarandakou A, Sikiotis K, et al. A comparative study of serum alpha-beta A immunoreactive inhibin and tumor-associated antigens CA125 and CEA in ovarian cancer. *Anticancer Res* 1996;16(6B):3827.

115. Burger HG, Robertson DM, Cahir N, et al. Characterization of inhibin immunoreactivity in post-menopausal women with ovarian tumours. *Clin Endocrinol (Oxf)* 1996;44(4):413.

116. Lambert-Messerlian GM, Steinhoff M, Zheng W, et al. Multiple im-

munoreactive inhibin proteins in serum from postmenopausal women with epithelial ovarian cancer. *Gynecol Oncol* 1997;65(3):512.

117. Burger HG, Baillie A, Drummond AE, et al. Inhibin and ovarian cancer. *J Reprod Immunol* 1998;39:77.

118. Menon U, Riley SC, Thomas J, et al. Serum inhibin, activin and follistatin in postmenopausal women with epithelial ovarian carcinoma. *BJOG* 2000;107(9):1069–1074.

119. Seifer DB, Schneyer AL. Multiple immunoreactive inhibin proteins in serum from postmenopausal women with epithelial ovarian cancer. *Gynecol Oncol* 1997;65(3):512.

120. Welt CK, Lambert-Messerlian G, Zheng W, et al. Presence of activin, inhibin, and follistatin in epithelial ovarian carcinoma. *J Clin Endocrinol Metab* 1997;82(11):3720.

121. Michiel DF, Oppenheim JJ. Cytokines as positive and negative regulators of tumor promotion and progression. *Semin Cancer Biol* 1992; 3(1):3.

122. Suzuki M, Ohwada M, Aida I, et al. Macrophage colony-stimulating factor as a tumor marker for epithelial ovarian cancer. *Obstet Gynecol* 1993;82(6):946.

123. Suzuki M, Ohwada M, Sato I, et al. Serum level of macrophage colony-stimulating factor as a marker for gynecologic malignancies. *Oncology* 1995;52(2):128.

124. Price FV, Chambers SK, Chambers JT, et al. Colony-stimulating factor-1 in primary ascites of ovarian cancer is a significant predictor of survival. *Am J Obstet Gynecol* 1993;168(2):520.

125. Gadducci A, Ferdeghini M, Castellani C, et al. Serum macrophage colony-stimulating factor (M-CSF) levels in patients with epithelial ovarian cancer. *Gynecol Oncol* 1998;70(1):111.

126. Woolas RP, Xu FJ, Jacobs IJ, et al. Elevation of multiple serum markers in patients with stage I ovarian cancer. *J Natl Cancer Inst* 1993; 85(21):1748.

127. Suzuki M, Kobayashi H, Ohwada M, et al. Macrophage colony-stimulating factor as a marker for malignant germ cell tumors of the ovary. *Gynecol Oncol* 1998;68(1):35.

128. Salman T, el-Ahmady O, Sawsan MR, et al. The clinical value of serum TPS in gynecological malignancies. *Int J Biol Markers* 1995; 10(2):81.

129. Shabana A, Onsrud M. Tissue polypeptide-specific antigen and CA 125 as serum tumor markers in ovarian carcinoma. *Tumour Biol* 1994; 15(6):361.

130. Sliutz G, Tempfer C, Kainz C, et al. Tissue polypeptide specific antigen and cancer associated serum antigen in the follow-up of ovarian cancer. *Anticancer Res* 1995;5(3):1127.

131. Tempfer C, Hefler L, Haeusler G, et al. Tissue polypeptide specific antigen in the follow-up of ovarian and cervical cancer patients. *Int J Cancer* 1998;79(3):241.

132. Hasholzner U, Baumgartner L, Stieber P, et al. Significance of the tumour markers CA 125 II, CA 72–4, CASA and CYFRA 21–1 in ovarian carcinoma. *Anticancer Res* 1994;14:2743.

133. Tempfer C, Hefler L, Heinzl H, et al. CYFRA 21–1 serum levels in women with adnexal masses and inflammatory diseases. *Br J Cancer* 1998; 78(8):1108.

134. Inaba N, Negishi Y, Fukasawa I, et al. Cytokeratin fragment 21–1 in gynaecologic malignancy: comparison with cancer antigen 125 and squamous cell carcinoma-related antigen. *Tumour Biol* 1995;16(6): 345.

135. Gadducci A, Ferdeghini M, Cosio S, et al. The clinical relevance of serum CYFRA 21–1 assay in patients with ovarian cancer. *Int J Gynecol Cancer* 2001;11(4):277.

136. Peters-Engl C, Medl M, Ogris E, et al. Tumour-associated trypsin inhibitor (TATI) and cancer antigen 125 (CA125) in patients with epithelial ovarian cancer. *Anticancer Res* 1995;15(6B):2727.

137. Medl M, Ogris E, Peters-Engl C, et al. TATI (tumour-associated trypsin inhibitor) as a marker of ovarian cancer. *Br J Cancer* 1995;71(5): 1051.

138. Venesmaa P, Stenman UH, Forss M, et al. Pre-operative serum level of tumour-associated trypsin inhibitor and residual tumour size as prognostic indicators in Stage III epithelial ovarian cancer. *Br J Obstet Gynaecol* 1998;105(5):508.

139. Baak JPA, Path FRC, Hermsen MAJA, et al. Genomics and proteomics in cancer. *Eur J Cancer* 2003;39(9):1199–1215.

140. Schummer M, Ng WV, Bumgarner RE, et al. Comparative hybridiza-

tion of an array of 21 500 ovarian cDNAs for the discovery of genes overexpressed in ovarian carcinomas. *Gene* 1999;238(2):375–385.

141. Hough CD, Sherman-Baust CA, Pizer ES, et al. Large-scale serial analysis of gene expression reveals genes differentially expressed in ovarian cancer. *Cancer Res* 2000;60(22):6281–6287.

142. Mok SC, Chao J, Skates S, Wong K-K, et al. Prostasin, a potential serum marker for ovarian cancer: identification through microarray technology. *J Natl Cancer Inst* 2001;93(19):1458–1464.

143. Kim JH, Skates SJ, Uede T, et al. Osteopontin as a potential diagnostic biomarker for ovarian cancer. *JAMA* 2002;287(13):1671–1679.

144. Wasinger VC, Cordwell SJ, Cerpa-Poljak A, et al. Progress with gene-product mapping of the mollicutes: *Mycoplasma genitalium*. *Electrophoresis* 1995;16:1090–1094.

145. Wilkins MR, Sanchez JC, Gooley AA, et al. Progress with proteome projects: why all proteins expressed by a genome should be identified and how to do it. *Biotechnol Genet Eng Rev* 1996;13:19–50.

146. Reynolds T. For proteomics research, a new race has begun. *J Natl Cancer Inst* 2002;94:552–554.

147. Wilkins MR, Sanchez JC, Williams KL, et al. Current challenges and future applications for protein maps and post-translational vector maps in proteome projects. *Electrophoresis* 1996;17:830–838.

148. Banks RE, Dunn MJ, Hochstrasser DF, et al. Proteomics: new perspectives, new biomedical opportunities. *Lancet* 2002;356(9243): 1749–1756.

149. Mills GB, Bast RC Jr, Srivastava S. Future for ovarian cancer screening: novel markers from emerging technologies of transcriptional profiling and proteomics. *J Natl Cancer Inst* 2001;93(19):1437–1439.

150. Ardekani AM, Hitt B, Brown MR, et al. A high throughput proteomic approach to serum marker development for discrimination between ovarian cancer patients and unaffected individuals. *Proc Soc Gynecol Oncol* 2001;32:102(abst).

151. Petricoin EF III, Ardekani AA, Hitt BA, et al. Use of proteomic patterns in serum to identify ovarian cancer. *Lancet* 2002;359(9306): 572–577.

152. Diamandis EP. Proteomic patterns in serum and identification of ovarian cancer. *Lancet* 2002;360(9327):169–170.

153. Elwood M. Proteomic patterns in serum and identification of ovarian cancer. *Lancet* 2002;360(9327):170.

154. Pearl DC. Proteomic patterns in serum and identification of ovarian cancer. *Lancet* 2002;360(9327):169–170.

155. Petricoin EF III, Mills GB, Kohn EC, et al. Proteomic patterns in serum and identification of ovarian cancer *Lancet* 2002;360(9327): 170–171.

156. Rockhill B. Proteomic patterns in serum and identification of ovarian cancer. *Lancet* 2002;360(9327):169.

157. Hakala A, Kacinski BM, Stanley ER, et al. Macrophage colony-stimulating factor 1, a clinically useful tumour marker in endometrial adenocarcinoma: comparison with CA 125 and the aminoterminal propeptide of type III procollagen. *Am J Obstet Gynecol* 1995;173(1):112.

158. Patsner B, Orr JW Jr, Mann WJ Jr. Use of serum CA 125 measurement in posttreatment surveillance of early-stage endometrial carcinoma. *Am J Obstet Gynecol* 1990;162(2):427.

159. Takeshima N, Shimizu Y, Umezawa S, et al. Combined assay of serum levels of CA125 and CA19–9 in endometrial carcinoma. *Gynecol Oncol* 1994;54(3):321.

160. Gadducci A, Ferdeghini M, Prontera C, et al. A comparison of retreatment serum levels of four tumor markers in patients with endometrial and cervical carcinoma. *Eur J Gynaecol Oncol* 1990;11(4):283.

161. Tomas C, Risteli J, Risteli L, et al. Use of various epithelial tumor markers and a stromal marker in the assessment of cervical carcinoma. *Obstet Gynecol* 1991;77(4):566.

162. Kurihara T, Mizunuma H, Obara M, et al. Determination of a normal level of serum CA125 in postmenopausal women as a tool for preoperative evaluation and postoperative surveillance of endometrial carcinoma. *Gynecol Oncol* 1998;69(3):192.

162a. Price FV, Chambers SK, Carcangiu ML, et al. CA 125 may not reflect disease status in patients with uterine serous carcinoma. *Cancer* 1998;82(9):1720.

163. Kato H, Torigoe T. Radioimmunoassay for tumour antigen of human squamous cell carcinoma. *Cancer* 1977;40:1621.

164. Lozza L, Merola M, Fontanelli R, et al. Cancer of the uterine cervix: clinical value of squamous cell carcinoma antigen (SCC) measurements. *Anticancer Res* 1997;17:525.

165. Ngan HY, Cheung AN, Lauder IJ, et al. Prognostic significance of serum tumour markers in carcinoma of the cervix, *Eur J Gynaecol Oncol* 1996;17(6):512.

166. Crombach G, Scharl A, Vierbuchen M,, et al. Detection of squamous cell carcinoma antigen in normal squamous epithelia and in squamous cell carcinomas of the uterine cervix. *Cancer* 1989;63(7):1337.

167. Duk JM, van Voorst Vader PC, ten Hoor KA, et al. Elevated levels of squamous cell carcinoma antigen in patients with a benign disease of the skin. *Cancer* 1989;64(8):1652.

168. Bolger BS, Dabbas M, Lopes A, et al. Prognostic value of preoperative squamous cell carcinoma antigen level in patients surgically treated for cervical carcinoma. *Gynecol Oncol* 1997;65(2):309.

169. Duk JM, Groenier KH, de Bruijn HW, et al. Pre-treatment serum squamous cell carcinoma antigen: a newly identified prognostic factor in early-stage cervical carcinoma. *J Clin Oncol* 1996;14(1):111.

170. Massuger LF, Koper NP, Thomas CM, et al. Improvement of clinical staging in cervical cancer with serum squamous cell carcinoma antigen and CA 125 determinations. *Gynecol Oncol* 1997;64(3):473.

171. Scambia G, Benedetti Panici P, Foti E, et al. Squamous cell carcinoma antigen: prognostic significance and role in the monitoring of neoadjuvant chemotherapy response in cervical cancer. *J Clin Oncol* 1994;12(11):2309.

172. Takeshima N, Hirai Y, Katase K, et al. The value of squamous cell carcinoma antigen as a predictor of nodal metastasis in cervical cancer. *Gynecol Oncol* 1998;68(3):263.

173. Gaarenstroom KN, Bonfrer JM, Kenter GG, et al. Clinical value of re-treatment serum Cyfra 21–1, tissue polypeptide antigen, and squamous cell carcinoma antigen levels in patients with cervical cancer. *Cancer* 1995;76(5):807.

174. Hong JH, Tsai CS, Chang JT, et al. The prognostic significance of pre- and posttreatment SCC levels in patients with squamous cell carcinoma of the cervix treated by radiotherapy. *Int J Radiat Oncol Biol Phys* 1998;41(4):823.

175. Gocze PM, Vahrson HW, Freeman DA. Serum levels of squamous cell carcinoma antigen and ovarian carcinoma antigen (CA 125) in patients with benign and malignant diseases of the uterine cervix. *Oncology* 1994;51(5):430.

176. Kim BG, Kim JH, Park SY, et al. Relationship between squamous cell carcinoma antigen levels and tumour volumes in patients with cervical carcinomas undergoing neoadjuvant chemotherapy. *Gynecol Oncol* 1996; 63(1):105.

177. Pectasides D, Economides N, Bourazanis J, et al. Squamous cell carcinoma antigen, tumor-associated trypsin inhibitor, and carcinoembryonic antigen for monitoring cervical cancer. *Am J Clin Oncol* 1994; 17(4):307.

178. Rose PG, Baker S, Fournier L, et al. Serum squamous cell carcinoma antigen levels in invasive cervical cancer: prediction of response and recurrence. *Am J Obstet Gynecol* 1993;168(3 Pt 1):942.

179. Hung YC, Shiau YC, Chang WC, et al. Early predicting recurrent cervical cancer with combination of tissue polypeptide specific antigen (TPS) and squamous cell carcinoma antigen (SCC). *Neoplasma* 2002;49(6):415–417.

180. Bonfrer JM, Gaarenstroom KN, Korse CM, et al. Cyfra 21–1 in monitoring cervical cancer: a comparison with tissue polypeptide antigen and squamous cell carcinoma antigen. *Anticancer Res* 1997;17:2329.

181. Ferdeghini M, Gadducci A, Prontera C, et al. Determination of serum levels of different cytokeratins in patients with uterine malignancies. *Anticancer Res* 1994;4:1393.

182. Sproston AR, Roberts SA, Davidson SE, et al. Serum tumour markers in carcinoma of the uterine cervix and outcome following radiotherapy. *Br J Cancer* 1995;72(6):1536.

183. Tsai SC, Kao CH, Wang SJ. Study of a new tumour marker, CYFRA 21–1, in squamous cell carcinoma of the cervix, and comparison with squamous cell carcinoma antigen. *Neoplasma* 1996;43(1):27.

184. Bonfrer JM, Gaarenstroom KN, Kenter G, et al. Prognostic significance of serum fragments of cytokeratin 19 measured by Cyfra 21–1 in cervical cancer. *Gynecol Oncol* 1994;55(3 Pt 1):371.

185. Kainz C, Sliutz G, Mustafa G, et al. Cytokeratin subunit 19 measured by CYFRA 21–1 assay in follow-up of cervical cancer, *Gynecol Oncol* 1995;56(3):402.

186. Nasu K, Etoh Y, Yoshimatsu J, et al. Serum levels of cytokeratin 19 fragments in cervical cancer. *Gynecol Obstet Invest* 1996;42(4):267.

187. Ferdeghini M, Gadducci A, Annicchiarico C, et al. Serum CYFRA

188. Callet N, Cohen-Solal Le Nir CC, Berthelot E, Pichon MF. Cancer of the uterine cervix: sensitivity and specificity of serum Cyfra 21.1 determinations. *Eur J Gynaecol Oncol* 1998;19(1):50.

189. Duk JM, Aalders JG, Fleuren GJ, et al. Tumor markers CA 125, squamous cell carcinoma antigen, and carcinoembryonic antigen in patients with adenocarcinoma of the uterine cervix. *Obstet Gynecol* 1989;73(4):661.

190. Borras G, Molina R, Xercavins J, et al. Tumour antigens CA19,9, CA125, and CEA in carcinoma of the uterine cervix. *Gynecol Oncol* 1995;57(2):205.

191. Avall-Lundqvist EH, Sjovall K, Nilsson BR, et al. Prognostic significance of pretreatment serum levels of squamous cell carcinoma antigen and CA 125 in cervical carcinoma. *Eur J Cancer* 1992;28A(10): 1695–702.

192. Duk JM, de Bruijn HW, Groenier KH, et al. Adenocarcinoma of the uterine cervix, Prognostic significance of pre-treatment serum CA 125, squamous cell carcinoma antigen, and carcinoembryonic antigen levels in relation to clinical and histopathologic tumour characteristics. *Cancer* 1990;65(8):1830.

193. Leminen A, Alftan H, Stenman UH, et al. Chemotherapy as initial treatment for cervical carcinoma: clinical and tumor marker response. *Acta Obstet Gynecol Scand* 1992;71(4):293.

194. Lam CP, Yuan CC, Jeng FS, et al. Evaluation of carcinoembryonic antigen, tissue polypeptide antigen, and squamous cell carcinoma antigen in the detection of cervical cancers. *Chung Hua I Hsueh Tsa Chih* (Taipei) 1992;50(1):7–13.

195. Gaarenstroom KN, Kenter GG, Bonfrer JMG, et al. Can initial serum Cyfra 21–1, SCC antigen, and TPA levels in squamous cell cervical cancer predict lymph node metastases or prognosis? *Gynecol Oncol* 2000;77(1):164–170.

196. Bae SN, Namkoong SE, Jung JK, et al. Prognostic significance of pretreatment squamous cell carcinoma antigen and carcinoembryonic antigen in squamous cell carcinoma of the uterine cervix. *Gynecol Oncol* 1997;64(3):418.

197. Scambia G, Benedetti Panici P, Foti E, et al. Multiple tumour marker assays in advanced cervical cancer: relationship to chemotherapy response and clinical outcome. *Eur J Cancer* 1996a;32A(2):259.

198. Sproston AR, Roberts SA, Davidson SE, et al. Serum tumour markers in carcinoma of the uterine cervix and outcome following radiotherapy. *Br J Cancer* 1995;72(6):1536.

199. Pras E, Willemse PHB, Canrinus AA, et al. Serum squamous cell carcinoma antigen and CYFRA 21–1 in cervical cancer treatment. *International Journal of Radiation Oncology, Biology, Physics* 2002; 52(1):23–32.

200. Nam JH, Chang KC, Chambers JT, et al. Urinary gonadotropin fragment, a new tumor marker. III, Use in cervical and vulvar cancers. *Gynecol Oncol* 1990;38(1):66.

201. Carter PG, Iles RK, Neven P, et al. Measurement of urinary beta core fragment of human chorionic gonadotropin in women with vulvovaginal malignancy and its prognostic significance. *Br J Cancer* 1995; 71(2):350.

202. Scambia G, Testa U, Panici PB, et al. Interleukin-6 serum levels in patients with gynecological tumors. *Int J Cancer* 1994;57(3):318.

203. Scambia G, Testa U, Benedetti Panici P, et al. Prognostic significance of interleukin 6 serum levels in patients with ovarian cancer. *Br J Cancer* 1995;71(2):354.

204. Schroder W, Ruppert C, Bender HG. Concomitant measurements of interleukin-6 (IL-6) in serum and peritoneal fluid of patients with benign and malignant ovarian tumors. *Eur J Obstet Gynecol Reprod Biol* 1994;56(1):43.

205. Plante M, Rubin SC, Wong GY, et al. Interleukin-6 level in serum and ascites as a prognostic factor in patients with epithelial ovarian cancer. *Cancer* 1994;3(7):1882.

206. Tempfer C, Zeisler H, Sliutz G, et al. Serum evaluation of interleukin 6 in ovarian cancer patients. *Gynecol Oncol* 1997;66(1):27.

207. Maccio A, Lai P, Santona MC, et al. High serum levels of soluble IL-2 receptor, cytokines, and C reactive protein correlate with impairment of T cell response in patients with advanced epithelial ovarian cancer. *Gynecol Oncol* 1998;69(3):248.

208. Barton DP, Blanchard DK, Michelini-Norris B, et al. Serum soluble interleukin-2 receptor alpha levels in patients with gynecologic can-

cers: early effect of surgery. *Am J Reprod Immunol* 1993;30(2–3): 202.

209. Ferdeghini M, Gadducci A, Prontera C, et al. Serum soluble interleukin-2 receptor assay in epithelial ovarian cancer. *Tumour Biol* 1993; 14(5):303.

210. Hurteau JA, Woolas RP, Jacobs IJ, et al. Soluble interleukin-2 receptor alpha is elevated in sera of patients with benign ovarian neoplasms and epithelial ovarian cancer. *Cancer* 1995;76(9):1615.

211. Gadducci A, Ferdeghini M, Malagnino G, et al. Elevated serum levels of neopterin and soluble interleukin-2 receptor in patients with ovarian cancer. *Gynecol Oncol* 1994;52(3):386.

212. Pavlidis NA, Bairaktari E, Kalef-Ezra J, et al. Serum soluble interleukin-2 receptors in epithelial ovarian cancer patients. *Int J Biol Markers* 1995;10(2):75.

213. De Bruijn HW, ten Hoor KA, van der Zee AG. Serum and cystic fluid levels of soluble interleukin-2 receptor-alpha in patients with epithelial ovarian tumors are correlated. *Tumour Biol* 1998;19(3):160.

214. Gadducci A, Ferdeghini M, Castellani C, et al. Serum levels of tumor necrosis factor (TNF), soluble receptors for TNF (55- and 75-kDa sTNFr), and soluble CD14 (sCD14) in epithelial ovarian cancer. *Gynecol Oncol* 1995b:(2):184.

215. Grosen EA, Granger GA, Gatanaga M, et al. Measurement of the soluble membrane receptors for tumor necrosis factor and lymphotoxin in the sera of patients with gynaecologic malignancy. *Gynecol Oncol* 1993;50(1):68.

216. Scambia G, Benedetti Panici P, Baiocchi G, et al. CA 15–3 serum levels in ovarian cancer. *Oncology* 1988;45(3):263.

217. Bast RC Jr, Knauf S, Epenetos A, et al. Coordinate elevation of serum markers in ovarian cancer but not in benign disease. *Cancer* 1991; 68(8):1758.

218. Scambia G, Benedetti Panici P, Perrone L, et al. Serum levels of tumour associated glycoprotein (TAG 72) in patients with gynecologic malignancies. *Br J Cancer* 1990;62(1):147.

219. Negishi Y, Iwabuchi H, Sakunaga H, et al. Serum and tissue measurements of CA72–4 in ovarian cancer patients. *Gynecol Oncol* 1993; 48(2):148.

220. Hasholzner U, Baumgartner L, Stieber P, et al. Clinical significance of the tumour markers CA 125 II and CA 72–4 in ovarian carcinoma. *Int J Cancer* 1996; 69(4):329.

221. Guadagni F, Roselli M, Cosimelli M, et al. CA 72–4 serum marker—a new tool in the management of carcinoma patients. *Cancer Invest* 1995;13(2):227.

222. Schutter EM, Sohn C, Kristen P, et al. Estimation of probability of malignancy using a logistic model combining physical examination, ultrasound, serum CA 125, and serum CA 72–4 in postmenopausal women with a pelvic mass: an international multicenter study. *Gynecol Oncol* 1998; 69(1):56.

223. Gocze PM, Szabo DG, Than GN, et al. Occurrence of CA 125 and CA 19–9 tumor-associated antigens in sera of patients with gynaecologic, trophoblastic, and colorectal tumors. *Gynecol Obstet Invest* 1988; 25(4):268.

224. Kobayashi H, Ohi H, Fujii T, et al. Characterisation and clinical usefulness of CA130 antigen recognised by monoclonal antibodies, 130–22 and 145–9, in ovarian cancers. *Br J Cancer* 1993a;67(2):237.

225. Xu FJ, Yu YH, Li BY, et al. Development of two new monoclonal antibodies reactive to a surface antigen present on human ovarian epithelial cancer cells. *Cancer Res* 1991;51(15):4012.

226. Xu FJ, Yu YH, Daly L, et al. OVX1 radioimmunoassay complements CA-125 for predicting the presence of residual ovarian carcinoma at second-look surgical surveillance procedures. *J Clin Oncol* 1993; 11(8):1506.

227. Berek JS, Bast RC Jr. Ovarian cancer screening. The use of serial complementary tumor markers to improve sensitivity and specificity for early detection. *Cancer* 1995; 76[10 Suppl]:2092.

228. Woolas RP, Conaway MR, Xu F, et al. Combinations of multiple serum markers are superior to individual assays for discriminating malignant from benign pelvic masses. *Gynecol Oncol* 1995;59(1): 111.

229. Devine PL, McGuckin MA, Ramm LE, et al. Serum mucin antigens CASA and MSA in tumors of the breast, ovary, lung, pancreas, bladder, colon, and prostate, A blind trial with 420 patients. *Cancer* 1993; 72(6):2007.

230. McGuckin MA, Layton GT, Bailey MJ, et al. Evaluation of two new assays for tumor-associated antigens, CASA and OSA, found in the serum of patients with epithelial ovarian carcinoma—comparison with CA125. *Gynecol Oncol* 1990;37(2):165.

231. Ward BG, McGuckin MA, Ramm LE, et al. The management of ovarian carcinoma is improved by the use of cancer-associated serum antigen and CA 125 assays. *Cancer* 1993;71(2):430.

232. Kierkegaard O, Mogensen O, Mogensen B, et al. Predictive and prognostic values of cancer-associated serum antigen (CASA) and cancer antigen 125 (CA 125) levels prior to second-look laparotomy for ovarian cancer. *Gynecol Oncol* 1995;59(2):251.

233. Meisel M, Straube W, Weise J, et al. A study of serum CASA and CA 125 levels in patients with ovarian carcinoma. *Arch Gynecol Obstet* 1995;256(1):9.

234. Tholander B, Taube A, Lindgren A, et al. Pretreatment serum levels of CA-125, carcinoembryonic antigen, tissue polypeptide antigen, and placental alkaline phosphatase, in patients with ovarian carcinoma, borderline tumors, or benign adnexal masses: relevance for differential diagnosis. *Gynecol Oncol* 1990;39(1):16.

235. Panza N, Pacilio G, Campanella L, et al. Cancer antigen 125, tissue polypeptide antigen, carcinoembryonic antigen, and beta-chain human chorionic gonadotropin as serum markers of epithelial ovarian carcinoma. *Cancer* 1988;61(1):76.

236. Hording U, Toftager-Larsen K, Dreisler A, et al. CA 125, placental alkaline phosphatase, and tissue polypeptide antigen in the monitoring of ovarian carcinoma, A comparative study of three different tumor markers. *Gynecol Obstet Invest* 1990;30(3):178.

237. Flyvbjerg A, Mogensen O, Mogensen B, et al. Elevated serum insulin-like growth factor–binding protein 2 (IGFBP-2) and decreased IGFBP-3 in epithelial ovarian cancer: correlation with cancer antigen 125 and tumor-associated trypsin inhibitor. *J Clin Endocrinol Metab* 1997;82(7):2308.

238. Høgdall CK, Mogensen O, Tabor A, et al. The role of serum tetranectin, CA 125, and a combined index as tumor markers in women with pelvic tumors. *Gynecol Oncol* 1995;56(1):22.

239. Høgdall CK, Høgdall EV, Hording U, et al. Pre-operative plasma tetranectin as a prognostic marker in ovarian cancer patients. *Scand J Clin Lab Invest* 1993;53(7):741.

240. Høgdall CK, Hording U, Norgaard-Pedersen B, et al. Serum tetranectin and CA-125 used to monitor the course of treatment in ovarian cancer patients. *Eur J Obstet Gynecol Reprod Biol* 1994;57(3):175.

241. Høgdall CK, Høgdall EV, Hording U, et al. Use of tetranectin, CA-125 and CASA to predict residual tumor and survival at second- and third-look operations for ovarian cancer. *Acta Oncologica* 1996;35(1): 63.

242. Udagawa Y, Aoki D, Ito K, et al. Clinical characteristics of a newly developed ovarian tumour marker, galactosyltransferase associated with tumour (GAT). *Eur J Cancer* 1998;34(4):489.

243. Nozawa S, Udagawa Y, Ito K et al. [Clinical significance of galactosyltransferase associated with tumor (GAT), a new tumor marker for ovarian cancer—with special reference to the discrimination between ovarian cancer and endometriosis.] *Gan To Kagaku Ryoho* 1994; 21(4):507.

244. Hilgers J, Kenemans P. The utility of lipid-associated sialic acid (LASA or LSA) as a serum marker for malignancy. A review of the literature. *Tumour Biol* 1992;13(3):121.

245. Petru E, Sevin BU, Averette HE, et al. Comparison of three tumor markers—CA-125, lipid-associated sialic acid (LSA), and NB/70K—in monitoring ovarian cancer. *Gynecol Oncol* 1990;38(2):181.

246. Suzuki M, Ohwada M, Tamada T. Clinical value of sialyl SSEA-1 antigen in patients with ovarian cancer. *Gynecol Oncol* 1990;36(3): 371.

247. Kobayashi H. Kawashima Y. Clinical usefulness of serum sialyl SSEA-1 antigen levels in patients with epithelial ovarian cancer. Comparative effectiveness of sialyl SSEA-1 and CA 125. *Gynecol Obstet Invest* 1990;30(1):52.

248. Iwanari O, Miyako J, Date Y, et al. Differential diagnosis of ovarian cancer, benign ovarian tumor and endometriosis by a combination assay of serum sialyl SSEA-1 antigen and CA125 levels. *Gynecol Obstet Invest* 1990;29(1):71.

249. Obermair A, Tempfer C, Hefler L, et al. Concentration of vascular endothelial growth factor (VEGF) in the serum of patients with suspected ovarian cancer. *Br J Cancer* 1998;77(11):1870.

250. Castelli M, Battaglia F, Scambia G, et al. Immunosuppressive acidic protein and CA 125 levels in patients with ovarian cancer. *Oncology* 1991;48(1):13.

251. Scambia G, Foti E, Ferrandina G, et al. Prognostic role of immunosuppressive acidic protein in advanced ovarian cancer. *Am J Obstet Gynecol* 1996b;175(6):1606.

252. Diamandis EP, Yousef GM, Soosaipillai AR, et al. Human kallikrein 6(zyme/protease M/neurosin): a new serum biomarker of ovarian carcinoma. *Clinical Biochemistry* 2000;33(7):579–583.

253. Yousef GM; Diamandis EP. Expanded human tissue kallikrein family—a novel panel of cancer biomarkers. *Tumour Biol* 2002;23(3):185–192.

254. Lo SS, Cheng DK, Ng TY, et al. Prognostic significance of tumour markers in endometrial cancer. *Tumour Biol* 1997;18(4):241.

255. Matorras R, Rodriguez-Escuderoi FJ, Diez J, et al. Monitoring endometrial adenocarcinoma with a four tumor marker combination, CA 125, squamous cell carcinoma antigen, CA 19,9 and CA 15,3. *Acta Obstet Gynecol Scand* 1992;71(6):458.

256. Tomas C, Penttinen J, Risteli J, et al. Serum concentrations of CA 125 and aminoterminal propeptide of type III procollagen (PIIINP) in patients with endometrial carcinoma. *Cancer* 1990;66(11):2399.

257. Ota Y, Inaba N, Shirotake S, et al. Enzyme immunoassay for placental protein 4 (PP4) and its possible diagnostic significance in patients with genital tract cancer. *Arch Gynecol Obstet* 1990;247(3):139–147.

258. Hareyama H, Sakuragi N, Makinoda S, et al. Serum and tissue measurements of CA72-4 in patients with endometrial carcinoma. *J Clin Pathol* 1996;49(12):967.

259. Xu Y, Gaudette DC, Boynton JD, et al. Characterization of an ovarian cancer activating factor in ascites from ovarian cancer patients. *Clin Cancer Res* 1995;1(10):1223.

260. Ferdeghini M, Gadducci A, Prontera C, et al. Serum soluble interleukin-2 receptor (sIL-2R) assay in cervical and endometrial cancer. Preliminary data. *Anticancer Res* 1993;13(3):709.

CHAPTER 8

Cancer Prevention Strategies

Paul F. Engstrom and Frank L. Meyskens, Jr.

Prevention is the ideal method of cancer control. Cancer prevention research seeks to identify the preventable causes of cancer, both positive and negative, and to reduce cancer incidence by effective application of prevention strategies in target populations (1). Three major approaches to cancer prevention currently exist.

Primary Prevention

Primary prevention focuses on reducing risk of cancer in normal asymptomatic individuals. Epidemiologic studies provide evidence that environmental factors such as chemicals, viruses, and radiation exposure play an important role in cancer incidence. It is estimated that 70% to 80% of all cancer is attributable to environmental risk factors, and that elimination of these factors could have a profound positive effect on cancer incidence and mortality (2). Cancer prevention strategies that minimize exposure to known causative agents should reduce cancer incidence. Reduction to exposure to carcinogens in tobacco smoke is an example of an effective primary preventive strategy. Similarly, limits placed on occupational exposure to chemical carcinogens such as asbestos and benzene represent an obvious and undoubtedly effective means of reducing cancer incidence. Unfortunately, for the majority of malignancies, including the gynecologic epithelial cancers, a single physical or chemical etiologic factor has not been identified, thereby limiting the application of exposure-based prevention strategies.

Another type of exposure-based strategy relies on dietary modification. It is possible to reduce suspected cancer-promoting constituents such as mutagens and fat or to en-

hance the intake of putative preventive agents such as fiber and perhaps affect cancer incidence (3). However, owing to the influence of countless variables such as bioavailability, metabolism, heredity, lifestyle, and period of exposure, the ability to predict the combined impact of various dietary constituents on cancer risk reduction is limited (4). There is convincing evidence from the epidemiology literature that adult obesity increases the risk of postmenopausal endometrial cancer (5). However, it is unlikely that dietary intervention studies can be mounted that would test the hypothesis that reduced calories in adolescence or middle age could reduce the mortality of this type of cancer. Chemoprevention has been a successful strategy of primary prevention in some common epithelial cancers; for example, tamoxifen for women at risk for breast cancer and finasteride for men at risk for prostate cancer (see below). *Chemoprevention* is a term coined more than 15 years ago by Sporn and Roberts (6) to describe the novel approach of reducing cancer risk in susceptible individuals by administering a specific natural or synthetic chemical compound to reverse, suppress, or delay the process of carcinogenesis. The definition of chemoprevention does not include food compounds ingested as a normal diet. For example, beta-carotene consumed in fruits and vegetables is not considered chemoprevention, but rather is subsumed under the field of diet and cancer (7). When provided at high doses, e.g., pills (i.e., used as a drug), beta-carotene or other single-nutrient therapy is considered to be chemoprevention.

Secondary Prevention

Secondary prevention is utilized to detect a preneoplastic process or a neoplasia at the earliest stages through screening or by utilizing a therapy/chemoprevention to reverse a preneoplastic lesion; for example, the use of calcium to reduce adenomatous polyps in the large bowel.

The natural history of cervical cancer with its long preinvasive stage and the availability of a simple test, the Papani-

Paul F. Engstrom: Department of Medicine, Temple University School of Medicine; and Population Science Division, Fox Chase Cancer Center, Philadelphia, PA 19111

Frank L. Meyskens, Jr.: Department of Medicine and Biological Chemistry, University of California at Irvine, Orange, CA 92715.

colaou smear, makes cervical cancer ideal for screening. The National Cancer Institute (NCI) recommends that women have Pap smears annually beginning at the age that they become sexually active. After three annual normal, or negative, smears, screening every 3 years is appropriate. Recent studies (8) emphasize that cervical cancer screening should continue beyond 65 years of age if women have not received regular prior screening. Eddy (9) has calculated that screening at least every 3 years from age 20 to 75 years of age will reduce the mortality of invasive cervical cancer by approximately 90%. Koss (10) has determined that the false-negative error rate in the primary screening process, given the current technology, can probably never be reduced below 5% (11). In his laboratory, approximately 25% of Pap smears were randomly rescreened and the false-negative rate was 3.9% (range 2.6% to 5.1%) over an 11-year period. An additional 1% to 2% of false-positive cases are picked up when there is systematic rereview of cases of prior negative smears in women returning with an abnormal smear. Some investigators have recommended that women who test positive for human papillomavirus (HPV) have more intensive screening including colposcopy because of the known association of carcinoma in situ and invasive cancer with HPV types 16, 18, 31, and 35 (12). The new Bethesda system for reporting results of smears of the uterine cervix should make the cytologic report a medical consultation (13). Under this new reporting system, the adequacy of the smear is stated, a primary assessment as to normal or other is determined, and a descriptive diagnosis of benign abnormalities, precancerous lesions, and invasive cancer is clearly stated in the report. Sensitivity to the cultural biases of subpopulations toward health (14) and the use of a single-visit approach to diagnosis and treatment of cervical cancer (15) may facilitate the effectiveness of screening in medically underserved women.

The techniques available for diagnosing endometrial cancer or ovarian cancer in asymptomatic women are far from ideal. The routine Papanicolaou smear is inadequate, and endometrial biopsy techniques have a sensitivity that ranges from 85% to 93% in the presence of vaginal bleeding (16). At this time, neither the American Cancer Society nor the NCI recommends the routine use of cytologic endometrial sampling as a routine screening test in perimenopausal and postmenopausal women with no symptoms (13). Although pelvic ultrasound and CA-125 tumor markers are used to diagnose cancer in women with a pelvic mass, these tests lack specificity and sensitivity for screening asymptomatic women. Based on a MEDLINE search, Carlson et al. (17) determined that the positive predictive value (PPV) of an abnormal ultrasound test is less than 1% for women at average risk and 2% for women with a history of ovarian cancer in one relative. The PPV of a positive CA-125 is 3% in women at average risk and 10% in women with one relative with ovarian cancer. There is general consensus that screening for ovarian cancer with ultrasound or CA-125 is not recommended for premenopausal and postmenopausal women without a family history of cancer or in women with a family history in one or more relatives without evidence of a hereditary cancer syndrome (18). Women from a family with one of the rare hereditary ovarian cancer syndromes should be referred to a specialized screening and counseling service for follow-up and evaluation (19).

Tertiary Prevention

Tertiary prevention seeks to decrease morbidity of established disease. The best example is the use of antiestrogen to prevent second breast cancer in women or cis-retinoic acid to delay second oral squamous-cell cancer in men and women with head and neck cancer. Some investigators have stretched tertiary prevention to include therapy that prevents metastasis; for example, the use of antiangiogenic treatments in patients with early-stage lung cancer.

This chapter stresses the scientific rationale for cancer chemoprevention, the planning and execution of chemoprevention trials, a description of potential cancer prevention agents, and a discussion of clinical trials in progress as it relates to gynecologic cancer prevention. The chapter ends with a discussion of future directions for chemoprevention of gynecologic cancer.

TUMOR CELL BIOLOGY

As the understanding of tumor cell biology expands, the development of general approaches to chemoprevention based on broad modification of overall exposure levels or diet is giving way to more refined and potentially more effective pharmacologic interventions. It is this understanding of the cellular transformation systems and the regulatory changes that are associated with abnormal growth and proliferation that will form the basis for designing new, effective chemoprevention agents (20).

Rather than a single initiating event, multiple changes in the cell genome acting in concert are required for the development of human cancer (21). Normal cells undergo initiation, promotion, clonal expansion, and progression in a stepwise process to transform into a malignant neoplasm (Fig. 8.1). If the carcinogenic factor is not detoxified or the damaged DNA is inadequately excised, initiation occurs with the conversion of a normal cell to its transformed counterpart. Initiation is a common event, but in the absence of a promoter, most initiated cells remain repressed during an individual's lifetime and never continue further through the subsequent stages of cancer development. The long latency period that characterizes human cancer is probably due to the requirement for multiple initiating or promoting events.

The next step in the multistage process of carcinogenesis is promotion, where repression of the initiated transformed cell is negated and the induction of cellular proliferation and hyperplasia occurs. Increased tumor incidence and/or shortened latency period to tumor appearance are the hallmarks of tumor promotion. Many chemical promoting agents modulate a designated receptor molecule or stimulate a ligand that modifies a specific region of DNA. Protein kinase C is the principal cellular receptor for the tumor promoter 12-O-tetradecanolylphorbol-13 acetate (TPA) (22). Endogenous steroid hormones probably function like tumor promoters over the lifetime in humans. These promoter receptor complexes alter genomic expression and select proliferative capabilities leading to clonal expansion. The number and type of genetic alterations that occur during initiation will influence the probability of initiated cells transforming into malignancy with each repeated cell replication. Promotion does not involve specific molecular changes in DNA structure, but rather affects the expression of the genome. Continued exposure to a promoting agent is necessary for the initiated cell to replicate, undergo clonal expansion, and proceed into the stage of progression. In the unique situation where an oncogenic virus infects the cell by its integration into the host genome, the stage of promotion is frequently bypassed with direct entry into the progression process.

Unlike initiation and promotion, which are substantially influenced by events external to the target cell, the factors that drive progression are largely the result of endogenous changes in the expanded clone of preneoplastic cells. Genetic changes in the mutated cells such as inactivation of tumor-suppressor genes and activation of proto-oncogenes result in alterations in growth control, defects in terminal differentiation, enhanced metastatic potential, and resistance to cytotoxicity (23). Some recent epidemiologic data suggest that progression may be affected by diet and tobacco carcinogens as well (24). The accumulation of genetic alterations that characterize progression from normal to neoplastic tissue has been delineated for colon cancer (25) and for hepatocellular carcinoma (26). The *p53* tumor-suppressor gene is mutated in malignant tumors of the lung, breast, brain, bladder, bowel, and liver. Normal *p53* function transiently arrests the cell cycle in G_1 or irreversibly results in programmed cell death (apoptosis); loss of *p53* activity can provide a distinct selective advantage to human tumors (27). During tumor progression, angiogenesis allows the tumor to grow beyond 1 to 2 mm in size. Eventually, the tumor cells will metastasize to distant tissues by disseminating through the vascular system.

INTRAEPITHELIAL NEOPLASIA

Intraepithelial neoplasia (IEN) is a noninvasive lesion that is generally recognized as moderate to severe dysplasia; it is on the causal pathway from normal tissue to cancer. It is further characterized by genetic abnormalities, loss of cellular control function, and some of the phenotypic hallmarks of invasive cancer. Cervical intraepithelial neoplasia (CIN) 2-3 is a prototypic example because it is a near-obligate cancer precursor, a risk marker for cancer, and a disease that requires surveillance (Pap smears) and treatment intervention (traditionally surgical excision) (28).

The term *dysplasia* is often used to refer to the morphologic alterations that characterize intraepithelial neoplasia: increased nuclear size, altered nuclear shape, increased nuclear stain uptake, nuclear pleomorphism, increased mitoses, altered mitoses, and disordered or absent maturation. Two of the major factors affecting the rate of progression of intraepithelial neoplasia are the cellular mutation rate, which is enhanced by environmental carcinogens, and the cellular proliferation rate, which is enhanced by agents that include sex hormones, inducers of chronic inflammation, and irritant chemicals that stimulate reactive hyperproliferation. Thus, a possible chemoprevention strategy for intraepithelial neoplasia in humans is to develop drug or drug combinations that will block mutagenic carcinogens and/or prevent epithelial hyperproliferation. Figure 8.1 integrates the concept of carcinogenesis, intraepithelial neoplasia, and cancer prevention.

FIELD CARCINOGENESIS

In 1953, Slaughter et al. (29) described multiple independent premalignant foci progressing concurrently and at different rates to form multiple second primary tumors (SPTs). He coined the term *field cancerization* for this process, which reflects an effect of carcinogenic exposure on a large epithelial surface or field. Other examples include solar ultraviolet radiation of the skin, bile acids and fatty acids in the colon, HPV infection of the anogenital and oral areas, and tobacco smoke carcinogens delivered to large areas of the upper aerodigestive tract and subsequently found in the bladder and cervix (30,31). The clinical magnitude of this problem is best illustrated by the 4% to 7% annual incidence of second primary tumors in patients with primary carcinoma of the head and neck and lung (32). According to field carcinogenesis theory, primary tumors and related SPTs result from progression of commonly initiated, although genetically different, premalignant lesions. Chung et al. (33) analyzed *p53* mutations in 31 patients with primary head and neck cancers and related STPs. Molecular support for the independent origin of the tumors is provided by two types of *p53* discordance: (a) the occurrence of *p53* mutations in one but not the other related primary tumor in 16 cases; and (b) the specifically distinct mutations of *p53* in primary tumors and SPTs in five cases.

MARKERS OF CARCINOGENESIS

Biomarkers are targets of assays that monitor critical aspects of the relevant tumor biology in a defined tumor system (34). Biomarkers have been proposed for use as surrogates or intermediate endpoints to the traditional clinical trial endpoints such as clinical response or cancer-related mortality

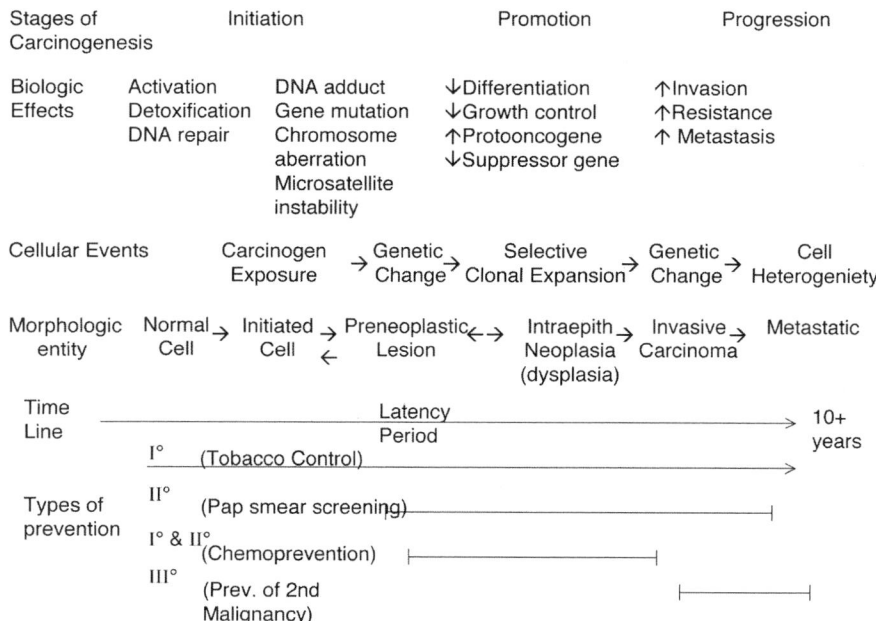

FIG. 8-1. Relationship of cancer causality and biology to prevention. The figure integrates hypothetical stages of carcinogens and biological effects commonly identified in animal models with cellular and morphological events that characterize many human epithelial neoplasms. These biological and pathological events have been superimposed on a theoretical time line that depicts a 10-year latency period. Examples of types of prevention (primary I°, secondary II°, or tertiary III°) are depicted. Thus, tobacco prevention/cessation is an effective intervention in patients at risk or with diagnosed epithelial neoplasms of the uterine cervix. On the other hand, Pap smear screening will identify women with IEN or early cancer. However, chemoprevention therapy has a narrower window of efficacy; for example, tamoxifen interrupts or reverses the progression of dysplasia or DCIS to invasive cancer and delays the appearance of a second breast cancer in the contralateral breast. (Based on schemas from Refs. 20, 21, and 22.)

because these traditional endpoints in prevention trials require protracted follow-up (35). Biomarkers have a number of applications for the management of individuals with cancer or at risk for cancer. A single biomarker or panels of individual biomarkers may be used to provide a clear picture of the state of cancer progression. Biomarker analysis can be used in a variety of other cancer-related applications, including risk or susceptibility assessment, early detection, prognostic determination, and disease progression. Ideally, a suitable biomarker should (a) be detectable in small tissue specimens that permit serial biopsies of the same site; (b) be expressed differently in normal than in high-risk or premalignant sites and in accordance with carcinogenic changes; (c) be subject to modulation by chemoprevention agents; and (d) have a low rate of spontaneous change (36).

Some biochemical or molecular events meet this definition, but to date no marker has been validated (i.e., shown to be a surrogate for a subsequent cancer outcome).

Table 8.1 is one classification schema for intermediate endpoint biomarkers (37). Traditionally, precancerous lesions such as polyps, leukoplakia, keratosis, or epithelial tissue dysplasia have served as macroscopic or microscopic evidence of the late stages of the carcinogenesis process. Elevated micronuclei in the aerodigestive tract and altered or increased proliferation markers such as proliferating cell nuclear antigen (PCNA) in the colon are consistent findings in high-risk individuals; however, studies to date indicate that measurement of both markers is associated with technical problems, possibly due to sampling error and random or spontaneous marker changes. In an attempt to find more specific markers, investigators are beginning to utilize molecular genetic techniques, such as those described by Fearon and Vogelstein (25), in the development and progression of dysplastic lesions leading to invasive colon carcinoma. One of these markers, *p53* mutation, is associated with an early stage of carcinogenesis in the aerodigestive tract, breast, and skin but marks later stage carcinogenesis in the colon and bladder.

A number of specialized biomarkers have been developed as targets for cancer prevention strategies. The lung cancer autocrine growth factor, gastrin-releasing peptide, appears to be critical to human fetal lung development and is found at only low levels of expression in normal individuals but at elevated levels in bronchial secretions and urine samples in smokers as well as in patients with resected lung cancers (38). The activity of the prostaglandin biosynthetic cascade has been used to monitor the effects of nonsteroidal antiinflammatory agents on epithelial tissue (39). Ornithine decar-

TABLE 8.1. *Candidate endpoint biomarkers*

Morphologic
  Uterine hyperplasia
  Colorectal adenoma
  Cervical intraepithelial neoplasm
  Prostatic intraepithelial neoplasm
  Ovarian microadenoma and epithelial invagination
  Nuclear morphometry; DNA ploidy
  Apoptosis TUNEL
Proliferation
  S-phase fraction
  Ki 67, MiB-1 antibody expression
  Proliferating cell nuclear antigen (PCNA)
  Bromdimyundine uptake
  DNA cytometry or immunohistochemical labeling
Differentiation
  Cell markers; e.g. keratin 17, vimentin
  Altered cell surface antigen expression
  Mucin or apomucin
  Cytokeratin
  Mn antigen
Genetic/Regulation
  Gene expression; e.g., *c-myc, c-ras*
  Growth factor; e.g., transforming growth factor-b
  Tumor suppressor; e.g., *p53*
  Loss of heterozygosity
  Microsatelites, RER
  DNA methylation
Biochemical
  Hormone level/metabolism
  ODC activity
  PSA
  HPV expression (16,18)

Source: Refs. 37 and 95.

boxylase (ODC) and polyamine levels are sensitive monitors of difluoromethylornithine (DFMO) intervention (40). The activity of the Phase II detoxification enzymes glutathione S-transferase and epoxide hydroxylase has served as an indicator of increased tissue risk for carcinogenesis and also as a model system for the study of anticarcinogens such as oltipraz (41).

Four areas of investigation appear particularly promising for the development of markers of cervical carcinogenesis (42). Investigators at the M. D. Anderson Hospital have studied the response of CIN (43,44) to DFMO and have found that subtle proliferative changes occur early, including a spatial dysregulation of epidermal growth-factor receptor (EGFR) expression (45). Second, Stanbridge and Liao and their coworkers (46,47) have identified a new marker, the Mn antigen, which seems to correlate with stages of progression. They have recently published a series of papers that show that this marker is an early diagnostic marker of cervical dysplasia and may be particularly valuable as an adjunct to cytologic diagnosis of atypical squamous cells of undetermined significance (ASCUS) and atypical glandular cells of undetermined significance (AGUS). Third, persistence of HPV has been shown to be an indicator of persistent disease

and so its detection (or absence) may be a useful marker of therapeutic effect (48,49). Finally, the profiling of differentially expressed genes in human primary cervical cancer by complementary DNA expression array opens up a broad vista of new markers to explore (50). A recent important advance has been the development of a model of human CIN in severe combined immunodeficiency (SCID) mice that should provide a useful experimental approach to the study of the biology of this lesion (51). Much work is necessary to validate the performance of these biochemical indicators as markers for high-risk individuals and surrogates for cancer activity. Once investigators have overcome the logistical and technical difficulties in obtaining and testing samples from the disease site under study, more specific markers of carcinogenesis may become available for future chemoprevention trials (52).

IDENTIFICATION OF CANDIDATE CHEMOPREVENTION AGENTS

The identification of agents with potential chemopreventive capacities is based on epidemiologic observation and laboratory animal studies (53). The initial agents used in chemoprevention were suggested by epidemiologic studies in which compounds that occur naturally in the diet were shown to be associated with decreased cancer incidence (e.g., vitamin A, selenium, and vitamin E) (1). More than 1,000 agents have been reported to inhibit the process of carcinogenesis; however, the number of compounds that have been thoroughly evaluated and advanced to clinical trials is much smaller.

The specific chemopreventive activities and structures are grouped into three general classes: antiproliferation, carcinogen-blocking agents, and antioxidants.

Antiproliferation Agents

Antiproliferatives comprise a diverse group of compounds including DFMO, antihormones, calcium, and retinoids. Decarboxylation of ornithine by the rate-limiting enzyme ornithine decarboxylase (ODC) is required for the biosynthesis of polyamines such as putrescine, spermine, and spermidine. Polyamines form noncovalent interactions with macromolecules such as nucleic acids and proteins, suggesting a necessary role in cellular proliferation and differentiation (54). DFMO alkylates ODC irreversibly, preventing conversion of ornithine to putrescine. Preclinical studies have established that DFMO has chemopreventive activity in several mouse and rat systems (55). Clinical studies have established the dose-limiting side effects of DFMO to include diarrhea, anemia, leukopenia, thrombocytopenia, and loss of hearing acuity. However, lower nontoxic doses may produce measurable lowering of the polyamine content in the bowel and prostate without the appearance of side effects (40).

One of the most widely studied antihormonal agents is

tamoxifen. Several mechanisms have been postulated for tamoxifen's antitumor effect, including (a) competition with estradiol for receptor sites in the nucleus, thereby leading to estrogen blockade; (b) modulation of the production of transforming growth factor-α and transforming growth factor-β, which are involved in cell proliferation; and (c) increase in sex hormone–binding globulin, thereby decreasing free-estrogen availability (56). Based on evidence in adjuvant trials of women with early-stage breast cancer that demonstrated a 38% reduction in new primary breast cancers with tamoxifen in comparison with placebo (57), the agent was proposed for primary prevention in women at high risk for breast cancer. Other effects of tamoxifen in the chemoprevention setting include potential beneficial effects on osteoporosis and atherosclerosis, but the development of second primary tumors of the uterus and liver is of concern (58).

Finasteride is a 5-α-reductase inhibitor that blocks the conversion of testosterone to dihydrotestosterone, which in turn is the major androgenic compound within the prostate gland. Preclinical studies have established a beneficial effect in reducing prostatic hypertrophy and in inhibiting human prostatic cancer cell lines. In a national trial, finasteride decreased benign prostatic hypertrophy in adult males with minimal or no toxicity (59). The initial analysis of the randomized double-blind placebo-controlled trial of finasteride for the prevention of prostatic carcinoma shows a 24.8% reduction in prevalence over a 7-year period (18.4% occurrence in the finasteride group versus 24.4% in the placebo group); however, the finasteride-treated men experienced more tumors of Gleason grade 7, 8, 9, or 10 (37%) than did the placebo group (22.2%). The investigators conclude that finasteride prevents or delays the appearance of prostatic cancer, but this possible benefit must be weighted against sexual side effects and the increased risk of high-grade prostatic cancer (60).

The retinoids include natural vitamin A (retinol) and the synthetic derivative fenretinoid (4-hydroxy-phenylretinamid, 4HPR). The retinoids control cell growth and differentiation at the level of gene expression through interaction with nuclear receptors (61). Preclinical studies demonstrate chemopreventive activity with the retinoids in mammary gland, bladder, and skin (62). Retinoids inhibit the proliferation and progression stages of carcinogenesis (63). They induce terminal differentiation in selected cells, stimulate intracellular communication, and are immunostimulants. Fenretinide (4-HPR) stimulates programmed cell death (apoptosis) (64,65). However, potential dose-related toxicity has been associated with the retinoids (i.e., vitamin A and its analogues accumulate in the liver and cause hepatic damage). They can also cause eye damage, and most relevant to the prevention of gynecologic cancers, they are teratogens. Several clinical trials using retinoids are underway or have been completed. 13-Cis-retinoic acid will suppress or reverse oral leukoplakia (66) and second primaries of the upper aero-digestive tract (67). Topical tretinoin 0.372% will reverse low-grade uterine cervical moderate dysplasia (68).

The chemopreventive potential of calcium was first shown by its protective effect against proliferation in the colon of patients at high risk for cancer (69). A total dose of 2,000 mg elemental calcium per day is the likely efficacious and nontoxic dose that can be recommended for people at risk for bowel cancer (70). A recently completed trial (71) demonstrated that calcium supplementation will delay or prevent adenomatous polyp formation in patients with previous colorectal cancer.

Blocking Agents

Carcinogen-blocking agents act by preventing the conversion of a procarcinogen into the active carcinogen. Examples include the inhibition of nitrosocarcinogen formation by ascorbic acid, α-tocopherol, and the phenols (72). However, the agents with the most potential in this class are agents that enhance carcinogen-detoxifying enzymes, especially the Phase II metabolic enzymes including glutathione s-transferases. Tallalay (73) has emphasized the desirability of selecting chemopreventive agents that induce mostly Phase II metabolic enzymes as opposed to compounds that induce both Phase I mixed-function oxidases and Phase II enzymes. Compounds whose chemopreventive activities fall into this classification include indoles, flavones, phenolic compounds, beta-carotene, ascorbic acid, vitamin E, selenium, oltipraz, and ellagic acid. Oltipraz [5-(2-pyrazinyl)-4-methyl-12-dithiol-3-thione] is a synthetic dithiolthione used to treat schistosomiasis in which glutathione depletion is fatal to the worm. The effects on the mammalian host are to increase glutathione levels and the activities of several Phase II detoxification enzymes including the glutathione S-transferases (74). In preclinical studies, oltipraz administered orally increases liver glutathione levels and induces enzymes involved in electrophile detoxification (i.e., glutathione s-transferases, epoxide hydrolase, and NAD(P)H quinone oxyreductase) (41,75). In Phase I clinical studies, oltipraz has low toxicity that includes photosensitivity, heat intolerance, altered taste, and gastrointestinal discomfort (76).

Antioxidants

The third class of inhibitors are the antioxidants such as beta-carotene, curcumin, N-acetyl-L-cystene, the nonsteroidal antiinflammatory drugs (NSAIDs), and polyphenols. These agents directly trap electrophilic sites on activated carcinogens, scavenge oxygen-free radicals, and organic-free radicals and terminate lipid peroxidation (77). Agents that enhance the Phase II metabolizing enzymes indirectly elevate the electrophile trapping potential by increased glutathione production and induction of the enzyme glutathione peroxidase. Antioxidant mechanisms may be both antimutagenic and antiproliferative (55).

Aspirin and the other NSAIDs inhibit the enzyme cyclooxygenase-2 (COX-2), which catalyzes the first step in conversion of arachidonic acid to the prostaglandins prostacycline and thromboxanes. The primary chemopreventive effect of cyclooxygenase inhibition is thought to be related to changes in tissue levels of these important biologic modifiers that play a role in cell proliferation, neoplasia, and immune response (78). In animal efficacy screens, the NSAIDs were active in rat colon, rat mammary gland, mouse bladder, and mouse skin, as well as in 1,2-dimethylhydrazine (DMH)–induced colon tumors in mice (55). Although preliminary clinical studies showed a response to high doses, sulindac in standard dose had no effect on colorectal adenomatous polyps in patients with familial adenomatous polyposis (79). However, daily use of aspirin 325 mg was associated with a significant reduction of colorectal adenomas in patients with previous colorectal cancer (80). Celecoxib, a specific COX-2 inhibitor, is approved by the Federal Food and Drug Adminiatration (FDA) for the management of adenomas in patients with familial adenomatous polyposis based on a phase III trial reported by Steinbach et al. (81). Although epidemiologic case-control studies suggest that aspirin or NSAIDs may reduce the risk of death from colon cancer, the only prospectively randomized control study of aspirin in male physicians failed to show an effect on colon cancer incidence and mortality (82). In clinical trials, beta-carotene has not been effective in preventing skin cancer (83), bowel polyps (84), or lung cancer deaths in U.S. or Finnish smokers (85,86).

With a better understanding of tumor cell biology, including an understanding of the changes in cellular genetics and a better understanding of proto-oncogenes and tumor-suppressor genes and their proteins, it may be possible to develop specific agents to target specified steps in the process of carcinogenesis (87). It may also become possible through the use of molecular genetics to identify the cancer-prone phenotype or genotype and thus target the intervention to those individuals at greatest risk of having the disease develop as well as those likely to respond to the drug in question. For instance, work on glutathione S-transferase μ indicates that people who inherit the null genotype are at greater risk for smoking-related cancers, but that they could also be the best candidates for therapy with blocking agents that enhance carcinogen-detoxifying enzymes (88).

The rationale for using a combination of chemopreventive agents is to increase efficacy and to reduce toxicity. As shown in Figure 8.2, the carcinogenic process could theoretically be interrupted or influenced by combining agents that affect different pathways; that is, decrease mutagenesis, increase differentiation, or increase apoptosis (89). Several combinations have shown synergism; that is, the inhibitory potency of the combination of agents is greater than the sum of the potencies of single agents. Synergistic chemopreventive activity has been reported for DFMO and piroxicam in rat colon (90) and 4-HPR and tamoxifen in rat mammary gland (91).

CHEMOPREVENTION TRIALS

Although oncologists' experience with chemotherapy treatment trials has helped in the design of chemoprevention research, there are key differences between these approaches. The differences relate primarily to the choice of agent or agents, the population under study, the study endpoints, and the relative risk/benefit of drug efficacy and toxicity. In contrast to treating individuals with the diagnosis of cancer, where significant toxicity is accepted, chemoprevention trials focus on individuals who do not have symptoms and where toxicity of any type tends to be unacceptable. Study subjects may be healthy individuals deemed to be at increased risk because of genetic susceptibility, lifestyle factors, exposure to known carcinogens, or preexisting medi-

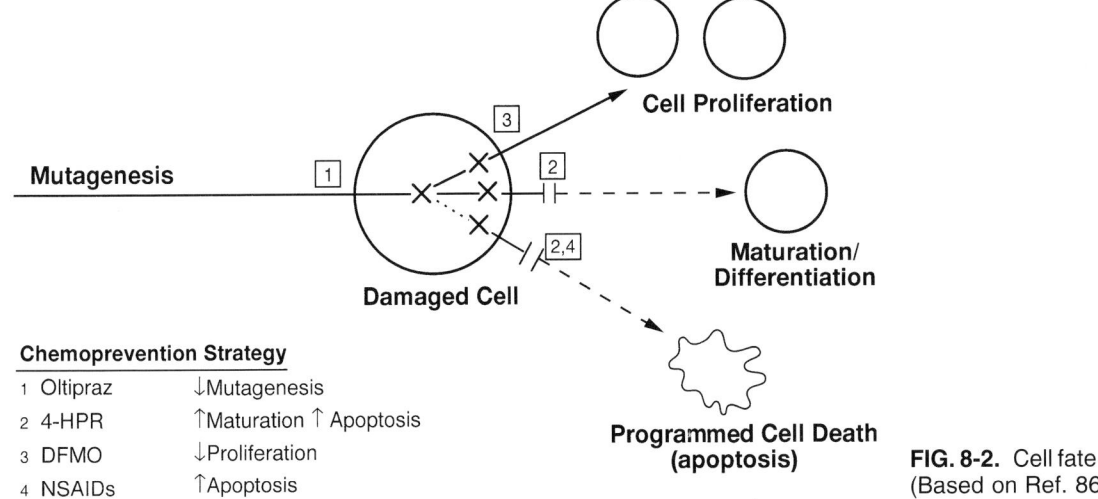

Chemoprevention Strategy

1	Oltipraz	↓Mutagenesis
2	4-HPR	↑Maturation ↑ Apoptosis
3	DFMO	↓Proliferation
4	NSAIDs	↑Apoptosis

FIG. 8-2. Cell fate and chemoprevention. (Based on Ref. 86.)

cal conditions that predispose to cancer. Another candidate population is composed of individuals with a previous diagnosis of cancer who are at increased risk for recurrence in the form of a second primary tumor or individuals with precancerous conditions. Recruitment to chemoprevention trials generally requires widespread community advertising and the collaboration of primary care and other nononcology specialists who have access to high-risk individuals, particularly ethnic minority populations (92). Compliance to chemoprevention interventions may decrease over time because these are healthy individuals who do not have a disease as a motivation for compliance in the trial, the duration of the intervention is frequently lengthy and requires maintenance of high enthusiasm over a long period of time, and because prevention trials involve medication plus complex behavioral and lifestyle changes (93).

As with cancer chemotherapy studies, clinical trials in chemoprevention can be classified as Phase I, II, or III (94). Phase I trials are primarily toxicity-pharmacokinetic studies of an agent after initial preclinical animal studies indicate useful activity. The objective of this phase is to assess incidence and significance of toxicity and to verify the effect on tissue biomarkers as well as to establish drug pharmacokinetics, tissue distribution, interactions, and metabolism. Phase II studies are conducted to establish activity using intermediate endpoint biomarkers rather than an invasive cancer endpoint. The size of the population for Phase II trials depends on the number of participants necessary to detect a statistically significant change in the study's chosen intermediate endpoint. After short-term activity is established, a Phase IIb or III trial is conducted to establish long-term efficacy in reducing cancer incidence. Phase III trials typically require thousands of subjects and 5 to 10 years or more to complete (95).

Table 8.2 is a list of NCI-sponsored randomized chemoprevention studies (64,71). Perhaps the most important study is the Breast Cancer Prevention Trial (P-1), which was implemented by the National Surgical Adjuvant Breast and Bowel Project (NSABP) (96). Tamoxifen reduced the risk of invasive breast cancer by 49% (two-sided $p <.00001$),

with a cumulative incidence through 69 months of follow-up of 43.4 versus 22.0 per 1,000 women in the placebo and tamoxifen groups, respectively. The decreased risk occurred over all age groups studied, among women with a history of lobular carcinoma or atypical hyperplasia, and in all categories of predicted 5-year risk. Tamoxifen also reduced the risk of noninvasive breast cancer by 50% (two-sided $p <.002$). Tamoxifen reduced the occurrence of estrogen receptor–positive tumors; however, no difference was observed in the occurrence of estrogen receptor–negative tumors. Secondary endpoints included no change in the annual rate of ischemic heart disease; a reduction in hip, radius, and spine fractures; an increase in endometrial cancer; and an increase in rates of stroke, pulmonary embolism, and deep vein thrombosis. The new NSABP chemoprevention trial, P-2, will compare the toxicity, risks, and benefits of the selected estrogen receptor modulator (SERM) raloxifen with those of tamoxifen.

SCIENTIFIC BASIS OF CHEMOPREVENTION IN GYNECOLOGIC CANCERS

A single scientific basis for a chemoprevention strategy in gynecologic cancers vis-à-vis a unifying hypothesis such as smoking-related damage in aerodigestive cancers is not possible because known etiologic and regulatory factors in cervical, ovarian, and endometrial cancers are quite different. Additionally, the types of studies done in the three cancers offer different levels of evidence. Only in cervical cancers have meaningful clinical prevention trials been done; therefore, the majority of the information about gynecologic cancers and prevention discussed here will relate to that malignancy. Sufficient information about ovarian cancer and etiologic factors has been gathered to allow a discussion of current and future issues regarding prevention.

CERVICAL, VAGINAL, AND VULVAR CANCER

Background

A unified approach to the scientific basis of chemoprevention in cervical cancer is shown in Figure 8.3. Prema-

TABLE 8.2. *Randomized chemoprevention trials (other than gynecologic cancer)*

Study Population	Intervention	No. of Subjects	Endpoint	Result	RR (95% CI)
High-risk women	Tamoxifen	13,388	Breast cancer	+	0.51 (0.39–0.66)
Men and women	Retinol	2,297	Skin scc	+	0.74 (0.56–0.99)
Resected adenoma patients	Ca^{2+}	930	Colon adenomas	+	0.81 (0.67–0.99)
Elderly patients	Selenium	1,312	Skin scc	NS	1.10 (0.95–1.20)
Linxian population	Retinol + zinc	29,584	All cancers	NS	1.00 (0.89–1.11)
Male physicians	β-carotene	22,071	All cancers	NS	0.98 (0.91–1.06)
High-risk males	Finasteride	18,000	Prostatic cancer	+	0.75 (0.64–0.81)
Finnish smokers	β-carotene	29,133	Lung cancer	—	1.16 (1.02–1.33)
Shipyard workers/smokers	β-carotene + retinol	18,314	Lung cancer	—	1.28 (1.04–1.57)

RR, relative risk; scc, squamous-cell carcinoma.
Source: Refs. 64 and 71.

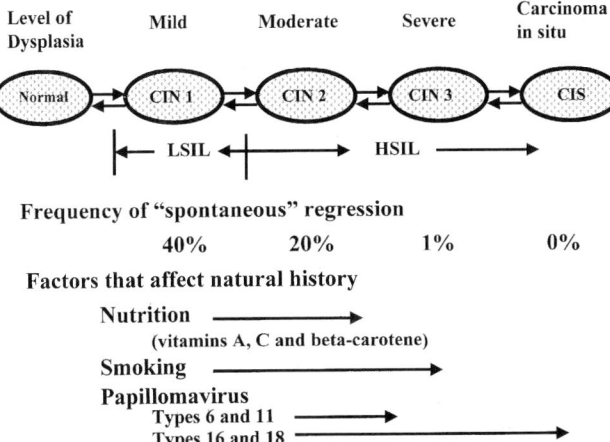

FIG. 8-3. Factors affecting cervical cancer carcinogenesis. The natural history of cervical cancer initiation, promotion, and progression is complex. The transition from one level to the next is not inevitable and a real "spontaneous" remission rate is evident that decreases in frequency as the lesion progresses. Both human papillomaviruses and mutagenic products from tobacco (e.g., cigarette smoking) play a role. Inflammation, other viruses, and nutrition also are likely to be involved in affecting the outcome.

lignant changes form a continuum divided into low- and high-grade squamous intraepithelial lesion (SIL) or cervical, vaginal, or vulvar intraepithelial neoplasia (CIN) 1, 2, and 3, which is largely equivalent to the older nosology of mild, moderate, and severe dysplasia (97). These lesions can persist, regress, or progress to an invasive malignancy. For the purposes of discussion of the carcinogenic process, we find the designation CIN to be most relevant because this classification takes into account colposcopic, cytologic, and biopsy results, whereas the SIL designation represents the reporting of Papanicolaou smears using the Bethesda system of cytologic grading (11). The phenotypic expression of the disease process as represented by histologic changes, its interaction with biologic features such as HPVs, and risk conveyed by various epidemiologic factors such as nutrient status and smoking are primarily represented and shown in relationship to the generalized carcinogenesis process. CIN is an excellent example of the potential to develop intermediate markers of cancer risk, which is a topic discussed extensively by us and others (98,99). For example, changes in cellular retinoid-binding proteins may be a feature of disease progression (100).

Etiologic Factors

In other histologic types of cancer, heritable or acquired changes in genes are a prominent feature of the disease process (25); to date, such alterations have not been a consistently described feature of cervical cancer development. The location of a family at heritable risk for cervical, vaginal,

or vulvar cancer would be an important contribution since analysis might allow identification of genes important to the development of these cancers. A number of external risk factors such as exposure to HPV, cigarette smoking, and nutrient deficiencies contribute to the development of CIN and cervical, vaginal, or vulvar cancer (101–104).

A remarkable achievement in the last decade has been the convincing demonstration evolving from experimental, clinical, and epidemiologic studies that HPVs are important in the development of cervical, vaginal, or vulvar cancer (30,105,106). In particular, HPV isotypes 6 and 11 appear to be present but unintegrated in CIN 1 and 2, whereas types 16 and 18 can become integrated and fully transform cervical epithelial cells (107). Epidemiologic studies have now clearly demonstrated that certain subtypes of HPV are the major risk factor for cervical cancer, with high relative risks for subtypes 16 and 18 and lower risks for subtypes 6 and 11 (30). The recent identification of subtype variants of HPV 16 that have different potential for oncogenicity should also refine the population of women at high risk (108,109). This is particularly germane to the current discussion inasmuch as HPVs express two transformation proteins (E_6 and E_7) that bind different important regulatory gene products, retinoblastoma (RB) protein and p53, respectively (110, 111). The binding and inactivation of these two tumor-suppressor gene products probably contribute to the increased proliferation seen in CIN, a status that conveys an increased chance for carcinogenic damage, mutation, and, consequently, progression of the disease (112). p53 may play a unique role in cervical carcinogenesis as well (113). This gene is polymorphic at amino acid 72 of the protein that it encodes. Storey et al. (114) have found that the arginine form of p53 is more susceptible to degradation by the HPV E_6 protein than is the proline variant. These investigators also report that patients with two copies of the arginine variant have a sevenfold higher risk of developing cervical cancer than individuals with the proline form. Other researchers, however, dispute these claims (115). Recent work by a number of laboratories also suggests that loss of heterozygosity in chromosomes 3p, 4p, 4q, and 11q is a common event during cervical carcinogenesis and that other and to be discovered tumor-suppressor genes are involved (116).

Evidence strongly implicates smoking as an independent risk factor in the development of cervical cancer (4). Two lines of evidence support this supposition: biological/biochemical and epidemiologic. First, the mucous secretions of the uterine cervix among smokers contains nicotine and cotinine as well as mutagenic activity (117). Second, a series of epidemiologic investigations suggests that cigarette smoking usage is related to CIN and cervical cancers: Sood (118) has done a careful meta-analysis of the subject and estimates that the available studies suggest a 42% to 46% increase in cervical cancer among smokers even after controlling for age and number of sexual partners. One study suggests that smoking has a greater effect on later stages of the carcinogenic process; risk for CIN 3, but not 2, increased with the number of cigarettes smoked per day (119). In a 10-year prospective study of cervical dysplasia, tobacco smoking was associated with a two- to fourfold increased risk of CIN 3 and invasive cancer in those women also infected with oncogenic HPV (120). Experience in patients with other cancers indicates that patients can be successfully encouraged to stop smoking. Because the cost of a physician-delivered smoking-cessation message is low and the potential benefits high, this preventive approach should be more commonly adopted in everyday practice.

The question of the role of diet and nutrition in the etiology of cervical, vaginal, or vulvar cancer is not yet resolved (121,122). Based on metabolic and epidemiologic data, insufficient intake of riboflavin, folic acid, vitamin A, beta-carotene, and vitamin C may convey an increased risk for CIN and cervical cancer. The status of vitamin nutriture also seems to have a role in the development of CIN and cervical cancer as determined by various epidemiologic studies (123–125) Vitamins A, C, and E, beta-carotene, and folic acid have a protective role. Individuals who have low dietary intake of these nutrients or who have low serum levels are at increased risk for CIN and cervical cancer. The relationship seems particularly strong for beta-carotenes and vitamin C.

Although the clinical natural history of CIN and cervical cancer has been known for quite some time and detailed since the advent of colposcopy, the biology of the disease process has been little studied until recently; largely limited by the unavailability of an appropriate model or experimental human systems. Although cell lines of cervical cancer are widely available (e.g., HeLa), CIN lines are only recently being developed. The effect of HPV on epithelial cell lines has been examined and transformation occurs under appropriate conditions (107). Additionally, retinoids enhance the nutriture of HPV-infected epithelial cells in culture (126).

Chemoprevention Trials

The biology and epidemiology of CIN provides ample opportunities for preventive strategies. Despite the increasing incidence of the disease throughout the world, especially in Latin America and the Indian subcontinent, the number of active prevention trials with intervention intent has been limited (127). The status of currently completed studies is provided in Table 8.3.

Folic Acid

Epidemiologic studies have indicated that a deficiency in folate might play a role in the etiology of cervical cancer. Several reports suggested a protective role for folate in the etiology of cervical neoplasms (128–130). Whitehead et al. (131) demonstrated that supplementation with 10 mg of daily oral folic acid reversed the megaloblastic features observed on Papanicolaou smears taken from users of oral contraceptives. Because the cytologic changes were not associated with evidence of systemic folate deficiency, these investigators postulated the existence of localized folate deficiency in the cervix as a result of oral contraceptive use. Subsequently, Butterworth et al. (128) investigated the possibility of a relationship between folate and oral contraceptives and CIN. Their initial study in oral contraceptive users demonstrated a statistically significant improvement of CIN 1 and CIN 2 in subjects treated with 10 mg of folic acid orally for 3 months. This study also reported a statistically significant lower mean red blood cell (RBC) folate concentration in oral contraceptive users compared with nonusers. Even lower RBC folate concentration levels were seen in oral contraceptive users with CIN compared with oral contraceptive users without CIN. However, two large randomized intervention trials have conclusively demonstrated that supplementation with folic acid does not enhance regression of CIN 1 and 2 over a 3- to 6-month time period (132,133). Both trials used subjects who already had a premalignant condition (CIN) and did not address whether folate deficiency corrected prior to the development of histologic changes would alter the eventual outcome; future trials will need to be designed differently to address this critical question. For example, women without CIN seen in a sexually transmitted disease clinic might be a good study population.

Retinoids

Retinoids are potent stimulators of the cellular response and affect the biologic functions of a variety of organs and tissues. Both in vitro and in vivo, retinoids modulate the growth of normal epithelial cells; in general slowing or inhibiting proliferation and enhancing differentiation and maturation of cells and tissues (61,134) Many epidemiologic studies have demonstrated a protective effect of vitamin A

TABLE 8.3. *Randomized clinical trials of chemoprevention of cervical cancer*

Target Completed Studies	Agent	Phase	No. of Cases	Results	Reference
CIN 1–2	Folic acid	III	335	No effect on regression rate	132
CIN 1–2	Folic acid	III	331	No effect on regression rate	133
CIN 2–3	Retinoic acid (topical)	III	301	Increased rate of regression of CIN 2 but not 3	68
CIN 1–2	β-carotene	III	69	No effect on regression rate	138
CIN 2–3	β-carotene	III	125	No effect on regression rate	139

against smoking-related tumors including cervical dysplasia and cancer (135). These observations supported the notion that vitamin A may affect the natural history of CIN and cervical malignancy (136).

Two main types of natural vitamin A exist: the precursor form as the carotenoids like beta-carotene, which are found in green leafy vegetables, and the preformed vitamin A, usually in the form of retinal, retinol, and retinyl ester, which is found in fish, liver, and fortified milk. The natural vitamin A compound, beta-carotene, has the advantage of not possessing the teratogenic toxicity profile of some of its synthetic counterparts. Manetta et al. completed a nonrandomized Phase II clinical trial in 30 women with mild to moderate dysplasia who took 30 mg of beta-carotene daily for 6 months (137). Sixty percent of the cervical lesions had regressed at 3 months, 70% at 6 months, and 33% at 12 months. After adjusting for patients with complete responses who dropped out of the study at 6 months, they estimated a true response of 43%. However, several large Phase III studies of beta-carotene supplementation in CIN have been completed and have shown no effect on regression (138, 139).

We conducted a series of preclinical studies using synthetic *trans*-retinoic acid (RA) and explored the feasibility of an optimal local delievery method to the uterine cervix (140,141). The device consisted of a cervical cap and collagen sponge insert within which the RA was placed. A Phase I trial was carried out, and a toxic dose was defined. The distribution of responses in the Phase I study suggested a dose-response effect (142,143). Based on this experience, the next lower dose, which was well tolerated, was chosen for use in a subsequent Phase II investigation. A Phase II trial including 20 patients demonstrated an encouraging complete clinical response rate of 50% for CIN (144). On the basis of these results, we designed and completed a randomized Phase III trial of topical RA in placebo cream versus placebo cream in patients with CIN 2 and 3. The investigation involved 301 participants and was carefully conducted, with comparison of endpoint to entry biopsy as the definitive comparison (68); the key results from the trial are shown in Table 8.4. RA increased the regression rate of moderate but

not severe dysplasia. Early experience with another retinoid (RII retinamide) given orally appears to be favorable as well (145).

Future Directions

Several other chemopreventive agents are also in clinical trial. These include the oral polyamine synthesis inhibitor difluoromethylornithine (DFMO) and fenretinide (4-HPR); both of these compounds have demonstrated substantial activity as inhibitors of carcinogenesis in many preclinical systems (55,146). Early studies with DFMO indicate that it can reduce polyamine levels in humans (68,147). Fenretinide 200 mg/day was not active compared to placebo in the treatment of high-grade cervical intraepithelial neoplasia (CIN 2 or 3) (148). Newer techniques to visualize the cervix such as three-dimensional light scattering may provide investigators with a more sensitive tool to quantify dysplastic cells in the epithelium (149).

The recent development of experimental models of cervical epithelium should allow more rapid understanding of the biology of CIN (150). The basic biology of HPV infection of cervical cells points toward several potential novel approaches (126). The most prominently being discussed is the development of an HPV-directed vaccine (151–153). These include blocking of the inactivation of *Rb* and *p53* by E_6 and E_7 using synthetic peptide inhibitors and vaccination against the HPV utilizing cytolytic T-lymphocyte recognition of E_6 and E_7 protein presented in association with class I molecules. Additionally, mediation of transforming growth factors may be important (126). In a Phase I clinical trial, a lipidated epitope of HPV 76–E_7 converted $CD8^+$ T-lymphocyte (CTL) response from unreactive to reactive in two of three evaluable patients with refractory cervical cancer (154). Several strategies are currently being explored to treat early-stage cervical cancer utilizing the immune system of the patient to detect and destroy cancer cells (tertiary prevention). Immune and antiviral responses to HPV 16 have been observed in Phase I clinical trials after vaccination of women with CIN lesions directly with an HLA-A-2–binding HPV 16 peptide (155). Another strategy is based on immunization of patients with their own dendritic cells; these dendritic cells can be generated in culture and loaded with a viral protein expressed by their tumor. After reinfusion back into the patient, these dentritic cells activate T cells so that they recognize and destroy the tumor (156).

Primary prevention of cervical cancer theoretically became possible when papillomavirus-like particles were created in the laboratory (157). Virus-like particles are devoid of DNA and are noninfectious. However, they mimic the natural structure of the virion and generate a potent immune response (158). Koutsky et al. (159) reported the results of a double-blind study which assigned women aged 16 to 23 years who were negative for HPV 16 DNA antibodies to placebo or HPV 16 virus-like particle vaccine given at day

TABLE 8.4. *Comparison of endpoint to entry biopsy in participants with CIN*

Dysplasia	Intervention	Regression[a]	Other[b]
Moderate	Retinoic acid	32 (43%) $p = .04$	43
	Placebo	18 (27%)	48
Severe	Retenoic acid	10 (25%) NS	30
	Placebo	16 (31%)	35

[a] Complete biopsy response (or endocervical curettage if biopsy not available).
[b] No response of CIN upstages.
NS = not specified
Source: Ref. 39.

0, month 2, and month 6. Biopsy tissue was evaluated for CIN and HPV 16 DNA. After 17.4 months median follow-up, the incidence of HPV 16 infection was 3.8 per 100 women years in the placebo group and 0 per 100 women years in the vaccine group (100% efficacy). Furthermore, all nine cases of HPV 16–related CIN occurred in the placebo group.

Nearly 20 types of HPV have been associated with cervical, vaginal, or vulvar cancer, and vaccination against one type will not protect against infection caused by another. It has been estimated that if types 16, 18, 31, 33, and 45 were included in a vaccination program, there would be an 85% decline in the risk of cancer, and a 45% to 70% decrease in the frequency of abnormal Pap smear attributable to HPV (160). Furthermore, if all sexually active women who are at risk for HPV were targeted, there would be a consequent favorable effect on neoplasms of the vulva and penis (161). It is premature to calculate the cost/benefit ratio of HPV vaccination; however, it would have a substantial effect on health system costs. Moreover, if the benefits of HPV vaccine are realized, especially in Third World countries, its effect could rival the benefit that hepatitis B vaccine has had on hepatitis and hepatocellular cancer in Taiwan (162).

ENDOMETRIAL CANCER

Endometrial carcinoma is the most common invasive gynecologic cancer in U.S. women, with approximately 40,100 new cases occurring in 2003 (163). However, the last three decades of the twentieth century have witnessed a 25% decrease in incidence and mortality from this disease. This favorable downturn almost certainly relates to the decreased use of unopposed estrogen replacement therapy. The initial case-control report of an association between estrogen replacement therapy and endometrial cancer appeared in 1975 (164). A number of confirmatory studies indicated that the risk of developing endometrial cancer increased with the duration of use, and that the risk could persist for more than 10 years after discontinuation (165,166). It was also known that progestational agents could successfully treat early endometrial cancer and could reverse the hyperplasia induced by estrogen therapy. The randomized controlled study of postmenopausal estrogen/progestin intervention (PEPI trial) (167) showed conclusively that combining a progestin with estrogen blocked the formation of endometrial hyperplasia and invasive carcinoma.

More recently, medical investigators have identified an association between endometrial cancer and the antiestrogen tamoxifen. Fornander et al. (168) reported in 1989 that second primary endometrial cancers occurred with a relative risk of 6.4 in patients treated as part of a randomized Swedish study of adjuvant breast cancer utilizing 40 mg of tamoxifen daily for 2 to 5 years. The NSABP B-14 trial comparing tamoxifen to placebo as adjuvant therapy for women with

node-negative estrogen receptor–positive breast cancer showed the hazard of developing endometrial cancer in 1,400 patients was 1.6 per 1,000 per year (58). There is conflicting evidence as to whether tamoxifen is associated with high-grade lesions that are potentially life threatening or whether the majority of the cases are a more low-grade superficial carcinoma (169). In the first analysis of the Breast Cancer Prevention Trial, where 13,400 subjects were randomized to tamoxifen versus a placebo for at least 5 years, the 50% reduction in invasive and preinvasive breast carcinoma in the tamoxifen arm was partially offset by a 10% increase in stage I endometrial cancer (96).

The estrogen-like effects in the uterus occur because tamoxifen binds AP-1 estrogen receptor ligands in endometrium cell nuclei, which stimulates c-*myc* and c-*fos* expression (170). For this reason, clinical investigators plan to study other SERMs in order to identify agents with less estrogenic effect on the uterus and, therefore, less risk of endometrial cancer. Raloxifene, a second-generation SERM, is approved for prophylaxis against postmenopausal osteoporosis and reportedly does not have an estrogenic effect on the uterus.

In addition to dose and duration of estrogen, other risk factors for endometrial cancer include obesity, high-fat diet, and reproductive factors such as nulliparity, early menarche, and late menopause. Women with the hereditary nonpolyposis colon cancer (HNPC) genetic abnormality have a tenfold increased risk of endometrial cancer compared with the general population and a cumulative lifetime risk of endometrial cancer of 20% (171).

Routine screening of women for endometrial cancer is not of any proven benefit. No screening test has been proven to be sufficiently acceptable or to decrease mortality (16). The Pap test used successfully for screening for cervical cancer lacks sensitivity for detection of endometrial cancer to be used as a screening technique (172). Because of the risk for endometrial hyperplasia and invasive adenocarcinoma in women taking tamoxifen, annual pelvic and rectal examinations have been recommended for these patients along with transvaginal sonography to detect endometrial hyperplasia (173). Although a portion of the women on the Breast Cancer Prevention Study were randomized to annual screening with transvaginal ultrasound and annual endometrial sampling, there were not sufficient cases to establish the benefits of this strategy.

OVARIAN CANCER

Background

A model for ovarian carcinoma carcinogenesis is shown in Figure 8.4. Primary prevention of ovarian cancer may well be approachable (174). In contrast to cervical cancer, there are considerable data suggesting involvement of a fa-

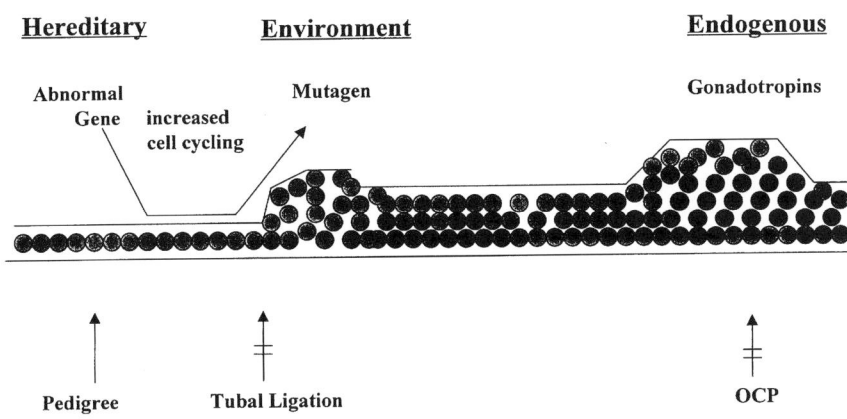

Hereditary **Environment** **Endogenous**

FIG. 8-4. Factors affecting ovarian carcinoma carcinogenesis. Three major features probably contribute to the development of ovarian cancer: abnormal genes acquired through hereditary, exogenous mutagens (e.g., talc or other), and uninterrupted exposure to gonadotropins. These three factors lead to a hyperproliferative state of the germinal epithelium; acquired genetic damage occurs more readily, and transformation occurs. An appreciation of the hereditable risk (pedigree), abrogation of mutagen exposure, and decreased gonadotropin levels should lead to a decreased risk for ovarian cancer.

milial or genetic component (175). Classic genetic pedigree studies have demonstrated three ovarian cancer syndromes with incomplete penetrance and variable prognosis. More recently, the *BRCA1* gene has been shown to segregate in a high proportion of families with a high risk of breast and ovarian cancers. Identification of women at a higher risk for ovarian cancer based on pedigree analysis and/or genetic linkage to *BRCA1* should allow identification of a cohort of women for preventive intervention.

There also are clearly a number of external factors including oral contraceptives and tubal ligation and perhaps other factors that mediate disease risk (176). In almost all systems, excess or inappropriate proliferation is a critical and necessary component in the early pathogenesis of cancer. Epidemiologic data strongly support a protective role of oral contraceptives against the development of ovarian cancer (177, 178), including preparations with low doses of hormones (179). Only a limited number of studies have examined the effect of hormone replacement therapy on ovarian cancer development. In the largest investigation reported to date, a cohort study of 44,241 participants in the Breast Cancer Detection and Demonstration Project (329 cases of ovarian cancer), estrogen-only (but not combined estrogen-progesterone) use was associated with a modest increased relative risk of ovarian cancer (180). A large prospective cohort study of 3,000,537 women (1,511 deaths from ovarian cancer) showed that mortality rates from ovarian cancer were significantly increased in overweight and obese women who have never used hormone replacement therapy (181). These observations suggest that uninterrupted ovulation plays a role in ovarian carcinogenesis either through repeated damage to the germinal epithelium during ovulation (without physiologic rest), increased gonadotropin levels, or both.

Tubal ligation or hysterectomy protects against the development of ovarian cancer (182); implying that access of a carcinogen or other factor to the ovary has been blocked. All six epidemiologic studies have shown a protective effect of tubal ligation against ovarian cancer development. To date, only talc has been implicated as a potential carcinogen

(183). It would be of considerable interest to conduct an epidemiologic study of the relationship of HPV exposure, other viruses, and ovarian cancer, but this has not yet been reported.

The evidence for other cultural factors having a role in ovarian cancer carcinogenesis is unsupported (184). Fertility drug usage and a high-fat diet and milk ingestion may have some role, but the positive associations are weak (185–187).

Prevention Studies

A biologic model for ovarian carcinogenesis in which hereditable genetic changes, inappropriate proliferation, and exposure to low doses of a carcinogen play a role is useful in developing an approach to the prevention of ovarian cancer.

Thorough pedigrees on all women with a clinical or family history of ovarian or breast cancer should be obtained (188). Information about prostatic cancer in male relatives should also be collected because an association with this hormone-dependent cancer may exist as well. Depending on the risk assessed by analysis of the disease genealogy and age of the woman, oral contraception, tubal ligation, or oophorectomy may be considered. The evidence supporting these approaches as preventive strategies is substantial. Many studies have demonstrated a decrease in ovarian cancer risk in women who take oral contraceptives (189). The reduction in risk increases with duration of usage, approaching 40% to 50% after 5 years, and occurs among both nulliparous and multiparous women. Importantly, a recent study indicates that this protective effect is conveyed by low-dose oral contraceptives as well (179). Narod et al. (190) evaluated 270 women with a *BRCA1* or *BRCA2* mutation and 161 of their sisters in a case-control study. The adjusted odds ratio for ovarian cancer associated with any past use of oral contraceptives was 0.5, and the risk decreased with prolonged duration of use. However, there is insufficient evidence to determine if chronic tamoxifen therapy will delay or prevent ovarian cancer (191). Several studies have suggested that tubal ligation reduces the risk for ovarian cancer; the

Nurse's Health Study demonstrated a 33% decrease in risk of ovarian cancer among women who underwent tubal sterilization (182). In this regard, the results of a randomized study of the effects of ethinyl estradiol, the oral contraceptive Triphasil, levonorgestrel (a progestin), or placebo on the ovarian epithelium of the primate macaques is of considerable interest (192). Apoptosis in the ovarian epithelium was increased sixfold in the progestin-treated group, whereas a lesser effect was seen in the oral contraceptive–treated group. No change from baseline was seen in the control or estrogen-treated group. If these results can be verified in human populations, then the development of a safe chemopreventive agent for women at high risk for ovarian cancer may be possible.

Prophylactic oophorectomy is a subject of some controversy. It has been estimated that 700 prophylactic oophorectomies would need to be performed in average-risk women to prevent one case of ovarian cancer (193). A person's age, medical history, reproductive plan, and proximity to menopause must be considered when trying to make an informed decision. In general, women older than age 50 years are encouraged to undergo the procedure, since the risk of ovarian cancer increases with age. Women who are less than age 50 years but greater than 40 years old should be counseled on the risk and benefits associated with surgical menopause and subsequent hormone replacement, as well as the risk of developing ovarian cancer based on their pedigree. Women who are being operated on for bowel cancer, especially if they are carriers of the HNPCC gene, should have a prophylactic hysterectomy and oophorectomy (194). Women with one of the three hereditary ovarian cancer syndromes should strongly consider oophorectomy at age 35 years or at the completion of childbearing (195). Rebbeck et al. (196) studied 551 women with disease-associated germline *BRCA1* or *BRCA2* mutations. They determined the incidence of ovarian cancer in 259 who had prophylactic oophorectomy and 292 matched controls who had not undergone the procedure. Of the women who had surgery, six (2.3%) received a diagnosis of stage I ovarian cancer at the time of the procedure and two developed peritoneal carcinoma 3.8 and 8.6 years after bilateral oophorectomy. Among the controls, 58 women (19.9%) developed ovarian cancer with a mean follow-up of 8.8 years. Kauff et al. (197) followed 170 *BRCA* carriers for an average of 2 years. They observed one peritoneal cancer among 98 women who chose salpingo-oophorectomy versus five ovarian/peritoneal cancers in 72 women with intact ovaries. In these genetically predisposed women, prophylactic oophorectomy reduces epithelial ovarian cancer (and breast cancer), although they should be counseled about the small risk of abdominal carcinomatosis (198). Schrag et al. performed an interesting decision analysis in order to determine the effect of prophylactic oophorectomy on life expectancy on women with *BRCA1–2* mutations. Their analysis suggested that a woman could delay oophorectomy until she was 40 years old with minimal loss of life expectancy (199).

Chemoprevention

Epidemiologic studies suggest that the use of the oral contraceptive pill for 5 years will significantly reduce the risk of developing ovarian cancer (189). This decreased risk can be observed for at least 10 years after discontinuing the pill. The most likely mechanism of action is by decreasing the frequency of ovulation and, thus, the mutagenic effects of cellular proliferation and entrapment of the ovarian epithelium within the stroma. There has been no randomized study of oral contraceptives with ovarian dysplasia or cancer as an endpoint.

Recent studies by Rodriguez-Burford et al. (200) show that acetylsalicylic acid, acetaminophen, and a COX-2 inhibitor separately can decrease the growth of fully transformed human epithelial ovarian cancer cells. In contrast to bowel cancer cells, the human epithelial ovarian cancer cells expressed COX-1 and COX-2 at low levels, suggesting that acetaminophen may be exerting its effects through a non–COX-2–dependent mechanism such as decreased ovulation (201).

DePalo et al. completed a preliminary analysis of women with T1-T2 breast cancer who were randomized to oral 4-hydroxyfenretinide or placebo (202). Six cases of ovarian cancer were diagnosed in the placebo versus none in the treated group ($p = .02$). Long-term follow-up has shown no significant difference between the two groups once the intervention was stopped. However, fenretinide and its derivatives continue to have considerable appeal; further studies should clarify the role that this vitamin A derivative may play in the chemoprevention of ovarian cancer (203). The Gynecologic Oncology Group and the Ovarian SPORE (Special Program of Research Excellence) investigators have set up a Clinical Trials Group to study chemoprevention agents in patients who are scheduled to undergo prophylactic oophorectomy. Investigators await the discovery of a recognizable intraepithelial neoplastic condition that can be diagnosed clinically in high-risk women (204).

Future Considerations

Despite the problems associated with active preventive intervention, these approaches should be the linchpin to lowering morbidity and mortality from ovarian carcinoma. Early detection through population-based screening has not proven to be effective in the management of ovarian cancer, and despite aggressive operative approaches and intensive chemotherapy, the 5-year survival rate remains less than 35%. Advances in the molecular genetics of ovarian cancer and the application of proteomic analysis to serum screening for ovarian cancer biomarkers (205) may allow clinicians to identify those women who are high or imminent risk for malignancy and therefore appropriate candidates for active preventive interventions.

REFERENCES

1. Greenwald P, Nixon DW, Malone WF, et al. Concepts in cancer chemoprevention research. *Cancer* 1990;65:1483.
2. Doll R, Peto R. *The causes of cancer: quantitative estimates of avoidable risk of cancer in the United States today.* Oxford, UK: Oxford University Press, 1981.
3. Vargas PA, Alberts DS. Primary prevention of colorectal cancer through dietary modification. *Cancer* 1992;70:1229.
4. Albanes D. Caloric intake, body weight and cancer: a review. *Nutr Cancer* 1987;9:199–217.
5. LeMarchand L. Anthropometry, body composition and cancer. In: Micozzi M, Moon T, eds. *Macronutrients: investigating their role in cancer.* New York: Marcel Dekker, 1992:321.
6. Sporn MB, Roberts AB. Role of retinoids in differentiation and carcinogenesis. *J Natl Cancer Inst* 1984;73:1381.
7. Willett WC, MacMahon B. Diet and cancer—an overview. *N Engl J Med* 1984;310:633.
8. Mandelblatt J, Gopaul I, Wistreich M. Gynecological care of elderly women: another look at Papanicolaou smear testing. *JAMA* 1986;256:367.
9. Eddy DM. Screening for cervical cancer. *Ann Intern Med* 1990;113:214.
10. Koss LG. Cervical (Pap) smear: new directions. *Cancer* 1993;71:1406.
11. Koss LG. The new Bethesda system for reporting results of smears of the uterine cervix. *J Natl Cancer Inst* 1990;82:988.
12. Koss LG. Cytologic and histologic manifestations of human papilloma virus infection of the female genital tract and their clinical significance. *Cancer* 1987;60:1942.
13. Averette HE, Steren A, Nguyen HN. Screening in gynecologic cancers. *Cancer* 1993;72:1043.
14. McPhee SJ, Stewart S, Brock KC, et al. Factors associated with breast and cervical cancer screening practices among Vietnamese American women. *Cancer Detect Prev* 1997;21:510.
15. Burger RA, Monk BJ, Van Nostrand KM, et al. Single-visit program for cervical cancer prevention in high-risk population. *Obstet Gynecol* 1995;86:491.
16. Pritchard KI. Screening for endometrial cancer: is it effective? *Ann Intern Med* 1989;110:177.
17. Carlson KJ, Skates SJ, Singer DE. Screening for ovarian cancer. *Ann Intern Med* 1994;121:124.
18. Ovarian cancer: screening, treatment and followup. NIH Consensus Statement 1994 Apr 5–7;12:1.
19. ACOG Committee Opinion: Committee on Gynecologic Practice. Genetic risk and screening techniques for epithelial ovarian cancer. 1992(December):No. 117.
20. Meyskens FL. Thinking about cancer causality and chemoprevention. *J Natl Cancer Inst* 1988;80:1278.
21. Shields PG, Harris CC. Molecular epidemiology and the genetics of environmental cancer. *JAMA* 1991;266:681.
22. Weinstein BI. Cancer prevention: recent progress and future opportunities. *Cancer Res* 1991;51:5080.
23. Jen J, Kim H, Plantadosi S, et al. Allelic loss of chromosome 18q and prognosis in colorectal cancer. *N Engl J Med* 1994;331:213.
24. Giovannucci E, Stampfer M, Colditz G, et al. Relationship of diet to risk of colorectal adenoma in men. *J Natl Cancer Inst* 1992;84:91.
25. Fearon ER, Vogelstein B. A genetic model for colorectal tumorigenesis. *Cell* 1990;61:759.
26. Sugimura T. Multistep carcinogenesis: a 1992 perspective. *Science* 1992;258:603.
27. Kunzler KW, Vogelstein B. Clinical implications of basic research: cancer therapy meets p53. *N Engl J Med* 1994;331:49.
28. O'Shaughnessy JA, Kelloff GJ, Gordon GB, et al. Treatment and prevention of intraepithelial neoplasia: an important target for accelerated new agent development. *Clin Cancer Res* 2002;8:314–346.
29. Slaughter DP, Southwide HW, Smejkal W. Field cancerization in oral stratified squamous epithelium: clinical implications of multicentric origin. *Cancer* 1953;6:963.
30. Koutsky L. Role of epidemiology in defining events that influence transmission and natural history of anogenital papillomavirus infections. *J Natl Cancer Inst* 1991;83:978.
31. Lippman SM, Benner SE, Hong WK. Cancer chemoprevention. *J Clin Oncol* 1994;12:851.
32. Lippman SM, Hong WK. Not yet standard: retinoids versus second primary tumor. *J Clin Oncol* 1993;11:1204.
33. Chung KY, Mukhopadhyay T, Kim J, et al. Discordant p53 gene mutations in primary head and neck cancers and corresponding second primary cancers of the upper aerodigestive tract. *Cancer Res* 1993;53:1676.
34. Mulshine JL, Jett M, Cuttitta F, et al. Scientific basis for cancer prevention intermediate cancer markers. *Cancer* 1993;72:978.
35. Schatzkin A, Gail M. The promise and peril of surrogate endpoints in cancer research. *Nat Rev/Cancer* 2002;21:19–27.
36. Armstrong WB, Taylor TH, Meyskens FL Jr. Point: Surrogate endpoint biomarkers are likely to be limited in their usefulness in the development of cancer chemoprevention agents against sporadic cancers. *Cancer Epidemiol Biomarkers Prev* 2003;12:589–592.
37. Kelloff GJ, Hawk ET, Crowell JA, et al. Strategies for identification and clinical evaluation of promising chemoprevention agents. *Oncology* 1996;10:1471.
38. Aguayo SM, King TE, Sherritt KM, et al. Urinary levels of bombesin-like peptides in asymptomatic cigarette smokers: a potential risk marker for smoking-related diseases. *Cancer Res* 1992;52:2727.
39. Karmali RA. Prostaglandins and cancer. *Prostaglandins Med* 1980;5:11.
40. Meyskens FL Jr, Gerner EW, Emerson S, et al. Effect of alpha-difluoromethylornithine on rectal mucosal levels of polyamines in a randomized, double-blinded trial for colon cancer prevention. *J Natl Cancer Inst* 1998;90(16):1212–1218.
41. Clapper ML, Everley LC, Strobel LA, Townsend AJ, Engstrom PF. Coordinate induction of glutathione s-transferase α, μ, and π expression in murine liver after a single administration of oltipraz. *Mol Pharmacol* 1994;45:489.
42. Vlastos AT, Schottenfeld D, Fallen M. Biomarkers and their use in cervical cancer chemoprevention. *Crit Rev Oncol Hematol* 2003;46:261–273.
43. Boiko IV, Mitchell MF, Pandey DK, et al. DNA image cytometric measurement as a surrogate endpoint biomarker in a phase I trial of alpha-difluoromethylornithine for cervical intraepithelial neoplasia. *Cancer Epidemiol Biomarkers Prev* 1997;6:849.
44. Hu W, Mitchell MF, Boiko IV, et al. Progressive dysregulation of proliferation during cervical carcinogenesis as measured by MPM-2 antibody staining. *Cancer Epidemiol Biomarkers Prev* 1997;6:711.
45. Boiko IV, Mitchell MF, Hu W, et al. Epidermal growth factor receptor expression in cervical intraepithelial neoplasia and its modulation during an alpha-difluoromethylornithine chemoprevention trial. *Clin Cancer Res* 1998;6:1383.
46. Brewer CA, Liao SY, Stanbridge EJ. A study of biomarkers in cervical carcinoma and clinical correlation of the novel biomarker, Mn. *Gynecol Oncol* 1996;63:337.
47. Liao SY, Stanbridge EJ. Expression of the Mn antigen in cervical Papanicolaou smears is an early diagnostic biomarker of cervical dysplasia. *Cancer Epidemiol Biomarkers Prev* 1996;5:549.
48. Ho GY, Burk RD, Klein S, et al. Persistent genital human papillomavirus infection as a risk factor for persistent cervical dysplasia. *J Natl Cancer Inst* 1993;87;1365.
49. Kadish AS, Ho GY, Burk RD, et al. Lymphoproliferative responses to human papillomavirus type 16 protein E6 & E7: outcome of HPV infection and associated neoplasia. *J Natl Cancer Inst* 1997;89:1285.
50. Shim C, Zhang W, Rhee CM, et al. Profiling of differentially expressed genes in human primary cervical cancer by complementary DNA expression array. *Clin Cancer Res* 1998;4:3045.

51. Taylor, JA, Tewari K, Liao SY, et al. Immunohistochemical analysis, human papillomavirus DNA detection, hormonal manipulation, and exogenous gene expression of normal and dysplastic human cervical epithelium in severe combined immunodeficiency mice. *J Virol* 1999; 73(6):5144–5148.

52. Kelloff GJ, O'Shaughnessy JA, Gordon GB, et al. Counterpoint: because some surrogate endpoint biomarkers measure the neoplastic process, they will have high utility in the development of cancer chemotherapeutic agents against sporadic cancers. *Cancer Epidemiol Biomarkers Prev* 2003;12:593–596.

53. Meyskens FL Jr. Biology and intervention of the premalignant process. *Cancer Bull* 1991;43:475.

54. Pegg AE, McCann PP. Polyamine metabolism and function. *Am J Physiol* 1982;243:212.

55. Kelloff GJ, Boone CW, Crowell JA, et al. Chemopreventive drug development: perspectives and progress. *Cancer Epidemiol Biomarkers Prev* 1994;3:85.

56. Jordan CV. Role of tamoxifen in the long-term treatment and prevention of breast cancer. *Oncology* 1988;2:19.

57. Fisher B, Costantino J, Redmond C, et al. A randomized clinical trial evaluating tamoxifen in the treatment of patients with node negative breast cancer who have estrogen-receptor positive tumors. *N Engl J Med* 1989;320:479.

58. Fisher B, Costantino JP, Redmond CR, et al. Endometrial cancer in tamoxifen-treated breast cancer patients; findings from national surgical adjuvant breast and bowel project (NSABP) B-14. *J Natl Cancer Inst* 1994;86:527.

59. Gornley GJ, Stoner E, Bruskewitz RC, et al. The effect of finasteride in men with benign prostatic hyperplasia. *N Engl J Med* 1992;327: 1185.

60. Thompson, IM, Goodman PJ Tangen CM, et al. The influence of finasteride on the development of prostate cancer. *N Engl J Med* 2003; 349:215–224.

61. Sun SY, Lotan R. Retinoids and their receptors in cancer development and chemoprevention. *Crit Rev Oncol Hematol* 2002;41:41–55.

62. Moon RC, Mehta RG. Chemoprevention of experimental carcinogenesis in animals. *Prev Med* 1989;18:576.

63. Meyskens FL Jr. Clinical trials of retinoids as differentiation inducers. In: Waxman S, Rossi GB, Takaku F, eds. *The status of differentiation therapy in cancer*. New York: Raven Press, 1987:349.

64. Lippman SM, Lee LJ, Sabicki AL. Cancer chemoprevention: progress and promise. *J Natl Cancer Inst* 1998;90:1514.

65. Hill DL, Grubbs CJ. Retinoids and cancer prevention. *Annu Rev Nutr* 1992;12:161.

66. Hong WK, Endicott J, Itri LM, et al. 13-cis-retinoic acid in the treatment of oral leukoplakia. *N Engl J Med* 1986;315:1501.

67. Hong WK, Lippman SM, Itri LM, et al. Prevention of second primary tumors with isotretinoin in squamous-cell carcinoma of the head and neck. *N Engl J Med* 1990;323:795.

68. Meyskens FL, Surwit E, Moon TE, et al. Enhancement of regression of cervical intraepithelial neoplasia II (moderate dysplasia) with topically applied all-*trans*-retinoic acid: a randomized trial. *J Natl Cancer Inst* 1994;86:539.

69. Lipkin M, Newmark H. Effect of dietary calcium on colonic epithelial-cell proliferation in subjects at high risk for familial colonic cancer. *N Engl J Med* 1985;313:1381.

70. Lipkin M, Friedman E, Winawer SI, Newmark H. Colonic epithelial cell proliferation in responders and nonresponders to supplemental dietary calcium. *Cancer Res* 1989;49:248.

71. Baron JA, Beach M, Mandel JS, et al. Calcium supplements for the prevention of colorectal adenomas. *N Engl J Med* 1999;340:101–107.

72. Wattenberg LW. Chemoprevention of cancer. *Cancer Res* 1985; 45:1.

73. Talalay P. The role of enzyme induction in protection against carcinogenesis. In: Wattenberg LW, Lipkin M, Boone CW, Kelloff GJ, eds. *Cancer chemoprevention*. Boca Raton, FL: CRC Press, 1992: 469.

74. Ansher SS, Dolan P, Bereding E. Biochemical effects of dithiolthiones. *Food Chem Toxicol* 1986;24:405.

75. Kensler TW, Groopmen JD, Roebuck BD. Chemoprotection by oltipraz and other dithiolethiones. In: Wattenberg L, Lipkin M, Boone CW, Kelloff GJ, eds. *Cancer chemoprevention*. Boca Raton, FL: CRC Press, 1992:205.

76. Benson AB. Oltipraz: a laboratory and clinical review. *J Cell Biochem* 1993;17:278.

77. Garewal H, Meyskens FL Jr, Killen D, et al. Response of oral leukoplakia to beta-carotene. *J Clin Oncol* 1990;8:1715.

78. Earnest DL, Hixson IJ, Alberts DS. Piroxicam and other cyclooxygenase inhibitors: potential for cancer prevention. *J Cell Biochem Suppl* 1992;161:156.

79. Giardiello FM, Yang VW, Hylend LM, et al. Primary chemoprevention of familial adenomatous polyposis with sulindac. *N Engl J Med* 2002;346:1054–1059.

80. Sandler RS, Halabi S, Baron JA, et al. A randomized trial of aspirin to prevent colorectal adenomas in patients with previous colorectal cancer. *N Engl J Med* 2003;348:883–899.

81. Steinbach G, Lynch PM, Phillips RKS, et al. The effect of celecoxib, a cyclooxygenase-2 inhibitor, in familial adenomatous polyposis. *N Engl J Med* 2000;342:1946–1952.

82. Giovannucci E, Rimm EB, Stampfer MJ. Aspirin use and the risk of colorectal cancer and adenoma in male health professionals. *Ann Intern Med* 1994:121:241–246.

83. Greenberg ER, Baron JA, Stukel TA, et al. A clinical trial of beta carotene to prevent basal-cell and squamous-cell cancers of the skin. *N Engl J Med* 1990;323:789.

84. Greenberg ER, Baron JA, Tostenson TD, et al. A clinical trial of antioxidant vitamins to prevent colorectal adenoma. *N Engl J Med* 1994;331:141.

85. The Alpha-Tocopherol, Beta Carotene Cancer Prevention Study Group. The effect of vitamin E and beta carotene on the incidence of lung cancer and other cancers in male smokers. *N Engl J Med* 1994;330:1029.

86. Omenn GS, Goodman GE, Thornquist MD, et al. Effects of a combination of beta carotene and vitamin A on lung cancer and cardiovascular disease. *N Engl J Med* 1996; 334:1150–1155.

87. Hong WK, Lippman SM. Cancer chemoprevention. *J Natl Cancer Inst Monogr* 1995;17:49.

88. Seidegard J, Pero RW, Markowitz NM, et al. Isoenzyme(s) of glutathione transferase (class Mu): the susceptibility to lung cancer: a follow-up study. *Carcinogenesis* 1990;11:33.

89. Kelloff GJ, Hawk ET, Karp JE. Progress in clinical chemoprevention. *Semin Oncol* 1997;24:241.

90. Reddy BS, Nagini J, Tokumo K, et al. Chemoprevention of colon carcinogenesis by concurrent administration of piroxicam, a nonsteroidal anti-inflammatory drug with α-difluoromethylornithine, an ornithine decarboxylase inhibitor in diet. *Cancer Res* 1991; 51:4528.

91. Ratko TA, Detrisac CJ, Driger NM, et al. Chemopreventive efficacy of combined retinoid and tamoxifen treatment following surgical excision of a primary mammary cancer in female rats. *Cancer Res* 1989; 49:4472.

92. Omenn GS, Goodman G, Grizzle J, et al. Recruitment for the β-carotene and retinol efficacy trial (CARET) to prevent lung cancer in smokers and in asbestos-exposed workers. *West J Med* 1992;156: 540.

93. Engstrom PF. Specific compliance issues in an antiestrogen trial of women at risk for breast cancer. *Prev Med* 1991;20:125.

94. Goodman GE. The clinical evaluation of cancer chemoprevention agents: defining and contrasting phase I, II, and III objectives. *Cancer Res* 1992;52:2752.

95. Szarka CE, Grana G, Engstrom P. Chemoprevention of cancer. In: Ozols RF, Eisenberg B, Kinsella TJ, eds. *Current problems in cancer*. St. Louis: Mosby–Year Book, 1994:1.

96. Fisher B, Costantino JP, Wickerham DL, et al. Tamoxifen for prevention of breast cancer: report of the national surgical adjuvant breast and bowel project P-1 study. *J Natl Cancer Inst* 1998;90:1371.

97. The Bethesda System for Reporting Cervical/Vaginal Cytologic Diagnoses: revised after the second National Cancer Institute Workshop, April 29–30, 1991. *Acta Cytol* 1993;37:115.

98. Meyskens FL Jr. Biomarker intermediate endpoints and cancer prevention. *J Natl Cancer Inst Monogr* 1992;13:177.

99. Mitchell MF, Hittelman WN, Hong WK, Lotan R, Schottenfeld D. The natural history of cervical intraepithelial neoplasia: an argument

for intermediate endpoint biomarkers. *Cancer Epidemiol Biomarkers Prev* 1994;3:619.

100. Hillemanns P, Tannnous-Khuri L, Koulos JP, et al. Localization of cellular retinoid-binding proteins in human cervical intraepithelial neoplasia and invasive carcinoma. *Am J Pathol* 1992;141:973.

101. Brinton LA. Editorial commentary: smoking and cervical cancer—current status. *Am J Epidemiol* 1990;131:958.

102. de Vet HC, Sturmans F. Risk factors for cervical dysplasia: implications for prevention. *Public Health* 1994;108(4):241.

103. Kitchener HC. The role of human papillomavirus in the genesis of cervical cancer. *Cancer Treat Res* 1994;70:29.

104. Schafer A, Friedmann W, Mieelke M, et al. The increased frequency of cervical dysplasia-neoplasia in women infected with the human immunodeficiency virus is related to the degree of immunosuppression. *Am J Obstet Gynecol* 1991;164:593.

105. Goff BA, Muntz HG, Bell DA, Wertheim I, Rice LW. Human papillomavirus typing in patients with Papanicolaou smears showing squamous atypia. *Gynecol Oncol* 1993;48:384.

106. Schiffman MH, Bauer HM, Hoover RN, et al. Epidemiologic evidence showing that human papillomavirus infection causes most cervical intraepithelial neoplasia. *J Natl Cancer Inst* 1993;85:958.

107. Munoz N, Bosch FX, de Sanjose S, Shah, KV. The role of HPV in the etiology of cervical cancer. *Mutat Res* 1994;305:293.

108. Xi LF, Koutsky LA, Galloway DA, et al. Genomic variation of human papillomavirus type 16 and risk for high grade cervical intraepithelial neoplasia. *J Natl Cancer Inst* 1997;89:796.

109. Hildesheim A, Schiffman M, Bromley C, et al. Human papillomavirus type 16 variants and risk of cervical cancer. *J Natl Cancer Inst* 2001; 93:315–318.

110. DeCaprio JA, Ludlow JW, Figge J, et al. SV40 large tumour antigen forms a specific complex with the product of the retinoblastoma susceptibility gene. *Cell* 1988;53:275.

111. Werness P, Levine AJ, Howley PM. Association of human papillomavirus types 16 and 18 E6 proteins with p53. *Science* 1990;248:76.

112. Kadish AS, Hagan RJ, Ritter DB, et al. Biologic characteristics of specific human papillomavirus types predicted from morphology of cervical lesions. *Hum Pathol* 1992;11:1262.

113. zur Hausen H. Papillomavirus and p53. *Nature* 1998;393:217.

114. Storey A, Thomas M, Kalita A, et al. Role of p53 polymorphism in the development of human papillomavirus–associated cancer. *Nature* 1998;393:229.

115. Helland A, Langerod A, Johnsen H, Olsen AO, Skovland E, Borresen-Dale AL. p53 polymorphism and risk of cervical cancer. *Nature* 1998; 396:530; discussion 532.

116. Larson AA, Liao SY, Stanbridge EJ, et al. Genetic alterations accumulate during cervical tumorigenesis and indicate a common origin for multifocal lesions. *Cancer Res* 1997;57:4171.

117. Holly EA, Cress RD, Ahn DK, et al. Detection of mutagens in cervical mucus in smokers and nonsmokers. *Cancer Epidemiol Biomarkers Prev* 1993;2:223.

118. Sood AK. Cigarette smoking and cervical cancer: meta-analysis and critical review of recent studies. *Am J Prev Med* 1991;7:208.

119. Ho GY, Kadish AS, Burk RD, et al. HPV 16 and cigarette smoking as risk factors for high-grade cervical intra-epithelial neoplasia. *Int J Cancer* 1998;78:281.

120. Castle PE, Wacholder S, Lorincz AT, et al. A prospective study of high-grade cervical neoplasia risk among human papillomavirus-infected women. *J Natl Cancer Inst* 2002;94:1406–1414.

121. Liu T, Soong SJ, Wilson NP, et al. A case control study of nutritional factors and cervical dysplasia. *Cancer Epidemiol Biomarkers Prev* 1993;2:525.

122. Potischman N, Hoover RN, Brinton LA, et al. The relations between cervical cancer and serological markers of nutritional status. *Nutr Cancer* 1994;21:193.

123. Basu J, Palan PR, Vermund SH, et al. Plasma ascorbic acid and beta-carotene levels in women evaluated for HPV infection, smoking, and cervix dysplasia. *Cancer Detect Prev* 1991;15:165.

124. Batieha AM, Armenian HK, Norkus EP, et al. Serum micronutrients and the subsequent risk of cervical cancer in a population-based nested case-control study. *Cancer Epidemiol Biomarkers Prev* 1993;2: 335.

125. Brock KE, Berry G, Mock PA, et al. Nutrients in diet and plasma and risk of in situ cervical cancer. *J Natl Cancer Inst* 1988;80: 580.

126. Batova A, Danielpour D, Pirisi L, Creek KE. Retinoic acid induces secretion of latent transforming growth factor β_1 and β_2 in normal and human papillomavirus type 16–immortalized human keratinocytes. *Cell Growth Differ* 1992;3:763.

127. Follen M, Meyskens FL Jr, Atkinson EN, et al. Why most randomized phase II cervical cancer chemoprevention trials are uninformative: lessons for the future. *J Natl Cancer Inst* 2001;93:1293–1296.

128. Butterworth CE Jr, Hatch KD, Gore H, et al. Improvement in cervical dysplasia associated with folic acid therapy in users of oral contraception. *Am J Clin Nutr* 1982;35:73.

129. Butterworth CE Jr, Hatch KD, Macaluso M, et al. Folate deficiency in cervical dysplasia. *JAMA* 1992;267:528.

130. Ran JY, Li XF, Rau HL, Wang LY, Herbert V. Selective folate deficiency in one but not another cell line: despite normal red-cell folate, folate therapy reduced cervical dysplasia and hyperploidy in women using oral contraceptives. *Blood* 1990;76:114a.

131. Whitehead N, Reyner F, Lindenbaum J. Megaloblastic changes in the cervical epithelium: association with oral contraceptive therapy and reversal with folic acid. *JAMA* 1973;226:1421.

132. Butterworth CE Jr, Hatch KD, Soong SJ, et al. Oral folic acid supplementation for cervical dysplasia: a clinical intervention trial. *Am J Obstet Gynecol* 1992;166:803.

133. Childers JM, Chu J, Voight L, et al. Chemoprevention of cervical cancer with folic acid: a phase III SWOG intergroup study. *Cancer Epidemiol Biomarkers Prev* 1995;45:489.

134. Lotan R. Effects of vitamin A and its analogs (retinoids) on normal and neoplastic cells. *Biochim Biophys Acta* 1980;605:33.

135. Singh VN, Gaby SK. Premalignant lesions: role of antioxidant vitamins and β-carotene in risk reduction and prevention of malignant transformation. *Am J Clin Nutr* 1991;53:386S.

136. Kahn MA, Jenkins RG, Tolleson WH, et al. Retinoic acid inhibition of human papillomavirus type 16–mediated transformation of human keratinocytes. *Cancer Res* 1993;53:905.

137. Manetta A, Schubbert T, Chapman J, et al. β-Carotene treatment of cervical intraepithelial neoplasia. *Cancer Epidemiol Biomarkers Prev* 1996;5:929.

138. Romney SL, Ho GY, Palan PR, et al. Effects of beta-carotene and other factors on outcome of cervical dysplasia and human papillomavirus infection. *Gynecol Oncol* 1997:65:483.

139. Keefe KA, Schell MJ, Brewer C, et al. A randomized, double-blind, Phase III trial using oral beta-carotene supplementation for women with high-grade cervical intraepithelial neoplasia. *Cancer Epidemiol Biomarkers Prev* 2001;10:1029–1035.

140. Dorr RT, Surwit EA, Meyskens FL Jr, et al. In vitro retinoid binding and release from a collagen sponge material in a simulated intravaginal environment. *J Biomaterials* 1982;16:839.

141. Meyskens FL Jr, Graham V, Chvapil M, et al. A Phase I trial of beta-all-trans-retinoic acid for mild or moderate intraepithelial cervical neoplasia delivered via a collagen sponge and cervical cap. *J Natl Cancer Inst* 1983;71:921.

142. Surwit EA, Graham V, Droegemueller W, et al. Evaluation of topically applied trans-retinoic acid in the treatment of cervical intraepithelial lesions. *Am J Obstet Gynecol* 1982;143:821.

143. Weiner SA, Surwit EA, Graham VE, Meyskens FL, Jr. Phase I trial of topically applied trans-retinoic acid in cervical dysplasia—clinical efficacy. *Invest New Drugs* 1986;4:241.

144. Graham V, Surwit ES, Weiner S, Meyskens FL Jr. Phase II trial of beta-all-trans-retinoic acid for intraepithelial cervical neoplasia delivered via a collagen sponge and cervical cap. *West J Med* 1986;145: 192.

145. Chen RD. Chemoprevention of cervical cancer—intervention study of cervical precancerous lesions by retinamide II and riboflavin. *Chung Hua Chung Liu Tsa Chih* 1993;15:272.

146. Kelloff GJ, Boone CW, Steele VE, et al. Progress in cancer chemoprevention: perspectives on agent selection and short-term clinical intervention trials. *Cancer Res* 1994;54:2015s.

147. Mitchell MF, Tortolero L, Lee IJ, et al. Phase I dose de-escalation trial of alpha-difluoromethylornithine in patients with grade 3 cervical intraepithelial neoplasia. *Clin Cancer Res* 1998;4:303.

148. Follen M, Atkinson EN, Schottenfeld D, et al. A randomized clinical

trial of 4-hydroxy-phenylretinamide for high grade squamous intraepithelial lesions of the cervix. *Clin Cancer Res* 2001;7:3356–3365.

149. Arifler D, Guilland M, Carraro A, et al. Light-scattering from normal and dysplastic cervical cells at different epithelial depths: finite-difference time-domain modeling with a perfectly matched layer boundary condition. *J Biomed Opt* 2003;8:484–494.

150. Darwiche N, Celli G, Sly L, et al. Retinoid status controls the appearance of reserve cells and keratin expression in mouse cervical epithelium. *Cancer Res* 1993;53:2287.

151. Khan SA. Cervical cancer, human papillomavirus and vaccines. *Clin Oncol (R Coll Radiol)* 1993;5:386.

152. Lowy DR, Schiller JT. Papillomaviruses and cervical cancer: pathogenesis and vaccine development. *J Natl Cancer Inst Monogr* 1998;23:27.

153. Roche JK, Crum CP. Local immunity and the uterine cervix: implications for cancer-associated viruses. *Cancer Immunol Immunother* 1991;33:203.

154. Steller MA, Garski KJ, Murakami M, et al. Cell-mediated immunological responses in cervical and vaginal cancer patients immunized with a lipidated epotype of human papillomavirus type 16 E7. *Clin Cancer Res* 1998;4:2103.

155. Muderspach L, Wilcznyski S, Roman L, et al. A phase I trial of HPV peptide vaccine for women with high grade cervical and vulvar intraepithelial neoplasia who are HVP-16 positive. *Clin Cancer Res* 2000;6:3406–3416.

156. Eiben GL, Velder MP, Kast WM. The cell-mediated immune response to human papilloma virus into cervical cancer: implications for immunotherapy. *Adv Cancer Res* 2002;86:113–148.

157. Zhou J, Sun XY, Stenzel DJ, Frazer IH. Expression of vaccinia recombinant HPV-16 L-1 and L-2 ORF protein in epithelial cells is sufficient for assembly of HPV virion-like particles. *Virology* 1991; 185: 251–257.

158. Harro CD, Pang YY, Roden RB, et al. Safety and immunogenicity trial in adult volunteers of a human papilloma virus 16 L-1 virus-like particles vaccine *J Natl Cancer Inst* 2001;93:284–292.

159. Koutsky LA, Ault KA, Wheeler CM, et al. A controlled trial of a human papillomavirus type 16 vaccine. *N Engl J Med* 2002;347: 1645–1651.

160. Walboomers JM, Jacob MV, Manos MM, et al. Human papilloma virus is a ncessary cause of invasive cervical cancer world wide. *J Pathol* 1999;189:12–19.

161. Crum CP. Editorial. The beginning of the end for cervical cancer? *N Engl J Med* 2002;347:1703–1705.

162. Huang K, Lin S. Nationwide vaccination: a success story in Taiwan. *Vaccine* 2000;18(1):S35–S38.

163. Jemal A, Murray T, Samuels A, et al. Cancer statistics, 2003. *CA Cancer J Clin* 2003;53:5–26.

164. Smith DC, Prentice R, Thompson DJ, et al. Association of exogenous estrogen and endometrial carcinoma. *N Engl J Med* 1975;293:1164.

165. Antunes CM, Stolley PD, Rosenshein NB, et al. Endometrial cancer and estrogen use: report of a large case-control study. *N Engl J Med* 1979;300:9.

166. Shapiros S, Kelly JP, Rosenberg L, et al. Risk of localized and widespread endometrial cancer in relation to recent and discontinued use of conjugated estrogens. *N Engl J Med* 1985;313:969.

167. Anonymous. Effects of hormone replacement therapy on endometrial histology in postmenopausal women: the postmenopausal estrogen/progestin intervention (PEPI) trial. *JAMA* 1996;275:370.

168. Fornander T, Rutquist LE, Cedumask B, et al. Adjuvant tamoxifen early breast cancer: occurrence of new primary cancer. *Lancet* 1989; 1:117.

169. Barakat RR. Tamoxifen and endometrial neoplasia. *Clin Obstet Gynecol* 1996;39:629.

170. Yang NN, Venugopalan M, Haridar S, et al. Identification of an estrogen response element activated by metabolites of 17 beta-estradiol and raloxifene. *Science* 1996;273:1222.

171. Watson P, Vasen HF, Mechlin JP, et al. The risk of endometrial cancer in hereditary non-polyposis colorectal cancer. *Am J Med* 1994;96: 516.

172. Burk JR, Lehman HF, Wolf FS. Inadequacy of Papanicolaou smear in the detection of endometrial cancer. *N Engl J Med* 1974;291:191.

173. Varner RE, Sparks JM, Cameron CD, et al. Transvaginal sonography

of the endometrium in post-menopausal women. *Obstet Gynecol* 1991; 78:195.

174. Grimes DA. Primary prevention of ovarian cancer [editorial]. *JAMA* 1993;270:2855.

175. Easton DF, Bishop DT, Ford D, et al. Genetic linkage analysis in familial breast and ovarian cancer: results from 214 families. The Breast Cancer Linkage Consortium. *Am J Hum Genet* 1993;52: 678.

176. Fathalla MF. Factors in the causation and incidence of ovarian cancer. *Obstet Gynecol Surv* 1972;27:751.

177. Bosetti C, Negri E, Trichopoulos D, et al. Long-term effects of oral contraceptives on ovarian cancer risk. *Int. J Cancer* 2002;102: 262–265.

178. Hankinson SE, Colditz GA, Hunter DJ, et al. A quantitative assessment of oral contraceptive use and risk of ovarian cancer. *Obstet Gynecol* 1992;80:708.

179. Rosenblatt KA, Thomas DB, Norman EA, et al. High-dose and low-dose combined oral contraceptives: protection against epithelial ovarian cancer and the length of the protective effect. *Eur J Cancer* 1992; 28:1872.

180. Lacey JV. Menopausal hormone replacement therapy and risk of ovarian cancer. *JAMA* 2002;288:334.

181. Rodriguez C, Calle EE, Fakhrabadi D, et al. Body mass index, height and the risk of ovarian cancer mortality in a prospective cohort of postmenopausal women. *Cancer Epidemiol Biomarkers Prev* 2002; 11:822–828.

182. Hankinson SE, Hunter DJ, Colditz GA, et al. Tubal ligation, hysterectomy, and risk of ovarian cancer. *JAMA* 1993;270:2813.

183. Harlow BL, Cramer DW, Bell DA, et al. Perineal exposure to talc and ovarian cancer risk. *Obstet Gynecol* 1992;80:19.

184. Shu XO, Gao T, Yuan JM. Dietary factors and epithelial ovarian cancer. *Br J Cancer* 1989;59:92.

185. Cramer DW, Willett WC, Bell DA, et al. Galactose consumption and metabolism in relation to the risk of ovarian cancer. *Lancet* 1989;2: 66.

186. Mettlin CJ, Piver MS. A case-control study of milk-drinking and ovarian cancer risk. *Am J Epidemiol* 1990;132:871.

187. Spirtas R, Kaufman SC, Alexander NJ. Fertility drugs and ovarian cancer: red alert or red herring? *Fertil Steril* 1993;59:291.

188. Trimble EL, Karlan BY, Lagasse LD, Hoskins WJ. Diagnosing the correct ovarian cancer syndrome. *Ovarian Cancer Syndromes* 1991; 78:1023.

189. Whittemore AS, Harris R, Itnyre J, et al. Characteristics relating to ovarian cancer risk: collaborative analysis of 12 US case-control studies. II. Invasive epithelial ovarian cancers in white women. *Am J Epidemiol* 1992;136:1184.

190. Narod SA, Resch H, Moslehi R, et al. Oral contraceptives and the risk of hereditary ovarian cancer. *N Engl J Med* 1998;339:424.

191. Cook LS, Weiss NS, Schwarz SM, et al. Population-based study of tamoxifen therapy and subsequent ovarian endometrial and breast cancers. *J Natl Cancer Inst* 1995;87:1343.

192. Rodriguez GC, Walmer DK, Cline M, et al. Effect of progestin on the ovarian epithelium of macaques: cancer prevention through apoptosis? *J Soc Gynecol Invest* 1998;5:271.

193. American College of Obstetricians and Gynecologists: Prophylactic Oophorectomy, ACOG Technical Bulletin 111, Washington, DC, ACOG, 1987.

194. Lynch HT, Smyrk TC. Hereditary colorectal cancer. *Semin Oncol* 1999;26:478–484.

195. Struewing JP, Watson P, Easton DF, et al: Prophylactic oophorectomy in inherited breast/ovarian cancer families. *J Natl Cancer Inst Monogr* 1995;33–35.

196. Rebbeck TR, Lynch HT, Neuhausen SL, et al. Prophylactic oophorectomy in carriers of BRCA1 or BRCA2 mutations. *N Engl J Med* 2002; 346:1616–1622.

197. Kauff ND, Satagopan JM, Robson ME, et al. Risk-reducing salpingo-oophorectomy in women with a BRCA1 mutation. *N Engl J Med* 2002;346:1609–1615.

198. Tobacman J, Greene M, Tucker U, et al. Intra-abdominal carcinomatosis after prophylactic oophorectomy in ovarian cancer-prone families. *Lancet* 1982;2:795.

199. Schrag D, Kuntz KM, Garber JE, et al. Decision analysis: effects of

prophylactic mastectomy and oophorectomy in life expectancy among young women with BRCA1 or BRCA2 mutations. *N Engl J Med* 1997;336:1465.

200. Rodriguez-Burford C, Barnes MN, Oelschlager DK. Effects of nonsteroidal anti-inflammatory agents (NSAIDs) on ovarian carcinoma cell lines: preclinical evaluation NSAIDs as chemopreventive agents. *Clin Cancer Res* 2002;8:202–209.

201. Mills GB. Editorial: Mechanisms underlying chemoprevention of ovarian cancer. *Clin Cancer Res* 2002;8:7–10.

202. Depalo G, Mariam L, Camerini T, et al. Effect of fenretinide on ovarian carcinoma occurrence. *Gynecol Oncol* 2002;86:24–27.

203. Veronesi U, Decensi A. Retinoids for ovarian cancer prevention: laboratory data sets the stage for thoughtful clinical trials. *J Natl Cancer Inst* 2001;93:486–489.

204. Brewer MA, Johnson K, Follen M, et al. Prevention of ovarian cancer: intraepithelial neoplasia. *Clin Cancer Res* 2003;9:20–30.

205. Ardekani A, Fishman D, Fusaro V, et al. Use of proteomic patterns in serum to identify ovarian cancer. *Lancet* 2002;359:572–577.

CHAPTER 9

Clinical Trials Methodology and Biostatistics

Brian Bundy and Mark Brady

This chapter focuses on the issues involved in the design and execution of randomized clinical trials (RCTs) in gynecologic oncology. Phase I and II trials are included because they are important research efforts that precede most RCTs. Statistical jargon and mathematical notation are avoided as much as possible. This chapter is an overview of this very expansive topic. More elaborate presentations of these issues can be found in dozens of books dedicated to the subject of RCTs; for example, see to name only a few: Redmond and Colton (1), Piantadosi (2), Meinert (3), Buyse (4), or Pocock (5).

The RCTs discussed in this chapter are primarily treatment trials that evaluate patients with a specific malignancy. In general, an RCT is any experiment that has humans as subjects and attempts to reduce the impact of a specific disease by testing an intervention. For cancer trials, the intervention may be applied at any point in the natural history of the disease from before carcinogenesis to the end result. RCTs that evaluate methods for the detection of cancer in a subclinical state (i.e., asymptomatic) are called screening trials. This early detection could mean diagnosing the disease in an earlier stage (e.g., the use of mammography in the detection of breast cancer) or in a premalignant state (e.g., the use of a Papanicolaou smear in the detection of cervical intraepithelial neoplasia). In such trials, the treatments available for those diagnosed in both the intervention and the control group are the same and are not being evaluated per se. However, the alternative hypothesis is based on the theory that the treatments are much more effective if administered early enough in the disease process. Chemoprevention trials represent another type of RCT with the purpose of reducing the occurrence of cancer. This approach usually enrolls high-risk, but disease-free, individuals to be treated with either the experimental agent or a placebo control. These trials require extremely large numbers of people and a substantial follow-up time so that enough incident cases can be observed for a meaningful comparison.

This chapter will not discuss in detail nonexperimental studies (also called observational studies) that address the etiology of cancer in humans. There are three broad categories of such studies: cohort, case-control, and cross sectional. The cohort study establishes a defined group of individuals and classifies them according to their exposure status (which can include environmental or lifestyle factors). The individuals are then followed for the occurrence of the disease that is under study. The case-control study identifies individuals on the basis of disease status and then ascertains their history of exposure. Measuring exposure could be as simple as questioning the individuals regarding certain exposures or may involve a more sophisticated assessment such as analyzing their blood for biologic markers. Though the case-control study is more susceptible to several methodologic flaws, it has been quite successful at times. For example, the deleterious effect of exogenous estrogens on perimenopausal women was indicated by more than a dozen case-control studies published from 1975 to 1985 (6). The cross-sectional study measures disease status and exposure for a population that is defined in a specific period of time. Newly diagnosed cases, as well as prevalent cases, are included. Such studies can be accomplished much more quickly than the first two types but are less popular because of the considerable potential of having methodologic flaws.

This chapter begins with some historical highlights from medical research. This synopsis is intended to provide a sense of how the concepts of an RCT matured from an intuition-based practice of medicine to the sophisticated evidence-based medicine used today. The subsequent sections describe components of an RCT that have dominated our discussions with clinical investigators over the years.

Brian Bundy: Department of Biostatistics, Roswell Park Cancer Institute, Buffalo, New York 14263

Mark Brady: Gynecology Oncology Group Statistical and Data Center, Roswell Park Cancer Institute, Buffalo, New York 14263

HISTORICAL PERSPECTIVE

Clinicians make treatment recommendations daily. These recommendations arise from culling information from standardized clinical guidelines, published reports, expert opinions, or personal experiences. The synthesis of information from these sources into a particular recommendation for an individual patient is based on a clinician's personal judgment. But what constitutes reliable and valid information worthy of consideration? Clinicians have long recognized that clinical trials are important sources of empirical evidence for shaping clinical judgment.

The Greek physician Hippocrates in the fifth century B.C. had a profound influence in freeing medicine from superstitions. He rejected the notion that diseases were of divine origin. Rather he postulated that diseases originated from natural causes that could be determined from observing environmental factors like diet, drinking water, or local weather. He also proposed the revolutionary concept that a physician could predict the course of a disease after carefully observing a sufficient number of cases. Despite these insights, medicine continued frequently to consist of a mixture of herbal concoctions, purging, bloodletting, and astrology.

In the Middle Ages, Avicenna (AD 980 to 1037) wrote his *Cannon of Medicine*, a work considered to be the preeminent source of medical and pharmaceutical knowledge of its time. In his writings, Avicenna proposed some rules for testing clinical interventions. First, he points to the need to experiment in humans since "testing a drug on a lion or horse might not prove anything about its effect on man." Also, he describes the basic experiment as observing pairs of individuals with uncomplicated forms of the disease. Finally, he emphasizes the need for careful observation of the times of action and reporting the reproducibility of effects (7).

Early trials frequently lacked a concurrent comparison group. For example, Lady Mary Wortley-Montague, in 1721, urged King George I to commute the sentences of six inmates from the Newgate prison if they agreed to participate in a smallpox inoculation trial (7). The prisoners were inoculated with smallpox matter from a patient with a naturally occurring form of the disease. Since these individuals remained free of smallpox, this was considered evidence supporting treatment by inoculation. Later, the results of this trial were considered somewhat less compelling, though, when it was discovered that some of these inmates might have been exposed to smallpox prior to the trial (3). Without a proper control group, it can be difficult to interpret the efficacy of the intervention. There are frequently many factors, both known and unknown, that influence response.

John Haygarth demonstrated the importance of controlling for assessment biases in 1800. At that time, magnetic healing rods were commonly used to relieve pain due to chronic rheumatism (3). He treated five patients on 2 consecutive days, once with sham wooden rods and once with genuine magnetic rods. He noted that four individuals reported pain relief and one experienced no relief regardless of which rods were used.

It had long been appreciated that there is a potential for misguided inference about the effectiveness of a treatment when it is compared to either historical controls or concurrent controls. The apparent benefits attributed to a new treatment might in fact be biases due to differences in patient characteristics between treatment groups. One of the earliest clinical trials to attempt to address this bias was reported in 1898 by Johannes Fibiger (8). Four hundred and eighty-four patients admitted to his clinic with diphtheria were given either standard care or diphtheria serum twice daily. The treatment was determined by the day of admission and alternated from day to day (9).

By the 1940s, the modern concept of treatment randomization was adapted from the field of agriculture. Corwin Hinshaw (10), using a coin toss, and later Bradford Hill (11), using random numbers in sealed envelopes, established the role of randomization in clinical trials. The unpredictable and spontaneous remissions exhibited by patients with pulmonary tuberculosis motivated Hinshaw. Although methodologic principles guided Hill, the short supply of streptomycin after World War II provided the opportunity to use randomization as an equitable way to distribute the drug (12).

One of the first randomized clinical trials in the study of gynecologic malignancies was initiated in 1948 (13). This trial compared ovarian irradiation to standard treatment for breast cancer. Initially, shuffled sealed envelopes were used to designate treatment. However, this procedure was later changed because of administrative difficulties so that treatment depended on the woman's date of birth.

Despite these methodologic advances, the inadequate justification for selecting one medical procedure over another one caused a contemporary physician to express his frustration:

> Early in my medical career I was appalled at the "willy-nilly" fashion by which treatment regimens slipped in and out of popularity. How many operations that I was trained to do or medicines that I was instructed to give because of somebody's conviction they were beneficial passed into oblivion for no apparent reason, only to be replaced by others of equally dubious worth? (14).

The first randomized clinical trial at the National Cancer Institute (NCI) was begun in 1955 (15). This trial involved 65 evaluable patients with acute leukemia from four different institutions. The trial incorporated many elements that should be part of any modern clinical trial: uniform criteria for response assessment, a randomized comparison of two treatment regimens, and a complete accounting of all patients entered. The published report included considerations for such issues as patient selection bias and the study's impact on the patient's welfare (16). The first NCI randomized clinical trial in solid tumors followed shortly thereafter and was organized by the Eastern Group for Solid Tumor

Chemotherapy (17). By 1998, there were 12 NCI-sponsored cooperative groups, and the annual funding for these groups was approximately $90 million.

In the late 1950s, most patients with gynecologic cancers were included incidentally in small trials to screen new agents for broad-range activity. The first NCI-sponsored group to organize trials specifically for gynecologic malignancies was the Surgical Ovarian Adjuvant Group. This group was formed in the late 1950s, initiated a few trials, and then disbanded in 1964. Starting in 1963, the Surgical Endometrial Adjuvant Group was one of the earliest efforts toward a multidisciplinary group. This cooperative group included gynecologic surgeons, medical oncologists, pathologists, radiation oncologists, and biostatisticians. It was from this group that the Gynecologic Oncology Group (GOG) was eventually formed in 1970 to deal with a broader range of gynecologic malignancies (18). Over the following 10 years, the field of gynecologic oncology matured. Board certification procedures for gynecologic oncologists were developed, fellowship programs were initiated in the comprehensive cancer centers, and a professional society for gynecologic oncologists was formed.

OBJECTIVES

In clinical oncology research, where the disease is often fatal, the ultimate purpose of a research program is to develop a treatment plan that puts the patients into a disease-free state, reduces the risk of cancer recurrence, and allows patients to return to their normal lifestyle within a reasonable period of time. The objectives of a particular clinical trial are more specific and less grandiose. A clinical trial attempts to answer a precisely defined set of questions with respect to the effects of a particular treatment(s) (4). These questions (objectives) form the foundation on which the rest of the trial is built. The objective typically incorporates three elements: the treatments to be evaluated, the ''yardstick'' to be used to measure treatment benefit (see Endpoints section below), and a brief description of the target population (see Eligibility Criteria section below). These three elements (i.e., ''what'', ''how,'' and ''who'') should be stated in the most precise, clear, and concise terms possible.

The choice of experimental therapy to be evaluated in a randomized clinical trial is not always easy. Both a plethora of new therapies or combinations and the absence of innovative concepts make for difficult choices. The former is problematic since many malignancies in gynecologic oncology are relatively uncommon. Definitive clinical trials may require 4 to 5 years to accrue a sufficient number of patients even in a cooperative group setting. This time frame limits the number of new therapies that can be evaluated. The absence of new therapies is a problem since substantial increases in patient benefit are less likely to be observed in trials that merely alter doses or schedules of already acceptable therapies. An open dialogue among expert investigators remains the most effective approach for establishing the objectives of any clinical trial.

Endpoints

The endpoint of a trial is some measurable entity of the patient's disease process that will reflect the treatment's effectiveness. An endpoint is also referred to as an outcome. A study may assess more than one endpoint, but in these instances, the endpoint of primary interest should be clearly specified. The primary endpoint can also be a composite measure of multiple outcomes. Some studies assessing quality of life aggregate the scores from several related dimensions that are considered components of a larger concept called quality of life.

Primary Endpoints

The primary endpoint that will reflect the effectiveness of the experimental therapy is not always obvious. The concepts that should guide the selection of the primary endpoint are clearness and meaningfulness. Clear endpoints have an unambiguous cause and effect relationship with the disease process. The meaningfulness of an outcome is judged from the patient's perspective; that is, the primary outcome should have direct relevance to the patient.

It is not always possible for a single endpoint to be clear and meaningful. For example, avoiding death is extremely relevant to the patient with a gynecologic malignancy. Therefore, survival time is a very meaningful endpoint for randomized trials involving these patients. However, some patients will not only receive the study treatment, but also other cancer therapies. Survival time may not be a clear endpoint in this case because of the potential influences of factors, particularly cancer therapies, that are external to the study. An analysis of trials comparing nonplatinum to platinum regimens in patients with advanced ovarian cancer speculated that these trials may have underestimated the effect of platinum. The reason is that many patients who were not randomized to the platinum regimen eventually received platinum (19). For this reason, progression-free interval (PFI) is often considered a more appropriate endpoint in these trials. The objective of a particular study may be to compare explicitly immediate therapy versus delayed therapy. In this case, survival time may be the only meaningful endpoint.

Endpoints may be classified as categorical (e.g., clinical response), continuous (e.g., serum CA-125 values), or time-to-event (e.g., survival time), which is a combination of the first two. A time-to-event endpoint includes both time (a continuous measure) and censoring status (categorical measure). The data type influences the methods of analysis.

Measurement Errors

The susceptibility of an outcome to measurement errors is an important consideration when choosing an endpoint.

Both random and systematic errors are components of measurement error. To define these terms, take, for example, the measurement of some biologic marker from a single patient's serum. There are three quantities that need to be introduced. The first quantity is the *true value* of the biologic marker contained in the sample (μ) that is unknown. The second is an *aggregate measure* of the biologic marker in the sample; the resulting value if it were possible to perform the laboratory procedure a multitude of times so that all variability of the measuring process was eliminated from the combined measure. Statisticians call this the expected value and algebraically denote it as E[X]. The third quantity is the observed and *recorded value* (x), which in most settings is measured once. Random error is the difference between the recorded value and the aggregate measure (i.e., x − E[X]). Systematic error is the difference between the aggregate measure and the true value (i.e., E[X] − μ). Systematic error is also called measurement bias. The random error plus the systematic error is equal to the total measurement error (i.e., x − μ). A more relevant example is measuring PFI in an RCT of ovarian cancer where the clinic workloads and the patient's personal commitments affect scheduling of follow-up visits. This fluctuation introduces random error, but not systematic error, to the endpoint. In contrast, an investigator that uses rising levels of CA-125 to define progression when progression is supposed to be based on clinical indicators is artificially shortening PFI and, therefore, likely introducing systematic error. Unlike the scheduling variation, increasing the number of patients enrolled by such an investigator will not attenuate the problem but rather intensifies its effect. Random error can be controlled by increasing the number of measurements taken (i.e., sample size); systematic error cannot be controlled in this way.

When there are recognized sources of error, it is important that the study design implement procedures to avoid or minimize their effect. Differential measurement bias represents the most catastrophic error in a clinical trial and occurs when the degree of bias differs between the treatment groups. In such cases, a comparison of the endpoint, subject to differential measurement bias, between the groups is invalid. For example, a trial that has the patients in one treatment group being evaluated every month (1-month group), whereas the other treatment group is evaluated every 3 months (3-month group) will introduce differential measurement bias in measuring PFI. The 3-month group will tend to have longer PFI than the 1-month group. Attention to potential biases due to different evaluation schedules is particularly important when PFI is compared in two groups receiving different treatment modalities (e.g., surgery vs radiation therapy).

Surrogate Endpoints

Surrogate endpoints essentially have no direct clinical relevance to the patient. Instead, surrogate endpoints are intermediate events in the etiologic pathway to other events that do have a direct relevance to the patient (20). The ideal surrogate endpoint is an early necessary precursor to a clinically relevant event. In addition, the ideal surrogate endpoint must follow the point of impact by the treatments being evaluated along the disease pathway. An example of a less than ideal surrogate endpoint is tumor response. There are biologic scenarios in which an agent could be ineffective in substantially reducing the primary tumor burden but quite effective in reducing micrometastases to distant organs. It is noteworthy that surrogate endpoints are sometimes justified on the basis of an analysis that demonstrates a statistical correlation between the surrogate and a relevant endpoint. However, although a correlation is a necessary condition, it is not a sufficient condition to justify using a particular surrogate as an endpoint in a clinical trial.

The reasons most frequently cited for making a surrogate endpoint the primary endpoint include reduction in study duration, decreased expense, or convenience. In advanced ovarian cancer trials, disease status assessed via reassessment laparotomy following treatment is regarded by some as a surrogate endpoint (21). Those patients with no pathologic evidence of disease are more likely to experience longer survival. The principal drawback to this endpoint is that patients may refuse reassessment surgery after completing treatment or it may become medically contraindicated. Even among highly motivated and very persuasive investigators, the percentage of patients not reassessed is typically greater than 15%. In these individuals, the surrogate endpoint is unknown.

Primary Endpoints in Gynecologic Oncology

In general, PFI is both a meaningful and clear endpoint in early and locally advanced gynecologic oncology trials. Survival time is considered the best choice in recurrent disease or distantly metastatic disease. The endpoint progression-free survival (PFS) is preferred to PFI but differs only slightly in meaning. The difference resides with the time measurement of patients dying without documented disease progression. For such patients, their PFIs are censored at the time of their death but their PFSs end at their death and are considered events. The concern with using PFI is that the death of these patients may be related to the disease but was not clinically evident (i.e., no autopsy performed). Another possibility is that the patient may have had a recurrence but was considered lost to follow-up by the clinic except for learning indirectly of the patient's death. Finally, deaths attributable to the treatment would be essentially ignored in evaluating PFI. It has become standard practice in ovarian and cervical cancer trials to use PFS instead of PFI. The word *survival* is substituted for *interval* (i.e., PF*S* vs PF*I*) to underscore that death is counted as an event regardless of the cause.

The primary endpoint has been controversial in trials of patients with recurrent cervical cancer. Historically, some trials have been designed with clinical response as the primary endpoint. However, in recent GOG trials with these patients, such as GOG Protocol #179 (A Randomized Phase III Study of Cisplatin Versus Cisplatin Plus Topotecan Versus MVAC in Stage IVB, Recurrent or Persistent Squamous Cell Carcinoma of the Cervix), survival time is considered the primary endpoint. The rationale for this choice arises in part from the observations that treatments that have demonstrated an improvement in the frequency of response did not induce a benefit in survival time (22). Although salvage therapies may have distorted the cause-effect relationship, the distortion is probably, at best, minimal since there are so few known treatments that have demonstrated an ability to influence survival time of patients with recurrent cervical cancer (i.e., median survival: 8.5 months).

In summary, the ideal endpoint provides reasonable assurance that inference about the causal relationship between the intervention and the endpoint is valid. The ideal endpoint has no or negligible systematic measurement error. Convenient and easy to measure outcomes are preferred. Unfortunately, in some diseases, these features are not available simultaneously. Some strategies for addressing various sources of biases are addressed later in the chapter (see Other Design Considerations).

ELIGIBILITY CRITERIA

The eligibility criteria serve two purposes in a clinical trial. The immediate purpose is to define those patients with a particular disease, clinical history, and personal and medical characteristics that may be considered for enrollment into the clinical trial. The subsequent purpose of eligibility criteria comes after the clinical trial is completed and the results are available. Physicians must then decide whether the results are applicable to their patient. A physician may consider the trial results to be applicable when the patient meets the eligibility criteria of the published study. Unfortunately, this principle is problematic. The necessary sampling procedure for selecting patients for the study (i.e., a random sample of all patients) has never been applied in clinical trials to our knowledge. Moreover, the principle ignores the fact that extrapolation is an inherent part of medical practice.

Within the general population there is a target population that includes those patient for whom the results of the trial are intended to apply (e.g., advanced endometrial cancer with no prior systemic cytotoxic therapies). Although an investigator can typically specify an idealized definition for the target population, additional practical issues also frequently need to be considered. For example, it is frequently debated whether or not to include patients with extra-ovarian papillary serous tumors into studies that target advanced ovarian cancer patients. Clinical investigators generally argue for the need to study a ''pure'' study population and ignore the fact that their treatment decisions for patients with extraovarian tumors frequently come from the results of

trials involving only patients with advanced ovarian cancer. Ideally, the size of a subgroup represented in a study should be in proportion to their presence in the target population (see Ethics section below). The degree to which a study sample reflects the target population determines the generalizability or external validity of the study results. Generalizability should be a driving force when determining the eligibility criteria. It is a serious indictment of a study's eligibility criteria if physicians frequently extrapolate the results to patients that would not have been eligible for the trial that produced the results.

The ideal situation is when each patient who meets the eligibility criteria of a clinical trial is asked to participate. This is seldom possible, since not all physicians who treat such patients participate in the study. Also, not all patients wish to be involved in a clinical trial. Impediments in traveling to a participating treatment center further reduce the target population. The source population is the subset of patients in the target population who have access to the study. Figure 9.1 displays the various sources restricting entry of patients to a clinical trial.

Restricted access to the study may contribute a biased sample from the target population, which is referred to as selection bias. For example, participating investigators at university hospitals might tend to enroll disproportionately more patients with ovarian cancer who have undergone very aggressive initial debulking surgeries than their counterparts at community hospitals.

A potentially useful approach for determining the necessity of a particular eligibility criterion is to identify clearly its function. There are four distinct functions that an eligibility criterion may serve: benefit-morbidity equipoise (safety), homogeneity of benefit (scientific), logistic and regulatory considerations (23).

Criteria for benefit-morbidity equipoise, or safety, are frequently imposed to eliminate patients for whom the risk of adverse effects from treatment are not commensurate with the potential for benefit (see Ethics section below). This concern can manifest in two ways. First, in oncology trials, there is often some concern that study treatments may be too toxic for those with compromised bone marrow reserves or kidney function. These patients are frequently excluded from trials because of the very likely possibility of a life-threatening adverse event. Second, even otherwise healthy cancer patients may be eliminated from the study because the antipated benefit is not sufficient to warrant any increase in the risk of a serious adverse event. For example, chemoradiation after hysterectomy is normally considered to be excessive treatment for a patient with stage IA cervical cancer since even without this treatment the risk of relapse is relatively small but the morbidity of this combined modality following hysterectomy may be substantial. Therefore, eligibility criteria that eliminate these patients may be justified.

Eligibility criteria may be warranted when there is a scientific or biologic rationale for a variation in treatment benefit

Sequential reduction of patient population

Forces reducing available patients

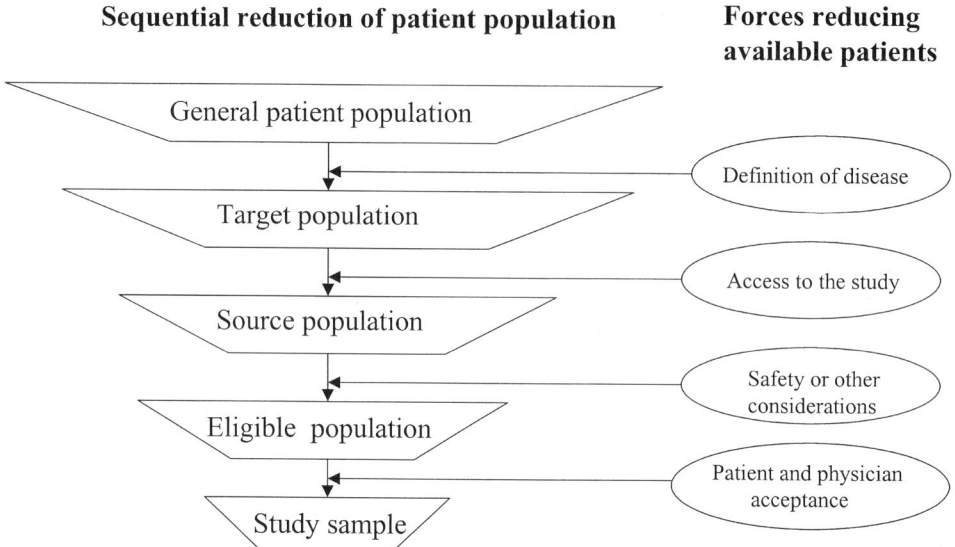

General patient population

Target population

Definition of disease

Source population

Access to the study

Eligible population

Safety or other considerations

Study sample

Patient and physician acceptance

FIG. 9.1. Sequential reduction of patient population.

across patient subgroups. There is no scientific reason to expect that the effect of treatment is entirely homogeneous across all subgroups of patients included in the study. The effect of a new therapy may be expected to have such dramatic inconsistencies across the entire spectrum of the target population that statistical power is compromised (23). One example of this type of exclusion criterion is found in GOG Protocol 152 [A Phase III Randomized Study of Cisplatin (NSC#119875) and Taxol (Paclitaxel) (NSC#125973) with Interval Secondary Cytoreduction versus Cisplatin and Paclitaxel in Patients with Suboptimal Stage III & IV Epithelial Ovarian Carcinoma]. This study is designed to assess the value of secondary cytoreductive surgery in patients with stage III ovarian cancer. All patients entered into this study are scheduled to receive three courses of cisplatin and paclitaxel. After completing this therapy, they are then randomized to either three additional courses of chemotherapy or interval secondary cytoreductive surgery followed by three additional courses of chemotherapy. Eligibility is restricted to patients with suboptimal (>1 cm of residual disease) stage III ovarian cancer. That is, the eligibility criteria exclude patients with microscopic disease since there is no scientific reason to expect interval debulking would be of any value to patients with no gross residual disease.

Clinical investigators frequently misconstrue the rationale for eligibility criteria to impose eligibility restrictions that promote homogeneity in patient prognoses. The desire to attain a study population with homogeneous risk is a common reason for excessive eligibility criteria. However, the concept is both unattainable and overemphasized. This notion may arise from an investigator's attempt to duplicate the experimental method conducted in the laboratory. It is standard practice in laboratory experiments on animals to use inbred strains in an effort to control genetic variability.

In large-scale clinical trials, this approach seldom has merit in light of the cost to generalizability. Eligibility criteria can be broadened in order to enhance generalizability. For example, GOG Protocol 165 [A Randomized Comparison of Radiation Plus Weekly Cisplatin versus Radiation plus PVI (Protracted Venous Infusion) 5-FU in Patients with Stage II-B,III-B and IV-A Carcinoma of the Cervix] includes patients with no surgical sampling of the paraaortic lymph nodes. Previous GOG trials required sampling of these nodes. However, there is no evidence or sound biologic justification to support the notion that the relative treatment benefit for the nonsurgical group is substantially different from that for the surgically staged. This is not to say whether or not surgical staging is itself beneficial.

Eligibility criteria can be justified on the basis of logistic considerations. For example, a study that requires frequent clinic visits for proper evaluation or toxicity monitoring may restrict patients who are unable to arrange reliable transportation. The potential problem with such a restriction is how it is structured. A criterion requiring that the patient have a car at her disposal is probably too restrictive in advanced cervical cancer since patients from this target population tend toward poorer socioeconomic status (SES) and may not have access to private transportation. Such a restriction will erode the generalizability of the trial by oversampling those with higher SES and may prolong study accrual. The more complicated the criterion becomes, the more likely that it will become problematic and function ineffectively. In general, complicated eligibility restrictions should be avoided.

Eligibility criteria based on regulatory considerations include those institutional and governmental regulations that require a signed and witnessed informed consent and study approval by the Institutional Review Board at the center where the patient is seeking treatment. These restrictions are required in most research settings and are not subject to the investigator's discretion. Regardless, these restrictions have the potential of eroding the trial's generalizability.

Recognizing each criterion's function is a valuable exercise in ensuring that the eligibility criteria are legitimate and minimal. Each criterion in a clinical trial should serve at least one of the four functions: benefit-morbidity equipoise, homogeneity of benefit, logistic and regulatory considerations. It is a worthwhile exercise to review each eligibility criterion in a study proposal to determine the function being served.

Currently, many biostatisticians believe that eligibility criteria in oncology trials tend to be too restrictive and complicated (23,24). Overly restrictive or complex eligibility criteria hamper accrual, prolong the study's duration, and delay the reporting of results. The Medical Research Council has demonstrated that it is possible to conduct trials with simple and few eligibility criteria (25). The ICON3 (International Collaborative Ovarian Neoplasms) trial compares a standard carboplatin or cisplatin, doxorubicin (Adriamycin) and cyclophosphamide regimen to paclitaxel plus carboplatin in women with newly diagnosed ovarian cancer. This trial has six eligibility criteria, three of which are for safety: (a) fit to receive, and no clear contraindication to, chemotherapy; (b) absence of sepsis; and (c) bilirubin less than twice the normal level for the center. This is in sharp contrast to GOG Protocol 162 [A Phase III Randomized Trial of Cisplatin (NSC #119875) with Paclitaxel (NSC #125973) Administered by Either 24-Hour Infusion or 96-Hour Infusion in Patients with Selected Stage III and Stage IV Epithelial Ovarian Cancer], which compares two different paclitaxel infusion durations in patients with advanced ovarian cancer and has 34 eligibility criteria.

CLINICAL TRIAL DESIGNS

The traditional approach to identifying and evaluating new treatment strategies has relied on evidence from Phase I, II, and III clinical trials. Each of these study designs stems from very distinct study objectives.

Phase I Trials

The purpose of a Phase I trial is to determine an acceptable dose or schedule of a new therapy as determined by toxicity and/or pharmacokinetics. A Phase I trial marks the first use of a new experimental agent in humans. Most Phase I trials escalate the dose or schedule of the new agent after either a prespecified number of consecutive patients have been successfully treated or within an individual as each dose is determined to be tolerable. The usual Phase I trial of a cytotoxic drug attempts to balance the delivery of the greatest dose intensity against an acceptable risk of dose-limiting toxicity (DLT). The conventional approach increases the dose after demonstrating that a small cohort of consecutive patients

(three to six) is able to tolerate the regimen. However, once an unacceptable level of toxicity occurs (e.g., two or three patients experiencing DLT), the previously acceptable dose level is used to treat a few additional patients in order to provide additional evidence that the current dose has an acceptably low risk of DLT. If this dose is still regarded as being acceptable, it becomes the dose and schedule studied in subsequent Phase II trials, and it is referred to as the maximum tolerated dose (MTD). Owing to the limited number of patients involved in a Phase I trials, outcome measures such as response and survival are not the primary interest in these studies. When these outcomes are reported, they are considered to be anecdotal evidence of treatment activity. Eligibility criteria for Phase I trials in oncology typically limit accrual to patients who have failed conventional treatments.

The development of a conventional Phase I strategy has been primarily ad hoc. Alternative strategies to identify the MTD have recently been proposed. The primary motivation for these newer strategies is to reduce the number of patients treated at therapeutically inferior doses and to reduce the overall size of the study. One of these alternatives implements a bayesian approach, and is referred to as the continual reassessment method (CRM) (26). It has the attractive feature of determining the dose level for the next patient based on the toxicity experience from the previously treated patients. Although the traditional approach has been criticized for treating too many patients at subtherapeutic doses and providing unreliable estimates of the MTD, CRM has been criticized for tending to treat too many patients at doses higher than the MTD (27). Refinements to CRM have been proposed (28) and have been found to have good properties when compared to alternative dose-seeking strategies (29). Another family of designs, termed the accelerated titration design (ATD), allows doses to be escalated within each patient and incorporates toxicity or pharmacologic information from each course of therapy into the decision of whether to escalate further or not (30). Both the CRM and ATD designs can provide significant advantages over the conventional Phase I design.

Phase II Trials

Once a dose and schedule for a new regimen has been deemed to be acceptable, a reasonable next step is to seek evidence that the new regimen is worthy of further evaluation in a particular patient population. The principal goal of a Phase II trial is to quantify prospectively the activity of the new therapy. Since a Phase II trial treats more patients at the MTD than in a Phase I trial, it also provides an opportunity to assess toxicities more reliably. A Phase II trial is often referred to as a drug-screening trial because it attempts judiciously to identify active agents worthy of further study in much the same way that a clinician screens a patient for further evaluation. The study should have adequate sensitivity to detect active treatments and adequate specificity for rejecting inactive treatments. A Phase II trial may evaluate a single new regimen or incorporate randomization to evaluate several new therapies or treatment schedules simultaneously. However, a concurrent control arm is rarely included in randomized Phase II trials since these trials are too small to draw a reliable inference about relative therapeutic efficacy of the experimental treatments.

Phase II trials can have a single-stage or multistage design. In a single-stage design, a fixed number of patients are treated with the new therapy. The goal of the single-stage design is to achieve a predetermined level of precision in estimating the endpoint. Although precision is one important goal in cancer trials, there is also a concern for minimizing the number of patients treated with inferior regimens. For this reason, many Phase II cancer trials use multistage designs. Multistage designs implement interim analyses of the data and apply predetermined rules to assess whether there is sufficient evidence to warrant continuing the trial. These rules, which are established prior to initiating the study, tend to terminate those trials with regimens having less than the desired activity, and tend to continue to full accrual those trials with regimens having at least a minimally acceptable level of activity. Two-stage designs that minimize the expected sample size when the new treatment has a clinically uninteresting level of activity have been proposed (31). These designs are often appropriate for trials involving a small number of clinics. However, Phase II trials in the cooperative group setting demand more flexibility in specifying when the interim analysis will occur. This is due to the significant administrative and logistic overhead of coordinating a considerable number of clinics. Modifications to the optimal design that do not require that the interim analyses occur after a precise number of patients are entered are useful in the cooperative group setting (32).

Regardless of the measure of treatment efficacy, most designs treat toxicity as merely a secondary observation. This approach is not likely to be appropriate in Phase II trials of very aggressive treatments, such as high-dose chemotherapy with bone marrow support. In these trials, stopping rules that explicitly consider both response and the cumulative incidence of certain toxicities may be more appropriate (33–35). Bayesian designs that permit continuous monitoring of both toxicity and response have also been proposed (36).

The procession from Phase I to Phase III is a typical research path for evaluating a new therapy in humans. However, this research paradigm may not always be appropriate, and all three elements (i.e., "what", "how," and "who") of a Phase II trial (see Objectives section above) have been challenged. It may be justifiable to eliminate strict Phase II testing of a new combination of known active agents if the combination is known to be safe and there is no antagonism anticipated between the agents, especially if the Phase III

trial includes a futility analysis (see Data Monitoring section below). Another challenge to the paradigm is directed at whether patients who have failed first-line therapy represent a fair test of a promising treatment plan. If the subsequent Phase III trial of the therapy will ultimately be used in newly diagnosed patients, it seems questionable whether first-line therapy failures represent the proper Phase II study population. Finally, clinical response has been a classic measure of activity in Phase II oncology clinical trials because the chronologic proximity of treatment and response strengthens the evidence for inferring cause and effect. However, response is a surrogate endpoint, and is almost certainly not an ideal one, especially in trials of patients with cervical cancer. Additionally, new treatments that exhibit a different mode of action from the traditional cytotoxic drugs (e.g., antiangiogenesis drugs) may make response unsuitable. PFI and survival time have been proposed to assess treatment efficacy in Phase II trials (37). There are many issues that come to bear on whether the conventional research paradigm is always appropriate. A thoughtful discussion among experts should precede all clinical research endeavors.

Phase III Trials

The goal of a Phase III trial is to determine prospectively and definitively the effects of a new therapy relative to a standard therapy in a well-defined population of patients. Phase III trials are also used to determine an acceptable standard therapy when there is no prior consensus on the appropriate standard therapy. Some Phase III trial methodologies, such as randomization and blocking, have origins in comparative laboratory experiments. However, in clinical trials, the experimental unit is a human being and, consequently, there are two very important distinctions. First, each individual must be informed of the potential benefits as well as the risks and must freely consent to participate before enrollment into the study (see Ethics section below). Second, an investigator has very limited control over the patient's environment during the observation period. This later distinction can have a profound statistical implication (see Primary Endpoints).

The strict definition of a Phase III trial does not necessitate concurrent controls (i.e., prospectively enrolled patients assigned the standard treatment) or randomization (i.e., random treatment allocation). However, these two features are almost synonymous with Phase III trials today. The principal drawback from inferring treatment differences from a historically controlled trial is that the treatment groups may differ in a variety of characteristics that are not apparent. Differences in outcome, which are in fact due to differences in characteristics between the groups, may be erroneously attributed to the treatment. Although mathematic models are often used to adjust for some potential biases, one can only adjust for factors that have been recorded accurately and consistently from both samples. Shifts in medical practice over time, differences in the definition of the disease, eligibility criteria, follow-up procedures, or recording methods can all contribute to a differential bias (see Endpoints section above). Unlike random error, this type of error cannot be reduced by increasing the sample size. Moreover, the undesirable consequences of moderate biases may be exacerbated with larger sample sizes. When a trial includes concurrent controls, the definition of disease and the eligibility criteria can be applied consistently to both treatment groups. Also, the standard procedures for measuring the endpoint can be uniformly applied to all patients. Inclusion of prospectively treated controls within the clinical trial requires a method of assigning the treatments to patients. Randomization and its benefits are discussed in the section on Other Design Considerations below.

It is useful to distinguish Phase III objectives as having an efficacy, equivalency, or noninferiority design consideration. An efficacy design is characterized by the search for new therapies that provide a therapeutic advantage over the current standard of care. An equivalency trial seeks to demonstrate that two treatments can be considered to be sufficiently similar on the basis of outcome that one can be reasonably substituted for the other. Noninferiority trials seek to identify new treatments that reduce toxicity, patient inconvenience, or treatment costs without significantly compromising efficacy.

Efficacy Trials

Efficacy designs are used very commonly in oncology trials. Examples include trials that assess the benefit of adding chemotherapy to radiation for the treatment of early-stage cervical cancer or trials that compare standard versus dose-intense platinum regimens for treating ovarian cancer. In each of these cases, the trial seeks to augment the standard of care in order to attain a better treatment response. From the outset of these trials, it is recognized that the treatment benefit may be accompanied by an increased risk of toxicity, inconvenience, or financial cost. However, it is hoped that the benefits will be sufficiently large to offset these concerns. Suppose treatment A is the standard of care for a particular target disease population. The quantitative difference between this treatment with respect to a particular outcome can be described on a horizontal axis as in Figure 9.2. If we are reasonably certain that the difference between treatments is less than zero (left of 0), then we would consider treatment A to be better. On the other hand, if the treatment difference is greater than zero (right of 0), then we would conclude that the new treatment, B, is better. Furthermore, we can use dotted lines to demarcate on this graphic a region in which the difference between A and B is small enough to warrant no clinical preference for A or B. Consider the results from a trial expressed as the estimated difference between treatments and the corresponding 95% or 99% confidence interval superimposed on this graph. The $(1 - \alpha)$% confidence interval depicts the values of the treatment difference that are consistent with the data such that they cannot be rejected when testing at the α level. An inconclusive trial is characterized by having such broad confidence intervals that the data cannot distinguish between A being preferred and B being preferred (Fig. 9.2). This is a typical consequence of a small trial. On the other hand, if the confidence interval entirely excludes the region where A is better than B, then we can conclude that B is significantly better than A (Fig. 9.2). Note that in this case the lower boundary of the confidence interval may extend into the region of clinical indifference, but the entire confidence interval must not include the region below (left of) zero difference.

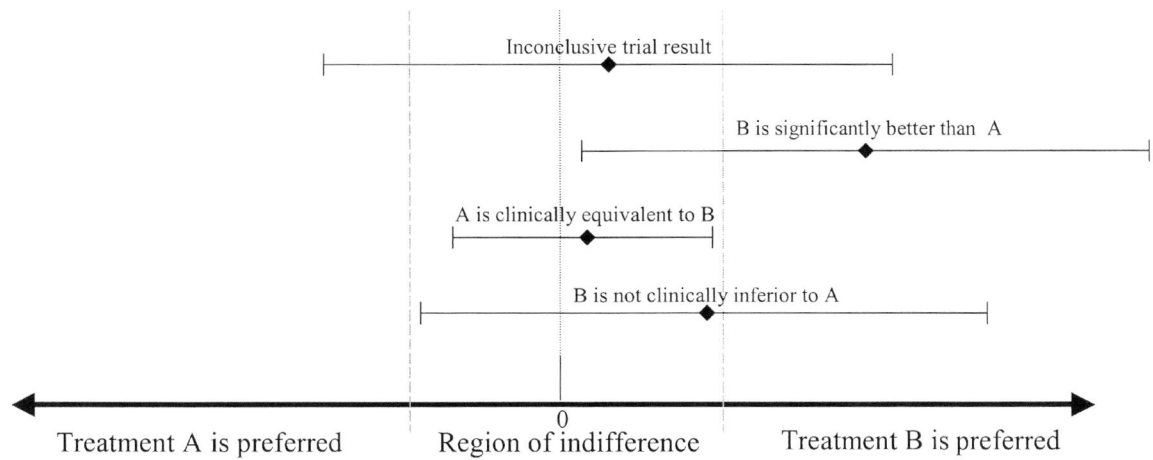

Difference between treatment A and B

FIG. 9.2. Graphic representation of the point estimates and confidence intervals describing the results from four hypothetical trials.

Equivalency Trials

The equivalency study design is perhaps a misnomer since it is actually impossible to generate enough data from any trial to claim definitively that the two treatments are equivalent. Instead, an investigator typically defines the limits for treatment differences that can be interpreted as being clinically irrelevant. If it is a matter of opinion for what differences can be considered to be clinically irrelevant, this issue can become a major source for controversy in the final interpretation of the trial results. Survival or progression-free survival endpoints are seldom used in cancer equivalency trials; however, bioequivalency designs are sometimes used for drug development. For example, if one agent is known to influence a particular biologic marker, then it may be desirable to design a trial to determine whether a new agent is as effective at modifying the expression of this biomarker. In this case, an investigator has some notion about the acceptable range of activity that can be considered to be clinically biologically equivalent. These studies are designed so that within tolerable limits, the treatments can be considered equivalent.

Notice that the results from the inconclusive trial in Figure 9.2 cannot be interpreted as demonstrating equivalency. Even though the estimated difference between the treatments is nearly zero, the confidence interval cannot rule out treatment differences that would lead to preferring A or B. Caution should be exercised in interpreting the results from studies that conclude "therapeutic equivalency" when only a small difference between treatments with regard to the outcome is observed that is declared not to be statistically significant. Even results from moderately large trials, which indicate therapeutic equivalence, may in fact be due to inadequate statistical power to detect clinically relevant differences.

Noninferiority Trials

A noninferiority study design may be considered when the currently accepted standard treatment is associated with significant toxicity and a new and less toxic treatment becomes available. The goal of this type of study is to demonstrate that substituting the new treatment for the current standard treatment does not compromise efficacy appreciably (38–41). Referring to Figure 9.2, the trial seeks to provide sufficient evidence to be reasonably certain that the difference between treatments A and B lies above the lower boundary of the indifference region. This lower boundary is often called the "noninferiority margin." The justification for the noninferiority margin selected in a particular study is often controversial. If this margin is set too low, then the study has an unacceptably high probability of recommending an inferior treatment. If it is too high, then the trial utilizes too many clinical and financial resources.

In order to select an appropriate margin of noninferiority, it is important to recognize that even though a noninferiority trial may explicitly compare only two treatments, implicitly there is a third treatment to be considered. Suppose that several historical studies indicate that treatment A is better than a placebo for treating a specific disease. In this case, the goal of a noninferiority study is to demonstrate that a new experimental treatment, B, does not significantly compromise efficacy when compared to currently accepted active control treatment, A. However, it must also demonstrate that B would have been better than a placebo if it had it been included in the current trial. In other words, the current trial will directly estimate the effectiveness of B relative to A, but it must also indirectly consider the effectiveness of B relative to the previous control treatment (placebo in this case). This indirect comparison relies on obtaining a reliable and unbiased estimate of the effectiveness of the current active control to the previous control from previous trials. Sometimes the margin of noninferiority is expressed as a proportion of the effectiveness of A relative to the previous standard treatment. For example, a noninferiority study could be designed to have a 95% chance of properly classifying a new treatment as being inferior if it is only half as effective as A. Some investigators may decide that they do not want to give up any of the benefit attributed to the current standard. In this case, the margin of noninferiority is set to zero, and this design is comparable to an efficacy trial design.

Obtaining reliable estimates for the effectiveness of the currently accepted active standard treatment can be a very troublesome aspect of noninferiority oncology trials. For example, cisplatin 75 mg/m^2 and paclitaxel 135 mg/m^2 infused over 24 hours was the first platinum-taxane combination to demonstrate activity in the treatment of advanced ovarian cancer (41a). Subsequently, several trials were conducted to assesses whether carboplatinum could be safely substituted for cisplatinum (42–44) or whether Taxotere could be substituted for paclitaxel (45). No trial has assessed the effectiveness of cisplatin added to a fixed dose of paclitaxel. Even worse, a meta-analysis that compared non–cisplatinum regimens to cisplatinum-containing regimens indicated that there was no significant treatment effect on overall survival attributable to adding cisplatin (45a). Moreover, there has been some controversy about the size of benefit provided by paclitaxel (46).

OTHER DESIGN CONSIDERATIONS

Randomization

There are several design features that may be considered for Phase III trials. Some are more pertinent than others to gynecologic oncology trials. The most important feature to be considered is randomization. A study with this feature has several scientific advantages. First, both the known and unknown prognostic factors tend to be distributed similarly across the treatment groups. Second, a potential source of differential selection bias is eliminated. This bias occurs when there is an association between treatment choice and prognosis. It need not be intentional. When a physician's interest in a trial or a patient's decision to participate in the trial depends on the assigned treatment, a nonrandom association between treatment and prognosis can be introduced. Third, it provides the theoretical underpinning for the significance test (47). In other words, the probability of a false-positive trial as stated in the study design is justified with randomization (see Sample Size section below). In short, randomization is the most effective method to form patient groups that are comparable.

It is sometimes argued that since many factors that influence prognosis are known, perhaps other approaches to allocating treatments can be considered and mathematic models used to adjust for imbalances in prognosis. However, the conclusions from this type of trial must be conditioned on the acceptability of the modeling assumptions. Results from these studies can polarize the medical community. They frequently provide enough evidence for those who already support the conclusions but insufficient evidence for those who are skeptical. For example, paclitaxel and platinum is currently the standard first-line treatment for advanced ovarian cancer in the United States. Following treatment, though, there is some disagreement regarding the value of reassessment (second-look) surgery. Those patients undergoing reassessment surgery and found to have residual disease frequently receive immediate preemptive second-line therapy despite the fact that the clinical value of reassessment surgery has never been subjected to a randomized trial. However, a nonrandomized comparison of surgery versus no surgery, adjusted for several prognostic factors, indicated that there was no benefit from reassessment surgery in women with optimal stage III ovarian cancer (48). Ardent supporters of reassessment surgery are not convinced, but others believe that this study decisively shifts the burden of proof onto those who support second-look surgery.

Kunz and Oxman (49) have compared the results from overviews of randomized and nonrandomized clinical trials that evaluated the same intervention. They reported that the non-randomized studies tended to overestimate the treatment effect from the randomized trials by 76% to 160%. Schutz et al. (50) compared 33 randomized controlled trials that had inadequate concealment of the pregenerated random treatment assignments to those studies that had adequate concealment. They found that those with inadequate concealment tended to overestimate the treatment effect (relative odds) by 40%. Some investigators do not appreciate the importance of concealment and will go to considerable lengths to subvert it (51). When the randomization technique requires pregenerated random treatment assignments, one must guarantee that the investigators enrolling patients have no access to the assignment lists.

The patient-physician relationship can occasionally be challenged by introducing the concept of treatment randomization (52). Patients may prefer a sense of confidence from their physicians regarding the "best" therapy for them. However, physicians involved in an RCT must honestly acknowledge that the best therapy is unknown and that an RCT is preferred to continued ignorance. One survey of 600 women seen in a breast clinic suggests that 90% of women prefer their doctor to admit uncertainty about the best treatment option rather than give them false hope (53).

Randomization Techniques

The simplest approach to randomization is to assign treatments based on a coin flip, sequential digits from random number tables, or computerized pseudo–random number generators. Each individual has the same probability of being allocated to a particular study treatment regardless of when they enter the study. Although this approach is simple, the statistical efficiency of the analyses can be enhanced by constraining the randomization so that each treatment is allocated an equal number of times. Permuted block randomization is sometimes used in order to promote equal treatment-group sizes. A block is created by shuffling a fixed number of cards for each treatment and then assigning the patients according to the random order of the deck. After completing each block, there are an equal number of patients assigned to the treatment groups. For example, consider a trial comparing treatments A and B. There are six possible ways the deck will be ordered when the block size is four: AABB, ABBA, BBAA, BABA, ABAB, and BAAB. A sufficient number of assignments for an RCT can be created by randomly selecting a series of blocks from the six distinct possibilities. There are three features of blocked randomization that may be problematic. First, the probability of a particular treatment being allocated is not the same throughout the study, as in simple randomization. Taking the example above, every fourth treatment is predetermined by the previous three allocations. Second, the use of small blocks in a single-institution study may undermine concealment and allow an investigator to deduce the next treatment. This potential problem can be corrected by continually changing the block size throughout the assignment list. Third, large block sizes can subvert the benefits of blocking. As block sizes increase, the procedure resembles simple randomization.

The statistical efficiency of the study can be further enhanced by stratifying patients into groups with similar prognoses and using separate lists of blocked treatments for each stratum. This procedure is called stratified block randomization. It is worth noting that using simple randomization within strata would defeat the purpose of stratification, since this is equivalent to simple randomization. Likewise, trials that stratify on too many prognostic factors are likely to have many uncompleted treatment blocks at the end of the study, which also defeats the intent of blocking (54).

When it is desirable to balance on more than a few prognostic factors, an alternative is dynamic randomization; a particular type being minimization. Whereas stratified block randomization will balance treatment assignments within each combination of the various factor levels, minimization tends to balance treatments in each factor separately. Each time a new patient is entered into the study, the number of individuals who share any of the prognostic characteristics of the new patient is tabulated. A metric, which measures the imbalance of these factors among the study treatments, is computed as if the new patient were allocated to each of the study treatments in turn. The patient is then allocated to the treatment that would favor the greatest degree of balance. In the event that the procedure indicates equal preference for two or more possible treatment allocations, simple randomization is used.

Masking Treatment

Blinding

Blinding is a mechanism to prevent the patient or physician from knowing which treatment is being used. In a single-blinded study, the patient is unaware of which of possibly several known treatments she is receiving. A double-blinded study results in a situation in which neither the patient nor the healthcare provider is aware of that information. One purpose of blinding is to avoid measurement bias, particularly differential measurement bias (see Endpoints section above). Such bias subjectivity occurs when the value of a measurement is influenced by the knowledge of which treatment is being received (see Historical Perspective section above). This bias can occur when the measurement of an endpoint is subjective. Most methods for assessing pain are subjective and require double blinding to ensure a valid study.

Oncology trials frequently do not implement blinding for several reasons. Sometimes, it is rather difficult to blind treatments when various treatment modalities are used (e.g., surgery vs radiation therapy or intravenous vs oral administrations), when good medical practice is jeopardized (e.g., special tests are required to monitor toxicity), or when it is logistically difficult (e.g., evaluating physician must be kept isolated from the treatment of the patient). In the absence of blinding, great care should be taken that the method of measuring the endpoint is precisely stated in the protocol and consistently applied to each patient. Trials that assess relief from symptoms or quality of life should give serious consideration to treatment blinding.

Schulz et al. (55) have reviewed 110 randomized clinical trials published between 1990 and 1991 in four journals devoted to the fields of obstetrics and gynecology. Thirty-one of these trials reported being double-blinded. However, blinding seemed to be compromised in at least three of the trials. Schultz et al. conclude that blinding should have been used more often despite the frequent impediments.

Placebo

A placebo is an inert treatment that is usually self-administered (e.g., in tablet form). Placebos blind the patient and also, usually, the physician to the knowledge of whether they are receiving the active or inert treatment. Placebos are frequently used in trials where there is no accepted standard treatment and the endpoint is susceptible to measurement bias. The use of a placebo is also important when the endpoint can be affected by the patient's psychologic response to the knowledge of receiving therapy combined with a belief that the therapy is effective. This phenomenon is aptly named the ''placebo effect.'' In such circumstances, the use of a placebo provides a treatment to control comparison that measures only the therapeutic effect. Note that the placebo effect is a distinctly different type of measurement bias from those that have been previously discussed.

GOG Protocol 137 [A Randomized Double-Blinded Trial of Estrogen Replacement Therapy versus Placebo in Women with Stage I or II Endometrial Adenocarcinoma (IND #43,226)] is a randomized double-blinded comparison of estrogen replacement therapy versus a placebo in women who have had a total abdominal hysterectomy and bilateral salpingo-oophorectomy for early-stage endometrial cancer. One primary reason for the use of a placebo in this trial was the potential for differential measurement bias being introduced by the physician monitoring patients on estrogens much more closely.

Sham procedures are similar to placebos in their function but require a more active role on the part of the investigator. The sham procedure is one that mimics the experimental procedure under study (excluding the therapeutic portion) to the extent that patients are blinded to whether they received the real procedure. Careful ethical considerations must precede the use of a placebo or sham procedure in any clinical trial (56).

Special Designs

Factorial Designs

Factorial designs assess two or more treatments, each being delivered at two or more levels within the same trial. The term *factorial* arises from historical terminology in which the treatments were referred to as factors. The total number of factor combinations being studied is the product of the number of levels for each factor or treatment. For example, a trial that evaluates treatment A at three levels and treatment B at two levels is called a 3-by-2 (denoted 3×2) factorial design. The advantage of this design is that the effectiveness of two treatments (i.e., A and B) is evaluated simultaneously. When the relative effects due to the various levels of A are independent of the levels of B, a factorial design provides a significant reduction in the required sample size when compared to trials that study A and B separately.

TABLE 9.1. *A schematic of a 2 × 2 factorial design*

		Factor A	
		No	Yes
Factor B	No	not A and not B	A
	Yes	B	A and B

The simplest form of this type of trial is the 2 × 2 factorial that includes four distinct treatment regimens: A, B, A and B, and not A and not B (Table 9.1). This study design provides two estimates of the effect of A. One estimate of the effect of A arises from comparing the group who received only A to those who received not A and not B and the second estimate arises from comparing those who received A and B to those who received only B. When there is no interaction between factors, these two estimates can be pooled into a single estimate for the effect of A, which is often called the main or the marginal effect of A. A similar approach can be applied for estimating the effect of B.

An interaction exists when the effect due to one of the factors (i.e., treatment A) depends on the level of the other factor (treatment B). A test for homogeneity compares these two estimates to determine whether the data support the hypothesis of no interaction. Reliable tests of interaction require a relatively large number of patients in each of the four treatment groups. This testing, in turn, reduces the advantage of the factorial design over two separate studies. Attention to the power of such tests is an important part of interpreting the study results (2,57,58).

Crossover Designs

In crossover trials, each patient receives a sequence of treatments and the individual's response is recorded after each treatment. Patients are usually randomized to one of the various possible sequences in which the treatments can be given. Crossover designs are rarely used in gynecologic oncology because the traditional endpoints are nonreversible events (e.g., first recurrence). This situation is in contrast to many acute illnesses where the endpoint can be measured many times owing to the cyclic nature of the illness (e.g., allergic reaction).

The simplest form of this study design is the two-treatment crossover design. Half of the patients receive treatment A, are evaluated, and then cross over to receive B and are evaluated again. The other half of the patients reverse the order of treatments, receiving B first and then A. The phrase "two-period design" is also used in this context to indicate the two spans of time in which each treatment is given and evaluated. Unlike other parallel designs, the crossover trial creates a treatment comparison within each patient. The purpose of a crossover design is to eliminate from the treatment comparison the component of variation due to differences in patient's inherent chance of response. Typically, the vari-

ability between individuals is considerably larger than the variability of repeated measurements from the same individual. The crossover design exploits this feature to improve sensitivity to treatment differences.

Crossover studies are susceptible to carryover effects. From the example above, a carryover effect is when the effect of treatment A is different when it follows treatment B compared to when it precedes treatment B. If this phenomenon is due to some interaction of the two treatments, a washout period between the two periods may be appropriate to eliminate this effect. The effect of a particular treatment may also depend on whether it is given relatively early or late in relation to the onset of the illness. This effect is called a treatment-by-period interaction. From a statistical standpoint, these effects create much the same problems as interactions in the factorial designs (see above).

Tailored Therapy

The recent advances in molecular biology have created an exponential increase in host and tumor factors (i.e., biomarkers) that may some day not only guide but dictate cancer therapy. The term *predictive factor* has become part of the vernacular of oncology to refer to a biomarker with this property and to distinguish it from a prognostic factor. The term has been defined in the literature (59), and more recently statisticians have begun considering how to design studies of predictive factors (60). A prognostic factor is defined as any characteristic of the host, or the disease, that can distinguish important differences in the risk of relapsing and/or dying of the disease. Often a patient's prognostic factors influence treatment recommendations in a rough fashion. For example, the most aggressive therapy is often recommended to patients with poor prognoses without strong evidence that it is more effective than a more conservative therapeutic approach (e.g., high-dose chemotherapy with autologous stem cell support).

Part A of Table 9.2 displays the "expected" outcome in terms of relative risk for a hypothetical prognostic factor (for simplicity, the factor has two states: present or absent) and two treatment regimens. The table indicates that the prognostic factor is associated with a one-third reduction in risk regardless of which treatment is given. In this situation, both the factor and the treatment have a multiplicative effect on risk with no interaction. A prognostic factor differentiates risk of the disease regardless of the therapy (even in the case of no therapy). In contrast, part B of Table 9.2 displays a hypothetical predictive factor having no prognostic value. What sets the purely predictive factor apart is that there is no multiplicative effect of either the factor when using therapy C or multiplicative effect of treatment E over C when the factor is absent. Rather, the risk reduction occurs only when treatment E is used in the presence of the factor; this is termed an interaction and is the essence of a predictive factor. Implicit in a potential predictive factor is usually

TABLE 9.2. *A theoretical example of relative risk associated with a prognostic and predictive factor within two different treatment regimens*

A. Prognostic

Prognostic factor	Treatment	
	E	C
Present (25% prevalence)	0.533 (0.667)	0.667
Absent	0.80 (1.0[a])	1.0[a]
Total	0.733	0.917

B. Predictive

Prognostic factor	Treatment	
	E	C
Present (25% prevalence)	0.50	1.0
Absent	1.0	1.0[a]
Total	0.875	1.0

[a] By definition the relative risk is expressed in terms of a reference group.

some biologic theory about the mechanism of action of treatment E in the presence of the factor. Unlike the indirect influence that a prognostic factor has on treatment decisions, a predictive factor dictates the use of one therapy over another (presuming the interaction is of sufficient magnitude). As indicated in Table 9.2 part B, the clear choice for a patient with the factor present is treatment E, whereas there is no compelling reason for administering treatment E over C to the patient without the factor.

The most celebrated predictive factor in oncology is HER-2/*neu* expression in breast cancer and the use of trastuzumab (Herceptin) (61). HER-2/*neu* was originally identified as a prognostic factor. Subsequently, HER-2/*neu* was also recognized as a predictive factor after trastuzumab was shown to be effective in patients with breast cancer expressing HER-2/*neu*. In gynecologic oncology, estrogen and progesterone receptor status has often been considered to be a predictive factor for hormonal therapy in endometrial cancer but the empirical evidence is weak (62). Chemosensitivity assays that were once hoped to become a major and effective therapeutic strategy are nothing more than potential predictive factors. The unique feature of a chemosensitivity assay is its compelling nature to be predictive. Results of such trials have oftentimes been disappointing because the assays were only prognostic. More precisely, the assay indicated that the patient's disease was sensitive (or resistant) to cytotoxic therapy rather than predictive of outcome for the agent used in the assay. In addition, many chemosensitivity trials were flawed in design because a substantial proportion of the patients in the control group received the same therapy as they would have if they were assigned to the assay-directed regimen (63). Some of these assays maintained popularity for an excessive period of time owing in part to less than optimally designed trials that could have dispelled their usefulness.

The need to design optimal clinical trials of predictive factors is critical now more than ever.

Sargent and Allegra (60) discuss issues involved in designing clinical trials of tumor markers (specifically predictive factors). Their suggestions include embedding the testing of such factors (possibly two or more) within a prospective therapeutic clinical trial and increasing the sample size goal to address both questions. To fully assess a predictive factor requires sufficient data both to complete the four cells displayed in part B of Table 9.2 and have sufficient power to perform statistical tests that will distinguish the predictive component of a factor from its prognostic component. The sample size required is primarily driven by the substantially larger sample sizes needed to detect interactions (58). The sample size requirement is also influenced by the prevalence of the factor. Prevalence of a factor that differs substantially from 50% will require considerably larger sample sizes than if there were equal probability of the factor being present or absent. It seems unrealistic to assume that an experimental agent, and the predictive factor that might indicate its use, would be ready for investigation in a large prospective clinical trial at the same time. If the experimental agent is being investigated in an RCT prior to the development of a potential predictive factor, the ideal plan is to conduct the trial and collect and store high-quality specimens until the predictive factor presents itself. It is important to realize that the potential for an important predictive factor to be discovered retrospectively in the completed trial is not diminished even if the therapeutic trial is negative (i.e., accepting the null hypothesis). In fact, a negative trial is very likely (i.e., low statistical power) in a situation illustrated by Table 9.2 part B, where the analysis addressing the benefit of treatment E over C is essentially conducted on the "Total" row without knowledge of the four table cells.

Hypothesis Test

A hypothesis is a conjecture based on prior experiences that leads to refutable predictions (64). A hypothesis is frequently framed in the context of either a null or an alternative hypothesis. The null hypothesis postulates that the study treatment does not influence an outcome measure. The premise of the alternative hypothesis is that a particular, well-defined treatment approach will influence the outcome to some degree. These hypotheses cast the purpose of the trial into a clear framework, such that the probabilities of errors associated with the statistics-based decision, to be applied at the end of the trial, can be quantified. Prospectively quantifying the acceptable levels for these errors provides the underpinning for determining the design and sample size of a particular trial (see Sample Size section below). Most RCTs include at least one hypothesis test of the treatment effect on the primary endpoint.

Table 9.3 displays the "correctness" of the two possible decisions that will be made based on whether the null or

TABLE 9.3. *The correctness of the two possible decisions to be made at the completion of the RCT for various states of reality as expressed by the null and alternative hypotheses*

| | Unknown state of reality for relative risk (RR)[a] | | |
Decision	H_0: $1 \leq RR$	H_a: $2/3 \leq RR < 1$	H_a: $RR < 2/3$
Accept H_0	Correct (true negative)	Correct?	Incorrect (type II error)
Reject H_0	Incorrect (type I error)	Incorrect?	Correct (true positive)

H_0, null hypothesis; H_a, alternative hypothesis.

[a] Relative risk is the risk of failure of the experimental group to control group.

alternative hypotheses are true. The test statistic, a function of the data generated from the study, provides a formalized way to make the decision. In general, the difference in the endpoint between treatments is algebraically denoted as Δ. The algebra of statistics uses Greek letters to represent the "unknown" parameters needed to specify the endpoint (random variable, in general) distribution. In a trial, the statistical design and analysis plan usually focuses on one of these parameters. Specifically, there are three statistical entities that stem from this focal parameter: first, the estimator of the difference between the parameter values for the two groups to be compared under the alternative hypothesis; second, the test that is optimal for detecting a difference in the parameter values; third, the definition of what difference will be considered clinically important to detect (discussed in detail below). A typical RCT in gynecologic oncology would consider the primary endpoint to be a time-to-event, say PFS, and therefore, the unknown parameter of interest is usually the relative risk (RR) of progression between treatment groups. In this text, we will freely interchange Δ and RR. In Table 9.3, the minimum, clinically important RR is two-thirds. This is a one-sided hypothesis conveying the point that the alternative hypothesis includes only increases in the PFS of the experimental group to be clinically relevant. For each state of reality, there is a correct and an incorrect decision. The probability of a type I error (α level) is the chance of rejecting the null hypothesis when it is true and the probability of a type II error (statistical term: β level) is the chance of accepting the null hypothesis when the alternative is true. The more common way of expressing this second error is the statistical power ($1 - \beta$), the probability of the complement to type II error.

Appropriate sizes of the type I and II errors are determined as part of the study design. Frequently, a statistician makes an initial selection, but it is important that the investigators approve the choice and feel free to pose alternative values if the initial choices seem to be unsuitable. In most RCTs, the errors are 0.05 for type I error and 0.10 to 0.20 for type II errors (statistical power of 0.90 to 0.80). The magnitudes of these errors reflect the consequences of making one error versus the other. Committing the type I error might be disastrous if it means discontinuing the use of a control treatment that is well tolerated and substituting an experimental ther-

apy that is very toxic (but in reality no better). In such a case, committing the type II error would not be considered to be as troubling as committing a type I error, and therefore, an α level of 0.05 and a β level of 0.20, the latter being four times larger than the former, may be appropriate. However, suppose the experimental therapy is much less toxic and very convenient for the patient to receive, but at the same time, there may be concerns that it may not be as effective as the control treatment (see Equivalency and Noninferiority Trials). In such trials, it is much more important to control the type II errors (missing a loss in efficacy when the experimental therapy is inferior).

Choosing a minimum, clinically important difference is as critical to the hypothesis test as the type I and II errors. Stringently controlling these errors, but at the same time choosing a large and overly optimistic effect size (Δ), is counterproductive. In Table 9.3, the reality may be that the relative risk is in the range: $2/3 \leq RR < 1$ (second column of Table 9.3). If 2/3 is the minimum, clinically important difference, the correctness of the decision is as stated without the question mark. By choosing an overly optimistic RR, owing to a lack of patients or finances, both decisions in the second column of the table are incorrect for a certain portion of the range. More importantly, the type II error is not controlled for clinically important differences. GOG studies of optimal stage III disease traditionally used a RR of 2/3. However, some have suggested that even a RR of 0.76 is clinically important (65). To ensure a high probability of correctly classifying an active experimental treatment requires a realistic choice of the minimal RR, or in general, Δ.

p-Value

Some researchers are overly fond of using *p*-values when presenting results; at times, statisticians play the role of the conservative physician cautiously prescribing a significance test only when it is appropriate. There is a general concern that the *p*-value is overused, even abused, and overemphasized in clinical studies. A common misconception is that the *p*-value is the probability that the null hypothesis is true. The null hypothesis is either true or false, and so it is therefore not subject to a probability statement.

Misconceptions about the *p*-value (or significance level)

may arise in part from a poor distinction between the *p*-value and the α level (the type I error) of a study (66). The α level is the probability of the test statistic rejecting the null hypothesis when it is true. It is set during the design phase of the study, and is unaltered by the results obtained. The *p*-value results from a statistical test on the observed data. It is the probability of the observed result or a more extreme result, given the null hypothesis is true. R.A. Fisher, who is credited with developing the concept of the *p*-value, suggested that it be used as a measure of credibility for the null hypothesis. J. Neyman and K. Pearson developed the notion of acceptance and rejection regions for the null hypothesis based on a critical value. Consequently, type I and II errors were spawned. Fisher was very much against using this ''black and white'' approach to measure the evidence of the true state of reality.

The *p*-value is problematic because it confounds the relative treatment benefit and the amount of data (sample size) (67). Suppose two trials studying the same disease and the same treatments yield the same *p*-value but one study is four times larger than the other. The *p*-value can be equal when the estimate of the relative treatment benefit from the smaller trial is approximately two times that in the larger trial. Assuming both were well-designed studies, one should have much more confidence in the estimate of the benefit from the larger trial. In short, the *p*-value tells us little about the size of the treatment effect.

Important clinical differences and statistically significant differences do not correspond as frequently as they should. A large meta-analysis may result in a statistically significant difference that is not to be considered important clinically. Meta-analysis refers to a formal and comprehensive statistical analysis of a complete, or close to complete, set of randomized trials that have a consistent experimental regimen and a common control regimen. The purpose for such an analysis may include the desire to overcome publication bias, to obtain an estimate of the average treatment effect, and/or to resolve apparent conflicts in the results of several trials (68). Conversely, the literature contains many small trials with nonsignificant results that are underpowered and cannot rule out clinically important differences (69).

A *p*-value of 0.050 is not necessarily a compelling result. Suppose a trial is properly designed using a statistical power of 90%, a type I error of 5% (a two-tail test), and a minimal, clinically important difference (Δ). The trial is properly executed and the *p*-value equals precisely 0.05. The relative benefit between treatment groups would be approximately 60% of the specified Δ (66). Ironically, this statistically significant estimate of the treatment benefit itself is not in the range of clinically important differences. Furthermore, suppose that after reviewing this study the investigators agree that the result is clinically important and that the next study should be designed to detect such a difference. It may be surprising that the size of the current trial is wholly inadequate to detect such a difference. To be precise, suppose the

observed difference in the current trial was the true difference and one wanted to confirm the results in a second trial (same regimens and sample size), then there is no better than a flip of a coin chance (50:50) of a significant difference in the second trial (66). These results are perhaps counterintuitive, but they emphasize the shortcomings of overinterpreting *p*-values. Furthermore, the meaning of a significant *p*-value is diminished considerably when associated with one test in a series of hypothesis tests conducted on data from a single RCT.

Sample Size

The primary goal in an RCT is either to estimate some parameter (estimator) or to conduct a hypothesis test (test statistic). The precision of either an estimator or a test statistic is a direct consequence of the size of the study population (sample size).

In the case of estimation, the larger the number of patients in the RCT, the more precise the estimator is in estimating the unknown parameter. The precision of an estimator is most simply expressed through the use of a confidence interval. In the case of the normal distribution, the width of the confidence interval is directly proportional to the standard error of the average. The formula for standard error reveals that the width of the confidence interval is indirectly proportional to the square root of the sample size. This relationship is approximately true for most estimators. However, for estimators that involve comparisons (e.g., estimator of relative risk), the confidence interval is affected by the number of patients in each of the treatment groups. In essence, the precision of the estimate is only as good as the smallest treatment group.

In the vast majority of RCTs, the sample size is based on one or more formal hypothesis tests to be conducted. These hypothesis tests arise from determining the most efficient way of comparing two distributions, or sometimes comparing the parameter that best indicates the central tendency of the distributions. The formula that will drive the decision is called the test statistic. Parameters arise from making a priori assumptions about the distributional structure of the endpoint (e.g., assuming the endpoint is normally distributed with unknown mean and variance). A more relevant example involves the endpoint response as a binary outcome; in this case, the parameter of interest is the unknown probability of response in both the control and the experimental groups, and a reasonable test statistic becomes the difference in the percentage of responses in one group minus the percentage from the other group.

There are five elements that need to be addressed to determine the sample size for a hypothesis test: (a) the test statistic employed; (b) the probability of rejecting the null hypothesis when it is true (type I error, or α level) and the consideration of whether it is important to detect departures from the null hypothesis in both directions (i.e., one-sided vs two-sided test); (c) the probability of not rejecting the null hypothesis when the alternative is true (type II error or β level); (d) the smallest difference considered clinically important, Δ, to detect; and (e) the anticipated value of the parameter or the distribution for one of the treatment groups.

An example will help to illustrate this point. Suppose it is decided to use tumor response as the endpoint in an RCT where the results could be displayed in a 2×2 table, and the test statistic will be the z-score (the difference in the proportion responding divided by the standard error of that difference). Furthermore, it is decided to set $\alpha = 0.05$, and detecting increases in the frequency of response is all that is of interest (one-sided test). Continuing, it is decided to set $\beta = 0.10$ (i.e., statistical power is 0.90), $\Delta = 15\%$ (the difference in the probability of response), and the frequency of response in the control group is anticipated to be 30%. Such a trial would require 354 patients in total, 177 in each treatment group. The degree to which one desires small α, β, and Δ for an RCT is the degree to which the sample size is increased.

There are legitimate concerns over the distributional assumptions in the sample-size determination above; specifically, the fact that the test statistic chosen is based on the tenuous assumption that each patient has the same chance of responding to treatment is a concern. In reality, there is a fair amount of heterogeneity among patients, and therefore, a more conservative test statistic, namely, Fisher's "exact" test, is more appropriate. This test is a nonparametric statistic, which means it does not require assuming any distributional structure and, therefore, has no parameters to estimate. Sample sizes based on this test statistic are somewhat larger than those based on the z-score described above. For example, in the hypothetical RCT described above, the sample size would be 380 patients (an increase of 26) owing to eliminating any assumptions about the distributional structure. This is a small increase in the sample size, and is considered an excellent trade-off to accommodate the heterogeneity among patients.

Most RCTs in gynecologic oncology include a hypothesis test of time-to-event endpoint (e.g., PFS, survival time). Determining an appropriate sample size for such a hypothesis is dramatically simplified by the assumption of proportional hazards. Consider survival time for simplicity: the hazard function is the probability of dying in the next moment after any particular point in time in the observation period, having survived at least to that point in time. This has been referred to as the force of mortality. One must make the assumption that the ratio of the two unknown hazard functions that arise from the two treatment groups is an unknown constant. There is no requirement that the hazard rate, and thus the survival distribution, has any particular structure. This single-parameter structure is referred to as a semiparametric model. The sample size for testing the difference in survival stems from this single parameter. The *total number of deaths*

required for a specified α, β, and Δ when the two treatment groups will be the same size is:

$$D = \frac{4(Z_{1-\alpha} + Z_{1-\beta})^2}{\log^2(\Delta)}$$

$Z_{1-\alpha}$ and $Z_{1-\beta}$ are the $1-\alpha$ and $1-\beta$ quantiles, respectively, from the standard normal deviation and Δ is the smallest clinically important hazard ratio to detect (70). If proportional hazards is a valid assumption, then an appropriate statistical test procedure is described by Mantel (71).

Table 9.4 provides the number of events required, based on the above formula, for $\alpha = 0.05$ (one-tailed test), $\beta = 0.10$ and 0.20, and RR = 0.5, 0.6, 0.667, 0.7, and 0.8 (relative hazard: the ratio of the experimental group hazard rate divided by the control group hazard rate). Notice the dramatic increase in the required number of events as one chooses smaller and smaller differences to detect. It is important to understand that the total sample size is larger than the number of deaths (or whatever events are associated with the endpoint) given in Table 9.4. To calculate the total sample size requires determining the proportion of patients that will have died at the time of the final analysis (element five from the list above). The proportion should be divided into the number of events from Table 9.4 to arrive at the total sample size. For example, in designing a two-arm RCT with survival as the endpoint, one decides to set $\alpha = 0.05$ (one-tail test), $\beta = 0.2$ (i.e., statistical power: 0.80), and $\Delta = 0.667$. Table 9.4 indicates that 150 deaths must be observed before conducting the test. Suppose now this is an early-stage cervical cancer trial in which we expect only 10% to have died when final analysis is conducted. Assuming no patients are lost to follow-up, the total sample-size goal would be 1,500 (150/0.10) patients. Now suppose the study involves recurrent cervical cancer patients, 90% of whom will have died when final analysis is conducted. This trial requires a total sample size of only 167 (150/0.90) patients, but it is based on exactly the same α, β, and Δ as the early-stage cervical cancer study.

Although relative hazards are often considered to be a very appropriate parameter to summarize the difference between two treatment groups, it is not obvious how the value

TABLE 9.4. *The net sample size (number of events) required to attain an α level of 0.05 (one-sided test), and the indicated statistical power and relative risk with equal size treatment groups*

Relative risk (RR)	Statistical power (1 − β)	
	0.80	0.90
0.50	51	71
0.60	95	131
0.667	150	208
0.70	194	269
0.75	299	414
0.80	497	688

translates into absolute differences at a particular time point on the graph. Clinical investigators often prefer to think in terms of absolute differences when discussing what is the smallest important difference to be used in designing the RCT. Assuming proportional hazards, the absolute difference in risk, Δ_{Abs}, is expressed by the following formula, which can be easily evaluated with a hand calculator:

$$\Delta_{Abs} = S_C(t)^\Delta - S_C(t)$$

In this formula, $S_C(t)$ is the survival rate at time t, and Δ is the hazard ratio of the experimental group to the control group. In the cervical cancer example, if the 3-year survival rate for the control group in the early-stage RCT is 90%, then a relative hazard of 0.667 would result in a difference of 3.2% at 3 years. In the recurrent disease RCT, if the survival rate is 10% at 3 years, then the difference would be 11.5%. In most situations, designing a trial in early-stage cervix cancer using a relative hazard of 0.667 would be considered to be too small of an improvement to be clinically important.

Data Monitoring

Data monitoring can be classified into three categories: administrative, quality control, and endpoint monitoring. Observing extremely poor accrual in a trial that questions the feasibility of completing the trial is an example of administrative monitoring. Any evaluation of an actively accruing trial that addresses whether the study will produce valid results is quality control monitoring. Endpoint monitoring is when comparisons are made of the endpoints between treatment groups. This last category is the only one that attempts to test the hypothesis earlier than the formal end of the trial. Although much of the statistical methodology for data monitoring was published 20 or more years ago, formal plans for data monitoring have become routine and expected in RCT designs only in the last several years. The most uncomplicated situation occurs when an ongoing trial provides incontrovertible evidence that one of the treatments is inferior. In this situation, the need to close the trial (or the arm using the inferior treatment) becomes essential. The challenge in a data monitoring plan is the definition of "incontrovertible evidence." The sophistication of data monitoring statistical methods and the formality associated with Data Monitoring Committee stem from a simple premise that knowledge of benefit (or harm) of an experimental treatment accumulates slowly over time. Many trials can be monitored because patients are enrolled over a period of years and differences in patient outcome may emerge between treatment groups before other patients are even enrolled. Endpoint monitoring was initially driven by the ethics of do no harm (see Ethics section below). However, endpoint monitoring has expanded to include terminating a trial because of the lack of improvement among the experimental group. Continuing the trial in this situation is not as much an ethical di-

lemma as a poor use of investigator's resources. This type of data monitoring is referred to as futility analysis. The term is ideal in that it conveys the thought that continuing the trial in the hopes of seeing a significant improvement is futile in the experimental group when compared to the control group. The remaining discussion involves the more common data monitoring for dramatic differences.

The cost in monitoring endpoints (for the purpose of stopping the trial) is subtle and influences the characteristics of the hypothesis tests. Most physicians' understanding of statistics comes from frequentist theory and fixed sample size designs. Fixed sample size designs to test a hypothesis can be described as conducting the test statistic once after completing the collection of a prespecified number of observations (see Hypothesis Test section above). Data monitoring for the purpose of stopping the trial early, thus varying the sample size, is in direct conflict with fixed sample size methods. The specific problem is the rule established to declare significance (i.e., rejecting the null hypothesis) for a one-time, end of the trial test is no longer correct when conducting the test multiple times over the active accrual period. Figure 9.3 is a theoretical illustration of how defining statistical significance is a by-product of how often the emerging data is to be analyzed. The line graphs display the changing p-value over the trial period for 20 fictitious RCTs when there is no difference in the effect of treatment (i.e., the null hypothesis is true). The thick lines are associated with declaring "significance"; the critical boundary for continual monitoring is the horizontal line and the critical region for the single test at the completion of the study is the vertical line. Visually, the rule is if the line touches the boundary, "significance" is declared. Note the vertical boundary identifies only 1 trial in 20 (1/20 or 5% error) as "significant," but the horizontal line (continual monitoring) identifies four additional "significant" trials under [(1 + 4]/20 or 25% error). This is a fivefold increase in the type I error since all 20 trials were simulated under the null hypothesis. Figure 9.3 dramatically illustrates why interim monitoring rules must be more stringent (i.e., significance level must be smaller) than what would be used if no data monitoring occurred. Notice that the four additional lines that touch the horizontal boundary return to a nonsignificant p-value by the end of the trial. This is an illustration that the act of monitoring is not what causes the increase in the type I error but rather it is closing the trial early and declaring "significance."

Data monitoring has a much greater impact than changing the rules for declaring "significance"; it also changes the meaning of the p-value and confidence interval estimates. Even the fixed sample size p-value calculated in a trial that achieves the entire sample size but had data monitoring is technically incorrect. However, most investigators ignore this fact to avoid the complexity that would result by providing adjusted p-values. Also, data monitoring affects the estimation of the statistical parameters. The estimator associated

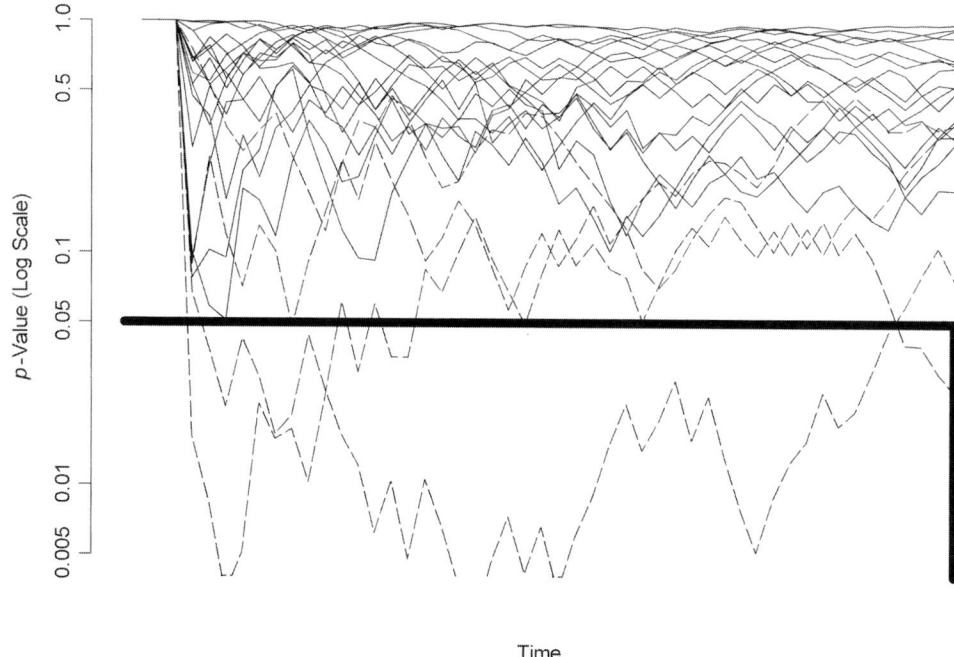

FIG. 9.3. Continual monitoring of 20 trials' conventional significance level under null hypothesis.

with the hypothesis being tested is biased when interim stopping rules are in use. For example, a trial that is stopped early owing to extreme improvement in the survival rate among the experimental group will likely provide overly optimistic estimates of the reduction in the mortality rate. Another cost to data monitoring is that early stopping of a trial may preclude answering all the research questions that were going to be addressed in the study. An example is the Women's Health Initiative (The RECT component: Estrogen plus Progestin in healthy postmenopausal women with an intact uterus) (72). This trial was terminated early in the follow-up phase because of the alarming increase in breast cancer risk in the treated group and the lack of any evidence of reducing coronary heart disease events. As part of the decision to terminate the study by the data and safety monitoring board, the blind was broken. All study participants were made aware of the deleterious effects so that they could discontinue use. What has and will become an issue is whether any endpoint analysis after additional follow-up will be valid because of the massive crossover that has likely occurred.

There has been a considerable amount of methodologic research in monitoring data in the fashion described here over the last 20 years (73–87). The most notable has been the development of the alpha spending function by DeMets and Lan (88). They were the first to use the analogy of (and metaphors from) spending money to data monitoring of endpoints, or more specifically, type I error. Withdrawing money from a bank account (noninterest bearing) extends the analogy in some nice ways, such as: There is a limit to the funds, the more one withdraws early on, the less there

is available later on, and one can make many withdrawals but the amount of each withdrawal must be small. These are all features of the alpha spending function. One distinction is clear in that the spending function needs to be stated in advance as part of the statistical design of the trial. DeMets and Lan were able to take several multiple testing procedures developed many years earlier (89,90) and describe them as different spending functions. The original procedures required that the number of times that data are formally evaluated be specified in advance and the timing of the "looks" be equally spaced on the information fraction scale. This is not necessary with the DeMets and Lan method. Figure 9.4 displays several spending functions differing by the amount spent early on in the trial versus later. One might choose to design a trial to spend early in the trial (e.g., Pocock spending function) because there is a considerable amount of evidence available from other studies to suggest the experimental therapy is superior to the standard. Alternatively, when designing a trial where there is little knowledge about the activity of an experimental therapy, one may opt to wait until the trial has a much larger sample size before spending the type I error (e.g., O'Brien and Fleming spending function). The thought behind such a strategy would be that only a large sample size will convince the practitioners to embrace a new standard if the trial is positive in favor of the experimental regimen.

Little has been said about futility analysis in this section. It should be mentioned that whereas early stopping rules for dramatic differences (as described above) have an impact on the type I error of the trial, futility analysis impacts the type II error adversely, or in other words, reduces the statisti-

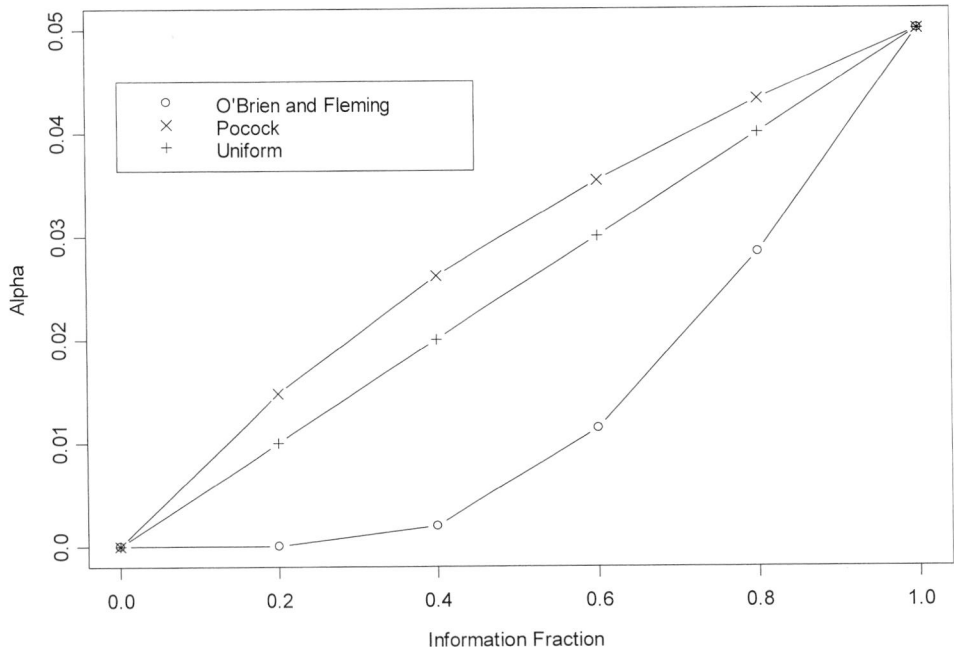

FIG. 9.4. Spending functions.

cal power. Often a simple rule for stopping based on futility is if the experimental group has a worse outcome to any degree when compared to the control group. In such a case, the null hypothesis is accepted. Such was the case in GOG Protocol 165 [A Randomized Comparison of Radiation Plus Weekly Cisplatin versus Radiation plus PVI (Protracted Venous Infusion) 5-FU in Patients with Stage II-B, III-B and IV-A Carcinoma of the Cervix). The GOG Data Monitoring Committee closed Protocol 165 based on a futility analysis.

Ideally, investigators should have a thorough understanding of the options and the consequences of monitoring clinical trials. It is only then that they will be able to provide guidance to the statistician in order to implement the optimal monitoring plan for the trial under design that is ethical, efficient, and valid.

Ethics

Historically, there have been many personal views expressed regarding the appropriateness of clinical studies involving human beings. Specifically, Claude Bernard, in 1865, wrote: ''Medicine by its nature is an experimental science, but it must apply the experimental method systematically.'' Prior to World War II, clinical trials tended to be small, and, therefore, they did not attract significant debate. However, at the Nuremberg Trials following World War II, it became apparent that Nazi physicians and military officials had performed strange and cruel experiments on war prisoners. These egregious violations of ethical conduct horrified the world and led to the development of the first international codes of ethics for human experimentation. Most notable of these is the Nuremberg Code, which was adopted

in 1947. These ethical standards were intended not only to apply to war crimes, but to human experimentation in general (91). The Nuremberg Code advanced ten principles (2):

1. Voluntary consent of the subject.
2. The study should yield worthwhile results unavailable by other means.
3. The design should reflect the current state of knowledge from animal studies or other empirical studies.
4. The study procedures should be conducted so as to avoid unnecessary injury or suffering.
5. No deaths or disabling injury can be expected to result from the study procedures.
6. The risk to the subject should be consistent with the study benefits.
7. Appropriate precautions must be taken to protect subjects from any harm.
8. The study should be planned, executed, and reported by qualified individuals.
9. Consent to participate is an ongoing process, which the individual can revoke at any time.
10. The assessment of risk and benefit is a continuous process. An investigator is obliged to terminate the trial when the risk of injury is imminent.

Unfortunately, at the time these codes were adopted, they had very little practical influence on the practices of human experimentation within the U.S. medical community. Many investigators considered them to be unrelated to clinical trials (92). Also, some important issues were not addressed in these guidelines, such as the inclusion of individuals who are mentally or physically unable to provide an informed consent.

Based on the standards set forth at the Nuremberg Trials, The World Medical Association (WMA), at its 18th Assembly held in Helsinki, Finland, 1964, adopted recommendations to guide physicians who participate in medical research involving human subjects. This document has become known as the Helsinki Declaration (93). It has been subsequently amended several times and most recently at the 48th General Assembly, Somerset West, Republic of South Africa, 1996. The current guidelines state, "medical progress is based on research that ultimately must rest in part on experimentation involving human subjects." It stresses that the risks to an individual incurred through participation in a research trial must be balanced against the potential benefits. Although all subjects must be adequately informed of the goals, procedures, anticipated benefits, and potential hazards, ultimately, responsibility for the human subjects must always rest with a medically qualified person and never with the research subjects themselves. Finally, in research involving human beings, "the interests of science and society should never take precedence over considerations related to the well-being of the subject" (93).

A few years after the Helsinki Declaration was adopted, Henry Beecher published an article that identified 22 clinical trials with serious deficiencies in clinical ethics. Each trial violated one or more of the principles advanced in the Helsinki Declaration and endangered the health or the life of the subjects (94). Many of these studies were conducted at prominent U.S. university medical schools, and many were either federally funded or funded by well-known pharmaceutical companies. In order to explain why an investigator would participate in these studies, Beecher suggested that the pressures for career advancement and promotion might have influenced ambitious physicians. Shortly afterward, the Tuskegee and Willowbrook incidents captured national attention. In the first incident, the U.S. Public Health Service monitored 201 men in Tuskegee, Alabama, with advanced syphilis to assess the natural history of the disease. This study continued despite the availability of an effective treatment. In the second incident, mentally handicapped children at the Willowbrook Hospital in New York State were intentionally infected with viral hepatitis.

In reaction to these incidents, the U.S. Congress established the National Commission for the Protection of Human Subjects of Biomedical and Behavioral Research by passing the National Research Act of 1974. The purpose of this commission was to investigate the ethical problems in clinical research. This Act also mandated that all research studies funded entirely or in part by the federal government be reviewed by Institutional Review Boards (IRBs). The commission described the role of the IRBs and provided ethical guidelines for research involving human subjects. These guidelines are presented in the Commission's 1978 Belmont Report. There are three important ethical principles for clinical research articulated in this report: respect for persons, beneficence, and justice.

The principle of respect for persons acknowledges that autonomous individuals, who are properly informed, should be free to exercise self-determination. At the same time, it recognizes that not all individuals are capable of self-determination and these persons must be protected (95,96). The informed-consent process arises from this principle. The principle of beneficence acknowledges that there is often a potential for both benefit and harm to the subjects of clinical research. This principle not only requires that there be a favorable balance toward benefit, but that the potential for harm be minimized and justified. The principle of justice requires that the burdens and benefits of research be distributed fairly. An injustice occurs when one group bears a disproportionate burden of research, whereas another reaps a disproportionate share of its benefits. Therefore, those obstacles, such as study eligibility criteria, which tend to limit access to clinical trials, must be appropriately justified or else eliminated (see Eligibility Criteria section above).

The actualization of these principles can be controversial. For example, some investigators have noted that there is a natural tension between the science and practice of medicine. On one hand, physicians have an uncompromisable covenant of loyalty and fidelity with their patients. This obliges the physician to exercise his or her best judgment in making treatment recommendations for each individual. The "randomized clinical trial routinely asks physicians to sacrifice the interests of their patients for the sake of the study" (97). On the other hand, there are many diseases in which the best available treatment is not known, or worse, the recommended treatment is based on limited scientific data and hunches that may be ineffective or even harmful. Historical examples include bezoar stone as a general antidote, bloodletting or purging for dysentery (7), thalidomide for sedation of pregnant women, and antiarrhythmic drugs following a myocardial infarction (98).

Dichotomizing the role of a physician as either caregiver or scientist is problematic. These roles should be viewed as part of a continuum that requires balance.

The tension between the interdependent responsibilities for providing personal and compassionate care, as well as scientifically sound and valid treatment, is intrinsic to the practice of medicine today. This tension is structurally part of the medical profession's covenant with the human community, not merely the expression of an individual physician-investigator's disordered intentions (99).

The trouble with the alternative viewpoint is that "medical progress is a noble goal but surely that does not sanctify the currently accepted experimental method or render it obligatory" (100). Not every medical issue is amenable to an experimental study. The efficacy of penicillin and the hazards of smoking were recognized without subjecting them to the rigors of a randomized clinical trial. Even among those issues that can be studied, it is not always clear that they should be. There certainly are many instances when clinical trials have been initiated in the absence of an ethical consensus (101,102).

This dichotomized view of the physician's role arises from his or her responsibility to both the individual patient and the community. However, clinical trials are not the only instance in which ethical consideration of the individual and the collective ethics can conflict. For example, it may be in the best interest of an individual always to be operated on by the most experienced surgeon, but society requires that inexperienced surgeons gain experience for future patients (103). The rising cost of health care also makes it necessary to weigh frequently the needs of the individual against the community's resources. This dichotomy in the physician's role leads to an artificial double standard, one for the practitioner and another for the investigator. Physicians who are not involved in clinical trials are no less obligated to inform their patients of treatment alternatives, as well as of the potential risks and benefits of each alternative. Also, respect for a patient's right to self-determination is appropriate regardless of whether the patient is involved in a clinical trial (2).

Another controversy in clinical trials occurs when a new therapeutic approach consists of the standard therapy augmented with a promising new drug. The experimental therapy is frequently associated with more risks than the standard approach. The justification for the randomized trial arises from the uncertainty over whether the additional risks may be offset by the benefits of new treatment. However, when given a choice between standard therapy and randomization, some patients with a generally fatal disease prefer to refuse randomization and "take their chances" with the experimental treatment outside the study. In this case, some investigators are reluctant to expose a patient to the risks of an unproven therapy *outside* of a clinical trial. It has been suggested that this provides another example of when clinical trials "violate the physician-patient relationship, forcing investigators to use patients instead of treating them as individuals" (52). Markman (104) has proposed another twist on this same issue. When paclitaxel was first being evaluated in ovarian cancer trials (in 1990), the supply of the drug was limited and it was not generally available outside of a clinical trial. The only chance a patient had to receive paclitaxel in front-line therapy was to accept randomization. In this case, the patient's choice was to receive standard therapy or consent to a randomized trial in return for a 50:50 chance of getting the experimental therapy.

There are ethical considerations that must be addressed at every point throughout a study beginning with its design. "An experiment is ethical or not at its inception; it does not become ethical *post hoc*" (94). The study must begin with clear and meaningful objectives that are worthy of investigation. Studies that address unimportant issues cannot be ethically justified. The study methods and design follow directly from these objectives. Since a study needs to be both scientifically and ethically justified, the investigators involved in the study must be both technically and humanely competent (2). Technical competence implies an appropriate level of education, knowledge, certification, and experience, whereas humanistic competence implies both compassion and empathy. The execution of the study must be devoid of scientific misconduct. Scientific misconduct includes any behavior that compromises the validity of the findings or violates the rights of the subjects who participate in the study (105). Since misconduct can arise from either fraud or incompetence, constant vigilance is the only countermeasure.

Since those physicians not involved in the study base their judgments about the internal and external validity of the study on summaries, all publications must be prepared accurately, completely, and objectively.

The enactment of the Health Insurance Portability Accountability Act (HIPAA) requires stringent criteria to ensure the health information privacy of patients. This legislation, which all institutions and investigators must abide by, has added a complicating factor to the carrying out of clinical trials. Not only are longer consent forms for participation in clinical trials required, but greater efforts to safeguard the identity and privacy of the patients are mandatory. This legislation applies not only to clinical record information and protocol studies regarding patients' treatment, but also to the handling of tissues or specimens and institutional research databases. All clinical investigators must carefully review the HIPAA requirements and make sure that all safeguards are in place to comply with this mandate. Institutions throughout the United States are allocating significant amounts of funding and personnel to ensure full compliance with HIPAA. For more information regarding HIPAA regulations, the reader is directed to (www.hhs.gov/ocr/hipaa

REFERENCES

1. Redmond CK, Colton T. *Biostatistics in clinical trials. The Wiley reference series in biostatistics.* Chichester, NY: John Wiley and Sons, 2001:xx, 501.
2. Piantadosi S. *Clinical trials: a methodologic perspective.* New York: John Wiley and Sons, 1997.
3. Meinert CL, Tonascia S. *Clinical trials: design, conduct and analysis.* New York: Oxford University Press, 1986.
4. Buyse ME, Staquet MJ, Sylvester RJ. *Cancer clinical trials, methods and practice.* New York: Oxford University Press, 1984.
5. Pocock SJ, Simon R. Sequential treatment assignment with balancing for prognostic factors in the controlled clinical trial. *Biometrics* 1975; 31:103–115.
6. Kelsey JL, Hildreth NG. *Breast and gynecologic cancer epidemiology.* Boca Raton, FL: CRC Press, 1983.
7. Bull JP. The historical development of clinical therapeutic trials. *J Chronic Dis* 1959;10:218–248.
8. Fibiger J. Om Serumbehandling af difteri. *Hospitalstidende* 1898;6: 765–769.
9. Hrobjartsson A, Gotzsche PC, Gluud C. The controlled clinical trial turns 100 years: Fibiger's trial of serum treatment of diphtheria. *Br Med J* 1998;317:1243–1245.
10. Hinshaw H, Feldman W. Evaluation of chemotherapeutic agents in clinical tuberculosis: a suggested procedure. *Am Rev Tuberc* 1944; 50:202–213.
11. Medical Research Council Streptomycin in Tuberculosis Trials Committee. Streptomycin treatment for pulmonary tuberculosis. *Br Med J* 1948;ii:769–782.
12. Yoshioka A. Use of randomisation in the Medical Research Council's

clinical trial of streptomycin in pulmonary tuberculosis in the 1940's. *Br Med J* 1998;317:1220–1223.

13. Paterson R, Russell M. Clinical trials in malignant disease. Breast cancer: value of radiation of the ovaries. *J Faculty Radiol* 1959;10:130–133.

14. Fisher B. Winds of change in clinical trials—from Daniel to Charlie Brown. *Control Clin Trials* 1982;4:65–73.

15. Frei E III, Holland JF, Schneiderman MA, et al. A comparative study of two regimens of combination chemotherapy in acute leukemia. *Blood* 1958;13:1126–1148.

16. Gehan EA, Schneiderman MA. Historical and methodolgic developments in clinical trials at the National Cancer Institute. *Stat Med* 1990;9:871–880.

17. Zubrod CG, Schneiderman M, Frei E III, et al. Appraisal of methods for the study of chemotherapy of cancer in man: comparative therapeutic trial of nitrogen mustard and thiophosphoramide. *J Chronic Dis* 1960;11:7–33.

18. Lewis GC, Blessing J, Kellner JR. Clinical trials in gynecology oncology: Cooperative Group Research. In: Griffiths CT, Fuller AF, eds. *Gynecology oncology.* Boston: Martinus Nijhoff, 1983:333–384.

19. Advanced Ovarian Cancer Trialists Group. Chemotherapy in advanced ovarian cancer; an overview of randomised clinical trials. *Br Med J* 1991;303:884–893.

20. Fleming TR, DeMets DL. Surrogate end points in clinical trials: are we being misled? *Ann Intern Med* 1996;125:605–613.

21. Creasman WT. Second-look laparotomy in ovarian cancer. *Gynecol Oncol* 1994;55(3 Pt 2):S122–S127.

22. Omura GA, Blessing JA, Vaccarello L, et al. Randomized trial of cisplatin versus cisplatin plus mitolactol versus cisplatin plus ifosfamide in advanced squamous carcinoma of the cervix: a Gynecology Oncology Group Study. *J Clin Oncol* 1997;15:165–171.

23. George SL. Reducing patient eligibility criteria in cancer clinical trials. *J Clin Oncol* 1996;14:1364–1370.

24. Begg CB, Engstrom PF. Eligibility and extrapolation in cancer clinical trials. *J Clin Oncol* 1987;5:962–968.

25. ICON Group T. Paclitaxel plus carboplatin versus standard chemotherapy with either single-agent carboplatin or cyclophosphamide, doxorubicin, and cisplatin in women with ovarian cancer: the ICON3 randomised trial. *Lancet* 2002;360:505–515.

26. O'Quigley J, Pepe M, Fisher L. Continual reassessment method: a practical design for phase I clinical trials in cancer. *Biometrics* 1990;46:33–48.

27. Korn EL, Midthune D, Chen TT, et al. A comparison of two phase I trial designs. *Stat Med* 1994;13:1799–1806.

28. Goodman SN, Zahurak ML, Piantadosi S. Some practical improvements in the continual reassessment method for phase I studies. *Stat Med* 1995;14:1149–1161.

29. Ahn C. An evaluation of phase I cancer clinical trial designs. *Stat Med* 1998;17:1537–1549.

30. Simon R, Freidlin B, Rubinstein L, et al. Accelerated titration designs for phase I clinical trials in oncology. *J Natl Cancer Inst* 1997;89:1138–1147.

31. Simon R. Optimal two-stage designs for phase II clinical trials. *Control Clin Trials* 1989;10:1–10.

32. Chen TT, Ng TH. Optimal flexible designs in phase II clinical trials. *Stat Med* 1998;17:2301–2312.

33. Conaway MR, Petroni GR. Designs for the phase II trials allowing for a trade off between response and toxicity. *Biometrics* 1996;52:1375–1386.

34. Bryant J, Day R. Incorporating toxicity considerations into the design of two-stage phase II clinical trials. *Biometrics* 1995;51:1372–1383.

35. Jennison C, Turnbull BW. Group sequential tests for bivariate response: interim analyses of clinical trials with both efficacy and safety endpoints. *Biometrics* 1993;49:741–752.

36. Thall P, Simon R, Estey E. New statistical strategy for monitoring safety and efficacy in single-arm clinical trials. *J Clin Oncol* 1996;14:296–303.

37. Emrich LJ. Required duration and power determinations for historically controlled studies of survival times. *Stat Med* 1989;8:153–160.

38. Wiens B. Choosing an equivalence limit for noninferiority or equivalence studies. *Control Clin Trials* 2002;23:2–14.

39. Rothmann M, Li N, Chen G, et al. Design and analysis of non-inferiority mortality trials in oncology. *Stat Med* 2003;22:239–264.

40. Senn S. Inherent difficulties with active control equivalence studies. *Stat Med* 1993;12:2367–2375.

41. Durrleman S, Simon R. Planning and monitoring of equivalence studies. *Biometrics* 1990;46:329–336.

41a. McGuire WP, Hoskins WT, Brady MF, et al. Cyclophosphamide and cisplatin compared with paclitaxel and cisplatin in patients with stage III and stage IV ovarian cancer *N Engl J Med* 1996;334(1):1–6.

42. du Bois A, Luck HJ, Meier W, et al. A randomized clinical trial of cisplatin/paclitaxel versus carboplatin/paclitaxel as first-line treatment of ovarian cancer. *J Natl Cancer Inst* 2003;95:1320–1329.

43. Neijt JP, Engelholm SA, Tuxen MK, et al. Exploratory phase III study of paclitaxel and cisplatin versus paclitaxel and carboplatin in advanced ovarian cancer. *J Clin Oncol* 2000;18:3084–3092.

44. Ozols RF, Bundy BN, Greer BE, et al. Phase III study of carboplatin and paclitaxel compared to cisplatin and paclitaxel in patients with "optimally" resected stage III ovarian cancer: A Gynecology Oncology Group Trial. *J Clin Oncol* 2003;21:3194–3200.

45. Vasey PA. Role of docetaxel in the treatment of newly diagnosed advanced ovarian cancer. *J Clin Oncol* 2003;21:136–144.

45a. Advanced Ovarian Cancer Trialists Group. Chemotherapy in advanced ovarian cancer: an overview of randomised clinical trials. *Brit Med J* 1991;303:884–893.

46. Sandercock J, Parmar MK, Torri V, Qian W. First-line treatment for advanced ovarian cancer: paclitaxel, platinum and the evidence. *Br J Cancer* 2002;87:815–824.

47. Byar DP, Simon RM, Friedewald WT, et al. Randomized clinical trials. Perspectives on some recent ideas. *N Engl J Med* 1976;295:74–80.

48. Greer G, Bundy BN, Ozols RF, et al. Implications of second-look laparotomy (SLL) in the context of Gynecologic Oncology Group (GOG) Protocol 158: a non-randomized comparison using an explanatory analysis. *Soc Gynecol Oncol* 2003;88:156.

49. Kunz R, Oxman A. The unpredictability paradox: review of empirical comparisons of randomised and non-randomised clinical trials. *Br Med J* 1998;317:1185–1190.

50. Schulz KF, Chalmers I, Hayes RJ, Altman DG. Empirical evidence of bias. Dimensions of methodological quality associated with estimates of treatment effects in controlled trials. *JAMA* 1995;273:408–412.

51. Schulz KF. Subverting randomization in controlled trials. *JAMA* 1995;274:1456–1458.

52. Emanuel EJ, Patterson WB. Ethics of randomized clinical trials. *J Clin Oncol* 1998;16:365–371.

53. Ellis PM, Coates AS. Ethics of randomized clinical trials. *J Clin Oncol* 1998;16:2570.

54. Therneau TM. How many stratification factors are "too many" to use in a randomization plan? *Control Clin Trials* 1993;14:98–108.

55. Schulz KF, Grimes DA, Altman DG, Hayes RJ. Blinding and exclusions after allocation in randomized contolled trials: survey of published parallel group trials in obstetrics and gynaecology. *Br Med J* 1996;312:742–744.

56. Rothman KJ, Michels KB. The continuing unethical use of placebo controls. *N Engl J Med* 1994;331:394–398.

57. Xiang AH, Sather HN, Azen SP. Power considerations for testing an interaction in a 2 x k factorial design with failure time outcome. *Control Clin Trials* 1994;15:489–502.

58. Peterson B, George SL. Sample size requirements and length of study for testing interactions in a 2 x k factorial design when time-to-failure is the outcome. *Control Clin Trials* 1993;14:511–522.

59. Henderson IC, Patek AJ. The relationship between prognostic and predictive factors in the management of breast cancer. *Breast Cancer Res Treat* 1998;52:261–288.

60. Sargent D, Allegra C. Issues in clinical trial design for tumor marker studies. *Semin Oncol* 2002;29:222–230.

61. Ross JS, Fletcher JA. The HER-2/neu oncogene: prognostic factor, predictive factor and target for therapy. *Semin Cancer Biol* 1999;9:125–138.

62. Creasman WT, Soper JT, McCarty KS Jr, et al. Influence of cytoplasmic steroid receptor content on prognosis of early stage endometrial carcinoma. *Am J Obstet Gynecol* 1985;151:922–932.

63. Von Hoff DD, Sandbach JF, Clark GM, et al. Selection of cancer chemotherapy for a patient by an in vitro assay versus a clinician. *J Natl Cancer Inst* 1990;82:110–116.

64. Last JM. *A Dictionary of Epidemiology*. New York: Oxford University Press, 1995.

65. Alberts DS, Liu PY, Hannigan EV, et al. Intraperitoneal cisplatin plus intravenous cyclophosphamide versus intravenous cisplatin plus intravenous cyclophosphamide for stage III ovarian cancer. *N Engl J Med* 1996;335:1950–1955.

66. Goodman SN. p Values, hypothesis tests, and likelihood: implications for epidemiology of a neglected historical debate. *Am J Epidemiol* 1993;137:485–499.

67. Lang JM, Rothman KJ, Cann CI. That confounded p-value. *Epidemiology* 1998;9:7–8.

68. Stangl DK, Berry DA. *Meta-analysis in medicine and health policy*. New York: Marcel Dekker, 2000.

69. Machin D, Stenning SP, Parmar MKB, et al. Thirty years of Medical Research Council randomized trials in solid tumors. *Clin Oncol* 1997; 9:100–114.

70. Schoenfeld DA. Sample-size formula for the proportional-hazards regression model. *Biometrics* 1983;39:499–503.

71. Mantel N. Evaluation of survival data and two new rank order statistics arising in its consideration. *Cancer Chemother Rep* 1966;50:163–170.

72. Rossouw JE, Anderson GL, Prentice RL, et al. Risks and benefits of estrogen plus progestin in healthy postmenopausal women: principal results rom the Women's Health Initiative randomized controlled trial. *JAMA* 2002;288:321–333.

73. Gail MH, DeMets DL, Slud EV. *Simulation Studies on Increments of the Two-sample Logrank Score Test for Survival Time Data, With Application to Group Sequential Boundaries. Survival Analysis.* Institute of Mathematical Statistics (Hayward), 1982:287–301.

74. Lan KKG, DeMets DL. Discrete sequential boundaries for clinical trials. *Biometrika* 1983;70:659–663.

75. Jennison C, Turnbull, BW. Repeated confidence intervals for group sequential trials. *Control Clin Trials* 1984;5:33–45.

76. Whitehead J. Supplementary analysis at the conclusion of a sequential clinical trial. *Biometrics* 1986;42:461–471.

77. Goldman AI. Issues in designing sequential stopping rules for monitoring side effects in clinical trials. *Control Clin Trials* 1987;8: 327–337.

78. Lan KKG, Wittes, J. The B-value: a tool for monitoring data. *Biometrics* 1988;44:579–585.

79. Freedman LS, Spiegelhalter DJ. Comparison of Bayesian with group sequential methods for monitoring clinical trials. *Control Clin Trials* 1989;10:357–367.

80. Armitage P. Comparison of Bayesian with group sequential methods for monitoring clinical trials. *Control Clin Trials* 1991;12:345–350.

81. Lan GKK, Zucker DM. Sequential monitoring of clinical trials: the role of information and brownian motion. *Stat Med* 1993;12:753–765.

82. Todd S, Whitehead J, Facey KM. Point and interval estimation following a sequential clinical trial. *Biometrika* 1996;83:453–461.

83. Lachin JM. Group sequential monitoring of distribution-free analyses of repeated measures. *Stat Med* 1997;16:653–668.

84. Choi SC, Lee, YJ. Interim analyses with delayed observations in clinical trials. *Stat Med* 1999;18:1297–1306.

85. Troendle JF, Yu KF. Conditional estimation following a group sequential clinical trial. Ccommunications in statistics. *Theory and Methods* 1999;28:1617–1634.

86. Bautista OM, Bain RP, Lachin JM. A flexible stochastic curtailing procedure for the log-rank test. *Stat Med* 2000;21:428–439.

87. Christensen E. Effective randomized clinical trial design: sequential analysis. *J Hepatol* 2003;38:550–551.

88. DeMets D, Lan GKK. The alpha spending function approach to interim analysis. In: Thall PF, ed. R*ecent advances in clinical trial design and analysis*. Boston: Kluwer Academic Publishers, 1995: 1–28.

89. Pocock SJ. Group sequential methods in the design and analysis of clinical trials. *Biometrika* 1977;64:191–199.

90. O'Brien PC, Fleming, TR. A multiple testing procedure for clinical trials. *Biometrics* 1979;35:549–556.

91. Katz J. The Nuremberg Code and the Nuremberg Trial: a reappraisal. *JAMA* 1996;276:1662–1666.

92. Faden RR, Lederer SE, Moreno JD. US medical researchers, the Nuremberg Doctors Trial, and the Nuremberg Code. *JAMA* 1996;276: 1667–1671.

93. World Medical Association. Declaration of Helsinki: recommendations guiding medical doctors in biomedical research involving human subjects (revised: 1975, 1983, 1989, 1996), 1964.

94. Beecher HK. Ethics and clinical research. *N Engl J Med* 1966;274: 1354–1360.

95. Michels R. Are research ethics bad for our mental health? *N Engl J Med* 1999;340:1427–1430.

96. Capron AM. Ethical and human-rights issues in research on mental disorders that may affect decision-making capacity. *N Engl J Med* 1999;340:1430–1434.

97. Hellman S, Hellman DS. Of mice but not men: problems of the randomized clinical trial. *N Engl J Med* 1991;324:1585–1589.

98. Epstein AE, Hallstrom AP, Rogers WJ, et al. Mortality following ventricular arrhythmia suppression by encainide, flecainide and moricizine after myocardial infaction: the original design concept of the Cardiac Arrhythmia Suppression Trial (CAST). *JAMA* 1993;270: 2451–2455.

99. Roy DJ. Controlled clinical trials: an ethical imperative. *J Chronic Dis* 1986;39:159–162.

100. Mackillop WJ, Johnston PA. Controlled clinical trials: an ethical imperative. *J Chronic Dis* 1987;40:363.

101. Adami H, Baron J, Rothman K. Ethics of a prostate cancer screening trial. *Lancet* 1994;343:958–960.

102. Noonan E. Ethicists fault mental health researchers over use of 'date-rape drug' on test subjects. Buffalo, NY: *Buffalo News* 1999:A–8.

103. Armitage P. Attitudes in clinical trials. *Stat Med* 1998;17:2675–2683.

104. Markman M. Ethical difficulties with randomized clinical trials involving cancer patients: examples from the field of gynecologic oncology. *J Clin Ethics* 1992;3:193–195.

105. Shapiro MF, Charrow RP. Scientific misconduct in investigational drug trials. *N Engl J Med* 1985;312:731–736.

CHAPTER 10

Diagnostic Imaging Techniques in Gynecologic Oncology

S.M. Ascher, C. Cooper, L. Scoutt, I. Imaoka, and H. Hricak

APPLICATIONS VERSUS INDICATIONS FOR IMAGING IN GYNECOLOGIC CANCER

Advances in ultrasound (US), computed tomography (CT), magnetic resonance imaging (MRI), and positron emission tomography (PET) have created great possibilities for imaging of the female genital tract. This chapter addresses the role of diagnostic imaging in evaluating gynecologic malignancy and attempts to differentiate applications (i.e., what is possible) from indications (i.e., what is necessary). As with any changing technologic arena, imaging strategies are not static and require ongoing updating and reevaluation.

The objectives of imaging in gynecologic cancer are straightforward: tumor detection, tumor diagnosis including image-guided percutaneous biopsy, staging, and follow-up. Monitoring treatment response and differentiating tumor recurrence from postirradiation and/or postoperative changes are also important.

IMAGING MODALITIES

Ultrasound

US is considered to be the initial imaging modality of choice in the work-up of most pelvic disorders. Currently,

S.M. Ascher: Department of Radiology, Georgetown University Hospital, Washington, DC 20007

C. Cooper: Department of Radiology, Georgetown University Hospital, Washington, DC 20007

L. Scoutt: Department of Radiology, Yale–New Haven Hospital, New Haven, Connecticut 06510

I. Imaoka: Department of Radiology, Tenri Hospital, Nara, Japan 6328552

H. Hricak: Department of Radiology, Memorial–Sloan Kettering Cancer Center, New York, New York 10021

the accepted roles of US in the evaluation of a woman with a suspected gynecologic malignancy include characterization of adnexal masses to differentiate benign from malignant ovarian masses, identification of endometrial abnormalities in women with intermenstrual or postmenopausal bleeding in order to assess for endometrial carcinoma, and detection of primary or recurrent gestational trophoblastic disease in women with elevated serum beta human chorionic gonadotropin (β-hCG) levels. Additionally, US is also used to detect and biopsy recurrent tumor masses or metastases and to guide drainage of postoperative fluid collections such as lymphoceles, seromas, or abscesses. Rarely, US may be used to guide biopsy of a primary pelvic tumor in a woman who presents with stage III disease when a histologic diagnosis is required to initiate chemotherapy. The role of US in screening high-risk patient populations for ovarian or endometrial carcinoma remains controversial.

Ultrasound offers many advantages: It is relatively inexpensive, widely available, provides multiplanar imaging, and is without known risk. However, US has many limitations as well: It is operator dependent and image quality may be significantly degraded by large patient body habitus and bowel gas. The best spatial and soft tissue resolution is provided by Transvaginal ultrasound (TVS) but at the cost of a significant decrease in the size of the field of view. Hence, US is not as useful as either CT or MR in assessing the local extent or distal spread of pelvic malignancies.

Computed Tomography

CT is the primary imaging modality for evaluating the overall extent of gynecologic malignancy and for detecting persistent and recurrent pelvic tumors. CT staging is more accurate than clinical staging in locally advanced disease and in cancers with a high propensity for lymphatic or peritoneal

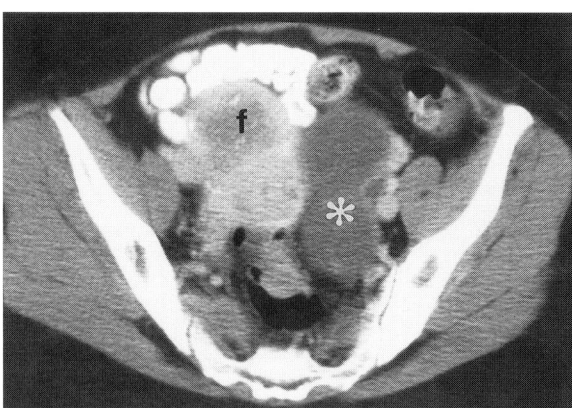

FIG. 10.1. Ovarian cancer. Oral and intravenous contrast-enhanced CT shows a left ovarian carcinoma (*asterisk*). Incidental note is made of uterine fibroids (f).

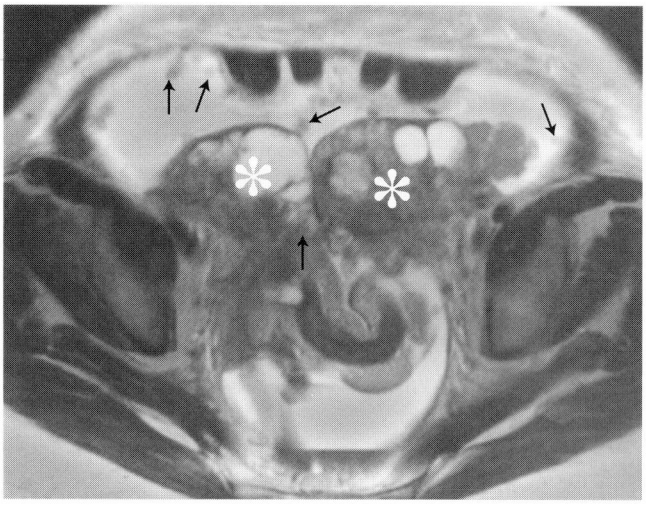

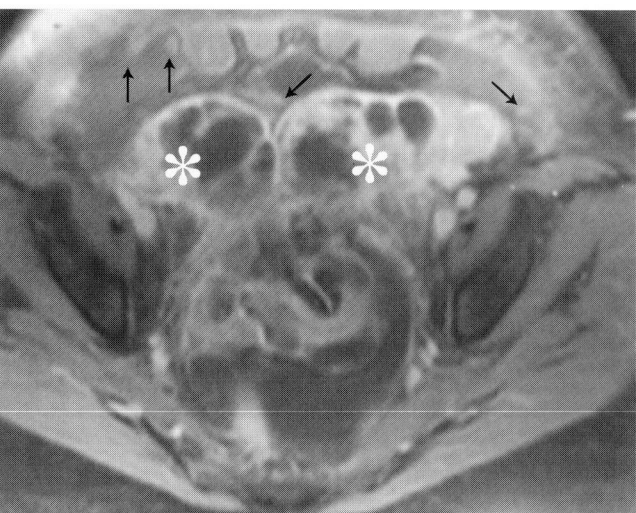

FIG. 10.2. Stage IIIB ovarian carcinoma. (**A**) MRI axial T2- and (**B**) axial contrast-enhanced fat-suppressed T1-W images show complex cystic and solid bilateral adnexal masses (*asterisks*, **A, B**). Small <2 cm peritoneal metastases are also demonstrated (*arrows*, **A, B**). Note the complex ascites with a fluid-fluid level (a, **A**).

metastases. CT surveys of the brain, chest, and upper abdomen provide information about extrapelvic disease. CT-guided biopsy can confirm metastatic spread of disease to the peritoneal cavity or retroperitoneum.

Advantages of CT include ready availability, short scanning times, and high spatial resolution (Fig. 10.1). The advent of multidetector CT (MDCT) using continuous spiral (helical) acquisitions and multirow detector arrays (4-, 8-, 12, and 16-slice systems) allows faster scanning with higher image quality. Rapid technologic advances in MDCT include the ability to obtain submillimeter slice thickness, multiphasic contrast studies (such as arterial and venous phase enhancement after a single injection), CT angiography, endoluminal ''fly-through'' techniques (as used in CT colonoscopy), and rapid three-dimensional (3-D) reconstructions. Small and difficult to access masses are more readily biopsied using CT fluoroscopy (1). Disadvantages of CT include the use of ionizing radiation, degradation of image quality by body habitus or metallic hip prosthesis, and the morbidity and mortality associated with iodinated contrast agents. Despite technical improvements, CT remains of limited utility in characterizing very-early-stage disease.

Magnetic Resonance Imaging

There is substantial evidence supporting the usefulness of MRI in staging gynecologic malignancies. MRI has been shown to be superior to CT in the workup of uterine and cervical cancers (2–5), and recent reports suggest that it may be useful in the evaluation of ovarian cancer as well (5a) (Fig. 10.2). In addition, there is evidence that MRI can differentiate radiation fibrosis from recurrent tumor (6,7). The accuracy of MR assessment of lymph node invasion is similar to that of CT; both rely on size criteria to detect lymphadenopathy (8). In addition, MR-guided biopsies are also gaining wider clinical acceptance.

Although MRI is still relatively expensive, it is cost minimizing in some clinical settings by limiting or eliminating the need for more expensive and/or more invasive diagnostic or surgical procedures (9–11). There are at least three cost-minimizing indications for MRI in the evaluation of women with gynecologic malignancy: (a) the staging of invasive cervical carcinoma as an adjunct to clinical examination; (b) the preoperative management of women with endometrial cancer (12); and (c) the characterization of adnexal lesions when ultrasonography and clinical examination are indeterminate (9–11). In addition, a meta-analysis of imaging and endometrial cancer found that MRI was the best modality for multifactorial assessment (12).

Advantages of MRI include superb spatial and tissue contrast resolution, absence of ionizing radiation, multiplanar capability, and fast (i.e., breathhold and breathing-independent) techniques. MRI is the modality of choice for patients with allergies to iodinated intravenous contrast media or impaired renal function. It is contraindicated in patients with pacemakers, cochlear implants, certain vascular clips, metallic objects in the eye, and neural stimulators. Also, some patients may experience claustrophobia, causing difficulty in completing the examination.

Positron Emission Tomography

With the most commonly used glucose analog, 2-[^{18}F]-fluoro-2-deoxy-D-glucose (FDG), PET exploits the accelerated rate of glycolysis common to neoplastic cells to image tumors (13). That is, PET takes advantage of the biochemical changes associated with malignancy that often precede, or are more specific than, the structural changes visualized by more conventional means (Fig. 10.3). PET does not have the same spatial resolution as CT or MRI, but image fusion techniques that overlay PET images onto other cross-sectional images can be obtained. Most recently, PET-CT scanners became commercially available and allow both modalities to be performed on a single machine equipped with both PET and CT detectors (Fig. 10.4B–D). Because PET requires specialized instrumentation and a local source of positron emitters, it is not as widely available as other modalities.

Most work to date with PET and gynecologic malignancy has focused on cervical cancer and ovarian cancer (14–17), and although FDG PET predominates, work with carbon 11 is promising.

Excretory Urography

The use of excretory urography in the evaluation of gynecologic malignancies has been on the decline in recent years; it is neither sensitive nor accurate in delineating tumor extent and bladder invasion (18,19). Today, cross-sectional examinations provide similar and, in many instances, additional information.

Barium Enema

Barium enema in the workup of gynecologic pelvic cancers is also on the decline. If barium enema is used, signs of bowel involvement include fixation and tethering of the bowel wall, irregular serrations at the mass–colon interface, an annular defect from circumferential involvement, and mucosal ulceration and fistulization from complete transmural invasion. Unfortunately, these signs are not specific for involvement from gynecologic cancer (20). In fact, barium enema has a low positive yield when used in the routine evaluation of women with gynecologic malignancy—it is

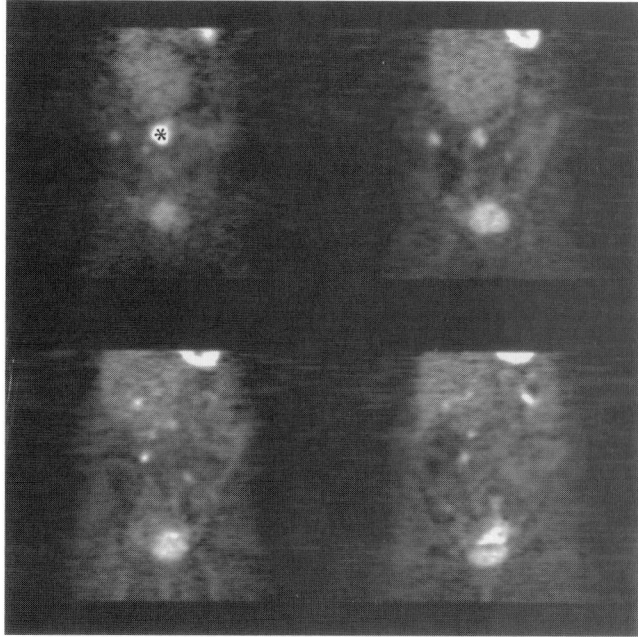

A

B

FIG. 10.3. Stage IV ovarian carcinoma. Coronal FDG PET images (**A, B**) show abnormal uptake in a large omental mass (*asterisk*), left hemipelvis (*arrow*), and multiple small omental, nodal, hepatic, and splenic metastases. Surgery confirmed widespread poorly differentiated papillary serous adenocarcinoma. (Courtesy of Steven Larson, M.D., Memorial Sloan–Kettering Cancer Center, New York, NY.)

useful only in the workup of women with advanced disease (21,22). Cross-sectional imaging has the advantage of providing information about structures surrounding the bowel and, thus, eliminates the need to infer this information indirectly from findings on barium enema.

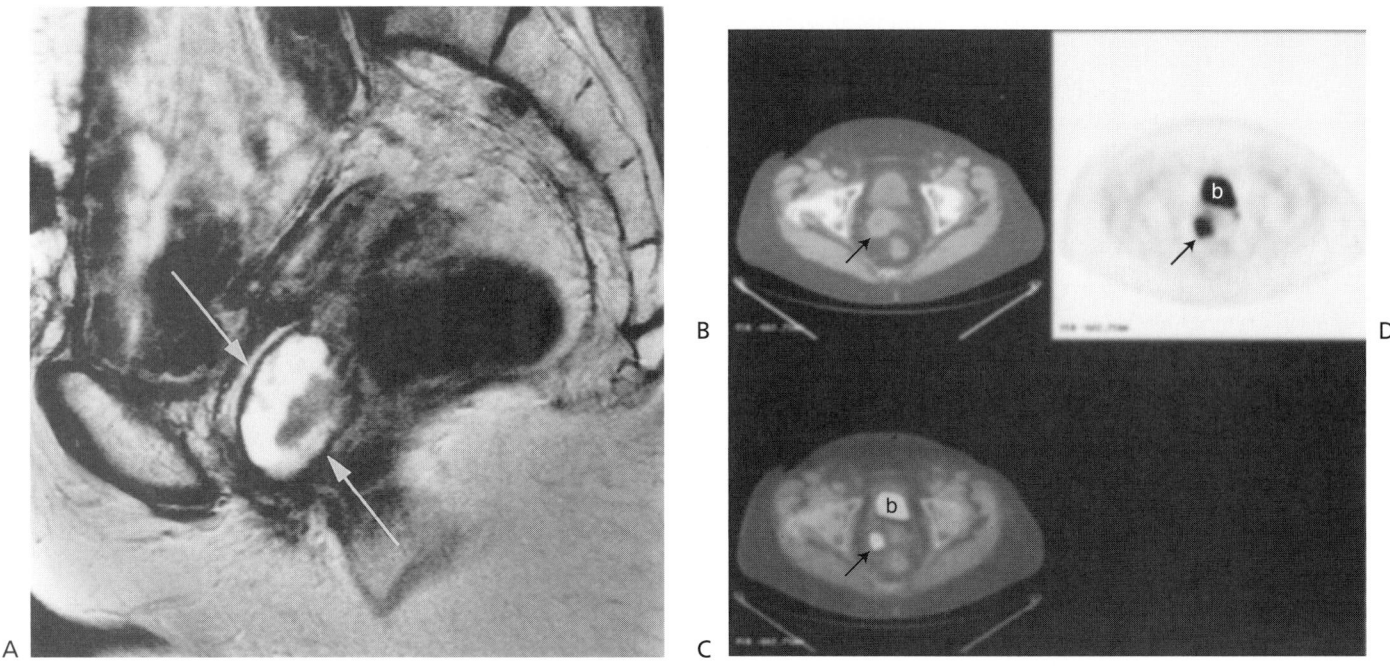

FIG. 10.4. Recurrent cervical cancer. **A:** Sagittal T2-W image shows a high signal intensity complex mass (*arrows*, **A**) at the vaginal stump consistent with tumor recurrence. In another patient with cervical cancer treated with radiation, axial (**B**) CT and (**C**) FDG PET and images show a soft tissue mass (*arrow*, **B**) and a "hot spot" (*arrow*, **C**) in the pelvis. Since these images are acquired at the same location, they can be combined. The resultant (**D**) PET-CT image provides accurate localization of tumor recurrence (*arrow*, **D**). Accumulation of FDG in the urinary bladder is normal (b, **C**, **D**). (Images **B**, **C**, and **D**, courtesy of Dr. Yeung, Memorial Sloan–Kettering Cancer Center, New York, NY.)

EXAMINATION TECHNIQUES AND NORMAL ANATOMY

Ultrasound

State of the art ultrasound evaluation of the female pelvis require a transvaginal approach. By placing the transducer closer to the organs of interest, less penetration of the US beam is necessary and a higher frequency probe can be used. The use of a higher frequency transducer, typically 5.0 to 7.5 MHz, results in significantly improved spatial resolution and fewer imaging artifacts in comparison to transabdominal imaging but at the cost of a smaller field of view. Hence, transabdominal imaging must be considered to be an important complementary imaging technique if the mass is larger than the TVS field of view, if the ovaries are displaced out of the pelvis, if the ovaries are not visualized because of the presence of bowel gas, or to evaluate important ancillary findings such as hydronephrosis, ascites, peritoneal/hepatic implants, and liver metastases. Transabdominal imaging also provides a better overall view of the pelvis and the relationship of structures to the pelvic side wall and bladder.

Patients undergoing TVS are examined with an empty bladder in the supine position with the knees flexed and the hips slightly elevated and externally rotated. A gel-filled condom is placed over the 5.0- to 7.5-MHz probe, which is inserted into the vagina following application of an external lubricant. Transabdominal pelvic imaging is performed with a 3.5- to 5.0-MHz curved array transducer using the distended urinary bladder as an acoustic window.

Sonohysterography (SHG) is a recently developed technique that is increasingly performed to better evaluate the endometrium. With this technique, sterile saline is infused into the endometrial cavity under continuous endovaginal ultrasound guidance. The sterile saline distends the endometrial cavity separating the anterior and posterior endometrial layers and outlining the endometrial surface. A baseline TVS examination is initially performed. After insertion of a single-hinged speculum, the cervix is cleansed with Betadine and a 5 to 7F catheter is threaded through the cervical os. The catheter should be flushed with saline prior to insertion to remove any air in the lumen. The speculum is removed and the endovaginal probe reinserted. Under continuous ultrasound imaging, 10 to 60 mL of sterile saline is slowly infused and images are obtained in both sagittal (long axis) and transverse (short axis) planes (23–25). If a balloon catheter is utilized, it should be deflated at the end of the procedure to allow complete visualization of the lower uterine segment. Antibiotic prophylaxis can be considered in patients who normally take prophylactic antibiotics prior to dental work. Premedication with nonsteroidal antiinflammatory agents will minimize uterine cramping. Contraindications to SHG include hematometria and acute pelvic inflammatory disease. Recently, 3-D sonohysterography has been described. This technique reduces operator dependence and length of examination time and has been reported to provide significant additional information in the majority of patients (26).

Normal Uterus

Both sagittal and transverse views of the uterus should be obtained. The normal myometrium is homogeneous and intermediate in echotexture. Anechoic tubular structures separating the outer one-third from the inner two-thirds of the myometrium represent the arcuate vessels, which are seen to best advantage on color flow imaging. The internal os can be recognized as a slight constriction of the uterine contour. Anechoic nabothian cysts are commonly seen in the cervix. Uterine volume is calculated using the formula 1/2 (L × W × D). The endometrium should be measured at the thickest part of the endometrial stripe in the uterine fundus on a midline sagittal image, and by convention is always reported as a double-layer measurement. The normal endometrium is highly echogenic. However, the thickness and echotexture of the endometrium varies with the hormonal status of the patient. At the end of the menses, the endometrial stripe is brightly echogenic and measures approximately 2 to 3 mm. During the proliferative stage, the endometrium becomes less echogenic and thickens, reaching a maximum of 8 mm. Near ovulation, a trilaminar appearance has been described. The central thin echogenic line represents a reflective artifact and/or mucus and secretions between the anterior and posterior layers of the endometruim. Subjacent is the relatively hypoechoic functionalis layer. The surrounding deeper basalis layer remains echogenic. Following ovulation, the functionalis layer becomes thicker and more echogenic during the secretory phase such that the entire stripe may reach 15 mm in thickness and is more uniformly echogenic just prior to menstruation (27,28). In some patients, the innermost layer of myometrium is relatively hypoechoic immediately subjacent to the endometrium and is termed the subendometrial halo. The subendometrial halo is less commonly visualized in postmenopausal women. Neither the subendometrial halo nor fluid or debris within the endometrial cavity should be included in measurements of the endometrial stripe (Fig. 10.5). At SHG, the endometrium should be homogeneous, symmetric, and regular without mass effect. The sum of the width of the two layers should not exceed the maximum acceptable width for the patient's hormonal status (1–3 mm).

The uterine artery originates from the internal iliac artery. Pulse Doppler examination will demonstrate a high impedance waveform characterized by an early diastolic notch and relatively little diastolic flow. Only minor changes occur in the uterine artery waveform during the menstrual cycle.

In postmenopausal women, the uterine corpus shrinks until it approximates the length of the cervix. The endometrium atrophies and should appear as a thin, regular echo-

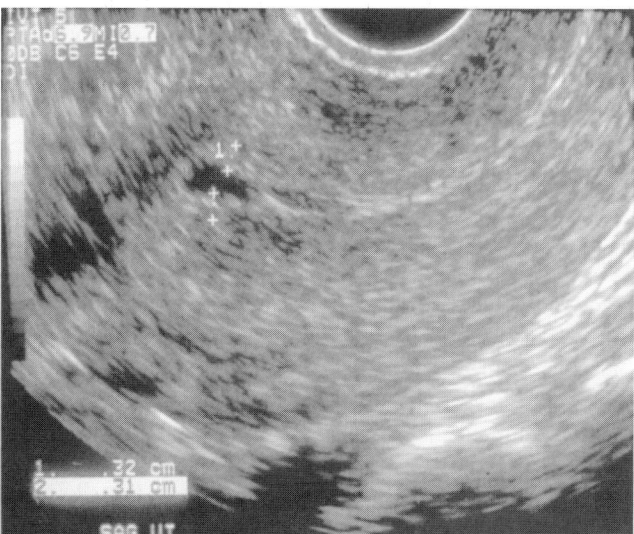

FIG. 10.5. Normal uterus. Fluid and/or debris within the endometrial cavity should not be included in measurements of the endometrial stripe. The endometrial width is reported as the sum of the anterior and posterior endometrial layers (calipers).

genic line <5 mm in width (29) (Fig.10.6). In women taking hormonal replacement therapy (HRT), less uterine and endometrial atrophy occurs (30,31). Women taking sequential HRT are best examined following withdrawal bleeding and the progesterone phase of their cycle when the endometrium is expected to be at the thinnest.

Normal Ovaries

The US appearance of the ovaries also changes with the patient's hormonal status. The premenopausal ovary has a relatively homogeneous outer cortex with a more echogenic

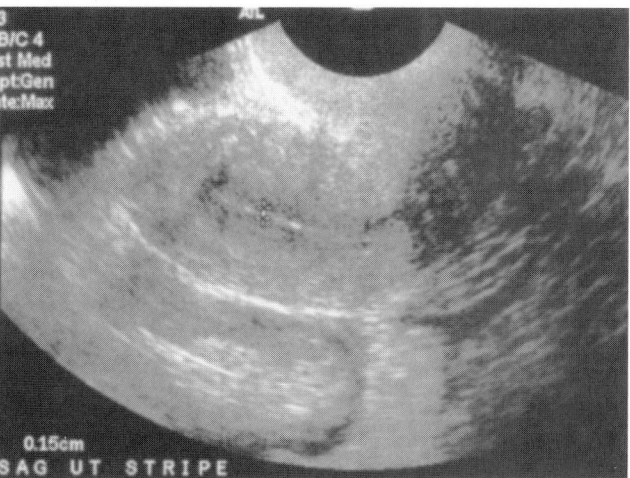

FIG. 10.6. Normal postmenopausal uterus. Note small size of uterine corpus and thin, regular endometrial stripe (calipers).

central medulla. Small anechoic cysts or follicles are common. At ovulation, one follicle becomes dominant, reaching a maximum diameter of 2.0 to 2.5 cm. Following ovulation, the corpus luteum develops. The corpus luteum may contain debris or hemorrhage and often involutes, appearing to be crenated just prior to menstruation. The ovaries atrophy with menopause and contain fewer cysts. Therefore, they may be more difficult to visualize with ultrasound. In women taking HRT, less ovarian atrophy will occur and follicles will continue to develop. Doppler evaluation of ovarian blood flow is best performed during days 3 to 7 of the menstrual cycle. The ovary undergoing ovulation in a given cycle demonstrates a relatively high-velocity, low-resistance waveform with continuous forward diastolic flow. The contralateral ovary will typically demonstrate a higher resistance low-velocity arterial waveform with either very low or no diastolic flow.

Computed Tomography

Techniques

CT studies of the pelvis require contrast opacification of the distal small bowel and colon. In some centers, patients receive 500 mL of a 2% barium solution the evening preceding the examination and an additional 500 mL 45 minutes before scan to fill small-bowel loops in the pelvis. In other protocols, the patient receives 600 to 1000 mL of dilute oral contrast at least 1 hour before the examination coupled with a 200-mL dilute contrast enema. Iodinated intravenous contrast is used to opacify the bladder and ureters, to differentiate contrast-filled blood vessels from adjacent lymph nodes, to enhance the myometrium, to visualize the endome-

trial cavity, and to delineate hypodense tumor boundaries from contiguous normal organ parenchyma.

Helical CT and more recently MDCT are becoming the standard of care in many hospital and outpatient settings. Optimal intravenous contrast enhancement for these faster scanners requires a mechanical power injector to administer 100 to 120 mL of 60% contrast agent at a rate of 2 mL/s or more. Scan parameters including injection rates, scan delays, and collimation vary for single-slice and MDCT studies. With MDCT, it is easy to obtain multiphasic contrast examinations with arterial and delayed venous phase images. Increased radiation exposure for multiple passes must be balanced with the likelihood of increased clinical yield. Image displays are likewise variable. For example, studies obtained at 2.5 mm collimation may be reconstructed to 5-mm slices to facilitate film-based reading. Increasingly, however, the enormous data sets generated by MDCT studies require sophisticated software and computer work stations to exploit fully this technology (1).

Normal Uterus and Pelvic Structures

CT examinations display the uterine corpus as a triangular or ovoid soft tissue mass behind the urinary bladder. The cervix is more rounded. On noncontrast scans, secretions within the endometrial canal are seen as centrally located decreased attenuation. With the improved temporal resolution of helical CT, the vagina, cervix, and uterine corpus can be differentiated based on both morphologic and enhancement characteristics (Fig. 10.7). Following bolus intravenous contrast administration, the myometrium in the corpus enhances to a greater degree than that of the cervix, and this allows better delineation of the endometrium. At the

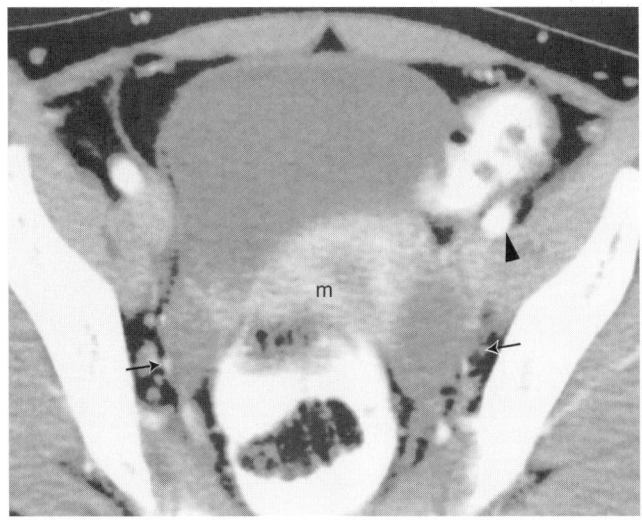
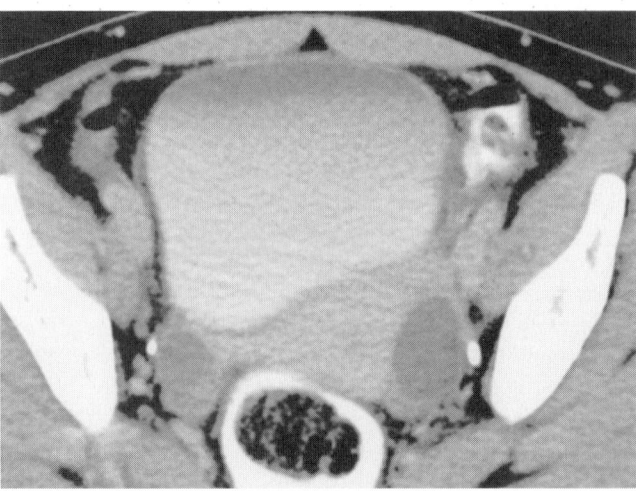

A

B

FIG. 10.7. Normal ovary and uterus on helical CT. **A:** Bolus contrast-enhanced axial image shows the normally enhancing uterine corpus myometrium (m) surrounding the lower attenuation endometrial canal. Note both ovaries (*arrows*), with associated functional cysts and densely enhancing external iliac arteries (*arrowheads*). **B:** On delayed images, the endometrium is isodense with the myometrium.

level of the fornix, the vagina has a flat rectangular or crescentic shape. The broad and round ligaments can be seen coursing laterally and anteriorly, respectively. Occasionally, the uterosacral ligaments are depicted as arc-like structures extending from the cervix to the sacrum.

Normal Ovaries

In the premenopausal patient, the normal ovaries are routinely seen, usually posterolateral to the uterine corpus (Fig. 10.7B). Their uniform soft tissue density is punctuated by small cystic regions representing follicles. In the postmenopausal patient, the ovaries are small and less readily detected.

Magnetic Resonance Imaging

Techniques

It is recommended that patients fast for 4 to 6 hours before the MR examination or be given an antiperistaltic (e.g., 1.0 mg glucagon intramuscularly). The routine use of bowel contrast agents is controversial, but some investigators advocate the administration of varying amounts (typically 400 to 600 mL) of oral contrast 10 to 40 minutes prior to the examination (32). When an oral contrast agent is used, the antiperistaltic is given just before scanning to optimize image quality (33). Gadolinium chelates (0.1 mmol/kg) are administered intravenously to opacify vessels, to highlight tumor interfaces, to assess lymph node status, to detect fistulas, and to identify locoregional and distant metastases. Patients are usually scanned in the supine position, with the bladder empty at the beginning of the study.

Using a high field strength (≥1 tesla) system and a phased-array surface coil, high-resolution T2-weighted images are obtained in under 5 minutes using fast-spin echo technique (T2W FSE) (34–37). Recently, parallel imaging has been gaining momentum. Parallel imaging allows faster acquisition of T2W FSE sequences by a factor of 2 or twice the spatial resolution for a given acquisition time. Although there are even faster imaging techniques [e.g., breath-hold FSE and breathing-independent half Fourier acquisition single-shot turbo spin echo (HASTE)], they do not have the same spatial resolution as fast-spin echo and therefore cannot replace T2W FSE for evaluating the primary tumor and extent of disease. (Fig. 10.8) (34,38). However, these heavily T2-weighted sequences (e.g., RARE, HASTE) are particularly attractive for performing MR urography (MRU) (Fig. 10.9) as an adjunct to T2W FSE images (39,40).

Normal Uterus and Pelvic Structures

Pelvic anatomy is exquisitely demonstrated on MRI scans. On T1-weighted sequences, the normal pelvic musculature and viscera demonstrate homogeneous low to medium signal intensity (Fig. 10.10). Cortical bone demonstrates low signal

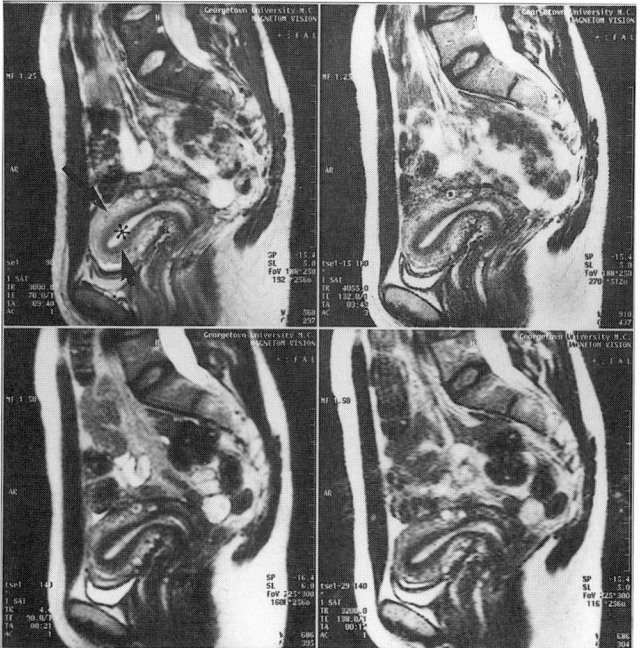

FIG. 10.8. Normal uterus on MRI. The normal uterus as imaged by four different T2-W sequences [conventional spin echo (acquisition time = 9:40 min), upper left; fast spin echo (acquisition time = 3:43 min), upper right; half Fourier single-shot turbo spin echo (acquisition time = 0.21 min), lower left; and breath-hold fast spin echo (acquisition time = 0.17 min), lower right) demonstrates normal zonal anatomy; high–signal intensity endometrium (*asterisk*); low–signal intensity junctional zone (*short arrow*), and intermediate–signal intensity myometrium (*long arrow*). Fast sequences improve patient tolerance and decrease imaging times.

intensity owing to immobile protons, and fatty marrow is high in signal intensity. Similarly, intrapelvic fat demonstrates increased signal intensity. It is the contrast resolution afforded by T2 weighting, however, that is the basis for the strength of MR in pelvic imaging. On these sequences, the uterus, cervix, and vagina exhibit distinct layers of different signal intensity—the so-called zonal architecture (Figs. 10.8 and 10.11 to 10.13). The endometrium images with high signal intensity, usually higher than subcutaneous fat. The peripheral myometrium is intermediate in signal intensity, being higher in signal intensity than striated muscle. Interposed between these two layers is a narrow band of decreased signal intensity, the junctional zone, which corresponds to the innermost myometrium. Its signal properties reflect its lower water content, compared with the remainder of the myometrium, which may be a function of its decrease in extracellular matrix/unit volume (41,42). The three zones seen on MR images are not comparable to the different zones seen on US (43). The width of the endometrium (both leaflets) varies with the menstrual cycle (44,45). In postmenopausal women not receiving exogenous hormones, uterine zonal anatomy is indistinct, and the endometrium typically measures less than 3 mm (44).

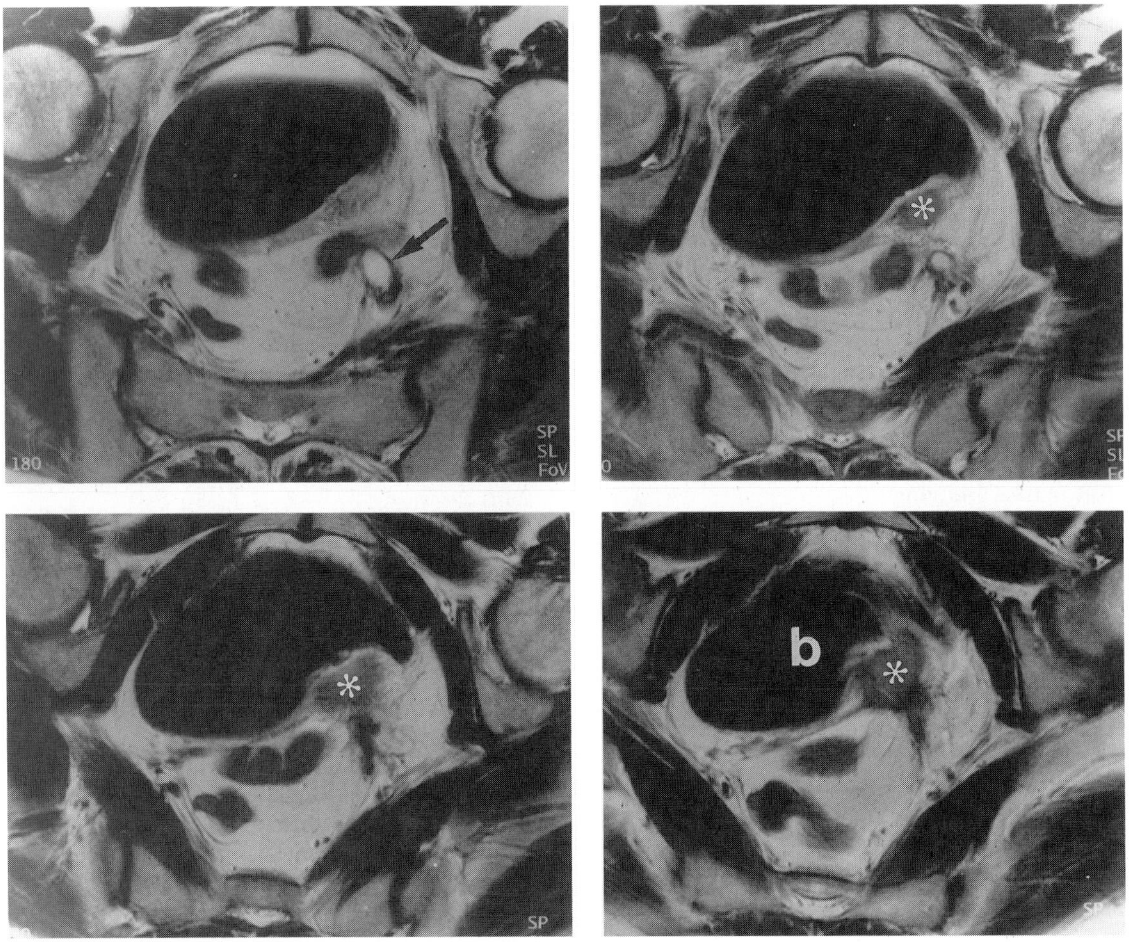

FIG. 10.9. MR urography. **A:** Sequential axial T2-W sequences show a dilated ureter (*arrow,* upper left, **A**) encased by a focus of recurrent cervical cancer (*asterisks,* upper right and lower right and left, **A**). Note that the recurrent disease indents and invades the urinary bladder (b). **B:** Maximum-intensity projection MR urogram in the same patient shows the dilated intrarenal collecting system and ureter.

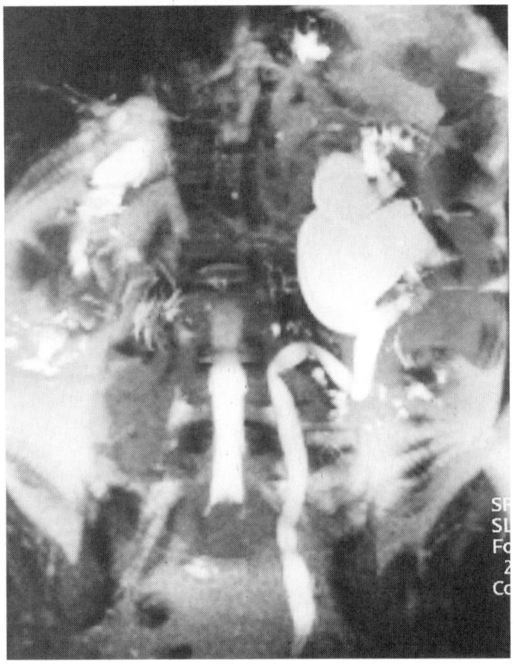

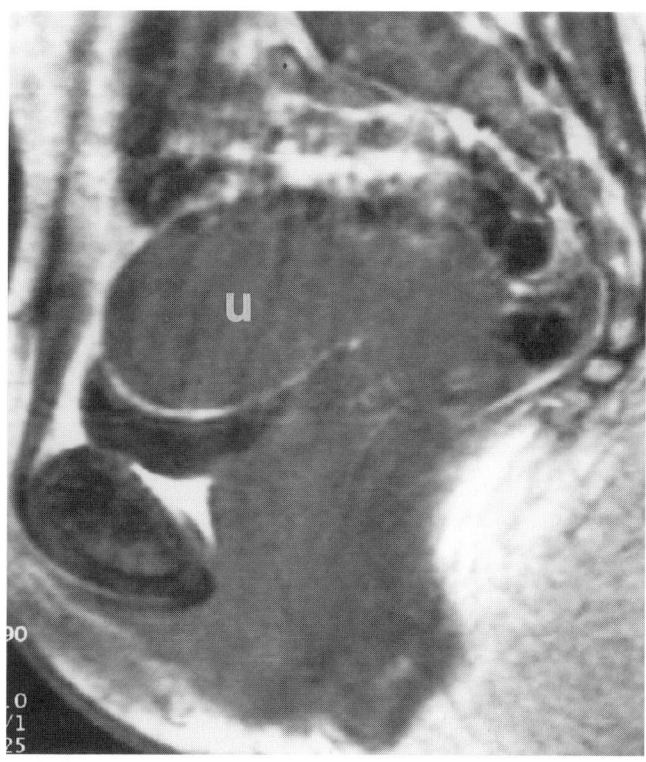

FIG. 10.10. Normal uterus on MRI. Sagittal T2-W image shows the normal intermediate–signal intensity uterus (u).

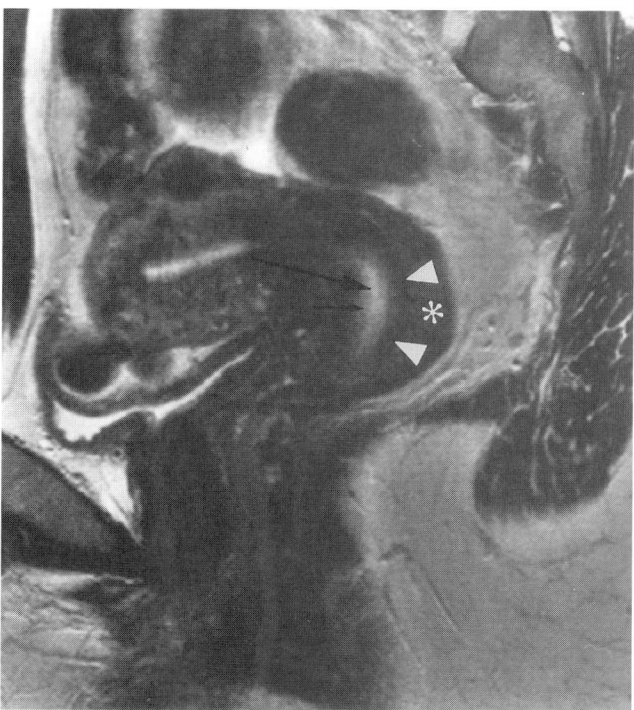

FIG. 10.11. Normal cervix on MRI. Sagittal T2-W sequence shows normal cervical zonal anatomy: high-signal intensity of the endocervical canal (*long arrow*); intermediate-signal intensity of the endocervical mucosal folds (*short arrow*); low-signal intensity of the fibrocervical stroma (*arrowheads*); and intermediate signal intensity of the cervical myometrium (*asterisk*).

The cervix also demonstrates zonal architecture on T2-weighted sequences. There is an inner area of high signal intensity, which is believed to represent epithelium and mucus; a middle area of predominantly low signal intensity, which is believed to represent fibrous stroma with a higher cell count or more nuclei; and an outer area of medium signal intensity, which is believed to represent fibrous stroma with a lower cell count or fewer nuclei and a high degree of vascularity (46,47) (Figs. 10.11 and 10.12). The use of pelvic surface coils has revealed yet another cervical layer: interposed between the high–signal intensity endocervical canal and the low–signal intensity fibrocervical stroma is a feathery layer of intermediate signal intensity, which is thought to represent the mucosal folds or plicae palmatae (Fig. 10.11) (37). T2-weighted images of the vagina reveal two zones (Fig. 10.13), the bright vaginal mucosa and the intermediate–signal intensity vaginal wall. The low–signal intensity ligamentous structures are identified by their anatomic location.

Following the administration of intravenous gadolinium chelates, the zonal anatomy of the uterus is demonstrated on T1-weighted images (Fig. 10.13). The endometrium and outer myometrium enhance to a greater extent than the junctional zone. Similarly, the inner cervical mucosa and outer smooth muscle enhance more than the fibrocervical stroma. The parametrial tissues, vaginal wall, and submucosa also enhance after intravenous contrast administration.

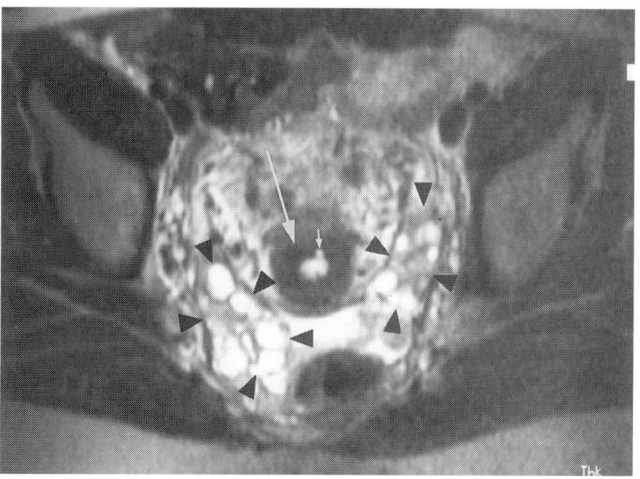

FIG. 10.12. Normal ovaries. Axial T2-W MR image shows high–signal intensity follicles (*arrowheads*) bilaterally. A nabothian cyst (*short arrow*) is seen within the fibrocervical stroma (*long arrow*).

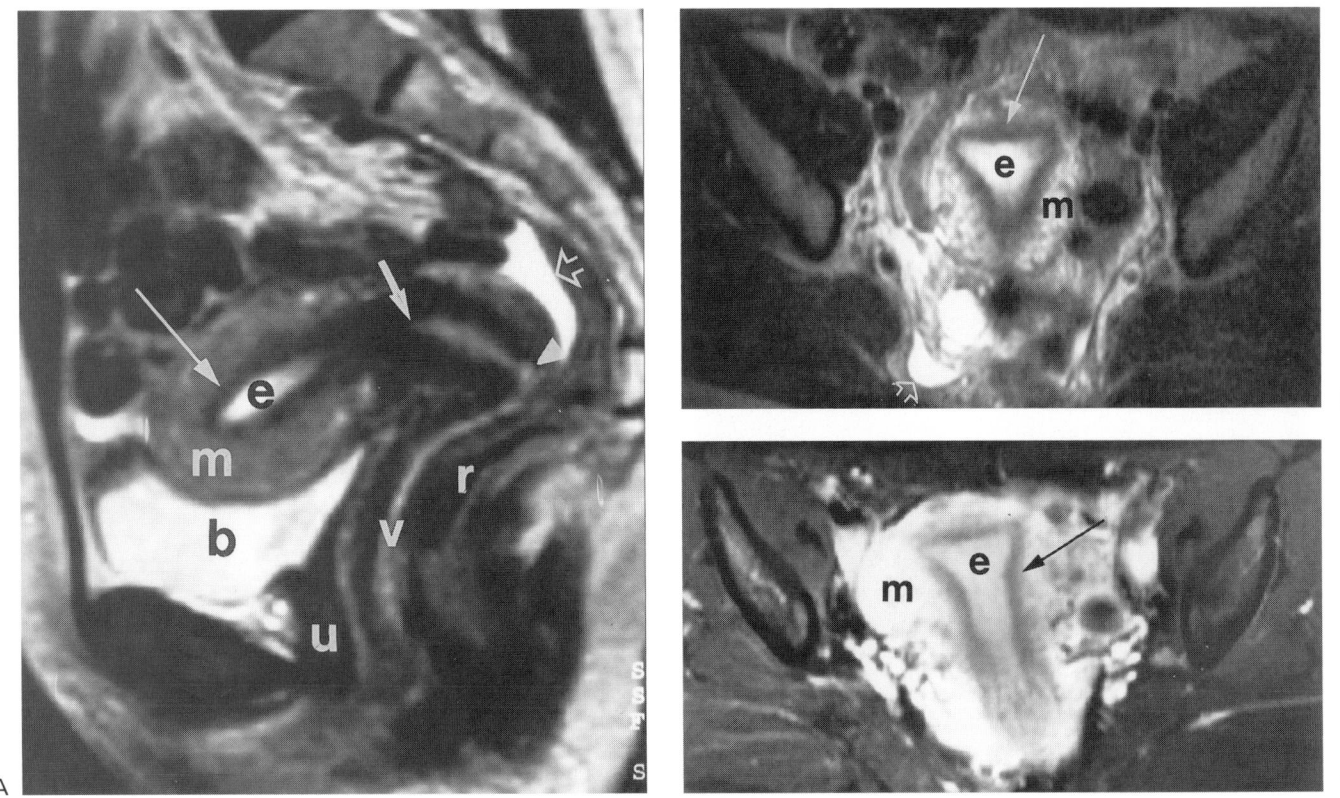

FIG. 10.13. Normal uterus and vagina. **A:** Sagittal, **(B)** axial T2-, and **(C)** postcontrast T1-W MR images from three different patients show the endometrium (e) of the uterine corpus separated from the myometrium (m) by the junctional zone (*long arrow*). The cervix extends from the internal os (*short arrow*) to the external os (*arrowhead*), which protrudes into the vagina (v). The vagina (v) is positioned between the bladder (b) and urethra (u) anteriorly and the rectum (r) posteriorly. Fluid is seen in the cul-de-sac (*open arrow*). Note that, after contrast, uterine zonal anatomy normally not seen on T1-W images becomes apparent.

Normal Ovaries

The normal MR appearance of the ovaries varies depending on the pulse sequence used. On T1-weighted images, the ovaries display homogeneous low to medium signal intensity, whereas on T2-weighted images, the follicles become brighter than the surrounding stroma (Fig. 10.12). The normal fallopian tubes are not routinely imaged because of their small size and tortuous course.

CERVICAL CANCER

Detection and Characterization

Ultrasound

Early cervical carcinoma is difficult to detect with either transabdominal or transvaginal sonography. However, recent work with high-frequency 20-MHz miniature intracervical US probes is promising. These probes are able to detect early cancers (invasion >5 mm) (48,49). In patients with more advanced cervical cancer, the cervix will appear to be enlarged and irregular on TVS. Occasionally a hypoechoic

mass mimicking a cervical myoma may be observed. (Fig. 10.14). If tumor obstructs the endocervical canal, hydrometra and/or hematometra will be present (Fig 10.14B).

The uterine cervix, parametrium, vagina, pelvic sidewall, rectum, and posterior bladder wall can sometimes be visualized to better advantage on transrectal ultrasound (TRUS). Cervical cancers are usually hypoechoic or isoechoic masses with ill-defined margins. The limited field of view of TRUS may preclude full assessment of the extent of a large tumor, the pelvic side wall, and pelvic lymph nodes (50).

Computed Tomography

In patients with cervical cancer, CT is of greatest utility in the evaluation of advanced disease. The primary tumor may appear on CT as cervical enlargement as well as a discrete low-attenuation or peripherally enhancing cervical mass. These regions of decreased attenuation are a function of tumor necrosis/ulceration and/or inherent differences in the attenuation between tumor and normal cervical tissue (Fig. 10.15). Distinguishing tumor from the normal cervix is often problematic, as half of cervical tumors are isodense

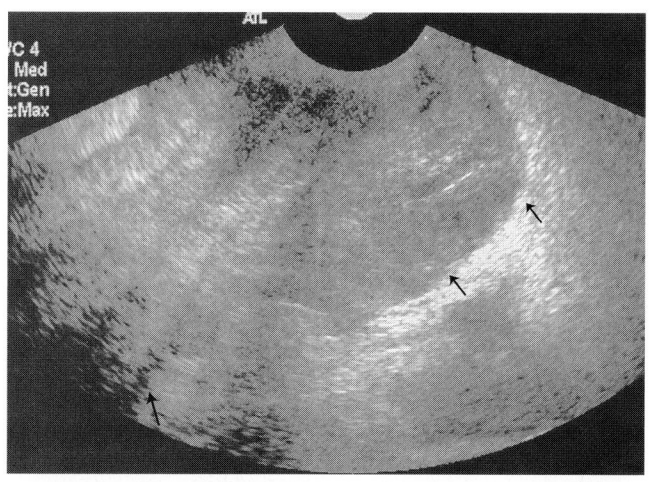
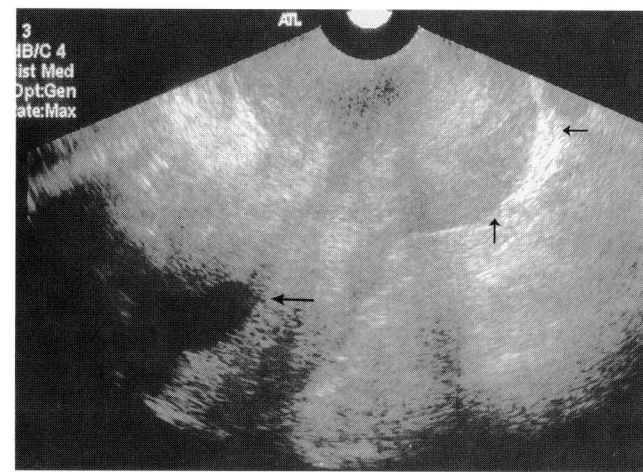
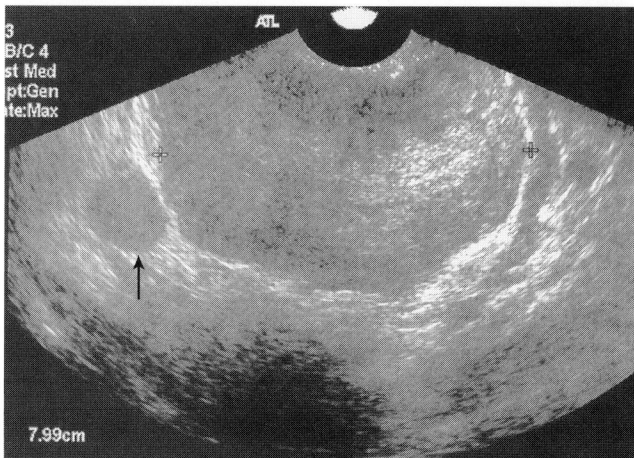

FIG. 10.14. Cervical carcinoma. A: Sagittal image demonstrating marked enlargement and heterogeneity of the cervix (short arrows). The margins are irregular and the endocervical canal is distorted and obscured by the mass. The uterus is slightly retroverted (*long arrow*). B: Sagittal image, which includes the uterus, demonstrating hydrometra (*long arrow*) as well as the cervical mass (*short arrows*). C: Transverse image through the large cervical mass (calipers) also demonstrates an enlarged right paracervical lymph node (*arrow*).

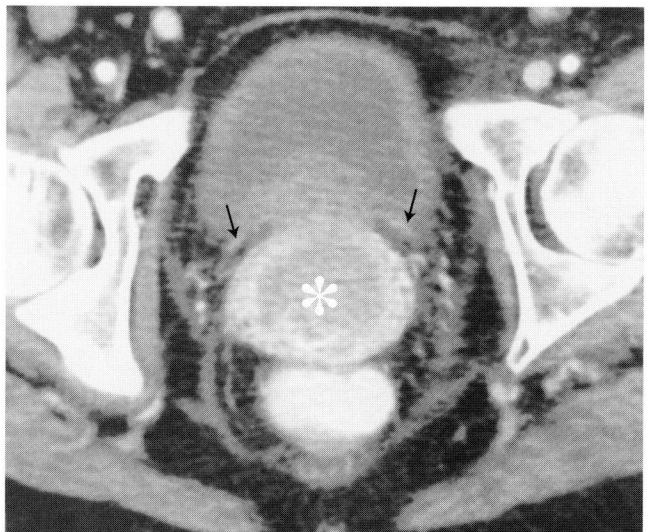

FIG. 10.15. Cervical cancer. Contrast-enhanced axial CT shows a low-attenuation cervical cancer (*asterisk*). Fat planes surrounding the distal ureters *(arrows)* are preserved.

to normal stroma on CT (2). Early parametrial invasion is not reliably detected by CT. Obstruction of the endocervical canal by cervical tumor can result in uterine enlargement with a fluid-filled endometrial cavity (Fig. 10.16) (51).

Magnetic Resonance Imaging

The ever-increasing body of literature on MRI and cervical cancer suggests that MRI is superior to US or CT for delineating the primary tumor site, tumor dimensions, and extent of disease. These MRI advantages are primarily due to the superior soft tissue contrast between tumor and normal tissue and the ability to define the tumor in the orthogonal plane (52,53). On T2-weighted images, the characteristic feature of cervical cancer is an intermediate–signal intensity mass. Tumor signal intensity is usually greater than the normal low–signal intensity fibrocervical stroma (Fig. 10.17).

On T1-weighted images, tumors are usually isointense with the normal cervix and may not be visible. Intravenous contrast highlights tumor heterogeneity and aids in the differentiation of viable tumor from debris and necrosis (54). Additionally, contrast helps to evaluate bladder and rectal

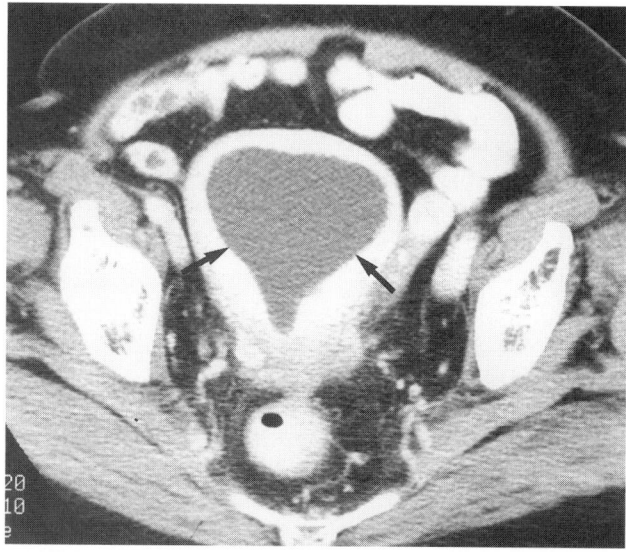

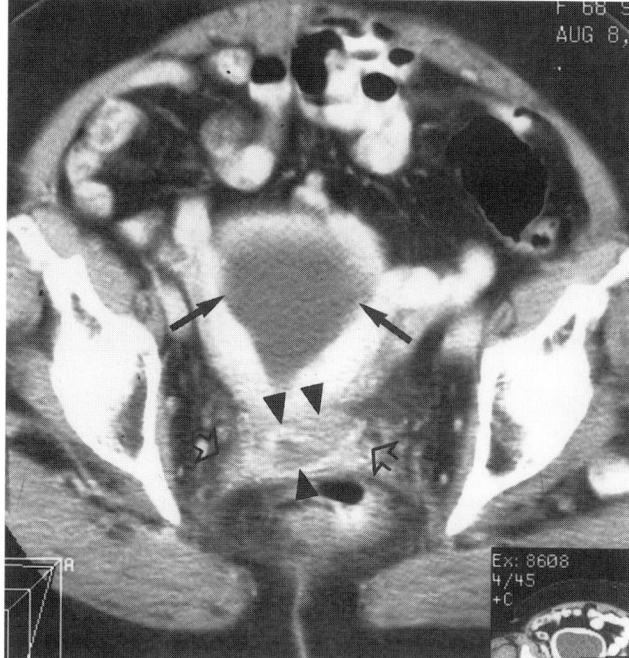

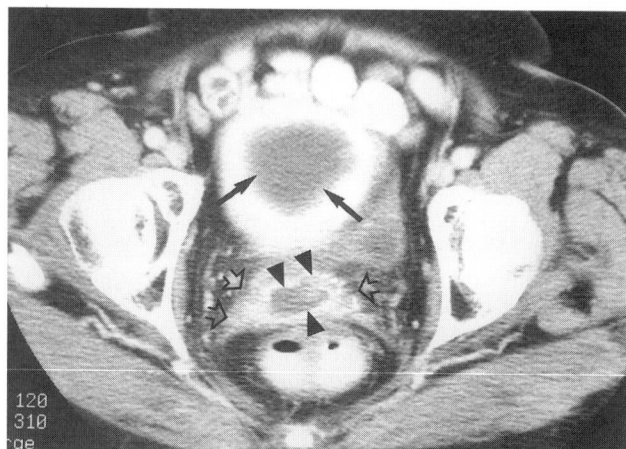

FIG. 10.16. Stage IIB cervical cancer. **(A, B):** Contiguous contrast-enhanced axial helical CT scans through the pelvis. **C:** a reconstructed paracoronal CT image shows hydrometro-colpos (*arrows*) secondary to a low-attenuation cervical carcinoma (*arrowheads*, **B, C**). There is also stranding of the parametrial fat (*open arrows*, **B, C**), suggesting parametrial invasion. Note that acquiring the data helically allows for high-quality reconstructions.

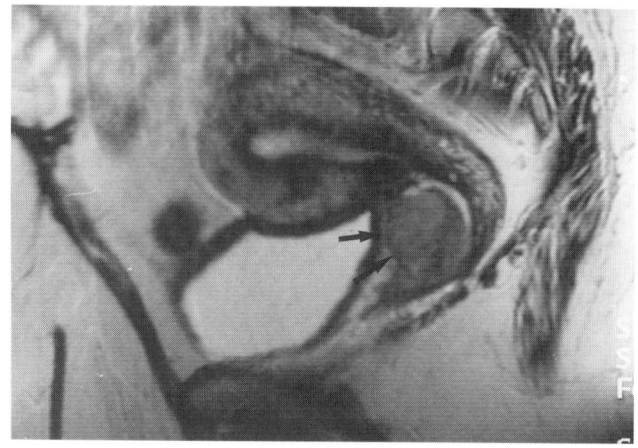

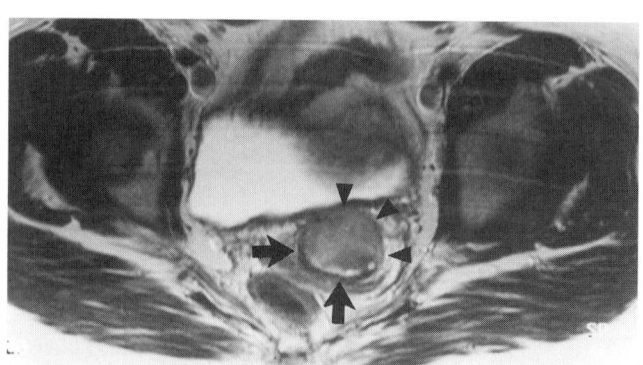

FIG. 10.17. Stage IB versus IIB cervical cancer. **A:** Sagittal T2-W MR image shows a high–signal intensity mass (*arrows*, **A**) in the anterior cervical lip bulging the normal cervical outline. **B:** Axial T2-W MR image shows intact low signal intensity cervical stroma on the right and posterior aspect of the cervix (*arrows*, **B**); whereas there has been full-thickness stromal invasion of the left and anterior aspect of the cervix (*arrowheads*, **B**). The parametrial invasion is controversial in this case because of the regular tumor margin and no discrete parametrial mass.

involvement. When dynamic contrast enhancement is used, the following MRI characteristics of cervical cancer can be seen. Early, within 60 seconds following a bolus of gadolinium chelate, the primary tumor exhibits increased enhancement relative to the normal cervical stroma. With time, this difference becomes less marked. On delayed images, the tumor may be isointense or hypointense to the cervical stroma (55). Dynamic imaging may improve detection of small lesions and assessment of stromal invasion (55,56). Signal intensity versus time curves, however, do not appear to make a significant contribution to the evaluation of tumor aggressiveness (57). Intravenous gadolinium is recommended for evaluating cervical cancer in selected cases, such as estimation of tumor necrosis prior to institution of therapy and suspected advanced disease involving the bladder and/or rectum.

In contrast to squamous-cell cervical carcinoma, adenoma malignum, a rare form of cervical adenocarcinoma, is depicted as a high–signal intensity multicystic lesion on T2-weighted sequences. The tumor extends from the endocervical glands to the deep cervical stroma and may mimic nabothian cysts. On postcontrast images, solid portions within the tumor enhance, which is a feature that may help distinguish adenoma malignum from nabothian cysts (58).

Positron Emission Tomography

There have been several encouraging studies of FDG PET in women with cervical cancer. Rose et al. (59) found in 32 patients that radioisotope was taken up in 91% of cervical tumors, and compared to surgical staging, FDG PET had a sensitivity of 72% and a specificity of 92% for detecting paraaortic lymphadenopathy. Another group of investigators reported on 23 women with cervical cancer who underwent FDG PET: 11 women with newly diagnosed cervical cancer and 12 women with clinically suspected recurrent disease (16). Primary tumor was correctly demonstrated by FDG PET in 10 of the 11 women with newly diagnosed disease—although parametrial invasion could not be assessed. It also identified locoregional and distant lymph node metastases and unsuspected lung metastases in three patients. In the women with clinically suspicious recurrent disease, FDG accumulation paralleled the findings on CT scan.

Although both of these studies report on a limited number of patients, they suggest that FDG is not only taken up by primary cervical lesions, but has the potential for detecting lymph node metastases and distant metastases that may be missed by conventional imaging studies. This detection ability is especially important for lymph node metastases, since size is the sole criterion for identifying lymphadenopathy on other cross-sectional modalities. Detection of both nodal and distant metastases may have profound therapeutic and prognostic significance because recent work has shown that radiation treatment alone is less effective in patients with

advanced cervical cancer than if chemotherapy is included (60–62).

Staging

Recommendations for diagnostic evaluation of tumor staging derive from the International Federation of Gynecology and Obstetrics (FIGO) clinical staging system and are based on findings from physical examination, colposcopy, lesion biopsies, chest radiography, cystoscopy, sigmoidoscopy, intravenous urography (IVU), and barium enema. When compared with surgical staging, clinical FIGO staging is flawed, with a reported error rate of 17% to 67%. These sobering statistics primarily reflect failure to identify parametrial extension (53,63–65). Furthermore, clinical FIGO staging does not include evaluation of lymph node metastases. The staging accuracy for barium enema and IVU are dismal, with both tests being positive in only advanced disease (21). Whereas hydronephrosis or a nonfunctioning kidney can be detected with IVU, excretory urography is insensitive to tumor extent (66,67). CT is more accurate than IVU in demonstrating the exact site of ureteral obstruction and the entire course of a hydroureter even in the absence of renal function (67,68). Although cross-sectional imaging is not mandated by FIGO, many women are referred for CT or MRI to define extent of disease.

Ultrasound

Transabdominal sonography plays a limited role in the staging of cervical cancer and is inferior to other cross-sectional modalities. Although the improved spatial resolution achieved with TVS and TRUS is helpful in the evaluation of tumor size and locoregional extent, poor contrast resolution impedes differentiation between tumor and normal adjacent cervical, uterine, parametrial, and vaginal tissue (69,70). Sonographic findings in parametrial invasion include irregularity or loss of the normal cervical contour (70,71). Pelvic sidewall involvement is diagnosed on US by a parametrial soft tissue mass or tumor extension to the sidewall and/or encasement of the iliac vessels (70,71). Bladder invasion is suggested by loss of the fat plane between cervix and bladder and direct extension of the tumor mass through the bladder wall. Lymph nodes may also be detected (Fig. 10.14C).

Diagnostic Value

One study reports an overall accuracy of 83% for TRUS staging of cervical cancer (70). The accuracy increases to 87% for parametrial involvement, with a sensitivity of 78% and a specificity of 89% (71). Unfortunately, these results have not been confirmed, limiting enthusiasm for this modality. Most agree that the contrast resolution and field of view with US is too limited to allow evaluation of the parametria. The modest performance of all US modalities, combined with the inability to assess lymph node status completely, particularly distant lymph node chains, limits its usefulness in the workup of patients with cervical cancer.

Computed Tomography

Conventional CT has been used extensively for evaluating cervical cancer, and its strengths and limitations are well known. Intravenous contrast is essential to delineate the interfaces of tumor, normal cervical stroma, and myometrium and to differentiate normal parauterine fat margins from irregular hypodense borders caused by tumor infiltration. The impact of advances in CT technology on the workup of cervical cancer is under investigation (72).

CT staging criteria are derived from FIGO staging (Table 10.1).

Stage I

CT staging attempts to differentiate tumor confined to the cervix (stage I) from tumor that has invaded the parametria (stage IIB). Tumor confined to the cervix does not alter the normal smooth, well-defined, cervical contour, periureteral fat planes are preserved, and there is no prominent stranding of the parametria or parametrial soft tissue mass (Fig. 10.15).

Stage II

Described CT criteria for parametrial invasion (stage IIB) include irregularity or effacement of the lateral cervical margins, thick parametrial soft tissue stranding, an eccentric soft-tissue mass, and obliteration of the normal periureteral fat planes. Diagnosis of early parametrial invasion is problematic on CT as irregular cervical margins and prominent parametrial soft tissue can be simulated by parametritis associated with previous uterine curettage or cervical conization. Loss of the periureteral fat plane around the pelvic ureter is the only reliable finding of parametrial tumor extension but indicates advanced disease (Fig. 10.16) (67,73). Intravaginal tumor (stage IIA) is best staged by clinical examination (74).

Stage III

Stage IIIB tumors involving the pelvic sidewall appear as irregular soft tissue strands extending to the piriformis and/or levator ani and/or obturator internus muscles. Alternatively, confluent soft tissue masses may envelop the pelvic sidewall musculature and iliac vessels. A fat plane of 3 mm or less between a parametrial mass and the pelvic sidewall suggests stage IIIB disease, since clinicians consider tumors to involve the sidewall if they are unable to interpose their fingers between the tumor and sidewall during pelvic examination under anesthesia (51). Detection of hydronephrosis or lymphadenopathy by CT also indicates stage IIIB disease (Fig. 10.18).

Stage IV

CT criteria for urinary bladder or rectal invasion (stage IVA) include focal loss of the normal perivesical/perirectal

TABLE 10.1. *Corresponding CT findings for staging of carcinoma of the cervix*

Stage 0		No tumor present
Stage I	IA	No tumor present
	IB	No tumor present or tumor does not alter cervical contour
Stage II	IIA	Thickening of vaginal wall (upper two-thirds)
	IIB	Irregular lateral cervical margin parametrial mass or strands
		Obliteration of periureteral fat
Stage III	IIIA	Thickening of vaginal wall (lower third)
	IIIB	Tumor extends to obturator internus, piriformis, levator ani muscles
		Dilated ureter
Stage IV	IVA	Thickening, nodularity, serration of bladder or rectal wall
		Obliteration of perivesical or perirectal fat
	IVB	Tumor in distant organs

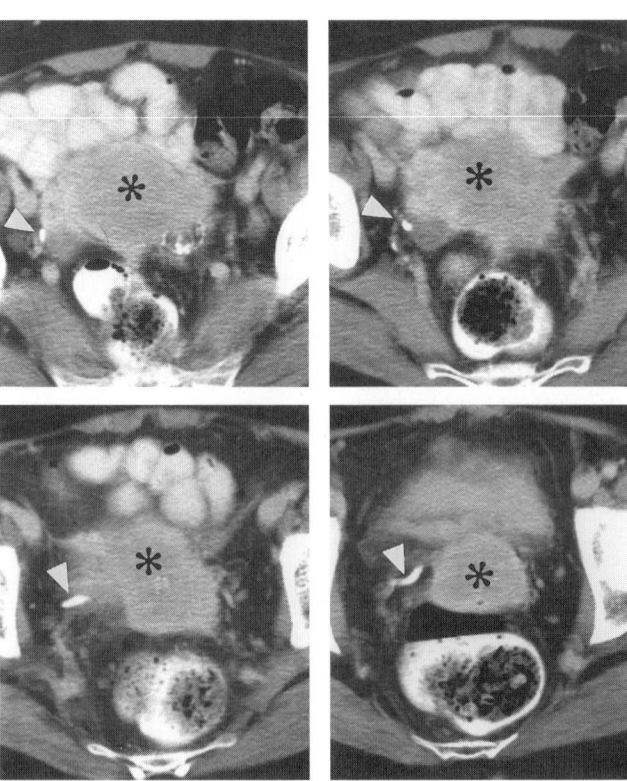

FIG. 10.18. Stage IIIB cervical cancer. Sequential contrast-enhanced CT scans show a low-density cervical mass extending into uterine body (*asterisk*). Note that the left periureteral fat is obliterated and a discrete left ureter is no longer seen. (*Arrowhead:* uninvolved right ureter.)

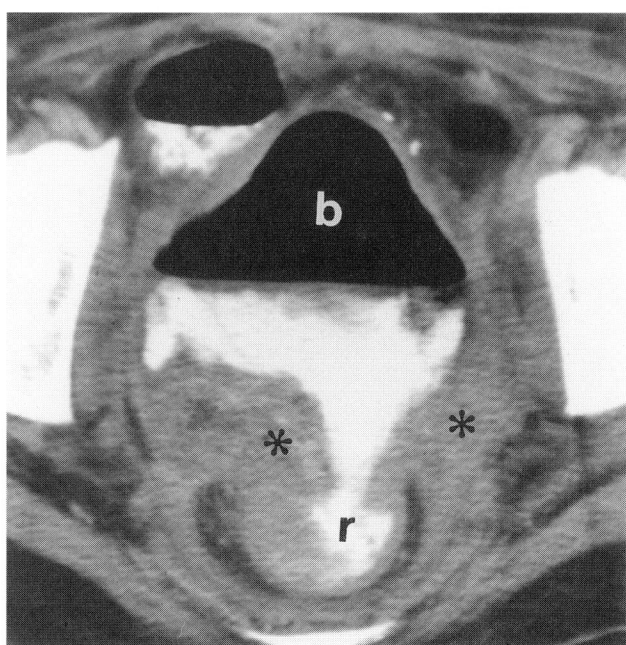

FIG. 10.19. Stage IVA cervical cancer with a vesicovaginal and rectovaginal fistula. CT scan shows a large irregular soft tissue mass (*asterisks*). The large fistulous tract between the bladder (b), mass, and rectum (r) is clearly outlined by contrast agent.

fat plane accompanied by asymmetric wall thickening, nodular indentations or serrations along the bladder or rectal walls, an intraluminal tumor mass, or a vesicovaginal fistula (Fig. 10.19) (74,75). Early invasion of the bladder or rectum is not reliably detected by CT.

Lymph Nodes

Although the FIGO system does not include lymph node status, the presence of lymphadenopathy affects prognosis. Detection of enlarged paraaortic or inguinal lymph nodes by CT is considered to be an extrapelvic tumor extension and correlates with stage IVB disease. Lymph nodes greater than 1 cm in the short axis are considered to be pathologically enlarged. Adenopathy with central necrosis is associated with a high likelihood of metastatic disease (76). Lymph node enlargement may also be secondary to benign inflammatory or reactive hyperplasia. Conversely, normal-sized lymph nodes may contain microscopic tumor foci. CT-guided biopsy and/or PET-CT can be useful to assess further patients with suspected nodal disease.

Diagnostic Value

The overall accuracy of conventional CT staging for cervical cancer ranges from 63% to 88% (2,3,67,74). For assessing parametrial invasion, accuracy varies from 55% to 80% (2,3,73,77), and both false-positive and false-negative diag-

noses occur. For example, in patients with clinical stage IB disease, a false-positive CT diagnosis of parametrial invasion leads to overstaging. On the other hand, 12% to 33% of patients with clinical stages IIB to IIIB disease are understaged by CT because microscopic tumor involvement of the pelvic sidewall, bladder, lymph nodes, or omentum cannot be detected (63,67,74). Nonetheless, CT is a valuable complement to clinical staging because of its accuracy in detecting advanced disease. In fact, 92% of stage IIIB through stage IVB lesions are accurately staged with CT (67). In the detection of lymphadenopathy, helical CT is similar to MR, with a sensitivity of 65%, specificity of 97%, and overall accuracy of 90% (76).

Magnetic Resonance Imaging

MR staging criteria are derived from FIGO staging conventions (Table 10.2).

Stage I

An intact area of low signal intensity, representing normal peripheral fibrous cervical stroma, is a reliable indication that the tumor is confined to the cervix (stage IB) (Fig. 10.17) (3,52,53,78).

Stage II

MRI determination of parametrial tumor extension (stage IIB) includes both morphologic and tissue signal alterations. Criteria include an irregular lateral cervical margin, prominent parametrial strands, eccentric parametrial enlargement, loss of parametrial fat planes on T1-weighted images, and/or abnormal high-signal tumor extending through the

TABLE 10.2. *Corresponding MRI findings (T2-W or contrast-enhanced T1-W images)*

Stage 0		No tumor present
Stage I	IA	No tumor present
	IB	Partial or complete disruption of low–SI stromal ring with intact tissue surrounding tumor
Stage II	IIA	Segmental disruption of low–SI vaginal wall (upper two-thirds)
	IIB	Complete disruption of low–SI stromal ring with tumor extending into parametrium
Stage III	IIIA	Segmental disruption of low–SI vaginal wall (lower third)
	IIIB	Tumor extends to obturator internus, piriformis, levator ani muscles Dilated ureter
Stage IV	IVA	Signal loss of low–SI bladder or rectal wall
	IVB	Tumor in distant organs

SI, signal intensity.

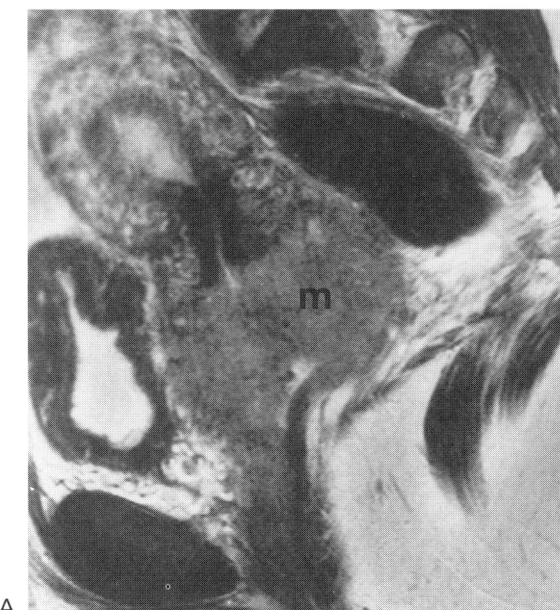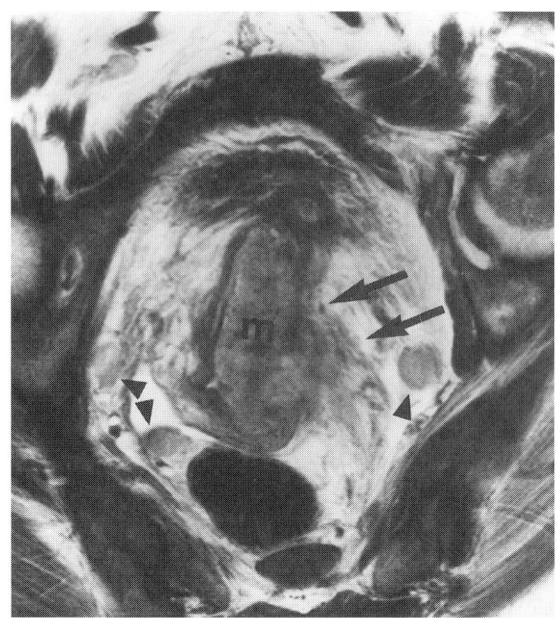

FIG. 10.20. Stage IIB cervical cancer with adenopathy. **A:** Sagittal and **(B)** oblique T2-W MR images show the bulky high–signal intensity tumor mass occupies the entire cervix (m). Note that tumor invasion extends beyond the cervical stroma (*arrows*, **B**). Intermediate–signal intensity metastatic lymph nodes are seen bilaterally (*arrowheads*, **B**).

low–signal intensity ring of fibrocervical stroma into the parametria or cardinal-uterosacral ligaments on T2-weighted images (Fig. 10.20) (3,52,53,78). Vaginal tumor involvement (stage IIA or IIIA) is recognized by segmental disruption of the low–signal intensity wall on T2-weighted images (Fig. 10.21A) (52,79).

Stage III

MRI criteria for pelvic sidewall extension (stage IIIB) are tumor extending beyond the lateral margins of the cardinal ligaments and loss of the normal low-signal intensity of the piriformis, levator ani, or obturator internus muscles on T2-weighted images (52). The presence of hydronephrosis also indicates stage IIIB disease.

Stage IV

In stage IVA disease, there is segmental loss of the normal low–signal intensity wall of the bladder or rectum. This is best seen on T2-weighted (Fig. 10.21) and/or contrast-enhanced T1-weighted images.

Diagnostic Value

The reported overall accuracy of MR staging for cervical cancer is 76% to 89% (3,19,52,53,80,81). In the evaluation of disease that is FIGO stage IB or higher, the reported staging accuracy is 95%, with a sensitivity of 92% and a specific-

ity of 100% (53). Approximately 5% to 15% of patients are understaged because microscopic tumor is not detected, and 9% to 14% of patients are overstaged because of false-positive findings (52,53). For parametrial extension, the overall accuracy of MRI has been reported to be 84% to 96% (3,19,52,53,73,78,80–82). In fact, one of the strengths of MRI is in the ability to exclude parametrial invasion with confidence. The negative predictive value (NPV) for parametrial invasion is 95%, making MRI extremely useful in the selection of appropriate surgical candidates. Identifying patients with full-thickness stromal invasion but no gross parametrial invasion, however, remains problematic (52). The positive predictive value (PPV) for identification of parametrial invasion is a modest 67%. The reported accuracy for identification of invasion of the pelvic sidewall is 95%, and the rate for invasion of the urinary bladder and rectal wall is 87% to 100% (52,80,83). In detection of pelvic lymph node involvement, MR studies parallel CT, with an overall accuracy of 72% to 93%, a sensitivity of 50% to 64%, and a specificity of 90% to 95% (2,3,53,73,81,84).

In general, the use of intravenous contrast does not improve staging accuracy for patients with cervical cancer (54, 80,82,85). The reported overall staging accuracy of contrast-enhanced images is 57% to 77% compared to 79% to 85% for combined unenhanced T1- and T2-weighted images (54, 80,82,85). Gadolinium contrast administration, therefore, is reserved for cases of advanced disease when the diagnosis of adjacent tissue invasion or fistula formation is uncertain (54,86). Recent investigations have evaluated dynamic contrast-enhanced MRI, and this technique compares favorably

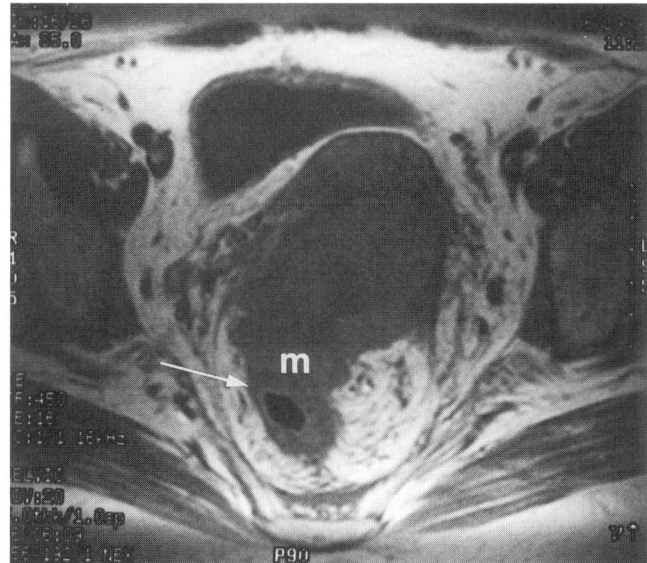

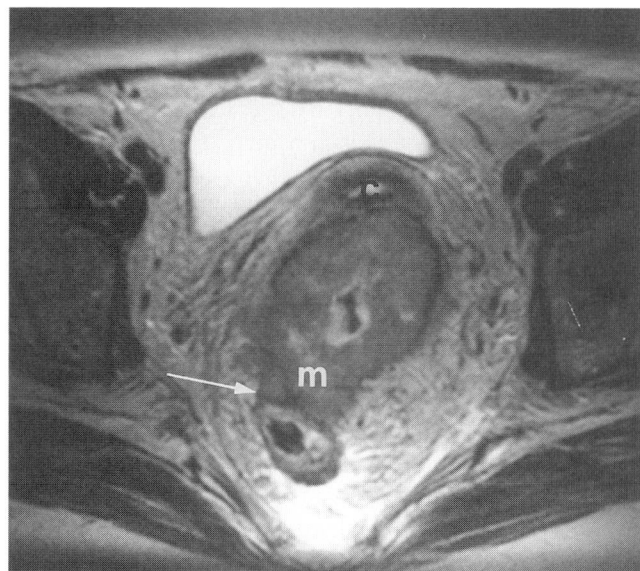

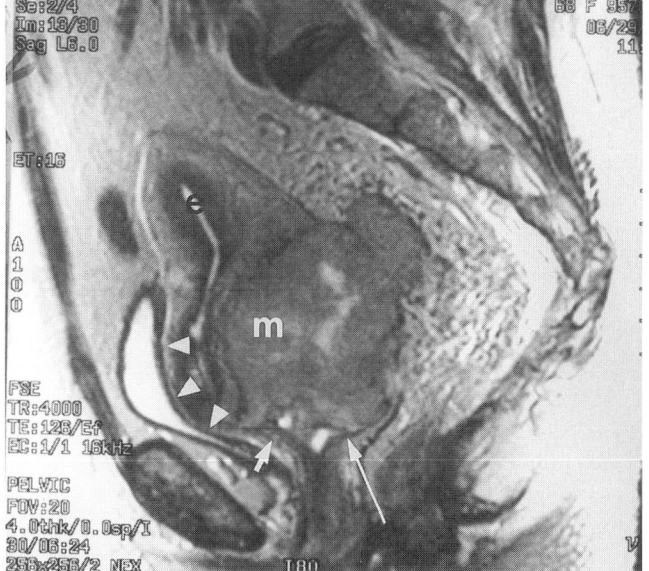

FIG. 10.21. Stage IVA cervical cancer. **A:** Axial T1-, and **(B)** axial T2-, and **(C)** sagittal T2-W MR images show a large tumor mass (m) of the posterior cervix. The mass invades the perirectal fat and extends to the rectum but spares the muscularis (*arrow*, **A, B**). On the sagittal image (**C**), the tumor is seen invading the vaginal lumen separating both the anterior (*short arrow*) and posterior (*long arrow*) vaginal walls. The presence of a preserved fat plane between the cervix and anterior vaginal fornix and bladder wall (*arrowheads*) excludes the presence of bladder invasion. Note the intact endometrium (e, **C**) and endocervical canal (c, **B**) pushed anteriorly by the mass. (Courtesy of Eric K. Outwater, M.D., University of Arizona Medical Center, Tuscon, AZ.)

with conventional T2-weighted and postcontrast T1-weighted sequences. Specifically, the accuracy of dynamic contrast-enhanced, T2-weighted, and postcontrast T1-weighted imaging for detecting stromal invasion is 78%, 61%, and 39%, respectively (55).

Surface coil imaging (e.g., endovaginal, endorectal, or phased-array coil) results in higher spatial resolution than conventional body coil imaging. When compared with body coil images, endorectal coil images provide greater anatomic detail and highlight the tissue planes between tumor and normal structures (87,88). Whether these imaging improvements change patient management, however, is controversial. Results from one study indicated that the use of an endorectal coil improved accuracy in detecting parametrial invasion. Accuracy with the endorectal coil was 95% versus 79% accuracy achieved with a body coil (87). Other studies,

however, have found no statistically significant difference in overall staging accuracy between the endorectal coil and the phased-array coil or between the phased-array coil and the body coil (89% vs 89% and 91% vs 89%, respectively). Nor was it possible to prove a significant difference in accuracy for detecting parametrial invasion (93% vs 96% and 95% vs 94%, respectively) (19,81).

Positron Emission Tomography

See section on Detection and Characterization above.

Modality Comparisons and Recommendations

MRI outperforms clinical and conventional CT staging for cervical cancer. In one study, the overall accuracy for cervical cancer staging was 70% for clinical evaluation, 63% for CT, and 83% for MRI (3). MRI is also superior to clinical examination and CT in the determination of parametrial extension; accuracy for MRI was 92% compared with 78% for clinical assessment and 70% for CT (3). In a follow-up study, it was found that MRI was superior to CT in tumor detection (sensitivity of 75% vs 51%), in parametrial evaluation (accuracy of 87% vs 80%), and in overall tumor staging (accuracy of 77% vs 69%) (2). Moreover, when pretreatment MRI is used to guide clinical management decisions, it has been shown to help minimize costs. In a study by Hricak et al. (9), the use of MR findings to guide treatment decisions in women with cervical cancer greater than 2 cm in diameter resulted in a decrease in the number of diagnostic tests ordered and a decrease in the number of invasive procedures performed. In fact, therapy based on MR findings led to a net cost savings of $401 for all patients and $449 for patients with stage IB disease.

A multiinstitutional trial (American College of Radiology Imaging Network #6651) comparing state of the art MRI and multidetector CT in women with cervical cancer presumed to be operable has recently closed. Analysis of that data will provide practice guidelines for this patient population. In the meantime, MRI appears to be the modality of choice for the preoperative evaluation of women with cervical cancer. MRI should be performed in women with (9,73,89):

1. Primary tumor with a transverse diameter greater than 2 cm on clinical examination
2. Primary tumor that is endocervical or predominantly infiltrative and cannot be accurately assessed clinically
3. Primary tumor in patients who are pregnant or have concomitant uterine lesions, making assessment by other means difficult

Monitoring Therapy and Detecting Recurrent Cervical Cancer

Ultrasound

TRUS has a role, albeit small, in the evaluation of recurrent cervical cancer and for biopsy guidance in selected patients (90,91). Reports from one study indicate that in about 25% of cases, TRUS provides information that is complementary to that obtained from CT. TRUS is most likely to be helpful in patients with small-volume recurrence in areas of previous irradiation (90). Unfortunately, differentiation between radiation fibrosis and recurrent disease cannot be made on the basis of tissue appearance or Doppler vascularity alone. Furthermore, because of its limited field of view, TRUS is not useful in the assessment of the cephalic extent of tumor, abnormalities of the upper urinary tract, or the presence of extrapelvic metastases (90). However, hydronephrosis is easily detected by transabdominal imaging, which can also serve to guide stent placement. Both TRUS and

TVS also have an important role, complementary to CT and MR, in detecting complications of therapy or advanced disease such as lymphoceles, fistulae, or abscesses.

Computed Tomography

CT has been used extensively to monitor patients with a history of cervical cancer and plan subsequent therapy (64, 67,92–94). Serial CT scans provide an objective measure of tumor response to radiation therapy or chemotherapy in nonsurgical candidates. Compared with its use for initial staging, CT has higher sensitivity and specifity and a lower false-negative rate when used for the detection of recurrent disease (64,93).

Recurrent tumor is often found central in the pelvis, in the surgical bed, vaginal cuff, or the preserved cervix. Distinctive CT features of recurrent pelvic tumor include asymmetry, soft tissue mass with hypodense tumor foci, compression and invasion of adjacent organs, and tumor extension to the pelvic sidewall, the iliopsoas muscle, or the innominate bone. Involvement of the rectum or bladder may result in fistula formation. CT is useful in defining the site of ureteral obstruction, which is common in patients with recurrent disease (95). Pelvic and paraaortic nodal metastases are often present (94).

Radiation therapy changes in the intact uterus are characterized by bilateral parametrial "whiskers" or poor definition and irregularity of the parametria without pelvic sidewall extension. Other classic radiation-induced changes on CT are thickening of the perirectal fascia, widening of the presacral space, a thick-walled bladder and rectum, a diffuse increase in the density of fat in the posterior pelvis, and thickening of small-bowel loops in the pelvic inlet (96). A major limitation of CT is the inability to differentiate reliably postradiation or postsurgical fibrosis from recurrent tumor (64,67,93).

In patients with equivocal findings, CT-guided fine-needle aspiration or core biopsy is an accurate way to differentiate recurrent tumor from posttreatment changes (96). In some cases, however, dense fibrous tissue surrounding nests of tumor cells may lead to a false-negative biopsy.

Because of extensive pelvic radiation therapy as well as improved CT imaging techniques, detection of recurrent disease outside the pelvis is increasing (97). CT is useful for assessment of metastases to solid organs (particularly the liver and adrenal glands), the peritoneum and omentum, the pulmonary parenchyma, and osseous spread.

Magnetic Resonance Imaging

Recurrent or residual cervical cancer demonstrates intermediate-signal on T1-weighted images and heterogeneous high-signal intensity on T2-weighted images, whereas uninvolved cervical stroma retains its low-signal intensity (Fig. 10.22A) (98–101). Lesions larger that 1 cm are accurately

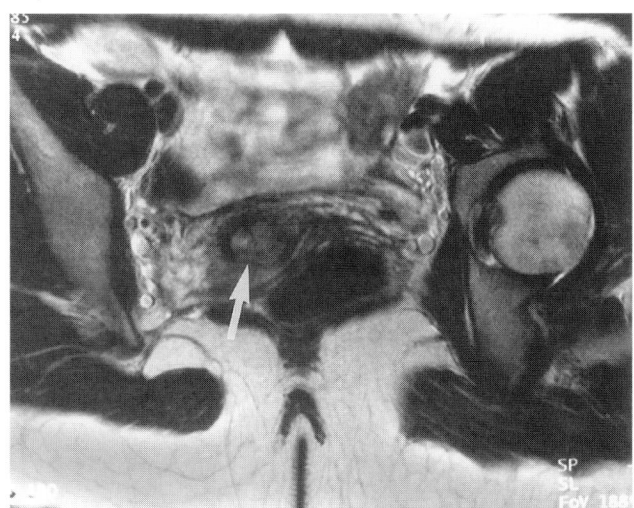
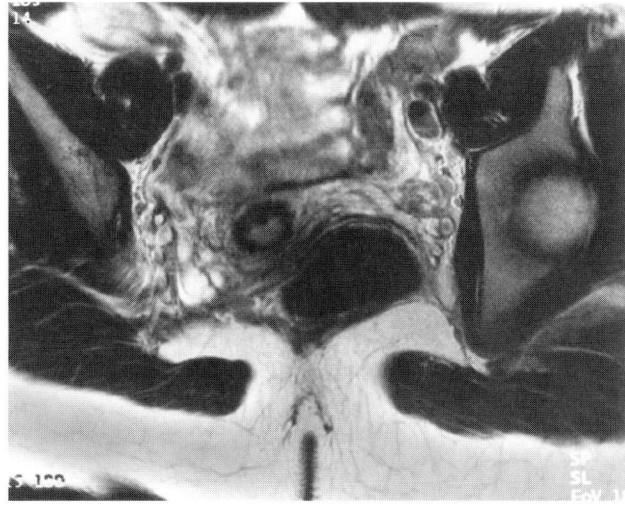

FIG. 10.22. Cervical cancer before and after radiation therapy. Axial T2-W MR image prior to radiation therapy (**A**) shows tumor enlarging the cervical canal and invading the cervical stroma (*arrow*, **A**). Axial T2-W MR image after radiation therapy (**B**) shows reconstitution of normal cervical anatomy.

depicted, but small lesions are more difficult to assess because of partial volume averaging. On T2-weighted images, tumor extension into the rectum and/or bladder is indicated by disruption of the low–signal intensity walls of these structures. The appearance of pelvic sidewall involvement is similar to that described earlier for the extension of a primary tumor.

Following gadolinium chelate administration, recurrent or residual tumor shows variable enhancement, which may lead to overstimulation or underestimation of the extent of disease. The value of intravenous contrast is to highlight bladder and rectal invasion, fistulae, and necrotic lymph nodes (102).

MRI is proving to be a promising modality for monitoring and predicting response to radiation therapy and/or chemotherapy (103–106). Accuracy rates are reported to range from 78% to 90% (100,107). An early (2 to 3 months posttreatment) and significant decrease in both T2 signal intensity and tumor burden are predictive of a favorable result (98). A large tumor volume and replacement of cervical stroma by carcinoma predict a poor response (108,109). Reports suggest that dynamic contrast-enhanced MRI may reflect tumor-tissue perfusion or angiogenesis and may be used to predict prognosis (110,111).

MRI is the most successful modality for differentiating recurrent tumor from posttreatment fibrosis secondary to irradiation, chemotherapy, and/or surgery (6,101). In a patient with a history of remote radiation therapy (>1 year), radiation-induced changes tend to be of low-signal intensity on both T1- and T2-weighted images, whereas recurrent tumor tends to be of moderate- to high-signal intensity on T2-weighted sequences. In this situation (remote radiation treatment), the difference in signal intensity between post treatment fibrosis and recurrent tumor is statistically significant

(Fig. 10.4A) (6), and a sensitivity of 86% and a specificity of 94% have been reported for detection of recurrent cervical cancer (112). Contrast enhancement may further aid in the detection of recurrent cervical cancer since recurrent tumor shows early enhancement compared with benign conditions. The accuracy of dynamic contrast-enhanced MRI for identifying recurrent disease approaches 85% compared to 64% to 68% for unenhanced T2-weighted images (7,113).

Positron Emission Tomography (Fig. 10–4B–D)

See section on Detection and Characterization above.

ENDOMETRIAL CARCINOMA

Detection and Characterization

Ultrasound

Endometrial atrophy is the most common cause of postmenopausal bleeding (114,115). Other causes include endometrial hyperplasia, polyps, submucosal fibroids, and endometrial carcinoma. Since approximately 10% of women with postmenopausal bleeding will be diagnosed with endometrial carcinoma, this diagnosis must be excluded in all perimenopausal or postmenopausal women presenting with abnormal vaginal bleeding (114,115). Endometrial biopsy and/or dilation and curettage (D and C) have traditionally been the gold standard for histologic diagnosis of endometrial pathology. However, if routine endometrial sampling is done in all women with postmenopausal bleeding, only one of every ten samples would be expected to be positive. In addition, significant sampling error has been reported with false-negative rates ranging from 2% to 6% (116–121). In order to decrease unnecessary endometrial biopsies, screening patients with postmenopausal bleeding with TVS or SHG has been advocated (122–128). Numerous trials in women with postmenopausal bleeding have been conducted to establish a threshold value for endometrial thickness below which endometrial pathology is unlikely. Cut-off values of 4 and 5 mm are most widely accepted (122,123). Above this level, endometrial sampling is suggested not only because of increased posttest probability of endometrial carcinoma but also because of the inability of TVS and/or SHG to differentiate accurately between benign and malignant causes of endometrial thickening (124,129–132). In the largest published series to date, a meta-analysis of 35 articles including 5,892 women, Smith-Bindman et al. (123) reported that using a cut-off of 5 mm for endometrial thickness, 96% of women with endometrial cancer had an abnormal TVS. In this series, a woman with a 10% pretest probability of endometrial carcinoma and a negative TVS had a posttest probability of endometrial carcinoma of only 1%. They concluded that TVS is highly accurate in identifying a subgroup of patients at extremely low risk, obviating the need for endometrial sampling in these patients.

In general, endometrial thickness greater than 4 or 5 mm is used as the sole ultrasound criterion for determining whether or not endometrial sampling is warranted in postmenopausal patients. However, the specificity of this criterion is low, ranging from 59% to 63% (123,133). In women taking HRT, the specificity is even lower, as HRT increases endometrial thickness. However, since the pretest probability of endometrial carcinoma is also likely increased, the same cut-off value is generally used. In woman on sequential HRT regimens, scanning should be performed after the progesterone part of the cycle when the endometrium is expected to be at its thinnest. Investigators have attempted to correlate the echo texture of the endometrium with histology in order to increase specificity. Cancers tend to be more heterogeneous, endometrial hyperplasia more homogenous and echogenic, whereas cystic areas are more often associated with polyps, cystic endometrial hyperplasia, or tamoxifen use (134–136). Observation of an irregular endometrial mass suggests endometrial carcinoma (Fig. 10.23). However, there is considerable overlap of these morphologic features. The most specific US finding for endometrial carcinoma is invasion of the myometrium or disruption of the subendometrial halo by an endometrial mass (Fig. 10.24). On sonohysterography, endometrial carcinoma is most commonly depicted as a broad-based, irregular mass (137). Difficulty in distending the endometrial cavity has also been described (138). Recently, 3-D SHG has been reported to be more accurate than either TVS or 2-D sonohysterography for the diagnosis of endometrial carcinoma. Endometrial volume and thickness has been reported to be higher in patients with postmenopausal bleeding and endometrial carcinoma (139). Additionally, this technique has been reported to be more accurate in detecting myometrial and cervical invasion by endometrial carcinoma (140).

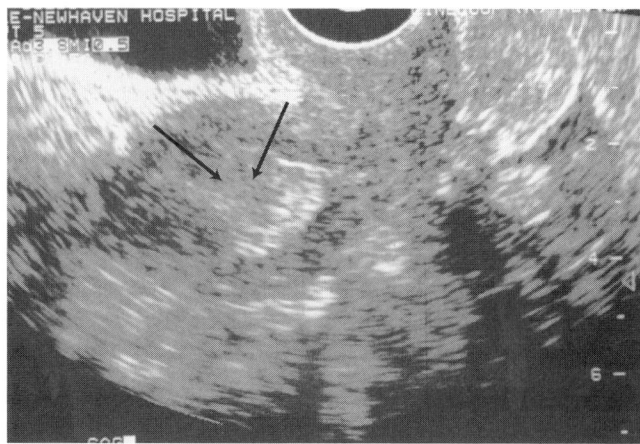

FIG. 10.23. Endometrial carcinoma. Sagittal image of the uterus demonstrates a thick endometrial stripe. Note irregular hypoechoic mass in the uterine fundus (*arrows*).

Doppler US has not been shown to be useful in distinguishing benign from malignant endometrial pathology as a wide range of peak systolic velocity and resistivity index is reported for benign and malignant endometrial pathology (141). However, benign endometrial polyps are more likely to have a single feeding vessel, whereas cancers more often have numerous feeding vessels and generalized increased vascularity (142) (Fig. 10.25).

Computed Tomography

High-quality pelvic CT in patients with endometrial carcinoma requires good bowel opacification with oral and rectal contrast. Intravenous contrast injection serves to enhance normal myometrium and delineate endometrial and myometrial tumor (92,94,143,144). On contrast-enhanced CT scans, endometrial tumor is seen as a hypodense mass relative to

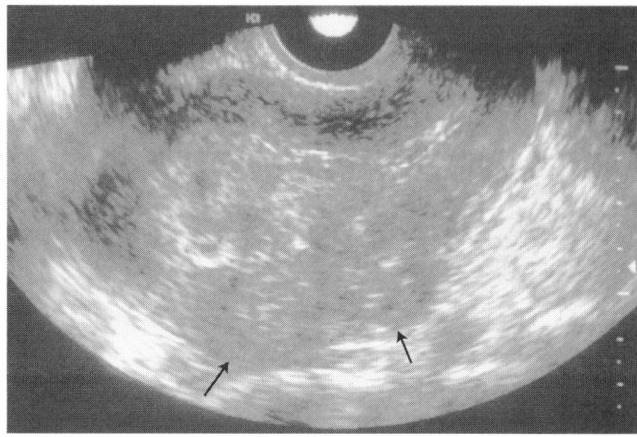

FIG. 10.24. Stage IC endometrial carcinoma. Note invasion (>50%) of myometrium (*arrows*) by asymmetric extension of more echogenic endometrial mass.

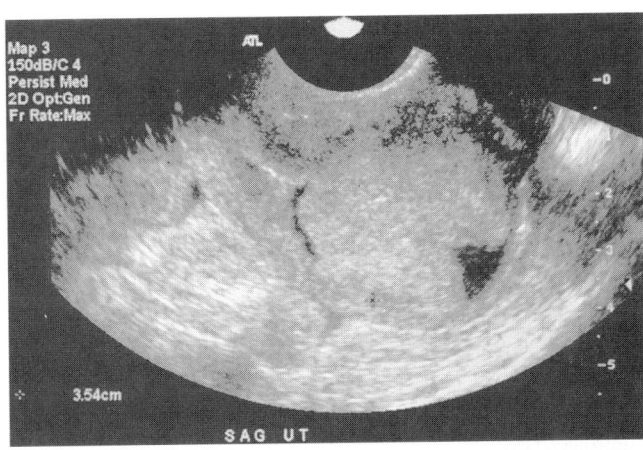
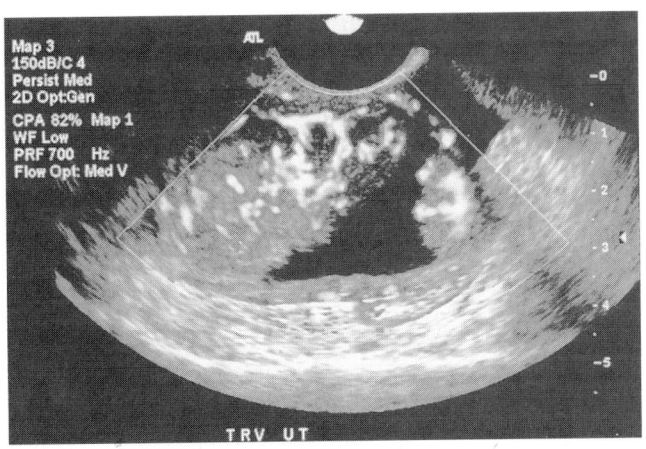

FIG. 10.25. Endometrial carcinoma—SHG. **A:** Fluid within the endometrial cavity outlines a large, irregular, broad based endometrial mass (calipers). **B:** Note marked vascularity of the mass on power Doppler imaging.

normal myometrium (Fig. 10.26). Occasionally, it is difficult to determine the origin of a pelvic mass on an axial CT scan. In these cases, reformatting the axial data set into the sagittal and/or coronal planes may be helpful.

Magnetic Resonance Imaging

On unenhanced T1-weighted images, endometrial carcinoma is isointense with the normal endometrium, and small tumors do not expand the canal. Therefore, these cancers usually go undetected. With larger tumors, the endometrium

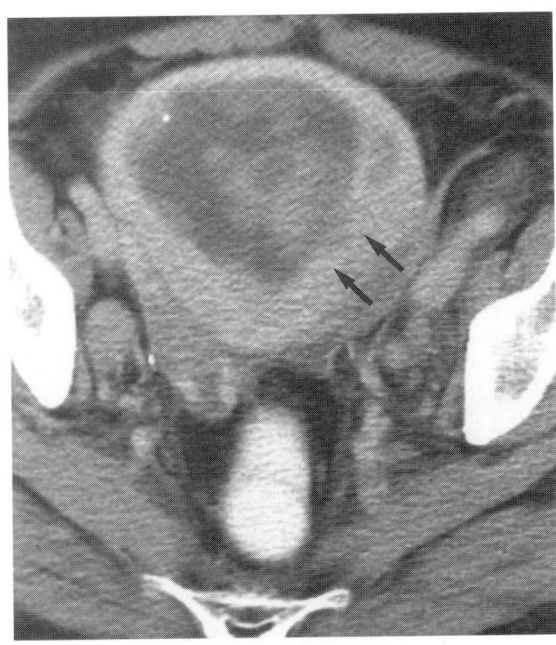

FIG. 10.26. Endometrial cancer. Contrast-enhanced CT scan shows enlarged uterus with a dilated, fluid-filled endometrial cavity. Heterogeneously enhancing tumor invades the myometrium (*arrows*).

is thickened and may be lobulated or irregular. Although endometrial cancer may demonstrate high-signal intensity on T2-weighted sequences, it is more typically heterogeneous (Fig. 10.27) and may even be low in signal intensity. The MR appearance of endometrial carcinoma is not specific and can also be seen with uterine fluid (hematometra or pyometra), submucosal degenerating leiomyoma, endometrial hyperplasia, polyps, and blood clots (145).

Most MR reports describe the appearance of endometrial adenocarcinomas, but there have been a few reports on the appearance of uterine sarcomas, which are seen as heterogeneous, medium– to high–signal intensity masses. The high–signal intensity components on both T1- and T2-weighted images reflect tumor necrosis with associated hemorrhage (145,146).

Routine use of intravenous contrast is necessary for state of the art MR evaluation of endometrial carcinoma. Following intravenous contrast administration, there is early enhancement of endometrial cancer relative to the normal endometrium, allowing identification of small tumors, even those contained by the endometrium, to be made. Contrast-enhanced images also differentiate viable tumor from necrosis, providing a more accurate measurement of tumor volume. Similarly, the distinction between tumor and endometrial fluid is obvious after gadolinium chelate administration; the former enhances, whereas the latter does not. The dynamic contrast-enhanced appearance of endometrial cancer has been described in a number of reports. Tumor conspicuity was more pronounced on dynamic enhanced images than on standard postcontrast T1-weighted images, although the tumors themselves enhanced heterogeneously (Fig. 10.27) (144,148,149).

Staging

Endometrial carcinomas are typically diagnosed by endometrial biopsy or dilation and curettage (D and C), with

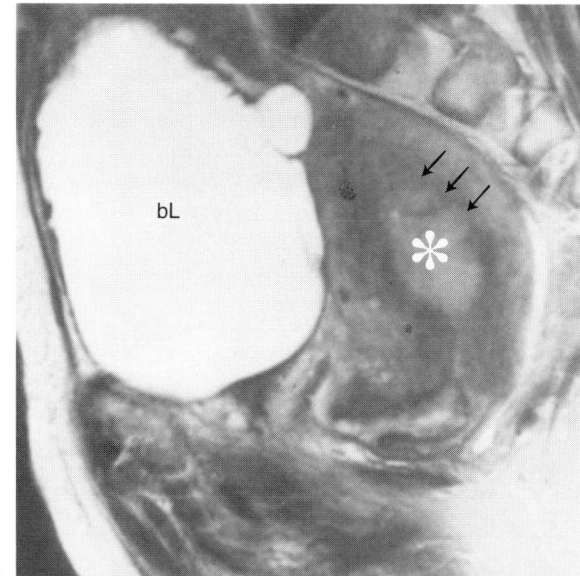

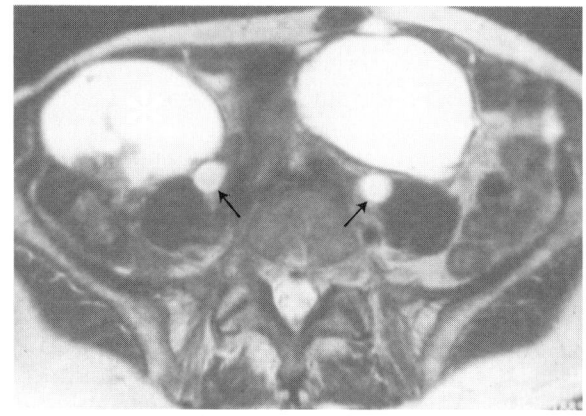

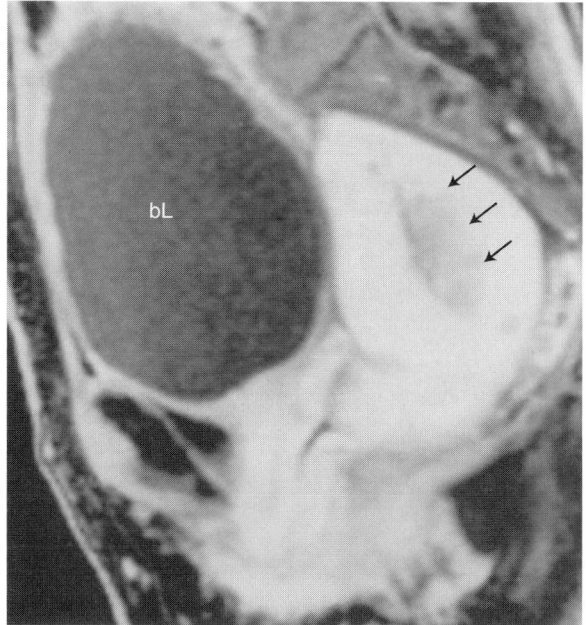

FIG. 10.27. Stage III endometrial cancer. **A:** Sagittal T2-, (**B**) axial T2-, and (**C**) sagittal contrast-enhanced fat-suppressed T1-W images in a woman with endometrial cancer. Abnormal heterogeneous signal distends the endometrial canal (*asterisk*, **A**). The posterior superior junctional zone is indistinct, suggesting myometrial invasion (*arrow*, **A**). In addition to the uterine abnormality there are bilateral complex cystic ovarian masses (*asterisks*, **B**) and bilateral hydroureters (*arrows*, **B**). Following contrast administration, there is increased conspicuity of the tumor–myometrial interface (*arrows*, **C**) confirming myometrial invasion. At surgery, endometrial cancer metastatic to the ovaries was found. (bL, urinary bladder)

imaging being reserved to evaluate extent of disease (4,5,54, 145,150–152). Imaging criteria for staging of endometrial cancer are based on the FIGO classification.

Ultrasound

The role of ultrasound in staging endometrial carcinoma is limited to evaluating stage I disease by assessing the depth of myometrial invasion. According to the FIGO classification, stage IA indicates tumor confined to the endometrium; stage IB indicates tumor invading less than one-half of the myometrium; stage IC indicates tumor invading more than one-half of the myometrium. For endometrial carcinoma to be considered stage IA by US criteria, the myometrial/endometrial interface should be smooth and regular and the hypoechoic subendometrial halo, if present, should be regular, symmetric, and uninterrupted. Myometrial invasion is documented when the tumor mass disrupts the subendometrial halo or extends into the subjacent myometrium (Fig. 10.24). TVS has been reported to have a sensitivity of 77% to 100%, a specificity of 65% to 93%, and an overall accuracy of

60% to 76% in assessing these three degrees of myometrial invasion (153–157). Understaging can occur with microscopic or minimal myometrial invasion. In addition, assessment of myometrial invasion is more difficult when the myometrium is thinned or distorted by fibroids (153). In the largest meta-analysis published to date, Kinkel et al. (157) reported that contrast-enhanced MRI is the most accurate imaging method for staging endometrial carcinoma.

Computed Tomography

CT staging criteria for endometrial carcinoma have been well described (Table 10.3.)

Stage I

In stage I disease, the tumor may reside solely within the endometrial cavity as a diffuse, circumscribed, vegetative, or polypoid mass; or it may invade the adjacent myometrium (Fig. 10.26). The latter finding usually corresponds to invasion of greater than one-third to one-half of the myometrium

TABLE 10.3. *Corresponding CT findings for staging of endometrial carcinoma*

Stage I	
IA	Normal myometrium enveloping central low-attenuation tumor
IB	Normal myometrium enveloping central low-attenuation tumor
	<50% myometrial invasion
IC	Normal myometrium enveloping central low-attenuation tumor
	50% myometrial invasion
Stage II	Central low-attenuation tumor extends into cervix
Stage III	
IIIA	Irregular uterine configuration
	Parametrial or pelvic sidewall extension
	Adnexal mass
IIIB	Thickening of vaginal wall
IIIC	Regional lymph nodes >1 cm in diameter
Stage IV	
IVA	Thickening, serration of bladder or rectal wall
	Obliteration of perivesical or perirectal fat
IVB	Tumor masses in distant organs or anatomic sites

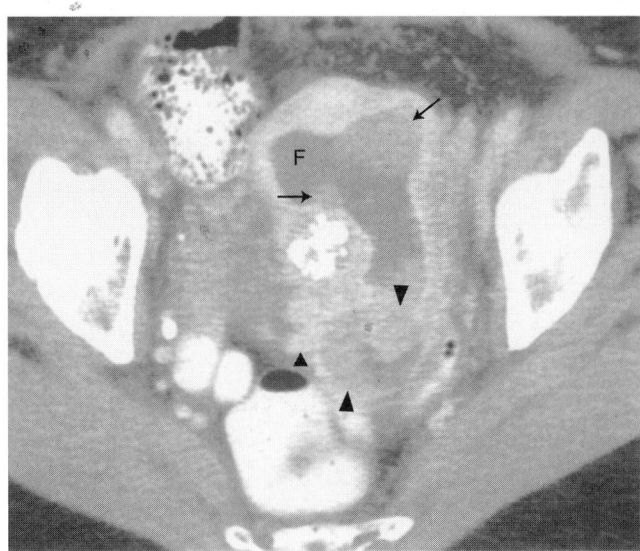

FIG. 10.28. Stage II endometrial cancer. Contrast-enhanced CT scan shows an enlarged uterine cavity with fluid (f) and tumor masses *(arrows)*. Tumor extends into the cervical canal *(arrowheads)*. A calcified myoma is also present.

(144). Tumor may also occlude the cervical os or vagina, resulting in uterine obstruction. In these instances, CT demonstrates an enlarged uterus with a distended, fluid-density endometrial cavity surrounded by contrast-enhanced myometrium of varying thickness (Fig. 10.26). Demonstration of intrauterine gas usually indicates a necrotic neoplasm rather than a pyometra, gas introduced by curettage or endometrial biopsy, or a fistula secondary to uterine invasion by an adjacent tumor (158).

Stage II

In stage II disease, there is endometrial tumor involvement of the cervix, which is characterized on CT as cervical enlargement greater than 3.5 cm in diameter and heterogeneous low-attenuation areas within the fibromuscular cervical stroma (Fig. 10.28) (92).

Stage III

On CT, parametrial extension is indicated by loss of the periureteral fat. Pelvic sidewall involvement is indicated by the depiction of less than 3 mm of intervening fat between the soft tissue mass and the pelvic sidewall (65). Fallopian tube and ovarian involvement are also consistent with stage III disease.

Stage IV

Pathologically enlarged lymph nodes and distant metastases are detected in the usual manner.

Diagnostic Value

CT is widely used for the staging of endometrial cancer (92,93,143,144). Its greatest clinical impact is in confirming parametrial and sidewall extension in stage III tumors and in detecting pelvic lymphadenopathy. Stage III tumors may be upstaged if extrapelvic metastases are depicted on CT studies (92,94). The accuracy of CT in patients with stage III or IV disease is 83% to 86% (92,94). For patients with stage I or II disease, CT accuracy is more variable: 58% to 92% (5,92,94). A report from the largest series to date to evaluate conventional CT detection of myometrial invasion with both dynamic and delayed images indicates an overall accuracy of 76% (143). Others have reported accuracy rates of 67% for delayed images (5). In one recent study, helical CT had a specificity of 42% for detection of deep myometrial invasion (stage IC) and a sensitivity of only 25% for cervical involvement (159).

Limitations of CT include a tendency to understage endometrial carcinoma because of failure to detect microscopic parametrial, lymph node, bowel, or bladder invasion (92,94). It is difficult to differentiate a leiomyoma from a uterine sarcoma with CT. CT is also particularly unreliable in the determination of myometrial invasion in elderly women with atrophic myometrium and a polypoid tumor in the endometrial cavity (94,143,144).

Currently, the role of CT in the workup of a patient with endometrial malignancy includes assessment of the depth of myometrial invasion, staging patients with an equivocal pelvic examination or a medical contraindication to surgical staging, screening for nodal or peritoneal metastases, and biopsy confirmation of stage III or stage IV disease (92,94, 143,144).

Magnetic Resonance Imaging

Most MR scans in women with endometrial cancer are performed after diagnostic D and C, and it is important to recognize post–D and C hemorrhage, which can be seen as a linear focal signal void. The results of at least one study indicate that this finding does not interfere with MR staging evaluation of the uterus (Table 10.4) (160).

Stage I

The MRI correlates of surgical FIGO subdivisions for stage I tumors have been described. Tumors are considered to be confined to the endometrium (stage IA) when the junctional zone is preserved (Fig. 10.29). Alternatively, in cases without a visualized junctional zone, as is common in postmenopausal women, stage IA disease is characterized by a sharp tumor–myometrium interface. In stage IB disease, there is disruption of the junctional zone, with an irregular myometrial–endometrial interface, and/or there is increased–signal intensity tumor in the inner half of the myometrium with preservation of the outer myometrium. In contradistinction, stage IC disease is characterized by

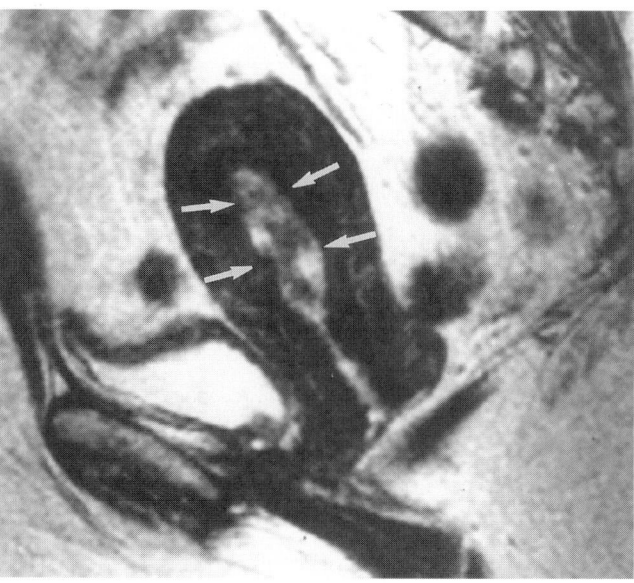

FIG. 10.29. Stage IA endometrial cancer in a patient receiving tamoxifen. Sagittal T2-W MR image shows a heterogeneous signal intensity mass within the uterine cavity (*arrows*). At pathology, a tamoxifen-related polyp complicated by a superficial endometrial cancer was found.

high–signal intensity tumor that extends into the outer myometrium with a thin, intact outer rim of normal myometrium.

Stage II

Stage II tumors are characterized by widening and expansion of the cervical canal, with associated heterogeneity of the cervical stroma. Assessment of the cervical involvement is facilitated by the multiplanar capabilities of MRI (Fig. 10.30) and dyamic contrast-enhanced sequences (151).

Stages III and IV

MRI can also be used to assess extrauterine spread. Extraserosal invasion (stage III) is depicted on T2-weighted images as high–signal intensity tumor extending beyond the outer uterine borders (Fig. 10.31) (145). Focal disruption of the normally low–signal intensity wall of the bladder or rectum signifies stage IVA disease (89). As with CT, size remains the criteria for determining lymph node involvement.

Diagnostic Value

Reports of the overall MR accuracy in staging of endometrial carcinoma range from 70% to 94% (54,145,150,161). Reports of accuracy in evaluation of myometrial invasion (on T2-weighted images) vary from 58% to 88% (145,147–150,162,163). Limitations of nonenhanced T2-weighted MR staging of endometrial carcinoma include difficulty in differentiating tumor from some benign entities,

TABLE 10.4. *Corresponding MRI findings (T2-weighted or contrast-enhanced T1-W images) for staging of endometrial carcinoma*

Stage 0	Normal or thickened endometrial stripe
Stage I	
IA	Thickened endometrial stripe with diffuse or focal abnormal signal intensity
	Endometrial stripe may be normal
	Intact junctional zone with smooth endometrial-myometrial interface
IB	Signal intensity of tumor extends into myometrium <50%
	Partial or full-thickness disruption of junctional zone with irregular endometrial–myometrial interface
IC	Signal intensity of tumor extends into myometrium >50%
	Full-thickness disruption of junctional zone
	Intact stripe of normal outer myometrium
Stage II	
IIA	Internal os and endocervical canal are widened
	Low signal of fibrous stroma remains intact
IIB	Disruption of fibrous stroma
Stage III	
IIIA	Disruption of continuity of outer myometrium
	Irregular uterine configuration
	Adnexal mass
IIIB	Segmental loss of hypointense vaginal wall
IIIC	Regional lymph nodes >1 cm in diameter
Stage IV	
IVA	Tumor signal disrupts normal tissue planes with loss of low signal intensity of bladder or rectal wall
IVB	Tumor masses in distant organs or anatomic sites

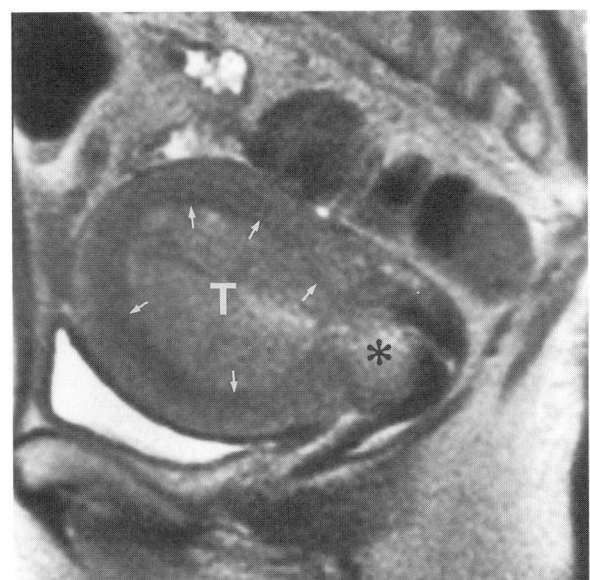
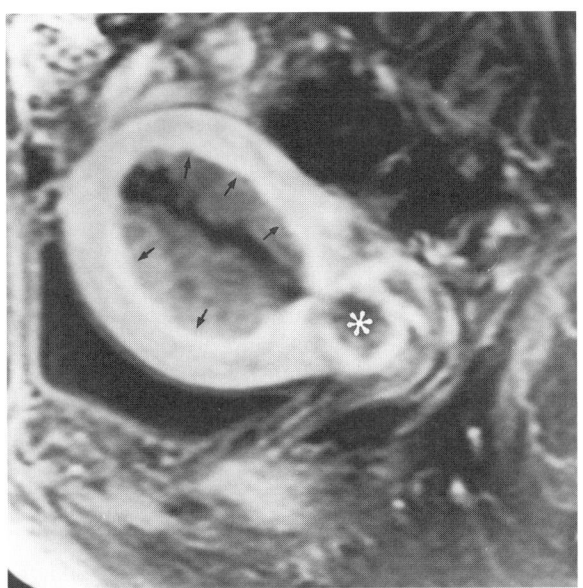

FIG. 10.30. Stage III endometrial cancer. **A:** Sagittal T2-W MR image shows a dilated tumor-filled endometrial cavity (T, **A**). **B:** Dynamic contrast-enhanced T1-W MR image provides better delineation of the tumor/myometrial interface (*arrows*, **A, B**). Note that tumor extends into cervical canal (*asterisk,* **A, B**). Ovarian involvement was also noted (not shown).

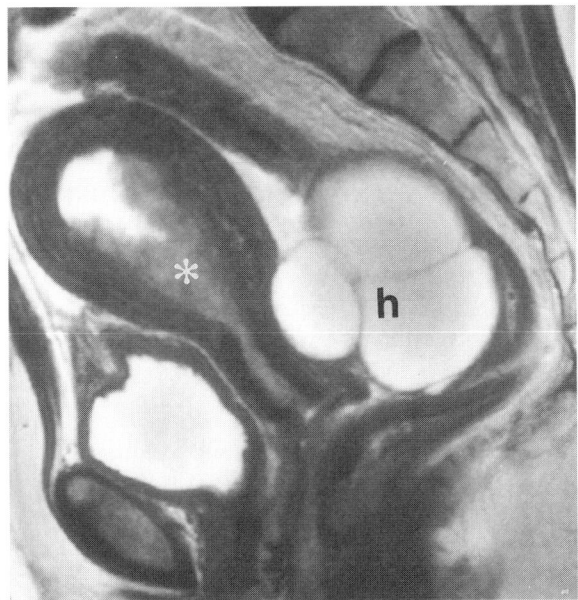
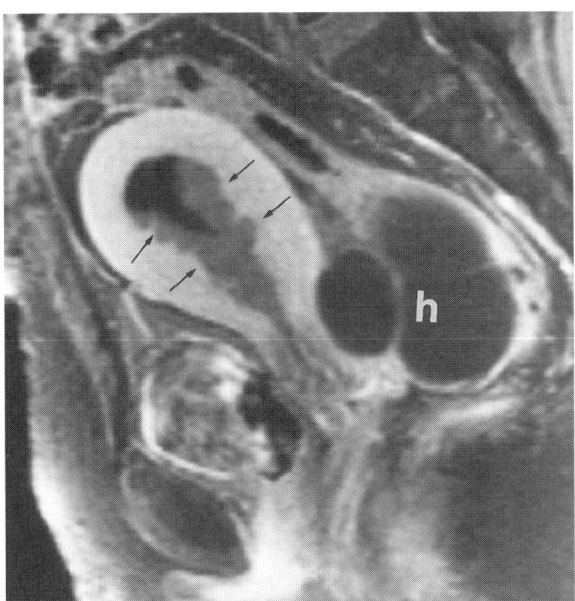

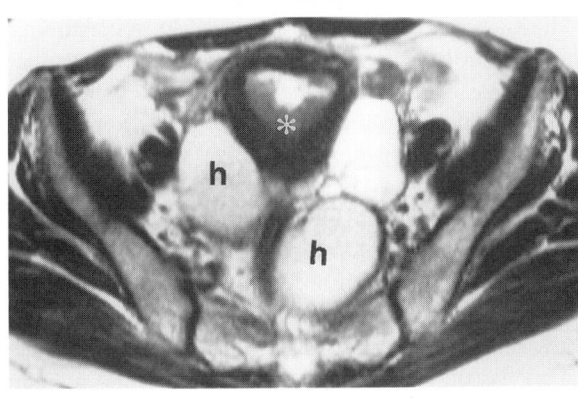

FIG. 10.31. Stage III clear-cell endometrial cancer. **A:** Sagittal T2- and **(B)** axial T2-W MR images show the uterine cavity contains an intermediate–signal intensity mass (*asterisks*, **A, B**) extending into the cervical canal. **C:** Sagittal T1-W MR images allow better delineation of the tumor/myometrial interface (*arrows*, **C**). Tumor involvement of the fallopian tubes has resulted in bilateral hydrosalpinx (h, **A, B, C**).

difficulty in determining myometrial invasion in postmenopausal women with poorly defined or absent junctional zones, and difficulty in detecting extrauterine spread.

These limitations have been at least partially overcome by the routine use of gadolinium chelates. Static contrast-enhanced MRI improves the accuracy of determining myometrial invasion to 68% to 78% (54,148,149,152,163,164). However, dynamic contrast-enhanced MRI is the best MR technique for detection of myometrial invasion, with an accuracy of 85% to 93% [significantly better than that of contrast-enhanced images (68% to 78%) or T2-weighted images (58% to 88%)] (97,148,149,165). In addition to increasing the conspicuity of the tumor–myometrial interface, the high tissue contrast allows accurate determination of cervical involvement as well. And although there are single-institution studies of highly resolved T2-weighted staging with a phased-array coil that report accuracy rates equal to those of dynamic contrast-enhanced imaging for the evaluation of myometrial and cervical invasion (166), to date, these have not been reproduced in multiintstitutional trials. Accuracy rates for the determination of cervical invasion are 82% to 91% (164,166).

Recommendations

Several studies suggest that MRI outperforms conventional CT in the assessment of depth of myometrial invasion (4,5). Two studies have reported that TVS is equivalent to T2-weighted MRI in evaluating myometrial invasion (68% to 69% vs 68% to 74%) (162,163), but contrast-enhanced MRI is superior to TVS (85% vs 68%) (163). A meta-analysis of studies reported between 1982 and 1997 showed significant differences in the accuracy of assessment of myometrial invasion among CT, TVS, and MRI. Contrast-enhanced MRI was significantly better than TVS and showed a trend toward better performance than CT (151). A follow-up meta-analysis and Bayesian analysis limited to detecting deep myometrial invasion also found contrast-enhanced MR to be superior to other modalities (97).

The imaging evaluation of patients with endometrial cancer is a function of physical examination, tumor type, and tumor stage. A chest radiograph is the only imaging study necessary in the majority of patients diagnosed with low-grade, clinical stage I tumors—that is, tumors that have a low pretest probability of extrauterine disease. However, transvaginal sonography is also reasonable to estimate myometrial invasion in patients with a low pretest probability of myometrial involvement. In patients with a high pretest probability of extrauterine disease (e.g., high tumor grade, aggressive cell type, suspicious physical examination, positive endocervical curettage, or elevated serum CA-125), more extensive imaging is indicated:

1. Dynamic contrast-enhanced MRI for multifactorial assessment to include myometrial invasion, extrauterine (e.g., cervical) extension, peritoneal disease, and lymphadenopathy.
2. CT or MRI to evaluate lymphadenopathy, with CT being used to biopsy suspicious lymph nodes.
3. Contrast-enhanced CT for detecting hematogenous abdominal disease—MRI, although less widely available, performs similarly.
4. MRI may also be helpful in patients with a large body habitus precluding adequate clinical assessment, patients with a contraindication to iodinated CT contrast, patients with medical contraindication to surgical staging, and patients with concomitant lesions (e.g, bulky and distorting fibroids) making clinical assessment difficult.

Monitoring Therapy and Detecting Recurrent Endometrial Cancer

Endometrial cancer tends to recur locally in women treated with surgery alone. The most common site of local recurrence is the vaginal cuff. Because the vaginal cuff is amenable to physical examination in the majority of patients, imaging is reserved for problem solving. For patients who fail radiation therapy, either alone or in combination with surgery, recurrences tend to be distant disease. In these cases, CT or MRI is usually performed. More recently, the usefulness of FDG PET for imaging endometrial cancer has been reported (14).

GESTATIONAL TROPHOBLASTIC DISEASE

The role of imaging in gestational trophoblastic disease (GTD) has been primarily to document metastatic disease at initial diagnosis or to evaluate persistent disease. No specific imaging findings allow differentiation of complete mole from invasive mole or choriocarcinoma (167–171).

Detection, Characterization, and Staging

Ultrasound

In patients with gestational trophoblastic neoplasia (GTN), TVS examination most commonly demonstrates a soft tissue mass distending the endometrial cavity. Typically, the mass is echogenic and heterogeneous, containing numerous cystic spaces (172–175) (Fig. 10.32A). In the case of complete hydatidiform mole, the small cystic spaces correspond to the hydropic villi (172,173). Hydropic degeneration of the placenta may have a similar US appearance. The mass is usually very vascular demonstrating increased vessel density and an abnormal uterine arterial waveform characterized by high peak systolic velocity and high diastolic blood flow (low RI) (176,177) (Fig. 10.32B). Irregularity of the border of the mass or asymmetric extension of the mass into the myometrium suggests myometrial invasion. The ovaries may become enlarged with numerous theca lutein cysts.

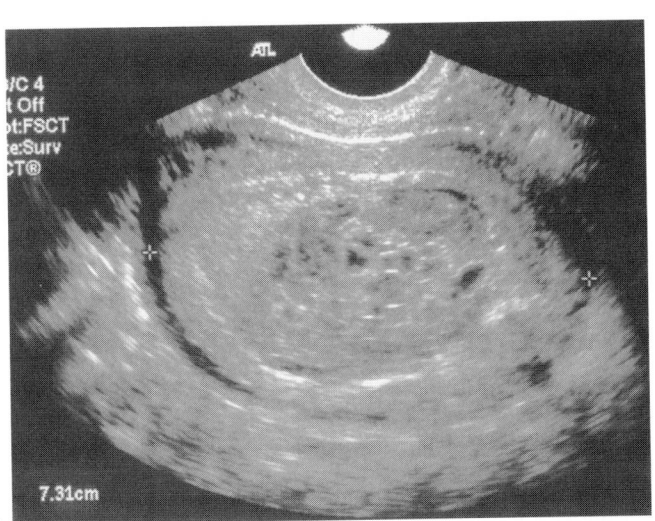
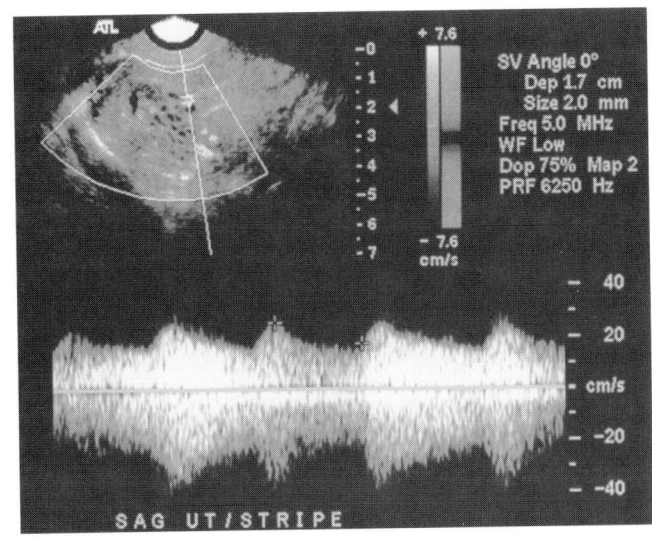

FIG. 10.32. Gestational trophoblastic neoplasia. **A:** Transverse view of the uterus demonstrates large heterogeneous mass containing numerous small cystic spaces and distending the endometrial cavity. **B:** Doppler interrogation reveals abundant flow characterized by a low-resistance arterial waveform pattern with high-velocity diastolic flow and low RI.

However, theca lutein cysts may not be detected in early stages of the disease (174). US can be helpful in assessing for recurrence of disease by documenting a persistent or recurrent endometrial mass. Occasionally, recurrence is manifested by the development of a uterine arteriovenous malformation without a discrete soft tissue mass. Successful treatment of a persistent mole with US-guided direct injection of methotrexate has been recently reported (178).

Computed Tomography

Uterine enlargement is the most common CT feature of GTD. Following administration of intravenous contrast, uterine enhancement is typically heterogeneous, and focal enlargement or irregular hypodense regions may be seen within the myometrium (179,180). These low-attenuation areas correspond to foci of hemorrhage and/or necrosis (180). Dynamic CT of the uterus can show contrast-enhanced vascular uterine lesions and dilated uterine vessels in the broad ligament (Fig. 10.33) (179). The extrauterine manifestations of GTD are well seen on CT. Bilateral ovarian enlargement due to multilocular theca lutein cysts can result in symptomatic torsion or hemorrhage (179,181). Locoregional spread is characterized by enhancing soft tissue nodules in the parametria and/or obliteration of the pelvic fat or muscle planes. Metastases to the lung, liver, and brain are vascular and prone to hemorrhage (179,181). Trophoblastic emboli to the lungs may produce symptoms of acute pulmonary embolism and occasionally result in large intravascular masses (179,182). The detection of unsuspected lung nodules helps identify high-risk patients who may fail initial methotrexate–folinic acid therapy.

Magnetic Resonance Imaging

On T2-weighted images, GTD is seen as a heterogeneous, predominantly high–signal intensity mass that obliterates normal uterine zonal anatomy (66). On T1-weighted images, it may be isointense or hyperintense to adjacent myometrium. The tumors are hypervascular, and enlarged vessels in the broad ligament and the uterus are depicted as signal voids on both T1- and T2-weighted images. Following contrast administration, the tumors are enhanced. MR angiography (e.g., 2-D time of flight or 3-D gadolinium-enhanced gradient echo sequences) highlights enlarged vessels. One group of investigators found that endometrial distention coupled with a uterine mass is more common in patients with primary molar disease than in patients with persistent GTD (167). Because it is possible with MRI to depict tumor that deeply invades the myometrium, it is particularly helpful in cases of invasive myometrial disease that spare the endometrium, a cause of nondiagnostic or false-negative D and Cs. MRI is also useful in the identification of extrauterine pelvic spread to the parametria, adnexa, and vaginal fornices (66). Theca lutein cysts may have a variable appearance on T1-weighted images but are high in signal on T2-weighted images (66). Despite the sensitivity of MRI in the detection of GTD, endometrial lesions with low levels (<700 mIU/ mL) of the β-subunit of β-hCG may not be depicted by MRI (US may be insensitive to these lesions as well) (183).

Another role of MRI in GTD is to monitor patients' responses to therapy. MR findings of regression of vascular abnormalities, development of intralesional hemorrhage, and return of normal uterine zonal anatomy parallel a favorable response to chemotherapy (66).

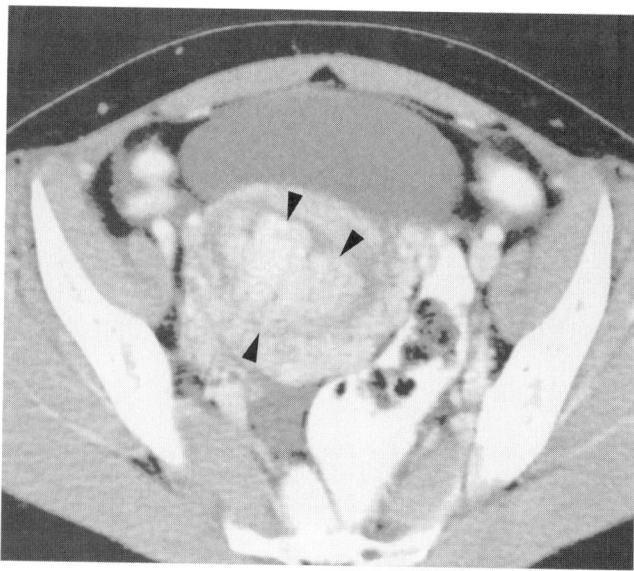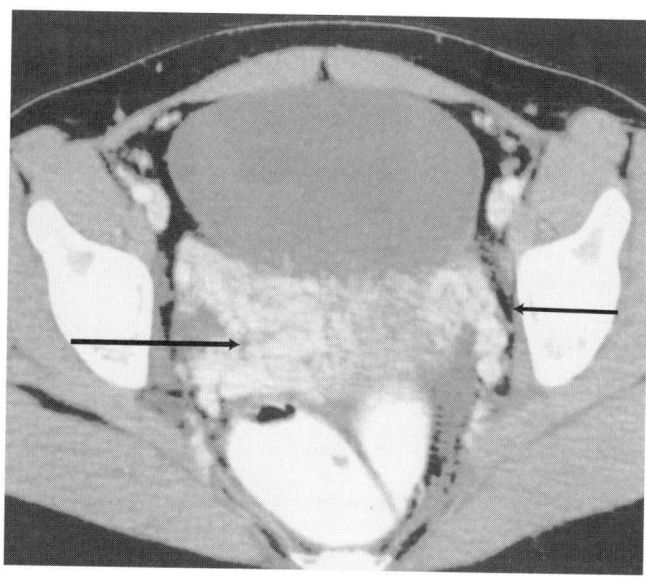

FIG. 10.33. Gestational trophoblastic disease. **A:** Contrast-enhanced CT of the pelvis in a woman with an elevated β-hCG shows a large enhancing vascular mass in the endometrial cavity *(arrowheads)*. **B:** A more caudal section shows bilateral tortuous dilated uterine vessels, highlighting the hypervascular nature of GTD *(arrows)*. The cervix *(asterisk)* is relatively hypovascular on bolus images.

Although there are as yet no published studies documenting the superiority of MRI for assessment of extrapelvic disease in patients with GTD, MRI is well suited for detecting hepatic and brain metastases.

OVARIAN CARCINOMA

Detection and Characterization

Ultrasound

Ultrasound has an important role in the detection and characterization of adnexal masses. US is an important component of screening programs for women at high risk for ovarian carcinoma and is considered to be the initial imaging modality of choice for characterizing an ovarian mass as being benign or malignant.

Whereas the 5-year survival rate for stages III and IV ovarian carcinoma is less than 15%, the 5-year survival rates for stages I and II disease are close to 90% and 70%, respectively (184). The overall 5-year survival rate for ovarian carcinoma is estimated to be approximately 50%, reflecting the fact that most patients do not become symptomatic until they have advanced disease. Hence, the clinical challenge is to diagnose ovarian carcinoma early when cure is possible but tumors are clinically silent. This challenge is made more difficult by the low prevalence of ovarian carcinoma in the general population. Therefore, efforts at screening patients for ovarian carcinoma have focused on high-risk populations. Risk factors include older age, high socioeconomic status, and factors that increase the number of ovulatory cycles such as early menarche, nulliparity, and late-onset

menopause (185–187). Having a first-degree relative with ovarian carcinoma significantly increases a woman's risk; reportedly from 1.4% to 5.0% (185–187). Approximately 10% of ovarian carcinomas are believed to be due to an inherited susceptibility. Three syndromes have been described: the breast/ovarian cancer syndrome; the Lynch 2 syndrome, or the hereditary nonpolyposis colorectal cancer syndrome; and hereditary site-specific ovarian cancer. In 1994, a National Institutes of Health (NIH) consensus conference (188) recommended that screening be offered to women with two or more first-degree relatives with ovarian carcinoma. It is also recommended that women with an inherited predisposition to ovarian cancer be screened (188–190). In practice, many women with a single first-degree relative are enrolled in screening programs.

Screening programs for ovarian cancer rely on physical examination, serologic markers, and endovaginal ultrasound. The serum CA-125 level is the most common serologic marker in widespread use. CA-125 is a glycoprotein expressed by 80% of epithelial tumors. However, it is expressed in only 20% to 50% of stage I ovarian carcinomas and rarely by mucinous cystadenocarcinomas. In addition, many benign conditions such as endometriosis, leiomyomata, and liver disease as well as other malignancies including pancreatic carcinoma may cause false-positive elevations of the serum CA-125 level (187,191,192). CA-125 titers are most useful in older patients or if rising particularly following remission of disease (187,191,192).

Numerous studies have reported on the potential role of ultrasound assessment of ovarian morphology and blood flow in screening for ovarian malignancy (190,193–200).

The results of these screening trials have consistently demonstrated that US detects more stage I ovarian carcinomas than CA-125 levels and physical examination (200). Nonetheless, very few stage I invasive carcinomas have been found in such screening programs; approximately 1 per 2000 women screened (187). In the Yale study (197), no stage I cancers have been detected, although two advanced ovarian carcinomas were found. In addition, 2 endometrial cancers, 11 breast cancers, and 1 colon cancer were found, prompting the recommendation that women at high risk for ovarian carcinoma be screened routinely for these malignancies as well. Only one study has demonstrated survival benefit of ovarian cancer screening trials. Van Nagell and colleagues (199) reported a decrease in case-specific ovarian cancer mortality with 93% 2-year and 84% 5-year survival in women with US-detected ovarian carcinoma.

Ultrasound is considered to be the initial imaging modality of choice to differentiate a benign from a malignant clinically suspected ovarian mass. Although a likely benign mass can be followed or removed by a general gynecologist, suspicion of a malignant ovarian mass initiates prompt referral to a gynecologic oncologist who can better perform the more complex therapeutic and staging cytoreduction surgery for ovarian carcinoma. Morphologic features remain the primary criteria for differentiating complex ovarian masses as being benign or malignant. Hence, TVS is the critical US imaging approach because of the improved spatial and soft tissue resolution afforded by the higher frequency endovaginal probe. Nonetheless, transabdominal ultrasound remains an important and complementary component of the US examination when a larger field of view is required; if a mass, for example, is displaced out of the pelvis or is so large that it is incompletely visualized by TVS. In addition, transabdominal imaging is required for evaluation of associated findings, such as ascites, peritoneal implants, or hydronephrosis. Such findings can be important not only to confirm the impression of malignancy but also for staging.

Numerous studies have reported that when strict US criteria and a pattern recognition approach for identification of benign ovarian masses are used, US examination has a near 95% to 99% NPV in excluding malignancy (201–207). Ultrasound features consistent with benign etiology include smooth, thin walls; few, thin septations; absence of solid components; or mural nodularity as well as pattern recognition for certain benign diagnoses. Simple cysts will be anechoic with a smooth, thin wall and posterior enhancement. Hemorrhagic cysts or endometriomas may contain uniform low-level echoes but should still demonstrate a smooth, thin wall and increased through transmission. The internal echogenicity may be quite complex and even irregular, especially in the case of hemorrhagic cysts. However, the appearance of the internal echoes will change over time and internal vascularity should never be noted. Several US patterns typical of dermoid cysts have been described including uniform increased echogenicity with posterior attenuation, echogenic

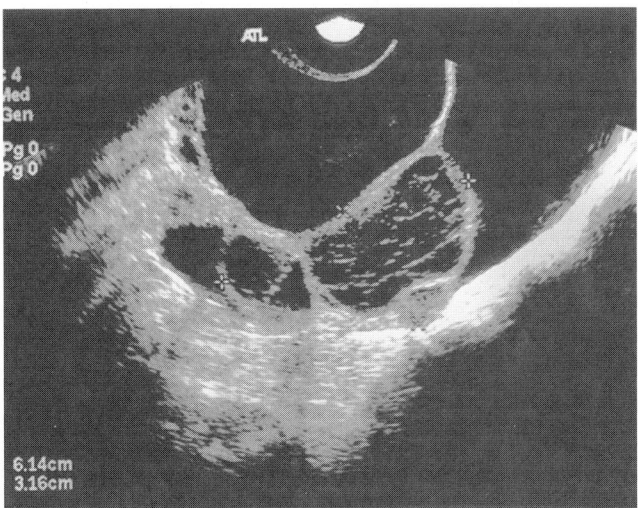

FIG. 10.34. Mucinous cystadenocarcinoma. Note large multilocular ovarian mass with numerous thick, irregular septations.

shadowing mural nodules, and layering with or without floating debris.

Conversely, mural nodules, mural thickening or irregularity, solid components, thick septations (>3 mm), and associated findings such as ascites, implants, and/or hydronephrosis suggest malignancy (Figs. 10.34 and 10.35). Such US descriptors have been reported to have a high sensitivity but lower specificity for malignancy (201–207). Some benign lesions such as hemorrhagic cysts, cystadenomas, or cystadenofibromas may have numerous thick septations and apparent mural nodules. Borderline tumors may have minimal findings. Scoring systems have been proposed to standardize evaluation of ovarian masses in an attempt to improve specificity (208–210). Using a stepwise logistic regression analysis to determine the most discriminating gray scale and Doppler sonographic features of malignancy, Brown et al. (210) reported that a multiparameter approach, which as-

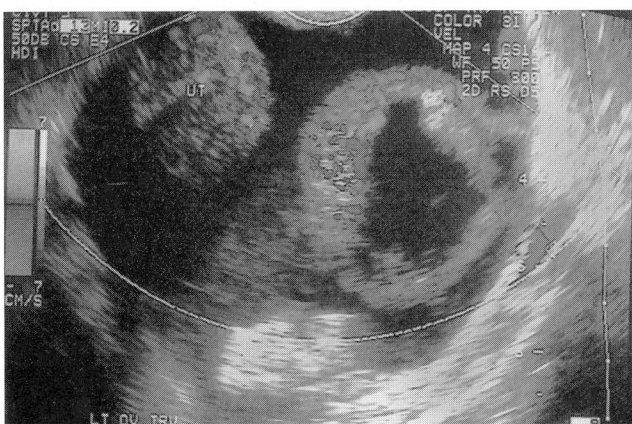

FIG. 10.35. Note irregular, thick walled left ovarian mass. The mass is highly vascular. Ascites is present. (See Color Plate.)

sessed for nonhyperechoic solid components, central blood flow on color Doppler, ascites, and thick septations, had a 93% sensitivity and specificity for malignancy. To achieve 100% sensitivity, specificity dropped to 86% in this study (210). However, Timmerman et al. (211) have reported similar findings and interobserver variability when readers used subjective criteria for evaluating ovarian masses. Solid ovarian masses are generally considered to be malignant (Fig. 10.36) despite the fact that Brenner's tumors, fibromas, and fibrothecomas are relatively common benign solid ovarian lesions. Furthermore, pedunculated fibroids, dermoids, and endometriomas can masquerade as solid ovarian lesions.

Color and pulse Doppler features are controversial, with some investigators considering blood flow characteristics to be merely confirmatory but others considering the Doppler examination to be a helpful discriminator (212–215). Tumor neovascularity is known to be characterized by an increased number of often tortuous vessels with arteriovenous shunts. Malignant neovascularity lacks the normal amount of smooth muscle cells in the vessel walls. Researchers had hoped that Doppler evaluation, which could potentially assess vascular compliance or resistance as well as vessel morphology, density, and distribution, would be helpful in characterizing ovarian masses. Although malignant ovarian lesions tend to demonstrate higher PSV and lower RI than benign masses, considerable overlap exists, and no discriminatory cut-off values are accepted (212–215). Similarly, although malignancies more often demonstrate increased vessel density and tortuosity, overlap exists, and rarely blood flow may not be demonstrable in a malignant lesion. Blood flow within an apparent solid area will help differentiate a true solid component from blood clot, but benign neoplastic papillary projections may have demonstrable flood flow. The role of intravenous contrast US evaluation of tumor vascularity with power and 3-D US has yet to be determined but may increase sensitivity in detection and characterization of small malignant-appearing vessels (215).

Computed Tomography

CT is the most commonly performed study for the preoperative evaluation of a suspected ovarian carcinoma. CT staging information may be useful in preoperative surgical planning, particularly if neoadjuvant chemotherapy is considered prior to debulking. In studies of adnexal lesions, the sensitivity, specificity, and accuracy of CT for characterizing benign versus malignant lesions is reported to be 89%, 96% to 99%, and 92% to 94%, respectively (216,217).

The CT features of ovarian cancer demonstrate varied morphologic patterns including a multilocular cyst with thick internal septations and solid mural or septal components, a partially cystic and solid mass, and a lobulated, papillary solid mass (Fig. 10.37). The outer border of the mass may be irregular and poorly defined, and amorphous, coarse calcifications and contrast enhancement may be seen in the cyst wall or soft tissue components (Fig. 10.38). Since the CT appearance of ovarian metastases is indistinguishable from a primary ovarian neoplasm, the stomach and colon should be carefully examined as potential primary tumor sites (Fig. 10.39) (218).

Magnetic Resonance Imaging

The role of MRI in patients with suspected or known ovarian carcinoma is still evolving. To optimize MRI detection and characterization of an adnexal mass, contrast-enhanced

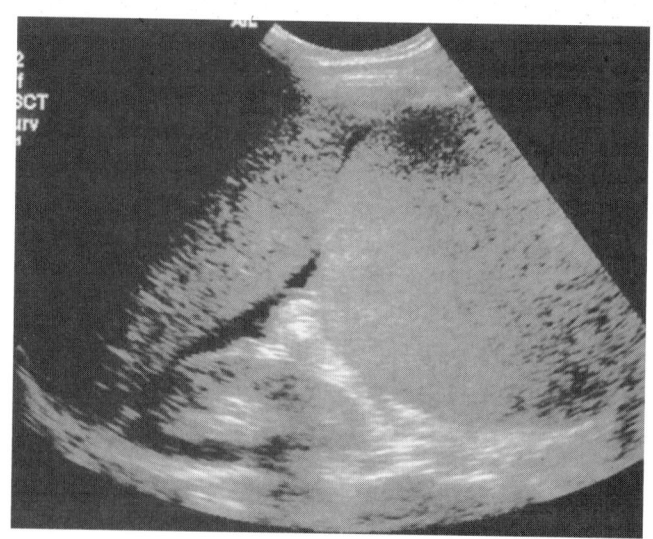
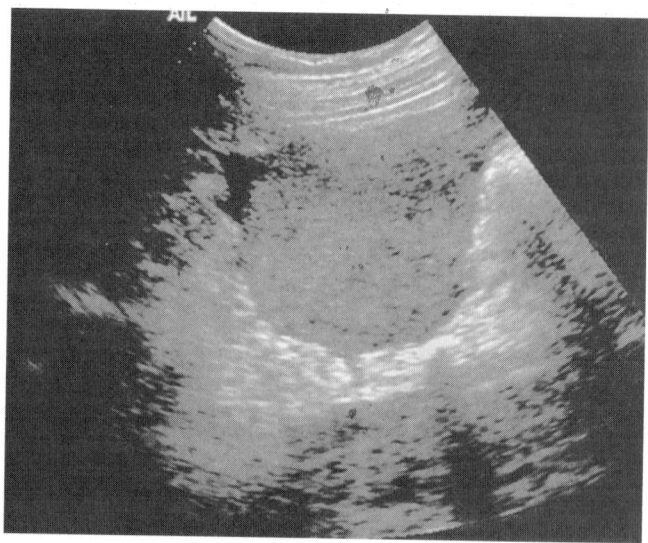

A

B

FIG. 10.36. A, B. Bilateral Krukenberg tumors. A 29-year-old woman presented with acute abdominal pain when 32 weeks pregnant. Transabdominal ultrasound demonstrated bilateral solid ovarian masses and ascites. Surgery revealed bilateral ovarian metastases from a primary gastric carcinoma.

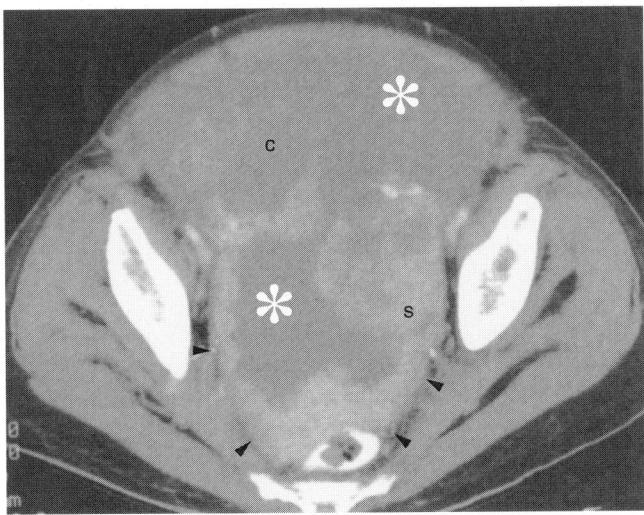

FIG. 10.37. Ovarian cancer. Contrast-enhanced CT shows bilateral ovarian masses with cystic (c) and solid (s) components. Thickened lobulated peritoneal tumor (*arrowheads*) and ascites *(asterisks)* are also evident.

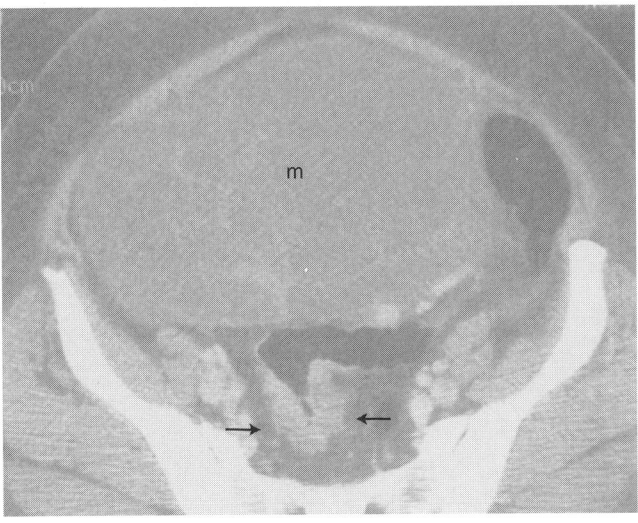

FIG. 10.39. Ovarian metastasis from colon cancer. Contrast-enhanced CT scan shows a large septated, predominantly cystic ovarian metastasis (m). The primary tumor is in the rectosigmoid colon *(arrows)*.

protocols and attention to eliminating, or at least limiting, bowel motion are needed. Additionally, imaging should be performed with a phased-array surface coil to maximize spatial resolution.

Primary and ancillary criteria have been proposed for the characterization of an adnexal mass as being malignant. In a study of 60 lesions (219), statistical analyses yielded the following five significant primary criteria for malignancy:

1. Size greater than 4 cm
2. Solid mass or large solid component (Fig. 10.40)
3. Wall thickness greater than 3 mm
4. Septal thickness greater than 3 mm and/or the presence of vegetations or nodularity (Fig. 10.41)
5. Necrosis

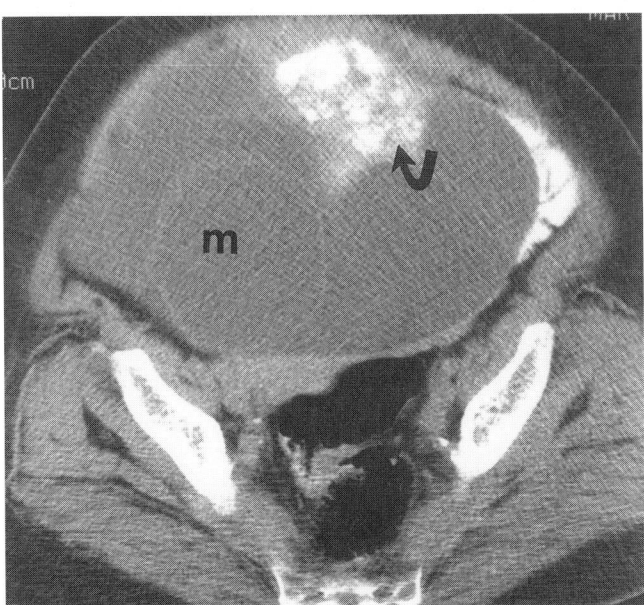

FIG. 10.38. Mucinous cystadenocarcinoma. Axial CT scan shows a large multiloculated low-attenuation mass (m) arising from the pelvis. Note the associated calcifications (*curved arrow*).

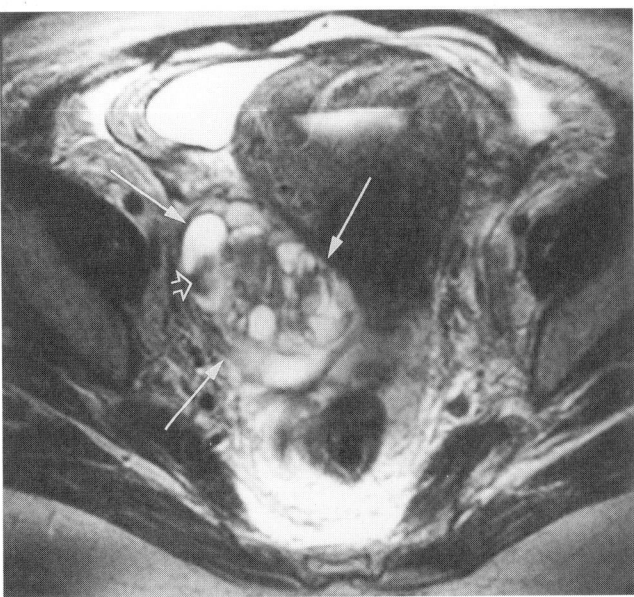

FIG. 10.40. Papillary serous cystadenocarcinoma. Axial T2-W MRI shows a mass replacing the right ovary. The mass contains both solid and cystic components (*arrows*). Note the large papillary projection within one of the cystic components (*open arrow*). (Courtesy of Eric K. Outwater, M.D., Arizona University Medical Center, Tucson, AZ.)

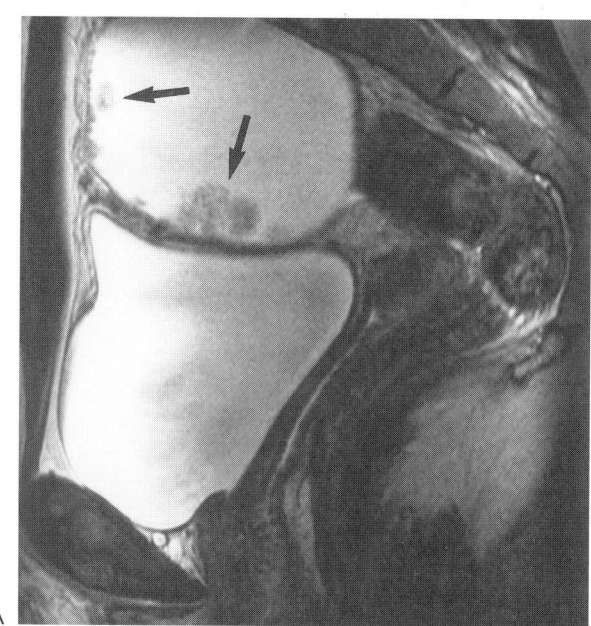
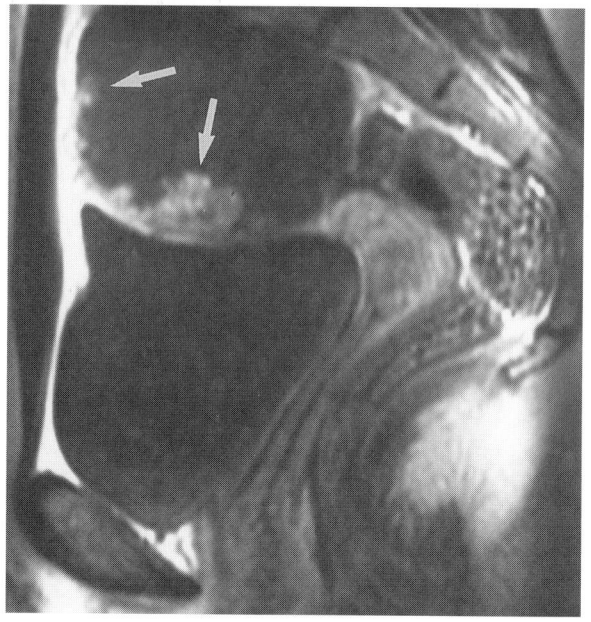

FIG. 10.41. Serous cystadenocarcinoma of low malignant potential. **A:** Sagittal T2- and **(B)** sagittal contrast-enhanced T1-W MR images show a cystic ovarian tumor with papillary projections (*arrows*, **A, B**). (Courtesy of Caroline Reinhold, M.D., Montreal General Hospital, Montreal, Quebec, Canada.)

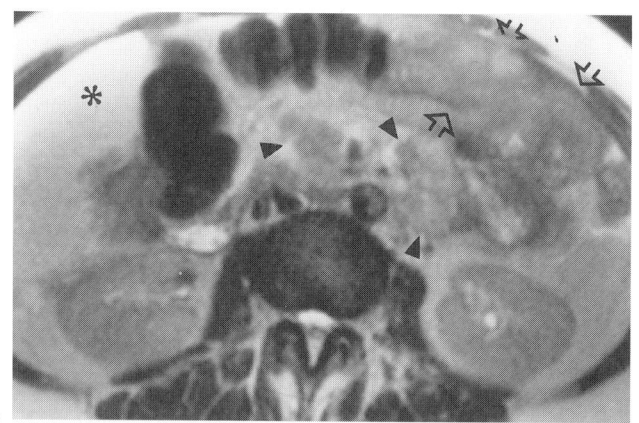
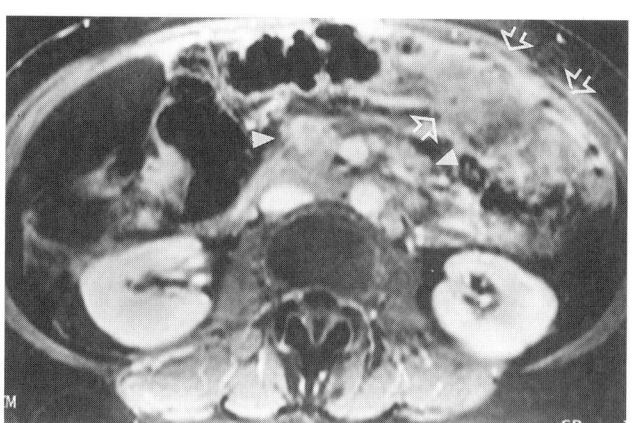
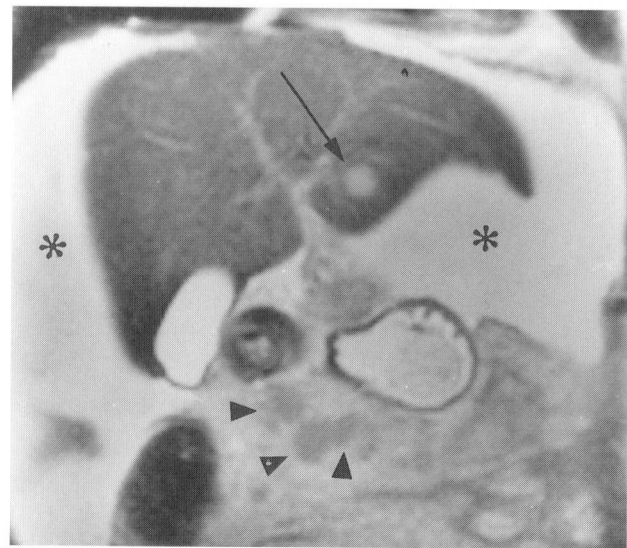

FIG. 10.42. Ovarian cancer dissemination. **A:** Axial T2- and **(B)** contrast-enhanced fat-suppressed T1-W MR images show an "omental cake" (*open arrows*, **A, B**) and multiple mesenteric metastases (*arrowheads*, **A, B**). **C:** Coronal T2-W image shows a high–signal intensity liver metastasis (*arrow*, **C**) in the left lobe. Large-volume ascites (*asterisks*, **A, C**) and mesenteric masses (*arrowheads*, **C**) are also demonstrated on the T2-W images.

Four ancillary criteria of malignancy were also statistically formulated:

1. Involvement of pelvic organs or sidewall
2. Peritoneal, mesenteric, or omental disease (Fig. 10.42)
3. Ascites (Fig. 10.42)
4. Adenopathy

When contrast-enhanced T1-weighted and unenhanced T1- and T2-weighted images were analyzed collectively, the presence of one or more of the five primary criteria, coupled with a single criterion from the ancillary group, correctly characterized 95% of malignant lesions (Figs. 10.40 and 10.41) (219). These rates reflect improvements in lesion characterization produced by the addition of intravenous contrast to the protocol and have been reproduced in other studies (5a,220). As with CT, disease metastatic to the ovary is often indistinguishable from primary ovarian cancer on MRI scans, and both the colon and stomach should be examined as potential primary tumor sites (218,221). The multiplanar capabilities of MRI make it easier to identify the origin of a mass, facilitating differentiation between ovarian and uterine pelvic tumors (Fig. 10.43).

Several studies have compared MR to CT and US for characterizing adnexal masses, with mixed results (5a,222, 223). One study found that low–field strength MRI is equivalent to CT for this determination, with accuracies of 86% and 92%, respectively (217). Another study suggests that TVS is superior to unenhanced MRI for lesion characterization (224), and yet another study indicates that the specificity of MR with intravenous contrast is higher than that of TVS (97% vs 69%) (222). Both TVS and MRI with intravenous contrast have high sensitivity (97% and 100%, respectively)

in the identification of solid components within an adnexal mass. MRI, however, shows higher specificity (98% vs 46%) (223). At present, the relatively high cost of MRI precludes its use as a screening modality, and studies suggest that MRI is most appropriately used for characterization of an adnexal lesion in cases where US and clinical examination are indeterminate (11,225).

Positron Emission Tomography

In the detection of ovarian cancer, FDG PET appears to be promising because of its potential to detect tumor prior to significant morphologic changes. This is important, as currently most patients with ovarian cancer present late in their disease owing to a lack of early imaging manifestations (Fig. 10.3). A study by Hubner et al. (226) found good correlation between PET and histologic findings in women with suspected ovarian cancer imaged prior to laparotomy. Specifically, the sensitivity, specificity, accuracy, PPV, and NPV of FDG PET were 83%, 80%, 82%, 86%, and 76%, respectively. Recently, the clinical significance of FDG PET to detect ovarian cancer and tumor spread was evaluated in 40 women with a suspicion of ovarian malignancy or recurrent disease scheduled for surgery (227). The results of preoperative PET were correlated with histologic diagnosis and intraoperative assessment of tumor spread. Primary or recurrent disease was predicted by PET with a sensitivity, specificity, and diagnostic accuracy of 90% for each. The PPV and NPV were 96% and 76%, respectively. PET did not perform as well in the detection of lymph node metastases, with a sensitivity, specificity, accuracy, PPV, and NPV of 72.7%, 92.3%, 86.4%, 80%, and 88.8%, respec-

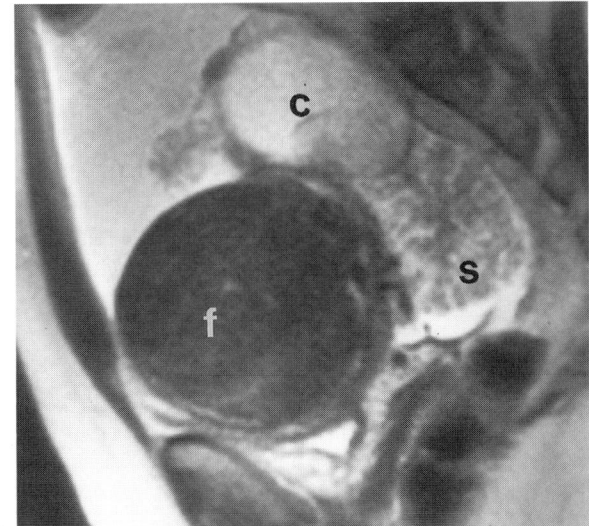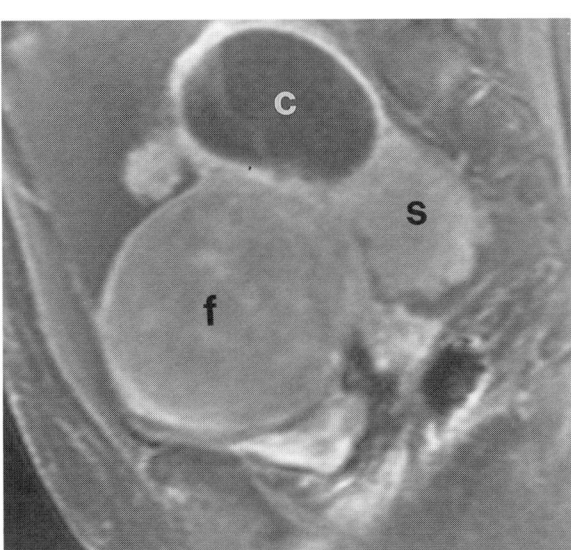

FIG. 10.43. Serous cystadenocarcinoma and uterine fibroid. **A:** Sagittal T2- and **(B)** contrast-enhanced fat-suppressed T1-W MR images show an ovarian cancer with both cystic (c, **A, B**) and solid papillary (s, **A, B**) components. MRI facilitates differentiation between the ovarian tumor and uterine fibroid (f, **A, B**).

tively—findings not dissimilar from those for CT or MRI. Peritoneal carcinomatosis was diagnosed when multiple foci of increased radionuclide uptake were identified that did not correlate to bowel and/or there was increased activity on the surface of the liver. For these determinations, PET had a 71% sensitivity, 100% specificity, 85% diagnostic accuracy, 100% PPV, and 76% NPV. The investigators concluded that PET is suitable for detecting ovarian malignancies, especially in patients with suspected recurrent disease, and may be helpful to monitor treatment response. Still, the poor spatial resolution of PET is problematic; however, PET-CT overcomes the spatial limitations of PET, especially in cases with equivocal findings.

Staging

Cross-sectional imaging is better accepted and more commonly used in the evaluation and staging of ovarian carcinoma than for other gynecologic malignancies. Imaging is an adjunct to surgical staging and is becoming a valuable tool in the detection of nonresectable disease. Furthermore, cross-sectional imaging is useful in the detection of intrahepatic disease, the presence of which may alter staging and therapy. Additionally, MRI and CT also provide a noninvasive mechanism to monitor treatment response. A barium enema may be helpful in identifying bowel involvement secondary to ovarian carcinoma, but it is not recommended as a routine procedure (228). Excretory urography is commonplace at many institutions, but is only abnormal in 12% to 18% of patients (228).

Ultrasound

Although MRI and CT are the primary cross-sectional imaging modalities used to stage ovarian carcinoma, peritoneal implants and ascites can occasionally be documented on careful ultrasound examination (Figs. 10.44 and 10.45). The specificity of US examination in documentating abdominal spread of disease has been reported to be slightly higher than CT and MRI (229). However, the sensitivity of US for the detection of small implants is lower than CT or MRI owing to relatively decreased spatial and soft tissue resolution (229,230).

Computed Tomography

CT clearly displays ovarian cancer that may abut or invade the uterine serosa and obscure the intervening parauterine fat plane. It is also useful in the detection of tumor involvement of the small and large bowel and the pelvic ureter and of metastases to the peritoneum, mesentery, gastrocolic ligament, greater omentum, liver, pelvic and paraaortic lymph nodes, and pseudomyxoma peritonei (231). CT detection of peritoneal implants depends on several factors including location, the presence or absence of surrounding ascites,

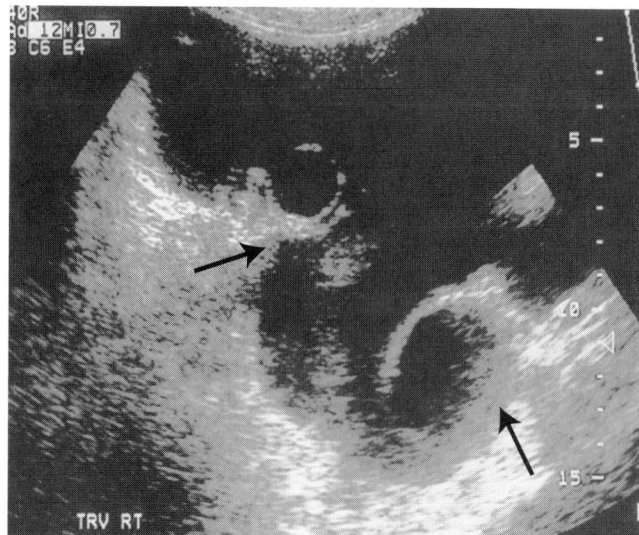

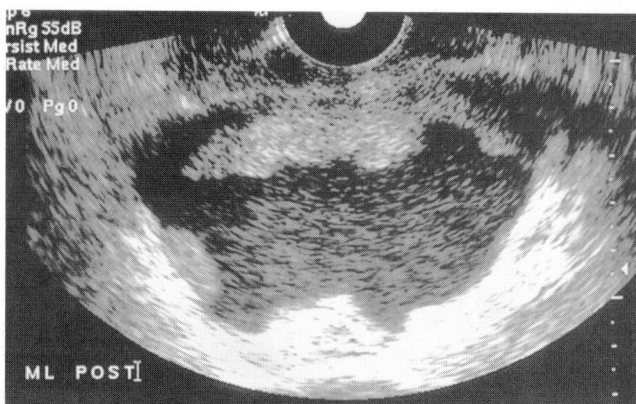

FIG. 10.44. Peritoneal spread of ovarian carcinoma. **A:** Note cystic metastases (*arrows*) along pelvic side wall made more visible by the presence of ascites. **B:** This patient with stage III ovarian carcinoma has more solid appearing peritoneal metastases. Echoes in the ascites indicates debris or hemorrhagic ascites.

and size. CT scans can identify psammomatous calcification in plaque-like peritoneal metastases from papillary serous cystadenocarcinoma of the ovary (232). The three sites most commonly involved are the right subphrenic space, the greater omentum, and the pouch of Douglas (Fig. 10.37) (231).

With conventional high-resolution scanners, peritoneal implants as small as 5 mm are detected in 50% of cases (230). With the increase in spatial resolution of MDCT, increased detection of peritoneal implants is likely.

Mesenteric metastases may appear on CT scans as either round or ill-defined soft tissue masses surrounded by contrast-filled small-bowel loops and mesenteric fat, or as thickened leaves of the mesentery caused by tumor coating peritoneal surfaces (Fig. 10.46). The most significant limitation of conventional CT in staging ovarian carcinoma is the inability to detect reliably serosal implants smaller than 10 mm,

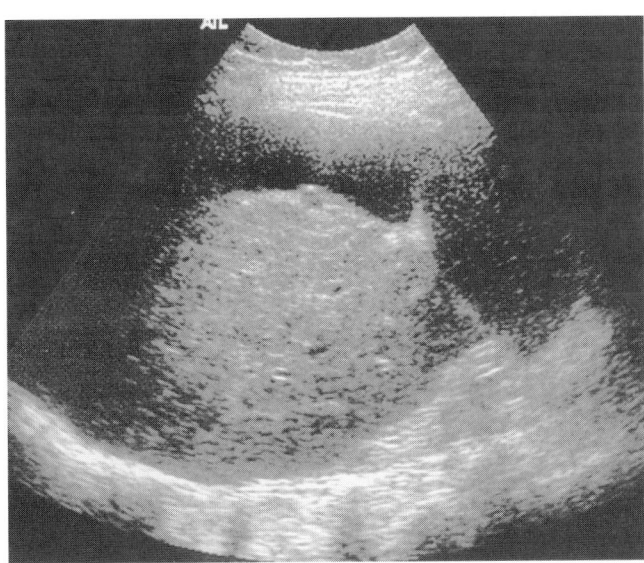

FIG. 10.45. Stage III ovarian carcinoma. Note small cystic implant on the surface of the liver. Ascites is present.

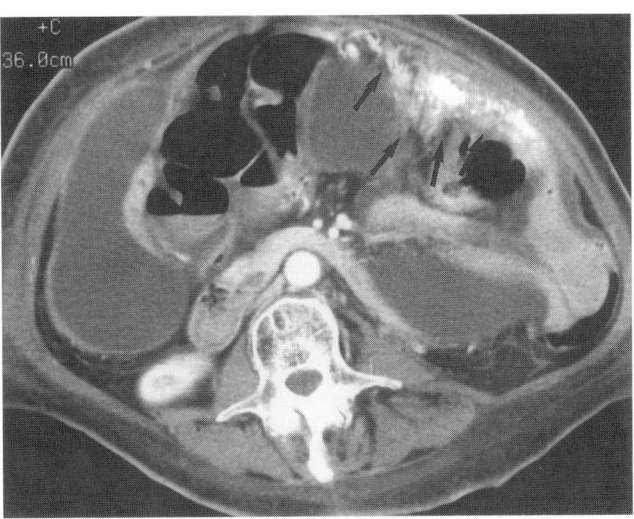

FIG. 10.47. Stage IIIC serous cystadenocarcinoma. Contrast-enhanced CT scan shows a large calcified "omental cake" (*arrows*). Peritoneal seeding is well seen in the setting of ascites and images as thickening of the peritoneum. (Courtesy of Cirrelda Cooper, M.D., Georgetown University Hospital, Washington, DC.)

especially in the absence of ascites. In fact, the sensitivity for these determinations is poor; only 14% to 27% (233, 234). Although ascites is a nonspecific finding, it is often associated with peritoneal tumor spread and aids CT visualization of small peritoneal implants (Fig 10.46)

Omental metastases are characterized as stranding or soft tissue nodules embedded in omental fat or the replacement of the omental fat with thick, nodular tumor ("omental cake") along the greater curvature of the stomach, in the gastrosplenic ligament, or anterior to the transverse colon and

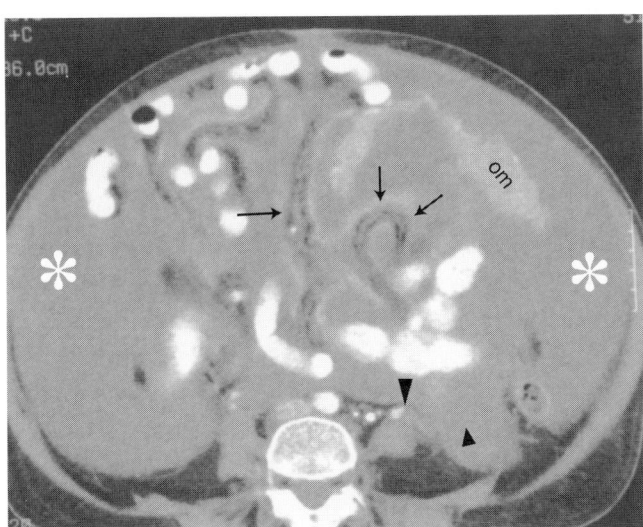

FIG. 10.46. Disseminated ovarian cancer. Contrast-enhanced CT shows tumor diffusely coating the small bowel mesentery (*arrows)* and an "omental cake" (om). Ascites (*asterisks*) delineates subtle posterior peritoneal implants-(*arrowheads*).

small bowel in the lower abdomen (Fig. 10.47) (103). The sensitivity of CT for detection of omental metastasis is reported to be 80% to 86% (233,234). Liver metastases on CT are most often capsular implants on the surface of the liver and less commonly hematogenous lesions in the parenchyma. Prominent hematogenous tumor spread to the liver should prompt careful attention to the bowel, as this pattern of spread may reflect an unsuspected gastrointestinal primary site. The least common CT findings are pelvic and inguinal lymphadenopathy or enlarged perirenal lymph nodes, representing tumor spread by the gonadal lymphatics. The sensitivity of CT for the detection of extrapelvic disease is approximately 95% to 100% for liver involvement and 50% to 60% for nodal involvement (233,234). Overall staging accuracy for CT has been reported to be 77% (233). It also has a high PPV for imaging bulky disease and is therefore useful for identifying patients with inoperable disease (233,234).

Magnetic Resonance Imaging

MRI is useful for the assessment of spread of ovarian tumor to the uterus, bladder, rectum, and pelvic sidewall, with accuracy ranging from 70% to 94% (233). Invasion is characterized by an interface of greater than 90% or direct soft tissue extension with irregular margins into adjacent structures (Fig. 10.2). Fat-suppressed contrast-enhanced sequences are used to depict intraabdominal disease (i.e., omental, peritoneal, and mesenteric metastases), which enhance and are bright against the low-signal intensity of intraabdominal fat (Fig. 10.48). With this technique, small lesions (1 cm) are conspicuous (5a).

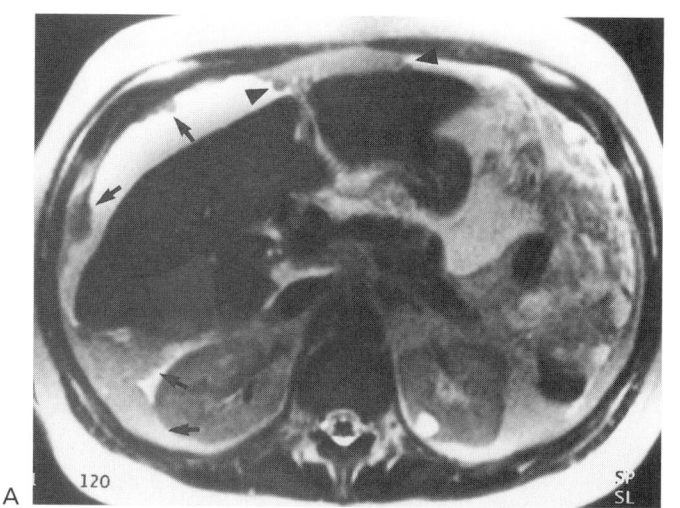 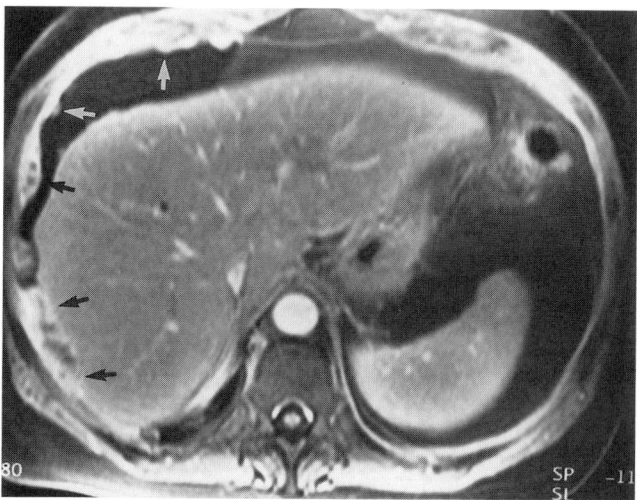

FIG. 10.48. Disseminated ovarian cancer. **A:** Axial T2- and **(B)** contrast-enhanced fat-suppressed T1-W MR images through the liver show peritoneal tumor implants along the right hemidiaphragm (*arrows*, **A, B**) and liver surface (*arrowheads*, **A**). Ascites facilitates the detection of small tumor deposits. The peritoneal nodules enhance (*arrows*, **B**).

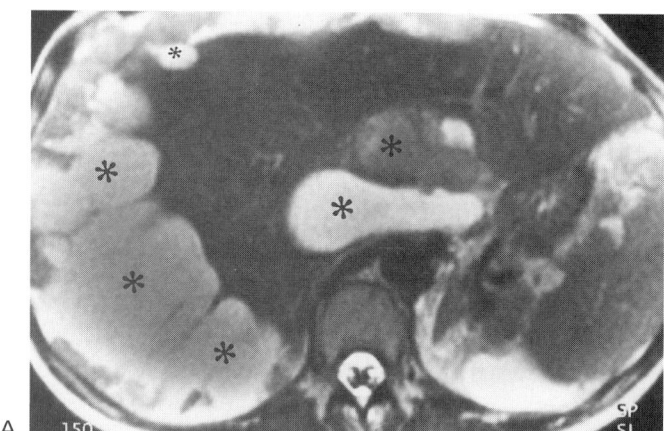

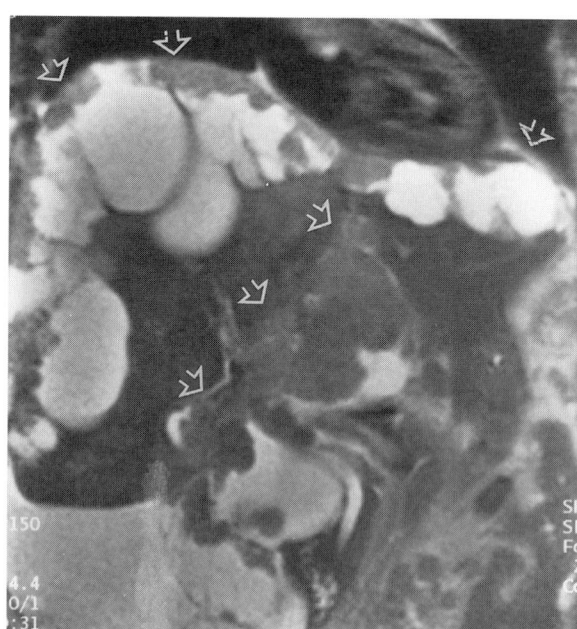

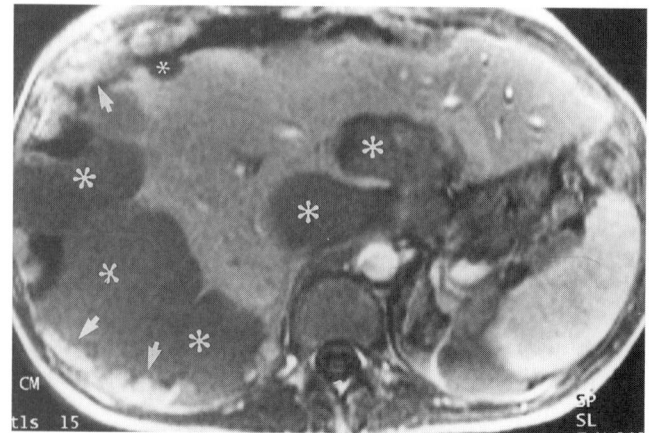

FIG. 10.49. Pseudomyxoma peritonei. **A:** Axial T2- and **(B)** postcontrast T1-W MR images show multiple complex cystic masses indenting the liver surface (*asterisks*, **A, B**). Note that the solid components of the tumor enhance (*arrows*, **B**). **C:** Coronal T2-W MR image demonstrates tumor within the subphrenic space, the ligamentum teres, and the hepatoduodenal ligament (*open arrows*, **C**).

The few prospective studies comparing contrast-enhanced CT and precontrast and postcontrast MR imaging found that MRI was at least equivalent and, in some cases, superior to CT for depiction of the internal architecture of ovarian tumors, showing the relationship between tumor and adjacent pelvic structures and delineating the intraabdominal extent of disease (Fig. 10.49) (5a). The overall staging accuracy of MRI in patients with ovarian malignancy is 75% to 78% (219,233).

Positron Emission Tomography

See section on Detection and Characterization above.

Identification of Persistent or Recurrent Ovarian Cancer

Imaging, especially US and CT, has been used to detect persistent or recurrent ovarian cancer and to document tumor response to subsequent therapy.

Ultrasound

US has the greatest sensitivity in detecting recurrent tumor in the pelvis or around the liver and right hemidiaphragm in the setting of ascites (235). However, the sensitivity of US in detecting microscopic disease, miliary peritoneal seeding, or macroscopic disease on the peritoneum and in the omentum with lesions less than 1 to 2 cm is poor (235, 236). Additionally, small, plaque-like lesions on the pelvic peritoneum or lesions high in the false pelvis are often missed on US (236).

Discrimination among absence of residual disease, microscopic disease, or minimal disease less than 2 cm also cannot be made on US studies, and they are not, therefore, sufficient to replace second-look laparotomy in making patient-management decisions (235). Despite these limitations, US can reliably confirm a clinical suspicion of gross macroscopic recurrent disease and is more accurate than clinical examination in detection of nonpalpable disease (235,236).

Computed Tomography

Although the use of CT allows assessment of more potential sites of tumor recurrence than US, it too has significant limitations. In the detection of persistent or recurrent ovarian cancer, the sensitivity of conventional CT is 51% to 84% and specificity is 81% to 93% (237–241). False-positive results are usually caused by misdiagnosis of adherent bowel loops as a tumor mass. The sensitivity of CT for disease detection is proportional to lesion size (237). Many studies report limitations in the detection of small (1 to 3 cm) tumor nodules in the mesentery and omentum and along peritoneal surfaces (237,239). Improved spatial imaging with MDCT will likely prove to be valuable in detecting subtle recurrence

and increase overall disease-detection accuracy (231,241). Nevertheless, a negative CT does not exclude microscopic disease or small tumor implants and thus cannot substitute for second-look laparotomy (237,239,241,242). Serum levels of the tumor-specific antigen CA-125 and PET can help to differentiate patients with small-volume disease and a ''negative'' CT from those with a true negative CT (239). CT-guided biopsy can be used to confirm suspected recurrence (239,242).

Magnetic Resonance Imaging

Few studies have compared state of the art contrast-enhanced fat-suppressed MRI to second-look laparotomy. Reports from early studies indicate that for detection of tumor recurrence in patients with treated ovarian cancer, the sensitivity of MRI is 78% to 81%, specificity is 88% to 93%, and accuracy is 86% to 88% (238,240). Reports from a subsequent study, using recurrent tumor size greater than 2 cm as indicative of inoperability, suggest that the accuracy of MRI is 82% for identification of patients who would not benefit from second-look surgery. The accuracy rate decreased to 38%, however, for lesions less than 2 cm in size (243).

For a complete abdominopelvic evaluation, both contrast-enhanced CT and MRI offer a comprehensive examination, albeit one that is limited in its detection of small tumor nodules. Both have comparable sensitivity, specificity, and accuracy (241).

Positron Emission Tomography

See section on Detection and Characterization above.

VAGINAL CANCER

US and conventional CT are limited in their assessment of the extent of early disease, although CT has been used to detect enlarged lymph nodes. Similarly, MRI may be used to screen for lymphadenopathy. Additionally, MRI criteria have been developed that correlate with FIGO staging schema. On T1-weighted images, vaginal tumors are isointense and are apparent only if they alter the vaginal contour (89). With progressive T2-weighting, tumors become brighter. Tumors confined to the vagina (stage I) may be occult on MRI, or there may be abnormal medium-signal intensity penetrating the vaginal wall. The surrounding perivaginal fat is preserved. With stage II disease, the normally high-signal intensity perivaginal fat is invaded by medium–signal intensity tumor. Tumor contiguous with the levator ani, obturator internus, or the piriformis muscle is diagnostic of pelvic sidewall invasion (stage III disease). MRI is particularly well suited for imaging stage IV disease (i.e., involvement of the bladder or rectum) by exploiting its multiplanar capabilities (Fig. 10.50). Vesicovaginal fistulae are made

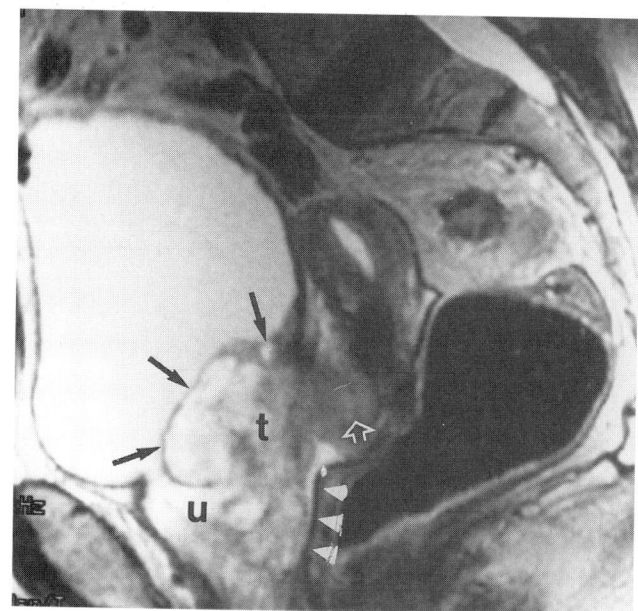
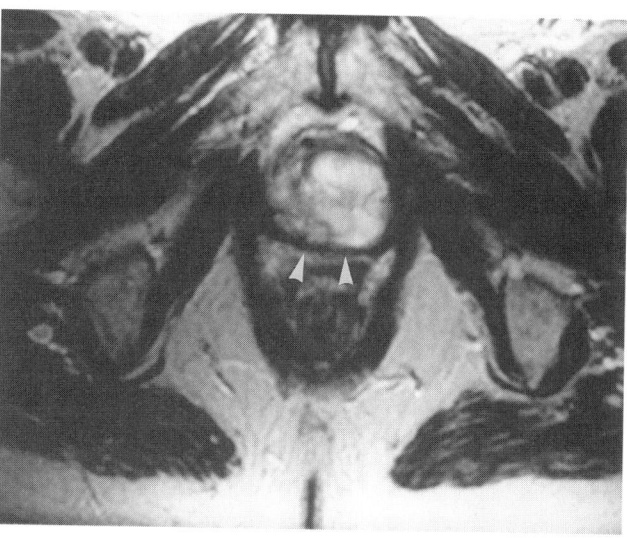

FIG. 10.50. Stage IV mucinous vaginal cancer. **A:** Sagittal and **(B)** axial T2-W MR images show a large high–signal intensity vaginal tumor (t, **A**) that invades the bladder trigone (*arrows*, **A**), the anterior lip of the cervix (*open arrow*, **A**), and the urethra (u, **A**). The posterior vaginal muscularis appears as a low–signal intensity line and is intact (*arrowheads*, **A, B**). (Courtesy of Eric K. Outwater, M.D., University of Arizona Medical Center, Tuscon, AZ.)

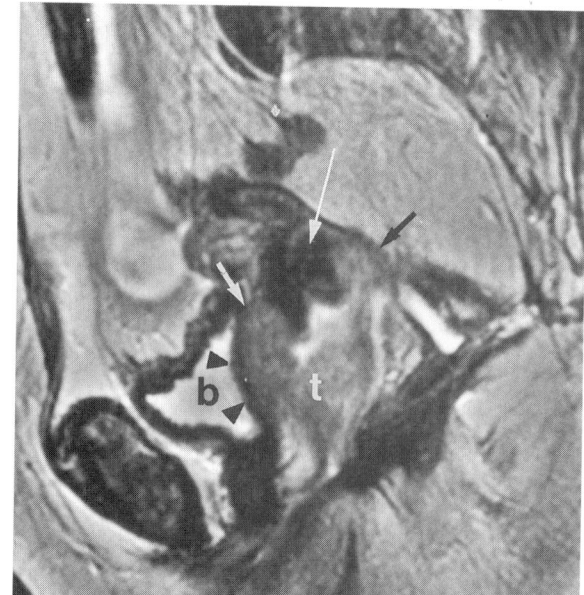
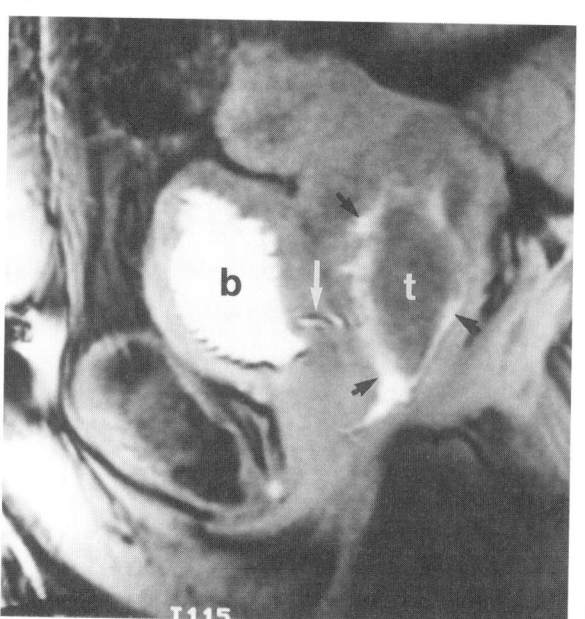

FIG. 10.51. Vaginal adenocarcinoma with a vesicovaginal fistula. **A:** Sagittal T2-W MR image shows the heterogeneous signal intensity vaginal tumor (t) extending into the anterior and posterior vaginal fornices (*short arrows*). Note the low signal intensity cervical stroma is relatively spared (*long arrow*). The large tumor also causes mass effect on the posterior wall (*arrowheads*) of the bladder (b). **B:** Sagittal gadolinium-enhanced fat-suppressed T1-W MR image just to the left of **A** shows contrast within the bladder (b). Gadolinium chelate (*short arrows*) is also seen within the vagina surrounding the tumor (t). Note the thin vesicovaginal tract in the bladder wall (*arrow*), representing the fistula. (Courtesy of Eric K. Outwater, M.D., University of Arizona Medical Center, Tuscon, AZ.)

more conspicuous via the administration of intravenous gadolinium chelates (Fig. 10.51) (86). However, MRI is imperfect as inflammatory changes or congestion of the vagina may appear similar to carcinoma (79).

VULVAR CANCER

Vulvar cancer is typically diagnosed and staged clinically. As with vaginal cancer, diagnostic imaging is usually limited to searching for deep pelvic lymphadenopathy in patients with inguinal lymph node metastasis. On CT, vulvar cancer appears as a soft tissue mass. On MRI, the tumor is intermediate-signal intensity on T1-weighted sequences, becoming progressively brighter with T2 weighting. In select cases, CT and MRI may be used to evaluate for tumor extension into adjacent structures (i.e., urethra) (89). MRI may also be used to differentiate recurrence from posttherapy changes, with the former becoming brighter on T2-weighted images, whereas the latter remains intermediate in signal intensity on T2-weighted sequences.

SUMMARY

Increased use of CT and MRI for staging gynecologic pelvic malignancies has led to a decline in the use of conventional and invasive radiologic studies such as intravenous urography and barium enema. In addition, transabdominal US is no longer used for primary cancer staging. Transvaginal US, however, in conjunction with Doppler US, is helpful in characterizing ovarian and endometrial masses, with TRUS being reserved for evaluating cervical cancer.

CT maintains a high-profile role in pelvic imaging because of its cost effectiveness, high spatial resolution, fast examination time, and wide availability. It ably detects enlarged lymph nodes and permits percutaneous biopsy of metastases and recurrent tumor. Conventional CT has been proved to be useful for primary staging of ovarian cancer, advanced cervical and endometrial cancers, and persistent and metastatic GTD and evaluation of recurrent pelvic malignancies. MDCT technology will likely further expand the utility of CT in the workup of patients with pelvic cancers, but clinical trials are needed.

MRI has been gaining favor for gynecologic pelvic cancer staging because of its superb contrast resolution and multiplanar imaging capabilities. It also has advantages over CT for patients allergic to iodinated intravenous contrast or with impaired renal function. Early reservations about MRI, vis-à-vis long scanning times and lack of oral and intravenous contrast, no longer apply. MRI shows excellent contrast resolution between tumor, cervical stroma, endometrium, myometrium, uterine ligaments, parametrial fat, and blood vessels. Most comparative studies show MRI to have advantages in local staging of clinical stage I and II cancers of the cervix and endometrium, and it has been shown to be cost minimizing in these situations. It may also be used for cases

of GTD when the uterus is being evaluated as the primary site of disease and to monitor response to therapy. In addition, MRI has utility for selected cases of vaginal cancer, especially to aid in detection of fistulae, and rivals CT for characterizing adnexal masses and staging primary ovarian neoplasms. It also plays an increasing role in the evaluation of recurrent ovarian cancer.

PET, especially PET-CT, is increasingly being used to evaluate gynecologic malignancies. Large multiinstitutional studies are needed before PET becomes a routine part of the imaging algorithms for gynecologic cancers.

FUTURE DIRECTIONS

Future innovations in gynecologic-oncology imaging will go beyond anatomy to focus on function. Specifically, functional imaging aims to provide *in vivo* cellular characterization and, ultimately, biologic signatures for both premalignant and malignant conditions. Functional technologies range in maturity: (a) reasonably established (e.g., MR spectroscopy), (b) less well developed (e.g., optical imaging), and (c) nascent technologies [e.g., electron paramagnetic resonance imaging (EPRI)]. These technologies will likely have a twofold impact on cancer incidence and mortality: (a) improvements in existing methods (e.g., optical imaging as an ''add on'' to conventional colposcopy for cervical cancer) and (b) development of new approaches to detect early or preinvasive cancers that traditionally have low survival rates and no proven early-detection algorithms (e.g., optical coherence tomography for surface epithelial ovarian cancer) (244).

Advances in functional imaging raise issues in data management and display. Image fusion, which marries anatomic and functional data, coupled with soft-copy display, will provide roadmaps for gynecologic cancer prevention and treatment.

ACKNOWLEDGMENTS

The authors wish to acknowledge the previous contributions made to this chapter by Jeffrey J. Brown and James W. Walsh.

REFERENCES

1. Ros PR, Ji H. Multisection (multi-detector) CT: Applications in the abdomen. *Radiographics* 2002;22:697–700.
2. Kim SH, Choi BI, Han JK, et al. Preoperative staging of uterine cervical carcinoma: comparison of CT and MRI in 99 patients. *J Comput Assist Tomogr* 1993;17:633–640.
3. Kim SH, Choi BI, Lee HP, et al. Uterine cervical carcinoma: comparison of CT and MR findings. *Radiology* 1990;175:45–51.
4. Kim SH, Kim HD, Song YS, et al. Detection of deep myometrial invasion in endometrial carcinoma: comparison of transvaginal ultrasound, CT, and MRI. *J Comput Assist Tomogr* 1995;19:766–772.
5a. Semelka RC, Lawrence PH, Shoenut JP, et al. Primary ovarian cancer: prospective comparison of contrast-enhanced CT and pre- and post-

contrast, fat-suppressed MR imaging with histologic correlation. *J Magn Reson Imaging* 1993;3:99–106.

5b. Varpula MJ, Klemi PJ. Staging of uterine endometrial carcinoma with ultra-low field (0.02T) MRI: a comparative study with CT. *J Comput Assist Tomogr* 1993;17:641–647.

6. Ebner F, Kressel HY, Mintz MC, et al. Tumor recurrence versus fibrosis in the female pelvis: differentiation with MR imaging at 1.5 T. *Radiology* 1988;166:333–340.

7. Kinkel K, Ariche M, Tardivon AA, et al. Differentiation between recurrent tumor and benign conditions after treatment of gynecologic pelvic carcinoma: value of dynamic contrast-enhanced subtraction MR imaging. *Radiology* 1997;204:55–63.

8. Dooms GC, Hricak H, Crooks LE, Higgins CB. Magnetic resonance imaging of the lymph nodes: comparison with CT. *Radiology* 1984;153:719–728.

9. Hricak H, Powell B, Yu KK, et al. Invasive cervical carcinoma: role of MR imaging in pretreatment work-up—cost minimization and diagnostic efficacy analysis. *Radiology* 1996;198:403–409.

10. Schwartz LB, Panageas E, Lange R, et al. Female pelvis: impact of MR imaging on treatment decisions and net cost analysis. *Radiology* 1994;192:55–60.

11. Yu KK, Hricak H. Can MRI of the pelvis be cost effective? *Abdom Imaging* 1997;22:597–601.

12. Hardesty LA, Sumkin JH, Nath ME, et al. Use of preoperative MR imaging in the management of endomertirial carcinoma: cost analysis. *Radiology* 2000;215:45–49.

13. Strauss LG, Conti PS. The application of PET in clinical oncology. *J Nucl Med* 1991;32:623–648.

14. Nakahara T, Fujii H, Ide M, et al. F-18 FDG Uptake in endometrial cancer. *Clin Nucl Med* 2001;26:82–83.

15. Reinhardt MJ, Ehritt-Braun C, Vogelgesang D, et al. Metastatic lymph nodes in patients with cervical cancer: Detection with MR imaging and FDG PET. *Radiology* 2001;218:776–782.

16. Grigsby PW, Dehdashti F, Siegel B. FDG-PET evaluation of carcinoma of the cervix. *Clin Positron Imaging* 1999;2:105–109.

18. Hillman BJ, Clark RL, Babbitt G. Efficacy of the excretory urogram in the staging of gynecologic malignancies. *AJR Am J Roentgenol* 1984;143:997–999.

19. Kim MJ, Chung JJ, Lee YH, et al. Comparison of the use of the transrectal surface coil and the pelvic phased-array coil in MR imaging for preoperative evaluation of uterine cervical carcinoma. *AJR Am J Roentgenol* 1997;168:1215–1221.

20. Gedgaudas RK, Kelvin FM, Thompson WM, Rice PP. The value of the preoperative barium-enema examination in the assessment of pelvic masses. *Radiology* 1983;146:609–613.

21. Griffin TW, Parker RG, Taylor WJ. An evaluation of procedures used in staging carcinoma of the cervix. *AJR Am J Roentgenol* 1976,127:825–829.

22. Pearl ML, Griffen T, Valea FA, Chalas E. The utility of pretreatment barium enema in women with endometrial carcinoma. *Gynecol Oncol* 1997;64:442–445.

23. Lev-Toaff AS. Sonohysterography: evaluation of endometrial and myometrial abnormalities. *Semin Roentgenol* 1996;31:288–298.

24. Sohaey R, Woodward P. Sonohysterography: technique, endometrial findings, and clinical applications. *Semin Ultrasound CT MR* 1999;20:250–258.

25. Goldstein SR: Saline infusion sonohysterography. *Clin Obstet Gynecol* 1996;39:248–258.

26. Lev-Toaff AS, Pinheiro LW, Bega, G, et al. Three-dimensional multiplanar sonohysterography. Comparison with conventional two-dimensional sonohysterography and X-ray hysterosalpingography. *J Ultrasound Med* 2001;20:295–306.

27. Lyons EA, Gratton D, Harrington C. Transvaginal sonography of normal pelvic anatomy. *Radiol Clin North Am* 1992;30:663–676.

28. Fleischer AC, Kalemeris GC, Entman SS. Sonographic depiction of the endometrium during normal cycles. *Ultrasound Med Biol* 1986;12:271–272.

29. Arger PH. Transvaginal ultrasonography in postmenopausal patients. *Radiol Clin North Am* 1992;30:759–767.

30. Levine D, Gosink BB, Johnson LA. Change in endometrial thickness in postmenopausal women undergoing hormone replacement therapy. *Radiology* 1995;197:603–608.

31. Lin MC, Gosink BB, Wolf SL, et al: Endometrial thickness after menopause: effect of hormone replacement. *Radiology* 1991;180:427–432.

32. Pels Rijcken TH, Davis MA, Ros PR. Intraluminal contrast agents for MR imaging of the abdomen and pelvis. *J Magn Reson Imaging* 1994;4:291–300.

33. Brown JJ, Duncan JR, Heiken JP, et al. Perfluoroctylbromide as a gastrointestinal contrast agent for MR imaging: use with and without glucagon. *Radiology* 1991;81:455–460.

34. Ascher SM. MR imaging of the female pelvis: the time has come. *Radiographics* 1998;18:931–945.

35. Gryspeerdt S, Van Hoe L, Bosmans H, et al. T2-weighted MR imaging of the uterus: comparison of optimized fast spin-echo and HASTE sequences with conventional fast spin-echo sequences. *AJR Am J Roentgenol* 1998:171:211–215.

36. Niitsu M, Tanaka YO, Anno I, Itai Y. Multishot echoplanar MR imaging of the female pelvis: comparison with fast spin-echo MR imaging in an initial clinical trial. *AJR Am J Roentgenol* 1997;168,651–655.

37. Smith RC, Reinhold C, McCauley TR, et al. Multicoil high-resolution fast spin echo MR imaging of the female pelvis. *Radiology* 1992;184:671–675.

38. Ascher SM, O'Malley J, Semelka RC, et al. T2-weighted MRI of the uterus: fast spin echo vs. breath-hold fast spin echo. *J Magn Reson Imaging* 1999;9:384–390.

39. Nolte-Ernsting CCA, Bücker A, Adam GB, et al. Gadolinium-enhanced excretory MR urography after low-dose diuretic injection: comparison with conventional excretory urography. *Radiology* 1998;209:147–157.

40. Rothpearl A, Frager D, Subramanian A, et al. MR urography: technique and application. *Radiology* 1995;194:125–130.

41. McCarthy S, Scott G, Majumdar S, et al. Uterine junctional zone: MR study of water content and relaxation properties. *Radiology* 1989;171:241–243.

42. Scoutt LM, Flynn SD, Luthringer DJ, et al. Junctional zone of the uterus: correlation of MR imaging and histologic examination of hysterectomy specimens. *Radiology* 1991;179:403–407.

43. Mitchell DG, Schonholz L, Hilpert PL, et al. Zones of the uterus: discrepancy between US and MR images. *Radiology* 1990;174:827.

44. Demas BE, Hricak H, Jaffe RB. Uterine MR imaging effects of hormonal stimulation. *Radiology* 1986;159:123–126.

45. McCarthy SM, Tauber C, Gore J. Female pelvic anatomy: MR assessment of variations during the menstrual cycle and with use of oral contraceptives. *Radiology* 1986;160:119–123.

46. deSouza NM, Hawley IC, Schwieso JE, et al. The uterine cervix on in vitro and in vivo MR images: a study of zonal anatomy and vascularity using an enveloping cervical coil. *AJR Am J Roentgenol* 1994;163:607–612.

47. Scoutt LM, McCauley TR, Flynn SD, et al. Zonal anatomy of the cervix: correlation of MR imaging and histologic examination of hysterectomy specimens. *Radiology* 1993;186:159–162.

48. Kikuchi A, Okai T, Kobayashi K, et al. Intracervcial US with a high-frequency miniature probe: a method for diagnosing early invasive cervical cancer. *Radiology* 1996;198:411–413.

49. Dubinsky TJ, Reed SD, Grieco V, Richardson ML. Intracervical sonographic-pathologic correlation: preliminary results. *J Ultrasound Med*. 2003;22:61–67.

50. Hawnaur JM, Johnson RJ, Carrington BM, Hunter RD. Predictive value of clinical examination, transrectal ultrasound and magnetic resonance imaging prior to radiotherapy in carcinoma of cervix. *Br J Radiol* 1998;71:819–827.

51. Ascher SM, Silverman PM. Applications of computed tomography in gynecologic diseases. *Urol Radiol* 1991;13:16–28.

52. Hricak H, Lacey CG, Sandles LG, et al. Invasive cervical carcinoma: comparison of MR imaging and surgical findings. *Radiology* 1988;166:623–631.

53. Togashi K, Nishimura D, Sagoh T, et al. Carcinoma of the cervix: staging with MR imaging. *Radiology* 1989;171:245–251.

54. Hricak H, Hamm B, Semelka RC, et al. Carcinoma of the uterus: use of gadopentetate dimeglumine in MR imaging. *Radiology* 1991;181:95–106.

55. Yamashita Y, Takahashi M, Sawada T, et al. Carcinoma of the cervix: dynamic MR imaging. *Radiology* 1992;182:643–648.

56. Seki H, Azumi R, Kimura M, Sakai K. Stromal invasion by carcinoma

of the cervix: assessment with dynamic MR imaging. *AJR Am J Roentgenol* 1997;168:1579–1585.

57. Postema S, Pattynama PMT, Van Rijswijk CSP, Trimbos JB. Cervical carcinoma: can dynamic contrast-enhanced MR imaging help predict tumor aggressiveness? *Radiology* 1999;210:217–220.

58. Doi T, Yamashita Y, Yasunaga T, et al. Adenoma malignum: MR imaging and pathologic study. *Radiology* 1997;204:39–42.

59. Rose PG, Adler LB, Rodriguez M, et al. Positron emission tomography for evaluating para-aortic lymph node metastasis in locally advanced cervical cancer before surgical staging: a surgico-pathologic study. *J Clin Oncol* 1999;17:41–45.

60. Keys HM, Bundy BN, Stehman FB, et al. Cisplatin, radiation and adjuvant hysterectomy compared with radiation and adjuvant hysterectomy for bulky stage IB cervical carcinoma. *N Engl J Med* 1999;340:1154–1161.

61. Morris M, Eifel PJ, Lu J, et al. Pelvic radiation with concurrent chemotherapy compared with pelvic and para-aortic radiation for high risk cervical cancer. *N Engl J Med* 1999;340:1137–1143.

62. Rose PG, Bundy BN, Watkins EB, et al. Concurrent cisplatin-based radiotherapy and chemotherapy for locally advanced cervical cancer. *N Engl J Med* 1999;340:1144–1153.

63. Villasanta U, Whitley NO, Haney PJ, Brenner D. Computed tomography in invasive carcinoma of the cervix: an appraisal. *Obstet Gynecol* 1983;62:218–224.

64. Walsh JW, Amendola MA, Hall DJ, et al. Recurrent carcinoma of the cervix: CT diagnosis. *AJR Am J Roentgenol* 1981;136:117–122.

65. Walsh JW, Vick CW. Staging of female genital tract cancer. In: Walsh JW, ed. *Computed tomography of the pelvis*. New York: Churchill Livingstone, 1985:163.

66. Hricak H, Demas BE, Braga CA, et al. Gestational trophoblastic neoplasm of the uterus: MR assessment. *Radiology* 1986;161:11–16.

67. Kilcheski TS, Arger PH, Mulhern CB Jr, et al. Role of computed tomography in the presurgical evaluation of carcinoma of the cervix. *J Comput Assist Tomogr* 1981;5:378–383.

68. Goldman SM, Fishman EK, Rosenshein NB, et al. Excretory urography and computed tomography in the initial evaluation of patients with cervical cancer: Are both examinations necessary? *AJR Am J Roentgenol* 1984;143:991–996.

69. Gitch G, Deutinger J, Rheinthaller A, et al. Cervical cancer: the diagnostic value of rectosonography for the judgment of parametrial invasion in regard to inflammatory stromal reaction. *Br J Obstet Gynaecol* 1993;100:696–697.

70. Innocenti P, Pulli F, Savino L, et al. Staging of cervical cancer: reliability of transrectal US. *Radiology* 1992;185:201–205.

71. Carter JR, Carson LF, Twiggs LB. Gynecologic oncology. In: Nyberg DA, Hill LM, Bohm-Velez M, Mendelson E, eds. *Transvaginal ultrasound*. St. Louis: Mosby, 1992:241.

72. Urban BA, Fishman EK. Helical (spiral) CT of the female pelvis. *Radiol Clin North Am* 1995;33:933–948.

73. Hricak H, Yu KK. Radiology in invasive cervical cancer. *AJR Am Roentgenol* 1996:167:1101–1108.

74. Walsh JW, Goplerud DR. Prospective comparison between clinical and CT staging in primary cervical carcinoma. *AJR Am J Roentgenol* 1981;137:997–1003.

75. Granberg S, Wikland M. Comparison between endovaginal and transabdominal transducers for measuring ovarian volume. *J Ultrasound Med* 1987;6:649–653.

76. Yang WT, Lam WWM, Yu MY, et al. Comparison of dynamic helical CT and dynamic MR imaging in the evaluation of pelvic lymph nodes in cervical carcinoma. *AJR Am J Roentgenol* 2000;175:759–766.

77. Yang WT, Walkden SB, Ho S, et al. Transrectal ultrasound in the evaluation of cervical carcinoma and comparison with spiral computed tomography and magnetic resonance imaging. *Br J Radiol* 1996;69:610–616.

78. Sironi S, Belloni C, Taccagni GL, DelMaschio A. Carcinoma of the cervix: value of MR in detecting parametrial involvement. *AJR Am J Roentgenol* 1991;156:753–756.

79. Chang YCF, Hricak H, Thurnher S, Lacey CG. Vagina: evaluation with MR imaging. Part II. neoplasms. *Radiology* 1988;169:175–179.

80. Hawighorst H, Schoenberg SO, Knapstein PG, et al. Staging of invasive cervical carcinoma and of pelvic lymph nodes by high resolution MRI with a phased-array coil in comparison with pathological findings. *J Comput Assist Tomogr* 1998;22:75–81.

81. Yu KK, Hricak H, Subak LL, et al. Preoperative staging of cervical carcinoma: phased array coil fast spin-echo versus body coil spin-echo T2-weighted MR imaging. *AJR Am J Roentgenol* 1998;171:707–711.

82. Scheidler J, Heuck AF, Steinborn M, et al. Parametrial invasion in cervical carcinoma: evaluation of detection at MR imaging with fat suppression. *Radiology* 1998;206:125–129.

83. Kim SH, Han MC. Invasion of the urinary bladder by uterine cervical carcinoma: evaluation with MR imaging. *AJR Am J Roentgenol* 1997;168:393–397.

84. Kim SH, Kim SC, Choi BI, Han MC. Uterine cervical carcinoma: evaluation of pelvic lymph node metastasis with MR imaging. *Radiology* 1994;190:807–811.

85. Sironi S, De Cobelli F, Scarfone G, et al. Carcinoma of the cervix: value of plain and gadolinium-enhanced MR imaging in assessing degree of invasiveness. *Radiology* 1993;188:797–801.

86. Outwater E, Schiebler ML. Pelvic fistulas: findings on MR images. *AJR Am J Roentgenol* 1993;160:327–330.

87. Kaji Y, Sugimura K, Kitao M, Ishida T. Histopathology of uterine cervical carcinoma: diagnostic comparison of endorectal surface coil and standard body coil MRI. *J Comput Assist Tomogr* 1994;18:785–792.

89. Carrington B, Hricak H. The uterus and vagina. In: Hricak H, Carrington BM, eds. *MRI of the pelvis: a text atlas*. London: Appleton & Lange, 1991:93.

90. Meanwell CA, Rolfe EB, Blackledge G, et al. Recurrent female pelvic cancer: assessment with transrectal ultrasonography. *Radiology* 1987;162:278–281.

91. Squillaci E, Salzini MC, Grandinetti ML, et al. Recurrence of ovarian and uterine neoplasms: diagnosis with transrectal US. *Radiology* 1988;169:355–358.

92. Balfe DM, Van Dyke J, Lee JKT, et al. Computed tomography in malignant endometrial neoplasms. *J Comput Assist Tomogr* 1983;7:677–681.

93. Franchi M, La Fianza A, Babilonti L, et al. Clinical value of computerized tomography (CT) in assessment of recurrent uterine cancers. *Gynecol Oncol* 1989;35:31–37.

94. Walsh JW, Goplerud DR. Computed tomography of primary, persistent, and recurrent endometrial malignancy. *AJR Am J Roentgenol* 1982;139:1149–1154.

95. Fulcher AS, O'Sullivan SG, Segreti EM, Kavanagh BD. Recurrent cervical carcinoma: Typical and atypical manifestations. *Radiographics* 1999;19:S103–S116.

96. Doubleday LC, Bernadino ME. CT findings in the perirectal area following radiation therapy. *J Comput Assist Tomogr* 1980;4:634–638.

97. Frei KA, Kinkel K, Bonel HM, et al. Prediction of deep myometrial invasion in patients with endometrial cancer: clinical utility of contrast-enhanced MR imaging—a meta-analysis and Bayesian analysis. *Radiology* 2000;216:444–449.

98. Flueckiger F, Ebner F, Poschauko H, et al. Cervical cancer: serial MR imaging before and after primary radiation therapy—a 2-year follow-up study. *Radiology* 1992;184:89–93.

99. Kim KH, Lee BH, Do YS, et al. Stage IIb cervical carcinoma: MR evaluation of effect of intraarterial chemotherapy. *Radiology* 1994;192:61–65.

100. Manfredi R, Maresca G, Smaniotto D, et al. Cervical cancer response to neoadjuvant therapy: MR imaging assessment. *Radiology* 1998;209:819–824.

101. Sugimura K, Carrington BM, Quivey JM, Hricak H. Postirradiation changes in the pelvis: assessment with MR imaging. *Radiology* 1990;175:805–813.

102. Semelka RC, Hricak H, Kim B, et al. Pelvic fistulas: appearances on MR images. *Abdom Imaging* 1997;22:91–95.

103. Cooper CR, Jeffrey RB, Silverman PM, et al. Computed tomography of omental pathology. *J Assist Tomogr* 1986;10:62–66.

104. Deleted in proof.

105. Hawnaur JM, Johnson RJ, Carrington BM, Hunter RD. Predictive value of clinical examination, transrectal ultrasound and magnetic resonance imaging prior to radiotherapy in carcinoma of cervix. *Br J Radiol* 1998;71:819–827.

106. Mayr NA, Tali ET, Yuh WTC, et al. Cervical cancer: application of MR imaging in radiation therapy. *Radiology* 1993;189:601–608.

107. Sironi S, Belloni C, Taccagni G, Del Maschio A. Invasive cervical

carcinoma: MR imaging after preoperative chemotherapy. *Radiology* 1991;180:719–722.

108. Amano M, Kato T, Anamo Y, Kumazaki T. Using MR imaging to predict and evaluate the response of invasive cervical carcinoma to systemic chemotherapy. *AJR Am J Roentgenol* 1998;171:1335–1339.

109. Mayr NA, Yuh WTC, Zheng J, et al. Prediction of tumor control in patients with cervical cancer: analysis of combined volume and dynamic enhancement pattern by MR imaging. *AJR Am J Roentgenol* 1998;170;177–182.

110. Hawighorst H, Knapstein PG, Knopp MV, et al. Uterine cervical carcinoma: comparison of standard and pharmacokinetic analysis of time-intensity curves for assessment of tumor angiogenesis and patient survival. *Cancer Res* 1998;58:3598–3602.

111. Mayr NA, Yuh WTC, Magnotta VA, et al. Tumor perfusion studies using fast magnetic resonance imaging technique in advanced cervical cancer: a new noninvasive predictive assay. *Int J Radiat Oncol Biol Phys* 1996;36:623–633.

112. Weber TM, Sostman DH, Spritzer CE, et al. Cervical carcinoma: determination of recurrent tumor extent versus radiation changes with MR imaging. *Radiology* 1995;194:135–139.

113. Yamashita Y, Harada M, Torashima M, et al. Dynamic MR imaging of recurrent postoperative cervical cancer. *J Magn Reson Imaging* 1996;1:167–171.

114. Brenner PF. Differential diagnosis of abnormal uterine bleeding. *Am J Obstet Gynecol* 1996;175:766–769.

115. Karlsson B, Granberg S, Hellberg P, Wikland M. Comparative study of transvaginal sonography and hysteroscopy for the detection of pathologic endometrial lesions in women with postmenopausal bleeding. *J Ultrasound Med* 1994;13:757–762.

116. Word B, Gravlee LC, Widerman GL. The fallacy of simple uterine curettage. *Obstet Gynecol* 1958;12:642–648.

117. Grimes DA. Diagnostic dilatation and curettage: a reappraisal. *Am J Obstet Gynecol* 1982;142:1–6.

118. Koonings PP, Moyer DI, Grimes DA. A randomized clinical trial comparing Pipelle and Tis-U-Trap for endometrial biopsy. *Obstet Gynecol* 1990;75:293–295.

119. Stock RJ, Kanbour A. Prehysterectomy curettage. *Obstet Gynecol* 1975;45:537–541.

120. Guido RS, Kanbour-Shakir A, Rulin MC, Christopherson WA. Pipelle endometrial sampling. Sensitivity in the detection of endometrial cancer. *J Reprod Med* 1995;40:553–555.

121. Hofmeister FJ. Endometrial biopsy: another look. *Am J Obstet Gynecol* 1974;118:773–777.

122. Karlsson B, Granberg S, Wikland M, et al. Transvaginal ultrasonography of the endometrium in women with postmenopausal bleeding—a Nordic multicenter study. *Am J Obstet Gynecol* 1995;172:1488–1494.

123. Smith-Bindman R, Kerlikowske K, Feldstein VA, et al. Endovaginal ultrasound to exclude endometrial cancer and other endometrial abnormalities. *JAMA* 1998;280:1510–1517.

124. Goldstein RB, Bree RL, Benson CB, et al. Evaluation of the woman with postmenopausal bleeding. Society of Radiologist in Ultrasound-Sponsored Consensus Conference Statement. *J Ultrasound Med* 2001;20:1025–1036.

125. Medverd JR, Dubinsky TJ. Cost analysis model: US versus endometrial biopsy in evaluation of peri- and postmenopausal abnormal vaginal bleeding. *Radiology* 2002;222:619–627.

126. Dubinsky TJ, Parvey HR, Maklad N. The role of transvaginal sonography and endometrial biopsy in the evaluation of peri- and postmenopausal bleeding. *AJR Am J Roentgenol* 1997;169:145–149.

127. Lev-Toaff AS, Toaff ME, Liu J-B, et al. Value of sonohysterography in the diagnosis and management of abnormal uterine bleeding. *Radiology* 1996;201:179–184.

128. Laifer-Narin S, Ragavendra N, Parmenter EK, Grant EG. False-normal appearance of the endometrium on coventional transvaginal sonography: comparison with saline hysterosonography. *AJR Am J Roentgenol* 2002;178:129–133.

129. Atri M, Nazarnia S, Aldis AE, et al. Transvaginal US appearance of endometrial abnormalities. *Radiographics* 1994;14:483–492.

130. Laifer-Narin SL, Ragavendra N, Lu DSK, et al. Transvaginal saline hysterosonography: characteristics distinguishing malignant and various benign conditions. *AJR Am J Roentgernol* 1999;172:1513–1520.

131. Dubinsky TJ, Stroehlein K, Abu-Ghazzeh Y, et al. Prediction of be-

132. Williams PL, Laifer-Narin SL, Ragavendra N. US of abnormal uterine bleeding. *Radiographics* 2003;23:703–718.

133. Langer RD, Pierce JJ, O'Hanlan KA, et al. Transvaginal ultrasonography compared with endometrial biopsy for the detection of endometrial disease. *N Engl J Med* 1997;337:1792–1798.

134. Sheth S, Hamper UM, Kurman RJ. Thickened endometrium in the postmenopausal woman: sonographic-pathologic correlation. *Radiology* 1993;187:135–139.

135. Hann, LE, Giess CS, Bach AM, et al. Endometrial thickness in tamoxifen-treated patients: correlation with clinical and pathological findings. *AJR Am J Roentgenol* 1997;168:657–661.

136. Hulka CA, Hall DA. Endometrial abnormalities associated with tamoxifen therapy for breast cancer: sonographic and pathologic correlation. *AJR Am J Roentgenol* 1993;160:809–812.

137. Dubinsky TJ, Stroehlein K, Abu-Ghazzeh Y, et al. Prediction of benign and malignant endometrial disease: hysterosonographic-pathologic correlation. *Radiology* 1999;210:393–397.

138. Affinito P, Palomba S, Pellicano M, et al. Ultrasonographic measurement of endometrial thickness during hormonal replacement therapy in postmenopausal women. *Ultrasound Obstet Gynecol* 1998;11: 343–346.

139. Bonilla-Musoles F, Raga R, Osborne NG, et al. Three dimensional hysterosonography for the study of endometrial tumors: comparison with conventional transvaginal sonography, hysterosalpingography, and hysteroscopy. *Gynecol Oncol* 1997;65:245–252.

140. Gruboeck K, Jurkovic D, Lawton F, et al. The diagnostic value of endometrial thickness and volume measurements by three-dimensional ultrasound in patients with postmenopausal bleeding. *Ultrasound Obstet Gynecol* 1996;8:272–276.

141. Sheth S, Hamper UM, McCollum ME, et al. Endometrial blood flow analysis in postmenopausal women: can it help differentiate benign from malignant causes of endometrial thickening? *Radiology* 1995; 195:661–665.

142. Sladkevicius P, Valentin L, Marsal K. Endometrial thickness and Doppler velocimetry of the uterine arteries as discriminators of endometrial status in women with postmenopausal bleeding: a comparative study. *Am J Obstet Gynecol* 1994;171:722–728.

143. Dore R, Moro B, D'Andrea F, et al. CT evaluation of myometrium invasion in endometrial carcinoma. *J Comput Assist Tomogr* 1987; 11:282–289.

144. Hamlin DJ, Burgener FA, Beecham JB. CT of intramural endometrial carcinoma: contrast enhancement is essential. *AJR Am J Roentgenol* 1981;137:551–554.

145. Hricak H, Stern JL, Fisher MR, et al. Endometrial carcinoma staging by MR imaging. *Radiology* 1987;162:297–305.

146. Shapeero LG, Hricak H. Mixed müllerian sarcoma of the uterus: MR imaging findings. *AJR Am J Roentgenol* 1989;153:317–319.

147. Ito K, Matsutomo T, Nakada T, et al. Assessing myometrial invasion by endometrial carcinoma with dynamic MRI. *J Comput Assist Tomogr* 1994;18:77–86.

148. Joja I, Asakawa M, Asakawa T, et al. Endometrial carcinoma: dynamic MRI with turbo-FLASH technique. *J Comput Assist Tomogr* 1996;20:878–887.

149. Seki H, Kimura M, Sakai K. Myometrial invasion of endometrial carcinoma: assessment with dynamic MR and contrast-enhanced Tl-weighted images. *Clin Radiol* 1997;52:18–23.

150. Hricak H, Rubinstein LV, Gherman GM, Karstaedt N. MR imaging evaluation of endometrial carcinoma: results of an NCI cooperative study. *Radiology* 1991;179:829–832.

151. Kinkel K, Yu KK, Kaji Y, et al. Radiological staging in patients with endometrial cancer: a meta-analysis. *Radiology* 1999: 212:711–718.

152. Sironi S, Colombo E, Villa G, et al. Myometrial invasion by endometrial carcinoma: assessment with plain and gadolinium-enhanced MR imaging. *Radiology* 1992;185:207–212.

153. DelMaschio A, Vanzulli A, Sironi S, et al. Estimating the depth of myometrial involvement by endometrial carcinoma: efficacy of transvaginal sonography vs MR imaging. *AJR Am J Roentgenol* 1993;160: 533–538.

154. Gordon AN, Fleischer AC, Reed GW. Depth of myometrial invasion in endometrial cancer: preoperative assessment by transvaginal ultrasonography. *Gynecol Oncol* 1990;39:321–327.

155. Teefey SA, Stahl JA, Middleton WD, et al. Local staging of endometrial carcinoma: comparison of transvaginal and intraoperative sonography and gross visual inspection. *AJR Am J Roentgenol* 1996;166:547–552.

156. Yamashita Y, Takahaski M, Sawada T, et al. Carcinoma of the cervix: dynamic MR imaging. *Radiology* 1992;182:643–648.

157. Kinkel K, Kaji Y, Yu KK, et al. Radiologic staging in patients with endometrial cancer: a meta-analysis. *Radiology* 1999;212:711–718.

158. Gross BH, Jafri SZH, Glazer GM. Significance of intrauterine gas demonstrated by computed tomography. *J Comput Assist Tomogr* 1983;7:842–845.

159. Hardesty LA, Sumkin JH, Hakim C, et al. The ability of helical CT to preoperatively stage endometrial carcinoma. *AJR Am J Roentgenol* 2001;176:603–606.

160. Ascher SM, Scoutt LM, McCarthy SM, et al. Uterine changes after dilation and curettage: MR imaging findings. *Radiology* 1991;80:433–435.

161. Seki H, Takano T, Sakai K. Value of dynamic MR imaging in assessing endometrial carcinoma involvement of the cervix. *AJR Am J Roentgenol* 2000;175:171–176.

162. DelMaschio A, Vanzulli A, Sironi S, et al. Estimating the depth of myometrial involvement by endometrial carcinoma: efficacy of transvaginal sonography vs MR imaging. *AJR Am J Roentgenol* 1993;160:533–538.

163. Minderhoud-Bassie W, Treurniet FEE, Koops W, et al. Magnetic resonance imaging (MRI) in endometrial carcinoma; preoperative estimation of depth of myometrial invasion. *Acta Obstet Gynecol Scand* 1995;74:827–831.

164. Yamashita Y, Mizutani H, Torashima M, et al. Assessment of myometrial invasion by endometrial carcinoma: transvaginal sonography vs. contrast-enhanced MR imaging. *AJR Am J Roentgenol* 1993;161:595–599.

165. Hulka CA, Hall DA. Endometrial abnormalities associated with tamoxifen therapy for breast cancer: sonographic and pathologic correlation. *AJR Am J Roentgenol* 1993;160:809–812.

166. Takahashi S, Murakami T, Narumi Y, et al. Preoperative staging of endometrial carcinoma: diagnostic effect of T2-weighted fast spin-echo MR imaging. *Radiology* 1998;206:539–547.

167. Barton JW, McCarthy SM, Kohorn EI, et al. Pelvic MR imaging finding in gestational trophoblastic disease, incomplete abortion, and ectopic pregnancy: are they specific? *Radiology* 1993;86:163–168.

168. Brandt KR, Coakley KJ. MR appearance of placental site trophoblastic tumor: a report of three cases. *AJR Am J Roentgenol* 1998;170:485–487.

169. Green CL, Angtuaco TL, Shah HR, Parmley TH. Gestational trophoblastic disease: a spectrum of radiologic diagnosis. *Radiographics* 1996;16:1371–1384.

170. Preidler KW, Luschin G, Tamussino K, et al. Magnetic resonance imaging in patients with gestational trophoblastic disease. *Invest Radiol* 1996;31:492–496.

171. Wagner BJ, Woodward PJ, Dickey GE. From the archives of the AFIP. Gestational trophoblastic disease: radiologic-pathologic correlation. *Radiographics* 1996:16:131–148.

172. Green CL, Angtuaco TL, Shah HR, Parmley TH. Gestational trophoblastic disease: a spectrum of radiologic diagnosis. *Radiographics* 1996;16:1371–1384.

173. Wagner BJ, Woodward PJ, Dickey GE. From the archives of the AFIP. Gestational trophoblastic disease: radiologic-pathologic correlation. *Radiographics* 1996;16:131–148.

174. Lazarus E, Hulka C, Siewert B, Levine D. Sonographic appearance of early complete molar pregnancies. *J Ultrasound Med* 1999;18:589–594.

175. Benson CB, Enest DR, Bernstein MR, et al. Sonographic appearance of first trimester complete hydatidiform moles. *Ultrasound Obstet Gynecol* 2000;16:188–191.

176. Dobkin GR, Berkowitz RS, Goldstein DP, et al. Duplex ultrasonography for persistent gestational trophoblastic tumor. *J Reprod Med* 1991;36:14–16.

177. Taylor KJ, Schwartz PE, Kohorn EI. Gestational trophoblastic neoplasia: diagnosis with Doppler US. *Radiology* 1987;165:445–448.

178. Su WH, Wang PH, Chang SP. Successful treatment of a persistent mole with myometrial invasion by direct injection of methotrexate. *Eur J Gynaecol Oncol* 2001;22:283–286.

179. Miyasaka M, Hachiya J, Furuya Y, et al. CT evaluation of invasive trophoblastic disease. *J Comput Assist Tomogr* 1984;9:459–462.

180. Rose PG. Hydatidiform mole: diagnosis and management. In: Yarbro JW, Bornstein RS, Mastrangelo MJ, MacFeem, eds. *Gestational trophoblastic neoplasia*. Philadelphia: WB Saunders, 1995:149–154.

181. Sanders C, Rubin E. Malignant gestational trophoblastic disease: CT findings. *AJR Am J Roentgenol* 1987;148:165–168.

182. Bagshawe KD, Garnett ES. Radiological changes in the lungs of patients with trophoblastic tumours. *Br J Radiol* 1963;36:673–679.

183. Kohorn EI, McCarthy SM, Taylor KJW. Nonmetastatic gestational trophoblastic neoplasia: role of ultrasonography and magnetic resonance imaging. *J Reprod Med* 1998;43:14–20.

184. Cannistra SA: Cancer of the ovary. *N Engl J Med* 1993;329:1550–1559.

186. Taylor KJW, Schwartz PE. Screening for early ovarian cancer. *Radiology* 1994;192:1–10.

187. Schwartz PE. Nongenetic screening of ovarian malignancies. *Obstet Gynecol Clin* 2001;28:1–13.

188. National Institutes of Health Consensus Development Conference Statement: Ovarian cancer: Screening, treatment, and follow-up. *Gynecol Oncol* 55:S4–S14, 1994.

189. Burke W, Daly M, Garber J, et al. Recommendations for follow-up care of individuals with an inherited predisposition to cancer: II. BRCA1 and BRCA2. *JAMA* 1997;277:997–1003.

190. Bourne TH, Whitehead MI, Campbell S, et al. Ultrasound screening for familial ovarian cancer. *Gynecol Oncol* 1991;43:92–97.

191. Bast RC Jr, Koug TJ, St John E, et al: A radioimmunoassay using a monoclonal antibody to monitor the course of epithelial ovarian cancer. *N Engl J Med* 1983;309:883–887.

192. Einhorn N, Sjovall K, Knapp RC, et al. Prospective evaluation of serum CA 125 levels for early detection of ovarian cancer. *Obstet Gynecol* 1992;80:14–18.

193. Campbell S, Bhan V, Royston P, et al: Transabdominal ultrasound screening for early ovarian cancer. *BMJ* 1989;299:1363–1367.

194. DePriest PD, Van Nagell JR Jr, Gallion HH, et al: Ovarian cancer screening in asymptomatic postmenopausal women. *Gynecol Oncol* 1993;51:205–209.

195. Bourne TH, Campbell S, Reynolds KM, et al: Screening for early familial ovarian cancer with transvaginal ultrasonography and colour flow imaging. *BMJ* 1993;306:1025–1029.

196. Van Nagell JR Jr, Gallion HH, Pavlik EJ, et al: Ovarian cancer screening. *Cancer* 1995;76:2086–2091.

197. Taylor KJW, Schwartz PE. Cancer screening in a high risk population: a clinical trial. *Ultrasound Med Biol* 2001;27:461–466.

198. Jacobs IJ, Skates SJ, MacDonald N, et al. Screening for ovarian cancer: a pilot randomized controlled trial. *Lancet* 1999;353:1207–1210.

199. Van Nagell JR, DePriest PD, Reedy MB, et al. The efficacy of transvaginal sonographic screening in asymptomatic women at risk for ovarian cancer. *Gynecol Oncol* 2000;77:350–356.

200. Troiano RN, Quedans-Case C, Taylor KJW. Correlation of findings on transvaginal sonography with serum CA125 levels. *AJR Am J Roentgenol* 1997;168:1587–1590.

201. Brown DL, Frates MC, Laing FC, et al. Ovarian masses: can benign and malignant lesions be differentiated with color and pulsed Doppler US? *Radiology* 1994;190:333–336.

202. Buy JN, Ghossain MA, Hugol D, et al. Characterization of adnexal masses: combination of color Doppler and conventional sonography compared with spectral Doppler analysis alone and conventional sonography alone. *AJR Am J Roentgenol* 1996;166:385–393.

203. DiSantis DJ, Scatarige JC, Kemp G, et al. A prospective evaluation of transvaginal sonography for detection of ovarian disease. *AJR Am J Roentgenol* 1993;161:91–94.

204. Mendelson EB, Bohm-Velez M. Transvaginal ultrasonography of pelvic neoplasms. *Radiol Clin North Am* 1992;230:703–734.

205. Jain KA. Prospective evaluation of adnexal masses with endovaginal gray-scale and duplex and color Doppler US: correlation with pathologic findings. *Radiology* 1994;191:63–67.

206. Stein SM, Laifer-Narin S, Johnson MB, et al. Differentation of benign and malignant adnexal masses: relative value of gray-scale, color Doppler, and spectral Doppler sonography. *AJR Am J Roentgenol* 1995;164:381–386.

207. Timor-Tritsch IE, Lerner JP, Monteagudo A, Santos R. Transvaginal ultrasonographic characterization of ovarian masses by means of color

flow-directed Doppler measurements and a morphologic system. *Am J Obstet Gynecol* 1993;168:909–913.

208. DePriest PD, Varner E, Powell J, et al. The efficacy of a sonographic morphology index in identifying ovarian cancer: a multi-institutional investigation. *Gynecol Oncol* 1994;55:174–178.

209. Kurjak A, Predanic M. New scoring system for prediction of ovarian malignancy based on transvaginal color Doppler sonography. *J Ultrasound Med* 1992;11:631–638.

210. Brown DL, Doubilet PM, Miller FH, et al. Benign and malignant ovarian masses; selection of the most discriminating gray-scale and Doppler sonographic features. *Radiology* 1998;208:103–110.

211. Timmerman D, Schwarzler P, Collins WP, et al. Subjective assessment of adnexal masses with the use of ultrasonography: an analysis of interobserver variability and experience. *Ultrasound Obstet Gynecol* 1999;13:8–10.

212. Hamper UM, Sheth S, Abbas FM, et al. Transvaginal color Doppler sonography of adnexal masses: differences in blood flow impedance in benign and malignant lesions. *AJR Am J Roentgenol* 1993;160:1225–1228.

213. Kurjak A, Predanic M, Kupesic-Urek S, Jukie S. Transvaginal color and pulsed Doppler assessment of adnexal tumor vascularity. *Gynecol Oncol* 1993;50:3–9.

214. Levine D, Feldstein VA, Babcock CJ, Filly RA. Sonography of ovarian masses: poor sensitivity of resistive index for identifying malignant lesions. *AJR Am J Roentgenol* 1994;162:1355–1359.

215. Fleischer AC, Brader KR. Sonographic depiction of ovarian vascularity and flow: current improvements and future applications. *J Ultrasound Med* 2001;20:241–250.

216. Buy JN, Ghossain MA, Sciot C, et al. Epithelial tumors of the ovary: CT findings and correlation with US. *Radiology* 1991;1178:811–818.

217. Ghossain MA, Buy JN, Ligneres C, et al. Epithelial tumors of the ovary: comparison of MR and CT findings. *Radiology* 1991;181:863–870.

218. Kim SH, Kim WH, Park KJ, et al. CT and MR findings of Krukenberg tumors: comparison with primary ovarian tumors. *Comput Assist Tomogr* 1996;20:393–398.

219. Stevens SK, Hricak H, Stern JL. Ovarian lesions: detection and characterization with gadolinium-enhanced MR imaging at 1.5 T. *Radiology* 1991;181:481–488.

220. Thurnher SA. MR imaging of pelvic masses in women: contrast-enhanced vs unenhanced images. *AJR Am J Roentgenol* 1992;159:1243–1250.

221. Ha HK, Baek SY, Kim SH, et al. Krukenberg's tumor of the ovary: MR imaging features. *AJR Am J Roentgenol* 1995;164:1435–1439.

222. Hata K, Hata T, Manabe A, et al. A critical evaluation of transvaginal Doppler studies, transvaginal sonography, magnetic resonance imaging and CA 125 in detecting ovarian cancer. *Obstet Gynecol* 1992;80:922–926.

223. Komatsu T, Konishi I, Mandai M, et al. Adnexal masses: transvaginal US and gadolinium-enhanced MR imaging assessment of intratumoral structure. *Radiology* 1996;198:109–115.

224. Jain KA, Friedman DL, Pettinger TW, et al. Adnexal masses: comparison of specificity of endovaginal US and pelvic MR imaging. *Radiology* 1993;186:697–704.

225. Outwater EK, Dunton CJ. Imaging of the ovary and adnexa: clinical issues and applications of MR imaging. *Radiology* 1995;194:1–18.

226. Hubner KF, McDonald TW, Niethammer JG, et al. Assessment of primary and metastatic ovarian cancer by positron emission tomography (PET) using 2-[18-F]deoxyglucose(2-[18F]FDG). *Gynecol Oncol* 1993;51:197–204.

227. Shroder W, Zimny C, Rudlowski C, et al. The role of 18 F-fluorodeoxyglucose positron emission tomography (18F-FDG PET) in diagnosis of ovarian cancer. *Int J Gynecol Cancer* 1999;9:117–122.

228. Buchsbaum HJ, Lifshitz S. Staging and surgical evaluation of ovarian cancer. *Semin Oncol* 1984;11:227–237.

229. Kurtz AB, Tsimikas JV, Tempany CMC, et al. Diagnosis and staging of ovarian cancer: comparative values of Doppler and conventional US, CT, and MR imaging correlated with surgery and histopathologic analysis—report of the Radiology Diagnostic Oncology Group. *Radiology* 1999;212:19–27.

230. Tempany CMC, Zou KH, Silverman SG, et al. Staging of advanced ovarian cancer: comparison of imaging modalities—report from the Radiological Diagnostic Oncology Group. *Radiology* 2000;215:761–767.

231. Buy JN, Moss AA, Ghossain MA, et al. Peritoneal implants from ovarian tumors: CT findings. *Radiology* 1988;169:691–694.

232. Mitchell DG, Hill MC, Hill S, Zaloudek C. Serous carcinoma of the ovary: CT identification of metastatic calcified implants. *Radiology* 1986;158:649–652.

233. Forstner R, Hricak H, Occhipinti KA, et al. Ovarian cancer: staging with CT and MR imaging. *Radiology* 1995;197:6l9–622.

234. Meyer JI, Kennedy AW, Friedman R, et al. Ovarian carcinoma: value of CT in predicting success of debulking surgery. *AJR Am J Roentgenol* 1995;165,875–878.

235. Murolo C, Constantini S, Foglia G, et al. Ultrasound examination in ovarian cancer patients. A comparison with second look laparotomy. *J Ultrasound Med* 1989;8:441–443.

236. Khan O, Cosgrove DO, Fried AM, Savage PE. Ovarian carcinoma follow-up: US versus laparotomy. *Radiology* 1986;159:111–113.

237. Goldhirsch A, Triller JK, Greiner R, et al. Computed tomography prior to second-look operation in advanced ovarian cancer. *Obstet Gynecol* 1983;62:630–634.

238. Low RN, Carter WD, Saleh F, Sigeti JS. Ovarian cancer: comparison of findings with perfluorocarbon-enhanced MR imaging, In-111–CYT-103 immunoscintigraphy, and CT. *Radiology* 1995;195:391–400.

239. Megibow AJ, Bosniak MA, Ho AG, et al. Accuracy of CT in detection of persistent or recurrent ovarian carcinoma: correlation with second-look laparotomy. *Radiology* 1988;166:341–345.

240. Prayer L, Kainz C, Kramer J, et al. CT and MR accuracy in the detection of tumor recurrence in patients treated for ovarian cancer. *J Comput Assist Tomogr* 1993;17:626–632.

241. Reuter KL, Griffin T, Hunter RE. Comparison of abdominopelvic computed tomography results and findings at second-look laparotomy in ovarian carcinoma patients. *Cancer* 1989;63:1123–1128.

242. Silverman PM, Osborne M, Dunnick NR, Bandy LC. CT prior to second-look operation in ovarian cancer. *AJR Am J Roentgenol* 1988;150:829–832.

243. Forstner R, Hricak H, Powell CB, et al. Ovarian cancer recurrence: value of MR imaging. *Radiology* 1995;196:715–720.

244. Chance B, Collins JM, Eckelman WC, et al. Report of the Joint Working Group on Quantitative In Vivo Functional Imaging in Oncology. *Acad Radiol* 1999 (*in press*).

Therapeutic Modalities and Related Subjects

CHAPTER 11

Perioperative and Critical Care

James J. Burke II, Janet L. Osborne, and Christopher K. Senkowski

Surgery remains the mainstay of treatment for women with gynecologic malignancies. Ultimately, outcomes of the surgical intervention rest with the gynecologic oncologist in concert with anesthesiologists, nursing staff, stomal therapists, physical therapists, pharmacists, social workers, and the social network/support of the patient as well as others. Careful assessment of the patient prior to surgery can lead to improved outcomes and minimize surprises in the postoperative period. Should the need arise, prudent consultation with other medical specialists prior to or following surgery can further enhance patient care, and result in better outcomes.

We have divided the chapter into two sections: preoperative care/risk recognition and postoperative care/critical care. Within each section, clinical information has been arranged by organ system and recommendations are based upon evidence (if available). The critical care section provides basic, yet practical, information for the reader so that co-management of the critically ill gynecologic oncology patient with an intensivist may be seamless.

PREOPERATIVE RISK ASSESSMENT

Initial Preoperative Evaluation

When patients are found to have a gynecologic malignancy (or suspicion is high as in the case of an adnexal mass), hopefully, they are referred to a gynecologic oncologist for

James J. Burke II: Department of Gynecology and Obstetrics. Division of Gynecologic Oncology, Mercer University School of Medicine, Memorial Health University Medical Center (Savannah), Savannah, Georgia 31404

Janet L. Osborne: Department of Obstetrics and Gynecology, Division of Gynecologic Oncology, Medical College of Wisconsin, Froedtert Memorial Lutheran Hospital, Milwaukee, Wisconsin 53228

Christopher K. Senkowski: Department of Gynecology and Obstetrics, Division of Gynecologic Oncology and Department of Surgery, Mercer University School of Medicine, Memorial Health University Medical Center (Savannah), Savannah, Georgia 31404

consultation and ultimate treatment. During this meeting, the gynecologic oncologist should take a thorough history, assessing for co-morbid conditions, which may impact perioperative risk [1]. Similarly, a thorough physical examination, looking for signs of diseases of which the patient is unaware, will aid in finding diseases that can impact surgical outcome. Review of accompanying medical records and radiographs is important. Ultimately, those patients who will benefit from surgery will be identified and will be deemed operative candidates, operative candidates who need further evaluation from specialists prior to surgery, or inoperable candidates. Subsequent discussions should focus on the course of treatment. If surgical, the planned operative procedure should be described to the patient in nonmedical terminology. Attendant risks of the procedure should be described to the patient as well as alternatives for therapy (if they exist). The length of time for the operation and length of anticipated hospital stay should be estimated for the patient and her family. These elements of the treatment plan constitute *informed consent,* and should be documented in the medical record by the physician at the initial consultation. Preferably, this "consenting" should be done before the patient is in the preoperative holding area on the day of her surgery. Should further evaluation be needed from a specialist (e.g., a cardiologist or a pulmonologist), a letter outlining the proposed surgical intervention should be sent to the consultant.

Ideally, laboratory data will be dictated by findings from the history and physical examination. However, most institutions have a "battery" of required laboratory testing prior to surgical intervention. A logical review of laboratory testing is available and we refer the reader to this review [2]. Table 11.1 shows recommendations for laboratory testing prior to surgery, the incidences of abnormalities, which influence changes in surgical management, and the indications for each test. Further, minimal evaluation for specific co-morbid disease states will be presented in the following sections of this chapter.

If the patient's condition requires the possibility of a stoma(s) (colostomy or urostomy), consultation with an enter

TABLE 11.1. *Recommended preoperative laboratory assessments with indications for testing*

Test	Incidence of abnormalities that influence management (%)	Indications
Hemoglobin	0.1	Anticipated major blood loss or symptoms of anemia
White blood cell count	0.0	Symptoms which suggest infection, myeloproliferative disorder, or myelotoxic medications
Platelet count	0.0	History of bleeding diathesis, myeloproliferative disorder, or myelotoxic medications
Prothrombin time	0.0	History of bleeding diathesis, chronic liver disease, malnutrition, recent or long-term antibiotic use
Partial thromboplastin time	0.1	History of bleeding diathesis
Electrolytes	1.8	Known renal insufficiency, CHF, medications which affect electrolytes
Renal function	2.6	Age >50 years, hypertension, cardiac disease, major surgery, diabetes, medications which affect renal function
Glucose	0.5	Obesity or known diabetes
Liver function tests	0.1	No indication. Consider albumin measurement for major surgery or chronic illness
Urinalysis	1.4	No indication
Electrocardiogram	2.6	Age >50 years, known CAD, diabetes, or hypertension
Chest radiograph	3.0	Age >50 years, known cardiac or pulmonary disease, symptoms or exam suggesting cardiac or pulmonary disease.

CHF, congestive heart failure; CAD, coronary artery disease.
Adapted from Smetana GW, Macpherson DS. The case against routine preoperative laboratory testing. *Med Clin N Am* 2003; 87 : 7–40, with permission.

ostomal therapist for marking of the planned stoma(s) should be considered. During this visit, the therapist will take into account the location of the patient's "waist," how she wears her clothing, the types of clothing she wears, and the location of the future stoma when she stands or sits. In addition, the therapist can initiate education on the function and care of the stoma(s).

Should the proposed surgery result in a marked change of body image or possible sexual dysfunction (e.g., exenteration, radical vulvectomy, or vaginal reconstruction), consultation with prior patients who have successfully recovered from similar operations may be warranted. In addition, these patients may benefit from psychologic counseling prior to their surgery.

Assessment of Cardiac Risk

Any gynecologic oncologist must be aware of the underestimation of cardiac disease in women when evaluating cardiac risk preoperatively. In the last decade, a great deal of literature has been published on this subject. In 2001, the National Heart, Lung and Blood Institute (NHLBI) launched the Heart Truth Project to promote education about heart disease among women (3). Statistics have shown that only one of three primary physicians correctly cited coronary artery disease as a leading cause of death in women. Similarly, studies have demonstrated that women are less often counseled on cardiac risk factors, less often prescribed lipid-lowering medications, less often offered invasive procedures and less often prescribed cardiac rehabilitation. Further, compared to men, women who had a myocardial infarction (MI) had a greater interval from onset of pain until arrival at hospital, were less likely to be treated with thrombolytics and beta-blocking agents, were less often evaluated with invasive methods, had higher rates of reinfarction, and had greater mortality (3).

In the assessment of perioperative risk, cardiac risk factors are certainly one of the top concerns for clinicians. There have been a number of reviews and different systems created for the purposes of assessing cardiac risk for patients undergoing noncardiac surgery (4–7). Realize that approximately 1 in 12 patients (>65 years old) will have significant coronary artery disease (8). It is estimated that over 30% of patients undergoing major elective surgery have at least one cardiac risk factor (9).

Cardiac risk indices have been published by at least 10 different investigators (10). Goldman et al. published the Multifactorial Index of Cardiac Risk (MICR) in 1977 (11). This risk index was the first, large, prospective multivariate analysis of patients undergoing noncardiac surgery. They used definite endpoints of cardiac death, ventricular tachycardia, pulmonary edema, and myocardial infarction. The MICR involves nine independent risk factors to create a point risk index and predict morbidity and mortality (Tables 11.2 and 11.3). One weakness of this index is underestimating risk in vascular surgery patients. Nonetheless, these crite-

TABLE 11.2. *Multifactorial index of cardiac risk (MICR)*

Risk factor	Points
S3 gallop or increased jugular venous pressure	11
Myocardial infarction in previous 6 months	10
More than five premature ventricular ectopic beats per minute	7
Rhythm other than sinus or premature atrial contractions	7
Age > 70 years	5
Emergency non-cardiac operative procedure	4
Significant aortic stenosis	3
Poor general health status	3
Abdominal or thoracic surgery	3
Possible total	53

Adapted from Goldman L, Caldera DL, Nussbaum SR, et al. Multifactorial index of cardiac risk in noncardiac surgical procedures. *N Engl J Med* 1977;297:845–80.

ria have been validated and have stood the test of time. Others have tried to revise the index including Detsky et al. (12), who made it much more complicated, and Lee et al. (13) who simplified it, but added recommendations for preoperative testing. In response to a shift in the literature from calculation of risk with indices to clinical decision making, especially in regard to the need for preoperative evaluation, the American College of Cardiology/American Heart Association (ACC-AHA) guidelines were developed (14) (Fig. 11.1).

Clearly, the approach to the patient must include a careful history and physical examination. Initially, age greater than 70 years was thought to be a risk factor for cardiac morbidity, but a recent clinical trial showed no increased, independent risk for cardiac complications (15). Any prior history of cardiac disease such as angina, myocardial infarction (MI), arrhythmia, pulmonary edema, or valvular disease must be elaborated. Patients with unstable angina, recent myocardial infarction, class III-IV heart failure, decompensated congestive failure, or aortic stenosis present the highest risk. These patients will likely require further invasive testing. Those patients with a history of a prior MI, mild angina, class I-II heart failure, and compensated congestive heart failure (CHF) will fall into a lower tier for noninvasive evaluation (Figure 11.1).

TABLE 11.3. *Multifactorial index of cardiac risk (MICR), cardiac risk class, morbidity and mortality*

Cardiac risk (%)	Total points	Morbidity (%)	Mortality
Class I	0–5	0.7	0.2
Class II	6–12	5.0	1.6
Class III	12–25	11.5	2.3
Class IV	>26	22.2	55.6

Adapted from Goldman L, Caldera DL, Nussbaum SR, et al. Multifactorial index of cardiac risk in noncardiac surgical procedures. *N. Engl J Med* 1977;297:845–850.

In patients without overt cardiac risks, other factors are considered to be helpful for uncovering subclinical disease. Classically, these risk factors are smoking, hyperlipidemia, hypertension, and diabetes mellitus.

In 1996, the ACC-AHA published guidelines, which have recently been updated in 2002 (14). With the recent explosion in invasive, interventional techniques as well as the new data on beta blockade, the algorithm has been refocused (Fig. 11.1) The classification defines clinical predictors as major, intermediate, and minor. In addition, the guidelines now utilize functional capacity in terms of metabolic equivalents (METs), with a level <4 being considered poor. The ability to climb one flight of stairs or walk up a hill would classify the patient in the >4 group.

Testing available for further evaluation include both invasive and noninvasive methods. Echocardiography can predict postoperative CHF in patients with ejection fractions (EF) less than 35% (16). Unfortunately, echocardiography cannot reliably predict ischemia. However, echocardiography is quite useful in the evaluation of valvular diseases and for follow-up of patients with known left ventricular (LV) dysfunction.

Stress testing either by exercise or by chemical induction provides valuable information for perioperative ischemic risk. Nuclear scintigraphy with evaluation of perfusion defects has shown a positive predictive value of 12% to 16% and a negative predictive value of 99% (17). Dobutamine stress echocardiography has shown similar predictive values.

The algorithm provides a way to segregate patients who should have their surgery delayed for further cardiac evaluation because of a recent MI; who should have their CHF optimized; or who should optimize control of dysrhythmias. In selected patients, it may be that coronary revascularization, angioplasty, stent placement, or valve replacement is prudent before the planned noncardiac surgery.

The risks of reinfarction after a recent MI are clearly related to the timing of an event, which could precipitate an MI. However, these rates have been declining secondary to improved perioperative care. Reported reinfarction rates have dropped from 37% in patients undergoing surgery within 3 months following MI to more recent figures of 5% to 10%. The rates fall even further the longer the interval from the original MI, with rates of reinfarction being 2% to 3% in the 4 to 6 months following and 1% to 2% after 6 months (18).

Perioperative Beta Blockade

In 1996, a multicenter, randomized, placebo-controlled trial was published that evaluated the use of beta blockade with atenolol versus placebo in patients undergoing noncardiac surgery (19). Although no differences in perioperative mortality or MI were seen, the atenolol group had significantly fewer ischemic episodes (24% vs 39%). Furthermore, in a 2-year follow-up, the atenolol group had a decreased

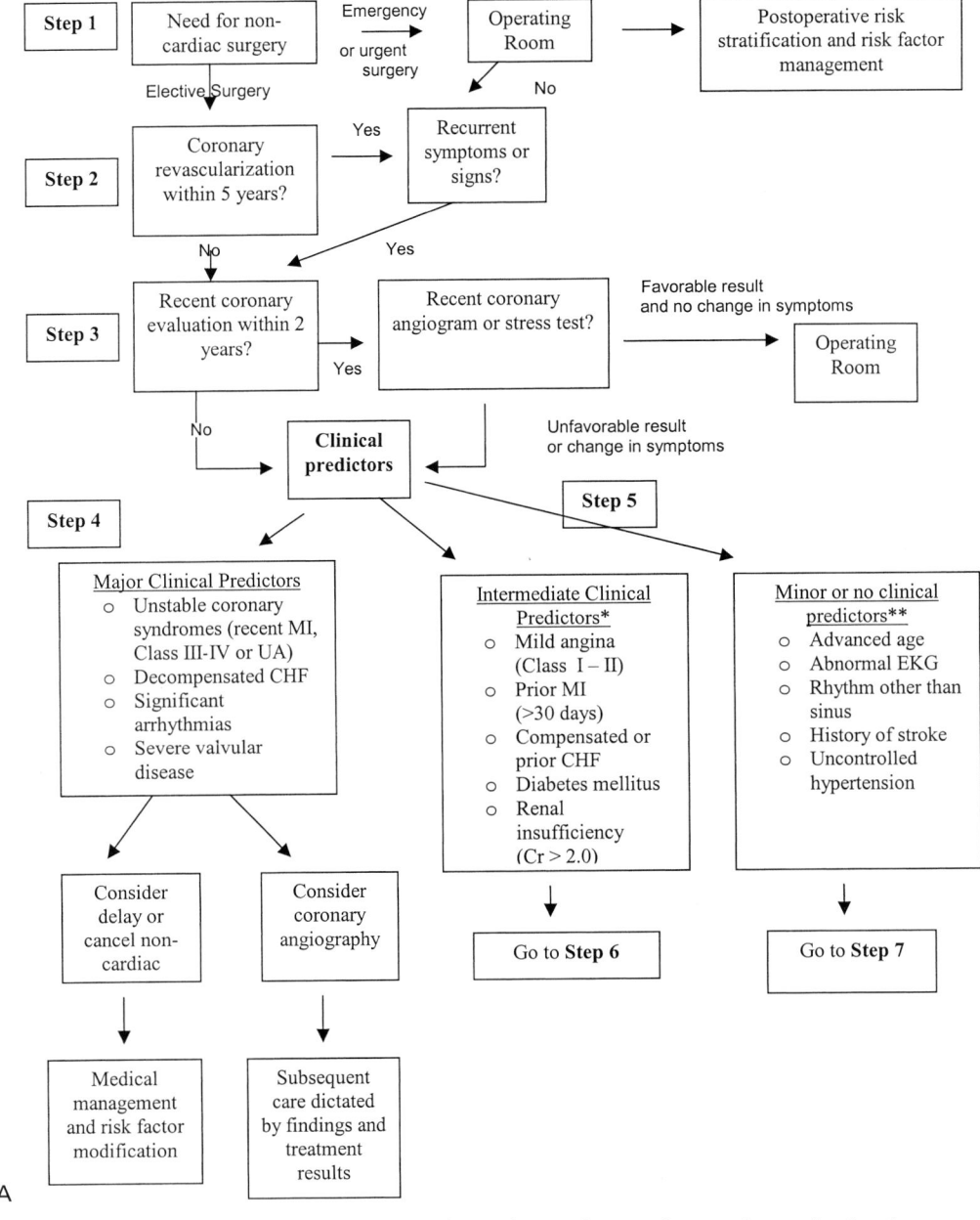

A

FIG. 11-1. A–C: ACC/AHA guideline update for perioperative cardiovascular evaluation for noncardiac surgery: a report of the American College of Cardiology/American Heart Association Task Force on Practice Guidelines (Committee to Update the 1996 Guidelines on Perioperative Cardiovascular Evaluation for Noncardiac Surgery). American College of Cardiology Web site. 2002. Available: www.acc.org/clinical/guidelines/perio/ update/periupdate_index.htm. Accessed Nov 15, 2002. MI, myocardial infarction; UA, unstable angina. (Adapted from Eagle KA, Berger PB, Calkins H, et al.) *(Figure continues.)*

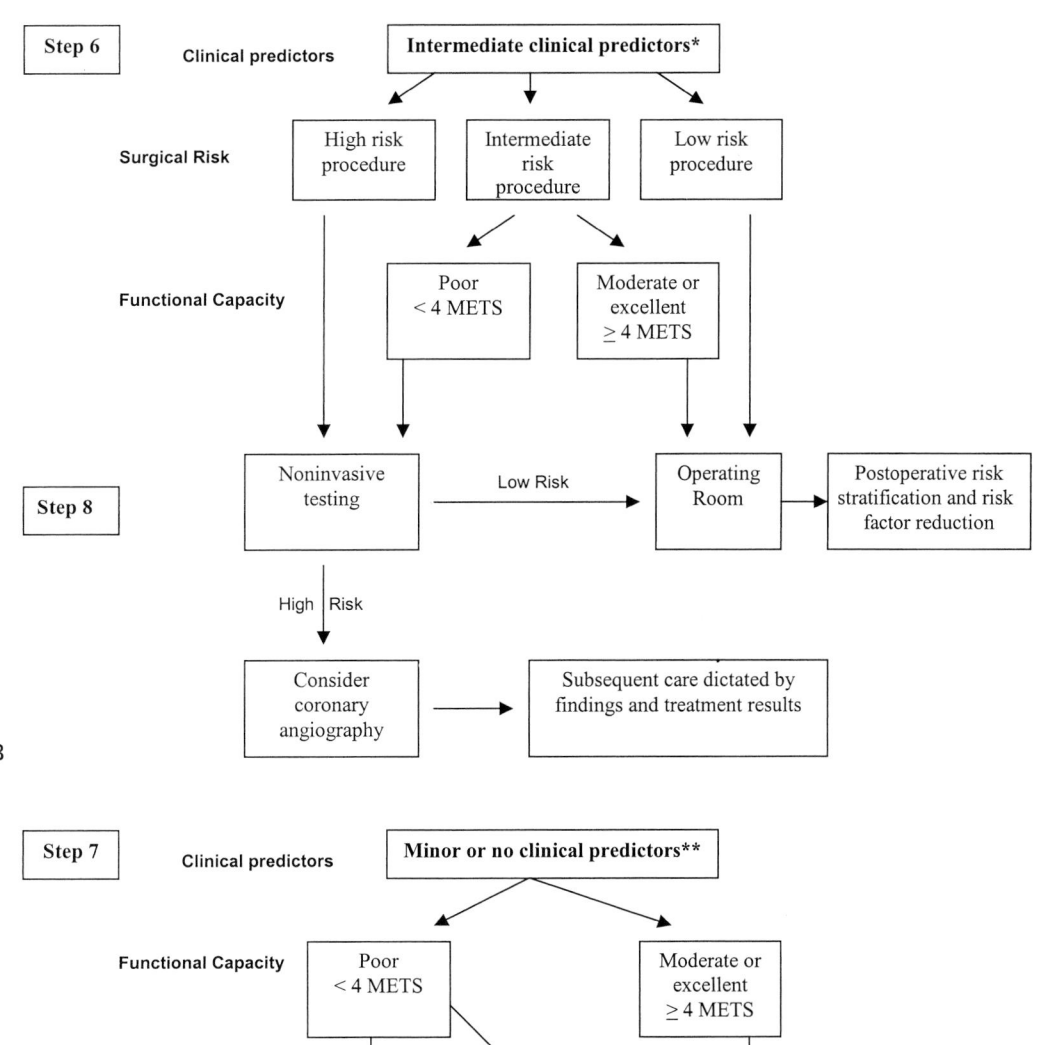

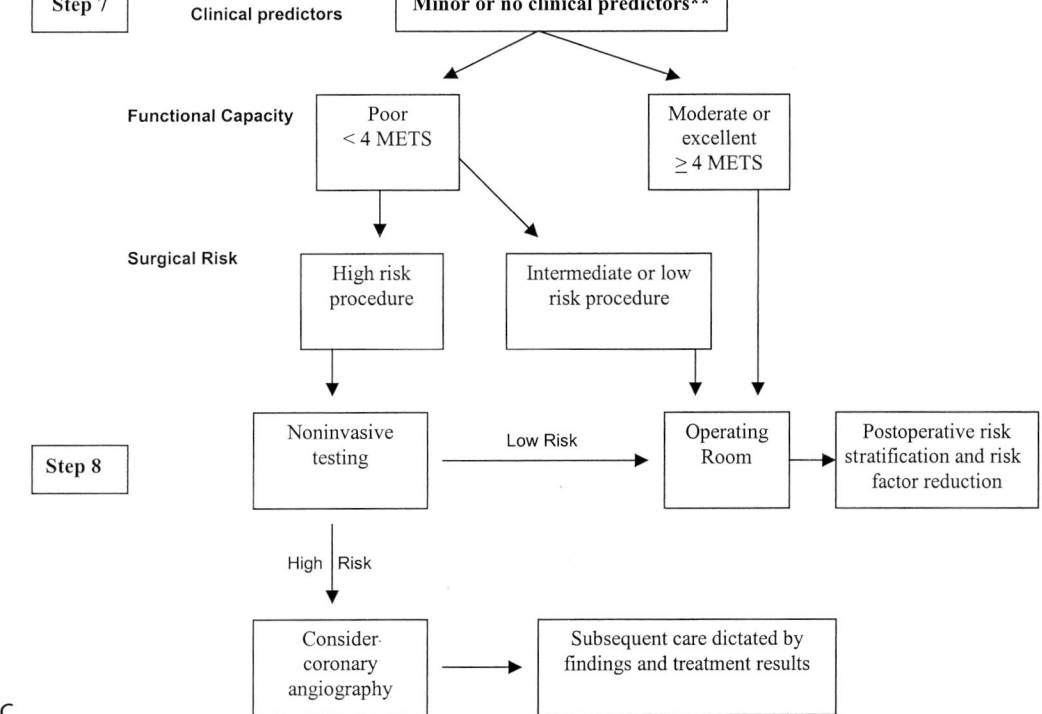

FIG. 11-1. Continued.

mortality (9 vs 21 deaths) and decreased number of cardiac events (16 vs. 32). Based on the findings of this study, patients with or at risk for coronary artery disease should receive preoperative and postoperative beta blockade.

Pulmonary Risk Assessment

Postoperative pulmonary complications represent a significant cause for morbidity and mortality in patients undergoing elective surgery. Approximately 25% of deaths within the early postoperative period (first week) are related to pulmonary issues. Pulmonary complications after major abdominal surgery range from 20% to 30% (20). Laparotomy results in a 45% decrease in vital capacity and a 20% reduction in functional residual capacity (FRC) (21). When the patient is in the supine position, FRC is reduced below alveolar closing volume (i.e., the volume at which point alveoli start closing) results in atelectasis (22).

When examining risk factors for postoperative pulmonary problems, a number of issues surface. General medical status (e.g., functional status, obesity, nutrition) is related to postoperative pulmonary complications (PPCs) (23). A history of congestive failure, renal failure, poor mental status, and immunosuppression are all associated with a higher PPC rate (24). Surgical issues such as the type of incision (thoracic and upper abdominal worse than midline or lower abdominal), duration of anesthetic (>2 hours), the use of a nasogastric tube (increased risk), and the use of parenteral (increased risk) versus epidural (decreased risk) analgesics are all correlated with PPC incidence (25).

In terms of direct pulmonary risk factors, the most common preexisting pulmonary disease is chronic obstructive pulmonary disease (COPD) (26). These patients retain carbon dioxide, have poor gas exchange, and have an increased residual volume. Smoking use, history of dyspnea, pneumonia and sleep apnea are other risk categories. Patients with asthma and other restrictive lung diseases (low FVC with normal FeV_1/FVC ratio) have minimal increased risk for PPC (27).

When interpreting the usual preoperative radiographic and laboratory values, several caveats must be kept in mind. A preoperative chest radiograph in normal adults has no predictive value other than providing essential baseline data for an at-risk patient. Arterial blood gas analysis in prospective trials has been shown not to be useful in providing risk stratification. However, it is useful in providing baseline data for patients with preexisting disease; that is, COPD (28). Preoperative pulmonary function tests (PFTs) have few supporting clinical trials other than in preparation for lung resection where they are clearly beneficial (29). A consensus statement was forwarded from the American College of Physicians in 1990 that recommended preoperative PFTs in the following settings: in patients with a history of smoking or dyspnea scheduled to undergo upper abdominal operations, coronary bypass, or lung resection; in patients with unex-

plained pulmonary disease; and in patients with planned extensive lower abdominal, head and neck, or orthopedic operations (30). It would appear from the data that PFTs are overutilized. In the case of major abdominal surgery in a patient with moderate to severe COPD, however, they may aid greatly in risk stratification and in providing baseline data.

Preoperative and perioperative strategies for reducing risk of PPCs include pulmonary expansion, smoking cessation, and optimization of gas exchange. Although preoperative and postoperative incentive spirometery has shown mixed results in reducing the rate of pulmonary complications, it continues to be widely recommended (31), and it should be considered as a preventive strategy for any patient undergoing laparotomy. In order to maximize patient compliance, preoperative counseling and education is necessary. Clearly, COPD must be optimized with control of infection and maximizing medical regimens. Reactive airway disease should be prevented with use of perioperative inhalation therapy such as beta agonists. Steroid therapy is generally reserved for patients already utilizing them as part of their medical regimen. These steroid-dependent patients will need stress-dose steroids to prevent insufficiency (see below). Prophylactic antibiotics are not indicated in COPD patients to prevent pulmonary infections.

Smoking-cessation programs have had an unclear effect on postoperative pulmonary complications (32). Although the data consist of poorly controlled trials, it appears that short-term abstinence (<8 weeks from the time of surgery) may actually increase the complication rate (33). Abstinence for greater than 10 weeks showed complication rates similar to nonsmokers (34). Unfortunately, the long-term success rates of smoking-cessation programs is low, and in the case of malignancy, the gynecologic oncologist rarely has the opportunity to delay the operation for 8 to 10 weeks.

Endocrinologic Risk Assessment

Diabetes

The incidence of diabetes is rising because of the obesity pandemic, the sedentary lifestyle of Americans, and the rapidly aging population (35). Interestingly, one-third to one-half of these patients are unaware that they have diabetes and are currently receiving no treatment. It is only during preoperative evaluation for elective surgery or acute hospitalization that most of those patients will be diagnosed (36). Understanding the basic physiology of diabetes and how it impacts perioperative risk is crucial for the surgeon.

There are two types of diabetes of concern for the surgeon. Type 1 diabetes occurs as a result of insulinopenia, with all type 1 diabetics being insulin dependent. In the absence of sufficient insulin, these patients are prone to ketosis. Type 1 diabetics account for approximately 10% of all diabetics. Type 2 diabetes occurs as a result of insulin resistance and impaired insulin secretion. Type 2 diabetics may be treated with diet alone, oral hypoglycemic agents, or insulin. These patients account for approximately 90% of all diabetics (37). Intraoperative as well as postoperative glycemic control is dictated by the type of diabetes a patient has.

When evaluating patients with diabetes for surgery, attention should be directed toward the long-term complications of diabetes, as these can impact perioperative risk. Most complications of diabetes are related to microvascular changes, such as diabetic retinopathy, neuropathy, nephropathy, and cardiovascular disease (38). In addition to a thorough history and physical examination, preoperative studies should include an electrocardiogram to rule out a prior ''silent'' MI (especially in patients with diabetes for than 10 years), serum creatinine and blood urea nitrogen and urinary analyses to assess renal function, and a hemoglobin A_{1c} to evaluate recent glycemic control. Should abnormalities be found, consultation with an appropriate specialist should be entertained (39). Ultimately, the type of diabetes, preoperative glycemic control, the extent and magnitude of the intended surgery, the elective or emergent nature of that surgery, and other co-morbid medical conditions will affect the metabolic changes these patients face intraoperatively and postoperatively.

The physiologic changes that diabetic patients encounter during surgery all result in a hyperglycemic state. The stress of surgery increases secretion of epinephrine, norepinephrine, cortisol, and growth hormone, all of which directly antagonize insulin action (40,41). In addition, gluconeogenesis and lipolysis are increased with mobilization of glucose precursors, and a net protein catabolism ensues. All of these factors affect ketosis and acidosis and require intraoperative glucose measurement, especially if the surgery last longer than 2 hours.

Although diabetic patients with vascular disease are at risk of silent postoperative MI and acute renal failure, postoperative infections (respiratory, urinary, and wound infections) account for about two-thirds of all postoperative complications and 20% of all postoperative deaths among diabetics undergoing surgery (42,43). Hyperglycemia has been shown to impair phagocytic function and chemotaxis of granulocytes when glucose levels are higher than 250 mg/dL (44). Other wound complications such as superficial wound dehiscence or fascial dehiscence are common among diabetic patients because of suppressed collagen synthesis by glucose levels higher than 200 mg/dL (45).

Although no prospective studies demonstrating better perioperative outcome from tight glycemic control in diabetics undergoing surgery have been done, several retrospective studies of diabetics undergoing cardiac surgery suggest a lower incidence of postoperative wound infections and complications (46–48). Similarly, a randomized prospective study of intensive insulin therapy (maintaining glucose levels between 80 and 110 mg/dL) versus conventional insulin therapy (glucose levels between 180 and 200 mg/dL) in critically ill postoperative patients demonstrated a 46% reduction in episodes of septicemia and a 34% reduction of in hospital mortality (49).

Glycemic control during surgery will depend upon the type of diabetes the patient has, the medications currently being utilized for treatment, the expected length of time that the patient will be nil per os (NPO), and the type of surgery the patient is having. Patients who are taking oral hypoglycemic agents for control should not take their morning dose on the day of surgery (because of the longer half-life of metformin and chlorpropamide, patients should be instructed to stop these medications 24 to 48 hours prior to surgery) (39). Table 11.4 shows recommendations for management of diabetic patients undergoing surgery (39).

Thyroid Disorders

When patients give history of hypothyroidism or hyperthyroidism during evaluation for surgery, thyroid-stimulating hormone (TSH) and thyroxine (T4) levels should be obtained. The primary objective is to determine if the patient

TABLE 11.4. *Management of diabetes mellitus during surgery*

Type	Minor surgery	Major surgery
Type I		
DM on insulin therapy	1/2–2/3 of usual a.m. insulin dose SQ	IV insulin infusion during surgery—frequent blood glucose monitoring necessary
Type II		
DM controlled with diet alone	No insulin during surgery	No insulin during surgery
DM controlled with oral medications	No insulin during surgery	Insulin may be required during surgery—frequent blood glucose monitoring may be required
DM poorly controlled with oral medications	Insulin may be required during surgery—frequent blood glucose monitoring may be required	IV insulin infusion during surgery—frequent blood glucose monitoring necessary

DM, diabetes mellitus; IV, intravenous; SQ, subcutaneous.
Adapted from Schiff RL, Welsh GA. Perioperative evaluation and management of the patient with endocrine dysfunction. *Med Clin N Am* 2003;87(1):175–192, with permission.

is euthyroid or mildly abnormal prior to surgical intervention so as to avoid the complications of myxedema or thyroid storm in the postoperative period.

Decisions to operate on patients with hypothyroidism will depend upon the level of hypothyroidism and the urgency of the surgery. Hypothyroidism can influence many physiologic functions such as myocardial function, respiration, gastrointestinal motility, hemostasis, and free water balance (39). Although there have been no prospective randomized studies looking at the surgical outcome of hypothyroid patients versus controls, several retrospective case-matched control studies have evaluated hypothyroid patients undergoing surgery. A study by Weinberg et al. demonstrated no differences between hypothyroid and euthyroid controls for perioperative complications. In addition, no differences in outcome were seen when hypothyroidism was stratified by thyroxine levels. The investigators concluded that patients with mild to moderate hypothyroidism should not be denied needed surgery in order to correct the metabolic problem. They further stated that insufficient numbers of patients with severe hypothyroidsim precluded recommendations for perioperative care of these patients (50). In another retrospective study, Ladenson reviewed perioperative complications among hypothyroid patients undergoing surgery, finding more intraoperative hypotension in noncardiac surgery, more heart failure in cardiac surgery, and more gastrointestinal and neuropsychiatric complications. They also noted that patients were unable to mount fever in the face of infection, although infection rates where not different. Further, no differences where found in the duration of hospitalization, perioperative arrhythmias, delayed anesthesia recovery, pulmonary complications, or mortality (51).

Patients with mild to moderate hypothyroidsim requiring urgent surgery may have it without delay. These patients may have more minor complications of ileus, postoperative delirium, or infection without fever. Patients with severe hypothyroidism (myxedema coma, decreased mentation, pericardial effusions, heart failure or very low levels of thyroxine) who are to undergo urgent/emergent surgery will need intravenous thyroxine and stress-dose glucocorticoids (see below) started prior to, during, and continued after surgery (52). Patients who develop seizures, coma, unexplained heart failure, hypothermia, prolonged ileus, or postoperative delirium should be evaluated for undiagnosed hypothyroidism or myxedematous coma (53–55).

Patients using thyroid replacement preparations can have their doses withheld during the immediate postoperative period until they are able to tolerate oral intake, as the half-life of these drugs is 5 to 9 days (39).

Most complications occurring in hyperthyroid patients undergoing surgery involve cardiac function, as T4 and T3 have a direct inotropic and chronotropic effect on the heart. Atrial fibrillation occurs in 10% to 20% of patients (56–59). The greatest perioperative risk for patients who have undiagnosed hyperthyroidism or who are inadequately treated is a rare, yet life-threatening, condition know as thyroid storm. Thyroid storm should be considered in any postoperative patient with fever, tachycardia, confusion, cardiovascular collapse, and death (60,61).

Patients with mild hyperthyroidism may have surgery with preoperative beta blockade. However, patients with moderate or severe disease should have surgery canceled until a euthyroid state is attained.

Thyrotoxic patients who require emergent/urgent surgery need premedication with antithyroid agents, beta blockade, and corticosteroids. Antithyroid medications include thionamides, propythiouracil (PTU), and iodine. Methimazole is a thionamide drug that blocks thyroid hormone synthesis and iodine blocks thyroid hormone release (62,63). Because adrenal reserve may be low in these patients, stress-dose steroids (see below) should be administered prior to and following surgery (64). Should thyroid storm occur, treatment with beta blockade, thionamides, iodine, and corticosteroids should be instituted. It is important to give the thionamides at least 1 hour prior to iodine administration to prevent uptake of iodine and synthesis of further hormone. Occasionally, supportive care in the ICU with correction of cardiac dysfunction and electrolyte abnormalities may be necessary (39).

Adrenal Suppression

Corticosteroids are used to treat a myriad of diseases, and it is not unusual to obtain a history from patients revealing steroid usage. It is important to ascertain the type of steroid used, the dosage prescribed, the duration of treatment, and whether or not a tapering schedule was used in stopping the medication.

Although some case series demonstrate biochemical evidence of hypothalamic-pituitary axis (HPA) suppression after exogenous steroid usage, none has demonstrated frank adrenal insufficiency, hypotension, and shock in surgical patients (65). However, recommendations for stress-dose steroids perioperatively have been made to prevent the occurrence of this life-threatening situation in patients with either "presumed" or documented HPA suppression. Giving stress-dose glucocorticoids needs to be weighed against the potential side effects of the drug (such as poor wound healing, fluid retention, and increased risk of infection) versus the benefits of supporting the HPA axis in a surgically stressed patient.

Three tiers of chronic glucocorticoid usage and subsequent HPA axis suppression have emerged. Several studies have shown that steroid equivalent to 5 mg of prednisone, as a single morning dose, alternate-day short-acting steroids given as a morning dose, and any dose of steroid given for less than 3 weeks seldom results in clinical suppression of the HPA and requires no stress-dose steroids perioperatively (66–68). However, patients who are chronically taking 20 mg prednisone (or equivalent) per day for more than 3 weeks

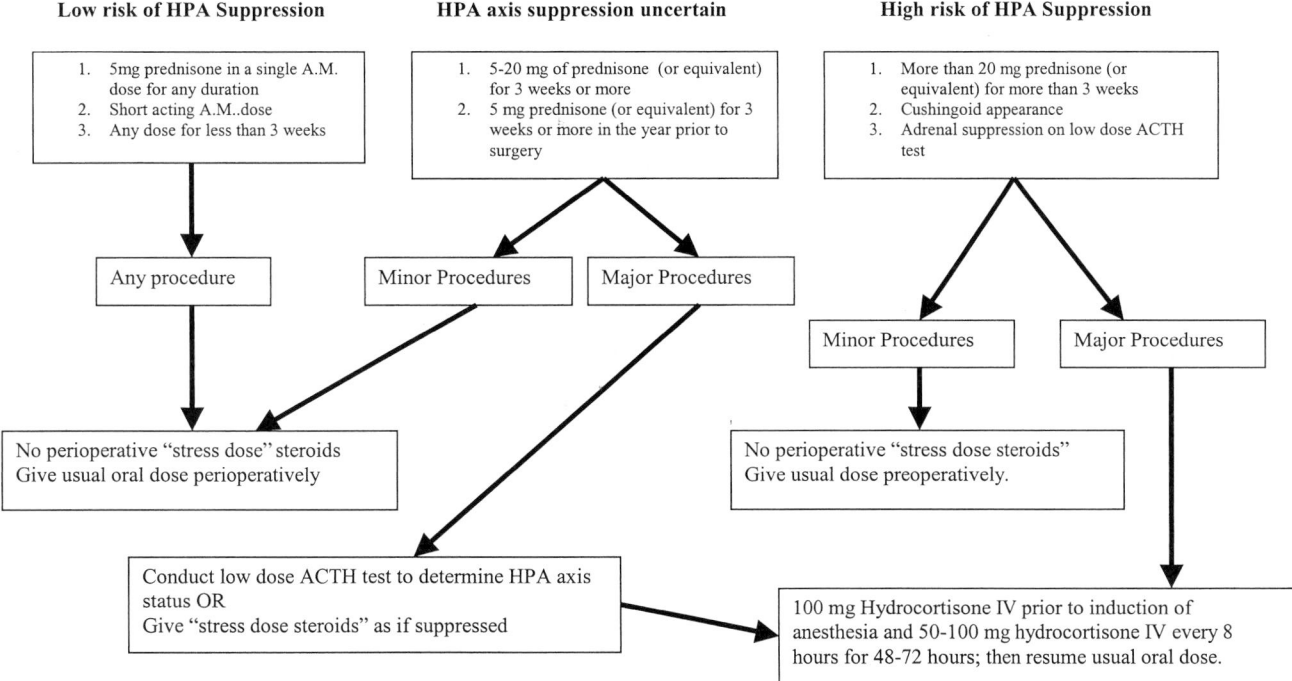

Low risk of HPA Suppression

1. 5mg prednisone in a single A.M. dose for any duration
2. Short acting A.M..dose
3. Any dose for less than 3 weeks

HPA axis suppression uncertain

1. 5-20 mg of prednisone (or equivalent) for 3 weeks or more
2. 5 mg prednisone (or equivalent) for 3 weeks or more in the year prior to surgery

High risk of HPA Suppression

1. More than 20 mg prednisone (or equivalent) for more than 3 weeks
2. Cushingoid appearance
3. Adrenal suppression on low dose ACTH test

Any procedure

Minor Procedures

Major Procedures

Minor Procedures

Major Procedures

No perioperative "stress dose" steroids
Give usual oral dose perioperatively

No perioperative "stress dose steroids"
Give usual dose preoperatively.

Conduct low dose ACTH test to determine HPA axis status OR
Give "stress dose steroids" as if suppressed

100 mg Hydrocortisone IV prior to induction of anesthesia and 50-100 mg hydrocortisone IV every 8 hours for 48-72 hours; then resume usual oral dose.

FIG. 11-2. Algorithm for stress-dose steroids. ACTH, adrenal corticotropin hormone; HPA, hypothalmus-pituitary-adrenal axis; IV, intravenous. (Adapted from Schiff RL, Welsh GA. Perioperative evaluation and management of the patient with endocrine dysfunction. *Med Clin North Am* 2003;87(1):175–192, with permission.)

or who appear clinically cushingoid require stress-dose steroids based upon the type of surgical stress (69) (Fig. 11.2). Patients whose steroid usage falls in between the first two tiers are more controversial and may require HPA testing to ascertain the functionality of the adrenal gland (70).

Renal Risk Assessment

Chronic kidney disease affects 8 million Americans, with most having a glomerular filtration rate (GFR) of less than 60 mL/min/1.73 m^2 (71). The most common form of renal failure facing the surgeon is acute renal failure (ARF) occurring during the postoperative period. This condition will be discussed below in the section on postoperative/critical care. However, with the aging population, increasing prevalence of diabetes and hypertension, and the advances in dialytic therapy, the number of patients living with end-stage renal disease (ESRD) is increasing. Therefore, surgeons must be cognizant of the potential perioperative risks associated with these patients.

The causes of ESRD are predominantly diabetes and hypertension, which account for 68% of patients with ESRD (72). As such, patients with these underlying diseases tend to have other co-morbid conditions such as coronary artery disease and peripheral vascular disease. Obviously, patients with ESRD have problems with fluid balance, electrolyte levels, and acid-base management. Furthermore, with reduced or absent renal function, these patients metabolize drugs such as antibiotics, anesthetics, and analgesics poorly. Finally, patients with ESRD are immunocompromised and are more susceptible to infections postoperatively. Taking this complex picture into consideration, the morbidity rate among ESRD patients undergoing surgery is 54% (range 12% to 64%) and the mortality rate is 4% (range 0% to 47%) (73).

Evaluation of ESRD patients undergoing surgery should focus on three areas: cardiac evaluation, fluid and electrolyte management and anemia, and bleeding diatheses. Of course, glycemic control for diabetics and blood pressure control for hypertensives is obvious. Cardiac disease is the leading cause of death among ESRD patients (72,74). Unfortunately, a large proportion of these patients have asymptomatic coronary artery disease (23% to 40%) (75,76), with 75% of diabetics being asymptomatic (77,78). Therefore, these patients need formal cardiac clearance from a cardiologist prior to surgical intervention.

ESRD patients who are dependent upon dialysis will need to be euvolemic prior to surgery. Thus, communication with the patient's nephrologist is paramount. Details about the operation should be discussed, with planned preoperative dialysis (without heparin 24 hours prior to surgery) and postoperative dialysis on the day of surgery for large intraoperative fluid loads. Electrolytes should be monitored in the immediate postoperative period, with hyperkalemia being aggressively managed with dialysis or medically if necessary. Hyperkalemia may be treated with glucose and insulin, which will drive the Na,K-ATPase pump resulting in an increase of intracellular potassium and a lowering of extracellular potassium. Ten milliliters of calcium gluconate can afford cardioprotection and membrane stabilization in patients with abnormal electrocardiograms (ECGs). Finally, 40 g of sodium polystyrene sulfonate (Kionex, Kexaylate) dissolved in 80 mL of sorbitol may be given orally or alternatively, 50 to100 g in 200 mL of water may be given rectally as a retention enema by inserting a Foley catheter into the rectum and filling the balloon. These administrations should be repeated every 2 to 4 hours until the potassium level is in a normal range (see section below on Potassium Derangements). Caution with use of this resin in postoperative patients is urged as intestinal necrosis can occur (79).

Patients with ESRD usually receive erythropoietin to maintain hemoglobin levels. In urgent situations, transfusion of blood is necessary to maintain hemoglobin prior to and during surgery. Uremic patients may have platelet dysfunction resulting in bleeding (80). If a patient has demonstrated prior bleeding because of uremic platelet dysfunction, these patients must be treated with 1-deamino-8-D-arginine vasopressin (dDAVP) intravenously or intranasally and with cryoprecipitate to prevent bleeding during surgery (81). In addition, patients may be treated with intravenous conjugated estrogens (0.6 mg/kg) if they are given 4 to 5 days prior to surgery (82).

Drug administration in ESRD must be done judiciously with careful attention to the pharmacokinetics of particular drugs. Multiple guidelines exist that can direct drug dose reductions for patients with ESRD (83).

Hepatic Risk Assessment

The incidence of liver disease in gynecologic oncology is not known. However, patients may present with a history of cirrhosis or acute or chronic hepatitis in conjunction with a gynecologic malignancy. Awareness of liver disorders and how they impact the perioperative risk is necessary to avoid unnecessary morbidity and mortality.

As mentioned earlier, thorough preoperative evaluation of patients includes a comprehensive history and physical examination, with further laboratory testing based upon historical and physical findings. Routine testing of liver function in asymptomatic patients rarely yields abnormal levels or changes in perioperative management (2). However, patients with histories of jaundice, blood transfusions, the use of alcohol or other recreational drugs, hepatitis, or physical findings of icterus, hepatosplenomegaly, palmar erythema, or spider nevi should be tested to rule out occult or active liver diseases (84).

Patients with acute hepatitis (viral or alcohol induced) should have surgery delayed until the acute phase of the disease process has passed and liver function tests have returned to normal. The older literature has demonstrated mortality rates of 0% to 58% in this patient group (84). Contrarily, patients with chronic hepatitis tolerate surgery well with no mortality (85,86).

Surgical risk in patients with cirrhosis of the liver is significant and correlates directly with the Child-Turcotte classification (Table 11.5). This system takes into consideration five components, three of which are subjective. Nonetheless, for predicting operative outcome, this system is quite reproducible and has been validated in a number of studies (87–90). Postoperative mortality rates have been shown to be 10% in Child class A and 30% and 80%, respectively, for Child classes B and C (87, 89). Patients with cirrhosis of the liver also have coagulopathies, which need to be corrected prior to surgery. Vitamin K administration, fresh frozen plasma, or cryoprecipitate may be administered to correct the prothrombin time to within 3 seconds of normal. Figure 11.3 presents an algorithm for patients with liver disease facing surgery (84).

Finally, selection of medications in patients with hepatic dysfunction needs to be done judiciously. Patients with liver dysfunction are particularly susceptible to anesthetic effects such as changes in hepatic metabolism of medications and changes in hepatic blood flow. Alterations in the type and the dose of an agent are necessary to avoid postoperative hepatic dysfunction and hepatitis. Postoperative pain management with narcotic agents needs to be reduced by as much as 50% to account for the altered hepatic metabolism in these patients (91).

TABLE 11.5. *Child-Turcotte classification and operative mortality*

Group designation	A (minimal)	B (moderate)	C (advanced)
Serum bilirubin (mg/dL)	<2.0	2.0–3.0	>3.0
Serum albumin (g/dL)	>3.5	3.0–3.5	<3.0
Ascites	None	Easily controlled	Poorly controlled
Neurologic disorder	None	Minimal	Advanced, coma
Nutrition	Excellent	Good	Poor, wasting
Operative Mortality	10%	30%	80%

Adapted from Child CG, Turcotte JG. Surgery and portal hypertension. In: Child CG, ed. *The liver and portal hypertension.* Philadelphia: WB Saunders, 1964:50, with permission.

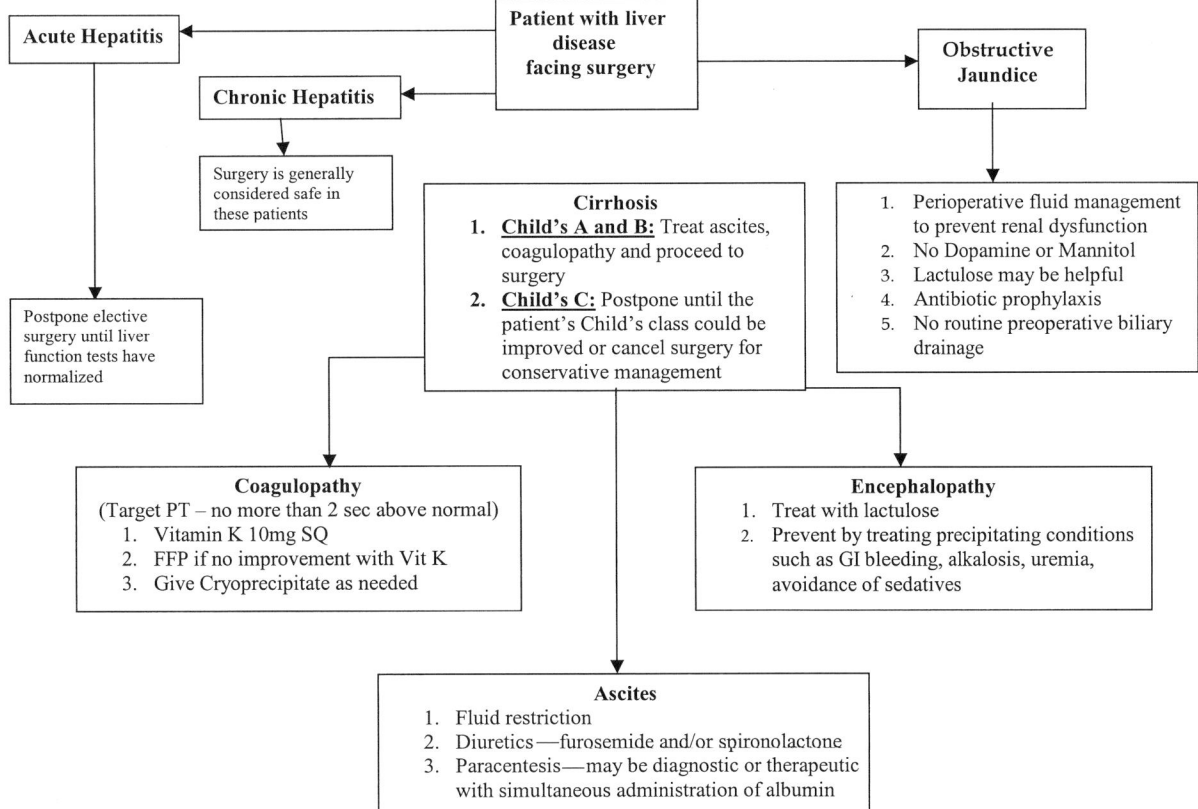

FIG. 11-3. Perioperative assessment of the patient with liver disease. FFP, fresh frozen plasma. (From Rizvon MK, Chou CL. Surgery in the patient with liver disease. *Med Clin North Am* 2003;87:211–227, with permission.)

Preoperative Nutritional Assessment

Clearly, the status of nourishment plays an important role in the way patients respond to the various stresses of their cancer care. The broader consideration of nutrition in gynecologic cancer patients is discussed in Chapter 35. The intent of this section is to present the concepts of preoperative nutritional evaluation and nutritional support of the gynecologic oncology patient. Early refeeding in the postoperative patient as well as enteral and parenteral nutritional support in the critically ill gynecologic patient will be discussed later.

The prevalence of malnutrition among cancer patients has been shown to be quite high (92,93). In addition, a direct correlation between the level of malnutrition and surgical outcome has been demonstrated (94,95). Specific rates of malnutrition among gynecologic oncology patients have been described. Tunca showed a high prevalence of severe protein malnutrition among ovarian cancer patients without gastrointestinal involvement. However, he was unable to demonstrate malnutrition among other gynecologic cancer sites (96). Orr and colleagues have shown increased rates of malnutrition with increasing stages of cervical cancer among patients (97). Recently, Santoso et al. demonstrated that 54%

of their patients admitted to the gynecologic oncology ward (medical and surgical admissions) demonstrated malnutrition. Most of their patients had cervical or uterine carcinomas, were obese, and were admitted for major abdominal surgeries (98). The question remains: how best to assess patients for nutritional status and what intervention(s) can correct deficiencies, producing improved postoperative outcomes?

Simply attaining a history of weight loss (amount and over what duration) can identify patients who may be malnourished, especially if the weight loss is greater than 10% of the patient's normal weight (99). However, recalled weights may be inaccurate and require corroboration of family members or comparison to prior recorded weights (100). Other important historical elements, which may identify patients who are at risk, are the type and/or duration of any "diets," recent surgical interventions, radiation or chemotherapy treatment, nausea or vomiting, and a history of alcohol or drug abuse (101).

Other methods for assessing nutritional status include body measurements and laboratory values. Table 11.6 lists these measures of nutritional depletion. The anthropometric measurements assess fat stores (the triceps skinfold) and pro-

TABLE 11.6. *Measurement of nutritional depletion*

Parameters	Depletion		
	Mild	Moderate	Severe
Triceps skin fold (TSF) % Standard	50–90	30–50	<30
Mid-arm muscle circumference (MAMC) % Standard	80–90	70–80	<70
Albumin g/dL	3.0–3.4	2.1–3.0	<2.1
Total lymphocyte count (TLC) Cmm	1200–1500	800–1200	<800
Weight loss, % initial			
In 1 week	<1	1–2	>2
In 1 month	<2	2–5	>5
In 3 months	<5	5.0–7.5	>7.5
In 6 months	<7.5	7.5–10.0	>10.0

tein stores (mid arm circumference). The resulting measurements are compared to standard tables of these measurements and a percentage is calculated to arrive at the level of depletion (or nourishment). Although the measurements are quite easy to obtain, there is a lack of standardization of measurement techniques, which can introduce error and produce inaccurate assessments of nutritional status. Total lymphocyte count is calculated by multiplying the percentage of lymphocytes, determined in the differential by the total white blood cell count. Several conditions can affect the percentage of lymphocytes, such as infection or recent chemotherapy or radiation administration, producing artificially low levels of lymphocytes and inaccurate nutritional assessments. A serum albumin level is usually included in most complete metabolic profiles. Because the half-life of serum albumin is 20 days, levels can give a picture of the patient's visceral protein stores over longer periods of time. However, the plasma level of serum albumin can be affected by the patient's volume status and events that increase catabolism, all of which may interfere with the clinical usefulness of this assessment method (102).

Several schemes have been developed to combine several of the measures in Table 11.6 and correlate them to surgical outcomes. The prognostic nutritional index (PNI) has been studied the most (98,103). This index combines the triceps skinfold, the serum albumin and transferrin levels, and delayed hypersensitivity response to mumps, tuberculin, and *Candida* antigens. Because it requires measurements of immune response, it is a cumbersome index to complete and probably has little clinically utility. Serum albumin emerges as the single test with the most predictive value of poor operative outcome due to malnutrition. Santoso and colleagues found that albumin levels correlated with the PNI and predicted longer lengths of stay for hospitalized, malnourished patients (98). Gibbs et al., through the National Veterans Affairs Surgical Risk Study, found that albumin levels less than 2.1 mg/dL were associated with an increased surgical morbidity from 10% to 65% (especially in predicting sepsis and major infections), as well as an increased 30-day mortality from 1% to 29% (104). Further, Delgado-

Rodriguez and colleagues showed that lower levels of serum albumin were predictive of longer lengths of stay, increased rates of nosocomial infections and in-hospital deaths among a general surgical population. This group of investigators also correlated their outcome measures to lower levels of high-density lipoprotein-cholesterol fractions (105).

Finally, studies have shown that experienced clinicians are able to assess nutritional status subjectively, as well as objective laboratory or anthropometric measures, merely by obtaining a history and examining the patient (106,107).

Since the mid 1980s several trials of total parenteral nutrition (TPN) to correct deficiencies preoperatively in order to improve operative outcomes were done. This controversial practice was called into question and ultimately answered with several prospective, randomized trials, which defined patients who would benefit from such repletion. The largest trial, the Veterans Affairs Cooperative Study, randomized 395 mostly male, surgical (abdominal or noncardiac thoracic surgeries) patients to receive at least seven days of preoperative and 3 days of postoperative TPN or to receive no perioperative nutritional supplementation. The TPN group had a greater number of infectious complications, mostly among patients classified as borderline or mildly malnourished compared to the unfed patients (14.1% vs 6.4%). However, a subset of severely malnourished patients derived benefit from lower operative complication rates (5% vs 43%, $p = .03$) without incurring an increase in infectious complications. The overall 30- and 90-day mortality rates where not different between the groups (108). A similar study by Bozzetti et al. randomized severely malnourished patients undergoing resection of gastric or colonic malignancies to 10 days of preoperative TPN and 9 days of postoperative TPN or no supplementation. His group showed that noninfectious, postoperative complication rates were lower among the TPN group versus the unfed control group (12% versus 34%, $p = .02$) (109). Although the method of nutritional assessment was different in these two studies, it is clear that patients assessed to be severely malnourished should be considered for preoperative TPN prior to abdominal surgery.

PREPARATION FOR SURGERY

Infection Prophylaxis

Surgical site infections account for nearly 40% of nosocomial infections in surgical patients and are a significant source of postoperative morbidity resulting in longer hospital stays and increased cost (110,111). Patient and operative environmental factors influence surgical infection rates. The goal of preoperative skin preparation is to reduce the risk of surgical site infection by reducing the microbial count to a subpathogenic level in a time-efficient and atraumatic manner. Whole-body scrubs or showers with antiseptic agents such as chlorhexidine or povidone-iodine prior to surgery reduce bacterial counts on the skin although this practice has not been shown to reduce wound infection rates (112,113). Patients undergoing surgery should simply be instructed to bathe or shower normally the night or morning prior to surgery, removing any debris from the skin surface.

Inappropriate hair removal techniques can traumatize the skin and provide an opportunity for colonization of microorganisms. It has long been shown that shaving the operative site increases infection rates, with the risk increasing the longer the interval between shaving and surgery (114–117). In one study, surgical site infection rates were 5.6% in patients who were shaved compared to 0.6% for those who did not shave or use a depilatory (116). Hair is generally sterile and therefore does not need to be removed unless the hair around the incision will interfere with the operation. When hair removal is necessary the simplest and least irritating method of hair removal is an electric or battery-powered clipper with a disposable head (110, 118).

New Prophylactic antimicrobials play a large role in reducing the rates of surgical site infections and should be used in clean-contaminated or contaminated operations, which include most procedures performed by gynecologic oncologists. Factors that increase the risk of postoperative infection in women undergoing radical pelvic surgery include longer duration of surgery, extremes of age, increased blood loss, anemia, poor nutritional status, the presence of tumor, prior pelvic irradiation, diabetes, obesity, peripheral vascular disease, and a history of post-surgical infection (110,119). A meta-analysis of 25 prospective randomized trials of antibiotic prophylaxis in women undergoing abdominal hysterectomy found that patients not receiving antibiotic prophylaxis had infection rates of 21.2% compared to 9% in those receiving any antimicrobial agent ($p = .00001$). Although this article established the necessity of prophylactic antibiotic use, the optimal regimen has not been defined (120).

Prophylactic antibiotics should provide coverage consistent with the microbial mileu most likely to be encountered. In gynecologic oncology surgery, potential infecting organisms are coliforms, enterococci, streptococci, clostridia, and bacteroides. In order to achieve and maintain effective tissue levels, parenteral antibiotics should be given 30 to 45 min-

utes prior to skin incision as a loading dose. For patients weighing >70 kg, the dosage should be doubled (i.e., cefotetan 2 g IV). Repeat doses should be given intraoperatively for surgeries lasting longer than 3 hours or when blood loss exceeds 1000 mL (121). Repeat doses postoperatively are unnecessary and subject the patient to the potential emergence of resistant organisms. Cephalosporins are the most frequently used antimicrobials for prophylaxis in gynecologic surgery. In the American Society of Health System Pharmacists (ASHP) guidelines on antimicrobial prophylaxis in surgery, cefazolin is recommended for gynecologic procedures (121). However, in a randomized, double-blind clinical trial Hemsell and colleagues reported that the risk of a major surgical site infection was significantly higher in patients undergoing hysterectomy who received cefazolin as compared to cefotetan for prophylaxis (122). A single dose of cefotetan has also been shown to be superior to cefazolin in elective clean-contaminated operations that last longer that 3 hours (123). Cefotetan has a plasma elimination half-life between 3.0 and 4.6 hours and is active against a wider variety of gram-negative aerobic and anaerobic species than cefazolin, making it an excellent, cost-effective choice for antibiotic prophylaxis in longer radical gynecologic operations. Cefotetan or cefmetazole are also recommended for prophylaxis prior to colorectal surgery (121).

Bowel Preparation

It is generally accepted that full mechanical bowel preparation is indicated when intestinal injury or bowel resection is anticipated. The ''clean'' bowel has a lower bacterial load and therefore a reduced chance of spilling fecal material, which potentially contaminates the wound and peritoneal cavity. Mechanical bowel preparation has several advantages unrelated to the risk of infection. It facilitates palpation of the entire colon during laparotomy. It may prevent mechanical disruption of the anastomosis by the passage of hard feces. Removal of solid material from the gastrointestinal tract prior to laparoscopy may improve exposure and lessen the chance of injury from manipulation of a heavy and distended feces-laden colon with the relatively traumatic laparoscopic grasping instruments.

Historically, clearing the colon in preparation for surgery was a complicated procedure requiring several days of clear liquid diet, cathartics, enemas, and preoperative hospitalization. The introduction of polyethylene glycol (PEG) electrolyte solution in the early 1980s revolutionized bowel preparation (124,125). PEG is an isoosmotic solution with especially designed electrolyte concentrations that result in virtually no net absorption of ions or water, and large volumes can be administered without significant fluid or electrolyte alterations. Several randomized studies have demonstrated that bowel cleansing with PEG can be performed safely as an outpatient preparation prior to colorectal surgery without increasing complication rates (126,127). Bowel preparation with PEG has some disadvantages. It requires oral intake of 4 L of a salty-tasting solution over a relatively short period of time. Many patients experience nausea, vomiting, and abdominal bloating and discomfort and are unable to drink the required volume.

Sodium phosphate is an osmotic cathartic that provides quality bowel cleansing while avoiding the need to ingest a large volume of solution (128,129). Generally, two 45-mL doses are taken 4 hours apart with at least three glasses of clear liquid with each dose. Colonic cleansing with this method may cause intravascular volume contraction in some patients. A randomized, blinded study showed that rehydration with a carbohydrate-electrolyte ''sport'' drink resulted in significantly less intravascular volume contraction as compared to rehydration with water (130). A meta-analysis of eight blinded studies which compared sodium phosphate to PEG for colonoscopy preparation suggest that sodium phosphate is an effective, better tolerated, and less costly regimen (131). Comparisons between these two preparations have also been studied in patients undergoing colorectal surgery with similar results (129,132). The use of sodium phosphate is not recommended for patients with renal insufficiency, symptomatic CHF, and liver failure with ascites (133). Hyperphosphatemia, hypernatremia, hypocalcemia, and hypokalemia have been reported after bowel preparation with sodium phosphate, but generally without clinical significance (129,131,134,135). However, serious and fatal metabolic derangements have been reported, and caution should be used in elderly patients or when prescribing multiple dose regimens (133,134,136–138).

Although regarded as being essential in preventing complications of colorectal surgery, the necessity of mechanical bowel cleansing has been disputed recently. Since 1992 at least five prospective randomized trials suggest that elective colon and rectal surgery may be performed safely without mechanical bowel preparation. All patients in these trials received systemic antibiotics. Brownson and colleagues randomized 179 patients to either preparation with PEG or no mechanical preparation. Surprisingly, patients who received preparation experienced a significant increase in intraabdominal infection and anastomotic leak. There was no difference in wound infection rates (139). Santos compared a 5-day regimen with no preparation and found a significantly increased rate of both wound infection and anastomotic dehiscence in prepped patients, whereas three other large studies found no differences between their study groups that included patients undergoing elective left colonic or rectal resection (140–143). At first glance, this appears to be overwhelming evidence to abandon this practice: However, all of these trials are greatly underpowered with a 60% or greater chance that a type II error occurred (144,145). In a recent survey of members of the American Society of Colon and Rectal Surgeons, essentially all routinely used mechanical bowel preparation, although 10% questioned its importance. Of the 515 surgeons who responded to the questionnaire,

47% routinely used sodium phosphate, 32% routinely used PEG, and 14% alternated between the two agents (146).

The importance of appropriate antimicrobial prophylaxis in patients undergoing colorectal surgery is well established (147,148). Numerous studies have compared different antibiotic regimens with broad-spectrum coverage against intestinal flora. Although no single regimen was consistently found to be superior, some regimens appeared to be inadequate (e.g., metronidazole, doxycycline, and piperacillin) as single agents. A single dose administered before the operation was as effective as prophylaxis that was continued into the immediate postoperative period (148). There is little evidence to suggest that oral antimicrobial agents offer additional benefit in the presence of parenteral prophylaxis. The ASHP guidelines on antimicrobial prophylaxis recommend 2 g of cefoxitin, cefotetan, or cefmetazole given intravenously at induction of anesthesia for colorectal surgery patients (121).

Blood Transfusion Prophylaxis

Medications associated with increased bleeding risks need to be stopped prior to surgery. Elderly patients are more likely to be taking daily aspirin, nonsteroidal anti-inflammatory medications, platelet aggregation inhibitors, and anticoagulants. It will take approximately 4 days after warfarin therapy is discontinued for the international normalized ratio (INR) to reach 1.5 for those patients with INR levels between 2.0 and 3.0. Most patients do not need to be covered with heparin therapy preoperatively unless the reason for anticoagulant therapy is an acute venous or arterial thromboembolism within 1 month of surgery (149). Patients also need to be asked about over-the-counter drug and dietary supplement usage. *Ginkgo biloba*, garlic supplements, and vitamin E have antiplatelet activity and may enhance bleeding risk (150). If possible, anemia should be corrected preoperatively. The use of recombinant human erythropoietin with concurrent iron and folic acid supplementation 2 to 3 weeks preoperatively has been shown to reduce allogeneic blood transfusions in patients undergoing elective surgery (151). It has been estimated that 60% of all blood transfused in the Untied States is given to surgical patients. Transfusion rates of approximately 5% have been reported for patients undergoing abdominal hysterectomy for benign disease (152). Radical procedures performed for the treatment of gynecologic malignancies are associated with an estimated blood loss of 1,000 mL or greater. Transfusion rates for patients undergoing radical hysterectomy have been reported as high as 80% (153). There is a growing demand by patients for better information about their care, risks involved, and alternatives available. Transfusion-associated risks should be explained to the patient as part of routine preoperatively counseling. The risk of transfusion-transmitted infection of human immunodeficiency virus, hepatitis B virus, and hepatitis C virus from red blood cell transfusion is estimated at 1:971,000 units, 1:81,000 units, and 1:813,000 units, respectively (154). Although these rates have significantly decreased in the last decade with the introduction of new screening technologies, transmission of other agents, bacterial contamination, transfusion reactions, increased infection complications, and immunosuppression remain risks of allogeneic blood transfusion (155–157). Increasing awareness of these adverse effects has prompted both physicians and patients to search for alternatives to the use of donor blood in the perioperative period.

Since the mid 1980s preoperative autologous blood donation (PABD) has been utilized in order to avoid allogeneic blood transfusion in patients undergoing elective surgery where excessive blood loss is anticipated. Although this practice decreases homologous blood use, 15% of autologous donors will still receive allogeneic transfusions, and 40% of units collected are not used and must be discarded (158). Furthermore PABD greatly increases the likelihood of any transfusion being necessary and is not without medical risks. Severe reactions during autologous donation occurred at a rate of 0.32% per unit collected and 0.75% per donor. Serious incidents during blood collection which required hospitalization were 12 times more likely in PABD compared to allogeneic donors (159). Transfusion to the wrong recipient, bacterial contamination, febrile nonhemolytic reactions, and allergic reactions have also been reported with autologous transfusion (160). The cost effectiveness of PABD has been found to be poor and has steadily deteriorated over the decade (160–162).

Acute normovolemic hemodilution (ANH) is an autologous blood-procurement strategy that is equivalent to PABD in reducing allogeneic transfusion needs. Its clinical utility has been extensively studied in patients undergoing radical prostatectomy, total joint replacement, and more recently major colorectal surgery. During ANH, blood is procured in the holding or operating room and replaced with colloid and crystalloid until a target hematocrit level of 28% is reached or blood volume of 2,000 mL is removed (163). ANH obviates the costs of blood testing, storage, or wastage because all blood collected during ANH is returned to the patient before the end of surgery. It is simple to perform and more convenient for the patient. Since the blood is collected at point-of-care there is no possibility for clerical error or contamination. ANH has been shown to be a cost effective yet underutilized strategy to reduce allogeneic blood transfusions (161–164).

Special Considerations for Obese Patients

Coexisting medical disorders, including coronary artery disease, hypertension, obesity, hypoventilation, and obstructive sleep apnea syndromes, adult-onset diabetes mellitus, pulmonary hypertension, gastroesophageal reflux, impaired cardiac function, and hypercoagulability are common in morbidly obese patients and contribute to increased perioperative morbidity and mortality. These co-morbidities may not have been previously diagnosed and symptoms may not manifest themselves until the patient undergoes physiologic stress related to surgery. For example, baseline pulmonary function studies of markedly obese patients demonstrate mild hypoxemia; decreased vital capacity, tidal volume, and expiratory reserve volume; increased resistance; and ventilation-perfusion inequalities (165). During the postoperative period, severe hypoxemia may occur secondary to sedation, pain, immobility, atelectasis, and anemia, leading to cardiac arrhythmia or ischemia (166). A thorough preoperative medical evaluation is necessary to detect coexisting disease and minimize surgical risk. A comprehensive review of the pathophysiology associated with morbid obesity is beyond the scope of this chapter, and we direct the reader elswhere for a thorough review (167).

Surgery in morbidly obese patients poses many challenges for teams on both sides of the surgical drape. The primary concern of the anesthesiologist is gaining adequate control of the airway. The combined problems of increased aspiration risk, rapid oxygen desaturation caused by decreased functional residual capacity, baseline hypoxemia, and increased oxygen demand, in addition to technical difficulties due to anatomic fat deposits, make intubation a high-risk procedure. An awake, fiberoptic-assisted intubation is often the technique of choice for obtaining an airway. Extubation should be delayed until the patient is fully awake and ideally sitting upright. There are technical operating room and instrumentation issues, which need to be addressed as well. Standard operating tables, stretchers, and hospital beds have weight limits, which have prompted specifically designed wider and sturdier models for the obese patient. Staff and patient safety during transfer of the patient from the operating table to the bed or gurney is also a concern in the extremely obese patient and must be taken into consideration. Proper retractors and extra long instruments are essential and may not be available in all hospitals. Although these practical considerations are ostensibly mundane, failure to prepare will obviate a successful outcome, add frustration to all involved, and possibly put the patient at risk.

Recent reports in the gynecologic oncology literature suggest performing panniculectomy to improve exposure of the peritoneal cavity and pelvic structures (168–170). Although this is a relatively straightforward procedure, it does require some experience and planning for optimal results. Hospital credentialing of surgical privileges may require the involvement of a plastic surgeon or proctoring until proficiency is demonstrated. In addition, since panniculectomy is considered a cosmetic procedure, many insurers may require prior authorization with documentation of medical necessity. Further discussions of the technique of panniculectomy will be presented in Chapter 12.

CRITICAL CARE AND POSTOPERATIVE MANAGEMENT

Cardiovascular Issues

Monitoring Issues

There are many tools at the hands of the modern-day clinician when it comes to monitoring the cardiovascular function of the patient. Clinical examination, heart rate, blood pressure, and ECG are a few. In the critical care setting, the addition of the arterial catheter, central venous pressure, and pulmonary artery catheter increases sophistication. Most patients in the intensive care unit (ICU) can be managed with simple clinical parameters. Fluid status can be assessed by daily weights, pulse rate, blood pressure, and urine output. Continuous ECG monitoring is helpful for detecting arrhythmias and ischemia. Central venous pressure (CVP) is often used for assessment of volume status and a crude estimation of cardiac function. If a patient has a central line then a port can be continuously transduced for CVP. It is a common mistake among novices to evaluate a single reading of CVP rather than reviewing the trend. When the CVP is correlated with volume status, the resulting graph is a scatter graph (i.e., no correlation). There is only correlation over time and in response to, for example, fluid challenges, transfusion, or therapy. One must remember that the CVP is a pressure measurement and not the desired measurement of volume (preload). Therefore, only crude estimations of fluid status can be made. When the status of a patient's cardiac output or fluid state is unclear, a pulmonary artery (PA) catheter (e.g., Swan-Ganz catheter) may be helpful.

These catheters are placed via a central vein (subclavian or jugular) as a central line. The catheter has a balloon-tipped transducer and is "floated" into the pulmonary artery. Waveforms of the right ventricle, pulmonary artery, and pulmonary capillary wedge pressure (PCWP) are directly visualized as the catheter progresses through the heart (Fig. 11.4), and confirmed placement is verified by chest radiograph (Fig.11.5). Complications of placement include pneumothorax, arrhythmia, line sepsis (2%), and rarely pulmonary artery rupture. The PA catheter allows the measurement of cardiac output and oxygen delivery and estimation of preload by obtaining the pulmonary artery occlusive pressure (PAOP) or PCWP, the "wedge."

A number of formulas for calculation of hemodynamic parameters are crucial in utilizing the PA catheter for the care of the critically ill patient (Table 11.7). Assessment of preload is desirable for determining fluid administration or diuretic requirements for patients. The ideal measure of preload would be left ventricular end-diastolic volume; however since this is unobtainable with current technology, intensivists settle for "the wedge" as an estimation. By inflating the balloon placed in the pulmonary artery, a direct column of standing fluid exists between the left atrium, through the pulmonary vasculature, and back to the balloon (transducer). The PAOP can be measured and is a crude reflection of left atrial pressure. If the PAOP is elevated, the preload is

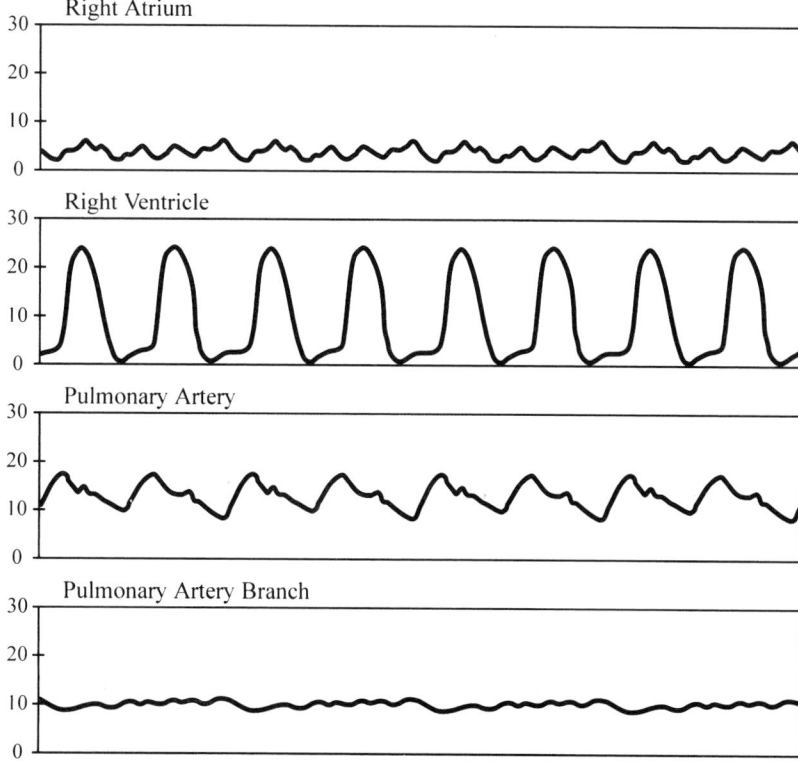

FIG. 11-4. Pulmonary artery catheter wave form readings as the catheter passes through the heart into the pulmonary artery. Y-axis is reading in millimeters of mercury (mm Hg).

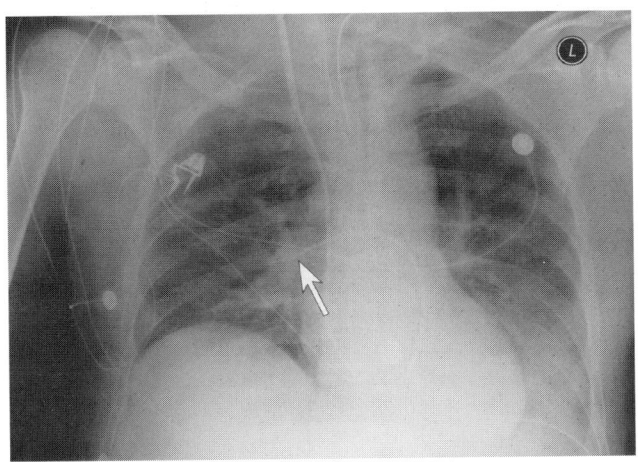

FIG. 11-5. Chest radiograph showing proper placement of pulmonary artery catheter in the pulmonary artery (*arrow* shows tip of pulmonary catheter).

adequate (or excessive), and if it is low, the patient may be volume depleted. These measurements, as previously mentioned with CVP, are dynamic and trend is important. For example, if the PAOP is low and a fluid bolus is given, the PAOP should increase if the diagnosis of volume depletion was correct.

Thermodilution techniques are used to calculate the cardiac output by injecting saline via a proximal port in the PA catheter and measuring the thermal changes at the distal tip of the PA catheter. By combining the preload assessment provided by the PAOP and the calculated cardiac output, differentiation between volume depletion and cardiogenic disease states can be made (see section on shock below). Newer PA catheters have been developed that can calculate right ventricular ejection fraction.

By taking a blood sample from the tip of the PA catheter, the most desaturated blood in the body is retrieved. In normal circulation, the blood from the superior vena cava and the

TABLE 11.7. *Hemodynamic formulas*

Cardiac output (CO) = stroke volume (SV) × heart rate (HR) [4–8 L/min]
Cardiac index (CI) = CO/body surface area (BSA)
Systemic vascular resistance (SVR) = Mean arterial pressure (MAP) – Central venous pressure (CVP) × 80/CO
[800–1200 dyne/s/cm^{-5}/m^2]
Arterial O_2 content (CaO_2) = (1.36) (hemoglobin) (oxygen saturation) + 0.003 (partial pressure of oxygen)
[20 mL O_2/dL]
O_2 delivery (DO_2) = CO × CaO_2 × 10
[600–1000 mL O_2/min]
O_2 availability (O_2AVI) = CI × CaO_2 × 10
[500–600 mL/min/m^2]
O_2 extraction ratio = (CaO_2 – CvO_2)/CaO_2
[25%]

Values in [ ] are normal values.

inferior vena cava mix and the blood from the coronary sinus is added to give a sample known as the mixed venous blood. By evaluating the oxygen saturation of this blood, oxygen delivery can be calculated (Table 11.7). This measurement is perhaps the most important function of the PA catheter, and current technology allows this function to be continuous via an infrared sensor at the tip of the PA catheter. For example, if oxygen delivery is determined to be low, there are only three situations that can be influenced by the clinician: increase cardiac output (with fluid, chronotropes, or inotropes), increase the hemoglobin, or increase the oxygen saturation. In a patient with a major operation and medical comorbidities, the measurement of a normal oxygen delivery provides reassurance to the clinician that end organs are being perfused.

Calculation of the systemic vascular resistance (SVR) is also possible with a PA catheter. Because the SVR is a calculated value and not directly measured, inaccuracies are inherent and overinterpretation of this value is cautioned. Rather than relying on the calculated SVR, the clinician should have complete understanding of the measured blood pressure and cardiac output and the ramifications therein to make therapeutic decisions (the SVR combines the two previously mentioned, measured variables).

In one study of ovarian cancer patients undergoing cytoreductive surgery, 18% of patients had indications for PA catheter use (171). Because of the issues of volume status in these patients, PA catheter placement for postoperative fluid management may be especially helpful.

Acute Postoperative Myocardial Infarction

MI usually manifests with acute chest discomfort, elevated cardiac enzymes, and ECG changes. Dyspnea, diaphoresis, nausea, and anxiety may also be associated. Risk factors that increase mortality from postoperative MI include female gender, advanced age, tachycardia, hypotension, and CHF (172). Treatment includes ICU monitoring with continuous ECG monitoring and supplemental oxygen, aspirin 325 mg immediately, sublingual nitroglycerin, and morphine sulfate as needed until pain resolves. Beta-blockers have been shown to decrease mortality by decreasing fatal arrhythmias and are also part of early treatment regimen. An evaluation for heparin therapy or thrombolytics can be made in consultation with a cardiologist.

Congestive Heart Failure

Patients with known CHF will be risk stratified, as previously mentioned, before major elective surgery. However in the postoperative setting, CHF will present in a number of ways (173). Patients with CHF are in a continuous hypervolemic state, and issues of fluid balance (strict ''ins'' and ''outs'') will be paramount during the perioperative period. In difficult cases, insertion of a PA catheter can be very helpful. Judicious fluid administration guided by the PAOP as well as selective use of inotropic support for augmentation of the cardiac output will aid the clinician in a successful outcome in these difficult patients (174).

Inotropes and Vasopressors

A variety of hemodynamically active drugs are available to support the cardiovascular function of patients in the perioperative period (175). In the broadest sense, they can be categorized as vasopressors, which elevate blood pressure, and inotropes, which enhance cardiac output (Table 11.8) (176). When faced with a patient in whom oxygen delivery is low and an increase in cardiac output is desired, inotropes such as dopamine or dobutamine should be used. Dopamine, at lower doses, activates dopaminergic receptors and increases circulation in mesenteric, cerebral, and renal vascular beds. At intermediate doses, dopamine stimulates beta-receptors in the heart and peripheral circulation. This activation causes tachycardia, increasing stroke volume and cardiac output. Increasing cardiac output in this fashion also increases demands for myocardial oxygen and could precipitate angina or an MI (177). At high doses, dopamine acts as an alpha agonist causing vasoconstriction. Dobutamine is a β_1 agonist with much greater inotropic effect than dopamine and causes peripheral arterial vasodilation, decreasing afterload (this dilation is abrupt and can cause hypotension in some patients). It is the drug of choice for severe heart failure.

Epinephrine is a potent sympathomimetic with varying effects based on the dose. The drug has beta-mimetic effects at lower doses and alpha-mimetic effects at higher doses. Epinephrine causes an acute increase in myocardial oxygen demand and is mainly reserved for cardiac arrest or severe circulatory failure. Norepinephrine and phenylephrine are pure alpha-mimetic agents, utilized for vasoconstriction (neurogenic shock). In most situations of shock, fluid resuscitation is preferred to administration of alpha agents. Although these agents will give a false sense of security that the blood pressure is normal, one must remember that the vasoconstriction underperfuses capillary beds, leading to an increased incidence of renal hypoperfusion (renal failure), splanchnic hypoperfusion (resulting in translocation of gut flora), and a myriad of other problems.

Vasopressin has emerged as an option similar to epinephrine with some important differences. This antidiuretic hormone in high doses provides potent vasoconstriction and leads to improved cerebral and coronary blood flow in shock states. Unlike epinephrine, there is less increase in myocardial oxygen demand and less propensity for inducing arrhythmias.

Amrinone (or inamrinone) is a phosphoesterase inhibitor that provides a positive inotropic effect on cardiac musculature while causing vasodilation. It is used in refractory cardiac failure.

Valvular Disease

In a recent study, approximately 4% of patients undergoing elective, noncardiac surgery were found to have clinically significant valvular disease. Important considerations in perioperative management are directed at patients with aortic stenosis and the level of associated ventricular failure. In addition these patients need endocarditis antibiotic prophylaxis (Table 11.9). Aortic stenosis (AS) is an independent risk factor for poor operative outcome, as previously mentioned (178). Patients with severe AS need valve replacement before elective surgery, whereas patients with mild to moderate AS need careful anesthetic control of blood pressure. Some patients may need intraoperative, continuous transesophageal echocardiography (179). The presence of aortic regurgitation, mitral stenosis, and mitral regurgitation require assessment of left ventricular function for the presence of congestive heart failure. Treatment and support will be related to support of ventricular function. Recently, the American Heart Association revised their recommendations for antibiotic prophylaxis for endocarditis (180). The common antibiotic regimens for endocarditis prophylaxis are presented in Table 11.9 for patients with anatomic cardiac defects and for whom risk is highest for the development of

TABLE 11.8. *Vasopressors: effects and dosage*

Drug	Systemic vasodilation	Systemic vasoconstriction	Inotropic effect	Chronotropic effect	Dysrhythmias	Dosing
Dopamine	+	0 to +++	++	+++	++	0.5–5 μg/kg/min for low range 5–10 mid range 10–20 high range
Dobutamine	++	0 to +	++++	++	+	2.5–20 μg/kg/min
Epinephrine	++	+++	++++	+++	+++	0.5–10 μg/min
Norepinephrine	0	++++	++	0	+	0.5–20 μg/min
Phenylephrine	0	+++	0	0	0	20–200 μg/min
Vasopressin	0	+++	0	0	0	0.04–0.12 U/min
Amrinone	++	0	++++	+	+	Load 0.75 mg/kg Maintenance 5–15 μg/kg/min

0, no effect; '+', slight effect *to* ++++, strong effect.

TABLE 11.9. *Antibiotic regimens for endocarditis prophylaxis in high- and moderate-risk patients undergoing genitourinary/gastrointestinal procedures*

Patient type	Antibiotic	Regimen
High-risk patients[a]	Ampicillin plus gentamicin	Ampicillin 2.0 g IM/IV plus 1.5 mg/kg (not to exceed 120 mg) within 30 minutes of starting procedure; 6 hours later, ampicillin 1.0 g IM/IV or amoxicillin 1.0 g orally
High-risk[a] patients allergic to ampicillin/amoxicillin	Vancomycin plus gentamicin	Vancomycin 1.0 g IV over 1–2 hours plus gentamicin 1.5 mg/kg IM/IV (not to exceed 120 mg); complete injection/infusion within 30 minutes of starting procedure
Moderate-risk patients[b]	Ampicillin or amoxicillin	Ampicillin 2.0 g IM/IV 30 minutes of starting procedure or amoxicillin 2.0 g orally 1 hour before procedure
Moderate-risk patients[b] allergic to ampicillin/amoxicillin	Vancomycin	Vancomycin 1.0 g IV over 1–2 hours; complete infusion within 30 minutes of starting procedure

[a] High-risk patients, prosthetic cardiac valves; previous history of bacterial endocarditis; complex cyanotic heart disease (e.g., tetralogy of Fallot); surgically constructed systemic pulmonary shunts or conduits.

[b] Moderate-risk patients; other congenital cardiac malformations; acquired valvar dysfunction; hypertrophic cardiomyopathy; mitral valve prolapse with valvar regurgitation and/or thickened leaflets.

IM, intramuscular; IV, intravenous.

endocarditis after extended gastrointestinal or genitourinary operations.

Arrhythmias

Whenever an arrhythmia occurs in the postoperative setting, myocardial ischemia must first be ruled out (181). If ECG and cardiac enzyme measurement are normal, an electrolyte or metabolic derangement or drug toxicity exists. Fortunately, most arrhythmias in the postoperative period are transient and self-resolving. Asymptomatic arrhythmias, except in the preoperative period (Table 11.2), are generally of little clinical significance. Hypercapnea, hypoxemia, hypokalemia, acidosis, inadequate analgesia, and anemia can all promote cardiac arrhythmias. Supraventricular tachycardia is the most common rhythm disturbance seen in the postoperative period (182). Treatment with cardizem or a betablocker is usually effective after correction of the underlying etiology. One significant new development has been the use of amiodarone as first-line treatment of acute-onset atrial fibrillation. Its usage has been associated with a lower incidence of recurrent atrial fibrillation (183).

Pulmonary Issues

Ventilator Management

The ability to provide ventilatory support to the surgical patient has been a tremendous advance in postoperative care. Mechanical ventilators have enabled oncologic surgeons to perform major operations for aggressive control of lesions that were once considered to be unresectable. Although preemptive preoperative therapies attempt to avoid postoperative mechanical ventilation, some patients will require this therapy. Mechanical ventilation must be thought of as providing two functions: ventilation and oxygenation. However, these two functions must be separated and applied independently to each particular situation. A more difficult concept for residents and fellows to understand is that ventilation has nothing to do with oxygenation. Many patients decompensate on the ward despite supplemental oxygen and a 100% oxygen saturation because tidal volumes were low and the patient was not ventilating.

When contemplating mechanical ventilation, one must ask two questions. Is the patient able to oxygenate her tissues adequately and can she ventilate adequately to maintain normal P_{CO_2} and acid-base function? Adequate oxygenation can be determined by measurement of oxygen saturation and arterial P_{O_2}. Targets are generally an O_2 saturation >92% or P_{O_2} greater than 65 mm Hg. Poor oxygenation may be caused by fluid overload, depressed mental status, underlying pulmonary disease, or shunt. Evaluation of the arterial blood gas will also give a pH and P_{CO_2} measurement. Patients may hypoventilate for a number of reasons. Postoperative pain may prohibit deep inspiration. Conversely, overuse of pain medication may depress the level of consciousness leading to fewer and poorer respirations. Atelectasis, pneumonia, and poor pulmonary compliance all lead to difficulties in ventilation. Finally, a bronchial mucous plug or a pneumothorax will lead to life-threatening ventilatory compromise. A respiratory rate greater than 35 per minute or a P_{CO_2} greater than 55 mm Hg are accepted indications for intubation and mechanical ventilation.

When intubating patients, the size of the endotracheal tube must be considered, as this may impact removal of mechanical ventilation. The larger the tube, the less resistance and the easier it will be for the patient to participate in "weaning" trials to discontinue ventilatory support (184). Typical recommendations are an 8.5-mm tube for women and a 9.0-mm tube for men.

Traditionally, there are pressure-cycled ventilators and volume-cycled ventilators. Pressure-cycled ventilators are used routinely in neonatal ICU patients because overinflation can be dangerous to neonates. In the adult ICU, most ventilators are volume cycled; meaning that the clinician sets the tidal volume, and regardless of the pressures necessary to give the volume, the volume will be delivered. In patients in whom pulmonary compliance is reduced [i.e., a stiff lung or acute respiratory distress syndrome (ARDS)] efforts at controlling pressure are important. When setting the ventilator, a number of decisions must be made. The mode of delivery, tidal volume and rate will determine ventilation, whereas the FIO_2 and pulmonary end-expiratory pressure (PEEP) will determine oxygenation.

Mode

There are a number of ventilator modes. The first developed was controlled mechanical ventilation (CMV), where the tidal volume and rate are set and that is exactly what the patient receives; no more and no less. This mode is very good for patients under general anesthesia or who are paralyzed. However, this mode is very disturbing to the patient who wishes to participate, however slightly, in her own ventilation. This mode has evolved into the current assist/control mode (A/C) whereby the patient is guaranteed the fixed rate and tidal volume but can also trigger breaths in between with a similar tidal volume. In addition, the machine will synchronize the breath when the patient triggers such a breath. This mode provides complete rest for the patient by performing all the work of breathing and is generally used for patients in the immediate postoperative period or for patients whose organ failure or ongoing sepsis is a more pressing concern.

Intermittent mandatory ventilation (IMV) is a mode whereby the clinician sets a rate and a tidal volume, which the machine delivers. Any breath initiated by the patient is delivered in relation to the amount of effort the patient puts forth, meaning a strong effort gives the patient a large breath and a meager effort a smaller one. This is sometimes called a weaning mode. The patient is given full support with rate and tidal volume until she is stronger. The rate is slowly turned down, allowing the patient more frequent, spontaneous breaths until extubation. Synchronized IMV (SIMV) ensures that a machine-delivered breath does not stack onto a patient-initiated breath.

Pressure support ventilation (PSV) is a mode where patient-initiated breaths are given support from the ventilator only during the beginning of ventilation (inspiratory phase). The support is meant to help the patient overcome the large amount of resistance present in the valves of the machine, the ventilator circuit, and the endotracheal tube. By titrating PSV to the spontaneous tidal volume produced by the patients, one can fully or partially support patient breathing and overcome the work of breathing. This mode of ventilation is important during the ''weaning'' process.

Work of Breathing

When conceptualizing the job of the ventilator, the different types of work must be defined (185). In addition to the physiologic work of breathing that all humans do on a daily basis, huge work loads are imposed from the resistance of the ventilator equipment (e.g., breathing through a straw analogy). Finally, there is the pathologic work of breathing from the pneumonia, the incision etc. The intent of mechanical ventilation during disease states is to assume the last two types of ''work'' so that the patient may convalesce. As a patient improves and the pathologic work has been removed, then the patient should be able to resume normal, physiologic work.

More Advanced Modes of Ventilation

With advanced circuitry and computer microprocessors, newer ventilator modes have been developed. Pressure-regulated volume control (PRVC) has largely replaced AC ventilation (ACV). PRVC provides the same function as AC while preventing overinflation. Recent data have shown that preventing overinflation (or stretch) of alveoli prevents trauma and a decreased incidence of ARDS (186). PRVC delivers the same tidal volume but changes the flow rate to prevent high pressures by measuring the pressure on a breath-to-breath basis. Volume control (VC ventilation) is a mode whereby a tidal volume target is set and the ventilator continually titrates the amount of PSV to provide this volume. This mode has been termed ''autowean'' or ''weekend'' mode because as the patient gets stronger, she will be able to meet the tidal volume setting. In situations where difficulties in ventilation are encountered such as ARDS, hypercarbia, and acidosis, pressure control (PC) is used. This mode is similar to the neonatal pressure-cycled ventilator where the maximum pressure is set and the flow rate is decreased but the inspiratory time is lengthened to achieve proper ventilation. Airway pressure release ventilation (APRV), high-frequency jet ventilation, and inverse ratio ventilation are other advanced modes beyond the scope of this chapter.

Setting the Ventilator

Initial ventilator settings require a rate of 12 to 14 breaths per minute with a tidal volume of 6 to 8 cc/kg. This is a departure from the traditional 12 cc/kg, which has been determined to result in greater alveolar trauma and increased risk for the development of ARDS (187). After initial setting of the ventilator, measurements of pH, PO_2, PCO_2, from arterial blood gas, are used to make further ventilator adjustments.

Oxygenation

Oxygenation is controlled by two settings, FIO_2 and PEEP. The inspired oxygen content can easily be controlled on the ventilator, keeping oxygen saturation greater than 92%. Inspired oxygen levels greater than 60% are considered to be potentially toxic, with such levels leading to pathologic changes similar to ARDS with acute inflammation and fibroproliferative changes. Human studies are few and have only examined effects on normal lungs, whereas no studies have clearly delineated the toxic effects of high oxygen levels in patients with underlying pulmonary disease (188). If it is necessary to have oxygen concentrations above 60%, the recommendation is to wean these levels as soon as possible. PEEP is another mechanism for improving oxygenation. In normal physiology, the glottis closes before full expiration creating a PEEP of approximately 4 cm H_2O and is termed physiologic PEEP. When ventilating patients, the addition of 5 cm H_2O PEEP is used as a baseline and is increased if added oxygen delivery is required. Increasing PEEP is the preferred method for improving oxygenation in postsurgical patients as opposed to increasing the F_{IO_2}. Postsurgical patients have atelectasis and shunting secondary to operative pain and anesthesia. The addition of PEEP recruits collapsed alveoli, improving oxygenation and lung compliance. However, the use of PEEP must be balanced by potential adverse effects, which include decreased cardiac output and the risk for barotrauma. Civetta et al. have shown that PEEP levels of 30 to 40 mm H_2O are easily tolerable in most patients; however, few clinical situations present in which patients need levels of PEEP this high (189).

Weaning from Ventilator

Multiple opinions exist on the techniques of weaning patients from mechanical ventilation, and no prospective randomized trial has proven one method to be superior to another (190). T-piece trials, spontaneous breathing trials, SIMV, and PSV are just a few. The best method of weaning is a treatment pathway agreed upon by clinicians, nurses, and respiratory therapists. Before discontinuing mechanical ventilation, the disease process that required ventilation should have resolved and patients should have proper mental status and the ability to generate a cough. Copious secretions are often an initial reason not to consider weaning or extubation. Criteria for extubation, whether on T-piece or minimal PSV, have traditionally included a respiratory rate less than 35, a P_{CO_2} less than 50 mm Hg, and a negative inspiratory force (NIF) greater than −20 cm H_2O.

Acute Respiratory Distress Syndrome

ARDS is a condition that has been well recognized and extensively studied (191). It is a form of refractory hypoxemia that can be elicited by a number of insults. In 1994, a consensus of American and European Intensivists defined the criteria for ARDS and a lesser form deemed acute lung injury (ALI) (192). Criteria include (a) acute onset after de-

fined insult; (b) bilateral diffuse infiltrates on chest radiograph; (c) no evidence of left atrial hypertension, CHF or a PAOP less than or equal to 18 mm Hg; and most importantly (d) impaired oxygenation. Impaired oxygenation was classified as ALI if the Pa_{O_2}/F_{IO_2} ratio was ≥300 mm Hg and ARDS if the Pa_{O_2}/F_{IO_2} ratio was ≥200 mm Hg. Post mortem examination of lungs with ARDS shows atelectasis, edema, inflammation, hyaline membrane deposition, and fibrosis. The mortality of ARDS is 30% to 40%. Treatment of these severely hypoxemic patients consists of mechanical ventilatory support with F_{IO_2} and PEEP. Because of alveolar damage, ventilation/perfusion mismatch occurs, resulting in a worsening shunt fraction and increasing dead space. As the pathologic process continues, not only does oxygenation become difficult but so also does ventilation as a result of decreased pulmonary compliance. The end result is a hypercapneic state and respiratory acidosis.

The recent ARDS NET trial comparing high tidal volume to achieve normocapnia with low tidal volumes to prevent barotrauma has shown significantly improved survival with the low volume protective strategy (186). Current strategies employ tidal volumes of 6 cc/kg and accept elevated PCO_2 levels (permissive hypercapnea).

The last 15 years have seen the elucidation of a number of systemic factors that are released upon physiologic insult (193). For example, cytokines, leukotrienes, endothelial adhesion molecules, and interleukins are useful in the defense of the organism, but systemically detrimental when activated by certain disease states. Investigations of the multiple organ dysfunction syndrome (MODS) where sequential organ failure leads to patient death has given significant credibility to the hypothesis that the lung may be the first organ system susceptible to these circulating inflammatory mediators (194). The pulmonary endothelium is acutely sensitive to circulating cytokines and is the first to manifest damage. In addition to supportive treatment for ARDS, operative injuries, or postoperative complications (e.g., intraabdominal abscess, anastomotic leak) must be sought and ruled out aggressively. ARDS is the result of some inciting cause and does not arise de novo as a primary problem.

Pneumonia

Pneumonia is a significant complication in postsurgical patients. Patients requiring mechanical ventilation are particularly susceptible to pneumonia [ventilator acquired pneumonia (VAP)] with rates as high as 30% after 72 hours of ventilation. The mortality rate from VAP ranges from 25% to 50%. The pathogens are often gram negative and resistant to multiple antibiotics. High clinical suspicion and aggressive treatment of VAP is crucial. An exhaustive review of this complicated and serious topic by Chastre and Fagon is recommended for further reading (195).

Pulmonary Embolism and Deep Venous Thrombosis Prophylaxis

The prevention of venous thromboembolism is an important component of perioperative management of the gynecologic oncology patient. The American College of Chest Physicians consensus statement published in 1998 reviews the data exhaustively and provides recommendations (196). Risk factors include age greater than 40 years, prolonged immobility, prior deep venous thrombosis (DVT), cancer diagnosis, major surgery, obesity, CHF, MI, stroke, indwelling femoral catheter, inflammatory bowel disease, estrogen use, nephrotic syndrome, and hypercoagulable states. The incidence of DVT in large groups of general surgical patients is around 20% and increases to 30% in patients with cancer diagnoses. The incidence of pulmonary embolism (PE) is 1.6% with a fatal PE rate of 0.9%. In trials comparing low-dose unfractionated heparin (LDUH) with no therapy in general surgical patients, the DVT rate was decreased from 25% to 8%. These studies also produced a 50% decrease in rate of fatal PE (196). Comparisons of low molecular weight heparin (LMWH) versus unfractionated heparin have shown equal efficacy. LMWH may have less bleeding complication (mostly wound hematomas) and greater ease of use with once daily dosing.

Sequential pneumatic compression devices (PCDs) are attractive for patients at risk for bleeding complications. In trials comparing PCD with LDUH, both have shown efficacy. Elastic stockings (Ted's hose) and aspirin usage are not currently recommended as DVT prophylaxis. Recently, studies have shown d-dimer positivity with DVT and PE, but the presence of any released blood or hematoma (i.e., any postoperative patient) makes the d-dimer positivity nonspecific. In the surgical patient, a negative d-dimer makes DVT or PE highly unlikely; however, a positive test is essentially useless.

Patients at low risk (age less than 40 years, no risk factors, and minor surgery) need no prophylaxis, but early ambulation is encouraged. Moderate risk patients (minor surgery in patient with risk factors, major surgery with no risk factors) should receive PCD, LMWH, or LDUH, with equal results. High-risk patients require LWMH in addition to PCD.

Diagnosis of DVT is performed by duplex ultrasonography, and treatment is with either heparinization to 1.5 times control prothrombin time or therapeutic doses of LMWH. Diagnosis of PE was traditionally made by pulmonary arteriogram. This practice has recently been abandoned because dynamic contrast-enhanced computerized tomography has better sensitivity. Once diagnosis is confirmed, the patient is anticoagulated with IV heparin or LMWH. Ultimately, the patient is converted to coumadin therapy for at least 3 months in the case of DVT and 6 months in the case of PE.

Fluid and Electrolyte Issues

Understanding fluid and electrolyte physiology in gynecologic oncology is paramount because of the underlying disease processes that face the gynecologic oncologist and the ultimate, radical surgical interventions that are needed to treat them. These treatments result in great fluid shifts perioperatively, requiring careful attention to input of fluids (volume and content/type) as well as output from renal and gastrointestinal sources, insensible sources, and drains. Since extensive discussions of these topics can be found elsewhere, this section will present a brief review of normal fluid and electrolyte physiology and discuss strategies for fluid resuscitation and correction of electrolyte deficiencies.

Total body water (TBW) can be calculated by various methods and varies directly with the amount of adipose or lean tissue present in an individual patient. TBW estimates, therefore, must be adjusted based on the adiposity of the patients. In women, TBW accounts for approximately 60% of a patient's weight. TBW is distributed into extracellular fluid (ECF) and intracellular fluid (ICF), with the ECF being further divided into intravascular (one-quarter of the ECF) and interstitial (three-quarters of the ECF) compartments. The ECF accounts for approximately one-third of the TBW, whereas ICF accounts for two-thirds (197,198). Direct measurement of the ECF and TBW are possible with the resulting difference being an estimated ICF. Table 11.10 describes the body fluid compartments and their contributions to body weight. Despite these arbitrary compartments (and concentration differences between compartments, which are discussed below), water flows freely across all compartments. Thus, a derangement in one compartment will result in a compensatory change in another (199).

The electrolyte composition of the various compartments is different. Sodium is the predominant cation in the ECF and potassium is the predominant cation of the ICF. Table 11.11 describes the various concentrations of electrolytes in the various fluid compartments. Because of the Donnan principle of equilibration, the content of cations and anions in the interstitial compartment is slightly higher than the intravascular compartment. This principle describes the unique relation between solutions of permeable and impermeable complex anions when these anions are unevenly distributed across a semipermeable membrane. Water on the

TABLE 11.10. *Body fluid compartments*

Total body water	Body weight (%)	Total body water (%)
Total	60	100
Intracellular	40	67
Extracellular	20	33
Intravascular	5	8
Interstitial	15	25

From Wait RB, Kahng KU, Dresner LS. Fluid and electrolytes and acid-base balance. In: Greenfield LJ, Mulholland M, Oldham KT, et al. eds. *Surgery: scientific principles and practice.* 2nd ed. Philadelphia: Lippincott–Raven Publishers, 1997:242–266, with permission.

TABLE 11.11 *Electrolyte concentrations in the various fluid compartments*

| | | Extracellular fluid | |
	Plasma	Interstitial fluid	Intracellular fluid
Cations			
Na$^+$	140	146	12
K$^+$	4	4	150
Ca^{2+}	5	3	10^{-7}
Mg^{2+}	2	1	7
Anions			
Cl$^-$	103	114	3
HCO$_3^-$	24	27	10
SO$_4^{2-}$	1	1	—
HPO$_4^{3-}$	2	2	116
Protein	16	5	40
Organic anions	5	5	—

From Wait RB, Kahng KU, Dresner LS. Fluid and electrolytes and acid-base balance. In: Greenfield LJ, Mulholland M, Oldham KT, et al. eds. *Surgery: scientific principles and practice.* 2nd ed. Philadelphia: Lippincott–Raven Publishers, 1997:242–266, with permission.

other hand, as mentioned earlier, freely equilibrates between the compartments (199).

Effective circulating volume (ECV) is a term used to describe the portion of the ECF that perfuses the organs of the body and affects baroreceptors (see below). In healthy patients, the ECV equates to the intravascular volume/compartment. But in disease states that increase "third spacing" such as sepsis (leaky capillaries), ascites due to intraabdominal metastasis, or bowel obstruction with resulting edema and transudation, the interstitial compartment increases at the expense of the intravascular compartment, decreasing the ECV (197).

The osmotic activity of a fluid compartment is affected by the component ions and is described in milliosmoles (mOsm). Normal serum osmolality (in the ECF, of course) averages 290 mOsm/kg of H$_2$O. Osmoreceptors in the hypothalamus respond to small changes in serum osmolality, increasing or decreasing secretion of antidiuretic hormone

(ADH) and modifying the thirst response. These receptors are responsible for the day-to-day fine tuning of fluid balance. Baroreceptors, on the other hand, in the intrathoracic vena cava, the atria, the aortic arch, the carotid arteries, and the renal parenchyma, sense volume changes by changes in pressure. These receptors begin a cascade of mediators such as aldosterone, atrial natriuretic peptide (ANP), prostaglandins, and the renin-angiotensin system, which ultimately result in changes of water and sodium balance mediated through the kidneys. These baroreceptors have little to do with the day-to-day fluid management and require intravascular losses of 10% to 20% to initiate activity (199).

The goal of fluid resuscitation is to maintain the ECV and return the patient to a homeopathic state. Many gynecologic oncology procedures are lengthy and can result in large blood losses requiring immediate intraoperative replacement. In addition, following procedures where evacuation of large amounts of ascites has occurred and/or "peritoneal stripping" has left denuded surfaces, these patients may have large fluid shifts into the interstitial compartment requiring large volumes of fluid to maintain the ECV. Finally, losses are not water alone and include electrolytes and clotting factors, which may need repletion. Selecting fluids to administer to a given patient is akin to selecting the correct intravenous medication to give; not *all* fluids are for *all* patients. The physician should understand the amount of daily maintenance fluid and electrolytes required by patients, calculate losses (fluid and electrolytes), determine ongoing fluid and electrolyte losses, and replace them with the appropriate fluid and electrolyte combinations. It is easy to fall into the trap of giving all patients an 8-hour rate (125 mL/hour) of maintenance fluid. However, an octogenarian, even with normal cardiac and renal function weighing 50 kg, does not need that much maintenance fluid. "Formulas" for calculating appropriate maintenance fluid requirements exist (199), but calculating 30 to 40 mL/kg/day, depending upon body frame size, is a much simpler and quicker estimate of maintenance fluid requirements for patients.

In general, the normal maintenance requirement of sodium is 1 to 2 mEq/kg/day and for potassium 0.5 to 1.0 mEq/

TABLE 11.12. *Electrolyte content of commonly used intravenous electrolyte solutions*

| Solution | Electrolyte concentration (mEq/L) | | | | | |
	Na$^+$	K$^+$	Ca^{2+}	Mg^{2+}	Cl$^-$	HCO^{3-}
Lactated Ringer's solution	130	4	4	—	109	28
0.2% NaCl	34	—	—	—	34	—
0.33% NaCl	56	—	—	—	56	—
0.45% NaCl	77	—	—	—	77	—
0.9% NaCl	154	—	—	—	154	—
3.0% NaCl	513	—	—	—	513	—
5.0% NaCl	855	—	—	—	855	—

Adapted from Wait RB, Kahng KU, Dresner LS. Fluid and electrolytes and acid-base balance. In: Greenfield LJ, Mulholland M, Oldham KT, et al. eds. *Surgery: scientific principles and practice.* 2nd ed. Philadelphia: Lippincott–Raven Publishers, 1997:242–266, with permission.

kg/day. Table 11.12 lists the various intravenous (IV) fluid preparations available for fluid resuscitation. Which fluid to be used is controversial and driven, in more instances, by "dogma," varying from physician-to-physician and institution-to-institution rather than by evidence. Controversy over which fluid type to use in fluid resuscitation continues to this day. Several meta-analyses have shown no advantage of colloid over crystalloid for resuscitation in surgical patients (200–207). Almost all studies have shown that administered colloid leaks from the intravascular compartment to the interstitial compartment in several hours, decreasing the ECV and requiring further administration of colloid (200–207). The use of colloid has been shown to be advantageous in conditions of hypoproteinemia or malnourished states where patients require plasma volume expansion and cannot tolerate large amounts of fluid (207).

Most of the time patients are given isotonic solutions, such as lactated Ringer's solution, to cover perioperative losses. In the immediate postoperative course, patients are given their maintenance fluid requirements in addition to the immediate intraoperative losses. It is helpful to convert all losses to equivalents of crystalloid to determine fluid rates. For example, to replace 500 mL of blood loss, one would give 1500 mL of isotonic fluid, a ratio of 3 mL of crystalloid to 1 mL of blood loss. It is traditional to replace one-half of the intraoperative losses in the first 24 hours, with the rest being replaced during the ensuing several days. Other intraoperative losses, which need to be accounted for, are the insensible losses which occur through evaporation from the incision (5 to 10 mL/kg/hour of operation) and from the anesthesia circuit and ascites.

Sodium Derangements

Hyponatremia is the most common electrolyte abnormality seen in postoperative patients and is caused by excess free water rather than a depletion of sodium. Increases in free water absorption are mediated by a self-limited, physiologic increase in the secretion of ADH in response to the stress of surgery. Serum sodium levels rarely fall below 130 mEq/L, but may be further exacerbated by intravenous administration of large volumes of hypotonic solutions (i.e., 0.2%, 0.33, 0.45% sodium solutions). Other disease states can result in a hyperosmolar condition, resulting in a hyperosmolar ECF, causing fluid to shift from the ICF and lowering the sodium levels. These conditions include hyperglycemia, mannitol ethylene glycol or ethanol ingestion, and uremia. For each increase of 180 mg/dL of glucose above 100 mg/dL, there is a concomitant decrease in the serum sodium of 5 mEq/L (198). In addition, during situations where potassium is low, there is a compensatory exchange of sodium for potassium, resulting in hyponatremia. In either of these prior cases, total body sodium does not change. Finally, patients with hyperproteinemia or hyperlipidemia may have falsely low sodium values, which result from errors in the laboratory measurement of sodium. This *pseudohyponatremia* does not result in any symptoms of hyponatremia (199).

The symptoms of hyponatremia are driven by cellular water intoxication and are related to the central nervous system (CNS) (e.g., lethargy, headaches, confusion, delirium, weakness, muscle cramps). The rate at which hyponatremia occurs also determines the symptoms. Chronic hyponatremia tends to be asymptomatic, whereas acute drops in the serum sodium (levels 120 to 130) result in the symptoms listed above. Correction of hyponatremia must be done carefully to avoid central pontine myelinolysis, which results in the "locked-in syndrome."

Because most hyponatremia is related to dehydration (low ECV), simple correction of this state will increase the sodium plasma level. If the patient has a high ECV [such as the syndrome of inappropriate antidiuretic hormone (SIADH) secretion] or is in an edematous state, free water restriction should normalize the sodium level. However, if patients have symptoms of hyponatremia, aggressive replacement of sodium is prudent should the duration of the hyponatremia be determined to be no longer than 48 hours. Hyponatremic states longer than 48 hours increase the risk of central pontine myelinolysis. Chronic cases need replacement at rates not to exceed 0.5 mEq/L/hour. Acute cases may be replaced at rates of 5 mEq/L/hour.

Hypernatremia is an uncommon finding and is related to large volumes of free water loss (through insensible routes such as breathing, sweating, and ventilation), diabetes insipidus, adrenal hyperfunction, or ingestion or administration of increased sodium solutions. Again, the symptoms are predominantly CNS oriented because of brain cell dehydration. Symptoms rarely occur until serum sodium levels exceed 160 mEq/L. In addition, the rapidity at which the derangement occurs determines the symptoms manifested. Treatment is carefully done with replacement of free water. Replacement too rapidly can cause cerebral edema and herniation. Patients with chronic hypernatremia need free water administration, which decreases the serum sodium no faster than 0.7 mEq/L.

Potassium Derangements

Whereas sodium is the major extracellular cation, potassium is the major intracellular cation by a ratio of 30:1. The intracellular potassium concentrations tend to be relatively constant, whereas the extracellular concentrations vary depending upon renal function/excretion. The majority of potassium secretion occurs in the distal tubule and the collecting duct of the nephron. Secretion is stimulated by increased urine flow, increased sodium delivery, high potassium levels, alkalosis, aldosterone, vasopressin, and beta-adrenergic agonists. Insulin causes potassium to move into cells (as previously mentioned), reducing the extracellular concentration of potassium. Serum potassium levels are further affected by the acid-base status of patients. In alkalotic states, the potassium shifts into cells in exchange for hydrogen ions, whereas in acidotic states the exchange is opposite.

The predominant reason for hyperkalemia in a postoperative patient is renal dysfunction or failure. When these patients become critically ill, serum potassium concentrations can increase by 0.3 to 0.5 mEq/L/day in noncatabolic patients and 0.7 mEq/L/day in catabolic patients. It is important to rule out a spuriously elevated level secondary to hemolysis at the time of the blood draw either from too small a gauge of needle or simply from the application of the tourniquet and squeezing (199).

Hyperkalemia changes the membrane potential established by differences between the intracellular and extracellular mileu. This increased concentration has deleterious effects on cardiac muscle function, causing peaked T waves, flattened P waves, prolonged QRS complexes, and deep S waves on the ECG and possibly resulting in ventricular fibrillation and cardiac arrest. Skeletal musculature is also affected with paresthesias and weakness, which can progress to a flaccid paralysis.

Treatment for hyperkalemia has been outlined in the section on renal risk factors. The mainstay is saline diuresis unless ECG changes are present, then infusion of calcium gluconate can be lifesaving. Utilization of 25 to 50 g of glucose and 10 to 20 units of regular insulin can drive potassium intracellularly and transiently lower plasma levels. Ultimately, definitive therapy relies upon increased excretion of potassium. For each gram of sodium polystyrene sulfonate (Kayexalate) (given in the doses previously mentioned) used either orally or rectally, 0.5 mEq of potassium will be removed. Finally, in patients not responding to these therapies or patients with renal failure, hemodialysis may be indicated.

Hypokalemia is caused by decreased intake, increased gastrointestinal losses (vomiting, diarrhea, fistulae), excessive renal losses (metabolic alkalosis, magnesium deficiency, hyperaldosteronism), a shift of potassium into the intracellular space (acute or uncompensated metabolic alkalosis, glucose and insulin administration, catecholamines), or any combination thereof. A reduction of serum potassium by 1 mEq/L represents a total body deficiency of about 100 to 200 mEq. [Remember that total exchangeable potassium is approximately 3,000 mEq with the majority being intracellular and thus the majority of the loss (199).] Symptoms of hypokalemia cause ECG changes with flattening of the T waves, depression of S-T segments, prominent U waves, and prolongation of the Q-T interval. Treatment is accomplished by replacement of potassium either orally or intravenously depending upon the severity of symptoms and whether or not the patient is able to take oral preparations. Intravenous replacement of potassium can be done at approximately 10 mEq/hour and should not be more concentrated than 40 mEq/L. If less fluid is desired, 20 mEq can be placed in 100 mL, but administration should not exceed 40 mEq/ hour (199).

Magnesium Derangements

Most magnesium in the body is confined to the intracellular space and bone. Less than 1% of total body magnesium is in the serum. Of the magnesium in the serum, 60% is ionized, 25% is protein bound, and 15% is complexed with nonprotein anionic species (199). Magnesium is absorbed in the small intestine, directed by levels of vitamin D, and filtered by the kidney for excretion. Approximately 40% of renally excreted magnesium is reabsorbed in the ascending loop of Henle. Loop diuretics, hypermagnesemia, hypercalcemia, acidosis, and phosphate depletion result in increased excretion of magnesium.

Patients with renal failure and receiving magnesium containing antacids or laxatives can become hypermagnesemic. In addition, patients with acidosis and dehydration may become hypermagnesemic. Patients present with CNS depression, loss of deep tendon reflexes, and ECG changes (prolonged P-R interval and QRS complex) in the face of elevated magnesium levels (greater than 8 mg/dL). As levels rise, patients will develop coma, respiratory failure, and/or cardiac arrest. Acute treatment of hypermagnesemia is slow IV infusion of 5 to 10 mEq of calcium. Because the etiology of this condition is usually renal failure, withholding magnesium-containing preparations may be all that is necessary. In severe instances, hemodialysis is required.

In gynecologic oncology patients, the overwhelming reason for hypomagnesemia is a history of cisplatin administration. However, other conditions such as hypoparathyroidism, malabsorptive states, chronic loop diuretic use and the diuretic phase of acute renal failure can cause hypomagnesemia. Symptoms are similar to hypocalcemia with muscle weakness, fasciculations, tetany, hypokalemia, and ECG changes (Q-T prolongation, torsades de pointes). Treatment can be accomplished with oral preparations in less acute situations. However, large doses may produce diarrhea, worsening the situation. Intravenous boluses of 2 to 3 g followed by infusions of 1 to 2 mEq/kg/day can be utilized for patients with severe symptoms.

Calcium Derangements

Almost all the calcium in the body is in bone, stored as hydroxyapatite crystals, and provides a supply that can be exchanged to the serum. Calcium homeostasis is controlled by parathyroid hormone (PTH), controlling intestinal absorption of calcium, renal excretion of calcium, and exchange of calcium from the bone. In the serum, calcium exists in three phases: 45% as an ionized form, which is responsible for most of the physiologic function of calcium; 40% in a protein bound form, bound mostly to albumin; and 15% in a nonionized form, complexed with nonprotein anions that do not easily dissociate. A serum total calcium level is usually obtained when assessing calcium homeostasis, as measurement of ionized calcium is cumbersome. The total calcium levels change by 0.8 g/dL for each 1 g/dL change of albumin (up or down) (199).

In gynecologic oncology patients with hypercalcemia, the underlying malignancy is usually the etiologic agent. Hypercalcemia may be caused by direct bony involvement, or more commonly, secretion of PTH-like peptides and/or other humoral factors, which increase serum calcium levels. Other reasons for hypercalcemia include primary, secondary, or tertiary hyperparathyroidism, thiazide diuretic use, or lithium usage (199,208). Patients present with muscle fatigue, weakness, confusion, coma, ECG changes (shortening of the Q-T interval), nausea, and vomiting. The goal of treatment is to increase calcium excretion and stop bone turnover in order to decrease serum total calcium. Initial measures include vigorous hydration (200 mL/hour) with 0.9% or 0.45% saline solutions. Furosemide or other loop diuretics may be helpful in patients with borderline cardiac function or in patients with fluid overload. If the underlying malignancy is a breast carcinoma, patients may respond to high doses of steroids to reduce calcium levels. Other pharmacologic agents have been developed to stop bone resorption and reduce serum calcium levels. Calcitonin (4 IU/kg every 12 hours via subcutaneous or intramuscular injection) has a rapid onset of action and works by interfering with osteoclast maturation at several points (208). However, the duration of response is usually about 48 hours because of downregulation of calcitonin receptors by osteoclasts. Bisphosphonates have emerged as the drug of choice for treatment of hypercalcemia in malignancy. These agents work by inhibiting osteoclast activity and survival. The nitrogen-containing bisphosphonates are the most potent. Pamidronate (approved in 1991) and zoledronic acid (approved in 2001) are utilized in the United States. Another agent, ibandronate, is utilized in Europe, but has not been approved for use in the United States. Zoledronic acid is the current drug of choice because of its proven superiority over pamidronate (209). The effective dose of zoledronic acid is 4 mg infused over 15 minutes and dosed every 3 to 4 weeks. Serum calcium levels return to normal in approximately 10 days and duration of response lasts approximately 40 days (210). Surgical resection is the treatment of choice for primary, secondary, or tertiary hyperparathyroidism (199, 208).

Hypocalcemia is caused by hypoparathyroidism, hypomagnesemia, pancreatitis, and malnutrition. Patients present with tetany, hyperactive deep tendon reflexes, a positive Chvostek sign, positive Trousseau sign, and ECG changes (prolonged Q-T interval, prolonged S-T segment). Low levels of calcium may be present because of low albumin levels, but these levels do not affect the ionized portion of calcium and usually do not cause symptoms. Symptomatic hypocalcemia can be treated with intravenous infusion of either calcium gluconate or calcium chloride at a rate not to exceed 50 mg/min. Calcium chloride dissociates into the ionized form of calcium more readily and is the treatment of choice to raise serum ionized calcium level.

Acid-Base Disturbances

Optimum cellular function requires a very narrow range of pH for chemical reactions to occur normally. Several buffering systems exist within the body to maintain this optimum pH. The predominant buffering system is the carbonic acid-bicarbonate buffering system. Derangements in the concentration of bicarbonate (HCO_3^-) or in concentrations of carbon dioxide (CO_2) result in acid-base disorders. Because the kidneys control excretion/generation of bicarbonate and the lungs exchange CO_2, these organs play a central role in the compensation of any acid-base disorder. Therefore, four situations arise in acid-base balance: metabolic acidosis and alkalosis and respiratory acidosis and alkalosis. Compensatory mechanisms exist in each situation in order to blunt the effect on pH (Table 11.13).

Metabolic Acidosis

Most clinically significant metabolic acidosis occurs with a net loss of bicarbonate either due to direct loss or when consumption is greater than generation. Situations where extra renal losses of bicarbonate occur include diarrhea, gastrointestinal fistulae, and urinary diversions (ureterosigmoidostomy or ureteroileostomy, which result in reabsorption of NH_4Cl from urine). Certain disease states result in the production of organic acids (ketoacidosis and lactic acidosis), which consume bicarbonate and outpace the renal com-

TABLE 11.13. *Concentrations of HCO_3 and pCO_2 in primary acid-base derangements and the compensatory response*

Disorder	pH	Primary		Compensatory Response	
		HCO_3^-	P_{CO_2}	HCO_3^-	P_{CO_2}
Metabolic acidosis	↓	↓			↓
Metabolic alkalosis	↑	↑			↑
Respiratory acidosis	↓		↑	↑	
Respiratory alkalosis	↑		↓	↓	

Adapted from Wait RB, Kahng KU, Dresner LS. Fluid and electrolytes and acid-base balance. In: Greenfield LJ, Mulholland M, Oldham KT, et al. eds. Surgery: scientific principles and practice. 2nd ed. Philadelphia: Lippincott–Raven Publishers, 1997:242–266, with permission.

pensatory mechanisms. Similarly, overdoses of certain drugs (e.g., aspirin) or ingestion of toxins (e.g., ethylene glycol, methanol) consume bicarbonate and outpace the renal compensatory mechanisms. Renal acidosis occurs when the intrinsic acid-excreting function of the kidney malfunctions, resulting in retention of acid and consumption of bicarbonate without concomitant regeneration of bicarbonate. These are classified as renal tubular acidosis (RTA I, distal tubule dysfunction; or RTA-II, proximal tubule dysfunction). Cardiac effects are the major findings in metabolic acidosis (peripheral arteriolar dilation, decreased cardiac contractility, and central venous constriction). Other manifestations of metabolic acidosis include gastric distention, abdominal pain, nausea, and vomiting. In surgical patients, lactic acidosis is the primary cause of metabolic acidosis and results from tissue hypoperfusion. Therefore, treatment should be aimed at increasing tissue perfusion with fluid and blood administration. The use of bicarbonate is best reserved for patients with other, not easily reversible causes of metabolic acidosis. Older patients and patients with cardiovascular disease may benefit from administration of bicarbonate. Administration should be instituted when the pH is 7.1 to 7.2. One or two ampules of bicarbonate (approximately 55 mEq/amp) can be administered intravenously, with further administrations being dictated by the pH obtained from an arterial blood gas measurement. In diabetic ketoacidosis, treatment with insulin and glucose infusion should not only reverse the acidosis but also treat the hyperglycemia.

Metabolic Alkalosis

Sustained metabolic alkalosis is an uncommon clinical entity and is related to renal dysfunction. Loss of HCl is the most common reason for an increase in extracellular bicarbonate. This situation occurs with prolonged nausea and vomiting or prolonged nasogastric suctioning of gastric contents. As acid is removed from the gastrointestinal tract, a net gain of bicarbonate occurs. Other situations that can result in a metabolic alkalosis include volume contraction, exogenous administration of bicarbonate or bicarbonate precursors (citrate, lactate, or calcium carbonate), hypokalemia, hypercalcemia, hypochloremia, excess mineralocorticoid usage, and high PCO_2. Patients rarely present with symptoms, as metabolic alkalosis occurs gradually. However, in patients who develop this situation acutely, most symptoms are CNS oriented (e.g., confusion, stupor, coma, muscle fasiculations, tetany). Correction of the underlying disease state usually corrects the metabolic alkalosis. Repletion of electrolyte abnormalities and infusion of appropriate fluids (chloride containing) restore volume and result in normal renal excretion of excess bicarbonate.

Respiratory Acidosis

A depression of the pH occurs when there is hypoventilation. This occurs secondary to airway obstruction, COPD, depression of the respiratory center, impaired excursion of the thorax, or inappropriate ventilatory management in the mechanically ventilated patient. Development of symptoms depends upon the chronicity or acute nature of the event. If chronic, most patients have no symptoms. If it is an acute change, drowsiness, restlessness, headache, or development of a flapping tremor may occur. Treatment of this condition is aimed at the underlying cause of the hypoventilation. In chronic conditions, the hypoxemia, and subsequent hypercapnia, resulting from the hypoventilation, may be the sole drive for the patient's respirations. Correction of the hypoxemia may further worsen the respiratory acidosis and must be considered. In general, correction of the PCO_2 must be done slowly because reequilibration of cerebral bicarbonate concentration lags behind systemic changes (199).

Respiratory Alkalosis

Respiratory alkalosis occurs when the PCO_2 decreases with hyperventilation. Hyperventilation may occur because of hypoxia, drugs, decreased lung compliance, and mechanical ventilation. With drops in the arterial PO_2, the peripheral chemoreceptors (in the carotid and aortic body) sense this change and result in hyperventilation to increase arterial PO_2 with a resulting decrease in PCO_2. Because of renal compensatory mechanisms, this condition is usually asymptomatic. However, in acute situations, patients may have a sensation of breathlessness, dizziness, nervousness with altered levels of consciousness and tetany. Treatment of underlying hypoxia should address the hyperventilation. If acute symptoms are present, having the patient rebreathe expired air should temporarily relieve the symptoms.

Postoperative Nutritional Issues

As mentioned earlier, the full consideration of nutrition in the gynecologic oncology patient is presented in Chapter 35. In this section, we will discuss early refeeding in the postoperative gynecologic oncology patient, indications for enteral nutrition, and total parenteral nutrition (TPN).

Although malnutrition has been shown to be prevalent among gynecologic oncology patients (98), many patients are adequately nourished, undergo surgery uneventfully, and have return of bowel function in 2–5 days while simultaneously resuming oral intake. Recently, several prospective randomized trials have been conducted that demonstrate the utility of early refeeding in the postoperative period. In these studies, patients in the early feeding group were fed on the first postoperative day, with 90% or more tolerating diets. The underlying malignancies, types of operations, and complications occurred at similar rates between the early refeeding and the "traditionally fed" patients in all the studies. The placement of nasogastric tubes (NGTs) for intolerance of diet was low among the studies (less than 10% incidence).

Finally, length of hospital stay was shorter among the earlier fed patients (211–216).

The use of the enteral route is preferred in sustaining or repleting patients in the postoperative period after extensive procedures. Enteral nutrition utilizes normal physiologic absorptive mechanisms, maintains gut epithelial integrity, and reduces infectious morbidity (217, 218). Studies on nutrition have found that the splanchnic circulation and support of the mucosal integrity of the small bowel may prevent progression to multiorgan dysfunction syndrome MODS (see below). Specifically, the intestinal mucosa will atrophy secondary to lack of luminal nutrients and intermittent activation of the destructive cytokine pathways and/or intermittent translocation of bacteria into the blood stream will occur. These events result in "priming" neutrophils, which ultimately leads to a fullblown systemic inflammatory response causing organ damage. A number of well-designed randomized trails have compared early enteral feeds to total parenteral nutrition (TPN) in patients with pancreatitis, major elective surgery, and trauma (217, 218). All these studies have shown a clear benefit for early enteral feeding, with a decrease in infectious complications (218).

Although considered a nonessential amino acid in nourished, healthy patients, glutamine has emerged as an essential amino acid in patients who are stressed and critically ill. This amino acid has been shown to be an important component in maintaining enterocyte integrity and has now been added to most enteral preparations (101,217,218).

Enteral feeds may be given in a variety of fashions and each is associated with its own type and number of complications. Intragastric feeds may be accomplished with NGTs, oral-gastric tubes, or percutaneous gastrostomy tubes (PEGs). Intragastric feeding has the advantage of utilizing the stomach as a reservoir for bolus feeding. In addition, stretching of the stomach stimulates the biliary-pancreatic axis, which may be trophic to the small bowel. Finally, the gastric secretions mix with the feeding material and decrease the osmolarity, thus reducing the incidence of diarrhea. The main disadvantage of this route of enteral feeding is the increased risk of gastric overdistention with high residual amounts of feeding material and the increased risk of aspiration pneumonia (217). Enteral feeds may also be accomplished through the placement of nasal tubes, which are positioned into the pylorus, duodenum or jejunum (such as Dobhoff tubes). These tubes have the advantage of being placed (or migrating) more distal in the upper gastrointestinal tract, greatly reducing the risk of aspiration. These types of tubes are preferred in patients who require long-term ventilation. Because of advances in endoscopic instrumentation, many of the tubes can be placed via this method. At the time of laparotomy, gastrostomy, or jejunostomy, tubes (such as a Stamm or Witzel tube) may be placed. These have the advantage of being placed at the time of major abdominal surgery under direct visualization/palpation. The techniques are described in other texts (217,219). Several enteral feeding preparations are available, but vary from hospital to hospital depending upon formulary make-up. The use of the enteral route is contraindicated in patients with mechanical intestinal obstructions, and for these patients, nutritional support can be accomplished through the parenteral route.

TPN took forefront in nutritional sustenance and replacement in the 1980s. The basic premise of TPN is to provide dietary precursors to maintain anabolic function. TPN can be broken into three components of replacement: glucose and lipid preparations for normal or increased energy expenditures and amino acid preparations for protein synthesis. Because of the higher osmolar load presented by these preparations, central venous access is necessary for administration. Subclavian, internal jugular, or peripherally inserted central catheters (PICCs) will need to be placed, and they present the first of several potential complications associated with TPN administration. At the time of placement, pneumothorax, intubation of arterial structures, air embolism, or cardiac arrhythmias may occur. Later complications include the possibility of infection at the skin entrance site or line sepsis. Should these infectious complications occur, removal of the catheter and antibiotic administration will be necessary (101).

The Harris-Benedict equation is utilized to calculate basal energy expenditure (BEE) for patients and approximates the BEE of a sedentary, fasting, nonstressed individual (220).

$$BEE = 666 + [9.6 \times weight\ (kg)]$$
$$+ [1.7 \times height\ (cm)] - [4.7 \times age\ (yr)]$$

Because stress of disease and surgical intervention need to be considered, "stress factors" have been developed and are multiplied by the BEE to arrive at kilocalories per day. Stress level multipliers are: 1.2 for a resting individual, 1.3 for an ambulatory individual or moderate stress (e.g., SIRS, sepsis), and 1.5 for severe stress/burn patients.

After calculation of caloric requirements, the composition of the TPN solution to be administered should be determined. Because there are many different types of TPN preparations available, consultation with the nutrition team or pharmacists in an individual hospital is necessary to arrive at the desired solution.

In aerobic situations, glucose is the primary substrate for energy expenditure. It provides 3.4 kcal/g and is usually given in a concentrated form in order to provide 70% of the calculated calories. The remaining 30% of calories is provided by lipid preparations. Not only does this component have denser caloric content (provide 9 kcal/g), but administration precludes the development of a fatty acid deficiency. Adjustment of the composition of TPN may be necessary depending upon the disease state (e.g., more contribution of kilocalories from fat vs carbohydrate in a ventilated patient because of the respiratory quotient of fat vs glucose).

Protein requirements are provided by amino acid solutions

TABLE 11.14. *Visceral proteins utilized as indicators for nutritional status during nutritional repletion*

Protein	Normal range	Half-life (days)	Levels low in	Levels high in
Albumin	3.5–5.4 g/dL	18	Liver disease, pregnancy, overhydration, nephrotic syndrome	Dehydration
Transferrin	200–400 mg/dL	8	Chronic infection, chronic inflammation, liver disease, iron overload, nephrotic syndrome	Iron deficiency, pregnancy
Prealbumin	20–40 mg/dL	2	Liver disease, inflammation, surgery, nephrotic syndrome	
Retinol-binding protein (RBP)	3–6 mg/dL	0.5	Liver disease, hyperthyroidism, zinc deficiency, nephrotic syndrome	Renal insufficiency

and are determined by the patient's age, sex, nutritional status, ongoing stress and co-morbid conditions. In general, 25% of protein requirements are obtained by normal oral intake. The remaining protein comes from breakdown of serum and organic proteins. Thus, periods of prolonged malnutrition, with decreased protein intake, and increased stress of disease will lead to breakdown of visceral protein. An estimate of maintenance protein requirements is 1 g nitrogen/kg of body weight. In situations of increased stress, the patient may need 1.2 to 1.5 g/kg in order to maintain and/or replace protein losses. Table 11.14 shows serum protein measurements and their respective half-lives, which are useful for determining anabolic versus catabolic response to TPN treatment. Another method to assess nitrogen balance (positive or negative) is (200):

Nitrogen balance

$$= \text{protein inake}/6.25 - (\text{urinary urea nitrogen} + 4)$$

The amount of protein intake is divided by 6.25 to give the grams of nitrogen taken in. The urinary urea nitrogen is expressed in grams based upon a 24-hour collection. The correction factor of 4 is meant to adjust for the grams of nitrogen lost in the stool or non–urea nitrogen losses.

In addition to these three main components of TPN, daily requirements of vitamins, trace elements, and insulin are necessary to maintain/regain nourishment. Again, these preparations vary by hospital formulary and need consultation with resident pharmacists.

The rate of infusion of TPN needs to be titrated upward to take into account the large glucose load that the patient will be receiving. This lower rate allows the pancreas time to increase insulin secretion in order to meet the glucose load being presented. Similarly, the rate of infusion needs to be decreased when TPN is being stopped to prevent hypoglycemia. During TPN administration, blood glucose measurements by finger stick are required so that hyperglycemia is avoided. For the first several days, measurement of serum electrolytes, with adjustments being made daily, is necessary.

As previously mentioned, complications from venous access are some of the drawbacks of TPN administration. Other complications include metabolic derangements, which most often are mild but need correcting as soon as they are identified, abnormalities of liver function tests, the clinical significance of which is unclear (101), and cholelithiasis/cholecystitis secondary to gallbladder sludge.

Renal Issues

Acute renal failure (ARF) or hospital-acquired renal insufficiency (HARI) continues to be a common problem among postsurgical patients. Although the incidence of HARI is 1.5 patients per 1000 admitted, the impact of HARI on morbidity and mortality is quite high (mortality averages 45%, but may exceed 80% if dialysis is required). The best methods for preventing HARI are reducing risk factors and reversing the condition by early detection and intervention (221).

When HARI presents in the postoperative patient, causes can be divided into three parts: prerenal, renal, or postrenal (inflow, parenchymal, and outflow). The function of glomeruli to create the urinary filtrate depends upon adequate renal perfusion and represents the prerenal component. If the renal mean arterial pressure (MAP) falls below 80 mm Hg, perfusion of the glomeruli decreases (some disease states require the renal MAP to be higher for adequate perfusion). Many situations can decrease renal MAP and include anesthetics, atherosclerotic emboli, decreased vascular resistance, hypotension, intravascular volume contraction, mechanical ventilation, sepsis, and any form of shock. Autoregulation of the glomeruli can be disrupted by nonsteroidal antiinflammatory drugs (NSAIDs), angiotensin-converting enzyme inhibitors (ACE inhibitors), calcium channel blockers (diltiazem or verapamil), and endotoxins produced by gram-negative sepsis.

Renal parenchymal damage occurs most commonly in the postoperative patient because of prolonged hypotension or direct injury from inflammatory responses initiated by sepsis. In general, if the hypoperfusion is corrected quickly, reversible azotemia, creatinine elevation, and decreased urine output may be the only manifestations. However, prolonged hypoperfusion can cause acute tubular necrosis (ATN), which results in sloughing of renal tubular cells into the tubular lumen and obstruction. In addition the production of Tamm-Horsfall proteins form coarse granular casts, inciting an intense inflammatory response, further injuring the renal parenchyma (222,223). Other agents that can induce ATN include aminoglycoside antibiotics and iodinated contrast media. Approximately 15% of patients who receive aminoglycosides will have nephrotoxicity, and serum levels of these antibiotics need to be carefully monitored (224). Iodinated contrast media, used in multiple radiographic procedures, induces ATN by impairing nitric oxide production and increasing free radical formation (225,226). Diabetic patients with creatinine clearance rates less than 50 mL/minute are at particularly high risk (227).

The final reason for ARF in the postoperative gynecologic oncology patient is outflow obstruction. Because of the radical pelvic procedures performed by gynecologic oncologists, ureteral injury is possible and needs to be excluded early in the evaluation of patients with ARF. Prompt reversal of the obstruction can further limit renal damage.

In general, expected postoperative urinary output should be maintained at 0.5 mL/kg of weight per hour. Most oliguria can be treated with intravascular expansion in the first 24 to 48 hours postsurgery. Hypoperfusion of the renal parenchyma must be avoided to prevent ATN from occurring. The definition of ARF is not standardized, but includes rising serial creatinine measurements, urine output less than 400 mL/24 hours, or, in drastic situations, the initiation of dialysis (221). Once diagnosed, calculating the fractional excretion of sodium (FENa) or chloride can help to discern between prerenal causes or renal causes (hypoperfusions versus ATN). The formula is presented below (221):

FENa = [urine Na level × serum Cr level]

/ [serum Na level × urine Cr level] × 100%

If the FENa is less than 1% and the urine specific gravity is greater than 1.025, the diagnosis is hypoperfusion. However, if ischemia has occurred, the FENa will be greater than 4% and the urine specific gravity will fall to 1.010 because of tubular damage and loss of renal concentrating mechanisms. One cannot calculate FENa in patients who have received diuretics or hyperosmotic agents (e.g., mannitol or contrast media). If prerenal and renal causes of low urine output have been excluded, ultrasonography may be useful in evaluating for outflow obstruction.

Once the underlying causes for HARI have been eliminated (e.g., hypoperfusion, obstruction, sepsis), only time can be offered as treatment. Therapies such as low-dose dopamine, furosemide, or mannitol administration or atrial natriuretic peptide use have not demonstrated prevention of or improved recovery from HARI (228–233). Dialysis remains the only intervention that can support patients until return of renal function. Indications for dialysis include (a) hyperkalemia, metabolic acidosis, or volume expansion that cannot be controlled; (b) symptoms of uremia or encephalopathy; or (c) platelet dysfunction inducing a bleeding diasthesis (221).

Shock

Definition

Shock is defined in its simplest terms as a decrease in tissue perfusion—a decrease below the lowest metabolic needs of the tissue bed. This usually results in a depletion of stored energy and an increase in anaerobic metabolism with a buildup of lactic acid in addition to other toxic waste products. Hypotension is incorrectly thought of as a defining component of shock. Hypotension often leads to hypoperfusion, but the hypotensive patient is not in shock until evidence of hypoperfusion occurs. Various types of shock exist.

Hemorrhagic Shock

The first thought for a surgeon managing a postoperative patient who manifests signs and symptoms of shock is hemorrhage. Hypovolemic shock secondary to inadequate preload can be the result of excessive or ongoing blood loss or inadequate replacement or both. Certainly after radical debulking procedures or major extirpative procedures, the potential for postoperative hemorrhage exists. Tachycardia, hypotension, and oliguria are typical clinical signs. In the face of these clinical signs, the surgeon should have high suspicion for active bleeding and be preparing to return the patient to the operating room for correction. Measurement of hemoglobin or hematocrit can be normal in the setting of acute blood loss since a decrease in red cells is accompanied by a decrease in mass. Once fluid is given for resuscitation, dilution will occur and the hemoglobin/hematocrit will fall. With invasive monitoring, the CVP will be low, as will cardiac output and the PAOP. As the stroke volume decreases to inadequate amounts, the heart compensates by increasing the heart rate in order to maintain cardiac output. The treatment in these cases is aggressive volume resuscitation and control of ongoing blood loss. The controversy between resuscitation with colloid (albumin, plasma) or crystalloid (normal saline or lactated Ringer's solution) has been mentioned earlier in the chapter. However, The Cochrane evidence-based review on this subject has proclaimed no benefit for colloid and perhaps an increased mortality with colloid (as well as cost). Recently, a large multicenter Australian study has begun in an attempt to shed more light on this subject, and its results are anticipated. As mentioned earlier, the ratio of crystalloid replacement to blood loss is 3 to 1 (3 cc crystalloid for each estimated 1-cc loss of blood). Blood products including packed red blood cells and fresh frozen plasma (in the case of a coagulopathy) are also indicated.

Endpoints of resuscitation include normalization of serum lactic acid and base deficit. Measurement of the base deficit via an arterial blood gas analysis has become an effective means for following response to resuscitation. Following large operations where patients are admitted to the ICU and where large, expected fluid shifts occur, the base deficit should be monitored serially until it has returned to normal.

If a patient has a worsening base deficit (i.e., becomes more negative), then a search for other problems, such as ongoing hemorrhage, subacute anastamotic leak(s), or tissue ischemia, must be made and be addressed before the base deficit will normalize. The base deficit should normalize within the first 24 hours after surgery.

In the case of continued or rapid bleeding, the obvious course of treatment is reoperation. A number of options are now available intraoperatively in these situations. Obvious bleeders are controlled and ligated. Raw surfaces can be coagulated or treated with fibrin sealants. Damage-control packing has been shown to increase survival in the direst situations. Massive transfusion, defined as greater than 1.5 blood volumes, presents a number of additional problems. These patients will have a dilutional coagulopathy, hypocalcemia, and hyperkalemia. After six to eight red blood cell transfusions have been given in rapid fashion for massive bleeding, some would advocate empiric fresh frozen plasma and platelets. Platelet transfusion is indicated for a platelet count <50,000 in the actively bleeding patient. Attention to delivery of warm transfusions is critical as hypothermia and acidosis will promote coagulopathy and worsening in bleeding. Once any of the ''lethal triad'' is manifested then the operation needs to be quickly terminated even if this means damage-control packing and transport to an ICU setting.

Cardiogenic Shock

A patient with adequate preload who shows signs of poor perfusion secondary to poor cardiac output is categorized as being in cardiogenic shock.. The etiology may be a decrease in contractility (secondary to myocardial infarction) or an increase in afterload (severe hypertension). Typically, ''pump failure'' results in decreased stroke volume and back-up of fluid into the pulmonary circulation. This leads to pulmonary edema and decreased oxygen delivery. The most common provocation for pump failure is the overadministration of fluid in a patient with compromised ventricular function. Treatment consists of diuresis and optimization of cardiac output without increasing myocardial oxygen demand (a difficult task). In the case where significant failure has led to hypotension, dopamine and dobutamine are usually the drugs of choice. The usage of these drugs has been discussed previously. Digoxin is commonly used for increasing contractility, but its effects are minor in the acute setting. In addition to inotropic support, correction of electrolyte disturbances (particularly potassium, calcium, and magnesium), maintenance of proper systemic oxygen saturation, and analgesia are important factors in decreasing myocardial stress.

Septic Shock

Septic shock has commonly been defined as hypotension related to infection with eventual organ failure secondary to hypoperfusion despite adequate fluid resuscitation. This definition has changed with that of SIRS and is discussed below. Sepsis is defined as a subset of patients with SIRS who have a documented infectious process and is included in the discussion below.

Infectious Disease Issues

Infections in the critically ill patient population are a significant cause of morbidity and mortality. Approximately 45% of ICU patients will have an infection and approximately half of those infected will have acquired the infection while in the ICU (234). Nosocomial infections are commonly associated with complications of medical or surgical therapy. Patients in the ICU are particularly vulnerable to invading microbes because of decreased host defenses, the presence of indwelling catheters and lines, which lowers the inoculum needed to cause infection and provide portals of entry, and the high incidence of resistant bacterial isolates found in ICUs (234,235). Initial therapy involves identifying and eradicating the source of infection and promptly initiating empirical antibiotic therapy aimed at multi-drug–resistant gram-negative and gram-positive organisms. If an intraabdominal or intapelvic source is suspected, empiric antibiotic therapy should include anaerobic coverage. Appropriate antibiotic classes include carbapenems, extended-spectrum penicillins, fluoroquinolone-metronidazole, aminoglycoside-metronidazole, or clindamycin combinations (236). Chapter 31 discusses the management of infections in the gynecologic cancer patient; therefore, information here is limited to infections pertaining to the critically ill patient.

Fungal Infections

Systemic fungal infections are a significant cause of morbidity and mortality in patients admitted to the ICU. A nonspecific and variable presentation makes the diagnosis of systemic candidal infection difficult. Risk factors that have been associated with candidemia include treatment with multiple antibiotics for extended periods, the presence of central venous catheters, the use of TPN, abdominal surgery, prolonged ICU stay, and compromised immune status (237). There are no data supporting prophylactic use of antifungals for all ICU patients; however, the International Conference for the Development of a Consensus on the Management and Prevention of Severe Candidal Infections recommends the use of fluconazole 400 mg/day for the high-risk, nonneutropenic patient who has received antibiotics for more than 14 days, has intravascular lines, is receiving hyperalimentation, has Candida species isolated from two or more sites, and has undergone complicated abdominal surgery (238). Fluconazole has excellent activity against C. albicans, but infections caused by Candida species other than C. albicans are better treated with amphotericin B (239).

Abdominal Infections

The diagnosis of an intraabdominal source of infection can be difficult in critically ill patients. Symptoms such as abdominal pain and peritoneal signs may not be apparent in patients who are obtunded or sedated and on a ventilator. Fever and leukocytosis may be absent in 35% and 55% of peritoneal infections, respectively (240). Ultrasonography is a useful diagnostic test that can be performed in the ICU and may assist with therapeutic intervention as well. It is extremely sensitive for evaluations of the pelvis and right upper quadrant, but evaluation of the entire abdomen can be limited by bowel gas, surgical dressings, and operator experience. For many of these reasons, a computed tomographic (CT) scan is the preferred study for the evaluation of patients with suspected intraabdominal infection. To avoid misdiagnosing fluid-filled bowel as a possible abnormal fluid collection, it is essential that contrast agents be used when conducting these studies. CT also has limitations, especially when used in the critically ill population. The presence of renal insufficiency precludes the use of intravenous contrast, and ileus or bowel obstruction may prevent complete opacification of the gastrointestinal tract (241). Diagnostic laparoscopy can be performed in the ICU with minimal anesthesia and is a safe, accurate, and cost-effective alternative to laparotomy when managing suspected intraabdominal processes (242,243).

Once identified, an intraabdominal abscess must be fully evacuated and the source controlled. Radiologically, assisted percutaneous drainage has become the preferred method for treating most abscesses located in the abdomen and pelvis. For well-delineated unilocular fluid collections, percutaneous drainage has a success rate better than 90% (244). Percutaneous drainage of complex abscesses or those with an enteric communication have a lower success rate, but remain a reasonable alternative of treatment for the high-risk patient (245,246). In some cases, surgery may be the only appropriate lifesaving intervention. Timely laparotomy in the critically ill patient with diffuse peritonitis allows for peritoneal toilet, debridement of infected and necrotic tissue, and control or repair of the source.

Sepsis and Systemic Inflammatory Response Syndrome

Inflammation is the body's initial response to tissue injury produced by chemical, mechanical, or microbial stimuli. Inflammation is an exceedingly complex cellular and humoral response involving interaction between the complement, kinin, coagulation, and fibrolytic cascades. The goal of inflammation is to enhance the movement of nutrients and phagocytic cells to the injury site in order to prevent invasion of microbes and limit the extension of injury. As a local response, this is beneficial, but appropriate regulation is necessary to prevent a pathologic, exaggerated systemic response, which is clinically identified as SIRS. The mediator

TABLE 11.15. *Definitions for systemic inflammatory response and sepsis (SIRS)*

SIRS	Two or more of the following in the setting of a known cause of inflammation: Temperature >38°C or <36°C Pulse >90 Respirations > 20/min or $PaCO_2$ < 32 mm Hg WBC count > 12,000 or < 4000 cells/mm^3 or > 10% band forms
Sepsis	SIRS due to known infection
Severe sepsis	Sepsis with evidence of organ dysfunction, hypoperfusion, or hypotension
Septic shock	Sepsis with hypotension despite adequate fluid resuscitation

Adapted from 1991 American College of Chest Physicians/Society of Critical Care Medicine Consensus Conference definitions.

response in SIRS can be divided into four phases based on the cytokine/cellular response: induction, triggering of cytokine synthesis, evolution of cytokine cascade, and elaboration of secondary mediators leading to cellular injury. The three most important mediators operating in SIRS appear to be tumor necrosis factor-α (TNF-α), interleukin-1 (IL-1), and interleukin-6 (IL-6) (235).

In 1992, the American College of Chest Physicians and the Society of Critical Care Medicine published definitions for SIRS and sepsis (Table 11.15) with the goal of standardizing terminology to aid clinicians in the diagnosis and treatment and to aid in the interpretation of research in this field (247). Many have criticized that the 1992 consensus definitions are too nonspecific to be of utility. In 2001, a group of experts reconvened and expanded the list of signs and symptoms of sepsis to reflect clinical bedside experience (248). In addition to the original criteria, altered mental status, oliguria, skin mottling, coagulopathy, hypoxemia, hyperglycemia in the absence of diabetes, thrombocytopenia, and altered liver function tests can also be used to establish the diagnosis of sepsis (249).

Sepsis with acute organ dysfunction (severe sepsis) is a complex condition that represents a major challenge to the critical care team and carries a crude mortality rate of 28% to 50% (250). Gram-negative and gram-positive organisms as well as fungi cause systemic sepsis and septic shock (251). Early recognition is crucial to patient survival because mortality rates are exceedingly high if the full clinical picture of shock and organ dysfunction develops. Septic shock is divided into an early hyperdynamic state and a late hypodynamic state.

Low systemic vascular resistance, splanchnic vasoconstriction, and increased cardiac output characterize the hyperdynamic phase of shock. Venous capacitance is increased and results in diminished effectiveness of the circulating blood volume. Aggressive volume resuscitation must be provided to restore preload and ventricular filling. These patients are best managed in an ICU with the placement of an arterial line, a PA catheter, and a bladder catheter. Initial therapy also includes prompt initiation of broad-spectrum antibiotics based on the probable source of infection. Laboratory tests of immediate concern include arterial blood gas determinations, creatinine, electrolytes, lactic acid, coagulation panel, and a complete blood count. Cultures should be obtained as soon as possible as well. Oxygenation and ventilation should be optimized with mechanical ventilation if indicated. If hypotension persists after optimization of the PCWP, the use of pressors or inotropic agents may be necessary. Surgical debridement or manipulation of infected material should not be performed until the patient has been stabilized.

In the hypodynamic phase of septic shock, hypotension results from cardiac output deterioration. The patient is often cool, mottled, oliguric, diaphoretic, and confused. The etiology of the hypodynamic cardiovascular response to sepsis may be inadequate volume resuscitation, underlying cardiac disease, or myocardial dysfunction associated with sepsis. This is a state of gross decompensation and is associated with greater mortality.

Numerous clinical trials have attempted to find specific agents that could modulate the underlying disease process in sepsis. Candidate therapies included agents that target mediators of inflammatory response, agents that boost the immune system, and prostaglandin inhibitors, but none was shown to be beneficial until recently. The Recombinant Human Activated Protein C Worldwide Evaluation in Severe Sepsis (PROWESS) study is the first clinical trial to show a clinically significant reduction in the 28-day all-cause mortality rate due to severe sepsis (252). This multicenter, prospective, double-blind, placebo-controlled study enrolled 1690 patients, who were randomized to treatment with a continuous infusion of drotrecogin alfa (activated) at a dose of 24μg/kg/hour for a total of 96 hours or placebo. Drotrecogin alfa (activated) is a recombinant form of human activated protein C, an endogenous protein with antithrombotic, profibrinolytic, and antiinflammatory properties that is frequently deficient in sepsis (253). Eligible patients were 18 years of age or older with a documented or a highly suspicious source of infection, at least three of the SIRS criteria, and evidence of acute end-organ dysfunction, including shock, severe hypoxia, oliguria, or acidosis for less than 24 hours. Patients began treatment within 24 hours of meeting study criteria. Drotrecogin alfa (activated) has significant anticoagulant properties; therefore, patients at high risk of or from bleeding were excluded, as well as those who were pregnant or breastfeeding, have human immunodeficiency virus infection with CD4 cell count ≤50/mm^3, weighed >35kg, had a transplanted organ other than a kidney, or were expected to die from non–sepsis-related disease within 1 month. The study was stopped at the second interim analysis because of a statistically significant reduction in mortality in the treatment arm. The mortality rate was 30.8% in the placebo group and 24.7% in the treatment arm, a reduction in relative risk of death of 19.4%, and an absolute reduction in risk of death of 6.1% ($p = .005$). Serious bleeding complications were higher in the drotrecogin alfa (activated) group despite exclusion of patients considered at higher risk of bleeding from being on study (3.5% vs 2.0%, $p = .06$). The Food and Drug Administration has approved drotrecogin alfa (activated) for the treatment of patients with sepsis who have a high risk of death. In light of the increased bleeding risk, appropriate patient selection for treatment with drotrecogin alfa (activated) should be an important consideration (254).

In addition to the use of drotrecogin alfa (activated), other management strategies have also been shown in randomized, controlled trials to reduce mortality associated with severe sepsis. These include limiting the tidal volume to 6 to 7 mL/kg ideal body weight for patients requiring mechanical ventilation for ARDS, early goal-directed therapy with hemodynamic interventions in order to balance systemic oxygen delivery with oxygen demand, the use of moderate-dose corticosteroids (hydrocortisone 200 to 300 mg and fludrocortisone 50 μg daily) for 7 days in patients with refractory septic shock, and maintaining tight blood sugar control with a goal of serum glucose levels between 80 and 110 mg/dL (255). These therapies are not mutually exclusive and optimal patient management may require a combination of approaches. Some of these strategies vary dramatically from traditional approaches and will require education and established protocols to incorporate them safely into practice.

Multiple Organ Dysfunction Syndrome

MODS can be defined as the development of progressive physiologic dysfunction of two or more organ systems after an acute threat to systemic homeostasis (248). Inciting factors are diverse and include SIRS, sepsis, massive trauma, burns, ischemia, and reperfusion injury. Consensus has not been reached as to the criteria used to define this clinical syndrome; that is, which organ systems are important or the degree of physiologic derangement necessary to constitute dysfunction. Pulmonary dysfunction is common and typically develops early in the course of SIRS or sepsis. Renal dysfunction initially is a prerenal azotemia unless the initial insult promoted a sudden oliguric acute tubular necrosis. Hyperbilirubinemia is the earliest marker of hepatic dysfunction. Gastrointestinal abnormalities include ileus, stress ulcers, diarrhea, and mucosal atrophy. The platelet count has been used as a surrogate marker of the hematologic system. Cardiac function is often measured by the degree of hypotension or the need for vasopressors. Deterioration of the nervous system is manifested by encephalopathy and peripheral neuropathies. The treatment of MODS is support of individual organ function and aggressive therapies aimed at correcting the underlying process. Mortality is related to the number of dysfunctional systems and is greater than 80% once four organ systems fail (256).

TABLE 11.16. *The sequential organ failure assessment (SOFA) score*

Variables	SOFA score				
	0	1	2	3	4
Respiratory: Pao$_2$/Fio$_2$, mm Hg	>400	≤400	≤300	≤200[a]	≤100[a]
Coagulation: platelets × 10^3/μL[b]	>150	150	100	50	20
Liver bilirubin, mg/dL[b]	<1.2	1.2–1.9	2.0–5.9	6.0–11.9	>12.0
Cardiovascular hypotension	No hypotension	Mean arterial pressure <70 mm Hg	Dop ≤5 or Dob (any dose)[c]	Dop >5, Epi 0.1, or Norepi 0.1[c]	Dop >15, Epi >0.1, or Norepi >0.1[c]
Central nervous system Glasgow Coma Scale score	15	13–14	10–12	6–9	<6
Renal creatinine, mg/dL or urine output, mL/d	<1.2	1.2–1.9	2.0–3.4	3.5–4.9 or <500	>5.0 or <200

Norepi, norephinephrine; Dob, dobutamine; Dop, dopamine; Epi, epinephrine; Fio$_2$, fraction of inspired oxygen; Pao$_2$–partial pressure oxygen.
[a] Values are with respiratory support.
[b] To convert bilirubin from mg/dL to μmol/L, multiply by 17.1.
[c] Adrenergic agents administered for at least 1 hour (doses given are in μg/kg per minute).
From Ferreira FL, Bota DP, Bross A, et al. Serial evaluation of the SOFA score to predict outcome in critically ill patients. *JAMA* 2001;286:1754–1758, with permission.

The Acute Physiology and Chronic Health Evaluation (APACHE) II provides population-based estimates of mortality for the day of ICU admission (257). Organ failure scores, such as the Sequential Organ Failure Assessment (SOFA), can help assess organ dysfunction over time and are useful to evaluate morbidity. Independent of the initial value, an increase of the SOFA score (Table 11.16) during the first 48 hours of an ICU admission predicts a mortality rate of at least 50% (258). It is important to note that these and other outcome prediction models were designed as tools to be used in critical care research in order to stratify patients by severity of illness. They are not particularly useful for making decisions for individual patients, nor have they been validated for this purpose.

Withdrawal of Life-sustaining Treatment

The decision to withdraw or withhold life-sustaining treatment is among the most difficult for patients, families, and health professionals to make. The ethical aspect of foregoing treatment resides in the legal and ethical right of the patient to self-determination. Unfortunately the majority of critically ill patients are unable to speak for themselves when decisions to limit treatment are considered; therefore, careful attention must be paid to previously expressed wishes and the input of surrogate decision makers. If a medical power of attorney is not in place, some states stipulate who the surrogate will be by a legal hierarchy. The ethical basis for identification of an appropriate surrogate is primary if none of the preceding legal bases apply. In this situation, the physician and other health care providers have the responsibility

to help identify the person or persons who have knowledge of the patient's values and preferences in order to assist with medical decisions on the patient's behalf. This process can become difficult in circumstances when family members or others close to the patient are in disagreement as to who should be the surrogate or what the patient would prefer. In these cases, health care providers should be knowledgeable of applicable legal directives and their ethical responsibility to act in their patient's best interest. Consultation with the institution's ethics committee may be helpful in trying to reach consensus (259). Although not responsible for the patient's death, those close to the patient often are left with feelings of guilt and anxiety in addition to their bereavement. It is important that the health care providers support the family both before and after the decision to withhold or withdrawal life-sustaining treatment has been made.

End of life care of patients in the ICU requires a dramatic paradigm shift in attitude and interventions from intensive rescue-type care to intensive palliative care. When considering the array of interventions that may be discontinued or held, physicians and surrogates should focus on clearly articulating the goals of care. For example, a goal for survival until the patient's important loved ones can gather to say their good-byes may justify short-term continuation of ventilator support. If the only goal is patient comfort, then such treatment should be stopped. The withdrawal of life-sustaining treatment is a clinical procedure and deserves the same preparation and expectation of quality as other medical procedures. Honest, caring, and culturally sensitive communication with the patient's loved ones and patient, if competent, should include explanations of how therapies will be withdrawn, what symptoms are expected, strategies to assess and ensure the patient's comfort, and information about the expected survival after interventions are withdrawn. Informed consent should be documented along with a formulated plan for withdrawing care (260). Adequate analgesia and sedation should be prescribed to relieve symptoms of pain, dyspnea, and anxiety during the dying process. Intravenous opioids and shorter acting benzodiazepines are the drugs of choice. The clinician's primary goal should be to prevent suffering and ensure the patient's comfort even if doing so unintentionally hastens the patient's death.

Neurologic Issues

The critically ill patient is invariably anxious, stressed, confused, uncomfortable, or in pain from immobility, wounds, preexisting disease, infection, invasive medical interventions, and routine nursing care such as airway suctioning, repositioning, or dressing changes. The restlessness and distress often associated with critical illness must be quelled with analgesia, sedation, and neuromuscular blockade as a last resort. The Society of Critical Care Medicine and ASHP clinical practice guidelines for sedation, analgesia, and neuromuscular blockade of the critically ill adult were revised in 2002. This comprehensive document is available online at www.ashp.org (261,262).

Analgesia

Maintaining an optimal level of comfort and safety for critically ill patients is a universal goal for all involved in their care. Unrelieved pain contributes to inadequate sleep and agitation. Pain may contribute to pulmonary dysfunction through localized guarding and generalized muscle rigidity that restricts movement of the chest wall and diaphragm. Unrelieved pain also evokes a stress response characterized by tachycardia, increased myocardial oxygen consumption, hypercoagulability, immunosuppression, and persistent catabolism (263). The combined use of effective analgesia and sedation may ameliorate the stress response and diminish pulmonary complications in postoperative critically ill patients. A comprehensive overview of pain management is covered in Chapter 33; therefore, only key aspects of pain management applicable to the patients in the ICU will be addressed.

Pharmacologic therapies include opioids, NSAIDs, and acetaminophen. ASHP guidelines recommend fentanyl, hydromorphone, and morphine given as a continuous infusion or scheduled doses rather than "as needed." Fentanyl has the most rapid onset and shortest duration, but repeated dosing may cause accumulation and prolonged effects. Fentanyl may also be administered via a transdermal patch to hemodynamically stable patients with more chronic analgesic needs. Morphine has a quick onset, but longer duration of action, so intermittent doses may be given. However, morphine causes

histamine release, which contributes to hypotension, especially in a hemodynamically unstable patient. Hydromorphone's duration of action is similar to morphine, but lacks an active metabolite or histamine release, making it an ideal drug for continuous infusion and for use in patients who cannot tolerate hypotension. Meperidine has an active metabolite that causes neuroexcitation including apprehension, tremors, delirium, and seizures so its use is not recommended in critically ill patients who may need repeated doses. The characteristics of analgesics and sedatives commonly used in ICU patients are summarized in Table 11.17.

Sedation

Sedatives are commonly used adjuncts for the treatment of anxiety and agitation. The physical environment of the ICU, limited ability to communicate, sleep deprivation, and medical circumstances precipitating the ICU admission are contributing factors creating anxiety in critically ill patients. Efforts to reduce anxiety, including frequent reorientation, provision of adequate analgesia, and optimization of the environment, may be supplemented with sedatives. Agitation is also common in ICU patients; however, not all patients with anxiety will exhibit agitation. Sedatives reduce the stress response and improve tolerance to routine ICU procedures. They may be necessary to facilitate mechanical ventilation. Generally, sedatives should be administered intermittently to determine the dose needed to achieve the sedation goal. Benzodiazepines are sedatives and hypnotics that cause anterograde amnesia, but lack analgesic properties. Midazolam has a rapid onset and short duration of effect with single doses, making it ideal for treating acutely agitated patients or for brief sedation with invasive procedures. Lorazepam has a slower onset but fewer potential drug interactions because of its metabolism via glucuronidation (Table 11.17).

Propofol is an intravenous general anesthetic that has sedative and hypnotic properties at lower doses. Like the benzodiazepines, propofol has no analgesic properties. Propofol has a rapid onset and short duration of sedation once discontinued. Propofol is a phospholipid emulsion that provides 1.1 kcal/mL from fat and should be counted as a caloric source. Long-term infusions may result in hypertriglyceridemia and monitoring is recommended after 2 days of use (261). Physiologic dependence and potential withdrawal symptoms have been described in ICU patients who have been exposed to more than 1 week of sedative or narcotic therapy, including the use of propofol (264).

Neuromuscular Blockade

Neuromuscular blocking agents (NMBAs) can be used to facilitate mechanical ventilation, to manage intracranial pressure in head trauma, to ablate muscle spasms, and to decrease oxygen consumption only when all other means to accomplish these aims have failed (262). Pancuronium is a

TABLE 11.17. *Characteristics of selected analgesics and sedatives frequently used in critically ill patients*

Agent	Indication	Active metabolites (effect)	Adverse effects	Intermittent dose (IV)[a]	Infusion dose range
Fentanyl	Pain	No metabolite, patient accumulates	Rigidity with high doses	0.35–1.5 μg/kg q 0.5–1 h	0.7–10 μg/kg/h
Hydromorphone	Pain	None	—	10–30 μg/kg q 1–2 h	7–15 μg/kg/h
Morphine	Pain	Yes (sedation)	Histamine release	0.01–0.15 mg/kg q 1–2 h	0.07–0.5 mg/kg/h
Ketorolac	Pain	None	GI bleeding, renal	15–30 mg q 6 h; decrease if >65 yr; avoid >5 day use	—
Midazolam	Acute agitation	Yes (prolonged sedation)	—	0.02–0.08 mg/kg q 0.5–2 h	0.04–0.2 mg/kg/h
Lorazepam	Sedation	None	Solvent-related acidosis/renal failure in high doses	0.02–0.06 mg/kg q 2–6 h	0.01–0.1 mg/kg/h
Propofol	Sedation	None	Elevated triglycerides	—	5–80 μg/kg/min
Haloperidol	Delirium	Yes (EPS)	QT interval prolongation	0.03–0.15 mg/kg q 0.5–6 h	0.04–0.15 mg/kg/h

[a] EPS =, extrapyramidal symptoms. More frequent doses may be needed for acute management in mechanically ventilated patients.

long acting NMBA that is effective for up to 90 minutes after intravenous bolus dose of 0.06 to 0.1 mg/kg. It can be used as a continuous infusion by adjusting the dose to the degree of neuromuscular blockade that is desired. Since pancuronium is vagolytic, 90% of patients will have an increase in heart rate of greater than ten beats per minute. For patients who cannot tolerate an increase in heart rate, vecuronium can be used. If neuromuscular blockade is necessary for patients with significant hepatic or renal failure, cisatracurium or atracurium should be used. Patients receiving any NMBA should be assessed using electronic twitch monitoring with a goal of adjusting the blockade to achieve one or two twitches. Before initiating neuromuscular blockade, patients should be adequately medicated with sedative and analgesic drugs as it is difficult to assess pain and anxiety after NMBAs are given.

Acute quadriplegic myopathy syndrome, also referred to as postparalytic quadriparesis, is a clinical triad of acute paresis, myonecrosis with increased creatine phosphokinase concentration, and abnormal electromyography that is related to prolonged exposure to NMBAs (265). This is a devastating complication of NMBA therapy and one of the reasons that indiscriminate use of these agents is discouraged. Increased risk of acute quadriplegic myopathy is associated with the concurrent use of corticosteroids; drug "holidays" may decrease the risk (262).

ICU Syndrome/Delirium

The ICU syndrome, first reported in the 1960s, describes a range of psychological disturbances exhibited by many critically ill patients (266). Other designations commonly used are ICU psychosis and postoperative delirium. The ICU syndrome has been defined as an altered emotional state occurring in a highly stressful environment that may manifest itself in a variety of psychologic reactions including fear, memory disturbance, anxiety, confusion, withdrawal, despair, agitation, and disorientation. Sleep deprivation, noise, constant light exposure, restriction of movement, limited ability to communicate, as well as the patient's preadmission mental state and coping ability have all been reported as causative factors of ICU syndrome. Current medical literature challenges this concept and argues that what is being called ICU syndrome or psychosis is diagnostic of delirium and not due to the ICU environment per se. Concerns have been raised that using the term *ICU syndrome* implies that confusion can be expected in the ICU setting and may reduce the vigilance necessary to recognize delirium and identify and treat the physiologic disturbances leading to it (267). Delirium is found in as many as 80% of critically ill patients and is associated with longer ICU admissions and increased mortality (268,269).

Delirium in the ICU setting is commonly caused by metabolic disturbances, hypoxia, electrolyte imbalances, alcohol or drug withdrawal, acute infection, and medications (Table 11.18) (267,270). Many drugs have anticholinergic properties that can exert an additive effect causing neurotoxicity, especially in elderly patients. Anticholinergic-related delirium can be differentiated from other causes of delirium if the mental status clears after administration of the cholinesterase inhibitor physostigmin. Delirium presents in both a hypoactive and hyperactive form. Hypoactive delirium, which is

TABLE 11.18. *Commonly used ICU drugs associated with delirium*[a]

Anesthetics	Anticonvulsants	Cimetidine[b]
Lidocaine	Carbamazepine	Corticosteroids[b]
Propofol	Phenobarbital	Digoxin[b]
	Phenytoin	
Antibiotics		Narcotic analgesics
Amphotericin B	Antihypertensives	Fentanyl
Aztreonam	Diltiazem	Meperidine[b]
Cephalosporins	Enalapril	Morphine
Ciprofloxacin	Hydralazine	
Doxycycline	Methyldopa	Nitroprusside
Imipenem	Propranolol	Phenylephrine
Metronidazole	Verapamil	Procainamide[b]
Penicillins		Scopolamine[b]
Tobramycin	Atropine[b]	Tricyclic antidepressants[b]

[a] Listing is not intended to be all inclusive.
[b] Drugs known to have significant anticholinergic properties.

associated with the worst prognosis, is characterized by psychomotor retardation, represents more global cerebral dysfunction, and is manifested by a calm appearance, inattention, and obtundation in extreme cases. Hyperactive delirium is more easily recognized by agitation and combative behaviors. Elderly patients may pose a particular diagnostic challenge when delirium is superimposed on baseline dementia.

The medical management of delirium consists of finding and treating underlying medical conditions and then controlling any behavioral disturbances if necessary. Neuroleptic drugs are the first-line agents for the treatment of delirium due to causes other than alcohol withdrawal syndrome, which is managed with benzodiazepines. Haloperidol is the neuroleptic of choice because it has minimal anticholinergic or hypotensive effects. A dose of 2 to 10 mg intravenously can be given every 20 to 30 minutes until agitation resolves. Once the delirium is controlled, scheduled doses every 4 to 6 hours consisting of 25% of necessary loading doses can be used and tapered off over several days. A continuous infusion can also be used (Table 11.17). Patients receiving repeat doses of haloperidol should be monitored for electrocardiographic changes. Extrapyramidal side effects such as rigidity, tremor, or facial tics can be managed with diphenhydramine hydrochloride (261).

REFERENCES

1. Dean MM, Finan MA, Kline RC. Predictors of complications and hospital stay in gynecologic cancer surgery. *Obstet Gynecol* 2001; 97(5 pt 1):721–724.
2. Smetana GW, Macpherson DS. The case against routine preoperative laboratory testing. *Med Clin North Am* 2003;87:7–40.
3. National Institutes of Health, National Heart, Lung, and Blood Institute. Women's Heart Health: Developing a National Health Education Action Plan. NIH Publication No. 01–2963, Sep 2001.
4. Hollenberg SM. Preoperative cardiac risk assessment. *Chest* 1999; 115[5 Suppl]:51–57.
5. Freeman WK, Gibbons RJ, Shub C. Preoperative assessment of cardiac patients undergoing noncardiac surgical procedures. *Mayo Clin Proc* 1989;64:1105–1117.
6. Romero L, de Virgilio C. Preoperative cardiac risk assessment: an updated approach. *Arch Surg* 2001;136:1370–1376.
7. Cerino M, Nattel S, Boucher Y, et al. Preoperative and long-term cardiac risk assessment. Predictive value of 23 clinical descriptors, 7 multivariate scoring systems and quantitative dipyridamole imaging in 360 patients. *Ann Surg* 1992;216:192–204.
8. Eagle KA, Boucher CA. Cardiac risk of noncardiac surgery. *N Engl J Med* 1989;321:1330–1332.
9. Blaustein AS. Preoperative and perioperative management of cardiac patients undergoing noncardiac surgery. *Cardiol Clin* 1995;13: 149–161.
10. Cohn SL, Goldman L. Preoperative risk evaluation and perioperative management of patients with coronary artery disease. *Med Clin North Am* 2003:111–136.
11. Goldman L, Caldera DL, Nussbaum SR, et al. Multifactorial index of cardiac risk in noncardiac surgical procedures. *N Engl J Med* 1977; 297:845–850.
12. Detsky AS, Abrams HB, McLaughlin JR, et al. Predicting cardiac complications in patients undergoing noncardiac surgery. *J Gen Intern Med* 1986;1:211–219.
13. Lee TH, Marcantonio ER, Mangione CM, et al. Derivation and prospective validation of a simple index for prediction of cardiac risk of major noncardiac surgery. *Circulation* 1999;100:1043–1049.
14. Eagle KA, Berger PB, Calkins H, et al. ACC/AHA guideline update for perioperative cardiovascular evaluation for noncardiac surgery: a report of the American College of Cardiology/American Heart Association Task Force on Practice Guidelines (Committee to Update the 1996 Guidelines on Perioperative Cardiovascular Evaluation for Noncardiac Surgery). American College of Cardiology Web site. 2002 Available: www.acc.org/clinical/guidelines/perio/ update/ periupdate_sendindex.htm. Accessed Nov 15, 2002.
15. Shammash JB, Ghali WA. Preoperative assessment and perioperative management of the patient with nonischemic heart disease. *Med Clin North Am* 2003;87:137–152.
16. Halm EA, Browner WS, Tubau JF, et al. Echocardiography for assessing cardiac risk in patients having noncardiac surgery. *Ann Intern Med* 1996;125:433–441.
17. Ferreira MJ. The role of nuclear cardiology for preoperative risk assessment prior to noncardiac surgery. *Rev Port Cardiol* 2001;19[Suppl 1]:163–169.
18. Ashton CM, Petersen NJ, Wray, NP, et al. The incidence of perioperative myocardial infarction in men undergoing noncardiac surgery. *Ann Intern Med* 1993;188:504–510.
19. Mangano DT, Layug EL, Wallace A, et al. Effect of atenolol on mortality and cardiovascular morbidity after noncardiac surgery. *N Engl J Med* 1996;335:1713–1720.

20. Fisher BW, Majumdar SR, McAlistar FA. Predicting pulmonary complications after nonthoracic surgery: a systematic review of blinded studies. *Am J Med* 2002;112:219–225.

21. Mitchell CK, Smoger SH, Pfeifer MP, et al. Multivariate analysis of factors associated with postoperative pulmonary complications following general elective surgery. *Arch Surg* 1998;133:194–198.

22. Beecher HK. Effect of laparotomy on lung volumes: demonstration of a new type of pulmonary collapse. *J Clin Invest* 1933;12:651–666.

23. The VA Total Parenteral Nutrition Cooperative Study Group. Perioperative total parenteral nutrition in surgical patients. *N Engl J Med* 1991;325:525–532.

24. Arozullah AM, Khuri SF, Henderson WG, et al. Development and validation of a multifactorial risk index for predicting postoperative pneumonia after major noncardiac surgery. *Ann Intern Med* 2001; 135:847–857.

25. Smetana GW. Preoperative pulmonary evaluation. *N Engl J Med* 1999;340:937–944.

26. Wong DH, Weber EC, Shell MJ, et al. Factors associated with postoperative pulmonary complications in patients with severe chronic obstructive pulmonary disease. *Anesth Analg* 1995;80:276–284.

27. Arozullah AM, Conde MV, Lawrence VA. Preoperative evaluation of postoperative pulmonary complications. *Med Clin North Am* 2003; 87:153–173.

28. Latimer RG, Dickman M, Day WC, et al. Ventilatory patterns and pulmonary complications after upper abdominal surgery determined by preoperative and postoperative computerized spirometry and bloods gas analysis. *Am J Surg* 1971;122:622–632.

29. Celli BR, Rodriguez KS, Snider GL. A controlled trial of intermittent positive pressure breathing, incentive spirometry, and deep breathing exercises in preventing pulmonary complications after abdominal surgery. *Am Rev Respir Dis* 1984;130:12–15.

30. Ferguson GT, Enright PL, Buist AS, et al. Office spirometry for lung health assessment in adults: a consensus statement from the National Lung Health Education Program. *Respir Care* 2000;45:513–530.

31. De Nino LA, Lawrence VA, Averyt EC, et al. Preoperative spirometry and laparotomy: blowing away dollars. *Chest* 1997;111:1536–1541.

32. Bluman LG, Mosca L, Newman N, et al. Preoperative smoking habits and postoperative pulmonary complications. *Chest* 1998;113:883–889.

33. Moller AM, Villebro N, Pedersen P, et al. Effect of preoperative smoking intervention on postoperative complications: a randomized clinical trial. *Lancet* 2002;359:114–117.

34. Nakagawa M, Tanaka H, Tsukuma H, et al. Relationship between the duration of the preoperative smoke-free period and the incidence of postoperative pulmonary complications after pulmonary surgery. *Chest* 2001;120:705–710.

35. Harris MI, Flega KM, Cowie CC, et al. Prevalence of diabetes, impaired fasting glucose, and impaired glucose tolerance in U.S. adults. *Diabetes Care* 1998;21:518–524.

36. Guyuron B, Raszewskie R. Undetected diabetes and the plastic surgeon. *Plast Reconstr Surg* 1990;86:471–474.

37. Hoogwerf BJ. Postoperative management of the diabetic patient. *Med Clin North Am* 2001;85(5):1213–1228.

38. Walter DP, Gatling W, Houston AC, et al. Mortality in diabetic subjects: an eleven year follow-up of a community-based population. *Diabet Med* 1994;11:968–973.

39. Schiff Rl, Welsh GA. Perioperative evaluation and management of the patient with endocrine dysfunction. *Med Clin North Am* 2003;87:175–192.

40. Hirsch IB, McGill JB. Role of insulin in management of surgical patients with diabetes mellitus. *Diabetes Care* 1990;13:980–981.

41. Hirsch IB, McGill JB, Cryer PE. Perioperative management of surgical patints with diabetes mellitus. *Anesthesiology* 1991;74:346–359.

42. DiPalo S, Ferrari G, Castoldi R, et al. Surgical septic complications in diabetic patients. *Acta Diabetol Latina* 1988;25:49–54.

43. Schiff Rl, Emanuele MA. The surgical patient with diabetes mellitus: guidelines for management. *J Gen Intern Med* 1995;10:154–161.

44. Gallacher SJ, Thomason F, Fraser WD, et al. Neutrophil bactericidal function in diabetes mellitus: evidence for association with blood glucose control. *Diabet Med* 1995;12:916–920.

45. Scherpereel PA, Travernier B. Perioperative care of diabetic patients. *Eur J Anesthesiol* 2001;18:277–294.

46. Furnary AP, Zerr KJ, Grunkemeier GL. Continuous intravenous insulin infusion reduces the incidence of deep sternal wound infection in diabetic patients after cardiac surgical procedures. *Ann Thorac Surg* 1999;67:352–362.

47. Golden SH, Peart-Vigilance C, Kao WHL. Perioperative glycemic control and the risk of infectious complications in a cohort of adults with diabetes. *Diabetes Care* 1999;22:1408–1414.

48. Pompocelli JJ, Baxter JK, Babineau TJ, et al. Early postoperative glucose control predicts nosocomial infection rate in diabetic patients. *JPEN J Parenter Enter Nutr* 1998;22:77–81.

49. Van Den Berghe G, Wouters P, Weekers F, et al. Intensive insulin therapy in critically ill patients. *N Engl J Med* 2001;345:1359–1367.

50. Weinberg AD, Brennan MD, Gorman CA. Outcome of anesthesia and surgery in hypothyroid patients. *Arch Intern Med* 1983;143:893–897.

51. Ladenson PW, Levin AA, Ridgway EC, et al. Complications of surgery in hypothyroid patients. *Am J Med* 1984;77(2):261–266.

52. Bennett-Guerrero E, Kramer DC, Schwinn DA. Effect of chronic and acute thyroid reduction on perioperative outcome. *Anesth Analg* 1997; 85:30–36.

53. Appoo JJ, Morin JF. Severe cerebral and cardiac dysfunction associated with thyroid decompensation after cardiac operations. *J Thorac Cardiovasc Surg* 1997;114:496.

54. Catz B, Russell S. Myxedema, shock and coma. *Arch Intern Med* 1961;108:407–417.

55. Holvey DN, Goodner CJ, Nicoloff JT, el al. Treatment of myxedema coma with intravenous thyroxine. *Arch Intern Med* 1964;113:89–96.

56. Forfar JC, Muir AL, Sawrers SA, et al. Abnormal left ventricular function in hyperthyroidism. *N Engl J Med* 1982;307:1165–1170.

57. Klein I, Ojamaa K. Mechanisms of disease: thyroid hormone and the cardiovascular system. *N Engl J Med* 2001;344:501–509.

58. Sawin CT, Geller A, Wolf PA. Low serum thyrotropin concentration as a risk factor for atrial fibrillation in older patients. *N Engl J Med* 1994;331:1249–1252.

59. Woeber KA. Thyrotoxicosis and the heart. *N Engl J Med* 1992;327:94–97.

60. Strube PJ. Thyroid storm during beta-blockade. *Anaesthesia* 1984;39:343–346.

61. McArthur JW, Rawson RW, Means JH, et al. Thyrotoxic crisis. *JAMA* 1947;132:868.

62. Baez A Aguayo J, Varrie M, et al. Rapid preoperative preparation in hyperthyroidism. *Clin Endocrinol* 1991;35:439–442.

63. Roti E, Robuschi G, Gardini E, et al. Comparison of methimazole and saturated solution of potassium iodide in early treatment of hyperthyroidism in Graves' disease. *Clin Endocrinol* 1988;28:305–314.

64. Mazzaferri EL, Skillman TG. Thyroid storm: a review of 22 episodes with special emphasis on the use of guanethidine. *Arch Intern Med* 1969;124:684–690.

65. Salem M, Rainsh RE, Bromberg J, et al. Perioperative glucocorticoid coverage: a reassessment 42 years after the emergence of a problem. *Ann Surg* 1994;219:416–425.

66. Ackerman GL, Nolan CM. Adrenocortical responsiveness after alternate-day corticosteroid therapy. *N Engl J Med* 1968;278:405–409.

67. Fauci AS. Alternate-day corticosteroid therapy. *Am J Med* 1978;64:729–731.

68. LaRochelle GE, LaRochelle AG, Ratner RE, et al. Recovery of the hypothalamic-pituitary-adrenal (HPA) axis in patients with rheumatic disease receiving low-dose prednisone. *Am J Med* 1993;95:258–264.

69. Christy NP. Corticosteroid withdrawal. In: Bardin CW, ed. *Current therapy in endocrinology and metabolism*. 3rd ed. New York: BC Decker, 1988:113.

70. Tordjman R, Jaffe A, Grazas N, et al. The role of the low dose (1 microgram) adrenocorticotropin test in the evaluation of patients with pituitary diseases. *J Clin Endocrinol Metab* 1995;80:1301–1305.

71. NKF-K/DOQI Clinical Practice Guidelines for Chronic Kidney Disease: evaluation, classification and stratification. *Am J Kidney Dis* 2000;37[Suppl 1]:S1–S266.

72. United States Renal Data System. USRDS 2001 Annual data report: atlas of end-stage renal disease in the United States. Bethesda, MD: National Institute of Health, National Institute of Diabetes and Kidney Diseases, 2001.

73. Kellerman PS. Perioperative care of the renal patient. *Arch Intern Med* 1994;154(15):1674–1688.

74. Foley RN, Parfrey PS, Sarnack MJ. Clinical epidemiology of cardio-

176. Guidelines for cardiopulmonary resuscitation and emergency cardiac care. Emergency Cardiac Care Committee and Subcommittees, American Heart Association. Part III. Adult advanced cardiac life support. *JAMA* 1992;268:2199–2241.

177. Chiolero R, Flatt J-P, Revelly J__P, Jequier E. Effects of catecholamines on oxygen consumption and oxygen delivery in critically ill patients. *Chest* 1991;100:1676–1684.

178. Raymer K, Yang H. Patients with aortic stenosis: cardiac complications in non-cardiac surgery. *Can J Anaesth* 1998;45:855–859.

179. Torsher LC, Shub C, Rettke SR, Brown DL. Risk of patients with severe aortic stenosis undergoing noncardiac surgery. *Am J Cardiol* 1998;81:448–452.

180. Dajani AS, Taubert KA, Wilson W, et al. Prevention of bacterial endocarditis. *Circulation* 96:358–366. 1997.

181. Christians KK, Wu B, Quebbeman EJ, et al. Postoperative atrial fibrillation in noncardiothoracic surgical patients. *Am J Surg* 2001;182:713–715.

182. Balser JR, Martinez EA, Winters BD, et al. Beta-adrenergic blockade accelerates conversion of postoperative supraventricular tachyarrhythmias. *Anesthesiology* 1998;89:1052–1059.

183. Roy D, Talajic M, Dorian P, et al. Amiodarone to prevent recurrence of atrial fibrillation. *N Engl J Med* 2000;342:913–920.

184. Bersten AD, Rutten AJ, Vedig AE: Additional work of breathing imposed by endotracheal tubes, breathing circuits, and intensive care ventilators. *Crit Care Med* 1989;21:1333–1337.

185. Banner MJ, Jaeger MJ, Kirby RR. Components of the work of breathing and implications for monitoring ventilator-dependent patients. *Crit Care Med* 1994;22:515–518.

186. Stewart T, Meade M, Cook D, et al. The Pressure and Volume-Limited Ventilation Strategy Group (1998). Evaluation of a ventilation strategy to prevent barotrauma in patients at high risk for acute respiratory distress syndrome. *N Engl J Med* 1998;338:356–361.

187. Amoto M, Barbas C, Medeiros D, et al. Effect of a protective-ventilation strategy on mortality in the acute respiratory distress syndrome. *N Engl J Med* 1998:338:347–354.

188. Lodat, R. Oxygen toxicity. *Crit Care Clin* 1990;6:749–765.

189. Kirby R, Downs J, Civetta J, et al. High level positive end expiratory pressure (PEEP) in acute respiratory insufficiency. *Chest* 1975;67:156–163.

190. Dries D. Weaning from mechanical ventilation. *J Trauma* 1997;43:372–384.

191. Bulger E, Jurkovich G, Gentilello L, et al. Current clinical options for the treatment and management of acute respiratory distress syndrome. *Crit Care Rev* 2000;48:562–572.

192. Bernard G, Artigas A, Brigham, KL, et al. Report of the American-European Consensus Conference on acute respiratory distress syndrome: definitions, mechanisms, relevant outcomes, and clinical trial coordination. Consensus Committee. *J Crit Care* 1994;9:72–81.

193. Luce J. Acute lung injury and the acute respiratory distress syndrome. *Crit Care Med* 1998;26:369–376.

194. Marshall J, Cook D, Christou N, et al. Multiple organ dysfunction score: a reliable descriptor of a complex clinical outcome. *Crit Care Med* 1995;23:1638–1652.

195. Chastre J, Fagon JY. Ventilator-associated pneumonia. *Am J Respir Crit Care Med* 2002;165:867–903.

196. Clagett P, Anderson F, Geerts W, et al. Prevention of venous thromboembolism. *Chest* 1998;(114):531S–560S.

197. Pestana C. *Fluids and electrolytes in the surgical patient.* 4th ed. Baltimore: Williams & Wilkins, 1989.

198. Vanatta JC, Fogelman MJ, eds. *Moyer's fluid balance: a clinical manual.* 2nd ed. Chicago: Year Book, 1976.

199. Wait RB, Kahng KU, Dresner LS. Fluids and electrolytes and acid-base balance. In: Greenfield LJ, Mulholland M, Oldham KT, et al., eds. *Surgery: scientific principles and practice.* 2nd ed. Philadelphia: Lippincott–Raven Publishers, 1997:242–266.

200. Lowe RJ, Moss GS, Jilek J, et al. Crystalloid versus colloid in the etiology of pulmonary failure after trauma. A randomized trial in man. *Surgery* 1977;81:676–683.

201. Virgilio RW, Rice CL, Smith DE, et al. Crystalloid versus colloid resuscitation: is one better? A randomized clinical study. *Surgery* 1979;85:129–139.

202. Weinstein PD, Doerfler ME. Systemic complications of fluid resuscitation. *Crit Care Clin* 1992;8:439–448.

203. Metildi LA, Shackford SR, Virgilio RW, et al. Crystalloid versus colloid in fluid resuscitation of patients with severe pulmonary insufficiency. *Surg Gynecol Obstet* 1984;158:207–212.

204. Rizoli SB. Crystalloids and colloids in trauma resuscitation: a brief overview of the current debate. *J Trauma* 2003;54[5 Suppl]:S82–S88.

205. Alderson P, Schierhout G, Roberts I, et al. Colloids versus crystalloids for fluid resuscitation in critically ill patients. *Cochrane Database Syst Rev* 2000;(2):CD000567.

206. Choi PT, Yip G, Quinonez LG, et al. Crystalloids vs. colloids in fluid resuscitation: a systematic review. *Crit Care Med* 1999;27:200–210.

207. Roberts JS, Bratton SL. Colloid volume expanders. Problems, pitfalls and possibilities. *Drugs* 1998;55:621–630.

208. Berenson JR. Treatment of hypercalcemia of malignancy with bisphosphonates. *Semin Oncol* 2002;29[Suppl 21]:12–18.

209. Mundy GR: Hypercalcemia. In: *Bone remodeling and its disorders.* 2nd. London, Martin Dunitz, 1999:107–122.

210. Major P, Lortholary A, Hon J, et al. Zolendronic acid is superior to pamidronate in the treatment of hypercalcemia of malignancy: a pooled analysis of two randomized, controlled clinical trials. *J Clin Oncol* 2001;19:558–567.

211. Pearl ML, Frandina M, Mahler L, et al. A randomized controlled trial of a regular diet as the first meal in gynecologic oncology patients undergoing intraabdominal surgery. *Obstet Gynecol* 2002;100:230–234.

212. Pearl ML, Valea FA, Fischer M, et al. A randomized controlled trial of early postoperative feeding in gynecologic oncology patients undergoing intra-abdominal surgery. *Obstet Gynecol* 1998;92:94–97.

213. Cutillo G, Maneschi F, Franchi M, et al. Early feeding compared with nasogastric decompression after major oncologic gynecologic surgery: a randomized study. *Obstet Gynecol* 199;93:41–45.

214. MacMillan SL, Kammerer-Doak D, Rogers RG, et al. Early feeding and the incidence of gastrointestinal symptoms after major gynecologic surgery. *Obstet Gynecol* 2000;96:604–608.

215. Steed HL, Capstick V, Flood C, et al. A randomized controlled trial of early versus ''traditional'' postoperative oral intake after major abdominal gynecologic surgery. *Am J Obstet Gynecol* 2002;186:861–865.

216. Schilder JM, Hurteau JA, Look KY, et al. A prospective controlled trial of early potoperative oral intake following major abdominal gynecologic surgery. *Gynecol Oncol* 1997;67:235–240.

217. Souba WW, Austen WG Jr. Nutrition and metabolism. In: Greenfield LJ, Mulholland M, Oldham KT, et al., eds. *Surgery: scientific principles and practice.* 2nd ed. Philadelphia: Lippincott–Raven Publishers, 1997:42–67.

218. Marik PE, Zaloga GP. Early enteral nutrition in acutely ill patients: a systematic review. *Crit Care Med* 2001;29;2264–2270.

219. Morrow CP, Curtin JP. *Gynecologic cancer surgery.* New York: Churchill Livingstone, 1996:194–205.

220. Blackburn GL, Bistrian BR, Moini BS, et al. Nutritional and metabolic assessment of the hospitalized patient. *JPEN J Parenter Enter Nutr* 1977;1:11–22.

221. Edwards BF. Postoperative renal insufficiency. *Med Clin North Am* 2001;85:1241–1254.

222. Klausner JM, Paterson IS, Goldman G, et al. Postischemic renal injury is mediated by neutrophils and leukotrienes. *Am J Physiol* 1989;256(5 pt 2):F794–F802.

223. Kribben A, Edelstein CL, Schrier RW. Pathophysiology of acute renal failure. *J Nephrol* 1999;12[Suppl 2]:S142–S151.

224. Prins JM, Buller HR, Kuijper EJ, et al. Once versus thrice daily gentamicin in patients with serious infections. *Lancet* 1993;341:335–339.

225. Murphy SW, Barrett BJ, Parfrey PS. Contrast nephropathy. *J Am Soc Nephrol* 2000;11:177–182.

226. Rudnick MR, Berns JS, Cohen RM, et al. Contrast media-associated nephrotoxicity. *Semin Nephrol* 1997;17:15–26.

227. McCullough PA, Wolyn R, Rocher LL, et al. Acute renal failure after coronary intervention: Incidence, risk factors and relationship to mortality. *Am J Med* 1997;103:368–375.

228. Baldwin L, Henderson A, Hickman P. Effect of postoperative low-dose dopamine on renal function after elective major vascular surgery. *Ann Intern Med* 1994;120:744–747.

229. Dishart MK, Kellum JA. An evaluation of pharmacological strategies for the prevention and treatment of acute renal failure. *Drugs* 2000;59:79–91.

230. Lassnigg A, Donner E, Grubhofer G, et al. Lack of renoprotective effects of dopamine and furosemide during cardiac surgery. *J Am Soc Nephrol* 2000;11:97–104.

231. Marik PE, Iglesias J. Low-dose dopamine does not prevent acute renal failure in patients with septic shock and oliguria. NORASEPT II Study Investigators. *Am J Med* 1999;107:387–390.

232. Sirivella S, Gielchinsky I, Parsonnet V. Mannitol, furosemide and dopamine infusion in postoperative renal failure complicating cardiac surgery. *Ann Thorac Surg* 2000;69:501–506.

233. Allgren RL, Marbury TC, Rahman SM, et al. Anaritide in acute tubular necrosis. Auriculin Anaritide Acute Renal Failure Study Group. *N Engl J Med* 1997;336:828–834.

234. Vincent JL, Bihari DJ, Suter PM, et al. The prevalence of nosocomial infection in intensive care units in Europe. Results of the European Prevalence of Infection in Intensive Care (EPIC) Study. EPIC International Advisory Committee. *JAMA* 1995;274:639–644.

235. Solomkin JS. Antibiotic resistance in postoperative infections. *Crit Care Med* 2001;29:N97–N99.

236. Stafford RE, Weigelt JA. Surgical infections in the critically ill. *Curr Opin Crit Care* 2002;8:449–452.

237. Wright WL, Wenzel RP. Nosocomial Candida. Epidemiology, transmission, and prevention. *Infect Dis Clin North Am* 1997;11:411–425.

238. Edwards JE, Jr., Bodey GP, Bowden RA, et al. International Conference for the Development of a Consensus on the Management and Prevention of Severe Candidal Infections. *Clin Infect Dis* 1997;25:43–59.

239. Kam LW, Lin JD. Management of systemic candidal infections in the intensive care unit. *Am J Health Syst Pharm* 2002;59:33–41.

240. Crabtree TD, Pelletier SJ, Antevil JL, et al. Cohort study of fever and leukocytosis as diagnostic and prognostic indicators in infected surgical patients. *World J Surg* 2001;25:739–744.

241. Gazelle GS, Mueller PR. Abdominal abscess. Imaging and intervention. *Radiol Clin North Am* 1994; 32:913–932.

242. Pecoraro AP, Cacchione RN, Sayad P, et al. The routine use of diagnostic laparoscopy in the intensive care unit. *Surg Endosc* 2001;15:638–641.

243. Kelly JJ, Puyana JC, Callery MP, et al. The feasibility and accuracy of diagnostic laparoscopy in the septic ICU patient. *Surg Endosc* 2000;14:617–621.

244. Oglevie SB, Casola G, vanSonnenberg E, et al. Percutaneous abscess drainage: current applications for critically ill patients. *J Intensive Care Med* 1994;9:191–206.

245. D'Harcour JB, Boverie JH, Dondelinger RF. Percutaneous management of enterocutaneous fistulas. *AJR Am J Roentgenol* 1996;167:33–38.

246. Goletti O, Lippolis PV, Chiarugi M, et al. Percutaneous ultrasound-guided drainage of intra-abdominal abscesses. *Br J Surg* 1993;80:336–339.

247. Davies MG, Hagen PO. Systemic inflammatory response syndrome. *Br J Surg* 1997;84:920–935.

248. American College of Chest Physicians/Society of Critical Care Medicine Consensus Conference. Definitions for sepsis and organ failure and guidelines for the use of innovative therapies in sepsis. *Crit Care Med* 1992;20:864–874.

249. Levy MM, Fink MP, Marshall JC, et al. 2001 SCCM/ESICM/ACCP/ATS/SIS International Sepsis Definitions Conference. *Crit Care Med* 2003;31:1250–1256.

250. Angus DC, Linde-Zwirble WT, Lidicker J, et al. Epidemiology of severe sepsis in the United States: analysis of incidence, outcome, and associated costs of care. *Crit Care Med* 2001;29:1303–1310.

251. Brun-Buisson C, Doyon F, Carlet J. Bacteremia and severe sepsis in adults: a multicenter prospective survey in ICUs and wards of 24 hospitals. French Bacteremia-Sepsis Study Group. *Am J Respir Crit Care Med* 1996;154:617–624.

252. Bernard GR, Vincent JL, Laterre PF, et al. Efficacy and safety of recombinant human activated protein C for severe sepsis. *N Engl J Med* 2001;344:699–709.

253. Pastores SM. Drotrecogin alfa (activated): a novel therapeutic strategy for severe sepsis. *Postgrad Med J* 2003;79:5–10.

254. Morris PE, Light RB, Garber GE. Identifying patients with severe sepsis who should not be treated with drotrecogin alfa (activated). *Am J Surg* 2002;184:S19–S24.

255. Vincent JL, Abraham E, Annane D, et al. Reducing mortality in sepsis: new directions. *Crit Care* 2002;6[Suppl 3]:S1–S18.

256. Vincent JL, de Mendonca A, Cantraine F, et al. Use of the SOFA score to assess the incidence of organ dysfunction/failure in intensive care units: results of a multicenter, prospective study. Working group on "sepsis-related problems" of the European Society of Intensive Care Medicine. *Crit Care Med* 1998;26:1793–1800.

257. Knaus WA, Draper EA, Wagner DP, et al. APACHE II: a severity of disease classification system. *Crit Care Med* 1985;13:818–829.

258. Ferreira FL, Bota DP, Bross A, et al. Serial evaluation of the SOFA score to predict outcome in critically ill patients. *JAMA* 2001;286:1754–1758.

259. Way J, Back AL, Curtis JR. Withdrawing life support and resolution of conflict with families. *BMJ* 2002;325:1342–1345.

260. Luce JM, Alpers A. Legal aspects of withholding and withdrawing life support from critically ill patients in the United States and providing palliative care to them. *Am J Respir Crit Care Med* 2000;162:2029–2032.

261. Society of Critical Care Medicine and American Society of Health-System Pharmacists. Clinical practice guidelines for the sustained use of sedatives and analgesics in the critically ill adult. *Am J Health Syst Pharm* 2002;59:150–178.

262. Society of Critical Care Medicine and American Society of Health-System Pharmacists. Clinical practice guidelines for sustained neuromuscular blockade in the adult critically ill patient. *Am J Health Syst Pharm* 2002;59:179–195.

263. Epstein J, Breslow MJ. The stress response of critical illness. *Crit Care Clin* 1999;15:17–33.

264. Cammarano WB, Pittet JF, Weitz S, et al. Acute withdrawal syndrome related to the administration of analgesic and sedative medications in adult intensive care unit patients. *Crit Care Med* 1998;26:676–684.

265. Lacomis D, Giuliani MJ, Van Cott A, et al. Acute myopathy of intensive care: clinical, electromyographic, and pathological aspects. *Ann Neurol* 1996;40:645–654.

266. McKegney FP. The intensive care syndrome. The definition, treatment and prevention of a new "disease of medical progress." *Conn Med* 1966;30:633–636.

267. McGuire BE, Basten CJ, Ryan CJ, et al. Intensive care unit syndrome: a dangerous misnomer. *Arch Intern Med* 2000;160:906–909.

268. Ely EW, Gautam S, Margolin R, et al. The impact of delirium in the intensive care unit on hospital length of stay. *Intensive Care Med* 2001;27:1892–1900.

269. Ely EW, Inouye SK, Bernard GR, et al. Delirium in mechanically ventilated patients: validity and reliability of the confusion assessment method for the intensive care unit (CAM-ICU). *JAMA* 2001;286:2703–2710.

270. Webb JM, Carlton EF, Geehan DM. Delirium in the intensive care unit: are we helping the patient? *Crit Care Nurs Q* 2000;22:47–60.

CHAPTER 12

Surgical Principles in Gynecologic Oncology

Dennis S. Chi and Donald G. Gallup

The management of most human cancers involves multimodal therapy, and this is especially true for female genital malignancies. Although some early gynecologic cancers can be eradicated by surgery alone, and chemotherapy as a single modality can often cure gestational trophoblastic malignancies, the optimal treatment for the majority of gynecologic malignancies requires surgery combined with chemotherapy and/or irradiation.

In this chapter, surgery is discussed both as a separate discipline and as an integral part of multimodal therapeutic planning. Although specific operations and relatively new surgical techniques are described for some disease sites, many procedures are addressed more completely in surgical texts and atlases to which the reader is referred (1–3). The role of surgical intervention in the treatment of gynecologic cancers is addressed herein with a more philosophic approach than would be taken in a surgical atlas. However, select illustrations and tips are included that have enabled us to approach various radical procedures more rapidly and safely. The major goal of this chapter is to give the reader an appreciation and understanding of the surgical principles of the subspecialty of gynecologic oncology.

TECHNICAL ASPECTS OF SURGERY

Many physicians who practice the art and science of surgery tend to focus on the technical craft of the specialty only when teaching young surgeons. At other times, we are acutely aware that the most difficult part of our practice is the decision of whether or not to utilize surgical therapy. Preoperative and postoperative management is also demanding since therapy must be tailored for individual patients

Dennis S. Chi: Gynecology Service, Department of Surgery, Memorial Sloan-Kettering Cancer Center, New York, New York 10021

Donald G. Gallup: Department of Gynecologic Oncology, Memorial Medical Center, Savannah, Georgia 31403

depending not only on their specific disease but also on their overall medical status. Owing to the significance of these pressing issues, we often take for granted the many years of preparation and experience in the craft of surgery.

Mastering the skills of surgery involves a thorough understanding of proper technique. It also requires frequent and consistent practice to keep surgical maneuvers well honed. For the student, this means actual practice in tying knots, manipulating instruments, and suturing. For the accomplished surgeon, it means that a sufficient case load must be maintained to ensure adequate practice of the technical art of the specialty. The surgeon should also keep abreast of new suture materials, instruments, and technical developments.

Anatomy

There is no substitute for a detailed knowledge of the anatomy of the pelvis and abdomen. The physician who pursues gynecologic oncology as a career must be completely familiar with the pelvis, abdomen, retroperitoneum, and the lymphatic drainage of the female genital tract. No amount of surgical skill or knowledge of cancer therapy can compensate for the lack of this knowledge.

Lymphatic drainage from the cervix follows the uterine arteries and cardinal ligaments to the pelvic lymph nodes that include the external iliac, internal iliac (hypogastric), and obturator node groups (Fig. 12.1). From these pelvic lymph nodes, the drainage proceeds superiorly through the common iliac lymph nodes and then up to the paraaortic nodes.

The lymphatic drainage from both the uterine corpus and the ovaries follows one of three routes (Fig. 12.1): (a) along the uterine arteries in the broad ligaments to the pelvic nodes, (b) in channels following the round ligaments to the inguinal lymph nodes, or (c) along the ovarian lymphatics in the infundibulopelvic ligaments directly up to the paraaortic nodes.

The anatomy of the paraaortic lymph nodes has been well

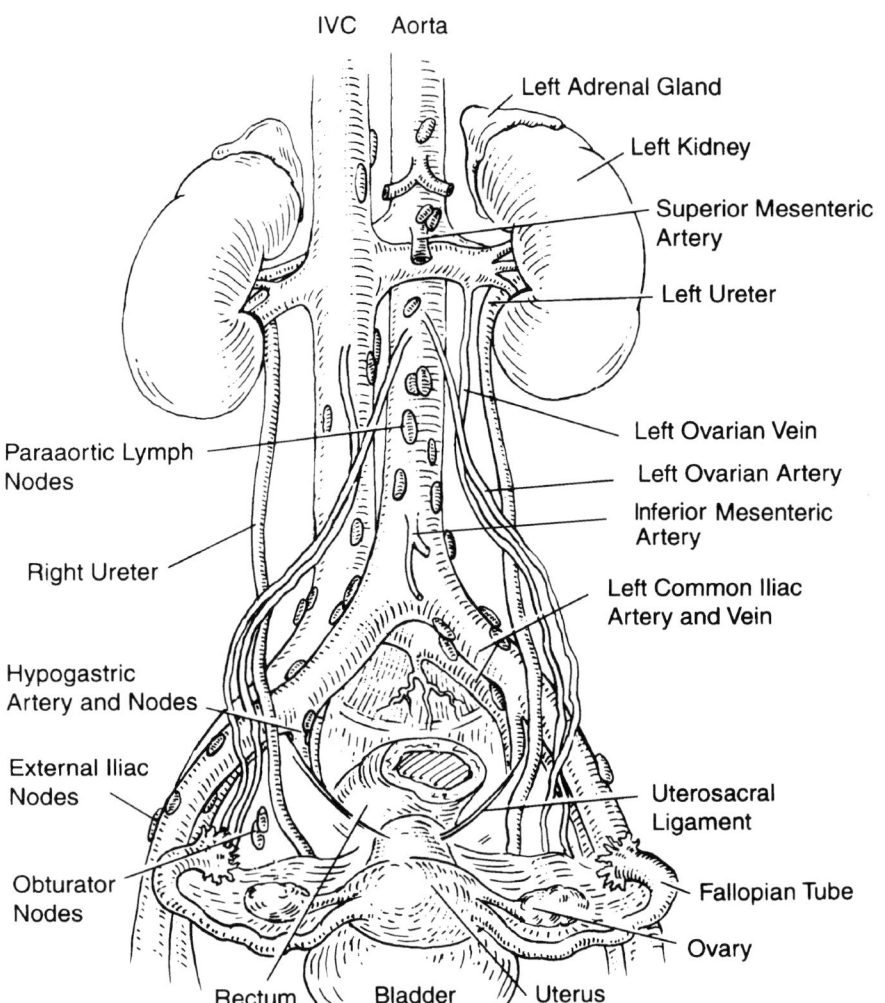

FIG. 12-1. The pelvic and paraaortic lymph nodes and their relationship to the major retroperitoneal vessels.

described by Fowler and Johnson (4). The paraaortic lymph nodes are part of the lumbar lymph node group. There are three subgroups: preaortic, retroaortic, and lateral aortic (right and left). The preaortic group drains the abdominal part of the gastrointestinal tract down to the mid rectum, whereas the retroaortic group has no special area of drainage. The lateral group receives lymphatic drainage from the iliac lymph nodes, ovaries, and other pelvic viscera (apart from the alimentary tract), and therefore it is this group of nodes that is sampled in the surgical staging of gynecologic malignancies.

There are typically 15 to 20 lateral aortic nodes per side. They are located adjacent to the aorta, anterior to the lumbar spine, extending bilaterally to the medial margins of the psoas major muscles, and up to the diaphragmatic crura (4). The lateral nodes usually dissected in gynecologic oncology span the region from the aortic bifurcation up to either the inferior mesenteric artery (IMA) or the renal veins.

The first major blood vessel encountered during a caudad-to-cephalad paraaortic node dissection is the IMA (Fig. 12.1). The IMA originates from the anterior surface of the

aorta approximately 3 to 4 cm above the aortic bifurcation. Next, the right and left ovarian arteries arise from their respective sides of the aorta about 5 to 6 cm above the bifurcation (Fig. 12.1). The right ovarian vein inserts into the right side of the inferior vena cava (IVC) approximately 1 cm below the right renal vein. The left ovarian vein does not insert directly into the IVC, but rather follows a path close to the left ureter inserting into the left renal vein lateral to the left border of the aorta. Three to four pairs of lumbar arteries and veins arise from the posterior surfaces of the aorta and IVC, respectively.

Patient Positioning

Patient positioning for radical gynecologic oncology procedures is often critical in improving exposure, particularly in obese patients. For women undergoing radical hysterectomy or a proposed supralevator exenteration, the patient can be placed in "jackknife" position that vastly improves exposure (Fig. 12.2) (2). The exaggerated lithotomy position is often used for improved access to the upper anterior vagina

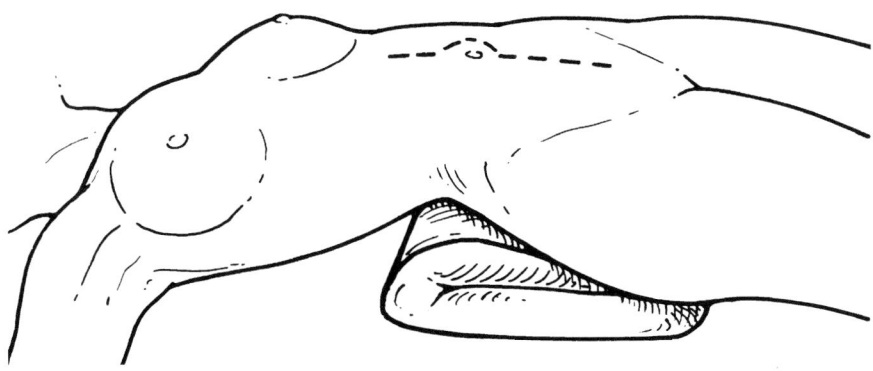

FIG. 12-2. The "jackknife" position. Two or three rolled sheets are placed underneath the hips. The table is tilted to a 30° Trendelenburg position, and the foot of the table is lowered. A midline incision can be used and extended above the umbilicus on the left or right. (Reprinted with permission from Gallup DG, Talledo OE. *Surgical atlas of gynecologic oncology.* Philadelphia: WB Saunders, 1994;66.)

(Fig. 12.3) (2). This modified lithotomy position can be useful in patients undergoing vesicovaginal fistula repairs, Schauta radical vaginal hysterectomy, or anterior exenteration. In the latter circumstance, the patient will need to be repositioned if a perineal approach is needed.

Abdominal Incisions

Abdominal incisions in gynecologic oncology vary with the indication for the procedure, associated preoperative conditions (such as the presence of ascites or bowel obstruction), suspicion of upper abdominal pathology, and the presence of a previous abdominal scar. Incisions for surgery for gynecologic oncology patients should be highly individualized. Three basic incisions are used for intraperitoneal exposure (Fig. 12.4) (2). Additionally, extraperitoneal access to the pelvic and paraaortic nodes can be achieved through a J-shaped incision (5) or a sunrise incision (6).

Transverse incisions offer the advantages of being the best cosmetic incisions for pelvic surgery while also being the least painful, resulting in less interference with postoperative pulmonary function. In addition, compared to vertical incisions, transverse incisions are allegedly stronger and allow better exposure to the pelvic sidewalls. Many gynecologic oncologists use transverse incisions when performing a radical hysterectomy or pelvic exenteration.

In performing the Maylard incision, it is recommended that the deep inferior epigastric vessels be isolated, sectioned, and ligated prior to dividing the rectus muscle (Fig. 12.5) (2). Occasionally, the pelvic surgeon will make a Pfannenstiel incision and find it inadequate. When more exposure is needed, the appropriate maneuver is to convert the Pfannenstiel to a Cherney-type incision. This conversion can be accomplished by dissecting the rectus muscles from the pyramidalis muscles and the anterior rectus sheath and then transecting the rectus tendons at their insertion into the pubic bone.

Lymph Node Dissection

The surgical technique used to dissect the pelvic and paraaortic lymph nodes involves either a transperitoneal or extraperitoneal approach. The approach utilized is generally dictated by the primary site of disease and the planned accompanying procedure. In cases of endometrial and ovarian carcinoma where the anticipated procedure includes a hysterectomy and/or surgical debulking, the approach is invariably transperitoneal. However, in the pretreatment surgical staging of patients with advanced-stage cervical cancer, the transperitoneal approach has been associated with significant radiation-induced intestinal morbidity due to postoperative adhesion formation (7). Therefore, current clinical

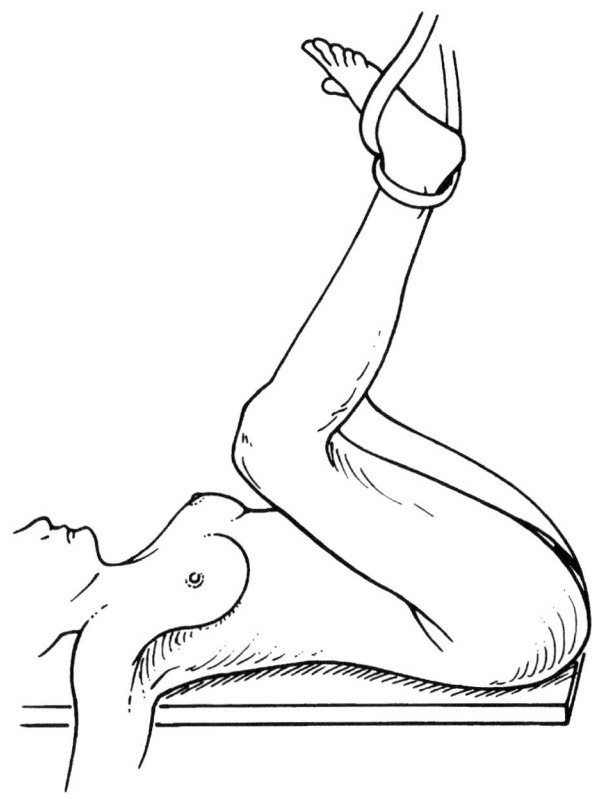

FIG. 12-3. The exaggerated lithotomy position. The table is placed in about a 15° Trendelenburg position. The buttocks protrude over the end of the table. In this position, the anterior vaginal wall will appear perpendicular to the surgeon's line of vision. (Reprinted with permission from Gallup DG, Talledo OE. *Surgical atlas of gynecologic oncology.* Philadelphia: WB Saunders, 1994:196.)

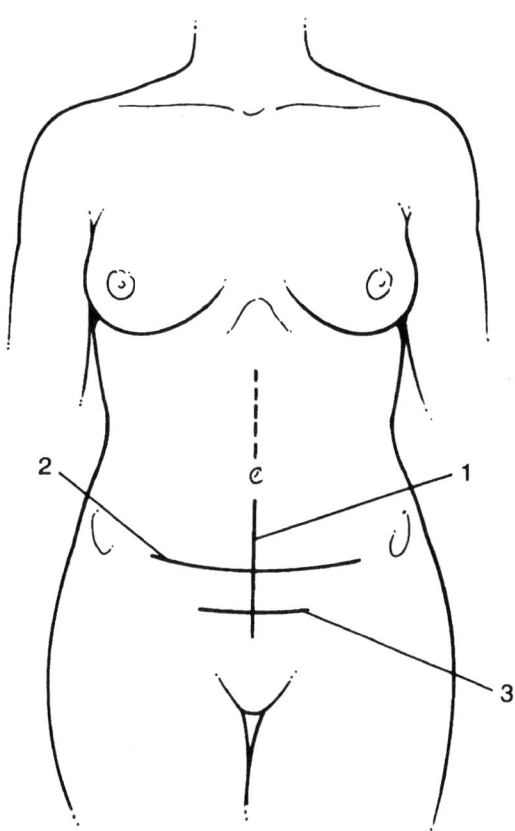

FIG. 12-4. Entry into the abdominal cavity can be made by three basic incisions: (1) the midline incision; (2) the transverse Maylard-type incision from anterior-superior iliac spine to anterior-superior iliac spine; and (3) the Pfannenstiel incision. The latter is not an incision for radical pelvic surgery, but it can be converted to a Cherney-type incision for improved exposure. For the patient who has some type of transverse incision, and for whom later exposure of the upper abdominal cavity is necessary, a midline upper abdominal incision can be separately used. (Reprinted with permission from Gallup DG, Talledo OE. *Surgical atlas of gynecologic oncology.* Philadelphia: WB Saunders, 1994:44.)

trials that require pretreatment surgical staging recommend that the lymph node sampling be performed via the extraperitoneal approach or by operative laparoscopy (8).

Pelvic Lymph Node Dissection

Whether a transperitoneal or extraperitoneal approach is used, most surgeons initially remove pelvic nodes by excising the loose areolar tissue over the external iliac vessels (Fig. 12.6) (2). The genitofemoral nerve courses laterally to the external iliac artery and should be identified and preserved prior to excising the lymphatic tissue. Mobilization and retraction of the external iliac vessels allows access to the obturator space. The obturator nodes are most easily teased away from the nerve and vessels if one begins the dissection caudad (Fig. 12.7) (2).

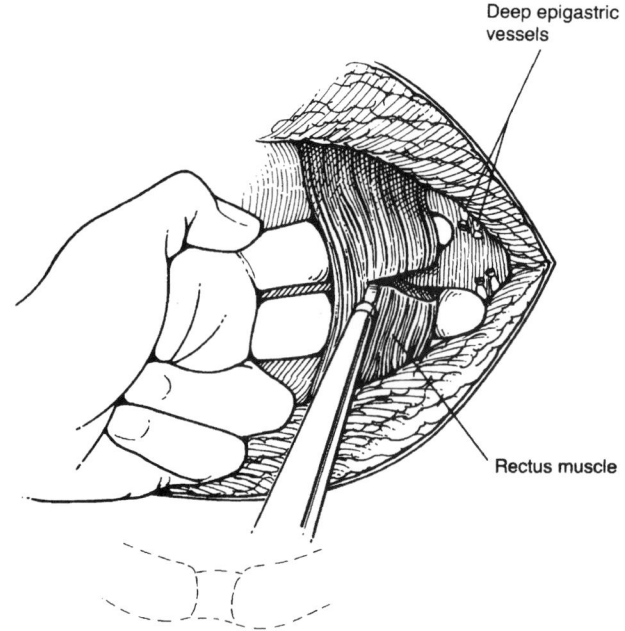

FIG. 12-5. The Maylard incision. A transverse incision has been made from the anterior-superior iliac spine to the opposite anterior-superior iliac spine. The fascia has been incised transversely. The deep inferior epigastric vessels are located on the lateral and posterior borders of the rectus muscle. They are bluntly dissected from this position by the finger of the operator, isolated, clamped, sectioned, and tied. Only after they are tied should the rectus muscle be incised. This can be done with the Bovie. (Reprinted with permission from Gallup DG, Talledo OE. *Surgical atlas of gynecologic oncology.* Philadelphia: WB Saunders Co., 1994:45.)

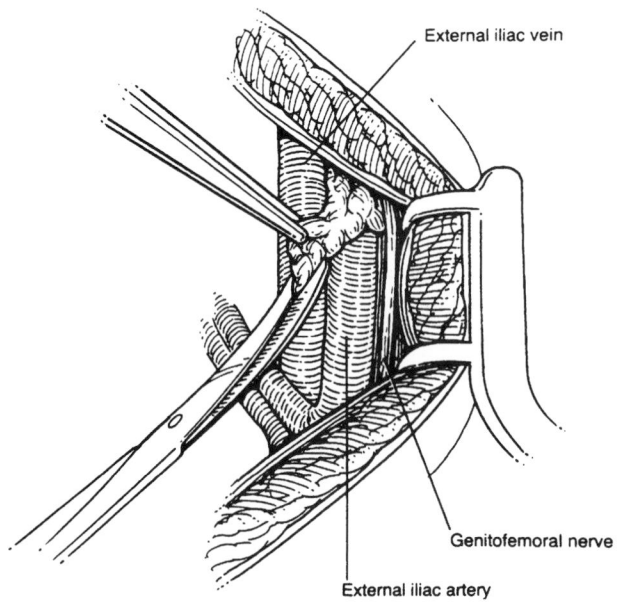

FIG. 12-6. Starting at the bifurcation of the common iliac vessels, the loose areolar tissue over the vein is excised from cephalad to caudad. Clips should be used at the bifurcation of the common iliac to avoid troublesome bleeding. (Reprinted with permission from Gallup DG, Talledo OE. *Surgical atlas of gynecologic oncology.* Philadelphia: WB Saunders, 1994:57.)

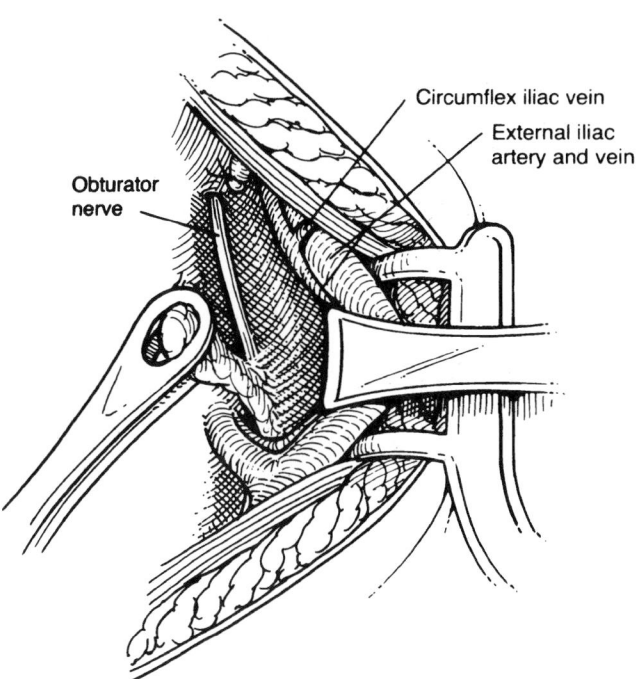

FIG. 12-7. A vein retractor is used to retract the external iliac veins anterior and lateral to expose the obturator space. Lymphatic tissue is gently teased from the psoas muscle. The entire lymphatic bundle is clamped, sectioned at its caudal end, and ligated at the pelvic sidewall. With the use of the Singley forceps, the lymphatic bundle is bluntly dissected from the obturator nerve and mobilized superiorly. Often, the obturator vein and artery must be sacrificed to obtain access to tissue posterior and lateral to the nerve. Once the tissue is mobilized superiorly, all areolar tissue is cleaned off the hypogastric vessels to the level of the bifurcation of the common iliac artery. The large tissue bundle is clamped and removed en bloc. A tie or clips may be used at the level of the bifurcation. (Reprinted with permission from Gallup DG, Talledo OE. *Surgical atlas of gynecologic oncology.* Philadelphia: WB Saunders, 1994:58.)

Transperitoneal Approach to the Paraaortic Nodes

The transperitoneal approach to the paraaortic lymph nodes can be accomplished by either the direct or the lateral approach. With the direct approach, the dissection begins with an incision in the peritoneum directly over the common iliac arteries and aorta. The lateral approach starts with an incision in the lateral paracolic gutters with subsequent medial reflection of the right and/or left colon. The advantage of the direct approach is that it involves less dissection of the intestine and ureter, whereas one of its main disadvantages is that it is associated with a greater degree of difficulty in exposing the left paraaortic nodes. Consequently, many surgeons sample the right paraaortic lymph nodes via the direct approach and use the lateral approach for the left-sided nodes (9).

With the direct approach to the right paraaortic nodes, an incision is made in the peritoneum overlying the right common iliac artery (Fig. 12.8). The incision is carried up over the aorta to the level of the duodenum. If the nodal dissection is to be carried out only to the level of the IMA, the duodenum is not mobilized. Using blunt dissection, the ureter and ovarian vessels are identified and mobilized laterally. The lymphatic tissue lateral to the right common iliac artery is elevated and the caudal end is clipped and divided. The dissection then proceeds in a caudad-to-cephaldad direction. A plane is created between the IVC and the lymphatic pedicle. The majority of the right paraaortic nodes overlie the IVC and they are generally easily dissected off the vessel. However, there is a fairly constant small vein within the lymphatics anterior to the IVC that inserts just above its bifurcation. If care is not taken to identify and ligate this so-called "fellow's" vein early in the dissection, it can easily be torn with resultant heavy bleeding (1). When the most cephaldad extent of the dissection is reached, the pedicle is clipped and divided (Fig. 12.9).

If the nodes above the IMA need to be sampled, the third portion of the duodenum is mobilized by bilaterally incising the peritoneum around it and then sharply dissecting the areolar tissue underneath (4). The superior portion of the peritoneal incision can be carried up as high as the ligament of Treitz, which can also be divided if needed. Inferiorly, the peritoneal incision is extended over the right ureter around the cecum and up along the right paracolic gutter to mobilize the small bowel mesentery and part of the right colon (Fig. 12.10) (4). The small bowel can then be put into a bowel bag outside the abdomen for further exposure. The

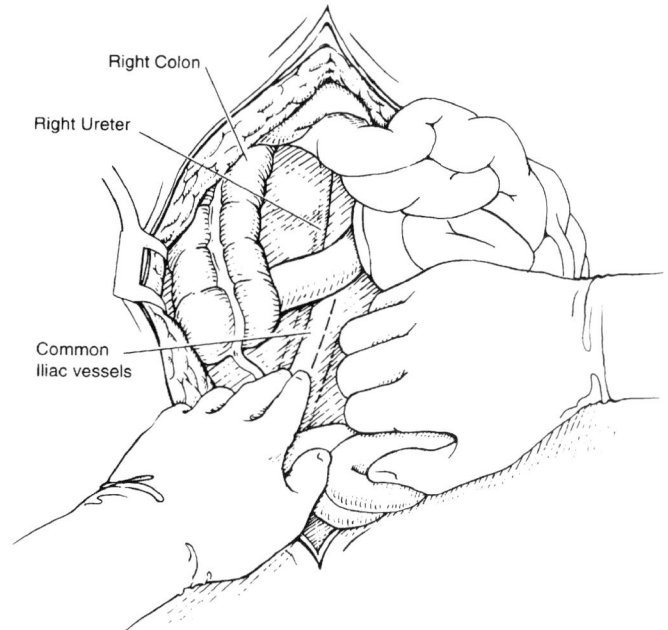

FIG. 12-8. The small bowel is elevated out of the pelvis placing the mesentery on gentle traction. The right ureter and common iliac artery are identified and the peritoneum overlying the artery is incised.

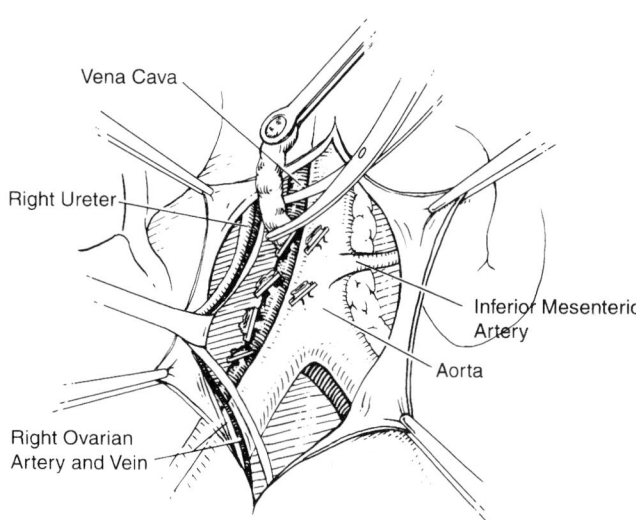

FIG. 12-9. The specimen is dissected in a cephaldad direction. Hemostatic clips are used on either side of the developing pedicle as it is mobilized and divided and also at the most cephaldad extent of the dissection before the specimen is removed.

duodenum is retracted superiorly allowing identification and ligation of the right ovarian artery and vein. The lymphatic tissue can then be safely dissected off of the right side of the aorta and the anterior surface of the IVC up to the level of the renal veins.

The left paraaortic lymph nodes may be removed through the same peritoneal incision. Sharp dissection is used to identify the left common iliac artery, left side of the aorta, IMA, left ureter, and left psoas muscle (Fig. 12.11). The ureter is again mobilized laterally. The lymphatic tissue lateral to the left common iliac artery and aorta is then removed in a caudad-to-cephaldad direction. The left paraaortic lymph nodes lie lateral and partially behind the aorta. In sampling these nodes, judicious use of vascular clips will help prevent troublesome bleeding from the lumbar vessels. Safe removal of the lymph nodes above the IMA requires identification and division of the left ovarian artery and vein and occasionally ligation of the inferior mesenteric artery and vein.

To remove right-sided paraaortic nodes via the lateral approach, the right paracolic gutter is incised along the line of Toldt (Fig. 12.12). The peritoneum is elevated off the psoas muscle and the incision is extended up to the hepatic flexure of the colon. Using sharp and blunt dissection, the right colon

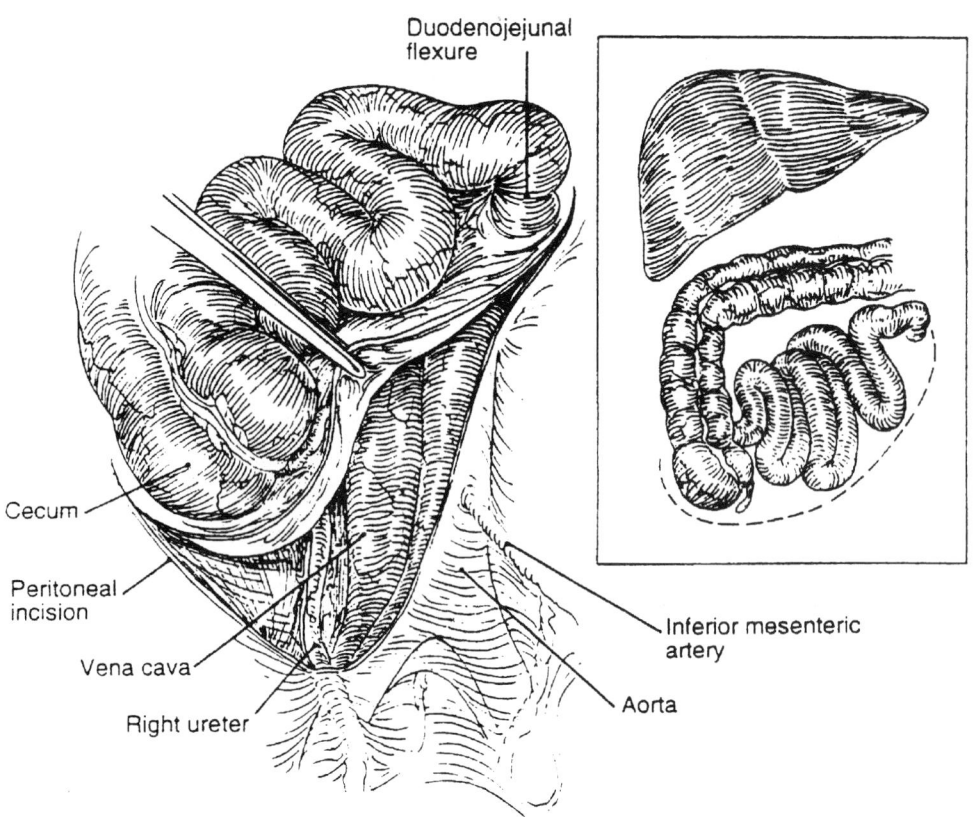

FIG. 12-10. Extended peritoneal incision. The peritoneal incision is extended over the right ureter around the cecum and the cephalad along the right paracolic gutter. This allows for mobilization of the small bowel mesentery as well as the ascending colon. (Reprinted with permission from Fowler JM, Johnson PR. Transperitoneal para-aortic lymphadenectomy. *Oper tech gynecol surg* 1996;1:9.)

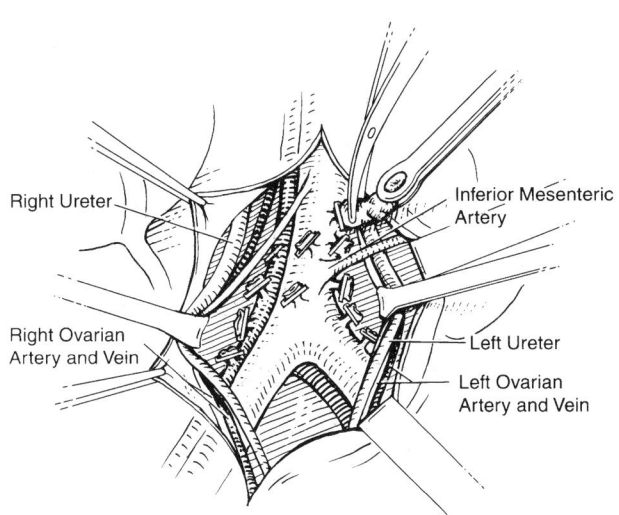

FIG. 12-11. Removal of the left paraaortic nodes through the same peritoneal incision. The dissection also proceeds in a cephalad direction, again using hemostatic clips on the lateral and medial margins. Care should be taken to avoid injury to the inferior mesenteric artery that arises approximately 3 to 4 cm above the aortic bifurcation.

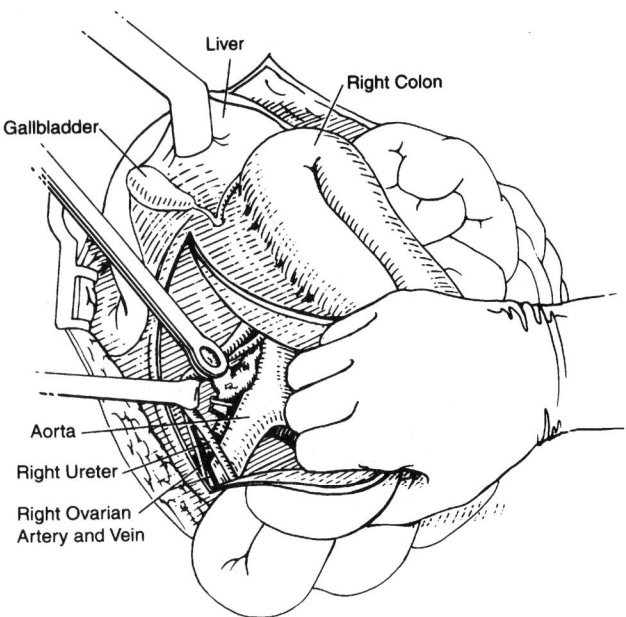

FIG. 12-13. With the ureter and ovarian vessels identified, the dissection begins at the right common iliac artery and proceeds cephalad up to the third portion of the duodenum.

is reflected medially. The ureter and ovarian vessels can be identified attached to the undersurface of the relected peritoneum. They may be left attached or mobilized laterally for better exposure. Further medial mobilization of the colon exposes the IVC and aorta. With the essential structures

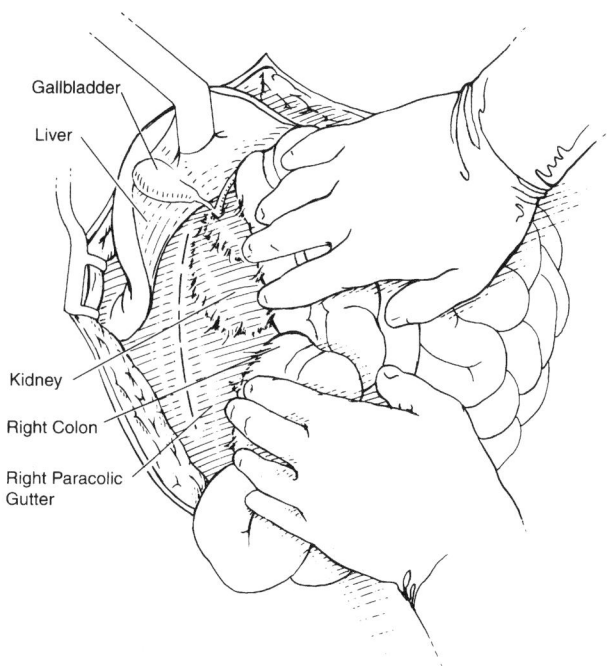

FIG. 12-12. The right paracolic gutter is exposed by medial traction on the ascending colon. The gutter is incised along the line of Toldt.

identified, the lymphatic tissue can then be dissected as previously described in a caudad-to-cephalad direction up to the third portion of the duodenum (Fig. 12.13).

If the lymph nodes above the IMA need to be sampled, the Kocher maneuver is used to reflect the duodenum medially. The peritoneum lateral to the convexity of the C-curve of the duodenum is incised and the second portion of the duodenum is then dissected off of the IVC. For further exposure, the peritoneal incision along the line of Toldt may need to be extended cephaldad to mobilize completely the hepatic flexure of the colon (Fig. 12.14). The right ovarian artery and vein are identified and divided. The right-sided paraaortic lymph nodes are then able to be dissected off of the IVC and right aorta up to the level of the renal vessels.

The lateral approach to the left paraaortic lymph nodes is accomplished in a similar fashion by incising along the line of Toldt and mobilization of the left colon medially (Fig. 12.15). Again, the ureter and ovarian vessels are identified on the undersurface of the reflected peritoneum, and they may be left attached or mobilized laterally for better exposure (Fig. 12.16). After further mobilization of the left colon and identification of the aorta and the IMA, the left-sided nodes are removed in a caudad-to-cephalad direction (Fig. 12.17). Sampling of the nodes above the IMA requires mobilization of the splenic flexure of the colon, division of the left ovarian artery and vein, and occasionally ligation of the inferior mesenteric artery and vein.

Extraperitoneal Approach to the Paraaortic Nodes

The extraperitoneal approach to the paraaortic lymph nodes by means of a supraumbilical transverse ''sunrise''

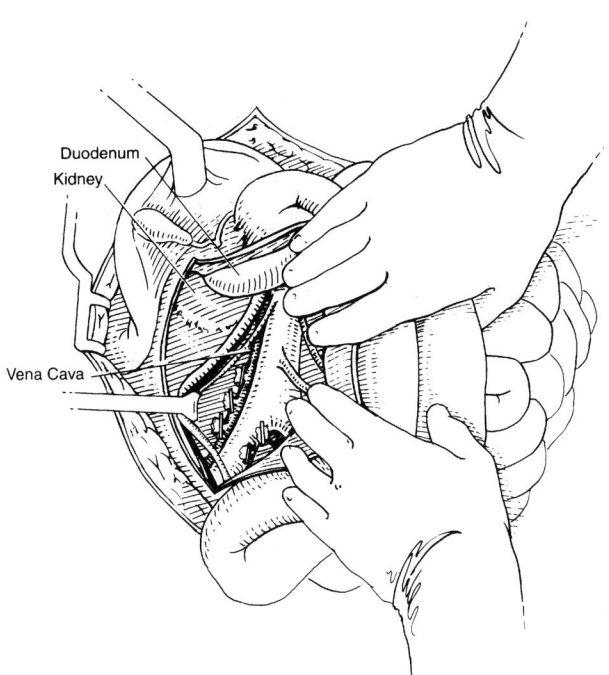

FIG. 12-14. The Kocher maneuver can be used to gain access to the lymph nodes above the IMA. The peritoneum lateral to the convexity of the C-curve of the duodenum is incised and the second portion of the duodenum is then dissected off of the IVC. The common bile duct and pancreatic duct enter the second portion of the duodenum posteromedially. For further exposure, the incision along the line of Toldt can be extended cephalad to mobilize completely the hepatic flexure of the colon.

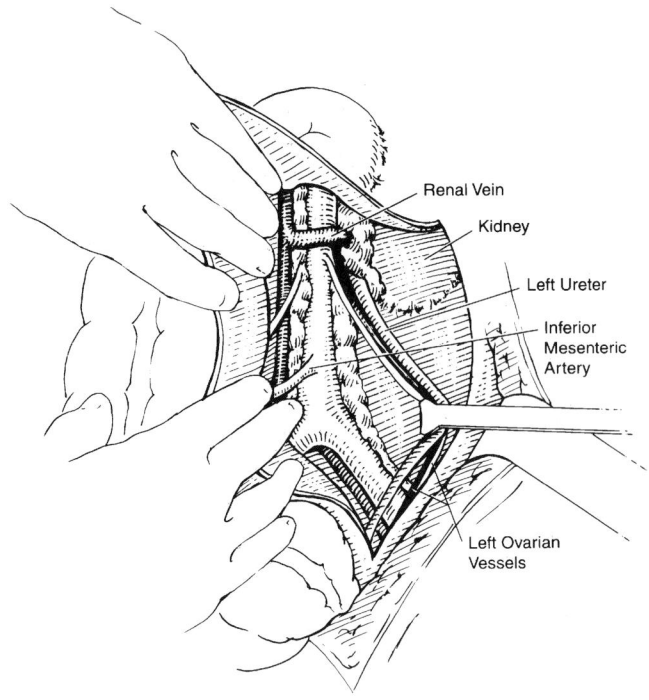

FIG. 12-16. Using sharp and blunt dissection, the left colon can be mobilized medially exposing the left ureter, ovarian vessels, and aorta.

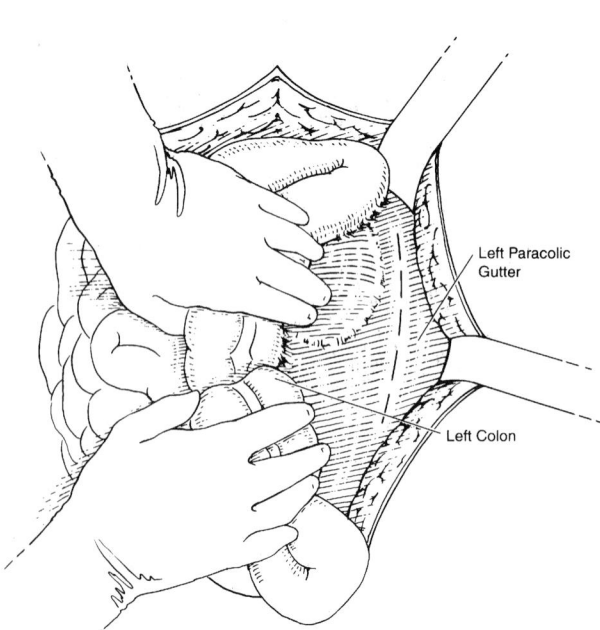

FIG. 12-15. The lateral approach to the left paraaortic nodes is accomplished by retracting the descending colon medially and incising along the line of Toldt.

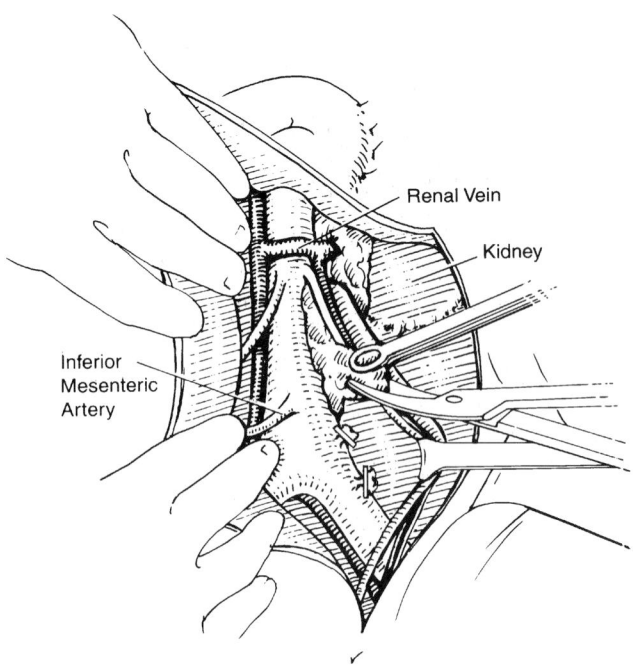

FIG. 12-17. Dissection begins at the left common iliac artery and proceeds cephalad using hemostatic clips. Care should be taken to avoid injury to the inferior mesenteric artery that arises approximately 3 to 4 cm above the aortic bifurcation.

incision was initially described by Gallup and colleagues (6). The skin incision is made 6 cm above the umbilicus in the midline and is carried laterally and caudad to the level of the iliac crests bilaterally (Fig. 12.18) (2).

The fascia is incised transversely. The rectus muscles are dissected off of the anterior-lying fascia cephalad and caudad. The right rectus muscle is transected. The right transversus muscle is then identified and transected caudally and laterally. The hand of the operator is inserted deep into the incision until the right psoas muscle and external iliac vessels are palpated. The peritoneum is then bluntly dissected from caudad and lateral to cephalad and medial, separating it from the underlying common iliac vessels until the great vessels are exposed (Fig. 12.19) (2). If the peritoneum is inadvertently entered, it must be closed immediately.

After identification of the right ureter and ovarian vessels, the right paraaortic nodes can be removed. In thin patients,

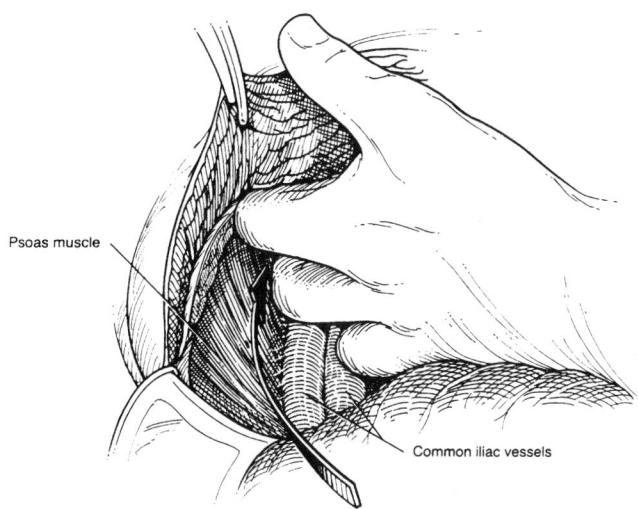

FIG. 12-19. With the rectus and transversus muscles transected, the operator's hand is inserted caudad until the psoas muscle and external iliac vessels are palpated. The peritoneum is then bluntly dissected from caudad and lateral to cephalad and medial, separating it from the underlying common iliac vessels until the aorta and vena cava are exposed. (Reprinted with permission from Gallup DG, Talledo OE. *Surgical atlas of gynecologic oncology.* Philadelphia: WB Saunders, 1994:121.)

the left paraaortic nodes may be able to be removed through a right abdominal approach. However, if exposure is difficult, the left rectus and transversus muscles can be transected and the peritoneum mobilized medially in a similar fashion to gain access to the left paraaortic nodes.

Laparoscopic Lymph Node Dissection

Pelvic node and paraaortic lymph node dissections are being done at a few centers via operative laparoscopy (10–12). Numerous reports have demonstrated the benefits of the minimal-access approach. However, there are still concerns regarding the long-term effects, and ongoing, prospective clinical trials will help answer many of the remaining questions regarding safety and efficacy (13). Laparoscopic lymph node dissections are discussed in greater detail in Chapter 13.

Radical Hysterectomy

In performing a radical hysterectomy, one of the most troublesome areas is intraoperative bleeding from the lateral cardinal ligament, which is also known as the "web." In order to have better access and exposure in this area, the surgeon can release the uterus posteriorly in the earlier steps of the procedure. The six classic spaces are developed prior to sectioning the uterosacral ligaments. With maximal mobility of the uterus achieved, the ureter is unroofed from the tunnel of tissue that contains the uterine vessels and its

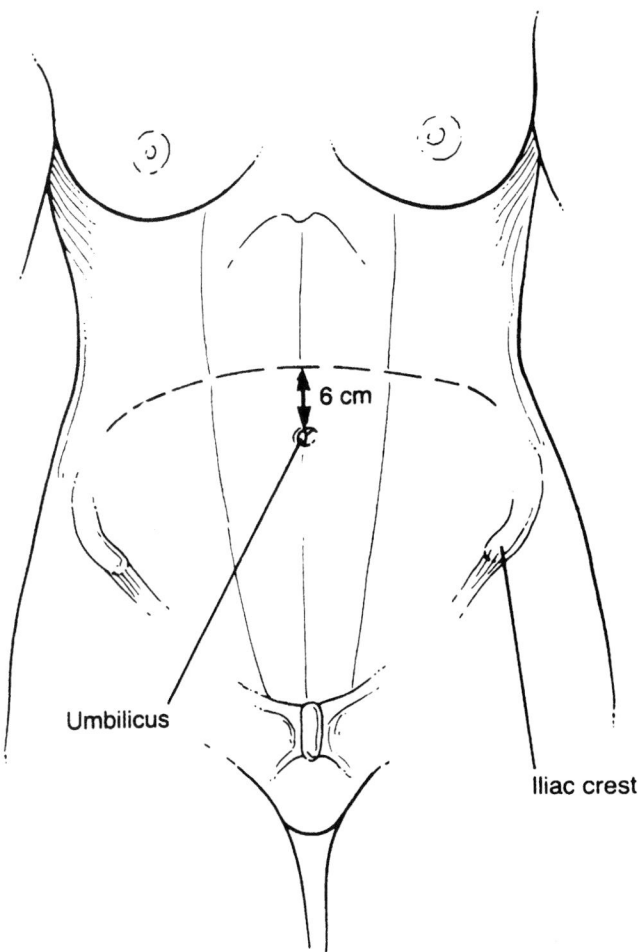

FIG. 12-18. The "sunrise" incision. In the center, the incision is approximately 6 cm above the umbilicus. The incision is carried laterally in a downward fashion to the level of the iliac crests. (Reprinted with permission from Gallup DG, Talledo OE. *Surgical atlas of gynecologic oncology.* Philadelphia: WB Saunders, 1994:118.)

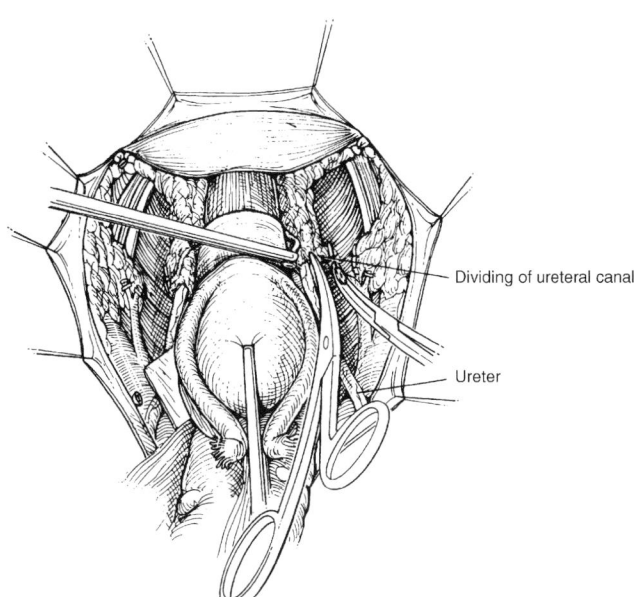

FIG. 12-20. Dissection of the ureter from the parametrium is begun. The ureteral canal is unroofed by placing traction on the medial stump of the uterine vessels. Because of the rich blood supply from anastomosis of vessels in this area, a clamp-cut technique is often used. (Reprinted with permission from Gallup DG, Talledo OE. *Surgical atlas of gynecologic oncology.* Philadelphia: WB Saunders, 1994:79.)

branches (Fig. 12.20). Once the ureter is unroofed, removal of any remaining cardinal ligament is accomplished with the ureter pulled laterally. To ensure that adequate vaginal margins are obtained, right-angle clamps are placed proximal to the level of resection of the specimen (Fig. 12.21). The pelvic lymphadenectomy can be done prior to or following the radical hysterectomy. The use of closed suction drains is advocated by many, although some avoid their use.

Ovarian Cancer Debulking

Ovarian malignancy often presents with large pelvic masses filling the pelvis. An initial incision over the lateral pelvic sidewall just anterior to the external iliac artery will allow adequate visualization of the ureter and the ovarian vessels (Fig. 12.22). The paracolic gutters can be incised cephalad along the avascular line of Toldt for more adequate exposure of the retroperitoneal space. To avoid further troublesome hemorrhage with large adnexal masses, if a hysterectomy is part of the planned procedure, the uterine vessels can be separately isolated and divided similar to a modified radical hysterectomy. When the anatomy is distorted by peritoneal implants, the ureters may need to be followed down to the tunnel and retracted laterally prior to removal of the uterus.

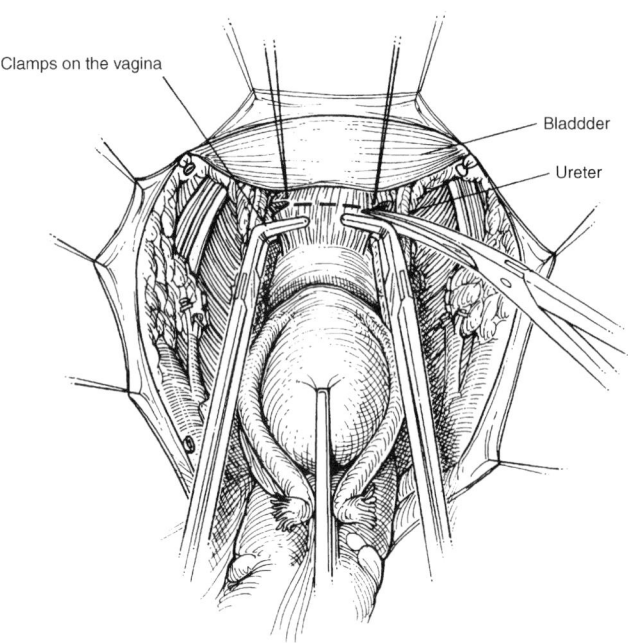

FIG. 12-21. The vaginal angles are clamped and sectioned after placing right-angle clamps across the proximal vagina. Note the vaginal incision is made caudad to these clamps. (Reprinted with permission from Gallup DG, Talledo OE. *Surgical atlas of gynecologic oncology.* Philadelphia: WB Saunders, 1994:81.)

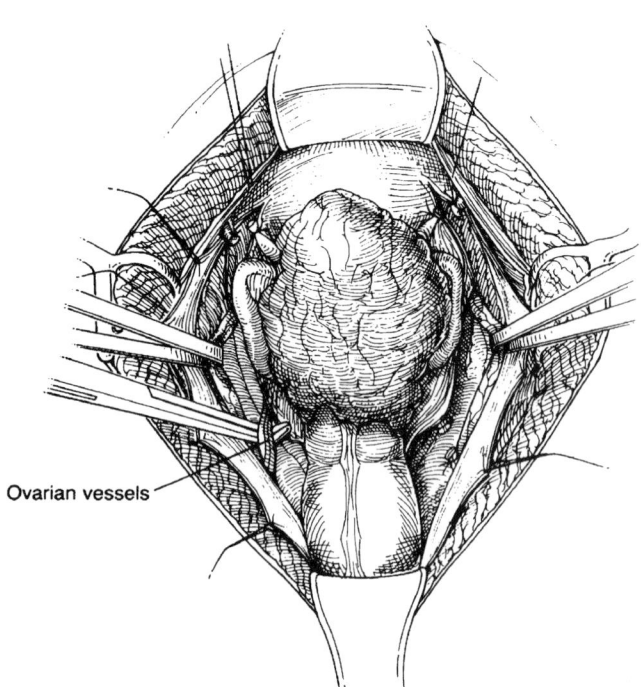

FIG. 12-22. The ovarian vessels are skeletonized and divided at the pelvic brim. Early control of these vessels will help reduce blood loss during the later dissection. The ureter can be mobilized off the medial leaf of the broad ligament and retracted laterally on a Penrose drain or vessel loop. (Reprinted with permission from Gallup DG, Talledo OE. *Surgical atlas of gynecologic oncology.* Philadelphia: WB Saunders, 1994:92.)

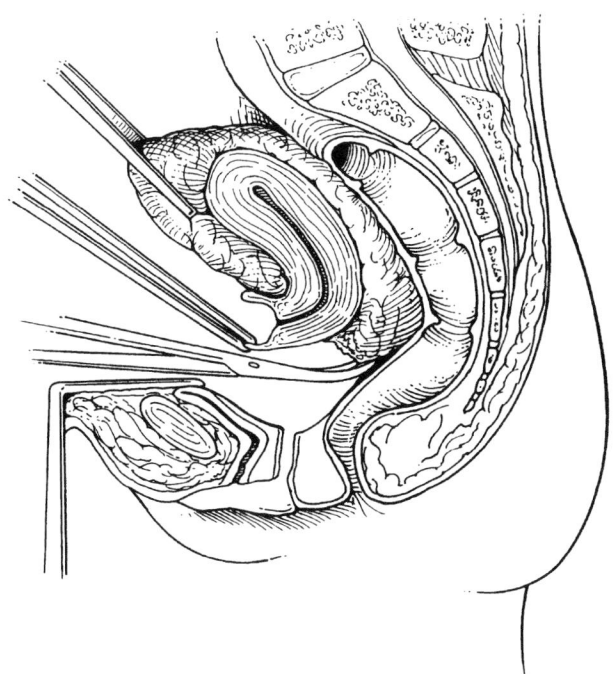

FIG. 12-23. The posterior vaginal wall is grasped and retracted cephalad. The uterus can now be sharply dissected off of the rectosigmoid. (Reprinted with permission from Gallup DG, Talledo OE. *Surgical atlas of gynecologic oncology.* Philadelphia: WB Saunders, 1994:103.)

In cases where ovarian tumors are densely adherent to or involve the rectosigmoid, a reverse hysterectomy can often help identify the rectovaginal plane. Once the uterine vessels are ligated bilaterally, the vagina is incised anteriorly below the level of the cervix. The posterior vagina is incised after elevating the anterior vaginal flap. The vaginal angles are ligated and the posterior vaginal wall is grasped with Kocher clamps and retracted cephalad (Fig. 12.23). The cardinal and uterosacral ligaments are then clamped and sectioned.

Continent Urinary Diversion

Over the past decade, interest in performing continent urinary diversions for patients with gynecologic malignancies has emerged. Most gynecologic oncologists will use a modification of the Indiana (14) or Miami (15) pouch. Poor candidates for continent urinary diversion include those with crippling arthritis or those psychologically unable to tolerate frequent self-catheterization of the pouch.

A modification of these pouches was recently described by King (2). The colon is transected just proximal to the hepatic flexure (Fig. 12.24). The colon is then detubularized by a longitudinal incision along the tinea. The continent mechanism is created by two maneuvers. First, the terminal ileal segment is tapered down over a #14 French Foley catheter by using a gastrointestinal anastomosis (GIA) stapling device along the antimesenteric border of the ileum. The

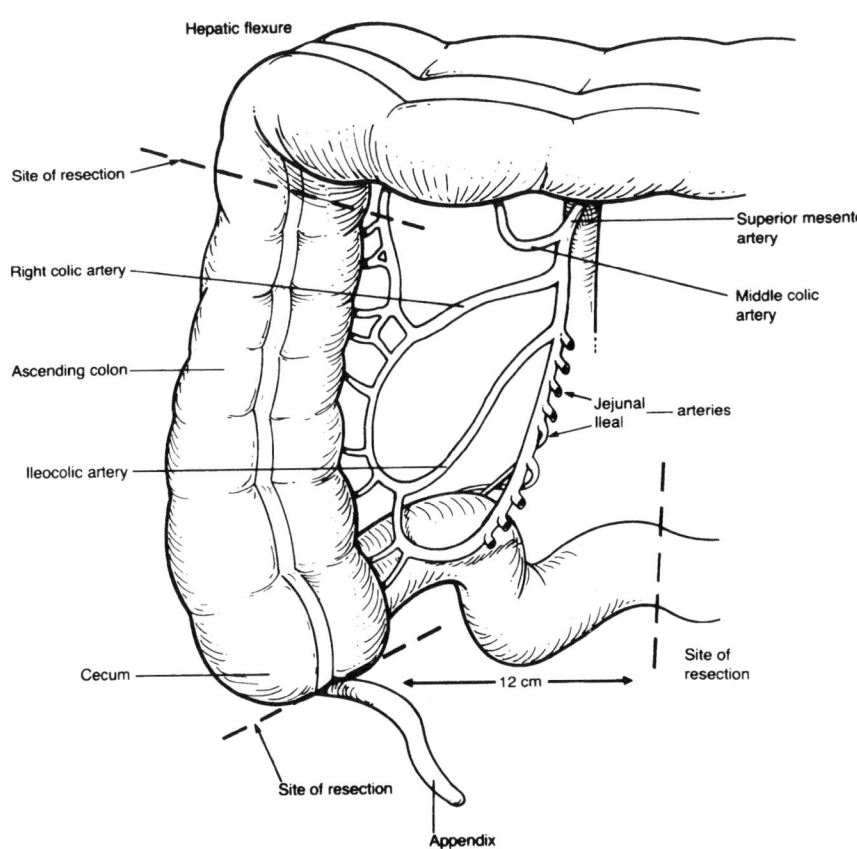

FIG. 12-24. The anatomic location and vascularity of the right colon segment utilized for formation of the continent urinary pouch. Illustrated are the anatomic sites of division for creation of the continent pouch. The ascending colon is divided distal to the right colic artery. The terminal ileum is divided approximately 12 cm from the ileocecal valve. The resection can be accomplished with the use of surgical staplers or by intestinal clamps. If the appendix is present, it should be removed. The ileocecal segment has a rich blood supply derived from the right colic artery and the ileocolic artery. If one is performing the Miami pouch type of urinary diversion, the transverse colon would be divided distal to the middle colic artery. (Reprinted with permission from Gallup DG, Talledo OE. *Surgical atlas of gynecologic oncology.* Philadelphia: WB Saunders,1994:186.)

second maneuver is to plicate the ileocecal valve by placing concentric purse-string sutures of 0 silk or polypropylene around it. The ureters are then implanted under direct vision (Fig. 12.25) (2). After closing the pouch, the ileal stoma can be brought out in several areas of the abdominal wall (Fig. 12.26) (2). Some use the umbilicus as the exit site. The ureteral stents can exit the abdomen via the ileal stoma or through separate incisions in the pouch and abdominal wall.

The use of a Penrose drain and a cecostomy tube for irrigation to remove mucus is optional.

Abdominal Closure

With the advent of more recently published closure methods and newer suture materials, the vertical, allegedly stronger, paramedian incision is unnecessary. A midline in-

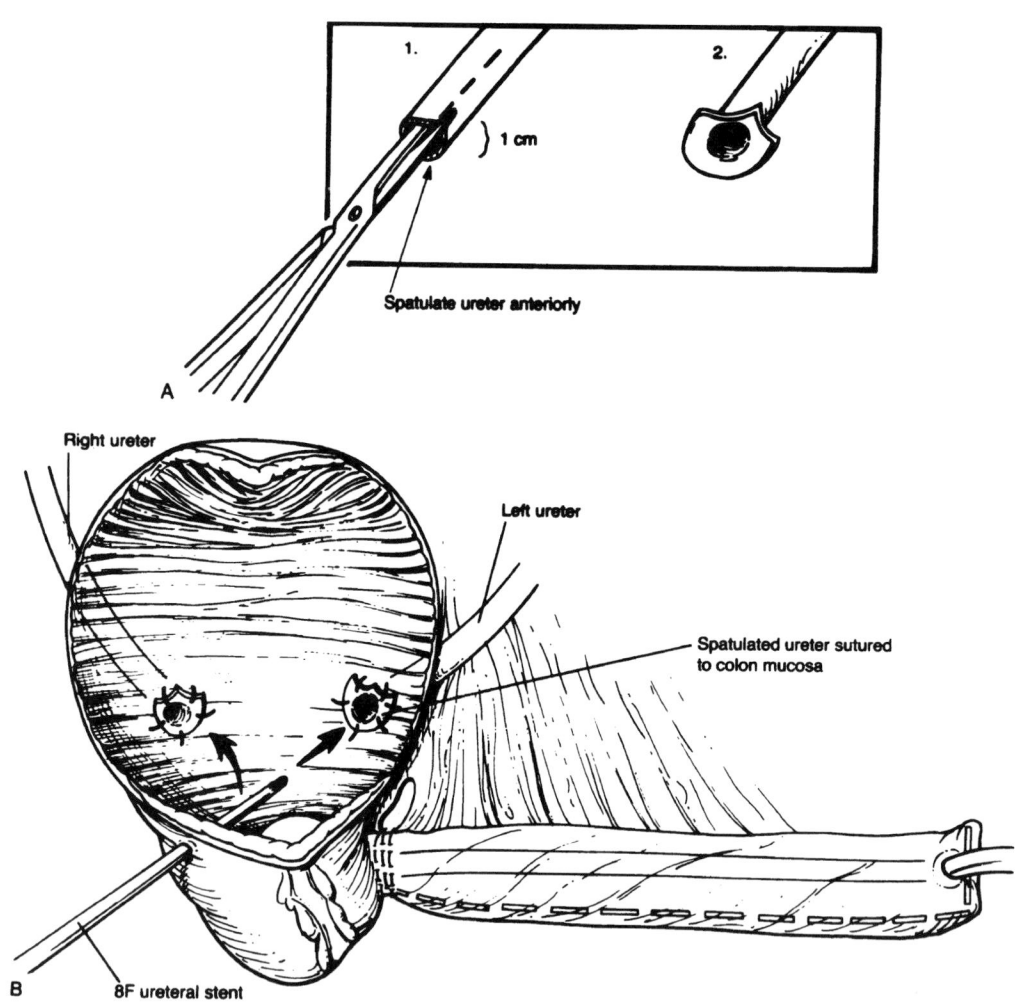

FIG. 12-25. A, B: Prior to beginning the continent diversion, the ureters have been transected (usually at the pelvic brim) and mobilized so that they are able to be brought to the area where the continent pouch will be located without tension. If necessary, the left ureter can be brought through or under the mesentery of the colon to facilitate its placement into the urinary pouch. An appropriate site is selected on what will be the posterior wall of the pouch, and a long thin clamp is used to perforate the colon and pull the ureter through. An approximately 1-cm segment of ureter is brought into the pouch. For ease of ureterointestinal anastomosis, the ureter should be secured posteriorly to the pouch by suturing the adventitial tissue of the ureter to the seromuscular layers of the pouch with three or four permanent 3-0 sutures. The ureter is spatulated to increase the lumen diameter. The ureter is sutured directly to the colon and is not tunneled. We use 4-0 polyglycolic suture. This is a full-thickness approximation of the colon and ureter. Once both ureters have been sutured into the pouch, two #8 French ureterointestinal stents or long pediatric feeding tubes are placed retrograde into the renal pelvis. If a feeding tube is used, it should be sutured to the ureter with 4-0 chromic to ensure against displacement due to ureteral peristalsis. Note the three concentric sutures at the ileocecal valve. (Reprinted with permission from Gallup DG, Talledo OE. *Surgical atlas of gynecologic oncology.* Philadelphia: WB Saunders, 1994:191.)

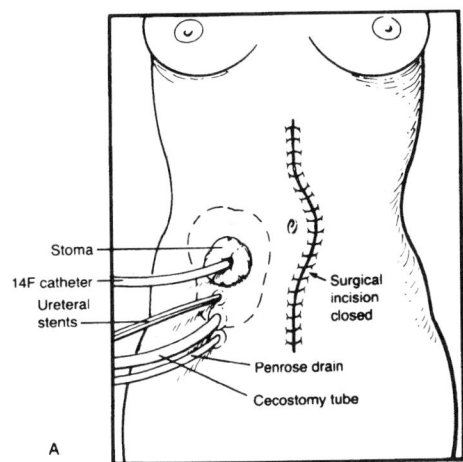

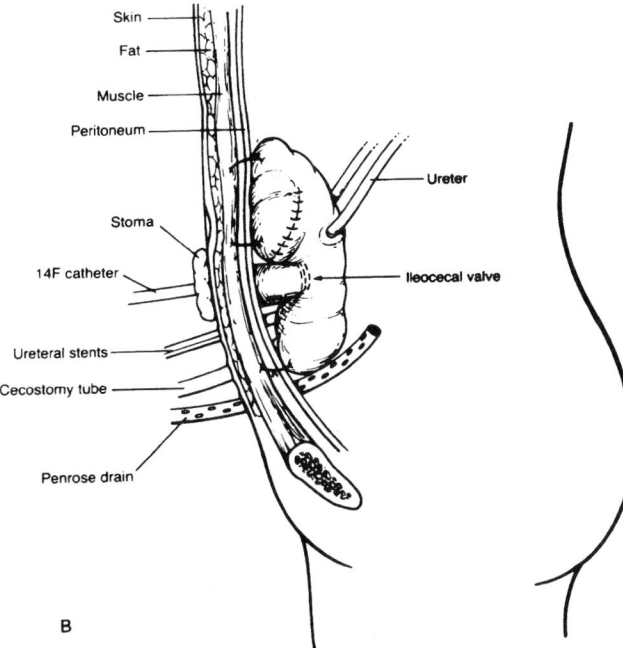

FIG. 12-26. A, B: the site for the ileal stoma is selected on the anterior abdominal wall and then incised through all abdominal tissue layers. The stoma is created for catheterization and the #14 French catheter should exit the pouch through this stoma. It is critical that the ileal segment be at a 90° angle with the abdominal wall so that catheterization is a "straight shot." The pouch may be sutured to the abdominal wall to accomplish this. All stents and drainage tubes are brought out through the anterior abdominal wall and secured. The pouch may also be anchored posteriorly (i.e., to the sacrum). (Reprinted with permission from Gallup DG, Talledo OE. *Surgical atlas of gynecologic oncology.* Philadelphia: WB Saunders, 1994:193.)

cision is preferable in modern-day gynecologic oncology. It is the least hemorrhagic of all incisions, and rapid entry is feasible. Exposure is excellent, and minimal nerve damage occurs.

In the past, many surgeons have advocated the relatively

time-consuming Smead-Jones closure (16). However, in the 1980s, it was noted that midline incisions could be safely closed with a running, mass closure. In 1989, Gallup and associates (17) reported on 210 patients, most of whom were at high risk for evisceration, who had midline incisions closed with a running, mass closure using #2 monofilament polypropylene suture. No eviscerations occurred. Since that publication, several gynecologic oncology services have published excellent results using monofilament absorbable or monofilament permanent sutures in a running, mass closure method (18–21).

Figure 12.27 illustrates a popular technique utilizing an absorbable suture (2). Eviscerations using this technique almost never occur.

Management of Select Surgical Complications

No matter how experienced and skillful a surgeon is, surgical complications are unavoidable. The obvious goal is to keep the complications to a minimum while expeditiously diagnosing and correcting those that inevitably occur. Patients who undergo surgery for gynecologic malignancies are at risk for a variety of complications. This section will

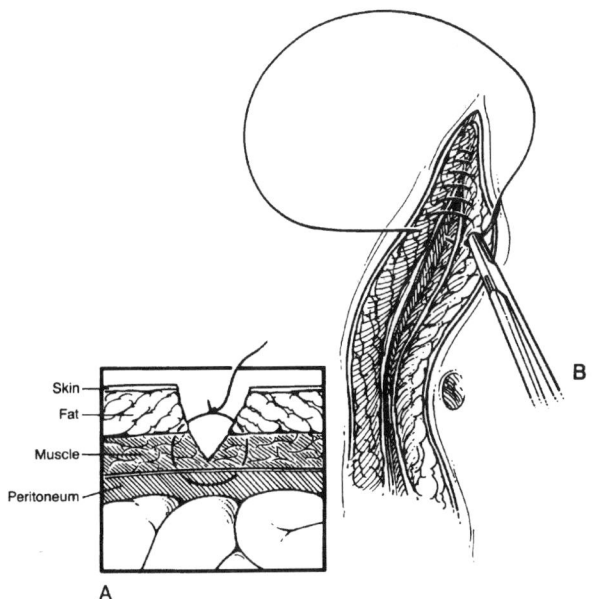

FIG. 12-27. A running #1 delayed absorbable suture (Maxon or PDS) is used to close midline incisions. One suture is started from the cephalad end. The knots are buried. The sutures are placed approximately 1 cm apart. **A:** The sutures are placed at least 2 cm from the fascial edge. The suture bite should include anterior fascia, a portion of the muscle, and the posterior fascia. The peritoneum is included if it is easily located. **B:** When the midpoint is reached from the cephalad and caudad ends, the sutures are tied and the knot buried. Six throws are used for each knot. (Reprinted with permission from Gallup DG, Talledo OE. *Surgical atlas of gynecologic oncology.* Philadelphia: WB Saunders, 1994:51.)

review the management of incisional hernias, lymphocysts, and colostomy complications such as parastomal hernias and stomal retraction.

Incisional Hernias

The principles of hernia repair include (a) dissection of the hernia sac from the subcutaneous fat, rectus margin, and peritoneal margin; (b) excision of the redundant peritoneal sac; and (c) primary closure with a monofilament permanent suture with or without the placement of a synthetic mesh prosthesis (polypropylene).

The skin and subcutaneous fat are cleared off of the anterior rectus sheath and hernia sac for about 3 to 4 cm in all directions. To help identify the various tissue planes, opening of the sac can be delayed until the boundaries of the hernia have been delineated. The sac can then be opened to dissect off any underlying bowel or omentum and to identify the margins of the fascial ring. After the sac is excised, the peritoneal edge is then trimmed back to healthy tissue.

If the fascial edges come together with moderate traction, it can be closed primarily with a mass closure technique using permanent monofilament suture. However, if the fascial defect of the hernia is greater than 4 cm or excessive traction is needed for primary closure, a polypropylene mesh may be required to reinforce the repair (1). To place the mesh, the fascia and peritoneum beneath the rectus muscle are dissected widely around the margins of the defect to allow primary closure of the peritoneum. The mesh is then placed and sutured into place laterally between the posterior fascia and the rectus muscle without entering the peritoneum. The remaining rectus fascia is then closed over the mesh.

Lymphocysts

Most lymphocysts are small, asymptomatic, and clinically insignificant. However, large lymphocysts can produce serious consequences such as venous obstruction, ureteral obstruction, leg edema, and pain. The diagnosis of a pelvic lymphocyst can be made most easily by pelvic ultrasound or computed tomographic (CT) scan, although occasionally a large, tense cyst can be palpated on physical examination.

Large or symptomatic pelvic lymphocysts can almost always be managed by percutaneous drainage with a pigtail catheter placed under CT or ultrasound guidance (22). If percutaneous drainage fails, instilling a sclerosing solution such as povidone-iodine or ethanol may eliminate the cyst (23,24). Refractory lymphocysts may require surgical marsupialization to ensure continued intraperitoneal drainage.

Parastomal Hernias

Some degree of parastomal hernia is common with end colostomies. Most hernias should be managed conservatively with special care of appliances and girdles because

they are usually harmless to the patient and surgical repair is associated with a significant risk of recurrence.

If the parastomal hernia causes significant problems, such as interference with the wearing of an appliance or unacceptable cosmetic problems, two options for surgical correction are available: local repair with or without support of a synthetic mesh and relocation of the stoma.

With a local repair, the stoma with the adjacent skin is dissected free down to the fascia. The hernia is identified, repaired, and closed in a fashion similar to that described earlier for incisional hernias. If the hernia is large, mesh (Marlex, Gore-Tex) may be required for repair or the stoma can be relocated to a higher midrectus position, to the umbilicus, or to the opposite side of the abdomen (1).

Stomal Retraction

A retracted stoma can lead to stomal stenosis, a parastomal abscess, or sinus formation. Operative revision is generally required. This can be accomplished locally by mobilization of the stoma down into the peritoneal cavity to obtain enough length to make a new, tension-free stoma. When sufficient length cannot be obtained in this manner, a laparotomy may be required to mobilize the colon or the stoma may need to be moved to another site.

SURGICAL MANAGEMENT OF GYNECOLOGIC CANCER

The gynecologic oncologist must be able to evaluate the woman with a genital tract malignancy, direct her management, perform the necessary surgical procedures, and supervise her postoperative care. A patient who is managed by a surgeon who is not a gynecologic oncologist may receive an operative procedure that is inappropriate or inadequate. McGowan and associates (25) reviewed the intraoperative evaluation of 291 women with primary ovarian cancer. Ninety-seven percent of the patients who underwent surgery by a gynecologic oncologist received complete staging operations, but only 52% and 35% had adequate operations by an obstetrician-gynecologist or a general surgeon, respectively.

Two British studies retrospectively analyzed the outcomes of over 1800 patients with ovarian cancer (26,27). Both studies found on multivariate analysis that patients' survival was adversely impacted when their initial operation was performed by a general surgeon as opposed to a gynecologic surgeon. These results are similar to those obtained by Nguyen et al. in a national survey of ovarian carcinoma (28). Eisenkop and colleagues analyzed the outcomes of 263 patients with stages IIIC and IV ovarian carcinoma (29). When the primary surgery was performed by gynecologic oncologists, as compared to general obstetricians-gynecologists and general surgeons, the rate of optimal cytoreduction was significantly higher, the operative mortality substantially lower, and the median survival significantly longer. In the three decades since the establishment of gynecologic oncology as a subspecialty, cancer therapy has become increasingly sophisticated and complex, and it is difficult for any one physician to master all the skills necessary for treating gynecologic malignancies. More often, we must use multimodal therapy and be involved in multidisciplinary care. There are many medical and radiation oncologists who have specialized in gynecologic cancer and they are integral members of the multidisciplinary team. The Gynecologic Oncology Group (GOG), with its emphasis on multidisciplinary research, has demonstrated the effectiveness of such an approach.

Another important factor in providing optimal patient care is the environment in which gynecologic oncology is practiced. The facilities used by the gynecologic oncologist should offer state of the art radiation therapy and chemotherapy. Patients should receive care tailored to the type and extent of their disease and not determined by the limitations of the available facilities.

Mortality rates for complex oncologic procedures, such as pelvic exenteration, have been demonstrated to be significantly lower in hospitals where the procedures are performed with a relatively high volume as compared to those in which the procedures are performed infrequently (30). A recent meta-analysis performed by Bristow and colleagues evaluated 81 studies involving 6885 patients with advanced ovarian cancer (31). This study demonstrated a 50% increase in median survival if patients primary surgery was performed at an "expert" center compared to less experienced centers.

Early Diagnosis and Prevention

There is a role for early diagnosis and prevention in virtually all female genital cancers. The management of a patient with an abnormal Papanicolaou (Pap) smear allows the gynecologic oncologist to use limited surgery to prevent the development of an invasive malignancy of the cervix or vagina. Guided by colposcopy, the surgeon can employ traditional surgical excision, laser surgery, cryotherapy, or a loop electrosurgical excision procedure (LEEP) to preserve function and prevent cancer. Preinvasive lesions of the vulva can be diagnosed and managed by laser or local excision, thereby potentially avoiding progression to invasive disease and its associated extensive surgical therapy.

The proper management of endometrial hyperplasia can prevent the subsequent development of endometrial cancer. Optimal management requires individualization of treatment. Complex hyperplasia without atypia in a premenopausal patient indicates the need for medical therapy with progesterone, but a similar problem in a postmenopausal patient may indicate the need for a hysterectomy. Atypia in either case requires consideration of hysterectomy to prevent the development of endometrial cancer. It is essential that the gynecologic oncologist recognize the significance of these cancer precursors.

No diagnostic test or early symptoms reliably herald the onset of ovarian or tubal cancer, and no preinvasive lesion has been identified. The only method of prevention for these cancers is surgical removal of the tubes or ovaries before cancer develops. Although quite rare, women can be identified who may have as high as a 40% lifetime risk of developing ovarian cancer. These are women who have a family history of ovarian cancer (site-specific cancer), who have a family history of breast and ovarian cancer, or who are members of a Lynch II family. These cancer-prone families are described in Chapter 2. These syndromes are seen infrequently, and rigid criteria must be fulfilled before the diagnosis can be made. For women who fall into one of these high-risk categories, surgical removal of the tubes and ovaries (and the uterus in Lynch II families) should be considered after childbearing is complete (32,33). Before that time, close monitoring is essential.

The decision to remove the ovaries and fallopian tubes to prevent ovarian cancer is generally accepted for the postmenopausal patient who undergoes an exploratory pelvic operation or a hysterectomy for benign disease. The removal of the fallopian tubes and ovaries represents little additional surgery, and although the chance of the disease in any woman is quite low, prevention is worthwhile because of the lack of an effective screening modality combined with the devastating effects of ovarian and fallopian tube cancer. However, removal of the ovaries and fallopian tubes in premenopausal women is controversial. For a patient younger than 40 years of age, it seems advisable not to recommend removal of the fallopian tubes and ovaries unless she has a familial risk of ovarian cancer. Between the ages of 40 and 50 years, the pros and cons should be carefully discussed with the patient, and her wishes must be taken into account.

Diagnosis and Staging

The diagnosis of any gynecologic cancer requires a surgical biopsy. The manner in which the histologic diagnosis is obtained varies with the disease and the clinical situation. A punch biopsy or an instrument biopsy may be sufficient for the diagnosis of an invasive cancer of the vulva, vagina, or cervix, but an excisional biopsy is necessary for the diagnosis of microinvasive or preinvasive cancer. A fine-needle aspiration biopsy for cytologic analysis may be adequate for establishing the extent of spread of a cancer, but not for providing histologic cell type and grade for the primary diagnosis. The histologic diagnosis of ovarian or fallopian tube carcinoma requires surgical exploration.

The current International Federation of Gynecology and Obstetrics (FIGO) staging system of gynecologic cancers requires surgical staging for vulvar, endometrial, and ovarian cancer. Cervical cancer remains a clinically staged disease, although many centers use surgical staging (by laparotomy or laparoscopy) for treatment planning. No official FIGO staging exists for fallopian tube cancer or uterine sarcomas, but fallopian tube cancers are usually staged on the basis of surgical and pathologic findings similar to ovarian carcinoma. Table 12.1 lists the current methods of staging for the various gynecologic malignancies.

The initial surgical procedure in a patient with known or suspected gynecologic cancer should be performed by a trained gynecologic oncologist because the accuracy of diagnosis and staging significantly influences subsequent therapy. As stated earlier, McGowan and coworkers (25) have demonstrated that ovarian cancer staging operations performed by general obstetricians-gynecologists or general surgeons are inadequate much more frequently than if the operation is performed by a gynecologic oncologist. These investigators also found that 66% of patients who underwent a staging operation in a university hospital had adequate operations compared with roughly 50% in community hospitals. Young and colleagues (34) reported excellent survival in patients with early ovarian cancer, but stressed that these data were applicable only to patients with adequate surgical staging.

In addition to the anatomic site and stage of disease, the plan of therapy for most gynecologic malignancies is also influenced by the histologic cell type and histologic grade (differentiation) of the cancer. The cooperation of the surgeon, pathologist, and cytologist cannot be overemphasized in the diagnosis and staging of cancer. It is the surgeon's responsibility to provide the pathologist or cytologist with a complete clinical history and an indication of what he or she hopes to learn from the anatomic specimen. Without this communication, the pathologist and cytologist will be unable to provide the information needed to direct the clinical care of the patient. Both the pathologist and the cytologist must be sure that the surgeon is aware of any special handling that is necessary for a particular specimen. There is no excuse for misinterpretation of a tissue or cytologic specimen because of a failure in communication.

Surgery as Primary Therapy

Surgery is usually the treatment method of choice for preinvasive diseases of the vulva, vagina, and cervix, for which local excision is both diagnostic and curative. Surgical margins should clear only gross and microscopic disease; removal of large areas of normal tissue is not required. For microinvasive lesions of these organs, wide local excision with a 1- to 2-cm normal tissue margin is appropriate.

Localized disease, such as stage I through stage III vulvar cancer, stage I vaginal cancer, and stages IB and IIA cervical cancer, are usually managed by an en bloc radical resection of the primary tumor and regional lymphadenectomy. In these surgical procedures, the operations themselves are designed to be curative without adjunctive therapy unless high-risk conditions are identified. As described in Chapter 20, there is a trend toward more conservative therapy for vulvar cancer. This allows preservation of normal tissues and prevents some of the disfigurement usually associated with this surgery. Surgery may be curative without adjuvant therapy for other cancers as well, including early-stage endometrial cancer, stage IA ovarian cancer, and early sarcomas of the uterus.

Findings at surgery may indicate the need for additional treatment. This therapy is usually called adjuvant therapy. It is administered because of the potential for occult spread of disease based on a surgical finding (e.g., positive lymph nodes). The use of adjuvant therapy requires that information be available to allow the selection of patients with a high risk of recurrence. These risk groups are defined for each disease site in the appropriate chapters of this book.

Surgery Combined with Other Therapies

In some cancers of the female genital system, surgery is the cornerstone of treatment but is not curative when used alone. Primary cytoreduction of gross disease is vital in advanced ovarian and fallopian tube cancer, but it is of little benefit without adjunctive therapy. Chemotherapy after surgery is a vital and necessary part of the treatment regimen for these cancers. For patients with clinical stage I or II endometrial cancer who have high-grade cancer or deep myometrial penetration, surgical removal of the uterus is an extremely important part of therapy. However, depending on the histopathologic findings of the surgical specimens, additional regional radiotherapy and/or chemotherapy may be indicated. It is the responsibility of the gynecologic oncologist to coordinate surgical therapy with chemotherapy and/or radiation therapy to ensure that the patient receives optimal care.

Surgery as Salvage Therapy

Occasionally, surgical resection can be curative in patients who have failed other therapies. These surgical procedures are almost always extensive and produce some limitation of function. After the failure of other therapies, radical surgery may be the patient's last chance of survival. The classic examples of this situation are vulvar, vaginal, cervical, or

TABLE 12.1. *FIGO staging of gynecologic cancers*

Site	Staging
Vulva	Surgical and pathologic staging
Vagina	Clinical staging
Cervix	Clinical staging
Corpus (endometrium)	Surgical and pathologic staging
Corpus (sarcoma)	None (most use modified clinical endometrial cancer staging)
Fallopian tube	None (most use modified surgical and pathology staging)
Ovary	Surgical and pathologic staging
Gestational trophoblastic	FIGO staging (clinical) NIH classification WHO classification (risk-oriented)

NIH, National Institutes of Health; WHO, World Health Organization.

uterine cancers that have failed primary surgery and irradiation or irradiation alone. In such cases, pelvic exenteration with removal of virtually all pelvic tissues may offer the only possibility for a cure. Five-year survival rates of 23% to 61% have been reported after pelvic exenteration (35–37).

The possibility of cure with pelvic exenteration is not without cost. The loss of the bladder and the rectum often requires permanent stomas, and sexual function is impaired or lost in many patients. For some patients, reconstructive techniques can prevent the need for stomas and may also restore sexual function. These procedures are described in detail in Chapter 22. During the last three decades, improvements in initial surgery and radiation therapy along with refinements in selection criteria have made operations like pelvic exenteration infrequent (38). Today, most patients experience distant failure rather than regional failure, and they are therefore not candidates for attempts at curative pelvic exenteration.

Surgery as salvage therapy may also play an important role in the management of ovarian, fallopian tube, and some endometrial cancers. For patients who have failed initial therapy and chemotherapy, second attempts at cytoreduction may be beneficial, provided that reasonable salvage therapy is available (39–41).

Surgery for Metastatic Disease

In selected cases, distant metastases from gynecologic tumors may be curable by surgical resection, or the resection may produce a prolonged disease-free interval. Fuller and colleagues (42) reported on 15 patients who underwent pulmonary resection of distant metastases from a variety of gynecologic malignancies. They reported a 5-year survival rate of 36% and a 10-year survival rate of 26%. Patients with solitary metastases had a median survival of 64 months, with a median survival of 48 months for those with multiple metastases. Levenback and associates (43) reported their experience with 45 patients who underwent pulmonary resection of metastases from uterine sarcomas. From the date of the pulmonary resection, the 5-year survival rate was 41%, with a 10-year survival rate of 35%. They found a statistically improved chance of survival for patients who developed pulmonary metastases 1 year or longer from their original therapy and for those with unilateral metastases. There was no statistical difference in survival based on the number of nodules (in one lung), the size of the lesion, the age of the patient, or the use of postresection adjunctive therapy. However, the small numbers of patients in this study precluded adequate evaluation of these factors.

Resection of intraabdominal or pelvic disease may offer palliation by removal of tumor bulk or may allow chemotherapy or irradiation a greater chance of eradicating disease. Resection of tumors that have a poor blood supply often leaves behind smaller tumors with a better blood supply that are more amenable to treatment with chemotherapy or irra-

diation. Resection of bulk disease also increases the number of residual tumor cells that enter the active cell cycle, in which they may be more responsive to these adjunctive therapies. The availability of new techniques for intraoperative electron beam irradiation or intraoperative brachytherapy may result in more utility for resection of distant and regional metastatic disease.

There is increasing evidence that salvage therapy in ovarian and fallopian tube cancers is likely to be effective only in patients with minimal residual disease. Secondary cytoreduction or resection of regional and distant metastases may play an important role in the treatment of these patients. Recent reports have demonstrated promising results with surgical resection of isolated metastases to the parenchyma of the liver and spleen (44,45).

Surgical Procedures for Specialized Care

Surgical placement of indwelling intravenous access systems allows patients to receive chemotherapy and nutritional supplements and to have necessary blood samples drawn with relative ease and comfort. Placement of these devices, usually semipermanent subcutaneous systems, is safe, contributes to the patient's well-being, and allows for more effective therapy.

The use of intracavitary therapy requires the temporary or semipermanent placement of chest tubes or intraperitoneal access devices. Results of many studies confirm that peritoneal access or vascular access devices placed totally beneath the skin have a low infection rate and a low rate of malfunction (46,47). Implanted arterial infusion devices are being evaluated in research studies to allow direct infusion of therapeutic agents into a tumor mass by means of the arterial system. This therapy often requires intraabdominal surgery to place the device into the appropriate portion of the vascular system.

Surgery for Reconstruction

Reconstructive surgery may be performed at the time of resection of the cancer, as a delayed procedure, or as required therapy to correct a complication of treatment. Vulvar reconstruction is usually done at the time of initial resection and may involve the use of free skin grafts, rotational flaps of adjacent skin and fat tissue, or myocutaneous grafts from the thigh, buttocks, or anterior abdominal wall. Vaginal reconstruction may also be performed, usually as a planned, delayed phase of reconstruction. Vaginal reconstruction requires free skin grafts or myocutaneous flaps depending on the size of the defect and whether or not there has been previous irradiation of the vaginal bed. The techniques of vulvar and vaginal reconstruction are explained in detail in Chapter 22.

Reconstruction as therapy for complications of treatment may be required for the closure of defects from improper wound healing, radiation necrosis, or tissue loss after extravasation of chemotherapeutic agents. Although free skin grafts may be used to reconstruct surgical wound disruption or tissue loss due to chemotherapy extravasation, radiation necrosis usually requires the use of myocutaneous flaps because of a lack of adequate blood supply in the area of the injury. Specific reconstructive techniques are discussed in more detail in Chapter 20.

Surgery for Palliation

Surgery for palliation may involve resection of tumor to relieve symptoms, or it may involve diversion or bypass of portions of the gastrointestinal or urinary tract to prolong life and provide comfort. Surgical procedures may also be used to provide pain relief by interrupting sensory nerve transmissions. Surgical removal of tumor bulk to provide palliation has been discouraged by many authorities. They point out that without effective adjunctive therapy, tumor regrowth occurs quickly and the surgical procedure proves to be futile. Although this may be true in most cases, the gynecologic oncologist should not uniformly dismiss the concept of surgical palliation. A surgical procedure to provide relief of symptoms is usually considered a failure if the tumor regrows in 6 to 12 months. However, palliative administration of a chemotherapeutic agent for 6 to 12 months is considered to be successful if there is minor tumor shrinkage or stabilization of disease despite the side effects of the chemotherapy. As a surgeon, the gynecologic oncologist must remember that a surgical procedure with limited risk and a reasonable recovery period may provide as much relief as 6 to 12 months of palliative chemotherapy or a course of palliative irradiation. The difficult decision about when to employ surgical palliation requires astute surgical judgment and a realistic assessment of the patient's condition and wishes.

Palliative surgery is more frequently used to relieve specific dysfunctions, such as obstruction of the urinary or intestinal tract. Relief of urinary tract obstruction may be accomplished by ureteroneocystostomy or by urinary conduit depending on the location of the obstruction and the location or extent of disease. A urinary conduit can provide immediate and permanent relief to the patient who has a ureterovaginal, vesicovaginal, or urethrovaginal fistula. It may also provide relief of urinary obstruction, which will prolong life and allow for the administration of additional chemotherapy or irradiation. The judgment of the surgeon and the desires of the patient become essential factors in this decision process. For the patient who is miserable because of constant urinary leakage or who may benefit from additional therapy, the decision to perform a urinary diversion is quite simple. If diversion is done to prolong life, however, the decision must be weighed carefully. For a patient who has a limited life expectancy or is in uncontrollable pain, performing a urinary diversion may do more harm than good.

The gynecologic oncologist must also consider the relative benefits of nonsurgical urinary diversion, such as placement of a ureteral stent or a percutaneous nephrostomy. For many patients, percutaneous nephrostomy is a better choice than surgical intervention. This is particularly true if the aim is to employ adjunctive chemotherapy or irradiation or if a surgical procedure is not feasible because of medical conditions or other surgical considerations. Unfortunately, a percutaneous nephrostomy cannot help the patient with a fistula because the nephrostomy will not totally divert the urine.

Placement of a ureteral stent, by cystoscopy or antegrade through a percutaneous nephrostomy, is usually better and safer than urinary diversion for the relief of obstruction. Current technology allows the placement of stents that can be left in place for months and can be changed easily over a guide wire by means of the cystoscope.

Intestinal obstruction threatens the patient's quality of life, and the decision of whether to perform an intestinal diversion is usually easy. Deciding whether the operation is feasible can be more difficult. For the patient with localized disease, a diverting colostomy or an intestinal bypass is usually possible and is not very difficult. For the patient with intraabdominal carcinomatosis, the decision is more complex. The surgeon may not be able to determine the extent of intestinal involvement preoperatively and may have difficulty deciding whether the surgical procedure will benefit the patient.

Pothuri and colleagues (48) recently evaluated 68 palliative operations performed on 64 patients with recurrent ovarian cancer and intestinal obstruction. In 84% of cases, a corrective surgical procedure was able to be performed, whereas no corrective surgical procedure was possible for the remaining 16%. Of the 57 cases where corrective surgery was possible, 71% were successfully palliated: defined as the ability to tolerate a regular or low-residue diet at least 60 days postoperatively. If surgery resulted in successful palliation, median survival was 11.6 months compared to 3.9 months for all other patients.

THE FUTURE OF GYNECOLOGY ONCOLOGY

As of 1999, the subspecialty of gynecologic oncology is over a quarter of a century old. From a cadre of farsighted individuals with a variety of training backgrounds, a cohesive subspecialty has developed with consistent standards of training, a system of certification, and recognition in the medical community. None of this has come easily, and we owe a great deal to that first generation of gynecologic oncologists.

Several current issues are affecting the future role of gynecologic oncology within the medical community. Our relationship with our parent specialty of obstetrics and gynecology is being reexamined, as well as our ties with general surgery and urology, specialties with which we often seem even more closely allied. As technologic advances occur, we are becoming more integrated with the specialties of medical oncology and radiation oncology. Although we remain primarily surgeons, and surgery remains our principal mode of therapy, it is critical to emphasize the integrated multidisciplinary management of the patient with gynecologic cancer.

The benefits of multidisciplinary care were recently highlighted in a clinical announcement by the National Cancer Institute (NCI) concerning concurrent chemoradiation for cervical cancer (49). In each of five randomized Phase III trials of women with various stages of cervical cancer, the addition of chemotherapy to radiotherapy was found to provide a significant survival benefit (8,50–53). The risk of death from cervical cancer was decreased by 30% to 50% with the multimodality approach.

Changes in Surgical Therapy

If the past decade is any indication of the future, significant changes in the technology of surgery can be expected to occur as we proceed through the new millennium. New materials, new surgical instruments, and new devices will be invented, and many of these will make surgical treatment better. Certainly, laparoscopic surgery appears to have made a significant impact on our specialty as well as on the other surgical specialties.

Innovative methods of supportive care will be developed to further the technical capabilities that we now possess, such as computerized anesthesia machines and transesophageal ultrasound. Anesthetic agents will become better and safer, to be joined by a new generation of antibiotics and cardiovascular medications. We will be able to treat the older patient surgically with relative safety, which is especially important because of the increased incidence of cancer in the elderly and because of the advancing age of our population. Our responsibilities include staying abreast of these advances and judiciously integrating them into our practices.

Changes in the Indications for Surgery

Early diagnosis will change the indications for surgery and the types of procedures that should be done. We will be able to treat more patients with less disfigurement and with greater preservation of function. A larger proportion of patients will present with early disease, allowing surgery to be used more frequently for definitive cure.

Better adjunctive therapies will increase the importance of initial surgical therapy. More patients will benefit from surgical cytoreduction to minimize disease. The availability of effective irradiation and chemotherapeutic regimens will make adjuvant therapy feasible in more cases, and it will become more important for us to identify risk groups who are likely to develop recurrent disease after surgery.

Multidisciplinary Therapy and Primary Care

In outlining the extent of surgical training required for the gynecologic oncologist, the founders of this discipline were

careful to include adequate training that would enable the gynecologic oncologist to become an accomplished abdominopelvic surgeon. The gynecologic oncologist must be trained to perform the gynecologic, gastrointestinal, and urologic surgery necessary to manage gynecologic cancer and its potential complications. As stated by John L. Lewis, Jr. (54), in reference to pelvic exenteration by a team of gynecologists, general surgeons, and urologists, ''Even when the surgery was successful, the postoperative care required committee meetings and its outcome was often less than successful.''

These same founders realized that, although training can produce a qualified surgical oncologist, the complete care of the cancer patient requires knowledge of the basic biologic, physical, and pharmacologic principles of radiation therapy and chemotherapy. This does not mean that the gynecologic oncologist must be a radiation oncologist or a medical oncologist, but it does demand that he or she know enough to ensure proper integration of all therapeutic modalities. Throughout the United States, this collaboration in the care of patients with gynecologic cancer has produced multidisciplinary teams of gynecologic oncologists, radiation oncologists, medical oncologists, and pathologists who provide state of the art cancer care. The GOG, a national cooperative research group, has demonstrated how this multidisciplinary approach to gynecologic oncology research can be achieved.

Despite the emphasis on multidisciplinary care, the gynecologic oncologist should maintain active involvement during all aspects of a patient's care. The principle of being the patient's physician until she is either cured or dies of her disease has been an integral part of our subspecialty and must be maintained. The constant involvement of the gynecologic oncologist through all phases of cancer treatment ensures optimal integration of surgery, irradiation, and chemotherapy. The patient receives continuity of care and the reassurance of a physician who is involved at each stage of her therapy and follow-up.

CONCLUSION

After three decades, the gynecologic oncologist has emerged as a surgical oncologist for women. The specialist has sufficient familiarity with radiation oncology and medical oncology to ensure the proper integration of all modalities of treatment, and he or she is able to apply surgical skills for primary therapy, secondary therapy, reconstruction, and palliation. The gynecologic oncologist stands in the obstetrics and gynecology community but has one foot in the community of surgeons.

The emergence of cooperative research groups, particularly the GOG, has allowed a generation of gynecologic oncologists to develop superior clinical research skills. These skills must be continually stressed in the training of young oncologists and as an integral part of the practice of our subspecialty. A growing number of young oncologists are receiving additional training in basic research. This is vital for the continued development of the subspecialty and for progress toward the prevention and care of gynecologic cancers. Our position in the arena of clinical practice is well established, and we must now establish ourselves equally well as scientists and surgical researchers.

REFERENCES

1. Morrow CP, Curtin JP, eds. *Gynecologic cancer surgery*. New York: Churchill Livingstone, 1996.
2. Gallup DG, Talledo OE, eds. *Surgical atlas of gynecologic oncology*. Philadelphia: WB Saunders, 1994.
3. Levine DA, Barakat RR, Hoskins WJ. *Atlas of procedures in gynecologic oncology*. London: Martin Dunitz, 2003.
4. Fowler JM, Johnson PR. Transperitoneal para-aortic lymphadenectomy. *Oper Tech Gynecol Surg* 1996;1:8.
5. Berman ML, Lagasse LD, Watring WG, et al. The operative evaluation of patients with cervical cancer by an extraperitoneal approach. *Obstet Gynecol* 1977;50:658.
6. Gallup DG, King LA, Messing MJ, Talledo OE. Paraaortic lymph node sampling by means of an extraperitoneal approach with a supraumbilical transverse "sunrise" incision. *Am J Obstet Gynecol* 1993;169:307.
7. Weiser EB, Bundy BN, Hoskins WJ, et al. Extraperitoneal versus transperitoneal selective paraaortic lymphadenectomy in the pretreatment surgical staging of advanced cervical carcinoma: a Gynecologic Oncology Group study. *Gynecol Oncol* 1989;33:283.
8. Rose PG, Bundy BN, Watkins EB, et al. Concurrent cisplatin-based chemoradiation for locally advanced cervical cancer: *New Engl J Med* 1999;340:1144.
9. Chi DS, Hoskins WJ. Sampling para-aortic lymph nodes in gynecologic cancers. *CME J of Gynecol Oncol (in press)*.
10. Childers JM, Hatch K, Surwit EA. The role of laparoscopic lymphadenectomy in the management of cervical carcinoma. *Gynecol Oncol* 1992;47:38.
11. Recio FO, Piver MS, Hempling RE. Pretreatment transperitoneal laparoscopic staging in pelvic and paraaortic lymphadenectomy in large (≥ 5 cm) stage IB2 cervical carcinoma: report of a pilot study. *Gynecol Oncol* 1996;63:333.
12. Abu-Rustum NR, Chi DS, Sonoda Y, et al. Transperitoneal laparoscopic pelvic and para-aortic lymph node dissection using the argon-beam coagulator and monopolar instruments: an 8-year study and description of technique. *Gynecol Oncol* 2003;89:504.
13. Chi DS. Laparoscopy in gynecologic malignancies. *Oncology* 1999; 13:773.
14. Rowland RG, Mitchell ME, Bihrle R, et al. Indiana continent urinary reservoir. *J Urol* 1987;137:1136.
15. Penalver MA, Benjany DE, Averette HE, et al. Continent urinary diversion in gynecologic oncology. *Gynecol Oncol* 1989;34:274.
16. Wallace D, Hernandez W, Schlaerth JB, et al. Prevention of abdominal wound disruption utilizing the Smead-Jones closure technique. *Obstet Gynecol* 1980;56:226.
17. Gallup DG, Talledo OE, King LA. Primary mass closure of midline incisions with a continuous running monofilament suture in gynecologic patients. *Obstet Gynecol* 1989;73:1.
18. Gallup DG, Nolan TE, Smith RP. Primary mass closure of midline incisions with a continuous polyglyconate monofilament absorbable suture. *Obstet Gynecol* 1990;76:872.
19. Montz FJ, Creasman WT, Eddy G, DiSaia PJ. Running mass closure of abdominal wounds using absorbable looped suture. *J Gynecol Surg* 1991;7:107.
20. Orr JW, Orr PF, Barrett JM, et al. Continuous or interrupted fascial closure: a prospective evaluation of No. 1 Maxon suture on 402 gynecologic procedures. *Am J Obstet Gynecol* 1990;163:1485.
21. Sutton G, Morgan S. Abdominal wound closure using a running, looped monofilament polybutester suture: comparison to Smead-Jones closure in historic controls. *Obstet Gynecol* 1992;80:650–654.
22. Conte M, Benedetti-Panici P, Guarglia L, et al. Pelvic lymphocele following radical paraaortic and pelvic lymphadenectomy for cervical carcinoma: incidence rate and percutaneous management. *Obstet Gynecol* 1990;76:268.
23. Gilliland JD, Spies JB, Brown SB, et al. Lymphoceles: percutaneous treatment with povidone-iodine sclerosis. *Radiology* 1989;171:227.
24. Akhan O, Cekirge S, Özmen M, Besim A. Percutaneous transcatheter ethanol sclerotherapy of postoperative pelvic lymphoceles. *Cardiovasc Intervent Radiol* 1992;15:224.
25. McGowan L, Lesher LP, Norris HJ, Barnett M. Misstaging of ovarian cancer. *Obstet Gynecol* 1985;65:568.
26. Kehoe S, Powell J, Wilson S, Woodman C. The influence of the operating surgeon's specialisation on patient survival in ovarian cancer. *Br J Cancer* 1994:70;1014.
27. Woodman C, Baghdady A, Collins S, Clyma JA. What changes in the organisation of cancer services will improve the outcome for women with ovarian cancer? *Br J Obstet Gynecol* 1997;104:135.
28. Nguyen HN, Averette HE, Hoskins W, et al. National survey of ovarian carcinoma, part V. The impact of physician's specialty on patient's survival. *Cancer* 1993;72:3663.
29. Eisenkop SM, Spirtos NM, Montag TW, et al. The impact of subspecialty training on the management of advanced ovarian cancer. *Gynecol Oncol* 1992;47:203.
30. Begg CB, Cramer LD, Hoskins WJ, Brennan MF. Impact of hospital volume on operative mortality for major cancer surgery. *JAMA* 1998; 280:1747.
31. Bristow RE, Tomacruz RS, Armstrong DK, et al. Survival effect of maximal cytoreductive surgery for advanced ovarian carcinoma during the platinum era: a meta-analysis. *J Clin Oncol* 2002;20:1248.
32. Kauff ND, Satagopan JY, Robson ME, et al. Risk reducing salpingo-oophorectomy in women with a BRCA1 or BRCA2 mutation. *N Engl J Med* 2002;346:1609.
33. Rebbeck TR, Lynch HT, Neuhausen SL, et al. Prophylactic oophorectomy in carriers of BRCA1 or BRCA2 mutations. *N Engl J Med* 2002; 346:1616.
34. Young RC, Walton LA, Ellenberg SS, et al. Adjuvant therapy in stage I and stage II epithelial ovarian cancer: results of two prospective randomized trials. *N Engl J Med* 1990;332:1021.
35. Lawhead RA, Clark GC, Smith DH, et al. Pelvic exenteration for recurrent or persistent gynecologic malignancies: a 10-year review of the Memorial Sloan-Kettering Cancer Center Experience (1972–1981). *Gynecol Oncol* 1989;33:279.
36. Morley GW, Hopkins MP, Lindenauer SM, et al. Pelvic exenteration, University of Michigan: 100 patients at 5 years. *Obstet Gynecol* 1989; 74:934.
37. Matthews CM, Morris M, Burke TW, et al. Pelvic exenteration in the elderly patient. *Obstet Gynecol* 1992;79:773.
38. Chi DS, Gemignani ML, Curtin JP, Hoskins WJ. Long-term experience in the surgical management of cancer of the uterine cervix. *Semin Surg Oncol* 1999;17:161.
39. Eisenkop SM, Friedman RL, Spirtos NM. The role of secondary cytoreductive surgery in the treatment of patients with recurrent epithelial ovarian carcinoma. *Cancer* 2000;88:144.
40. Scarabelli C, Gallo A, Carbone A. Secondary cytoreductive surgery for patients with recurrent epithelial ovarian carcinoma. *Gynecol Oncol* 2001;83:504.
41. Chi DS, McCaughtry K, Schwabenbauer S, et al. Identification of prognostic factors for survival following secondary cytoreductive surgery in patients with recurrent epithelial ovarian carcinoma. *Gynecol Oncol* 2003;8:247.
42. Fuller AF, Scannell JG, Wilkins W Jr. Pulmonary resection for metastases from gynecologic cancers: MGH experience, 1943–1982. *Gynecol Oncol* 1985;22:174.
43. Levenback C, Rubin SC, McCormack PM, et al. Resection of pulmonary metastases from uterine sarcomas. *Gynecol Oncol* 1992;45:202.
44. Chi DS, Fong Y, Venkatraman ES, Barakat RR. Hepatic resection for metastatic gynecologic carcinomas. *Gynecol Oncol* 1997;66:45.
45. Gemignani ML, Chi DS, Gurin CC, et al. Splenectomy in recurrent epithelial ovarian cancer. *Gynecol Oncol* 1999;72:407.
46. Davidson SA, Hoskins WJ, Rubin SC, et al. Intraperitoneal chemotherapy: analysis of complications with an implanted subcutaneous port and catheter system. *Gynecol Oncol* 1991;41:101.

47. Makhija S, Leitao M, Sabbatini P, et al. Complications asociated with intraperitoneal chemotherapy catheters. *Gynecol Oncol* 2001;81:77.

48. Pothuri B, Vaidya A, Aghajanian C, et al. Palliative surgery for bowel obstruction in recurrent ovarian cancer: an updated series. *Gynecol Oncol* 2003;89:306.

49. National Cancer Institute. Clinical announcement regarding concurrent chemoradiation for cervical cancer. February 22, 1999.

50. Whitney CW, Sause W, Bundy BN, et al. Randomized comparison of fluorouracil plus cisplatin versus hydroxyurea as an adjunct to radiation therapy is stage IIB-IVA carcinoma of the cervix with negative para-aortic lymph nodes: a Gynecologic Oncology Group and Southwest Oncology Group study. *J Clin Oncol* 1999;17:1339.

51. Morris M, Eifel PJ, Lu J, et al. Pelvic radiation with concurrent chemotherapy compared with pelvic and para-aortic radiation for high risk cervical cancer. *N Engl J Med* 1999;340:1137.

52. Keys HM, Bundy BN, Stehman FB, et al. Cisplatin, radiation, and adjuvant hysterectomy compared with radiation and adjuvant hysterectomy for bulky stage IB cervical carcinoma. *N Engl J Med* 1999;340: 1154.

53. Peters WA, Liu PY, Barrett R, et al. Concurrent chemotherapy and pelvic radiation therapy compared with pelvic radiation therapy alone as adjuvant therapy after radical surgery in high-risk early-stage cancer of the cervix. *J Clin Oncol* 2000;18:1606.

54. Lewis JL Jr. Training of the gynecologic oncologist. In: Coppleson M, ed. *Gynecologic oncology: fundamental principles and clinical practice.* Edinburgh: Churchill Livingstone, 1981;4.

CHAPTER 13

Laparoscopic Surgery in Gynecologic Cancer

Daniel F. Dargent, Marie Plante, and Yukio Sonoda

Laparoscopy became a regular feature in the practice of gynecology during the 1960s. Although it played a role in the early detection of pelvic, mainly ovarian, malignancies (1), the concept of using it in the management of gynecologic cancer did not emerge until the late 1980s.

Urologists were the first to consider whether endoscopy could play a role in the management of pelvic tumors. The first report was published in 1980 by Hald and Rasmussen (2). These Danish urologists used an instrument derived from the Carlens mediastinoscope for assessing the iliac nodes in patients affected by urinary bladder or prostatic cancer. The tip of the instrument was placed in direct contact with the iliac vessels after digital preparation was made through a short inguinal incision. Small samples were taken from the tissues surrounding the vessels using forceps introduced through the instrument. The decision to perform radical surgery, which is only of benefit for node-negative patients, was made according to the result of the endoscopic assessment.

When laparoscopic surgery was pioneered in patients affected by gynecologic cancer, the rationale was similar: By assessing the pelvic lymph nodes in patients affected by cervical cancer, candidates for vaginal radical hysterectomy (VRH) could be determined (3). The technique was also similar except that the laparoscope was used instead of direct endoscopy.

THE EARLY YEARS (1987–1992): RETROPERITONEAL LAPAROSCOPIC PELVIC LYMPHADENECTOMY

The first laparoscopic pelvic assessments were performed through two separate inguinal incisions. The view obtained

of the pelvic sidewall was much wider than the view obtained with the mediastinoscope, and node sampling was easier with an instrument introduced through a separate port. After a dozen attempts, the technique was refined and required only a suprapubic midline incision. This approach, panoramic retroperitoneal pelviscopy, was first described in a monograph published in 1989 by Dargent and Salvat (4) and reported the data of 107 procedures. Thereafter, the data for 200 patients' operations performed between December 1986 and February 1991 were detailed in the classic textbook edited by Nichols and published in 1993 (5).

There was some criticism during the 5 years following the initial description of laparoscopic lymphadenectomy. Critics were concerned about operative risks, the limited area of dissection, and oncologic risks (two abdominal implants noted among the first 200 operations), but the main obstacle was cultural in nature. The surgical anatomy of the retroperitoneal space was unfamiliar to the gynecologic surgeon, especially when viewed through a laparoscope. It was only after Querleu (6) devised the transumbilical transperitoneal laparoscopic approach did the concept of the "oncolaparoscopy" begin to grow.

THE MATURATION PERIOD: 1992–2003

In June 1989, Querleu (6) presented his first report on laparoscopic transumbilical transperitoneal lymphadenectomy as a staging procedure for patients affected by cervical cancer. The technique used was the routine laparoscopic technique: Both broad ligaments were opened using a peritoneal incision made alongside the axis of the iliac vessels, allowing dissection and retrieval of the pelvic nodes under laparoscopic guidance. The data on the first 39 operations were published in 1991 in the *American Journal of Obstetrics and Gynecology* (7).

Months after Querleu's publication, Childers and Surwit (8) published the first two American cases—both patients with endometrial cancer. They added a paraaortic sampling

Daniel F. Dargent: Claude Bernard University, Lyon, France 69437

Marie Plante: Laval University, Quebec City, Canada 00126

Yukio Sonoda: Memorial Sloan–Kettering Cancer Center, New York, New York 10021

to the pelvic lymphadenectomy. The operation was completed with a transvaginal hysterectomy. After the publication of these cases, the concept of laparoscopically assisted surgical staging emerged. That same year, the use of the laparoscope in the management of cervical cancer was reported (9). The "oncolaparoscopic" movement began by (a) applying this new concept to malignancies other than endometrial cancer, (b) increasing the thoroughness of the staging dissection, and (c) combining staging with the preparation for radical vaginal surgery with a progressive move to purely laparoscopic radical surgery.

The transition of laparoscopy-assisted surgical staging from endometrial cancer to cervical cancer was not unexpected. The first reports did not clearly indicate the rationale for the laparoscopic staging, but only demonstrated that the staging was feasible and probably safe (9,10). Subsequently, surgeons began to distinguish the different roles of laparoscopy between early- and advanced-stage disease (11,12). The use of laparoscopic surgery in the management of ovarian cancer was first reported in 1973 (13); however, it was not until 1990 that laparoscopic management of ovarian cancer was first reported (14). Except for the concept of laparoscopic restaging for incidental adnexal cancers (15), this application remains the most questionable. Endoscopy, specifically inguinoscopy, has also been introduced into the management of vaginal and vulvar cancers (16). With time, laparoscopy may find a place in the management of all gynecologic malignancies.

The extent of laparoscopic staging has gone through a pendular development. In its earliest form, laparoscopic lymphadenectomy was limited to the interiliac area (4). The laparoscopic pelvic lymphadenectomy described by Querleu (7) soon progressed to the common iliac area and then to the inframesenteric aortic area (8). Beginning in 1993 (17, 18), the infrarenal paraaortic nodes were included in laparoscopic dissection, and thereafter Possover et al. (19) described laparoscopic suprarenal retrocrural dissection. It was around this time that the concept of sentinel node biopsy emerged as a procedure that could potentially eliminate the need for systemic dissection. This concept has been combined with laparoscopy to produce a convenient method for carrying out this type of biopsy (20).

Laparoscopy-assisted radical surgery and purely laparoscopic radical surgery were foreseeable developments from the concept of laparoscopic staging. Laparoscopically assisted surgical staging was being established during a period when the use of laparoscopically assisted vaginal hysterectomy was commonplace for benign conditions (21). Thus, it was a natural extension of laparoscopically assisted vaginal hysterectomy to apply it to the treatment of endometrial cancer (8). The use of laparoscopy in the management of cervical cancer was initiated by combining laparoscopically assisted surgical staging with the Schauta radical vaginal hysterectomy (3). Descriptions of the laparoscopically assisted vaginal radical hysterectomy, or celio-Schauta, began

appearing in the early 1990s (22–24), and soon after, series using this new procedure began to appear in the literature (25,26). In spite of this, the use of the laparoscopically assisted vaginal radical hysterectomy remains limited because of the lack of training of most gynecologic surgeons in the field of advanced vaginal surgery. As more surgeons are familiar with the abdominal approach to radical hysterectomy, the use of laparoscopy resulted in the development of laparoscopic radical hysterectomy, which was also initially described in early 1990s by Canis (27) and Nezhat (10). Conceptually, this approach is easier to grasp by those more familiar with the abdominal approach, as witnessed by the growing number of publications demonstrating its feasibility and safety (28–30). Laparoscopy has recently also been employed to perform pelvic exenteration (31).

OTHER DEVELOPMENTS AND THE QUESTIONS THEY RAISE

The most radical operation in the gynecologic surgery repertoire, the pelvic exenteration, can be carried out with a laparoscope (31). The next development in the field of laparoscopy may come from robotics. "Light" robots that employ voice commands to maneuver the laparoscope are already being used by some. They allow extra freedom for instrument manipulation. The "heavy" robots employ instruments with seven degrees of motion to perform the most delicate gestures in the tightest of spaces without any tremor. The biggest drawbacks of these robots are the cost and size. For the experienced laparoscopic surgeon, these "heavy" robots have yet to demonstrate an obvious benefit except for fine suturing in which the robot excels. Thus, these robots may eventually be employed when laparoscopic suturing is required; that is, during reconstruction operations following exenterative surgery. As the use of robots grows, these procedures will undoubtedly be further developed.

The future of laparoscopic extirpative surgery is a second point of discussion. The data available on total laparoscopic or laparoscopically assisted radical surgery seem to be comparable to those of open surgery. The radical nature of the surgeries can be preserved with laparoscopy. In general, the operative time is increased, but the blood loss is generally diminished and the postoperative morbidity is improved. However, good level-one evidence regarding the use of laparoscopy is not yet available in the field of gynecologic cancer surgery. During the emergence of laparoscopy, improvements in open abdominal surgery have also occurred. Newer technologies (i.e., Ligasure, Tyco; Biclamp, Erbe, Tubingen, Germany) and better analgesics decrease blood loss, operative time, and postoperative pain for open surgery. Only through well-designed randomized trials will the better surgical approach be determined.

The future of laparoscopically assisted surgical staging is the third point open to discussion. There are no doubts about its feasibility and safety. One can, in spite of the absence of direct manual sensation, assess the peritoneal cavity and the retroperitoneal spaces with the same accuracy as through an open incision. One may also argue the visual assessment is better thanks to the optical magnification. On the other hand, if doubts exist about the benefits of laparoscopy in extirpative surgery, they do not exist in the specific field of surgical staging. Laparoscopy paralleled with xiphopubic laparotomy or J-shaped large side incisions that were the standard in the past and is a more acceptable surgical staging procedure. However, in spite of its obvious benefits, laparoscopic staging has been challenged. A recent randomized trial has demonstrated that surgically staged patients with cervical cancer had a worse survival irrespective of the surgical approach used (open surgery or laparoscopy) (32). The results of this trial are largely biased (see below), but one has to recognize surgical staging has an excellent potential to separate the good and the poor prognostic cases without necessarily improving life expectancy. In the future, prognostic information obtained from newer procedures, such as the sentinel node biopsy, or from the molecular analysis of the tumor itself could replace the information obtained from imaging and surgical staging.

BASIC ELEMENTS OF LAPAROSCOPIC SURGERY

Laparoscopic surgery is usually performed via CO_2 insufflation to create a pneumoperitoneum. There are several techniques used to enter the abdomen for laparoscopic procedures. "Closed" laparoscopy, employing a Veress needle followed by blind insertion of the first trocar, is favored by many laparoscopic surgeons. Others prefer direct "blind" trocar insertion. Although the use of disposable trocars with retractable blades for direct trocar insertion appears to be safer than the use of metal reusable trocars with sharp point tips, the obvious potential danger of these closed techniques is the risk of bowel or vascular injuries. This is of particular concern since the majority of complications following laparoscopic surgery are related to trocar insertion (33). Conversely, the "open" technique where the fascia and the peritoneum are surgically opened and the trocar inserted under direct visualization is considered by many to be the safest access technique.

CO_2 Laparoscopy: Closed Versus Open Technique

Bonjer et al. (34) reviewed the literature and compared data between 12,444 open laparoscopic cases and 489,335 closed laparoscopic cases. Rates of visceral and vascular injuries were 0.083% and 0.075%, respectively, after closed laparoscopy and 0.048% and 0.0%, respectively, after open laparoscopy ($p = .002$). Mortality rates were 0.003% for the closed and 0.0% for the open laparoscopic technique ($p = NS$). In another randomized trial of blind versus open laparoscopy for laparoscopic cholecystectomy, the major complication rate was 4.0% in the blind group and 1.3% in the open group, respectively ($p < .05$). Minor complications occurred in 6.7% of patients in both groups (35). In a large series of 2,000 cases performed for general surgerical procedures, there was no vascular injury and only one bowel injury with the open laparoscopic technique (36). Perone (37) published a series of 585 cases of laparoscopy using a simplified open technique. There were no technical failures or major complications despite the fact that nearly 30% of the patients had undergone previous laparoscopy or laparotomy.

Decloedt et al. (38) performed laparoscopic surgery in patients with gynecologic malignancies and reported only a 1% complication rate for the open laparoscopic technique despite the fact that a high proportion of the patients had previous major surgery and/or radiation therapy. In another study of patients who underwent operations for pelvic masses, it was noted that all the vascular injuries occurred during direct trocar insertion in patients without prior abdominal surgery; Dottino et al. now routinely use an open technique in all their cases (39). Altogether the data seem to indicate that the open laparoscopic technique is safer than closed laparoscopy. A recent large series, however, comparing 8,324 cases of direct laparoscopic entry versus 1,562 cases of open laparoscopy for gynecologic procedures did not show a difference in the rate of major complications. In fact, there were more conversions to laparotomy in the open technique group (40).

In patients with prior abdominal surgery, using midline incisions, Childers et al. (41) proposed the use of a Veress needle in the left upper quadrant to insufflate first the abdomen prior to the trocar entry. Also, in cases where the risk of injury appears to be high because of prior abdominal surgery, smaller 5- or 7-mm trocars may be used to enter the abdomen, as opposed to the traditional 10- to 12-mm trocars. Choosing the lateral flank, rather than the midline subumbilical area, as an entry site may also be useful. This can potentially decrease the risk of damaging bowel loops that could be adherent under the anterior abdominal wall from prior surgeries.

Gasless Laparoscopy

With hopes of decreasing tumor cell spillage, gasless laparoscopy was developed in the early 1990s (42). The gasless system involves lifting the abdominal wall using an abdominal wall-lifting device. Valveless ports and conventional instruments or laparoscopic instruments can be used without gas leak (43,44). Several devices have been developed that avoid the use of CO_2 to distend the abdomen. Two devices frequently used are the Laparolift retraction system (Origin Medsystems, Menlo Park, CA) and the Abdo-lift (Karl Storz, Tuttingen, Germany).

Theoretically, gasless laparoscopy has numerous advantages over traditional CO_2 laparoscopy: It avoids the problem of CO_2 leakage as well as difficulties associated with creating and maintaining adequate CO_2 pressure. Indeed, high-pressure irrigation and large-volume suction devices can be used without losing the CO_2 gas, which when lost, can seriously impair adequate visibility. Gasless laparoscopy can also avoid the potential for infectious particles contaminating the CO_2 insufflation gas and the problem of lowering the body temperature (45), thus avoiding potential risks of metabolic and hemodynamic instability from CO_2 insufflation (46). In patients for whom general anesthesia and CO_2 pneumoperitoneum are contraindicated, gasless laparoscopy can be used as it does not significantly increase the intraabdominal pressure. The procedure can also be performed under epidural anesthesia, and has been successfully performed during pregnancy (47–52).

Galen et al. (44) performed 80 gynecologic procedures using gasless laparoscopy. They compared gasless laparoscopically assisted vaginal hysterectomy with 150 laparoscopically assisted vaginal hysterectomies performed with CO_2 pneumoperitoneum. They concluded that the Laparolift retraction system satisfactorily maintained visualization during the entire procedure, including the vaginal portion of the surgery. In another series of 49 laparoscopic gynecologic surgeries performed with gasless laparoscopy, the success rate was 90%. It allowed the surgical team to use the vaginal and laparoscopic approaches simultaneously (53). In Thailand, Tintara et al. performed 40 gynecologic procedures using gasless laparoscopy and reported no surgical complications. They considered the operative field to be virtually the same as that of the CO_2 pneumoperitoneum except in morbidly obese patients (54).

Tintara et al. also recently published a series comparing 31 gasless laparoscopic hysterectomies (GLHs) with 31 total abdominal hysterectomies (55). The operating time was longer by almost 1 hour, but blood loss, hospital stay, and convalescence were lower in the GLH group (55). Comparable results were also reported by others (56). Conversely, a clinical trial of 30 cases looking at the measure of visualization as primary outcome concluded that exposure with conventional laparoscopy using pneumoperitoneum is superior to that offered by gasless laparoscopy (57).

Data in gynecologic oncology are limited. A gasless pelvic lymphadenectomy has been reported by one team (43); the operators retrieved 45 lymph nodes and found this approach to be satisfactory. On the other hand, Johnson and Sibert (58) reported a randomized comparison of gasless versus CO_2 laparoscopy for tubal ligation and reported markedly increased technical difficulty with the gasless approach. Another group conducted a randomized comparison of gasless and CO_2 laparoscopy in 57 patients undergoing infertility surgery (59). Six patients in the gasless group had to be converted to CO_2 pneumoperitoneum because of inadequate exposure. The operators concluded that times to achieve exposure and close incisions were longer, and exposure and ease of surgery were worse in the gasless group. They found no advantages to this procedure over the conventional CO_2

approach (59). In a randomized prospective study, postoperative pain appeared to be similar for both techniques in patients undergoing laparoscopic tubal ligation (60).

Currently, gasless laparoscopy is not as widely used as CO_2 laparoscopy and the data on the former procedure are more limited. However, the technique does merit further evaluation in oncology patients, particularly because of the concerns that CO_2 pneumoperitoneum may increase tumor spread (see the section on port-site metastasis below).

PORT-SITE METASTASIS

There has been increasing concern among surgical oncologists about the apparent increased rate of port-site metastases following laparoscopic procedures. The reported rate of abdominal wall recurrences from two large studies following traditional abdominal surgery was 1% to 1.5% (61,62). In the last few years, as laparoscopic procedures have become more popular in oncology patients, there have been several reports in the literature of port-site metastases following laparoscopic surgery for a variety of cancers.

Schaeff et al. (63) conducted a literature review of port-site metastasis and found 164 reported cases from 90 publications, including 29 cases in gynecologic procedures. Wang et al. (64) recently conducted a similar MEDLINE search and found that the rate of port-site metastasis in ovarian cancer varies between 1.1% and 13.5%. Initial reports in gynecologic oncology surgery suggested that patients with adenocarcinomas of the ovaries with ascites and peritoneal seeding were at highest risk for port-site metastasis. Although most reports suggest that port-site metastases occur in advanced-stage cancer and poorly differentiated tumors, thus being an indicator of tumor virulence, there have been worrisome reports of low-stage and well-differentiated tumors causing postlaparoscopy tumor seeding (63). Borderline tumors (64), squamous-cell cancers of the cervix (65, 66), and adenocarcinomas of the endometrium have also been reported to metastasize to port sites (67).

The time period between the laparoscopic surgery and the appearance of port-site metastasis varies between 1 week and 3 years (67). Of concern, a number of port-site metastases have been documented to develop very rapidly after laparoscopic procedures; as early as 1 to 2 weeks. Timely referral for staging and definitive treatment becomes very important, as delays in referral have been shown to increase the rate of port-site metastasis and worsen prognosis. Several measures have been recommended to decrease the risk of port-site metastasis. These include thorough irrigation of the port-sites (68), the use of large volumes of saline for lavage of the abdominal cavity (69) and of the port-sites (64), slow abdominal wall deflation, the use of a wound protector, and the use of a specimen bag to retrieve the specimen (70).

Clearly, morcellation of suspicious solid tumors should be avoided at all cost, and according to Canis et al., if the abdominal wall is protected with a bag and the tumor is not morcellated, the incidence of trocar-site metastasis is approximately 1% (71). To reduce further the risk of trocar-site metastasis, some laparoscopic surgeons recommend re-section of the laparoscopic ports in a full-thickness fashion at the time of the staging laparotomy; ideally within 1 week of the laparoscopic surgery (72–74). Van Dam et al. also recommend closing all the layers of the trocar sites at the end of the laparoscopic procedure; that is, the peritoneum, the rectus sheath, and the skin. Indeed, in their study, they noted that trocar-site metastasis developed in 58% of their patients with only the skin closure of the trocar site compared to 2% of patients with closure of all layers (74).

The causes of port-site metastasis seem to be multifactorial: gas used, local trauma, tumor manipulation, biologic properties of the tumor, and individual surgical skills (63). Wang et al. (64) have identified a number of risk factors associated with port-site metastasis: ovarian cancer, adenocarcinoma histology, peritoneal carcinomatosis, the presence of ascites, and diagnostic or palliative procedures performed for malignancy. Based on a review of experimental data, Canis et al. concluded that the risk of dissemination following laparoscopic surgery is increased when a large number of malignant cells are present. For that reason, they suggested that adnexal tumors with external vegetations and bulky lymph nodes should be considered as contraindications to CO_2 laparoscopy (75). Other reported etiologies of port-site recurrence include trauma to the port site from frequent removal of instruments, tumor seeding from removal of the specimen through the port, and potential leakage of ascites (63,64). Trocar-site hematomas seem also to favor the rapid growth of tumor implants.

In an animal model, it was demonstrated that pneumoperitoneum itself may play an important role in the etiology of port-site metastasis (76). Others are concerned about the use of CO_2, as it may increase tumor-cell spillage and implantation (77). Local immune suppression and growth-factor secretion may also be involved (78). Recent data from animal studies suggest that the underlying immune or metabolic status of the host has a marked independent effect on tumor spread and implantation (79).

Owing to concerns regarding the potential increased risk of tumor dissemination associated with CO_2 laparoscopy, some experts advocate the use of gasless laparoscopy. An animal model comparing gasless laparoscopy, CO_2 laparoscopy, and laparotomy was performed to study peritoneal tumor growth and abdominal wall metastasis. The study concluded that CO_2 insufflation promotes tumor growth in the peritoneum and is associated with greater abdominal wall metastasis than gasless laparoscopy. They also found that direct contact between a solid tumor and the port site enhances local tumor growth (77). Other studies in rats have also shown that CO_2 may have an effect on growth stimulation on tumor cells (80) and CO_2 insufflation results in tumor dissemination during laparoscopy, leading to port-site metastasis (81). In these rat models, it appears that gasless lap-

aroscopy may reduce the risk of wound metastasis following laparoscopic surgery for cancer (82). Conversely, using an ovarian cancer xenograft animal model, two recent studies from the same investigators seem to indicate that CO_2 laparoscopy has a minor impact on visceral metastasis and survival and has no deleterious effect on tumor growth compared to gasless laparoscopy (83,84). Similar results have been shown in humans. Abu-Rustum et al. retrospectively reviewed patients with persistent metastatic intraabdominal peritoneal or ovarian cancer at time of second-look surgery. There was no difference in overall survival between patients who underwent laparoscopy or laparotomy; thus, they concluded that CO_2 pneumoperitoneum did not appear to reduce overall survival (85). In fact, a higher rate of port-site metastasis with gasless laparoscopy has been reported in some series (86). In a large review of 2,593 laparoscopic procedures on 1,288 women all with malignant disease, Abu-Rustum et al., identified 7 patients who developed a trocar-related subcutaneous implant. However, there were no "isolated" trocar-related implants noted, and all seven patients had synchronous metastasis or carcinomatosis. They argued that subcutaneous implantation should not be routinely used as an argument against laparoscopy (87).

Despite the above data, it is still controversial as to whether the use of gasless laparoscopy will reduce the risk of port-site metastasis. Some argue that the risk of tumor dissemination is just as great with gasless laparoscopy (64, 81,88). Others argue that the surgical technique and the thorough lavage of the port site are probably more important than the use of CO_2 (89). Reymond et al. (89) claim that gasless laparoscopy is not the solution to the problem since numerous port-site metastases have been reported after thoracoscopy where CO_2 insufflation was not used. In their opinion, the surgeon's role in seeding tumor cells is important and can be decreased by avoiding excessive tumor manipulation and frequent replacement of trocars. Variation in surgeons' techniques may explain the large differences in the reported incidence of port-site metastasis (0% to 21%). Meticulous surgical technique and the use of preventive measures will keep the incidence of port-site metastasis to about 1%, which is comparable to that seen with open laparotomy (89).

LAPAROSCOPIC MANAGEMENT OF PELVIC MASSES

A growing body of literature indicates that the laparoscopic management of pelvic masses is safe and effective. It significantly reduces the length of hospital stay, operative morbidity, and overall postoperative recuperation time. Despite careful preoperative evaluation, it appears to be inevitable that some of those masses will turn out to be malignant. Proper management and following strict surgical guidelines is very important in achieving optimal results.

Large series reported that among all patients approached

TABLE 13.1. *Reports in the literature concerning laparoscopic management of pelvic masses*

Authors (ref.)	No. of ovarian malignancies/no. of laparoscopies for pelvic masses	%
Nezhat et al., 1992 (90)	4/1,011	0.40
Hulka et al., 1992 (91)	55/13,739	0.40
Canis et al., 1994 (92)	19/757	2.5
Blanc et al., 1994 (93)	78/5,307	1.4
Marana et al., 1995 (94)	2/949	0.21
Wenzl et al., 1996 (95)	108/16,601	0.65
Yuen et al., 1997 (96)	0/102	0
Hidlebaugh et al., 1997 (97)	8/405 ~	2.0
Guglielmina et al., 1997 (98)	34/803	4.2
Malik et al., 1998 (99)	11/292	3.7
Dottino et al., 1999 (39)	17/160	10.6
Sadik et al., 1999 (100)	2/220	1.0
Ulrich et al., 2000 (101)	10/211	4.7
Serur et al., 2001 (102)	7/100	7.0
Mettler et al., 2001 (103)	6/493	1.2
Mendilcioglu et al., 2002 (104)	2/61	3.3
Havrileski et al., 2003 (105)	8/396	2.0

[a]Surveys from the American Association of Gynecologic Laparoscopists (AAGL), from France, and from Austria.

laparoscopically for pelvic masses, the overall rate of malignancy is low (Table 13.1) (39,90–105). The rate varies greatly among the studies according to the preoperative selection criteria used and the study design. It is also interesting that the rate of malignancy reported since 1997 seems to be higher. This may be explained by the fact that more surgeons are becoming comfortable with invasive laparoscopic techniques and thus are more likely to approach high-risk pelvic masses laparoscopically.

Preoperative Selection

In 1994, Canis et al. (92) published an extensive, retrospective, 12-year analysis with long-term follow-up of 757 patients from 1980 to 1991. All patients had ovarian masses and were managed by laparoscopy. They followed a strict set of criteria to select cases for laparoscopic management. The complete preoperative investigation included a pelvic sonogram, CA-125 measurement, and pelvic examination. Obviously malignant or suspicious masses were managed with laparotomy. The others underwent a laparoscopic evaluation, which included a peritoneal cytologic testing, cyst puncture, and endocystic evaluation, also referred to as "cystoscopy." At laparoscopy, if a malignant mass was encountered or was considered to be highly suspicious, an immediate midline laparotomy was performed. Following this algorithm, their rate of inadvertent malignancy was 2.5% (19 of 757), including 12 borderline and 7 invasive cancers. Additionally, 27 masses were falsely diagnosed as being malignant (3.6%), which means that these patients had an unnecessary laparotomy. Based on that experience, Canis et al. consider laparoscopic management of pelvic masses to be safe and reliable (92).

Although it is generally agreed that by careful preoperative and intraoperative assessment most cancers can be adequately diagnosed and properly managed, the preoperative evaluation is frequently of limited value and cannot discriminate a benign mass from a malignant mass. Benacerraf et al. (106) used sonography to study 100 women undergoing laparotomy for ovarian masses; sonography was misleading in 15% of cases. Guglielmina et al. (98) reviewed their experience with laparoscopic management of over 800 ovarian cysts and concluded that neither ultrasound nor laparoscopic evaluation can accurately predict the exact nature of an adnexal mass. Even when carefully conducted, preoperative investigation cannot accurately detect all ovarian cancers (99). Maiman et al. (107) noted that four of the so-called "benign" characteristics were present in 31% of the pelvic masses found to be malignant. According to Nezhat et al. (90), neither the CA-125 level, pelvic ultrasound, nor peritoneal cytologic testing had sufficient specificity to predict malignancy.

Laparoscopic Approach

In general, the laparoscopic management for pelvic masses is considered to be safe and effective. There are several reported advantages to this approach: shorter hospital stay, decreased postoperative pain and recovery time, less adhesion formation, decreased hospital cost, and lower complication rate. The failure rate of laparoscopy in removing pelvic masses is low (< 5%) (10,107,108).

In a randomized trial, Yuen et al. (96) compared laparoscopy with laparotomy in the management of ovarian masses in 102 patients. Exclusion criteria included masses suspicious for malignancy and lesion diameter greater than 10 cm. Their data showed that inadvertent cyst rupture was frequent in both groups and operative time was comparable. The laparoscopic approach was associated with significant reductions in operative morbidity, postoperative pain, required analgesia, hospital stay, and recovery period. Those findings were confirmed by others (14,108–110). Recently, Jennings et al. (111) reported a significantly decreased length of hospital stay without an adverse effect on the surgical complication rate in patients undergoing operations in a gynecologic oncology unit.

Concerns Regarding Laparoscopic Management of Pelvic Masses

There are several concerns regarding the laparoscopic management of benign-appearing pelvic masses. These include failure to diagnose malignancy; underestimation of the extent of disease; tumor spillage from rupture of the masses; inability to perform complete staging, implying another surgery for the patient; and most importantly, long delays before a staging procedure or definitive treatment that can adversely affect the ultimate prognosis of the patient (39,112). The risk of port-site metastasis has been discussed extensively above.

Intraoperative Frozen Section

The management of any pelvic mass, either by laparoscopy or by laparotomy, should include access to accurate frozen section, so the necessary procedure can be performed immediately. In one large series, the overall accuracy of frozen section was 92.7% (113). However, in a collected series of over 11,000 laparoscopies for ovarian cysts, Lehner et al. (112) reported that frozen section was obtained at the time of laparoscopy in only 34% of cases. Frozen section was obtained in 40% of cases in Maiman et al.'s survey of Society of Gynecologic Oncologists (SGO) members (107). Also of interest in the latter study is that the average age of patients with invasive cancers was 44 years, and 29% of these tumors were borderline. Ovarian cancer is thus not uncommon in perimenopausal women, and surgeons should always keep a high index of suspicion. Most surgeons consider availability of frozen section at the time of laparoscopy mandatory, even in younger women, so that a staging procedure can be performed without delay when indicated (39, 90,112,114,115).

Tumor Spillage

It remains controversial as to whether intraoperative tumor spillage carries a poorer prognosis. Some surgeons have noted that preoperative tumor rupture or the presence of ascites may worsen the prognosis (42), whereas others did not find any difference in survival among stage I patients with intraoperative spillage (114). Mettler et al. (116) found

that tumor propagation does not occur in ruptured stage I cases if definitive surgery is performed within 1 week. According to others, the grade of the tumor and the presence of ascites in stage I cancer of the ovary is more important in relation to survival than is rupture of the ovarian capsule at surgery (117,118). Nevertheless, all pelvic masses should be considered to be potentially malignant and, consequently, all efforts should be made to avoid rupture.

Delayed Staging

Maiman et al. (107) surveyed SGO members with regard to their management of ovarian neoplasms later found to be malignant. The response rate from members was 42% and 42 cases of ovarian malignancy were reported. In that survey, immediate staging had been performed in 17% of cases, delayed in 71% (median, 36 days), and not performed in 12%. The investigators raised significant concerns with regard to the negative outcome of some laparoscopically managed ovarian cancers, particularly as it related to the significant number of patients who were not restaged and to the delay between the initial procedure and the definitive treatment. They concluded that delays of more than 4 weeks had a negative impact on patient outcome.

Blanc et al. (119) conducted a similar multiinstitutional French survey and recorded 5,307 ovarian lesions treated laparoscopically, of which 1.4% were malignant. Staging of cancer cases was performed immediately in 25% of the cases, delayed in 58% (median 78 days), and not performed in 16%. In those who had delayed staging, 22.4% were upstaged.

Kindermann et al. (115) also sent a questionnaire to 273 German departments of obstetrics and gynecology with a response rate of 46%. They collected a total of 192 ovarian cases managed laparoscopically. Overall, 16% of borderline stage IA and 39% of malignant stage IA tumors (based on laparoscopy) had spread of disease identified at staging laparotomy. In 92% of cases, capsule rupture and tumor morcellation with intraabdominal spillage occurred at laparoscopy. Endoscopy bags were used in only 7.4% of ovarian cancer cases. In patients staged more than 8 days after initial laparoscopy, nearly 75% of cases were upstaged (20% to stage IC and 53% to stages II-III). Most disturbing, trocarsite metastasis was identified in 52% of patients with stages IC-III at initial laparoscopy if definitive surgery was delayed more than 8 days.

Leminen et al. (120) reported on eight patients who had their staging laparotomy after laparoscopic surgery within a mean of 17 days (range 7 to 29). In four patients, the disease had spread from a localized to an advanced stage during the delay. They concluded that laparoscopic surgery of ovarian masses later found to be malignant can cause considerable and rapid spread of the disease. Hopkins et al. reported a similar experience with three young women who had laparoscopic removal of what appeared to be benign lesions. All three underwent reexploration within 3 weeks, yet trocar-site metastasis and intraabdominal tumor spread had already occurred (73).

Finally, Lehner et al. (112) sent a questionnaire to all gynecology departments in Austria regarding laparoscopic management of ovarian masses later found to be malignant. Of the 70 cancers identified, 48 patients underwent an immediate laparotomy to complete surgery, 24 had a laparotomy within 17 days (median 9.9 days), and 24 patients had delays of more than 17 days (median 47.7 days). The cut-off of 17 days was chosen arbitrarily. Only 10% of malignant tumors were reported using an endoscopy bag. They found that patients in whom definitive surgery was delayed more than 17 days were more likely to be upstaged (odds ratio of 5.3 for borderline tumors and 9.2 for invasive cancers). In a multivariate analysis, delay of more than 17 days was an independent prognostic factor for stage of disease in borderline cases. This was not statistically significant in the cases of invasive ovarian cancer. The study does not provide data as to whether survival was subsequently affected by the upstaging.

The above studies emphasize that poor surgical technique and delayed definitive surgery when managing ovarian masses by laparoscopy can have a very serious impact on patients' survival. It also underscores the fact that, because of the subsequent upstaging, a number of patients will likely be subjected to adjuvant chemotherapy, which they may not have otherwise needed.

COMPREHENSIVE MANAGEMENT OF SUSPICIOUS PELVIC MASSES

Dottino et al. (39) challenged the concept that patients with a suspicious pelvic mass should necessarily undergo laparotomy. In their study, they purposely approached all the pelvic masses referred to their oncology unit by laparoscopy regardless of the suspicion of malignancy except when there was evidence of gross metastatic disease (i.e., "omental cake") or masses extending above the umbilicus. All masses were sent for immediate frozen-section analysis. Despite the fact that the majority of the masses were considered to be suspicious for malignancy preoperatively, 87% of the masses were in fact benign and 88% were successfully managed by laparoscopy. Not surprisingly, compared with other series (Table 13.1) (39,90–105), a higher proportion of the masses turned out to be malignant (10.6%), but most of them were managed laparoscopically following oncologic standards. If debulking was deemed to be best performed by laparotomy, the laparoscopy was converted to an open case. In many instances, adequate surgery could be completed by laparoscopy. Long-term data on overall outcome and survival following laparoscopic surgery for ovarian cancer are not available.

Canis et al. (114) also suggest performing a diagnostic laparoscopy regardless of the ultrasonographic appearance

of the pelvic mass, although they recommend an immediate laparotomy for staging of cancer cases. They also reiterate the importance of frozen-section analysis to decide appropriate definitive treatment. When indicated, they consider restaging of cancers as an "oncologic emergency." Quinlan et al. (110) included complex masses and septated cysts in their selection criteria. Laparoscopy by trained laparoscopists can be used to evaluate adnexal masses in women with risk factors for ovarian cancer with a low complication rate and reduced hospital stay (121).

Borderline tumors often present as multilocular lesions on sonogram and may have elevated CA-125 levels. Darai et al. (122) reported a series of 43 borderline tumors of which 34 were approached by laparoscopy. Of those, 27 were completely managed by laparoscopy. There were four recurrences, three of which occurred in patients who had ovarian cystectomies only. They concluded that laparoscopic management of borderline tumors is feasible, but ovarian cystectomies are associated with a higher risk of recurrence.

It would thus appear that even though suspicious masses have traditionally been managed by laparotomy, laparoscopic management of high-risk pelvic masses can be successfully performed in an oncology referral population if there is expertise in operative laparoscopy, availability of immediate and accurate pathologic evaluation, and appropriate further treatment where indicated. In many cases, having an oncologist skilled in advanced laparoscopic procedures allows laparoscopic completion of the staging procedure. However, when skilled assistance is unavailable, it is best to terminate the laparoscopic procedure after a cancer diagnosis and promptly to refer the patient for definitive surgery. As stated by Alvarez et al. (123), "accuracy is more important than immediacy."

According to the literature, laparoscopy for the management of pelvic masses can eliminate the need for unnecessary laparotomy in most cases. Statistically, the majority of them will be benign and can be adequately managed laparoscopically, and most of the recent investigators conclude that laparoscopy is a safe approach for the treatment of adnexal masses (Table 13.1) (39,90–105). However, the above data clearly demonstrate that delayed staging and definitive treatment can have a negative impact on patient outcome more than the laparoscopic procedure itself. When appropriate referral for a staging operation is made in a timely fashion, ideally within 2 weeks, it is unlikely that disease progression will occur (115,123). Moreover, until proven otherwise, ovarian masses should always be considered to be potentially malignant. Thus, surgeons should be technically meticulous in order to minimize the risk of ovarian cyst rupture and spillage, and specimens should always be retrieved intact through an endobag to reduce the risk of trocar-site metastasis. With advances in laparoscopic surgical technique, suspicious ovarian masses can be approached laparoscopically as long as a plan is in place for appropriate staging and treatment by laparotomy or laparoscopy (39).

LAPAROSCOPIC EXTRAPERITONEAL STAGING: PELVIC AND AORTIC LYMPH NODE DISSECTIONS

Laparoscopy enables visual assessment, sampling, and systematic dissection of the lymph nodes located in the extraperitoneal space along the pelvic sidewall and in the paraaortic area. Both direct and indirect transumbilical approaches are discussed.

Transumbilical Transperitoneal Laparoscopic Lymphadenectomies

The transumbilical transperitoneal technique for laparoscopic lymphadenectomy remains the most popular approach employed by gynecologists. This in part has to do with the familiarity of gynecologists with this indirect approach. The setup is essentially the same as for routine laparoscopy. The ports are placed in a similar configuration as that used for traditional pelvic laparoscopy (Fig. 13.1). The size of the ports will depend on the instruments that are to be employed. When paraaortic lymphadenectomy is to be performed, it is helpful to place the lateral ports slightly more cephalad avoiding the abdominal wall vasculature, and an additional port in the left upper quadrant may be required to assist with retraction of the intestines.

Pelvic Dissection

The surgeon intending to perform a pelvic dissection stands on the patient's left side. The video monitor is placed at the foot of the operating table. The peritoneum is divided along the pelvic brim between the round ligament and the infundibulopelvic (IP) ligament, which are best left undivided until the dissection is finished. Prior to opening the peritoneum, the umbilical ligament is located, which is seen as an oblique peritoneal fold on the posterior surface of the abdominal wall. By following this "Ariadne's thread" from front to back, once the broad ligament is opened, it is easy to identify the superior vesical artery and its ventral continuation, the umbilical ligament. The superior vesical artery is the first surgical landmark in the pelvic dissection. Retracting it medially enables one to open the paravesical space and free the pelvic sidewall. This exposes the external iliac vessels at the point where they cross Cooper's ligament. In obese patients whose anatomic structures are covered with fatty tissue, it is recommended to locate Cooper's ligament first. This can be identified by palpation with a blunt instrument on the posterior surface of the pubis, lateral to the umbilical ligament—much the same way a blind person seeks the edge of the pavement with a cane.

Prior to dissection, one must identify the major vascular landmarks including the common, external, and internal iliac vessels. The dissection starts with grasping the tissues located anterior to the external iliac vessels and gently placing them on traction. A second instrument can then be used to dissect the connective fibers and lymphatic channels joining the node-bearing tissues to the surrounding structures (Fig. 13.2). In 20% of cases, an accessory obturator vein will be found in the obturator nodal tissue and insert on the inferior surface of the external iliac vein; blunt dissection is generally enough to free the nodal tissue from this structure. Once the nodes are freed from beneath the vein and the obturator nerve is exposed, the external iliac vein is traced back to the bifurcation of the common iliac vessels.

The next step is to dissect the node-bearing tissues located

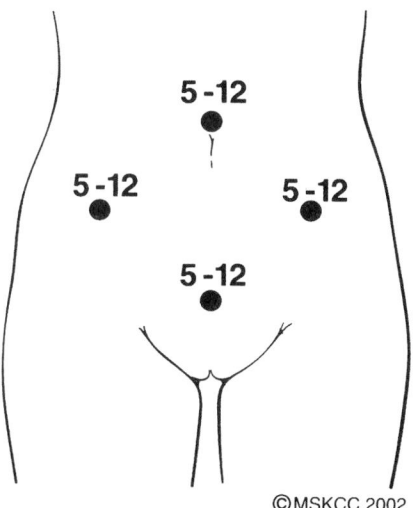

FIG. 13.1. Transperitoneal trocar placement for laparoscopic lymphadenectomy.

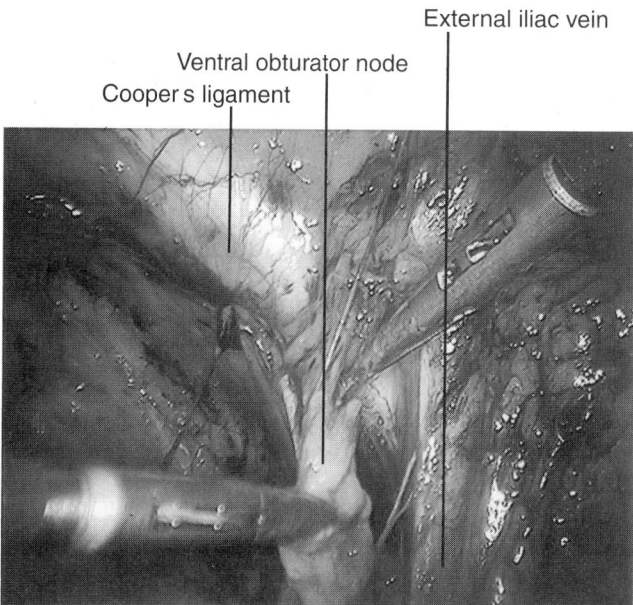

FIG. 13.2. Pelvic laparoscopic lymphadenectomy. The pelvic lymphadenectomy is initiated. Picture of the ventral part of the right pelvic sidewall. (See Color Plate.)

between the external iliac vessels and the psoas muscle. One starts ventrally at the level of the origin of the circumflex artery and continues dorsally to the level of the common iliac artery. At that point, it is often necessary to make a lateral peritoneal incision in order to reflect the ileocecal junction upward on the right side and the sigmoid colon on the left side. The ureter is identified at the level at which it crosses the iliac vessels. If the IP ligament has not been divided and the posterior sheet of the broad ligament is intact, the ureter remains attached to its natural support. Both are pushed medially. The pararectal space is then opened. The node-bearing tissues alongside the inferior aspect of the common iliac artery and posterior aspect of the internal iliac artery are exposed.

Dissection techniques and the sequence of which the landmarks are identified vary from surgeon to surgeon. The most basic technique of dissection is recommended; that is, grasping the nodes with grasping forceps and employing blunt dissection to separate the node-bearing tissue from the underlying structures. Such a technique (Fig. 13.2) requires skill, but once this skill is acquired, less blood loss is involved. Only the resistant structures, that is, the blood vessels, must be controlled before being divided, and these are few if the dissection is performed in the correct tissue planes. Needless to say, other techniques exist that can yield comparable results.

Removal of the nodes can be accomplished by (a) gathering them (e.g., in the uterovesical space) and extracting them at the end of the procedure using an extracting bag; or (b) using a specialized nodal extractor such as the Coelio-Extractor (Groupe Lepine, Lyon, France) to deliver the nodes without contaminating the abdominal wall.

Querleu (7) was the first to provide data describing the feasibility and safety of transumbilical transperitoneal laparoscopic pelvic dissection. There were 39 procedures performed on patients with cancer of the cervix, stage IB to IIB, and the mean duration of the procedure was 80 minutes. No conversion to laparotomy was required. The mean node count was 8.7 (range 3 to 22). Positive nodes were found in 5 patients who were subsequently treated with radiotherapy, and the remaining 34 patients underwent either an abdominal radical hysterectomy or a VRH. All patients were followed for 5 years (124), and the 5-year survival rate was similar to the survival of a historical group of patients who underwent standard abdominal radical hysterectomy. Patients were matched for age, stage, and therapy. Childers and coworkers (9) reported the experience from 18 patients with cervical cancer who were initially managed with laparoscopy. Five patients had immediate abdominal radical hysterectomy and 13 were subsequently treated with radiotherapy. No complications were observed. The duration of the staging procedure was 75 to 175 minutes for the patients assessed prior to radiotherapy. The mean number of lymph nodes was 31.4 (range 17 to 37) for patients submitted to abdominal radical hysterectomy. One year later, Childers et al. (125) provided

data for 53 patients with endometrial cancer. All the patients underwent laparoscopic assessment, and 29 underwent pelvic lymphadenectomy plus aortic sampling. Three intraoperative complications occurred (one pneumothorax, one transection of the ureter, and one bladder injury) and three postoperative complications (two patients had a postoperative ileus and one patient had significant atelectasis). The issue was addressed again 5 years later (126) in 125 patients. The rate of complications did not vary. However, the rate of conversion to laparotomy dropped from 8% (2 of 25) to 0% (0 of 100), whereas the operative time decreased from 196 minutes to 128 minutes ($p < .02$) and the hospital stay from 3.2 days to 1.8 days ($p < .0001$).

Aortic Dissection

Two techniques have been described for performing an aortic dissection with the laparoscope. In the first (9), the setup is the same as the one used for the pelvic dissection. Two details differ: The video monitor is put on the side of the patient opposite the side where the surgeon stands; and the video camera is turned clockwise 90 degrees, so that the axis of the aorta appears to be horizontal. The intestines are pushed under the diaphragmatic areas. The dorsal peritoneum is opened longitudinally alongside the axis of the aorta. The upper peritoneal flap is developed upward. The right ovarian vessels and the right ureter are identified and pushed laterally. The nodal tissue on the ventral aspect of the vena cava is removed followed by that in the interaorticocaval space. Finally, the nodes from the anterior aspect of the aorta are removed. The origin of the inferior mesenteric artery is identified, and the nodes lying on the left side of the aorta are mobilized and delivered.

In the second technique (18), the surgeon stands between the patient's legs with the monitor at the head of the bed. The dorsal peritoneum is opened transversely alongside the axis of the right common iliac vessels. The upper peritoneal flap is pushed cranially at the same time as the last ileal loop. The right gonadal vessels are identified at the level of the third portion of the duodenum. After having mobilized and divided the ovarian vessels, one finds the left renal vein and begins the dissection that is performed alongside the anterior aspect of the vena cava and then continued in the interaorticocaval space, alongside the ventral aspect of the aorta, and, finally, alongside the left aspect of the aorta. Gaining access to the retroaortic and retrocaval spaces necessitates mobilizing the vessels laterally and medially in order to clear out each of the spaces in two steps. The lumbar arteries and veins a represent major danger during this final part of the dissection.

Since 1993, many series have appeared in the literature describing laparoscopic lymphadenectomy (11,12,17, 127–136). Most have included data from an inframesenteric dissection as well. Summarizing the larger series (Table 13.2) (7,11,12,17,27,127–137), one can assume that the

TABLE 13.2. *Selected series of laparoscopic pelvic and/or inframesenteric lymph node dissection*

Author (ref.)	Year	No. of patients	Disease site	Mean pelvic nodes	Mean inframesenteric nodes
Querleu et al. (7)	1991	39	Cervix	8.7	–
Childers et al. (17)	1993	61	Gyn	–	6.3
Spirtos et al. (128)	1995	40	Endometrium	20.8	7.9
Su et al. (131)	1995	38	Cervix	15	–
Hatch et al. (12)	1996	37	Cervix	35	11
Chu et al. (11)	1997	67	Cervix	26.7	8
Possover et al. (127)	1998	150	Gyn	26.8	7.3
Vidaurreta et al. (132)	1999	84	Cervix	18.5	–
Dottino et al. (129)	1999	94	Gyn	11.9	3.7
Renaud et al (133)	2000	57	Cervix	27	3
Altgassen et al. (134)	2000	108	Cervix	21.0–24.3	5.1–10.6
Scribner et al. (130)	2001	103	Endometrium	18.1	11.9
Vergote et al. (135)	2002	41	Cervix	–	6
Spirtos et al. (27)	2002	78	Cervix	23.8	10.3
Schlaerth et al. (137)	2002	69	Cervix	32.1	12.1
Abu-Rustum et al. (136)	2003	114	Gyn	10.7	5.7

Gyn, cervical, endometrial, and ovarian tumors.

mean number of pelvic nodes retrieved laparoscopically was 21 and the mean number of aortic nodes was 8. This number is close to the number of nodes retrieved by laparotomy (138). Comparative studies confirm that the numbers are approximately the same (29,139). Fowler et al. (140) addressed the fact that 25% of the pelvic nodes were still present at laparotomy after the patient underwent a laparoscopic lymphadenectomy; however, no patients with negative nodes at laparoscopy had positive nodes at laparotomy.

The thoroughness of laparoscopic lymphadenectomy has been demonstrated by the recent GOG study (137). In this series in which laparoscopic pelvic and paraaortic lymphadenectomy was immediately followed by laparotomy, the mean number of retrieved pelvic nodes was 32.1 (16.6 on the left side and 15.5 on the right side). In spite of this large number, the results were judged to be incomplete in 6 of the 40 patients who subsequently underwent laparotomy after laparoscopic lymphadenectomy. The objective of laparoscopic lymphadenectomy should be to remove the nodes at risk for spread of disease. The rarity of pelvic sidewall recurrences in node-negative patients managed without a complete lymphadenectomy suggests that laparoscopy enables us to remove the significant nodes. If a criterion to judge the adequacy of the procedure had to be selected, photographic records taken at the end of the laparoscopic procedure would provide the best means to this end. In the GOG study, the result was judged to be inadequate in three of the patients whose photographic records were reviewed by two independent observers. If clearly identifying the dorsal part of the obturator nerve and lumbosacral nerve is required (Figs. 13.3 to 13.5), the risk of missing positive pelvic nodes is very low, at least in cases of cervical and endometrial cancer.

Lymphadenectomy is one of the cornerstone procedures in gynecologic oncology. The development of the laparoscopic lymphadenectomy has opened the door for the use of mini-

mally invasive surgery in the management of gynecologic malignancies. The benefits of the procedure alone are difficult to assess since in most of the reported series the procedure is combined with additional operations. This makes it difficult to assess the role of laparoscopic lymphadenectomy either in duration of surgery, appraising intraoperative or postoperative complications, and duration of hospital stay. In Querleu et al.'s inaugural series (7), the procedure was discontinued in 1 of 14 patients owing to an anesthetic problem. One case of intraoperative bleeding was controlled

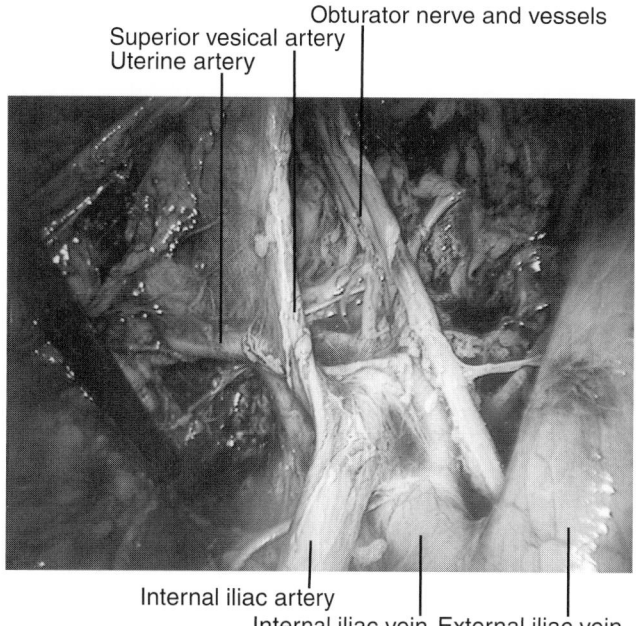

FIG. 13.3. Pelvic laparoscopic lymphadenectomy. The pelvic lymphadenectomy is complete. Picture of the dorsal part of the right pelvic sidewall. (See Color Plate.)

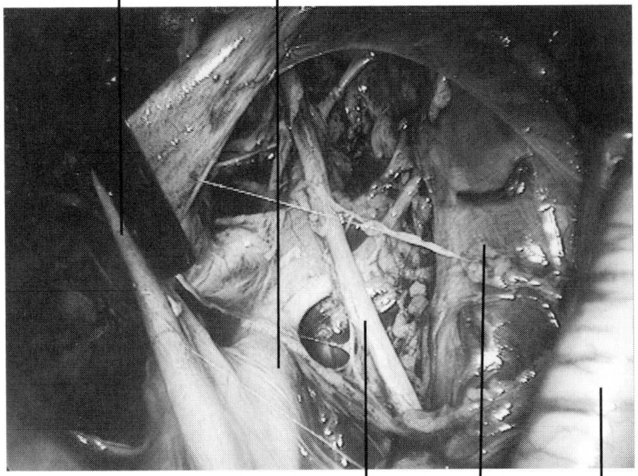

External iliac vein   Internal iliac vein

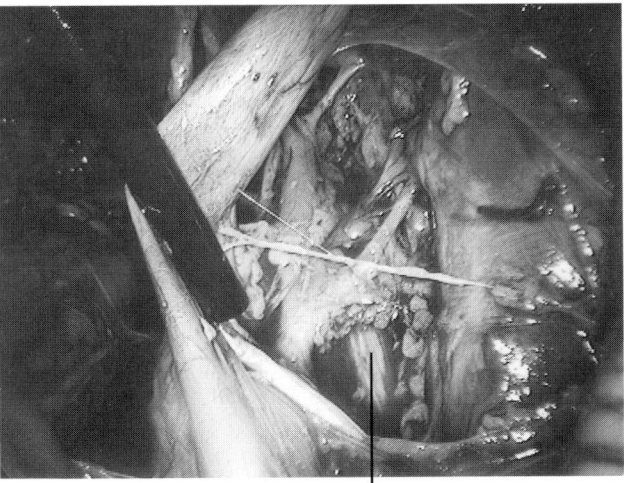

Obturator nerve Psoas muscle

External iliac artery

FIG. 13.4. Pelvic laparoscopic lymphadenectomy. The pelvic lymphadenectomy is complete. Same view as Figure 13.2, but the external iliac vein has been pushed medially. (See Color Plate.)

laparoscopically, and all patients except one were discharged the day after the procedure. Possover et al. (127) reported ten major vessel injuries were registered among 150 procedures (four vena cava, two right renal vein, two external iliac vein, one internal iliac vein, and one internal iliac artery). A conversion to laparotomy was necessary in four of these cases. The mean hospital stay for the 26 patients submitted to

Lumbosacral nerve

FIG. 13.5. Pelvic laparoscopic lymphadenectomy. The pelvic lymphadenectomy is complete. Same view as Figure 13.3, but the external iliac vein and the obturator nerve have been pushed medially. The lumbosacral nerve is visible; this, more than the lymph node count, is proof that the pelvic lymphadenectomy has been done thoroughly. (See Color Plate.)

lymphadenectomy for pure staging was 3.2 days. Dottino et al. (129) reviewed 94 cases of laparoscopic lymphadenectomies of which three required conversion. There was one vascular injury, one case of densely adherent nodal tissue that was felt to be laparoscopically unresectable, and one case of a bulky cervical tumor making laparoscopy difficult. Thirty patients had laparoscopic lymphadenectomy alone and the mean hospital stay was 3.6 days; however, this number included a group of patients who received postoperative chemotherapy. Patients who did not receive chemotherapy were discharged in 1.7 days. Scribner et al. (130) reviewed their first 103 laparoscopic lymphadenectomies. Laparoscopy was completed in 70.9% of patients, with obesity, adhesions, and intraperitoneal disease being the main reasons for not being able to complete the laparoscopic procedure. Three procedural complications included a bladder laceration, a ureteral injury, and one vessel injury at trocar insertion. Other operative procedures were performed and direct correlation with the lymphadenectomy was not mentioned. These studies do seem to imply that laparoscopic lymphadenectomy is feasible with an acceptable complication rate.

Childers, Querleu, and their early followers initially limited the surgical effort to the right inframesenteric area. Consequently, the mean lymph node yield was about eight (Table 13.2) (7,11,12,17,27,127–137). This number is not much different from the number reported with dissection at laparotomy (138). It is now known from studies like those published by Benedetti-Panici et al. (141) that the actual number of nodes is around 20 if the dissection is continued to the level of the left renal vein. Michel et al. (142) reports that, in cervical cancer involving aortic nodes, the involvement on the left side of the aorta is 72% (23 of 32) and involves the supramesenteric level in 25% of cases (8 of 32). Because of these findings, the aortic dissection must be extended to the left side and to the level of the left renal vein.

As the need to perform a systematic infrarenal dissection became more evident, data regarding this procedure under transumbilical transperitoneal laparoscopic guidance began to appear for adnexal cancers (15). Possover et al. (127) also performed such operations in selected cases (ovarian cancer and uterine cancer with high risk of metastasis). When comparing the infrarenal lymphadenectomy to the inframesenteric lymphadenectomy, Kohler et al. (143) demonstrated that this could be performed safely. This extended paraaortic lymphadenectomy only took an additional 31 minutes on average and significantly increased the mean node counts from 9.0 to 19.6. A report from the same group (144) indicates that the greatest dangers are not in the higher part of the dissection, but they are lower where tributaries to the anterior aspect of the vena cava are found in the area of the bifurcation of the vena cava in 58.0% of cases versus 19.6% in the area between the bifurcation and the inferior mesenteric artery and 0.9% of cases in the area between the inferior mesenteric artery and the right ovarian vein. Furthermore, it appears that if need be dissection higher than the left renal vein is feasible. Possover et al. (19) attempted this in patients with stage IIIB cervical cancer, transecting at first the left paracolic peritoneum and the left phrenicocolic ligament and mobilizing medially the colonic flexure, left kidney and adrenal gland, tail of pancreas, and spleen. The median number of retrieved nodes was ten. No intraoperative or postoperative complications occurred.

Extraperitoneal Laparoscopic Pelvic Lymphadenectomy

Laparoscopic pelvic lymphadenectomy can be performed using the direct extraperitoneal approach. Historically, this approach was the first method described. Although it is no longer routinely used, one remaining application may be laparoscopic preparation for vaginal radical trachelectomy. The direct extraperitoneal approach had the advantage of completely avoiding the ''other surface'' of the peritoneum and thus minimizing the risk of postoperative adhesions potentially impairing the fertility. This risk, however, appears to be low with the indirect transumbilical approach, and the direct approach does have two drawbacks: (a) loss of time (approximately 15 minutes); and (b) potential for postoperative collections, that is, hematomas, abscesses, lymphoceles (which may be preventable by creating a peritoneotomy at the end of the dissection).

In spite of the above disadvantages to the direct approach to the pelvic extraperitoneal spaces, this approach may be useful in cases where the pelvic cavity is not accessible or not easily accessible such as in pregnancy more than 16 weeks or when severe postoperative adhesions are present. This approach starts with a blind digital preparation of the preperitoneal space. It is also possible to obtain access to the correct space under direct optical guidance through a 10-mm incision thanks to the new laparoscopic trocars that have a cutting tip (Endotip, Storz, Tuttingen, Germany) or accommodates a cutting and transparent punch (Visiport, Tyco; Optiview, Ethicon, Cincinnati, Ohio).

Midline Suprapubic Access

Midline suprapubic access is obtained through an incision made 3 to 4 cm above the pubis. The surgeon stands across from the pelvic sidewall to be dissected and handles the trocar obliquely in order to get access directly to the iliopubic bone at an equal distance from the midline and the external iliac vessels. Once the bone is located, the extraperitoneal space is insufflated and the ancillary trocars can be placed (at 5 to 6 cm from each other on a vertical line running perpendicular to the pubis at 3 to 4 cm lateral to the midline). Cooper's ligament leads to the external iliac vessels that can be traced in ideal conditions from the femoral ring to the bifurcation of the common iliac artery.

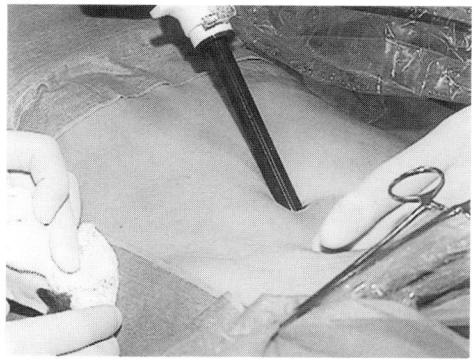

FIG. 13.6. Umbilical extraperitoneal laparoscopic approach. The instrument used is the Visiport (US Surgical Corporation Norwalk, CT). (See Color Plate.)

Transumbilical Access

Getting direct access to the extraperitoneal spaces while using a transumbilical microincision (Fig. 13.6) can be obtained using the same technique one uses for routine transumbilical laparoscopy. One only has to use the previously mentioned dissecting trocars (see above) and stop the sharp dissection once the fascia parietalis is opened; that is, before entering the peritoneal serosa. Once the fascia is opened, the CO_2 insufflation begins, and one proceeds to use the laparoscope as a blunt dissector until the symphysis pubis is reached. After using a fine-needle puncture to check the retroperitoneal channel one has created on the midline (Fig. 13.7), a 10- to 20-mm trocar is introduced in the midline that will accommodate the laparoscopic scissors that are used to prepare the posterior surface of the abdominal wall up to the level of McBurney's point. Care must be taken not to dissect too close to the muscle (staying posterior to the inferior epigastric vessels) and not too close to the serosa (acci-

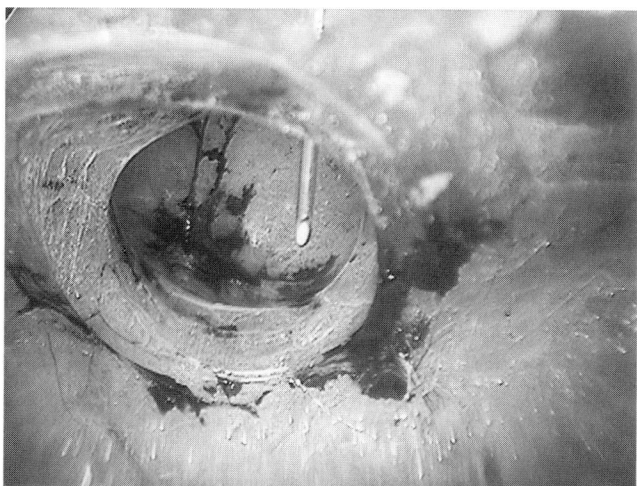

FIG. 13.7. Umbilical extraperitoneal laparoscopic approach. A spinal needle is introduced in the midline in the extraperitoneal space before the ancillary instruments are put in place. (See Color Plate.)

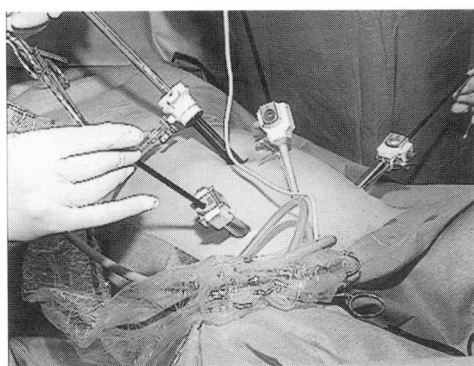

FIG. 13.8. Umbilical extraperitoneal laparoscopic approach. Position of laparoscopic trocar and ancillary trocars. (See Color Plate.)

dental peritoneotomy makes the continuation of the surgery very difficult if not impossible). Having prepared the posterior surface of the abdominal wall on both sides, the setup is exactly the same as that used for routine laparoscopy (Fig. 13.8). The access to the retropubic space is ideal, but access to the iliac vessels is limited by the adherent nature of the peritoneum to the abdominal wall, particularly at the level of the inguinal canals. In order to mobilize this, division of the round ligaments is required at the most distal point where they disappear into the inguinal canals (Fig. 13.9). Once the ligaments are divided and the peritoneum developed dorsally, the view obtained of the pelvic sidewall is similar to that seen in the transumbilical transperitoneal approach. The only difference is the superior vesical arteries and umbilical ligaments now run dorsally since the bladder has been detached from the abdominal wall and reflected dorsally.

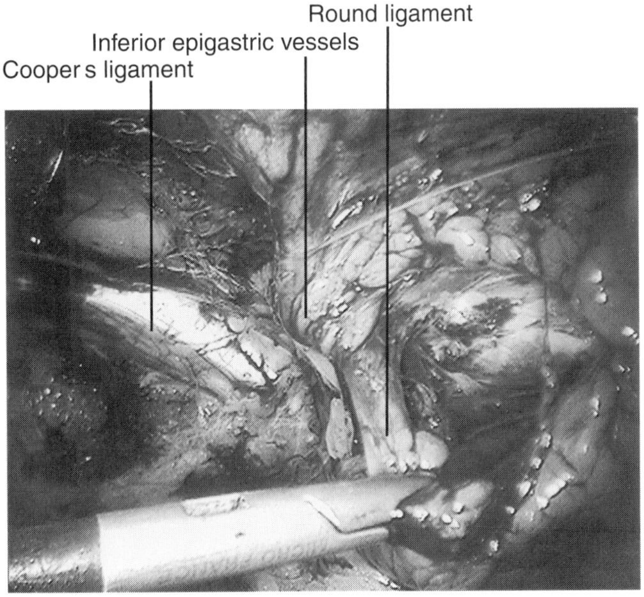

Round ligament
Inferior epigastric vessels
Cooper s ligament

FIG. 13.9. Umbilical extraperitoneal laparoscopic approach. The round ligament on the right side is freed before being divided. (See Color Plate.)

Sentinel Node Biopsy

The use of the sentinel node (SN) concept in the clinical management of epithelial malignancies started in the 1970s. The urologist Cabanas (145) proposed replacement of full inguinofemoral dissection that was traditionally combined with radical surgery for penile cancer with only a biopsy of the so-called sentinel node (SN). The use of the new technique spread rapidly beginning in the early 1990s. In gynecologic oncology, the first application was in vulvar cancer (146), but this was soon followed by its application in cervical cancer (20,147–162) and endometrial cancer (161,162). Numerous opinions about techniques of injection, methods of dissection, modality of pathologic assessment, and, even more, the practical use of the end results have been put forth. The only point that gives rise to quasiunanimity is that the laparoscope is a tool perfectly suitable for SN biopsy technique in the field of cervical cancer. Table 13.3 (20,147–153, 155–158,160,163,164) summarizes the literature concerning the use of SN biopsy in early cervical carcinoma. The data should be interpreted carefully because of the different techniques employed between one team and the other.

The SN injection is started by injecting the normal tissues surrounding the tumor. The size of the needle is ideally 21 gauge. The injection must not be too deep and not too superficial (Fig. 13.10). A ''learning curve effect'' does exist with this technique. Many factors may contribute to the discrepancies in the literature such as the nature of the injected medium: either a blue dye (Lymphazurin or Patent Blue Violet) or radioisotopic colloidal particles. The blue dyes have to be used at an appropriate dilution and in appropriate quantity. The isotope used for the radioisotopic technique is generally technetium 99m, but the colloidal particles vary in nature and size (2 to 80 nm), which contributes to variability in the transit time and number of detected nodes. No matter

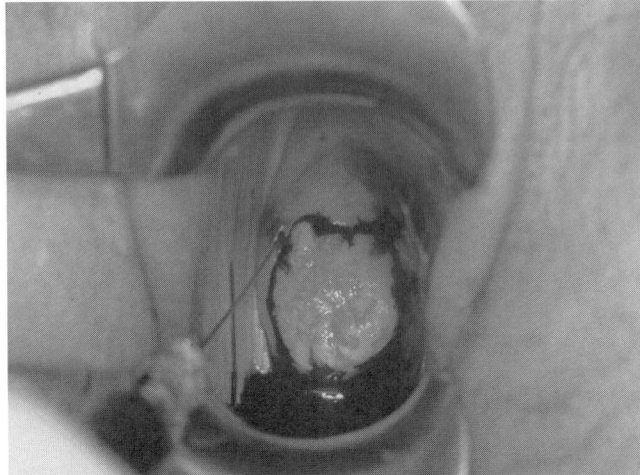

FIG. 13.10. Injection of the dye. The dye is injected into the tissue surrounding the tumor. The sentinel lymph node procedure should only be used for early-stage cancers. (See Color Plate.)

TABLE 13.3. Reports in the literature concerning sentinel node biopsy in early cervical cancer

Author (ref.)	No. of Patients	FIGO Stage	Injection technique	Surgical technique	SN detection/ no. of patients (%)	Average No. of SNs	Pathologic Assessment	No. of SN-positive patients (%)	No. of SN false-negative patients (%)
Echt, 1999 (147)	13	IB	B	Laparotomy	2 (15)	1.5	H & E	2 (100)	0
Medl, 2000 (148)	3	NS	B	Laparotomy	3 (100)	–	NS	3 (100)	0
O'Boyle, 2000 (149)	20	IB-IIA	B	Laparotomy	12 (60)	1.9	H & E	4 (33)	0[a]
Dargent, 2000 (20)	69[b]	IA2-IB1	B	Laparoscopy	59 (85)[b]	1.1 b	H & E	6 (10)[b]	0
Verheijen, 2000 (151)	10	IB	B and R	Laparotomy	8 (80)	1.8	IHC	1 (12)	0
Kamprath, 2000 (150)	18	I-II	R	Laparoscopy	16 (88)	–	–	1 (6)	0
Lantzsch, 2001 (157)	14	IB1	R	Laparotomy	13 (93)	2	IHC	1 (8)	0
Malur, 2001 (155)	50	I-IV	B and R	Laparoscopy	39 (78)[c]	2	H & E	5 (13)	1 (3)[d]
Levenback, 2002 (163)	39	I-IIA	B and R	Laparotomy	39 (100)	4.7	IHC	8 (20)	1 (3)
Barranger, 2003 (153)	13	IA-IIA	B and R	Laparoscopy	12 (92)	1.7	IHC	2 (15)	0
Lambaudie, 2003 (152)	12	IA2-IB1	B and R	Laparoscopy	11 (92)	1.7	IHC	2 (18)	1 (9)[e]
Buist, 2003 (156)	25	I-IIA	B and R	Laparoscopy	25 (100)	2.3	IHC	9 (36)	1 (4)
Plante, 2003 (158)	70	IA-IIA	B and R	Laparoscopy	61 (87)[f]	1.9	IHC	8 (11)	0
Dargent, 2003 (160)	139[g]	IA2-IB1	B	Laparoscopy	125 (90)[g]	1.1[g]	H & E	18 (14)	0
Dargent, 2004 (164)	29	IA2-IB1	B	Laparoscopy	29 (100)	2	IHC	5 (17)	3 (10)

B, blue dye; R, radioactive isotope; H&E, hematoxylin and eosin; NS, not significant; IHC, immunohistochemistry

[a]One pN1 patient among the eight patients with no SN detected (149).

[b]Sixty-nine pelvic sidewalls assessed in 35 patients.

[c]Detection rate: 55,5% with B alone, 76% with R alone, and 90% with B and R.

[d]Four pN1 patients among the eleven patients with no SN detected (155).

[e]one metastasis in one node of the only patient with no SN detected.

[f]Detection rate: 79% with B alone, 93% with R alone, and 93% with B and R

[g]One hundred and thirty-nine pelvic sidewalls assessed in 70 patients.

what the radioisotopic colloid used, the detection rate is generally higher and the number of detected nodes greater with the radioisotopic technique. It appears that the combination of blue dye and isotopes is the most accurate. The result of the radioisotopic injection can be assessed 3 hours after a lymphoscintigraphy (Fig. 13.11). The result of the blue dye injection is assessed at the time of surgery, which is performed soon after injection.

The surgery is performed in the usual fashion for laparoscopic pelvic surgery; usually within 12 hours of injection of the colloidal radioisotope and immediately after the injection of the blue dye. The procedure starts with the transperitoneal assessment. If the injection has been done correctly, the blue channels are located through the dorsal leaf of the broad ligament and traced from the center of the pelvis to the pelvic sidewall. The isotopic detection probe demonstrates where the injected nodes are situated (level of radioactivity ten or more times higher than the basic level). In order to dissect the nodes, the pelvic peritoneum is opened alongside the external iliac vessel axis, and the broad ligament is opened. Some surgeons, in particular those who use an isotope, immediately search for the SNs, whereas others first identify the blue channels and trace them to the SNs. Tech-

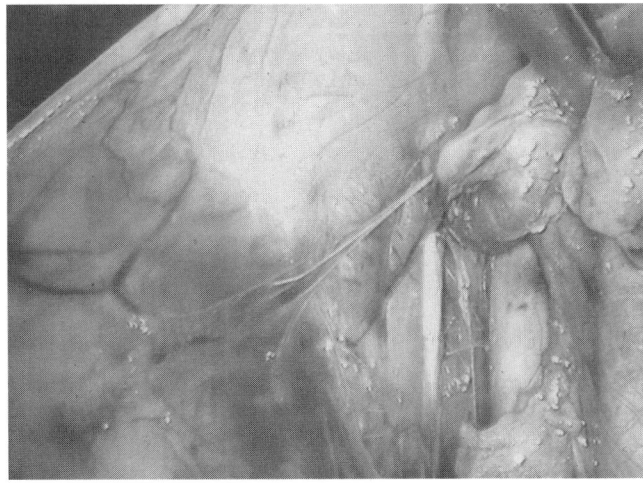

FIG. 13.12. Dissection of the sentinel node. The main lymphatic channel crosses the umbilical ligament and ends in a node situated between the external iliac vein and the obturator nerve. (See Color Plate.)

nique plays a major role in the chances for success, and may explain the variations in the "SN detection rate." It also may explain the great variations in the number and the topography of the detected nodes.

The use of blue dye will demarcate one or more lymphatic channels at the base of broad ligament. They run parallel to the uterine artery, cross the obliterated obturator artery, and end in a node situated in the so-called interiliac area; that is, at the bifurcation to the common iliac artery either medial or dorsal to the external iliac vein (Fig. 13.12) or between it and the external iliac artery. One node is usually found (or two or three juxtaposed micronodes). However, in 5% of the cases, injected nodes are found in two distant basins. At least one node should be found on each pelvic sidewall. In approximately 15% of cases (Fig. 13.13), the SN is located either in the region of the internal iliac artery or in the common iliac and/or low aortic area. Such results are usually observed when the dissection is performed by first identifying the blue lymphatic channels.

The results are quite different when isotopes are used. The number of SNs is higher. Reports generally do not specify if these more numerous nodes are found on one side only or on both sides. However, detected nodes are often found in distant basins. This means that the sensitivity of the isotopic technique is higher than the sensitivity of the blue dye technique. But this questions the specificity and even challenges the concept itself. Since SN dissection with a radioisotope may include multiple anatomic areas, it may tend to resemble a systematic dissection more than a true "sentinel node" biopsy.

Pathologic assessment of the SN can be performed by various techniques. Frozen section has been criticized because of the higher rate of false negatives. It does have the advantage of immediate answers in patients with metastasis

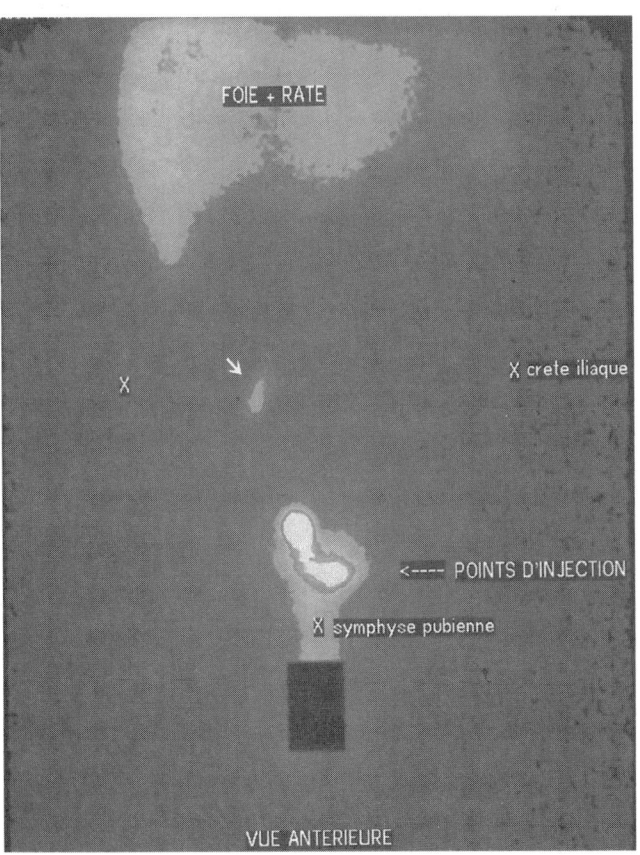

FIG. 13.11. Lymphoscintigraphy. One hot spot only is visible. No sentinel lymph node was detected on the left side. The sentinel lymph node on the right side was a common iliac node. (See Color Plate.)

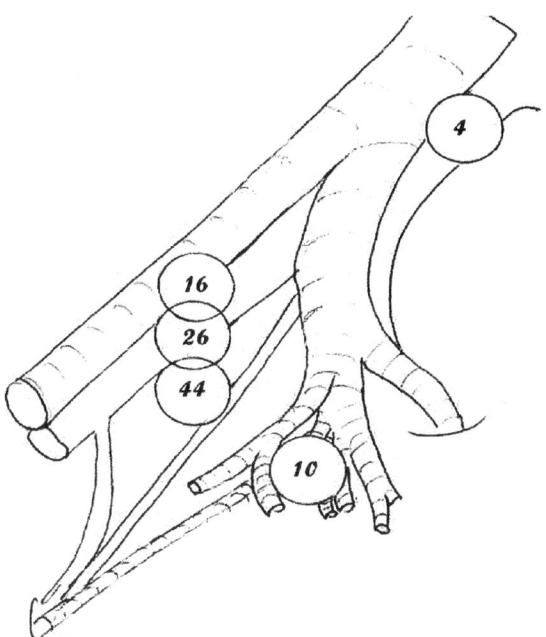

FIG. 13.13. Topography of sentinel node location. The most common place where the sentinel node is situated is at the contact of the external iliac vein, ventral to the origin of the uterine artery.

to the SN (no false positive). The classic unilevel sectioning after paraffin embedment and the hematoxylin and eosin (H&E) staining are the most widely used techniques. Micrometastasis, however, can be missed. Multilevel sectioning may help minimize this problem. The literature concerning the topic is very confusing. Ideally, the best technique is serial sectioning of the entire node with all slides being stained and assessed, but this is unrealistic. The semiserial sectioning entails examining slides at 40- to 200-μm (depending on institutional protocol) intervals. Even the so-called micromicrometastasis can thus be identified. Using immunostains can improve the sensitivity. The most common antibodies used in the current practice are those directed toward the cytokeratins. Very small clusters of epithelial cells (Fig. 13.14) and isolated epithelial cells can be identified that were previously impossible to identify after the standard H&E staining. However, if true serial sectioning is not employed, these epithelial cells can be missed as well. Molecular biology analysis for cytokeratins or human papillomavirus (HPV) may provide the highest sensitivity. Each group has its own personal technique, and this explains the great variability of the rate of positive and false-negative SNs reported in the literature. With the unilevel sectioning and classic H&E staining, the rate of SN positive is, in cervical cancer stage I B1, approximately 15%, and the rate of false-negative varies between 0% and 17%. Both rates are much higher if semiserial sectioning and immunostaining are used both for the assessment of the SN and the non-SN. In the Marchiole series (165), the rate of SN positivity

increased from 10.3% (3 of 29) to 27.5% (5 of 29) using semiserial sectioning and cytokeratin AE1 and AE3 immunostaining. However, the rate of false negative was also increased to 37% as three of the five micrometastases were discovered in non-SNs with the SNs being uninvolved. This questions the role of SN biopsy in the clinical management of early cervical cancer.

The goal of the SN concept is avoiding systematic dissection in patients who do not have node metastasis. This goal is reached if one does not consider micrometastasis as being clinically relevant. However, in spite of the fact that the clinical significance of micrometastasis is not clearly established, it seems oncologically safer to remove nodes that could be involved. On the other hand, laparoscopy makes systematic dissection a relatively safe and acceptable procedure that may be no more morbid than a laparoscopic SN biopsy. A reasonable strategy may include (a) laparoscopy with SN biopsy, (b) frozen sections of the SN, and (c) systematic dissection if the frozen section is negative. In the cases where either the SN biopsy or other nodes have metastasis, chemoradiation can be given. The risk for radiation enteritis is minimized by the decreased adhesion formation after laparoscopy.

The concept of SN biopsy has been tested in advanced cervical carcinoma. The detection rate is low, and the clinical value is only theoretical. In endometrial cancer, several publications (162,166,167) demonstrate similarities with the early cervical cancer model. Injections of the cervix give better results than injections of the fundus (166), which give rise to a larger amount of diffusion and results in a higher false-negative rate (50% in one of the published series) (162). Laparoscopy can also be used with SN biopsy in endometrial cancer. However, SN biopsy may not have the impact

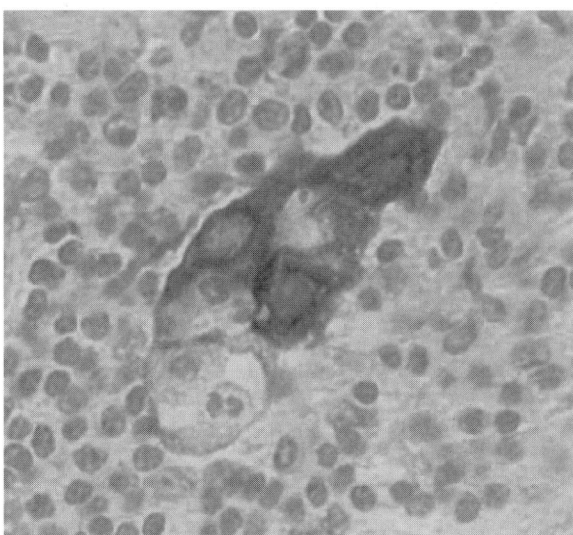

FIG 13–14. Micrometastasis. Immunohistochemistry can be used to identify micrometastasis in the sentinel lymph node. (See Color Plate.)

on the current management of endometrial cancer as it does with cervical cancer. In ovarian, tubal, and peritoneal cancers, the application of the SN concept is not to be likely applicable.

Extraperitoneal Laparoscopic Aortic Lymphadenectomy

Unlike pelvic lymphadenectomy, the use of the extraperitoneal approach to laparoscopically remove the aortic nodes followed the introduction of the transperitoneal technique. Transperitoneal laparoscopic aortic lymphadenectomy still remains the more common approach employed by the majority of gynecologic oncologists. However, this innovative extraperitoneal approach does have several advantages when compared to the transperitoneal technique and has gained increasing popularity.

An extraperitoneal approach to the aorta is begun by using a 3-cm incision made at McBurney's point (or at the point exactly opposite on the left side of the patient). The contralateral nodes can be removed using a one-sided approach. The left-sided approach is preferred for several reasons, which will be illustrated below. The successive layers of the abdominal wall are transected, including the parietal fascia, leaving the parietal peritoneum intact. Insertion of a transperitoneal laparoscopic trocar is recommended so that the area where the extraperitoneal dissection starts can be visualized to prevent entry into the peritoneal cavity. Once the parietal fascia is opened, the surgeon's forefinger is introduced into the extraperitoneal space and develops the retroperitoneal space along the psoas muscle and common iliac artery. With gentle blunt dissection, the peritoneal sac is elevated off the underlying structures. The second landmark is the iliac crest, which is followed laterally in order to open the inferior part of the side. At this time, a laparoscopic trocar with a pneumostatic tool (Blunt Tip Auto Suture, Norwalk, CT) is introduced.

Once the extraperitoneal space has been adequately developed, insufflation begins and the gas from the peritoneal cavity is drained, the extraperitoneal laparoscopic assessment can begin. This trocar accommodates one laparoscopic forceps, which is used to develop the extraperitoneal spaces to the level of the lower ribs. A second ancillary trocar is introduced in the infracostal area in the midaxillary line.

The video monitor is placed on the opposite side of the table from the surgeon as he or she seeks the first landmark (Fig. 13.15): the fascia of the psoas muscle. Detaching the peritoneum from the muscle reveals the second landmark, the ureter (Fig. 13.16); and then the third landmark, the ovarian vein, a fragile structure that must be handled carefully. After pushing the peritoneum medially, the common iliac vessels can be identified and the aortic dissection can begin. The lower aspect of the dissection is shown (Fig. 13.17).

The lateral aspect of the aorta is approached in a caudal to cranial direction. At the level of the origin of the inferior

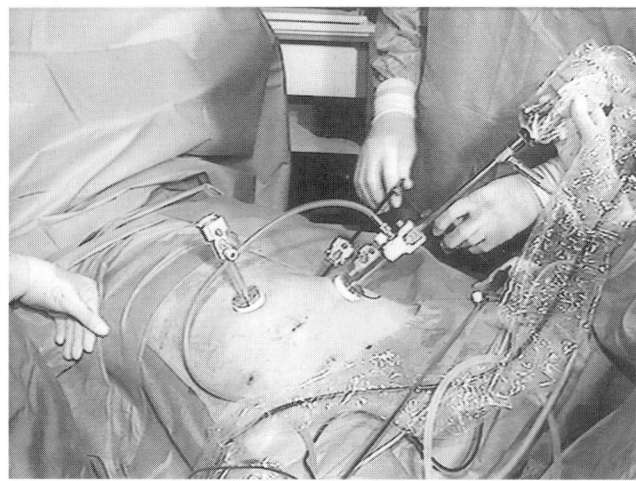

FIG. 13.15. Left-sided extraperitoneal laparoscopic approach. Position of laparoscopic trocar and ancillary trocars (the extraperitoneal approach is preceded by a transumbilical transperitoneal approach; the umbilical trocar is left in place after exsufflation). (See Color Plate.)

mesenteric artery, the dissection becomes more difficult owing to the presence of the lower mesenteric autonomic nervous plexus. There are no drawbacks in dividing this plexus in a woman. Once the nervous plexus is divided and the ventrolateral aspect of the aorta is freed up, the dissection is continued cranially up to the level of the left renal vein. This is the superior limit of the dissection of the left paraaortic lymph nodes. The anterior aspect of the completed dissection is shown (Fig. 13.18).

If one starts with the right-sided dissection, it is easy to remove the nodal tissue on the anterior aspect of the vena cava and the interaorticocaval space where the right lateroaortic nodes lie. However, the difficulty lies in reaching the left lateral aspect of the aorta. This is largely due to the

Left ureter

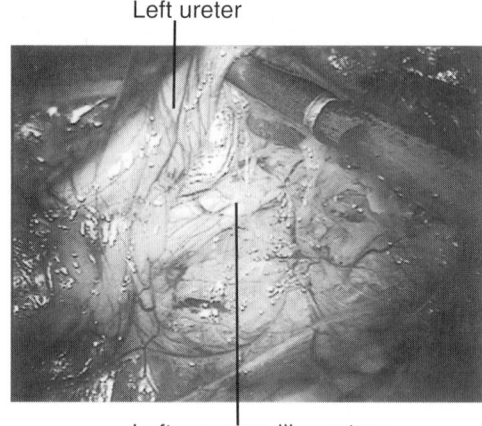

Left common iliac artery

FIG. 13.16. Left-sided extraperitoneal laparoscopic approach. The left ureter is pushed ventrally. The left common iliac artery is visible. (See Color Plate.)

Aorta

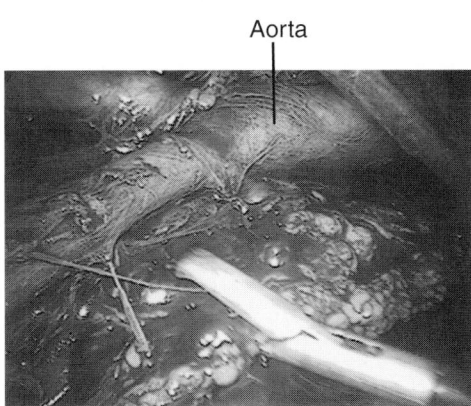

FIG. 13.17. Left-sided extraperitoneal laparoscopic approach. Picture taken at the end of the common iliac and lower aortic dissection. (See Color Plate.)

noncompressible nature of the aorta. Conversely, if dissection is started on the left side, exposing the right lateral aspect of the aorta can be simplified by dissecting from beneath the aorta. Hence, it is recommended to start with the left side and move to the right side only if difficulties arise. When comparing the unilateral to the bilateral approach, the total node counts of a unilateral left-sided approach have been shown to be comparable to those from a bilateral extraperitoneal approach and a transperitoneal approach; however, the right-sided node counts are significantly decreased compared to the bilateral approach (168).

During the unilateral left-sided technique, the separation of the left aortic nodes is performed either cranially to caudally or vice versa. The nodes are located between the artery and the psoas muscle. Separating these structures reveals the lumbar sympathetic chain and the vertebral vessels. Once the left aortic lymph nodes have been retrieved, attention now moves to the retroaortic space. The aorta is separated from the common ventral vertebral ligament. The aim of this maneuver is to remove the few nodes lying in the retroaortic space while exposing the nodes on the right side of the aorta

Aorta

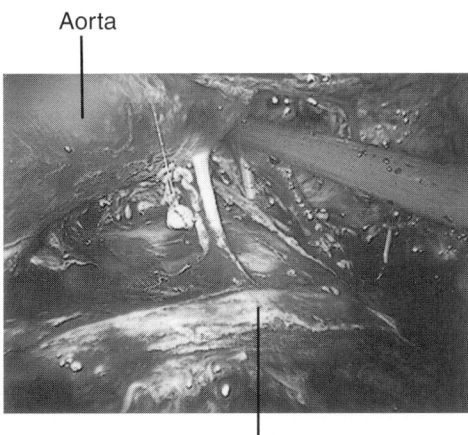

Sympathetic chain

FIG. 13.19. Left-sided extraperitoneal laparoscopic approach. Picture taken at the beginning of the retroaortic dissection: the lumbar arteries and veins are visible. (See Color Plate.)

and the interaorticocaval space. This dissection can be made in the spaces located between the successive lumbar arteries (Fig. 13. 19) but access to the interaorticocaval space is limited. It is better to divide the collaterals of the aorta: the fifth lumbar arteries in all cases and the fourth if needed. Division of these lumbar vessels opens the retroaortic space and simplifies the removal of the right aortic nodes (Fig. 13.20). The additional exposure allows the right laterocaval nodes to be removed via the retrocaval or the precaval routes. Dissection of these nodes is usually only performed for a right ovarian tumor. Thus, except for cases of ovarian cancer, there is no need to proceed this far if the caval dissection appears from the left side to be dangerous (owing to the distribution of the vertebral veins).

Reports on this particular approach are relatively sparse in the gynecologic oncology literature and have been limited

Inferior mesenteric artery

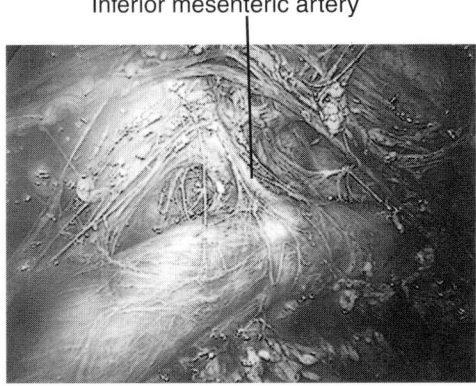

FIG. 13.18. Left-sided extraperitoneal laparoscopic approach. Picture taken at the end of the aortic dissection. (See Color Plate.)

Aorta

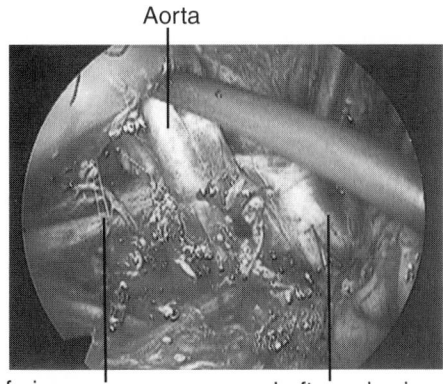

Inferior vena cava   Left renal vein

FIG. 13.20. Left-sided extraperitoneal laparoscopic approach. Picture taken after the lumbar arteries and veins have been divided and the interaorticocaval space appeared: the junction of the left renal vein and inferior vena cava is visible. (See Color Plate.)

to patients with cervical cancer. Vasilev and McGonigle (169) were the first to publish data on laparoscopic extraperitoneal paraaortic lymphadenectomy using a left-sided approach in humans. They reported an average of five nodes in four cases; the dissection was limited to the inframesenteric area. In a larger series, Querleu et al. used this technique to perform an infrarenal aortic dissection, and by doing such, the mean node count rose to 20.7 (170).

Recently, Sonoda et al. (171) reported on 111 patients with locally advanced cervical cancer who underwent surgical staging. This comprises the largest series to date using this novel approach for the management of locally advanced cervical cancer. In this study, 30 patients were found to have positive nodes. The mean duration of the procedure was 157 ± 46 minutes and the average number of nodes was 19. The mean postoperative stay was 2 days. Perioperative complications occurred in 14 patients. The majority of these complications were symptomatic lymphoceles that occurred in 11 patients: Eight of these lymphoceles were drained under radiologic guidance, two required a catheter placed under anesthesia, and one required laparoscopic drainage. In the final 37 patients, marsupialization of the peritoneum was performed to drain the retroperitoneal fluid into the peritoneal cavity. No further symptomatic lymphoceles were observed after adopting this maneuver. There were two retroperitoneal hematomas and one bowel obstruction from a trocar-site hernia. Only two patients in the series required a reoperation for a complication. Of the 30 patients with positive nodes, only the patient who had a trocar-site hernia that required small bowel resection developed radiation enteritis. This is consistent with the finding that the laparoscopic extraperitoneal approach is associated with less adhesion formation in the radiation field (172). The benefits of surgical staging of locally advanced cervical cancer remain controversial, and procedure-related morbidity must be taken into consideration. Thirty (27%) of 111 patients in this series were found to have positive lymph nodes in spite of negative imaging studies and received extended field radiation with or without chemotherapy. However, the overall survival was still significantly worse in this group of patients with positive aortic nodes.

The subject of surgical staging for locally advanced cervical cancer remains controversial and has been prospectively studied in only one small randomized trial (32). The primary objective of this study was to determine percentage of improvement in detection of paraaortic node metastasis with survival being secondary. Unfortunately, the study was closed prematurely because both a significantly worse progression-free and overall survival were identified in the group undergoing surgical staging. Treatment after the staging procedure was inconsistent and biased, thus tainting the conclusions on survival. Additionally, there was a background of unfavorable characteristics facing the surgically staged group. In general, the surgically staged patients were of higher stage, had larger tumor size, and fewer received

concurrent chemoradiation as compared to the patients who were clinically staged. These differences in variables did not reach statistical significance, but this was most likely due to the small sample size. In spite of this randomized prospective trial, the controversy on surgical staging for locally advanced cervical cancer still exists. Until definitive conclusions on the optimal management of locally advanced cervical cancer are reached, extraperitoneal laparoscopic aortic lymphadenectomy appears to be a reasonable approach for these patients when surgical staging is employed.

LAPAROSCOPIC ASSISTANCE TO RADICAL SURGERY AND LAPAROSCOPIC RADICAL SURGERY

Laparoscopy can be used to assist extirpative transvaginal surgery or it can be used to perform the entire operation, after which the specimen is removed transvaginally.

Laparoscopically Assisted Vaginal Hysterectomy and Laparoscopic Hysterectomy

The concept of laparoscopic assistance to vaginal hysterectomy emerged in 1984 (21) as a procedure for the management of benign conditions. Its use for the management of endometrial cancer was naturally foreseeable. The main contraindication to the vaginal approach in endometrial cancer was the inability to assess the ovaries and tubes, the peritoneal serosa, and the retroperitoneal spaces. This was made possible by using laparoscopic assessment of the pelvis before undertaking the hysterectomy. Laparoscopically assisted vaginal hysterectomy (LAVH) includes five types, which are listed here, and whose descriptions can be found elsewhere (173):

- Type 0: Laparoscopy is only used to assess the pelvic cavity and the organs it includes.
- Type 1: Laparoscopic management of inflammatory peritoneal adhesions and control of the round ligaments and infundibulopelvic ligaments.
- Type 2: Laparoscopic preparation and division of the uterine arteries.
- Type 3: Laparoscopic management of the paracervical ligaments.
- Type 4: Laparoscopic transection of the vagina, transvaginal extraction of the specimen, and laparoscopic closure of the vagina.

Type 4 LAVH corresponds to the total laparoscopic hysterectomy first described by Reich (174). This technique as well as others has been used in the field of endometrial cancer. Childers et al. (8) were the first to report on the combined use of laparoscopy with vaginal hysterectomy for the treatment of early-stage endometrial cancer. This group later reported on a series of 59 patients with clinical stage I endometrial cancer who were staged by this new procedure (125).

Their technique included an inspection of the intraperitoneal cavity, intraperitoneal washings, and LAVH. Patients with preoperative grade 2 or 3 tumors or grade 1 tumors with greater than 50% myometrial invasion underwent laparoscopic pelvic and paraaortic lymphadenectomy. Six patients had intraperitoneal disease. Two patients could not undergo laparoscopic lymphadenectomy secondary to obesity, and two patients required conversion to laparotomy for intraoperative complications. These reports stimulated the interest in laparoscopic management of endometrial cancer.

Laparoscopically Assisted Vaginal Radical Hysterectomy

The introduction of laparoscopy into the realm of gynecologic oncology was first proposed as a means of expanding the use of VRH for the management of cervical cancer. The laparoscope was to perform the lymphadenectomy before the radical hysterectomy, which was entirely done through the vaginal approach. Subsequently, the concept of laparoscopically assisted vaginal radical hysterectomy (LAVRH) appeared with variations in the degree of laparoscopic preparation for the vaginal part of the surgery with the ultimate development being the total laparoscopic radical hysterectomy.

Vaginal Radical Hysterectomy After Laparoscopic Staging

Type 0 LAVRH, although not discussed here, combines pelvic lymphadenectomy as previously described and a VRH whose description can be found elsewhere (175).

The first large series of LAVRH (5) reported on type 0 LAVRH. The technique was used until June 1992. At that time (unpublished data), the series included 95 cases. The mean duration of the laparoscopic staging was 60.4 ± 25.8 minutes. The Schauta-Stoeckel technique (less radical) was used in 28 cases and the Schauta-Amreich technique (more radical) was used in 67 cases. The mean duration of the surgery was 74 ± 31 minutes and 89 ± 26 minutes, respectively. No perioperative complication was observed with the Schauta-Stoeckel technique, whereas six complications were observed with the Schauta-Amreich technique: one cystotomy, four ureterotomies, and one proctotomy (all repaired immediately with no postoperative complications). Only one patient required reoperation for postoperative bleeding after a Schauta-Amreich procedure. Only 14 patients received transfusions. Among the 28 patients who underwent the Schauta-Stoeckel operation, 8 suffered from urinary bladder problems but only 1 had persistent dysuria after 6 months. Among the 67 patients who underwent the Schauta-Amreich procedure, 27 suffered the same bladder problems and 10 had persistent dysuria after 6 months.

Laparoscopic Vaginal Radical Hysterectomy

As with LAVH, there are different techniques between the two extremes of the spectrum; that is, laparoscopy for staging purposes only and laparoscopy for the entire procedure. The techniques first described were highly radical comparable to types 3 and 4 abdominal radical hysterectomy (ARH). A less radical approach appears to be possible leading to surgery like type 2 ARH. Laparoscopically assisted vaginal radical trachelectomy (LVRT) is a conservative modification of this less radical LAVRH.

Supraradical Laparoscopically Assisted Vaginal Radical Hysterectomy

Since 1992 a series (12,22,25,26,176) of reports have been published describing a variant of techniques of LAVRH that could be designated as type 3, and that involved preparation of the parametrium during the laparoscopic step. The common feature of these techniques was the quest for radicalness that was made possible by the laparoscope. In fact, one of the technical difficulties of the radical vaginal approach is the clamping of the parametrium close to the pelvic sidewall due to the obliquity of the latter to the former; this is in contrast to the oblique angle along which the "vaginal" surgeon naturally works. Alternatively, using an ipsilateral iliac laparoscopic port, one can operate in the plane of the pelvic sidewall, and using endoscopic staplers, bipolar cauterization, the argon-beam coagulator, or other devices, the surgeon can divide the parametrium at its lateral insertion. As a consequence, the operative specimen (Fig. 13.21) is very large; that is, identical to type 3 ARH. It can even be extended (26) by the addition of a piece of the "posterior parametrium"; that is, uterosacral ligaments, which are easily divided during laparoscopy.

In 1993, Kadar (176) reported an operative time of 10 hours. However, the postoperative course was uneventful

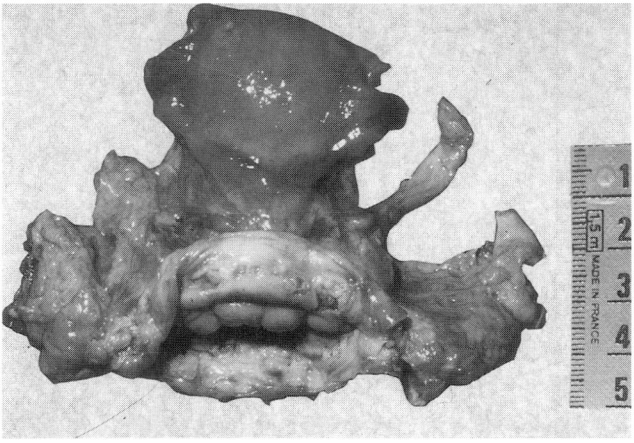

FIG. 13.21. Specimen of supraradical LAVRH (distal celio-Schauta). (See Color Plate.)

and the patient went back to work after 3 weeks. The operative time for the second patient was 8 hours. The blood loss was 2 L, and the postoperative pyelogram revealed a transection of the left ureter, which was reimplanted by laparotomy. Pulmonary embolism and vesicovaginal fistula occurred after the reoperation. Roy et al. (25) reported on 25 cases with a mean duration of the operation of 270 minutes. Two conversions to laparotomy occurred, one for an external iliac vein injury and the second for a cystotomy. One other cystotomy was repaired transvaginally. Five patients received a transfusion. These data were similar to those collected in a comparative group of 27 patients who underwent ARH. In the series of 37 cases reported by Hatch et al. (12), the mean operative time was 225 minutes. Two intraoperative bladder injuries and one large bowel injury occurred. Two postoperative ureterovaginal fistulas developed. Four patients required blood transfusion. When compared to a matched series of 30 patients treated by ARH, the mean operative time was significantly longer for LAVRH, but blood loss, rate of transfusion, and mean hospital stay were significantly lower for LAVRH. Martin (177) reported on Dargent's experience in 28 patients from June 1992 to June 1994. The mean duration of the operation was 204 minutes. Four complications occurred during the transvaginal portion of the surgery: one bladder injury, two ureteral injuries, and one internal iliac vein collateral injury. The first three injuries were repaired transvaginally. The bleeding complication was managed by laparoscopic reexploration, and eight patients received blood transfusions. During the postoperative course, a surgical reexploration was necessary in three instances: one for bleeding, one for incisional dehiscence, and one for intestinal obstruction. Fourteen patients suffered from bladder problems, and one had persistent dysuria after 6 months. Schneider et al. (26) reported a series of 33 patients. The mean operative time was 295 minutes. Three patients sustained injury to the bladder, one patient had injury to the left ureter, and another patient had an injury to the left internal iliac vein. Blood transfusions were necessary in four women.

Since 1999 a larger series has been compiled demonstrating that the oncologic outcomes are at an acceptable level. Operative complications are less frequent, which may be due to the "learning curve effect" as well as the trend toward less radical surgery. The standard operation of today ends up with an operative specimen that is similar to type 2 ARH (Fig. 13.22), but this is combined with laparoscopic paracervical lymphadenectomy to preserve the radical nature.

Modified Laparoscopically Assisted Vaginal Radical Hysterectomy

Laparoscopic Step. The route used for introducing the laparoscope can be either transperitoneal or extraperitoneal. Pelvic lymphadenectomy is performed first and then "para-

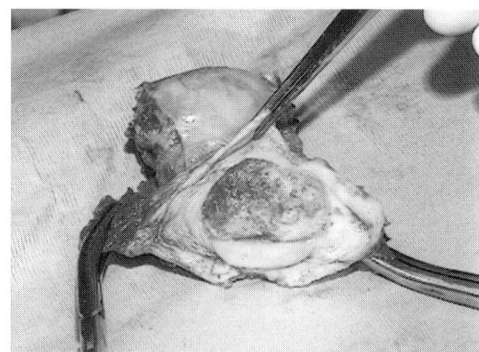

FIG. 13.22. Specimen of modified LAVRH (proximal celio-Schauta). (See Color Plate.)

cervical cellulolymphadenectomy." Paracervical cellulolymphadenectomy consists of removing all the lymph node–bearing tissues located in the vasculonervous web making up the lateral part of the paracervical ligament. It is a multistep procedure.

First, the "deep obturator nodes" (nodes located underneath the obturator nerve) are removed, which completely opens up the paravesical space, reveals the origin of the obturator vessels, and exposes the ventral surface of the paracervical ligament.

The dorsal aspect of the paracervix is exposed in the second step. The pararectal space opens when pushing the posterior sheet of the broad ligament, to which the ureter is attached, medially. Following the ureter ventrally, one arrives at the point where the ureter crosses the uterine artery. Starting from this point, the pararectal space is developed as far as the sacrospinous muscle. The fatty tissues lying between the ventral aspect of the sacrum, the lateral aspect of the rectum, and the medial aspect of the pelvic sidewall are removed. During this part of the procedure, one must proceed carefully owing to the confined nature of the pararectal space, especially on the left side where the presence of the left common iliac vein poses an added obstacle.

Once the two aspects of the paracervical ligament are exposed, the fatty tissue among the paracervical vascular network must be removed. This can be done by using the grasping and dissecting forceps similar to the technique that is recommended for pelvic dissection. This technique is better suited to paracervical dissection for which the use of scissors is dangerous. Another solution could be using a vacuum curette as recommended by Hockel (178) for open dissection. It is perfectly possible to adapt this technique to laparoscopic dissection, but with the disadvantage of working in a gasless environment.

The last step of the paracervical dissection is cleaning out the retrovascular area (i.e., the space located lateral to the common iliac vessels and medial to the psoas muscle). The lymph node–bearing tissues located in this space are quite abundant. One must take care not to injure the collateral vasculature from the common iliac vessels to the psoas muscle. Once the deepest part of the obturator nerve and the lumbosacral nerve crossing the sacroiliac joint have been identified, the procedure is completed (Figs. 13.2 to 13.4).

Since paracervical cellulolymphadenectomy has been performed, there is no need to divide the cardinal ligament at the level of its origin. The division can be performed in the mid part and is easiest when performed transvaginally. This is the rationale of the technique of LVRH recommended by Dargent and Querleu.

Transvaginal Step. The transvaginal portion of the Dargent and Querleu LAVRH simulates the modified VRH described by Stoeckel. In both, the paracervical ligaments are divided at an intermediate level. However, the technique differs in that no paravaginal incisions are used in the Dargent and Querleu LAVRH. Stoeckel made two incisions: one on each side of the patient.

The first step of the transvaginal operation is the formation of the vaginal cuff. A series of Kocher forceps is put onto the vaginal mucosa following a circular line located at the level of the junction between the upper and the middle thirds. Traction is exerted on the forceps, creating an internal vaginal prolapse. The two sheets of the vaginal fold raised by the traction are separated from each other by injection with saline midway between each traction forceps. The outside sheet of the fold is then divided. The division is gradually made outside a line drawn by exerting appropriate traction on each pair of forceps. The pressure on the scalpel blade must be released as soon as the saline drop appears, so as not to enter the opposite sheet of the fold. This full-thickness incision (incision of the three layers of the vaginal wall) is made only on the anterior and posterior aspects of the developed vaginal cuff (Fig. 13.23). Only the skin is incised on the dorsolateral aspects (between three and four o'clock and between eight and nine o'clock), so that the relationship between the vaginal cuff and the paracervical ligaments is maintained.

Once separated from the remainder of the vagina, the cuff

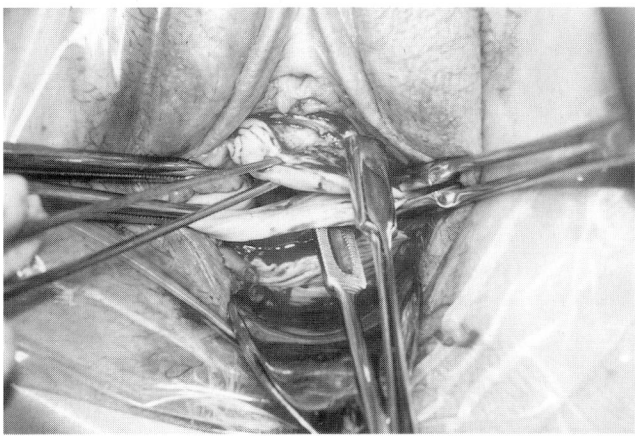

FIG. 13.24. Technique of modified LAVRH. Closing the vaginal cuff with Chroback forceps. (See Color Plate.)

is taken into strong grasping forceps that are aligned in a frontal plane (Fig. 13.24). It is retracted dorsally in order to free the ventral aspect of the vaginal cuff at the same time as the ventral aspect of the uterus and surrounding tissues (i.e., paracervical and parametrial ligaments). The bladder floor and terminal ureter are attached to these structures and must be separated from them. The vesicovaginal space is carefully developed in the midline so as not to injure the bladder, which is very close to the tips of the grasping forceps. Caution must be taken because of the condensation of the cellular tissue joining the bladder floor to the vagina. This condensation raises a pseudoaponeurotic coronal structure named the supravaginal septum, which must be perforated (Fig. 13.25) to reach the appropriate space. Once the midline intervisceral space has been opened, the bladder pillars can be approached.

The bladder pillars are divided in two steps. Initially, the pillar is separated into the lateral and medial parts by opening the caudal brim of the pillar at an equal distance from its

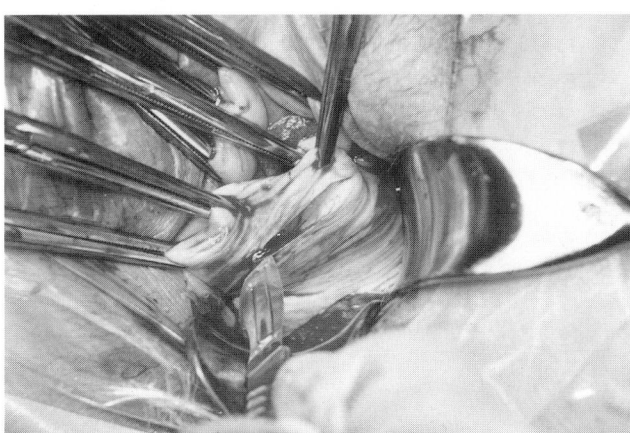

FIG. 13.23. Technique of modified LAVRH (proximal celio-Schauta). Incision of the vagina. (See Color Plate.)

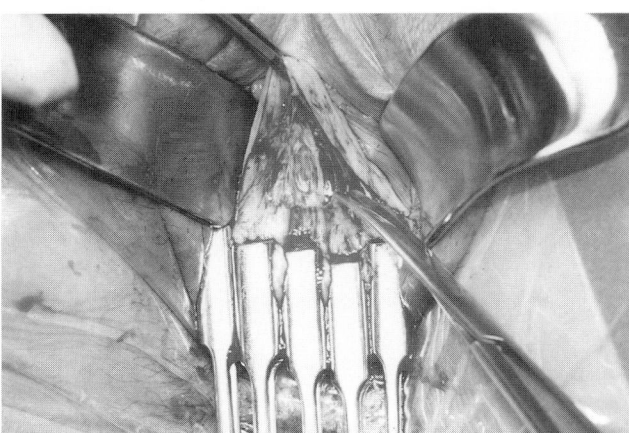

FIG. 13.25. Technique of modified LAVRH. Opening the vesicovaginal space. (See Color Plate.)

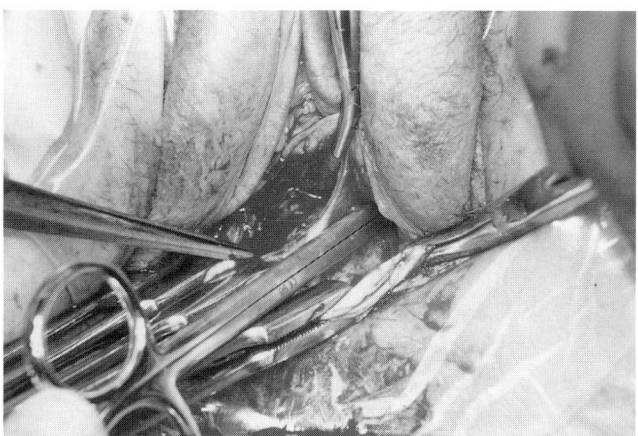

FIG. 13.26. Technique of modified LAVRH. Opening the paravesical space on the left side of the patient. (See Color Plate.)

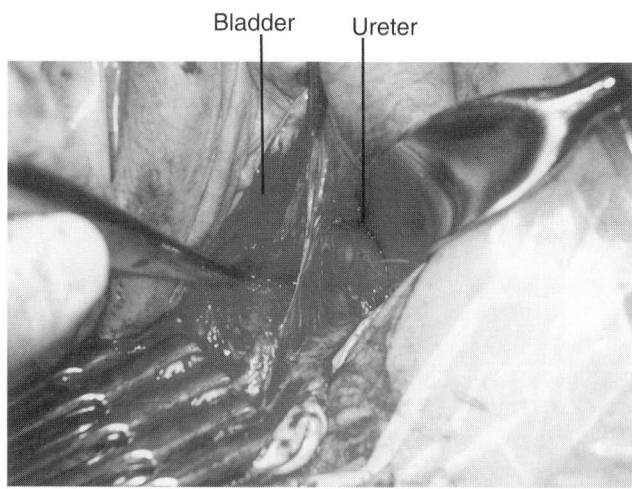

FIG. 13.28. Technique of modified LAVRH. The location where the ureter enters the bladder floor is visible. The medial fibers of the bladder pillar can be cut. (See Color Plate.)

two sides and two extremities. After opening, the scissors are pushed laterally (Fig. 13.26). One ensures that the instrument is placed lateral to the ureter by palpating and feeling the "plop." These fibers are divided after stapling or bipolar cauterization (Fig. 13.27), making the paravesical space wider. A bigger retractor is put in place and the knee of the ureter appears in the deepest part. Once the knee of the ureter has been identified, the medial fibers (Fig. 13.28) of the pillar can be divided. This division exposes the ventral aspect of the juxtauterine part of the paracervical ligament. The paraisthmic window (the inferior brim of which is the superior brim of the paracervical ligament) is identified by palpation. The arch of the uterine artery is located inside it. The afferent branch of the arch is isolated (Fig. 13.29) and dissected upward as far as the level of the knee of the ureter. Then the dissection is pushed further laterally inside the knee of the ureter and the artery is cut close to its origin.

Freeing the dorsal aspect of the vaginal cuff is easier than freeing its ventral aspect. The grasping forceps are retracted

ventrally. The pouch of Douglas is opened in the midline and the rectal pillars are divided; that is, the sacrouterine ligaments or, more precisely, the medial part of them (i.e., the rectouterine peritoneal folds). Once these ligaments have been divided, the dorsal aspect of the paraisthmic windows is palpated. Their inferior brim corresponds to the superior brim of the paracervical ligaments.

A right-angle dissector is pushed from back to front through the parauterine ligament. Opening the dissector frees the upper brim of the paracervical ligament. This is done while dividing the paracolpos; that is, the expansion that the paracervix sends to the vagina. This division is done by deepening the dorsolateral incision in the vagina and pushing

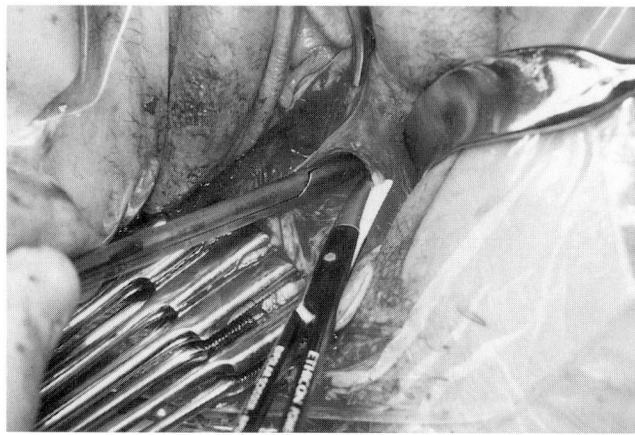

FIG. 13.27. Technique of modified LAVRH. Dividing the lateral fibers of the bladder pillar on the left side of the patient. (See Color Plate.)

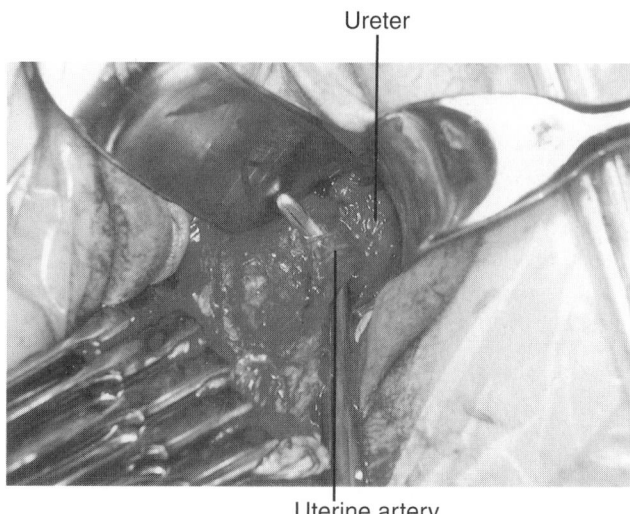

FIG. 13.29. Technique of modified LAVRH. The medial fibers of the bladder pillar have been divided; the arch of the uterine artery is demonstrated. (See Color Plate.)

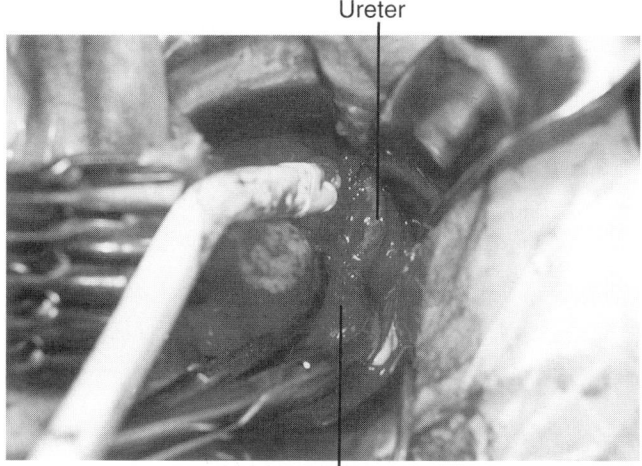

Ureter

Paracervical ligament

FIG. 13.30. Technique of modified LAVRH. Two clamps are put on the paracervical ligament, the distal one being just underneath the tip of the knee of the ureter. (See Color Plate.)

it laterally while controlling the bleeders encountered during this action.

Now that the dorsal and ventral aspects of the paracervical ligaments are both exposed with the superior and inferior brims, they can be divided. Two clamps are placed on each ligament, the most lateral being just at the contact of the tip of the knee of the ureter (Fig. 13.30).

Once the two paracervical ligaments have been divided, the operation can be completed without difficulty.

Sardi (179) reported on 47 patients who underwent a procedure closer to type 0 LAVRH than to type 3. After 4 years, the overall survival was 100% for stage IA, 88% for stage IB1, and 85% for stage IB2. Sardi suggested that 20 cases were needed to obtain the minimum skill to perform LAVRH. Renaud (133) reviewed the charts of 102 patients affected by cervical cancer who had laparoscopic lymphadenectomy followed by VRH or trachelectomy in 91 of them (stage IA in 77%, IB1 in 17%, and IIA in 6%). There were two intraoperative complications due to laparoscopy and four due to VRH; however, only one postoperative complication was considered to be major (an abscess which required surgical drainage). With a median follow-up of 36 months, there were four recurrences in 91 patients. Three of the intraoperative and postoperative complications occurred in the first 25 cases compared to four in the following 77 cases. Querleu (180) used personal interview and a standardized questionnaire in 60 of 95 patients who underwent LAVRH in order to assess the impact of the paracervical lymphadenectomy on late urinary bladder dysfunction. No difference was found between the patients operated before and after introduction of the new procedure. However, the paracervical dissection apparently failed to prevent the pelvic recurrences observed in the patients who had cancers 2

cm or greater. Six of 14 patients with tumors 2 cm or greater recurred with no difference being observed between those who underwent paracervical lymphadenectomy and those who did not. Conversely, only one recurrence was observed in the group of 81 patients affected by a tumor less than 2 cm. The uselessness of a very large surgery in small tumors is demonstrated in the Dargent's series (unpublished data). Among 216 patients affected by cervical cancer stages pIA2 and pIB1 who underwent LAVRH between December 1986 and May 2002, the actuarial 5-year disease-free survival was 94.2%. No recurrence was observed in the 144 patients with stage pIA and stage pIB1 <2 cm large cancers. Conversely, among the 72 patients affected by stage pIB1 ≥2 cm, the addition of a paracervical dissection was likely to decrease the risk of recurrence, which was as high as 18.9% during the first 3 years. Among the 53 patients followed during 3 years or more, the number of early recurrences were 3 of 11 after a proximal radical hysterectomy, 4 of 23 with a distal radical hysterectomy, and 3 of 19 with a proximal radical hysterectomy combined with a laparoscopic paracervical dissection. Hertel (181) reported on 200 patients with cervical cancer stages IA to IIIA treated in Jena using LAVRH, and confirmed that the incidence of complications decreased significantly when comparing the first half with the second half of the series (65% of the complications in the first half vs 35% in the second). This decrease could be linked to improvement in the technique (182,183). It could also be due to a change in the surgical radicality. In the reported series, the VRH was either performed according to the Schauta-Stoeckel technique that is similar to type 2 radical hysterectomy (102 cases) or according to a more extensive original technique (98 cases) described by Possover (184). At the time of the report, no change in the indications was formally introduced, but after having identified three independent risk factors for recurrence [TNM stage (IB2 or greater), lymph node metastasis, and lymphovascular space involvement], the investigators decided not to use LAVRH for high-risk cases and to reserve it only for low-risk cases. This resulted in a projected 98% 5-year overall survival rate, even when the more patient-friendly Schauta-Stoeckel technique was used (average duration of the surgery 298 minutes vs 371; $p = .0001$).

Laparoscopic Vaginal Radical Trachelectomy

Radical trachelectomy is a conservative variant of radical hysterectomy for young patients affected by early invasive cancer on the superficial aspect of the cervix. This operation was devised by the Romanian gynecologist Aburel using a laparotomy. None of his patients ever became pregnant. Postoperative adhesions, excessive tissue removal, and inaccurate isthmovaginal suturing were the probable causes for the lack of pregnancies in his patients. Using the laparoscopic vaginal approach allows successful outcomes.

The operation proceeds the same way as LAVRH. The

arch of the uterine artery is identified, and the uterine artery must be preserved. Once the arch is identified, the afferent branch is followed laterally, ensuring that no lymph node is located along its course (if so, this node is removed). Once this dissection has been completed, the dorsal aspect of the paracervical ligament and its superior and inferior brims are cleared. The paracervical ligament is then divided at the same level that it is divided in LAVRH. The clamps are put in place taking care not to compromise the uterine artery. The uterine artery collaterals going to the lateral fornix and to the cervix (cervicovaginal arteries) are controlled and divided. At this stage, the most important difference from LAVRH occurs: The uterus is divided 5 mm below the isthmus (Fig. 13.31), which is generally easy to locate owing to the previous dissections that have freed its anterior, posterior, and lateral aspects. The specimen is sent to the laboratory for assessment of its superior margin by frozen section. The cavity is sounded and a dilator is inserted to widen the canal and facilitate the reconstruction.

Once the results of the frozen section determine negative margins, the reconstruction is undertaken. Initially, the pouch of Douglas is closed with a circular running suture, including the posterior aspect of the supraisthmic part of the uterus and taking the stumps of the paracervical ligaments that reattach the uterus to its natural support. Isthmic cerclage, using the same suture used for the conventional prophylaxis of miscarriage, is then performed. Finally, the isthmovaginal suturing is performed using two Sturmdorf stitches approximating the vaginal mucosa and the isthmic mucosa with great care—the previous dilation facilitates this crucial step of the operation. The reconstruction is completed by three interrupted stitches in each lateral part and eventually results in a new os (Fig. 13.32).

The data on laparoscopic vaginal radical trachelectomy are sparse. After the first presentation made by Dargent et al. (185) in 1994, Schneider et al. (186) published two cases and then Shepherd (187) reported ten cases. The patients all had invasive cancer stage IB1 <2 cm in diameter. No complications were reported. Six pregnancies occurred after

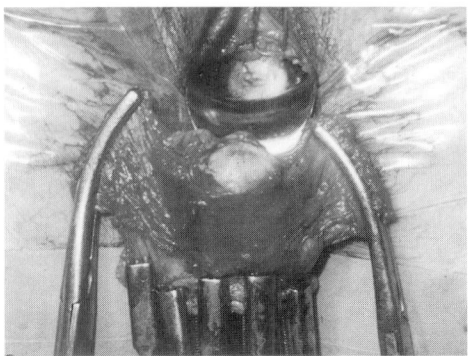

FIG. 13.31. Specimen of LVRT. The radicality is the same as in the modified LAVRH. The transected uterine isthmus is visible. (See Color Plate.)

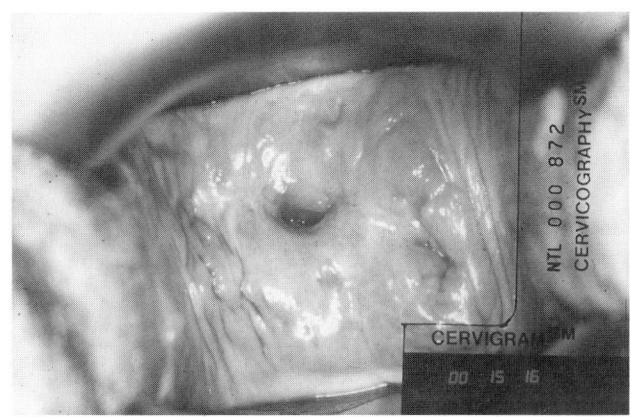

FIG. 13.32. Postoperative picture after LVRT. The contour of the cervix has disappeared but the uterine orifice remains patent. (See Color Plate.)

surgery and three live infants were delivered. One septic abortion occurred at 18 weeks and there were no recurrences. Roy and Plante (188) reviewed their first 31 cases in 1998. Most of the patients were stage IA and stage IB1 <2 cm in diameter. Only two patients had lesions >2 cm. Four complications required laparotomy: two external iliac vessel injuries during the laparoscopic step of the operation, one episode of intraoperative bleeding, and one bladder injury during the transvaginal step. Seven pregnancies occurred and four births were registered, one of them at 25 weeks of gestation. One recurrence was observed among the 26 patients followed for more than 6 months (median follow-up 25 months). The patient had a stage IIA 3-cm squamous cancer. Covens et al. (189) compared 31 patients treated with laparoscopic vaginal radical trachelectomy for stage IB1 cervical cancer <2 cm with two control groups, one matched and the other one unmatched (541 patients). The 2-year actuarial recurrence-free survival rates were 95%, 100%, and 98%, respectively. The cumulative actuarial conception rate at 12 months was 40%.

Dargent's experience was reviewed in May 2002 (190). Of the 96 patients with a follow-up of 1 to 15 years, one secondary cancer was observed (bilateral suprarenal gland cancer in a patient treated for neuroendocrine cancer of the cervix) and as well as four recurrences. The retrospective univariate analysis demonstrated that the maximal tumor diameter (≥ 2 cm) and the depth of infiltration (≥ 1 cm) were the only two significant factors of risk. The chance of recurrence was 0 for the small tumors, 19% for the tumors ≥ 2 cm (n = 21), and 25% for the tumors ≥ 2 cm with a depth of infiltration ≥ 1 cm (n = 19). The obstetric outcomes (unpublished data) were assessed at the same time. Forty-seven patients attempted to become pregnant, of which 36 succeeded and 11 did not (3 because of male factors). The 55 pregnancies ended with 11 early miscarriages, 8 late miscarriages, and 36 live births. No recurrences were reported in the 61 patients from Shepherd (191), Schlaerth (192), and

Burnett (193). However, Morice (194) reported the first central pelvic recurrence after radical trachelectomy. The tumor was 21 mm large, and the proximal tumor-free margin was only 4 mm. The recurrence developed on the isthmus 26 months after the surgery. Bernardini (195) reported on the obstetric outcomes of 30 patients attempting to become pregnant after radical trachelectomy, of which 18 succeeded and 12 did not. Among the 22 registered pregnancies, 3 resulted in first-trimester abortion and 1 in an induced 17-week abortion after rupture of the membranes. Of the 18 pregnancies lasting past the seventeenth week, all resulted in a viable birth, but 6 occurred at or before 36 weeks of gestation.

One might assume, from summarized data, that laparoscopic vaginal radical trachelectomy provides the same chances for survival as either VRH or ARH. The question remains, however, as to whether the operation is acceptable for tumors >2 cm in which the risk of recurrence is significant. There is no question about the absolute contraindication when the proximal tumor-free margin is too short (less than 10 mm). With regard to reproductive outcome, the main problem is miscarriage. Dargent's early experience suggests that cervical closure performed by the Saling method (196) at the end of the first trimester of pregnancy could improve the efficacy of the cerclage placed at the time of the initial procedure.

Laparoscopic Radical Hysterectomy

Laparoscopic radical hysterectomy was first introduced by Canis et al. (27) and shortly thereafter by Nezhat et al. (1992) (10). These two early cases were limited to stage IA2 tumors; however, as experience grew, the procedure was applied to larger tumors (197,198).

Spirtos soon described a standardized technique to perform what was termed a laparoscopic type 3 radical hysterectomy (199). He separated this operation into eight components: (a) right and left aortic lymphadenectomy, (b) right and left pelvic lymphadenectomy, (c) development of the paravesical and pararectal spaces, (d) ureteral dissection, (e) ligation and dissection of the uterine artery, (f) development of the vesicouterine and rectovaginal spaces, (g) resection of the parametria, and (h) resection of the upper vagina. All the steps are carried out with the laparoscope, including the vaginal closure. Spirtos uses staplers for transecting the parametria and an argon-beam coagulator for dissection of the uterine artery, ureter, and paravaginal tissue and to open the vagina. Other American surgeons have found this technique to be successful (29). However, the procedure can be performed with basic bipolar coagulation as well (200).

The duration of the first operative attempt on a 30-year-old patient with stage IA2 squamous cervical cancer (depth of infiltration 4 mm) was 8 hours (27). The postoperative course was uneventful. In the Nezhat's (197) series of seven patients published in 1993, the operating time was 315 minutes. One procedure was finished through laparotomy. No

serious complications occurred postoperatively. Sedlacek (201) reported 14 patients with stage IB cancer. Operative time was 7 hours. Four bladder injuries occurred and four ureterovaginal or vesicovaginal fistulas were observed postoperatively. Average blood loss was 334 mL versus 1,380 mL in a comparative series of patients treated by abdominal radical hysterectomy. In Spirtos' initial experience (199), all operations were completed laparoscopically. The average operation time was 253 minutes. No patient was transfused and there were no intraoperative or postoperative complications. In 1998, Canis (202) reported a study of 41 laparoscopic radical hysterectomies performed between November 1989 and September 1996. The mean duration of the procedure was 270 minutes. There were no major operative or postoperative complications. Only one patient required a blood transfusion. At 8 to 80 months of follow-up, no recurrence was observed (12 stage IA2, 24 stage IB, and five stage II).

When compared to ARH, total laparoscopic radical hysterectomy has been shown to be feasible, safe, and associated with low morbidity. Abu-Rustum et al. (29) compared a group of patients who underwent a laparoscopic radical hysterectomy with pelvic lymphadenectomy to a group of patients managed with laparotomy. Patient age, body mass index, stage, histology, and mean pelvic lymph node counts were similar in both groups. Although the median operative time for the laparoscopic procedure was significantly longer (360 vs 285, $p < .01$), the estimated blood loss and hospital stay were significantly less.

Recently, follow-up data on the oncologic outcomes have been reported. In the largest series to date, Spirtos et al. (28) reported on 78 consecutive patients who underwent laparoscopic radical hysterectomy with aortic and pelvic lymphadenectomy. The average operative time was 205 minutes (150 to 430 minutes) and the average blood loss was 225 mL (range 50 to 700 mL). With a mean follow-up of 66.8 months ($\pm$ 1.78 months), the estimated 5-year disease-free survival was 89.7% and the estimated 5-year overall survival was 93.6%. Similar survival data have been reported by other groups performing laparoscopic radical hysterectomy (203). Pomel et al. reported a 5-year survival rate of 96% in 50 patients with stages IA2 and IB1 cervical cancers treated with laparoscopic radical hysterectomy (203). Laparoscopic radical hysterectomy appears to be a reasonable option for patients with early-stage cervical cancer.

Laparoscopic Pelvic Exenteration

Using the laparoscope to assess the feasibility of pelvic exenteration was addressed for the first time by Plante (204) and subsequently reported by Köhler (205). Pomel (31) extended the procedure by actually performing a total laparoscopic pelvic exenteration with a small incision to create an ileal conduit and the diverting ileostomy. The operative time was 9 hours, and the postoperative course was uneventful.

One can imagine that the complementary reconstruction will eventually be performed with a closed abdomen as well!

LAPAROSCOPY AND CANCER OF THE CERVIX

Although more than a century has passed since the first radical hysterectomy was performed by Clark (206), the role of surgery in the management of cervical cancer still remains a matter for debate. It is generally accepted that early cases can be managed using surgery or radiotherapy. Advanced cases must be treated using radiotherapy. The controversy arises from the many discrepancies existing among the definition of early and advanced cases. For some experts, the concept of ruling out surgery in the management of bulky but resectable tumors appears to be inappropriate considering that these tumors are less likely to be cured by radiotherapy. What should be the place of laparoscopic surgery in this controversial area of management? For simplification, the question will be addressed separating tumors <4 cm from tumors ≥4 cm and greater.

Early Stages

Surgery and radiotherapy produce comparable survival in the treatment of early cervical cancer (207). Even if the question of cost effectiveness is not clearly settled, the majority of gynecologic oncologists have a preference for surgery, especially in young patients whose ovarian function can be preserved. Data obtained from the extensive use of radical surgery have demonstrated that the chances for cure depend in large part on the state of regional lymph nodes (208,209). For tumors <4 cm in diameter, the 5-year disease-free survival is approximately 90% as long as the nodes are negative and approximately 60% if one or two nodes are involved. Disease-free survival drops to 15% if three or more nodes are involved. The opportunity to identify nodal spread is one of the advantages of a surgical versus a radiotherapeutic approach. However, when nodal spread is discovered after surgery is completed, it only serves to help adjust adjuvant therapy that has a low efficacy (62,210–212). Knowledge of lymph node status before the onset of radiotherapy is obviously better. Here lies the first indication for laparoscopy—the assessment of the regional lymph nodes to help decide on treatment modalities.

Staging

If accepted, the concept of pretherapeutic laparoscopic staging raises a series of practical questions, which we will try to answer in the order they appear in daily practice.

Prelaparoscopic Imaging

The sensitivity and specificity of computed tomographic (CT) scanning are approximately 60% and 85%, respectively (213). Lymphangiography has a slightly better accuracy, but it cannot be easily obtained in many centers. CT scanning [and/or magnetic resonance imaging (MRI)] must be performed in every case, and if enlarged nodes are detected, they must be assessed by guided biopsy. If the biopsy reveals metastatic involvement, there is no point in performing a laparoscopy. If the biopsy is negative, laparoscopy should be undertaken.

Sentinel Node Biopsy

Although SN biopsy does not replace systematic lymphadenectomy, it deserves to be implemented in all cases. The first reason is that there are no false positives. Since involved lymph nodes can lead to altered therapy, the information is priceless. For the pathologist, identification of the node(s) at greatest risk for metastasis may help minimize the false-negative rate. The final (and possibly the best) reason for performing SN biopsy is that the scientific community needs more data and should encourage surgicopathologic studies regarding this matter.

Management of Bulky Nodes

Even if prelaparoscopic imaging does not suggest suspicious lymph nodes, it is still possible to encounter an obviously metastatic node. Freeing such a node laparoscopically is technically possible (127) even if vascular adhesions exist. One should, however, refrain from undertaking this dissection because of the hazard of tumor dissemination from nodal rupture. Two options for management are suggested: (a) referring the patient to the radiotherapist after having documented the metastatic involvement by fine-needle aspiration or (b) opening the abdomen and performing nodal debulking.

Pelvic Versus Pelvic and Aortic Lymphadenectomy

In the cases where the pelvic lymph nodes appear to be uninvolved neither at prelaparoscopic imaging, laparoscopic assessment, nor at frozen section (frozen sections done on the SN and on the other pelvic nodes), the question is whether an aortic dissection has to be added. The risk of involvement of the aortic nodes is small if the pelvic nodes are negative (214) Therefore, we assume that aortic dissection is not indicated. If pelvic node involvement is found at the time of the initial laporoscopic staging, one should perform a paraaortic dissection using the same approach—the transumbilical transperitoneal one. If the pelvic node involvement is discovered at final pathology (no frozen sections during the initial procedure or a false negative of the frozen section: 20% to 40% of the cases), aortic dissection is performed at a second surgery. We recommend using the left-side extraperitoneal approach to do this. The dissection has to be extended up to the level of the left renal vein because isolated supramesenteric metastasis can exist (142).

Proposed Algorithms

Many opinions exist as to the exact role of lymphadenectomy in the management of early cervical cancers. The lymphadenectomy itself clearly plays a role in prognosis as nodes are found to be apparently free. Radiotherapy given as adjuvant treatment to the pN1 patients decreases the chance of recurrence; however, it can produce iatrogenic complications such as radiation enteritis, which is increased if radiation follows surgical dissection (207). Taking these facts into account, some oncologists abort surgery as soon as they know that lymph node involvement exists. Others may proceed with radical surgery in spite of nodal disease, and in such cases, these surgeons deny any value to laparoscopic staging. The former group may have interest in laparoscopic staging, but the question remains of how to adopt this in the pN1 cases. The proposed algorithms (Figs. 13.33 and 13.34) represent a compromise taking into account the truth in surgical dissection for the patients with limited nodal involvement and the necessity of radiotherapy in all pN1 cases. If bulky nodes are noted at laparoscopy, debulking probably is useful (215,216), but it appears to be safer to do such by laparotomy.

If the nodes appear to be endoscopically normal but are involved on frozen section, the decision depends essentially on the number of involved nodes. If this number is less than three, radical surgery is a reasonable choice. We prefer performing it by laparotomy for safety (and rapidity) reasons. If the number of positive lymph nodes exceeds two, primary chemo-radiotherapy is the best option, and we recommend aborting the radical hysterectomy.

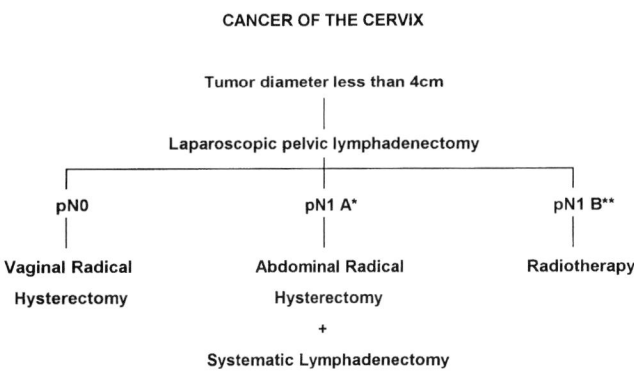

CANCER OF THE CERVIX

Tumor diameter less than 4cm

Laparoscopic pelvic lymphadenectomy

pN0 — pN1 A* — pN1 B**

Vaginal Radical Hysterectomy

Abdominal Radical Hysterectomy
+
Systematic Lymphadenectomy

Radiotherapy

* pN1A = 1 or 2 Positive Lymph Nodes

** pN1B = 3 or more Positive Lymph Nodes

FIG. 13.34. Algorithm for laparoscopy in early cervical cancer (2).

If the nodes are normal, radical surgery is the treatment of choice. The laparoscopically assisted and the purely laparoscopic radical hysterectomies are offered as alternatives to classic ARH.

Laparoscopic Assistance to Radical Surgery

After deciding to use the laparoscopic approach for performing radical hysterectomy, one must decide between the various forms of laparoscopic assistance to VRH and purely laparoscopic radical hysterectomy. The data concerning both types of approaches have been addressed in the previous sections of this chapter. We favor the combined approach for three reasons. The first is the purely laparoscopic approach requires a large degree of manipulation of the tumor; whereas, in laparoscopically assisted operation, there is no tumor manipulation during the laparoscopic step and the tumor is protected inside the vaginal cuff at the beginning of the vaginal step. The second reason is the vaginal approach allows easy management of the juxtauterine tissues, especially the vesicovaginal spaces, bladder pillars, and parametrium. Additionally, delineation of the vaginal cuff is much more precise using the vaginal route. The third and most important reason favoring the mixed approach is that this is good training for performing radical vaginal trachelectomy.

Advanced Cases and Recurrences

Radiotherapy given for advanced cervical cancers fails in two of three cases because of extrapelvic recurrences. These recurrences arise mostly in the abdominal cavity either extraperitoneally (aortic nodes) or intraperitoneally. One way of tackling this problem could be to give systematic extended-field radiotherapy. However, a prospective study (217) in which extended-field radiotherapy was given either routinely or after lymphangiographic selection did not yield the expected results. Moreover, extended-field radiotherapy in-

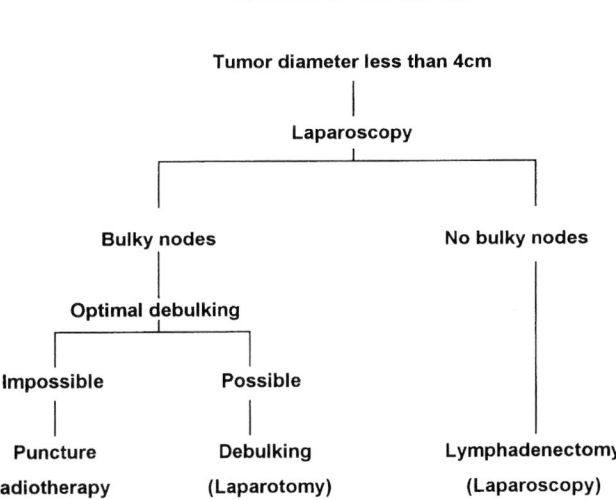

CANCER OF THE CERVIX

Tumor diameter less than 4cm

Laparoscopy

Bulky nodes — No bulky nodes

Optimal debulking

Impossible — Possible

Puncture Radiotherapy

Debulking (Laparotomy)

Lymphadenectomy (Laparoscopy)

FIG. 13.33. Algorithm for laparoscopy in early cervical cancer (1).

cludes a risk of severe complications close to 20% (218). Thus, the indications for its use must be limited to appropriately selected cases.

Staging laparotomy was devised as an answer to the question of selection of the indications for extended-field radiotherapy. It has some success in spite of its drawbacks, which include intraoperative and postoperative complications and enhanced risk of radiation enteritis because of peritoneal adhesions resulting from surgery. A GOG study (219) demonstrated that an extraperitoneal approach decreases these drawbacks, and laparoscopy may produce an even better result.

Laparoscopic staging of advanced cervical cancer can be performed using the classic transumbilical transperitoneal approach, which enables the surgeon to assess the peritoneal cavity and perform pelvic and aortic dissections. A more conservative approach could be limiting dissection to the pelvic area and going further only in the cases where the pelvic nodes are involved. Another approach entails using transumbilical laparoscopy only for assessing the peritoneal cavity and guiding digital preparation preceding extraperitoneal aortic dissection (discussed above). Most important in the selection of extended-field radiotherapy are (a) peritoneal cytology and (b) the status of the aortic nodes. The status of the pelvic lymph nodes does not alter pelvic radiation fields. This highlights the benefits of the combination of transumbilical laparoscopy and extraperitoneal dissection. It is the ideal way to perform laparoscopic staging in the management of advanced cervical cancer (Fig. 13.35). The benefits of this staging should not be overestimated since using laparoscopy in place of laparotomy only avoids the deleterious effects of operative adhesions but does not increase survival.

An additional benefit of pretherapeutic laparoscopy is the possibility of performing ovarian transposition for patients less than 40 or 45 years of age. Studies demonstrate that laparoscopic transposition is both feasible and effective (220).

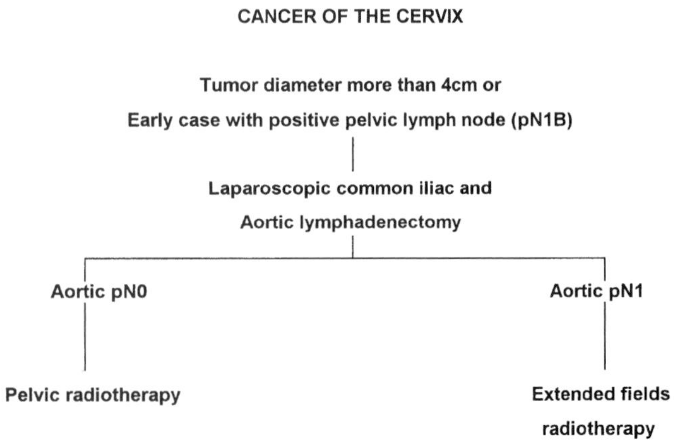

CANCER OF THE CERVIX

Tumor diameter more than 4cm or

Early case with positive pelvic lymph node (pN1B)

|

Laparoscopic common iliac and

Aortic lymphadenectomy

|

Aortic pN0   Aortic pN1

Pelvic radiotherapy   Extended fields

radiotherapy

FIG. 13.35. Algorithm for laparoscopy in advanced cervical cancer.

An additional indication for combined laparoscopic assessment is selection for pelvic exenteration in patients diagnosed with pelvic recurrence of cervical cancer (204,205). Both positive peritoneal cytology and positive aortic nodes are contraindications to exenteration. As previously mentioned, it is advantageous to identify these findings without having to perform a laparotomy.

LAPAROSCOPIC SURGERY AND ENDOMETRIAL CANCER

No disputes exist with regard to the place of surgery in the treatment of endometrial cancer. Hysterectomy and bilateral salpingo-oophorectomy are part of all traditional treatment protocols. Total hysterectomy has been traditionally performed through an open approach to assess completely the peritoneal cavity and perform lymph node sampling or lymphadenectomy. Vaginal hysterectomy has been used in the management of endometrial cancers in certain situations (221). However, the vaginal route does not allow for the evaluation of the peritoneal cavity or the retroperitoneal lymph nodes. Minimally invasive surgery has become increasingly popular in the management of gynecologic malignancies. With the development of improved instruments and surgeons' skills, laparoscopic surgeons began to perform more complicated procedures including sampling of the retroperitoneal lymph nodes.

Using a combined laparoscopic and vaginal approach, all the procedures required for endometrial cancer surgery can be accomplished. Complete assessment of the peritoneal surfaces and retroperitoneal dissection is possible. Thus, the addition of laparoscopy transforms the basic transvaginal hysterectomy into an oncologic complete operation. Minimally invasive management of endometrial cancer is appealing, and does not require long training. This explains why the use of LAVH in the treatment of endometrial cancer gained popularity long before LAVRH in the treatment of cervical cancer.

Feasibility studies concerning minimally invasive surgery in endometrial cancer are becoming more numerous. In addition to the two series mentioned earlier (42,125), there are other reports (224–226) that confirm the previous data. However, we are still awaiting the results of well-designed prospective randomized trials. In the joint series of Querleu and Dargent (unpublished observations), 111 laparoscopic staging procedures for endometrial cancer from January 1987 to June 1998 were reviewed. Laparoscopy was associated with node dissection only in 6.0%, with vaginal hysterectomy only in 13.5%, and with both node dissection and vaginal hysterectomy in 75.0% of the cases. Conversion to laparotomy was necessary in 5.55% of the cases. The mean operative time was 157 + 51 minutes. Two intestinal injuries and two bladder injuries occurred, which were repaired without subsequent problems. No complications occurred during the postoperative period. Infectious morbidity was 3%. Seven symptomatic lymphocysts and two tumoral implants (one umbilical and one perineal episiotomy) were observed.

The advantages of LAVH have been illustrated when compared to abdominal hysterectomy for the management of early-stage endometrial cancer. In a retrospective review of 320 patients, Gemignani et al. (227) demonstrated that LAVH was associated with a decreased hospital stay, fewer complications, and resulted in less overall hospital charges. Others have also demonstrated significantly lower hospital costs when patients with early endometrial cancer are managed by laparoscopy (139), but total costs may be higher when surgeons' fees are added (228).

Patients who undergo laparoscopic surgery seem to report a higher level of satisfaction with laparoscopy when compared to patients treated with total abdominal hysterectomy. They benefit from a shorter recovery time and are able to return to work and full activity more quickly (228).

Laparoscopic lymph node sampling seems to be comparable to the traditional laparotomy approach. In a comparison of the two techniques, Boike et al. (229) demonstrated that there was no significant difference in the number of lymph nodes obtained. Recurrence rates also appear to be comparable in retrospective studies, and survival of women with early-stage endometrial cancer does not appear to be compromised by laparoscopy (228).

The combined laparoscopic and vaginal approach to the management of endometrial cancer has been prospectively compared to the abdominal approach in several small studies. Malur et al. (230) compared 37 patients treated by a laparoscopic and vaginal approach to 33 patients treated by laparotomy. All patients underwent pelvic and aortic lymph node dissection except for patients with well-differentiated tumors that invaded to less than the inner third of the myometrium. There was no difference in the mean Quetelet index (QI), mean number of lymph nodes, and mean operation time. The laparoscopic group did have less blood loss, fewer transfusions, and shorter hospital stay. With a mean follow-up of 16.5 (2 to 43) and 21.6 (2 to 48) months for the laparoscopic and laparotomy groups, respectively, the recurrence-free and overall survival were not significantly different (97.3% vs 93.3% and 83.9% vs 90.9%, respectively). Other small prospective trials have demonstrated the association of laparoscopy with less blood loss and shorter hospital stay in the management of endometrial cancer (231).

Since obesity is a major risk factor for the development of endometrial cancer, many patients will present with a high QI. Performing a staging procedure in an obese patient can be difficult, but may not be an absolute contraindication. Scribner et al. (232) reported on their experience of laparoscopic pelvic and paraaortic lymphadenectomy in the obese patient. In 55 patients, laparoscopic staging was completed in 44% of patients with a QI $\geq$35 compared to a completion rate of 82% in patients with a QI <35 ($p = .004$). In spite of this difference, Scribner et al. concluded that obesity is not an absolute contraindication to laparoscopic staging. Similarly, the same investigators studied the surgical management of a group of patients 65 years or older with endometrial cancer. Although the operating room time and transfusion rate were significantly higher in the patients managed by laparoscopy compared to laparotomy, laparoscopy was associated with decreased hospital stay, less postoperative ileus, and less infectious complications with comparable blood loss and node counts. Scribner et al. concluded that older age was not an absolute contraindication to laparoscopic staging (233).

The issue of retrograde seeding with the use of a uterine manipulator has been addressed by Sonoda et al. (234) In a retrospective study of 377 patients with early-stage endometrial cancer treated with either LAVH or total abdominal hysterectomy (TAH), the investigators found that patients in the LAVH group had a significantly higher incidence of positive peritoneal washings (10.3% vs 2.8%, $p = .002$). The two groups did not differ in known prognostic factors; thus, Sonoda et al. hypothesized that this finding may be caused by the routine use of an intrauterine manipulator during the LAVH procedure in this series. A subsequent report by Vergote et al. (235) similarly reviewed their experience with endometrial cancer patients treated with either LAVH or TAH. At their institution, the use of a uterine manipulator was not routinely used, and no difference in positive peritoneal cytology was observed. Although LAVH with intrauterine manipulation may be associated with an increased incidence of positive peritoneal cytology, this finding alone does not appear to have a detrimental clinical impact (236).

Laparoscopic surgery for the management of endometrial cancer undoubtedly has its limitations. Large fibroid uteri that cannot be removed without morcellation should not be operated on using laparoscopic surgery if endometrial cancer is present. Placing such unusual situations aside, the preliminary results for the use of laparoscopy are encouraging. Given this, the GOG is conducting a large prospective trial to determine the equivalency in terms of cancer outcome of LAVH with surgical staging compared to the traditional laparotomy approach. A quality of life instrument is included in this study and should provide additional information regarding laparoscopic management. However, until the results from this trial are available, many still consider the abdominal approach to represent the standard of care.

LAPAROSCOPY IN OVARIAN CANCER

Laparoscopy can be used in several different ways in the management of ovarian cancer depending on the stage of the disease and the anticipated goals of the procedures.

Advanced Ovarian Cancer

In patients with advanced ovarian cancer characterized by ascites, carcinomatosis, and omental cake, optimal surgical debulking may not be feasible even by laparotomy. Unfortunately, there is no perfect tool to determine preoperatively whether patients can be optimally debulked surgically. CT scan often underestimates the extent of the disease; in particular the extent and location of carcinomatosis. Nelson et al. have proposed a set of criteria that appears to predict accurately the inability to debulk patients surgically (237). They found that CT scan was highly sensitive for detection of ascites and mesenteric and omental diseases, but was poor for detection of liver involvement, omental attachment to the spleen, gallbladder fossa disease, and peritoneal nodules <2 cm (237). In the early 1990s, Schwartz et al. pioneered the concept of neoadjuvant chemotherapy in patients with advanced disease with the goals of chemoreducing the tumor bulk and then using surgical debulking for those who show a good response to the chemotherapy (238,239). Recent studies suggest that quality of life is improved with this approach (240). However, other malignancies, particularly of gastrointestinal (GI) origin (such as colon, pancreas, stomach, and others), can mimic ovarian cancer. In some series, up to 20% of patients with presumed advanced ovarian cancer had a GI primary malignancy (241) due in part to inconclusive cytologic examination of ascitic fluid. Some, however, have argued that it is extremely accurate and helpful (242).

In cases where the diagnosis remains unclear, histologic confirmation of an ovarian primary malignancy is critical before initiation of chemotherapy. However, an adequate biopsy specimen cannot always be safely obtained under radiologic guidance. This is where laparoscopy becomes a valuable diagnostic tool. Indeed, the laparoscopic exploration of the abdominal cavity allows the surgeon to determine whether the disease can be optimally surgically debulked or not. If so, then a laparotomy can be performed to complete the surgery. If not, an adequate tissue specimen can be obtained for histologic confirmation. In a recent series of 18 patients with ovarian cancer explored laparoscopically, 7 (40%) were found to have unresectable disease and were spared a laparotomy. In the remaining patients, a laparotomy was performed and complete debulking was accomplished (243). However, the diagnostic laparoscopic procedure can have some pitfalls: First, the presence of a large amount of ascites may lead to a reduced visibility; second, the GI anatomy can be distorted, the colon and/or small bowel may be adherent to the anterior abdominal wall or omentum, which may increase the risk of bowel injury. An open laparoscopic approach may be preferable in such cases, although a recent large trial does not seem to indicate that open laparoscopy reduces the risk of major complications (40). Finally, the issue of trocar-site implantation remains controversial, particularly in patients with adenocarcinoma, ascites, and carcinomatosis (see section on port-site metastasis above). However, when trocar sites are carefully closed after the procedure and the chemotherapy initiated within 1 week, the risk of trocar-site metastasis can be reduced substantially (244,245). In cases of advanced ovarian cancer, laparoscopy appears to be a good triage method to select out patients who would not benefit from a laparotomy and can thus be spared the associated morbidity.

Second-look Surgery

For those who perform second-look evaluation following first-line chemotherapy, laparoscopy may be a valuable approach to reduce the morbidity of the procedure. The magnification of the view allows a good evaluation of the peritoneal surfaces; in particular the costodiaphragmatic recessus and pelvic cul-de-sac. However, laparoscopy may be less accurate in the prerenal and porta hepatis regions as well as in the root of the mesentery where small implants may go unnoticed. It is reassuring that the rate of negative evaluations and the rate of recurrences in patients with negative laparoscopic second looks are equivalent to those described in studies of second-look assessment by laparotomy (246). Conversely, in a prospective comparative study, a French group found the laparoscopic second-look evaluation suboptimal when compared to the abdominal approach, mainly because of the presence of adhesions that appeared to limit the thoroughness of the evaluation (247). In that study, the positive predictive value was 100%, but the negative predictive value was 86% (two false-negative cases) (247). Clearly, if residual tumor implants are readily confirmed at laparoscopy, then a laparotomy can be avoided in those patients. In patients with negative laparoscopic evaluation, it remains uncertain if laparotomy is more accurate, particularly in patients with diffuse adhesions. Large randomized trials are not available to answer this important question.

In terms of morbidity, a pilot study from the Memorial Sloan–Kettering Cancer Center demonstrated that the laparoscopic approach results in less morbidity, shorter operating time, shorter hospital stay, less blood loss, and lower total hospital charges (248). In a series of 150 cases, Husain et al. also concluded that the complication rate of the laparoscopic approach is low and that it is a safe approach even in patients who had a prior abdominal surgery (246). Clough et al. have also reported similar findings (247). Concerns about the effect of CO_2 pneumoperitoneum on the risk of tumor dissemination have been raised (see section on gasless laparoscopy above). However, a recent study including 131 patients operated on by laparoscopy does not seem to indicate that laparoscopic surgical procedures with CO_2 pneumoperitoneum reduce overall survival of patients with metastatic intraabdominal carcinoma of ovarian/peritoneal origin (85). Finally, in the context of second-look surgery, laparoscopy may be used to place intraperitoneal (IP) catheters under direct laparoscopic guidance in patients found to have residual disease at the time of the second-look operation (249).

Staging Procedure in Early-stage Disease

On occasions, despite thorough preoperative investigation, patients are operated on for a presumed benign ovarian mass, yet an unexpected diagnosis of ovarian cancer occurs on final pathology, or the operating surgeon does not feel comfortable completing the staging procedure. In such situations, a complete surgical staging at a second surgery should be performed to determine the true stage. This information is critical for recommendations of adjuvant chemotherapy. Roughly, in presumed stage I disease, the chances of finding more advanced disease is in the range of 20% to 30% and the most frequent site of metastasis are the lymph nodes (250,251). Laparoscopy may be an excellent alternative to complete the staging in such cases since a complete pelvic and paraaortic node sampling, an infracolic omentectomy, and a complete peritoneal assessment (with or without contralateral bilateral salpingo-oophorectomy and vaginal hysterectomy in older women) can be safely performed laparoscopically (252–255). Early studies showed that the morbidity of the laparoscopic procedure is low and the results are accurate (252–255). In the early 1990s, Querleu et al. even demonstrated that a complete laparoscopic infrarenal lymph node dissection could be accomplished in the context of restaging ovarian or fallopian tube cancers (15). In a more recent study including 46 cases, infrarenal lymphadenectomies were performed laparoscopically (143). The morbidity was low and the investigators noted that the number of lymph nodes obtained was doubled compared to the number of lymph nodes obtained by the more frequently performed inframesenteric lymphadenectomy (143). Although there are no randomized trials comparing both approaches, it would appear that a comprehensive laparoscopic restaging of patients with early-stage ovarian cancer is feasible, is accurate, and the morbidity is lower compared to the same procedure done by laparotomy. However, this procedure should only be performed by experienced and skilled laparoscopists capable of performing advanced and complex oncologic laparoscopic procedures.

With regard to borderline tumors, the value of a restaging procedure is controversial since the prognosis of patients with presumed stage I disease is excellent, and the value of adjuvant treatment is questionable even in more advanced disease. In a series of 56 patients refered with suspected stage IA disease, only 4 (7%) were upstaged (256). Conversely, in a recent series of 30 patients who underwent complete laparoscopic staging for presumed ovarian cancer, 26.6% of patients were upstaged as a result of the staging procedure (257). However, all the patients are alive with the exception of only one patient who developed a recurrence (257). The investigators concluded that whenever staging of a patient with a borderline tumor is considered, laparoscopy appears to be the method of choice since the procedure is accurate, the complication rate and the morbidity are low, and, very importantly, the incidence of infertility in young patients is minimized (257). It would appear, however, that laparoscopic ovarian cystectomy only for borderline tumor is associated with a higher risk of recurrence compared to a complete oophorectomy (122).

Laparoscopic Surgical Management of Early-stage Ovarian Cancer

It is uncommon for gynecologic oncologists knowingly to operate on a woman with ovarian cancer laparoscopically unless it is to determine the resectablility of patients with advanced disease (see section above). Thus, in most instances, the ovarian cancer is diagnosed inadvertently at the time of surgery for a presumed benign ovarian mass. There are two options: (a) complete the surgery laparoscopically or (b) convert to a laparotomy.

In experienced hands, the surgery can technically be completed laparoscopically, particularly when the cancer appears to be limited to the ovary and when there is no evidence of gross metastatic disease (39). In a recent series reported by Havrilesky et al., the ovarian malignancies discovered at the time of laparoscopy for pelvic masses were managed laparoscopically, and this was not associated with an adverse outcome (105). Conversely, when faced with the discovery of an ovarian malignancy, another option is simply to convert the laparoscopy to a laparotomy to complete the surgery (102,258). According to Canis et al., laparoscopic surgery is becoming the standard treatment approach for the management of benign adnexal masses, whereas laparotomy remains the gold standard for the treatment of malignant tumors (101). Having a gynecologic oncologist on standby is probably the ideal situation so that proper surgery can be completed immediately to avoid delay. It is thus extremely important always to inform patients explored laparoscopically for a pelvic mass of the possibility of a laparotomy if an ovarian malignancy is discovered.

Whether or not laparoscopy compromises outcome in patients managed laparoscopically for a pelvic mass compared with patients managed by laparotomy is not clear (259). Unfortunately, there are no prospective randomized trials with a large number of patients and long-term follow-up to answer this very important question. There are several uncertainties that are still not well answered with regard to the safety and efficacy of minimally invasive surgery in early-stage ovarian cancer (260). Until such solid data are available, oncologists should remain very cautious with regard to the use of laparoscopy in the management of suspicious complex adnexal masses and early-stage ovarian cancer. Caution should be used when counseling such patients. First and foremost, minimal access surgery should not compromise outcome, particularly for patients with early-stage disease, who have an excellent prognosis.

There are a few troubling reports of trocar-site recurrences following laparoscopic surgery. For instance, an isolated abdominal wall metastasis has been reported in a women operated on for early-stage ovarian cancer 10 years earlier (261). Port-site metastasis at the trocar site of a previous endocholecystectomy performed 7 months prior to abdominal surgery for advanced ovarian cancer has also been reported; the metastasis appeared after completion of platinum-based chemotherapy (262). These two reports suggest that cancer cells can probably be trapped at the level of trocar sites and remain dormant for several years. Trocar-site metastasis may also be only the tip of the iceberg. Indeed, CT scan may show more extensive spread, either tracking within the abdominal wall, or associated with intraabdominal carcinomatosis (263). Huang et al. also recently reported that port-site metastasis that appears during chemotherapy or after adequate chemotherapy is associated with a very poor prognosis (264). So trocar-site metastasis associated with laparoscopic surgery is a very serious condition and all efforts should be made to reduce its occurrence.

Despite the above, the risk of malignancy in patients operated on for presumed benign pelvic masses is relatively low (Table 13.1) (39,90–105) but will always be present despite adequate and thorough preoperative evaluation. So, the majority of women will benefit from the minimally invasive laparoscopic approach, which is clearly associated with lower morbidity and cost. In the event of a malignancy discovered at the time of surgery, clear mechanisms have to be in place to minimize the risk of tumor dissemination, particularly at the level of trocar sites: appropriate surgical technique to prevent tumor spillage (such as avoidance of cyst puncture or morcellation, the use of an endobag, proper closure of trocar sites), conversion to immediate laparotomy if satisfactory surgery cannot be adequately completed laparoscopically, and rapid referral to proper centers either to complete surgery or for adjuvant chemotherapy. Proper teaching following strict oncologic and surgical principles is thus essential to promote safe laparoscopic surgery (265). If strict guidelines are followed, in the end, women will benefit from minimally invasive laparoscopic surgery for the management of benign masses, and outcome should not be jeopardized for those found to have a malignancy discovered inadvertently.

VIDEOENDOSCOPIC SURGERY AND CANCER OF THE VULVA AND VAGINA

Surgery for the management of cancers of the vaginal and/or vulva includes lymph node dissection. For cancers of the upper half of the vagina, the management is similar to that of patients with cervical cancers. Open surgery is the standard, but laparoscopically assisted vaginal radical surgery can be used as well (266). The best indication for laparoscopy may be for the reoperation of the patients with incidental cervical cancer discovered at simple hysterectomy. This "Schauta sine utero" (267) seems to be safer than the classic open restaging. In a series of 17 patients managed between 1987 and 2003, no recurrence was observed among the four patients considered as being free of disease after laparoscopic vaginal restaging versus one of four patients who underwent only laparoscopic restaging and one of three patients who underwent abdominal restaging and were considered to be disease free (D.F.D., unpublished data).

For the cancers of the lower half of the vagina and cancers of the vulva, inguinofemoral dissection combined with or without pelvic dissection should be performed. The inguinofemoral lymphadenectomy has two major drawbacks (268): (a) wound drainage, which increases the length of the hospital stay, and (b) leg edema, which can be a very disabling sequela. Using separate incisions, the rate of these complications has decreased (269) but they still occur, which explains the current interest in SN biopsy introduced in 1994 by Levenback (146). Many oncologists currently refrain from performing systematic dissection if the SN biopsy is negative. The presence of micrometastasis can be a source of recurrences (270,271), and they probably cannot be completely ruled out by assessment of the SN alone. For such reasons, we recommend a systematic dissection using the videoendoscopic approach, which seems to be safe and simultaneously less morbid.

Videoendoscopic Inguinofemoral Dissection or Inguinoscopy

Videoendoscopic inguinofemoral dissection was performed for the first time in July 1994 (16). The technique was initially developed from the technique devised by Suzanne et al. (272) for axillary dissection. There is infiltration of the triangle of Scarpa with 200 mL of saline with lidocaine and epinephrine, followed by liposuction, widening of the liposuction orifice, and introduction of the laparoscopic trocar. CO_2 insufflation then enables dissection with the aid of two ancillary trocars. The advantage of presurgical liposuction is a clear operative field from the onset. However, the hazards of preoperative infiltration and blind liposuction (seeding of tumor cells by unrecognized trauma of involved lymph nodes) led to discontinuation of the use of this technique and moving to direct and gasless videoendoscopic dissection.

The first step of direct endoscopic dissection involves creating a tunnel starting from the tip of the triangle of Scarpa and undermining up to the level of the arch of the saphenous vein. A 1.5-cm transverse incision is made at the point where the sartorius muscle crosses the adductor magnus muscle. The subcutaneous fascia is crossed and the tunnel is continued up medially using scissors under the protection of a luminous retractor (the laryngoscope is the most cost-effective tool). Once the level of the saphenous vein is reached, the scissors are opened to widen the tunnel. The Laparofan (Origin Braun) is put in the prepared space and linked to the Laparolift (Origin Medsystems, Menlo Park, CA). The videoendoscopic portion of the surgery can then be initiated.

As soon as the triangle of Scarpa is opened, the laparoscope is introduced through an adapted rubber sheath that prevents obscuring of the lens. The first landmark is generally the accessory saphenous vein, which goes vertically to the arch of the great saphenous vein (its direction is not vertical but oblique medially to lateral landmarks). Identifying this vein leads to the arch and then to the inguinal ligament and, finally, to the femoral fascia. The femoral fascia must be opened in order to skeletonize the medial surface of the femoral vessels to the level of the femoral ring where the Cloquet's node is located. The dissection is performed using forceps and scissors introduced through ancillary 5-mm openings made on each side of the midline. The saphenous vein and most of its collaterals can usually be preserved. The adipose pads and lymph nodes are retrieved after widening one of the ancillary openings. At the end of the dissection, all the node-bearing tissue medial to the femoral vessels must be removed including the space located in front of the pubic bone. There is no need to dissect lateral to the femoral vessels.

Indications and Results

Inguinofemoral dissection is indicated for all surgically managed cancers of the vulva and lower half of the vagina. In clitoral and low vaginal cancers, bilateral dissections are required and pelvic lymphadenectomy is recommended. For cancers located on the lateral part of the vulva, ipsilateral groin dissection is considered to be adequate if the nodes are uninvolved (by intraoperative assessment using frozen section or postoperative assessment by permanent section). Contralateral groin dissection and pelvic dissection are not to be considered necessary.

Videoendoscopic groin dissection has the same indications; however, it should not be performed in the presence of obvious metastatic involvement. Such cases should be handled with standard open dissection. Similarly, if nodal involvement is detected during the procedure, conversion to the open technique is recommended. Finally, if nodal involvement is only detected on final report, reoperation with resection of the scar is indicated.

Between July 1994 and July 1996, Dargent (16) performed 15 dissections using the videoendoscopic technique assisted by liposuction. The last patient, who had a vulvar cancer with two positive lymph nodes that were not detected preoperatively, had an inguinal recurrence that appeared a few days after the surgery. The likely source of this recurrence may have been unrecognized seeding of tumor cells from traumatized metastatic nodes. This technique was discontinued and replaced by the gasless technique described earlier. The new technique was used for 13 additional dissections between July 1996 and December 1997. The mean operative time was 88 minutes for the first technique versus 78 minutes for the second. Neither postoperative wound drainage nor inferior limb edema was observed in the patients who underwent the videoendoscopic dissection regardless of the technique. The mean number of nodes was seven for the first technique and six for the second. An inguinal recurrence arising in a missed positive node was noted 6 months after the surgery. This recurrence was treated by

surgical resection. The patient was without evidence of disease one year later.

CONCLUSIONS

The most difficult question to answer is the actual benefit both the patient and the surgeon garner from the use of laparoscopic surgery rather than classic open surgery. For extirpative surgery, this benefit remains purely hypothetical as there is a paucity of level one evidence on this subject. The GOG has launched a trial to assess the advantages of laparoscopic surgery in the management of endometrial cancer. A French group has done the same for the management of early cervical cancer. Both organizations have met similar difficulties in enrolling patients owing to the public awareness that laparoscopic surgery is more patient friendly. This concept may deter patients from participating in randomized trials that could result in patients foregoing laparoscopy for laparotomy. However, without such randomized trials, the questions surrounding the laparoscopic approach, which include quality of life, will never be answered. The only truly recognized improvement is radical trachelectomy. Although no births were reported after the initial attempts of the pioneers using an abdominal approach, one birth was reported by the new supporters of the older method (273). This one success is in contrast to the numerous births reported after the laparoscopic vaginal operation. In regard to the staging surgery, laparoscopically assisted staging surgery greatly reduces the morbidity without sacrificing accurate assessment of disease spread. A brief operative procedure and hospitalization can now provide definitive information upon which appropriate treatment can be prescribed. Here may be the future of laparoscopic oncosurgery. However, even with this indication where the superiority to open surgery looks clear, we still require prospective evidence upon which it can be justified.

REFERENCES

1. De Brux JA, Dupre-Froment J, Mintz M. Cytology of the peritoneal fluids sampled by coelioscopy or by cul de sac puncture, its value in gynecology. *Acta Cytol* 1968;12:395–405.
2. Hald T, Rasmussen F. Extraperitoneal pelvioscopy: a new aid in staging of lower urinary tract tumors. A preliminary report. *J Urol* 1980; 124:245–248.
3. Dargent D. A new future for Schauta's operation through pre-surgical retroperitoneal pelviscopy. *Eur J Gynecol Oncol* 1987;8:292–296.
4. Dargent D, Salvat J. Envahissement ganglionnaire pelvien: place de la pelviscopie rétropéritonéale. In: Dargent D, Salvat J, eds. *L'envahissement ganglionnaire pelvien.* Paris: Medsi McGraw-Hill, 1989.
5. Dargent D, Arnould P. Percutaneous pelvic lymphadenectomy under laparoscopic guidance. In: Nichols D, ed. *Gynecologic and obstetrics surgery.* St. Louis: Mosby, 1993:583.
6. Querleu D. Laparoscopic lymphadenectomy. Presented at the Second World Congress of Gynecologic Endoscopy, Clermont-Ferrand, France, June 5–8, 1989.
7. Querleu D, Leblanc E, Castelain B. Laparoscopic pelvic lymphadenectomy in the staging of early carcinoma of the cervix. *Am J Obstet Gynecol* 1991;164:579–583.
8. Childers JM, Surwit EA. Combined laparoscopic and vaginal surgery

for the management of two cases of stage I endometrial cancer. *Gynecol Oncol* 1992;45:46–48.

9. Childers JM, Hatch K, Surwit EA. The role of laparoscopic lymphadenectomy in the management of cervical carcinoma. *Gynecol Oncol* 1992;47:38–41.

10. Nezhat CR, Burrell MO, Nezhat FR, et al. Laparoscopic radical hysterectomy with paraaortic and pelvic node dissection. *Am J Obstet Gynecol* 1992;166:864–866.

11. Chu KK, Chang SD, Chen FP, Soong YK. Laparoscopic surgical staging in cervical cancer—preliminary experience among Chinese. *Gynecol Oncol* 1997;64:49–53.

12. Hatch KD, Hallum AV III, Nour M. New surgical approaches to treatment of cervical cancer. *J Natl Cancer Inst Monogr* 1996;21:71–75.

13. Bagley CM Jr, Young RC, Schein PS, et al. Ovarian carcinoma metastatic to the diaphragm—frequently undiagnosed at laparotomy. A preliminary report. *Am J Obstet Gynecol.* 1973;116:397–400.

14. Reich H, McGlynn F, Wilkie W. Laparoscopic management of stage I ovarian cancer. *J Reprod Med* 1990;35:601–604.

15. Querleu D, LeBlanc E. Laparoscopic infrarenal paraaortic lymph node dissection for restaging of carcinoma of the ovary or fallopian tube. *Cancer* 1994;73:1467–1471.

16. Mathevet P. Laparoscopic surgery in the management of gynecological cancer: vulvar and vaginal cancers. In: Querleu D, Childers J, Dargent D, eds. *Laparoscopic surgery in gynecologic oncology.* Oxford, UK: Blackwell Science, 1999:170–175.

17. Childers JM, Hatch KD, Tran AN, Surwit EA. Laparoscopic paraaortic lymphadenectomy in gynecologic malignancies. *Obstet Gynecol* 1993;82:741–747.

18. Querleu D. Laparoscopic paraaortic node sampling in gynecologic oncology: a preliminary experience. *Gynecol Oncol* 1993;49:24–29.

19. Possover M, Krause N, Drahonovsky J, Schneider A. Left-sided suprarenal retrocrural para-aortic lymphadenectomy in advanced cervical cancer by laparoscopy. *Gynecol Oncol* 1998;71:219–222.

20. Dargent D, Martin X, Mathevet P. Laparoscopic assessment of the sentinel lymph node in early stage cervical cancer. *Gynecol Oncol* 2000;79:411–415.

21. Semm K *Operationslehre für endoskopische abdominal Chirurgie—Operativ Pelviscopie.* Stuttgart: Schattauerpub, 1984.

22. Dargent D, Mathevet P. Radical laparoscopic vaginal hysterectomy. *J Gynecol Obstet Biol Reprod (Paris)* 1992;21:709–710.

23. Querleu D. Laparoscopically assisted radical vaginal hysterectomy. *Gynecol Oncol* 1993;51:248–254.

24. Querleu D. Radical hysterectomies by the Schauta-Amreich and Schauta-Stoeckel techniques assisted by celioscopy. *J Gynecol Obstet Biol Reprod (Paris)* 1991;20:747–748.

25. Roy M, Plante M, Renaud MC, Tetu B. Vaginal radical hysterectomy versus abdominal radical hysterectomy in the treatment of early-stage cervical cancer. *Gynecol Oncol* 1996;62:336–339.

26. Schneider A, Possover M, Kamprath S, et al. Laparoscopy-assisted radical vaginal hysterectomy modified according to Schauta-Stoeckel. *Obstet Gynecol* 1996;88:1057–1060.

27. Canis M, Mage G, Wattiez A, et al. Does endoscopic surgery have a role in radical surgery of cancer of the cervix uteri? *J Gynecol Obstet Biol Reprod (Paris)* 1990;19:921.

28. Spirtos NM, Eisenkop SM, Schlaerth JB, Ballon SC. Laparoscopic radical hysterectomy (type III) with aortic and pelvic lymphadenectomy in patients with stage I cervical cancer: surgical morbidity and intermediate follow-up. *Am J Obstet Gynecol* 2002;187:340–348.

29. Abu-Rustum NR, Gemignani ML, Moore K, Sonoda Y, et al. Total laparoscopic radical hysterectomy with pelvic lymphadenectomy using the argon-beam coagulator: pilot data and comparison to laparotomy. *Gynecol Oncol* 2003;91:402–409.

30. Pomel C, Atallah D, Le Bouedec G, et al. Laparoscopic radical hysterectomy for invasive cervical cancer: 8-year experience of a pilot study. *Gynecol Oncol* 2003;91:534–539.

31. Pomel C, Rouzier R, Pocard M, et al. Laparoscopic total pelvic exenteration for cervical cancer relapse. *Gynecol Oncol* 2003;91:616–618.

32. Lai CH, Huang KG, Hong JH, et al. Randomized trial of surgical staging (extraperitoneal or laparoscopic) versus clinical staging in locally advanced cervical cancer. *Gynecol Oncol* 2003;89:160–167.

33. Bateman BG, Kolp LA, Hoeger K. Complications of laparoscopy—operative and diagnostic. *Fertil Steril* 1996;66:30–35.

34. Bonjer HJ, Hazebroek EJ, Kazemier G, et al. Open versus closed establishment of pneumoperitoneum in laparoscopic surgery. *Br J Surg* 1997;84:599–602.

35. Cogliandolo A, Manganaro T, Saitta FP, Micali B. Blind versus open approach to laparoscopic cholecystectomy: a randomized study. *Surg Laparosc Endosc* 1998;8:353–355.

36. Rice JG, McCall JG, Wattchow DA. Improving the ease and safety of laparoscopy: a technique for open insertion of the umbilical trocar. *Aust N Z J Surg* 1998;68:664–665.

37. Perone N. Laparoscopy using a simplified open technique. A review of 585 cases. *J Reprod Med* 1992;37:921–924.

38. Decloedt J, Berteloot P, Vergote I. The feasibility of open laparoscopy in gynecologic-oncologic patients. *Gynecol Oncol* 1997;66:138–140.

39. Dottino PR, Levine DA, Ripley DL, Cohen CJ. Laparoscopic management of adnexal masses in premenopausal and postmenopausal women. *Obstet Gynecol* 1999;93:223–228.

40. Chapron C, Cravello L, Chopin N, et al. Complications during set-up procedures for laparoscopy in gynecology: open laparoscopy does not reduce the risk of major complications. *Acta Obstet Gynecol Scand.* 2003;82:1125–1129.

41. Childers JM, Brzechffa PR, Surwit EA, et al. Laparoscopy using the left upper quadrant as the primary trocar site. *Gynecol Oncol* 1992;50:221–225.

42. Sjovall K, Nilsson B, Einhorn N. Different types of rupture of the tumor capsule and the impact on survival in early ovarian carcinoma. *Int J Gynecol Cancer* 1994;4:333–336.

43. Bojahr B, Lober R, Straube W, Kohler G. Gasless laparoscopic-assisted radical vaginal hysterectomy with lymphadenectomy for cervical carcinoma. *J Am Assoc Gynecol Laparosc* 1996;3:S4.

44. Galen DI, Jacobson A, Weckstein LN, et al. Gasless laparoscopy for gynecology. *J Am Assoc Gynecol Laparosc* 1995;2:S68.

45. Hill DJ, Maher PJ, Wood EC. Gasless laparoscopy—useless or useful? *J Am Assoc Gynecol Laparosc* 1994;1:265–268.

46. Chang FH, Soon YK, Lee CL, et al. Laparoscopic removal of a large leiomyoma using airlift gasless laparoscopy. *J Am Assoc Gynecol Laparosc* 1996;3:S7.

47. Akira S, Yamanaka A, Ishihara T, et al. Gasless laparoscopic ovarian cystectomy during pregnancy: comparison with laparotomy. *Am J Obstet Gynecol* 1999;180:554–557.

48. Pelosi MA. Gasless laparoscopy under epidural anesthesia during pregnancy. *J Am Assoc Gynecol Laparosc* 1995;2:S75.

49. Tanaka H, Futamura N, Takubo S, Toyoda N. Gasless laparoscopy under epidural anesthesia for adnexal cysts during pregnancy. *J Reprod Med* 1999;44:929–932.

50. Schmidt T, Nawroth F, Foth D, et al. Gasless laparoscopy as an option for conservative therapy of adnexal pedical torsion with twin pregnancy. *J Am Assoc Gynecol Laparosc* 2001;8:621–622.

51. Romer T, Bojahr B, Schwesinger G. Treatment of a torqued hematosalpinx in the thirteenth week of pregnancy using gasless laparoscopy. *J Am Assoc Gynecol Laparosc* 2002;9:89–92.

52. Stepp KJ, Tulikangas PK, Goldberg JM, et al. Laparoscopy for adnexal masses in the second trimester of pregnancy. *J Am Assoc Gynecol Laparosc.* 2003;10:55–59.

53. D'Ercole C, Cravello L, Guyon F, et al. Gasless laparoscopic gynecologic surgery. *Eur J Obstet Gynecol Reprod Biol* 1996;66:137–139.

54. Tintara H, Leetanaporn R, Getpook C, et al. Simplified abdominal wall-lifting device for gasless laparoscopy. *Int J Gynaecol Obstet* 1998;61:165–170.

55. Tintara H, Choobun T, Geater A. Gasless laparoscopic hysterectomy: a comparative study with total abdominal hysterectomy. *J Obstet Gynaecol Res* 2003;29:38–44.

56. Li B, Hao J, Gao X, et al. Gynecological procedures under gasless laparoscopy. *Chin Med J* 2001;114:514–516.

57. Lukban JC, Jaeger J, Hammond KC, et al. Gasless versus conventional laparoscopy. *N J Med.* 2000;97:29–34.

58. Johnson PL, Sibert KS. Laparoscopy. Gasless vs. CO_2 pneumoperitoneum. *J Reprod Med* 1997;42:255–259.

59. Goldberg JM, Maurer WG. A randomized comparison of gasless laparoscopy and CO_2 pneumoperitoneum. *Obstet Gynecol* 1997;90:416–420.

60. Guido RS, Brooks K, McKenzie R, et al. A randomized, prospective comparison of pain after gasless laparoscopy and traditional laparoscopy. *J Am Assoc Gynecol Laparosc* 1998;5:149–153.

61. Hughes ES, McDermott FT, Polglase AL, Johnson WR. Tumor recurrence in the abdominal wall scar tissue after large-bowel cancer surgery. *Dis Colon Rectum* 1983;26:571–572.
62. Reilly WT, Nelson H, Schroeder G, et al. Wound recurrence following conventional treatment of colorectal cancer. A rare but perhaps underestimated problem. *Dis Colon Rectum* 1996;39:200–207.
63. Schaeff B, Paolucci V, Thomopoulos J. Port site recurrences after laparoscopic surgery. A review. *Dig Surg* 1998;15:124–134.
64. Wang PH, Yuan CC, Lin G, et al. Risk factors contributing to early occurrence of port site metastases of laparoscopic surgery for malignancy. *Gynecol Oncol* 1999;72:38–44.
65. Pastner B, Damien M. Umbilical metastasis from a stage IB cervical cancer after laparoscopy: a case report. *Fertil Steril* 1992;58:1248–1249.
66. Wang PH, Yuan CC, Chao KC, et al. Squamous cell carcinoma of the cervix after laparoscopic surgery. A case report. *J Reprod Med* 1997;42:801–804.
67. Wang PH, Yen MS, Yuan CC, et al. Port site metastasis after laparoscopic-assisted vaginal hysterectomy for endometrial cancer: possible mechanisms and prevention. *Gynecol Oncol* 1997;66:151–155.
68. Childers JM, Aqua KA, Surwit EA, et al. Abdominal-wall tumor implantation after laparoscopy for malignant conditions. *Obstet Gynecol* 1994;84:765–769.
69. Umpleby HC, Fermor B, Symes MO, et al. Viability of exfoliated colorectal carcinoma cells. *Br J Surg* 1984;71:659–663.
70. Jeon HM, Kim JS, Lee CD, et al. Late development of umbilical metastasis after laparoscopic cholecystectomy for a gallbladder carcinoma. *Oncol Rep* 1999;6:283–287.
71. Canis M, Mage G, Botchorishvili R, et al. Laparoscopy and gynecologic cancer: is it still necessary to debate or only convince the incredulous? *Gynecol Obstet Fertil* 2001;29:913–918.
72. Morice P, Viala J, Pautier P, et al. Port-site metastasis after laparoscopic surgery for gynecologic cancer. A report of six cases. *J Reprod Med* 2000;45:837–840.
73. Hopkins MP, von Gruenigen V, Gaich S. Laparoscopic port site implantation with ovarian cancer. *Am J Obstet Gynecol* 2000;182:735–736.
74. van Dam PA, DeCloedt J, Tjalma WA, et al. Trocar implantation metastasis after laparoscopy in patients with advanced ovarian cancer: can the risk be reduced? *Am J Obstet Gynecol* 1999;181:536–541.
75. Canis M, Botchorishvili R, Wattiez A, et al. Cancer and laparoscopy, experimental studies: a review. *Eur J Obstet Gynecol Reprod Biol* 2000;91:1–9.
76. Cavina E, Goletti O, Molea N, et al. Trocar site tumor recurrences. May pneumoperitoneum be responsible? *Surg Endosc* 1998;12:1294–1296.
77. Bouvy ND, Giuffrida MC, Tseng LN, et al. Effects of carbon dioxide pneumoperitoneum, air pneumoperitoneum, and gasless laparoscopy on body weight and tumor growth. *Arch Surg* 1998;133:652–656.
78. Neuhaus SJ, Texler M, Hewett PJ, Watson DI. Port-site metastases following laparoscopic surgery. *Br J Surg* 1998;85:735–741.
79. Mathew G, Watson DI, Ellis TS, et al. The role of peritoneal immunity and the tumour-bearing state on the development of wound and peritoneal metastases after laparoscopy. *Aust N Z J Surg* 1999;69:14–18.
80. Jacobi CA, Sabat R, Bohm B, et al. Pneumoperitoneum with carbon dioxide stimulates growth of malignant colonic cells. *Surgery* 1997;121:72–78.
81. Mathew G, Watson DI, Ellis T, et al. The effect of laparoscopy on the movement of tumor cells and metastasis to surgical wounds. *Surg Endosc* 1997;11:1163–1166.
82. Watson DI, Mathew G, Ellis T, et al. Gasless laparoscopy may reduce the risk of port site metastasis following laparoscopic tumor surgery. *Arch Chir* 1997;132:166–168.
83. Lecuru F, Agostini A, Camatte S, et al. Impact of pneumoperitoneum on visceral metastasis rate and survival. Results in two ovarian cancer models in rats. *Br J Obstet Gynaecol* 2001;108:733–737.
84. Lecuru F, Agostini A, Camatte S, et al. Impact of pneumoperitoneum on tumor growth. *Surg Endosc* 2002;16:1170–1174.
85. Abu-Rustum NR, Sonoda Y, Chi DS, et al. The effects of CO2 pneumoperitoneum on the survival of women with persistent metastatic ovarian cancer. *Gynecol Oncol* 2003; 90:431–434.
86. Agostini A, Robin F, Aggerbeck M, et al. Influence of peritoneal factors on port-site metastases in a xenograft ovarian cancer model. *Br J Obstet Gynaecol* 2001;108:809–812.
87. Abu-Rustum NR, Rhee EH, Chi DS, et al. Subcutaneous tumor implantation after laparoscopic procedures in women with malignant disease. *Obstet Gynecol* 2004;103:480–487.
88. Bouvy ND, Marquet RL, Jeekel H, Bonjer HJ. Impact of gas(less) laparoscopy and laparotomy on peritoneal tumor growth and abdominal wall metastases. *Ann Surg* 1996;224:694–700.
89. Reymond MA, Schneider C, Kastl S, et al. The pathogenesis of port-site recurrences. *J Gastrointest Surg* 1998;2:406–414.
90. Nezhat F, Nezhat C, Welander CE, Benigno B. Four ovarian cancers diagnosed during laparoscopic management of 1011 women with adnexal masses. *Am J Obstet Gynecol* 1992;167:790–796.
91. Hulka JF, Parker WH, Surrey MW, Phillips JM. Management of ovarian masses. AAGL 1990 survey. *J Reprod Med* 1992;37:599–602.
92. Canis M, Mage G, Pouly JL, et al. Laparoscopic diagnosis of adnexal cystic masses: a 12-year experience with long-term follow-up. *Obstet Gynecol* 1994;83:707–712.
93. Blanc B, Boubli L, D'Ercole C, Nicoloso E. Laparoscopic management of malignant ovarian cysts: a 78 case national survey. Part 1: preoperative and laparoscopic evaluation. *Eur J Obstet Gynecol Reprod Biol* 1994;56:177–180.
94. Marana R, Vittori G, Porpora MG, et al. Laparoscopic treatment of ovarian cysts in women under 40 years of age. *J Am Assoc Gynecol Laparosc* 1995;2:S20.
95. Wenzl R, Lehner R, Husslein P, Sevelda P. Laparoscopic surgery in cases of ovarian malignancies: an Austria-wide survey. *Gynecol Oncol* 1996;63:57–61.
96. Yuen PM, Yu KM, Yip SK, et al. A randomized prospective study of laparoscopy and laparotomy in the management of benign ovarian masses. *Am J Obstet Gynecol* 1997;177:109–114.
97. Hidlebaugh DA, Vulgaropulos S, Orr RK. Treating adnexal masses. Operative laparoscopy vs. laparotomy. *J Reprod Med* 1997;42:551–558.
98. Guglielmina JN, Pennehouat G, Deval B, et al. Treatment of ovarian cysts by laparoscopy. *Contracept Fertil Sex* 1997;25:218–229.
99. Malik E, Bohm W, Stoz F, et al. Laparoscopic management of ovarian tumors. *Surg Endosc* 1998;12:1326–1333.
100. Sadik S, Onoglu AS, Gokdeniz R, et al. Laparoscopic management of selected adnexal masses. *J Am Assoc Gynecol Laparosc* 1999;6:313–316.
101. Ulrich U, Paulus W, Schneider A, Keckstein J. Laparoscopic surgery for complex ovarian masses. *J Am Assoc Gynecol Laparosc* 2000;7(3):373–380.
102. Serur E, Emeney PL, Byrne DW. Laparoscopic management of adnexal masses. *JSLS* 2001;5:143–151.
103. Mettler L, Jacobs V, Brandenburg K, et al. Laparoscopic management of 641 adnexal tumors in Kiel, Germany. *J Am Assoc Gynecol Laparosc* 2001;8:74–82.
104. Mendilcioglu I, Zorlu CG, Trak B, et al. Laparoscopic management of adnexal masses. Safety and effectiveness. *J Reprod Med.* 2002;47:36–40.
105. Havrilesky LJ, Peterson BL, Dryden DK, et al. Predictors of clinical outcomes in the laparoscopic management of adnexal masses. *Obstet Gynecol* 2003;102:243–251.
106. Benacerraf BR, Finkler NJ, Wojciechowski C, Knapp RC. Sonographic accuracy in the diagnosis of ovarian masses. *J Reprod Med* 1990;35:491–495.
107. Maiman M, Seltzer V, Boyce J. Laparoscopic excision of ovarian neoplasms subsequently found to be malignant. *Obstet Gynecol* 1991;77:563–565.
108. Hidlebaugh DA, Vulgaropulos S, Orr R. Trends in oophorectomy by laparoscopic versus open techniques. *J Am Assoc Gynecol Laparosc* 1996;3:S17–S18.
109. Parker WH, Levine RL, Howard FM, et al. A multicenter study of laparoscopic management of selected cystic adnexal masses in postmenopausal women. *J Am Coll Surg* 1994;179:733–737.
110. Quinlan DJ, Townsend DE, Johnson GH. Laparoscopic removal of adnexal masses. *Mt Sinai J Med* 1999;66:31.
111. Jennings TS, Dottino P, Rahaman J, Cohen CJ. Results of selective use of operative laparoscopy in gynecologic oncology. *Gynecol Oncol* 1998;70:323–328.
112. Lehner R, Wenzl R, Heinzl H, et al. Influence of delayed staging

laparotomy after laparoscopic removal of ovarian masses later found malignant. *Obstet Gynecol* 1998;92:967–971.

113. Rose PG, Rubin RB, Nelson BE, et al. Accuracy of frozen-section (intraoperative consultation) diagnosis of ovarian tumors. *Am J Obstet Gynecol* 1994;171:823–826.

114. Canis M, Botchorishvili R, Kouyate S, et al. Surgical management of adnexal tumors. *Ann Chir* 1998;52:234–248.

115. Kindermann G, Maassen V, Kuhn W. Laparoscopic preliminary surgery of ovarian malignancies. Experiences from 127 German gynecologic clinics. *Geburtshilfe Frauenheilk* 1995;55:687–694.

116. Mettler L, Semm K, Shive K. Endoscopic management of adnexal masses. *J Soc Laparoendosc Surg* 1997;1:103–112.

117. Dembo AJ, Davy M, Stenwig AE, et al. Prognostic factors in patients with stage I epithelial ovarian cancer. *Obstet Gynecol* 1990;75:263–273.

118. Sevelda P, Dittrich C, Salzer H. Prognostic value of the rupture of the capsule in stage I epithelial ovarian carcinoma. *Gynecol Oncol* 1989;35:321–322.

119. Blanc B, D'Ercole C, Nicoloso E, Boubli L. Laparoscopic management of malignant ovarian cysts: a 78 case national survey. Part 2: follow-up and final treatment. *Eur J Obstet Gynecol Reprod Biol* 1995;61:147–150.

120. Leminen A, Lehtovirta P. Spread of ovarian cancer after laparoscopic surgery: report of eight cases. *Gynecol Oncol* 1999;75:387–390.

121. Ripley D, Golden A, Fahs MC, Dottino P. The impact of laparoscopic surgery in the management of adnexal masses. *Mt Sinai J Med* 1999;66:31–34.

122. Darai E, Teboul J, Walker-Combrouze F, et al. Borderline ovarian tumors: a series of 43 patients. *Contracept Fertil Sex* 1997;25:933–938.

123. Alvarez RD, Kilgore LC, Partridge EE, et al. Staging ovarian cancer diagnosed during laparoscopy: accuracy rather than immediacy. *South Med J* 1993;86:1256–1258.

124. Querleu D, Leblanc E. Laparoscopic modified radical hysterectomy in laparoscopic surgery. In: Querleu D, Childers J, Dargent D, eds. *Laparoscopic surgery in gynaecological oncology.* Oxford, UK: Blackwell Science, 1999:49–52.

125. Childers JM, Brzechffa PR, Hatch KD, Surwit EA. Laparoscopically assisted surgical staging (LASS) of endometrial cancer. *Gynecol Oncol* 1993;51:33–38.

126. Melendez TD, Childers JM, Nour M, et al. Laparoscopic staging of endometrial cancer: the learning experience. *J Soc Laparoendosc Surg* 1997;1:45–49.

127. Possover M, Krause N, Plaul K, et al. Laparoscopic para-aortic and pelvic lymphadenectomy: experience with 150 patients and review of the literature. *Gynecol Oncol* 1998;71:19–28.

128. Spirtos NM, Schlaerth JB, Spirtos TW, et al. Laparoscopic bilateral pelvic and paraaortic lymph node sampling: an evolving technique. *Am J Obstet Gynecol* 1995;173:105–111.

129. Dottino PR, Tobias DH, Beddoe A, et al. Laparoscopic lymphadenectomy for gynecologic malignancies. *Gynecol Oncol* 1999;73:383–388.

130. Scribner DR Jr, Walker JL, Johnson GA, et al. Laparoscopic pelvic and paraaortic lymph node dissection: analysis of the first 100 cases. *Gynecol Oncol* 2001;82:498–503.

131. Su TH, Wang KG, Yang YC, et al. Laparoscopic para-aortic lymph node sampling in the staging of invasive cervical carcinoma: including a comparative study of 21 laparotomy cases. *Int J Gynaecol Obstet* 1995;49:311–318.

132. Vidaurreta J, Bermudez A, di Paola G, Sardi J. Laparoscopic staging in locally advanced cervical carcinoma: a new possible philosophy? *Gynecol Oncol* 1999;75:366–371.

133. Renaud MC, Plante M, Roy M. Combined laparoscopic and vaginal radical surgery in cervical cancer. *Gynecol Oncol* 2000;79:59–63.

134. Altgassen C, Possover M, Krause N, et al. Establishing a new technique of laparoscopic pelvic and para-aortic lymphadenectomy. *Obstet Gynecol* 2000;95:348–352.

135. Vergote I, Amant F, Berteloot P, et al. Laparoscopic lower para-aortic staging lymphadenectomy in stage IB2, II, and III cervical cancer. *Int J Gynecol Cancer* 2002;12:22–26.

136. Abu-Rustum NR, Chi DS, Sonoda Y, et al. Transperitoneal laparoscopic pelvic and para-aortic lymph node dissection using the argon-beam coagulator and monopolar instruments: an 8-year study and description of technique. *Gynecol Oncol* 2003;89:504–513.

137. Schlaerth JB, Spirtos NM, Carson LF, et al. Laparoscopic retroperitoneal lymphadenectomy followed by immediate laparotomy in women with cervical cancer: a Gynecologic Oncology Group study. *Gynecol Oncol* 2002;85:81–88.

138. Gallup DG, King LA, Messing MJ, Talledo OE. Paraaortic lymph node sampling by means of an extraperitoneal approach with a supraumbilical transverse "sunrise" incision. *Am J Obstet Gynecol* 1993;169:307–311.

139. Spirtos NM, Schlaerth JB, Gross GM, et al. Cost and quality-of-life analyses of surgery for early endometrial cancer: laparotomy versus laparoscopy. *Am J Obstet Gynecol* 1996;174:1795–1799.

140. Fowler JM, Carter JR, Carlson JW, et al. Lymph node yield from laparoscopic lymphadenectomy in cervical cancer: a comparative study. *Gynecol Oncol* 1993;51:187–192.

141. Benedetti-Panici P, Maneschi F, Scambia G, et al. Lymphatic spread of cervical cancer: an anatomical and pathological study based on 225 radical hysterectomies with systematic pelvic and aortic lymphadenectomy. *Gynecol Oncol* 1996;62:19–24.

142. Michel G, Morice P, Castaigne D, et al. Lymphatic spread in stage Ib and II cervical carcinoma: anatomy and surgical implications. *Obstet Gynecol* 1998;91:360–363.

143. Kohler C, Tozzi R, Klemm P, Schneider A. Laparoscopic paraaortic left-sided transperitoneal infrarenal lymphadenectomy in patients with gynecologic malignancies: technique and results. *Gynecol Oncol* 2003;91:139–148.

144. Possover M, Plaul K, Krause N, Schneider A. Leftsided laparoscopic para-aortic lymphadenectomy: anatomy of the ventral tributaries of the infrarenal vena cava. *Am J Obstet Gynecol* 1998;179:1295–1297.

145. Cabanas RM. An approach for the treatment of penile carcinoma. *Cancer* 1977; 39:456–466.

146. Levenback C, Burke TW, Gershenson DM, et al. Intraoperative lymphatic mapping for vulvar cancer. *Obstet Gynecol* 1994;84:163–167.

147. Echt ML, Finan MA, Hoffman MS, et al. Detection of sentinel lymph nodes with lymphazurin in cervical, uterine, and vulvar malignancies. *South Med J* 1999;92:204–208.

148. Medl M, Peters-Engl C, Schutz P, et al. First report of lymphatic mapping with isosulfan blue dye and sentinel node biopsy in cervical cancer. *Anticancer Res* 2000;20:1133–1134.

149. O'Boyle JD, Coleman RL, Bernstein SG, et al. Intraoperative lymphatic mapping in cervix cancer patients undergoing radical hysterectomy: a pilot study. *Gynecol Oncol* 2000;79:238–243.

150. Kamprath S, Possover M, Schneider A. Laparoscopic sentinel lymph node detection in patients with cervical cancer. *Am J Obstet Gynecol* 2000;182:1648.

151. Verheijen RH, Pijpers R, van Diest PJ, et al. Sentinel node detection in cervical cancer. *Obstet Gynecol* 2000;96:135–138.

152. Lambaudie E, Collinet P, Narducci F, et al. Laparoscopic identification of sentinel lymph nodes in early stage cervical cancer: prospective study using a combination of patent blue dye injection and technetium radiocolloid injection. *Gynecol Oncol* 2003;89:84–87.

153. Barranger E, Grahek D, Cortez A, et al. Laparoscopic sentinel lymph node procedure using a combination of patent blue and radioisotope in women with cervical carcinoma. *Cancer* 2003;97:3003–3009.

154. Rhim CC, Park JS, Bae SN, Namkoong SE. Sentinel node biopsy as an indicator for pelvic nodes dissection in early stage cervical cancer. *J Korean Med Sci* 2002;17:507–511.

155. Malur S, Krause N, Kohler C, Schneider A. Sentinel lymph node detection in patients with cervical cancer. *Gynecol Oncol* 2001;80:254–257.

156. Buist MR, Pijpers RJ, van Lingen A, et al. Laparoscopic detection of sentinel lymph nodes followed by lymph node dissection in patients with early stage cervical cancer. *Gynecol Oncol* 2003;90:290–296.

157. Lantzsch T, Wolters M, Grimm J, et al. Sentinel node procedure in Ib cervical cancer: a preliminary series. *Br J Cancer* 2001;85:791–794.

158. Plante M, Renaud MC, Tetu B, et al. Laparoscopic sentinel node mapping in early-stage cervical cancer. *Gynecol Oncol* 2003;91:494–503.

159. van Dam PA, Hauspy J, Vanderheyden T, et al. Intraoperative sentinel node identification with technetium-99m–labeled nanocolloid in patients with cancer of the uterine cervix: a feasibility study. *Int J Gynecol Cancer* 2003;13:182–186.

160. Dargent D, Enria R. Laparoscopic assessment of the sentinel lymph nodes in early cervical cancer. Technique—preliminary results and future developments. *Crit Rev Oncol Hematol* 2003;48:305–310.

161. Gargiulo T, Giusti M, Bottero A, et al. Sentinel lymph node (SLN) laparoscopic assessment early stage in endometrial cancer. *Minerva Ginecol* 2003;55:259–262.

162. Burke TW, Levenback C, Tornos C, et al. Intraabdominal lymphatic mapping to direct selective pelvic and paraaortic lymphadenectomy in women with high-risk endometrial cancer: results of a pilot study. *Gynecol Oncol* 1996;62:169–173.

163. Levenback C. Lymphatic mapping and sentinel node identification in patients with cervix cancer undergoing radical hysterectomy and pelvic lymphadenectomy. *J Clin Oncol* 2002;20:688–893.

164. Dargent D, Marchiole P, Buenerd A, Mathevet P. Is the absence of metastases, including micrometastases, in the sentinel nodes predictive of the absence of metastases in the other regional nodes in early stage cervical cancer patients? Society of Gynecologic Oncologists, San Diego, February 7–11, 2004. Abstract #58.

165. Marchiole PA, Buenerd A, Scoazec JY, et al. The sentinel node biopsy is not accurate in predicting nodal status in patients with early cervical carcinoma. Cancer 2004 (in press).

166. Holub Z, Jabor A, Kliment L. Comparison of two procedures for sentinel lymph node detection in patients with endometrial cancer: a pilot study. *Eur J Gynaecol Oncol* 2002;23:53–57.

167. Pelosi E, Arena V, Baudino B, et al. Pre-operative lymphatic mapping and intra-operative sentinel lymph node detection in early stage endometrial cancer. *Nucl Med Commun* 2003;24:971–975.

168. Dargent D, Ansquer Y, Mathevet P. Technical development and results of left extraperitoneal laparoscopic paraaortic lymphadenectomy for cervical cancer. *Gynecol Oncol* 2000;77:87–92.

169. Vasilev SA, McGonigle KF. Extraperitoneal laparoscopic para-aortic lymph node dissection. *Gynecol Oncol* 1996;61:315–320.

170. Querleu D, Dargent D, Ansquer Y, et al. Extraperitoneal endosurgical aortic and common iliac dissection in the staging of bulky or advanced cervical carcinomas. *Cancer* 2000;88:883–891.

171. Sonoda Y, Leblanc E, Querleu D, et al. Prospective evaluation of surgical staging of advanced cervical cancer via a laparoscopic extraperitoneal approach. *Gynecol Oncol* 2003;91:326–331.

172. Occelli B, Narducci F, Lanvin D, et al. De novo adhesions with extraperitoneal endosurgical para-aortic lymphadenectomy versus transperitoneal laparoscopic para-aortic lymphadenectomy: a randomized experimental study. *Am J Obstet Gynecol* 2000;183:529–533

173. Donnez J, Nisolle M. *An atlas of operative laparoscopy and hysteroscopy.* 2nd ed. Boca Raton, FL: CRC Press–Parthenon, 2001.

174. Reich HJ, De Caprio J, McGlynn F. Laparoscopic hysterectomy. *J Gynecol Surg* 1989;5:213.

175. Dargent D, Mathevet P. Radical vaginal hysterectomy in the primary management of invasive cervical cancer. In: Rubin S, Hoskins W, eds. *Cervical cancer and preinvasive neoplasia.* New York: Raven Press, 1996:207.

176. Kadar N, Reich H. Laparoscopically assisted radical Schauta hysterectomy and bilateral laparoscopic pelvic lymphadenectomy for the treatment of bulky stage IB carcinoma of the cervix. *Gynaecol Endosc* 1993;2:135.

177. Martin X. Hysterectomie elargie laparoscopico-vaginale dans le traitement des cancers du col uterin. *These Medecine Lyon* October 1997; 191.

178. Hockel M, Konerding MA, Heussel CP. Liposuction-assisted nerve-sparing extended radical hysterectomy: oncologic rationale, surgical anatomy, and feasibility study. *Am J Obstet Gynecol* 1998;178: 971–976.

179. Sardi J, Vidaurreta J, Bermudez A, di Paola G. Laparoscopically assisted Schauta operation: learning experience at the Gynecologic Oncology Unit, Buenos Aires University Hospital. *Gynecol Oncol* 1999; 75:361–365.

180. Querleu D, Narducci F, Poulard V, et al. Modified radical vaginal hysterectomy with or without laparoscopic nerve-sparing dissection: a comparative study. *Gynecol Oncol* 2002;85:154–158.

181. Hertel H, Kohler C, Michels W, et al. Laparoscopic-assisted radical vaginal hysterectomy (LARVH): prospective evaluation of 200 patients with cervical cancer. *Gynecol Oncol* 2003;90:505–511.

182. Possover M, Stober S, Plaul K, Schneider A. Identification and preservation of the motoric innervation of the bladder in radical hysterectomy type III. *Gynecol Oncol* 2000;79:154–157.

183. Possover M. Technical modification of the nerve-sparing laparoscopy-assisted VRH type 3 for better reproducibility of this procedure. *Gynecol Oncol* 2003;90:245–247.

184. Possover M, Krause N, Kuhne-Heid R, Schneider A. Laparoscopic assistance for extended radicality of radical vaginal hysterectomy: description of a technique. *Gynecol Oncol* 1998;70:94–99.

185. Dargent D, Brun JL, Remy I. Pregnancies following radical trachelectomy for invasive cervical cancer. *Gynecol Oncol* 1994;52:105(abst).

186. Schneider A, Krause N, Kuhne-Heid R, et al. Laparoscopic paraaortic and pelvic lymph node excision—initial experiences and development of a technique. *Zentralbl Gynakol* 1996;118:498–504.

187. Shepherd JH, Crawford RA, Oram DH. Radical trachelectomy: a way to preserve fertility in the treatment of early cervical cancer. *Br J Obstet Gynaecol* 1998;105:912–916.

188. Roy M, Plante M. Pregnancies after radical vaginal trachelectomy for early-stage cervical cancer. *Am J Obstet Gynecol* 1998;179: 1491–1496.

189. Covens A, Shaw P. Is radical trachelectomy a safe radical hysterectomy for early-stage IB carcinoma of the cervix. *Cancer* 1999;86: 2273–2279.

190. Dargent D, Franzosi F, Ansquer Y, et al. Extended trachelectomy relapse: plea for patient involvement in the medical decision. *Bull Cancer* 2002;89:1027–1030.

191. Shepherd JH, Mould T, Oram DH. Radical trachelectomy in early stage carcinoma of the cervix: outcome as judged by recurrence and fertility rates. *Br J Obstet Gynaecol* 2001;108:882–885.

192. Schlaerth JB, Spirtos NM, Schlaerth AC. Radical trachelectomy and pelvic lymphadenectomy with uterine preservation in the treatment of cervical cancer. *Am J Obstet Gynecol* 2003;188:29–34.

193. Burnett AF, Roman LD, O'Meara AT, Morrow CP. Radical vaginal trachelectomy and pelvic lymphadenectomy for preservation of fertility in early cervical carcinoma. *Gynecol Oncol* 2003;88:419–423.

194. Morice (Gynecol Oncol 2004; in press).

195. Bernardini M, Barrett J, Seaward G, Covens A. Pregnancy outcomes in patients after radical trachelectomy. *Am J Obstet Gynecol* 2003; 189:1378–1382.

196. Saling E. Early total occlusion of os uteri prevents habitual abortion and premature deliveries. *Z Geburtshilfe Perinatol* 1981;185: 259–261.

197. Nezhat CR, Nezhat FR, Burrell MO, et al. Laparoscopic radical hysterectomy and laparoscopically assisted vaginal radical hysterectomy with pelvic and paraaortic node dissection. *J Gynecol Surg* 1993;9: 105–120.

198. Sedlacek TV, Campion MJ, Hutchins RA, Reich H. Laparoscopic radical hysterectomy: a preliminary report. *J Am Assoc Gynecol Laparosc* 1994;1(4, Part 2):S32.

199. Spirtos NM, Schlaerth JB, Kimball RE, et al. Laparoscopic radical hysterectomy (type III) with aortic and pelvic lymphadenectomy. *Am J Obstet Gynecol* 1996;174:1763–1767.

200. Canis M, Wattiez A, Mage G, et al. Laparoscopic radical hysterectomy for cervical cancer. In: Querleu D, Childers J, Dargent D, eds. *Laparoscopic surgery in gynaecological oncology.* Paris: Blackwell Science, 1999:70–77.

201. Sedlacek TV. Laparoscopic radical hysterectomy: the next evolutionary step in the treatment of invasive cervical cancer. *J Gynecol Tech* 1995;1:223.

202. Canis M, Dauplat J, Pomel C, et al. Laparoscopic radical hysterectomy for cervical cancer. Results about 41 cases IGCS. *Int J Gynecol Cancer* 1997;7:3(abst).

203. Pomel C, Atallah D, Bouedec GL, et al. Laparoscopic radical hysterectomy for invasive cervical cancer: 8-year experience of a pilot study. *Gynecol Oncol* 2003;91:534–539.

204. Plante M, Roy M. Operative laparoscopy prior to a pelvic exenteration in patients with recurrent cervical cancer. *Gynecol Oncol* 1998;69: 94–99.

205. Kohler C, Tozzi R, Possover M, Schneider A. Explorative laparoscopy prior to exenterative surgery. *Gynecol Oncol* 2002;86:311–315.

206. Clark VG. A more radical method of performing hysterectomy for cancer of the uterus. *Bull Johns Hopkins Hosp* 1895:120–124.

207. Landoni F, Maneo A, Colombo A, et al. Randomised study of radical

surgery versus radiotherapy for stage Ib-IIa cervical cancer. *Lancet* 1997;350:535–540.

208. Alvarez RD, Potter ME, Soong SJ, et al. Rationale for using pathologic tumor dimensions and nodal status to subclassify surgically treated stage IB cervical cancer patients. *Gynecol Oncol* 1991;43:108–112.

209. Delgado G, Bundy B, Zaino R, et al. Prospective surgical-pathological study of disease-free interval in patients with stage IB squamous cell carcinoma of the cervix: a Gynecologic Oncology Group study. *Gynecol Oncol* 1990;38:352–357.

210. Fiorica JV, Roberts WS, Greenberg H, et al. Morbidity and survival patterns in patients after radical hysterectomy and postoperative adjuvant pelvic radiotherapy. *Gynecol Oncol* 1990;36:343–347.

211. Soisson AP, Soper JT, Clarke-Pearson DL, et al. Adjuvant radiotherapy following radical hysterectomy for patients with stage IB and IIA cervical cancer. *Gynecol Oncol* 1990;37:390–395.

212. Thomas GM, Dembo AJ. Is there a role for adjuvant pelvic radiotherapy after radical hysterectomy in early stage cervical cancer? *Int J Gynecol Cancer* 1993;3:193.

213. Dargent D, Salvat J. Valeur des méthodes non invasives dans l'appréciation de l'état des ganglions ilio-pelviens et lombo-aorticques. In: Dargent D, Salvat J, eds. *L'envahissement ganglionnaire pelvien.* Paris: Medsi McGraw-Hill, 1989:55.

214. Berman ML, Bergen S, Salazar H. Influence of histological features and treatment on the prognosis of patients with cervical cancer metastatic to pelvic lymph nodes. *Gynecol Oncol* 1990;39:127–131.

215. Hacker NF, Wain GV, Nicklin JL. Resection of bulky positive lymph nodes in patients with cervical carcinoma. *Int J Gynecol Cancer* 1995;5:250–256.

216. Cosin JA, Fowler JM, Chen MD, et al. Pretreatment surgical staging of patients with cervical carcinoma: the case for lymph node debulking. *Cancer* 1998;82:2241–2248.

217. Haie C, Pejovic MH, Gerbaulet A, et al. Is prophylactic para-aortic irradiation worthwhile in the treatment of advanced cervical carcinoma? Results of a controlled clinical trial of the EORTC radiotherapy group. *Radiother Oncol* 1988;11:101–112.

218. Cunningham MJ, Dunton CJ, Corn B, et al. Extended-field radiation therapy in early-stage cervical carcinoma: survival and complications. *Gynecol Oncol* 1991;43:51–54.

219. Weiser EB, Bundy BN, Hoskins WJ, et al. Extraperitoneal versus transperitoneal selective paraaortic lymphadenectomy in the pretreatment surgical staging of advanced cervical carcinoma (a Gynecologic Oncology Group study). *Gynecol Oncol* 1989;33:283–289.

220. Johnson PL, Sibert KS. Laparoscopy. Gasless vs. CO_2 pneumoperitoneum. *J Reprod Med* 1997;42:255–259.

221. Chan JK, Lin YG, Monk BJ, et al. Vaginal hysterectomy as primary treatment of endometrial cancer in medically compromised women. *Obstet Gynecol* 2001;97(5 Pt 1):707–711.

222. Dargent D. Imaging and endoscopy in management of endometrial carcinoma. *Giorn It Oncol* 1995;3:149.

223. Creasman WT, Morrow CP, Bundy BN, et al. Surgical pathologic spread patterns of endometrial cancer. A Gynecologic Oncology Group study. *Cancer* 1987;60:2035–2041.

224. Bidzinski M, Mettler L, Zielinski J. Endoscopic lymphadenectomy and LAVH in the treatment of endometrial cancer. *Eur J Gynaecol Oncol* 1998;19:32–34.

225. Holub Z, Voracek J, Shomani A. A comparison of laparoscopic surgery with open procedure in endometrial cancer. *Eur J Gynaecol Oncol* 1998;19:294–296.

226. Mettler L. Indications for laparoscopic surgery in cases of gynecological malignancies (endometrial cancer). *Int Surg* 1996;81:266–270.

227. Gemignani ML, Curtin JP, Zelmanovich J, et al. Laparoscopic-assisted vaginal hysterectomy for endometrial cancer: clinical outcomes and hospital charges. *Gynecol Oncol* 1999;73:5–11. .

228. Eltabbakh GH, Shamonki MI, Moody JM, Garafano LL. Laparoscopy as the primary modality for the treatment of women with endometrial carcinoma. *Cancer* 2001;91:378–387.

229. Boike G, Lurain J, Burke J. A comparison of laparoscopic management of endometrial cancer with traditional laparotomy. *Gynecol Oncol* 1994;52:105.

230. Malur S, Possover M, Michels W, Schneider A. Laparoscopic-assisted vaginal versus abdominal surgery in patients with endometrial cancer—a prospective randomized trial. *Gynecol Oncol* 2001;80:239–244.

231. Fram KM. Laparoscopically assisted vaginal hysterectomy versus abdominal hysterectomy in stage I endometrial cancer. *Int J Gynecol Cancer* 2002;12:57–61.

232. Scribner DR Jr, Walker JL, Johnson GA, et al. Laparoscopic pelvic and paraaortic lymph node dissection in the obese. *Gynecol Oncol* 2002;84:426–430.

233. Scribner DR Jr, Walker JL, Johnson GA, et al. Surgical management of early-stage endometrial cancer in the elderly: is laparoscopy feasible? *Gynecol Oncol* 2001;83:563–568.

234. Sonoda Y, Zerbe M, Smith A, et al. High incidence of positive peritoneal cytology in low-risk endometrial cancer treated by laparoscopically assisted vaginal hysterectomy. *Gynecol Oncol* 2001;80:378–382.

235. Vergote I, De Smet I, Amant F. Incidence of positive peritoneal cytology in low-risk endometrial cancer treated by laparoscopically assisted vaginal hysterectomy. *Gynecol Oncol* 2002;84:537–538.

236. Sonoda Y, Luken DW, Chi DS, et al. The significance of positive peritoneal cytology in clinical early-stage endometrial cancer patients treated by laparoscopically assisted vaginal hysterectomy. Society of Gynecologic Oncologists. San Diego, February 7–11, 2004. Abstract #108.

237. Nelson BE, Rosenfield AT, Schwartz PE. Preoperative abdominopelvic computed tomographic prediction of optimal cytoreduction in epithelial ovarian carcinoma. *J Clin Oncol*.1993;11:166–172.

238. Schwartz PE, Chambers JT, Makuch R. Neoadjuvant chemotherapy for advanced ovarian cancer. *Gynecol Oncol* 1994;53:33–37.

239. Schwartz PE, Rutherford TJ, Chambers JT, et al. Neoadjuvant chemotherapy for advanced ovarian cancer: long-term survival. *Gynecol Oncol* 1999;72:93–99.

240. Chan YM, Ng TY, Ngan HY, Wong LC. Quality of life in women treated with neoadjuvant chemotherapy for advanced ovarian cancer: a prospective longitudinal study. *Gynecol Oncol* 2003;88:9–16.

241. Plante M, Renaud MC, Roy M. Flaws in the use of neoadjuvant chemotherapy in advanced ovarian cancer. In: 8th Biennial Meeting of the International Gynecologic Cancer Society, Bologna: Monduzzi Editore, 2001:197.

242. Schwartz PE, Zheng W. Neoadjuvant chemotherapy for advanced ovarian cancer: the role of cytology in pretreatment diagnosis. *Gynecol Oncol* 2003;90:644–650.

243. Ben David Y, Bustan M, Shalev E. Laparoscopy as part of the evaluation and management of ovarian and cervix neoplasms. *Harefuah* 2001;140:464–467.

244. van Dam PA, DeCloedt J, Tjalma WA, et al. Trocar implantation metastasis after laparoscopy in patients with advanced ovarian cancer: can the risk be reduced? *Am J Obstet Gynecol.* 1999;181(3):536–541.

245. Ansquer Y, Leblanc E, Clough K, et al. Neoadjuvant chemotherapy for unresectable ovarian carcinoma: a French multicenter study. *Cancer* 2001;15:91:2329–2334.

246. Husain A, Chi DS, Prasad M, et al. The role of laparoscopy in second-look evaluations for ovarian cancer. *Gynecol Oncol* 2001;80:44–47.

247. Clough KB, Ladonne JM, Nos C, et al. Second look for ovarian cancer: laparoscopy or laparotomy? A prospective comparative study. *Gynecol Oncol* 1999;72:411–417.

248. Abu-Rustum NR, Barakat RR, Siegel PL, et al. Second-look operation for epithelial ovarian cancer: laparoscopy or laparotomy? *Obstet Gynecol* 1996;88(4 Pt 1):549–553.

249. Anaf V, Gangji D, Simon P, Saylam K. Laparoscopical insertion of intraperitoneal catheters for intraperitoneal chemotherapy. *Acta Obstet Gynecol Scand* 2003;82:1140–1145.

250. Soper JT, Johnson P, Johnson V, et al. Comprehensive restaging laparotomy in women with apparent early ovarian carcinoma. *Obstet Gynecol* 1992;80:949–953.

251. Faught W, Le T, Fung Kee Fung M, et al.Early ovarian cancer: what is the staging impact of retroperitoneal node sampling? *J Obstet Gynaecol Can* 2003;25:18–21.

252. Chu KK, Chen FP, Chang SD. Laparoscopic surgical procedures for early ovarian cancer. *Acta Obstet Gynecol Scand* 1995;74:391–392.

253. Amara DP, Nezhat C, Teng NN, et al. Operative laparoscopy in the management of ovarian cancer. *Surg Laparosc Endosc* 1996;6:38–45.

254. Childers JM, Lang J, Surwit EA, Hatch KD. Laparoscopic surgical staging of ovarian cancer. *Gynecol Oncol* 1995;59:25–33.

255. Pomel C, Provencher D, Dauplat J, et al. Laparoscopic staging of early ovarian cancer. *Gynecol Oncol* 1995;58:301–306.

256. Land R, Perrin L, Nicklin J. Evaluation of restaging in clinical stage 1A low malignant potential ovarian tumours. *Aust N Z J Obstet Gynaecol.* 2002;42:379–382.

257. Querleu D, Papageorgiou T, Lambaudie E, et al. Laparoscopic restaging of borderline ovarian tumours: results of 30 cases initially presumed as stage IA borderline ovarian tumours. *Brit J Obstet Gynaecol* 2003;110:201–204.

258. Biran G, Golan A, Sagiv R, et al. Conversion of laparoscopy to laparotomy due to adnexal malignancy. *Eur J Gynaecol Oncol* 2002;23: 157–160.

259. Canis M, Botchorishvili R, Manhes H, et al. Management of adnexal masses: role and risk of laparoscopy. *Semin Surg Oncol* 2000;19: 28–35.

260. Theodoridis TD, Bontis JN. Laparoscopy and oncology: where do we stand today? *Ann N Y Acad Sci.* 2003;997:282–291.

261. Haughney RV, Slade RJ, Brain AN. An isolated abdominal wall metastasis of ovarian carcinoma ten years after primary surgery. *Eur J Gynaecol Oncol* 2001;22:102.

262. Carlson NL, Krivak TC, Winter WE 3rd, Macri CI. Port site metastasis of ovarian carcinoma remote from laparoscopic surgery for benign disease. *Gynecol Oncol* 2002;85:529–531.

263. Viala J, Morice P, Pautier P, et al. CT findings in two cases of port-site metastasis after laparoscopy for ovarian cancer. *Eur J Gynaecol Oncol* 2002;23:293–294.

264. Huang KG, Wang CJ, Chang TC, et al. Management of port-site metastasis after laparoscopic surgery for ovarian cancer. *Am J Obstet Gynecol* 2003;189:16–21.

265. Canis M, Rabischong B, Houlle C, et al. Laparoscopic management of adnexal masses: a gold standard? *Curr Opin Obstet Gynecol* 2002; 14:423–428.

266. Magrina JF, Walter AJ, Schild SE. Laparoscopic radical parametrectomy and pelvic and aortic lymphadenectomy for vaginal carcinoma: A case report. *Gynecol Oncol* 1999;75:514–516.

267. Kohler C, Tozzi R, Klemm P, Schneider A. "Schauta sine utero": technique and results of laparoscopic-vaginal radical parametrectomy. *Gynecol Oncol* 2003;91:359–368.

268. DiSaia PJ, Creasman WJ. Invasive carcinoma of the vulva. In: DiSaia PJ, Creasman WJ, eds. *Clinical gynecologic oncology.* 4th ed. New York: Mosby, 1993:263.

269. Lin JY, DuBeshter B, Angel C, Dvoretsky PM. Morbidity and recurrence with modifications of radical vulvectomy and groin dissection. *Gynecol Oncol* 1992;47:80–86.

270. Terada KY, Shimizu DM, Wong JH. Sentinel node dissection and ultrastaging in squamous cell cancer of the vulva. *Gynecol Oncol* 2000;76:40–44.

271. Tamussino KF, Bader AA, Lax SF, et al. Groin recurrence after micrometastasis in a sentinel lymph node in a patient with vulvar cancer. *Gynecol Oncol* 2002;86:99–101.

272. Suzanne F, Emering C, Wattiez A, et al. Axillary lymphadenectomy by lipo-aspiration and endoscopic picking. Apropos of 72 cases. *Chirurgie* 1997;122:138–142.

273. Rodriguez M, Guimares O, Rose PG. Radical abdominal trachelectomy and pelvic lymphadenectomy with uterine conservation and subsequent pregnancy in the treatment of early invasive cervical cancer. *Am J Obstet Gynecol* 2001;185:370–374.

CHAPTER 14

Biologic and Physical Aspects of Radiation Oncology

Carlos A. Perez, James A. Purdy, Zuofeng Li, and E.J. Hall

HISTORICAL PERSPECTIVE

The biologic effects of ionizing radiations were recognized shortly after Roentgen (1) discovered x-rays in 1895 and Marie and Pierre Curie reported their discovery of radium in 1898 (2). The first patient treated with x-ray therapy was reported in 1899, following which clinical radiation therapy had an exciting growth in the early 1920s. From 1913 through 1930, numerous reports were published on the use of irradiation: namely, intracavitary radium for the treatment of carcinoma of the uterine cervix. As noted by Janeway (3), Wickham began his work in this field in 1906 and published results of the treatment of 1,000 cases in 1912 (4). Kroenig (5) published an introduction to the use of radioactivity in gynecology, but although he may have done pioneer work in the field, it was the reports of Bumm (6) and Doederlein (7) at Halle in 1913, along with others (8), that furnished great impetus to the treatment of cancer of the uterus with radium. By 1934, Coutard (9) had developed a protracted, fractionated dose scheme that remains the basis for current radiation therapy, and in 1936, Paterson (10) published results of the treatment of cancer with x-rays, including that of the uterine cervix. With time, the use of ionizing radiation was refined, and treatment planning and delivery became more accurate and reproducible. X-ray generators operating at 800 to 1,000 kV were used for medical purposes as early as 1932: these were followed by cyclotrons, synchrocyclotrons, betatrons, bevatrons, linear accelerators, and nuclear reactors. Radioisotopes such as ^{60}Co, ^{137}Cs, ^{196}Au, ^{192}Ir, ^{125}I, and recently, ^{103}Pd and ^{252}Cf have supplemented brachytherapy techniques.

Carlos A. Perez, James A. Purdy, and Zuofeng Li: Department of Radiation Oncology, Washington University School of Medicine, St. Louis, Missouri 63108

E.J. Hall: Center for Radiological Research, Columbia University, New York, New York 10032

RADIATION ONCOLOGY IN CANCER MANAGEMENT

Radiation oncology is a clinical and scientific specialty devoted to the management of patients with cancer (and occasionally some benign diseases) by ionizing radiation, alone or combined with other modalities, investigation of the biologic and physical basis of radiation therapy, and training of professionals in the field.

The aim of radiation therapy is to deliver a precisely measured dose of irradiation to a defined tumor volume with as minimal damage as possible to surrounding normal tissues, resulting in eradication of the tumor, prolongation of survival, and a high quality of life at competitive cost. In addition to curative efforts, irradiation plays a major role in cancer management in the effective palliation or prevention of symptoms of the disease: Bleeding is eliminated, pain can be alleviated, luminal patency restored, skeletal integrity preserved, and organ function reestablished with minimal morbidity in a variety of clinical circumstances (11).

PRESCRIPTION OF IRRADIATION AND TREATMENT PLANNING

The clinical use of irradiation is a complex process involving many professionals and multiple interrelated functions (Fig.14.1). The aim of therapy should be defined before treatment as either curative or palliative. In the palliation of primary tumors, relatively high doses of irradiation (sometimes 75% to 80% of curative dose) may be required to control the tumor for the expected survival period of the patient.

The prescription of irradiation is based on the following factors:

1. Evaluation of the full *extent of the tumor* (staging) by whatever means available, including imaging, nuclear medicine, ultrasound, and other studies.

KEY STAFF FUNCTION IN RADIATION THERAPY

	KEY STAFF	SUPPORTIVE ROLE
1. CLINICAL EVALUATION	Rad. Oncologist	
2. THERAPEUTIC DECISION	Rad. Oncologist	
3. TARGET VOLUME LOCALIZATION		
Tumor Volume	Rad. Oncologist	Sim. Tech./Dosimetrist
Sensitive Critical Organs	Rad. Oncologist	Sim. Tech./Dosimetrist
Patient Contour	Dosimetrist	Sim. Tech./Dosimetrist
4. TREATMENT PLANNING		
Beam Data Computerization	Physicist	
Computation of Beams	Physicist	Dosimetrist
Shielding Blocks, Treatment Aids, etc.	Dosimetrist/ Mold Room Tech.	Rad. Oncologist/ Physicist
Analysis of Alternate Plans	Rad. Oncologist/ Physicist	Dosimetrist
Selection of Treatment Plan	Rad. Oncologist/ Physicist	
Dose Calculation	Dosimetrist	Physicist
5. SIMULATION/VERIFICATION OF TREATMENT PLAN	Rad. Oncologist/ Sim. Tech.	Dosimetrist/ Physicist
6. TREATMENT		
First Day Setup	Rad. Oncologist/ Physicist/ Therapy Techs.	Dosimetrist/ Physicist
Localization Films	Rad. Oncologist/ Therapy Techs.	
Dosimetry Checks/ Initial Chart Review	Physicist/ Rad. Oncologist	Dosimetrist/ Chief Tech.
Repositioning/Retreatment	Therapy Techs.	Dosimetrist/ Chief Tech.
7. PERIODIC EVALUATION (During Treatment)		
Tumor Response/Tolerance	Rad. Oncologist	Nurses/RTTs
8. FOLLOW-UP EVALUATION	Rad. Oncologist	Nurses

FIG. 14.1. Functions involved in radiation therapy. (From Radiation Oncology in Integrated Cancer Management: Report of the Inter-Study Council for Radiation Oncology. Inter-Study Council for Radiation Oncology, 1986, with permission.)

2. Knowledge of the *pathologic characteristics* of the disease, including potential areas of spread, that may influence choice of therapy (e.g., rationale for elective irradiation of the lymphatics in the pelvis).

3. Definition of *goal of therapy* (cure or palliation).

4. Selection of appropriate *treatment modalities*, which may be irradiation alone or combined with surgery, chemotherapy, or both. The choice may have a significant impact on the volume treated and the doses of radiation delivered.

5. Determination of the *optimal dose and fractionation of radiation and volume* to be treated, which depends on the anatomic location, histologic type, stage and other characteristics of the tumor, and the normal structures (organs at risk) in the region.

6. Periodic *evaluation* of the patient's general condition, tumor response, and status of the normal tissues treated during and after therapy.

The radiation oncologist must work closely with the gynecologic and/or medical oncologist to integrate the various modalities and with the physics, treatment planning, and dosimetry staffs to ensure the greatest possible accuracy and practicality in the design of treatment plans and computation of dose distributions. The ultimate responsibility for treatment decisions and the technical execution of the radiation therapy, as well as its consequences, will always rest with the radiation oncologist (12).

It should be stressed that different doses of radiation are required for a given probability of tumor control that depends on the initial number of clonogenic cells present. Therefore, varying radiation doses are delivered to certain portions of the tumor (periphery vs central portion) or in cases in which all gross tumor has been surgically removed (13). From the standpoint of cell burden, a clinical tumor can be considered to encompass several compartments: (a) macroscopic, visible, or palpable; (b) microextensions into

DEFINITION OF "VOLUMES" IN RADIATION THERAPY

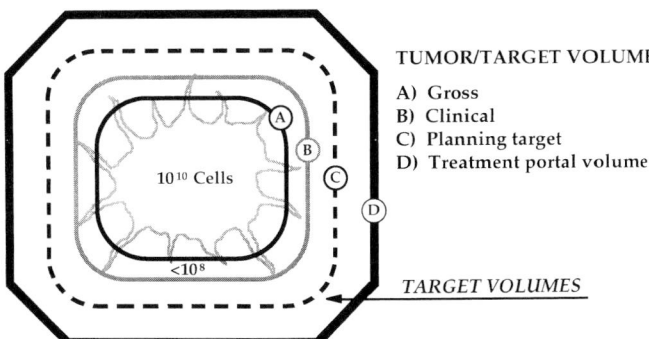

TUMOR/TARGET VOLUME

A) Gross
B) Clinical
C) Planning target
D) Treatment portal volume

TARGET VOLUMES

FIG. 14.2. Schematic representation of "volumes" in radiation therapy. The treatment portal volume includes the gross tumor volume, potential areas of local and regional microscopic disease around the tumor (clinical), and a margin of surrounding normal tissue (planning). (From Perez CA, Purdy JA. Rationale for treatment planning in radiation therapy. In: Levitt SH, Khan FM, Potish RA, eds. *Levitt and Tapley's technological basis of radiation therapy: practical clinical applications.* 2nd ed. Philadelphia: Lea & Febiger, 1992. Modified in: Perez CA, Brady LW, Roti Roti JL. Overview. In: Perez CA, Brady LW, eds. *Principles and practice of radiation oncology.* 3rd ed. Philadelphia: Lippincott–Raven Publishers, 1998:1, with permission.)

adjacent tissues; and (c) subclinical disease, presumed to be present but not detectable even under the microscope. These various targets have been defined according to International Commission on Radiation Units (ICRU) Report No. 50 as gross tumor volume (GTV), all known gross disease including abnormally enlarged regional lymph nodes: clinical target volume (CTV), which encompasses the GTV plus regions considered to harbor potential microscopic disease: planning target volume (PTV) provides a margin around the CTV to allow for variation in treatment setup, breathing motion, or other anatomic motion during treatment, but does not include beam characteristics (penumbra) (Fig. 14.2) (14). The treatment portals must adequately cover all three compartments in addition to a margin to compensate for geometric inaccuracies during daily irradiation exposure. Sensitive structures within the irradiated volume, such as the bladder or the rectum in the pelvis, should be clearly identified, and the maximum doses to be delivered to them must be specified. The concept of organs at risk (OAR) within the irradiated volume have been further defined in ICRU Bulletin No. 62 (Fig. 14.3) (15).

Simulation with conventional or three-dimensional (3-D) simulators is necessary in most instances to identify accurately the tumor volume and sensitive structures and to document the configuration of the portals and target volume to be irradiated. *Treatment aids,* such as shielding blocks, molds, masks, immobilization devices, and compensators, are ex-

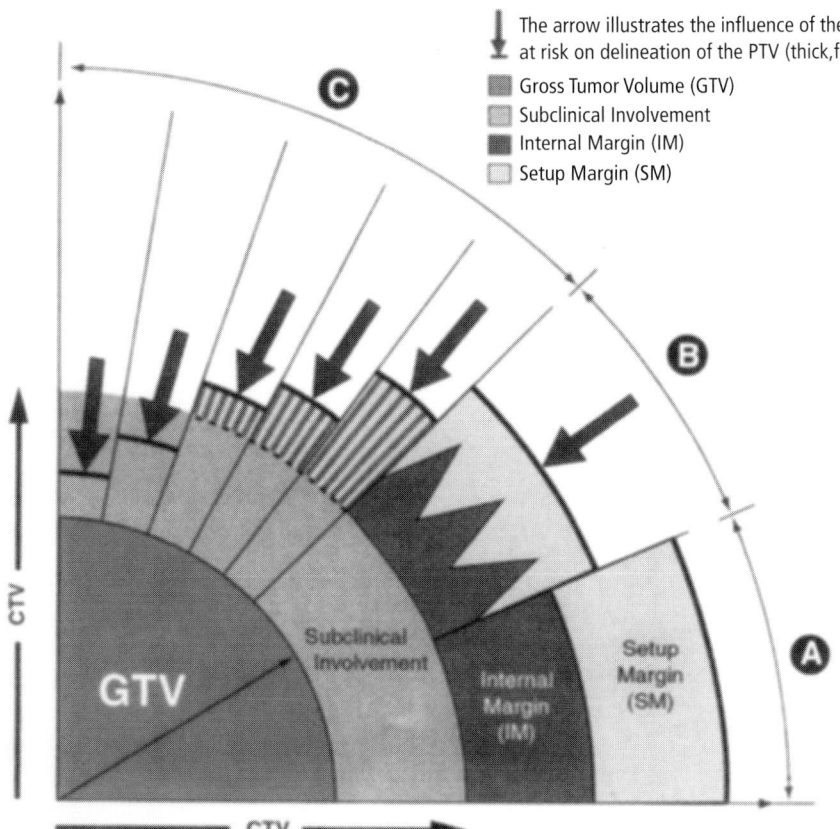

The arrow illustrates the influence of the organs at risk on delineation of the PTV (thick, full line).

- Gross Tumor Volume (GTV)
- Subclinical Involvement
- Internal Margin (IM)
- Setup Margin (SM)

FIG. 14.3. Schematic representations of the relations between the different volumes (GTV, CTV, PTV, and PRV) in different clinical scenarios. (From International Commission on Radiological Units and Measurements. Report No. 62 Prescribing, Recording, and Reporting Photon Beam Therapy [Supplement to ICRU Report 50]. Bethesda, MD: International Commission of Radiation Units and Measurements, 1999, with permission.)

tremely important elements in treatment planning and delivery of optimal dose distribution. *Repositioning* and *immobilization* are critical since the only effective irradiation is that which strikes the clonogenic tumor cells. Therefore, in fractionated irradiation, accurate setup should be such that the patient will maintain the desired position during every daily treatment. Devices such as the Alpha Cradle, plaster casts, thermoplastic molds, bite blocks, and arm boards are invaluable in assisting technologists in patient positioning. *Treatment planning and dosimetry* procedures are valuable tools that assist the radiation oncologist and physicist in achieving optimal irradiation of the target volume with relative sparing of surrounding normal tissues. Treatment is delivered with external beams (photons, electrons, protons), with intracavitary or interstitial radiation sources, or with combinations of various modalities. Accuracy is periodically assessed with portal (localization) films: on-line verification monitoring is under investigation (16).

Suit and associates (17) reviewed various recent technologic developments that through more precise treatment planning and delivery techniques reduce the volume irradiated and improve dose distributions, which should enhance therapeutic outcome.

STRUCTURE OF THE ATOM

The atom may be thought of as consisting of a centrally located core (the nucleus) surrounded by small orbiting particles (the electrons). The overall dimension of the atom is about 10^{-10} m, and the nucleus is about 10^{-14} m. Nearly all of the mass of the atom is contained in the nucleus, which is composed of protons and neutrons, known collectively as nucleons. A proton carries a positive electrical charge equal in magnitude to the charge of the electron: collectively, the protons constitute the electrical charge of the nucleus. A neutron has a slightly larger mass than a proton and has no electrical charge. Electrons, which are negatively charged, have a rest mass about 2,000 times smaller than that of either a proton or a neutron and thus contribute very little mass to an atom (3).

Electrical charges of opposite signs attract one another by an electrostatic force, whereas charges of the same sign repel one another. The negatively charged electrons are thus bound to the positively charged nucleus and can be considered to revolve around it like planets revolving around the sun. Niels Bohr quantitated this planetary model in 1913 with his theory, in which he postulated that the electrons are confined to specific orbits at specific distances from the nucleus. When an electron moves to an orbit closer to the nucleus, energy is released: conversely, for the electron to move farther away from the nucleus, energy must be supplied. Electron orbits are grouped into shells in which only a certain maximum number of electrons is allowed, given by the relationship $2n^2$, where n is an integer specific to each shell and is called the *principal quantum number*. Two electrons can exist in the first shell, 8 in the second, 18 in the third, and so on. Historically, the shells are labeled by letters of the alphabet, with K being the shell closest to the nucleus, L the next, and so forth. Modern physics has replaced the simplistic orbiting electron model of Bohr with an abstract model of diffuse electron clouds that represent probability functions of the electron's position. However, to understand radiologic physics, the simple model of a nucleus composed of protons and neutrons and surrounded by electrons is sufficient.

The atom of an element is specified by its atomic number, denoted by the symbol Z, and its mass number, denoted by the symbol A. The atomic number is equal to the number of protons in the nucleus, and the mass number is equal to the number of nucleons (protons and neutrons) in the nucleus. Hence, A minus Z is equal to the number of neutrons, denoted by the symbol N, within the nucleus. In addition, each element has an associated chemical symbol, (e.g., Co for cobalt). When these definitions are used, the standard notation to specify an atom is $_{Z}^{A}X$, as illustrated by $_{27}^{60}Co$, which is a radioactive isotope of the element cobalt that has an atomic number of 27 (i.e., 27 protons) and a mass number of 60 (i.e., 60 nucleons or 27 protons and 33 neutrons).

Isotopes of an element, such as $_{27}^{58}Co$, $_{27}^{59}Co$, and $_{27}^{60}Co$, have the same atomic number but different numbers of neutrons and, therefore, different mass numbers. Isotopes have the same chemical properties but have different physical properties. Atoms such as $_{27}^{60}Co$ and $_{28}^{60}Ni$, which have the same mass number but different numbers of protons and neutrons, are called *isobars*. Atoms such as $_{27}^{57}Co$ and $_{26}^{56}Fe$, which have the same number of neutrons but different atomic and mass numbers, are called *isotones*.

To complete the picture of atomic structure, the concept of binding energy of an electron must be considered. An electron in an inner shell of an atom is attracted to the nucleus by a force greater than that which the nucleus exerts on an electron farther away. To move an electron from one shell to another farther away (a process called *excitation*) or to remove it completely from the atom (*ionization*), energy must be supplied. Specifically, the energy required to remove an electron completely from an atom is termed the *binding energy* of the electron.

TYPES OF IRRADIATION

The most commonly used radiations in clinical radiation therapy are x-rays, γ-rays and electrons. Protons, neutrons, and other heavier particles have been employed in more experimental treatments.

X-rays and γ-rays are forms of electromagnetic radiation, similar to heat and light, but with a much smaller wavelength. X-rays and γ-rays have the same physical and biologic properties: the different names reflect their different origins. Gamma rays arise from within the nucleus, which means that in practice they are mostly emitted from radioactive isotopes. X-rays arise from outside the nucleus, which means that they are produced by bombardment of a target with high-speed electrons.

Quantum physics allows x-rays and γ-rays to be represented as a stream of photons or pockets of energy. The photon energy (E) is related to the frequency (v) of radiation by the expression

$$E = hv$$

where h is a constant known as Planck's constant. As the wavelength gets shorter, the frequency increases and the photon energy increases. Although x-rays and γ-rays have the same nature as radio waves, heat, and light, they have a shorter wavelength and thus a larger photon energy. This allows them to break chemical bonds and produce biologic effects.

Alpha particles are equivalent to the nucleus of helium, which has two protons and two neutrons. They have a large mass, are positively charged, and are stopped by a few sheets of paper or a few centimeters of air.

Beta particles are negatively charged electrons and are more penetrating than alpha particles, but they are stopped by a few millimeters of aluminum. These particles can transverse a few millimeters in tissue (about 4 mm/1 MV maximum energy).

Protons carry a positive electrical charge equal in magnitude to the charge on the electron. They can be accelerated to high energies (100 to 300 MeV) by a device such as a *cyclotron* or *synchrotron*. The synchrotron has the advantage of simple energy variability, whereas the cyclotron is capable of higher beam intensity.

Neutrons have a mass similar to that of protons, but carry no net electrical charge. They are produced by acceleration of a charged particle, such as a proton or deuteron, to high energies and bombardment of suitable target material, such as beryllium (cyclotron-produced neutrons). Neutrons are also emitted as a by-product of the fission of heavy radioactive atoms in nuclear reactors.

UNITS USED IN RADIATION THERAPY

The *roentgen* (R), the unit for exposure, was also defined at the second International Congress of Radiology in 1928. The definition has been modified slightly by subsequent congresses, but the basic concept remains the same. The roentgen is that amount of x radiation or γ radiation that causes the associated corpuscular emission per 0.001293 g of air to produce, in air, ions carrying one electrostatic unit of charge (esu) of either sign. The value 0.001293 g is the mass of 1 cm^3 of air at 0°C and 760 mm Hg pressure; "associated corpuscular emission" refers to the Compton and pair-production electrons set in motion by the interactions between the incident photons and the air molecules. By conversion of units, the roentgen can be expressed as follows:

$$1 \text{ R} = 2.58 \times 10^{-4} \text{ C/kg air}$$

With the advent of SI units, the roentgen is no longer used to designate a radiation unit, and SI unit for exposure is coulombs per kilogram (C/kg), which is equivalent to approximately 3,876 R (Table 14.1).

Kerma, an acronym for the kinetic energy released in the material, represents the transfer of energy from the photons to the directly ionizing particles (step 1). The subsequent transfer of energy from the directly ionizing particles to the medium (step 2) is represented by the absorbed dose and is defined in terms of the energy deposited by the radiation beam as it passes through the medium. The SI unit for kerma is joule per kilogram (J/kg), which is called *gray* (Gy) (Table 14.1).

The *rad* represents the absorption of 0.01 J/kg of the absorbing material (1 rad = 0.01 J/kg). The rad has now been replaced with the SI unit for absorbed dose (1 J/kg), which is called *gray* (Gy) (Table 14.1). By conversion of units, the gray can be expressed as follows:

$$1 \text{ Gy} = 1 \text{ J/kg} = 1 \text{ cGy} = 100 \text{ rad}$$

Activity, which describes the radioactivity of a sample and is denoted by the symbol A, is defined as the total number of disintegrations per unit of time interval and is given by the following relationship:

$$A = \frac{N}{t} = \gamma N$$

The decay constant equation given above can be expressed in terms of activity:

$$A = A_0 e^{-\lambda t}$$

where A is the activity at time t and A_0 is the initial activity. The *curie* (Ci), a unit of activity, is equal to 3.7×10^{10} disintegrations per second, the approximate number of decays per second by 1 g of ^{226}Ra. The *becquerel* (Bq), the

TABLE 14.1. *SI units for radiation therapy*

Quantity	SI Unit (Name)	Non-SI Unit	Conversion Factor
Exposure	C kg^{-1}	roentgen (R)	1 C $kg^{-1} \approx$ 3876 R
Absorbed dose, kerma	J kg^{-1} [gray (Gy)]	rad	1 Gy = 100 rad
Dose equivalent	J kg^{-1} [sievert (Sv)]	rem	1 Sv = 100 rem
Activity	s^{-1} [becquerel (Bq)]	curie	1 Bq = 2.7×10^{-11} Ci

SI unit for activity, is equal to one disintegration per second (Table 14.1).

$$1 \text{ Bq} = 1 \text{ dps} = 2.7 \times 10^{-11} \text{ Ci} = 2.7 \times 10^{-8} \text{ mCi}$$

or in terms of megabecquerels (Mbq)

$$1 \text{ mCi} = 37 \text{ Mbq}$$

INTERACTION OF RADIATION WITH MATTER

When an x-ray photon enters a thin layer of matter, it is possible that it will pass through without interaction, or it may interact (usually with the atomic electrons) in one of several ways: for the radiations used in radiation therapy the dominant process is the *Compton effect*.

The Compton effect is the interaction of a photon with a loosely bound orbital electron in which part of the incident photon's energy is transferred as kinetic energy to the electron and the remaining energy is carried away by another photon, which thus has less energy than the incident one (Fig. 14.4). The binding energy of the electron is small compared with the incident photon's energy. The energy of the Compton-scattered photon is equal to the difference between the energy of the incident photon and the energy transferred to the electron. If the incoming photon's energy is low (e.g., 100 keV), very little energy is transferred to the electron. As the photon's energy increases, a greater proportion of the energy is transferred to the electron, so the scattered photon necessarily retains a smaller proportion of the incident energy. The photon may be scattered at any angle with respect to the direction of the incident photon, but the Compton electron is confined to angles between 0 and 90 degrees with respect to the direction of the incident photon. If the incoming photon's energy is low, the distribution of the scattered photons is isotropic—equal in all directions. The scatter angles decrease for photons and electrons as the incident

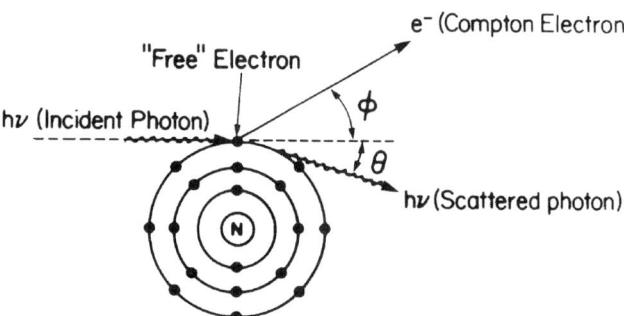

FIG. 14.4. Schematic drawing illustrating the process of the Compton effect. The incident photon interacts with one of the atom's outer electrons, and the energy is shared between the ejected electron and a scattered photon. (From Purdy JA. Principles of radiologic physics, dosimetry, and treatment planning. In: Perez CA, Brady LW, eds. *Principles and practice of radiation oncology.* 3rd ed. Philadelphia: Lippincott–Raven Publishers, 1998, with permission.)

photon's energy increases (e.g., at megavoltage photon energies, both are scattered predominantly in the forward direction).

The probability that a photon will interact with a target atom via the Compton process (σ_c/ρ) depends on the energy of the incoming photon, generally decreasing as the energy of the photon is increased. The probability of a Compton interaction is nearly independent of the atomic number of the absorber and is directly proportional to the number of electrons per gram. This is important in radiation therapy because, as a consequence, when conventional radiations are used to treat a region of the body where bone is involved, the absorbed dose is the same in bone as in soft tissue. If lower energy x-rays are used, as was the case in the 1930s, the Compton process is not the dominant absorption process, and there is preferential absorption in bone since dose depends on the Z of the absorber.

BIOLOGIC EFFECTS OF IONIZING RADIATIONS

Radiations are said to be ionizing if they can ionize atoms or molecules through which they pass (i.e., they are able to knock bound electrons out of orbit).

As already described, the first step in the absorption of x-rays or γ-rays in biologic material results in the photon giving up part or all of its energy to produce a fast-moving recoil electron. This electron may then interact with DNA, the principal target in the cell, by one of two processes: direct or indirect action (Fig. 14.5). In direct action, the electron results in an ionization in the DNA strand, causing a break. This process accounts for only about one-third of the damage produced by x-rays or γ-rays, but is the dominant process for more densely ionizing radiations, such as γ particles or neutrons. Tissues are composed largely of water: thus the most likely reaction is for the fast electron to interact with a water molecule to produce a variety of species, the most important of which is the hydroxyl radical (˙OH). Free radicals carry no electrical charge, but are highly reactive because they have an unpaired electron in the outer shell. They also have a relatively long half-life (10^{-5} second), so they can diffuse some distance to the DNA and cause a break. It is estimated that hydroxyl radicals formed within a distance equal to double the radius of the DNA double helix can diffuse to the DNA and cause biologically significant damage. This process accounts for about two-thirds of the damage produced by x-rays or γ-rays and is that component of the biologic effect that can be modified by chemical sensitizers and protectors. The initial DNA damage leads to a cascade of biologic events (Fig. 14.6) that results in lethality when the cell attempts to divide (mitotic death) or results in programmed cell death (apoptosis).

DNA Breaks and Chromosomal Aberrations

Strong circumstantial evidence exists that DNA is the principal target for all biologic effects of radiation. There is

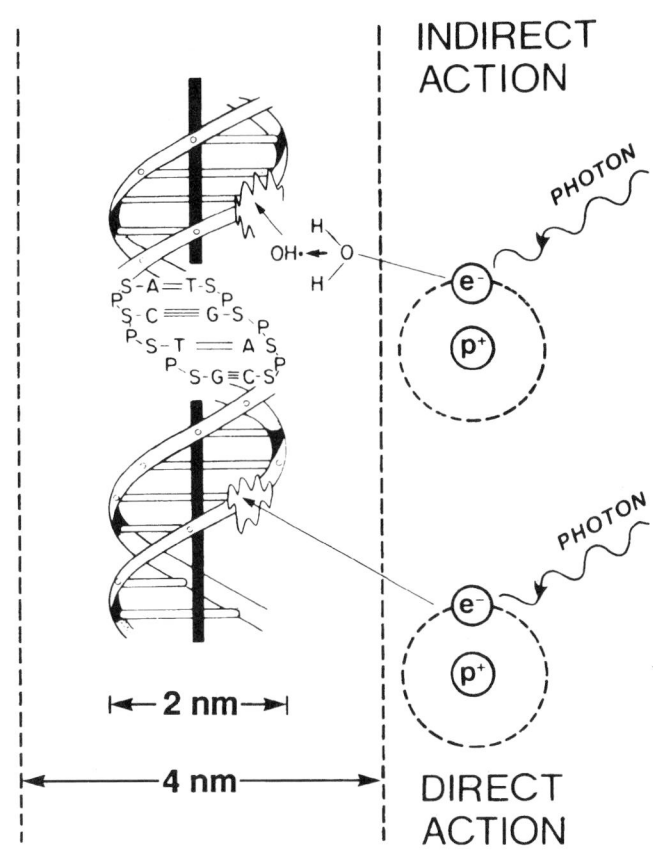

FIG. 14.5. The direct and indirect actions of radiation. The structure of DNA is shown schematically: the letters S, P, A, T, G, and C represent sugar, phosphorus, adenine, thymine, guanine, and cytosine, respectively. In direct action, a secondary electron resulting from absorption of an x-ray photon interacts with the DNA to produce an effect. In indirect action, the secondary electron interacts with, for example, a water molecule to produce an OH' radical, which in turn produces the damage to the DNA. It is estimated that free radicals produced in a cylinder with a radius of 20 Å (2 nm) can affect the DNA. Indirect action is dominant for sparsely ionizing radiation, such as x-rays. (From Hall EJ. *Radiobiology for the radiologist*. 4th ed. Philadelphia: JB Lippincott Co, 1994.)

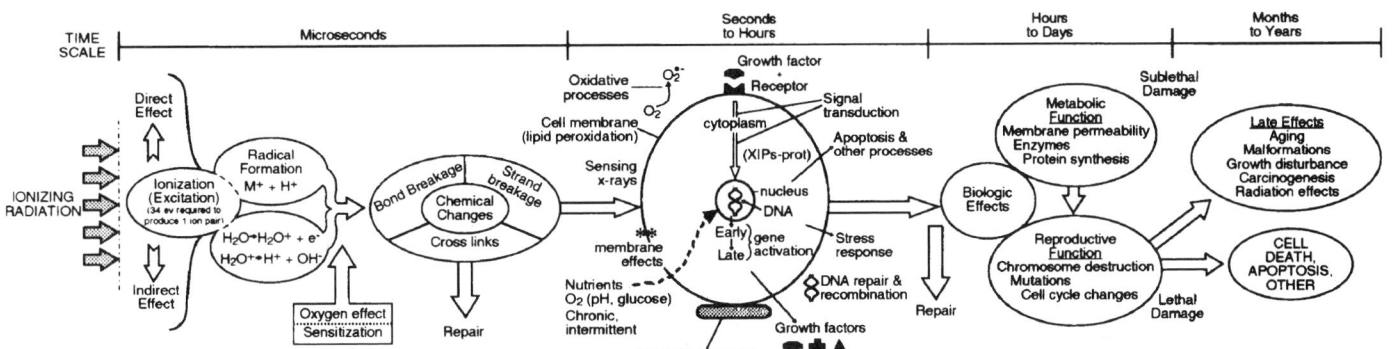

FIG. 14.6. Schematic representation of the various processes that take place after irradiation of an organism. (Modified from Perez CA, Thomas PRM. Radiation therapy: basic concepts and clinical implications. In: Sutow WW, Fernbach DJ, Vietti TJ, eds. *Clinical pediatric oncology*. 3rd ed. St. Louis: Mosby, 1984. In: Perez CA, Brady LW, Roti Roti JL. Overview. In: Perez CA, Brady LW, eds. *Principles and practice of radiation oncology*. 3rd ed. Philadelphia: Lippincott–Raven Publishers, 1998:33, reprinted with permission.)

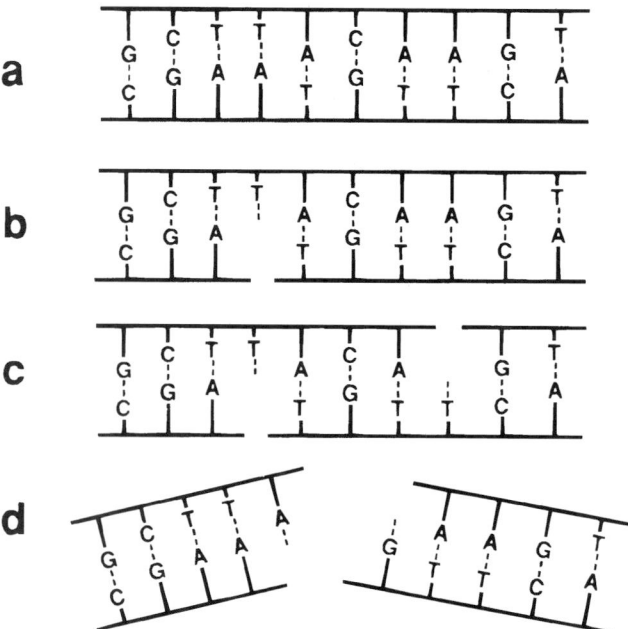

FIG. 14.7. Diagrams of single- and double-strand DNA breaks caused by radiation. **A:** Two-dimensional representation of the normal DNA double helix. The base pairs carrying the genetic code are complementary (i.e., adenine pairs with thymine, guanine pairs with cytosine). **B:** A break in one strand is of little significance because it is readily repaired, using the opposite strand as a template. **C:** Breaks in both strands, if well separated, are repaired as independent breaks. **D:** If breaks occur in both strands and are directly opposite or separated by only a few base pairs, this may lead to a double-strand break, where the chromatin snaps into two pieces. (Courtesy of Dr. John Ward) (From Hall EJ. *Radiobiology for the radiologist.* 4th ed. Philadelphia: JB Lippincott Co, 1994.)

clear evidence that the sensitive site(s) for radiation-induced cell killing is in the nucleus as opposed to the cytoplasm (18). (a) It has been demonstrated that cells are killed by radioactive tritiated thymidine incorporated into the DNA. (b) Certain analogs of thymidine, particularly halogenated pyrimidines, are selectively incorporated into DNA in place of thymidine. This substitution increases the radiosensitivity of mammalian cells, which is proportional to the amount of chemical incorporated. Substituted deoxyuridines, which are not incorporated into DNA, have no effect on cellular radio-sensitivity. (c) Factors that modify cell lethality, such as variation in the type of radiation, oxygen concentration, or dose rate, also affect the production of chromosomal damage in a quantitatively and qualitatively similar fashion. (4) A correlation has been demonstrated between nucleic acid volume and radiosensitivity.

DNA consists of two strands that form a double helix, with each strand being composed of deoxynucleotides, the sequence of which must be complementary. A break in a single strand, caused by either the direct or indirect effects illustrated in Figure 14.5, has little biologic consequence since the break can be repaired using the opposite strand as a template. However, if breaks occur in both strands that are directly opposite, or separated by only a few base pairs, a double-strand break (DSB) occurs, and the piece of chromatin snaps in two (Fig. 14.7).

There is good evidence that most of the important biologic effects of ionizing radiations are a direct consequence of the rejoining of two DSBs. Figure 14.8 illustrates two ways in which a DSB in each of two chromosomes may rejoin. In the top half of the figure, the two broken chromosomes rejoin in such a way that a dicentric fragment and an acentric fragment are formed. This exchange-type aberration is lethal to the cell: the fragment with a centromere will be lost during

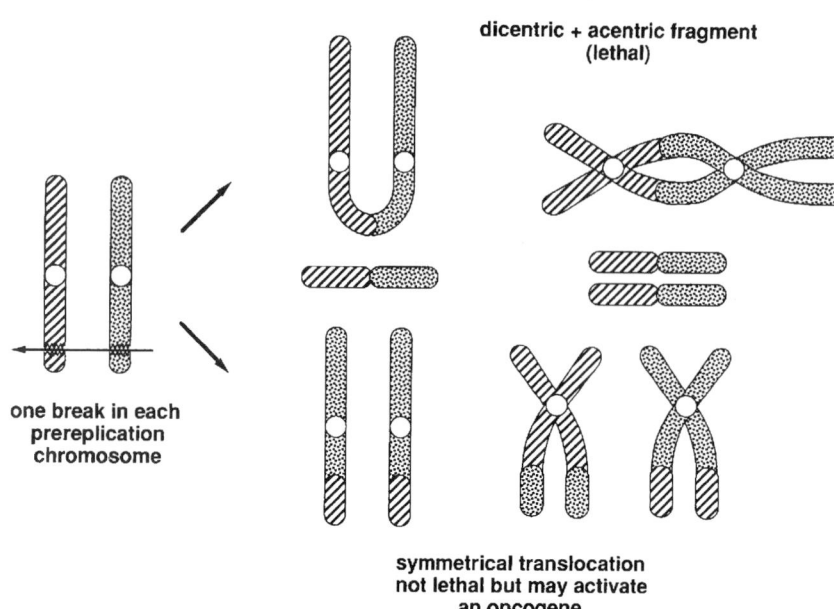

dicentric + acentric fragment (lethal)

one break in each prereplication chromosome

symmetrical translocation not lethal but may activate an oncogene

FIG. 14.8. Most biologic effects of radiation are due to the incorrect joining of breaks in two chromosomes. For example, the two broken chromosomes may recombine to form a dicentric (a chromosome with two centromeres) and an acentric fragment (a fragment with no centromere). This is a lethal lesion resulting in cell death. Alternatively, the two broken chromosomes may exchange broken ends, called symmetrical translocation, which does not lead to death of the cell, but in a few special cases activates an oncogene by moving it from a quiescent to an active site.

cell division, whereas the aberrant chromosome with two centromeres will make a normal mitosis impossible. Aberrations of this type represent the principal mechanism whereby radiation kills cells. Note that breaks in *two* chromosomes are necessary for an exchange-type aberration. The two breaks can be produced by a single electron track (Fig. 14.8), in which case the probability of an interaction is proportional to dose (i.e., doubling the dose doubles the yield of aberrations). On the other hand, the two chromosomal breaks may result from two separate electrons, in which case the probability of an interaction increases with the dose (19) (i.e., doubling the dose makes an aberration four times as likely). In practice, both possibilities occur, so that the yield of chromosomal aberrations is a linear-quadratic function of dose:

$$\text{Aberration yield} = \alpha D + \beta D^2$$

This linear-quadratic relationship is ubiquitous in radiation biology for all biologic effects of γ-rays and x-rays. Scoring dicentric aberrations can be used as a biologic dosimeter. If someone is suspected of being exposed accidentally to a large dose of radiation, a sample of blood can be taken, the peripheral lymphocytes may be stimulated to divide, and the incidence of dicentric aberrations scored. This observation accurately reflects the average total body dose. The lowest dose that can be assessed conveniently is about 25 cGy.

As shown in Figure 14.8, it is possible for the breaks in the two chromosomes to rejoin as shown in the lower portion of the figure. This leads to a symmetric translocation that is quite compatible with cell viability. However, it represents a rearrangement of genetic material and, in a few instances, leads to a malignant change. For example, Burkitt's lymphoma and some types of leukemia result from a translocation that either moves an oncogene from a quiescent to an active chromosomal site or results in a fusion gene. This is one of the most likely mechanisms for radiation-induced carcinogenesis, which is discussed later.

Effects of Radiation on Cells

In many cells, radiation-induced lethality is not instantaneous, because cells continue to function and even undergo several divisions before biologic death occurs. Noncycling lymphocytes, thymocytes, and hematopoietic cells have been shown to undergo interphase cell death without progressing through the mitotic phase of the cell cycle (20). Two patterns of morphologic changes are associated with cell death in mammalian cells (21). *Cell necrosis*, which is degenerative, is the most usual type of cell damage. Necrotic cell death results from the collapse of cellular metabolism and depletion of its adenosine triphosphate storage (20). The final events of necrosis involve membrane rupture, loss of lysosomal enzymes, degradation of nuclear chromatin, and karyolysis (21). The other process of radiation-induced cell death is *apoptosis* (programmed cell death), which is charac-

terized by chromatin condensation and segmentation, fragmentation of the nucleus into apoptotic bodies, cell shrinkage, and loss of cellular contact with neighboring cells (22, 23). Apoptosis occurs spontaneously in various solid tumors (24) and contributes to the balance between tumor cell gain and cell loss. Fuks and Weichselbaum (21) summarized concepts on radiation-induced cellular lesions, repair of radiation damage, role of genes and enzymes in genetic control of radiation damage repair, stress genes induced by ionizing radiation, and growth factors and cytokines that modulate response of mammalian cells to ionizing radiation.

Within minutes after irradiation, signal transduction pathways, mediated by protein kinase C and tyrosine kinase, are stimulated (25). This stimulation is probably critical to induction of many genes and proteins, including early-response genes, which, in turn, activate other genes, including those for tumor necrosis factor, fibroblast growth factor, and transforming growth factor-β (26). In addition, new proteins, such as tissue plasminogen activator, are synthesized. It is theorized that this cascade of gene activation and transcription and protein synthesis is related to key cellular functions that permit the cell to survive a dose of radiation.

Apoptosis

Apoptosis, or programmed cell death, a phenomenon distinct from necrosis, was first described in 1972 by Kerr and colleagues (27). Dewey and associates (28) published a thorough review of radiation-induced apoptosis and its relevance to radiation therapy. The general hypothesis is that apoptosis is programmed by specific signals in the cell that cause an endonuclease to cleave DNA at internucleosomal sites.

Apoptosis is detected by histologic evaluation of membrane blebbing and chromatin condensation, by flow cytometry using fluorescent nucleotides and terminal transferase to detect fragmented DNA by detecting apoptotic cells, which are usually very small with characteristic profiles of right-angle and forward light scattering, or by using DNA fluorochrome to detect a decrease in fluorescence as small DNA fragments diffuse from the cell that is undergoing apoptosis (23,29). Several oncogenes, cytokines, and growth factors have been reported to play a role in promoting or reducing radiation-induced apoptosis.

Apoptosis, frequently seen within 4 to 6 hours after irradiation, occurs spontaneously and is enhanced by x irradiation as observed *in vivo* in the intestinal crypt and salivary and lacrimal glands with nondividing cells and nondividing lymphocytes. Apoptotic cells are eliminated very rapidly *in vivo*, making it difficult to quantify apoptosis in this setting. In contrast, this cell death mechanism is easy to quantify *in vitro* because apoptotic cells persist in culture for many hours. In cell lines susceptible to apoptosis, this process sometimes occurs early, before cells enter mitosis, or later, after the cells divide. Late apoptosis may be associated with mitotically linked death and, in fact, may be triggered by

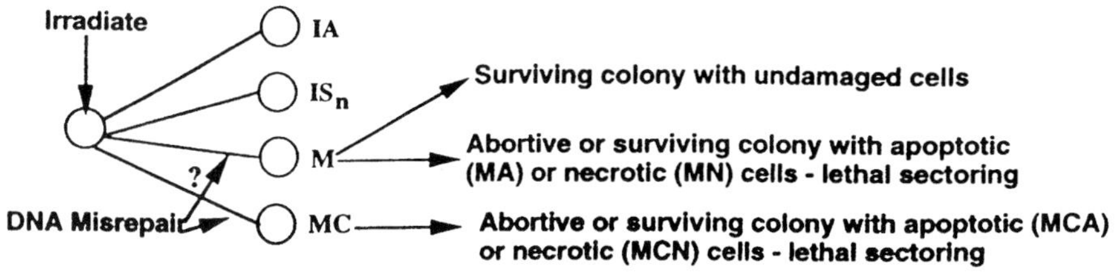

FIG. 14.9. Schematic diagram to illustrate possible fates of an irradiated cell that should be studied as genetic expression is modulated. The question mark refers to whether or not DNA misrepair could result in MN or MA without the irradiated cell having manifested a chromosomal aberration(s). IA, apoptosis before division: IS_n, cellular senescence: M, apoptosis or necrosis occurs after the cell divides: MC, apoptosis or necrosis with chromosomal aberrations. (Reprinted from Dewey WC, Ling CC, Meyn RE. Radiation-induced apoptosis: relevance to radiotherapy. *Int J Radiat Oncol Biol Phys* 1995:33:781, with permission from Elsevier.)

chromosomal aberrations. Apoptosis may be quite important for clinically relevant doses of fractionated irradiation, even if it causes a relatively small reduction in clonogenic survival. However, this requires that cells be recruited into the apoptotic-susceptible fraction after each dose fraction. Figure 14.9 illustrates possible fates of an irradiated cell.

Hellman and Weichselbaum (30) noted that apoptosis is an important mechanism of cell death following irradiation. It appears that with progression of certain tumors, spontaneous and therapy-related apoptosis occurs less frequently. The apoptotic response to irradiation can be modified by cytokines to protect normal tissues or to induce tumor cell killing. Tumor necrosis factor increases apoptosis following irradiation in some tumors, whereas protecting the hematopoietic compartment, possibly by blocking apoptosis (31). Another mechanism of reversible loss of proliferative capacity induced by irradiation is necrosis, which occurs with high doses of irradiation and is a major mechanism seen with large dose fractions, such as in stereotactic irradiation. In carcinoma of the cervix, tumor proliferation is associated with apoptosis and tumor size, which correlate with tumor progression, and are thus predictive of treatment outcome (32).

Cell Survival Curves

The relevant endpoint in radiation therapy is reproductive death, which is the loss of a cell's reproductive integrity or loss of unlimited proliferative capacity. A tumor cell may be physically and morphologically intact and may be able to carry out metabolic functions and even go through one or more divisions, but if its ability to divide indefinitely is removed, it is reproductively dead (33). A cell that retains reproductive integrity and is able to proliferate indefinitely is said to be clonogenic (18).

A cell survival curve is the relationship between the fraction of cells surviving and the dose of radiation delivered. A cell survival curve can be obtained for cells cultured *in vitro* where the cells are obtained from a wide variety of tumors or normal tissues. Survival curves *in vivo* can be

obtained for a number of transplantable tumors in laboratory animals and for a variety of self-renewing normal tissues, such as the skin or intestinal epithelium.

Because cell lethality results largely from chromosomal aberrations, it is not surprising that the shape of the cell survival curve is linear-quadratic, just like that for chromosomal aberrations (Fig. 14.10). At low doses, cell killing is dominated by the single-event (α) component, interpreted to be due to chromosomal aberrations caused by a single charged particle. At higher acute doses, cell lethality is largely due to multiple events—chromosomal aberrations resulting from breaks caused by separate electrons.

In practice, radiation therapy is almost always delivered either continuously at a low dose rate (as in intracavitary treatments) or as multiple small daily doses delivered over several weeks (as in external beam irradiation). The effective cell survival curve is then an extension of the initial slope because single breaks caused by individual electrons may repair before a second break is formed, which could interact to produce a lethal exchange-type aberration.

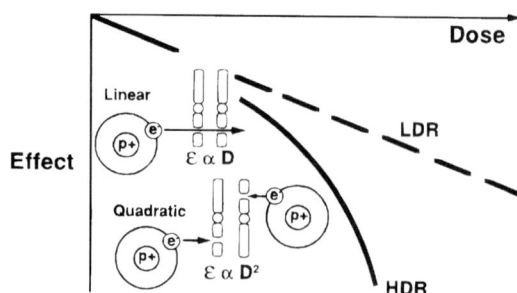

FIG. 14.10. Cell killing by radiation is largely due to aberrations caused by breaks in two chromosomes. The dose-response curve for high-dose rate (HDR) irradiation is linear-quadratic: the two breaks may be caused by the same electron (dominant at low doses) or by two different electrons (dominant at higher doses). For low-dose rate (LDR) irradiation, where radiation is delivered over a protracted period, the principal mechanism of cell killing is by the single electron. Consequently, the LDR survival curve is an extension of the low-dose region of the HDR survival curve.

Tumor Regrowth Assay

The effect of irradiation on a tumor can be quantitated by tumor regrowth measurements that will be proportional to the cell killing, repair, and repopulation induced by each dose of irradiation in comparison to nonirradiated control tumors. Growth delay can be expressed as the time taken after irradiation for the tumor to regrow to the size it was at the time of irradiation.

Tumor regression after irradiation is a complex phenomenon, and is the result of four mechanisms: cell killing, rate of dead cell removal (cell loss), apoptosis (cell actively participates in cell death by providing molecules and energy involved in the process), and the proliferation of surviving cells. The delay after which a biologically nonviable cell will physically die is correlated with a cell turnover rate of the tumor, whereas the efficiency of clearance of dead cells is linked with the tumor architecture (34). A frequently used endpoint, TCD_{50}, is the irradiation dose at which 50% of tumors are locally controlled.

Sensitivity to Radiation and Cell Proliferative Cycle

Several investigators have demonstrated experimentally that the sensitivity of cells to radiation and to most chemotherapeutic agents varies depending on the phase of the proliferative cycle the cell is in at the time it is exposed to the physical or chemical event (35,36).

Following a single dose of irradiation, the cell-age distribution of surviving cells changes as a result of two factors: (a) preferential killing of cells in the more sensitive phases of the proliferative cycle, leading to an increase in the percentage of viable cells in more resistant phases; and (b) a temporary premitotic cell cycle block that prevents the progression of proliferating cells through the cell cycle. The duration of this block varies with the phase of the cycle and the cells under consideration.

Terasima and Tolmach (36) showed that synchronized HeLa cells in culture irradiated with a single dose of 3 Gy were more sensitive to radiation during late G_1 and late G_2 phases and more resistant during early G_1, and Sinclair (35) reported that Chinese hamster cells are more sensitive during mitosis and are particularly resistant during the latter part of the S phase. Clonogenic cells out of cycle (G_0) may be affected by irradiation depending on the individual sensitivity of the cell, but the effects of irradiation are apparent only when the cell reverts to a proliferating cycle and goes through one or more mitoses. The prospects for exploiting cell reassortment (synchronization) in the treatment of cancer has raised great hopes that have not been fulfilled, probably due to the great heterogeneity of tumor and normal cells (36) and the lack of specific knowledge about the cell cycle in humans.

RADIATION EFFECTS ON THE EMBRYO AND FETUS

Limited experience regarding pelvic irradiation in pregnant women, usually for therapeutic purposes, has been described. The number of patients is small, whereas the doses are large and not accurately known. However, in reviewing the literature, Dekaban (37) proposed the following generalizations: (a) Even therapeutic doses of several Gy delivered to the embryo within the first 2 to 3 weeks of gestation are not likely to cause severe abnormalities, although a considerable number of embryos may be resorbed or aborted. This is often referred to as the "all or nothing effect": either the embryo is killed or it develops normally. (b) Irradiation between 4 and 11 weeks of gestation produces severe abnormalities in most organs in surviving fetuses. (c) Irradiation between 11 and 16 weeks of gestation frequently produces stunted growth, microcephaly, and mental retardation, as well as other abnormalities of the eye, skeleton, and genitals. The same pattern is seen following irradiation at 16 to 20 weeks of gestation, but to a milder degree. (d) Irradiation after 30 weeks of gestation is unlikely to produce gross structural abnormalities, but could cause some functional disabilities.

More precise information concerning the effects of radiation comes from two sources where the doses are known more precisely and cover a wider range. These are studies in laboratory animals (mainly rats and mice) and the study of survivors of the atomic bombings of Hiroshima and Nagasaki.

Animal Studies

Animal studies show that irradiation during preimplantation (up to about 10 days in the human) may result in embryonic death, but does not produce malformations. Irradiation during organogenesis, the period when organs and limbs are forming by cellular differentiation (10 days to 6 weeks in the human), leads to a wide range of gross malformations and, if the dose is large enough, may also result in neonatal death (i.e., death at or about the time of birth). Irradiation during this period may also cause temporary growth retardation, where the offspring is smaller than normal at birth but recovers by the time it becomes an adult. The major deleterious deletion effect observed in animals from irradiation during the fetal period is permanent growth retardation.

Studies of Japanese Survivors of the Atomic Bomb

About 1,600 children were irradiated *in utero* at Hiroshima and Nagasaki when those cities were bombed in World War II. The principal effects observed were microcephaly and severe mental retardation, often occurring together. Mental retardation was not observed following irradiation before 8 weeks of gestation and was most common

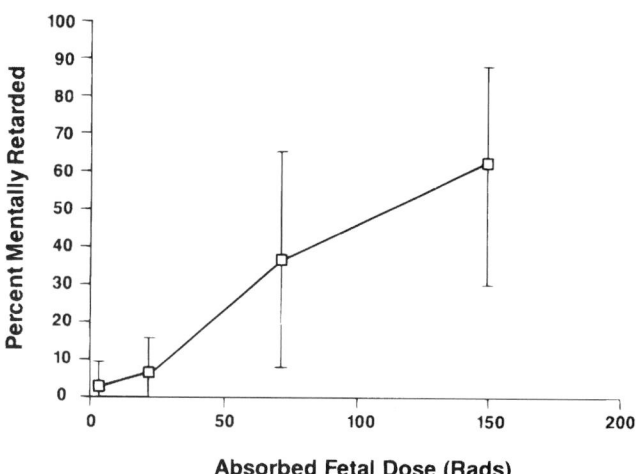

FIG. 14.11. The frequency of severe mental retardation as a function of dose among those exposed to atomic bomb radiation at Hiroshima and Nagasaki at 8 to 15 weeks of gestational age. The vertical bars represent 90% confidence intervals. The data are consistent with a linear relation between risk and dose, with a slope of 40% per Gray. On the other hand, the data are also consistent with a threshold of about 2 Gy. (Redrawn from Otake M, Schull WJ. In utero exposure to A-bomb radiation and mental retardation: a reassessment. *Br J Radiol* 1984:57:409–414. In: Hall EJ. *Radiobiology for the radiologist.* 4th ed. Philadelphia: JB Lippincott Co, 1994, with permission.)

following irradiation at 8 to 15 weeks of gestation, where the risk appeared to increase linearly, with dose giving rise to a risk estimate of 40% per Gy. The data are consistent with a threshold of about 20 cGy, which seems likely since the mechanism of the effect is thought to be due to killing of cells as they migrate from their place of birth to their site of function. Other studies indicate a loss of IQ that amounts to about 30 points per Gy (Fig. 14.11). Mental retardation was also observed following irradiation at 16 to 25 weeks of gestation, but the risk was lower by a factor of four than at 8 to 15 weeks.

The risks of radiation exposure according to stage of gestation are summarized in Table 14.2 (38). Figure 14.12 summarizes the deleterious effects of radiation on the developing embryo from the various data sources: animal studies, the Japanese atomic bomb survivors, and patients exposed medically. In summary, exposure to radiation during the first 10 days following conception may lead to the loss of the embryo and is unlikely to result in a viable abnormal child. To be safe, the entire period from 10 days to 25 weeks must be considered to be potentially dangerous for the production of anomalies by a radiation exposure of 10 to 20 cGy or more, with the 8- to 15-week period being the most sensitive for severe mental retardation, which is the best documented effect in humans. The later fetal period appears to be resistant to radiation effects. The risk of radiation therapy during pregnancy may be acceptable, particularly if the maximum fetal dose is limited to less than 0.1 Gy (38).

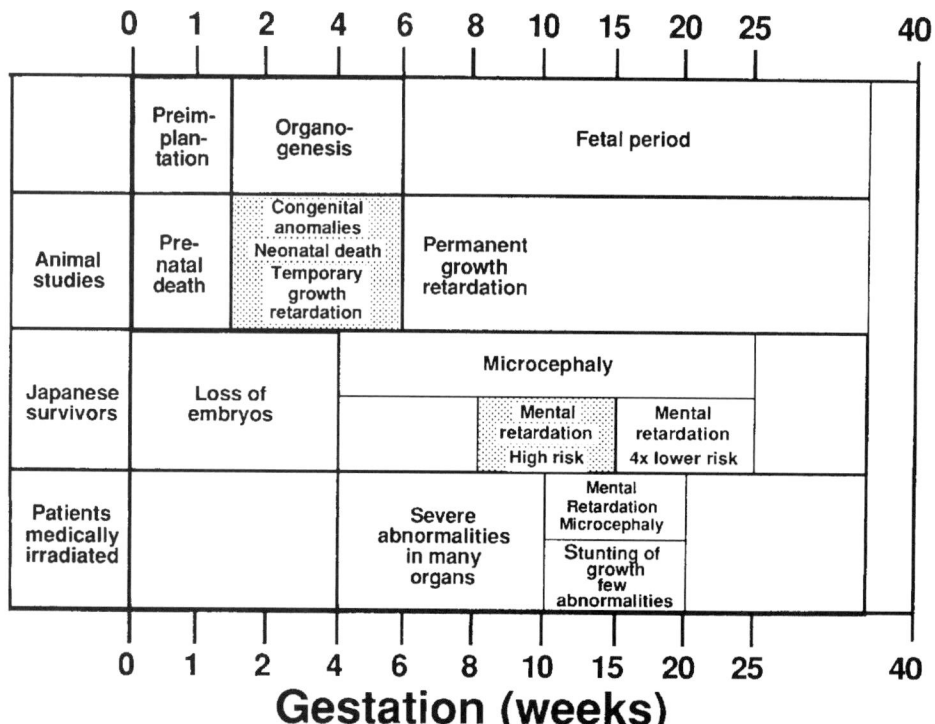

FIG. 14.12. Summary of the effects of radiation on the developing embryo and fetus from three principal sources: medical radiation, laboratory animal studies, and survivors of the atomic bomb attacks on Nagasaki and Hiroshima. The animal studies indicate a wide range of structural abnormalities during organogenesis, whereas the principal effect observed in humans is reduced head diameter with or without severe mental retardation. (Modified from Hall EJ. *Radiobiology for the radiologist.* 4th ed. Philadelphia: JB Lippincott Co, 1994.)

TABLE 14.2. *Radiation exposure risks in terms of stage of gestation*

Stage	Days Postconception	Threshold (Gy)	Primary Risk(s)
Preimplantation		0.1	Lethality (50% risk at 1 Gy)
Embryonic	950	0.050.1	Malformations, growth retardation, small head size (40% risk at 0.5 Gy)
Early fetal	51105	0.12	Small head size, mental retardation, and growth retardation (40% per Gy)
Midfetal	106175	0.5	Small head size, growth retardation
Late fetal	>175	0.5	Growth retardation

Source: Sneed PK. Comments on "Fetal dose evaluation during breast cancer radiotherapy." *Breast Dis* 1999;9:409, with permission.

Acute Effects of Whole-Body Irradiation

After irradiation, a prodromal syndrome may develop within a few hours. In most mammals, three types of syndromes can be identified depending on the dose: (a) cerebrovascular, occurring at high doses (100 Gy), with death occurring in hours as a result of neurologic and cardiovascular injury; (b) gastrointestinal, noted with doses of 5 to 12 Gy, with death occurring in a matter of days, associated with extensive bloody diarrhea and destruction of the gastrointestinal mucosa; and (c) bone marrow or hematopoietic, with doses of 2.5 to 5.0 Gy, with death occurring within several weeks after exposure due to depletion of the bone marrow, infection, and bleeding. The mean lethal dose for humans is approximately 4 Gy.

DELETERIOUS EFFECTS OF RADIATION AND RADIATION PROTECTION

The deleterious effects of radiation include heritable effects caused by mutations in irradiated germ cells and cancer or leukemia due to changes induced in somatic cells.

Heritable Effects

Radiation does not result in new, bizarre mutations, but increases the incidence of the spectrum of mutations that occur spontaneously in a population. Almost all we know about radiation-induced heritable effects comes from animal experiments. In particular, massive experiments involving millions of mice have been used to estimate the risk of heritable effects of radiation. The doubling dose is that required to double the spontaneous mutation rate, or it is the dose required to produce an incidence of mutations equal to the spontaneous rate. Based on the mouse data, the best estimate for the doubling dose in humans is 1 Gy. It is believed that the incidence of mutations approximates a linear function of dose (i.e., if the dose is doubled, the number of induced mutations will also double). Children of the survivors of Hiroshima and Nagasaki have been carefully studied for over 40 years. No significant excess of heritable effects has been observed: the results are consistent with the mouse data, which leads to the conclusion that estimates based on the

mouse data are conservative. The International Commission on Radiological Protection estimates that, for a radiation-exposed working population, the probability per capita for radiation-induced hereditary disorders is 0.6×10^{-2} per sievert (Sv). This is based on the doubling dose (1 Gy) for mutations plus a very approximate allowance for multifactorial diseases.

Cancer and Leukemia

There are many examples of radiation-induced cancer and leukemia in humans. The experience includes patients exposed to medical irradiation and early workers exposed occupationally, as well as survivors of the atom bomb attacks on Hiroshima and Nagasaki. A long latent interval often exists between exposure to radiation and the appearance of a related malignancy. Leukemias may occur 5 to 7 years after irradiation, whereas solid tumors may take 40 years or more to develop. Regardless of the age at time of exposure, radiation-induced malignancies tend to appear at the same age as spontaneous malignancies of the same type. *In utero* irradiation from an obstetric x-ray examination results in a 1.4-fold increased risk of childhood malignancy per 0.01 to 0.02 Gy (39).

Both radiation carcinogenesis and hereditary effects are considered to be stochastic: that is, the probability of an effect increases with dose, with no threshold, but the severity of the effect does not vary with dose. For the general population, the National Council on Radiation Protection (NCRP) suggests a risk estimate of excess cancer mortality of 10×10^{-2}/Sv for high doses and 5×10^{-2}/Sv for low doses and low dose rates. It is important to note that this is an average figure. Young children are much more sensitive, while mature adults are much less sensitive (40).

The risk of second malignancies after radiation therapy is a controversial subject. One of the reasons for the uncertainty is that patients undergoing radiation therapy are often at high risk of a second cancer because of lifestyles and/or genetic predisposition: this factor is more dominant than the radiation risk. The only reliable estimates come from two instances where surgery is an equal option, or the case of radiation therapy for Hodgkin's disease, whereas the inci-

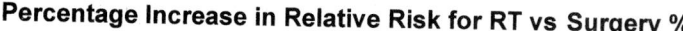

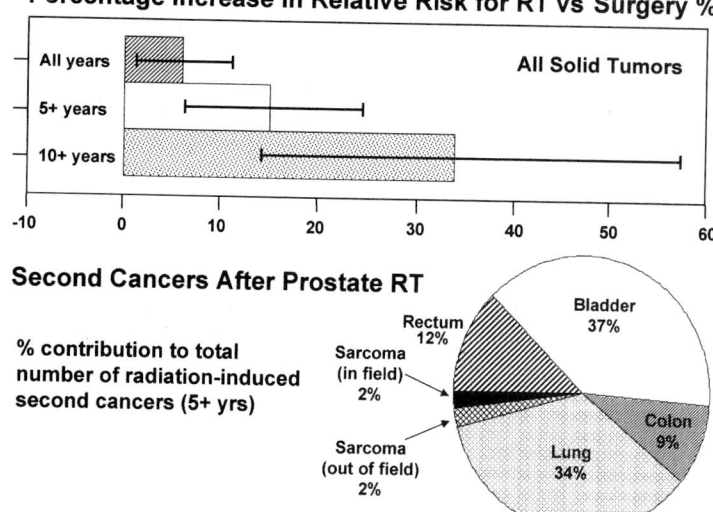

FIG. 14.13. Incidence and sites of second cancers in men with carcinoma of the prostate treated with radiation therapy. (From Brenner DJ, Curtis RE, Hall EJ, et al. Second malignancies in prostate patients after radiotherapy compared with surgery. *Cancer* 2000:88:398. Copyright © 2000 American Cancer Society. Reprinted by permission of Wiley-Liss Inc., a subsidiary of John Wiley & Sons, Inc.)

dence of breast cancer after radiation therapy of young women is too high to be missed (41–43).

The largest and best controlled study compares second cancers in men treated for prostatic cancer with radiation therapy versus surgery (42). In patients surviving 10 years after treatment, 1 in 70 developed an excess second malignancy. These included sarcomas in heavily irradiated tissue, as well as carcinomas in nearby organs such as the bladder, rectum, colon, or even the lung. The distribution is shown in Figure 14.13.

Radiation Protection

Radiation protection has two objectives. One is to prevent clinically significant deterministic effects by adhering to dose limits below the apparent or practical threshold. Deterministic effects include damage to tissues (e.g., a cataract) in which the severity of the effect increases with dose above a certain threshold that below which the effect is not seen. The second objective is to limit the risk of stochastic effects (cancer and heritable effects) to a reasonable level in relationship to societal needs and benefits gained (44). Because there is no threshold, there is no dose at which the risk is zero. In relation to stochastic effects, the relevant quantity to control is the *effective dose*, which is defined as the product of measured dose and two factors, the radiation weighting factor (W_R) and the tissue weighting factor (W_T). The radiation weighting factor is designed to take into account the quality of the radiation, but is essentially 1 for all radiations used routinely in radiation therapy and can be ignored. The tissue weighting factor is important when only part of the body is exposed and takes into account the different sensitivities of various tissues to stochastic effects. For example, only the dose to the gonads is relevant to heritable effects, whereas the dose to, for example, bone marrow, thyroid, breast (in females), colon, and lung is important for

the induction of cancer or leukemia. In contrast, the head and extremities are relatively resistant. If dose is measured in grays, the effective dose is in sieverts. It is important to recognize that the permissible limits refer to effective dose, which is not necessarily the same as the dose registered by a radiation monitor, especially if some part of the body is shielded.

For individuals occupationally exposed who must, therefore, wear a radiation monitor and be over 18 years of age, the NCRP recommends that the cumulative effective dose should not exceed 10 mSv × age (in years), but 50 mSv is allowed in any 1 year. In practice, the maximum permissible effective dose is 10 mSv/year, although an occasionally higher limit is allowable. This is designed to limit the risk of stochastic effects (i.e., cancer and heritable effects) to a reasonable level. ''Reasonable'' is defined as a risk of death comparable to safe industries. The lens of the eye is allowed 150 mSv/year, whereas the hands and feet are allowed 500 mSv/year to limit the risk of deterministic effects. In the case of a pregnant worker occupationally exposed, the embryo/fetus should not receive more than 0.5 Sv/month after the pregnancy is declared. Members of the general public are limited to doses one-tenth the occupational limits.

The most effective way to minimize radiation exposure to personnel involved in intracavitary gynecologic applications is to use a computer-controlled remote afterloading device, which essentially eliminates radiation exposure to nurses and technical staff.

FACTORS AFFECTING BIOLOGIC EFFECTS OF IONIZING RADIATIONS

Linear Energy Transfer and Relative Biologic Effectiveness

When radiation is absorbed in biologic material, ionization and excitation occur along the tracks of individual charged particles in a pattern that depends on the type of radiation involved (photons give rise to fast electrons, particles carrying a negative electric charge and having very small mass, whereas neutrons give rise to recoil protons, particles also carrying unit electric charge but having a mass nearly 2,000 times greater than that of the electron). As a result, the primary events may be sparsely or densely ionizing (low or high linear energy transfer radiations).

Linear energy transfer (LET) is an expression of the energy transfer per unit length of the particle track (keV/μm of unit density material) (Fig. 14.14). The LET of an ionizing particle depends basically on the energy and charge possessed by the particle: the greater the charge and the smaller the velocity, the higher the LET. This varying rate of energy released in an absorber is expressed as different biologic effects in living cells. Although objections have been raised to the definition of LET, since in some circumstances it can be misleading, it is useful as a simple way to indicate the quality of various types of radiation. For instance, ^{60}Co γ-rays and 250-kVp x-rays have unique LET values of about 0.3 and 2.0 keV/μm, respectively. The value for 14-MeV neutrons is 12 keV/μm, and for heavy charged particles, it is 100 to 2,000 keV/μm (18).

Relative biologic effectiveness (RBE) is defined as the ratio of the dose required for a given radiation to produce the same biologic effect induced by 250-kV x-rays. Because x-ray and neutron survival curves have different shapes, with the x-ray survival curve having an initial shoulder, whereas the neutron curve is exponential with regard to dose, the resultant RBE will depend on the level of biologic damage (and therefore the dose) chosen (18). ^{60}Co has an RBE of about 0.95 (45) and neutrons have an RBE of approximately 2.3 (46).

The RBE is a very complex quantity, and depends on the radiation quality (LET, irradiation dose, number of dose fractions, dose rate, and biologic system or endpoint use). As the LET increases, the RBE will decrease, so that for 15-MeV neutrons, the RBE is about 1.6. *Therapeutic gain factor* has been defined as the ratio of the RBE for the tumor divided by the RBE of the normal tissues. It should always be larger than unity.

Oxygen Enhancement Effect

Well-oxygenated cells are more sensitive to irradiation than hypoxic cells. The oxygen enhancement ratio (OER) is the ratio of the doses needed to achieve the same biologic effect (the hypoxic effect divided by fully hypoxic effect) by various types of radiations. For the oxygen effect to be observed, the oxygen must be present during or within milliseconds after the radiation exposure because it acts at the free radical level (18). After radiation exposure, these free radicals break chemical bonds, initiating the final expression of biologic damage. If oxygen is present, it reacts with the free radical R·, producing RO_2, an organic peroxide that is a nonrestorable form of the target material: that is, the reaction results in a change in the chemical composition of the material exposed to the radiation. If oxygen were not present, many of the ionized target molecules could repair themselves and recover the ability to function normally (18). A small amount of oxygen will potentiate the effect of irradiation. Experiments have shown that a concentration of oxygen of about 2% will make the radiation response virtually indistinguishable from that obtained under normal aeration conditions, and further increases of oxygen tension will not affect the slope of the survival curve (Fig. 14.15, *inset*).

For low LET radiations, such as x-rays or γ-rays, the OER at high doses is between 2.5 and 3.0: that is, the radiation dose required to produce a given biologic effect is about three times as large in the absence of oxygen as in its presence. For 2.5-MeV α-rays, the OER is 1. There is some evidence that the OER has a smaller value of about 2 at lower doses, on the order of the typical dose per fraction in clinical radiation therapy (18). This would correspond to the linear, or α, component of the linear-quadratic dose-response relationship. For high LET, densely ionizing radiations such as α particles, the survival curve does not have an initial shoulder, and the OER is 1, implying that there is no oxygen enhancement effect: for neutrons, the OER has an intermediate value of approximately 1.6.

Growing tumors rapidly develop a hypoxic population of cells because of inadequate vascular supply and poor diffusion of oxygen. Increasing cellular oxygen tension enhances the radiation sensitivity of cells, and hypoxia decreases it (Fig. 14.15). Gray (71) was the first to postulate that the oxygen effect might be important in radiation therapy because malignant tumors frequently have a significant population of hypoxic cells.

Thomlinson and Gray (48) demonstrated that all tumor cords with a radius in excess of 200 μm had a necrotic center, that no tumor cord with a radius smaller than 160 μm showed evidence of necrosis, and that the thickness of the sheaths of actively growing tumor cells never exceeded 180 μm. It appeared that tumor cells could proliferate and

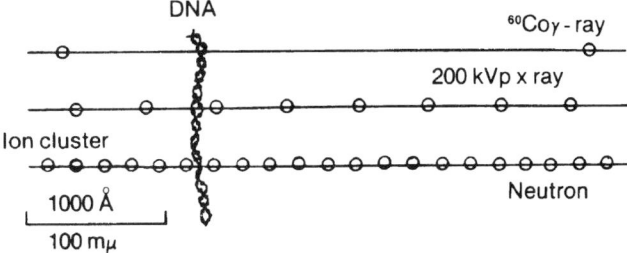

FIG. 14.14. Schematic representation of linear energy transfer for various ionizing particles and x-rays. Neutrons have a large number of ionizations and are recognized as high-LET particles. (Modified from Young MEJ. *Radiological physics.* 2nd ed. London: HK Lewis, 1967, with permission.)

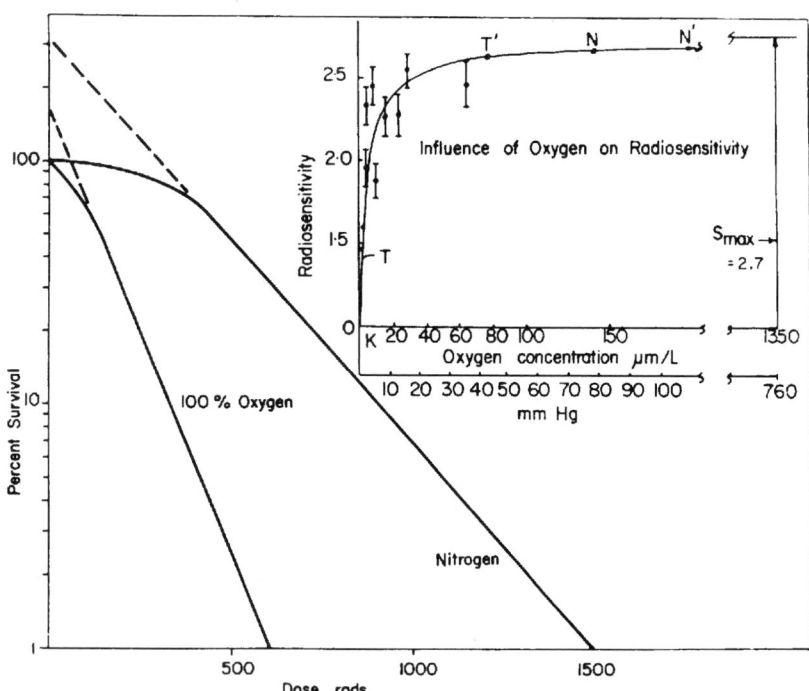

FIG. 14.15. Influence of oxygen tension on radiosensitivity according to Deschner and Gray (330). Survival curve for human embryo liver cells in tissue culture irradiated with and without oxygen. (From Johns HE, Cunningham JR. *The physics of radiology.* 3rd ed. Springfield, IL: Charles C Thomas, 1972, with permission.)

grow actively only if they were close to a supply of oxygen or nutrients. Thus, up to 150 μm from a capillary the cells are well oxygenated. There is a marginal zone of hypoxic cells, and at a greater distance, an area of anoxic necrotic cells. The hypoxic viable cells more significantly affect the radiosensitivity of the tumor. Several animal tumors have shown proportions of hypoxic cells ranging from 1% to 25% (18). Inadequately oxygenated cells, even as few as 1%, have a substantial impact on the radiosensitivity of a tumor, increasing the dose of irradiation necessary to eradicate it (Fig. 14.16).

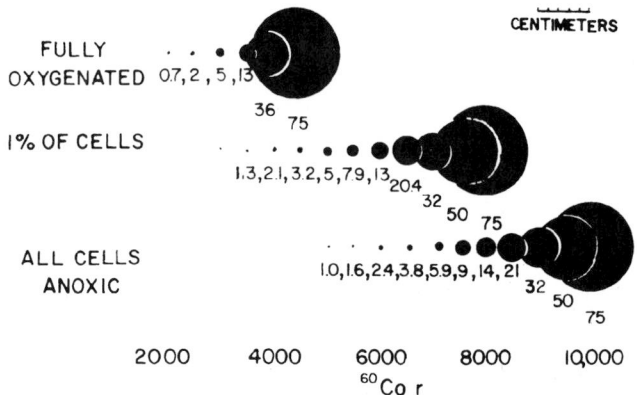

FIG. 14.16. Doses of radiation necessary to yield 90% tumor cure with lesions of different size depending on whether they are well oxygenated or hypoxic (Hewitt's data). Note that a dose of radiation two to three times higher is necessary in the presence of hypoxia. (From Fowler JF, Margan RL, Wood CAP. Biological and physical advantages and problems of neutron therapy. *Br J Radiol* 1963:36:79, with permission.)

Wouters and Brown (49) postulated that the fraction of tumor cells at intermediate oxygen levels is more important than radiobiologically hypoxic cells in determining the response of human tumors to fractionated radiation therapy. Oxygen electrode and nitroimidazole-binding studies suggest that tumors contain a significant fraction of cells at intermediate oxygen levels.

The hypoxia described by Thomlinson and Gray, which is diffusion-limited, has been called chronic hypoxia. Regions of hypoxia also develop in tumors as a result of the temporary closing of a particular blood vessel. This has been termed acute hypoxia.

At the moment at which a dose of radiation is delivered, a proportion of the tumor cells may be hypoxic, but if the radiation is delayed until a later time, a different group of cells may be hypoxic. The occurrence of acute hypoxia was postulated in the 1970s by Brown (49a) and later demonstrated unequivocally in rodent tumors by Chaplin and his colleagues (50,51).

It was postulated that if patients are irradiated by breathing oxygen, under pressure in a sealed chamber (3 to 4 atm), an increased response would be obtained in the hypoxic cells: if normal tissue is well oxygenated, the increase in radiosensitivity with hyperbaric oxygen would be minimal, so that a given dose of radiation would have a greater relative effect on the tumor than on normal cells (52). Several clinical trials dealing with tumors of the head and neck, cervix, bladder, and other sites have been reported by Churchill-Davidson and associates (53) and van den Brenk (52), with encouraging but inconclusive results. Although the incidence of complications was somewhat greater, appropriate adjustment in dose and fractionation showed no significant enhancement of skin or mucosal reactions or permanent damage to other normal tissues (54).

Treating cancer patients in a high-pressure oxygen tank is technically challenging and restricts the number of radiation fractions delivered. It is also dangerous, since human tissue is flammable at 3 atm of oxygen: as witnessed by astronauts who died in a fire in an oxygenated capsule. A more recent concept is to use nicotinamide, a vitamin B3 analog, to overcome transient hypoxia caused by the intermittent closing down of blood vessels and carbogen breathing to overcome chronic hypoxia. This is the basis of the Accelerated, Hyperfractionated, Carbogen Breathing, and Nicotinamide (ARCON) trials underway in Europe (55). The radiation delivery is also accelerated to avoid tumor proliferation and hyperfractionated to minimize damage to late-responding tissues.

Hypoxia has a wider importance in oncology than contributing to resistance to killing by x-rays. Hypoxia accelerates malignant progression leading to a more aggressive tumor. It has been shown in the laboratory that hypoxia leads to genomic instability, upregulation of bcl, downregulation of p53, and stimulation of vascular endothelial growth factor (56).

These molecular studies are supported by at least two clinical results. First, in advanced carcinoma of the cervix, local control as well as survival was poorer in patients whose tumors were hypoxic as judged by measurements with an Eppendorf probe (PO_2 <10 mm Hg) regardless of whether the treatment was irradiation or surgery (57). Second, a clinical study of patients with soft-tissue sarcoma showed a clear correlation between distant metastatic spread and hypoxia, which was judged by measurements with an Eppendorf probe (58).

Reoxygenation

In many animal tumor systems, it has been demonstrated that a proportion of hypoxic cells become oxygenated following a dose of irradiation. The oxygen status of cells in a tumor is not static but dynamic and constantly changing (18). The phenomenon of reoxygenation is illustrated in Figure 14.17, which demonstrates that initial doses of irradiation to a mixed cell population will preferentially kill aerated cells. Immediately after irradiation, the majority of surviving cells will be hypoxic, but if sufficient time is allowed before the next radiation dose, the process of reoxygenation will restore the proportion of hypoxic cells to about 15%. Repeating this process several times will progressively decrease the number of hypoxic cells, enhancing the response of the tumor to subsequent doses of irradiation. The time sequence for reoxygenation varies for tumors and normal tissues but, in general, is a few days. The process of reoxygenation is complete within 24 hours of a fractionated x-ray treatment.

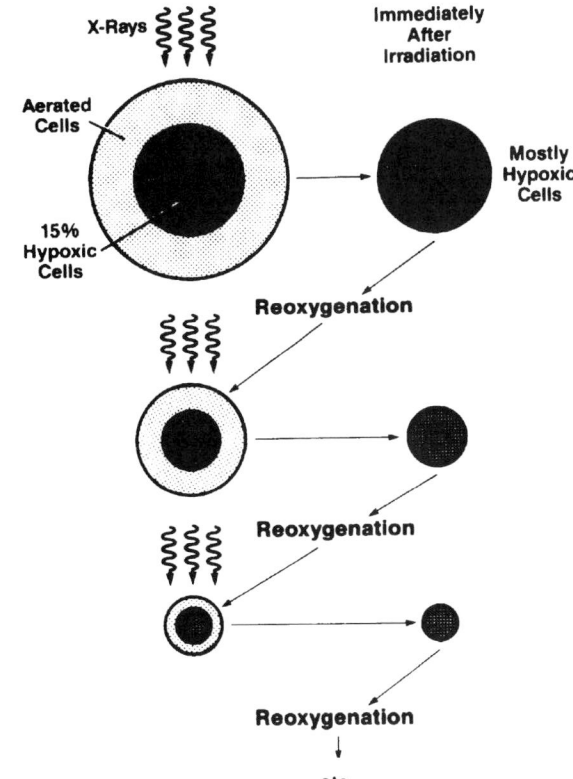

FIG. 14.17. The process of reoxygenation. Tumors contain a mixture of aerated and hypoxic cells. A dose of x-rays kills a greater proportion of aerated than hypoxic cells because they are more radiosensitive. Immediately after irradiation, most cells in the tumor are hypoxic, but the preirradiation pattern tends to return because of reoxygenation. If the radiation is given in a series of fractions sufficiently separated in time for reoxygenation to occur, the presence of hypoxic cells does not greatly influence the response of the tumor. (From Hall EJ. *Radiobiology for the radiologist.* 4th ed. Philadelphia: JB Lippincott Co, 1994.)

Although reoxygenation is not completely understood, it is postulated that as a large proportion of viable aerated cells are sterilized, the demand for oxygen diminishes, and that it would be possible for the oxygen to diffuse larger distances and reach cells that were previously hypoxic. However, aerated cells will not always die promptly, and it is unlikely that the demand for oxygen would decrease in such a short time. Revascularization of the tumor as cells are destroyed may be another mechanism for improved oxygenation. Although reoxygenation cannot be measured in human tumors, it is presumed to occur with multifraction irradiation.

Denekamp and Joiner (59) experimentally calculated the amount of reoxygenation that would be considered effective in a course of fractionated irradiation. They concluded that even a small amount (25%) of reoxygenation may be adequate with 30 small fractions of 2 Gy, but more extensive reoxygenation is necessary to overcome the influence of hypoxic cells with 6 large fractions of 6 Gy.

Radiation Sensitizers

Various drugs have been developed that selectively increase the effect of ionizing radiation on tumor cells. Mechanisms of action of radiosensitizers potentially include:

1. Suppression of intracellular sulfhydryl or other endogenous radioprotective substances
2. Radiation-induced formation of cytotoxic substances from the radiolysis of the sensitizer
3. Inhibition of radiation cellular repair processes
4. Sensitization by structural incorporation of thymine analogs into intracellular DNA
5. Oxygen-like sensitization with electron-affinic compounds, which experimentally have produced enhancement of x irradiation effects in ratios of 1.2 to 1.4 in hypoxic cells (60)

Hypoxic Cell Sensitizers

A number of hypoxic cell radiosensitizers have been synthesized and tested in experimental conditions, and some have been tested in clinical trials. The structures of three of these are shown in Figure 14.18. These compounds are ''oxygen mimics'': the vital difference between these drugs and oxygen, on which their success depends, is that the sensitizers are not rapidly metabolized by the cells in the tumor through which they diffuse. Because of this, they can penetrate further than oxygen and reach hypoxic cells more remote from the blood supply. Misonidazole produced appreciable radiosensitization with cells in culture, as well as in animal studies. However, the dose that could be used clinically was suboptimal because of peripheral neuropathy,

which proved to be limiting. More than 20 randomized clinical trials have been performed in Europe and the United States, with uniformly disappointing results except for a local control benefit in certain subgroups of patients.

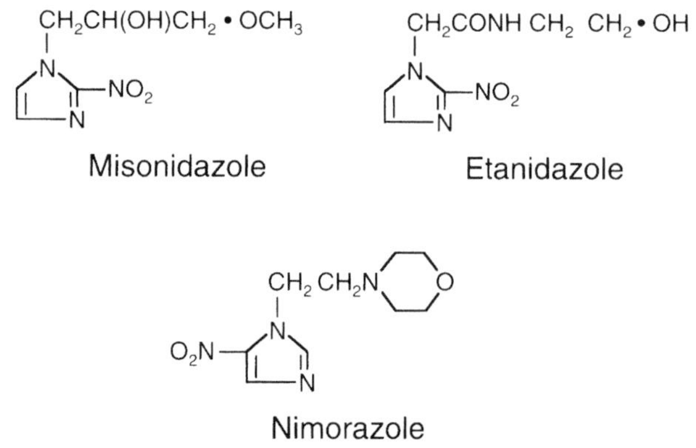

Spurred by the promise of misonidazole in the laboratory, a less toxic drug, etanidazole, was developed. Its lower neurotoxicity is a function of a shorter half-life *in vivo* plus a lower partition coefficient, so that it penetrates poorly into nerve tissue and does not cross the blood−brain barrier. However, controlled clinical trials by the Radiation Therapy Oncology Group (RTOG) in the United States and a multicenter consortium in Europe showed no benefit for etanidazole when added to conventional radiation therapy (61,62).

By contrast, nimorazole is a 5-nitroimidazole that is less effective as a radiosensitizer than either misonidazole or etanidazole but is much less toxic, so that very large doses could be given. In a Danish head and neck trial, this compound produced a significant improvement in both locoregional control and survival compared with radiation therapy alone in patients with supraglottic and pharyngeal carcinoma (63). This compound has not been tried elsewhere. It is interesting to note that Overgaard and colleagues performed a meta-analysis in which they identified 10,602 patients treated in 82 randomized clinical trials involving hyperbaric oxygen, chemical sensitizers, carbogen breathing, or blood transfusions. Tumor sites included the bladder, uterine cervix, central nervous system, head and neck, and lung (64).

Overall, local tumor control was improved by 4.6%, survival by 2.8%, and the complication rate increased by only 0.6%. The largest number of trials involved head and neck tumors, which also showed the greatest benefit. It was also concluded that the problem of hypoxia may be marginal in most adenocarcinomas and most important in squamous cell carcinomas.

Bioreductive Drugs

Research efforts have turned from attempts to radiosensitize hypoxic cells to producing compounds that specifically kill cells deficient in oxygen. The first compound is a triazine-di-N-oxide, known as tirapazamine (TPZ), synthesized by Standford Research International. This compound is believed to be activated by the enzyme cytochrome P-450 and is selectively toxic to hypoxic cells, having little or no effect on aerated cells at the concentrations used. Figure 14.19 shows survival curves for cells treated with tirapazamine under aerated and hypoxic conditions. TPZ is not a radiosensitizer as used but is designed to be used as an adjunct to radiation, with the radiation killing the aerated cells and the drug killing the radioresistant hypoxic cells. However, little clinical research has been done except for one RTOG Phase II trial. The reason for lack of interest may be the reported side effects of nausea and severe muscle cramping. The situation is quite different in the case of combinations of TPZ and chemotherapy agents. A Phase III trial has been

FIG. 14.18. The structure of misonidazole, etanidazole, and nimorazole, the three hypoxic cell radiosensitizers used most widely in clinical trials. Misonidazole and etanidazole are 2-nitroimidazoles: nimorazole is a 5-nitroimidazole. Misonidazole and etanidazole are equally active as radiosensitizers, but etanidazole is less neurotoxic because it has a short half-life and is hydrophilic. Nimorazole is less active but very much less toxic than either misonidazole or etanidazole, so that larger doses are tolerable.

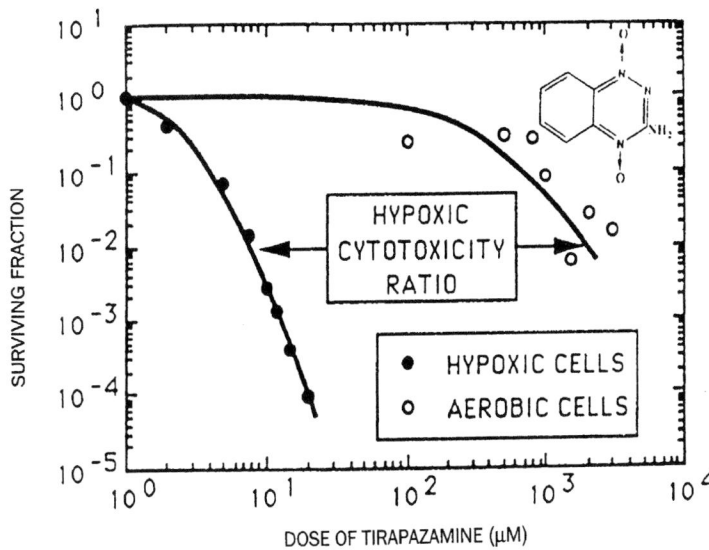

FIG. 14.19. Dose-response curves for Chinese hamster cells exposed for 1.5 hours to graded concentrations of SR 4233 (tirapazamine) under aerated and hypoxic conditions. Cells deficient in oxygen are killed preferentially. The hypoxic cytoxicity ratio (defined as the ratio of drug concentrations under aerated and hypoxic conditions required to produce the same cell survival) is variable between different cell lines. For Chinese hamster cells shown, the ratio is about 100: for cells of human origin, the ratio is somewhat smaller—closer to 20. Tirapazamine is an organic nitroxide synthesized by Stanford Research International. Its structure is shown in the inset. (Courtesy of Dr. J. Martin Brown.)

completed comparing cisplatin alone or cisplatin combined with TPZ for advanced non–small cell lung cancer. There was a doubling of response rates and an increase in survival in patients receiving the combined treatment without any corresponding increase in toxicity (65).

Amifostine (Ethyol)

Amifostine [WR-2721 (S-2-[3-aminopropylamino]-ethyl dihydrogen phosphorothioate, Ethyol, US Bioscience, West Conshohocken, PA)] is one of over 3,000 compounds developed to protect soldiers from total-body irradiation in the event of a nuclear attack (66). It has now found potential application in cancer therapy.

Amifostine is an inactive prodrug that is dephosphorylated to the active, free thiol species, WR 1065, in tissue by cell membrane–bound and capillary alkaline phosphatase. The higher specific activity of the membrane-bound enzyme in normal tissue versus tumor tissue promotes rapid transport of the active thiol metabolite into the normal cell, with limited uptake in cancer cells. The higher pH and higher activity of capillary alkaline phosphatase in normal tissue also contribute to the preferential uptake of WR 1065 by normal cells. Possible mechanisms of protection by WR 1065 include scavenging oxygen free radicals, direct intracellular binding to and subsequent detoxification of the active species of alkylating and platinum compounds, prevention or reversal of cisplatin-DNA adduct formation, induction of hypoxia, and alterations in intracellular glutathione and polyamine levels.

The recommended schedule of amifostine is a 15-minute IV infusion administered 15 to 30 minutes prior to radiation therapy. Although an optimal dose has not been defined, amifostine is generally given at the maximum tolerated dose ranging from 740 to 910 mg/m^2.

Pharmacokinetic studies in humans have shown that, fol-

lowing IV administration at a dose of 740 to 910 mg/m^2, amifostine is rapidly cleared from the plasma and taken up into normal tissues with an α half-life of <1 minute and a β half-life of <10 minutes. Within 5 to 10 minutes after completion of a 15-minute infusion, more than 90% of the parent drug is cleared from the plasma. The uptake varies considerably between different tissues.

The dose-limiting toxicities of amifostine include nausea, vomiting, and hypotension. However, the emesis and hypotension can be moderated through the preadministration of IV fluids, dexamethasone (20 mg IV in adults), and ondansetron (0.15 mg/kg IV) within 1 hour prior to radiation therapy. Amifostine administered on a daily times five schedule at 825 mg/m^2 with cisplatin and radiation therapy can result in hypocalcemic effects.

Amifostine has been approved by the United States Federal Drug Administration as a radioprotector (67). A modest goal is to use a radioprotector to reduce the troublesome side effects of radiation therapy. The RTOG has conducted a Phase III randomized clinical trial that demonstrated the efficacy of amifostine in reducing xerostomia in head and neck cancer patients receiving radiation therapy without prejudice to early tumor control (68). The drug was administered daily 30 minutes before each dose fraction in a multifraction regimen. Three months after treatment, the incidence of xerostomia was significantly reduced in patients treated with amifostine. There was an improvement in the patients' assessments of such symptoms as dry mouth and difficulty in eating or speaking and in the need for fluids and oral comfort aids. There was no difference in locoregional tumor control between patients who received the radioprotector and those who did not. In a study conducted in Japan with 37 patients with cervical cancer treated with amifostine before irradiation and compared with a later cohort of 46 patients treated with irradiation alone, some protective effects were observed with amifostine (69). More recently, a study by the Gynecologic Oncology Group (GOG) in patients with cervical cancer who received 340 to 910 mg/m^2 amifostine before cisplatin and whole-pelvic irradiation suggested that, in comparison with historical controls, the amifostine-treated patients had less radiation toxicity than control patients (70).

Other Modifiers of Radiation Response Used in Clinical Practice

Several approaches have been used to enhance the therapeutic ratio in radiation therapy:

1. *Perfluorocarbons.* These agents are administered in emulsion (they are insoluble in water) in sufficient concentrations, coupled with inhalation of 95% to 100% oxygen, to enhance oxygen transport and release it in the presence of low oxygen tension (71,72). Their potential application in the treatment of patients with cancer is under evaluation.

2. *Halogenated pyrimidines.* The halogenated pyrimidines, 5-iododeoxyuridine (IUdR) and 5-bromodeoxyuridine (BUdR), are very similar to the normal DNA precursor thymidine, but with a halogen substituted in place of the methyl group. These compounds, incorporated into the DNA chain in place of thymidine, weaken the structure of the DNA and make cells more susceptible to damage by photons or ultraviolet light. These drugs have been used in small groups of patients without definite proof of efficacy. Although tumor responses were reported to be good, normal tissue damage was unacceptable. A particularly promising application of halogenated pyrimidines may be in conjunction with low-dose rate brachytherapy since it may be possible to maintain a high concentration of the compounds for the time of the implant, and the sensitizing effect is as great at low- as at high-dose rates (18).

3. *Cytotoxic agents.* Drugs such as actinomycin D, doxorubicin, mitomycin C, 5-fluorouracil, cyclophosphamide, cisplatin, methotrexate, bleomycin, paclitaxel, gemcitabine, and others have been shown to interact with radiation to maximize tumor cell killing. In some instances, increased normal tissue reactions have been observed.

4. *Radioprotectors.* A number of cysteamine derivatives and cyclophosphate derivatives of cysteamine have been demonstrated to be radioprotectors. Sulfhydryl compounds are efficient radioprotectors against sparsely ionizing radiations by scavenging free radicals: the compounds block radical formation by competing with oxygen, facilitating the chemical restitution of the original target molecule. The protective effect of sulfhydryl compounds tends to parallel the oxygen effect, being maximal for low LET and minimal for densely ionizing radiations. The protective effect can be expressed as the dose-reduction factor, which represents the ratio of the dose of irradiation in the presence of the drug over the dose of irradiation in the absence of the drug neces-

sary to produce a given level of lethality. These compounds have been shown to protect normal tissues more effectively than tumors from the effects of irradiation and some chemotherapeutic agents (73).

5. *Hyperthermia.* Heat at temperatures above 42.5°C has been shown to kill cells by itself and to enhance the effects of irradiation and numerous cytotoxic agents. Heat selectively kills cells that are chronically hypoxic, nutritionally deficient, and have a low pH—characteristics shared by tumor cells in comparison with the better-oxygenated and better-nourished normal cells. Furthermore, heat preferentially kills cells in the S phase of the proliferative cycle, which are known to be relatively resistant to irradiation (36, 74).

Radiosensitivity and Radiocurability

Radiosensitivity expresses the response (degree and speed of regression) of the tumor to irradiation. *Radiocurability* refers to the eradication of tumor at the primary or regional site and reflects a direct effect of the irradiation, which may not parallel the patient's ultimate outcome.

At least four concepts potentially explain the differences in radiosensitivity of tumors:

1. *Hypoxia.* It is possible that the less responsive tumors either have a high hypoxic fraction and/or fail to reoxygenate during fractionated irradiation (75). It is difficult to prove that hypoxia is important in conventional radiation therapy, and some question its importance in view of the limited success of neutron therapy or hypoxic cell radiosensitizers (76,77).
2. *Proportion of clonogenic cells.* Proliferating cells are more radiosensitive.
3. *Inherent radiosensitivity of tumor cells.* Fertil and Malaise (78) and Deacon and associates (79) established a positive correlation between the steepness of the initial slope of the oxiccell survival curve for human tumor cells and their response to radiation. The magnitude of differences between cell lines at low doses is sufficient to explain the range of curability observed clinically (75).
4. *Repair of radiation damage.* Repair of sublethal damage (split dose) is found in almost all tumor cell lines (80). Potentially lethal damage (PLD) has been noted to vary considerably from one cell line to another and has been reputed by Weichselbaum and Little (81) to correlate with clinical radiocurability, with less curable tumors showing the greatest degree of PLD recovery.

There is no significant correlation between the responsiveness of a tumor to irradiation and its radiocurability: thus, a tumor may be radiosensitive and yet incurable, or relatively radioresistant and still curable by irradiation alone or in combination with other modalities. For instance, a slowly responding adenocarcinoma of the cervix has a good probability of being cured by radiation therapy. Conversely, a patient with a malignant lymphoma may have complete regression of the tumor after a few fractions of irradiation and still have a limited chance of cure.

Probability of Tumor Control

It is axiomatic in radiation therapy that higher doses of irradiation increase tumor control, and numerous dose-response curves in a variety of tumors have been published. As Fletcher (82) pointed out, dose-response curves can be elicited only when a group of homogeneous tumors is given a range of radiation doses, indicating that tumor control is a probabilistic event. For every increment of radiation dose, a certain fraction of cells will be killed. Therefore, the total number of surviving cells will be proportional to the initial number present and the fraction killed with each dose (82). Thus, various levels of irradiation will yield different probabilities of tumor control depending on the number of clonogenic cells present. For subclinical disease in carcinomas of the cervix or endometrium, doses of 45 to 50 Gy will sterilize the disease in over 90% of patients (83). *Subclinical disease* has been referred to as deposits of tumor cells that are too small to be detected clinically and even microscopically but, if left untreated, may subsequently evolve to clinically apparent tumor. Microscopic evidence of tumor, such as at the surgical margin, should not be regarded as subclinical disease. Cell aggregates greater than $10^6/cm^3$ or higher are required for the microscopic detection. Therefore, these volumes must receive more radiation—in the range of 60 to 65 Gy in 6 to 7 weeks for epithelial tumors. Clinically palpable tumors require even higher doses (82,84).

Baclesse (85,86) popularized the concept of different radiation doses for various portions of the tumor proportional to cell burden. Radiation administered through smaller portals to gross disease is considered a ''boost,'' but this is not a ''boost'' in a biologic sense because it is necessary to obtain a probability of control roughly equivalent to that of subclinical aggregates (82). Portals that are progressively reduced in size (''shrinking field'' technique) are used to administer progressively higher doses of radiation to the central portion of the tumor, where more clonogenic cells (presumably hypoxic) are present, in comparison with lower doses that would be required to eradicate the disease in the periphery, where a lesser number of better-oxygenated tumor cells are presumably present. The same is true for the combination of brachytherapy to treat cervical cancers to higher doses and external irradiation to treat parametrial tissues and pelvic lymph nodes.

EXTERNAL BEAM RADIATION THERAPY EQUIPMENT

In the simplest radiation therapy machine, the kilovoltage x-ray machine, electrons are accelerated by an electric field produced by high voltage generated in a transformer applied directly between the filament (cathode) and the x-ray target (anode). The potential difference (kilovolt peak, kVp) can be varied and metal filters added to absorb lower energy photons, thus changing the penetrability (or quality) of the x-ray beam. The combination of a variable kilovolt peak and different filtration provides the capability of generating multiple effective energy x-ray beams from the same machine. The degree of penetrability is used to categorize the unit as a contact, superficial, or orthovoltage (deep therapy) x-ray machine. A detailed review of these types of treatment machines is provided by Biggs et al. (87).

A superficial unit is an x-ray machine that operates at potentials of 50 to 150 kilovoltage (kVp) and 5 to 10 milliamperes (mA) current. Added beam filtration (1 mm Al to 1 mm Al + 0.25 mm Cu) produces half-value layers (HVLs) of 1 to 8 mm of aluminum. Attached cones are typically used: lead masks are used to define irregular fields. The source to surface distance (SSD) is typically 15 or 20 cm. These machines are used primarily to treat skin lesions.

An orthovoltage x-ray machine is functionally similar to a superficial x-ray machine but operates at a kVp. Most orthovoltage machines operate in the 200 to 300 kVp range with tube currents of 10 to 20 mA. With the use of added filters, such as the *Thoreaus filter* (a combination filter consisting of sheets of tin, copper, and aluminum arranged with highest atomic number always closest to the x-ray target so that the higher energy characteristic x-rays are absorbed by the lower-Z metal), HVLs of 1 to 4 mm copper are common. Fields are usually defined by detachable cones: lead masks are used to define irregular fields. The SSD is typically 50 cm. Few of these machines are still used clinically.

After World War II, the development of supervoltage and isotope teletherapy units drastically altered the course of radiation therapy. The development of nuclear reactors allowed manmade production of radioactive nuclides such as cobalt-60, which emitted high-energy photons (γ-rays) in sufficient amounts and at a reasonable price for commercial use in radiation therapy. The decay of ^{60}Co produces two γ-rays having energies of 1.17 and 1.33 MeV, respectively. The high specific activity of ^{60}Co permits the fabrication of small, high-activity sources, typically 1.5 to 2.0 cm in diameter. The first cobalt-60 teletherapy machine was loaded with its ^{60}Co source in August 1951 in the Saskatoon Cancer Clinic in Canada, and the first patient was treated on November 8 of that year (88). A detailed review of cobalt-60 teletherapy machines is provided by Glasgow (89).

The advantages of a cobalt-60 teletherapy machine include the relative constancy of beam output, predictability of decay because of a well-defined half-life, and lack of day-to-day output fluctuations typically found in electrical machines. Isocentric ^{60}Co machines, such as the Theratronics International Ltd. Theratron-780 and Theratron-1000 have a source-to-axis distance (SAD) of 80 or 100 cm, respectively. Source activities vary from about 5,000 to 13,000 Ci and yield exposure rates of 150 to 250 R/min at 1 meter

(Rmm). Maximum field sizes of 40 × 40 cm at a treatment distance of 100 cm are available on newer machines. The $d_{1/2}$ in tissue (the depth at which the dose has been reduced to 50% of the d_{max} value) is about 10 cm. Most ^{60}Co machines still in use are isocentric units. As shown in Figure 14.20, isocentric units allow the radiation beam to be positioned about an axis of rotation at different angular orientations. Isocentric units simplify the setup of the second and subsequent portals of a multifield treatment and provide the capability for moving beam or rotational (arc) therapy. The number of ^{60}Co teletherapy units in clinical use in the United States continues to decline as a result of the lower depth dose compared with high-energy photon beams from linear accelerators, the relatively poor field flatness for large fields, the need to replace the ^{60}Co source approximately every 4 to 5 years, strict Nuclear Regulatory Commission requirements, and costly licensing fees.

The medical linear accelerator (also called a "linac") has become the dominant radiation therapy treatment unit and accounts for more than 80% of all operational megavoltage treatment units in the industrialized world (90). The first linear accelerator (8 MV) for medical use became operational in 1953 at the Radiation Research Center of the Medical Research Council at Hammersmith Hospital in London (91). Shortly thereafter, Ginzton and co-workers (92) at Stanford developed a 6-MV medical linear accelerator. Since then, advances in accelerator design and construction have been continuous (90). The linear accelerator uses high-frequency electromagnetic waves to accelerate electrons to high energy through a microwave accelerator structure. The high-energy electron beam is made to strike a metal target, producing a penetrating *bremsstrahlung* x-ray beam. If the x-ray target is removed, the accelerated electrons can exit the treatment head and be used for treatment. This type of machine is called a multimodality linear accelerator: it typically provides two or three x-ray beams (6, 10, and 18 MV) and multiple electron beam energies (e.g., 6 to 25 MeV). Modern

medical linear accelerators are designed so that the source of radiation can rotate around a horizontal axis (gantry axis). As the gantry rotates, the collimating axis moves in a vertical plane. The *isocenter* is the point of intersection of the collimator axis and the gantry axis (Fig. 14.21).

The *accelerator structure* in a low-energy (4 to 6 MeV) linear accelerator is typically mounted vertically in the treatment head along with the components associated with producing, controlling, and monitoring the x-ray beam. The accelerated electrons proceed in a straight line and strike a target producing bremsstrahlung x-rays. The *magnetron* and associated electronics, along with the wave guide necessary to transmit the radio frequency power from the magnetron to the accelerator structure, are all situated within a gantry or connecting stand. In high-energy medical linear accelerators, the accelerating structure is much longer and is placed horizontally (or at some angle with respect to the horizontal), requiring that the electrons be bent through a suitable angle, usually 90 to 270 degrees between the accelerating structure and the x-ray target. This is enabled by the beam transport system, which consists of an achromatic focusing bending magnet and steering and focusing coils. Modern multimodality linear accelerators usually produce two or three different x-ray beams of widely separated energy from the same accelerator structure in addition to multiple electron beam energies. At the exit window of the accelerating structure, the high-energy electrons emerge in the form of a pencil beam of about 2 to 3 mm in diameter.

Modern linear accelerators are now equipped with multileaf collimators (MLCs) (Fig. 14.22A) and asymmetric jaws (Fig. 14.22B) to facilitate field shaping and abutted field radiation techniques. The asymmetric jaw feature allows each set of jaws to open and close independently of the opposing jaw. The MLC leaves (small blocks) are typically carried on two opposed carriages that transport the leaves in unison. The leaves have individual computer-assigned positons. MLC systems were originally designed to replace

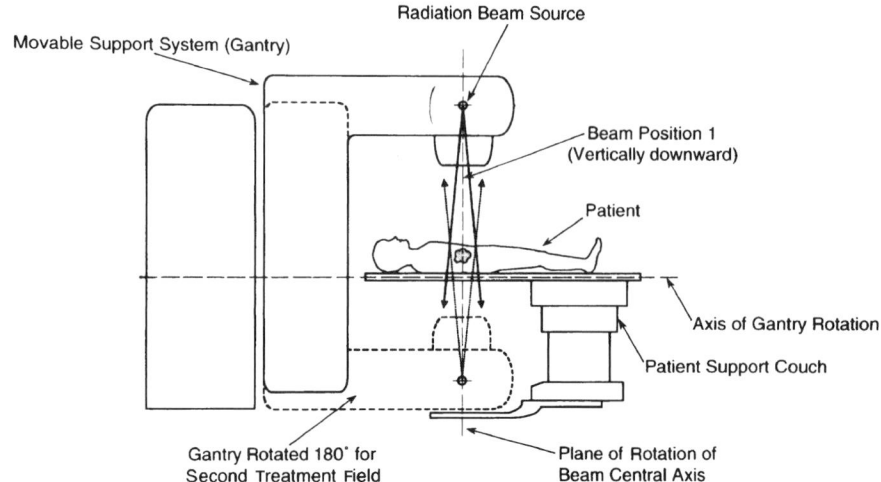

Radiation Beam Source

Movable Support System (Gantry)

Beam Position 1 (Vertically downward)

Patient

Axis of Gantry Rotation

Patient Support Couch

Gantry Rotated 180° for Second Treatment Field

Plane of Rotation of Beam Central Axis

FIG. 14.20. Example of multifield radiation therapy using parallel opposed beams with an isocentrically mounted radiation source.

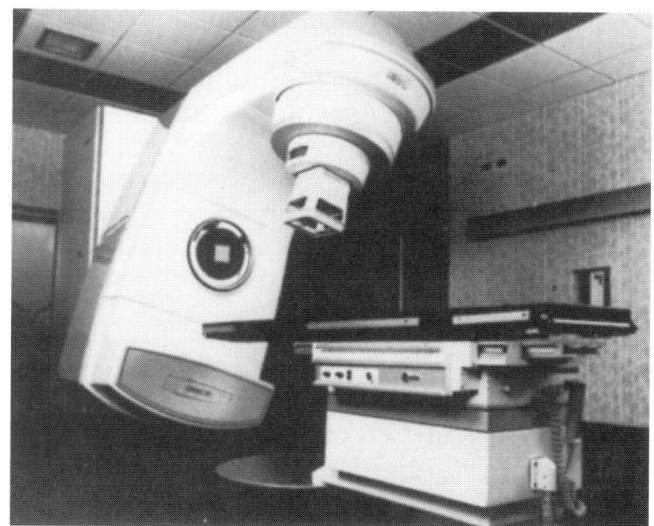

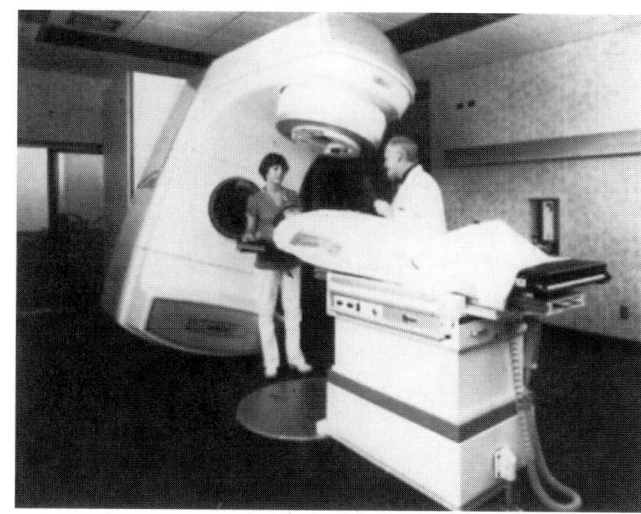

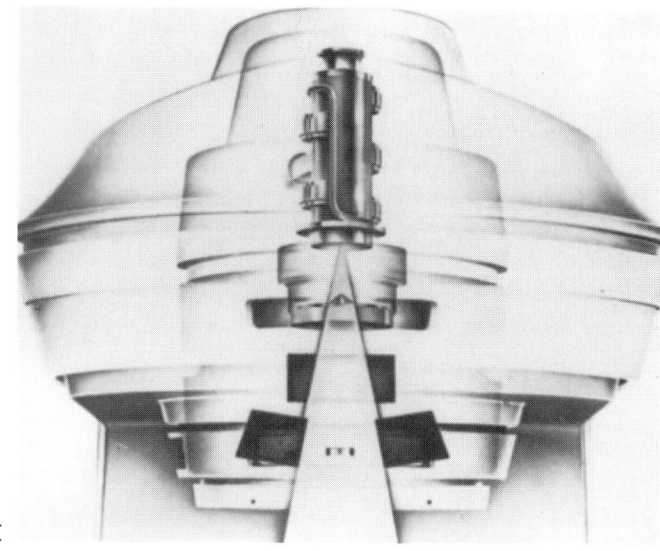

FIG. 14.21. Isocentrically mounted medical linear accelerator. **A:** With electron applicator. **B:** Patient setup for x-ray therapy. **C:** In-line radiation head. (From Karzmark CJ, Nunan CS, Tanabe E. *Medical electron accelerators*. New York: McGraw-Hill, 1993, with permssion.)

poured blocks, but they also provide the capability for intensity-modulated radiation therapy (IMRT) in which the beam intensity is modulated using computer optimization techniques (93).

The microtron, credited to Veksler (94), is an electron accelerator that combines the basic principles of the electron linear accelerator and the cyclotron. In the *circular microtron*, the electrons are accelerated as they pass through a microwave cavity and move in a uniform magnetic field where they describe circular trajectories of increasing radii. Adjustments are made to the cavity voltage, frequency, and magnetic field so that the electrons always encounter the electrical field of the microwave cavity in phase. A second configuration, called a *racetrack microtron*, uses two D-shaped magnet pole pieces that are separated by a fixed distance within which is a multicavity accelerator structure. This configuration provides much higher energy than the circular microtron. It uses a multicavity (typically six) accel-

erating structure rather than a single cavity between the separated pole pieces and provides energy gains of 5 MeV per orbit. Exiting beam energies range from 5 to 50 MeV for electrons and photons. The performance specifications of the microtron are similar to those of a typical medical linear accelerator; however, a few institutions use microtrons clinically.

The use of proton beams for radiation therapy is credited to Wilson, who, in 1946, pointed out the superior dose distribution provided by protons (95). Details on the history and development of proton beam therapy is provided in reviews by Miller (96), Moyers (97), and in the text by Breuer and Smit (98). The principal components of a radiation therapy *proton accelerator* are the accelerator, a beam transport system for guiding the beam to one or more treatment rooms, and a beam delivery system to direct and shape the beam for individual patient treatments. In most existing or proposed proton treatment facilities, either a cyclotron or a synchro-

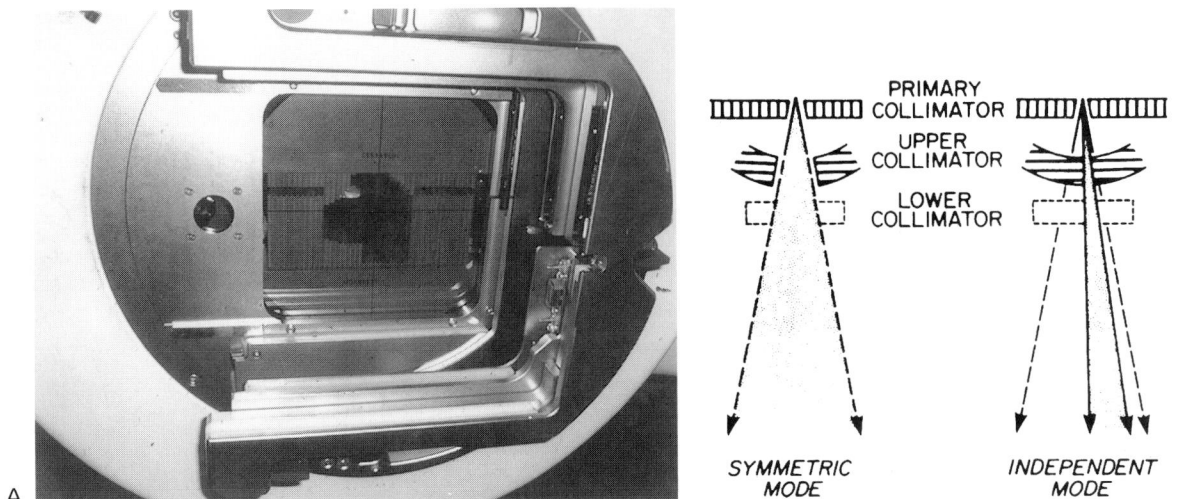

FIG. 14.22. A: Multileaf collimator. (Courtesy of Varian Associates, Palo Alto, CA.). **B:** Treatment technique for breast cancer using independent collimators. (From Purdy JA, Klein EE. External photon beam dosimetry and treatment planning. In: Perez CA, Brady LW, eds. *Principles and practice of radiation oncology.* 3rd ed. Philadelphia: Lippincott–Raven Publishers, 1998:281, with permission.)

tron is used for the proton accelerator. The synchrotron has the advantage of simple energy variability, whereas the cyclotron is capable of higher beam intensity.

The basic absorption characteristics of protons allow highly conformal radiation dose distributions. Protons traverse relatively straight paths through a tissue medium, slowing down continuously by interactions with surrounding electrons and by occasional nuclear interactions. This results in depth-dose characteristics that show an approximately constant dose over most of the beam range but rising to a sharp *Bragg peak* at the end of range as shown in Figure 14.23.

Superposition of monoenergetic proton beams allows the customization of depth-dose characteristics for individual patients through the generation of spread out Bragg peaks that cover the target and drop sharply to zero dose a few millimeters beyond the target.

The RBE of protons is indistinguishable from that of 250-kV x-rays, as is the OER (18). The main advantage of the proton beam is physical, since the dose deposited by monoenergetic protons increases slowly with depth and reaches a short maximum near the end of the particle range in the Bragg peak region. The beam has sharp edges with little side scatter, and the dose falls to zero after the Bragg peak. A proton beam energy of 250 MeV penetrates approximately 38 cm of water and is adequate for most radiation therapy applications. Beam intensity must be adequate to overcome losses in the beam delivery system and provide tolerable treatment times considering patient motion and facility throughput. Beam spreading is accomplished by scattering foil systems or dynamic beam scanning systems. With appropriate treatment planning, it is possible to deliver high radiation doses to deep-seated tumors with relative sparing

of normal tissues. Protons have primarily been used to treat pituitary and base of skull tumors and uveal melanomas.

Two proton clinical facilities are presently operating within the United States, including Loma Linda University Medical Center (99) and the recently opened Northeast Proton Therapy Center (NPTC) at the Massachusetts General Hospital. Institutions outside the United States that provide proton treatments included the Gustav Werner Institute in Upsala, Sweden; the Institute for Theoretical and Experimental Physics in Moscow; and a 1-GeV synchrocyclotron is used for proton treatment at the Joint Institute for Nuclear Research in Dubai; the National Institute for Radiological Science in Chiba, Japan; the Particle Radiation Medical Center in Tsukuba, Japan; and the Paul Scherrer Institute in Villigen, Switzerland (97).

Fast neutrons were first used for radiation therapy at the Berkeley Laboratory in California in the late 1930s. However, because of severe undesirable effects on normal tissues, their use was discontinued: later an interest in these particles was rekindled in both Europe and the United States. Most neutron radiation therapy over the past several decades was performed either with nuclear physics cyclotrons that were only marginally suitable for radiation therapy applications (because of their low-energy, stationary and fixed collimators, and non–hospital-based location), or with machines manufactured specifically for radiation therapy that did not meet modern standards (i.e., low energy, low output, unreliable). Modern neutron therapy machines, with proton and deuteron energies of about 50 MeV, produce neutron beams with depth-dose characteristics equivalent to about 6-MV x-rays.

Neutrons can be produced by acceleration of deuterons to an energy of 300 keV directed onto a tritium target (14-

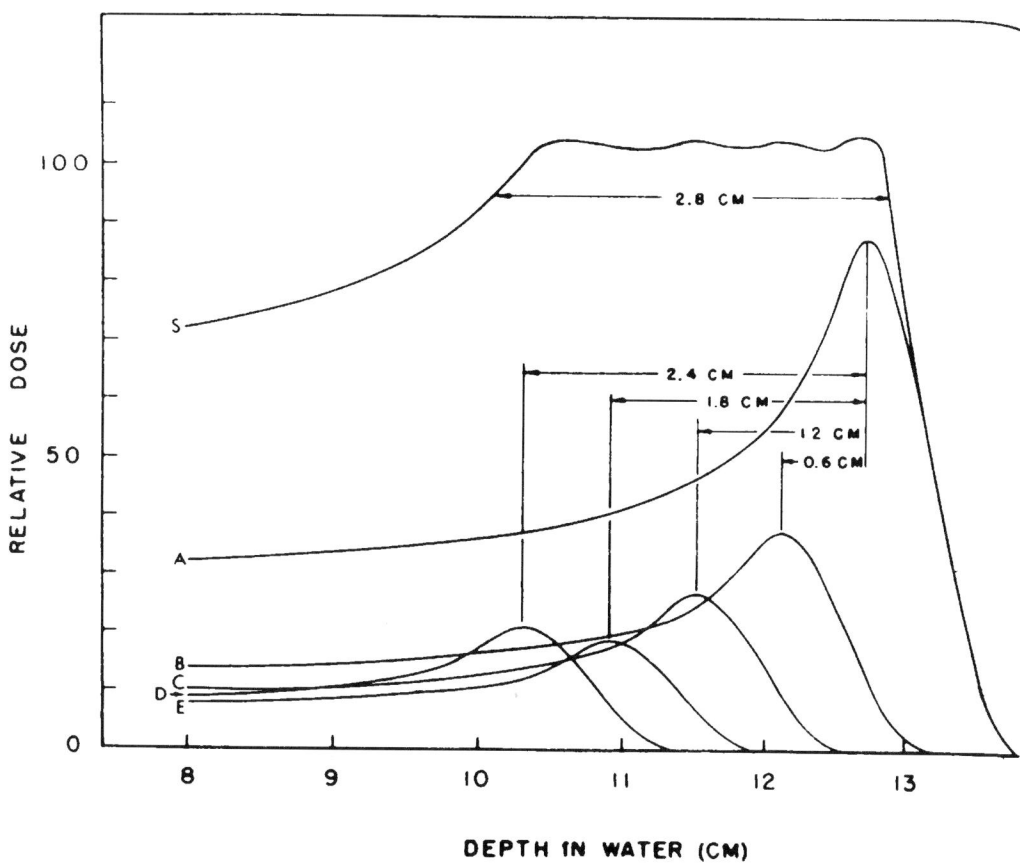

FIG. 14.23. Illustration of the way in which the Bragg peak for a proton beam can be spread out. Curve *A* is the depth-dose distribution for the primary beam of 160-MeV protons at the Harvard cyclotron. Beams of lower intensity and shorter range, as illustrated by curves *B, C, D,* and *E,* can be added to give a composite curve, *S,* which results in a uniform dose over 2.8 cm. (From Hall EJ. *Radiobiology for the radiologist.* 4th ed. Philadelphia: JB Lippincott Co, 1994.)

MeV neutrons are produced). They can also be produced using a cyclotron to accelerate positively charged particles, such as protons or deuterons to high energies until the particle is extracted from the accelerator and made to impinge on a beryllium (Be) target. The proton-Be reaction is most commonly used in modern isocentric neutron therapy machines. The main reasons that this reaction is preferred over deuteron-Be are that proton accelerators are much smaller and less expensive than deuteron accelerators per average neutron energy, and proton beams are much easier to bend around the gantry of an isocentric unit. For example, to obtain neutron beams having a penetration comparable to 6-MV X-rays, the deuterons must be accelerated to energy of about 50 MeV. In the United States, several proton-Be high-energy cyclotrons especially designed for hospital use have been used to treat a large number of patients. A deuteron-Be superconducting cyclotron design at Harper Hospital in Detroit takes advantage of the fact that the neutron yield for the deuteron-Be reaction is about five times that of proton-Be (100). Using superconducting technology, the entire cyclotron is small enough to be rotated around the patient iso-centrically, eliminating the need for bending the deuteron beam around a rotating gantry.

Several clinical trials have been reported using neutrons, usually mixed with photons, to treat patients with locally advanced carcinoma of the uterine cervix: improved pelvic tumor control and acceptable morbidity were observed (101).

Simulators

The conventional radiation therapy simulator mimics the functions and motions of a radiation therapy unit and uses a diagnostic x-ray tube to simulate the radiation properties of the treatment beam (Fig. 14.24A) (102). A simulator allows the beam direction and the treatment fields to be determined to encompass the target volume and to spare normal structures from excessive radiation. Radiographic visualization of internal structures in relation to external landmarks allows special shielding devices to be constructed. Gantry arms are rigid enough to support heavy shielding blocks and simulated electron cones: couch widths are similar to therapy

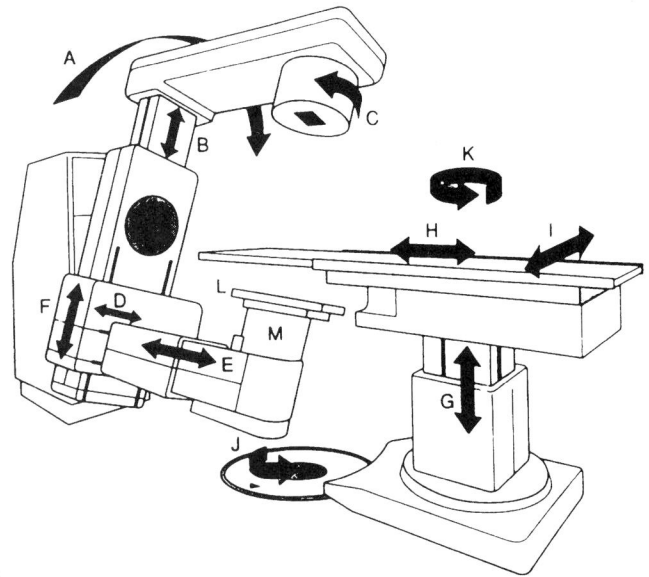

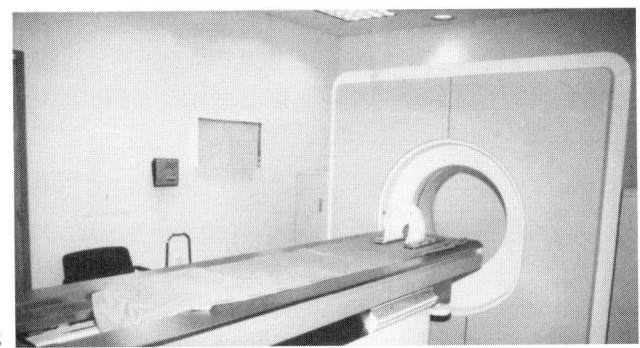

FIG. 14.24. A: The basic components and motions of a radiation therapy simulator: A, gantry rotation; B, source-axis distance; C, collimator rotation; D, image intensifier (lateral); E, image intensifier (longitudinal); F, image intensifier (radial); G, patient table (vertical); H, patient table (longitudinal); I, patient table (lateral); J, patient table rotation about isocenter; K, patient table rotation about pedestal; L, film cassette; M, image intensifier. Motions not shown include field size delineation, radiation beam diaphragms, and source–tray distance. (From Van Dyk J, Mah K. Simulators and CT scanners. In: Williams JR, Thwaites DI, eds. *Radiotherapy physics.* New York: Oxford Medical Publications, 1993, Figure 7.3 (p. 118). Reprinted by permission of Oxford University Press.) **B:** 3-D simulator that is basically a modified CT scanner with a flat couch suite for treatment planning.

unit couch widths, and operating consoles feature digital displays of parameters and programmable settings for SAD, gantry angles, and field sizes. Most simulators are equipped with x-ray fluoroscopy to expedite field setup and beam angulations, and some units feature automatic exposure control for improved radiographic techniques.

The latest feature on conventional simulators uses the imaging device to record transmitted beam intensities as the simulator gantry rotates (103). The resulting reconstructed images are analogous to conventional computed tomo-graphic (CT) images. This is typically referred to as a simulator with single CT scan capability. This type of unit suffers from slow scan speed (which is not adequate for volumetric scans required for 3-D planning), and the image quality is not comparable to that provided by modern spiral CT scanners.

Limitations of conventional simulators prompted the development of the 3-D simulator, a CT scanner with features designed for radiation therapy interfaced with a work station having advanced radiation therapy planning software features, which allows 3-D treatment planning (Fig. 14.24B) (103). A 3-D simulator introduces the concept of virtual simulation whereby the generation and comparison of beam's eye view (BEV) digitally reconstructed radiographs can be done in the absence of the patient. A recent advance in their development is the large-bore (85-cm) CT scanner developed specifically for radiation oncology applications (104). This device allows 3-D simulation of complex treatment techniques, for example, tangential breast irradiation, that have been difficult to set up because of the diagnostic CT scanner bore size limitation.

Electron Beams

Electron beam characteristics are distinctly different from those of megavoltage x-ray beams (Fig. 14.25). The central axis percentage depth dose (PDD) falls off rapidly, and the maximum range (expressed in centimeters) of electrons in tissue is approximately one-half of their megaelectron volt (MeV) energy (e.g., 12-MeV electrons have a range of about 6 cm). Electrons lose about 2 MeV of energy for each centimeter of tissue transversed. Because electron beams are available on linear accelerators in relatively small (3 to 4 MeV) energy intervals, the radiation oncologist must know the lesion depth accurately to select the correct energy. Normally, the 80% or 90% depth isodose curve is used to encompass the target volume: the 80% isodose curve usually envelops a depth of tissue in centimeters about one-third of the electron energy.

In selecting the proper field size to use to encompass the tumor volume, the radiation oncologist must consider the constriction on the central axis of the 80% isodose line in relation to the bulging of the percentile isodose curves at the edge of the field caused by electrons scattering out of the field (Fig. 14.25).

Lack of understanding of the physical characteristics of radiation beams can lead to unsatisfactory clinical results. For instance, Stehman and colleagues (105) reported on a GOG protocol randomizing 58 patients with carcinoma of the vulva to be treated with inguinal femoral lymph node dissection or electron beam radiation therapy (50 Gy at 3-cm depth). The study was closed prematurely after accessing 52 evaluable patients when, on follow-up, 5 of 27 failures (18.5%) were noted in the radiation therapy group in contrast to no failures in the surgical group. The concerns of many radiation oncologists were considered in a report by Koh

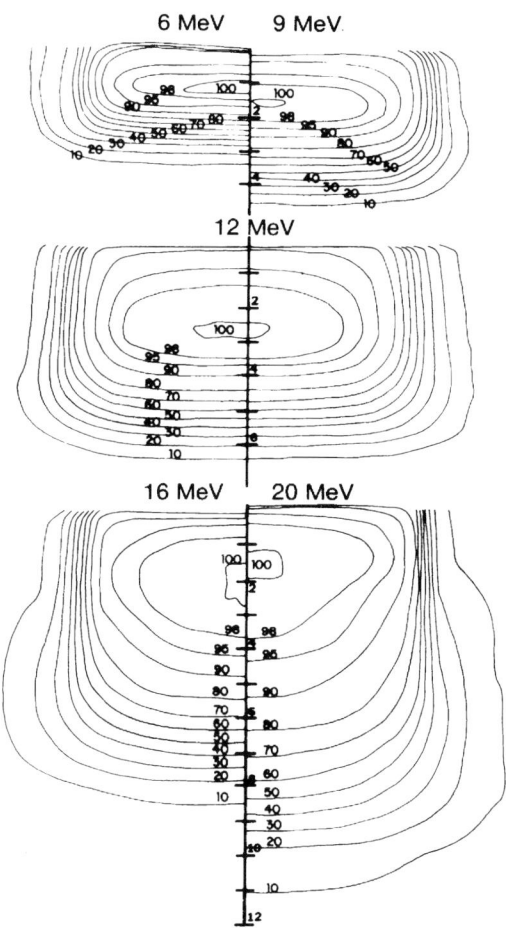

FIG. 14.25. Electron beam central axis isodose curves for a 10-cm × 10-cm field at 100-cm SSD. These data are for the Varian Clinac 20 at the Department of Radiation Oncology, Washington University in St. Louis. (From Glasgow GP, Purdy JA. External beam dosimetry and treatment planning. In: Perez CA, Brady LW, eds. *Principles and practice of radiation oncology*. 2nd ed. Philadelphia: JB Lippincott Co, 1992: 208–245.)

and associates (106) in which it was determined that the depth of the inguinal femoral nodes ranged from 3 to 18 cm (107). Therefore, inadequate radiation dose distributions possibly resulted in the unfavorable outcome with elective groin node irradiation as delivered in the randomized study.

NEW RADIATION MODALITIES

In addition to photons, electrons, protons, and neutrons, other radiation modalities have been investigated in clinical radiation oncology. The physical and biologic characteristics of these modalities are compared in Figure 14.26.

Negative Pi-Mesons

Pi-mesons, or pions, are intermediate in size between electrons and protons. They occur in nature as "nuclear glue"

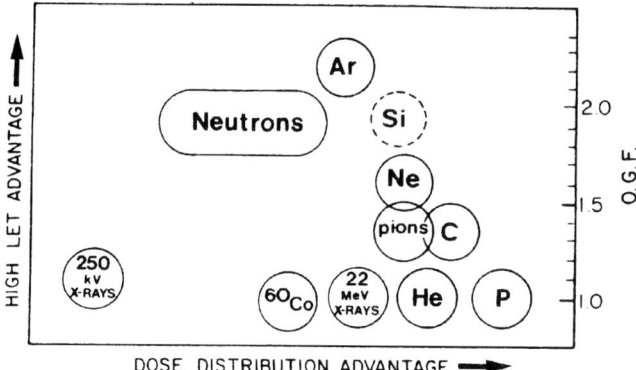

FIG. 14.26. The advantages of the various new radiation modalities compared with conventional 250-kV x-rays. ^{60}Co teletherapy units, x-rays from a linear accelerator or a betatron, high-energy helium ions, and high-energy protons result in a progressive improvement in the dose distribution that can be achieved. This allows improved localization of dose within the target volume, whereas minimizing the dose to the transit normal tissues. The biologic properties of these radiations do not differ significantly from 250-kV x-rays: therefore, they share none of the presumed advantages associated with a high LET.

Neutrons enjoy the advantages of high LET, such as lowered oxygen enhancement ratio and reduced repair of sublethal and potentially lethal damage, as well as reduced variation of radiosensitivity as a function of phase of the cell cycle. They are similar to photons in dose distribution. The depth doses for lower energy cyclotron-produced beams, such as Hammersmith (16 MeV d$^+$Be), are poorer than for ^{60}Co, whereas for higher energy beams, such as the new generation of hospital-based cyclotrons using the p$^+$Be process and with energies of 50 to 70 MeV, the depth doses are comparable to megavoltage x-rays from a linear accelerator.

Negative pi-mesons combine some advantages of high LET with improved dose distribution, but the edges to the beam are not as sharp as for protons or heavy charged particles. Carbon and neon ions in a 10-cm spread-out Bragg peak give good dose distributions but little advantage of high LET. Argon ions give the biggest high LET advantage, greater than for neutrons, but because they break up so readily, they can be used only for relatively shallow depths. Silicon is perhaps the best compromise for a heavy ion: it combines an excellent dose distribution with high-LET advantages that equal those of neutrons. (From Hall EJ. *Radiobiology for the radiologist*. 3rd ed. Philadelphia: JB Lippincott Co, 1988.)

since protons and neutrons are thought to be held together in the atomic nucleus by the mutual exchange of pi-mesons. Pions may be positive, negative, or neutral, but in all cases, they are unstable, with a lifetime of only 2.54×10^{-8} second (18). A limited number of patients were treated with pions at Los Alamos, New Mexico, but no clinical results have been reported.

Heavy Ions

With increasing mass, there is a rapid rise in the energy that an ion must possess to have sufficient range to be of practical use in radiation therapy. At the present time, the only machine in the world capable of producing heavy ions for biomedical applications is located at the University of California at Berkeley. Heavy ions are directly ionizing charged particles, with constant energy in the entrance plateau and a great deal of energy deposited at the Bragg peak region. The depth of the peak depends on the energy of the particles. The narrow Bragg peak is spread with a ridge filter consisting of an absorber of variable thickness moved rapidly in a direction perpendicular to the beam direction. Helium, carbon, and neon high- and low-energy beams have been used for the treatment of some patients. No results in gynecologic tumors have been published.

Helium Ions

The physical properties of helium ions are similar to those of protons, with a well-defined range and a large proportion of the energy deposited near the end of the range in the Bragg peak region. However, the helium ion must have four times higher energy to have the same range as the proton. Thus, 600-MeV helium ions and 150-MeV protons both have a range in water of about 16 cm. As with protons, most of the applications of helium ions have been in the treatment of pituitary tumors. A few patients with pancreatic or pelvic tumors have been treated.

Radioimmunoglobulins

The development of monoclonal antibodies against tumor cells, reported by Kohler and Milstein (108), allowed mass production of antibodies of predetermined specificity. Radioisotopes have been attached to antibodies to enhance the destruction of tumor cells. This has the advantage, in comparison with toxins or drugs, that the isotope only has to be in close proximity to neoplastic cells to radiate them. Goldenberg and associates (109) described imaging of large tumors with polyclonal anti–carcinoembryonic antigen antibodies labeled with [131]I. These trials were further developed by Order (110), who used ^{131}I antiferritin polyclonal antibodies for treatment of hepatoma. This technology has also been used for the treatment of malignant lymphomas and melanomas. Order (110) reported that the use of antiovarian labeled radioimmunoglobulin increased survival in mice carrying an ovarian carcinoma: however, no clinical trials in gynecologic tumors have been reported. More recently, ^{90}Y, a pure β-emitter of relatively high energy (0.9 MeV), has replaced [131]I (111).

RADIATION DOSIMETRY

In 1928, at the second International Congress of Radiology, the ionization of air (called "exposure") was adopted as the quantitative measurement of radiation to be used for describing a photon beam (112). As the beam passes through air or other materials, it creates ion pairs through the ionization process. The number of ion pairs collected in an electric field in air (or ionization current) is a measure of the quantity of radiation passing through the air.

The *roentgen* is the amount of x radiation or γ radiation such that the associated corpuscular emission per 0.001293 g of air produces ions carrying one electrostatic unit of charge (esu) of either sign. This definition for the unit for exposure was established at the 1928 Congress (112) and was modified slightly by subsequent congresses, but the basic concept remains the same. The value 0.001293 g is the mass of 1 cm^3 of air at 0°C and 760 mm Hg pressure; "associated corpuscular emission" refers to the Compton and pair-production electrons set in motion by the interactions between the incident photons and the air molecules. By conversion of units, the roentgen is defined as 1 R = 2.58 $\times$ 10^{-4} C/kg of air. The SI unit for exposure is coulombs per kilogram (C/kg) of air. According to the definition, the electrons produced in a specified volume must spend all their energies by ionization in air, and the total charge must be measured. However, because some electrons produced inside the specified volume create ion pairs outside the volume and some electrons produced outside the volume contribute ionization inside the specified volume, the gain and loss of ion pairs (electronic equilibrium) must be the same for the definition of the roentgen to be satisfied.

Small ionization chambers (so-called thimble chambers) are typically used to measure exposure. The chambers measure the ionization produced, which is then converted to exposure in roentgens by use of an exposure calibration factor assigned to the chamber by a calibration laboratory, such as the American Association of Physicists in Medicine (AAPM) Accredited Dosimetry Calibration Laboratories.

Dosimetry Calibration Laboratories

Treatment machine calibration in terms of exposure is still common for superficial and orthovoltage x-ray machines. However, beyond about 3 MeV, the definition of the roentgen cannot be applied. To overcome this dilemma, the ICRU introduced the concept of *absorbed dose*, which is defined in terms of the energy deposited by the radiation beam as it passes through a medium. Its unit, the rad or centigray (cGy), represents the absorption of 0.01 J/kg of the medium (1 cGy = 0.01 J/kg). The SI unit for absorbed dose is 1 J/kg, which is called the *gray* (Gy) (1 Gy = 100 rad). The absorbed dose concept is best understood by considering the interaction of a beam of radiation passing through an absorbing medium as a two-stage process. The first step occurs when the energy carried by the photons is transformed into kinetic energy of high-speed electrons. The second step occurs as these electrons are slowed down, depositing their energy in the medium. *Kerma*, an acronym for kinetic energy released in the matter, represents the transfer of energy from the indirectly ionizing photons to the directly ionizing electron particles (step 1). The subsequent transfer of energy from the directly ionizing particles to the medium (step 2) consists of the absorbed dose.

High-energy treatment machine calibrations are performed using a calibrated thimble chamber as a Bragg-Gray cavity, and the ionization readings are converted to absorbed dose. Details of the calibration procedure for high energy photon and electron beams are given in the 1983 AAPM protocol (113).

External Beam Dosimetry Parameters

Radiation dose distributions are seldom measured directly in a patient. Instead the distributions are calculated using dosimetry data measured in water or other tissue-equivalent material. The most commonly used parameters are discussed in this section.

Percentage depth dose (PDD) is the ratio, expressed as a percentage, of the absorbed dose on the central axis at depth, d, to the absorbed dose at a reference point, d_o. PDD is affected by a number of parameters, including the d, d_o, field size, SSD, and radiation beam energy (or quality). Field shape and added beam collimation can also affect the central axis depth-dose distribution. Published reports show varying depth-dose characteristics for different types of accelerators operating at the same nominal energy (26,114). These variations can be attributed to differences in energy of the electrons striking the x-ray target, the type of x-ray target and flattening filter material, and the materials and geometry of the collimating system.

Photon beam PDD increases with increasing energy, increasing SSD, and increasing field size. Figure 14.27 shows

that the depth of the 50th percentile isodose at central axis increases from 13.8 cm for 4-MV x-rays to over 22 cm for 25-MV x-rays (115). The depth of maximum dose varies from 1 cm for 4-MV x-rays to over 3.5 cm for 25-MV x-rays. However, the depth of maximum dose position is not unambiguously defined by the energy of the x-ray beam, but is dependent on the treatment head design of the particular machine and field size.

The PDD at the surface and in the build-up region for megavoltage photon beams depends significantly on geometric variables such as SSD, field size, distance between the skin and the collimator, and the presence or absence of a secondary blocking tray (116). Examples of measured build-up region depth-dose data for photon energies ranging from ^{60}Co γ-rays to 25-MV x-rays are presented in Figure 14.28.

The *tissue-air ratio* (TAR) is the ratio of the absorbed dose at a given point in a phantom to the absorbed dose that

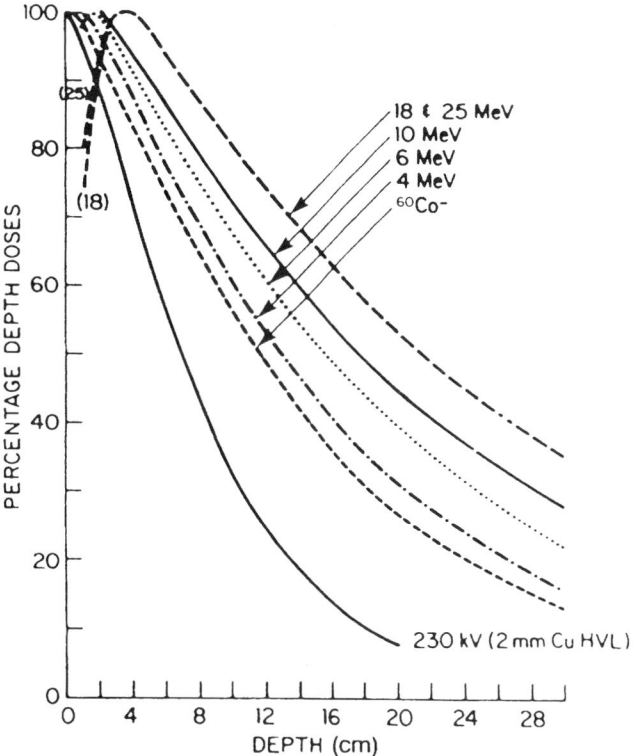

FIG. 14.28. Typical x-ray or photon beam central-axis percentage depth-dose curves for a 10-cm × 10-cm beam for 230 kV (2 mm Cu HVL) at 50 cm SSD, ^{60}Co and 4 MV at 80 cm SSD, and 6 MV, 10 MV, 18 MV, and 25 MV at 100 cm SSD. The last two beams coincide at most depths but do not coincide in the first few millimeters of the build-up region. The 4-MV, 6-MV, 18-MV, and 25-MV data are for the Varian Clinac 4, 6, 20, and 35 units, respectively, at the Department of Radiation Oncology, Washington University in St. Louis. (From Cohen M, Jones DEA, Greene D. Central axis depth dose data for use in radiotherapy. *Br J Radiol* 1972:11:21, with permission.)

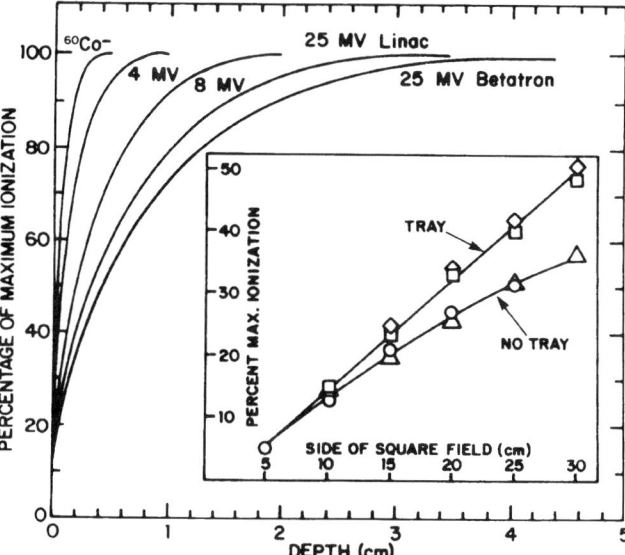

FIG. 14.27. Examples of percentage depth-dose curves in the build-up region for photon energies ranging from ^{60}Co to 25-MV x-rays. (From Velkley DE, Manson DJ, Purdy JA, et al. Build-up region of megavoltage photon radiation sources. *Med Phys* 1975:2:14–19, with permission.)

would be measured at the same point but in the absence of the phantom (dose in free space), with all other conditions of the irradiation (e.g., collimator, distance from the source) being equal. TAR depends on depth, field size, and beam quality, but is assumed to be independent of the distance from the source (112). The TAR at the depth of maximum dose is called the *peakscatter factor* or *backscatter factor*.

The concepts of *tissue-phantom ratio* (TPR) and *tissue-maximum ratio* (TMR) were proposed for high-energy radiation as an alternative to TAR in response to arguments raised against the use of in-air measurements for photon beams with a maximum energy greater than 3 MeV (117, 118). The TPR is intended to be analogous to the TAR but has the advantage that the reference dose is directly measurable over the entire range of x-rays and γ-rays in use, so there is no problem obtaining a value for the dose in free space when the depth for electronic build-up is great. The TMR definition is similar to the definition of TPR except that the reference depth is just large enough to provide maximum dose build-up at that point.

For a given field size, the *output factor* (OF) is defined as the ratio of the dose rate at the depth of maximum dose for the given field size to that for a reference field size (usually 10×10 cm) at its d_{max}. Thus, the dose rate for any field size is simply its OF multiplied by the reference field dose rate. The customary method for specifying OFs for rectangular x-ray fields is to determine an equivalent square field based on data published by the *British Journal of Radiology* (118) or on an area/perimeter calculation (119). Dose calculations to tumor/target volumes in a patient are performed using parameters such as OF, PDD, and TAR.

The radiation oncologist refers to relevant doses using the following terms (Fig. 14.29).

Backscatter dose refers to the dose contributed by scattered photons and secondary electrons produced in the absorber and scattered back to the surface. *Skin dose* or *surface dose* is the amount of radiation dose received by the most superficial layers of the skin. The surface dose is typically significant only for superficial or orthovoltage energies at which the maximum dose is at the skin. For high-energy x-rays or γ-rays, the *point of maximum dose* is some distance below the skin: the dose to that point for a given field is referred to as the *maximum dose* or, at some institutions, the *given dose*.

The *tumor dose* can be specified with the following terms: ICRU reference point dose, the dose delivered to the center of the PTV; minimal tumor dose, the lowest dose delivered to the PTV; in general maximum tumor dose, the highest dose in the PTV (it may be no more than 10% to 15% over the minimum dose with adequate treatment planning); and mean tumor dose, the average dose administered to the PTV.

Exit dose is the amount of dose that is received at the exit surface of the patient. The actual dose received by the tissues at or near the exit surface will be less than that calculated from the standard depth dose data as it neglects the fact that in many situations there is insufficient material beyond the exit surface to provide the total scatter dose.

Integral dose is the total dose delivered (total energy absorbed) over the entire volume or to the body of the patient. The unit of integral dose is the rad-gram or megarad-gram.

Isodose Curves and Dose Profiles

An *isodose curve* represents points of equal dose. A set of such curves, normally given in 10% increments normalized to the dose at the reference depth, can be plotted on a chart referred to as an *isodose chart* to give a visual representation of the dose distribution in a single plane. Figure 14.30 illustrates typical isodose curves for common γ-ray and x-ray energies showing the relative uniformity of the beams at depth and the dose distributions in the penumbra region (16). Beam parameters such as source size, flattening filter, field size, and SSD play an important role in the shape of the isodose curve. For example, ^{60}Co units,

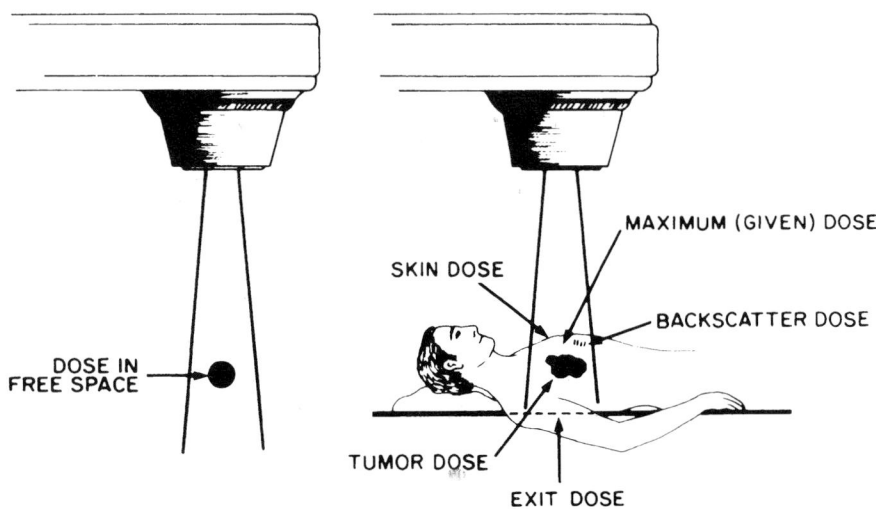

FIG. 14.29. Types of doses commonly used in radiation therapy. (See text for detailed explanation.) (Modified from Perez CA, Thomas PRM. Radiation therapy: basic concepts and clinical implications. In: Sutow WW, Fernbach DJ, Vietti TJ, eds. *Clinical pediatric oncology.* 3rd ed. St. Louis: CV Mosby, 1984, reprinted with permission from Elsevier.)

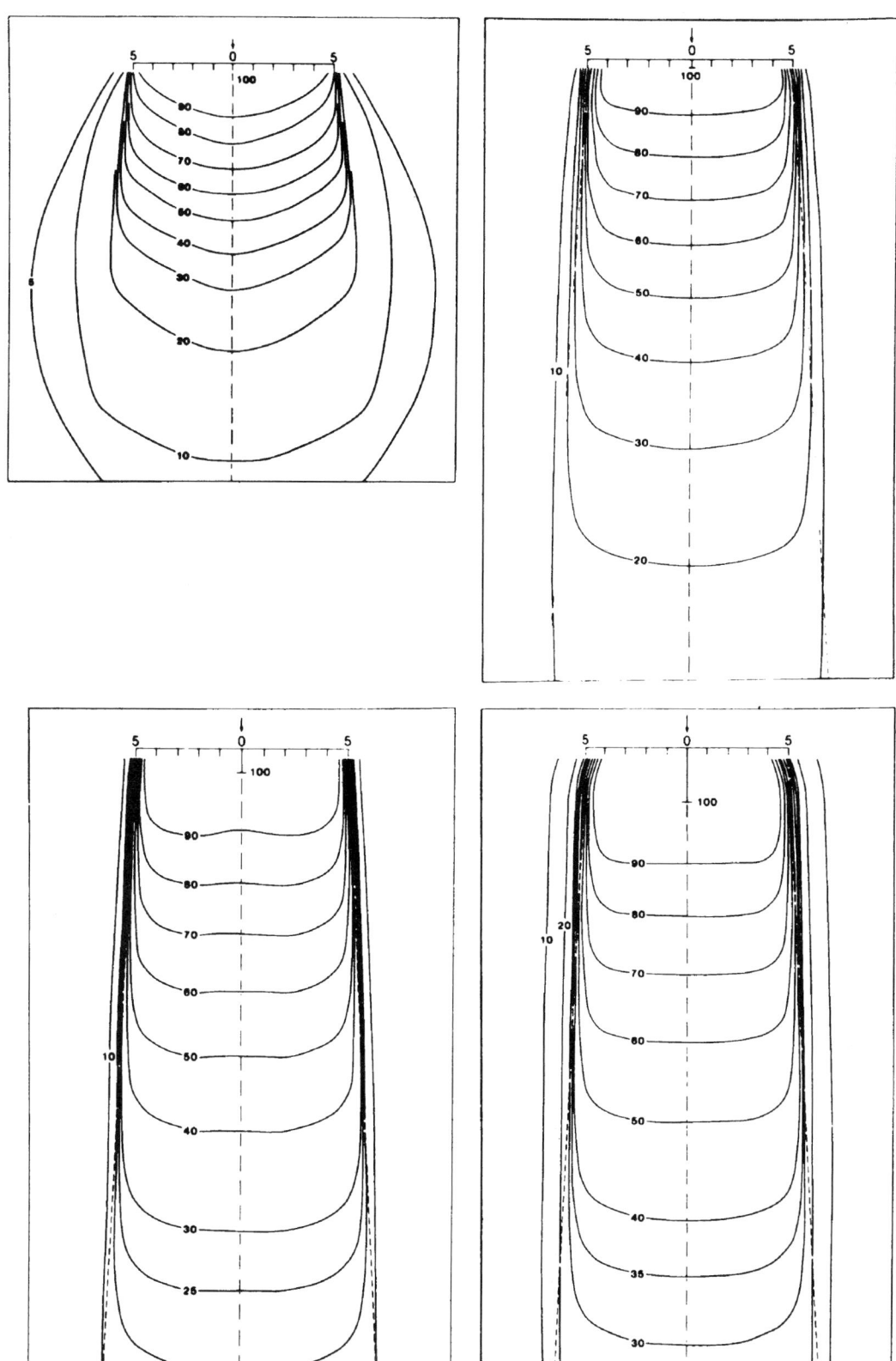

FIG. 14.30. Isodose distributions for different quality radiation. **A:** 200 kVp, SSD = 50 cm, HVL = 1 mm Cu, field size = 10 × 10 cm. **B:** ^{60}Co, SSD = 80 cm, field size = 10 × 10 cm. **C:** 4-MV x-rays, SSD = 100 cm, field size = 10 × 10 cm. **D:** 10-MV x-rays, SSD = 100 cm, field size = 10 × 10 cm. (From Khan FM. *The physics of radiation therapy.* 2nd ed. Baltimore: Williams & Wilkins, 1994, with permission.)

owing to source size and design, exhibit a large penumbra near the beam edge: their isodose distributions are rounded toward the source. Linear accelerator isodose distributions can exhibit "horns" (i.e., greater penetrability away from the central axis, with some portions of the curves rounded away from the beam target). The greater intensity of some of these beams off the central axis must be considered carefully.

A *dose profile* is a representation of the dose in an irradiated volume as a function of spatial position along a single plane (Fig. 14.31). Dose profiles are particularly well suited to demonstrate field flatness and penumbra. The data are typically given as ratios of doses normalized to the dose on the central axis. The profiles are called off-axis factors (OAFs) or off-center ratios (OCRs) and may be measured in air with only a build-up cap or in a phantom at selected depths. The in-air OAF gives only the variation in primary beam intensity; the in-phantom OCR shows the added effect of phantom scatter.

A *wedge field isodose distribution* is generated by the use of wedge filters (generally constructed of brass or steel) placed in the beam. The wedge filter causes a progressive decrease in intensity across the field, causing the isodose distribution to have a planned asymmetry. The *wedge angle* is the angle the isodose curve subtends with a line perpendicular to the central axis at a specific depth and for a specific field size. In the past, the definition has been based on the 50th percentile isodose curve and, more recently, the 80th percentile isodose curve. The wedge angle is a function of field size and depth. The *wedge factor* is the ratio of the dose measured in a tissue-equivalent phantom at the depth of maximum build-up on the central axis with the wedge in place to the dose at the same point with the wedge removed.

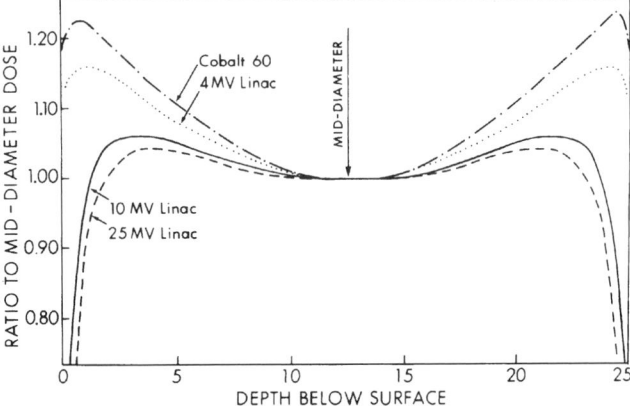

FIG. 14.31. Dose profile of various pelvic diameters used in anteroposterior and posteroanterior portals with different photon energies. With photons below 10 MV, higher integral doses are delivered to the bladder and rectum. (From Perez CA, Purdy JA, Korba A, et al. High-energy x-ray beams in the management of head and neck and pelvic cancers. In: Kramer S, ed. *High-energy photons and electrons.* New York: John Wiley and Sons, 1976, with permission.)

THREE-DIMENSIONAL CONFORMAL RADIATION THERAPY

Three-dimensional radiation treatment planning (3-D RTP) systems are now standard practice in radiation oncology departments. These advanced planning systems provide BEV displays, allowing the treatment planner a viewpoint from the perspective of the source of radiation looking out along the axis of the radiation beam, similar to that obtained when viewing simulation radiographs (120,121). High-quality digitally reconstructed radiographs (DRRs) are also characteristic of these advanced systems. Most modern systems also provide a room eye view (REV) display that allows optimal positioning of a treatment beam isocenter and quick review of the target volume coverage by a specific 3-D isodose volume (122). In addition, dose-volume histograms (DVHs) provide a means of rapid assessment of the treatment plan dose distribution (123). DVHs provide a complete summary of the entire 3-D dose matrix, showing the amount of target volume or critical structure receiving more or less than a specified dose level. However, because they do not provide spatial dose information, they do not replace the other methods of dose display, but only complement them.

3-D planning emphasizes the delineation of the image-based GTV, CTV, PTV, and critical OAR for the individual patient, requiring the radiation oncologist to account for microscopic disease uncertainty and patient setup and organ movement uncertainties. The reader is referred to ICRU Reports 50 and 62 (14,15) and the articles by Purdy (124,125) for details regarding GTV, CTV, and PTV nomenclature and methodology.

Three dimensional conformal radiation therapy (3-D CRT) treatment plans often use multiple radiation beams and may be shaped using MLCs to conform to the target volume. To improve the conformality of the dose distribution, conventional beam modifiers (e.g., wedges and/or compensating filters) are sometimes used. This form of 3-D CRT can be referred to as "conventional 3-D CRT" to avoid confusion with IMRT, which can potentially achieve greater conformality by modulating the radiation beam fluence across the PTV (94).

Intensity-Modulated Radiation Therapy

With IMRT, the beam intensity (fluence) is optimized using computer algorithms that consider the target and normal tissue dimensions and user-defined constraints such as PTV and OAR dose coverage and dose-volume limits. The beam intensity is proportional to the target thickness as assessed from a BEV as the beam is angled around the patient. Where the target is "thicker," the beam fluence is higher: where it is thinner or where there is an organ at risk to be avoided, the intensity is lower. The IMRT planning process is sometimes referred to as *inverse planning*. It should be noted that the term *forward treatment planning* is now being used to describe the planning of traditional 3-D CRT, and it is also occasionally used in conjunction with IMRT when computer optimization algorithms are not utilized in planning IMRT.

Over the past decade, a variety of techniques have been explored for delivering IMRT (93). At this time, none of the techniques has emerged as being clearly superior.

Mackie et al. (126) first proposed an approach called "tomotherapy" in which intensity-modulated photon therapy is delivered using a rotating slit beam. A temporally modulated slit MLC is used to move leaves rapidly in or out of the slit. The radiation source and the collimator continuously revolve around the patient, similar to that of a CT unit. Either the patient is translated between successive rotations (serial tomotherapy) or during rotation (helical tomotherapy).

A commercial slit collimator (called MIMiC) of the type proposed by Mackie et al. (126) has been built by the NOMOS Corporation (Sewickey, PA) and incorporated into their serial tomotherapy IMRT system, known as Peacock (127). The MIMiC is mounted to an unmodified linear accelerator, and treatment is delivered to a narrow slice (1.6 or 3.2 cm wide) of the patient using arc rotation. The beamlets are turned on and off by driving the MIMiC leaves out and in the beam path, respectively, as the gantry rotates around the patient. An indexing device is used to adjust precisely the position of the patient on the couch after each rotational arc is exposed (Fig. 14.32). A complete treatment is accomplished by sequential delivery to adjoining slices.

In the helical tomotherapy IMRT system, the dose is delivered using a narrow MLC similar to MIMiC and small linear

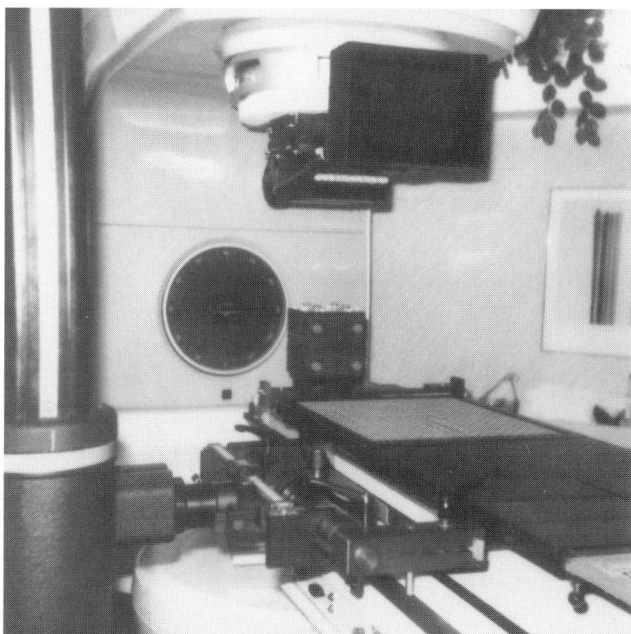

FIG. 14.32. Serial arc IMRT device with small MLC (MIMiC) and comphor attached to the head of 6-MeV accelerator and indexing device to adjust the position precisely.

accelerator mounted in a modified CT scanner gantry. The radiation is delivered while the patient is moved through the gantry in the same way as a spiral CT study is conducted. The original proposal included a CT system mounted on the same gantry to allow the simultaneous acquisition of a kilovoltage CT verification scan study (Fig. 14.33). A system using megavoltage CT has been clinically implemented at the University of Wisconsin (128) and other units have been installed in the United States and Canada.

A conventional MLC, used in a dynamic mode, provides a full-field approach to IMRT as opposed to the slit-beam approach of tomotherapy. For a fixed gantry position, the opening formed by each pair of opposing MLC leaves is swept across the target volume under computer control with the radiation beam on to produce the desired fluence profiles. The setting of the leaf pair opening and its speed for each MLC leaf pair are determined by a technique first introduced by Convery and Rosenbloom (129). This IMRT approach is referred to as *sliding window* or *dynamic multileaf collimation* (DMLC).

A second conventional MLC IMRT approach uses a sequence of static MLC fields (typically called *segments*) that are set up at selected orientations of the gantry under computer control. When the MLC leaves come to a stop at each prescribed segment position, the radiation beam is turned on. This IMRT method is referred to as *step-and-shoot* or *segmental multileaf collimation* (SMLC). The leaf sequences can be determined by methods such as the one suggested by Bortfeld et al. (130). Most medical linear accelerator manufacturers are now providing SMLC IMRT capability.

A third MLC approach, called intensity modulated arc therapy (IMAT) (131) employs a combination of dynamic multileaf collimation and arc therapy. The shape of the field formed by the MLC changes continuously during gantry rotation. Multiple superimposing arcs are used, and the field shape for a specific gantry angle changes from one arc to the next appropriately so that the cumulative fluence distribution of all arcs generates the desired distribution.

In almost all of these significantly different treatment delivery approaches, the underlying principles of optimization are similar, although the specifics may be quite different.

As the clinical use of IMRT becomes more widespread, it is important that the radiation oncology team stay fully aware that ensuring the safety and accuracy of this new modality is more difficult than with the conventional 3-D CRT process. Therefore, it is essential that the radiation oncology team maintain a strong commitment to a rigorous quality assurance program when this new treatment modality is implemented in the clinic.

Several single institutions (99,132,133) and one cooperative group, the RTOG (134), have reported their early clinical experience in the use of 3-D CRT and/or IMRT for several treatment sites with encouraging results. These reports have generated significant enthusiasm for the treatment of

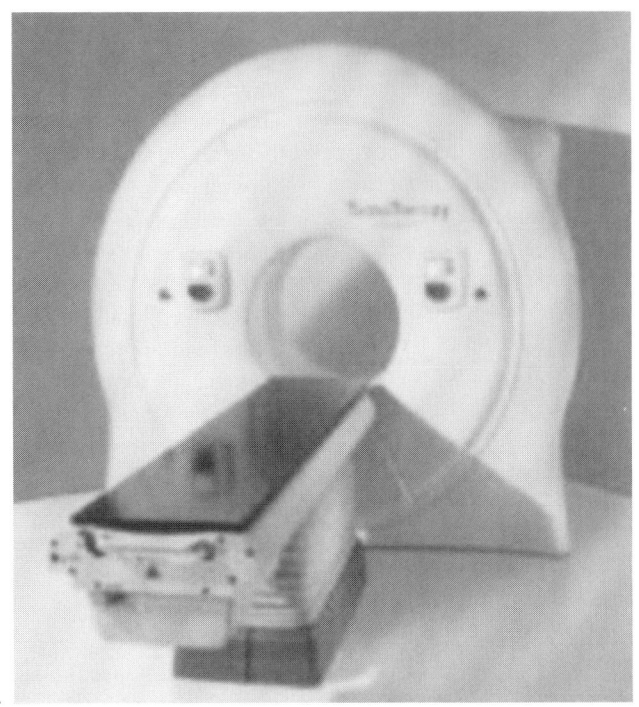

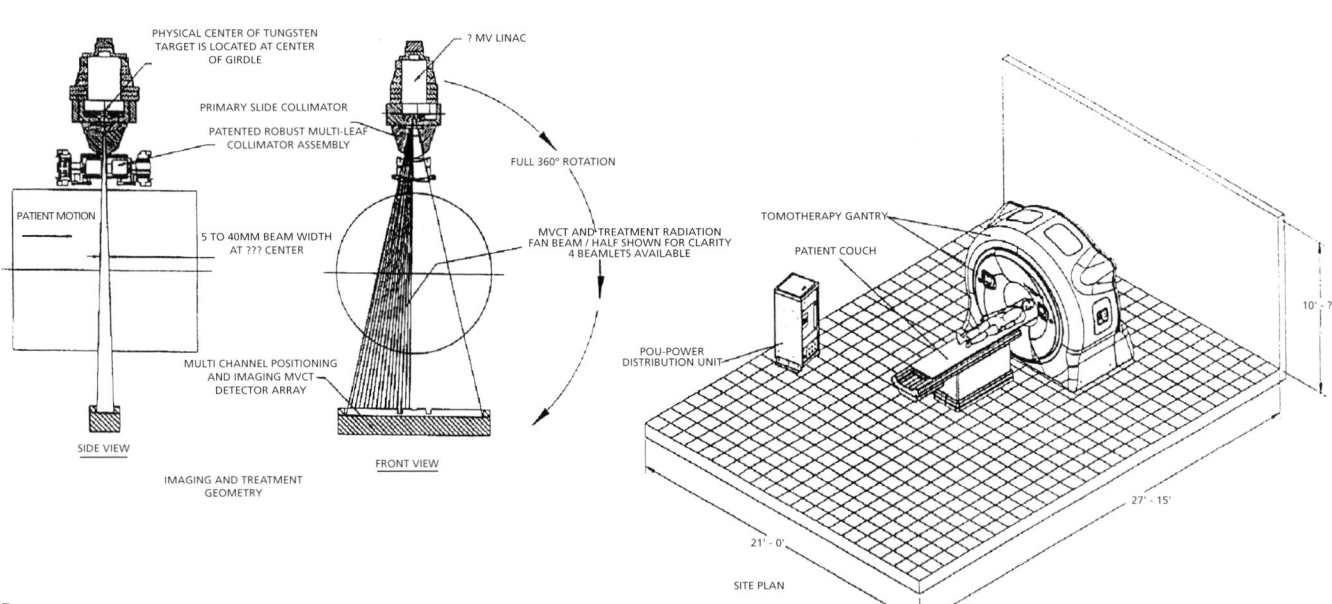

FIG. 14.33. A: Helical tomotherrapy device commercially available for IMRT. **B:** Diagrammatic representation of the device. (Courtesy of TomoTherapy Inc, Madison, WI.)

patients with cancer using these new technologies (see Chapter 18).

Portelance and colleagues (135) carried out CT scan studies of 10 patients with cervical cancer: target and critical structures were delineated and IMRT, as well as conventional planning with two- and four-field techniques, were compared. Treatment planning was done with prescription of 45 Gy in 25 fractions to the uterus and pelvic and paraaortic lymph nodes. Normalization of all IMRT plans to obtain

a full coverage of the cervix with the 95% isodose curve was performed (Fig. 14.34A). The volume of small bowel receiving the prescribed dose (45 Gy) with IMRT technique was with four fields, $11.01 \pm 5.67\%$; seven fields, $15.05 \pm 6.76\%$; and nine fields, $13.56 \pm 5.30\%$ (Fig. 14.34B). These were all significantly better than with two-field ($35.58 \pm 13.84\%$) and four-field ($34.24 \pm 17.82\%$) conventional techniques ($p <.05$). The fraction of rectal volume receiving a dose greater than the prescribed dose was for four fields,

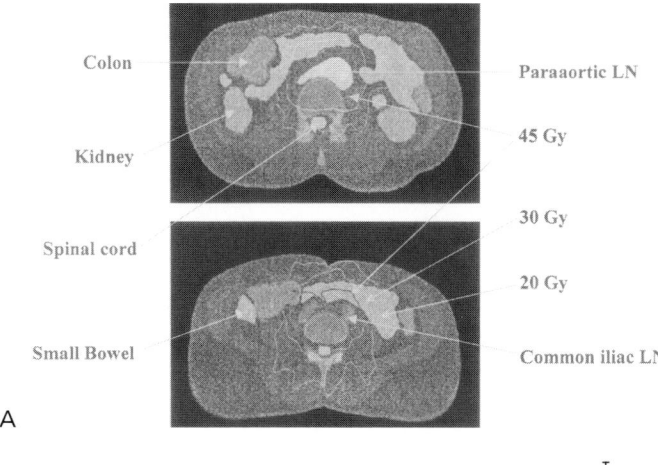

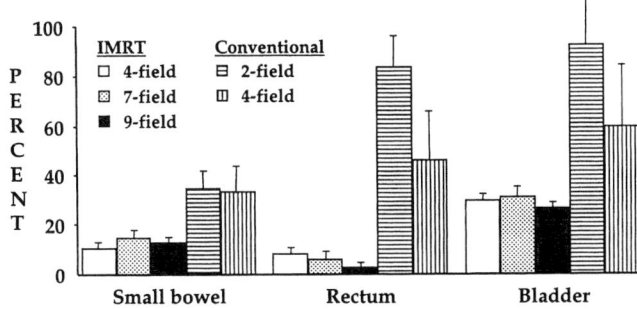

FIG. 14.34. **A:** Axial views of intensity modulated radiation therapy dose distribution. **B:** The functional volume of the small bowel, rectum, and bladder receiving ≥45 Gy with intensity-modulated radiation therapy and conventional techniques when 100% of the target volume (uterus) receives ≥95% of the prescription dose (45 Gy). (Reprinted from Portelance L, Chao KSCC, Grigsby PW, et al. Intensity-modulated radiation therapy (IMRT) reduces small bowel and bladder doses in patients with cervical cancer receiving pelvic and para-aortic irradiation. *Int J Radiat Oncol Biol Phys* 2001:51: 261–266, with permission from Elsevier.)

8.55 ± 4.64%; seven fields, 6.37 ± 5.19%; nine fields, 3.34 ± 3.0%; in contrast to 84.01 ± 18.37 with two-field and 46.37 ± 24.97% with four-field conventional technique ($p < .001$). The fractional volume of bladder receiving the prescribed dose and higher was as follows: for four fields, 30.29 ± 4.64%; seven fields, 31.66 ± 8.26%; and nine fields, 26.91 ± 5.57%. Volume was significantly larger with the two-field (92.89 ± 35.26%) and with the four-field (60.48 ± 31.80%) techniques ($p < .05$).

Kavanagh and co-workers (136) reported on the clinical outcomes of a small cohort of stages IIB-IVA cervix cancer patients with intercurrent medical illness or severe tumor-related anatomic distortion that limited the ability to deliver a high brachytherapy dose. These patients were treated with IMRT to provide a simultaneous boost dose to the primary tumor at the time of external beam treatment to a larger

pelvic field given in conventional fractions. The toxicity of IMRT or early tumor responses were not described.

Mundt and associates (137) treated 40 patients with gynecologic cancer with pelvic IMRT. After customized immobilization, all patients underwent contrast-enhanced CT, and a target volume was contoured consisting of the upper vagina, parametria, uterus (if present), and presacral and pelvic lymph nodes. The clinical target volume was expanded by 1 cm to create a PTV: seven- or nine-field, 6-MV coplanar IMRT plans were generated for all patients. Acute toxicities were compared with 35 patients previously treated with conventional whole pelvic radiation therapy. Whole pelvic IMRT plans provided excellent PTV coverage with considerable sparing of the surrounding normal tissues (Fig. 14.35A and B). On average, 98.1% of the PTV received the prescription dose. The average percentage of the PTV

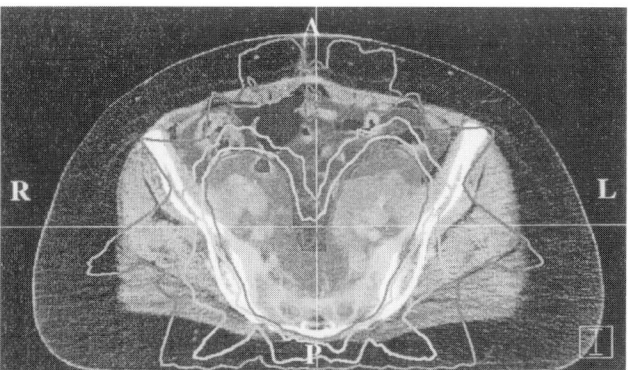

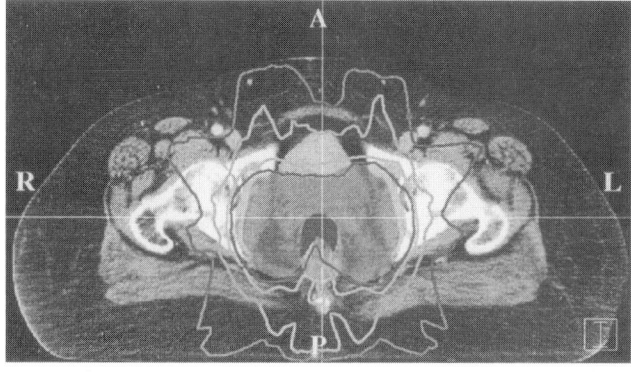

FIG. 14.35. **A:** Isodose curves from a whole pelvic intensity modulated radiation therapy plan superimposed on an axial CT slide through the upper pelvis. The small bowel and PTV are shaded in orange and green, respectively. Highlighted are the 100% (red), 90% (green), 70% (light blue), and 50% (dark blue) isodose curves. **B:** Isodose curves from a whole pelvic intensity-modulated radiation therapy plan superimposed on an axial CT slide through the lower pelvis. The bladder, rectum, and PTV are shaded in yellow, light blue, and green, respectively. Highlighted are the 100% (red), 90% (green), 70% (light blue), and 50% (dark blue) isodose curves. (Reprinted from Mundt AJ, Lujan AE, Rotmensch J, et al. Intensity-modulated whole pelvic radiotherapy in women with gynecologic malignancies. *Int J Radiat Oncol Biol Phys* 2002: 52:1330, with permission from Elsevier.)

receiving 110% and 115% of the prescription dose was 9.8% and 0.2%, respectively. IMRT was well tolerated, and no patient developing grade 3 toxicity. Grade 2 acute gastrointestinal toxicity was less common in the pelvic IMRT group (60%) versus 91% with conventional radiation therapy ($p = .002$). Moreover, the percentage of whole pelvis IMRT and whole pelvis radiation therapy patients requiring no or only infrequent antidiarrheal medications was 75% and 34%, respectively ($p = .001$). Although less grade 2 genitourinary toxicity was seen in the pelvic IMRT group (10% versus 20%), this difference was not statistically significant ($p = .22$).

RADIOACTIVITY

Radiation Decay

Radioactive elements decay by emitting one or more of three distinct types of radiation: α particles, having a positive electrical charge; β particles, having a negative charge and γ-rays, having no charge. An α particle is a helium nucleus, β particles are electrons, and γ-rays are a form of electromagnetic radiation similar to x-rays but originating from within the nucleus of the atom. In addition to α and β particles and γ-rays, various other particles, the so-called elementary particles, have been detected.

A large nucleus in the atom is not as stable as a small nucleus. Consequently, a nuclide having too many protons in relation to the number of neutrons is said to have an unfavorable N to Z ratio and decays to reach a stable configuration.

Mathematics of Radiation Decay

Activity describing the radioactivity of a sample and denoted by the symbol A is the total number of disintegrations per unit of time. The curie (Ci), a unit of activity, is equal to 3.7×10^{10} disintegrations per second, the approximate number of decays per second by 1 g of ^{226}Ra. The becquerel (Bq), the name for the SI unit for activity, is equal to one disintegration per second.

The decay constant of a radioactive nucleus is the fraction of the total number of atoms that decay per unit of time and is denoted by the symbol λ.

Knowing the decay constant λ and the initial radioactivity A_0, a radioisotope's activity at a later time (t) can be calculated using the exponential decay equation

$$A(t) = A_0 \cdot e^{-\lambda \cdot t}$$

The half-life of a radionuclide is the time required for the number of radioactive atoms in a particular sample to decrease by one-half. The half-life, $T_{1/2}$, is related to the decay constant by $T_{1/2} = 0.693/\lambda$. The average life, T_a, of a radioactive nuclide is related to the decay constant and the half-life by $T_a = 1/\lambda = 1.44\ T_{1/2}$. The average life represents the time period that a hypothetical source would need, if it retained its original activity for that time period and then suddenly decayed to zero activity, to produce the same number of disintegrations as produced over an infinite time period by the source if it decayed exponentially.

Modes of Radiation Decay

Gamma decay occurs when a nucleus undergoes a transition from a higher to a lower energy level. In this process, a high-energy photon called a γ-ray is emitted. As previously indicated, γ-rays are identical to the x-rays emitted by excited atoms, except γ-rays originate from within the nucleus and x-rays originate from outside the nucleus. Half-lives for decay are usually very short, typically 10^{-15} second.

Internal conversion is closely related to γ decay. Instead of emitting a γ-ray, the excess energy from the excited nucleus is transferred to an electron in one of the inner atomic shells, causing ejection of the electron from the atom with subsequent emission of characteristic x-rays. The probability of internal conversion occurring increases as the atomic number increases.

In β decay, a neutron within the nucleus is converted into a proton, and an electron and an antineutrino are emitted, or a proton is converted into a neutron, and a positron and a neutrino are emitted. The positron is a positively charged particle with the same mass and spin as the electron, and is considered to be the the antiparticle of the electron. In β decay, the emitted particles may vary in kinetic energy, but rarely exceeds 3 MeV. Half-lives for β decay are long compared with γ decay half-lives, varying from seconds to years.

α decay occurs when the ratio of neutrons to protons is low in nuclides with atomic numbers above 82. As indicated earlier, the emitted particle in α decay is a helium nucleus (two protons and two neutrons). Half-lives in α decay range from 10^{-3} to 10^{10} years.

Of the 103 elements known currently (evidence of elements 104 to 109 now exists), the first 92 occur naturally. The remaining 11 elements have been produced artificially. In general, the elements with high atomic numbers tend to be radioactive: in fact, all but one of the elements with an atomic number above 82 (lead) are radioactive ($^{209}_{93}$Bi is stable).

Daughter Nuclides and Radioactive Equilibrium

Radioactive nuclides undergo successive transformations through α and β decay in which the parent nuclide produces a radioactive product called the *daughter nuclide* (112). When the half-life of the parent nuclide is longer than the half-life of the daughter nuclide, an equilibrium condition results. When this occurs, the ratio of the activity of the daughter nuclide to the activity of the parent nuclide becomes constant, and the apparent decay rate of the daughter nuclide will be controlled by the parent nuclide's decay rate.

Two types of radioactive equilibrium are transient equilibrium and secular equilibrium. Transient equilibrium is established when the parent nuclide's half-life is not much greater than the daughter nuclide's half-life. In secular equilibrium, the half-life of the parent nuclide is much greater than that of the daughter nuclide.

Physical Aspects of Brachytherapy

Brachytherapy (*brachy* from the Greek for "short distance") consists of placing sealed radioactive sources very close to or in contact with the target tissue. Because the absorbed dose falls off rapidly with increasing distance from the sources, high doses may be safely delivered to a well-localized target region over a short time. *Implantation* is the procedure of surgically inserting radioactive sources or applicators designed to hold them. The *implant* is the completed assembly of sources and applicators.

Brachytherapy Techniques

Brachytherapy techniques vary according to the following:

1. *Surgical approach:* whether the sources are inserted into body cavities, directly into tissues, or applied on top of skin or a mucosal surface.
2. *Length of treatment time:* whether the sources are removed after a precalculated treatment time or left in the patient forever.
3. *Location and timing of source loading:* whether the sources are inserted into the patient in the operating room or after surgery in the patient's hospital room.
4. *Method of loading sources:* whether done manually or using a robotic unit (afterloader).
5. *Rate at which dose is delivered:* whether the prescribed radiation doses are delivered over days or minutes.

Intracavitary, Interstitial, and Mold Therapy

Based on surgical approach, implantation technques may be broadly characterized as intracavitary, interstitial, or surface-dose applications. *Intracavitary insertion* consists of positioning applicators designed to hold a number of sources into a body cavity in proximity to the target tissue. Intracavitary treatment using tandem and colpostat applicators (Fig. 14.36) is almost universally used in definitive radiation therapy of advanced cervix cancer. All intracavitary implants are *temporary implants*, which are removed from the patient as soon as the prescribed dose has been delivered [24 to 72 hours after insertion for a low-dose rate (LDR) implant]. *Interstitial brachytherapy* consists of surgically implanting small radioactive sources directly into the target tissues. A *permanent interstitial implant* remains in place and is not removable: the initial source strength is chosen so that the

prescribed dose is fully delivered only when the implanted radioactivity has decayed to a negligible level. Permanent implants are useful in treating localized malignancies. Temporary interstitial implants, in which the treatment time is used to control the total dose delivered, are widely used in the treatment of localized gynecologic malignancies. *Surface-dose applications* (sometimes called *plesiocurietherapy* or *mold therapy*) consist of an applicator containing an array of radioactive sources designed to deliver a uniform dose distribution to a skin or mucosal surface. The vaginal cylinder is the most commonly used intracavitary surface-dose applicator in gynecologic brachytherapy.

Preloaded and Afterloaded Brachytherapy

Temporary implant technology can also be classified according to the method used to introduce, or load, the radioactive sources into the implant site. The preloaded or "hot source" technique consists of positioning the radioactive sources in the implant site during the operative procedure. For an intracavitary insertion, applicators into which the appropriate sources have been preloaded are inserted into the patient. For interstitial brachytherapy, radioactive needles with trocar points (Fig. 14.37) are inserted directly into the target tissue. Radiation exposure to operating room personnel and to the hands and fingers of the radiation oncologist has been nearly eliminated by use of modern afterloading techniques, which were first introduced in the United States by Henschke (138) and Suit (139). These techniques consist of inserting nonradioactive applicators into the patient during the operative procedure and then afterloading the radioactive sources into the patient after she has returned to her room. For intracavitary therapy, tube-like sources of ^{137}Cs ("intracavitary tubes" in Fig. 14.37) are manually inserted into plastic sleeves or inserts, which are introduced into the vaginal and uterine applicators. The process of performing a manually afterloaded interstitial implant is illustrated in Figure 14.38. During the procedure, flexible plastic tubes or hollow metal needles are inserted through the target tissue. After the patient has returned to her room, ribbons consisting of radioactive ^{192}Ir seeds encapsulated in nylon ribbons (Fig. 14.38) are inserted into the hollow applicators. The plastic tubes or metal needles are crimped or capped to hold the radioactive sources in place.

Remote Afterloading Brachytherapy. After the sources are manually loaded into the patient, they remain throughout the entire treatment period. This will give radiation exposure to nursing and other inpatient staff responsible for the care of the patient. This radiation exposure can be greatly reduced or eliminated by the use of remote afterloading technology. A remote afterloading system consists of a pneumatically or motor-driven source transport system for robotically transferring radioactive material between a shielded safe and the treatment applicator (140). Transfer tubes connect the applicator to the shielded safe. By pressing a button located

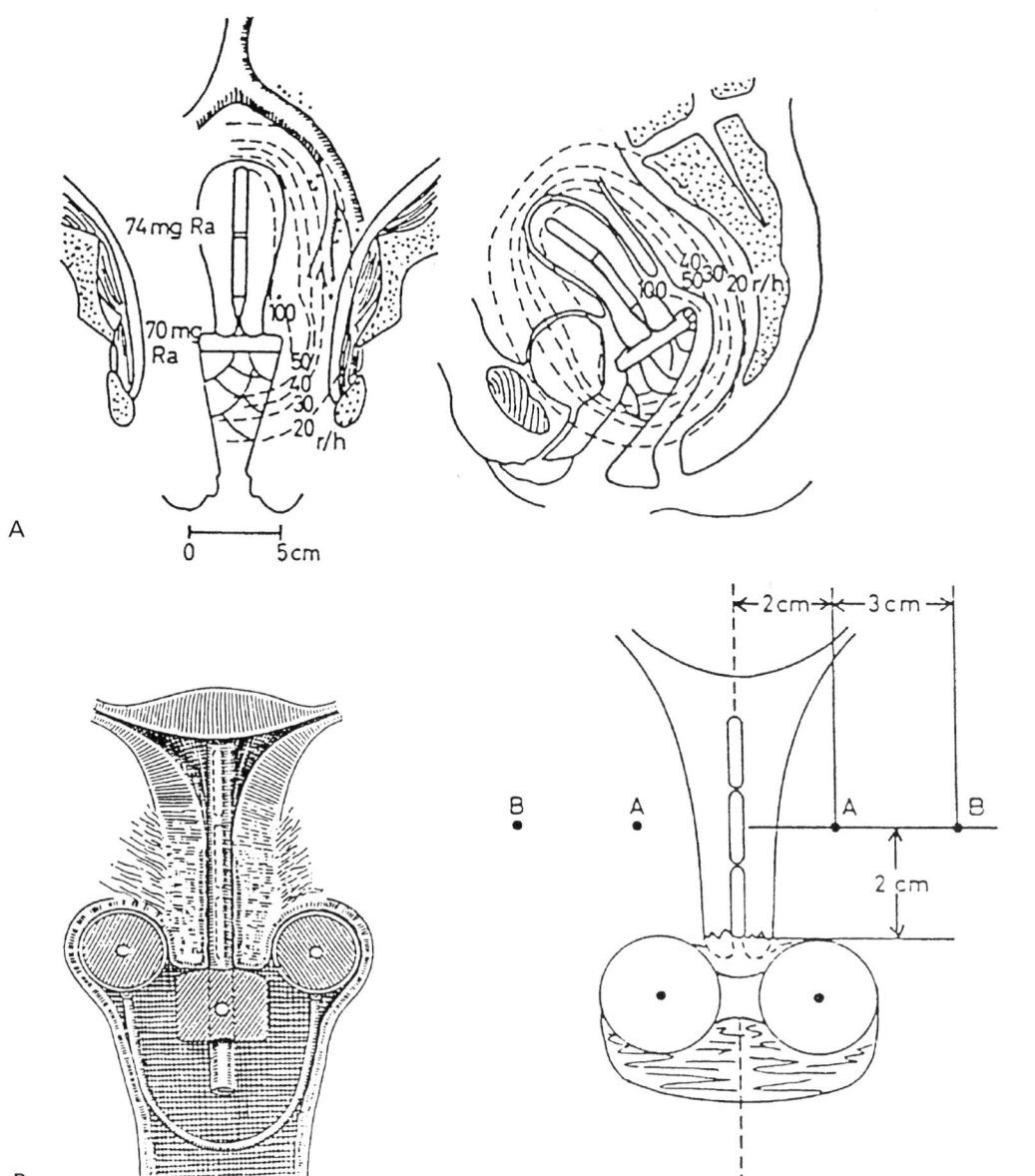

FIG. 14.36. A: The Stockholm system. The intrauterine rod-shaped applicator is loaded with 53 to 88 mg radium (74 mg in the example shown). The vaginal applicator usually consists of a flat box containing 60 to 80 mg radium (70 mg in the example shown), but in special cases, other forms of vaginal applicators may be used. Classically, the two applicators are not fixed to each other, but fixed or semifixed combinations have been developed. The vaginal applicator is held against the cervix and lateral fornices by careful and systematic gauze packing. Typically, two or three applications are given at 3-week intervals, each application lasting for 27 to 30 hours. (From Walstam R. The dosage distribution in the pelvis in radium treatment of carcinoma of the cervix. *Acta Radiol* 1954:42:237, with permission.) **B:** The Paris system. Typical radium application for a treatment of cervical carcinoma consisting of three individualized vaginal sources (one in each lateral fornix and one central in front of the cervical os) and one intrauterine source made of three radium tubes (in so-called tandem position). The active length of the sources is usually 16 mm, their linear activity being between 6 and 10 mg/cm, and their strength between 10 and 15 mg of radium. The total activity used is one of the lowest in use for such treatments and implies a typical application duration of 6 to 8 days. Typically, the ratio of the total activity of the vaginal sources to the total activity of the uterine sources should be 1 (with variations between 0.66 and 1.5). (From Pierquin B. *Precis de curietherapie, endocurietherapie et plesiocurietherapie.* Paris: Masson, 1964, with permission.) **C:** The Manchester system. Definitions of points A and B in the classical Manchester system are found in the text. In a typical application, the loading of intrauterine applicators varied between 20 and 35 mg of radium and between 15 and 25 mg of radium for each vaginal ovoid. The resultant treatment time to get 8,000 R at point A was 140 hours. (From Meredith WJ. *Radium dosage: the Manchester system.* Edinburgh: Livingstone, 1967, with permission.)

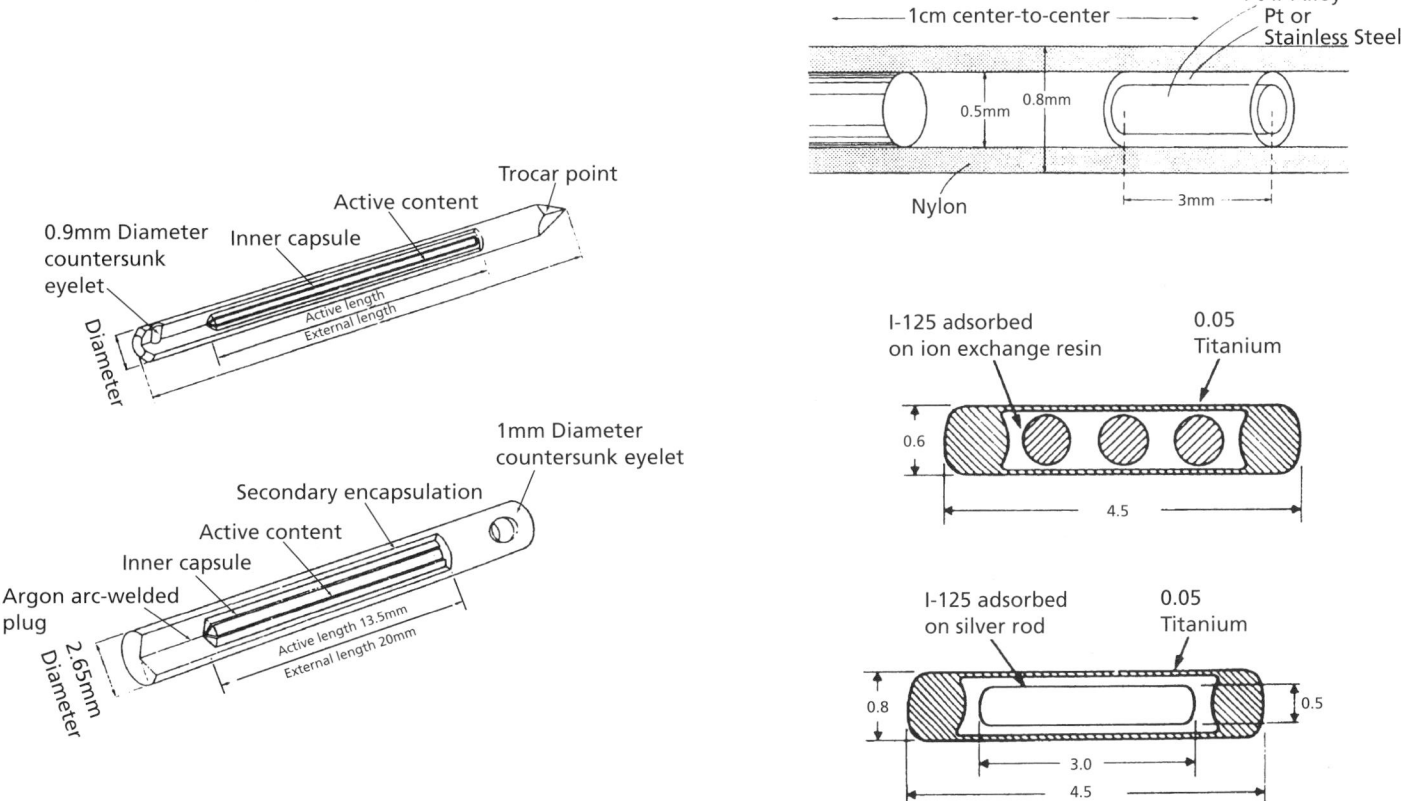

FIG. 14.37. Commonly used types of sealed low-dose rate brachytherapy sources. **Left:** (a) ^{137}Cs CDCS A-type needle used for nonafterloading interstitial implants. The source is encapsulated in about 0.5 mm of stainless steel. (b) ^{137}Cs CDCS J-type tube used for intracavitary brachytherapy. (Reproduced with permission of Amersham International PLC.) **Upper Right:** ^{192}Ir interstitial sources encapsulated in 0.8-mm–diameter nylon tubing. The inner cylinder represents the active Ir-Pt core of the individual seed, which is encapsulated in either 0.1 mm of Pt or 0.2 mm of stainless steel. (From Anderson LL, Nath R, Weaver KA, et al. *Interstitial brachytherapy: physical, biological, and clinical considerations.* New York: Raven Press, 1990, with permission.) **Lower Right:** ^{125}I interstitial sources. (a) Model 6702 seed contains no radiopaque marker and is used for temporary implantation. (b) Model 6711 seed, commonly used for permanent implants, contains ^{125}I adsorbed on a radiopaque silver rod. (Reproduced with permission of Amersham International PLC.)

outside the patient's room, the source retracts into the shielded safe, allowing the nurse or other healthcare worker exposure-free access to the patient. After the visitor leaves the room and closes the door, the sources are transported back into treatment position and treatment resumes. Most remote afterloaders are equipped with a timer that automatically retracts the source when the programmed treatment time, corrected for gaps and interruptions, has been administered. The use of these devices is reviewed in more detail later in this chapter.

Low-Dose Rate and High-Dose Rate Brachytherapy. In addition to classifying implants according to surgical approach, method of source loading, and duration, the rate at which absorbed dose is delivered to the prescription point is an important parameter. According to ICRU Report No. 38, dose rates of 40 to 200 cGy/h (0.4 to 2 Gy/h) are referred to as low-dose rate (LDR) (141). To deliver clinically useful

total doses of 10 to 70 Gy, treatment times of 24 to 144 hours are required, which limits the practice of LDR brachytherapy to inpatients. The total source strength loaded into LDR implants results in relatively low exposure rates around the patient. Even with manual afterloading techniques, good-quality nursing and medical care can be administered without exceeding regulatory limits on exposure of personnel. The majority of the accumulated clinical brachytherapy experience consists of retrospective studies of patients treated with LDR techniques.

A high-dose rate (HDR) implant uses prescription dose rates in excess of 20 cGy/min (12 Gy/h). Modern HDR remote afterloaders contain sources capable of delivering substantially higher dose rates: treatment times are usually only a few minutes. HDR brachytherapy differs significantly from LDR brachytherapy with respect to dose response, level of technical and logistical complexity required, patient safety

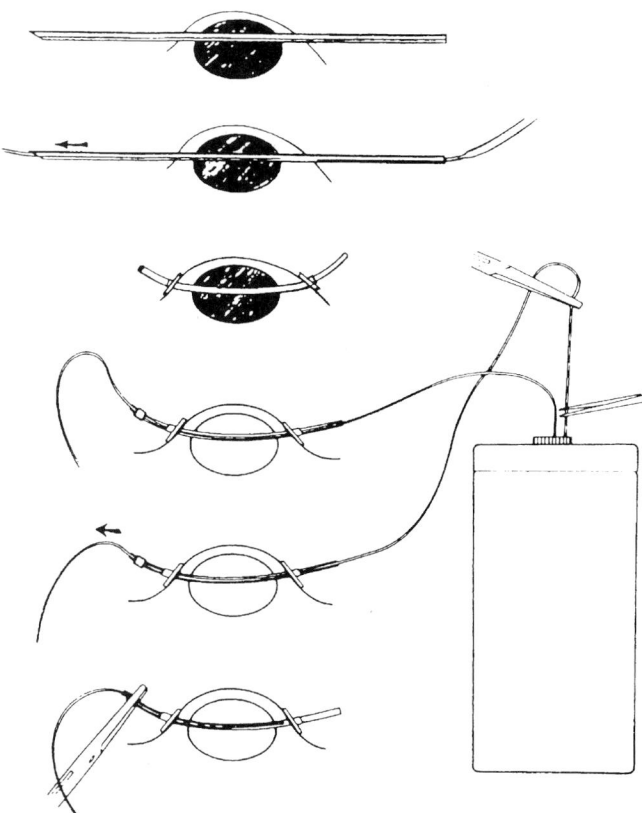

FIG. 14.38. Step-by-step procedure used to perform a manually afterloaded interstitial implant using ^{192}Ir seeds encapsulated in a nylon ribbon. The external diameters of the catheters and needles used as applicators range from 1.5 to 1.9 mm. (From Hilaris BS, Nori D, Anderson LL. *An atlas of brachytherapy.* New York: Macmillan, 1988, with permission.)

issues, and socioeconomic considerations. A heavily shielded vault and remote afterloading device are essential components of an HDR brachytherapy facility. HDR brachytherapy is an outpatient procedure delivered in discrete fractions at daily or weekly intervals, much like external beam irradiation.

Radioactive Sources for Brachytherapy

The important physical properties of the radionuclides commonly used in radiation therapy are listed in Table 14.3. Properties such as photon energy, half-life, radiation output per unit activity, specific activity (Ci/g), and toxicity play a critical role in defining the clinical applications appropriate for each isotope.

Photon energy of brachytherapy sources used in management of gynecologic patients is of less importance than in external beam irradiation. Absorbed dose varies approximately inversely with the square of the distance for sources that emit photons with energies greater than 100 keV (inverse square law). Only for very low-energy sources, such as ^{103}Pd and ^{125}I, does the depth-dose curve significantly

deviate from inverse-square law. These sources are not suitable for intracavitary therapy because tissue attenuation limits the dose that can be delivered to the target volume periphery. Although penetration in tissue is independent of photon energy above 100 keV, the HVL in lead (a measure of radiation protection–shielding cost) rises steeply with energy. Because of their nearly identical depth-dose characteristics to radium 226, artificial brachytherapy radionuclides (e.g., ^{137}Cs) with mean photon energies in excess of 100 keV are referred to as *radium substitutes*.

Classically, radium substitutes with half-lives of a few days such as ^{222}Rn and ^{198}Au were used for permanent implants. Currently, longer lived but very-low-energy photon emitters are used for permanent implantation (e.g., ^{103}Pd and ^{125}I), although ^{198}Au is still used for its dosimetric and dose-rate advantages.

Because of practical and theoretical limits on how much ^{137}Cs and ^{226}Ra can be concentrated into a small pellet (low specific activity), these isotopes are not useful for HDR brachytherapy. ^{192}Ir and ^{60}Co, both of which have large neutron capture cross sections and have very high specific activities, are the radionuclides currently used for HDR brachytherapy.

Radium and Radon

Radium 226 (^{226}Ra) was the first radionuclide used in clinical brachytherapy. Clinical use of radium has rapidly declined because of safety concerns. However, because of its years of therapeutic use, it is the standard against which therapy and dosimetry with substitute radioisotopes have been compared. ^{226}Ra has a half-life of 1,620 years. The γ-rays from radium and its decay products range in energy from about 0.05 to 2.4 MeV, with an average energy of about 0.8 MeV. The maximum β-ray energy is about 3.26 MeV.

^{226}Ra sources consist of a radium salt (sulfate) mixed with filler (usually barium sulfate) and are contained in cylindrical cells, which were placed in needles or tubes (similar to those in Fig. 14.37) with platinum walls 0.5- and 1.0-mm thick, respectively. Radium tubes were typically 22 mm long and contain from 5 to 25 mg of radium in 15-mm active length. Full-intensity needles popularized in the Manchester system of dosimetry typically have 0.66 mg of radium per centimeter: half-intensity needles have 0.33 mg of radium per centimeter, and quarter-intensity needles have 0.165 mg of radium per centimeter. Needles with 1.0 and 0.5 mg of radium per centimeter have also been used. Indian club needles have one "hot" end; dumbbell needles have two hot ends, usually with 1.0 mg of radium per centimeter between the ends. In addition to knowing the activity per unit active length of a source, it is necessary to state its total activity, total physical length, active length, source diameter, and wall filtration.

^{222}Rn (radon), with a half-life of 3.83 days, is a gas produced when radium decays: it was the first radioisotope used

TABLE 14.3. *Physical properties and uses of brachytherapy radionuclides*

Element	Isotope	Energy (MeV)	Half-life	HVL-lead (mm)	Source form	Clinical Application
Obsolete Sealed Sources of Historic Significance						
Radium	^{226}Ra	0.83 (avg)	1,626 years	16	Radium salt encapsulated in tubes and needles	LDR intracavitary and interstitial
Radon	^{222}Rn	0.83 (avg)	3.83 days	16	Radon	Permanent interstitial Temporary molds
Currently Used Sealed Sources						
Cesium	^{137}Cs	0.662	30 years	6.5	Cesium salt encapsulated in tubes and needles	LDR intracavitary and interstitial
Iridium	^{192}Ir	0.397 (avg)	74 days	6	Seeds in nylon ribbon Encapsulated source on steel cable	LDR temporary interstitial HDR interstitial and intracavitary
Cobalt	^{60}Co	1.25	5.26 years	11	Encapsulated spheres	HDR intracavitary
Iodine	^{125}I	0.028	59.6 days	0.025	Seeds	Permanent interstitial
Palladium	^{103}Pd	0.020	17 days	0.013	Seeds	Permanent interstitial
Gold	^{196}Au	0.412	2.7 days	6	Seeds	Permanent interstitial
Strontium	^{90}Sr-^{90}Y	2.24 MeV βmax	28.9 years		Plaque	Superficial ocular lesions
Developmental Sealed Sources						
Americium	^{241}Am	0.060	432 years	0.12	Tubes	LDR intracavitary
Ytterbium	^{169}Yb	0.093	32 days	0.48	Seeds	LDR temporary interstitial
Californium	^{252}Cf	2.4 (avg) neutrons	2.65 years			
Samarium	^{145}Sm	0.043	340 days	0.060	Seeds	LDR temporary interstitial
Unsealed Radioisotopes Used for Radiopharmaceutical Therapy						
Strontium	^{89}Sr	1.4 MeV βmax	51 days		SrC12 IV solution	Diffuse bone metastases
Iodine	^{131}I	0.61 MeV βmax 0.364 MeV g	8.06 days		Capsule NaI oral solution	Thyroid cancer
Phosphorus	^{32}P	1.71 MeV βmax	14.3 days		Chromic phosphate colloid instillation	Ovarian cancer seeding: peritoneal surface
					Na$_2$PO$_3$ solution	Polycythemia vera, chronic leukemia

LDR, low-dose rate; HDR, high-dose rate.

for permanent implants. The radon gas was extracted from ^{226}Ra decay and encapsulated in gold seeds, which were used in brachytherapy for many years. Because of hazards to patients and personnel posed by radon gas from ruptured seeds or ruptured radium sources, ^{222}Rn seeds and ^{226}Ra needles are no longer manufactured in the United States. With the development of nuclear technology after World War II, numerous other radioisotopes have been developed as radium or radon substitutes (Table 14.3).

Cobalt 60

Cobalt 60 (^{60}Co) is produced from thermal neutrons captured by ^{59}Co. The subsequent decay to ^{60}Ni releases two highly energetic γ-rays (1.17 and 1.33 MeV), but ^{60}Co has a relatively short half-life (5.26 years). ^{60}Co tubes and needles were used for brachytherapy during the 1960s and 1970s. Because of its high specific activity, ^{60}Co spherical pellets are used for HDR intracavitary therapy in some centers.

Cesium 137

Cesium 137 (^{137}Cs), a fission by-product, is a popular radium substitute because of its 30-year half-life. Its single γ-ray (0.66 MeV) is less penetrating (HVL$_{Pb}$ = 0.65 cm) than the γ-rays from radium (HVL$_{Pb}$ = 1.4 cm) or ^{60}Co (HVL$_{Pb}$ = 1.1 cm). Modern ^{137}Cs intracavitary tubes (Fig. 14.37) are the mainstay for intracavitary treatment of gynecologic malignancies. The radioactive material is distributed in insoluble glass microspheres, which produce far less hazard from ruptured sources than does the radon gas in a radium tube. Modern ^{137}Cs tubes usually have about a 2.65-mm external diameter with lengths of about 21 mm and active lengths between 14 and 20 mm depending on the vendor's design. A number of source designs are available for interstitial and intracavitary remote afterloaders. [137]Cs needles are available as replacements for [226]Ra needles in nonafterloading interstitial implants: however, their use has rapidly declined in favor of more popular afterloading systems.

Iridium 192

Iridium 192 (^{192}Ir), which has a 74-day half-life and lower energy γ-rays (average γ-ray energy, 0.4 MeV), is the most widely used source for temporary interstitial implants (142). In the United States, ^{192}Ir is available as seeds (0.5-mm diameter by 3 mm long). The seeds are encapsulated in a 0.8-mm diameter nylon ribbon and are usually spaced at 1-cm center-to-center intervals (Fig. 14.38). A manual afterloading system was developed by Henschke (138) at Memorial Hospital in New York. In addition to "double-ended" flexible catheters, which require fixation at both the distal and proximal skin surfaces, a variety of single-ended (often called "blind-ended") catheters requiring fixation only at the proximal skin surface are available. Guides are available as rigid steel or flexible plastic needles, which can be inserted through the skin surface using an obturator or flexible plastic catheters, which can be placed operatively. In addition to eliminating radiation exposure hazards in the operating room, ^{192}Ir ribbons can be trimmed to the appropriate active length for each catheter. In addition, ^{192}Ir ribbons can be used in conjunction with remote afterloaders. Finally, high-intensity ^{192}Ir sources are used in the latest generation single-stepping source HDR remote afterloading devices (140,143–146).

Gold 198, Iodine 125, and Palladium 103

Insoluble gold198 ([198]Au) seeds, with a 2.7-day half-life and a 0.412-MeV γ-ray, are still used to perform permanent implants in the classic LDR regimen. However, iodine 125 (^{125}I) seeds, which emit γ-rays and x-rays with energies below 0.0355 MeV, are readily shielded by a few tenths of a millimeter of lead ($HVL_{Pb} = 0.002$ cm). The encapsulation of ^{125}I in a 0.5-mm titanium external tube about 4.5 mm long with welds on each end and a metallic (silver rod) radiopaque marker in the middle produces a highly anisotropic sealed source (147) (Fig. 14.37). Ruptured seeds damaged during the implant procedure can leak ^{125}I, which follows the iodine metabolic pathway in the body and is preferentially absorbed by the thyroid. Careful inspection and leak tests of ^{125}I seeds before and after the implant procedure are required, particularly when seeds are reused several times.

Palladium 103 ([103]Pd), produced from thermal neutron capture in [102]Pd, is a newer alternative to ^{125}I for permanent implants. [103]Pd emits 20- to 23-keV characteristic x-rays and has a shorter half-life (17 days vs 60 days). Because treatment is delivered at threefold higher dose rates, [103]Pd is theoretically more effective in controlling tumors with high mitotic activity (148). The anisotropy of the dose around the seed is slightly less than that for ^{125}I seeds, although the isodoses exhibit more rapid spatial gradients than those from [125]I.

Radiopharmaceuticals

Iodine 131 (^{131}I), phosphorus 32 (^{32}P), strontium 89 (^{89}Sr), and samarium 153 ([153]Sm) with 8.05-day, 14.3-day, 50-day, and 46.3 hours half-lives, respectively, are commonly used unsealed radiopharmaceuticals. [131]I treatment of the thyroid uses energetic β-rays, ranging in energy from 69 to 192 keV, to deliver about 90% of the dose: only about 10% of the dose comes from the emitted 80 to 637 keV γ-rays. [32]P, a pure β emitter with a maximum β-ray energy of 1.71 MeV, is used as sodium phosphate to treat blood diseases such as polycythemia vera. Chromic phosphate is used as a colloidal suspension in intracavitary instillations (usually 15 mCi for intraperitoneal instillations).

Strontium 90

Strontium 90 (^{90}Sr), a fission by-product with a half-life of 28.9 years, decays to yttrium 90 (^{90}Y), which decays in 64 hours to [90]Zr. [90]Y, a β emitter with a maximum β energy of 2.27 MeV, is widely used as a sealed source to treat shallow lesions, such as those of the skin or eye. [90]Y (as powdered yttrium oxide, plastic exchange beads, or glass microspheres) is used to treat carcinoma of the liver. Strontium 89 is provided by bombarding yttrium 89 with neutrons. It decays to stable yttrium 89. [89]Sr has a physical half-life of 50.6 days. It decays by beta-particle emission to yttrium 89 with the maximum energy of the beta particles of 1.46 MeV and an average of 0.42 MeV. It does not undergo γ decay.

Strontium 89, an analog of calcium, concentrates in osteoblastic bone cancer lesions (149).

Following intravenous injection, ionic ^{89}Sr is rapidly cleared from the blood, and about 50% of the injected activity is deposited in bone where it remains for as long as 100 days. Normal bone appears to take up a small fraction of the administered activity where it is retained for a much shorter time. Urinary excretion is the primary method of elimination of unabsorbed [89]Sr. Administration in the United States is typically 4 mCi for IV administration in the treatment of painful bone metastases.

Samarium 153 ([153]Sm)

Samarium 153 Lexidronam is a therapeutic agent consisting of radioactive [153]Sm and a tetraphosphonate chelator, ethylenediamine tetramethylenephosphonate (EDTMP). [153]Sm is produced in high yield and purity by neutron irradiation of isotopically enriched samarium 152 oxide. [153]Sm has a half-life of 46 hours (1.9 days). The primary radiation emission is beta with a maximum energy of 0.81 MeV and mean of 0.23 MeV. The beta particle of [153]Sm-EDTMP penetrates an average of 3.1 mm of soft tissue and 1.7 mm in bone. For the photon emission, specific γ-ray (103 kV) constant for [153]Sm is 0.46 R/mCi-h at 1 cm (1.24×10^{-5} mSv/MBq-h at 1 m), and this delivers 28% of the dose.

[153]Sm-EDTMP has an affinity for bone, concentrates in areas of bone turnover, and binds to hydroxyapatite. Quadramet (Berlex Laboratories, Wayne, NJ) accumulates in osteoblastic lesions at a greater rate than in normal bone with a lesion to normal bone ratio of approximately 5.82. The mechanism of action of Quadramet in relieving pain of bone metastases is not well known, but is assumed to be the result of destruction of tumor cells in the bone. Quadramet is formulated as a sterile, nonpyrogenic, clear, colorless to light amber isotonic solution for intravenous administration. The recommended dose of Quadramet is 1 mCi/kg (37 MBq/kg) administered intravenously over a period of 1 to 2 minutes through a secure indwelling catheter and followed with a saline flush. Caution should be exercised when the dose is determined in a very thin or very obese patient.

In a study of 19 patients during the first 30 minutes, radioactivity in the blood decreased by 15% of the injected dose with a half-life of 5.5 minutes. During the first 6 hours, 34.5% ($\pm 15.5\%$) of the radioactive [153]Sm-EDTMP was excreted in the urine. Less than 1% of the dose injected remained in the blood 5 hours after injection. Overall, the greater number of metastatic lesions, the less radioactivity excreted.

Developmental Radionuclides

Several new isotopes, which emit low-energy photons in the 40 to 100 keV range, are under development and investigation for use in sealed-source brachytherapy. These include ytterbium 169 ([169]Yb) (150,151), americium 241 ([241]Am) (152), and samarium 145 ([145]Sm) (153). In this photon energy range, sources give rise to depth doses in tissue qualitatively similar to those of conventional radium-substitute isotopes, which closely approximate inverse-square law falloff. In contrast, ultra-low-energy sources such as [103]Pd and ^{125}I have depth-dose characteristics significantly less penetrating than that predicted by inverse-square law. The photons emitted by [169]Yb and [241]Am sources, averaging 93 and 60 keV, respectively, interact with water largely by approximately elastic Compton interactions, giving rise to multiple scattered photons, which compensates for attenuation of primary photons. However, unlike higher energy radium-substitute photons, these low-energy photons interact photoelectrically in lead and other shielding materials, offering the prospect of effectively shielding critical structures with thin foils of

metal. Unlike ^{137}Cs and ^{192}Ir, which require 2 to 5 mm of tungsten shielding to produce a twofold dose reduction, these new isotopes make possible customization of shielding to improve clinical outcome of individual patients (152). Investigators at Yale (154) have developed a preloaded [241]Am LDR intracavitary system resembling the Stockholm applicator system. Samuels and associates (155) treated a small series of cervical cancer patients with recurrences following definitive radiation therapy with shielded [241]Am plaques, demonstrating the feasibility and utility of the customized internal shielding strategy. Because of the low energy of the emitted photons and high atomic number of [241]Am, self-absorption is extremely high. This dictates a source design with a large surface to volume ratio, resulting in a bulky source with a minimum diameter of about 1 cm, which limits the use of [241]Am to intracavitary therapy (154,156).

[145]Sm interstitial seeds, encapsulated in titanium of the same dimensions as currently available ^{125}I seeds, have been developed by Fairchild and coworkers (153) at the Brookhaven National Laboratory. This isotope emits photons with an average energy of 43 keV, which is slightly higher than that of [125]I. Besides improved radiation protection and more flexible internal shielding, an important biologic rationale for use of [145]Sm and other intermediate-energy isotopes is radiosensitization of tumor cells that have incorporated halogenated thymidine analogs, such as iodeoxyuridine (IUdR) and bromodeoxyuridine (BUdR), into their DNA (157). These halogenated thymidine analogs are preferentially incorporated into actively proliferating cells (i.e., tumor rather than normal tissue cells) and are known to be potent radiosensitizers. In vitro studies demonstrate that, by using low-energy brachytherapy sources emitting photons just above the K-absorption edge of iodine (33.2 keV), additional radiosensitization results from Auger electron cascades arising from photoelectric absorption of 40- to 60-keV photons by the incorporated iodine atoms. Because of the limited range of the Auger electrons, this additional cytotoxic enhancement is highly localized to cells with significant IUdR or BUdR uptake.

[169]Yb has a number of characteristics that warrant its continued investigation as a brachytherapy isotope (150,151, 158). It decays by electron capture, producing x-rays and γ-rays ranging from 49.8 to 307.7 keV (average 93 keV) with a half-life of 32 days. In addition to enhanced radiation protection and local shielding capabilities ($\text{HVL}_{Pb} = 0.2$ mm), its nonradioactive precursor, [168]Yb, has an extremely large neutron-capture cross section, making activity concentrations as large as 10 Ci/mm^3 possible. Unlike [241]Am or ^{125}I, miniaturized [169]Yb interstitial and intracavitary sources can be easily constructed for LDR brachytherapy. Potentially, high-intensity [169]Yb sources could be used to deliver HDR intraoperative brachytherapy treatments in lightly shielded operating rooms, thereby broadening the clinical indications of brachytherapy. Permanent implantation with this isotope

may not be practical since the 308-keV photon line may pose a significant radiation safety hazard.

Brachytherapy Dosimetry and Specification of Source Strength

Unsealed radioisotopes, including those commonly used in therapeutic applications, are usually quantified in terms of true or contained activity (i.e., the number of atoms decaying or disintegrating per second). Despite frequent use of activity-type units such as the millicurie, curie, and becquerel, sealed brachytherapy sources are almost never specified in terms of contained activity for the purpose of dose calculation or treatment prescription. Sealed brachytherapy sources are calibrated and specified in terms of the radiation output (in centigrays per hour) along the transverse bisector (the axis perpendicular to and bisecting the long axis of the source), as illustrated in Figure 14.39. Source strength is specified in terms of air kerma rate (dose rate to air) at a 1-m distance from the source measured as if the source and detector were surrounded by a vacuum. The resultant quantity, air kerma strength, is defined as the product of the air kerma rate and the square of the distance and is denoted by the symbol S_K. The units ascribed to air kerma strength in clinical practice are $\mu Gy \cdot m^2 \cdot h^{-1}$ or $cGy \cdot cm^2 \cdot h^{-1}$. Larger units, $cGy \cdot m^2 \cdot h^{-1}$, are often used in conjunction with high-intensity HDR sources. These units are related by 1 $\mu Gy \cdot m^2 \cdot h^{-1} = 1 \, cGy \cdot cm^2 \cdot h^{-1} = 10-4 \, cGy \cdot m^2 \cdot h^{-1}$. Use of these units in clinical practice has been endorsed by the ICRU (141), the AAPM (159), and the American Endocurietherapy Society (160).

A number of older quantities remain in use (161). ^{137}Cs tubes, ^{192}Ir seeds, and other radium substitutes are frequently specified in terms of the quantity equivalent mass of radium,

with units of mgRaEq. The strength of a given source in mgRaEq is the mass (in milligrams) of ^{226}Ra encapsulated by 0.5 mm of platinum that gives the same transverse-axis radiation output or air kerma strength as the given source. A 1-mgRaEq source of ^{137}Cs or ^{192}Ir has an air kerma strength, S_K, of 7.23 $cGy \cdot cm^2 \cdot h^{-1}$. Equivalent mass of radium simply describes the radiation output of a source as a multiple of that of a 1-mg ^{226}Ra needle. Apparent activity, usually associated with units of millicuries, is the air kerma strength of a source relative to the output of a hypothetical 1-mCi point source consisting of the same radionuclide as the given source. Historically, apparent activity was used to quantify the strength of permanent implant sources such as ^{125}I.

The use of a dosimetric quantity, such as exposure or absorbed dose, to quantify and prescribe brachytherapy treatments was introduced in Manchester, England, in the 1930s. Regardless of the quantities chosen to prescribe brachytherapy, computation and isodose display of the dose distribution within and around the implanted volume are now essential elements of current standard of practice. The process of calculating the dose distribution for an implant is called treatment planning and usually relies on digital computers equipped with specialized treatment-planning software. The mathematical model used to calculate absorbed dose rate, given the source locations, internal construction, isotope, and strength is called the dose-calculation algorithm. The most widely used basic algorithm, the isotropic point source model, has been in clinical use since the 1920s:

$$\dot{D}(r) = S_K \cdot \overline{(\mu_{en} / \rho)}\,^{med}_{air} \cdot \frac{T(r)}{r^2}$$

$D(r)$ is the dose rate (in centigrays per hour) at distance r (in centimeters) from the point source, and $(\mu_{en}/\rho)^{med}_{air}$ is the mass-energy absorption coefficient ratio used to convert dose in air (used for source calibration) to dose in the medium surrounding the source. The factor $T(r)$ describes the effect of the surrounding medium on dose distribution and reflects the competition between attenuation of primary photons and build-up of scattered photons. For radium substitute isotopes, $T(r) \approx 1$ for distances up to 5 cm. Inverse-square law, represented by the $1/r^2$ term, dominates the dose distribution. This simple one-dimensional model is almost universally used for interstitial seed sources with photon energies above 300 keV and was generalized to extended sources (e.g., ^{137}Cs intracavitary tubes) by Sievert (162) in 1921. Dose measurements using thermoluminescent dosimeters (TLDs) (163) and Monte Carlo photon transport (MCPT) calculations (164,165) have shown this algorithm to be accurate within 5% for single sources containing radium-substitute isotopes surrounded by a homogeneous medium.

The simple analytic models, described in the previous paragraph, are not sufficiently accurate for clinical use either in the 60- to 100-keV energy range (^{241}Am and ^{169}Yb) or in the 30-keV energy range of low-energy permanent implant

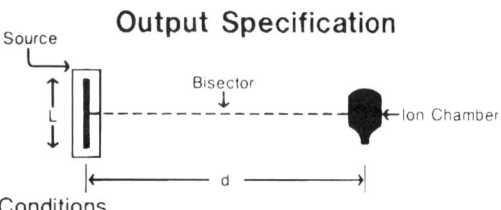

Output Specification

Conditions
1. Large distance d >> source and detector dimensions
2. Free in space
   - measured in air
   - corrected for air attenuation
   - corrected for scattering from air, walls, etc.

FIG. 14.39. Schematic diagram showing the experimental setup used to establish standards of brachytherapy source strength. It is the basis of source specification in terms of apparent activity, equivalent mass of radium, and the quantity endorsed by most advisory groups, air kerma strength, S_K. The measurement distance (d) must be large enough relative to source and ion chamber dimensions to ensure that the inverse-square law is valid.

sources. Inaccurate dosimetry has been a serious barrier to accumulation of consistent clinical experience with ^{125}I permanent implantation: the dose rate per apparent milicuries at 1 cm has changed by nearly a factor of two since its introduction in 1964 (165). In the 40 years since then, low-energy brachytherapy dosimetry has been placed on a firm foundation by validation and acceptance of two quantitative dosimetry methods, TLD solid water phantom dosimetry and MCPT dosimetry calculations (145). Acceptance for clinical treatment planning of absorbed dose rates directly measured by TLDs is largely, but not exclusively, due to the results of the interstitial brachytherapy dosimetry contract sponsored by the National Cancer Institute (163). This contract involves a collaboration between three groups (Yale, University of California at San Francisco, and Memorial Sloan-Kettering), collectively known as the Interstitial Collaborative Working Group (ICWG). Each group independently measured the dose distributions around ^{125}I and ^{192}Ir seeds, correcting for many sources of experimental error (energy dependence, directional anisotropy, self-attenuation, and positional errors). The data sets were critically compared and a final set of dosimetry data endorsed in the ICWG final report (163). At -1 to 5-cm distances, interinvestigator agreement was within 5%. Later, this work was extended to encompass other published measurements, and MCPT and a final set of two-dimensional data for ^{125}I, [103]Pd, and ^{192}Ir interstitial sources were developed and endorsed for clinical use by Task Group 43 of the AAPM (166). TLD measurements have been used to characterize the dosimetric properties of [241]Am[213] and [169]Yb (158).

In parallel with the introduction of TLD dose measurement techniques, Williamson and colleagues (145,165,167) have developed and validated MCPT simulation as a reliable and accurate dosimetry tool in brachytherapy. MCPT simulation is a numerical solution to a fundamental theoretical method of characterizing the absorbed dose distribution in a complex system of sources and applicators—that of radiation transport theory. Input to the model includes a detailed 3-D geometric model of the source, applicators, and tissue heterogeneities along with a cross-sectional library, which quantitatively describes the photon attenuation and scattering processes that give rise to transport and absorption of ionizing radiation within the system. The output includes absorbed dose rates or detector responses at designated locations in the system. MCPT calculations have been used to calculate two-dimensional dose-rate distributions about sources, to characterize shielded vaginal applicators dosimetrically, and to assess systematically the effects of different shielding materials near brachytherapy sources. Comparison of MCPT calculations and TLD measurements shows excellent agreement (2% to 3%) between the two approaches. It is expected that the use of detailed dosimetry will improve our understanding of many important dosimetric effects neglected by conventional dose-calculation models, including applicator attenuation and shielding, inter-source and applicator attenuation, and the effect of tissue composition heterogeneities on low-energy source dose distributions. Other Monte Carlo calculation software packages, such as MCNP and EQS4 (168,169) have since been used to calculate values of dosimetric parameters of newly developed brachytherapy sources, including low-energy ^{125}I and [103]Pd seeds, β-emitting intravascular brachytherapy sources, and ^{192}Ir sources used in HDR remote afterloaders. These later software packages typically utilize more complete radiation transport modeling in the inclusion of electron transport, therefore providing the potential of more accurate calculations at extremely short distances (submillimeter) from the source or near heterogeneous tissue interfaces.

Clinical Applications of Brachytherapy

A detailed description of multiple brachytherapy techniques is available in other textbooks (170), and specific details are described in the pertinent anatomic chapters of this textbook.

Preoperative and Postoperative Implant Care

It is extremely important for gynecologic and radiation oncologists to assess the condition of the patient the day of the brachytherapy procedure and to log in the chart detailed instructions for nursing personnel, including test results to be obtained, medications to be administered, preparation procedures for the operating room, and radiation safety measures. Clear postoperative orders are necessary, including time of removal of radioactive sources, appropriate medications, and radiation safety precautions.

Removal of Implants

Applicators in intracavitary insertions or small interstitial implants of the vagina/vulva can be removed in the patient's room, although parametrial or more extensive interstitial implants may need to be removed in a treatment room. Bleeding at the time of needle or catheter removal is infrequent, but when it occurs, it may cause the patient or the assisting staff to panic. Firm and steady pressure with a finger or a compress over the bleeding point for several minutes is usually adequate treatment; occasionally, suturing with absorbable catgut may be necessary.

The afterloading nylon tubing is more easily removed. For radiation protection, it is advisable initially to uncrimp the metallic buttons and carefully remove the radioactive sources, which are accounted for and immediately placed in a portable safe or shielded cart. Then, each individual tube is removed by cutting one end and pulling the other one.

After all needles or tubes are removed, the implanted site may be gently palpated to verify that all implant materials have been removed. The patient should be surveyed, and after the radioactive sources are taken out of the room, ambient exposure rates should be measured to ensure that all radioactive sources have been safely transferred to the radioactive source storage area.

Dose Rate

Figure 14.40 summarizes the dose-rate effect in terms of repair and redistribution (18). For acute exposures at high-dose rate, the survival curve has a significant initial shoulder. As the dose rate is lowered and the treatment time protracted, more sublethal damage can be repaired during the exposure. Subsequently, the survival curve becomes progressively shallower (D_0 increases), and the shoulder tends to disappear. There is a point at which all sublethal damage is repaired, resulting in a limiting slope. However, in at least some cell lines, a further lowering of the dose rate allows cells to progress through the cycle and accumulate in G_2, which is a radiosensitive phase. Here, the cell survival curve becomes steeper again (the so-called inverse dose-rate effect). Further reduction in dose rate will allow cells to pass through the G_2 block and divide. Proliferation may occur during the radiation exposure if the dose rate is low enough and exposure time is long compared with the length of the mitotic cycle. Further reduction in biologic effect may occur as the dose rate is progressively lowered because cell proliferation will tend to balance or exceed cell death.

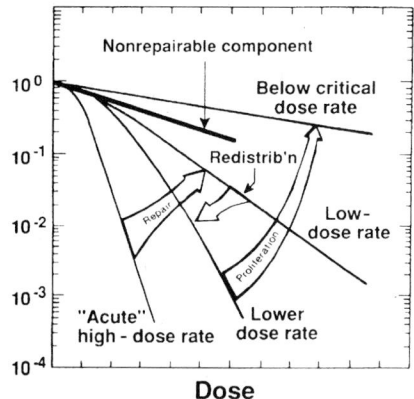

FIG. 14.40. The dose-rate effect due to repair of sublethal damage, redistribution in the cycle, and cell proliferation. The dose-response curve for acute exposures is characterized by a broad initial shoulder. As the dose rate is reduced, the survival curve becomes progressively shallower as more and more sublethal damage is repaired, but cells are "frozen" in their positions in the cycle and do not progress. As the dose rate is lowered further and for a limited range of dose rates, the survival curve steepens again because cells can progress through the cycle to pile up at a block in G_2, a radiosensitive phase, but still cannot divide. A further lowering of dose rate allows cells to escape the G_2 block and divide: cell proliferation may then occur during the protracted exposure, and survival curves become shallower as cell birth from mitosis offsets cell killing from irradiation. (Based on the ideas of Joel Bedford. In: Hall EJ. *Radiobiology for the radiologist.* 4th ed. Philadelphia: JB Lippincott Co, 1994.)

The dose rate at which irradiation is delivered may significantly influence the biologic response to a given dose, particularly in the case of sparsely ionizing radiations, such as r-rays and γ-rays (18). Three main biologic processes are involved in the dose-rate effect:

1. Repair of sublethal damage, which occurs when radiation is delivered at a low-dose rate and the treatment time is extended to a point that it is comparable to the repair half-time. As the dose rate is reduced, more sublethal damage is repaired because the radiation injury is spread out over a longer period.
2. Cell proliferation, which occurs during the course of protracted radiation exposure if the dose rate is low enough or the cell cycle time is short enough.
3. Redistribution and accumulation of cells throughout the proliferative cycle. With a low-dose rate, proliferation decreases, because cells are arrested and accumulate in G_2, which is a relatively radiosensitive phase of the cycle. As a result, cell killing may be greater at a lower dose rate.

With the advent of moderate-dose rate and HDR remote-control afterloading devices, emphasis on the biologic effects of irradiation dose rate has increased. The so-called dose-rate effect is most dramatic between 0.1 Gy/min and 1 Gy/min (18). Dutreix (171) reviewed the role of dose rate on biologic effects as assessed by the ability of the cell to repair radiation damage (α/β ratio) and the repair kinetics (repair time constant). The biologic effect achieved by a given radiation dose decreases as the dose rate diminishes, chiefly as a result of the increase in cell repair that occurs during continuous prolonged irradiation because cell proliferation is virtually negligible in the range of treatment times used in curietherapy (171). Dutreix (171) states that variation of the isoeffect dose occurs mainly in the range of medium-dose rates (1 to 10 Gy/h), and it vanishes at a very high-dose rate because cell repair is negligible during the short treatment time. At a very low dose rate, because the cell killing is caused only by direct lethal events considered independent of the dose rate, cell repair is also negligible. The induction of sublethal injury is relatively slow compared with the rate of repair, and cell killing by accumulation of sublethal injury remains minimal. The dose-rate effect in clinical brachytherapy (172) was described initially by Green and Paterson, as reported by Ellis (173). The historical isoeffect curve for interstitial implants with radium needles showed that a significant increase in dose was necessary to achieve the same normal tissue tolerance when overall time was increased from 2 to 10 days. The validity of Paterson's curve was questioned by Pierquin and associates (174), who used the same dose of 70 Gy with treatment times ranging from 3 to 8 days for the treatment of head and neck tumors with ^{192}Ir implants. However, a retrospective analysis of the Paris data by Mazeron and colleagues (175) clearly shows that both tumor control and normal tissue necrosis varied with implant time and therefore with dose rate. A complication in the analysis of these data arises from the fact that dose rate varies with implant size when iridium wires of equal activity are used, so that small tumors are treated at a low-dose rate and large tumors at a high-dose rate.

Hall and Brenner (176) published a review of radiobiologic effects and clinical relevance of dose rate. Included were several important concepts, including the following: (a) Based on laboratory data, it may be possible to design schedules with a pulse width of several minutes and a pulse interval of about 1 hour to achieve cell killing equivalent to that obtained with continuous 30 Gy in 60 hours (0.5 Gy/h). (b) From radiobiologic data, the linear-quadratic equation can be used to estimate the equivalency of HDR and LDR exposures with a variety of fractionation schedules (remembering that a lower number of fractions may result in enhanced late effects).

Special consideration should be given to the effect of HDR brachytherapy on normal tissues. Thus, the tumor dose must be adjusted (15% to 40% decrease depending on fractionation) in comparison with that delivered with conventional low-dose rates (177) The biologically effective doses may be estimated by use of the linear quadratic equations:

$$E = \alpha \cdot D + \beta \cdot d \cdot D$$

where it is assumed that all sublethal damage is repaired, D is the total dose in grays, and d is the dose per fraction in grays. Then the target organ repair half time is known as $T_{1/2}$, and let $\mu = 0.693/T_{1/2}$ be the repair constant,

$$E = \alpha \cdot D + \beta \cdot \frac{2\left(1 - \dfrac{1 - e^{-\mu \cdot t}}{\mu \cdot t}\right)}{\mu \cdot t} D^2$$

Based on these equations and knowledge of the ratio α/β for a given tissue type, it is possible to estimate the equivalent total doses or dose per fraction between two brachytherapy treatment schedules—either low-dose rate or high-dose rate technique (178,179).

Low- and High-Dose Rate Remote-Control Afterloading

Remote afterloading brachytherapy for interstitial and intracavitary applications is being used with increasing frequency for both LDR and HDR implants. Anderson (180) reviewed the developmental aspects of remote afterloading. The characteristics of several commercially available systems are described in Table 14.4. More details are given in a report by Glasgow and associates (140).

Low-Dose Rate Remote Afterloading

Advantages of LDR remote-control afterloading include reduced radiation exposure to hospital personnel, improved control of isodose distributions, low probability of misplacing or losing sources, less source preparation work for the source curator, medical and nursing staff not rushed by fear of exposure while caring for the patient, and source loading, unloading, and recording performed automatically.

LDR units use ^{137}Cs or ^{192}Ir, whereas HDR systems are built for either ^{60}Co or ^{192}Ir sources. LDR applications do not require shielded rooms, whereas specially shielded rooms are necessary for HDR procedures (^{60}Co or ^{192}Ir).

After the empty applicators are placed in the patient, the sources are loaded under pneumatic/mechanical control through hollow tubes connected to the applicators by a remotely activated system. A sorting and selection device and transport train for the sources are available. Safety mechanisms for checking correct connection of the applicator and the position of the sources are integral components of the system. Most units produce a hard copy of the treatment at completion of the procedure. Equipment for remote-control afterloading brachytherapy is available for multiple anatomic sites and applications.

With remote afterloading equipment for gynecologic use, the isodose distributions obtained with standard 2-cm cesium tubes and the Fletcher-Suit-Delclos tandem, ovoids, and vaginal cylinders should be reproduced (181). Wilkinson and associates (182) and Jones and colleagues (183) described the use of Selectron afterloading equipment to simulate the Manchester system for intracavitary therapy, and Dean and coworkers (184) described its use with the Newcastle system. More recently, Grigsby and colleagues (185) have adapted the Selectron to Fletcher-Suit tandems and Delclos vaginal applicators.

Results of therapy with LDR remote afterloading implants are generally not compared with the results obtained with manual afterloading systems since there are no significant changes in isotopes or dose rates. Battermann and Szabol (186) described similar local tumor control and complications for remote-control afterloading and the previously used manual afterloading when the same treatment policies were used.

Low- and Medium-Dose Rate Brachytherapy

Uterine Cervix

Initially, three systems for intracavitary brachytherapy in carcinoma of the uterine cervix were developed: the Paris, the Stockholm, and the Manchester systems (Fig. 14.36). The systems differed in the type of applicator used, strength of the source, and time of administration. All systems use an intrauterine applicator, or tandem, and some type of vaginal applicator. In the United States, most systems used are derivations of the Manchester technique.

The use of a colpostat or vaginal cylinder with the largest clinically indicated diameter will yield the highest tumor

TABLE 14.4. *Features of some popular remote afterloading systems*

System	Manufacturer or Vendor	No. of Sources	No. of Channels	Radioisotopes and Nominal Activities	LDR	HDR	Applicator Intracavitary	Applicator Interstitial
Afterloading Buchler	Buchler GmbH, Germany	1 (oscillating)	3 (uses 2 additional stationary sources)	0.1 Ci ^{137}Cs; 4 Ci ^{137}Cs; 10 Ci ^{192}Ir; 1.2 Ci ^{60}Co	Yes	Yes	Yes	Yes
Curietron	CIS-US, France	6	6	0.5 Ci ^{137}Cs	Yes	Yes	Yes	Yes
Curietron-192	CIS-US, France	20-LDR; 2-HDR	20	0.001 Ci ^{192}Ir[a]; 10 Ci ^{192}Ir	Yes	Yes	Yes	Yes
Gamma Med II	Isotopen Technik Dr. Sauerwein GmbH, Germany	1 (stepping)	2	10 Ci ^{192}Ir	No	Yes	Yes	No
Gamma Med II	IsotopenTechnik Dr. Sauerwein GmbH, Germany	1 (stepping)	12	10 Ci ^{192}Ir	No	Yes	Yes	Yes
Gamma Med IIi	IsotopenTechnik Dr. Sauerwein GmbH, Germany	1 (stepping)	24	10 Ci ^{192}Ir	No	Yes	Yes	Yes
Selectron (LDR)	Nucletron Engineering BV, Netherlands	48 pellet sources per channel	3 or 6	0.01–0.04 Ci[a] per pellet; 2.2 Ci ^{137}Cs	Yes	No	Yes	No
Selectron (HDR)	Nucletron Engineering BV, Netherlands	20	3	0.01–0.5 Ci per source; 12 Ci ^{60}Co	No	Yes	Yes	No
Micro Selectron (LDR)	Nucletron Engineering BV, Netherlands	45 ribbons	15	0.001 Ci ^{192}Ir[a]; 0.001 Ci ^{137}Cs[a]	Yes	No	Yes	Yes
Micro Selectron (HDR)	Nucletron Engineering BV, Netherlands	1	18	10 Ci ^{192}Ir	No	Yes	Yes	Yes
Vari-Source	Varian Associates			Ci ^{192}Ir		Yes	Yes	Yes

LDR, low dose rate; HDR, high-dose rate.

[a] Nominal activity; user selects desired activity.

dose at the depth for a given mucosal dose. When the strength of the sources to be placed in the vaginal colpostats is selected, it is extremely important to keep in mind the surface dose because excessive irradiation to the vaginal mucosa (maximum 150 Gy total dose to the proximal and 90 to 100 Gy total dose to the distal vagina) may result in severe mucosal atrophy, fibrosis, and vaginal stenosis or necrosis (187).

In a review of 274 patients with cervical cancer treated with irradiation alone, Au and Grigsby (188) reported 11% grade 1 and 2 and 4% grade 3 sequelae with LDR brachytherapy doses in the range of 150 Gy. Also, they noted that the grade 3 complication rate increased from about 3% to 5% to 6% when the dose rate was increased from 175 cGy/h to 350 cGy/h and to 9% with 700 cGy/h (Fig. 14.41A). With HDR brachytherapy, the projected grade 3 tolerance dose varied from 30 Gy in two fractions to 50 to 60 Gy in five

fractions computing single ovoid surface dose or all source dose (Fig.14.41B).

Longer tandems will result in improved doses delivered to the lateral parametrium and the pelvic lymph nodes (189).

Manchester System. The Manchester intracavitary system, introduced by Tod and Meredith (190) in 1938, was the first applicator and loading system designed to meet certain dosimetric specifications. It used a dosimetric field quantity (total dose at point A) to prescribe treatment rather than milligram hours. Point A was defined as being 2 cm above the mucous membrane of the lateral vaginal fornix and 2 cm lateral to the center of the uterine canal. Allegedly, this area corresponded to the paracervical triangle, in the medial edge of the broad ligament, where the uterine vessels cross the ureter. A subsequent arbitrary convention defined point A as being 2 cm above the external cervical os and 2 cm lateral to the midline. Yet another definition located point A 2 cm above the distal end of the lowest source in the

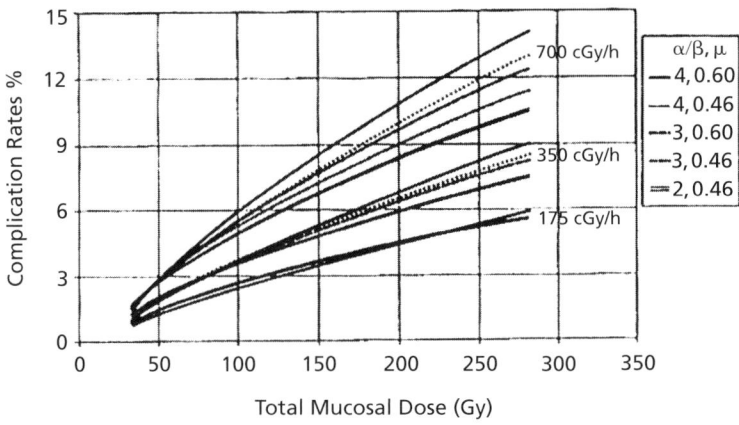

A

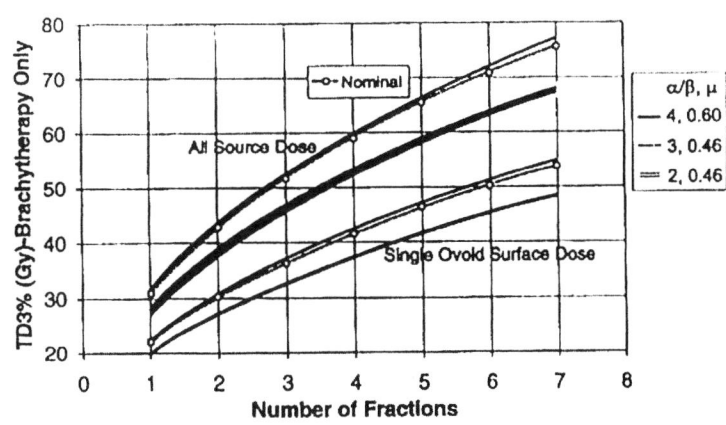

B

FIG. 14.41. A: Complication rates over selected dose rates at 1.75, 3.50, and 7.00 Gy/h, showing increasing sensitivities to total mucosa dose (higher gradient) and to α/β and μ (wider spread) as dose rate increases. B: Grade 3 complication TD3 for fractionated HDR schemes based on BED. The TD3 limits are shown in brachytherapy all source dose and single ovoid surface dose. (Reprinted from Au SP, Grigsby PW. The irradiation tolerance dose of the proximal vagina. *Radiother Oncol* 2003:67:77, with permission from Elsevier.)

cervical canal and 2 cm lateral to the tandem. Batley and Constable (191) illustrated how these different definitions affected the dose to point A (Fig. 14.42). The two most vulnerable points in the pelvis were thought to be (a) the vaginal mucosa and (b) the rectovaginal septum, opposite the cervix. Point B was established at the same level as point A, 5 cm from the midline: this point was near the obturator lymph nodes and gave an indication of the lateral throw-off dose.

The Manchester applicators consisted of a rubber intra-uterine tandem and two ellipsoid "ovoids" that conformed to the isodose curves from ^{226}Ra tubes positioned on the long axis of the applicator (Fig. 14.36C). The applicators were intended to be used with ^{226}Ra tubes of 2.2-cm length, - mm platinum (Pt) filtration, and active length between 1.0 and 1.5 cm. The small, medium, and large ovoid diameters were 2.0, 2.5, and 3.0 cm, respectively, and are the same as Fletcher's small, medium, and large colpostats. The pre-loaded ovoids contained no shielding and relied on extensive anterior and posterior packing (1.0- to 1.5-cm thick) to spare bladder and rectal tissues. The ovoid dimensions and appli-cator loadings were designed to ensure that:

1. Point A dose rate, about 0.53 Gy/h in modern units, re-mained constant for all allowed applicator loadings and combinations.

2. Vaginal contribution to point A was limited to 40% of the total dose.
3. Rectal dose should be 80% or less of the dose at point A; this rectal dose can usually be achieved by careful packing.

Small, medium, and large ovoids were loaded with 17.5, 20.0, and 22.5 mg of radium, respectively, to compensate for the greater source-to-point A treatment distances with the larger ovoids. The point B dose, determined largely by inverse-square law, was calculated by the formula 9 Gy to point B for every 4,000 mgh administered.

In the absence of external beam treatment, a total point A exposure of 8,000 R (72.8 Gy) in 144 hours split between two applications was traditionally prescribed. Because the point A dose rate is constant, whether the application con-tains 60 or 80 mg of ^{226}Ra, point A prescription amounts to using time, not milligram hours, as the factor that quantifies treatment. In contrast to the Paris and Stockholm systems, which prescribed a fixed number of milligram hours, equiv-alent Manchester treatment regimens could deliver from 8,400 to 11,200 mgh depending on the length of the tandem and the diameter of the colpostats (190,192).

Fletcher Applicator System. The Fletcher applicators ad-hered to the basic Manchester design, with many improve-ments, including internal shielding consisting of 3- to 5-mm

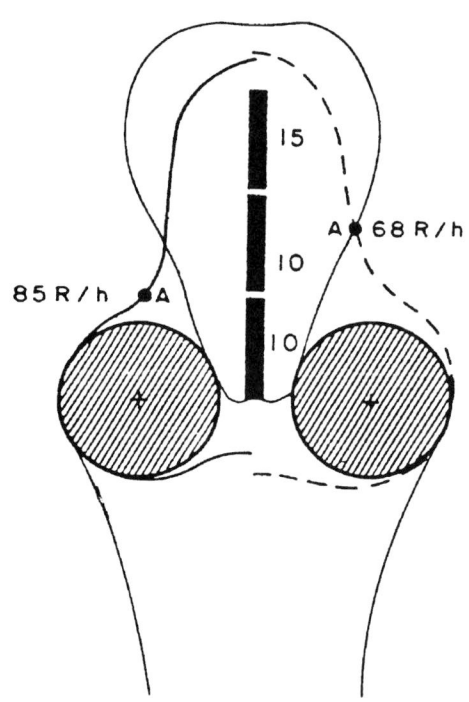

FIG. 14.42. Diagram showing the position of point A when the cervix protrudes between the ovoids. The position of point A is no longer the same using the original and newer definitions. The newer definition (point A, 2 cm above distal end of lowest cervical source and 2 cm lateral to midline) results in point A lying at a higher dose level, resulting in decreased time of insertion. (From Batley F, Constable WC. The use of the "Manchester system" for treatment of cancer of the uterine cervix with modern afterloading radium applicators. *J Can Assoc Radiol* 1967:18:396, with permission.)

thick tungsten in the medial, anterior, and posterior faces of the colpostat, which reduces the dose adjacent to the ovoids by 40% to 50% (189). Afterloading capability was incorporated into the Fletcher applicator by Suit and colleagues (139). The rectal shield subtends 180 degrees, and the bladder shield subtends 150 degrees (Fig. 14.43). The 3M Fletcher-Suit-Delclos colpostat and the traditional Fletcher-Suit rectangular-handled applicator both have shields of significantly different shape, thickness, and position that decrease the dose to the bladder trigone and the anterior rectal wall without decreasing the irradiation to the uterosacral and broad ligaments. The Fletcher colpostat has a diameter of 2.0 cm that can be increased to 2.5 or 3.0 cm by use of small and large slip-on plastic caps. At Washington University, the 2-cm–diameter Fletcher ovoids have a surface dose of 6.3 cGy/mgh and are loaded with ^{137}Cs 20-mgRaEq sources. If plastic caps are used with the regular ovoids, the surface dose with 2.5 cm ovoids is 4.2 cGy/mgh, and it is 3.0 cGy/mgh with 3.0 cm ovoids. Therefore, 25- or 30-mgRaEq sources are inserted. When a colpostat with the largest diameter consistent with the patient's anatomy is used, the dose to the vaginal mucosa in relation to doses delivered at larger

distances can be minimized. The Fletcher loadings in small, medium, and large colpostats (15, 20, and 25 mg, respectively) are similar to those of the Manchester system. When the source strength is increased to compensate for increased source-to-prescription point distance, the time required to deliver a fixed dose remains approximately constant. Because the radioactive sources are distributed over the longest possible tandem, penetration is maximized and a smaller dose is delivered to the uterine mucosa in relation to doses administered at distances on the order of 2 cm. Because of the similarity of Fletcher loadings (55 to 85 mg) to Manchester loadings, point A dose rates are nearly independent of the loading.

The tandems, about 6 mm in diameter, are available in three curvatures. A flange or stopper is used to keep the uterine tandem in the selected position: a keeled flange can be used to avoid rotation of the tandem. A special yoke was designed to maintain the position between the intrauterine tandem and the colpostats (193). In general, the loading in the tandem is with 20–10–10 mgRaEq ^{137}Cs sources.

When the effects of the intrauterine tandem and the contralateral colpostat are included, applicator shielding reduces midline rectal and bladder doses by 10% to 20% in relationship to conventional treatment-planning calculations, which ignore shielding and include only the effects of source encapsulation. When an applicator-source combination is used that differs from that on which one's clinical experience is based, critical structures can be overdosed and the tumor undertreated if dosimetric differences are ignored. The dosimetric features and dose prescriptions for the Fletcher system have been described in detail elsewhere (82,194).

The total number of milligram hours prescribed depends on (a) the total dose (in centigrays) desired at point A (according to tumor stage or volume), (b) the number and strength of sources inserted in the tandem and vaginal colpostats, (c) the number of insertions performed (one or two), and (d) the whole-pelvis dose delivered with external irradiation.

Although the intrauterine tandem and the colpostats are inserted independently, ideally, the tandem should be in the midline or as nearly as possible equidistant from the lateral pelvic wall, crossing the mid long axis of the ovoids, and the vaginal colpostats should be symmetrically positioned against the cervix in relation to the tandem (Fig. 14.44A). Ideally, the tandem should be placed along the sagittal axis of the pelvis and equidistant from the pubis and the sacral promontory (Fig. 14.44B) as allowed by the geometry of the patient and the tumor to avoid overdosage to the bladder, rectosigmoid, or either ureter.

It is extremely important when applicators are purchased to examine the design, to obtain radiographs to identify the position of the shielding (195), and to take dosimetric measurements after determining the diameter and thickness of the walls of the applicator to determine exactly the dose distribution around the applicators (194,196).

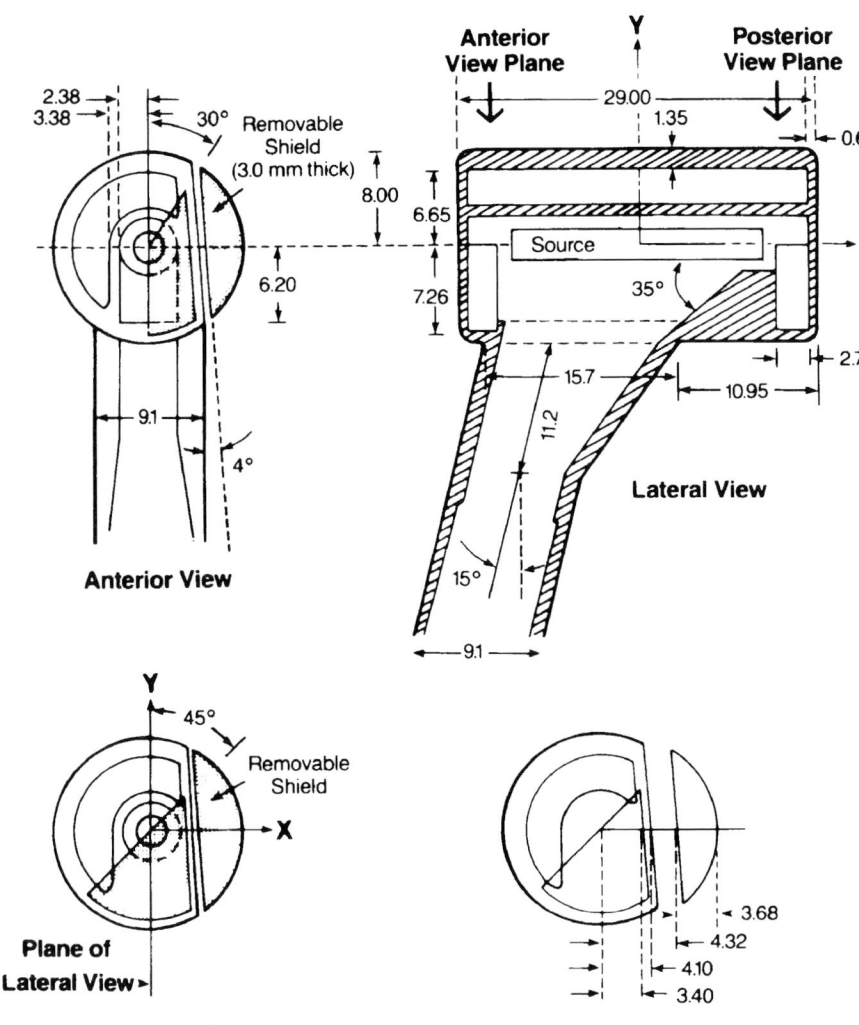

FIG. 14.43. Detailed structure of the Fletcher-Suit-Delclos colpostat marketed by 3M Corporation. The body of the applicator consists of stainless steel with 3-mm–thick tungsten alloy shields. The removable medial shields are inset into a 2-cm outer diameter nylon cap (not shown) that allows the applicator to be converted to a shielded Delclos minicolpostat. The shape of the shields is patterned after the original Fletcher design. All dimensions are described elsewhere (323). (From Delclos L, Fletcher GH, Sampiere V, et al. Can the Fletcher gamma ray colpostat system be extrapolated to other systems? *Cancer* 1978;41:970. Copyright © 1978 American Cancer Society. Reprinted by permission of Wiley-Liss Inc., a subsidiary of John Wiley & Sons, Inc.)

Because there is no universal intracavitary system that can be applied to all patients and because patients' anatomies vary, as do tumor morphologies and vaginal extension, it is imperative to have available several applicators with tandems of various lengths and curvatures, as well as colpostats of different diameters and design.

Weeks and associates (197,198) and Schoeppel and colleagues (199) described specially constructed plastic after loading Fletcher-Suit colpostats that can be used for CT treatment planning in gynecologic tumors. They eliminate the artifacts produced by metallic applicators on CT scans. The dose output of the loaded colpostat is 2% higher than that of the standard metallic applicators. In the direction of maximum thickness of shielding, the transmission rate is approximately 50% compared with 70% for the standard applicator. The plastic applicator was used on several patients with satisfactory results. Since these applicators do not contain high atomic–number materials such as tungsten and steel, they do not cause artifacts on CT or magnetic resonance (MRI) images that obscure patient anatomy. Ap-

plication of these CT/MRI–compatible applicators allows image-based treatment planning and evaluation of 3-D radiation dose distribution relative to the patient anatomy as visible on CT and MRI images.

With recent advances in molecular imaging technology, the use of positron emission tomography/(PET/FDG) imaging for the intracavitary brachytherapy treatment of cervical cancer was evaluated at Washington University (200,201). These preliminary studies demonstrated the feasibility and accuracy of PET/FDG–based treatment planning for intracavitary brachytherapy treatments using the Fletcher-Suit–type applicators, and indicated the potential for more accurate tumor definition relative to the applicators and improved tumor coverage by the radiation dose.

Minicolpostats. When the vagina is narrow or if there is distortion of the anatomy because of tumor in the cervix or vagina, it is not always possible to insert regular ovoids. Minicolpostats have a diameter of 1.6 cm and a flat inner surface to allow their insertion in patients for whom the only alternative would be a protruding vaginal source in the

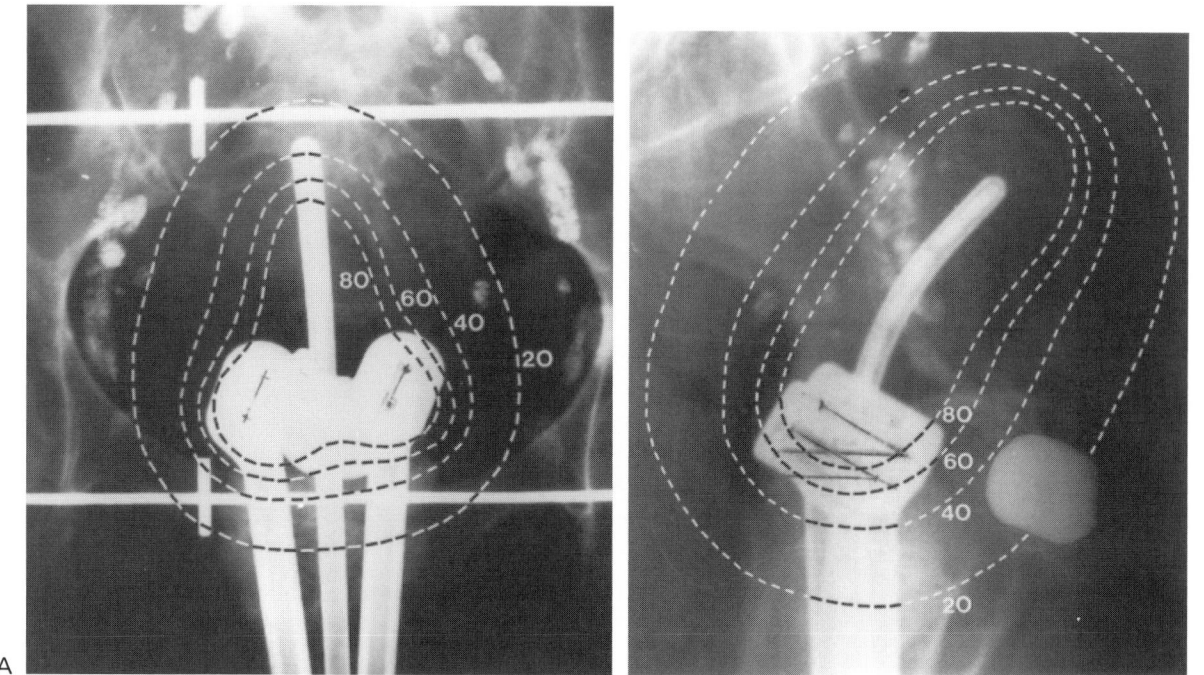

FIG. 14.44. A: Anteroposterior view of intracavitary insertion for carcinoma of the uterine cervix. **B:** Lateral view of same implant. Isodose curves (cGy/h) are superimposed. (From Perez CA, Grigsby PW, Williamson JF. Clinical applications of brachytherapy I: low dose-rate. In: Perez CA, Brady LW, eds. *Principles and practice of radiation oncology.* 3rd ed. Philadelphia: Lippincott–Raven Publishers, 1998: 487, with permission.)

tandem (202). Some miniovoids have no shielding: thus, the surface dose is significantly higher than with regular ovoids (at Washington University, with 3M cesium sources, the surface dose is 9.9 cGy/mgh in the miniovoids in contrast to 6.3 cGy for the 2-cm–diameter ovoids), and they are usually loaded with 10-mg sources. The dose at the top and bottom of a minicolpostat is about one-third of the dose at the lateral surface. The 3M miniovoids have internal shielding. However, phantom measurements have not demonstrated a significant decrease in dose for the newer minicolpostats with rectal shielding for a source separation of 3 cm, which potentially could allow undue user confidence in the doses delivered (203).

Kuske and associates (203), in dosimetry studies that compared TLDs in phantom with computer-calculated doses, reported that the dose to point A, bladder, and rectum with the minicolpostats is approximately 10% higher than with the regular ovoids. Because of the decreased capacity of the vaginal vault, packing may be more difficult, which results in the bladder and rectum being in closer proximity to the cesium sources. Despite using 10-mgRaEq sources in the miniovoids and decreasing the total exposure by 10%, the tandem in the minicolpostat system contributes an 8% higher dose to point A and the surrounding structures than with the regular colpostats.

Evaluating the results of therapy for 99 patients with carcinoma of the cervix on whom miniovoids were used, Kuske

and colleagues (203) noted a 15% incidence of grade 3 complications compared with 8% observed in a group of 194 patients treated during the same period with regular (2 cm) colpostats ($p = .08$).

Henschke Applicator. Other applicators, such as the Henschke applicator, are commercially available (195). With the Henschke applicator, the basic configuration of the ovoids is hemispheric, with the sources inserted parallel to the lateral wall of the vaginal vault and the intrauterine tandem. Three ovoid diameters and various tandems are available. Although this applicator's configuration conforms better to a narrow vaginal vault, the radioactive sources are parallel to the long axis of the bladder and the rectum and do not have any shielding, thus potentially delivering a higher dose to these organs. Delclos and colleagues (195) emphasized that the dosimetry with the Fletcher colpostats is unique and that treatment techniques and tables derived for this applicator should not be used with other applicators because their use might result in significantly higher doses to the vagina, bladder, or rectum. Figure 14.45 illustrates the differences in doses delivered with the Fletcher and the Henschke applicators to the bladder or rectum for a normalized dose of 70 Gy to point A. Users should familiarize themselves with the dosimetric aspects of these devices.

Interstitial Implants. Metallic needles containing ^{226}Ra, ^{60}Co, or ^{137}Cs, or afterloading metallic guides, or Teflon catheters for insertion of ^{192}Ir wires or seeds, have been

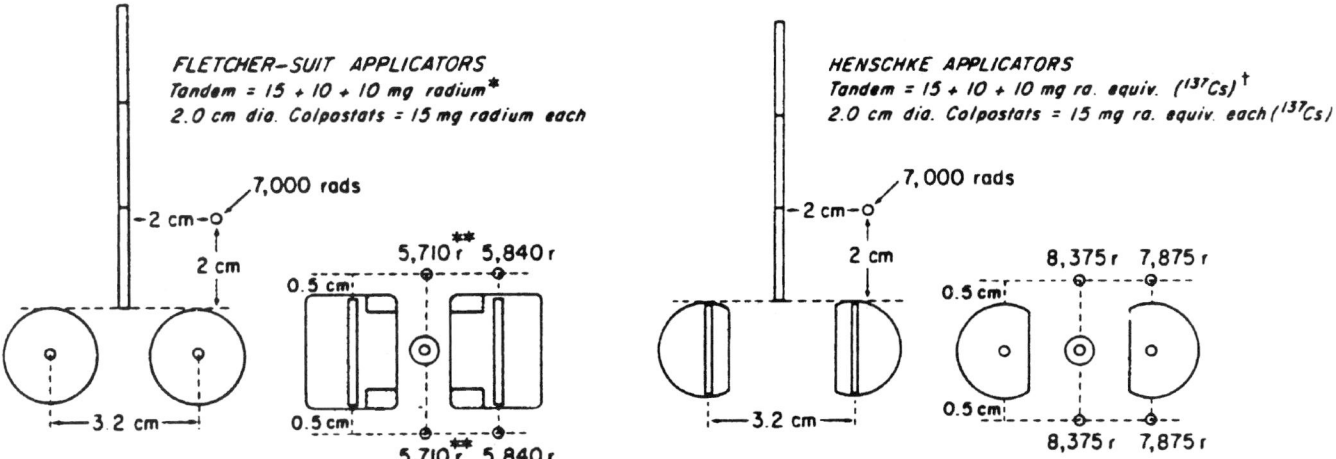

FIG. 14.45. Comparison of doses delivered by Fletcher or Henschke colpostats to a plane 0.5 cm anterior and 0.5 cm posterior to the poles of the colpostats with the dose normalized at 70 Gy to point A. It is obvious that the number of milligram hours (mgh) must be reduced in the Henschke system to bring the dose to the bladder and rectum more in line with that obtained with the Fletcher applicator. (From Delclos L, Fletcher GH, Sampiere V, et al. Can the Fletcher gamma ray colpostat system be extrapolated to other systems? *Cancer* 1980:41:970. Copyright © 1980 American Cancer Society. Reprinted by permission of Wiley-Liss Inc., a subsidiary of John Wiley & Sons, Inc.)

implanted in the parametrium to increase the parametrial dose after the use of conventional external and intracavitary irradiation or in the cervix using a transvaginal or transperineal approach (sometimes in lieu of intracavitary insertions when the cervical canal cannot be identified) (204).

The procedure is similar to that followed for intracavitary insertions. The cervix should always be held firmly with a tenaculum. For implants in the cervix itself, the needles or nylon catheters with metallic guides (5 to 6 cm long) are inserted straight, about 1.2 cm apart, following the position of the uterus (which can be verified with a finger in the rectum) in a single- or double-circle arrangement. If a single circle is used, full-intensity sources (0.66 mgReEq/cm) are required. If a double circle is implanted, the central one should have half-intensity sources (usually four), and the periphery should have full-intensity sources. At Washington University, parametrial Teflon catheters (with metallic guides), usually 12 to 15 cm long, are inserted through the vaginal fornices. A double-plane or volume implant usually can be placed in each parametrium. The catheters are implanted starting at 1 o'clock on the patient's left side and at 11 o'clock on the right and are directed parallel to the coronal plane of the patient and 5 to 10 degrees lateral toward the pelvic wall. The peripheral plane should be placed 1.2 to 1.5 cm lateral to the medial plane, and the catheters should be inserted in the same fashion, about 10 degrees lateral from the midline.

Care should be exercised to avoid insertion of the needles in the bladder unless it is necessary in order to cover the tumor volume. The operator should keep in mind the expected anatomic location of the major pelvic vessels, especially veins (since arteries are more difficult to pierce).

If the uterosacral ligament area is to be implanted, the catheters are directed 5 to 10 degrees posteriorly. In general, about six to eight catheters can be easily implanted in each parametrium (Fig. 14.46). It is preferable to implant the interstitial catheters alone, without vaginal colpostats or cylinders, to prevent displacement or enhanced penetration of the needles/catheters. Gentle packing with iodoform gauze will keep the needles/catheters in place. Cystoscopy and a careful rectal examination at the completion of the procedure will help to identify any misplaced needles/catheters, which should be withdrawn or reinserted immediately.

Results reported by several investigators using interstitial LDR brachytherapy in locally advanced uterine carcinoma are shown in Table 14.5 (205–208). HDR interstitial implants have also been used with satisfactory results (209).

Several investigators (210–215) have developed methods that allow the postimplant dose distribution calculation of these implants based on CT images of the patient anatomy and also facilitate the use of CT images in guiding the insertion of needles and catheters into the target volume, so that dose distributions optimal in target coverage and dose homogeneity may be achieved. With the general availability of commercial treatment-planning systems that provide such

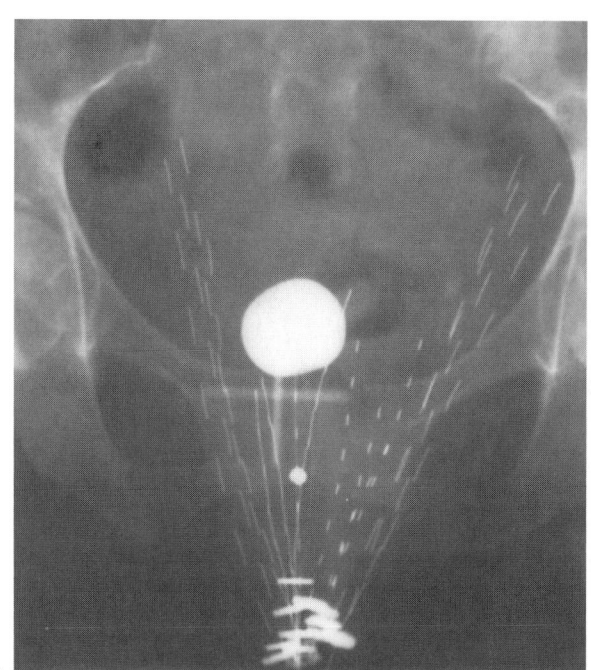
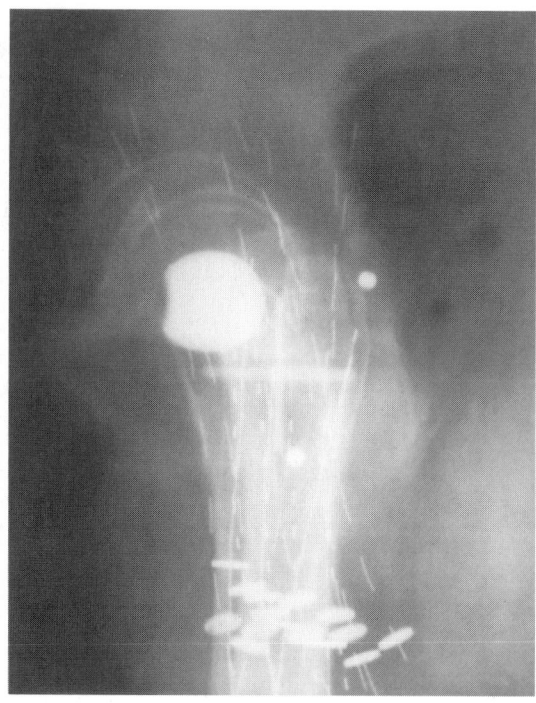

A

B

FIG. 14.46. Anteroposterior **(A)** and lateral **(B)** radiographs of the pelvis showing bilateral parametrial implant (with sources extending into vaginal walls) for extensive carcinoma of the uterine cervix. Upper radiopaque marker indicates position of the cervix. Lower radiopaque marker denotes distal margin of vaginal tumor extension. (From Perez CA, Grigsby PW, Williamson JF. Clinical applications of brachytherapy I: low dose-rate. In: Perez CA, Brady LW, eds. *Principles and practice of radiation oncology.* 3rd ed. Philadelphia: Lippincott–Raven Publishers, 1998:487, with permission.)

capabilities, image-guided interstitial brachytherapy has become a very useful modality for selected patients.

Templates. A variety of templates have been designed over the years to more easily place radioactive sources and to obtain more homogeneous doses in the cerivx, vagina, or parametrial tissues.

Syed-Neblett templates. Several Syed-Neblett templates have been devised and are primarily used for gynecologic tumors. They consist of two Lucite plates joined by six screws that tighten to grasp as many as 38 afterloading, hollow, stainless steel needles. The needles are designed to hold

[192]Ir seeds encapsulated in nylon ribbons. Six additional needles fit into the grooves of a 2-cm–diameter plastic vaginal cylinder that is placed inside an opening in the middle of the template. These needles are arranged in concentric circles or arcs with a spacing of 1 cm between adjacent needles (Fig. 14.47).

A 4 × 10–cm area can be implanted in a butterfly distribution. The 17-gauge needles supplied with the templates are 20 cm long, but they can be shortened to treat more shallow areas. The vaginal cylinder has a central opening for placement of a tandem if desired.

TABLE 14.5. *Summary of results with external beam and interstitial brachytherapy template for locally advanced (IIB, IIIB) cervical carcinoma*

Study	Reference	No. of Patients	Local Recurrence (%)	Complications (%)
Feder et al., 1978	324	35	14 (40)	3 (9)
Aristizabal et al., 1985	205	118	30 (25)	25 (21)
Martinez et al., 1985	207	37	6 (16)	2 (5.4)
Gaddis et al., 1983	206	51	17 (33)	8 (16)
Ampuero et al., 1983	19	24	9 (38)	7 (29)
Total		265	76 (29)	45 (17)

Source: Perez CA, Grigsby PW, Williamson JF. Clinical applications of brachytherapy I: low dose-rate. In: Perez CA, Brady LW, eds. *Principles and practice of radiation oncology.* 3rd ed. Philadelphia: Lippincott–Raven Publishing Co, 1998:487–560, with permission.

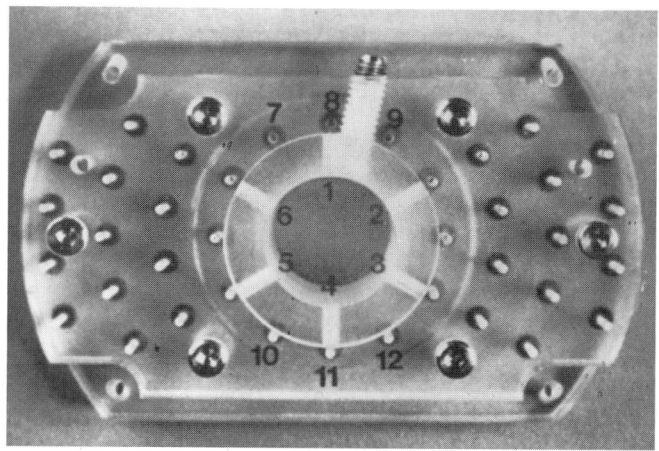

FIG. 14.47. Syed-type perineal template used for interstitial parametrial irradiation. (Reprinted by permission of the publisher from Aristizabal SA, Valencia A, Ocampo G, et al. Interstitial parametrial irradiation in cancer of the cervix stage IIB-IIIB. *Endocurietherapy/Hyperthermia Oncol* 1985:1:42. Copyright 1985 Endocurietherapy Research Foundation.)

A urethral template has two concentric rings with a total of 17 needles with the same 1-cm spacing as the rectal template. A cylindrical volume with either a 2- or 4-cm diameter is implanted with this template. It is a single plate with no machine screws to other plates. A Foley urethral catheter is inserted through the central opening to drain the urinary bladder. Potish and Williamson (216) have reviewed the clinical and dosimetric considerations of using large templates.

Martinez universal perineal interstitial template. The Martinez universal perineal interstitial template (MUPIT) applicator was designed to treat locally advanced or recurrent tumors in the prostatic, anorectal, perineal, and gynecologic areas. The device consists of two acrylic cylinders, one that can be placed in the vagina and the other in the rectum, an acrylic template with an array of holes that allows placement of the metallic guides in the tissues to be implanted, and a cover plate (Fig. 14.48). The cylinders are placed in the vagina or rectum or both and fastened to the template so that a fixed geometric relationship among the tumor volume, normal structures, and source placement is preserved throughout the course of the implantation. When the MUPIT device is used, no intracavitary sources are inserted, except in some patients requiring an intrauterine tandem (beyond the volume treated with the interstitial sources).

Molds. Individually tailored brachytherapy molds, instead of standard intracavitary applicators, may be used to achieve optimal dose distribution, particularly when there is disruption of the anatomy. Initially, the configuration of the anatomic area to be molded is determined with a liquid plaster cast to form a negative plaster mold. Then the mold is constructed from plastic or acrylic. Computations for the dose desired are carried out, and optimal placement of the

sources is determined. Small holes are drilled in the mold to contain the nylon ribbons or catheters with the radioactive sources or the rigid radium (or cesium) needles. These techniques have been extensively described by Paterson (217) and Fletcher (82).

Acrylic molds have been used for the treatment of vaginal and uterine cervix lesions. Lichter and colleagues (218) described the use of thermoplastic vaginal molds for this purpose. The locations of the channels for insertion of the sources and for a central tandem (if desired) are determined by the topography of the tumor. The central tandem can be placed in the uterus or the vagina, through the vaginal mold, and locked into position.

Endometrium

Carcinoma of the endometrium may grow irregularly into the uterine cavity and produce a deformity of the lumen of the uterus resulting from (a) exophytic tumor, (b) thickening of the uterine wall caused by myometrial infiltration, or (c) uterine enlargement. It is important to determine the size and shape of the uterus, which can be accomplished by rotating the uterine sound and measuring the width and depth of the uterine cavity as well as by bimanual palpation or hysterogram. Special care should be taken to avoid a perforation: if perforation occurs, packing with Heyman capsules should not be performed at that time. However, a carefully inserted tandem may be used, avoiding the site of perforation. Ultrasound may help in ascertaining the exact position of the tandem. Rutledge and Delclos (219) also cautioned against rupture (splitting) of the cervix, which may be caused by excessive careless dilatation. Uterine packing with capsules was originally described by Heyman and colleagues (220) in 1934.

In addition to the metallic and plastic standard Heyman capsules, afterloading Heyman-Simon capsules are commercially available in 6-, 8-, and 10-mm diameters and 2- to 3-cm lengths. They have the advantage of decreasing exposure to the operators and facilitating better verification of the position of the sources in the uterus before loading. Inactive metallic guides and, later, ^{137}Cs sources are inserted.

When capsules are used, it is convenient to insert an afterloading tandem to cover the lower uterine segment because doing so permits more flexibility in the loading to obtain improved coverage of this portion of the uterus and the cervical canal. Afterloading colpostats should be used routinely to irradiate the vaginal cuff.

It is critical to record the order of insertion of the capsules (by numbers that are printed on each capsule), so that removal is done in the reverse order of insertion. Otherwise, the capsules may become jammed, making removal more difficult. Ideally, a minimum of four capsules should be inserted. If fewer are allowed by the size of the endometrial cavity, it may be better to just insert an afterloading tandem.

The dose of irradiation delivered with this system is some-

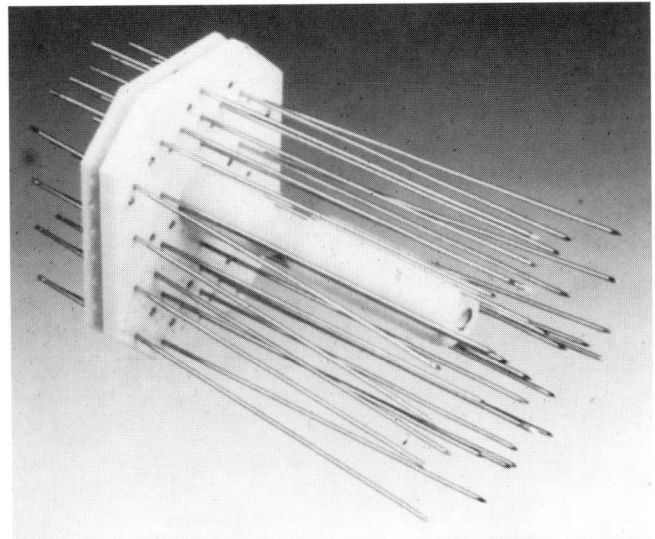

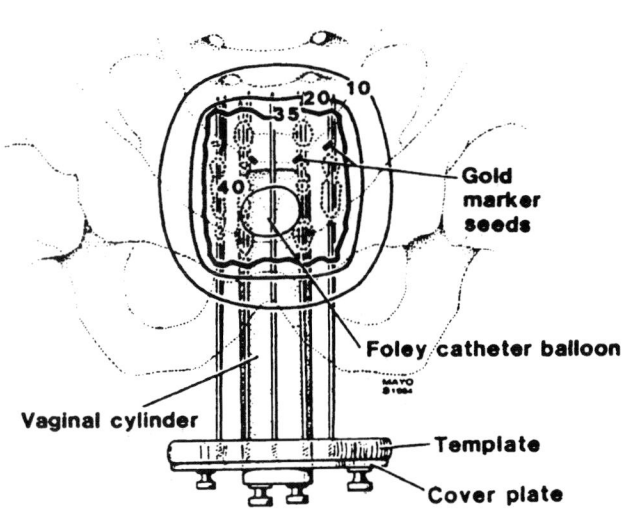

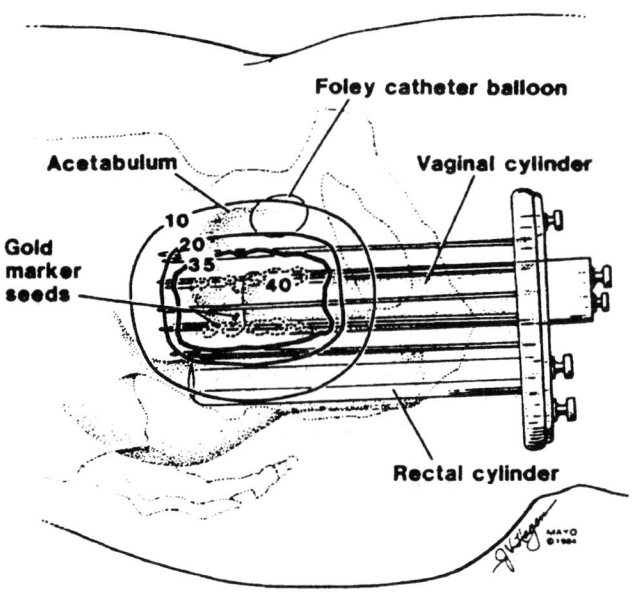

FIG. 14.48. A: Martinez Universal Perineal Interstitial Template (MUPIT). (Courtesy of Dr. Alvaro Martinez, William Beaumont Hospital, Detroit, Michigan.) **B:** Diagrammatic representation in coronal and sagittal planes of same template. (Reprinted from Martinez A, Edmundson GK, Cox RS, et al. Combination of external beam irradiation and multiple-site perineal applicator [MUPIT] for treatment of locally advanced or recurrent prostatic, anorectal, and gynecologic malignancies. *Int J Radiat Oncol Biol Phys* 1985:11: 391–398, with permission from Elsevier.)

what empirically derived, and only estimates of dose administered to the serosa of the uterus can be offered. At Washington University, in preoperative insertions, 3,500 mgh is used in the uterine cavity: however, cavities larger than 8 cm receive doses of approximately 4,000 mgh. Doses of 60 to 65 Gy to the mucosal surface of the vagina are delivered (1,900 to 2,000 mgh) with 2-cm–diameter vaginal ovoids. Grigsby and colleagues (221) reported higher survival and fewer pelvic recurrences and distant metastases in patients with stage I poorly differentiated endometrial carcinoma when doses higher than 3,500 mgh were delivered to the uterus. A lesser beneficial impact was noted in moderately differentiated tumors.

For postoperative irradiation in endometrial carcinoma, if no preoperative irradiation was delivered, afterloading colpostats are used to deliver 60 to 70 Gy to the vaginal mucosa

(1,800 to 2,000 mgh) in patients with moderately or poorly differentiated tumors even in the absence of deep myometrial invasion. When there is deep myometrial invasion (>50%), regardless of the histologic features, the intracavitary therapy is combined with external irradiation (20 Gy whole pelvis and additional 30 Gy to parametria with midline shielding). If a preoperative implant was performed, only external irradiation is administered as outlined.

Vagina, Vulva, and Female Urethra

The indications for and techniques of interstitial therapy for carcinomas of the vagina, vulva, and urethra have been discussed elsewhere (222). These areas are potentially vulnerable to severe complications because of the lower tolerance of the surrounding tissues to irradiation and because they are exposed to the constant irritation of perspiration, urine, and, occasionally, feces: therefore, it is important to minimize irradiation to the surrounding normal areas.

The use of interstitial implants ideally should be limited to a volume encompassing 75% or less of the circumference of the vagina, particularly when the lesion involves the posterior wall and rectovaginal septum. The remaining normal tissues should be kept away from the implanted area as much as possible, with the judicious use of gauze packing, cylinders, or templates. Two rolls of gauze are placed on top of and between the thighs, so that when the legs are brought down from the lithotomy position (in which the implant is done), the inside surfaces of the thighs are separated as much as possible from the radioactive sources.

Vaginal Applicators. Afterloading vaginal cylinders have a central hollow metallic cylinder, in which the sources are placed, and plastic rings of varying diameter, 2.5 cm in length, which are inserted over the cylinder. Domed cylinders are used to irradiate the vaginal cuff homogeneously when indicated. Delclos and coworkers (202) recommend that a short cesium source be used at the top to obtain a uniform dose around the dome because a lower dose is noted at the end of the linear cesium sources. Some cylinders have lead shielding to protect selected portions of the vagina. A flange with a keel is placed over the tandem after the last plastic cylinder has been inserted to secure the system in place and avoid rotation. When any type of vaginal applicator is used, the surface dose must be determined in addition to the tumor dose.

Perez and coworkers (223) designed and constructed a vaginal applicator that incorporates two ovoid sources and a central tandem that can be used to treat the entire vagina (alone or in combination with the uterine cervix). The applicator has vaginal apex caps and additional cylinder sleeves that allow for increased dimensions (Fig. 14.49). The average surface dose rate around the 2-cm ovoids is about 1.2 Gy/h, and in the 2.5-cm–diameter vaginal cylinder it is 1 Gy/h, with usual loading of 20-mgRaEq ^{137}Cs sources in the ovoids and 10- to 15-mgRaEq ^{137}Cs sources in the cylinder (Fig. 14.49D). The tandem in the uterus can be used when clinically indicated with standard loadings depending on the depth of the uterus (20–10–10 or 20–10 mgRaEq). When the uterine tandem and vaginal cylinder are used, the strength of the sources in the ovoids should always be 15 mgRaEq. The vaginal cylinder or uterine tandem never carries an active source at the level of the ovoids. The acronym MIRA-LVA (Mallinckrodt Institute of Radiology Afterloading Vaginal Applicator) describes the device.

Rectovaginal Septum

When needles or stainless steel guides are being implanted for tumors of the posterior vaginal wall, the rectal ampulla is kept distended with a 30-mL Foley catheter to minimize irradiation of the opposite rectal wall. It is important to assess the anatomy of the rectum. When the catheters are inserted in the thin rectovaginal septum, one finger (covered with a second glove) should be inserted in the rectum to ensure that the catheters do not protrude beyond the rectal mucosa. If protrusion occurs, the catheters should be withdrawn and reinserted in a satisfactory position.

Proximal Female Urethra

An open-bladder implant technique similar to that described by Battermann and Boon (224) for carcinoma of the bladder may be used for proximal urethral lesions that extend into the bladder neck. This procedure allows direct visualization of tumor extension into the bladder.

After a lower abdominal incision, the bladder is opened to visualize the tumor area in the bladder neck and urethra. Plastic carriers that consist of a hollow part and a thinner leading end are used. The tubes penetrate the abdominal wall, are tunneled in the bladder muscle through the bladder wall, and penetrate the abdominal wall again. This technique ensures good fixation of the tubes and thus the position of the radioactive sources. The catheters should be placed in such a way that removal is feasible without a second laparotomy, although in more complex cases, one may be necessary. Dummy sources are introduced in the carriers to visualize the length of the source to be used while the bladder is still open. After the bladder is closed, the position of the sources is checked, and then the abdomen is closed. A Foley catheter is placed for drainage. After film localization, the dose distribution is determined. The carriers are connected to the MicroSelectron, and the radioactive phase of the procedure is started. The tubes are well tolerated and, after completion of irradiation, can be removed easily. For bladder tumors, a dose of 40 Gy is given by brachytherapy at a dose rate of 0.3 to 0.5 Gy/h. All patients receive preoperative external irradiation to prevent tumor seeding during operation (30 Gy). Similar techniques are applicable to proximal urethral lesions.

Vulva/Distal Urethra

Vulvar or distal urethral tumors can be treated with brachytherapy techniques. The patient is placed in the lithotomy position and single, double-plane, or volume implants can be designed around the urethra or in the vulvar labia. It is helpful to place carefully #8 or #10 Hegar dilator in the urethra during the procedure for orientation of the planes of the implant. If the proximal urethra is involved, the radioactive sources must be inserted to reach the bladder. When the procedure is completed, the Hegar dilator is withdrawn. Cystoscopy is performed to ascertain the position of the catheters in the bladder, and an indwelling catheter is inserted. If there is intravesical bleeding, periodic irrigation of the bladder is necessary while the implant is in place (every 4 hours), and it is preferable to leave the catheter in place for a few days (up to 1 week) to avoid clot formation and bladder neck obstruction. When the vulva is involved, the sources

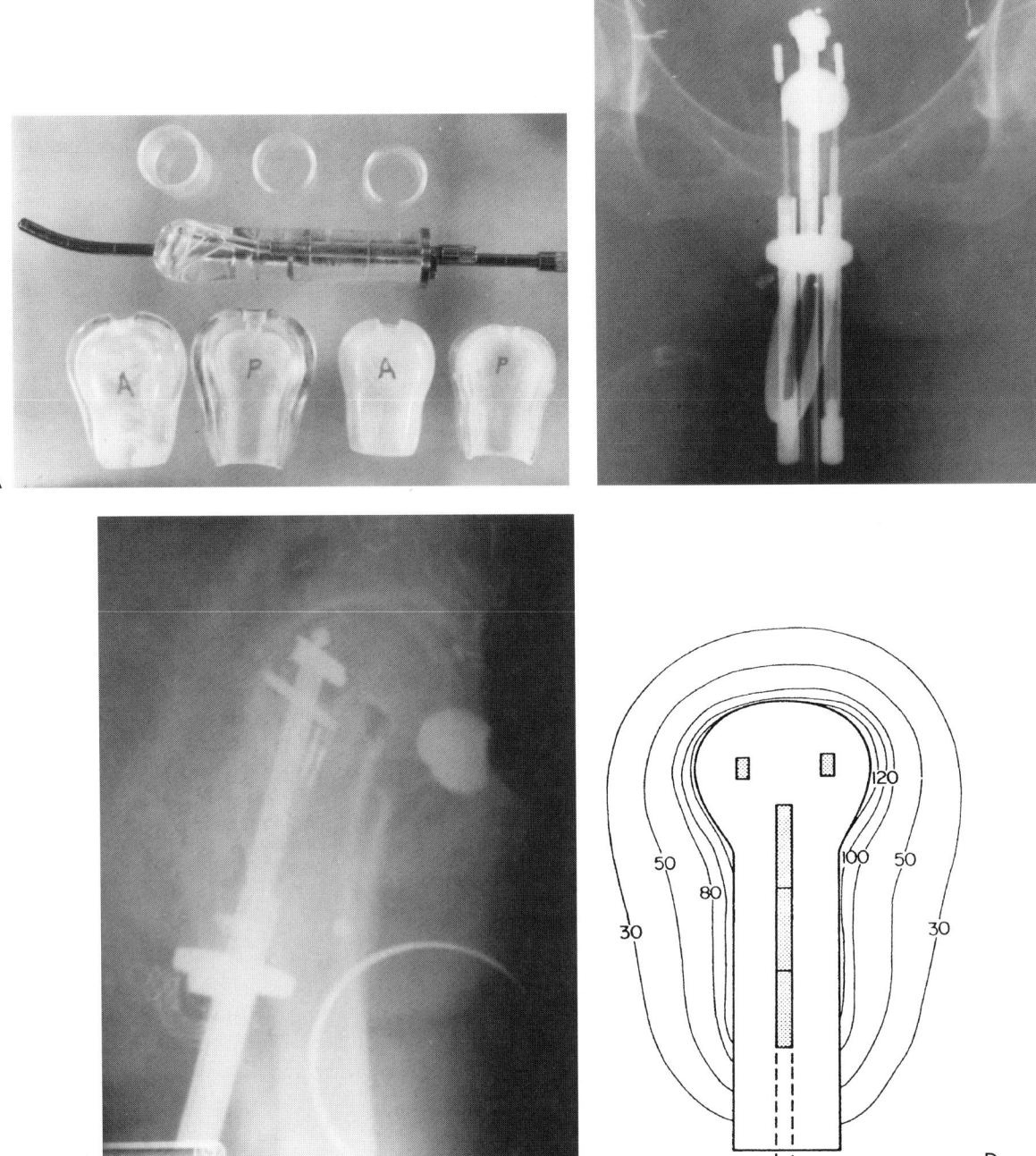

FIG. 14.49. A: MIRALVA applicator with plastic sleeves to increase diameter of vaginal cylinder, afterloading tandem, and plastic caps (*A, P*) of different sizes to increase diameter of vaginal cuff portion of applicator. Anteroposterior **(B)** and lateral **(C)** radiographs depicting position of MIRALVA applicator for treatment of patient with vaginal recurrence of a carcinoma of the uterine cervix previously treated with radical hysterectomy. **D:** Isodose curves of MIRALVA applicator. (Reprinted from Perez CA, Slessinger E, Grigsby PW. Design of an afterloading vaginal applicator [MIRALVA]. *Int J Radiat Oncol Biol Phys* 1990:18:1503, with permission from Elsevier.)

must protrude into the perineum. If the tumor extends into the vagina, an intravaginal cylinder with some sources may be necessary to increase the dose to the vaginal mucosa (Fig. 14.50). The design of the implant, placement of the radioactive sources, and tumor doses are similar to those for comparable lesions in the vagina.

High-Dose Rate Brachytherapy in Carcinoma of Cervix

According to ICRU Report No. 38, HDR brachytherapy delivers doses higher than 20 cGy/min (12 Gy/h or higher) (141). Advantages of HDR remote afterloading include: Radiation exposure of medical and nursing personnel is vir-

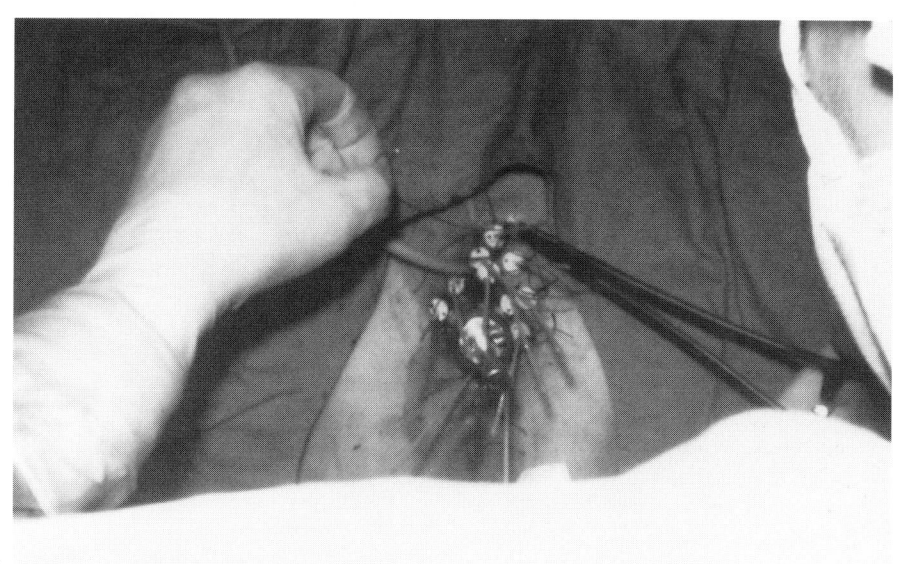

A

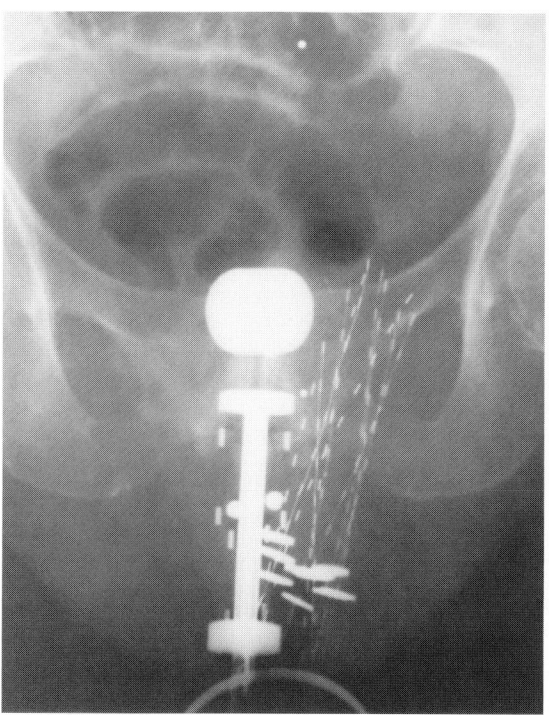

B

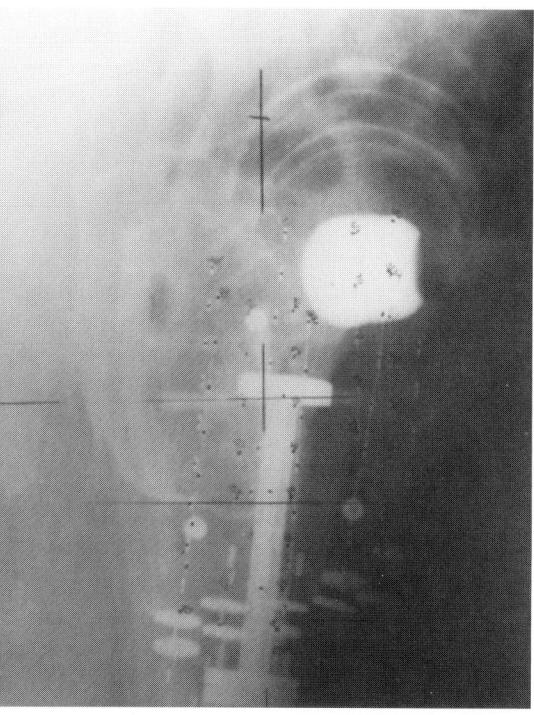

C

FIG. 14.50. A: Patient at completion of interstitial implant and intracavitary insertion with stainless steel guides for ^{192}Ir tubing and Delclos vaginal cylinder. Bladder catheter is in place. The metallic buttons on the plastic catheters are being sutured to the skin to secure the position of the implant. Anteroposterior **(B)** and lateral **(C)** radiographs of implant for urethral tumor with left paraurethral extension. (From Perez CA, Grigsby PW, Williamson JF: Clinical applications of brachytherapy I: low dose-rate. In: Perez CA, Brady LW, eds. *Principles and practice of radiation oncology.* 3rd ed. Philadelphia: Lippincott–Raven Publishers, 1998:487, with permission.)

tually eliminated: patient immobilization time is short, and complications resulting from prolonged bedrest, such as pulmonary emboli, are eliminated: general anesthesia is avoided, and patient discomfort is decreased: treatment planning and dosimetry are more exact, and optimization is possible: and treatment can be performed on an outpatient basis without the need of an operating room, thus reducing healthcare costs.

Fractionation and adjustment of total dose are crucial factors in lowering the frequency of complications without compromising the results of therapy with HDR systems (225–227). Warmelink and associates (228), using the extrapolative response dose model, proposed fractionation schemes for high-dose rates, based on experience derived from LDR brachytherapy. Orton and colleagues (229) noted that the dose ratio of HDR to LDR for equivalent biologic effects is 0.5 to 0.6. In a survey involving brachytherapy practice in a large number of institutions, they noted that frequently four to six HDR fractions were used. Dose per fraction greater than 7 to 7.5 Gy resulted in a significantly higher incidence of sequelae.

Petereit and Pearch (230) analyzed fractionation schedules reported in HDR intracavitary brachytherapy literature and attempted to correlate these to the treatment outcomes reported. They were not able to identify a dose-response relationship from this study. It was proposed this lack of apparent dose-response relationship may be due to the lack of detailed description in the fractionation schedule reporting in the literature, and that future HDR publications should provide accurate fractionation details for each stage of disease, while reporting actuarial complication rates.

High-dose rate afterloading brachytherapy is used in the treatment of patients with gynecologic malignancies for curative intent (231–233). In the United States, there has been increased use of HDR remote afterloading intracavitary brachytherapy for carcinoma of the cervix and endometrium (234,235). The subject is discussed in more depth in Chapter 22.

High-Dose Rate Brachytherapy in Endometrial Carcinoma

Nori and associates (236) noted that, for dose rates between 1 and 2 Gy/min to point A, there is a linear relationship between total dose and fractionation dose. This relationship correlates the total dose to point A and fractionation with local tumor control and complications for HDR and LDR brachytherapy (237).

Nori and associates (236) and Mandell and colleagues (238) reported on 330 patients treated postoperatively with HDR remote afterloading brachytherapy to the vaginal vault for stage I and II endometrial carcinoma at high risk for pelvic recurrence (i.e., deep myometrial invasion, high histologic grade, extrauterine tumor extension). The total vaginal vault dose was 21 Gy to a depth of 0.5 cm given in three

TABLE 14.6. *Survival and recurrence results in endometrial cancer patients treated at Memorial Hospital with high-dose rate brachytherapy*

	Total no. of Patients	5-Year Survival (%)	Pelvic Recurrence (%)
-1965 (mainly surgery only)			
Stage I	536	70	
Stage II	24	46	22
-1976 (irradiation and surgery)			
Stage I	247	92	
Stage II	22	82	2.7

Source: Nori D, Hilaris BS, Batata M, et al. Remote afterloading in cancer management. II. Clinical applications of remoteafter loaders. In: Hilaris BS, Batata MA, eds. *Brachytherapy oncology —1983.* New York: Memorial Sloan-Kettering Cancer Center, 1983:101–118, with permission.

fractions at 2-week intervals. Additional external beam pelvic irradiation was given to higher risk patients (40 Gy to the midplane of the pelvis with four-field technique). The total pelvic/vaginal recurrence rate was 2.7%, with a 3.7% incidence of vaginal complications, none of which required surgical correction. The 5-year survival rate was 92% for stage I and 82% for stage II disease. A nonrandomized comparison of their results with surgery alone or combined with irradiation is shown in Table 14.6.

Sorbe and colleagues (239) treated 366 patients with stage I endometrial carcinoma with preoperative HDR remote afterloading brachytherapy (275 patients) or irradiation alone (91 patients). All patients received six intracavitary fractions in 8 days with 5 to 12 Gy per fraction. External irradiation was given to all medically inoperable patients and to operable patients with high-risk factors at the time of surgery. The dose of HDR intracavitary irradiation per fraction was the most important factor in the development of complications, local tumor control, and residual disease in the uterus. Their recommendation is to deliver six fractions of 5 to 8 Gy per fraction for preoperative and medically inoperable patients with stage I endometrial cancer.

Peschel and associates (240) reported their experience with 103 patients with stage I carcinoma of the endometrium treated with HDR remote afterloading techniques in addition to surgery. The tumor control rate in the vaginal apex was 99%. Severe complications were noted in 6% of patients treated with external irradiation and remote afterloading brachytherapy. McCormick et al. recently reviewed this subject (241).

Dose Specification in Gynecologic Intracavitary Therapy

In this section, the physical relationships between point A dose and milligram hours prescription are reviewed (242).

Alternatively, minimum dose to a predefined target volume could be used as the basis of treatment prescription: however, this volume is difficult to define using currently available imaging technology. The lack of accurate dose computation algorithms that account for applicator shielding is another factor mitigating against the use of minimum tumor dose as a prescription criterion. Knowledge of tumor control and complications incidence, in terms of milligram hours (82) and dose at fixed reference points relative to the applicator (141,190), remains the basis of intracavitary treatment prescription.

The conceptual significance of point A has been obscured by the widespread current practice of defining point A as being 2 cm superior to the cervical os rather than 2 cm superior to the lateral vaginal fornix, as originally specified by Tod and Meredith (190). In practice, the os is radiographically demarcated by the tandem collar or the inferiormost aspect of the caudal intrauterine source, whereas the lateral fornix is indicated by the colpostat surface. Because the vertical position of the colpostat in relation to the caudal aspect of the tandem varies significantly with each patient, the distance between the "revised" point A and the vaginal sources will vary, giving large fluctuations in the dose rate. This phenomenon is illustrated in the study by Potish and Gerbi (243) of 90 Fletcher intracavitary applications in which they compared dose rates calculated on the basis of the classic and revised point A definitions. Revised point A dose rates were both higher and much more variable than their classic counterparts. The classic values are nearly independent of the applicator loading and have a mean value (0.52 Gy • h⁻¹) very close to that predicted by the Manchester system.

The ICRU introduced the concept of *reference volume* (isodose surface) to report and compare intracavitary treatments (141). Reference volume describes the tissue encompassed by a reference isodose surface. This reference volume is described by three dimensions: the height (d_h), which is the maximum dimension along the intrauterine source and is measured in the oblique frontal plane containing that source: the width (d_w), which is the maximum dimension perpendicular to the intrauterine source measured in the same plane: and the thickness (d_t), which is the maximum dimension perpendicular to the intrauterine source and is measured in the oblique sagittal plane containing that source (Fig. 14.51) (141). An absorbed dose level of 60 Gy (both external and intracavitary) is recommended by ICRU Report No. 38 as the reference level for LDR therapy.

Potish (244) analyzed the effect of applicator geometry on classic dose specification parameters in 90 Fletcher-Suit intracavitary applications for cervical cancer. He identified five significant factors: milligrams in colpostats, milligrams in tandem, lateral displacement of colpostats in frontal plane, vertical separation between the colpostats and tandem sources, and anteroposterior displacement of the colpostats in relationship to the tandem. Applicator/source geometry

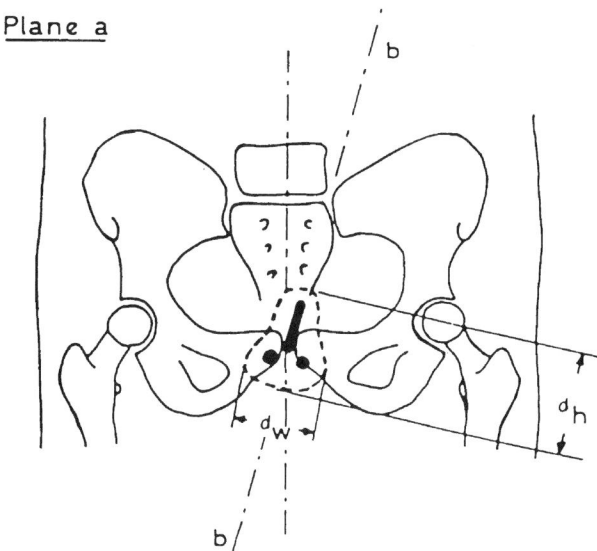

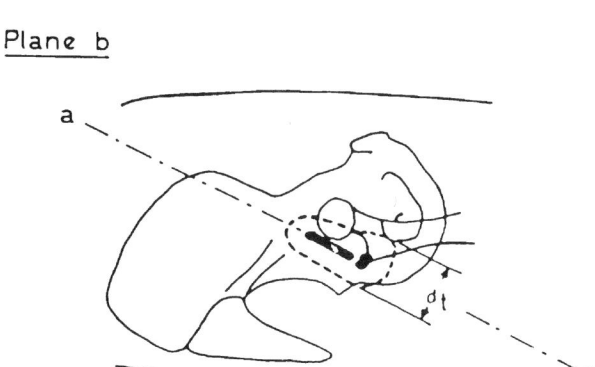

FIG. 14.51. Geometry for measurement of the size of the pear-shaped ICRU reference isodose surface (*broken line*) in a typical treatment of cervical carcinoma using one rod-shaped uterine applicator and two vaginal applicators. *Plane a* is the "oblique" frontal plane that contains the intrauterine device. The oblique frontal plane is obtained by rotation of the frontal plane around a transverse axis. *Plane b* is the "oblique" sagittal plane that contains the intrauterine device. The oblique sagittal plane is obtained by rotation of the sagittal plane around the AP axis. The height (d_h) and width (d_w) of the reference volume are measured in *plane a* as the maximal sizes parallel and perpendicular to the uterine applicator, respectively. The thickness (d_t) of the reference volume is measured in *plane b* as the maximal size perpendicular to the uterine applicator. (From International Commission on Radiation Units and Measurements. Report 38: dose and volume specification for reporting intracavitary therapy in gynecology. Bethesda, MD: International Commission on Radiation Units, 1985:10, with permission.)

had little effect on the product of ICRU volume specification, but it greatly influenced the individual ICRU components and "traditional" dose calculation points.

Katz and Eifel (245) measured various distances between intracavitary applicators and normal structures for approximately 400 patients treated at M.D. Anderson Cancer Center between 1990 and 1994 in an effort to quantify the M.D.

Anderson criteria for acceptable implant geometry and to relate these parameters to treatment outcome. The distances measured included those between tandem and sacrum; tandem and the pubis; cervical markers and ovoid surfaces; tandem and posterior surfaces of ovoids; and posterior ovoid surface and vaginal packing posterior extension on lateral radiograph films. From the AP radiograph film they measured the distance between tandem axis, and patient midline was obtained. Corresponding doses to reference points were reviewed. They reported narrow ranges for all these distances measured from the retrospective reviews of patient films and correspondingly narrow ranges of doses to reference points.

Crook and associates (246) and Esche with the same group (247), using computerized dosimetry, correlated the volume of the reference isodose, defined as the product of the three orthogonal ICRU dimensions, with milligram hours and external irradiation using the Fletcher system. This reference volume was directly proportional to milligram hours and doses of external irradiation to the pelvis over 30 Gy but did not depend appreciably on moderate changes in source geometry (247). The investigators described a close correlation between treatment sequelae and reference doses to various critical organs (246).

The relationship among milligram hours, point A dose, and ICRU reference volume can be clarified by examination of the volumetric characteristics of an intracavitary implant by a dose volume histogram (DVH). DVHs conveniently summarize complex 3-D dose distributions in an easily assimilable unidimensional format by ignoring the spatial location of each dose level.

Eisbruch and colleagues (248) studied the relationship between the volume of reference isodose surfaces, administered mgRaEq-h, and the product of the ICRU orthogonal dimensions for 204 intracavitary implants as digitized from orthogonal simulation radiographs. They found that the commonly used practice of estimating relative volume contained within isodose surfaces by the ICRU Report No. 38 orthogonal dimensions product is unsatisfactory. In addition, isodose surface volumes could be estimated accurately knowing only the mgRaEq-h despite large variations in underlying implant geometry from patient to patient. Prescribing intracavitary therapy by mgRaEq-h or its derivative, total reference air kerma, is equivalent to requiring that each isodose curve surface expand during the treatment to encompass a specified volume. Constraining the mgRaEq-h delivered, therefore, serves to limit the volume of tissue irradiated to high doses. To a first approximation, the volume $V(M,D)$ encompassed by the isodose surface taken to dose D with an administration of M mgRaEq-h is:

$$V(M,D) \propto [M/D]^{3/2}$$

Other points of dose calculation described in ICRU Report No. 38 (141) (lymphatic trapezoid and pelvic wall reference points) are not used in everyday practice. Although it is logical that the dose rates and volumetric distribution between external and intracavitary therapy may give rise to different biologic effects on tumor and normal tissues, sufficient data are not available to introduce correction factors into dose prescription systems to quantify these effects. When external beam and intracavitary therapy are combined, the time-dose schedule of the entire treatment should be reported.

Reference Points Related to Organs at Risk

In addition to prescription of intracavitary therapy to achieve local tumor control, a means of quantifying absorbed dose delivered to therapy-limiting normal structures, such as bladder and rectum, is needed. Many different reference points have been proposed. The bladder and rectal reference points proposed by Chassagne and Horiot (249) are illustrated in Figure 14.52. The bladder reference point is outlined by a Foley catheter with 7 mL of radiopaque fluid in the balloon. The catheter is pulled downward to bring the balloon against the bladder neck and urethra. On lateral radiographs, the reference point is obtained by drawing an anteroposterior line through the center of the balloon and projecting it where it crosses the posterior surface of the balloon. The reference point for the rectal dose is obtained on the lateral radiograph at a point where an anteroposterior line drawn from the lower end of the intrauterine source (or from the middle of the intravaginal sources) crosses the rectal wall, which is arbitrarily displaced 5 mm posterior to the vaginal wall. The vaginal wall is identified by an intravaginal mold or by opacification with packing gauze soaked in radiopaque (40% iodine) material.

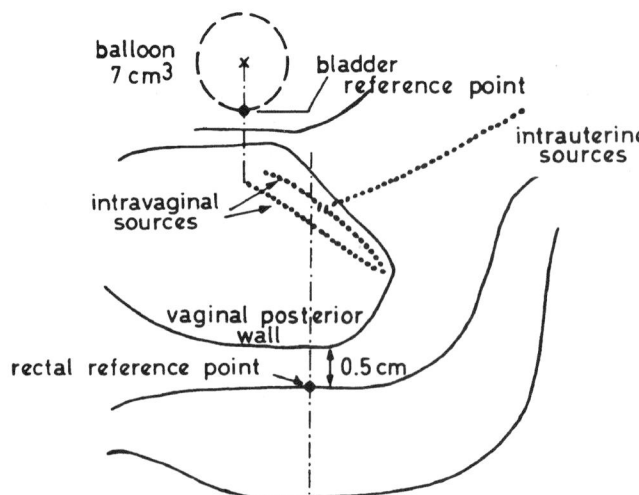

FIG. 14.52. Reference points for bladder and rectal brachytherapy doses proposed by ICRU. (From International Commission on Radiation Units and Measurements. Report 38: dose and volume specification for reporting intracavitary therapy in gynecology. Bethesda, MD: International Commission on Radiation Units, 1985:11, with permission.)

Using CT/MRI–compatible intracavitary applicators, it is possible to outline the critical organs such as rectum and bladder, and evaluate the 3-D dose distributions that they receive from the treatments. Several investigators (250–253) have reported significantly higher maximum bladder and rectum doses, as determined from these 3-D dose distributions, compared with the traditionally reported reference bladder and rectal doses that are evaluated based on planar radiographic films.

Radiation Safety and Quality Assurance in Brachytherapy

The biologic effects of radiation depend not only on dose but also on the type of radiation. The dosimetric quantity in relation to radiation protection is the dose equivalent, H, and is given by the product of the absorbed dose and the quality factor for the radiation. The quality factor is used to equate the biologic effects in tissues produced by different types of radiations. The SI unit for both dose and dose equivalent is joule/kilogram, and, as mentioned earlier, the name for the SI unit of dose equivalent is the sievert (Sv). If the dose is expressed in rad (cGy), the unit for dose equivalent is the rem.

The amount of natural radiation exposure that individuals receive depends on the geographic location in which they live. Also, the human body is naturally radioactive, containing minute quantities of radioactive ^{40}K and ^{226}Ra and trace amounts of other radioisotopes, and contributes 24 mrem to an individual's dose equivalent. Generally, these so-called background radiations produce dose equivalents of 100 to 200 mrem per year. In addition to background radiation, the population is exposed to radiation from various other manmade medical and nonmedical sources.

It is extremely important in the use of brachytherapy to formulate and strictly observe radiation safety procedures at each institution. The safety of personnel, patients, and visitors is based on three basic factors: (a) *time* of radiation exposure as short as possible, (b) *distance* as great as practically allowed between the radioactive sources and the operator, and (c) *shielding* to diminish radiation exposure to all concerned. Furthermore, careful quality control procedures should be followed in the prescription and calculation of doses, preparation, calibration, and handling of radioactive sources and verification of treatment parameters.

Protection Against Radiation from Brachytherapy Sources

This subject has been dealt with in detail in the pertinent NCRP Reports (254). A brief review is presented here.

Storage: Radiation source storage safes, which are lead lined and have lead-filled drawers, are commonly used. Particular attention should be paid to the following consider-

ations when a storage safe is chosen: adequacy of shielding, distribution of sources, and time required for personnel to remove and return sources to the safe. In addition, a radium storage area must be ventilated to a direct filtered exhaust to the outdoors because of possible radon leaks. A sink for cleaning source applicators with a filter or trap to prevent loss of sources should be provided.

Source Preparation: All brachytherapy source preparation should be performed behind a barrier that adequately shields the individual. Typically, a protective L-block shield constructed of lead and having a lead glass viewing window is used. Sources should never be picked up directly with the hands. Instead, long forceps should be used to provide as much distance as possible between the source and the individual's hands.

Source Inventory: A well-defined procedure must be in place to maintain accountability for all sources.

Source Transportation: Sources should be transported in lead containers or leaded carts. The thickness of lead needed depends on the source type and the amount of material.

Leak Testing: Sources must be tested for leaks periodically (typically, every 6 months). Methods of leak-testing a sealed source are reviewed in NCRP Report 40 (254).

At the Department of Radiation Oncology at Washington University, formal quality assurance procedures for brachytherapy have been established to minimize treatment errors. For temporary implants, source loadings are usually prescribed after the physician has reviewed the orthogonal dummy source localization radiographs. The prescription is written on a form that is given to the brachytherapy source curator and specifies the configuration of source strengths for intracavitary treatment or the array of active lengths and linear activity if iridium wires or seed ribbons are used for interstitial techniques. Treatment duration is generally determined after the computer planar isodose rate distributions are reviewed and double-checked with "hand calculations." The source curator documents the preparation of sources in a treatment logbook, on a source inventory sheet that is to be posted on the patient's door, and on a magnetic source inventory board in the radioactive source room. If iridium is used, the vendor's lot identification code is also documented. A well-type dose calibrator is used to verify the source activity (Berkeley). When manual intracavitary afterloading is used, the various cesium tubes are color coded to ensure prompt patient loading. The attending physician or resident (after verifying the source loading) and the source curator load the applicator in the patient. The loading time is documented by the physician, and the curator or physicist measures the radiation exposure levels around the patient and arranges lead shields appropriately. The nursing staff is actively involved in checking every 3 to 4 hours that applicators or sources have not become dislodged over the course of treatment. Procedures for emergency source removal are indicated.

The attending physician or resident is responsible for the unloading of the implant. The physician counts the sources as they are removed and places them in a lead carrier. After the sources are removed, the patient is surveyed to ensure that no sources remain in the patient or in the patient's room. The unloading time is documented, and all radiation warning signs are removed from the patient's door. The source curator checks that all sources have been recovered and returns the sources to their designated storage area. The magnetic inventory board is revised to show that the sources have been returned to the storage area. Additionally, source recovery is documented in the source logbook.

Nuclear Regulatory Commission Regulations

Nuclear Regulatory Commission regulations require that all brachytherapy procedures be carried out by authorized users and that specific procedures be followed (255).

Radiation Safety in the Operating Room

When radioactive sources are prepared in the operating room, a workbench with shielding should be placed in one corner so that during the final preparation of the radioactive materials, no one except the brachytherapy technician preparing them is exposed to radiation. The workbench is designed with a frontal working area with an L-shaped lead screen to protect the trunk, lower extremities, and medial aspect of the arms. In addition, a leaded glass screen reduces exposure to the eyes.

Behind the barrier, there should be a lead well to store the remaining radioactive material while the individual needles, wires, grains, or seeds are being prepared for insertion into the patient. The radioactive sources are immediately placed in the storage well of the workbench and brought into the operating room. The bench is covered with sterile drapes.

Sterilization of the radioactive sources is done by soaking the radium or cesium needles in a germicidal solution such as Cydex. Gold grain magazines and iridium wires are sterilized by gas.

When using radioactive sources, the operating surgeon, assistants, and anesthesiologist work behind individual lead barriers. Exposure to the eyes and hands can be reduced only by distance and by dexterity gained through experience. All radioactive sources should be handled with long instruments. Because most procedures are performed with afterloading techniques, exposure to the fingers during manipulation is minimal.

The details of protective procedures used during the preparation and transportation of radioactive materials and the regulations governing them have been described in detail by various investigators, including Pierquin and associates (256) and Nath et al. (257).

Dose, Time, and Fractionation in Radiation Therapy

The biologic effect of a given dose of radiation on a tissue or tumor depends not only on the total dose but also on the number of fractions and the overall time in which it is delivered. What is observed can be explained in terms of the four "Rs" of radiobiology:

1. Repair of sublethal damage and potentially lethal damage
2. Repopulation of cells between fractions
3. Redistribution of cells throughout the cell cycle (partially because of radiation-induced synchrony)
4. Reoxygenation observed after one or more exposures to radiation

In general, fractionation of irradiation spares acute reactions because of repair of sublethal damage and compensatory proliferation in the epithelium of the skin or mucosa, which accelerates at 2 or 3 weeks after initiation of therapy. Normal tissues behave as actively proliferating cells for expression of acute reactions but as slowly proliferating cells in the manifestation of late injury (258).

The choice of optimal dose/time/fractionation schedules for various tumors should be individualized depending on cell kinetic characteristics and clinical observations (259). Fowler (260) published theoretic considerations based on a series of assumptions of the values used in the linear-quadratic equation with a time factor in which he attempted to predict the optimal dose fractionation schedules for tumors with various cell-doubling times. He concluded that optimal overall times primarily depend on the doubling time of the tumor cells and the intrinsic radiosensitivity, α (assumed to be proportional to α/β). Short overall times are required for tumors with a low α/β ratio or fast proliferation. For median potential doubling times of 5 days and median radiosensitivity, overall times of 2.5 to 4.0 weeks would be optimal. More slowly proliferating tumors (such as most gynecologic tumors) should be treated with longer overall times. Fowler believes that five fractions per week are preferable to three fractions because there is less log cell killing with the latter schedule (about one log for all except overall time of 1 or 2 weeks). He stressed that clinical trials should be carried out to select logically appropriate dose-time schedules. Flow cytometry and other *in vitro* techniques to assess tumor radiosensitivity in biopsy specimens may be helpful in this endeavor.

Altered Fractionation

Without solid biologic basis and out of empiricism and convenience, the "standard" fractionation for radiation therapy has evolved into five weekly fractions. Other fractionation schedules have been proposed that deliver several fractions daily or use a split-course regimen. The various types of schedules are shown in Figure 14.53, and the characteristics of hyperfractionation, accelerated fractionation,

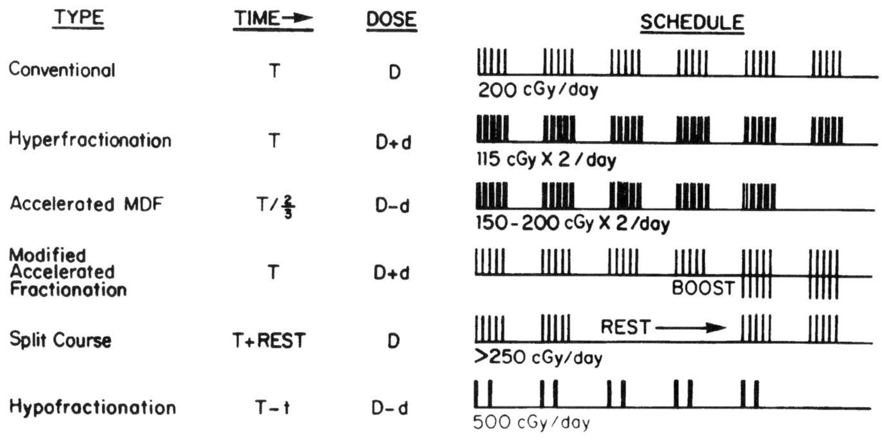

TYPE	TIME→	DOSE	SCHEDULE
Conventional	T	D	200 cGy/day
Hyperfractionation	T	D+d	115 cGy X 2 / day
Accelerated MDF	T/$\frac{2}{3}$	D-d	150-200 cGy X 2/day
Modified Accelerated Fractionation	T	D+d	BOOST
Split Course	T+REST	D	REST → >250 cGy/day
Hypofractionation	T-t	D-d	500 cGy/day

FIG. 14.53. Various types of fractionation schedules used in radiation therapy. (From Perez CA, Brady LW, Roti Roti JL. Overview. In: Perez CA, Brady LW, eds. *Principles and practice of radiation oncology.* 3rd ed. Philadelphia: Lippincott–Raven, 1998:1, with permission.)

or split-course schedules, as well as potential advantages or disadvantages, are summarized in Table 14.7.

The advantages of prolonging the time for a course of therapy are: (a) it spares acute reactions because compensatory proliferation in skin or mucosa accelerates at 2 or 3 weeks after starting a course of daily irradiation; (b) it allows better reoxygenation in tumors during fractionated therapy; and (c) it avoids the use of large doses per fraction (greater than 2 or 3 Gy) that may cause greater normal tissue damage later. On the other hand, the disadvantages are: (a) tumor cells may proliferate, thus making ultimate cure less likely (for the same tumor dose); (b) it is inconvenient for patients; and (c) there is less efficiency in the operation of the department.

When multiple daily fractionation is used, biologic studies suggest that a minimum of 4 and preferably 6 or even 8 hours should be allowed between fractions to allow maximum repair of normal late-responding tissues (261,262).

With *accelerated fractionation,* several fractions of radiation (two or three) are given daily over a shorter total period. The indication for such a protocol is a rapidly growing tumor in which significant repopulation may occur during prolonged treatment. In practice, some reduction in total dose or a rest interval must be allowed because acutely responding normal tissues cannot tolerate the accelerated schedule. These schedules appear to be preferable for use with hypoxic cell sensitizers or other chemical modifiers of radiation response that require the presence of a high concentration of the compound in the tumor at the time of radiation exposure.

With *hyperfractionation,* a larger number of smaller than conventional dose fractions are given daily. The total dose administered daily is usually 10% to 15% greater than with standard fractionation: the total period of time is unchanged, and the total dose administered is higher than with standard fractionation. The goal of hyperfractionation is to achieve the same incidence of late effects on normal tissue that is observed with a comparable conventional regimen, whereas increasing the probability of tumor control (262).

TABLE 14.7. *Comparison of various external beam irradiation fractionation schedules*

	Conventional	Split-Course	Accelerated (Multiple Daily Fractions)	Hyperfractionation
Indication, in tumors, of growth rate	Average	Average or slow	Rapid	Slow (with large cell loss factors)
Normal tissue effects, acute	Standard	Standard or greater	Greater	Standard or greater
Normal tissue effects, late	Standard	Greater	Standard (if complete repair of sublethal occurs) or greater	Lower
Advantages		Shorter actual treatment time (fewer fractions)	Destroys more tumor cells; prevents tumor cell repopulation; less overall treatment time	(?)Lower oxygen enhancement ratio with small doses; spares late damage; allows reoxygenation; allows stem cell repopulation
Disadvantages		May permit tumor repopulation		More fractions

Source: Perez CA, Brady LW, Roti Roti JL. Overview. In: Perez CA, Brady LW, eds. *Principles and practice of radiation oncology.* 3rd ed. Philadelphia: Lippincott–Raven, 1998, with permission.

Although there are no data for human tumors, Withers and associates (258) believe it is reasonable to postulate that tumors with an actively dividing clonogenic population will respond like acutely reacting normal tissues, whereas those with slowly dividing clonogens would mimic slowly reacting normal tissues.

Accelerated Repopulation

Hermens and Barendsen (263) showed that accelerated repopulation of tumor cells occurred following irradiation. Withers and associates (264) summarized the results of irradiation of human head and neck cancer and suggested that the same phenomenon of accelerated proliferation could be seen. The effectiveness of a course of fractionated irradiation depends on the killing by individual fractions as well as on the rate of proliferation of surviving cells between irradiation fractions. Neoadjuvant chemotherapy might also lead to increased proliferation of surviving tumor cells after partial regression of the lesion, which could result in decreased cell killing by subsequent fractionated irradiation. The total dose of irradiation to produce a 50% probability of tumor control must be increased when fractionation is prolonged beyond 4 weeks because of repopulation of surviving cells, which may result in improved nutrition of those cells following early shrinkage of the tumor due to the initial irradiation fractions. In carcinoma of the uterine cervix, Fyles et al. (265) and Perez et al. (266) estimated that the dose of irradiation should be increased by 0.6 Gy for every day of interruption or prolongation of the overall treatment time beyond 7 weeks.

Isoeffect Graphs

In 1944, Strandqvist (267) published a classic monograph describing the results of treatment of 280 patients with skin cancer (squamous-cell and basal-cell carcinoma). An isoeffect line was drawn, plotting total dose against overall time, both on log scales, which resulted in a straight line with a slope of 0.22. This indicates that dose and time are related by a simple power function:

$$\text{Total dose} \propto (\text{overall time})^{0.22}$$

He also produced a graph for various degrees of radiation reaction on the skin, ranging from erythema to necrosis, which all had a slope of 0.33.

Analysis of a vast body of data on skin cancer by Cohen (268) demonstrated that, in general, the slope of the isoeffect curve for tumor curability is less steep than that for normal tissue reactions, in contrast to Strandqvist, whose limited data indicated that they were the same. Furthermore, as stated earlier, tolerance of normal tissues is strongly related to the volume irradiated.

The major contribution of Ellis (269) was to point out that

"overall time" in the Strandqvist and Cohen plots included different numbers of fractions as well. He separated out these two parameters and showed that number of fractions was much more important than overall time. For example, 60 Gy in 6 weeks in 30 fractions given five times weekly would not result in the same normal tissue damage as the same dose in the same time given in only 18 fractions, three fractions per week.

Clinical Observations on Dose-Time and Tumor Control

Different fractionation schedules have been shown to affect therapeutic outcome with low LET radiations (photons and electrons). Fowler and coworkers (270), in experiments using a mammary murine adenocarcinoma, demonstrated that with different fractionated schedules of x irradiation there was an optimal time (about 10 days) to obtain tumor control in about 50% of the animals with the various schedules. With a shorter time, only the multiple daily fraction schedule (nine fractions) was effective. If a longer period was allowed (18 days), the probability of tumor control decreased even with multiple-fraction schedules (15 fractions) because of tumor proliferation. Fowler (271), on the other hand, showed no significant impact of fractionation on tumor control or survival in mice irradiated with neutrons.

There is a potential impact of modifying the overall time by split course when the daily fractions of radiation administered are higher than conventional (administration of 2.5 to 3.0 Gy tumor dose for 10 fractions, 2 or 3 weeks' rest, and administration of a second course similar to the first one for a total of 50 or 60 Gy). The RTOG reported no therapeutic advantage of this regimen in carcinoma of the uterine cervix (272). The tumor control and survival rates were comparable to those obtained with conventional fractionation. If anything, the late effects were slightly greater with the split-course regimen.

In contrast, reports published by the University of Florida on patients with carcinoma of the uterine cervix treated to definitive doses of radiation therapy with conventional fractionation but with a rest period halfway through the course of therapy showed that some groups of patients in the split-course regimen exhibited lower tumor control and survival (273). This is most probably a result of the repopulation of clonogenic surviving cells in the tumor during the rest period.

Clinical Observations on Dose-Time and Normal Tissue Effects

Several studies have been implemented in a variety of human tissues in an effort to determine the dose-time relationship. Figure 14.54 illustrates the tolerance limits for several organs. Examples of the effects of different fractionation

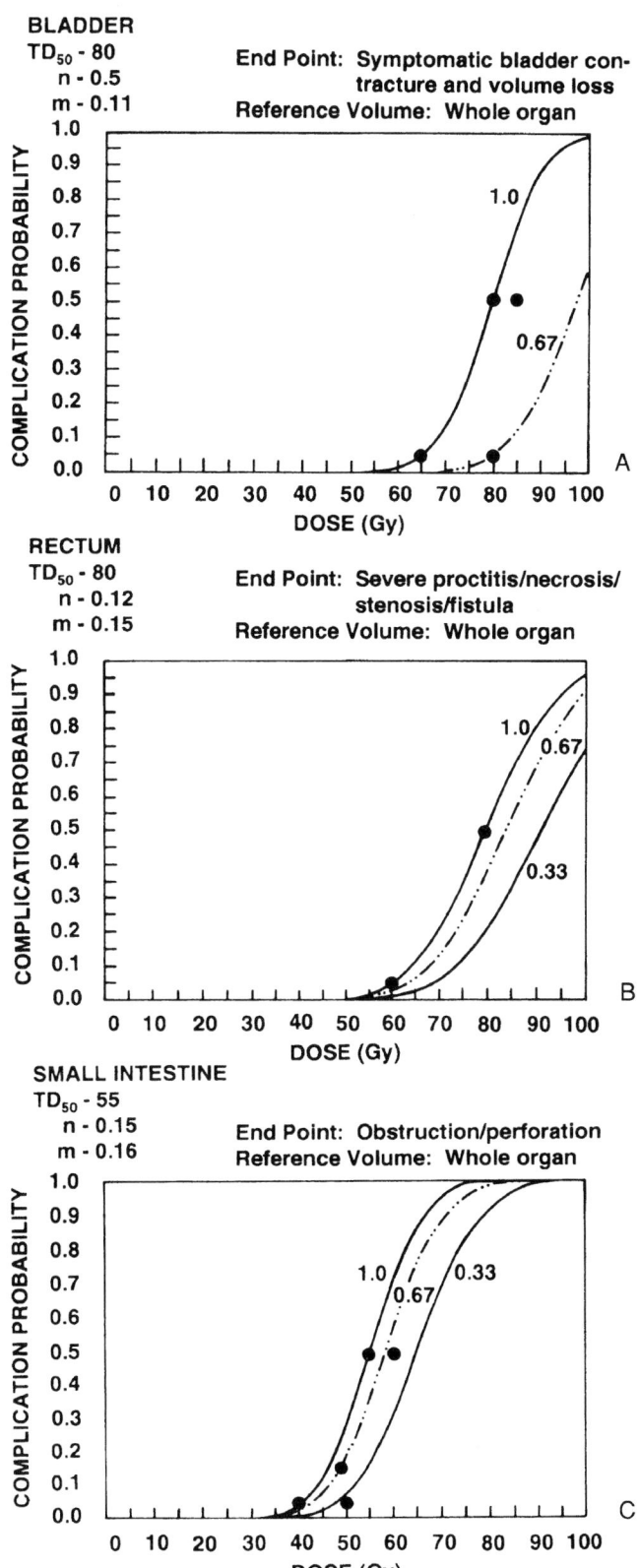

FIG. 14.54. Normal-tissue radiation tolerance: **(A)** Bladder. **(B)** Rectum. **(C)** Small intestine. (Reprinted from Burman C, Kutcher GJ, Emami B, et al. Fitting of normal tissue tolerance data to an analytic function. *Int J Radiat Oncol Biol Phys* 1991: 21:123–135, with permission from Elsevier.)

schedules and normal tissue effects have been reported for several organs.

Singh (274) noted more serious late complications (12 in 24 patients) after five weekly doses of 5.8 Gy in patients with stage III carcinoma of the uterine cervix using equal nominal standard doses in radiation equivalent therapy (ret units) (time-dose factor of 66) when compared with patients receiving 2 Gy daily, five times per week (none in 24 patients). Eight patients in each group developed proctitis lasting over 6 months.

Meoz and associates (275) reported on 30 patients with advanced pelvic malignancies who were treated with three once per week doses of 10 Gy that were preceded by 4 g/m^2 of misonidazole. There were five major complications (three bowel obstructions, one bowel perforation, and one vesicovaginal fistula), which is considered excessive for palliative treatment.

In contrast, Spanos and colleagues (276) reported on a Phase II study of daily multifraction split-course irradiation in 142 patients (half had recurrent or metastatic disease in the pelvis only and the other half had associated extrapelvic metastases) who received 3.7 Gy per fraction given twice daily for 2 consecutive days, repeated at 3- to 6-week intervals for a total of three courses, aiming to a total tumor dose of 44.4 Gy. The dose was based on linear-quadratic equation considerations of acute and late effects, assuming an α/β ratio of 10 for acute and 4 for late effects. Twenty-seven patients survived more than 1 year: there were only two recorded cases of grade 3 lower gastrointestinal tract toxicity.

RTOG has conducted several clinical trials with either hyperfractionated or accelerated fractionation schedules in a variety of tumors and normal tissues. We must wait for some time for the late effects on normal tissues to manifest themselves before drawing definite conclusions about the safety of these altered fractionation schedules.

The effect of dose fractionation on normal tissue effects has been emphasized by experimental and clinical observations on late effects in animals and patients treated with single-dose intraoperative radiation therapy. Doses of 10 to 15 Gy have an effect five times or greater than the same amount of irradiation given in 2-Gy fractions (277). Osteosarcoma occurred in 21% (8 of 38) of the dogs that received doses greater than 25 Gy intraoperatively. However, only one of four dogs that received 25-Gy intraoperative irradiation combined with 50-Gy external beam irradiation developed a tumor, and none occurred at doses below this level. LeCouteur and associates (278) reported severe peripheral neuropathy in dogs receiving doses of intraoperative irradiation of approximately 20 Gy, whereas dogs treated with less than 15 Gy did not have evidence of neuropathy. Likewise, Shaw and coworkers (279) noted peripheral neuropathy in 32% of 50 patients who received intraoperative irradiation as a component of therapy for primary or recurrent pelvic cancer: the development of neurotoxicity was more common with doses of 15 to 25 Gy than with doses of 10.0 to 12.5 Gy.

Linear-Quadratic Equation (α/β Ratio)

Besides the isoeffect concepts previously discussed, more recent formulations based on dose survival models have been proposed to evaluate the biologic equivalence of various doses and fractionation schedules. These assumptions are based on a linear-quadratic survival curve represented by the equation:

$$Log_e\ S = \alpha D + \beta D^2$$

in which αD represents the linear, nonreparable component of log cell killing, and βD^2 represents a component of cell killing that is a quadratic function of dose because it involves multiple events, as described earlier (Fig. 14.55). The dose at which the two components of cell killing are equal constitutes the α/β ratio.

The overall effect of many small fractions is to amplify the dominance of the α component. The β effect is then unimportant because repair will be almost complete. The more radiocurable tumors have higher α values than the less curable tumors.

The shape of the dose survival curves with photons differs for acutely and slowly responding normal tissues, although this is not observed with neutrons (Fig. 14.56). The severity of the late effects changes more rapidly with a variation in the size of dose per fraction when a total dose is selected to

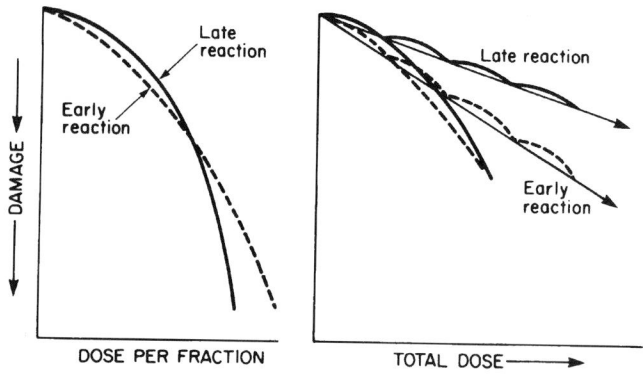

FIG. 14.56. Difference in cell survival curves for acute and late radiation effects with single or multifractionated doses of irradiation. (Reprinted from Fowler JF. Fractionation and therapeutic gain. In: Steel GG, Adams GE, Peckham MT, eds. *Biological basis of radiotherapy.* Amsterdam: Elsevier Science, 1983:181, with permission from Elsevier.)

yield equivalent acute effects. With a decreasing size of dose per fraction, the total dose required to achieve a certain isoeffect increases more for late-responding tissues than for acutely responding tissues. Thus, in hyperfractionated regimens, the tolerable dose would be increased more for late effects than for acute effects. Conversely, if large doses per fraction are used, the total dose required to achieve isoeffects in late-responding tissues would be reduced more for late effects than for acute effects. In general, acutely reacting tissues have a high α/β ratio (between 6 and 15 Gy), whereas those tissues involved in late effects have a low α/β ratio (1 to 5 Gy). Some of these values for normal tissues and tumors are summarized in Table 14.8.

Two treatment regimens can be compared with the following formula:

$$\frac{Dr}{Dx} = \frac{\alpha/\beta + dx}{\alpha/\beta + dr}$$

in which Dr = known total dose (reference dose)
Dx = new total dose (with different fractionation schedule)
dr = known fractionation (reference)
dx = new fractionation schedule.

An example of use of this formula is as follows: Suppose 50 Gy in 25 fractions is delivered to yield a given biologic effect. If one assumes that the subcutaneous tissue is the limiting parameter (late reaction), it is desirable to know what the total dose to be administered will be using 4-Gy fractions. Assume α/β = 5 Gy.

Using the above formula,

$$Dx = Dr\frac{\alpha/\beta + dr}{\alpha/\beta + dx}$$

Thus,

$$Dx = 50\ Gy\ \frac{5 + 2}{5 + 4} = 39\ Gy$$

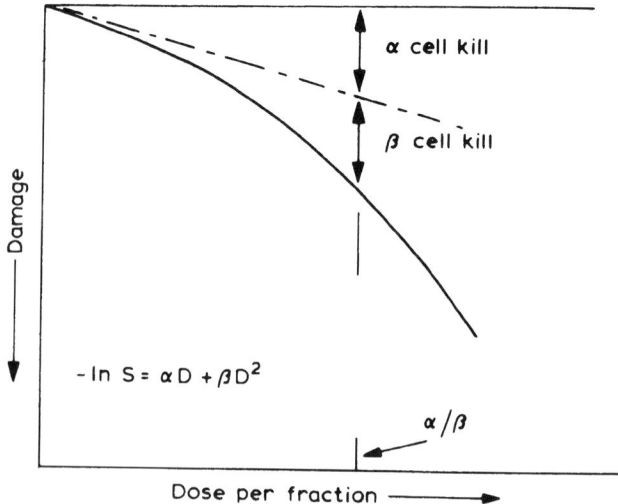

FIG. 14.55. At a dose equal to the α/β ratio, the log cell kill due to the α process (nonreparable) is equal to that due to the β process (reparable injury): α/β is thus a measure of how soon the survival curve begins to bend over significantly. (Reprinted from Fowler JR. Fractionation and therapeutic gain. In: Steel GG, Adams GE, Peckham MJ, eds. *Biological basis of radiotherapy.* Amsterdam: Elsevier Science, 1983: 181–194, with permission from Elsevier.)

TABLE 14.8. α/β *ratios for human normal tissues and tumors*

Tissue or Organ	Endpoint	α/β (Gy)[a]
Early reactions		
Skin	Erythema	8.8–12.3
Mucosa	Desquamation	11.2
Oral mucosa	Mucositis	815
Late reactions		
Skin/vasculature	Telangiectasia	2.6–2.8
Subcutis	Fibrosis	1.7
Muscle/vasculature/cartilage	Impaired shoulder movement	3.5
Nerve	Brachial plexopathy	~2 to <3.6[b]
	Optic neuropathy	1.6
Spinal cord	Myelopathy	<3.3
Eye	Corneal injury	2.9
Bowel	Stricture/perforation	3.9
Lung	Pneumonitis	3.3
	Fibrosis (radiologic)	3.1
Head and neck	Various late effects	3.5–3.8
Oral cavity and oropharynx	Various late effects	0.8
Tumors		
Head and neck		
Larynx		14.5[b]
Vocal cord		~13
Oropharynx		~16[b]
Buccal mucosa		6.6
Tonsil		7.2
Nasopharynx		16
Skin		8.5[b]
Melanoma		0.6
Liposarcoma		4

[a] Studies related to these data may be found in the original publication.
[b] Reanalysis of original published data.
Source: Compiled by Bentzen and Thames (unpublished). See also Thames HD, Bentzen SM, Turesson I, et al. Time-dose factors in radiotherapy: a review of the human data. *Radiother Oncol* 1990;19:219. (Modified from Joiner MC, van der Kogel AJ. The value of α/β. In: Steel GG, ed. *Basic clinical radiobiology.* 2nd ed. London: Arnold, 1997;111, with permission.)

Yaes (280) proposed a modification of the linear-quadratic isoeffect model in which the effect of proliferation is taken into account for multiple daily fractionation schedules. The proposed isoeffect relationship involves the fraction size and the total dose of irradiation and predicts higher isoeffect doses for small dose fractions.

Linear-quadratic models may be used to calculate the α/β ratio in some clinical situations (178). For instance, Bentzen and associates (281), in 163 patients receiving postmastectomy irradiation (36.6 Gy in 12 fractions, two fractions per week, or 40.92 Gy in 22 fractions, five fractions per week), analyzed the occurrence of impaired shoulder movement resulting from fibrosis. The α/β ratio was estimated at 3.5 Gy.

Effects of Irradiation on Abdominal and Pelvic Normal Tissues

Chronologically, the effects of irradiation have been categorized as *acute* (first 6 months), *subacute* (second 6 months), or *late*, when they are observed, after 6 months (282). The gross manifestations depend on the kinetic properties of the cells (slow or rapid renewal), architecture of the tissues (serial or parallel), volume of tissue irradiated, the dose, and fractionation of irradiation given.

No correlation has been established between the incidence and severity of acute reactions and late effects. Withers and colleagues (258) compiled data depicting isoeffect lines for acute or late effects in several organs. The slopes for late reactions were steeper than for acute effects, and the doses required for acute effects did not correlate with those for late effects. This may be due to the difference in the cell survival (curves) for acute or late effects (Fig. 14.56) (283).

Factors enhancing propensity to radiation injury may include the general and nutritional condition of the patient, hygiene, superimposed infection, or trauma (physical or chemical). Combining irradiation with surgery or cytotoxic agents frequently modifies the tolerance of normal tissues to a given dose of radiation (Fig. 14.57), which may necessitate adjustments in treatment planning.

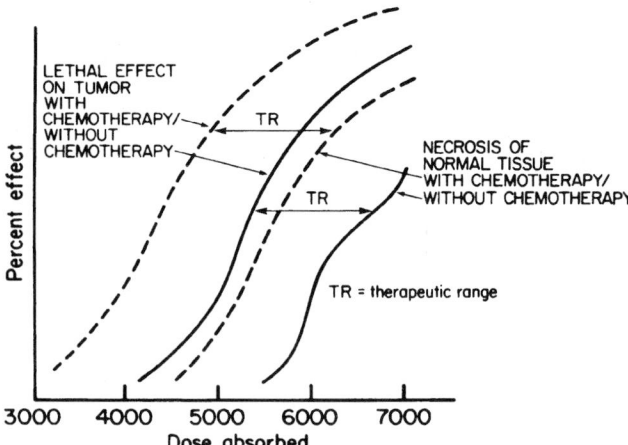

FIG. 14.57. Theoretic curves for tumor control and complications as a function of radiation dose both with and without chemotherapy. TR = Therapeutic range, or the difference between tumor control and complication frequency. (Reprinted from Perez CA, Thomas PRM. Radiation therapy: basic concepts and clinical implications. In: Sutow WW, Fernbach DJ, Vietti TJ, eds. *Clinical pediatric oncology.* 3rd ed. St. Louis: Mosby, 1984:167, with permission from Elsevier.)

Although most of the information concerning the effects of radiation on normal tissues is fragmentary and, in general, incomplete, several reviews have been published (226,284): the most comprehensive was published by Rubin and Casarett (282) more than 30 years ago and later updated by Emami et al. (285). Significant changes in those organs commonly irradiated in the treatment of gynecologic tumors are discussed briefly in the following sections.

Skin

Depending on the type of radiation and energy used and the area treated, different exposure doses of radiation are necessary to produce skin changes. These effects evolve from erythema to dry desquamation, moist desquamation, and ulceration with necrosis and are more frequently seen with lower energy and orthovoltage equipment. With ^{60}Co, high-energy x-rays, neutrons, and high-energy electrons, subcutaneous fibrosis is more frequently observed.

In general, single doses ranging from 6 Gy (superficial machine) to 7.5 Gy (orthovoltage machines) are necessary to produce erythema. With low-energy x-ray fractionated doses (2 Gy per day), erythema is usually noted after 20 Gy and with ^{60}Co or 4- to 6-MV x-rays after higher doses. Dry desquamation appears with doses over 50 Gy delivered with megavoltage equipment. Skin ulceration or necrosis may appear with doses over 65 Gy.

With moderate doses of radiation (up to 60 Gy), there is transient epilation from which the patient usually recovers in 3 to 6 months. The other skin appendages, as well as the fingernails, follow the same recovery pattern. It has been shown that these effects may be enhanced by the combination of irradiation and some chemotherapeutic agents, particularly actinomycin D and doxorubicin (Adriamycin). It is also well known that chemotherapy can "recall" radiation reactions after the radiation therapy has been completed and the original reaction subsides (286). With larger doses of radiation (>60 Gy), permanent epilation, as well as depopulation of sebaceous and sweat glands, may be observed.

Chronic and late effects are characterized by atrophy of the epidermis, epilation with loss of hair follicles and sebaceous and sweat glands, telangiectasia, occasional hyperpigmentation, and areas of hyperkeratosis. Large doses of irradiation may produce necrosis and ulceration with complete denudation of the skin, vascular degeneration, fibrosis, and associated inflammation. Split- or full-thickness skin grafts may not be successful after doses of 60 Gy. In this case, a skin graft with a vascular pedicle is required.

Small and Large Intestine

It is common to observe watery diarrhea with intermittent abdominal cramping starting in the second or third week of abdominal or pelvic irradiation. Increased peristalsis, disturbance of the absorption mechanisms, and a decreased transit time also occur (287). When the rectum is included in the irradiated volume, there is rectal discomfort, tenesmus, and mucus, sometimes mixed with blood, in the stools.

Despite a rapid cell turnover, small bowel mucosal changes have been associated with necrosis of proliferating epithelial cells in the crypts of Lieberkühn, degeneration of endothelial cells, edema of the submucosal connective tissues, inflammatory cell infiltration, and sometimes leakage of erythrocytes (288). If the dose of radiation is large enough, it may cause temporary or permanent ulceration. This type of lesion may be associated with either fibrosis and stenosis or perforation with fistula formation. In general, doses of 60 Gy are necessary to produce this more advanced radiation damage to the small bowel (Fig. 14.58) and the entire rectosigmoid. Recent careful dosimetric analyses have shown that limited volumes of the rectum can tolerate doses of about 75 Gy (external beam and brachytherapy) with an acceptable morbidity (Fig. 14.59) (289).

Doxorubicin and 5-fluorouracil enhance radiation effects in the intestine more than other cytotoxic agents (290).

Liver

Clinical and pathologic studies have shown that the liver is not a radioresistant organ. The clinical course and liver changes depend on the dose of irradiation and are characterized by liver enlargement and varying amounts of ascites (291). Laboratory studies frequently show abnormal liver function tests, but the alkaline phosphatase test has been the most reliable single laboratory study (291). Ogata and coworkers (292) described postirradiation changes in hepatic

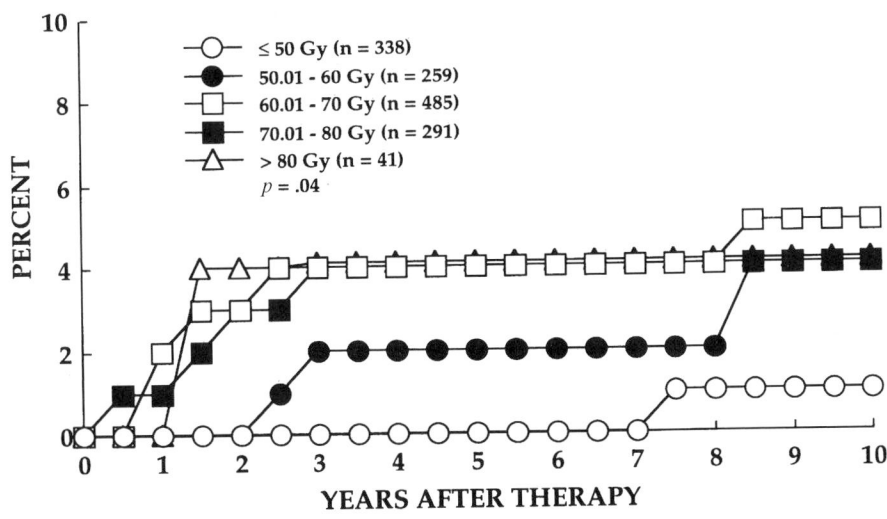

FIG. 14.58. Actuarial rate of severe small bowel sequelae correlated with total dose to lateral pelvic nodes in carcinoma of uterine cervix (Mallinckrodt Institute of Radiology). (Reprinted from Perez CA, Grigsby PW, Lockett MA, et al. Radiation therapy morbidity in carcinoma of the uterine cervix: dosimetric and clinical correlation. *Int J Radiat Oncol Biol Phys* 1999:44:855, with permission from Elsevier.)

vessels, particularly in the centrolobar vein branches of three patients in whom part of the liver was irradiated during treatment of lung tumors. Ingold and associates (291) reported similar findings in a group of 40 patients receiving irradiation alone to the entire liver during the treatment of disseminated ovarian carcinoma or malignant lymphoma. No damage was observed with doses below 30 Gy. After doses of 35 to 40 Gy, almost half of the patients showed radiation damage, and with doses over 40 Gy, 75% of the patients developed radiation hepatitis (291). Lower doses are reported to produce hepatitis when administered concomitantly with cytotoxic drugs. Hepatic cell necrosis and connective tissue proliferation within the lumen of small efferent veins, without preexisting thrombosis, have been described.

Kidney

Functional changes have been described after exposure of the kidney to irradiation. Symptoms of acute radiation

nephritis, which usually appear within 6 months of irradiation with doses in the range of 20 to 23 Gy in 3 to 5 weeks, are lassitude, headaches, shortness of breath, vomiting, nocturia, and leg edema (293). Both systolic and diastolic pressures can be elevated. Urinary output is adequate, and urinalysis shows albuminuria and low specific gravity. Gross hematuria never occurs, although epithelial and hyaline casts are seen, and red blood cells may be observed on microscopic examination. A normocytic, normochromic anemia may appear. Renal function studies are abnormal, and the blood urea nitrogen (BUN) level is elevated. Grave prognostic signs are generalized edema and a BUN over 100 mg/100 mL. Blood pressure alone is not a reliable prognostic sign, but increasing hypertension associated with progressive anemia and a rising BUN level is ominous (293).

Chronic nephritis usually appears about 18 months or later after exposure to radiation. The clinical course is slow, with progressive anemia, arterial hypertension, and impairment of renal function. Some patients may not have manifestations

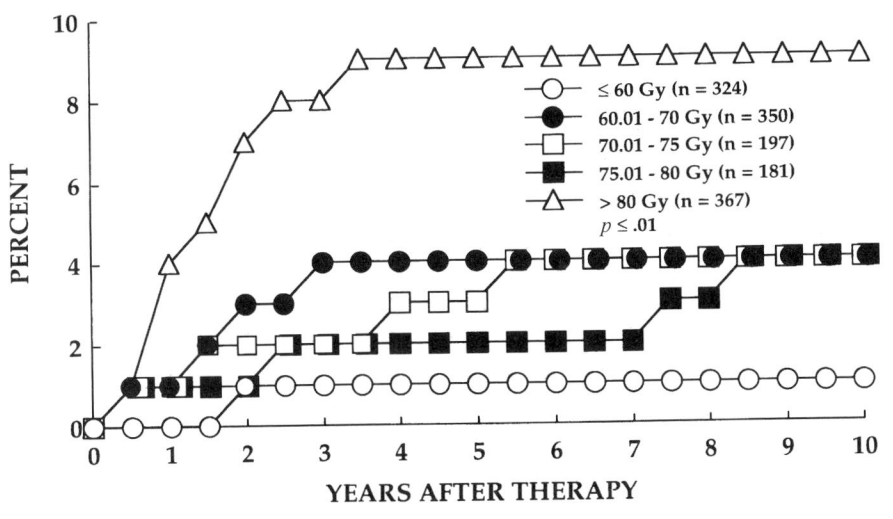

FIG. 14.59. Actuarial rate of severe rectum-rectosigmoid sequelae correlated with total dose to rectum in carcinoma of uterine cervix (Mallinckrodt Institute of Radiology). (Reprinted from Perez CA, Grigsby PW, Lockett MA, et al. Radiation therapy morbidity in carcinoma of the uterine cervix: dosimetric and clinical correlation. *Int J Radiat Oncol Biol Phys* 1999:44:855, with permission from Elsevier.)

of acute nephritis, and the first manifestations of renal damage are decreased specific gravity of the urine and albuminuria. The BUN level may be elevated. Anemia is always present. Renal function studies show decreased blood flow and filtration rates. Intravenous pyelograms may show good excretion of contrast material, but the kidneys are small.

Rather uncommon is the development of malignant hypertension, which is manifested by severe hypertensive encephalopathy, throbbing headaches, papilledema, retinitis, and hemorrhages. These side effects usually appear after a latent period of 18 to 24 months, and the absence of acute renal failure or severe renal impairment suggests a different pathophysiologic mechanism (293). Albuminuria may be present, but the urine is otherwise normal. Renal function is preserved until the terminal phase.

Patients with chronic radiation nephritis may die of chronic uremia or renal failure, malignant hypertension, cerebral vascular accident, or congestive heart failure secondary to increased blood pressure. However, hypertension caused by unilateral nephritis can be reversed after nephrectomy if it is performed early enough.

Bladder

Acute and transient radiation cystitis may be observed with moderate doses of irradiation (>30 Gy) and usually requires no specific treatment. However, with higher doses, more severe symptoms of cystitis develop, which may require treatment. Congestion of the mucosa and swelling of the bladder wall are noted. Significant spasm of the bladder musculature, which may be improved with administration of smooth muscle relaxants, may also occur. It is important to rule out the presence of a concomitant bacterial infection, which may exacerbate the symptoms. Urinalysis and urine cultures obtained under sterile conditions, when indicated, should be obtained before institution of antibiotic therapy.

With doses above 60 Gy to the entire bladder, chronic cystitis and occasionally hematuria may be observed (because of telangiectasis in the bladder mucosa). With higher doses, more severe chronic cystitis, fibrosis, and decreased bladder capacity, as well as vesicovaginal fistula, may occur. Studies have demonstrated that with doses below 75 to 80 Gy to limited volumes of the bladder, the incidence of grade 3 or 4 complications is 5% or less, whereas with higher doses, a greater incidence of sequelae is noted (Fig. 14.60) (289,294).

Ovaries

Ovarian irradiation has been shown to reduce significantly the urinary excretion of estrogens: serum gonadotropins will be elevated if permanent damage has occurred. In women treated with doses of 1 to 2 Gy, which may be equivalent to the scattered irradiation dose that some patients could receive during the treatment of a thoracic or abdominal malignancy, some transient effects on the granulosa cells have been observed, and menstruation may be temporarily irregular. With larger doses that cause greater injury to the granulosa cells, there may be no recovery. The oocyte degenerates, and the follicle becomes atrophic. After small doses of radiation in both the testes and ovaries, numerous chromosomal abnormalities are observed in germ cells, even for prolonged periods (295). Because there are no stem cells in the ovary analogous to the type A spermatogonia of the male, radiation damage of the follicles may result in permanent sterility. Small doses of radiation (as low as 3 Gy) may produce appreciable cellular killing in the ovary: with larger doses, menopausal symptoms and sterility may be produced (296).

The dose necessary to castrate a woman depends on her age: a larger dose is required during the period of more active follicular proliferation. A single dose of 6.5 to 8.0 Gy or fractionated doses of 15 to 20 Gy (depending on age) are known to produce permanent castration and sterility in most patients. Midline oophoropexy has been used in young

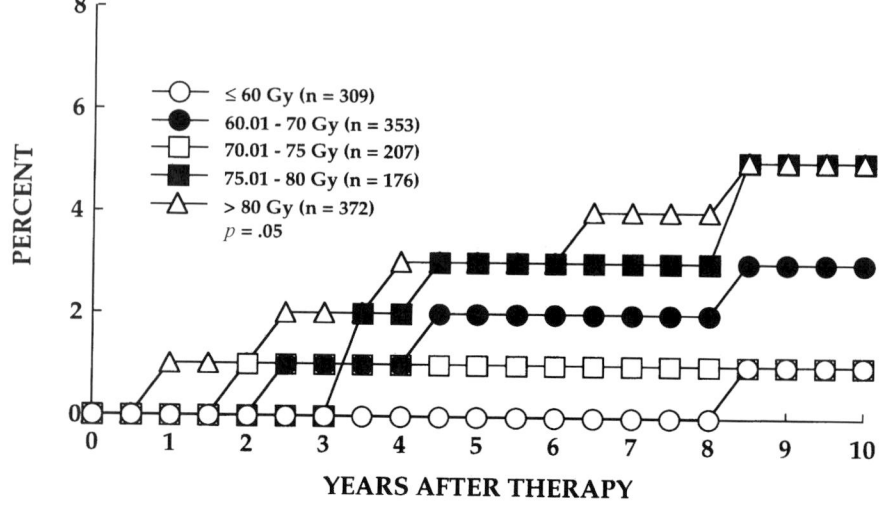

FIG. 14.60. Actuarial rate of severe urinary sequelae correlated with total dose to bladder in carcinoma of uterine cervix (Mallinckrodt Institute of Radiology). (Reprinted from Perez CA, Grigsby PW, Lockett MA, et al. Radiation therapy morbidity in carcinoma of the uterine cervix: dosimetric and clinical correlation. *Int J Radiat Oncol Biol Phys* 1999;44:855, with permission from Elsevier.)

women treated with irradiation for Hodgkin's disease in an effort to spare the ovaries.

Bone Marrow

The acute effects of irradiation on the bone marrow are usually observed after whole-body irradiation, and they mostly result from direct cell killing. Within a few hours after a large dose of radiation, there is prompt reduction in the number of lymphocytes and, consequently, the white blood count. A significant drop in lymphocytes has been found in humans after a single dose of as little as 0.25 Gy total-body irradiation because of the marked sensitivity of circulating lymphocytes to interphase irradiation. The lymphocyte count will remain low for a week, and if the dose of radiation is not lethal, slow repopulation may be seen after this time. However, local-field irradiation may also induce transient lymphopenia, which is thought to be the result of irradiation of the lymphocytes circulating through the vascular bed and may not be indicative of bone marrow reserve depletion. The granulocyte decrease is noted a day after radiation exposure, and the lowest value is reached after about a week. This is due to the killing of stem cells and lack of repopulation. After sublethal doses of radiation, the granulocytes do not return to normal for at least 2 to 3 weeks, and it is during this period that death from bone marrow depression during acute radiation sickness occurs. Thrombocytopenia caused by radiation effects on the platelets leads to hemorrhages in these patients with ecchymosis, hematemesis, and melena, which complicate fluid and electrolyte imbalance during the first and second week after exposure. The circulating red cells are extremely radioresistant. Chronic irradiation, however, may give rise to protracted anemia, because erythropoietic tissue seems to have less ability to recover from radiation damage than granulopoietic tissue.

More permanent chronic changes are noted even when small segments of the bone marrow are irradiated to doses over 30 Gy, and recovery may take up to 18 months or longer in a proportion of patients with good reparative capacity. Fatty infiltration of the bone marrow, vascular degeneration, and fibrosis, which prevent repopulation, are noted (297). As the volume of bone marrow irradiated increases, so does the dose required to prevent regeneration. These changes are more prominent in patients who have received bone marrow–depressing chemotherapeutic agents or those treated with these drugs after radiation therapy and older patients (298). Special care should be exercised for patients receiving combination therapy or retreatment after irradiation or chemotherapy: frequent white blood cell and platelet counts are necessary, particularly if the bone marrow is infiltrated with malignant cells.

Peripheral Nerves

Although radiation-induced lumbosacral plexopathy is a rare complication of pelvic irradiation, Georgiou and colleagues (299) reported four cases among 2,410 patients treated to the pelvis for carcinoma of the cervix or endometrium. All patients received external beam and intracavitary irradiation. The total calculated dose to the lumbosacral plexus was approximately 73 Gy. Lumbosacral or pelvic nerve neuropathy has been observed in patients with single-dose intraoperative irradiation to doses of 15 to 25 Gy (300, 301).

Combination of Irradiation with Other Therapeutic Modalities

Steel and associates (302) summarized the biologic basis of combined modality therapy as spatial cooperation (different compartments of efficacy), additivity of antitumor effect by two or more agents, and nonoverlapping toxicity.

Irradiation and Surgery

The main combinations of surgery and radiation therapy revolve around preoperative, postoperative, and intraoperative radiation therapy; the use of surgery or irradiation alone to treat the primary disease and lymph node metastases; or less than conventional surgery followed by irradiation for regional subclinical disease. Some types of tumors are indications for combined surgery and radiation therapy, including those with low cure rates with either modality alone, those with great potential for recurrence or residual disease after surgery, and those at risk for lymphatic invasion. Preservation of function and desire to enhance cosmesis are also indications for combined therapy.

The combination of surgery and radiation therapy has produced neither dramatic nor substantial improvement in the survival of patients with cancer. This may be due in part to the lack of analysis of reasons for locoregional failure and to the potential for disseminated metastases. Failure to demonstrate the real value of combined surgery-radiation therapy is probably also related to indiscriminate application of combined management to all patients, including inappropriate groups, such as those in whom disease is too advanced locally and regionally and those who have substantial potential for disseminated disease at the time of initial treatment.

The rationale for preoperative radiation therapy relates to its potential ability to eradicate subclinical disease beyond the margins of the surgical resection, to diminish tumor implantation by decreasing the number of viable cells within the operative field, to sterilize lymph node metastases outside the operative field, to decrease the potential for dissemination of clonogenic tumor cells that might produce distant metastases, and to increase the possibility of resectability. Tumor cells can be disseminated beyond the operative field (outside the subsequently irradiated volume) during surgery, and surgical trauma may interfere with the vascular supply of the tissues, thereby rendering hypoxic the residual tumor cells within the postoperatively irradiated volume. The main disadvantage of preoperative irradiation is that it may interfere with normal healing of the tissues affected by the radiation. Such interference, however, is minimal when the radiation doses are below 45 to 50 Gy in 5 weeks.

The rationale for postoperative irradiation is based on the fact that it is possible to treat any residual tumor in the operative field (a) by destroying subclinical foci of tumor cells following the surgical procedure, (b) by eradicating adjacent subclinical foci of cancer (including lymph node metastases), and (c) by delivering higher doses than can be achieved with preoperative irradiation, with the greater dose being directed to the volume of high risk or known residual disease. The potential disadvantage of postoperative irradiation is that a delay is imposed on the initiation of radiation therapy until wound healing is completed. Theoretic and experimental evidence suggests that the radiation effect may be impaired by vascular changes produced in the tumor bed by surgery. Experimental data suggest that preoperative irradiation may be more effective than postoperative irradiation.

Irradiation and Chemotherapy

Chemotherapy alone or combined with irradiation may be used in several settings. In primary chemotherapy, the modality is used (a) as definitive treatment, (b) as part of the primary lesion treatment (even if later followed by other local therapy), and (c) when the primary tumor response to the initial treatment is the key identifier of systemic effects. Adjuvant chemotherapy is used as an adjunct to other local modalities as part of the initial curative treatment. Frei (303) proposed the term *neoadjuvant chemotherapy* when this modality is used in the initial treatment of patients with local tumors before surgery or irradiation.

The effects of combined radiation therapy–chemotherapy can be described as independent, additive, or interactive. Chemotherapy and irradiation can be administered sequentially or concomitantly.

Administration of chemotherapy before irradiation produces some cell killing and reduction in the number of cells to be eliminated by the irradiation. The use of chemotherapy during radiation therapy has a strong rationale because it could interact with the local treatment (additive and even supraadditive action) and could also affect subclinical disease early in treatment. Nevertheless, it must be remembered that the combination of modalities may enhance normal tissue toxicity (Fig. 14.57). Chemotherapy after irradiation, as an adjuvant, has been used primarily for control of subclinical disease.

When combination therapy (i.e., irradiation and cytotoxic drugs) is chosen, it is important to assess (a) the effectiveness of concomitant or sequential administration of two methods of therapy, (b) the toxicity of combined modalities, and (c) the salvage rate for patients failing initial treatment with a single modality. In combined treatment, when new agents with inherent toxicity are added, results may be inferior to those with a combination involving fewer agents. Toxicity may lower tumor control because (a) the added toxicity may require lowering the doses of the effective agents, which will decrease response rate and (b) initial increased fatal toxicity will prevent some dying patients from demonstrating tumor response that could have been observed had they survived. Overall survival may be compromised as well. In locally advanced carcinoma of the cervix, several reports have documented improved tumor control and survival (Chapter 22).

Hyperthermia

Interest in the clinical application of hyperthermia is encouraged by biologic reports that indicate that there may be a significant advantage to the use of heat combined with irradiation and cytotoxic drugs to enhance the killing of tumor cells (74,304). The clinical use of heat has been hampered by a lack of adequate equipment to deliver heat in deep-seated and even large superficial lesions and of thermometry techniques that provide reliable information on heat distribution in the target tissues. However, significant progress has been made in technologic advances in the field (305).

In vitro and *in vivo* biologic experiments strongly suggest that heat may be more damaging to tumors than to normal tissues for several reasons: (a) chronically hypoxic cells may have an increased sensitivity to heat (they are at least as thermosensitive as oxygenated cells); (b) cells with a low pH (<6.8) that are metabolically deprived (tumor cells) are more heat sensitive; (c) heat affects cells in S phase, which are known to be resistant to irradiation (36); and (d) blood flow in the tumor is reduced (74). Heat causes a greater degree of mitotic delay than irradiation, and this factor may affect the distribution of cells in the cell cycle after exposure to heat or x-rays. Dewey and associates (74) pointed out that the response of the tumor may be affected by physiologic changes associated with lowering of the blood flow and oxygen tension produced by hyperthermia.

The biologic rationale for combining hyperthermia and irradiation in the treatment of cancer rests on two biologic mechanisms: radiosensitization and direct hyperthermia cytotoxicity. It can be hypothesized that hypoxic cells in the center of a tumor are relatively radioresistant but thermosensitive, whereas well-vascularized peripheral portions of the tumor are more sensitive to irradiation. This premise supports the use of combined irradiation and heat because hyperthermia is especially effective against centrally located hypoxic cells and irradiation eliminates the tumor cells in the periphery of the tumor, where heat is less effective.

About 30% to 75% of patients with large gynecologic tumors have recurrences at the primary site, and many have regional lymph node recurrences. Both patterns of failure could be improved if effective radiation sensitizers were developed. An area in which hyperthermia may be quite useful, perhaps alone at high temperatures (45°C) or at 43°C combined with moderate doses of irradiation (about 40 Gy), is in the treatment of patients with recurrences following definitive radiation therapy (60 to 70 Gy). Also, large epithelial tumors or specific histologic lesions (melanomas, soft tissue sarcomas, neurogenic tumors) that are not usually controlled with irradiation alone (because of tolerance of surrounding normal tissues) potentially could be more efficaciously treated with definitive doses of irradiation (65 to 75 Gy) and heat. Hypothetically, this combination would enhance the biologic effects of irradiation on the tumor without increasing morbidity in the normal tissues. Furthermore, the effects of hypoxic sensitizers combined with irradiation or cytotoxic drugs can be enhanced by the administration of heat.

Whole-body hyperthermia has been used for the treatment of disseminated disease, either alone or with chemotherapeutic agents. It may have potential value not only in the treatment of overt metastatic disease but also as an adjuvant, combined with chemotherapy, for the treatment of micrometastases.

Power Deposition in Hyperthermia

The physical agents employed to administer clinical hyperthermia are (a) electromagnetic fields at very high microwave frequencies (300 to 2,450 MHz), (b) "low-frequency" microwaves (60 to 120 MHz), (c) electromagnetic fields at radiofrequencies (0.1 to 27 MHz), and (d) ultrasound at frequencies of 0.3 to 3 MHz. The main characteristics of these modalities are summarized in Table 14.9.

Temperature elevations with radiofrequency (RF) electric fields may be produced through conductive, dielectric, or inductive heating. Conductive or resistive heating refers to heating with RF currents that are driven between pairs of opposing external electrodes: the resulting power deposition is effected through collisions of moving ions with tissue molecules. With dielectric or capacitative heating, the power is deposited in tissue through the interaction of the electrical fields produced by electrodes with a dielectric medium. Inductive heating refers to tissue heating with RF "eddy current" induced by the RF magnetic fields produced in the tissue by an external coil applicator surrounding the tissue. Ultrasound is generated by conversion of electric voltage charges into mechanical forces in motion in a piezoelectric crystal.

Interstitial Hyperthermia

Interstitial hyperthermia can be performed with coaxial microwave antennas, by RF electric current, or with "hot source" techniques (i.e., inductively heated ferromagnetic seeds or resistant wires).

Interstitial microwave hyperthermia may be produced through the use of coaxial microwave antennas inserted in Teflon catheters (tubes) implanted in the tissue volume of interest. Generally, the frequency required is 300 to 915 MHz. The heating pattern of a coaxial antenna operating at microwave frequencies is ellipsoidal, coincident with the antenna axis. At 915 MHz, the heating length is approximately 3.5 cm, and the lateral reach is about 1 cm from the antenna. A major problem with the design of microwave antennas is the so-called dead space at the distal end of the antenna. The clinical significance is that, in certain situations, the volume of implant has to be significantly longer than tumor volume at the expense of normal tissue.

Microwave antennas are usually placed in plastic catheters

TABLE 14.9. *Physical agents and techniques for local hyperthermia*

	Microwaves		RF Electric and Magnetic Fields		Ultrasound
	External (waveguide cavities)	Interstitial (coaxial antennas)	External (plates, coils)	Interstitial (needle arrays)	External (piezoelectric crystal transducers)
Frequency range	300–2,450 MHz	300–1,000 MHz	0.1–27 MHz	0.1–1.0 MHz	0.3–3.0 MHz
Area coverage	10–400 cm²[a]	Implant volume (20–1,000 cm³)	10–200 cm²[a]	Implant volume (20–1,000 cm³)	5–75 cm²[a]
Therapeutic depth	Up to 3 cm (muscle)		Up to 8 cm (muscle)		Up to 6 cm (muscle)
Power required	20–300 W[a]	10–200 W	20–400 W[a]	10,200 W	10,100 W[a]
Suitable for heating	Tumors in superficial muscle; in muscle behind fat or bone	Tumors in any volume that can be implanted	Tumors in superficial muscle or muscle behind fat (coils)	Tumors in any volume that can be implanted	Tumors in muscle; in muscle behind fat; deep-seated tumors (multiple beams)
Unsuitable for heating	Deep-seated tumors	Tumor in volumes that cannot be surgically invaded	Tumors in muscle behind fat (plates)	Tumors in volumes that cannot be surgically invaded	Tumors behind (or near) bone or air cavities

RF, radiofrequency.
[a] Single applicator or pair of plates.
Source: Perez C, Emami B, Nussbaum GH. Clinical experience with external local hyperthermia in treatment of superficial malignant tumors. *Front Radiat Ther Oncol* 1984;18:83, with permission.

inserted to hold the ^{192}Ir sources used for brachytherapy. Hence, the volume heated by an application of interstitial hyperthermia is usually the implant volume (20 to 100 cm^3).

Intracavitary Microwave Antennas. Intracavitary microwave antennas are used to deliver local hyperthermia to tumor sites in and adjacent to hollow viscera or cavities, such as in gynecologic (vagina, cervix, and uterus) and genitourinary (prostate, bladder, and urethra) systems. Temperatures of 42°C can be achieved for lengths of about 5 cm with effective penetration of about 0.5 cm around the applicator.

Radiofrequency. Interstitial heating with RF electric fields is essentially resistive heating produced by currents driven between electrically connected arrays of metallic needles (or between an intracavitary electrode and a needle array). The connected respective needle arrays constitute flat or curved electrodes in vivo. The slabs of tissue between respective pairs of adjacent arrays can all be heated simultaneously either by connecting alternate arrays together to form a circuit with two "multiplane" electrodes (i.e., arrays 1, 3, 5, and so on, as one electrode; arrays 2, 4, 6, and so on, as the second electrode) or by heating only one slab at any instant but sweeping rapidly back and forth (via electronic switching) through successive pairs of "single-plane" electrodes. Either of these techniques permits the entire implanted volume to be heated in a single application. The frequencies used in such applications are typically 0.1 to 1.0 MHz. The power required is usually 10 to 200 W.

Deep Hyperthermia

Electromagnetic or ultrasound devices are used for depositing heat at depth and are sometimes used to treat patients with gynecologic malignancy. The electromagnetic devices for heating deep-seated tumors use low-frequency (<100 MHz) microwaves or 8 to 27 MHz RF to overcome problems with attenuation that are present at higher frequencies (306). Ultrasound devices use lower frequencies (1 to 2 MHz) and shorter wavelengths (<1 cm): therefore, in principle, they could be more precisely defined than external electromagnetic devices. However, they often are not very useful for heating deep-seated tumors because of problems with reflections at interfaces (e.g., air-containing cavities, bone) and coupling.

Thermometry

At present, direct and continuous monitoring of temperatures in clinical hyperthermia with invasive probes constitutes the only reliable method of thermal treatment verification. Clinical temperature probes should be able to measure temperature to both an accuracy and precision of 0.1°C in phantoms for calibration and 0.2°C when used *in vivo*. Reference thermometers and other devices used for calibration should be able to establish temperature to within 0.02°C by National Institute of Standards and Technology (NIST) calibrated mercury-in-glass thermometers and by NIST traceable highly stable thermistor probes. The basic principles of thermometry were reviewed by Samulski (307) in AAPM Monograph No. 16.

Invasive thermometers fall into three basic categories: electrically conducting, minimally conducting, and nonconducting (optical) probes. They are typically designed to fit in 20- to 29-gauge plastic tubes or hypodermic needles.

Conducting probes include standard thermistor and thermocouple sensors with metallic leads. Standard thermistors have a sensor that is a semiconductor, the resistance of which decreases with increasing temperature. The temperature-dependent parameter is the resistivity of the semiconductor material. Thermocouple sensors use the junction between these two similar metals. Redistribution of charge across the junction leads to the establishment of a potential difference of known temperature dependence.

Nonconducting (optical) probes use sensors composed of gallium arsenide or a mixture of two rare earth phosphors. The "leads" of both optical probes are optical fibers. Gallium arsenide (GaAs), designed by Christensen (308), is a semiconductor for which the "band gap" (the energy separation of electrons in the conduction and valence bands) is a known function of temperature. In the rare earth biphosphor probe developed by Wickersheim (309), a pulse of incident light excites both phosphor materials, causing them to fluoresce.

Noninvasive thermometry is currently the subject of considerable research and is not likely to be commercially available in the near future. Techniques being evaluated include infrared thermography, microwave thermography (radiometry), and ultrasound reconstruction (to provide mappings of temperature-dependent ultrasound velocity or absorption).

Results with Hyperthermia

Deep (Regional) Hyperthermia. Reports from single-institution studies and an RTOG Phase I-II study indicate that, although temperatures exceeding 42°C could be obtained in 10% to 20% of patients, in only a minority of the sessions could the temperature be maintained long enough to achieve the desired goal of heating the tumor to at least 42°C. Incomplete heating was usually the result of local pain and discomfort (reported incidence of 30% to 70%) or systemic stress (10% to 25%) (310–313). Pelvic heating is limited by local pain (28% to 68% of sessions), discomfort or anxiety (6% to 23%), or cardiac symptoms (5% to 13%) (306,311,312, 314). In an RTOG study (84-01) there were four grade 4 toxicities in 54 patients, three of which were attributable to the catheter used for temperature monitoring and one that resulted from unrecommended surgery following maximum-dose irradiation (310).

Petrovich and associates (311) summarized the results in 353 patients treated with regional hyperthermia for a variety of pelvic and abdominal tumors. In most instances, heat was combined with irradiation, except in 42 patients who received chemotherapy. Complete response was observed in 35 patients (10%) and partial response in 59 (17%). Complete response was noted in 12% of patients receiving irradiation in addition to heat compared with 2% of those treated with heat alone. Treatment tolerance was good in 149 patients (42%), fair in 112 (32%), poor in 62 (18%), and not recorded in 30 (8%). Pain during the heat session was observed in 123 patients (35%). Cardiovascular symptoms were noted in 10 patients (3%), anxiety reaction in 6 (2%), and claustrophobia in 4 (1%). Ten patients (3%) developed blisters in the hyperthermia-treated areas.

Hornback and associates (315) described a nonrandomized study of microwave hyperthermia (433 MHz) and irradiation that yielded improved pelvic tumor control (72%) in 79 patients with stage IIIB carcinoma in comparison with previously irradiated historic controls (53%). However, 5-year survival rates were comparable in both groups (22% to 30%).

Sharma and colleagues (316) reported a 70% disease-free survival rate at 18 months in 20 patients with stage IIB-III carcinoma of the uterine cervix treated with irradiation and hyperthermia in comparison with a 50% disease-free survival rate in 22 patients treated with irradiation alone. The grade 3 complication rate (8%) was similar in both groups.

Interstitial Hyperthermia. The experience with interstitial hyperthermia has been more limited than with external applicators. The RTOG conducted a prospective randomized trial (RTOG 84-19) to evaluate the efficacy of interstitial irradiation alone versus interstitial thermoirradiation: no significant difference in local tumor control was observed (317).

Gynecologic tumors have occasionally been treated with interstitial thermoirradiation. In 14 patients with stage III and IV cervical carcinoma reported on by Vora and coworkers (318), there were eight complete responses and one partial response. Five of eight complete responders were alive without any tumor at follow-up, which ranged from 6 to 47 months.

Intracavitary Hyperthermia. Li and colleagues (319) described the design and heating patterns of 915-MHz and 2,450-MHz applicators for intracavitary therapy of carcinoma of the uterine cervix. Vaginal and cervical heating were done separately, one to three times, to temperatures of 43.5°C to 45°C. The applicators were used in three patients with stage IIB and IIIB cervical carcinoma who were treated with radiation therapy. Results of therapy were not described.

PHOTODYNAMIC THERAPY

In 1966, Lipson and coworkers (320) reported on the treatment of a patient with recurrent breast cancer with a hematoporphyrin derivative for fluorescence detection of tumor tissue that would localize exposure of the tumor to light. A comparison of photodynamic therapy and ionizing radiation is shown in Table 14.10.

Photodynamic therapy involves the interaction of a sensitizer, light, and oxygen. The ground-state sensitizer is excited by the absorption of light and can subsequently react through a free radical mechanism or, alternatively, via a spin-state transition involving reactive singlet oxygen. Both pathways yield potentially cytotoxic compounds, although the singlet oxygen process is thought to be predominant in photodynamic therapy (321). The deactivation of activated sensitizer to ground state can also occur with either liberation of heat or emission of a photon (the latter process is called fluorescence or phosphorescence depending on the spin state of the excited sensitizer). The hematoporphyrin photosensitizer is a complex mixture of porphyrins produced by the acetic acid–sulfuric acid treatment of hematoporphyrin, which in turn is manufactured commercially by the degradation of hemoglobin. Photofrin 2 is taken up by the reticuloendothelial system. Highest levels and longest retention are seen in the liver, spleen, kidney, and adrenals. The tumor to normal tissue ratio is 20 to 1 in the brain, 6 to 1 in the liver, and 1 to 1 in the skin. The compound can be retained in the skin for up to 8 weeks, and cutaneous photosensitivity is the only known side effect, which can be prevented by avoiding exposure to sunlight. It is advised that the drug not be used in patients with compromised hepatic function because the

TABLE 14.10. *Comparison of photodynamic therapy and ionizing irradiation*

Criterion	Photodynamic Therapy	Irradiation
Cellular damage	Polysystem	DNA
Tumor death	Somatic, vascular	Reproductive
Latency	Immediate	Delayed
Anoxia	Reduces effect	Reduces effect
Mutagenicity	No	Yes
Therapeutic ratio	Tumor selectively damaged	Normal tissue repair
Retreatment limits	Apparently none	Cumulative tolerance dose
Fractionation	? No benefit	Beneficial
Dose-rate effects	Probably no	Yes

Source: Perez CA, Brady LW, Roti Roti JL. Overview. In: Perez CA, Brady LW, eds. *Principles and practice of radiation oncology.* 3rd ed. Philadelphia: Lippincott–Raven, 1998: 178, with permission.

TABLE 14.11. *Photodynamic therapy results*

Study	Reference	No. of Patients/Sites	Dose	Response (%) CR	Response (%) PR/SR	Comments
Bladder						
Benson	325	4	Focal 150 J/cm²	100		TIS; recur elsewhere in bladder
Tsuchiya et al.	326	8	Focal 120360 J/cm²	100		Ta-T2; recur at 618 months
Hisazumi	250	9/36	Focal 50300 J/cm²	50	19	Ta, T1 lesions; all CR <2 cm
Prout et al.	327	19/50	Focal 100200 J/cm²	24	50	Ta, T1, TIS lesions
Benson	325	10	Whole bladder 2545 J/cm²	60	20	TIS or TIS + 2
Gynecologic						
Rettenmaier et al.	328	6/9	2040 J/cm²	22	44	Lesions of vagina, perineum
Corti et al.	329	7/7	60240 J/cm²	71	29	Vaginal/vault lesions
Ward	322	5/5		40	60	CR durable at 10, 12 months
McCaughan	45	5/5	Variable	100		Superficial tumor eradicated for 515 months

CR, Clinical complete response; PR/SR, partial or significant response.
Source: Perez CA, Brady LW, Roti Roti JL. Overview. In: Perez CA, Brady LW, eds. *Principles and practice of radiation oncology.* 3rd ed. Philadelphia: Lippincott–Raven, 1998, with permission.

liver is the primary metabolic and excretory organ for porphyrins and the site of highest accumulation of these compounds after injection.

These compounds, which selectively localize in the tumor, are photochemically activated over a relatively narrow frequency range of light at a wavelength with appropriate tissue penetration. Hematoporphyrin absorbs light most strongly in the ultraviolet/visible blue region around 400 nm, with other less-prominent peaks seen at or near 500, 540, and 580 nm. In the clinic, red light (630 nm) is most frequently used because it has deeper tissue penetration, although the excitation band is less prominent. The penetration of red light in tissue is a complex phenomenon that depends on many factors, including tissue density, organ pigmentation, blood flow, surface geometry, and tissue interfaces. Photodynamic therapy with this light may produce tumor necrosis at a depth of 3 to 7 mm. Photodynamic therapy requires adequate light to produce effective photosensitization: the energy and wavelength are dictated by the photochemical properties of the photosensitizer, the biologic and physical characteristics of the tumor, and the mode of light delivery used. The amount of light energy delivered is generally expressed in joules and represents the product of light output or power in watts (joules/second) and the length of light exposure in seconds. Laser systems for use in clinical photodynamic therapy include argon-pumped dye laser and pulsed metal–vapor laser, which yield 4 to 5 W of usable light (322).

Tumor destruction by photodynamic therapy in vivo has been ascribed to both direct cytotoxicity of tumor cells and indirect cytotoxicity, possibly resulting from damage to small blood vessels that supply the tumor.

Association between loss of cellular viability and inhibition of membrane transport, as well as localization of hematoporphyrin derivative fluorescence in a membrane fraction, suggest that membrane targets are involved in cellular inactivation by photodynamic therapy (322). Other types of cellular injury have been reported, but plasma membrane damage and mitochondrial injury appear to be the most critical for cellular destruction. DNA damage might be less pronounced than other cytotoxic effects occurring elsewhere in the cell.

Treatment appears to be effective to a depth of approximately 5 mm depending on dose delivered, concentration of sensitizer injected, and type of light delivery. Lesions thicker than 5 mm may need several external treatments or interstitial techniques. Photodynamic therapy has been used with encouraging results in some patients with malignant tumors in various locations, including carcinoma of the urinary bladder and some gynecologic malignancies (Table 14.11).

REFERENCES

1. Roentgen WC. On a new kind of rays (preliminary communication). Translation of a paper read before the Physikalische-medicinischen Gesellschaft of Wurzburg on December 28, 1895. *Br J Radiol* 1931; 4:32.
2. Curie P, Curie M, Bemont G. Sur une nouvelle substance fortemont

radioactive contenue dans la pechblende (note presented by M. Becquerel). *Compt Rend Acad Sci (Paris)* 1898:127:1215.

3. Janeway HH. The treatment of uterine cancer by radium. *Surg Gynecol Obstet* 1919;29:242.

4. Wickham L, Degrais P. *Radium therapie, cancer de l'uterus.* 2nd ed. Paris: 1912.

5. Kroenig B. Roentgen rays, radium and mesothorium in the treatment of uterine fibroids and malignant tumors. *Am J Obstet* 1914;69:205.

6. Bumm E. Ueber die Erfolge der Roentgen und Mesothorium Behandlung beim Uteruskarcinom. Deutsche Gesellsch f. Gynaek, Halle, 1913.

7. Doederlein A. Roentgen-Mesothorium Behandlung bei Myom und Carcinom des Uterus. *Surg Gynecol Obstet* 1913;18:428.

8. Degrais P. Radium therapie du cancer du col de l'uterus. *Ann de Gynecol et d'obstet* 1915;xi:609. *Surg Gynecol Obstet* 1915;22:298.

9. Coutard H. Principles of x-ray therapy of malignant diseases. *Lancet* 1934;2:1.

10. Paterson R. The radical x-ray treatment of the carcinomata. *Br J Radiol* 1936;9:671.

11. Radiation Oncology in Integrated Cancer Management: Report of the Inter-Study Council for Radiation Oncology. Inter-Study Council for Radiation Oncology, 1986.

12. Perez CA. The critical need for accurate treatment planning and quality control in radiation therapy. *Int J Radiat Oncol Biol Phys* 1977; 2:815.

13. Fletcher GH. Implications of the density of clonogenic infestations in radiotherapy. *Int J Radiat Oncol Biol Phys* 1986;12:1675.

14. International Commission on Radiation Units and Measurements. Report No. 50: Prescribing, recording, and reporting photon beam therapy. Bethesda, MD: International Commission on Radiation Units and Measurements, 1993.

15. International Commission on Radiological Units and Measurements. Report No. 62: Prescribing, recording, and reporting photon beam therapy (Supplement to ICRU Report 50). Bethesda, MD: International Commission of Radiation Units and Measurements, 1999.

16. Graham ML, Cheng AY, Geer LY, et al. On-line fiber optic imaging: methods to analyze treatment variation in daily portal imaging. *Int J Radiat Oncol Biol Phys* 1991;20:613.

17. Suit HD, Becht J, Leong J, et al. Potential for improvement in radiation therapy. *Int J Radiat Oncol Biol Phys* 1988;14:777.

18. Hall EJ. *Radiobiology for the radiologist.* 4th ed. Philadelphia: JB Lippincott Co, 1994.

19. Ampuero F, Doss LL, Khan LM, Skipper B, Hilgers RD. The Syed-Neblett interstitial template in locally advanced gynecological malignancies. *Int J Radiat Oncol Biol Phys* 1983;9:1897.

20. Yamada T, Ohyama H. Radiation-induced interphase death of rate thymocytes is internally programmed (apoptosis). *Int J Radiat Biol* 1988;53:65.

21. Fuks Z, Weichselbaum RR. Radiation therapy. In: Mendelsohn J, Howley PM, Israel MA, et al., eds. *The molecular basis of cancer.* Philadelphia: WB Saunders, 1995:404.

22. Kerr JFR, Harmon BV. Definition and incidence of apoptosis: an historical perspective. In: Tomei LD, Cope FO, eds. *Apoptosis: the molecular basis of cell death.* Cold Spring Harbor, NY: Cold Spring Harbor Laboratory Press, 1991:5.

23. Wyllie AH, Kerr JFR, Currie AR. Cell death: the significance of apoptosis. *Int Rev Cytol* 1980;68:251.

24. Wyllie AH. The biology of cell death in tumours. *Anticancer Res* 1985;5:131.

25. Coleman CN. Beneficial liaisons: radiobiology meets cellular and molecular biology. *Radiother Oncol* 1993;28:1.

26. Chae HP, Jarvis LJ, Uckum FM. Role of tyrosine phosphorylation in radiation-induced activation of c-jun proto-oncogene in human lymphohematopoietic precursor cells. *Cancer Res* 1993;53:447.

27. Kerr JFR, Wyllie AH, Currie AR. Apoptosis: a basic biological phenomenon with wide-ranging implications in tissue kinetics. *Br J Cancer* 1972;26:239.

28. Dewey WC, Ling CC, Meyn RE. Radiation-induced apoptosis: relevance to radiotherapy. *Int J Radiat Oncol Biol Phys* 1995;33:781.

29. Chrest FJ, Buchholz MA, Kim YH, et al. Identification and quantitation of apoptotic cells following anti-CD3 activation of murine G_0 T-cells. *Cytometry* 1993;14:883.

30. Hellman S, Weichselbaum RR. Radiation oncology and the new biology. *Cancer J Sci Am* 1995;1:174.

31. Neta R, Oppenheim JJ. Radioprotection with cytokines: learning from nature to cope with radiation damage. *Cancer Cells* 1991;3:391.

32. Tsang RW, Fyles AW, Li Y-Q, et al. Tumor proliferation and apoptosis in human uterine cervix carcinoma I: correlations between variables. *Radiother Oncol* 1999;50:85.

33. Court Brown WM, Buckton KE, McLean AS. Quantitative studies of chromosome aberrations in man following acute and chronic exposure to x-rays and gamma rays. *Lancet* 1965;1:1239.

34. Tubiana M. The causes of clinical radioresistance. In: Steel GG, Adams GE, Peckham MJ, eds. *The biological basis of radiotherapy.* Amsterdam: Elsevier Science, 1983:13.

35. Sinclair WK. Cyclic x-ray responses in mammalian cells in vitro. *Radiat Res* 1968;33:620.

36. Terasima T, Tolmach LJ. Variations in several responses of HeLa cells to x-irradiation during division cycle. *Biophys J* 1963;3:11.

37. Dekaban AS. Abnormalities in children exposed to x-radiation during various stages of gestation: tentative timetable of radiation to the human fetus. I. *J Nucl Med* 1968;9:471.

38. Sneed PK. Comments on "Fetal dose evaluation during breast cancer radiotherapy." *Breast Dis* 1999;9:409.

39. Doll R, Wakeford R: Risk of childhood cancer from fetal irradiation. *Br J Radiol* 1997;70:130.

40. International Commission on Radiological Protection: Recommendations, Annals of the ICRP Publication 60. Oxford, England, Pergamon Press, 1990.

41. Boice JD Jr, Engholm G, Kleinman RA, et al. Radiation dose and second cancer risk in patients treated for cancer of the cervix. *Radiat Res* 1988;116:3.

42. Brenner DJ, Curtis RE, Hall EJ, et al. Second malignancies in prostate patients after radiotherapy compared with surgery. *Cancer* 2000;88:398.

43. Travis LB, Curtis RE, Boice JD Jr: Late effects of treatment for childhood Hodgkin's disease. *N Engl J Med* 1996;335:352.

44. National Council on Radiation Protection and Measurements. Report No. 116: Limitation of exposure to ionizing radiation. Bethesda, MD: NCRP, 1993.

45. Hall EJ. The relative biological efficiency of x-rays generated at 220 kVp and gamma radiation from a cobalt 60 therapy unit. *Br J Radiol* 1961;34:313.

46. Fowler JF, Margan RL. Symposium on pretherapeutic experiments with fast neutrons and x-rays on tumour and normal tissue in the rat. *Br J Radiol* 1963;36:115.

47. Brown JM. Evidence for acute hypoxic cells in mouse tumours, and a possible mechanism of reoxygenation. *Br J Radiol* 1979;52:650.

48. Thomlinson RH, Gray LH. The histological structure of some human lung cancers and the possible implications for radiotherapy. *Br J Cancer* 1955;9:539.

49. Wouters BG, Brown JM. Cells at intermediate oxygen levels can be more important than the "hypoxic fraction" in determining tumor response to fractionated radiotherapy. *Radiat Res* 1997;147:541.

50. Chaplin DJ, Durand RE, Olive PL: Acute hypoxia in tumors: implications for modifiers of radiation effects. *Int J Radiat Oncol Biol Phys* 1986;12:1279.

51. Chaplin DJ, Olive PL, Durand RE: Intermittent blood flow in a murine tumor: Radiobiological effects. *Cancer Res* 1987;47:597.

52. Van den Brenk HAS. Hyperbaric oxygen in radiation therapy. *Am J Roentgenol Radium Ther Nucl Med* 1968;102:8.

53. Churchill-Davidson I, Foster CA, Wiernik G, et al. The place of oxygen in radiotherapy. *Br J Radiol* 1966;39:321.

54. Henk JM, Smith CW. Radiotherapy and hyperbaric oxygen in head and neck cancer. *Lancet* 1977;1:104.

55. Kaanders JHAM, Pop LAM, Marres HAM, et al. Accelerated radiotherapy with carbogen and nicotinamide (ARCON) for laryngeal cancer. *Radiother Oncol* 1998;48:115.

56. Giaccia AJ, Brown JM, Wouters B, et al. Cancer therapy and tumor physiology. *Science* 1998;279:12.

57. Hockel M, Schlenger K, Aral B, et al. Association between tumor hypoxia and malignant progression in advanced cancer of the uterine cervix. *Cancer Res* 1996;56:4509.

58. Brizel DM, Scully SP, Harrelson JM, et al. Tumor oxygenation pre-

dicts for the likelihood of distant metastases in human soft tissue sarcoma. *Cancer Res* 1996;56:941.

59. Denekamp J, Joiner MC. The potential benefit from a perfect radiosensitizer and its dependence on reoxygenation. *Br J Radiol* 1982;55:657.

60. Stone RS. Neutron therapy and specific ionization. *Am J Roentgenol* 1948;59:771.

61. Coleman CN, Wasserman TH, Urtasun RC, et al. Final report of the phase I trial of the hypoxic cell radiosensitizer SR 2508 (etanidazole) Radiation Therapy Oncology Group 83–03. *Int J Radiat Oncol Biol Phys* 1990;18:389.

62. Eschwege F, Sancho-Garnier H, Chassagne D, et al. Results of a European randomized trial of Etanidazole combined with radiotherapy in head and neck carcinomas. *Int J Radiat Oncol Biol Phys* 1997;39:275.

63. Overgaard J, San Hansen H. Overgaard M, et al. Randomized double-blind phase III study of nimjarzaole as a hypoxic radiosensitizer of primary radiotherapy in supraglottic larynx and pharynx carcinoma. Results of the Danish Head and Neck Cancer Study (DAHANCA) protocol 5-85. *Radiother Oncol* 1998;46:135.

64. Overgaard J, Horsman MR: Modification of hypoxia-induced radioresistance in tumours by the use of oxygen and sensitizers. *Semin Radiat Oncol* 1996;6:10.

65. von Pawel J, con Roemeling R. Survival benefit from Tirazone (tirapazamine) and cisplatin in advanced non-small cell lung cancer (NSCLC) patients: final results from the international phase III CATAPULT-I trial. *Proc Am Soc Clin Oncol* 1998:17:454(abst).

66. Sweeney TR: *A survey of compounds from the antiradiations drug development program of the US Army Medical Research and Development Command.* Washington, DC, Walter Reed Army Institute of Research, 1979.

67. Wasserman T. Radioprotective effects of amifostine. *Semin Oncol* 1999;26[Suppl 7]:89.

68. Brizel D, Saner R, Wannemacher M, et al. Randomized phase III trial of radiation ± amifostine in patients with head and neck cancer. *Proc ASCO* 17, 1998.

69. Mitsuhashi N, Takahashi I, Takahashi M, et al. Clinical study of radioprotective effects of amifostine (YM-08310, WR-2721) on long-term outcome for patients with cervical cancer. *Int J Radiat Oncol Biol Phys* 1993;26:407.

70. Wadler S, Goldberg G, Fields A, et al. The potential role of amifostine in conjunction with cisplatin in the treatment of locally advanced carcinoma of the cervix. *Semin Oncol* 1996;23[Suppl 8]:64.

71. Gray LH. Radiobiologic basis of oxygen as modifying factor in radiation therapy. *Am J Roentgenol Radium Ther Nucl Med* 1961;85:803.

72. Song CW, Zhang WL, Pence DM, et al. Increased radiosensitivity of tumors by perfluorochemicals and carbogen. *Int J Radiat Oncol Biol Phys* 1985;11:1833.

73. Brizel DM, Wasserman TH, Henke M, et al. Phase III randomized trial of amifostine as a radioprotector in head and neck cancer. *J Clin Oncol* 2000;18:3339.

74. Dewey WC, Hopwood LE, Sapareto SA, Gerweck LE. Cellular responses to combinations of hyperthermia and radiation. *Radiology* 1977;123:463.

75. Steel GG, Peacock JH. Why are some human tumours more radiosensitive than others? *Radiother Oncol* 1989;15:63.

76. Dische S. Chemical sensitizers for hypoxic cells: a decade of experience in clinical radiotherapy. *Radiother Oncol* 1985;3:97.

77. Duncan W. A clinical evaluation of fast neutron therapy. In: Steel GG, Adams GE, Peckham MJ, eds. *The biological basis of radiotherapy.* Amsterdam: Elsevier Science, 1983:277.

78. Fertil B, Malaise EP. Inherent cellular radiosensitivity as a basic concept for human tumor radiotherapy. *Int J Radiat Oncol Biol Phys* 1981;7:621.

79. Deacon J, Peckham MJ, Steel GG. The radioresponsiveness of human tumours and the initial slope of the cell survival curve. *Radiother Oncol* 1984;2:317.

80. Elkind MM. DNA damage and cell killing: cause and effect. *Cancer* 1985;45:2123.

81. Weichselbaum RR, Little JB. The differential response of human tumours to fractionated radiation may be due to a post-irradiation repair process. *Br J Cancer* 1982;46:532.

82. Fletcher GH, ed. *Textbook of radiotherapy.* 3rd ed. Philadelphia: Lea & Febiger, 1980.

83. Fletcher GH. Keynote address: the scientific basis of the present and future practice of clinical radiotherapy. *Int J Radiat Oncol Biol Phys* 1983;9:1073.

84. Fletcher GH, Shukovsky LJ. The interplay of radiocurability and tolerance in the irradiation of human cancers. *J Radiol Electrol* 1975;56:383.

85. Baclesse F. Carcinoma of the larynx. *Br J Radiol* 1949;3:1.

86. Baclesse F. Roentgentherapy alone in the cancer of the breast. *Acta Unio Int Contra Cancrum* 1959;15:1023.

87. Biggs P, Ma CM, Doppke K, et al. Kilovoltage x-rays. In: Van Dyk J, ed. *The modern technology of radiation oncology.* Madison, WI: Medical Physics Publishing, 1999:287.

88. Robison RF. The race for megavoltage. *Acta Oncol* 1995;34:1055.

89. Glasgow CP. Cobalt-60 teletherapy. In: Van Dyk J, ed. *The modern technology of radiation oncology.* Madison, WI: Medical Physics Publishing, 1999:313.

90. Karzmark CJ, Nunan CS, Tanabe E. *Medical electron accelerators.* New York: McGraw-Hill, 1993.

91. Miller CW. Traveling-wave linear accelerator for x-ray therapy. *Nature* 1953;171:297.

92. Ginzton EL, Mallory KB, Kaplan HS. The Stanford medical linear accelerator. I. Design and development. *Stanford Med Bull* 1957;15:123.

93. Intensity Modulated Radiation Therapy Working Group. Intensity modulated radiation therapy: current status and issues of interest. *Int J Radiat Oncol Biol Phys* 2001;51:880.

94. Veksler VJ. A new method for acceleration of relativistic particles. *Dokl Akad Nauk SSSR* 1944;43:329.

95. Wilson RW. Radiological use of fast protons. *Radiology* 1946;47:487.

96. Miller DW. A review of proton beam radiation therapy. *Med Phys* 1995;22:1943.

97. Moyers MF: Proton therapy. In: Van Dyk J, ed. *The modern technology of radiation oncology.* Madison, WI: Medical Physics Publishing, 1999;823.

98. Breuer H, Smit BJ. *Proton therapy and radiosurgery.* Berlin: Springer-Verlag, 2000.

99. Coutrakon G, Bauman M, Lesyna D, et al. A prototype beam delivery system for the proton medical accelerator at Loma Linda. *Med Phys* 1991;18:1093.

100. Maughan RL, Powers WE. A superconducting cyclotron for neutron radiation therapy. *Med Phys* 1994;21:779.

101. Maor MH, Gillespie BW, Peters LJ, et al. Neutron therapy in cervical cancer: results of a phase III RTOG study. *Int J Radiat Oncol Biol Phys* 1988;14:885.

102. Van Dyk J, Munro PN. Simulators. In: Van Dyk J, ed. *The modern technology of radiation oncology.* Madison, WI: Medical Physics Publishing, 1999:95.

103. Van Dyk J, Taylor JS. CT simulators. In: Van Dyk J, ed. *The modern technology of radiation oncology.* Madison, WI: Medical Physics Publishing, 1999;131.

104. Garcia-Ramirez JL, Mutic S, Dempsey JF, et al. Performance evaluation of an 85-cm-bore x-ray computed tomography scanner designed for radiation oncology and comparison with current diagnostic CT scanners. *Int J Radiat Oncol Biol Phys* 2002;52:1123.

105. Stehman FB, Bundy BN, Thomas G, et al. Groin dissection versus groin radiation in carcinoma of the vulva: a Gynecologic Oncology Group study. *Int J Radiat Oncol Biol Phys* 1992;24:389.

106. Koh W-J, Chiu M, Stelzer KJ, et al. Femoral vessel depth and the implications for groin node radiation. *Int J Radiat Oncol Biol Phys* 1993;27:969.

107. Petereit DG, Mehta MP, Buchler DA, Kinsella TJ. Inguinofemoral radiation of N0,N1 vulvar cancer may be equivalent to lymphadenectomy if proper radiation technique is used. *Int J Radiat Oncol Biol Phys* 1993;27:963.

108. Kohler G, Milstein C. Continuous cultures of fused cells secreting antibody of predefined specificity. *Nature* 1975;256:495.

109. Goldenberg DM, DeLand F, Kim E, et al. Use of radiolabeled antibodies to carcinoembryonic antigen for the detection and localization of diverse cancers by external photoscanning. *N Engl J Med* 1978;298:1384.

110. Order SE. Presidential address: systemic radiotherapy in the new frontier. *Int J Radiat Oncol Biol Phys* 1990;18:981.

111. Goffman TE, Raubitschek A, Mitchell JB, Glatstein E. The emerging biology of modern radiation oncology. *Cancer Res* 1990;50:7735.

112. Johns HE, Cunningham JR. *The physics of radiology*. 4th ed. Springfield, IL: Charles C Thomas, 1983.

113. American Association of Physicists in Medicine, Task Group 21: Radiation Therapy Committee. A protocol for the determination of absorbed dose from high energy photon and electron beams. *Med Phys* 1983;10:741.

114. Joint Working Party of the British Institute of Radiology and the Hospital Physicists' Association. Central axis depth dose data for use in radiotherapy. *Br J Radiol* 1983[Suppl 17] (entire issue).

115. Purdy JA. The application of high energy x-rays and electron beams in radiotherapy. *IEEE Trans Nucl Sci NS* 1979;26:1833.

116. Velkley DE, Manson DJ, Purdy JA, Oliver GD Jr. Build-up region of megavoltage photon radiation sources. *Med Phys* 1975;2:14.

117. Holt JG, Laughlin JS, Moroney JP. The extension of the concept of tissue-air (TAR) to high energy x-ray beams. *Radiology* 1970;96:437.

118. Karzmark CJ, Deubert A, Loevinger R. Tissue-phantom ratios: an aid to treatment planning. *Br J Radiol* 1965;38:185.

119. Khan FM. *The physics of radiation therapy*. 2nd ed. Baltimore: Williams & Wilkins, 1994.

120. Goitein M, Abrams M, Rowell D, et al. Multi-dimensional treatment planning: II. Beam's eye view, back projection, and projection through CT sections. *Int J Radiat Oncol Biol Phys* 1983;9:789.

121. Grant W III. Experience with intensity modulated beam therapy delivery. In: Palta J, Mackie TR, eds. *Teletherapy: present and future*. College Park, MD: Advanced Medical Publishing, 1996:793.

122. Purdy JA, Harms WB, Matthews JW, et al. Advances in 3-dimensional radiation treatment planning systems: room-view display with real time interactivity. *Int J Radiat Oncol Biol Phys* 1993;27:933.

123. Drzymala RE, Mohan R, Brewster L, et al. Dose-volume histograms. *Int J Radiat Oncol Biol Phys* 1991;21:71.

124. Purdy JA. Dose-volume specification and reporting. In: Shiu AS, Mellenberg DE, eds. *General practice of radiation oncology physics in the 21st century*. Madison, WI: Medical Physics Publishing, 2000;3.

125. Purdy JA. Dose-volme specification: New challenges with intensity-modulated radiation therapy. *Semin Radiat Oncol* 2002;12:199.

126. Mackie TR, Holmes T, Swerdloff S, et al. Tomotherapy: A new concept for the delivery of dynamic conformal radiotherapy. *Med Phys* 1993;20:1709.

127. Carol MP. Integrated 3D conformal planning/multivane intensity modulating delivery system for radiotherapy. In: Purdy JA, Emami B, eds. *3D radiation treatment planning and conformal therapy*. Madison, WI: Medical Physics Publishing, 1995:435.

128. Ruchala KJ, Olivera GH, Kapatoes JM, et al. Megavoltage CT image reconstruction during tomotherapy treatments. *Phys Med Biol* 2000; 45:3545.

129. Convery DJ, Rosenbloom ME: The generation of intensity-modulated fields for conformal radiotherapy by dynamic collimation. *Phys Med Biol* 1992;37:1359.

130. Bortfeld T, Kahler DL, Waldron TJ, et al. X-ray field compensation with multileaf collimation. *Int J Radiat Oncol Biol Phys* 1994;28:723.

131. Yu CX: Intensity modulated arc therapy with dynamic multileaf collimation: An alternative to tomotherapy. *Phys Med Biol* 1995;40:1435.

132. Chao KSC, Ozyigi G, Tran BN, et al. Patterns of failure in patients receiving definitive and postoperative IMRT for head and neck cancer. *Int J Radiat Oncol Biol Phys* 2003;55:312.

133. Hanks GE, Schultheiss TE, Hanlon AL, et al. Optimization of conformal radiation treatment of prostate cancer: report of a dose escalation study. *Int J Radiat Oncol Biol Phys* 1997;37:543.

134. Michalski JM, Purdy JA, Winter K, et al. Preliminary report of toxicity following 3D radiation therapy for prostate cancer on 3DOG/RTOG 9406, Level III (79.2 Gy). *Int J Radiat Oncol Biol Phys* 2000;46:391.

135. Portelance L, Chao KS, Grigsby PW, et al. Intensity modulated radiation therapy (IMRT) reduces small bowel, rectum and bladder doses in patients with cervical cancer receiving pelvic and para-aortic irradiation. *Int J Radiat Oncol Biol Phys* 2001;51:261.

136. Kavanagh BD, Schefter TE, Wu Q, et al. Clinical application of intensity-modulated radiotherapy for locally advanced cervical cancer. *Semin Radiat Oncol* 2002;12:260..

137. Mundt AJ, Lujan AE, Rotmensch J, et al. Intensity-modulated whole pelvic radiotherapy in women with gynecologic malignancies. *Int J Radiat Oncol Biol Phys* 2002;52:1330.

138. Henschke UK, Hilaris BS, Mahan GD. Afterloading in interstitial and intracavitary brachytherapy. *Am J Roentgenol* 1963;90:386.

139. Suit HD, Moore EB, Fletcher GH, et al. Modifications of Fletcher ovoid system for afterloading using standard sized radium tubes (milligram and microgram). *Radiology* 1963;81:126.

140. Glasgow GP, Bourland JD, Grigsby PW, et al. Remote afterloading technology: report of the American Association of Physicists in Medicine Task Group No. 41. New York: American Institute of Physics, 1993.

141. International Commission on Radiation Units and Measurements. Report No. 38: Dose and volume specification for reporting intracavitary therapy in gynecology. Bethesda, MD: International Commission on Radiation Units, 1985:1.

142. Glasgow GP, Dillman LT. Specific γ-ray constant and exposure rate constant of ^{192}Ir. *Med Phys* 1979;6:49.

143. Daskalov GM, Loffler E, Williamson JF: Monte Carlo–aided dosimetry of a new high dose rate brachytherapy source. *Med Phys* 1998; 25:2200.

144. Wang R. Sloboda RS: Monte Carlo dosimetry of the VariSource high dose rate ^{192}Ir source. *Med Phys* 1998;25:415.

145. Williamson JF. Recent advances in brachytherapy dosimetry. In: Smith AR, ed. *Radiation therapy physics*. Berlin: Springer-Verlag, 1995:247.

146. Williamson JF, Li Z: Monte Carlo aided dosimetry of the microselectron pulsed and high-dose rate ^{192}Ir sources. *Med Phys* 1995;22:809.

147. Ling CC, Huang DY, Barnett C. Improved dose distributions with customized I-125 source loading in temporary interstitial implants. *Int J Radiat Oncol Biol Phys* 1988;15:769.

148. Ling CC. Permanent implants using Au-198, Pd-103, and I-125: radiobiological considerations based on the linear quadratic model. *Int J Radiat Oncol Biol Phys* 1992;23:81.

149. Porter AT, McEwan AJB, Powe JE, et al. Results of randomized phase III trial to evaluate the efficacy of strontium-89 adjuvant to local external beam irradiation in the management of endocrine resistant metastatic prostate cancer. *Int J Radiat Oncol Biol Phys* 1993;25:805.

150. Mason DL, Battista JJ, Barnett J, Porter AT. Ytterbium-169: calculated physical properties of a new radiation source for brachytherapy. *Med Phys* 1992;19:695.

151. Perera H, Williamson JF, Li Z, et al. Dosimetric characteristics, air-kerma strength calibration and verification of Monte Carlo simulation for a new Ytterbium-169 brachytherapy source. *Int J Radiat Oncol Biol Phys* 1994;28:953.

152. Nath R, Gray L. Dosimetry studies on prototype ^{241}Am sources for brachytherapy. *Int J Radiat Oncol Biol Phys* 1987;13:897.

153. Fairchild RG, Kalef-Erza J, Packer S, et al. Samarium-145: a new brachytherapy source. *Phys Med Biol* 1987;32:847.

154. Nath R, Peschel RE, Park CH, Fischer JJ. Development of an ^{241}Am applicator for intracavitary irradiation of gynecologic cancers. *Int J Radiat Oncol Biol Phys* 1988;14:969.

155. Samuels M, Peschel RE, Papadopoulos D, et al. A feasibility study of intracavitary americium-241 for recurrent pelvic malignancies. *Endocurietherapy Hyperthermia Oncol* 1991;7:131.

156. Nath R, Gray L, Park CH. Dose distributions around cylindrical ^{241}Am sources for a clinical intracavitary applicator. *Med Phys* 1987;14:809.

157. Nath R, Bongiorni P, Rossi PI, Rockwell S. Enhancement of IUdR radiosensitization by low energy photons. *Int J Radiat Oncol Biol Phys* 1987;13:1071.

158. Piermattei A, Arcovito G, Azario L, et al. Experimental dosimetry of ^{169}Yb seeds prototype 6 for brachytherapy treatment. *Phys Med* 1992 ; 8:163.

159. Nath R, Anderson L, Jones D, et al. *Specification of brachytherapy source strength: a report by Task Group 32 of the American Association of Physicists in Medicine*. New York: American Institute of Physics, 1987.

160. Williamson JF, Anderson LL, Grigsby PW, et al. American Endocurietherapy Society recommendations for specification of brachytherapy source strength. *Endocurietherapy Hyperthermia Oncol* 1993;9:1.

161. Williamson JF, Nath R. Clinical implementation of AAPM Task Group 32 recommendations on brachytherapy source strength specification. *Med Phys* 1991;18:439.

162. Sievert RM. Die Intensitätsverteilung der primaren—Strählung in der Nähe medizinischer Radiumpräparate. *Acta Radiol* 1921;1:89.

163. Anderson LL, Nath R, Weaver KA, et al. Interstitial brachytherapy: physical, biological, and clinical considerations. New York: Raven Press, 1990.

164. Williamson JF. Monte Carlo and analytic calculation of absorbed dose near ^{137}Cs intracavitary sources. *Int J Radiat Oncol Biol Phys* 1988; 15:227.

165. Williamson JF. Comparison of measured and calculated dose rates in water near I-125 and Ir-192 seeds. *Med Phys* 1991;18:776.

166. Nath R, Anderson L, Luxton G, Weaver K, et al. Dosimetry of interstitial brachytherapy sources: recommendations of the AAPM Radiation Therapy Committee Task Group 43. *Med Phys* 1995;22:209.

167. Williamson JF, Ezzell GA, Olch A, Thomadsen BR. Quality assurance for high dose-rate remote afterloading brachytherapy. In: Nag S, ed. *Textbook on high-dose rate brachytherapy.* Armonk, NY: Futura Publishing, 1994:147.

168. Capote R, Mainegra E, Lopez E: Anisotropy function for 192Ir low-dose rate brachytherapy sources: an EGS4 Monte Carlo study. *Phys Med Biol* 2001;46:1487.

169. Chibani O, Li XA: Monte Carlo dose calculations in homogeneous media and at interfaces: A comparison between CEPTS, EGSnrc, MCNP, and measurements. *Med Phys* 2002;29:835.

170. Perez CA, Brady LW, Halperin EC, Schmitt-Ullrich R, eds. *Principles and practice of radiation oncology.* 4th ed. Baltimore: Lippincott Williams & Wilkins, 2003.

171. Dutreix J. Expression of the dose rate effect in clinical curietherapy. *Radiother Oncol* 1989;15:25.

172. Orton CG. Time-dose factors (TDFs) in brachytherapy. *Br J Radiol* 1974;47:603.

173. Ellis F. *Time and dose relationships in radiation biology as applied to radiotherapy.* Brookhaven National Laboratory, BNL50203 (C-57), 1969:313.

174. Pierquin B, Chassagne D, Baillet F, Paine CH. Clinical observations on the time factor in interstitial radiotherapy using Iridium 192. *Clin Radiol* 1973;24:506.

175. Mazeron J-J, Lusinchi A, Marinello G, et al. Interstitial radiation therapy for squamous cell carcinoma of the tonsillar region: the Creteil experience (1971–1981). *Int J Radiat Oncol Biol Phys* 1985;12:895.

176. Hall EJ, Brenner DJ. The dose-rate effect revisited: radiobiological considerations of the importance in radiotherapy. *Int J Radiat Oncol Biol Phys* 1991;21:1403.

177. Orton CG, Cohen L. A unified approach to dose-effect relationships in radiotherapy. I. Modified TDF and linear quadratic equations. *Int J Radiat Oncol Biol Phys* 1988;14:549.

178. Dale RG. The application of the linear-quadratic dose-effect equation to fractionated and protracted radiotherapy. *Br J Radiol* 1985;58:515.

179. Ling CC, Burman C, Chui CS, et al. Conformal radiation treatment of prostate cancer using inversely-planned intensity modulated photon beams produced with dynamic multileaf collimation. *Int J Radiat Oncol Biol Phys* 1996;35:721.

180. Anderson LL. Remote afterloading in cancer management. I. Afterloader design and optimization potential. In: Hilaris BS, Batata MA, eds. *Brachytherapy oncology—1983.* New York: Memorial Sloan-Kettering Cancer Center, 1983:93.

181. Perez CA, Grigsby PW, Williamson JF. Clinical applications of brachytherapy I: low dose-rate. In Perez CA, Brady LW, eds. *Principles and practice of radiation oncology.* 3rd ed. Philadelphia: Lippincott–Raven Publishers, 1998:487.

182. Wilkinson JM, Moore CJ, Notley HM, Hunter RD. The use of Selectron afterloading equipment to simulate and extend the Manchester system for intracavitary therapy of the cervix uteri. *Br J Radiol* 1983; 56:409.

183. Jones D, Notley H, Hunterk R. Geometry adopted by Manchester radium applicators and Selectron afterloading applicators in intracavitary treatment for carcinoma cervix uteri. *Br J Radiol* 1987;60:481.

184. Dean E, Lambert G, Dawes P. Gynaecological treatments using the Selectron remote afterloading system. *Br J Radiol* 1988;61:1053.

185. Grigsby PW, Williamson JF, Perez CA. Source configuration and dose rates for the Selectron afterloading equipment for gynecologic applications. *Int J Radiat Oncol Biol Phys* 1992;24:321.

186. Battermann JJ, Szabol B. Preliminary results of radiation therapy for carcinoma of the uterine cervix, using the Selectron afterloading ma-

chine. In: Mould RF, ed. *Brachytherapy 2.* Netherlands: Nucletron International BV, 1989:229.

187. Hintz BL, Kagan AR, Chan P, et al. Radiation tolerance of the vaginal mucosa. *Int J Radiat Oncol Biol Phys* 1980;6:711.

188. Au SP, Grigsby PW. The irradiation tolerance dose of the proximal vagina. *Radiother Oncol* 2003:67:77.

189. Fletcher GH. Cervical radium applicators with screening in the direction of bladder and rectum. *Radiology* 1953;60:77.

190. Tod MC, Meredith WJ. A dosage system for use in the treatment of cancer of the uterine cervix. *Br J Radiol* 1938;11:809.

191. Batley F, Constable WC. The use of the "Manchester system" for treatment of cancer of the uterine cervix with modern afterloading radium applicators. *J Can Assoc Radiol* 1967;18:396.

192. Tod MC, Meredith WJ. Treatment of cancer of the cervix uteri: a revised "Manchester method." *Br J Radiol* 1953;26:252.

193. Delclos L. Afterloading interstitial irradiation techniques. In: Levitt SH, Khan FM, Potish RA, eds. *Levitt and Tapley's technological basis of radiation therapy: practical clinical applications.* Philadelphia: Lea & Febiger, 1992:123.

194. Haas JS, Dean RD, Mansfield CM. Dosimetric comparison of the Fletcher family of gynecologic colpostats, 1950–1980. *Int J Radiat Oncol Biol Phys* 1985;11:1317.

195. Delclos L, Fletcher GH, Sampiere V, Grant WH III. Can the Fletcher gamma ray colpostat system be extrapolated to other systems? *Cancer* 1978;41:970.

196. Saylor WL, Dillard M. Dosimetry of ^{137}Cs sources with Fletcher-Suit gynecological applicator. *Med Phys* 1976;3:117.

197. Weeks KJ, Dennett MS. Dose calculation and measurements for a CT compatible version of the Fletcher applicator. *Int J Radiat Oncol Biol Phys* 1990;18:1191.

198. Weeks KJ, Schoeppel SL, Pruss K, et al. A computed tomography-compatible afterloading Fletcher-Suit-Delclos colpost with adjustable shielding. *Endocurietherapy Hyperthermia Oncol* 1989;5:169.

199. Schoeppel SL, Fraass BA, Hopkins MP, et al. A CT-compatible version of the Fletcher system intracavitary applicator: clinical application and 3-dimensional treatment planning. *Int J Radiat Oncol Biol Phys* 1989;17:1103.

200. Malyapa RS, Mutic S, Low DA, et al. Physiologic FDG-PET three-dimensional brachytherapy treatment planning for cervical cancer. *Int J Radiat Oncol Biol Phys* 2002;54:1140.

201. Mutic S, Grigsby PW, Low DA, et al. PET-guided three-dimensional treatment planning of intracavitary gynecologic implants. *Int J Radiat Oncol Biol Phys* 2002;52:1104.

202. Delclos L, Fletcher GH, Moore EB, et al. Minicolpostats, dome cylinders, other additions and improvements of the Fletcher-Suit afterloadable system: indications and limitations of their use. *Int J Radiat Oncol Biol Phys* 1980;6:1195.

203. Kuske RR, Perez CA, Jacobs AJ, et al. Mini-colpostats in the treatment of carcinoma of the uterine cervix. *Int J Radiat Oncol Biol Phys* 1988; 14:899.

204. Prempree T. Parametrial implant in stage IIIB cancer of the cervix. III. A 5-year study. *Cancer* 1983;52:748.

205. Aristizabal SA, Valencia A, Ocampo G, et al. Interstitial parametral irradiation in cancer of the cervix stage IIB-IIIB. *Endocurietherapy Hyperthermia Oncol* 1985;1:41.

206. Gaddis O Jr, Morrow CP, Klement V, et al. Treatment of cervical carcinoma employing a template for transperineal interstitial ^{192}Ir brachytherapy. *Int J Radiat Oncol Biol Phys* 1983;9:819.

207. Martinez A, Edmundson GK, Cox RS, et al. Combination of external beam irradiation and multiple-site perineal applicator (MUPIT) for treatment of locally advanced or recurrent prostatic, anorectal, and gynecologic malignancies. *Int J Radiat Oncol Biol Phys* 1985;11:391.

208. Syed AMN, Puthawala AA, Tansey LA, et al. Temporary iridium-192 implantation in the management of carcinoma of the prostate. In: Hilaris BS, Batata MA, eds. *Brachytherapy oncology—1983.* New York: Memorial Sloan-Kettering Cancer Center, 1983:83.

209. Demanes DJ, Rodriguez RR, Bendre DD, et al. High dose rate transperineal interstitial brachytherapy for cervical cancer: high pelvic control and low complication rates. *Int J Radiat Oncol Biol Phys* 1999; 45:105.

210. Eisbruch AE, Johnston CM, Martel MK, et al. Customized gynecologic interstitial implants: CT-based planning, dose evaluation, and

optimization aided by laparotomy. *Int J Radiat Oncol Biol Phys* 1998: 40:1087.

211. Erickson B, Albano K, Gillin M: CT-guided interstitial implantation of gynecological malignancies. *Int J Radiat Oncol Biol Phys* 1996; 36:699.

212. LaVigne M, Schoeppel SL, McShan DL. The use of CT-based 3-D anatomical modeling in the design of customized perineal templates for interstitial gynecologic implants. *Med Dosimetry* 1991;16:187.

213. Li Z, Palta JR, Mitchell TP, et al. Virtual simulation and CT-based planning of interstitial GYN brachytherapy. *Med Phys* 1999;26:1077.

214. Marsh LH, Robertson JM, McShan DL. Simplified method for three-dimensional evaluation of interstitial brachytherapy applications. *Med Dosimetry* 1994;19:203.

215. Stock RG, Chan K, Terk CM, et al. A new technique for performing Syed-Neblett template interstitial implants for gynecological malignancies using transrectal-ultrasound guidance. *Int J Radiat Oncol Biol Phys* 1997;37:819.

216. Potish RA, Williamson JF. Clinical and physical aspects of interstitial template therapy in gynecological malignancy. In: Levitt SH, Khan FM, Potish RA, eds. *Technological basis of radiation therapy: practical and clinical applications.* 2nd ed. Philadelphia: Lea & Febiger, 1992:155.

217. Paterson R. *The treatment of malignant disease by radiotherapy.* 2nd ed. Baltimore: Williams & Wilkins, 1963.

218. Lichter AS, Dillon MB, Rosenshein NB, Suit HD. The use of custom molds for intracavitary treatment of carcinoma of the cervix. *Int J Radiat Oncol Biol Phys* 1978;4(9,10):873.

219. Rutledge FN, Delclos L. Adenocarcinoma of the uterus. In: Fletcher GH, ed. *Textbook of radiotherapy.* 3rd ed. Philadelphia: Lea & Febiger, 1980:798.

220. Heyman J, Reuterwall O, Benner S. The Radiumhemmet experience with radiotherapy in cancer of the corpus of the uterus: classification, method of treatment and results. *Acta Radiol* 1941;11:11.

221. Grigsby PW, Perez CA, Kuten A, et al. Clinical stage I endometrial cancer: results of adjuvant irradiation and patterns of failure. *Int J Radiat Oncol Biol Phys* 1991;21:379.

222. Perez CA, Camel HM, Galakatos AE, et al. Definitive irradiation in carcinoma of the vagina: long-term evaluation of results. *Int J Radiat Oncol Biol Phys* 1988;15:1283.

223. Perez CA, Slessinger E, Grigsby PW. Design of an afterloading vaginal applicator (MIRALVA). *Int J Radiat Oncol Biol Phys* 1990;18: 1503.

224. Battermann JJ, Boon TA. Interstitial therapy in the management of T2 bladder tumors. *Endocurietherapy Hyperthermia Oncol* 1988;4:1.

225. Huilgol NG, Mehta AR, Kulkarni V, et al. Hypofractionated external radiation with high and low dose rates in the treatment of advanced cancer of the cervix. *Int J Radiat Oncol Biol Phys* 1988;14:577.

226. Lacassagne A, Gricouroff G. *Action of radiation on tissues: an introduction to radiotherapy.* New York: Grune & Stratton, 1958.

227. Teshima T, Chatani M, Hata K, Inoue T. High-dose rate intracavitary therapy for carcinoma of the uterine cervix. II. Risk factors for rectal complication. *Int J Radiat Oncol Biol Phys* 1988;14:281.

228. Warmelink C, Ezzell G, Orton C. Use of a time-dose-fractionation model to design high dose-rate fractionation schemes. In: Mould RF, ed. *Brachytherapy 2.* Amsterdam: Nucletron International BV, 1989: 41.

229. Orton CG, Seyedsadr M, Somnay A. Comparison of high and low dose rate remote afterloading for cervix cancer and the importance of fractionation. *Int J Radiat Oncol Biol Phys* 1991;21:1425.

230. Petereit DG, Pearcey R: Literature analysis of high dose rate brachytherapy fractionation schedules in the treatment of cervical cancer: Is there an optimal fractionation schedule? *Int J Radiat Oncol Biol Phys* 1999;46:259.

231. Jacobs H. Experiences with interstitial HDR afterloading therapy in genital and breast cancer. In: Vahrson H, Rauthe G, eds. *High dose rate afterloading in the treatment of cancer of the uterus, breast and rectum.* Baltimore: Urban & Schwarzenberg, 1988:258.

232. Rattka P. Experience in the treatment of cancer of the cervix using HDR brachytherapy in Gliwice. In: Mould RF, ed. *Brachytherapy 2.* Leersum, The Netherlands: Nucletron International BV, 1989:296.

233. Rauthe G, Vahrson H, Giers G. Five-year results and complications in endometrium cancer: HDR afterloading versus conventional radium therapy. In: Vahrson H, Rauthe G, eds. *High dose rate afterloading*

in the treatment of cancer of the uterus, breast and rectum. Baltimore: Urban & Schwarzenberg, 1988:240.

234. Fu KK, Phillips TL. High-dose-rate versus low-dose-rate intracavitary brachytherapy for carcinoma of the cervix. *Int J Radiat Oncol Biol Phys* 1990;19:791.

235. Nag S, Orton C, Young D, et al. The American Brachytherapy Society survey of brachytherapy practice for carcinoma of the cervix in the United States. *Gynecol Oncol* 1999;73:111.

236. Nori D, Hilaris BS, Batata MA, et al. Remote afterloading in cancer management. II. Clinical applications of remote afterloaders. In: Hilaris BS, Batata MA, eds. *Brachytherapy oncology—1983.* New York: Memorial Sloan-Kettering Cancer Center, 1983:101.

237. Arai T. Relationship between total isoeffect dose and number of fractions for the treatment of uterine cervical carcinoma by high dose rate intracavitary irradiation: working party on the use of radionuclides and afterloading techniques in the treatment of cancer of the uterus. London: High Dose Workshop, 1978.

238. Mandell L, Dattatreyudu N, Anderson L, Hilaris B. Postoperative vaginal radiation in endometrial cancer using a remote afterloading technique. *Int J Radiat Oncol Biol Phys* 1985;11:473.

239. Sorbe B, Frankendal B, Risberg B. Intracavitary irradiation of endometrial carcinoma stage I by a high dose rate afterloading technique. *Gynecol Oncol* 1989;33:135.

240. Peschel RE, Healey GA, Smith RJ, et al. High dose rate remote afterloading for endometrial cancer. *Endocurietherapy Hyperthermia Oncol* 1989;5:209.

241. McCormick TC, Cardenes H, Randall ME: Early-stage endometrial cancer: Is intravaginal radiation therapy alone sufficient therapy? *Brachytherapy* 2003;1:61.

242. Potish RA, Deibel FC, Khan FM. The relationship between milligram-hours and dose to point A in carcinoma of the cervix. *Radiology* 1982; 145:478.

243. Potish RA, Gerbi BJ. Role of point A in the era of computerized dosimetry. *Radiology* 1986;158:827.

244. Potish RA. The effect of applicator geometry on dose specification in cervical cancer. *Int J Radiat Oncol Biol Phys* 1990;18:1513.

245. Katz A, Eifel PJ. Quantification of intracavitary brachytherapy parameters and correlation with outcome in patients with carcinoma of the cervix. *Int J Radiat Oncol Biol Phys* 2000;48:1417.

246. Crook JM, Esche BA, Chaplain G, et al. Dose-volume analysis and the prevention of radiation sequelae in cervical cancer. *Radiother Oncol* 1987;8:321.

247. Esche BA, Crook JM, Isturiz J, Horiot J-C. Reference volume, milligram-hours and external irradiation for the Fletcher applicator. *Radiother Oncol* 1987;9:255.

248. Eisbruch AE, Williamson JF, Dickson R, et al. Estimation of tissue volume irradiated by intracavitary implants. *Int J Radiat Oncol Biol Phys* 1993;25:733.

249. Chassagne D, Horiot JC. Propositions pour une definition commune des points de reference en curietherapie gynecologique. *J Radiol Electrol Med Nucl* 1977;58:371.

250. Hayata Y, Dougherty TJ, eds. *Lasers and hematoporphyrin derivative in cancer.* Tokyo: Igaku-Shoin, 1983.

251. Ling CC, Shell MC, Working KR, et al. CT-assisted assessment of bladder and rectum dose in gynecological implants. *Int J Radiat Oncol Biol Phys* 1987;13:1577.

252. Schoeppel SL, Ellis JH, LaVigne ML, et al. Magnetic resonance imaging during intracavitary gynecologic brachytherapy. *Int J Radiat Oncol Biol Phys* 1992;23:169.

253. Schoeppel SL, LaVigne M, Martel MK, et al. Three-dimensional treatment planning of intracavitary gynecologic implants: Analysis of ten cases and implications for dose specification. *Int J Radiat Oncol Biol Phys* 1994;28:277.

254. National Council on Radiation Protection and Measurements. Report no. 40: Protection against radiation from brachytherapy sources. Bethesda, MD: NCRP, 1974.

255. United States Nuclear Regulatory Commission. Medical use of byproduct material. Title 10, Chapter 1, Part 35, Code of Federal Regulations. Washington, DC: US Government Printing Office, 1988.

256. Pierquin B, Wilson J-F, Chassagne D. Radiation protection and the organizational plan of a brachytherapy department. In: Pierquin B, Wilson J-F, Chassagne D, eds. *Modern brachytherapy.* New York: Masson, 1987:43.

257. Nath R, Anderson Meli JA, et al. Code of practice for brachytherapy physics: Report of the APM Radiation Therapy Committee Task Group No. 56. American Association of Physicists in Medicine. *Med Phys* 1997;24:1557.

258. Withers HR, Thames HD, Peters LJ. Differences in fractionation response of acutely and late responding tissues. In: Karcher KH, et al., eds. *Progress in radio-oncology II.* New York: Raven Press, 1982: 287.

259. Cox JD. Fractionation: a paradigm for clinical research in radiation oncology. *Int J Radiat Oncol Biol Phys* 1987;13:1271.

260. Fowler JF. How worthwhile are short schedules in radiotherapy? A series of exploratory calculations. *Radiother Oncol* 1990;18:165.

261. Fowler JF. The linear quadratic formula and progress in fractionated radiotherapy: a review. *Br J Radiol* 1989;62:679.

262. Withers HR, Peters LJ, Thames HD, Fletcher GH. Hyperfractionation. *Int J Radiat Oncol Biol Phys* 1982;8:1807.

263. Hermens AF, Barendsen GW. Changes in cell proliferation characteristics in a rat rhabdomyosarcoma before and after x-irradiation. *Eur J Cancer* 1969;5:173.

264. Withers HR, Taylor JMF, Maciejewski B. The hazard of accelerated tumor clonogen repopulation during radiotherapy. *Acta Oncol* 1988; 27:131.

265. Fyles A, Keane TJ, Barton M, et al. The effect of treatment duration in the local control of cervix cancer. *Radiother Oncol* 1992;25:273.

266. Perez CA, Grigsby PW, Castro-Vita H, et al. Carcinoma of the uterine cervix. I. Impact of prolongation of overall treatment time and timing of brachytherapy on outcome of radiation therapy. *Int J Radiat Oncol Biol Phys* 1995;32:1275.

267. Strandqvist M. Studien uber die kumulative Wirkung der Rontgenstrahlen bie Fraktionierung. *Acta Radiol Suppl (Stockh)* 1944;55:1.

268. Cohen L. Clinical radiation dosage. II. Interrelation of time, area and therapeutic ratio. *Br J Radiol* 1949;22:706.

269. Ellis F. Is NSD-TDF useful to radiotherapy? *Int J Radiat Oncol Biol Phys* 1985;11:1685.

270. Fowler JF, Denekamp J, Page AL, et al. Fractionation with x-rays and neutrons in mice: response of skin and C3H mammary tumours. *Br J Radiol* 1972;45:237.

271. Fowler JF. La Ronde: radiation sciences and medical radiology. *Radiother Oncol* 1983;1:1.

272. Marcial VA, Amato D, Marks RD, et al. Split-course versus continuous pelvis irradiation in carcinoma of uterine cervix: a randomized prospective clinical trial of the Radiation Therapy Oncology Group. *Int J Radiat Oncol Biol Phys* 1983;9:431.

273. Parsons JT, Thar TL, Bova FJ, Million RR. An evaluation of split-course irradiation for pelvic malignancies. *Int J Radiat Oncol Biol Phys* 1980;6:175.

274. Singh K. Two regimens with the same TDF but differing morbidity used in the treatment of stage III carcinoma of the cervix. *Br J Radiol* 1978;51:357.

275. Meoz RT, Spanos WJ, Doss L, et al. Misonidazole combined with large-fraction pelvic irradiation in the treatment of patients with advanced pelvic malignancies: preliminary report of an ongoing RTOG phase I-II study. *Am J Clin Oncol* 1983;6:417.

276. Spanos W Jr, Perez CA, Marcus S, et al. Effect of rest interval on tumor and normal tissue response: a report of phase III study of accelerated split course palliative radiation for advanced pelvic malignancies (RTOG-8502). *Int J Radiat Oncol Biol Phys* 1993;25:399.

277. Powers BE, Gillette EL, McChesney SL, et al. Bone necrosis and tumor induction following experimental intraoperative irradiation. *Int J Radiat Oncol Biol Phys* 1989;17:559.

278. LeCouteur RA, Gillette EL, Powers BE, et al. Peripheral neuropathies following experimental intraoperative radiation therapy (IORT). *Int J Radiat Oncol Biol Phys* 1989;17:583.

279. Shaw EG, Gunderson LL, Martin JK, et al. Peripheral nerve and ureteral tolerance to intraoperative radiation therapy: clinical and dose-response analysis. Consensus Meeting on Phase III Trials in Intraoperative Radiation Therapy, Philadelphia, July 10–11, 1987.

280. Yaes RJ. Linear-quadratic model isoeffect relations for proliferating tumor cells for treatment with multiple fractions per day. *Int J Radiat Oncol Biol Phys* 1989;17:901.

281. Bentzen SM, Overgaard M, Thames HD. Fractionation sensitivity of a functional endpoint: impaired shoulder movement after postmastectomy radiotherapy. *Int J Radiat Oncol Biol Phys* 1989;17:531.

282. Rubin P, Casarett GW. *Clinical radiation pathology.* Vols 1 and 2. Philadelphia: WB Saunders, 1968.

283. Berkjis CC. *Pathology of irradiation.* Baltimore: Williams & Wilkins, 1971.

284. Ilic S, Ristic B. Five-year results with HDR afterloading cervix cancer: dependence on fractionation and dose. *Strahlenther Onkol* 1988; 82[Suppl]:139.

285. Emami B, Lyman J, Brown A, et al. Tolerance of normal tissue to therapeutic irradiation. *Int J Radiat Oncol Biol Phys* 1991;21:109.

286. Cassady JR, Richter MP, Piro AJ, Jaffe N. Radiation-Adriamycin interactions: preliminary clinical observations. *Cancer* 1975;36:946.

287. Ratzkowski E, Hochman A. Gastrointestinal function after abdominal cobalt irradiation. *Acta Radiol (Ther)* 1968;7:417.

288. Schlea CC, Stoddard DH: Californium isotopes proposed for intracavitary and interstitial radiation therapy with neutrons. *Nature* 1965; 206:1058.

289. Perez CA, Fox S, Lockett MA, et al. Impact of dose in outcome of irradiation alone in carcinoma of the uterine cervix: analysis of two different methods. *Int J Radiat Oncol Biol Phys* 1991;21:885.

290. Phillips TL, Wharam MD, Margolis LW. Modification of radiation injury to normal tissues by chemotherapeutic agents. *Cancer* 1975; 35:1678.

291. Ingold JA, Reed GB, Kaplan HS, Bagshaw MA. Radiation hepatitis. *Am J Roentgenol Radium Ther Nucl Med* 1965;93:200.

292. Ogata K, Hozawa K, Yoshika M, et al. Hepatic injury following irradiation: a morphologic study. *Tokushima J Exp Med* 1963;9:240.

293. Luxton RW, Kunkler PB. Radiation nephritis. *Acta Radiol* 1962;2: 169.

294. Cohen M, Jones DEA, Greene D. Central axis depth dose data for use in radiotherapy. *Br J Radiol* 1972;11:8.

295. Blood AD, Tijo JH. In vivo effects of diagnostic x-irradiation on human chromosomes. *N Engl J Med* 1964;270:1341.

296. Zuckerman S. The sensitivity of the gonads to radiation. *Clin Radiol* 1965;16:1.

297. Knospe WH, Blom J, Crosby WH. Regeneration of locally irradiated bone marrow. I. Dose dependent long-term changes in the rate, with particular emphasis upon vascular and stromal reaction. *Blood* 1966; 28:398.

298. Sacks EL, Goris ML, Glatstein E, et al. Bone marrow regeneration following large field radiation: influence of volume, age, dose, and time. *Cancer* 1978;42:1057.

299. Georgiou A, Grigsby PW, Perez CA. Radiation induced lumbrosacral plexopathy in gynecologic tumors: clinical findings and dosimetric analysis. *Int J Radiat Oncol Biol Phys* 1993;26:479.

300. Garton GR, Gunderson LL, Webb MJ, et al. Intraoperative radiation therapy in gynecologic cancer: update of the experience at a single institution. *Int J Radiat Oncol Biol Phys* 1997;37:839.

301. Gemignani ML, Alektiar KM, Leitao M, et al. Radical surgical resection and high-dose intraoperative radiation therapy (HDR-IORT) in patients with recurrent gynecologic cancers. *Int J Radiat Oncol Biol Phys* 2001;50:687.

302. Steel GG, Adams GE, Horwich A, eds. *The biological basis of radiotherapy.* Amsterdam: Elsevier Science, 1989.

303. Frei E III. What's in a name: neoadjuvant. *J Natl Cancer Inst* 1989; 80:1088.

304. Dewhirst MW, Sim DA. Estimation of therapeutic gain in clinical trials involving hyperthermia and radiotherapy. *Int J Hyperthermia* 1986;2:165.

305. Perez CA, Emami B. Clinical trials with local (external and interstitial) irradiation and hyperthermia: current and future perspectives. *Radiol Clin North Am* 1989;27:525.

306. Myerson RJ, Leybovich L, Emami BN, et al. Phantom studies and preliminary clinical experience with the BSD 2000. *Int J Hyperthermia* 1991;7:937.

307. Samulski TV. Current technologies for invasive thermometry. In: Paliwal BR, Hetzel FW, Dewhirst MW, eds. *Biological, physical and clinical aspects of hyperthermia.* New York: American Association of Physicists in Medicine, 1988:168.

308. Christensen DA. A nonperturbing temperature probe using semiconductor band edge shift. *J Bioeng* 1977;1:541.

309. Wickersheim KA. A new fiberoptic thermometry system for use in medical hyperthermia. *SPIE Proc* Sept 14, 1986:Vol 713.

310. Emami B, Myerson RJ, Scott C, et al. Phase I/II study, combination of

radiotherapy and hyperthermia in patients with deep-seated malignant tumors: report of a pilot study by the Radiation Therapy Oncology Group. *Int J Radiat Oncol Biol Phys* 1991;20:73.

311. Petrovich Z, Langholtz B, Gibbs FA, et al. Regional hyperthermia for advanced tumors: a clinical study of 353 patients. *Int J Radiat Oncol Biol Phys* 1989;16:601.

312. Sapozink MD, Gibbs FA Jr, Egger MJ, Stewart JR. Regional hyperthermia for clinically advanced deep-seated pelvic malignancy. *Am J Clin Oncol* 1986;9:162.

313. Uehara S, Omagari J. Deep local and regional hyperthermia with annular phased array. *Strahlenther Onkol* 1989;165:715.

314. Gibbs FA Jr. Regional hyperthermia in the treatment of cancer. In: Paliwal BR, Hetzel FW, Dewhirst MW, eds. *Biological, physical and clinical aspects of hyperthermia. Medical Physics Monograph No. 16.* New York: American Association of Physicists in Medicine, 1988: 330.

315. Hornback NB, Shupe RE, Shidnia H, et al. Advanced stage IIIB cancer of the cervix treatment by hyperthermia and radiation. *Gynecol Oncol* 1986;23:160.

316. Sharma S, Patel FD, Sandhu APS, et al. A prospective randomized study of local hyperthermia as a supplement and radiosensitizer in the treatment of carcinoma of the cervix with radiotherapy. *Endocurietherapy Hyperthermia Oncol* 1989;5:151.

317. Emami B, Scott C, Perez CA, et al. Phase III study of interstitial thermoradiotherapy compared with interstitial radiotherapy alone in the treatment of recurrent or persistent human tumors: a prospectively controlled randomized study by the Radiation Therapy Oncology Group. *Int J Radiat Oncol Biol Phys* 1996;34:1097.

318. Vora NL, Luk KH, Forell B, et al. Interstitial local current field hyperthermia for advanced cancers of the cervix. *Endocurietherapy Hyperthermia Oncol* 1988;4:97.

319. Li DJ, Chou CK, Luk KH, et al. Design of intracavitary microwave applicators for the treatment of uterine cervix carcinoma and its preliminary clinical applications. In: Sugahara T, Saito M, eds. *Hyperthermic oncology 1988.* Vol 1. London: Taylor & Francis, 1989:604.

320. Lipson RL, Baldes EJ, Olsen EM. Hematoporphyrin derivative for detection and management of cancer. Proceedings of the IX International Cancer Congress, 1966.

321. DeLaney TF, Glatstein EJ. Photodynamic therapy: theory and practice. 31st ASTRO Scientific Meeting, Refresher Course No. 108, 1989.

322. Doiron DR, Gomer CJ, eds. *Porphyrin localization and treatment of tumors.* New York: Alan R. Liss, 1984.

323. Williamson JF. Dose calculations about shielded gynecological colpostats. *Int J Radiat Oncol Biol Phys* 1990;19:167.

324. Feder BH, Syed AMN, Neblett D. Treatment of extensive carcinoma of the cervix with the "transperineal parametrial butterfly": a preliminary report on the revival of Waterman's approach. *Int J Radiat Oncol Biol Phys* 1978;4:735.

325. Benson RC. Laser photodynamic therapy for bladder cancer. *Mayo Clin Proc* 1986;61:859.

326. Tsuchiya A, Obara N, Miwa M, et al. Hematoporphyrin derivative and laser photoradiation in the diagnosis and treatment of bladder cancer. *J Urol* 1983;130:79.

327. Prout GR Jr, Lin CW, Benson R Jr, et al. Photodynamic therapy with hematoporphyrin derivative in the treatment of superficial transitional-cell carcinoma of the bladder. *N Engl J Med* 1987;317:1251.

328. Rettenmaier MA, Berman ML, DiSaia PJ, et al. Gynecologic uses of photoradiation therapy. *Prog Clin Biol Res* 1984;170:767.

329. Corti L, Tomio L, Maluta S, et al. Recurring gynaecologic cancer treated with photodynamic therapy. *Photochem Photobiol* 1987;46: 949.

330. Deschner EE, Gray LH. Influence of oxygen tension on x-ray–induced chromosomal damage in Ehrlich ascites tumor cells irradiated in vitro and in vivo. *Radiat Res* 1959;11:115.

CHAPTER 15

Principles of Chemotherapy in Gynecologic Cancer

Michael A. Bookman

HISTORICAL OVERVIEW OF CANCER CHEMOTHERAPY

The first report of a drug-mediated tumor response was noted over 125 years ago using Fowler's solution (arsenic trioxide in potassium bicarbonate) in patients with Hodgkin's disease and leukemia (1). Arsenic compounds had been used for various medicinal purposes for over 2000 years, and it was not surprising that they were tested in patients with cancer. Cyclic hematologic toxicity was observed following arsenic administration in normal individuals and patients with leukemia (2), establishing a close association between tumor response and host toxicity that still exists today. Cumulative dose-limiting toxicity (arsenic poisoning) was also described following expanded utilization of arsenic in chronic myelogenous leukemia (3), coinciding with a transition toward radiation therapy for the management of leukemia and lymphoma around 1940.

The term *chemotherapy* has been attributed to Paul Ehrlich, a Nobel laureate physician and bacteriologist, who developed *in vivo* rodent models of infection, including the introduction in 1910 of Salvarsan, an organic arsenical originally used to cure syphilis and still used in the management of trypanosomiasis. His early *in vivo* modeling also encouraged the development of inbred transplantable rodent tumors, thereby establishing a paradigm that has been widely adopted for screening new antitumor agents.

Although the topical vesicant properties of sulfur mustard received much attention during World War I, multiple systemic effects, including leukopenia, bone marrow aplasia, and mucosal ulceration, emerged with further study, and would ultimately have greater importance. Cancer chemo-

therapy, in the traditional sense, began with the demonstration that nitrogen mustard had reproducible activity against transplanted lymphoma in mice, prompting clinical trials as early as 1942 (4). However, owing to World War II, much of the research remained classified until 1946. Following the demonstration by Farber in 1948 that aminopterin, an antifolate, could induce temporary remission in childhood leukemia (5), antimetabolites became the next major category of agents to be developed, and were ultimately associated with cures in women with choriocarcinoma (6). Research during the 1940s also included the Nobel Prize–winning observations of Huggins and others (7) regarding the antitumor effect of estrogens in prostatic cancer.

Between 1945 and 1965, many important chemotherapeutic agents, such as actinomycin D, cyclophosphamide, 5-fluorouracil, vinca alkaloids, and progestogens, were developed and demonstrated to have antitumor activity in clinical trials. Between 1965 and 1975, the pace of new drug discovery and development continued. During this period, cisplatin was shown to have activity in testicular and ovarian tumors, and doxorubicin, bleomycin, etoposide, and tamoxifen entered our clinical arsenal. This was followed by identification of analogs, such as carboplatin, idarubicin, and vinorelbine, with antitumor activity similar to the parent compound but with a reduction in nonhematologic toxicity. The 1990s and beyond have brought important new agents into clinical practice, including the taxanes (paclitaxel and docetaxel), camptothecins (topotecan and irinotecan), nucleoside analogs (gemcitabine and capecitabine), alternative organoplatinums (oxaliplatin), an inhibitor of the proteasome complex (bortezomib), and a minor groove DNA alkylating agent (ecteinascidin).

Attention has also been directed at alternative formulations of standard agents, including liposomal or polymer-based encapsulation, protein conjugation, or lipid solubilization, to modify drug disposition and tumor targeting. In

Division of Medical Science, Fox Chase Cancer Center, Philadelphia, Pennsylvania 19111

addition, conventional agents have been utilized for regional (intraperitoneal) administration, prolonged intravenous infusion, continuous oral administration, high-dose therapy with hematopoietic progenitor cell support, and weekly low-dose therapy, each with the goal of maximizing tumor drug exposure, but with a variable impact on host toxicity and clinical outcomes.

With the availability of multiple agents, each with a different molecular target, mechanism of action, pattern of resistance, and spectrum of host toxicity, we have also seen expanded utilization of multidrug combinations, as well as the incorporation with radiation. The use of adjuvant therapy has been greatly expanded in selected clinical situations, and we have begun to see applications of chemoprevention.

Nonetheless, the majority of advanced tumors eventually demonstrate broad resistance to conventional cytotoxic chemotherapy, and there has been renewed interest in novel biologic and immunologic approaches with non–cross-resistant mechanisms. In addition, with greater understanding of the mechanisms associated with drug resistance, newer agents have been developed that may partially reverse the resistant phenotype through blockade of specific pathways, such as the drug efflux pump MDR-1. Exploration of the biologic mechanisms associated with tumor invasion, metastasis, and angiogenesis has led to the development of metalloproteinase inhibitors and antiangiogenesis reagents. As basic research in molecular biology uncovers specific genetic and growth-regulatory factors associated with tumorigenesis, targeted small molecules have been developed that modulate a number of intracellular pathways. These include inhibition of protein tyrosine kinases associated with specific growth-factor receptors and downstream components of signal transduction pathways, cyclin-dependent kinases associated with cell cycle progression, as well as interference with posttranslational protein modifications, such as farnesylation of the *ras* oncogene and other intracellular targets (8,9).

TUMOR BIOLOGY IN RELATIONSHIP TO CHEMOTHERAPY

Tumor Growth and Cellular Kinetics

Many of the principles of modern chemotherapy are derived from knowledge of the growth characteristics of normal and tumor tissues. Each tissue has an innate capacity for growth that is regulated by internal and external factors. The growth characteristics of tumors differ from normal tissues, and the exploitation of these differences has provided the historical basis for utilization of radiation and chemotherapy.

The cellular kinetics of normal tissues also explains many of the toxicities associated with chemotherapeutic agents. All normal tissues, particularly during fetal development and variably during adult life, possess the capacity for cellular division and growth. Three categories of proliferative activity predominate: *static, expanding,* and *renewing.*

The *static* population generally includes well-differentiated cells that rarely undergo cell division after an initial period of proliferation during fetal life. Typical of this group are striated muscle and neurons, with oocytes representing a specialized subcategory.

The *expanding* population of normal tissues retains the capacity to grow, but in their adult state, they are normally quiescent. Under stress, especially after injury, a proliferative burst is followed by return to quiescence. Typical of this pattern of growth are the components of liver parenchymal tissue, including hepatocytes, bile duct epithelium, and vascular endothelium.

The *renewing* cell population is in a continuous proliferative state with ongoing cell division balanced by cell loss and terminal differentiation. Typical renewing populations include the bone marrow, epidermis, gastrointestinal epithelium, and spermatocytes.

The patterns of normal cell growth partially explain some of the toxic effects of cytotoxic therapy and why some tissues are commonly spared (10). Renewing cell populations with constant turnover are most sensitive to acute injury from chemotherapy or irradiation. This is reflected by the frequent occurrence of bone marrow suppression, mucositis, and azoospermia during cytotoxic drug treatment, with relative sparing of nonproliferative compartments, such as brain, muscle, bone, and oocytes. However, even nondividing tissues can experience late chronic effects related to DNA damage following radiation therapy or chemotherapy.

Unregulated growth of cancer cells occurs because of altered growth-factor signaling and/or disruption of checkpoint mechanisms that exist in normal cells. Despite a capacity for continuous growth, the actual process of cancer cell division is not more rapid than division in normal cells.

Programmed cell death, or apoptosis, has emerged as a major mechanism for regulating growth. Furthermore, it is known that certain oncogenes, like c-*myc* and *bcl-2*, and tumor-suppressor genes (antioncogenes), like *Rb* and *p53*, are central to the regulation of apoptosis. Expression of these genes can alter the sensitivity of cancer cells to treatment with chemotherapy and radiation. For instance, overexpression of functional *bcl-2* and nonfunctional *p53* genes can render tumor cells resistant to a number of chemotherapeutic agents (11), suggesting that efforts to restore apoptotic signaling may improve chemosensitivity.

Antioncogenes, such as *Rb* or *p53*, contribute to growth restraint in normal cells. This has specific relevance to gynecologic malignancies, because the E7 protein from the papillomaviruses involved in cervical cancer can inhibit *Rb* and allow cell cycle release (12). In addition, the E6 protein from the same viruses can increase the degradation of *p53*, which also allows increased cell proliferation.

In contrast to cancer, in all normal populations an equilibrium is reached between cell loss or death and new cell production. In a renewing system, there is extensive cell turnover. In static systems, there is very little cell division and correspondingly reduced cell loss. The failure of balanced cell growth is one aspect that differentiates tumors from normal tissues.

Gompertzian Tumor Growth

During initial cell divisions, tumor growth seems to follow an exponential pattern. As the tumor grows larger, the rate of growth slows. This pattern of exponential growth with exponential growth retardation and is known as gompertzian growth (Fig. 15.1). As the tumor mass increases, the time required to double the tumor volume also increases. The kinetic explanation for this apparent paradox is illustrated in Figure 15.2, showing the effect of exponential growth by comparing the number of cells in the tumor mass with the number of doublings (13). In accordance with gompertzian kinetics, exponential growth is not strictly maintained throughout the entire growth history. For example, if a skilled radiologist recognized a 0.5-cm tumor on a chest radiograph, or a clinician palpated a 1-cm tumor mass, we might assume that the tumor had been detected quite early. Unfortunately, the tumor has already undergone at least 30

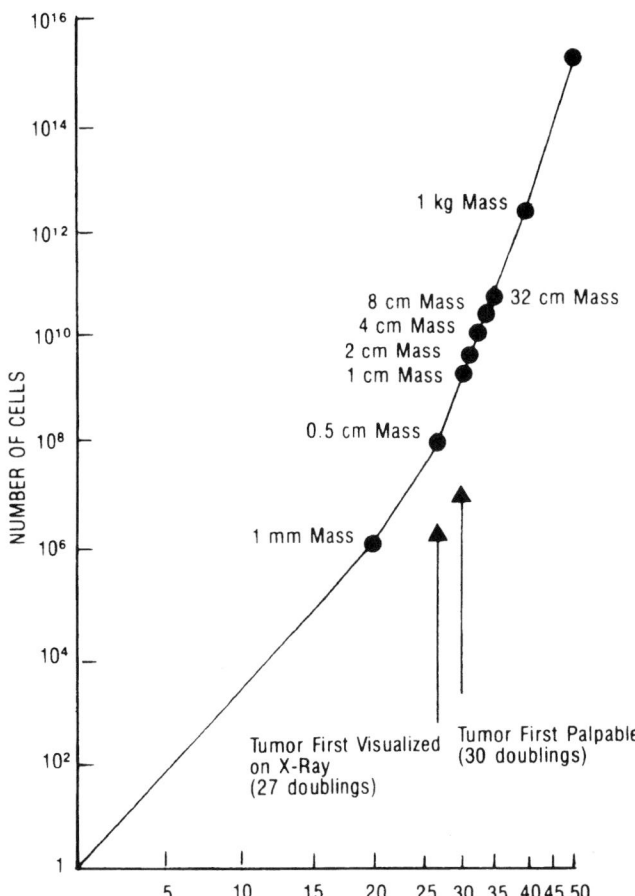

FIG. 15.2. Theoretical tumor doubling curve assumes exponential tumor growth. The vertical axis is the number of cells, and the horizontal axis is the number of doublings.

doublings prior to detection (Fig. 15–2). If we adjust for ongoing cell loss, the number of actual cell doublings would be much greater. The model also suggests other conclusions of clinical relevance. First, metastatic disease may occur well before obvious evidence of the primary lesion. Second, at later stages of tumor growth, a small number of doublings can produce a marked change in the size of the tumor with an increased potential for adverse clinical consequences. For instance, a 1-cm mass (at least 30 prior doublings) becomes a 4-cm mass after just two more doublings.

Limited information exists regarding the actual doubling times of human tumors *in vivo* (14,15), as summarized in Table 15.1. To be included for this type of analysis, tumors were relatively circumscribed and serially measurable by radiographic imaging, often as pulmonary metastases, representing a selective sample. It is clear that embryonal tumors, lymphomas, and mesenchymal tumors have shorter doubling times than adenocarcinomas or squamous-cell carcinomas. In addition, metastases generally have faster doubling times than their corresponding primary lesions. The average doubling time observed in human tumors is approximately 50 days, with a broad range.

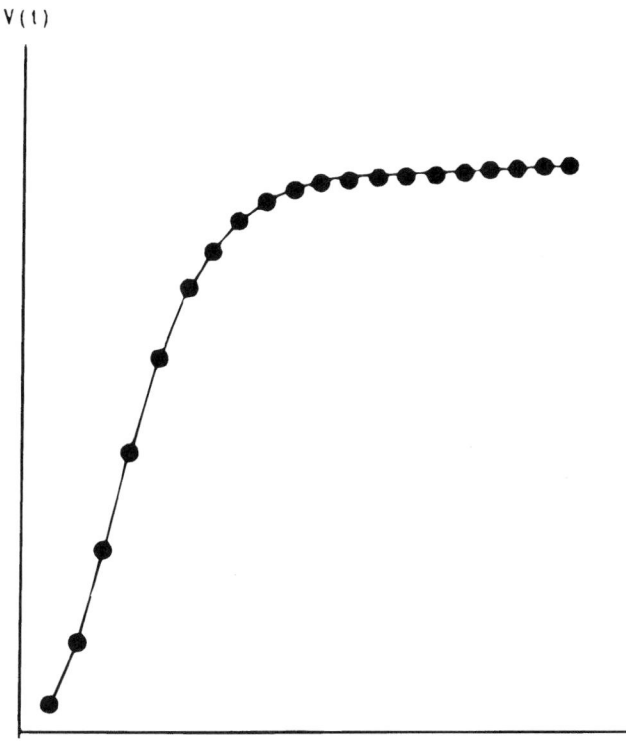

FIG. 15.1. Hypothetical gompertzian tumor growth curve. Exponential tumor growth with exponential growth retardation. The vertical axis is tumor volume, and the horizontal axis is time.

TABLE 15.1. *Doubling times of human tumors*

Tumor histology	Patients (n)	Doubling time (mean ± 2 SD, days)
Embryonal tumors (lung metastases)	76	27 ± 5
Lymphomas	51	29 ± 6
Malignant mesenchymal tumors	87	41 ± 7
Squamous-cell carcinomas (lung metastases)	51	58 ± 9
Squamous-cell carcinomas (primary tumors)	97	82 ± 14
Adenocarcinomas (lung metastases)	134	83 ± 12
Adenocarcinomas (primary tumors)	34	166 ± 48

Cell Cycle Kinetics

The kinetics of individual tumor cells is also important in understanding tumor growth. Figure 15.3 is a schematic view of the cell cycle. Cells can remain in a noncycling postmitotic compartment (G_0) for extended periods of time,

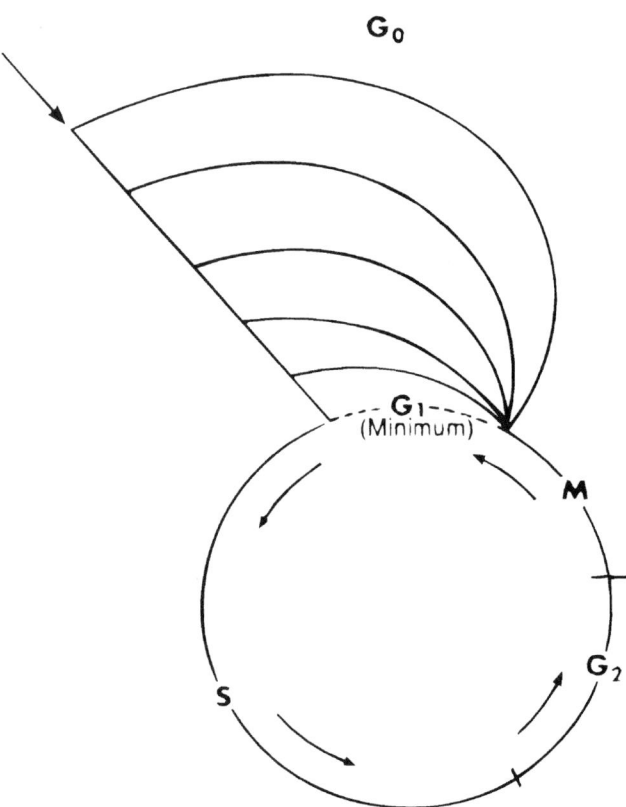

FIG. 15.3. Phases of the cell cycle, beginning with M (mitosis) and proceeding through G_1 (postmitotic phase), S (DNA synthetic phase), and G_2 (premitotic phase). As G_1 becomes progressively longer, it is known as G_0.

but retain the ability to reenter active cycling when triggered by growth factors or other local signals. The point of entry, or first gap phase (G_1), can be of variable length and associated with diverse cellular activities, including protein and RNA synthesis, DNA repair, and cell growth. After passing the first checkpoint in G_1, the cell enters the DNA synthetic phase (S), during which a complete copy of the cellular DNA is created through replication. The second gap phase (G_2) provides another opportunity for checkpoint control before entering active mitosis (M), during which the nuclear membrane disappears and the chromosomes condense (prophase) and align (metaphase) in conjunction with the appearance of the mitotic apparatus, consisting of microtubules, centrioles, and the kinetochore. Mitotic alignment is associated with one final checkpoint prior to actual separation (anaphase), followed by dissolution of the mitotic apparatus (telophase) and creation of daughter cells through cytokinesis. The postmitotic period (G_1) is variable, and cells can further differentiate, enter a noncycling state (G_0), or initiate another cycle.

Cell cycle events have important implications for the patient, tumor, and cancer therapist. Most chemotherapeutic agents disrupt DNA, RNA, or protein synthesis. Rapidly proliferating cells (i.e., short G_1) are most sensitive to chemotherapy, whereas cells that slowly proliferate (i.e., G_0 or long G_1) are generally less sensitive. Nondividing cells, such as the differentiated elements of a mature teratoma, may occupy space and contribute to tumor bulk and symptoms, but are relatively insensitive to chemotherapy.

Cell cycle times may be estimated by performing labeled mitotic curves *in vivo* or *in vitro*, and appear to be relatively similar for many solid tumors, with cycle times ranging from 10 to 31 hours (16). Compared with the tremendous variation in human tumor doubling times, this is a relatively narrow range, suggesting that the primary reason for variations in clinical tumor growth cannot be ascribed to variations in the cell cycle.

Growth fraction and programmed cell death also influence the overall tumor growth rate and response to therapy. The growth fraction is the proportion of tumor cells that are actively cycling. In a typical solid tumor, only a fraction of the cells are rapidly proliferating, primarily those that are most proximal to small blood vessels. With the marked heterogeneity of human tumors at a microscopic level, growth fractions are quite variable, ranging from 25% to 95%. Although it may seem paradoxical, cell loss is very high in human tumors, ranging from 70% to more than 95%, and small changes in cell loss could produce major changes in overall tumor growth (17).

Log Cell Kill

In principle, the rational use of chemotherapy relies on basic concepts of cellular kinetics, but the translation from preclinical models to solid tumors has been challenging. In animals, the curability of transplanted tumors is inversely proportional to the tumor cell number, size, and timing of treatment initiation. In part, this is the result of important tumor-host interactions, such as the time required to establish a blood supply. However, this is also an illustration of first-order cell-kill kinetics, whereby a constant fraction of exposed cells are killed, rather than a constant number. Using first-order kinetics, a single treatment for a tumor weighing 1 g (approximately 10^9 cells) might yield 90% cell kill and would only decrease the tumor population by one log, leaving 10^8 viable cells. Without further treatment, the tumor would grow back at a constant rate, with only a modest delay in lethality. Only when the log cell kill is very large (>99%) and the therapies are repetitive, can chemotherapy be cura-

tive. Although certain unusual cancers, such as choriocarcinoma, can be cured with a single application of a single drug, most human cancers are intrinsically less sensitive, and more sophisticated therapeutic techniques are needed to achieve adequate tumor response. This is one reason why multidrug combinations have been developed. In addition, chemotherapy is usually distributed over multiple cycles to allow for host recovery and achieve the cumulative cell kill required for tumor regression and cure.

It is thought that prolonged survival or cure can be achieved only when the cell population is reduced to between 10^1 and 10^4 cells. In most circumstances, cell burdens of this size are not clinically detectable. This realization has led to the use of adjuvant chemotherapy in the early stages of cancer, where microscopic residual disease is suspected.

TABLE 15.2. *Relationship of chemotherapy agents to intracellular targets and cell cycle progression*

Process	Classification	Cell cycle arrest	Cellular targets and mechanisms	Examples
Inhibition of nucleotide synthesis and metabolism	Antimetabolites and nucleoside analogs	G_1, S	Thymidylate synthase, thymidylate phosphorylase, dihydrofolate reductase, ribonucleotide reductase	6-Mercaptopurine, methotrexate, 5-fluorouracil, cytarabine, gemcitabine, hydroxyurea
Inhibition of DNA synthesis and repair	Topoisomerase inhibition	S	Stabilization of DNA-topoisomerase (I and II) cleavable complex	Topotecan, irinotecan, doxorubicin, etoposide
Direct DNA damage	Alkylating agents and related compounds	G_1, G_2, S	DNA adduct formation, free radical production, strand breakage	Radiation, bleomycin, cisplatin, carboplatin, oxaliplatin, doxorubicin, mitomycin C, nitrogen mustard, nitrosoureas, ecteinascidin
Mitotic apparatus and microtubule dynamics	Antimicrotubule reagents	M	Dysregulation of tubulin polymerization, microtubule function, and signaling through associated proteins	Vincristine, vinblastine, vinorelbine, colchicine, paclitaxel, docetaxel, epothilones
Mitotic checkpoint control	Cell cycle agents	G_1, S, G_2, M	Cyclin-dependent kinases	Flavopiridol
Transmembrane and intracellular signal transducion	Signal transduction modulators	G_0, G_1, S, G_2	Epidermal growth factor receptors, vascular endothelial growth factor and receptors, associated tyrosine kinases, bcl-2, protein kinase-C, hormone receptors, aromatase, integrin, apoptosis induction, activation or restoration of p53	Trastuzumab, bevacizumab, cetuximab, erlotinib, gefitinib, bryostatin, tamoxifen, anastrazole, *p53* gene therapy
Gene regulation	DNA methylation	NA	Gene methylation status, DNA methyltransferase	Azacytidine
Protein processing	Farnesylation inhibitors	NA	Posttranslational protein modifications	Tipifarnib, bisphosphonates
Protein degradation	Proteasome inhibitors	NA	Inhibition of the proteasome complex and clearance of ubiquinated proteins	Bortezomib

It has also been used to rationalize the continuation of active chemotherapy for several cycles beyond clinical evidence of tumor remission.

Cell Cycle Specificity

Chemotherapeutic agents have complex mechanisms of action and can affect tumor cells through multiple pathways. Nevertheless, certain anticancer drugs are known to be proliferation dependent and cell cycle specific. Other drugs are cycle nonspecific, and are capable of killing in all phases of the cell cycle, generally without dependence on the proliferative rate. Examples of cycle-nonspecific drugs include alkylating agents, particularly nitrogen mustard, which are effective against a variety of solid tumors, including those with low growth fractions. Cell cycle–specific agents depend on the proliferative fraction of the tumor and phase of the cell cycle. A typical example is hydroxyurea, which inhibits ribonucleotide reductase. Not surprisingly, cell cycle–specific drugs tend to be more effective against tumors with a high proliferative rate and growth fractions. The interaction of specific cytotoxic agents with the cell cycle is summarized in Table 15.2.

PHARMACOLOGIC PRINCIPLES OF CHEMOTHERAPY

General pharmacologic principles should be considered by the physician in selecting and managing anticancer agents, including their mechanisms of action, absorption, distribution, metabolism, and excretion. Each of these factors may influence the effectiveness and/or toxicity of chemotherapy, and can be of particular importance in the development of combination regimens. A detailed discussion of the pharmacology of individual chemotherapeutic agents is provided in Chapter 16.

Absorption

Different routes of administration and absorption influence drug selection. Drugs may be given orally, intravenously, intramuscularly, intraarterially, or intraperitoneally. Selection of the route of administration depends on solubility, requirements for drug activation, local tissue tolerance, feasibility for an individual patient, and optimal tumor drug exposure, which is estimated as the area under the concentration-time curve (AUC) for the drug and active metabolites. The ultimate effectiveness of any chemotherapeutic agent depends on optimizing the AUC at critical tumor sites. However, there are no established techniques for noninvasive measurement of active drug concentration at these critical sites, and we are forced to extrapolate tumor drug exposure from preclinical models and plasma concentrations over time. Promising research in magnetic resonance spectroscopy and positron emission tomography may soon provide

clinically relevant information on drug distribution and tumor metabolism using selected agents.

Distribution and Transport

The extent of drug binding to serum proteins, as well as physical properties, such as lipid solubility, diffusion, and molecular weight, or requirement for active membrane transport, may have an impact on tumor drug exposure. Delivery may also be impaired by factors such as hypoxia, local redox potential, high tumor interstitial pressures, or reduced vascularity, perhaps best exemplified by hypoxic areas within large necrotic lesions. In addition, some areas of the body, particularly the brain, are actively protected from drug exposure, and can serve as pharmacologic tumor sanctuaries, where sequestered cancer cells may survive otherwise curative systemic therapy. Although uncommon with solid tumors that disrupt the blood-brain barrier, this was a common problem in acute leukemia until effectively managed with intrathecal drug delivery and/or high peak plasma levels. In addition to achieving local delivery, most drugs must be internalized within tumor cells to achieve cytotoxicity. Internalization can be accomplished by passive diffusion, active transport, pinocytosis, or receptor-mediated endocytosis.

Biotransformation

Some agents, such as cyclophosphamide, ifosfamide, and capecitabine, are administered as prodrugs and must undergo metabolism to the active form either in the liver, tumor, or other host tissues. For many of these agents, intraperitoneal or intraarterial administration would be ineffective, as it would achieve high local concentrations without an opportunity for hepatic activation.

Drug Excretion

Drug inactivation, elimination, or excretion can dramatically influence cumulative exposure, which significantly affects antitumor activity and host toxicity. Inactivation and excretion of chemotherapeutic agents occurs primarily by the liver, kidneys, and body tissues, with lesser elimination through the stool. Any impairment of normal liver or kidney function can disturb drug metabolism and excretion. The clinician must be extremely careful if either of these organs is functionally impaired (18). Guidelines exist for modifying drug doses for patients with renal impairment (19), including dosing parameters for patients on dialysis receiving individual drugs, such as carboplatin (20). However, owing to the rapid introduction of new drugs, clinicians are urged to consult updated compendiums (21), the drug prescribing information, and online database resources.

Modifications of drug doses may also be required for patients with liver disease, particularly for paclitaxel, docetaxel, doxorubicin, and the vinca alkaloids (vincristine, vinblastine, and vinorelbine), which are primarily metabolized in the liver and/or excreted in the bile. Excessive toxicity may occur with doses that would ordinarily be acceptable, and guidelines for treating patients with impaired liver function should be consulted. However, variability in nonhepatic clearance and compensatory host adaptations, such as increased renal clearance, make these recommendations less rigid than those provided for patients with renal dysfunction. For example, dose reduction of etoposide in the setting of biliary obstruction remains controversial and may not be required (22).

In some cases, organ dysfunction may be reversible, such as hydronephrosis associated with retroperitoneal adenopathy or biliary obstruction from periportal adenopathy. In these circumstances, organ function should be monitored and drug doses adjusted on a cycle-by-cycle basis to account for changes in clearance. Finally, the toxicity of many drugs can be enhanced in patients with advanced physiologic age or impaired nutritional status. In these circumstances, a low serum creatinine level may not accurately reflect underlying renal function, and a decreased serum albumin level could increase effective drug exposure as a consequence of a reduction in protein binding. Guidelines for initial dose adjustment in this situation have not been established, and careful monitoring of toxicity is required.

Drug Interactions

During routine care, patients may receive a variety of drugs, including antiemetics, antihistamines (H1 and H2), steroids, nonsteroidal antiinflammatory agents, anticoagulants, narcotics, and antiinfective agents. In addition, adult patients are frequently receiving medication to manage underlying conditions, such as diabetes, hypertension, and elevated cholesterol. In view of the number and diversity of medications in common use, it is somewhat surprising that most drug interactions with cytotoxic chemotherapy appear to be of little consequence. However, prospective studies of chemotherapy administration in noncancer volunteers are impractical, and many potential interactions have not been fully explored. In addition, the occurrence of excessive hematologic and/or nonhematologic toxicity in an individual patient treated with chemotherapy is usually attributed directly to the chemotherapy, and managed with treatment modifications rather than ascribed to a potential drug interaction.

In some instances, interactions may be critical, and some of the more important drug interactions are listed in Table 15.3. Particular attention should be placed on drugs that could alter renal function, such as aminoglycoside antibiotics, nonsteroidal antiinflammatory agents, and diuretics in patients with reduced fluid intake. Typical of *in vivo* interactions relevant in gynecologic cancer chemotherapy are the displacement of methotrexate from its transport protein by aspirin or sulfonamides, suppression of pseudocholinesterase by alkylating agents with increased apnea duration during succinylcholine-assisted general anesthesia, impairment of doxorubicin clearance by preadministration of paclitaxel, and impairment of paclitaxel clearance by preadministration of cisplatin.

TABLE 15.3. *Physiologic and pharmacologic interactions in cancer chemotherapy*

Interaction	Cause and/or agent	Impact
Alterations in renal clearance	Obstruction, renal dysfunction, hypovolemia, hypotension, non-steroidals, nephrotoxins (aminoglycosides, cisplatin)	Decreased clearance of methotrexate and carboplatin
Alterations in biliary excretion	Biliary obstruction	Decreased clearance of doxorubicin, mitoxantrone, vincristine, vinblastine, etoposide, paclitaxel
Microsomal activation	Hepatic dysfunction	Impaired activation of cyclophosphamide and ifosfamide
Carrier protein displacement	Sulfonamide, salicylates, phenytoin	Increased methotrexate toxicity from higher unbound drug levels
Altered intestinal absorption	Oral antibiotics (neomycin)	Decreased absorption of methotrexate
Decreased metabolism	Allopurinol	Delayed clearance of 6-mercaptopurine
Cholinesterase inhibition	Cyclophosphamide, glucocorticoids	Decreased clearance of succinylcholine
Monoamine oxidase inhibition	Procarbazine	Neurotoxicity and seizures from tricyclic antidepressants and phenothiazines
MDR-1 (P-170) competition	Natural products and other substrates, including verapamil, cyclosporine, tamoxifen	Increased toxicity from natural products (doxorubicin, vincristine)
Induction of CYP-3A4	Glucocorticoids, barbiturates, rifampin	Increased activation of cyclophosphamide
Inhibition of CYP-3A4	Ketoconazole, itraconazole, fluconazole, erythromycin	Decreased metabolism of substrates (potentially significant)
Substrate for CYP-3A4	Cyclophosphamide, ifosfamide, paclitaxel, docetaxel, etoposide, vincristine, vinblastine, tamoxifen, gefitinib	Decreased metabolism of other substrates (usually not clinically significant)

Increased attention has been focused on drug metabolism and potential interactions at the level of cytochrome P450 (CYP) isozymes, particularly CYP-3A4, which is potentially linked to the metabolism of nearly half of all pharmaceutical agents (23). These interactions are guided by several common principles. Drugs that are *substrates* for the same isozyme may competitively inhibit metabolism, but these interactions are usually not of clinical consequence. Drugs that *directly inhibit* CYP isozymes without being a substrate for that isozyme are more likely to have clinical consequences. In this regard, itraconazole, ketoconazole, and fluconazole can inhibit CYP-3A4 at low concentrations, and erythromycin can inhibit CYP-3A4 via covalent binding and inactivation. Other drugs act as *inducers* of CYP isozymes by increasing gene expression or protein levels, such as glucocorticoids, barbiturates, and rifampin, which can increase the net activity of CYP-3A4, resulting in decreased concentrations of susceptible compounds. In addition, many drugs that interact with CYP-3A4 are natural products and may also interact with the MDR-1 multidrug resistance transporter P-170 (see below). Among the anticancer agents that are substrates for CYP-3A4 are cyclophosphamide, ifosfamide, docetaxel, etoposide, paclitaxel (also CYP-2C8), vincristine, vinblastine, tamoxifen, and gefitinib (24). CYP-2C9 and CYP-2D6 are inhibited by imatinib, and doxorubicin can inhibit CYP-2D6. Cyclosporine and verapamil can increase concentrations of doxorubicin and etoposide, probably through blockade of the P-170 drug efflux pump.

Owing to the diversity and rapid adoption of new chemotherapy and nonchemotherapy compounds, information regarding drug interactions is best obtained from updated compendiums (21), online databases (e.g., http://www.medicalletter.com or http://www.micromedex.com or http://www.drug-interactions.com), or the drug manufacturer.

DRUG RESISTANCE AND TUMOR CELL HETEROGENEITY

The curative potential of chemotherapy is limited by the emergence of drug resistance, which can be either intrinsic or acquired, and may involve one drug or multiple agents (pleiotropic resistance). Of interest, tumors with intrinsic or primary drug resistance to natural products often arise from duct cells or cells lining excretory organs (25). These cells, which normally detoxify, transport, and excrete a wide variety of toxic compounds, may retain these normal functions after transformation, manifesting as chemoresistance. With few exceptions, attempts to differentiate prospectively drug-responsive tumors from their resistant counterparts using morphologic, cytogenetic, immunologic, or molecular biologic techniques have not yet been successful. However, within the next few years, high-throughput molecular profiling by gene expression or proteomic array is expected to identify patterns that are predictive of tumor resistance or response to specific chemotherapeutic agents.

The presence of intrinsic drug resistance is inferred based on clonal survival of tumor populations after initial chemotherapy exposure. Solid tumors are thought to consist of a mixture of clonal variants with different mutations and patterns of resistance. Following repetitive cycles of chemotherapy, a process of clonal selection can occur, enriching for resistant populations, even while there could be a reduction in clinical tumor volume associated with elimination of more sensitive tumor elements. From a clinical perspective, the end result of this process is indistinguishable from acquired resistance, which develops from cumulative mutations, or phenotypic alterations, over a period of time. However, acquired resistance is more likely to have a reversible component that could influence the timing and selection of subsequent chemotherapy. The most well-documented specific example is amplification of the dihydrofolate reductase (DHFR) gene, which is associated with acquired resistance to methotrexate (26). DHFR gene amplification is not generally observed prior to methotrexate exposure, and can be reversed in the absence of drug exposure.

From the perspective of gynecologic oncology, there are two major patterns of drug resistance that emerge with continued treatment. The first is broad-based multidrug, or pleiotropic, drug resistance that has been associated with overexpression of MDR-1 (P-170 glycoprotein) and/or other membrane-associated transport proteins (27,28). This multidrug resistance phenotype has maximal impact on natural products and their analogs, including the anthracyclines, vinca alkaloids, and taxanes. The second is resistance to alkylating agents, especially platinum compounds, mediated through a completely different set of cellular mechanisms, including increased glutathione production, damage tolerance, and capacity for DNA repair.

Mechanisms of Multidrug Resistance

The best characterized mechanism of pleiotropic drug resistance is overexpression of the *MDR-1* gene and its product, the P-170 glycoprotein, an energy-dependent transmembrane efflux pump (29,30). After exposure to a potential P-170 substrate, tumor cells will develop cross resistance to a variety of structurally and functionally unrelated agents derived from natural products. This pleiotropic resistance is associated with increased drug efflux and a net lowering of intracellular drug concentration. Although relatively uncommon in ovarian cancer (31,32), with increased utilization of natural products, including taxanes, etoposide, and liposomal doxorubicin, this pattern of resistance may become more prevalent. Mutations in the β-tubulin subunit have been associated with paclitaxel resistance in preclinical models, but this does not appear to be a common mechanism in the clinical setting (33), and expression of MDR-1 has been more frequently observed as a potential marker of resistance (29).

Other chemotherapeutic agents are not substrates for P-170 and remain unaffected by increased expression. For example, several cell lines with multidrug resistance mediated by P-170 demonstrated increased uptake, phosphorylation, and sensitivity to gemcitabine, a nucleoside analog, which could be reversed by verapamil, an inhibitor of MDR-1 (30). This has potential implications for optimal timing, sequence, and combination of agents in the clinical setting.

Other energy-dependent transporter proteins have been identified in drug-resistant cell lines that do not overexpress MDR-1. These include the multidrug resistance–associated protein (MRP), which is representative of a family of canalicular multispecific organic anion transport (cMOAT) proteins (34). Similar to MDR-1, these proteins include multiple transmembrane domains, but appear to have more broad tissue distribution and greater association with intracellular membrane–bound compartments. Another member of the family with relevance to gynecologic cancer is the Breast Cancer Resistance Protein (BCRP) or adenosine triphosphate–binding cassette protein G2 (ABCG2) that dimerizes to form a membrane-associated energy-dependent drug efflux pump responsible for atypical multidrug resistance following exposure to mitoxantrone or camptothecins, including topotecan. Overexpression of BCRP has been documented in ovarian cancer cells resistant to topotecan (35).

Strategies to Overcome Alkylating Agent Resistance

Human ovarian cell lines resistant to alkylating agents, cisplatin, and irradiation contain elevated levels of cellular glutathione (GSH). Using resistant cell lines, it has been possible to demonstrate a restoration of drug sensitivity by exposure to the synthetic amino acid buthionine sulfoximine (BSO), which inhibits gamma-glutamylcysteine synthetase, causing GSH depletion (36). The exact mechanism by which GSH and other thiol compounds modulate cytotoxicity is unknown, although they can interfere with the formation of DNA-platinum adducts (37). There is also evidence of increased drug metabolism through GSH-linked transferases, which can vary for specific platinum compounds (38), and which may also contribute to cisplatin-mediated nephrotoxicity (39). Although clinical trials of BSO with melphalan have documented an 80% to greater than 90% reduction in tumor-associated GSH levels (40,41), this approach has not yet been demonstrated to improve the outcomes of platinum-based therapy.

In view of the prominent role of thiols in mediating a subset of platinum resistance, a sterically hindered platinum complex (ZD0473) was developed with the expectation that it would favor interacting with DNA rather than glutathione or metallothioneins (42). A Phase II trial in recurrent ovarian cancer documented response rates of 8.4% in platinum-resistant disease and 32.4% in platinum-sensitive disease similar to expectations with cisplatin or carboplatin (43). Of interest, there was no documented peripheral neuropathy or nephrotoxicity even in this group of patients with prior platinum

therapy, implicating thiol reactions in the generation of these nonhematologic toxicities.

Enhanced capacity for DNA repair can play a role in drug resistance to alkylating agents and cisplatin. Human ovarian cancer cell lines resistant to melphalan demonstrate increased ability to repair melphalan damage, and this phenotype can be reversed by aphidicolin, a potent inhibitor of alpha and beta DNA polymerase (44). Increased damage tolerance is another mechanism that contributes to resistance, and is perhaps best illustrated by the mismatch repair system. Errors in DNA replication following platinum adduct formation can be detected by the postreplicative DNA mismatch repair system, which contains several well-characterized genes, including *MLH1* and *MSH2*. Of note, cellular attempts to repair platinum alkylation by this mechanism are not successful as the repair is directed at the nascent daughter DNA strand rather than the platinated parental strand. Eventually, abortive attempts at repair are associated with apoptotic cell death. Thus, loss of mismatch repair can actually promote cell survival by ignoring DNA damage in noncritical areas of the genome and has emerged as another mechanism of drug resistance. Loss of *MLH1* or other mismatch repair genes is not uncommon in ovarian cancer and appears to increase after exposure to carboplatin or cisplatin (45).

Oxaliplatin is one of several diaminocyclohexane (DACH) platinum derivatives that forms platinum adducts that differ in three-dimensional structure from the more established diamine compounds, such as cisplatin and carboplatin (46). As a consequence of these structural differences, oxaliplatin adducts are not detected by the mismatch repair system (47), and there was hope that oxaliplatin would retain clinical activity in patients with platinum-resistant tumors. However, in Phase II studies, the response rate among ovarian cancer patients with less than a 6-month platinum-free interval was less than 7% (48,49).

Agent-Specific Mechanisms of Resistance

A number of specific alterations have been identified in the setting of individual drugs (Table 15.4). For example, DHFR gene amplification was demonstrated in a patient with methotrexate-resistant ovarian cancer who had localized DHFR gene copies on an abnormally staining region of chromosome 4q (50). Methotrexate resistance has also been associated with defects in polyglutamation, limiting intracellular methotrexate accumulation (51).

The action of nucleoside analogs, such as gemcitabine (2, 2-difluorodideoxycytidine), is dependent on active membrane transport for uptake, which is followed by double phosphorylation and potential incorporation in DNA. This complex process offers several opportunities for development of resistance, such as decreased activity of specific nucleoside transport proteins or reduced phosphorylation by depletion of deoxycytidine kinase (52). In addition, the main enzymatic target of phosphorylated gemcitabine, the M2

TABLE 15.4. *Specific mechanisms of tumor drug resistance*

Mechanism	Examples	Specific target or effects
Impaired activation	5-Fluorouracil	Reduced levels of thymidylate synthase, thymidylate phosphorylase, or dihydropyrimidine dehydrogenase
	Methotrexate	Reduced intracellular polyglutamation
	Doxorubicin	Low P450 enzymes
	Cyclophosphamide, ifosfamide	Decreased microsomal function
	Gemcitabine	Decreased deoxycytidine kinase
Increased drug efflux	Natural products	Increased MDR-1 (P-170)
	Topotecan, mitoxantrone	Increased BCRP (ABCG2)
Increased drug inactivation	Alkylating agents, cisplatin	Elevated glutathione and other cellular thiols
Accelerated DNA repair	Alkylating agents, cisplatin, radiation	Induction of DNA repair enzymes
Increased damage tolerance	Alkylating agents, cisplatin, radiation	Loss of DNA mismatch repair
Transport defects	Melphalan	Reduced carrier-mediated uptake
	Gemcitabine	Decreased nucleoside transporter
Target alterations	Methotrexate	DHFR gene amplification
	Vincristine, paclitaxel	Altered β-tubulin binding
	Hydroxyurea, gemcitabine	Decreased ribonucleotide reductase
	Glucocorticoids	Decreased receptor binding
	Camptothecins	Decreased topoisomerase-I
	Anthracyclines, etoposide	Decreased topoisomerase-II

subunit of ribonucleotide reductase, can undergo gene amplification in resistant cell lines (53) similar to the primary mechanism of resistance to hydroxyurea, an inhibitor of ribonucleotide reductase. Of interest, sensitivity to gemcitabine can actually be increased severalfold by prior exposure to flavopiridol, an inhibitor of cyclin-dependent kinase activity, which has been shown to accelerate catabolism of the M2 subunit protein through the proteasome complex (54). Increased levels of target gene expression or protein, including thymidylate synthase, thymidylate phosphorylase, and dihydropyrimidine dehydrogenase, have also been associated with resistance to 5-fluorouracil in colon cancer, and have been correlated with clinical outcomes following 5-fluorouracil treatment (55,56). Even a superficial analysis of these specific examples would suggest potential strategies for screening of tumor tissue to guide the selection of optimal chemotherapy regimens, providing a basis for the application of tissue, gene, and protein arrays.

Tumor Heterogeneity and Assays of Chemotherapy Response

Solid tumors have traditionally been considered to be a homogeneous collection of clonally derived cells with similar features, but it is now clear that tumors are composed of subpopulations with diverse biologic characteristics. Through genetic instability and regulatory processes, such as gene methylation, these subpopulations may exhibit different kinetic properties, angiogenic potential, receptor content, immunogenicity, and susceptibility to chemotherapy. In addition, there can be variability in the potential for metastatic spread among cells that appear to be similar at a morphologic and genetic level (57). Recognition of tumor heterogeneity has altered our understanding of tumor behavior with implications for multiagent and multimodality treatment programs.

Following the development of model systems for screening new anticancer compounds, it is not surprising that attention was focused on the process of screening actual human tumor cells for sensitivity and resistance to chemotherapy agents (58). A variety of methods have been developed utilizing clonogenic survival, ^{3}H-thymidine incorporation, vital dye exclusion, treatment of transplanted tumor xenografts, and colorimetric analysis of adenosine triphosphate levels. Although there is relatively good correlation between high-level resistance to individual agents demonstrated *in vitro* and lack of a clinical response *in vivo*, it is more difficult to predict sensitivity to specific agents, or to guide the utilization of drug combinations (59), reflecting tumor cell heterogeneity, assay complexity, and other clinical variables. A nonrandomized Phase II trial in recurrent epithelial ovarian cancer has suggested good correlation between *ex vivo* assay sensitivity and clinical response (60). Wider adoption of these approaches will need to address the lack of prospective randomized data, as well as the complexities of obtaining and shipping fresh tumor tissue, delay in receiving assay results, and substantial nonreimbursed financial costs. In addition, with the rapid development of gene expression and proteomic arrays, it is possible that adequate predictions can be obtained from profiling existing frozen tumor specimens, as opposed to assays on fresh tumor biopsies.

Dose Intensity

The dose and frequency of drug administration can contribute to the overall effectiveness of a treatment regimen, as well as the spectrum and severity of host toxicity. Dose intensity is a standardized measure of the amount of drug administered over time, most commonly expressed as mg/m^2/week. A series of retrospective studies in ovarian cancer (61) suggested a correlation between actual delivered dose intensity and clinical outcomes.

Prospective randomized trials were undertaken to evaluate critically the dose-intensity hypothesis. For example, in a Phase III study performed by the Gynecologic Oncology Group in advanced ovarian carcinoma (GOG-97), 485 patients were randomized to a combination of standard or dose-intense cyclophosphamide and cisplatin, while adjusting the total number of cycles on each arm to achieve equivalent cumulative dosing. Outcomes were similar in the two groups, providing no evidence that a doubling of dose intensity would produce significant improvements in either disease-free or overall survival in advanced ovarian cancer (62).

Delivered dose intensity is limited by cumulative nonhematologic (cisplatin) or hematologic (carboplatin) toxicity. Although multiple cycles of high-dose carboplatin and paclitaxel can be safely administered with support from hematopoietic progenitor cells and growth factors, there is no evidence (from small nonrandomized studies) that a two- to threefold increase in carboplatin dose intensity and cumulative dose delivery is associated with a substantial improvement in clinical outcomes (63), and it is unlikely that this will be further evaluated.

Preclinical studies demonstrate a sigmoidal relationship between dose and tumor response. This is characterized by a *lag phase* and lower *threshold* for observing benefit; a *linear phase*, where increases in dose are matched by improved efficacy; and a *plateau*, where toxicity continues to increase but there is no incremental improvement in response. In highly responsive tumors (e.g., choriocarcinoma, dysgerminoma), the entire dose-response curve is shifted to the left, with the result that standard chemotherapy doses are already situated near the upper plateau, and further dose increases are unlikely to achieve any improvement in clinical outcomes. In resistant tumors (e.g., previously treated cervical cancer), the curve is shifted to the right, and is also flattened, reducing the maximal potential benefit of dose-intense therapy. For heterogeneous tumors with sensitive and resistant populations, such as epithelial ovarian cancer, it is unlikely that increased dose intensity would achieve long-term clinical benefit. However, lower than standard doses are potentially suboptimal, and arbitrary dose reductions or delays for nonphysiologic factors should be avoided. True dose-intense regimens have not been demonstrated to improve long-term clinical outcomes in women with gynecologic cancer, with the possible exception of recurrent germ-cell tumors.

GENERAL PRINCIPLES OF CHEMOTHERAPY

Primary Treatment Recommendations

Although certain general principles guide the clinician in choosing the appropriate classes of drugs or combinations,

the decision to use these agents *at all* must be considered carefully. The critical factors involved in formulating a recommendation are reviewed in Table 15.5.

Natural History

Antineoplastic agents should be used only in patients whose malignancy has been established histologically, with consideration of the expected natural history, based on the primary tumor site, extent of disease, and rate of progression. Individual factors that could have an impact on tolerance for therapy must be evaluated in the context of treatment goals, including physiologic age (as reflected by vital organ function), general health, performance status, desire for treatment, and the presence of underlying illness. Prior history, including any previous cancer treatment and residual functional impairment, as well as patterns of recurrence, should also be considered. Finally, the emotional, social, and financial concerns of the patient and family must be respected. Recommendations and goals should be presented to the patient and family in conjunction with a reasonable analysis of potential risks and benefits, which contributes to the process of informed consent, and which should be followed by sharing of written information for future reference.

Clinical Assessment

Chemotherapy should not be instituted unless the physician is prepared to monitor tumor response (if applicable) carefully while managing expected and unexpected toxici-

TABLE 15.5. *Important considerations before using antineoplastic drugs*

Natural history of the malignancy
- Biopsy proof of malignancy
- Identification of primary site
- Rate of progression or grade
- Stage of disease, patterns of spread

Patient characteristics
- Physiologic age, nutritional status, performance status
- Vital organ function; bone marrow reserve
- Comorbid conditions
- Extent of previous treatment

Supportive Care
- Adequate facilities to evaluate, monitor, and treat potential drug toxicities
- Emotional, social, and financial status; support from family
- Collaboration with referring physician

Treatment Goals
- Parameters to monitor objective response to treatment
- Potential benefits
  - Curative intent
  - Improved or sustained quality of life
  - Control of disease
  - Palliation of symptoms

ties. If proper facilities are not readily available, and the decision is made to begin therapy, the patient should be referred to a physician or facility that can provide integrated care.

In view of the potential for serious toxicity, it is desirable to have some objective means of measuring tumor response by physical examination, radiographic imaging, and/or analysis of serum tumor markers. However, it is not uncommon to administer multiple cycles of adjuvant or postoperative chemotherapy without any direct means of documenting tumor response. In these circumstances, the physician should be alert for any clinical evidence of tumor recurrence or progression during treatment. In patients with evaluable disease, continued administration of chemotherapy requires verification of ongoing benefit.

Expectations

The likelihood of achieving long-term benefit influences the choice of treatment and the acceptance of potential toxicity. Primary and recurrent tumors (following surgical resection or radiation without prior chemotherapy) can generally be grouped according to the likelihood of achieving a durable response. Most importantly, there are a group of tumors for which chemotherapy has been curative in the majority of patients, including choriocarcinoma and ovarian germ-cell tumors. These patients should be treated aggressively with curative intent. Toxicity in this setting is acceptable, assuming that it is reversible, as the probability of long-term survival is high.

Other more common cancers, such as advanced epithelial ovarian carcinoma, have high response rates to primary therapy (exceeding 75%), with prolongation of disease-free and median overall survival, but with only a modest improvement in overall mortality. Patients with these tumors usually benefit from therapy in terms of extended survival or quality-adjusted survival, and they should receive primary treatment at full doses unless contraindicated.

A third group of cancers, including advanced endometrial and cervical carcinoma, have lower response rates to chemotherapy (typically 30%) with limited improvement in overall survival. Treatment with an initial course of therapy is reasonable, with careful monitoring of toxicity and response, and consideration of alternative therapy in the event of progressive disease.

Other tumors, including uterine leiomyosarcoma, are more resistant to primary therapy, achieving a low frequency of objective response without prolongation of survival. In this setting, the use of chemotherapy should be restricted and particular emphasis placed on including these patients in well-structured clinical trials to evaluate innovative treatments.

The decision to embark on antineoplastic drug therapy is obviously complex. Optimal patient care demands careful review of the multiple factors affecting therapy to maximize any opportunity for improving survival and quality of life.

Management of Recurrent Disease

Patients with recurrent or progressive disease after prior systemic chemotherapy are much less likely to achieve long-term benefit from additional treatment. This is due to the tendency for drug resistance to evolve within the tumor and the impact of prior therapy and/or progressive disease on performance status and vital organ function. As such, treatment goals are usually palliative, with attention to quality of life and control of symptoms. In this population, the frequency of stable disease usually exceeds the objective response rate. With appropriate chemotherapy regimens that avoid cumulative toxicity, patients without further disease progression may remain on therapy for prolonged periods of time with an acceptable quality of life. Outside of a clinical trial, most patients are best managed with single-agent chemotherapy with regular assessment of ongoing response and routine management of toxicity. However, patients with epithelial ovarian cancer and a prolonged treatment-free interval of greater than 2 years generally receive reinduction with a front-line platinum-based combination. Although there is no established role for dose-intense multiagent chemotherapy with or without hematopoietic support in this setting, selected patients with recurrent germ-cell tumors can be managed aggresively with curative intent.

Choice of Specific Chemotherapeutic Regimens

After the decision to use chemotherapy has been made, the appropriate regimen must be selected. The physician is aided in this task by the results of randomized trials and evolving standards of care, including published practice guidelines. However, not every patient can receive "standard" therapy because of idiosyncratic reactions, vital organ dysfunction, prior treatment, or other factors. Practical individualized decisions are facilitated by the logical grouping of chemotherapeutic agents in several classes with similar pharmacologic properties, mechanisms of action, and spectrum of toxicity. The most important classes are the alkylating agents (including platinum), antimetabolites, antitumor antibiotics, antimicrotubule agents, nucleoside analogs, and hormones.

Primary Therapy

With the diversity of agents currently available, a number of platinum-based combinations have been developed and evaluated in the management of gynecologic cancer, and some combination regimens have been widely adopted as "standard of care" for primary management of advanced-stage or recurrent disease. Phase III trials have demonstrated the superiority of specific regimens, such as paclitaxel and either cisplatin (64) or carboplatin (65) in ovarian cancer, paclitaxel, cisplatin, and doxorubicin with granulocyte colony-stimulating factor (G-CSF) in endometrial cancer (66), as well as cisplatin with either paclitaxel (67) or topotecan in cervical cancer (68). However, other Phase III trials in epithelial ovarian cancer have suggested that sequential therapy with platinum followed by paclitaxel may offer similar long-term outcomes (69,70).

In fact, none of the standard combinations for advanced ovarian, endometrial, or cervical cancer has been directly compared to sequential therapy with the best active single agents, and the superiority of combination therapy has not been fully established. Although the initial frequency of tumor response is often increased with combination therapy, long-term outcomes such as overall survival and symptom-adjusted quality of life can be similar for patients who receive optimal sequential therapy with single agents. This is primarily related to the advanced stage of disease at the time of initial treatment with systemic chemotherapy and the lack of curative therapy for the majority of patients. As such, if individual patient circumstances contraindicate the use of a standard combination regimen, it remains a reasonable option to begin therapy with one of the active single agents. In addition to their application as primary therapy for advanced disease, combinations can also be employed as adjuvant therapy for patients with early-stage disease at increased risk for recurrence and for patients whose disease recurs more than 2 years after initial therapy.

Adjuvant chemotherapy refers to the initial use of systemic chemotherapy after surgery and/or radiation therapy has been performed with curative intent and there is no evidence of residual disease. Adjuvant chemotherapy is considered if the subsequent risk for recurrence after initial definitive therapy is relatively high (generally greater than 20%), but it is not routinely recommended when the risk of recurrence is less than 10%. In the adjuvant therapy of epithelial ovarian cancer, long-term results from randomized trials have documented a reduction in the risk of recurrence after platinum-based chemotherapy (71,72). However, in carefully staged patients (to exclude occult advanced-stage disease), it has been difficult to establish an advantage in overall survival.

Concurrent chemotherapy with radiation (chemoradiation) refers to the use of chemotherapy to sensitize tumor to the effects of radiation delivered with curative intent. This has been most extensively studied in the primary management of locally advanced cervical cancer, where platinum-based chemoradiation has been proven to be superior to radiation alone (73). In general, the duration of chemotherapy coincides with the duration of external beam radiation. Although the preferred weekly dose of cisplatin might appear to be low, these regimens can exceed the overall dose-intensity of cisplatin when used to treat advanced disease, and patients require monitoring to avoid cumulative toxicity and treatment interruptions.

Neoadjuvant chemotherapy generally refers to the use of chemotherapy in the management of locally advanced disease in situations where it would be difficult or impractical to perform immediate surgery or radiation. Following a response to initial chemotherapy, there is an expectation that morbidity associated with the overall treatment program can be minimized in conjunction with a reduction in radiation treatment volume or extent of surgery. This approach is most often considered in advanced cervical cancer, where high initial response rates to neoadjuvant therapy have been observed. However, the long-term benefit of this approach has not been established. Neoadjuvant therapy is also a consideration in advanced ovarian cancer, particularly in patients with large-volume ascites, pleural effusions, diffuse small-volume disease, or comorbidities that might increase surgical risk. Although generally responsive to platinum-based therapy, it has been difficult to conduct randomized neoadjuvant trials owing to comorbidities in the target population, the desire to establish a definitive tissue diagnosis, and the bias toward initial cytoreductive surgery.

Monitoring of Tumor Response

Generally accepted criteria for evaluation of response are necessary to facilitate treatment decisions and comparisons among different regimens. Several standards have been used, including those developed by the World Health Organization (WHO). However, in 2000, an international working group including the European Organization for Research and Treatment of Cancer (EORTC), the National Cancer Institute of Canada (NCIC), and the National Cancer Institute (NCI) of the United States developed, validated, and published new Response Evaluation Criteria in Solid Tumors (RECIST), which have subsequently been widely adopted within clinical trials (74). RECIST is based on the prospective designation of at least one "target lesion" that measures at least 2 cm in one dimension, as well as "nontarget lesions" that are used to corroborate response. Radiographic imaging by helical computed tomography (CT) or magnetic resonance imaging (MRI) are the preferred techniques to monitor tumor response, and the same technique that is used for initial assessment should be used for subsequent measurements. The use of physical examination is restricted to cutaneous lesions or superficial adenopathy that can be directly measured. The omission of findings on bimanual pelvic examination posed a particular challenge for monitoring regional disease in patients with gynecologic tumors, and the criteria were subsequently modified by GOG to include pelvic lesions measurable by physical examination, as summarized in Table 15.6.

The summary response designation within RECIST integrates the findings from target and nontarget lesions, as well as serum tumor markers (if applicable). Serum tumor markers are not sufficient to declare response, but if initially elevated, must normalize to designate a complete response. International criteria to declare disease progression on the basis of a serial elevation in CA-125 have been widely adopted

TABLE 15.6. *Overall Disease Response Categories (RECIST)*

Complete response (CR)[a]	Disappearance of all *target*[c] and *nontarget* lesions and normalization of tumor marker levels (if appropriate)
Partial response (PR)	Disappearance of all *target* lesions without progression of *nontarget* lesions, without appearance of new lesions, and persistence of abnormal tumor marker levels -*Or*-At least a 30% decrease in the sum LD of *target* lesions (taking as reference the baseline sum LD) without progression of *nontarget* lesions or appearance of new lesions. *Note:* In the case where the only *target* lesion is a solitary pelvic mass measured by physical exam (not radiographically measurable), a 50% decrease in the LD is required.
Progressive disease (PD)	At least a 20% increase in the sum LD of *target* lesions, taking as reference the smallest sum LD recorded since the start of treatment, or the appearance of one or more new lesions, or progression of any *nontarget* lesion. *Note:* In the case where the only *target* lesion is a solitary pelvic mass measured by physical exam (not radiographically measurable), a 50% increase in the LD is required.
Stable disease (SD)[b]	Neither sufficient shrinkage of *target* lesions to qualify for PR nor sufficient increase to qualify for PD, taking as reference the smallest sum LD since the start of treatment. No appearance of new lesions (*target* or *nontarget*).

[a] To be assigned PR or CR, changes in tumor measurements must be confirmed by repeat assessments no less than 4 weeks after the criteria for response are first met. The duration of overall response is measured from the time that criteria are met for CR or PR (whichever status is recorded first) until the first date that recurrence or PD is objectively documented, taking as reference for PD the smallest measurements recorded since the treatment started.

[b] In the case of SD, follow-up measurements must have met the SD criteria at least once after study entry at a minimum interval (in general, not less than 6 to 8 weeks) that is defined in the study protocol. SD is measured from the start of the treatment until the criteria for disease progression are met, taking as reference the smallest measurements recorded since the treatment started.

[c] All measurable lesions up to a maximum of five lesions per organ and ten lesions in total, representative of all involved organs, should be identified as *target* lesions and recorded and measured at baseline. *Target* lesions should be selected on the basis of their size (lesions with the longest diameter) and their suitability for accurate repeated measurements (either by imaging techniques or clinically). All other lesions (or sites of disease) should be identified as *nontarget* lesions and should also be recorded at baseline. Measurements of these lesions are not required, but the presence or absence of each should be noted throughout follow-up.

Measurable lesions: lesions that can be accurately measured in at least one dimension with longest diameter $\geq$20 mm using conventional techniques or $\geq$10 mm with spiral CT scan.

Nonmeasurable lesions: all other lesions, including small lesions (longest diameter <20 mm with conventional techniques or <10 mm with spiral CT scan); i.e., bone lesions, leptomeningeal disease, ascites, pleural/pericardial effusion, inflammatory breast disease, lymphangitis cutis/pulmonis, cystic lesions, and also abdominal masses that are not confirmed and followed by imaging techniques.

(75,76), but there is incomplete agreement on criteria to define a partial response during treatment (77). Overall, RECIST is more detailed and specific than previous response criteria, and is also more demanding of the clinical team and radiologist, particularly if there are a large number of target and nontarget lesions.

A *complete response* refers to the complete disappearance of all objective evidence of tumor and a resolution of all signs and symptoms referable to the tumor. Complete regressions of cancer are generally those associated with a prolongation of survival. A *partial response* refers to at least a 30% decrease in the sum of the longest diameter of all measurable lesions. Usually, this would be accompanied by some degree of subjective improvement and the absence of any new le-

sions during treatment. Partial remissions are generally accompanied by improved well-being for a period of time, but are not expected to improve overall survival. A variety of terms have been used to designate lesser responses (e.g., minor response, objective regression), but these are rarely associated with any significant clinical benefit. *Progressive disease* is defined as a 20% or greater increase in the sum of the longest diameter of all measurable lesions or the appearance of new lesions. *Stable disease* is the term applied to patients without measurable tumor response or progression fitting one of the prior criteria. Disease stabilization is an acceptable goal in the setting of palliative therapy for recurrent disease provided that symptoms have not progressed and the patient can tolerate continued therapy.

TABLE 15.7. *CTCAE grading of myelosuppression*

Element	Grade[a]			
	1	2	3	4
Leukocytes (per mm^3)	LLN–3,000	<3,000–2,000	<2,000–1,000	<1,000
Granulocytes (per mm^3)	<2,000–1,500	<1,500–1,000	<1,000–500	<500
Hemoglobin (g/dL)	LLN–10.0	<10.0–8.0	<8.0–6.5	<6.5
Platelets (per mm^3)	LLN–75,000	<75,000–50,000	<50,000–25,000	<25,000

LLN, lower limit normal (institutional).

[a] Common Terminology Criteria for Adverse Events (CTCAE), version 3.0, Cancer Therapy Evaluation Program, National Cancer Institute, 10 JUN 2003 (http://ctep.info.nih.gov/reporting/ctc.html).

Changes in the volume of ascites or pleural fluid are not usually considered in the measurement of response, as a number of factors unrelated to cancer can influence third-space fluid accumulation, such as nutritional status, renal function, and treatment-related toxicity. However, appearance of a new fluid collection with cytologic verification would represent progressive disease. Similarly, the appearance of new symptoms, such as a partial small bowel obstruction, does not always indicate progression of disease, but could be related to prior surgery, irradiation, chemotherapy, or infection. In general, it is preferable to base decisions regarding treatment on objective measures of response as described rather than subjective findings or symptoms.

Toxicity Assessment, Dose Modification, and Supportive Care

Chemotherapeutic regimens are universally toxic, with a narrow margin of safety, and it is often necessary to adjust doses individually in accordance with patient tolerance. Initial chemotherapy dosing is based on body surface area, weight, renal function, and hepatic function, using guidelines from clinical trials. However, there are a number of other factors that could further influence host tolerance, including nutritional status, performance status, extent of disease, prior therapy, third-space fluid accumulations, metabolic polymorphisms, and uncharacterized drug interactions. Current dose algorithms generally fail to address these factors, although emerging pharmacodynamic and pharmacogenetic research may improve our ability to perform individualized dose calculations in the future. As such, it is necessary to use host toxicity as an indication of general drug metabolism, with ongoing modifications to avoid serious acute and cumulative toxicity.

The Cancer Therapy Evaluation Program (CTEP) of the National Cancer Institute has developed a detailed and comprehensive set of guidelines for the description and grading of acute and chronic organ-specific toxicity in collaboration with the Food and Drug Administration (FDA), international cooperative groups, and the pharmaceutical industry. Most clinical research protocols have incorporated these criteria, which are also applicable to the grading of toxicity for standard chemotherapy regimens outside of a clinical trial. The current version of the Common Terminology Criteria for

TABLE 15.8. *Representative drug dose modifications*

Category (timing)	Parameters	CTCAE grade	Dose or schedule modifications
Granulocytes (day of therapy)	> 1,500/mm^3	0, 1	Full doses of all drugs.
	< 1,500/mm^3	2, 3, 4	Delay until recovered. If already delayed, reduce dose by one level or add G-CSF.
Platelets (day of therapy)	WNL	0	Full doses of all drugs.
	< LLN to 75,000/mm^3	1	Delay until recovered.
	< 75,000/mm^3	2	Delay until recovered. If already delayed, reduce dose by one level.
Granulocytes (cycle nadir)	> 1,000/mm^3	0, 1, 2	Full doses of all drugs.
	< 500/mm^3 for ≥7 days	4	Reduce dose by one level. If already reduced, add G-CSF.
	< 1000/mm^3 with fever	3, 4	Reduce dose by one level. If already reduced, add G-CSF.
Platelets (cycle nadir)	≥ 50,000/mm^3	3	Full doses of all drugs.
	< 50,000/mm^3 with bleed	3, 4	Reduce doses by one level.
	< 25,000/mm^3	4	Reduce doses by one level.

CTC, common toxicity criteria; G-CSF, granulocyte colony-stimulating factor; LLN, lower limit normal; WNL, within normal limits.

Adverse Events (CTCAE) is available in electronic format from CTEP (http://ctep.info.nih.gov). Basic hematologic parameters have been summarized in Table 15.7.

In view of the narrow safety margin for chemotherapy, it is important that all orders be reviewed by a nurse and pharmacist with oncology experience. Height, weight, calculation of body surface area, pertinent laboratory values, and methods of dose calculation should be clearly indicated and verifiable. Pretemplated orders encourage systematic review and can reduce the risk of error. In addition, it is preferable to have predefined dose levels to account for expected treatment modifications rather than relying on percentage-based modifications. For example, it is not always obvious if a percentage refers to the degree of dose reduction or the amount of drug to be administered, which becomes compounded over multiple cycles, with the potential for more than one modification. One convenient method of structured dose modification is illustrated in Table 15.8. With this approach, modifications for the subsequent course of therapy are implemented according to the degree (grade), duration, and timing of toxicity experienced during the preceding course. Although treatment can be delayed on a week-by-week basis to allow for recovery, delays of greater than 2 weeks should be avoided through dose modification and utilization of hematopoietic growth factors. With expanded utilization of combination regimens, it is also helpful to know the patterns of toxicity associated with individual drugs, as it might be appropriate to modify one component rather than an entire regimen.

MANAGEMENT OF TOXICITY

Bone Marrow Toxicity

Bone marrow toxicity is the most common dose-limiting side effect associated with cytotoxic drugs, and neutropenia is the most common manifestation of bone marrow toxicity, occurring 7 to 14 days after initial drug treatment and persisting for 3 to 10 days. CTCAE grading criteria are summarized in Table 15.7. For purposes of dose modification, the absolute neutrophil count (ANC) is preferred over total white blood count, as this more accurately reflects dose tolerance and risk of infection, which parallels the duration of grade 4 neutropenia (ANC $\leq 500/mm^3$). Dose-limiting thrombocytopenia is less common than neutropenia, but has become more frequent with wider utilization of carboplatin. A systematic approach to management of hematologic toxicity can help to reduce the risk of error and facilitate overall compliance with a treatment regimen (Table 15.8).

Radiation, alkylating agents (e.g., melphalan, carboplatin), and other DNA-damaging agents (e.g., nitrosoureas, mitomycin C), can have cumulative long-term effects on the bone marrow. Most other agents, including the taxanes and topotecan, show no evidence of cumulative toxicity and can be administered for many cycles without dose modification.

In view of the frequent occurrence of neutropenia, and the risk of infectious complications, utilization of G-CSF or granulocyte-macrophage colony-stimulating factor (GM-CSF) has increased. Although these agents promote more rapid granulocyte recovery, avoiding potential complications and facilitating the maintenance of dose intensity, their use has not been shown to improve long-term survival for patients with advanced gynecologic tumors compared to conservative management with dose reduction and cycle delay. In addition, G-CSF and GM-CSF are not effective in the management of thrombocytopenia and may actually increase the degree of thrombocytopenia by diversion of immature marrow elements; a particular problem after multiple cycles of carboplatin. Recombinant megakaryocyte growth factor is an option to maintain platelet counts (78). However, current treatment programs are not associated with a high frequency of complicated grade 4 thrombocytopenia, and the value of aggressive support would appear to be limited.

Moderate degrees of anemia are quite common in cancer patients receiving chemotherapy, which may contribute to chronic fatigue. With increased recognition of bloodborne viral pathogens and limited supplies of banked blood, frequent transfusions are not practical or recommended, and many patients will adapt to chronic anemia with minimal symptoms. The availability of recombinant erythropoietin has provided a safe and effective alternative for the management of anemia associated with chemotherapy (79), and should be considered on a case-by-case basis, although financial costs at the recommended dose and schedule can be greater than the intermittent use of blood products (80).

Gastrointestinal Toxicity

Most anticancer agents are associated with some degree of nausea, vomiting, and anorexia. There are three major categories of nausea and vomiting: *anticipatory*, occurring prior to actual administration of chemotherapy; *acute-onset*, beginning within 1 hour of chemotherapy administration and persisting for less than 24 hours; and *delayed*, beginning more than 1 day after chemotherapy administration and persisting for several days. Prophylactic management of these adverse effects improves patient acceptance and facilitates completion of therapy with full doses on schedule.

The antiemetic regimen is tailored to the emetogenic potential of the regimen, which reflects the incorporation of specific drugs, as well as the dose and schedule of drug administration. Mild nausea and vomiting can often be managed effectively with H-1 antihistamines (diphenhydramine), phenothiazines (prochlorperazine or thiethylperazine), butyrophenones (haloperidol), steroids (dexamethasone or methylprednisolone), benzamides (metoclopramide), or benzodiazepines (lorazepam). These are likely to be sufficient with drugs such as bleomycin, paclitaxel, vinca alkaloids, 5-fluorouracil, methotrexate, or mitomycin C.

For drugs with more severe emetogenic potential, including cisplatin, carboplatin, cyclophosphamide, or dactinomycin, a more aggressive prophylactic regimen is required. In general, these patients should receive a 5-hydroxytryptamine (5-HT3) receptor antagonist, such as ondansetron or granisetron, prior to chemotherapy and repeated at 8- to 12-hour intervals. Both compounds are also available in an oral formulation, which has been helpful in the management of delayed and/or chronic nausea after chemotherapy, or nausea associated with multiday oral chemotherapy regimens. Longer acting 5-HT3 antagonists have also become available, including dolasetron, which requires only a single intravenous or oral dose prior to chemotherapy. As a group, the 5-HT3 antagonists have been quite effective in controlling severe emesis with few side effects, but are more expensive than prochlorperazine (81). Alternative approaches include metoclopramide, which can cause sedation, diarrhea, and, occasionally, extrapyramidal reactions. Chronic nausea and vomiting can be a particular problem after several cycles of cisplatin and occasionally, carboplatin (82). The mechanism is poorly understood, and symptoms can be difficult to control with currently available medications, prompting the use of extended steroid administration, cannabinoids, or repeated dosing with 5-HT3 receptor antagonists.

Anticipatory nausea and vomiting can become a significant problem during repeated cycles of chemotherapy, as patients associate environmental cues (such as odor, carpeting, or paint colors) with nausea. In addition to behavioral modification, it can sometimes be modulated by pretreatment with antiemetics and amnesic drugs, such as benzodiazepines, administered orally at home prior to arriving at the treatment center. Lorazepam (0.05 mg/kg) can also be given by slow intravenous push 1 hour before therapy, with doses being continued as needed every 4 hours for up to six doses (83). Unfortunately, this particular schedule produces significant sedation and can be used only in hospitalized patients or outpatients with independent transportation.

Diarrhea, oral stomatitis, esophagitis, and gastroenteritis are also problems. Patients with significant oral or esophagogastric symptoms may be managed with oral viscous lidocaine (2%) or other topical anesthetics or a slurry of sucralfate, which can bind to ulcerated mucosa. In refractory cases, patients should be screened for secondary infectious complications, such as candidiasis and herpes simplex. Noninfectious secretory diarrhea is a dose-limiting toxicity associated with irinotecan, and is generally managed with prophylactic antimotility agents and intravenous hydration, with utilization of octreotide in severe cases. Diarrhea can also result from diffuse mucosal injury following administration of doxorubicin, 5-fluorouracil, methotrexate, and other agents. In the setting of chemotherapy, patients are also at increased risk for infectious diarrhea, and screening for *Clostridium difficile* is appropriate.

Alopecia

Scalp alopecia is one of the most emotionally taxing side effects of chemotherapy. Aside from long-lasting alopecia that follows cranial irradiation, it is almost always reversible, but it can be a major deterrent to successful chemotherapy. Total scalp alopecia is particularly common with drugs like doxorubicin and paclitaxel, and there is generally some degree of partial alopecia with cisplatin, carboplatin, cyclophosphamide, vinca alkaloids, and 5-fluorouracil. In a minority of cases, patients treated with paclitaxel will also experience loss of eyelashes, eyebrows, and other body hair, which can be particularly distressing. A variety of physical techniques have been devised to minimize alopecia, including scalp tourniquets and ice caps designed to decrease scalp blood flow. Although partially effective, they are rarely successful with extended chemotherapy.

Skin Toxicity

Skin toxicities that occur during chemotherapy include allergic or hypersensitivity reactions, skin hyperpigmentation, photosensitivity, radiation recall reactions, nail abnormalities, folliculitis, palmar-plantar erythrodysesthesia (PPE, hand-foot syndrome), and local extravasation necrosis. Many of these are drug specific and self limited, but occasionally they may be dose limiting.

PPE is a reversible but painful erythema, scaling, swelling, or ulceration involving the hands and feet. This occurs more often with chronic oral or intravenous medications, weekly treatment regimens, and formulations that increase drug circulation time, such as prolonged oral etoposide, weekly and continuous-infusion 5-fluorouracil, capecitabine, and polyethylene glycol (PEG)–liposomal doxorubicin (Doxil), where it has emerged as a major dose-limiting toxicity (84).

Extravasation necrosis is a serious complication seen after tissue infiltration of vesicant drugs such as doxorubicin, dactinomycin, mitomycin C, and vincristine (85,86). These drugs should always be administered through a freely flowing intravenous line with careful monitoring. Caution is also required during utilization of central venous ports, as malfunctions in the needle, hub, or tubing can be associated with gradual extravasation that will not be apparent for several hours (87). Any suspected infiltration should prompt immediate removal of the intravenous line and application of ice packs to the infiltrated area every 6 hours for 3 days. Small series have reported a limited experience with local infiltration or topical application of steroids, *n*-acetylcysteine, dimethylsulfoxide (DMSO), and hyaluronidase with variable results, and recommendations are imprecise. However, a single systemic dose of dexrazoxane, a topoisomerase II catalytic inhibitor, appears to offer specific protection against injury from anthracyclines, including doxorubicin and daunorubicin (88). Skin necrosis from some extravasations may eventually require surgical debridement and skin grafting.

Neurotoxicity

Peripheral neuropathy is the most common neurotoxicity encountered in gynecologic oncology, and is a particular risk with continued administration of cisplatin, paclitaxel, vinca alkaloids, and hexamethylmelamine (89,90). Although less common with carboplatin, it can still occur, particularly in combination with paclitaxel. Peripheral neuropathy generally begins with symptoms of parasthesia accompanied by loss of vibratory and position sense in longer nerves associated with the feet and hands. It then progresses to functional impairment, with gait unsteadiness and loss of fine motor coordination, such as trouble buttoning clothes and writing. This is closely followed by loss of deep tendon reflexes and eventual development of motor weakness. With paclitaxel and other nonplatinum agents, this is almost always reversible, but may require several months posttherapy for substantial improvement. In more severe cases, accompanied by neuronal injury or demyelination, recovery may require active neuronal regeneration over an extended period of time.

Neuropathy can become clinically apparent after two to three courses of therapy, with mild symptoms that resolve between cycles. Careful questioning and examination may reveal subtle findings at an earlier stage, and functional assessments have been developed that demonstrate good concordance with actual neuropathy (91). Most importantly, if related to cisplatin, neuropathy can continue to progress after therapy has been discontinued owing to ongoing axonal demyelination and loss, with long-term persistence of symptoms. Cisplatin has also been associated with permanent ototoxicity, and at higher doses, with loss of color vision (92) and autonomic neuropathy. Patients with underlying neurologic problems, such as diabetes, alcoholism, or carpal tunnel syndrome, are particularly susceptible. All patients who receive potentially neurotoxic therapy, especially cisplatin and paclitaxel, should be routinely queried regarding proprioception and fine motor tasks and examined for loss of vibratory sense, high-frequency hearing, and deep tendon reflexes.

Amifostine has been reported to reduce the frequency and severity of platinum-mediated neuropathy (93) and is being evaluated as a treatment to promote resolution of established neuropathy. However, a nonrandomized study in patients receiving cisplatin and paclitaxel in combination with amifostine failed to achieve a targeted reduction in the incidence of neuropathy (94). Widespread substitution of carboplatin for cisplatin has reduced, but not eliminated, the risk of clinical neuropathy and ototoxicity.

Other neurotoxicities include acute and chronic encephalopathies, usually associated with intrathecal chemotherapy, acute cerebellar syndromes, autonomic dysfunction, inappropriate secretion of antidiuretic hormone (SIADH), and cranial nerve paresis. Of particular relevance to the gynecologic cancer population, an acute reversible metabolic encephalopathy has been well described in association with ifosfamide (95), and attributed to the toxic metabolite chloroacetaldehyde. Of note, this syndrome can potentially be prevented by infusion of methylene blue (96), which may act

through inhibition of monoamine oxidase activity with reduced chloroacetaldehyde formation in the liver (97).

Genitourinary Toxicity

Renal toxicity is a well-recognized side effect of cisplatin (98), with implication of specific local metabolites (39) even though only a small fraction of cisplatin is cleared by renal excretion. In contrast, carboplatin undergoes extensive renal clearance with little risk of toxicity. Indeed, with increased substitution of carboplatin for cisplatin, and with a reduction in overall cisplatin dose intensity, there has been a decline in clinical familiarity with cisplatin-mediated nephrotoxicity. Careful attention to hydration status and saline-driven urinary output before, during, and immediately after therapy is required to reduce the risk associated with this serious complication (99).

Another troublesome side effect is hemorrhagic cystitis, which can be seen with cyclophosphamide or ifosfamide, attributed to the metabolite acrolein. With moderate-dose cyclophosphamide, this complication can be prevented by maintaining high urinary output, which reduces overall urothelial exposure to the toxic metabolites. However, patients receiving combination regimens often have reduced oral intake postchemotherapy, and selected patients receiving cyclophosphamide might benefit from supplemental intravenous hydration. The risk of cystitis is essentially 100% with ifosfamide, even with aggressive hydration, but this can be prevented with simultaneous administration of mesna, which binds and neutralizes acrolein in the urine (100).

Hypersensitivity Reactions

Increased utilization of paclitaxel, a natural product with poor solubility, has focused attention on the risk of hypersensitivity reactions (HSR). For intravenous administration, paclitaxel is formulated in Cremephor-EL, a mixture of polyoxyethylated castor oil and dehydrated alcohol, which has been associated with mast cell degranulation and clinical HSR. Over 80% of reactions occur within minutes during either the first or second cycle of drug administration and can usually be managed with prophylactic medication (corticosteroids, histamine H1/H2 blockade) followed by rechallenge beginning at a lower rate of infusion (101,102). Similar reactions have been reported with docetaxel and Doxil.

With improved survival and an increased utilization of second-line therapy, patients can also experience more traditional allergic reactions to selected chemotherapy agents. Carboplatin, an organoplatinum compound, has emerged as a major source of late allergic reactions. These occur most often during the second cycle of a second course of therapy, suggesting a process of antigen recall and priming of the immune response (103). Patients receiving a second course of carboplatin-based therapy should be closely monitored for early signs of hypersensitivity to avoid more serious reactions. Unlike the situation with paclitaxel, carboplatin reactions are not readily prevented or circumvented with prophylactic medication, although strategies for desensitization have been reported (104).

Other Significant Toxicities

A comprehensive discussion of all potential toxicities for currently available chemotherapeutic agents is beyond the scope of this chapter, and additional information is available in other chapters. Nevertheless, a variety of other important toxicities are occasionally encountered in regimens commonly used in gynecologic oncology. These include cardiac toxicity from cumulative doxorubicin exposure, radiation recall vasculitis from doxorubicin, pulmonary fibrosis from bleomycin, gonadal dysfunction in premenopausal women from alkylating agents, and secondary acute leukemia from the chronic administration of alkylating agents, particularly melphalan in ovarian cancer.

DEVELOPMENTAL CHEMOTHERAPY

Background

The identification, evaluation, and regulatory approval of effective drugs for cancer treatment is a long, complicated, and expensive process. Of note, it has been argued that the expanded availability of only 17 existing generic chemotherapeutic agents would substantially improve worldwide mortality from cancer (105). However, most cases of advanced disease remain incurable with current treatments, and the search for new agents remains a high priority. Promising candidates are identified and prioritized through preclinical screening (106), utilizing derivatives of previously defined active agents or established drug classes or new compounds engineered to interact with a specific target. In addition, there continues to be broad screening of natural products isolated from terrestrial and marine sources (107). Some evidence of antitumor activity during screening must be demonstrated before clinical trials are undertaken. Thus far, all useful antitumor agents have demonstrated antitumor activity using *in vitro* or *in vivo* screening systems.

These traditional approaches are being increasingly challenged by the large number of new genes and potential targets identified through molecular biology, genomics, and proteomics. Principles of genomic libraries, solid-phase organic synthesis (108), and combinatorial chemical library generation (109) have been adopted by the pharmaceutical industry to promote high-throughput screening (110). As new targets are identified, a large number of related compounds can be created, beginning with lead natural products or known reagents (111), and then screened for improved target binding and/or inhibition of target function (112). Substantial bioinformatics resources are required to manage and analyze the large amount of data generated from these pro-

cesses, but the accumulation of gene expression and proteomic data can facilitate "pre-discovery" modeling of potential targets and reagents prior to making decisions about actual development. To some extent, these processes have evolved in parallel, as it is clear that agents generated from a library or a database will still require some form of biologic validation prior to entering complex and expensive clinical studies.

After antitumor activity has been identified, the new agent must be formulated for human use and produced in sufficient quantities to support clinical trials. This is never a trivial achievement, as was evident from the natural supply limitations and formulation problems encountered in early trials with paclitaxel (113) and the camptothecins (114). Clinical-grade material is then subjected to detailed preclinical toxicology tests in animals. These toxicology trials are done in several animal species and may explore different schedules of drug administration to provide a basis for clinical development. As such, they are time consuming, complex, and expensive.

After all of the steps of preclinical testing are completed, new agents can enter clinical evaluation. As such, clinical trials are the primary means utilized to evaluate new agents in a systematic manner. All physicians and patients are urged to consider participation in clinical trials, which are available for almost all diagnoses and treatment circumstances. Sponsors of clinical trials include the NCI in collaboration with individual institutions and national groups, such as the Gynecologic Oncology Group (GOG), as well as the pharmaceutical industry, and individual institutions.

Clinical Trials

Detailed rationale and methodology for clinical trials design has been covered in other sections. This material is provided to highlight key concepts related to investigational drug development.

Phase I Trials

Phase I trials are typically first-in-human studies for new compounds and employ a dose- and/or schedule-escalating design to determine the dose-limiting toxicity (DLT), maximally tolerated dose (MTD), and pharmacokinetic parameters applicable to each regimen. In the most common model, accrual is suspended when more than one DLT event occurs within a dose level (two of six patients), as this would generally exceed predefined limits for the MTD. Modifications of the standard dose-escalation schema have been developed to enroll fewer patients at lower dose levels with greater dose increments between successive dose levels in the absence of toxicity. As the MTD is approached, the dose level increments are reduced and accrual can be expanded. These newer methods aim to minimize the number of patients treated at very low (nonefficacious and nontoxic) doses, whereas providing greater precision for estimating the MTD and DLT at higher doses (115).

Tumor response is not a primary endpoint within a Phase I trial, which will typically include patients representing a variety of primary tumor types and multiple prior therapies. Comprehensive analysis of aggregate Phase I data, often from multiple trials, will generally determine a dose, schedule, and disease site profile for evaluation in Phase II studies. However, with the increased number and diversity of compounds that merit early testing, it is also important to prioritize these studies carefully within the limited clinical resources that are available.

Phase I studies can also serve to evaluate novel combinations of investigational and/or commercially available drugs to establish feasibility and tolerability of the proposed regimen before embarking on larger trials. In certain situations, such as epithelial ovarian cancer, disease-specific Phase I trials may enroll newly diagnosed patients without prior therapy, as the experimental combinations generally incorporate other known active agents, such as platinum and paclitaxel.

Phase II Trials

After the recommended dose and schedule have been defined, the regimen can receive focused evaluation in patients with a specific cancer diagnosis, usually in the setting of measurable disease after one prior chemotherapy regimen. Phase II trials are designed and powered based on a surrogate endpoint that is thought to reflect clinical benefit, such as response rate, disease stabilization rate, biologic (tumor marker) response rate, or the proportion of patients alive and progression free at a specific time interval. Although each of these endpoints may reflect antitumor activity, they are viewed as surrogate endpoints in comparison with overall survival or quality-adjusted survival, which provide a true measure of clinical benefit. In general, each Phase II trial tests a single hypothesis, such as response rate, to determine if the new agent or regimen crosses a threshold based on historical data in the same patient population with an appropriate degree of power (type II or β error) and precision (type I or α error). Through this process, new agents are "selected" for further development based on historical controls. In order to conserve patient resources and minimize the number of patients who might receive ineffective therapy, most Phase II studies utilize a multistage accrual design with early-stopping parameters, as proposed by Gehan (116) and modified by Simon (117).

Although most Phase II trials are single-arm nonrandomized studies, there are circumstances where randomized Phase II evaluations are appropriate (118–120). Randomized Phase II trials allocate patients among two or more treatment arms to minimize potential differences in prognostic factors or other variables. Each arm is then independently tested against the same historical threshold value. Using this approach, one or both arms can be "selected" for further clinical development. Such randomized trials are generally underpowered for direct comparison of response rate and survival between each arm owing to the limited number of patients. Examples include looking at two different schedules of drug administration with comparative analysis of toxicity and noncomparative reporting of response data to facilitate the selection of experimental arms for future studies. This approach has been utilized to select between two different schedules of topotecan administration in recurrent ovarian cancer (121).

Phase III Trials

If a promising regimen is identified for further testing, it then moves toward a Phase III randomized trial, in which it is directly compared with an existing standard regimen in a particular clinical setting, as defined by the type of cancer and stage at enrollment. Phase III trials generally require a minimum of 150 patients per arm to provide adequate *precision* for the comparison of primary study endpoints while avoiding false-positive conclusions (type I or α error) and adequate *power* to detect a difference while avoiding a false-negative result and potentially missing a true advantage of one arm over the other (type II or β error). In keeping with current drug registration guidelines of the FDA, the primary endpoint of most Phase III trials is a true measure of clinical benefit, such as overall survival or quality-adjusted survival, with secondary endpoints of progression-free survival, response rate, and toxicity.

Owing to the large number of uniformly staged and treated patients required for a Phase III trial, such studies are best conducted through a national clinical trials organization, such as GOG. To minimize potential sources of bias, Phase III trials frequently stratify patients into groups according to key prognostic variables prior to randomization, such as stage or extent of residual disease, as well as other minor variables, such as location of the treating institution. Verification of patient diagnosis, stage of disease, eligibility, treatment delivered, and tumor response can further improve the reliability of results reported from clinical trials.

FDA Approval and Postmarketing Studies

Following a successful Phase III trial, or a group of trials, a sponsor can apply to the FDA for marketing approval for a specific disease indication. This triggers a detailed review of clinical trials and pharmaceutical data by the Oncology Drug Advisory Committee (ODAC), which then issues a recommendation to the FDA, followed by formal review and a decision by the FDA, which may grant approval or request additional data. In the United States, all marketing requires approval for at least one specific indication by the FDA. The average time from initial drug discovery to application for an FDA-approved indication is 10 to 12 years, involving considerable expense and effort, as noted above. Supplemental Phase IV, or postmarketing, studies can be required by the FDA as part of the approval process, or performed by the sponsor to evaluate alternative drug formulations, or resolve questions regarding dose, schedule, or toxicity. In addition, Phase IV studies may involve substitution of the new agent in combination chemotherapeutic regimens already established for the disease. These studies are not commonly employed in the development of new chemotherapeutic regimens, but can provide confirmatory "postmarketing" evidence of safety and efficacy.

Development of Combination Regimens

With some notable exceptions, such as choriocarcinoma and childhood Burkitt's lymphoma, single agents are not sufficient to achieve prolonged survival or cure. Development of combination regimens has been accelerated by our knowledge of cell killing, pharmacokinetics, molecular targets, tumor heterogeneity, and drug resistance. Combinations can approach maximal cell kill by including drugs with minimal overlap of toxicities, such that antitumor effects can be summed but the toxicities dispersed. Combinations are also more likely to demonstrate activity against heterogeneous tumor populations, and effective combinations would prevent the emergence of drug resistance. However, in practice, it may also encourage greater resistance among surviving cell fractions.

Cumulative hematologic or nonhematologic toxicity limits the dose and duration of therapy that can be safely administered with specific single agents, such as doxorubicin, cisplatin, carboplatin, bleomycin, and mitomycin. Protective agents, such as amifostine (122) and dexrazoxane (123), together with growth factors, novel schedules of drug administration, and new formulations may overcome some of these limitations.

No direct evidence currently exists to indicate whether optimal combinations should utilize sequential single agents, doublets, or triplets. Utilization of single agents generally precludes any biologic interaction between the various components of a treatment regimen, but permits administration of each agent at the full active dose. The use of sequential doublets generally permits higher doses of individual drugs, compared to a triplet regimen, but over a smaller number of cycles with each agent. Doublets have the potential advantage of sequentially introducing more than one regimen with a different mechanism of action and/or pattern of resistance, which has been postulated to prevent the emergence of drug resistance.

Development of combination chemotherapy has been guided by several principles (Table 15.9). However, much of the reported experience has been derived from empiric combinations evaluated in conventional Phase I dose-escalating trials. Ideally, each of the drugs employed in a new combination should have independent activity as a single

TABLE 15.9. *Principles of combination chemotherapy*

Each component should have:
- Activity against the target tumor as a single agent
- A different mechanism of action and cellular target
- A biochemical basis for additive or synergistic effects in combination with at least one of the other agents
- No evidence of antagonistic interactions
- Distinct patterns of resistance to discourage the emergence of drug-resistant phenotypes

Optimal dose, schedule, and sequence of drug administration should be determined from preclinical data and early clinical trials to maximize tumor response and minimize host toxicity. Minimal overlap of nonhematologic toxicity is desirable to maintain safely full therapeutic doses of each component over multiple cycles.

agent, as verified in Phase II studies. Generally, drugs that can produce complete remissions are preferred to agents that produce only partial regressions, but complete remissions are uncommon in previously treated patients with recurrent disease. An attempt should be made to use drugs with minimal overlap of toxicities to avoid excessive dose reduction. Although this may broaden the range of toxicities encountered with each combination, it avoids cumulative and serious toxicity within individual organ systems. Bone marrow recovery usually proves to be the most dominant factor in cycle timing, and in practice, cycles of most combinations can be repeated every 3 to 4 weeks.

Several of these strategies are currently under evaluation in epithelial ovarian cancer based on preclinical models that have suggested an advantage for combinations with platinum, which has been attributed to inhibition of DNA repair (Table 15.10). Each of the selected agents (topotecan, gemcitabine, and Doxil) has also demonstrated independent activity against recurrent ovarian cancer, adding to the overall potential benefit of the combination. Ultimately, it remains to be established through well-designed Phase III trials if utilization of these newer combinations can be successfully translated into improved long-term clinical outcomes.

Drug Interactions, Scheduling, and Sequence

Drugs should be used in their optimal dose and schedule. However, new combinations have the potential to alter the pharmacokinetics, bioavailability, toxicity, and efficacy of individual components based on substrate-dependent effects, such as a reduction in nucleotide pools or altered metabolism. Therefore, the optimal dose and schedule for individual agents within a combination might differ from their use as single agents, and regimen development would benefit from preclinical models and Phase I trials with pharmacodynamic endpoints.

The impact of sequence variations using platinum with either paclitaxel or topotecan has been explored in Phase I clinical trials with somewhat surprising results. For example,

TABLE 15.10. *Representative agents for development of combination regimens*

Agent	Cellular target	Mechanism of action	Schedule-dependent effects	Patterns of resistance	Interaction with platinum
Platinum	DNA	DNA adduct formation	Independent	↑GSH ↑DNA repair ↑Damage tolerance ↓Accumulation	NA
Paclitaxel	β- tubulin	↑Tubulin aggregation	Dependent (toxicity)	↑MDR-1 (P-170) β- tubulin mutations	↓Heme toxicity ↑Neuropathy
Topotecan	Topoisomerase-I	Stabilize DNA-topoisomerase complex	Dependent (efficacy)	↓Topoisomerase-I ↑BCRP (ABCG2)	↑Heme toxicity
Gemcitabine	Ribonucleotide reductase, DNA, nucleotide pool	↓DNA synthesis ↓Nucleotide pools Masked chain termination	Dependent (metabolism)	↑Ribonucleotide reductase	↑Heme toxicity
Doxil	Topoisomerase-II	↓DNA synthesis	Prolonged clearance	↑MDR-1 (P-170)	↑Heme toxicity

NA = Not applicable

prior administration of cisplatin can delay subsequent clearance of paclitaxel when administered as a 24-hour infusion (124). The mechanism for this effect is unknown, but is not attributable to platinum-mediated renal dysfunction. Instead, it has been postulated to occur following cisplatin-mediated inhibition of cytochrome P-450 mixed-function oxidases that participate in paclitaxel metabolism. This enzymatic effect is not shared by carboplatin, and prior carboplatin exposure has not been demonstrated to interfere with clearance of paclitaxel. However, most combinations with carboplatin have utilized a shorter (3-hour) paclitaxel infusion, which would tend to blunt the impact of sequencing. Earlier preclinical models had demonstrated enhanced cytotoxicity when paclitaxel was administered prior to cisplatin and antagonism by the reverse sequence (125,126). Thus, the schedule ultimately adopted in clinical practice (paclitaxel followed by cisplatin) is both less toxic and potentially more efficacious. Although this would appear to be firmly grounded in science, it is more likely due to practical considerations owing to the risk of acute paclitaxel HSR, which can require interruption of treatment in approximately 5% of cases, and it was more practical to administer the carboplatin after it was clear that the patient had already tolerated the paclitaxel.

A different pattern of was observed with sequences of platinum and topotecan. Preclinical models have consistently favored the sequence of platinum followed by topotecan, which has been postulated to interfere with repair of platinum-mediated DNA damage. In a Phase I clinical trial, treatment with cisplatin on day 1 was associated with increased bone marrow toxicity compared with the reverse sequence (127). In this instance, the sequence recommended for further clinical evaluation was clearly more toxic, but may also have greater antitumor efficacy.

Even with a single drug, the schedule of administration can have a significant impact on host toxicity and potential

efficacy (Table 15.11). Early studies with paclitaxel utilized an arbitrary 24-hour infusion, which was selected to reduce the risk of hypersensitivity reactions. Preclinical data suggested that prolonged exposure (96 hours) might have greater efficacy, prompting a Phase I trial (128). Owing to increased bone marrow and mucosal toxicity, the MTD was lowered, and the frequency of serious neuropathy was reduced. However, the 96-hour regimen was not demonstrated to have significant activity in patients with recurrent ovarian cancer (129). A prior randomized trial had documented equivalent efficacy of a 3-hour infusion compared with a 24-hour infusion in recurrent ovarian cancer (130), reinforcing a clinical shift toward the convenient 3-hour schedule, which achieved a higher MTD, primarily due to a marked decrease in bone marrow toxicity, but with an increased incidence of neuropathy. This was followed by Phase I evaluation of a weekly low-dose 1-hour infusion, which was almost devoid of serious toxicity, including a decreased incidence of alopecia, with maintenance of clinical efficacy (131). Thus, the optimal preclinical regimen (96-hour exposure) was superseded in the clinical setting by an unexpected series of observations from empiric Phase I trials, yielding decreased toxicity, improved convenience, and the potential for increased efficacy.

With topotecan, a different relationship was defined (Table 15.11). Initial studies utilized an inconvenient daily infusion for 5 consecutive days, which was based on preclinical data suggesting that prolonged exposure would be more efficacious. This 5-day regimen achieved a 33% response rate in a GOG Phase II trial in recurrent platinum-sensitive ovarian cancer with expected dose-limiting neutropenia and thrombocytopenia (132). This was followed by the evaluation of single 24-hour infusion once every 3 weeks, achieving only a 7% response rate in a similar population (133). An attempt to define an intermediate 3-day regimen achieved only a 14% response rate (134). Topotecan was also evalu-

TABLE 15.11. *Impact of paclitaxel and topotecan infusion duration and schedule on toxicity and efficacy*

Dose and schedule			Dose-limiting toxicities				
Infusion duration (h)	Dose interval (wk)	Single-agent unit dose (mg/m^2/d)	Neutropenia	Mucositis	Alopecia	Neuropathy	Antitumor efficacy
Paclitaxel							
96	3–4	80–120	+++	++	+++	+	+++
24	3	135	++	0	+++	++	+++
3	3	175	+	0	+++	+++	+++
1	1	80	0	0	+	+	+++
Topotecan							
21	4	0.40	+++	0	0	0	+++
5	3–4	1.25	+++	0	0	0	+++
3	3	2.00	+++	0	0	0	++
1	3	8.50	+++	0	0	0	±
1	1	1.75	++	0	0	0	±
1	1	4.0	+	0	0	0	UA

UA, underevaluation.

ated as a prolonged intravenous infusion for 21 days to maximize the duration of exposure (135). Although conducted in a different patient population, the overall response rate (35%) was similar to the 5-day regimen, and once again, there was equivalent hematologic toxicity without dose-limiting non-hematologic toxicity. Finally, a randomized Phase II trial conducted by the NCIC and EORTC determined that the 5-day schedule was more appropriate for further clinical development owing to limited activity of an experimental weekly schedule (121). However, this has been challenged on the grounds of inadequate dosing for the weekly regimen, which clearly has reduced hematologic toxicity, and studies are ongoing to evaluate a revised weekly treatment program. In this situation, changes in drug schedule, over a wide range, were associated with substantial differences in efficacy, but without any change in the spectrum or severity of host toxicity, with the exception of reduced hematologic toxicity on the weekly schedule. Thus, each new agent needs to be independently evaluated in the appropriate clinical setting to select the optimal dose and schedule for cancer treatment.

Regional Chemotherapy

Although most chemotherapy is administered by the systemic route, there are unique situations in which the regional use of chemotherapy has been studied. If primary tumors or their metastases are anatomically confined to specific organs or particular regions of the body, or if unique pharmacokinetic circumstances exist that favor regional clearance, there is a theoretical rationale for regional chemotherapy. Intraarterial drug administration has been studied in a variety of circumstances, including cervical cancer, localized recurrence of rectal carcinoma, and intracarotid therapy for head and neck cancer. Local complications are potentially serious, including arterial thrombosis, wound slough, lymphedema, and osteonecrosis caused by the shared arterial blood supply

between the tumor and neighboring normal tissues. These experimental approaches may achieve higher response rates, but have not yet demonstrated an improvement in long-term outcomes.

Intracavitary chemotherapy has been used for tumors confined to the peritoneum, pleura, or pericardium. The rationale for this approach is based on the fact that clearance from a body cavity is delayed compared to the systemic circulation, achieving more prolonged exposure to higher regional concentrations of active agents. This technique has been most extensively studied in ovarian cancer, with evaluation of many agents, including 5-fluorouracil, doxorubicin, cisplatin, carboplatin, cytarabine, melphalan, etoposide, and paclitaxel (136,137). Phase I studies have uniformly demonstrated a pharmacologic advantage favoring the intraperitoneal compartment. However, penetration of peritoneal tumor nodules by passive diffusion is limited by fibrotic adhesions, tumor encapsulation, and high interstitial pressures as a consequence of intratumoral capillary leak without functional lymphatic drainage. As such, the major role for intracavitary chemotherapy is presumed to be in patients with minimal residual disease.

Cisplatin has been established as the intraperitoneal drug of choice in ovarian cancer, achieving a laparotomy-confirmed response rate of greater than 32% at doses between 50 and 150 mg/m^2, using systemic thiosulfate rescue at the higher dose levels (138). One long-term analysis reported an actuarial 2-year survival rate of 74% for patients with minimal residual disease treated with a variety of intraperitoneal therapies (139), although this may partially reflect the biology of small-volume disease, which can also be managed effectively with observation followed by systemic therapy. A Phase II trial of intraperitoneal paclitaxel demonstrated a 61% pathology-confirmed complete response rate among 28 assessable patients with initial microscopic disease (140). However, only 1 of 31 patients (3%) with greater than microscopic disease achieved a complete response, emphasizing the limitations of drug access and penetration by diffusion from the peritoneal space. In contrast to cisplatin, paclitaxel was poorly absorbed from the peritoneal compartment, suggesting that patients might benefit from combined intravenous and intraperitoneal administration to optimize tumor drug exposure.

Based on pilot Phase II data with a combined intraperitoneal regimen (141), a Phase III trial has completed accrual for patients with optimally debulked stage III ovarian cancer comparing intravenous cisplatin and paclitaxel against an experimental combination of intraperitoneal cisplatin, intraperitoneal paclitaxel, and supplemental intravenous paclitaxel. Preliminary analysis has revealed a modest improvement in progression-free survival at the expense of increased hematologic and nonhematologic toxicity (142), primarily attributable to the relatively high dose of intraperitoneal cisplatin. This has prompted reconsideration of intraperitoneal carboplatin, and pilot studies have been initiated to define the optimal dose of intraperitoneal carboplatin in combination with paclitaxel in anticipation of future Phase III trials.

REFERENCES

1. Lissauer A. Zwei Falle von Leucaemie. *Berl Klin Wochenschr* 1865; 2:403.
2. Cutler EG, Bradford EH. Action of iron, cod-liver oil, and arsenic on the globular richness of the blood. *Am J Med Sci* 1878;75:74–84.
3. Kandel EV, LeRoy GV. Chronic arsenical poisoning during the treatment of chronic myeloid leukemia. *Arch Intern Med* 1937;60:846–866.
4. Gilman A. The initial clinical trial of nitrogen mustard. *Am J Surg* 1963;105:574–578.
5. Farber S, Diamond LK, Mercer RD, et al. Temporary remissions in acute leukemia in children produced by folic acid antagonist, 4-aminopteroylglutamic acid (aminopterin). *N Engl J Med* 1948;238:787.
6. Hertz R, Ross GT, Lipsett MB. Primary chemotherapy of nonmetastatic trophoblastic disease in women. *Am J Obstet Gynec* 1963;86:808–814.
7. Huggins C, Hodges CV. Studies on prostatic cancer. The effect of castration, of estrogen and of androgen injection on serum phosphatases in metastatic carcinoma of the prostate. *Cancer Res* 1941;1:293.
8. Adjei AA. Blocking oncogenic Ras signaling for cancer therapy. *J Natl Cancer Inst* 2001;93:1062–1074.
9. Haluska P, Dy GK, Adjei AA. Farnesyl transferase inhibitors as anticancer agents. *Eur J Cancer* 2002;38:1685–1700.
10. Cell kinetics and the chemotherapy of cancer. *Cancer Chemother Rep* 1971;2:23.
11. Lotem J, Sachs L. Regulation by bc-12, c-myc and p53 of susceptibility to induction of apoptosis by heat shock and chemotherapy compounds in differentiation-competent and -defective myeloid leukemic cells. *Cell Growth Differ* 1993;4:41–47.
12. Scheffner M, Munger K, Byrne JC, Howley PM. The state of the p53 and retinoblastoma genes in human cervical carcinoma cell lines. *Proc Natl Acad Sci U S A* 1991;88:5523–5527.
13. Collins VP, Loeffler RK, Tivey H. Observations on growth rates of human tumors. *AJR Am J Roentgenol* 1956;76:988–1000.
14. Charbit A, Malaise EP, Tubiana M. Relationship between the pathological nature and the growth rate of human tumors. *Eur J Cancer* 1971;7:307–315.
15. Baserga R. The relationship of the cell cycle to tumor growth and control of cell division: a review. *Cancer Res* 1965;25:581–595.
16. Tannock I. Cell kinetics and chemotherapy: a critical review. *Cancer Treat Rep* 1978;62:1117–1133.
17. Steel GG. Cell loss as a factor in the growth rate of human tumors. *Eur J Cancer* 1967;3:381–387.
18. Powis G. Effect of human renal and hepatic disease on the pharmacokinetics of anticancer drugs. *Cancer Treat Rev* 1982;9:85–124.
19. Bennett WM, Singer I, Golper T, et al. Guidelines for drug therapy in renal failure. *Ann Intern Med* 1977;86:754–783.
20. Motzer RJ, Niedzwiecki D, Isaacs M, et al. Carboplatin-based chemotherapy with pharmacokinetic analysis for patients with hemodialysis-dependent renal insufficiency. *Cancer Chemother Pharmacol* 1990; 27:234–238.
21. *United States Pharmacopeia*. USP DI oncology drug information. 2nd ed. Rockville, MD: Association of American Cancer Centers, 1998.
22. Hande KR, Wolff SN, Greco FA, et al. Etoposide kinetics in patients with obstructive jaundice. *J Clin Oncol* 1990;8:1101–1107.
23. Tanaka E. Clinically important pharmacokinetic drug-drug interactions: role of cytochrome P450 enzymes. *J Clin Pharm Ther* 1998; 23:403–416.
24. Kivisto KT, Kroemer HK, Eichelbaum M. The role of cytochrome P450 enzymes in the metabolism of anticancer agents: implications for drug interactions. *Br J Clin Pharmacol* 1995;40:523–530.
25. Fojo AT, Ueda K, Slamon DJ, et al. Expression of multidrug resistance gene in human tumors and tissues. *Proc Natl Acad Sci U S A* 1987; 84:265–269.
26. Nunberg JH, Kaufman RJ, Schimke RT, et al. Amplified dihydrofolate reductase genes are localized to a homogeneously staining region in a single chromosome in a methotrexate-resistant Chinese hamster ovary cell line. *Proc Natl Acad Sci U S A* 1978;75:5553–5556.
27. Fojo AT, Whang-Peng J, Gottesman MM, et al. Amplification of DNA sequences in human multidrug-resistant KB carcinoma cells. *Proc Natl Acad Sci U S A* 1985;82:7661–7665.
28. Ling V, Thompson LH. Reduced permeability in CHO cells as a mechanism of resistance to colchicine. *J Cell Physiol* 1974;83:103–116.
29. Yusuf RZ, Duan Z, Lamendola DE, et al. Paclitaxel resistance: molecular mechanisms and pharmacologic manipulation. *Curr Cancer Drug Targets* 2003;3:1–19.
30. Bergman AM, Pinedo HM, Talianidis I, et al. Increased sensitivity to gemcitabine of P-glycoprotein and multidrug resistance-associated protein-overexpressing human cancer cell lines. *Br J Cancer* 2003; 88:1963–1970.
31. Schondorf T, Scharl A, Kurbacher CM, et al. Amplification of the mdr1-gene is uncommon in recurrent ovarian carcinomas. *Cancer Lett* 1999;146:195–199.
32. Rubin SC, Finstad CL, Hoskins WJ, et al. Expression of P-glycoprotein in epithelial ovarian cancer: evaluation as a marker of multidrug resistance. *Am J Obstet Gynecol* 1990;163:69–73.
33. Lamendola DE, Duan Z, Penson RT, et al. Beta tubulin mutations are rare in human ovarian carcinoma. *Anticancer Res* 2003;23:681–686.
34. Belinsky MG, Bain LJ, Balsara BB, et al. Characterization of MOAT-C and MOAT-D, new members of the MRP/cMOAT subfamily of transporter proteins. *J Natl Cancer Inst* 1998;90:1735.
35. Maliepaard M, van Gastelen MA, de Jong LA, et al. Overexpression of the BCRP/MXR/ABCP gene in a topotecan-selected ovarian tumor cell line. *Cancer Res* 1999;59:4559–4563.
36. Green JA, Vistica DT, Young RC, et al. Potentiation of melphalan cytotoxicity in human ovarian cancer cell lines by glutathione depletion. *Cancer Res* 1984;44:5427–5431.
37. Sadowitz PD, Hubbard BA, Dabrowiak JC, et al. Kinetics of cisplatin binding to cellular DNA and modulations by thiol-blocking agents and thiol drugs. *Drug Metab Dispos* 2002;30:183–190.
38. Daubeuf S, Balin D, Leroy P, Visvikis A. Different mechanisms for gamma-glutamyltransferase–dependent resistance to carboplatin and cisplatin. *Biochem Pharmacol* 2003;66:595–604.
39. Hanigan MH, Lykissa ED, Townsend DM, et al. Gamma-glutamyl transpeptidase-deficient mice are resistant to the nephrotoxic effects of cisplatin. *Am J Pathol* 2001;159:1889–1894.
40. O'Dwyer PJ, Hamilton TC, LaCreta FP, et al. Phase I trial of buthionine sulfoximine in combination with melphalan. *J Clin Oncol* 1996; 14:249–256.
41. Bailey HH, Ripple G, Tutsch KD, et al. Phase I study of continuous-infusion L-S,R-buthionine sulfoximine with intravenous melphalan. *J Natl Cancer Inst* 1997;89:1789–1796.
42. Holford J, Beale PJ, Boxall FE, et al. Mechanisms of drug resistance

to the platinum complex ZD0473 in ovarian cancer cell lines. *Eur J Cancer* 2000;36:1984–1990.

43. Gore ME, Atkinson RJ, Thomas H, et al. A phase II trial of ZD0473 in platinum-pretreated ovarian cancer. *Eur J Cancer* 2002;38: 2416–2420.

44. Masuda H, Ozols RF, Lai GM, et al. Increased DNA repair as a mechanism of acquired resistance to cis-diamminedichloroplatinum (II) in human ovarian cancer cell lines. *Cancer Res* 1988;48: 5713–5716.

45. Aebi S, Kurdihaidar B, Gordon R, et al. Loss of DNA mismatch repair in acquired resistance to cisplatin. *Cancer Res* 1996;56:3087–3090.

46. Raymond E, Chaney SG, Taamma A, Cvitkovic E. Oxaliplatin: a review of preclinical and clinical studies. *Ann Oncol* 1998;9: 1053–1071.

47. Vaisman A, Varchenko M, Umar A, et al. The role of hMLH1, hMSH3, and hMSH6 defects in cisplatin and oxaliplatin resistance: correlation with replicative bypass of platinum-DNA adducts. *Cancer Res* 1998;58:3579–3585.

48. Piccart MJ, Green JA, Lacave AJ, et al. Oxaliplatin or paclitaxel in patients with platinum-pretreated advanced ovarian cancer: a randomized phase II study of the European Organization for Research and Treatment of Cancer Gynecology Group. *J Clin Oncol* 2000;18: 1193–1202.

49. Fracasso PM, Blessing JA, Morgan MA, et al. Phase II study of oxaliplatin in platinum-resistant and refractory ovarian cancer: a Gynecologic Group Study. *J Clin Oncol* 2003;21:2856–2859.

50. Trent JM, Buick RN, Olson S, et al. Cytologic evidence for gene amplification in methotrexate-resistant cells obtained from a patient with ovarian adenocarcinoma. *J Clin Oncol* 1984;2:8–15.

51. Cowan KH, Jolivet J. A methotrexate-resistant human breast cancer cell line with multiple defects, including diminished formation of methotrexate polyglutamates. *J Biol Chem* 1984;259:10793–10800.

52. Obata T, Endo Y, Murata D, et al. The molecular targets of antitumor 2'-deoxycytidine analogues. *Curr Drug Targets* 2003;4:305–313.

53. Zhou B, Mo X, Liu X, et al. Human ribonucleotide reductase M2 subunit gene amplification and transcriptional regulation in a homogeneous staining chromosome region responsible for the mechanism of drug resistance. *Cytogenet Cell Genet* 2001;95:34–42.

54. Jung CP, Motwani MV, Schwartz GK. Flavopiridol increases sensitization to gemcitabine in human gastrointestinal cancer cell lines and correlates with down-regulation of ribonucleotide reductase M2 subunit. *Clin Cancer Res* 2001;7:2527–2536.

55. Johnston PG, Lenz HJ, Leichman CG, et al. Thymidylate synthase gene and protein expression correlate and are associated with response to 5-fluorouracil in human colorectal and gastric tumors. *Cancer Res* 1995;55:1407–1412.

56. Salonga D, Danenberg KD, Johnson M, et al. Colorectal tumors responding to 5-fluorouracil have low gene expression levels of dihydropyrimidine dehydrogenase, thymidylate synthase, and thymidine phosphorylase. *Clin Cancer Res* 2000;6:1322–1327.

57. Fidler IJ, Kripke ML. Metastasis results from preexisting variant cells within a malignant tumor. *Science* 1977;197:893–895.

58. Kern DH, Weisenthal LM. Highly specific prediction of antineoplastic drug resistance with an in vitro assay using suprapharmacologic drug exposures. *J Natl Cancer Inst* 1990;82:582–588.

59. Cortazar P, Johnson BE. Review of the efficacy of individualized chemotherapy selected by in vitro drug sensitivity testing for patients with cancer. *J Clin Oncol* 1999;17:1625–1631.

60. Nagourney RA, Brewer CA, Radecki S, et al. Phase II trial of gemcitabine plus cisplatin repeating doublet therapy in previously treated, relapsed ovarian cancer patients. *Gynecol Oncol* 2003;88:35–39.

61. Levin L, Hryniuk W. Dose intensity analysis of chemotherapy regimens in ovarian cancer. *J Clin Oncol* 1987;5:756–767.

62. McGuire WP, Hoskins WJ, Brady MF, et al. Assessment of dose-intensive therapy in suboptimally debulked ovarian cancer: a Gynecologic Oncology Group study. *J Clin Oncol* 1995;13:1589–1599.

63. Schilder RJ, Gallo JM, Millenson MM, et al. Phase I trial of multiple cycles of high-dose carboplatin, paclitaxel, and topotecan with peripheral-blood stem-cell support as front-line therapy. *J Clin Oncol* 2001; 19:1183–1194.

64. McGuire WP, Hoskins WJ, Brady MF, et al. Cyclophosphamide and cisplatin compared with paclitaxel and cisplatin in patients with stage III and stage IV ovarian cancer. *N Engl J Med* 1996;334:1–6.

65. Ozols RF, Bundy BN, Greer BE, et al. Phase III trial of carboplatin and paclitaxel compared with cisplatin and paclitaxel in patients with optimally resected stage III ovarian cancer: a Gynecologic Oncology Group study. *J Clin Oncol* 2003;21:3194–3200.

66. Fleming GF, Brunetto VL, Cella D, et al. Phase III trial of doxorubicin plus cisplatin with or without paclitaxel plus filgrastim in advanced endometrial carcinoma: a Gynecologic Oncology Group study. *J Clin Oncol (in press)*.

67. Moore DH, Blessing JA, McQuellon RP, et al. Phase III study of cisplatin with or without paclitaxel in stage IVB, recurrent or persistent squamous cell carcinoma of the cervix: a Gynecologic Oncology Group study. *J Clin Oncol (in press)*.

68. Long HJ, Bundy BN, Grendys EC, et al. Randomized phase III trial of cisplatin (P) vs cisplatin plus topotecan (T) vs MVAC in stage IVB, recurrent or persistent carcinoma of the uterine cervix: a Gynecologic Oncology Group study. *Gynecol Oncol (in press)*.

69. Muggia FM, Braly PS, Brady MF, et al: Phase III randomized study of cisplatin versus paclitaxel versus cisplatin and paclitaxel in patients with suboptimal stage III or IV ovarian cancer: a Gynecologic Oncology Group study. *J Clin Oncol* 2000;18:106–115.

70. The International Collaborative Ovarian Neoplasm (ICON) Group. Paclitaxel plus carboplatin versus standard chemotherapy with either single-agent carboplatin or cyclophosphamide, doxorubicin, and cisplatin in women with ovarian cancer: The ICON3 randomised trial. *Lancet* 2002;360:505–515.

71. Young RC, Brady MF, Nieberg RK, et al. Adjuvant treatment for early ovarian cancer: a randomized phase III trial of intraperitoneal ^{32}P or cyclophosphamide-cisplatin. A Gynecologic Oncology Group study. *J Clin Oncol (in press)*.

72. Trimbos JB, Vergote I, Bolis G, et al. EORTC-ACTION collaborators. European Organisation for Research and Treatment of Cancer—Adjuvant ChemoTherapy in Ovarian Neoplasm. Impact of adjuvant chemotherapy and surgical staging in early-stage ovarian carcinoma: European Organisation for Research and Treatment of Cancer—Adjuvant ChemoTherapy in Ovarian Neoplasm trial. *J Natl Cancer Inst* 2003; 95:113–125.

73. Rose PG, Bundy BN, Watkins EB, et al. Concurrent cisplatin-based radiotherapy and chemotherapy for locally advanced cervical cancer. *N Engl J Med* 1999;340:1144–1153.

74. Therasse P, Arbuck SG, Eisenhauer EA, et al. New guidelines to evaluate the response to treatment in solid tumors. European Organization for Research and Treatment of Cancer, National Cancer Institute of the United States, National Cancer Institute of Canada. *J Natl Cancer Inst* 2000;92:205–216.

75. Rustin GJ, Marples M, Nelstrop AE, et al. Use of CA-125 to define progression of ovarian cancer in patients with persistently elevated levels. *J Clin Oncol* 2001;19:4054–4057.

76. Vergote I, Rustin GJ, Eisenhauer EA, et al. Re: new guidelines to evaluate the response to treatment in solid tumors [ovarian cancer]. Gynecologic Cancer Intergroup. *J Natl Cancer Inst* 2000;92: 1534–1535.

77. Rustin GJ. Use of CA-125 to assess response to new agents in ovarian cancer trials. *J Clin Oncol* 2003;21[10 Suppl]:187–193.

78. Fanucchi M, Glaspy J, Crawford J, et al. Effects of polyethylene glycol-conjugated recombinant human megakaryocyte growth and development factor on platelet counts after chemotherapy for lung cancer. *N Engl J Med* 1997;336:404–409.

79. Del Mastro L, Venturini M, Lionetto R, et al. Randomized phase III trial evaluating the role of erythropoietin in the prevention of chemotherapy-induced anemia. *J Clin Oncol* 1997;15:2715–2721.

80. Barosi G, Marchetti M, Liberato NL. Cost-effectiveness of recombinant human erythropoietin in the prevention of chemotherapy-induced anaemia. *Br J Cancer* 1998;78:781–787.

81. Bonneterre J, Chevallier B, Metz R, et al. A randomized double-blind comparison of ondansetron and metoclopramide in the prophylaxis of emesis induced by cyclophosphamide, fluorouracil, and doxorubicin or epirubicin chemotherapy. *J Clin Oncol* 1990;8:1063–1069.

82. du Bois A, Vach W, Kiechle M et al: Pathophysiology, severity, pattern, and risk factors for carboplatin-induced emesis. *Oncology* 1996; 53[Suppl 1]:46–50.

83. Friedlander ML, Sims K, Kearsely JH. Impairment of recall improves tolerance of cytotoxic chemotherapy. *Lancet* 1983;2:686.

84. Muggia FM, Hainsworth JD, Jeffers S. Phase II study of liposomal

doxorubicin in refractory ovarian cancer: antitumor activity and toxicity modification by liposomal encapsulation. *J Clin Oncol* 1997; 15: 987–993.

85. Dunagin WG. Dermatologic toxicity. *Semin Oncol* 1982;9:14–22.

86. Kassner E. Evaluation and treatment of chemotherapy extravasation injuries. *J Pediatr Oncol Nurs* 2000;17:135–148.

87. Schulmeister L, Camp-Sorrell D. Chemotherapy extravasation from implanted ports. *Oncol Nurs Forum* 2000;27:531–538.

88. Langer SW, Sehested M, Jensen PB. Treatment of anthracycline extravasation with dexrazoxane. *Clin Cancer Res* 2000;6:3680–3686.

89. Verstappen CC, Heimans JJ, Hoekman K, Postma TJ. Neurotoxic complications of chemotherapy in patients with cancer: clinical signs and optimal management. *Drugs* 2003;63:1549–1563.

90. Quasthoff S, Hartung HP. Chemotherapy-induced peripheral neuropathy. *J Neurol* 2002;249:9–17.

91. Calhoun EA, Welshman EE, Chang CH, et al. Psychometric evaluation of the Functional Assessment of Cancer Therapy/Gynecologic Oncology Group—Neurotoxicity (Fact/GOG-Ntx) questionnaire for patients receiving systemic chemotherapy. *Int J Gynecol Cancer.* 2003;13:741–748.

92. Wilding G, Caruso R, Lawrence TS, et al. Retinal toxicity after high-dose cisplatin therapy. *J Clin Oncol* 1985;3:1683–1689.

93. Mollman JE, Glover DJ, Hogan WM, Furman RE. Cisplatin neuropathy. Risk factors, prognosis, and protection by WR-2721. *Cancer* 1988;61:2192–2195.

94. Moore DH, Donnelly J, McGuire WP, et al. Limited access trial using amifostine for protection against cisplatin- and three-hour paclitaxel–induced neurotoxicity: A phase II study of the Gynecologic Oncology Group. *J Clin Oncol* 21;2003:4207–4213.

95. Nicolao P, Giometto B. Neurological toxicity of ifosfamide. *Oncology* 2003;65[Suppl 2]:11–16.

96. Pelgrims J, De Vos F, Van den Brande J, et al. Methylene blue in the treatment and prevention of ifosfamide-induced encephalopathy: report of 12 cases and a review of the literature. *Br J Cancer.* 2000; 82:291–294.

97. Aeschlimann C, Cerny T, Kupfer A. Inhibition of (mono)amine oxidase activity and prevention of ifosfamide encephalopathy by methylene blue. *Drug Metab Dispos* 1996;24:1336–1339.

98. Arany I, Safirstein RL. Cisplatin nephrotoxicity. *Semin Nephrol* 2003; 23:460–464.

99. Santoso JT, Lucci JA 3rd, Coleman RL, et al. Saline, mannitol, and furosemide hydration in acute cisplatin nephrotoxicity: a randomized trial. *Cancer Chemother Pharmacol* 2003;52:13–18.

100. Andriole GL, Sandlund JT, Miser JS, et al. The efficacy of mesna as a uroprotectant in patients with hemorrhagic cystitis receiving further orazaphosphorine chemotherapy. *J Clin Oncol* 1987;5:799–803.

101. Bookman MA, Kloth DD, Kover PE, et al. Short-course intravenous prophylaxis for paclitaxel-related hypersensitivity reactions. *Ann Oncol* 1997;8:611–614.

102. Weiss RB, Donehower RC, Weirnik PH, et al. Hypersensitivity reactions from Taxol. *J Clin Oncol* 1990;8:1263–1268.

103. Markman M, Kennedy A, Webster K, et al. Clinical features of hypersensitivity reactions to carboplatin. *J Clin Oncol* 1999;17:1141.

104. Rose PG, Fusco N, Smrekar M, et al. Successful administration of carboplatin in patients with clinically documented carboplatin hypersensitivity. *Gynecol Oncol* 2003;89:429–433.

105. Sikora K, Advani S, Koroltchouk V, et al. Essential drugs for cancer therapy: a World Health Organization consultation. *Ann Oncol* 1999; 10:385–390.

106. Grever MR, Schepartz S, Chabner BA. The National Cancer Institute: cancer drug discovery and development program. *Semin Oncol* 1992; 19:622–638.

107. Cragg GM, Newman DJ, Weiss RB. Coral reefs, forests, and thermal vents: the worldwide exploration of nature for novel antitumor agents. *Semin Oncol* 1997;24:156–163.

108. Brocchini S. Combinatorial chemistry and biomedical polymer development. *Adv Drug Deliv Rev* 2001;53:123–130.

109. Geysen HM, Schoenen F, Wagner D, Wagner R. Combinatorial compound libraries for drug discovery: an ongoing challenge. *Nat Rev Drug Discov* 2003;2:222–230.

110. Leonard KA, Deisseroth AB, Austin DJ. Combinatorial chemistry in cancer drug development. *Cancer J.* 2001;7:79–83.

111. Breinbauer R, Manger M, Scheck M, Waldmann H. Natural product guided compound library development. *Curr Med Chem* 2002;9: 2129–2145.

112. Batra S, Srinivasan T, Rastogi SK, Kundu B. Identification of enzyme inhibitors using combinatorial libraries. *Curr Med Chem* 2002;9: 307–319.

113. Wani MC, Taylor HL, Wall ME, et al. Plant antitumor agents. VI. The isolation and structure of Taxol, a novel antileukemic and antitumor agent from *Taxus brevifolia. J Am Chem Soc* 1971;93: 2325–2327.

114. Wall ME, Wani MC, Cook CE, et al. Plant antitumor agents. I. The isolation and structure of camptothecin, a novel alkaloidal leukemia and tumor inhibitor from *Camptotheca accuminata. J Am Chem Soc* 1966;88:3888–3890.

115. Babb J, Rogatko A, Zacks S. Cancer phase I clinical trials: efficient dose escalation with overdose control. *Stat Med* 1998;17:1103–1120.

116. Gehan EA. The determination of the number of patients required in a preliminary and follow-up trial of a new chemotherapeutic agent. *J Chronic Dis* 1961;13:346–353.

117. Simon R. Optimal two-stage designs for phase II clinical trials. *Controlled Clin Trials* 1989;10:1.

118. Estey EH, Thall PF. New designs for phase 2 clinical trials. *Blood* 2003;102:442–448.

119. Steinberg SM, Venzon DJ. Early selection in a randomized phase II clinical trial. *Stat Med* 2002;21:1711–1726.

120. Strauss N, Simon R. Investigating a sequence of randomized phase II trials to discover promising treatments. *Stat Med* 1995;14:1479–1489.

121. Hoskins P, Eisenhauer E, Beare S, et al. Randomized phase II study of two schedules of topotecan in previously treated patients with ovarian cancer: a National Cancer Institute of Canada Clinical Trials Group study. *J Clin Oncol* 1998;16:2233–2237.

122. Mollman JE, Glover DJ, Hogan WM, Furman RE. Cisplatin neuropathy. Risk factors, prognosis, and protection by WR-2721. *Cancer* 1988;61:2192–2195.

123. Swain SM, Whaley FS, Gerber MC, et al. Cardioprotection with dexrazoxane for doxorubicin-containing therapy in advanced breast cancer. *J Clin Oncol* 1997;15:1318–1332.

124. Rowinsky EK, Gilbert M, McGuire WP, et al. Sequences of Taxol and cisplatin: a phase I and pharmacologic study. *J Clin Oncol* 1991; 9:1692–1703.

125. Rowinsky EK, Citardi M, Noe DA, Donehower RC. Sequence-dependent cytotoxicity between cisplatin and the antimicrotubule agents Taxol and vincristine. *J Cancer Res Clin Oncol* 1993;119:737–743.

126. Jekunen AP, Christen RD, Shalinsky DR, Howell SB. Synergistic interaction between cisplatin and Taxol in human ovarian carcinoma cells in vitro. *Br J Cancer* 1994;69:299–306.

127. Rowinsky EK, Kaufmann SH, Baker SD, et al. Sequences of topotecan and cisplatin: Phase I, pharmacological and in vitro studies to examine sequence dependence. *J Clin Oncol* 1996;14:3074–3084.

128. Wilson WH, Berg SL, Bryant G, et al. Paclitaxel in doxorubicin-refractory or mitoxantrone-refractory breast cancer: a phase I/II trial of 96-hour infusion. *J Clin Oncol* 1994;12:1621–1629.

129. Markman M, Rose PG, Jones E, et al. Ninety-six-hour infusional paclitaxel as salvage therapy of ovarian cancer patients previously failing treatment with 3-hour or 24-hour paclitaxel infusion regimens. *J Clin Oncol* 1998;16:1849–1851.

130. Eisenhauer EA, ten Bokkel Huinink WW, Swenerton KD, et al. European-Canadian randomized trial of paclitaxel in relapsed ovarian cancer: high-dose versus low-dose and long versus short infusion. *J Clin Oncol* 1994;12:2654–2666.

131. Fennelly D, Aghajanian C, Shapiro F, et al. Phase I and pharmacologic study of paclitaxel administered weekly in patients with relapsed ovarian cancer. *J Clin Oncol* 1997;15:187–192.

132. McGuire WP, Blessing JA, Bookman MA, et al: Topotecan has substantial antitumor activity as first-line salvage therapy in platinum-sensitive epithelial ovarian carcinoma: A Gynecologic Oncology Group Study. *J Clin Oncol* 2000;18:1062–1067.

133. Markman M, Blessing JA, Alvarez RD, et al: Phase II evaluation of 24-h continuous infusion topotecan in recurrent, potentially platinum-sensitive ovarian cancer: A Gynecologic Oncology Group study. *Gynecol Oncol* 2000;77:112–115.

134. Miller DS, Blessing JA, Lentz SS, McMeekin DS. Phase II evaluation of three-day topotecan in recurrent platinum-sensitive ovarian carci-

noma: a Gynecologic Oncology Group study. *Cancer* 2003;98: 1664–1669.

135. Hochster H, Wadler S, Runowicz C, et al: Activity and pharmacodynamics of 21-day topotecan infusion in patients with ovarian cancer previously treated with platinum-based chemotherapy: New York Gynecologic Oncology Group. *J Clin Oncol* 1999;17:2553–2561.

136. Markman M. Intraperitoneal antineoplastic drug delivery: rationale and results. *Lancet Oncol* 2003;4:277–283.

137. Myers C. The clinical setting and pharmacology of intraperitoneal chemotherapy: an overview. *Semin Oncol* 1985;12:12.

138. TenBokkel Huinink WW, Dubbelman R, Aartsen E, et al. Experimental and clinical results with intraperitoneal cisplatin. *Semin Oncol* 1985;12:43–46.

139. Howell SB, Zimm S, Markman M, et al. Long-term survival of advanced refractory ovarian carcinoma patients with small-volume disease treated with intraperitoneal chemotherapy. *J Clin Oncol* 1987; 5:1607–1612.

140. Markman M, Brady MF, Spirtos NM, et al. Phase II trial of intraperitoneal paclitaxel in carcinoma of the ovary, tube, and peritoneum: a Gynecologic Oncology Group Study. *J Clin Oncol* 1998;16: 2620–2624.

141. Rothenberg ML, Liu PY, Braly PS, et al. Combined intraperitoneal and intravenous chemotherapy for women with optimally debulked ovarian cancer: results from an intergroup phase II trial. *J Clin Oncol* 2003;21:1313–1319.

142. Armstrong DK, Bundy BN, Baergen R, et al: Randomized phase III study of intravenous (IV) paclitaxel and cisplatin versus IV paclitaxel, intraperitoneal (IP) cisplatin and IP paclitaxel in optimal stage III epithelial ovarian cancer (OC): a Gynecologic Oncology Group trial (GOG 172). *Proc An Meet Am Soc Clin Oncol* 2002;21:201a (abst 803).

CHAPTER 16

Pharmacology and Therapeutics in Gynecologic Cancer

David S. Alberts, Lisa M. Hess, Daniel D. Von Hoff, and Robert T. Dorr

The determinants of effective cancer drug therapies include drug disposition, tumor kinetics, and drug resistance. These factors profoundly influence the cytotoxicity of each anticancer drug and must be considered in designing therapeutic regimens. These principles are discussed in Chapter 15. In this chapter, we elaborate the basic and clinical pharmacology of cancer chemotherapeutic and biologic agents and provide a limited discussion of cytotoxic, molecularly targeted, antiangiogenesis, and modulating/supportive care drugs useful in the treatment of patients with gynecologic cancer.

DETERMINANTS OF EFFECTIVE DRUG THERAPIES

Drug Disposition Factors

The term *pharmacokinetics* describes the time course of drug disposition in body fluids and tissues through the use of mathematical models. These models use an equation or set of equations to describe the concentration versus time profile of a specific drug after administration into the body. The models are often illustrated by box diagrams, with each box or compartment corresponding to a region of the body, although the compartments may not represent real anatomic regions. A drug is considered to be uniformly distributed within a compartment if its concentration within tissues has reached homogeneity.

Pharmacokinetic models may be useful in predicting the plasma or tissue concentrations of drugs in the body after any one of several routes or methods of drug administration. The simplest model has one compartment into which the drug is assumed to be instantaneously introduced, and elimination occurs by one linear route. The disappearance of the drug from this compartment can be described by a straight line if plotted on semilogarithmic graph paper. As discussed by Tozer (1), no one-compartment pharmacokinetic model can be used to describe the disposition of commonly used anticancer drugs; nevertheless, the one-compartment pharmacokinetic model lends itself to an understanding of the concept of plasma half-life (i.e., $t_{1/2}$), which represents the time required for the concentration of a drug at any point on the plasma concentration · time elimination curve to achieve half its value. This constant may be applied repeatedly, so that, for instance, only 25% of the drug remains in two half-lives. The equation for plasma half-life that can be applied to any linear plasma concentration-time elimination curve is as follows: $t_{1/2}z = 0.693$/slope of the linear elimination curve (i.e., λ_z or rate constant for that part of the curve). Unfortunately, the terminal half-life of a drug is often a poorly reproducible parameter because it is highly dependent on plasma levels, often at the limit of drug assay sensitivity.

Pharmacokinetic Models

The pharmacokinetics of virtually all anticancer drugs require two- or three-compartment models for their mathematic description. These models are commonly referred to as biphasic or triphasic models (i.e., two or three phases observed on semilogarithmic plots). Conceptually, the one-compartment model relates to a drug that remains confined

David S. Alberts: Departments of Medicine, Pharmacology and Public Health, Arizona Cancer Center, College of Medicine, University of Arizona, Tucson, Arizona 85724

Lisa M. Hess: Department of Medicine, Arizona Cancer Center, University of Arizona, Tucson, Arizona 85724

Daniel D. Von Hoff: Department of Medicine, Arizona Cancer Center, College of Medicine, University of Arizona, Tucson, Arizona 85724

Robert T. Dorr: Department of Pharmacology, Arizona Cancer Center, College of Medicine, University of Arizona, Tucson, Arizona 85724

to the intravascular space after intravenous injection, and the two- or three-compartment model allows the pharmacokinetic description of anticancer drugs whose ultimate targets are beyond the intravascular space in tumor tissues. On a physiologic basis, the first and second phases of a biphasic or triphasic pharmacokinetic model represent the distribution of the anticancer drug after intravenous injection into the plasma compartment and tissues, respectively. The second and third phases of these models represent drug metabolism and excretion (i.e., elimination from the body through metabolism and renal or extrarenal excretion).

Drug Clearance and AUC Concepts

Wisdom dictates using the simplest mathematical model that can provide the "best" fit of the actual plasma concentration · time data using nonlinear least squares regression. After the mathematic model is selected, it is possible to generate the important pharmacokinetic parameters that describe the disposition of a specific anticancer drug within the body. Besides the determination of the terminal-phase plasma half-life (i.e., half-life related to the second or third phase of the biphasic or triphasic plasma concentration · time data), the area under the plasma disappearance curve ($AUC_0\infty$) and total body plasma clearance (Cl_T) are the most significant and clinically useful pharmacokinetic parameters.

Although the height of an anticancer drug's peak plasma level correlates with peak dose and the degree of its associated normal tissue toxicity, the drug's plasma AUC tends to correlate with its ultimate antitumor activity and normal tissue side effects. For example, when an identical dose of melphalan (0.6 mg/kg) is administered first orally and then intravenously 1 month later, because of its poor oral availability, the melphalan plasma AUC after the oral dose would be only one-third of that after the intravenous dose (Fig. 16.1). As would be anticipated, the equivalent intravenous dose of melphalan was associated with a twofold to threefold deeper nadir in granulocytes and a greater than twofold increase in objective response rates in various cancer types (e.g., myeloma).

The plasma AUC (in mg/mL · hour) can be estimated through the use of a pharmacokinetic model or measured directly by plotting the drug's plasma concentrations against time on semilogarithmic graph paper. Then, it is possible to calculate the areas of successive trapezoids wherein the upper surface of the trapezoid is a line that connects two successive plasma concentration data points. By convention, when the plasma AUC is measured in this way, the terminal part of the AUC is ignored (i.e., that part extending from the last drug concentration data point).

After the plasma AUC has been determined, it is possible to derive the anticancer drug's total body clearance rate based on the following formula: $Cl_T = dose (mg)/AUC (mg/mL · hour)$. The resulting Cl_T is measured in units of milli-

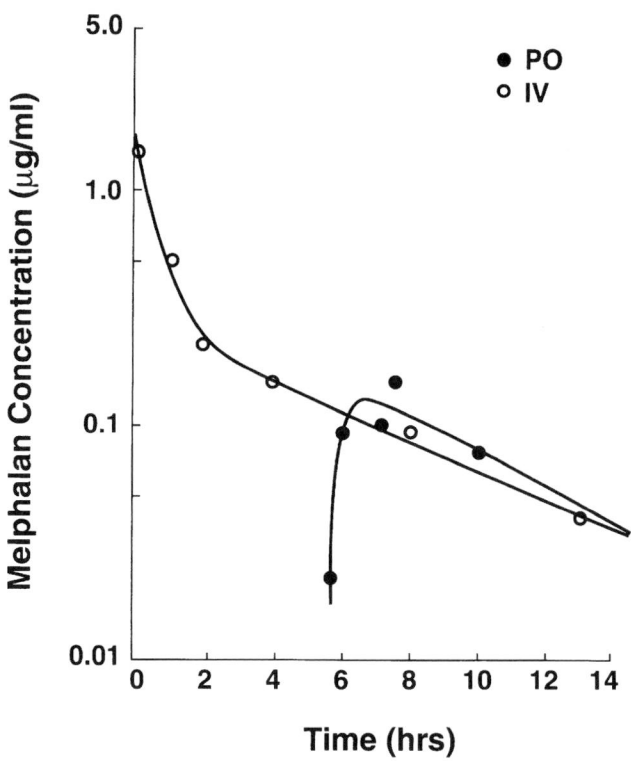

FIG. 16.1. Plasma disappearance curves for intravenous and oral (tablets) melphalan (0.6 mg/kg) in a patient with ovarian cancer. The melphalan plasma AUC associated with the bolus oral dose was only one-third of that associated with the intravenous dose. (Reprinted with permission from Alberts DS, Chang SY, Chen HS, et al.. Oral melphalan kinetics. *Clin Pharmacol Ther* 1979;26:737.)

liters or liters per minutes or hours with normalization to the body surface area. The total body clearance of an anticancer drug depends on the drug's dose and plasma AUC and represents the rate at which the drug is eliminated from the entire body. The drug's total body clearance is made up of the combination of renal clearance (Cl_R) plus nonrenal clearance (Cl_{NR}). The renal clearance of a drug can be calculated by the following equation: $Cl_R = Ae_c/AUC$, where Ae_c is the total amount of the unchanged drug that is excreted. For many drugs, renal clearance is proportional to creatinine clearance. In a patient with severe renal impairment, if the nonrenal clearance is unaltered, the total body clearance is diminished significantly. This phenomenon is observed in patients with relatively severe renal impairment who receive drugs like methotrexate and carboplatin, both of which are eliminated mainly through renal excretion.

Volume of Distribution

The volume of distribution (Vd) of an anticancer drug is another important pharmacokinetic parameter that relates the drug plasma concentration (measured at the time of administration through extrapolation of the terminal phase of the concentration-time curve to 0 time) to the total amount of drug in the body. Thus, Vd_{area} represents the volume of distribution of a drug in the terminal phase of its elimination from the body. The volume of distribution in the terminal phase can be derived using the following equation: $Vd_{area} = dose/AUC \cdot slope (\lambda_z)$, where λ_z is the rate constant in the terminal phase of a biphasic or triphasic elimination curve.

Linear and Nonlinear Kinetics

Although linear pharmacokinetic models are extremely useful with respect to concept formation and the study of the pharmacokinetics of anticancer drugs administered in relatively normal dose ranges, the pharmacokinetics of an anticancer drug given to maximally tolerated doses may exhibit deviations from the normal linear behavior. As discussed by Collins and Dedrick (see reference 259), there are at least two explanations for nonlinear kinetics. First, nonlinearity may be caused by changes in drug excretion at high doses. For example, at extremely high doses of methotrexate (i.e., 7 to 8 g/m^2), the drug load outstrips the renal tubular secretion capacity. Second, nonlinearity may be observed for drugs that depend almost completely on elimination through a specific degradative enzyme system (e.g., antimetabolites). Drugs like arabinosyl cytosine and 5-fluorouracil administered in high doses may overcome the capacity of their respective degradative enzymes with a resultant decrease in their total body clearance rates and plasma levels that are more than proportionate to their doses.

Intraperitoneal Drug Pharmacokinetics

Intraperitoneal drug administration has become an increasingly important therapeutic strategy in the management of patients with advanced ovarian cancer who have minimal residual intraperitoneal disease after primary or secondary exploratory laparotomies. Two large Phase III trials in the Gynecologic Oncology Group (GOG) and the Southwest Oncology Group (GOG-104 and GOG-114) comparing various combination, cisplatin-based chemotherapeutic regimens administered intravenously (IV) or intraperitoneally (IP) have documented significant survival advantages for the intraperitoneal cisplatin treatment arms (2,3). Most recently, in GOG-172, an intraperitoneal regimen (intravenous paclitaxel on day 1 and 2, intraperitoneal cisplatin on day 2, and intraperitoneal paclitaxel on day 8) was associated with a 28% reduction in the risk of recurrence as compared to the intravenously administered regimen (intravenous paclitaxel plus cisplatin) ($p = .01$) (4). Survival data were not available from this trial as of the time of publication of this chapter. The intraperitoneal arm of this GOG trial was piloted in an intergroup Phase III trial led by the Southwest Oncology Group (SWOG-9619), which documented the longest median progression-free survival (33 months) as compared to the same dose administered intravenously of any prior U.S.

cooperative group study in women with stage III optimally debulked disease (5). Despite the superior activity of this intravenous paclitaxel/intraperitoneal cisplain-paclitaxel regimen evaluated in GOG-172 and SWOG-9619, there was significantly more myelotoxicity and peripheral neuropathy in comparison to a standard intravenous paclitaxel (135 mg/m^2 by 24-hour infusion) and cisplatin (75 mg/m^2 on day 2) regimen.

The intraperitoneal administration of cisplatin in women with stage III optimal residual disease has been shown to be associated with an incremental improvement in survival of 18 months as compared with intravenous cisplatin ($p = .02$) (2). This increase in survival is similar to that which was achieved when intravenous cisplatin was initially added to primary combination chemotherapeutic regimens for the treatment of this disease (6). Of considerable interest, the intraperitoneal cisplatin/intravenous cyclophosphamide arm of this study was associated with significantly less grade 4 neutropenia and grade 2 or greater tinnitus and clinical hearing loss related to the much lower peak plasma levels achieved after intraperitoneal dosing.

The incremental increase in cisplatin efficacy associated with intraperitoneal administration likely results from the delivery of approximately 20-fold greater concentrations of cisplatin to the intraperitoneal space than are achievable with intravenous administration. Anticancer drugs with known activity against ovarian cancer that undergo slow clearance from the intraperitoneal space into the systemic circulation without causing significant chemical peritonitis are the favored intraperitoneal compounds. Clearly, paclitaxel falls into this category. Intraperitoneal administration of this large taxane molecule results in 1,000-fold greater concentration in the intraperitoneal space than is achievable with intravenous administration (7). In contrast, cisplatin undergoes rapid clearance from the systemic circulation after administration by the intraperitoneal route. Another active intraperitoneal drug, fluorodeoxyuridine (3 g/day for 3 consecutive days every 3 weeks), has limited systemic circulation because it undergoes rapid hepatic extraction and elimination by degradative enzymes.

As with intravenous administration of anticancer drugs, the drug clearance rate from the intraperitoneal space is the most useful pharmacokinetic parameter for comparing drugs that are administered by the intraperitoneal route in the treatment of ovarian cancer. The peritoneal clearance rate can be calculated by dividing the drug dose by its intraperitoneal concentration · time product, which must be measured with repeated intraperitoneal fluid content sampling. Intraperitoneal drugs with slow clearance rates are favored because they result in prolonged exposure of the intraperitoneal tumor bed to high concentrations of anticancer drug. It is also possible to assess the pharmacokinetic characteristics of drug doses by comparing their peak intraperitoneal concentration with peak plasma concentration after intraperitoneal dosing or comparing their intraperitoneal concentration · time product

(AUC$_{IP}$) with their plasma concentration · time products after intraperitoneal dosing. Virtually all commonly used drugs administered intraperitoneally in patients with ovarian cancer have peak or concentration · time product ratios of more than 20. In some cases, the ratio can be much greater (e.g., ratio for paclitaxel is 150 to 800).

Except for drugs whose cytotoxicity depends on continuous exposure (i.e., arabinosyl cytosine and methotrexate), drugs used by the intraperitoneal route should be administered relatively rapidly in at least 2 L of peritoneal dialysate and remain within the peritoneal space without removal. For schedule-independent drugs, it is important to maintain high concentrations as long as possible within the intraperitoneal space to improve efficacy. It is of considerable interest that as the intraperitoneal dialysate volume decreases, a drug's intraperitoneal clearance rate increases rapidly. Thus, large volumes of intraperitoneal fluid increase the chances for uniform drug distribution throughout the intraperitoneal space and optimize the intraperitoneal clearance rates.

Ultimately, the effectiveness of intraperitoneal therapy depends on the inherent cytotoxic potency of the individual agent and its ability to penetrate from the outer surface to the inner core of intraperitoneal tumors. The degree of tumor penetration depends on the chemical structure of the compound and its molecular weight. There is an inverse relationship between molecular weight and tumor penetration. The higher the molecular weight of the anticancer drug, the lower the tumor penetration. One advantage of cisplatin over carboplatin as an intraperitoneal agent is its lower molecular weight. Los and colleagues (8) have demonstrated in intraperitoneal ovarian cancer animal studies that it requires almost 10 times more intraperitoneal carboplatin than cisplatin to achieve similar intratumoral concentrations; however, there is renewed interest to develop intraperitoneal carboplatin–intraperitoneal and intravenous paclitaxel regimens to reduce the potential for cisplatin-paclitaxel–induced peripheral neuropathy (see Special Applications, in Carboplatin section below).

CLINICAL PHARMACOLOGY OF ACTIVE DRUGS AGAINST GYNECOLOGIC CANCERS

We discuss below in alphabetical order the clinical pharmacology of cytotoxic, biologic and modulating/supportive care drugs with demonstrated activity against gynecologic cancers. We also include several of the recently Food and Drug Administration (FDA)–approved drugs for other indications that may prove active against gynecologic cancers.

Cytotoxic Agents

Altretamine

Chemistry

Altretamine (hexamethylmelamine, Hexalen), a synthetic cytotoxic antineoplastic s-triazine derivative, has FDA approval for treatment of persistent or recurrent ovarian cancer after first-line chemotherapy with cisplatin or other alkylating agents. The drug also exhibits antitumor activity against breast cancer, lymphomas, small-cell carcinoma of the lung, and endometrial and cervical cancer. The empiric formula of altretamine is $C_9H_{18}N_6$ (molecular weight = 210.28).

Mechanism of Action

The mechanism of action of altretamine is not completely elucidated. Although it bears structural similarity to and cross reactivity with triethylene-melamine, a classic alkylating agent, evidence demonstrating altretamine to be an alkylating agent is inconclusive. Altretamine does not consistently demonstrate cross resistance with classic alkylating agents used in rodent tumors or in human cancer treatment, but its clinical antitumor spectrum resembles that of an alkylating agent. Altretamine is inactive against most common murine and human tumor cell lines in vitro. Rutty and Connors (9,10) presented definitive evidence that metabolic activation of altretamine is necessary for its cytotoxic activity. It is extensively demethylated in vivo in the presence of liver enzymes and these N-methylolmelamine derivatives are more cytotoxic than the parent compound (10). Additional studies have shown that the reactive methyl intermediates, formed during altretamine N-demethylations, covalently bind to tissue macromolecules, including DNA, and that the cytotoxicity against certain human solid tumor cells in vitro is dependent on the metabolic formation of the reactive intermediates or their direct addition to cell culture incubate (11).

Drug Disposition

Altretamine is practically insoluble in water and, therefore, it has only been administered orally in clinical studies, precluding absolute bioavailability studies. After administration of altretamine to laboratory animals by any route, urinary recovery of parent drug was very low (<1%), and urinary recovery of total dose or total radioactivity after administration of ^{14}C-labeled drug was as high as 90%. Ames (11) determined that the bioavailability of the parent compound in rabbits after oral administration was 25% of that obtained after intravenous administration. Moreover, after giving the rabbits labeled altretamine by stomach tube, 85% of labeled drug equivalents was recovered in the urine. The high rate of recovery suggests efficient gastrointestinal absorption.

The urinary recovery and bioavailability data demonstrate that altretamine is well absorbed after oral administration and that the drug is extensively metabolized regardless of route of administration. The low bioavailability of intact altretamine is due to first-pass metabolism rather than to poor absorption.

After oral administration in doses of 120 to 300 mg/m^2, peak plasma levels, measured by gas chromatographic assay, from 0.2 to 20.8 mg/L are reached between 0.5 and 5.0 hours. The terminal-phase plasma half-life ranges from 4.7 to 10.2 hours (12). The interpatient variability of AUCs, ranging from 1.2 to 60.1 mg/L · h, is most likely due to the differences in the rate at which the drug is metabolized.

Administration and Dosage

The recommended dose for altretamine as a single agent for use in the palliative treatment of patients with ovarian cancer is 260 mg/m^2/day, orally, for 14 to 21 consecutive days in a 28-day cycle (13). The total daily doses should be given as four divided oral doses after meals and at bedtime. Compliance to this regimen in a small group of patients with relapsed ovarian cancer has been documented to be over 95% (14). There is no pharmacokinetic information on this dosing regimen and the effect of food on altretamine bioavailability in humans. In combination regimens, altretamine is typically used at a dose of 150 mg/m^2/day for 7 to 14 days of monthly cycles (15,16).

Altretamine should be temporarily discontinued for 14 days or longer and subsequently restarted with a 20% to 25% dose reduction for any of the following side effects: gastrointestinal intolerance unresponsive to symptomatic measures; leukocyte count less than 2,000/mm^3 or granulocyte count less than 1,000/mm^3; platelet count less than 75,000/mm^3; or progressive neurotoxicity. If neurologic symptoms fail to stabilize on the reduced-dose schedule, altretamine should be discontinued.

Side Effects and Toxicities

Altretamine is administered at a dose of 260 mg/m^2 (single agent) or 150 mg/m^2 (in combination) on an intermittent schedule and is relatively well tolerated. Single-agent data for this drug are available for 1,014 patients (17). With high, continuous daily dosing, nausea and vomiting were the dose-limiting toxic effects, and a form of reversible peripheral neurotoxicity occurred occasionally. Myelosuppression was mild to moderate. Leukocyte and platelet counts usually recovered within 1 week of therapy discontinuation.

In a study of 395 patients with advanced ovarian cancer treated with altretamine-containing combination regimens with or without cisplatin, no additional effect of altretamine on the incidence or severity of neurotoxicity could be demonstrated (18). Peripheral neuropathy and central nervous system symptoms are more likely to occur in patients receiving continuous, high-dose daily altretamine administered on an intermittent schedule than in those receiving moderate doses. Neurologic toxicity reverses after the drug is discontinued. Pyridoxine should not be used concomitantly with altretamine to reduce neurotoxicity because clinical trials data suggest it may inhibit cytotoxic activity. Concurrent administration of altretamine and antidepressants of the monoamine oxidase (MAO) inhibitor class may cause severe orthostatic hypotension. Cimetidine, an inhibitor of microsomal drug metabolism, increased altretamine's half-life and toxicity in a rat model.

In two recent Phase II studies of single-agent altretamine, at a dose of 260 mg/m^2 for 14 to 21 days of each monthly cycle, the most common toxicity was grade 2 to 3 nausea (23%) (19,20). In a consolidation therapy Phase II trial, only three patients (4%) experienced any grade 4 toxicity: granulocytopenia (two patients) and anxiety/depression (one patient). The most common grade 3 toxicities were malaise, fatigue, or lethargy in seven patients (7%) and nausea in six patients (6%). Aside from these, there were no other grade 3 or 4 toxicities that occurred in more than 5% of patients (19).

With continuous high-dose daily drug administration, nausea and vomiting of gradual onset occur frequently. Although in most instances these symptoms are controllable with antiemetics, the severity sometimes requires altretamine dose reduction or, rarely, discontinuation.

Data from three large clinical trials demonstrated that altretamine can be added to full therapeutic doses of cyclophosphamide, doxorubicin, and cisplatin (CHAP) without evidence of increased hematologic toxicity (21–23). Leukopenia below 3,000 cells/mm^3 occurred in fewer than 15% of the patients on a variety of intermittent- or continuous-dose altretamine regimens. Fewer than 1% had leukopenia below 1,000 cells/mm^3. When given in high doses over a 21-day course, nadirs of leukocyte and platelet counts were reached by 3 to 4 weeks, and normal counts were observed by 6 weeks. With continuous administration, nadirs are reached in 6 to 8 weeks.

Bleomycin

Chemistry

Bleomycin (Blenoxane), an antineoplastic, is a mixture of complex glycopeptides originally isolated from a strain of the fungus *Streptomyces verticillis*. The primary components are bleomycins A$_2$ and B$_2$. The family of bleomycin glycopeptides have a relatively high molecular weight and are quantitated in units of cytotoxic activity (i.e., roughly 1 U/1 mg of polypeptide protein). Bleomycin is used as palliative treatment in patients with advanced cervical (24) and vulvar cancers. Other clinical indications include squamous-cell carcinomas of the head and neck, lymphomas, and testicular carcinoma. The molecular formula of bleomycin A$_2$ is C$_{55}$H$_{84}$N$_{17}$O$_{21}$S$_3$ (molecular weight = 1,414) and the molecular formula of bleomycin B$_2$ is C$_{55}$H$_{84}$N$_{20}$O$_{21}$S$_2$ (molecular weight = 1,425).

Mechanism of Action

Although the exact mechanism of action is unknown, a key to its activity is the isolation of native compounds from

S. verticillis as coordinated Cu(II) complexes, which are inactive as antitumor agents. When complexed with ferrous iron, bleomycin becomes a potent oxidase, producing DNA strand breaks by oxygen free radicals. Its unique mechanism of action is schedule dependent and cell cycle dependent for the G_2 phase.

The oxygen radicals produced by the bleomycin-iron complex bound to DNA primarily cause single-strand breaks and a lesser degree of double-strand breaks. There is a subsequent release of base propenals of all four DNA bases: guanine, thymine, adenine, and cytosine. These modified free bases result from cleavage of the deoxyribose sugar at the 3'-4' bond. There is an apparent specificity for the release of thymine and for DNA binding at guanine-rich sequences in actively transcribed genes (25). The linker regions of DNA between nucleosomes comprise an important site for specific strand cleavage by bleomycin (26). Several mechanisms have been theorized to explain the development of resistance to bleomycin. Less important mechanisms appear to include DNA repair, membrane alterations, and decreased drug accumulation. The primary mechanism probably involves metabolic inactivation of bleomycin by a cytosolic hydrolase, which is in the cysteine proteinase family. The enzyme inactivates bleomycin by replacing a terminal amine with a hydroxyl group. The distribution of bleomycin hydrolase appears to explain some of the relative resistance and sensitivity to bleomycin in normal tissues. Normal tissues with high intrinsic hydrolase activities, such as the liver, spleen, intestine, and bone marrow, are not targets for bleomycin's toxic effects. In contrast, lung tissues and skin have low levels of hydrolase activity and are particularly susceptible to bleomycin-induced toxicity. However, there appears to be no direct correlation between hydroxylase levels in tumor cells and bleomycin-induced cytotoxicity (26). The development of other methods of bleomycin metabolism by tumor cells may be responsible for the emergence of drug resistance (27).

Drug Disposition

Bleomycin is eliminated predominantly by urinary excretion. This accounts for 45% to 62% of a dose after 24 hours. In the blood, the drug is rapidly cleared, and two phases of elimination are apparent. As a practical point, this means that over 95% of a dose has been completely eliminated by 24 hours (about six half-lives) (28). If administered by an intracavitary route, a large percentage of a bleomycin dose is absorbed, and the fractional systemic bioavailability is about 45% for intrapleural or intraperitoneal injections. The drug appears to efflux more slowly from the peritoneal cavity. This suggests that there is significantly greater local drug retention in the intraperitoneal space. This may explain some of the drug's unique efficacy by intracavitary administration (29,30). An increased exposure to drug in these local compartments is also reflected by the tenfold higher drug levels achieved with intraperitoneal or intrapleural therapy than with equivalent intravenous dosing.

Renal insufficiency markedly alters bleomycin elimination (31,32). This effect becomes most pronounced in patients with creatinine clearance values less than 25 to 35 mL/min (31). In these patients, the volume of distribution is unaltered at about 20 L, but the half-life varies as the inverse exponent of creatinine clearance. Thus, significant bleomycin dose reductions are required in all patients with reduced renal function.

Dosage

Bleomycin (in combination with cisplatin and etoposide or vinblastine) is used most commonly by bolus intravenous administration at dosages of as high as 30 mg/week for up to 12 weeks in the treatment of patients with germ-cell tumors of ovary. These 30-mg doses often are associated with delayed febrile episodes that can be inhibited successfully with a morning dose of dexamethasone or prednisone.

Bleomycin continues to be used commonly by continuous intravenous infusion at dosages of 10 mg/m²/day for 4 consecutive days, with courses repeated every 4 weeks. This schedule has been proven to be successful in the treatment of women with metastatic cervical cancer. Total bleomycin doses should usually not exceed 400 mg to avoid serious pulmonary toxicity.

Bleomycin can also be administered by the intramuscular route in doses of 15 to 30 mg. Absorption appears to be complete, and because of its lack of vesicant activity, the intramuscular route has been proven to be extremely safe (33).

Side Effects and Toxicities

Bleomycin's dose-limiting side effect is pulmonary toxicity, which occurs in approximately 10% of treated patients and in rare instances can result in death. The likelihood of lung damage increases with advanced age, chest irradiation (34), hyperoxia during surgical anesthesia (35,36), renal insufficiency, and cumulative doses greater than 400 U. However, pulmonary toxicity is variable and may occur in younger patients following low cumulative doses. Bleomycin-induced lung damage presents as pneumonitis with dry cough, dyspnea, and rales and may progress within weeks to pulmonary fibrosis. Bleomycin should be discontinued at the first clinical signs of lung toxicity. Acute pneumonitis is often responsive to corticosteroid therapy; however, there is no effective therapy for the chronic pulmonary fibrosis that may result for bleomycin therapy (37).

Recently, evidence from preclinical models of bleomycin-induced pulmonary thrombosis has documented that pretreatment with amifostine can abrogate this dose-limiting toxicity (38,39).

Bleomycin is nonmyelosuppressive (a factor that facilitates its use in combination chemotherapeutic regimens). Mucocutaneous toxicities, including mucositis, are the primary acute side effects of bleomycin. Manifestations of cutaneous reactions include hyperpigmentation, erythema, rash, striae, pruritus, thickening of the nail beds, and, in rare instances, scleroderma (40). Fever, chills, and alopecia are common. Mild nausea, vomiting, and anorexia may also occur, but are typically self-limiting. Infrequent side effects include headache, pain at tumor site, and anaphylactoid reactions. An idiosyncratic reaction consisting primarily of mucositis and skin rash has also been reported (41).

Special Precautions

Bleomycin should be used with extreme caution in patients with significant renal impairment or compromised pulmonary function; frequent radiographs are recommended. Because up to 70% of a bleomycin dose is eliminated by renal excretion, the bleomycin dose should be reduced for individuals with severe renal insufficiency. Unfortunately, there are no prospectively evaluated dosing nomograms for bleomycin dose adjustment. An empiric dose-adjustment formula has been described (31). The percentage dose reductions that are indicated by applying this formula to a "normal" creatinine clearance (CrCl) of 120 mL/min and a fractional urinary drug excretion of 0.45 are: CrCl >35 mL/min, no dose reduction required; CrCl = 20 mL/min, 50% dose reduction; CrCl = 15 mL/min, 52% dose reduction; CrCl = 10 mL/min, 55% dose reduction; and CrCl = 5 mL/min, 60% dose reduction. This is only a general guide, and it has not been clinically validated in a prospective study or retrospective analysis. Patients over 65 years of age may be at increased risk of developing orthostatic hypotension, especially when the recommended rate of intravenous infusion is exceeded.

Drug Interactions

Nephrotoxic drugs may significantly reduce the rate of bleomycin clearance and thus increase toxicity. Yee and co-workers (42) observed markedly reduced bleomycin clearance in children who had received six courses of a regimen including cisplatin (cumulative dose 300 mg/m²). In another case report, fatal bleomycin pulmonary toxicity occurred in a patient with cisplatin-induced acute renal failure (43). Similar toxic interactions should be anticipated for combinations of bleomycin with other nephrotoxic drugs, such as aminoglycosides, amphotericin, or cyclosporine.

Special Applications

Because of its nonvesicant nature, bleomycin has been administered by a number of nonvascular routes, including intramuscular (33), subcutaneous (44), and, most significantly, intrapleurally for the management of malignant effu-

sions. When compared with tetracycline, intrapleurally administered bleomycin, 60 to 120 U, had greater therapeutic benefit for the management of malignant pleural effusions (29,30). When compared with tetracycline, intrapleurally administered bleomycin 60 to 120 U had greater therapeutic benefit as evidenced by a longer time to effusion recurrence (46 vs 32 days, $p = .037$) and a lower 3-month effusion recurrence rate (30% vs 53%, $p = .047$). Because toxicities were similar for both therapies, bleomycin was selected as the preferred intrapleurally administered therapy for malignant pleural effusions (30).

There is evidence that a cytosolic hydrolase in the cysteine protein family inactivates bleomycin by replacing a terminal amine with a hydroxyl group. The distribution of bleomycin hydrolase appears to explain some of the relative resistance and sensitivity to bleomycin in normal tissues. Normal tissues with high intrinsic hydrolase activities, such as the liver, spleen, intestine, and bone marrow, are not targets for bleomycin's toxic effects. In contrast, lung tissues and skin have low levels of hydrolase activity and are particularly susceptible to bleomycin-induced toxicity. However, there appears to be no direct correlation between hydroxylase levels in tumor cells and bleomycin-induced cytotoxicity (26). The development of other methods of bleomycin metabolism by tumor cells may be responsible for the emergence of drug resistance (27).

Capecitabine

Chemistry

Capecitabine (Xeloda) is an orally administered antineoplastic agent. In patients with metastatic breast cancer, capecitabine in combination with docetaxel is indicated after failure of prior anthyracycline-containing chemotherapy, and monotherapy is indicated for those who are resistant to paclitaxel and are resistant to anthyracycline-containing chemotherapy (or further anthyracycline-containing chemotherapy is not indicated). Capecitabine is a fluoropryrimidine carbamate prodrug form of 5'-deoxy-5-fluorouridine (5'-DFUR) that is enzymatically converted to 5-flurouracil (5-FU) in vivo. Its chemical name is 5'-deoxy-5-fluoro-N-[(pentyloxy) carbonyl]-cytidine and its molecular weight is 359.35.

Mechanism of Action

Capecitabine itself is inactive, but after absorption in the gastrointestinal tract is metabolized to 5-FU by three enzymes: carboxylesterase, which converts capecitabine to 5'-deoxy-5-fluorocytidine in the liver; is converted to 5'-deoxy-5-fluorouridine by cytidine deaminase in the liver and tumor tissue; and thymidine phosphorylase, which in many cases is highly expressed in tumors, completes the final step of conversion to 5-FU. Theoretically, capecitabine therapy is likely to be most effective in patients with tumors that express high concentrations of thymidine phosphorylase (resulting in greater 5-FU being generated in the tumor) and low concentrations of dihydropyrimidine dehydrogenase (which rapidly breaks down 5-FU) (45). 5-FU acts as a false pyrimidine or antimetabolite ultimately to inhibit the formation of the DNA-specific nucleoside base thymidine. The metabolites of 5-FU, 5-fluoro-21-deoxyuridine-5′-monophosphate (FdUMP) and 5-fluorouridine triphosphate (FUTP), inhibit thymidylate synthase (FdUMP) and are incorporated into cellular RNA (FUTP). DNA synthesis and function is inhibited by the incorporation of FdUNP into cellular DNA (46).

Drug Disposition

After oral administration, capecitabine reaches peak blood levels in about 1.5 hours, and peak 5-FU levels are reached at about 2 hours. Food reduces the rate and extent of absorption for both capecitabine and 5-FU. Plasma protein binding is not dose dependent and is less than 60% for capecitabine and its metabolites. Capecitabine (95.5% of administered dose) and its metabolites are excreted in urine. Capecitabine has no effect on the pharmacokinetics of docetaxel or vice versa. The precise pharmacokinetics of capecitabine have been difficult to establish, which is thought to be due to the large interindividual and intraindividual variation in expression of the enzyme dihydropyrimidine dehydrogenase (45).

Administration and Dosage

Capecitabine is available as 150- and 500-mg tablets for oral use. The recommended dose is 2500 mg/m^2 daily to be administered as two doses: 1250 mg/m^2 in the morning and 1,250 mg/m^2 in the evening for 2 weeks followed by a 1-week rest (21-day cycle). Because of the high rate of grade 2 or greater capecitabine-induced palmar-plantar erythrodysesthesia (PPE), recommendations have been made to reduce the starting dose to 2,000 mg/m^2 daily. It should be taken with water within 30 minutes after a meal. The same dosage of capecitabine should be used when combined with docetaxel, which should be administered at 75 mg/m^2 as a 1-hour infusion on day 1 of the 21-day cycle. Premedication (per docetaxel labeling) should be started prior to docetaxel administration for patients receiving the combination therapy.

Side Effects and Toxicities

The only side effect that occurs more frequently with capecitabine than with intravenous 5-FU is PPE (15% to 20% of patients). The other more common side effects of capecitabine include diarrhea (40%) and nausea and vomiting (30% to 40%). Grade 3 hyperbilirubinemia occurred in 15.2% and grade 4 in 3.9% of patients in the clinical safety database of Xeloda. Of those patients experiencing grades 3 and 4

hyperbilirubinemia, many (64% and 71%, respectively) had liver metastases at baseline, and 57.5% and 35.5% had elevations in alkaline phosphatase or transaminases, respectively. Other less common side effects include myelosuppression (less frequent than with IV 5-FU), leukopenia, and cardiotoxicity. In general, capecitabine is relatively well tolerated.

Special Precautions

Because capecitabine is administered orally, patients should be informed how to monitor their toxicity symptoms and be instructed to maintain the prescribed dosing regimen. Capecitabine has been shown to alter coagulation parameters in patients undergoing treatment concomitantly with coumarin-derivative anticoagulants (e.g., warfarin) (45). Therefore, patients taking oral coumarin-derivative anticoagulant therapy should be monitored regularly with regard to coagulation parameters (international normalized ratio or prothrombin time). Patients over the age of 80 years and those with mild to moderate liver dysfunction should also be closely monitored.

Carboplatin

Chemistry

Carboplatin (Paraplatin) is an alkylating agent that is approved by the Food and Drug Adminstration for the treatment of patients with advanced ovarian cancer of epithelial origin. It is also active against metastatic endometrial and cervical cancer. Carboplatin has a molecular formula of $C_6H_{12}N_2O_7Pt$ and a molecular weight of 371.25. Its chemical name is platinum, diammine[1,1-cyclobutane-dicarboxylato(2-)0,0′]-,(SP-4-2). The water solubility of carboplatin (14 mg/mL) is approximately 10 times that of cisplatin.

Mechanism of Action

Carboplatin, like cisplatin, produces an equal number of predominantly interstrand DNA cross links rather than DNA-protein cross links, causing equivalent lesions and biologic effects. The differences in potencies appear to be related to the aquation rate, which is 14 mg/mL for carboplatin, as compared to 1 mg/mL for cisplatin. It covalently binds to DNA with preferential binding to the N-7 position of guanine and adenine (46). Like cisplatin, carboplatin must first undergo sequential losses of the nonamine carboxylato ligands. Although this process proceeds readily with the loss of the chlorides in cisplatin, the rate of leaving or "opening" of the carboxylato moieties in carboplatin is much slower (47). The molar potency of carboplatin in creating DNA lesions and cytotoxicity was observed to be roughly 2% of cisplatin *in vitro* and 25% to 33% of cisplatin *in vivo* (48, 49). A more striking difference is the markedly delayed onset of peak cross linking for carboplatin compared with cisplatin. With carboplatin, maximal DNA cross linking occurs 18 hours after exposure compared with 6 to 12 hours for cisplatin (49). In addition, carboplatin-induced DNA cross links appear to have a slower rate of resolution than cisplatin-induced cross links. This slower onset and offset of carboplatin cross linking is believed to be a direct result of a slow rate of monofunctional adduct formation or a slower rate of conversion of monoadducts to cross links. Despite the pharmacokinetic differences between carboplatin and cisplatin, Phase III studies and meta-analyses of clinical studies reveal equivalent activity between carboplatin and cisplatin in all prognostic subgroups of ovarian cancer patients (50,51).

Harrap (52) described nuclear protein phosphorylation after treatment with both cisplatin and carboplatin. These events appear to correlate with cell killing (53). Carboplatin reacts with two sites on DNA to produce cross links, as has been observed with cisplatin (54). The formation of DNA adducts results in the inhibition of DNA synthesis and function and inhibits transcription (46). These lesions involve a bifunctional platinum adduct to a single-strand DNA. This may produce transcriptional miscoding and an inhibition of DNA synthesis. It is possible that the cytotoxic effects of carboplatin are the result of binding to nuclear and cytoplasmic proteins. Carboplatin-induced cytotoxicity is not cell cycle phase specific, but it can be maximized by exposing cells in S phase to the drug.

Drug Disposition

The pharmacokinetics of carboplatin differ significantly from those of cisplatin. Table 16.1 shows that the plasma clearance of carboplatin is biphasic and slower than that of cisplatin, with a much higher percentage of drug being excreted in the urine. Unlike cisplatin, relatively little carboplatin is bound to plasma proteins. The major route of elimination of carboplatin is glomerular filtration and tubular secretion. There is little or no true metabolism of the drug. The carboxylato bonds in carboplatin are slowly hydrolyzed to yield transient aquated intermediates. These activated platinum species are believed to lead directly to irreversible adducts to DNA or protein. Overall, the rate of hydrolysis of carboplatin is significantly slower than that of cisplatin, leading to much slower reactivity with DNA (55). Because

TABLE 16.1. *Carboplatin pharmacokinetics*

Cumulative 24-h urinary excretion	65% (if creatinine clearance >60 mL/min)
In vitro half-life (H$_2$O)	~24 h
Plasma half-life	
β phase (free drug)	180 min
Protein-bound drug	>5 days
Volume of distribution	16–20 L
Protein binding	30% (slow equilibration)

as much as 65% of a carboplatin dose is excreted in the urine, significant dose adjustments are recommended for patients with creatinine clearance values less than 60 mL/min.

Carboplatin is widely distributed in body fluids and achieves good penetration into pleural effusions and ascites fluid (56,57). Pharmacokinetic studies in patients receiving continuous carboplatin infusions show that, although total platinum levels increase over the course of the infusion, free or active platinum levels can decrease from 78% on day 1 to 38% on day 4 of a 4-day infusion.

Administration and Dosage

Carboplatin is usually administered as a brief infusion over 15 minutes or longer in a solution of 0.9% sodium chloride or 5% dextrose in water. The drug is typically diluted in 500 mL of fluid and infused IV over 15 to 30 minutes to 1 hour without further hydration (58,59). Carboplatin also has been administered as a continuous 24-hour IV infusion for 1, 4, or 5 days or as a continuous IV infusion for 21 days.

The Calvert equation is the most frequently used formula for carboplatin dosing, inasmuch as it requires minimal calculations, results in predictable levels of myelosuppression, and prevents underdosing or overdosing in patients with excellent or poor renal function, respectively (60). The Calvert formula appears below along with general guidelines for selecting the specific carboplatin AUC.

$$\text{Carboplatin total dose(mg)} = \text{AUC(mg/mL} \cdot \text{min)} \times [\text{GFR(mL/min)} + 25]$$

AUC = 7, when carboplatin is used as a single agent in patients with good bone marrow reserve; 6, when carboplatin is used in combination regimens in patients with good bone marrow reserve or when used as a single agent in patients who have had prior moderate chemotherapy; and 4, when carboplatin is used as a single agent in patients with prior heavy chemotherapy exposure.

Glomerular filtration rate (GFR) can be determined by measuring creatinine clearance (i.e., [^{51}Cr]-ethylenediamine-tetraacetic acid) for all patients or estimated creatinine clearance for patients who have had no prior cisplatin exposure or have not had cisplatin for at least 2 months prior to carboplatin dose determination.

As an example, if the desired carboplatin AUC is 6 for a patient with an estimated creatinine clearance (CrCl) of 75 mL/min, the total carboplatin dose would equal 6 × (75 + 25), or 600 mg.

As noted above, the Calvert formula uses the following estimate of carboplatin clearance: Cl = GFR + 25. Although the method may be optimal (61), isotopic determination of the GFR as measured by [^{51}Cr]-ethylenediamine-tetraacetic acid (^{51}Cr-EDTA) is a costly, invasive procedure and the estimated creatinine clearance is often substituted for the GFR. A commonly used method for estimating creatinine clearance is the Cockroft-Gault equation (62):

$$CrCl = 0.85 \times (140 - age) \times Wt(kg) / 0.72 \times Scr(mg/dL)$$

(CrCl as calculated by the above equation is reduced by 15% for women; Scr = serum creatinine.)

Both the Cockroft-Gault calculation of creatinine clearance and creatinine clearance based on a 24-hour urine collection result in a systematic underestimation of the carboplatin AUC by approximately 10% (63–65). This level of bias may be deemed to be acceptable in view of the clinical utility of substituting creatinine clearance for GFR.

The Calvert formula has been prospectively evaluated by Sorenson et al. (66) in 24 previously untreated ovarian cancer patients and was found to predict more accurately carboplatin exposure than calculation of dose based on body surface area. The AUC of carboplatin as calculated by the Calvert formula accurately predicted the level of myelosuppression as determined by the relative decrease in the platelet count (66).

The recommendation dosage for single-agent carboplatin in ovarian cancer patients with good bone marrow reserve, based on body surface area, is 360 mg/m² given intravenously every 4 weeks. Because renal excretion is the primary route of carboplatin elimination, the carboplatin dose must be reduced for patients with compromised kidney function. The drug manufacturer's package insert recommends carboplatin doses of 250 and 200 mg/m² for patients with creatinine clearances of 41 to 59 and 16 to 40 mL/min, respectively.

The most frequently used primary chemotherapeutic regimen for advanced ovarian cancer is a combination of paclitaxel (175 mg/m² by 3-hour IV infusion) followed by carboplatin (at a targeted AUC of 5 or 6 by 30- to 60-minute IV infusion) every 21 days (if blood counts are adequate) for six cycles (67).

Side Effects and Toxicities

Although the activity is comparable to cisplatin, carboplatin is better tolerated, as measured by toxicity [e.g., low incidence of alopecia (68)] and quality of life analysis (50). The usual dose-limiting toxicity of carboplatin is bone marrow suppression, particularly thrombocytopenia (69). Leukopenia and anemia also occur but are less severe. Nonetheless, transfusions may be needed by 20% of all patients receiving carboplatin (70).

The platelet nadir is achieved 3 weeks after an IV bolus injection, and recovery is generally complete 4 to 5 weeks after dosing. However, patients with poor bone marrow reserve from previous chemotherapy or radiation therapy can have more profound thrombocytopenia and leukopenia with carboplatin treatment. Cell depletion may persist for several weeks after dosing.

Nausea and vomiting induced by carboplatin is much less severe than with cisplatin and rarely lasts beyond 24 hours. In a recent study of 943 ovarian cancer patients randomized to carboplatin, only 9% experienced greater than grade 2 nausea and/or vomiting (68). Emesis can usually be blocked entirely with aggressive therapy using antiemetic drug combinations (71). Diarrhea has been reported in only 6% of patients and constipation in 3% of carboplatin-treated patients (70).

Nephrotoxicity has been reported with carboplatin, but it is much less common and less severe than with cisplatin. In a large review, transient elevations in serum creatinine and blood urea nitrogen were described in 7% and 16% of patients, respectively (70). Measured creatinine clearances dropped in 25% of patients, and a slight increase in uric acid was described in the same percentage of patients. However, there can be a significant loss of serum electrolytes, including potassium (16% of patients) and magnesium (37%). Serum calcium is only rarely decreased after carboplatin (70).

A few cases of carboplatin-induced hematuria have been described. Hepatic enzyme elevations occasionally occur with carboplatin (70). Alkaline phosphatase was transiently increased in 36% of patients and serum glutamic oxaloacetic transaminase (SGOT) or serum glutamic pyruvic transaminase (SGPT) in about 15% of patients. Serum bilirubin levels are rarely elevated (4%) (70).

Neurotoxicity is uncommon after carboplatin and was described in only 25 of 428 (6%) patients treated on a variety of schedules for different tumor types (70). Mild paresthesias have been reported in a few patients receiving cumulative carboplatin doses of more than 1.6 g/m² (69). Unlike cisplatin, these peripheral nerve toxicities rarely produce any disabling symptoms. In most cases, no neurotoxicity was attributed to the drug.

Ototoxicity does not appear to be problematic with carboplatin, and only 8 of 710 (1.1%) patients have described clinical hearing deficits, mainly tinnitus (70). However, if pretreatment and serial audiometric tests are performed, as many as 15% of the patients may have some decrease in audio acuity. Fortunately, ototoxicity from carboplatin sometimes improves after therapy is halted. Like cisplatin, greater ototoxicity from carboplatin can be expected in patients with preexisting hearing loss or in those concurrently being given other ototoxic drugs, such as aminoglycosides.

Other rare carboplatin toxicities include alopecia (2% of patients), mucositis (2%), skin rash (1.7%), injection-site irritation without extravasation necrosis (0.4%), and a flu-like syndrome (1.3%) (70). The same study described alterations in taste sensation. Skin disorders from carboplatin treatment may appear as an erythematous rash in exposed areas and do not occur in all patients who had developed similar rashes on cisplatin (69).

Although carboplatin-associated hypersensitivity reactions rarely occur when the drug is administered as part of an initial chemotherapeutic regimen, subsequent administration of carboplatin in the setting of second-line or salvage therapy is associated with an increased risk of hypersensitivity. It has been estimated that over 25% of patients who receive more than six courses of platinum-based (i.e., cisplatin or carboplatin) chemotherapy develop sensitivity to carboplatin (72). The onset of symptoms may occur during the carboplatin infusion or up to 3 days after drug administration. Mild reactions consist of localized itching and erythema, primarily of the palms and soles, and/or facial flushing, whereas severe reactions can cause diffuse erythema, tachycardia, wheezing, facial edema, chills, rigors, throat and chest tightness, dyspnea, vomiting, alterations in blood pressure (both hypotension and hypertension), and, in extreme cases, respiratory arrest. Mild cases may respond to IV diphenhydramine (50 mg) or oral diphenhydramine (25 to 50 mg every 4 to 6 hours) and additional courses of carboplatin can be administered. Severe hypersensitivity reactions typically necessitate the discontinuance of carboplatin; however, some patients are able to receive additional courses of carboplatin with administration of corticosteroids for several days prior to carboplatin administration. Hypersensitivity reactions may also occur when carboplatin is administered by the intraperitoneal route (73).

Platinum-based chemotherapy (either cisplatin or carboplatin) has been shown to increase the risk of leukemia in ovarian cancer patients (74) Following carboplatin-based chemotherapy, the estimated relative risk of leukemia is 6.5 (95% confidence interval, 1.1 to 9.4). The relative risk increases as a function of both cumulative dose and duration of treatment. Patients who receive 4,000 mg or greater of carboplatin have a relative risk of 7.6 of developing leukemia, whereas patients who receive more than 12 months of carboplatin-based chemotherapy have a relative risk of 7.0. Although radiation therapy alone does not increase the risk of leukemia, radiation therapy administered in combination with platinum-based chemotherapy is associated with a significantly higher risk of leukemia than platinum-based chemotherapy without radiation ($p = .006$). The average time to onset of secondary leukemia is 4 years after the diagnosis of ovarian cancer. Although the potential benefits of platinum-based chemotherapy for ovarian cancer far outweigh the risk of secondary leukemia, the dose-dependent leukemogenic potential of platinum-based chemotherapy should be considered during its administration to patients with early-stage disease.

With the high doses of carboplatin used in autologous bone marrow transplantation programs, other severe toxicities may occur. These include hepatotoxicity (both hepatitis and cholestasis) and severe renal dysfunction (56,75). Nausea, vomiting, and electrolyte wasting are also more profound with high-dose carboplatin treatments. In addition, other unusual toxic effects may occur. These include hemorrhagic colitis, optic neuritis, and interstitial pneumonitis.

As noted below (see Drug Interactions), paclitaxel ameliorates carboplatin-induced thrombocytopenia.

Drug Interactions

Although the pharmacokinetics of carboplatin is not altered by coadministration of paclitaxel, patients who receive combination chemotherapy with carboplatin plus paclitaxel experience less thrombocytopenia than would be predicted if carboplatin was administered as a single agent (63,76). The relationship between free platinum exposure and thrombocytopenia following carboplatin/paclitaxel chemotherapy can be described by a sigmoid maximum effect model (63). In that the degree of neutropenia appears to be unaffected by coadministration of paclitaxel and carboplatin, this pharmacodynamic interaction is believed to occur at the megakaryocyte level (76).

The cytoprotective agent amifostine reduces carboplatin-induced thrombocytopenia (77) but also extends the plasma half-life of carboplatin (78). In a randomized trial of carboplatin with or without amifostine, the median platelet nadir of patients treated with carboplatin 500 mg/m^2 was 88,000/μL, whereas the nadir in patients who received amifostine 910 mg/m^2 was 127,000/μL ($p = .023$) (77). Pharmacokinetic studies have shown that amifostine administered just before the carboplatin infusion and 2 to 4 hours thereafter is associated with a significant increase in the terminal half-life of the ultrafiltrable platinum species (e.g., in patients with a creatinine clearance less than 80 mL/min the platinum half-life increased from 4.2 to 5.6 hours with the addition of amifostine). In patients with good renal function, the impact of the increase in terminal half-life was associated with a minimal effect on the AUC. However, patients with impaired renal function experienced significant increases in the AUC of the ultrafiltrable platinum species (78).

Special Applications

Patients with advanced ovarian cancer have been treated with intraperitoneal carboplatin in doses ranging from 200 to 650 mg/m^2 (79). Response rates have ranged from 10% to greater than 50%, with the higher response rates being observed in patients with minimal residual disease and no prior chemotherapy. These response rates are comparable with those observed with intraperitoneal cisplatin; however, cisplatin may be a better choice for intraperitoneal platinum therapy in that it is associated with less systemic toxicity (i.e., myelosuppression) and appears to have significantly better penetration into tumor masses (80,81).

Because of its relative lack of nonhematologic side effects, carboplatin has become the platinum analog of choice for bone marrow transplantation regimens. A regimen developed at Loyola University that consists of high-dose carboplatin combined with cyclophosphamide, mitoxantrone, and autologous bone marrow support was selected for an intergroup Phase III study of high-dose versus standard-dose chemotherapy for ovarian cancer patients with low-volume, persistent disease following primary chemotherapy (GOG-164). Although this study was closed in May 1999 because of inadequate patient accrual, the high-dose regimen was well tolerated among the 24 patients entered to the trial. With adequate hydration and mannitol diuresis to prevent nephrotoxicity, nonhematologic side effects were predominantly mucositis, ototoxicity, and diarrhea (75).

Cisplatin

Chemistry

Cisplatin (Platinol, *cis*-diamminedichloroplatinum) is a primary drug in the treatment of advanced cancer of the ovary, cervix, and endometrium. It has the molecular formula $PtCl_2H_6N_2$ (molecular weight = 300.1). It is a planar inorganic heavy metal complex containing a central atom of platinum surrounded by two chloride atoms and two ammonia molecules in the *cis* position. It is soluble in water at a concentration of 1 mg/mL. Only the *cis*-isomer is therapeutically active.

Mechanism of Action

Cisplatin's interaction with DNA is probably its primary mode of action. The antitumor effect of cisplatin has been correlated with binding to DNA and the production of intrastructural cross links and formation of DNA adducts, similar to carboplatin (54,82). Intrastrand cisplatin adducts can cause changes in DNA conformation that may affect DNA replication (83). Platinum DNA adduct levels have been measured in patients' leukocytes and correlated with clinical response (82).

Mechanisms of cisplatin drug resistance is an area of concentrated research. Methods by which tumor cells may develop resistance to platinum agents include decreased drug accumulation, increased glutathione levels, enhanced DNA repair, and increased capacity to tolerate DNA damage (84, 85). Platinum resistance is related to expression of excision repair proteins, one of which (ERCC-1) has been identified as playing a critical role in the synergy of gemcitabine and cisplatin. A recent Phase II trial suggests that gemcitabine may reverse cisplatin resistance, as gemcitabine-cisplatin combination therapy was active in platinum-resistant ovarian cancer patients (86). Mechanisms of resistance also include the increased inactivation of thiol-containing proteins such as glutathione and glutathione-related enzymes, a deficiency in mismatch repair enzymes (e.g., hMHL1, hMSH2), and decreased drug accumulation due to alterations in cellular transport (46).

Drug Disposition

Cisplatin demonstrates a triphasic disappearance curve with a $t_{1/2\alpha}$ of 20 minutes, a $t_{1/2\beta}$ of 48 to 70 minutes, and a terminal-phase half-life of 24 hours (87). The first two phases of disappearance represent clearance of free drug from the plasma, and the third phase is probably removal of drug from the plasma proteins. The ratio of cisplatin to total free platinum in plasma has a great deal of interpatient variability; from 0.5 to 1.1 after a dose of 100 mg/m². Three hours after a bolus injection and 2 hours after a 3-hour infusion, 90% of the plasma protein is bound to the platinum in cisplatin, not the cisplatin itself. The complexes between albumin and platinum are slowly eliminated with a minimum half-life of 5 days or more (88). Ninety percent of the drug is removed by renal mechanisms (i.e., glomerular filtration and tubular secretion), and less than 10% is removed by biliary excretion. Fecal excretion appears to be insignificant. Platinum is present in tissues for as long as 180 days after the last administration. There is a potential for accumulation of ultrafilterable platinum plasma concentrations whenever cisplatin is administered on a daily basis but not when dosed on an intermittent schedule.

Administration and Dosage

Cisplatin may be administered intravenously or intraperitoneally. Cisplatin should be mixed only in solutions containing 0.9% or more sodium chloride, because drug stability is directly related to the concentration of the salt. When admixed with dextrose-containing solutions, by chromatographic analysis, the drug appears to be relatively unstable, with decomposition evident by 2 hours (89). Platinum also can form significant, colored complexes if directly admixed with mannitol and stored for 2 to 3 days (90). Short-term (<24 hour) admixtures, however, have been successfully used. Needles or intravenous sets containing aluminum should not be used in the preparation or administration of cisplatin, because this drug rapidly reacts with aluminum, resulting in a loss of drug potency and the formation of a black precipitate (91).

To protect against nephrotoxicity, it is critical that a high urinary output be maintained during cisplatin therapy. Several methods of accomplishing this have been recommended; however, the most widely practiced method involves prehydration and mannitol diuresis (92). If cisplatin is administered in a hospital setting, patients should receive hydration with 1 to 2 L of fluid prior to cisplatin. Mannitol diuresis is accomplished by diluting the cisplatin in 2 L of normal saline containing 37.5 g of mannitol. The solution is then infused over 6 to 8 hours. Adequate hydration and urinary output should be maintained during the next 24 hours. A safe outpatient procedure using concurrent mannitol that appears to prevent serious nephrotoxicity has also been reported (93). The desired dose of cisplatin plus 50 g mannitol is diluted to 1 L with 5% dextrose plus 0.45% sodium chloride, USP. This solution may then be infused at a rate of no greater than 1 mg/min. For patients with known cardiac disease, the dose may be placed in 200 mL of a 10% mannitol solution and infused at a rate of no greater than 1 mg/min. This is followed by 200 mL of additional 10% mannitol. An alternative is to add the drug to 400 mL of 10% mannitol that is then brought up to a 1-L volume with normal saline containing 3 g of magnesium sulfate and administered intravenously over 1 hour (94).

Intraperitoneal (IP) cisplatin was administered in the following method in a Phase III intergroup study (INT 0051) of IP cisplatin/IV cyclophosphamide versus IV cisplatin/IV cyclophosphamide (2). A totally implantable device (intravenous port) was surgically placed in the intraperitoneal space at least 2 days before cisplatin administration. Alternatively, a Tenckhoff catheter was used to access the intraperitoneal space during each cisplatin administration. If an implantable device was used, the peritoneal cavity was accessed by inserting a 19-gauge Huber-point needle through the skin into the port following a povidone-iodine (Betadine) prep of the skin. Before cisplatin infusion, the peritoneal cavity was drained as completely as possible (if an effusion was present) via the catheter. Cisplatin was mixed in 2 L of normal saline and then warmed to body temperature. The 2-L cisplatin solution was instilled as rapidly as possible into the intraperitoneal space via the catheter. Instillation typically required 30 to 60 minutes. If the flow rate was judged to be slow, a blood pressure cuff was placed around the infusion bag and inflated to 100 mm Hg to increase the flow. The cisplatin solution was allowed to remain in the intraperitoneal cavity (i.e., the fluid was not drained). Concurrent with the start of IP cisplatin administration, the patient received hydration in the form of at least 1 L normal saline with 3 g $MgSO_4$ and 40 g mannitol. Subsequent hydration with 1 L normal saline was performed at the investigator's discretion. When administered as a single agent, the standard dosing regimen for cisplatin is 75 to 100 mg/m^2 every 21 to 28 days; when used in combination with other agents, the dose should be reduced to 50 to 75 mg/m^2. A commonly used regimen for primary chemotherapy of ovarian cancer is paclitaxel 135 mg/m^2 by 24-hour IV infusion followed by cisplatin 75 mg/m^2 every 21 days for six cycles (95). It is not possible to use a 3-hour paclitaxel infusion schedule in combination with cisplatin because of excessive neurotoxicity (96).

Retrospective analysis by Levin and Hryniuk (97) strongly suggests that the cisplatin efficacy against ovarian cancer is directly correlated with cisplatin dose intensity (i.e., mg/m^2/wk). Typical high-dose regimens include 20 mg/m^2 daily for 5 days repeated every 3 weeks, 100 to 120 mg/m^2 IV every 3 to 4 weeks, or 100 mg/m^2 on day 1 and day 8 repeated every 20 days (98,99). Holleran and DeGregorio (100) prepared an excellent review of high-dose (200 mg/m^2/course) cisplatin. Dose-limiting toxicities with the higher dose regimens include severe, relatively irreversible neurotoxicity and myelosuppression. Responses have been seen in conventional-dose cisplatin-refractory patients, but they generally are of relatively short duration.

Side Effects and Toxicities

Dose-related nephrotoxicity is the major dose-limiting toxicity of cisplatin. It is manifested by renal tubular damage resulting in an elevation of the BUN or serum creatinine. The peak detrimental effect on renal function usually occurs between the tenth and twentieth days after treatment. The renal damage is usually reversible. Patients concomitantly receiving gentamicin and cephalothin have been shown to be at greater risk of developing acute renal failure (101).

Madias and Harrington (102) have characterized the renal damage of cisplatin as being similar to mercury nephrotoxicity. Pathologically, renal tubular necrosis, degeneration, and interstitial edema without glomerular changes are observed. Although clinically overt renal toxicity may be common, it is usually reversible. However, some degree of long-term damage is likely. The renal-protective effect of hydration and mannitol is well established in animals and humans, and renal impairment can be prevented (93).

Ototoxicity, manifested by high-frequency hearing loss (above the frequency of normal speech), may be seen in as many as 30% of patients treated with cisplatin (103). Hearing impairment may be dose related and can be unilateral or bilateral. Occasional tinnitus (but not vestibular dysfunction) has been reported. The ototoxicity may be partially reduced by adequate hydration and the use of mannitol diuresis. Fleming and colleagues (103) have demonstrated that patients with lower than average threshold before chemotherapy with cisplatin were more likely to experience greater threshold shifts.

Neurotoxicity can be a dose-limiting side effect of cisplatin, particularly with high-dose regimens (104). The range of cisplatin-induced neurologic deficits include peripheral sensory neuropathy, ototoxicity, autonomic neuropathy manifested by orthostatic hypotension and gastric paresis, Lhermitte's syndrome, and rarely focal encephalopathy, often accompanied by cortical blindness. Peripheral neuropathy is by far the most common cisplatin-induced neurotoxicity. Neurotoxicity is dose dependent, with symptoms typically developing after cumulative doses of 300 mg/m^2 or greater. A review of published literature (105) found that neurotoxicity occurred in 85% of patients at cumulative doses of 300 mg/m^2 or greater, but occurred in only 15% of patients who had received a cumulative dose below this level. Initial symptoms are usually numbness and tingling in the distal fingers and toes. If cisplatin is continued, proximal extension of the peripheral neuropathy occurs, and the sense of joint position becomes impaired, resulting in more severe neurologic symptoms, including ataxia, gait disturbances, loss of manual dexterity, and wheelchair dependency. Symptoms may begin and progress up to 4 or more months after discontinuation of cisplatin. In 30% to 50% of patients, cisplatin neuropathy is irreversible.

Early clinical data suggest that a number of investigational agents may ameliorate cisplatin-induced neurotoxicity

(104). Agents that have been associated with positive pre-clinical results include ORG2766 (106), an ACTH analog, and the sulfhydryl-based compounds amifostine and glutathione. Only amifostine has been associated with a significant reduction of grades 2 and 3 neurotoxicity in the setting of an adequately designed Phase III trial (107). Further development of a neuroprotective agent, such as amifostine, could significantly enhance the clinical effectiveness of cisplatin, enabling dose-intensive therapy and greater cumulative doses to be delivered to more patients with sensitive tumors. In 2003 the GOG initiated a Phase III trial of low-dose, intravenous bolus amifostine three times weekly to reverse grade 2 or greater peripheral neuropathy (GOG-192).

Symptomatic hypomagnesemia frequently occurs with cisplatin. In a study to determine the effects of magnesium supplementation on cisplatin-induced hypomagnesemia, the administration of magnesium (oral and intravenous) with cisplatin to one group of patients produced less renal tubular damage and no compromise in efficacy than that seen in a group not supplemented with magnesium (108).

Without adequate antiemetic therapy, most patients who receive cisplatin experience nausea and vomiting. This reaction may be severe and usually starts within the first hour after treatment and may persist for 24 to 48 hours. Delayed nausea and vomiting, lasting from 3 to 5 days, also may occur. The combination of a 5-HT3 inhibitor (e.g., ondansetron or granisetron) with dexamethasone (10 to 40 mg IV) has reduced the incidence of severe nausea and vomiting by as much as 75% (109). Delayed nausea and vomiting can be eradicated by continuation of oral low-dose dexamethasone (with or without a 5-HT3 inhibitor) for the first 5 days after platinum treatment (110). Other less effective antiemetic regimens to prevent cisplatin-induced nausea and vomiting include prochlorperazine, dexamethasone, and lorazepam; metoclopramide and dexamethasone; metoclopramide and methylprednisolone; or metoclopramide and lorazepam (71, 111).

Anaphylactic hypersensitivity reactions consisting of tachycardia, wheezing, hypotension, and facial edema occurring within a few minutes of IV administration have occurred occasionally after a dose of cisplatin given to previously treated patients (112,113). These hypersensitivity reactions have been controlled with corticosteroids, epinephrine, or antihistamines. Wiesenfeld and colleagues (114) reported successful retreatment with cisplatin after apparent allergic reactions in two patients. *In vivo* and *in vitro* tests in one patient could not demonstrate an immunologic basis for the initial reaction. Both patients were successfully rechallenged with cisplatin after only diphenhydramine pretreatment. This suggests a nonallergic cause of the acute hypersensitivity reactions occasionally seen with platinum.

Myelosuppression occurs in 25% to 30% of patients receiving the recommended dose, and is more pronounced at higher doses. Coombs-positive hemolytic anemia also occurs as a result of cisplatin treatment. Cisplatin-induced ane-mia has been shown to respond to recombinant erythropoietin (115).

Drug Interactions

When cisplatin is given in combination with other agents, the order of drug sequence can affect the severity of drug-induced myelosuppression. Rowinsky and Donehower (116) conducted a Phase I study of sequential escalating doses of paclitaxel and cisplatin therapy and determined that myelosuppression was more severe when cisplatin administration preceded paclitaxel than when given after paclitaxel. Another Phase I study was conducted to evaluate the effects of drug sequence of treatment with cisplatin in combination with topotecan (117). This study also found a significantly higher incidence of myleosupporession when cisplatin was administered first.

Cisplatin-induced nephrotoxicity should be considered whenever this agent is given prior to or in combination with other cytotoxic drugs that are cleared by renal elimination (e.g., bleomycin, ifosfamide, etoposide, methotrexate). Cisplatin reduces the renal clearance of these agents, resulting in an increased accumulation of these drugs. Yee and co-workers (42) observed markedly reduced bleomycin clearance in children who had received six courses of a regimen including cisplatin (cumulative dose 300 mg/m^2). In another case report, fatal bleomycin pulmonary toxicity occurred in a patient with cisplatin-induced acute renal failure (43).

Cisplatin is directly inactivated by mesna and amifostine (46). The FDA has approved amifostine to reduce the cumulative renal toxicity associated with repeated administration of cisplatin in patients with advanced ovarian cancer. In a Phase III randomized study of ovarian cancer patients, amifostine treatment, prior to IV cisplatin plus cyclophospham, did not appear to reduce cisplatin's anticancer activity (118). However, there are only limited data in other chemotherapeutic settings, and the FDA recommends that amifostine should not be administered to patients in settings where chemotherapy could produce a significant survival advantage or cure except in a clinical trial (119).

Special Applications

The efficacy of cisplatin can be increased significantly in patients with stage III, optimal disease (i.e., <1 cm^2 residual tumor) epithelial ovarian cancer when it is administered by the intraperitoneal (IP) route as part of a primary, combination chemotherapy regimen. A pivotal Phase III intergroup trial (INT 0051) performed by members of the SWOG Gynecologic Oncology Group (GOG), and Eastern Cooperative Oncology Group (ECOG) determined that the IP administration of cisplatin 100 mg/m^2 (plus cyclophosphamide 600 mg/m^2 every 3 weeks for six cycles) was associated with a highly significant 8-month increase in overall survival as compared with the standard treatment arm (IV cisplatin 100 mg/m^2 plus IV cyclophosphamide 600 mg/m^2 every 3 weeks for six cycles) in patients with advanced, optimal ovarian cancer. The intraperitoneal arm was also associated with a significant reduction in the incidence of granulocytopenia, clinical hearing loss, and neurotoxicity (2). A Phase III study conducted by the GOG (GOG-172) was recently completed that compared IV paclitaxel plus IV cisplatin to IV paclitaxel followed by IP cisplatin plus IP paclitaxel on day 8. Despite the higher incidence of toxicity in the IP arm, the preliminary results demonstrate a 0.73 risk of recurrence in the IP arm as compared to the standard IV therapy (4). Although immature, survival data also showed a trend favoring the IP arm. This study supports the findings of the two previous randomized trials that also demonstrated an improvement in outcome with IP therapy.

Intraperitoneal therapy is not recommended for patients who have suboptimal cytoreductive surgery (i.e., >1 cm in largest diameter of a tumor nodule), because IP cisplatin (as well as other cytotoxic agents) only penetrates a few millimeters into tumor plaques (8).

Multiple Phase III studies have shown that cisplatin-based chemotherapy as an adjunct to radiation therapy improves survival in cervical cancer patients (14,120–122).

Cyclophosphamide

Chemistry

Cyclophosphamide (Cytoxan, Neosar, CTX, CPM, and Endoxan) is an alkylating agent that before the advent of paclitaxel was used in the primary chemotherapy of advanced, epithelial-type ovarian and endometrial cancer. At this time, it is uncommonly used in the treatment of gynecologic cancers because og the more effective agents currently available (e.g., paclitaxel). It is occasionally used in the third-line treatment of ovarian cancer and as a second-line agent in the treatment of choriocarcinoma. It is a cyclic phosphamide ester of nitrogen mustard and is referred to chemically as 2-[bis-(2-chloroethyl)amino]tetrahydro-2H-1,3,2,-oxazaphosphorine 2-oxide monohydrate. Its molecular weight is 279.1. The monohydrate is un-ionized and lipid soluble; in normal saline or water, it is soluble to a maximum of 4% at room temperature.

Mechanism of Action

Cyclophosphamide, a bifunctional substituted nitrogen mustard, was synthesized in 1958 in an attempt to achieve greater selective toxicity for tumor tissue. The N-methyl moiety of nitrogen mustard is replaced with a cyclic phosphamide group, resulting in a stable, inactive compound. The bis-(2-chloroethyl) group cannot ionize until the cyclic phosphamide is opened at the phosphorus-nitrogen linkage. Activation of cyclophosphamide is a multistep process.

The liver microsomal P450 mixed-function oxidase system converts the parent drug to 4-hydroxycyclophosphamide. This metabolite exists in equilibrium with the acyclic tautomer, aldophosphamide. These compounds may be further oxidized by hepatic aldehyde oxidase to the inactive metabolites of carboxyphosphamide and 4-ketocyclophosphamide. Nonenzymatic conversion to the cytotoxic compounds of phosphoramide mustard and acrolein occurs in susceptible peripheral tissues.

Most of the alkylating agents, like cyclophosphamide, are bifunctional, which facilitates their reaction with two cellular molecules. Accordingly, they can cross link the two opposite strands of DNA to give an interstrand cross link, react with two sites on the same strand (intrastrand cross link), or cross link DNA to protein. The latter type of lesion is generally considered to be innocuous, but the relative significance of the other cross links is still in contention. DNA intrastrand cross links are more frequent than interstrand cross links and are more often considered to be the critical lesions.

These two classes can be differentiated by the structure of the cross links in DNA. Generally, the entire mustard is involved in the cross link, with the two mustard ''arms'' linked usually to the N7 position of guanine. Because these guanines can be separated by several bases in DNA, the linkages represent particularly bulky lesions.

Drug Disposition

After IV administration, approximately 15% of the drug is excreted unchanged in the urine and the remainder as metabolites. The plasma half-life of the parent compound after doses of 6 to 80 mg/kg appears to range from 4.0 to 6.5 hours (123,124). Approximately 50% of the alkylating metabolites (but not parent drug) are bound to plasma proteins.

Although cyclophosphamide is exclusively excreted by the kidney, because of the un-ionized nature of the intact drug molecule, tubular reabsorption is avid. Hepatic inactivation appears to be the major mechanism of active drug elimination. The mean renal clearance of intact drug is approximately 11 mL/min, or 15% of creatinine clearance, but renal elimination remains the major route of disposition of the more polar, less lipid-soluble metabolites (125). There can be significantly prolonged retention of active (alkylating) metabolites in patients with severe renal failure, and doses should be adjusted accordingly.

Dosage

Cyclophosphamide is active in many different types of malignancies. The dosing schemes are numerous and depend on the particular disease. Two general categories of treatment schedules exist. In the method generally used to treat ovarian and endometrial cancers, an intermediate dose (600 to 1,000 mg/m^2) is given all at once over a short period.

This treatment approach usually involves other drugs, such as cisplatin, carboplatin, or doxorubicin, whose additive toxic effects must be considered in selecting the dose and frequency of cyclophosphamide administration. Adequate hydration for 72 hours before and following high-dose treatment with cyclophosphamide is recommended to reduce cyclophosphamide-induced hemorrhagic cystitis (126).

Side Effects and Toxicities

Myelosuppression consisting primarily of leukopenia is the usual dose-limiting toxic effect of cyclophosphamide. Both the nadir and time of bone marrow recovery are rapid at 8 to 14 and 18 to 21 days, respectively. Although this drug has long been considered to be "platelet sparing," significant thrombocytopenia can also occur at very high doses (>1.5 g/m^2).

Acute, sterile hemorrhagic cystitis is an infrequent toxic manifestation but is occasionally dose limiting. It is understandably more common in poorly hydrated or renally compromised patients. The onset of this complication may be delayed from 24 hours to several weeks. It is detected by gross hematuria or a microscopic hematuria of greater than 20 erythrocytes per high-power field. The bleeding may persist but is usually transient. Prophylactic hydration with intake of at least 3 L/day appears to offer the best protection. With continued therapy, patients characteristically develop a fibrotic "small bladder," and urinary frequency may become a permanent problem. There is a definite increase in the risk of bladder cancer in these patients. The availability of the sulfhydryl mesna as a prophylactic treatment of patients at high risk for developing cyclophosphamide-induced cystitis has almost completely eliminated this side effect.

A syndrome of inappropriate antidiuretic hormone (SIADH), or "water intoxication," has been reported after cyclophosphamide treatment. This is more common with IV doses greater than 50 mg/kg and is both a limitation to and consequence of fluid loading (127).

Alopecia occurs to some degree in all patients receiving cyclophosphamide and is significant in at least half of all patients treated. Regrowth of hair may occur even with continuing treatment.

Gastrointestinal problems are more common with high doses given orally. Anorexia, nausea, and vomiting are all common reactions, but they are usually controlled with IV antiemetic regimens.

A rare pulmonary toxic effect has been reported with a pneumonitis picture similar to "busulfan lung." The typical clinical presentation is that of an interstitial pneumonitis, usually occurring after long-term and continuous low-dose therapy (128). The onset of symptoms is insidious. Pathologically, there can be alveolitis with eventual fibrosis and atypical type II pneumocytes. Steroids may be beneficial.

Other toxic effects include testicular atrophy, sometimes with reversible oligospermia and azoospermia. Amenorrhea also has been reported. As with all alkylating agents, drug-induced congenital abnormalities are possible.

Karchmer and Hansen (129) described a patient with a "tongue-burning" sensation, urticaria, and hypotension during a bolus injection. The subsequent cyclophosphamide injection in this patient produced a classic anaphylactic reaction even though an antihistamine had been injected prophylactically. The patient was resuscitated, and subsequent treatment was switched to chlorambucil without further incident.

With high-dose therapy used for bone marrow transplant (120 to 180 mg/kg), cyclophosphamide-associated cardiac toxicity has been reported (130).

Special Precautions

It is important to keep the patient well hydrated during cyclophosphamide therapy to reduce the potential for hemorrhagic cystitis. It is advisable to administer at least 1 L of additional IV fluids (usually normal saline) to assure an adequate urine volume to excrete the cyclophosphamide metabolite acrolein, which can otherwise alkylate bladder mucosa and cause hemorrhagic cystitis. The patient should be instructed to drink at least eight glasses of fluid daily during the 2 days after cyclophosphamide administration. In patients prone to developing cystitis, consider administering prophylactic IV mesna, a sulfhydryl-containing compound that can neutralize acrolein.

Drug Interactions

Cyclophosphamide must be metabolized to be active. Although some cyclophosphamide may be activated by phosphatases and phosphamidases peripherally, most of the drug is metabolized by microsomal enzymes in the liver (131, 132). These enzymes may be activated by drugs like phenobarbital or inhibited by drugs like proadifen (SKF 525A). Because active and toxic metabolites are generated by the reactions of these enzymes and cyclophosphamide, many potential drug interactions may exist.

Barbiturates and other inducers of hepatic microsomal enzymes, such as phenytoin and chloral hydrate, may increase the rate of hepatic conversion of cyclophosphamide to its toxic metabolites. Similarly, cyclophosphamide may block the metabolism of barbiturates, increasing sedative effects. Although the clinical significance of these reactions is not clear, cyclophosphamide toxicity may be increased by the H$_2$-histamine blocker cimetidine (133). Cimetidine, but not ranitidine, may increase cyclophosphamide's myelotoxicity through an increase in the concentration · time product of its active metabolites (e.g., 4-hydroxycyclophosphamide and phosphoramide mustard) (134). Thus, H$_2$-blockers like ranitidine may be safer to use than cimetidine when high doses of cyclophosphamide are administered.

Dactinomycin

Chemistry

Dactinomycin (actinomycin D, ACT-D, Cosmegen) has been proven to be active in the treatment of patients with germ-cell tumors of the ovary and endometrium and of gestational trophoblastic disease (135–137). It has a molecular weight of 1,255 and an empiric formula of $C_{62}H_{86}N_{12}O_{16}$. The drug is an antitumor antibiotic isolated from *Streptomyces parvulus*. The molecular structure includes two peptide loops linked to a three-ring chromophoric phenoxazone ring system (actinocin). The drug is highly soluble in water, forming an amber- to gold-colored solution.

Mechanism of Action

Dactinomycin becomes anchored into or around a purine-pyrimidine base pair in DNA by intercalation. DNA-dependent ribosomal RNA synthesis and new messenger RNA synthesis is inhibited. The peptide loops appear to allow tight drug binding to DNA because the actinocin (phenoxazone) moiety alone is inactive. This can occur adjacent to any G-C pair in DNA.

Bound dactinomycin molecules dissociate very slowly from DNA owing to electrostatic interactions of the cyclic peptide rings with each strand of the DNA double helix. This process, which stabilizes the intercalative interaction, appears to be crucial for cytotoxicity.

Dactinomycin on a molar basis is one of the most potent antineoplastic agents available. The drug possesses some hypocalcemic activity, similar to mithramycin. Although maximal cell killing is observed in the G_1 phase, the cytotoxic action is thought to be primarily cell cycle nonspecific. Actively proliferating cells are more sensitive than quiescent cells to the lethal effects of the drug (138).

In that dactinomycin is a natural product, it is not surprising that the primary mode of tumor cell resistance to dactinomycin is mediated through overexpression of P-glycoprotein (139).

Drug Disposition

Tattersall and colleagues (140) studied the pharmacokinetics of radiolabeled [^{3}H]dactinomycin in patients, and the drug appeared to be only minimally metabolized and was concentrated in nucleated cells. There was a greater drug uptake into bone marrow than in plasma. Drug penetration into the central nervous system was not observed. Urinary and fecal recovery totaled only 30% each after 9 days, and there was significant drug retention in lymphocytes and granulocytes. This may explain the prolonged terminal plasma half-life of 36 hours observed after single dactinomycin doses. There appears to be little metabolism because approximately 90% of excreted drug is collected as the intact

molecule. Some monolactone forms of dactinomycin are recovered in the urine.

Using a more specific radioimmunoassay, a much shorter dactinomycin half-life is described ($t_{1/2\alpha} = 0.78$ minutes, $t_{1/2\beta} = 3.5$ hours) (141). The discrepancies between these and Tattersall's findings reflect the differences in the assays used.

Administration and Dosage

Dactinomycin is administered intravenously by slow IV push or, preferably, into the tubing of a freely running IV solution. A 5- to 10-mL flush of 5% dextrose in water (D_5W) or normal saline is recommended before and after IV push administration to assure vein patency and to flush any remaining drug from the tubing.

Dactinomycin is commonly given intravenously in short "pulse" doses of 500 $\mu g/m^2$ daily for as long as 5 days in adults. The dose for each 2-week cycle should not exceed 15 $\mu g/kg/day$ or 400 to 600 $\mu g/m^2/day$ for 5 days.

A wide variety of dosing regimens have been employed. Several clinical studies have documented equal efficacy and toxicity for single-dose dactinomycin regimens (142,143). In nonmetastatic gestational trophoblastic cancer, a single IV dose of 1.25 mg/m^2 every 14 days produced a 99% remission rate after four courses of therapy (143). Compared with five divided doses of 500 $\mu g/m^2/day$, the single-dose method produced slightly greater mild to moderate toxic effects.

Side Effects and Toxicities

Bone marrow depression is the usual dose-limiting toxic effect of dactinomycin. It is usually manifested 7 to 10 days after dosing. All blood elements are affected, but primarily the platelets and leukocytes are depressed. Combined with gastrointestinal reactions, myelosuppression appears to be dose limiting as well as dose dependent (144). Immunosuppression is another well-known effect of dactinomycin. Patients should not receive this drug during viral infection because of the risk of developing disseminated disease.

Severe gastrointestinal consequences, such as vomiting, can occasionally represent the acute dose-limiting toxic effects of dactinomycin. Vomiting can persist for 4 to 20 hours, but it can be controlled by combination antiemetic regimens (145). Mucositis can also be severe. It is characterized by severe oral ulcerations and diarrhea in 30% of patients.

Reversible alopecia may occur with dactinomycin. A variety of other skin manifestations have been reported, including acneiform changes, erythema, and hyperpigmentation.

Dactinomycin is toxicologically similar to the anthracyclines and characteristically interacts with radiation therapy, producing delayed "radiation recall" skin damage. Previously irradiated or even irritated skin may become reddened and inflamed after drug administration. Frank necrosis is sometimes reported. Oral ulcers may also develop after radiation therapy. These reactions may occur months after radiation therapy. Experimentally, radiation therapy given after dactinomycin does not produce this effect.

Dactinomycin potentiates pulmonary radiation and decreases radiation tolerance by at least 20%. Reintroduction of dactinomycin following pulmonary radiation has resulted in fatal pulmonary fibrosis (146).

As noted in the "Special Precautions" section below, dactinomycin is highly ulcerogenic if extravasated.

Special Precautions

Dactinomycin is extremely damaging to soft tissue and every effort should be made to assure vein patency during administration. Extravasations characteristically result in immediate pain and swelling followed by indolent, poorly healing necrotic ulcers (145).

Dactinomycin is highly potent and is typically dosed in micrograms per kilogram. Doses must be calculated and prepared carefully to prevent inadvertent overdosage of this drug. No specific antidote to overdosage is known, although granulocyte colony-stimulating factors may be useful.

Dactinomycin is a potent immunosuppressant and can inhibit the effectiveness of vaccinations given after drug administration. The drug also produces radiation recall skin and soft tissue damage if given after ionizing radiation.

Docetaxel

Chemistry

Docetaxel (Taxotere) is a semisynthetic analog of paclitaxel and has an FDA-approved indication for locally advanced or metastatic breast cancer after failure of prior chemotherapy. It is also FDA approved for locally advanced or metastatic non–small-cell lung cancer after failure of prior platinum-based chemotherapy. It also has shown marked antitumor activity against a variety of solid tumors, including both platinum-sensitive and platinum-refractory epithelial ovarian cancer (147,148). The natural component of docetaxel is 10-deacetyl baccatin III, which is extracted from the needles of the European yew tree (*Taxus baccata* L.) (148). Docetaxel has a molecular weight of 861.9 and the empirical formula $C_{43}H_{53}NO_{14} \cdot 3H_2O$. Unlike paclitaxel, which uses a polyoxyl compound (Cremophor) as a diluent, docetaxel is formulated in Tween 80 and alcohol.

Mechanism of Action

In a manner similar to paclitaxel, docetaxel promotes microtubule assembly and inhibits the depolymerization of tubulin. However, compared with paclitaxel, the microtubules formed by docetaxel are more slowly reversible and there are differential effects on tau binding sites and on microtubule-associated proteins. Docetaxel-induced stabilization of microtubules halts cellular division in M phase, thereby preventing cell replication (149).

Drug Disposition

The pharmacokinetics of docetaxel when administered as an IV infusion lasting from 1 to 24 hours have been investigated in a number of studies (150). When administered as a typical 1-hour infusion at doses of 70 to 100 mg/m², pharmacokinetics reveals triphasic elimination with a plasma AUC of 3.13 to 4.83 mg/mL/h, a peak plasma concentration of 2.57 to 3.67 μg/mL, and a terminal-phase plasma half-life of 13.6 hours. There is very limited renal excretion of docetaxel; the 24-hour urinary excretion was 1.4% of the dose administered. Plasma drug clearance was determined to be 21.3 L/h/m² (151).

Administration and Dosage

All patients receiving docetaxel should be premedicated with oral corticosteroids such as dexamethasone 16 mg/day (e.g., 8 mg BID) for 3 days beginning 1 day prior to docetaxel administration in order to reduce fluid retention and the risk of hypersensitivity reactions.

Docetaxel is commercially available in single-dose 20- and 80-mg vials with accompanying diluent vials. Both the docetaxel vials and the diluent vials should stand at room temperature for approximately 5 minutes prior to mixing. The entire contents of the diluent vial should be aseptically transferred to the docetaxel vial and the resulting contents should be gently rotated for 15 seconds to promote complete mixture. The resulting concentration of docetaxel is 10 mg/mL. Foam may be present owing to the Tween 80; however, it should largely dissipate within a few minutes. The infusion solution is prepared by aseptically withdrawing the proper amount of docetaxel with a calibrated syringe and adding it to a 250-mL infusion bag or bottle containing either 0.9% sodium chloride or 5% dextrose solution to produce a final concentration of 0.3 to 0.9 mg/mL. The infusion solution should be mixed by manual rotation and inspected for particulate formation and/or discoloration. Solutions that are cloudy or that contain particulate matter should be discarded.

The recommended dose of docetaxel for salvage chemotherapy of breast cancer is 60 to 100 mg/m² IV as a continuous 1-hour infusion every 3 weeks. For non–small-cell lung cancer, the recommended dose is 75 mg/m² IV as a continuous 1-hour infusion every 3 weeks. The optimal dosing schedule for docetaxel in gynecologic cancers is presently undefined. A 100-mg/m² dose administered as a 1-hour infusion every 3 weeks has been used in Phase II trials (149). Other tolerable docetaxel dose schedules that have been identified in Phase I studies are: 50 mg/m²/day on days 1 and 8 every 3 weeks; 70 to 90 mg/m² by 24-hour continuous IV infusion every 3 weeks; 80 to 100 mg/m² by 6-hour infusion every 3 weeks; 14 mg/m²/day for 5 days by 1-hour infusion every 21 days (152); and 30 to 35 mg/m^2 weekly (153,154). Docetaxel has been administered in combination with cisplatin using the following schedule: docetaxel 85 to 100 mg/m^2 as a 1-hour IV infusion followed (3 hours after completion) by cisplatin 75 mg/m^2 as a 3-hour IV infusion, with cycles being repeated every 3 weeks (155).

The docetaxel dose should be reduced for patients with moderate liver impairment (see Special Precautions section below).

Side Effects and Toxicities

The major dose-limiting toxicity of docetaxel is neutropenia, which is noncumulative and generally resolves within 7 to 8 days. The combined results of early Phase II studies of docetaxel (without steroid premedication) in ovarian cancer revealed that at a dose level of 100 mg/m^2 every 3 weeks, over 90% of patients developed grades 3 to 4 neutropenia, with febrile neutropenia occurring in 8% to 44% of patients (156). The incidence of other grade 3 to 4 toxicities were stomatitis 0% to 5%, diarrhea 6% to 20%, dermatitis 4% to 8%, acute hypersensitivity reactions 7% to 12%, and fluid retention 8% to 12%. Other docetaxel-induced side effects include alopecia, anemia, neurosensory effects (paresthesia, dysesthesia, pain), and asthenia (152).

In early Phase II studies, slow-onset (i.e., after three to five courses), cumulative fluid retention leading to peripheral or generalized edema with possible development of pleural effusion and/or ascites was a common dose-limiting toxicity. However, a 5-day premedication regimen with corticosteroids, starting the day before docetaxel administration, significantly reduces this side effect. In a retrospective analysis, severe fluid retention occurred in 20% of patients who received no premedication compared with 5% of patients who received steroid prophylaxis. Additionally, the percentage of patients who discontinued treatment secondary to fluid retention was reduced from 32% to 2% ($p < .00001$) with the use of a 5-day corticosteroid regimen (152). Steroid prophylaxis also reduces the incidence and severity of dermatologic side effects and hypersensitivity reactions.

The spectrum of docetaxel-induced hypersensitivity reactions is less severe than that associated with paclitaxel. In the absence of prophylactic medication, mild hypersensitivity reaction as characterized by flushing, rash, and pruritus occurs in approximately 5% of docetaxel administrations. Moderate reactions with dyspnea and/or slight hypertension occur in 8% of treatments, and severe reactions (with bronchospasm, angioedema, and/or severe hypertension) occur in less than 2% of docetaxel administrations (157). Initial symptoms of hypersensitivity to docetaxel therapy generally occur within minutes of the start of the first or second course of docetaxel and resolve rapidly with interruption of the infusion. Patients can be successfully rechallenged with docetaxel therapy following medication with corticosteroids, antihistamines, and H$_2$-agonists.

Dermatologic toxicities typically appear as maculopapular eruptions and desquamation generally localized to the extremities. Nail changes, including onycholysis, may also occur. Skin changes are largely self-limiting and may be alleviated with glycerin/chlorhexidine ointment or oral pyridoxine. This side effect can often be prevented with prophylactic oral steroids and H$_1$- and H$_2$-agonists (158). Recurrent skin toxicity refractory to oral prophylactic medication and pyridoxine therapy may respond to local hypothermia during docetaxel administration (159).

Special Precautions

Patients with impaired liver function have a significant reduction in docetaxel clearance and an increased risk of life-threatening side effects. Analysis of the overall safety database revealed that patients with moderately impaired liver function (defined as transaminase levels more than 1.5 times the upper limit of normal and alkaline phosphatase more than 2.5 times the upper limit of normal) have a 27% reduction in docetaxel clearance and a 38% increase in the area under the concentration-time curve (152). When compared with patients with normal liver function, patients with at least moderately impaired liver function had a significantly greater incidence of febrile neutropenia (40% vs 16%) and toxic death (20% vs 1.4%). Grades 3 to 4 nausea/vomiting, stomatitis, and thrombocytopenia were also increased in patients with impaired liver function (152).

The recommended docetaxel dose level for a patient with moderate hepatic impairment (defined as transaminases between 1.5 and 3.5 times the upper limit of normal and an alkaline phosphatase between 2.5 and 6.0 times the upper limit of normal) is 75 mg/m^2 over 1 hour. No safe docetaxel dose can be recommended for patients with greater than moderate liver impairment (160).

Special Applications

Verschraegen and colleagues (161) have published preliminary evidence that patients with ovarian cancer may respond to docetaxel even though they have had progression of their disease on paclitaxel. They noted a partial response rate of 37.5% in eight eligible patients. A recent Phase II study conducted by the GOG of 60 patients with paclitaxel-resistant ovarian and peritoneal carcinoma observed responses in 22.4% of patients, with 5.2% achieving complete response and 17.2% achieving partial response (at a dose of 100 mg/m^2 IV over 1 hour every 21 days) (162). However, the 75% incidence of grade 4 neutropenia in this study suggests that further study is needed to determine the appropriate dose and schedule.

Doxorubicin

Chemistry

Doxorubicin (Adriamycin), a primary agent in the treatment of metastatic endometrial cancer and advanced ovarian cancer, is an anthracycline antibiotic obtained from *Streptomyces peucetius* var. *caesius*. It has a molecular weight of 580. The doxorubicin structure includes a water-soluble basic reducing amino sugar, daunosamine, linked by a glycosidic bond to carbon atom number 7 on the D-ring of the water-insoluble chromophore aglycone, adrimycinone.

Structural changes in the side groups of doxorubicin alter antitumor potency and pharmacokinetic properties. The aglycone is inactive, and modifications in the amino sugar substituents can also alter antitumor or toxic potency (163).

In DNA, the amino sugar projects into the minor groove and can interact electrostatically with negatively charged phosphate groups in the DNA strand to stabilize the aglycone moiety. Doxorubicin can also form complexes with iron or copper by means of the hydroquinone moieties (164). Metaliron doxorubicin complexes may contribute to cardiotoxicity by enhancing redox cycling of the quinone moiety to produce membrane-damaging oxygen free radicals (165).

Doxorubicin hydrochloride is freely soluble in water, slightly soluble in normal saline, and very slightly soluble in alcohol.

Doxorubicin also is commercially available in a polyethylene glycol (PEG)–coated (pegylated, Stealth) liposomal form (see Liposomal Encapsulated Doxorubicin section below).

Mechanisms of Action

DNA Binding. The anthracyclines, including doxorubicin, probably have several modes of action. The anthracycline portion of the molecule appears to intercalate between stacked nucleotide pairs in the DNA helix by means of P-P–type bonds (166). The drug may also bind ionically around certain base pairs of DNA (adlineation). The overall effect of this is interference with nucleic acid synthesis, specifically an inhibition of DNA synthesis (167). However, preribosomal RNA synthesis is also affected by the drug binding to DNA, preventing DNA-directed RNA and DNA transcription (168).

Mechanisms other than intercalation may also contribute to the antitumor effect of the doxorubicin molecule. The contribution of alkylation to antitumor effects has not been established.

Free-Radical Formation. Oxygen free-radical intermediates containing an unpaired electron can be formed by doxorubicin. This can react rapidly with oxygen to form superperoxide, and with hydrogen peroxide, highly reactive hydroxyl radicals can form. These radicals damage membrane lipids by peroxidation, break DNA strands by attacking ribose-phosphate bonds, and directly oxidize purine or pyrimidine bases, thiols, and amines (165,169). Free-radical mechanisms have most often been associated with cardiotoxicity.

Doxorubicin appears to be active in all phases of the cell cycle, and although maximally cytotoxic in S phase, it is not phase specific (170). Cells exposed to lethal doxorubicin concentrations in G_1 can proceed through S phase but are then blocked and die in G_2. Higher concentrations can also produce an S-phase blockade (171).

Inhibition of DNA Topoisomerase II. Topoisomerases are enzymes capable of covalent binding to DNA, forming transient breaks in one strand (TOPO-I) or two strands (TOPO-II). This activity is highly phase dependent for G_2, and in the case of TOPO-II, normally mediates strand passage to facilitate DNA condensation or decondensation (172). Doxorubicin and other DNA intercalators inhibit the strand-passing activity of TOPO-II by increasing and stabilizing the initial enzyme-DNA (cleavable) complexes. This leads to protein-linked DNA double-strand breaks that are roughly proportional to the cytotoxic potency of the drug *in vitro* (173).

Drug Disposition

Doxorubicin pharmacokinetics is usually described using a two-compartment or three-compartment open model. The drug is rapidly distributed in body tissues, and about 75% of the drug is bound to plasma proteins, principally albumin (174). In the blood, the free doxorubicin fraction depends on the hematocrit, with more free drug being available in patients with a reduced hematocrit (175). The avid binding to DNA is believed to explain the prolonged terminal elimination half-life of 30 to 40 hours, the large apparent volume of distribution of up to 28 L/kg, and the incomplete (50%) total recovery of drug in urine, bile, and feces (176). Human tissues with high drug concentrations (in descending order) include liver, lymph nodes, muscle, bone marrow, fat, and skin (177). The drug does not distribute into the central nervous system.

There is a significant distribution of doxorubicin into human breast milk (178). Doxorubicin levels of 0.24 μM and 0.2 μM of doxorubicinol have been measured in human milk. They produce cumulative AUCs in breast milk of 9.9 and 16.5 μM · hour, respectively. Both of these values were greater than concurrent plasma AUC values. However, doxorubicin does not appear consistently to pass the placenta. Except for one study reporting low drug levels in placental blood of 0.78 to 1.19 nmol/g and no drug in cord blood plasma, several other trials detected no drug in amniotic fluid after doxorubicin administration to pregnant patients (179–181).

Doxorubicin is extensively metabolized and eliminated primarily as glucuronide conjugates of the parent aglycone or its hydroxylated congener doxorubicinol (176,182). The conjugated metabolites are exclusively excreted in the bile and feces. Overall, biliary excretion accounts for about 40%

of an administered dose (183). Approximately 42% of the biliary drug is parent doxorubicin, 22% is doxorubicinol, and 36% is other metabolites (183). Only 5% to 10% of the administered drug is excreted in the urine as doxorubicin (40%), doxorubicinol (29%), and other metabolites (31%).

In liver disease, patients with cholestasis have delayed doxorubicin clearance and experience exaggerated toxic reactions from standard doses (184). However, hepatoma patients with cirrhosis or simple hepatocellular enzyme elevation appear to have normal doxorubicin clearance and toxic effects from standard doses (185).

Although obesity reduces clearance of doxorubicin in adult cancer patients (186), there were no differences in doxorubicin toxicity between normal, mildly obese, and obese patients.

There is some evidence that repeated doxorubicin dosing alters pharmacokinetics (187,188). In these reports, doxorubicin levels were lower after repeated dosing, which suggests increased drug clearance. However, because neither toxicity nor response rates are altered, the clinical significance of these observations has not been established. Age may also be a factor. In one trial, the highest clearances of doxorubicin were observed in the younger patients (189). These observations suggest that higher peak doxorubicin levels may be achieved in older patients.

The hepatic extraction ratio for doxorubicin in humans is 0.45 to 0.50, and systemic drug levels are about 25% lower with intraarterial administration compared with IV dosing (190). Several studies have shown that the pharmacokinetics of intraarterial drug is similar to those after IV doses (177, (191). The relatively low hepatic extraction rate and similar overall disposition patterns provide little pharmacokinetic rationale for intraarterial administration as a means of localizing doxorubicin effects to the liver (192).

Administration and Dosage

Short IV push infusions and IV bolus injections have been used with doxorubicin. A slow IV push over several minutes with constant monitoring of the patient and blood return can help minimize the chance of serious tissue damage occurring because of extravasation. A 5- to 10-mL flush of normal saline or D_5W before and after administration is strongly recommended to test vein patency and flush any remaining drug from the tubing. Alternatively, injection into the side port of a running IV infusion has also been recommended. The patient should be asked to report immediately any change in sensation during the administration. Old venipuncture sites or infusion sites previously used for administering blood, antibiotics, or other medications should not be used to administer doxorubicin. Heparin locks (unless recently inserted) are not recommended because the drug is chemically incompatible with sodium heparin.

Continuous IV infusion of doxorubicin appears significantly to lessen cardiotoxicity if infusion durations are 96

hours or longer (193). However, prolonged infusions increase the incidence and severity of stomatitis and dermatologic reactions. Administration through tunneled central venous catheters or indwelling vascular access ports is mandatory for all prolonged infusions. Careful patient and site monitoring are required because doxorubicin extravasation from central vascular access devices can occur.

Numerous dosing schedules have been reported. The individual doxorubicin dose depends on clinical variables, including the cumulative dose administered to date and the potential for interaction with other drugs or radiation (Table 16.2). As a single agent, doses of 60 to 75 mg/m² as a single intravenous injection have been used and repeated no more often than every 3 weeks. An alternative scheme uses 20 to 30 mg/m² given daily for 3 consecutive days and repeated in 3 weeks (194). When used in combination therapy, the most commonly used dosage is 40 to 60 mg/m² given as a single intravenous injection every 21 to 28 days.

Both the dose and rate of dosing (dose intensity) can have therapeutic impacts for different agents and tumors (195). Clinical studies with doxorubicin show that greater dose intensity is associated with enhanced response rates in breast cancer (196). The doses compared in this trial were 70 mg/m² every 21 days for eight cycles versus 35 mg/m² every 21 days for 16 cycles.

Dose adjustments are required in a number of clinical settings (Table 16.3), specifically in the case of hyperbilirubinemia. A 50% dose reduction is indicated if plasma bilirubin concentration is 1.2 to 3.0 mg/dL, and the dose must be reduced by 75% if plasma bilirubin concentration reaches 3.1 to 5.0 mg/dL.

Side Effects and Toxicities

The single acute dose-limiting toxicity for doxorubicin is bone marrow suppression. The most commonly seen dose-limiting toxicity is leukopenia, with a nadir at 10 to 14 days.

TABLE 16.2. *Intravenous dosing guidelines for doxorubicin*

Dose (mg/m²)[a]	Intravenous method	Schedule	Average cumulative tolerable dose[c] (mg/m²)
60–75[b]	Bolus	Every 3 weeks	550
30	Bolus	3 successive days, every 3 weeks	550
20	Bolus	Weekly	750
60	96-h infusion	Every 3–4 weeks	1,000

[a] Lower doses should be administered to patients with hepatobiliary dysfunction and for poor bone marrow reserve or performance status.

[b] Allows for greater dose intensity in breast cancer.

[c] Represents average total cumulative dose tolerated without clinical evidence of doxorubicin cardiotoxicity.

TABLE 16.3. *Modifications of doxorubicin doses*[a]

Condition	Recommended dose modification
Prior doxorubicin	Limit total cumulative lifetime dose (by IV bolus) to 550 mg/m² (209)
Prior chest radiation therapy	Reduce total dose limit to 300–350 mg/m²
Obesity	Base dose on ideal body weight (186)
Hepatobiliary dysfunction	Reduce dose for elevated serum bilirubin (Give 50% of dose for serum bilirubin of 1.2–1.9 μg/dL, and give 25% of dose for serum bilirubin ≥3.0 mg/dL) (184) Use indocyanine green disappearance rate as an indicator of doxorubicin clearance
Infusion method	Greater cumulative (total) dose may be afforded by weekly bolus doses or continuous (96-h) infusions[b] (193)

[a] Average safe cumulative doxorubicin dose is 750 mg/m² using standard infusion schedules.

[b] Average safe cumulative doxorubicin dose is 1,000 mg/m² when administered with a 96-h infusion schedule.

Other hematologic toxicities, such as anemia and thrombocytopenia, have been reported, but they are rare and generally less severe. Recovery from myelosuppression is usually prompt, with resolution often within about 1 week after the nadir.

Doxorubicin is known to produce local skin and deep-tissue damage at the site of inadvertent extravasations (197, 198). Ulcers may result after 33% of extravasations. The lesions undergo a slow, indolent expansion and occasionally involve tendons and other deep structures. They characteristically do not heal and are associated with prolonged local drug retention (199). Reilly and colleagues (197) recommend early surgical debridement, with skin grafting and tendon repair for serious infiltrations. Numerous pharmacologic antidotes have been evaluated, but few have demonstrated unequivocal clinical efficacy. The application of cold, topical dimethylsulfoxide is recommended (200).

Etcubanas and Wilbur (201) and Souhami and Feld (202) reported other unusual injection-site reactions. The most common reaction consists of an erythematous streak up the vein (i.e., flare reaction). It is usually associated with delayed urticaria and pruritus. Symptoms rarely last more than 1 hour with or without treatment with antihistamines and glucocorticosteroids.

Cardiac consequences from the drug have included acute effects, such as a rare pericarditis-myocarditis syndrome or electrophysiologic aberrations, and a total-dose–related cardiomyopathy (203,204). Nonspecific electrocardiographic changes during infusion or immediately afterward may be seen. These include T-wave flattening, ST depression, supraventricular tachyarrhythmias, and extra systolic contractions (205). These conduction abnormalities are generally transient, not associated with severe morbidity, and do not require dose modification.

Cardiomyopathy from doxorubicin is dose related. It presents initially as a clinical syndrome identical to classic congestive heart failure. It is usually irreversible, but symptoms can be managed with standard medical therapy involving digitalis, glycosides, and diuretics. Potential risk factors for doxorubicin cardiotoxicity include cumulative doses greater than 550 mg/m², prior mediastinal irradiation (≥20 Gy), age greater than 70 years, and preexisting cardiovascular diseases, such as prior myocardial infarction or long-standing hypertension (206). Anthracycline-induced cardiomyopathy can also occur 4 to 20 years after the drug is stopped at standard dose limits (207). The administration of anthracyclines incorporated into liposomes is one method that may significantly reduce the risk of cardiac toxicity (see Liposomal Encapsulated Doxorubicin section below) (208).

At total doses under 500 mg/m², the incidence of cardiomyopathy is less than 1%; between 501 and 600 mg/m², 11% are affected; and the incidence is 30% for doses above 600 mg/m². In a retrospective cardiotoxicity study of 4,018 patient records, Von Hoff and associates (209) described an overall incidence of 2.2% for doxorubicin-induced congestive heart failure. In this analysis, there was no influence of performance status, sex, race, and tumor type on the incidence of cardiomyopathy. However, elderly patients were at greater risk even after adjustment for the normally decreased cardiac function in this group. The major determinants were the dose, the schedule of administration, and the age of the patient. A weekly doxorubicin dosing schedule was associated with significantly less congestive heart failure than an every-3-weeks dosing schedule. Continuous IV infusions over 96 hours also can significantly lessen doxorubicin cardiotoxicity (210).

Dexrazoxane (Zinecard) is a chemoprotective agent with an FDA-approved indication for reducing doxorubicin-associated cardiomyopathy in women with metastatic breast cancer who have received a cumulative doxorubicin dose of ≥300 mg/m² and who, in their physician's opinion, would benefit from further doxorubicin therapy (see Modulating Agents section below).

There is evidence that doxorubicin is a radiosensitizing or "radiomimetic" agent and can cause reactivation of tissue reactions in areas previously irradiated (211,212). Radiation recall reactions have also been reported in areas of previous drug infiltration. A particularly sensitive area for serious recall toxicity is the esophagus (213).

Other toxic effects are observed in rapidly proliferating normal tissues. These include marked alopecia in all hairy body areas. Stomatitis may occur at high doses and is more pronounced when the drug is given on consecutive days. It generally begins in the sublingual and lateral tongue regions as a burning sensation with noticeable erythema. The initial inflammation typically progresses to ulceration after a few days. Anal fissures or proctitis have been rarely reported. Nausea and vomiting are common but of moderate intensity. Diarrhea is rare with consecutive daily dosing, and the emetic effects are generally limited to the first day of treatment. Hyperpigmentation of the skin, especially the nail beds, may occur. Longitudinal banding corresponding to individual injections also has been reported (214). Conjunctivitis and excessive tearing lasting several days have been described. Also, a case of probable doxorubicin-induced hypertensive encephalopathy has been reported (215).

Extravasations of doxorubicin are known to cause severe ulceration and soft tissue necrosis (197,198). Vein patency should be assured before injection and constantly monitored during administration.

As discussed later in this chapter, pegylated liposomal encapsulation dramatically alters the pharmacokinetic profile of doxorubicin and, hence, the drug's toxicity profile.

Drug Interactions

Doxorubicin is believed to interact with numerous other drugs. Most of these effects have been described only in experimental systems, and their clinical significance is, therefore, unknown. However, several potentially significant interactions have been described in cancer patients. Altered doxorubicin disposition is postulated with α-interferon, and substantial doxorubicin dose reductions are required (216). The combination of doxorubicin with H_2-antihistamines, such as ranitidine or cimetidine, may also increase toxicities significantly and necessitate drug dose reduction (93).

Special Applications

Doxorubicin has been investigationally administered intrapleurally to patients with malignant pleural effusions (217). Doses of 30 mg were diluted in 20 mL of saline and administered by paracentesis needle as a bolus. Eight of 11 patients responded to doxorubicin, including one complete response. This response rate was superior to nitrogen mustard or tetracycline. Toxicity included pain or fever in 20% of patients and nausea or vomiting in 45% of patients. No alopecia or hematologic toxicity was reported. Markman and colleagues (218) combined doxorubicin (3 mg) with cytarabine (61 mg) and cisplatin (100 mg/m²) in the treatment of seven cancer patients with malignant pleural effusions. Two ovarian cancer patients responded, and no significant systemic toxicities were reported. All injections were given in 250 mL of saline, and aggressive hydration was given to counteract cisplatin nephrotoxicity.

Etoposide

Chemistry

Intravenous etoposide (VP-16) is used commonly in combination chemotherapy regimens for the treatment of patients with germ-cell tumors of the ovary (137). Oral etoposide has activity as a salvage agent for refractory or recurrent ovarian cancer (219). It is a semisynthetic epipodophyllotoxin derived from the root of *Podophyllum* (the May apple plant, or mandrake). The chemical name is demethylepipodophyllotoxin 9-[4,6-O-(R)-ethylidene-β-D-glucopyranoside]. Etoposide has the molecular formula of $C_{29}H_{32}O_{13}$ and a molecular weight of 588.58. It is highly soluble in methanol and chloroform, slightly soluble in ethanol, and sparingly soluble in water. Because of poor water solubility, the commercial drug is dissolved in an ethanol-based cosolvent system.

Etoposide was originally synthesized from *P. embodi* (220). Structure-activity studies show that the hydroxyl group at the C-4′ position is required for activity and that alterations at this site can dramatically affect activity.

Mechanism of Action

There is marked schedule dependence for etoposide cell killing, and cytotoxic effects are maximal in G_2 phase (221). There is also some activity against cells in late S phase, and the drug can halt cell cycle traverse at the S-G_2 interphase (222).

Etoposide produces protein-linked DNA strand breaks by inhibiting DNA TOPO-II enzymes (223). This normal mammalian enzyme mediates double-strand–passing activities in G_2 phase to condense or decondense supercoiled DNA (224). Drug-induced inhibition of TOPO-II is an energy-dependent process that is influenced by dose and duration of exposure.

Etoposide does not bind directly to DNA, but rather stabilizes a transition form of the DNA–TOPO-II complex (223). The number of single and double DNA strand breaks reflects the cytotoxic dose-response curve (225). Etoposide and intercalative drugs such as doxorubicin "poison" TOPO-II enzymes by stabilizing an otherwise transient form of TOPO-II covalently linked with DNA (173). Normal TOPO-II strand-passing activity is thereby blocked, and cell progression out of G_2 phase is halted (172,226). The production of cytotoxicity by etoposide may ultimately involve chromosomal breaks characterized as sister chromatid exchanges (227).

Another postulated etoposide mechanism involves microsomal activation to reactive intermediates capable of generating oxygen free radicals (225). Nucleoside transport is also inhibited at high drug concentrations, but whether this makes a major contribution to the antitumor effect is unknown (228).

Drug Disposition

A two-compartment open pharmacokinetic model appears to describe adequately etoposide disposition in cancer patients (229). The terminal half-life of the drug appears to be about 7 hours and is independent of the dose, route, or method of administration (230). Renal excretion appears to account for about 30% of overall drug elimination. Forty-two to 66% of radiolabeled drug is recovered in the urine, of which less than half is parent etoposide.

With standard doses of etoposide, no drug is detectable in the cerebrospinal fluid (CSF), and even after doses of 400 to 800 mg/m^2, CSF levels were less than 2% of concurrent plasma levels (231). Despite the low distribution of drug into the CSF, mean levels of 1.4 μg/g (range undetectable to 5.9 μg/g) have been measured in brain tumor tissue (232). The drug also distributes into myometrial carcinoma and normal myometrium, achieving levels 50% of those in the blood (233).

Biliary secretion of parent drug accounts for 2% or less of the dose, although fecal recovery of drug and metabolites is variable, ranging from 1.5% to 16.3% (234). However, patients with obstructive jaundice excrete a larger fraction of the dose in urine (46%) than do unaffected patients (35%), which suggests that there is a slight decrease in hepatic drug metabolism with a commensurate increase in renal clearance (231).

The plasma protein binding of etoposide is normally high, averaging 95% in typical patients (235). The free (unbound) fraction of etoposide can vary from 6% to 37% among patients. Patients with increased bilirubin or decreased albumin may have an increase in the free fraction even though systemic clearance is unaltered (235). Myelosuppression may also be commensurately increased in these patients.

Other conditions that may decrease etoposide clearance include prior cisplatin therapy, obesity, and elevated alkaline phosphatase levels (236).

The absolute oral bioavailability of etoposide gelatin capsules ranges from 25% to 74%, with a mean of 48% (237). Some patients experience a 30% change in overall bioavailability (both increased and decreased) with repeat dosing. Neither food nor other chemotherapeutic agents appear to alter etoposide absorption (238). Wide variations in peak levels and AUC values were also described in this trial.

Administration and Dosage

Etoposide must be diluted prior to use with either 0.5% dextrose or 0.9% sodium chloride to give a final concentration of 0.2 to 0.4 mg/mL. Etoposide should be given by IV infusion over a 30- to 60-minute period. Severe hypotension may occur if the drug is given too rapidly. Although not a vesicant, extravasation of the drug should be avoided (239). Examine all solutions for fine precipitates; mix before use. Precipitation may occur if the solution is prepared 0.4 mg/

mL. Continuous infusions of etoposide have been used as a means of enhancing efficacy because of its phase-specific mode of antitumor action. Most infusions have used 5-day courses, although 72-hour infusions have also been employed (240,241).

Oral administration of etoposide capsules may be useful if patient compliance is high, and low-emetogenic drug regimens are used. The capsules may be taken all at once to achieve the desired dose. Neither food nor other chemotherapeutic drugs appear to alter oral absorption of the drug (238). The GOG has investigated multiple trials of oral etoposide at various dosing regimens. Based on a cumulative review of these trials and schedules, it was found to be active in platinum-resistant ovarian cancer patients (overall response rate 26.8%; 7.3% clinical complete remission rate) and in platinum-sensitive patients (overall response rate 34.1%; 14.6% clinical complete remission rate) (242). One of these trials that demonstrated activity used an oral etoposide dosing schedule of 50 mg/m^2/day for 21 days every 28 days with dose escalation to 60 mg/m^2/day when feasible (243). Studies using similar oral etoposide dosing schedules in patients with cervical cancer and endometrial cancer failed to show significant activity in these tumor types (219,244–246).

The variety of doses and schedules that have been used with etoposide are presented in Table 16.4. General principles of dosing include more frequent administration to take advantage of cell cycle–dependent cytotoxicity, an approximate doubling of oral doses due to 50% bioavailability for the gelatin capsules, and significant dose reductions for combinations of etoposide with other myelosuppressive drugs or for patients with poor bone marrow reserve or poor performance status. In general, etoposide doses can be repeated every 3 to 4 weeks depending on the leukocyte count. A pharmacokinetic study in patients with obstructive jaundice showed that no significant dose reductions are needed if renal function is normal (247).

Side Effects and Toxicities

Side effects and toxicities for oral and intravenous administration of etoposide as a single agent are similar. The principal toxicity of etoposide is dose-related and dose-limiting bone marrow suppression. Leukopenia and thrombocytopenia occur, but leukopenia consistently predominates, with a nadir at approximately 16 days and with recovery usually beginning by days 20 to 22.

Gastrointestinal complaints of nausea, vomiting, or anorexia are usually minor and are more frequent with the oral preparations (248). Other adverse effects include alopecia in 20% to 90% of patients, headache, fever, and hypotension (249). Severe hypotension can occur if the drug is infused too rapidly (<30 minutes) (234). Stomatitis has been infrequently reported. Rare instances of generalized allergic reactions and anaphylaxis have occurred (250). A few episodes

TABLE 16.4. *Intravenous and oral dosing schedules for etoposide*

Administration method	Dose		Repeat dosing interval (wks)	Clinical application
	mg/m²/day	Days		
Short single-dose IV infusion	200–250	1	7	Single agent, small-cell lung cancer
Short multiple-dose IV infusion	100	1–5	3–4	Testicular cancer
	100	1, 3, 5	3–4	With other drugs
	45	1–7	3	Phase I
Continuous IV infusion	125	1–5	4	Phase I, single agent
	30	1–5	4	With cisplatin in advanced cancer
	80	1–5	4	Phase I, good-risk patients
	50	1–5	4	Poor-risk patients
	125	1–3	4	Adult patients with advanced cancer (240)
	500	1 (24-h)	3	Small-cell lung cancer
Oral	160	1–5	3–4	Small-cell lung cancer
	50	1–21	4	Ovarian cancer (243)

of cardiotoxicity, including myocardial infarction and congestive heart failure, have been described (251). Immune suppression appears to be minimal with this drug (249).

Bronchospasm with severe wheezing has been rarely observed and has usually been responsive to antihistamines and glucocorticosteroids.

Chemical phlebitis also has been associated with etoposide, although the reaction is most likely related to solubilizers in the diluent. Diluted solutions of etoposide are not vesicants. For inadvertent extravasations of highly concentrated etoposide solution, hyaluronidase may be effective (252).

Neurotoxicity has been rarely reported with etoposide. This has consisted of somnolence and fatigue in 3% of patients and peripheral neuropathy in less than 1% of patients. However, the drug may exacerbate preexisting neuropathy caused by vincristine (253). Predisposing factors included advanced age, impaired nutritional status, and poor performance status. Degradation of myelin lamellae has been observed in affected nerves.

Special Applications

Despite preclinical data showing peritonitis with intraperitoneal injections, combinations of etoposide and cisplatin have been administered safely by the intraperitoneal route. Barakat et al. (254) performed a Phase II study of three courses of intraperitoneal cisplatin 100 mg/m² plus etoposide 200 mg/m² as consolidation therapy in patients with stages II to IV epithelial ovarian cancer with negative second-look surgeries. When compared with a similar group of contemporaneous patients who did not receive consolidation therapy, the disease-free survival distribution between the two groups (using the log-rank test) was found to be significant ($p = .03$) in favor of consolidation therapy (254). European researchers have used a combination of etoposide 350 mg/m² IP, followed by cisplatin 200 mg/m² IP with IV sodium thiosulfate (4 g/m² bolus, followed by 12 g/m² over

6 hours) protection every 4 weeks for four to six cycles in ovarian cancer patients with either no residual disease or minimal residual disease at second-look surgery. The regimen was fairly well tolerated, although there was one study-related patient death from a bowel perforation and resulting complications. Other major clinical complications were nausea, vomiting, and the formation of intraabdominal adhesions. Grade 3 to 4 leukopenia and thrombocytopenia occurred in 30% and 6% of cycles, respectively (255).

Etoposide in combination with other chemotherapeutic agents and autologous stem-cell rescue is often used in salvage therapy for germ-cell tumors or metastatic trophoblastic disease. Two commonly used regimens are bleomycin, etoposide, and cisplatin (BEP) and ifosfamide, carboplatin, and etoposide (ICE) (256,257).

5-Fluorouracil and Floxuridine

Chemistry

5-Fluorouracil (5-FU) is a fluorinated pyrimidine differing from the normal DNA substrate, uracil, by a fluorinated number 5 carbon (chemically, 5-fluoro-2,4(1H,3H)-pyrimidinedione). 5-FU has activity as a second-line agent in advanced ovarian and cervical cancers and, in combination with cisplatin, is used as an adjunct to radiation therapy in women with locally advanced cervical cancer. Floxuridine (FUDR) is highly similar to its prodrug, 5-FU. The discussion of FUDR in this chapter will be limited to its special application as an intraperitoneally administered agent for salvage therapy for ovarian cancer. 5-FU is light sensitive and precipitates at low temperatures or, occasionally, with prolonged standing at room temperature. It has the molecular formula of $C_4H_3FN_2O_2$ and a molecular weight of 130.08.

Mechanism of Action

5-FU acts as a false pyrimidine or antimetabolite ultimately to inhibit the formation of the DNA-specific nucleoside base thymidine. There are at least three mechanisms of action: inhibition of thymidylate synthase by 5-fluoro-21-deoxyuridine-5′-monophosphate (FdUMP), the active metabolite of 5-FU; incorporation of 5-fluorouridine triphosphate (FUTP) into cellular RNA; and incorporation of FUTP into cellular DNA (258). 5-FU is a cell cycle phase-specific agent with cytotoxic effects seen maximally in S phase.

Drug Disposition

There is disagreement over whether 5-FU is eliminated by a two-compartment or three-compartment model (259–261). Fraile and associates (262) demonstrated that plasma levels of 5-FU after oral administration are quite erratic. Schaaf and colleagues (263) documented that the pharmacokinetic characteristics of 5-FU are nonlinear. Doubling of the dose was accompanied by a decrease in nonrenal clearance. The half-life from the high dose was twice as long as that for the low dose of 5-FU. Their data were compatible with a product-inhibition model. Yoshida and coworkers (264) found positive correlations between the dose and serum steady-state levels (C_{SS}) and areas under the concentration-time curves (AUC). Patients who developed toxic reactions had greater C_{SS}s and AUCs. However, there were no correlations between serum levels and patient response to therapy.

5-FU and FUDR are extensively metabolized in the liver (hepatic metabolism can detoxify up to 80% of the total dose). However, there is no absolute documentation that patients with impaired liver function require dose reductions of 5-FU (265); however, patients should be monitored as they may be at increased risk of toxicity. As much as 15% of a dose may be found intact in the urine by 6 hours, with 90% of this excreted in the first hour. Depressed renal function does not generally require dosage adjustment for 5-FU.

5-FU distributes to all areas of body water by simple diffusion. Significant quantities of the drug may enter the central nervous system, and after 15 mg/kg given IV, CSF levels of 6 to 8×10^{-6} M are obtained after 30 minutes. These levels persist for several hours and slowly subside. Although distribution to brain tissue is less rapid, abnormal areas, such as those with neoplasms, may more readily take up drug.

5-FU achieves high and persistent levels in effusions after IV administration. Hepatic administration through the portal vein or artery also achieves high concentrations in the liver parenchyma and produces relatively low systemic levels.

Santini and colleagues (266) showed that therapeutic monitoring of 5-FU levels in patients with head and neck cancer can be used to improve the therapeutic index of the drug (i.e., less toxicity with maximal efficacy).

Administration and Dosage

Doses of 5-FU to be given by the IV push route do not require further dilution from the commercial solution. Vein patency should be assured before giving a dose, with a 5-to 10-mL flush of normal saline or D_5W and another flush after the dose to rinse the remaining drug from the tubing. For short infusion (less than 24 hour), the rate of administration is not critical, and the dose should be given at a rate compatible with the particular vein selected. The patient should be continuously monitored to guard against extravasation. Most doses can be conveniently given over 1 to 2 minutes in this fashion.

Continuous infusions (over 4 to 5 days) may maximize efficacy of this cycle-specific drug and lessen hematologic toxicity (267,268). Infusions of the drug may be added to a convenient volume of D_5W or normal saline, and each reconstituted daily dose can be administered over 24 hours. Commonly, the daily dose of the drug is added to 1 L, although volume is not critical.

Regimens reported for the use of 5-FU include the use of a loading dose, weekly IV bolus, continuous infusions over 4 to 5 days or over 6 weeks, and oral dosing. The dosing of 5-FU should be based on lean body weight (i.e, exclude fat and edematous weight from calculations) (269,270).

5-FU may be administered intravenously as a bolus, rapid injection on a monthly (425 to 450 mg/m² IV on days 1 to 5 every 28 days) or a weekly schedule (500 to 600 mg/m² every week for 6 weeks every 8 weeks), or continuous IV infusion (24-hour infusion 2400 to 2600 mg/m² every week; 96-hour infusion 800 to 1000 mg/m²/day; or 120-hour infusion 1000 mg/m²/day on days 1 to 5 every 21 to 28 days) (46). Oral doses of up to 15 to 20 mg/kg/day for 5 to 8 days have been used (271). However, the efficacy of oral 5-FU has not been confirmed at this time (see Capecitabine section above for a discussion of the oral prodrug of 5-FU).

The loading dose scheme calls for one course of 400 to 500 mg/m² (12 mg/kg; maximum of 800 mg) daily for 5 days every 28 days given as a single daily bolus injection or as a 4-day continuous infusion. This is followed by a weekly maintenance regimen. Horton and co-researchers (272) and Jacobs and co-workers (273), however, strongly associated the use of the loading dose with significant morbidity and occasional fatalities, and suggested that it offers no greater antitumor efficacy over a weekly bolus injection of 15 mg/kg given IV.

Maintenance 5-FU dosing regimens include the following: 200 to 250 mg/m² (6 mg/kg) every other day for 4 days, repeated in 4 weeks (if toxicity has resolved); or 500 to 600 mg/m² (15 mg/kg), given IV weekly as a continuous infusion or bolus injection (with and without the loading dose).

By continuous infusion, higher daily doses have been successfully used, and many investigators have reported lessened hematologic toxicity and enhanced efficacy. Most of a dose is eliminated by the liver and the remainder by the kidney. Therefore, marked dysfunction in either system probably requires a dose reduction.

There are two commonly used dosing regimens for 5-FU combined with leucovorin: 370 mg/m²/day of 5-FU for 5 days plus leucovorin given as a continuous infusion of 500 mg/m^2/day, beginning 24 hours before the first dose of 5-FU and continuing for 12 hours after completion of therapy; or 5-FU given at doses of 500 to 1,000 mg/m^2 every 2 weeks, preceded by calcium leucovorin at a dose of 20 mg/m^2 given as a 10-minute infusion (274,275).

Phase III studies performed by the GOG, SWOG, and Radiation Therapy Oncology Group have documented the efficacy of cisplatin/5-FU chemotherapy as an adjunct to radiation therapy in women with high-risk cervical cancer (14,121,276). The regimen used in the SWOG study was cisplatin 70 mg/m^2 by 2-hour IV infusion on day 1 of radiation followed by 5-FU 1,000 mg/m^2/day by 96-hour continuous infusion on days 1 to 4 every 3 weeks for four cycles, with the first and second cycles given concurrently with radiation therapy (121). The addition of concurrent cisplatin-based therapy to radiation therapy significantly improved progression-free and overall survival in this study; however, no definitive study has compared cisplatin versus cisplatin/5-FU as an adjunct to radiation therapy for cervical cancer, and the relative importance of 5-FU remains to be addressed.

Side Effects and Toxicities

The most pronounced and dose-limiting toxic effects of 5-FU are on the normal, rapidly proliferating tissues of the bone marrow and the lining of the gastrointestinal tract. Some nausea and vomiting can be expected. These adverse effects may respond relatively well to antiemetic treatment. Stomatitis, however, is usually an early sign of impending severe toxicity that may become evident after 5 to 8 days of therapy. Symptoms include soreness, erythema, or ulceration of the oral cavity or dysphagia. Other reported gastrointestinal symptoms are diarrhea, proctitis, and esophagitis.

Leukopenia, primarily granulocytopenia, and thrombocytopenia occur with a nadir at 9 to 14 days for the granulocytes and 7 to 14 days for platelets. Patients who are poor candidates for 5-FU therapy are those with a total leukocyte count of 2,000/mm^3 or less or platelet count of 100,000/mm^3 or less or those with poor nutritional status at the outset of therapy.

Some degree of alopecia is expected, although hair regrowth has occurred even when successive doses are given. Partial loss of nails and hyperpigmentation of the nail beds and other body areas (e.g., face, hands) have been reported. These may resemble the hyperpigmentation seen in Addison's disease. A maculopapular rash may occur on the extremities and sometimes the trunk. The rash is usually reversible. Sunlight may heighten or initiate many dermatologic reactions to 5-FU.

PPEs have been reported with very long continuous infusion 5-FU (over several weeks). This has been reported in 42% to 82% of patients in various series. The syndrome is progressive and disrupts treatment (277). This has encouraged the development of prodrugs of 5-FU, such as 5'-deoxy-5-fluorouridine, capecitabine, BOF-A2, ftorafur, UFT, and

S-1 (278,279). Although there is no indicated treatment for PPE, the incidence has been reduced to a few percentage points by limiting 5-FU continuous infusion durations to 21 days with at least 1 additional week off drug. Possible therapies that have yet to be evaluated in clinical trials include DMSO, systemic corticosteroids, and pyridoxine (vitamin B$_6$) (280,281).

Hyperpigmentation over the veins used for 5-FU administration has been observed (282). In one the veins remained patent, but there was marked darkening of the skin immediately over the vein.

5-FU may also cause an acute cerebellar syndrome that can persist beyond the period of actual treatment (149,283). Neurotoxicity may be evidenced by headache, minor visual disturbances, cerebellar ataxia, or all three. This is a rare complication. The neurotoxic metabolite is probably fluorocitrate.

Cardiotoxicity is a rare but potentially serious toxicity attributable to 5-FU. The incidence of cardiotoxicity may vary from 1.2% to 18.0% of patients (284), and includes cases of myocardial infarction, angina, dysrhythmias, cardiogenic shock, sudden death, and electrocardiographic changes. The mechanism producing 5-FU–induced cardiotoxicity is unknown.

Special Precautions

5-FU should never be given to pregnant women. 5-FU may increase the cortisone requirement in patients who have had an adrenalectomy (e.g., for breast cancer), and consideration should be given to increased doses of cortisone for patients receiving 5-FU.

Because dihydropyrimidine dehydrogenase is the rate-limiting enzyme in the metabolism of 5-FU, patients with a familial deficiency of dihydropyrimidine dehydrogenase (familial pyrimidinemia) should not receive 5-FU. The administration of 5-FU to patients with this enzyme deficiency has led to severe toxicity and even death (285,286).

Accidental splashing of 5-FU on the skin or eyes of personnel should be treated with immediate irrigation with saline solution or water. There have been no long-term sequelae of these accidents (287).

Because of the alkaline nature of the drug, admixture with any acidic agents (amino acids, penicillin, multivitamins, insulin, tetracycline) represents a theoretic incompatibility.

Special Applications

FUDR, a closely related analog of 5-FU, has efficacy as a salvage agent when administered as an intraperitoneal agent to stage III ovarian cancer patients with minimal residual disease (i.e., <1 cm) following second-look surgery. A SWOG study utilized intraperitoneal FUDR (3 g/day for 3 days every 3 weeks for six courses) as a salvage regimen in this patient population and documented a median overall survival of 38 months (288). Additionally, 69% of study patients had not progressed 12 months after receiving intraperitoneal FUDR. Because the majority of the intraperitoneal FUDR dose is extracted during "first pass," it is relatively well tolerated, although grade 4, uncomplicated neutropenia was observed in 14% of patients (288). Because of the favorable 1-year progression-free survival in this study, a subsequent Phase I-II trial was conducted by the SWOG (80). The researchers recommend that the regimen of IP FUDR + IP cisplatin (or IP FUDR with both platinums) be tested in a Phase III trial in comparison to IP cisplatin (80).

Speyer and colleagues (289) investigated intraperitoneal 5-FU in patients with ovarian and colon carcinomas. Using a Tenckhoff catheter, patients received repeated 36-hour courses of eight 2-L exchanges, each 4 hours long, or a 3- to 5-day course of single, daily 2-L instillations. 5-FU concentrations ranged from 10^{-6} M (130 µg/L) to 8×10^{-3} M (1 g/L).

The procedure was relatively well tolerated locally, although there were two instances of catheter-related bacterial peritonitis that were easily managed. Concentrations of 4×10^{-3} M for 36 hours caused mucositis, pancytopenia, and alopecia. The systemic toxicities were quite severe with the highest dose tested (8×10^{-3} M). Pharmacokinetic studies revealed first-order drug elimination, with an intraperitoneal half-life of 72 to 112 minutes. Intraperitoneal drug levels were 300-fold greater than simultaneous plasma levels. Intraperitoneal 5-FU administration appears to produce high drug concentrations with minimal systemic toxicity. Objective responses were documented in two of seven patients studied in this Phase I investigation. The investigators recommended further intraperitoneal 5-FU investigation at initial drug concentrations of 4×10^{-3} M (500 mg/L) for 36 hours (289).

Suhrland and Weisberger (290) used intracavitary 5-FU to manage malignant pleural effusions from carcinoma of the breast and lung tumors and to control malignant ascites from ovarian carcinoma. Approximately 38% of the patients responded to a single intracavitary dose of 2 to 3 g. For pericardial effusions, doses of 500 to 1,000 mg were used. Repeat dosing was not necessary. Patients with pleural effusions also tended to respond better than those with ascites. Although side effects were minimal in this study, some systemic toxicity was consistently produced.

Gemcitabine

Chemistry

Gemcitabine (Gemzar) is a relatively new chemotherapeutic agent that was approved by the FDA in 1995 for treatment of patients with advanced pancreatic cancer based on an increase in survival and clinical benefit (improvement in pain and performance status). The combination of gemcitabine plus cisplatin also is FDA approved and is considered standard therapy for patients with advanced non–small-cell lung cancer. Gemcitabine has demonstrated significant activity in advanced ovarian cancer patients and is active against refractory ovarian cancer and cervical cancer, as well as other solid tumors (291–295). Gemcitabine is a synthetic nucleoside analog with a structure that is highly similar to deoxycitidine and cytosine arabinoside (ara-C). Gemcitabine HCl is 2'-deoxy-2',2'-difluorocytidine monohydrochloride (β isomer). The empiric formula for gemcitabine is $C_9H_{11}F_2N_3O_4 \cdot HCl$ and the agent has a molecular weight of 299.66.

Mechanism of Action

Gemcitabine is a prodrug and undergoes multiple phosphorylations by deoxycytidine kinase at the intracellular level to form the active diphosphate and triphosphate metabolites. The triphosphate is incorporated into DNA as a fraudulent base pair. Following the insertion of gemcitabine, one additional deoxynucleotide is added to the end of the DNA chain before replication is terminated. This process is known as "masked chain termination" and prevents exonucleases from excising off the fraudulent base pair (296, 297). The diphosphate inhibits ribonucleotide reductase and thereby depletes the deoxynucleotide pools that are necessary for DNA synthesis and repair (298). Inactivation of gemcitabine occurs when the drug is metabolized by cytidine deaminase (both intracellulary and extracellulary) to form difluorodeoxyuridine (299).

Drug Disposition

Following administration of gemcitabine 1,000 mg/m^2 by 30-minute IV infusion, the parent compound undergoes rapid clearance in a diphasic manner. The plasma half-life and clearance are dose, age, and gender dependent. Gemcitabine pharmacokinetics were evaluted in 353 patients with varied solid tumors using short infusions (<70 minutes) and long infusions (70 to 285 minutes) at various total doses (500 to 3600 mg/m^2) (300). There is a three- to fourfold interpatient variability in pharmacokinetics. As noted above, gemcitabine is metabolized intracellularly by deoxycytidine kinase to form the active diphosphate and triphosphate metabolites. The drug is inactivated both intracellularly and extracellularly by cytidine deaminase to form difluorodeoxyuridine (dFdU). Of the administered gemcitabine dose, 99% is excreted in the urine either as the parent compound (<10%) or as dFdU (301,302).

Dutch researchers have performed a pharmacokinetic schedule-finding study of gemcitabine plus cisplatin. Gemcitabine 800 mg/m^2 was administered as a 30-minute infusion either 4 hours before, 24 hours before, 4 hours after, or 24 hours after administration of cisplatin 50 mg/m^2 by 1-hour IV infusion. Neither of the dosing schedules that used a 4-hour interval between drug administrations resulted in significant pharmacokinetic or pharmacologic differences. However, when gemcitabine was administered 24 hours before cisplatin, there was a twofold decrease in the plasma AUC of platinum. Furthermore, when the order of the drugs was reversed (i.e., cisplatin was administered 24 hours before gemcitabine), there was a 1.5-fold increase in the concentration-time product of the active triphosphate metabolite of gemcitabine within white blood cells. On the basis of these results, the investigators are conducting a Phase II study of the cisplatin/gemcitabine combination wherein cisplatin is administered 24 hours prior to gemcitabine (303).

Administration and Dosage

Gemcitabine should be diluted in 0.9% sodium chloride to a concentration of no greater than 40 mg/mL (higher drug concentrations may result in incomplete dissolution). Gemcitabine is generally administered as a 30-minute IV infusion at a dose of 1,000 mg/m^2; infusion durations of greater than 60 minutes are associated with dose-limiting flu-like symptoms (304).

The standard dosing schedule used for treatment of pancreatic cancer is 1,000 mg/m^2 by 30-minute IV infusion once weekly for 7 weeks for cycle 1 followed by a 1-week rest and then 1,000 mg/m^2 once weekly for 3 weeks followed by a 1-week rest for subsequent cycles (305).

Multiple Phase II studies of single-agent gemcitabine in refractory/recurrent ovarian cancer have used a dosing schedule of 800 to 1,250 mg/m^2 once weekly for 3 weeks followed by a week of rest; however, doses above 1,000 mg/m^2 may be associated with higher toxicity (291,295,306).

In vitro studies have shown synergism between gemcitabine and cisplatin in a variety of human cancer cell lines (307,308). It is believed that this synergism is primarily the result of increased platinum-DNA adduct formation (308). As noted (see Drug Disposition section above), the interval between cisplatin and gemcitabine administration can affect both pharmacokinetic and pharmacologic parameters (303). This combination appears to be especially promising for patients with advanced ovarian cancer. Several Phase II studies have been conducted in previously untreated ovarian cancer patients using a dosing schedule of cisplatin (75 to 100 mg/m^2) on day 1 followed by gemcitabine 1,250 mg/m^2 days 1 and 8 (293,309,310). Others have performed Phase II studies of gemcitabine plus cisplatin for patients with relapsed ovarian cancer after prior platinum-based chemotherapy and have determined that cisplatin 30 mg/m^2 plus gemcitabine 600 to 750 mg/m^2 on days 1 and 8 every 21 days is an active and tolerable regimen that demonstrated activity in platinum-resistant patients (86,311).

Side Effects and Toxicities

Gemcitabine-induced toxicity is highly schedule dependent; small daily doses are associated with greater toxicity than large doses administered on a weekly basis (312). The dose, schedule and duration of infusion of gemcitabine directly affects the toxicity profile (312). Infusion durations of greater than 60 minutes are associated with increased myelosuppression and hepatic toxicity, whereas the administration of small daily doses results in dose-limiting flu-like symptoms (299,304). When gemcitabine is administered using the standard weekly dosing schedule, therapy is generally well tolerated and bone marrow suppression is the major dose-limiting toxicity.

Analysis of safety data from 22 completed clinical trials in which gemcitabine was administered on a weekly basis to 979 patients revealed that neutropenia was the most significant hematologic side effect. Six percent of patients experienced grade 4 neutropenia and an additional 20% experienced grade 3 neutropenia. Grade 4 leukopenia was experienced by less than 1% of patients. Decreases in white blood cell counts were noncumulative, short-lived, and rarely resulted in complications. Only 6 of 979 patients (1.1%) developed severe infections, and no patient developed a life-threatening infection. Grades 3 and 4 anemia were experienced by 6.8% and 1.3% of patients, respectively, and only 2 of the 979 patients discontinued gemcitabine secondary to anemia. Grades 3 and 4 thrombocytopenia occurred in 4.1% and 1.1% of patients, respectively. Less than 1% of patients received platelet transfusions and only four patients (0.4%) discontinued therapy on account of thrombocytopenia (312).

Gemcitabine is associated with a low incidence of hepatic toxicity. Grade 3 elevations in alkaline phosphatase, alanine aminotransferase (ALT), or aspartate aminotransferase (AST) occurred in less than 8% of patients. Grade 4 elevations in these liver enzymes occurred in 2% or less of patients. Grade 3 or 4 increases in bilirubin occurred in 1.8% and 0.8% of patients, respectively. It is noteworthy that one-third of patients in this study population had documented liver metastases (312).

Clinically significant renal toxicity rarely occurs with gemcitabine therapy. However, rare cases of hemolytic uremic syndrome have been reported with gemcitabine therapy. The incidence is believed to be approximately 0.6% (312, 313).

Other nonhematologic toxicities that were reported in more than 5% of patients were nausea/vomiting (64.3% overall, 17.1% grade 3, 1.2% grade 4), fever (37.3% overall, 0.7% severe), edema (greater than 20% of patients), flu-like symptoms (18.9%, 0.9% severe), cutaneous reactions (24.8%, 0.2% severe), alopecia (14.1%, 0.4% severe), diarrhea (12.1%, 0.7% severe), somnolence (9.1%, 0.9% severe), infection (8.7%, 1.1% severe), mucositis (8.4%, 0.2% severe), constipation (7.8%, 0.7% severe), and dyspnea (7.7%, 1.2% severe). Nausea and vomiting rarely were dose limiting and only two (0.2%) patients discontinued gemcitabine therapy because of nausea. Fever was a fairly frequent toxicity and sometimes occurred in the absence of flu-like symptoms or infection. Subcutaneous edema, including peripheral edema and facial edema, occurred in a significant number of patients. Edema was generally mild to moderate in nature; few patients (0.6%) discontinued gemcitabine because of this side effect, and the edema resolved after drug discontinuation. Flu-like symptoms consisted of headache, back pain, chills, myalgia, asthenia, and anorexia and were generally short lived. Paracetamol was reported to provide relief to some patients. Cutaneous reactions consisted of erythema in mild cases (15.5%) and dry desquamation, vesiculation, and/or pruritus in moderate cases (9.1%). Only one patient developed severe cutaneous toxicity that was characterized as moist desquamation and ulceration. Dyspnea (with or without bronchospasm) occurs in less than 10% of patients following gemcitabine administration. This toxicity generally occurs within a few hours of treatment and resolves within 6 hours (312).

Fatal pulmonary toxicity (acute respiratory distress syndrome) has been reported as a rare side effect of gemcitabine therapy (314). Symptoms include progressive dyspnea, tachypnea, marked hypoxemia, and bilateral interstitial infiltrates consistent with pulmonary edema. Some patients have responded to the termination of gemcitabine therapy and treatment with corticosteroids and diuretics. Prior radiation therapy to the mediastinum may be a risk factor for gemcitabine-induced pulmonary edema (314,315).

Possible incompatibilities between gemcitabine solutions and other drug solutions have not been studied.

Ifosfamide

Chemistry

In combination with cisplatin, ifosfamide (IFEX, Holoxan) is a commonly used drug for the first-line treatment of patients with advanced cancer of the cervix, and in combination chemotherapy, it is a second-line treatment for patients with advanced cancer of the ovary (316,317). It also has activity in advanced or recurrent endometrial cancer (318). Chemically, ifosfamide is 3-(2-chloroethyl)-2-[(2-chloroethyl)amino]-tetrahydro-2H-1,3,2-oxazaphosphorine-2-oxide, and is chemically related to the nitrogen mustards and a structual analog of cyclophosphamide. It differs only in the position of one of the two chloroethyl groups, which is transposed to the endocyclic (ring) nitrogen in ifosfamide. The molecular formula is $C_7H_{15}Cl_2N_2O_2P$, and the compound has a molecular weight of 261.1.

Mechanism of Action

Ifosfamide is a metabolically activated alkylating agent. Like cyclophosphamide, it must first undergo hydroxylation by microsomal (mixed-function oxidase) enzyme systems (319). The activation of ifosfamide occurs more slowly than that of cyclophosphamide, and there is quantitatively greater oxidation of the chloroethyl side chains with ifosfamide. This leads to a greater production of chloracetaldehyde, a possible neurotoxin.

The activation process generates highly reactive metabolites, particularly 4-hydroxyifosfamide, which are capable of cellular uptake and, ultimately, covalent binding to protein and to DNA (320). Metabolites can spontaneously break down to yield the bladder irritant acrolein and the active alkylating moiety, ifosforamide mustard. Cross linking of DNA strands proceeds from ifosforamide mustard, but acrolein binds nonspecifically and covalently to bladder epithelium. The DNA–cross-link distance is greater for ifosfamide (seven atoms) compared with cyclophosphamide (five atoms). Furthermore, the aziridine forms more slowly and is less reactive since it lacks a positive charge (321). Chain scission of DNA and inhibition of thymidine uptake also occur with ifosfamide. The primary mechanism of alkylation is not cell cycle specific.

Drug Disposition

The pharmacokinetics of ifosfamide appears to be qualitatively similar to those of cyclophosphamide. Creaven and co-workers (322) found a plasma half-life of radiolabeled ifosfamide (5,000 mg/m^2) of 13.8 hours, with 82% urinary (radioactivity) recovery.

The plasma decay pattern appears to be biexponential (two-compartment model) for large bolus doses and monoexponential (one-compartment model) with fractionated doses. In contrast to single-dose pharmacokinetics studies, Allen and associates (323) found that with sequential daily administration of 2,400 mg/m^2/day for 3 days, there is monoexponential plasma decay with a half-life of 6.9 hours and a metabolized urinary recovery fraction of 72.8%, in contrast to the biexponential decay (plasma half life 15.2 hours) of a single-bolus dose of ifosfamide (5,000 mg/m^2). This finding suggests that the metabolic disposition of the drug may be dose dependent. These half-lives are approximately twice those reported for cyclophosphamide. Of note, a longer ifosfamide half-life may be seen in obese patients who are more than 20% over ideal body weight. The renal clearance rate of ifosfamide is about twice that for cyclophosphamide: 21.3 versus 10.7 mL/min in bolus dosing and 18.7 versus 10.7 mL/min with fractionated doses. Only about half of an ifosfamide dose is metabolized compared with about 90% for cyclophosphamide. This reflects a substantial difference in the metabolic clearance capacity for the two analogs. Although more intact (inactive) ifosfamide than cyclophosphamide is renally excreted, urinary alkylating activity persists longer with ifosfamide.

Creaven and co-workers (322) demonstrated that because unchanged ifosfamide, but not metabolites, penetrates the blood-brain barrier, alkylating activity in the CSF may occur but is probably negligible.

Administration and Dosage

Ifosfamide is reconstituted by the addition of sterile water to the vial, which should be shaken to dissolve. Ifosfamide may be further diluted to a concentration of 0.6 to 29.0 mg/mL in 5% dextrose or 0.9% sodium chloride. It is administered intravenously, usually by a short infusion. Ifosfamide may also be administered by slow IV push in a 75-mL minimal volume of sterile saline solution but not water and infused over at least 30 minutes or by continuous infusion over 5 days. Large single doses of ifosfamide produce much more toxicity than fractionated schedules, which are therefore preferred in solid-tumor treatment regimens. Adequate hydration of the patient before and for 72 hours after ifosfamide therapy is recommended to reduce the incidence of drug-induced hemorrhagic cystitis. The use of a concurrent prophylactic agent for hemorrhagic cystitis, such as mesna (Mesnex), is required to prevent severe hematuria from high-dose ifosfamide. At least 2 L of fluid each day is recommended to produce a copious urine output.

Continuous infusions of ifosfamide over 24 hours have also been given every 3 weeks (324). Mesna can be given concurrently in the same infusion container or as a 4-hour intermittent IV bolus (325,503). However, renal toxicities may be increased with the single, large infusions. Extravasation of the drug should not cause tissue necrosis, but one case report has been described (325a).

The FDA-approved dose for testicular cancer is 1,200 mg/m^2/day for 5 consecutive days every 21 days. Other dosage schedules include 2,000 mg/m^2 IV continuous infusion on days 1 to 3 every 21 days as part of the MAID regimen (mesna, Adriamycin, infosfamide, dacarbazine) for soft tissue sarcoma; 1,000 mg/m^2 on days 1 and 2 every 28 days as part of the ICE regimen (ifosfamide, carboplatin, etoposide) for non-Hodgkin's lymphoma; and 1,000 mg/m^2 on days 1 to 3 every 21 to 28 days as part of the TIC regimen (paclitaxel, ifosfamide, carboplatin) for head and neck cancer (46).

A Phase II study evaluated ifosfamide (1500 mg/m^2 IV over 1 hour, days 1 to 3) with mesna in combination with paclitaxel (175 mg/m^2, IV over 3 hours on day 1) and cisplatin (75 mg/m^2 IV over 2 hours on day 2) as first-line therapy in advanced, suboptimally debulked epithelial ovarian cancer patients (326). This regimen was associated with an 85% objective response rate and a median overall survival of 52.8 months in 22 patients with stage III or IV disease. A regimen of paclitaxel (175 mg/m^2), ifosfamide (5,000 mg/m^2), and cisplatin (75 mg/m^2 or 50 mg/m^2 in irradiated patients) every 21 days in 45 recurrent or persistent cervical cancer patients was associated with a 67% objective response rate (327).

Morgan and colleagues (328) evaluated several IV push and infusion dose schedules in non–small-cell lung cancer: 700 to 900 mg/m^2/day by IV push for 5 days repeated every 3 weeks; 700 to 1000 mg/m^2/day for 5 days repeated every 3 weeks plus 1 g/day of oral ascorbic acid; 4 g/m^2 slow infusion repeated every 3 weeks; and 900 mg/m^2 by IV push weekly. There appeared to be less hematuria produced with the sequential 5-day schedule with concomitant ascorbic acid.

Rodriguez and colleagues (329) described a 47% response rate in leukemia patients with continuous infusions of ifosfamide at 1,200 mg/m^2/day given for 5 days. Significant genitourinary toxicity was not encountered, and myelosuppression predominated as the dose-limiting toxicity. In combination with other cytotoxic drugs, such as doxorubicin or lomustine (CCNU), a single IV push dose of 1,000 mg/m^2 (not to exceed 12,500 g total) has been recommended.

Side Effects and Toxicities

Creaven and associates (322) reviewed the clinical toxicity of ifosfamide given as a large bolus injection (200 to 10,000 mg/m^2) and in a fractionated 3-day (2,400 mg/m^2/day) schedule. Urinary tract toxicity is the dose-limiting factor with both schedules. The clinical hallmark is hemorrhagic cystitis, which is caused by excretion of active alkylating metabolites into the urinary bladder. Vigorous hydration with oral and intravenous fluids and concomitant mesna are needed to prevent serious ifosfamide-induced bladder damage. Hydration may also overcome the antidiuretic effects of this drug. Nelson and colleagues (325) used IV furosemide (20 to 40 mg) to maintain adequate urine flow in a Phase I study of ifosfamide. Diuretic responses usually occurred within 1 hour.

Symptoms of dysuria and urinary frequency appear to parallel those of hematuria. The onset of symptoms is 1 to 2 days after injection, with an average duration of 9 days (range 1 to 41 days) (330). Dose-related ifosfamide-induced nephrotoxicity was detected by elevation of the BUN, producing a subsequent dose-related uremia in 66% of patients receiving 150 mg/kg. Other lesions seen at autopsy (four of seven patients) included evidence of acute tubular necrosis and pyelonephritis. At low daily doses, granular cylindruria was seen in all patients; denoting marked tubular damage. The cylindruria cleared within 10 days of drug discontinuance (330). DeFronzo and co-researchers (331) also described glomerular dysfunction and a Fanconi-type picture in a patient treated with ifosfamide. Prior cisplatin therapy may also increase ifosfamide-induced nephrotoxicity (332,333).

Nausea and vomiting appear to be common and are more severe after a rapid injection of large ifosfamide doses. Emesis typically begins within a few hours of administration and persists an average of 3 days (range 1 to 28 days) (330).

Hematologic toxicity from ifosfamide usually involves only a mild to moderate degree of leukopenia in most patients. In a review by Creaven and co-workers (322), significant thrombocytopenia was not encountered for any of the dose schedules used.

Lethargy and confusion are seen with high doses of ifosfamide and may be caused by the chloracetaldehyde metabolite. Nelson and associates (325) observed that this lasted from 1 to 8 hours, was spontaneously reversible, and was related to the passage of intact drug into the central nervous system (CNS). Seizures, ataxia, stupor, and weakness have been reported after ifosfamide. These effects may be increased by concomitant neurotoxic drugs, such as certain antiemetics, tranquilizers, narcotics, and antihistamines. There is a single case report of nonconvulsive status epilepticus associated with ifosfamide therapy. The patient responded to discontinuation of the ifosfamide and phenytoin therapy (334). Although alkylating metabolites appear to penetrate the blood-brain barrier, the levels achieved are too low to be useful in the treatment of CNS tumors (322).

Alopecia is usually seen with ifosfamide, especially when large bolus doses are used. In a study by Van Dyk et al. (330), the average onset of maximal hair loss was 19 days (range 11 to 32 days) after the start of treatment.

Hepatic enzyme elevations have been described in some patients. The elevations in alkaline phosphatase and serum transaminase are transient and typically resolve rapidly without sequelae.

Special Precautions

The patient must be kept well hydrated during ifosfamide therapy to reduce the potential for hemorrhagic cystitis. The use of mesna given intravenously or orally is required to prevent hemorrhagic cystitis. Table 16.5 outlines the recommended mesna schedule for ifosfamide uroprotection.

Patients who have received previous or concurrent therapy with radiation or cytotoxic drugs may require significant ifosfamide dosage reductions. Dose reductions should also be considered for patients with impaired renal function and/or serum albumin concentrations below 3.5 g/dL.

Drug Interactions

Several drug interactions are possible with ifosfamide. Because the compound undergoes hepatic activation by microsomal enzymes, induction is potentially possible by pretreatment with various enzyme-inducing drugs, such as phenobarbital, phenytoin, and chloral hydrate.

Nephrotoxic drugs like cisplatin may significantly increase ifosfamide renal damage (332). Other drug interactions reported for cyclophosphamide that may also occur with ifosfamide include reactions with metabolic alteration of H_2-antihistamines, such as cimetidine.

Irinotecan

Chemistry

Irinotecan (CPT-11, Camptosar), a TOPO-I inhibitor, is a water-soluble semisynthetic derivative of camptothecin, a natural product extracted from the stem wood of the *Camptotheca acuminata* tree that has significant antitumor activity. It was approved by the FDA in 1998 for treatment of patients with progressive metastatic colon or rectal cancer following 5-FU therapy. Early clinical development of camptothecin was halted because of severe, unpredictable hemorrhagic cystitis, vomiting, and myelosuppression. Subsequently, irinotecan was formulated as a prodrug to have greater water solubility, increased antitumor activity, and less toxicity than the parent compound. Its chemical name is (4S)-4,11-diethyl-4-hydroxy-9-[(4-piperidino-piperidino)carbonyloxy]-1H-pyrano[3',4':6,7]indolizino[1,2-b]quinoline-3,14(4H,12H) dione hydrochloride trihydrate. This drug has a molecular weight of 677.19 and the empirical formula is $C_{33}H_{38}N_4O_6 \cdot HCl \cdot 3H_2O$.

Mechanism of Action

Irinotecan's cytotoxicity is believed to be related to the inhibition of TOPO-I, an enzyme necessary for DNA replication (224). Irinotecan is activated to the active metabolite, SN-38, by the liver (335). Irinotecan and SN-38 bind to the transient TOPO-I–DNA complex, stabilize the complex, and thereby promote DNA single-strand breaks. These strand breaks prevent DNA replication and result in cell death (224, 335). Current research suggests that the cytotoxicity of irinotecan is due to DNA damage produced during DNA synthesis. Mammalian cells cannot repair these double-strand breaks.

Drug Disposition

Pharmacokinetic studies performed by Rothenberg et al. (336) have determined that when irinotecan is administered as a 90-minute IV infusion at dose ranges of 50 to 180 mg/m^2, the plasma terminal-phase half-life for irinotecan (total) was 7.9 ± 2.8 hours, 6.3 ± 2.2 hours for irinotecan (lactone), and 11.5 ± 3.8 hours for SN-38 (the active metabolite). The time of peak plasma concentration for irinotecan

TABLE 16.5. *Dosing schedules for mesna combined with ifosfamide*

Route of mesna administration	Dose (mg/kg) as a percentage of ifosfamide dose at times before and after ifosfamide		
	15 min before	4 h after	8 h after
Intravenous	20%	20%	20%
Oral[a]	Not recommended; use IV route	0%	0%

[a] For highly reliable patients with total emetic control, mesna solution can be diluted 1:1 to 1:10 in carbonated cola drinks or in chilled fruit juices (e.g., apple, grape, tomato, and orange juice) and administered orally.

was at infusion end, whereas the time of peak concentration for total SN-38 varied from 30 to 90 minutes after completion of the infusion. Plasma clearance was unrelated to dose, with a mean clearance of 15.3 ± 3.5 L/h/m^2 for the total and 45.6 ± 10.8 L/h/m^2 for the lactone. At the 150-mg/m^2 dose, the following pharmacokinetics parameters were observed: peak plasma concentration, 1.97 μg/mL for total irinotecan; 0.83 μg/mL for the lactone form; and 36.7 ng/mL for total SN-38; and concentration-time product (AUC) 8.44 μg · h/mL for total irinotecan, 2.81 μg · h/mL for the lactone form, and 409.8 ng · h/mL for total SN-38. Renal excretion was not a major route of drug elimination.

Abigerges et al. (337) determined in their pharmacokinetic study of irinotecan (100 to 700 mg/m^2 by 30-minute IV infusion) that the plasma disposition of irinotecan was biphasic or triphasic. The mean plasma terminal-phase half-life, volume of distribution, and total body clearance of irinotecan were 14.2 ± 0.9 hours, 157 ± 8 L/m^2, and 15 ± 1 L/m^2/h, respectively. Both the irinotecan and SN-38 concentration-time product (AUC) increased linearly with dose. At the 350-mg/m^2 dose level, the irinotecan and SN-38 AUCs were 34.0 ± 4.1 μg · h/mL and 451 ± 100 ng · h/mL, respectively. The plasma terminal-phase half-life of SN-38 was 13.8 ± 1.4 hours.

Administration and Dosage

The appropriate dose of irinotecan should be diluted with 500 mL of dextrose (5%) to a final concentration of 0.12 to 1.1 mg/mL and administered IV over 90 minutes (336). Alternatively, French investigators have administered irinotecan by diluting the appropriate amount of drug in 250 mL of 0.9% sodium chloride solution and delivering the drug IV over 30 minutes (337).

In the United States, the recommended dose for irinotecan therapy in colon cancer patients is 125 mg/m^2 weekly by 90-minute infusion for 4 weeks followed by a 2-week rest. In Europe, the recommended dose is 300 to 350 mg/m^2 by 90-minute infusion every 21 days. The U.S. schedule has been used in three Phase II clinical trials, wherein irinotecan displayed modest activity in cervical cancer patients (338–340). When administered as a single dose every 3 weeks, a 240-mg/m^2 dose is recommended (336,341). French investigators have determined that a 600-mg/m^2 30-minute IV infusion every 3 weeks can be administered if drug-induced diarrhea is aggressively managed by high-dose loperamide (e.g., up to 16 mg/day); however, these investigators recommended a dose level of 350 mg/m^2 every 3 weeks until further experience is gained with higher dose levels (337).

Side Effects and Toxicities

Diarrhea and neutropenia are the major dose-limiting toxicities associated with irinotecan (336,337,341). Other moderate to severe toxicities associated with irinotecan therapy include anemia, dehydration (secondary to diarrhea), nausea, vomiting, anorexia, abdominal cramping, cumulative asthenia, thrombocytopenia, renal insufficiency, elevations in liver transaminases, and alopecia.

The diarrhea associated with irinotecan appears to be due to two separate mechanisms. The diarrhea that may occur during irinotecan infusion is highly responsive to atropine therapy and, therefore, appears to be related to cholinergic activity. However, the subacute diarrhea that develops 2 to 3 weeks after irinotecan therapy is refractory to anticholinergic agents. The most effective treatment for the subacute diarrhea is institution of therapy with antimotility agents (i.e., loperamide or diphenoxylate hydrochloride with atropine sulfate) at the first signs of increased intestinal motility (e.g., loose bowels). If left untreated, subacute diarrhea can rapidly progress to grade 4 toxicity. This life-threatening diarrhea is refractory to antidiarrheal therapy and generally lasts for 5 to 7 days. Patients with grade 4 diarrhea should be hospitalized and receive supportive care with IV fluids and electrolyte replacement (336).

Special Precautions

As described above (see Side Effects and Toxicities section), irinotecan can induce grade 4 diarrhea that is refractory to antidiarrheal medication. Patients who are receiving irinotecan must be monitored carefully for early symptoms of increased intestinal motility and should receive antimotility therapy (e.g., up to 16 mg/day loperamide) as soon as initial symptoms of diarrhea appear. A low level of glucuronidation in the biliary system has been associated with the development of severe diarrhea in some patients (342).

Special Applications

The TOPO-I inhibitor irinotecan also has been shown to have activity against advanced cervical cancer. Cottu and colleagues (343) reported response rates in patients with relapsed cervical cancer ranging from 20% to 22%. The GOG reported a response rate of 13.3% (6 of 45) in patients with advanced cervical cancer with no prior chemotherapy (339). No responses were reported in second-line (after resistance to cisplatin) treatment in a Phase II study of 16 patients (338). However, Verschraegen et al. (340) reported a 21% response rate in the same patient population (n = 42). Reviews by Eisenhauer and Vermorken (344) and Verschraegen et al. (345) have reported response rates ranging from 13% to 24%. The combination of irinotecan (60 mg/m^2 90-min IV on days 1, 8, and 15) followed by cisplatin (60 mg/m^2 on day 8) administered every 3 weeks, has demonstrated activity in a recent Phase II trial of first-line treatment of cervial cancer, with a 1-year disease-free and overall survival of 26.7 and 65.1%, respectively (346).

Liposomal Encapsulated Doxorubicin

Chemistry

Liposomal doxorubicin (Doxil, Caelyx) has an FDA-approved indication for treatment of patients with metastatic, refractory ovarian cancer and AIDS-related Kaposi's sarcoma. Doxorubicin HCl, which is the established name for (8S,10S)-10-[(3-amino-2,3,6-trideoxy-α-L-lyxohexopyranosyl)oxy]-8-glycolyl-7,8,9,10-tetrahydro- 6,8,11-trihydroxy-1-methoxy-5,12-naphthacenedione hydrochloride, has a molecular weight of 579.99 and the molecular formula $C_{27} H_{29} NO_{11} \cdot HCl$. The liposomal carriers are composed of N-(carbonyl-methoxypolyethylene glycol 2000)-1,2-distearoyl-sn-glycero-3-phosphoethanolamine sodium salt (MPEG-DSPE), 3.19 mg/mL; fully hydrogenated soy phosphatidylcholine (HSPC), 9.58 mg/mL; and cholesterol, 3.19 mg/mL. Greater than 90% of the drug is encapsulated in the liposomes. The liposomal encapsulation of doxorubicin dramatically alters the pharmacokinetic and toxicity profiles of the drug.

Mechanism of Action

The mechanism of action of doxorubicin is discussed previously (see Doxorubicin section). Liposomes are microscopic vesicles composed of a phospholipid bilayer that are capable of encapsulating active drugs. The liposomes of the encapsulated form of doxorubicin are formulated with surface-bound methoxypolyethylene glycol (MPEG), a process often referred to as pegylation, to protect liposomes from detection by the mononuclear phagocyte system (MPS) and to increase blood circulation time (347).

Drug Disposition

Liposomal doxorubicin is associated with a much longer plasma half-life, slower plasma clearance, and reduced volume of distribution than free doxorubicin. In a pharmacokinetics study performed in six patients with solid tumors, the area under the plasma disappearance curve was 1.0 mg/L · hour versus 609 mg/L · hour when 25 mg/m^2 of doxrubicin was administered as free drug or as a pegylated liposomal form, respectively. The initial half-life was 0.07 versus 3.2 hours and the terminal half-life was 8.7 versus 45.2 hours for the free and liposomal forms of doxorubicin, respectively. Additionally, the steady-state volume of distribution was 254 L versus 4.1 L for the free and liposomal forms, respectively (348). Liposomal encapsulation of doxorubicin has also been shown to result in fourfold to 16-fold increases in tumor-tissue drug concentrations relative to that achieved following administration of the free form.

Administration and Dosage

Liposomal doxorubicin must be diluted in 250 mL of 5% dextrose prior to administration. Because liposomal doxorubicin contains no preservative or bacteriostatic agent, aseptic technique must be strictly observed. Liposomal doxorubicin may be administered as an IV infusion over 30 to 60 minutes. In that liposomal doxorubicin is not a vesicant, extravasation of the drug is not a critical concern. For ovarian cancer patients, liposomal doxorubicin should be administered at a dose of 50 mg/m^2 (every 4 weeks) at an initial rate of 1 mg/min to reduce the risk of infusion reactions. The rate may be increased to a 60-minute infusion if no adverse events are noted. The recommended dose in AIDS-related Kaposi's sarcoma patients is 20 mg/m^2 over 30 minutes, once every 3 weeks, for as long as patients respond and tolerate treatment.

Side Effects and Toxicities

Unlike the parent drug, liposomal doxorubicin is not a vesicant and is associated with minimal cardiotoxicity, alopecia, and nausea/vomiting. However, the liposomal encapsulation results in acute infusion reactions, and an increased rate of PPE and stomatitis (349). PPE is a dose-limiting toxicity that can occur in 26% of patients who receive 50 mg/m^2 every 4 weeks (350). Stomatitis is a second dose-limiting toxicity associated with liposomal doxorubicin. Current methods to prevent PPE and stomatitis include dose reduction and discontinuation (grade 1—redose. If patient has experienced previous grade 3 or 4 toxicity, delay the treatment by 2 weeks until resolution to grades 0 to 1 and reduce dose by 25% before returning to orginal dose level; grades 2 to 4—delay up to 2 weeks until resolved, if no resolution to grades 0 to 1, discontinue; grades 3 to 4—after delay and resolution to grades 0 to 1, decrease dose by 25%, if no resolution, discontinue). To help relieve pain from PPE, topical wound care, elevation, and cold compresses may be used as supportive care (281). Topical DMSO has been used to treat skin extravations (99% DMSO four times daily up to 14 days), but has yet to be evaluated in a randomized trial (280). Other possible therapies that have yet to be evaluated in clinical trials include systemic corticosteroids and pyridoxine (vitamin B$_6$) (281).

Infusion-related reactions occur in less than 10% of patients treated with liposomal doxorubicin and are most common during the first course of treatment. Symptoms may include flushing, shortness of breath, facial swelling, headache, chills, back pain, tightness in the chest and throat, and hypotension. Alopecia has been observed in only 15% of ovarian cancer patients treated with liposomal doxorubicin.

Melphalan

Chemistry

Melphalan (Alkeran, L-phenylalanine mustard, L-PAM) is a phenylalanine derivative of nitrogen mustard that acts as a bifunctional alkylating agent. Melphalan is FDA approved for the chemotherapy of patients with multiple myeloma. The agent's molecular formula is $C_{13}H_{18}Cl_2N_2O_2$ and its molecular weight is 305.2. It is known chemically as 4-[bis(2-chloroethyl)amino]-L-phenylalanine. Melphalan is water insoluble and previously was only commercially available in a 2-mg tablet form. However, a parenteral formulation was approved by the FDA in 1993. Melphalan for injection is supplied as a freeze-dried powder in single-use vials containing 50 mg melphalan and 20 mg povidone. A vial of sterile diluent (10 mL) is also supplied.

Mechanism of Action

Melphalan is an alkylating agent of the bischloroethylamine type. Its cytotoxicity appears to be related to the extent of its interstrand cross linking with tumor-cell DNA, probably by binding at the N^7 position of guanine (351). The cross-helical base pairing causes strain and possible rupture of the double-stranded DNA backbone.

Melphalan is relatively stable in media containing high concentrations of chloride ions and at acid pH (351). It has a relatively short *in vitro* half-life in plasma of approximately 2 hours owing to the rapid hydroxylation of the chloroethyl groups of the molecule. Melphalan may form a reactive immonium ion that can alkylate or hydroxylate the monohydroxy and dihydroxy metabolites. Monohydroxy melphalan possesses only 2% of the cytotoxicity of the parent compound, and the dihydroxy derivative is inactive (352).

Melphalan is usually transported into cells by two amino acid–transporting systems: the sodium-independent system that transfers leucine and a monovalent cation-dependent system similar to that which transfers alanine, serine, or cysteine (353). Melphalan efflux from cells appears to be sodium independent, to be stimulated by amino acids in the extracellular medium, and to occur by a simple diffusion mechanism.

Drug Disposition

Melphalan has extremely variable systemic availability after oral administration. In the average patient, approximately one-third of an administered dose of melphalan can be recovered from plasma after a bolus oral dose. The range of systemic availability after oral dosing varies from none to over 90%. The terminal-phase plasma half-life of orally administered melphalan is approximately 90 minutes, and the 24-hour urinary excretion rate averages 11% (354). Melphalan penetration into cerebrospinal fluid is low. Plasma protein binding ranges from 60% to 90%, and approximately 30% is irreversibly bound to plasma proteins.

Studies of melphalan metabolism, using an isolated perfused rat liver model and *in vitro* rat microsomal enzyme preparations, have documented insignificant hepatic biotransformation (355).

Two groups of investigators have reported that the systemic availability of melphalan is increased if the drug is administered in the fasting state. The presence of a large meal appears to enhance melphalan degradation at the alkaline pH found in the upper small bowel before systemic absorption (356,357).

Patients with multiple myeloma receiving intravenously administered melphalan achieved longer durations of survival than those receiving the oral formulation. Furthermore, a significantly lower dose of intravenously administered drug was associated with life-threatening leukopenia and infectious complications compared with the oral formulation (357).

Administration and Dosage

The usual IV dose is 16 mg/m² (15- to 20-minute infusion), administered at 2-week intervals for four doses, then at 4-week intervals. The oral agent dose is 6 mg/day for 2 to 3 weeks, followed by up to 4 weeks without treatment. As a single agent, one-time IV doses of 1 mg/kg repeated at 4- to 6-week intervals are generally well tolerated. Although the manufacturer reports equal effects from intravenous or oral doses, bioavailability differences and the potential for lessened hepatic clearance of IV doses suggest IV dosing at reduced levels. In a surgical adjuvant setting for ovarian carcinoma, melphalan has been used in large cyclic doses of 1 mg/kg given IV over 8 hours and repeated in 4 weeks (358). The apparently equivalent therapeutic results with intravenous and oral dosing are surprising in light of the reported poor oral absorption of the compound.

Side Effects and Toxicities

Compared with other standard alkylating agents, melphalan is relatively well tolerated after oral administration. Except for dose-limiting bone marrow suppression (i.e., neutropenia, thrombocytopenia, anemia), other acute side effects are uncommon and include infrequent nausea and vomiting and, rarely, skin rash and pulmonary toxicity (359). Melphalan is characterized by its potential to cause cumulative bone marrow damage, as expressed by profound and prolonged depression of neutrophils and platelets. There is a slow reduction in peripheral leukocyte and platelet counts to their nadirs at 28 to 35 days after drug administration followed by a 14- to 21-day recovery period.

Acute nonlymphocytic leukemia has been reported in patients with multiple myeloma and ovarian cancer after prolonged melphalan therapy. In one Swedish study of 474 patients with ovarian carcinoma, there were four cases of acute nonlymphocytic leukemia among 12 patients who received 800 mg or more of melphalan (360). An evaluation of the relationship between alkylating agents and leukemic disorders in 3,363 one-year survivors of ovarian cancer revealed that the 10-year cumulative risk of acquiring leukemia was 11.2% after treatment with melphalan and 5.4% after cyclophosphamide treatment (361). The risk of developing leukemia after melphalan and cyclophosphamide treatment was significantly higher than in matched patient groups who received no chemotherapy. These data suggest that, to reduce the leukemia risk, the total dose of melphalan should not exceed 600 mg.

Special Applications

One major impediment to the success of cancer chemotherapy is the rapid development of drug resistance as manifested clinically by short objective responses and subsequent, progressive tumor growth despite aggressive chemotherapy. Several mechanisms have been postulated to explain this relatively universal phenomenon.

Wang and Tew (362) presented evidence that the development of tumor resistance *in vitro* to alkylating agents is associated with concurrent elevation of intracellular glutathione–S-transferase concentrations. Knowledge of this drug-resistance mechanism may provide a clinically useful approach to its reversal. Ozols and colleagues (363) demonstrated that buthionine sulfoximine (BSO), a specific inhibitor of intracellular sulfhydryl-independent glutathione synthesis, reverses established resistance to melphalan *in vitro* and *in vivo* in two human ovarian cancer cell lines. Two Phase I studies have shown that BSO can be combined safely with melphalan, with a resulting depletion of glutathione levels in peripheral blood lymphocytes and tumor biopsies to less than 10% and 20% of baseline values, respectively (364,365). Phase II trials of melphalan plus BSO are being conducted in ovarian cancer and melanoma (365).

Melphalan therapy has been used in autologous bone marrow transplantation. A series of studies have been reported for high-dose (120 to 225 mg/m^2) IV administered melphalan against adult melanoma, breast, and colon cancers (366, 367). Although the resulting high response rates appear to be promising, most have been partial, and survival advantages have not yet been established. In general, these high doses of melphalan have been tolerated relatively well, with diarrhea and stomatitis becoming severe and dose-limiting at doses greater than 200 mg/m^2.

Because ovarian cancer remains confined to the intraperitoneal space for most of its natural history, there has been increasing interest in the intraperitoneal administration of cytotoxic drugs to patients with minimal residual intraperitoneal disease (i.e., plaques <1 cm in diameter) after aggressive cytoreductive surgery or primary chemotherapy. Melphalan is an extremely attractive drug for administration by the intraperitoneal route in patients with ovarian cancer (368, 369). Melphalan exhibits a high degree of *in vitro* cytotoxicity as compared with other standard chemotherapeutic agents when tested against fresh human ovarian cancer tumors at drug concentrations achievable by intraperitoneal administration (368). In addition to its high degree of cytotoxicity, melphalan's high molecular weight ensures a relatively low clearance from the peritoneal space.

In a Phase I dose-finding study, Howell and co-workers (369) showed that an intraperitoneal melphalan dose of 70 mg/kg was tolerated, with only moderate leukopenia (median nadir 2,000 cells/μL) and thrombocytopenia (median nadir 69,000 platelets/μL) and no evidence of peritoneal irritation. The peak peritoneal concentration averaged 93-fold greater than the plasma concentration, and total drug exposure for the peritoneal cavity averaged 63-fold greater than that for the plasma.

Methotrexate

Chemistry

Methotrexate is an active drug in the first-line treatment of gestational choriocarcinoma, chorioadenoma destruens, and hydatidiform mole. It is used in the prophylaxis and treatment of meningeal leukemia, and is used in combination with other agents for the treatment of breast cancer, epidermoid cancers of the head and neck, advanced mycosis fungoides, advanced non-Hodgkin's lympoma, lung cancer, and metastatic squamous-cell cancer of the cervix. Methotrexate is a cell cycle–specific antifolate analog, which differs from folic acid in two substitutions: an amino group for a hydroxyl in the pteridine portion of the molecule and a methyl group on the amino nitrogen between the pteridine nucleus and the benzoyl group of 4-amino-10-methyl folic acid. Chemically, methotrexate is N-[4-[[(2,4-diamino-6-pteridinyl)methyl]-benzoyl]-L-glutamic acid. It is a weak acid with a molecular weight of 454.45 and a molecular formula of $C_{20}H_{22}N_8O_5$. It is only slightly soluble in water and alcohol. Sodium methotrexate is water soluble and is used in injectable preparations.

Mechanism of Action

Free intracellular methotrexate tightly binds to dihydrofolate reductase, blocking the reduction of dihydrofolate to tetrahydrofolic acid, the active form of folic acid. As a result, thymidylate synthetase and various steps in de novo purine synthesis that require 1-carbon transfer reactions are halted. This in turn arrests DNA, RNA, and protein synthesis.

Amino acid syntheses blocked by methotrexate include those requiring 1-carbon transfer, such as the conversion of glycine to serine and homocysteine to methionine. Experimental studies have shown that thymidylate synthetase is inhibited at methotrexate concentrations of 10^{-8} M or less, but inhibition of purine synthesis requires concentrations of 10^{-7} M or greater (370).

Methotrexate undergoes a variable degree of polyglutamation intracellularly. The polyglutamated forms of the drug are positively charged and do not readily pass through cell membranes. Methotrexate polyglutamates form an intracellular pool of active drug that is retained for long periods, sometimes months, after a single dose (371). The ability of tumor cells to add t-glutamyl residues to methotrexate may be a key determinant of antitumor activity.

The effects of methotrexate are rapidly reversible as free methotrexate leaves the cells. The normal intracellular levels of dihydrofolate are very low (10^{-8} M) but increase greatly after methotrexate administration.

Resistance to methotrexate may develop as a result of elevated dihydrofolate reductase activity or defective transport of methotrexate into malignant cells. Increased dihydrofolate reductase enzyme levels may also result from amplification of the dihydrofolate reductase gene, a process associated with homogeneously staining regions of chromosomes and an unstable inheritance mediated by double minutes or extra chromosomal DNA fragments (372). Certain quinazolines have been shown to be effective inhibitors of thymidylate synthetase and may be useful clinically in overcoming this type of resistance (373). In vitro studies and clinical experimentation with high-dose therapy indicate that a major mechanism of resistance is probably secondary to decreased cellular uptake.

Methotrexate is classified as a cell cycle phase–specific antimetabolite with activity mostly in S phase. Experimentally, methotrexate synchronizes tumor cells in S phase about 36 to 72 hours after administration (374).

The enhanced toxic effect on tumors compared with normal tissue from high-dose methotrexate with leucovorin rescue may be a result of bypassing normal carrier-mediated cell membrane transport of methotrexate. Leucovorin and its metabolite, 5-methyltetrahydrofolate, share a common influx transport site with methotrexate. There appear to be at least two active transport carrier systems involved in the influx and efflux of methotrexate and folates (375). If normal cells are rescued with calcium leucovorin, methotrexate can then exert a relatively greater toxic effect on the tumor cells. Selective rescue of normal cells may be mediated by a slower rate of DNA synthesis relative to the tumor cell or to tissue-specific differences in transmembrane transport.

Drug Disposition

Orally administered methotrexate is rapidly but incompletely absorbed from the gastrointestinal tract. It reaches peak blood levels in approximately 1 hour. Approximately 50% to 60% of the drug in the blood is bound to plasma proteins. Methotrexate is widely distributed to body tissues. In conventional doses, methotrexate is excreted unchanged in the urine. In high doses, it is partially metabolized to 7-hydromethotrexate, which is only slightly soluble in acidic solutions. About 1% to 11% of a dose is excreted as the 7-hydroxy metabolite, and this may comprise as much as 35% of the drug level in the terminal elimination phase. Only about one-third of an oral dose is absorbed, but intramuscular absorption is almost 100% (376).

The hepatic extraction coefficient for methotrexate appears to be very low and intraarterial hepatic doses show metabolism and pharmacokinetics similar to IV doses (377). Methotrexate is both filtered at the glomerulus and actively secreted by the renal tubule. Drugs that interfere with renal excretion of weak acids, such as probenecid, sulfinpyrazone, and salicylates, may be expected to reduce the rate of methotrexate excretion. Probenecid has been used successfully in one study to produce a prolonged elevation of plasma methotrexate levels from otherwise low doses of methotrexate (378).

Plasma decay of methotrexate levels have been reported to be biphasic and possibly triphasic. Huffman and associates (379) reported half-lives after a 30 mg/m^2 dose to be triphasic: 0.750 ± 0.11, 3.49 ± 0.55, and 26.99 ± 4.44 hours, respectively. Stoller and colleagues (380) reported a biphasic plasma decay for high-dose therapy of 2.06 ± 0.16 and 10.4 ± 1.8 hours. Wang and co-researchers (381) reported age-dependent biphasic elimination of high-dose methotrexate.

Patients with pleural effusions may accumulate methotrexate that slowly distributes from this compartment back into the plasma to increase systemic exposure and the risk of toxicity (382). Effusions should be drained before administration of methotrexate.

Administration and Dosage

Methotrexate may be given by the oral, intramuscular, intravenous (intravenous infusion or push), intraarterial, or intrathecal routes. For treatment of neoplastic disease, oral administration of low-dose methotrexate is preferred owing to the rapid absorption of the tablet form of the agent. Methotrexate has been given by numerous dosing schedules. The usual starting doses are adjusted based on clinical response and hematologic monitoring. In general, methotrexate is administered orally or intramuscularly in doses of 15 to 30 mg daily for a 5-day course. Courses are usually repeated for three to five times as required, with rest periods of 1 or more weeks between courses until toxicities subside (383). Leucovorin is indicated following treatment with higher doses of methotrexate to diminish toxicity.

If the IV formulation is administered, the dose should be reduced by 50% for patients with renal insufficiency (BUN $\geq$30 mg/L). Similar dose reductions should be made for the oral form, although no specific guidelines are available. Methotrexate administration is contraindicated in patients with a creatinine clearance less than 40 mL/min and/or a serum creatinine greater than 2 mg/dL.

Side Effects and Toxicities

Hematologic effects of methotrexate include leukopenia, thrombocytopenia, and anemia. They occur rapidly and depend on the dose and schedule used. The nadir of hemoglobin depression occurs after 6 to 13 days and of reticulocyte at 2 to 7 days, with rebound between 9 and 19 days.

Leukocyte nadir occurs within 4 to 7 days, followed by partial recovery and then, in rare instances, a second decrease in the leukocyte counts occurs during days 12 to 21. The platelet nadir is reached in 5 to 12 days. Hypogammaglobulinemia may also occur after methotrexate administration.

Nausea, vomiting, and anorexia are usually the earliest gastrointestinal symptoms. Gingivitis, glossitis, pharyngitis, stomatitis, and ulcerations with bleeding of the mucosal membranes of the mouth or other portions of the gastrointestinal tract may occur. If ulcerative stomatitis or diarrhea occurs, methotrexate therapy must be interrupted to prevent severe hemorrhagic enteritis or intestinal perforation.

Hepatotoxicity is more common in patients receiving high-dose therapy and in those receiving frequent small doses. Hepatocellular injury is indicated in liver function tests by a rise in serum glutamic oxaloacetic transaminase (SGOT) and serum glutamic pyruvic transaminase (SGPT), usually within the first 12 hours. Prothrombin times may rise with a decrease in plasma factor VII activity, and indirect hyperbilirubinemia may develop. All of these usually return to normal within 1 week. Hepatocytes appear to be protected by fractionated high-dose methotrexate treatments with leucovorin rescue if treatments are administered at intervals of less than 1 week. This may be due to leucovorin activity remaining from prior doses. Various pathologic hepatic changes can occur, including atrophy, necrosis, fatty changes, fibrosis, and cirrhosis. Liver biopsy is the only reliable means of assessing the degree of methotrexate hepatotoxicity.

Dermatologic side effects include erythematous rashes, pruritus, urticaria, folliculitis, vasculitis, photosensitivity, depigmentation, or hyperpigmentation. Alopecia may occur, with several months being required for regrowth.

CNS effects include dizziness, malaise, and blurred vision. Encephalopathy also has been reported. Intrathecal administration has been followed by increased CSF pressure, convulsions, paresis, and a syndrome resembling the Guillain-Barré syndrome (384). Deaths have been reported after intrathecal therapy.

Renal failure may occur in patients receiving methotrexate, especially in high doses. This risk may be decreased by alkalinization of the urine to increase methotrexate solubility and by giving large quantities of fluid.

Other reactions rarely reported include chills and fever, osteoporosis, and pulmonary reactions, mainly fibrosis (385).

Drug Interactions

Potential drug interactions have been postulated to occur with other protein-bound drugs, such as salicylates, sulfonamides, phenytoin, and p-aminobenzoic acid. These drugs displace methotrexate from its protein-binding site in the blood, causing an increase in the levels of the free drug. However, the overall degree of binding is probably not high enough for major displacement interactions.

Antibiotics used in gut sterilization may also alter methotrexate pharmacokinetics in humans, eliminating the slow phase of excretion (386). Salicylates and probenecid may also compete with methotrexate for renal tubular secretion and increase its serum half-life.

Ethyl alcohol may increase the possibility of methotrexate-induced hepatotoxicity. Oral anticoagulants, such as warfarin, may be greatly potentiated by methotrexate. Methotrexate may alter the liver metabolism of these drugs.

There are several drug interactions described for methotrexate with other chemotherapeutic agents. For example, a clinically significant interaction between methotrexate and L-asparaginase involves the administration of methotrexate 3 to 24 hours before L-asparaginase. The methotrexate treatment is believed to block protein synthesis and reduce asparaginase toxicities, allowing larger doses to be given. Some sequential methotrexate combinations may produce enhanced therapeutic activity. For example, methotrexate given 4 to 9 hours before 5-FU may produce enhanced antitumor activity in breast cancer, but with a commensurate increase in toxic effects (132,387). The mechanism of this interaction involves a significant increase in 5-FU for at least 3 hours (387). The reverse sequence decreases therapeutic activity (388).

Methotrexate activity is enhanced, and thus toxicity increased, when it is used with aspirin, penicillins, nonsteroidal antiinflammatory agents, cephalosporins, or phenytoin. These agents inhibit the renal excretion of methotrexate (46).

Special Applications

Very high doses of methotrexate have been administered for a variety of tumors. Although leucovorin rescue reduces toxicity, it is still not certain that high-dose therapy is superior to more conventional dosing without rescue. Specific dosing schemes vary, but a high dose of methotrexate is usually administered intravenously and followed by calcium leucovorin 24 to 36 hours after initiation of therapy to prevent toxicity. Table 16.6 presents specific dosing recommendations.

The dose range of methotrexate with leucovorin rescue is 100 mg/m^2 to 10 g/m^2 given every 1 to 3 weeks. The lower end of this dosing spectrum has been administered in four divided oral doses over a 24-hour period. Most frequently, the dose is given by IV infusion in 1 to 2 L of fluid as a rapid infusion or over 6 to 24 hours. Higher peak methotrexate levels occur with more rapid IV infusions, and this may be theoretically more efficacious. There does not appear to be a clinical difference in toxicity between rapid and prolonged infusions. Only the 500- and 1,000-mg vials with no preservative should be used for this purpose. Further dilution of methotrexate is necessary and can be accomplished with normal saline or D$_5$W.

TABLE 16.6. *Determination of leucovorin dose for high-dose methotrexate (50–250 mg/kg over 6 h) regimens[a]*

Plasma methotrexate concentration at 48 h (M)	Leucovorin administration	
	mg/m² of leucovorin every 8 h	No. of doses of leucovorin
$<5 \times 10^{-7}$	15	7
5×10^{-7}	15	8
1×10^{-6}	100	8
2×10^{-6}	100	8

[a] Plasma methotrexate concentration at 96 h should be determined also. If the plasma concentration at 96 h is $\geq 5 \times 10^{-6}$ M, the previously used leucovorin regimen should be continued until the plasma methotrexate concentration is $\leq 5 \times 10^{-7}$ M. All patients should also be prehydrated for 12 h to establish an alkaline diuresis using 1.5 L/m² of fluid containing 10 mEq of bicarbonate and 20 mEq of KCl (pH of urine should be 7.0).

High-dose methotrexate has been associated with reversible nephrotoxicity. At high concentrations, methotrexate may precipitate in the renal tubule, causing tubular dilatation and damage. The pK_a of methotrexate is 5.4. When the urine pH is near this value, methotrexate exists predominantly in its insoluble form and is likely to precipitate. Renal toxicity may be prevented by increasing urine alkalinity and flow. Sodium bicarbonate (3 g every 3 hours for 12 hours before therapy) is usually sufficient to induce an alkaline urine in adults. The sodium bicarbonate should be continued with frequent urine pH checks during the therapy and for 48 hours after the dose has been delivered. Methotrexate serum levels are useful in predicting toxic reactions and appropriately adjusting rescue doses of leucovorin (389,390). High-dose methotrexate with rescue is complicated and potentially extremely toxic. Only experienced teams using carefully designed protocols should attempt this treatment. Immediate methotrexate levels should be readily available. Fatal renal or hematologic reactions have occurred at major treatment centers despite the prophylactic precautions described (391).

Mitomycin

Chemistry

Mitomycin (Mutamycin, mitomycin C) is a purple antibiotic isolated from *Streptomyces caespitosus* that is indicated for disseminated adenocarcinoma of the stomach or pancreas in combination with other agents and as palliative treatment. It has also has been proven to be useful in combination chemotherapy as a third-line agent in the treatment of advanced cervical cancer. Its chemical name is [1*a*R]-6-amino-8-[[(aminocarbonyl)oxy]methyl]- 1,1*a*,2,8,8*a*,8*b*-hexahydro-8*a*-methoxy-5- methylazirino[2′,3′:3,4]-pyrrolo[1,2-*a*]indole-4,7-dione, and it has a molecular weight of

334. Mitomycin is heat stable, is soluble in water and other organic solvents, and has a unique absorption peak at 365 nM (392). In solution, it is slowly inactivated by visible but not ultraviolet light. It is very unstable in acidic and highly basic conditions. The aziridine and carbamate groups on mitomycin are necessary for alkylating activity but not for antibacterial activity. The compound is activated by reduction of the quinone moiety, which releases a methanol residue from the molecule. This allows the aziridine ring to open, exposing an electrophilic carbon at C_1 (alkylating site). The second (cross-linking) site for alkylation is exposed at C_{10} after an enzymatic or chemically mediated loss of the carbamate side chain.

Mechanism of Action

Mitomycin is activated *in vivo* to an alkylating agent that cross links complementary DNA strands, halting DNA synthesis. DNA is the major site of mitomycin activity, although at extremely high concentrations, RNA synthesis may also be affected. The active metabolites of mitomycin resulting from reduction of the quinone moiety yield an opened aziridine ring exposing the primary alkylating site at C_1. A second alkylating site at C_{10} is exposed with the enzymatic loss of the carbamate side chain (393). The molecular site of DNA binding has been identified at the N_2 and O_6 positions of adjacent guanines in the minor groove of DNA (394).

Activation of the drug can be mediated by chemical reducing agents, by microsomal enzymes, or even by brief exposure to an acidic pH. The extent of DNA binding appears to be related to the guanine and cytosine content of the particular DNA. Cytotoxicity probably results directly from DNA synthesis inhibition secondary to alkylation.

Oxygen free radicals may also contribute to the cytotoxicity of mitomycin by producing DNA strand breaks (395). Oxygen free radicals are produced by cyclic redox reactions of the quinone moiety. Mitomycin's cytotoxic action is not cell cycle phase–specific, but cytotoxic effects are maximized if cells are treated in late G_1 and early S phase. In addition to the direct cytotoxic effects of the drug, mitomycin also causes chromosomal aberrations (mutagenic activity), and in experimental systems, it is a potent carcinogen and teratogen.

Kennedy and co-workers (396) described selective activation of mitomycin by hypoxic cells, suggesting some drug selectivity for hypoxic tumors. Resistance to mitomycin involves an increase in specific cytosolic proteins (possibly a glutathione transferase) and collateral resistance with anthracyclines and dactinomycin (397,398). The latter type of multidrug resistance is mediated by P-glycoprotein expression, with resultant enhanced drug efflux, as observed in mitomycin C–resistant L-1210 cells (399).

Drug Disposition

Mitomycin is cleared rapidly from the vascular compartment. Peak serum concentrations of about 1 μg/mL are typically achieved after IV bolus doses of 10 mg/m^2 (400). Less than 10% of the dose is excreted into the urine, and this is complete within a few hours after administration. Mitomycin also has been detected in the bile and feces, although animal studies demonstrate that the highest drug levels occur in the kidneys. Detectable levels were also found in muscle, lung, intestine, stomach, and eye, but not in the brain, spleen, or liver (392).

The primary means of mitomycin elimination is by liver metabolism, but the specific enzymes responsible are unknown. However, the enzymes responsible for metabolism do not appear to involve the P450 mixed-function oxide family. *In vitro* studies demonstrate drug inactivation on contact with tissue preparations from the spleen, liver, kidney, brain, and heart. This inactivation is further augmented by anaerobic conditions (392).

There is no detectable change in mitomycin pharmacokinetics in patients with altered hepatic function nor when other drugs, including furosemide, are given concurrently (400,401). Schilcher and colleagues (402) showed that the pharmacokinetics of mitomycin do not change after the administration of high doses.

Mitomycin distribution into bile and ascites fluids has been quantitated in patients receiving standard IV doses. The maximum biliary level of 0.5 μg/mL was achieved after 2 hours and was five- to eightfold higher than simultaneous plasma levels during the elimination phase (403). Mitomycin also rapidly penetrates into ascites fluid and reaches maximal concentrations of 0.05 μg/mL 1 hour after administration. This distribution represents about 40% of the total plasma exposure. The drug also appears to slightly concentrate in cervical tissues after IV administration (404).

With intraarterial administration, the hepatic extraction of mitomycin averages only 23% (405). The calculated relative advantage for hepatic arterial infusions is only 2.5- to 3.6-fold greater than for other methods.

Administration and Dosage

Sterile water (10 mL) should be added to each 5-mg vial of mitomycin and shaken gently to dissolve. Mitomycin should be administered intravenously to avoid extravasation of the drug. If extravasation occurs, severe local tissue necrosis may occur (406). The drug is usually given by a slow IV push, with continuous patient monitoring to lessen the chance of extravasation. Short infusions in 100 to 150 mL of D$_5$W or normal saline have also been used. Vein patency should be checked before the administration of any dose, using 5 to 10 mL of fluid that does not contain the drug. The same procedure should follow the dose. This flushes any remaining drug from the tubing and the venipuncture site.

The recommended dose of mitomycin used as a single agent is 20 mg/m^2 given IV every 6 to 8 weeks. In combination with other myelosuppressive drugs, mitomycin doses are typically limited to 10 mg/m^2 every 6 to 8 weeks. Bolus doses greater than 20 mg/m^2 produce severe toxicity without greatly enhancing efficacy.

Repeat dosing of mitomycin should be based on adequate marrow recovery, including leukocytes, platelets, and erythrocytes. Leukocyte count should return to 4,000/mm^3 and platelet count to 100,000/mm^3.

An ambulatory continuous infusion of mitomycin has been administered at 0.75 mg/m^2/day for consecutive 50-day dosing (407). A dosing regimen of 3 mg/m^2/day for 5 days every 4 to 6 weeks has also been used (407). These regimens are believed to deliver greater dose intensity by reducing myelosuppression. Intraarterial perfusion doses of 20 mg/m^2 have been given every 6 to 8 weeks (408).

Side Effects and Toxicities

Bone marrow suppression involving platelets, leukocytes, and erythrocytes is the most serious toxicity, and it can continue for 3 to 8 weeks after drug administration is halted (392). Myelosuppression, particularly anemia, can be cumulative. This has been minimized by keeping total lifetime doses under 50 to 60 mg/m^2.

Gastrointestinal disturbances in the form of nausea, vomiting, and anorexia occasionally develop. These reactions are usually not severe and have an onset within 1 to 2 hours after administration. They may persist for several hours. Stomatitis may also occur, but it is generally not severe.

Renal toxicity detected by increasing serum BUN and creatinine levels with glomerular dysfunction is occasionally seen. This does not appear to be dose- or treatment-duration related, and it is usually not severe. However, mitomycin can also induce a microangiopathic hemolytic anemia with progressive renal failure (hemolytic-uremic syndrome) and cardiopulmonary decompensation. This disease is fatal within 3 to 4 weeks of diagnosis, although the onset is typically delayed for months after mitomycin administration (409). The incidence of this toxic effect may approach 10% among patients given large cumulative doses (409). In one series, renal complications from mitomycin developed in 1.6% of 63 patients receiving a total dose of 50 mg/m^2 or less, 11% of 37 patients receiving 50 to 69 mg/m^2, and 28% of 18 patients receiving total doses greater than 70 mg/m^2 (410). This suggests that a threshold for inducing microangiopathic hemolytic anemia may be a cumulative dose of about 50 mg/m^2 of mitomycin. Signs of the disease include thrombocytopenia, circulating schistocytes, and acute renal failure. Histopathologic examinations of the kidneys reveal fibrin thrombi in arterioles, tubular atrophy, and widespread glomerular necrosis. There are now several cases of successful treatment with serial transfusions over protein A columns (411).

Veno-occlusive disease of the liver has been reported after high-dose mitomycin therapy and autologous bone marrow transplantation (412). Signs include progressive hepatic dysfunction, abdominal pain, and ascites. Although this rarely has been observed with low-dose therapy, it appears to be much more frequent after high-dose regimens.

Alopecia may occur after mitomycin therapy, but it is usually not severe. Rarely, purple bands in the nail beds correspond to sequential doses of the drug. Lethargy or weakness may occur and can last from several days to 3 weeks. Fatigue and some drowsiness or confusion have also been observed. Dose-related skin reactions and fever with drug administration are occasionally seen.

Severe soft tissue ulcers may also be expected if the drug escapes the vein during administration. Mitomycin extravasation injuries can result in chronic ulcers that can expand over months (406). Particularly distressing aspects of some mitomycin extravasations include the delayed (3 to 4 months) and sometimes distal occurrence of a soft tissue ulceration after uneventful injections in a peripheral vein (413,414). In animals, the only effective antidote to mitomycin skin reactions was topical DMSO (99% DMSO). Mitomycin extravasations may be empirically treated with topical application of 1.5 mL of DMSO every 6 hours for 14 days (415).

Interstitial pneumonia thought to be secondary to mitomycin has been reported for a small number of patients. These patients showed rapid improvement after treatment with corticosteroids (416).

Special Precautions

Myelosuppression may be cumulative with successive doses of mitomycin and may necessitate dose reductions. Careful monitoring of blood counts is critical. Serious local ulceration may occur if the drug is delivered outside the vein. Extravasation of mitomycin must be avoided.

Clinically significant antitumor drug synergy in humans has yet to be described for mitomycin, although it is probably at least additive in several drug combinations, including the FAM regimen (5-FU, doxorubicin, mitomycin) used in gastrointestinal cancer, the MOB regimen [mitomycin, vincristine (Oncovin), bleomycin] used in carcinoma of the uterine cervix, and megestrol acetate in patients with advanced breast cancer.

Special Applications

Mitomycin and intraperitoneal hyperthermia were combined to treat prophylactically patients with gastric cancer (417). Mitomycin (8 to 100 μg/mL) was administered continuously in bags containing 2,000 mL of heated (40 to 45°C) saline solution. The total perfusion was 8 to 12 L over 50 to 60 minutes, comprising a mitomycin C dose of 64 to 100 mg. Low peak plasma levels (0.1 μg/mL) were produced, and approximately 39% of the administered dose was retained intraperitoneally. The half-lives of mitomycin C in the perfusate are 10 to 17 minutes (α) and 70 to 120 minutes

(β) (418). Serum protein levels decreased significantly during and after the procedure, indicating that serum protein reaccumulates in the peritoneal space.

Mitomycin (5 to 10 mg) has also been given every 28 days combined with cisplatin (100 mg/m^2) using the intraperitoneal route. Mitomycin was always given 1 week after cisplatin, and the dose was diluted in 2 L of normal saline. In 11 patients with malignant peritoneal mesothelioma, 5 of 8 previously untreated patients had reduced fluid reaccumulation lasting from 2 to 32 months (median 5 months) (218). The major toxic reaction was pain, and catheter failure was related to the intraperitoneal mitomycin.

Oxaliplatin

Chemistry

Oxaliplatin (Eloxatin, diaminocyclohexane platinum, DACH platinum) is a third-generation platinum with the molecular formula $C_8H_{14}N_2O_4Pt$ and the chemical name of cis-[(1R,2R)-1,2-cyclohexanediamine-N,N'][oxalato(2-)-O,O']platinum, and it has a molecular weight of 397.3. Oxaliplatin is an organoplatinum complex in which the platinum atom is complexed with 1,2-diaminocyclohexane (DACH) and with an oxalate ligand as a leaving group. Oxaliplatin is slightly soluble in water (6 mg/mL), slightly soluble in methanol, and practically insoluble in ethanol and acetone. It is FDA approved for second-line treatment in metastatic colorectal cancer in combination with fluoropyrimidines.

Mechanism of Action

Oxaliplatin binds to DNA in a manner similar to cisplatin, in that it binds to repeating deoxyguanosines d(GpG) in a single DNA strand. It reacts with DNA to produce intrastrand cross links (>90%) at adenine-guanine d(ApC) sites and to produce intrastrand cross links (<5%) with guanosines of opposing DNA strands $(dG)_2$ (46,126). This results in inhibition of DNA synthesis, function, and transcription. Oxaliplatin reacts more rapidly with DNA to form these interlinks and intralinks (e.g., within 15 minutes) than the other platinum agents (12 hours for cisplatin and over 24 hours for carboplatin) (126). Furthermore, unlike the other platinum-DNA adducts, mismatch repair enzymes are unable to recognize the adducts formed by oxaliplatin because of their bulkier size (46).

Drug Disposition

In a summary of pharmacokinetic studies, plasma platinum C_{max} values have been shown to be in the range of 2.59 to 3.22 μg/mL, and mean AUC_{0-48h} in the range of 50.4 to 71.5 μg/ mL · hour after an oxaliplatin dose of 130 mg/m^2 (2-hour infusion) (419). Intrapatient and interpatient variability was moderate to low (23% and 6%, respectively) (420). In

1-hour infusion studies, mean plasma platinum C_{max} and AUC_{0-24h} increased in a dose-dependent fashion up to 180 mg/m^2. The pharmacokinetics of platinum in ultrafiltrate after administration of oxaliplatin are triphasic and characterized by short α (0.28 hour) and β (16.3 hours) distribution phases, which are followed by a long terminal γ phase (273 hours) (419). Oxaliplatin is primarily cleared from plasma by renal excretion (53.8%) and covalent tissue binding. Clearance is not affected by age, gender, or hepatic impairment (419).

Administration and Dosage

Reconstitute oxaliplatin by adding 10 mL sterile water for each 50-mg vial, or dextrose (5%). The solution must be further diluted in 250 to 500 mL of 5% dextrose prior to administration. The infusion line should be flushed with D_5W prior to administration of any concomitant medication (420). Premedication with antiemetics is recommended.

The recommended dose for metastatic colorectal cancer is as follows: on day 1 of every 2-week cycle, oxaliplatin (85 mg/m^2) is generally administered intravenously with leucovorin (200 mg/m^2) over 120 minutes at the same time in two separate bags using a Y-line, followed by 5-FU (400 mg/m^2 IV bolus), followed by 5-FU (600 mg/m^2) in 500 mL D_5W as a 22-hour continuous infusion. On day 2, the patient should receive leucovorin (200 mg/m^2) over 120 minutes at the same time in two separate bags using a Y-line, followed by 5-FU (400 mg/m^2 IV bolus), followed by 5-FU (600 mg/m^2) in 500 mL D_5W as a 22-hour continuous infusion.

In Phase II trials for gynecologic cancers, the recommended dose of oxaliplatin is 130 mg/m^2 intravenously over 2 hours every 21 days (421,422).

Side Effects and Toxicities

Oxaliplatin produces dose-limiting peripheral neuropathy and gastrointestinal and hematologic adverse events. Neurotoxic symptoms usually resolve within a week of stopping therapy; however, symptom intensity is cumulative with repeated courses of oxaliplatin (126,420,423). Other common adverse events include mild leukopenia and mild to moderate thrombocytopenia. Nausea and vomiting are common, and antiemetic prophylaxis is required with oxaliplatin therapy.

Unlike other platinum-containing agents, oxaliplatin is not associated with nephrotoxicity. Alopecia has not been reported with oxaliplatin.

Special Applications

Oxaliplatin is an agent with substantial activity in platinum-sensitive ovarian cancer patients previously treated with cisplatin. Bougnoux and colleagues (424) noted two complete and eight partial responses in 24 patients who were platinum sensitive (41.7% response rate). Similar findings

were seen in a more recent phase II study, which also saw a 42% response rate in platinum-sensitive patients (425). Chollet and colleagues (426) studied similar populations of patients and noted six responses in 13 platinum-sensitive patients (46%) and a 17% response rate (3 of 18 patients) in platinum-resistant patients. Recent Phase II studies have seen only minimal activity in platinum-resistant patients (less than 6% response rate) (421,425).

Paclitaxel

Chemistry

Paclitaxel (Taxol) is one of the most commonly used drugs in oncology, with FDA approval for primary or salvage therapy for epithelial ovarian cancer, as salvage therapy for metastatic breast cancer, in second-line treatment of AIDS-related Kaposi's sarcoma, and in the treatment of non–small-cell lung cancer. It is also active against a variety of other solid tumors, including cervical and endometrial cancer (427,428). It is a diterpene plant product derived from the bark of the Pacific yew, *Taxus baccata.* It has a molecular weight of 853.9, is insoluble in water, and has an empiric formula of $C_{47}H_{51}NO_{14}$. Its chemical name is 5β,20-epoxy-1,2α,4,7β,10β,13α-hexahydroxytax-11-en-9-one4,10-diacetate 2-benzoate 13-ester with (2R,3S)-N-benzoyl-3-phenylisoserine.

Mechanism of Action

Paclitaxel acts as a mitotic spindle poison. In a manner contrary to known mitotic spindle inhibitors, such as colchicine and podophyllotoxin, paclitaxel promotes assembly of microtubules and stabilizes them, preventing depolymerization. This inability to depolymerize microtubules prevents cellular replication (116).

Drug Disposition

Early pharmacokinetic studies using standard doses and a 24-hour infusion suggested that paclitaxel pharmacokinetics were linear; however, with short infusions and/or high dose levels, paclitaxel's nonlinear pharmacokinetics become readily apparent (160). The nonlinearity is due to saturable distribution, metabolism, and elimination. Terminal elimination half-life is largely dependent on the dose and administration schedule. At a dose level of 175 mg/m^2 with a 3-hour infusion, mean pharmacokinetic parameters of paclitaxel include the following: plasma $t_{1/2\alpha}$, 16 minutes; plasma $t_{1/2\beta}$, 140 minutes; plasma $t_{1/2\gamma}$, 18.75 hours; plasma clearance, 12.69 L/h/m^2; plasma AUC, 16.81 μmol/L · hour; 48-hour urinary excretion, <10% of dose; and 48-hour fecal excretion, 70% of dose (160).

Clearance is rapid and not due to urinary excretion; the major route of paclitaxel elimination is believed to be via hepatic metabolism and subsequent biliary excretion (429). About 70% to 80% of the drug is eliminated by fecal excretion.

Administration and Dosage

All patients undergoing paclitaxel therapy should receive premedication to prevent severe hypersensitivity reactions. A recommended regimen is dexamethasone (either 20 mg orally the night before treatment and the morning of treatment or 20 mg IV 30 minutes before paclitaxel delivery) plus diphenhydramine (50 mg) and famotidine (20 mg) IV 30 minutes before chemotherapy (430). For the majority of patients, administration of dexamethasone 20 mg IV 30 to 60 minutes before paclitaxel is sufficient and has beeb proven to be effective in preventing hypersensitivity reactions.

Paclitaxel is commercially available as an injection concentrate in 30-mg (5 mL), 100-mg (16.7 mL), and 300-mg (50 mL) multidose vials. Before infusion, paclitaxel must be diluted with 0.9% sodium chloride, 5% dextrose, 5% dextrose and 0.9% sodium chloride injection, or 5% dextrose in Ringer's injection to a final concentration of 0.3 to 1.2 mg/mL. The solution is stable for up to 27 hours at room temperature. Paclitaxel should be administered through an in-line filter with a microporous membrane not greater than $0.22\ \mu$ to remove particulates that are present in paclitaxel solutions. Although particulate formation does not indicate loss of drug potency, solutions exhibiting excess particulate matter formation should be discarded. Because of the possibility of leaching of phthalate plasticizers with paclitaxel solutions, only nonpolyvinylchloride (such as polyethylene or polyolefin) IV administration sets should be used.

As a result of an unacceptable level of severe hypersensitivity reactions in early Phase I studies (most likely related to the Cremaphor EL vehicle), a 24-hour infusion schedule and a premedication regimen with corticosteroids and histamine H_1- and H_2-antagonists were used in all Phase II and III clinical trials conducted in the United States from 1987 to 1992. Later clinical studies established that a 3-hour paclitaxel infusion schedule can be administered safely without a significant increase in major hypersensitivity reactions and that the shortened infusion schedule is associated with significantly less grade 4 neutropenia than the 24-hour infusion (i.e., 71% vs 18% for the 24- and 3-hour infusions, respectively) (431). Follow-up studies have determined that a 1-hour infusion schedule also is feasible; however, infusion durations less than 1 hour are associated with a prohibitively high rate of hypersensitivity reactions (432).

There were early concerns that the shorter infusion schedules might be associated with a decline in efficacy. However, results from GOG-158, a Phase III, randomized study in women with optimal disease, advanced ovarian cancer, revealed that paclitaxel 175 mg/m² by 3-hour infusion combined with carboplatin (targeted AUC of 7.5) (arm II) had similar activity with less toxicity than paclitaxel 135 mg/m²

by 24-hour infusion plus cisplatin 75 mg/m² (arm I) (433). Median progression-free survival and overall survival were 19.4 and 48.7 months, respectively, for arm I (paclitaxel-cisplatin) compared with 20.7 and 57.4 months, respectively, for arm II (paclitaxel-carboplatin). Because of its ease of administration and lower toxicity profile (cisplatin plus short-infusion paclitaxel is associated with dose-limiting neurotoxicity), the recommended primary chemotherapy regimen for advanced ovarian cancer is paclitaxel 175 mg/m² by 3-hour infusion plus carboplatin (targeted AUC of 6.0 to 7.5) every 21 days for six cycles (433). Although this generally is a well-tolerated regimen, neurosensory toxicity and prolonged thrombocytopenia can prove to be dose limiting. The FDA-approved regimen for first-line treatment of ovarian cancer is paclitaxel 135 mg/m² over 24 hours plus cisplatin 75 mg/m² every 21 days for six cycles or paclitaxel 175 mg/m² over 4 hours plus cisplatin 75 mg/m².

The FDA-approved recommended regimen for salvage therapy for patients with platinum-refractory ovarian cancer is paclitaxel 135 or 175 mg/m² administered IV over 3 hours every 3 weeks, but the optimal regimen has not clearly been established. Paclitaxel has been administered by various other schedules during investigational studies in patients with solid tumors, including 135 to 250 mg/m² as a 24-hour continuous infusion every 3 weeks; 212 to 225 mg/m² as a 6-hour infusion every 3 weeks; 30 mg/m² as a 1-hour infusion daily for 5 days every 3 weeks; 30 mg/m² as a 6-hour infusion daily for 5 days every 3 weeks; 120 to 140 mg/m² as a 96-hour infusion every 3 weeks; and 150 mg/m² as a 120-hour infusion every 3 weeks (116).

Special Precautions

Before the institution of standard prophylactic medications, the incidence of major hypersensitivity reactions associated with paclitaxel therapy approached 25% to 30%. With premedication, the incidence of severe hypersensitivity reactions has decreased to less than 2%. The majority of paclitaxel-induced hypersensitivity reactions can be categorized as grade 1, with symptoms of dyspnea with bronchospasm, urticaria, and hypotension. Major sensitivity reactions usually occur within the first 10 minutes after the first or second dose of paclitaxel (116). Minor symptoms of flushing and rashes are not predictive of the future development of severe manifestations (116,431). According to National Cancer Institute guidelines for paclitaxel administration, emergency equipment must be available and medical personnel should be in attendance during paclitaxel infusion, especially during the first 15 minutes of the first and second courses. Vital signs should be periodically monitored during the first several hours of drug infusion. The paclitaxel infusion should be discontinued immediately if symptoms of a major hypersensitivity reaction occur (including respiratory distress, hypotension, generalized urticaria, and angioedema). Severe hypersensitivity reactions may be treated with IV epinephrine, IV diphenhydramine, IV fluids, and nebulized beta-agonists. Steroid therapy may be helpful in the resolution of recurrent symptoms (434). There is strong evidence that patients who develop major hypersensitivity reactions may be successfully retreated with slow, low-dose infusions of paclitaxel after premedication with multiple high doses of corticosteroids and antihistamines (435).

Drug Interactions

Paclitaxel therapy appears to modify the hematologic toxicity associated with platinum agents. Rowinsky et al. (436) conducted a Phase I study of sequential escalating doses of paclitaxel and cisplatin therapy and determined that myelosuppression was more severe when paclitaxel was administered immediately after cisplatin therapy than when given prior to cisplatin.

Concomitant medications that contain substrates or inhibitors of hepatic enzymes, principally cytochrome P450 isoenzymes CYP_2C_8 and CYP_3A_4, may increase paclitaxel clearance, and caution should be exercised when administering paclitaxel. In a study by Chang et al. (437), the pharmacokinetics of paclitaxel were significantly altered by the concomitant use of anticonvulsants (i.e., phenytoin, carbamazapine, and phenobarbital), and the maximum tolerated doses of paclitaxel in malignant glioma patients were 360 mg/m^2 for those on anticonvulsant therapy versus 240 mg/m^2 for those not receiving anticonvulsants. There was also a significant difference in paclitaxel metabolite and toxicity profiles between the two groups. Central neurotoxicity, rather than neutropenia, was the dose-limiting toxicity in patients on anticonvulsant therapy who received paclitaxel at a dose greater than 350 mg/m^2.

Special Applications

Paclitaxel is a particularly promising agent for intraperitoneal administration, in that this route of drug delivery results in a more than 3-log increased exposure of the peritoneal cavity relative to systemic circulation. Additionally, potentially cytotoxic levels of paclitaxel remain in the peritoneal cavity for 5 to 7 days following intraperitoneal (IP) administration, and thus weekly intraperitoneal treatment results in continuous drug exposure (438). A Phase II study in women with ovarian, fallopian, or peritoneal cancer and small-volume residual disease following primary chemotherapy has shown that IP paclitaxel has significant activity as evidenced by a 61% surgically defined complete response rate (439). Recent Phase II and Phase III trials of IP paclitaxel in stage III, optimal ovarian cancer patients conducted by the SWOG and the GOG have demonstrated a progression-free and overall survival benefit to IP therapy (4,5). Combined IP/IV therapy with cisplatin and paclitaxel remains a promising strategy for the treatment of ovarian cancer (4,440,441).

Paclitaxel has demonstrated activity against both endome-

trial and cervical cancers (442). Woo and colleagues (443) reported a 43% response rate to paclitaxel (95% CI: 6% to 80%) in seven patients with advanced, progressive, or recurrent endometrial cancer following platinum analog treatment. A GOG study noted a 14.3% complete and 21.4% partial response rate in 28 evaluable patients with endometrial cancer not previously treated with chemotherapy (444). Leukopenia was the most prominent side effect noted. A response rate of 37% (95% CI: 16% to 62%) was reported in 19 patients pretreated with cisplatin, doxorubicin, and cyclophosphamide (445). A GOG phase II trial of paclitaxel (3-hour infusion of 200 mg/m^2 every 21 days or 175 mg/m^2 for patients with prior pelvic radiation therapy) found a 27.3% response rate (95% CI: 15% to 42.8%) in 44 persistent or recurrent endometrial cancer patients who failed prior chemotherapy (428).

A GOG Phase II trial of single-agent paclitaxel in advanced cervix cancer has demonstrated a response rate of 31% (427). Trials of combination cisplatin-paclitaxel (IV paclitaxel 175 mg/m^2 by 3-hour infusion followed by cisplatin 75 mg/m^2) in metastatic and recurrent cervical cancer show moderate activity (47% response rate; 95% CI: 30% to 65%) (446). A similar response rate (45%) was seen in another Phase II trial of first-line therapy of advanced cervical cancer (IV paclitaxel 135 mg/m^2 by 24-hour infusion followed by cisplatin 75 mg/m^2 every 28 days) (447).

Topotecan

Chemistry

Topotecan (Hycamtin, topotecan hydrochloride) was approved by the FDA in 1996 for treatment of ovarian cancer patients after failure of primary chemotherapy. It is also indicated in the treatment of small-cell lung cancer after failure of first-line chemotherapy. Topotecan is a semisynthetic analog of camptothecin. The parent compound is derived from the bark of an ornamental tree native to Asia, *Camptotheca acuminata*. Sodium camptothecin was studied in clinical trials in the late 1960s through the early 1970s. However, clinical development of this agent was halted despite evidence of a variety of tumor responses because of severe and unpredictable toxicities (e.g., myelosuppression and hemorrhagic cystitis) (448). Topotecan and other camptothecin analogs (e.g., irinotecan) have been formulated in an effort to overcome unacceptable toxicities and to increase cytotoxicity and water solubility. Topotecan incorporates a stable basic side chain at the 9-position of the A-ring of 10-hydroxycamptothecin, which increases aqueous solubility. The molecular weight is 457.9 (the HCl salt) and the formula is $C_{23}H_{23}N_3O_5 \cdot HCl$ (the free base has a molecular weight of 421.5). The chemical name of topotecan is (S)-10-[(dimethylamino)methyl]-4-ethyl-4,9-dihydroxy-1H-pyrano[3',4':6,7] indolizino [1,2-b]quinoline-3,14-(4H,12H)-dione monohydrochloride.

Mechanism of Action

In a manner similar to camptothecin, topotecan's cytotoxicity results from the inhibition of TOPO-I, an enzyme that induces reversible single-strand breaks during DNA replication. Camptothecin analogs bind with and stabilize the transient TOPO-I–DNA complex, preventing religation of the single-strand breakage. The interaction of the ternary topotecan–TOPO-I–DNA complex with replication enzymes results in double-strand DNA breaks and cellular death. Topotecan exists in a pH-dependent equilibrium as both a closed lactone ring and a hydroxy acid; the hydroxy acid is formed by hydrolysis of the lactone ring. The active lactone form predominates at a pH below 7.0, and at a pH of 6.0, over 80% of topotecan exists in the lactone form. Slow reaction kinetics studies have shown that the hydroxy acid is inactive and only the closed lactone bonds with the TOPO-I–DNA complex (335).

Drug Disposition

After IV administration, plasma pharmacokinetics show that the lactone form, which is active as an inhibitor of TOPO-I, is rapidly converted to the hydroxy acid form. At the end of a brief infusion, approximately half of the dose administered exits as hydroxy acid (449). One hour after administration, less than 30% of the dose remains in the lactone form. Topotecan does not inhibit TOPO-II.

Both forms of topotecan are subject to rapid biphasic elimination. In a summary of pharmacokinetics studies, the mean half-life of topotecan lactone was only 3.0 hours (range 1.2 to 4.9 hours) (335). Binding to plasma proteins is approximately 35%. Renal excretion appears to account for 40% to 70% of drug clearance (46,126).

When topotecan was administered as a weekly 24-hour IV infusion of 1 to 2 mg/m^2, the plasma steady-state concentration and the AUC increased linearly with dose. The lactone to total drug concentration ratio was constant, which suggests that the total drug concentration may be used as a measure of active lactone exposure with weekly, long infusions (450). Additionally, comparison of day 1 pharmacokinetics values with blood counts showed that both the topotecan AUC and lactone AUC were predictive of the level of neutrophil reduction on days 15, 22, and 29 using the sigmoid E_{max} model (450). This led the investigators to suggest that topotecan-induced myelosuppression is noncumulative and that elimination probably remains unchanged with repeat dosing in individual patients. Other studies have also found a correlation between the topotecan AUC and level of neutropenia (449,451).

Limited sampling models for topotecan pharmacokinetics have been proposed that may facilitate tailoring of topotecan drug doses in individual patients and large pharmacodynamic studies of topotecan (452,453). Plasma concentrations of the lactone and hydroxy acid forms of topotecan at 2 hours, after a 30-minute infusion, reliably predicted the lactone form AUC, the hydroxy acid AUC, the total topotecan AUC, and the clearance rate.

Administration and Dosage

Each 4-mg vial of topotecan should be reconstituted with 4 mL of sterile water. The resulting solution can be further diluted with either 0.9% sodium chloride or 5% dextrose. Because the active lactone form of topotecan is subject to a pH-dependent hydrolysis to the inactive hydroxy acid, consideration should be given to maintenance of an acidic pH during drug infusion. When the topotecan lactone is dissolved in 5% dextrose, only approximately 10% is converted to the hydroxy acid (449). Because the product does not contain an antibacterial preservative, it should be used immediately once constituted.

Parenteral topotecan has been administered by IV infusions varying in length from 30 minutes to 21 days (335). As discussed below, the dosing schedule has a profound effect on the maximum tolerated dose (MTD).

An oral formulation has been evaluated in murine tumor models and in Phase I-II trials. It has been associated with excellent bioavailability and similar efficacy as compared with parenteral topotecan in four of the five murine tumor models tested (454). In early phase human trials, oral topotecan is well tolerated and active in second-line therapy of ovarian cancer and small-cell lung cancer, and is associated with less neutropenia than the intravenous formulation (455–457).

The standard FDA-approved dosing regimen is 1.5 mg/m^2/day × 5 days by 30-minute IV infusion every 21 days, for a minimum of four courses owing to delayed tumor response, as tolerated (in the absence of tumor progression). However, this dosing schedule is associated with a more than 80% incidence of grade IV neutropenia. Many oncologists, therefore, use a dose of 1.25 mg/m^2/day for 5 days and/or administer prophylactic G-CSF.

In Phase I studies, the MTD of topotecan was highly dependent on the length of infusion schedules; longer infusions were generally associated with lower MTDs. The estimated MTD of topotecan when administered as a 30-minute, 72-hour, and 120-hour continuous infusion is 22.5 mg/m^2, 1.6 mg/m^2/day (4.8 mg/m^2 total), and 0.68 mg/m^2/day (3.4 mg/m^2 total), respectively. As a continuous 21-day infusion administered every 28 days, the MTD of topotecan appears to be 0.5 mg/m^2/day (10.5 mg/m^2/cycle) (335,458,459). More recently, a weekly dosing schedule has been developed that appears to maintain antitumor activity without causing severe myelosuppression (460,461).

Side Effects and Toxicities

Toxicity data are available from a Phase III, randomized study of topotecan 1.5 mg/m^2/day for 5 days every 21 days versus paclitaxel 175 mg/m^2 IV over 3 hours every 21 days in ovarian cancer patients with progressive or recurrent disease following primary platinum-based chemotherapy (462). Neutropenia was the predominant toxicity in this study: 79% of patients experienced grade 4 neutropenia, 25% of patients experienced febrile neutropenia, and 5% of patients developed sepsis [two patients (2%) died of sepsis]. The onset of grade 4 neutropenia was on days 9 through 15 of a chemotherapy cycle and it did respond to G-CSF therapy. Thrombocytopenia also occurred frequently: 50% of patients experienced grades 3 to 4 thrombocytopenia (25% experienced grade 4). Grade 4 anemia occurred in 3.6% of patients.

The most common nonhematologic toxicities were cumulative, dose-related alopecia (76%) and nausea/vomiting (10% grades 3 to 4), which was amenable to antiemetic therapy. Other frequent toxicities were fatigue (41%), constipation (43%), diarrhea (40%), abdominal pain (27%), fever in the absence of neutropenia (29%), stomatitis (24%), dyspnea (24%), and asthenia (22%) (462).

Although the results of this study described in the above paragraphs led to an FDA approval of topotecan as salvage therapy for patients with ovarian cancer with a recommended dose level of 1.5 mg/m^2/day for 5 days, it is important to note that the patients in this European study had only received one prior platinum-based chemotherapeutic regimen, and that most had received cisplatin (not carboplatin) and none had received prior paclitaxel. In general, topotecan-induced myelosuppression is more severe in patients who have previously received carboplatin and/or multiple prior chemotherapeutic regimens. For this reason, many clinicians use an initial topotecan dose of 1.25 mg/m^2/day and/or administer prophylactic G-CSF.

Special Precautions

Because topotecan has a high rate of renal excretion and a modest hepatic clearance, a clinical study was conducted to evaluate the impact of renal and hepatic dysfunction on toxicity in patients undergoing treatment with topotecan on a daily × 5 dosing schedule (463,464). Pharmacokinetic analyses showed clear correlations between creatinine clearance and plasma clearance of both topotecan and topotecan lactone (r^2 = 0.65, p <.0001). Although the standard dose for patients with good renal function is 1.5 mg/m^2/day × 5 days, this study determined that the recommended starting dose for patients with moderate hepatic dysfunction (creatinine clearance of 20 to 39 mL/min) was 0.75 mg/m^2. The investigators urged extreme caution with topotecan administration in patients with more profound renal insufficiency and recommend further dose reductions for heavily pretreated patients (463). Hepatic insufficiency did not appear to exacerbate hematologic toxicity (463). Nonhematologic toxicity appeared to be unaffected by either renal or hepatic insufficiency.

Drug Interactions

Drug sequence of the paclitaxel/topotecan combination had no apparent impact on hematologic toxicities or pharmacologic behavior (465). However, drug sequence of the cisplatin/topotecan combination did have a significant impact on toxicity and topotecan pharmacokinetics. Prior administration of cisplatin significantly reduced the clearance of topotecan (possibly as a result of subclinical nephrotoxicity) and increased hematologic toxicity (466). In GOG-182, carboplatin was administered on day 3 of a daily × 3 topotecan administration schedule, because administration of carboplatin on day 1 was associated with excessive neutropenia and thrombocytopenia (467).

There has been interest in sequential administration of topotecan (TOPO-I inhibitor) with TOPO-II inhibitors (e.g., doxorubicin, etoposide). The rationale is that administration of a TOPO-I inhibitor would induce upregulation of TOPO-II in tumor cells and thus enhance cytotoxicity. One clinical/translational study of topotecan (0.17 to 1.05 mg/m^2/day as a 72-hour continuous infusion on days 1 to 3) followed by etoposide (75 or 100 mg/m^2/day as a 2-hour infusion daily on days 8 to 10) failed to show reliable downregulation of TOPO-I and upregulation of TOPO-II following administration of topotecan (468). Although significant clinical activity was observed in this Phase I study in patients with various solid tumors, the investigators concluded that the toxicity and translational research results did not support a significant synergistic advantage of this combination. Another study of the TOPO-I and TOPO-II inhibitor combination therapy (IV topotecan 0.5 mg/m^2 per day for 5 days and oral etoposide 50 mg twice daily for 7 days of every 21-day cycle, with dose escalation of topotecan 0.75 and 1.0 mg/m^2) found the combination to be safe and effective in small-cell lung cancer patients; however, the incidence of grades 3 to 4 neutropenia was 25%, and two patients died from neutropenic sepsis (469).

TOPO-I is a biochemical mediator of radiosensitization in cultured mammalian cells by camptothecin derivatives (470). There are in vitro and in vivo data suggesting that topotecan may have activity as a radiation-sensitizing agent (471). However, this apparent synergistic relationship remains to be explored in clinical trials.

Special Applications

Phase I trials of intraperitoneal (IP) topotecan have demonstrated the feasibility of IP administration and the favorable toxicity profile (472,473). Pharmacokinetic studies revealed that the pharmacologic advantage associated with IP administration of topotecan (expressed as the ratio of the peritoneal to plasma AUC) was 31.2 (473). In a Netherlands study, patients were treated with escalating doses (5 to 30 mg/m^2 every 21 days). The dose-limiting toxicity was acute hypotension, chills, and fever at the 30-mg/m^2 dose level

(472). The University of California, San Diego study treated patients with escalating doses from 2 to 4 mg/m^2 every 21 days. The MTD of intraperitoneal topotecan was determined to be 4 mg/m^2 every 21 days and the recommended dose for further Phase II study was 3 mg/m^2. The dose-limiting toxicity was neutropenia. Other toxicities included anemia, vomiting, fever, and abdominal pain (473).

Vinblastine Sulfate

Chemistry

Vinblastine (Velban) is used in the treatment of germ-cell tumors of the ovary (474) and has demonstrated activity in early clinical trials of cervical, endometrial, and ovarian cancers (474,475). In combination with other agents, it has also demonstrated activity in early trials of ovarian cancer (476). Vinblastine, is the sulfate salt of an alkaloid isolated from *Vinca rosea* (periwinkle). It is structurally related to vincristine, another alkaloid isolated from the same plant. Vinblastine sulfate is a white to off-white crystalline powder that is freely soluble in water, soluble in methane, and slightly soluble in ethanol. Its empiric formula is $C_{46}H_{58}N_4O_9 \cdot H_2SO_4$, and it has a molecular weight of 909.07.

Mechanism of Action

Vinblastine binds to tubulin and inhibits microtubule assembly. This inhibition prevents mitotic spindle formation and results in an accumulation of cells in metaphase (477).

Vinblastine is considered cell cycle phase specific for mitosis; however, the cytotoxic effect probably occurs in S phase and is expressed only in M phase. At high doses, direct effects may be expressed in S and G_1 phases. Vinblastine may be assumed to have stathmokinetic (cell cycle arrest) effects similar to vincristine.

Drug Disposition

After IV administration, vinblastine is rapidly cleared from the plasma and concentrated in various tissues. The apparent volume of distribution for the central compartment is quite large (three to four times the blood volume). Vincristine and vindesine approximate total body water in their distributions. There is a triphasic vinblastine elimination pattern, with average half-lives of 3.7 minutes, 1.6 hours, and 24.8 hours, respectively (478). The drug also localizes in platelet and leukocyte fractions of whole blood (479). A radiolabeled drug study has shown that urinary elimination accounts for approximately 33% of the total vinblastine radioactivity, with 21% appearing in the stool; both after 72 hours (479). A large portion of the radiolabel was retained in the body: 73% remained at 6 days after dosing. Apparently,

insufficient amounts of the drug pass the blood-brain barrier to produce an effective concentration in the central nervous system. Vinblastine is partially metabolized in the liver. Most of the drug is, therefore, ultimately excreted intact in the bile or the urine. Toxicity may be increased if there is obstructive liver disease, and doses should be greatly reduced.

Administration and Dosage

The solution for administration is usually prepared by adding 10 mL of sodium chloride solution (which may be preserved with phenols or benzyl alcohol) to the 10-mg vial. The use of other solutions is not generally recommended. The resultant solution has a concentration of 1 mg/mL and a pH of 3.5 to 5.0. Solutions prepared with preserved sodium chloride injection may be stored in the refrigerator (protected from light) for 28 days without significant loss of potency.

Vinblastine is usually given by the IV push technique, with the total dose being delivered over approximately 1 minute. This is usually accomplished by slowly pushing the dose through the injection site of a running IV infusion. Alternatively, the drug may be given directly into the vein. If this method is followed, the double-needle technique should be used: Do not use the same needle to withdraw the dose from the vial that is used for the direct injection into the vein. Vinblastine is very irritating and should not be given intramuscularly or subcutaneously. Vein patency should be checked before drug administration by flushing with a small quantity of normal saline or D_5W. After the dose has been given, the site should be flushed again to assure that all of the drug has been delivered into the vein.

Vinblastine has been given by several dosing schemes. The dose depends on the protocol being followed, condition of the patient, other drugs or irradiation being used, and individual patient response. Usually, the drug is given no more frequently than once every week. In general, the dosage range is 3.8 to 18.5 mg/m^2 when used in combination with other agents. Patients are customarily started at a low dose and worked up in 1.8- to 1.9-mg/m^2 increments depending on the degree of resulting leukopenia (e.g., the dose should not be increased beyond the dose at which the white cell count reaches 3,000 cells/mm^3) (478). The dosage ranges for the indicated use of vinblastine are 6 mg/m^2 IV on days 1 and 15 as part of the doxorubicin-bleomycin-vinblastine-dacarbazine regimen (Hodgkin's disease) and 0.15 mg/kg IV on days 1 and 2 as part of the cisplatin-vinblastine-bleomycin regimen (testicular cancer) (46).

Side Effects and Toxicities

The major toxic effect of vinblastine is a dose-related bone marrow depression. This is more frequent and severe than with the close structural analog, vincristine. Dose-related leukopenia occurs with a nadir of 4 to 10 days and with recovery occurring over another 7 to 14 days. Because of the relatively predictable nadir, it may be possible to administer vinblastine cautiously as often as every 7 to 10 days. Thrombocytopenia typically occurs; however, with standard dosing regimens, serious platelet depressions are infrequent. Erythrocytes are usually only slightly depressed.

Nausea and vomiting occur rarely with vinblastine therapy and are at least partially responsive to antiemetics. Severe stomatitis is occasionally observed. Gastrointestinal symptoms, which may be related to neurotoxicity, include constipation, adynamic ileus, and abdominal pain, especially if high doses (>20 mg) are used. These side effects are rarely seen with doses of less than 10 mg. Prophylactic stool softeners may prevent constipation. Generalized muscle and tumor pain are commonly experienced by patients receiving vinblastine, especially in high doses (480).

Neurotoxicity associated with vinblastine occurs less frequently than with vincristine and usually occurs in patients on prolonged therapy or in those receiving high individual doses. Symptoms include paresthesias, peripheral neuropathy, depression, headache, malaise, jaw pain, urinary retention, tachycardia, orthostatic hypotension, or convulsions. Vocal cord paralysis and cranial nerve paralysis have also been reported (481).

Extravasations of vinblastine may result in local soft tissue necrosis. Treatment with subcutaneously administered hyaluronidase is recommended (200).

Other side effects include a reversible and mild alopecia, rashes, and photosensitivity reactions. Transient hepatitis has also been reported on the continuous-infusion regimen.

There have been several reports of a Raynaud's phenomenon associated with vinblastine or bleomycin in treating testicular cancer. The reaction consists of a delayed presentation of a cold feeling in the hands with physical evidence of cyanosis (482). Ginsberg and co-workers (483) demonstrated a case of vinblastine-associated syndrome of inappropriate antidiuretic hormone (ADH) secretion, which was previously thought to occur only with vincristine.

The drug is well documented as a teratogen in humans, and as with most anticancer drugs, usage in pregnancy is strongly contraindicated (484).

Special Precautions

Avoid extravasation of vinblastine. If extravasation occurs, stop the administration of the remaining drug immediately. Dorr and Alberts (485) favor injection of a corticosteroid into the infiltration site with sodium chloride to dilute the drug. Only minor tissue damage has occurred when vinblastine extravasation was treated with 50 to 500 mg of hydrocortisone sodium succinate. This is followed by cold compresses to minimize spread of the reaction.

Liver disease may alter the elimination of vinblastine and necessitate a dosage reduction. Neurotoxicity may be more frequent in patients with underlying neurologic problems or those who are weak or cachectic at the start of treatment.

Vinblastine solution is topically irritating and has caused corneal irritation when inadvertently splashed in the eyes. Protective precautions should be used by all persons working with the drug.

Vinorelbine

Chemistry

Vinorelbine (Navelbine) is a third-generation semisynthetic vinca alkaloid that has been commercially available in the United States since 1994 for treatment of non–small-cell lung cancer. Vinorelbine also appears to have significant activity in breast cancer patients (486,487) and moderate activity in patients with cervical or ovarian cancer (488,489), as well as other tumor types (490). It has a molecular formula of $C_{45}H_{54}N_4O_8 \cdot 2C_4H_6O_6$ and a molecular weight of 1079.12. Vinorelbine's structure differs from that of the parent compounds, vincristine and vinblastine, in that it contains a nine-member (rather than eight-member) catharanthine ring (491). Its chemical name is 3′,4′-didehydro-4′-deoxy-C′-norvincaleukoblastine[R-(R*,R*)-2,3-dihydroxybutanedioate-(1:2)(salt)].

Mechanism of Action

Like other vinca alkaloids, vinorelbine is classified as a "spindle poison" since it interacts with tubulin with resulting inhibition of microtubule assembly and cellular division during mitosis (492). Vinelorbine blocks cell cycle progression specifically in G_2 and M phases (126).

Drug Disposition

The pharmacokinetics of vinorelbine show large interpatient variability and are best described by a triphasic model. Following IV administration of a 30-mg/m² dose, a peak plasma level of 1,000 ng/mL is achieved, but the plasma level declines to 100 ng/mL within 2 hours. Vinorelbine rapidly binds to platelets (78% of total dose) and plasma proteins (13.5%), and only 1.7% is available as free drug (492). The drug readily diffuses into other tissues, and has a large volume of distribution (75.61 L/kg). The terminal half-life is approximately 45 hours (493).

The primary means of vinorelbine clearance appears to be hepatic metabolism. Approximately 18% and 46% is recovered in the urine and feces, respectively; however, recovery was incomplete in pharmacokinetic studies (494,495).

Administration and Dosage

Vinorelbine is a vesicant and requires careful administration. The drug should be diluted in a syringe or IV bag to a concentration of 1.5 to 3.0 mg/mL (syringe) or 0.5 to 2 mg/mL (IV bag). When using a syringe or IV bag, vinorelbine should be diluted with dextrose (5%) or sodium chloride (0.9%). When using an IV bag, it may also be diluted with sodium chloride (0.45%), Ringer's injection, or lactated Ringer's injection. Diluted vinorelbine should be administered over 6 to 10 minutes into a side port of a free-flowing IV line closest to the IV bag. Following vinorelbine administration, the vein should be flushed with at least 75 to 125 mL of IV solution. Longer IV infusions (e.g., 20 minutes) are associated with a higher incidence of phlebitis (496).

Vinorelbine solution is incompatible with fluorouracil, mitomycin, and thiotepa. It is also incompatible with several antibiotics (including a number of cephalosporins, amphotericin B, ampicillin, piperacillin, and trimethoprim-sulfamethoxazole), acyclovir, furosemide, ganciclovir, methylprednisolone, and sodium bicarbonate (497).

Vinorelbine is generally administered at a dose of 30 mg/m^2 every week. This dosing schedule has been used in combination chemotherapeutic regimens; however, the recommended dosing schedule in combination with cisplatin (100 mg/m^2 every 4 weeks) is weekly administration of vinorelbine at a dose of 25 mg/m^2. Attempts to increase vinorelbine dose intensity using a daily × 3 every 21 days dosing schedule with or without G-CSF have not been successful (498, 499). However, Weiss et al. (500) have reported that continuous infusion of vinorelbine at doses of 8 to 10 mg/m^2/day with concurrent administration of G-CSF results in a twofold increase in vinorelbine dose intensity without increasing toxicity.

Side Effects and Toxicities

The primary dose-limiting toxicity of vinorelbine is myelosuppression, chiefly granulocytopenia (36% of patients, <500 cells/mm^3). A safety summary of data from North American clinical trials reported that when vinorelbine was administered at a dose of 30 mg/m^2/week to patients with breast cancer and non–small-cell lung cancer, 64% of patients experienced grades 3 to 4 granulocytopenia, 50% experienced grades 3 to 4 leukopenia, and 9% developed grades 3 to 4 anemia. Despite the high incidence of granulocytopenia, most events were uncomplicated, and only 7% of patients required hospitalization for fever and/or infection. The death rate due to sepsis was 1% to 2%. Myelosuppression was noncumulative, and the incidence of grades 3 and 4 granulocytopenia declined during later cycles of vinorelbine therapy. The granulocyte nadir typically occurred on day 14 of treatment, with recovery of the granulocyte count within 7 days (501).

Vinorelbine therapy is frequently associated with transient increases in liver enzymes, especially alkaline phosphatase. Virtually all patients experience a rise in alkaline phosphatase, with approximately 25% developing grade 3 toxicity and an additional 2% experiencing grade 4 elevations. In-

creases in AST and ALT also occur in more than half of all patients. However, most patients with liver enzyme increases remain asymptomatic and do not require dose modification of vinorelbine. Total bilirubin also can be elevated: 10% of patients experience some degree of increased bilirubin, with 2% experiencing grade 4 elevation. Because of the high incidence of liver and bone metastases in the study population (breast cancer and non–small-cell lung cancer patients), the proportion of these toxicities that is directly attributable to vinorelbine therapy is unknown (501).

Other common toxicities associated with vinorelbine when administered as a single agent at a dose of 30 mg/m^2/week by a 20-minute IV infusion include nausea (38% overall, 2% severe), vomiting (17% overall, 2% severe), constipation (31%, 3% severe), asthenia (29%, 5% severe), injection-site reactions (26%, 2% severe), anorexia (15%, 1% severe), diarrhea (15%, 1% severe), stomatitis (14%, 0% severe), pain (13%, 2% severe), paresthesia (13%, <1% severe), fever (11%, 1% severe), and alopecia (10%, <1% severe) (501). Vinorelbine-induced nausea and vomiting are generally mild and are readily controlled with standard antiemetic medication (501). Injection-site reactions include erythema, warmth, pain, and phlebitis. Repeated administration of vinorelbine can result in discoloration of the vein. As discussed above, shortening the injection duration to 6 to 10 minutes significantly reduces the incidence of injection-site reactions (496).

Injection-site pain and pain of unspecified etiology has been reported with administration of vinorelbine as a single agent (501). Additionally, acute tumor pain has been reported in several cancer patients who received treatment with vinorelbine plus a platinum-containing agent (either carboplatin or cisplatin) (502,503).

Pulmonary toxicity is an infrequent side effect of vinorelbine. Approximately 5% of patients experience dyspnea. Some cases of dyspnea are characterized by rapid onset during administration and resolve with bronchodilator therapy. Other cases occur usually within 1 hour of vinorelbine infusion and are characterized by life-threatening progressive dyspnea and the development of interstitial infiltrates (501, 504). The co-administration of mitomycin may increase the pulmonary toxicity of vinorelbine (504).

Rare side effects of vinorelbine include pancreatitis, PPE (with prolonged infusions), paralytic ileus, and syndrome of inappropriate ADH secretion (505–508).

Special Precautions

Vinorelbine extravasation can result in severe local irritation, tissue necrosis, and phlebitis. If extravasation occurs, the injection should be halted immediately and any remaining portion of the dose should be injected into a different vein. Specific antidotes for vinorelbine extravasation have not been studied; however, vinblastine extravasation reactions may be ameliorated with the use of corticosteroid injections followed by cold compresses (485).

Drug Interactions

In that vinca alkaloids are metabolized by the cytochrome P450 3A system, coadministration of strong P450 inhibitors, such as erythromycin and ketoconazole, could potentially reduce vinorelbine clearance and increase toxicity (509, 510). Doxorubicin and etoposide also are metabolized by the P450 system, and coadministration of these drugs with vinorelbine could potentially affect vinorelbine metabolism (509).

Mitomycin is known to exacerbate vinca alkaloid–induced pulmonary toxicity (511), and the combination of high-dose vinorelbine (50 mg/m^2 on days 1 and 21) plus mitomycin (15 mg/m^2 on day 1) has been associated with life-threatening acute pulmonary toxicity characterized by rapid onset of severe, progressive dyspnea and the development of bilateral interstitial infiltrates (504).

The combination of paclitaxel and vinorelbine has been associated with severe neurotoxicity including grade 4 motor neuropathy, irreversible ototoxicity, and vocal cord paresis (512,513). In one report of clinical experience in five patients with preexisting, mild to moderate, paclitaxel-induced sensory neuropathy, the combination of vinorelbine 25 to 30 mg/m^2 followed by paclitaxel 150 mg/m^2 by 3-hour infusion every 2 weeks resulted in severe, slowly reversing motor neuropathy in all five patients. Four of the five patients required the use of a wheelchair (512).

Special Applications

On a well-tolerated weekly dose schedule for vinorelbine, Bajetta and colleagues (514) noted four partial responses and one complete response in 31 patients (24 platinum-resistant, four platinum-sensitive, five with undetermined sensitivity) for an overall response rate of 15% (95% CI of 5.1, 37.9%). A Phase II trial (vinorelbine 30 mg/m^2 weekly infusion) in persistent or recurrent ovarian cancer found a 29% objective response rate; granulocytopenia was a dose-limiting but manageable toxicity (489). This is consistent with previous findings of a 21% response rate in the population of heavily pretreated and platinum-resistant ovarian cancer patients (514).

Molecularly Targeted Agents

Erlotinib

Chemistry

Erlotinib (OSI-774, Tarceva), an experimental agent, is a tyrosine kinase inhibitor (specifically, HER-1/EGFR) that has the potential for inhibiting tumor-cell growth of a variety of tumors. Phase I and II studies have demonstrated activity in advanced non–small-cell lung cancer, ovarian cancer, pancreatic, and head and neck squamous-cell cancer (515). A number of phase III trials have been completed in non–small-cell lung cancer and others are in development and ongoing (ovarian and pancreatic cancer).

Drug Disposition

Erlotinib is rapidly absorbed after administration, with peak plasma levels occurring at 4 hours. Plasma levels increase with dose, but daily administration does not cause unexpected drug accumulation (516). Up to 95% of erlotinib is bound to plasma proteins. It is primarily metabolized by CYP$_3$A$_4$, which suggests that concomitant treatment with potent CYP$_3$A$_4$ inhibitors (e.g., ketaconazole, systemic antifungals, erythromycin) may affect the metabolism of erlotinib (516).

Administration and Dosage

Erlotinib is administered orally. Clinical trials have found a 150-mg/day dose to be active with manageable toxicity levels, and have recommended this dose for future clinical trials. When administered at 200 mg/day, diarrhea is dose limiting.

Side Effects and Toxicities

The dose-limiting toxicities associated with erlotinib include diarrhea and rash; however, at a dose of 150 mg/day, diarrhea can be effectively managed with loperamide. Other less common toxicities include headache, nausea and vomiting, and mucositis (515). It can be administered as a single agent, and has an additive effect on antitumor activity when combined with cisplatin, doxorubicin, gemcitabine, or low-dose paclitaxel without an associated increase in toxicity (517).

Gefitinib

Chemistry

Gefitinib (ZD1839, Iressa), an epidermal growth factor receptor–specific tyrosine kinase (EGFR-TK) inhibitor, is approved by the FDA for the treatment of advanced non–small-cell lung cancer. It is currently under investigation for its potential role in the treatment of gynecologic malignancies that express the EGFR. Gefitinib has been and is currently being evaluated in preclinical and early-phase studies of ovarian, endometrial, and cervical cancer (518–520). The chemical name of gefitinib is 4-quinazolinamine-N-3-chloro-4-fluorophenyl)-7-methoxy-6-[3-4-morpholinpropoxy]. It has the molecular formula $C_{22}H_{24}C1FN_4O_3$ and a molecular weight of 446.9.

Mechanism of Action

Although the exact mechanism is not fully understood, gefitinib inhibits EGFR-TK, which results in the inhibition of mitogenic and antiapoptotic signals (46).

Drug Disposition

Gefitinib is absorbed slowly; peak plasma levels are obtained within 3 to 7 hours of administration and steady-state plasma levels are achieved within 10 days. Gefitinib is primarily eliminated by metabolism and excretion in feces. The half-life is approximately 48 hours.

Administration and Dosage

Gefitinib is administered orally at a daily dose of 250 mg. Higher doses have been associated with greater toxicity; however, doses up to 500 mg/day may be considered for patients who receive concomitant treatment with potent CYP_3A_4 inhibitors (e.g., rifampicin, phenytoin). When higher doses are administered, the patient should be carefully monitored for adverse events and clinical response.

Side Effects and Toxicities

The most common adverse events associated with the 250-mg/day dose include diarrhea (67%), rash (54%), acne (33%), dry skin (26%) nausea (18%), and anorexia (10%); however, in only 2% of all cases were side effects dose limiting. Although rare (1%), interstitial lung disease (ILD) has been observed in patients taking gefitinib, with up to 33% of these cases being fatal. Patients who have an acute onset or worsening of pulmonary symptoms (dyspnea, cough, fever) should discontinue gefitinib treatment until a diagnosis of ILD is ruled out. Patients taking coumarin-derived anticoagulants should be monitored closely for changes in clotting parameters, as bleeding events have occurred with gefitinib treatment.

Imatinib

Chemistry

Imatinib mesylate (STI-571, Gleevec) is used in the treatment of patients with Philadelphia chromosome–positive chronic myeloid leukemia (CML), and it is also indicated for the treatment of patients with Kit (CD-117)–positive unresectable and/or metastatic malignant gastrointestinal stromal tumors. Imatinib is currently under investigation for its potential role in the treatment of gynecologic tumors expressing c-ABL, c-KIT, and platelet-derived growth factor receptor-β (PDGFR-β). A recent evaluation of 52 ovarian serous carcinomas found they express c-ABL (71%) and PDGFR-β (81%), but fewer (26% of high-grade vs 0% low-grade tumors) express c-KIT (518). Imatinib's chemical designation is 4-[(4-methyl-1-piperazinyl)methyl]-N-[4-methyl-3-[[4-(3-pyridinyl)-2-pyrimidinyl]amino]-phenyl]benzamide methanesulfonate. It has the molecular formula of $C_{29}H_{31}N_7O \cdot CH_4SO_3$ and a molecular weight of 589.7.

Mechanism of Action

Imatinib is a protein–tyrosine kinase inhibitor. It inhibits receptor tyrosine kinases for platelet-derived growth factor (PDGF), stem-cell factor (SCF), and c-KIT and inhibits PDGF- and SCF-mediated cellular events. Through this inhibition, it inhibits proliferation and induces apoptosis in cells that express an activating c-KIT mutation and in Bcr-Abl–positive cell lines.

Drug Disposition

Imatinib is quickly absorbed, with C_{max} being obtained 2 to 4 hours after adminstration. The half-life of the drug is approximately 18 hours, and the half-life of the active metabolite, the N-desmethyl derivative, is approximately 40 hours. Roughly 95% of imatinib binds to plasma proteins, primarily to albumin and $(\alpha)_1$-acid glycoprotein. Similar to other molecularly targeted agents, imatinib is largely metabolized by the CYP_3A_4 enzyme. Elimination is in the feces (68%) and the urine (13%), predominantly as metabolites (80% feces, 95% urine) (522). Although clearance may increase with body weight, the interpatient variability (40%) makes it unnecessary to adjust dose for body weight and/or age. Owing to this variability, it is important to monitor the patient for any treatment-related toxicity.

Administration and Dosage

Imatinib is administered orally at a recommended dosage of 400 or 600 mg daily. In CML patients in accelerated phase or blast crisis without severe adverse drug reactions, the dose may be increased (400 to 600 mg or 600 mg to 800 mg) in the case of disease progression, failure of response within 3 months, or loss of a previous hematologic response.

Side Effects and Toxicities

Patients taking imatinib often experience edema (71% any grade, 12% grade 3/4). The most frequent grade 3/4 side effects in patients with CML (myeloid blast crisis) treated with imatinib include hemorrhage (19%), musculoskeletal pain (9%), rash (5%), headache (5%), nausea (4%), vomiting (4%), diarrhea (4%), and abdominal pain (6%) (522). Most events related to fluid retention (e.g., rapid weight gain, pleural effusion, pulmonary edema) are manageable by interrupting imatinib treatment or by diuretic and other supportive care treatments.

Trastuzumab

Chemistry

Trastuzumab (Herceptin) is a DNA-derived monoclonal antibody to the human epidermal growth factor receptor 2 protein (HER-2). Trastuzumab should be used in patients who have had their tumor evaluated for HER-2/neu overexpression. Treatment is indicated in metastatic breast cancer patients who overexpress HER-2. The HER-2/neu receptor is present in some ovarian (523), cervical (524), and endometrial cancers (525). A Phase II study conducted by the GOG of single-agent trastuzumab found a 7.3% response rate in patients with recurrent or refractory ovarian and peritoneal carcinoma (2+ and 3+ HER-2 overexpression), suggesting its low clincal value in this cohort of patients (526).

Mechanism of Action

The activity of trastuzumab is related to its ability to inhibit the proliferation of tumor cells that overexpress HER-2. Trastuzumab is a mediator of antibody-dependent cellular cytotoxicity, which is preferentially exerted on cancer cells that overexpress HER-2.

Drug Disposition

When using the recommended loading dose of 4 mg/kg followed by a weekly maintenance dose of 2 mg/kg, the average half-life is 5.8 days, with serum steady-state concentrations being reached between 16 and 32 weeks. Combination therapy with paclitaxel results in an increase in mean serum concentrations and decreased clearance of trastuzumab.

Administration and Dosage

Trastuzumab should be reconstituted with 20 mL of bacteriostatic water to yield 21 mg/mL trastuzumab and should be used within 28 days. If the patient is hypersensitive to benzyl alcohol, trastuzumab should be reconstituted with sterile water and used immediately. The initial dose of trastuzumab is 4 mg/kg administered intravenously over 90 minutes. The weekly maintenance dose is 2 mg/kg administered over 30 minutes (if initial dose was well tolerated).

Side Effects and Toxicities

The most serious side effects of trastuzumab include cardiomyopathy, hypersensitivity reactions, pulmonary events, and neutropenia. However, the most common events include fever, diarrhea, infections, chills, cough, headache, rash, and insomnia.

Estrogen Receptor/Progesterone Receptor–targeted Agents

Anastrozole

Chemistry

Anastrozole (Arimidex) is FDA approved for the adjuvant treatment of postmenopausal patients with estrogen receptor positive (ER +) breast cancers following tamoxifen therapy. Chemically, it is 1,3-benzenediacetonitrile, $\alpha,\alpha,\alpha',\alpha'$-tetramethyl-5-(1H-1,2,4-triazol-1-ylmethyl). It has a molecular formula of $C_{17}H_{19}N_5$ and a molecular weight of 293.4.

Mechanism of Action

Anastrozole is a nonsteroidal aromatase inhibitor that prevents the peripheral conversion of androgens (androstenedione and testosterone) to estrogens (estrone, estrone sulfate, and estradiol) (46). Anastrozole has a significant effect on serum estradiol; as low as 1 mg/day has caused estradiol levels to be undetectable (527). In patients receiving 5 and 10 mg of anastrozole, there was no effect on adrenal corticosteroids or aldosterone.

Drug Disposition

Following oral administration, anastrozole is well absorbed into the systemic circulation and not affected by food ingestion. Pharmacokinetics are linear and not affected by repeated dosing. Anastrozole has been shown to have fewer side effects and a significant survival advantage as compared to megestrol acetate in the treatment of postmenopausal patients with breast cancer (528).

Administration and Dosage

Anastrozole is administered orally at a dose of 1 mg/day.

Side Effects and Toxicities

When compared in a controlled clinical study to megestrol acetate, the principal side effect of anastrozole was diarrhea (occurred in 8.4% vs 2.8% of patients treated with megestrol acetate). In general, it is very well tolerated, with the most frequent side effects (any grade) being asthenia (18%), nausea (18%), headache (14%), hot flushes (13.2%), and pain (10%).

Special Applications

It is hypothesized that anastrozole may play a role on a molecular level in the endometrium. Most endometrioid carcinomas are associated with endometrial hyperplasia and are estrogen receptor (ER) and progesterone receptor (PR) positive. In addition to ER/PR status, there is a progressive increase in the expression of the protein pS2 from normal to hyperplastic to well-differentiated carcinoma (529). Aromatase inhibition may be able to alter the course of disease by preventing the endometrium from being exposed to estrogen. This may in turn alter the expression of the pS2 protein as there is a strong association between ER/PR expression and expression of pS2 protein (529). Aromatase activity has been demonstrated in both ER/PR–positive and ER/PR–negative endometrial carcinomas (530). Although much research has yet to be done, one Phase II trial demonstrated minimal activity in an unselected population of recurrent endometrial carcinoma patients (531).

Medroxyprogesterone

Chemistry

The chemical name of medroxyprogesterone acetate is pregn-4-ene-3,20-dione,17-(acetyloxy)-6-methyl-,(6α)-. Its empirical formula is $C_{24}H_{34}O_4$, with a molecular weight of 386.53. Medroxyprogesterone acetate therapy has been evaluated for potential therapeutic use in women with atypical endometrial hyperplasia and stage I endometrial adenocarcinoma who wish to preserve fertility with some success (532, 533), and has demonstrated activity when used with other agents in advanced or recurrent endometrial cancer (534, 535).

Tamoxifen

Chemistry

Tamoxifen citrate (Nolvadex) is a nonsteroidal agent with antiestrogenic properties. It is indicated for the treatment of metastatic breast cancer and as adjuvant treatment in node-positive breast cancer in postmenopausal patients. Tamoxifen competes with estrogen for binding sites, which explains its increased effectiveness in ER + tumors. Chemically, tamoxifen is (Z)2-[4-(1,2-diphenyl-1-butenyl) phenoxy]-N,N-dimethylethanamine 2-hydroxy-1,2,3-propanetricarboxylate (1:1), and has a molecular weight of 563.62.

Mechanism of Action

Tamoxifen is a nonsteroidal agent that has antiestrogenic properties in the breast and ovary, but acts like an estrogen agonist in the endometrium and bone (536,537). It may exert its antitumor effects by binding the estrogen receptors. Because of this mechanism, it is most beneficial in the treatment of ER + tumors.

Drug Disposition

Peak plasma concentrations (average 40 ng/mL) take place approximately 5 hours after dosing. The decline in plasma concentrations is biphasic with a terminal elimination half-life of about 6 days. Steady-state concentrations for tamoxifen are achieved in about 4 weeks after initiation of therapy. Tamoxifen is extensively metabolized, with N-desmethyl tamoxifen being the major metabolite. Approximately 65% of the administered dose is eliminated in the feces within 2 weeks (522).

Administration and Dosage

Tamoxifen is available in 10- and 20-mg tablets for oral administration. The recommended dosage is 20 to 40 mg/day; when the higher daily dose is prescribed, it should be divided into two doses of 20 mg (morning and evening).

Side Effects and Toxicities

Tamoxifen causes estrogenic changes of the vaginal and cervical squamous epithelium and increases the incidence of cervical and endometrial polyps (538). It is associated with an increased risk of uterine malignancies (endometrial adenocarcinoma and uterine sarcoma). Other serious adverse events associated with tamoxifen treatment include stroke, deep vein thrombosis, and pulmonary embolism. A discussion weighing the benefits versus the risks should take place prior to treatment with tamoxifen; however, the benefits have been determined to outweigh the risks in women who take tamoxifen to reduce the risk of breast cancer recurrence (522). The National Adjuvant Breast and Bowel Project (NSABP P-1) found a higher incidence of the following side effects for tamoxifen versus placebo, respectively: vaginal discharge (54.7 vs 34%); cold sweats (21.4% vs 14.8%); hot flashes (77.7% vs 65.1%); night sweats (66.8% vs 54.9%); and genital itching (47.1% vs 38.3%) (539).

Special Applications

About 5% of ovarian cancers express hormonal receptors, a factor supporting the investigation of tamoxifen in the treatment of ovarian malignancies. It has demonstrated activity in patients with platinum-refractory ovarian cancer, with response rates ranging from 13% to 17% (with some complete responses), and with durations ranging from 4.4 months to more than 5 years (540–543). In the series by Hatch and colleagues (542), patients with ovarian cancer who had complete or partial responses on tamoxifen were more likely to have a ER + tumor (89% ER +) than those who had stable disease or progression on tamoxifen (59% had elevated ER). The favorable toxicity profile of tamoxifen makes it an ideal agent to consider in patients with refractory ovarian cancer.

Antiangiogenesis Agents

Angiogenesis is the process by which new blood vessels are sprouted from preexisting ones. Endothelial cells must migrate, proliferate, and assemble into tubes during this process. In normal tissues, blood vessel growth is tightly controlled by numerous angiogenesis-stimulating factors and angiogenesis-inhibiting factors. Vascular endothelial growth factor (VEGF) and platelet-derived endothelial-cell growth factor (PD-ECGF) are two of the most extensively studied growth factors that appear to function primarily as angiogenesis-stimulating factors. Other growth factors and cytokines, such as basic fibroblast growth factor (bFGF), have multiple functions in addition to angiogenesis stimulation (544). Naturally occurring factors that suppress angiogenesis include angiostatin, endostatin, interferon-α, interferon-β, interferon-γ, interleukin-1, interleukin-12, platelet factor-4, thrombospondin-1, 1,2-methoxyestradiol, tissue inhibitor metalloproteinases (TIMPs), and, at high concentrations, tumor necrosis factor-α (545).

In the early 1970s, Folkman (546) pioneered the study of tumor angiogenesis with his observation that the growth of tumor nodules to a diameter of greater than 1 to 2 mm required neovascularization of the tumor. He hypothesized that pharmacologic suppression of tumor angiogenesis could induce tumor dormancy. Further research has shown that formation of new blood vessels within tumor nodules results in an exponential increase in tumor cell growth, the transition from hyperplasia to malignancy parallels the induction of neovascularization, and tumor angiogenesis is a prerequisite for metastatic spread (544,547–549). Additionally, blood vessel density of tumors has been shown to be a potentially important new prognostic factor in multiple human neoplasms, including cancers of the ovary and cervix and endometrium (550–554).

Obviously, this is a very brief discussion of tumor angiogenesis. The reader is referred to several recent reviews on angiogenesis inhibition and its potential for cancer treatment (545,555–558). Several angiogenetic agents that have FDA approval for various indications that may have potential for the treatment of gynecologic cancers are briefly discussed below.

Bevacizumab

Bevacizumab (Avastin) is recombinant humanized monoclonal Ig G1 antibody that is designed to inhibit angiogenesis through targeting VEGF. This chemopreventive strategy is fairly tumor specific. It is currently under investigation in non–small-cell lung, breast, prostatic, renal-cell, and a variety of other malignancies. In 2003, a Biologics License Application was filed with the the FDA and it was approved for treatment for first-line metastatic colorectal cancer in combination with 5-FU–based chemotherapy. Although no trials have yet been conducted in gynecologic malignancies, ovarian, endometrial and cervical cancers have been shown to express VEGF-A (559–561). Future clinical research will likely evaluate the use of bevacizumab in these gynecologic malignancies.

Thalidomide

Thalidomide (Thalomid) is an antiangiogenic agent that is indicated for the treatment of cutaneous manifestations of erythema nodosum leprosum (ENL). However, thalidomide has been used in the treatment of various advanced malignancies and has demonstrated possible activity in ovarian and papillary-serous peritoneal carcinoma (562). Thalidomide has the chemical name α-(N-phthalimido)glutarimide. The molecular structure is $C_{13}H_{10}N_2O_4$, and it has a molecular weight of 258.2.

Although the exact mechanism of action is not fully characterized, the immunologic effects of thalidomide may be related to suppression of excessive tumor necrosis factor-α (TNF-α) production and downmodulation of selected cell surface adhesion molecules involved in leukocyte migration (563).

Thalidomide is an oral agent, which is supplied in 50-mg gelatin capsules. When used in chemotherapeutic regimens, the dose of thalidomide is generally titrated up to 400 mg/day as an evening dose (46). When used in a pilot study of ovarian and peritoneal carcinoma, daily thalidomide was initiated at 200 mg, with doses increasing by 100 mg per day every 2 weeks until response or tolerance (562).

Thalidomide is teratogenic and should not be used at any time during pregnancy. Latex condoms should be used by sexually active males using the drug because thalidomide is present in semen. The most common side effects include somnolence, peripheral neuropathy, dizziness, neutropenia, rash, and HIV viral load increase.

MODULATING AGENTS/SUPPORTIVE CARE DRUGS USED IN THE TREATMENT OF GYNECOLOGIC CANCERS

Defining approaches to improve the therapeutic index of cancer chemotherapy, such that tumor-cell kill is enhanced while toxicity to normal cells is minimized remains a fundamental goal of cancer treatment. A major limiting factor in successful cancer therapy is the ability of the tumor to develop resistance to the drugs used for treatment. A second fundamental problem faced by the oncologist treating patients with chemotherapy are the acute and chronic toxic effects of the drugs to the normal tissues. One approach that holds promise for the improvement of the therapeutic index is the concept of modulation, or the use of drugs with little or no cytotoxic activity to modulate the efficacy of standard anticancer drugs. Modulating agents can be divided into three main classes based on their ability to (a) protect host tissue from the toxic effects of the cancer drugs, (b) potentiate anticancer drugs, and (c) reverse acquired drug resistance. In this section, we discuss agents with chemoprotective abilities used with chemotherapy in the treatment of gynecologic cancers. The drugs outlined are not meant to be fully inclusive and the reader is referred to Tew et al.

(564) for a complete review on the subject of modulation of anticancer drug activities.

Chemoprotective Agents

Amifostine

Chemistry

Amifostine (Ethyol) is, to date, the most extensively developed broad-spectrum cytoprotective agent. Originally developed as a radioprotective compound, amifostine was selected from a series of over 4,400 synthetic thiol derivatives developed by the U.S. Army as having the most effective radioprotective effects and best safety profile (565). Subsequently, an extensive number of studies have demonstrated that amifostine selectively protects normal, but not tumor, tissue from the toxicities induced by radiation therapy and chemotherapy (564,566,567). Amifostine is FDA approved and indicated to reduce the cumulative renal toxicity associated with repeat cisplatin administration in patients with advanced ovarian cancer or non–small-cell lung cancer. More recently, it was FDA approved for chronic, three times weekly dosing, 15 to 20 minutes prior to daily radiation therapy in patients with head and neck cancer. Chemically, it is 2-[(3-aminopropyl)amino]ethanethiol dihydrogen phosphate (ester), its empiric formula is $C_5H_{15}N_2O_3PS$, and it has a molecular weight of 214.22.

Mechanism of Action

Amifostine is an inactive prodrug that is dephosphorylated to the active, free thiol species, WR1065, at the tissue site by cell membrane–bound and capillary alkaline phosphatase. The higher specific activity of the membrane-bound enzyme in normal tissue versus tumor tissue promotes rapid transport of the active thiol metabolite into the normal cell, with negligible transport into the cancer cells. The higher pH and higher activity of capillary alkaline phosphatase in normal tissue also contribute to the preferential uptake of WR1065 by normal cells (568). A number of mechanisms of protection by WR1065 have been reported, including scavenging of oxygen free radicals, direct intracellular binding to and subsequent detoxification of the active species of alkylating and platinum compounds, prevention or reversal of cisplatin-DNA adduct formation, induction of hypoxia, and alterations in intracellular glutathione and polyamine levels.

In addition to protecting normal cells from the cytotoxic effects of chemotherapy, amifostine has been shown to stimulate bone marrow progenitor cells (569) and sensitize tumor cells both *in vitro* and *in vivo* to the cytotoxic effects of anticancer agents, including nitrogen mustard, paclitaxel, melphalan, and carboplatin (78,570–572). Thus, amifostine is unique in that it is the only known modulating agent that may improve the therapeutic index for antitumor agents by dual mechanisms; that is, decreasing toxicity to normal tissue and potentiating tumor-specific cytotoxicity.

Drug Disposition

Pharmacokinetic studies in humans have shown that following IV administration at a dose of 740 or 910 mg/m^2, amifostine is rapidly cleared from the plasma and taken up into normal tissues with an α half-life of less than 1 minute and a β half-life of less than 10 minutes (573). Within 5 to 10 minutes after completion of a 15-minute infusion, greater than 90% of the parent drug is cleared from the plasma. A terminal elimination phase with a half-life of 48 minutes has also been reported (574). However, the plasma levels were very low during the elimination phase, and repeat dosing with amifostine at 2-hour intervals did not lead to increasing peak values at the end of each infusion.

Analyses of the human pharmacokinetics of WR1065 and the symmetric disulfide WR33278 following a single dose or three doses of amifostine (740 or 910 mg/m^2) 15 minutes before and 2 and 4 hours after chemotherapy have also been reported (574). WR1065 is rapidly cleared from the plasma by fast uptake into the tissues and conversion to disulfides. The initial half-life of 0.18 hour is followed by a slower, second phase with a half-life of 7.3 hours, where only low plasma levels are present. The final half-life of the disulfides ranged from 8.4 to 13.4 hours, and these metabolites were detectable 24 hours after treatment. As such, the disulfides may serve as an exchangeable pool of WR1065. After repeat dosing with amifostine, peak levels of WR1065 were increased, but peak levels of the disulfides were slightly decreased. This may suggest a change in the uptake or elimination of WR1065 or a saturation of the disulfide formation.

Amifostine changes the pharmacokinetics of carboplatin in humans, resulting in a longer, final half-life of ultrafiltrable platinum species in patients with a normal creatinine clearance, and a small increase in the AUC value (78). One can speculate that amifostine's effect on carboplatin pharmacokinetics may increase the efficacy of carboplatin in patients, similar to what has been observed in tumor-bearing mice. The effect of amifostine on the pharmacokinetics of cisplatin is minor, resulting in an increase of the final half-life of ultrafiltrable platinum but not unchanged cisplatin (575).

Administration and Dosage

The originally recommended schedule of amifostine was as a 15-minute IV infusion administered 15 to 30 minutes before chemotherapy; however, more recent studies have documented a markedly lower incidence of both hypotension and emesis when amifostine is administered by rapid IV bolus (576). Although an optimal dose has not been defined, amifostine is generally given at the MTD ranging from 740 to 910 mg/m^2.

Special Applications

Amifostine has been shown in a number of clinical trials to protect against cisplatin-induced nephrotoxicity and neurotoxicity and cyclophosphamide-induced hematotoxicity (566). Results of a randomized, multicenter Phase III trial of cyclophosphamide (1,000 mg/m^2) and cisplatin (100 mg/m^2) with or without amifostine (910 mg/m^2) every 3 weeks for six cycles in advanced epithelial ovarian cancer patients confirmed that pretreatment with amifostine reduces the cumulative renal, hematologic, and neurologic toxicities of the chemotherapy regimen (118). Final analysis of 242 patients (122 received amifostine) revealed that amifostine pretreatment yielded significant protection against the toxic effects of cisplatin. Twenty-six percent of patients (31 of 120) on the chemotherapy-alone arm compared with 10% of patients (12 of 122) pretreated with amifostine had treatment-limiting renal, neurologic, or ototoxicity requiring discontinuation of cisplatin treatment ($p = .001$). No patients on the amifostine arm discontinued therapy because of nephrotoxicity compared with seven patients on the chemotherapy-alone arm ($p = .008$). Significant hematoprotection also was observed, including a 53% reduction in the percentage of patients experiencing neutropenia-associated events ($p = .019$) and a 62% reduction in the total incidence of neutropenia-associated events ($p = .005$). The latter resulted in a 61% reduction in the number of days in the hospital ($p = .019$) and a 61% reduction in days on antibiotics ($p = .031$). No difference in survival was observed at a 41-month median follow-up period between patients on either arm of the study, suggesting that amifostine does not reduce the antitumor efficacy of chemotherapeutic treatment.

Results from a study in breast cancer patients receiving high-dose chemotherapy with autologous bone marrow support showed that amifostine treatment of bone marrow cells prior to *ex vivo* purging with 4-hydroxycyclophosphamide (4-HC) resulted in a significant decrease in time to leukocyte engraftment from 36 days (4-HC alone) to 26 days ($p = .032$) (577). Additionally, those patients treated with amifostine required significantly fewer platelet transfusions and days of antibiotic therapy. Results of a randomized Phase II trial of carboplatin plus amifostine versus carboplatin alone in patients with advanced solid tumors indicated that amifostine can reduce the cumulative thrombocytopenia resulting from carboplatin treatment (77).

Side Effects and Toxicities

The dose-limiting toxicities of amifostine include nausea, vomiting, and arterial hypotension. However, the emesis and hypotension can be reduced to relatively mild toxicities through rapid IV bolus administration together with the pre-administration of IV fluids, dexamethasone (20 mg IV in adults), and ondansetron (0.15 mg/kg IV) within 1 hour prior to chemotherapy (578). Amifostine administered on a daily

$\times$ 5 schedule at 825 mg/m^2, with cisplatin and radiation therapy, can result in hypocalcemic effects; however, these doses are no longer used in clinical trials. Wadler (579) reported that amifostine in extremely high doses can lead to a cumulative effect on decreased serum ionized calcium levels, which is mediated by direct inhibition of parathyroid hormone (PTH) activity. Administration of oral calcium with vitamin D supplements and frequent monitoring of serum ionized calcium levels are recommended for patients treated with the higher doses of amifostine, cisplatin, and radiation therapy.

Special Applications

The complications associated with IV administration have led to the ongoing development of amifostine for subcutaneous (SC) administration at 200 mg/m^2 three times weekly. The SC administration of amifostine has been evaluated in a number of preclinical and clincial studies; safety and efficacy studies have been conducted and are ongoing (580–583).

Dexrazoxane

Dexrazoxane (Zinecard), a metal-chelating agent, belongs to the bis-dioxopiperazine family, and was originally designed as a potential antitumor agent. Although early clinical trials failed to provide significant evidence of cytotoxic activity (584), an observation was made that the drug caused a marked increase in the urine clearance of iron and zinc (585). These findings, coupled with preclinical studies that showed that dexrazoxane and other chelating agents could prevent the acute myocardial damage induced by anthracyclines (586) without reducing the antitumor effect of the drugs (587) led to the use of dexrazoxane as a cardioprotective agent. Animal studies have shown that dexrazoxane can offer significant protection against anthracycline-induced cardiotoxicity, and dexrazoxane was most effective when given from 30 minutes before to 15 minutes after doxorubicin (588). Subsequent studies demonstrated that the degree of cardioprotection elicited by dexrazoxane is dependent on the dose of the anthracycline and the severity of the cardiomyopathy (589). Results from the initial clinical study of dexrazoxane in patients with metastatic breast cancer were encouraging and confirmed those of the preclinical studies. Speyer et al. (590) conducted a randomized trial of FAC (fluorouracil 500 mg/m^2, doxorubicin 50 mg/m^2, cyclophosphamide 500 mg/m^2) versus FAC plus dexrazoxane 1,000 mg/m^2, administered as an IV bolus injection 30 minutes before FAC therapy. Pretreatment with dexrazoxane offered significant protection against doxorubicin-induced cardiotoxicity as assessed by clinical examination, radionuclide scan of left ventricular ejection fraction, and endomyocardial biopsy. Patients receiving dexrazoxane received higher cumulative doses of doxorubicin, and significantly fewer of these patients were removed from the study because of cardiotoxicity.

Chemistry

Dexrazoxane is an FDA-approved chemoprotective agent that reduces the severity and incidence of cardiomyopathy in women with metastatic breast cancer undergoing doxorubicin therapy. Dexrazoxane is specifically indicated for women who have received a cumulative dose of 300 mg/m^2 or greater and who, in their physician's opinion, would benefit from further doxorubicin therapy. It is chemically known as (S)-4,4'-(1-methyl-1,2-ethanediyl)bis-2,6-piperazinedione, has the molecular formula $C_{11}H_{16}N_4O_4$, and has a molecular weight of 268.28.

Mechanism of Action

The proposed mechanism by which dexrazoxane reduces cardiotoxicity is through chelation of free or loosely bound iron by the hydrolyzed form of the drug (591). This prevents the binding of anthracyclines to intracellular iron and subsequent formation of toxic free radicals.

Administration and Dosage

Dexrazoxane must be reconstituted with 0.167 M (M/6) sodium lactate to give a concentration of 10 mg dexrazoxane for each milliliter of sodium lactate. It may be further diluted with either 0.9% sodium chloride or 5.0% dextrose to a concentration range of 1.3 to 5.0 mg/mL in intravenous infusion bags. It should be given slow IV push or rapid drip IV infusion. Dexrazoxane should be administered no less than 30 minutes before doxorubicin, and the recommended dose ratio of dexrazoxane to doxorubicin is 10:1 (i.e., dexrazoxane 500 mg/m^2:doxorubicin 50 mg/m^2).

Side Effects and Toxicities

Although randomized studies have shown that myelosuppression was slightly greater in patients pretreated with dexrazoxane, this does not appear to be clinically significant. In addition to dose-limiting granulocytopenia, other toxicities associated with the drug include mild nausea/vomiting and alopecia.

A number of studies in patients with advanced breast cancer have confirmed the protective effects of dexrazoxane against anthracycline-induced cardiotoxicity (592,593). Additionally, dexrazoxane was shown to have a significant cardioprotective effect in pediatric patients treated up to a cumulative doxorubicin dose of 410 mg/m^2 (594).

Special Applications

In addition to the cardioprotection indication for dexrazoxane, there are a number of other potential applications for this agent (595). Of particular interest, relative to the treatment of gynecologic malignancies, is the finding that dexrazoxane can enhance the effects of cisplatin in both drug-sensitive and drug-resistant human ovarian cancer cell lines.

Leucovorin

Leucovorin (folinic acid, citrovorum factor) was the original chemoprotective agent employed to overcome high-dose methotrexate-induced bone marrow toxicity (596,597). Leucovorin can serve as a substitute for the endogenous reduced-folate cofactor (N^5,N^{10}-methylene tetrahydrofolate) that is diminished by methotrexate. Thus, leucovorin can "rescue" cells by replenishing intracellular reduced-folate pools and preventing methotrexate toxicity via blockade of thymidine synthesis. Leucovorin acts in a dose- and time-dependent fashion and must be given within 48 hours of methotrexate in order to elicit its rescue effects.

Leucovorin is also a successful modulatory agent used clinically to potentiate the antitumor activity of 5-FU (564). Leucovorin can enhance the DNA toxicity induced by 5-FU through the formation of a stable tertiary complex of 5,10-methylene tetrahydrofolate, thymidylate synthase, and fluorodeoxyuridine monophosphate. Compared with 5-FU alone, this combination has been shown to produce higher response rates and, in some cases, longer survival for patients with metastatic gastrointestinal malignancies (598). The combination of 5-FU and leucovorin currently is being tested extensively in other malignancies, including metastatic breast cancer (599). A complete review of leucovorin as a modulating agent is beyond the scope of this chapter and the reader is referred to a number of excellent reviews on this topic (564,600).

Mesna

Mesna (Mesnex) is used clinically as the specific chemoprotective agent against bladder toxicity resulting from oxazophosphorine-based alkylating agents, such as cyclophosphamide and ifosfamide. It is sodium-2-mercaptoethane sulfone, with the molecular formula $C_2H_5NaO_3S_2$ and a molecular weight of 164.18.

Mechanism of Action

Mesna inactivates the protein-reactive aldehyde, acrolein metabolite of ifosfamide and cyclophosphamide, which accumulates in the urinary bladder and results in dose-limiting urotoxicity (252). Plasma conversion of mesna to its inactive disulfide metabolite, dimesna, allows for the pretreatment and simultaneous administration of mesna as a urinary protector for ifosfamide and cyclophosphamide (high dose). Following renal filtration and secretion, dimesna is converted back to the active parent compound by glutathione reductase, which is subsequently delivered to the bladder. The mesna free sulfydryl groups in the urinary bladder can directly complex to and thus neutralize acrolein, in addition to potentially blocking acrolein formation in the urinary tract (601). The metabolic characteristic of mesna should preclude any potential protection to tumors. Indeed, there is no clinical evidence that mesna co-administration with ifosfamide results in decreased antitumor activity. However, mesna has been shown to prevent the cytotoxicity of platinum agents when given simultaneously with them in *in vitro* models. As such, careful scheduling of mesna is warranted for clinical trials using ifosfamide in combination with platinum compounds. Additionally, mesna should not be given simultaneously with cisplatin.

Drug Disposition

Proper scheduling of mesna has been based on pharmacokinetic analysis, which showed that mesna and dimesna have relatively short half-lives of approximately 1 hour and that peak urinary thiol accumulation following IV or oral mesna occurs at 1 and 3 hours, respectively (602). Because the half-life of mesna is much shorter than that of acrolein, it must be administered beyond the completion of ifosfamide.

Administration and Dosage

Mesna is available as an IV injection and in 400-mg tablets. For IV administration, it should be diluted to obtain a final concentration of 20 mg/mL. The diluted solution is stable for 24 hours at room temperature. The approved schedule for IV administration of mesna is as a bolus dose (20% of the ifosfamide dose) prior to ifosfamide and two additional doses 4 and 8 hours after ifosfamide treatment (317). A combination of IV and oral mesna has been used more recently to simplify outpatient ifosfamide therapy. The oral dose of mesna is usually twice that of the IV dose, based on a 50% urinary bioavailability of oral mesna. Oral doses of 3 g/m^2 have been well tolerated in patients; however, nausea was observed in healthy volunteers receiving oral doses greater than 2 g/m^2. Goren (603) reviewed the dosing schedules and incidence of hematuria in 47 clinical studies in which oral mesna was administered to 1,986 patients who received greater than 6,475 courses of ifosfamide. Compilation of the data showed that a variety of doses and schedules of oral and IV mesna were effective at preventing hemorrhagic cystitis in patients treated with a number of different ifosfamide regimens. Although an optimal dose and schedule of mesna has not been established, adequate protection against ifosfamide-induced cystitis can be achieved using an initial IV dose of mesna that is equal to 20% of the ifosfamide dose, followed by two oral doses of mesna, each equal to 40% of the ifosfamide dose.

Side Effects and Toxicities

The most common side effects of mesna include headache, injection site reactions, flushing, dizziness, nausea, vomiting, flu-like symptoms, and coughing. Patients may develop hematuria (up to 6%) when adminstered ifosfamine plus mesna; a urine sample should be evaluated for hematuria each day prior to ifosfamide therapy.

Special Applications

The superiority of mesna as a chemoprotectant against ifosfamide- and cyclophosphamide-induced bladder toxicity has been demonstrated in a number of clinical trials (317). In a comparative study of patients treated with ifosfamide at a dose of 2 g/m^2/day for 5 days, only 20% of the patients treated with mesna (400 mg/m^2) exhibited hematuria compared with 60% of those treated with N-acetylcysteine (NAC, 1.5 g/m^2) (603). Similar results were reported by Munshi et al. (605), wherein 4.2% of patients treated with mesna developed hematuria compared with 27.9% of NAC patients. In a Phase II trial of ifosfamide and mesna in patients with platinum/paclitaxel–refractory ovarian cancer, there were no documented episodes of hemorrhagic cystitis, but one patient experienced treatment-related microscopic hematuria (316).

Subcutaneous administration of mesna is also being explored as an alternative to IV and oral dosing (606). Patients with gynecologic cancers receiving ifosfamide were treated with an initial IV dose of mesna at 20% of the ifosfamide dose. A subcutaneous infusion of mesna was given approximately 30 minutes after the completion of the ifosfamide infusion. A total dose of mesna equal to 40% of the ifosfamide dose was infused at a rate of 4 mL/hr over 8 hours. The subcutaneous infusion of mesna was well tolerated, and no episodes of gross hematuria were observed.

REFERENCES

1. Tozer N. Pharmacokinetics concepts basic to cancer chemotherapy. In: Ames MM, Powis G, Covach JS, eds. *Pharmacokinetics of anticancer agents in humans.* New York: Elsevier, 1983:1–27.
2. Alberts DS, Liu PY, Hannigan EV, et al. Intraperitoneal cisplatin plus intravenous cyclophosphamide versus intravenous cisplatin plus intravenous cyclophosphamide for stage III ovarian cancer [comment]. *N Engl J Med* 1996;335:1950–1955.
3. Markman M, Bundy BN, Alberts DS, et al. Phase III trial of standard-dose intravenous cisplatin plus paclitaxel versus moderately high-dose carboplatin followed by intravenous paclitaxel and intraperitoneal cisplatin in small-volume stage III ovarian carcinoma: an intergroup study of the Gynecologic Oncology Group, Southwestern Oncology Group, and Eastern Cooperative Oncology Group. *J Clin Oncol* 2001; 19:1001–1007.
4. Armstrong DK, Bundy BN, Baergen R, et al. Randomized phase III study of intravenous (IV) paclitaxel and cisplatin versus IV paclitaxel, intraperitoneal (IP) cisplatin and IP paclitaxel in optimal stage III epithelial ovarian cancer (OC): a Gynecologic Oncology Group trial (GOG 172). *Proc ASCO* 2002:803.
5. Rothenberg ML, Liu PY, Braly PS, et al. Combined intraperitoneal and intravenous chemotherapy for women with optimally debulked

ovarian cancer: results from an intergroup phase II trial. *J Clin Oncol* 2003;21:1313–1319.

6. Omura G, Blessing JA, Ehrlich CE, Miller, A, et al. A randomized trial of cyclophosphamide and doxorubicin with or without cisplatin in advanced ovarian carcinoma. A Gynecologic Oncology Group study. *Cancer* 1986;57:1725–1730.

7. Markman M. Intraperitoneal therapy of ovarian cancer. *Semin Oncol* 1998;25:356–360.

8. Los G, Mutsaers PH, van der Vijgh WJ, et al. Direct diffusion of cis-diamminedichloroplatinum(II) in intraperitoneal rat tumors after intraperitoneal chemotherapy: a comparison with systemic chemotherapy. *Cancer Res* 1989;49:3380–3384.

9. Rutty CJ, Connors TA. In vitro studies with hexamethylmelamine. *Biochem Pharmacol* 1977;26:2385–2591.

10. Rutty CJ, Connors TA, Nguyen Hoang N, et al. In vivo studies with hexamethylmelamine. *Eur J Cancer* 1978;14:713–720.

11. Ames MM, Powis G, Kovach JS, Eagan RT. Disposition and metabolism of pentamethylmelamine and hexamethylmelamine in rabbits and humans. *Cancer Res* 1979;39:5016–5021.

12. D'Incalci M, Bolis G, Mangioni C, et al. Variable oral absorption of hexamethylmelamine in man. *Cancer Treat Rep* 1978;62:2117–2119.

13. Markman M, Blessing JA, Moore D, et al. Altretamine (hexamethylmelamine) in platinum-resistant and platinum-refractory ovarian cancer: a Gynecologic Oncology Group phase II trial. *Gynecol Oncol* 1998;69:226–229.

14. Morris M, Eifel PJ, Lu J, et al. Pelvic radiation with concurrent chemotherapy compared with pelvic and para-aortic radiation for high-risk cervical cancer. *N Engl J Med* 1999;340:1137–1143.

15. Frasci G, Comella G, Comella P, et al. Carboplatin (CBDCA)-hexamethylmelamine (HMM)-oral etoposide (VP-16) first-line treatment of ovarian cancer patients with bulky disease: a phase II study. *Gynecol Oncol* 1995;58:68–73.

16. Kristensen GB, Baekelandt M, Vergote IB, Trope C. A phase II study of carboplatin and hexamethylmelamine as induction chemotherapy in advanced epithelial ovarian carcinoma. *Eur J Cancer* 1995;31A:1778–1780.

17. Division of Cancer Treatment N. Annual Report to the Food and Drug Administration. Hexamethylmelamine (NSC 13875; IND #954). Washington, DC: U.S. Government Printing Office, 1988.

18. van der Hoop RG, van der Burg ME, ten Bokkel Huinink WW, et al. Incidence of neuropathy in 395 patients with ovarian cancer treated with or without cisplatin. *Cancer* 1990;66:1697–1702.

19. Rothenberg ML, Liu PY, Wilczynski S, et al. Phase II trial of oral altretamine for consolidation of clinical complete remission in women with stage III epithelial ovarian cancer: a Southwest Oncology Group trial (SWOG-9326). *Gynecol Oncol* 2001;82:317–322.

20. Keldsen N, Havsteen H, Vergote I, et al. Altretamine (hexamethylmelamine) in the treatment of platinum-resistant ovarian cancer: a phase II study. *Gynecol Oncol* 2003;88:118–122.

21. Bruckner HW, Cohen CJ, Feuer E, Holland JF. Modulation and intensification of a cyclophosphamide, hexamethylmelamine, doxorubicin, and cisplatin ovarian cancer regimen. *Obstet Gynecol* 1989;73(3 Pt 1):349–356.

22. Edmonson JH, Wieand HS, McCormack GW. Role of hexamethylmelamine in the treatment of ovarian cancer: where is the needle in the haystack? *J Natl Cancer Inst* 1988;80:1172–1173.

23. Hainsworth JD, Jones HW 3rd, Burnett LS, et al. The role of hexamethylmelamine in the combination chemotherapy of advanced ovarian cancer: a comparison of hexamethylmelamine, cyclophosphamide, doxorubicin, and cisplatin (H-CAP) versus cyclophosphamide, doxorubicin, and cisplatin (CAP). *Am J Clin Oncol* 1990;13:410–415.

24. Baker LH, Opipari MI, Wilson H, et al. Mitomycin C, vincristine, and bleomycin therapy for advanced cervical cancer. *Obstet Gynecol* 1978;52:146–150.

25. Mirabelli CK, Huang CH, Crooke ST. Role of deoxyribonucleic acid topology in altering the site/sequence specificity of cleavage of deoxyribonucleic acid by bleomycin and talisomycin. *Biochemistry* 1983;22:300–306.

26. Dorr RT. Bleomycin pharmacology: mechanism of action and resistance, and clinical pharmacokinetics. *Semin Oncol* 1992;19[2 Suppl 5]:3–8.

27. Sebti SM, Jani JP, Mistry JS, et al. Metabolic inactivation: a mechanism of human tumor resistance to bleomycin. *Cancer Res* 1991;51:227–232.

28. Alberts DS, Chen HS, Liu R, et al. Bleomycin pharmacokinetics in man. I. Intravenous administration. *Cancer Chemother Pharmacol* 1978;1:177–181.

29. Ostrowski MJ. Intracavitary therapy with bleomycin for the treatment of malignant pleural effusions. *J Surg Oncol Suppl* 1989;1:7–13.

30. Ruckdeschel JC, Moores D, Lee JY, et al. Intrapleural therapy for malignant pleural effusions. A randomized comparison of bleomycin and tetracycline. *Chest* 1991;100:1528–1535.

31. Crooke ST, Comis RL, Einhorn LH, et al. Effects of variations in renal function on the clinical pharmacology of bleomycin administered as an IV bolus. *Cancer Treat Rep* 1977;61:1631–1636.

32. Crooke ST, Luft F, Broughton A, et al. Bleomycin serum pharmacokinetics as determined by a radioimmunoassay and a microbiologic assay in a patient with compromised renal function. *Cancer* 1977;39:1430–1434.

33. Oken MM, Crooke ST, Elson MK, et al. Pharmacokinetics of bleomycin after IM administration in man. *Cancer Treat Rep* 1981;65:485–489.

34. Samuels ML, Johnson DE, Holoye PY, Lanzotti VJ. Large-dose bleomycin therapy and pulmonary toxicity. A possible role of prior radiotherapy. *JAMA* 1976;235:1117–1120.

35. Ingrassia TS 3rd, Ryu JH, Trastek VF, Rosenow EC 3rd. Oxygen-exacerbated bleomycin pulmonary toxicity. *Mayo Clin Proc* 1991;66:173–178.

36. Katz EJ, Andrews PA, Howell SB. The effect of DNA polymerase inhibitors on the cytotoxicity of cisplatin in human ovarian carcinoma cells. *Cancer Commun* 1990;2:159–164.

37. Maher J, Daly PA. Severe bleomycin lung toxicity: reversal with high dose corticosteroids. *Thorax* 1993;48:92–94.

38. Nici L, Calabresi P. Amifostine modulation of bleomycin-induced lung injury in rodents. *Semin Oncol* 1999;26[2 Suppl 7]:28–33.

39. Nici L, Santos-Moore A, Kuhn C, Calabresi P. Modulation of bleomycin-induced pulmonary toxicity in the hamster by the antioxidant amifostine. *Cancer* 1998;83:2008–2014.

40. Kerr LD, Spiera H. Scleroderma in association with the use of bleomycin: a report of 3 cases. *J Rheumatol* 1992;19:294–296.

41. Haerslev T, Avnstorp C, Joergensen M. Sudden onset of adverse effects due to low-dosage bleomycin indicates an idiosyncratic reaction. *Cutis* 1993;52:45–46.

42. Yee GC, Crom WR, Champion JE, et al. Cisplatin-induced changes in bleomycin elimination. *Cancer Treat Rep* 1983;67:587–589.

43. Bennett WM, Pastore L, Houghton DC. Fatal pulmonary bleomycin toxicity in cisplatin-induced acute renal failure. *Cancer Treat Rep* 1980;64:921–924.

44. Crooke ST, Bradner WT. Bleomycin, a review. *J Med* 1976;7:333–428.

45. Gerbrecht BM. Current Canadian experience with capecitabine: partnering with patients to optimize therapy. *Cancer Nursing* 2003;26:161–167.

46. Chu E, DeVita VT. *Physicians' Cancer Chemotherapy Drug Manual 2003*. Sudbury, MA: Jones and Bartlett Publishers, 2003.

47. Horacek P, Drobnik J. Interaction of cis-dichlorodiammineplatinum (II) with DNA. *Biochim Biophys Acta* 1971;254:341–347.

48. DeNeve W, Valeriote F, Tapazoglou E, et al. Discrepancy between cytotoxicity and DNA interstrand crosslinking of carboplatin and cisplatin in vivo. *Invest New Drugs* 1990;8:17–24.

49. Micetich KC, Barnes D, Erickson LC. A comparative study of the cytotoxicity and DNA-damaging effects of cis-(diammino)(1,1-cyclobutanedicarboxylato)-platinum(II) and cis-diamminedichloroplatinum(II) on L1210 cells. *Cancer Res* 1985;45:4043–4047.

50. du Bois A, Luck HJ, Meier W, et al. Carboplatin/paclitaxel versus cisplatin/paclitaxel as first-line chemotherapy in advanced ovarian cancer: an interim analysis of a randomized phase III trial of the Arbeitsgemeinschaft Gynakologische Onkologie Ovarian Cancer Study Group. *Semin Oncol* 1997;24[5 Suppl 15]:S15–44–S15–52.

51. Aabo K, Adams M, Adnitt P, et al. Chemotherapy in advanced ovarian cancer: four systematic meta-analyses of individual patient data from 37 randomized trials. Advanced Ovarian Cancer Trialists' Group. *Br J Cancer* 1998;78:1479–1487.

52. Harrap KR. Preclinical studies identifying carboplatin as a viable cisplatin alternative. *Cancer Treat Rev* 1985;12[Suppl A]:21–33.

53. Wilkinson R, Cox PJ, Jones M, et al. Selection of potential second generation platinum compounds. *Biochem J* 1978;60:851.

54. Zwelling LA, Kohn KW. Mechanism of action of cis-dichlorodiammineplatinum(II). *Cancer Treat Rep* 1979;63:1439–1444.

55. Gaver RC, George AM, Deeb G. In vitro stability, plasma protein binding and blood cell partitioning of 14C-carboplatin. *Cancer Chemother Pharmacol* 1987;20:271–276.

56. Shea TC, Flaherty M, Elias A, et al. A phase I clinical and pharmacokinetic study of carboplatin and autologous bone marrow support. *J Clin Oncol* 1989;7:651–661.

57. Van Echo DA, Egorin MJ, Whitacre MY, et al. Phase I clinical and pharmacologic trial of carboplatin daily for 5 days. *Cancer Treat Rep* 1984;68:1103–1114.

58. Horwich A, Dearnaley DP, Duchesne GM, et al. Simple nontoxic treatment of advanced metastatic seminoma with carboplatin. *J Clin Oncol* 1989;7:1150–1156.

59. Misset B, Escudier B, Leclercq B, et al. Acute myocardiotoxicity during 5-fluorouracil therapy. *Intensive Care Med* 1990;16:210–211.

60. Calvert AH, Newell DR, Gumbrell LA, et al. Carboplatin dosage: prospective evaluation of a simple formula based on renal function. *J Clin Oncol* 1989;7:1748–1756.

61. Martino G, Frusciante V, Varraso A, et al. Efficacy of 51Cr-EDTA clearance to tailor a carboplatin therapeutic regimen in ovarian cancer patients. *Anticancer Res* 1999;19:5587–5591.

62. Cockroft DW, Gault MH. Prediction of creatinine clearance for serum creatinine. *Nephron* 1976;16:31.

63. Belani CP, Kearns CM, Zuhowski EG, et al. Phase I trial, including pharmacokinetic and pharmacodynamic correlations, of combination paclitaxel and carboplatin in patients with metastatic non–small-cell lung cancer. *J Clin Oncol* 1999;17:676–684.

64. Calvert AH, Boddy A, Bailey NP, et al. Carboplatin in combination with paclitaxel in advanced ovarian cancer: dose determination and pharmacokinetic and pharmacodynamic interactions. *Semin Oncol* 1995;22[5 Suppl 12]:91–98; Discussion 99–100.

65. Okamoto H, Nagatomo A, Kunitoh H, et al. Prediction of carboplatin clearance calculated by patient characteristics or 24-hour creatinine clearance: a comparison of the performance of three formulae. *Cancer Chemother Pharmacol* 1998;42:307–312.

66. Sorensen BT, Stromgren A, Jakobsen P, Jakobsen A. Dose-toxicity relationship of carboplatin in combination with cyclophosphamide in ovarian cancer patients. *Cancer Chemother Pharmacol* 1991;28:397–401.

67. Neijt JP, du Bois A. Paclitaxel/carboplatin for the initial treatment of advanced ovarian cancer. *Semin Oncol* 1999;26[1 Suppl 2]:78–83.

68. The International Collaborative Ovarian Neoplasm G. Paclitaxel plus carboplatin versus standard chemotherapy with either single-agent carboplatin or cyclophosphamide, doxorubicin, and cisplatin in women with ovarian cancer: the ICON3 randomised trial [Comment]. *Lancet* 2002;360:505–515.

69. Calvert AH, Harland SJ, Newell DR, et al. Early clinical studies with cis-diammine-1,1-cyclobutane dicarboxylate platinum II. *Cancer Chemother Pharmacol* 1982;9:140–147.

70. Canetta R, Rozencweig M, Carter SK. Carboplatin: the clinical spectrum to date. *Cancer Treat Rev* 1985;12[Suppl A]:125–136.

71. Plezia PM, Alberts DS, Kessler J, et al. Immediate termination of intractable vomiting induced by cisplatin combination chemotherapy using an intensive five-drug antiemetic regimen. *Cancer Treat Rep* 1984;68:1493–1495.

72. Markman M, Kennedy A, Webster K, et al. Clinical features of hypersensitivity reactions to carboplatin. *J Clin Oncol* 1999;17:1141.

73. Shukunami K, Kurokawa T, Kawakami Y, et al. Hypersensitivity reactions to intraperitoneal administration of carboplatin in ovarian cancer: the first report of a case. *Gynecol Oncol* 1999;72:431–432.

74. Travis LB, Holowaty EJ, Bergfeldt K, et al. Risk of leukemia after platinum-based chemotherapy for ovarian cancer. *N Engl J Med* 1999;340:351–357.

75. Stiff PJ, McKenzie RS, Alberts DS, et al. Phase I clinical and pharmacokinetic study of high-dose mitoxantrone combined with carboplatin, cyclophosphamide, and autologous bone marrow rescue: high response rate for refractory ovarian carcinoma. *J Clin Oncol* 1994;12:176–183.

76. Calvert AH. A review of the pharmacokinetics and pharmacodynamics of combination carboplatin/paclitaxel. *Semin Oncol* 1997;24[1 Suppl 2]:S2–85–S2–90.

77. Budd GT, Ganapathi R, Adelstein DJ, et al. Randomized trial of carboplatin plus amifostine versus carboplatin alone in patients with advanced solid tumors. *Cancer* 1997;80:1134–1140.

78. Korst AE, van der Sterre ML, Eeltink CM, et al. Pharmacokinetics of carboplatin with and without amifostine in patients with solid tumors. *Clin Cancer Res* 1997;3:697–703.

79. Markman M, Reichman B, Hakes T, et al. Evidence supporting the superiority of intraperitoneal cisplatin compared to intraperitoneal carboplatin for salvage therapy of small-volume residual ovarian cancer. *Gynecol Oncol* 1993;50:100–104.

80. Muggia FM, Jeffers S, Muderspach L, et al. Phase I/II study of intraperitoneal floxuridine and platinums (cisplatin and/or carboplatin). *Gynecol Oncol* 1997;66:290–294.

81. DeGregorio MW, Lum BL, Holleran WM, et al. Preliminary observations of intraperitoneal carboplatin pharmacokinetics during a phase I study of the Northern California Oncology Group. *Cancer Chemother Pharmacol* 1986;18:235–238.

82. Reed E, Ozols RF, Tarone R, et al. Platinum-DNA adducts in leukocyte DNA correlate with disease response in ovarian cancer patients receiving platinum-based chemotherapy. *Proc Natl Acad Sci U S A* 1987;84:5024–5028.

83. Rice JA, Crothers DM, Pinto AL, Lippard SJ. The major adduct of the antitumor drug cis-diamminedichloroplatinum(II) with DNA bends the duplex by approximately equal to 40 degrees toward the major groove. *Proc Natl Acad Sci U S A* 1988;85:4158–4161.

84. Perez RP. Cellular and molecular determinants of cisplatin resistance. *Eur J Cancer* 1998;34:1535–1542.

85. Reed E. Platinum-DNA adduct, nucleotide excision repair and platinum based anti-cancer chemotherapy. *Cancer Treat Rev* 1998;24:331–344.

86. Rose PG, Mossbruger K, Fusco N, et al. Gemcitabine reverses cisplatin resistance: demonstration of activity in platinum- and multidrug-resistant ovarian and peritoneal carcinoma. *Gynecol Oncol* 2003;88:17–21.

87. DeConti RC, Toftness BR, Lange RC, Creasey WA. Clinical and pharmacological studies with cis-diamminedichloroplatinum (II). *Cancer Res* 1973;33:1310–1315.

88. Gensia Sicor Pharmaceuticals I. Cisplatin Package Insert. 2000.

89. Earhart RH. Instability of cis-dichlorodiammineplatinum in dextrose solution. *Cancer Treat Rev* 1979;6:1105.

90. Eshaque M, McKay MJ, Theophande T, et al. p-Mannitol platinum complexes. *Wadley Med Bull* 1976;7:338.

91. Prestayko AW, Cadiz M, Crooke ST. Incompatibility of aluminum-containing IV administration equipment with cis-dichlorodiammineplatinum(II) administration. *Cancer Treat Rep* 1979;63:2118–2119.

92. Hayes DM, Cvitkovic E, Golbey RB, et al. High dose cis-platinum diamine dichloride: amelioration of renal toxicity by mannitol diuresis. *Cancer* 1977;39:1372–1381.

93. Rainey JM, Alberts DS. Safe, rapid administration schedule for cis-platinum-mannitol. *Med Pediatr Oncol* 1978;4:371–375.

94. Brock J, Alberts DS. Safe, rapid administration of cisplatin in the outpatient clinic. *Cancer Treat Rep* 1986;70:1409–1414.

95. McGuire WP, Hoskins WJ, Brady MF, et al. Cyclophosphamide and cisplatin compared with paclitaxel and cisplatin in patients with stage III and stage IV ovarian cancer. *N Engl J Med* 1996;334:1–6.

96. Connelly E, Markman M, Kennedy A, et al. Paclitaxel delivered as a 3-hr infusion with cisplatin in patients with gynecologic cancers: unexpected incidence of neurotoxicity. *Gynecol Oncol* 1996;62:166–168.

97. Levin L, Hryniuk WM. Dose intensity analysis of chemotherapy regimens in ovarian carcinoma. *J Clin Oncol* 1987;5:756–767.

98. Bonomi P, Blessing JA, Stehman FB, et al. Randomized trial of three cisplatin dose schedules in squamous-cell carcinoma of the cervix: a Gynecologic Oncology Group study. *J Clin Oncol* 1985;3:1079–1085.

99. Gandara DR, Wold H, Perez EA, et al. Cisplatin dose intensity in non-small cell lung cancer: phase II results of a day 1 and day 8 high-dose regimen. *J Natl Cancer Inst* 1989;81:790–794.

100. Holleran WM, DeGregorio MW. Evolution of high-dose cisplatin. *Invest New Drugs* 1988;6:135–142.

101. Gonzalez-Vitale JC, Hayes DM, Cvitkovic E, Sternberg SS. Acute renal failure after cis-dichlorodiammineplatinum(II) and gentamicin-cephalothin therapies. *Cancer Treat Rep* 1978;62:693–698.

102. Madias NE, Harrington JT. Platinum nephrotoxicity. *Am J Med* 1978; 65:307–314.

103. Fleming S, Peppard S, Ratanatharathorn V, et al. Ototoxicity from cis-platinum in patients with stages III and IV previously untreated squamous cell cancer of the head and neck. *Am J Clin Oncol* 1985; 8:302–306.

104. Alberts DS, Noel JK. Cisplatin-associated neurotoxicity: can it be prevented? *Anticancer Drugs* 1995;6:369–383.

105. Cersosimo RJ. Cisplatin neurotoxicity. *Cancer Treat Rev* 1989;16: 195–211.

106. Stengs CH, Klis SF, Huizing EH, Smoorenburg GF. Protective effects of a neurotrophic ACTH(4–9) analog on cisplatin ototoxicity in relation to the cisplatin dose: an electrocochleographic study in albino guinea pigs. *Hear Res* 1998;124:108–117.

107. Rose PG. Amifostine cytoprotection with chemotherapy for advanced ovarian carcinoma. *Semin Oncol* 1996;23[4 Suppl 8]:83–89.

108. Willox JC, McAllister EJ, Sangster G, Kaye SB. Effects of magnesium supplementation in testicular cancer patients receiving cis-platin: a randomised trial. *Br J Cancer* 1986;54:19–23.

109. Morrow GR, Hickok JT, Rosenthal SN. Progress in reducing nausea and emesis. Comparisons of ondansetron (Zofran), granisetron (Kytril), and tropisetron (Navoban). *Cancer* 1995;76:343–357.

110. Latreille J, Pater J, Johnston D, et al. Use of dexamethasone and granisetron in the control of delayed emesis for patients who receive highly emetogenic chemotherapy. National Cancer Institute of Canada Clinical Trials Group. *J Clin Oncol* 1998;16:1174–1178.

111. Kris MG, Gralla RJ, Tyson LB, et al. Controlling delayed vomiting: double-blind, randomized trial comparing placebo, dexamethasone alone, and metoclopramide plus dexamethasone in patients receiving cisplatin. *J Clin Oncol* 1989;7:108–114.

112. Khan A, Hill JM, Grater W, et al. Atopic hypersensitivity to cis-dichlorodiammineplatinum(II) and other platinum complexes. *Cancer Res* 1975;35:2766–2770.

113. Von Hoff DD, Slavik M, Muggia FM. Allergic reactions to cis platinum [Letter]. *Lancet* 1976;1:90.

114. Wiesenfeld M, Reinders E, Corder M, et al. Successful re-treatment with cis-dichlorodiammineplatinum(II) after apparent allergic reactions. *Cancer Treat Rep* 1979;63:219–221.

115. Abels RI. Use of recombinant human erythropoietin in the treatment of anemia in patients who have cancer. *Semin Oncol* 1992;19[3 Suppl 8]:29–35.

116. Rowinsky EK, Donehower RC. Paclitaxel (Taxol). *N Engl J Med* 1995;332:1004–1014.

117. de Jonge MJ, Loos WJ, Gelderblom H, et al. Phase I pharmacologic study of oral topotecan and intravenous cisplatin: sequence-dependent hematologic side effects. *J Clin Oncol* 2000;18:2104–2115.

118. Kemp G, Rose P, Lurain J, et al. Amifostine pretreatment for protection against cyclophosphamide-induced and cisplatin-induced toxicities: results of a randomized control trial in patients with advanced ovarian cancer. *J Clin Oncol* 1996;14:2101–2112.

119. Schuchter LM, Hensley ML, Meropol NJ, Winer EP, American Society of Clinical Oncology C, Radiotherapy Expert P. 2002 update of recommendations for the use of chemotherapy and radiotherapy protectants: clinical practice guidelines of the American Society of Clinical Oncology. *J Clin Oncol* 2002;20:2895–2903.

120. Keys HM, Bundy BN, Stehman FB, et al. Cisplatin, radiation, and adjuvant hysterectomy compared with radiation and adjuvant hysterectomy for bulky stage IB cervical carcinoma. *N Engl J Med* 1999; 340:1154–1161.

121. Peters WA 3rd, Liu PY, Barrett RJ 2nd, et al. Concurrent chemotherapy and pelvic radiation therapy compared with pelvic radiation therapy alone as adjuvant therapy after radical surgery in high-risk early-stage cancer of the cervix. *J Clin Oncol* 2000;18:1606–1613.

122. Rose PG, Bundy BN, Watkins EB, et al. Concurrent cisplatin-based radiotherapy and chemotherapy for locally advanced cervical cancer. *N Engl J Med* 1999;340:1144–1153.

123. Bagley CM Jr, Bostick FW, DeVita VT Jr. Clinical pharmacology of cyclophosphamide. *Cancer Res* 1973;33:226–233.

124. Struck RF, Alberts DS, Horne K, et al. Plasma pharmacokinetics of cyclophosphamide and its cytotoxic metabolites after intravenous versus oral administration in a randomized, crossover trial. *Cancer Res* 1987;47:2723–2726.

125. Cohen JL, Jao JY, Jusko WJ. Pharmacokinetics of cyclophosphamide in man. *Br J Pharmacol* 1971;43:677–680.

126. Dorr RT, Von Hoff DD. *Cancer Chemotherapy Handbook*. 2nd ed. Norwalk, CT: Appleton & Lange; 1994.

127. DeFronzo RA, Braine H, Colvin M, Davis PJ. Water intoxication in man after cyclophosphamide therapy. Time course and relation to drug activation. *Ann Intern Med* 1973;78:861–869.

128. Topilow AA, Rothenberg SP, Cottrell TS. Interstitial pneumonia after prolonged treatment with cyclophosphamide. *Am Rev Respir Dis* 1973;108:114–117.

129. Karchmer RK, Hansen VL. Possible anaphylactic reaction to intravenous cyclophosphamide. Report of a case. *JAMA* 1977;237:475.

130. Braverman AC, Antin JH, Plappert MT, et al. Cyclophosphamide cardiotoxicity in bone marrow transplantation: a prospective evaluation of new dosing regimens. *J Clin Oncol* 1991;9:1215–1223.

131. Connors TA, Cox PJ, Farmer PB, et al. Some studies of the active intermediates formed in the microsomal metabolism of cyclophosphamide and isophosphamide. *Biochem Pharmacol* 1974;23:115–129.

132. Wiemann MC, Cummings FJ, Kaplan HG, et al. Clinical and pharmacological studies of methotrexate-minimal leucovorin rescue plus fluorouracil. *Cancer Res* 1982;42:3896–3900.

133. Dorr RT, Soble MJ, Alberts DS. Interaction of cimetidine but not ranitidine with cyclophosphamide in mice. *Cancer Res* 1986;46: 1795–1799.

134. Struck RF, Alberts DS, Plezia PM, et al. Effect of the antiulcer drug ranitidine on the pharmacokinetics and hematologic toxicity of cyclophosphamide and its cytotoxic metabolites in patients. *Proc AACR* 1988;29:187(abst).

135. Homesley HD. Single-agent therapy for nonmetastatic and low-risk gestational trophoblastic disease. *J Reprod Med* 1998;43:69–74.

136. Harris NL, Brenner DE, Anthony LB, et al. The influence of ranitidine on the pharmacokinetics and toxicity of doxorubicin in rabbits. *Cancer Chemother Pharmacol* 1988;21:323–328.

137. Williams SD. Ovarian germ cell tumors: an update. *Semin Oncol* 1998;25:407–413.

138. Schwartz HS. Some determinants of the therapeutic efficacy of actinomycin D (NSC-3053), adriamycin (NSC-123127), and daunorubicin (NSC-83142). *Cancer Chemother Rep* 1974;58:55–62.

139. Knutsen T, Mickley LA, Ried T, et al. Cytogenetic and molecular characterization of random chromosomal rearrangements activating the drug resistance gene, MDR1/P-glycoprotein, in drug-selected cell lines and patients with drug refractory ALL. *Genes Chromosomes Cancer* 1998;23:44–54.

140. Tattersall MH, Sodergren JE, Dengupta SK, et al. Pharmacokinetics of actinoymcin D in patients with malignant melanoma. *Clin Pharmacol Ther* 1975;17:701–708.

141. Brothman AR, Davis TP, Duffy JJ, Lindell TJ. Development of an antibody to actinomycin D and its application for the detection of serum levels by radioimmunoassay. *Cancer Res* 1982;42:1184–1187.

142. Blatt J, Trigg ME, Pizzo PA, Glaubiger D. Tolerance to single-dose dactinomycin in combination chemotherapy for solid tumors. *Cancer Treat Rep* 1981;65:145–147.

143. Petrilli ES, Twiggs LB, Blessing JA, et al. Single-dose actinomycin-D treatment for nonmetastatic gestational trophoblastic disease. A prospective phase II trial of the Gynecologic Oncology Group. *Cancer* 1987;60:2173–2176.

144. Philips RS, Schwartz HS, Sternberg SS, Tan CTC. The toxicity of actinomycin D. *Ann N Y Acad Sci* 1970;89:348.

145. Frei E 3rd. The clinical use of actinomycin. *Cancer Chemother Rep* 1974;58:49–54.

146. Cohen IJ, Loven D, Schoenfeld T, et al. Dactinomycin potentiation of radiation pneumonitis: a forgotten interaction. *Pediatr Hematol Oncol* 1991;8:187–192.

147. Francis P, Schneider J, Hann L, et al. Phase II trial of docetaxel in patients with platinum-refractory advanced ovarian cancer. *J Clin Oncol* 1994;12:2301–2308.

148. Gelmon K. The taxoids: paclitaxel and docetaxel. *Lancet* 1994;344: 1267–1272.

149. Gottlieb JA, Luce JK. Cerebellar ataxia with weekly 5-fluorouracil administration. *Lancet* 1971;1:138–139.

150. Bruno R, Sanderink GJ. Pharmacokinetics and metabolism of Taxotere (docetaxel). *Cancer Surv* 1993;17:305–313.

151. Aapro MS. Phase I and pharmacokinetic study of RP 56976 in a new ethanol-free formulation of Taxotere. *Ann Oncol* 1992;3:208.

152. Von Hoff DD. The taxoids: same roots, different drugs. *Semin Oncol* 1997;24[4 Suppl 13]:S13–3–S13–10.

153. Maisano R, Mare M, Zavettieri M, et al. Is weekly docetaxel an active and gentle chemotherapy in the treatment of metastatic breast cancer? *Anticancer Res* 2003;23:1923–1926.

154. Stemmler HJ, Gutschow K, Sommer H, et al. Weekly docetaxel (Taxotere) in patients with metastatic breast cancer. *Ann Oncol* 2001;12:1393–1398.

155. Pronk LC, Schellens JH, Planting AS, et al. Phase I and pharmacologic study of docetaxel and cisplatin in patients with advanced solid tumors. *J Clin Oncol* 1997;15:1071–1079.

156. Kaye SB, Piccart M, Aapro M, et al. Phase II trials of docetaxel (Taxotere) in advanced ovarian cancer—an updated overview. *Eur J Cancer* 1997;33:2167–2170.

157. Wanders J, Schrijvers D, Bruntsch U, et al. The EORTC-ECTG experience with acute hypersensitivity reactions (HSR) in Taxotere studies. *Proc ASCO* 1993;12:73(abst).

158. Galindo E, Kavanagh J, Fossella F, et al. Docetaxel (Taxotere) toxicities: analysis of a single institution experience with 168 patients (623 courses). *Proc Am Soc Clin Oncol* 1994;13:164.

159. Zimmerman GC, Keeling JH, Lowry M, et al. Prevention of docetaxel-induced erythrodysesthesia with local hypothermia. *J Natl Cancer Inst* 1994;86:557–558.

160. Eisenhauer EA, Vermorken JB. The taxoids. Comparative clinical pharmacology and therapeutic potential. *Drugs* 1998;55:5–30.

161. Verschraegen CF, Kudelka AP, Steger M, et al. Randomized phase II study of two dose levels of docetaxel in patients with advanced epithelial ovarian cancer who have failed paclitaxel chemotherapy. *Proc ASCO* 1997;16:381(abst).

162. Rose PG, Blessing JA, Ball HG, et al. A phase II study of docetaxel in paclitaxel-resistant ovarian and peritoneal carcinoma: a Gynecologic Oncology Group study. *Gynecol Oncol* 2003;88:130–135.

163. Henry DW. Structure-activity relationships among daunorubicin and Adriamycin analogs. *Cancer Treat Rep* 1979;63:845–854.

164. Hasinoff BB, Davey JP. Adriamycin and its iron(III) and copper(II) complexes. Glutathione-induced dissociation; cytochrome c oxidase inactivation and protection; binding to cardiolipin. *Biochem Pharmacol* 1988;37:3663–3669.

165. Myers CE, Gianni L, Simone CB, et al. Oxidative destruction of erythrocyte ghost membranes catalyzed by the doxorubicin-iron complex. *Biochemistry* 1982;21:1707–1712.

166. Di Marco A, Zunino F, Silverstrini R, et al. Interaction of some daunomycin derivatives with deoxyribonucleic acid and their biological activity. *Biochem Pharmacol* 1971;20:1323–1328.

167. Painter RB. Inhibition of DNA replicon initiation by 4-nitroquinoline 1-oxide, Adriamycin, and ethyleneimine. *Cancer Res* 1978;38:4445–4449.

168. Driscoll JS, Hazard GF Jr, Wood HB Jr, Goldin A. Structure-antitumor activity relationships among quinone derivatives. *Cancer Chemother Rep* 1974;4:1–362.

169. Goodman J, Hochstein P. Generation of free radicals and lipid peroxidation by redox cycling of Adriamycin and daunomycin. *Biochem Biophys Res Commun* 1977;77:797–803.

170. Kim SH, Kim JH. Lethal effect of Adriamycin on the division cycle of HeLa cells. *Cancer Res* 1972;32:323–325.

171. Ritch PS, Occhipinti SJ, Cunningham RE, Shackney SE. Schedule-dependent synergism of combinations of hydroxyurea with Adriamycin and 1-beta-D-arabinofuranosylcytosine with Adriamycin. *Cancer Res* 1981;41:3881–3884.

172. Glisson BS, Ross WE. DNA topoisomerase II: a primer on the enzyme and its unique role as a multidrug target in cancer chemotherapy. *Pharmacol Ther* 1987;32:89–106.

173. Tewey KM, Chen GL, Nelson EM, Liu LF. Intercalative antitumor drugs interfere with the breakage-reunion reaction of mammalian DNA topoisomerase II. *J Biol Chem* 1984;259:9182–9187.

174. Eksborg S, Ehrsson H, Ekqvist B. Protein binding of anthraquinone glycosides, with special reference to Adriamycin. *Cancer Chemother Pharmacol* 1982;10:7–10.

175. Piazza E, Broggini M, Trabattoni A, et al. Adriamycin distribution in plasma and blood cells of cancer patients with altered hematocrit. *Eur J Cancer Clin Oncol* 1981;17:1089–1096.

176. Benjamin RS, Riggs CE Jr, Bachur NR. Plasma pharmacokinetics of Adriamycin and its metabolites in humans with normal hepatic and renal function. *Cancer Res* 1977;37:1416–1420.

177. Lee YT, Chan KK, Harris PA, Cohen JL. Distribution of Adriamycin in cancer patients: tissue uptakes, plasma concentration after IV and hepatic IA administration. *Cancer* 1980;45:2231–2239.

178. Egan PC, Costanza ME, Dodion P, et al. Doxorubicin and cisplatin excretion into human milk. *Cancer Treat Rep* 1985;69:1387–1389.

179. D'Incalci M, Broggini M, Buscaglia M, Pardi G. Transplacental passage of doxorubicin. *Lancet* 1983;1:75.

180. Karp GI, von Oeyen P, Valone F, et al. Doxorubicin in pregnancy: possible transplacental passage. *Cancer Treat Rep* 1983;67:773–777.

181. Roboz J, Gleicher N, Wu K, et al. Does doxorubicin cross the placenta? *Lancet* 1979;2:1382–1383.

182. Bachur NR. Adriamycin (NSC-123127) pharmacology. *Cancer Chemother Rep* 1975;6:153.

183. Riggs CE Jr, Benjamin RS, Serpick AA, Bachur NR. Bilary disposition of Adriamycin. *Clin Pharmacol Ther* 1977;22:234–241.

184. Benjamin RS. A practical approach to Adriamycin (NSC-123127). *Cancer Chemother Rep* 1975;6:191.

185. Chan KK, Chlebowski RT, Tong M, et al. Clinical pharmacokinetics of Adriamycin in hepatoma patients with cirrhosis. *Cancer Res* 1980;40:1263–1268.

186. Rodvold KA, Rushing DA, Tewksbury DA. Doxorubicin clearance in the obese. *J Clin Oncol* 1988;6:1321–1327.

187. Gessner T, Robert J, Bolanowska W, et al. Effects of prior therapy on plasma levels of Adriamycin during subsequent therapy. *J Med* 1981;12:183–193.

188. Morris RG, Reece PA, Dale BM, et al. Alteration in doxorubicin and doxorubicinol plasma concentrations with repeated courses to patients. *Ther Drug Monit* 1989;11:380–383.

189. Robert J, Hoerni B. Age dependence of the early-phase pharmacokinetics of doxorubicin. *Cancer Res* 1983;43:4467–4469.

190. Garnick MB, Ensminger WD, Israel M. A clinical-pharmacological evaluation of hepatic arterial infusion of Adriamycin. *Cancer Res* 1979;39:4105–4110.

191. Bern MM, McDermott W Jr, Cady B, et al. Intraaterial hepatic infusion and intravenous Adriamycin for treatment of hepatocellular carcinoma: a clinical and pharmacology report. *Cancer* 1978;42:399–405.

192. Chen HS, Gross JF. Intra-arterial infusion of anticancer drugs: theoretic aspects of drug delivery and review of responses. *Cancer Treat Rep* 1980;64:31–40.

193. Legha SS, Benjamin RS, Mackay B, et al. Reduction of doxorubicin cardiotoxicity by prolonged continuous intravenous infusion. *Ann Intern Med* 1982;96:133–139.

194. Creasey WA, McIntosh LS, Brescia T, et al. Clinical effects and pharmacokinetics of different dosage schedules of Adriamycin. *Cancer Res* 1976;36:216–221.

195. Hryniuk W, Levine MN. Analysis of dose intensity for adjuvant chemotherapy trials in stage II breast cancer. *J Clin Oncol* 1986;4:1162–1170.

196. Carmo-Pereira J, Costa FO, Henriques E, et al. A comparison of two doses of Adriamycin in the primary chemotherapy of disseminated breast carcinoma. *Br J Cancer* 1987;56:471–473.

197. Reilly JJ, Neifeld JP, Rosenberg SA. Clinical course and management of accidental Adriamycin extravasation. *Cancer* 1977;40:2053–2056.

198. Rudolph R, Stein RS, Pattillo RA. Skin ulcers due to Adriamycin. *Cancer* 1976;38:1087–1094.

199. Dorr RT, Dordal MS, Koenig LM, et al. High levels of doxorubicin in the tissues of a patient experiencing extravasation during a 4-day infusion. *Cancer* 1989;64:2462–2464.

200. Dorr RT. Antidotes to vesicant chemotherapy extravasations. *Blood Rev* 1990;4:41–60.

201. Etcubanas E, Wilbur JR. Uncommon side effects of Adriamycin (NSC-123127) [Letter]. *Cancer Chemother Rep* 1974;58:757–758.

202. Souhami L, Feld R. Urticaria following intravenous doxorubicin administration. *JAMA* 1978;240:1624–1626.

203. Lefrak EA, Pitha J, Rosenheim S, et al. Adriamycin (NSC-123127) cardiomyopathy. *Cancer Chemother Rep* 1975;6:203.

204. Lenaz L, Page JA. Cardiotoxicity of Adriamycin and related anthracyclines. *Cancer Treat Rev* 1976;3:111–120.

205. Rinehart JJ, Lewis RP, Balcerzak SP. Adriamycin cardiotoxicity in man. *Ann Intern Med* 1974;81:475–478.

206. Minow RA, Benjamin RS, Gottlieb JA. Adriamycin (NSC-123127) cardiomyopathy—an overview with determinants of risk factors. *Cancer Chemother Rep* 1975;6:195.

207. Steinherz LJ, Steinherz PG, Tan CT, et al. Cardiac toxicity 4 to 20 years after completing anthracycline therapy. *JAMA* 1991;266:1672–1677.

208. Speyer J, Wasserheit C. Strategies for reduction of anthracycline cardiac toxicity. *Semin Oncol* 1998;25:525–537.

209. Von Hoff DD, Layard MW, Basa P, et al. Risk factors for doxorubicin-induced congestive heart failure. *Ann Intern Med* 1979;91:710–717.

210. Bielack SS, Erttmann R, Winkler K, et al. Doxorubicin: effect of different schedules on toxicity and anti-tumor efficacy. *Eur J Cancer Clin Oncol* 1989;25:873–882.

211. Donaldson SS, Glick JM, Wilbur JR. Adriamycin activating a recall phenomenon after radiation therapy [Letter]. *Ann Intern Med* 1974;81:407–408.

212. Greco FA, Brereton HD, Kent H, et al. Adriamycin and enhanced radiation reaction in normal esophagus and skin. *Ann Intern Med* 1976;85:294–298.

213. Newburger PE, Cassady JR, Jaffe N. Esophagitis due to Adriamycin and radiation therapy for childhood malignancy. *Cancer* 1978;42:417–423.

214. Priestman TJ, James KW. Adriamycin and longitudinal pigmented banding of fingernails [Letter]. *Lancet* 1975;1(7920):1337–1338.

215. Patterson AHG. Hypertensive reaction to Adriamycin [Letter]. *Cancer Treat Rep* 1978;62:1269.

216. Sarosy GA, Brown TD, Von Hoff DD, et al. Phase I study of alpha 2-interferon plus doxorubicin in patients with solid tumors. *Cancer Res* 1986;46:5368–5371.

217. Kefford RF, Woods RL, Fox RM, Tatersall MH. Intracavitary Adriamycin, nitrogen mustard and tetracycline in the control of malignant effusions: a randomized study. *Med J Aust* 1980;2:447–448.

218. Markman M, Howell SB, Green MR. Combination intracavitary chemotherapy for malignant pleural disease. *Cancer Drug Deliv* 1984;1:333–336.

219. Rose PG, Blessing JA, Buller RE, et al. Prolonged oral etoposide in recurrent or advanced non-squamous cell carcinoma of the cervix: a Gynecologic Oncology Group study. *Gynecol Oncol* 2003;89:267–270.

220. Keller-Juslen C, Kuhn M, Stahelin H, von Wartburg A. Synthesis and antimitotic activity of glycosidic lignan derivatives related to podophyllotoxin. *J Med Chem* 1971;14:936–940.

221. Misra NC, Roberts DW. Inhibition by 4′-demethyl-epipodophyllotoxin 9-(4,6-O-2-thenylidene-beta-D-glucopyranoside) of human lymphoblast cultures in G2 phase of the cell cycle. *Cancer Res* 1975;35:99–105.

222. Krishan A, Paika K, Frei E III. Cytofluorometric studies on the action of podophyllotoxin and epipodophyllotoxins (VM-26, VP-16–213) on the cell cycle traverse of human lymphoblasts. *J Cell Biol* 1975;66:521–530.

223. Ross W, Rowe T, Glisson B, et al. Role of topoisomerase II in mediating epipodophyllotoxin-induced DNA cleavage. *Cancer Res* 1984;44:5857–5860.

224. Chen AY, Liu LF. DNA topoisomerases: essential enzymes and lethal targets. *Annu Rev Pharmacol Toxicol* 1994;34:191–218.

225. Wozniak AJ, Ross WE. DNA damage as a basis for 4′-demethylepipodophyllotoxin-9-(4,6-O-ethylidene-beta-D-glucopyranoside) (etoposide) cytotoxicity. *Cancer Res* 1983;43:120–124.

226. Smith PJ, Anderson CO, Watson JV. Predominant role for DNA damage in etoposide-induced cytotoxicity and cell cycle perturbation in human SV40-transformed fibroblasts. *Cancer Res* 1986;46:5641–5645.

227. Chatterjee S, Trivedi D, Petzold SJ, Berger NA. Mechanism of epipodophyllotoxin-induced cell death in poly(adenosine diphosphate-ribose) synthesis-deficient V79 Chinese hamster cell lines. *Cancer Res* 1990;50:2713–2718.

228. Wozniak AJ, Glisson BS, Hande KR, Ross WE. Inhibition of etoposide-induced DNA damage and cytotoxicity in L1210 cells by dehydrogenase inhibitors and other agents. *Cancer Res* 1984;44:626–632.

229. Allen LM, Creaven PJ. Comparison of the human pharmacokinetics of VM-26 and VP-16, two antineoplastic epipodophyllotixin glucopyranoside derivatives. *Eur J Cancer* 1975;11:697–707.

230. D'Incalci M, Farina P, Sessa C, et al. Pharmacokinetics of VP16–213 given by different administration methods. *Cancer Chemother Pharmacol* 1982;7:141–145.

231. Hande KR, Wedlund PJ, Noone RM, et al. Pharmacokinetics of high-dose etoposide (VP-16–213) administered to cancer patients. *Cancer Res* 1984;44:379–382.

232. Stewart DJ, Richard MT, Hugenholtz H, et al. Penetration of VP-16 (etoposide) into human intracerebral and extracerebral tumors. *J Neurooncol* 1984;2:133–139.

233. D'Incalci M, Sessa C, Rossi C, et al. Pharmacokinetics of etoposide in gestochoriocarcinoma. *Cancer Treat Rep* 1985;69:69–72.

234. Creaven PJ, Newman SJ, Selawry OS, et al. Phase I clinical trial of weekly administration of 4′-demethylepipodophyllotoxin 9-(4,6-O-ethylidene-beta-D-glucopyranoside) (NSC-141540; VP-16-213). *Cancer Chemother Rep* 1974;58:901–907.

235. Stewart CF, Arbuck SG, Fleming RA, Evans WE. Changes in the clearance of total and unbound etoposide in patients with liver dysfunction. *J Clin Oncol* 1990;8:1874–1879.

236. Pfluger KH, Schmidt L, Merkel M, et al. Drug monitoring of etoposide (VP16-213). Correlation of pharmacokinetic parameters to clinical and biochemical data from patients receiving etoposide. *Cancer Chemother Pharmacol* 1987;20:59–66.

237. Smyth RD, Pfeffer M, Scalzo A, Comis RL. Bioavailability and pharmacokinetics of etoposide (VP-16). *Semin Oncol* 1985;12[1 Suppl 2]:48–51.

238. Harvey VJ, Slevin ML, Joel SP, et al. The effect of food and concurrent chemotherapy on the bioavailability of oral etoposide. *Br J Cancer* 1985;52:363–367.

239. Dorr RT, Alberts DS. Skin ulceration potential without therapeutic anticancer activity for epipodophyllotoxin commercial diluents. *Invest New Drugs* 1983;1:151–159.

240. Bennett CL, Sinkule JA, Schilsky RL, et al. Phase I clinical and pharmacological study of 72-hour continuous infusion of etoposide in patients with advanced cancer. *Cancer Res* 1987;47:1952–1956.

241. Steward WP, Thatcher N, Edmundson JM, et al. Etoposide infusions for treatment of metastatic lung cancer. *Cancer Treat Rep* 1984;68:897–899.

242. Ozols RF. Oral etoposide for the treatment of recurrent ovarian cancer. *Drugs* 1999;58[Suppl 3]:43–49.

243. Rose PG, Blessing JA, Mayer AR, Homesley HD. Prolonged oral etoposide as second-line therapy for platinum-resistant and platinum-sensitive ovarian carcinoma: a Gynecologic Oncology Group study. *J Clin Oncol* 1998;16:405–410.

244. Morris M, Brader KR, Burke TW, et al. A phase II study of prolonged oral etoposide in advanced or recurrent carcinoma of the cervix. *Gynecol Oncol* 1998;70:215–218.

245. Rose PG, Blessing JA, Lewandowski GS, et al. A phase II trial of prolonged oral etoposide (VP-16) as second-line therapy for advanced and recurrent endometrial carcinoma: a Gynecologic Oncology Group study. *Gynecol Oncol* 1996;63:101–104.

246. Rose PG, Blessing JA, Van Le L, Waggoner S. Prolonged oral etoposide in recurrent or advanced squamous cell carcinoma of the cervix: a Gynecologic Oncology Group study. *Gynecol Oncol* 1998;70:263–266.

247. Hande KR, Wolff SN, Greco FA, et al. Etoposide kinetics in patients with obstructive jaundice. *J Clin Oncol* 1990;8:1101–1107.

248. Rozencweig M, Von Hoff DD, Henney JE, Muggia FM. VM 26 and VP 16-213: a comparative analysis. *Cancer* 1977;40:334–342.

249. Anonymous. Epipodophyllotoxin VP 16213 in treatment of acute leukaemias, haematosarcomas, and solid tumours. *BMJ* 1973;3:199–202.

250. Dombernowsky P, Nissen NI, Larsen V. Clinical investigation of a new podophyllum derivative, epipodophyllotoxin, 4′-demethyl-9-(4,6-O-2-thenylidene-D-glucopyranoside) (NSC-122819), in patients with malignant lymphomas and solid tumors. *Cancer Chemother Rep* 1972;56:71–82.

251. Aisner J, Whitacre M, VanEcho DA, et al. Doxorubicin, cyclophosphamide and VP16–213 (ACE) in the treatment of small cell lung cancer. *Cancer Chemother Pharmacol* 1982;7:187–193.

252. Dorr RT. Chemoprotectants for cancer chemotherapy. *Semin Oncol* 1991;18[1 Suppl 2]:48–58.

253. Thant M, Hawley RJ, Smith MT, et al. Possible enhancement of vincristine neuropathy by VP-16. *Cancer* 1982;49:859–864.

254. Barakat RR, Almadrones L, Venkatraman ES, et al. A phase II trial of intraperitoneal cisplatin and etoposide as consolidation therapy in patients with stage II-IV epithelial ovarian cancer following negative surgical assessment. *Gynecol Oncol* 1998;69:17–22.

255. van Rijswijk RE, Hoekman K, Burger CW, et al. Experience with intraperitoneal cisplatin and etoposide and i.v. sodium thiosulphate protection in ovarian cancer patients with either pathologically complete response or minimal residual disease. *Ann Oncol* 1997;8:1235–1241.

256. Fields KK, Elfenbein GJ, Lazarus HM, et al. Maximum-tolerated doses of ifosfamide, carboplatin, and etoposide given over 6 days followed by autologous stem-cell rescue: toxicity profile. *J Clin Oncol* 1995;13:323–332.

257. Lotz JP, Andre T, Donsimoni R, et al. High dose chemotherapy with ifosfamide, carboplatin, and etoposide combined with autologous bone marrow transplantation for the treatment of poor-prognosis germ cell tumors and metastatic trophoblastic disease in adults. *Cancer* 1995;75:874–885.

258. Rustum YM. Biochemical rationale for the 5-fluorouracil leucovorin combination and update of clinical experience. *J Chemother* 1990;2[Suppl 1]:5–11.

259. Collins JM, Dedrick RL. Pharmacokinetics of anticancer drugs. In: Chabner BE, ed. *Pharmacologic principles of cancer treatment.* Philadelphia: WB Saunders; 1982:73.

260. Collins JM, Dedrick RL, King FG, et al. Nonlinear pharmacokinetic models for 5-fluorouracil in man: intravenous and intraperitoneal routes. *Clin Pharmacol Ther* 1980;28:235–246.

261. McDermott BJ, van den Berg HW, Murphy RF. Nonlinear pharmacokinetics for the elimination of 5-fluorouracil after intravenous administration in cancer patients. *Cancer Chemother Pharmacol* 1982;9:173–178.

262. Fraile RJ, Baker LH, Buroker TR, et al. Pharmacokinetics of 5-fluorouracil administered orally, by rapid intravenous and by slow infusion. *Cancer Res* 1980;40:2223–2228.

263. Schaaf LJ, Dobbs BR, Edwards IR, Perrier DG. Nonlinear pharmacokinetic characteristics of 5-fluorouracil (5-FU) in colorectal cancer patients. *Eur J Clin Pharmacol* 1987;32:411–418.

264. Yoshida T, Araki E, Iigo M, et al. Clinical significance of monitoring serum levels of 5-fluorouracil by continuous infusion in patients with advanced colonic cancer. *Cancer Chemother Pharmacol* 1990;26:352–354.

265. Floyd RA, Hornbeck CL, Byfield JE, et al. Clearance of continuously infused 5-fluorouracil in adults having lung or gastrointestinal carcinoma with or without hepatic metastases. *Drug Intell Clin Pharm* 1982;16:665–667.

266. Santini J, Milano G, Thyss A, et al. 5-FU therapeutic monitoring with dose adjustment leads to an improved therapeutic index in head and neck cancer. *Br J Cancer* 1989;59:287–290.

267. Lokich JJ, Ahlgren JD, Gullo JJ, et al. A prospective randomized comparison of continuous infusion fluorouracil with a conventional bolus schedule in metastatic colorectal carcinoma: a Mid-Atlantic Oncology Program Study. *J Clin Oncol* 1989;7:425–432.

268. Moertel CG, Schutt AJ, Reitemeier RJ, Hahn RG. A comparison of 5-fluorouracil administered by slow infusion and rapid injection. *Cancer Res* 1972;32:2717–2719.

269. Moertel CG. Chemotherapy of gastrointestinal cancer. *N Engl J Med* 1978;299:1049–1052.

270. Reitemeier RJ, Moertel CG. Comparison of 5-flourouracil in treating patients with advanced carcinoma of the large intestine. *Cancer Chemother Rep* 1962;1962:87.

271. Nadler SH. Oral administration of fluorouracil. A preliminary trial. *Arch Surg* 1968;97:654–656.

272. Horton J, Olson KB, Sullivan J, et al. 5-FU in cancer: an improved regimen. *Ann Intern Med* 1970;73:897.

273. Jacobs EM, Reeves WJ Jr, Wood DA, et al. Treatment of cancer with weekly intravenous 5-fluorouracil. Study by the Western Cooperative Cancer Chemotherapy Group (WCCCG). *Cancer* 1971;27:1302–1305.

274. Bruckner HW, Glass LL, Chesser MR. Dose-dependent leucovorin efficacy with an intermittent high-dose 5-fluorouracil schedule. *Cancer Invest* 1990;8:321–326.

275. Doroshow JH, Multhauf P, Leong L, et al. Prospective randomized comparison of fluorouracil versus fluorouracil and high-dose continuous infusion leucovorin calcium for the treatment of advanced measurable colorectal cancer in patients previously unexposed to chemotherapy. *J Clin Oncol* 1990;8:491–501.

276. Whitney CW, Sause W, Bundy BN, et al. Randomized comparison of fluorouracil plus cisplatin versus hydroxyurea as an adjunct to radiation therapy in stage IIB-IVA carcinoma of the cervix with negative para-aortic lymph nodes: a Gynecologic Oncology Group and Southwest Oncology Group study. *J Clin Oncol* 1999;17:1339–1348.

277. Curran CF, Luce JK. Fluorouracil and palmar-plantar erythrodysesthesia. *Ann Intern Med* 1989;111:858.

278. Malet-Martino M, Martino R. Clinical studies of three oral prodrugs of 5-fluorouracil (capecitabine, UFT, S-1): a review. *Oncologist* 2002;7:288–323.

279. Malet-Martino M, Jolimaitre P, Martino R. The prodrugs of 5-fluorouracil. *Curr Med Chem Anti-Cancer Agents* 2002;2:267–310.

280. Lopez AM, Wallace L, Dorr RT, et al. Topical DMSO treatment for pegylated liposomal doxorubicin-induced palmar-plantar erythrodysesthesia. *Cancer Chemother Pharmacol* 1999;44:303–306.

281. Nagore E, Insa A, Sanmartin O. Antineoplastic therapy-induced palmar plantar erythrodysesthesia ('hand-foot') syndrome. Incidence, recognition and management. *Am J Clin Dermatol* 2000;1:225–234.

282. Hrushesky WJ. Serpentine supravenous 5-fluorouracil (NSC-19893) hyperpigmentation. *Cancer Treat Rep* 1976;60:639.

283. Boileau G, Piro AJ, Lahiri SR, Hall TC. Cerebellar ataxia during 5-fluorouracil (NSC-19893) therapy. *Cancer Chemother Rep* 1971;55:595–598.

284. Cianci G, Morelli MF, Cannita K, et al. Prophylactic options in patients with 5-fluorouracil–associated cardiotoxicity. *Br J Cancer* 2003;88:1507–1509.

285. Diasio RB, Beavers TL, Carpenter JT. Familial deficiency of dihydropyrimidine dehydrogenase. Biochemical basis for familial pyrimidinemia and severe 5-fluorouracil-induced toxicity. *J Clin Invest* 1988;81:47–51.

286. Lu Z, Zhang R, Diasio RB. Population characteristics of hepatic dihydropyrimidine dehydrogenase activity, a key metabolic enzyme in 5-fluorouracil chemotherapy. *Clin Pharmacol Ther* 1995;58:512–522.

287. Curran CF, Luce JK. Accidental acute exposure to fluorouracil. *Oncol Nurs Forum* 1989;16:468.

288. Muggia FM, Liu PY, Alberts DS, et al. Intraperitoneal mitoxantrone or floxuridine: effects on time-to-failure and survival in patients with minimal residual ovarian cancer after second-look laparotomy—a randomized phase II study by the Southwest Oncology Group. *Gynecol Oncol* 1996;61:395–402.

289. Speyer JL, Sugarbaker PH, Collins JM, et al. Portal levels and hepatic clearance of 5-fluorouracil after intraperitoneal administration in humans. *Cancer Res* 1981;41:1916–1922.

290. Suhrland LG, Weisberger AA. Intracavitary 5-fluorouracil in malignant effusions. *Arch Intern Med* 1965;116:431.

291. Fowler WC Jr, Van Le L. Gemcitabine as a single-agent treatment for ovarian cancer. *Gynecol Oncol* 2003;90:S21–S23.

292. Hansen SW, Tuxen MK, Sessa C. Gemcitabine in the treatment of ovarian cancer. *Ann Oncol* 1999;10[Suppl 1]:51–53.

293. Belpomme D, Krakowski I, Beauduin M, et al. Gemcitabine combined with cisplatin as first-line treatment in patients with epithelial ovarian cancer: a phase II study. *Gynecol Oncol* 2003;91:32–38.

294. Zarba JJ, Jaremtchuk AV, Gonzalez Jazey P, et al. A phase I-II study of weekly cisplatin and gemcitabine with concurrent radiotherapy in locally advanced cervical carcinoma. *Ann Oncol* 2003;14:1285–1290.

295. Markman M, Webster K, Zanotti K, et al. Phase 2 trial of single-agent gemcitabine in platinum-paclitaxel refractory ovarian cancer. *Gynecol Oncol* 2003;90:593–596.

296. Huang P, Chubb S, Hertel LW, et al. Action of 2′,2′-difluorodeoxycytidine on DNA synthesis. *Cancer Res* 1991;51:6110–6117.

297. Plunkett W, Huang P, Gandhi V. Preclinical characteristics of gemcitabine. *Anticancer Drugs* 1995;6[Suppl 6]:7–13.

298. Heinemann V, Xu YZ, Chubb S, et al. Inhibition of ribonucleotide reduction in CCRF-CEM cells by 2′,2′-difluorodeoxycytidine. *Mol Pharmacol* 1990;38:567–572.

299. Abbruzzese JL, Grunewald R, Weeks EA, et al. A phase I clinical, plasma, and cellular pharmacology study of gemcitabine. *J Clin Oncol* 1991;9:491–498.

300. Eli Lilly and Company. Gemzar (Gemcitabine HC) for Injection. Prescribing Information; 2003.

301. Allerheiligen S, Johnson R, Hatcher B, et al. Gemcitabine pharmacokinetics are influenced by gender, body surface area, amd duration of infusion. *Proc ASCO* 1994;13:136(abst).

302. Storniolo AM, Allerheiligen SR, Pearce HL. Preclinical, pharmacologic, and phase I studies of gemcitabine. *Semin Oncol* 1997;24[2 Suppl 7]:S7–2–S7–7.

303. van Moorsel CJ, Kroep JR, Pinedo HM, et al. Pharmacokinetic schedule finding study of the combination of gemcitabine and cisplatin in patients with solid tumors. *Ann Oncol* 1999;10:441–448.

304. O'Rourke TJ, Brown TD, Havlin K, et al. Phase I clinical trial of gemcitabine given as an intravenous bolus on 5 consecutive days. *Eur J Cancer* 1994;30A:417–418.

305. Hui YF, Reitz J. Gemcitabine: a cytidine analogue active against solid tumors. *Am J Health Syst Pharm* 1997;54:162–170; Quiz 197–198.

306. D'Agostino G, Amant F, Berteloot P, et al. Phase II study of gemcitabine in recurrent platinum- and paclitaxel-resistant ovarian cancer. *Gynecol Oncol* 2003;88:266–269.

307. Bergmann AM, Ruiz van Haperen VM, Veerman G, et al. Synergistic interaction between cisplatin and gemcitabine in vitro. *Clin Cancer Res* 1996;2:521.

308. van Moorsel CJ, Pinedo HM, Veerman G, et al. Mechanisms of synergism between cisplatin and gemcitabine in ovarian and non-small cell lung cancer cell lines. *Br J Cancer* 1999;80:981.

309. Bauknecht T, Hefti A, Morack G, et al. Gemcitabine combined with cisplatin as first-line treatment in patients 60 years or older with epithelial ovarian cancer: a phase II study. *Int J Gynecol Cancer* 2003; 13:130–137.

310. Nogue M, Cirera L, Arcusa A, et al. Phase II study of gemcitabine and cisplatin in chemonaive patients with advanced epithelial ovarian cancer. *Anticancer Drugs* 2002;13:839–845.

311. Nagourney RA, Brewer CA, Radecki S, et al. Phase II trial of gemcitabine plus cisplatin repeating doublet therapy in previously treated, relapsed ovarian cancer patients. *Gynecol Oncol* 2003;88:35–39.

312. Aapro MS, Martin C, Hatty S. Gemcitabine—a safety review. *Anticancer Drugs* 1998;9:191–201.

313. Serke S, Riess H, Oettle H, Huhn D. Elevated reticulocyte count—a clue to the diagnosis of haemolytic-uraemic syndrome (HUS) associated with gemcitabine therapy for metastatic duodenal papillary carcinoma: a case report. *Br J Cancer* 1999;79:519–521.

314. Pavlakis N, Bell DR, Millward MJ, Levi JA. Fatal pulmonary toxicity resulting from treatment with gemcitabine. *Cancer* 1997;80:286–291.

315. Sauer-Heilborn A, Kath R, Schneider CP, Hoffken K. Severe non-haematological toxicity after treatment with gemcitabine. *J Cancer Res Clin Oncol* 1999;125:637–640.

316. Markman M, Kennedy A, Sutton G, et al. Phase 2 trial of single agent ifosfamide/mesna in patients with platinum/paclitaxel refractory ovarian cancer who have not previously been treated with an alkylating agent. *Gynecol Oncol* 1998;70:272–274.

317. Sutton G. Ifosfamide and mesna in epithelial ovarian carcinoma. *Gynecol Oncol* 1993;51:104–108.

318. Sutton GP, Blessing JA, DeMars LR, et al. A phase II Gynecologic Oncology Group trial of ifosfamide and mesna in advanced or recurrent adenocarcinoma of the endometrium. *Gynecol Oncol* 1996;63: 25–27.

319. Allen LM, Creaven PJ. Activation of the antineoplastic drug isophosphamide by rat liver microsomes. *J Pharm Pharmacol* 1972;24: 585–586.

320. Allen LM, Creaven PJ. Interaction of mechlorethamine and isophosphamide with bovine serum albumin and rat liver microsomes. *J Pharm Sci* 1973;62:854–856.

321. Boal JH, Williamson M, Boyd VL, et al. 31P NMR studies of the kinetics of bisalkylation by isophosphoramide mustard: comparisons with phosphoramide mustard. *J Med Chem* 1989;32:1768–1773.

322. Creaven PJ, Allen LM, Cohen MH, Nelson RL. Studies on the clinical pharmacology and toxicology of isophosphamide (NSC-109724). *Cancer Treat Rep* 1976;60:445–449.

323. Allen LM, Creaven PJ, Nelson RL. Studies on the human pharmacokinetics of isophosphamide (NSC-109724). *Cancer Treat Rep* 1976;60: 451–458.

324. Stuart-Harris RC, Harper PG, Parsons CA, et al. High-dose alkylation therapy using ifosfamide infusion with mesna in the treatment of adult advanced soft-tissue sarcoma. *Cancer Chemother Pharmacol* 1983; 11:69–72.

325. Nelson RL, Creaven PJ, Cohen MH, Fossieck BE Jr. Phase I clinical trial of a 3-day divided dose schedule of ifosfamide (NSC 109724). *Eur J Cancer* 1976;12:195–198.

325a. Mateu J, Alzamora M, Franco M, Buisan MJ. Ifosfamide extravasation. *Ann Pharmacother* 1994;28:1243.

326. Papadimitriou CA, Kouroussis C, Moulopoulos LA, et al. Ifosfamide, paclitaxel and cisplatin first-line chemotherapy in advanced, suboptimally debulked epithelial ovarian cancer. *Cancer* 2001;92: 1856–1863.

327. Zanetta G, Fei F, Parma G, et al. Paclitaxel, ifosfamide and cisplatin (TIP) chemotherapy for recurrent or persistent squamous-cell cervical cancer. *Ann Oncol* 1999;10:1171–1174.

328. Morgan LR, Harrison EF, Hawke JE, et al. Toxicity of single- vs. fractionated-dose ifosfamide in non–small cell lung cancer: a multicenter study. *Semin Oncol* 1982;9[4 Suppl 1]:66–70.

329. Rodriguez V, McCredie KB, Keating MJ, et al. Isophosphamide therapy for hematologic malignancies in patients refractory to prior treatment. *Cancer Treat Rep* 1978;62:493–497.

330. Van Dyk JJ, Falkson HC, Van der Merwe AM, Falkson G. Unexpected toxicity in patients treated with iphosphamide. *Cancer Res* 1972;32: 921–924.

331. DeFronzo RA, Abeloff M, Braine H, et al. Renal dysfunction after treatment with isophosphamide (NSC-109724). *Cancer Chemother Rep* 1974;58:375–382.

332. Goren MP, Wright RK, Pratt CB, et al. Potentiation of ifosfamide neurotoxicity, hematotoxicity, and tubular nephrotoxicity by prior cis-diamminedichloroplatinum(II) therapy. *Cancer Res* 1987;47: 1457–1460.

333. Hacke M, Schmoll HJ, Alt JM, et al. Nephrotoxicity of cis-diamminedichloroplatinum with or without ifosfamide in cancer treatment. *Clin Physiol Biochem* 1983;1:17–26.

334. Bhardwaj A, Badesha PS. Ifosfamide-induced nonconvulsive status epilepticus. *Ann Pharmacother* 1995;29:1237–1239.

335. Creemers GJ, Lund B, Verweij J. Topoisomerase I inhibitors: topotecan and irinotecan. *Cancer Treat Rev* 1994;20:73–96.

336. Rothenberg ML, Kuhn JG, Burris HA 3rd, et al. Phase I and pharmacokinetic trial of weekly CPT-11. *J Clin Oncol* 1993;11:2194–2204.

337. Abigerges D, Chabot GG, Armand JP, et al. Phase I and pharmacologic studies of the camptothecin analog irinotecan administered every 3 weeks in cancer patients. *J Clin Oncol* 1995;13:210–221.

338. Irvin WP, Price FV, Bailey H, et al. A phase II study of irinotecan (CPT-11) in patients with advanced squamous cell carcinoma of the cervix. *Cancer* 1998;82:328–333.

339. Look KY, Blessing JA, Levenback C, et al. A phase II trial of CPT-11 in recurrent squamous carcinoma of the cervix: a Gynecologic Oncology Group study. *Gynecol Oncol* 1998;70:334–338.

340. Verschraegen CF, Levy T, Kudelka AP, et al. Phase II study of irinotecan in prior chemotherapy-treated squamous cell carcinoma of the cervix. *J Clin Oncol* 1997;15:625–631.

341. Rowinsky EK, Grochow LB, Ettinger DS, et al. Phase I and pharmacological study of the novel topoisomerase I inhibitor 7-ethyl-10-[4-(1-piperidino)-1-iperidino]carbonyloxycamptothecin (CPT-11) administered as a ninety-minute infusion every 3 weeks. *Cancer Res* 1994; 54:427–436.

342. Gupta E, Lestingi TM, Mick R, et al. Metabolic fate of irinotecan in humans: correlation of glucuronidation with diarrhea. *Cancer Res* 1994;54:3723–3725.

343. Cottu PH, Extra JM, Lerebours F, et al. Clinical activity spectrum of irinotecan. *Bull Cancer* 1998;Spec No:21–5.

344. Eisenhauer EA, Vermorken JB. New drugs in gynecologic oncology. *Curr Opin Oncol* 1996;8:408–414.

345. Verschraegen CF. Irinotecan for the treatment of cervical cancer. *Oncology (Huntingt)* 2002;16[5 Suppl 5]:32–4.

346. Chitapanarux I, Tonusin A, Sukthomya V, et al. Phase II clinical study of irinotecan and cisplatin as first-line chemotherapy in metastatic or recurrent cervical cancer. *Gynecol Oncol* 2003;89:402–407.

347. Alza Corporation. DOXIL (doxorubicin HCl liposome injection) package insert; 2001.

348. Gabizon A, Catane R, Uziely B, et al. Prolonged circulation time and enhanced accumulation in malignant exudates of doxorubicin encap-

sulated in polyethylene-glycol coated liposomes. *Cancer Res* 1994;54:987–992.

349. Alberts DS, Garcia DJ. Safety aspects of pegylated liposomal doxorubicin in patients with cancer. *Drugs* 1997;54[Suppl 4]:30–35.

350. Gordon AN, Fleagle JT, Guthrie D, et al. Recurrent epithelial ovarian carcinoma: a randomized phase III study of pegylated liposomal doxorubicin versus topotecan. *J Clin Oncol* 2001;19:3312–3322.

351. Chang SY, Evans TL, Alberts DS. The stability of melphalan in the presence of chloride ion. *J Pharm Pharmacol* 1979;31:853–854.

352. Goodman GE, Chang SE, Alberts DS. The antitumor activity of melphalan and its hydrolysis products. *Proc AACR* 1980;21:1207(abst).

353. Goldenberg GJ, Lam HY, Begleiter A. Active carrier-mediated transport of melphalan by two separate amino acid transport systems in LPC-1 plasmacytoma cells in vitro. *J Biol Chem* 1979;254:1057–1064.

354. Alberts DS, Chang SY, Chen HS, et al. Oral melphalan kinetics. *Clin Pharmacol Ther* 1979;26:737–745.

355. Evans TL, Chang SY, Alberts DS, et al. In vitro degradation of L-phenylalanine mustard (L-PAM). *Cancer Chemother Pharmacol* 1982;8:175–178.

356. Alberts DS, Peng YM, Fisher B. Minimal mephalan (LPAM) systemic availability (SA): a potential cause for failure of adjuvant breast cancer trials. *Proc ASCO* 1984;3:C149(abst).

357. Bosanquet AG, Gilby ED. Pharmacokinetics of oral and intravenous melphalan during routine treatment of multiple myeloma. *Eur J Cancer Clin Oncol* 1982;18:355–362.

358. Rutledge F. Chemotherapy of ovarian cancer with melphalan. *Clin Obstet Gynecol* 1968;11:354–366.

359. Taetle R, Dickman PS, Feldman PS. Pulmonary histopathologic changes associated with melphalan therapy. *Cancer* 1978;42:1239–1245.

360. Einhorn N. Acute leukemia after chemotherapy (melphalan). *Cancer* 1978;41:444–447.

361. Greene MH, Harris EL, Gershenson DM, et al. Melphalan may be a more potent leukemogen than cyclophosphamide. *Ann Intern Med* 1986;105:360–367.

362. Wang AL, Tew KD. Increased glutathione-S-transferase activity in a cell line with acquired resistance to nitrogen mustards. *Cancer Treat Rep* 1985;69:677–682.

363. Ozols RF, Louie KG, Plowman J, et al. Enhanced melphalan cytotoxicity in human ovarian cancer in vitro and in tumor-bearing nude mice by buthionine sulfoximine depletion of glutathione. *Biochem Pharmacol* 1987;36:147–153.

364. Bailey HH, Ripple G, Tutsch KD, et al. Phase I study of continuous-infusion L-S,R-buthionine sulfoximine with intravenous melphalan. *J Natl Cancer Inst* 1997;89:1789–1796.

365. O'Dwyer PJ, Hamilton TC, LaCreta FP, et al. Phase I trial of buthionine sulfoximine in combination with melphalan in patients with cancer. *J Clin Oncol* 1996;14:249–256.

366. Lazarus HM, Gray R, Ciobanu N, et al. Phase I trial of high-dose melphalan, high-dose etoposide and autologous bone marrow re-infusion in solid tumors: an Eastern Cooperative Oncology Group (ECOG) study. *Bone Marrow Transplant* 1994;14:443–448.

367. Weaver CH, Bensinger WI, Appelbaum FR, et al. Phase I study of high-dose busulfan, melphalan and thiotepa with autologous stem cell support in patients with refractory malignancies. *Bone Marrow Transplant* 1994;14:813–819.

368. Alberts DS, Young L, Mason N, Salmon SE. In vitro evaluation of anticancer drugs against ovarian cancer at concentrations achievable by intraperitoneal administration. *Semin Oncol* 1985;12[3 Suppl 4]:38–42.

369. Howell SB, Pfeifle CE, Olshen RA. Intraperitoneal chemotherapy with melphalan. *Ann Intern Med* 1984;101:14–18.

370. Zaharko DS, Fung WP, Yang KH. Relative biochemical aspects of low and high doses of methotrexate in mice. *Cancer Res* 1977;37:1602–1607.

371. Jolivet J, Schilsky RL, Bailey BD, et al. Synthesis, retention, and biological activity of methotrexate polyglutamates in cultured human breast cancer cells. *J Clin Invest* 1982;70:351–360.

372. Alt FW, Kellems RE, Bertino JR, Schimke RT. Selective multiplication of dihydrofolate reductase genes in methotrexate-resistant variants of cultured murine cells. 1978. *Biotechnology* 1992;24:397–410.

373. Calvert AH, Jones TR, Jackman AL, et al. 2-Amino-4-hydroxyquinaz-

374. Weinstein G, Newburger A, Troner M. Cell kinetic synchronization of human malignant melanoma (MM) with low-dose methotrexate (MTX) in vivo. *Proc AACR* 1979;20:403(abst).

375. Chello PL, Sirotnak FM, Dorick DM. Alterations in the kinetics of methotrexate transport during growth of L1210 murine leukemia cells in culture. *Mol Pharmacol* 1980;18:274–280.

376. Campbell MA, Perrier DG, Dorr RT, et al. Methotrexate: bioavailability and pharmacokinetics. *Cancer Treat Rep* 1985;69:833–838.

377. Ignoffo RJ, Oie S, Friedman MA. Pharmacokinetics of methotrexate administered via the hepatic artery. *Cancer Chemother Pharmacol* 1981;5:217–220.

378. Aherne GW, Piall E, Marks V, et al. Prolongation and enhancement of serum methotrexate concentrations by probenecid. *BMJ* 1978;1:1097–1099.

379. Huffman DH, Wan SH, Azarnoff DL, Hogstraten B. Pharmacokinetics of methotrexate. *Clin Pharmacol Ther* 1973;14:572–579.

380. Stoller RG, Jacobs SA, Drake JC, et al. Pharmacokinetics of high-dose methotrexate (NSC-740). *Cancer Chemother Rep* 1975;6:91.

381. Wang YM, Sutow WW, Romsdahl MM, Perez C. Age-related pharmacokinetics of high-dose methotrexate in patients with osteosarcoma. *Cancer Treat Rep* 1979;63:405–410.

382. Evans WE, Pratt CB. Effect of pleural effusion on high-dose methotrexate kinetics. *Clin Pharmacol Ther* 1978;23:68–72.

383. Ben Venue Laboratories I. Methotrexate Injection, USP. Package Insert. 2000.

384. Bleyer WA, Drake JC, Chabner BA. Neurotoxicity and elevated cerebrospinal-fluid methotrexate concentration in meningeal leukemia. *N Engl J Med* 1973;289:770–773.

385. Everts CS, Westcott JL, Bragg DG. Methotrexate therapy and pulmonary disease. *Radiology* 1973;107:539–543.

386. Creaven GB, Morgan RG. Alteration of methotrexate (MTX) pharmacokinetics by gut sterilization in man. *Proc AACR* 1975;16:134(abst).

387. Cadman E, Heimer R, Davis L. Enhanced 5-fluorouracil nucleotide formation after methotrexate administration: explanation for drug synergism. *Science* 1979;205:1135–1137.

388. Bowen D, White JC, Goldman ID. A basis for fluoropyrimidine-induced antagonism to methotrexate in Ehrlich ascites tumor cells in vitro. *Cancer Res* 1978;38:219–222.

389. Stoller RG, Hande KR, Jacobs SA, et al. Use of plasma pharmacokinetics to predict and prevent methotrexate toxicity. *N Engl J Med* 1977;297:630–634.

390. Stoller RG, Kaplan HG, Cummings FJ, Calabresi P. A clinical and pharmacological study of high-dose methotrexate with minimal leucovorin rescue. *Cancer Res* 1979;39:908–912.

391. Von Hoff DD, Penta JS, Helman LJ, Slavik M. Incidence of drug-related deaths secondary to high-dose methotrexate and citrovorum factor administration. *Cancer Treat Rep* 1977;61:745–748.

392. Crooke ST, Bradner WT. Mitomycin C: a review. *Cancer Treat Rev* 1976;3:121–139.

393. Lown JW, Weir G. Studies related to antitumor antibiotics. Part XIV. Reactions of mitomycin B with DNA. *Can J Biochem* 1978;56:269–304.

394. Tomasz M, Chowdary D, Lipman R, et al. Reaction of DNA with chemically or enzymatically activated mitomycin C: isolation and structure of the major covalent adduct. *Proc Natl Acad Sci U S A* 1986;83:6702(abst).

395. Dusre L, Covey JM, Collins C, Sinha BK. DNA damage, cytotoxicity and free radical formation by mitomycin C in human cells. *Chem Biol Interact* 1989;71:63–78.

396. Kennedy KA, Rockwell S, Sartorelli AC. Preferential activation of mitomycin C to cytotoxic metabolites by hypoxic tumor cells. *Cancer Res* 1980;40:2356–2360.

397. Matsumoto S, Shigeoka T, Takakura Y, et al. Cellular interaction and in vitro antitumor effect of various mitomycin C prodrugs in mitomycin C-resistant L1210 leukemia cell lines. *Chem Pharm Bull (Tokyo)* 1987;35:3792–3799.

398. Taylor CW, Brattain MG, Yeoman LC. Occurrence of cytosolic protein and phosphoprotein changes in human colon tumor cells with the development of resistance to mitomycin C. *Cancer Res* 1985;45:4422–4427.

399. Dorr RT, Liddil JD, Trent JM, Dalton WS. Mitomycin C resistant

L1210 leukemia cells: association with pleiotropic drug resistance. Biochem Pharmacol 1987;36:3115–3120.

400. van Hazel GA, Scott M, Rubin J, et al. Pharmacokinetics of mitomycin C in patients receiving the drug alone or in combination. *Cancer Treat Rep* 1983;67:805–810.

401. Verweij J, den Hartigh J, Stuurman M, et al. Relationship between clinical parameters and pharmacokinetics of mitomycin C. *J Cancer Res Clin Oncol* 1987;113:91–94.

402. Schilcher RB, Young JD, Ratanatharathorn V, et al. Clinical pharmacokinetics of high-dose mitomycin C. *Cancer Chemother Pharmacol* 1984;13:186–190.

403. den Hartigh J, McVie JG, van Oort WJ, Pinedo HM. Pharmacokinetics of mitomycin C in humans. *Cancer Res* 1983;43:5017–5021.

404. Malviya VK, Young JD, Boike G, et al. Pharmacokinetics of mitomycin-C in plasma and tumor tissue of cervical cancer patients and in selected tissues of female rats. *Gynecol Oncol* 1986;25:160–170.

405. Hu E, Howell SB. Pharmacokinetics of intraarterial mitomycin C in humans. *Cancer Res* 1983;43:4474–4477.

406. Argenta LC, Manders EK. Mitomycin C extravasation injuries. *Cancer* 1983;51:1080–1082.

407. Lokich J, Perri J, Fine N, et al. Mitomycin C: phase I study of a constant infusion ambulatory treatment schedule. *Am J Clin Oncol* 1982;5:443–447.

408. Tseng MH, Luch J, Mittelman A. Regional intra-arterial mitomycin C infusion in previously treated patients with metastatic colorectal cancer and concomitant measurement of serum drug level. *Cancer Treat Rep* 1984;68:1319–1324.

409. Hanna WT, Krauss S, Regester RF, Murphy WM. Renal disease after mitomycin C therapy. *Cancer* 1981;48:2583–2588.

410. Valavaara R, Nordman E. Renal complications of mitomycin C therapy with special reference to the total dose. *Cancer* 1985;55:47–50.

411. Lesesne JB, Rothschild N, Erickson B, et al. Cancer-associated hemolytic-uremic syndrome: analysis of 85 cases from a national registry. *J Clin Oncol* 1989;7:781–789.

412. Lazarus HM, Gottfried MR, Herzig RH, et al. Veno-occlusive disease of the liver after high-dose mitomycin C therapy and autologous bone marrow transplantation. *Cancer* 1982;49:1789–1795.

413. Johnston-Early A, Cohen MH. Mitomycin C-induced skin ulceration remote from infusion site. *Cancer Treat Rep* 1981;65:529.

414. Wood HA, Ellerhorst-Ryan JM. Delayed adverse skin reactions associated with mitomycin-C administration. *Oncol Nurs Forum* 1984;11:14–18.

415. Olver IN, Aisner J, Hament A, et al. A prospective study of topical dimethyl sulfoxide for treating anthracycline extravasation. *J Clin Oncol* 1988;6:1732–1735.

416. Chang AY, Kuebler JP, Pandya KJ, et al. Pulmonary toxicity induced by mitomycin C is highly responsive to glucocorticoids. *Cancer* 1986;57:2285–2290.

417. Koga S, Hamazoe R, Maeta M, et al. Prophylactic therapy for peritoneal recurrence of gastric cancer by continuous hyperthermic peritoneal perfusion with mitomycin C. *Cancer* 1988;61:232–237.

418. Fujimoto S, Shrestha RD, Kokubun M, et al. Pharmacokinetic analysis in intraperitoneal hyperthermic perfusion using mitomycin C in far-advanced gastric cancer. *Gan To Kagaku Ryoho* 1989;16:2411–2415.

419. Graham MA, Lockwood GF, Greenslade D, et al. Clinical pharmacokinetics of oxaliplatin: a critical review. *Clin Cancer Res* 2000;6:1205–1218.

420. Sanofi-Synthelabo. Eloxatin (Oxaliplatin for injection) Package Insert. 2002.

421. Fracasso PM, Blessing JA, Morgan MA, et al. Phase II study of oxaliplatin in platinum-resistant and refractory ovarian cancer: a Gynecologic Group study. *J Clin Oncol* 2003;21:2856–2859.

422. Fracasso PM, Blessing JA, Wolf J, et al. Phase II evaluation of oxaliplatin in previously treated squamous cell carcinoma of the cervix: a Gynecologic Oncology Group study. *Gynecol Oncol* 2003;90:177–180.

423. Gamelin E, Gamelin L, Bossi L, Quasthoff S. Clinical aspects and molecular basis of oxaliplatin neurotoxicity: current management and development of preventive measures. *Semin Oncol* 2002;29[5 Suppl 15]:21–33.

424. Bougnoux P, Dieras V, Petit T, et al. A multicenter phase II study of oxaliplatin (OXA) as a single agent in platinum (PT) and/or taxanes

425. Dieras V, Bougnoux P, Petit T, et al. Multicentre phase II study of oxaliplatin as a single-agent in cisplatin/carboplatin +/− taxane-pretreated ovarian cancer patients. *Ann Oncol* 2002;13:258–266.

426. Chollet P, Bensmaine MA, Brienza S, et al. Single agent activity of oxaliplatin in heavily pretreated advanced epithelial ovarian cancer. *Ann Oncol* 1996;7:1065–1070.

427. Curtin JP, Blessing JA, Webster KD, et al. Paclitaxel, an active agent in nonsquamous carcinomas of the uterine cervix: a Gynecologic Oncology Group Study. *J Clin Oncol* 2001;19:1275–1278.

428. Lincoln S, Blessing JA, Lee RB, Rocereto TF. Activity of paclitaxel as second-line chemotherapy in endometrial carcinoma: a Gynecologic Oncology Group study. *Gynecol Oncol* 2003;88:277–281.

429. Dorr RT. Pharmacology of the taxanes. *Pharmacotherapy* 1997;17:96S–104S.

430. Markman M, Kennedy A, Webster K, et al. Paclitaxel-associated hypersensitivity reactions: experience of the gynecologic oncology program of the Cleveland Clinic Cancer Center. *J Clin Oncol* 2000;18:102–105.

431. Eisenhauer EA, ten Bokkel Huinink WW, Swenerton KD, et al. European-Canadian randomized trial of paclitaxel in relapsed ovarian cancer: high-dose versus low-dose and long versus short infusion. *J Clin Oncol* 1994;12:2654–2666.

432. Tsavaris NB, Kosmas C. Risk of severe acute hypersensitivity reactions after rapid paclitaxel infusion of less than 1-h duration. *Cancer Chemother Pharmacol* 1998;42:509–511.

433. Ozols RF, Bundy BN, Greer BE, et al. Phase III trial of carboplatin and paclitaxel compared with cisplatin and paclitaxel in patients with optimally resected stage III ovarian cancer: a Gynecologic Oncology Group study. *J Clin Oncol* 2003;21:3194–3200.

434. Rowinsky EK, Eisenhauer EA, Chaudhry V, et al. Clinical toxicities encountered with paclitaxel (Taxol). *Semin Oncol* 1993;20[4 Suppl 3]:1–15.

435. Peereboom DM, Donehower RC, Eisenhauer EA, et al. Successful re-treatment with Taxol after major hypersensitivity reactions. *J Clin Oncol* 1993;11:885–890.

436. Rowinsky EK, Gilbert MR, McGuire WP, et al. Sequences of Taxol and cisplatin: a phase I and pharmacologic study. *J Clin Oncol* 1991;9:1692–1703.

437. Chang SM, Kuhn JG, Rizzo J, et al. Phase I study of paclitaxel in patients with recurrent malignant glioma: a North American Brain Tumor Consortium report. *J Clin Oncol* 1998;16:2188–2194.

438. Francis P, Rowinsky E, Schneider J, et al. Phase I feasibility and pharmacologic study of weekly intraperitoneal paclitaxel: a Gynecologic Oncology Group pilot study. *J Clin Oncol* 1995;13:2961–2967.

439. Markman M, Brady MF, Spirtos NM, et al. Phase II trial of intraperitoneal paclitaxel in carcinoma of the ovary, tube, and peritoneum: a Gynecologic Oncology Group Study. *J Clin Oncol* 1998;16:2620–2624.

440. Alberts DS, Markman M, Armstrong D, et al. Intraperitoneal therapy for stage III ovarian cancer: a therapy whose time has come! *J Clin Oncol* 2002;20:3944–3946.

441. Markman M, Kulp B, Peterson G, et al. Second-line therapy of ovarian cancer with paclitaxel administered by both the intravenous and intraperitoneal routes: rationale and case reports. *Gynecol Oncol* 2002;86:95–98.

442. Thigpen T, Vance RB, Khansur T. The platinum compounds and paclitaxel in the management of carcinomas of the endometrium and uterine cervix. *Semin Oncol* 1995;22[5 Suppl 12]:67–75.

443. Woo HL, Swenerton KD, Hoskins PJ. Taxol is active in platinum-resistant endometrial adenocarcinoma. *Am J Clin Oncol* 1996;19:290–291.

444. Ball HG, Blessing JA, Lentz SS, Mutch DG. A phase II trial of paclitaxel in patients with advanced or recurrent adenocarcinoma of the endometrium: a Gynecologic Oncology Group study. *Gynecol Oncol* 1996;62:278–281.

445. Lissoni A, Zanetta G, Losa G, et al. Phase II study of paclitaxel as salvage treatment in advanced endometrial cancer. *Ann Oncol* 1996;7:861–863.

446. Papadimitriou CA, Sarris K, Moulopoulos LA, et al. Phase II trial of paclitaxel and cisplatin in metastatic and recurrent carcinoma of the uterine cervix. *J Clin Oncol* 1999;17:761–766.

(TX) pretreated advanced ovarian cancer (AOC): final results. *Proc ASCO* 1999;18:368(abst).

447. Piver MS, Ghamande SA, Eltabbakh GH, O'Neill-Coppola C. First-line chemotherapy with paclitaxel and platinum for advanced and recurrent cancer of the cervix—a phase II study. *Gynecol Oncol* 1999; 75:334–337.

448. Slichenmyer WJ, Rowinsky EK, Donehower RC, Kaufmann SH. The current status of camptothecin analogues as antitumor agents. *J Natl Cancer Inst* 1993;85:271–291.

449. Rowinsky EK, Grochow LB, Hendricks CB, et al. Phase I and pharmacologic study of topotecan: a novel topoisomerase I inhibitor. *J Clin Oncol* 1992;10:647–656.

450. O'Dwyer PJ, LaCreta FP, Haas NB, et al. Clinical, pharmacokinetic and biological studies of topotecan. *Cancer Chemother Pharmacol* 1994;34[Suppl]:S46–S52.

451. Stewart CF, Baker SD, Heideman RL, et al. Clinical pharmacodynamics of continuous infusion topotecan in children: systemic exposure predicts hematologic toxicity. *J Clin Oncol* 1994;12:1946–1954.

452. Minami H, Beijnen JH, Verweij J, Ratain MJ. Limited sampling model for area under the concentration time curve of total topotecan. *Clin Cancer Res* 1996;2:43–46.

453. van Warmerdam LJ, Verweij J, Rosing H, et al. Limited sampling models for topotecan pharmacokinetics. *Ann Oncol* 1994;5:259–264.

454. McCabe FL, Johnson RK. Comparative activity of oral and parenteral topotecan in murine tumor models: efficacy of oral topotecan. *Cancer Invest* 1994;12:308–313.

455. von Pawel J, Gatzemeier U, Pujol JL, et al. Phase II comparator study of oral versus intravenous topotecan in patients with chemosensitive small-cell lung cancer. *J Clin Oncol* 2001;19:1743–1749.

456. Clarke-Pearson DL, Van Le L, Iveson T, et al. Oral topotecan as single-agent second-line chemotherapy in patients with advanced ovarian cancer. *J Clin Oncol* 2001;19:3967–3975.

457. Gore M, Oza A, Rustin G, et al. A randomised trial of oral versus intravenous topotecan in patients with relapsed epithelial ovarian cancer. *Eur J Cancer* 2002;38:57–63.

458. Stevenson JP, Scher RM, Kosierowski R, et al. Phase II trial of topotecan as a 21-day continuous infusion in patients with advanced or metastatic adenocarcinoma of the pancreas. *Eur J Cancer* 1998;34: 1358–1362.

459. Von Hoff DD, Burris HA 3rd, Eckardt J, et al. Preclinical and phase I trials of topoisomerase I inhibitors. *Cancer Chemother Pharmacol* 1994;34[Suppl]:S41–S45.

460. Rowinsky EK. Weekly topotecan: an alternative to topotecan's standard daily × 5 schedule? *Oncologist* 2002;7:324–330.

461. Morris RT. Weekly topotecan in the management of ovarian cancer. *Gynecol Oncol* 2003;90:S34–S38.

462. ten Bokkel Huinink W, Gore M, Carmichael J, et al. Topotecan versus paclitaxel for the treatment of recurrent epithelial ovarian cancer. *J Clin Oncol* 1997;15:2183–2193.

463. O'Reilly S, Rowinsky EK, Slichenmyer W, et al. Phase I and pharmacologic study of topotecan in patients with impaired renal function. *J Clin Oncol* 1996;14:3062–3073.

464. O'Reilly S, Rowinsky E, Slichenmyer W, et al. Phase I and pharmacologic studies of topotecan in patients with impaired hepatic function. *J Natl Cancer Inst* 1996;88:817–824.

465. O'Reilly S, Fleming GF, Barker SD, et al. Phase I trial and pharmacologic trial of sequences of paclitaxel and topotecan in previously treated ovarian epithelial malignancies: a Gynecologic Oncology Group study. *J Clin Oncol* 1997;15:177–186.

466. Rowinsky EK, Kaufmann SH, Baker SD, et al. Sequences of topotecan and cisplatin: phase I, pharmacologic, and in vitro studies to examine sequence dependence. *J Clin Oncol* 1996;14:3074–3084.

467. Gordon AN, Hancock KC, Matthews CM, et al. Phase I study of alternating doublets of topotecan/carboplatin and paclitaxel/carboplatin in patients with newly diagnosed, advanced ovarian cancer. *Gynecol Oncol* 2002;85:129–135.

468. Hammond LA, Eckardt JR, Ganapathi R, et al. A phase I and translational study of sequential administration of the topoisomerase I and II inhibitors topotecan and etoposide. *Clin Cancer Res* 1998;4: 1459–1467.

469. Mok TS, Wong H, Zee B, et al. A Phase I-II study of sequential administration of topotecan and oral etoposide (toposiomerase I and II inhibitors) in the treatment of patients with small cell lung carcinoma. *Cancer* 2002;95:1511–1519.

470. Chen AY, Choy H, Rothenberg ML. DNA topoisomerase I-targeting

drugs as radiation sensitizers. *Oncology (Huntingt)* 1999;13[10 Suppl 5]:39–46.

471. Rave-Frank M, Glomme S, Hertig J, et al. Combined effect of topotecan and irradiation on the survival and the induction of chromosome aberrations in vitro. *Strahlenther Onkol* 2002;178:497–503.

472. Hofstra LS, Bos AM, de Vries EG, et al. A phase I and pharmacokinetic study of intraperitoneal topotecan. *Br J Cancer* 2001;85: 1627–1633.

473. Plaxe SC, Christen RD, O'Quigley J, et al. Phase I and pharmacokinetic study of intraperitoneal topotecan. *Invest New Drugs* 1998;16: 147–153.

474. Long HJ 3rd, Rayson S, Podratz KC, et al. Long-term survival of patients with advanced/recurrent carcinoma of cervix and vagina after neoadjuvant treatment with methotrexate, vinblastine, doxorubicin, and cisplatin with or without the addition of molgramostim, and review of the literature. *Am J Clin Oncol* 2002;25:547–551.

475. Gebbia V, Testa A, Borsellino N, et al. Cisplatin and vinorelbine in advanced and/or metastatic adenocarcinoma of the endometrium: a new highly active chemotherapeutic regimen. *Ann Oncol* 2001;12: 767–772.

476. Aravantinos G, Bafaloukos D, Fountzilas G, et al. Phase II study of docetaxel-vinorelbine in platinum-resistant, paclitaxel-pretreated ovarian cancer. *Ann Oncol* 2003;14:1094–1099.

477. Noble RR, Beer CT. Experimental observations concerning the mode of action of vinca alkaloids. In: Wih S, ed. *The vinca alkaloids in the chemotherapy of malignant disease.* Alburcham, UK: John Sherrat & Sons; 1968:4.

478. Velban (vinblastine sulfate for injection, USP). In: *Physicians Desk Reference.* 55th ed. Montvale, NJ: Medical Economics, 2001.

479. Owellen RJ, Hartke CA. The pharmacokinetics of 4-acetyl tritium vinblastine in two patients. *Cancer Res* 1975;35:975–980.

480. Lucas VS, Huang AT. Vinblastine-related pain in tumors. *Cancer Treat Rep* 1977;61:1735–1736.

481. Brook J, Schreiber W. Vocal cord paralysis: a toxic reaction to vinblastine (NSC-49842) therapy. *Cancer Chemother Rep* 1971;55:591–593.

482. Teutsch C, Lipton A, Harvey HA. Raynaud's phenomenon as a side effect of chemotherapy with vinblastine and bleomycin for testicular carcinoma. *Cancer Treat Rep* 1977;61:925–926.

483. Ginsberg SJ, Comis RL, Fitzpatrick AV. Vinblastine and inappropriate ADH secretion. *N Engl J Med* 1977;296:941.

484. Cohlan SW, Kitay D. The teratogenic effect of vincaleukoblastine in the pregnant rat. *J Pediatr* 1965:541.

485. Dorr RT, Alberts DS. Vinca alkaloid skin toxicity: antidote and drug disposition studies in the mouse. *J Natl Cancer Inst* 1985;74:113–120.

486. Blajman C, Balbiani L, Block J, et al. A prospective, randomized Phase III trial comparing combination chemotherapy with cyclophosphamide, doxorubicin, and 5-fluorouracil with vinorelbine plus doxorubicin in the treatment of advanced breast carcinoma. *Cancer* 1999; 85:1091–1097.

487. Llombart-Cussac A, Pivot X, Rhor-Alvarado A, et al. First-line vinorelbine-mitoxantrone combination in metastatic breast cancer patients relapsing after an adjuvant anthracycline regimen: results of a phase II study. *Oncology* 1998;55:384–390.

488. Morris M, Brader KR, Levenback C, et al. Phase II study of vinorelbine in advanced and recurrent squamous cell carcinoma of the cervix. *J Clin Oncol* 1998;16:1094–1098.

489. Burger RA, DiSaia PJ, Roberts JA, et al. Phase II trial of vinorelbine in recurrent and progressive epithelial ovarian cancer. *Gynecol Oncol* 1999;72:148–153.

490. Peacock NW, Burris HA, Dieras V, et al. A phase I trial of vinorelbine in combination with mitoxantrone in patients with refractory solid tumors. *Invest New Drugs* 1998;16:37–43.

491. Mangeney P, Andriamialisoa RZ, Lallemand JY. 5′ Nor-anhydrovinblastine, prototype of a new class of vinblastine derivatives. *Tetrahedron* 1979;35:2175.

492. Johnson SA, Harper P, Hortobagyi GN, Pouillart P. Vinorelbine: an overview. *Cancer Treat Rev* 1996;22:127–142.

493. Marquet P, Lachatre G, Debord J, et al. Pharmacokinetics of vinorelbine in man. *Eur J Clin Pharmacol* 1992;42:545–547.

494. Wargin WA, Lucas VS. The clinical pharmacokinetics of vinorelbine (Navelbine). *Semin Oncol* 1994;21[5 Suppl 10]:21–27.

495. Leveque D, Jehl F. Clinical pharmacokinetics of vinorelbine. *Clin Pharmacokinet* 1996;31:184–197.

496. Lozano M, Muro H, Triguboff E, et al. A randomized trial for effective prevention of Navelbine (NVB) related phlebitis. *Proc ASCO* 1995; 14:535(abst).

497. Trissel LA, Martinez JF. Visual, turbidimetric, and particle-content assessment of compatibility of vinorelbine tartrate with selected drugs during simulated Y-site injection. *Am J Hosp Pharm* 1994;51: 495–499.

498. Gershenson DM, Burke TW, Morris M, et al. A phase I study of a daily x3 schedule of intravenous vinorelbine for refractory epithelial ovarian cancer. *Gynecol Oncol* 1998;70:404–409.

499. Havlin KA, Ramirez MJ, Legler CM, et al. Inability to escalate vinorelbine dose intensity using a daily x3 schedule with and without filgrastim in patients with metastatic breast cancer. *Cancer Chemother Pharmacol* 1999;43:68–72.

500. Weiss AJ, Sabol J, Lackman RD. Concurrent administration of vinorelbine with recombinant human granulocyte colony-stimulating factor: an effective method of increasing dose intensity. Am *J Clin Oncol* 1999;22:38–41.

501. Hohneker JA. A summary of vinorelbine (Navelbine) safety data from North American clinical trials. *Semin Oncol* 1994;21[5 Suppl 10]: 42–46; Discussion 46–47.

502. Gebbia V, Testa A, Valenza R, et al. Acute pain syndrome at tumour site in neoplastic patients treated with vinorelbine: report of unusual toxicity. *Eur J Cancer* 1994;30A:889.

503. Kornek GV, Kornfehl H, Hejna M, et al. Acute tumor pain in patients with head and neck cancer treated with vinorelbine. *J Natl Cancer Inst* 1996;88:1593.

504. Raderer M, Kornek G, Hejna M, et al. Acute pulmonary toxicity associated with high-dose vinorelbine and mitomycin C. *Ann Oncol* 1996;7:973–975.

505. Raderer M, Kornek G, Scheithauer W. Re: Vinorelbine-induced pancreatitis: a case report. *J Natl Cancer Inst* 1998;90:329.

506. Hoff PM, Valero V, Ibrahim N, et al. Hand-foot syndrome following prolonged infusion of high doses of vinorelbine. *Cancer* 1998;82: 965–969.

507. Liebmann J, Friedman K. Adynamic ileus in a patient with non–small-cell lung cancer after treatment with vinorelbine. *Am J Med* 1996; 101:658–659.

508. Garrett CA, Simpson TA Jr. Syndrome of inappropriate antidiuretic hormone associated with vinorelbine therapy. *Ann Pharmacother* 1998;32:1306–1309.

509. Budman DR. Vinorelbine (Navelbine): a third-generation vinca alkaloid. *Cancer Invest* 1997;15:475–490.

510. Zhou-Pan XR, Seree E, Zhou XJ, et al. Involvement of human liver cytochrome P450 3A in vinblastine metabolism: drug interactions. *Cancer Res* 1993;53:5121–5126.

511. Ozols RF, Hogan WM, Ostchega Y, Young RC. MVP (mitomycin, vinblastine, and progesterone): a second-line regimen in ovarian cancer with a high incidence of pulmonary toxicity. *Cancer Treat Rep* 1983;67:721–722.

512. Parimoo D, Jeffers S, Muggia FM. Severe neurotoxicity from vinorelbine-paclitaxel combinations. *J Natl Cancer Inst* 1996;88:1079–1080.

513. Tibaldi C, Pazzagli I, Berrettini S, De Vito A. A case of ototoxicity in a patient with metastatic carcinoma of the breast treated with paclitaxel and vinorelbine. *Eur J Cancer* 1998;34:1133–1134.

514. Bajetta E, Di Leo A, Biganzoli L, et al. Phase II study of vinorelbine in patients with pretreated advanced ovarian cancer: activity in platinum-resistant disease. *J Clin Oncol* 1996;14:2546–2551.

515. Herbst RS. Erlotinib (Tarceva): an update on the clinical trial program. *Semin Oncol* 2003;30[3 Suppl 7]:34–46.

516. Hidalgo M, Bloedow D. Pharmacokinetics and pharmacodynamics: maximizing the clinical potential of erlotinib (Tarceva). *Semin Oncol* 2003;30[3 Suppl 7]:25–33.

517. Akita RW, Sliwkowski MX. Preclinical studies with erlotinib (Tarceva). *Semin Oncol* 2003;30[3 Suppl 7]:15–24.

518. Sewell JM, Macleod KG, Ritchie A, et al. Targeting the EGF receptor in ovarian cancer with the tyrosine kinase inhibitor ZD 1839 ("Iressa"). *Br J Cancer* 2002;86:456–462.

519. Simpson BJ, Bartlett JM, Macleod KG, et al. Inhibition of transforming growth factor alpha (TGF-alpha)–mediated growth effects in ovarian cancer cell lines by a tyrosine kinase inhibitor ZM 252868. *Br J Cancer* 1999;79:1098–1103.

520. Medical Research and Communications Group ZP. ZD1839: Investigator's Brochure, Edition 3; 1999.

521. Schmandt RE, Broaddus R, Lu KH, et al. Expression of c-ABL, c-KIT, and platelet-derived growth factor receptor-beta in ovarian serous carcinoma and normal ovarian surface epithelium. *Cancer* 2003; 98:758–764.

522. PDR Electronic Library, Vol 6.0.0a. In: *Thomas Medical Economics*, 2003.

523. Hellstrom I, Goodman G, Pullman J, et al. Overexpression of HER-2 in ovarian carcinomas. *Cancer Res* 2001;61:2420–2423.

524. Bellone S, Palmieri M, Gokden M, et al. Selection of HER-2/neu-positive tumor cells in early stage cervical cancer: implications for Herceptin-mediated therapy. *Gynecol Oncol* 2003;91:231–240.

525. Santin AD, Bellone S, Gokden M, et al. Overexpression of HER-2/neu in uterine serous papillary cancer. *Clin Cancer Res* 2002;8: 1271–1279.

526. Bookman MA, Darcy KM, Clarke-Pearson D, et al. Evaluation of monoclonal humanized anti-HER2 antibody, trastuzumab, in patients with recurrent or refractory ovarian or primary peritoneal carcinoma with overexpression of HER2: a phase II trial of the Gynecologic Oncology Group. *J Clin Oncol* 2003;21:283–290.

527. Plourde PV, Dyroff M, Dukes M. Arimidex: a potent and selective fourth-generation aromatase inhibitor. *Breast Cancer Res Treat* 1994; 30:103–111.

528. Buzdar AU, Jonat W, Howell A, et al. Anastrozole versus megestrol acetate in the treatment of postmenopausal women with advanced breast carcinoma: results of a survival update based on a combined analysis of data from two mature phase III trials. Arimidex Study Group. *Cancer* 1998;83:1142–1152.

529. Koshiyama M, Yoshida M, Konishi M, et al. Expression of pS2 protein in endometrial carcinomas: correlation with clinicopathologic features and sex steroid receptor status. *Int J Cancer* 1997;74:237–244.

530. Watanabe K, Sasano H, Harada N, et al. Aromatase in human endometrial carcinoma and hyperplasia. Immunohistochemical, in situ hybridization, and biochemical studies. *Am J Pathol* 1995;146:491–500.

531. Rose PG, Brunetto VL, VanLe L, et al. A phase II trial of anastrozole in advanced recurrent or persistent endometrial carcinoma: a Gynecologic Oncology Group study. *Gynecol Oncol* 2000;78:212–216.

532. Kobiashvili H, Charkviani L, Charkviani T. Organ preserving method in the management of atypical endometrial hyperplasia. *Eur J Gynaecol Oncol* 2001;22:297–299.

533. Imai M, Jobo T, Sato R, et al. Medroxyprogesterone acetate therapy for patients with adenocarcinoma of the endometrium who wish to preserve the uterus-usefulness and limitations. *Eur J Gynaecol Oncol* 2001;22:217–220.

534. Thigpen JT, Brady MF, Alvarez RD, et al. Oral medroxyprogesterone acetate in the treatment of advanced or recurrent endometrial carcinoma: a dose-response study by the Gynecologic Oncology Group. *J Clin Oncol* 1999;17:1736–1744.

535. Bafaloukos D, Aravantinos G, Samonis G, et al. Carboplatin, methotrexate and 5-fluorouracil in combination with medroxyprogesterone acetate (JMF-M) in the treatment of advanced or recurrent endometrial carcinoma: a Hellenic Cooperative Oncology Group study. *Oncology* 1999;56:198–201.

536. Jordan VC, Assikis VJ. Endometrial carcinoma and tamoxifen: clearing up a controversy. *Clin Cancer Res* 1995;1:467–472.

537. Bilimoria MM, Assikis VJ, Jordan VC. Should adjuvant tamoxifen therapy be stopped at 5 years? *Cancer J Sci Am* 1996;2:140.

538. Varras M, Polyzos D, Akrivis C. Effects of tamoxifen on the human female genital tract: review of the literature. *Eur J Gynaecol Oncol* 2003;24:258–268.

539. Day R. Quality of life and tamoxifen in a breast cancer prevention trial: a summary of findings from the NSABP P-1 study. National Surgical Adjuvant Breast and Bowel Project. *Ann N Y Acad Sci* 2001; 949:143–150.

540. Ahlgren JD, Ellison NM, Gottlieb RJ, et al. Hormonal palliation of chemoresistant ovarian cancer: three consecutive phase II trials of the Mid-Atlantic Oncology Program. *J Clin Oncol* 1993;11:1957–1968.

541. Gelmann EP. Tamoxifen for the treatment of malignancies other than breast and endometrial carcinoma. *Semin Oncol* 1997;24[1 Suppl 1]: S1–65–S1–70.

542. Hatch KD, Beecham JB, Blessing JA, Creasman WT. Responsiveness

of patients with advanced ovarian carcinoma to tamoxifen. A Gynecologic Oncology Group study of second-line therapy in 105 patients. *Cancer* 1991;68:269–271.

543. Markman M, Iseminger KA, Hatch KD, et al. Tamoxifen in platinum-refractory ovarian cancer: a Gynecologic Oncology Group Ancillary Report. *Gynecol Oncol* 1996;62:4–6.

544. Strohmeyer D. Pathophysiology of tumor angiogenesis and its relevance in renal cell cancer. *Anticancer Res* 1999;19:1557–1561.

545. Malonne H, Langer I, Kiss R, Atassi G. Mechanisms of tumor angiogenesis and therapeutic implications: angiogenesis inhibitors. *Clin Exp Metastasis* 1999;17:1–14.

546. Folkman J. Tumor angiogenesis: therapeutic implications. *N Engl J Med* 1971;285:1182–1186.

547. Folkman J, Watson K, Ingber D, Hanahan D. Induction of angiogenesis during the transition from hyperplasia to neoplasia. *Nature* 1989; 339:58–61.

548. Gimbrone MA Jr, Leapman SB, Cotran RS, Folkman J. Tumor dormancy in vivo by prevention of neovascularization. *J Exp Med* 1972; 136:261–276.

549. Srivastava A, Laidler P, Davies RP, et al. The prognostic significance of tumor vascularity in intermediate-thickness (0.76–4.0 mm thick) skin melanoma. A quantitative histologic study. *Am J Pathol* 1988; 133:419–423.

550. Abulafia O, Triest WE, Sherer DM. Angiogenesis in primary and metastatic epithelial ovarian carcinoma. *Am J Obstet Gynecol* 1997; 177:541–547.

551. Alvarez AA, Krigman HR, Whitaker RS, et al. The prognostic significance of angiogenesis in epithelial ovarian carcinoma. *Clin Cancer Res* 1999;5:587–591.

552. Cooper RA, Wilks DP, Logue JP, et al. High tumor angiogenesis is associated with poorer survival in carcinoma of the cervix treated with radiotherapy. *Clin Cancer Res* 1998;4:2795–2800.

553. Kaku T, Hirakawa T, Kamura T, et al. Angiogenesis in adenocarcinoma of the uterine cervix. *Cancer* 1998;83:1384–1390.

554. Kaku T, Kamura T, Kinukawa N, et al. Angiogenesis in endometrial carcinoma. *Cancer* 1997;80:741–747.

555. Sauer G, Deissler H. Angiogenesis: prognostic and therapeutic implications in gynecologic and breast malignancies. *Curr Opin Obstet Gynecol* 2003;15:45–49.

556. Paley PJ. Angiogenesis in ovarian cancer: molecular pathology and therapeutic strategies. *Curr Oncol Rep* 2002;4:165–174.

557. Sieczkiewicz GJ, Hussain M, Kohn EC. Angiogenesis and metastasis. *Cancer Treat Res* 2002;107:353–381.

558. Folkman J. Seminars in Medicine of the Beth Israel Hospital, Boston. Clinical applications of research on angiogenesis. *N Engl J Med* 1995; 333:1757–1763.

559. Gadducci A, Viacava P, Cosio S, et al. Vascular endothelial growth factor (VEGF) expression in primary tumors and peritoneal metastases from patients with advanced ovarian carcinoma. *Anticancer Res* 2003; 23:3001–3008.

560. Holland CM, Day K, Evans A, Smith SK. Expression of the VEGF and angiopoietin genes in endometrial atypical hyperplasia and endometrial cancer. *Br J Cancer* 2003;89:891–898.

561. Gaffney DK, Haslam D, Tsodikov A, et al. Epidermal growth factor receptor (EGFR) and vascular endothelial growth factor (VEGF) negatively affect overall survival in carcinoma of the cervix treated with radiotherapy. *Int J Radiat Oncol Biol Phys* 2003;56:922–928.

562. Abramson N, Stokes PK, Luke M, et al. Ovarian and papillary-serous peritoneal carcinoma: pilot study with thalidomide. *J Clin Oncol* 2002; 20:1147–1149.

563. Celgene Corporation. Thalomid (thalidomide): Balancing the Benefits and Risks, 1998.

564. Tew KD, Houghton PJ, Houghton JA. *Preclincial and clinical modulation of anticancer drugs*. Boca Raton, FL: CRC Press; 1993.

565. Davidson DE, Grenan MM, Sweeney TR. Biological characteristics of some improved radioprotectors. In: Brady LW, ed. *Radiation sensitizers*. New York: Masson, 1980:309.

566. Schucter LM, Glick JH. The current status of WR2721 (Amifostine): a chemotherapy and radiation therapy protector. In: De Vita VT, Hellman S, Rosenberg SA, eds. *Biologic therapy of cancer updates*. Philadelphia: JB Lippincott Company, 1993:1.

567. Yuhas JM. Biological factors affecting the radioprotective efficacy

pf S-2-[3-aminopropylamino] ethylphosphorothioic acid (WR 2721). *Radiat Res* 1980;44:632.

568. Calabro-Jones PM, Aguilera JA, Ward JF, et al. Uptake of WR-2721 derivatives by cells in culture: identification of the transported form of the drug. *Cancer Res* 1988;48:3634–3640.

569. List AF, Heaton R, Glinsmann-Gibson B, Capizzi RL. Amifostine stimulates formation of multipotent and erythroid bone marrow progenitors. *Leukemia* 1998;12:1596–1602.

570. Millar JL, McElwain TJ, Clutterbuck RD, Wist EA. The modification of melphalan toxicity in tumor bearing mice by s-2-(3-aminopropylamino)-ethylphosphorothioic acid (WR 2721). *Am J Clin Oncol* 1982;5:321–328.

571. Taylor CW, Wang LM, List AF, et al. Amifostine protects normal tissues from paclitaxel toxicity while cytotoxicity against tumour cells is maintained. *Eur J Cancer* 1997;33:1693–1698.

572. Valeriote F, Tolen S. Protection and potentiation of nitrogen mustard cytotoxicity by WR-2721. *Cancer Res* 1982;42:4330–4331.

573. Shaw LM, Glover D, Turrisi A, et al. Pharmacokinetics of WR-2721. *Pharmacol Ther* 1988;39:195–201.

574. Korst AE, Eeltink CM, Vermorken JB, van der Vijgh WJ. Pharmacokinetics of amifostine and its metabolites in patients. *Eur J Cancer* 1997;33:1425–1429.

575. Korst AE, van der Sterre ML, Gall HE, et al. Influence of amifostine on the pharmacokinetics of cisplatin in cancer patients. *Clin Cancer Res* 1998;4:331–336.

576. Wagner W, Radmard A, Schonekaes KG. A new administration schedule for amifostine as a radioprotector in cancer therapy. *Anticancer Res* 1999;19:2281–2283.

577. Shpall EJ, Stemmer SM, Hami L, et al. Amifostine (WR-2721) shortens the engraftment period of 4-hydroperoxycyclophosphamide-purged bone marrow in breast cancer patients receiving high-dose chemotherapy with autologous bone marrow support. *Blood* 1994;83: 3132–3137.

578. Gall HE, Eeltink CM, Vermorken JB. Nursing protocol for effective administration of amifostine. *Eur J Cancer* 1995;31A:S286.

579. Wadler S, Haynes H, Beitler JJ, et al. Management of hypocalcemic effects of WR2721 administered on a daily times five schedule with cisplatin and radiation therapy. The New York Gynecologic Oncology Group. *J Clin Oncol* 1993;11:1517–1522.

580. Bonner HS, Shaw LM. New dosing regimens for amifostine: a pilot study to compare the relative bioavailability of oral and subcutaneous administration with intravenous infusion. *J Clin Pharmacol* 2002;42: 166–174.

581. Koukourakis MI, Kyrias G, Kakolyris S, et al. Subcutaneous administration of amifostine during fractionated radiotherapy: a randomized phase II study. *J Clin Oncol* 2000;18:2226–2233.

582. Penz M, Kornek GV, Raderer M, et al. Subcutaneous administration of amifostine: a promising therapeutic option in patients with oxaliplatin-related peripheral sensitive neuropathy. *Ann Oncol* 2001;12:421–422.

583. Cassatt DR, Fazenbaker CA, Kifle G, Bachy CM. Subcutaneous administration of amifostine (ethyol) is equivalent to intravenous administration in a rat mucositis model. *Int J Radiat Oncol Biol Phys* 2003; 57:794–802.

584. Creighton AM, Hellmann K, Whitecross S. Antitumour activity in a series of bisdiketopiperazines. *Nature* 1969;222:384–385.

585. Von Hoff DD, Howser D, Lewis BJ, et al. Phase I study of ICRF-187 using a daily for 3 days schedule. *Cancer Treat Rep* 1981;65: 249–252.

586. Herman EH, Ferrans VJ. Reduction of chronic doxorubicin cardiotoxicity in dogs by pretreatment with (+/-)-1,2-bis(3,5-dioxopiperazinyl-1-yl)propane (ICRF-187). *Cancer Res* 1981;41:3436–3440.

587. Wadler S, Green MD, Muggia FM. Synergistic activity of doxorubicin and the bisdioxopiperazine (+)-1,2-bis(3,5-dioxopiperazinyl-1-yl)-propane (ICRF 187) against the murine sarcoma S180 cell line. *Cancer Res* 1986;46:1176–1181.

588. Green MD, Alderton P, Gross J, et al. Evidence of the selective alteration of anthracycline activity due to modulation by ICRF-187 (ADR-529). *Pharmacol Ther* 1990;48:61–69.

589. Imondi AR, Della Torre P, Mazue G, et al. Dose-response relationship of dexrazoxane for prevention of doxorubicin-induced cardiotoxicity in mice, rats, and dogs. *Cancer Res* 1996;56:4200–4204.

590. Speyer JL, Green MD, Kramer E, et al. Protective effect of the bispiperazinedione ICRF-187 against doxorubicin-induced cardiac toxicity

in women with advanced breast cancer. *N Engl J Med* 1988;319: 745–752.

591. Blum RH, Walsh C, Green MD, Speyer JL. Modulation of the effect of anthracycline efficacy and toxicity by ICRF-187. *Cancer Invest* 1990;8:267–268.

592. Swain SM, Whaley FS, Gerber MC, et al. Cardioprotection with dexrazoxane for doxorubicin-containing therapy in advanced breast cancer. *J Clin Oncol* 1997;15:1318–1332.

593. Venturini M, Michelotti A, Del Mastro L, et al. Multicenter randomized controlled clinical trial to evaluate cardioprotection of dexrazoxane versus no cardioprotection in women receiving epirubicin chemotherapy for advanced breast cancer. *J Clin Oncol* 1996;14:3112–3120.

594. Wexler LH, Andrich MP, Venzon D, et al. Randomized trial of the cardioprotective agent ICRF-187 in pediatric sarcoma patients treated with doxorubicin. *J Clin Oncol* 1996;14:362–372.

595. Von Hoff DD. Phase I trials of dexrazoxane and other potential applications for the agent. *Semin Oncol* 1998;25[4 Suppl 10]:31–36.

596. Bertino JR. ''Rescue'' techniques in cancer chemotherapy: use of leucovorin and other rescue agents after methotrexate treatment. *Semin Oncol* 1977;4:203–216.

597. Kamen BA, Winick NJ. High dose methotrexate therapy: insecure rationale? *Biochem Pharmacol* 1988;37:2713–2715.

598. Erlichman C. Fluorouracil and leucovorin for metastatic colorectal cancer. *J Chemother* 1990;[2 Suppl 1]:38–40.

599. Zaniboni A, Arcangeli G, Meriggi F, et al. Low-dose 6-S leucovorin and 5-fluorouracil as salvage treatment in metastatic breast cancer. *Proc ASCO* 1994;13:91(abst).

600. Kobayashi K, Schilsky RL. Update on biochemical modulation of chemotherapeutic agents. *Oncology (Huntingt)* 1993;7:99–106, 109; Discussion 110–114, 117.

601. Brock N, Pohl J, Stekar J, Scheef W. Studies on the urotoxicity of oxazaphosphorine cytostatics and its prevention—III. Profile of action of sodium 2-mercaptoethane sulfonate (mesna). *Eur J Cancer Clin Oncol* 1982;18:1377–1387.

602. Burkert H. Clinical overview of mesna. *Cancer Treat Rev* 1983; 10[Suppl A]:175–181.

603. Goren MP, McKenna LM, Goodman TL. Combined intravenous and oral mesna in outpatients treated with ifosfamide. *Cancer Chemother Pharmacol* 1997;40:371–375.

604. Legha S, Papadopoulos N, Plager C, et al. A comparative evaluation of the uroprotective effect of mercaptoethane sulfonate (mesna) and N-acetylcysteine (NAC) in sarcoma patients treated with ifosfamide. *Proc ASCO* 1990;9:1205(abst).

605. Munshi NC, Loehrer PJ Sr, Williams SD, et al. Comparison of N-acetylcysteine and mesna as uroprotectors with ifosfamide combination chemotherapy in refractory germ cell tumors. *Invest New Drugs* 1992;10:159–163.

606. Markman M, Kennedy A, Webster K, et al. Continuous subcutaneous administration of mesna to prevent ifosfamide-induced hemorrhagic cystitis. *Semin Oncol* 1996;23[3 Suppl 6]:97–98.

CHAPTER 17

Hormones and Human Malignancies

Amir A. Jazaeri, G. Larry Maxwell, and Laurel W. Rice

Hormones have been linked to several of the most commonly occurring human malignancies, including the breast, endometrium, ovary, and colon. The ability of hormones to stimulate cellular proliferation, leading to random genetic errors, is the basis by which these peptides promote the development of human neoplasia. The laboratory investigation of the pathways and mechanisms by which hormones affect their biologic responses is an exploding area of research, largely as a result of the tremendous potential for translational research and improved patient care. This chapter will review the relationship between hormones and human malignancies, specifically as they relate to risk, prevention, and treatment.

HORMONE RECEPTOR PATHWAYS AND MECHANISMS

Overview

Steroid hormones are involved in a variety of growth and developmental processes and exert their physiologic effects by binding to their respective receptors. Steroid hormone receptors are part of the ligand-activated nuclear transcription factor superfamily whose members also include glucocorticoid, mineralocorticoid, androgen, thyroid, retinoid, progesterone (PR), and estrogen (ER) receptors (1). In the inactive state, these receptors are bound to repressor/chaperone complexes within the cytoplasm. Upon binding to their respective ligands, the receptor-ligand complex undergoes dimerization followed by nuclear localization (leading to the name "nuclear receptor"). Inside the nucleus the steroid hormone-receptor complex binds to specific DNA sequences called response elements (2). Also participating in this interaction are nuclear receptor coactivators and corepressors, as well as the general transcription machinery (3). The net result of these interactions is the transcriptional activation or repression of hormone-responsive genes.

Steroid Hormone Biosynthesis

Although a detailed description of steroid biosynthesis is beyond the scope of this chapter, a brief overview is presented (Fig. 17.1) to highlight targets of therapeutic intervention. The rate-limiting and irreversible reaction in steroid synthesis is the conversion of cholesterol to pregnenolone by the P450-linked side chain–cleaving enzyme P450-ssc (4). In the ovary, this reaction is regulated by follicle-stimulating hormone (FSH) and luteinizing hormone (LH) via cAMP and protein kinase A (PKA) signaling (5). This leads to increased production of androgen intermediates, androstenedione, and testosterone that are then converted by the P450-aromatase enzyme to estrone and estradiol (E2), respectively. The expression of P450-aromatase enzyme is not limited to the ovaries; its expression and action in a variety of tissues lead to local E2 production in these tissues (6). This local E2 biosynthesis may be especially significant in men and postmenopausal women, where ovarian hormone production is lacking. Furthermore, high levels of locally synthesized E2 have been implicated in breast carcinogenesis (7).

Examination of the transcription patterns of the gene encoding aromatase *CYP19* has revealed tissue-specific promoter usage. Promoter I.1 is used in the placenta; I.4 in adipose tissue, bone, and skin; and promoter II in breast cancer (CA), endometriosis, and ovarian CA (8). The transcripts generated from these promoters are translated into the same protein. However, the presence of tissue-specific promoters has raised the possibility of developing tissue-

Amir A. Jazaeri; MD Anderson Cancer Center, Houston, Texas 77030

G. Larry Maxwell: Walter Reed Army Medical Center, Division of Gynecologic Oncology, Washington, DC 20307

Laurel W. Rice: University of Virginia Health System, Obstetrics and Gynecology, Division of Gynecologic Oncology, Charlottesville, Virginia 22908

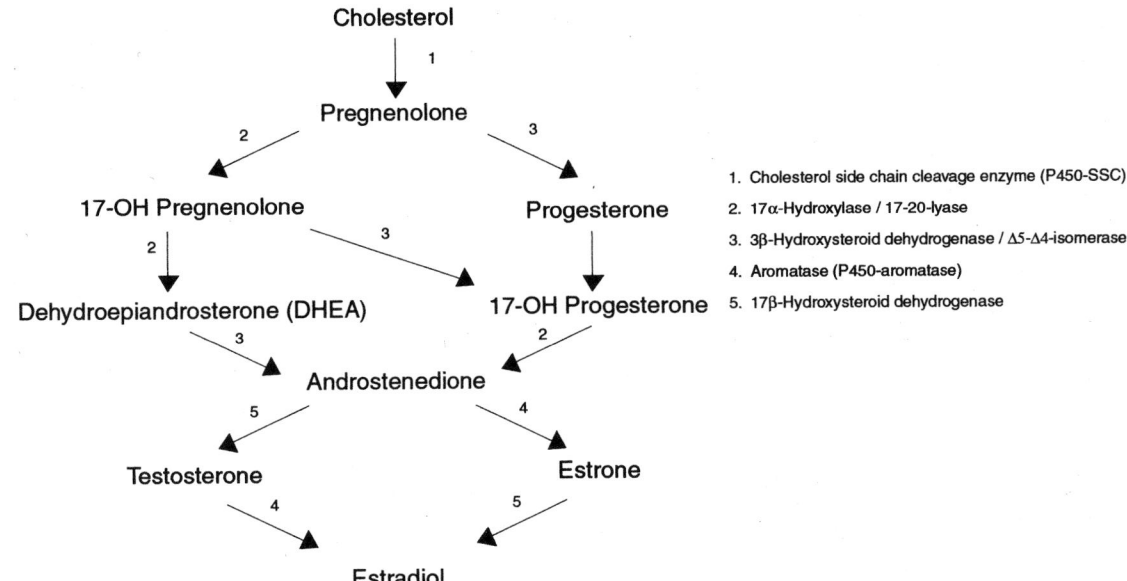

1. Cholesterol side chain cleavage enzyme (P450-SSC)
2. 17α-Hydroxylase / 17-20-lyase
3. 3β-Hydroxysteroid dehydrogenase / Δ5-Δ4-isomerase
4. Aromatase (P450-aromatase)
5. 17β-Hydroxysteroid dehydrogenase

FIG. 17.1. Steroid hormone biosynthesis. Notice the important role of aromatase in the conversion of androgens to E2s.

selective aromatase inhibitors. Such agents would be able to block E2 in breast CA, for example, without affecting estrogenic pathways in bones (6).

Steroid Hormone Receptor Structure

Steroid receptors are composed of six functional domains (Fig. 17.2) (9). The A/B domain is highly variable among the different members of this family and contains within it the hormone-independent activating-1 (AF-1) domain. The C region consists of the DNA-binding domain (DBD) and is relatively conserved. Within the central DBD two zinc fingers target the receptors to their corresponding hormone-response elements. The DBD binds as a dimer with each monomer recognizing half of the palindromic DNA sequence of the response element. The D domain is a peptide linker that connects the DBD to the ligand-binding domain (LBD). The E region is a multifunctional domain and contains amino acids involved in ligand binding, receptor dimerization, nuclear localization, coactivator/corepressor interaction, and ligand-dependent activating function (AF-2). The F region is a variable extension of the E region.

Estrogen Receptors

The two main isoforms of the human E2 receptors (ERs) are ER-α and ER-β. ER-α is encoded by the *ESR1* gene, which maps to the 6q25.1 locus. This isoform was the only known ER until 1996 when a second isoform, now known as ER-β, was discovered. Estrogen receptor-β is encoded by the *ESR2* gene located on chromosome 14q23 (10). The human ERs exhibit 96% and 58% homology in their DBD

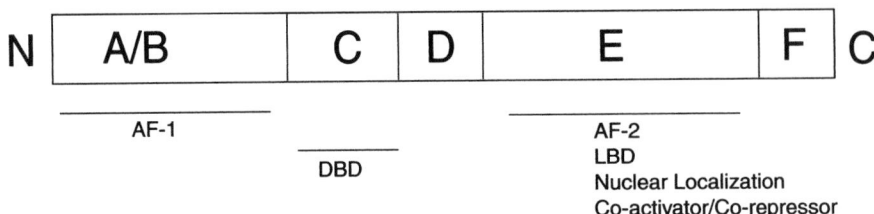

AF-1

DBD

AF-2
LBD
Nuclear Localization
Co-activator/Co-repressor

FIG. 17.2. Functional domains common to steroid receptors. The A/B domain is highly variable among the different members of this family and contains the hormone-independent activating-1 or AF-1 domain. The C region consists of the DNA-binding domain (DBD). The D domain is a peptide linker that connects the DBD to the ligand-binding domain (LBD). The E region is a multifunctional domain and contains the LBD as well as amino acids involved in receptor dimerization, nuclear localization, coactivator/corepressor interaction, and ligand-dependent activating function (AF-2). The F region is a variable extension of the E region.

and LBD, respectively, whereas the other domains show relatively little similarity. These structural differences result in distinct ligand affinities and physiologic properties. For example, raloxifene has a significantly higher affinity for ER-α, and genistein, a naturally occurring phytoestrogen, has a 30-fold higher affinity for ER-β compared to ER-α *in vitro*. Furthermore, tamoxifen and raloxifene exhibit partial agonist activities after binding to ER-α, whereas they act as pure antagonists when bound to ER-β (11). This is thought to result from distinct conformational changes induced by ligand binding in the two receptors (12).

ER-α is the predominant ER isoform in some tissues including the breast, uterus, and pituitary gland, whereas ER-β has notably higher expression in ovarian granulosa cells, prostate gland, gastrointestinal tract, endothelial cells, and parts of the nervous system (13,14). However, in many tissues, some expression of both receptors is observed. As noted above, ER-α and ER-β have been shown to have unique physiologic properties. In addition, they are capable of forming ER-α/ER-β heterodimers and thus influencing each other's function (15). In this context, ER-β has been shown to function as a dominant inhibitor of ER-α (16). Therefore, it is likely that normal physiologic function in E2-responsive tissues relies on the relative expression ratio of ER-α and ER-β in those tissues. There is evidence to suggest that perturbations of the normal ER-α to ER-β ratio correlate with neoplastic states. Cancers of the ovary, colon, and endometrium are all characterized by a relative loss of the normally predominant ER subtype when compared to normal tissue (17–20). Whether these changes predispose to or are a result of carcinogenesis remains to be elucidated. The development of ER-α, ER-β, and double knockout mice (ERKO, βERKO, and αβERKO, respectively) has helped with the identification of each receptor's physiologic role in their target organs (21). These findings are summarized in Table 17.1.

Both ER-α and ER-β have several isoforms resulting from exon deletions owing to alternative splicing (22–24). In addition, an alternative transcriptional start site for the *ESR2* gene results in "long" and "short" forms of ER-β that differ by 43 amino acids in the N-terminus of the proteins (23,25). Several of these ER-α and ER-β "splice-variants" have been demonstrated to poccess altered hormone-binding and/or transcriptional properties. Some can act in a dominant negative fashion by dimerizing with the wild-type receptors and interfering with their function *in vitro* (23). The *in vivo* physiologic or pathophysiologic significance of these variants awaits further clarification.

In addition to the above-described classic nuclear receptor mechanism of action, ER-α and ER-β have been shown to regulate transcription by interacting with other transcription factors (26,27). This mechanism involves protein-protein interaction and does not require DNA binding. One example of this type of interaction is the influence of ERs on the transcriptional activity mediated by the components of the activating protein-1 (AP-1) pathway jun and fos (27). In the presence of ER-α, E2 stimulates AP-1–dependent transcription, whereas tamoxifen and raloxifene inhibit it. In contrast, ER-β produces the opposite effect, with estradiol inhibiting and tamoxifen and raloxifene stimulating AP-1–mediated transcription. An additional mechanism of ER action involves "cross-talk" with growth factors including insulin-like growth factor-1 (IGF-1), epidermal growth factor (EGF), and transforming growth factor-β (TGF-β) (28,29). EGF can mimic the effects of E2 on the reproductive tract. This effect is dependent on ER-α since it can be blocked by ER antagonists and is absent in ERKO mice despite an intact EGF-signaling cascade (28,30). One mechanism for this cross-talk involves signal transduction from growth-factor receptors via the ras/raf/mitogen-activated protein kinase (MAPK) intermediaries culminating in the phosphorylation and activation of ER's AF-1 domain (31). More recently, the PI 3′K (phosphatidylinositol 3-kinase)/AKT cascade has been identified as another pathway that plays a significant role in the initiation of ER activity (32). In this signaling cascade, phosphoinositol 3,4,5-triphosphate (PIP3) is gener-

TABLE 17.1. *Summary of findings from estrogen-receptor knockout mice experiments*

Organ	Phenotype		
	αERKO	βERKO	αβERKO
Pituitary gland	High LH	None	High LH
Ovary	Hemorrhagic cysts, high estrogen and testosterone due to high LH, anovulatory	Reduced ovulation	Anovulatory, "sex-reversed" follicles with Sertoli-like cells
Endometrium	Estrogen insensitive, no growth or induction of estrogen-responsive genes	Normal growth and response to estrogen	Estrogen insensitive, no growth or induction of estrogen-responsive genes
Breast	No pubertal development	Normal development and lactation	No pubertal development

LH, luteinizing hormone.

ated by PI 3′K, and acts as a second messenger to recruit and activate downstream targets, including the serine/threonine protein kinase B (AKT) (33,34). AKT activation results in cell survival and inhibition of apoptosis (35). In normal tissue, this pathway is kept in check by a phosphatase called PTEN. PTEN is a tumor suppressor that negatively regulates the PI 3′K/AKT pathway by dephosphorylating PIP3. The activation of the PI 3′K/AKT pathway is particularly relevant in endometrial adenocarcinoma (36–41) where up to 80% of malignancies and 55% of premalignant lesions have been shown to harbor PTEN mutations (40,42). PI 3′K and AKT have been shown to stimulate ER-α expression and bring about its activation (via phosphorylation of AF-1) in the absence of E2 (43,44). Most investigations of the growth factor–ER cross-talk have involved ER-α. However, similar interaction involving ER-β is currently being investigated.

Progesterone Receptors

The effects of progesterone are mediated by two progesterone receptor (PR) proteins, PRA and PRB. The two PR proteins are products of the same gene, *PGR*, which has been mapped to chromosome 11q22-q23. These isoforms result from transcription from alternative promoters (45). The two PR forms are identical except that PRB has an additional 164 amino acids contained at its N-terminus compared to PRA. This unique region of PRB contains a transcription-activating functional domain, AF-3, in addition to AF-1 and AF-2, which are common to PRA (46). The two PRs exhibit differences in function that are cell context and promoter dependent. For example, PRB uniformly exhibits progestin-dependent transactivation in various cell types examined. Howeve, PRA's transcriptional activity is cell and response element specific. When tested on simple progestin-response elements (PREs), PRA and PRB display similar transactivational activity. However, PRA's activity is reduced or abolished on more complex response elements (47). In addition, PRA has been shown to act in a dominant negative fashion, antagonizing the transcriptional activity of not only PRB, but also other nuclear receptors such as the glucocorticoid, mineralocorticoid, androgen, and estrogen receptors (48).

In general, most tissues express equal levels of the two PR isoforms. However, differential expression can be observed as each promoter is regulated independently. For example, in the endometrium, stromal cells express predominantly PRA throughout the menstrual cycle, whereas the epithelial cells switch from PRA to PRB during the early secretory phase (49). It has been hypothesized that dysregulation of the normal PRA to PRB ratio may lead to disordered proliferation or neoplasia. In support of this hypothesis, PRA knockout (PRAKO) mice exhibit endometrial hyperplasia mediated by PRB following exposure to progestins (50). Similar studies using PRB knockout (PRBKO) mice have shown that PRA is sufficient for eliciting progesterone's reproductive responses in the ovary and the uterus. In contrast,

PRB is required to elicit normal proliferative responses of the mammary gland to progesterone (50). Finally, changes in PR isoform relative or overall expression have been described in endometrial, ovarian, and breast cancers (19,51, 52). The significance of these alterations awaits further investigation.

HORMONES AS RISK FACTORS FOR HUMAN MALIGNANCIES

Endogenous Hormones and Modulation of Cancer Risk

Obesity

The prevalence of obesity, defined as a body mass index (BMI) >30, has become an epidemic health care issue, affecting 20% of Americans and approximately 35% of eastern Europeans. When overweight patients (BMI >25) are included, the prevalence of this problem in the United States approaches 56% (53). In women with endometrial CA, obesity is a co-morbid condition in up to 40% cases (54,53). Obesity has been associated with a two- to fivefold increase in endometrial CA risk in both premenopausal and postmenopausal women (53,55). A recent case-control study performed by the American Cancer Society reported that the in CA death rates were 62% higher for morbidly obese women compared to normal-sized women. Specifically, the relative risk of CA-related mortality was significantly increased among obese women with breast CA (RR 1.63, 95% CI 1.44 to 1.85) and colon CA (RR 1.33, 95% CI 1.17 to 1.51). In patients with cervical and ovarian CA, a moderate (RR <2) yet significantly increased risk was observed. Uterine CA was most strongly associated with death: Women with BMI >40 had an RR of CA-related mortality of 6.25 (95% CI 3.75 to 10.42) (53,56). The results of recent epidemiologic studies have prompted the International Agency for Research on Cancer (IARC) to recommend avoidance of weight gain in order to minimize the risk of cancers of the colon, breast, and endometrium (53,57).

The relationship between obesity and endometrial carcinoma has been the most clearly elucidated. Progesterone deficiency, related to oligoovulation or anovulation, is one of the major risk factors for endometrial cancer in obese premenopausal women. The endometrium is chronically stimulated by unopposed E2, inducing neoplastic changes.

In both premenopausal and postmenopausal women, excess weight frequently results in increased androgen production, which decreases hepatic production of sex hormone–binding protein (SHBG). Reducing SHBG increases bioavailable estrogens, including estrane. Obesity is also associated with greater bioavailability of estradiol (E2), but this effect is noted only among postmenopausal women. In premenopausal women, negative feedback of estradiol on FSH, a stimulator of ovarian estradiol synthesis and aromatase activity, helps maintain constant estradiol levels throughout the menstrual cycle. Peripheral conversion of androgens in premenopausal women is subsequently limited by decreased FSH and aromatase activity. Endometrial CA risk, therefore, does not appear to be directly related to plasma E2 levels prior to menopause.

Obesity may also induce insulin resistance, which can lead to elevated levels of IGF-1. Progestin deficiency, frequently accompanying obesity, can also lower levels of IGF binding protein (IGF-BP1), resulting in increased levels of IGF-1. The unregulated increase in serum IGF-1 provides a stimulus for continuous growth of the endometrium. Hyperinsulinemia can also lead to a reduction in SHBG. Hyperinsulinemia induces LH-mediated hypersecretion of ovarian androgens leading to oligoovulation and the polycystic ovary syndrome (PCOS), a disease process highly correlated with risk of endometrial CA.

In obese postmenopausal women, peripheral conversion of androgens is an important source of serum estrogens. Elevated FSH levels typically present in postmenopausal women also contribute to the estrogenic state by the stimulation of aromatase activity. The increase in endogenous unopposed estrogens among obese postmenopausal women leads to the observed increased risk of developing endometrial carcinoma (53,58).

Perinatal Estrogen Levels

An association between perinatal exogenous estrogen exposure and an increased risk of CA in the offspring suggests that CA risk may be modulated *in utero*. The synthetic nonsteroidal estrogen diethylstilbestrol (DES) was administered during pregnancy to over 2 million women in the 1940s through the 1960s. Subsequently, DES was banned by the Food and Drug Administration (FDA) due to its teratogenic effects on limb bud development. Epidemiologic studies later revealed that there was a higher incidence of clear cell adenocarcinoma of the vagina and cervix in seemingly normal offspring of mothers who ingested DES prenatally (53, 59,60). In a laboratory setting, DES has been found to induce gynecologic carcinomas in developmentally exposed rodents (53,61). Mice treated neonatally with DES on days 1 to 5 have a 90% to 95% incidence of endometrial carcinoma at 18 months of life (62). These data strongly implicate a direct role of estrogen exposure, even early in development, in gynecologic carcinogenesis.

The increased incidence of gynecologic CA associated with antenatal DES exposure would suggest that the developing fetus or neonate is particularly susceptible to the epigenetic effects of estrogen. Investigators recently evaluated the carcinogenic potential of neonatal exposure for another E2 compound, genistein, a naturally occurring phytoestrogen found in many soy products. In this study, treated mice received equivalent estrogenic doses of DES, genistein, or placebo on days 1 to 5. At 18 months, the incidence of uterine adenocarcinomas was 31% for DES and 35% for genistein,

suggesting that estrogenic compounds, other than DES, may be carcinogenic if exposure occurs early during development (53,63).

A growing body of evidence suggests that elevated perinatal levels of endogenous estrogen also may lead to an increased risk of CA in the offspring (53,64). High birth weight, which is an indirect measurement of perinatal endogenous estrogen (53), is associated with an increased risk of breast CA in the newborn's adulthood (65). This increased breast CA risk is even more dramatic in twins, where the levels of perinatal estrogen are more pronounced compared to singleton pregnancies (53,66). Neonatal conditions, such as neonatal jaundice or prematurity, which are associated with increased estrogen, are also associated with a significantly increased risk of breast CA. In contrast, preeclampsia, a condition characterized by low E2 levels during pregnancy, is associated with a decreased risk of breast CA in the newborn's adulthood.

Exogenous Hormones and Modulation of Cancer Risk

Breast

Hormone Replacement Therapy

Women with No History of Breast Cancer. Multiple epidemiologic investigations have evaluated the relationship between hormone replacement therapy (HRT) and breast CA. In a meta-analysis of 51 studies of 52,705 women with breast CA and 108,411 women without breast CA, the Collaborative Group on Hormonal Factors in Breast Cancer (CGHFBC) determined that the risk of developing breast CA is increased in women using HRT, especially among women with >5 years of use (RR 1.3, 95% CI 1.21 to 1.49). The cumulative incidence of breast CA was 45 per 1,000 women between the ages of 50 and 70 years, and the use of HRT for >5 years was associated with an estimated cumulative excess of two breast CAs for every 1,000 users. The increased risk of breast CA associated with prolonged HRT was greater for women with low weight or body mass index. Breast CA diagnosed in women who had a history of HRT tended to be less advanced clinically compared to women with a negative history of use (67). The Breast Cancer Detection Demonstration Project, a cohort study with 46,355 postmenopausal women, 2,082 of whom were diagnosed with incident cases of breast CA, reported that women who had taken unopposed E2 had a 1.2-fold (95% CI 1.0 to 1.4) increase in breast CA risk, whereas women taking combination E2 and progestin regimens had a 1.4-fold (95% CI 1.1 to 1.8) increased risk. Breast CA risk was significantly elevated only in recent users with a BMI <24 (68). Finally, a recently reported case-control study involving 1,897 women with breast CA revealed that women using combination HRT had a statistically higher risk of breast CA (OR 1.24, 95% CI 1.07 to 1.45) than women taking unopposed E2 (OR 1.06, 95% CI 0.97 to 1.15) (69).

The Women's Health Initiative (WHI), a randomized, double-blind, placebo-controlled trial, recently reported the interim analysis of 8,506 women who received continuous combination HRT (0.625 mg of conjugated equine estrogen plus 2.5 mg of medroxyprogesterone acetate) versus 8,102 women prescribed placebo. The Data and Safety Monitoring Board for the trial recommended early cessation of this trial arm secondary to the observed adverse effects. Interim results from the WHI study revealed that the risk of coronary heart disease (HR 1.29, 95% CI 1.02 to 1.63), stroke (HR 1.41, 95% CI 1.07 to 1.85), and pulmonary embolism (HR 2.13, 95% CI 1.39 to 3.25) were all significantly elevated in patients receiving continuous combination HRT. The observed increased risk of breast CA (HR 1.26, 95% CI 1.0 to 1.59) was similar to results from the aforementioned observational studies (70). The results from the estrogen-only arm are unavailable at this time.

Women with a History of Breast Cancer. There is apprehension among physicians to prescribe HRT to women with a positive personal history of breast CA. The theoretical concern has been that exogenous hormones may stimulate the growth of dormant microscopic disease and ultimately lead to a decreased disease-free interval and survival.

Several case-control studies have reported that the rates of breast CA recurrence among survivors taking HRT vary from 3% to 7% (71–73) and do not appear significantly to diverge from stage-specific population rates of recurrence. In a case-control study by DiSaia et al. (74), 41 sporadic breast CA patients taking HRT were matched to controls according to age, stage, and socioeconomic status. A majority of the patients had early-stage disease. Recurrences were detected in 12 patients with stage I disease, 1 with stage II, and 2 with stage III. No evidence of increased disease recurrence was noted among the patients receiving HRT. In a subsequent analysis by the same investigators, 125 sporadic breast CA survivors receiving HRT were compared to 363 control subjects matched according to age at diagnosis, stage of breast CA, and year of diagnosis. The analysis revealed that the risk of death was lower among the breast CA patients receiving HRT (OR 0.28, 95% CI 0.11 to 0.71) According to the American College of Obstetricians and Gynecologists, the projected absolute lifetime risk for non-HRT users is approximately 10 cases of breast CA per 100 women. This risk would increase to 12 cases per 100 women using unopposed E2 and 14 cases per 100 women using combined E2 and progestin (75). Data from a prospective, randomized trial are not available.

Oral Contraceptives

Since their introduction in the 1960s, over 200 million women throughout the world have taken oral contraceptives (OCs). The CGHFBC performed a meta-analysis of 54 epidemiologic studies on 53,297 women with breast CA and 100,239 women without breast CA. Women who were cur-

rent users or who had used OCs in the previous 10 years were at an increased risk of breast CA (RR 1.24, 95% CI 1.15 to 1.33). In women taking OCs, the breast CA that developed was less advanced than that diagnosed in women with no history of OC use (76). Because the results from this meta-analysis reflected data from studies completed over the prior 25 years, the Women's Contraceptive and Reproductive Experiences (Women's CARE) Study was initiated in an effort to provide a more contemporary analysis of the relationship between OCs and breast CA risk (77). In this case-control study, a total of 4,574 women with breast CA and 4,682 controls were compared. The RR was 1.0 (95% CI 0.8 to 1.3) for current OC use and 0.9 (95% CI 0.8 to 1.0) for previous use, suggesting that among women 35 to 64 years of age, current or former OC use is not associated with a significantly increased risk of breast CA.

Women with BRCA *Mutations.* In the meta-analysis by the CGHFBC, the increased risk of breast CA associated with OC use was not influenced by a family history of breast CA (76). However, a three-fold increased risk of breast CA was observed among women taking OCs who had a positive family history of breast CA. This increased risk was observed only in women using high–estrogen potency formulations before 1975 (78). A subsequent matched case-control study by Narod et al. revealed that among *BRCA1* carriers, an increased risk of early-onset breast CA was evident in women who used OCs prior to 1975 (OR 1.42, 95% CI 1.17 to 1.75), used OCs prior to age 30 years (OR 1.29, 95% CI 1.09 to 1.52), or who used OCs for 5 or more years. Despite the increased risk associated with OC usage among *BRCA1* carriers, an increased risk of breast CA was not observed among women with a *BRCA2* carrier status (79). In *BRCA1* carriers, the protective effects of OC against ovarian CA must be weighed against the possible increased risk of OC use and breast CA.

Ovary

Hormone Replacement Therapy

Women with No History of Ovarian Cancer. Recently, several well-designed case-control and cohort studies have evaluated the relationship between HRT and ovarian carcinoma. The American Cancer Society's Cancer Prevention Study II found that after accounting for oral contraceptive pill (OC) use and parity, postmenopausal women using HRT had higher rates of ovarian CA–related deaths compared to nonusers (RR 1.51, 95% CI 1.16 to 1.96). The increased mortality risk was most notable for women using HRT for 10 or more years and persisted for up to 29 years after HRT cessation (80). This study is limited by the lack of information regarding estrogen and progestin potency. Another cohort study of 44,241 former participants in the Breast Cancer Detection Demonstration Project identified 329 women who developed ovarian CA during follow-up. Multivariant analysis revealed an increased association of estrogen-only HRT with ovarian CA (RR 1.6, 95% CI 1.2 to 2.0) after accounting for age, menopause type, and OC use (81). In contrast, an increased risk of ovarian CA was not noted among women who used estrogen and progestin. A Swedish case-control trial evaluated 655 case subjects with ovarian CA and 3,819 control subjects. An increased risk of ovarian CA was noted among women with a history of either estrogen (OR 1.43, 95% CI 1.02 to 2.00) or estrogen with sequentially added progestins (OR 1.54, 95% CI 1.15 to 2.05), particularly with hormone use exceeding 10 years. However, the use of estrogen with continuously added progestin was *not* associated with an increased risk of ovarian CA when compared to nonusers (82). The latter two studies suggest that HRT regimens containing both E2 and progestin may not have the increased risk of ovarian CA observed with E2 therapy alone. However, the WHI recently identified, in women taking continuous combined HRT, an HR of 1.58 (95% CI 0.77 to 3.24) for developing invasive ovarian carcinoma (83). The importance of the presence or absence of progesterone in HRT, as well as the type and potency, remains to be clearly elucidated.

Women with a History of Ovarian Cancer. Only one randomized controlled clinical trial exists evaluating the risk of ovarian CA recurrence in patients receiving HRT. This study was designed to detect a 20% difference in survival between the two treatment groups. In this study, 130 patients less than 59 years of age with invasive ovarian CA were randomized to continuous E2 HRT or no supplementation. The median disease-free interval for women receiving HRT versus not was 34 months and 27 months, respectively, not reaching statistical significance (84).

Oral Contraceptives

Multiple epidemiologic studies have revealed that OCs are *NOT* a risk factor for ovarian cancer, but rather a means of prevention (see below).

Endometrium

Hormone Replacement Therapy

Women with No History of Endometrial Cancer. Multiple case-control and cohort studies also have suggested that the risk of endometrial CA is elevated among patients receiving unopposed estrogen. A meta-analysis of 30 studies indicated that the summary RR of endometrial CA was 2.7 for patients receiving unopposed estrogen (85). The use of unopposed estrogen also has been shown to be associated with the development of endometrial hyperplasia. In the Postmenopausal E2/Progestin Intervention (PEPI) trial, 875 patients were randomized to receive one of five regimens: (a) placebo; (b) conjugated equine E2 (CEE), 0.625 mg/d; (c) CEE, 0.625 mg/d plus continuous medroxyprogesterone (MPA) 2.5

mg/d; (d) CEE, 0.625 mg/d plus MPA, 10 mg for 12 days each month; or (e) CEE, 0.625 mg/d plus micronized progesterone (MP), 200 mg/d for 12 days per month. Patients receiving unopposed estrogen had a significantly increased risk of atypical adenomatous endometrial hyperplasia (34% vs 1%) (86).

The addition of progestin to HRT has been shown to eliminate the increased risk of hyperplasia associated with unopposed E2. Although progestins have been associated with the effective treatment of endometrial hyperplasia, the data supporting the protective effects of progestins in HRT are limited. Many of the initial HRT regimens combining progestin and estrogens utilized the progestin for 7 days a month (87). Subsequent studies have recommended prolongation of the progestin component to at least 10 days each month. A case-control study of 832 endometrial CA patients and 1,114 controls in Washington State revealed that patients using a combined regimen of estrogen combined with progestin (0.625 mg/d CEE, 2.5 mg/d MPA) had a significantly lower relative risk (RR 1.4, 95% CI 1.0 to 1.9) of endometrial CA compared to patients who had taken unopposed estrogen (RR 4.0, 95% CI 3.2 to 5.1). However, patients receiving less than 10 days of cyclic progestin had an RR that was much higher (RR 3.1, 95% CI 1.7 to 5.7) than patients receiving 10 to 21 days of cyclic progestin (RR 1.3, 95% CI 0.8 to 2.2). Patients using either regimen of cyclic combination HRT had a increased risk of endometrial CA when these cyclic regimens of combination HRT were taken for a duration exceeding 5 years (cyclic progestin <10 days /month, RR 3.7, 95% CI 1.7 to 8.2; cyclic progestin 10 to 21 days each month, RR 2.5, 95% CI 1.1 to 5.5) (88). Subsequent data from the same investigators suggested that the use of a continuous progestin HRT regimen may actually be protective against endometrial CA (89). The largest case-control study of continuous HRT involved 79 case subjects and 88 control subjects and revealed that the RR of patients receiving continuous HRT was 1.07 (95% CI 0.80 to 1.43) (90). Data from the WHI indicated that the HR for EEC was 0.81 (95% CI, 0.48 to 1.36) in patients receiving continuous HRT with an average follow-up of 5.6 years (83).

There has recently been some suggestion that the degree of endometrial CA risk reduction may be dependent on the type of progestin used in the continuous HRT regimen. A Swedish case-control study found that patients with a continuous HRT involving testosterone-derived progestins (i.e., norhisterone, norhisterone acetate, levonorgestrel, lynestrenol) were associated with a lower RR of endometrial CA than those patients whose regimens involved progesterone-derived progestins (i.e., medroxyprogesterone) (91). Data from the Continuous Hormones as Replacement Therapy (CHART) study found no evidence of endometrial hyperplasia in participants who received norethindrone acetate (a testosterone-derived progestin). In this clinical trial, 1,265 patients were randomized to placebo versus one of eight treatment groups involving either various doses of unopposed ethinyl estradiol or various combinations of ethinyl estradiol plus norethindrone. Approximately 1,134 endometrial biopsies were performed over a 2-year follow-up period among women who received the combination HRT regimen; 1,232 biopsies were performed in the women given unopposed E2. As the doses of unopposed ethinyl estradiol were increased, there were increased percentages of subjects with endometrial hyperplasia. There were no cases of hyperplasia noted among the subjects who received different doses of the testosterone-derived progestin norethindrone. The protective effect was noted even among patients randomized to receive doses of norethindrone as low as 0.2 mg (86). In contrast, the PEPI trial identified hyperplasia on a surveillance endometrial biopsy in 3 of 339 patients who received E2 with a progesterone-derived progestin. Further studies are needed to determine if the degree of endometrial CA risk is influenced by the progestational activity of the progestin.

Women with a History of Endometrial Cancer. The use of E2 among patients with endometrial CA is controversial. *In vitro* treatment of Ishikawa endometrial CA cells with estrogen upregulates ER expression and augments growth in endometrial CA cells (92,93). However, *in vivo* growth of residual microscopic endometrial CA in patients has not been proven to date. Four retrospective cohort studies have evaluated patients with early-stage endometrial CA receiving E2 postoperatively. Creasman and colleagues (94) evaluated 221 patients with stage I disease of which 47 patients received postoperative HRT and 174 patients did not. Patients receiving HRT were followed for a median of 26 months. Regression analysis revealed that there was no increased risk of recurrent disease associated with HRT use even when adjusting for age, tumor grade, myometrial lymph node status, and peritoneal cytology. A subsequent study by Lee and colleagues (95) compared the outcomes of 44 low-risk endometrial CA patients (stage IA/IB G_1/G_2 disease) who received HRT following treatment to 99 patients who received no HRT. There were no recurrences observed among the endometrial CA patients receiving HRT for a median duration of 64 months. Investigators from the University of California, Irvine, have also failed to demonstrate an increased risk of recurrent disease associated with postoperative HRT (96). In the first study, investigators evaluated 123 women with surgical stages I and II endometrial CA. Sixty-one women received postoperative estrogen, and the mean duration of follow-up was 40 months. The disease-free interval was not significantly shortened among the patients receiving E2 (96). The second study was a retrospective cohort study that involved 75 patients with stages I-III disease who received HRT (51% E2 only, 49% E2 with added progestin) postoperatively. This group of patients was then matched according to decade of age at diagnosis and stage of disease to a group of endometrial CA patients in the study cohort not receiving HRT. Both groups were comparable in terms of parity, tumor grade, depth of myometrial invasion, histology, lymph node status, surgical treatment, concurrent

morbidities, and postoperative radiation. The patients receiving HRT were followed for a mean interval of 83 months and patients not receiving HRT were followed for a comparable interval of 69 months. Patients using HRT had a longer disease-free interval compared to nonhormone users. Among the 150 patients, only 8 patients had stage III disease (97).

In a Committee Opinion by the American College of Obstetricians and Gynecologists Committee of Gynecologic Practice, the members announced that "the decision to use HRT in these women [endometrial CA patients] should be individualized on the basis of potential benefit and risk to the patient" (98). The Gynecologic Oncology Group initiated a multicenter randomized controlled trial aimed at an enrollment of 2,100 patients with stages I and II endometrial CA. The study was closed after enrollment of 1,200 patients because accrual decreased sharply after the publication of the results of the WHI. With the closure of this GOG protocol, the safety of exogenous estrogen use in women who have undergone surgical management of endometrial CA may never be fully ascertained.

Oral Contraceptives

Multiple epidemiologic studies have revealed that OCs are *NOT* a risk factor for endometrial cancer, but rather a means of prevention (see below).

Selective Estrogen Receptor Modulators

The antiestrogen tamoxifen has been used in the adjuvant therapy of advanced breast CA for years and has recently been evaluated as a chemopreventive agent in patients at a high risk for developing this malignancy. Tamoxifen increases the risk of second primary malignancies at other sites. A randomized controlled trial involving 2,729 women performed by the Stockholm Breast Cancer Study Group revealed patients given tamoxifen (40 mg daily) had a nearly sixfold increased risk of endometrial CA and a threefold increased risk of gastrointestinal CA (53,99). These findings were confirmed in the National Surgical Adjuvant Breast and Bowel Project (NSABP). In this study, 2,843 patients with node-negative invasive breast CA were randomized to receive tamoxifen (40 mg daily) or placebo. The RR of endometrial CA in patients receiving tamoxifen was 7.5 (CI 1.7 to 32.7) (100) compared to placebo (53). When the population-based rates of endometrial CA from another NSABP trial (B-06) and data from the Surveillance, Epidemiology, and End Results (SEER) Program were used in the calculation of risk, the RR of endometrial CA associated with tamoxifen use was 2.3 and 2.2, respectively. In addition, the average annual HR during follow-up was only 1.6/1000 in the group receiving tamoxifen (53,100), suggesting that routine screening would not be cost effective.

Other selective estrogen receptor modulators (SERMs) are being evaluated as adjuvant treatment for breast CA in an attempt to avoid the increased risk of secondary malignancies while maintaining the same or greater effectiveness. Results from the Multiple Outcomes of Raloxifene Evaluation (MORE) study indicate that patients receiving raloxifene had a lower incidence of breast CA without any increase in endometrial CA risk (53,101). However, the primary endpoint in this investigation was risk reduction of fracture in postmenopausal women with osteoporosis. Several other SERMs are under investigation. The results of ongoing clinical trials will confirm these preliminary findings and establish the applicability of this contemporary generation of SERMs.

Colon

Hormone Replacement Therapy

Multiple epidemiologic studies have revealed that HRT is *NOT* a risk factor for colon cancer, but rather protects against this malignancy (see below).

Oral Contraceptives

Multiple epidemiologic studies have revealed that OCs are NOT a risk factor for colon cancer, but rather protect against this malignancy (see below).

Selective Estrogen Receptor Modulators

In vitro evidence has revealed that both tamoxifen and raloxifene are effective in reducing cell proliferation and viability of colon CA cell lines, suggesting a possible application in the prevention of colon CA (102). Unfortunately, the available epidemiologic evidence is limited and controversial regarding the issue of tamoxifen's effects on colorectal CA risk. A meta-analysis by the Stockholm Breast Cancer Study Group analyzed 4,914 postmenopausal women participating in one of three Scandinavian clinical trials evaluating adjuvant tamoxifen: the Stockholm Trial, the Danish Breast Cancer Group Trial, and the South-Swedish Trial (99). The joint analysis of these three trials revealed that adjuvant tamoxifen therapy in breast CA patients increased the risk of colorectal CAs (RR 1.9, 95% CI 1.1 to 1.3) (99). In contrast, findings from the National Surgical Adjuvant Breast and Bowel Project (NSABP) B-14 and the Surveillance Epidemiology and End Results Program (103) have failed to confirm an increased risk of colorectal CA among patients receiving adjuvant tamoxifen therapy. Additional epidemiologic trials are needed to resolve the issue of adjuvant tamoxifen therapy and the risk of secondary sporadic colorectal CAs.

Although some epidemiologic evidence suggests that tamoxifen may be associated with an increased risk of sporadic colorectal CA, SERMs have been used in the treatment of desmoid tumors associated with hereditary colorectal CA. Colorectal CA includes two main mechanisms of inheritance: familial adenomatous polyposis (FAP) and hereditary nonpolyposis colorectal CA (HNPCC). Desmoid tumors are fibroaponeurotic tumors that occur rarely in the general population but can be found in 12% to 17% of patients with FAP (104). Tamoxifen has been shown to have growth inhibition in desmoid tumor cell lines in an E2-independent mechanism (105). According to the practice guidelines of the Standard Task Force of Colon and Rectal Surgeons, high-dose tamoxifen (120 mg/d) and other SERMs may be used in the treatment of aggressive desmoid tumors. This recommendation is weak (level III) and based on limited descriptive European case series (106,107). The use of tamoxifen in the prevention or treatment of the primary colorectal CA is not advocated.

Phytoestrogens

Increased rates of breast, colon, ovarian, and endometrial CA are found in Western societies. Phytoestrogens are possible dietary mediators of increased CA risk that are subdivided into two groups: isoflavonoids and lignans. Isoflavonoids are compounds with inherent estrogenic activity that can lead to low IGF expression and inhibition of aromatase and growth factors, resulting in a possible chemoprotective effective in the breast. Lignans are compounds formed from plant lignan precursors by intestinal microflora. Both isoflavonoids and lignans are found in foods such as whole grain rye bread, soybeans, and red clover. Studies suggest that the development period during which the isoflavonoid is ingested is important in modulation of future CA risk. Ingestion of soy before or during adolescence may decrease the risk of future breast CA. However, there is no convincing evidence indicating that soy or other isoflavanoids are protective against breast CA or colon CA if ingested during adulthood (53,108). There is a paucity of data regarding the association between isoflavanoids and other CAs affecting women. A case-control study using a Hawaiian group revealed that the high consumption of soy products in adults significantly decreased the risk of endometrial CA even after accounting for confounding influences (53,109). Large population-based studies are need to determine the effects of isoflavonoids on specific CA risk, particularly since they are becoming a more common component of the American diet.

Consumption of whole grain products, berries, fruits, and vegetables can stimulate production of lignans, which can be indirectly measured via urinary enterolactone. Although women with breast CA have significantly lower levels of urinary enterolactone, it is unknown whether higher levels of enterolactone are protective against breast CA or whether they are a marker for an unknown chemoprotective compound associated with a healthier diet. High enterolactone production has been associated with inhibition of colon CA in animal models, but elevated levels have not been confirmed to be protective against colon CA in humans (53, 108). In contrast, obesity as well as increased dietary fat intake are associated with decreased levels of urinary lignan, suggesting the increased risk of CA associated with obesity may be in part related to lignan production.

HORMONES AND THE PREVENTION OF HUMAN CANCERS

Chemoprevention can be defined as the use of specific natural or synthetic chemical agents to reverse, suppress, or prevent the progression toward malignancies. Human carcinogenesis proceeds through multiple discernible stages of molecular and cellular alterations, thus providing the scientific rationale for clinical CA chemoprevention. The necessary requirements for evaluation of chemoprevention include (a) identification of high-risk individuals based on family history and/or genetic mutations, (b) identification of putative surrogate endpoints or biomarkers for CA, and (c) the possibility that relatively nontoxic agents may decrease the risk of a given malignancy. Prospective clinical trials are mandatory for evaluating potential strategies for preventing human malignancies.

Breast Cancer Chemoprevention

Selective Estrogen Receptor Modulators

Reducing the incidence of breast CA has the potential to provide a major impact on the morbidity of the disease and its treatment, cost to the individual and to society, and overall CA mortality. Epidemiologic studies indicate that E2-mediated events play a role in the development of breast CA. Tamoxifen, a SERM, has been utilized as a chemopreventive agent for breast CA in four randomized prospective placebo-controlled clinical trials. Raloxifene, a second-generation SERM, was investigated in the Multiple Outcomes of Raloxifene Evaluation (MORE) trial, in which the primary endpoint was risk reduction of fracture in postmenopausal women with osteoporosis; the incidence of breast CA was a secondary endpoint. These five studies are reviewed and summarized below.

Chemoprevention Clinical Trials

Breast Cancer Prevention Trial. In 1992, the National Cancer Institute in collaboration with the NSABP initiated the Breast Cancer Prevention Trial (BCPT, P-1) (110). The primary goal was to determine whether tamoxifen administered for 5 years prevented breast CA in women at high risk, including women 60 years of age or older and women 35 to 59 years old with a 5-year predicted risk of breast CA of at least 1.66%, or with a history of lobular carcinoma *in situ* (LCIS). Risk was estimated using the Gail model (111). Each of the 13,388 women enrolled was randomly assigned to

receive tamoxifen 20 mg/d or placebo. The median follow-up time was 54.6 months, with 175 cases of invasive breast CA in the placebo group compared with 89 in the tamoxifen group (RR 0.51; 95% CI 0.39 to 0.66; $p < .00001$). Tamoxifen reduced the incidence of ER-positive tumors by 69%, but there was no difference in the incidence of ER-negative tumors.

Italian Tamoxifen Prevention Study. This double-blind placebo-controlled, randomized trial began recruitment in October 1992 and ended in July 1997 and included healthy women aged 35 to 70 years of age (112). The trialist and data-monitoring committee ended recruitment because 26% of women dropped out of this study; 5,408 women were randomized to receive tamoxifen 20 mg/d or placebo for 5 years. Women were allowed to take HRT. The primary endpoints were reduction in the frequency and mortality of breast CA. At a median follow-up of 46 months, 19 CAs were diagnosed in the tamoxifen arm and 22 among women in the placebo arm ($p = .6$). An update was reported in 2002 (113). At 81.2 months of follow-up, 45 of 2,708 women receiving placebo and 34 of 2,700 women receiving tamoxifen developed breast CA (OR 0.76; 95% CI 0.47 to 1.60). The difference was not statistically significant ($p = .215$). Among women who used HRT either at baseline or during the study, breast CA was diagnosed in 17 of 791 receiving placebo and 6 of 793 receiving tamoxifen ($p = .022$).

Royal Marsden Hospital Chemoprevention Trial. This trial was initiated in 1986 as a preliminary pilot study for the International Breast Cancer Intervention Study (IBIS-I) (114). The aim of this study was to assess whether tamoxifen would prevent breast CA in healthy women at increased risk for the disease based on family history only. Each participant had at least one first-degree relative under the age of 50 years with breast CA, one first-degree relative with bilateral breast CA, or one affected first-degree relative of any age and another affected first-degree or second-degree relative. Women were allowed to take HRT during this study. Randomization of 2,494 women between the ages of 30 and 70 years to tamoxifen 20 mg/d or placebo occurred. The median follow-up was 70 months, and 2,471 of the women were analyzed. The frequency of breast CA was the same for women receiving tamoxifen and placebo (tamoxifen = 34, placebo = 36; RR 1.06, CI 0.7 to 1.7), and there appeared to be no interaction between the use of HRT and the effect of tamoxifen on breast CA occurrence. An update of this trial reported 75 cases of breast CA in the placebo group compared to 62 in the tamoxifen group (OR 0.83, 95% CI 0.58 to 1.16) (115,116).

International Breast Cancer Intervention Study. Randomization occurred to tamoxifen 20 mg/d or placebo for 7,152 women aged 35 to 70 years and at high risk for breast CA (117). Eligible women had risk factors for breast CA indicating at least a twofold relative risk among those aged 45 to 70 years, a fourfold relative risk among those aged 40 to 44 years, and a tenfold relative risk among those aged

35 to 39 years. The women enrolled in this study were at moderately increased risk of developing breast CA, with 60% of the study cohort having a 10-year risk ranging from 5% to 10%. The IBIS-I investigators used a model to predict the absolute 10-year risk of developing breast CA, but the details of their model have not been published. The use of HRT was permitted, and approximately 40% of women used such therapy at some point during the trial. The primary endpoint was the incidence of breast CA, including ductal carcinoma *in situ* (DCIS). At a median follow-up of 50 months (7,139 women analyzed), 69 women in the tamoxifen group compared to 101 women in the placebo group developed breast CA (overall 32% reduction in breast CA rate; 95% CI 8 to 50; $p = .01$). The risk of developing ER-positive invasive tumors was reduced by 31%, but there was no reduction in the risk of ER-negative tumors. There was no difference in the incidence of breast CA among women taking HRT during the study. However, among women who received HRT before the trial, 21 cases of breast CA developed in the placebo group and 9 in the tamoxifen group (OR 0.43, 95% CI 0.80 to 6.06).

Multiple Outcome of Raloxifene Evaluation. The MORE study was a multicenter randomized double-blind trial of raloxifene 60 or 120 mg/d or placebo for 3 years, with the primary endpoint of rate of fracture in postmenopausal women with osteoporosis (118). Breast CA incidence was a secondary endpoint. A total of 7,705 women, at least 2 years postmenopausal and no older than 80 years of age, were enrolled. Women who were taking E2 during the previous 6 months were excluded, and 12.3% of women reported a family history of breast CA. There were 27 cases of invasive breast CA in the placebo group compared to 13 in the raloxifene group (RR 0.24; 95% CI 0.13 to 0.44; $p < .001$). There was no difference in breast cancer incidence between the two doses of raloxifene. Raloxifene reduced the risk of invasive ER-positive breast CA by 90% (RR 0.10; 95% CI 0.04 to 0.24), but did not reduce the risk of ER-negative breast CA. Four-year results from this study have now been reported (119). These results, with extension to 4 years after initiation of the trial, are consistent with the results based on the 3-year follow-up. The MORE trial was not designed to evaluate invasive breast CA as a primary endpoint. In addition, women in this trial were at lower risk of breast CA compared with women in the BCPT. Further study of raloxifene is indicated, and at this time, this SERM cannot be recommended for chemoprevention outside of a clinical trial.

Summary of the Tamoxifen Chemoprevention Trials. The Royal Marsden and Italian studies failed to confirm the results of the BCPT, a reduction in the incidence of ER-positive breast CA in women taking tamoxifen. An updated report from the Italian Tamoxifen Prevention Study found a reduction in the incidence of ER-positive breast CA among a subgroup of women. The results of the IBIS-I study confirmed that tamoxifen reduces the risk of breast CA. Numer-ous methodologic differences exist between the BCPT and European trials in trial design, trial implementation, and characteristics of the women studied. It is probable that both the Royal Marsden and Italian trials would fail to detect an overall effect for tamoxifen among the populations studied. Both of these trials were statistically less powerful and smaller than the BCPT, with fewer person-years of follow-up and fewer reported events. As well, the risk of breast CA among women in these trials was lower than the BCPT. The FDA approved the use of tamoxifen for breast CA risk reduction in women aged 35 years or older with a 5-year risk of 1.66% or greater.

In January 2003, Cuzick et al. (116) published an overview of the above breast CA chemoprevention trials. The results are summarized in Figure 17.3. Tamoxifen reduced the incidence of ER-positive breast CAs by 48% (95% CI 36 to 58; $p < .0001$), with no reduction in the incidence of ER-negative breast CAs. Age had no effect on the degree of breast CA reduction. The rates of endometrial CA increased in all the tamoxifen prevention trials (consensus RR 2.4; 95% CI 1.5 to 4.0; p, .0005); no increase in endometrial CA was observed with the use of raloxifene. Venous thromboembolic events were increased in all the tamoxifen prevention studies (RR 1.9; 95% CI 1.4 to 2.6; $p < .0001$), with similar results seen in the MORE study. Overall, there was no effect on all-cause mortality in the tamoxifen prevention trials (hazard ratio 0.90; 95% CI 0.70 to 1.17; $p = .44$). The investigators concluded that the evidence clearly shows that tamoxifen can reduce the risk of ER-positive breast CA.

The STAR Trial (Study of Tamoxifen and Raloxifene), powered to demonstrate superior efficacy or equivalence of either tamoxifen (20 mg/d) or raloxifene (60 mg/d) in reducing the incidence of primary breast CA, was opened to accrual on July 1, 1999. Risk assessments have been performed on 107,855 women and 12,637 have been randomized to either SERM for 5 years. The trial will recruit a total of 22,000 postmenopausal women whose projected 5-year risk of developing breast CA is 1.66% or higher as determined by the Gail model. Eligible women include postmenopausal women 35 years of age or older with no prior history of invasive breast CA or DCIS. Postmenopausal women with a history of LCIS who are aged 35 years or older are also eligible. The STAR Trial is scheduled to report outcomes in 2007.

Aromatase Inhibitors

Aromatase inhibitors (AIs) are being considered for use in breast CA chemoprevention. In contrast to SERMs, which are competitive inhibitors of E2 at its receptor, AIs suppress plasma E2 levels by inhibiting or inactivating aromatase, the enzyme responsible for the synthesis of E2s from androgenic substrates. This class of compounds has effectively challenged tamoxifen for use as adjuvant therapy in postmenopausal women with ER-positive breast CAs, who comprise

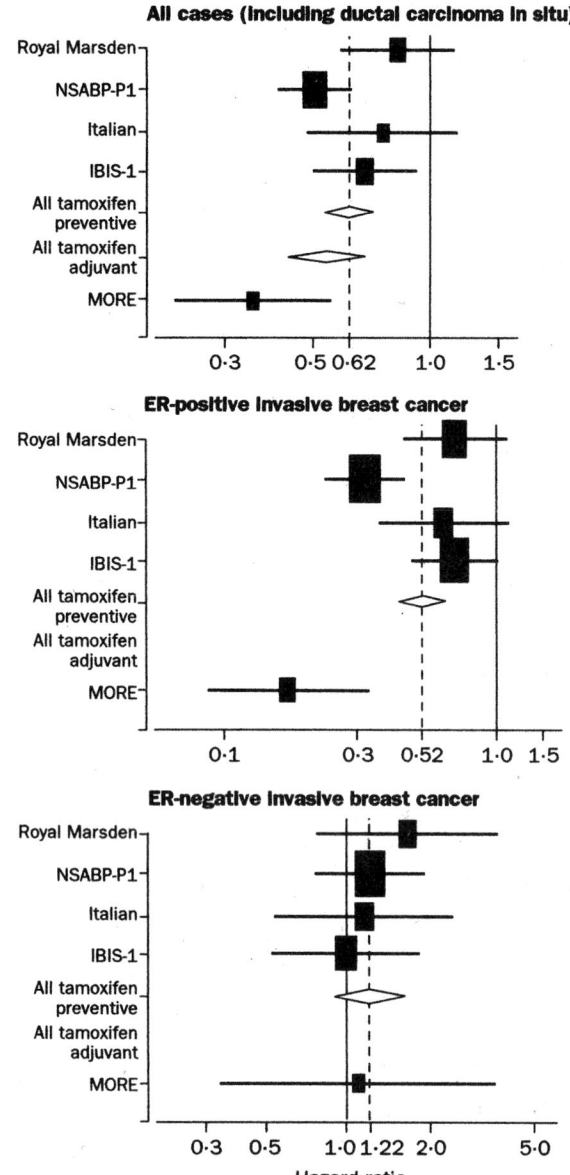

FIG. 17.3. Incidence of breast cancer. Note that the scale for the hazard ratio on the horizontal axis is different for each section of the figure. (Reprinted with permission from Cuzick J, Powles T, Veronesi U, et al. Overview of the main outcomes in breast-cancer prevention trials. *Lancet* 2003;361: 296–300.)

the majority of patients with breast CA. Evaluating women with early-stage breast CA, the ATAC (Arimidex, Tamoxifen Alone or in Combination) Trialists' Group found that the incidence of contralateral invasive breast CA was lower in those receiving the third-generation AI [anastrozole (Arimidex)] when compared to tamoxifen after a median of 33 months of follow-up (see below). By extrapolation, Arimidex might reduce the early incidence of breast CA to an even greater extent than tamoxifen and thus have potential in breast CA chemoprevention (113,120). The long-term ef-

fects of profound E2 suppression in postmenopausal women are unknown, and careful monitoring for bone demineralization and other potential problems is essential.

Prophylactic Oophorectomy

The potential role for oophorectomy as chemoprevention (decreased E2 levels) for breast CA in premenopausal women is an area of active investigation. In genetically uncharacterized premenopausal women, oophorectomy is associated with a 50% reduction in breast CA incidence, but also incurs the associated negative effects of a surgically induced early menopause (121,122). In this patient population, where the overall incidence of breast CA is one in eight, it is not standard practice to offer oophorectomy for breast CA prevention. However, in premenopausal women with germline *BRCA1* and *BRCA2* mutations, the cumulative lifetime risk (to 70 years of age) of invasive breast CA is 60% to 85%, allowing for more serious consideration for prophylactic oophorectomy as a chemoprevention. The prevalence of germline *BRCA1* or *BRCA2* in the general population is 0.1% to 0.2%, contributing to a small fraction of all cases of breast CA but as many as 10% of cases diagnosed in women younger than 40 years of age and approximately 75% of familial cases. Two recent publications support the practice of recommending prophylactic oophorectomy after the completion of childbearing in premenopausal women (123,124). Kauff et al., in a prospective study, reported on 170 carriers of *BRCA* mutations with a mean follow-up of 24.2 months, 98 of whom underwent prophylactic salpingo-oophorectomy (123). A 70% risk reduction in breast CA incidence was identified. Rebbeck et al., in a multicenter retrospective analysis, reported on 551 carriers of *BRCA* mutations with 11 years of follow-up, 259 of whom underwent a prophylactic salpingo-oophorectomy. A 53% risk reduction in breast CA incidence was identified (124). The reduced risk of a subsequent diagnosis of breast CA in women with *BRCA* mutations, after salpingo-oophorectomy, confirms an earlier report of a 47% reduction in this patient population (125).

Phytochemicals

Phytochemicals with potential anticancer properties span a wide range of chemical types and activities. Their presence, concentration, and bioavailibilty in any of thousands of plant species used by humans are variably and incompletely documented. Several studies have specifically examined the effects of vegetables and fruit intake on breast CA risk. These studies suggest a protective effect of vegetable intake, particularly those rich in carotenoids. Beta-carotene intake has been associated with lower breast CA risk in several studies (126–128). High dietary fiber intake has also been associated with a lower risk of breast CA (129). The multiplicity of phytochemical actions at different sites in the process of tumorogenesis complicates the investigative effort needed for the development of chemopreventive agents from this class of compounds.

Endometrial Cancer Chemoprevention

Chemoprevention strategies for EEC have been based on the observation that exposure to E2, with insufficient progestational stimulation, predisposes women to EC and its precursor lesion, atypical endometrial hyperplasia. Whereas marked obesity, the use of exogenous E2, early menarche, and diabetes have been identified as risk factors for the development of EC, only early menarche has been associated with serous carcinoma, as well as its precursor lesion, endometrial intraepithelial carcinoma (EIC) (130). This observation, as well as other investigational work, supports the existence of a dualistic model for endometrial carcinogenesis, where atypical endometrial hyperplasia and EC are E2 related and endometrial intraepithelial carcinoma (EIC) and serous carcinoma are E2 unrelated. Further delineation of E2-independent pathways of endometrial carcinogenesis will be necessary to develop chemoprevention strategies for serous carcinoma, which accounts for a minority of endometrial CAs, but a disproportionate number of endometrial CA deaths. Chemoprevention strategies for EEC, because of its clear association with E2, have been more easily identified, and are described below.

Continuous Combined Hormone Replacement Therapy

Premature termination of one comparison (continuous combined HRT: daily conjugated equine E2 0.625 mg and medroxyprogesterone acetate 2.5 mg) in the Women's Health Initiative primary prevention trial occurred because cardiovascular disease and breast CA were increased, recognizing that colorectal CA, endometrial CA, and osteoporotic fractures were reduced (131). The reduction seen in the incidence of EEC with continuous HRT is in agreement with case-control studies that have documented a reduction in the incidence of this malignancy in women taking continuous combined HRT (88,89,91).

Oral Contraceptives

There is substantial evidence that ever-use of OCs reduces the risk of EEC by approximately 50% (132). Numerous epidemiologic studies demonstrate that the reduced risk depends on the duration of OC use. The risk is reduced by 20% with 1 year of use, 40% with 2 years of use, and 60% with 4 or more years of use (133).

A preliminary analysis of the Centers for Disease Control (CDC) Cancer and Steroid Hormone (CASH) Study attempted to characterize the protective effect of specific oral contraceptive formulations on EEC risk by comparing 187

endometrial CA cases with 1,320 controls (134). The CASH Study determined that continuous OC formulations provided protective effects (RR 0.4, 95% CI 0.2 to 0.9), whereas sequential OCs did not (RR 2.1, 95% CI 0.8 to 5.8). Similarly, in the World Health Organization (WHO) Collaborative Study of Neoplasia and Steroid Contraceptives, 132 cases of EEC and 835 matched controls were evaluated to determine the protective effects of OCs on endometrial CA. Investigators found that the risk of EEC was decreased among women who had a history of combination OC use (OR 0.53, 95% CI 0.29 to 0.97) (135). In both the CASH and the initial WHO study, combination OC formulations were not categorized according to the potency of estrogen and progestin, thereby preventing an assessment of the effects on EEC risk according to the potency of the hormonal components.

In order to understand better the protective effects of combination OCs, two case-control studies have attempted to evaluate progestin and estrogen potency of OC formulations in relation to EEC risk. Following further enrollment of patients in the WHO Collaborative Study of Neoplasia and Steroid Contraceptives, investigators reported an analysis of 220 cases of EEC and 1,537 controls (136). In this study, a lower risk of EEC was observed with high–progestin potency OC formulations compared with low-progestin potency. Although the number of patients using high-potency progestin was very small in this study, the results suggested that high–progestin potency OC formulations could be more protective against EEC. A second case-control study evaluated 316 cases and 501 controls from women in the King or Pierce counties of Washington State. Among these women, the relative risk for women who had used a high–progestin potency OC (RR 0.3, 95% CI 0.1 to 0.9) was as low as the relative risk for women using a low-potency progestin (RR 0.2, 95% CI 0.1 to 0.8) (53). These results did not find a potency-dependent protective effect and suggested that the progestin potency was adequate to achieve a protective effect against endometrial CA in most combination OC formulations. The methods of classifying progestin potency were the same in both the WHO Study and the Washington State study, thereby eliminating differences in classification as a reason for the different findings from these two studies. Details regarding the specific OCs taken by case and control subjects were not reported in the Washington State study. The OC formulations used in the second WHO study contained progestins that are no longer used in OCs marketed in the United States. Extrapolation of the data from these two studies to the protective effects of contemporary OC formulations is therefore difficult. Case-control studies using OC formulations with progestins currently used in contemporary formulations are needed to resolve the controversy of progestin dosage and EEC risk.

A population-based national case-control study from Sweden indicated that the subsequent use of HRT did not modify the long-term protective effect of previous OC use (137).

Intrauterine Devices

Seven studies have reported the relationship between previous copper or nonmedicated intrauterine device (IUD) use and endometrial CA (138–144). In all but one study, previous IUD use was associated with a decreased risk of EEC. The one study in which this relationship was not validated was based on research in China, where the steel ring IUD was utilized, suggesting that this type of IUD is not protective against this malignancy (143). The landmark Cancer and Steroid Hormone Study of the CDC was one of the studies to report significant protection against EEC (138). The majority of the articles reported subgroup analyses regarding factors such as type of IUD and duration/timing of use. In general, no consistent pattern emerged from the articles to suggest that length or timing of use or type of IUD was associated with an increase or decrease in the risk of EEC (145).

The levonorgestrel-releasing IUD was investigated by Gardner and colleagues in women taking tamoxifen as adjuvant therapy for breast CA (146). This preliminary investigation, which included 122 women, randomized 64 patients to the IUD group and 58 patients to the no-IUD group. The investigators did an outpatient hysteroscopic assessment with endometrial sampling at entry and after 12 months. A uniform decidual response was seen in all women with the IUD in place. Similar histologic patterns were identified in both groups at baseline and after 12 months. A statement about the effect of this device on the incidence of EEC in women taking tamoxifen cannot be made, but warrants further prospective evaluation.

Phytochemicals

The effect of dietary phytochemical consumption on endometrial CA risk is not clearly delineated. Levi et al. found a strong negative association between beta-carotene and vitamin C intake and endometrial carcinoma among Swiss women, but no clear effect was seen in similar studies in China and the United States (147–149). Barbone et al. demonstrated a protective effect of carotene intake on endometrial CA (150). Zheng found a weak negative correlation between endometrial CA and plant food intake in the Iowa Women's Health Study (151). As is the case with breast CA, further investigative efforts are necessary to establish the role of phytochemicals in the prevention of endometrial CA.

Ovarian Cancer Chemoprevention

Whereas efforts to improve the survival of ovarian cancer patients continue to focus on the development of more effective systemic therapies, the prevention of ovarian CA is an area of increasing interest. As is the case with breast CA, assessment of prevention efforts must be analyzed by genetic predisposition. In genetically uncharacterized U.S. women,

the lifetime risk of developing ovarian CA is approximately 1.5%. *BRCA1* mutations increase the risk to 30% to 60%, whereas women who harbor a mutant *BRCA2* gene have an estimated risk of 10% to 30% (152). Precancerous lesions have not been well defined for ovarian CA, although phenotypic changes have recently been described (153). Future chemoprevention trials in ovarian CA have the potential to utilize biochemical markers of transformation, including cell cycle progression and apoptosis, as surrogate endpoint markers (154,155). Although hysterectomy alone, as well as tubal ligation, has been associated with a decreased risk of developing ovarian CA, this chapter will focus on chemoprevention.

Oral Contraceptives

The ability of OCs to reduce the risk of ovarian CA has been extensively studied, and it is estimated that there is an overall reduction in risk approximating 40% (132). The adjusted odds ratio for ever-use of OCs has consistently been shown to be between 0.6 and 0.7 (156–158). The degree of protection and the length of protection appear to be associated with the duration of OC usage. Prolonged risk reduction has been reported when OCs are used longer than 4 to 6 years, and minimal benefit has been observed if utilization is restricted to a period of 6 months to 2 years (159–162). One of the largest case-control studies to date is the CDC Cancer and Steroid Hormone Study. In this study, 546 women with ovarian CA and 4,228 control subjects from eight population-based CA registries were compared. Women with a history of OC use had a 40% reduced risk of epithelial ovarian CA (RR 0.6, 95% CI 0.5 to 0.7) when compared to women with no history of OC use. This protective effect was evident with as little as 3 months of OC use and continued for up to 15 years following discontinuation of OC use. OC-mediated risk reduction was independent of the histologic type of ovarian CA (163).

It has been estimated that more than half of all ovarian CAs in the United States could be prevented from developing by OC usage for at least 4 to 5 years (157,158,164). The protective effect of OCs appears to be consistent across races, as John et al. demonstrated a reduction in risk of 0.6 in African-American women with OC use of 6 years or more (165). The estrogen/progestin content of any particular OC and how it relates to protection against ovarian CA needs further investigation. Ness et al. demonstrated an identical risk reduction for OCs with high-estrogen/high-progesterone content when compared with low-estrogen/low-progesterone–content pills (166). Schildkraut et al., in an observational study, recently reported that low-progesterone OC formulations were associated with a significantly higher risk of ovarian CA when compared with high–progesterone potency OC formulations (167).

The lifetime risk of ovarian CA is approximately 45% in *BRCA1* carriers and 25% among *BRCA2* carriers (168). In women carrying *BRCA1* or *BRAC2* mutations, Modan and colleagues concluded that OCs did not protect against ovarian CA in Israeli Jewish women. However, Narod and colleagues showed that the use of OCs in Jewish and non-Jewish women with *BRCA* mutations was strongly protective against this malignancy, with an odds ratio of 0.44 (95% CI 0.28 to 0.68) (169,170). Important differences exist between the two studies—most notably that the controls in the Narod et al. study were all mutation carriers, whereas in the Modan et al. study, only 1.7% of the controls carried the mutation. The use of OCs as a chemopreventive agent against ovarian CA should be considered in *BRCA* carriers.

Little is known about the mechanism of the protective effect of OCs against ovarian CA, although it has been postulated that a major mechanism of OCs protection relates to a decrease in ovulatory cycles. There are data to suggest that an increased rate of apoptosis in aberrant epithelial cells secondary to the progestational component may also play an important role. Recently, Rodriguez and colleagues examined the effect on ovarian epithelium of levonorgesterol in 130 ovulatory macaque monkeys (171). They demonstrated significantly increased apoptotic cell counts in the ovarian epithelium of animals exposed to progesterone, leading to the hypothesis that progestin-induced apoptosis of the ovarian epithelium is responsible for the chemopreventive effect of OCs.

Colon Cancer Chemoprevention

Colorectal CA is the fourth most common CA and the second most common cause of CA death in the United States. In the year 2000, there were an estimated 50,400 new cases of colon CA and 16,200 cases of rectal CA diagnosed in U.S. women; approximately 24,600 and 3,900 women died from these disorders, respectively (172).

Hormone Replacement Therapy

Two recent meta-analyses have calculated an approximate one-third reduction in the risk of colon CA among current or recent users of HRT compared with about a 10% to 20% reduction among ever-users versus never-users of HRT (173, 174). Although Nanda et al. determined that rectal CA was not related to HRT usage, Grodstein et al. determined a reduction in risk for ever-users versus never-users (RR 0.81, 95% CI 0.72 to 0.92). Both meta-analyses are limited by lack of consistent and accurate reporting on type of HRT, as well as lack of control for potential confounders, such as diet, site of CA, family history, or screening. Adenomatous polyps precede colorectal CAs by a decade or more, thus any association between their presence and HRT is of obvious interest. Two case-control studies have found a protective effect of HRT on the development of adenomatous polyps (175,176). The prospective Nurses' Health Study reported a decreased risk of large adenomatous polyps for current

users (RR 0.74, 95% CI 0.55 to 0.99), whereas there was no association between small adenomatous polyps and HRT (177).

The WHI, a randomized controlled primary prevention trial in which 16,608 postmenopausal women aged 50 to 79 years with an intact uterus at baseline were recruited by 40 U.S. clinical centers in 1993 to 1998, confirmed what other observational studies have suggested: a reduction in the incidence of colorectal CA in those women taking combined estrogen and progesterone therapy. In 8,506 women prescribed estrogen and progesterone, with a placebo control group of 8,102 women, a hazard ratio of 0.63 with a nominal 95% CI of 0.43 to 0.92 was observed. Colorectal CA rates were reduced by 37% (10 vs 16 per 10,000 person-years) (131,177).

There are several hypotheses regarding a protective effect of HRT on the risk of colorectal CA, including alteration of the predominant ER isoform, as well as E2's ability to decrease production of secondary bile acids.

Oral Contraceptives

The relationship between OCs and colorectal CA has not been clearly delineated. Recently, a large case-control study was conducted in northern Italy between the years 1985 and 1992, with 709 cases of colorectal CA and 992 control subjects (178). Ever-use of OCs versus never-use through use of a multiple logistic regression was associated with a reduced risk of colorectal CA (RR 0.58, 95% CI 0.36 to 0.92). Further, there was a suggestion that duration of use (i.e., more than 2 years) was associated with increased protection. More recently, the Nurses' Health Study cohort identified 502 cases of colorectal CA among participants between 1980 and 1992 (179). Among women using OCs, use for 6 or greater years was associated with a 40% reduction in risk of colorectal CA (RR 0.60, 95% CI 0.40 to 0.89). The trend for the duration effect was statistically significant ($p = .02$). Several smaller studies, all with serious limitations in study design and/or execution, have reported varying results regarding the relationship between OCs and colorectal CA.

HORMONES AND THE TREATMENT OF HUMAN CANCERS

Whereas the role of hormones in the treatment of human malignancies has been most extensively examined in the management of breast carcinoma, the potential to exploit hormone-signaling pathways in the management of other malignancies, affecting both men and woman, is rapidly becoming a reality. As our understanding of both the molecular biology of CA and of the human genome expands, targeted therapeutics, including hormonal manipulation, will undoubtably assume a more critical role in the management of human malignancies.

Breast

Overview

When considering hormonal treatment (HT) of breast CA, it is important to distinguish between premenopausal women, in whom the primary source of estrogen is the ovaries, and postmenopausal women, in whom aromatization of androgens in the peripheral tissue is the major source of estrogen production. In premenopausal women, removal of the ovaries via surgical or radiologic ablation, or inhibition of ovarian estrogen production with a gonadotropin-releasing hormone (GnRH) analog, results in marked decrease in estrogen levels. SERMs, most notably tamoxifen, are a treatment option for both premenopausal and postmenopausal women with ER-positive disease; they reduce tumor cell proliferation by binding to and blocking the activation of ERs. In premenopausal women, treatment with tamoxifen plus ovarian ablation may provide added benefit by decreasing estrogen levels through two complementary mechanisms (180). AIs interfere with estrogen production by targeting the peripheral aromatization of androgens. Owing to the high level of ovarian estrogen in premenopausal women, AIs offer little clinical benefit in this patient population. In contrast, in postmenopausal women, in whom peripheral tissue production of estrogen is responsible for the majority of circulating estrogen, AIs are a likely choice in the selection of HT. As more than 80% of breast CA cases occur in woman over the age of 50 years, the following discussion will focus on endocrine treatments for postmenopausal women with hormonally responsive tumors.

Adjuvant Hormonal Therapy for Early-stage Breast Cancer

Tamoxifen prescribed for approximately 5 years after surgery to patients with early, ER-positive breast CA is the current standard of adjuvant therapy worldwide. The Early Breast Cancer Trialists' Collaborative Group (EBCTCG) conducted a meta-analysis to assess recurrence and mortality rates among randomized trials of women wth primary breast CA who received adjuvant tamoxifen therapy or placebo. Table 17.2 details the reduction in recurrence and mortality,

TABLE 17.2. *Hormone receptor status: effect on response rate in early-stage disease*

Receptor Status	N	Reduction in Recurrence % (95% CI)	Reduction in Mortality % (95% CI)
ER$^+$, PgR$^+$	7,000	37 ($\pm$6)	16 ($\pm$8)
ER$^+$, PgR$^-$	2,000	32 ($\pm$12)	18 ($\pm$14)
ER$^-$, PgR$^+$	602	23 ($\pm$24)	9 ($\pm$28)
ER$^-$, PgR$^-$	2,000	1 ($\pm$14)	1 ($\pm$14)

All patients were treated with tamoxifen.
Early Breast Cancer Trialists Collaborative Group. *Lancet* 1998;351:1451–1467.

stratified by ER and PR status, revealing that women with hor-mone receptor–positive tumors experience a more significant improvement in both endpoints. Conversely, women with hormone receptor–negative tumors received little, if any, benefit from HT (180). Furthermore, the EBCTCG established that hormone receptor–positive women receiving tamoxifen demonstrated a 21%, 28%, and 50% reduction in recurrence and a 14%, 18%, and 28% reduction in mortality in the treatment groups of 1 year, 2 years, and approximately 5 years, respectively, with consistent benefits across various tamoxifen dosing regimens (20 to 40 mg/d) (180). Although the efficacy of tamoxifen in the adjuvant setting has been established, the toxicity profile of this agent, including an increased risk of EEC and thromboembolic events, has prompted investigative efforts into alternative therapies.

AIs are indicated for the treatment of advanced breast CA in women in whom ovarian function has ceased due to either menopause or ablative maneuvers, including surgery, radiation, or GnRH analogs. Third-generation–specific AIs, which include anastrozole (Arimidex), letrozole (Femara), and exemestane (Aromasin), are now available in the United States and are approved for the treatment of metastatic breast CA. Only recently was anastrozole alone approved (2002) as adjuvant treatment for early breast CA. The ATAC trial included 9,366 postmenopausal women with operable, early, invasive breast CA who had completed primary treatment and were candidates for adjuvant HT. The data demonstrated superior efficacy of anastrozole when compared to tamoxifen in improving disease-free survival in postmenopausal women with hormone receptor–positive or unknown early-stage breast CA. Disease-free survival was significantly longer for patients on anastrazole alone than for those who received tamoxifen alone (HR 0.83, 95% CI 0.71 to 0.96; *p*, .013) or the combination of both (0.81, 95% CI 0.70 to 0.94; *p*, .006). The combination was not significantly different from tamoxifen alone (HR 1.02, 95% CI 0.89 to 1.18; *p*, .8) (120). The disease-free survival estimates at 3 years were 89.4%, 87.4%, and 87.2% on anastrazole, tamoxifen, and the combination, respectively. Incidence of contralateral breast cancer was significantly lower with anastrazole than with tamoxifen (odds ratio 0.42 [0.22–0.79], *p* = 0.007). After publication of the ATAC data, the American Society of Clinical Oncology (ASCO) Health Services Research Committee suggested that a 5-year course of tamoxifen remain the standard adjuvant HT pending updated data from the ATAC trial and other trials of third-generation AIs in the adjuvant setting (181). The panel further suggested that it would be reasonable for a patient to be treated with anastrazole if there was a history of cardiovascular disease or thromboembolic events or if the patient developed complications or intolerable side effects attributable to tamoxifen.

Goss et al. conducted a double-blind placebo-controlled trial evaluating the effectiveness of 5 years of letrozole in 5,187 postmenopausal women with early-stage breast CA who had completed 5 years of tamoxifen therapy (182). The estimated 4-year disease-free survival rates were 93% for the letrozole group and 87% for the control group ($p < 0.001$), suggesting that in this subset of breast cancer patients, AI therapy after tamoxifen provides a survival advantage. Further investigation into combination adjuvant therapy will be needed to confirm this survival advantage.

Hormonal Therapy for Metastatic Breast Cancer

Regression of advanced breast CA as a result of prophylactic oophorectomy in premenopausal women was first described in 1896 (183). In unselected series of premenopausal women with metastatic breast CA, a 30% to 40% response with oophorectomy has been identified, whereas in ER-positive tumors, a 50% to 60% response has been noted.

Endocrine therapy for postmenopausal women with advanced hormonally responsive breast CA is based on the observation that greater than three-fourths of these patients respond to HT, whereas only 11% of patients with hormone receptor–negative tumors show a response. Tamoxifen has been the gold standard of first-line HT for metastatic breast CA since the 1970s. Previous trials in which tamoxifen was compared with other endocrine agents including diethylstilbestrol, progestins, androgens, other antiestrogens, and first- and second-generation AIs consistently failed to show superiority of any of these agents to tamoxifen as first-line HT in hormonally responsive metastatic breast CA. These trials were underpowered, and most of them were not blinded, but their results were interpreted as suggesting that tamoxifen provided the maximal possible endocrine control of breast CA. Recently, multicenter double-blind trials of third-generation AIs as first-line therapy in metastatic postmenopausal hormonally responsive breast CA have refuted this hypothesis. Mouridsen et al. compared tamoxifen to letrozole in 907 women with a median follow-up of 18 months. Letrozole was associated with a longer time to disease progression than tamoxifen (9.4 vs 6.0 months; $p = .0001$) (184). Two trials compared tamoxifen to anastrozole, with conflicting results. Nabholtz and colleagues found that anastrozole provided longer time to disease progression compared to tamoxifen (11.1 vs 5.6 months; $p = .005$) (185). Bonnetterre et al., in a similarly designed study, failed to confirm these findings; anastrozole was as effective as tamoxifen, but not superior (186). Exemestane is presently being compared to tamoxifen, with results being unavailable at this time. In summary, letrozole is superior to tamoxifen as first-line therapy in hormonally responsive metastatic postmenopausal breast CA and anastrozole is convincingly at least as effective.

Endometrium

Hormonal Treatment of Endometrioid Endometrial Cancer

The median survival of women with advanced or recurrent endometroid endometrial cancer (EEC) is less than 1 year.

TABLE 17.3. *Endometrioid endometrial carcinoma clinical estimates*

	Grade 1	Grade 2	Grade 3	Total
Estimated new cases 2003 (SEER)	12,030	17,243	10,827	40,100
Estimated deaths 2003	2,040	2,924	1,836	6,800
% of cases with deep myometrial invasion	10%	20%	42%	22%
Extrauterine spread at diagnosis	10.40%	26.00%	59.60%	21.80%
5-year survival (all stages)	87%	75%	58%	68%

Utilizing the best chemotherapeutic regimen available, the complete response rate in those patients with advanced stage EEC is only 22%. Histologic grade is known to be a predictor of stage and survival, with grade 3, poorly differentiated CAs portending a higher risk of extrauterine disease, thus poorer survival. Estimates from the SEER data registry for 2003 for both incidence and mortality are provided in Table 17.3. Carcangiu et al. evaluated 183 patients with EEC, establishing a correlation between the International Federation of Gynecology and Obstetrics (FIGO) grade and hormone receptor expression (187). The recognized association of higher grade with lower ER/PR expression carries implications for the use of HT in advanced EEC. A majority of advanced cases of EEC are grade 3 lesions, limiting the use of HT in this patient population.

Advanced or Recurrent Endometrioid Endometrial Cancer

Progestational Agents

The use of progestational agents in women with advanced or recurrent EEC has been under investigation for several decades. Several different types of progestational agents have been investigated, including hydroxyprogesterone caproate (Delatutin), medroxyprogesterone acetate (MPA, Provera), and megestrol acetate (Megace). A majority of studies evaluating this treatment modality have included small numbers of patients with no stratification for well-recognized predictors of response. In the last decade, several studies with larger patient sample size, clearer eligibility criteria, and clearer definition of response and toxicity have evaluated the effectiveness of progestational agents in the treatment of advanced or recurrent EEC. The Gynecologic Oncology Group (GOG), in GOG protocol 48, evaluated unselected patients with advanced or recurrent EEC. An overall response rate (MPA 50 mg three times daily) of 18%

(32 complete and 26 partial responses among 331 patients with measurable disease) and median progression-free and overall survival times of 4.0 and 10.5 months, respectively, was identified (188). In another GOG protocol, 299 eligible women with advanced or recurrent EEC were randomized to receive either oral MPA 200 mg/d or oral MPA 1,000 mg/d until unacceptable toxicity or disease progression (189). Among the 145 patients receiving the low-dose regimen, there were 25 (17%) complete responses and 11 (8%) partial responses; 109 patients (75%) demonstrated no response. Among the 154 patients receiving the high-dose regimen, there were 14 (9%) complete responses and 10 (6%) partial responses; 130 patients (84%) had no response. The overall response rates (complete plus partial; 25% and 16% for low- and high-dose regimens, respectively) favored the low-dose regimen. The median progression-free survival time was 3.2 months for the low-dose regimen and 2.5 months for the high-dose regimen. There was an association, including patients receiving both dosing regimens of MPA, between response and histologic grade, with well-differentiated tumors responding more frequently than poorly differentiated lesions. The response rates were 37% (22 of 59 patients), 23% (26 of 113), and 9% (12 of 127) for those with grade 1, 2, or 3, respectively. As well, there was a noteworthy correlation between response and receptor content. The response rate was 8% (7 of 86 patients) for patients who were PR-negative and 37% (17 of 46) for patients who were PR-positive ($p < .001$). The response rate was 7% (4 of 55) for patients who were ER-negative and 26% (20 of 77) for patients who were ER-positive ($p = .005$). An association between receptor status and tumor grade was established. The median concentrations of PRs were 79.0, 18.0, and 7.2 fmol/mg cytosol protein for grades 1, 2, and 3 tumors, respectively. The median concentrations of ERs were 36, 13, and 9.9 fmol/mg cytosol protein for grades 1, 2, and 3 tumors, respectively. These associations were both statistically significant. After tumor grade was adjusted for, PR concentration remained an important predictor of survival. In summary, the overall response rate for the progestational agents in women with advanced or recurrent EEC is relatively low. However, many women with advanced or recurrent EEC present at an advanced age with significant medical co-morbidities, both of which limit cytotoxic chemotherapy as a viable option. Hormonal therapy, specifically progestational agents, remains a therapeutic alternative for this patient population, particularly in those women who can predictably expect a higher response based on grade and receptor content.

Combination Chemotherapy and Progestational Agents

Combining chemotherapy with hormonal therapy is an area of active research. Pinelli and colleagues prospectively treated 13 advanced EEC patients with carboplatinum 300 mg/mm^2 every 4 weeks for six cycles. Additionally, Megace 80 mg/day for 3 weeks followed by tamoxifen 40 mg/d for 3 weeks was prescribed. The Megace alternated with the tamoxifen every 3 weeks. A complete response was obtained in 30% of patients, a partial response in 46%, stable disease in one patient, and disease progression in two patients (190). The GOG is presently evaluating, in a prospective fashion, the role of combination cytotoxic chemotherapy and HT in the treatment of advanced or recurrent EEC.

Selective Estrogen Receptor Modulators

SERMs have been and continue to be investigated for HT of EEC. Tamoxifen was studied by the GOG in a Phase II study of patients with advanced or recurrent EEC. At a dose of 20 mg twice daily, only 10% of 68 patients demonstrated objective response, but response occurred more commonly in grades 1 and 2 tumors (23% and 14%, respectively) compared to grade 3 tumors (3%) (191). From pooled reports of eight other studies including 257 patients, 22% of patients with advanced EEC responded to tamoxifen, but the range was wide in that that it was from 0 to 53% (192). Tamoxifen appears to increase PR, making it theoretically an agent that may be synergistic with progestational therapy. In one small pilot study of 20 patients with recurrent or metastatic poorly differentiated endometrial CA, tamoxifen at 10 mg twice daily was given for 5 days followed by MPA 50 mg twice daily on days 6 to 25 (193). One patient had a complete response, and 10 patients had stable disease for greater than 8 weeks. The median duration of response for those with stable disease was 4 months. In a study comparing MA with MA plus tamoxifen, the Eastern Cooperative Group reported that response rates to MA (20%) were not different from those to the combination (19%), and concluded that the combination offered no clinical advantage (194). The GOG found a 27% response rate to sequential MA and tamoxifen (MA 160 mg/day for 3 weeks alternating with tamoxifen 40 mg/day for 3 weeks), and have included this regimen in its large Phase III study comparing systemic chemotherapy with hormonal therapy.

Other SERMs are also under investigation, including raloxifene and its metabolite, LY353381.HCl. LY353381 (arzoxifene) is a third-generation SERM. First-generation SERMs, such as tamoxifen, have mixed estrogenic agonist and antagonist activity, whereas second-generation SERMs, such as raloxifene, have more selective E2 antagonism. LY353381 is a potent E2 antagonist in mammary and uterine tissues, with enhanced bioavailability and antiestrogenic activity compared with raloxifene. The potential for LY353381 to have activity in patients with EEC prompted McKeekin and colleagues to initiate a Phase II, open-labeled study with arzoxifene at 13 centers nationwide (195). Secondary endpoints included the duration, overall survival, and assessment of the safety of the drug. Patients with measurable recurrent/advanced EC not amenable to curative therapies were eligible if either the primary tumor or recurrent tumor was ER positive and/or PR positive. If receptor status could not be determined, patients with well-differentiated or moderately differentiated EEC were also permitted. Prior use of salvage chemotherapy was not allowed; however, prior use of progestins was permitted and patients were stratified by prior exposure to progestational agents. Patients received arzoxifene 20 mg/day PO, and were treated for at least 8 weeks in the absence of disease progression or unacceptable toxicity. Thirty-four patients received treatment. Twenty-six patients were ER positive and 22 were PR negative. Nine (1 complete response + 8 partial responses) of 29 patients responded (31%, CI 25 to 51%), with a median duration of response of 13.9 months. Two additional patients had stable disease for >6 months. The median progression-free interval was 3.7 months (CI 1.9 to 6.6 months) for all 29 patients. Toxicity was minimal with no grades 3 and 4 toxic effects. The investigators concluded that arzoxifene demonstrated a high response rate, with the longest median duration of response reported in a Phase II trial of this patient population. Burke and Walker reported on two Phase I studies evaluating the safety and pharmacokinetics of single and multiple doses of arzoxifene. As well, two multi-institutional Phase II trials were completed on 100 women with metastatic or recurrent EEC treated with arzoxifene. They identified no serious adverse events in the single-dose Phase I study, the principal side effect being hot flashes in 5 of 15 healthy volunteers. In the second Phase I study, conducted in 32 women with metastatic breast cancer, 1 patient had a serious, possibly drug-related adverse reaction (pulmonary embolism). The two multiinstitutional trials demonstrated significant activity at 20 mg/day in patients with metastatic or recurrent endometrial cancer. Observed clinical response rates were 25% and 31%, with a median response duration of 19.3 and 13.9 months, respectively. Progression of the disease was stabilized in a substantial number of women. Toxicity was mild except for two cases of pulmonary embolism that might have been drug related. The researchers concluded that further investigation is warranted to verify these preliminary response rates and the clinical significance of the stable disease cases, as well as to compare clinical outcomes with those in progestin-treated women (196). The ease of administration and extremely favorable toxicity profile make this an agent warranting further evaluation. Investigation continues into the role of SERMs in the treatment of women with advanced or recurrent EC.

Aromatase Inhibitors

Anastrozole and letrozole are active, highly selective non-steroidal competitive inhibitors of the enzyme aromatase. It has been shown that significant amounts of aromatase are found in endometrial CA, with low amounts being present in the surrounding normal endometrial tissue. Rose et al. recently found in 23 patients that anastrozole (Arimidex) at 1 mg a day for 28 days has minimal activity, with only a 9% partial response rate and a progression-free interval of

1 to 6 months in women with advanced EEC (197). The National Cancer Institute of Canada is currently conducting a Phase II study evaluating letrozole, a third-generation aromatase inhibitor, in women with advanced or recurrent endometrial CA.

Antigonadotropins

Antigonadotropins, such as danazol, antagonize pituitary gonadotropin release and limit adrenal and estrogen production. Danazol has yet to be clinically tested in patients with endometrial CA. However, in vitro studies have shown it to inhibit endometrial tumor cell migration (similar to MPA) and inhibit invasive activity (not demonstrated by MPA) (198,199). The clinical effects of danazol on endometrial hyperplasia have been evaluated (200). Of 15 patients with pathologically proven hyperplasia, all were successfully converted to atrophic endometriums by day 90 of danazol 400 mg/day. Given the perceived low toxicity of danazol in comparison to conventional chemotherapy, the lack of effective agents in this disease, and a theoretical rationale for its activity in endometrial CA, a Phase II trial has been initiated by the GOG (GOG-0180).

Adjuvant Therapy for Endometrioid Endometrial Cancer

The use of progestational agents as adjuvant therapy for stages I and II EEC has been investigated by von Minckwitz and colleagues (201). They conducted a randomized trial of 388 patients with early-stage EEC who received either MPA (n = 133) or tamoxifen (n = 121) orally for 2 years or were observed only (n = 134) after surgical therapy. After 56 months of follow-up, no benefit was observed from adjuvant progestin or tamoxifen therapy after surgical treatment in early-stage EEC. However, given the low frequency of recurrence in this patient population, larger randomized studies are needed to evaluate fully the role of progestational agents as adjuvant therapy in early EEC.

Progestational Agents as Primary Therapy for Endometrioid Endometrial Cancer

Several small series have retrospectively reported on the use of progestational agents alone, not preceded by hysterectomy, in the treatment of patients with EEC, either because of the desire to maintain fertility or because of co-morbid conditions. No randomized controlled studies exists evaluating progestational agents in either clinical scenario. Montz and colleagues, in a prospective pilot study, reported on the use of the progesterone IUD in women with presumed stage IA, grade 1 EEC, who were at significant risk for perioperative morbidity (202). Twelve patients were followed for 36 months after the placement of the progesterone IUD, with endometrial biopsies every 3 months. Prior to enrollment, each patient underwent radiographic imaging in an attempt to rule out evidence of myometrial invasion, and as well underwent hysteroscopy prior to the placement of the IUD. Follow-up endometrial biopsies were negative in 7 of 11 patients at 6 months and in 6 of 8 patients at 12 months. This treatment modality warrants further investigation.

Ovary

Several investigators have established that hormone receptors are expressed in epithelial ovarian CA, and that significant alterations occur with malignant transformation (203). Rao and Slotman reviewed 45 series, including 2,508 ovarian CA patients, and reported that 67% of tumors expressed ER and 47% expressed PR (204). Recently, one investigation found that the expression of the ERs and PRs correlated with long-term survival in invasive ovarian CA; the ER⁻PR⁺ phenotype predicted a more favorable tumor biology and long-term survival (205). However, multiple studies investigating the relationship between hormone receptor status in ovarian CA and prognostic factors, including disease-free interval and survival, have not produced consistent results. The ambiguous results in studies evaluating receptor status and survival in ovarian CA patients are due to several factors, including small numbers with heterogeneous groups of patients, different receptor assay methods, and heterogeneity in the receptor content within one tumor population.

A large number of hormonal agents have been evaluated in the treatment of ovarian CA, including SERMs, E2, progestogens, androgens, AIs, and gonadotropin-releasing hormone (GnRH) agonists. Progestin therapy in patients with advanced ovarian CA has a global response rate of 8% to 15% (204,206). One of the most widely studied compounds in this clinical setting is tamoxifen. Preclinical studies have confirmed that tamoxifen inhibits ovarian cell growth *in vitro*, providing rationale for the use of this agent in the treatment of ovarian CA. Several studies have evaluated the activity of single-agent tamoxifen in the treatment of advanced ovarian CA (Table 17.4) (207–224). Perez-Garcia and Carrasco reviewed the literature evaluating single-agent tamoxifen in the treatment of patients with advanced ovarian CA, most of whom were heavily pretreated and refractory

TABLE 17.4. *Tamoxifen therapy for advanced ovarian cancer*

Study (reference)	No. of evaluable patients	Median no. of lines prior CT (%)	Dose (mg/n)	No. of patients responding (%) OR	CR	PR	SD
Hatch et al. (210)	105	1 (100)	20/12	18 (17)	10 (10)	8 (8)	40 (38)
Marth et al. (213)	65[a]	1 (24) ≥2 (74)	30–40/24	4 (6)	2 (3)	2 (3)	50 (77)
Landoni et al. (212)	55	NS	40/24	0	0	0	19 (35)
Osborne et al. (214)	51	0 (2) 1 (41) 2 (57)	20/12[b]	1 (2)	0 (0)	1 (2)	5 (9)
Gennatas et al. (208)	50	0 (50) 1–2 (50)	20/12	28 (56)	2 (4)	26 (52)	NS
Rolski et al. (217)	47	1–4	40/24	3 (6)	1 (2)	2 (4)	22 (47)
Quinn (216)	40	1	20/12	9 (23)	5 (13)	4 (10)	12 (30)
Jager et al. (211)	33	NS (≥1)	30/24	0 (0)	0 (0)	0 (0)	2 (6)
Weiner et al. (224)	31	3	10/12[b]	3 (10)	1 (3)	2 (6)	6 (19)
Van der Velden et al. (223)	16	1	20/12	2 (13)	2 (13)	0 (0)	6 (38)
	14	2 or 3	20/12	0 (0)	0 (0)	0 (0)	4 (29)
Ahlgren et al. (207)	29	1 (50) ≥2 (50)	20/12[b]	5 (17)	2 (7)	3 (10)	18 (62)
Shirey et al. (29)	23	NS(≥1)	20–40/24	0 (0)	0 (0)	0 (0)	19 (83)
Slevin et al. (221)	22	2	20/12	0 (0)	0 (0)	0 (0)	1 (5)
Pagel et al. (215)	21	NS	NS	8 (38)	1 (5)	7 (3)	12 (57)
Hamerlynck et al. (209)	18	NS	20/12	1 (6)	0 (0)	1 (6)	2 (11)
Schwartz et al. (219)	13	≥2	10/12	1 (8)	0 (0)	1 (8)	4 (31)
Rowland et al. (218)	9	1–3	20/24	0 (0)	0 (0)	0 (0)	NS
Van der Vange et al. (222)	6	2	20/12	1 (17)	0 (0)	1 (17)	1 (17)
Total	648			84 (13.0)	26 (4.0)	58 (9.0)	223 (37.9)[c]

Note, OR, overall response; CR, complete response; PR, partial response; SD, stable disease; NS, not stated; CT, chemotherapy.

[a] Only evaluable patients are included (but prior CT lines refer to the whole population).

[b] With a loading dose of 100 mg/24 h during 1 day (Osborne et al. [214], 40 mg/24 h during 7 days (Weiner et al. [224]), and 40 mg/24 h during 30 days (Ahlgren et al. [207]).

[c] Calculated over the number of patients included in trials that report these data.

to chemotherapy (225). A total of 648 patients were included with an overall response rate (ORR) of 13% (95% CI 10.4 to 15.6, range 0 to 56), including a 4% complete response rate and a 9% partial response rate. In 38% of patients, stable disease was noted. These results are not entirely dissimilar from those seen with progestins. The role of GnRH agonists in the management of refractory ovarian CA has been evaluated in multiple studies and has been summarized by Paskeviciute and colleagues (226). In this study, GnRH agonists induced an overall objective response in 8.5% of refractory ovarian CA patients with disease stabilization in 23% of these women.

Comparing chemotherapy alone to chemotherapy and hormonal therapy primarily in patients with advanced ovarian CA has been carried out by several investigators. However, these studies had small patient sample size and were not randomized controlled studies. Schwartz and colleagues evaluated cisplatinum and doxorubicin, with or without tamoxifen after initial surgery, without finding significant overall survival (OS) or progression-free survival (PFS) differences between both groups (227). Emons and colleagues randomized 135 patients with advanced ovarian CA to receive the GnRH triptorelin, or placebo, following surgery and chemotherapy, until the patient's death or termination of the trial. There were no significant differences in OS or PFS between the groups, with documented gonadotropin suppression (228). At least four randomized studies comparing chemotherapy and MPA or a GnRH versus chemotherapy alone in ovarian CA patients have been reported. These studies contain many of the same flaws as noted throughout this discussion, namely, small sample size and no stratification for optimal versus suboptimal surgical status, menopausal status, and histologic status.

Combining cytotoxic chemotherapy and tamoxifen or other hormonal agents as salvage therapy for patients with advanced ovarian CA is an area of investigation that warrants further study (229).

As previously stated, in patients with ovarian CA, receptor status does not reproducibly correlate with prognostic factors, including survival or disease-free interval. However, receptor status may be useful in predicting response to hormonal agents. Although several investigators have approached this question, results are not conclusive. The ascertainment of receptor status as a predictor of hormonal activity in ovarian CA will require a randomized clinical trial comparing hormonal activity in patients expressing hormone receptors versus those with no receptor expression, controlling for the many variables recognized as important prognosticators in ovarian CA.

Colon

The clinical data available evaluating the relationship between hormones and colon CA relate primarily to hormones as risk factors for the development of this common human malignancy. There is a plethora of data in colon CA cell lines regarding the effect of hormonal agents on cell growth, as well as cell death. To date, there are no clinical studies evaluating the treatment of colon CA, either in the adjuvant setting or otherwise, with hormonal agents.

REFERENCES

1. Evans RM. The steroid and thyroid hormone receptor superfamily. *Science* 1988;240:889–895.
2. O'Malley BW, Tsai SY, Bagchi M, et al. Molecular mechanism of action of a steroid hormone receptor. *Recent Prog Horm Res* 1991; 47:1–24; Discussion 24–26.
3. Molenda HA, Kilts CP, Allen CP, Tetel M. Nuclear receptor coactivator function in reproductive physiology and behavior. *Biol Reprod* 2003;69:1449–1457.
4. Miller WL. Molecular biology of steroid hormone synthesis. *Endocr Rev* 1988;9:295–318.
5. Channing CP, Tsafriri A. Mechanism of action of luteinizing hormone and follicle-stimulating hormone on the ovary in vitro. *Metabolism* 1977;26:413–468.
6. Simpson ER, Dowsett M. Aromatase and its inhibitors: significance for breast cancer therapy. *Recent Prog Horm Res* 2002;57:317–338.
7. Pasqualini JR, Chetrite G, Blacker C, et al. Concentrations of estrone, estradiol, and estrone sufate and evaluation of sulfatase and aromatase activities in pre- and postmenopausal breast cancer patients. *J Clin Endocrinol Metab* 1996;81:460–1464.
8. Davis SR. Minireview: aromatase and the regulation of estrogen biosynthesis—some new perspectives. *Endocrinology* 2001;142: 4589–4594.
9. Kumar V, Green S, Stack G, et al. Functional domains of the human estrogen receptor. *Cell* 1987;51:941–951.
10. Mosselman S, Polman J, Dijkema R. ER beta: identification and characterization of a novel human estrogen receptor. *FEBS Lett* 1996; 392: 49–53.
11. Barkhem T, Carlsson B, Nilsson Y, et al. Differential response of estrogen receptor alpha and estrogen receptor beta to partial estrogen agonists/antagonists. *Mol Pharmacol* 1998;54:105–112.
12. Christensen DJ, Gron H, Norris JD, et al. Estrogen receptor (ER) modulators each induce distinct conformational changes in ER alpha and ER beta. *Proc Natl Acad Sci U S A* 1999;96:3999–4004.
13. Kuiper GG, Carlsson B, Grandien K, et al. Comparison of the ligand binding specificity and transcript tissue distribution of estroen receptors alpha and beta. *Endocrinology* 2000;138:863–870.
14. Taylor AH, Al-Azzawi F. Immunolocalisation of oestrogen receptor beta in human tissues. *J Mol Endocrinol* 2000;24:145–155.
15. Pace P, Taylor J, Suntharalingam S, et al. Human estrogen receptor beta binds DNA in a manner similar to and dimerizes with estrogen receptor alpha. *J Biol Chem* 1997;272:25832–25838.
16. Hall JM, McDonell DP. The estrogen receptor beta-isoform (ERbeta) of the human estrogen receptor modulates Er alpha transcriptional activity and is a key regular of the cellular response to estrogens and antiestrogens. *Endocrinology* 1999;140:5566–5578.
17. Brandenberger AW, Tee MK, Jaffe RB. Estrogen receptor alpha (Er-alpha) and beta (ER-beta) mRNAs in normal ovary, ovarian serous cystadenocarcinoma and ovarian cancer cell lines: down-regulation of ER-beta in neoplastic tissues. *J Clin Enocrinol Metab* 1998;83: 1025–1028.
18. Foley EF, Jazaeri AA, Shupnik MA, et al. Selective loss of estrogen receptor beta in malignant human colon. *Cancer Res.* 2000;60: 245–248.
19. Jazaeri AA, Nunes KJ, Dalton MS, et al. Well-differentiated endometrial adenocarcinomas and poorly differentiated mixed mullerian tumors have altered ER and PR isoform expression. *Oncogene* 2001; 20:6965–6969.
20. Pujol P, Rey JM, Nirde P, et al. Differential expression of estrogen receptor-alpha and -beta messenger RNAs as a potential marker of ovarian carcinogenesis. *Cancer Res* 1998;58:5367–5373.
21. Hewitt S, Korach KS. Oestrogen receptor knockout mice: roles for

oestrogen receptors alpha and beta in reproductive tissues. *Reproduction* 2003;125:143–149.

22. Jazaeri O, Shupnik MA, Jazaeri AA, Rice LW. Expression of estrogen receptor alpha mRNA and protein variants in human endometrial carcinoma. *Gynecol Oncol* 1999;74:38–47.

23. Ogawa S, Inoue S, Watanabe T, et al. Molecular cloning and characterization of human estrogen receptor betacx: a potential inhibitor of estrogen action in human. *Nucleic Acids Res* 1998;26:3505–3512.

24. Zhang QX, Hilsenbeck SG, Fuqua SA, Borg A. Multiple splicing variants of the estrogen receptor are present in individual human breast tumors. *J Steroid Biochem Mol Biol* 1996;59:251–260.

25. Leygue E, Dotzlaw H, Lu B, et al. Estrogen receptor beta: mine is longer than yours? *Clin Endocrinol Metab* 1998;83:3754–3755.

26. Galien R, Garcia T. Estrogen receptor impairs interleukin-6 expression by preventing protein binding on the NF-kappaB site. *Nucleic Acids Res* 1997;25:2424–2429.

27. Paech K, Webb P, Kuiper GG, et al. Differential ligand activation of estrogen receptors ERalpha and ERbeta at API sites. *Science* 1997;277:1508–1510.

28. Ignar-Trowbridge DM, Nelson KG, Bidwell MC, et al. Coupling of dual signaling pathways: epidermal growth factor action involves the estrogen receptor. *Proc Natl Acad Sci U S A* 1992;89:4658–4662.

29. Lee AV, Weng CN, Jackson JG Yee D. Activation of estrogen receptor-mediated gene transcription by IGF-I in human breast cancer cells. *Endocrinology* 1997;152:39–47.

30. Curtis SW, Washburn T, Sewall C, et al. Physiological coupling of growth factor and steroid receptor signaling pathways: estrogen eceptor knockout mice lack estrogen-like response to epidermal growth factor. *Proc Natl Acad Sci U S A* 1996;93:12626–12630.

31. Bunone G, Briand PA, Miksicek RJ, Picard D. Activation of the unliganded estrogen receptor by EGF involves the MAP kinase pathway and direct phosphorylation. *EMBO J* 1996;15:2174–2183.

32. Migliaccio A, Castoria G, Di Domenico M, et al. Sex steroid hormones act as growth factors. *J Steroid Biochem Mol Biol* 2002;83:31–35.

33. Stephens L, Anderson K, Stokoe D, et al. Protein kinase B kinases that mediate phosphatidylinositol 3,4:5-trisphosphate-dependent activation of protein kinase B. *Science* 1998;279:710–714.

34. Delcommenne M, Tan C, Gray V, et al. Phosphoinositide-3-OH kinase-dependent regulation of glycogen synthase kinase 3 and protein kinase B/AKT by the integrin-linked kinase. *Proc Natl Acad Sci USA* 1998;95:11211–11216.

35. Datta SR, Brunet A, Greenberg ME. Cellular survival: a play in three Akts. *Genes Dev* 1999;13:2905–2927.

36. Matsushima-Nishiu M, Unoki M, Ono K, et al. Growth and gene expression profile analyses of endometrial cancer cells expressing exogenous pten. *Cancer Res* 2001;61:3741–3749.

37. Bussaglia E, del Rio E, Matias-Guiu X, Prat J. PTEN mutations in endometrial carcinomas: a molecular and clinicopathologic analysis of 38 cases. *Hum Pathol* 2000;31:312–317.

38. Yaginuma Y, Yamashita T, Ishiya T, et al. Abnormal structure and expression of PTEN/MMAC1 gene in human uterine cancers. *Mol Carcinog* 2000;27:110–116.

39. Maxwell GL, Risinger JI, Gumbs C, et al. Mutation of the PTEN tumor supressor gene in endometrial hyperplasias. *Cancer Res* 1998;58:2500–2503.

40. Mutter GL, Lin MC, Fitzgerald JT, et al. Altered PTEN expression as a diagnostic marker for the earliest endometrial precancers. *J Natl Cancer Inst* 2000;92:924–930.

41. Risinger JI, Hayes K, Maxwell GL, et al. PTEN mutation in endometrial cancers is associated with favorable clinical and pathologic characteristics. *Clin Cancer Res* 1998;4:3005–3010.

42. Mutter GL, Lin MC, Fitzgerald JT, et al. Altered PTEN expression as a diagnostic marker for the earliest endometrial precancers. *J Natl Cancer Inst* 2000;92:924–930.

43. Campbell RA, Bhat-Nakshatri P, Patel NM, et al. Phosphatidylinositol 3-kinase/AKT-mediated activation of estrogen receptor alpha: a new model for anti-estrogen resistance. *J Biol Chem* 2001;276:9817–9824.

44. Martin MB, Franke TF, Stoica GE, et al. A role for Akt in mediating the estrogenic functions of epidermal growth factor and insulin-like growth factor I. *Endocrinology* 2000;141:4503–4511.

45. Kastner P, Krust A, Turcotte B, et al. Two distinct estrogen-regulated promoters generate transcripts encoding the two functionally different human progesterone receptor forms A and B. *EMBO J* 1990;9:1603–1614.

46. Sartorius CA, Melville MY, Hovland AR, et al. A third transactivation function (AF3) of human progesterone receptors located in the unique N-terminal segment of the B-isoform. *Mol Endocrinol* 1994;8:1347–1360.

47. Graham JD, Clarke CL. Expression and transcriptional activity of progesterone receptor A and progesterone receptor B in mammalian cells. *Breast Cancer Res* 2002;4:187–190.

48. Huse B, Verca SB, Matthey P, Rusconi S. Definition of negative modulation domain in the human progesterone receptor. *Mol Endocrinol* 1998;12:1334–1342.

49. Mote PA, Balleine RL, McGowan EM, Clarke CL. Heterogeneity of progesterone receptors A and B expression in human endometrial glands and stroma. *Hum Reprod* 2002;3[15 Suppl]:48–56.

50. Conneely OM, Mulac-Jericevic B, DeMayo F, et al. Reproductive functions of progesterone receptors. *Recent Prog Horm Res* 2002;57:339–355.

51. Arnett-Mansfield RL, deFazio A, Wain GV, et al. Relative expression of progesterone receptors A and B in endometrioid cancers of the endometrium. *Cancer Res* 2001;61:4576–4582.

52. Mote PA, Bartow S, Tran N, Clarke CL. Loss of co-ordinate expression of progesterone receptors A and B is an early event in breast carcinogenesis. *Breast Cancer Res Treat* 2002;72:163–172.

53. Voigt LF, Deng Q, Weiss NS. Recency, duration, and progestin content of oral contraceptives in relation to the incidence of endometrial cancer (Washington, USA). *Cancer Causes Control* 1994; 5:227–233.

54. Bianchini F, Kaaks R, Vainio H. Overweight, obesity, and cancer risk. *Lancet Oncol* 2002;3:565–574.

55. Bergstrom A. Overweight as an avoidable cause of cancer in Europe. *Int J Cancer* 2001;91:421–430.

56. Calle EE, Rodriguez C, Walker-Thurmond K, Thun MJ. Overweight, obesity, and mortality from cancer in a prospectively studied cohort of U.S. adults. *N Engl J Med* 2003;348:1625–1638.

57. Weight control and physical activity. *IARC handbooks of cancer prevention 6.* 2002.

58. Kaaks R, Lukanova A, Kurzer MS. Obesity, endogenous hormones, and endometrial cancer risk: a synthetic review. *Cancer Epidemiol Biomarkers Prev* 2002;11:1531–1543.

59. Herbst AL. Adenocarcinoma of the vagina. Association of maternal stilbestrol therapy with tumor apearance in young women. *N Engl J Med* 1971;284:878–881.

60. Herbst AL, Cole P, Colton T, et al. Age-incidence and risk of diethylstilbestrol-related clear cell adenocarcinoma of the vagina and cervix. *Am J Obstet Gynecol* 1977;128:43–50.

61. McLachlan JA, Newbold RR, Bullock BC. Long-term effects on the female mouse genital tract associated with prenatal exposure to diethylstilbestrol. *Cancer Res* 1980;40:3988–3999.

62. Newbold RR, Bullock BC, McLachlan JA. Uterine adenocarcinoma in mice following developmental treatment with estrogens: a model for hormonal carcinogenesis. *Cancer Res* 1990;50:7677–7681.

63. Newbold RR, Banks EP, Bullock B, Jefferson WN. Uterine adenocarcinoma in mice treated neonatally with genistein. *Cancer Res* 2001; 61:4325–4328.

64. Ekbom A. Growing evidence that several human cancers may originate in utero. *Semin Cancer Biol* 1998;8:237–244.

65. Michels KB, Trichopoulos D, Robins JM , et al. Birthweight as a risk factor for breast cancer. *Lancet* 1996;348:1542–1546.

66. Kaijser M, Lichtenstein P, Granath F , et al. In utero exposures and breast cancer: a study of opposite-sexed twins. *J Natl Cancer Inst* 2001;93:60–62.

67. Collaborative Group on Hormonal Factors in Breast Cancer. Breast cancer and hormone replacement therapy: collaborative reanalysis of data from 51 epidemiological studies of 52,705 women with breast cancer and 108,411 women without breast cancer. *Lancet* 1997;350:1047–1059.

68. Schairer C. Menopausal estrogen and estrogen-progestin replacement therapy and breast cancer risk. *JAMA* 2002;283:485–491.

69. Ross RK. Effect of hormone therapy on breast cancer risk: estrogen versus estrogen plus progestin. *J Natl Cancer Inst* 2000;92:328–332.

70. Writing Group for the Women's Health Initiative Investigators. Risks and benefits of estrogen plus progestin in healthy postmenopausal

women. Principal results from the Women's Health Initiative random-ized controlled trial. *JAMA* 2002;288:321–333.

71. Eden JA. A case-control study of combined continuous estrogen-pro-gestin replacement therapy among women with a personal history of breast cancer. *Menopause* 1995;2:67–72.

72. Bluming AZ. Hormone replacement therapy in women with previ-ously treated primary breast cancer: update III (abstract 131a). *Proc Am Soc Clin Oncol* 1997;16A:463.

73. Vassilopoulou-Sellin R, Asmar L, Hortobagyi GN, et al. Estrogen replacement therapy after localized breast cancer: clinical outcome of 319 women followed prospectively. *J Clin Oncol* 1999;17:1482–1487.

74. DiSaia PJ, Brewster WR, Ziogas A, Anton-Culver H. Breast cancer survival and hormone replacement therapy: a cohort analysis. *Am J Clin Oncol* 2000;23:541–545.

75. ACOG Committee opinion: Estrogen replacement therapy in women with previously treated breast cancer. Washington, DC: American College of Obstetricians and Gynecologists, 1994.

76. Collaborative Group on Hormonal Factors in Breast Cancer. Breast cancer and hormonal contraceptives: collaborative reanalysis of indi-vidual data on 53,297 women with breast cancer and 100,239 women without breast cancer from 54 epidemiological studies. *Lancet* 1996;347:1713–1727.

77. Marchbanks PA, McDonald JA, Wilson HG, et al. Oral contraceptives and the risk of breast cancer. *N Engl J Med* 2002;346:2025–2032.

78. Grabick DM. Risk of breast cancer with oral contraceptive use in women with a family history of breast cancer. *JAMA* 2000;284:1791–1798.

79. Narod SA, Dube MP, Klijn J, et al. Oral contraceptives and the risk of breast cancer in BRCA1 and BRCA2 mutation carriers. *J Natl Cancer Inst* 2002;94:1773–1779.

80. Rodriguez C, Patel AV, Calle EE, et al. Estrogen replacement therapy and ovarian cancer mortality in a large prospective study of US women. *JAMA* 2001;285:1460–1465.

81. Lacey JV Jr., Mink PJ, Lubin JH, et al. Menopausal hormone replace-ment therapy and risk of ovarian cancer. *JAMA* 2002;288:334–341.

82. Riman T. Hormone replacement therapy and the risk of invasive epi-thelial ovarian cancer in Swedish women. *J Natl Cancer Inst* 2002;94:497–504.

83. Anderson GL, Judd HL, Klaunitz AM, et al. Effect of estrogen plus progestin on gynecologic cancers and associated diagnostic proce-dures. *JAMA* 2003;290:1739–1748.

84. Guidozzi F, Daponte A. Estrogen replacement therapy for ovarian carcinoma survivors: a randomized controlled trial. *Cancer* 1999;86:1013–1018.

85. Grady D. Hormone replacement therapy and endometrial cancer risk: a meta-analysis. *Obstet Gynecol* 1995;85:302–313.

86. Speroff L, Rowan J, Symons J, et al. The comparative effect on bone density, endometrium, and lipids of continuous hormones as replace-ment therapy (CHART study). A randomized controlled trial. *JAMA* 1996;276:1397–1403.

87. Flowers CE. Mechanisms of uterine bleeding in postmenopausal pa-tients receiving estrogen alone or with a progestin. *Obstet Gynecol* 1983;61:135–143.

88. Beresford SA, Weiss NS, Voigt LF, McKnight B. Risk of endometrial cancer in relation to use of oestrogen combined with cyclic progesta-gen therapy in postmenopausal women. *Lancet* 1997;349:458–461.

89. Hill DA, Weiss NS, Beresford SA, et al. Continuous combined hor-mone replacement therapy and risk of endometrial cancer. *Am J Obstet Gynecol* 2000;183:1456–1461.

90. Pike MC, Peters RK, Cozen W, et al. Estrogen-progestin replacement therapy and endometrial cancer. *J Natl Cancer Inst* 1997;89:1110–1116.

91. Weiderpass E, Adami HO, Baron JA, et al. Risk of endometrial cancer following estrogen replacement with and without progestins. *J Natl Cancer Inst* 1999;91:1131–1137.

92. Holinka CF, Hata H, Kuramoto H, Gurpide E. Responses to estradiol in a human endometrial adenocarcinoma cell line (Ishikawa). *J Setroid Biochem* 1986;24:85–89.

93. Farnell YZ, Ing NH. The effects of estradiol and selective estrogen receptor modulators on gene expression and messenger RNA stability in immortalized sheep endometrial stromal cells and human endome-

trial adenocarcinoma cells. *J Setroid Biochem Mol Biol* 2003;84:453–461.

94. Creasman WT, Henderson D, Hinshaw W, Clarke-Pearson DL. Estro-gen replacement therapy in the patient treated for endometrial cancer. *Obstet Gynecol* 1986;67:326–330.

95. Lee RB. Estrogen replacement therapy following treatment for stage I endometrial carcinoma. *Gynecol Oncol* 1990;67:189–191.

96. Chapman JA. Estrogen replacement in surgical stage I and II endome-trial cancer survivors. *Obstet Gynecol* 1996;175:1195–2000.

97. Suriano KA, McHale M, McLaren CE, et al. Estrogen replacement therapy in endometrial cancer patients: a matched control study. *Ob-stet Gynecol* 2001;97:555–560.

98. ACOG committee opinion. Hormone replacement therapy in women treated for endometrial cancer. Number 234, May 2000 (replaces num-ber 126, August 1993). *Int J Gynaecol Obstet* 2001;73:283–284.

99. Rutqvist LE, Johansson H, Signomklao T, et al. Adjuvant tamoxifen therapy for early stage breast cancer and second primary malignancies. Stockholm Breast Cancer Study Group. *J Natl Cancer Inst* 1995;87:645–651.

100. Fisher B, Costantino JP, Redmond CK, et al. Endometrial cancer in tamoxifen-treated breast cancer patients: findings from the National Surgical Adjuvant Breast and Bowel Project (NSABP) B-14. *J Natl Cancer Inst* 1994;86:527–537.

101. Ettinger B, Black DM, Mitlak BH, et al. Reduction of vertebral frac-ture risk in postmenopausal women with osteoporosis treated with raloxifene: results from a 3-year randomized clinical trial. Multiple Outcomes of Raloxifene Evaluation (MORE) Investigators. *JAMA* 1999;282:637–645.

102. Picariello L, Fiorelli G, Martineti V. Growth response of colon CA cell lines to selective estrogen receptor modulators. *Anticancer Res* 2003;23:2419–2424.

103. Newcomb PA, Solomon C, White E. Tamoxifen and risk of large bowel CA in women with breast CA. *Breast Cancer* 1999;53:271–277.

104. Church J, Simmang C on behalf of the Collaborative Group of the Americas on Inherited Colorectal CA and the Standards Committee of the American Society of Colon and Rectal Surgeons. Practice pa-rameters for the treatment of patients with dominantly inherited colo-rectal CA (familial adenomatous polyposis and hereditary nonpolypo-sis colorectal cancer). *Dis Colon Rectum* 2003;46:1001–1012.

105. Serpell JW, Paddle-Ledinek JE, Johnson WR. Modification of growth of desmoid tumors in tissue culture by anti-oestrogenic substances: a preliminary report. *Aust N Z J Surg* 1996;66:457–463.

106. Bus PJ, Verspaget HW, van Krieken JH. Treatment of mesenteric desmoid tumors with the antioestrogenic agent toremifene: case histo-ries and an overview of the literature. *Eur J Gastroenterol Hepatol* 1999;11:1179–1183.

107. Kadmon M, Moslein G, Buhr HJ Herfarth C. Desmoid tumors in patients with familial adenomatous polyposis (FAP). Clinical and therapeutic observations from the Heidelberg polyposis register. *Chir-urg* 1995;66:997–1005.

108. Adlercreutz H. Phyto-oestrogens and cancer. *Lancet Oncol* 2002;3:364–373.

109. Goodman MT, Wilkens LR, Hankin JH, et al. Association of soy and fiber consumption with the risk of endometrial cancer. *Am J Epidemiol* 1997;146:294–306.

110. Fisher B, Costantino JP, Wickerham DL, et al. Tamoxifen for preven-tion of breast cancer: report of the National Surgical Adjuvant Breast and Bowel Project P-1 Study. *J Natl Cancer Inst* 1998;90:1371–1388.

111. Gail MH, Brinton LA, Byar DP, et al. Projecting individualized proba-bilities of developing breast cancer for white females who are being examined annually. *J Natl Cancer Inst* 1989;81:1879–1886.

112. Veronesi U, Maisonneuve P, Costa A, et al. Prevention of breast cancer with tamoxifen: preliminary findings from the Italian random-ized trial among hysterectomised women. *Lancet* 1998;352:93–97.

113. Veronesi U, Maisonneuve P, Sacchini V, et al. Tamoxifen for breast cancer among hysterectomised women. *Lancet* 2002;359:1122–1124.

114. Powles T, Eeles R, Ashley S, et al. Interim analysis of the incidence of breast cancer in the Royal Marsden Hospital tamoxifen randomised chemoprevention trial. *Lancet* 1998;352:98–101.

115. Chlebowski RT, Col N, Winer EP, et al. American Society of Clinical Oncology technology assessment of pharmacologic interventions for breast cancer risk reduction including tamoxifen, raloxifene, and aro-matase inhibition. *J Clin Oncol* 2002;20:3328–3343.

116. Cuzick J, Powles T, Veronesi U, et al. Overview of the main outcomes in breast-cancer prevention trials. *Lancet* 2003;361:296–300.

117. Cuzick J, Forbes J, Edwards R, et al. First results from the International Breast Cancer Intervention Study (IBIS-I): a randomised prevention trial. *Lancet* 2002;360:817–824.

118. Cummings SR, Eckert S, Krueger KA, et al. The effect of raloxifene on risk of breast cancer in postmenopausal women: results from the MORE randomized trial. Multiple Outcomes of Raloxifene Evaluation. *JAMA* 1999;281:2189–2197.

119. Cauley JA, Norton L, Lippman ME, et al. Continued breast cancer risk reduction in postmenopausal women treated with raloxifene: 4-year results from the MORE trial. Multiple outcomes of raloxifene evaluation. *Breast Cancer Res Treat* 2001;65:125–134.

120. Baum M. Budzar AU, Cuzick J, et al. Anastrazole alone or in combination with tamoxifen versus tamoxifen alone for adjuvant treatment of postmenopausal women with early breast cancer: first results of the ATAC randomised trial. *Lancet* 2002;359:2131–2139.

121. Parazzini F, Braga C, La Vecchia C, et al. Hysterectomy, oophorectomy in premenopause, and risk of breast cancer. *Obstet Gynecol* 1997;90:453–456.

122. Satagopan JM, Offit K, Foulkes WD, et al. The lifetime risks of breast cancer in Ashkenazi Jewish carriers of BRAC1 and BRAC2 mutations. *Cancer Epidemiol Biomarkers Prev* 2001;10:467–473.

123. Kauff ND, Satagopan JM, Robson ME, et al. Risk-reducing salpingo-oophorectomy in women with a BRCA1 or BRCA2 mutation. *N Engl J Med* 2002;346:1609–1615.

124. Rebbeck TR, Lynch HT, Neuhausen SL, et al. Prophylactic oophorectomy in carriers of BRCA1 or BRCA2 mutations. *N Engl J Med* 2002; 346:1616–1622.

125. Rebbeck TR, Levin AM, Eisen A, et al. Breast cancer risk after bilateral prophylactic oophorectomy in BRCA1 mutation carriers. *J Natl Cancer Inst* 1999;91:1475–1479.

126. Buring JE, Hennekens CH. Beta-carotene and cancer chemoprevention. *J Cell Biochem Suppl* 1995;22:226–230.

127. Howe GR, Hirohata T, Hislop TG, et al. Dietary factors and risk of breast cancer: combined analysis of 12 case-control studies. *J Natl Cancer Inst* 1990;82:561–569.

128. Van't Veer P, Kolb CM, Verhoef P, et al. Dietary fiber, beta-carotene and breast cancer: results from a case-control study. *Int J Cancer* 1990;45:825–828.

129. Shankar S, Lanza E. Dietary fiber and cancer prevention. *Hematol Oncol Clin North Am* 1991;5:25–41.

130. Sherman M, Sturgeon S, Brinton L, et al. Endometrial cancer risk factors differ by histopathologic type. *Mod Pathol* 1995;8:97A(abst).

131. Rossouw JE, Anderson GL, Prentice RL, et al. Risks and benefits of estrogen plus progestin in healthy postmenopausal women: principal results from the Women's Health Initiative randomized controlled trial. *JAMA.* 2002;288:321–333.

132. Prentice RL, Thomas DB. On the epidemiology of oral contraceptives and disease. *Adv Cancer Res* 1987;49:285–401.

133. Schlesselman JJ. Oral contraceptives and neoplasia of the uterine corpus. *Contraception* 1991;43:557–579.

134. Oral contraceptive use and the risk of endometrial cancer. The Centers for Disease Control Cancer and Steroid Hormone Study. *JAMA* 1983; 249:1600–1604.

135. The WHO Collaborative Study of Neoplasia and Steroid Contraceptives. Depomedroxyprogesterone acetate (DMPA) and risk of endometrial cancer. *Int J Cancer* 1991;49:186–190.

136. Rosenblatt KA, Thomas DB. Hormonal content of combined oral contraceptives in relation to the reduced risk of endometrial carcinoma. The WHO Collaborative Study of Neoplasia and Steroid Contraceptives. *Int J Cancer* 1991;49:870–874.

137. Weiderpass E, Adami HO, Baron JA, et al. Use of oral contraceptives and endometrial cancer risk (Sweden). *Cancer Causes Control* 1999; 10:277–284.

138. Castellsague X, Thompson WD, Dubrow R. Intra-uterine contraception and the risk of endometrial cancer. *Int J Cancer* 1993;54: 911–916.

139. Hill DA, Weiss NS, Voigt LF, Beresford SA. Endometrial cancer in relation to intra-uterine device use. *Int J Cancer* 1997;70:278–381.

140. Parazzini F, La Vecchia C, Moroni S. Intrauterine device use and risk of endometrial cancer. *Br J Cancer* 1994;70:672–673.

141. Rosenblatt KA, Thomas DB. Intrauterine devices and endometrial cancer. *Contraception* 1996;54:329–332.

142. Salazar-Martinez E, Lazcano-Ponce EC, Lira-Lira GG, et al. Reproductive factors of ovarian and endometrial cancer risk in a high fertility population in Mexico. *Cancer Res* 1999;59:3658–3662.

143. Shu XO, Brinton LA, Zheng W, et al. A population-based case-control study of endometrial cancer in Shanghai, China. *Int J Cancer* 1991; 49:38–43.

144. Sturgeon SR, Brinton, LA Berman ML, et al. Intrauterine device use and endometrial cancer risk. *Int J Epidemiol* 1997;26:496–500.

145. Hubacher D, Grimes DA. Noncontraceptive health benefits of intrauterine devices: a systematic review. *Obstet Gynecol Surv* 2002;57: 120–128.

146. Gardner FJ, Konje JC, Abrams KR, et al. Endometrial protection from tamoxifen-stimulated changes by a levonorgestrel-releasing intrauterine system: a randomised controlled trial. *Lancet* 2000;356: 1711–1717.

147. Levi F, La Vecchia C, Gulie C, Negri E. Dietary factors and breast cancer risk in Vaud, Switzerland. *Nutr Cancer* 1993;19:327–335.

148. Potischman N, Swanson CA, Brinton LA, et al. Dietary associations in a case-control study of endometrial cancer. *Cancer Causes Control* 1993;4:239–250.

149. Shu XO, Zheng W, Potischman N, et al. A population-based case-control study of dietary factors and endometrial cancer in Shanghai, People's Republic of China. *Am J Epidemiol* 1993;137:155–165.

150. Barbone F, Austin H, Patridge EE. Diet and endometrial cancer: a case-control study. *Am J Epidemiol* 1993;137:393–403.

151. Zheng W, Kushi LH, Potter JD, et al. Dietary intake of energy and animal foods and endometrial cancer incidence. The Iowa women's health study. *Am J Epidemiol* 1995;142:388–394.

152. Shaw PA, Deavers MT, Mills GB. Clinical characteristics of genetically determined ovarian CA. In: Vogel IVG, ed. *Management of patients at high risk for breast CA.* Cambridge, MA: Blackwell Science 2001:94–107.

153. Salazar H, Godwin AK, Daly MB, et al. Microscopic benign and invasive malignant neoplasms and a cancer-prone phenotype in prophylactic oophorectomies. *J Natl Cancer Inst* 1996;88:1810–1820.

154. van Hoeven KH, Ramondetta L, Kovatich AJ, et al. Quantitative image analysis of MIB-1 reactivity in inflammatory, hyperplastic, and neoplastic endocervical lesions. *Int J Gynecol Pathol* 1997;16:15–21.

155. Williams GT, Smith CA. Molecular regulation of apoptosis: genetic controls of cell death. *Cell* 1993;74:777–779.

156. Ness RB, Grisso JA, Vergona R, et al. Oral contraceptives, other methods of contraception, and risk reduction for ovarian cancer. *Epidemiology* 2001;12:307–312.

157. Stanford JL. Oral contraceptives and neoplasia of the ovary. *Contraception* 1991;43:543–556.

158. Whittemore AS. Characteristics relating to ovarian cancer risk: collaborative analysis of 12 US case-control studies. II. Invasive epithelial ovarian cancers in white women. Collaborative Ovarian Cancer Group. *Am J Epidemiol* 1992;136:1184–1203.

159. Gross TP, Schlesselman JJ, Stadel BV, et al. The risk of epithelial ovarian cancer in short-term users of oral contraceptives. *Am J Epidemiol* 1992;136:46–53.

160. Parazzini F, La Vecchia C, Negri E, et al. Oral contraceptive use and the risk of ovarian cancer: an Italian case-control study. *Eur J Cancer* 1993;27:594–598.

161. Rosenberg L, Palmer JR, Zauber AG, et al. A case-control study of oral contraceptive use and invasive epithelial ovarian cancer. *Am J Epidemiol* 1994;139:654–661.

162. Hartge P, Whittemore AS, Itnyre J, et al. Rates and risks of ovarian cancer in subgroups of white women in the United States. The Collaborative Ovarian Cancer Group. *Obstet Gynecol* 1994;84:760–764.

163. The Cancer and Steroid Hormone Study of the Centers for Disease Control and the National Institute of Child Health and Human Development: The risk of ovarian cancer associated with oral-contraceptive use. *N Engl J Med* 1987;316:650–655.

164. Hankinson SE, Colditz GA, Hunter DJ, et al. A quantitative assessment of oral contraceptive use and risk of ovarian cancer. *Obstet Gynecol* 1992;80:708–714.

165. John EM, Colditz GA, Hunter DJ. Characteristics relating to ovarian cancer risk: collaborative analysis of seven U.S. case-control studies.

Epithelial ovarian cancer in black women. Collaborative Ovarian Cancer Group. *J Natl Cancer Inst* 1993;5:142–147.

166. Ness RB, Grisso JA, Klapper J, et al. Risk of ovarian cancer in relation to estrogen and progestin dose and use characteristics of oral contraceptives. SHARE Study Group. Steroid Hormones and Reproductions. *Am J Epidemiol* 2000;152:233–241.

167. Schildkraut JM, Calingaert B, Marchbanks PA, et al. Impact of progestin and estrogen potency in oral contraceptives on ovarian cancer risk. *J Natl Cancer Inst* 2002;94:32–38.

168. Ford D, Easton DF, Stratton M, et al. Genetic heterogeneity and penetrance analysis of the BRCA1 and BRCA2 genes in breast cancer families. *Am J Hum Genet* 1998;62:676–689.

169. Modan B, Hartge P, Hirsh-Yechezkel G, et al. Parity, oral contraceptives, and the risk of ovarian cancer among carriers and noncarriers of a BRCA1 or BRCA2 mutation. *N Engl J Med* 2001;345:235–240.

170. Narod SA, Risch H, Moslehi R, et al. Oral contraceptives and the risk of hereditary ovarian cancer. Hereditary Ovarian Cancer Clinical Study Group. *N Engl J Med* 1998;339:424–428.

171. Rodriguez GC, Grisso JA, Klapper J, et al. Effect of progestin on the ovarian epithelium of macaques: cancer prevention through apoptosis? *J Soc Gynecol Invest* 1998;5:271–276.

172. Greenlee RT, Murray T, Bolden S, Wingo PA. Cancer statistics, 2000. *CA Cancer J Clin* 2000;50:7–33.

173. Grodstein F, Newcomb PA, Stampfer MJ. Postmenopausal hormone therapy and the risk of colorectal cancer: a review and meta-analysis. *Am J Med* 1999;106:574–582.

174. Nanda K, Bastian LA, Hasselblad V, Simel DL. Hormone replacement therapy and the risk of colorectal cancer: a meta-analysis. *Obstet Gynecol* 1999;93:880–888.

175. Peipins LA, Newman B, Sandler RS. Reproductive history, use of exogenous hormones, and risk of colorectal adenomas. *Cancer Epidemiol Biomarkers Prev* 1997;6:671–675.

176. Potter JD, Bostick RM, Grandits GA, et al. Hormone replacement therapy is associated with lower risk of adenomatous polyps of the large bowel: the Minnesota Cancer Prevention Research Unit Case-Control Study. *Cancer Epidemiol Biomarkers Prev* 1996;10:779–784.

177. Grodstein F, Martinez ME, Platz EA, et al. Postmenopausal hormone use and risk for colorectal cancer and adenoma. *Ann Intern Med* 1998;128:705–712.

178. Fernandez E, La Vecchia C, D'Avanzo B, et al. Oral contraceptives, hormone replacement therapy and the risk of colorectal cancer. *Br J Cancer* 1996;73:1431–1435.

179. Martinez ME, Grodstein F, Giovannucci E, et al. A prospective study of reproductive factors, oral contraceptive use, and risk of colorectal cancer. *Cancer Epidemiol Biomarkers Prev* 1997;6:1–5.

180. Tamoxifen for early breast cancer: an overview of the randomised trials. Early Breast Cancer Trialists' Collaborative Group. *Lancet* 1998;351:1451–1467.

181. Winer EP, Hudis C, Burstein HJ, et al. American Society of Clinical Oncology technology assessment on the use of aromatase inhibitors as adjuvant therapy for women with hormone receptor-positive breast cancer: status report 2002. *J Clin Oncol* 2002;20:3317–3327.

182. Goss PE, Ingle JN, Martino S, et al. A ranomized trial of letrozole in postmenopausal women after five years of tamoxifen therapy for early-stage breast cancer. *N Engl J* 2003;349:1793–1802.

183. Beatson CT. Inoperable cases of carcinoma of the mamma. *Lancet* 1896;162–165.

184. Mouridsen H, Gershanovich M, Sun Y, et al. Superior efficacy of letrozole versus tamoxifen as first-line therapy for postmenopausal women with advanced breast cancer: results of a phase III study of the International Letrozole Breast Cancer Group. *J Clin Oncol* 2001;19:2596–2606.

185. Nabholtz JM, Buzdar A, Pollak M, et al. Anastrozole is superior to tamoxifen as first-line therapy for advanced breast cancer in postmenopausal women: results of a North American multicenter randomized trial. Armidex Study Group. *J Clin Oncol* 2000;22:3758–3767.

186. Bonneterre J, Thurlimann B, Robertson JF, et al. Anastrozole versus tamoxifen as first-line therapy for advanced breast cancer in 668 postmenopausal women: results of the Tamoxifen or Arimidex Randomized Group Efficacy and Tolerability study. *J Clin Oncol* 2000;22:3748–3757.

187. Carcangiu ML, Chambers JT, Voynick IM, et al. Immunohistochemical evaluation of estrogen and progesterone receptor content in 183 patients with endometrial carcinoma. Part I: Clinical and histologic correlations. *Am J Clin Pathol* 1990;94:247–254.

188. Thigpen JT, Blessing JA, DiSaia PJ, et al. A randomized comparison of doxorubicin alone versus doxorubicin plus cyclophosphamide in the management of advanced or recurrent endometrial carcinoma: a Gynecologic Oncology Group study. *J Clin Oncol* 1994;12:1408–1414.

189. Thigpen JT, Brady MF, Alvarez RD, et al. Oral medroxyprogesterone acetate in the treatment of advanced or recurrent endometrial carcinoma: a dose-response study by the Gynecologic Oncology Group. *J Clin Oncol* 1999;17:1736–1744.

190. Pinelli DM, Fiorica JV, Roberts WS, et al. Chemotherapy plus sequential hormonal therapy for advanced and recurrent endometrial carcinoma: a phase II study. *Gynecol Oncol* 1996;60:462–467.

191. Thigpen T, Brady MF, Homesley HD, et al. Tamoxifen in the treatment of advanced or recurrent endometrial carcinoma: a Gynecologic Oncology Group Study. *J Clin Oncol* 2001;19:364–367.

192. Moore TD, Phillips PH, Nerenstone SR, Cheson BD. Systemic treatment of advanced and recurrent endometrial carcinoma: current status and future directions. *Clin Oncol* 1991;9:1071–1088.

193. Kline RC, Freedman RS, Jones LA Atkinson EN. Treatment of recurrent or metastatic poorly differentiated adenocarcinoma of the endometrium with tamoxifen and medroxyprogesterone acetate. *Cancer Treat Rep* 1987;71:327–328.

194. Schinella RA, Yeap BY, Weiner LM, et al. Megestrol and tamoxifen in patients with advanced endometrial cancer: an Eastern Cooperative Oncology Group Study (E4882). *Am J Clin Oncol* 2001;24:43–46.

195. McMeekin DS, Gordon A, Fowler J, et al. A phase II trial of arzoxifene, a selective estrogen response modulator, in patients with recurrent or advanced endometrial cancer. *Gynecol Oncol* 2003;1:64–69.

196. Burke TW, Walker CL. Arzoxifene as therapy for endometrial cancer. *Gynecol Oncol* 2003;90:S40–S46.

197. Rose PG, Brunetto VL, VanLe L, et al. A phase II trial of anastrozole in advanced recurrent or persistent endometrial carcinoma: a Gynecologic Oncology Group study. *Gynecol Oncol* 2003;78:212–216.

198. Fujimoto J, Ichigo S, Hori M, et al. Progestins and danazol effect on cell-to-cell adhension, and E-cadherin and alpha- and beta-catenin mRNA expressions. *Steroid Biochem Mol Biol* 1996;57:275–282.

199. Ueda M, Fujii H, Yoshizawa K, et al. Effects of sex steroids and growth factors on migration and invasion of endometrial adenocarcinoma SNG-M cells in vitro. *Jpn J Cancer Res* 1996;87:524–533.

200. Soh E, Sato K. Clinical effects of danazol on endometrial hyperplasia in menopausal and postmenopausal women. *Cancer* 1990;66:983–988.

201. von Minckwitz G, Loibl S, Brunnert K, et al. Adjuvant endocrine treatment with medroxyprogesterone acetate or tamoxifen in stage I and II endometrial cancer—a multicentre, open, controlled, prospectively randomized trial. *Eur J Cancer* 2002;38:2265–2271.

202. Montz FJ, Bristow RE, Bovicelli A, et al. Intrauterine progesterone treatment of early endometrial cancer. *Am J Obstet Gynecol* 2002;186:651–657.

203. Li AJ, Baldwin RL, Karlan BY. Estrogen and progesterone receptor subtype expression in normal and malignant ovarian epithelial cell cultures. *Am J Obstet Gynecol* 2003;189:22–27.

204. Rao BR, Stolman BJ. Endocrine E role in ovarian cancer. *Cancer* 1996;3:309–326.

205. Munstedt K, Steen J, Knauf AG, et al. Steroid hormone receptors and long term survival in invasive ovarian cancer, *Cancer* 2000;89:1783–1791.

206. Schwartz PE. The role of hormonal therapy in the management of ovarian cancer. In: Gershenson DM, McQuire WP, eds. *Ovarian cancer: controversies in management.* New York: Churchill Livingstone, 1998:325–341.

207. Ahlgren JD, Ellison NM, Gottlieb RJ, et al. Hormonal palliation of chemoresistant ovarian cancer: three consecutive phase II trials of the Mid-Atlantic Oncology Program. *J Clin Oncol* 1993;11:1957–1968.

208. Gennatas C, Dardoufas C, Karvouni H, et al. Phase II trial of tamoxifen in patients with advanced epithelial ovarian cancer. *Proc Am Soc Clin Oncol* 1996;15:782.

209. Hamerlynck JV, Vermorken JB, Van der Burgh ME. Tamoxifen therapy in advanced ovarian cancer. *Proc Am Soc Clin Oncol* 1985;4:15(abst).

210. Hatch KD, Beechan JB, Blessing JA, Creasman WT. Responsiveness

of patients with advanced ovarian cancer to tamoxifen: a Gynecologic Oncology Group study. *Cancer* 1991;68:269–271.

211. Jager W, Sauerbrei W, Beck Maassen V, et al. A randomized comparison of triptorelin and tamoxifen as treatment of progressive ovarian cancer. *Anticancer Res* 1995;15:2639–2642.

212. Landoni F, Bonazzi C, Regallo M, et al. Antiestrogen as last-line treatment in epithelial ovarian cancer. *Chemioterapia* 1985;4[Suppl 2]:1059–1060.

213. Marth C, Sorheim N, Kaern J, Trope C. Tamoxifen in the treatment of recurrent ovarian carcinoma. *Int J Gynecol Cancer* 1997;7:256–261.

214. Osborne RJ, Malik ST, Slevin ML, et al. Tamoxifen in refractory ovarian cancer: the use of a loading dose schedule. *Br J Cancer* 1988; 57:115–116.

215. Pagel J, Rose C, Thorpe S, Hald I. Treatment of advanced ovarian carcinoma with tamoxifen: a phase II trial. *Proc 2nd Eur Conf Clin Oncol* 1983;42 (abstract).

216. Quinn MA. *Hormonal therapy of ovarian cancer.* London: Royal College of Obstetricians and Gynaecologists, 1987:383–393.

217. Rolski J, Pawlicki M. Evaluation of efficacy and toxicity of tamoxifen in patients with advanced chemotherapy resistant ovarian cancer. *Ginekol Pol* 1998;69:586–589.

218. Rowland K, Bonomi P, Wilbanks G, et al. Hormone receptors in ovarian cancer. *Proc Am Soc Clin Oncol* 1985;4:117(abst C-456).

219. Schwartz PE, Keating G, MacLusky N, et al. Tamoxifen therapy for advanced ovarian cancer. *Obstet Gynecol* 1982;59:583–588.

220. Shirley DR, Kavanagh JJ, Gershenson DM, et al. Tamoxifen therapy of epithelial ovarian cancer. *Obstet Gynecol* 1985;66:575–578.

221. Slevin ML, Harvey VJ, Osborne RJ, et al. A phase II study of tamoxifen in ovarian cancer. *Eur J Cancer Clin Oncol* 1986;22:309–312.

222. Van der Vange N, Greggi S, Burger C, et al. Experience with hormonal therapy in advanced epithelial ovarian cancer. *Acta Oncol* 1995;34: 813–820.

223. Van der Velden J, Gitsch G, Wain GV, et al. Tamoxifen in patients with advanced epithelial ovarian cancer. *Int J Gynecol Cancer* 1995; 5:301–305.

224. Weiner SA, Alberts DS, Surwitt EA, et al. Tamoxifen therapy in recurrent epithelial ovarian carcinoma. *Gynecol Oncol* 1987:27: 208–213.

225. Perez-Garcia JL, Carrasco EM. Tamoxifen therapy for ovarian cancer in the adjuvant and advanced settings: systematic review of the literature and implications for future research. *Gynecol Oncol* 2002;84: 201–209.

226. Paskeviciute L, Roed H, Engelholm S. No rules without exception: long-term complete remission observed in a study using a LH-RH agonist in platinum-refractory ovarian cancer. *Gynecol Oncol* 2002; 86:297–301.

227. Schwartz PE, Chambers JT, Kohorn EI, et al. Tamoxifen in combination with cytotoxic chemotherapy in advanced epithelial ovarian cancer. A prospective randomized trial. *Cancer* 1989;63:1074–1078.

228. Emons G, Ortmann O, Teichert HM, et al. Luteinizing hormone-releasing hormone agonist triptorelin in combination with cytotoxic chemotherapy in patients with adanced ovarian carcinoma. A prospective double blind randomized trial. Decapeptyl Ovarian Cancer Study Group. *Cancer* 1996;78:1452–1460.

229. Benedetti Panici P, Greggi S, Amoroso M, et al. A combination of platinum and tamoxifen in advanced ovarian cancer failing platinum-based chemotherapy: results of Phase II study. *Int J Gynecol Cancer* 2001;11:438–444.

CHAPTER 18

Innovative Twenty-first Century Therapies

Eric K. Rowinsky, Arno J. Mundt, and Nadeem R. Abu-Rustum

The convergence of a plethora of recently acquired information about specific molecular abnormalities that "drive" the malignant phenotype coupled with profound advances in biomedical technology have ushered in a new era of abundant novel systemic and radiotherapeutic options to treat patients with gynecologic malignancies. It has also brought about many challenges for clinical investigators. For example, as novel anticancer therapeutics are developed, prioritization of these therapies for efficient allotment of clinical trial resources, identification of patients whose malignancies most likely express the molecular constituents resembling the true target, and derivation of relevant endpoints for both screening and assessment will be critical to their successful incorporation into our therapeutic armamentarium (1).

In this chapter, several promising novel systemic therapeutics and advances in the delivery of radiotherapy, particularly intensity modulated radiation therapy (IMRT), which are likely to make incremental improvements in outcome and therapeutic indices for patients with gynecologic malignancies will be discussed. This chapter will not include information on agents targeting malignant angiogenesis, which are reviewed in Chapter 16.

In addition to medical and radiotherapeutic advancements, this chapter will address some of the ongoing innovations in minimally invasive surgery relating to gynecologic oncology. Laparoscopic applications in selected oncologic disorders and the surgical techniques for laparoscopic lymphadenectomy, radical hysterectomy, and radical vaginal trachelectomy will be described. The role of laparoscopic sentinel lymph node detection will be summarized, and the current status of robotically assisted minimally invasive gynecologic surgery will be addressed.

SYSTEMIC THERAPIES: ADVANCES IN THE TWENTY-FIRST CENTURY

The number of rationally designed, target-based systemic therapeutics undergoing development is unprecedented, as shown in Table 18.1. The cellular processes that are specifically being targeted for therapeutic development are those that principally confer autonomy, which is the hallmark of the malignant phenotype. Novel targets include those that are involved in aberrant signal transduction, cell cycle dysregulation, evasion of apoptosis, sustained angiogenesis, tissue invasion, metastasis, and immune tolerance (2–4). Based on the results of preclinical studies and early clinical trials to date, more selective therapeutics are likely to result in less cytotoxicity to normal tissues and, hence, more "breathing room" to maximize the therapeutic indices of multiagent regimens. Therefore, it is expected that the development of therapeutic agents that can differentiate between malignant and normal tissues will more readily achieve high therapeutic indices. However, since most new targets for antiproliferative therapies have not yet been validated in clinical practice, prioritizing the long list of rationally designed, target-based therapeutics entering clinical evaluations so that those with a high potential for improving clinical outcome are accurately identified for further study is a formidable challenge.

PROLIFERATIVE SIGNAL TRANSDUCTION ELEMENTS AS THERAPEUTIC TARGETS

The broad term *signal transduction* refers to the means by which regulatory molecules that govern the fundamental

Eric K. Rowinsky: Institute for Drug Development, Cancer Therapy and Research Center, Department of Medicine, University of Texas Health Science Center at San Antonio, Texas 78229

Arno J. Mundt: Departments of Radiation and Cellular Oncology, University of Chicago, Chicago, Illinois 60637

Nadeem R. Abu-Rustum: Minimally Invasive Surgery, Gynecology Service, Department of Surgery, Memorial Sloan–Kettering Cancer Center, New York, New York 10021

TABLE 18.1. *Common targets and therapeutics under development as anticancer approaches*

General target	Specific target	Therapeutic
Growth signal transduction	Growth-factor receptors (e.g., ErbB, insulin growth factor, c-kit)	Anti-receptor antibodies Small-molecule inhibitors of receptor tyrosine kinases Antiligand antibodies
	Ras	Small-molecule inhibitors of farnesyltransferase ASON (K-Ras, H-Ras, N-Ras)
	Raf	ASONs Small-molecule inhibitors
	MAPK	Small-molecule inhibitors
	Rapamycin-sensitive and PI 3′K/Akt pathways	Rapamycin analogs Small-molecule inhibitors against mTOR, PI 3′K, akt, p70^{s6k}
Death-survival equilibrium	Bcl-2	ASONs TRAIL agonist ligands
	TRAIL and other death receptors	TRAIL agonist antibodies
	Survival proteins	Therapeutics targeting survivin, clusterin, others
Epigenetic mechanisms	Histone deacetylation	HDAC inhibitors
	Histone methylation	Methyltransferase inhibitors and ASONs
Cell cycle control	Cyclin-dependent kinases (CDKs)	Small-molecule kinase inhibitors (e.g., flavopyridol)
	Checkpoint kinases 1 and 2	Small-molecule kinase inhibitors
Protein degradation	Heat shock protein (Hsp-90)	Geldanamycin derivatives
	Ubiquitin-proteasome degradation pathway	Proteasome inhibitors Ubiquitin ligase inhibitors

processes of cell growth, differentiation, and survival (e.g., extracellular hormones, growth factors, and cytokines, which are specialized proteins) communicate and induce responses within cells, resulting in the tight coordination of proliferative and other essential processes among various tissues. Cell signaling is extremely complex, with a wide array of components interacting through cascades of chemical signals arranged in overlapping networks (5,6). These networks, consisting of parallel tracks and intricate interconnections, enhance the robustness and diversity of signaling, and permit fine tuning, amplification, and diminution of output, which may not be accomplished as efficiently by simpler linear cascades. However, the inherent redundancy and complexity of networks also confer protection against toxins, thereby decreasing the likelihood that any therapeutic manipulation against a single element will be highly successful unless the element significantly contributes to the tumor's proliferative advantage.

Targeting aberrant and/or overactive proliferative cell-signaling elements is perhaps the most important of ongoing developmental therapeutic endeavors against cancer since aberrations in signal transduction processes have been consistently demonstrated to enhance proliferation, invasiveness, metastasis, and angiogenesis, and confer shortened survival and poor response to nonspecific cytotoxic modalities (5–7). Furthermore, the development of therapeutics against

such processes is projected to yield broadly generalizable results since most malignancies, including gynecologic cancers, possess at least one aberrant signaling element that confers a proliferative or survival advantage (5–7). The most common aberrations are those involving "loss of protein function" but others result in "gain of function" or unchecked, autonomous, or constitutive activity of elements that normally regulate cell signaling (2,5,6,8). In contrast to the situations represented by chronic myelogenous leukemia and gastrointestinal stromal-cell tumors, in which single aberrations, such as a *bcr-abl* translocation or a c-*kit* mutation, are the principal drivers of tumor proliferation and successful targeting results in profound cytoreductive effects, most malignancies possess multiple aberrations, several of which confer a proliferative advantage (2,9,10). However, targeting any one specific "driver" in a tumor that has multiple relevant aberrations may result in therapeutic efficacy, the magnitude of which relates to the importance of the driver itself and its contribution to the tumor's proliferative and/or surival advantage. Nevertheless, even if the overall efficacy achieved by targeting only one of many drivers may be somewhat limited, the innate importance of many types of signaling elements, several of which are shown in Figure 18.1, as well as the selectivity of their cognate therapeutics, may impart minimal toxicity and high therapeutic indices, rendering the agent attractive for clinical use.

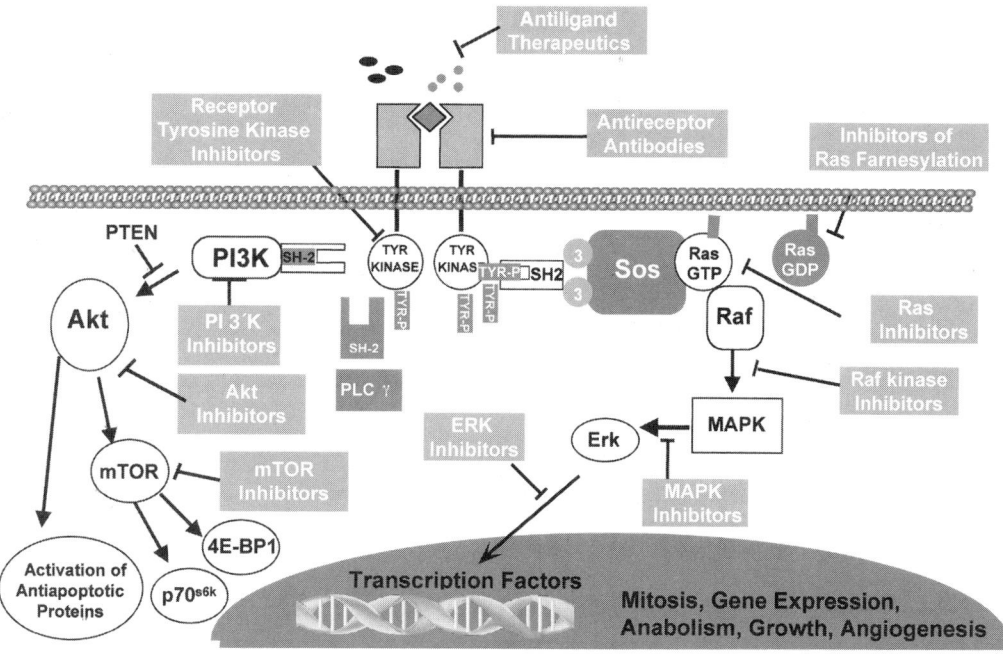

FIG. 18.1. Schematic representation of critical signal transduction pathways and pathway elements that are being targeted with therapeutic strategies consisting of small molecules, antibodies, ASONs, and other novel approaches.

Targeting the ErbB Receptor Family

Most current developmental efforts directed against signal transduction processes involve either membrane receptors or elements that comprise downstream signaling cascades. With regard to signal transduction receptors, developmental efforts are predominantly being directed against receptor tyrosine kinases (RTKs) and G-protein receptors (GPCRs), which have secondary relay systems that permit signal amplification, diversification, and cross-talk (5,6,8). The complexity of signal transduction networks and the challenges related to the development of therapeutics against these intricate systems are exemplified by the complex structural and functional aspects of the ErbB receptor family and related downstream processes, as well as the multifactoral determinants of each specific signal. The overexpression and/or constitutive activation of ErbB receptors favor cell proliferation, invasiveness, angiogenesis, and resistance to both chemotherapy and radiotherapy (3,5,6,8). Members of the ErbB receptor family include ErbB1 (also called EGFR or HER-1), ErbB2 (HER-2 or neu), ErbB3 (HER-3), and ErbB4 (HER-4), which are commonly overexpressed, overactive, or aberrant in ovarian and other epidermoid gynecologic malignancies (8–18). In addition to the extracellular domain of the ErbB that binds to growth factors and serves as a target for therapeutic antibodies, the ErbB receptor comprises a transmembrane domain and intracellular portions that consist of an RTK domain and a domain that regulates RTK activity (Fig. 18.2) (5,6,8,11,12). Ligand binding induces conformational changes in the receptor, which in turn acti-

vates the RTK, thereby facilitating dimerization with other ErbB receptors (5,6,8,10–17). Following dimerization, conformational changes result in phosphorylation or "activation" of specific tyrosine residues. Activated ErbB receptors in turn phosphorylate or activate specific downstream signaling elements, thereby transducing mitogenic and other types of signals in the cell.

The specificity and potency and, in essence, the diversity of intracellular signals are determined, in part, by the effectors of ErbB, as well as by the identity of the ligand, dimer, and specific structural determinants of the receptors. However, the principal determinant is the vast array of phosphotyrosine-binding (PTB) proteins that associate with the C-terminal "downstream docking" tail of each ErbB receptor after engagement into dimeric complexes (5,6,8, 10–17). Whether a specific site is autophosphorylated, and hence which signaling proteins are engaged, is determined by many factors, including the identity of the ligand and the specific heterodimer partner.

The diversity of signals generated through the ErbB receptor family is largely determined by the amino acid sequences of the C-terminal domains of the receptors (11–17). These critical sequences, which contain tyrosine residues that undergo phosphorylation, represent docking sites for various proteins involved in signal transduction. Docking sites are provided for proteins that recognize specific phosphotyrosine residues in the context of their surrounding amino acids. Each ErbB receptor displays a distinct pattern of C-terminal autophosphorylation sites. At least for ErbB2, which does

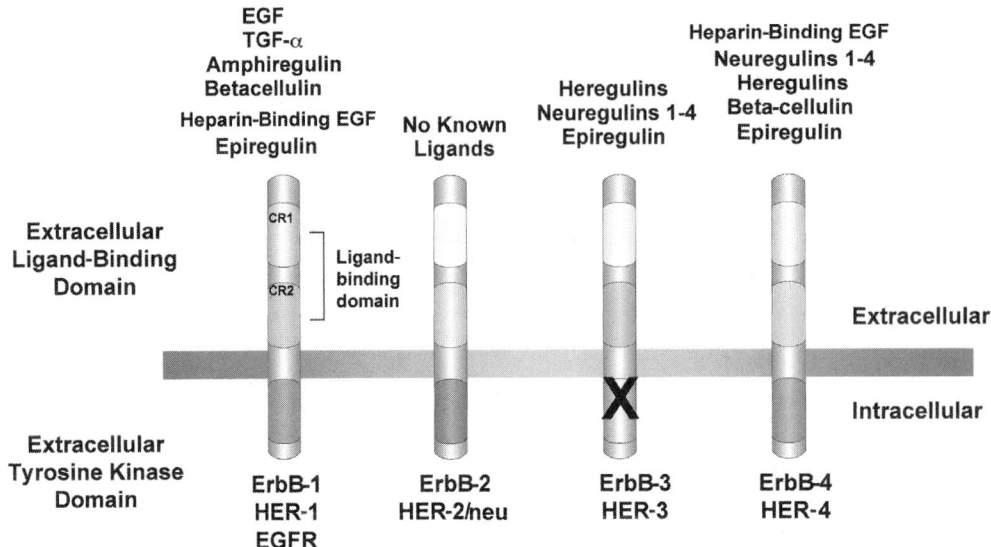

FIG. 18.2. Structure of ErbB family receptors and their cognate ligands. The receptor consists of three domains: a ligand-binding extracellular domain containing two cysteine-rich regions (CR1 and CR2), a transmembrane domain, and an intracellular domain containing a tyrosine kinase region.

not have a direct activating ligand, PTB sites are essential for the transforming properties of the receptor. It is now evident that there is a great deal of overlap in the signaling pathways activated by the four ErbB receptors. For example, the mitogen-activated protein kinase (MAPK) signaling pathway is an invariable target of all ErbB family members. There are also many examples of preferential modulation of specific pathways such as the presence of multiple binding sites for the regulatory subunit of phosphatidylinositol 3-kinase (PI 3′K) on ErbB3 and ErbB4 that render these receptors the most efficient activators of the PI 3′K "cell survival" pathway (13–15). Signals arising from the simultaneous activation of linear cascades, including the MAPK, stress-activated protein kinase cascade (SAPK), protein kinase C, and PI 3′K pathways are integrated in the nucleus into distinct transcriptional programs, the culmination of which is the net cellular response.

The principal process by which ErbB signaling is turned off is ligand-mediated receptor endocytosis, and the kinetics of this processes are often understated with regard to the overall magnitude of signaling (5,6,11,18). The kinetics of signal degradation is determined in part by the composition of the receptors. For ErbB, ligand stimulation results in rapid endocytosis and lysosomal degradation of both the receptor and ligand. ErbB1 receptors are more likely to be degraded via endosome formation and hydrolysis, whereas the other ErbB receptors are relatively endocytosis impaired and are more often recycled (5,6,18). The rapid endocytosis and degradation of the activated ErbB receptor attenuate the signal generated at the cell surface in response to growth factor stimulation. The specific mode and site of degradation are also determined in part by the composition of the dimer. For

example, ErbB1 homodimers are processed primarily to the lysosome, ErbB3 molecules are constitutively recycled, and heterodimerization with ErbB2 decreases the rate of endocytosis and increases recycling of its partners (5,6,18). ErbB2 homodimers, which are stable in the environment of the endosomal vacuole, are rapidly tagged with ubiquitin and processed for digestion, resulting in relatively weak signals, whereas ErbB2 heterodimers are unstable in the endosome, resulting in a lower rate of degradation and a higher rate of receptor recirculation. Networks also integrate heterologous signals from other networks and systems. In the case of ErbB, heterologous signals, including those induced by hormones, neurotransmitters, lymphokines, and stress inducers, are integrated into downstream messengers (6). These interactions are mediated by protein kinases that directly phosphorylate the ErbB receptors, thereby affecting their kinase activity or endocytic transport. One type of *trans*-regulatory mechanism involves the activation of GPCRs, such as those for lysophosphatidic acid, thrombin, and endothelin. Agonists of GPCRs may result in a net increase of tyrosine phosphorylation of ErbB1 and ErbB2 by increasing the intrinsic kinase activity or inhibiting the phosphatase activity of the receptor. By a poorly defined mechanism, these agonists can also activate matrix metalloproteinases, which can then cleave membrane-tethered ErbB ligands (such as heparin binding-EGF), thereby freeing them to bind to ErbBs. Activation of GPCRs may also activate Src family kinases, which leads to phosphorylation of tyrosine residues on the intracellular domains of ErbB. These activities can subsequently trigger events downstream of ErbB1, possibly contributing to the mitogenic potential of heterologous agonists. Interconnections between other signaling pathways help to integrate and coordinate cellular responses to extracellular stimuli.

The ErbB receptor family and related signaling network provide enormous signaling diversity at many levels, including ligand specificity, receptor partnering, providing scaffolding sites for effector signaling proteins and substrate specificity for their kinase activities, receptor degradation, and integration of heterologous signals (5,6,8,11–18). In addition, diversity between different types of cells and tissues can exist, depending on the expression levels and the preferred stoichiometry for interactions of the receptors and ligands. Taken together, it is clear that ErbB receptors couple to specific downstream pathways with differing efficiencies, thus affording an astonishing range of signaling possibilities. The particular cellular response to ErbB stimulation is a function of the cellular context, as well as the specific ligand and ErbB dimer. This has been shown best for mitogenic and transforming responses; homodimeric receptor combinations are less mitogenic and transforming than the corresponding heterodimeric combinations, and ErbB2-containing heterodimers are the most potent. For example, neither ErbB2 nor ErbB3 alone can be activated by ligand, and the ErbB2-ErbB3 heterodimer is the most transforming and mitogenic receptor complex.

Current Therapeutic Efforts Against the ErbB Receptor Family

Targeting ErbB2 with monoclonal antibodies [trastuzimab (Genentech Inc., South San Francisco, CA)] has resulted in impressive clinical activity, albeit limited to patients with breast cancer whose tumors have amplified ErbB2, resulting in overexpression of the target that drives tumor proliferation (6,19,20). However, trastuzimab has been associated with minimal activity in patients with advanced ovarian carcinoma, which commonly expresses ErbB2 (21). The lack of prominent activity despite receptor expression is likely due to the fact that *HER-2/neu* gene amplification, which is a prominent driver of proliferation in breast cancer, is uncommon in other malignancies. Many other therapeutics that specifically target ErbB2, such as small-molecule RTK inhibitors [TAK-165 (Takeda, Osaka, Japan), CP724,714 (Pfizer Inc., Groton, CT)] and monoclonal antibodies targeting ErbB-containing heterodimers [2C4 (Genentech)], are under development (8,22,23). Still other investigational agents bind to the extracellular domain of ErbB subfamily members including antibodies that specifically bind to ErbB1 [e.g., cetuximab (IMC-225; Imclone Systems Inc., New York, NY), EMD72000 (Merck KGaA, Darmstadt, Germany), ABX-EGF (Abgenex Inc., Freemont, CA), h-R3 (National Institute of Oncology, Havana, Cuba), MDX-447 (Medarex Inc., Annandale, NJ)] or small molecules that competitively and reversibly inhibit the TK activity of ErbB1 [e.g., gefitinib (AstraZeneca London, UK; erlotinib (OSIP Inc., Melville, NY)] or multiple ErbB receptor subfamilies [e.g., GW572016 (Glaxo SmithKline, Middlesex, UK)] that inhibit RTK of ErbB1 and ErbB2) (8,22–25).

Still other small molecules form irreversible covalent linkages with cysteine residues in the RTK domains of several types of ErbB receptors. For example, CI-1033 is an irreversible inhibitor of all four ErbB family member RTKs, and a Phase II study in patients with advanced ovarian cancer is in progress, whereas EKB-569 irreversibly inhibits the TK activity of both ErbB1 and ErbB2 (8,22–25). The relative therapeutic merits of antibodies versus small molecules, inhibitors of a single ErbB RTK versus multiple RTKs, and reversible receptor binding versus irreversible receptor binding are not known, but antibodies do result in rapid receptor internalization and degradation. In clinical evaluations in non–small-cell lung, colorectal, renal, head and neck, and ovarian carcinomas, largely in unscreened patients with regard to the target or in those patients whose tumors express ErbB1 as determined by immunohistochemistry, low rates of objective tumor regression have been observed (8,22,23). Few studies have been performed to date in gynecologic malignancies; however, epidermoid carcinomas of gynecologic origin commonly express all ErbB receptor targets, but the role of ErbB as a driver of proliferation is not known. In an early Phase II study of erlotinib in previously treated patients with ErbB-expressing ovarian carcinoma, 3 (10%) of 30 heavily pretreated subjects had major (partial) responses and 15 (50%) had stable disease as their best response (26), and clinical trials are ongoing with many of the aforementioned agents. For the most part, these nonrandomized clinical evaluations with signal transduction inhibitors were not designed to assess robustly the degree to which these agents affect several other clinically relevant endpoints, such as the rate of tumor growth, time to tumor progression, survival, and improvement in tumor-related symptoms. Other important challenges will be to discern which patients have the highest likelihood of responding to ErbB-targeted therapies based on the biologic features of their tumors and the optimal means to develop combination therapy.

Targeting the MAPK Pathway (Ras/Raf/MEK)

Following activation of membrane-bound members of the Ras family of small GPCRs, proliferative signals are relayed to downstream intracellular signaling elements along the MAPK pathway, most prominently the Raf family kinases, which in turn trigger MEK/extracellular signal–regulated kinase (ERK1/ERK2) (27–29). Likewise, Ras can directly relay survival signals via activation of the PI 3′K "cell survival" or antiapoptotic pathway (28,29). Ras activation through the MAPK pathway modulates the activity of nuclear transcription factors such as Fos, Jun, and AP-1, which regulates the transcription of genes that are required for proliferation (30–33).

MAPK is the convergence point for a broad array of signals from membrane receptors, and the network of phosphorylation-mediated signals emanating from MAPKs is equally expansive. Functional MAPK circuits are three-tiered kinase modules (30–33). The Raf-1-MEK-ERK module is employed ubiquitously in the transduction of cell type–specific growth and differentiation signals from RTKs and GPCRs. Signaling through MAPK mediates inflammatory and stress responses to stimuli such as cytokines, FasL, and tumor necrosis factor (TNF), whereas the SAPK pathway transduces these signals, and is involved with growth, differentiation, and cellular stresses induced by oxidation and DNA damage. The MAPK pathway does not function in isolation but instead it is integrated into other cellular signaling networks that impact upon MAPK signaling. Since cells are almost always receiving multiple stimuli, response outputs represent the integration of many signaling pathways, and a slight shift in signal balance can alter transcriptional profiles and influence cell cycle commitment, as well as the balance between cell survival and apoptosis. Corresponding to the prominence of MAPKs in numerous signaling events, perturbations in the MAPK signaling pathway can have profound pathologic consequences. Therapeutic efforts are currently being directed at several components of the MAPK pathway; however, the Raf-1-MEK-ERK module appears to be most relevant at this time.

Targeting Raf

Since the Raf family of signaling elements is immediately downstream of Ras, which has not been successfully targeted by inhibitors of Ras farnesylation and antisense oligonucleotides (ASONs) to date, and the first committed step in the MAPK pathway and Raf mutations are associated with proliferative and transforming properties, Raf has become an important target for therapeutic development. The Raf family is composed of three related serine/threonine protein kinases, Raf-1, A-Raf, and B-Raf, which act, in part, as downstream effectors of the Ras signaling. Raf-1 is ubiquitous, whereas B-Raf is found mainly in neural tissue, and A-Raf is most abundant in urogenital organs, including the ovary, kidney, testes, and prostate. B-Raf and A-Raf, like Raf-1, are Ras effectors, but the specificity of their activity is not well understood. Raf mutations have also been recently described, and it appears that mutated B-Raf, which has elevated kinase activity and transforming properties, occurs in 66% of malignant melanoma and at a lower frequency in a wide variety of human cancers. Furthermore, Raf may play a broader role in tumorigenesis, as it can be activated independently of Ras by protein kinase C-α and promotes the expression of the multidrug resistance gene (mdr1) (34–36). Activated Ras interacts directly with the amino-terminal regulatory domain of the Raf kinase, resulting in a cascade of reactions that include direct activation of MEK (34–36). The serine-threonine kinase, Raf-1, the best-characterized downstream effector of Ras, is activated in a number of steps, including phosphorylation, recruitment to the plasma membrane, and binding to activated Ras (30–33). Additional

steps, including interactions with other proteins, are required, although these steps are less well defined. Following activation, Raf-1, in turn, activates mitogen-activated ERK kinase (MEK) through phosphorylation of two separate serines. Raf-1 is the protein product of the c-raf proto-oncogene.

Since Raf kinase is the first committed step in the MAPK pathway, it is an attractive target for therapeutic development, and its successful inhibition may block signals from a diverse array of growth stimuli. Furthermore, there is a large body of experimental data indicating that inhibition of Raf kinase can reverse the phenotype of Ras-transformed cells and block tumor growth. Moreover, decreased tumorogenicity has been demonstrated in cell lines in which the activation of MEK, the protein that Raf normally activates, is disrupted owing to various mutations. Several types of approaches to targeting Raf, including antisense oligonucleotides and small molecules, are being evaluated. ISIS 5132 (CGP 69846A; ISIS Pharmaceuticals Inc., Carlsbad, CA) is a 20-base phosphorothioate ASON designed to hybridize to the 3′ untranslated sequences of the c-raf-1 gene (37–39). Binding of ISIS 5132 to Raf-1 mRNA promotes RNAaseH-mediated mRNA degradation and reduced Raf-1 protein synthesis in a nucleotide sequence-specific and concentration-dependent fashion. ISIS-5132 inhibits both the expression of c-Raf mRNA and the proliferation of ovarian, lung, colon, cervical, prostatic, and colon carcinoma cell lines (34,37, 38). Acute toxicities include fever; fatigue; transient, asymptomatic prolongation of activated partial thromboplastin time, and activation of alternate complement activation and have been ascribed to the phosphorothioate backbone. Disease-directed Phase II evaluations of ISIS-5132 as both a single agent and component of multiagent regimens are being performed (34,39). Another approach involves the use of small-molecule inhibitors of Raf. BAY 43–9006 (Bayer Corporation Pharmaceutical Division, West Haven, CT), a small-molecule inhibitor belonging to a class of compounds defined as bis-aryl ureas that was designed to specifically target Raf kinase, inhibits the ATP-binding site of Raf kinase and is active in growth factor receptor overexpressing and mutated K-ras–bearing cell lines (34,40,41). The importance of therapeutics that effectively target cells driven by ras mutations cannot be overstated since ras mutations occur in 30% of human malignancies and since cells with the predominant mutation, K-ras, are not effectively targeted by farnesyltransferase inhibitors owing to alternative prenylating pathways that confer drug resistance. Ras mutations drive growth signals downstream through Raf and other MAPK signaling elements. BAY 43–9006 is active in cell lines with Ras activation through mutation or through overexpression of growth factor receptors. Prominent antitumor activity in human colon, pancreatic, lung, and ovarian cell lines has been reported (34, 40,41). BAY 43–9006 has demonstrated potent growth-inhibitory activity against HCT 116 colon (mutant K-ras), MIA PaCa-2 pancreatic (mutant K-ras),

H460 non–small cell lung (mutant *K-ras*), and SKOV-3 ovarian (*wild type-ras*) carcinomas. In early clinical trials, stomatitis, vomiting, diarrhea, skin rash (erythema, folliculitis, dry skin, desquamation), and hand-foot syndrome have been reported, whereas moderate lymphopenia and anemia have been the most common hematologic toxicities (34). Antitumor activity has been noted in a wide range of tumor types in Phase I evaluations, and broad Phase II evaluations are ongoing (34).

Targeting MEK

MEK [also called MAPK kinase (MAPKK)] is a dual-specificity kinase in that it activates ERK by phosphorylating both tyrosine and threonine residues. Two related genes code for MEK1 and MEK2 (30–33). Both MEK proteins play critical roles in the Ras signaling pathways. However, MEK1 and MEK2 differ in ERK-binding affinities and, possibly, in their abilities to activate ERK. In the mitogen-activated Ras/Raf/MEK/ERK cascade, Raf usually activates the dual-specific serine threonine and tyrosine kinases MEK1 and MEK2, which then activate ERK1 and ERK2. MEK has not been identified as an oncogene product in human malignancies; however, it is a critical point of convergence that integrates input from a variety of protein kinases through Ras. In addition, Ras is very restricted in its substrate specificity, with the MAPKs being the sole known substrates of importance. Therefore, MEK is a target of great interest for the development of oncologic therapeutics. CI-1040 (Pfizer), an orally administered selective small-molecule inhibitor of MEK, significantly inhibited the growth of a variety of human cancer cell lines and xenografts (42,43). Importantly, antitumor activity, which has been related to levels of MAPK expression, has been achieved without notable toxicity. In Phase I trials, inhibition of phosphorylation of ERK, which is downstream of MEK, has been documented. Diarrhea and fatigue appear to be the principal toxicities. CI-1040 is entering Phase II trials in a number of solid malignancies.

Targeting ERK

In mammalian cells, there are two closely related genes that code for extracellular signal-regulated kinases ERK1 and ERK2. Following activation, ERKs enter the nucleus of cells where they become phosphorylated and in turn activate transcription factors, which leads to the expression of genes involved in growth and differentiation (30–33). Although no direct inhibitors of ERK are currently in clinical development, the kinase is actively being pursued as a strategic target for therapeutic development.

Signaling Through the PI 3′K/Akt/PTEN Pathway

Cellular survival is an active ''decision'' that is monitored continuously and regulated by signals that promote either survival or programmed cell death, which is termed apoptosis. These signals relay information about the availability of growth and survival factors, supply of nutrients and oxygen, cellular stress, and genomic integrity, and activate death receptors. Sufficiently positive signals enable survival and repair under conditions of limited cellular or genomic damage. Nonetheless, it is essential that irreparable DNA damage lead to apoptosis to prevent the propagation of deleterious mutations. However, a wide variety of amplified, overexpressed, and aberrant signaling elements in the PI 3′K/Akt/PTEN pathway result in unchecked proliferative, anabolic, and survival signals in many types of malignancies (44–46).

PI 3′K phosphorylates phosphoinositides, phosphoinositidites, which in turn generate 3-phosphorylated phospholipids (PI3Ps) that act as membrane tethers for proteins with pleckstrin homology (PH) regions, such as Akt and phosphoinositide-dependent kinase-1 (PDK1). Binding of Akt to membrane PI3Ps causes the translocation of Akt to the plasma membrane, bringing Akt into contact with PDK1, which is responsible for phosphorylation events that are necessary to activate Akt. Akt is the focal point for survival signals from growth and survival factor receptors (44–47). Akt, when phosphorylated or activated, inhibits apoptosis by phosphorylating many substrates, including apoptosis effectors such as FKHR, GSK-3, and caspase-9. The PI 3′Ks, Akt, and PDK1 are important in the regulation of many cellular processes including proliferation, carbohydrate metabolism, and motility, and there is emerging evidence that these kinases are important components of the molecular mechanisms of disease such as cancer, diabetes, and chronic inflammation (46,47).

The dominant survival function of Akt is suggested by the frequent and causal role of activating mutations of several components of the Akt pathway in the development of many types of cancer (44,45). Growth-factor RTKs, integrin-dependent cell adhesion, and GCPRs activate PI 3′K both directly and indirectly through adaptor molecules. The tumor-suppressor oncogene *PTEN,* which is responsible for the production of the tumor-suppressor phosphatase PTEN, is a negative regulator of Akt activation. Deletions or mutations of *PTEN* in many cancers, particularly endometrial, ovarian, and breast carcinomas and high-grade astrocytomas, allow genomically compromised cells to survive and accumulate further DNA damage, which in turn leads to neoplastic transformation (44,48). Furthermore, hyperactivity of PI 3′K or Akt, which results in the relay of survival and anabolic signals, has been described in many types of cancers (44). Additionally, persistent signaling through the PI 3′K/Akt pathway by stimulation of the insulin-like growth-factor receptor appears to be a mechanism of resistance to inhibitors of ErbB1 and ErbB2 (49,50). Therefore, this pathway is an attractive target for therapeutic development, as such agents might inhibit proliferation and reverse the repression of apoptosis and the resistance to cytotoxic therapy in cancer cells. Although many efforts are being directed at developing specific inhibitors of PI 3′K, PDK1, and Akt, these efforts have largely resulted in nonspecific kinase inhibitors. However, therapeutics directed against signaling elements downstream of PI 3′K and Akt, such as molecular target of rapamycin (mTOR) and the antiapoptotic protein Bcl-2, appear to be more fruitful and are undergoing clinical development (7).

Signaling through mTOR-Dependent and Rapamycin-Sensitive Pathways

mTOR (also called FRAP, RAFT1, and RAPT1) is a member of a recently identified family of protein kinases called phosphoinositide-3 kinase–related kinases (PIKKs), which preferentially link proliferative stimuli to cell cycle progression and nutrient utilization (7, 51,52). mTOR, which plays a critical role in the transduction of proliferative signals mediated through the PI 3′K/Akt signal transduction pathway, regulates the initiation of protein translation by altering the phosphorylation states of the translational regulator eukaryotic initiation factor 4E-binding protein (4E-BP1) and a 70-kD S6 kinase known as $p70^{s6k}$ (Fig. 18.3).

Targeting mTOR

Inhibition of mTOR function abolishes the proliferative and nutrient utilization signals mediated through the PI 3′K/

Akt signaling pathway and results in cell cycle arrest in cancer cell lines (7,51,52). Therefore, inhibition of mTOR has the potential to inhibit tumor growth, and it has become a target for the development of novel cancer therapeutics currently in early stages of development. One such agent, rapamycin, a macrolide fungicide isolated from *Streptomyces hygroscopicus,* is a specific inhibitor of mTOR that exerts potent antimicrobial, immunosuppressant, and antineoplastic actions (7,51). Because of its profound immunosuppressive actions, rapamycin was initially developed and received regulatory approval for prevention of allograft rejection following organ transplantation. However, impressive antiproliferative activity occurs following treatment of a diverse range of experimental tumors. Experimental tumors with aberrations of signaling elements that activate the PI 3′K pathway, such as *PTEN* mutations and hyperactivation of PI 3′K and Akt, are especially sensitive to inhibition of mTOR via rapamycin treatment (7,53,54).

The antiproliferative effects of rapamycin and rapamycin analogs appear to be due to their ability to bind to the intracellular immunophilin FKBP-12, and the complex then binds to and inhibits the activity of mTOR (7,51,52). The inhibition of mTOR blocks the activation of 4E-BP1, $p70^{s6k}$, and other translational modulators (Fig. 18.4), which in turn

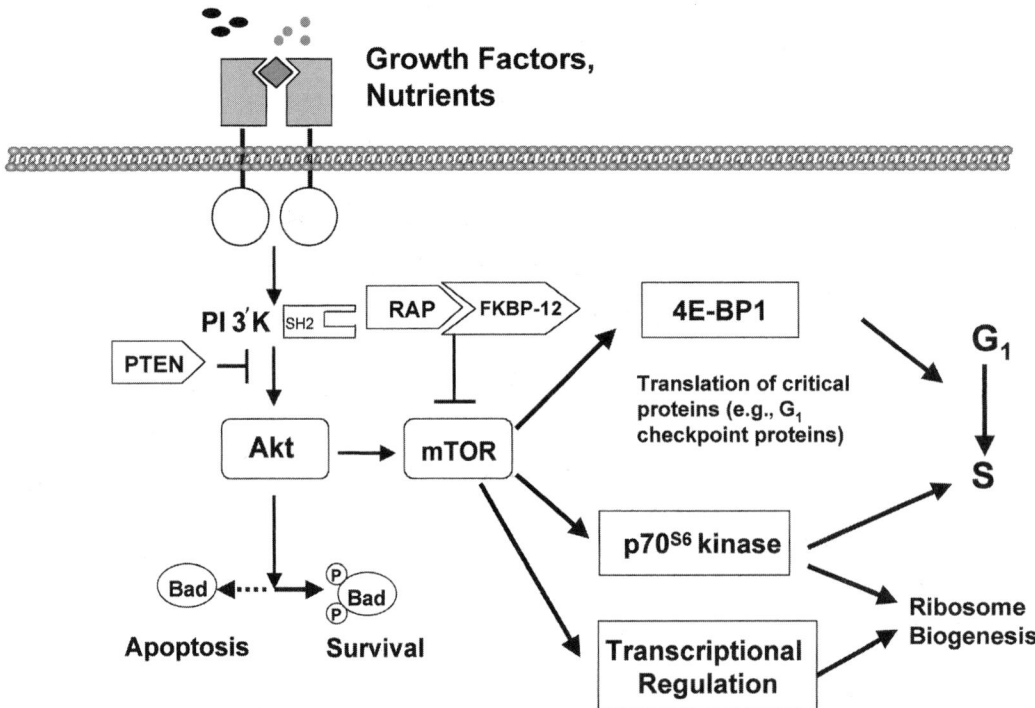

FIG. 18.3. Rapamycin-sensitive signal transduction pathway. Growth factors and nutrients induce signaling along several pathways including the PI 3′K cell survival pathway, which relay proapoptotic signals downstream, as well as growth-stimulatory signals downstream through mTOR. Rapamycin (RAP) and RAP analogs bind to the immunophilin FK506 binding protein-12 (FKBP-12). The RAP–FKBP-12 complex blocks the kinase activity of mTOR, which in turn inhibits 4E-BP1, $p70^{s6k}$, and other translational regulators. The inhibition of 4E-BP1 and $p70^{s6k}$ decreases ribosomal biosynthesis and the translational of mRNA of specific proteins essential for cell cycle progression from G_1 to S phase.

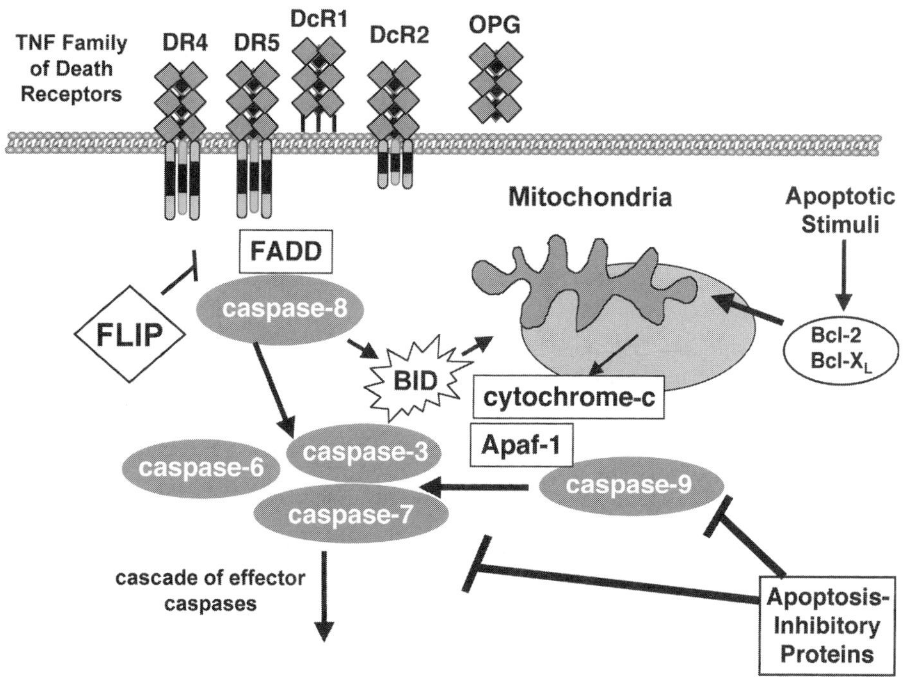

FIG. 18.4. Schematic representation of intrinsic and extrinsic pathways of apoptosis. The intrinsic pathway is mediated by Bcl-2 family members at the mitochondria that release cytochrome-c and activate the pro-apoptotic protein apoptotic protease activating factor-1 (Apaf-1) and the cascade of caspases. The extrinsic pathway is mediated by the TNF family of receptors at the cellular membrane. TNFR, tumor necrosis family receptor; DD, death domain; DED, death effector domains; FADD, Fas-associated death domain; BAX, Bax protein.

inhibits the synthesis of proteins required for cell cycle traverse from G_1 to S and ribosomal biosynthesis. However, the poor solubility and chemical stability of rapamycin preclude its administration on a variety of dose schedules, and several rapamycin analogs that are more amenable to parenteral administration, such as CCI-779 (Wyeth Ayerst, Philadelphia, PA), RAD001 (Novartis, Basel, Switzerland), and AP23573 (Ariad Pharmaceuticals, Cambridge, MA), are under development (7,55). The toxicities of CCI-779, which is the furthest along in clinical development, are similar to those caused by rapamycin (e.g., mild cytopenias, fatigue, and elevations of serum triglycerides, liver functions), and regression of several types of advanced cancers (e.g., breast, renal, and lung carcinomas and soft tissue sarcoma) has been reported. Clinical evaluations in patients with endometrial and ovarian carcinomas are ongoing.

REGULATORS OF APOPTOSIS AS ANTICANCER TARGETS

Enhancing or restoring apoptotic mechanisms to improve the effectiveness of chemotherapy, irradiation, and hormone therapy, particularly in malignancies with deficiencies in apopototic triggering mechanisms, is the objective in developing a wide range of therapeutic strategies. Rationally derived therapeutics directed at the regulation of the Bcl-2 family members that are the principal components of the intrinsic pathway of apoptosis are in late clinical trials, whereas strategies aimed at targeting the TNF receptor (TNFR) family via the extrinsic pathway of apoptosis are in earlier developmental stages.

There is a hierarchical organization to the pathways of cellular apoptosis. The final common biochemical pathway that executes apoptotic cell death requires the activation of a family of tightly regulated intracellular cysteine proteases called caspases. Caspases induce enzymatic activation of many proteins involved in apoptosis, most importantly other caspase family members, leading to a cascade of proteolysis downstream with autoactivation of other caspases. Caspase-3, caspase-6, caspase-7, caspase-8, and caspase-9 have a well-described function in cell death pathways. The downstream caspases mediate cellular destruction of "housekeeping" cellular functions through cleavage of protein kinases and other signal transduction proteins, cytoskeletal proteins, chromatin-modifying proteins, repair protein, and inhibitory subunits of endonucleases.

The activation of upstream caspases is mediated by the intrinsic and extrinsic pathways of apoptosis (Fig. 18.4). Although these pathways appear to be linked, each pathway utilizes a separate upstream caspase family member to regulate the activation of caspase-3 and other downstream caspases.

Targeting the Intrinsic Pathway of Apoptosis

The intrinsic pathway is a mitochondrial membrane–dependent pathway mediated by the Bcl-2 family of proteins (56). The *bcl-2* gene was originally identified as the chromosomal breakpoint of the translocation of a portion of chromosome 18 to 14 in follicular B-cell non-Hodgkin's lymphoma, and its protein belongs to a superfamily of apoptosis regulatory gene products, which may be death antagonists (Bcl-2,

Bcl-X$_L$, Bcl-2, Bfl-1, and Mcl-1) or death agonists (Bax, Bak, Bcl-X$_s$, Bad, Bid, Bik, Bim, and Hrk) (57). The ratio of death antagonists to agonists, as well as the interactions of these proteins, determines whether a cell will respond to an apoptotic signal. This death/life balance is mediated, at least in part, by the selective and competitive dimerization of antagonists and agonists (58). Many of the proapoptotic and antiapoptotic members of this regulatory family, such as Bax, act at the level of the outer mitochondrial membrane (56). Following mitochondrial membrane disruption, cytochrome-c and other protease activators (including caspase-2, caspase-3, and caspase-9) and apoptosis-inducing factors (apoptosis protease activating factor-1; Apaf-1) are released. Cytochrome-c, along with deoxyadenosine triphosphate, binds to and changes the conformation of the Apaf-1 complex, which results in the activation of caspase-9. The dynamic equilibrium between proapoptotic and antiapoptotic proteins determines the susceptibility of the cell to apoptotic death. Many novel therapeutic agents that perturb this dynamic equilibrium may enhance the effectiveness of chemotherapy, irradiation, and hormone therapy.

Targeting Bcl-2

Targeting the Bcl-2 antiapoptotic protein, which is over-expressed and dysfunctional in many common human malignancies, including several gynecologic cancers, along with the pivotal role of Bcl-2 in regulating apoptosis following apoptotic stimuli from anticancer therapeutics, makes Bcl-2 an attractive target for therapeutic intervention (59–61). Oblimersen sodium (G3139, Genasense; Genta, Berkeley Heights, NJ) is an 18-mer phosphorothioate AOSN directed at the first six codons of the human Bcl-2 open reading frame. ASONs hybridize to the complementary sequence present on the target mRNA, followed by RNaseH-mediated degradation of mRNA. Modifications of the phosphate backbone of the ASON, such as phosphorothioate substitutions, resist degradation and permit stability in the plasma and intracellular environment. Extensive preclinical investigations indicate that oblimersen sodium treatment leads to sequence-specific and dose-dependent degradation of Bcl-2 mRNA with subsequent inhibition of Bcl-2 protein expression *in vitro* and *in vivo* (62,63). Furthermore, several lines of evidence indicate that oblimersen sodium treatment enhances the effectiveness of other therapeutic modalities including cytotoxic therapeutics. Normal and aberrant Bcl-2 expression mediates resistance to apoptosis to a broad spectrum of chemotherapeutic agents including alkylating agents, antimetabolites, mitomycin, irinotecan, and taxanes, and Bcl-2 ASON treatment markedly enhances the antitumor effectiveness of many of a wide variety of agents, particularly the taxanes and alkylating agents (64,65). The antimicrotubule agents, including taxanes and vinca alkaloids, also lead to hyperphosphorylation of the Bcl-2 protein, decreased hetero-

dimerization with Bax, and increased apoptosis, all of which appear to be enhanced when oblimersen sodium is combined with these antimicrotubule agents (64,65).

The feasibility of administering oblimersen sodium alone or in combination with various chemotherapeutic agents is currently being evaluated. The principal toxicities of oblimersen sodium administered either as a protracted intravenous infusion or subcutaneously include hyperglycemia, transient hepatic transaminase elevations, fever, fatigue, thrombocytopenia, leukopenia, and local inflammation at the injection site. The early observations of clinical activity against lymphomas and leukemias with oblimersen sodium administered as a single agent may be due to the pivotal role that Bcl-2 expression has in the etiology of these disorders and provide ''proof of principle'' that Bcl-2 inhibition may restore apoptosis in tumors in which Bcl-2 regulation is aberrant. In many other malignancies, however, Bcl-2 expression may not be fundamental to cell survival except in the presence of external apoptotic stimuli such as chemotherapy and irradiation.

Although none is in clinical development, peptide and small-molecule inhibitors of Bcl-2-bax heterodimer fomation have been described (66,67). One small-molecule inhibitor, HA14–1, which was discovered using a computer screening strategy based on the predicted structure of the Bcl-2 protein surface, binds to a surface pocket of the Bcl-2 protein (67). Such work may ultimately lead to a series of small-molecule therapeutics that replace Bcl-2 antisense strategies. Several agents targeting other components of the intrinsic pathway of apoptosis are in preclinical development. These include AOSNs directed at Bcl-X$_L$ and anti-apoptotic regulatory proteins such as clusterin, survivin, and TRPM-2 and other therapies directed at enhancing the expression of the antiapoptotic protein Bax, including inhibition of the proteosome and/or ubiquitin pathway and Bax gene transfection (68–71) (see section on Targeting Regulators of Protein Trafficking below).

Targeting the Extrinsic Pathway of Apoptosis

The extrinsic pathway of apoptosis refers to the activation of caspase-8 as a result of apoptosis, inducing ligands that bind to the TNFR family. The TNFR protein complex includes the receptors TNFR1, Fas (Apo1), DR3 (Apo2), DR4 [TNF-related apoptosis-inducing ligand (TRAIL) R1], DR5 (TRAILR2), or DR6 bundled with an intracytoplasmic death domain protein and critical adaptor proteins (72). Critical adaptor proteins, particularly TRADD or FADD (TNF-α or Fas-associated death domain protein, respectively), mediate intracytoplasmic signals from the receptor using death domain proteins to interact with the receptor and death effector domains to interact with procaspase-8 (73–75). The proteins engage proteases and cleave the N-terminal of caspase-8, thereby activating the caspase cascade.

Targeting TRAIL Receptors

There are several homeostatic mechanisms for the regulation of cell death in the extrinsic pathway. Decoy receptors for Fas ligands and TRAIL (TRAIL R3/DcR1 and TRAIL R-4/DcR2) compete for ligand and modulate apoptotic signals. Moreover, several intracellular proteins interact with death domain proteins to inhibit the signal transduction of apoptosis and include the protein silencer of death domains and FAP1, which may represent a mechanism of resistance to Fas-inducing apoptosis (76). In addition, members of the death-effect domain family (e.g., FLIP) compete with pro-caspase-8 for the binding with FADD and inhibit apoptosis (72). Dysregulation of these mediators may lead to malignant transformation. Mutations or deletions in the FAS gene have been found in cells from patients with many types of malignancies. It is likely that the intrinsic and extrinsic apoptotic pathways are linked at many critical juncture points. For example, abrogation of TRAIL-mediated apoptosis occurs in some cancer cell lines secondary to overexpression of Bcl-2 family proteins, whereas TNF-α–mediated expression of nuclear factor-κB (NF-κB) activates several Bcl-2 family genes that have antiapoptotic functions (77,78).

TNF, which has the potential to induce apoptosis in tumor cells and mediates inflammatory processes, is the prototypic ligand for the TNFR family (79). TNF-α and Fas ligands are not candidates for drug therapy owing to their nonspecific activation of multiple TNFRs and their causality of septic shock and fulminant hepatic failure in animals (80). In contrast, recombinant soluble human TRAIL is a candidate for clinical development based on the potential to induce apoptosis in a broad spectrum of human cancer cell lines, but not in normal cells *in vitro* (81–83). Moreover, antitumor activity without toxicity has been observed in xenograft models. The selectivity of TRAIL in mediating apoptosis in tumor cells and not normal cells has not been elucidated, but the overexpression of death receptors and/or a relative absence of decoy receptors in tumor cells have been proposed as explanations. However, preclinical studies demonstrating apoptosis in human hepatic cells *in vitro* raised concerns about clinical evaluations. Recent evidence indicates that different versions of recombinant soluble human TRAIL may exhibit a different propensity for hepatocytic toxicity. Recombinant soluble human TRAIL is undergoing late-stage preclinical and toxicologic evaluations prior to entry into the clinic (84).

Monoclonal antibodies with agonist-like properties at the DR4 and DR5 sites may represent alternate strategies for the induction of apoptosis via the extrinsic pathway. Following antibody-antigen complex formation, caspase activation and apoptosis induction occur, resulting in tumor regression in several xenograft models (85,86). The affinity for DR4 binding appears to be less important for agonist activity than the specific binding site on the receptor (85). This implies that the specific agonist site exists within the receptor, and suggests that widely divergent results may be obtained with different antibodies directed to the same target DR4 (85). Clinical investigations of humanized antibodies directed against DR4 have begun.

TARGETING REGULATORS OF PROTEIN TRAFFICKING

Targeting the Heat Shock Protein Complex

Since the structure and function of proteins are highly dependent on the maintenance of their precise three-dimensional structure, targeting chaperone proteins, which are responsible for protein folding, is a logical therapeutic strategy against cancer (87,88). Geldanamycin analogs target the ATP-binding site of the heat shock protein 90 (Hsp-90), an abundant and highly conserved chaperone protein that plays an important role in the generation, regulation, and degradation of signaling elements and other critical proteins. Proteins that are folded by Hsp-90 include the cyclin-dependent kinases (CDK4 and CDK6), focal adhesion kinases that are involved in integrin signaling, components of the MAPK and PI 3′K pathways, raf-1, 3-phosphoinositide-dependent kinase-1, and the proangiogenic hypoxia-inducible factor HIF-1α. The first Hsp-90 inhibitor to enter clinical trials, 17-(allylamino)-17-demethoxygeldanamycin (17AAG), is a less toxic derivative of geldanamycin, whose development was terminated because of unacceptable hepatotoxicity (89).

Targeting the Ubiquitin-Proteasome Protein Degradation Pathway

The principal mechanism that is responsible for intracellular protein degradation is the ubiquitin-proteasome pathway (91,92). This pathway "tags" protein substrates with poly-ubiquitin chains, marking them for degradation to peptides and free ubiquitin. It is modulated by a proteasome, which is a large multimeric protease that is found in all eukaryotic cells. Many important proteins, such as the cyclins, cyclin-dependent kinase inhibitors, and transcription factors (e.g., NF-κB) are tagged by the ubiquitin-proteasome pathway, and therefore it plays a critical role in neoplastic growth and metastasis. Inhibiting the proteosome perturbs the cyclic degradation of these critical proteins, resulting in the accumulation of cyclin-dependent kinase inhibitors and ultimately cell cycle arrest and apoptosis. Several inhibitors of the proteasome pathway have recently been identified, including dipeptide boronate derivatives (93,94). Bortezomib (formerly known as PS-341; Velcade, Millennium Pharmaceuticals, Cambridge, MA), a peptidyl boronic acid and highly selective inhibitor of the chymotryptic site within the 20S proteasome, has recently received regulatory approval for treating patients with drug-refractory multiple myeloma (93,94). Bortezomib is a cell-permeable molecule that reversibly inhibits the proteasome and blocks cell division in the G_2/M phase of the cell cycle, leading to cytotoxicity via apoptosis. The agent also inhibits the degradation of wild-type p53 and stabilizes p21, which induces G_1 arrest by inhibiting cyclin D-dependent, E-dependent, and A-dependent kinases and activating NF-κB. In preclinical studies, bortezomib has demonstrated broad anticancer activity, with toxicity being related to the degree of proteasomal inhibition. These studies predicted that severe toxicity would occur when proteasomal activity is inhibited by at least 70% to 80%, and therefore the achievement of this magnitude of proteasomal inhibition is an objective in clinical trials. Broad clinical evaluations of bortezomib in patients with gynecologic and other solid malignancies are ongoing. Based on impressive activity in preclinical studies when bortezomib is combined with a wide variety of cytotoxic agents, clinical evaluations of relevant combination regimens are also being performed.

TARGETING EPIGENETIC DNA MODIFICATIONS

Targeting processes that result in posttranslational or epigenetic modifications in histone proteins associated with DNA is a strategic approach to novel therapeutic development (95,96). To date, therapeutic targeting focuses on covalent modifications made in the amino-terminal tails of histones, which package eukaryotic DNA into units that are folded into chromatin fibers. Highly conserved histone proteins (H1, H2A, H2B, H3, and H4) and the nucleosomes they form with DNA are the basic blocks of eurkaryotic chromatin, the organization of which determines the expression of any particular gene (96–98).

Nucleosomes form the basic repeating unit of chromatin and consist of DNA wrapped around a histone octomer that is in turn formed by four histone partners: an H3-H4 tetramer and two H2A-H2B dimers. Extending out from the nucleo-some are the charged amino-terminal tails of the histones. The tail of histone H4 appears to extend into the adjacent nucleosome to interact with the H2A-H2B complex, indicating that the histone tails might regulate higher order chromatin structure. Indeed, the amino acid histone tail domains are targets for various posttranslational modifications, including acetylation, methylation, phosphorylation ADP-ribosylation, and ubiquitination (Fig. 18.5). How the code is established and maintained remains to be determined, but many modification sites are close enough to each other that modification of a histone tail by one enzyme might influence the rate and efficiency at which subsequent enzymes use the newly modified tails as substrates. In essence, interfering with these modifications modulates histone-associated proteins and gene expression. Covalent modifications of core histone tails by histone acetyltransferases (HATs), histone methyltransferases (HMTs), kinases, and especially histone deacetylases (HDACs) regulate gene expression (95,96).

Targeting Histone Deacetylases

HATs catalyze the acetylation of the ε-NH2 group on lysine residues with histone tails leading to transcriptional activation, whereas HDACs function in opposition by deacetylating lysine residues and inducing transcriptional repression through chromatin condensation (96,97). Transcriptional aberrations may be among the leading contributors to the conference of the neoplastic phenotype, which is the case in acute promyelocytic leukemia, in which aberrant transcriptional repression mediated by HDACs is a common mechanism utilized by oncoproteins. Alterations in chromatin structure can impact on normal cell differentiation and lead to malignant tumor formation. Furthermore, the fact that HDAC inhibitors are active against a wide variety of cancers *in vitro* and in xenograft models, and that defects

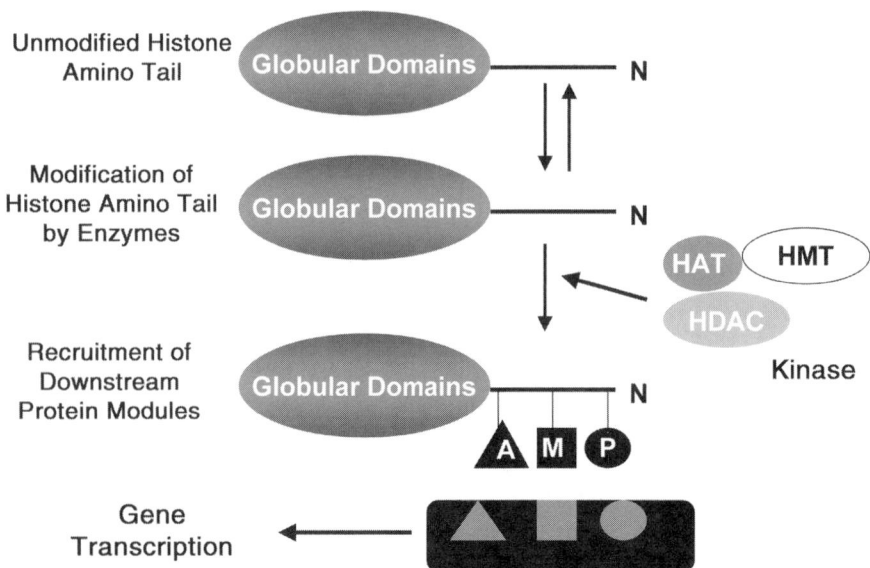

FIG. 18.5. Covalent posttranslational modifications on the histone amino tail domain. Pictured are the enzymes HAT, HDAC, HMT, and kinases that covalent modify histones. HAT, histone acetyltransferase; HDAC, histone deaceyltransferase; HMT, histone methyltransferase; A, acetyl group; M, methyl group; P, phosphate.

in the acetylation machinery occur in most epithelial and hematologic malignancies, suggests that the pharmacologic inhibition of HDAC may have broad therapeutic ramifications. In preclinical investigations, many structurally diverse compounds have been shown to bind to HDAC; promote histone acetylation; induce cell cycle arrest, differentiation, or apoptosis; and possess prominent antitumor activity. HDAC inhibitors that are under development as anticancer therapeutics include (a) short-chain fatty acids (e.g., butyrates); (b) hydroxamic acids [e.g., trichostatin A, suberoylanilide hydroxamic acid (SAHA; Aton Pharmaceutics, New York, NY), oxamflatin, LAH-824, and LBH-589 (Novartis)]; (c) benzamides (e.g., MS-275); and (d) cyclic peptides (e.g., depsipeptide, trapoxin A, apicidin). The early results of Phase I studies, particularly of hydroxamic acid derivatives, have demonstrated antitumor activity and clinical benefit at doses below the MTD.

At a more fundamental level, it will be important to gain an understanding of the nature of the molecular basis of the selectivity of HDAC inhibitors in altering gene transcription, and whether there are differences in the biologic function of different HDACs. Furthermore, it will be helpful to understand why normal cells are apparently more resistant to the apoptotic effects of HDAC inhibitors, as well as the role of nonhistone substrates of HDACs, such as transcription factors, in the suppression of cell growth. This knowledge will undoubtedly contribute to both the further understanding of the process of transformation and the development of effective agents to treat various cancers.

NOVEL CYTOTOXIC COMPOUNDS

A number of novel cytotoxic agents with unique mechanisms of action are being evaluated in patients with ovarian cancers in an effort to identify therapeutics that would not be cross resistant with taxane and platinating compounds.

Ecteinascidin-743

Ecteinascidin-743 (ET-743; Pharmamar, Madrid, Spain), a tetrahydroisoquinoline alkaloid isolated from the marine ascidian *Ecteinascidia turbinata,* is a DNA minor-groove interactive agent with specific affinity toward guanine-cytosine–rich sequences (98,99). ET-743–guanine adducts are formed only in double-strand DNA and these adducts are reversible upon DNA denaturation. Nuclear magnetic resonance and x-ray crystallographic studies have demonstrated that two of three subunits (A and B) bind to nucleic acids in the minor groove of DNA, but subunit C, which lacks DNA-binding capabilities, acts as a molecular hinge that facilitates binding of ET-743 to critical nuclear proteins (98–102). In essence, ET-743's dual affinity for DNA and proteins produces DNA–ET-743–protein cross links. Recent studies have also indicated that ET-743 interacts with nuclear histones and transcription factors such as E2F1,

c-fos, NF-y, and SP-1. Additionally, ET-743 perturbs cell cycle progression and induces G_1 arrest, S phase delay, and G_2/M arrest. These cell cycle effects have been observed in p53 mutated cell lines, suggesting that the cell cycle arrest induced by ET-743 is not dependent on p53. ET-743 does not inhibit topoisomerase I and II, but does interact with cellular microtubules and disorganizes intermediate filament bundles.

ET-743 is of particular interest for development in gynecologic malignancies because it has been demonstrated consistently to enhance the cytotoxic effects of platinating agents (102). In contrast to apoptosis mediated by platinating agents, ET-743–mediated apoptosis following the induction of DNA damage is enhanced by the nucleotide excision repair pathway and inhibited by the mismatch repair pathway (102). Tumor cells that are resistant to platinum compounds because of the upregulation of the nucleotide excision repair pathway are therefore likely to be sensitive to ET-743, and the combination of both agents may be more effective than either agent alone. ET-743 has also demonstrated substantial antiproliferative activity against a wide variety of hematologic and solid tumors cancers *in vitro*, with IC_{50} values ranging from 1 pM to 10 nM. These investigations, as well as studies conducted in the human tumor cloning assay, indicate that the antiproliferative effects of ET-743 are several-fold higher with continuous than short-term treatment. ET-743 has also displayed substantial antiproliferative effects in both murine and human tumor xenografts, including those derived from human melanoma, breast, ovarian, renal, lung, and prostatic cancers. In addition, the agent has demonstrated antiproliferative activity similar to cisplatin and paclitaxel against various human ovarian tumor xenografts (103).

In early clinical evaluations, antitumor activity has been particularly notable in patients with soft tissue sarcoma and breast cancer refractory to anthracyclines and patients with ovarian cancer resistant to platinum agents and taxanes (101, 104). The principal toxicities of ET-743 include reversible transaminitis, emesis, and myelosuppression; however, these adverse effects appear to be less common on intermittent divided-dose schedules.

TLK-286

TLK-286 (TELCYTA, Telik, Palo Alto, CA) is a small-molecule prodrug that is metabolically activated by glutathione S-transferase P1–1 (GST P1–1) to release an alkylating nitrogen mustard moiety (105,106). The enzyme GST P1–1 is overexpressed in ovarian, breast, lung, and many other human malignancies, and enzyme activity in tumors appears to relate to resistance to commonly used chemotherapeutic drugs, particularly alkylating agents. Following intracellular uptake of TLK-286, drug activation, and DNA damage, tumor cells undergo apoptosis. Myelosuppression is the principal toxicity of the agent. In a Phase II study of TLK-286 in patients with recurrent advanced ovarian carcinoma, 31 of 36 patients were evaluable for efficacy and one patient experienced a complete response, three patients had partial responses, and 12 patients had stable disease as their best response (107). The objective response rate was 15% in patients whose diseases progressed after second-line therapy and 13% in patients whose tumors progressed following two to four lines of treatment. A randomized Phase III trial is underway in patients with advanced ovarian cancer whose disease has progressed following platinum-based chemotherapy and one second-line treatment.

Antimicrotubule Agents

Several natural products, which are structurally dissimilar to the taxanes, share their mechanism of action, and show comparable activities, have been identified and several are in clinical evaluations. Rhazinilam, like paclitaxel, originates from tree bark; however, it is the first nontaxane identified that induces cold-stable tubulin polymerization *in vitro* and microtubule bundling in cells (108). Unlike paclitaxel, rhazinilam is capable of inducing tubulin polymerization in the cold, but its polymerized product is unstable. In contrast, discodermolide, which has been isolated from a marine sponge, polymerizes tubulin *in vitro* more potently and rapidly than does paclitaxel (109,110). Discodermolide-induced microtubules are stable following treatment with calcium and cold temperature, which typically depolymerize tubulin, and are composed of very short microtubules instead of tubulin spirals. In addition, discodermolide appears to be active in cancer cells with mulitdrug resistance conferred by overexpression of P-glycoprotein and related resistance proteins (109,110), and nanomolar concentrations are active in cancer cells with taxane resistance being conferred by the overexpression of P-glycoprotein and other resistance proteins or tubulin mutations. Interestingly, discodermolide and paclitaxel have demonstrated therapeutic synergism in preclinical studies (111). The natural product itself (XAA296; Novartis) is currently being evaluated in early clinical investigations.

Another class of natural products—the epothilones—which are 16-member macrolides derived from myxobacterium, also stabilize tubulin, favoring net polymerization (112–115). The epothilones induce the formation of microtubules that are long, rigid, and resistant to destabilization by cold temperature and calcium. The epothilones are at least as potent as taxanes and induce mitotic arrest and microtubule bundling. Similar to discodermolide, the epothilones exert prominent cytotoxic activity in tumors with multidrug resistance conferred by overexpression of P-glycoprotein and associated resistance proteins. Experimental studies have also indicated that the epothilones and taxanes differ in terms of resistance conferred by point mutations in β-tubulin; however, the significance of tubulin mutations in conferring clinical resistance to antimicrotubule agents is

not clear. Several members of the epothilone B family, particularly epothilone B itself (EPO-0906; Novartis) and the epothilone B analog BMS-247550 (Bristol Myers Squibb, Princeton, NJ), have demonstrated impressive activity against human xenografts of ovarian, breast, and colorectal cancers, some of which are clearly resistant to various taxanes. A Phase II trial of EPO-0906 in patients with ovarian cancer refractory to platinating agents has recently been completed and preliminary data indicate a modest degree of activity (116) Several other epothilone B and D analogs are also undergoing broad clinical evaluations.

The marine soft coral–derived natural products sarcotidicytins A and B and eleutherobin also promote tubulin polymerization in a manner analogous to that of the taxanes, but they appear to be much weaker substrates for P-glycoprotein (117). However, other marine-derived, microtubule-stabilizing cytotoxins, such as laulimalide and isolaulimalide, are poorer substrates for P-glycoprotein and other multidrug resistance proteins (118). Because the epothilones, discodermolide, and eleutherobin competitively inhibit paclitaxel binding to microtubules, a common pharmacophore, which may enable the development of hybrid constructs with more desirable biologic characteristics, has been identified (119).

Targeting Mitotic Kinesins

Although tubulin is the most abundant protein component of the mitotic spindle apparatus, many additional proteins, such as mitotic kinesins, play critical roles in the mechanics of mitosis and in progression through the premitotic cell cycle checkpoint. Kinesins are motor proteins that translate chemical energy released by the hydrolysis of adenosine triphosphate (ATP) into mechanical force for movement along microtubules, transport of a wide variety of cargoes, and the intracellular organization of the mitotic spindle and other microtubule-containing structures (120–122).

The mitotic kinesins are a subgroup of kinesin motor proteins that function exclusively in mitosis in proliferating cells (122). During mitosis, different, highly specialized mitotic kinesins play critical roles in various aspects of mitotic spindle assembly, including the establishment of spindle bipolarity, spindle pole organization, chromosomal alignment and segregation, and regulation of microtubule dynamics. The establishment of mitotic spindle bipolarity is among the earliest events in spindle assembly, and it requires the function of a specific kinesin motor protein KSP (also known as Eg5), which has no known role outside of mitosis (123).

The expression profiles of KSP mRNA in normal tissues are consistent with preferential expression of KSP in proliferating cells relative to normal adjacent tissue. As essential elements in mitotic spindle assembly and function, KSP and mitotic kinesins provide attractive targets for intervention into the cell cycle. A therapeutic targeting KSP may prove to be equally or more efficacious as the taxanes and vinca alkaloids without the potential for neurotoxicity or other side effects associated with interference with tubulin function in nondividing cells. Furthermore, combinations of therapeutics targeting KSP and tubulin dynamics may exhibit additive or synergistic cytotoxicity. SB-715992 (Glaxo SmithKline; Cytokinetics, South San Francisco, CA), a polycyclic, nitrogen-containing heterocycle, is the first KSP-targeting therapeutic to enter clinical trials (124). The compound, which is 10,000-fold more selective for KSP relative to other members of the kinesin superfamily, has been shown to block assembly of a functional mitotic spindle, thereby causing cell cycle arrest in mitosis and subsequent cell death.

RADIATION THERAPY: ADVANCES IN THE TWENTY-FIRST CENTURY

Radiation therapy has been used in the treatment of gynecologic malignancies for over a century (125). Over the years, numerous technologic advancements have been introduced, notably megavoltage energy machines, high-dose–rate brachytherapy and computed tomography–based treatment planning. These innovations have markedly improved the quality and delivery of radiation in gynecologic patients.

Despite such advancements, the basic approach to the planning and delivery of radiation in gynecology patients has remained essentially unchanged. After determining the site to be treated, a limited number of treatment fields (typically two to four) are selected. Select variables (e.g., beam energy, weighting) are altered iteratively to produce a treatment plan that irradiates the target tissues while avoiding, as best as possible, the nearby normal tissues. Fields are shaped with customized blocks to reduce further the dose to neighboring normal tissues.

Intensity-modulated Radiation Therapy

In recent years, a novel approach to the planning and delivery of radiation has been introduced, which is known as intensity-modulated radiotherapy (IMRT) (126,127). IMRT provides the ability to conform the dose to the shape of the target in three dimensions, thereby sparing the nearby normal tissues. Enthusiasm is rapidly increasing for IMRT in the United States. In a recent survey (128), 32% of radiation oncologists stated that they currently use IMRT in their clinics, with 80% having adopted it only in the last 1 to 2 years. Moreover, >90% of IMRT nonusers plan to adopt it in the near future. Favorable reports have also appeared in the media regarding IMRT (129,130).

To date, most attention has been focused on prostatic and head and neck cancers (131–134). In these sites, IMRT has been shown to result in lower rates of complications by reducing the volume of normal tissues irradiated. Promising outcomes have also been reported using IMRT as a means of escalating doses in these patients. Of the radiation oncologists surveyed by Mell et al. (132), 15% stated they have

treated a gynecologic patient with IMRT. In fact, a strong rationale exists for its use in gynecologic patients. Standard approaches result in the irradiation of considerable volumes of normal tissues exposing patients to a wide range of sequelae (139,140). Sparing of normal tissues with IMRT may not only reduce the risk of untoward toxicity, but also allows the use of higher than conventional doses in select patients (137,138). IMRT may also provide a means of treating cervical cancer patients unable to undergo brachytherapy, improving their chance of cure (139).

IMRT and Inverse Planning

IMRT is an advanced form of three-dimensional conformal radiotherapy that utilizes computer-optimized intensity-modulated beams to generate highly conformal dose distributions (140). Although first used in the 1990s, the concepts underlying IMRT are not new. In fact, IMRT was first proposed by Takahashi in the 1960s (141). However, its implementation in clinical practice had to await the development of sophisticated computerized optimization programs (142).

Unlike conventional approaches, IMRT planning is an inverse process whereby the treatment planner delineates the target and normal tissues directly on a planning computed tomography (CT) scan (143). Specific dose-volume constraints are entered for the target and normal tissues and the optimization program generates a treatment plan that best satisfies these goals. This approach is distinguished from the trial-and-error forward conventional planning method. Inverse planning is clearly a powerful tool. Whereas conventional approaches result in an acceptable plan, inverse planning generates the optimal one.

During the optimization process, each beam is divided into small "beamlets" whose intensity is varied until the desired dose distribution is obtained (143). The resultant intensity profile of each beam is quite complex and could not be determined manually (Fig. 18.6). In contrast, conventional approaches use beams of uniform intensity. Although beam intensity can be modulated manually by various treatment aids, for example, wedges and compensators, they are not modulated to the extent as in IMRT.

When cast into the patient, the intensity-modulated beams result in highly conformal dose distributions. Such dose distributions are nearly always superior to those achieved with conventional planning, particularly in complex shaped targets (143,147). IMRT plans are distinguished by rapid dose gradients outside the target, resulting in considerable sparing of neighboring normal tissues (140). An example IMRT plan in a gynecologic patient is shown in Figure 18.7.

Intensity-modulated beams are delivered using a linear accelerator equipped with a multileaf collimator whose "leaves" (typically 0.5 to 1.0 cm in width) move in and out of the beam's path under computer control (140,143). The longer the leaves remain open at a particular position, the

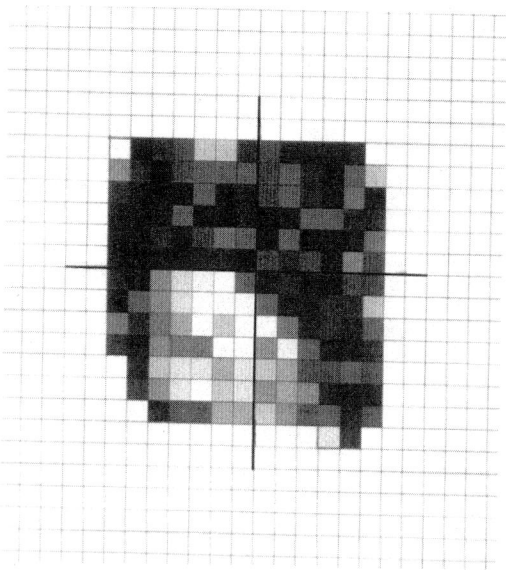

FIG. 18.6. Intensity profile of a treatment beam in a patient treated with IMRT.

greater the intensity of radiation. At some centers, modulated beams are delivered using compensators (143).

IMRT Process

The IMRT process begins with simulation. Unlike in conventional approaches, a contrast-enhanced planning CT scan is performed, typically using a CT simulator. Thin slices (3 to 5 mm) are used, encompassing the entire region of interest. Attention is focused on optimal patient immobilization, given the rapid dose gradients in IMRT plans (140). At the University of Chicago, an upper and lower body alpha cradle is fabricated and indexed to the treatment table for intensity-modulated whole pelvic radiation therapy (IM-WPRT) pa-

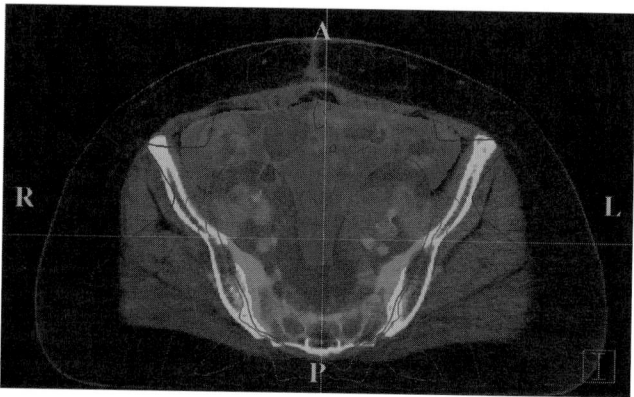

FIG. 18.7. Example of an IMRT plan in a patient with a gynecologic malignancy. High-dose isodose lines conform to the lateral iliac lymph nodes and posterior presacral region, reducing the dose to the centrally placed bowel.

tients (144,145). Patients are simulated in the supine position (145). Recent data, however, have suggested a benefit to prone positioning (146). Bladder, rectal, oral, and intravenous contrast are administered to ensure optimal visualization of the target and normal tissues (144,145). Intravenous contrast is necessary because the pelvic vessels serve as surrogates for the lymph nodes. A vaginal marker is placed to identify the vaginal cuff. Treatment planning continues with target and tissue delineation. Two targets are delineated on the planning CT: a gross target (GTV) and a clinical target (CTV) volume (147). The GTV consists of all visualizable tumor (primary and other sites). The primary tumor is often poorly visualized even when contrast is used. Ongoing work is evaluating the incorporation of other imaging modalities, for example, magnetic resonance (MR) imaging and positron emission tomography (PET) (148), into the planning process.

The CTV in an individual patient is a function of the site treated. In women receiving adjuvant IM-WPRT, the CTV consists of the upper vagina, parametria, presacral region, and pelvic lymph nodes (common, internal, and external iliacs) (144,145). Contrast-enhanced vessels are included with a 0.5- to 1.0-cm margin to cover the pelvic lymph nodes. In patients with an intact uterus, the entire uterus is included. If more comprehensive volumes are treated, the CTV may also include the paraaortic (149) and/or inguinal (150) lymph nodes. The CTV is uniformly expanded at most centers by 1 cm in three dimensions, creating a planning target volume (PTV) to account for setup uncertainty and organ motion (144,145).

Normal tissues contoured on the planning CT scan include the bladder, rectum, and small bowel. The bone marrow within the iliac crests is outlined in IM-WPRT patients at our center, particularly when chemotherapy is planned (151, 152). Recent data have suggested that delineation of the active (red) marrow is possible by incorporating a technetium 99m scan in the planning process (153). Depending on the site treated, other normal structures may include the kidneys (153a) and femoral heads (150).

IMRT planning continues with dose specification. First, the prescription dose is selected. In most IM-WPRT patients, 45 Gy is delivered in 1.8-Gy daily fractions (144,145). Given the inherent inhomogeneities of IMRT planning, larger fractions are not recommended. More complicated dose prescriptions are used in women undergoing a simultaneous integrated boost (SIB) (154,155). If the whole abdomen is treated, 30 Gy in 150-cGy daily fractions is recommended (153a).

A more challenging task is the specification of dose-volume constraints for the PTV and normal tissues. Such constraints serve as input parameters in the inverse planning optimization process and are often entered in the form of dose-volume histograms (DVH) (143). Priority is given to PTV coverage. However, in all IMRT plans, a small percentage of the PTV will receive below the prescription dose. A reasonable approach is to cover ≥98% of the PTV with the prescription dose (144,145). Input parameters for the normal tissues are less intuitive. The parameters used in IM-WPRT patients treated at our center were derived empirically over a number of years (Table 18.2). Recent publications from other centers have included their dose-volume constraints (149).

Albeit many aspects of IMRT planning are automated, one must still select the number of beams, beam angles, and energy. Typically, seven or nine equally spaced coplanar beams are used (51.4- and 40.0-degree increments, respectively) delivered with 6-MV photons in patients treated with IM-WPRT (144, 145). Fewer beams result in poorer conformity; more beams do not improve the overall quality of the plan (144). At other centers, other beam configurations are used (153a). In the future, beam number and configuration may also be included in the optimization process (161).

Using inverse planning, the treatment-planning computer generates a dose distribution that best satisfies the input constraints. At most centers, a number of potential plans are generated by varying the input parameters. Plan evaluation is a time-consuming process. Each plan is evaluated qualitatively slice-by-slice for dose conformity and the presence of hot and cold spots. Each plan is also evaluated quantitatively by assessing the PTV and normal tissue DVHs. At our center, an IM-WPRT plan is acceptable only if ≥98% of the PTV receives the prescription dose. Cold spots are only acceptable along the periphery of the PTV. Cold spots are never acceptable within the CTV, particularly within the GTV (144).

Given the inherent inhomogeneity of IMRT, a long-standing policy at our center in IM-WPRT patients has been to accept plans with up to 20% and 2% of the PTV receiving 110% and 115% of the prescription dose, respectively (144). With newer planning software, however, the PTV receiving 110% and 115% of the prescription dose in recent patients have been, on average, 11.5% and 0.2%, respectively (157). If brachytherapy is planned, care is taken to avoid hot spots along the anterior rectal and posterior bladder walls.

Less is known about what makes a normal tissue DVH acceptable. Normal tissue DVHs in IMRT plans will be superior to those seen in conventional plans (144). However, although the DVH of a tissue may appear better, it does not necessarily follow that a clinically significant difference will result. Only with careful follow-up of patients treated with IMRT will this question be answered (158). Both before and during IMRT, rigorous quality assurance is essential. A full discussion of quality assurance procedures is beyond the scope of this text and interested readers are referred elsewhere (140). Several quality assurance procedures including independent monitor unit checks and verification of calculated IMRT dose distributions using both phantom and film dosimetry have been proposed.

Preclinical Data

Numerous investigators have compared IMRT and conventional planning in gynecologic patients. Of note, most have focused on women undergoing pelvic irradiation in an attempt to reduce the volume of small bowel irradiated. These studies are summarized in Table 18.3.

Roeske et al. (144) compared conventional WPRT and IM-WPRT plans in ten gynecologic patients at the University of Chicago. The CTV consisted of the upper vagina, parametria, uterus (if present), and pelvic lymph nodes, and was expanded by 1 cm, creating a PTV. Although PTV coverage was similar, the volume of small bowel receiving the prescription dose in the IMRT plans was decreased by a factor of two (17.4% vs 33.8%; $p = .0005$) compared with conventional approaches. The volumes of rectum and bladder irradiated were also reduced by 23%. Other investigators have reported reductions in the small bowel irradiated using IMRT planning ranging from 40% to 70% (159) (Table 18.3). Marked reductions in the volume of bladder and rectum irradiated have also been reported (161).

Lujan et al. (151) demonstrated that IM-WPRT planning could also be used to minimize the volume of pelvic bone marrow irradiated. Bone marrow (within the iliac crests) was contoured in ten women and added as a constraint in the planning process. Although the volume receiving 10 Gy was slightly increased, IMRT planning reduced the bone marrow volume treated at all dose levels above 15 Gy. Of note, the addition of bone marrow as a constraint did not compromise PTV coverage or spare other normal tissues.

TABLE 18.2. *Input planning parameters for IM-WPRT patients—University of Chicago*

	Goal (Gy)	Volume below goal (%)	Minimum (Gy)	Maximum (Gy)
PTV	45	3	42.8	47.3
Organ	Limit (Gy)	Volume above limit (%)	Minimum (Gy)	Maximum (Gy)
Bladder	35.1	40	27.9	42.8
Rectum	35.8	54	27.5	42.8
Small bowel	38.1	0	8.2	42.8

IM-WPRT, intensity-modulated whole pelvic radiation therapy; PTV, planning target volume.

TABLE 18.3. *Comparative planning studies for IM-WPRT versus conventional WPRT*

WPRT study (ref)	Tumor	n	CTV-PTV margin (cm)	↓Volume receiving prescription dose IM-WPRT vs conventional		
				Bowel	Bladder	Rectum
Roeske et al. (20)	C,E	10	1	↓50%	↓23%	↓23%
Ahamad et al. (38)	C,E	10	0, 1.0, 0.5[a]	↓63%[b]	NS	NS
			0.5, 1.5, 1[a]	↓47%[b]	NS	NS
			1.0, 2.0, 1.5[a]	↓40%[b]	NS	NS
Chen et al. (36)	C,E	7	1	↓70%	↓[c]	↓[c]
Selvaraj et al. (37)	NS	7	NS	↓51%[d]	↓31%[d]	↓66%[d]

IM-WPRT, intensity-modulated whole pelvic radiation therapy; WPRT, whole pelvic; CTV, clinical target volume; PTV, planning target volume; C, cervical cancer; E, endometrial cancer; NS, not stated.

[a] Around lymph nodes, anterior to vaginal vault, posterior to vaginal vault.
[b] Reduction in absolute volume receiving >90% of the prescription dose.
[c] Data not shown.
[d] Reduction in percent volume receiving ≥30 Gy.

Several investigators have evaluated IMRT planning in gynecologic patients treated with more comprehensive fields. In ten advanced cervical cancer patients undergoing pelvic plus paraaortic RT, Portelance et al. (153) noted significant reductions in the small bowel, bladder, and rectum using IMRT planning compared to conventional two- or four-field approaches. Hong et al. (153a) evaluated IMRT planning in ten endometrial cancer patients undergoing whole abdomen radiation therapy (WART). PTV coverage was improved with IMRT planning, particularly near the kidneys (under the conventional blocks). Moreover, the volume of pelvic bones (and thus bone marrow) receiving 21 Gy or higher was reduced by 60%.

Two recent series have focused on gynecologic patients treated with pelvic-inguinal RT. In vulvar cancer patients, Garofalo et al. (150) reported that IMRT planning reduced the volume of all normal tissues irradiated, including the small bowel, bladder, rectum, and bone marrow. Of particular note, the dose to the femoral heads was also significantly reduced. In contrast, Gilroy et al. (162) noted that higher doses to the pelvic tissues and greater setup complexity were seen with IMRT. However, the sole goal of this study was to reduce the dose to the femoral heads. No attempt was made to spare the small bowel and other pelvic tissues.

Several investigators have evaluated IMRT as a means to deliver higher than conventional doses in gynecology patients. Lujan and colleagues (154) found that dose escalation was feasible using an SIB technique in patients with involved pelvic nodes, without compromising normal tissue sparing. Mutic et al. (148) proposed a PET-guided SIB approach to irradiate involved paraaortic lymph nodes in advanced cervical cancer patients. In their exploratory study, 59.4 Gy could be delivered to PET-positive paraaortic nodes, while still maintaining acceptable doses to the normal tissues. Kavanagh et al. (155,163) presented an SIB technique to treat the primary tumor and/or involved lymph nodes to

higher dose in cervical cancer patients undergoing IM-WPRT.

IMRT as an alternative for brachytherapy has also been discussed (139,164). In cervical cancer patients unable to receive brachytherapy, Roeske et al. (165) found that a total dose of 75 Gy or higher was feasible with IMRT. Select patients could receive doses as high as 81 Gy to the residual tumor. Low et al. (166) proposed a technique known as applicator-guided IMRT as a replacement for brachytherapy. As envisioned, an applicator would be placed in the cervix to localize the tumor and reproducibly position the bladder and rectum during treatment. MRI and/or PET imaging would be used to delineate the tumor and treatment would be delivered with HDR dose schedules.

Clinical Studies

Outcome data in gynecologic patients treated with IMRT remain limited. Mundt et al. (167,168) have provided a series of detailed analyses of acute gastrointestinal (GI) toxicity in IM-WPRT patients. In a recent analysis (168), acute gastrointestinal GI sequelae were compared in 40 IM-WPRT and 35 conventional WPRT. The groups were well-balanced in terms of tumor site, stage, surgery, radiation dose, and chemotherapy. IM-WPRT was associated with less grade ≥2 acute GI toxicity (60% vs 91%; $p = .002$) than conventional WPRT. Moreover, the percentage of IM-WPRT and WPRT patients requiring no (or only infrequent) antidiarrheal medications was 75% and 34%, respectively ($p = .001$). Although less urinary toxicity (10% vs 20%) was observed, this difference failed to reach statistical significance ($p = .22$).

Mundt et al. (157) recently evaluated chronic GI toxicity in a cohort of 30 IM-WPRT patients with a median follow-up of 19.6 months (range 8 to 33 months). Compared to

WPRT patients treated in the year prior, IM-WPRT patients experienced less chronic GI sequelae (11.1% vs 50.0%; $p = .001$). On multivariate analysis controlling for age, stage, chemotherapy, surgery, and length of follow-up, IMRT was correlated with less chronic GI toxicity ($p = .01$; OR 0.16, 95% CI 0.04, 0.67).

Brixey et al. (152) compared the acute hematologic toxicity in women undergoing IM-WPRT versus WPRT. Whereas sequelae were infrequent in RT-alone patients, WPRT patients treated with chemotherapy developed more grade $\geq$2 leukopenia (60% vs 31.2%; $p = .08$) and a lower white blood cell count nadir (2.8 vs 3.6; $p = .05$) than IM-WPRT patients treated with chemotherapy. The WPRT patients also developed a lower absolute neutrophil count nadir (1874 vs 2669; $p = .04$). Of note, these benefits were realized although bone marrow was not entered as a constraint in the planning process, but was simply spared owing to the highly conformal nature of the IM-WPRT plans.

Kavanagh et al. (155) treated seven advanced cervical cancer patients with IM-WPRT with a SIB to the primary tumor and/or involved pelvic nodes. All patients also received weekly cisplatin. Treatment was well tolerated except in two patients who developed grade 3 acute GI toxicity. All patients achieved a complete response even though one could not undergo brachytherapy. Unfortunately, no analysis of long-term toxicity or tumor control was provided.

Pelvic control in 60 IM-WPRT patients at the University of Chicago has been recently analyzed. Most patients (65%) had early-stage cervical or endometrial cancers. The IM-WPRT dose was 45 Gy; 33 also received brachytherapy. At a median follow-up of 22.5 months, 4 patients failed in the pelvis, for a 2-year actuarial pelvic control of 89.8%. All four pelvic failures were in locally advanced/recurrent patients and occurred within the GTV. One patient failed simultaneously in the CTV in the lateral pelvis. None of the early-stage patients failed in the pelvis. Moreover, no failures in any patient occurred outside the CTV, suggesting that IMRT planning did not adversely impact on pelvic control.

Issues/Concerns

Several important issues and concerns exist regarding IMRT in general and gynecologic IMRT in particular. First, implementation of IMRT requires a considerable capital investment in terms of new software and hardware (140). A significant investment in time is also required. New approaches and procedures for nearly every aspect of treatment planning and delivery must be learned and adopted. Recent changes, however, in IMRT reimbursement recognize these investments in time and capital needed for adoption and routine use of IMRT.

A more fundamental concern is that, despite promising preliminary data, IMRT remains a new, unproven technol-

ogy. Most outcome data in gynecology (and in other sites) consist of relatively small series with limited follow-up. Moreover, most focus solely on toxicity, not on long-term tumor control. Whether improved dose distributions achieved with IMRT planning truly translate into improved patient outcome remains to be determined. Concerns have also been raised regarding the mutagenic potential of IMRT given the spread of low dose to a larger volume of normal tissues (169). These concerns can only be allayed by careful, long-term observation of IMRT patients.

Finally, no consensus guidelines exist regarding how any aspect of gynecologic IMRT planning and delivery should be performed. To ensure optimal treatment outcomes, standards are needed. To this end, the Gynecologic IMRT Working Group was recently formed consisting of 45 institutions in the United States, Canada, Europe, and Asia. The group is in the process of developing a consensus statement on IM-WPRT planning in gynecologic patients. Such guidelines will not only help individual clinicians interested in adopting gynecologic IMRT but also aid cooperative groups in the development of prospective trials. Only with carefully designed prospective trials will the full potential of IMRT in gynecology be realized.

ADVANCES IN MINIMALLY INVASIVE SURGERY

Minimally invasive and laparoscopic surgery for gynecologic oncology is discussed in detail in other chapters and a summary of recent advances will be presented here. The utility of advanced operative laparoscopy in gynecologic oncology expanded following advancements in laparoscopic retroperitoneal surgery, particularly pelvic and aortic lymphadenectomy. The performance of a laparoscopic retroperitoneal dissection opened the door for more advanced laparoscopic gynecologic cancer applications and operations including the revival of radical vaginal surgery (169) and the complete laparoscopic management and staging of selected patients with a variety of gynecologic malignancies. The potential oncologic effects of laparoscopy and pneumoperitoneum will continue to be debated (170) until the results of ongoing prospective randomized trials in malignant disease are available.

Laparoscopic Pelvic and Aortic Lymph Node Dissection in Gynecologic Malignancies

Laparoscopic surgical staging with pelvic and aortic lymph node dissection for gynecologic cancers was initially reported from France by Querleu (172). Since this initial report many investigators have adopted the laparoscopic transperitoneal and extraperitoneal surgical approach for cervical cancer and other gynecologic malignancies where a retroperitoneal node dissection is indicated and continue to modify the technical details of the procedure. It is well estab-

TABLE 18.4. Summary of laparoscopic pelvic and aortic lymph node dissection complications in the management of gynecologic malignancies (selected series utilizing the transperitoneal approach in the majority of cases with total N ≥30)

Study (ref)	N	PLN	PAN	ORT	HD	Complications
Querleu et al. (172)	39	8.7	—	90	1	1 vascular 1 hematoma 1 pneumoperitoneum
Spirtos et al. (177)	40	20.8	7.9			2 vascular 2 DVT 2 intestinal obstruction
Su et al. (178)	38	15	—	77	—	1 vascular 1 ureteral
Chu et al. (175)	67	26.7	8	93	2	1 vascular
Possover et al. (179)	150	26.8	7.3			10 vascular 2 lymphedema 2 nerve injury 3 intestinal
Vidaurreta et al. (180)	84	18.5	—	108	1–2	1 vascular 2 lymphocele
Dottino et al. (181)	94	11.9	3.7			1 vascular
Querleu et al. (182)	53	With common iliac	20.7	126	1–2	1 ureteral
Altgassen et al. (183)	108	21–24.3	5.1–10.6	Aortic: 35–73 Pelvic: 61–70	—	3 vascular 1 hemorrhage 2 nerve injury 3 intestinal obstruction
Scribner et al. (184)	103	23.2	6.8			1 vascular (fatal) 1 ureteral 1 DVT 2 pulmonary embolus (1 fatal)
Schlaerth et al. (185)	67	32.1	12.1	209	6.3 with radical hysterectomy	7 vascular 1 ureteral 1 hematoma
Vergote et al. (176)	42	—	6			1 DVT I UVF
Spirtos et al. (186)	84	23.8	10.3			2 lymphocyst 1 hematoma
Abu-Rustum et al. (173)	114	10.3	5.3			3 intestinal 4 infectious 1 DVT

N, number of patients; PLN, mean pelvic lymph nodes; PAN, mean aortic lymph nodes; DVT, deep vein thrombosis; VF, ureterovaginal fistula; ORT, mean operating room time in minutes; HD, mean hospital stay in days.

lished at this point that transperitoneal or extraperitoneal laparoscopic pelvic and aortic lymph node dissection for gynecologic malignancies, in selected patients, is feasible, yields similar pathologic specimen results as the open approach, and is associated with low morbidity (173). Furthermore, this minimally invasive surgical approach may provide valuable information that may not be available by clinical staging techniques. For example, in cervical cancer, CT was able to detect retroperitoneal nodal metastasis in only 17% to 57% of patients staged laparoscopically (174–176). Table 18.4 (172,173,175–186) summarizes selected reports on complications and outcome of laparoscopic pelvic and aortic lymph node dissection in the management of gynecologic malignancies. It is evident from these data that the minimally invasive approach is feasible with a low complication rate in multiple centers worldwide.

Technique for Transperitoneal Laparoscopic Staging with Aortic and Pelvic Lymph Node Dissection for Gynecologic Malignancies

There are numerous variations on techniques available to perform laparoscopic pelvic and paraaortic lymphadenectomy for cervical cancer. This is a summary of the transperitoneal approach using monopolar electrosurgical instruments or the argon beam coagulator (173). The instruments needed usually include the following:

1. 5-mm trocars ×2, 10-mm blunt port (open laparoscopy), and 5/12-mm trocar (Fig. 18.8).
2. 10-mm argon beam coagulator set at 70 W with gas flow rate at 3 to 4 L/min
3. 5-mm graspers ×2, 10-mm lymph node spoon
4. 5- and 10-mm laparoscopic clip appliers

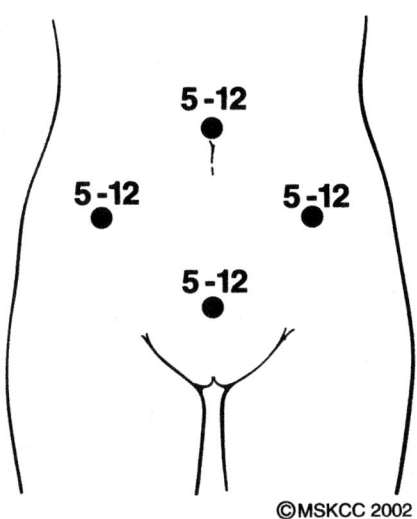

FIG. 18.8. 5–12-mm transperitoneal trocar placement for laparoscopic pelvic lymphadenectomy and total laparoscopic radical hysterectomy.

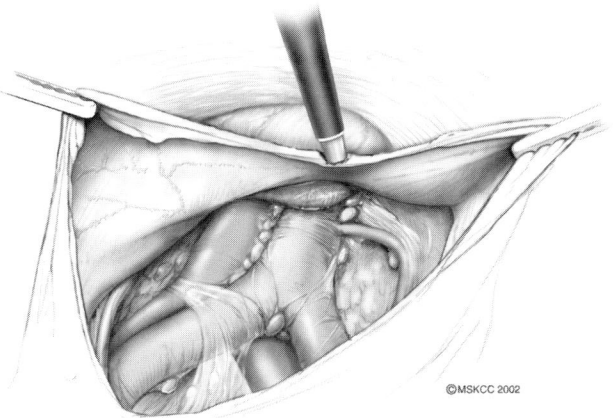

FIG. 18.9. Transperitoneal laparoscopic paraaortic lymph node dissection: initial retroperitoneal incision.

5. Suction irrigation

6. 4 × 8 gauze

The paraaortic lymph node dissection is usually performed first. The patient is placed in the dorsal lithotomy position with the legs in the universal Allen stirrups. A Foley catheter is inserted. Open laparoscopic technique is performed, and the blunt port is inserted in the umbilicus. Five-millimeter trocars are placed medial to the iliac crest, usually 1 cm superior and 1 cm medial, avoiding the abdominal wall vasculature. A 5/10- or 5/12-mm trocar is placed in the suprapubic area. Preoperative bowel prep is usually performed, and the patient is offered epidural anesthesia. Epidural anesthesia may facilitate bowel contraction by sympathetic blockade and may facilitate exposure. The patient is placed in the steep Trendelenburg position. Orogastric intubation is preferred.

Bilateral Paraaortic Lymphadenectomy

The camera is placed in the suprapubic port and the surgeon stands on the patient's right-hand side. The surgeon operates with the argon beam coagulator placed in the umbilical region and a 5-mm grasper in the left hand through the right lower quadrant 5-mm trocar. The assistant stands on the patient's left side holding the camera with the left hand and the suprapubic port and holding a grasper through the left lower quadrant 5-mm trocar. The right paraaortic lymph node dissection is performed first.

The argon beam coagulator is used to incise the retroperitoneum over the right common iliac artery. The incision is extended cephalad to the level of the duodenum (Fig. 18.9).

The incision is then extended caudal over the sacrum. Two leaves of peritoneum are developed. The surgeon and the assistant will first focus on the right lateral leaf to identify the edge of the vena cava, the psoas muscle, and the right ureter (Fig. 18.10).

Once the right ureter and the psoas muscle have been identified, the duodenum is then identified and protected, and the nodal dissection is started from the edge of the right common iliac artery and continues cephalad to the desired level, usually to the level of the duodenum near the insertion of the right ovarian vein into the vena cava (Fig. 18.11). Clips are used as needed.

Following completion of the right paraaortic lymph node dissection, the left paraaortic nodes are approached. The transperitoneal retroperitoneal incision may have to be extended horizontally below the duodenum toward the left renal vein insertion. The inferior mesenteric artery (IMA) is identified and protected. The left common iliac artery is identified and protected. The surgeon's left hand grasper is

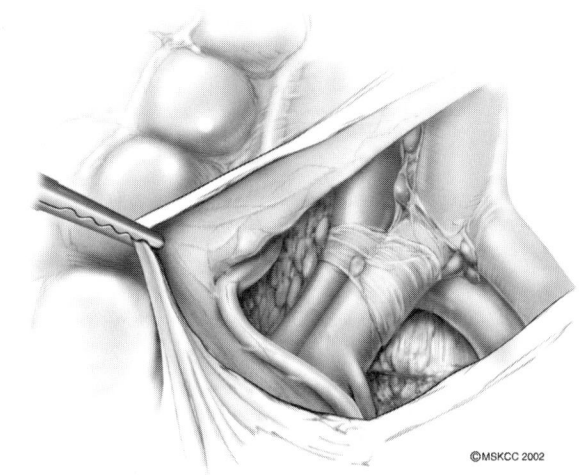

FIG. 18.10. Identifying the right ureter and inferior vena cava.

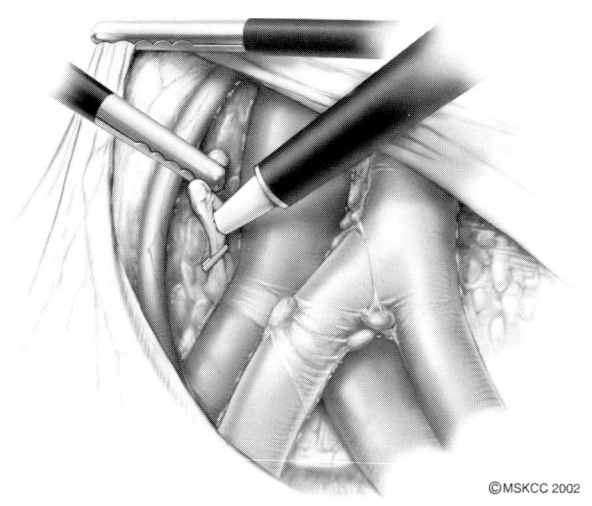

FIG. 18.11. Removal of right paraaortic and paracaval lymph nodes.

used to elevate the IMA, and then using blunt dissection, the left psoas muscle and ureter are identified in the window below the IMA. The assistant then grasps the lymph nodes just laterally to the left common iliac artery and lower aorta and the surgeon proceeds with removing those lymph nodes (Fig. 18.12).

Interaortocaval lymph nodes can also be removed with this approach. If the supramesenteric/infrarenal left-sided nodes are to be removed, the incision below the duodenum has to be extended laterally to the vicinity of the renal vessels. The nodal dissection is carried just lateral to the edge

of the aorta superior to the IMA. This will complete the bilateral paraaortic lymph node dissection (Fig. 18.13).

To complete the dissection, the incision is extended further over the left common iliac vein, and lymph nodes just below the aortic bifurcation are removed over the left common iliac vein.

Following completion of the paraaortic lymph node dissection, if an omentectomy is needed, such as for staging of adnexal or corpus cancer, the omentectomy is performed through the same setup. A 10-mm vessel-sealing device, such as the Atlas Ligasure, (Valleylab, Boulder, CO) is used from the lateral ports. This will require placement of 10-mm ports instead of 5-mm ports; therefore, if an omentectomy is anticipated, the 10-mm ports would be placed at the beginning of the procedure instead of 5-mm ports. The omentectomy is then performed in the usual manner with the Ligasure starting from the lateral edge of the omentum on either side. The omentum is removed at the end of the case with an endobag.

After completion of the procedure in the upper abdomen, attention is drawn to the pelvis. The camera is switched back to the umbilicus. The surgeon stands on the patient's left-hand side and the assistant stands on the patient's right-hand side. The assistant holds the camera with the left hand and a grasper with the right hand through the right lower quadrant trocar. The surgeon operates with the right hand through the suprapubic port with the argon beam coagulator (ABC) or the grasper in the left hand through the left lower quadrant trocar.

Bilateral Pelvic Lymphadenectomy

The pelvic lymphadenectomy is started by developing the paravesical and pararectal spaces. The round ligament is di-

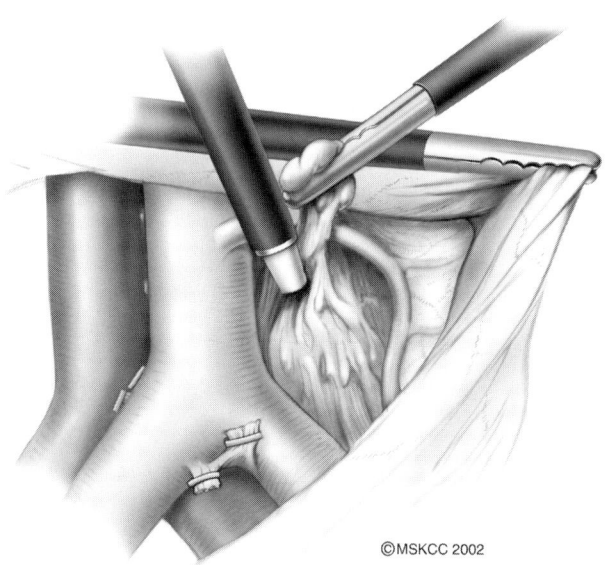

FIG. 18.12. Removal of left paraaortic lymph nodes.

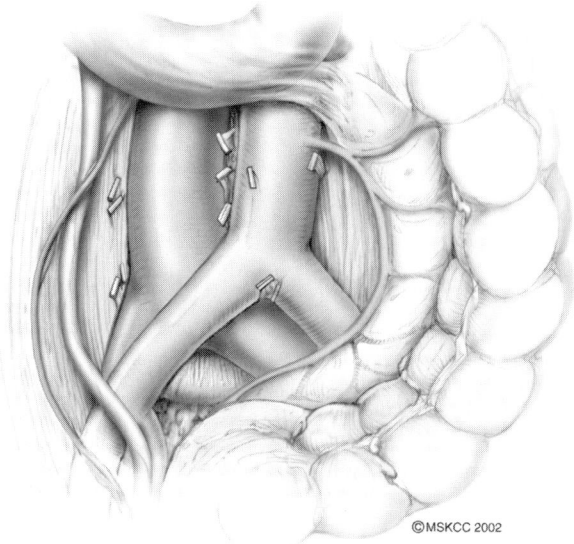

FIG. 18.13. Completed transperitoneal paraaortic lymph node dissections.

Following complete development of the pararectal and paravesical spaces and keeping the ureter medially, the lymph node dissection is started. The lymph node dissection is usually started over the distal common iliac artery on the right side and carried to the level of the deep circumflex iliac vessels. The psoas muscle is identified. The genitofemoral nerve is protected the lymph nodes between the genitofemoral nerve and the surface of the right external iliac artery and vein are removed. The dissection is usually carried from the psoas medially (Fig. 18.16). The deep circumflex iliac vessels are protected.

Then the obturator nerve is identified. The obturator vessels are protected, and the lymph node package just below the external iliac vein is grasped. The edge of the vein is cleared and dissected laterally, and the lymph node package between the inferior edge of the right external iliac vein and the superior edge of the obturator nerve is grasped and dissected sharply. This package is usually removed fairly easily; however, note should be taken of the possibility of an anastomotic obturator vein that can be inserting into the distal part of the external iliac vein. This vein should be protected. Once this nodal package is removed, lymph nodes around and below the obturator nerve can be removed. Hypogastric nodes can now be removed from the proximal part of the umbilical ligament and near the uterine artery origin. The iliac vessels can then be dissected from the psoas muscle and pulled medially, and the obturator space is exposed through the lateral approach to ensure removal of all nodal tissue, particularly in the proximal part just lateral to the common iliac artery (Fig. 18.17). The same is done on the contralateral side.

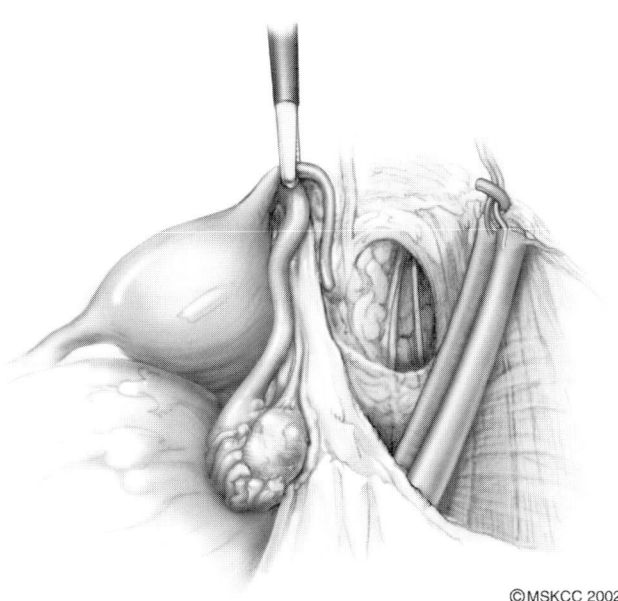

©MSKCC 2002

FIG. 18.14. Opening of right paravesical space.

vided with the ABC. The umbilical ligament is isolated. A retroperitoneal incision between the round ligament and the umbilical ligament parallel to the umbilical ligament is performed and extended just to the reflection of the interior abdominal wall. The umbilical ligament is then placed on traction medially, and using the ABC, the paravesical space is developed to expose the external iliac vessels, the obturator area and the obturator internus muscle, and the pubic bone (Fig. 18.14).

Then the retroperitoneal incision is extended over the psoas muscle parallel to the infundibulopelvic (IP) ligament. The IP ligament is pulled medially. The ureter is visualized and protected and the hypogastric vessel is identified. The pararectal space is developed (Fig. 18.15).

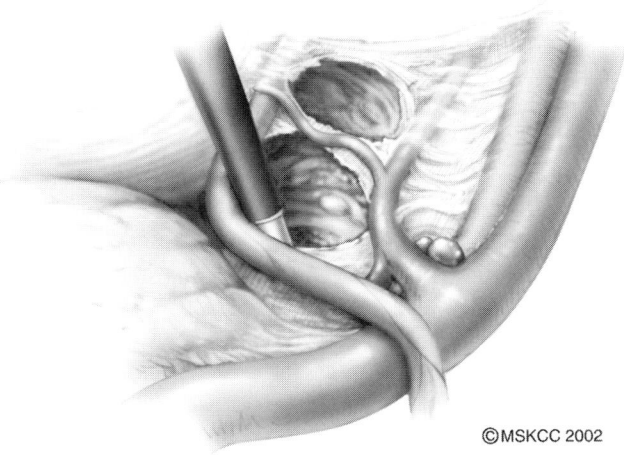

©MSKCC 2002

FIG. 18.15. Opening of right pararectal space.

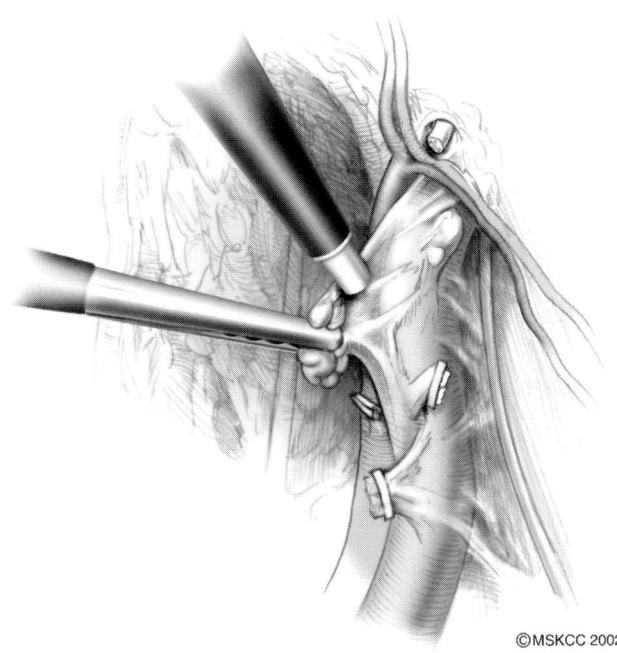

©MSKCC 2002

FIG. 18.16. Removal of right external iliac lymph nodes.

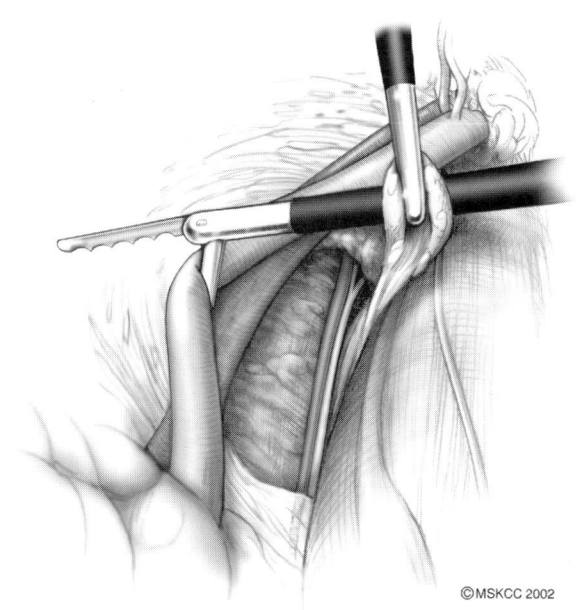

FIG. 18.17. Lateral approach to right obturator and common iliac lymph nodes between the psoas muscle and the external iliac vessels.

Peritoneal biopsies can be taken as needed. Pelvic washings are also done as needed. It may be helpful to have a 4 × 8 gauze placed in the patient during the dissection to facilitate dissection and ensure hemostasis.

Laparoscopic Pelvic Lymphadenectomy with Laparoscopically Assisted Radical Vaginal Hysterectomy

The radical vaginal hysterectomy (Schauta) for treatment of early cervical cancer was historically associated with a reduction in postoperative mortality when compared to the abdominal Wertheim radical hysterectomy. However, with the popularization of complete bilateral pelvic lymphadenectomy in the 1940s as an important component in the surgical management of cervical cancer, the Schauta vaginal operation became less popular, particularly in the United States, as it is not feasible to perform the pelvic lymphadenectomy via the vaginal route. European surgeons, however, have maintained the principles of radical vaginal surgery, and pioneers such as Daniel Dargent are credited with reviving radical vaginal surgery for cervical cancer through a combined laparoscopic retroperitoneal pelvic lymphadenectomy and radical vaginal hysterectomy (170,187). This approach became more popular among gynecologic oncologists interested in minimally invasive surgery, and the laparoscopically assisted radical vaginal hysterectomy is now commonly performed by many institutions for the surgical management of selected patients with early cervical cancer. This approach provides the potential benefits of laparoscopy and maintains

a previously accepted oncologic procedure for the treatment of cervical cancer. In the recently published large series of 200 patients by Hertel et al. (188), major intraoperative injury occurred in 6% of cases including seven ureteral injuries, four vascular injuries, and one intestinal injury. In addition, 14 (7%) patients sustained cystotomy. Postoperative severe complications occurred in 8% of cases including ureterostenosis (3.5%), reexploration (3.5%), and urinary fistula (1%). Blood transfusion was necessary in 19.2% of cases with a median of 2 blood units being transfused. Table 18.5 (188–199) summarizes selected publications on laparoscopically assisted radical vaginal hysterectomy.

Laparoscopic Pelvic Lymphadenectomy with Radical Vaginal Trachelectomy

This operation is a major innovation in the surgical therapy of early cervical cancer. Although the concept of a radical abdominal trachelectomy was described and performed on women with cervical cancer by Aburel in Rumania in the last century (200,201), the abdominal procedure did not become popular, and fertility-sparing surgery in cervical cancer remained limited to conization for women with very early lesions and a strong desire to retain reproductive function. The radical vaginal approach to trachelectomy was developed by Professor Daniel Dargent in 1987 in France (202). It is a modification of the radical vaginal hysterectomy with two main purposes: treat early cervical cancer and preserve uterine morphology and reproductive function. One of the main advantages in learning to perform radical vaginal hysterectomy is that the experience gained allows the surgeon to offer radical trachelectomy to selected young women with early invasive cervical cancer who wish to preserve their fertility (192). To date, several series are available in the English literature to document feasibility and safety, and many healthy births have been documented in women treated for early cervical cancer with this approach, including a case of pregnancy after radical trachelectomy and pelvic irradiation (203). The general eligibility criteria for radical vaginal trachelectomy include women less than 40 years old with a very strong desire to preserve fertility, no clinical evidence of impaired fertility, lesion size less than 2 cm, International Federation of Gynecology and Obstetrics (FIGO) stage IA-IB1 lesions, no involvement of the upper endocervical canal, and negative regional lymph nodes (204).

In a recent series of 96 radical trachelectomies performed between April 1987 and May 2002 at Hôspital Edouard Herriot in Lyon, France, one second cancer (bilateral suprarenal glands cancer) and four recurrences were observed (205). The retrospective unifactorial analysis demonstrated that the maximal tumoral diameter (2 cm or more) and the depth of infiltration (1 cm or more) were the only two significant factors of risk. Age less than 30 years and the presence of lymphovascular space involvement were

TABLE 18.5. *Summary of reports on laparoscopic pelvic and aortic lymph node dissection with laparoscopic assisted radical vaginal hysterectomy for apparent early stage cervical cancer*

Study (ref)	N	LN	ORT	HD	Complications	Recurrence
Querleu (189)	8	12.6	281	4.1	No major	2
Kadar (190)	8	30.9	–	3	1 reexploration	0
Garza-Leal (191)	3	22	–	7	No major	0
Roy et al. (192)	25	27	270	7	1 vascular 2 cystotomy 1 abscess 1 hematoma	0
Primicero et al. (193)	17	14	–	–	No major	–
Schneider et al. (194)	33	27.2	295	11	1 vascular 3 cystotomy 1 ureteral	1
Hatch et al. (195)	37	46	225	3	2 cystotomy 2 UVF 11% transfusion	–
Sardi et al. (196)	47	17	267	4	1 ureteral 1 abscess 1 hematoma	4
Renaud et al. (197)	57	30	270	5	3 cystotomy 1 vascular 1 abscess 1 hematoma 4% transfusion	2
Querleu et al. (198)	95	18	228		18% severe urinary symptoms	7
Park et al. (199)	52	27.7 pelvic 22.1 paraaortic	380	–	4 ureteral	
Hertel et al. (188)	200	22 pelvic 8 paraaortic	333	14	Major intraoperative 6% and postoperative 8%	Pelvic 20 Pelvic and distant 4 Distant 13

N, number of patients; LN, mean pelvic and aortic lymph nodes; ORT, mean operating room time in minutes; HD, mean hospital stay in days; UVF, ureterovaginal fistula.

likely to be risk factors, but the level of statistical significance was not reached. Histology other than squamous, infiltration of the parametrium, and involvement of the vaginal cuff had no prognostic impact. The chances for recurrence were 19% for patients affected by a tumor 2 cm or more and 25% for patients affected by a tumor 2 cm or more with a depth of infiltration 1 cm or more (205).

Table 18.6 (196,202,204–212) summarizes selected publications on radical vaginal trachelectomy.

Technique for Radical Vaginal Trachelectomy

A laparoscopic pelvic lymphadenectomy with or without paraaortic node dissection is completed, and multiple frozen sections are obtained from selected nodal packages and any suspicious nodes. Once all frozen sections are negative, the vaginal component is started.

Cystoscopy and the insertion of bilateral temporary retrograde ureteral catheters are at the surgeon's discretion. The catheters may help identify the ureters in difficult cases and

are removed at the end of the procedure. If there is concern of ureteral injury, the catheter can be changed over a guide wire to a double-J stent. The stent may be left in place for 4 to 6 weeks.

The radical vaginal trachelectomy is begun by delineating an adequate vaginal margin (usually 1 to 2 cm). Eight Kocher clamps are placed circumferentially around the cervix on the vaginal mucosa. A dilute solution of vasopressin is used to liberally inject the vaginal mucosa between the Kocher clamps (Fig. 18.18). This step helps separate the planes of dissection.

The assistants place two Brieski vaginal wall retractors at the 2 and 10 o'clock positions. A scalpel is now used to circumferentially incise the vaginal mucosa. The lateral incisions are shallow and the anterior and posterior incisions are deep. The shallow lateral incisions allow traction to be put on the parametria and pulled downward.

The Kocher clamps can now be removed, and the anterior and posterior vaginal mucosa can be folded over the ectocervix. The Krobach clamps are aligned horizontally to keep the ectocervix covered (Fig. 18.19).

TABLE 18.6. *Summary of laparoscopic pelvic and/or aortic lymph node dissection with radical vaginal trachelectomy*

Study (ref)	Nᵃ	LN	ORT	HD	Birth	Complications	Recurrence
Dargent et al. (202)	28	–	–	–	3	None	1 aortic LN
Roy and Plante (204)	30	–	285	4	4	4	1 local
Shepherd et al. (206)	10	–	–	–	3	–	1 local
Covens et al. (207)	32	–	180	1	3	6% transfusion 3% infectious 3% non-infectious	1 local
Renaud et al. (197)	34	26	260	4	–	2 vascular 1 cystotomy 1 hematoma	1 local 1 distant
Dargent et al. (208)	47	–	129	7	13	6% transfusion 1 cystotomy 5 reexplored	1 local 1 distant
Shepherd et al. (209)	30	–	–	–	9	6% transfusion	–
Dargent et al. (205)	96					–	–
Covens (210)	81		180	1	18		4 2 pelvic 3 non pelvic
Schlaerth et al. (211)	12	23	–	3.2	2	2 cystotomy	none
Burnett et al. (212)	21	22	318	3	3	1 hematoma 3 transient neuropathy 1 lymphocyst	none

N, number of patients; LN, mean pelvic and aortic lymph nodes; ORT, mean operating room time in minutes; HD, mean hospital stay in days.

ᵃ Some patients may be reported more than once.

The posterior cul-de-sac can now be sharply entered (Fig. 18.20). This allows the uterosacral ligaments to be isolated and the inferior portion of this ligament can be divided. By releasing the posterior attachments, there is greater uterine descensus, which is helpful for the more difficult anterior dissection.

The anterior portion of the dissection begins by sharply developing the vesicouterine space. The posterior vaginal retractor is removed, and the downward traction is placed on the specimen with the Krobach clamps. During this portion of the procedure, the surgeon should keep the axis of

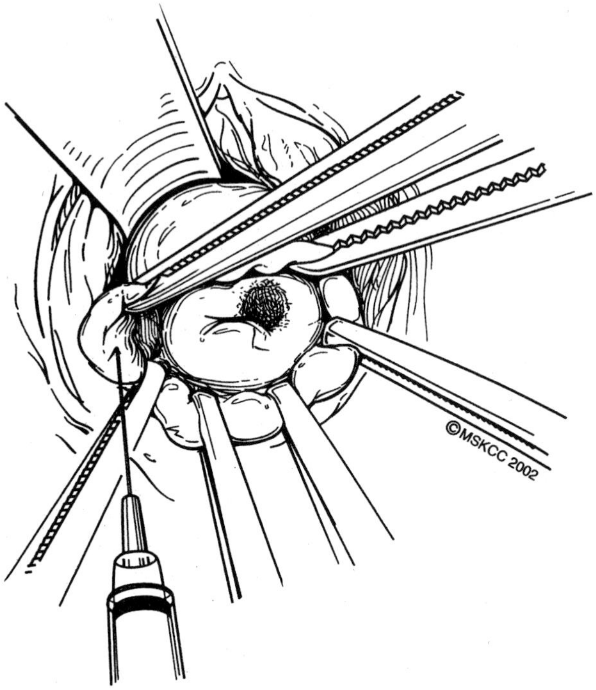

FIG. 18.18. Preparing the vaginal margin.

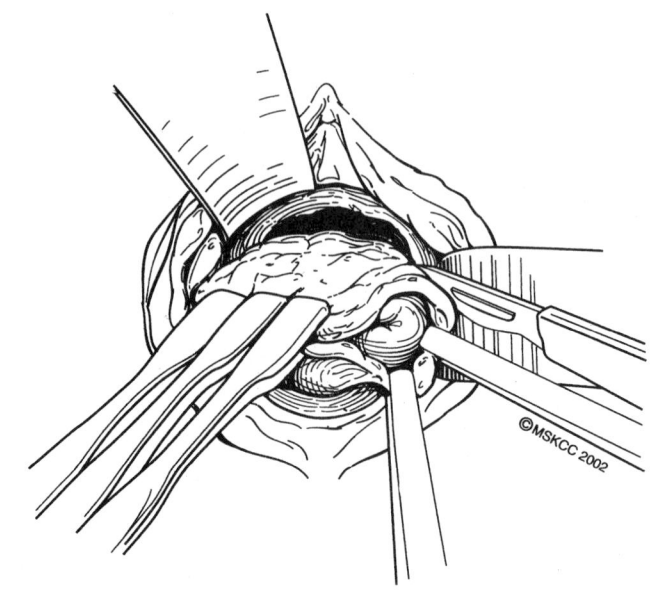

FIG. 18.19. Incising the vaginal mucosa.

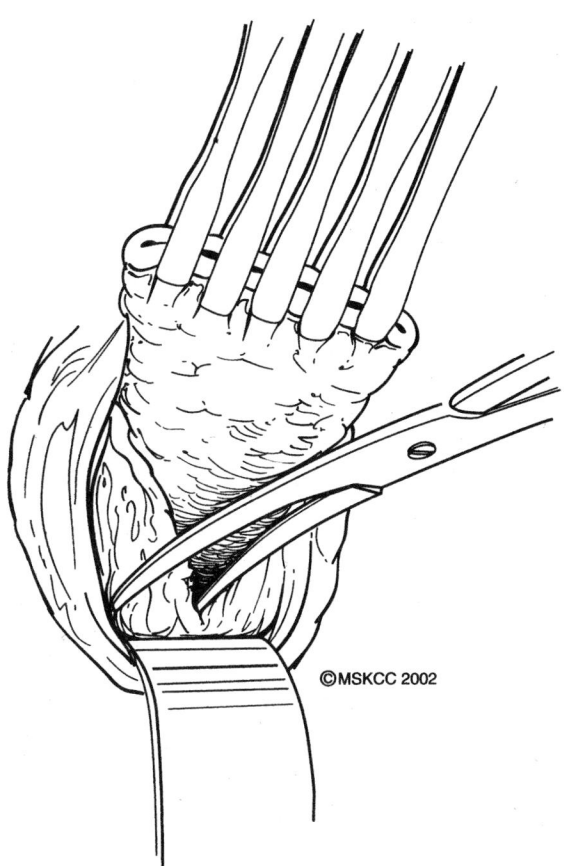

FIG. 18.20. Posterior colpotomy.

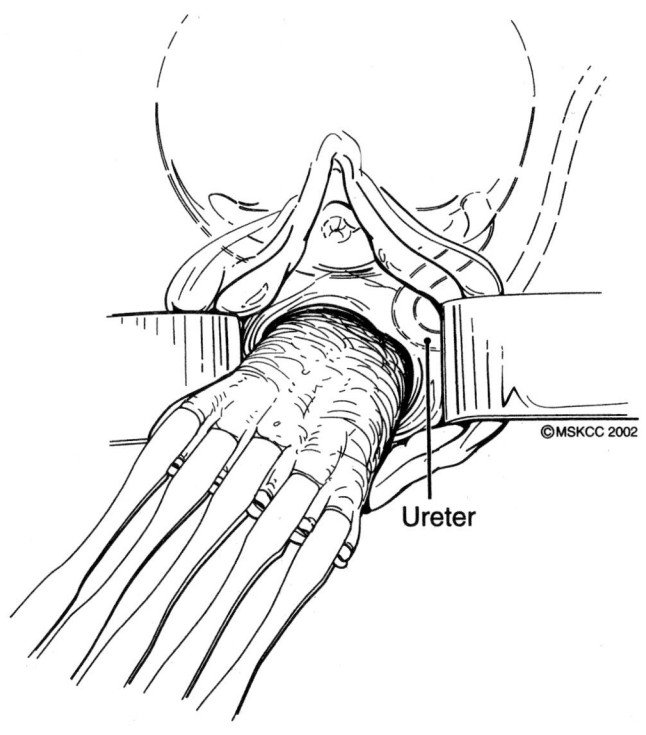

FIG. 18.21. Identifying the ureter.

the scissors perpendicular to the axis of the vagina. This maneuver helps avoid tunneling into the bladder. Once the vesicouterine space is developed, the paravesical spaces must be opened. The left paravesical space is opened by placing two Kocher clamps on the vaginal mucosa at the 1 and 3 o'clock positions. By doing such, a small dimple is noted in between the two Kocher clamps. The Metzenbaum scissors are used to gently spread this dimple, tunnel under the vaginal mucosa, and enter the left paravesical space. The tissue between the paravesical and vesicouterine spaces is the left bladder pillar. The knee of the left ureter can now be palpated in the left bladder pillar (Fig. 18.21).

The inferior aspect of the left bladder pillar can now be transected. This frees the knee of the left ureter and allows it to be pushed superiorly. After doing such, two curved Heaney camps can be placed across the parametrium to obtain an adequate margin. The parametrium is now divided between the two clamps, and the pedicle is secured with a suture ligature. The cervicovaginal branch of the left uterine artery is doubly clamped, divided, and secured with a suture ligature (Fig. 18.22).

The procedures of opening the paravesicle space, dividing the inferior aspect of the bladed pillar, and dividing the parametrium and cervicovaginal branch of the uterine artery are

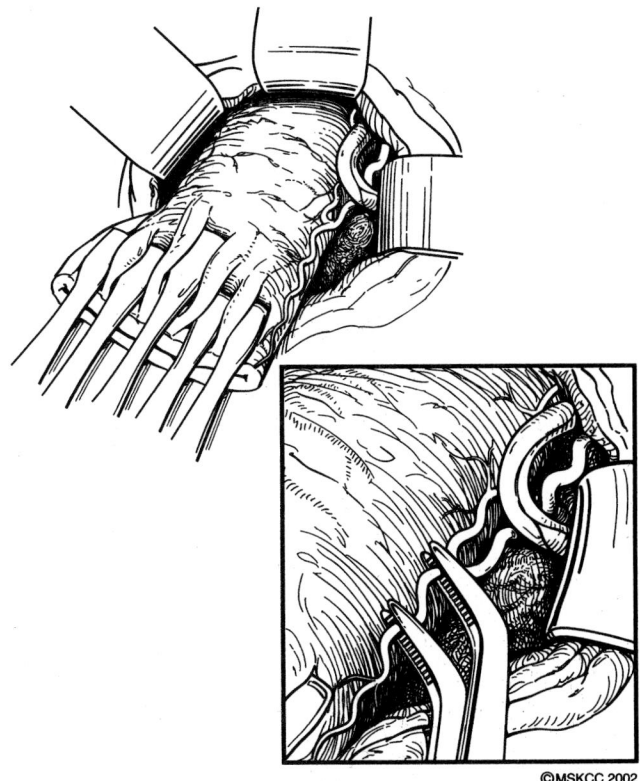

FIG. 18.22. Ligating the paracervical vessels.

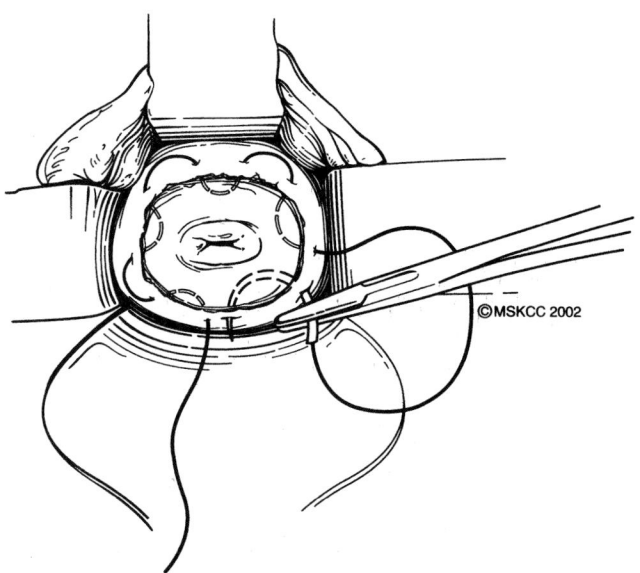

FIG. 18.23. Inserting permanent cerclage.

repeated on the right side. Once the branches of the uterine artery have been secured, the cervix can be amputated. An endocervical and endometrial curettage is performed, and frozen section analysis is performed on the endocervical margin and endocervical/endometrial curettage. It is preferable to leave 1 cm of cervical stump to place a cerclage with a permanent suture (Fig. 18.23).

The vaginal mucosa can now be reapproximated to the cervical stump to complete the vaginal portion of the procedure. Laparoscopy is the final step in the procedure to assure pelvic hemostasis.

Laparoscopic Pelvic Lymphadenectomy with Total Laparoscopic Radical Hysterectomy

The total laparoscopic radical hysterectomy has been the subject of controversy and debate in the gynecologic oncology community. A laparoscopic radical hysterectomy with pelvic and aortic lymph node dissection was first reported by Nezhat et al. in 1992 (213). However, Spirtos is credited for the development, standardization, and popularization of this operation in the United States (186,214). This technically challenging procedure was initially received with caution by gynecologic oncologists, who for decades have utilized the abdominal radical hysterectomy as the traditional approach. No randomized trials are available so far to compare these two surgical approaches; however, more than 150 patients have so far been reported with encouraging results. Comparison to laparotomy was recently reported in a pilot series in which 19 patients were offered the laparoscopic approach and the procedure was completed laparoscopically in 17 patients (89.5%) (173). Two patients, in the beginning of the study, underwent conversion to laparotomy: one because of parametrial bleeding and one because of pelvic adhesions and cystotomy. Mean body mass index was 23.1 (range 18–30) and mean pelvic lymph node count was 25.5 (range 15–39), and one patient (5.3%) had positive nodes. Mean estimated blood loss was 301 mL (range 75–1500 mL) compared to 693 mL in the laparotomy group ($p < .01$), mean operating time was 371 min (range 230–600 min) compared to 295 min in the laparotomy group ($p < .01$), and mean hospital stay was 4.5 days (range 3–11 days) compared to 9.7 days in the laparotomy group ($p < .01$). There were no ureteral injuries or fistula formation, and all patients remain clinically disease free with short follow-up. It appeared from

TABLE 18.7. *Summary of reports on laparoscopic radical hysterectomy and pelvic lymphadenectomy with or without paraaortic aortic lymphadenectomy*

Study (ref)	N[a]	PLN	ORT	EBL	LOS	Complications	Recurrence
Nezhat et al. (213,215)	7	22	315	30–250	2.1	None	None
Sedlacek et al. (216,217)	14	16	420	334	5.5	1 VVF, 1 ureteral injury	–
Ting (218)	4	8	330–480	150–500	–	None	–
Osterzenski (219)	6	–	280	–	2–6	1 hydronephrosis	–
Spirtos et al. (214)	10	18.3	253	300	3.2	None	–
Kim and Moon (220)	18	22	363	619	–	None	–
Hsieh et al. (221)	8	–	–	–	6.5	None	1 distant
Spirtos et al. (186)	78	23.8	205	250	2.9	1.3% transfusion, 3 cystotomies, 1 UVF, 1 DVT, 5 conversion	8(10.3%)
Lee and Huang (222)	12	19.2	235	428	6.8	2 transfusion	None at 1 year
Abu-Rustum et al. (171)	19	25.5	371	301	4.5	1 transfusion, 2 conversion, 1 fever	None

N, number of patients; DVT, deep vein thrombosis; LN, mean pelvic and aortic lymph nodes; ORT, mean operating room time in minutes; HD, mean hospital stay in days; VVF, vesicovaginal fistula; UVF, ureterovaginal fistula.
[a] Some patients may be reported more than once.

these and other data that the total laparoscopic radical hysterectomy with pelvic lymphadenectomy for selected patients with stage I cervical cancer is feasible, safe, and associated with a low morbidity. Estimated blood loss and postoperative hospitalization appear to be shorter than historical controls, at the cost of a longer operating time. The largest series reported so far by Spirtos et al. (186) describes 78 consecutive patients all with early cervical cancer and a Quetelet body mass index <35 who underwent the procedure. In all, 94% of the procedures were completed laparoscopically with an average operative time of 205 minutes and an average blood loss of 225 mL, with only one patient (1.3%) requiring transfusion. There was one ureterovaginal fistula documented. The average lymph node count was 34, with 11.5% of patients having positive lymph nodes. Three patients (3.8%) had close or positive surgical margins and 5.1% have recurred with a minimum of 3-year follow-up.

Table 18.7 (171,186,213–222) summarizes reports on laparoscopic radical hysterectomy with pelvic and aortic lymphadenectomy.

Technique of Total Laparoscopic Radical Hysterectomy with Pelvic Lymphadenectomy

The technique described differs from the laparoscopically assisted vaginal approach in that the entire operation is per-

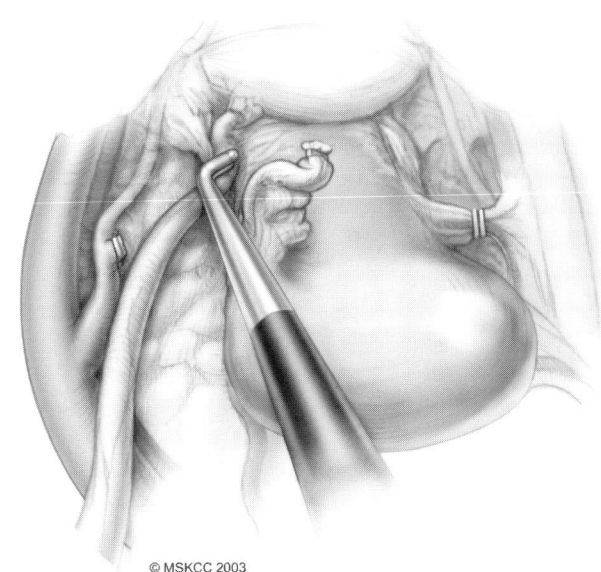

FIG. 18.25. The medial edge of the divided uterine vessels is pulled medially and the ureter is unroofed with the ABC and endoscopic right-angle dissector with clips placed as needed

formed laparoscopically and the only vaginal component to the operation is the removal of the hysterectomy specimen.

Cystourethroscopy and insertion of bilateral temporary ureteral catheters or stents are placed at the surgeon's discretion. In addition, the insertion of a uterine manipulator is optional.

A four-trocar transperitoneal approach was usually used for these procedures. Three accessory 5–12-mm trocars were then placed under direct visualization medial to the iliac crest and in the suprapubic area (173).

A transperitoneal pelvic and paraaortic lymphadenectomy is performed as previously described.

For the total laparoscopic radical hysterectomy, the uterine vessels are stapled with a vascular endoscopic stapler (United States Surgical Corporation, AutoSuture Multifire Endo GIA 30–2.0) at their origin from the hypogastric vessels (Fig. 18.24) or sealed with the endoscopic vessel-sealing system (Ligasure, Valleylab Boulder, CO). The bladder flap is dissected sharply and pushed caudal using the ABC. A vaginal probe (Apple Medical, Marlboro, MA) facilitates the dissection by stretching the vaginal fornix. The medial edge of the divided uterine vessels is then pulled medially and the ureter is unroofed with the ABC, with an endoscopic right-angle dissector with clips being placed as needed (Fig. 18.25). A posterior cul-de-sac peritoneal incision is then made and the rectovaginal septum developed (Fig. 18.26). The uterosacral ligaments are divided or stapled and the remaining parametria and paracolpos is divided (Figs. 18.27 and 18.28). Anterior colpotomy is then performed using the ABC guided by the vaginal probe and the incision extended

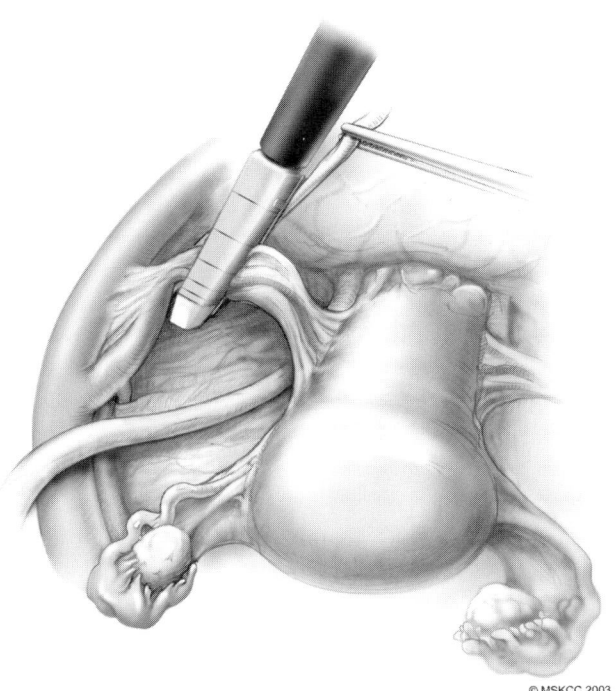

FIG. 18.24. The uterine vessels are stapled with a vascular endoscopic stapler (AutoSuture Multifire Endo GIA 30–2.0; United States Surgical Corporation, Norwalk, CT) at the origin from the hypogastric vessels.

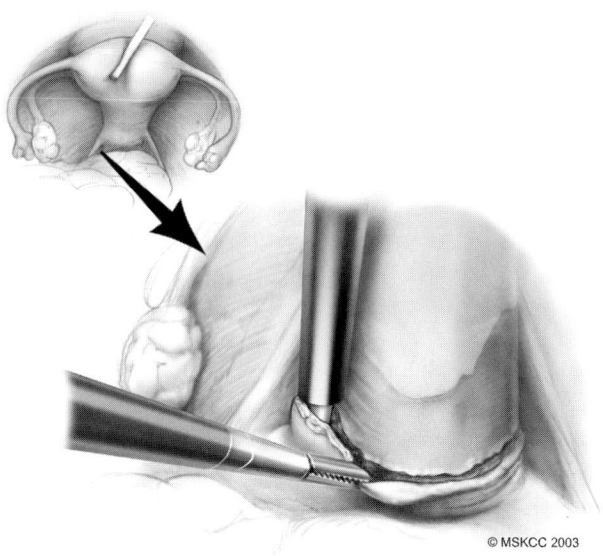

FIG. 18.26. A posterior cul-de-sac peritoneal incision is made with the ABC and the rectovaginal septum is developed.

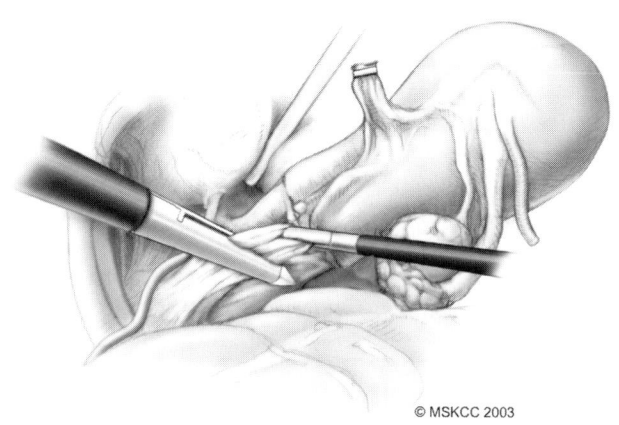

FIG. 18.28. The remaining parametria and paracolpos are divided by the endoscopic stapler.

circumferentially (Figure 18.29). The specimen is removed vaginally. The vaginal cuff is then closed in the anteroposterior posterior direction using the Endostich (United States Surgical Corporation) with absorbable suture in a running manner (Fig. 18.30). The port sites are closed to secure fascia approximation. The ureteral catheters are usually removed at the completion of the operation or prior to discharge.

Laparoscopic Sentinel Lymph Node Detection in Gynecologic Malignancies

Regional lymph node involvement is an important prognostic indicator in patients with a variety of solid tumors. In gynecologic neoplasms, regional lymph node metastasis

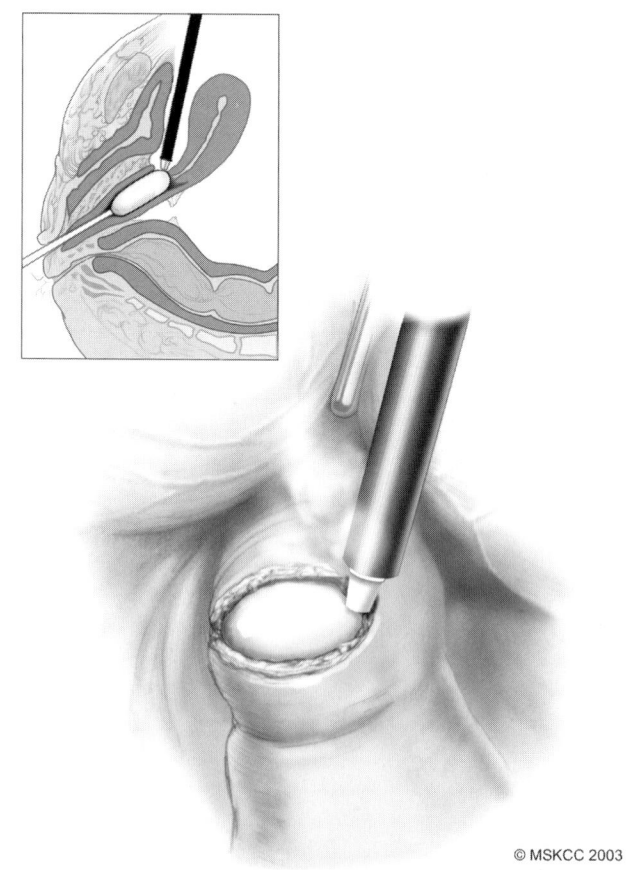

FIG. 18.29. Anterior colpotomy is performed using the ABC, guided by the nonconducting vaginal probe, and the incision extended circumferentially.

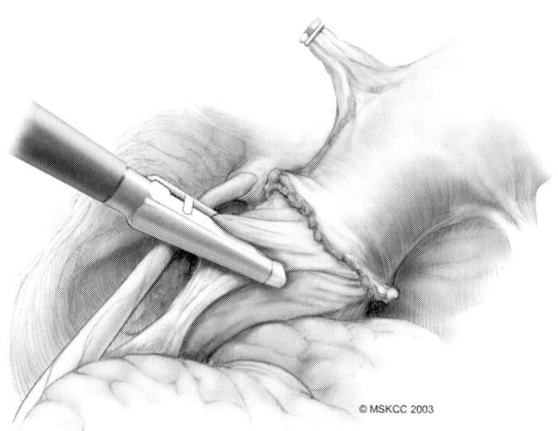

FIG. 18.27. The uterosacral ligaments are divided or stapled.

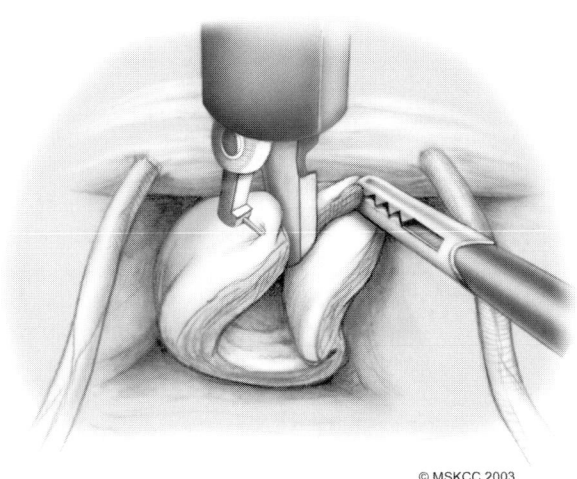

© MSKCC 2003

FIG. 18.30. The vaginal cuff is closed anterior to posterior using the Endostich (United States Surgical Corporation, Norwalk, CT) in a running manner.

TABLE 18.8. *Summary of laparoscopic sentinel lymph node detection in women with cervical cancer*

Study (ref)	No. of patients	Injection technique	Detection rate (%)	False negative (%)
Dargent et al. (223)	35	Blue dye	85	0
Kamprath et al. (224)	18	Radioisotope	89	0
Malur et al. (225)	50 (46 laparoscopic)	Mixed	78	1.6
Barranger et al. (226)	13	Blue dye and radioisotope	92	0
Buist et al. (227)	25	Blue dye and radioisotope	10	11
Lambaudie et al. (228)	12	Blue dye and radioisotope	92	8.3

is a predictor of survival in patients with apparent early cancers of the vulva, cervix, ovary, and uterus. Conventional lymph node dissection in gynecologic malignancies is occasionally associated with considerable morbidity including wound complications, infection, lymphedema, and vascular complications. In addition, the detection of nodal metastasis may dramatically alter the overall oncologic treatment plan, which ultimately may result in an overall improvement in outcome. Delay in delivering the necessary treatment due to complications related to the nodal dissection may be avoided if the necessary information can be obtained with a minimally invasive approach.

Intraoperative lymphatic mapping and sentinel lymph node dissection were designed as a minimally invasive alternative to routine elective lymph node dissection. In patients with primary cutaneous melanoma and breast carcinoma, this has become an acceptable standard of care. However, in gynecologic malignancies, radical resection of vulvar and cervical cancers along with comprehensive lymphadenectomy remains the standard of care. Intraoperative lymphatic mapping and sentinel node identification have the potential to improve the therapeutic index of treatment of patients with gynecologic malignancies, improved detection of lymph node metastases, and reduced surgical morbidity.

Two different approaches are currently used to identify sentinel lymph nodes: lymphatic mapping with dye and lymphoscintigraphy. Sentinel lymph node detection with the combined technique (preoperative lymphoscintigraphy with technetium 99m–labeled colloid and blue dye) appears to result in the highest detection rate in vulvar and cervical cancer. In these tumors, the injection site is more easily accessible, and nodal metastasis commonly follows a stepwise anatomic nodal drainage. Thus, sentinel lymph node identifi-

cation is potentially more feasible. In addition, the utility of novel pathologic techniques such as histopathologic ultrastaging, step sectioning, and immunohistochemistry staining may help increase the accuracy and rate of detection of metastatic disease and possibly alter management.

Table 18.8 (223–228) summarizes results of laparoscopic sentinel lymph node detection in women with cervical cancer.

Sentinel node detection in endometrial cancer is even more challenging since the injection site is potentially variable and access to the endometrial cavity requires either hysteroscopy, laparoscopy, or laparotomy. Recently, laparoscopic sentinel node detection during laparoscopy-assisted vaginal hysterectomy with bilateral salpingo-oophorectomy and bilateral systematic pelvic lymphadenectomy was attempted. Radioactive isotope injection was performed 24 hours before surgery and blue dye injection was performed just before surgery in the cervix at 3, 6, 9, and 12 hours. Sentinel nodes were detected unilaterally and bilaterally in the pelvis in similar frequency. Paraaortic evaluation was not uniformly performed (229). The role of sentinel node detection in ovarian cancer remains undetermined.

Undoubtedly, the detection of the sentinel lymph nodes is one of the significant surgical advances in clinical cancer research, which may have a global and widespread impact on our understanding of tumor spread, overall oncologic care, and patient outcomes.

Robotically Assisted Laparoscopic Surgery

The etymology of the word *robot* is from Czech (*robota*) meaning compulsory labor. The term was first introduced in Karel Capel's play *Rossum's Universal Robots* in Prague in 1921 (230).

Industry has used mechanical robots successfully for fine, delicate, repetitive tasks for decades. Recently, robots have been introduced into clinical medicine and surgery. The initial devices in the 1980s were used for stereotactic biopsies and neurosurgery; however, currently, more advanced systems are routinely being used in cardiac, thoracic, orthopedic, urologic, general, and gynecologic surgery.

Voice activation of some types of equipment in the operating room, such as the laparoscope or the light source, has also become commonly available, and advances in computer software have allowed a computer controller to translate a surgeon's movements from the handles located in a console to the robotic arms that hold the surgical instruments. This remote console may be placed away from the surgical field.

Telerobotic surgery refers to the utilization of a surgical system in which the robot is manipulated by input devices under the surgeon's control and the surgeon may be remote from the operating room. The approved telerobotic devices in the United States that are used in gynecologic surgery are the da Vinci System (Intuitive Surgical, Mountainview, CA) and the Computer Motion AESOP (automated endoscopic system for optimal positioning) system. The ease of accomplishing difficult tasks and the potential advantages over traditional laparoscopy are partly due to the increased number of degrees of freedom, the vividness of the three-dimensional imaging, band filtration with more precision, and less tremor. In addition, the sitting position provides improved ergonomics and comfort by recreating the eye-hand motor axis.

On the other hand, the potential disadvantages of the current models are size and weight, limitation in surgical field, cost, limited trocar and energy source options, and absence of haptics (no sense of force feedback from the instruments).

Animal trials in telerobotic surgery have demonstrated favorable results. Robotic technology has the potential to make laparoscopic microsuturing easier. Robotics has been used to perform uterine horn reanastomosis in a live porcine model, and this application appeared to be safe in creating laparoscopic microsurgical anastomoses with adequate lumen patency rates achieved during the acute phase and at 4-week follow-up (231). In another pilot animal study, the feasibility and safety of using a robotic device, Zeus, to perform complex gynecologic surgery such as adnexectomy and hysterectomy in ten female pigs were undertaken. After 1 week of observation, the animals were sacrificed and the surgical site was explored. The procedures were uneventful and no complications were noted. The researchers concluded that this technology has the potential to be used for more complex gynecologic procedures (232).

Clinical experience in gynecology is limited and there are few published clinical trials. The initial trials have focused on laparoscopic microsuturing such as that performed during coronary bypass surgery or tubal anastomosis. Preliminary results have demonstrated that laparoscopic coronary bypass surgery with the internal mammary artery can be achieved. In an initial study to compare robotic versus human laparoscopic camera control, the AESOP system was utilized in 50 patients undergoing routine gynecologic endoscopic sur-

gical procedures. The elimination of the camera holder allowed two surgeons to perform complex laparoscopic surgery faster than without the robotic arm (233).

Robotic surgery in gynecology appeared to be useful and applicable in performing laparoscopic microsurgical tubal reanastomosis after tubal sterilization. Eight patients with previous laparoscopic tubal sterilization who requested tubal reanastomosis underwent laparoscopic tubal reanastomosis using a remote-controlled robot. The robot, with three-dimensional vision, allows the surgeon to perform ultraprecise manipulations with intraabdominal articulated instruments while providing the necessary degrees of freedom (234). Microsurgical applications in gynecologic general surgery (robotic tubal reanastomosis) appear to be acceptable indications for this technology (235).

Recently, a case series of 11 patients reporting the use of robotic surgery for performing hysterectomy and bilateral salpingo-oophorectomy demonstrated feasibility and safety. Four trocars were used: one for the camera, two for the robotic arms controlled by the operating surgeon from the surgeon's console, and an additional port for use by the surgical assistant. All patients tolerated the procedure and recovered satisfactorily (236). The da Vinci Surgical System has also been used to perform an endoscopic ovarian transposition. The ovaries were mobilized on their respective infundibulopelvic ligaments and sutured to the ipsilateral pericolic gutters (237). Trials and pilot investigations of telerobotic surgery in gynecologic oncology are ongoing, and it appears that its utilization will be limited to applications in which the current device can be used in part of the operation to perform a specific highly precise task such as fine suturing or dissection.

This technology will undoubtedly improve with full integration into new operating room systems, additional degrees of freedom, small-size devices, easier use, and improved optics and surgical instrumentation.

From investigations in nongynecologic applications, it appears that the results of robotic-assisted surgery compare favorably with those of conventional laparoscopy with respect to mortality, complications, and length of stay. Robotic-assisted surgery, in the pilot phase, appears to be safe and effective, and its role in surgery will likely expand as the technology evolves; however, there are currently no data to justify the routine use of these systems in terms of patient outcomes or reduced complications (238).

REFERENCES

1. Rowinky EK. The challenges of developing therapeutics that target signal transduction in patients with gynecological and other malignancies. *J Clin Oncol* 2003;21[10 Suppl]:175–186.
2. Hanahan D, Weinberg RA. The hallmarks of cancer. *Cell* 2000;100: 57–70.
3. Nam N-H, Parang K: Current targets for anticancer drug discovery. *Curr Drug Targets* 2003;4:159–179, 2003.

4. Lane D. The promise of molecular oncology. *Lancet* 1998;351[Suppl 2]:17–20.

5. Oved S, Yarden Y. Signal transduction: molecular ticket to enter cells. *Nature* 2002;416:133–136.

6. Yarden Y, Sliwkowski MX. Untangling the ErbB signalling network. *Nat Rev Mol Cell* Biol. 2001;2:127–137.

7. Hidalgo M, Rowinsky EK. The rapamycin-sensitive signal transduction pathway as a target for cancer therapy. *Oncogene* 2000;19: 6680–6686.

8. Rowinsky EK. Targeting signal transduction: The erbB receptor family as a target for therapeutic development against cancer. In: *Horizons in cancer therapeutics: from bench to bedside.* Meniscus Education Institute, West Conshohocken, PA, 2001:2:3–36.

9. Demetri GD, von Mehren M, Blanke CD, et al. Efficacy and safety of imatinib mesylate in advanced gastrointestinal stromal tumors. *N Engl J Med.* 2002;347:472–480.

10. Kantarjian H, Sawyers C, Hochhaus A, et al. Hematologic and cytogenetic responses to imatinib mesylate in chronic myelogenous leukemia. *N Engl J Med* 2002;346:645–652.

11. Schlessinger. Cell signaling by receptor tyrosine kinases. *Cell* 2000; 103:211–225.

12. Walker RA. The erbB/HER type 1 tyrosine kinase receptor family. *J Pathol* 1998;185:234–235.

13. Simon MA. Receptor tyrosine kinases: specific outcomes from general signals. *Cell* 2000;103:13–15.

14. Daly RJ. Take your partners, please: signal diversification by the erbB family of receptor tyrosine kinases. *Growth Factors* 1999;16: 255–263.

15. Riese DJ II, Stern DF. Specificity within the EGF family/ErbB receptor family signaling network. Bioassays 1998;20:41–48.

16. Olayioye MA, Neve RM, Lane HA, Hynes NE. The ErbB signaling network: receptor heterodimerization in development and cancer. *EMBO J* 2000;19:3159–3167.

17. Riese DJ II, van Raaij TM, Plowman GD, et al. The cellular response to neuregulins is governed by complex interactions of the erbB receptor family. *Mol Cell Biol* 1995;15:5770–5776.

18. Shtiegman K, Yarden Y. The role of ubiquitylation in signaling by growth factors: implications to cancer. *Semin Cancer Biol* 2003;13: 29–40.

19. Baselga J, Albanell J, Molina MA, Arribas J. The ErbB receptor family: a therapeutic target for cancer. *Trends Mol Med* 2002;8[Suppl 4]: S19–S26.

20. Ranson M, Sliwkowski MX. Perspectives on anti-HER monoclonal antibodies. *Oncology* 2002;63[Suppl 1]:17–24.

21. Bookman MA, Darcy KM, Clarke-Pearson D, et al. Evaluation of monoclonal humanized anti-HER2 antibody, trastuzumab, in patients with recurrent or refractory ovarian or primary peritoneal carcinoma with overexpression of HER2: a phase II trial of the Gynecologic Oncology Group. *J Clin Oncol* 2003;21:283–290.

22. Arteaga C. Targeting HER1/EGFR: a molecular approach to cancer therapy. *Semin Oncol.* 2003;30[Suppl 7]:3–14.

23. Arteaga C. Overview of epidermal growth factor receptor biology and its role as a therapeutic target in human neoplasia. *Semin Oncol* 2002; 5[Suppl 14]:3–9.

24. Fry DW. Site-directed irreversible inhibitors of the erbB family of receptor tyrosine kinases as novel chemotherapeutic agents for cancer. *Anticancer Drug Des* 2000;15:3–16.

25. Greenberger LM, Discafani C, Wang Y-F, et al. EKB-569: a new irreversible inhibitor of EGFR tyrosine kinase for the treatment of cancer. *Clin Cancer Res* 2000;6[Suppl]:4544s (abst).

26. Finkler N, Gordon A, Crozier M, et al. Phase 2 evaluation of OSI-774, a potent oral antagonist of the EGFR-TK in patients with advanced ovarian cancer. *Proc Am Soc Clin Oncol* 2001;20:208a(abst).

27. Magee T, Marshall C. New insights into the interaction of Ras with the plasma membrane. *Cell* 1999;98:9–12.

28. Sebolt-Leopold JS. Development of anticancer drugs targeting the MAP kinase pathway *Oncogene* 2000;19:6594–6599.

29. Lopez-Ilasaca M, Crespo P, Pellici PG, et al. Linkage of G protein–coupled receptors to the MAPK signaling pathway through PI3-kinase gamma. *Science* 1997;275:394–397.

30. Lewis TS, Shapiro PS, Ahn NG. Signal transduction through MAP kinase cascades. *Adv Cancer Res* 1998;74:49-139.

31. Ichijo H. From receptor to stress-activated MAP kinases. *Oncogene* 1999;18:6087–6093.

32. Cobb MH. MAP kinase pathways. *Prog Biophys Mol Biol* 1999;71: 479–500.

33. Herrera R, Sebolt-Leopold JS. Unraveling the complexities of the Raf/MAP kinase pathway for pharmacological intervention. *Trends Mol Med* 2002; 8[Suppl 4]:S27–S31.

34. Beerham M, Patnaik A, Rowinsky EK. Regulation of c-Raf-1: therapeutic implications. *Clin Adv Hematol Oncol* 2003;1:476–481.

35. Kolch W, Heidecker G, Kochs G, et al. Protein kinase C α activates RAF-1 by direct phosphorylation. *Nature* 1993;364:249–252.

36. Cronwell MM, Smith DE. A signal transduction pathway for activation of the mdr1 promotor involves the proto-oncogene C-raf kinase. *J Biol Chem* 268:153467–15350, 1993.

37. Phillips F, Mullen P, Monia BP, et al. Association of c-Raf expression with survival and its targeting with antisense oligonucleotides in ovarian cancer. *Br J Cancer* 2001;85:1753–1758.

38. Monia BP, Johnston JF, Geiger T, et al. Antitumor activity of a phosphorothioate antisense oligodeoxynucleotide targeted against C-raf kinase. *Nat Med* 1996:2:668–675.

39. Oza AM, Swenerton K, Faught W, et al.: Phase II study of CGP 69846A (ISIS 5132) in recurrent epithelial ovarian cancer: an NCIC clinical trials group study (NCIC IND.116). *Gynecol Oncol* 2003;89: 129–133.

40. Lyons JF, Wilhelm S, Hibner B, Bollag G. Discovery of a novel raf kinase inhibitor. *Endocr Relat Cancer* 2001;8:219–225.

41. Wilhelm S, Chien DS. BAY 43–9006: preclinical data. *Curr Pharm Des* 2002;8:2255–2257.

42. Sebolt-Leopold JS. Development of anticancer drugs targeting the MAP kinase pathway. *Oncogene* 2000;19:6594–6599.

43. Sebolt-Leopold JS, Dudley DT, Herrera R, et al. Blockade of the MAP kinase pathway supresses growth of colon tumors in vivo. *Nat. Med* 1999;5:810–816.

44. Vivanco I, Sawyers CL: The phosphatidylinositol 3-kinase AKT pathway in human cancer. *Nat Rev Cancer* 2002;2:489–501.

45. Cantley LC. The phosphoinositide 3-kinase pathway. *Science* 2002; 296:1655–1657.

46. Stein RC. Prospects for phosphoinositide 3-kinase inhibition as a cancer treatment. *Endocr Relat Cancer* 2001;8:237–248.

47. Stein RC, Waterfiedl MD: PI3-kinase inhibition: a target for drug development? *Mol Med Today* 2000;6:347–357.

48. Konopka B, Paszko Z, Janiec-Jankowska A, Goluda M. Assessment of the quality and frequency of mutations occurrence in *PTEN* gene in endometrial carcinomas and hyperplasias. *Cancer Lett* 2002;178: 43–51.

49. Chakravarti A, Loeffler JS, Dyson NJ. Insulin-like growth factor receptor I mediates resistance to anti-epidermal growth factor receptor therapy in primary human glioblastoma cells through continued activation of phosphoinositide 3-kinase signaling. *Cancer Res* 2002;62: 200–207.

50. Lu Y, Zi X, Zhao Y, et al. Insulin-like growth factor-I receptor signaling and resistance to trastuzumab (Herceptin). *J Natl Cancer Inst* 2001;19:1852–1857.

51. Schmelzle T, Hall MN. TOR, a central controller of cell growth. *Cell* 2000;13:103:253–262.

52. Rohde J, Heitman J, Cardenas ME. The TOR kinases link nutrient sensing to cell growth. *J Biol Chem.* 2001;276:9583–9586.

53. Podsypanina K, Lee RT, Politis C, et al. An inhibitor of mTOR reduces neoplasia and normalizes p70/S6 kinase activity in Pten +/- mice. *Proc Natl Acad Sci U S A* 2001;98:10320–10325.

54. Neshat MS, Mellinghoff IK, Tran C, et al. Enhanced sensitivity of PTEN-deficient tumors to inhibition of FRAP/mTOR. *Proc Natl Acad Sci U S A* 2001;98:10314–10319.

55. Mita MM, Mita A, Rowinsky EK. Mammalian target of rapamycin: a new molecular target for breast cancer. *Clin Breast Cancer* 2003; 4:126–137.

56. Hockenbery D, Nunez G, Milliman C, et al. Bcl-2 is an inner mitochondrial membrane protein that blocks programmed cell death. *Nature* 1990;348:334.

57. Reed JC. Bcl-2 and the regulation of programmed cell death. *J Cell Biol* 1994;124:1–6.

58. Korsmeyer SJ. Regulators of cell death. *Trends Genet* 1995;11: 101–105.

59. Tsujimoto Y, Finger LR, Yunis J, et al. Cloning of the chromosome breakpoint of neoplastic B cells with the t(14;18) chromosome translocation. *Science* 1984;226:1097–1099.

60. Krajewska M, Krajewski S, Epstein JI, et al. Immunohistochemical analysis of bcl-2, bax, bcl-X, and mcl-1 expression in prostate cancers. *Am J Pathol* 1996;148:1449–1457.

61. Silvestrini R, Veneroni S, Daidone MG, et al. The Bcl-2 protein: a prognostic indicator strongly related to p53 protein in lymph node-negative breast cancer patients. *J Natl Cancer Inst* 1994;86:499–504.

62. Jansen B, Schlagbauer-Wadl H, Brown BD, et al. Bcl-2 antisense therapy chemosensitizes human melanoma in SCID mice. *Nat Med* 1998;4:232–234.

63. Gleave M, Tolcher A, Miyake H, et al. Progression to androgen independence is delayed by adjuvant treatment with antisense Bcl-2 oligodeoxynucleotides after castration in the LNCaP prostate tumor model. *Clin Cancer Res* 1999;5:2891–2898.

64. Haldar S, Chintapalli J, Croce CM. Taxol induces bcl-2 phosphorylation and death of prostate cancer cells. *Cancer Res* 1996;56:1253–1255.

65. Miayake H, Tolcher A, Gleave ME. Chemosensitization and delayed androgen-independent recurrence of prostate cancer with the use of antisense Bcl-2 oligodeoxynucleotides. *J Natl Cancer Inst* 2000;92:34–41.

66. Wang JL, Zhang ZJ, Choksi S, et al. Cell permeable Bcl-2 binding peptides: a chemical approach to apoptosis induction in tumor cells. *Cancer Res* 2000;60:1498–1502.

67. Wang JL, Liu D, Zhang ZJ, et al. Structure-based discovery of an organic compound that binds Bcl-2 protein and induces apoptosis of tumor cells. *Proc Natl Acad Sci U S A* 2000;97:7124–7129.

68. Miyake H, Hara S, Zellweger T, et al. Acquisition of resistance to Fas-mediated apoptosis by overexpression of clusterin in human renal-cell carcinoma cells. *Mol Urol* 2001;5:105–111.

69. Zellweger T, Miyake H, Cooper S, et al. Antitumor activity of antisense clusterin oligonucleotides is improved in vitro and in vivo by incorporation of 2′-O-(2-methoxy)ethyl chemistry. *J Pharmacol Exp Ther* 2001;298:934–940.

70. Li B, Dou QP. Bax degradation by the ubiquitin/proteasome-dependent pathway: involvement in tumor survival and progression. *Proc Natl Acad Sci U S A* 2000;97:3850–3855.

71. Strobel T, Swanson L, Korsmeyer S, et al. BAX enhances paclitaxel-induced apoptosis through a p53-independent pathway. *Proc Natl Acad Sci U S A* 1996;93:14094–14099.

72. Zapata JM, Pawlowski K, Haas E, et al. A diverse family of proteins containing tumor necrosis factor receptor-associated factor domains. *J Biol Chem* 2001;276:24242–24252.

73. Chinnaiyan AM, Tepper CG, Seldin MF, et al. FADD/MORT1 is a common mediator of CD95 (Fas/APO-1) and tumor necrosis factor receptor-induced apoptosis. *J Biol Chem* 1996;271:4961–4965.

74. Chinnaiyan AM, Prasad U, Shankar S, et al. Combined effect of tumor necrosis factor-related apoptosis-inducing ligand and ionizing radiation in breast cancer therapy. *Proc Natl Acad Sci U S A* 2000;97:1754–1759.

75. Pan G, O'Rourke K, Chinnaiyan AM, et al. The receptor for the cytotoxic ligand TRAIL. *Science* 1997;276:111–113.

76. Jiang Y, Woronicz JD, Liu W, Goeddel DV. Prevention of constitutive TNF receptor 1 signaling by silencer of death domains. *Science* 1999;283:543–546.

77. Hinz S, Trauzold A, Boenicke L, et al. Bcl-XL protects pancreatic adenocarcinoma cells against CD95- and TRAIL-receptor–mediated apoptosis. *Oncogene* 2000;19:5477–5486.

78. Munshi A, Pappas G, Honda T, et al. TRAIL (APO-2L) induces apoptosis in human prostate cancer cells that is inhibitable by Bcl-2. *Oncogene* 2001;20:3757–3765.

79. Havell EA, Fiers W, North RJ. The antitumor function of tumor necrosis factor (TNF), I. Therapeutic action of TNF against an established murine sarcoma is indirect, immunologically dependent, and limited by severe toxicity. *J Exp Med* 1998;167:1067–1085.

80. Ashkenazi A, Pai RC, Fong S, et al. Safety and antitumor activity of recombinant soluble Apo2 ligand. *J Clin Invest* 1999;104:155–162.

81. Chinnaiyan AM, Prasad U, Shankar S, et al. Combined effect of tumor necrosis factor-related apoptosis-inducing ligand and ionizing radiation in breast cancer therapy. *Proc Natl Acad Sci U S A* 2000;97:1754–1759.

82. Ogasawara J, Watanabe-Fukunaga R, Adachi M, et al. Lethal effect of the anti-Fas antibody in mice. *Nature* 1993;364:806–809.

83. Walczak H, Miller RE, Ariail K, et al. Tumoricidal activity of tumor necrosis factor-related apoptosis-inducing ligand in vivo. *Nat Med* 1999;5:157–163.

84. Lawrence D, Shahrokh Z, Marsters S, et al. Differential hepatocyte toxicity of recombinant Apo2L/TRAIL versions. *Nat Med* 2001;7:383–385.

85. Chuntharapai A, Dodge K, Grimmer K, et al. Isotype-dependent inhibition of tumor growth in vivo by monoclonal antibodies to death receptor 4. *J Immunol* 2001;166:4891–4898.

86. Ichikawa K, Liu W, Zhao L, Wang Z, et al. Tumoricidal activity of a novel anti-human DR5 monoclonal antibody without hepatocyte cytotoxicity. *Nat Med* 2001;7:954–960.

87. An WG, Schnur RC, Neckers L, Blagosklonny MV. Depletion of p185erbB2, Raf-1 and mutant p53 proteins by geldanamycin derivatives correlates with antiproliferative activity. *Cancer Chemother Pharmacol* 1997;40:60–64.

88. Munster PN, Tong W, Schwartz L, et al. Phase I trial of 17-(allylamino)-17-demethoxygeldanamycin (17-AAG) in patients with advanced solid malignancies. *Proc Am Soc Clin Oncol* 2001;20:327a(abst).

89. Wilson RH, Takimoto CH, Agnew EB, et al. Phase I pharmacologic study of 17-(allylamino)-17-demethoxygeldanamycin (AAG) in adult patients with advanced solid tumors. *Proc Am Soc Clin Oncol* 2001;20:325a(abst).

90. Young JC, Moarefi I, Hart LF. HSP-90: a specialized but essential protein folding tool. *J Cell Biol* 2001;154:267–273.

91. Read MA, Neish AS, Luscinskas RW, et al. The proteasome pathway is required for cytokine-induced endothelial-leukocyte adhesion molecule expression. *Immunity* 1995;2:493–506.

92. Palombella VJ, Rando OJ, Goldberg AL, Maniatis T. The ubiquitin-proteasome pathway is required for processing the NF-κB1 precursor protein and the activation of NF-κB. *Cell* 1994;78:773–785.

93. Cusack JC. Rationale for the treatment of solid tumors with the proteasome inhibitor bortezomib. *Cancer Treat Rev* 2003;1[Suppl]:21–31.

94. Adams J. Potential for proteasome inhibition in the treatment of cancer. *Drug Discov Today* 2003;8:307–315.

95. Brown R, Strathdee G. Epigenomics and epigenetic therapy of cancer. *Trends Mol Med* 2002;8[Suppl]:S43–S48.

96. Marks P, Rifkind RA, Richon VM, et al. Histone deacetylases and cancer: causes and therapies. *Nat Rev Cancer* 2001;1:194–202.

97. Kalebic T. Epigenetic changes: potential therapeutic targets. *Ann N Y Acad Sci* 2003;983:278–285.

98. van Kesteren Ch, de Vooght MM, Lopez-Lazaro L, et al. Yondelis (trabectedin, ET-743): the development of an anticancer agent of marine origin. *Anticancer Drugs* 2003;14:487–502.

99. Garcia-Rocha M, Garcia-Gravalos MD, Avila JL: Characterisation of antimitotic products from marine organisms that disorganise the microtubule network: ecteinascidin 743, isohomohalichondrin and LL-15. *Br J Cancer* 1996;73:875–883.

100. Mantovani R, La Valle E, Bonfanti M, et al. Effect of ET-743 on the interaction between transcription factors and DNA. *Ann Oncol* 1998;9:534a(abst).

101. Scotto KW. ET 743: more than just an innovative mechanism of action. *Anticancer Drugs* 2002;13:S3–S6.

102. D'Incalci M, Colombo T, Ubezio P, et al. The combination of yondelis and cisplatin is synergistic against human tumor xenografts. *Eur J Cancer* 2003;39:1920–1926.

103. Minuzzo M, Marchini S, Broggini M, et al. Interference of transcriptional activation by the antineoplastic drug ecteinascidin-743. *Proc Natl Acad Sci U S A* 2000;97:6780–6784.

104. Colombo N, Capri G, Bauer J, et al. Phase II and pharmacokinetic study of 3-hr infusion of ET-743 in ovarian cancer patients failing platinum-taxanes. *Proc Am Soc Clin Oncol* 2002;21:221a(abst 880).

105. Townsend DM, Shen H, Staros AL, et al. Efficacy of a glutathione S-transferase pi-activated prodrug in platinum-resistant ovarian cancer cells. *Mol Cancer Ther* 2002;1:1089–1095.

106. Rosen LS, Brown J, Laxa B, et al. Phase I study of TLK286 (glutathione S-transferase P1–1 activated glutathione analogue) in advanced refractory solid malignancies. *Clin Cancer Res.* 2003;9:1628–1638.

107. Kavanagh JJ, Spriggs D, Bookman M, et al. Phase 2 study of TLK286 (GSTpi-1 activated glutathione analog) in patients with platinum and

paclitaxel refractory/resistant advanced epithelial ovarian cancer. *Eur J Cancer* 2002:38:A100a(abst).

108. David B, Sevenet T, Morgat M, et al. Rhazinilam mimics the cellular effects of taxol by different mechanisms of action. *Cell Motil Cytoskeleton*. 1994;28:317–326

109. Jordan MA. Mechanism of action of antitumor drugs that interact with microtubules and tubulin. *Curr Med Chem Anticancer Agents* 2002;2:1–17.

110. Kowalski RJ, Giannakakou P, Gunasekera SP, et al. The microtubule-stabilizing agent discodermolide competitively inhibits the binding of paclitaxel (Taxol) to tubulin polymers, enhances tubulin nucleation reactions more potently than paclitaxel, and inhibits the growth of paclitaxel-resistant cells. *Mol Pharmacol* 1997;52:613–622.

111. Martello LA, McDaid HM, Regl DL. Taxol and discodermolide represent a synergistic drug combination in human carcinoma cell lines. *Clin Cancer Res.* 2000;6:1978–1987.

112. Wartmann M, Altmann KH. The biology and medicinal chemistry of epothilones. *Curr Med Chem Anticancer Agents* 2002;2:123–148.

113. Abraham J, Agrawal M, Bakke S, et al. Phase I trial and pharmacokinetic study of BMS-247550, an epothilone B analog, administered intravenously on a daily schedule for five days. *J Clin Oncol* 2003; 21:1866–1873.

114. Verrills NM, Flemming CL, Liu M, et al. Microtubule alterations and mutations induced by desoxyepothilone B: implications for drug-target interactions. *Chem Biol* 2003;10:597–607.

115. Lee FY, Borzilleri R, Fairchild CR, et al. BMS-247550: a novel epothilone analog with a mode of action similar to paclitaxel but possessing superior antitumor efficacy. *Clin Cancer Res* 2001;7:1429–1437.

116. Kaye SB, Oza A, Gore, M. Preliminary results from a phase II trial of EPO906 in patients with advanced refractory ovarian cancer. *Eur J Cancer* 2002;38:127a(abst).

117. Long BH, Carboni JM, Wasserman AJ, et al. Eleutherobin, a novel cytotoxic agent that induces tubulin polymerization, is similar to paclitaxel (Taxol). *Cancer Res* 1998;58:1111–1115.

118. Pryor DE, O'Brate A, Bilcer G, et al. The microtubule stabilizing agent laulimalide does not bind in the taxoid site, kills cells resistant to paclitaxel and epothilones, and may not require its epoxide moiety for activity. *Biochemistry* 2002;41:9109–9115.

119. Ojima I, Chakravarty S, Inoue TA. Common pharmacophore for cytotoxic natural products that stabilize microtubules. *Proc Natl Acad Sci U S A* 1999;96:4256.

120. Vale RD, Milligan RA. The way things move: looking under the hood of molecular motor proteins. *Science* 2000;288:88–95.

121. Goldstein LS, Philip AV. The road less traveled: emerging principles of kinesin motor utilization. *Annu Rev Cell Dev Biol* 1999;15: 141–183.

122. Wood KW, Cornwell WD, Jackson JR. Past and future of the mitotic spindle as an oncology target. *Curr Opin Pharmacol* 2001;4:370–377.

123. Blangy A, Lane HA, d'Herin P, et al. Phosphorylation by p34cdc2 regulates spindle association of human Eg5, a kinesin-related motor essential for bipolar spindle formation in vivo. *Cell* 1995;83: 1159–1169.

124. Chu Q, Holen KD, Rowinsky EK, et al. A phase I study to determine the safety and pharmacokinetics of IV administered SB-715992, a novel kinesin spindle protein (KSP) inhibitor, in patients (pts) with solid tumors. *Proc Am Soc Clin Oncol* 2003;22:131a(abst).

125. Cleaves M. Radium: With a preliminary note on radium rays in the treatment of cancer. *Med Rec* 1903;64:1719–1723.

126. Leibel SA, Fuks Z, Zelefsky MJ: Intensity-modulated radiotherapy. *Cancer J* 2002;8:164–171.

127. Nutting C, Dearnaley DP, Webb S. Intensity modulated radiation therapy: a clinical review. *Br J Radiol* 2000;73:459–466.

128. Mell LK, Roeske JC, Mundt AJ. Survey of intensity modulated radiotherapy use in the United States. *Cancer* 2003;98:204–208.

129. Carmichael M, Murdock J, Rappleye C. "Your next . . . ." *Newsweek,* June 24, 139:64–66, 2002.

130. Brown E. Cancer in the crosshairs. *Forbes,* October 28, 170:351–364, 2002.

131. Teh BS, Mai WY, Augsburger ME, et al. Intensity modulated radiation therapy (IMRT) following prostatectomy: more favorable acute genitourinary toxicity profile compared to primary IMRT for prostate cancer. *Int J Radiat Oncol Biol Phys* 2001;49:465–471.

132. Zelefsky MJ, Fuks Z, Hunt M, et al. High-dose intensity modulated radiation therapy for prostate cancer: early toxicity and biochemical outcome in 772 patients. *Int J Radiat Oncol Biol Phys* 2002;53: 1111–1119.

133. Chao KS, Ozyigit G, Tran BN, et al. Patterns of failure in patients receiving definitive and postoperative IMRT for head-and-neck cancer. *Int J Radiat Oncol Biol Phys* 2003;55:312–319.

134. Eisbruch A, Kim HM, Terrell JE, et al. Xerostomia and its predictors following parotid-sparing irradiation of head-and-neck cancer. *Int J Radiat Oncol Biol Phys* 2001;50:695–672.

135. Perez CA, Breaux S, Bedwinek JM, et al. Radiation therapy alone in the treatment of carcinoma of the uterine cervix. II. Analysis of complications. *Cancer* 1984;54:235–246.

136. Corn BW, Lanciano RM, Greven KM. Impact of improved irradiation technique, age, and lymph node sampling on the severe complication rate of surgically staged endometrial cancer patients: a multivariate analysis. *J Clin Oncol* 1994;12:510–517.

137. Stock RG, Chen AS, Flickinger JC, et al. Node-positive cervical cancer: impact of pelvic irradiation and patterns of failure. *Int J Radiat Oncol Biol Phys* 1995;31:31–36.

138. Mundt AJ, Murphy KT, Rotmensch J, et al. Surgery and postoperative radiation therapy in FIGO Stage IIIC endometrial carcinoma. *Int J Radiat Oncol Biol Phys* 2001;50:1154–1160.

139. Mundt AJ, Roeske JC. Could intensity modulated radiation therapy (IMRT) replace brachytherapy in the treatment of cervical cancer? *Brachytherapy J* 2002;1:195–196.

140. Intensity Modulated Radiation Therapy Collaborative Working Group. Intensity modulated radiotherapy: current status and issues of interest. *Int J Radiat Oncol Biol Phys* 2001;51:880–914.

141. Takahashi S. Conformation radiotherapy. Rotation techniques as applied to radiography and radiotherapy of cancer. *Acta Radiol Diagn (Stockh)* 1965;242:1.

142. Brahme A. Optimization of stationary and moving beam radiation therapy technique. *Radiother Oncol* 1998;12:129.

143. Purdy JA. 3D treatment planning and intensity-modulated radiation therapy. *Oncology* 1999;13:155–168.

144. Roeske JC, Lujan A, Rotmensch J, et al. Intensity-modulated whole pelvic radiation therapy in patients with gynecologic malignancies. *Int J Radiat Oncol Biol Phys* 2000;48:1613–1621.

145. Mundt AJ, Roeske JC, Lujan AE. Intensity modulated radiation therapy in gynecologic malignancies. *Med Dosim* 2002;27:131.

146. Adli M, Mayr NA, Kaiser HS, et al. Does prone positioning reduce small bowel dose in pelvic radiation with intensity-modulated radiotherapy for gynecologic cancer? *Int J Radiat Oncol Biol Phys* 2003; 57:230–238.

147. International Commission on Radiation Units and Measurements (ICRU): Report Number 50: Prescribing, recording, and reporting photon beam therapy. Washington, DC: ICRU; 1993.

148. Mutic S, Malyapa RS, Grigsby PW, et al. PET-guided IMRT for cervical carcinoma with positive para-aortic lymph nodes–a dose-escalation treatment planning study. *Int J Radiat Oncol Biol Phys* 2003;55:28–35.

149. Portelance L, Chao KS, Grigsby PW, et al. Intensity-modulated radiation therapy (IMRT) reduces small bowel, rectum, and bladder doses in patients with cervical cancer receiving pelvic and para-aortic irradiation. *Int J Radiat Oncol Biol Phys* 2001;51:261–266.

150. Garofalo M, Lujan AE, Roeske JC, Mundt AJ: Intensity modulated radiation therapy in the treatment of vulvar carcinoma. Presented at the 88th Annual Meeting of the Radiologic Society of North America, Chicago, December 1–6, 2002.

151. Lujan AE, Mundt AJ, Yamada SD, et al. Intensity-modulated radiation therapy as a means of reducing dose to bone marrow in gynecologic patients receiving whole pelvic radiation therapy. *Int J Radiat Oncol Biol Phys* 2003;57:516–521.

152. Brixey CJ, Roeske JC, Lujan AE, et al. Impact of intensity-modulated radiation therapy on acute hematologic toxicity in women with gynecologic malignancies. *Int J Radiat Oncol Biol Phys* 2002;54: 1388–1396.

153. Roeske JC, Lujan AE, Mundt AJ. Incorporation of SPECT bone marrow imaging into IMRT planning in gynecology patients undergoing IM-WPRT. Presented at the 6th International Conference on Dose, Time and Fractionation. Madison, WI, September 23–26, 2001.

153a. Hong L, Alektiar K, Chui C, et al. IMRT of large fields: whole abdomen irradiation. *Int J Radiat Oncol Biol Phys* 2002;54:278–289.

154. Lujan AE, Mundt AJ, Roeske JC. Sequential versus simultaneous boost in the female pelvis using intensity modulated radiation therapy. Presented at the 43rd Annual Meeting of the American Association of Physicists in Medicine, Salt Lake City, July 22–26, 2001.

155. Kavanagh B, Schefter TE, Wu Q, et al. Clinical application of intensity modulated radiotherapy for locally advanced cervical cancer. *Semin Radiat Oncol* 2002;12:260–271.

156. Pugachev A, Xing L: Computer-assisted selection of coplanar beam orientations in intensity-modulated radiation therapy. *Phys Med Biol* 2001;46:2467.

157. Mundt AJ, Mell LK, Roeske JC. Preliminary analysis of chronic gastrointestinal toxicity in gynecology patients treated with intensity modulated whole pelvic radiation therapy. *Int J Radiat Oncol Biol Phys* 2003;56:1354–1360.

158. Roeske JC, Bonta D, Lujan AE, Mundt AJ: Dose volume histogram analysis of acute gastrointestinal toxicity in gynecologic patients undergoing intensity modulated whole pelvic radiation therapy. Radiother Oncol *(in press)*.

159. Chen Q, Izadifar S, King S. Comparison of IMRT with 3-D CRT for gynecologic malignancies. *Int J Radiat Oncol Biol Phys* 2001;51: 332a(abst).

160. Selvaraj RN, Gerszten K, King GC. Conventional 3D versus intensity modulated radiotherapy for adjuvant treatment of gynecologic malignancies: a comparative study of dose-volume histograms and the potential impact on toxicities. *Int J Radiat Oncol Biol Phys* 2001;51: 218a(abst).

161. Ahamad A, D'Souza W, Salehpour M. Intensity modulated radiation therapy for post-hysterectomy pelvic radiation: selection of patients and planning target volume. *Int J Radiat Oncol Biol Phys* 2002;54: 42a(abst).

162. Gilroy JS, Amdur RJ, Louis DA. Irradiating the inguinal nodes without breaking a leg. *Int J Radiat Oncol Biol Phys* 2002;54;68a(abst).

163. Schefter TE, Kavanagh BD, Wu Q. Technical considerations in the application of intensity-modulated radiotherapy as a concomitant integrated boost for locally advanced cervix cancer. *Med Dosim* 2002; 27:177a(abst).

164. Alektiar K. Could intensity modulated radiation therapy (IMRT) replace brachytherapy in the treatment of cervical cancer? *Brachytherapy J* 2002;1:194–195.

165. Roeske JC, Mundt AJ: A feasibility study of IMRT for the treatment of cervical cancer patients unable to receive intracavitary brachytherapy. *Med Phys* 2000;27:1382–1383.

166. Low DA, Grigsby PW, Dempsey JF, et al. Applicator-guided intensity modulated radiation therapy. *Int J Radiat Oncol Biol Phys* 2002;52: 1400–1406.

167. Mundt AJ, Roeske JC, Lujan AE, et al. Initial clinical experience with intensity-modulated whole pelvis radiation therapy in women with gynecologic malignancies. *Gynecol Oncol* 2001;456–463.

168. Mundt AJ, Lujan AE, Rotmensch J, et al. Intensity-modulated whole pelvic radiotherapy in women with gynecologic malignancies. *Int J Radiat Oncol Biol Phys* 2002;52:1330–1337.

169. Hall EJ, Wuu CS. Radiation-induced second cancer: the impact of 3D-CRT and IMRT. *Int J Radiat Oncol Biol Phys* 2003;56:83.

170. Dargent D. A new future for Schauta's operation through presurgical retroperitoneal pelviscopy. *Eur J Gynaecol Oncol* 1987;8:292–296.

171. Abu-Rustum NR, Gemignani ML, Moore K, et al. Total laparoscopic radical hysterectomy with pelvic lymphadenectomy using the argon-beam coagulator: pilot data and comparison to laparotomy. *Gynecol Oncol.* 2003;91:402–409.

172. Querleu D, Leblanc E, Castelain B. Laparoscopic pelvic lymphadenectomy in the staging of early carcinoma of the cervix. *Am J Obstet Gynecol* 1991;164:579–581.

173. Abu-Rustum NR, Chi DS, Sonoda Y, et al. Transperitoneal laparoscopic pelvic and para-aortic lymph node dissection using the argon-beam coagulator and monopolar instruments: an 8-year study and description of technique. *Gynecol Oncol.* 2003;89:504–513.

174. Childers JM, Hatch K, Surwit EA. The role of laparoscopic lymphadenectomy in the management of cervical carcinoma. *Gynecol Oncol.* 1992;47:38–43.

175. Chu KK, Chang SD, Chen FP, Soong YK. Laparoscopic surgical staging in cervical cancer—preliminary experience among Chinese. *Gynecol Oncol* 1997;64:49–53.

176. Vergote I, Amant F, Berteloot P, Van Gramberen M. Laparoscopic lower para-aortic staging lymphadenectomy in stage IB2, II, and III cervical cancer. *Int J Gynecol Cancer* 2002;12:22–26.

177. Spirtos NM, Schlaerth JB, Spirtos TW, et al. Laparoscopic bilateral pelvic and para-aortic lymph node sampling: an evolving technique. *Am J Obstet Gynecol* 1995;173:105–111.

178. Su TH, Wang KG, Yang YC, et al. Laparoscopic para-aortic lymph node sampling in the staging of invasive cervical carcinoma: including a comparative study of 21 laparotomy cases. *Int J Gynaecol Obstet* 1995;49:311–318.

179. Possover M, Krause N, Plaul K, et al. Laparoscopic para-aortic and pelvic lymphadenectomy: experience with 150 patients and review of the literature. *Gynecol Oncol* 1998;71:19–28.

180. Vidaurreta J, Bermudez A, di Paola G, Sardi J. Laparoscopic staging in locally advanced cervical carcinoma: a new possible philosophy? *Gynecol Oncol* 1999;75:366–371.

181. Dottino PR, Tobias DH, Beddoe A, et al. Laparoscopic lymphadenectomy for gynecologic malignancies. *Gynecol Oncol* 1999;73: 383–388.

182. Querleu D, Dargent D, Ansquer Y, et al. Extraperitoneal endosurgical aortic and common iliac dissection in the staging of bulky or advanced cervical carcinomas. *Cancer* 2000;88:1883–1891.

183. Altgassen C, Possover M, Krause N, et al. Establishing a new technique of laparoscopic pelvic and para-aortic lymphadenectomy. *Obstet Gynecol* 2000;95:348–352.

184. Scribner DR Jr, Walker JL, Johnson GA, et al. Laparoscopic pelvic and para-aortic lymph node dissection: analysis of the first 100 cases. *Gynecol Oncol* 2001;82:498–503.

185. Schlaerth JB, Spirtos NM, Carson LF, et al. Laparoscopic retroperitoneal lymphadenectomy followed by immediate laparotomy in women with cervical cancer: a gynecologic oncology group study *Gynecol Oncol* 2002;85:81–88.

186. Spirtos NM, Eisenkop SM, Schlaerth JB, Ballon SC. Laparoscopic radical hysterectomy (type III) with aortic and pelvic lymphadenectomy in patients with stage I cervical cancer: surgical morbidity and intermediate follow-up. *Am J Obstet Gynecol* 2002;187:340–348.

187. Dargent D, Mathevet P. Schauta's vaginal hysterectomy combined with laparoscopic lymphadenectomy. *Baillieres Clin Obstet Gynaecol* 1995;9:691–705.

188. Hertel H, Kohler C, Michels W, et al. Laparoscopic-assisted radical vaginal hysterectomy (LARVH): prospective evaluation of 200 patients with cervical cancer. *Gynecol Oncol* 2003;90:503–504.

189. Querleu D. Laparoscopically assisted radical vaginal hysterectomy. *Gynecol Oncol.* 1993;51:248–254.

190. Kadar N. Laparoscopic vaginal radical hysterectomy: an operative technique and its evolution. *Gynaecol Endosc* 1994;3:109–122.

191. Garza-Leal J. Vaginally assisted laparoscopic radical hysterectomy in Mexico. *J Am Assoc Gynecol Laparosc* 1994;1[4, Part 2]:S12.

192. Roy M, Plante M, Renaud MC, Tetu B. Vaginal radical hysterectomy versus abdominal radical hysterectomy in the treatment of early-stage cervical cancer. *Gynecol Oncol.* 1996;62:336–339.

193. Primicero M, Montanino-Oliva M, Casa A, Cirese E. Laparoscopic lymphadenectomy and vaginal radical hysterectomy for the treatment of cervical cancer. *J Am Assoc Gynecol Laparosc* 1996;3[Suppl]: S40–S41.

194. Schneider A, Possover M, Kamprath S, et al. Laparoscopy-assisted radical vaginal hysterectomy modified according to Schauta-Stoeckel. *Obstet Gynecol* 1996;88:1057–1060.

195. Hatch KD, Hallum AV 3rd, Nour M. New surgical approaches to treatment of cervical cancer. *J Natl Cancer Inst Monogr* 1996;21: 71–75.

196. Sardi J, Vidaurreta J, Bermudez A, di Paola G. Laparoscopically assisted Schauta operation: learning experience at the Gynecologic Oncology Unit, Buenos Aires University Hospital. *Gynecol Oncol* 1999; 75:361–365.

197. Renaud MC, Plante M, Roy M. Combined laparoscopic and vaginal radical surgery in cervical cancer. *Gynecol Oncol* 2000;79:59–63.

198. Querleu D, Narducci F, Poulard V, et al. Modified radical vaginal hysterectomy with or without laparoscopic nerve-sparing dissection: a comparative study. *Gynecol Oncol* 2002;85:154–158.

199. Park CT, Lim KT, Chung HW, et al. Clinical evaluation of laparoscopic-assisted radical vaginal hysterectomy with pelvic and/or paraaortic lymphadenectomy. *J Am Assoc Gynecol Laparosc* 2002;9: 49–53.

200. Aburel E. Sub-corporeal extended colpohysterectomy in therapy of incipient cancer of cervix. *C R Soc Fr Gynecol* 1957;27:237–243.

201. Aburel E. Proceedings: Extended abdominal exstirpation of cervix and isthmus in early stages of cervix carcinoma (carcinoma in situ and microcarcinoma). *Arch Gynakol* 1973;214:106–108.

202. Dargent D, Brun JL, Roy M, Remy I. Pregnancies following radical trachelectomy for invasive cervical cancer. *Gynecol Oncol* 1994;52: 105a(abst).

203. Martin XJ, Golfier F, Romestaing P, Raudrant D. First case of pregnancy after radical trachelectomy and pelvic irradiation. *Gynecol Oncol* 1999;74:286–287.

204. Roy M, Plante M. Pregnancies after radical vaginal trachelectomy for early-stage cervical cancer. *Am J Obstet Gynecol* 1998;179[6 Pt 1]: 1491–1496.

205. Dargent D, Franzosi F, Ansquer Y, et al. Extended trachelectomy relapse: plea for patient involvement in the medical decision. *Bull Cancer* 2002;89:1027–1030.

206. Shepherd JH, Crawford RA, Oram DH. Radical trachelectomy: a way to preserve fertility in the treatment of early cervical cancer. *Br J Obstet Gynaecol* 1998;105:912–916.

207. Covens A, Shaw P, Murphy J, et al. Is radical trachelectomy a safe alternative to radical hysterectomy for patients with stage IA-B carcinoma of the cervix? *Cancer* 1999;86:2273–2279.

208. Dargent D, Martin X, Sacchetoni A, Mathevet P. Laparoscopic vaginal radical trachelectomy: a treatment to preserve the fertility of cervical carcinoma patients. *Cancer* 2000;88:1877–1882.

209. Shepherd JH, Mould T, Oram DH. Radical trachelectomy in early stage carcinoma of the cervix: outcome as judged by recurrence and fertility rates. *Br J Obstet Gynaecol* 2001;108:882–885.

210. Covens A. Preserving fertility in early cervical cancer with radical trachelectomy. *Contemp OB/GYN* 2003; Feb:48–66.

211. Schlaerth JB, Spirtos NM, Schlaerth AC. Radical trachelectomy and pelvic lymphadenectomy with uterine preservation in the treatment of cervical cancer. *Am J Obstet Gynecol* 2003;188:29–34.

212. Burnett AF, Roman LD, O'Meara AT, Morrow CP. Radical vaginal trachelectomy and pelvic lymphadenectomy for preservation of fertility in early cervical carcinoma. *Gynecol Oncol* 2003;88:419–423.

213. Nezhat CR, Burrell MO, Nezhat FR, et al. Laparoscopic radical hysterectomy with paraaortic and pelvic node dissection. *Am J Obstet Gynecol* 1992;166:864–865.

214. Spirtos NM, Schlaerth JB, Kimball RE, et al. Laparoscopic radical hysterectomy (type III) with aortic and pelvic lymphadenectomy. *Am J Obstet Gynecol* 1996;174:1763–1767.

215. Nezhat CR, Nezhat FR, Burrell MO, et al. Laparoscopic radical hysterectomy and laparoscopically assisted vaginal radical hysterectomy with pelvic and paraaortic node dissection. *J Gynecol Surg* 1993;9: 105–120.

216. Sedlacek TV, Campion MJ, Hutchins RA, Reich H. Laparoscopic radical hysterectomy: a preliminary report. *J Am Assoc Gynecol Laparosc* 1994;1[4 Pt 2]):S32.

217. Sedlacek TV, Campion MJ, Reich H, Sedlacek T. Laparoscopic radical hysterectomy: a feasibility study. *Gynecol Oncol* 1995;56: 126a(abst).

218. Ting HC. Laparoscopic radical hysterectomy: a preliminary experience. *J Am Assoc Gynecol Laparosc* 1994;1[4 Pt 2]):S36.

219. Ostrzenski A. A new laparoscopic abdominal radical hysterectomy: a pilot phase trial. *Eur J Surg Oncol* 1996;22:602–606.

220. Kim DH, Moon JS. Laparoscopic radical hysterectomy with pelvic lymphadenectomy for early, invasive cervical carcinoma. *J Am Assoc Gynecol Laparosc* 1998;5:411–417.

221. Hsieh YY, Lin WC, Chang CC, et al. Laparoscopic radical hysterectomy with low paraaortic, subaortic and pelvic lymphadenectomy. Results of short-term follow-up. *J Reprod Med* 1998;43:528–534.

222. Lee CL, Huang KG. Total laparoscopic radical hysterectomy using Lee-Huang portal and McCartney transvaginal tube. *J Am Assoc Gynecol Laparosc* 2002;9:536–540.

223. Dargent D, Martin X, Mathevet P. Laparoscopic assessment of the sentinel lymph node in early stage cervical cancer. *Gynecol Oncol* 2000;79:411–415.

224. Kamprath S, Possover M, Schneider A. Laparoscopic sentinel lymph node detection in patients with cervical cancer. *Am J Obstet Gynecol* 2000;182:1648.

225. Malur S, Krause N, Kohler C, Schneider A. Sentinel lymph node detection in patients with cervical cancer. *Gynecol Oncol* 2001;80: 254–257.

226. Barranger E, Grahek D, Cortez A, et al. Laparoscopic sentinel lymph node procedure using a combination of patent blue and radioisotope in women with cervical carcinoma. *Cancer* 2003;97:3003–3009.

227. Buist MR, Pijpers RJ, van Lingen A, et al. Laparoscopic detection of sentinel lymph nodes followed by lymph node dissection in patients with early stage cervical cancer. *Gynecol Oncol* 2003;90:290–296.

228. Lambaudie E, Collinet P, Narducci F, et al. Laparoscopic identification of sentinel lymph nodes in early stage cervical cancer: prospective study using a combination of patent blue dye injection and technetium radiocolloid injection.*Gynecol Oncol* 2003;89:84–87.

229. Pelosi E, Arena V, Baudino B, et al. Preliminary study of sentinel node identification with 99mTc colloid and blue dye in patients with endometrial cancer. *Tumori* 2002;88:S9–S10.

230. Bann S, Khan M, Hernandez J, et al. Robotics in surgery. *J Am Coll Surg* 2003;196:784–795.

231. Margossian H, Garcia-Ruiz A, Falcone T, et al. Robotically assisted laparoscopic microsurgical uterine horn anastomosis. *Fertil Steril* 1998;70:530–534.

232. Margossian H, Falcone T. Robotically assisted laparoscopic hysterectomy and adnexal surgery. *J Laparoendosc Adv Surg Tech A* 2001; 11:161–165.

233. Mettler L, Ibrahim M, Jonat W. One year of experience working with the aid of a robotic assistant (the voice-controlled optic holder AESOP) in gynaecological endoscopic surgery. *Hum Reprod* 1998; 13:2748–2750.

234. Degueldre M, Vandromme J, Huong PT, Cadiere GB. Robotically assisted laparoscopic microsurgical tubal reanastomosis: a feasibility study. *Fertil Steril* 2000;74:1020–1023

235. Falcone T, Steiner CP. Robotically assisted gynaecological surgery. *Hum Fertil (Camb)* 2002;5:72–74.

236. Diaz-Arrastia C, Jurnalov C, Gomez G, Townsend C Jr. Laparoscopic hysterectomy using a computer-enhanced surgical robot. *Surg Endosc* 2002;16:1271–1273.

237. Molpus KL, Wedergren JS, Carlson MA. Robotically assisted endoscopic ovarian transposition. *JSLS* 2003;7:59–62.

238. Talamini MA. Robotic surgery: is it for you? *Adv Surg* 2002;36:1–13.

Disease Sites

CHAPTER 19

Pathogenesis and Diagnosis of Preinvasive Lesions of the Lower Genital Tract

Thomas C. Wright, Jr.

The high level of public and professional interest in various aspects of preinvasive lesions of the lower genital tract is due to many factors. Perhaps the most important is the marked increase over the last four decades in the number of patients in North America and Western Europe diagnosed with human papillomavirus (HPV)–associated disease. This increase is partly due to a heightened awareness of various clinical and pathologic manifestations of HPV infections and to the increased use of highly sensitive tests for the detection of HPV infections and cervical cancer precursors. In addition, a real increase in the prevalence of HPV infections appears to have taken place during this time.

HPV-associated genital tract disease is now the most commonly diagnosed sexually transmitted disease in the United States. Data compiled as part of the National Disease and Therapeutic Index, a national survey of office-based private practitioners, indicate that initial office visits for genital warts increased from approximately 60,000 in 1966 to almost 360,000 in 1986. However, the number of new cases has dropped in the United States over the last decade. In 1996, there were slightly under 200,000 initial visits for genital warts (Fig. 19.1) (1). It has been suggested that these numbers reflect only a small percentage of the total numbers of HPV cases, and that the prevalence of condyloma acuminatum in the United States among sexually active men and women between the ages of 15 and 49 years is 1.4 million cases (2).

Cervical cancer precursors also appear to have increased in prevalence over the last two decades in the United States and Western Europe. An increase in the incidence of high-grade cervical cancer precursors began to be detected in the early 1980s in white women under the age of 50 years in the United States according to the National Cancer Institute's Surveillance, Epidemiology, and End Results (SEER) program (3). In 1980, the incidence of carcinoma *in situ* of the cervix in white women under the age of 50 years was 27 per 100,000; by 1990, it had increased to 45 per 100,000 women. Currently, approximately 7% of all Papanicolaou (Pap) smears from the United States are diagnosed as having a cytologic abnormality, with wide variations depending on the characteristics of the population screened and the particular cytology laboratory being used (4). It has been estimated that approximately 1,100,000 women receive a cytologic result of low-grade cervical cancer precursors each year in the United States and another 2,750,000 have equivocal cytologic changes referred to as atypical squamous cells (5).

DEFINITIONS AND TERMINOLOGY OF PREINVASIVE LESIONS OF THE LOWER GENITAL TRACT

The terminology used to classify preinvasive lesions of the lower genital tract has changed many times over the last 50 years and is continuing to do so. Unfortunately, these changes, and the lack of a uniform terminology, have been an ongoing source of confusion for the clinician. Despite recent attempts to simplify the classification and make the terminology more uniform, as much controversy exists today as existed 30 years ago regarding the appropriate definitions of preinvasive lesions of the lower genital tract.

Cervix

Squamous Lesions

For more than a century, it has been recognized that invasive squamous cell carcinomas of the cervix are associated

Thomas C. Wright, Jr.: Division of Gynecological and Obstetrical Pathology, College of Physicians and Surgeons of Columbia University, New York, New York 10032

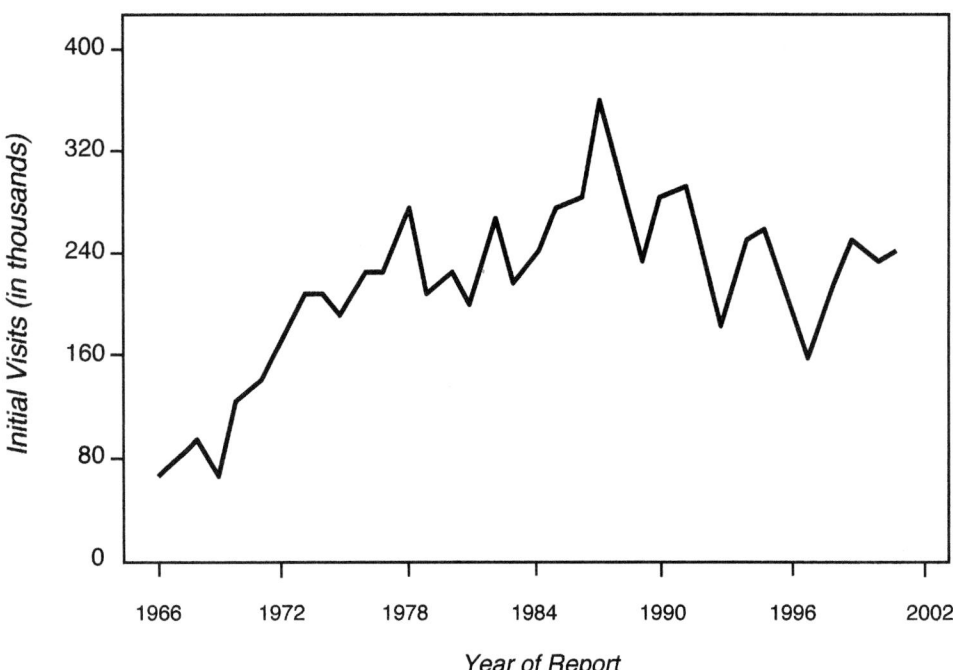

FIG. 19.1. Initial visits for genital warts in the United States. The graph represents the number of initial visits for genital warts to physicians' offices in the United States from 1966 to 2002. (Data are derived from the National Disease and Therapeutic Index.)

with lesions histologically and cytologically identical to invasive cervical carcinoma but that lack the capacity to invade the subepithelial stroma. Because of their unique spatial and temporal relationships with cervical cancer, these intraepithelial lesions were referred to as carcinoma *in situ*.

The spatial relationship between carcinoma *in situ* and invasive cancer was first mentioned by Sir John Williams in 1886 and subsequently by Cullen, Shauenstein, and Rubin, who remarked on the histologic features of the epithelium adjacent to invasive cervical carcinomas and suggested that these changes might represent a precursor lesion (6). The term *carcinoma in situ* was introduced by Schottlander and Kermauner to emphasize that the nonepithelial component probably represented the origin of the invasive component. The temporal relationship between carcinoma *in situ* and invasive cancer was identified by Smith and Pemberton, who observed that carcinoma *in situ* could precede the development of invasive cervical cancer by months or years. This temporal relationship was subsequently confirmed by others. The hypothesis that cervical cancer develops from preinvasive precursor lesions suggested that the development of cervical cancer could be prevented by the detection and treatment of precursor lesions, and formed the basis for the development of cytologic screening tests for cervical cancer. Carcinoma *in situ* was considered to be a highly significant lesion by most clinicians, and patients with this diagnosis were generally treated by hysterectomy. A definition for carcinoma *in situ* was formalized in exceptionally narrow terms in 1961 at the First International Conference on Exfoliative Cytology. Carcinoma *in situ* was defined as an epithelial lesion that "in the absence of invasion shows a surface lining

epithelium in which throughout its whole thickness no differentiation takes place" (7).

As exfoliative cytology came into widespread use for the detection of cervical cancer and carcinoma *in situ*, it became apparent that a wide spectrum of epithelial abnormalities of the cervix existed. These ranged from lesions in which the majority of the cells had the cytologic features of carcinoma *in situ* to lesions in which the extent and degree of atypia were much less. Cervical lesions that had features between those of normal cervical epithelium and carcinoma *in situ* were designated as *dysplasia* by Reagan and Hamonic in 1956 (8). The term *dysplasia* actually means an "abnormality of growth and development," and it was used to designate a proliferation of cytologically abnormal cells that superficially resemble those of the basal level of the epithelium but that also show nuclear atypia, changes in the nuclear-cytoplasmic ratio, and loss of normal polarity. Depending on the degree and thickness of the epithelial changes, dysplasia was frequently subdivided into mild, moderate, and severe forms; it was believed that these subdivisions reflected the relative potential of the lesions for developing into invasive carcinomas. Histologically, a key distinguishing feature of dysplasia was that the atypical cells did not extend through the full thickness of the epithelium or invade the basement membrane. In addition to the term *dysplasia*, lesions with this histology have been termed *basal cell hyperactivity* and *atypical hyperplasia*. Clinically, the importance of dysplasia was that it was considered to be a potentially reversible process. Dysplastic lesions were either ignored, followed, or treated depending on the views of the treating physician.

This initial classification of cervical cancer precursors was based solely on histology, and the histologic differences between dysplasia and carcinoma *in situ* were often quite subtle. Sometimes the only histologic difference between a severely dysplastic lesion and carcinoma *in situ* was the presence or absence of a single layer of flattened cells at the surface of the cervical epithelium. In several studies, it was demonstrated that pathologists could not reproducibly distinguish between severe dysplasia and carcinoma *in situ* (9). This led to the argument that the marked difference in the clinical management of the two types of lesions was inappropriate and that a classification of cervical cancer precursors based solely on histologic criteria should be abandoned (10). This line of reasoning fostered studies designed to characterize the biologic and pathologic parameters of different types of cervical cancer precursors and to determine the behavior of the different types of precursors during long-term follow-up.

In descriptive studies that used a variety of techniques to measure DNA synthesis (including electron microscopy, tissue culture, chromosome analysis, DNA ploidy analysis, and radioautography), it was reported that dysplastic lesions, carcinoma *in situ*, and invasive carcinoma formed a continuum rather than a series of discrete steps. In 1973, based on follow-up studies of patients with cervical cancer precursor lesions and studies of the biology of these lesions, Richart proposed that the term *cervical intraepithelial neoplasia* (CIN) be used to encompass all forms of cervical cancer precursor lesions, including dysplasia and carcinoma *in situ* (11). The CIN terminology divided cervical cancer precursor lesions into three groups or grades. CIN 1 corresponded to mild dysplasia, and CIN 2 corresponded to moderate dysplasia. Since studies had shown that pathologists could not reproducibly distinguish between severe dysplasia and carcinoma *in situ*, CIN 3 encompassed both of these lesions (9). The CIN terminology stressed the concept that all cervical cancer precursors formed a continuum and that lesions of all grades of severity had the potential to progress to invasive cancer if left untreated. Since the risk for progression of any individual lesion is unknown (i.e., by light microscopy it is impossible to categorize the lesions as to which will persist or progress), the CIN terminology emphasized that all ''precursor'' lesions should be treated. Inherent in this reasoning was the acknowledgment that appropriate treatment and eradication of precursors (irrespective of their histologic grade) eliminate or greatly reduce a patient's risk for subsequent development of invasive cervical cancer.

The CIN terminology provided information in a context that made approaches to clinical management straightforward and became the most widely used terminology for cervical cancer precursors. However, over the last 15 years, tremendous advances in our understanding of the pathogenesis of cervical cancer precursors have taken place. These advances have changed both our pathologic nomenclature and our approach to clinical management of cervical cancer precursor lesions. It is now clear that the CIN (continuum)

concept of cervical cancer precursor has certain limitations. For example, the spectrum of histologic changes grouped together as CIN is now recognized to represent two distinct biologic entities. One entity is a productive HPV infection rather than a neoplasm or cancer precursor. The characteristic histologic feature of a productive HPV infection is the presence of HPV cytopathic effect (e.g., koilocytosis with multinucleation, perinuclear halos, nuclear enlargement, and nuclear atypia). These productive HPV infections can be associated with any HPV type including ''low– or no–''oncogenic risk HPVs as well as ''high''–oncogenic risk HPV types. The other HPV-associated biologic entity should be considered to be an actual neoplasm or cancer precursor rather than simply a productive viral infection. These neoplasms, or ''true precursors,'' are invariably monoclonal and are usually associated with ''high-risk'' HPV types such as 16, 18, 31, 33, 35, 39, 45, 51, or 56. These lesions are also frequently aneuploid and often demonstrate specific loss of heterozygosity (LOH) at chromosomal loci that are observed in invasive cervical cancers (12,13).

These advances in our understanding of the biology of preinvasive lesions of the cervix have led to suggestions that the terminology used to refer to cervical cancer precursors be modified (14). The proposed terminologies abolish the three-tiered CIN 1, 2, and 3 classification and replace it with a two-tiered classification. To allow histopathologic findings to be easily correlated with cytologic findings, one of the proposed classifications follows that of the Bethesda System for cytologic diagnosis that uses the terms *high-grade squamous intraepithelial lesion* and *low-grade squamous intraepithelial lesion* to report cytologic diagnoses (15). In this proposed classification system, lesions previously classified as mild dysplasia, koilocytotic atypia, koilocytosis, flat condyloma, and CIN 1 are grouped together into a single entity termed *low-grade squamous intraepithelial lesion* (i.e., low-grade SIL, or LSIL), and lesions previously classified as CIN 2 and 3 are grouped together into a single entity termed *high-grade squamous intraepithelial lesion* (i.e., high-grade SIL, or HSIL). A similar modification of the CIN system of nomenclature was also suggested. In this modified scheme, CIN 1 was termed low-grade CIN 1 and CIN 2 and 3 were combined under the high-grade CIN 2,3 rubric.

In this chapter, we will use a two-tiered terminology (e.g., CIN 1 and CIN 2,3) because it is the most widely used terminology in the United States and was adopted for clinical guidelines at the 2001 Consensus Conference (16). However, two points should be emphasized about the use of any terminology for cervical cancer precursors. First, it is important to remember that the histologic appearance of a lesion does not unequivocally predict whether it represents a simple productive viral infection or a neoplasm. Although the majority of histologically high-grade lesions contain ''cancer-associated'' HPV types, are monoclonal proliferations, and are aneuploid, the converse is not true. Lesions that are histologically low grade are quite heterogeneous with respect to their associated HPV types, clonal status, and ploidy. Some histologically low-grade lesions can be classified as productive viral infections but others contain "cancer-associated" HPV types and have the biologic features of a precursor lesion. Therefore histologic appearance does not necessarily predict the biologic behavior of an individual lesion. Second, it must be emphasized that different terminologies are currently in use by different pathology laboratories around the world. For example, in 1994, the World Health Organization (WHO) recommended continued use of the dysplasia terminology, divided into mild (CIN 1), moderate (CIN 2), and severe (CIN 3) and carcinoma *in situ*, for cervical cancer precursors (17).

Glandular Lesions

Interest in glandular lesions of the cervix has been stimulated by an apparent increase in the number of women, especially those under the age of 35 years, who are being diagnosed with invasive adenocarcinoma of the cervix and glandular precursor lesions. Large series of women with invasive cervical cancers and cancer registries have demonstrated that the relative proportion of adenocarcinomas to squamous cell carcinomas of the cervix has been increasing over the last 3 decades. Most large series from the 1950s and 1960s reported that 95% of invasive cervical cancers were squamous cell carcinomas and only 5% were adenocarcinomas (18,19). However beginning in the 1970s, case series began reporting that 75% to 80% of invasive cervical cancers were squamous cell carcinomas and that 20% to 25% of cases were either adenocarcinomas, adenosquamous cell carcinomas, or undifferentiated carcinomas (20–23). This relative increase is clearly demonstrated by the clinical series of Shingleton et al. (24). During the 1974 to 1978 period, adenocarcinomas accounted for 7% of all cervical cancers, whereas by 1979 to 1980, they accounted for 19%. Similarly, cancer registries from the United States and Europe have reported that the ratio of adenocarcinomas to squamous cell carcinomas has increased over the same period (25–29). In the Finnish Cancer Registry, 6% of cervical cancers were classified as adenocarcinomas in 1953 to 1957, whereas by 1978 to 1982, 17% were classified as adenocarcinomas (26).

Cancer registries from the United States, Norway, and the United Kingdom have all reported an increase in the absolute incidence of invasive adenocarcinomas of the cervix in women 35 years of age or younger (25,27–30). It is important to note, however, that despite the increased incidence of invasive adenocarcinoma in young women and the clear increase in the relative proportions of adenocarcinomas to squamous cell carcinomas over the last three decades, the absolute number of invasive adenocarcinomas has not actually increased when women of all age groups are combined. Instead, the number of women with invasive squamous cell carcinomas has decreased, producing a relative increase.

The first indication that precursor lesions existed for invasive adenocarcinomas of the cervix was the description by Helper in 1952 of highly atypical endocervical cells lining architecturally normal endocervical glands adjacent to frankly invasive adenocarcinomas of the cervix (18). Freidell and Mckay subsequently described two additional patients with similar histologic findings and coined the term *adenocarcinoma in situ* (AIS) to refer to these glandular lesions that were histologically highly atypical but noninvasive (31). Inherent in the use of the term *adenocarcinoma in situ* to refer to these lesions was the acknowledgment that these lesions were precursors to invasive adenocarcinoma of the cervix. In addition to the highly atypical glandular lesions referred to as adenocarcinoma *in situ*, glandular lesions with a lesser degree of histologic abnormality than adenocarcinoma *in situ* are also found in the cervix. These low-grade glandular lesions have been referred to by a variety of terms including *endocervical dysplasia*, *atypical hyperplasia*, and more recently *endocervical glandular atypia* (14,32). By way of analogy to squamous lesions, some investigators have suggested that the term *cervical intraepithelial glandular neoplasia* (CIGN) be used to refer to all of these noninvasive glandular lesions (33). Using the cervical intraepithelial glandular neoplasia terminology, atypical hyperplasia is classified as either cervical intraepithelial glandular neoplasia grade 1 or 2 depending on the degree of cytologic atypia and mitotic activity present and adenocarcinoma *in situ* is classified as cervical intraepithelial glandular neoplasia grade 3 (33).

It is important to note that although there is considerable evidence indicating that adenocarcinoma *in situ* is a precursor for invasive adenocarcinoma of the cervix, there is little evidence to support such a role for the lower grade glandular abnormalities. Since the terms *endocervical dysplasia* and *cervical intraepithelial glandular neoplasia* imply a relationship between the low-grade lesions and adenocarcinoma *in situ* and invasive adenocarcinoma that is not documented, we prefer the use of the more noncommittal term *endocervical glandular atypia* to refer to the low-grade lesions that lack the features of adenocarcinoma *in situ* (14).

Vulva and Vagina

The terminology used for preinvasive lesions of the vulva and vagina has tended to parallel that used for the cervix. The original description used for preinvasive lesions of the vulva was made in 1912 by Bowen, who described a lesion of the thigh and buttock that he termed "precancerous dermatosis" (34). These lesions were grossly red and scaly and were characterized microscopically by significant cellular atypia. Clinically, they either persisted or recurred. Bowen believed that these lesions, which subsequently came to be called *Bowen's disease*, were precursors to invasive squamous cell carcinomas of the vulva. Since this original description, a number of other terms have been used for lesions with significant cellular atypia that lack invasion. These include erythroplasia of Queyrat, atypical hyperplasia, dysplasia, atypia, carcinoma *in situ*, carcinoma *in situ* simplex, and intraepithelial carcinoma.

The International Society for the Study of Vulvar Disease (ISSVD) proposed in 1976 that the term *carcinoma in situ* be used for variants of intraepithelial carcinoma and that the term *atypia* be used for less severe epithelial changes (35). Recently, the term *vulvar intraepithelial neoplasia* (VIN), together with a grade of 1 to 3, has been adopted for these lesions (36). Similarly, the term *vaginal intraepithelial neoplasia* (VAIN), together with a grade of 1 to 3, is widely used to describe preinvasive lesions of the vagina. It should be pointed out, however, that data that suggest a continuum between all grades of vulvar and vaginal preinvasive lesions and invasive squamous cell carcinoma at these sites are significantly less compelling than those for the cervix.

NATURAL HISTORY OF PREINVASIVE LESIONS OF THE LOWER GENITAL TRACT

Cervix

The concept that certain epithelial lesions are precursors of invasive squamous cell carcinoma of the cervix has received significant support from a variety of epidemiologic and long-term follow-up studies. Several different methods have been used to study the natural history of different types of cervical cancer precursors. When cytologic screening programs for cervical cancer were introduced to previously unscreened populations in the 1940s and 1950s, a large difference in the mean age of patients with invasive cervical cancer and patients with "dysplasia" became apparent (Table 19.1). In the study by Reagan and co-workers, the mean age of patients with "dysplasia" was 34 years, the mean age of patients with carcinoma *in situ* was 42 years, and the mean age of patients with invasive cancer was 48 years (37). Similar age distributions were observed by Patten in his studies (38). These data were interpreted to imply that it takes over 10 years for a dysplastic lesion to progress to carcinoma *in situ* and invasive cancer (39,40).

The most direct way to study the natural history of cervical cancer precursors is to study cervical lesions prospectively without therapeutic intervention. Before widespread acceptance of the fact that a high percentage of carcinoma *in situ* lesions inevitably progress to invasive cancer, patients with carcinoma *in situ* were followed prospectively in several studies. These studies, with all their attendant methodologic problems (including lack of standardized histologic criteria, small patient numbers, inadequate and short patient follow-up, and wide differences in results), form the basis of our estimates of the premalignant potential of carcinoma *in situ*. Now that the premalignant potential of carcinoma *in situ* is universally accepted, it would obviously be unethical to repeat these prospective follow-up studies of carcinoma *in situ* lesions using more contemporary methods.

In 1961, Kottmeier reported on a group of 31 women with carcinoma *in situ* who were followed for at least 12 years (41). Twenty-two (72%) of these women subsequently developed invasive cancer. Similarly, Koss and co-workers in 1963 reported a long-term follow-up study of 67 women with carcinoma *in situ* proved by biopsy (42). In this study, a lower frequency of progression was detected than in the study by Kottmeier (Table 19.2). Sixty-one percent of carcinoma *in situ* lesions persisted, and only 6% progressed to invasive cancer. However, the follow-up time was only 3 years.

A larger study of the natural history of carcinoma *in situ* was that of Green and Donovan from New Zealand (Table 19.2) (43). On the basis of a short-term follow-up study of patients with carcinoma *in situ*, it was initially proposed that carcinoma *in situ* either had a low malignant potential or took much longer than 20 years to develop into invasive cancer (44). However, on long-term follow-up of a group of 817 patients whose Pap smears reverted to normal, 12 patients (1.5%) subsequently developed invasive carcinoma. Of the group of 131 patients with persistently abnormal Pap smears (followed for 4 to 23 years), 29 (22%) developed invasive carcinoma of the cervix or vaginal vault and 90 (69%) had persistent carcinoma *in situ*. This and other follow-up studies clearly demonstrate that, once established, carcinoma *in situ* has a significant potential for progression to invasive cancer, and progression is usually a slow process that requires years.

Whether carcinoma *in situ*, once established, can spontaneously regress in the absence of therapy is controversial. Based on the studies of Kottmeier and Green, it would appear that, once established, carcinoma *in situ* only rarely regresses spontaneously (43,45). However, other follow-up studies have found that about one-third of carcinoma *in situ* lesions regress during follow-up (6). Evaluation of data obtained from the British Columbia population-based screening program suggests that the cumulative incidence of carcinoma *in situ* is significantly higher than the cumulative incidence of invasive cervical cancer (46). Similar data have been obtained from cytologic screening programs in Sweden. These cytologic data have been interpreted as indicating that many cases of carcinoma *in situ* regress spontaneously (46,47).

Many prospective studies have also followed the transi-

TABLE 19.1. *Age distribution of cervical cancer precursors*

Cytology	Mean age at diagnosis (yr)	
	Patten (78)	Reagan et al. (37)
Dysplasia	34.7	34
Slight	32	–
Moderate	35.7	–
Marked	38.4	–
Carcinoma *in situ*	42.3	41.5
Invasive cancer	51.7	48.2

TABLE 19.2. *Natural history of patients with cervical cancer precursors*

Reference	Patients (no.)	Diagnosis		Regression (%)	Persistence (%)	Progression (%)	Follow-up period (yr)
		Method	Actual				
Kottmeier (45)	31	Biopsy	CIS	–	–	72	>12
Koss et al. (42)	26	Biopsy	CIN 1, 2	39	15	46	0.5–7
	67	Biopsy	CIS	25	61	6	3
Green and Donovan (44)	576	Biopsy	CIS	–	–	0.17	1–12
McIndoe et al. (43)	131	Biopsy	CIS	8	69	22	1–28

CIS, carcinoma *in situ*; CIN, cervical intraepithelial neoplasia.

tions between different grades of CIN. These studies have obtained quite different estimates of the frequency of mild dysplasia, the likelihood of progression from low-grade to high-grade precursors, and the time required for this progression. The major reasons for the differences in results between these studies include the use of cervical biopsies rather than cytology to document the presence of an abnormality since these can remove small precursor lesions in their entirety, as well as differences in study design, and different criteria used to diagnose a given lesion.

The two most widely quoted follow-up studies are the historical cohort study from Toronto published by Holowaty et al. and the prospective clinical trials of Nasiell et al. The Toronto study utilized a historical cohort of women whose cervical cytology was evaluated at a single large laboratory in an era (1962 to 1980) during which CIN lesions were managed conservatively (48). Rates of regression and progression were estimated using actuarial methods and through linkage to the Ontario Cancer Registry. Both mild and moderate dysplasias were found to be more likely to regress than progress. The risk of mild dysplasia progressing to severe dysplasia or worse was approximately 1% per year. In contrast the risk of moderate dysplasia progressing was 16% at 2 years and 25% at 5 years (Table 19.3). The majority of

TABLE 19.3. *Natural history of dysplasia—Toronto Historical Cohort Study*

Progression	% Occurring at		
	2 yrs	5 yrs	10 yrs
Mild to moderate or worse	11	20	29
Mild to severe or worse	2	6	9
Moderate to severe or worse	16	25	32
Regression			
Mild to normal (×1)	44	74	88
Mild to normal (×2)	–	39	62
Moderate to normal (×1)	33	63	83
Moderate to normal (×2)	–	29	54

From Holowaty P, Miller AB, Rohan T, To T. Natural history of dysplasia of the uterine cervix. *J Natl Cancer Inst* 1999;91:252.

both mild and moderate dysplasias showed spontaneous clearance, and much of the clearance occurred within 2 years of diagnosis.

Nasiell and associates reported on 555 women with a single Pap smear that showed mild dysplasia who were followed colposcopically and cytologically without major treatment (49). Biopsies were performed in only 14% of these patients. In this series, 62% of the patients with a mean follow-up time of 39 months developed normal Pap smears, with apparent regression of their mild dysplasia. Persistent dysplasia occurred in 22% of the patients, with a mean follow-up of 52 months, and progression to severe dysplasia, carcinoma *in situ*, and invasive carcinoma occurred in 16% of the patients, with a mean follow-up of 48 months. Two patients who were lost to follow-up in this study subsequently developed invasive carcinoma, which was detected 79 and 125 months after a diagnosis of mild dysplasia. A number of other studies have investigated cohorts of women with moderate dysplasia. In a study of identical design to that used to study the biologic behavior of mild dysplasia, Nasiell et al. followed patients originally diagnosed cytologically as having moderate dysplasia. By life table analysis, progression to severe dysplasia, carcinoma *in situ*, and invasive carcinoma occurred in 33% of the patients after 12 or more years of follow-up (50).

Melnikow et al. performed a comprehensive meta-analysis of studies in which women with a cytologic result of SIL were followed (51). The analysis included 13,226 women with a cytologic result of LSIL who were followed for at least 6 months and had a median weighted follow-up of 29 months. There were 10,026 women with HSIL who had a median weighted follow-up of 25 months. The pooled estimates for regression to normal were 47% for LSIL and 35% for HSIL (Fig. 19.2). No evidence of a relationship between the proportion of subjects regressing to normal and the length of follow-up was observed. Rates of progression of LSIL were 7% at 6 months and 21% at 24 months. For HSIL, the 6- and 24-month pooled progression rates were 7% and 24%. The pooled progression rates for invasive cancer at 6 and 24 months for LSIL were 0.04% and 0.15%, repectively. For HSIL, they were 0.15% at 6 months and 1.44% at 24 months.

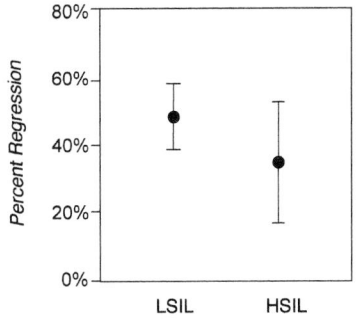
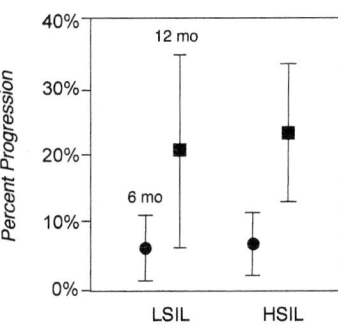

FIG. 19.2. Pooled estimates of the rates of spontaneous regression (**left panel**) of a cytologic diagnosis of LSIL and HSIL obtained from the literature. Pooled estimates of the rates of spontaneous progression of LSIL and HSIL after 6 months (*circles*) and 12 months (*squares*) are shown (**right panel**). Progression for HSIL is from CIN 2 to CIN 3 or carcinoma *in situ*. Bars represent 95% confidence intervals. (Modified with permission from Melnikow J, Nuovo J, Willan AR, et al. Natural history of cervical squamous intraepithelial lesions: a meta-analysis. *Obstet Gynecol* 1998;92:727.)

The natural history of untreated biopsy-confirmed CIN has been reviewed in a number of studies, most of which were conducted in the 1970s and 1980s. Table 19.4 provides a summary of the results of these different studies (52). The higher the grade of a lesion, the more likely it is to persist and the less likely it is to regress. Overall it appears that approximately 57% of CIN 1 will spontaneously regress in the absence of therapy, 32% persist as CIN, and 11% progress to carcinoma *in situ*. The rates of persistence and progression are greater for CIN 2,3. Forty-three percent of CIN 2 lesions regress, 35% persist, and 22% progress to carcinoma *in situ*. The equivalent rates for CIN 3 lesions were 32% regression, 56% persistence, and 12% progression to carcinoma *in situ*. Overall, the progression of all grades of CIN to invasive cancer in the published observational studies is 1.7%. The rate at which CIN progresses appears to be relatively slow. Using life-table analysis of data from a prospective follow-up study, Barron and Richart estimated that the mean transit time to carcinoma *in situ* from very mild dysplasia was 85 months, from mild dysplasia 58 months, from moderate dysplasia 38 months, and from severe dysplasia only 12 months (Fig. 19.3) (40).

Vulva

Studies on the natural history of VIN lesions are much fewer than for CIN. Partly because of the paucity of studies, the relationships between VIN and invasive squamous cell carcinoma of the vulva appear to be less straightforward than those documented between CIN and invasive squamous cell carcinoma of the cervix. Unlike the cervix, in which the

majority of carcinomas are associated with a CIN lesion, only a third of invasive vulvar squamous carcinomas have a coexisting VIN 3 lesion (53). Many textbooks state that the vast majority of patients with VIN do not subsequently develop invasive squamous carcinoma. In a review of six published follow-up studies, it was reported that only 16 of 330 patients (4.8%) with VIN progressed to invasive cancer (54). Solitary lesions in postmenopausal women had the highest risk of progression; multifocal lesions in women of reproductive age rarely progressed, although well-documented cases of young patients with VIN 3 who have developed cancer exist. In a series from Denmark, Hording et al. reported that only 4% of 73 women with VIN 3 developed invasive cancer during follow-up (median follow-up was 5 years) (55).

What is generally not emphasized is that most of the patients in these follow-up studies were treated for their VIN or followed for relatively short periods of time. This fact explains, in part, the low incidence of progression. For example, in a recent follow-up series of surgically untreated women with VIN, Herod et al. observed a very low rate of progression (56). In this series, 19 women with VIN (8 cases of VIN 1, 5 cases of VIN 2, and 6 cases of VIN 3) were followed without surgical treatment. None of the 19 women developed invasive disease during follow-up, but median length of follow-up was only 30 months. In a long-term follow-up study of women with VIN, Jones and Roland found that only 3% of 105 women with treated VIN developed invasive vulvar cancer. In contrast, of eight women

TABLE 19.4. *Natural history of CIN is dependent on lesional grade*

	% Regression	% Persist	Progress to CIS
CIN 1	57	32	11
CIN 2	43	35	22
CIN 3	32	56	12

From Mitchell MF, Tortolero-Luna G, Wright T, et al. Cervical human papillomavirus infection and intraepithelial neoplasia: a review. *J Natl Cancer Inst Monogr* 1996;21:17.

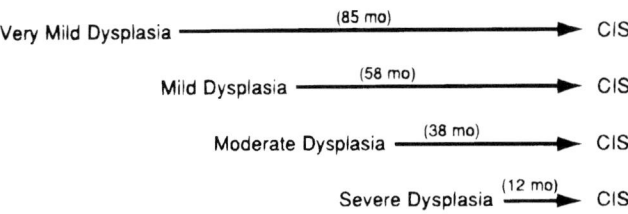

FIG. 19.3. Transition times from varying degrees of dysplasia to carcinoma *in situ*. (Adapted with permission from Barron BA, Richart RM. A statistical model of the natural history of cervical carcinoma II. Estimates of the transition from dysplasia to carcinoma in situ. *J Natl Cancer Inst* 1970;45:1025.)

between the ages of 28 and 73 years with biopsy-documented VIN 3 who were followed without further treatment, seven developed invasive squamous cell carcinoma of the vulva within 8 years of diagnosis (57).

RISK FACTORS FOR THE DEVELOPMENT OF LOWER GENITAL TRACT CANCERS AND PREINVASIVE LESIONS OF THE LOWER GENITAL TRACT

Cervix

Risk Factors

A large number of epidemiologic studies have analyzed risk factors for the development of cervical cancer and its precursors. Although the risk factors are similar for both cervical cancer and its precursors, the association with the risk factors is generally much stronger for cervical cancer than for precursor lesions. The major risk factors found in most studies are markers of sexual behavior such as number of sexual partners, early age of first pregnancy and first intercourse, sexually transmitted diseases, and parity. In addition, lower socioeconomic class, cigarette smoking, oral contraceptive use, and immunosuppression from any cause are associated with both cervical cancer and its precursors (Table 19.5).

It has been known for almost a century that cervical cancer has many of the characteristics of a sexually transmitted disease. The observations that the disease was much more frequent in married women than in celibate women, that it was more common in prostitutes and incarcerated women than in the general population, and that it was highly associated with a woman's lifetime number of male sexual partners

TABLE 19.5. *Risk factors for cervical cancer and its precursor lesions*

Demographic factors
Older age
Race (e.g., Black, Hispanic, American Indian)
Residence in selected parts of Africa, Asia, or Latin America
Low socioeconomic status
Low educational level

Behavioral and sexual factors
Large number of sexual partners
Early age at first coitus
Cigarette smoking
Long-term oral contraceptive use
Diet low in folate, carotene, vitamin C

Medical/gynecologic factors
Multiparity
Early age at first pregnancy
History of sexually transmitted diseases (especially herpes genitalis or HPV-associated lesions)
Infection with specific types of HPV
Lack of routine cytologic screening
Immunosuppression (any cause)

all argue for venereal transmission. The fact that a woman's risk was increased not only by the number of sexual partners that she had, but also by the number of sexual partners that her male partner or partners had, strengthens the epidemiologic evidence that cervical cancer behaves as a sexually transmitted disease (58). With so much evidence favoring the sexual transmission of cervical cancer, many investigators have searched for an etiologic agent among the known sexually transmitted diseases.

Over the past 100 years, virtually every known sexually transmitted infection has been suggested as the etiologic agent for cervical cancer and, in more recent times, for cervical cancer precursors. The list includes *Treponema pallidum, Trichomonas vaginalis, Candida albicans, Chlamydia trachomatis,* and the herpes simplex viruses (HSV). There is now considerable evidence for a role for both *C. trachomatis* and HSV as co-factors in the pathogenesis of HPV-associated cervical neoplasia. One recent case control study found that among HPV-infected women there was a twofold risk for cervical cancer associated with having antibodies to *C. trachomatis* (59). This risk is similar to the 2.5-fold increased risk observed with seroconversion in a prospective seroepidemiologic study (60). The prevalence of antibodies to HSV is also increased among women with cervical cancer. Smith et al. performed a pooled analysis of clinical samples from seven case-control studies of cervical cancer. After adjusting for HPV status and sexual behavior, HSV seropositivity was associated with an approximately twofold increased risk of cervical cancer (59). It has been suggested that both *C. trachomatis* and HSV act as co-factors in HPV-associated neoplasia, possibly through the induction of cervical inflammation (61).

Human Papillomavirus

Over the last 15 years, evidence has been accumulating rapidly to implicate HPV in the pathogenesis of cervical cancer and its preinvasive precursors. The first real evidence that linked HPV to cervical cancer came from Meisels and colleagues, who in 1977 recognized that the cells in acuminate genital warts were identical to cells in certain flat lesions considered to be cervical cancer precursors (62). These cells were characterized by nuclear enlargement with irregular nuclear outlines, hyperchromaticity, and the presence of perinuclear halos. They called cells with these features "koilocytes." This histologic linkage between acuminate warts and cervical cancer precursors suggested that an etiologic linkage might exist between HPV and cervical cancer since it had been known that acuminate genital warts were sexually transmitted and caused by HPV (63). Subsequently, it was shown that HPV could be found by electron microscopy in low-grade cervical cancer precursors (64). Further clarification of the role of HPV in producing lower anogenital tract cancers depended on the work of zur Hausen and others who were able to identify HPV DNA in genital tract lesions and, through the use of molecular cloning technology, to identify individual viruses, clone them from the lesions, and produce sufficient quantities of HPV DNA to enable them to apply hybridization technology to the study of HPV-induced lesions (65). The development of molecular probes for HPV DNA detection led to the demonstration that HPV DNA was present in the majority of cervical cancers as well as in most high-grade precursors and to the conclusion that HPV plays a critical role in the pathogenesis of female anogenital tract neoplasia (66).

There is also strong epidemiologic evidence for a causal association between HPV and cervical cancer and its precursors. It has now been shown that there is a consistently strong relationship between HPV infection and cervical neoplasia, that the temporal sequence between infection and the development of cancer is correct, that the association between HPV and cervical cancer is relatively specific, and that the epidemiologic findings are consistent with the natural history and biologic behavior of HPV infections and cervical cancer (66).

Studies that use sensitive molecular methods to detect and type HPV in cervical lesions have found that almost all cervical cancers and their precursors are associated with HPV DNA. For example, in a large study that analyzed over 1,000 invasive cervical cancers from all over the world using the polymerase chain reaction (PCR), high-risk types of HPV were identified in over 90% of the invasive cervical cancers (67). Moreover, the same types of HPV were identified in cancers from all different geographic locations. When cases initially classified as HPV DNA negative were retested with other PCR methods, high-risk HPV types were identified in almost all of them (68). This indicates that essentially all cervical cancers are caused by specific high-risk types of HPV.

Large case-control studies have identified HPV infection as a risk factor in the development of CIN and cervical cancer. For example, a recent pooled analysis of data from 11 case-control studies shows that HPV was detected in 1,739 of 1,918 patients with cervical cancer (91%) compared to 259 of 1,928 control women (13%). The pooled odds ratio for cervical cancer associated with any HPV type was 158 (69). In an earlier case-control study that used PCR to detect and type HPV DNA in 436 women with cervical cancer and 387 control women from Spain and Colombia, Bosch et al. found that when HPV DNA positivity was controlled for, the number of lifetime sexual partners, but not age at first intercourse, disappeared as a risk factor.

A number of prospective studies of colposcopically and cytologically negative women indicate that the temporal sequence between HPV infection and the development of cancer is what would be expected for a causal agent. HPV infection occurs first and then subsequently high-grade cervical cancer precursors or cancer occur. For example, in a study of colposcopically negative "high-risk" women enrolled from sexually transmitted disease clinics and methadone mainte-

nance clinics in New York City, the incidence of CIN was significantly higher in colposcopically and cytologically negative women who had HPV type 16 or 18 DNA detected in cervical secretions than in those who lacked HPV DNA (70). As might be predicted, persistent infection with high-risk types of HPV was much more closely linked with the subsequent development of CIN 2,3 than is detection of high-risk HPV DNA at a single visit.

Taken together, these epidemiologic studies clearly demonstrate that there is a strong and consistent association between specific types of HPV DNA and invasive cervical cancer and its precursor lesions, and that exposure to HPV precedes the development of cervical disease. When combined with the enormous body of molecular evidence demonstrating a role for HPV in the development of cervical cancer and CIN, these findings clearly indicate that HPV infection, acquired through sexual contact, is a "necessary cause" of both CIN and invasive cervical cancer (66,71). Based on these data, the International Agency for Research on Cancer (IARC) of the World Health Organization has classified HPV 16 and 18 as carcinogens in humans (72).

Smoking, Diet, and Oral Contraceptives

In addition to risk factors associated with sexual behavior, several other risk factors such as low socioeconomic class and cigarette smoking have also been associated with the development of cervical cancer (73,74). In a comprehensive review of the literature, Szarewski concluded that a positive association between cigarette smoking and the development of cervical cancer had been reported by the majority of studies designed to address this question (75). Several mechanisms could account for the association between cigarette smoking and cervical cancer. One is the secretion of cigarette smoke by-products, including nicotine and cotinine, in cervical mucus of tobacco users and women passively exposed to cigarette smoke (76). DNA adducts (e.g., structurally altered DNA sequences) are significantly more common in the cervical epithelium of smokers than in nonsmokers, and it has been suggested that the secretion of cigarette smoke by-products might have a direct mutagenic effect on the cervical epithelium (77). Another possible mechanism that could account for the association is the effect of cervical smoke by-products on local immune responses in the cervix. There is a reduction in the number of Langerhans cells in the cervices of smokers compared to nonsmokers, and this reduction may result in a decreased level of local immunity to HPV (78).

The use of combined oral contraceptives has also been found to be a risk factor for the development of cervical cancer and its precursors in some studies. A recent systematic review of the literature concluded that the relative risk of cervical cancer among women using oral contraceptives for less than 5 years, 5 to 9 years, and 10 or more years was 1.1, 1.6, and 2.2, respectively (79). The elevated risk observed after 5 or more years remained when the analysis was restricted to HPV-positive women. Other studies have suggested that oral contraceptive use may accelerate the progression of CIN from low-grade to high-grade or to invasive cancer (80). Associations between exogenous hormones and cervical disease could be explained by a number of mechanisms including direct promoting effects of estrogens and progestins on the HPV genome, as well as by indirect effects such as a reduction in blood folate levels that is occasionally observed in women on oral contraceptives (81). Whether an association exists between endogenous hormone levels and invasive cervical cancer is even more controversial. There is no association between age at menarche or age of menopause and the risk of invasive cervical squamous cell carcinoma, and it has been suggested that the strong association observed between early age of first parity and risk for cervical cancer reflects the risk of exposure to a sexually transmitted agent at an early age rather than an influence of endogenous hormones (82).

Only a few studies have focused on relationships between cervical cancer and diet, but some evidence suggests that a diet low in either vitamin A or C may be associated with an increased risk (83). Other studies have not detected an association between dietary intake of beta-carotene or retinol and CIN (83). A recent review of the role of antioxidant nutrients on cervical disease concluded that there are six studies that have properly controlled for HPV. In all six, an inverse relationship was observed between serum beta-carotene and cervical carcinogenesis (61). In studies that measured carotenoids other than beta-carotene, inverse associations between cervical neoplasia and serum lycopene and beta-carotene have been observed (61). Folate deficiency has also been considered to be a risk factor. A recent case-control study reported that folate deficiency enhances the effects of other risk factors such as parity, HPV 16 infection, and cigarette smoking on the development of CIN (84).

Immunosuppression

Immunosuppression is another risk factor for the development of both CIN and cervical cancer. In studies of patients with renal transplants, a relative risk of 13.6 has been reported for the development of cervical carcinoma *in situ* in transplant recipients compared to women in the general population (85). Over the last decade, it has become widely accepted that there is also an association between cervical disease and infection with the human immunodeficiency virus (HIV) (86,87). HPV infections are more prevalent and tend to be more persistent in HIV-infected women (88). Numerous studies have documented a higher prevalence of cervical neoplasia among HIV-infected women compared to various control groups of HIV-uninfected women (89,90). There also appears to be an increase in invasive cervical cancer. Among women in New York City, the standardized incidence ratio for cervical cancer is 9.2 times higher in

HIV-infected compared to HIV-noninfected women (91). It is clear that the invasive cervical cancers that do develop in HIV-infected women act aggressively and respond poorly to standard forms of therapy (92). Invasive cervical cancer was designated in 1993 as an AIDS case-defining illness by the Centers for Disease Control and Prevention (93).

HUMAN PAPILLOMAVIRUSES

Classification

Papillomaviruses are members of the A genus of the family Papovaviridae. This family of viruses includes the papillomaviruses, polyomavirus, and SV40 virus. They are all double-stranded DNA tumor viruses, but they are dissimilar in size, lack shared antigens, and have only limited DNA sequence homologies. However, as more is learned about their biologic properties, it is becoming apparent that the actions of the Papovaviridae on their target cells are similar.

The characteristic features of human papillomaviruses that set them apart from other members of the Papovaviridae are a double-stranded, circular DNA genome of 7,800 to 7,900 base pairs, a nonenveloped virion, and an icosahedral capsid composed of 72 capsomers that measures 45 to 55 nm in diameter. Papillomaviruses are widely distributed among mammals and are highly species specific. They are classified based on their species of origin and the extent of DNA relatedness between viral isolates. Human papillomaviruses are epitheliotropic. They infect epithelial cells of the skin and mucous membranes, often producing local epithelial proliferation or warts at the sites of infection. There has been only limited success in propagating HPV in either tissue culture.

Within a given species, many types and subtypes of papillomaviruses may exist. Since the capsid proteins of different papillomaviruses are antigenically similar, papillomaviruses are subdivided into genotypes and subtypes based on their extent of DNA relatedness as determined by DNA hybridization under stringent conditions rather than into serotypes based on structural antigenic features. In order to be classified as a distinct type, the E6, E7, and L1 gene sequences (about one-third of the genome) must differ by more than 10% from those of other known HPV types. In addition to types, there also are subtypes or variants of specific types, such as HPV 16. In order to be considered a subtype or variant, the sample viruses must differ by 2% to 5% from the original isolate. In humans, more than 100 types of papillomaviruses have been characterized. Although the different types are quite similar structurally, they have significant specificity with regard to the anatomic location of the epithelia that they infect and the type of lesions that they produce at the site of infection (94). For example, HPV types 1, 2, 4, 26, 27, 29, 41, and 57 are associated with common warts (verrucae vulgaris); types 1, 2, and 4 with deep plantar warts; and type 7; with common warts on the hands of meat handlers (butcher's warts). HPV types 5, 8, 9, 12, 14, and others are associated with flat warts and cancers in patients with epidermodysplasia verruciformis, which is a rare, heritable, lifelong skin disease characterized by the development of multiple flat warts throughout life. These warts may progress to skin cancer (95).

Over 30 types of HPVs that infect the anogenital tract have been described (Table 19.6). These different types of HPVs tend to be associated with different types of lesions. HPV 6 is also the most common HPV type found in association with exophytic condylomas of the male and female anogenital tract in adults (96,97). Most exophytic condylomas that are not associated with HPV 6 are associated with HPV 11. Exophytic condylomas are occasionally associated with HPV type 16 or 31, but are almost never found in association with HPV 18. In adults, cutaneous HPV types such as HPV 1 or 2 are seldom associated with exophytic condylomas. However, approximately one of five exophytic condylomata acuminata in children are associated with HPV 2, which is a common cutaneous HPV type (8). Small, raised, plaque-type warts on the penis are also commonly associated with HPV. The most common HPV types detected in small, slightly raised penile lesions are HPVs 6, 16, and 42.[99]

More than 80% of CIN lesions are found to be associated with HPV when sensitive, molecular methods are used to detect HPV DNA. CIN 1 is quite heterogeneous with regard to associated HPV types (100–102). CIN 1 can be associated with any of the anogenital HPV types that have been identified in women in the general population. Although the studies performed in the mid-1980s indicated that HPVs 6 and 11 were the predominant types of HPVs associated with CIN 1, subsequent studies have detected HPVs 6 and 11 in only 21% of CIN 1; HPVs 16 and 18, combined, are detected in about one of five CIN 1 lesions. More than one type of HPV is detected in about 10% of women with CIN 1.

In contrast to CIN 1, almost half of all CIN 2,3 lesions are associated with HPV 16 (79,100–102). The prevalence of HPV 16 in women with high-grade SIL (CIN 2,3) varies from 30% to 77% in different studies. A meta-analysis of the distribution of HPV types in CIN 2,3 lesions in the published literature concluded that HPV 16 is identified in 45% of all CIN 2,3 lesions, HPV 18 in 7.1%, and HPV 31 in 8.8% (Fig. 19.4) (79). Fifty-two percent of CIN 2,3 lesions are associated with either HPV 16 or 18. HPV types 33, 31, 58,

and 52 are the next most common types found in CIN 2,3. Multiple types of HPV are uncommonly detected in women with CIN 2,3 (101). The associations between specific types of HPVs and invasive cervical cancers are similar to those observed in women with CIN 2,3 (Fig. 19.4) (79). HPV 16 is the most common HPV type found in association with invasive cervical squamous cell carcinomas and HPV 18 is the second most common. All other types are much less commonly found.

Based on their associations with benign epithelial proliferations, high-grade cancer precursors, or invasive cancers of the vulva, vagina, anus, and cervix, HPVs have been categorized into three groups: "high-risk" viruses that are classified as "high-risk" because infection with these HPV types is associated with a high relative risk of cancer; "low-risk" viruses that are associated with a relatively low-risk of invasive cervical cancer; and "indeterminant risk" viruses that are occasionally associated with cervical cancer (Table 19.6) (69). It is important to recognize that all of the 30 different types of anogenital HPVs have been isolated from cervicovaginal secretions of women lacking any colposcopic or cytologic evidence of cervical disease. The most common HPV types detected in women with no cytologic evidence of cervical disease include high-risk types such as 16, 31, 51, 52, 58, and 56 (103–105).

Genomic Organization

The overall genomic organization of all sequenced HPV types is similar. The genome contains eight open reading frames (ORFs) that are transcribed from a single DNA strand as a polycistronic message (Fig. 19.5). OTFs are DNA segments that are transcriptional units and have the capacity to encode protein. The viral DNA can be divided into three regions. First, there is an upstream regulatory region (URR) of about 400 base pairs that contains a complex array of overlapping binding sites for a large number of different transcriptional activators and transcriptional repressors (106). These include keratinocytic-specific transcription factor 1 (KRF 1), activator protein 1 (AP 1), and nuclear factor (NF-I/CTF) as well as virally derived transcriptional factors. This region plays a role in regulating the production of viral proteins and infectious particles, and it potentially may play a central role in determining the host range of specific types of HPVs (106,107).

Downstream of the URR is the early region. The early region encodes for proteins that play a fundamental role in viral infection and replication. Within the early region are six ORFs designated E1, E2, E4, E5, E6, and E7. The E6 and E7 ORFs are important in the immortalizing and transforming functions of HPVs (108). E1 encodes two distinct proteins that are required for extrachromosomal DNA replication. The E1 protein of bovine papillomavirus has both an ATPase and a helicase function, and the E1 protein of HPV 11 has been shown to be an ATPase (109). The E2 protein

TABLE 19.6. *Classification of anogenital HPV types*

"Low-risk" types	6, 11, 40, 42, 43, 44, 53[a], 54, 61, 72, 81
"High-risk" types	16, 18, 31, 33, 35, 39, 45, 51, 52, 56, 58, 59, 68, 82
Possible high-risk types	26, 66, 73

[a] Classified as "low-risk" based on other data.
From Munoz N, Bosch FX, de Sanjose S, et al. Epidemiologic classification of human papillomavirus types associated with cervical cancer. *N Engl J Med* 2003;348:518.

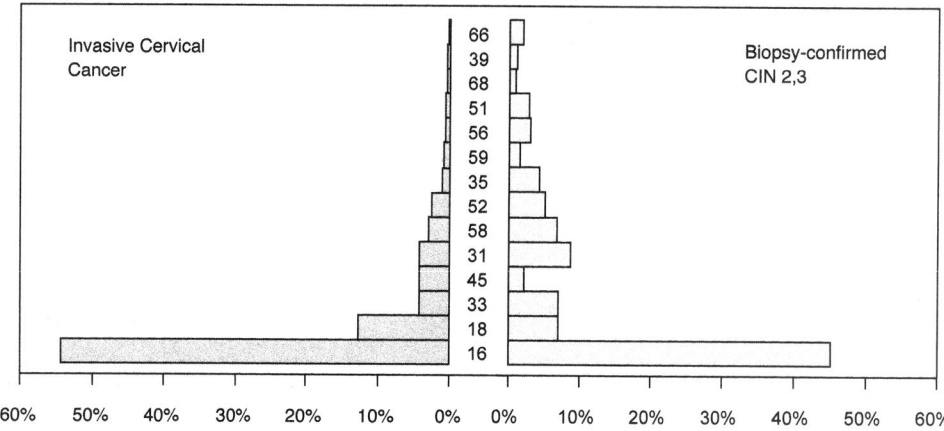

FIG. 19.4. Distribution of HPV types determined by PCR in cases of invasive cervical cancer and biopsy-confirmed CIN 2,3. (Modified with permission from Clifford GM, Smith JS, Aguado T, Franceschi S. Comparison of HPV type distribution in high-grade cervical lesions and cervical cancer: a meta-analysis. *Br J Cancer* 2003;89:101.)

has important transcriptional regulatory activities (110). Together with E1, E2 is also required for extrachromosomal DNA replication to occur, which is a fundamental role in viral infection and replication. E2 also acts as a key regulator of transcription of the E6 and E7 ORFs. The E4 protein has many characteristics of a structural viral protein and is similar to the protein products of the late region (65). Like the L1 and L2 capsid proteins, the E4 protein is expressed during the late stages of the viral life cycle, at a time when complete

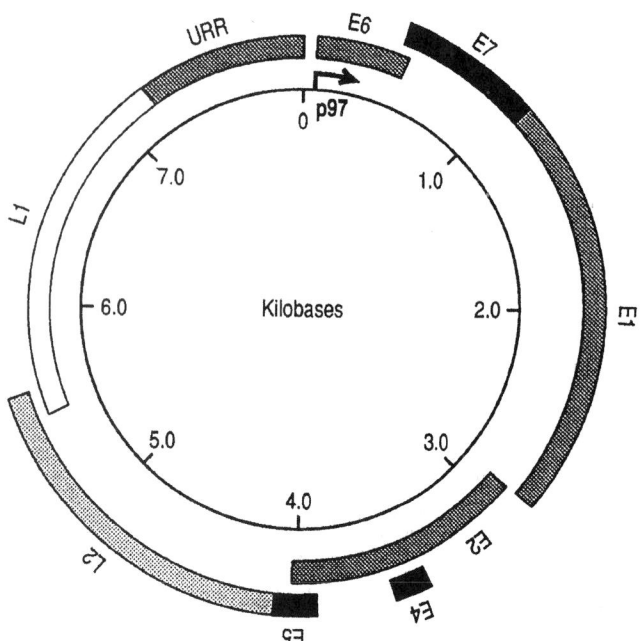

FIG. 19.5. Schematic of genomic organization of HPV. (Reprinted with permission from Wright TC, Ferenczy AF, Kurman RJ. Precancerous lesions of the cervix. In: Kurman RJ, ed. *Blaustein's pathology of the female genital tract.* 4th ed. New York: Springer-Verlag, 1994:229.)

virions are being produced. The E4 protein is thought to disrupt the normal intermediate filament matrix of infected epithelial cells and disrupt the cornified cell envelope. This is thought to facilitate the release of assembled virions from the infected epithelium and to produce the characteristic cytopathic infection (e.g., "koilocytosis") (111). E5 appears to play a role in the early course of infection. E5 stimulates cell growth by forming complexes with epidermal growth factor receptor, platelet-derived growth factor receptor, and colony-stimulating factor-1 receptor (112). Unlike E6 and E7 that are required for the development of cervical cancer, E5 is often lost during the development of cervical cancers.

The late region is downstream of the early region and includes two ORFs: L1, which encodes for the major capsid protein, and L2, which encodes for the minor capsid protein. The L1 major capsid protein is highly conserved among papillomaviruses of all species and serves as a convenient source of antigen for the production of antibodies to the papillomavirus. The minor capsid protein, L2, shows considerable sequence variation between different types of HPV and has been used as an antigen for the production of type-specific antibodies to HPV. Expression of L1 and L2 capsid proteins occurs late during the viral life cycle and coincides with the production of complete virions (111). Expression of L1 and L2 capsid proteins is posttranscriptionally regulated by cell-derived factors and occurs only in superficial and intermediate squamous epithelial cells. This explains, in part, why virion production and the resultant cytopathic effects of HPV infection are most pronounced in CIN 1 and in condyloma acuminatum, but are less common in CIN 2,3 and invasive cancer that contain fewer differentiated cells.

Life Cycle

The life cycle of HPV infections is tightly coupled with the differentiation of the stratified epithelium that is the target of infection. Unlike any other known virus families, infection requires access to the actively proliferating basal cells of the epithelium (Fig. 19.6) (113). This occurs usually at sites of microtrauma to the epithelium. Binding of HPV to the basal cells appears to involve interactions with cell surface–associated α_6-integrin that may act as the receptor for binding and entry into the cells (114). After HPV has entered into the basal cell, the viral genome undergoes limited replication. This results in approximately 50 copies of the HPV genome in individual basal cells at the site of infection. The viral genome remains in a circular episomal form that replicates in synchrony with cellular DNA replication (108). Viral gene expression is largely suppressed in the basal cells, although there appears to be limited expression of E5, E6, and E7, which are the "early" viral gene products. These early viral gene products stimulate the proliferation of the HPV-infected basal cells and their lateral expansion within the epithelium.

As the infected basal cells proliferate, they migrate from the basal/parabasal compartment to the suprabasal compartment. Epithelial cells that are not infected with HPV exit the cell cycle when leaving the basal/parabasal compartment. In contrast, HPV-infected cells reenter S phase, which results in amplification of the viral genome to thousands of copies per cell. As the cells reach the upper layers of the epithelium, the E1 and E4 proteins and viral capsid proteins are produced and infectious virions are assembled. Coincident with the assembly of large numbers of infectious virions, the typical HPV-associated cytopathic effects occur. The cytopathic effects are most prominent in the upper layers of the epithelium and include multinucleation, nuclear enlargement, hyper-

chromasia, and regions of perinuclear clearing or halos (i.e., koilocytes).

Transforming Functions

HPV E7 Oncoprotein

Characterization of the regions of the HPV genome responsible for the immortalizing and transforming functions indicates that both functions reside predominantly in the E6/E7 ORFs. The E6/E7 ORFs of HPVs 16 and 18 encode for several distinct proteins. The E7 protein is the major transforming and immortalizing activity of HPV (65,108). E7 is a small zinc-binding protein composed of approximately 100 amino acids that is phosphorylated in the native state and lacks enzymatic activity. Comparison of the amino acid sequences of the HPV 16 E7 protein with those of proteins made by related DNA-transforming viruses shows a high degree of similarity between this region and the conserved domains 1 and 2 of the adenovirus E1A polypeptides as well as the SV40 and polyoma large T antigens and the *myc* oncogene. The HPV 16 E7 gene product can cooperate with activated *ras* oncogenes for transformation and contains a consensus sequence for casein kinase II–mediated serine phosphorylation and a binding site for the product of the retinoblastoma (*Rb*) gene, as well as the structurally related "Rb-like pocket proteins," p130 and p107 (Fig. 19.7) (115). These proteins (Rb, p130, and p107) all play an important role in regulating cell proliferation.

Although the exact mechanism of action of E7 within cells has not been fully worked out, it is clear that the binding of

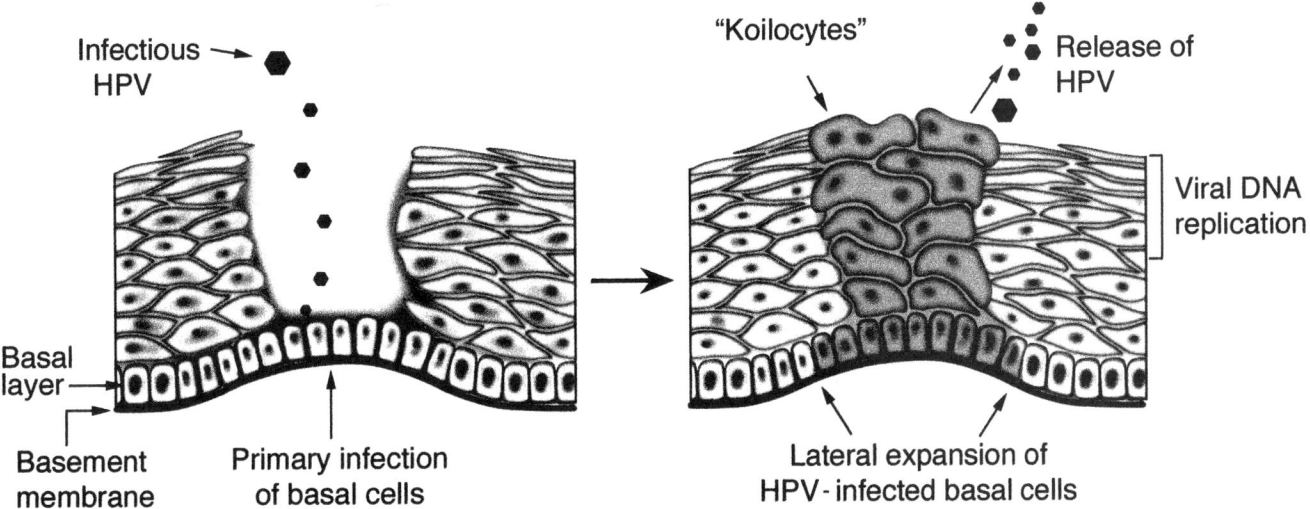

FIG. 19.6. Life cycle of HPV infections. HPV infects cells of the basal layer where it exists in a low copy number in episomal form. Basal cells infected with HPV have a proliferative advantage and expand laterally. As HPV-infected cells progress through the more differentiated layers of the epithelium, viral replication is turned on and large numbers of copies of HPV DNA are produced. Late genes, including the viral capsid, are produced in the most superficial layers of the epithelium and infectious virions are assembled. This produces the characteristic cytopathic effects of HPV (e.g., koilocytosis).

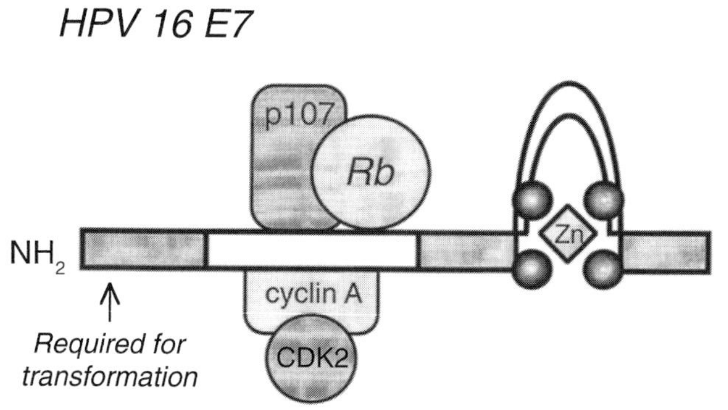

HPV 16 E7

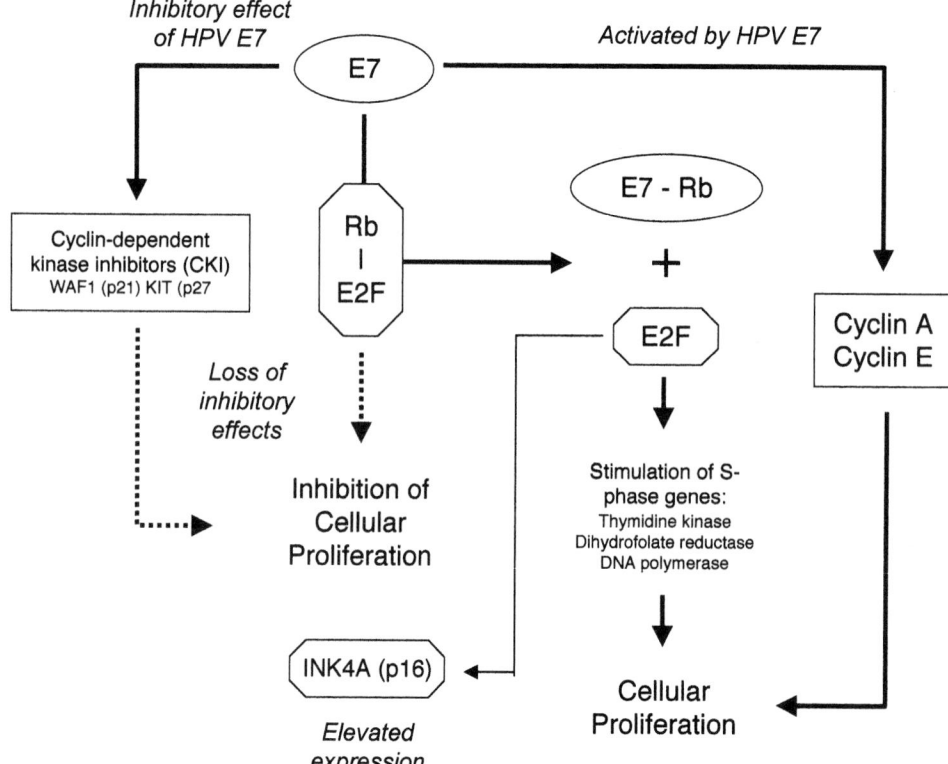

FIG. 19.7. HPV 16 E7 oncoprotein. (Reprinted with permission from Park TJ, Fujiwara H, Wright TC. Molecular biology of cervical cancer and its precursors. *Cancer* 1995;76:1902.)

the E7 protein to either Rb or the other Rb-like pocket proteins blocks the cell proliferation-inhibitory function of these endogenous tumor suppressors (Fig. 19.8) (65,108,115). When cells are not proliferating, Rb is bound to a cellular transcriptional factor called E2F. Binding of E7 to Rb releases E2F that results in the expression of a variety of cellular regulatory genes such as thymidine kinase and DNA polymerase. E7 also activates cyclins E and A and blocks the cellular proliferation-inhibiting activities of cyclin-dependent kinase inhibitors such as WAF1 (p21) and KIPI (p27). This end result of these activities is stimulation of

cell proliferation. Binding of E7 to Rb also results in the increased expression of a cyclin-dependent kinase inhibitor INK4A (p16). Increased expression of INK4A (p16) appears to be a good marker of HPV-induced neoplasia (116).

HPV E6 Oncoprotein

Like the HPV E7 protein, the E6 protein is a small zinc-binding protein (approximately 150 amino acids long) that lacks endogenous enzymatic activity and exerts its effects through binding to cell cycle–regulatory proteins (Fig. 19.9). The E6 proteins of high-risk HPV types have sequence homology with both adenovirus E1B protein and SV40 large T antigen. All of these proteins have the capacity to bind to an endogenous cellular protein known as p53 (115). The cellular p53 protein is a transcriptional activator that has features of both a tumor-suppressor gene and an oncogene. In noninfected cells, p53 levels increase in response to stress, cell or DNA damage, or aberrant cell proliferation signals. High levels of p53 induce expression of genes such as *WAF1/(p21)* that is a repressor of important G_1-specific cyclin-dependent kinases (CDKs) that are required for cell cycle progression. Therefore, in cells exposed to radiation, chemical mutagens, or other forms of stress, p53 levels become elevated, and this elevates the levels of proteins such as *WAF1/(p21)* that cause the cells to arrest in the G_1 phase of the cell cycle. This G_1 growth arrest is thought to provide an opportunity either for the cells to repair DNA damage

FIG. 19.8. Interactions between HPV 16 E7, Rb, E2F, and other proteins important in control of cellular proliferation.

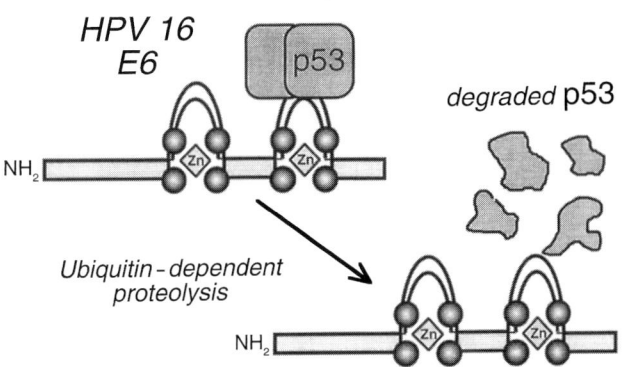

FIG. 19.9. HPV 16 E6 oncoprotein. The HPV 16 E6 protein can bind endogenous (i.e., cellular) p53 and cause it to undergo proteolytic degradation via a ubiquitin-dependent pathway. (Reprinted with permission from Park TJ, Fujiwara H, Wright TC. Molecular biology of cervical cancer and its precursors. *Cancer* 1995;76:1902.)

caused by the stress prior to the next round of DNA synthesis or for the cells to be eliminated through programmed cell death (*apoptosis*). Binding of HPV E6 to p53 results in the rapid proteolytic degradation of the bound p53 through an ubiquitin-dependent pathway (Fig. 19.9) (65,108,115). This reduces the amount of p53 present within the cell and causes a loss of the p53 repair mechanism. The net effect of this is a blockage of apoptosis and an increase in cellular proliferation (Fig. 19.10).

Role of Viral Integration in Transformation

In condylomas and most low-grade cervical cancer precursor lesions, HPV DNA exists as a closed circular form termed an *episome*. When the HPV genome is in the episomal form, the E2 ORF is physically intact, and transcription from the E6 and E7 ORFs is presumed to be well regulated. However, in some high-grade precursor lesions, almost all HPV 18–associated carcinomas, and 75% of HPV

16–associated carcinomas, the HPV genome becomes physically integrated into the host chromosomal DNA (117,118). Although integration is thought to be important in the transition of many cervical lesions from a premalignant to a malignant state, integration may not be an absolute requirement for malignancy. Some invasive cancers appear to contain only episomal HPV DNA sequences (117,119). Integration into the host chromosomal DNA appears to be a random event that does not lead to the consistent activation of specific cellular oncogenes. However, integration requires that the episomal viral genome break, and this break frequently leads to disruption of the E2 ORF (Fig. 19.11) (120). E2-derived proteins act as important regulators of the expression of the E6 and E7 ORFs (110). The E2 ORF encodes for three DNA-binding proteins that bind to a specific nucleotide sequence (ACCGN$_4$CGGT) in both the URR and in the E6 and E7 promotor. In most infected epithelia, E2 acts to inhibit transcription from the E6 and E7 ORFs (121). Disruption of the E2 ORF with retention of the E6 and E7 ORFs could result in the unregulated expression of the E6 and E7 ORFs and uncontrolled cell proliferation.

Role of Cellular Factors in Transformation

It is clear that the development of cervical cancer is a complex process that involves several steps and requires that both viral and cellular events take place. Simple infection with a specific HPV type is not sufficient for the development of anogenital tract cancer or its precursors. Numerous laboratories are actively studying the molecular and cellular events responsible for the transformation of cells by HPV and the development of cervical cancers. These studies are rapidly yielding new insights. Loss of heterozygosity (LOH) studies of primary cervical tumors indicate a high frequency of allelic loss on chromosomes 3p, 4p, 4q, and 11q (122). Nonrandom, cytogenetic deletions in the region of 3p14-p21 appear to be especially important and suggest that a tumor-

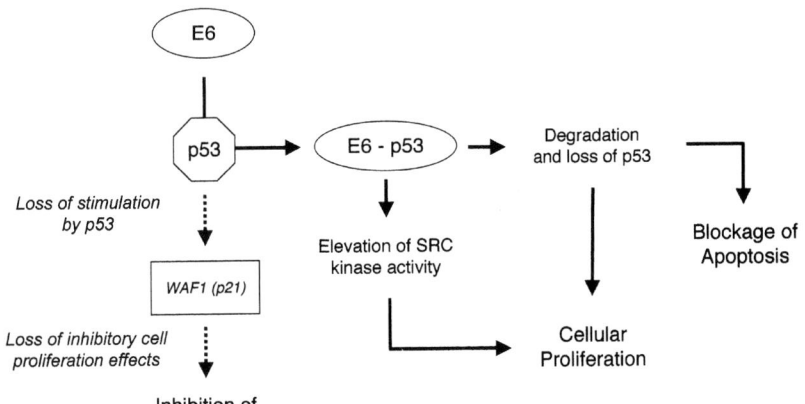

FIG. 19.10. Interactions between HPV 16 E6 and p53.

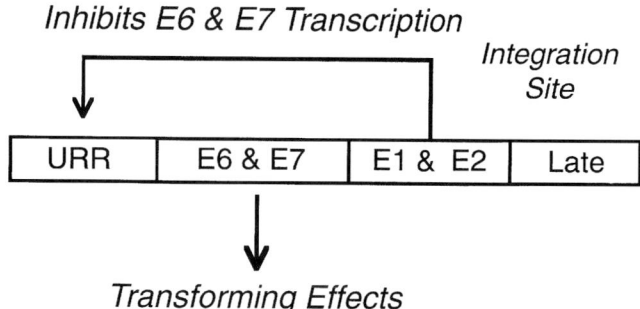

Inhibits E6 & E7 Transcription

Integration Site

URR	E6 & E7	E1 & E2	Late

Transforming Effects

FIG. 19.11. Effects of integration of the HPV circular DNA into the cellular genome. Integration physically disrupts the HPV DNA in the E1/E2 region. (Reprinted from Park TJ, Fujiwara H, Wright TC. Molecular biology of cervical cancer and its precursors. *Cancer* 1995;76:1902.)

suppressor gene important in cervical cancer may reside in this location (123).

Prevalence of HPV Infections

HPV Detection Methods

The prevalence of genital tract HPV infections and the frequency of exposure to HPV in the general population vary widely in different studies These variations are partly due to the different sensitivities of the methods used for detecting HPV infection and differences in the populations studied. Therefore, it is essential to understand the multiple molecular methods that can be used to detect HPV and their limitations. These include Southern blot and dot blot methods, PCR, and solution hybridization methods such as the Hybrid Capture 2 HPV DNA assays (Digene Corporation, Gaithersburg, MD). Each of these methods has advantages and disadvantages, and their sensitivity and specificity vary greatly (124).

Today, PCR methods are generally considered to be the gold standard for HPV DNA detection. PCR is extremely sensitive, and with currently well-established methods has the ability to detect and type all of the known anogenital HPV types. Currently, two different approaches are used to detect and type HPV DNA using PCR. One approach utilizes "type-specific" primers and the other utilizes "consensus" primers (124). "Type-specific" primers are designed to bind to specific DNA sequences found in only a single type of HPV. Therefore, these primers amplify only a single HPV type. In contrast, "consensus" primers are small oligonucleotides that bind to conserved DNA sequences that are present in many different types of HPVs. An advantage of consensus primers is that they allow many different types of HPVs to be identified using a single assay. For example, one of the most widely used consensus primers recognizes conserved sequences in the L1 ORF and amplifies more than 25 different types of anogenital HPVs (124). Although PCR is used

for many large epidemiologic studies, PCR is somewhat labor intensive and prone to contamination.

The commercially available, Food and Drug Administration (FDA)–approved, Hybrid Capture 2 HPV DNA assay has become the most widely used HPV DNA assay for clinical use (124). Hybrid Capture is a "second-generation" HPV test that is nonradioactive and uses chemiluminescence to detect a larger number of HPV types. Hybrid Capture 2 has an analytic sensitivity of 1 pg/mL of HPV DNA that corresponds to approximately 5,000 copies of HPV DNA. The Hybrid Capture 2 HPV DNA assay is designed to identify low-risk and high-risk HPV types separately. The low-risk probe mixture detects HPV types 6, 11, 42, 43, and 44. The high-risk probe mixture detects HPV types 16, 18, 31, 33, 35, 39, 45, 51, 52, 56, 58, 59, and 68. For most clinical indications, only the high-risk probe mixture is used for testing.

Prevalence of HPV in Women

In nonpregnant women with normal Pap smears, studies that used either PCR or Hybrid Capture 2 have detected HPV DNA in cervical samples in 4% to 43% of women (125–131). These appear, however, to be underestimations, since when multiple samples are taken over time, the cumulative prevalence in cytologically negative women is generally considerably higher (88,132,133). Based on these studies, it is clear that the prevalence of HPV infection in the general population is consistently higher than the prevalence of CIN by about one order of magnitude. The majority of women who are infected with HPV will never develop CIN 2,3 or cancer. As for cervical neoplasia, the independent risk factors for HPV DNA positivity are young age, high number of sexual partners, lower levels of education and income, and immunosuppression (71). For example, in a study from the Netherlands, the overall prevalence of HPV DNA positivity was 14% in women under the age of 35 years but was 5% in women 35 years of age or older (134). Other studies have shown a similar impact of age on the prevalence of high-risk HPV DNA positivity (Table 19.7).

Several points need to be emphasized with regard to HPV DNA prevalence studies. First, it is clear that the specific populations that are studied greatly affect the results. Adolescent, sexually active girls have a higher prevalence of HPV DNA positivity than do older women. Pregnancy increases the HPV DNA detection rate, as does the use of oral contraceptives in some studies (135). Second, the method of cervical sampling may influence the measured prevalence. A final point is that the detection of HPV DNA is often episodic rather than constant. Several studies have shown considerable variation in HPV DNA detection in individual women on a day-to-day basis (136,137). For example, in a study of HIV-seronegative, inner city middle-aged women enrolled in New York City, Sun et al. found that HPV DNA was detected in cervical samples using PCR in 31% of the

TABLE 19.7. *Prevalence of high-risk HPV DNA by age*

Country (ref.)	<25 yrs (%)	25–34 yrs (%)	35–44 yrs (%)	45+ yrs (%)
Netherlands (134)[a,c]	13	10	2	2
Costa Rica (218)[a,c]	10	6	3	3
Newfoundland (129)[b,d]	17	12	5	4
United Kingdom (219)[b,c]		3	3	5
France (220)[b,d]	21	20	13	11
United States (130)[b,c]	21	16	15	—

[a] Only women with negative Papanicolaou tests.
[b] All women (including those with and without abnormal Papanicolaou tests).
[c] Detected using PCR.
[d] High-risk HPV types detected using Hybrid Capture 2.

women at their first visit. However, after five scheduled visits 6 months apart, 73% of the women had been HPV DNA positive on at least one occasion (88). This variability appears to be due to episodic shedding of either free virus or virally infected cells from the cervical epithelium.

The prevalence of HPV-related anogenital infections appears to be increased during pregnancy and in immunosuppressed women. One study showed that the prevalence of HPV DNA positivity increased from the first to the third trimester, and that there was a dramatic reduction in prevalence during the postpartum period (138). Although few studies document differences in the prevalence of condylomata acuminata in pregnant patients, it is frequently stated that pregnancy is associated with an increase in the prevalence of genital warts and with an increase in the size of genital warts. It has been suggested that this is due to increased vascularity, perineal moisture, and hormonal stimulation. HPV infections appear to be particularly prevalent among HIV-infected women (139,140).

Transmission

Both genital and nongenital HPV appear to be transmitted predominantly through close personal contact, and transmission is facilitated by minor trauma at the site of inoculation. However, there continues to be considerable controversy as to how frequently anogenital HPV infections can be transmitted through vertical infection from mother to infant through autoinoculation or by contact with fomites.

Sexual Transmission

Since the time of the ancient Greeks and Romans, condylomata acuminata have been thought to be sexually transmitted. Ciuffo first demonstrated the transmission of warts using a cell-free filtrate of wart tissue in 1907. Since that initial demonstration, numerous studies have suggested that condylomata acuminata are sexually transmitted. The best data on the transmissibility and incubation period of genital warts are those of Oriel, who found that 60% of the sexual partners of patients with condylomas developed condyloma themselves (63). Similarly, Barrasso and associates reported that 64% of the male consorts of women with cervical HPV infections have histologic evidence of penile HPV infections (99). Age of the lesion appears to influence the infectivity of condylomata acuminata. Contact with a person whose genital warts have been present only a short time is more likely to result in transmission of the disease than contact with a person whose lesions have been present for a long time (141). In Oriel's study, the incubation period for HPV infection ranged from 3 weeks to 8 months, with an average of 3 months (63). In some cases, this incubation period can be much longer; there are occasional reports of women in whom genital warts have developed as long as 20 years after exposure. It should be pointed out that, clinically, it is often impossible to determine when a patient who develops condylomata acuminata was actually exposed to the virus.

Sexual transmission of HPV DNA positivity has also been documented in two studies of young women. In a study of 604 women attending a university, HPV DNA was detected by PCR in only 3% of women reporting no prior vaginal intercourse, 7% of women with one male sexual partner, 33% of women with two to four partners, and 53% of women with five or more male partners (142). In a prospective study that included virginal young women, Kjaer et al. found that only those women who initiated sexual activity became HPV DNA positive, and that the number of new partners was the most important determinant of HPV acquisition (143).

Perinatal and Fomite Transmission

It is clear from studies of small babies with anogenital warts, from studies of older children and adolescents who develop laryngeal papillomatosis, and from studies of squamous cell carcinomas of the conjunctiva and nose that nonsexual transmission of genital HPV types can occur. Studies of young children with genital condylomata acuminata have convincingly demonstrated that nonvenereal transmission occurs since approximately 17% of genital condylomas in this age group are associated with nongenital HPV types (98). Whether nonvenereal transmission in this setting occurs through contact with fomites or through heteroinoculation is presently unclear. HPV is relatively resistant to desiccation, and there are instances in which it appears that anogenital HPV types have been transferred through fomites (144,145). Another example of nonvenereal transmission is laryngeal papillomatosis. Laryngeal papillomatosis is an uncommon disorder characterized by the development of recurrent laryngeal papillomas that are associated with HPV type 6 or 11. The incidence of this uncommon disorder ranges from 0.4 to 1.1 per 100,000 (146). This disorder develops in older children and young adults and it has been suggested that the HPV infection is acquired either *in utero* or during birth.

HPV DNA has been detected in nasal and oropharyngeal swabs in neonates born to women who have genital HPV infections. PCR studies have detected HPV DNA in almost two-thirds of amniotic fluid samples from pregnant women with SIL (CIN) (147). In two comprehensive studies of vertical transmission, perinatal transmission of HPV occurred in 30% to 55% of infants born to mothers who had cervical HPV infections, and many of these infections persisted for over 6 weeks (148,149). These studies suggest that vertical transmission of HPV infections can occur, but it appears that vertically acquired HPV infection plays little role in the development of cervical neoplasia in adults. Similarly, transmission via fomites appears to occur, although it is probably an uncommon event and unlikely to account for a significant proportion of anogenital HPV infections in adults.

Association of HPV Types with Specific Lower Genital Tract Lesions

Outcome After Exposure

Exposure to a HPV of any type can result in three different outcomes (Fig. 19.12). Exposure can lead to no infection with HPV, produce a "latent HPV infection," or produce an HPV infection associated with a clinically observable lesion. Latent infections are defined as HPV infections that can be detected using molecular methods in patients lacking

gross or microscopic evidence of HPV infection. HPV infections that are associated with clinically observable lesions include a variety of entities that can be detected with the naked eye. These observable lesions include condylomata acuminata, flat condylomas, vulvar intraepithelial neoplasia, and invasive cancers. They also include lesions, sometimes referred to as *subclinical infections*, that are unassociated with macroscopic lesions or symptoms but can be detected either by colposcopy or peniscopy. All of these HPV infections are readily detected by microscopic examinations of the affected tissues since the cytopathic effects of HPV must be present for a diagnosis to be made. In contrast, latent infections cannot be detected by colposcopy or microscopic analysis of the affected tissue since the presence of latent virus is not associated with characteristic morphologic changes in the latently infected cells.

The concept of latent HPV infections arose from studies demonstrating the presence of HPV DNA in histologically normal tissues at some distance from clinically apparent lesions (150). However, the separation between latent HPV infections and HPV infections associated with clinically observable lesions is not as precise as previously thought. It is now apparent that HPV-associated lesions that are histologically low grade frequently spontaneous regress, and that women with latent HPV infections frequently develop clinically observable lesions over time. Moreover, prospective follow-up studies that have used sensitive and accurate typing methods have found that the detection of HPV DNA in women without clinically apparent lesions is variable, and that women can be classified as being latently infected at one visit, yet be classified as HPV DNA negative at a subsequent visit (88,137,151).

PATHOLOGY OF PREINVASIVE LESIONS OF THE LOWER GENITAL TRACT

Cervix

Localization of CIN

The use of colposcopy to identify CIN and careful microscopic studies of the distribution of CIN in conization and hysterectomy specimens have greatly increased our knowledge of the clinical appearance and distribution of CIN. Colposcopic and histologic mapping studies of the position of CIN have shown that the vast majority of lesions develop in a region of the cervix called the *transformation zone* (152, 153). At the time of menarche, most young women have some endocervical-type columnar epithelium present on the portio (vaginal portion) of the cervix. This endocervical-type epithelium appears to be salmon red to the naked eye and has been referred to as *cervical erosion, ectropion, cervical ectopy,* or *native columnar epithelium.* In response to a variety of stimuli including low pH, trauma, hormonal factors, and cervicovaginal infections, shortly after menarche, the columnar epithelium gradually becomes replaced by a

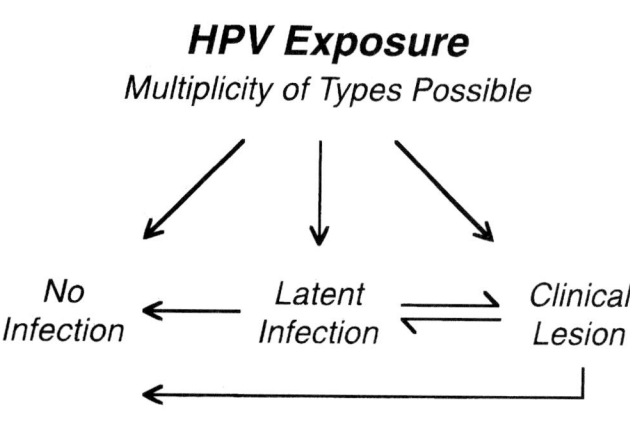

FIG. 19.12. Possible outcomes after exposure to HPV.

stratified squamous epithelium (Fig. 19.13). The replacement of columnar epithelium by a stratified squamous epithelium occurs by two different processes. One is called *squamous metaplasia* and the other is the direct ingrowth of squamous epithelium from the periphery of the portio, referred to as *epidermidization*. As these processes occur, the histologic junction between stratified squamous epithelium and endocervical-type columnar epithelium moves inward toward the external cervical os. By the age of 40 years, the entire portio is covered by mature squamous epithelium in most women.

The transformation zone is defined as the region of the cervix that lies between the original squamocolumnar junction and the current or anatomic squamocolumnar junction (Fig. 19.13). The transformation zone is of critical importance in cervical pathology and colposcopy because it is the site at which CIN usually develops as well as the major locus for cervical carcinomas. Although CIN often extends into the endocervical canal, it rarely extends out onto the native squamous epithelium of the portio (152). The mechanisms responsible for the restricted distribution of CIN on the cervix are unknown. CIN occurs twice as often on the anterior cervical lip as on the posterior lip, and it rarely involves the lateral cervical angles without involving either the anterior or posterior lip (154).

Origin of CIN

There are three potential cells of origin of CIN: the basal cells of the mature squamous epithelium of the portio, the basal cells of squamous metaplastic cells, and endocervical reserve cells. Since the majority of CIN arises in the transformation zone with one margin adjacent to the current squamocolumnar junction, it would appear that the cell of origin of the majority of CIN is the basal cell of squamous metaplasia. The recent demonstration that α_6-integrin is a possible receptor for HPV provides support this model since α_6-integrin is only expressed in basal cells and epidermal stem cells

(114). Over the years, there has been some controversy as to whether CIN develops from a single focus or cell and then enlarges centrifugally over the cervix, or whether it can develop as a field effect from multiple foci. Based on colposcopic observations, Coppleson suggested that CIN develops as a multicellular event and enlarges either by the coalescence of multiple foci or by transformation of adjacent normal cells (155). Other studies suggest that CIN develops from either a unicellular or a unifocal origin. A unicellular origin of CIN is supported by studies of the distribution of glucose-6-phosphatase in CIN lesions. Glucose-6-phosphatase is an X-linked enzyme marker. Individual cells of patients who are heterozygous for different isoenzymes express only a single form within an individual cell. Studies of the distribution of glucose-6-phosphatase in CIN lesions suggest that only a single isoenzyme is expressed within a lesion, indicating a unicellular origin (156,157). Chromosomal studies also support a unicellular origin (158).

These theories as to the origin of CIN were developed before it was realized that low-grade CIN 1 can be associated with different HPV types and may often represent a different biological entity than CIN 2,3. Since CIN 1 frequently develops from a latently infected cervical epithelium, is often associated with multiple types of HPVs, and has many of the features of a productive viral infection rather than a neoplasm, it might be predicted that these lesions would be polyclonal in origin. Using more modern molecular techniques, Park et al. have reported that CIN 1 associated with low– or no–oncogenic risk HPV types is typically polyclonal, whereas CIN 1 associated with ''cancer-associated'' HPV types is typically monoclonal, as are almost all CIN 2,3 lesions (159). This indicates that CIN 1 associated with low-risk or novel types of HPV is biologically different at its inception from lesions that are histologically low grade but associated with high-risk HPV types. There also are now data to suggest that some CIN 2,3 lesions develop de novo without a preexisting CIN 1 (160,161). In a study of 54

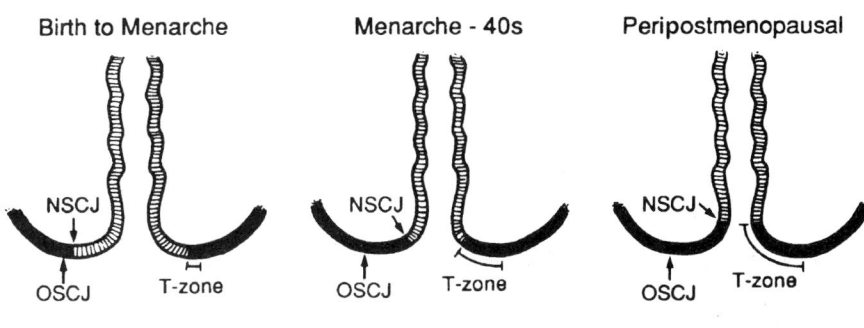

Birth to Menarche   Menarche - 40s   Peripostmenopausal

 = Squamous epithelium
 = Columnar epithelium
OSCJ = Original squamocolumnar junction
NSCJ = New squamocolumnar junction
T-zone = Region between original and new
         squamocolumnar junction

FIG. 19.13. The transformation zone.

cytologically negative women who were HPV 16 DNA positive, 17 (31%) developed CIN on follow-up and 41% of the incident cases were first identified as CIN 3 (161).

Microscopic Appearance of CIN

The two histologic hallmarks of CIN, regardless of grade, are the presence of nuclear atypia and aberrant cytoplasmic differentiation. Nuclear atypia in CIN can take many forms. In most cases, the nuclei become enlarged and an increase in the nuclear to cytoplasmic ratio occurs. The extent of nuclear enlargement usually varies from cell to cell, leading to an irregular appearance of the epithelium. Multinucleation also often occurs. The nuclei of cells in CIN are usually hyperchromatic, and the chromatin is coarsely clumped. The nuclear outline is sometimes irregular and angulated rather than round.

Aberrant cytoplasmic differentiation is also invariably found in CIN irrespective of grade. The normal, stratified, squamous epithelium of the cervix can be divided into three layers (Fig. 19.14). The basal layer is composed of a single layer of cells that is in contact with the basement membrane and serves to bind the epithelium to it. The parabasal layer is the proliferative compartment and is one to two cell layers thick. This is the site at which mitoses are observed in the normal cervix. As cells leave the parabasal layer, they become progressively more mature and develop cytoplasmic flattening. Squamous intraepithelial lesions have aberrant differentiation and deviate from this normal pattern. The extent and type of aberrant differentiation vary greatly from lesion to lesion. In the original CIN terminology, lesions were graded 1 to 3 based on the extent to which the epithelium was replaced by undifferentiated basaloid cells (11). Lesions were classified as follows: CIN 1 if the undifferentiated cells involved only the lower third of the epithelium

(Fig. 19.15A); CIN 2 if undifferentiated cells and mitoses were present up to two-thirds of the way through the epithelium (Fig. 19.15B); and CIN 3 if they extended through more than two-thirds of the epithelium (Fig. 19.15C).

In CIN 1, the HPV cytopathic effect is usually a prominent feature, and immature basaloid cells and mitotic figures are restricted to the lower third of the epithelium. The cytopathic

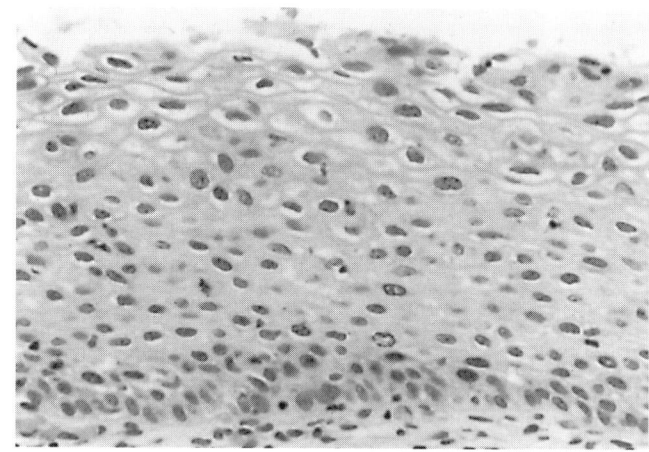

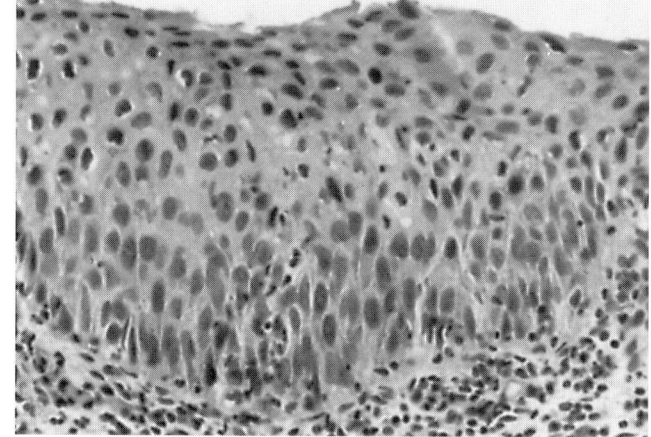

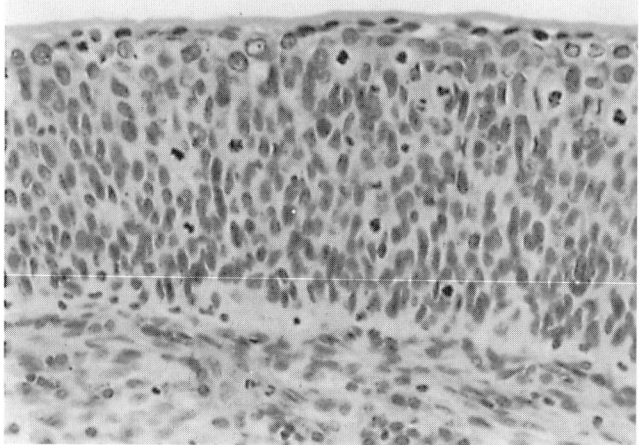

FIG. 19.15. Histology of **(A)** CIN 1, **(B)** CIN 2, **(C)** CIN 3.

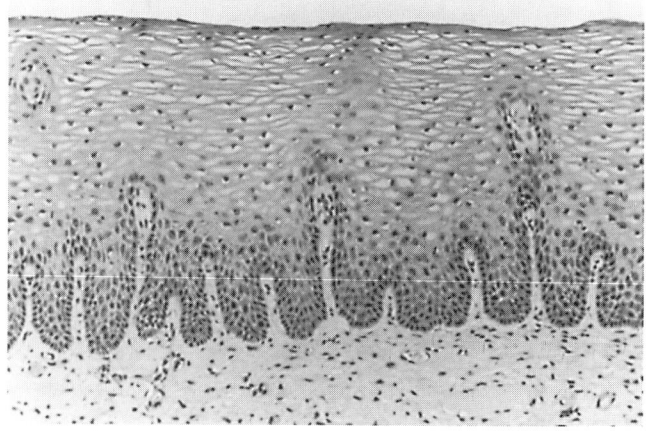

FIG. 19.14. Normal stratified squamous epithelium of the cervix.

effect of HPV can best be described as the formation of a region of perinuclear clearing or vacuolization (Fig, 19.16). Cells with a combination of nuclear atypia and perinuclear clearing were described by Koss and Durfee and are called *koilocytes*, a term derived from the Greek word *koilos*, which means hollow or empty (162). *In situ* hybridization techniques readily detect the presence of HPV DNA in koilocytes within tissue sections since these cells contain multiple copies of HPV DNA (Fig. 19.16). Electron microscopic studies have confirmed the presence of completely formed viruses in koilocytes (64). However, the presence of perinuclear clearing, or halos, in cells without significant nuclear atypia is seen in a variety of nonneoplastic disorders as well as HPV infections. These disorders include infections with *Trichomonas* organisms, *Gardnerella vaginalis*, and *Candida* organisms. In addition, perinuclear clearing can occasionally be a feature of the atrophic epithelial changes found in postmenopausal patients or in immature squamous metaplasia. Before the recognition that all CINs are associated with HPV infections, cervical condylomas and CIN 1 were generally classified as separate histopathologic entities. With the widespread application of HPV typing to cervical lesions, it has become evident that it is impossible to distinguish on histologic grounds alone between flat cervical condylomas and CIN 1 lesions associated with low–oncogenic risk HPV types and those associated with high–oncogenic risk HPV types (14). Since clinical and histologic criteria do not allow segregation of low-grade lesions on the basis of oncogenic potential, distinctions between flat cervical condylomas and low-grade CIN 1 lesions are no longer clinically meaningful and have been dropped from the Bethesda terminology.

Although HPV-induced cytopathic effects are often present, they are usually less prominent in CIN 2,3 than in CIN

1. CIN 2,3 are characterized by immature basaloid cells and mitotic figures that extend into the upper two-thirds of the epithelium. The immature basaloid cells usually have nuclear crowding, pleomorphism, and loss of normal cell polarity. Cytoplasm is usually minimal, which results in a high nuclear to cytoplasmic ratio. Also found in most high-grade lesions are abnormal mitotic figures (Fig. 19.17). Most squamous cell carcinomas of the cervix have chromosomal abnormalities, and many are aneuploid. This suggests that aneuploid precursor lesions are highly significant and may have the capacity to progress to an invasive carcinoma if left untreated. Support for such a hypothesis comes from studies that have documented that the percentage of CIN lesions that are aneuploid increases as the grade of the lesion increases (163). In one study that used an imaging system to measure the DNA content of Feulgen-stained cervical cells, it was found that 33% of mildly dysplastic lesions were aneuploid (163). The percentage of aneuploid lesions increased with increasing severity of the dysplasia to 75% of moderate dysplasia and 90% of severe dysplasia and carcinoma *in situ* lesions. Similar results have been obtained using other techniques to assess DNA content. The best histologic predictor of an aneuploid lesion is the presence of abnormal mitotic figures. Eighty-five percent of CINs with aneuploid DNA patterns contain abnormal mitotic figures (164).

Microscopic Appearance of Endocervical Glandular Atypia and Adenocarcinoma in Situ

Both endocervical glandular atypia and adenocarcinoma *in situ* of the endocervix are characterized by endocervical glands that are lined by atypical glandular cells and lack

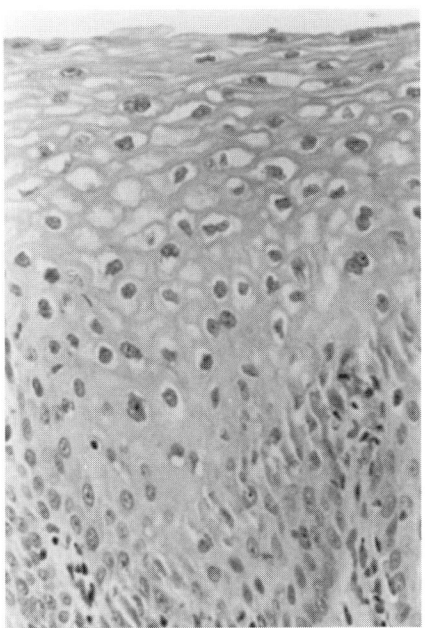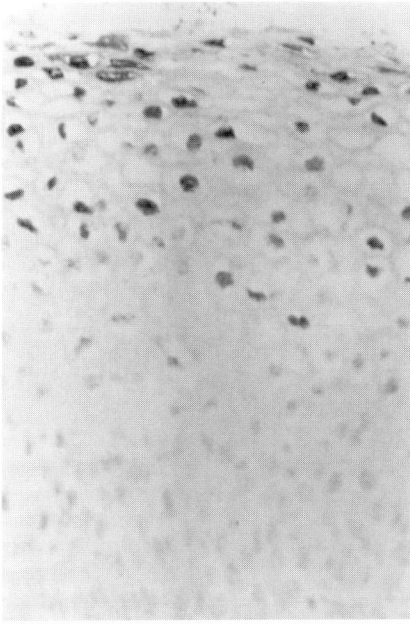

A,B

FIG. 19.16. A: CIN 1 lesions are characterized by the presence of cells with perinuclear halos and nuclear atypia. **B:** *In situ* hybridization of a CIN 1 lesion using probes for HPV 16/18 detects HPV DNA appearing as dark staining of the nuclei of the superficial cells.

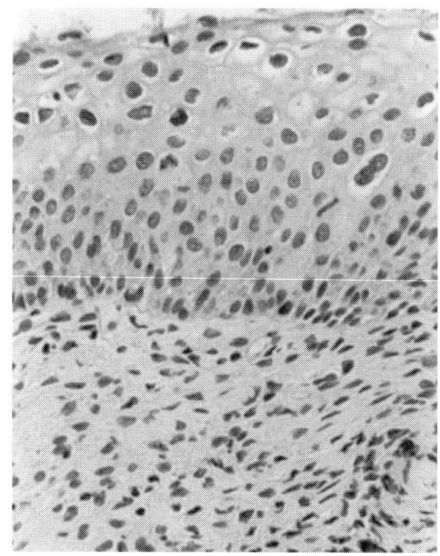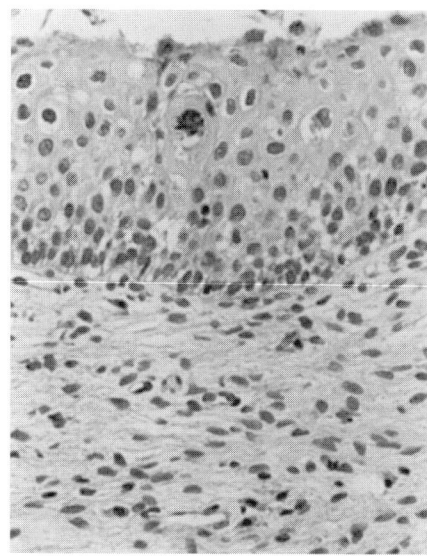

A,B

FIG. 19.17. Histology of **(A)** CIN 1 that lacks abnormal mitotic figures and **(B)** CIN 2,3 that is classified as high-grade because it contains abnormal mitotic figures.

evidence of stromal invasion (Fig. 19.18A). In both lesions, individual endocervical cells have many of the histologic and cytologic features of invasive adenocarcinoma. The atypical endocervical cells are enlarged with hyperchromatic, elongated nuclei (Fig. 19.18B). Characteristically, the chromatin pattern is coarse and granular. There is a reduction in the amount of cytoplasm and only minimal intracellular mucin is present. A characteristic feature of both endocervical glandular atypia and adenocarcinoma *in situ* is crowding of the cells and pseudostratification. Abrupt transitions between involved and uninvolved epithelium are frequently observed.

Endocervical glandular atypia and adenocarcinoma *in situ* are differentiated from each other by their relative degrees of mitotic activity and pseudostratification. Mitotic figures are quite common, and atypical mitotic figures are frequently observed in adenocarcinoma *in situ*. There is marked pseudostratification of the endocervical cells that form two or three cell layers. This results in cribriforming and complex papillary infoldings of the epithelium into the gland lumens. In contrast, mitotic figures are relatively uncommon in endocervical glandular atypia, and the atypical endocervical cells are not pseudostratified. Instead they form a single row of cells. Cribriforming and papillary infoldings are also infrequent in endocervical glandular atypia.

Architectural features are used to distinguish between adenocarcinoma *in situ* and invasive endocervical adenocarcinoma. Invasion is diagnosed when atypical glands extend beyond the depth of the normal, uninvolved, endocervical glands. This is usually approximately 5 to 6 mm from the surface (165). Features suggestive of invasion include desmoplasia or stromal reaction around the involved glands, exuberant gland budding, back-to-back glands, and papillary projections from the endocervical surface.

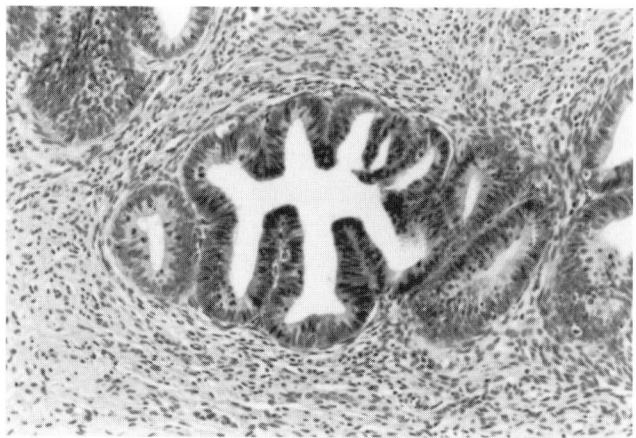

A

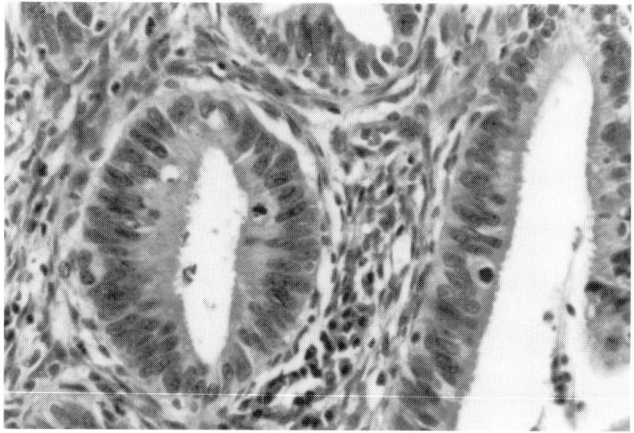

B

FIG. 19.18. Adenocarcinoma *in situ* of the cervix. **A:** Adenocarcinoma *in situ* is characterized by glands lined by atypical endocervical cells that frequently form papillary projections into the glandular lumen. **B:** At higher magnification, the endocervical cells are pseudostratified and there are numerous mitotic figures.

Vulva

Gross Appearance of Vulvar HPV-associated Lesions

Anogenital warts can be categorized into three separate types based on their gross appearances (166). One is a hyperplastic, cauliflower-like lesion called condyloma acuminatum. These raised exophytic lesions are pink to white and are found in moist areas such as the labia, perianal region, glans penis, inner aspect of the prepuce, and urethral meatus. Another is a small sessile plaque type of wart. These are most common on the penile shaft. The final type is a keratotic, verruca vulgaris–like wart.

Vulvar condylomas occur in women of all age groups but have a peak incidence from ages 20 to 24 years. They vary in size from small, easily treated lesions to large, inflamed masses that tend to recur after treatment (Fig. 19.19). A key feature of HPV infection of the lower female genital tract is that it often involves multiple sites and is multifocal. For example, 22% to 32% of female patients with vulvar condylomas will have concurrent cervical lesions (167,168). Therefore, it is essential that the entire lower genital tract be examined carefully in all patients with vulvar condylomas. Vulvar lesions with a typical gross appearance of condylomas are readily recognized and are rarely confused with other lesions. However, when the appearance is atypical, the

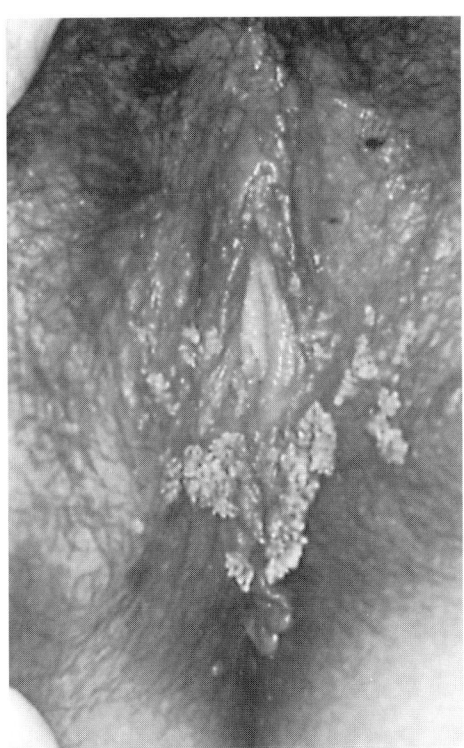

FIG. 19.19. Gross features of vulvar condyloma acuminatum. (Used with permission courtesy of Dr. D. Townsend, University of California. From Wright TC, Richart RM: Pathology quiz: condyloma acuminatum. *Contemp OB/GYN* 1990; 4:5.)

differential diagnosis can include almost any raised vulvar lesion, including condyloma latum, molluscum contagiosum, fibropapilloma, lymphoma, hidradenoma, and even verrucous carcinoma if the lesion is large. In atypical cases, a biopsy of the lesion is mandatory and usually diagnostic. The classic histologic features of condylomata acuminata are papillomatosis, acanthosis with hyperkeratosis, parakeratosis, and the presence of nuclear atypia with multinucleation and koilocytosis (Fig. 19.20). As mentioned previously, condylomata acuminata are usually associated with HPV types 6 and 11. HPV DNA can be detected by *in situ* hybridization in more than 90% of cases of condylomata acuminata (Fig. 19.20) (96).

Many patients have small genital epithelial lesions that are clinically suggestive of plaque-type anogenital warts and are better visualized after the application of 4% acetic acid but that histologically lack characteristic HPV-associated cytopathic effects. These lesions are particularly common in men and occur on the corona glandis and along each side of the frenulum of the penis. The term *pearly penile papules* has been used for these lesions (169). In women, a common mimic of condylomata acuminata is *micropapillomatosis labialis* (170). Micropapillomatosis labialis occurs at the introitus and appears as multiple, soft papillary projections that are characteristically bilateral and symmetric (Fig. 19.21). Although micropapillomatosis labialis can histologically be mistaken for an HPV-related lesion, multiple studies have failed to detect HPV DNA in a significant number of cases (170,171). Another common entity that is often confused with condyloma acuminatum, especially by pathologists, is benign fibropapilloma of the anogenital region.

Like CIN 2,3, VIN has been increasing in incidence over the last two decades (172–174). VIN usually presents as a slightly raised, sharply demarcated lesion that can be black, white, gray, red, or brown depending on the age, race, and complexion of the patient (Fig. 19.22). These lesions tend to be unifocal in older patients and multifocal in younger patients. The margins are often irregular, and the lesions vary in size from several millimeters to large, confluent lesions that involve the entire vulva. The majority of lesions are 1 to 3 cm in diameter. Most commonly, VIN develops on the labia minora, around the anus, and at the introitus (175). The clitoris and urethra are involved less commonly (172,175).

Bowenoid papulosis is considered by many to be a separate entity. It is a disease characterized by multiple small papules that are often violaceous and occasionally coalesce to form large plaques. The lesions develop on the vulvar skin and occasionally on the abdomen. Bowenoid papulosis is a disease of young women, with a peak incidence in the third decade. However, despite the relatively innocuous gross appearance of Bowenoid papulosis, this lesion is identical histologically to VIN 3. Invasive vulvar carcinoma may arise in untreated cases of Bowenoid papulosis.

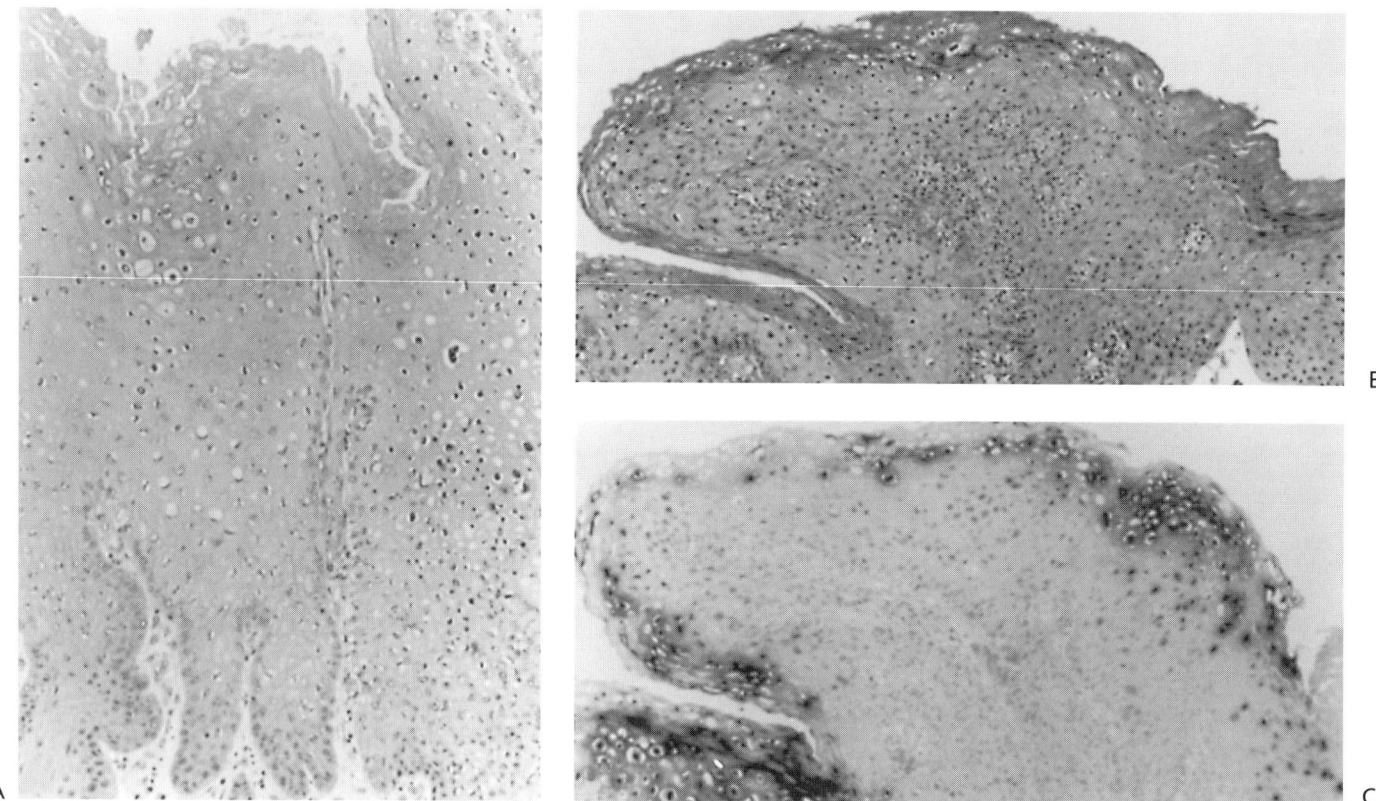

FIG. 19.20. A, B: Histology of condyloma acuminatum. **C:** *In situ* hybridization of a vulvar condyloma using probes for HPV 6/11.

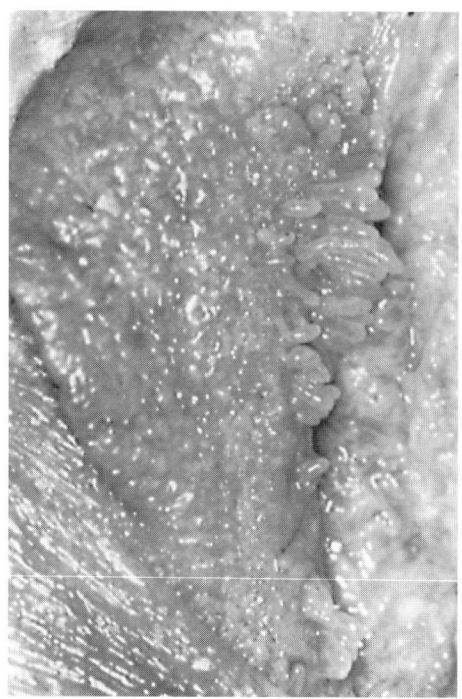

FIG. 19.21. Characteristic gross features of micropapillomatosis labialis. (Courtesy of Dr. Alex Ferenczy, Jewish General Hospital, McGill University, Montreal, Quebec, Canada.)

Microscopic Appearance of VIN

Microscopically, VIN lesions are similar to CIN lesions. The four major histologic features are increased numbers of undifferentiated cells with nuclear atypia, alterations in epidermal maturation with disorganization, parakeratosis and hyperkeratosis, and the presence of abnormal mitotic figures (Fig. 19.23) (176). VIN lesions are histologically graded on a scale of 1 to 3, using criteria identical to those used for the original CIN terminology for cervical cancer precursors. Nuclear atypia in VIN typically involves the basal and parabasal cell layers as well as cells in the upper, more differentiated cell layers in most cases. Nuclear size in VIN varies from small and hyperchromatic to pleomorphic and large. VIN lesions have recently been subdivided into three histopathologic types termed *warty*, *basaloid*, and *well-differentiated*. Each of these has distinctive clinical features (172,177). Separation into these three subtypes is based predominantly on nuclear size and the amount of cytoplasmic differentiation. In general, invasive vulvar cancers that are HPV DNA positive occur in younger women and are associated with the warty and basaloid variants of VIN. These two histopathologic types are histopathologically similar to CIN (177,178). Warty VIN is characterized by prominent HPV cytopathic effects in squamous cells residing in the superficial portions of the epithelium, the presence of parakeratosis and hyperkeratosis on the surface of the lesion,

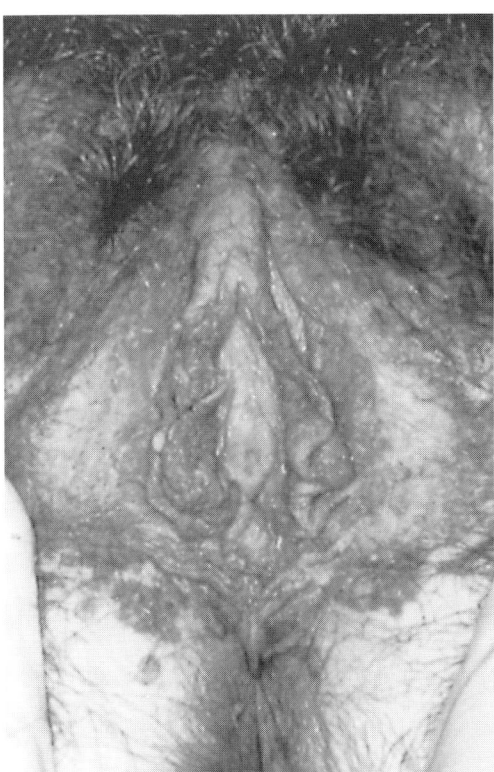

FIG. 19.22. Gross features of vulvar intraepithelial neoplasia. (Used with permission courtesy of Dr. D. Townsend, University of California. From Wright TC, Richart RM: Pathology quiz: condyloma acuminatum. *Contemp OB/GYN* 1990;4:5.)

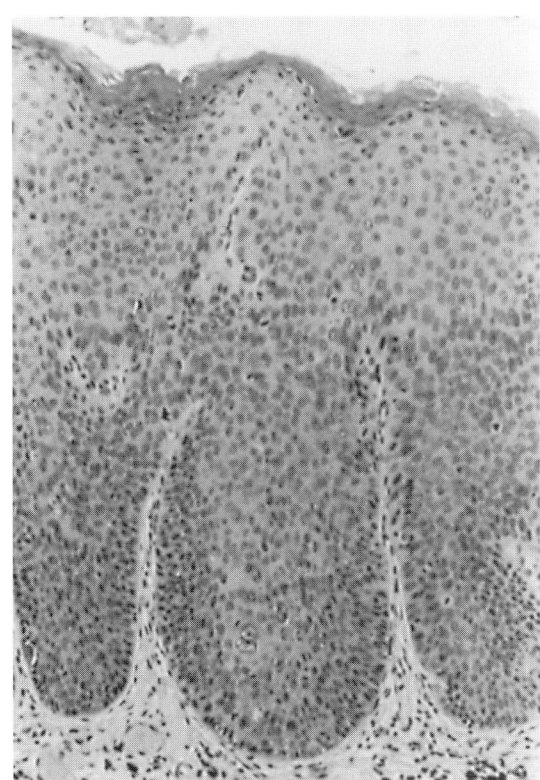

FIG. 19.23. Microscopic features of VIN 3.

and a surface architecture that typically has spikes and papillary projections. Cells with small, hyperchromatic nuclei and clear cytoplasmic halos termed ''cor ronds'' are also typical. The deeper (e.g., more basally located cells) cells have large, pleomorphic nuclei with coarsely clumped chromatin, and abnormal mitotic figures are commonly seen. Because of its verrucopapillary architecture and koilocytotic features, the histologic appearance of warty VIN is similar to that of many CIN 2,3 lesions.

The other histologic subtype of VIN that is frequently associated with HPV DNA–positive vulvar cancers in younger women is the basaloid type of VIN. Basaloid VIN is composed of small cells with limited amounts of cytoplasm that resemble the cells of carcinoma *in situ* of the cervix. These cells replace the full thickness of the epithelium. Atypical mitotic figures can be present in basaloid VIN, but tend to be less common than in warty VIN. The surface of basaloid VIN tends to be smooth and covered with a keratin layer.

In contrast to the warty and basaloid variants of VIN that are associated with HPV DNA–positive vulvar cancers in younger women, well-differentiated VIN is found in older women and tends to be associated with HPV DNA–negative invasive vulvar cancers (172,179). This type of VIN was originally referred to as carcinoma *in situ*, simplex type.

Well-differentiated VIN is composed of pleomorphic, large keratinocytes with minimal nuclear hyperchromasia and coarsely clumped chromatin. The characteristic feature is cells with large amounts of eosinophilic cytoplasm that occur at the tips of the rete pegs and frequently form keratin pearls. These lesions often occur adjacent to well-differentiated invasive vulvar cancers and are also often associated with either squamous hyperplasia or lichen sclerosis of the vulva (172).

These histologic variants, especially the warty and basaloid forms, are frequently found together in the same patient. Moreover, there are no data to suggest that histopathologic type has a significant impact on either rates of progression to invasive vulvar cancer or response to standard therapies. One additional point needs further clarification. Although the histologic distinction between cervical condyloma and CIN 1 is no longer thought to be possible, vulvar condyloma and VIN are still distinguished from one another. The reason for retaining this distinction for the vulva is that the vast majority of vulvar condylomas are caused by HPV 6 or 11, which are low–oncogenic risk HPV types (96). The development of invasive vulvar carcinoma from a preexisting condyloma acuminatum is an extremely rare event. Histologically, the distinction between vulvar condyloma and VIN is made on the basis of two features: the presence or absence of abnormal mitotic figures and the presence or absence of nuclear atypia that involve the basal and parabasal cell layers.

Vagina

Vaginal intraepithelial neoplasia (VAIN) lesions are generally white with sharp borders. They are best evaluated with colposcopy after the application of 4% acetic acid. In general, vascular changes are not striking in VAIN lesions, although punctation is occasionally seen. The histologic features of VAIN are identical to those of CIN and VIN.

CYTOLOGIC SCREENING FOR CERVICAL CANCER AND ITS PRECURSORS

Background

Cytologic evaluation of cells obtained from the cervix and vagina was first proposed by Dr. George Papanicolaou in the 1940s as a method for detecting cervical cancer and its precursors. Since those early studies, cervical cytology has proved to be the most efficacious and cost-effective method for cancer screening. The institution of communitywide Pap smear screening programs for detecting cervical abnormalities was followed by a dramatic reduction in both the incidence of and death rates from cervical cancer (46). This fact has perhaps been best documented in British Columbia, Canada, where a Pap smear screening program was instituted in the late 1950s on a provincewide basis using centralized facilities. The British Columbia screening program was widely supported, and it is estimated that more than half of the women at risk for developing cervical cancer received a Pap smear each year. Largely as a result of this screening program, the incidence of cervical cancer in British Columbia dropped from 25 cases per 100,000 women in 1954 to 8 cases per 100,000 women in 1984, and death rates from cervical cancer fell from a high of 13 cases per 100,000 in 1962 to 3 cases per 100,000 in 1983 (180). Similar results have been reported from Scandinavia and the United States.

Differences in the use of cervical cancer screening programs are responsible for the worldwide variations in the incidence of cervical cancer. Cervical cancer is the second most common female malignancy in the world and the most common female malignancy in the developing countries of Africa, Asia, and South America, where cytologic screening programs are not widely available (181). In contrast, cervical cancer is currently the thirteenth most common female malignancy in the United States, where cytology is in widespread use (182).

Accuracy of Cervical Cytology

Despite the proven effectiveness of cervical cytology in reducing the incidence of cervical cancer, over the last several years, the accuracy of cervical cytology has been questioned. Two factors need to be considered when assessing the accuracy of any diagnostic test including cervical cytology. One is whether the test is specific in detecting a given condition; the other is the sensitivity of the test for detecting

a given condition. Several large meta-analyses have been conducted that indicate that both the sensitivity and specificity of cervical cytology are lower than previously thought (183,184). The first of these was by Fahey et al., who estimated that the mean sensitivity of a conventional cervical cytology was 58% and the mean specificity was 69%, *when used in a screening setting* (Fig. 19.24) (183). The second meta-analysis was by Nanda et al., who considered different cytologic cut-offs and endpoints (184). When a cytologic cut-off of atypical squamous cells of undetermined significance (ASCUS) is used and the endpoint is biopsy-confirmed CIN 1 or worse, the average sensitivity of conventional cytology was 68% and the average specificity 75% (Fig. 19.24). When the cytologic cut-off was LSIL and the endpoint was biopsy-confirmed CIN 2,3 or worse, the average sensitivity was 81% and the specificity 77%.

A number of factors influence the false-negative rate of cervical cytology. Of key importance is the use of a proper technique for sampling the cervix (185,186). When cervical cytology was first introduced, only cells from the vaginal pool were sampled. It quickly became apparent that this method was inadequate, resulting in a high false-negative rate. In 1947, Ayre reported on the use of a wooden spatula to scrape cells from the surface of the cervix. Since the ma-

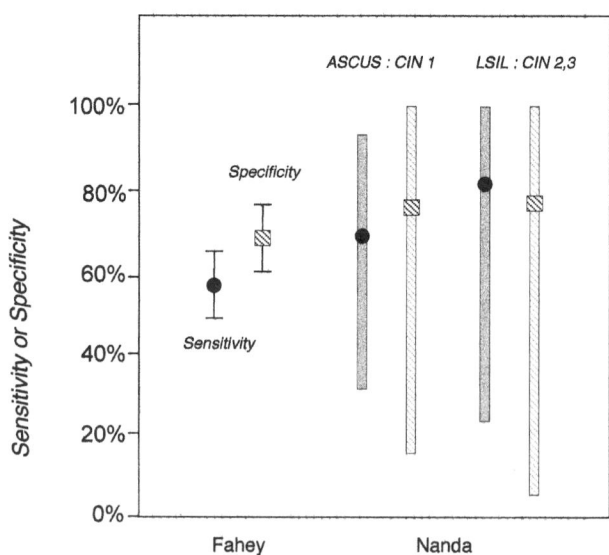

Performance of Conventional Papanicolaou Test

FIG. 19.24. Estimates of the sensitivity (*circles*) and specificity (*squares*) of conventional cervical cytology obtained from two meta-analyses (those of Fahey et al. *left side with bars showing 95% confidence intervals* and Nanda et al. *right side with bars representing range of values in different studies*). (Modified with permission from Fahey MT, Irwig L, Macaskill P. Meta-analysis of Pap test accuracy. *Am J Epidemiol* 1995; 141:680 and Nanda K, McCrory DC, Myers ER, et al. Accuracy of the Papanicolaou test in screening for and follow-up of cervical cytologic abnormalities: a systematic review. *Ann Intern Med* 2000;132:810.)

jority of CIN and cancers involve the transformation zone, spatulas were designed to sample this area. This approach had a lower false-negative rate than simple aspiration of cells from the vaginal pool. Sampling the endocervical canal also reduces the false-negative rate. This sample can be taken with an endocervical brush (e.g., cytobrush), one of the newer collection devices such as a cell broom, or a saline-moistened cotton-tipped applicator. The number of endocervical cells that are obtained with a cotton-tipped applicator is less than the number obtained with a cytobrush (187), and several studies have reported a higher CIN detection rate when cytobrushes are used (187,188). Other important factors for reducing the false-negative rate are the rapid fixation of cells to prevent artifactual changes secondary to air-drying and the use of a cytology laboratory with stringent quality control standards.

Although a false-negative rate of 20% for a cancer screening test appears to be unacceptably high, the test has been effective despite its limitations owing to the natural history of the disease, and the use of cervical cytology has reduced the incidence of cervical cancer by almost 80% in the United States over the last three decades (189). The effectiveness of cervical cytology is attributable to the fact that invasive cervical cancer requires an average of about 10 to 17 years to develop from a CIN 1 lesion and 5 to 10 years to develop from a carcinoma *in situ* lesion (14). If cervical cytology is performed on a routine basis, it is unlikely that a cervical neoplasm would not be detected while in a precursor stage, although such cases do rarely occur. The current screening recommendation from the American Cancer Society and the American College of Obstetricians and Gynecologists is that cervical cancer screening should be initiated approximately 3 years after the initiation of sexual intercourse, but no later than age 21 years (190,191). After 30 years of age, the interval between cervical cytology examinations can be extended to 2 to 3 years in women who have had three consecutive negative cervical cytology screening test results and who have no history of CIN 2,3, are not immunocompromised nor have a history of, DES exposure (190,191). There is currently no consensus as to when to stop screening. The American Cancer Society recommends that screening be discontinued in women 70 years and older with three documented negative screening tests within the preceding 10 years and no history of cervical cancer, DES exposure, or immunosuppression (191). The U.S. Preventive Services Task Force recommends discontinuing screening at age 65 years in women who have had adequate recent screening and who are not otherwise at high risk for cervical cancer (192). Routine screening is not recommended for women who have undergone a hysterectomy for benign indications and who have no prior history of CIN 2,3.

Obtaining an Optimal Cervical Cytology

To obtain an optimal cervical cytology, it is necessary to observe several simple guidelines. The patient should be instructed not to douche, wash her vagina, or have intercourse for 24 hours before obtaining the specimen. Cervical cytology should not be obtained during menses or less than 1 week after stopping intravaginal antibiotics or antifungal agents. Cervical cytology should be taken before a bimanual examination and using a minimal amount or no lubricant. It is preferable not to apply acetic acid to the cervix before the cervical cytology is taken. An Ayre-type spatula or cell broom type of device should be used and rotated around the cervix several times with firm pressure. A cytobrush is immediately placed in the external os, rotated 180 degrees only, and withdrawn. Cells obtained with the cytobrush and the spatula are placed on the same slide (Fig. 19.25). The sample is immediately fixed and labeled with the patient's name and date of birth. With the advent of government mandated work rules that limit the number of slides that a cytotechnologist can screen each day, most cytopathology laboratories in the United States request that a single slide technique be used for cervical cytology.

Liquid-based Cytology

Recently, liquid-based cytology has been introduced for cervical cytologic screening. With liquid-based cytology, the clinician obtains the sample from the cervix in the usual fashion using either an Ayre-type spatula and a cytobrush or one of the newer collection devices such as a cell broom. The sample is then transferred to a vial containing a liquid preservative fluid. The sample is sent to the cytology laboratory where a slide is prepared for evaluation. Two liquid-based cytology methods are currently available in the United States. One is the ThinPrep Pap Test, marketed by Cytyc Corporation, and the other is SurePath, marketed by TriPath Imaging. The ThinPrep method uses a filter method to collect a monolayer of epithelial cells and separate the epithelial cells from blood, mucus, and inflammatory debris. The SurePath method uses a density centrifugation method to enrich epithelial cells and reduce blood and inflammatory cells.

There are several advantages to liquid-based cytology. First, multiple clinical trials have demonstrated an increased detection of SIL for both methods, and both methods have FDA-approved labeling indicating that they detect significantly more cases of HSIL than does a conventional cervical cytology (193). Because of this improved sensitivity, the recent American Cancer Society screening recommendations direct that in women under the age of 30 years requiring screening, conventional cervical cytology should be performed at yearly intervals, whereas if liquid-based cytology is used, the screening interval should be every 2 years (191). Both of the commercially available methods also produce a reduction in the number of samples that have obscuring blood and inflammation, and both offer the advantage of providing residual cellular material that can be used for a variety of molecular tests (194). This is particularly useful for HPV DNA testing in women who have atypical squa-

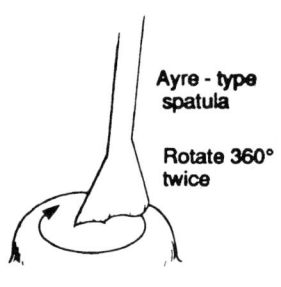

Ayre - type spatula

Rotate 360° twice

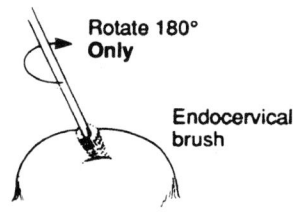

Rotate 180° Only

Endocervical brush

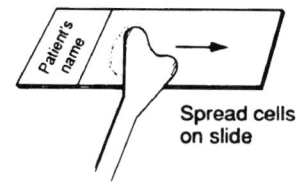

Patient's name

Spread cells on slide

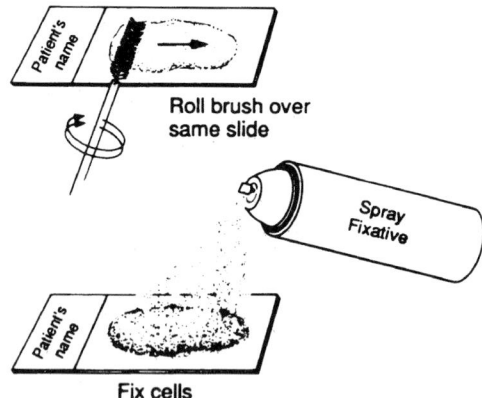

Patient's name

Roll brush over same slide

Spray Fixative

Patient's name

Fix cells

FIG. 19.25. Preferred procedure for obtaining a Pap smear.

TABLE 19.8. *The 2001 Bethesda System*

SPECIMEN ADEQUACY
Satisfactory for evaluation (*note presence/absence of endocervical transformation zone component*)
Unsatisfactory for evaluation (*specify reason*)
Specimen rejected/not processed (*specify reason*)
Specimen processed and examined, but unsatisfactory for evaluation of epithelial abnormality because of (*specify reason*)
GENERAL CATEGORIZATION (*Optional*)
Negative for intraepithelial lesion or malignancy
Epithelial cell abnormality
Other
INTERPRETATION/RESULT
Negative for Intraepithelial Lesion or Malignancy
Organisms
  Trichomonas vaginalis
  Fungal organisms morphologically consistent with *Candida* species
  Shift in flora suggestive of bacterial vaginosis
  Bacteria morphologically consistent with *Actinomyces* species
  Cellular changes consistent with herpes simplex virus
Other nonneoplastic findings (*optional to report; list not comprehensive*)
  Reactive cellular changes associated with inflammation (includes typical repair)
  Radiation
  Intrauterine contraceptive device
  Glandular cells' status posthysterectomy
  Atrophy
Epithelial Cell Abnormalities
Squamous cell
  Atypical squamous cell (ASC)
    of undetermined significance (ASC-US)
    cannot exclude HSIL (ASC-H)
  Low-grade squamous intraepithelial lesion (LSIL)
  High-grade squamous intraepithelial lesion (HSIL)
  Squamous cell carcinoma
Glandular cell
  Atypical glandular cells (AGC) (*specify endocervical, endometrial, or not otherwise specified*)
  Atypical glandular cells, favor neoplastic (*specify endocervical or not otherwise specified*)
  Endocervical adenocarcinoma *in situ* (AIS)
  Adenocarcinoma
Other (*list not comprehensive*)
  Endometrial cells in a woman ≥40 years of age

From Solomon D, Davey D, Kurman R, et al. The 2001 Bethesda System: terminology for reporting results of cervical cytology. *JAMA* 2002;287:2114.

---

mous cells of undetermined significance (ASC-US), the so-called "reflex HPV DNA testing" approach (195).

Terminology of Cytologic Reports

The Bethesda System terminology is used for reporting cervical cytology results in the United States. The Bethesda System underwent significant modifications in 2001 (Table 19.8) (15). The major features of the 2001 Bethesda System are that it requires (a) an estimate of the adequacy of the specimen for diagnostic evaluation; (b) a general categorization of the specimen as being either "negative for intraepi-

thelial lesion or malignancy," as having an "epithelial cell abnormality," or as "other" (i.e., having endometrial cells in a woman 40 years of age and older); and (c) a descriptive diagnosis that includes a description of epithelial cell abnormalities. This system provides clear criteria for determining whether a specimen is adequate for evaluation. In addition, the terminology closely correlates with histopathologic terminology. The terms *low-grade squamous intraepithelial lesion* (LSIL) and *high-grade squamous intraepithelial lesion*

TABLE 19.9. *Comparison of Papanicolaou, WHO, and Bethesda cervical cytology terminology*

Papanicolaou	WHO System	Bethesda System
Class I	Normal	Within normal limits
Class II	Atypical	Benign cellular changes (or) atypical squamous cells of undetermined significance
Class III	Dysplasia	Squamous epithelial cell abnormality
	Mild dysplasia	Low-grade squamous intraepithelial lesion (SIL)
	Moderate dysplasia	High-grade SIL
	Severe dysplasia	High-grade SIL
Class IV	Carcinoma *in situ*	High-grade SIL
Class V	Invasive squamous cell carcinoma	Squamous cell carcinoma
	Adenocarcinoma	Adenocarcinoma

(HSIL) are used to designate cytologic changes that correlate with CIN 1 and CIN 2,3, respectively. The way these terms correlate with the two previous terminologies utilized for reporting cervical cytology results is provided in Table 19.9. Direct cytologic-histologic correlation can be made, a fact that is an important feature for quality control in cytology laboratories. In addition, the Bethesda System attempts to separate epithelial changes secondary to inflammation or repair from those associated with cervical cancer precursors whenever possible. Nondiagnostic squamous cell abnormalities are included in a category of *atypical squamous cells* (ASC). ASC is used when a specimen has features suggestive, but not diagnostic, of an SIL. This category is further subdivided into two subcategories: atypical squamous cells of undetermined significance (ASC-US) and atypical squamous cells—cannot exclude HSIL (ASC-H). The risk of a woman with ASC-US of having biopsy-confirmed CIN 2,3 is approximately 7% to 17% and the risk of a woman with ASC-H is approximately 40% (16). Nondiagnostic glandular-cell abnormalities are included in a category of *atypical glandular cells* (AGC). This category is further subdivided into either not further classified or atypical glandular cells—favor neoplasia.

Cytologic Features of CIN

The features used to diagnose SIL cytologically are similar to those used to diagnose CIN in histopathologic specimens. These features include nuclear enlargement with an increase in the nuclear-cytoplasmic ratio, nuclear hyperchromaticity, irregular nuclear membranes, and multinucleation. Perinuclear clearing, or halos, are also commonly present. An example of normal superficial cells is shown in Figure 19.26A. In LSIL, cytologic changes are seen predominantly in superficial cells [i.e., more mature cell types (Fig. 19.26B)]. In HSIL, the cytologic changes are seen in intermediate and parabasal cells [i.e., less mature cell types (Fig. 19.26C)].

The prevalence of SIL varies greatly depending on the population studied. In student health clinics and sexually transmitted disease clinics, the prevalence of SIL is frequently more than 10% (196). In contrast, in the general population, the prevalence of LSIL is reported to be approximately 2% and the prevalence of HSIL is approximately 0.5% (197).

USE OF COLPOSCOPY

Over the last 25 years, colposcopy combined with colposcopically directed cervical biopsies has become the primary modality by which women with abnormal Pap smears are evaluated. Colposcopic examination consists of viewing the cervix with a long–focal length, dissecting-type microscope at a magnification of about 16× after a solution of dilute (4%) acetic acid has been applied to the cervix. The acetic acid solution acts to remove and dissolve the cervical mucus and causes CIN lesions to become whiter than the surrounding epithelium (acetowhite). This coloration allows the colposcopist to identify and biopsy epithelial lesions. In addition to allowing the detection of acetowhite areas, colposcopy also allows for the detection of blood vessel patterns that can indicate high-grade CIN lesions and the detection of invasive cancers. Colposcopy and appropriately directed biopsy have greatly facilitated the management of patients with preinvasive lesions of the cervix because they allow the clinician to rule out invasive cancer and determine the limits of preinvasive disease. Conservative ablative treatment modalities such as cryosurgery, laser ablation, and a loop electrosurgical excision procedure (LEEP) can then be used to treat preinvasive disease with success rates similar to those obtained with cone biopsies.

MANAGEMENT OF CYTOLOGIC ABNORMALITIES AND CIN

Overview

In 2001, the American Society for Colposcopy and Cervical Pathology sponsored a consensus workshop to develop guidelines for the management of women with cytologic abnormalities and biopsy-confirmed CIN. These guidelines incorporated not only the changes in terminology that took place as a result of the 2001 Bethesda Workshop, but also the

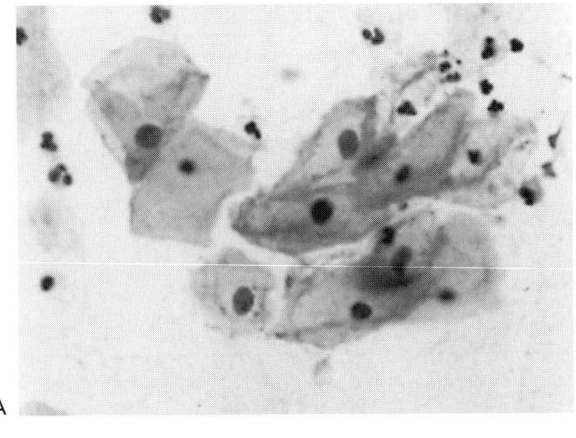

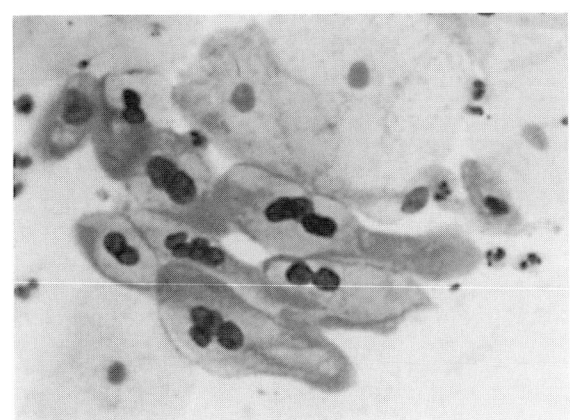

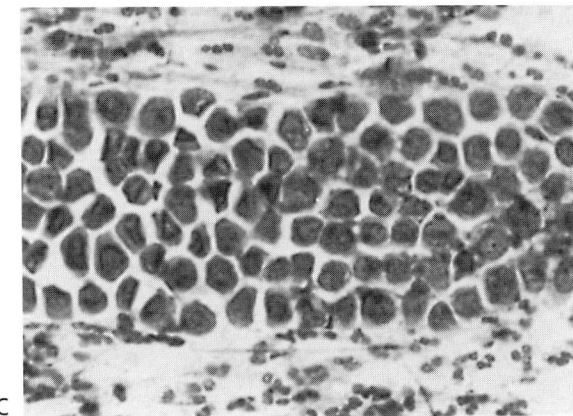

FIG. 19.26. Cervical cytology. **A:** Normal superficial cells. **B:** Low-grade SIL (CIN 1) in which the cells are multinucleated with slightly enlarged hyperchromatic nuclei and perinuclear halos. **C:** High-grade SIL (CIN 2, 3) with cells with high nucleocytoplasmic ratios.

findings of the large NCI-sponsored ASCUS/LSIL Triage Study (ALTS) (198). A unique feature of these guidelines is that not only are they evidence based, but each recommendation is accompanied by a grading of both the strength of the recommendation and the strength of the data supporting the recommendation. The complete recommendations and management algorithms are available on line at www. asccp.org.

Atypical Squamous Cells

A vexing group of patients for both clinicians and cytologists are those whose cervical cytology is atypical (i.e., not normal) but lacks the characteristic features of SIL or cancer. In the past, many cytology laboratories subdivided atypical smears into two categories: atypical, reparative-inflammatory changes (i.e., benign atypia); and atypical smears, suggestive but not diagnostic of CIN. The 2001 Bethesda System classifies specimens that have reparative-inflammatory changes as being "negative for intraepithelial lesion or malignancy." In the current terminology, only those specimens that have features suggestive of SIL should be classified as ASC. The number of cytologic specimens that are diagnosed as ASC varies greatly among different cytology laboratories and patient populations. The reported incidence of atypical Pap smears that fall into this category varies

greatly from under 1% to more than 10% (199). These differences reflect the difficulties encountered by cytologists in determining the significance of minor degrees of cytologic atypia and in reproducibly recognizing these changes. In the most recent report from the College of American Pathologists (CAP), the median ASC rate from reporting laboratories from the United States was 4.5% (4).

The clinical significance of an ASC result depends on a number of factors including the age of the patient, the patient's history, and the subclassification of the result (e.g., ASC-US or ASC-H). The prevalence of biopsy-confirmed CIN 2,3 found in women undergoing colposcopy for an ASC cytology is generally reported as being 5% to 17% (16). A study of 46,009 women undergoing routine cytologic screening in the Northern California Kaiser Permanente Medical Group found that 3.5% had a diagnosis of ASCUS (200). At colposcopy, 13% of these women were diagnosed with CIN 1, 7% with CIN 2,3, and one woman had invasive cervical cancer. In the large, multicenter ALTS study, 15% of the women referred with ASC were found to have biopsy-confirmed CIN 2,3 at the initial colposcopic examination and 20% had biopsy-confirmed CIN 1 (198). Overall, it appears that between one-third and one-half of all women diagnosed as having CIN 2,3 have ASC as their initial abnormal cervical cytologic result (201,202). Although the risk that a woman with ASC has invasive cervical cancer is quite low, about 1 per 1,000, the very large number of women with this cytologic interpretation (2.5 million annually) guarantees that each year approximately 2,500 women with invasive cervical cancer will have only equivocal results on their cervical cytology. Therefore, women with ASC-US need to receive some form of follow-up evaluation, but consideration should be given to preventing unnecessary inconvenience, anxiety, cost, and discomfort (16).

Atypical Squamous Cells of Undetermined Significance

Three methods are in widespread use for the management of women with ASC. These are immediate colposcopy, HPV DNA testing, and a program of repeat cervical cytology. A number of studies have directly compared the sensitivity and specificity of repeat cervical cytology and HPV DNA testing for identifying women with CIN 2,3 (16). In every single study, HPV DNA testing identified more cases of CIN 2,3 than did a single repeat cervical cytology, but referred approximately equivalent numbers of women for colposcopy. Moreover, cost-effectiveness modeling using mathematic models has demonstrated that HPV DNA testing for women with ASC-US is a highly attractive alternative to immediate colposcopy or a program of repeat cytology when the initial ASC-US cytology was obtained from a liquid-based sample or when a co-collected HPV test was taken at the time a conventional cytology was obtained (203). Based on this evidence, the 2001 ASCCP Consensus Conference concluded that although all three of the methods traditionally used to manage women with ASC-US (i.e., colposcopy, repeat cytology, and HPV DNA testing) are safe and effective, high-risk HPV DNA testing is the preferred approach to managing women with ASC-US whenever liquid-based cytology is used for screening or co-collection of a sample for HPV DNA testing can be performed (16). Figure 19.27 provides the algorithm recommended for the management of women with ASC-US. This algorithm is appropriate for women of all ages with ASC-US.

Data from ALTS indicate that the sensitivity for CIN 2,3 of HPV DNA testing is similar in all groups; far fewer older women are referred for colposcopy (31% of women 29 years and older) using this approach than are younger women (65% of women under 29 years of age) (204). Although the increased referral to colposcopy of younger women with ASC-US by HPV testing might seem to favor another approach for triage at younger ages, similar higher rates of repeat abnormal cytology at younger ages did not favor one triage program over another.

Atypical Squamous Cells—Cannot Exclude HSIL

The prevalence of biopsy-confirmed CIN 2,3 is considerably higher among women referred for the evaluation of an ASC-H cervical cytology than it is for women referred for the evaluation of ASC-US. CIN 2,3 is identified in 24% to 94% of women with ASC-H (16). Because of this high risk, the 2001 Consensus Guidelines recommend that all women with ASC-H be referred for a colposcopic evaluation. If CIN is not identified, a complete review of the original cytology as well as of all biopsies should be undertaken, and if the diagnosis does not change, the patient should be followed up utilizing either repeat cytology at 6 and 12 months or high-risk HPV DNA testing at 12 months (Fig. 19.28).

Low-grade Squamous Intraepithelial Lesions

As with ASC, there is considerable variation between populations and laboratories in the rate at which LSIL is reported. In 1996, the median rate of LSIL reported from the College of American Pathology survey was 1.6%, but rates as high as 7.7% have been reported from laboratories serving high-risk populations (4,205). A cytologic result of LSIL is a very specific indicator of the presence of high-risk types of HPV. In ALTS, 83% of the women referred for the evaluation of LSIL were high-risk HPV DNA–positive (206). However, a cytologic result of LSIL is a poor predictor of the grade of CIN that will be identified at colposcopy. CIN 2,3 is identified at colposcopy in 15% to 30% of women with LSIL on cervical cytology (197,201). Therefore, the 2001 Consensus Guidelines recommend that all women with a cytologic result of LSIL be referred for a colposcopic evaluation (Fig. 19.29) (207). This allows women with significant disease to be rapidly identified and reduces the risk of women being lost to follow-up. A diagnostic excisional procedure is not required when a woman with LSIL cytology is found to have an unsatisfactory colposcopic examination.

Because a cytologic result of LSIL appears to be less accurate in postmenopausal women with significant atrophy, follow-up without initial colposcopy is acceptable in these women, as is the use of a course of intravaginal estrogen followed by a repeat cytology. Invasive cervical cancer is extremely uncommon in adolescents, whereas a cytology result of LSIL is quite common. Therefore, follow-up without colposcopy is also acceptable for adolescents with LSIL.

High-grade Squamous Intraepithelial Lesions

The cytologic result of HSIL is uncommon, accounting for only about 0.5% of all cervical cytology results, and is associated with a significant risk for CIN 2,3 and invasive cervical cancer (4,197). Women with a cytologic result of HSIL have a 70% to 75% risk of having CIN 2,3 and a 1% to 2% risk of having invasive cervical cancer (207). Therefore, all women with a cytologic result of HSIL should be referred for a colposcopic evaluation (207. Subsequent management depends on whether or not the patient is pregnant, whether the colposcopic examination is satisfactory, and whether or not the patient is suitable for immediate excision (''see and treat''). Women referred for the evaluation of HSIL in whom the colposcopic examination is satisfactory

Management of Women with Atypical Squamous Cells of Undetermined Significance (ASC-US)

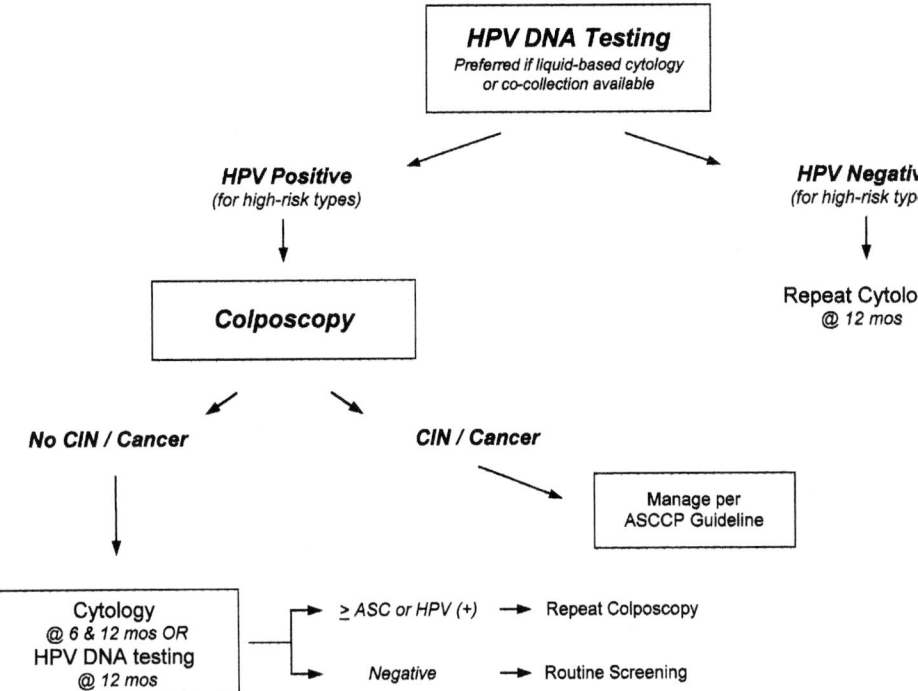

FIG. 19.27. 2001 Consensus Guidelines for the management of women with ASC-US. (Used with permission from the American Society of Colposcopy and Cervical Pathology.)

Management of Women with Atypical Squamous Cells: Cannot Exclude High-grade SIL (ASC - H)

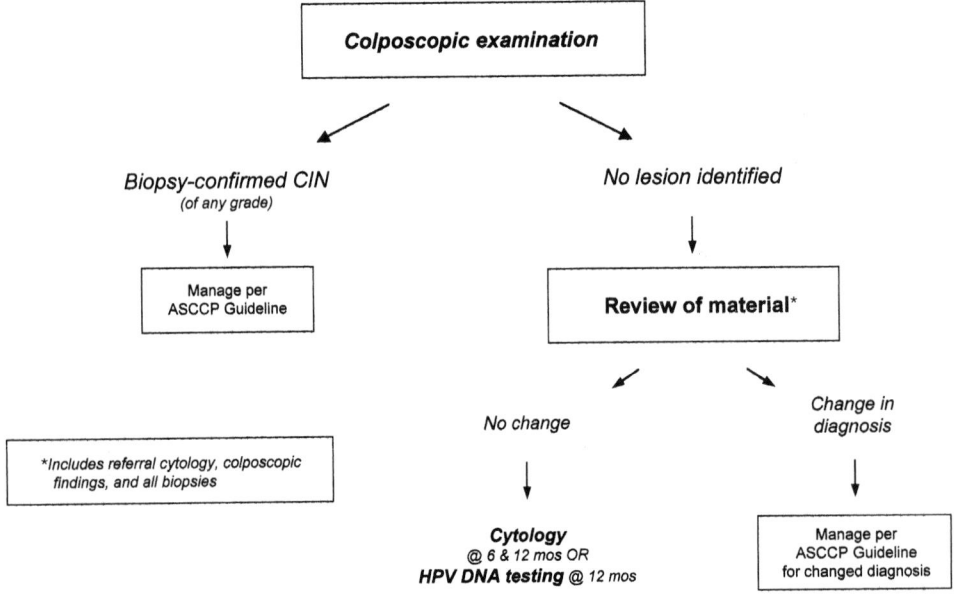

FIG. 19.28. 2001 Consensus Guidelines for the management of women with ASC-H. (Used with permission from the American Society of Colposcopy and Cervical Pathology.)

Management of Women with Low-grade Squamous Intraepithelial Lesions (LSIL)*

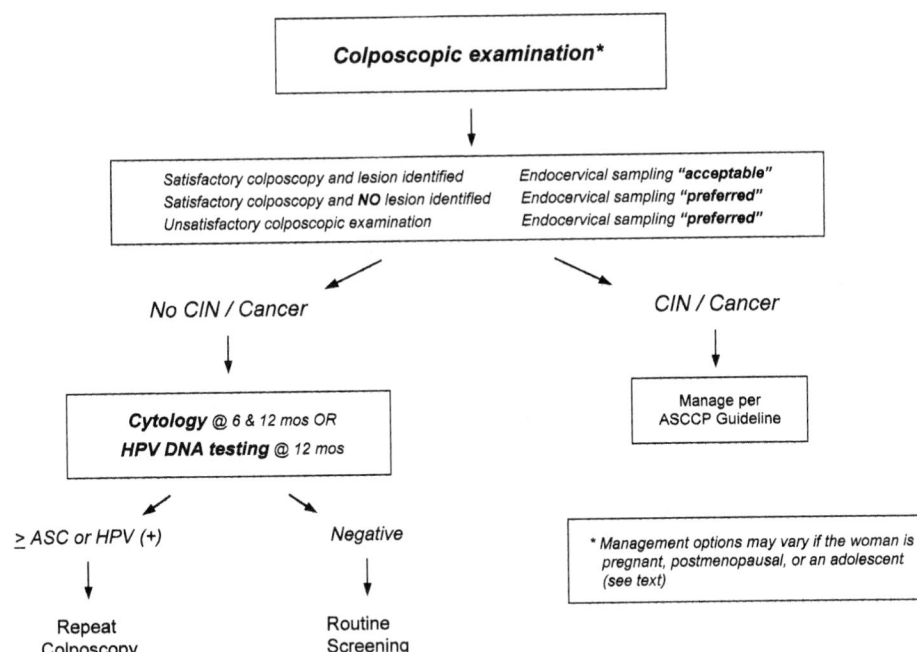

FIG. 19.29. 2001 Consensus Guidelines for the management of women with LSIL. (Used with permission from the American Society of Colposcopy and Cervical Pathology.)

and who are found to have no CIN or only CIN 1 have up to a 35% risk of having undetected CIN 2,3 (209). Therefore, it is recommended that a complete review of the original cytology as well as of all biopsies should be undertaken, and if the diagnosis does not change, the patient should undergo a diagnostic excisional procedure (16). Women with HSIL who have an unsatisfactory colposcopic examination also require a diagnostic excisional procedure.

Biopsy-confirmed CIN 1

Women with a histologically confirmed CIN 1 lesion represent a heterogeneous group. A number of studies have clearly demonstrated a high level of variability in the histologic diagnosis of CIN 1. In ALTS, only 43% of biopsies that were originally diagnosed as CIN 1 at the clinical centers were subsequently classified as CIN 1 by the reference pathology committee. Forty-one percent were downgraded to normal and 13% were upgraded to CIN 2,3 (209). Another issue is that a colposcopically directed biopsy only represents a sampling of a lesion and a diagnosis of CIN 1 does not preclude the existence of a CIN 2,3 lesion. Studies of women with CIN 1 on colposcopically directed biopsy who subsequently undergo loop electrosurgical excision have identified CIN 2,3 in up to 55% of the excised specimens (210). Therefore, a diagnosis of CIN 1 on a cervical biopsy does not necessarily indicate that an individual woman actually has CIN or that CIN 2,3 is not present. This heterogeneity is reflected in the natural history of untreated CIN 1 lesions. The majority of CIN 1 lesions spontaneously regress

but 11% have progressed to carcinoma *in situ* in prospective follow-up studies (52).

Because of the above considerations, the 2001 Consensus Guidelines state that the management options for women with biopsy-confirmed CIN 1 who have a satisfactory colposcopic examination include follow-up without treatment or treatment with the use of ablative (e.g., cryotherapy, electrofulguration, or laser ablation) or excisional modalities such as loop electrosurgical excision (207). It is important to perform an endocervical sampling in order to assure that an unsuspected lesion is not present in the endocervical canal. All treatment modalities are considered to be acceptable since randomized controlled clinical trials comparing cryotherapy, laser ablation, and LEEP for treating biopsy-confirmed CIN have reported no significant differences in either complication rates or success rates (211–213). A comprehensive review of controlled and randomized trials of various treatment modalities found no significant differences in outcomes after treatment in women with CIN with satisfactory colposcopic examinations (214).

However, because most CIN 1 lesions spontaneously regress in the absence of treatment, the 2001 Consensus Guidelines state that follow-up using a program of repeat cytology at 6 and 12 months or HPV DNA testing at 12 months is the *preferred* form of management. When follow-up is utilized, women with a repeat cytology result of ASC or greater or who are high-risk HPV DNA–positive should be referred to colposcopy. In settings where colposcopy is readily available, follow-up using a combination of cytology and colposcopy at 12 months is considered to be acceptable. Women who undergo cytologic or colposcopic regression during follow-up remain at risk for recurrent CIN and should be followed with repeat cytology at 12 months. When women have persistent CIN 1, the decision to treat the lesion should be based on both provider and patient preferences (207).

It is unusual to have biopsy-confirmed CIN 1 lesions in women with unsatisfactory colposcopic examinations. In one series of women with CIN 1 undergoing conization, a 10% rate of CIN 2,3 was observed. Therefore, it is recommended that women with biopsy-confirmed CIN 1 who have an unsatisfactory colposcopic examination undergo a diagnostic excisional procedure (207).

Biopsy-confirmed CIN 2,3

Women with a untreated histologically confirmed CIN 2,3 lesion are felt to have a significantly high risk of progressing to invasive cervical cancer to warrant routine treatment. Provided the colposcopic examination is satisfactory and there is no suggestion of invasive disease (e.g., by either colposcopy, cytology, or histology) both ablative or excisional treatment modalities are considered to be acceptable forms of treatment (207). In patients with recurrent CIN (either CIN 1 or CIN 2,3), it is preferred that an excisional treatment modality be used. A diagnostic excisional procedure is recommended for all women with biopsy-confirmed CIN 2,3 and an unsatisfactory colposcopic examination.

The risk of recurrent CIN 2,3 or invasive cancer after treatment remains elevated for many years after treatment. A large follow-up study from the United Kingdom reported that the cumulative risk of invasive cervical cancer was 5.8 per 1,000 after 8 years of follow-up, which is approximately 100 times higher than in women in the general population (215). The size of the original CIN 2,3 lesion appears to be an important determinant of the rate of recurrence. Large lesions have a higher failure rate than small lesions. The 2001 Consensus Guidelines recommend that after treatment for CIN 2,3, follow-up using either cytology or cytology and colposcopy be conducted at 4- to 6-month intervals until at least three negative cytology results are obtained. Annual cytology is recommended thereafter (207). High-risk HPV DNA testing performed at least 6 months after treatment is also considered to be an acceptable option. When CIN is identified at the margins or a diagnostic excisional procedure, it is preferred that the 4- to 6-month follow-up visit include a colposcopic examination and endocervical sampling. This is because in the majority of these cases, CIN will not be identified during subsequent follow-up (216, 217).

REFERENCES

1. 1997 Sexually Transmitted Disease Surveillance Report. Centers for Disease Control and Prevention, Atlanta, GA. http://www.cdc.gov/nchstp/dstd/Stats__Trends/1997__Surv__Rpt: Division of Sexually Transmitted Disease Prevention, United States Department of Health and Human Services, Public Health Service, Centers for Disease Control and Prevention, Atlanta GA., 1999 (vol 2000).
2. Koutsky LA, Kiviat NB. Human papillomaviruses. In: Holmes KK, Mardh P-A, Sparling PF, et al, eds. *Sexually transmitted diseases.* New York: McGraw-Hill, 1998;211–213.
3. Larsen NS. Invasive cervical cancer arising in young white females. *J Natl Cancer Inst* 1994;86:6.
4. Jones BA, Davey DD. Quality management in gynecologic cytology using interlaboratory comparison. *Arch Pathol Lab Med* 2000;124:672.
5. Results of a randomized trial on the management of cytology interpretations of atypical squamous cells of undetermined significance. *Am J Obstet Gynecol* 2003;188:1383.
6. Koss LG. *Diagnostic cytology and its histopathologic basis.* Vol 1. New York: JB Lippincott Co, 1992.
7. Weid GL. *Proceedings of the First International Congress on Exfoliative Cytology.* Philadelphia: JB Lippincott Co, 1961.
8. Reagan JW, Hamonic MJ. The cellular pathology in carcinoma in situ; a cytohistopathological correlation. *Cancer* 1956;9:385.
9. Cocker J, Fox H, Langley FA. Consistency in the histological diagnosis of epithelial abnormalities of the cervix uteri. *J Clin Pathol* 1968;21:67.
10. Richart RM. Natural history of cervical intraepithelial neoplasia. *Clin Obstet Gynecol* 1968;10:748.
11. Richart RM. Cervical intraepithelial neoplasia: a review. In: Sommers SC, ed. *Pathology annual.* Vol 8. East Norwalk, CT: Appleton-Century-Crofts, 1973.
12. Fu YS, Reagan JW. *Pathology of the uterine cervix, vagina, and vulva.* Philadelphia: WB Saunders, 1989.
13. Chung TK, Cheung TH, Lo WK, et al. Loss of heterozygosity at the short arm of chromosome 3 in microdissected cervical intraepithelial neoplasia. *Cancer Lett* 2000;154:189.
14. Wright TC, Ferenczy AF, Kurman RJ. Precancerous lesions of the cervix. In: Kurman RJ, ed. *Blaustein's pathology of the female genital tract.* New York: Springer-Verlag, 2002.
15. Solomon D, Davey D, Kurman R, et al. The 2001 Bethesda System: terminology for reporting results of cervical cytology. *JAMA* 2002;287:2114.
16. Wright TC Jr, Cox JT, Massad LS, et al. 2001 Consensus Guidelines for the Management of Women with Cervical Cytological Abnormalities. *JAMA* 2002;287:2120.
17. Scully RE, Bonfiglio TA, Kurman RJ, et al. *Histological typing of female genital tract tumors.* Berlin: Springer-Verlag, 1994.
18. Helper TK, Dockerty MB, Randall LM. Primary adenocarcinoma of the cervix. *Am J Obstet Gynecol* 1952;63:800.
19. Mikuta JJ, Celebre JA. Adenocarcinoma of the cervix. *Obstet Gynecol* 1969;33:753.
20. Anton-Culver H, Bloss JD, Bringman D, et al. Comparison of adenocarcinoma and squamous cell carcinoma of the uterine cervix: a population based epidemiologic study. *Am J Obstet Gynecol* 1992;166:1507.
21. Anderson GH, Benedet JL, LeRiche JC, et al. Invasive cancer of the cervix in British Columbia: a review of the demography and screening histories of 437 cases seen from 1985–1988. *Obstet Gynecol* 1992;80:1.
22. Davis JR, Moon LB. Increased incidence of adenocarcinoma of uterine cervix. *Obstet Gynecol* 1975;45:79.
23. Horowitz IR, Jacobson LP, Zucker PK, et al. Epidemiology of adenocarcinoma of the cervix. *Gynecol Oncol* 1988;31:25.
24. Shingleton HM, Gore H, Bradley DH, Soong S-J. Adenocarcinoma of the cervix. I. Clinical evaluation and pathologic features. *Am J Obstet Gynecol* 1981;139:799.
25. Eide TJ. Cancer of the uterine cervix in Norway by histologic type, 1970–1984. *J Natl Cancer Inst* 1987;79:199.
26. Leminen A, Paavonen J, Forss M, et al. Adenocarcinoma of the uterine cervix. *Cancer* 1990;65:53.
27. Peters RK, Chao A, Mack TM, et al. Increased frequency of adenocarcinoma of the uterine cervix in young women in Los Angeles county. *J Natl Cancer Inst* 1986;76:423.
28. Parazzini F, La Vecchia C. Epidemiology of adenocarcinoma of the cervix. *Gynecol Oncol* 1990;39:40.
29. Schwartz SM, Weiss NS. Increased incidence of adenocarcinoma of

the cervix in young women in the United States. *Am J Epidemiol* 1986;124:1045.

30. Chilvers C, Mant D, Pike MC. Cervical adenocarcinoma and oral contraceptives. *BMJ* 1987;295:1446.

31. Friedell GH, McKay DG. Adenocarcinoma in situ of endocervix. *Cancer* 1953;6:887.

32. Bousfield L, Pacey F, Young Q, et al. Expanded cytologic criteria for the diagnosis of adenocarcinoma in situ of the cervix and related lesions. *Acta Cytol* 1980;24:283.

33. Gloor E, Hurlimann J. Cervical intraepithelial glandular neoplasia (adenocarcinoma in situ and glandular dysplasia). A correlative study of 23 cases with histologic grading, histochemical analysis of mucins and immunohistochemical determination of the affinity for four lectins. *Cancer* 1986;58:1272.

34. Bowen JT. Precancerous dermatosis: a study of two cases of chronic atypical epithelial proliferation. *J Cutan Dis* 1912;30:241.

35. Friedrich EG. International Society for the Study of Vulvar Disease: new nomenclature for vulvar disease. *Obstet Gynecol* 1976;47:122.

36. Ridley CM, Frankman O, Jones ISC, et al. New nomenclature for vulvar disease: International Society for the Study of Vulvar Disease [Letter]. *Lancet* 1989;20:495.

37. Reagan JW, Hicks DJ, Scott RB. Atypical hyperplasia of uterine cervix. *Cancer* 1955;8:42.

38. Patten SF. *Diagnostic cytopathology of the uterine cervix*. Basel: Karger, 1978.

39. Barron BA, Richart RM. A statistical model of the natural history of cervical carcinoma based on a prospective study of 557 cases. *J Natl Cancer Inst* 1968;41:1343.

40. Barron BA, Richart RM. A statistical model of the natural history of cervical carcinoma. II. Estimates of the transition from dysplasia to carcinoma in situ. *J Natl Cancer Inst* 1970;45:1025.

41. Kottmeier HL. Evolution et traitment des epitheliomas. *Rev Fran Gynecol Obstet* 1961;56:821.

42. Koss LG, Stewart FW, Foote FW, et al. Some histological aspects of behavior of epidermoid carcinoma in situ and related lesions of the uterine cervix. *Cancer* 1963;16:1160.

43. McIndoe WA, McLean MR, Jones RW, Mullins PR. The invasive potential of carcinoma in situ of the cervix. *Obstet Gynecol* 1984;64:451.

44. Green GH, Donovan JW. The natural history of cervical carcinoma in situ. *J Obstet Gynecol Br Commonw* 1970;77:1.

45. Kottmeier H-L. Annual Report on the Results of Treatment in Carcinoma of the Uterus, Vagina and Ovary. International Federation of Gynecology and Obstetrics—Stockholm, 1976.

46. Miller AB. *Cervical cancer screening programmes: managerial guidelines*. Geneva: World Health Organization, 1992.

47. Ponten J, Adami H-O, Bergstrom R, et al. Strategies for global control of cervical cancer. *Int J Cancer* 1995;60:1.

48. Holowaty P, Miller AB, Rohan T, To T. Natural history of dysplasia of the uterine cervix. *J Natl Cancer Inst* 1999;91:252.

49. Nasiell K, Roger V, Nasiell M. Behavior of mild cervical dysplasia during long-term follow-up. *Obstet Gynecol* 1986;67:665.

50. Nasiell K, Nasiell M, Vaclavinkova V. Behavior of moderate cervical dysplasia during long-term follow-up. *Obstet Gynecol* 1983;61:609.

51. Melnikow J, Nuovo J, Willan AR, et al. Natural history of cervical squamous intraepithelial lesions: a meta-analysis. *Obstet Gynecol* 1998;92:727.

52. Mitchell MF, Tortolero-Luna G, Wright T, et al. Cervical human papillomavirus infection and intraepithelial neoplasia: a review. *J Natl Cancer Inst Monogr* 1996;21:17.

53. Buscema J, Stern J, Woodruff JD. The significance of the histological alterations adjacent to invasive vulvar carcinoma. *Am J Obstet Gynecol* 1987;156:212.

54. Roy M. VIN: latest management approaches. *Contemp OB/GYN* 1988;32:170.

55. Hording U, Junge J, Poulsen H, Lundvall F. Vulvar intraepithelial neoplasia. III. A viral disease of undetermined progressive potential. *Gynecol Oncol* 1995;56:276.

56. Herod JJ, Shafi MI, Rollason TP, et al. Vulvar intraepithelial neoplasia: long term follow up of treated and untreated women. *Br J Obstet Gynaecol* 1996;103:446.

57. Jones RW, Rowan DM. Vulvar intraepithelial neoplasia. III. A clinical study of the outcome in 113 cases with relation to the later development of invasive vulvar carcinoma. *Obstet Gynecol* 1994;84:741.

58. Bosch FX, Castellsague X, Munoz N, et al. Male sexual behavior and human papillomavirus DNA: key risk factors for cervical cancer in spain. *J Natl Cancer Inst* 1996;88:1060.

59. Smith JS, Munoz N, Herrero R, et al. Evidence for Chlamydia trachomatis as a human papillomavirus cofactor in the etiology of invasive cervical cancer in Brazil and the Philippines. *J Infect Dis* 2002;185:324.

60. Anttila T, Saikku P, Koskela P, et al. Serotypes of Chlamydia trachomatis and risk for development of cervical squamous cell carcinoma. *JAMA* 2001;285:47.

61. Castle PE, Giuliano AR. Genital tract infections, cervical inflammation, and antioxidant nutrients—assessing their roles as human papillomavirus cofactors. *J Natl Cancer Inst Monogr* 2003;29.

62. Meisels A, Roy M, Fortier M, Morin C. Condylomatous lesions of the cervix: morphologic and colposcopic diagnosis. *Am J Diagn Gynecol Obstet* 1979;1:109.

63. Oriel JD. Natural history of genital warts. *Br J Vener Dis* 1971;47:1.

64. Laverty CR, Russell P, Hills E, Booth N. The significance of noncondylomatous wart virus infection of the cervical transformation zone: a review with discussion of two illustrative cases. *Acta Cytol* 1978;22:195.

65. zur Hausen H. Papillomaviruses and cancer: from basic studies to clinical application. *Nat Rev Cancer* 2002;2:342.

66. Bosch FX, de Sanjose S. Human papillomavirus and cervical cancer—burden and assessment of causality. *J Natl Cancer Inst Monogr* 2003;3.

67. Bosch FX, Manos MM, Munoz N, et al. Prevalence of human papillomavirus in cervical cancer: a worldwide perspective. International Biological Study on Cervical Cancer (IBSCC) study group. *J Natl Cancer Inst* 1995;87:779.

68. Walboomers JM, Jacobs MV, Manos MM, et al. Human papillomavirus is a necessary cause of invasive cervical cancer worldwide. *J Pathol* 1999;189:12.

69. Munoz N, Bosch FX, de Sanjose S, et al. Epidemiologic classification of human papillomavirus types associated with cervical cancer. *N Engl J Med* 2003;348:518.

70. Ellerbrock TV, Chiasson MA, Bush TJ, et al. Incidence of cervical squamous intraepithelial lesions in HIV-infected women. *JAMA* 2000;283:1031.

71. Bosch FX, Lorincz A, Munoz N, et al. The causal relation between human papillomavirus and cervical cancer. *J Clin Pathol* 2002;55:244.

72. IARC. *Human papillomaviruses. IARC monographs on the evaluation of carcinogenic risks to humans*. Vol 64. Lyon: IARC, 1995.

73. Becker TM, Wheeler CM, McGough NS, et al. Sexually transmitted diseases and other risk factors for cervical dysplasia among Southwestern Hispanic and non-Hispanic white women. *JAMA* 1994;271:1181.

74. Brinton LA. Epidemiology of cervical cancer—an overview. In: Munoz N, Bosch FX, Shah K, Meheus A, eds. *The epidemiology of cervical cancer and human papillomavirus*. Vol 119. Lyon: IARC Scientific Publications, 1992.

75. Szarewski A, Cuzick J. Smoking and cervical neoplasia: a review of the evidence. *J Epidemiol Biostat* 1998;3:229.

76. McCann MF, Irwin DE, Walton LA, et al. Nicotine and cotinine in the cervical mucus of smokers, passive smokers, and nonsmokers. *Cancer Epidemiol Biomarkers Prevent* 1992;1:125.

77. Simons AM, Phillips DH, Coleman DV. Damage to DNA in cervical epithelium related to smoking tobacco. *BMJ* 1993;306:1444.

78. Barton SE, Maddox PH, Jenkins D, et al. Effect of cigarette smoking on cervical epithelial immunity: a mechanism for neoplastic change? *Lancet* 1988;2:652.

79. Clifford GM, Smith JS, Aguado T, Franceschi S. Comparison of HPV type distribution in high-grade cervical lesions and cervical cancer: a meta-analysis. *Br J Cancer* 2003;89:101.

80. Vessey MF. Exogenous hormones in the aetiology of cancer in women. *J R Soc Med* 1984;77:542.

81. de Villiers EM. Relationship between steroid hormone contraceptives and HPV, cervical intraepithelial neoplasia and cervical carcinoma. *Int J Cancer* 2003;103:705.

82. Bornstein J, Rahat MA, Abramovici H. Etiology of cervical cancer: current concepts. *Obstet Gynecol Surv* 1995;50:146.

83. Potischman N, Brinton LA. Nutrition and cervical neoplasia. *Cancer Causes Control* 1996;7:113.

84. Butterworth CEJ, Hatch KD, Macaluso M, et al. Folate deficiency and cervical dysplasia. *JAMA* 1992;267:528.

85. Porreco R, Penn I, Droegemueller W, et al. Gynecologic malignancies in immunosuppressed organ homograft recipients. *Obstet Gynecol* 1975;45:359.

86. Palefsky JM, Holly EA. Immunosuppression and co-infection with HIV. *J Natl Cancer Inst Monogr* 2003;41.

87. Kuhn L, Sun X-W, Wright TC. Human immunodeficiency virus infection and female lower genital tract malignancy. *Curr Opin Obstet Gynecol* 1999;11:35.

88. Sun XW, Kuhn L, Ellerbrock TV, et al. Human papillomavirus infection in HIV-seropositive women; natural history and variability of detection. *N Engl J Med* 1997;337:1343.

89. Massad LS, Ahdieh L, Benning L, et al. Evolution of cervical abnormalities among women with HIV-1: evidence from surveillance cytology in the women's interagency HIV study. *J Acquir Immune Defic Syndr* 2001;27:432.

90. Wright TC, Ellerbrock TV, Chiasson MA, et al. Cervical intraepithelial neoplasia in women infected with human immunodeficiency virus: prevalence, risk factors, and validity of Papanicolaou smears. *Obstet Gynecol* 1994;84:591.

91. Fordyce EJ, Wang Z, Kahn AR, et al. Risk of cancer among women with AIDS in New York City. *AIDS Public Policy J* 2000;15:95.

92. Maiman M. Management of cervical neoplasia in human immunodeficiency virus-infected women. *J Natl Cancer Inst* 1998;23:43.

93. Centers for Disease Control and Prevention. 1993 revised classification system for HIV infection and expanded surveillance case definition for AIDS among adolescents and adults. *MMWR* 1993;41:1.

94. de Villiers EM. Hybridization methods other than PCR: an update. In: Munoz N, Bosch FS, Shah KV, Meheus A, eds. *The epidemiology of human papillomavirus and cervical cancer*. Vol 119. Lyon: IARC Scientific Publications, 1992.

95. de Villiers EM. *Human papillomaviruses: reference chart*. Burlington, NC: Roche Biomedical Laboratories, 1988.

96. Felix JC, Wright TC. Analysis of lower genital tract lesions clinically suspicious for condylomata using in situ hybridization and the polymerase chain reaction for the detection of human papillomavirus. *Arch Pathol Lab Med* 1994;118:39.

97. Zhu WY, Leonardi C, Penneys NS. Polymerase chain reaction in detection of human papillomavirus DNA and types of condyloma acuminata. *Chin Med J* 1993;106:141.

98. Obalek S, Misiewicz J, Jablonska S, et al. Childhood condyloma acuminatum: association with genital and cutaneous human papillomaviruses. *Pediatr Dermatol* 1994;10:101.

99. Barrasso R. HPV related genital lesions in men. In: Munoz N, Bosch F, Shah K, Mehens A, eds. *The epidemiology of cervical cancer and human papillomavirus*. Vol 119. Lyon: IARC Scientific Publications, 1992.

100. Bergeron C, Barrasso R, Beaudenon S, et al. Human papillomaviruses associated with cervical intraepithelial neoplasia. Great diversity and distinct distribution in low- and high-grade lesions. *Am J Surg Pathol* 1992;16:641.

101. Lungu O, Sun XW, Felix J, et al. Relationship of human papillomavirus type to grade of cervical intraepithelial neoplasia. *JAMA* 1992; 267:2493.

102. Genest DR, Stein L, Cibas E, et al. A binary (Bethesda) system for classifying cervical cancer precursors: criteria, reproducibility, and viral correlates. *Hum Pathol* 1993;24:730.

103. Jacobs MV, Walboomers JM, Snijders PJ, et al. Distribution of 37 mucosotropic HPV types in women with cytologically normal cervical smears: the age-related patterns for high-risk and low-risk types. *Int J Cancer* 2000;87:221.

104. Liaw KL, Glass AG, Manos MM, et al. Detection of human papillomavirus DNA in cytologically normal women and subsequent cervical squamous intraepithelial lesions. *J Natl Cancer Inst* 1999;91:954.

105. Peyton CL, Gravitt PE, Hunt WC, et al. Determinants of genital human papillomavirus detection in a US population. *J Infect Dis* 2001;183:1554.

106. Turek LP. The structure, function, and regulation of papillomaviral genes in infection and cervical cancer. *Adv Viral Res* 1994;44:305.

107. Apt D, Chong T, Liu Y, Bernard HU. Nuclear factor 1 and epithelial cell-specific transcription of human papillomavirus type 16. *J Virol* 1993;67:4455.

108. Fehrmann F, Laimins LA. Human papillomaviruses: targeting differentiating epithelial cells for malignant transformation. *Oncogene* 2003;22:5201.

109. Bream GL, Ohmstede CA, Phelps WC. Characterization of human papillomavirus type 11 E1 and E2 proteins expressed in insect cells. *J Virol* 1993;67:2655.

110. Ustav E, Ustav M. E2 protein as the master regulator of extrachromosomal replication of the papillomaviruses. *Papillomavirus Rep* 1998; 9:145.

111. Doobar J. Late stages of the papillomvirus life cycle. *Papillomavirus Rep* 1998;9:119.

112. Hwang ES, Nottoli T, Dimaio D. The HPV16 E5 protein: expression, detection, and stable complex formation with transmembrane proteins in cos cells. *Virology* 1995;211:227.

113. zur Hausen H. Papillomaviruses causing cancer: evasion from host-cell control in early events in carcinogenesis. *J Natl Cancer Inst* 2000; 92:690.

114. Evander M, Frazer IH, Payne E, et al. Identification of the alpha6 integrin as a candidate receptor for papillomaviruses. *J Virol* 1997; 71:2449.

115. Munger K, Howley PM. Human papillomavirus immortalization and transformation functions. *Virus Res* 2002;89:213.

116. Klaes R, Friedrich T, Spitkovsky D, et al. Overexpression of p16(ink4a) as a specific marker for dysplastic and neoplastic epithelial cells of the cervix uteri. *Int J Cancer* 2001;92:276.

117. Cullen AP, Reid R, Campion M, Lorincz AT. Analysis of the physical state of different human papillomavirus DNAs in intraepithelial and invasive cervical neoplasia. *J Virol* 1991;65:606.

118. Das BC, Sharma JK, Gopalakrishna V, Luthra UK. Analysis by polymerase chain reaction of the physical state of human papillomavirus type 16 in cervical preneoplastic and neoplastic lesions. *J Gen Virol* 1992;73:2327.

119. Braun L, Mikumo R, Mark HF, Lauchlan S. Analysis of the growth properties and physical state of human papillomavirus type 16 genome in cell lines derived from primary cervical tumors. *Am Pathol* 1993; 143:832.

120. Choo K-B, Pan C-C, Han S-H. Integration of human papillomavirus type 16 into cellular DNA of cervical carcinoma: preferential deletion of the E2 gene and invariable retention of the long control region and the E6/E7 open reading frames. *Virology* 1987;161:259.

121. Scheffner M, Romanczuk H, Munger K, et al. Functions of human papillomavirus proteins. *Curr Top Microbiol Immunol* 1994;186:83.

122. Mitra AB, Murty VV, Li RG, et al. Allelotype analysis of cervical carcinoma. *Cancer Res* 1994;54:4481.

123. Larson AA, Kern S, Curtiss S, et al. High resolution analysis of chromosome 3p alterations in cervical carcinoma. *Cancer Res* 1997;57: 4082.

124. Iftner T, Villa LL. Human papillomavirus technologies. *J Natl Cancer Inst Monogr* 2003:80.

125. Cuzick J, Beverley E, Ho L, et al. HPV testing in primary screening of older women. *Br J Cancer* 1999;81:554.

126. Salmeron J, Lazcano-Ponce E, Lorincz A, et al. Comparison of HPV-based assays with Papanicolaou smears for cervical cancer screening in Morelos State, Mexico. *Cancer Causes Control* 2003;14:505.

127. Kuhn L, Denny L, Pollack A, et al. Human papillomavirus DNA testing for cervical cancer screening in low-resource settings. *J Natl Cancer Inst* 2000;92:818.

128. Belinson J, Qiao YL, Pretorius R, et al. Shanxi Province Cervical Cancer Screening Study: a cross-sectional comparative trial of multiple techniques to detect cervical neoplasia. *Gynecol Oncol* 2001;83: 439.

129. Ratnam S, Franco EL, Ferenczy A. Human papillomavirus testing for primary screening of cervical cancer precursors. *Cancer Epidemiol Biomarkers Prevent* 2000;9:945.

130. Kulasingam SL, Hughes JP, Kiviat NB, et al. Evaluation of human papillomavirus testing in primary screening for cervical abnormalities: comparison of sensitivity, specificity, and frequency of referral. *JAMA* 2002;288:1749.

131. Bauer HM, Ting Y, Greer CE, et al. Genital human papillomavirus infection in female university students as determined by a PCR-based method. *JAMA* 1991;265:472.

132. Wheeler CM, Greer CE, Becker TM, et al. Short-term fluctuations in the detection of cervical human papillomavirus DNA. *Obstet Gynecol* 1996;88:261.

133. Ho GY, Bierman R, Beardsley L, et al. Natural history of cervicovaginal papillomavirus infection in young women. *N Engl J Med* 1998; 338:423.

134. Melkert PW, Hopman E, van den Brule AJ, et al. Prevalence of HPV in cytomorphologically normal cervical smears, as determined by the polymerase chain reaction, is age-dependent. *Int J Cancer* 1993;53: 919.

135. Schneider A, Hotz M, Gissman L. Prevalence of genital HPV infections in pregnant women. *Int J Cancer* 1987;40:198.

136. Schneider A. HPV infection in women and their male partners. *Contemp OB/GYN* 1988;32:131.

137. Evander M, Edlund K, Gustafsson A, et al. Human papillomavirus infection is transient in young women: a population-based cohort study. *J Infect Dis* 1995;171:1026.

138. Fife KH, Katz BP, Roush J, et al. Cancer-associated human papillomavirus types are selectively increased in the cervix of women in the first trimester of pregnancy. *Am J Obstet Gynecol* 1996;174:1487.

139. Sun X-W, Ellerbrock RV, Lungu O, et al. Human papillomavirus infection in human immunodeficiency virus-seropositive women. *Obstet Gynecol* 1995;85:680.

140. Palefsky JM, Minkoff H, Kalish LA, et al. Cervicovaginal human papillomavirus infection in human immunodeficiency virus-1 (HIV)-positive and high-risk HIV-negative women. *J Natl Cancer Inst* 1999; 91:226.

141. Chaung T-Y. Condyloma acuminatum in Rochester, Minn, 1950–1978. I. Epidemiology and clinical features. *Arch Dermatol* 1984;1:20.

142. Burk RD, Ho GY, Beardsley L, et al. Sexual behavior and partner characteristics are the predominant risk factors for genital human papillomavirus infection in young women. *J Infect Dis* 1996;174:679.

143. Kjaer SK, Chackerian B, van den Brule AJ, et al. High-risk human papillomavirus is sexually transmitted: evidence from a follow-up study of virgins starting sexual activity (intercourse). *Cancer Epidemiol Biomarkers Prev* 2001;10:101.

144. Roden RB, Lowy DR, Schiller JT. Papillomavirus is resistant to desiccation. *J Infect Dis* 1997;176:1076.

145. Ferris DG, Batish S, Wright TC, et al. A neglected lesbian health concern: cervical neoplasia. *J Fam Pract* 1996;43:581.

146. Armstrong LR, Preston EJ, Reichert M, et al. Incidence and prevalence of recurrent respiratory papillomatosis among children in Atlanta and Seattle. *Clin Infect Dis* 2000;31:107.

147. Armbruster-Moraes E, Ioshimoto LM, Leao E, Zugaib M. Presence of human papillomavirus DNA in amniotic fluids of pregnant women with cervical lesions. *Gynecol Oncol* 1994;54:152.

148. Pakarian F, Kaye J, Cason J, et al. Cancer associated human papillomaviruses: perinatal transmission and persistence. *Br J Obstet Gynaecol* 1994;101:514.

149. Tenti P, Zappatore R, Migliora P, et al. Perinatal transmission of human papillomavirus from gravidas with latent infections. *Obstet Gynecol* 1999;93:475.

150. Ferenczy A, Mitao M, Nagai N, et al. Latent papillomavirus and recurring genital warts. *N Engl J Med* 1985;313:784.

151. Hildesheim A, Schiffman MH, Gravitt PE, et al. Persistence of type-specific human papillomavirus infection among cytologically normal women. *J Natl Cancer Inst* 1994;169:235.

152. Abdul-Karim FW, Fu YS, Reagan JW, Wentz WB. Morphometric study of intraepithelial neoplasia of the uterine cervix. *Obstet Gynecol* 1982;60:210.

153. Saito K, Saito A, Fu YS, et al. Topographic study of cervical condyloma and intraepithelial neoplasia. *Cancer* 1987;59:2064.

154. Richart RM. Colpomicroscopic studies of the distribution of dysplasia and carcinoma in-situ on the exposed portion of the human uterine cervix. *Cancer* 1965;18:950.

155. Coppleson M. The origin and nature of premalignant lesions of the cervix uteri. *Int J Gynecol Obst* 1970;8:539.

156. Park IJ, Jones HW. Glucose-6-phosphate dehydrogenase and the histogenesis of epidermoid carcinoma of the cervix. *Am J Obstet Gynecol* 1968;102:106.

157. Smith JW, Townsend DE, Spark RS. Genetic variants of glucose-6-phosphate dehydrogenase in the study of carcinoma of the cervix. *Cancer* 1971;28:529.

158. Spriggs AI, Bowey CE, Cowdell RH. Chromosomes of precancerous lesions of the cervix uteri. *Cancer* 1971;27:1239.

159. Park TW, Fujiwara H, Wright TC. Molecular biology of cervical cancer and its precursors. *Cancer* 1995;76:1902.

160. ter Haar-van Eck SA, Rischen-Vos J, Chadha-Ajwani S, Huikeshoven FJM. The incidence of cervical intraepithelial neoplasia among women with renal transplant in relation to cyclosporine. *Br J Obstet Gynaecol* 1995;102:58.

161. ter Harmsel B, Smedts F, Kuijpers J, et al. Relationship between human papillomavirus type 16 in the cervix and intraepithelial neoplasia. *Obstet Gynecol* 1999;93:46.

162. Koss L, Durfee GR. Unusual patterns of squamous epithelium of uterine cervix: cytologic and pathologic study of koilocytotic atypia. *Ann N Y Acad Sci* 1956;63:1245.

163. Fu YS, Huang I, Beaudenon S, et al. Correlative study of human papillomavirus DNA, histopathology and morphometry in cervical condyloma and intraepithelial neoplasia. *Int J Gynecol Pathol* 1988; 7:297.

164. Winkler B, Crum CP, Fujii T, et al. Koilocytotic lesions of the cervix: the relationship of mitotic abnormalities to the presence of papillomavirus antigens and nuclear DNA content. *Cancer* 1984;53:1081.

165. Anderson MC, Hartley RB. Cervical crypt involvement by intraepithelial neoplasia. *Obstet Gynecol* 1980;55:546.

166. Schneider A. Latent and subclinical genital HPV infections. *Papillomavirus Rep* 1990;1:2.

167. Ward KA, Houston JR, Lowry BE, et al. The role of early colposcopy in the management of females with first episode anogenital warts. *Int J STD AIDS* 1994;5:343.

168. Coker R, Desmond N, Tomlinson D, et al. Screening for cervical abnormalities in women with anogenital warts in an STD clinic: an inappropriate use of colposcopy. *Int J STD AIDS* 1994;5:442.

169. Ferenczy A, Richart RM, Wright TC. Pearly penile papules: absence of human papillomavirus DNA by the polymerase chain reaction. *Obstet Gynecol* 1991;78:118.

170. Bergeron C, Ferenczy A, Richart RM, Guralnick M. Micropapillomatosis labialis appears unrelated to human papillomavirus. *Obstet Gynecol* 1990;76:281.

171. Cone R, Beckman A, Aho M, et al. Subclinical manifestations of vulvar human papillomavirus infection. *Int J Gynecol Pathol* 1991; 10:26.

172. Kaufman RH. Intraepithelial neoplasia of the vulva. *Gynecol Oncol* 1995;56:8.

173. Sturgeon SR, Brinton LA, Devesa SS, Kurman RL. In situ and invasive vulvar cancer incidence trends (1973–1987). *Am J Obstet Gynecol* 1992;166:1482.

174. Iversen T, Tretli S. Intraepithelial and invasive squamous cell neoplasia of the vulva: trends in incidence, recurrence, and survival rate in Norway. *Obstet Gynecol* 1998;91:969.

175. McNally OM, Mulvany NJ, Pagano R, et al. VIN 3: a clinicopathologic review. *Int J Gynecol Cancer* 2002;12:490.

176. Wilkinson EJ. Premalignant and malignant lesions of the vulva. In: Kurman RJ, ed. *Blaustein's pathology of the female genital tract.* New York: Springer-Verlag, 1994.

177. Haefner HK, Tate JE, McLachlin CM, Crum CP. Vulvar intraepithelial neoplasia: age, morphological phenotype, papillomavirus DNA and coexisting invasive carcinoma. *Hum Pathol* 1995;26:147.

178. Park JS, Jones RW, McLean MR, et al. Possible etiologic heterogeneity of vulvar intraepithelial neoplasia. A correlation of pathologic characteristics with human papillomavirus detection by in situ hybridization and polymerase chain reaction. *Cancer* 1991;67:1599.

179. Wilkinson EJ. Premalignant and malignant tumors of the vulva. In: Kurman RJ, ed. *Blaustein's pathology of the female genital tract.* New York: Springer-Verlag, 1994.

180. Liu S, Semenciw R, Probert A, Mao Y. Cervical cancer in Canada: changing patterns in incidence and mortality. *Int J Gynecol Cancer* 2001;11:24.

181. Pisani P, Parkin DM, Bray F, Ferlay J. Estimates of the worldwide mortality from 25 cancers in 1990. *Int J Cancer* 1999;83:18.
182. Cervical cancer facts and figures—2003. American Cancer Society, 2003.
183. Fahey MT, Irwig L, Macaskill P. Meta-analysis of Pap test accuracy. *Am J Epidemiol* 1995;141:680.
184. Nanda K, McCrory DC, Myers ER, et al. Accuracy of the Papanicolaou test in screening for and follow-up of cervical cytologic abnormalities: a systematic review. *Ann Intern Med* 2000;132:810.
185. Dehner LP. Cervicovaginal cytology, false-negative results, and standards of practice. *Am J Clin Pathol* 1993;99:45.
186. Wilkinson EJ. Pap smears and screening for cervical neoplasia. *Clin Obstet Gynecol* 1990;33:817.
187. Koonings PP, Dickinson K, d'Ablaing G III, Schlaerth JB. A randomized clinical trial comparing the cytobrush and cotton swab for pap smears. *Obstet Gynecol* 1992;80:241.
188. Boon ME, Alons-van Kordelaar JJ, Rietveld-Scheffers PE. Consequences of the introduction of combined spatula and cytobrush sampling for cervical cytology. Improvements in smear quality and detection rates. *Acta Cytol* 1986;30:264.
189. Miller AB. Failures of cervical cancer screening. *Am J Public Health* 1995;85:795.
190. ACOG practice bulletin: clinical management guidelines for obstetrician-gynecologists. No. 45, August 2003. Cervical cytology screening (replaces committee opinion 152, March 1995). *Obstet Gynecol* 2003; 102:417.
191. Saslow D, Runowicz CD, Solomon D, et al. American Cancer Society guideline for the early detection of cervical neoplasia and cancer. *CA Cancer J Clin* 2002;52:342.
192. U.S. Preventive services task force. Guide to clinical preventive services. Washington, DC: U.S. Department of Health and Human Services, 2003.
193. Austin RM, Ramzy I. Increased detection of epithelial cell abnormalities by liquid-based gynecologic cytology preparations. A review of accumulated data. *Acta Cytol* 1998;42:178.
194. Vassilakos P, Saurel J, Rondez R. Direct-to-vial use of the autocyte prep liquid-based preparation for cervical-vaginal specimens in three European laboratories. *Acta Cytol* 1999;43:65.
195. Wright TC Jr, Lorincz A, Ferris DG, et al. Reflex human papillomavirus deoxyribonucleic acid testing in women with abnormal Papanicolaou smears. *Am J Obstet Gynecol* 1998;178:962.
196. Richart RM, Wright TC. Controversies in the management of low grade cervical intraepithelial neoplasia. *Cancer* 1993;71:1413.
197. Jones BA, Novis DA. Follow-up of abnormal gynecologic cytology: a College of American Pathologists Q-probes study of 16132 cases from 306 laboratories. *Arch Pathol Lab Med* 2000;124:665.
198. Solomon D, Schiffman M, Tarrone R. Comparison of three management strategies for patients with atypical squamous cells of undetermined significance: baseline results from a randomized trial. *J Natl Cancer Inst* 2001;93:293.
199. Solomon D. ALTS results. Personal communication, 2001.
200. Manos MM, Kinney WK, Hurley LB, et al. Identifying women with cervical neoplasia: using human papillomavirus DNA testing for equivocal Papanicolaou results. *JAMA* 1999;281:1605.
201. Lonky NM, Sadeghi M, Tsadik GW, Petitti D. The clinical significance of the poor correlation of cervical dysplasia and cervical malignancy with referral cytologic results. *Am J Obstet Gynecol* 1999;181: 560.
202. Kinney WK, Manos MM, Hurley LB, Ransley JE. Where's the high-grade cervical neoplasia? The importance of minimally abnormal Papanicolaou diagnoses. *Obstet Gynecol* 1998;91:973.
203. Kim JJ, Wright TC, Goldie SJ. Cost-effectiveness of alternative triage strategies for atypical squamous cells of undetermined significance. *JAMA* 2002;287:2382.
204. Sherman ME, Schiffman M, Cox JT, Group TA. Effects of age and HPV load on colposcopic triage: data from the ASCUS LSIL triage study (ALTS). *J Natl Cancer Inst* 2002;94:102.
205. Takezawa K, Bennett BB, Wilkinson EJ, et al. Squamous intraepithelial lesions of the cervix in a high-risk population. *J Lower Gen Tract Dis* 1998;2:136.
206. Human papillomavirus testing for triage of women with cytologic evidence of low-grade squamous intraepithelial lesions: baseline data from a randomized trial. The atypical squamous cells of undetermined significance/low-grade squamous intraepithelial lesions triage study (ALTS) group. *J Natl Cancer Inst* 2000;92:397.
207. Wright TC Jr, Cox JT, Massad LS, et al. 2001 consensus guidelines for the management of women with cervical intraepithelial neoplasia. *Am J Obstet Gynecol* 2003;189:295.
208. Brown FM, Faquin WC, Sun D, et al. LSIL biopsies after HSIL smears. Correlation with high-risk HPV and greater risk of HSIL on follow-up. *Am J Clin Pathol* 1999;112:765.
209. Stoler MH, Schiffman M. Interobserver reproducibility of cervical cytologic and histologic interpretations: realistic estimates from the ASCUS-LSIL triage study. *JAMA* 2001;285:1500.
210. Massad LS, Halperin CJ, Bitterman P. Correlation between colposcopically directed biopsy and cervical loop excision. *Gynecol Oncol* 1996;60:400.
211. Mitchell MF, Tortolero-Luna G, Cook E, et al. A randomized clinical trial of cryotherapy, laser vaporization, and loop electrosurgical excision for treatment of squamous intraepithelial lesions of the cervix. *Obstet Gynecol* 1998;92:737.
212. Alvarez RD, Helm CW, Edwards RP, et al. Prospective randomized trial of LLETZ versus laser ablation in patients with cervical intraepithelial neoplasia. *Gynecol Oncol* 1994;52:175.
213. Ferenczy A. Comparison of cryo- and carbon dioxide laser therapy for cervical intraepithelial neoplasia. *Obstet Gynecol* 1985;66:793.
214. Nuovo J, Melnikow J, Willan AR, Chan BK. Treatment outcomes for squamous intraepithelial lesions. *Int J Gynaecol Obstet* 2000;68: 25.
215. Soutter WP, de Barros Lopes A, Fletcher A, et al. Invasive cervical cancer after conservative therapy for cervical intraepithelial neoplasia. *Lancet* 1997;349:978.
216. Vedel P, Jakobsen H, Kryger-Baggesen N, et al. Five-year follow up of patients with cervical intra-epithelial neoplasia in the cone margins after conization. *Eur J Obstet Gynaecol Reprod Biol* 1993;50:71.
217. Moore BC, Higgins RV, Laurent SL, et al. Predictive factors from cold knife conization for residual cervical intraepithelial neoplasia in subsequent hysterectomy. *Am J Obstet Gynecol* 1995;173:361.
218. Herrero R, Hildesheim A, Bratti C, et al. Population-based study of human papillomavirus infection and cervical neoplasia in rural Costa Rica. *J Natl Cancer Inst* 2000;92:464.
219. Cuzick J, Szarewski A, Terry G, et al. Human papillomavirus testing in primary cervical screening. *Lancet* 1995;345:1533.
220. Clavel C, Masure M, Bory JP, et al. Human papillomavirus testing in primary screening for the detection of high-grade cervical lesions: a study of 7932 women. *Br J Cancer* 2001;89:1616.

CHAPTER 20

Vulva

David H. Moore, Wui-Jin Koh, William P. McGuire, and Edward J. Wilkinson

Malignant tumors of the vulva are rare in that they account for less than 5% of all cancers of the female genital tract. Consequently, many physicians who provide primary health care for women may never encounter a patient with vulvar cancer. Although an occasional patient will present without symptoms, the vast majority of women with vulvar cancer initially present with complaints such as irritation, pruritus, pain, or a mass lesion that does not resolve. The time interval between the onset of symptoms and the diagnosis of cancer is usually protracted by the patient, who ignores her symptoms or attempts a number of self-remedies, and the physician, who may prescribe empiric topical therapies without a proper physical examination or tissue biopsy confirmation. Jones and Joura evaluated the clinical events preceding the diagnosis of squamous-cell carcinoma of the vulva and found that 88% of patients had experienced symptoms for more than 6 months, 31% of women had three or more medical consultations prior to the diagnosis of vulvar carcinoma, and 27% had applied topical estrogen or corticosteroids to the vulva (1).

The vulva is covered by keratinized squamous epithelium, and expectedly the majority of malignant vulvar tumors are squamous-cell carcinomas. Consequently, our current understanding of the epidemiology, spread patterns, prognostic factors, and survival data for vulvar cancer is derived almost exclusively from retrospective observations and a few prospective studies of squamous-cell carcinomas. Malignant melanoma is the second most common cancer of the vulva. Although there is some consensus regarding the behavior and treatment of vulvar melanoma, its rarity precludes the conduct of prospective clinical trials. A number of other malignant tumors may also arise on the vulva including basal cell carcinoma, adenocarcinomas (derived from the Bartholin gland, eccrine sweat glands, Paget's disease, or ectopic breast tissue), and a host of very rare soft tissue sarcomas including leiomyosarcomas, malignant fibrous histiocytomas, liposarcomas, angiosarcomas, rhabdomyosarcomas, epithelioid sarcomas, and Kaposi's sarcomas. Finally, the vulva may be secondarily involved with malignant disease originating in the bladder, anorectum, or other genital organs.

The traditional therapeutic approach to vulvar cancer has been radical surgical excision of the primary tumor and inguinal-femoral lymph nodes. As our clinical understanding of this disease evolved, it became evident that survival could be improved with the administration of postoperative radiation therapy to selected patients at high risk for locoregional failure. More recent developments have included the administration of radiation therapy and concurrent chemotherapy in the postoperative setting and as primary therapy for locally advanced tumors not amenable to radical surgery. An individualized approach to vulvar cancer management, often employing multiple modalities in an effort to achieve excellent disease control with better cosmetic results and sexual function, is now the norm. These and other topics pertinent to the principles of management of women with vulvar cancer will be the subject of this chapter.

ANATOMY

The vulva consists of the external genital organs including the mons pubis, labia minora and majora, clitoris, vaginal vestibule, perineal body, and their supporting subcutaneous tissues (2). The vulva is bordered superiorly by the anterior

David H. Moore: Department of Obstetrics and Gynecology, Indiana University School of Medicine, Indianapolis, Indiana 46202

Wui-Jin Koh: Department of Radiation Oncology, University of Washington School of Medicine, Seattle, Washington 98109

William P. McGuire: The Harry and Jeanette Weinberg Cancer Institute at Franklin Square Hospital Center, Baltimore, Maryland 21237

Edward J. Wilkinson: Department of Pathology and Laboratory Medicine, University of Florida College of Medicine, Gainesville, FL 32610.

abdominal wall, laterally by the labiocrural fold at the medial thigh, and inferiorly by the anus. The vagina and urethra open onto the vulva. The mons pubis is a prominent mound of hair-bearing skin and subcutaneous adipose and connective tissue that is located anterior to the pubic symphysis. After puberty it is covered by coarse pubic hair. The labia majora are two elongated skin folds that course posterior from the mons pubis and blend into the perineal body. The skin of the labia majora is pigmented and contains hair follicles and sebaceous glands. The labia minora are a smaller pair of skin folds medial and parallel to the labia majora that extend inferiorly to form the margin of the vaginal vestibule. Superiorly, the labia minora separate into two components that course above and below the clitoris, fusing with those of the opposite side to form the prepuce and frenulum, respectively. The skin of the labia minora contains sebaceous glands, but is not hair bearing and has little or no underlying adipose tissue. The clitoris is supported externally by the fusion of the labia minora (prepuce and frenulum) and is approximately 2 to 3 cm anterior to the urethral meatus. It comprises erectile tissue organized into the glans, body, and two crura. The glans has a concentration of nerve endings important for normal sexual response. Two loosely fused corpora cavernosa form the body of the clitoris and extend superiorly from the glans, ultimately dividing into the two crura. The crura course laterally beneath the ischiocavernosus muscles and attach to the ischial rami.

The vaginal vestibule is situated in the center of the vulva and is demarcated circumferentially by the labia minora and inferiorly by the perineal body. Both the vagina and urethra open onto the vestibule. Anteriorly, numerous small vestibular glands are located beneath the vestibular mucosa and open onto its surface adjacent to the urethral meatus. The vestibular bulbs, a loose collection of bilateral erectile tissue covered superficially by the bulbocavernosus muscle, are located laterally. The Bartholin glands, two small mucus-secreting glands situated within the subcutaneous tissue of the posterior labia majora, have ducts opening onto the posterolateral portion of the vestibule. The perineal body is a 3- to 4-cm band of skin and subcutaneous tissue located between the posterior extension of the labia majora, separates the vaginal vestibule from the anus, and forms the posterior margin of the vulva.

The vulva has a rich blood supply derived primarily from the internal pudendal artery, which arises from the anterior division of the internal iliac (hypogastric) artery, and the superficial and deep external pudendal arteries, which arise from the femoral artery. The internal pudendal artery exits the pelvis and passes behind the ischial spine to reach the posterolateral vulva, where it divides into several small branches to the ischiocavernosus and bulbocavernosus muscles, the perineal artery, artery of the bulb, urethral artery, and dorsal and deep arteries of the clitoris. Both external pudendal arteries travel medially to supply the labia majora

and their deep structures. These vessels anastomose freely with branches from the internal pudendal artery.

Innervation of the vulva is derived from multiple sources and spinal cord levels. The mons pubis and upper labia majora are innervated by the ilioinguinal nerve (L1) and the genital branch of the genitofemoral nerve (L1–2). Either of these nerves may be easily injured during pelvic lymph node dissection with resulting paresthesias. The pudendal nerve (S2–4) enters the vulva in parallel with the internal pudendal artery and gives rise to several branches that innervate the lower vagina, labia, clitoris, perineal body, and their supporting structures.

The vulvar lymphatics run anteriorly through the labia majora, turn laterally at the mons pubis, and drain primarily into the superficial inguinal lymph nodes. Elegant lymphatic dye studies by Parry-Jones demonstrated that vulvar lymphatic channels do not extend lateral to the labiocrural folds and generally do not cross the midline unless the site of dye injection is at the clitoris or perineal body (3). Several small lymphatics may drain from the clitoris under the pubic symphysis directly into the pelvic nodes. Many of these observations have been substantiated by surgical-pathologic studies and sentinel lymph node mapping studies that will be discussed later.

The vulvar lymphatics drain to the superficial inguinal lymph nodes located within the femoral triangle formed by the inguinal ligament superiorly, the border of the sartorius muscle laterally, and the border of the adductor longus muscle medially. About ten superficial inguinal lymph nodes lie along the saphenous vein and its branches between Camper's fascia and the cribriform fascia overlying the femoral vessels (Fig. 20.1). The superficial nodes are located within the triangle formed by the inguinal ligament superiorly, the border of the sartorius muscle laterally, and the border of the adductor longus muscle medially (Fig. 20.2) (4). Lymphatic drainage proceeds from the superficial to the deep inguinal (or femoral) nodes, which are located beneath the cribriform fascia and medial to the femoral vein. There are usually three to five deep nodes, the most superior of which is Cloquet's node located under the inguinal ligament. The deep inguinal nodes drain superiorly into the medial portion of the external iliac nodes and then upward through the pelvic and aortic lymph node chains (Fig. 20.3).

EPIDEMIOLOGY

Most vulvar cancers occur in postmenopausal women, although more recent reports suggest a trend toward younger age at diagnosis (5,6). Observational studies have suggested associations between hypertension, diabetes mellitus, and obesity with vulvar carcinoma (7). However, it is not clear whether these represent independent risk factors or merely coexisting medical conditions common to the aging process. More recent analysis has not confirmed the prognostic significance of these diagnoses (8).

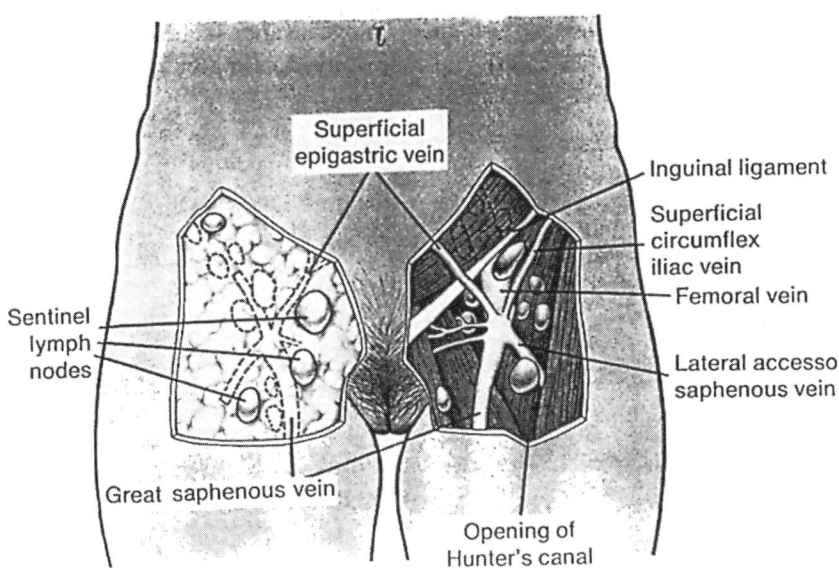

FIG. 20.1. The superficial inguinal lymph nodes comprise eight to ten subcutaneous nodes located between Camper's fascia and the cribriform fascia. These nodes are immediately adjacent to the saphenous vein and its branches. (Reprinted with permission from DiSaia PJ, Creasman WT, Rich WM. An alternative approach to early cancer of the vulva. *Am J Obstet Gynecol* 1979;133:825.)

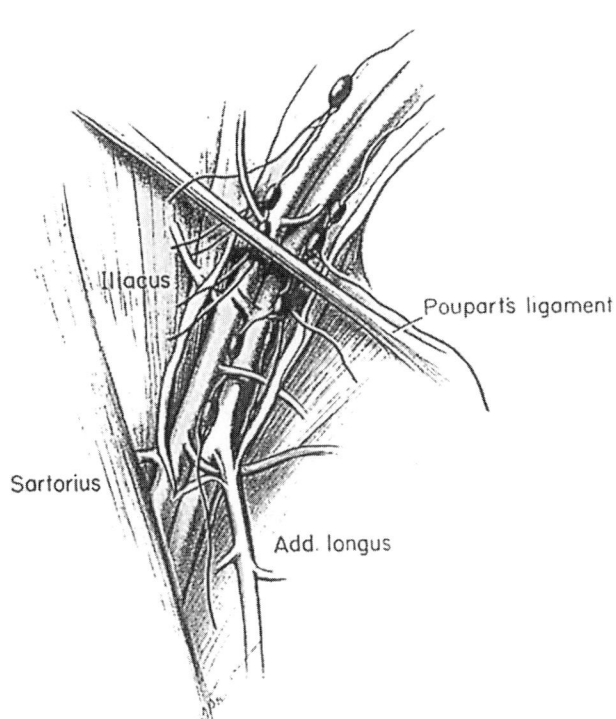

FIG. 20.2. Anatomic diagram of the right groin with the superficial structures removed demonstrates the saphenous vein and the boundaries of inguinal dissection—the sartorius muscle, inguinal ligament, and adductor longus muscle. (Reprinted with permission from Plentl AA, Friedman EA, eds. *Lymphatic system of the female genitalia.* Philadelphia: WB Saunders, 1971.)

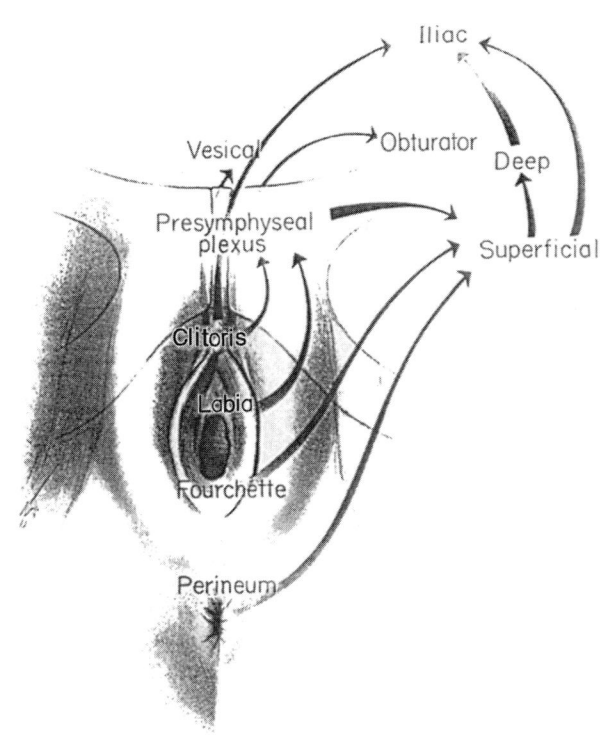

FIG. 20.3. The lymphatic drainage of the vulva initially flows to the superficial inguinal nodes then to the deep femoral and iliac groups. Drainage from midline structures may flow directly beneath the symphysis to the pelvic nodes. (Reprinted with permission from Plentl AA, Friedman EA, eds. *Lymphatic system of the female genitalia.* Philadelphia: WB Saunders, 1971.)

Several infectious agents have been proposed as possible etiologic agents in vulvar carcinoma, including granulomatous infections, herpes simplex virus, and human papillomavirus (HPV). Reports associating vulvar cancer with granuloma inguinale, lymphogranuloma venereum, or syphilis are largely historical and anecdotal (7). The observed coexistence of vulvar cancer with these granulomatous infections may only reflect such patients' risk for any sexually transmitted disease (8). Kaufman and colleagues identified serologic evidence of infection with herpes simplex virus type 2 and carcinoma *in situ* of the vulva in a small group of women (9). However, they were unable to isolate whole viral antigens, again suggesting an association with a sexually transmitted infection but failing to establish a direct causal link between the two.

Recent areas of investigation have focused on the neoplastic potential of human papillomaviruses (HPVs). Strong associations between vulvar condylomata and the later development of vulvar cancer have been identified (8). In addition, HPV DNA has been isolated from both invasive and carcinoma *in situ* lesions (10,11). HPV type 16 appears to be most common, but types 6 and 33 have also been identified (12,13). HPV DNA can be identified in approximately 70% to 80% of intraepithelial lesions, but is seen in only 10% to 50% of invasive lesions. HPV-related cancers may exhibit distinguishing clinical and histologic features, leading some to suggest a stratification scheme for vulvar cancers based on the presence or absence of an HPV association (14). Although much of the information linking past or current vulvar HPV infection with neoplastic transformation is enticing, the evidence for a causative relationship is presently inconclusive.

Brinton and colleagues conducted a case-control analysis and identified women with a history of genital condylomata, those with a previous abnormal Papanicolaou smear, and those who smoked as having an increased risk for vulvar cancer (8). Those who both smoked and had a history of genital warts had a 35-fold increase in risk when compared with women without these factors (Table 20.1). Chronic immunosuppression has also been linked to invasive vulvar tumors (5). HPV infection and nonspecific immune suppression may act as cofactors in the development of some vulvar cancers.

Both chronic vulvar inflammatory lesions, such as vulvar dystrophy or lichen sclerosus, and squamous intraepithelial lesions, particularly carcinoma *in situ*, have been suggested as precursors of invasive squamous cancers (Fig. 20.4). Carli et al. suggested a possible role of lichen sclerosus as a precursor to vulvar cancer based on their observation that 32% of vulvar cancer cases not HPV related were associated with lichen sclerosus (15). However, Hart and co-workers, in a large pathologic review, were unable to identify transitions from lichen sclerosus to vulvar cancer (16). In an observational study of women with carcinoma *in situ*, 7 of 8 untreated cases progressed to invasive carcinoma within 8 years, and 4 of 105 treated women presented with invasive tumors from 7 to 18 years later (17). Although some intraepithelial lesions regress spontaneously, it appears that a more significant number persist or progress to invasive cancer. Recent incidence analyses from the United States and Norway have identified a two- to threefold increase in carcinoma *in situ* lesions from the 1970s to the 1990s (18, 19). However, a concomitant rise in the incidence of invasive

TABLE 20.1. *Relative risks of* in situ *and invasive vulvar cancers by selected risk factors*

	In situ series			Invasive series		
	No. of cases	RR	95% CI	No. of cases	RR	95% CI
No. of sexual partners						
0–1	17	1.00		48	1.00	
2	11	2.78	0.9–8.3	17	1.22	0.6–2.5
3–4	23	2.33	0.9–6.0	28	3.32	1.6–7.1
5–9	23	5.08	1.7–14.8	11	1.50	0.6–3.9
≥10	22	2.74	0.9–7.9	8	0.83	0.3–2.5
Trend test	p = .03			p = .24		
Ever had an abnormal Pap smear						
No	64	1.00		90	1.00	
Yes	30	1.92	0.9–3.9	11	1.41	0.5–3.6
No previous Pap smear	2	0.37	0.1–1.9	10	2.46	0.9–6.7
Ever had genital warts						
No	73	1.00		105	1.00	
Yes	23	18.50	5.5–62.5	8	14.55	1.71–25.6
Current smoking status						
Nonsmoker	22	1.00		46	1.00	
Current smoker	55	4.65	2.2–10.0	48	1.19	0.6–2.2
Exsmoker	19	1.78	0.7–4.4	19	0.40	0.2–0.8

CI, confidence interval; RR, relative risk.
Reprinted with permission from Brinton LA, et al. Case-control study of cancer of the vulva. *Obstet Gynecol* 1990;75:864.)

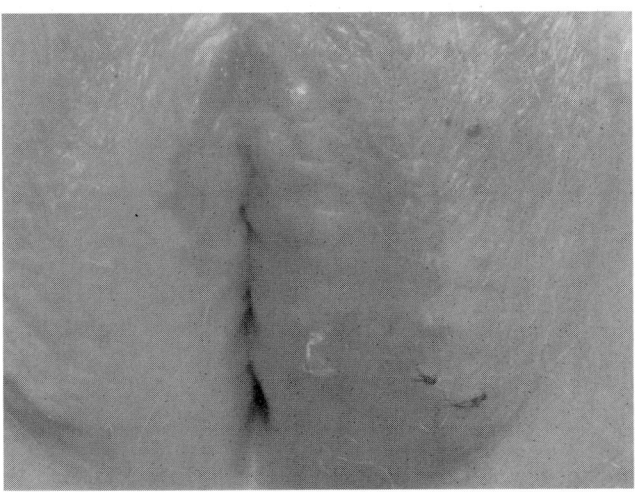

FIG. 20.4. This T1 lesion arose from a background of lichen sclerosus and demonstrates the typical irregular surface features and superficial ulceration of a squamous-cell carcinoma. The biopsy site is marked with a suture.

vulvar cancers has not yet been seen. This discrepancy leads to several alternative hypotheses: (a) affected women have not reached the age at which invasive lesions are seen; (b) aggressive treatment of preinvasive disease has prevented the development of invasive tumors; or (c) the causes of *in situ* and invasive lesions are not strongly related (19).

Trimble and colleagues have postulated that squamous carcinoma of the vulva may represent a final common endpoint of heterogeneous etiologic pathways (20). According to their studies, two histologic subtypes—with basaloid or warty features—are associated with HPV, whereas keratinizing squamous carcinomas are not. Furthermore, basaloid or warty carcinomas are associated with classic risk factors for cervical carcinoma, including age at first intercourse, lifetime number of sexual partners, prior abnormal Papanicolaou smears, smoking, and lower socioeconomic status. Keratinizing squamous carcinomas are weakly linked to these factors, and in some cases not at all. Flowers et al. have reported that mutations in the *p53* tumor-suppressor gene are more frequently found in HPV-negative vulvar carcinomas versus those associated with HPV (21). The *p53* tumor-suppressor gene has several key regulatory functions, including the control of cell growth and proliferation. The common denominator in the development of vulvar carcinoma appears to be functional inactivation of the *p53* tumor-suppressor gene either by genetic mutation in HPV-negative tumors or by inactivation through the expression of HPV gene products (22).

Mitchell et al. evaluated 169 women with invasive vulvar cancers and noted that second genital squamous neoplasms occurred in 13% of cases (23). The risk of a second primary tumor was significantly increased in cancer cases with HPV DNA, intraepithelioid growth pattern, or adjacent dysplasia. These observations support the concept that some squamous

lesions may be initiated by sexually transmitted viruses capable of producing neoplastic change within the entire field of the lower genital tract. The obvious clinical implication is that a patient with an established squamous lesion of the vulva, vagina, or cervix needs to be evaluated and monitored for new or coexistent lesions at other sites.

CLINICAL PRESENTATION

Most women with vulvar cancer present with pruritus and a recognizable lesion. Selecting the most appropriate site for biopsy in women with condylomata, chronic vulvar dystrophy, multifocal dysplasia, or Paget's disease can be difficult, and multiple biopsies may be required. Optimal management for any patient presenting with a suspicious lesion is to proceed directly to biopsy under local analgesia. Tissue biopsies should include the cutaneous lesion in question and contiguous underlying stroma, so that the presence and depth of invasion can be accurately assessed.

Although other techniques to facilitate the assessment of

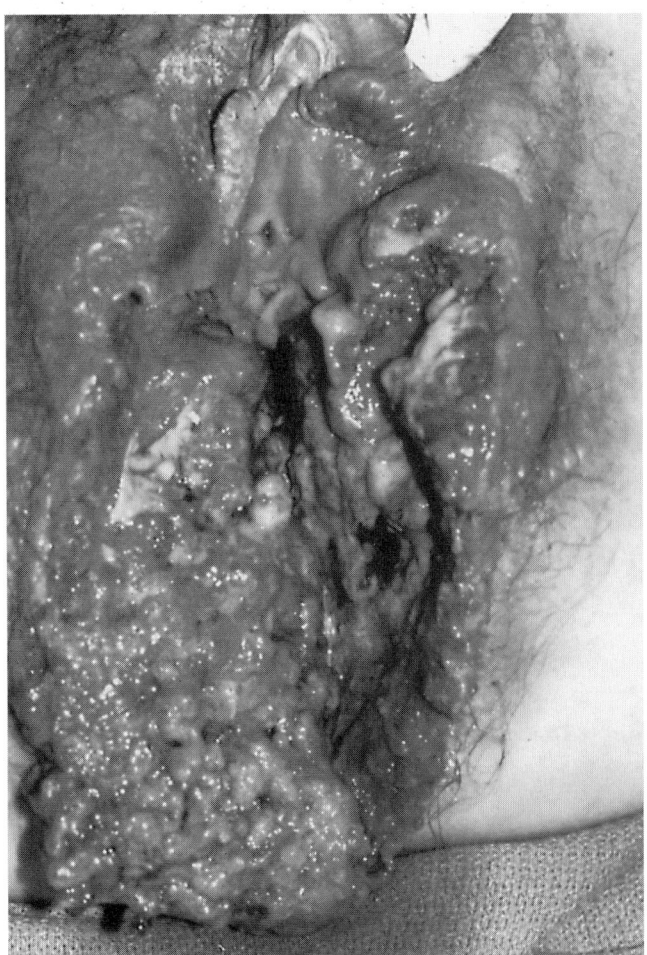

FIG. 20.5. This patient ignored symptoms and an obvious tumor for more than a year. Although uncommon, such late presentations occur. Therapy options are limited.

vulvar lesions (e.g., toluidine blue stain or exfoliative cytology) have been described, they are less accurate than, and should not be considered a substitute for, tissue biopsy. As noted previously, one of the greatest clinical pitfalls in the management of women with vulvar cancer is delay in diagnosis. The goals of immediate evaluation with outpatient biopsy are to provide an accurate and definitive diagnosis and to avoid delay in the planning of appropriate therapy. Unfortunately, some women ignore or deny obvious symptoms and lesions for long periods of time and present with advanced disease (Fig. 20.5). The presentation in such cases is generally dominated by local pain, bleeding, and surface drainage from the tumor. Metastatic disease in the groin lymph nodes or at distant sites may also be symptomatic.

DIAGNOSTIC EVALUATION

The evaluation of the patient with vulvar cancer must take into consideration the clinical extent of disease, the anticipated treatment plan, and the presence of coexisting medical illnesses. Initial evaluation should include a detailed physical examination with measurements of the primary tumor, assessment for extension to adjacent mucosal or bony structures, and possible involvement of the inguinal lymph nodes. Women with small cancers and clinically negative groin nodes require few diagnostic studies other than those for preoperative clearance. Additional radiographic and endoscopic studies should be considered for those with large primary tumors or suspected metastases. Potentially useful studies include barium enema, proctosigmoidoscopy, cystourethroscopy, computed tomographic (CT) scan, and intravenous pyelography. Fine-needle aspiration biopsy from sites of suspected metastases may eliminate the need for surgical exploration in some patients with advanced tumors. Because neoplasia of the female genital tract is often multifocal, evaluation of the vagina and cervix—including cervical cytologic screening—should always be performed in women with vulvar neoplasms.

STAGING SYSTEMS

The International Federation of Gynecology and Obstetrics (FIGO) adopted a modified surgical staging system for vulvar cancer in 1989, which remained relatively unchanged in their 1995 recommendations (Table 20.2) (24). The previous clinical system provided reliable information regarding the primary lesion but an inaccurate assessment of groin node involvement in 20% to 30% of cases. The frequent discrepancy between clinical staging and surgical-pathologic findings spurred the acceptance of the current surgical evaluation of the inguinal lymph nodes. The American Joint Committee on Cancer (AJCC) has published a TNM classification scheme that is correlated with the FIGO staging system (Table 20.3) (25). Tumor assessment is based on physical examination with endoscopy in cases of bulky disease. Nodal status is determined by the surgical evaluation of the groins. The presence or absence of distant metastases is based on an unspecified diagnostic workup tailored to the patient's clinical presentation.

A microinvasive substage (IA) is defined as tumors ≤2 cm in diameter and depth of invasion ≤1 mm. Prior attempts to define a microinvasive substage were hindered by the lack of uniformity in defining the techniques for measuring depth of invasion and the cutoff level for a depth of invasion that provided a reliably low risk of lymph node metastasis (26,27). The technique recommended by the International Society for the Study of Vulvar Disease and the International Society of Gynecologic Pathologists to assess depth of stromal invasion is to measure from the base of the epithelium at the nearest superficial dermal papillae to the deepest point of tumor penetration (28).

PATTERNS OF SPREAD

Vulvar cancers metastasize in three ways: (a) local growth and extension into adjacent organs, (b) lymphatic embolization to regional lymph nodes in the groin, and (c) hematogenous dissemination to distant sites. Objective clinical descriptions of local growth have been categorized in the TNM staging system (Table 20.3). These descriptive definitions are clinically useful in that local surgical resection with a wide margin is almost universally feasible in women with T1 or T2 tumors, occasionally possible in those with T3 lesions, and impossible in those with T4 tumors without resorting to an exenterative operation.

A more precise understanding of the lymphatic drainage of the vulva has been key to developing an individualized surgical approach to vulvar cancer. The lymphatic dye studies described by Parry-Jones demonstrated that the dermal lymphatic network of the vulva courses superiorly to the area of the mons pubis and then turns laterally to drain into the superficial lymph nodes of the ipsilateral groin (3). Lymphatic channels from the superficial group then perforate the cribriform fascia to the deep inguinal (femoral) nodes.

TABLE 20.2. *FIGO staging of vulvar carcinoma*

Stage	Clinical findings
0	Carcinoma *in situ;* intraepithelial carcinoma
I	Tumor confined to the vulva or perineum; 2 cm or less in greatest dimension; no nodal metastasis
IA	Stromal invasion ≤1 mm
IB	Stromal invasion >1 mm
II	Tumor confined to the vulva or perineum; more than 2 cm in greatest dimension; no nodal metastasis
III	Tumor of any size with adjacent spread to the urethra, vagina, or the anus or with unilateral regional lymph node metastasis
IVA	Tumor invades upper urethra, bladder mucosa, rectal mucosa, pelvic bone, or bilateral regional node metastases
IVB	Any distant metastasis, including pelvic lymph nodes

TABLE 20.3. *American Joint Committee on Cancer Staging (2002)*

Primary tumor (T)

TNM Categories	FIGO Stages	
TX		Primary tumor cannot be assessed
T0		No evidence of primary tumor
Tis	0	Carcinoma *in situ* (preinvasive carcinoma)
T1	I	Tumor confined to the vulva or to the vulva and perineum, 2 cm or less in greatest dimension
T1a	IA	Tumor confined to the vulva or to the vulva and perineum, 2 cm or less in greatest dimension, and with stromal invasion no greater than 1 mm[a]
T1b	IB	Tumor confined to the vulva or to the vulva and perineum, 2 cm or less in greatest dimension, and with stromal invasion greater than 1 mm[a]
T2	II	Tumor confined to the vulva or to the vulva and perineum, more than 2 cm in greatest dimension
T3	III	Tumor of any size with contiguous spread to the lower urethra and/or vagina or anus
T4	IVA	Tumor invades any of the following: upper urethra, bladder mucosa, rectal mucosa, or is fixed to the pubic bone

Regional lymph nodes (N)

NX		Regional lymph nodes cannot be assessed
N0		No regional lymph node metastasis
N1	III	Unilateral regional lymph node metastasis
N2	IVA	Bilateral regional lymph node metastasis

Distant metastasis (M)

MX		Distant metastasis cannot be assessed
M0		No distant metastasis
M1	IVB	Distant metastasis (including pelvic lymph node metastasis)

[a] The depth of invasion is defined as the measurement of the tumor from the epithelial-stromal junction of the adjacent most superficial dermal papilla to the deepest point of invasion.

Stage Grouping			
Stage 0	Tis	N0	M0
Stage I	T1	N0	M0
Stage IA	T1a	N0	M0
Stage IB	T1b	N0	M0
Stage II	T2	N0	M0
Stage III	T1	N1	M0
	T2	N1	M0
	T3	N0	M0
	T3	N1	M0
Stage IVA	T1	N2	M0
	T2	N2	M0
	T3	N2	M0
	T4	Any N	M0
Stage IVB	Any T	Any N	M1

Observations following cutaneous dye injection showed that lymphatic drainage from lateral sites was to the ipsilateral groin. No lymphatic channels were located beyond the labio-crural fold, and crossover drainage to the opposite groin was rare. Drainage from midline injections could be bilateral (29). Some channels from the clitoral area appeared to drain beneath the symphysis directly to the pelvic nodes. These anatomic descriptions confirmed the clinical impressions originally outlined by Way (Fig. 20.6) (30,31). More recent experience with intraoperative mapping has demonstrated that lymphatic drainage from most vulvar sites proceeds initially to a "sentinel" node located within the superficial

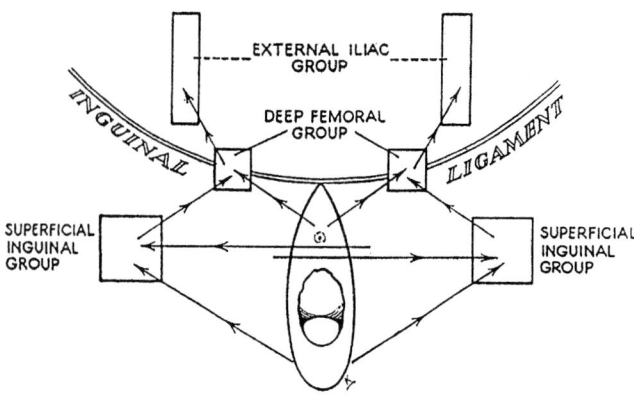

FIG. 20.6. Way's schematic representation of the potential routes of lymphatic spread from vulvar cancer based on his clinical observations. (Reprinted with permission from Way S. *Malignant disease of the female genital tract*. New York: Churchill Livingstone, 1951.)

inguinal group (32). However, aberrant channels coursing directly to deep inguinal, contralateral superficial inguinal, and pelvic lymph nodes were observed in a few cases. These infrequent anatomic variations may ultimately provide the explanation for unanticipated lymph node failure.

Inguinal node metastasis can be predicted by the presence of certain parameters, including lesion diameter ≥2 cm, poor differentiation, increasing depth of stromal invasion, and invasion of lymphovascular spaces (33). Clinically important observations regarding nodal metastases include the following: (a) the superficial inguinal nodes are the most common site of lymphatic metastasis; (b) in-transit metastases within the vulvar skin are exceedingly rare, suggesting that most initial lymphatic metastases represent embolic phenomena; (c) metastasis to the contralateral groin or deep pelvic nodes is unusual in the absence of ipsilateral groin metastases; and (d) nodal involvement generally proceeds in a stepwise fashion from the superficial inguinal to the deep inguinal and then to the pelvic nodes.

Spread beyond the inguinal lymph nodes is considered to be distant metastasis. This may occur as secondary or tertiary level lymphatic metastases to the pelvic/aortic nodes or as a result of hematogenous dissemination to more distant sites, such as bone, lung, or liver. Distant metastases are uncommon at initial presentation, and more often are seen in the context of recurrent vulvar cancer.

PATHOLOGY

Most vulvar malignancies arise within squamous epithelium, and of these tumors, squamous-cell carcinomas comprise the majority of tumors. Although the vulva does not have an identifiable transformation zone, as in the cervix, squamous neoplasms arise most commonly on the labia minora, clitoris, fourchette, perineal body, or medial aspects of the labia majora—areas in which keratinized stratified

squamous epithelia join with the nonkeratinized squamous mucosa of the vestibule.

Most vulvar squamous carcinomas arise within areas of epithelium involved by some recognized epithelial-cell abnormality. Approximately 60% of cases have adjacent vulvar intraepithelial neoplasia (VIN). In cases of superficially invasive squamous carcinoma of the vulva, the frequency of adjacent VIN approaches 85% (27,34). Lichen sclerosus, usually with associated squamous-cell hyperplasia and/or VIN of differentiated type, can be found adjacent to vulvar squamous-cell carcinoma in 15% to 40% of the cases. Granulomatous disease is also associated with vulvar squamous-cell carcinoma; however, this is not a commonly associated finding in the United States. Thus, vulvar squamous-cell carcinoma precursors can be considered in two distinct groups: those associated with human papillomavirus (VIN) and those that are not (e.g., those associated with lichen sclerosus, chronic granulomatous disease).

Vulvar Carcinomas

Squamous-Cell Carcinoma

The term *microinvasive carcinoma* is not recognized as being meaningful in reference to the vulva because there are no commonly agreed-on pathologic criteria established for this term. The International Society for the Study of Vulvar Disease (ISSVD) proposed a substage of FIGO stage I, stage IA, as a solitary squamous carcinoma of the vulva measuring 2 cm or less in diameter with clinically negative nodes, with depth of invasion 1 mm or less (28). This definition of stage IA vulvar carcinoma has been accepted by FIGO, the American Joint Committee on Cancer (AJCC), and the World Health Organization. The depth of invasion is specifically defined as the measurement from the epithelial stromal junction of the most superficial adjacent dermal papillae to the deepest point of invasion (26,35). Tumor thickness is defined as the measured distance from the overlying surface epithelium, or the bottom of the granular layer if the surface is keratinized, to the deepest point of invasion. These terms are specified by the International Society of Gynecological Pathologists (ISGP), the World Health Organization (37), FIGO (24), and the College of American Pathologists (CAP) (Fig. 20.7).

Stage I squamous carcinomas of the vulva, with a reported depth of invasion or thickness of 5 mm or more, have a lymph node metastasis rate of 15% or higher. Tumors with a depth of invasion or thickness of 3 mm have a lymph node metastasis rate averaging 12%. Therefore, a 3- or 5-mm tumor thickness is not acceptable as one considered to be superficial and of no or little risk of metastasis. Tumors with a depth of invasion of 1 mm or less carry minimal or no risk of lymph node metastasis (26,38).

The Gynecologic Oncology Group (GOG) correlated morphologic features of vulvar carcinoma with tumor inva-

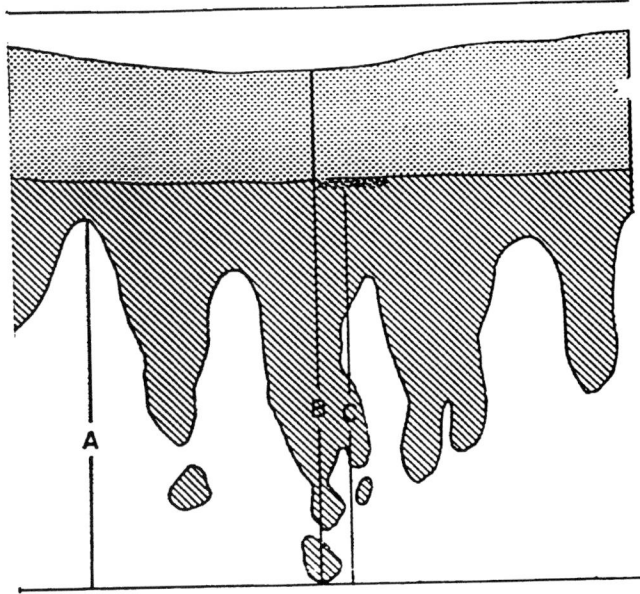

FIG. 20.7. Methods for measurement for vulvar superficially invasive carcinomas. **A:** Depth of invasion: the measurement from the epithelial stromal junction of the most superficial dermal papillae to the deepest point of invasion. This measurement is defined as the depth of invasion and is used to define stage IA vulvar carcinoma. The measurement **(B)** is the thickness of the tumor from the surface of the lesion to the deepest point of invasion. Measurement **(C)** is from the bottom of the granular layer to the deepest point of invasion. This is also defined as thickness of the tumor in cases in which there is a keratinized surface. The International Society of Gynecological Pathologists and the World Health Organization recommend that both the depth of invasion and thickness of tumor, as well as method of measurement, be defined in the pathology reports. (With permission by Edward J. Wilkinson, MD.)

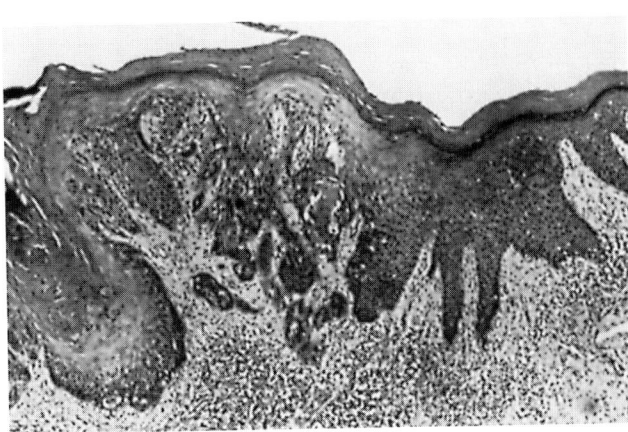

FIG. 20.8. Microinvasive carcinoma of the vulva. The lesion is less than 2 cm across and the depth of invasion is less than 1 mm, measured from the overlying surface epithelium.

sion. Their findings were remarkably similar to those of the ISSVD (39). Because the GOG study did not measure tumor depth by the standards currently defined by FIGO, a reported case with 1-mm invasion with lymph node metastasis cannot be considered as a FIGO stage IA tumor. The ISSVD and CAP have agreed on the definition of depth of invasion and thickness of tumor because considerable variations can exist among measurements from various superficial points in very superficial tumors of approximately 1 mm (Fig. 20.8) (26). There are significant differences between tumor depth of invasion and thickness when superficially invasive tumors are measured; vulvar epithelium can be up to 0.77 mm thick, which can significantly influence the difference between the depth of invasion and the measurement of tumor thickness (40). Tumors with invasion deeper than 1 mm can be readily measured by determining thickness, but tumors with surface ulceration may have a thickness, as measured from the surface, significantly less than the depth of invasion. With large tumors, thickness may be the only reliable measurement because of the lack of identifiable adjacent dermal papillae.

In addition to tumor stage and depth or thickness, other pathologic features include vascular space invasion, growth pattern of the tumor, grade of the tumor, and tumor type. Vascular space involvement can be defined as tumor within an endothelium-lined vascular space. Strict pathologic criteria require that the tumor be attached to the wall of an endothelium-lined vessel, but this is not observed in all cases. Vascular space involvement by squamous-cell carcinoma of the vulva is associated with a higher frequency of lymph node metastasis and a lower overall 5-year survival rate. No reliable methods unambiguously predict lymph node metastasis by quantitation of vascular space involvement by tumor.

Tumor growth pattern influences the rate of lymph node metastasis and survival. Three factors describe the growth pattern: confluent, compact (pushing pattern), and finger-like (or spray or diffuse) growth poorly differentiated. Confluent growth is defined as a tumor mass composed of interconnected tumor exceeding 1 mm in dimension (Fig. 20.9). Tumors with confluent growth, by definition, have a depth of invasion exceeding 1 mm. Confluent growth is characteristic of deeply invasive squamous-cell carcinomas that are associated with stromal desmoplasia, resulting in fibrovascular stromal changes adjacent to the interconnected cords of tumor. Compact (pushing: well differentiated) growth is squamous tumor growth that maintains continuity with the overlying epithelium and infiltrates as a well-defined and circumscribed tumor mass without islands of infiltrating tumor remote from the tumor mass. Tumors with compact growth typically have thickness of 5 mm or less and rarely invade vascular space. They are characteristically well differentiated, with the tumor cells resembling the squamous cells of the adjacent and overlying epithelium. There is usually minimal stromal desmoplasia, although there may be a lymphocytic inflammatory cell infiltrate. Finger-like (spray or diffuse growth: poorly differentiated) growth is characterized by a trabecular appearance with small islands

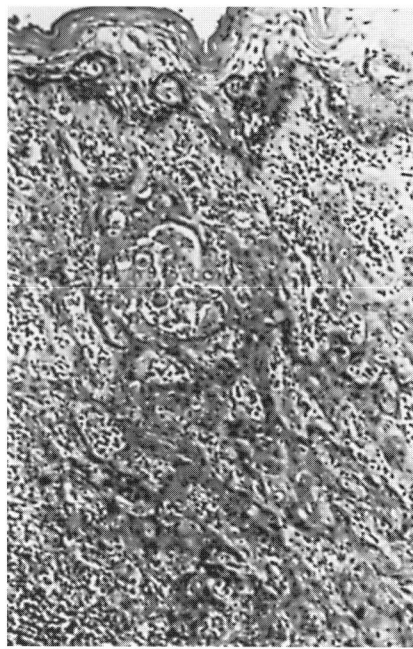

FIG. 20.9. Confluent pattern of invasion. The tumor has a trabecular pattern of growth associated with a marked chronic inflammatory stromal infiltrate. The tumor diameter exceeds 1 cm.

of poorly differentiated tumor cells found within the dermis or submucosa deeper than the bulk of the tumor mass. Tumors with this growth pattern are typically associated with a desmoplastic stromal response (Fig. 20.10) and a lymphocytic inflammatory-cell infiltrate. Vascular space involve-

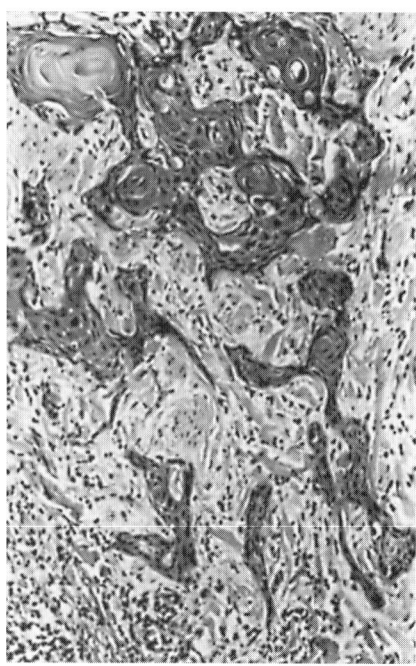

FIG. 20.10. Finger-like growth. The tumor forms small nests surrounded by a desmoplastic stroma.

ment is more commonly seen with this pattern of growth than with tumors with a compact pattern of growth (41). In tumors with a depth of invasion less than 5 mm, the finger-like pattern of growth is associated with a higher frequency of inguinofemoral lymph node metastasis.

In some cases, a single tumor may have both compact and finger-like growth patterns. Mixed patterns, in our experience, are more commonly encountered in frankly invasive vulvar carcinomas and are rarely seen in superficially invasive tumors. The GOG has referred to tumors with a compact pattern of growth as well differentiated and to tumors with the finger-like pattern of growth as poorly differentiated. Using this terminology, the GOG proposed the following grading system for vulvar squamous-cell carcinoma:

- Grade 1 tumors are composed of well-differentiated tumor and contain no poorly differentiated element.
- Grade 2 tumors contain both patterns, with the poorly differentiated portions making up one-third or less of the tumor.
- Grade 3 tumors also contain both components, with the poorly differentiated portion comprising more than one-third but less than one-half of the tumor.
- Grade 4 tumors have one-half or more of the tumor composed of the poorly differentiated elements (42).

The GOG has reported that tumors with grade 1 histology have little risk and that the risk of lymph node metastasis increases with higher grades.

An alternate grading system that has been generally accepted by pathologists is as follows: Grade 1 tumors have no undifferentiated cells, grade 2 tumors have undifferentiated cells but they comprise less than half the tumor, grade 3 tumors have undifferentiated cells comprising half or more of the tumor (43). The American Joint Committee on Cancer (AJCC) has offered the following grading: GX being grade not assessed, G1 being well differentiated, G2 moderately differentiated, G3 partially differentiated, G4 undifferentiated (44).

Tumors with a finger-like pattern of growth (poorly differentiated) lack laminin production compared with those that are well differentiated (45). Vulvar intraepithelial neoplasia also has associated laminin. This suggests that areas of tumor without laminin may be more active areas of tumor proliferation than areas with well-differentiated growth containing laminin. The absence of laminin in a questionable focus of invasion, as demonstrated by immunoperoxidase staining techniques, may support the diagnosis of invasion.

In a study of tumor-cell proliferation using MIB-1 immunohistochemistry, a monoclonal antibody related to the proliferation-related protein KI-67, which is applicable in formation-fixed paraffin-embedded tissue, Hendricks et al. demonstrated that, in well-differentiated tumors, MIB-1 expression was detected in the tumor cells near the dermal tumor interface but not in the tumor cells in the center of tumor foci or near the tumor epithelial surface (46). Poorly differentiated tumors demonstrated MIB-1 expression throughout the tumor-cell population. This difference in pattern of expression in MIB-1 was significantly related to survival and as a predictor of outcome appeared to be somewhat more reliable than tumor growth pattern alone. DNA ploidy analysis (i.e., diploid vs aneuploid) of vulvar carcinoma does not appear to have prognostic significance in regard to survival (47).

The ISGP Committee of Terminology for Non-Neoplastic Epithelial Disorders and Tumors and the CAP recommend that the following information be included in the pathology report of all excised vulvar squamous-cell carcinomas (48):

1. Depth of tumor invasion in millimeters
2. Thickness of the tumor in millimeters
3. Method of measurement of the depth of invasion and thickness
4. Presence or absence of vascular space (lymphatic) involvement by tumor
5. Diameter of the tumor measured from the specimen in the fresh or fixed state
6. Clinical measurement of the tumor diameter in the patient, if available

In a multivariate retrospective analysis of 39 cases of vulvar squamous carcinoma, in addition to clinical stage, and when corrected for treatment modality, pattern of tumor invasion, depth of tumor invasion, and lymph node status were all found to be significant prognostic factors. In addition, dermal desmoplasia associated with tumor invasion also had a suggestive association (47). Desmoplasia (a fibroblastic stromal tumor response) has been correlated with a higher risk of lymph node metastasis and poorer survival (49,50). Findings that did not correlate with survival were squamous-cell carcinoma type, vascular space involvement by tumor, adjacent VIN, tumor nuclear grade, or associated degree of inflammatory response (47).

Vulvar squamous-cell carcinomas of the basaloid and warty types, as well as VIN of all but the differentiated type, are recognized to be associated with human papillomavirus, primarily HPV 16. The HPV can be detected within the tumor cells by a variety of techniques, including polymerase chain reaction (PCR), hybrid capture, and in situ hybridization. A surrogate marker for high-risk HPV infection, p16INK 4, can be detected by employing immunohistochemical methods and is under study in regard to determining in cellular upregulation related to high-risk HPV. Approximately one-quarter (27% ± 9%) of the women with vulvar squamous carcinoma have anti–HPV 16 antibodies expressed serologically as IgG antibodies to HPV 16 virus as measured by enzyme-linked immunosorbent assay (ELISA) (51).

Squamous-cell carcinoma of the vulva, as well as VIN 3, overexpress p53 in approximately one-half of the cases and have evidence of p16 methylation in approximately two-thirds of the cases (52). However, p16 methylation appears to be an early event and a relatively frequent genetic change in vulvar neoplasia, whereas loss of pRb expression appears to be a late event, being identified in invasive squamous carcinoma but not in VIN (52).

Vulvar squamous-cell carcinomas may be of several histopathologic types that are generally classified as follows (53):

- Squamous-cell carcinoma of the usual type
  Keratinizing type
  Nonkeratinizing type
- Basaloid carcinoma (cloacogenic carcinoma)
- Warty (condylomatous) carcinoma
- Acantholytic squamous-cell carcinoma (adenoid squamous-cell carcinoma)
- Giant-cell squamous-cell carcinoma
- Spindle-cell carcinoma (may have sarcomatous-like stroma)
- Lymphoepithelial-like carcinoma
- Verrucous carcinoma
- Basal-cell carcinoma
  Adenoid basal-cell carcinoma
  Metatypical basal-cell carcinoma (basosquamous carcinoma)
  Sebaceous-cell carcinoma

Squamous-cell carcinomas of the keratinizing type have keratin pearls and/or dyskeratotic squamous cells. Squamous carcinomas that are associated with lichen sclerosus are usually of a keratinizing type, and approximately half of those tumors express p53, as does the associated differentiated VIN if present (54). These tumors, when associated with lichen sclerosus, are typically not associated with HPV. Nonkeratinizing squamous-cell carcinomas do not have significant areas of keratinization. These tumors may be associated with VIN and with HPV 16.

Basaloid squamous carcinomas have little differentiation and the tumor cells resemble epithelial basal cells. The tumor grows in cords and forms tumor clusters. The tumor is usually surrounded by a desmoplastic, hyalinized dermis. These tumors are typically associated with basaloid VIN, but may have warty VIN, and usually are associated with HPV 16 (55).

Warty (condylomatous) carcinomas have a keratinized papillomatous surface and usually have prominent intracellular bridges. When the tumor invades the dermis, the cell groups typically have squamous keratin pearls. The tumor cells have markedly atypical nuclei with nuclear pleomorphism, hyperchromasia, and multinucleation. The adjacent epithelium is involved with VIN that may be of warty or less commonly basaloid VIN in about two-thirds of the cases. These tumors are commonly associated with HPV 16 (55).

Acantholytic squamous-cell carcinoma (adenoid squamous-cell carcinoma; pseudoglandular squamous-cell carcinoma) refers to squamous-cell carcinomas with pseudoglandular features. These tumors are characterized by small gland-like spaces within a tumor that otherwise appears to be a poorly differentiated squamous-cell carcinoma. This tumor should be differentiated from adenosquamous carcinomas that contain an obvious adenocarcinoma component (56). Adenoid squamous carcinoma does not contain sialomucin, but adenosquamous carcinoma typically contains mucin within the adenocarcinoma component. Although there are few reported cases of adenoid squamous carcinoma of the vulva, these tumors may have a more aggressive clinical behavior.

Giant-cell squamous-cell carcinoma has multinucleated tumor giant cells intermixed within the squamous carcinoma (57). It may resemble amelanotic melanoma. Squamous-cell carcinoma with tumor giant cells does not contain S100 antigen, melanoma-specific antigen, or HMB-45 on immunoperoxidase staining, as usually present in malignant melanoma. These tumors do express low molecular weight keratin, similar to other squamous carcinomas, which also distinguishes them from melanoma. Electron microscopy is helpful if needed because this tumor has desmosomes and features of squamous carcinoma and lacks melanosomes or melanin, as seen in melanoma.

Spindle-cell squamous-cell carcinomas consist of poorly differentiated neoplastic epithelial cells that have an elongated spindle shape and may mimic a spindle-cell melanoma or a sarcoma (Fig. 20.11) (58). Squamous-cell carcinoma of the vulva may evoke a sarcoma-like stromal response that may be confused with a primary sarcoma (59). Spindle-cell squamous-cell carcinomas can be differentiated from sarcomas by immunoperoxidase techniques. Like other squamous-cell carcinomas, the spindle-cell variant contains keratin and lacks the antigens distinctive to sarcomas of various origin. S100 antigen and melanoma-specific antigen are usually immunoreactive in a spindle-cell melanoma and lacking in a spindle-cell squamous-cell carcinoma.

Lymphoepithelial-like carcinoma is relatively rare and has been observed predominantly in older women. Unlike the nasopharyngeal tumor of similar histologic appearance, in the vulva, this tumor is not related to Epstein-Barr virus, although very few cases have been reported to date (60). The tumor consists of neoplastic squamous cells intermixed with a prominent inflammatory component, consisting prominently of lymphocytes. The squamous cells usually are found in small groups within the inflammatory cell component; however, the neoplastic squamous cells may be isolated as single neoplastic cells surrounded by the intense lymphocytic infiltrate. The differential diagnosis includes unusual inflammatory conditions as well as lymphoma. Immunohistochemical studies demonstrate cytokeratin immunoreactive neoplastic squamous cells. The inflammatory cells are immunoreactive for LCA (CD-45), and both of these immunohistochemical studies may be of value to distinguish the cells present.

Verrucous Carcinoma

Verrucous carcinoma of the vulva typically presents as an exophytic-appearing growth that can be locally destructive. Clinically, it may resemble condyloma acuminatum. The so-called Buschke-Lowenstein giant condyloma is classified as a variant of verrucous carcinoma by the ISGP Committee on Non-Neoplastic Epithelial Disorders and Tumors and by the World Health Organization.

Microscopically, verrucous carcinoma is characterized by well-differentiated epithelial cells. The tumor growth pattern is characterized by a ''pushing'' tumor-dermis interface with minimal stroma between the acanthotic epithelium (Fig. 20.12). The surface is often hyperkeratotic, and there may be parakeratosis. Observed mitoses are characteristically normal. Within the dermis, a mild lymphocytic inflammatory-cell response is usually seen. Vascular space involvement by tumor is characteristically lacking. Because of its excellent prognosis, strict histologic criteria should be used in the diagnosis of verrucous carcinoma. Squamous carcinomas with focal verrucous features should not be described or diagnosed as verrucous carcinoma.

Verrucous carcinomas are characteristically diploid, unlike typical squamous-cell carcinomas of the vulva, which are usually aneuploid by DNA analysis. Verrucous tumors may be associated with HPV type 6 or its variants (61).

The major differential diagnosis of verrucous carcinoma includes keratoacanthomas, pseudocarcinomatous (pseudoepitheliomatous) hyperplasia, epithelioid sarcoma, and malignant rhabdoid tumor.

Basal-Cell Carcinoma and Variants

Basal-cell carcinoma is a relatively rare tumor comprising 2% to 4% of infiltrative neoplasms of the vulva. These tu-

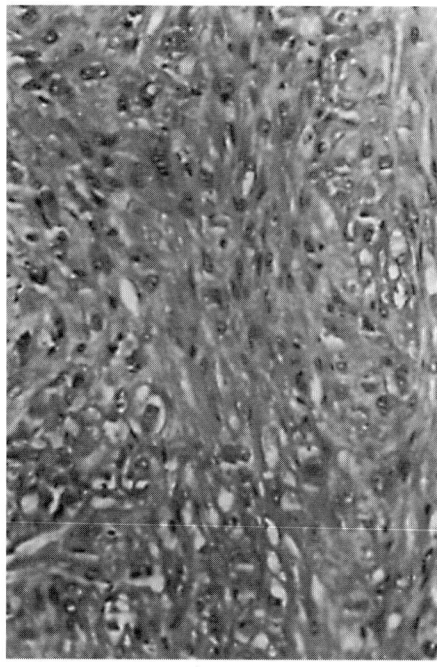

FIG. 20.11. Spindle-cell squamous carcinoma. The tumor cells have a spindle shape and poorly defined cell junctions.

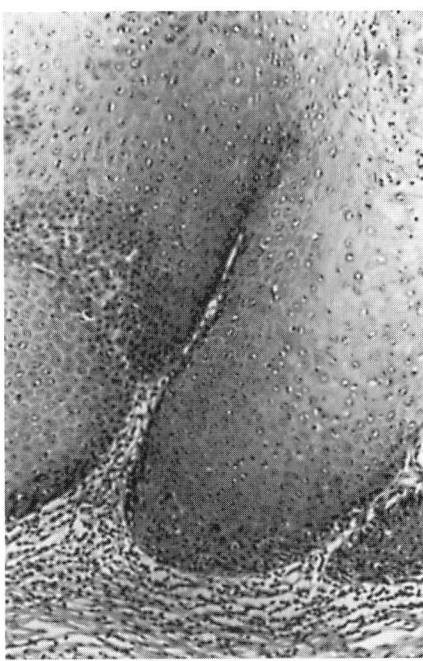

FIG. 20.12. Verrucous carcinoma. The epithelial cells are well differentiated, and the tumor has a "pushing border" with a delicate vascular core between the epithelial elements.

mors are most commonly found in elderly women. The surface of the tumor appears to be granular and is well circumscribed; on palpation, the tumor is characteristically very firm. Vulvar basal-cell carcinoma most commonly arises on the labia majora and is typically 2 cm or less in diameter; however, giant basal-cell carcinomas have been described (62).

The epithelial cells comprising basal-cell carcinoma are typically small and vary in form, with small hyperchromatic nuclei that may exhibit some nuclear pleomorphism. These tumors may have a variety of growth patterns (e.g., trabecular, insular), although peripheral nuclear palisading is a relatively consistent finding.

Metatypical basal-cell carcinoma is a variant of basal-cell carcinoma that usually occurs at mucocutaneous junctions. The term *basosquamous carcinoma* is applied to these tumors because of their microscopic features, which include basal-cell carcinoma intermixed with a squamous-cell carcinoma component. Nuclear pleomorphism is usually seen in metatypical basal-cell carcinoma and in the basal-cell and squamous-cell components of the tumor. The deeper tumor cells, close to the underlying stroma, have the greatest degree of nuclear pleomorphism and the more prominent squamous features. These tumors have a more aggressive clinical behavior than typical basal-cell carcinoma. A variant of vulvar basal-cell carcinoma, *adenoid basal-cell carcinoma,* has gland-like features (63).

The differential diagnosis of basal-cell carcinoma includes poorly differentiated squamous-cell carcinoma, Mer-

kel-cell tumor of the skin, and metastatic small-cell carcinoma. Squamous-cell carcinoma can be distinguished by its lack of characteristic basal-cell carcinoma growth patterns and the presence of intracellular bridges and keratin formations. Nuclear pleomorphism is typically much greater in squamous-cell carcinoma than in basal-cell carcinoma.

Sebaceous carcinoma of the vulva is a basosquamous-cell carcinoma with sebaceous differentiation. These tumors may be associated with VIN (64).

Merkel-Cell Tumors

Merkel-cell tumors are neuroendocrine tumors of the skin that morphologically resemble small-cell carcinomas of neuroendocrine type in other body sites. Merkel-cell tumors have been associated with squamous-cell carcinoma and vulvar intraepithelial neoplasia (65). Merkel-cell tumors are subclassified as carcinoid-like (trabecular), intermediate type, and small-cell (oat-cell) type. They are characteristically within the dermis, are infiltrative, and often involve vascular spaces. These tumors contain neuron-specific enolase and low molecular weight keratin; the keratin stains as a distinct perinuclear cytoplasmic dot. Dense core neurosecretory granules are seen by electron microscopy. These features differentiate Merkel-cell tumors from basal-cell or squamous-cell carcinomas. These tumors frequently have both regional lymph node and distant metastases and are associated with a poor prognosis.

Transitional-Cell Carcinoma

Transitional-cell carcinoma may be a primary tumor of the vulva, usually arising within Bartholin's gland. More commonly, transitional-cell carcinoma is metastatic to the vulva, having arisen within the bladder or urethra (66).

Microscopically, transitional-cell carcinomas are composed of relatively uniform cells; nuclear pleomorphisms may be marked in high-grade urothelial neoplasms. The cytoplasm is eosinophilic without apparent inclusions or keratin formations, although focal keratin formation may be seen. The tumors may exhibit papillary-like growth.

Adenocarcinoma and Carcinoma of Bartholin's Gland

Most primary adenocarcinomas of the vulva arise within Bartholin's gland. Adenocarcinomas may also arise from other glands or skin appendages of the vulva, including sweat glands and Skene's glands (67,68). Clear-cell adenocarcinoma arising in endometriosis has been reported in the groin (69). Invasive vulvar Paget's disease has given rise to adenocarcinoma (Fig. 20.13). Primary malignant tumors arising within Bartholin's gland include adenocarcinoma and squamous-cell carcinoma, which occur with approximately equal frequency and account for approximately 80% of all primary malignant tumors in this site.

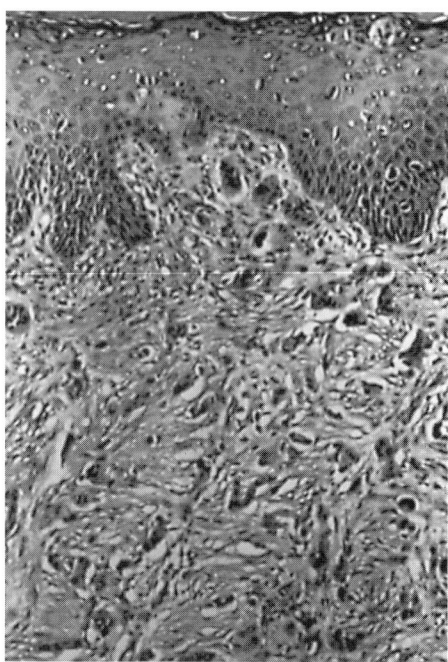

FIG. 20.13. Adenocarcinoma underlying Paget's disease. The adenocarcinoma is composed of small tumor clusters within the underlying dermis.

Adenoid cystic carcinomas comprise approximately 15% of all primary carcinomas, with adenosquamous carcinomas and transitional-cell carcinomas each comprising approximately 5% of the primary Bartholin's gland tumors (70).

Carcinoma of Bartholin's gland generally occurs in older women and is rare in women younger than 50 years of age. In clinical practice, it is generally advisable to biopsy an enlarged Bartholin's gland in a woman 50 years of age or older, especially if there is no known history of a prior Bartholin cyst. If a cyst is drained and a palpable mass persists, excision is indicated. Fine-needle aspiration of a Bartholin mass for cytologic evaluation may help to establish a positive diagnosis.

Primary carcinomas within Bartholin's gland are usually solid tumors and are often deeply infiltrative. A variety of histologic types of adenocarcinoma have been described within Bartholin's gland. Mucinous, papillary, and muco-epidermal tumor types have been described in addition to adenosquamous, squamous, and transitional-cell carcinoma. Adenocarcinoma of Bartholin's gland is typically immuno-reactive for carcinoembryonic antigen (CEA) (71). Histopathologic features that identify a carcinoma arising in Bartholin's gland include (a) recognizable transition from Bartholin's gland to tumor, (b) histologic tumor type must be consistent with origin from Bartholin's gland, and (c) the tumor must not be metastatic to Bartholin's gland.

These malignancies are characteristically deep and difficult to detect in their early growth. Approximately 20% of women with primary carcinoma of Bartholin's gland have metastatic tumor to the inguinofemoral lymph nodes at the time of primary tumor diagnosis.

Adenocarcinoma Arising in Skin Appendages Including Tumors of Sweat-Gland Origin

The labia majora were once thought to be within the milk line, but evidence supports that this is not the case (72,73). In humans, the milk line does not involve the vulva. The breast-like tumors found arise from specialized anogenital glands that reside in the intralabial sulci and are also thought to be the origin of papillary hidradenoma. Both benign and malignant breast-like tumors have been observed within the vulva (74). Fibroadenoma, intraductal papilloma, and lactating adenoma have been observed. Primary adenocarcinoma of the vulva may arise in specialized anogenital glands, which reside in the intralabial sulcus. These glands are believed to be the origin of papillary hidradenoma of the vulva, and may resemble breast tissue (43,72,73).

A variety of other skin appendage tumors have been reported in the vulva; however, the majority of these are benign tumors. Primary carcinomas of sweat gland origin are relatively rare within the vulva, comprising approximately 10% of all vulvar malignant tumors. A variety of sweat gland carcinomas have been described in this site, including eccrine adenocarcinoma, eccrine porocarcinoma, and clear-cell hidradenocarcinoma (68). Primary adenocarcinomas of apocrine gland origin have also been described arising within the vulva, and some of these have been associated with vulvar Paget's disease. These should be distinguished from the benign papillary hidradenoma, which typically arises in the intralabial papillary sulcus from specialized anogenital glands and contains a myoepithelial-cell population, distinguishing it from adenocarcinoma (43,72,73).

A mucinous enteric-like adenocarcinoma, resembling anorectal mucinous adenocarcinoma, has also been observed in the vulvar vestibule. These tumors usually also involve the distal vagina (75,76).

Adenosquamous Carcinoma

Adenosquamous carcinomas are epithelial tumors composed of both malignant squamous and gland-forming elements. Adenosquamous carcinomas account for approximately 5% of all tumors of Bartholin's gland. These tumors may be composed of a poorly differentiated squamous component mixed with cells bearing small glandular lumens containing mucin (27).

Adenoid Cystic Carcinoma

Adenoid cystic carcinoma arising within the vulva most commonly arises within Bartholin's gland and comprises approximately 15% of all carcinomas of Bartholin's gland. Microscopically, adenoid cystic carcinomas are composed of relatively uniform small cells with regular, round nuclei and minimal cytoplasm. The cord-like or "nested" arrangement contains gland-like lumens that include an acellular eosinophilic material (70). Electron microscopy has documented that this material is basement membrane–like material rather than a secretion. These tumors are therefore more properly considered to be a variant of squamous-cell carcinoma than adenocarcinoma.

Vulvar Paget's Disease

Vulvar Paget's disease is now recognized to be a heterogeneous group of intraepithelial neoplastic processes that have a similar clinical presentation, typically presenting as an eczematoid, red, weeping area on the vulva, often localized to the labia majora, perineal body, clitoral area, or other sites. In the vulva, Paget's disease typically occurs in older, postmenopausal white women, although it has also been described in a premenopausal woman. Because of its eczematoid appearance, it is not unusual for vulvar Paget's disease to be misdiagnosed as eczema or contact dermatitis. Wilkinson and Brown have recently proposed a classification of genital Paget's disease that divides this entity into two subsets: Paget's disease of cutaneous origin and Paget's disease of non-cutaneous origin (Table 20.4) (77).

Clinical Features

Vulvar Paget's disease is usually localized, but it can be extensive, involving most of the vulva as well as the perianal areas and the vaginal mucosa. In rare cases, it may involve the medial upper thighs and buttocks. Differences in clinical presentation may be identified that can assist in distinguishing cutaneous from noncutaneous Paget disease. Primary

TABLE 20.4. *Genital Paget's disease: histologic classification*

Primary cutaneous Paget's disease:
  Intraepithelial cutaneous Paget's disease
  Intraepithelial cutaneous Paget's disease with associated invasion
  Paget's disease of underlying adenocarcinoma of skin appendage or vulval glandular origin
Paget's disease of noncutaneous origin:
  Paget's disease secondary to anorectal adenocarcinoma
  Paget's disease secondary to urothelial neoplasia [pagetoid intraepithelial neoplasia (PUIN)]
      PUIN of intraepithelial urothelial neoplasia origin
      PUIN as a manifestation of urothelial carcinoma
  Paget's disease as a manifestation of other noncutaneous carcinoma (e.g., endocervical adenocarcinoma, endometrial adenocarcinoma, ovarian carcinoma)

Reprinted with permission from Wilkinson EJ, Brown HM. Vulvar Paget's disease of urothelial origin: a report of three cases and a proposed classification of vulvar Paget's disease. *Hum Pathol* 2002;33:549.

early cutaneous vulvar Paget's disease usually involves the labium majus. In more advanced cases, the lesion may extend onto the vulvar vestibule or involve the perianal skin by continuity. Paget's disease of urothelial origin (PUIN) primarily involves the periurethral area and may extend to the vulvar vestibule or vagina; it involves vulvar skin only in advanced cases. Primary anorectal Paget's disease primarily involves the perianal area in early cases.

Paget's disease of all types accounts for approximately 2% or less of all vulvar tumors. Intraepithelial Paget's disease of cutaneous origin is the most common. Intraepithelial cutaneous Paget's disease is found to have associated invasion of the Paget's cells in approximately 10% to 20% of cases. Cutaneous Paget's disease associated with underlying adenocarcinoma of skin appendages or vulvar glandular origin, such as Bartholin's gland adenocarcinoma, is relatively rare.

Perianal Paget's disease has a recognized association with anorectal adenocarcinoma. Paget's disease presenting as a manifestation of associated bladder or urethral transitional-cell carcinoma is well documented but is uncommon (77, 78). In these cases, the intraepithelial neoplasia cells are neoplastic transitional epithelial cells that have extended to the vulvar mucosa or skin without invading the underlying vulvar dermis. The term *pagetoid urothelial intraepithelial neoplasia* (PUIN) has been proposed by Wilkinson (77). This PUIN has also has been referred to as "pseudo-Paget's disease" (79) or pagetoid transitional-cell neoplasia (77). In such cases, total vulvectomy is not indicated because there is no associated underlying adenocarcinoma. The tumor cells are from the bladder and/or urethra, representing an intraepithelial transitional-cell neoplasm.

Microscopic Features

Typical Paget's disease is characterized by the presence of Paget's cells, which are found within the involved epithelium. A Paget's cell is relatively large with a prominent nucleus that typically has coarse chromatin and a prominent nucleolus. On hematoxylin and eosin staining, the cytoplasm is distinctly pale compared with the surrounding keratinocytes. The cytoplasm may be vacuolated or appear foamy and typically is somewhat basophilic. The Paget's cells are generally found in higher concentration near the basement membrane, but are also seen throughout the epithelium. These cells may be clustered together and may have an acinar or gland-like arrangement (Fig. 20.14).

Paget's disease of cutaneous, urothelial, or anorectal origin can be distinguished by immunohistochemical studies. Paget's cells of cutaneous origin and anorectal origin are rich in CEA (77). Paget's cells of cutaneous origin also express cytokeratin 7 (CK-7) and gross cystic disease fluid protein (GCDFP) (80). More than one-half of the cases may also express c-erB2 (HER-2/*neu*), but this was not found to influence metastasis risk (81,82). Paget's cells infrequently express CA-125, and estrogen receptor is generally negative

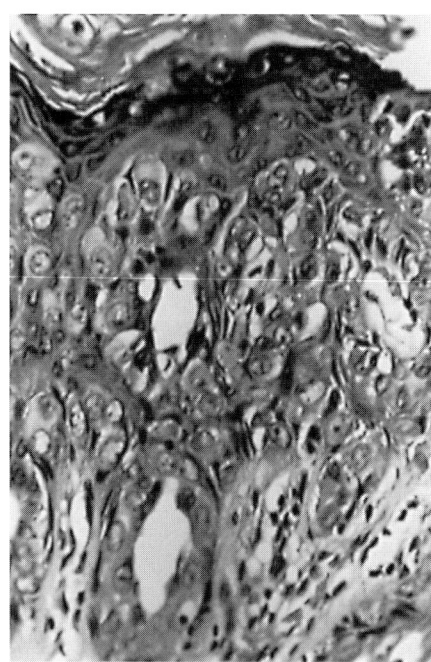

FIG. 20.14. Paget's disease. The large cells with prominent cytoplasm and large nuclei represent the intraepithelial Paget's cells. A few small gland-like intraepithelial structures are formed by the Paget's cells.

(82,83). Paget cells of anorectal origin typically do not express CK-7 or GCDFP, but do express CK-20, which is typically not expressed in cutaneous Paget's disease (77). Paget's disease of urothelial origin does not express CEA or GCDFP, may express CK-7 and/or CK-20, but does express Uroplakin III (77,84).

In some cases, Paget's disease may be associated with a distinctive squamous hyperplasia, or papillomatous hyperplasia, which must be distinguished from VIN. Immunohistochemical study for CK-7 is useful in many cases to identify the Paget's cells that are strongly CK-7 positive, whereas the adjacent normal or hyperplastic epithelial cells are negative (85). Paget's cells may be aneuploid or diploid by DNA ploidy analysis; however, prognosis does not appear to be influenced by DNA ploidy. Invasive Paget's disease with depth of invasion ≤1 mm has reportedly little risk for recurrence (82).

In addition to distinguishing the type of Paget's disease identified (i.e., cutaneous, anorectal, urothelial, or of other noncutaneous origin), the pathologist must distinguish other intraepithelial neoplastic processes that may have a similar microscopic appearance. Superficial spreading malignant melanoma, pagetoid vulvar intraepithelial neoplasia, pagetoid reticulosis, and clear-cell papulosis are the more common neoplasms that microscopically may resemble Paget's disease. These can be differentiated by immunoperoxidase techniques because melanomas do not express cy-

tokeratins, as seen in Paget's disease; they do, however, express S100 protein, HMB-45, and melan-A, which are absent in Paget's cells (86). Pagetoid VIN may microscopically resemble Paget's disease, but the cells of VIN do not express CEA, S100, or melan-A (77, 87). Pagetoid reticulosis, a cutaneous lymphoproliferative neoplastic process, is characterized by intraepithelial cells that express leukocyte common antigen, among other lymphoproliferative markers, but lack CEA or cytokeratins. Clear-cell papulosis is a localized proliferation of Toker's cells that are cutaneous Paget-like cells. Clear-cell papulosis is a rare condition that usually involves the skin of the lower abdomen and occurs most commonly in children, but has been described in the lower genital tract of men (88). Toker's cells, unlike Paget's cells, are typically tadpole shaped or caudate. They do, however, have immunohistochemical findings similar to cutaneous Paget's cells.

Vulvar Malignant Melanoma

Malignant melanoma of the vulva accounts for less than 10% of all primary malignant neoplasms on the vulva. This tumor occurs predominantly in white women, with approximately one-third of the cases occurring in women younger than 50 years of age and the peak frequency between the sixth and seventh decades. The tumor may arise from preexisting pigmented lesions or from normal-appearing skin. The tumor may be elevated or nodular, and although usually pigmented, amelanotic melanoma may resemble squamous carcinoma. In the clinical setting, the differential diagnosis includes atypical or large vulvar nevi and melanosis of the vulva (43,89).

Vulvar malignant melanomas may be subclassified into three specific categories: superficial spreading malignant melanoma, nodular melanoma, and acral lentiginous melanoma (90,91). Superficial spreading melanoma and nodular melanomas are most often reported (90,92). Histopathologic differentiation of these two types is based on identification of a superficial spreading component. Superficial spreading melanomas have radial growth involving four or more retia lateral to their vertical or infiltrative growth (43). Nodular melanomas show minimal or no radial growth. Superficial spreading malignant melanoma characteristically shows junctional melanocytes with radial growth, and a vertical growth pattern may be absent. The tumor cells are highly variable but are most commonly relatively large with nuclei showing minimal variation in size and containing prominent nucleoli (Fig. 20.15). These cells may or may not contain pigment. The form of the cells ranges from epithelioid to spindle shaped; in some cases, the spindle-cell type may predominate. The spindle cells may be relatively small with oval nuclei and elongated cytoplasm. They may infiltrate the adjacent dermis in cords and sheets.

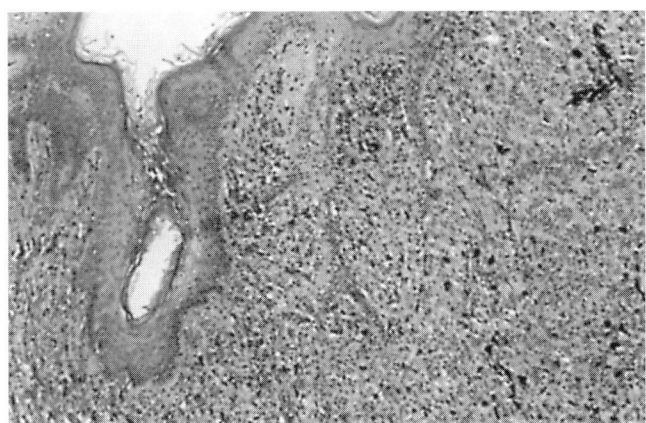

FIG. 20.15. Malignant melanoma. The tumor is within the dermis and contains dark melanin pigment. Junctional growth is seen within the overlying epithelial dermal junction.

Malignant melanoma typically contains S100 antigen, HMB-45, and melan-A and lacks CEA and cytokeratin. The microscopic differential diagnosis for superficial spreading malignant melanoma is primarily vulvar Paget's disease. Immunohistochemical techniques are essential in discriminating superficial spreading melanoma from Paget's disease (43,86). Nonpigmented nodular melanomas may mimic squamous-cell carcinoma or spindle-cell neoplasms of various types. In these circumstances, immunoperoxidase procedures are of great value because squamous-cell carcinomas do not contain the S100 protein or melan-A found in melanomas, and melanomas do not express cytokeratin (43).

The level of invasion and tumor thickness are essential measurements in evaluating malignant melanoma (92). The Clark level definitions were modified by Chung and colleagues (93). Measurements for vulvar melanomas can be applied as for skin, as described by Breslow (94), but within the vulvar vestibule and perineal area there is neither a keratin nor a granular layer, and modifications of this system must be used (93). Malignant melanomas that have a thickness of less than 0.75 mm have little or no risk for metastasis. Melanomas at Clark level 2 or thickness of 1.49 mm, or tumor volume of 100 mm^3, also correlate with good prognosis (95). A poor prognosis is correlated with Clark level 5, thickness >2 mm, or mitotic count exceeding 10/mm^2. Other microscopic prognostic factors include a minimal or absent inflammatory reaction and surface ulceration (92).

Vulvar melanoma has been described with associated with N-ras codon 12 mutations, as commonly seen in sun exposure–related melanomas; however, most mucosal melanomas not associated with sun exposure do not express N-ras exon 2 mutations (96).

Melanomas arising in the vulva may metastasize to other sites within the lower female genital tract, including the cervix, vagina, urethra, and rectum. Distant metastasis is common, particularly in the setting of recurrent melanoma.

Long-term survival is poor, approximately 5%, for patients with distant metastasis (91).

Vulvar Sarcomas

Leiomyosarcoma

Leiomyosarcoma is the most common primary vulvar sarcoma. It most commonly arises in the labia majora or Bartholin's gland area, although these tumors may arise in the clitoris and labia minora. The tumors are generally 5 cm in diameter or larger when first diagnosed and may be deep within the subcutaneous tissue. On microscopic examination, leiomyosarcomas are composed of interlacing spindle-shaped cells, sometimes with an epithelioid appearance. Microscopic criteria of leiomyosarcomas include infiltrating margins, moderate to severe nuclear atypia, and a mitotic figure count of five mitoses per 10 high-power fields or higher. A diagnosis of leiomyosarcoma may be made if three of the above four criteria are present, or if metastasis is present. Tumors that have only one or two of the above criteria, without metastasis or overt infiltration, can be classified as atypical leiomyomas, or smooth-muscle tumors of uncertain malignant potential; the risk of recurrence for these tumors is uncertain but significantly less that for those classified as leiomyosarcoma (97–99).

Malignant Fibrous Histiocytoma

Malignant fibrous histiocytoma arises from histiocytes with fibroblastic differentiation. It is considered the second most common sarcoma of the vulva and has its peak frequency in middle age. Malignant fibrous histiocytoma typically presents as a solitary mass that may appear somewhat brownish or pigmented, secondary to areas of focal hemorrhage within the tumor. On microscopic examination, the tumor is characterized by a complex interlacing cellular growth pattern with marked nuclear pleomorphism, including multinucleated cells and large bizarre cells. Abnormal mitotic figures may be apparent. Microscopic variants of this tumor include inflammatory, giant-cell, myxoid, and angiomatoid types (43,100). On immunoperoxidase study, these tumors contain α_1-antitrypsin and α_1-antichymotrypsin. Malignant fibrous histiocytoma typically has infiltrative margins and may involve the underlying fascia. Involvement of the fascia is associated with a higher risk of local spread and distant metastasis.

Epithelioid Sarcoma

Epithelioid sarcoma may arise within the labia majora, subclitoral area, and clitoris (101). Its microscopic features may resemble squamous carcinoma. Epithelioid sarcoma is usually relatively superficial, arising in and involving the reticular dermis, but may occur in deeper structures. On microscopic examination, the tumor is nodular and may have areas of necrosis. The tumor cells have an epithelioid appearance with eosinophilic cytoplasm, but there may be metaplastic components, including cartilage and bone. On immunohistochemical study, this tumor contains cytokeratin, which does not distinguish it from epithelial tumors, but is of value in differentiating it from other types of soft tissue tumors. Epithelioid sarcoma rarely metastasizes, although local recurrence is a risk. Differential diagnosis for this tumor includes squamous-cell carcinoma and malignant rhabdoid tumor, both of which are capable of distant metastasis and aggressive behavior (101). Immunoperoxidase studies have not been of value in differentiating epithelioid sarcoma from malignant rhabdoid tumor. The distinction is based primarily on microscopic features.

Malignant Rhabdoid Tumor

Malignant rhabdoid tumor has been described in the vulva and, like epithelioid sarcoma, may be relatively superficial and contain tumor cells with an epithelioid appearance with eosinophilic cytoplasm. Unlike epithelioid sarcoma, malignant rhabdoid tumors have relatively pleomorphic nuclei. Metaplastic elements are usually not present. Malignant rhabdoid tumor also has eosinophilic cytoplasmic inclusions, which are not present in epithelioid sarcoma. These inclusions give some of the cells the appearance of signet-ring cells. Electron microscopic evaluation of the rhabdoid tumor reveals that the eosinophilic inclusions are composed of intermediate filaments. Malignant rhabdoid tumor has a lobulated architecture but lacks necrosis or granulomatous features, which are often found in epithelioid sarcoma (101).

Other Sarcomas

Other rare primary sarcomas of the vulva include angiosarcoma, Kaposi's sarcoma, hemangiopericytoma, rhabdomyosarcoma, alveolar soft-part sarcoma, and liposarcoma (45,102). Sarcoma botryoides is a variant of rhabdomyosarcoma that may involve the vulva, but most cases arise within the vagina or base of bladder. Aggressive angiomyxoma, a locally aggressive but rarely metastatic sarcoma, has also been documented arising within the vulva (42). Kaposi's sarcoma and angiosarcoma should be differentiated from bacillary angiomatosis, which is a benign pseudoneoplastic infectious process (103).

Other Vulvar Malignancies

Malignant Schwannoma

Malignant schwannoma has been reported in the vulva, and approximately half of the cases are associated with neu-rofibromatosis. Most malignant schwannomas occur in women of reproductive age (104). This tumor is found primarily in the labia majora or minora, but may arise in other sites within the vulva. On microscopic examination, it is typically highly cellular and is composed of spindle cells with nuclear palisading. Metaplastic elements, such as cartilage, epithelial islands, and striated muscle, may be seen in approximately 50% of the cases. Malignant schwannoma is immunoreactive for S100 protein. In some cases, a nerve trunk can be identified adjacent to or within the tumor mass.

Yolk Sac Tumor

Yolk sac tumor (endodermal sinus tumor) is a rare germ cell tumor of the vulva, primarily arising in the labial or clitoral areas (105). The age range of patients is from just under 2 to 26 years. Distinctive microscopic features are similar to endodermal sinus tumor in the ovary, including the presence of Schiller-Duval bodies, distinctive globules that are periodic acid–Schiff (PAS) positive, and the presence of α-fetoprotein within the tumor, as demonstrated by immunoperoxidase technique.

Tumors Metastatic to the Vulva

Most tumors metastatic to the vulva occur in postmenopausal women, and in the majority of cases are also associated with tumor metastatic to additional sites. Metastasis commonly involves the labia majora, althought the labia minora, clitoris, introitus, and mons pubis may also be the first site identified. The clinical presentation is usually a nodule or mass. In some cases, the metastatic lesion may present as a Bartholin's gland mass (70). Vulvar pain, or an ulcer, may also herald a metastasis (106). Tumors metastatic to the vulva arise in the genital tract in approximately one-half of the cases. Primary sites include the cervix, vagina, endometrium, and ovary. Cervical carcinoma is the most common origin of metastasis. Metastasis from nongenital sites accounted for 44% of the secondary vulvar malignancies in a large series of 66 cases (106). Tumors arising in breast, rectum, colon, anus, bladder, pancreas, and lung were the predominant epithelial tumors, with melanoma and lymphoma being the predominant nonepithelial tumors. In 6 of the 66 reported cases, the primary tumor site could not be determined (106). Renal and gastric carcinomas, as well as neuroblastoma, may also metastatize to the vulva. Gestational choriocarcinoma can also involve the vulva. Tumors from the rectum, cervix, vagina, or urethra may also involve the vulva by contiguous growth (107). Contiguous involvement is commonly associated with metastasis to regional lymph nodes and widespread metastases.

PROGNOSTIC FACTORS

Prognosis has been most extensively evaluated in women with squamous-cell carcinomas. The major prognostic factors in vulvar cancer—tumor diameter, depth of tumor invasion, nodal spread, and distant metastasis—have been incorporated into the current FIGO staging system. These are clearly the most important predictors of tumor recurrence and death from disease (108–113). However, several additional features may be useful in refining the prognosis in smaller subsets of patients.

Wharton and colleagues suggested the concept of "microinvasive" carcinoma of the vulva in their 1975 report and proposed eliminating groin dissection for patients with small tumors that invaded <5 mm (68). A number of later reports confirmed that 10% to 20% of patients meeting these criteria had occult groin metastases, making the elimination of inguinal lymph node evaluation undesirable for these patients (114–117). Several investigators have further attempted to define a population of microinvasive tumors whereby the risk of inguinal metastasis is negligible (39,118–122). The consensus opinion is that only tumors with <1 mm invasion fulfill this requirement (17,39,59,123). This is reflected in the FIGO classification of tumors invading ≤1 mm into stage IA (24).

Risk of local recurrence, although clearly associated with tumor size and extent, is also related to the adequacy of the surgical resection margins. Heaps and co-workers, in their analysis of formalin-fixed tissue specimens, were able to demonstrate a sharp rise in the incidence of local recurrence for tumors with microscopic margins less than 8 mm (124). They suggested that this would correspond to a minimum margin of 1 cm in fresh, unfixed tissue.

The single most important prognostic factor in women with vulvar cancer is metastasis to the inguinal lymph nodes. The presence of inguinal node metastasis portends a 50% reduction in long-term survival (125,126). Because the clinical prediction of lymph node spread is inaccurate, node status is now determined via surgical biopsy. Prognostic issues that appear to be important in evaluating lymphatic involvement are (a) whether nodal spread is bilateral or unilateral, (b) the number of positive nodes, (c) the volume of tumor in the metastasis, and (d) the level of the metastatic disease. Multiple positive nodes, bilateral metastases, involvement beyond the groin, and bulky disease are associated with poor prognosis (38,127). Rutledge and colleagues have provided a detailed analysis of prognostic factors, including tumor size; tumor grade; FIGO stage; therapy aim (curative vs palliative); nodal status (groin, pelvic, Cloquet's); margin status (deep surgical, vaginal, lateral); patient age; site of lesion (clitoris or mons vs. labia); gross tumor appearance (ulcerative vs nonulcerative); clinical stage of tumor, nodes, metastasis; and patient medical status (128).

TREATMENT

Development of the radical vulvectomy with bilateral inguinofemoral lymphadenectomy during the 1940s and 1950s was a dramatic improvement over prior surgical options and greatly enhanced survival, particularly for women with smaller tumors and negative lymph nodes (129,130). The ability to resect vulvar tumors successfully eliminated prolonged survival marked by local and regional progression of disease and associated pain, drainage, and bleeding. Long-term survival of 85% to 90% can now be routinely obtained with radical surgery. However, radical surgery can be associated with postoperative complications such as wound breakdown and lymphedema.

More recently, surgical emphasis has evolved to an individualized approach for tumors at either end of the spectrum. Many gynecologists believe that smaller vulvar tumors can be acceptably managed by less-radical surgical approaches, and have proposed more limited resections for certain subsets considered to represent early or low-risk disease (59, 131,132). The obvious advantages of such an approach are retention of a significant portion of the uninvolved vulva, less operative morbidity, and fewer late complications. In contrast, radical surgery is frequently ineffective in curing patients with bulky tumors or positive groin nodes. Multimodality programs that incorporate radiation, surgery, and chemotherapy are now being investigated in women with these high-risk tumors based upon success with similar approaches in women with squamous cancers of the cervix (133–136). It seems fair to state that "quality" issues predominate at the lower end of the disease scale, whereas "survival" concerns are most important at the upper end. At present, there are limited curative treatment options for women who present with disseminated disease.

Microinvasive Tumors

Tumors demonstrating early invasion of the vulvar stroma (≤1 mm) have minimal risk for lymphatic dissemination. Excisional procedures that incorporate a 1-cm normal tissue margin are likely to provide curative results (137). Patients in this category represent the only subset for whom the status of the groin lymph nodes can be ignored. These so-called microcarcinomas tend to arise in younger patients with multifocal preinvasive disease and are commonly associated with HPV infections. Occult invasion in lesions thought to be intraepithelial is common (138,139). Consequently, the entire lower genital tract and vulva should be carefully evaluated before surgical resection of these lesions is attempted. The risk of vulvar recurrence or development of a new lesion at another vulvar site is significant. After primary therapy these patients should undergo frequent follow-up examinations.

Stage I and II Cancers

Traditional management of stage I and II vulvar cancer has been radical vulvectomy with bilateral inguinofemoral lymphadenectomy. The operation removes the primary tumor with a wide margin of normal skin, along with the remaining vulva, dermal lymphatics, and regional nodes. This approach provides excellent long-term survival and local control in approximately 90% of patients (140,141). Disadvantages of radical surgery include loss of normal vulvar tissue with alterations in appearance and sexual function, a 50% incidence of wound breakdown, a 30% incidence of groin complications (breakdown, lymphocyst, lymphangitis), and a 10% to 15% incidence of lower extremity lymphedema (142,143). Additional postoperative therapy, primarily irradiation, should be considered in the 10% to 20% of patients with positive nodes with the understanding that this will further increase the incidence of lymphedema (144).

In an effort to reduce morbidity and enhance psychosexual recovery, several groups have espoused a more limited surgical approach for women with small vulvar cancers (145, 146). Although some patients with T2 lesions have been treated in this manner, most have limited the conservative approach to women with T1 cancers. DiSaia and colleagues were the first to describe successful conservative resection of tumors measuring 1 cm or less with invasion of <5 mm (132). Additional reports have expanded this experience to include more patients with larger lesions and more significant invasion (Table 20.5) (59,147,148). The most common recommendation is to resect the primary lesion with a 1- to 2-cm margin of normal tissue and to carry the dissection to the deep perineal fascia. These operations should not be confused with the concept of excisional biopsy, which is used primarily as a diagnostic procedure.

Limited resection of the primary tumor is combined with a more conservative surgical approach to the groin, in which the ipsilateral superficial groin nodes are used as the sentinel group for lymphatic metastases (132,148,149). Bilateral superficial dissections are performed in patients whose tumors encroach on midline structures (clitoris or perineal body) (147). In patients with negative inguinal nodes, no further dissection or postoperative therapy is used. Patients with positive nodes can undergo additional nodal dissection of the deep nodes and the contralateral groin, or be treated with postoperative irradiation, or both. The risk of chronic groin complications and lymphedema is related to the extent of groin dissection (131). Patients with superficial and deep

lymphadenectomy followed by irradiation have the greatest likelihood of morbidity.

With limited resection, survival of 90% or better is attainable for patients with stage I vulvar carcinoma—with acceptable anatomic appearance and function. Critics of conservative surgical approaches cite several potential risks, including potential recurrence in retained vulvar skin, inadequate assessment of the groin nodes, inadequate surgical therapy in women with nodal spread, and the potential for leaving intransit skin metastases. Examination of the published experience using a selective approach to inguinal lymphadenectomy would suggest that unanticipated ipsilateral groin failure occurs in 3% to 5% of cases (Table 20.6), whereas contralateral groin failure is uncommon. Because randomized prospective evaluations of surgical therapy have not been performed, a critical comparison of radical vulvectomy and radical wide excision is not possible.

In an attempt to reduce treatment-related morbidity, yet retain the essential components of radical excision of the primary tumor plus groin lymph node assessment, some have introduced modifications of the classic radical operation. These include the use of "triple incision" techniques that separate the vulvectomy incision from the groin incisions, as well as those techniques that use a more limited dissection of the deep inguinal nodes (150). Others have recently begun to evaluate the potential for cutaneous lymphatic mapping to define and target the true sentinel groin nodes (151). Preliminary experience with both intraoperative lymphatic dye and radioisotope injections suggests that a sentinel node can often be identified in the groin (32,152,153). This early experience supports the concept that the assessment of lymphatic metastases can ultimately be reduced to the biopsy of one or two identifiable nodes (Fig. 20.16).

The concept of a "sentinel lymph node" was first introduced by Cabanas. Using lymphangiography for the clinical evaluation of penile carcinoma, he suggested that the sentinel lymph node was the first lymph node in the lymphatic pathway and the main site of metastasis (154). DiSaia and colleagues described the eight to ten superficial lymph nodes above the cribriform fascia as being "sentinel nodes." When these lymph nodes proved to be negative, the risk for metastasis to the deep inguinal or pelvic lymph nodes was negligible (132). In 1992, Morton et al. introduced the use of vital blue dye (isosulfan blue) to identify lymphatic drainage from malignant melanoma (155). Levenback utilized this intraoperative blue dye–staining technique for sentinel lymph node

TABLE 20.5. *Proposed criteria for conservative surgical resection*

Investigator (ref.)	Tumor diameter (cm)	Depth of invasion (mm)	Groin dissection
Wharton et al. (68)	<2	<5	None
DiSaia et al. (132)	<1	<5	Superficial
Berman et al. (59)	<2	<5	Superficial
Burke et al. (131)	Resectable	Any	Superficial
Stehman et al. (19)	<2	<5	Superficial

TABLE 20.6. *Unanticipated groin failure in patients with negative superficial lymphadenectomy*

Investigator (ref.)	No. of patients	%
Burke et al. (147)	4/76	5.2
Berman et al. (59)	0/50	0
Stehman et al. (148)	6/121	5.0
Total	10/247	4.1

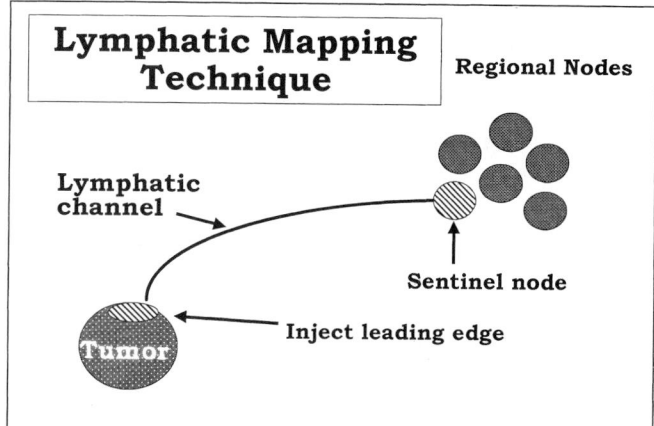

FIG. 20.16. Intraoperative lymphatic mapping is accomplished by injecting the leading edge of the visible tumor with isosulfan blue dye. The dye is taken up by the specific node that drains the tumor site. This "sentinel" node can be visually identified and separated from other nodes within the regional group. In concept, all tumors with nodal metastases can be detected by biopsy of the sentinel node.

identification in vulvar squamous-cell carcinoma (Fig. 20.17) (151). Further work has demonstrated that blue dye staining alone has relatively low sensitivity in identifying the sentinel lymph node, particularly among patients with midline primary tumors. Lymphoscintigraphy using radioactive technetium 99m administered shortly before surgery, combined with the intraoperative use of a hand-held gamma

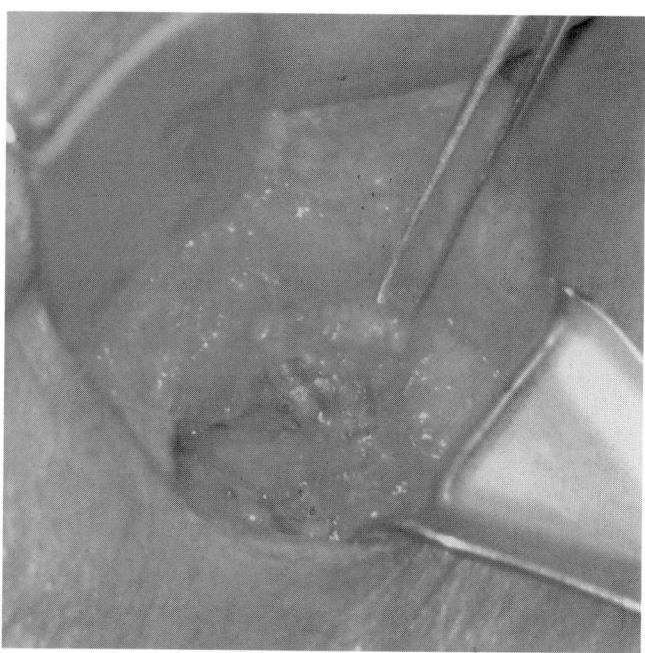

FIG. 20.17. Following isosulfan blue dye injection, sentinel lymph node biopsy is performed. In this case, the sentinel lymph node is easily identified by the visible presence of dye. (Photo courtesy of Charles Levenback, MD, Houston, TX).

probe, has significantly improved the sensitivity of sentinel lymph node identification (156).

Several studies have suggested that sentinel lymph node biopsy is a highly accurate procedure with a negative predictive value approaching 100% (157–160). In the largest series published to date, de Hullu and colleagues performed sentinel lymph node identification and biopsy in 59 women with primary vulvar carcinoma using the combination of intraoperative isosulfan blue dye staining plus preoperative lymphoscintigraphy (161). Only 60% of sentinel lymph nodes were visible with blue staining alone. With the addition of the hand-held gamma probe, sentinel lymph nodes were identified in 89% of groins dissected. Lymph node metastases were present in 27 groins, and all were detected using sentinel lymph node identification and biopsy. The negative predictive value of a negative sentinel lymph node was 100%. Although promising, these results await confirmation by a prospective randomized controlled trial before sentinel lymph node identification and biopsy may be considered to be part of the standard of surgical care for vulvar carcinoma.

In summary, therapy for women with stage I and II cancers must be individualized to the patient and her tumor. Radical vulvectomy provides excellent local control and long-term survival, but has significant morbidity and sexual function limitations. More conservative approaches appear to be safe in most stage I settings and may be applicable in some stage II patients. The surgical approach to the groin nodes is evolving. The accuracy of the superficial inguinal nodes (or the "sentinel" node identified by intraoperative mapping) as predictors of nodal spread is currently being evaluated. If these concepts prove to be suitably sensitive and specific, more extensive inguinal lymphadenectomy might be abandoned.

Stage III and IV Cancers

By definition, stage III tumors extend to adjacent mucosal structures or the inguinal lymph nodes. Many are bulky, but some are of limited volume yet are considered to be high stage because of their proximity to critical central structures. Some of these primary tumors can be curatively resected by radical operations, such as radical vulvectomy or some variation of pelvic exenteration and vulvectomy. However, recent therapeutic efforts have focused on combined-modality treatment programs involving sequenced radiation therapy or chemoradiation therapy and radical surgery. There are now ample data from retrospective series, and a few prospective trials, from which to conclude that vulvar cancers are radioresponsive and that function-sparing operations are feasible in selected patients with advanced disease who receive combined-modality treatment. A similar experience has been reported for patients with stage IVA tumors. Exenterative resection may also be considered for selected patients. Although occasional cures have been described with innovative combinations of surgery, irradiation, and chemotherapy, treatment of patients with stage IVB vulvar cancer should be considered palliative.

Node-Positive Cancers

An optimal management strategy for node-positive patients is yet to be defined. Two factors appear to be important in the management of regional disease: Radiation therapy can have a significant impact on controlling or eradicating small-volume nodal disease; and surgical resection of bulky nodal disease also improves regional control and probably enhances the curative potential of irradiation.

Patients who undergo bilateral inguinofemoral lymphadenectomy as initial therapy and are found to have positive nodes—particularly more than one positive node—are likely to benefit from postoperative irradiation to the groins and lower pelvis (144). Radiation therapy is superior to surgery in the management of patients with positive pelvic nodes. The morbidity of combining superficial and deep inguinal lymphadenectomy with irradiation is substantial. The highest incidences of chronic groin and extremity complications, primarily lymphedema, are seen in such cases.

Several management options are available for patients found to have positive nodes during the course of superficial lymphadenectomy when performed as a staging procedure: (a) no further surgical therapy may be performed; (b) the lymphadenectomy can be extended to include the ipsilateral deep nodes, the contralateral groin nodes, or both; or (c) postoperative irradiation can be added to any of these surgical options. Given the heterogeneity of vulvar cancer presentations, treatment individualization is necessary. If postoperative radiotherapy to the inguinal nodes is deemed necessary, it would be reasonable to limit resection to grossly positive nodes, thereby minimizing the likelihood of lymphedema following combined radical surgery and radiation. Postoperative radiation requires careful treatment planning using CT imaging to evaluate for any measurable residual and to determine appropriate groin node depth. Excellent local control and minimal morbidity have been achieved when selective inguinal lymphadenectomy and tailored postoperative adjuvant therapy were administered to carefully selected patients (147).

Recurrent Cancer

Regardless of initial treatment, vulvar cancer recurrences can be categorized into three clinical groups: local (vulva), groin, and distant. The reported experience with local recurrence on the vulva is surprisingly good. Recurrence-free survival can be obtained in up to 75% of cases when the recurrence is limited to the vulva and can be resected with a gross clinical margin (162,163). The observation that many of these vulvar recurrences occur at sites remote from the initial primary tumor or that they occur years after apparently successful primary treatment suggests that some recurrences

probably represent new primary tumors rather than the development of new disease. Recurrences in the groin are almost universally fatal. A few patients may be saved by resection of bulky disease and local irradiation. Patients who develop distant metastases are candidates for systemic cytotoxic therapy, which is largely palliative.

SURGICAL TECHNIQUES

Radical Vulvectomy and Bilateral Inguinofemoral Lymphadenectomy

Although a number of modifications have been described, the basic incisions for radical vulvectomy and bilateral lymphadenectomy can be described as being based on either a ''butterfly'' or ''longhorn'' approach. The butterfly incisions use convex ''wings'' over the groins and around the anus to facilitate closure of the defect (Fig. 20.18). The longhorn incisions were developed to limit skin resection over the groin in an attempt to reduce wound breakdown (Fig. 20.19) (164). The arcing superior incision is placed from the lateral margins of the groin dissection across the mons pubis. The lateral vulvar incisions are placed at the labiocrural folds because these topographic landmarks represent the most lateral location of the superficial vulvar lymphatics. The perianal incision is placed to allow resection of the perineal body. These incisions are taken to the level of

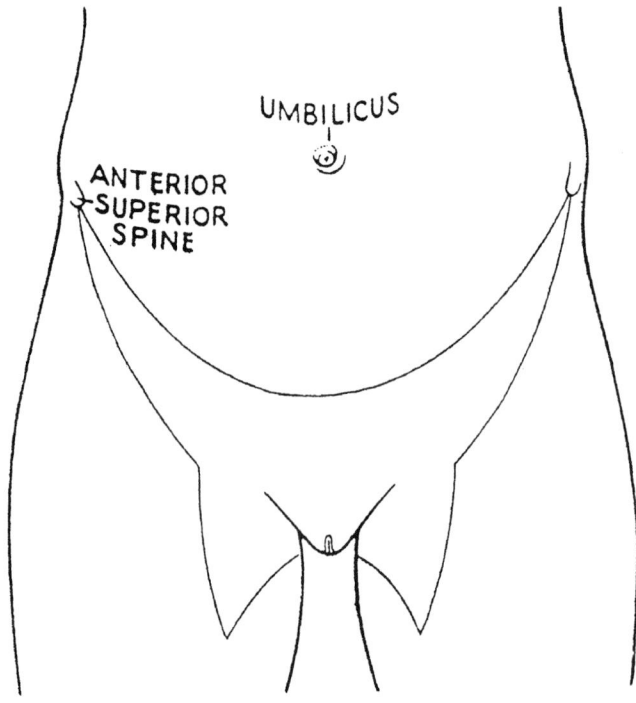

FIG. 20.18. ''Butterfly'' incisions for the superior portion of a radical vulvectomy with bilateral inguinofemoral lymphadenectomy. (Reprinted with permission from Way S. *Malignant disease of the female genital tract.* New York: Churchill Livingstone, 1951.)

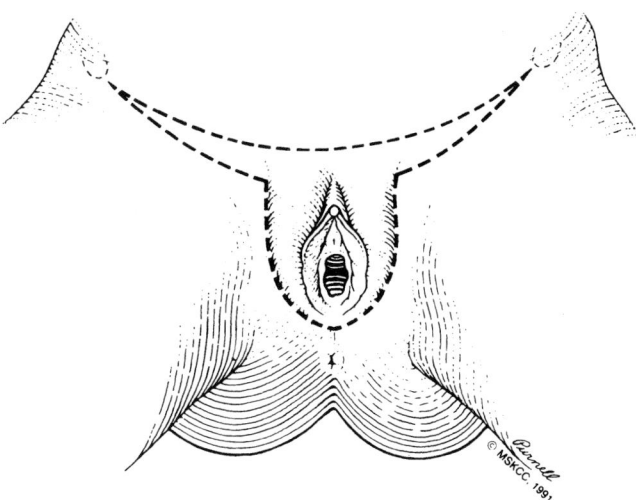

FIG. 20.19. Modified skin-sparing "longhorn" incisions for en bloc radical resection.

the deep inguinal and perineal fascia and permit en bloc removal of both superficial and deep groin nodes, the entire vulva, and an intervening skin bridge.

After removal of the specimen, the skin and mucosal edges are undermined to permit mobilization and primary closure with delayed absorbable suture. Some degree of tension at the suture lines is unavoidable, particularly in the perineal body and periurethral areas. Closed suction drains are usually placed in the groin sites to remove excess lymphatic and serous fluid accumulations and are usually removed when drain output is minimal (5 to 14 days).

Some degree of wound breakdown is seen in approximately 50% of patients (143). Local wound care results in satisfactory secondary healing in most of these cases. Lymphocyst formation is relatively common and frequently presents as a tense but nontender groin mass. Percutaneous needle drainage is usually sufficient, but occasionally replacement of a groin drain may be required. Inguinal cellulitis, lower extremity lymphangitis, and lymphedema are uncommon late sequelae. The incidence of these complications ise related to the extent of groin therapy and is highest in patients treated with superficial and deep lymphadenectomy along with groin irradiation.

Radical Wide Excision

Several names have been applied to the procedures used to resect small vulvar cancers: radical wide excision, radical local excision, wide local excision, modified radical vulvectomy, and hemivulvectomy. Regardless of the preferred nomenclature, the surgical procedure should be adequately defined and described. Surgical incisions are devised to allow for at least a 2-cm resection margin encompassing the primary lesion (Fig. 20.20). Dissection is carried to the deep perineal fascia. Recent data suggest that a 1-cm margin may be adequate for some tumors (142). If this information is verified by other studies, it will be most useful when planning the resection of tumors in close proximity to midline structures. Tumors that encroach on the anus or anal sphincters can be managed by radical wide excision with sphincter or flap repair, or they can be treated with combined-modality therapy as outlined in the section on radiation therapy below. Most radical wide excision sites can be closed primarily. In some patients, rhomboid flaps can be used to facilitate coverage of the vulvar defect (165). Some form of inguinal lymphadenectomy, performed through a separate incision, is generally combined with radical wide excision. The necessary extent of the groin dissection is an area of current investigation.

Ambulation is begun on the day of surgery. Perineal irrigation and air drying are started 24 hours after operation. The average hospital stay for patients undergoing radical wide excision is usually 3 days or less. Wound breakdown,

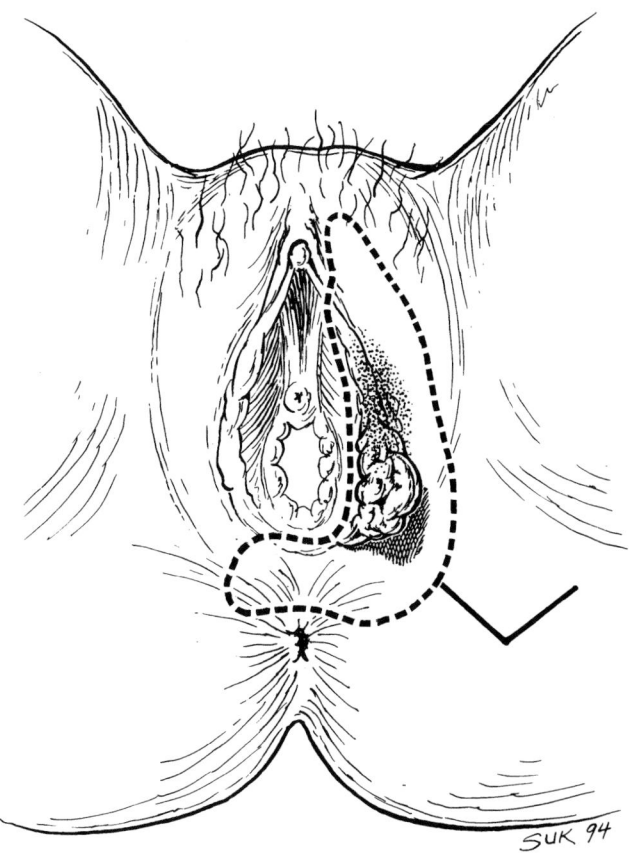

FIG. 20.20. Planned resection of a left labial squamous carcinoma and adjacent carcinoma *in situ* by radical wide excision. A 2-cm margin is outlined. Rhomboid flap repair using a V incision is anticipated. (Reprinted with permission from Burke TW, Morris M, Levenback C, et al. Closure of complex vulvar defects using local rhomboid flaps. *Obstet Gynecol* 1994;84:1044.)

usually of minor degree, is reported in approximately 15% of cases (59,131). The incidence and severity of groin complications are proportional to the extent of the lymphadenectomy.

Triple-Incision Techniques

As a radical operation, the three-incision technique represents an intermediate surgical procedure with radical vulvectomy and en bloc inguinofemoral lymphadenectomy at one end of the spectrum and radical wide excision at the other. For this approach, radical vulvectomy is accomplished using two elliptical incisions—an inner one circumscribing the vaginal introitus and vulvar vestibule and an outer one placed at the labiocrural folds and brought across the mons pubis and perineal body. When carried to the deep perineal fascia, this resection allows complete removal of the vulvar skin in a manner identical to that achieved with radical vulvectomy; however, bilateral inguinofemoral lymphadenectomy is accomplished via separate incisions parallel to the inguinal ligaments. The three-incision concept preserves the radicality of the vulvar resection while retaining skin over the groin. Consequently, the incidence of major wound breakdown is significantly reduced to approximately 15% to 20% of cases (150,166,167). As with other techniques, the incidence and severity of groin complications are related to the extent of the lymphadenectomy performed.

Inguinal Lymphadenectomy

Appropriate surgical management of the inguinal nodes is controversial and evolving. Precise recommendations are not possible because there is a wide range of treatment philosophy. Nevertheless, the surgical approaches to the groin lymph nodes can be readily defined and described.

Excisional Biopsy

Most preoperative diagnostic dilemmas related to enlarged groin nodes can be resolved simply and accurately using fine-needle aspiration biopsy. However, surgical removal of one or two lymph nodes may occasionally be considered in the management of women with vulvar cancer. Selective excision of groin lymph nodes may be considered when fine-needle aspiration biopsy results are negative or equivocal, or to remove bulky positive nodes before beginning a course of combined-modality therapy. A small incision is made over the palpable node and dissection is carried to the level of the lymph node mass. The involved node is freed from the adjacent subcutaneous tissues and removed. The incision is closed with skin staples or absorbable sutures. The decision to electively place a closed suction drain depends upon the extent of the dissection, the amount of subcutaneous free space, and surgeon preference. Most lymph node biopsies can be performed as outpatient procedures, and some can be accomplished under local anesthesia.

Superficial Inguinal Lymphadenectomy

Superficial inguinal lymphadenectomy involves the removal of the eight to ten lymph nodes that lie superficial to the cribriform fascia and surrounding the branches of the saphenous vein. This is a more meticulous and complete lymphatic dissection than that described for excisional biopsy. The anatomic boundaries of the superficial lymphatic dissection are the inguinal ligament superiorly, the border of the sartorius muscle laterally, and the border of the adductor longus muscle medially. The anterior limit is the superficial subcutaneous fascia (Camper's fascia), and the posterior limit is the cribriform fascia overlying the femoral artery, vein, and deep nodes.

The skin incision used to provide access to the groin is made parallel to the inguinal ligament approximately from a point overlying the adductor longus tendon laterally to a point below the anterosuperior iliac spine. The superficial subcutaneous fat is left attached to the skin to provide blood supply, but is separated from the underlying nodal tissue by dissecting inferiorly at the level of Camper's fascia. The lymphadenectomy specimen is developed by continuing the inferior dissection along the borders of the sartorius and adductor longus muscles. As the dissection proceeds, the specimen is mobilized off the cribriform fascia. Care should be taken to identify and individually ligate the vessels that perforate this fascia. The saphenous vein is encountered at the lower medial margin of the dissection, and whenever possible should be preserved to minimize the risk for postoperative lymphedema (Fig. 20.21). The dissected specimen is

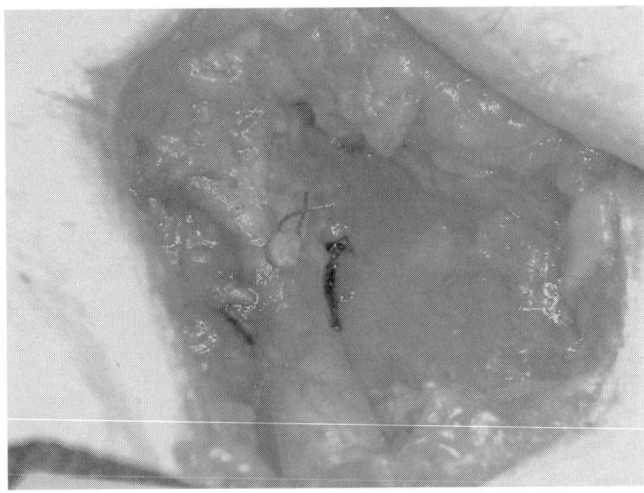

FIG. 20.21. The patient is undergoing superficial and deep dissection of the right groin nodes. At this point in the procedure, the saphenous vein, which is entering the surgical field from the right lower aspect, has been identified and preserved.

forwarded for pathologic assessment. The skin incision can be closed with either staples or absorbable sutures. A closed-suction drain is placed and removed when output is <25 mL per day.

Deep Inguinal (Femoral) Lymphadenectomy

The deep inguinal (femoral) lymph nodes lie medial to the femoral vein beneath the cribriform fascia. This space contains three to five nodes, the channels of which course beneath the inguinal ligament and continue in the pelvis as the external iliac nodal chain. The most superior deep inguinal node is known as Cloquet's node.

Surgical removal of the deep nodes is performed as an extension of a superficial lymphadenectomy rather than as an isolated procedure. The usual approach is to open the cribriform fascia along the sartorius muscle at the time of the superficial lymphadenectomy. The cribriform fascia is then mobilized medially as a part of the specimen. Once the superior aspect of the femoral vein is identified and exposed, the deep nodes are removed in continuity with the superficial nodes. Some surgeons then cover the exposed femoral vessels by removing the sartorius muscle from its insertion onto the anterior iliac spine and transposing the muscle over the femoral vessels by suturing the free edge of the muscle to the inguinal ligament.

Because all of the deep nodes are consistently located medial to the femoral vein, some surgeons have recommended eliminating the removal of the entire cribriform plate (168). They suggest opening the fascia medial to the vein and removing only the adjacent nodes. This modified approach to the deep nodes may help to reduce acute morbidity while providing a more definitive lymphatic resection. In a retrospective review of 194 patients undergoing various modifications of inguinofemoral lymphadenectomy, Rouzier et al. showed that techniques of groin node dissection that preserved the cribriform fascia and saphenous vein were associated with a decreased risk of postoperative morbidity without jeopardizing outcomes (169).

Surgical Resection for Recurrent Disease

The site, extent, and volume of recurrent vulvar cancer have important implications on both resectability and potential for cure. Recurrences can be categorized as local (vulva), groin, or distant (lung, bone, liver, brain). Surgical therapy plays a curative or palliative role in selected subsets of patients with recurrent disease (170).

Radical Wide Excision

As many as 75% of patients with recurrent disease limited to the vulva can be salvaged by radical wide excision or reexcision of the tumor (113,162,163). Surgical principles of recurrent vulvar tumors are identical to those for primary tumors: wide excision with a measured normal tissue margin of at least 2 cm. Particular attention is also focused on obtaining a clear deep margin. Because most patients have had prior operative therapy, primary closure of the vulvar defect is frequently more difficult. More complex reconstructive efforts may be needed to restore tissue integrity.

Pelvic Exenteration

Curative resection may still be possible when vulvar recurrence extends to the vagina, proximal urethra, or anus. Selected patients have achieved long-term survival after pelvic exenteration for such recurrences (83,171–173). The surgical approach in these cases should be individualized to the size and location of the recurrent tumor, prior therapies, and the age and overall health of the patient. Patients considered for pelvic exenteration should have a thorough preoperative evaluation to exclude the presence of regional and/or distant metastases. Frequently, anterior or posterior exenteration with an extended vulvar phase will provide excellent resection margins while allowing preservation of one major excretory system. The techniques used to perform the exenteration are identical to those routinely used for the treatment of women with recurrent cervical carcinoma. Unilateral gracilis flap repair may be combined with tailored exenteration to provide coverage for the surgical defect (174).

Resection of Groin Recurrence

Patients who develop groin recurrence are rarely curable. Untreated groin recurrence follows a particularly morbid course characterized by pain, bleeding, skin breakdown, and infection. Palliative treatment should be considered for these patients. Surgical resection should be viewed with caution in the previously irradiated patient. Cure is unlikely with resection alone, and wound healing is impaired. The debility caused by a combination of unresolved recurrence and surgical wound breakdown is worse than that of progressive recurrence alone. Patients who develop groin recurrence without a history of prior irradiation should be considered for surgical resection in combination with preoperative or postoperative radiation therapy. The surgical approach is limited to the removal of gross tumor to the extent feasible. The operative goal is to resect or debulk the recurrence to a small volume in the hope that subsequent irradiation will achieve regional control. Tumor reduction is especially difficult when the recurrence arises within the deep compartment or encases the femoral vessels. Extended survival is possible for the few patients who achieve control of recurrent disease in the groin and do not later manifest distant metastasis. Isolated groin recurrence is a rare event, so the data to support the efficacy of this treatment are anecdotal.

Vulvar Reconstruction

With careful planning and adequate tissue mobilization, most vulvar defects can be closed primarily with absorbable sutures. When large portions of the vulva have been resected, when tissue mobility is poor, or when radiation therapy has been administered previously, primary closure may not be feasible. Alternate tissue sources must be considered for these difficult cases.

Rhomboid Flaps

The rhomboid flap is a local tissue advancement flap that draws its blood supply from the subcutaneous vascular network. These flaps can be developed at any level of the vulva. Single or combination flaps can be designed to cover a wide variety of defects. The maximal practical flap size is approximately 4 cm². Rhomboid flaps are particularly useful in providing closure of large midline defects following the radical wide excision of periclitoral or perineal body tumors (165, 175,176).

The rhomboid flap is designed by marking a V-shaped incision adjacent to the tissue defect needing coverage (Fig. 20.22). Flap size should correspond to the measured size of the defect. The flap incision is carried approximately 1.0 to 1.5 cm into the subcutaneous tissue. The flap is then developed by dissection within the subcutaneous tissue. When the adjacent tissues have been undermined, the flap can be ro-

tated over the defect and sutured in place. Rhomboid flap repairs provide full-thickness padded coverage without tension.

Myocutaneous Flaps

Several types of myocutaneous flaps—gracilis, gluteus, tensor fascia lata, rectus abdominis—have been used to provide repair and reconstruction of large vulvar and groin defects (177–181). Myocutaneous flaps, unlike local advancement flaps, include a segment of muscle and receive their blood supply and innervation through a clearly defined neurovascular pedicle. These are large, thick tissue sources that are best suited for the reconstruction of substantial defects. Although each of the flaps listed has proponents and specific advantages, the widest degree of experience has been reported for gracilis flaps. A gracilis flap can be designed to cover virtually any vulvar defect (Fig. 20.23).

The gracilis muscle is a broad flat muscle that courses through the superficial portion of the medial thigh. It is a weak adductor whose absence produces little perceptible deficit. The flap design is initiated by drawing a line from the pubic tubercle to the medial femoral condyle. The gracilis muscle lies directly beneath this line. Flap size should be limited to a skin paddle of 6 to 8 cm × 10 to 12 cm. Smaller flaps have been associated with a lower incidence of necrosis and wound separation (174). The skin-paddle incisions are carried to the gracilis fascia. The distal muscle is identified and transected 2 to 3 cm beyond the edge of the skin paddle. The myocutaneous unit is then developed by continuing the dissection more proximally. The main vascular bundle is usually encountered approximately 7 cm below the pubic tubercle. If possible, this pedicle should be preserved; however, if additional mobility is required, this vascular pedicle

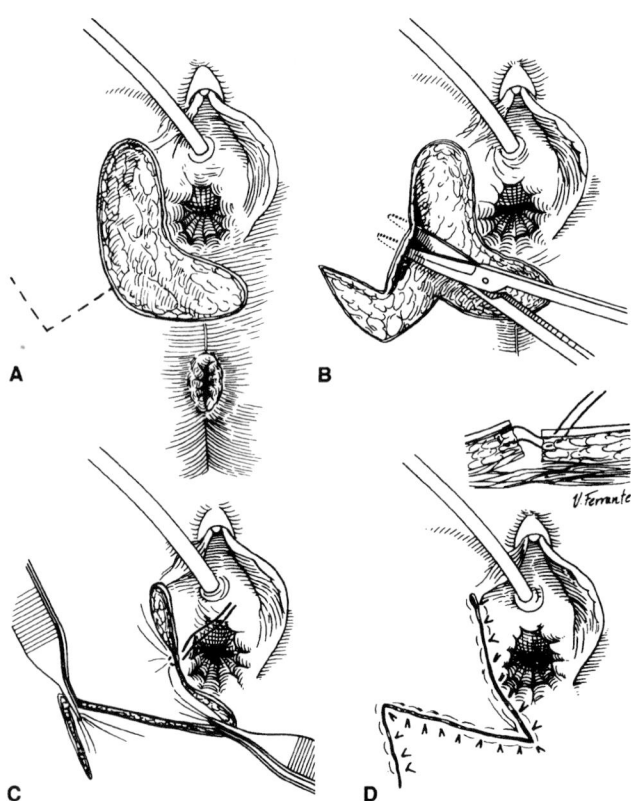

FIG. 20.22. Technique for a unilateral rhomboid-flap repair. **A:** The flap is outlined. **B:** A 1-cm-thick flap of skin and subcutaneous tissue is raised. The area is undermined. **C:** The flap is rotated, and stay sutures are placed. **D:** Completed repair.

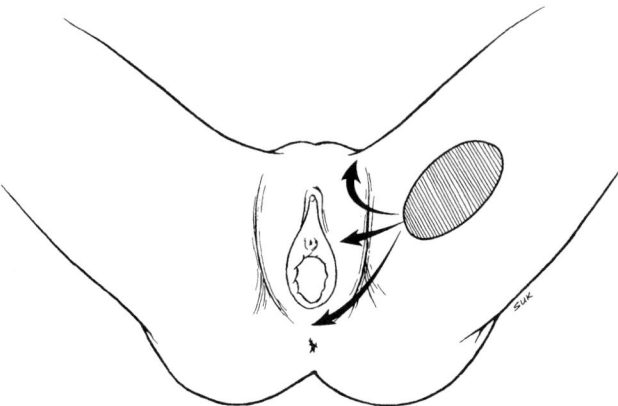

FIG. 20.23. Diagrammatic representation of possible external placements for a gracilis myocutaneous flap. These flaps can be used to reconstruct large defects of the groin, labium majus, or perineal body. (Reprinted with permission from Burke TW, et al.. Perineal reconstruction using single gracilis myocutaneous flaps. *Gynecol Oncol* 1995;57:223.)

may be sacrificed. Flap viability is thought to be retained through blood supply derived from the more proximal obturator branches. Once developed, the flap is mobilized through a subcutaneous tunnel to reach the perineum or groin. The flap can be trimmed and sutured into position.

RADIATION THERAPY

Early reports of severe local reactions and poor survival rates with primary radiation therapy of vulvar carcinomas led some previous investigators to conclude that radiotherapy had a very limited role in the curative management of these patients (182–184). The use of high doses of radiation alone, delivered with low-energy photons and electrons, in patients who were mostly poor surgical candidates, resulted in a suboptimal therapeutic window between tumor control probability and normal tissue complications (185). However, more contemporary experiences, emphasizing appropriate fractionation, attention to treatment planning detail, and recognition of vulvar and low pelvic radiation tolerance limits, have clearly demonstrated that relatively high doses of irradiation can be delivered safely. In selected patients, treatment of the vulva and/or regional lymph nodes improves locoregional control rates and survival rates and may even reduce overall treatment morbidity. Radiation therapy is now accepted as an important element in the multidisciplinary management of patients with locoregionally advanced disease in the vulva.

Treating Locally Advanced Disease in the Vulva

Following initial resection of a vulvar primary, various surgical-pathologic features have been identified that are associated with a higher risk of local recurrence. Podratz et al. reported a 24% incidence of vulvar recurrence in 71 patients with stage III carcinoma (113). Recurrence was correlated with tumor size and nodal status. Heaps et al. reported that a close surgical margin was the most powerful predictor of local recurrence in their patients (124). They observed 21 vulvar recurrences in 44 patients with tumor margins <8 mm (deep or at the skin surface) compared with no local recurrences in 91 patients with margins ≥8 mm (after fixation). Lymph-vascular space invasion and deep tumor

penetration are also associated with a greater and increased risk of recurrence (114,124,186). Although many local recurrences are controlled with additional surgery or irradiation, salvage surgery is often morbid, and local recurrences may provide additional opportunity for regional and distant tumor spread. Although no prospective trials of postoperative vulvar site radiotherapy have been completed, adjuvant radiation of the primary tumor bed in selected patients with close margins or other high-risk features likely improves local control (187).

Alternatively, in patients who present with more advanced primary tumors, radiation therapy may be delivered preoperatively. Advocates of this approach have listed several theoretical advantages for patients with locally advanced vulvar carcinomas:

1. Less radical resection of the vulva may be adequate to achieve local tumor control after preoperative treatment of the vulva with irradiation.
2. Tumor regression during radiation therapy may allow the surgeon to obtain adequate surgical margins without sacrificing important structures such as urethra, anus, and clitoris.
3. Radiation treatment alone may be sufficient to sterilize microscopic regional disease when the inguinal nodes are clinically normal and may mobilize fixed and matted nodes, facilitating subsequent surgical excision.

Although the published experiences with preoperative single-modality radiation therapy are small, several investigators have reported excellent responses and high local control rates after treatment of advanced tumors with relatively modest doses of radiation therapy followed by local resection (Table 20.7) (188–192). These reports provide emerging evidence that radiation can significantly debulk advanced local disease and allow for more conservative, viscera-sparing surgery without a loss of local control.

More recently, a number of published series have suggested the therapeutic benefit of concurrent chemoradiation, typically followed by limited surgical resection, in addressing locally advanced disease (Table 20.8) (41,66,136, 193–207). These trials were prompted by extrapolation from the excellent results reported with chemoirradiation of carcinoma of the anus (208,209). Typical regimens have included

TABLE 20.7. *Preoperative radiation therapy for treatment of locally advanced carcinoma of the vulva*

Investigator (ref.)	Year	No. of patients	Radiation dose (Gy)	No. with no tumor in surgical specimen (%)	Local recurrences (%)
Fairey et al. (190)	1985	7	55	?	1 (14)
Hacker et al. (191)	1984	8	44–54	4 (50)	1 (12)
Boronow (189)	1987	34	Ext beam 42.0–52.2 (± brachytherapy)	15 (44)	5 (15)
Jafari and Magalotti (192)	1981	4	30–42	4 (100)	0
Acosta et al. (188)	1978	14	36–55	5 (36)	1 (7)[a]

[a] Outside irradiation field.

TABLE 20.8. *Concurrent chemoirradiation in the management of locally advanced or recurrent carcinoma of the vulva*

Investigator (ref.)	No. of patients	Chemotherapy	Radiation dose (Gy)	No. with recurrent or persistent local disease after RT ± surgery (%)	Follow-up (months)
Moore et al. (136)	73	5-FU + CDDP	47.6	15 (21)	22–72
Cunningham et al. (194)	14	5-FU + CDDP	45.5	4 (29)	7–81
Landoni et al. (200)	58	5-FU + Mito	54	13 (22)	4–48
Lupi et al. (201)	31	5-FU + Mito	54	7 (23)	22–73
Whalen et al. (205)	19	5-FU + Mito	45.5	1 (5)	3–70
Eifel et al. (195)	12	5-FU + CDDP	40.5	5 (42)	17–30
Koh et al. (199)	20	5-FU ± CDDP or Mito	30.5	9 (45)	1–75
Akl et al. (206)	12[a]	5-FU + Mito	36	0	8–125
Russell et al. (41)	25	5-FU ± CDDP	47.7	6 (24)	4–52
Han et al. (207)	14	5-FU + Mito or CDDP	40–62	6 (43)	42–73
Scheistroen and Trope (203)	42	Bleomycin	45	39 (93)	7–60
Berek et al. (193)	12	5-FU + CDDP	44.5	0	7–60
Thomas et al. (204)	24	5-FU ± Mito	44.6	10 (42)	5–43
Evans et al. (196)	4	5-FU + Mito	25.7	2 (50)	20–29
Levin et al. (66)	6	5-FU + Mito	18.6	0	1–25
Iversen (197)	15	Bleomycin	15.4	11 (83)[b]	4

5-FU, 5-fluorouracil; Mito, mitomycin C; CDDP, cisplatin.
[a] All patients were N0.
[b] Most patients had unresectable, stage IV lesions.

combinations of irradiation and concurrent 5-fluorouracil plus cisplatin or mitomycin C. Most studies included small numbers of patients with various disease presentations, including patients with very advanced or recurrent lesions, and none of these experiences can be compared meaningfully with results of treatment with irradiation alone. Nonetheless, most investigators have observed impressive regressions of advanced lesions, suggesting that responses may be better than would be expected with irradiation alone. Randomized trials of the role of chemoirradiation have not been done and are likely nonfeasible given the small number of patients, and the heterogeneity of clinical presentations, with this disease. However, recent trials that demonstrated improved local control and survival when concurrent cisplatin-containing chemotherapy was added to radiation treatment of cervical cancers suggest that this approach may also be useful for women with other locally advanced lower genital tract neoplasms (133–135,210).

The most compelling data in support of concurrent chemoradiation in the management of locally advanced disease come from a large prospective Phase II trial performed by the Gynecologic Oncologic Group (GOG protocol 101). In this study, 71 evaluable patients with locally advanced T3 or T4 primary tumors who were deemed not resectable by standard radical vulvectomy underwent preoperative chemoradiation. Chemotherapy consisted of two cycles of 5-fluorouracil and cisplatin. Radiation was delivered to a dose of 47.6 Gy, using a planned split-course regimen, with part of the radiation given twice daily during the 5-fluorouracil infusion. Patients underwent planned resection of the residual vulvar tumor, or incisional biopsy of the original tumor site in the event of a complete clinical response, 4 to 8 weeks

after chemoradiotherapy. A complete clinical tumor response was noted in 33 of 71 (47%) patients. Following vulvar excision or biopsy, 22 patients (31%) were found to have no residual tumor in the pathologic specimen. In all, only 2 of 71 patients (3%) had unresectable disease after chemoradiation, and for only 3 patients was it not possible to preserve urinary and/or gastrointestinal continuity. With a median follow-up interval of 50 months, 11 patients (16%) have developed locally recurrent disease in the vulva (136). These results are all the more notable considering the relatively low dose of radiation used in these typically bulky, advanced tumors.

It is important to be cautious in designing aggressive treatment protocols for this group of patients, who are often elderly and with coexistent medical problems. Serious pulmonary toxicity has been observed in patients treated with bleomycin (197,202). In the largest published series of patients treated with mitomycin C and 5-fluorouracil, hematologic tolerance was acceptable, but the administered dose of mitomycin C was more conservative than what is usually used in the treatment of anal cancers (204).

The use of concurrent weekly cisplatin with radiation has been widely tested in patients with locally advanced cervical cancer and found to be therapeutically beneficial and well tolerated (133,135). In an attempt further to improve clinical and pathologic complete response, and ultimately local tumor control rates, the GOG has just initiated another prospective Phase II trial (GOG protocol 205), which combines weekly cisplatin with daily fractionated radiotherapy. Radiation will be given to a total dose of 57.6 Gy (representing a 20% dose escalation over that used in GOG 101) to the gross tumor volume using careful treatment planning and boost techniques, and the planned 2-week break specified in the previous trial has been eliminated.

Following chemoradiation for locally advanced disease, it remains undefined if surgery is necessary for those patients who achieve complete clinical response. In GOG 101, about 70% of patients who achieved complete clinical response were found to have no pathologic residual in the surgical specimen (136). At this point, we continue to recommend biopsies of the original tumor bed in patients who achieve complete clinical response. In those with residual disease after chemoradiation, surgical resection would be individualized and tailored to the extent and location of residuum.

Treatment of Regional Disease

Although radical inguinal lymphadenectomy has historically been considered the treatment of choice for regional management of invasive vulvar carcinoma, a number of retrospective studies have suggested that regional prophylactic radiation therapy is an effective method of preventing groin recurrences with minimal morbidity (211–213). In a review of 91 patients treated electively for cancers with primary drainage to the inguinal nodes, Henderson and colleagues observed only two failures after treatment with 45 to 50 Gy in 5 weeks, and both of these were outside the treatment fields (211). Complications were rare, with only one case of mild leg edema, which may not have been treatment related. In another review of patients treated for vulvar carcinomas, Petereit and colleagues found no difference in the groin recurrence rate for clinically negative inguinal nodes treated with radical lymphadenectomy or radiation therapy even though the irradiated patients had more advanced primary tumors (213). Leiserowitz and colleagues (130) had no groin recurrences in 23 patients with locally advanced, clinically N0 vulvar cancers after prophylactic treatment of the groins with concurrent chemoirradiation (214).

The GOG tried to define the optimal approach to clinically negative inguinal nodes in a trial that randomized patients between inguinal node irradiation and radical lymphadenectomy (followed by inguinopelvic irradiation in patients with positive nodes) after resection of the primary tumor (19). This study was closed after entry of only 58 patients when there appeared to be a higher rate of groin recurrence in the radiation treatment arm. However, this study has been criticized because the treatment protocol, which recommended combination photon and electron dosing to a depth of 3 to 4 cm, likely delivered an inadequate dose to the inguinal nodes (215,216).

Although the role of prophylactic radiotherapy in the undissected but high-risk groin remains controversial, there is strong evidence that adjunctive radiation therapy improves survival and regional tumor control in patients who are treated with radical inguinal node dissection—particularly those with clinically positive nodes. Retrospective studies suggested that patients with metastases to multiple nodes or

extranodal extension had an increased risk of groin recurrence after radical surgery and therefore may benefit from radiation therapy (217,218). However, the critical role of radiation therapy was not appreciated until 1986, when Homesley et al. published results of a prospective GOG trial in 114 patients with inguinal metastases (144). In that study, all patients underwent radical vulvectomy and inguinal lymphadenectomy. Patients who had positive inguinal nodes were randomized intraoperatively to receive either pelvic node dissection or postoperative irradiation to the pelvis and inguinal nodes. The trial was closed before the projected accrual goal because an interim analysis revealed a statistically significant overall survival advantage for the radiation treatment arm (p = .03). The differences between the 2-year survival rates of patients treated with radiation therapy versus pelvic dissection were most marked for patients with clinically positive nodes (59% vs 31%, respectively) and for those with two or more positive groin nodes (63% vs 37%, respectively). There was no significant difference in survival between the treatment groups for patients with only one microscopically positive node, although the investigators commented that the number of patients in this subset was insufficient for reliable analysis. The most striking difference in the patterns of recurrence for the two treatment groups was the much larger number of inguinal failures among patients who were treated with surgery alone (Fig. 20.24). These groin recurrences were rarely, if ever, salvageable. The vulva, regardless of tumor pathologic risk factors, was not included in the radiation treatment fields in this study, and approximately 9% of patients in both treatment arms had recurrences at the primary site at the time of the analysis, raising the question of whether selective radiation to the vulva might have decreased local recurrences.

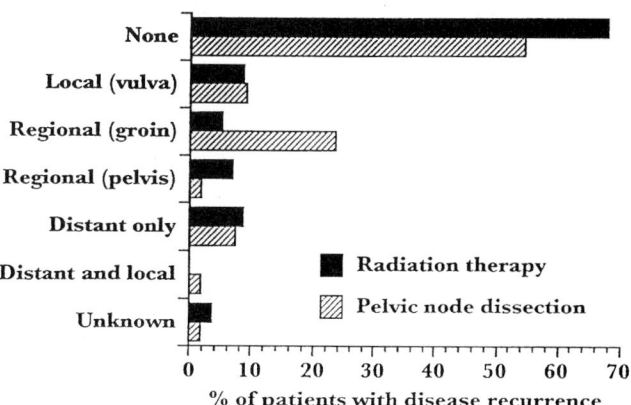

FIG. 20.24. Sites of disease recurrence in patients treated with adjuvant radiation therapy to the pelvis and inguinal region or with pelvic node dissection following radical vulvectomy and bilateral inguinal lymphadenectomy. (Modified with permission from Homesley HD, Bundy BN, Sedlis A, Adcock L. Radiation therapy versus pelvic node resection for carcinoma of the vulva with positive groin nodes. *Obstet Gynecol* 1986;68:733.)

Successful use of concurrent chemotherapy and radiation therapy following radical hysterectomy in patients with cervical cancer suggests that concurrent chemotherapy might be valuable for patients with node-positive vulvar cancer (134). Although a randomized trial was initiated to address the role of adjuvant chemoradiation following resection of node-positive tumors, the study was deemed nonfeasible and closed because of the relative rarity of these cancers and lack of patient accrual.

However, the role of preoperative chemoradiation has been assessed in patients who present with bulky, unresectable inguinal adenopathy. In the aforementioned GOG 101 study of preoperative chemoradiation for locoregionally advanced vulvar cancer, there was a cohort of 42 evaluable patients with N2 or N3 nodal disease that were deemed initially unresectable. Patients received 47.6 Gy of radiotherapy in split-course fashion with two concurrent cycles of 5-fluorouracil and cisplatin as previously described above. Three to 8 weeks later, planned inguinal-femoral lymph node dissection was performed. In only two patients (5%) did nodal disease remain unresectable. The surgical specimen showed histologic clearance of nodal disease in 15 patients (36%). At a median follow up of 78 months, only 1 of 37 (3%) patients who completed the full prescribed regimen of preoperative chemoradiation and bilateral inguinal-femoral node dissection relapsed in the groin (219). This study, although nonrandomized, provides further evidence of the efficacy of combined chemoradiotherapy in the management of locoregionally advanced vulvar cancer.

Radiation Therapy Technique

Techniques commonly used for treatment of vulvar carcinoma reflect the need to encompass the lower pelvic and inguinal nodes as well as the vulva while minimizing the dose to the femoral heads. One approach is to treat with an anterior field that encompasses the inguinal regions, lower pelvic nodes, and vulva and a narrower posterior field that encompasses the lower pelvic nodes and vulva but excludes the majority of the femoral heads. If the fields are evenly weighted to the mid plane of the pelvis using 6-MV photons, the contribution of the anterior field to the groin nodes (at 3- to 5-cm depth) will generally be 60% to 70% of the dose to the mid pelvis. The difference may be made up by supplementing the dose to the lateral groins with anterior electron fields of appropriate energy (Fig. 20.25). Kalnicki and associates described another technique using a partial transmission block, which also reduces the dose to the femoral heads (220). CT scans are used to determine the appropriate electron energy and to detect enlarged nodes that may not be appreciated on clinical examination. Gross disease in the groins or vulva may be boosted with *en face* electron fields. In some cases, interstitial implants or *en face* electron fields may be used to boost the dose to the primary site (221, 222). If radiation is directed to the regional nodes only, with

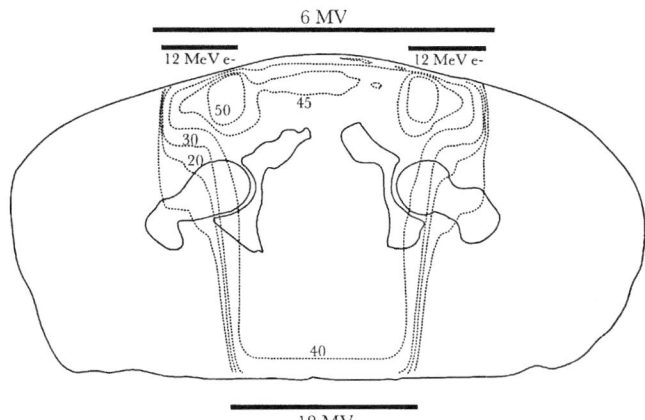

FIG. 20.25. The radiation dose to the femoral heads can be reduced by delivering part of the dose to inguinal nodes with appropriate-energy electron fields. In this example, a wide anterior 6-MV field encompasses the primary site as well as the inguinal and pelvic nodes. Electron fields are placed anteriorly to overlap slightly with the exit of a narrower posterior 18-MV field that encompasses the primary and pelvic nodes.

intentional sparing of the vulva, are must be taken to avoid a large "mid-line" block, which may lead to higher medial groin and vulvar failures (223).

Acute Complications of Radiation Therapy

Acute radiation reactions are brisk, and doses of 35 to 45 Gy routinely induce confluent moist desquamation. However, with adequate local care, this acute reaction usually heals within 3 to 4 weeks. Sitz baths, steroid cream, and treatment of possible superimposed *Candida* infection all help to minimize the discomfort. If the patient is sufficiently flexible, she may be placed in a frog-leg position during treatment to minimize the dose and ensuing skin reaction on the medial thighs; care must then be taken, however, to deliver an adequate dose to the vulvar skin. Although most patients will develop confluent mucositis by the fourth week of treatment, this is usually tolerated if the patient is warned in advance and assured that the discomfort will resolve after treatment is completed. Although a treatment break is occasionally required, delays should be minimized, because they may allow time for repopulation of tumor cells.

Late Complications of Radiation Therapy

Many factors add to the late morbidity of radiation treatment in patients with vulvar carcinoma. Patients with advanced vulvar carcinomas often are treated with radiation therapy following radical surgery, which may include extensive dissection of the inguinal and possibly pelvic nodes. Large ulcerative cutaneous lesions frequently have superimposed infection. Patients are often elderly and may have

TABLE 20.9. *Single-agent cytotoxics in squamous vulvar cancer*

Drug	Dose and schedule	No. of patients entered	Complete response	Partial response	Investigator (ref.)
Adriamycin	45 mg/m^2 IV q 3 weeks	4	0	3	Deppe et al. (228)
Bleomycin	15 mg IM twice weekly	11	2	3	Trope et al. (104)
Cisplatin	50 mg/m^2 q 3 weeks	22	0	0	Thigpen et al. (229)
Piperazinedione	9 mg/m^2 IV q 3 weeks	13	0	0	Thigpen et al. (229)
Mitoxantrone	12 mg/m^2 IV q 3 weeks	19	0	0	Muss et al. (230)
Etoposide	100 mg/m^2 IV days 1, 3, 5	18	0	0	Slayton et al. (231)

complicating medical conditions such as diabetes, multiple prior surgeries, and osteoporosis. The contribution of concurrent chemotherapy to local morbidity is not yet clearly defined, but may contribute to bowel and bone complications (224,225).

The incidence of lower extremity edema after inguinal irradiation alone is negligible (211,213,218,226). Although radiation therapy probably contributes to the incidence of peripheral edema following radical node dissection, no difference was evident in the GOG randomized study (144). However, the investigators admitted that evaluation of lymphedema was not a major consideration of the study and that the complication may have been underreported. Femoral head fractures have occasionally been reported in patients treated with irradiation to the inguinal nodes (191,204,211). Techniques that limit the dose to the femoral heads to less than 35 Gy should minimize the risk of this complication. It is not known whether severe osteoporosis contributes to femoral head complications. In general, with careful treatment planning technique, the risk of a major late complication following regional nodal radiation, either electively or adjuvant to lymph node dissection, is low (226). It has been suggested that concurrent chemotherapy may increase the risk, but this remains to be adequately substantiated (224).

The effects of radiation therapy on the long-term cosmesis and function of the vulva are poorly understood. Although treatment with irradiation and wide excision is becoming a more accepted alternative to radical vulvectomy for selected patients, and major complication rates appear to be acceptable, very little has been reported regarding more subtle late effects of such treatment in the vulva. Late effects are dose related. Although Frischbier and Thomsen reported a 24% incidence of late ulceration in a large number of patients treated primarily with electron-beam radiation therapy to the vulva, the relatively large dose per fraction (3 Gy/d) that was used probably contributed to this high incidence (227). Better information will become available only as treating physicians record and report the late cosmetic and functional results of treatment.

CHEMOTHERAPY

Data on the use of chemotherapeutic agents for the treatment of vulvar malignancies are limited; the incidence is

low, the majority of patients are cured with surgery with or without postoperative radiation therapy, and thus chemotherapy has been used primarily as a salvage therapy. Patients with advanced vulvar cancers tend to be older, making them poor candidates for cytotoxic therapy because of concomitant diseases that increase the likelihood for significant adverse effects. Furthermore, recurrent vulvar cancer often occurs in the setting of extensive prior surgery and/or radiation therapy, making tolerance to cytotoxic therapy poor. No single institution has a large enough patient population to allow adequate Phase II testing of cytotoxic agents.

Squamous Cell Carcinoma

Squamous carcinoma is the only cell type for which reproducible information exists on the value of cytotoxic therapy. Several drugs have undergone Phase II testing in squamous vulvar cancer (Table 20.9) (104,228–231). Only doxorubicin (Adriamycin) and bleomycin appear to have activity as single agents. Although methotrexate has been claimed to have activity, data are inadequate for confirmation. Cisplatin, a drug that has demonstrated broad activity in most gynecologic tumors (e.g., epithelial ovary, endometrial adenocarcinoma, endometrial mixed mesodermal tumors, and squamous carcinoma of the cervix), has notably little activity in vulvar and vaginal squamous tumors. This lack of activity, however, is based on treatment of refractory patients only. No trials of this agent as a presurgical cytoreductive regimen have been attempted. With the recent dramatic results obtained with concurrent cisplatin-based chemotherapy and radiation therapy in locally advanced squamous cancer of the cervix, one must consider a similar approach in the patient with locally advanced squamous cancer of the vulva.

Several drug combinations have also been used in squamous vulvar cancer. These combinations consisted principally of drugs without clear evidence of single-agent activity in Phase II studies. Nevertheless, these combinations have been evaluated as initial therapy for patients with inoperable disease. Significant responses have allowed operative intervention in some patients. Combinations used in vulvar squamous cancer are listed in Table 20.10 (40,232,233). As noted above, the significant response rates observed with primary chemotherapy in inoperable disease presentations and the poor response rates in refractory disease should lead investi-

TABLE 20.10. *Combination chemotherapy regimens in squamous vulvar cancer*

Regimen	Dose and schedule	No. of patients entered	Complete response	Partial response	Investigator (ref.)
Bleomycin	15 mg/m^2 cont. IV days 1–3	22[a]	2	4	Belinson et al. (233)
Vincristine	1.4 mg/m^2 IV day 3				
Mitomycin C	10 mg/m^2 IV day 3				
Cisplatin	60 mg/m^2 IV day 3				
Bleomycin	5 mg IM days 1–5	28[b]	3	15	Durrant et al. (232)
Methotrexate	15 mg PO days 1 and 4				
CCNU	40 mg PO days 5–7				
Bleomycin	5 mg IV days 1–6	1	1	0	Shimizu et al. (40)
Vincristine	1 mg IV day 6				
Mitomycin C	10 mg IV day 6				
Cisplatin	100 mg IV day 6				

[a] Five of 6ix responses with no prior therapy; 1 of 16 responses in refractory disease.
[b] No patient with prior radiation therapy or chemotherapy; responses were the same for primary therapy and recurrences; eight patients had resectable disease after chemotherapy.

gators to the earlier consideration of using cytotoxic therapy in stage III and IV vulvar cancers. Toxicity with these regimens has been reported as being tolerable, although some patient selection for good performance status was probably operational. In the one well-reported trial, 64% of patients had mucositis (21% severe), and infections or fever occurred in 35% (232). Bleomycin-induced lung disease was responsible for one death. Patients should be selected who are at lowest risk for chemotherapy-associated toxicity (i.e., no concomitant disease, normal organ function, younger age).

There are increasing reports of the concomitant use of cytotoxic therapy with irradiation, usually as primary therapy in advanced and inoperable disease (Table 20.8). This approach may have increased impetus based on recent reports from several large randomized trials demonstrating superior outcome for combined chemoirradiation over radiation therapy alone in locally advanced squamous cancer of the cervix (133–135,210). It is not possible from such study designs to comment specifically on the effects of chemotherapy on the disease. Nevertheless, these studies are cited because chemotherapy may have played a role in the end result. The largest experience was recently reported by the GOG, in which 73 patients with T3 or T4 cancers were treated with split-course radiation therapy with concomitant chemotherapy [cisplatin, 75 mg/m^2 on day 1, and 5-fluorouracil (5-FU), 1,000 mg/m^2/d on days 1 to 5]. Irradiation of the primary tumor in a split course was followed by resection of residual primary tumor and inguinofemoral nodes. Those patients with unresectable groin nodes received chemoirradiation to both the primary tumor and involved nodes. Seven patients never underwent surgery for various reasons. After chemoirradiation, 46% of patients were grossly tumor free. Of the 54% with gross residual disease, only five had positive margins at resection. Only 3% of the patients completing planned chemoirradiation and surgery had residual

unresectable disease, and in only three patients was it not possible to preserve urinary and/or gastrointestinal continence. Survival data from this study remain immature, but demonstrated that this approach is feasible with acceptable toxicity (primarily decreased wound healing and enhanced cutaneous reactions) and with a possible decrease in the need for more radical surgery (136). Landoni et al. treated 58 advanced primary and 17 recurrent disease patients with 5-FU (750 mg/m^2/d on days 1 to 5) and mitomycin C (15 mg/m^2 on day 1) at the beginning of each of two courses of irradiation separated by 2 weeks (total dose of 54 Gy). Primary chemoradiation was followed by wide local excision and inguinal lymphadenectomy. A total of 89% of patients completed planned radiation therapy and chemotherapy, and 72% underwent surgery. Response was noted in 80%, and pathologic complete response was observed in both primary and nodes in 31%. Three treatment-related deaths were also recorded (200). Lupi et al. treated 31 patients with mitomycin C and 5-FU using the same doses as in the previous study and split-course irradiation to only 36 Gy. Response was noted in 29 of 31 (94%) patients, but postoperative morbidity was noted in 65% and mortality in 14%. Of patients with positive inguinal nodes, 55% (five of nine) were rendered pathologically disease free at surgery. Recurrence was noted in 32%, and survival was not reported (201). Whalen et al. treated 19 patients with clinical stage III/IV vulvar carcinoma and clinically negative nodes with 45 to 50 Gy and 5-FU (1,000 mg/m^2/d continuous intravenous infusion over 96 hours weeks 1 and 5) and mitomycin C (10 mg/m^2 on day 1 only). A response rate of 90% and a local control rate of 74% were observed. Survival was not reported (205). Cunningham et al. treated 14 patients not candidates for radical vulvectomy with cisplatin (50 mg/m^2) and 5-FU (1,000 mg/m^2/d over 96 h) in combination with 50 to 65 Gy irradiation to vulva and bilateral groins and 45 to 50 Gy to the pelvis. Surgery was not performed in complete responders. There was a 64% complete-response rate and only one recurrence in that group, with mean follow-up of 36 months. All partial responders died of disease. Toxicity was moderate, with five patients requiring treatment delay due to desquamative reactions and one late bowel complication (194). Thomas and associates treated 33 patients with stage II, III, or IV disease: nine with definitive radiation therapy and chemotherapy as a preoperative adjuvant, nine with definitive radiation therapy and chemotherapy, and 15 with radiation therapy and chemotherapy after local recurrence following surgery. Chemotherapy consisted of infusional 5-FU given at a dose of 1,000 $mg/m^2/d$ over 4 to 5 days; six patients also received low-dose mitomycin C. Various doses and techniques of irradiation were used. Seven of nine patients treated with neoadjuvant therapy remained free of disease at 5 to 45 months; one after local excision of a vulvar recurrence. Of the nine patients receiving curative-intent radiation therapy and chemotherapy, six were alive without evidence of disease at 5 to 43 months. Of the 15 patients treated after recurrence, seven were alive without evidence of disease for 5 to 45 months. It is impossible to determine the role of chemotherapy in these patients, but it appears that combined-modality therapy offers the potential for long-term disease control without radical surgery (204).

RESULTS OF THERAPY

The overall results of therapy for women with squamous cancers of the vulva are excellent. Approximately two-thirds of patients present with early-stage tumors. Five-year survival rates of 80% to 90% are routinely reported for stage I and II disease (234). As anticipated, survival rates for patients with advanced disease are poor: 60% for stage III cases and 15% for stage IV (Fig. 20.26).

Several strategies to enhance survival for women with vulvar cancer are evident. High-risk patients can be educated and screened more consistently for the development of early cancer. Women with HPV infections, *in situ* vulvar disease, long smoking history, and other genital neoplasms are at risk for developing vulvar cancer. Careful screening targeted at women with these high-risk factors may lead to improvements in early diagnosis.

The survival rate for women with nodal spread is one-half that of women without nodal disease who have similarly sized primary tumors (Fig. 20.27). A more precise understanding of lymphatic flow and tumor spread might enable us to identify better those patients with subclinical metastases who now present with unanticipated groin or distant failure. Better treatment options for node-positive patients are needed, possibly multimodality therapy that incorporates irradiation, chemotherapy, or both with surgery.

MANAGEMENT OF OTHER VULVAR MALIGNANCIES

Because nonsquamous vulvar malignancies are exceedingly rare, relatively little definitive information is available regarding optimal treatment and long-term outcome. Most available information is derived from isolated case reports or small series spanning long periods of time.

Malignant Melanoma

Malignant melanoma is the second most common vulvar malignancy (91,93,235). Vulvar melanomas are most commonly seen in postmenopausal white women. Typical presentations include an asymptomatic pigmented lesion or an identified mass that may be painful or bleeding (Fig. 20.28). A definitive diagnosis is established by biopsy.

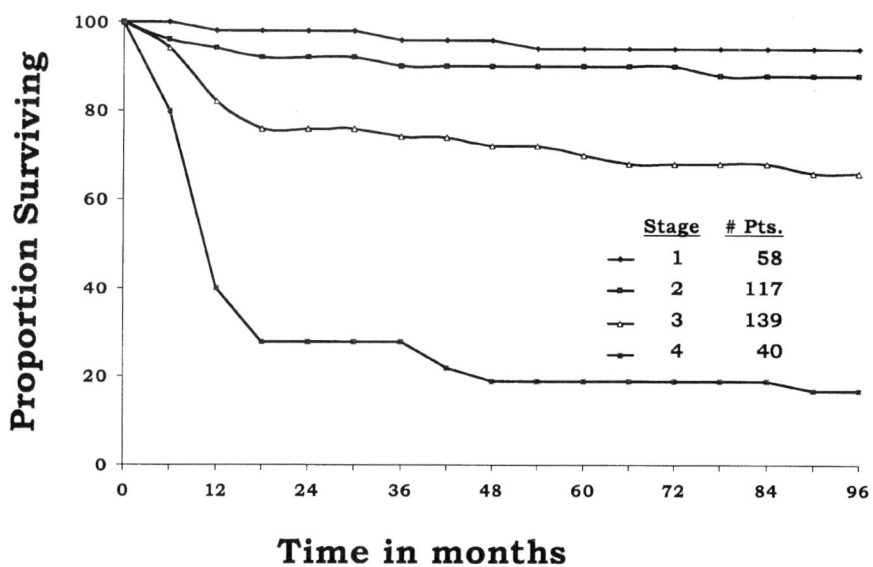

Stage	# Pts.
1	58
2	117
3	139
4	40

FIG. 20.26. Invasive squamous vulvar carcinoma. Survival by FIGO stage. (Patients treated at M.D. Anderson Cancer Center 1944–1990; data courtesy of F. N. Rutledge.)

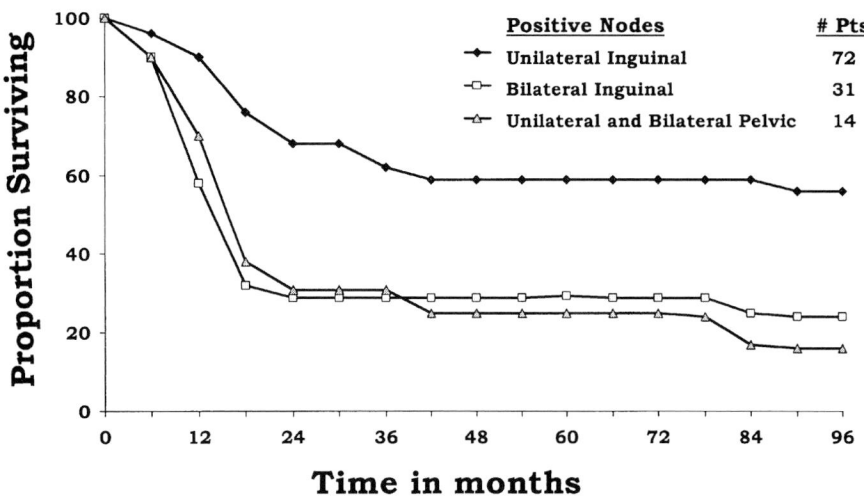

FIG. 20.27. Invasive squamous vulvar carcinoma. Survival of patients with positive nodes. (Data courtesy of F. N. Rutledge.)

Immunohistochemical staining for melanoma-specific antigen and S100 may be helpful in uncertain cases. Melanomas may arise from existing pigmented vulvar lesions or as new isolated primary tumors. Consequently, any pigmented vulvar lesion should be considered for biopsy. Melanomas are staged according to one of the three available microstaging systems, which base prognosis on either depth of local invasion or tumor thickness (Table 20.11). Inguinal lymphatic and distant metastases are frequent.

The primary treatment modality for vulvar melanoma is radical surgical excision. Radical vulvectomy with bilateral inguinofemoral lymphadenectomy has been the treatment of choice (93,235,236). Because most failures are distant, ultraradical local resection does not appear to enhance survival. As a result, more recent reviews recommend some form of hemivulvectomy or radical wide excision, with or without inguinal lymphadenectomy (237,238). Depth of invasion and the presence of ulceration are significant prognostic factors, and should be considered in treatment planning. Look et al. reported that none of the patients with lesion depth of ≤1.75 mm experienced a recurrence, and suggested that these patients could be treated with wide local excision. In contrast, all patients with lesion depth of >1.75 mm recurred despite radical tumor excision (239). Based on information derived from large series of patients with cutaneous melanomas at nongenital sites, regional lymphadenectomy should probably be considered a prognostic rather than a therapeutic procedure (240). Lymphadenectomy can be avoided in patients with superficial melanomas (level III), for whom the risk of metastatic disease is negligible. Sentinel lymph node identification and biopsy have been increasing applied to the surgical management of cutaneous malignant melanomas; however, data regarding sentinel lymph node biopsy for vulvar melanomas are insufficient.

Radiation therapy may be useful in enhancing local and regional control for some high-risk patients. Despite reported complete clinical response rates and local tumor control rates of 50% to 70% for patients with localized recurrences treated with radiation therapy, alone or in combination with hyperthermia, these modalities have rarely been used in the primary treatment of vulvar melanoma (241,242). Doses in the range of 40 to 50 Gy, delivered in fractions of 4 to 8 Gy (one to three weekly fractions), have been described as being more effective (243).

Systemic chemotherapy—in either an adjuvant or salvage setting—is considered to be palliative, but responses are truly rare and adverse effects may be significant. Biologic and immunologic approaches to the treatment of malignant melanoma are currently being evaluated. The Southwest Oncology Group reported their results of a randomized trial of an adjuvant allogeneic tumor vaccine in patients with

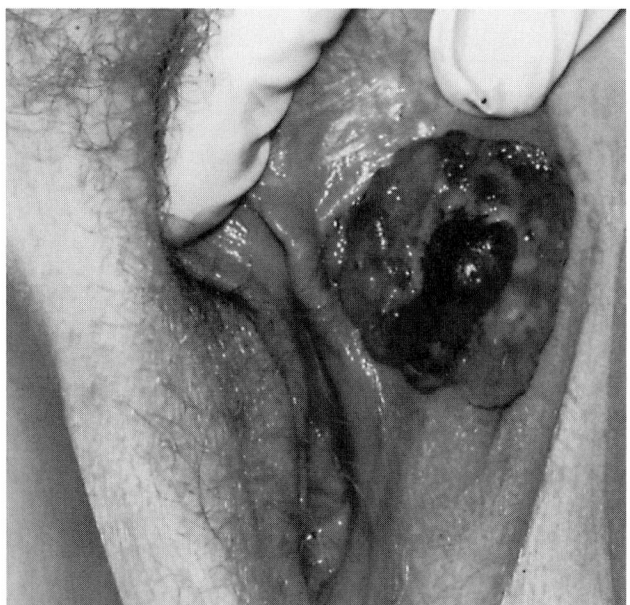

FIG. 20.28. Nodular, darkly pigmented malignant melanoma of the left labium majus.

TABLE 20.11. *Microstaging systems for vulvar melanomas*

Stage	Clark et al. (48)	Chung et al. (47)	Breslow (28)
I	Intraepithelial	Intraepithelial	<0.76 mm
II	Into papillary dermis	1 mm from granular layer	0.76–1.50 mm
III	Filling dermal papillae	12 mm from granular layer	1.51–2.25 mm
IV	Into reticular dermis	>2 mm from granular layer	2.26–3.00 mm
V	Into subcutaneous fat	Into subcutaneous fat	>3 mm

intermediate-thickness, node-negative melanoma. There was no evidence of improved disease-free survival among patients randomized to receive vaccine (244).

Overall survival rates in women with vulvar melanoma are approximately 50% (91,235,237). Patients with superficial lesions have an excellent chance for cure after surgical resection, but patients with deeper lesions or metastases at the time of diagnosis have a more limited prognosis. These patients are good candidates for investigational trials.

Verrucous Carcinoma

Verrucous carcinomas are locally invasive and rarely metastasize (245). Consequently, treatment by radical wide excision is usually curative (246). Local recurrence can occur, especially when the tumor has been inadequately resected. Although radiation therapy has been reported to cause anaplastic transformation in some cases of verrucous carcinoma, this finding has not been observed by others (247, 248).

Basal Cell Carcinoma

Basal cell carcinomas should be removed by excisional biopsy using a minimum surgical margin of 1 cm (249). Lymphatic or distant spread is exceedingly rare (250). Local recurrence may occur, particularly in tumors removed with suboptimal resection margins.

Adenocarcinoma

Patients presenting with apparent vulvar adenocarcinoma should first undergo an extensive clinical evaluation to determine whether the lesion in question represents a primary versus a metastatic tumor. Despite the paucity of data regarding the evaluation and treatment of vulvar adenocarcinoma, resection of localized disease by radical wide excision, hemivulvectomy, or radical vulvectomy seems appropriate (251). The incidence of groin node metastases is approximately 30% (252). Some form of inguinal lymphadenectomy should be included with primary surgical resection. Radiation therapy may have a role in enhancing local control for women with large primary tumors or inguinal metastases (24). The effectiveness of chemotherapy is unknown, although a single case report documents a response with pegylated liposomal doxorubicin (Doxil) in adenocarcinoma of the vulva (253).

Paget's Disease

Paget's disease is associated with an underlying invasive adenocarcinoma component in approximately 15% of cases (13,254,255). In addition, 20% to 30% of patients will have or will later develop an adenocarcinoma at another nonvulvar location (256,257). Observed sites of nonvulvar malignancies developing in patients with extramammary Paget's disease include breast, lung, colorectum, gastric, pancreas, and upper female genital tract. Screening and surveillance for tumors at these sites should be considered in all patients with Paget's disease.

Paget's disease should be resected with a wide margin. If underlying invasion is suspected, the deep margins should be extended to the perineal fascia. Some suggest careful assessment of the surgical margins using multiple frozen sections to ensure complete excision (258,259). This approach can be cumbersome and may not influence the long-term incidence of recurrence. Pierie et al. showed that patients with microscopic positive margins had a significantly higher rate of recurrence; however, with extended follow-up, all patients eventually recurred (260). Repeat local excision of recurrent disease is usually effective in the absence of invasion (261).

Vulvar Sarcomas

The specific histologic types of vulvar sarcoma are described in the pathology section above. All types of vulvar sarcoma are rare, but leiomyosarcoma, malignant fibrous histiocytoma, and rhabdomyosarcoma predominate (262, 263). Cures have occasionally been obtained with aggressive resection of either primary or locally recurrent disease. The results of regional and systemic therapy for leiomyosarcoma are disappointing. These patients are excellent candidates for clinical trials. Rhabdomyosarcoma seems to be more responsive to both chemotherapy and radiation. The current treatment of choice is to combine chemoradiation with limited surgical resection of residual disease (262,264).

Tumors Metastatic to the Vulva

Treatment of secondary vulvar tumors should be directed against the primary tumor. As with bulky vulvar cancers, a

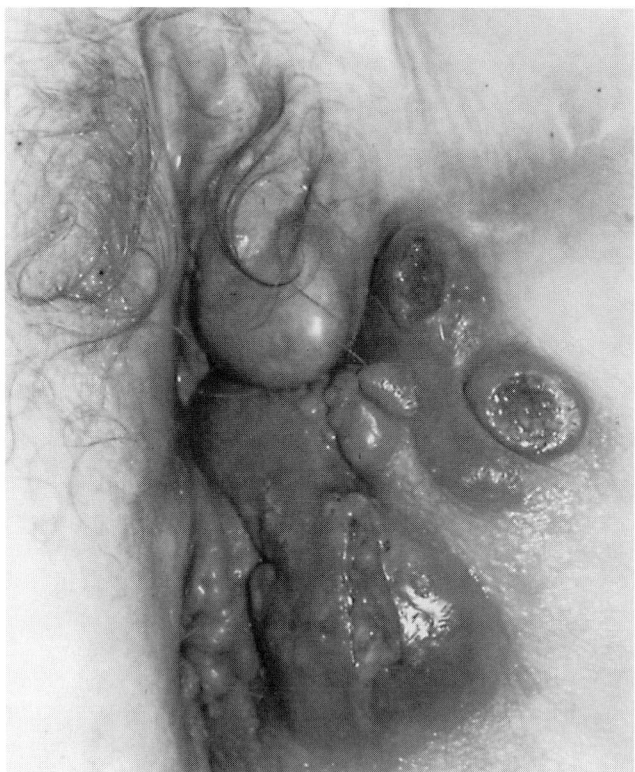

FIG. 20.29. Multiple in-transit lymphatic metastases from a cloacogenic carcinoma of the rectum. A large constricting lesion was evident on rectal examination.

multimodal approach seems to provide some opportunity for long-term survival along with enhanced local tumor control and organ preservation.

Cutaneous vulvar lymphatic metastases may occur as in-transit tumor emboli from anorectal tumors or as retrograde flow metastases when bulky tumors of the cervix or uterus obstruct the normal lymphatic drainage patterns (Fig. 20.29). These metastases are multiple and are often bilateral. Their histology reflects that of the primary tumor. Because this metastatic pattern is associated with advanced tumors, the primary tumor should be readily detectable by examination.

FUTURE DIRECTIONS

Vulvar cancer is an uncommon neoplastic disease and its relative rarity is a major obstacle in designing prospective randomized trials. Current trends in its management are focusing on a more individualized approach that emphasizes conservative vulvar surgical resection when feasible, the use of reconstructive procedures to preserve or restore vulvar function, potential reduction in groin complications through sentinel lymph node biopsy, and multimodality therapy for advanced or disseminated disease. Most data supporting these concepts are preliminary. Further investigation is likely to result in ongoing refinement of the criteria used to select patients for specific surgical procedures. The greatest gaps

in our present understanding of this disease and its treatment include (a) the uncertain role of infectious and epidemiologic factors in the development of the primary tumor; (b) the lack of consensus regarding the extent of groin dissection required to accurately assess lymphatic spread; (c) the lack of a well-defined management plan for patients with lymph node metastases; (d) the absence of proven systemic therapy for women with distant spread or recurrence; (e) scant information to evaluate the components and timing of combined-modality treatment; and (f) poor understanding of different forms of treatment on the psychosexual adjustment of patients. These all represent areas of current investigation. Additional clinical experience should help to establish a rational approach to therapy that maximizes the potential for cure while minimizing morbidity.

REFERENCES

1. Jones RW, Joura EA. Analyzing prior clinical events at presentation in 102 women with vulvar carcinoma: evidence of diagnostic delays. *J Reprod Med* 1999;44:766.
2. Warwick R, Williams PL, eds. *Gray's anatomy.* 35th ed. Philadelphia: WB Saunders, 1973.
3. Parry-Jones E. Lymphatics of the vulva. *J Obstet Gynecol Br Empire* 1963;70:751.
4. Plentl AA, Friedman EA, eds. *Lymphatic system of the female genitalia.* Philadelphia: WB Saunders, 1971.
5. Carter J, Carlson J, Fowler J, et al. Invasive vulvar tumors in young women: a disease of the immunosuppressed? *Gynecol Oncol* 1993;51:307.
6. Messing MJ, Gallup DG. Carcinoma of the vulva in young women. *Obstet Gynecol* 1995;86:51.
7. Franklin EW, Rutledge FD. Epidemiology of epidermoid carcinoma of the vulva. *Obstet Gynecol* 1972;39:165.
8. Brinton LA, Nasca PC, Mallin K, et al. Case-control study of cancer of the vulva. *Obstet Gynecol* 1990;75:859.
9. Kaufman RH, Dreesman GR, Burke J, et al. Herpes-virus–induced antigens in squamous-cell carcinoma in situ of the vulva. *N Engl J Med* 1981;305:483.
10. Ansink AC, Krul MRL, DeWeger RA, et al. Human papillomavirus, lichen sclerosus, and squamous cell carcinoma of the vulva: detection and prognostic significance. *Gynecol Oncol* 1994;52:180.
11. Downey GO, Okagaki T, Ostrow RS, et al. Condylomatous carcinoma of the vulva with special reference to human papillomavirus DNA. *Obstet Gynecol* 1988;72:68.
12. Bloss JD, Liao S-Y, Wilczynski SP, et al. Clinical and histologic features of vulvar carcinomas analyzed for human papillomavirus status: evidence that squamous cell carcinoma of the vulva has more than one etiology. *Hum Pathol* 1991;22:711.
13. Kurman RJ, Trimble CL, Shah KV. Human papillomavirus and the pathogenesis of vulvar carcinoma. *Curr Opin Obstet Gynecol* 1992;4:582.
14. Hording U, Junge J, Daugaard S, et al. Vulvar squamous cell carcinoma and papillomaviruses: indications for two different etiologies. *Gynecol Oncol* 1994;52:241.
15. Carli P, De Magnis A, Mannone F, et al. Vulvar carcinoma associated with lichen sclerosus: experience at the Florence, Italy vulvar clinic. *J Reprod Med* 2003;48:313.
16. Hart WR, Norris HJ, Helwig EB. Relation of lichen sclerosus et atrophicus of the vulva to development of carcinoma. *Obstet Gynecol* 1975;45:369.
17. Jones RW, Rowan DM. Vulvar intraepithelial neoplasia III: a clinical study of the outcome in 113 cases with relation to the later development of invasive vulvar carcinoma. *Obstet Gynecol* 1994;84:741.
18. Iversen T, Tretli S. Intraepithelial and invasive squamous cell neopla-

sia of the vulva: trends in incidence, recurrence, and survival rate in Norway. *Obstet Gynecol* 1998;91:969.

19. Stehman F, Bundy B, Thomas G, et al. Groin dissection versus groin radiation in carcinoma of the vulva: a Gynecologic Oncology Group study. *Int J Radiat Oncol Biol Phys* 1992;24:39.

20. Trimble CL, Hildesheim A, Brinton LA, et al. Heterogeneous etiology of squamous carcinoma of the vulva. *Obstet Gynecol* 1996;87:59.

21. Flowers LC, Wistuba II, Scurry J, et al. Genetic changes during multistage pathogenesis of human papillomavirus positive and negative vulvar carcinomas. *J Soc Gynecol Invest* 1999;6:213.

22. Hietanen SH, Kurvinen K, Syrjanen K, et al. Mutation of tumor suppressor gene p53 is frequently found in vulvar carcinoma cells. *Am J Obstet Gynecol* 1995;173:1477.

23. Mitchell MF, Prasad CJ, Silva EG, et al. Second genital primary squamous neoplasms in vulvar carcinoma: viral and histopathologic correlates. *Obstet Gynecol* 1993;81:13.

24. Creasman WT. New gynecologic cancer staging. *Gynecol Oncol* 1995;58:157.

25. Beahrs OH, Henson DE, Hutter RVP, et al., eds. *Manual for staging of cancer.* 4th ed. Philadelphia: JB Lippincott Co, 1992.

26. Wilkinson EJ. Superficial invasive carcinoma of the vulva. *Clin Obstet Gynecol* 1985;28:188.

27. Zaino RJ. Carcinoma of the vulva, urethra and Bartholin's gland. In: Wilkinson EJ, ed. *Pathology of the vulva and vagina: contemporary issues in surgical pathology.* Vol 9. New York: Churchill Livingstone, 1987;119.

28. Kneale BL. Microinvasive cancer of the vulva: report of the International Society for Study of Vulvar Disease Task Force, 7th Congress. *J Reprod Med* 1984;29:454.

29. Iversen T, Aas M. Lymph drainage from the vulva. *Gynecol Oncol* 1983;16:179.

30. Way S. The anatomy of the lymphatic drainage of the vulva and its influence on the radical operation of carcinoma. *Ann R Coll Surg Engl* 1948;187:3.

31. Way S. *Malignant disease of the female genital tract.* New York: Churchill Livingstone, 1951.

32. Levenback C, Burke TW, Morris M, et al. Potential applications of intraoperative lymphatic mapping in vulvar cancer. *Gynecol Oncol* 1995;59:216.

33. Homesley HD, Bundy BN, Sedlis A, et al. Prognostic factors for groin node metastasis in squamous cell carcinoma of the vulva (a Gynecologic Oncology Group study). *Gynecol Oncol* 1993;49:279.

34. Dvoretsky PM, Bonfiglio TA, Helmkamp F, et al. The pathology of superficially invasive thin vulvar squamous cell carcinoma. *Int J Gynecol Pathol* 1984;3:331.

35. Wilkinson EJ, Kneale B, Lynch PJ. Report of the ISSVD Terminology Committee. *J Reprod Med* 1986;1:973.

36. Wilkinson EJ, Rico MJ, Pierson KK. Microinvasive carcinoma of the vulva. *Int J Gynecol Pathol* 1982;1:29.

37. Scully RE, Bonfiglio TA, Kurman RJ, et al. *Histological typing of female genital tract tumors. World Health Organization international histological classification of tumors.* 2nd ed. New York: Springer-Verlag, 1994.

38. Curry SL, Wharton JT, Rutledge F. Positive lymph nodes in vulvar squamous carcinoma. *Gynecol Oncol* 1980;9:63.

39. Sedlis A, Homesley H, Bundy BN, et al. Positive groin lymph nodes in superficial squamous cell vulvar cancer. *Am J Obstet Gynecol* 1987;156:1159.

40. Shimizu Y, Hasumi K, Masubuchi K. Effective chemotherapy consisting of bleomycin, vincristine, mitomycin C and cisplatin (BOMP) for a patient with inoperable vulvar cancer. *Gynecol Oncol* 1990;36:423.

41. Russell AH, Mesic JB, Scudder SA, et al. Synchronous radiation and cytotoxic chemotherapy for locally advanced or recurrent squamous cancer of the vulva. *Gynecol Oncol* 1992;47:14.

42. Steeper TA, Rosai J. Aggressive angiomyxoma of the female pelvis and perineum. *Am J Surg Pathol* 1983;7:463.

43. Wilkinson EJ. Neoplastic diseases of the vulva. In: Kurman RJ, ed. *Blaustein's pathology of the female genital tract.* 4th ed. New York: Springer-Verlag, 1994:96.

44. American Joint Commission on Cancer. *Cancer staging manual.* 6th ed. Philadelphia: Lippincott–Raven Publishers, 2002.

45. Ehrmann RL, Dwyer IM, Yavner BA, Hannock WW. An immunoperoxidase study of laminin and Type IV collagen distribution in carcinoma of the cervix and vulva. *Obstet Gynecol* 1988;72:257.

46. Hendricks JB, Wilkinson EJ, Drew P, et al. Ki-67 expression in vulvar carcinoma. *Int J Gynecol Pathol* 1994;13:205.

47. Drew PA, Al-Abbadi MA, Orlando C, et al. Prognostic factors in carcinoma of the vulva: a clinicopathologic and DNA flow cytometric study. *Int J Gynecol Pathol* 1996;15:235.

48. Wilkinson, EJ. Protocol for the examination of specimens from patients with carcinomas and malignant melanomas of the vulva: a basis for checklists. Cancer Committee of the American College of Pathologists. *Arch Pathol Lab Med* 2000;124:51.

49. Ambros RA, Kallakury BVS, Malfetano J, Mihm MC Jr. Cytokine, cell adhesion receptor, and tumor suppressor gene expression in vulvar squamous carcinoma: correlation with prominent fibromyxoid stromal response. *Int J Gynecol Pathol* 1996;15:320.

50. Ambrose RM, Malfetano J, Mihm MC. Clinicopathologic features of vulvar squamous cell carcinomas exhibiting prominent fibromyxoid stromal response. *Int J Gynecol Pathol* 1996;15:137.

51. Carter JJ, Koutsky LA, Wipf GC, et al. The natural history of human papillomavirus type 16 capsid antibodies among a cohort of university women. *J Infect Dis* 1996;174:927.

52. Lerma E, Esteller M, Matis-Guiu X, et al. P16 methylation, pRb and P53 in squamous cell carcinoma of the vulva. *Mod Pathol* 1999;12:119A.

53. Steeper TA, Piscioli F, Rosai J. Squamous cell carcinoma with sarcoma-like stroma of the female genital tract: clinicopathologic study of four cases. *Cancer* 1983;52:890.

54. Yang B, Hart WR. Vulvar intra-epithelial neoplasia of the simplex (differentiated) type: a clinicopathologic study including analysis of HPV and p53 expression. *Am J Surg Pathol* 2000;24:429.

55. Kurman RJ, Toki T, Schiffman MH. Basaloid and warty carcinomas of the vulva: distinctive types of squamous cell carcinoma frequently associated with human papillomaviruses. *Am J Surg Pathol* 1993;17:133.

56. Underwood JW, Adcock LL, Okagaki T. Adenosquamous carcinoma of skin appendages (adenoid squamous cell carcinoma, pseudoglandular squamous cell carcinoma, adenoacanthoma of sweat gland of Lever) of the vulva: a clinical and ultrastructural study. *Cancer* 1978;42:1851.

57. Wilkinson EJ, Croker BP, Friedrich EG Jr, Franzini DA. Two distinct pathologic types of giant cell tumor of the vulva: a report of two cases. *J Reprod Med* 1988;33:519.

58. Copas P, Dyer M, Comas FV, Hall DJ. Spindle cell carcinoma of the vulva. *Diagn Gynecol Obstet* 1982;4:235.

59. Berman ML, Soper JT, Creasman WT, et al. Conservative surgical management of superficially invasive Stage I vulvar carcinoma. *Gynecol Oncol* 1989;35:352.

60. Niu W, Heller DS, D'Cruz C. Lymphoepithelioma-like carcinoma of the vulva. *J Lower Genital Tract Disease* 2003;7:184.

61. Rando RF, Sedlacek TV, Hunt J, et al. Verrucous carcinoma of the vulva associated with an unusual type 6 human papillomavirus. *Obstet Gynecol* 1986;67:70S.

62. Dudzinski MR, Askin FB, Fowler WC Jr. Giant basal cell carcinoma of the vulva. *Obstet Gynecol* 1984;63:57S.

63. Merino MJ, LiVolsi VA, Schwartz PE, Rudnicki J. Adenoid basal cell carcinoma of the vulva. *Int J Gynecol Pathol* 1982;1:299.

64. Jacobs DM, Sandles LG, LeBoit PE. Sebaceous carcinoma arising from Bowen's disease of the vulva. *Arch Dermatol* 1986;122:1191.

65. Bottles K, Lacey CG, Goldberg J, et al. Merkel cell carcinoma of the vulva. *Obstet Gynecol* 1984;63:61S.

66. Levin W, Goldberg G, Altaras M, et al. The use of concomitant chemotherapy and radiotherapy prior to surgery in advanced stage carcinoma of the vulva. *Gynecol Oncol* 1986;25:20.

67. Taylor RN, Lacey CG, Shuman MA. Adenocarcinoma of Skene's duct associated with a systemic coagulopathy. *Gynecol Oncol* 1985;22:250.

68. Wharton JT, Gallager S, Rutledge RN. Microinvasive carcinoma of the vulva. *Am J Obstet Gynecol* 1974;118:159.

69. Klein AE, Bauer TW, Marks KE, Belinson JL. Papillary clear cell adenocarcinoma of the groin arising from endometriosis. *Clin Orthop Relat Res* 1999;361:192.

70. Woolcott RJ, Henry RJ, Houghton CR. Malignant melanoma of the vulva: Australian experience. *J Reprod Med* 1988;33:699.

71. Nadji M, Ganji P. The application of immunoperoxidase techniques in the evaluation of vulvar and vaginal disease in the evaluation of the vulva and vagina. In: Wilkinson EJ, ed. *Contemporary issues in surgical pathology.* Vol 9. New York: Churchill Livingstone, 1987: 239.

72. Van der Putte SCJ. Mammary-like glands of the vulva and their disorders. *Int J Gynecol Pathol* 1994;13:150.

73. Van der Putte SCJ, van-Gorp HM. Cysts of mammary-like glands in the vulva. *Int J Gynecol Pathol* 1995;14:184.

74. Cho D, Buscema J, Rosenshein NB, et al. Primary breast cancer of the vulva. *Obstet Gynecol* 1985;66:79S.

75. Fox H, Wells M, Harris M, et al. Enteric tumors of the lower female genital tract: a report of three cases. *Histopathology* 1988;12:167.

76. Nagar HA, McKinney KA, Price JH, et al. Enteric epithelium progressing through dysplasia to adenocarcinoma within the vagina. *Eur J Surg Oncol* 1999;25:106.

77. Wilkinson EJ, Brown HM. Vulvar Paget disease of urothelial origin: a report of three cases and a proposed classification of vulvar Paget disease. *Hum Pathol* 2002;33:549.

78. Powell FC, Bjornsson J, Doyle JA, Cooper AJ. Genital Paget's disease and urinary tract malignancy. *J Am Acad Dermatol* 1985;13:84.

79. Malik S, Wilkinson EJ. Pseudopaget's disease of the vulva: a case report. *J Lower Genital Dis* 1999;3:201.

80. Chan TY, Alt SZ, Mandavilli SR, et al. Immunohistochemical analysis of Paget's disease of the vulva: implications for histogenetics and diagnosis. *Mod Pathol* 1999;12:114A.

81. Chen CH, Ji H, Suh KW, et al. Control of HPV-associated malignancies grown in liver with DNA vaccine. *Mod Pathol* 1999;112:53A.

82. Crawford D, Nimmo M, Thomson T, et al. Vulvar Paget's disease: prognostic factors. *Mod Pathol* 1999;12:114A.

83. Cavanagh D, Shepherd JH. The place of pelvic exenteration in the primary management of advanced carcinoma of the vulva. *Gynecol Oncol* 1982;13:318.

84. Brown HM, Wilkinson EJ. Uroplakin-III to distinguish vulvar Paget disease secondary to urothelial carcinoma. *Hum Pathol* 2002;33:545.

85. Brainard JA, Hart WR. Proliferative squamous cell lesions in anogenital Paget's disease. *Mod Pathol* 1999;12:113A.

86. Shah KD, Tabibzadch SS, Gerber MA. Immunohistochemical distinction of Paget's disease from Bowen's disease and superficial spreading melanoma with the use of monoclonal cytokeratin antibodies. *Am J Clin Pathol* 1987;88:689.

87. Raju RR, Goldblum JR, Hart WR. Pagetoid squamous cell carcinoma in situ (pagetoid Bowen's disease) of the external genitalia. *Int J Gynecol Pathol* 2003;22:127.

88. Chen YH, Wong TW, Lee JY. Depigmented genital extramammary Paget's disease: a possible histogenetic link to Toker's clear cells and clear cell papulosis. *J Cutan Pathol* 2001;28:105.

89. Sison-Torre EQ, Ackerman AB. Melanosis of the vulva: a clinical simulator of malignant melanoma. *Am J Dermatopathol* 1985;7:51.

90. Benda JA, Platz CE, Anderson B. Malignant melanoma of the vulva: a clinical pathologic review of 16 cases. *Int J Gynecol Pathol* 1986; 5:202.

91. Podratz KC, Gaffey TA, Symmonds RE, et al. Melanoma of the vulva: an update. *Gynecol Oncol* 1983;16:153.

92. Johnson TL, Kumar N, White CD. Prognostic features of vulvar melanoma: a clinicopathologic analysis. *Int J Gynecol Pathol* 1986;5: 110.

93. Chung AF, Woodruff JM, Lewis JL Jr. Malignant melanoma of the vulva: a report of 44 cases. *Obstet Gynecol* 1975;45:638.

94. Breslow A. Thickness, cross-sectional area and depth of invasion in the prognosis of cutaneous melanoma. *Ann Surg* 1970;172:902.

95. Beller U, Demopoulos RI, Bechnan EM. Vulvovaginal melanoma: a clinicopathologic study. *J Reprod Med* 1986;31:315.

96. Jiveskog S, Ragnarsson-Olding B, Platz A, Ringborg U. N-ras mutations are common in melanomas from sun-exposed skin of humans but rare in mucosal membranes or unexposed skin. *J Invest Dermatol* 1998;111:757.

97. Nielsen GP, Young RH. Mesenchymal tumors and tumor-like lesions of the female genital tract: a selective review with emphasis on recently described entities. *Int J Gynecol Pathol* 2001;20:105.

98. Nielsen GP, Rosenberg AE, Koerner FC, et al. Smooth-muscle tumors of the vulva: a clinicopathological study of 25 cases and review of the literature. *Am J Surg Pathol* 1996;20:779.

99. Nirenberg A, Ostor AG, Slavin J, et al. Primary vulvar sarcomas. *Int J Gynecol Pathol* 1995;14:55.

100. Taylor RN, Bottles K, Miller TR, et al. Malignant fibrous histiocytoma of the vulva. *Obstet Gynecol* 1985;66:145.

101. Perrone T, Swanson PE, Twiggs L, et al. Malignant rhabdoid tumor of the vulva: is distinction from epithelioid sarcoma possible? *Am J Surg Pathol* 1989;13:848.

102. LiVolsi VA, Brooks JJ. Soft tissue tumors of the vulva. In: Wilkinson EJ, ed. *Pathology of the vulva and vagina: contemporary issues in surgical pathology.* Vol. 9. New York: Churchill Livingstone, 1987: 209.

103. Cockerell CJ, LeBoit PE. Bacillary angiomatosis: a newly characterized, pseudoneoplastic, infectious, cutaneous vascular disorder. *J Am Acad Dermatol* 1990;22:501.

104. Trope C, Johnsson JE, Larsson G, et al. Bleomycin alone or combined with mitomycin C in treatment of advanced or recurrent squamous cell carcinoma of the vulva. *Cancer Treat Rep* 1980;64:639.

105. Ungerleider RS, Donaldson SS, Warnke RA, et al. Endodermal sinus tumor: the Stanford experience and the first reported case arising in the vulva. *Cancer* 1978;41:1627.

106. Neto AG, Deavers MT, Silva EG, Malpica A. Metastatic tumors of the vulva: a clinicopathologic study of 66 cases. *Am J Surg Pathol* 2003;27:799.

107. Levine RL. Urethral cancer. *Cancer* 1980;45:1965.

108. Boutselis JG. Radical vulvectomy for invasive squamous cell carcinoma of the vulva. *Obstet Gynecol* 1972;39:827.

109. Collins CG, Lee FYL, Lopez JJ. Invasive carcinoma of the vulva with lymph node metastases. *Am J Obstet Gynecol* 1971;109:446.

110. Iversen T, Aalders JG, Christensen A, et al. Squamous cell carcinoma of the vulva: a review of 424 patients, 1956–1974. *Gynecol Oncol* 1980;9:271.

111. Kurzl R, Messerer D. Prognostic factors in squamous cell carcinoma of the vulva: a multivariate analysis. *Gynecol Oncol* 1989;32:143.

112. Malfetano JH, Piver S, Tsukada Y, Reese P. Univariate and multivariate analyses of 5-year survival, recurrence, and inguinal node metastases in Stage I and II vulvar carcinoma. *J Surg Oncol* 1985;30:124.

113. Podratz KC, Symmonds RE, Taylor WF. Carcinoma of the vulva: analysis of treatment failures. *Am J Obstet Gynecol* 1982;143:340.

114. Binder SW, Huang I, Fu YS, et al. Risk factors for the development of lymph node metastasis in vulvar squamous carcinoma. *Gynecol Oncol* 1990;37:9.

115. Donaldson ES, Powell DE, Hanson MB, et al. Prognostic parameters in invasive vulvar cancer. *Gynecol Oncol* 1981;11:184.

116. Hacker NF, Berek JS, Lagasse LD, et al. Individualization of treatment for Stage I squamous cell vulvar carcinoma. *Obstet Gynecol* 1984; 63:155.

117. Parker RT, Duncan I, Rampone J, et al. Operative management of early invasive epidermoid carcinoma of the vulva. *Am J Obstet Gynecol* 1975;123:349.

118. Buscema J, Stern JL, Woodruff JD. Early invasive carcinoma of the vulva. *Am J Obstet Gynecol* 1981;140:563.

119. Chu J, Tamimi HK, Ek M, Figge D. Stage I vulvar cancer: criteria for microinvasion. *Obstet Gynecol* 1982;59:716.

120. Hoffman JS, Kumar NB, Morley GW. Microinvasive squamous carcinoma of the vulva: search for a definition. *Obstet Gynecol* 1983;61: 615.

121. Magrina JF, Webb MJ, Gaffey TA, et al. Stage I squamous cell cancer of the vulva. *Am J Obstet Gynecol* 1979;134:453.

122. Ross MJ, Ehrmann RL. Histologic prognosticators in Stage I squamous cell carcinoma of the vulva. *Obstet Gynecol* 1987;70:774.

123. Zucker PK, Berkowitz RS. The issue of microinvasive squamous cell carcinoma of the vulva: an evaluation of the criteria of diagnosis and methods of therapy. *Obstet Gynecol Surv* 1985;40:136.

124. Heaps JM, Fu YS, Montz FJ, et al. Surgical-pathologic variables predictive of local recurrence in squamous cell carcinoma of the vulva. *Gynecol Oncol* 1990;38:309.

125. Farias-Eisner R, Cirisano FD, Grouse D, et al. Conservative and individualized surgery for early squamous carcinoma of the vulva: the treatment of choice for Stage I and II (T1–2 N0–1M0) disease. *Gynecol Oncol* 1994;53:55.

126. Figge DC, Tamimi HK, Greer BE. Lymphatic spread in carcinoma of the vulva. *Am J Obstet Gynecol* 1985;152:387.

127. Hacker NF, Berek JS, Lagasse L, et al. Management of regional lymph

nodes and their prognostic influence in vulvar cancer. *Obstet Gynecol* 1983;61:408.

128. Rutledge FN, Mitchell MF, Munsell MF, et al. Prognostic indicators for invasive carcinoma of the vulva. *Gynecol Oncol* 1991;42:239.

129. Taussig FJ. Cancer of the vulva: an analysis of 155 cases. *Am J Obstet Gynecol* 1940;40:764.

130. Way S. Carcinoma of the vulva. *Am J Obstet Gynecol* 1960;79:692.

131. Burke TW, Stringer CA, Gershenson DM, et al. Radical wide excision and selective inguinal node dissection for squamous cell carcinoma of the vulva. *Gynecol Oncol* 1990;38:328.

132. DiSaia PJ, Creasman WT, Rich WM. An alternative approach to early cancer of the vulva. *Am J Obstet Gynecol* 1979;133:825.

133. Keys HM, Bundy BN, Stehman FB, et al. Cisplatin, radiation, and adjuvant hysterectomy compared with radiation and adjuvant hysterectomy for bulky stage IB cervical carcinoma. *N Engl J Med* 1999; 340:1154.

134. Peters WA, Liu PY, Barrett RJ, et al. Concurrent chemotherapy and pelvic radiation therapy compared with pelvic radiation therapy alone as adjuvant therapy after radical surgery in high-risk early-stage cancer of the cervix. *J Clin Oncol* 2000;18:1606.

135. Rose PG, Bundy BN, Watkins EB, et al. Concurrent cisplatin-based radiotherapy and chemotherapy for locally advanced cervical cancer. *N Engl J Med* 1999;340:1144.

136. Moore DH, Thomas GM, Montana GS, et al. Preoperative chemoradiation for advanced vulvar cancer: A phase II study of the Gynecologic Oncology Group. *Int J Radiat Oncol Biol Phys* 1998;42:1317.

137. Kelley JL III, Burke TW, Tornos C, et al. Minimally invasive vulvar carcinoma: an indication for conservative surgical therapy. *Gynecol Oncol* 1991;144:240.

138. Chafe W, Richards A, Morgan L, Wilkinson E. Unrecognized invasive carcinoma in vulvar intraepithelial neoplasia (VIN). *Gynecol Oncol* 1988;31:154.

139. Modesitt SC, Waters AB, Walton L, et al. Vulvar intraepithelial neoplasia III: occult cancer and the impact of margin status on recurrence. *Obstet Gynecol* 1998;92:962.

140. Morley GW. Infiltrative carcinoma of the vulva: results of surgical treatment. *Am J Obstet Gynecol* 1976;124:874.

141. Podratz KC, Symmonds RE, Taylor WF, et al. Carcinoma of the vulva: analysis of treatment and survival. *Obstet Gynecol* 1983;61:63.

142. Figge CD, Gaudenz R. Invasive carcinoma of the vulva. *Am J Obstet Gynecol* 1974;119:382.

143. Rutledge F, Smith JP, Franklin EW. Carcinoma of the vulva. *Am J Obstet Gynecol* 1970;106:1117.

144. Homesley HD, Bundy BN, Sedlis A, Adcock L. Radiation therapy versus pelvic node resection for carcinoma of the vulva with positive groin nodes. *Obstet Gynecol* 1986;68:733.

145. Hacker NF, Van der Velden J. Conservative management of early vulvar cancer. *Cancer* 1993;71:1673.

146. Iversen T, Abeler V, Aalders J. Individualized treatment of Stage I carcinoma of the vulva. *Obstet Gynecol* 1981;57:85.

147. Burke TW, Levenback C, Coleman RC, et al. Surgical therapy of T1 and T2 vulvar carcinoma: further experience with radical wide excision and selective inguinal lymphadenectomy. *Gynecol Oncol* 1995; 57:215.

148. Stehman FB, Bundy BN, Dvoretsky PM, Creasman T. Early Stage I carcinoma of the vulva treated with ipsilateral superficial inguinal lymphadenectomy and modified radical hemivulvectomy: a prospective study of the Gynecologic Oncology Group. *Obstet Gynecol* 1992; 79:490.

149. Morris JM. A formula for selective lymphadenectomy. *Obstet Gynecol* 1977;50:152.

150. Hacker NF, Leuchter RS, Berek JS, et al. Radical vulvectomy and bilateral inguinal lymphadenectomy through separate groin incisions. *Obstet Gynecol* 1981;58:574.

151. Levenback C, Burke TW, Gershenson DM, et al. Intraoperative lymphatic mapping for vulvar cancer. *Obstet Gynecol* 1994;84:163.

152. Barton DPJ, Berman C, Cavanagh D, et al. Lymphoscintigraphy in vulvar cancer: a pilot study. *Gynecol Oncol* 1992;46:341.

153. DeCesare SL, Fiorica JV, Roberts WS, et al. A pilot study utilizing intraoperative lymphoscintigraphy for identification of the sentinel lymph nodes in vulvar cancer. *Gynecol Oncol* 1997;66:425.

154. Cabanas RM. An approach for the treatment of penile carcinoma. *Cancer* 1977;39:456.

155. Morton D, Wen D, Cochran A. Management of early-stage melanoma by intraoperative lymphatic mapping and selective lymphadenectomy: an alternative to routine elective lymphadenectomy or 'watch and wait.' *Surg Oncol Clin North Am* 1992;1:247.

156. Makar APH, Scheistroen M, van den Weyngaert D, Trope CG. Surgical management of stage I and II vulvar cancer: the role of the sentinel node biopsy. *Int J Gynecol Cancer* 2001;11:255.

157. DeCicco C, Sideri M, Grana C, et al. Sentinel node biopsy in early vulvar cancer. *Br J Cancer* 2000;82:295.

158. Sliutz G, Reinthaller A, Lantzsch T, et al. Lymphatic mapping of sentinel nodes in early vulvar cancer. *Gynecol Oncol* 2002;84:449.

159. Levenback C, Coleman RL, Burke TW, et al. Intraoperative lymphatic mapping and sentinel node identification with blue dye in patients with vulvar cancer. *Gynecol Oncol* 2001;83:276.

160. Moore RG, Depasquale SE, Steinhoff MM, et al. Sentinel node identification and the ability to detect metastatic tumor to inguinal lymph nodes in squamous cell cancer of the vulva. *Gynecol Oncol* 2003;89: 475.

161. De Hulla JA, Hollema H, Piers DA, et al. Sentinel lymph node procedure is highly accurate in squamous cell carcinoma of the vulva. *J Clin Oncol* 2000;18:2811.

162. Hopkins MP, Reid GC, Morley GW. The surgical management of recurrent squamous cell carcinoma of the vulva. *Obstet Gynecol* 1990; 75:1001.

163. Piura B, Masotina A, Murdoch J, et al. Recurrent squamous cell carcinoma of the vulva: a study of 73 cases. *Gynecol Oncol* 1993;48:189.

164. Abitol MM. Carcinoma of the vulva: improvements in the surgical approach. *Am J Obstet Gynecol* 1973;117:483.

165. Burke TW, Morris M, Levenback C, et al. Closure of complex vulvar defects using local rhomboid flaps. *Obstet Gynecol* 1994;84:1043.

166. Burrell MO, Franklin EW III, Campion MJ, et al. The modified radical vulvectomy with groin dissection: an eight-year experience. *Am J Obstet Gynecol* 1988;159:715.

167. Siller BS, Alvarez RD, Conner WD, et al. T2/3 vulva cancer: a case-control study of triple incision versus en bloc radical vulvectomy and inguinal lymphadenectomy. *Gynecol Oncol* 1995;57:335.

168. Borgno G, Micheletti L, Barbero M, et al. Topographic distribution of groin lymph nodes: a study of 50 female cadavers. *J Reprod Med* 1990;35:1127.

169. Rouzier R, Haddad B, Dubernard G, et al. Inguinofemoral dissection for carcinoma of the vulva: effect of modifications of extent and technique on morbidity and survival. *J Am Coll Surg* 2003;196:442.

170. Buechler DA, Kline JC, Tynes JC, et al. Treatment of recurrent carcinoma of the vulva. *Gynecol Oncol* 1979;8:180.

171. Miller B, Morris M, Levenback C, et al. Pelvic exenteration for primary and recurrent vulvar cancer. *Gynecol Oncol* 1995;58:189.

172. Phillips B, Buchsbaum JH, Lifshitz S. Pelvic exenteration for vulvovaginal carcinoma. *Am J Obstet Gynecol* 1981;141:1038.

173. Thornton WN, Flanagan WL Jr. Pelvic exenteration in the treatment of advanced malignancy of the vulva. *Am J Obstet Gynecol* 1973; 117:774.

174. Burke TW, Morris M, Roh MS, et al. Perineal reconstruction using single gracilis myocutaneous flaps. *Gynecol Oncol* 1995;57:221.

175. Barnhill DR, Hoskins WJ, Metz P. Use of the rhomboid flap after partial vulvectomy. *Obstet Gynecol* 1983;62:444.

176. Helm CW, Hatch KD, Partridge EE, Shingleton HM. The rhomboid flap for repair of the perineal defect after radical vulvar surgery. *Gynecol Oncol* 1993;50:164.

177. Achauer BM, Braly P, Berman ML, DiSaia PJ. Immediate vaginal reconstruction following resection for malignancy using the gluteal thigh flap. *Gynecol Oncol* 1984;19:79.

178. Ballon SC, Donaldson RC, Roberts JA. Reconstruction of the vulva using a myocutaneous graft. *Gynecol Oncol* 1979;7:123.

179. Chafe W, Fowler WC, Walton LA, Currie JL. Radical vulvectomy with use of tensor fascia lata myocutaneous flap. *Am J Obstet Gynecol* 1983;145:207.

180. Patsner B, Hetzler P. Postradical vulvectomy reconstruction using the inferiorly based transverse rectus abdominis (TRAM) flap: a preliminary experience. *Gynecol Oncol* 1994;55:78.

181. Potkul RK, Barnes WA, Barter JF, et al. Vulvar reconstruction using a mons pubis pedicle flap. *Gynecol Oncol* 1994;55:21.

182. Ellis F. Cancer of the vulva treated by radiation. *Br J Radiol* 1949; 22:513.

183. Helgason NM, Hass AC, Latourette HB. Radiation therapy in carcinoma of the vulva. *Cancer* 1972;30:997.

184. Tod MC. Radium implantation treatment of carcinoma of vulva. *Br J Radiol* 1949;22:508.

185. Busch M, Wagener B, Duhmke E. Long term results of radiotherapy alone for carcinoma of the vulva. *Adv Ther* 1999;16:89.

186. Boyce J, Fruchter RG, Kasambilides E, et al. Prognostic factors in carcinoma of the vulva. *Gynecol Oncol* 1985;20:364.

187. Faul CM, Mirmow D, Huang Q, et al. Adjuvant radiation for vulvar carcinoma: improved local control. *Int J Radiat Oncol Biol Phys* 1997; 38:381.

188. Acosta AA, Given FT, Frazier AB, et al. Preoperative radiation therapy in the management of squamous cell carcinoma of the vulva: preliminary report. *Am J Obstet Gynecol* 1978;132:198.

189. Boronow RC, Hickman BT, Reagan MT, et al. Combined therapy as an alternative to exenteration for locally advanced vulvovaginal cancer: II. Results, complications and dosimetric and surgical considerations. *Am J Clin Oncol* 1987;10:171.

190. Fairey RN, MacKay PA, Benedet JL, et al. Radiation treatment of carcinoma of the vulva, 1950–1980. *Am J Obstet Gynecol* 1985;151: 591.

191. Hacker NF, Berek JS, Julliard GJF, Lagasse LD. Preoperative radiation therapy for locally advanced vulvar cancer. *Cancer* 1984;54:2056.

192. Jafari K, Magalotti M. Radiation therapy in carcinoma of the vulva. *Cancer* 1981;47:686.

193. Berek JS, Heaps JM, Fu YS, et al. Concurrent cisplatin and 5-fluorouracil chemotherapy and radiation therapy for advanced-stage squamous carcinoma of the vulva. *Gynecol Oncol* 1991;42:197.

194. Cunningham MJ, Goyer RP, Gibbons SK, et al. Primary radiation, cisplatin, and 5-fluorouracil for advanced squamous carcinoma of the vulva. *Gynecol Oncol* 1997;66:258.

195. Eifel PJ, Morris M, Burke TW, et al. Preoperative continuous infusion cisplatinum and 5-fluorouracil with radiation for locally advanced or recurrent carcinoma of the vulva. *Gynecol Oncol* 1995;59:51.

196. Evans LS, Kersh CR, Constable WC, Taylor PT. Concomitant 5-fluorouracil, mitomycin C, and radiotherapy for advanced gynecologic malignancies. *Int J Radiat Oncol Biol Phys* 1988;15:901.

197. Iversen T. Irradiation and bleomycin in the treatment of inoperable vulval carcinoma. *Acta Obstet Gynecol Scand* 1982;61:195.

198. Kalra JK, Grossman AM, Krumholz BA, et al. Preoperative chemoradiotherapy for carcinoma of the vulva. *Gynecol Oncol* 1981;12:256.

199. Koh WJ, Wallace HJ, Greer BE, et al. Combined radiotherapy and chemotherapy in the management of local-regionally advanced vulvar cancer. *Int J Radiat Oncol Biol Phys* 1993;26:809.

200. Landoni F, Maneo A, Zanetta G, et al. Concurrent preoperative chemotherapy with 5-fluorouracil and mitomycin C and radiotherapy (FUMIR) followed by limited surgery in locally advanced and recurrent vulvar carcinoma. *Gynecol Oncol* 1996;61:321.

201. Lupi G, Raspagliesi F, Zucali R, et al. Combined preoperative chemoradiotherapy followed by radical surgery in locally advanced vulvar carcinoma: a pilot study. *Cancer* 1996;77:1472.

202. Mäkinen J, Salmi T, Gronroos M. Individually modified treatment of invasive squamous vulvar cancer: 10-year experience. *Ann Chir Gynaecol* 1987;76[Suppl]:68.

203. Scheistroen M, Trope C. Combined bleomycin and irradiation in preoperative treatment of advanced squamous cell carcinoma of the vulva. *Acta Oncol* 1992;32:657.

204. Thomas G, Dembo A, DePetrillo A, et al. Concurrent radiation and chemotherapy in vulvar carcinoma. *Gynecol Oncol* 1989;34:263.

205. Whalen SA, Slater JD, Wagner RJ, et al. Concurrent radiation therapy and chemotherapy in the treatment of primary squamous cell cancer of the vulva. *Cancer* 1995;75:2289.

206. Akl A, Akl M, Boike G, et al. Preliminary results of chemoradiation as a primary treatment for vulvar carcinoma. *Int J Radiat Biol Phys* 2000;48:415.

207. Han SC, Kim DH, Higgins SA, et al. Chemoradiation as primary or adjuvant treatment for locally advanced carcinoma of the vulva. *Int J Radiat Oncol Biol Phys* 2000;47:1235.

208. Cummings B. Anal canal carcinomas. In: Meyer JL, Vaeth JM, eds. *Frontiers in radiation oncology.* Vol 26. Basel: Karger, 1992:131.

209. Rich TA, Ajani JA, Morrison WH, et al. Chemoradiation therapy for anal cancer: radiation plus continuous infusion of 5-fluorouracil with or without cisplatin. *Radiother Oncol* 1993;27:209.

210. Morris M, Eifel PJ, Lu J, et al. Pelvic radiation with concurrent chemotherapy compared with pelvic and paraaortic radiation for high-risk cervical cancer. *N Engl J Med* 1999; 340:1137.

211. Henderson RH, Parsons JT, Morgan L, Million R. Elective ilioinguinal lymph node irradiation. *Int J Radiat Oncol Biol Phys* 1984;10:811.

212. Kucera H, Weghaupt K. The electrosurgical operation of vulva carcinoma with postoperative irradiation of inguinal lymph nodes. *Gynecol Oncol* 1988;29:158.

213. Petereit D, Mehta M, Buchler D, Kinsella T. A retrospective review of nodal treatment for vulvar cancer. *Am J Clin Oncol* 1993;16:38.

214. Leiserowitz GS, Russell AH, Kinney WK, et al. Prophylactic chemoradiation of inguinofemoral lymph nodes in patients with locally extensive vulvar cancer. *Gynecol Oncol* 1997;66:509.

215. Eifel PJ. Vulvar carcinoma: radiotherapy or surgery for the lymphatics? *Front Radiat Ther Oncol* 1994;28:218.

216. Koh WJ, Chiu M, Stelzer KJ, et al. Femoral vessel depth and the implications for groin node radiation. *Int J Radiat Oncol Biol Phys* 1992;27:969.

217. Origoni M, Sideri M, Garsia S, et al. Prognostic value of pathological patterns of lymph node positivity in squamous cell carcinoma of the vulva stage III and IVA FIGO. *Gynecol Oncol* 1992;45:313.

218. Simonsen E, Nordberg UB, Johnsson JE, et al. Radiation therapy and surgery in the treatment of regional lymph nodes in squamous cell carcinoma of the vulva. *Acta Radiol Oncol* 1984;23:433.

219. Montana GS, Thomas GM, Moore DH, et al. Preoperative chemoradiation for carcinoma of the vulva with N2/N3 nodes: a Gynecologic Oncology Group study. *Int J Radiat Oncol Biol Physics* 2000;48: 1007.

220. Kalnicki S, Zide A, Malecki N, et al. Transmission block to simplify combined pelvic and inguinal radiation therapy. *Radiology* 1987;164: 578.

221. Carlino G, Parisi S, Montemaggi P, Pastore G. Interstitial radiotherapy with ^{192}Ir in vulvar cancer. *Eur J Gynaecol Oncol* 1984;5:183.

222. Miyazawa K, Nori D, Hilaris BS, Lewis JT. Role of radiation therapy in the treatment of advanced vulvar carcinoma. *J Reprod Med* 1983; 28:539.

223. Dusenbery KE, Carlson JW, LaPorte RM, et al. Radical vulvectomy with postoperative irradiation for vulvar cancer: therapeutic implications of a central block. *Int J Radiat Oncol Biol Phys* 1994;29:989.

224. Jenkins PJ, Montefiore DJ, Arnott SJ. Hip complications following chemoradiotherapy. *Clin Oncol* 1995;7:123.

225. Thomas G, Dembo A, Fyles A, et al. Concurrent chemoradiation in advanced cervical cancer. *Gynecol Oncol* 1990;38:446.

226. Katz A, Eifel PJ, Jhingran A, Levenback CF. The role of radiation therapy in preventing regional recurrences of invasive squamous cell carcinoma of the vulva. *Int J Radiat Oncol Biol Phys* 2003;57:409.

227. Frischbier HJ, Thomsen K. Treatment of cancer of the vulva with high-energy electrons. *Am J Obstet Gynecol* 1971;111:431.

228. Deppe G, Bruckner HW, Cohen CJ. Adriamycin treatment of advanced vulvar carcinoma. *Obstet Gynecol* 1977;50:13.

229. Thigpen JT, Blessing JA, Homesley HD, et al. Phase II trials of cisplatin and piperzinedione in advanced or recurrent squamous cell carcinomas of the vulva: a Gynecologic Oncology Group study. *Gynecol Oncol* 1986;23:358.

230. Muss HB, Bundy BN, Christopherson WA. Mitoxantrone in the treatment of advanced vulvar and vaginal carcinoma. *Am J Clin Oncol* 1989;12:142.

231. Slayton RE, Blessing JA, Beecham J, et al. Phase II trial of etoposide in the management of advanced or recurrent squamous cell carcinoma of the vulva and carcinoma of the vagina: a Gynecologic Oncology Group study. *Cancer Treat Rep* 1987;71:869.

232. Durrant KR, Mangione C, Lacave AJ, et al. Bleomycin, methotrexate, and CCNU in advanced inoperable squamous cell carcinoma of the vulva: a Phase II study of the EORTC Gynaecological Cancer Cooperative Group (GCCG). *Gynecol Oncol* 1990;37:359.

233. Belinson JL, Stewart JA, Richards A, et al. Bleomycin, vincristine, mitomycin C, and cisplatin in the management of gynecologic squamous-cell cancer. *Gynecol Oncol* 1985;20:387.

234. Kosary CL. FIGO stage, histology, histologic grade, age and race as prognostic factors in determining survival for cancers of the female gynecological system: an analysis of 1973–87 SEER cases of cancers of the endometrium, cervix, ovary, vulva and vagina. *Semin Surg Oncol* 1994;10:31.

235. Morrow CP, Rutledge FN. Melanoma of the vulva. *Obstet Gynecol* 1972;39:745.
236. Jaramillo BA, Ganjei P, Averette HE, et al. Malignant melanoma of the vulva. *Obstet Gynecol* 1985;66:398.
237. Phillips GL, Bundy BN, Okagaki T, et al. Malignant melanoma of the vulva treated by radical hemivulvectomy: a prospective study of the Gynecology Oncology Group. *Cancer* 1994;73:2626.
238. Trimble EL, Lewis JL Jr, Williams LL, et al. Management of vulvar melanoma. *Gynecol Oncol* 1992;45:254.
239. Look KY, Roth LM, Sutton GP. Vulvar melanoma reconsidered. *Cancer* 1993;72:143.
240. Balch CM. The role of elective lymph node dissection in melanoma: rationale, results, and controversies. *J Clin Oncol* 1988;6:163.
241. Emami B, Perez CA. Combination of surgery, irradiation, and hyperthermia in treatment of recurrences of malignant tumors. *Int J Radiat Oncol Biol Phys* 1987;13:611.
242. Singhal RM, Narayana A. Malignant melanoma of the vulva: response to radiation. *Br J Radiol* 1991;64:846.
243. Habermalz HJ, Fischer JJ. Radiation therapy of malignant melanoma: experience with high individual treatment doses. *Cancer* 1976;38:2258.
244. Sondak VK, Liu PY, Tuthill RJ. Adjuvant immunotherapy of resected, intermediate-thickness, node-negative melanoma with an allogeneic tumor vaccine: overall results of a randomized trial of the Southwest Oncology Group. *J Clin Oncol* 2002;20:2058.
245. Gallousis S. Verrucous carcinoma: report of three vulvar cases and a review of the literature. *Obstet Gynecol* 1972;40:502.
246. Japaze H, Dinh TV, Woodruff JD. Verrucous carcinoma of the vulva: study of 24 cases. *Obstet Gynecol* 1982;60:462.
247. Demian SDE, Bushkin FL, Echevarria RA. Perineural invasion and anaplastic transformation of verrucous carcinoma. *Cancer* 1973;32:395.
248. Proffitt SD, Spooner TR, Kosek JC. Origin of undifferentiated neoplasm from verrucous carcinoma of the oral cavity following irradiation. *Cancer* 1970;26:389.
249. Breen JL, Neubecker RD, Greenwald E, Gregorio CA. Basal cell carcinoma of the vulva. *Obstet Gynecol* 1975;46:122.
250. Hoffman MS, Roberts WS, Ruffolo EH. Basal cell carcinoma of the vulva with inguinal lymph node metastases. *Gynecol Oncol* 1988;29:113.
251. Copeland LJ, Sneige N, Gershenson DM, et al. Bartholin gland carcinoma. *Obstet Gynecol* 1986;67:794.
252. Leuchter RS, Hacker NF, Voet RL, et al. Primary carcinoma of the Bartholin gland: a report of 14 cases and a review of the literature. *Obstet Gynecol* 1982;60:361.
253. Huang GS, Juretzka M, Ciaravino G, et al. Liposomal doxorubicin for treatment of metastatic chemorefractory vulvar adenocarcinoma. *Gynecol Oncol* 2002;87:313.
254. Creasman WT, Gallager HS, Rutledge F. Paget's disease of the vulva. *Gynecol Oncol* 1975;3:133.
255. Parmley TH, Woodruff JD, Julian CG. Invasive vulvar Paget's disease. *Obstet Gynecol* 1975;46:341.
256. Hart WR, Millman RB. Progression of intraepithelial Paget's disease of the vulva to invasive carcinoma. *Cancer* 1977;40:2333.
257. Fanning J, Lambert L, Hale TM, et al. Paget's disease of the vulva: prevalence of associated vulvar adenocarcinoma, invasive Paget's disease, and recurrence after surgical excision. *Am J Obstet Gynecol* 1999;180:24.
258. Kodama S, Kaneko T, Saito M, et al. A clinicopathologic study of 30 patients with Paget's disease of the vulva. *Gynecol Oncol* 1995;56:63.
259. Stacy D, Burrell MO, Franklin EW III. Extramammary Paget's disease of the vulva and anus: use of intraoperative frozen-section margins. *Am J Obstet Gynecol* 1986;155:519.
260. Pierie JP, Choudry U, Muzikansky A, et al. Prognosis and management of extramammary Paget's disease and the association with secondary malignancies. *J Am Coll Surg* 2003;196:45.
261. Bergen S, DiSaia PJ, Liao SY, Berman ML. Conservative management of extramammary Paget's disease of the vulva. *Gynecol Oncol* 1989;33:151.
262. Hays DM, Shimada H, Raney RB, et al. Clinical staging and treatment results in rhabdomyosarcoma of the female genital tract among children and adolescents. *Cancer* 1988;61:1893.
263. Tavassoli FA, Norris HJ. Smooth muscle tumors of the vulva. *Obstet Gynecol* 1979;53:213.
264. Bell J, Averette H, Davis J, Toledano S. Genital rhabdomyosarcoma: current management and review of the literature. *Obstet Gynecol Surv* 1986;41:257.

CHAPTER 21

Vagina

Higinia R. Cardenes, Lawrence M. Roth, William P. McGuire, and Katherine Y. Look

ANATOMY

The vagina is a tubular structure lined by nonkeratinized squamous epithelium extending from the vestibule to the uterus. It lies dorsal to the bladder and ventral to the rectum. It averages 7.5 cm in length. Beneath the mucosa lies a submucosal layer of elastin and a double muscularis layer, which is highly vascularized with a rich innervation and lymphatic drainage. The muscularis layer is composed of smooth muscle fibers arranged circularly in the inner portion and longitudinally in the outer portion. The proximal vagina is supplied by the vaginal artery branch from the uterine or cervical branch of the uterine artery. It runs along the lateral wall of the vagina and anastamoses with the inferior vesical and middle rectal arteries from the surrounding viscera (1). The accompanying venous plexus, running parallel to the arteries, ultimately drains to the internal iliac vein. The lumbar plexus and pudendal nerve, with branches from sacral roots 2 to 4, provide innervation to the vaginal vault (Fig. 21.1).

The lymphatic drainage of the vagina is complex, consisting of an extensive inter-communicating network. Fine lymphatic vessels coursing through the submucosa and muscularis coalesce into small trunks running laterally along the walls of the vagina. The upper anterior vagina drains along cervical channels to the interiliac chain; the posterior vagina drains into the inferior gluteal, presacral, and anorectal nodes. The distal vaginal lymphatics drain into the inguinal and femoral nodes, and from there to the pelvic nodes. Lymphatic flow from lesions in the mid vagina may drain either way (2). However, because of the presence of inter-commu-

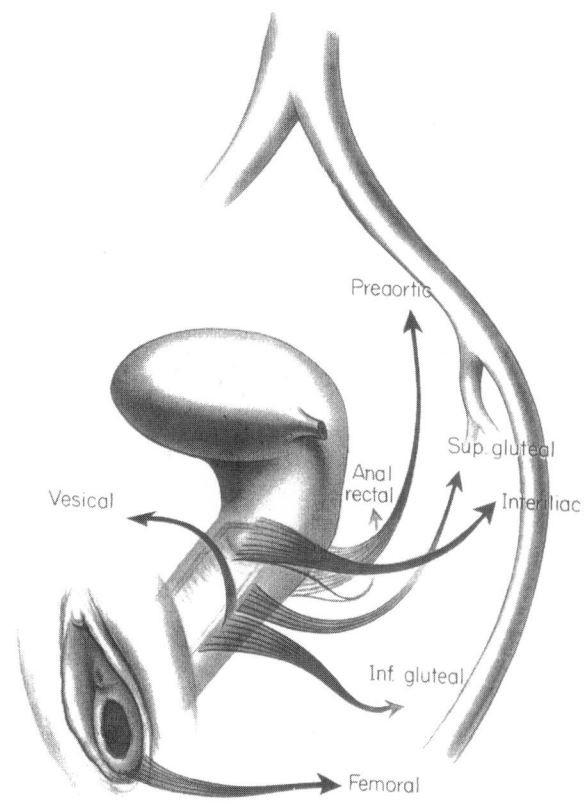

FIG. 21.1. Lymphatic drainage of the vagina. (Reprinted from Plentl AA, Friedman EA. Lymphatic system of the female genitalia. In: Plentl AA, Friedman EA, eds. *The morphologic basis of oncologic diagnosis and therapy.* Philadelphia: WB Saunders, 1971:55, Fig. 5–2. Used with permission.)

Higinia R. Cardenes: Department of Radiation Oncology, Indiana University School of Medicine, Indianapolis, Indiana 46202.

Lawrence M. Roth: Department of Surgical Pathology and Obstetrics & Gynecology, Indiana University School of Medicine, Indianapolis, Indiana 46202

William P. McGuire: Department of Medical Oncology, The Harry and Jeanette Weinberg Cancer Institute, Franklin Square Hospital Center, Baltimore, Maryland 21237

Katherine Y. Look: Section of Gynecologic Oncology, Indiana University School of Medicine, Indianapolis, Indiana 46202

nicating lymphatics along the terminal branches of the vaginal artery and near the vaginal wall, the external iliac nodes are at high risk even in lesions of the lower third of the vagina. Such a complex lymphatic drainage pattern has significant implications for therapeutic planning. Therefore, bilateral pelvic nodes should be considered to be at risk in any invasive vaginal carcinoma, and bilateral groin nodes should be considered to be at risk in those lesions involving the distal third of the vagina.

PATHOLOGY

Squamous-Cell Carcinoma

Squamous-cell carcinoma (SCC) represents about 80% to 90% of primary vaginal cancers. These tumors occur in older women, and are most often located in the upper, posterior wall of the vagina. According to the recommendations of the International Federation of Gynecology and Obstetrics (FIGO), a tumor of the vagina that involves the cervix or vulva should be classified as a primary cervical or vulvar cancer, respectively. Additionally, for a neoplasm to be considered a vaginal primary, there must not have been a cervical cancer for 5 years prior to the diagnosis (3). It may be difficult or impossible histologically to distinguish a primary vaginal SCC from recurrent cervical or vulvar disease.

Histologically, keratinizing, nonkeratinizing, basaloid, warty, and verrucous variants have been described. Tumors may also be graded as moderately or poorly differentiated. However, there is little correlation between tumor grade and survival (4). Most cases are moderately differentiated and nonkeratinizing. Well-differentiated tumors show prominent keratin or squamous pearl formation (Fig. 21.2). Rarely, poorly differentiated tumors have a spindle-cell appearance. Warty SCC has a papillary appearance with hyperkeratosis and koilocytosis. Verrucous carcinoma is a rare, distinct var-

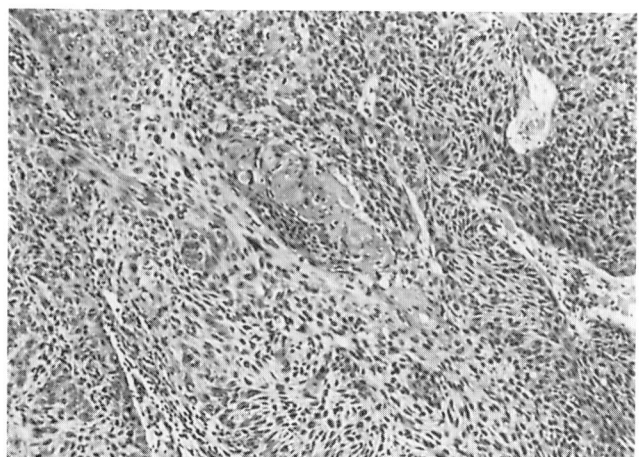

FIG. 21.2. Well-differentiated vaginal squamous-cell carcinoma with focal keratinization (*center*). (Courtesy of Dr. Deborah J. Gersell, St Louis, MO.)

iant of well-differentiated SCC, with a papillary growth pattern, pushing borders, bulbous pegs of acanthotic epithelium with little or no atypia, and surface maturation in the form of parakeratosis and hyperkeratosis without koilocytosis. Because of its well-differentiated character, the microscopic diagnosis of verrucous carcinoma may be difficult, especially if the biopsy is superficial (5).

Vaginal intraepithelial neoplasia (VAIN) is a precursor of SCC, and is graded from I to III depending upon the degree of nuclear atypia and crowding and the proportion of the epithelium involved. VAIN I typically involves the lower third to one-half of the epithelium, VAIN II one-half to two-thirds the thickness of the epithelium, and VAIN III more than three-fourths the thickness. Alternatively, VAIN can be classified as low or high grade. High-grade lesions indicate involvement of the outer third of the mucosa, and include carcinoma *in situ* (CIS), which encompasses the entire thickness of the epithelium. The true incidence of VAIN and its rate of progression to invasive carcinoma are unknown, ranging in several series from 9% to 28% (6–8).

Clear-Cell Adenocarcinoma and Vaginal Adenosis

Diethylstilbestrol (DES)–associated clear-cell adenocarcinoma (CCA) has a predilection for the upper third of the vagina and the exocervix. It is frequently located at or near the lower margin of the zone of glandular tissue in the vagina or cervix. Most CCAs are exophytic and superficially invasive (9). CCA is arranged in tubulocystic, solid, papillary, or mixed cell patterns, and is mainly composed of clear and hobnail-shaped cells (Fig. 21.3A,B). The clear cells are cuboidal or columnar with abundant glycogen-rich cytoplasm and distinct cell membranes. The hobnail cells have large atypical protruding nuclei rimmed by a small amount of cytoplasm.

Vaginal adenosis is a condition in which müllerian-type glandular epithelium is present after vaginal development is complete. Although adenosis is the most common histologic abnormality in women exposed to DES in utero, it is not strictly confined to this population. Adenosis is associated with 97% of vaginal and 52% of cervical CCAs. The glandular epithelium may replace the surface epithelium and/or form glands in the superficial stroma (10,11). The glandular epithelium undergoes progressive squamous metaplasia (10, 12) and ultimately only stromal nodules or pegs of immature squamous epithelium containing small mucin droplets may remain (13). A few CCAs have been detected among women under surveillance for adenosis (14). Atypical adenosis of tuboendometrial type appears to be a precursor lesion of CCA (15). Whether immature squamous metaplasia in adenosis is associated with an increased risk of vaginal intraepithelial neoplasia or SCC is controversial (11).

Other Adenocarcinomas

Only a few cases of *mucinous adenocarcinoma* have been described (16). Histologically, the tumors may resemble typ-

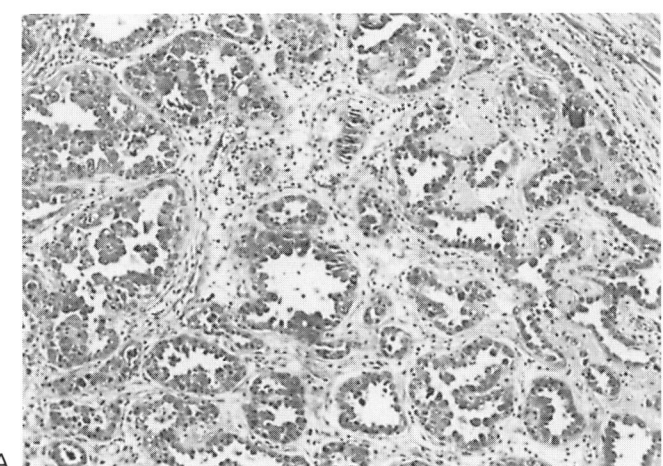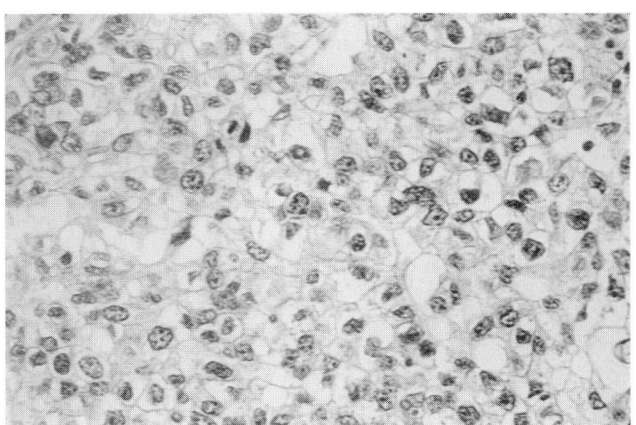

A   B

FIG. 21.3. A: Clear-cell adenocarcinoma with tubulocystic and papillary growth patterns. Hobnail cells predominate. **B:** Clear-cell adenocarcinoma with a solid growth pattern. Note the tumor cells with pleomorphic nuclei, clear cytoplasm, and distinct cell borders.

ical endocervical (17) or intestinal (18) adenocarcinoma. Some cases may be related to DES exposure (19). A relationship to vaginal adenosis has been described in a patient not exposed to DES (20). Rare cases of mucinous adenocarcinoma have been described in neovaginas (21,22).

Endometrioid adenocarcinoma of the vagina usually arises in endometriosis (23). *Mesonephric adenocarcinoma* is a rare variant that may arise from mesonephric duct remnants that are mostly situated deep in the lateral walls of the vagina (24). Primary *papillary serous adenocarcinoma* of the vagina has rarely been reported (25).

Melanoma

Melanoma is the second most common cancer of the vagina, accounting for 2.8% to 5.0% of vaginal neoplasms. The most common locations are the lower third and the anterior vaginal wall, although oftentimes it is multifocal (26–28). Grossly, these tumors are typically pigmented, and show considerable variation in size, color, and growth patterns, being polypoid or nodular in the majority of cases. Microscopically, they are composed of epithelioid cells, spindle cells, or nevus-like cells; melanin pigment is often present. Junctional activity is usually present. Poorly differentiated tumors may be difficult to distinguish from sarcoma or SCC. Premelanosomes may be identified by electron microscopy. Immunohistochemical stains are frequently positive for S100 protein, HMB-45, and melan-A. Tyrosinase and MART-1 are useful markers when S100 is negative or only focally positive. Tumor thickness correlates with prognosis, and may be measured by the method of Breslow (29).

Mesenchymal Tumors

Embryonal rhabdomyosarcoma (RMS) is a rare pediatric tumor. The botryoid variant, or sarcoma botryoides, is the

most common malignant vaginal tumor in infants and children (30). Ninty percent of cases occur in children younger than 5 years of age. Sarcoma botyroides has a characteristic gross appearance consisting of multiple gray-red, translucent, edematous, grape-like masses that fill the vagina, and may protrude from it. Microscopically, there is a zone of condensed round, or spindle, cells (the cambium layer) immediately beneath the intact vaginal epithelium. Elsewhere, the tumor is composed of small dark spindle-shaped cells, sparsely distributed in a myxoid stroma (Fig. 21.4). Some cells may show skeletal muscle differentiation, evidenced by intensely eosinophilic cytoplasm with cross striations. Inmmunohistochemical stains with antibodies directed against actin, desmin, or myoglobin facilitate the recognition of striated muscle differentiation.

Leiomyosarcoma is the most common vaginal sarcoma in adults (31). The frequency and behavior are uncertain be-

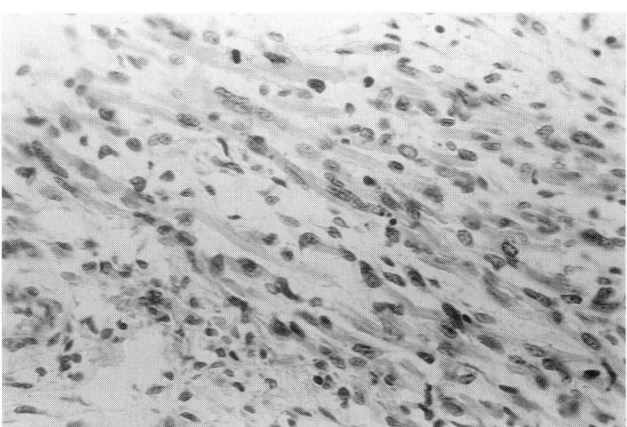

FIG. 21.4. Embryonal rhabdomyosarcoma. The tumor is composed of strap cells with atypical, elongated, often tandem, nuclei and edematous stroma.

cause of the variable histologic criteria used to distinguish benign and malignant smooth muscle tumors. It is currently recommended that smooth muscle tumors greater than 3 cm in diameter, with five or greater mitoses per 10 high-power fields (HPFs), moderate or marked cytologic atypia, and infiltrating margins be classified as leiomyosarcoma (32). The gross appearance varies greatly depending on cellularity, type, and extent of degenerative change and the amount of necrosis and hemorrhage (32). Microscopically, they are composed of interlacing bundles of spindle-shaped cells with blunt-ended nuclei and fibrillar cytoplasm. An epithelioid pattern or extensive myxoid change occurs uncommonly (32, 33). Because smooth muscle tumors vary from area to area, adequate sampling (one block/1 to 2 cm of tumor diameter) is essential for accurate diagnosis.

Other sarcomas that may occur in the vagina include *endometrioid stromal sarcoma*, which may arise in endometriosis (34–36); *alveolar soft part sarcoma* (37); *malignant fibrous histiocytoma* (38), a biphasic tumor interpreted as resembling synovial sarcoma (39) or *malignant mixed tumor* (40); angiosarcoma (41); *malignant peripheral nerve sheath tumor*; and *hemangiopericytoma* (42).

Malignant Lymphoma and Leukemia

Malignant lymphoma may be localized to the female genital tract or occur there as part of a widespread disease process (43,44). The majority of primary lymphomas involving the vagina are of the diffuse large B-cell type, but follicular lymphomas also occur. The histologic diagnosis depends on the identification of monomorphous, cytologically atypical, mitotically active lymphoid cells deeply penetrating the stroma. Characteristically, the mucosa is intact. The tumors typically express CD20. Patients with vaginal lymphomas characteristically present with vaginal bleeding. Those with primary lymphomas also have a mass on clinical examination. Leukemic infiltrates, especially granulocytic sarcoma, can be impossible to distinguish from lymphoma. Chloracetate esterase or myeloperoxidase stains may be helpful in some cases.

Uncommon Vaginal Tumors

Neuroendocrine small-cell carcinoma may occur in the vagina either in pure form or associated with squamous or glandular elements (45). A high proportion of these tumors show immunohistochemical or ultrastructural evidence of neuroendocrine differentiation (46). *Adenosquamous carcinoma* is an uncommon neoplasm of the vagina composed of an admixture of glandular and squamous elements (47). Tumors diagnosed as *carcinosarcomas* of the female genital tract appear to be metaplastic carcinomas, and should be treated as epithelial neoplasms, although the prognosis is poor. This tumor is rare in the vagina, and typically occurs in

postmenopausal women (48). Uncommonly, *yolk sac tumors* have been reported in the vagina (49,50).

EPIDEMIOLOGY AND ETIOLOGIC RISK FACTORS

Primary vaginal cancer is a rare entity. Most carcinomas found in the vagina represent metastasis from other primary gynecologic (cervix or vulva) and nongynecologic sites. Carcinoma of the vagina accounts for only 1% to 2% of all female genital neoplasias (4). Creasman et al. (51) published information in 1998 in the National Cancer Data Base (NCDB) report on 4,885 patients with primary diagnosis of vaginal cancer registered from 1985 to 1994. Approximately 92% of the patients were diagnosed with *in situ* or invasive SCC or adenocarcinomas, 4% with melanomas, 3% with sarcomas, and 1% with other or unspecified types of cancer. In the NCDB report, invasive carcinomas accounted for 72% of the carcinoma cases, or 66% of all vaginal cancers. *In situ* carcinomas accounted for 28%, SCC represented 79% of invasive vaginal carcinomas, and adenocarcinomas represented 14%.

Carcinoma of the vagina is considered to be associated with advanced age, with the peak incidence occurring in the sixth and seventh decades of life. However, vaginal cancer is increasingly being seen in younger women, possibly due to human papillomavirus (HPV) infection or other sexually transmitted diseases. Only about 10% of patients are 40 years of age or younger (52). In the NCDB report, only 1% of the carcinoma patients were less than 20 years old at the time of diagnosis, and over 80% of those patients had *in situ* lesions. As patient age increased, the number of invasive tumors increased, reaching a peak in patients aged 70 to 79 years. The percentage of *in situ* carcinomas decreased to only 11% in patients over 80 years old (51).

Squamous-Cell Carcinoma

Potential risk factors for SCC include prior history of cervical intraepithelial neoplasia (CIN), HPV infection, immunosuppression, and possibly previous pelvic irradiation. HPV is the likely etiologic agent of SCC and its precursor lesion, VAIN. HPV has been recovered from 80% of VAIN lesions and 60% of invasive SCC of the vagina (53,54). In a case-control study of VAIN and early-stage cancer of the vagina, Brinton et al. (6) reported a 2.9-fold increase in therapy for genital warts and a 3.8-fold increase in prior abnormal Papanicolaou (Pap) smears in patients with VAIN compared to controls. This association likely represents the sequelae of infection with high-risk HPV strains (HPV 16, 18, 31, and 33) (55). The process most commonly occurs in the upper vagina, and it is frequently multifocal. Approximately one-half of the lesions are associated with concomitant Cervical intraepithelial neoplasia (CIN) or vulvar intraepithelial neoplasia (7). In studies reporting on groups of women with VAIN and SCC of the vagina, the following risk factors have been identified: five or more sexual partners, sexual debut before age 17 years, smoking, low socioeconomic status, a history of genital warts, prior abnormal cytology, and prior hysterectomy (6,54).

Patients with previous cervical carcinoma have a substantial risk of developing vaginal carcinoma, presumably because these sites share exposure and/or susceptibility to endogenous or exogenous carcinogenic stimuli. Ten percent to 50% of patients with VAIN-CIS or invasive carcinoma of the vagina have undergone prior hysterectomy or radiotherapy (RT) for CIS or invasive carcinoma of the cervix (56–67). The interval from therapy for cervical cancer or preinvasive disease to the development of carcinoma of the vagina averages nearly 14 years, but there have been cases with the vaginal primary manifesting 50 years after therapy for cervical cancer (58,68).

It is controversial as to whether or not prior pelvic RT is a risk factor. Boice et al. (69) reported a 14-fold increase risk of cancer of the vagina in women previously irradiated. However, Lee et al. (70) did not find prior RT to be associated with an increase in risk. It is biologically plausible that there could be an apparent increase in risk given that prior pelvic RT would have likely been given for HPV-associated cervical carcinoma, and the antecedent HPV infection would increase the risk of SCC in the vagina. Such an association has led to the recommendation that patients treated for CIN or carcinoma of the cervix continue to undergo lifelong surveillance with vaginal cytologic evaluation even after hysterectomy (71). In addition, there is evidence that *in utero* exposure to DES doubles the risk of development of VAIN. The putative mechanism is an enlargement of the transformation zone at risk, which is then at risk for infection with HPV (72).

Clear-Cell Adenocarcinoma

An increased incidence of CCA of the vagina in young women related to *in utero* exposure to DES during the first 16 weeks of pregnancy was first reported in 1971 (73). Specific suggested mechanisms of carcinogenesis focus on the retention of nests of abnormal cells of müllerian duct origin, which, after stimulation by endogenous hormones during puberty, are promoted into adenocarcinomas. The median age at diagnosis in the DES-exposed patients is 19 years (73), whereas prior to this report, most patients with CCA of the vagina were elderly. The incidence of CCA in the exposed female population from birth to 34 years is estimated to be between 0.14 and 1.4 per 1,000. Approximately 90% of the patients had stage I-II disease at diagnosis (74, 75). Hicks and Piver noted that 60% of CCA patients had been exposed to DES or similar agents *in utero*, that most cases involved the anterior upper third of the vaginal wall, and that DES-associated CCA cases had been reported from ages 7 to 34 (76). Fortunately, the incidence of this tumor

has decreased in recent years, and may decrease even more since the practice of prescribing DES during pregnancy has been discontinued.

Melanoma

Trimble's examination of the Surveillance; Epidemiology and End Results (SEER) data on 30,295 melanomas found 51 vaginal melanomas (0.3% of all melanomas), with an annual incidence of 0.026 per 100,000 and a median age at diagnosis of 66.3 years (77). In the NCDB report by Creasman et al. (51), vaginal melanomas represented 4% of primary vaginal cancers.

Sarcomas

Sarcomas represent 3% of primary vaginal cancers, and are most common in adults, with leiomyosarcoma representing 50% to 65% of vaginal sarcomas (51). Malignant mixed müllerian tumor (MMMT, carcinosarcoma), endometrial stromal sarcoma, and angiosarcoma are less common. Embryonal rhabdomyosarcoma/sarcoma botryoides is a rare pediatric tumor. Prior pelvic RT is a risk factor, particularly for mixed mesodermal tumors and vaginal angiosarcomas. Unfortunately, most of the sarcomas are diagnosed at an advanced stage. Histopathologic grade appears to be the most important predictor of outcome (78).

NATURAL HISTORY

The majority (57% to 83%) of vaginal primaries occur in the upper third or at the apex of the vault, most commonly in the posterior wall; the lower third may be involved in as many as 31% of patients (56,58,79). Lesions confined to the middle third of the vagina are uncommon. The location of the vaginal carcinoma is an important consideration in planning therapy and determining prognosis. Vaginal tumors may spread along the vaginal walls to involve the cervix or the vulva. A lesion on the anterior wall may infiltrate the vesicovaginal septum and/or the urethra; those on the posterior wall may eventually involve the rectovaginal septum and subsequently infiltrate the rectal mucosa. Lateral extension toward the parametrium and paracolpal tissues is not uncommon in more advanced stages of the disease.

The issue of regional nodal metastasis, both the incidence of occult nodal disease and the anatomic pathways of lymphatic spread, are somewhat controversial. There does seem to be a significant risk of nodal metastasis for patients with disease beyond stage I. Although data on staging lymphadenectomy are sparse, two studies reported a significant incidence of nodal disease in early-stage vaginal carcinoma. In Al-Kurdis and Monaghan's series (80), the incidence of pelvic nodal metastasis was 14% and 32% for stages I and II, respectively, whereas in Davis et al.'s series (68), the incidence was 6% and 26% for stages I and II, respectively.

The incidence is expected to be higher for stage III, although no substantial data are available.

Distant metastasis may occur, primarily in patients with advanced disase at presentation, or those who recurred after primary therapy. In Perez et al.'s series (64), the incidence of distant metastasis was 16% in stage I, 31% in stage IIA, 46% in stage IIB, 62% in stage III, and 50% in stage IV.

CLINICAL PRESENTATION

Vaginal Intraepithelial Neoplasia –Carcinoma *in situ*

VAIN most often is asymptomatic (59). In modern practice, VAIN is usually detected by cytologic evaluation performed following hysterectomy as part of a surveillance strategy in patients with a history of CIN or invasive cervical carcinoma. In these cases, VAIN has a predilection for involvement of the upper vagina; likely secondary to a "field effect." A discharge may be present, but is likely secondary to superimposed vaginal infections. It should be noted that evidence-based guidelines do not support routine cytologic studies following hysterectomy for noncervical pathology. The American Cancer Society released guidelines in 2002 that said surveillance cytology in such patients is *not* necessary. Rather, surveillance cytology posthysterectomy should be limited to those patients with a prior history of CIN or invasive cervix cancer (81).

Invasive Squamous-Cell Carcinoma

In patients with invasive disease, irregular vaginal bleeding, often postcoital, is the most common presenting symptom followed by vaginal discharge and dysuria. Pelvic pain is a relatively late symptom generally related to tumor extent beyond the vagina (58,79). In a series of 84 patients with invasive carcinoma, including 55 with SCC, Tjalma et al. noted that 62% of patients had vaginal discharge, 16% had positive cytology, 13% had a mass, 4% had pain, and 2% had dysuria. Forty-seven percent of the lesions were located on the posterior wall and 24% on anterior wall; 29% had involvement of both walls (82). In 10% to 20%, no symptoms were reported, and the diagnosis was made by cytologic examination.

Other Histologies

The most common presenting symptom in patients with CCA is vaginal bleeding (50% to 75%) or abnormal discharge. More advanced cases may present with dysuria or pelvic pain (73). Cytology is abnormal in only 33% of cases. Therefore, in addition to four-quadrant cytology, Hanselaar et al. recommended palpation of the entire vaginal vault to assess for submucosal irregularity (83). The majority of CCA lesions are exophytic, superficially invasive in the

upper third of the vault near the cervix. Ninety-seven percent will be associated with mucosal adenosis (9,15,84).

Embryonal RMS, the most common malignant vaginal tumor in children, presents as a protruding, edematous grape-like mass. Ninety percent of these sarcomas present before the age of 5 years. The average age at presentation was 23.5 months in Maurer et al.'s series (85). In adults, symptoms most commonly noted were pain accompanied by a mass.

DIAGNOSTIC WORKUP

In general, in patients with suspected vaginal malignancy, thorough physical examination with detailed speculum inspection, digital palpation, colposcopic and cytologic evaluation, and biopsy constitute the most effective procedure for diagnosing primary, metastatic, or recurrent carcinoma of the vagina. In symptomatic patients, biopsy of any abnormal exophytic or endophytic lesion noted at the time of the examination is indicated. Examination under anesthesia is recommended for the thoroughness of evaluation of all of the vaginal walls and local extent of the disease, primarily if the patient is in great discomfort because of advanced disease, in order to obtain a biopsy. Biopsies of the cervix, if present, are recommended to rule out a primary cervical tumor. It is important that the speculum be slowly withdrawn from the vaginal fornix so that the total vaginal mucosa may be visualized.

The patient with a history of preinvasive or invasive carcinoma of the cervix found to have abnormal cytology following prior hysterectomy or RT should be offered colposcopy with application of acetic acid to the entire vault, followed by biopsies as indicated by areas of white epithelium, mosaicism, punctation, or atypical vascularity. It can be very helpful for the menopausal patient or the patient previously irradiated to use a short course of topically applied estrogen into the vaginal vault once or twice a week for 1 month prior to the colposcopy in order to foster epithelial maturation. Another method of identifying the area(s) most in need of biopsy would be, after application of acetic acid, to apply half-strength Schiller's iodine to determine if the Schiller-positive (nonstaining) areas correspond with the involved areas identified after acetic acid application.

STAGING

At present, primary malignancies of the vagina are all staged clinically. In addition to a complete history and physical examination, routine laboratory evaluations including complete blood cell count (CBC) with differential and platelets and assessment of renal and hepatic function should be undertaken. In order to determine the extent of disease, the following tests are allowed by International Federation of Gynecology and Obstetrics (FIGO) criteria: chest radiograph, a thorough bimanual and rectovaginal examination, cystoscopy, proctoscopy, and intravenous pyelogram. If the patient is in significant discomfort, the examination should be conducted under anesthesia, preferably by a radiation oncologist and gynecologic oncologist who will be involved in her ongoing care. However, it can be difficult even for the experienced examiner to differentiate between disease confined to the mucosa (stage I) and disease spread to the submucosa (stage II) (57,79). Cystoscopy and proctoscopy are generally performed on patients with symptoms or clinical findings suspicious for bladder or rectal infiltration, respectively.

Pelvic computed tomography (CT) scan is generally performed to evaluate inguinofemoral and/or pelvic lymph nodes, as well as extent of local disease. In patients with vaginal melanoma or sarcoma, chest, abdomen, and pelvic CT scans are often part of the workup. Magnetic resonance imaging (MRI) has emerged as a potentially important imaging modality in the evaluation of vaginal cancers, predominantly the T1-weighted with contrast and T2-weighted images (Fig. 21.5). An additional role of MRI is differentiation

of tumor from fibrotic tissue in patients with suspected recurrent vaginal carcinoma (86). In modern practice, for the majority of patients with disease volume and/or location requiring definitive RT to achieve cure, therapeutic planning will be guided by disease volume assessment utilizing CT and/or MRI even though such radiologic modalities are not "allowed" for purposes of staging.

The two commonly used staging systems for carcinoma of the vagina are the FIGO (Table 21.1) and the American Joint Commission on Cancer (TNM) classifications (87). According to FIGO guidelines, patients with tumor involvement of the cervix or vulva should be classified as primary cervical or vulvar cancers, respectively. Therefore, multiple biopsies of the cervix are mandatory to rule out a cervical primary. Perez et al. (88) proposed in 1973 that FIGO stage II vaginal cancer should be subdivided into stage IIA (tumor infiltrating the subvaginal tissues but not extending into the parametrium) and stage IIB (tumor infiltrating the parametrium but not extending to pelvic side walls). However, most

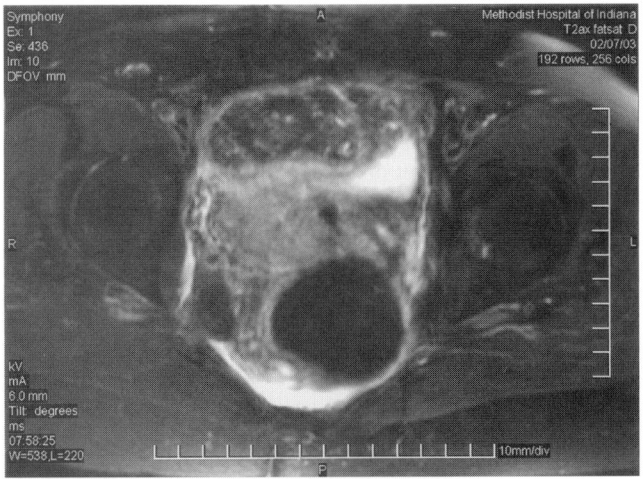

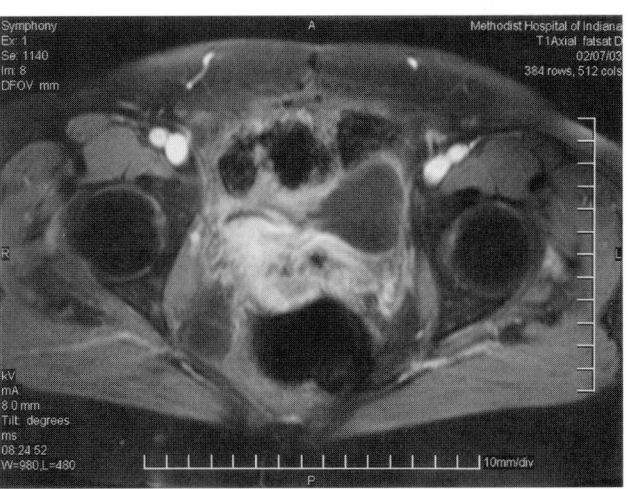

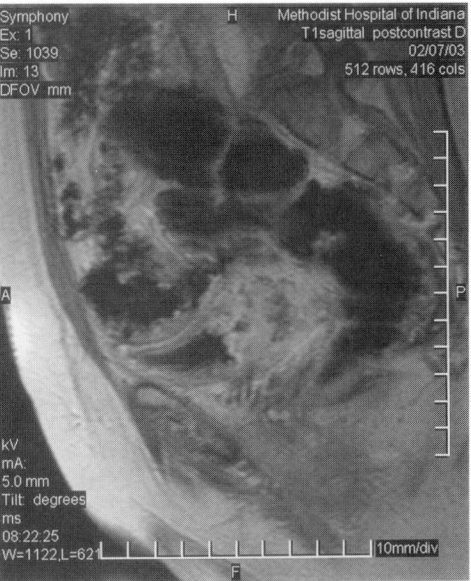

FIG. 21.5. MRI images of locally advanced vaginal cancer. **A:** T2 axial—fat saturation. **B:** T1 sagittal—fat saturation. **C:** T1 sagittal—postcontrast.

TABLE 21.1. *FIGO staging system for carcinoma of the vagina*

Stage	Description
0	Carcinoma *in situ*, intraepithelial neoplasia
I	Limited to the vaginal wall
II	Involvement of the subvaginal tissue but without extension to the pelvic sidewall
III	Extension to the pelvic sidewall
IV	Extension beyond the true pelvis or involvement of the bladder or rectal mucosa. Bullous edema as such does not permit a case to be allotted to stage IV
IVA	Spread to adjacent organs and/or direct extension beyond the true pelvis
IVB	Spread to distant organs

investigators do not use this classification, and there are few published data to support it (64,89).

PROGNOSTIC FACTORS INFLUENCING CHOICE OF TREATMENT

Invasive Squamous-Cell Carcinoma

As with most primaries, stage of disease is the dominant prognostic factor in terms of ultimate outcome (61–64, 90–98). In Creasman et al.'s report, the 5-year survival rate was 96% for patients with stage 0, 73% for stage I, 58% for stage II, and 36% for those with stage III-IV disease, respectively (51)[1]. In Perez et al.'s series, including 165 patients with primary vaginal carcinomas treated with definitive RT, the 10-year actuarial disease-free survival was 94% for stage 0, 75% for stage I, 55% for stage IIA, 43% for stage IIB, 32% for stage III, and 0% for those with stage IV (64).

The impact of lesion location has been controversial, with a series from Tarraza et al. (99) reporting that upper-third lesions develop local recurrences more frequently, and lower-third lesions develop a disproportionate number of sidewall and distant recurrences. However, a larger series failed to note any difference in site of recurrence based on primary lesion location (64). Several investigators (61,67, 100,101) have shown better survival and decreased recurrence rates for patients with cancers involving the proximal half of the vagina when compared with those in the distal half or those involving the entire length of the vagina. In addition, lesions of the posterior wall have a worse prognosis than those involving other vaginal walls (10-year recurrence rates of 32% and 19%, respectively) (61), which probably reflects the greater difficulty of performing adequate brachytherapy procedures in this location.

The prognostic importance of lesion size has been controversial, with an adverse impact being noted by Tjalma et al. (82) and Chyle et al. (61), which is contrary to Perez et al.'s findings (101). In the Chyle et al. series (61), lesions

measuring less than 5 cm in maximum diameter had a 20% 10-year local recurrence rate compared to 40% for those lesions larger than 5 cm. Similarly, in the Princess Margaret Hospital (PMH) experience, tumors larger than 4 cm in diameter fared significantly worse than smaller lesions (62). In the Perez et al. series (91), stage was an important predictor of pelvic tumor control and 5-year disease-free survival, but the size of the tumor in stage I patients was not a significant prognostic factor. However, in stage IIA disease, lower pelvic tumor control and survival were noted with tumors larger than 4 cm. In stages IIB and III, tumor size was not a significant prognostic factor, probably related to the difficulty in assessing size and the fact that higher doses of RT were delivered for larger tumors. Stock et al. (56) reported that disease volume, a likely surrogate for stage or lesion size, adversely impacted survival as well as local control.

Age was a significant prognostic factor in Urbanski et al.'s series (67), with 5-year survival of 63.2% for patients below the age of 60 years compared with 25% for those over 60 years of age (*p*<.001). Similar findings were reported by Eddy et al. (95). However, most of these series do not correct for death secondary to intercurrent disease in the elderly population. No statistical significance of age to survival was found in the series of Dixit et al. (96) and Perez et al. (91).

With regard to the histologic type and grade, several series (62,67,101) have shown the histologic grade to be an independent, significant predictor of survival. However, the histology of the tumor (SCC vs other) has not been found to be a prognostic factor for disease-free survival among the patients with invasive tumors.

Other Histologies

An increased propensity for distant metastases to the lung and supraclavicular nodes has been reported in patients with CCA (101). Stage, tubulocystic pattern, size less than 3 cm, and depth of invasion less than 3 mm were all noted to be associated with superior survival (9).

Vaginal melanoma has a higher propensity for development of distant metastases, and affected patients do more poorly than patients with SCC. A review by Reid et al. of 115 vaginal melanoma patients noted that depth of invasion and size of lesion (>3 cm) adversely impacted survival, but stage did not, perhaps because it was known for only 42 of the 115 patients in the series (28).

Patients with malignant mesenchymal tumors of the vagina do less well than those with invasive SCC. Specific, adverse prognostic factors for vaginal sarcoma identified by Tavassoli and Norris (32) included infiltrative versus pushing borders, high mitotic rate of five or more mitoses per 10 HPFs, size >3 cm in diameter, and cytologic atypia.

GENERAL MANAGEMENT: TREATMENT OPTIONS AND OUTCOME

Owing to its rarity, data concerning the natural history, prognostic factors, and treatment of vaginal carcinoma derive from small, retrospective studies. Most of the currently available literature in terms of radiotherapeutic and surgical techniques refers to primary SCC of the vagina. There is evidence that patients with early stage I, primarily with a lesion located in the upper or distal third of the vagina, and highly selected young women with stage II vaginal cancers can be successfully treated with surgery alone. However, few studies directly compare the two treatment modalities. Surgical resection generally requires a radical approach with urinary and fecal diversion in order to secure adequate margins, and therefore has largely been replaced by RT in order to maximize cure and improve quality of life. Furthermore, most patients are elderly, and a radical surgical approach is often not feasible. Local excision and partial and complete vaginectomy have given way to a more individualized approach that takes into consideration the patient's age, the extent of the lesion, and whether it is localized or multicentric. In younger patients with early-stage disease, treatment can also depend on the desire to preserve a functional vagina. In Stock et al.'s series (56), all 30 patients treated for primary carcinoma of the vagina that underwent radical vaginectomies or exenterative procedures completely lost vaginal function. Radical surgery in the past precluded vaginal function, but this situation has been improved significantly by the use of split-thickness grafts, intestinal segments, and myocutaneous flap reconstruction (104).

In most patients, the primary treatment modality is RT, as reported by the Society of Gynecologist Oncologists in practice guidelines published in 1998 (51). RT provides excellent tumor control in early and superficial lesions and with satisfactory functional results. This makes it imperative that RT techniques yielding optimal tumor control and functional results are utilized.

The site of tumor involvement at the time of diagnosis is often related to the gynecologic history. A significant percentage of patients with vaginal cancer have had previous hysterectomy for benign, premalignant, and malignant lesions, and a majority of these patients have tumors limited to the upper third of the vagina (56,66). This contrasts with patients who have not had a hysterectomy, among whom only 25% to 30% have lesions limited to the upper third of the vagina, partly because cancers that have spread to involve the cervix are often classified as cervical cancers.

Despite the acceptance of RT as the treatment of choice for this disease, in particular for patients with lesions involving the mid third of the vagina or stage II and greater, the optimal therapy for each stage is not well defined in the literature. Intracavitary and interstitial irradiation is used in small superficial stage I disease. A combination of external beam RT (EBRT) with intracavitary and/or interstitial brachytherapy with or without chemotherapy is used in more extensive stage I and stages II to IV disease. Data regarding the use of cytotoxic therapy in vaginal carcinomas are based on underpowered Phase II trials of various monotherapies

or extrapolated from SCC of the cervix, which has a similar biology.

Radiation Therapy Techniques

External Beam Radiotherapy

EBRT is advisable in patients with deeply infiltrating or poorly differentiated stage I lesions and in all patients with stages II to IVA disease. The treatment is generally delivered using opposed anterior and posterior fields (AP/PA). The pelvis receives between 20 and 45 Gy depending on the stage of the disease. This will be followed, in some cases, by bilateral pelvic sidewall boosts to 50 to 55 Gy. High-energy photons (>10 MV) are usually preferred. Treatment portals cover at least the true pelvis with 1.5- to 2.0-cm margin beyond the pelvic rim. Superiorly, the field extends to either L4-L5 or L5-S1 to cover the pelvic lymph nodes up to the common iliacs, and extends distally to the introitus to include the entire vagina. Lateral fields, if used, should extend anteriorly to adequately include the external iliac nodes, anterior to the pubic symphysis, and at least to the junction of S2-S3 posteriorly (Fig. 21.6).

In patients with tumors involving the middle and lower vagina with clinically negative groins, the bilateral inguinofemoral lymph node regions should be treated electively to 45 to 50 Gy. Planning CT is recommended to determine adequately the depth of the inguinofemoral nodes. A number of techniques have been used to treat the areas at risk without overtreating the femoral necks. Some of the most commonly used techniques include the use of unequal loading (2:1, AP/PA), a combination of low- and high-energy photons (4 to 6 MV, AP, and 15 to 18 MV, PA), or equally weighted beams with a transmission block in the central AP field, utilizing small AP photon or electron beams to deliver a daily boost to the inguinofemoral nodes. A technique has been developed and implemented at Indiana University that uses a narrow PA field to treat the pelvis and a wider AP field encompassing the pelvis and inguinofemoral nodes, with daily AP photon boost to the inguinal nodes being delivered using the asymmetric collimator jaws (105). Advantages of this technique include simplicity of setup and treatment (single isocenter, no need for transmission block), dose homogeneity, reduced dose to the femoral necks, low potential risk of nodal underdose, and elimination of dosimetric difficulties inherent in electron boosts (Fig. 21.7).

For patients with positive pelvic nodes, an additional boost to the areas of gross nodal disease, as defined by CT scan, should be given using small fields (similar to the parametrial boost with midline shielding) to deliver a total dose between 60 and 65 Gy with high-energy photons. In patients with clinically palpable inguinal nodes, additional doses of 15 to 20 Gy (calculated at a depth determined by CT scan) are necessary with reduced portals. This is generally

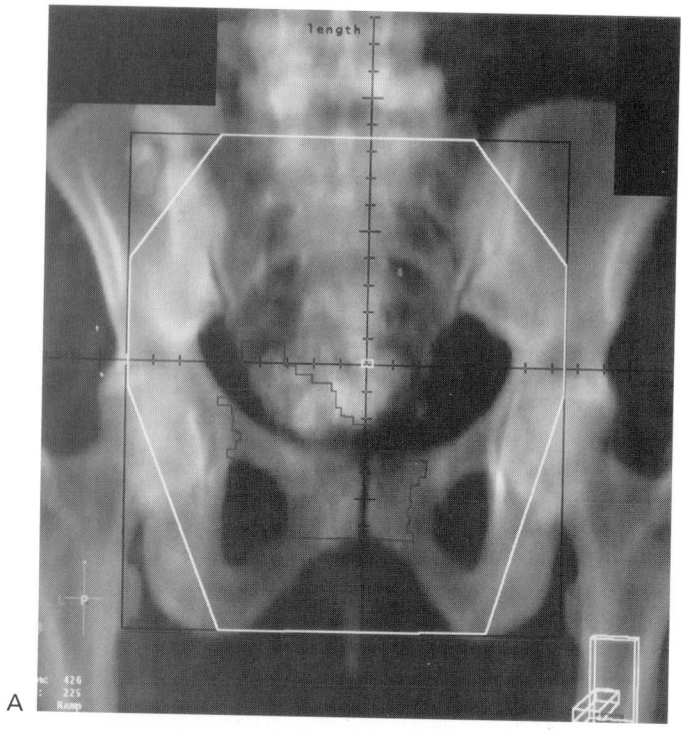

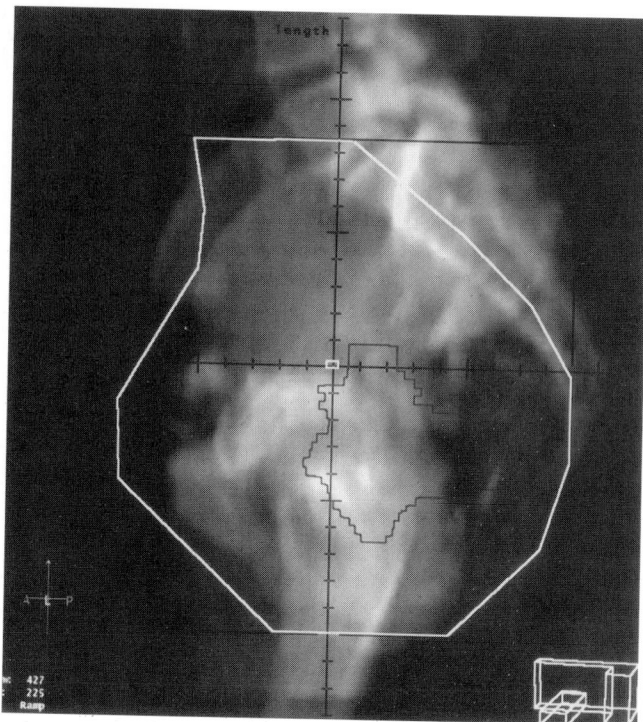

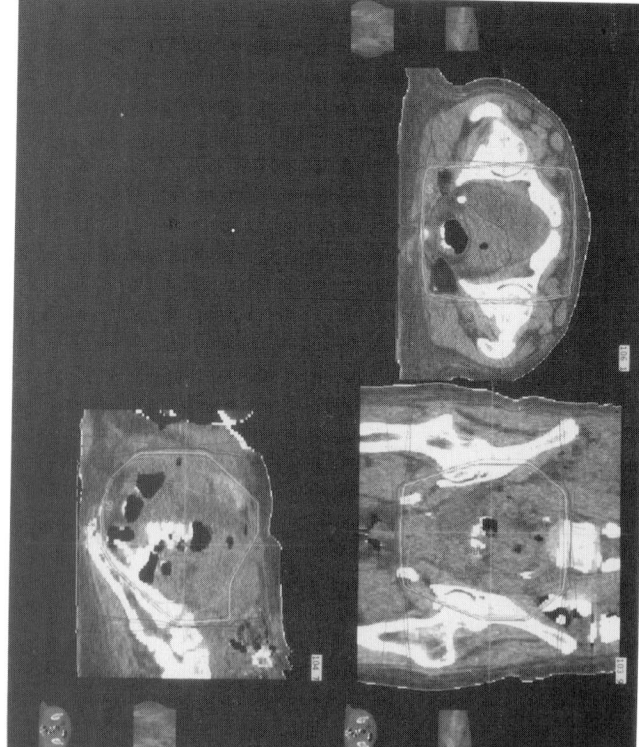

FIG. 21.6. Proximal-third vaginal cancer—squamous-cell carcinoma. Digital reconstructed radiographs (DRRs) AP/PA (**A**) and right/left lateral (**B**) whole pelvis fields. **C:** Axial, sagittal and coronal isodose distributions.

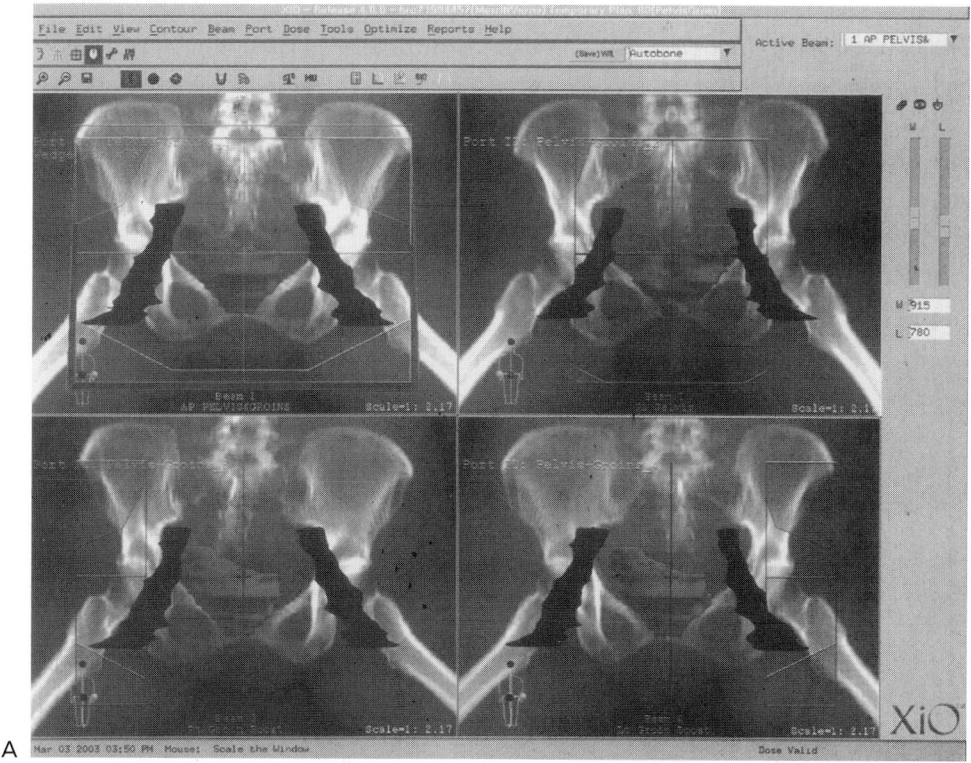

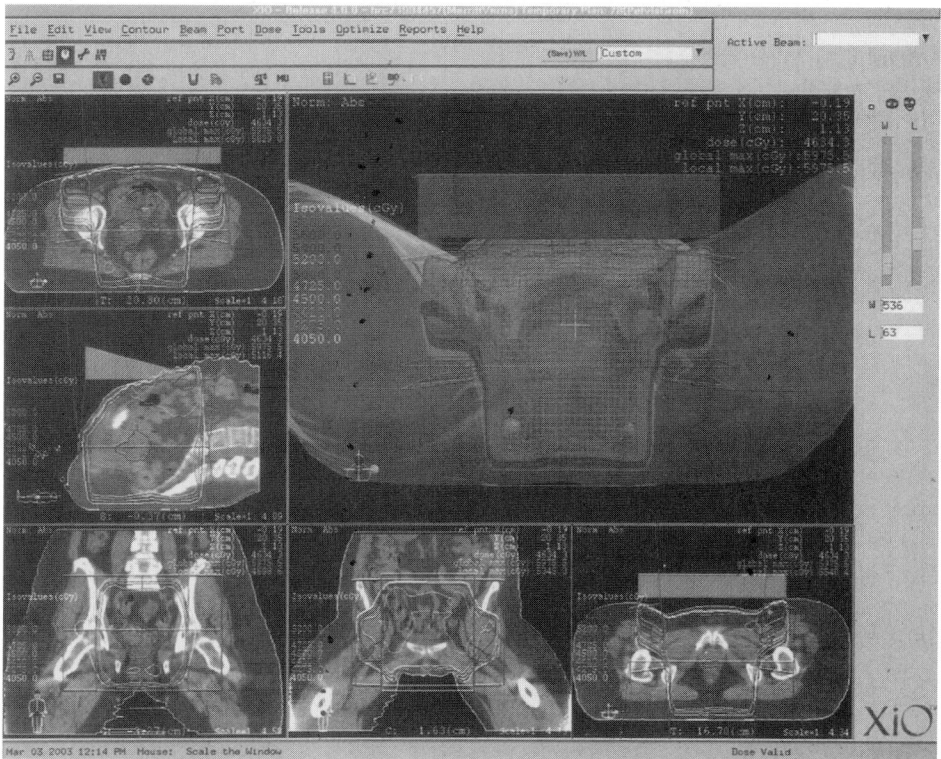

FIG. 21.7. Vaginal cancer with distal-third vaginal involvement—squamous-cell carcinoma. Technique for pelvic and inguinofemoral nodal irradiation. **A:** Digital reconstructed radiographs (DRRs) AP/PA and daily right and left inguinofemoral photon boost. **B:** Axial, sagittal, and coronal isodose distributions.

achieved by using low-energy photons or electron beam (12 to 18 MeV).

Low-Dose–Rate Intracavitary Brachytherapy

VAIN and small T1 lesions with less than a 0.5-cm depth can be adequately treated with intracavitary brachytherapy (ICB) alone. Low-dose–rate ICB (LDR-ICB) is performed using vaginal cylinders such as Burnett, Bloedorn, Delclos (106), or MIRALVA (Nucletron Veenendaal, The Netherlands) (107) loaded with cesium 137 (^{137}Cs) radioactive sources. The largest possible diameter that can be comfortably accommodated by the patient should be used to improve the ratio of mucosa to tumor dose, and eliminate vaginal rugations. In general, the vulva is sutured closed for the duration of the implant in order to secure the position of the applicators. Perez et al. (107,108) designed and constructed a vaginal applicator that incorporates two ovoid sources and a central tandem that can be used to treat the entire vagina (alone or in combination with the uterine cervix).

In patients with upper vagina lesions with less than a 0.5-cm depth of invasion, vaginal colpostats alone (after hysterectomy) or in combination with intrauterine tandem, loaded with ^{137}Cs sources similar to that used in treatment of cervical cancer, can be used to treat the proximal vagina to a minimum dose of 65 to 70 Gy, estimated to 0.5-cm depth, including the contribution of EBRT if given. When indicated, the remainder of the vagina can be treated by performing a subsequent implant using vaginal cylinders (generally 50 to 60 Gy prescribed to the vaginal surface). It is important to avoid the placement of a protruding source over the vulva, with the subsequent increased risk of complications. The use of LDR remote-control afterloading technology allows the reduction of radiation exposure to hospital personnel and optimization of the isodose distribution.

High-Dose–Rate Intracavitary Brachytherapy

High-dose–rate intracavitary brachytherapy (HDR-ICB) is typically performed with a 10-Ci single iridium 192 (^{192}Ir) source (Micro-Selectron HDR, Nucletron). The applicators are similar to those described for LDR-ICB.

Little information regarding HDR-ICB in the treatment of primary carcinoma of the vagina is available (66,109). Few patients have been treated, follow-up is short, publication bias is likely, and there is no agreement on treatment regimen. Generally, the number of insertions ranges from one to six (median three), with the dose per fraction ranging from 300 to 800 cGy (median 700 cGy). Nanavati et al. (109) reported 13 patients with primary vaginal cancer (5 stage I, 4 stage IIA, and 4 stage IIB) treated with external beam RT (45 Gy) and HDR-ICB (20 to 28 Gy in three to four fractions calculated at 0.5 cm from the surface of the applicator). All 13 patients had a complete response, and local control was achieved in 92% of the patients with a

median follow-up of only 2.6 years (range 0.7 to 5.2 years). The investigators did not observe any acute or chronic intestinal or bladder grade 3 or 4 toxicity. However, moderate to severe vaginal stenosis occurred in 46% of the patients. They recognize that "late-occurring toxicity could be missed at a medium follow-up of 2.6 years."

Many aspects remain unknown or not well understood in the use of HDR-ICB. These include the radiobiologic equivalency of HDR to LDR, fractionation schedule, total dose, specification of dose prescription, and how to combine HDR with EBRT and/or LDR brachytherapy. In addition, optimization approaches and methods of dose calculation, such as the inclusion of anisotropic corrections, are not well described in the sparse literature available to date (110,111). These factors could result in an increased incidence of severe complications, such as vaginal necrosis, and rectovaginal or vesicovaginal fistulas (112,113). In the opinion of the researchers, until further data are available with longer follow-up, as well as a better understanding of the physical and radiobiologic principles involved in the HDR-ICB, this should not be routinely used in the radiotherapeutic management of primary vaginal carcinoma. Given its excellent results and extensively documented long-term outcome and complications, we strongly encourage the continued use of LDR-ICB (61,62,64,91).

Interstitial Brachytherapy

Interstitial brachytherapy (ITB) is an important component in the treatment of more advanced primary vaginal carcinomas, typically in combination with EBRT and/or ICB. In the first place, a careful definition of the "target volume," which is the gross tumor volume (based on clinical, radiologic and operative findings) and a margin of adjoining normal tissue, is required. Other considerations include whether a permanent (^{198}Au or ^{125}I) or temporary implant (^{192}Ir) is optimal, the geometry of the implant (e.g., single or double plane or volume implant), source distribution, dose rate, and total dose, based upon tumor size, location, local extent, and proximity of normal structures (114). The principal advantages of temporary implants are readily controlled distribution of the radioactive sources and easier modification of the dose distribution. The main advantages of a permanent seed implant include relative safety/simplicity, easy applicability, cost effectiveness, and ability, in most cases, to be performed using local anesthesia. As a general rule, temporary implants are more commonly used in the curative treatment of larger gynecologic malignancies, whereas permanent implants are usually performed for smaller volume disease.

When performing an interstitial procedure, freehand implants or template systems designed to assist in preplanning and to guide and secure the position of the needles in the target volume can be employed. Popular commercially available templates include the Syed-Neblett device (SNIT)

(Alpha Omega Services, Bellflower, CA) (115), the modified Syed-Neblett (116), and the "MUPIT" (Martinez Universal Perineal Interstitial Template) (117). These templates generally consist of a perineal template, vaginal obturator, and 17-gauge hollow guides of various lengths that can be afterloaded with ^{192}Ir sources. The vaginal obturator is 2 cm in diameter and 12 or 15 cm in length with six to seven grooves on its surface for the placement of guide needles. It is centrally drilled so that it can allow the placement of a tandem to be loaded with ^{137}Cs sources. This makes it possible to combine an interstitial and intracavitary application simultaneously (Fig. 21.8).

The major advantage of these systems is greater control of the placement of the sources relative to tumor volume and critical structures owing to the fixed geometry provided by the template. In addition, improved dose-rate distributions are obtained by means of computer-assisted optimization of the source placement and strength during the planning and loading phase.

Owing to the inaccuracies of pelvic examination and close proximity of the rectum and bladder to the target volume, there exists a serious risk of either underdosing the target volume or causing bladder and rectal morbidity. In order to improve the accuracy of target localization and needle placement, several investigators have explored performing interstitial implant (ITI) under transrectal ultrasound (TRUS), CT, MRI-planned implants with endorectal coil, laparotomy, and laparoscopic guidance (118–120). Al-

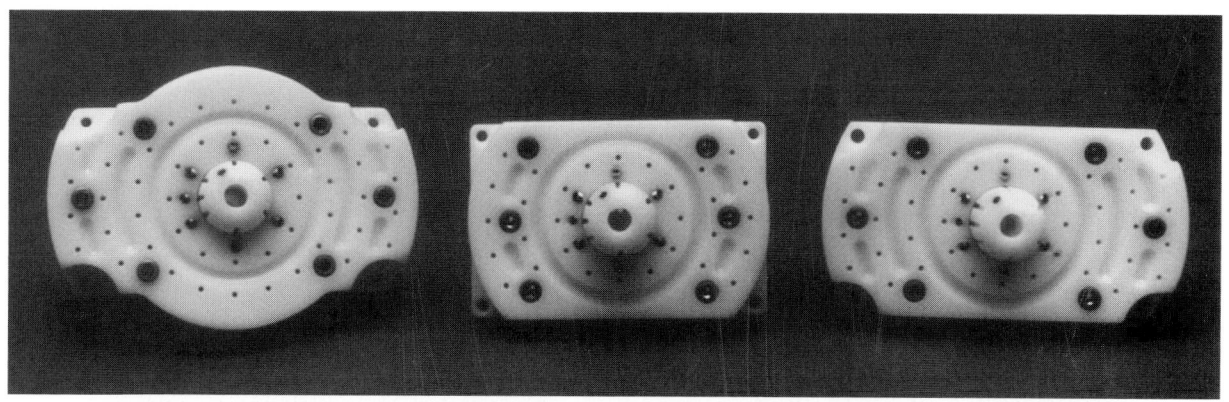

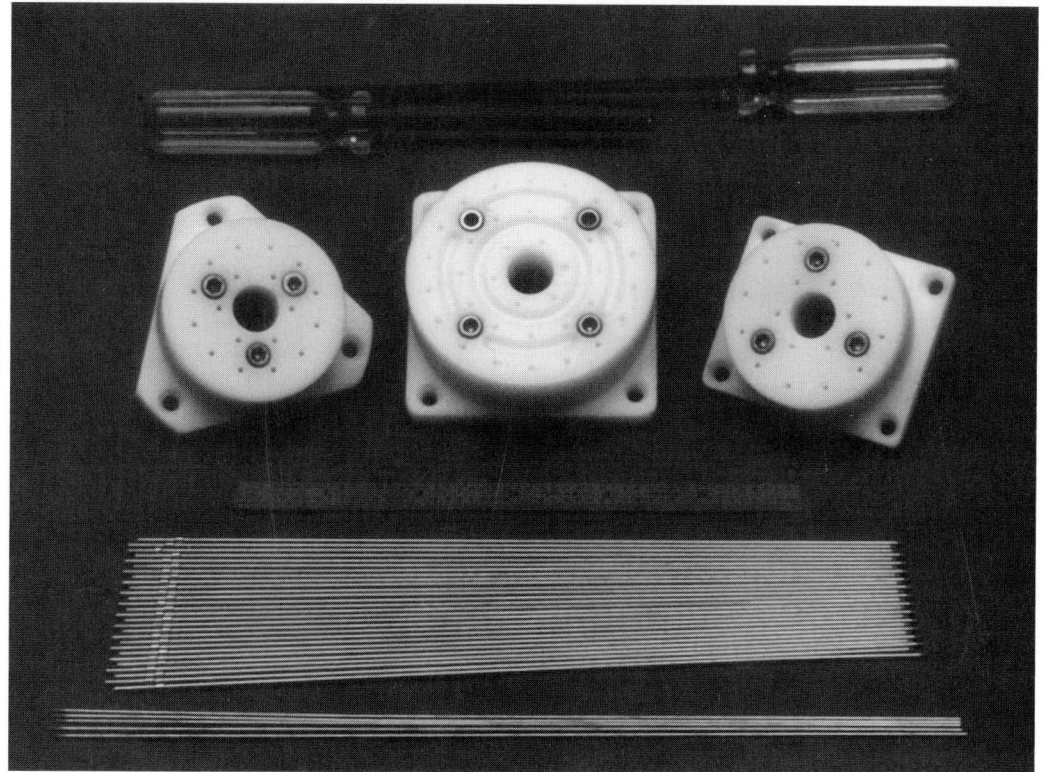

FIG. 21.8. A: Syed-Neblett and modified (**B**) templates. (Courtesy of Best Medical International.)

though laparotomy facilitates the displacement of bowel during the procedure by using slings or tissue expanders and/or lysis of adherent bowel (116), there is some degree of associated morbidity, such as ileus, bleeding, and increased operative time. Laparoscopy is a shorter and less invasive procedure. A real-time TRUS-guided Syed-Neblett template implantation technique was reported by Stock et al. (120). With this technique, invasive laparotomy/laparoscopy can often be avoided, providing an interactive, noninvasive technique allowing for highly accurate needle placement (120).

SQUAMOUS-CELL CARCINOMA: TREATMENT OPTIONS AND OUTCOME BY FIGO STAGES

FIGO Stage 0: VAIN-CIS

VAIN has been approached both surgically and medically by multiple investigators. Treatment options include local excision, partial or complete vaginectomy, laser vaporization, topical 5% fluorouracil (5-FU) administration, or ICB alone. Overall, the reported control rates are very similar among the different approaches, ranging from 48% to 100% for laser, 52% to 100% for colpectomy, 75% to 100% for topical 5-FU, and 83% to 100% for RT (Table 21.2) (51,61, 62,91,121–127,130–132,134). The degree of VAIN and the

age and general health of the patient are important treatment considerations. A therapy appropriate for CIS in a woman with good performance status and many anticipated years of life expectancy may not be appropriate for a woman with multiple co-morbid conditions who may succumb to one of her other illnesses before the CIS would be expected to progress to invasive carcinoma.

The anatomic constraints posed by the location of the vagina with the close proximity of the bladder and rectum led to the use of the CO_2 laser as a relatively noninvasive surgical approach (8,121–124). In a series of six patients, Stafl reported an 83% control rate with CO_2 laser if the involved mucosa was ablated to a depth of 1.5 to 2.0 mm (121). In a subsequent series of 36 patients, Townsend et al. achieved a 92% control rate; however, 32% of patients required more than one treatment, and follow-up was short (122). Jobson and Homesley suggested ablation of the entire vault to improve control rates (100%), and claimed that all 15 of their patients were able to resume coitus. However, of note, 26% required a second treatment, and follow-up averaged only 15 months (123). A subsequent series (8) noted less ideal control rates of 58% with laser vaporization. Hoffman et al. resorted to upper colpectomy in 32 patients, of whom 31 had undergone prior hysterectomy and 14 prior therapy for VAIN, and found a 28% risk of invasive disease (125). These

TABLE 21.2. *VAIN—carcinoma in situ—treatment approach and results*

Treatment modality/ investigator (ref.)	No. of patients	Comments	Outcome control
Laser therapy			
Stafl et al. (121)	6	Depth to 1.5–2.0 mm	LCR 83%
Townsend et al. (122)	36	32% had more than one treatment	LCR 92%
Jobson and Homesley (123)	15	26% required second treatment	LCR 100%
Julian et al. (124)	10	Used to effect colpectomy	LCR 80%
Hoffman et al. (8)	26	3 of 11 failures had invasive disease. Recommended excision. Not ideal	LCR 58%
Topical 5-FU			
Woodruff et al. (130)	9	1%–2% 5-FU q month	LCR 88%
Piver et al. (131)	8	20% 5-FU q day × 5 Could use 5% or 10%	LCR 75%
Petrilli et al. (132)	15	5% 5-FU BID × 5 days Repeat in 12 weeks	LCR 80%
Krebs (134)	31	1/3 applicator q week × 10 weeks	LCR 81%
Surgical excision			
Creasman et al. (51)	23		5-year survival 96%
(NCDB)			LCR 100%
Fanning et al. (126)	15	Used LEEP, one patient had cancer	66%
Robinson et al. (127)	46	CUSA—29 primaries	52%
Hoffman et al. (125)	32	CUSA—17 recurrent 28% invasive cancer of 23 with VAIN	LCR 83%
Irradiation			
Chyle et al. (61)	37		10-year DFS 83%
Kirkbride et al. (62)	14		10-year CSS 100%
Perez et al. (135)	20		10-year DFS 94%

CSS, Cause-specific survival; CUSA, cavitron ultrasonic aspirator; DFS, disease-free survival; LCR, local control rate; LEEP, loop electrosurgical excision procedure; NCDB, National Cancer Data Base; VAIN, vaginal intraepithelial neoplasia.

reports of invasive disease in the laser failures, and in patients who had undergone upper colpectomy for presumed VAIN, prompted some to begin to use the laser to effect colpectomy (124). Later series have used novel approaches with a loop electrosugical device (126) or the Cavitron ultrasonic aspirator (127) to effect partial colpectomy with satisfactory results, at least in the reporting investigator's hands. In a series of 52 patients reported by Diakomanolis et al., in which 28 underwent laser and 24 had partial colpectomy, results were found to be operator dependent, but they favored partial colpectomy for unifocal disease and laser ablation for multifocal disease (128). Overall, the control rates following laser vaporization range from 58% to 100% (8,121–124); however as many as one-quarter to one-third will require a second vaporization (122,123). Patients most likely to fail after vaporization are those with anatomic distortion caused by scarring (125). In general, patient acceptance is high and scarring minimal (129).

Although partial colpectomy has many advocates for focal VAIN without any prior history of pelvic RT, patients who had received prior pelvic RT for other gynecologic malignancies, wherein partial colpectomy would have high risk of fistula formation, may benefit from a medical approach with topical application of 5-FU. This acts by inciting a desquamation of the vaginal squamous epithelium, which later reepithelializes with presumably normal cells. Multiple schedules have been suggested since the first use of 5-FU, including monthly, daily, twice a day, and weekly administrations, with control rates ranging from 75% to 88% (130–134). However, we prefer the schedule suggested by Krebs et al. of one-third applicator weekly for 10 weeks (134). It is important that the perineal skin be protected with a topical ointment such as zinc oxide to prevent painful vulvar erosions regardless of which 5-FU application schedule is chosen.

Although partial or total vaginectomy has been considered by many to be an acceptable treatment, one of its main drawbacks is shortening or stenosis of the vagina, frequently with poor functional results. Hoffman (125) reported a 17% recurrence rate in a series of 32 patients with CIS of the vagina who underwent upper vaginectomy. In this series, 44% had received prior therapy, including laser vaporization, or topical 5-FU and local excision. Nine patients (28%) were found to have invasive cancer upon final pathologic examination. Four of 9 patients with invasive carcinoma showing more than 3.5-mm infiltration were treated subsequently with RT, 3 of whom remained free of disease. Of the five patients with less than 2-mm invasion, one received RT for local recurrence, and the remaining four patients were without disease after surgery alone. Of 23 patients with VAIN III, 19 (83%) remained without evidence of recurrence at a mean follow-up of 38 months. Overall, five of nine patients with microinvasive carcinoma required RT in addition to surgery, and only 72% of all patients treated with surgery remained free of disease at last follow-up (23 of 32). Hoffman et al.

(125) advocated upper vaginectomy with 1-cm margins when there were concerns about possible invasion, and when the lesion was confined to the upper one-third or one-half of the vagina. To minimize postoperative stenosis, Hoffman (125) recommended not closing the mucosa, using a dilator with estrogenic vaginal cream, and consideration of a skin graft. Prior RT is probably a contraindication to vaginectomy owing to significantly increased morbidity (125). Control rates of 66% to 100% following partial colpectomy effected either with a traditional surgical approach (125), with cavitational ultrasonic aspiration (CUSA) (127), or with the loop electrosurgical excision procedure LEEP (126) have been achieved.

RT has a long history of documented efficacy, and has a significantly better therapeutic ratio than other modalities (61,62,89,91). Using conventional LDR-ICB techniques, the entire vaginal mucosa should receive between 60 and 80 Gy in one or two implants (135). Perez et al. reported only one distal local failure in the 20 patients treated for CIS (135).

There have been some reports in the literature regarding the use of HDR-ICB for patients with VAIN III. Ogino et al. (136) reported six patients treated with HDR to a mean dose of 23.3 Gy (range 15 to 30 Gy), none of whom developed recurrent disease. Limited rectal bleeding and moderate to severe vaginal mucosa reactions were noted in patients treated to the entire length of the vagina. MacLeod et al. (137) used HDR-ICB to treat 14 patients with VAIN III with a dose of 34 to 45 Gy in 4.5- to 8.5-Gy fractions, achieving a local tumor control of 78.5%. With a median duration of follow-up of 46 months, two patients developed grade 3 vaginal toxicity. At the present time, no definite conclusions can be drawn from the limited data published in the literature regarding the use of HDR-ICB. Based on the excellent local control and functional results obtained with LDR-ICB, this remains, in our opinion, the treatment of choice when definitive RT is used.

Invasive Squamous-Cell Carcinoma

Surgical Approach: Outcomes

In general, SCC of the vagina has been treated with RT. However, several surgical series have reported acceptable to excellent outcomes in well-selected patients, with survival rates after radical surgery for stage I disease ranging from 75 to 100%. Cases in which surgery may be the preferred treatment include selected stage I-II patients, with lesions at the apex and upper third of the posterior or lateral vagina that could be approached with radical hysterectomy, upper vaginectomy, and pelvic lymphadenectomy providing adequate margins (56–58,68,79) and very superficial lesions that may be removed with wide local excision. Lesions in the lower third of the vagina would require vulvovaginectomy in addition to dissection of inguinofemoral node exenteration to achieve negative margins (56–58,79). If the margins are found to be close or positive after resection, adjuvant RT is recommended. However, for lesions at other sites, and those cases requiring more extensive resection, definitive RT is the treatment of choice, with isolated central failures offered exenteration (79).

In a review of the NCDB for cancers of the vagina, Creasman et al. noted superior survival in those undergoing surgery (51). However, they and Tjalma et al. (82) recognized that there may be bias in surgical series. Younger, healthier patients with better performance status are more likely to be offered radical surgery, whereas older patients with multiple co-morbid medical conditions are offered RT.

Ball and Bearman's series (57) included 58 patients: 27 stage I and 18 stage II disease. Twenty-seven patients were managed primarily with surgery, with an overall 78% 5-year survival rate; 84% in patients with stage I and a 63% rate in those with stage II disease, which is comparable to the results reported by Perez et al. in their RT series (64). Rubin et al. (79) reported 75 cases of vaginal cancer: 14 patients with stage I and 35 patients with stage II. RT was the primary modality used in this series; however, eight patients (five with stage I and three with stage II) underwent primary surgery with curative intent. Six of these eight patients survived 5 years, and the local control rate for stage I patients was 80%. However, only one patient with stage II was a long-term survivor. This surgical outcome compares unfavorably with the remaining patients in whom RT was the primary modality. In general, patients with lesions that could be encompassed by radical vulvovaginectomy with or without hysterectomy did better than those requiring exenteration. Rubin et al. (79) advocated that exenteration should be reserved for those with central failure after RT, or as primary therapy in those with disease not fixed to the bone. Davis et al. (68) reported on 52 patients with cancer of the vagina treated with surgery alone in a series that included 89 cases. In this nonrandomized series, an 85% 5-year survival rate was achieved in stage I patients compared to 65% in those treated with RT (68). Of 45 patients with stage II disease, 49% survived after surgery, 50% after RT, and 69% after surgery and RT.

Peters et al.'s series (92) included 86 vaginal carcinomas, with an overall survival rate of 56%. Most were treated with RT. However, 12 highly selected patients had surgery, with a 75% survival rate. The investigators suggested that vaginectomy with radical hysterectomy, if the uterus was still in place, should be limited to those with superficial disease because the closeness of the bladder and rectum limited the true radicality of surgical approaches. These same investigators also reported on a small series of six patients with stage I disease with apparent microinvasive carcinoma of the vagina and less than 3 mm of invasion, all of whom survived, with a median follow-up of 132 months (138). Gallup et al. (58) reported 28 cases, of which 57% were stage I-II lesions (only three patients had stage II), and of these, 83% survived. Most patients

in this series received RT; however, all three patients with stage I disease who were treated with surgery survived. Extent of surgery and median follow-up were not stated.

In the largest single-institution series reported to date by Stock et al. (56), of 100 patients with carcinoma of the vagina (including 85 with SCC), a 47% 5-year survival rate was achieved. In this series, 40 patients were treated with surgery alone, 47 with radiation alone, and 13 with combination therapy. Overall, 5-year survival was 47%. Survival for stage I patients was 56% when treated with surgery versus 80% for those who recieved RT, whereas for stage II patients, a 68% survival was seen versus a 31% survival in those who underwent RT (56). The investigators acknowledged that the apparent surgical superiority for stage II patients may have been due to selection bias in that those treated with RT alone were more likely to have had stage IIB disease with extensive paracolpos involvement, and those with lesser involvement were preferentially offered surgery. They advocated RT for stage II patients with extensive paracolpos. Stock et al. concluded that for upper-third vault lesions, radical hysterectomy and pelvic lymphadenectomy with upper vaginectomy should be offered to those with stage I lesions, with a consideration for wide local excisions, and postoperative RT for patients with small lesions. If there was extension to the paracolpos, RT should be recommended; however, in very well-selected patients, there might be a role for surgery.

Tjalma et al. reported on 55 cases of SCC of the vagina, including 27 cases with stage I and 12 with stage II disease, with a median follow-up of 45 months (82). Of the 27 cases with stage I disease, 26 underwent surgery, and 4 of them received some form of postoperative RT. A 91% 5-year survival rate was achieved for stage I disease. Surgery was a part of the primary management for 6 of the 12 patients with stage II disease. In the multviariate analysis, age and lesion size were the only prognostic factors. Tjalma et al. concluded that surgery should be considered part of the therapeutic approach for stage I and minimal stage II disease (82). However, as Stock et al. suggested (56), and later Creasman et al. (51) and Tjalma et al. (82) concurred, such apparent improvement in small surgical series may be secondary to a selection bias that "cherry picks" patients with better performance status and smaller lesions for surgery, whereas older patients with more co-morbid medical conditions and larger stage I-II lesions undergo RT.

Although several series have reported on primary surgical approaches, including exenterations for patients with advanced stage III-IV SCC, achieving control rates as high as 50% for highly selected patients (56–58,79), the number of patients treated in any single series is so small that in modern practice, primary exenteration for advanced disease would not be recommended as the preferred approach. Therefore, advanced-stage patients should receive definitive RT, probably in combination with concurrent chemotherapy, although the role of combined modality therapy is unknown.

With regard to the surgical technique, if a complete vaginectomy is to be undertaken, most experts have suggested a combined abdominoperineal approach, with the perineal incision in the pubocervicovesical fascia made beneath the urethra and above the rectum so as to avoid the hemorrhoidal plexus. Some have suggested that the perineal incision can be made before or after the abdominal incision to perform the radical abdominal resection. However, we would favor performing the abdominal incision, first mobilizing the bladder, urethra, and rectum down to the perineum, and dividing the paracolpos at the side wall, mobilizing the ureters, and harvesting the nodes such that if unresectable disease is found, the patient would be spared a perineal incision. Given the large defect that is left after surgical resection, placement of a gracilis myocutaneous flap allows not only coverage of the defect, but may serve as a neovagina in the sexually active woman (104,139).

Radiation Therapy Approach: Outcomes

Most investigators emphasize that brachytherapy alone is adequate for superficial stage I patients. Ninety-five percent to 100% local control has been achieved with intracavitary and interstitial techniques (56,63,64,67,101,138,140,141). Superficial lesions can be adequately treated with ICB alone using afterloading vaginal cylinders. Mucosal doses of 80 to 120 Gy are typically delivered, depending on the diameter of the cylinders, when prescribing 65 to 70 Gy at 0.5-cm depth beyond the vaginal surface (135). For lesions thicker than 0.5 cm at the time of implantation, it is advisable to combine ICB and ITB in order to deliver a tumor dose in the range of 65 to 70 Gy, calculated to the base of the lesion, limiting the proximal and distal vaginal mucosal doses to 140 and 100 Gy, respectively.

There are no well-established criteria regarding the use of EBRT in patients with stage I disease. Perez et al. (64, 91) did not find a significant correlation between the technique of irradiation used and the probability of local or pelvic recurrence, probably since the treatment technique varied based on tumor-related factors. There is general consensus that EBRT (20 to 50 Gy) is advisable for larger, more infiltrating or poorly differentiated tumors that may have a higher risk of lymph node metastasis. Chyle et al. (61) recommended EBRT in addition to brachytherapy for stage I disease to cover at least the paravaginal nodes, and, in larger lesions, to cover the external and internal iliac nodes. The 5-year survival for patients with stage I disease treated with RT alone ranges from 70% to 95%.

Patients with stage II disease are uniformly treated with EBRT followed either by ICB and/or ITB. Perez et al. (91) showed that in stage IIA, the local tumor control was 70% (37 of 53) in patients receiving brachytherapy combined with EBRT, compared with 40% (4 of 10) in patients treated with either brachytherapy or EBRT alone. In stage IIB, the locoregional control was also superior with combined EBRT and brachytherapy (61% vs 50%, respectively). Generally, 40–50 Gy is delivered to the whole pelvis, followed by an additional boost of 30–35 Gy given with brachytherapy. Patients with lesions limited to the upper third of the vagina can be treated with an intrauterine tandem and vaginal ovoids or cylinders. In patients with parametrial infiltration, a ''boost'' with EBRT and/or an interstitial implant is advisable to deliver a minimum tumor dose of 70–75 Gy and 55–60 Gy to the pelvic side wall. The 5-year survival for patients with stage II disease treated with RT alone ranges between 35% and 70% for stage IIA, and 35% and 60% for stage IIB. The results of several series published in the literature using different treatment approaches for stage I and II vaginal cancer are shown in Table 21.3 (51,56,57,61, 62,67,68,79,82,101).

Generally, patients with stage III and IVA disease will receive 45–50 Gy EBRT to the pelvis, and in some cases, additional parametrial dose with midline shielding to deliver up to 60 Gy to the pelvic side walls. Ideally, ITB brachytherapy boost is performed, if technically feasible, to deliver a minimum tumor dose of 75–80 Gy. If brachytherapy is not feasible, a shrinking-field technique can be used, with fields defined using the three-dimensional treatment planning capabilities to deliver a tumor dose around 65 Gy. The overall cure rate for patients with stage III disease is 30%-50%. Stage IVA includes patients with rectal or bladder mucosa involvement, or in most series, positive inguinal nodes. Although some patients with stage IVA disease are curable, many patients are treated palliatively with EBRT only. Pelvic exenteration can also be curative in highly selected stage IV patients with small-volume central disease. Table 21.4 (51,56,57,61,62,67,79,91,101) shows the treatment results with different therapeutic modalities, including four series that reported the use of primary surgery in highly selected patients with advanced disease. However, each of these series reported a far greater number of patients with similar stage disease treated with RT, which represents the preferred approach in contemporary practice (64,89).

Role of Chemotherapy and Radiation

The control rate in the pelvis for stages III-IV patients is relatively low, and about 70% to 80% of the patients have persistent disease or recurrent disease in the pelvis in spite of high doses of EBRT and brachytherapy. Failure in distant sites does occur in about 25% to 30% of the patients with locally advanced tumors, which is much less than pelvic recurrences. Therefore, there is a need for better approaches to the management of advanced disease such as the use of concomitant chemoradiotherapy. Agents such as 5-FU, mitomycin, and cisplatin have shown promise when combined

TABLE 21.3. *FIGO stage I–II vaginal cancer—treatment approach and results*

Treatment modality/ investigator (ref.)	No. of patients	Outcome-survival
Irradiation ± surgery		
Chyle et al. (61)	59 St I	10-year DFS 76%
	104 St II	10-year 69%
Creasman et al. (NCDB) (51)	169 St I	5-year survival 73%; 79% S + RT (47),[a] 63% RT (122)
	175 St II	5-year survival 58%; 58% S + RT (39), 57% RT (136)
Davis et al. (68)	19	5-year survival 100%; S + RT (5), 65% RT (14)
Kirkbride et al. (62)	40 St I	5-year survival 72%
	38 St II	5-year 70%
Kucera and Vavra (101)	16 St I	5-year 81%
	23 St II	5-year 43.5%
Perez et al. (91)	59 St I	10-year DFS 80%
	63 St IIA	10-year 55%
	34 St IIB	10-year 35%
Stock et al. (56)	8 St I	5-year 100%; S + RT, 80% RT
	35 St II	5-year 69% S + RT, 31% RT
Urbanski et al. (67)	33 St I	5-year survival 73%
	37 St II	5-year 54%
Radical surgery		**5-year survival**
Ball and Berman (57)	19 St I	84%
	8 St II	63%
Creasman et al. (NCDB) (51)	76 St I	90%
	34 St II	70%
Davis et al. (68)	25 St I	85%
	27 St II	49%
Rubin et al. (79)	5 St I	80%
	3 St II	33%
Stock et al. (56)	17 St I	56%
	23 St II	68%
Tjalma et al. (82)	26[b]	91%

CSS, Cause-specific survival; DFS, disease-free survival; LCR, local control rate; RT, radiotherapy; S, surgery; St, stage.

[a] The most common surgical procedure was wide local excision (64%). Seventy-seven percent of the patients were treated with external beam RT alone (37%) or in combination with brachytherapy (40%). Seventeen percent of the patients were treated with brachytherapy alone.

[b] Four patients received adjuvant radiation.

with RT, with complete response rates as high as 60% to 85% (142,143), but long-term results of such therapy have been variable. In these small studies, many of the patients had advanced (stage III) disease at the initiation of combined-modality therapy, perhaps explaining the lack of long-term disease control. Evans et al. (142) found no local recurrences, however, among patients achieving a complete response with RT and 5-FU plus mitomycin C (12 of 25 patients), with a median follow-up period of 28 months, suggesting that local control may be improved with combined-modality therapy since local failure is common with radiation alone in large-volume pelvic disease. The survival for the entire population was 56% (66% for patients with primary vaginal cancer). Only two patients had severe complications, although the investigators recognize that longer follow-up is probably required to assess the true incidence of late effects. More sobering are the data from Roberts et al. (143), who reported 67 patients with advanced cancers of the vagina, cervix, and vulva treated with concurrent 5-FU, cisplatin, and RT. Although 85% experienced a complete response, 61% of the cancers recurred, with a median time to recurrence of only 6 months and an overall survival at 5 years of 22%. Further, 9 of 67 patients (13%) developed severe late complications of which 8 required surgeries. Kersch et al. (144) reported that five of eight vaginal cancer patients achieved local control with combined-modality therapy. Studies of primary chemoradiation in primary vaginal cancer are small or heterogeneous populations including cervical and vulvar cancers, making it difficult truly to assess the role of combined-modality therapy in the management of locally advanced disease. No randomized trials comparing radiation with or without chemotherapy have been reported.

Further investigation is needed to determine the therapeutic efficacy of the concurrent chemoradiotherapeutic and the optimal chemotherapeutic regimen. Recently published data on locally advanced cervical cancer have demonstrated an advantage in locoregional control, overall survival, and disease-free survival for patients receiving cisplatin-based chemotherapy concurrently with RT (145–148). The only drug common to all the studies was cisplatin, suggesting it

TABLE 21.4. *FIGO stage III-IV vaginal cancer—outcome with radiation therapy with/without surgery*

Treatment modality/ investigator (ref.)	No. of patients	Outcome-survival
Irradiation ± surgery		
Chyle et al. (61)	55 St III	10-year DFS 47%
	16 St IV	10-year 27%
Creasman et al. (NCDB) (51)	180 St III-IV	5-year survival 36%; 60% S + RT (36), 35% RT (144)
Kirkbride et al. (62)	42ª St III-IV	5-year survival 53%
Kucera and Vavra (101)	46 St III	5-year survival 35%
	19 St IVA	5-year 32%
Perez et al. (91)	20 St III	10-year DFS 38%
	15 St IV	0%
Stock et al. (56)	9 St III	5-year DFS 0%
	8 St IV	0%
Urbanski et al. (67)	40 St III	5-year survival 22.5%
	15 St IVA	0%
Radical surgery		**5-year survival**
Ball and Berman (57)	2 St III	50%
Creasman et al. (NCDB) (51)	St III-IV, 211	47%
Rubin et al. (79)	2 St III	50%

CSS, Cause-specific survival; DFS, disease-free survival; LCR, local control rate; NCDB, National Cancer Data Base; RT, radiotherapy; S, surgery; St, stage.
ª Twenty patients stage III-IV were treated with chemotherapy (5-FU ± mitomycin C) and radiotherapy.

may be the only agent needed to improve radiation sensitivity. Based on these data, consideration should be given to a similar approach in patients with advanced vaginal cancer. Randomized trials comparing radiation therapy alone to chemoradiation therapy, however, are unlikely because of small patient numbers.

PATTERNS OF FAILURE IN SQUAMOUS-CELL CARCINOMA

Of patients recurring, at least 85% will have locoregional failure, and the vast majority of these recurrences will be confined to the pelvis and vagina. The rate of locoregional recurrence in stage I is approximately 10% to 20% versus 30% to 40% in stage II. The pelvic control rate for patients with stage III and stage IV is relatively low, and about 50% to 70% of the patients have recurrences or persistence in spite of well-designed RT. The median time to recurrence is 6 to 12 months. Tumor recurrence is associated with a dismal prognosis, with only a few long-term survivors after salvage therapy. Failure in distant sites alone or associated with locoregional failure does occur in about 25% to 40% of patients with locally advanced tumors (61,62,67,68,91, 101,149) (Table 21.5).

Potential Radiation Therapy–Related Factors Influencing Outcome

It is important to recognize that analysis of RT doses and techniques and their impact on local/pelvic tumor control is fraught with difficulty since the available data are retrospective and not the result of prospective randomized or dose-escalation studies. Andersen (60) has shown in a small series of 29 patients with primary carcinoma of the vagina that a combination of EBRT and brachytherapy was significantly better than brachytherapy alone, and the cure rate in patients receiving a total tumor dose of 70 Gy or more was significantly higher than that in patients receiving lower doses. In the Stanford experience (65), earlier stage and higher RT dose had a positive influence on survival. Nine of 16 patients receiving ≤75 Gy had recurrent disease versus 3 of 22 receiving >75 Gy. Larger series have not found a significant impact of the RT dose and recurrence rate, probably because larger tumors received higher EBRT and brachytherapy doses (61,91).

Perez et al. (64,91) reported increased tumor control in patients with stages IIA to IVA with EBRT and brachytherapy compared to patients receiving brachytherapy alone. In patients with stage I disease, no correlation was found between the technique of RT used and the incidence of local or pelvic recurrences. In addition, they suggested that doses in the range of 70 to 75 Gy to the primary tumor volume and 55 and 65 Gy to the medial parametria for patients with more advanced disease are necessary to optimize tumor and pelvic control. Furthermore, of 100 patients with primary tumors involving the upper and middle third of the vagina who received no elective irradiation to the groins, none developed metastatic inguinofemoral lymph nodes, which is in contrast to 3 of 29 (10%) patients with lower-third primaries and 1 of 20 patients with tumors involving the entire

TABLE 21.5. *Sites of recurrence*

Investigator (ref.)	No. of patients	Percentage of recurrence	Locoregional recurrence	Distant recurrence	Local + distant
Chyle et al. (61)	301	35%	21%	11%	3%
Davis et al. (68)	89	St I (23%)	18%	5%	
		St II (36%)	16%	20%	Not shown
Kirkbride et al. (62)	153	42%	32%	7%	3%
Kucera and Vavra (101)	110	24.5%	21%	4%	0.5%
Perez et al. (91)	212	St 0 (5%)	5%	0	0
		St I (22%)	8%	8%	5%
		St IIA (47%)	17%	13%	17%
		St IIB (71%)	15%	26%	29%
		St III (55%)	5%	20%	30%
		St IVA (73%)	27%	0	47%
		TOTAL: 42%	13%	12%	17%
Tabata et al. (149)	51	St 0-II (36%)	36%	0%	Not shown
		St III-IV (92%)	50%	42%	
Urbanski et al. (67)	125	53%	41%	8%	4%

St, stage.

length of the vagina. Of seven patients with initially palpable inguinal lymph nodes treated with doses in the range of 60 Gy, only one developed a nodal recurrence. The investigators recommended that elective RT of the inguinal lymph nodes should be carried out only in patients with primary tumors involving the lower third of the vagina.

Stock et al. (56) found a significant increase in local control and 5-year survival for patients receiving EBRT and brachytherapy compared to those treated with EBRT alone. The 5-year actuarial local control and survival in the EBRT and brachytherapy group were 44% and 50%, respectively, compared with 12% and 9%, respectively, in the EBRT alone group. However, these two groups were not evenly matched, with a large percentage of stage IV lesions in the EBRT alone group compared with the brachytherapy group.

Lee et al. (90) identified overall treatment time as the most significant treatment factor predicting pelvic tumor control in 65 patients with carcinomas of the vagina treated with definitive RT. If the entire course of RT, including EBRT and brachytherapy, was completed within 9 weeks, pelvic tumor control was 97% in contrast to only 57% when treatment time extended beyond 9 weeks ($p<.01$). Conversely, Perez et al. (91) did not find a significant impact of prolongation of treatment time on pelvic tumor control. Nevertheless, these investigators advocate completion of treatment within 7 to 9 weeks.

CLEAR-CELL CARCINOMA OF THE VAGINA

Since Herbst and Scully's first report (150) of seven adenocarcinomas arising in the vagina of adolescent females after *in utero* exposure to DES, there have been several reports limited to DES-related vaginal CCA (73,151–153). In 1979, Herbst et al. (152) reported 142 cases of stage I CCA of the vagina. An 8% risk of recurrence was seen after radical

surgery (N = 117), and an 87% survival was achieved. There was a 36% risk of recurrence after RT for stage I lesions; however, the investigators acknowledged that, in general, RT was reserved for large stage I lesions that involved more of the vault and were less amenable to surgical resection. As the majority of CCAs occur in the upper third of the vault, the largest series (152,154,155) addressing the surgical approach to these lesions have advocated radical hysterectomy, pelvic and paraaortic lymphadenectomy, and sufficient colpectomy to achieve negative margins. Senekjian et al. have also reported a series of exenterations done for CCA (156). However, there have also been efforts to attempt fertility-sparing radical resections (157,158) or more limited wide local excisions followed by some form of RT (154).

Senekjian et al. (154) reported a series of 219 stage I CCA cases with 92% overall 5-year survival rates and 88% 10-year survival rates, respectively, in 176 patients receiving conventional therapy (identical to 43 patients who had undergone local therapy). Of the 176 patients treated conventionally, 128 underwent radical hysterectomy and vaginectomy; 16 had the same operation followed by adjuvant RT; and 32 were treated with RT alone. Because of the risk of node metastases, 14 of 43 patients treated with local therapy underwent extraperitoneal pelvic lymphadenectomy. Of the 43 patients treated with local therapy, 9 had vaginectomy, 17 had local excision alone, 6 had brachytherapy alone, and 11 had combined local exicision and brachytherapy. The 10-year actuarial recurrence rate was an unsatisfactory 45% in those who underwent local excision alone versus only 16% if they had received conventional therapy and 27% if they had received local excision followed by RT. Senekjian et al. (154) advocated a combination of wide local excision and extraperitoneal node dissection followed by brachytherapy for patients desirous of fertility preservation.

In a subsequent report, Senekjian et al. (155) reviewed the experience with 76 cases with stage II CCA from the Registry for Research on Hormonal Transplacental Carcinogenesis. The overall 5- and 10-year survival rates were 83% and 65%, respectively. Of the 76 patients, 22 received surgery exclusively (either radical hysterectomy with vaginectomy, 13 patients, or exenterative type procedure, 9 patients), 38 received RT alone, 12 received combination therapy, and 4 underwent other approaches. Patients treated with primary RT achieved an 87% 5-year survival rate versus 80% for those treated with surgery and 85% for those receiving both treatments. The investigators concluded that most patients with stage II vaginal CCA should be treated with combination EBRT and brachytherapy; however, small, easily resectable lesions in the upper fornix might undergo resection, allowing better preservation of coital and ovarian function (155). Senekjian et al. (156) reported their experience of 20 pelvic exenterations for CCA of the vagina, including 13 for primary lesions and 7 for recurrent disease; they described a 72% success rate if the exenterations were done as part of primary therapy. They advocated reserving exenterative approaches for those who have failed RT in order to maximize quality of life for the greatest number of patients (156). There are few published reports regarding the use of systemic therapy for CCA. Fowler et al. (159) reported one complete and one partial response after treatment with melphalan (1 mg/kg qd × 5 days). Robboy et al. (103) reported responses in recurrent disease to both 5-FU and vinblastine.

MELANOMA OF THE VAGINA

Vaginal melanoma is an exceedingly rare entity. It accounts for 2% to 3% of all primary tumors of the vagina and approximately 0.5% of all malignant melanomas in females. Therefore, the number of patients with vaginal melanoma is too small to permit prospective controlled trials. Melanoma of the vagina, with its propensity to develop distant metastases and its lack of a recognized precursor lesion, has presented therapeutic challenges for surgeons. Investigators have reported small series with generally disappointing results irrespective of treatment modality (26,160–165). Because of the reputation of melanoma as a radioresistant tumor, it is not surprising that radical surgery has been considered to be the treatment of choice in operable patients. However, limited data are available which validate its efficacy. Although 75% 2-year survival has been achieved after radical excision in small series (165), most series report 5-year survival rates of 5% to 30% regardless of radicality of surgery (26–28,160,165).

Morrow and DiSaia, in their review of all genital melanoma, noted no long-term survivors after isolated wide local excision for vaginal melanoma; however, 3 of 19 patients survived following exenteration (27). In Chung et al.'s series of 19 patients, 7 were treated with radical surgery, including one exenteration and six radical vaginectomies, with or without hysterectomy, with an overall survival of 21%. All patients treated with wide local exicision developed recurrences (26). Similarly, Levitan et al. (164), in their review of the literature, argued that although the 2-year survival following radical surgery was better (20% to 40%) than with any other therapy, the 5-year survival rates were equally poor (average 8%) regardless of type of therapy. Furthermore, the incidence of distant recurrence was not influenced by the extent of surgical resection. Geisler et al. (162) published the Indiana University experience using pelvic exenteration for malignant melanomas of the vagina or urethra with more than 3 mm of invasion. None of the four patients included in this study had recurrences, and three patients remained alive with a minimum follow-up of 31 months. Conversely, Bonner et al. (160) reported nine cases of vaginal melanoma: Three received wide local excisions and six underwent radical surgery (including exenterations and radical vaginectomies with or without hysterectomies), with a 29% actuarial 5-year survival rate. All nine patients suffered locoregional recurrence. The investigators advocated that surgery alone was ineffective in obtaining local control, and that preoperative RT should be considered (160).

Reid et al. (28) reported an overall 17% 5-year survival rate in a report of 15 patients, including 13 who underwent surgery. In addition, they reviewed the literature, summarizing the results achieved in 115 patients with vaginal melanoma, and compared outcomes for the 55 patients who underwent some form of surgery, including the 24 treated conservatively with wide local excision or partial vaginectomy to the 31 treated with more radical excisions. No difference in survival or disease-free survival was found among the different surgical procedures (28). In a meta-analysis of essentially the same patient population (N = 119 patients), Van Nostrand et al. (165), after adding 8 of their own cases, reached different conclusions. They stated that radical surgery is recommended for patients with primary vaginal melanomas of less than 10 cm². In Van Nostrand et al.'s own series of eight patients with vaginal melanoma, including four treated conservatively and four undergoing radical surgery, the only long-term survivor was in the radical surgery group. In their review of the literature, comprising a total of 119 patients, there was 48% 2-year survival rate if treated with radical surgery (50 patients) versus only 20% if treated conservatively (69 patients) ($p < .005$). Therefore, Van Nostrand et al. advocated radical excision for those vaginal melanomas less than 10 cm² in area (165).

Not all surgeons support a radical resection approach. Buchanan et al. (161) performed a literature review of 66 cases reported since the publication of Reid et al. (28). Survival was influenced by tumor size, with a median survival time of 41 months of those with lesions <3 cm and 21 months in those with larger lesions. However, there was no statistically significant difference in median survival or 2- and 5-year survival among the various surgical strategies. Hence, many investigators have adopted Irvin et al.'s suggestion that if distant failure and death are expected, quality of life should be optimized by wide excision followed by RT to effect local control, while obviating the need for disfiguring radical surgery (163). In Irvin et al.'s series (163), all patients treated with wide local excision or brachytherapy alone developed recurrent disease locally, whereas those patients treated with radical surgical resection or with wide local excision followed by high-dose per fraction EBRT maintained locoregional control until death.

Recent retrospective data suggest that vaginal melanoma is reasonably radioresponsive and possibly radiocurable (163,166). In Petru et al.'s series (166) of 14 patients, the three long-term survivors received either primary RT after biopsy only or adjuvantly after local excision. Tumor size was found to be prognostically important, with 43% of patients with tumors ≤3 cm surviving longer than 5 years compared with 0% in patients with tumors >3 cm. The median overall survival was 10 months, and the 5-year disease-free survival and overall survival rates were 14% and 21%, respectively. The investigators concluded that prolonged local control could be obtained with RT as an adjunct to more limited surgery, or even with RT alone, primarily in patients with lesions ≤3 cm in diameter.

In summary, given that the high incidence of distant metastasis remains a major factor in limiting curability, a more conservative treatment approach might be more reasonable in selected patients. Patients with vaginal melanoma should probably be managed in a manner similar to that recommended for cutaneous lesions (167). Wide local excision with 1- to 2-cm margins should be the surgical treatment of choice for most primary vaginal melanomas since radical surgery has failed to improve long-term survival. The role of adjuvant RT is unclear, but it appears to improve survival in some series. The use of systemic chemotherapy and/or immunotherapy has been very disappointing in the limited published data (168).

SARCOMAS OF THE VAGINA

Sarcomas represent 3% of vaginal primaries (51) with leiomyosarcoma representing 50% to 65% of vaginal sarcomas. Unfortunately, most of the sarcomas are diagnosed at an advanced stage. Histopathologic grade appears to be the most important predictor of outcome (78). Most vaginal leiomyosarcomas arise from the posterior wall of the vagina. Radical surgical resection, such as posterior pelvic exenteration, offers the best chance for cure (51,169). The largest series on vaginal sarcomas reported to date included 17 cases, of which 35% had received prior RT. This series that included ten leiomyosarcomas, four malignant mixed müllerian tumors (MMMTs), and three other sarcoma types noted that all were resistant to chemotherapy, and all of the failures were first noted as pelvic recurrences. There were only three survivors seen, and all had undergone exenterative surgery.

The 5-year survival rate was 36% in patients with leiomyosarcoma and 17% in those with MMMT (31).

Vaginal MMMTs occur more commonly in postmenopausal women. In approximately half of the cases there is a history of prior pelvic RT (31,170). Despite surgery and adjuvant RT, patients usually do poorly, with a high incidence of local and distant recurrences. The treatment of choice is complete surgical resection, followed by EBRT and ICB in an attempt to decrease the local recurrence rate.

The roles of adjuvant chemotherapy and RT in vaginal sarcomas have not been clearly defined, primarily owing to limited patient numbers and even fewer data where chemotherapy was used as the primary treatment rather than as salvage therapy at recurrence. Adjuvant RT seems to be indicated in patients with high-grade tumors and locally recurrent low-grade sarcomas. According to Peters et al. (31) the most common site of failure is the pelvis. In 50% of patients with recurrence, it is the only site of failure. Extrapolating data from the Gynecologic Oncology Group (171) for uterine sarcomas and considering patterns of failure, patients with localized MMMTs would be appropriately treated with pelvic exenteration, or with more limited surgical resection followed by postoperative RT, unless the patient has received prior pelvic RT. Since patterns of failure suggest that local therapies only reduce the local recurrence rate and do not improve survival, consideration should be given to adjuvant treatments with agents that are active in similar tumors arising in the uterus. Agents found to be active in MMMT of the uterus include ifosfamide, cisplatin, and paclitaxel, although it remains unclear whether any combination of these agents is better than ifosfamide alone, which has produced the highest response rate among these agents.

Embryonal RMS of the vagina, the most common pediatric vaginal tumor, is such a rare lesion that no single institution has sufficient experience to identify superior therapeutic strategies. Rather, cooperative efforts through the Intergroup Rhabdomyosarcoma Study Group (IRSG) have demonstrated that the use of of multimodality therapy with wide local excision and cytotoxic chemotherapy with or without RT makes it possible to avoid exenterative surgery and optimize quality of life for these young patients (85,172–174).

Prior to the modern era of multimodality therapy, Hilgers reported that only 20% to 30% 5-year survival rates were achieved with the use of exenterative-type surgery alone (175). Later, several small series noted that 70% survival could be achieved if RT and combination cytotoxic chemotherapy including vincristine, actinomycin D, and cyclophosphamide (VAC) were given in addition to radical surgery (30,175,176).

In a series of reports from the IRSG, survival rates in excess of 85% have been achieved utilizing VAC chemotherapy and wide excision with or without adjuvant RT, sparing the great majority of patients from exenterative surgery (172–174,177,178). In a subsequent report, the IRSG summarized the outcome of 72 patients with embryonal RMS of the vagina treated on four IRSG trials. Over the course of the four IRSG trials, the need for radical resection decreased from 100% to 13%, with continued improvement in disease-free survival (179). Andrassy et al. suggested that after biopsy to document RMS, multiagent induction chemotherapy with doxorubicin, cisplatin, vincristine, actinomycin D, and cyclophosphamide should be utilized, then local resection undertaken, with radical resection being reserved for those with persistent or recurrent disease (179). In addition, several non-IRSG series have shown that combination chemotherapy with or without RT leads to sufficient tumor shrinkage, and that less radical resections can become feasible (177,178), allowing preservation of anatomy and function. Flamant et al. (177) reported 11 cases of vaginal RMS (8 stage I, 2 stage II, 1 stage III) in whom 100% survival was achieved with multimodality therapy. Eight patients received neoadjuvant chemotherapy, generally a VAC regimen, and all patients underwent brachytherapy (doses of 26 to 75 Gy), followed by maintenance chemotherapy and VAC alternating with VAD (vincristine, doxorubicin, dacarbazine). Seven patients underwent ovarian transposition in an attempt to preserve function. The investigators noted partial ovarian insufficiency in one patient without ovarian transposition. They recommended a brachytherapy at a total dose of approximately 50 to 60 Gy (177).

LYMPHOMAS OF THE VAGINA

Lymphomatous involvement of the vagina most often represents metastatic spread from another primary site. Although surgery including radical hysterectomy, pelvic lymphadenectomy, vaginectomy, and exenteration has been performed in the past, more recent reports suggest that combination RT and chemotherapy can achieve excellent results. Radical surgery in such patients then should be avoided, as lymphoma represents a systemic disease. Following biopsy, patients with lymphoma should be managed with combined chemoradiation. Extrapolation from patients with similar tumors arising in extranodal sites would suggest that RT has its primary role in preventing local recurrence in patients who present with bulky disease. In some patients who have a rapid and complete response to multiagent chemotherapy, RT may not be indicated since the combination of both modalities increseases the risk of second malignancies. Harris et al. noted in a clinicopathologic series of 25 lower genital tract lymphomas, including 4 vaginal lymphomas, that definitive local therapy prevented relapse (44). Prevot et al. (180) and Perren et al. (181) also advocated the use of less extensive surgery, with RT plus cytotoxic multiagent chemotherapy such as CHOP [cyclophosphamide, hydroxydaunomycin (doxorubicin), Oncovin (vinblastine), prednisone] or BACOP [bleomycin, Adriamycin (doxorubicin), cyclophosphamide, Oncovin (vinblastine), prednisone] for six cycles to effect local control with better preservation of fertility.

YOLK SAC (ENDODERMAL SINUS) TUMORS OF THE VAGINA

Prior to the use of multiagent cytotoxic chemotherapy, less than 25% of patients with yolk sac tumor (YST), or endodermal sinus tumor (EST), of the vagina survived. However, Young and Scully noted 100% survival in a small series of six patients who had received chemotherapy (182). The VAC regimen in conjunction with surgery or RT was advocated by Copeland et al. (183). Collins et al. (184) reported on the use of combination bleomycin, vinblastine, and platinum (BVP) for patients with EST of the vagina. Aartsen et al. (185) reported a successful pregnancy following surgery and chemotherapy. Most recently, Hwang et al. have reported two cases, one of which did well with partial vaginectomy followed by two years of VAC; however, the second one developed a central persistence following wide local excision and VAC, but was salvaged with bleomycin, etoposide, and platinum (BEP) (186). Given the excellent results that three to four cycles of BEP have achieved in malignant germ-cell neoplasms of the ovary (187), it is likely that BEP will become the preferred regimen for EST of the vagina used in conjunction with parital vaginectomy, as it requires less prolonged administration and is less oophorotoxic than VAC.

SALVAGE THERAPY

In general, the patient with recurrent cancer of the lower female genital tract presents a difficult clinical dilemma. Optimal therapy for patients with recurrent gynecologic cancer after potentially curative therapy has not been completely defined, partly owing to the difficulty of conducting prospective randomized trials in this heterogeneous population. It must be determined if the disease is amenable to curative salvage therapy, implying some reasonable chance of cure, or whether palliation is the primary goal. Treatment selection factors include primary therapy, extent of the disease at presentation, site of recurrence, extent of the recurrence, disease-free interval, evidence of metastatic disease, patient age, performance status, and coexisting medical conditions (Table 21.6). The presence of distant metastasis portends a poor prognosis, and although chemotherapy may result in objective responses and improvements in short-term survival, the current lack of curative systemic treatments focuses therapeutic attempts on symptom palliation and quality of life.

In most cases, only patients with small-volume local recurrences and no metastatic disease are curable (Table 21.7). Therefore, careful workup to establish extent of disease is crucial. When salvage therapies are contemplated, local recurrences should be confirmed by biopsy, and, when possible, parametrial recurrences should be documented pathologically. Pelvic sidewall involvement can almost always be diagnosed in the presence of a symptom triad of sciatic pain,

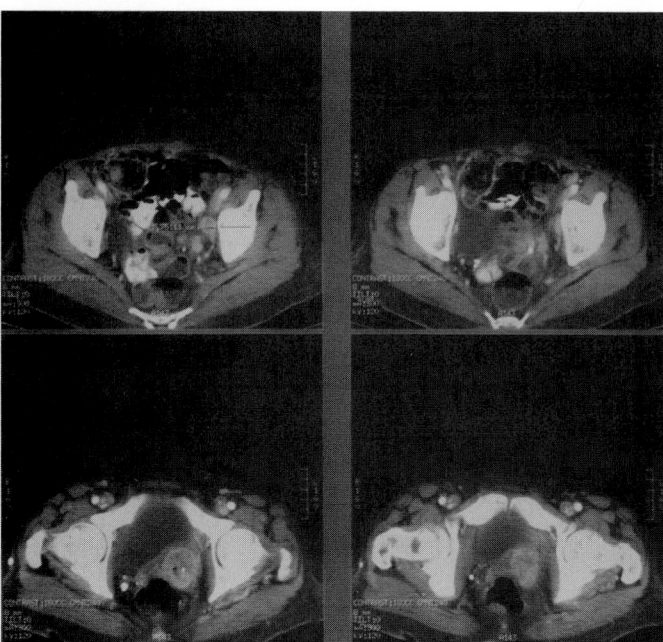

A1

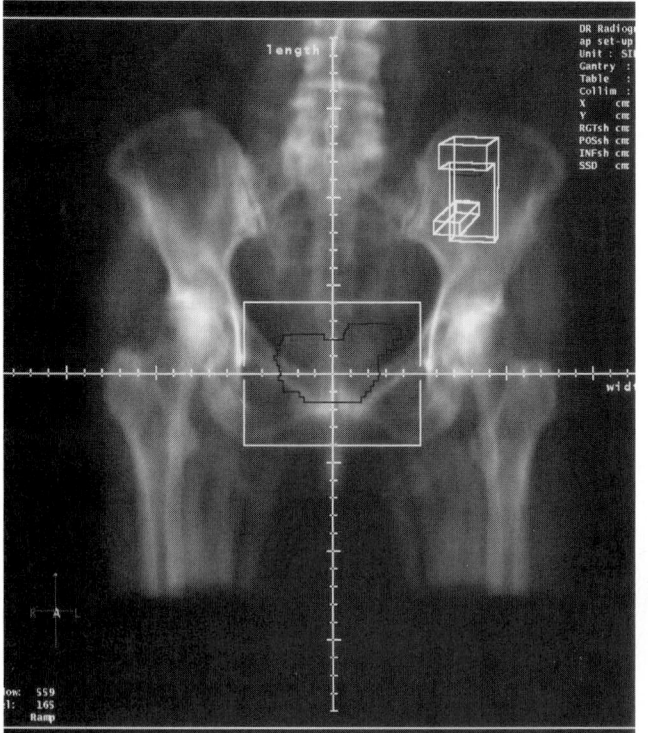

A2

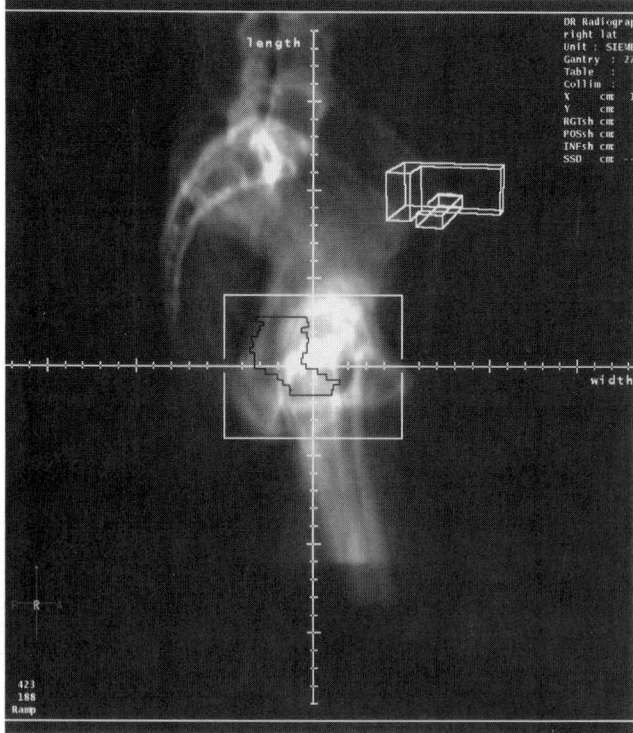

A3

FIG. 21.9. Interstitial plus endocavitary brachytherapy in a patient with locally advanced vaginal cancer. **A:** Planning CT scan (**A1**), AP (**A2**), and lateral (**A3**) DRRs demonstrating the reconstructed volume to be implanted. *(Figure continues.)*

leg edema, and hydronephrosis. It is important to evaluate for regional and/or distant metastasis by physical examination and imaging studies such as CT or MRI scans. More recently, the positron emission tomography (PET) scan has been used to document the extent of recurrent disease (188), but both false-positive and false-negative results have been reported.

Generally, patients with isolated pelvic or regional recur-rences after definitive surgery who have not received prior RT are managed with EBRT, often in conjunction with brachytherapy. Concurrent cisplatin-based chemotherapy may also be recommended. Salvage options for patients with central recurrence after definitive or adjuvant RT are limited to radical surgery, usually exenterative or, in selected pa-tients with small-volume disease, reirradiation using intersti-tial radiation implants or highly conformal three-dimen-

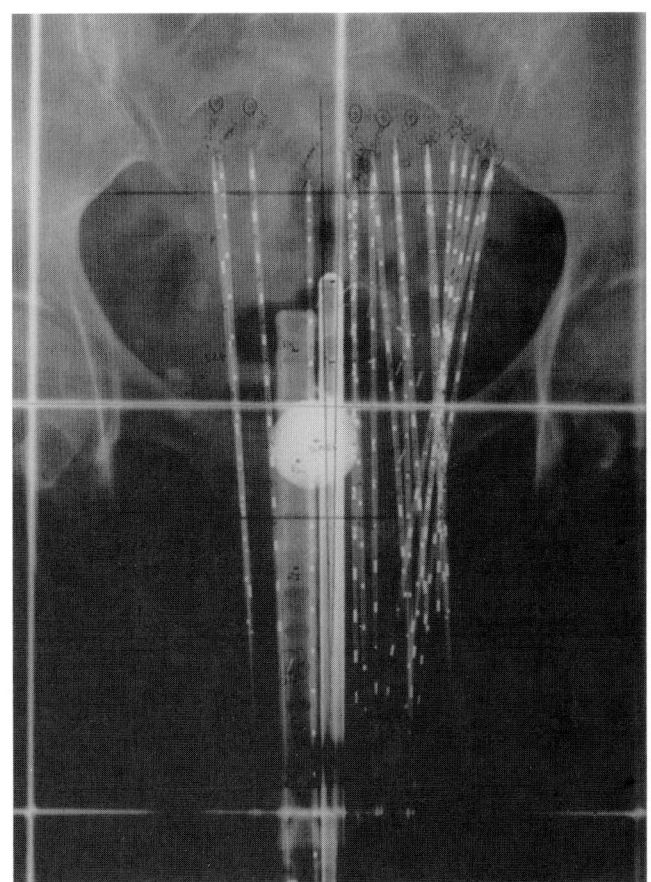

B1

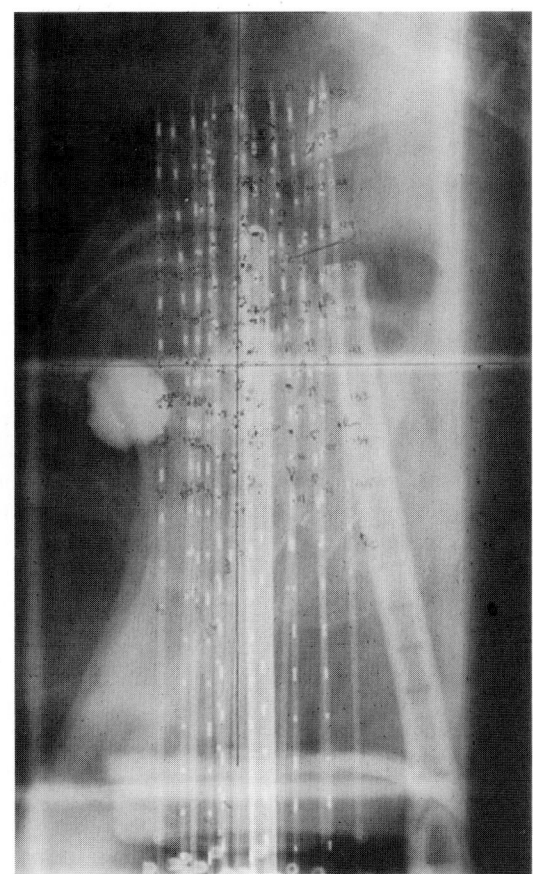

B2

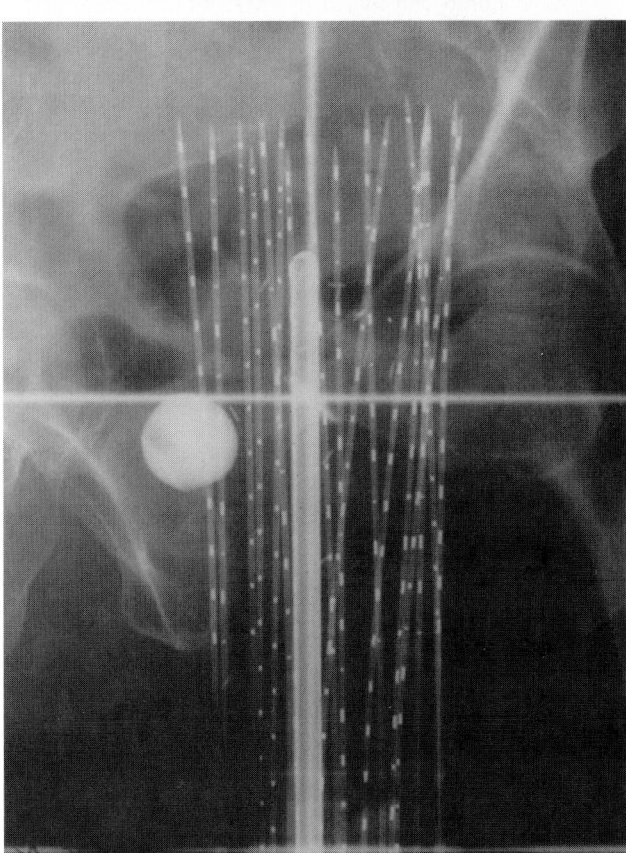

B3

FIG. 21.9. Continued. **B:** (**B1**) AP, (**B2**) lateral, and (**B3**) oblique radiographs of the implant.

sional EBRT. Response rates with chemotherapy are low and the impact on survival limited. Further, response to chemotherapy in central pelvic recurrences following RT tends to be less common than response at distant sites. Additionally, prior high-dose radiation therapy compromises bone marrow tolerance of many agents that are active in this tumor (e.g., ifosfamide and doxorubicin). However, chemotherapy-responsive patients can obtain meaningful palliation in many cases.

Surgical Considerations

Despite thorough clinical evaluation of patients considered to be excellent candidates for salvage surgery, this will be aborted in over 25% of the cases because of advanced disease found at the time of the exploratory laparotomy (189). Pelvic exenteration results in long-term functional and psychologic changes that have not been adequately studied (190). Surgical refinements have done much to improve body image changes associated with pelvic exenteration. The purposes of vaginal and perineal reconstruction following radical pelvic surgery for recurrent gynecologic cancer are primarily twofold: to restore or create vulvovaginal function, and thereby minimize the effects of surgical treatment on body image and normal sexual activity; and to minimize postoperative complications by transferring to the pelvic defect healthy tissue with a good blood supply (104,139). A detailed review of urinary diversion and pelvic reconstruction techniques is not within the scope of this chapter.

Radiation Therapy Considerations

Those patients who have not received prior RT should receive whole-pelvis EBRT followed, when feasible, by brachytherapy. Generally, the whole pelvis receives a dose of 40 to 50 Gy. Inguinofemoral lymph node regions should be included in patients with involvement of the distal third of the vagina or with vulvar recurrences. The gross tumor volume in the vagina, paravaginal tissues, and/or parametrium should receive an additional boost, preferably with an interstitial implant, to bring the total tumor dose to 75 to 80 Gy. The role of combined chemoradiotherapy in the management of patients with recurrent disease is unknown. Given the rarity of vaginal carcinoma and the heterogeneity within the population with recurrent disease, large randomized studies intended to answer this question will probably never be conducted. However, by extrapolation from the available data for locally advanced cervical and vulvar cancer (146–148,191), it seems that a combined-modality approach may improve the locoregional control and survival in patients with isolated pelvic recurrences.

Reirradiation in previously irradiated patients must be undertaken with extreme caution. However, selected patients who are medically inoperable, technically unresectable, or refuse to undergo exenterative surgery are appropriately considered for reirradiation to limited volumes. A variety of techniques is available, and the choice is based on patient and tumor-related factors, as well as the experience of the radiation oncologist. When using EBRT, multiple-beam arrangements utilizing three-dimensional treatment planning are favored. Only limited doses are possible, and the physician might consider a hyperfractionated regimen in an attempt to decrease the incidence of late toxicity.

In patients with small, well-defined vulvovaginal or pelvic recurrences, reirradiation using primarily interstitial techniques has been attempted with control rates between 50%

TABLE 21.6. *Advantages and disadvantages of salvage surgery and interstitial reirradiation*

Salvage therapy	Advantages	Disadvantages
Surgery	Ability to assess the extent of disease and act accordingly Applicable to larger volume recurrences	Perioperative morbidity and mortality, particularly after previous RT Prolonged hospitalization High rate of reoperation Expense Applicable only to selected patients with good performance status/good general condition Detrimental to patient self-image
Reirradiation	Little perioperative morbidity or mortality Little or no hospitalization for permanent implants unless laparotomy is required Relatively inexpensive Preserves structure and function in most patients Applicable to patients who are medically infirm or aged	Extent of disease difficult to assess in some cases Risk of late radiation injury Applicable only to small-volume recurrences if excessive complication rate is to be avoided

RT, radiotherapy
Reprinted with permission from Randall ME, Evans L, Greven KM, et al. Interstitial re-irradiation for recurrent gynecological malignancies: results and analysis of prognostic factors. *Gynecol Oncol* 1993;48:23–31.

and 75% and grade 3 or higher complication rates between 7% and 15% (192–196). The rationale, logistics, and selection of implant technique when performing an ITI have been reviewed earlier in the chapter. Permanent radioactive seed implants (e.g., ¹⁹⁸Au) in patients with small vaginal recurrences often provide long-lasting tumor control in elderly or medically debilitated patients previously treated with definitive doses of RT (Fig. 21.10). Advantages and disadvantages of surgery and reirradiation as salvage therapies are shown in Table 21.6 (193).

Other potential treatment options include the use of surgery and intraoperative RT (IORT), which allows direct visualization of the target volume and displacement and/or shielding of the surrounding normal tissues. Several ap-

proaches have been used. Intraoperative electron beam and HDR have been used for treatment of isolated central and nodal recurrences (197). However, the published series are generally small, including a wide spectrum of patients with different gynecologic malignancies, varying amounts of residual disease, and disparate initial therapies. The locoregional recurrence and distant metastasis rates after intraoperative radiotherapy (IORT) vary between 20% and 60% and 20% and 58%, respectively. The 3- to 5-year actuarial survival is poor, ranging from 8% to 25%. Grade 3 or higher toxicity has been reported in about 35% of patients (197, 198). In the Memorial Sloan–Kettering Cancer Center experience using radical surgical resection and HDR-IORT, patients with complete gross resection had a 3-year local con-

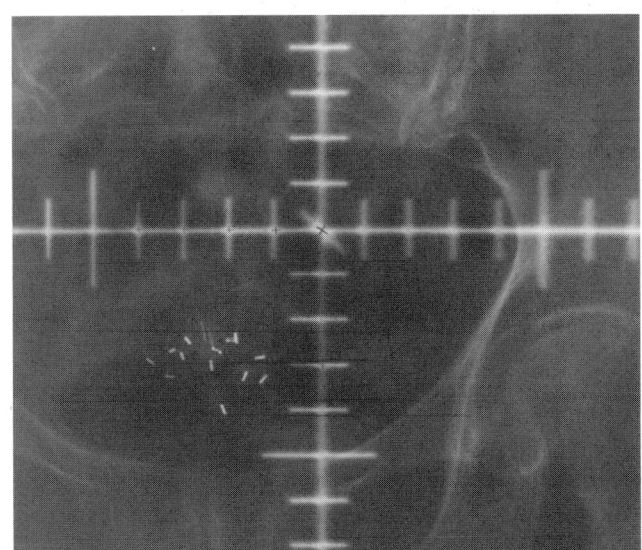

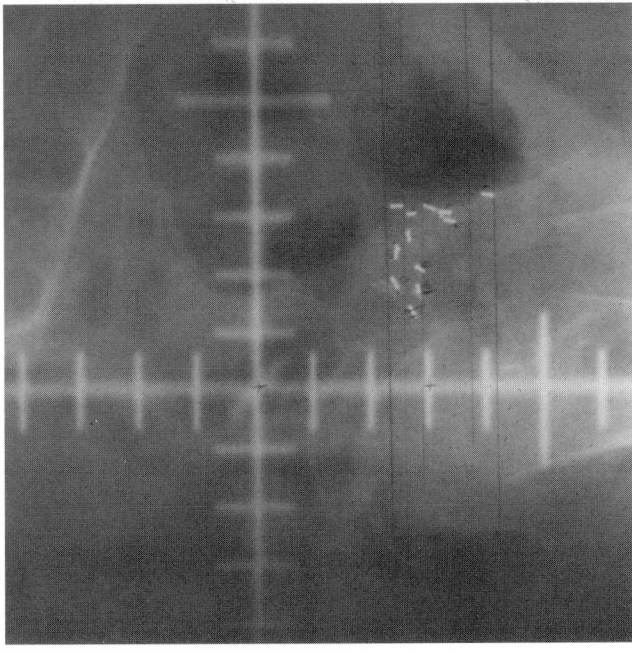

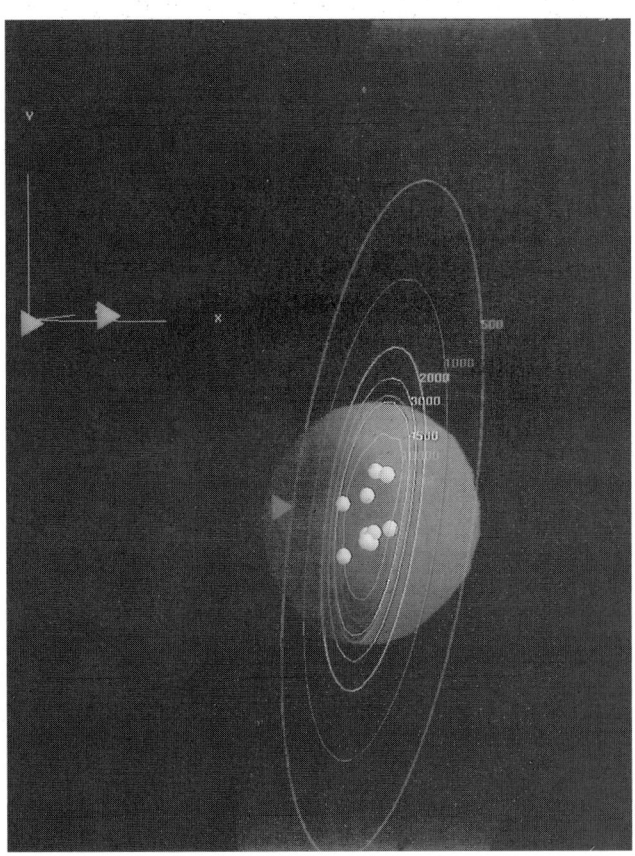

FIG. 21.10. A: AP radiograph of an interstitial ¹²⁵I permanent implant in a patient with recurrent vaginal carcinoma at the apex. **B:** Lateral radiograph. **C:** Three-dimensional reconstruction of the isodose distribution.

TABLE 21.7. *Salvage treatment of recurrence*

Investigator (ref.)	No. of patients	Percentage of recurrence	Locoregional recurrence	Salvage treatment	Patient status after salvage treatment
Chyle et al. (61)[a]	310	35%	64 (21%)	Not stated	Local: 5-year survival 20% Other: 5-year survival 4%
Davis et al. (68)	89	29%	13 (15%)	10 surgery 3 RT	4 alive NED All DOD
Kirkbride et al. 62)[b]	128	42%	43 (33.5%)	1 EBRT 3 brachytherapy 1 surgery	Not stated
Kucera and Vavra (101)	110	24.5%	23 (21%)	Not stated	
Stock et al. (56)	100	46%		4 surgery 1 ITI interstitial RT	Not stated
Urbanski et al. (67)	125	53%	51 (41%)	2 patients: pelvic exenteration 5 patients: CHT	DOD

CHT, Chemotherapy; DOD, dead of disease; EBRT, electron beam radiotherapy; ITI, interstitial implant; NED, no evidence of disease; RT, radiotherapy.

[a]Tumors that recurred locally had a better 5-year survival (20%) than those that recurred beyond the primary site (pelvic nodes, paraaortic nodes, and systemic disease) (4%). The patients who received additional surgery or RT fared better (30%, 5-year survival) than patients who either had no salvage treatment or received chemotherapy (4%, 5-year survival).

[b]One hundred and twenty-eight patients treated with RT alone; 43 patients had locoregional recurrences (31%, 24/78, in the group treated with EBRT + brachytherapy; 17%, 2/12, in the group treated with implant only; 45%, 17/38, in the group treated with EBRT alone). In the 26 patients treated with chemoradiotherapy there were 8 vaginal and 8 pelvic failures (62%) versus 22 vaginal and 8 pelvic failures in 91 patients treated with irradiation (33%). This probably reflects a selection bias, with more advanced stages of the disease receiving combined-modality therapy.

trol rate of 83% compared to 25% in patients with gross residual disease. Interestingly, most of the failures in the microscopic group were distant, perhaps indicating a potential role for adjuvant chemotherapy (199).

Hockel et al. (200) described a combined operative and radiotherapeutic treatment (CORT) for the treatment of recurrent gynecologic malignances infiltrating the pelvic side wall. The procedure involves gross complete resection of the tumor and a single plane interstitial implant. In order to improve the therapeutic index, well-vascularized tissue is transposed to the pelvis to protect the hollow organs and reduce the late effects of RT. Reconstruction of pelvic organs is performed as with exenteration. The tumor bed is irradiated postoperatively, days 10 to 14, using HDR brachytherapy. In a total of 48 patients treated with this technique, the overall severe complication rate was 33% at 5 years. The 5-year survival rate was 44%, and the absolute local control rate was 60% for the first 20 patients and 85% for the last 28 treated patients (200).

Stereotactic body radiotherapy (SBRT), also known as extracranial stereotactic radioablation (ESR), is a novel treatment paradigm that delivers a small number of high-dose fractions to extracranial targets using a linear accelerator with highly precise, accurate, and reproducible target localization based on the same principles as that of gamma-knife therapy. By means of better target localization and patient immobilization, smaller margins of normal tissue surrounding the gross tumor volume are required, which allows treatment complications to be minimized. Blomgren et al. (201) reported on 15 patients with 19 extrahepatic abdominal tu-

mors that had a mean survival of 17.7 months. The toxicity was more often self-limited except for four patients with gastrointestinal bleeding. They concluded that this treatment, which is noninvasive, painless, rapid, and does not require hospitalization, does not impair the quality of life are the patients when used properly.

TREATMENT COMPLICATIONS AND THEIR MANAGEMENT

The anatomic location of the vagina places the lower gastrointestinal and genitourinary tracts at greatest risk for complications after surgery or RT. Although in most of the retrospective series, the investigators comment on the nature of the complications encountered, little information is typically given regarding their prevention or manangement (56–58, 79,92,125). In modern oncology, survival rate is the primary endpoint in treatment evaluation, but the analysis of treatment complications and quality of life is of crucial importance. Clearly, the knowledge of common acute and late complications with standard RT and consideration of risk factors may improve the therapeutic ratio of RT for gynecologic malignancies in general and for vaginal cancer in particular (202).

The acute and chronic pathophysiology of vaginal RT has been well described by Grigsby et al. (203). As an immediate response to high-dose RT, there is loss of most or all of the vaginal epithelium, especially in areas in proximity to brachytherapy sources. Clinically, the severity of the acute effects (edema, erythema, moist desquamation, and confluent mucositis with or without ulceration) varies in intensity and duration depending upon patient age, hormonal status, tumor size, stage, RT dose, and personal hygiene. These effects usually resolve within 2 to 3 months after completion of therapy. In some patients, there is progressive vascular damage with subsequent ulcer formation and mucosal necrosis, which may require up to 8 months for healing. Chemotherapy concurrently with RT enhances the acute mucosal response to both EBRT and brachytherapy. The effects of chemotherapy on the incidence of late complications, if any, are unclear. Over time, most patients will develop some degree of vaginal atrophy, fibrosis, and stenosis. Telangiectasis is commonly seen in the vagina. Vaginal narrowing or shortening, paravaginal fibrosis, loss of elasticity, and reduced lubrication often result in dyspareunia. More severe complications include necrosis with ulceration that can progress to fistula formation (rectovaginal, vesicovaginal, urethrovaginal).

The RT tolerance limits of the entire vagina are ill defined given the variety of techniques employed for the treatment of vaginal cancers. An irradiation tolerance level of the proximal vagina was suggested by Hintz et al. (204) based on a study of 16 patients who received a maximum surface dose of 140 Gy, none of whom developed severe complications or necrosis of the upper vagina. Based on their previous observation of a patient who developed a vesicovaginal fistula after receiving a 150-Gy mucosal dose to the anterior vaginal wall, they recommended a tolerance dose level of 150 Gy (direct summation of EBRT dose and ICB) to the anterior upper vaginal mucosa. They also recommended keeping the total dose to the distal vagina less than 98 Gy. In addition, it was also observed that the posterior wall of the vagina is more prone to radiation injury than the anterior or lateral walls, and that the dose should be kept below 80 Gy in order to minimize the risk of rectovaginal fistula. Rubin and Casarett (205) suggested that the tolerance of the vaginal mucosa (TD 5/5: 5% necrosis within 5 years) is approximately 90 Gy for ulceration and more than 100 Gy for fistula formation. This tolerance limit has been specified as a direct summation of dosage given by LDR-ICB and EBRT in the treatment of cervical cancer. Within the low-dose-rate range, whether a correction for the brachytherapy dose rate is necessary remains controversial. In a more recent series from Washington University, the traditional LDR tolerance dose of 150 Gy to the mucosa of the proximal vagina was shown to yield a nominal 11% and 4% grades 1, 2, and 3 sequelae, respectively (206).

The incidence of grade 2 or higher complications has been reported to be 15% to 25%, with the average of severe complications (those requiring surgery for correction or necessitating hospitalization) being approximately 8% to 10%. Table 21.8 (56,61,62,67,79,91,92,101) shows the incidence of complications greater than grade 2 in several large series of vaginal cancer patients.

Host factors that may increase the risk of complications

TABLE 21.8. *Complications of therapy (>grade 2)*

Investigator (ref.)	No. of patients	Percentage of complications (>grade 2)
Chyle et al. (61)	310	19% actuarial at 20 years
Kirkbride et al. (62)	153	10%
Kucera and Vavra (101)	110	5.5%
Perez et al. (91)	212	13%
Peters et al. (92)	86	8%
Rubin et al. (79)	75	23%
Stock et al. (56)	100	16% actuarial at 10 years
Urbanski et al. (67)	125	13%

include prior pelvic surgery, pelvic inflammatory disease, immunosuppression status, collagen vascular disease, low body weight, patient age, significant smoking history, and co-morbid illness (e.g., diabetes, hypertension, and cardiovascular disease) (64,91).

Lee et al. (90) showed that the total dose to the primary site was the most significant factor predicting the development of a severe complication (9% in patients receiving ≤80 Gy as compared with 25% in those receiving higher doses). Perez et al. (64) reported an increase in the rate of severe complications with higher clinical stage, probably reflecting the higher doses delivered with EBRT and brachytherapy.

Ball et al. (57) reported on 58 patients with carcinoma of the vagina, including 30 who underwent surgery. There were four rectovaginal fistulae (one following RT and three after exenterative surgery) and two vesicovaginal fistulae (one following radical vaginectomy and the other following a recurrence, being managed with cystectomy and diversion). The single ureterovaginal fistula occurred after radical vaginectomy and partial cystectomy, and was managed with ureteroneocystotomy.

In Peters et al.'s report (92) of 86 vaginal primaries, there were two fistulae in the 57 patients who received primary RT. However, there was a 44% rate of fistula formation in the nine patients who underwent reirradiation after having previously received RT for an earlier cancer. Rubin et al. (79) reported a 23% incidence of complications after RT, including a 13% rate of fistula formation and a 10% rate of cystitis/proctitis. Although two patients developed fistulae following combination therapy, the investigators did not think that the rate of complications following combination therapy was greater than that seen following RT alone.

In Stock et al.'s series (56) of 100 patients with vaginal carcinoma, there was a 16% actuarial complication rate at 10 years. All patients undergoing vaginectomies or exenterations lost vaginal function. None of the patients was offered vaginal reconstruction in this series. The investigators emphasized that therapeutic options need to be individualized such that surgery is offered only to those most likely to benefit and least likely to suffer complications.

Treatment options for acute radiation vaginitis include daily vaginal douching with a diluted hydrogen peroxide/water mixture. This should continue for 2 to 3 months or until the mucosal reactions have subsided. Patients are then advised to continue douching once or twice per week for several months. Regular vaginal dilation is recommended as a way for patients to maintain vaginal health and good sexual function, although the compliance rate is low. The lack of resolution of vaginal ulceration or necrosis after several months of adequate therapy must be appropriately evaluated, considering the possibility of recurrent tumor. The use of topical estrogens following completion of RT appears to stimulate epithelial regeneration more than systemic estrogens.

Some patients with severe radiation sequelae, such as fistula formation, will respond to conservative treatment with antibiotics and periodic limited debridement of necrotic tissue. More recently, Delanian et al. (207) published a randomized trial demonstrating the effectiveness of the combination of pentoxifyllin and vitamin E in the regression of radiation-induced fibrosis.

Patients with more severe gastrointestinal or urinary late effects will require urinary or fecal diversion with possible delayed reanastomosis. Occasionally, repair of the fistula may be attempted by employing a myocutaneous graft in which the skin, subcutaneous fat, and muscle are mobilized using a vascular pedicle to maintain the blood supply to the pedicled graft (Martius flap), or by excision of the necrotic tissue with reestablishment of organ continuity (such as in the treatment of high rectovaginal fistula). A detailed review of the pathogenesis and management of potential late effects of treatment is not within the scope of this chapter, and may be found elsewhere in the textbook.

It is likely that improvements in modern practice such as advancements in surgical techniques (such as more generous use of myocutaneous flaps) (104,139), improved supportive care during the immediate postoperative stay, the use of more sophisticated RT field setting (three-dimensional conformal therapy) and treatment delivery, more accurate brachytherapy techniques, and dose calculations have the potential to lessen complication rates posttherapy regardless of which modality is used.

PALLIATIVE RADIATION THERAPY

At the present time, there is no curative option for patients who present with stage IVB disease. Many of these patients suffer from severe pelvic pain or bleeding. If vaginal bleeding is the main concern, ICB, if feasible, often offers a good symptom control with relatively low morbidity. For patients who have received prior RT, intracavitary doses in the range of 35 to 40 Gy to point A should be prescribed.

A short course of EBRT using high-dose fractionation schedules has been used, including single doses of 10 Gy per fraction, times three, with an interval of 4 to 6 weeks between courses, combined with misonidazole (RTOG clinical trial 79–05), resulting in significant palliation in selected patients with advanced gynecologic malignancies. The overall response rate was 41% for patients completing the three courses; however, the actuarial 45% incidence of grades 3 and 4 late gastrointestinal toxicity was unacceptable (208).

Spanos et al. (209) reported on a Phase II study (RTOG 85–02) of daily multifraction split-course EBRT in patients with recurrent or metastatic disease. The regimen consisted of 3.7 Gy per fraction given twice daily for 2 consecutive days and repeated at 3- to 6-week intervals for a total of three courses (tumor dose 44.4 Gy). Occasionally, this regimen was combined with an ICI (4,500 mgh), with a midline block in the last 14.4 Gy. Complete tumor response was noted in 15 patients (10.5%) and partial response in 32 (22.5%). In patients completing three courses of irradiation (59%), the rate of complete or partial response was 45%. Twenty-seven patients survived longer than 1 year. Late complications were significantly fewer, with a projected actuarial rate of 5% at 12 months.

In a subsequent Phase III Study (210), 136 patients were randomized between rest intervals of 2 versus 4 weeks between the split courses of RT. Decreasing the interval between courses did not result in a significant improvement in tumor response (34% vs 26%). More patients in the 2-week rest group completed the three courses of therapy, and not surprisingly, patients completing all three courses had a higher overall response rate than patients completing less than three courses (42% vs 5%) and a higher complete response rate (17% vs 1%). This schedule offers significant logistic benefits, and has been shown to result in good tumor regression and excellent palliation of symptoms (210). Spanos et al. (211) reported a trend toward increased acute toxicity in patients with shorter rest periods, but late toxicity was not significantly different in the two groups.

CHEMOTHERAPY IN ADVANCED RECURRENT VAGINAL CANCER

Given its rarity, most chemotherapy reports for treatment of metastatic disease in vaginal cancer are anecdotal or combined with reports of treatment of advanced or recurrent cervix cancer. Concurrent chemoradiation is frequently employed in clinical practice in the treatment of unresectable locoregionally advanced disease. Various chemotherapeutic agents have been used with limited success (142,143). Evans et al. (142) reported on seven patients with vaginal cancers who were treated with a combination of 5-FU 1,000 $mg/m^2/d$ for 4 days, mitomycin C 10 mg/m^2 day 1, and primary irradiation, receiving 2,000 to 6,500 cGy. All of the vaginal cancer patients responded, and 66% were alive with a median follow-up of 28 months.

Treatment of recurrent or metastatic disease is confined to a handful of Phase II clinical trials and anecdotal reports. In general, regimens that are active in cervical cancer are usually active in vaginal cancer. Thigpen et al. (212) reported the results of a Phase II trial of cisplatin 50 mg/m^2 every 3 weeks in 26 patients with advanced or recurrent vaginal cancer. There were 22 evaluable patients, 16 with SCC, 2 adenosquamous carcinoma, 1 CCC, 1 leiomyosarcoma, and 2 unspecified. Of the 16 SCC patients, there was 1 complete response (6.2%). It should be noted that these patients, for the most part, had received prior surgery and RT. Muss et al. (213) reported no responses in 19 evaluable patients who were treated with mitoxantrone 12 mg/m^2 every 3 weeks. Median survival of patients with vaginal cancer was 2.7 months. Other anecdotal reports of responses in trials that included advanced cervical cancer include a report by Long et al. (214) in which three patients with advanced vaginal SCC received treatment with methotrexate, vinblastine, doxorubicin, and cisplatin (MVAC). All three patients achieved a complete response of short duration. Patton et al. (215) reported the results of intraarterial chemotherapy with mitomycin C, bleomycin, cisplatin, and vincristine, including six patients with primary vaginal cancer and 40 patients with cervical cancer. Seventy-six percent responded to intraarterial chemotherapy and subsequently received primary RT. The report did not give details as to site of relapse impact on disease-free survival or overall survival.

At the present time, systemic treatment of advanced vaginal cancer outside of a clinical trial is purely anecdotal, although it might be reasonable to extrapolate from the experience reported with SCC of the cervix and vulva (145–148, 191). Although published response rates are low, standard therapy should include cisplatin alone or in conjunction with RT in patients with locoregionally advanced vaginal cancer.

SUMMARY AND CONCLUSIONS

The malignant histologies of the vagina are so rare that randomized clinical trials have not been undertaken. It is difficult to establish strong, evidence-based recommendations in such a rare disease as cancer of the vagina. Therefore, future progress will likely come from reports from single institutions. Most of the available data refer to the treatment of primary invasive SCC of the vagina, since this represents the most common histology. We would like to make the following management recommendations based on the available data.

Vaginal Intraepithelial Neoplasia

In patients with unifocal disease, partial colpectomy has come to be favored over laser vaporization, since there is an approximately 25% risk that there can be underlying invasive disease, and one-quarter to one-third of patients will require a second laser vaporization to effect long-term control. However, for patients who develop VAIN following radiation wherein colpectomy would be associated with a higher risk of fistulae development, there may be a role for

laser vaporization and/or topical 5-FU application. Intracavitary brachytherapy alone has provided satisfactory functional and local control results as well.

Invasive Squamous-Cell Carcinoma

Although RT can control many cases of vaginal cancer, local control remains a problem. The treatment of invasive SCC with RT should include the use of brachytherapy, with particular attention to a technique that ensures that the treatment volume is adequately covered. In larger tumors, the dose that is needed to achieve local control may well exceed the tolerance of surrounding normal tissues. Although not specifically proven for patients with vaginal primaries, the addition of chemotherapy (i.e., weekly cisplatin) as a radiosensitizing agent may help to improve these results if we extrapolate the strong evidence-based therapy in locally advanced cervical cancer. Although there are multiple series that demonstrate excellent results with radical surgery for well-selected early-stage patients, RT will continue to be the primary modality even for early-stage disease and for those elderly patients with multiple co-morbid conditions.

Clear-Cell Adenocarcinoma

It has been suggested that patients with early-stage disease may be offered fertility-sparing combined-modality local therapy with extraperitoneal node dissection and wide local excision followed by brachytherapy with acceptable local failure rates. However, advanced-stage disease would require primary RT. Patients who have completed childbearing would be best served by radical hysterectomy, colpectomy, and lymphadenectomy. Exenteration should be reserved for those patients who have isolated central failures following definitive RT.

Melanoma

The risk of distant metastases is high enough that most modern investigators have suggested that ultraradical surgery, although it might improve 2-year survival rates, has not led to an increase in long-term survival. Wide excision followed by RT to effect local control may obviate the need of disfiguring surgery in those likely destined to develop distant metastases.

Sarcoma

The work of the IRSG and others has proven that pediatric embryonal RMS of the vagina is best approached with induction multiagent-combination therapy, including VAC followed by local resection with or without brachytherapy, with radical surgery being reserved for those with persistent or recurrent disease. Patients with adult-onset vaginal sarcoma do not respond as well to chemotherapy, and the only long-term survivors are those who have been offered exenterative surgery.

REFERENCES

1. Sedlis A, Robboy SJ. Diseases of the vagina. In: Kurman RJ, ed. *Blaustein's pathology of the female genital tract.* 3rd ed. New York: Springer-Verlag, 1987:98–140.
2. Plentl AA, Friedman EA. Lymphatic system of the female genitalia. In: Plentl AA, Friedman EA, eds. *The morphologic basis of oncologic diagnosis and therapy.* Philadelphia: WB Saunders, 1971:51–74.
3. Zaino RJ, Robboy SJ, Kurman RJ. Diseases of the vagina. In: Kurman RJ, ed. *Blaustein's pathology of the female genital tract.* 5th ed. New-York: Springer-Verlag, 2002:151–206.
4. Herbst AL, Green TH Jr, Ulfelder H. Primary carcinoma of the vagina. *Am J Obstet Gynecol* 1970;106:210.
5. Vayrynen M, Romppanen T, Koskela E, et al. Verrucous squamous cell carcinoma of the female genital tract: Report of three cases and survey of the literature. *Int J Gynaecol Obstet* 1981;19:351.
6. Brinton LA, Nasca PC, Mallin K, et al. Case-control study of in situ and invasive carcinoma of the vagina. *Gynecol Oncol* 1990;38:49–54.
7. Aho MK, Vesterinen E, Meyer B, et al. Natural history of vaginal intraepithelial neoplasia. *Cancer* 1991;68:195–197.
8. Hoffman MS, Roberts WS, LaPolla JP, et al. Laser vaporization of grade 3 vaginal intraepithelial neoplasia. *Am J Obstet Gynecol* 1991; 165:1342–1344.
9. Herbst AL, Robboy SJ, Scully RE, et al. Clear-cell adenocarcinoma of the vagina and cervix in girls: analysis of 170 registry cases. *Am J Obstet Gynecol* 1974;119:713–724.
10. Antonioli DA, Burke L. Vaginal adenosis: analysis of 325 biopsy specimens from 100 patients. *Am J Clin Pathol* 1975;64:625.
11. Robboy SJ, Scully RE, Welch WR, Herbst AL. Intrauterine diethylstilbestrol exposure and its consequences: pathologic characteristics of vaginal adenosis, clear cell adenocarcinoma and related lesions. *Arch Pathol Lab Med* 1977;101:1.
12. Hart WR, Townsend DE, Aldrich JO, et al. Histopathologic spectrum of vaginal adenosis and related changes in stilbestrol-exposed females. *Cancer* 1976;37:763.
13. Robboy SJ, Prat J, Welch WR, Barnes AB. Squamous cell neoplasia controversy in the female exposed to diethylstilbestrol. *Hum Pathol* 1977;8:843.
14. Kaufman RH, Korhonen MO, Strama T, et al. Development of clear cell adenocarcinoma in DES-exposed offspring under observation. *Obstet Gynecol* 1982;59:68S.
15. Robboy SJ, Young RH, Welch WR, et al. Atypical vaginal adenosis and cervical ectropion: association with clear cell adenocarcinoma in diethylstilbestrol-exposed offspring. *Cancer* 1984;54:869–875.
16. Ebrahim S, Daponte A, Smith TH, et al. Primary mucinous adenocarcinoma of the vagina. *Gynecol Oncol* 2001;80:89.
17. Clement PB, Benedet JL. Adenocarcinoma in situ of the vagina: a case report. *Cancer* 1979;43:2479.
18. Fox H, Wells M, Harris M, et al. Enteric tumours of the lower female genital tract: a report of three cases. *Histopathology* 1988;12:167.
19. DeMars LR, Van Le L, Huang I, Fowler WC. Primary non–clear cell adenocarcinomas of the vagina in older DES-exposed women. *Gynecol Oncol* 1995;58:389.
20. Maassen V, Lampe B, Untch M, et al. Adenocarcinoma and adenosis of the vagina. On the histogenesis, diagnosis and therapy of a rare genital neoplasm. *Geburtshilfe Frauenheilkd* 1993;53:308.
21. Munkarah A, Malone JM Jr, Budey HD, Evans TN. Mucinous adenocarcinoma arising in a neovagina. *Gynecol Oncol* 1994;52:272.
22. Hiroi H, Yasugi T, Matsumoto K, et al. Mucinous adenocarcinoma arising in a neovagina using the sigmoid colon thirty years after operation: a case report. *J Surg Oncol* 2001;77:61.
23. Haskel S, Chen SS, Spiegel G. Vaginal endometrioid adenocarcinoma arising in vaginal endometriosis: a case report and literature review. *Gynecol Oncol* 1989;34:232.
24. Hinchey WW, Silva EG, Guarda LA, et al.. Paravaginal wolffian duct (mesonephros) adenocarcinoma: a light and electron microscopic study. *Am J Clin Pathol* 1983;80:539.
25. Riva C, Fabbri A, Facco C, et al. Primary serous papillary adenocarcinoma of the vagina: a case report. *Int J Gynecol Pathol* 1997;16:286.
26. Chung AF, Casey MJ, Flannery JT, et al. Malignant melanoma of the vagina: report of 19 cases. *Obstet Gynecol* 1980;55:720–727.
27. Morrow CP, DiSaia PJ. Malignant melanoma of the female genitalia: a clinical analysis. *Obstet Gynecol Surv* 1976;31:233–271.
28. Reid GC, Schmidt RW, Roberts JA, et al. Primary melanoma of the vagina. A clinicopathologic analysis. *Obstet Gynecol* 1989;74: 190–199.
29. Breslow A. Tumor thickness, level of invasion and node dissection in stage I cutaneous melanoma. *Ann Surg* 1975;182:572.
30. Copeland LJ, Gersheson DM, Saul PB, et al. Sarcoma botryoides of the female genital tract. *Obstet Gynecol* 1985;66:262–267.
31. Peters WA, Kumar NB, Andersen WA, Morley GW. Primary sarcoma of the adult vagina: a clinicopathologic study. *Obstet Gynecol* 1985; 65:699–704.
32. Tavassoli FA, Norris HJ. Smooth muscle tumors of the vagina. *Obstet Gynecol* 1979;53:689–693.
33. Chen KTK, Hafez GR, Gilbert EF. Myxoid variant of epithelioid smooth muscle tumor. *Am J Clin Pathol* 1980;74:350.
34. Berkowitz RS, Ehrmann RL, Knapp RC. Endometrial stromal sarcoma arising from vaginal endometriosis. *Obstet Gynecol* 1978;51: 34S.
35. Granai CO, Walters MD, Safaii H, et al. Malignant transformation of vaginal endometriosis. *Obstet Gynecol* 1984;64:592.
36. Ulbright TM, Kraus FT. Endometrial stromal tumors of extrauterine tissue. *Am J Clin Pathol* 1981;76:371.
37. O'Toole RV, Tutle SE, Lucas JG, Sharma HM. Alveolar soft part sarcoma of the vagina: an immunohistochemical and electron microscopic study. *Int J Gynecol Pathol* 1985;4:258.
38. Webb MJ, Symmonds RE, Weiland LH. Malignant fibrous hystiocytoma of the vagina. *Am J Obstet Gynecol* 1974;119:190.
39. Okagaki T, Ishida T, Hilgers RD. A malignant tumor of the vagina resembling synovial sarcoma: a light and electron microscopic study. *Cancer* 1976;37:2306.
40. Shevchuk MM, Fenoglio CM, Lattes R, et al. Malignant mixed tumor of the vagina probably arising in mesonephric nests. *Cancer* 1978; 24:214.
41. Prempree T, Tang CK, Hatef A, Forster A. Angiosarcoma of the vagina: a clinicopathologic report: a reappraisal of radiation treatment of angiosarcomas of the female genital tract. *Cancer* 1983;51:618.
42. Buscema J, Rosenshein NB, Taqi F, Woodruff JD. Vaginal hemangiopericytoma: a histopathological and ultrastructural evaluation. *Obstet Gynecol* 1985;66[Suppl 3]:82S.
43. Chorlton I, Karnei RF, King FM, et al. Primary malignant reticuloendothelial disease involving the vagina, cervix and corpus uteri. *Obstet Gynecol* 1974;44:735.
44. Harris NL, Scully RE. Malignant lymphoma and granulocytic sarcoma of the uterus and vagina: a clinicopathologic analysis of 27 cases. *Cancer* 1984;53:2229.
45. Kaminski JM, Anderson PR, Han AC, et al. Primary small cell carcinoma of the vagina. *Gynecol Oncol* 2003:88:451–455.
46. Ulich TR, Liao S-Y, Layfield L, et al. Endocrine and tumor differentiation markers in poorly differentiated small-cell carcinoids of the cervix and vagina. *Arch Path Lab Med* 1986;110:1054.
47. Sulak P, Barnhill D, Heller P, et al. Nonsquamous carcinoma of the vagina. *Gynecol Oncol* 1988;29:309.
48. Shibata R, Umezawa A, Takehara K, et al. Primary carcinosarcoma of the vagina. *Pathol Int* 2003;53:106.
49. Clement PB, Young RH, Scully RE. Extraovarian pelvic yolk sac tumours. *Cancer* 1988;62:620.
50. Handel LN, Scott SM, Giller RH, et al. New perspectives on therapy for vaginal endodermal sinus tumors. *J Urol* 2002;168:687–690.
51. Creasman WT, Phillips JL, Menck HR. The National Cancer Data Base report on cancer of the vagina. *Cancer* 1998;83:1033–1040.
52. Di Domenico A. Primary vaginal squamous cell carcinoma in the young patient. *Gynecol Oncol* 1989;35:185–187.
53. Okagaki T, Twiggs LB, Zachow KR, et al. Identification of human papillomavirus DNA in cervical and vaginal intraepithelial neoplasia with molecularly cloned virus-specific DNA probes. *Int J Gynecol Pathol* 1983;153:183.
54. Daling JR, Medeleine MM, Schwartz SM, et al. A population-based

study of squamous cell vaginal cancer: HPV and cofactors. *Gynecol Oncol* 2002;84:263–270.

55. Reeves WC, Brinton LA, Garcia M, et al. Human papilloma virus infection and cervical cancer in Latin America. *N Engl J Med* 1989; 320:1437–1441.

56. Stock RG, Chen ASJ, Seski J. A 30-year experience in the management of primary carcinoma of the vagina: analysis of prognostic factors and treatment modalities. *Gynecol Oncol* 1995;56:45–52.

57. Ball HG, Berman ML. Management of primary vaginal carcinoma. *Gynecol Oncol* 1982;14:154–163.

58. Gallup DG, Talledo OE, Shah KJ, Hayes C. Invasive squamous cell carcinoma of the vagina. A 14-year study. *Obstet Gynecol* 1987;69: 782–785.

59. Lenehan PM, Meffe F, Lickrish GM. Vaginal intraepithelial neoplasia: biologic aspects and management. *Obstet Gynecol* 1986;68:333–337.

60. Andersen ES. Primary carcinoma of the vagina. *Gynecol Oncol* 1989; 33:317–320.

61. Chyle V, Zagars GK, Wheeler JA, et al. Definitive radiotherapy for carcinoma of the vagina. *Int J Radiat Oncol Biol Phys* 1996;35: 891–905.

62. Kirkbride P, Fyles A, Rawlings GA, et al. Carcinoma of the vagina—experience at the Princess Margaret Hospital (1974–1989). *Gynecol Oncol* 1995;56:435–443.

63. Leung S, Sexton M. Radical radiation therapy for carcinoma of the vagina—impact of treatment modalities on outcome: Peter MacCallum Cancer Institute experience 1970–1990. *Int J Radiat Oncol Biol Phys* 1993;25:413–418.

64. Perez CA, Camel HM, Galakatos AE, et al. Definitive irradiation in carcinoma of the vagina: long-term evaluation and results. *Int J Radiat Oncol Biol Phys* 1988;15:1283–1290.

65. Spirtos NM, Doshi BP, Kapp DS, Teng N. Radiation therapy for primary squamous cell carcinoma of the vagina: Stanford University experience. *Gynecol Oncol* 1989;35:20–26.

66. Stock RG, Mychalczak B, Armstrong JG, et al. The importance of the brachytherapy technique in the management of primary carcinoma of the vagina. *Int J Radiat Oncol Biol Phys* 1992;24:747–753.

67. Urbanski K, Kojs Z, Reinfuss M, Fabisiak W. Primary invasive vaginal carcinoma treated with radiotherapy: analysis of prognostic factors. *Gynecol Oncol* 1996;60:16–21.

68. Davis KP, Stanhope CR, Garton GR, et al. Invasive vaginal carcinoma: analysis of early stage disease. *Gynecol Oncol* 1991;42: 131–136.

69. Boice JD, Engholm G, Kleinerman RA, et al. Radiation dose and second cancer risk in patients treated for cancer of the cervix. *Radiation Res* 1988;116:3–55.

70. Lee JY, Perez CA, Ettinger N, et al. The risk of second primaries subsequent to irradiation for cervix cancer. *Int J Radiat Oncol Biol Phys* 1982;8:207–211.

71. Manetta A, Guttrecht EL, Berman ML, DiSaia PJ. Primary invasive carcinoma of the vagina. *Obstet Gynecol* 1990;76:639–642.

72. Bornstein J, Adam E, Adler-Storthz K, et al. Development of cervical and vaginal squamous neoplasia as a late consequence of in utero exposure to diethylstilbestrol. *Obstet Gynecol Surv* 1988;43:15–21.

73. Herbst AL, Ulfelder H, Poskanzer DC. Adenocarcinoma of the vagina: association of maternal stilbestrol therapy with tumor appearance in young women. *N Engl J Med* 1971;284:878–881.

74. Melnick S, Cole P, Anderson D, et al. Rates and risks of diethylstilbestrol-related clear-cell adenocarcinoma of the vagina and cervix. *N Engl J Med* 1987;316:514–516.

75. Herbst AL, Anderson D. Clear cell adenocarcinoma of the vagina and cervix secondary to intrauterine exposure to diethylstilbestrol. *Semin Surg Oncol* 1990;6:343–346.

76. Hicks ML, Piver MS. Conservative surgery plus adjuvant therapy for vulvovaginal rhabdomyosarcoma, diethylstilbestrol clear cell adenocarcinoma of the vagina, and unilateral germ cell tumors of the ovary. *Obstet Gynecol Clin North Am* 1992;19:219–233.

77. Trimble EL. Melanomas of the vulva and vagina. *Oncology* 1996;10: 1017–1024.

78. Curtin JP, Saigo P, Slucher B, et al. Soft-tissue sarcoma of the vagina and vulva: a clinicopathologic study. *Obstet Gynecol* 1995;86: 269–272.

79. Rubin SC, Young J, Mikuta JJ. Squamous carcinoma of the vagina:

80. Al-Kurdi M, Monaghan JM. Thirty-two years experience in management of primary tumors of the vagina. *Br J Obstet Gynaecol* 1981; 88:1145–1150.

81. Saslow D, Runowicz CD, Solomon D, et al. American Cancer Society guideline for the early detection of cervical neoplasia and cancer. *CA Cancer J Clin* 2002;52:342–362.

82. Tjalma W, Monaghan JM, de Barros Lopes A, et al. The role of surgery in invasive carcinoma of the vagina. *Gynecol Oncol* 2001; 81:360–365.

83. Hanselaar AG, Van Leusen ND, DeWilde PC, et al. Clear cell adenocarcinoma of the vagina and cervix. A report of the central Netherlands registry with emphasis on early detection and prognosis. *Cancer* 1991; 67:1971–1978.

84. Robboy SJ, Welch WR, Young RH, et al. Topographic relation of cervical ectropion and vaginal adenosis to clear cell adenocarcinoma. *Obstet Gynecol* 1982;60:546–551.

85. Maurer HM, Beltangady M, Gehan EA. The Intergroup RMS Study I.A. Final Report. *Cancer* 1988;61:209–220.

86. Chang YCF, Hricak H, Thurnher S, Lacey CG. Vagina: evaluation with MR imaging. *Radiology* 1988;169:175–179.

87. American Joint Committee on Cancer (AJCC). Vagina. In: Greene FL, Page DL, Fleming ID, et al., eds. *AJCC cancer staging manual.* 6th ed. New York: Springer-Verlag, 2002:251–257.

88. Perez CA, Arneson AN, Galakatos A. Radiation therapy in carcinoma of the vagina. *Cancer* 1973;31:36–44.

89. Prempree T, Amommam R. Radiation therapy of primary carcinoma of the vagina. *Acta Radiol Oncol* 1985;24:51–56.

90. Lee WR, Marcus RB Jr, Sombeck MD, et al. Radiotherapy alone for carcinoma of the vagina: the importance of overall treatment time. *Int J Radiat Oncol Biol Phys* 1994;29:983–988.

91. Perez CA, Grigsby PW, Garipagaoglu M, et al. Factors affecting long-term outcome of irradiation in carcinoma of the vagina. *Int J Radiat Oncol Biol Phys* 1999;44:37–45.

92. Peters WA, Kumar NB, Morley GW. Carcinoma of the vagina. Factors influencing treatment outcome. *Cancer* 1985;55:892–897.

93. Chu AM, Beechinor R. Survival and recurrence patterns in the radiation treatment of carcinoma of the vagina. *Gynecol Oncol* 1984;19: 298–307.

94. MacNaught R, Symonds RP, Hole D, Watson ER. Improved control of primary vaginal tumors by combined external beam and interstitial brachytherapy. *Clin Radiol* 1986;37:29–32.

95. Eddy GL, Marks RD, Miller MC, Underwood PB. Primary invasive vaginal carcinoma. *Am J Obstet Gynecol* 1991;165:292–298.

96. Dixit S, Singhal S, Baboo HA. Squamous cell carcinoma of the vagina. A review of 70 cases. *Gynecol Oncol* 1993;48:80–87.

97. Delclos L. In: Levitt SH, Tapley N, eds. *Technological basis of radiation therapy practical clinical applications.* Philadelphia: Lea & Febiger, 1984:193–227.

98. Dancuart F, Delclos L, Wharton JT, et al. Primary squamous cell carcinoma of the vagina treated by radiotherapy: a failures analysis—the MD Anderson hospital experience 1955–1982. *Int J Radiat Oncol Biol Phys* 1988;14:745–749.

99. Tarraza MH Jr, Muntz H, Decain M, et al. Patterns of recurrence of primary carcinoma of the vagina. *Eur J Gynecol Oncol* 1991;12: 89–92.

100. Ali MM, Huang DT, Goplerud DR, et al. Radiation alone for carcinoma of the vagina. Variation in response related to the location of the primary tumor. *Cancer* 1996;77:1934–1939.

101. Kucera H, Vavra N. Radiation management of primary carcinoma of the vagina: clinical and histopathological variables associated with survival. *Gynecol Oncol* 1991;40:12–16.

102. Perez CA, Bedwinek JM, Breaux SR. Patterns of failure after treatment of gynecologic tumors. *Cancer Treat Rep* 1983;2:217.

103. Robboy SJ, Herbst AL, Scully RE. Clear cell adenocarcinoma of the vagina and cervix in young females: analysis of 37 tumors that persisted or recurred after primary therapy. *Cancer* 1974;34:606–614.

104. Magrina JF, Basterson BJ. Vaginal reconstruction in gynecologic oncology. A review of techniques. *Obstet Gynecol Surv* 1981;36:1–10.

105. Dittmer PH, Randall ME. A technique for inguinal node boosts using photon fields defined by asymmetric collimator jaws. *Radiother Oncol* 2001;59:61–64.

106. Delclos L, Fletcher GH, Moore EB, et al. Minicolpostats, dome cylinders, other additions and improvements of the Fletsher-Suit afterloadable system: indications and limitations of their use. *Int J Radiat Oncol Biol Phys* 1980;6:1195–1206.

107. Perez CA, Slessinger ED, Grigsby PW. Design of an afterloading vaginal applicator (MIRALVA). *Int J Radiat Oncol Biol Phys* 1990; 18:1503–1508.

108. Slessinger ED, Perez CA, Grigsby PW, Williamson JF. Dosimetry and dose specification for a new gynecological brachytherapy applicator. *Int J Radiat Oncol Biol Phys* 1992;22:1117–1124.

109. Nanavati PJ, Fanning J, Hilgers RD, et al. High-dose-brachytherapy in primary stage I and II vaginal cancer. *Gynecol Oncol* 1993;51: 67–71.

110. Gore E, Gillin MT, Albano K, Erikson B. Comparison of high dose-rate and low dose-rate dose distributions for vaginal cylinders. *Int J Radiat Oncol Biol Phys* 1995;31:165–170.

111. Li Z, Liu C, Palta JR. Optimized dose distribution of a high dose rate vaginal cylinder. *Int J Radiat Oncol Biol Phys* 1998;41:239–244.

112. Tyree WC, Cardenes H, Randall M, Papiez L. High-dose rate brachytherapy for vaginal cancer: learning from treatment complications. *Int J Gynecol Cancer* 2002;12:27–31.

113. Rutkowski T, Bialas B, Rembielak A, et al. Efficacy and toxicity of MDR versus HDR brachytherapy for primary vaginal cancer. *Neoplasma* 2002;49:197–200.

114. Hilaris BS, Nori D, Anderson LL. Brachytherapy treatment planning. *Front Radiat Ther Oncol* 1987;21:94–106.

115. Syed AMN, Puthawala AA, Neblett D, et al. Transperineal interstitial-intracavitary "Syed-Neblett" applicator in the treatment of carcinoma of the uterine cervix. *Endocuriether Hypertherm Oncol* 1986;2:1–13.

116. Disaia PJ, Syed N, Puthwala AA. Malignant neoplasia of the upper vagina. *Endocuriether Hypertherm Oncol* 1990;6:251–256.

117. Martinez A, Cox RS, Edmundson GK. A mutiple-site perineal applicator (MUPIT) for treatment of prostatic, anorectal and gynecologic malignancies. *Int J Radiat Oncol Biol Phys* 1984;10:297–305.

118. Corn BW, Lanciano RM, Rosenblum N, et al. Improved treatment planning for the Syed-Neblett template using endorectal-coil magnetic resonance and intraoperative (laparotomy/laparoscopy) guidance: a new integrated technique for hysterectomized women with vaginal tumors. *Gynecol Oncol* 1995;56:255–261.

119. Childers JM, Surwit EA. Current status of operative laparoscopy in gynecologic malignancies. *Oncology* 1993;7:47–57.

120. Stock RG, Chen K, Terk M, et al. A new technique for performing Syed-Neblett template interstitial implants for gynecological malignancies using transrectal-ultrasound guidance. *Int J Radiat Oncol Biol Phys* 1997;37:819–825.

121. Stafl A, Wilkinson EJ, Mattingly R. Laser treatment of cervical and vaginal neoplasia. *Am J Obstet Gynecol* 1977;128:128–134.

122. Townsend DE, Levine RU, Crum CP, Richart R. Laser therapy of vaginal intra-epithelial neoplasia with the carbon dioxide laser. *Am J Obstet Gynecol* 1982;143:565–568.

123. Jobson V, Homesley HD. Treatment of vaginal intraepithelial neoplasia with the carbon dioxide laser. *Obstet Gynecol* 1983;62:90–93.

124. Julian TM, O'Connell BJ, Gosewehr JA. Indications, techniques, and advantages of partial laser vaginectomy. *Obstet Gynecol* 1992;80: 140–143.

125. Hoffman MS, DeCesare SL, Roberts WS, et al. Upper vaginectomy for in situ and occult, superficially invasive carcinoma of the vagina. *Am J Obstet Gynecol* 1992;166:30–33.

126. Fanning J, Manahan KJ, McLean SA. Loop electrosurgical excision procedure for partial upper vaginectomy. *Am J Obstet Gynecol* 1999; 181:1382–1385.

127. Robinson JB, Sun CC, Bodurka-Bevers D, et al. Cavitational ultrasonic surgical aspiration for the treatment of vaginal intraepithelial neoplasia. *Gynecol Oncol* 2000;78:235–242.

128. Diakomanolis E, Rodolakis A, Boulgaris Z, et al. Treatment of vaginal intraepithelial neoplasia with laser ablation and upper vaginectomy. *Gynecol Obstet Invest* 2002;54:17–20.

129. Wright VC, Riopelle MA. Laser surgery for vaginal disease. In: *Gynecologic laser surgery. a practical handbook.* Houston: Biomedical Communications, 1986:155–160.

130. Woodruff JD, Parmley THE, Julian CG. Topical 5-fluorouracil in the treatment of vaginal carcinoma in situ. *Gynecol Oncol* 1975;3: 124–132.

131. Piver MS, Barlow JJ, Tsukada Y, et al. Postirradiation squamous cell carcinoma in situ of the vagina: treatment by topical 20% 5-fluorouracil cream. *Am J Obstet Gynecol* 1979;135:377–389.

132. Petrilli ES, Townsend DE, Morrow CP, Nakao CY. Vaginal intraepithelial neoplasia: biologic aspects and treatment with topical 5-fluorouracil and the carbon dioxide laser. *Am J Obstet Gynecol* 1980;138: 321–328.

133. Daly JW, Ellis GE. Treatment of vaginal dysplasia and carcinoma insitu with topical 5-fluorouracil. *Obstet Gynecol* 1980;55:350–352.

134. Krebs HB. Treatment of vaginal intraepithelial neoplasia with laser and topical 5-fluorouracil. *Obstet Gynecol* 1989;73:657–660.

135. Perez CA, Korba A, Sharma S. Dosimetric considerations in irradiation of carcinoma of the vagina. *Int J Radiat Oncol Biol Phys* 1977; 2:639–649.

136. Ogino I, Kitamura T, Okajima H, Matsubara S. High-dose-rate intracavitary brachytherapy in the management of cervical and vaginal intraepithelial neoplasia. *Int J Radiat Oncol Biol Phys* 1998;40: 881–887.

137. MacLeod C, Fowler A, Dalrymple C, et al. High-dose-rate brachytherapy in the management of high-grade intraepithelial neoplasia of the vagina. *Gynecol Oncol* 1997;65:74–77.

138. Peters WA, Kumar NB, Morley GW. Microinvasive carcinoma of the vagina: a distinct clinical entity? *Am J Obstet Gynecol* 1985;153: 505–507.

139. Burke TW, Morris M, Roh MS, et al. Perineal reconstruction using single gracilis myocutaneous flaps. *Gynecol Oncol* 1995;57:221–225.

140. Reddy S, Saxena VS, Reddy S, et al. Results of radiotherapeutic management of primary carcinoma of the vagina. *Int J Radiat Oncol Biol Phys* 1991;21:1041–1044.

141. Chu AM, Beechinor R. Survival and recurrence patterns in the radiation treatment of carcinoma of the vagina. *Gynecol Oncol* 1984;19: 298–307.

142. Evans LS, Kersh CR, Constable WC, Taylor PT. Concomitant 5-fluorouracil, mitomycin-C and radiotherapy for advanced gynecological malignancies. *Int J Radiat Oncol Biol Phys* 1988;15:901–906.

143. Roberts WS, Hoffman MS, Kavanagh JJ, et al. Further experience with radiation therapy and concomitant intravenous chemotherapy in advanced carcinoma of the lower female genital tract. *Gynecol Oncol* 1991;43:233–236.

144. Kersch CR, Constable W, Spaulding C, et al. A Phase I-II trial of multimodality management of bulky gynecologic malignancy. Combined chemoradiosensitization and radiotherapy. *Cancer* 1990;66: 30–34.

145. Keys HM, Bundy BN, Stehman FB, et al. Cisplatin, radiation and adjuvant hysterectomy compared with radiation and adjuvant hysterectomy for bulky stage IB cervical carcinoma. *N Engl J Med* 1999; 340:1154–1161.

146. Morris M, Eifel PJ, Lu J, et al. Pelvic irradiation with concurrent chemotherapy compared with pelvic and para-aortic radiation for the high-risk cervical cancer. *N Engl J Med* 1999;340:1137–1143.

147. Rose PG, Bundy BN, Watkins EB, et al. Concurrent cisplatin-based radiotherapy and chemotherapy for locally advanced cervical cancer. *N Engl J Med* 1999;340:1144–1153.

148. Whitney CW, Sause W, Bundy BN, et al. Randomized comparison of fluorouracil plus cisplatin versus hydroxyurea as an adjunct to radiation therapy in stage IIB-IVA carcinoma of the cervix with negative para-aortic lymph nodes: a Gynecologic Oncology Group and Southest Oncology Group Study. *J Clin Oncol* 1999;17:1339–1348.

149. Tabata T, Takeshima N, Nishida H, et al. Treatment failure in vaginal cancer. *Gynecol Oncol* 2002;84:309–314.

150. Herbst AL, Scully RD. Adenocarcinoma of the vagina in adolescence: a report of seven cases including six clear-cell carcinomas (so-called mesonephromas). *Cancer* 1970;25:745–757.

151. Herbst AL, Kurman RJ, Scully RE, Poskanzer DC. Clear cell adenocarcinoma of the genital tract in young females. Registry report. *N Engl J Med* 1972;287:1259.

152. Herbst AL, Norusis MJ, Rosenow PJ, et al. An analysis of 346 cases of clear cell adenocarcinoma of the vagina and cervix with emphasis on recurrence and survival. *Gynecol Oncol* 1979;7:111–122.

153. Herbst AL, Anderson D. Clear cell adenocarcinoma of the vagina and cervix secondary to intrauterine exposure to diethylstilbestrol. *Semin Surg Oncol* 1990;6:343–346.

154. Senekjian EK, Frey KW, Anderson D, Herbst AL. Local therapy in

stage I clear cell adenocarcinoma of the vagina. *Cancer* 1987;60:1319–1324.

155. Senekjian EK, Frey KW, Stone C, Herbst AL. An evaluation of stage II vaginal clear cell adenocarcinoma according to substages. *Gynecol Oncol* 1988;31:56–64.

156. Senekjian EK, Frey K, Herbst AL. Pelvic exenteration in clear cell adenocarcinoma of the vagina and cervix. *Gynecol Oncol* 1989;34:413–416.

157. Hudson CN, Crandon AJ, Baird PJ, Willcocks D. Preservation of reproductive potential in diethylstilbestrol-related vaginal adenocarcinoma. *Am J Obstet Gynecol* 1983;145:375–377.

158. Hudson CN, Findlay WS, Roberts H. Successful pregnancy after radical surgery for diethyl-stilboestrol (DES)–related vaginal adenocarcinoma. Case report. *Br J Obstet Gynaecol* 1988;95:818–819.

159. Fowler WC, Brantley JC, Edelman DA. Clear cell adenocarcinoma of the genital tract. *South Med J* 1979;72:15–17.

160. Bonner JA, Perez-Tamayo C, Reid GC, et al. The management of vaginal melanoma. *Cancer* 1988;62:2066-2072.

161. Buchanan DJ, Schlaerth J, Kuroaki T. Primary vaginal melanoma: thirteen-year disease free survival after wide local excision and review of recent literature. *Am J Obstet Gynecol* 1998;178:1177–1184.

162. Geisler JP, Look KY, Moore DA, Sutton GP. Pelvic exenteration for malignant melanomas of the vagina or urethra with over 3 mm of invasion. *Gynecol Oncol* 1995;59:338–341.

163. Irvin WP, Bliss SA, Rice LW, et al. Case report. Malignant melanoma of the vagina and locoregional control: radical surgery revisited. *Gynecol Oncol* 1998;71:476–480.

164. Levitan Z, Gordon AN, Kaplan AL, Kaufman RH. Primary malignant melanoma of the vagina: report of four cases and review of the literature. *Gynecol Oncol* 1989;33:85–90.

165. Van Nostrand K, Lucci J, Schell M, et al. Primary vaginal melanoma: improved survival with radical pelvic surgery. *Gynecol Oncol* 1994;55:234–237.

166. Petru E, Nagele F, Czerwenka K, et al. Primary malignant melanoma of the vagina: long-term remission following radiation therapy. *Gynecol Oncol* 1998;70:23–26.

167. Das Gupta T, D'Urso J. Melanoma of female genitalia. *Surg Obstet Gynecol* 1964;119:1074–1078.

168. Brand E, Fu YS, Lagasse LD, Berek JS. Vulvovaginal melanoma: report of seven cases and literature review. *Gynecol Oncol* 1989;33:54.

169. Hachi H, Ottmany A, Bougtab A, et al. Leiomyosarcoma of the vagina: a rare case. *Bull Cancer* 1997;84:215–217.

170. Neesham D, Kerdemelidis P, Scurry J. Case report. Primary malignant mixed mullerian tumor of the vagina. *Gynecol Oncol* 1998;70:303–307.

171. Hornback NB, Omura G, Major FJ. Observations on the use of adjuvant radiation therapy in patients with stage I and II uterine sarcoma. *Int J Radiat Oncol Biol Phys* 1986;12:2127–2130.

172. Hays DM, Shimada H, Raney RB Jr, et al. Sarcomas of the vagina and uterus: the Intergroup Rhabdomyosarcoma Study. *J Pediatr Surg* 1985;20:718–724.

173. Raney RB Jr, Gehan EA, Hays DM, et al. Primary chemotherapy with or without radiation and/or surgery for children with localized sarcoma of the bladder, prostate, vagina, uterus, and cervix: a comparison of the results in Intergroup Rhabdomyosarcoma Studies I and II. *Cancer* 1990;66:2072–2081.

174. Andrassy RJ, Hays DM, Raney RB, et al. Conservative surgical management of vaginal and vulvar pediatric rhabdomyosarcoma: a report from the Intergroup Rhabdomyosarcoma Study III. *J Pediatr Surg* 1995;30:1034–1037.

175. Hilgers RD. Pelvic exenteration for vaginal embryonal rhabdomyosarcoma. A review. *Obstet Gynecol* 1975;45:175–180.

176. Grosfeld JL, Smith JP, Clatworthy HW. Pelvic rhabdomyosarcoma in infants and children. *J Urol* 1972;107:673–675.

177. Flamant F, Gerbaulet A, Nihol-Fekete C, et al. Long-term sequelae of conservative treatment by surgery, brachytherapy and chemotherapy for vulvar and vaginal rhabdomyosarcoma in children. *J Clin Oncol* 1990;8:1847–1853.

178. Friedman M, Peretz BA, Nissenbaum M, Paldi E. Modern treatment of vaginal embryonal rhabdomyosarcoma. *Obstet Gynecol Surv* 1986;41:614–618.

179. Andrassy RJ, Wiener ES, RAney RB, et al. Progress in the surgical managment of vagina rhabdomyosarcoma: a 25 year review from the Intergroup Rhabdomyosarcoma Study Group. *J Pediatr Surg* 1999;34:731–734.

180. Prevot S, Hugol D, Andouin J, et al. Primary non-Hodgkins's maligant lymphoma of the vagina: report of threee cases and review of the literature. *Pathol Res Pract* 1992;188:78–85.

181. Perren T, Farrant M, McCarthy K, et al. Lymphomas of the cervix and upper vagina: a report of five cases and a review of the literature. *Gynecol Oncol* 1992;44:87–95.

182. Young RH, Scully RE. Endodermal sinus tumor of the vagina: a report of nine cases and review of the literature. *Gynecol Oncol* 1984;18:380–392.

183. Copeland LJ, Sneige N, Ordonez N, et al. Endodermal sinus tumor of the vagina and cervix. *Cancer* 1985;55:2558–2565.

184. Collins HS, Burke TW, Heller PB, et al. Endodermal sinus tumor of the infant vagina treated exclusively by chemotherapy. *Obstet Gynecol* 1989;73:507–509.

185. Aartsen EJ, Delamarre JFM, Gerretsen G. Endodermal sinus tumor of the vagina: radiation therapy and progeny. *Obstet Gynecol* 1993;81:893–895.

186. Hwang EH, Han SJ, Lee MK, et al. Clinical experience with conservative surgery for vaginal endodermal sinus tumor. *J Pediatr Surg* 1996;31:219–22.

187. Williams S, Blessing JA, Liao SY, et al. Adjuvant therapy of ovarian germ cell tumors cisplatin, etoposide, and bleomycin: a trial of the Gynecologic Oncology Group. *J Clin Oncol* 1994;12:701–706.

188. Sun SS, Chen TC, Yen RF, et al. Value of whole body 18F-fluoro-2-deoxyglucose positron emission tomography in the evaluation of recurrent cervical cancer. *Anticancer Res* 2001;21:2957–2961.

189. Miller B, Morris M, Rutledge E, et al. Aborted exenterative procedures in recurrent cervical cancer. *Gynecol Oncol* 1993;50:94–99.

190. Ratliff CR, Gershenson DM, Morris M, et al. Sexual adjustment of patients undergoing gracilis myocutaneous flap vaginal reconstruction in conjunction with pelvic exenteration. *Cancer* 1996;78:2229–2235.

191. Moore DH, Thomas GM, Montana GS, et al. Preoperative chemoradiation for advanced vulvar cancer. A Phase II study of the Gynecologic Oncology Group. *Int J Radiat Oncol Biol Phys* 1988;42:79–85.

192. Russell AH, Koh WJ, Markette K, et al. Radical reirradiation for recurrent or second primary carcinoma of the female reproductive tract. *Gynecol Oncol* 1987;27:226–232.

193. Randall ME, Evans L, Greven KM, et al. Interstitial re-irradiation for recurrent gynecological malignancies: results and analysis of prognostic factors. *Gynecol Oncol* 1993;48:23–31.

194. Wang X, Cai S, Ding Y, Wei K. Treatment of late recurrent vaginal malignancy after initial radiotherapy for carcinoma of the cervix: an analysis of 73 cases. *Gynecol Oncol* 1998;69:125–129.

195. Gupta AK, Vicini FA, Frazier AJ, et al. Iridium-192 transperineal interstitial brachytherapy for locally advanced or recurrent gynecological malignancies. *Int J Radiat Oncol Biol Phys* 1999;43:1055–1060.

196. Charra C, Roy P, Coquard R, et al. Outcome of treatment of upper third vaginal recurrences of cervical and endometrial carcinomas with interstitial brachytherapy. *Int J Radiat Oncol Biol Phys* 1998;40:421–426.

197. Haddock MG, Martinez-Monge R, Petersen IA, et al. Locally advanced primary and recurrent gynecologic malignancies. EBRT with or without IORT or HDR-IORT. In: Gunderson LL, Calvo F, Harrison LB, et al., eds. *Current clinical oncology: intraoperative irradiation: techniques and results.* New Totowa, NJ: Humana Press, 1999:397–419.

198. Garton GR, Gunderson LL, Webb MJ, et al. Intraoperative radiation therapy in gynecologic cancer: update of the experience at a single institution. *Int J Radiat Oncol Biol Phys* 1997;37:839–843.

199. Gemignani ML, Alektiar KM, Leitao M, et al. Radical surgical resection and high-dose intraoperative radiation therapy (HDR-IORT) in patients with gynecologic cancers. *Int J Radiat Oncol Biol Phys* 2001;50:687–694.

200. Hockel M, Schlenger K, Hamm H, et al. Five-year experience with combined operative and radiotherapeutic treatment of recurrent gynecologic tumors infiltrating the pelvic wall. *Cancer* 1996;77:1918–1933.

201. Blomgren H, Lax I, Goranson H, et al. Radiosurgery of tumors in the body: Clinical experience using a new method. *J Radiosurg* 1998;1:63–74.

202. Cardenes H, Song G, Randall M. Late sequelae of radiation therapy in the management of gynecological malignancies. Current medical literature. *Gynecol Oncol* 2001;2:1–10.

203. Grigsby PW, Russell A, Bruner D, et al. Late injury of cancer therapy on the female reproductive tract. *Int J Radiat Oncol Biol Phys* 1995; 31:1281–1299.

204. Hintz BL, Kagan AR, Gilbert HA, et al. Radiation tolerance of the vaginal mucosa. *Int J Radiat Oncol Biol Phys* 1980;6:711–716.

205. Rubin P, Casarett GW. The female tract genital. In: Rubin P, Casarett GW, eds. *Clinical Radiation Pathology*. Philadelphia: WB Saunders, 1986:396–342.

206. Au SP, Grigsby PW. The irradiation tolerance dose of the proximal vagina. *Radiother Oncol* 2003;67:77–85.

207. Delanian S, Porcher R, Balla-Mekias, Lefaix JL. Randomized, placebo-controlled trial of combined pentoxifylline and tocopherol for regression of superficial radiation-induced fibrosis. *J Clin Oncol* 2003; 21:2545–2550.

208. Spanos WJ, Wasserman T, Meoz R, et al. Palliation of advanced pelvic malignant disease with large fraction pelvic radiation and misonidazole: final Report of RTOG Phase I/II Study. *Int J Radiat Oncol Biol Phys* 1987;13:1479–1482.

209. Spanos WJ, Guse C, Perez CA, et al. Phase II study of multiple daily fractionations in the palliation of advanced pelvic malignancies. Preliminary report of the RTOG 85–02. *Int J Radiat Oncol Biol Phys* 1989;17:659–662.

210. Spanos WJ, Perez CA, Marcus S, et al. Effect of rest interval on tumor and normal tissue response. A report of Phase III study of accelerated split-course palliative radiation for advanced pelvic malignancies (RTOG 85-02). *Int J Radiat Oncol Biol Phys* 1993;25:399–403.

211. Spanos WJ, Clery M, Perez CA, et al. Late effect of multiple daily fraction palliation schedule for advanced pelvic malignancies (RTOG 85–02). *Int J Radiat Oncol Biol Phys* 1994;29:961–967.

212. Thigpen JT, Blessing JA, Homesley HD, et al. Phase II trial of cisplatin in advanced or recurrent cancer of the vagina: a Gynecologic Oncology Group study. *Gynecol Oncol* 1986;23:101–104.

213. Muss HB, Bundy BN, Christopherson WA. Mitoxantrone in the treatment of advanced vulvar and vaginal carcinoma: a Gynecologic Oncology Group study. *Am J Clin Oncol* 1989;12:142–144.

214. Long HJ 3rd, Cross WG, Wieand HS, et al. Phase II trial of methotrexate, vinblastine, doxorubicin, and cisplatin in advanced/recurrent carcinoma of the uterine cervix and vagina. *Gynecol Oncol* 1995;57: 235–239.

215. Patton TJ Jr, Kavanagh JJ, Delclos L. Five-year survival in patients given intra-arterial chemotherapy prior to radiotherapy for advanced squamous carcinoma of the cervix and vagina. *Gynecol Oncol* 1991; 42:54–59.

CHAPTER 22

Uterine Cervix

Marcus E. Randall, Helen Michael, Jan Ver Morken, and Fred Stehman

EPIDEMIOLOGY AND RISK FACTORS

Worldwide, cervical cancer is the third most common malignancy, and the second most common cancer (after breast cancer) in women (1). Nearly one-half million new cases occur each year (2). The majority of cases occur in developing countries without availability of routine Papanicolaou smear screening. Cervical cancer is the leading cause of death from cancer in developing countries (2). The highest incidence of the disease is seen in Central and South America, southern and eastern Africa, and the Caribbean (3).

There is a correlation between incidence and mortality in a given area, but Africa appears to have a disproportionately higher mortality (3). The incidence and mortality of this disease in North America have declined during the last half-century owing to both increased availability of Pap smear screening and a decrease in fertility rate. These declines in incidence have slowed in recent years, and there is a trend toward increasing incidence in some populations of white women in the United States (3). Cervical carcinoma is the sixth most common malignant tumor in women in the United States, but black and Hispanic women are disproportionately affected.

Cervical cancer is a sexually transmitted disease associated with chronic infection by oncogenic types of human papillomavirus (HPV). Therefore, risk factors for cervical cancer are the same as those for sexually transmitted disease,

including early age at onset of sexual activity, multiple pregnancies, and multiple sexual partners. Wives of patients who have penile cancer have an increased risk of cervical cancer later in life (4). An increased risk of cervical cancer has also been reported in association with long-term oral contraceptive use (5), but patients with this variable may also have other risk factors, such as increased sexual activity. Tobacco smoking is also a risk factor for cervical cancer (6). Patients infected with human immunodeficiency virus (HIV) are often also infected with HPV, and they have higher rates of cervical dysplasia and progression to invasive carcinoma than HIV-negative women (7). Anti-retroviral therapy does not affect HPV-related disease in HIV-infected patients (7).

ANATOMY

The uterus is a muscular, hollow organ located in the midplane of the pelvis, behind the bladder and in front of the rectum. Usually anteverted, its position may change with expansion of the bladder or the rectum. The fundus is partially covered by peritoneum. Its anterior and lateral surfaces are in contact with extraperitoneal connective tissue, and are related to the bladder and the broad ligaments.

The regions of the uterus are the corpus and the cervix. The cervix is separated from the corpus by a subtle constriction (the isthmus), and is divided into two regions: an upper, or supravaginal, portion above the ring, which contains the endocervical canal, and the vaginal portion, which projects into the vault.

The uterine corpus is attached to the surrounding structures in the pelvis by two pairs of ligaments: the broad and the round. The broad ligament is a double layer of peritoneum extending from the lateral margin of the uterus to the lateral wall of the pelvis. The fallopian tubes lie at the superior margin of the broad ligament, and are posterior to it. They enter the uterus in the posterolateral-fundal portions. The two layers of peritoneum forming the broad ligament enclose the extraperitoneal connective tissue, which is desig-

Marcus E. Randall: Professor, Department of Radiation Oncology, Indiana University School of Medicine, Indianapolis, Indiana 46202.

Helen Michael: Professor, Department of Pathology and Laboratory Medicine, Indiana University School of Medicine, Indianapolis, Indiana 46202.

Jan Ver Morken: Professor of Oncology, University of Antwerp, Antwerp, Belgium.

Fred Stehman: Professor and Chair, Department of Obstetrics and Gynecology, Indiana University School of Medicine, Indianapolis, Indiana 46202.

nated the parametrium as it reaches the uterus. Inferiorly, the broad ligament follows the plane of the pelvic floor, and ends medially in the upper portion of the vagina (8).

The round ligament is a true band of dense connective tissue and smooth muscle, and contains small vessels and nerves. It extends forward horizontally from its attachment in the anterolateral-fundal portion of the uterus to the lateral pelvic wall. The cord ascending from the lateral wall of the true pelvis crosses the pelvic brim and extends laterally. It exits the abdomen through the internal inguinal ring to traverse the inguinal canal and insert into the fascia of the labium majus.

The uterosacral ligaments are paired supports for the lower uterus, and consist of fibrous tissue with smooth muscle. They extend from the uterus to the sacrum, and run along the recto-uterine-peritoneal fields (8).

The cardinal ligaments, also called the transverse cervical ligaments (Mackenrodt's), consist of thickened connective tissue and fascia arising at the upper lateral margins of the cervix and inserting into the fascial covering of the pelvic diaphragm. These two pairs of ligaments, the uterosacrals and cardinals, provide most of the support for the uterus and cervix.

The uterus has a rich network of lymphatics that drain principally into the paracervical lymph nodes, from which they drain into the hypogastric lymph nodes and the external iliacs (of which the obturator nodes are the innermost component). The pelvic lymphatics drain into the common iliac and the periaortic lymph nodes. Lymphatics from the fundus pass laterally across the broad ligament, continuous with those of the ovary, ascending along the ovarian vessels into the periaortic lymph nodes. Some of the fundal lymphatics also drain into the external and internal common iliac lymph nodes.

The main arteries supplying the uterus are the uterine arteries, which originate from the anterior division of the hypogastric artery. The uterine artery lies on the inner wall of the true pelvis, passing medially and slightly forward on the fascia that covers the upper surface of the levator ani muscle in the lower margin of the broad ligament. In the parametrial tissue, enclosed by the peritoneal layers of the ligament, the uterine artery arches over the ureter about 1.5 cm from the uterus. On reaching the cervix, just above the lateral fornix of the vagina, it gives off a vaginal branch. The uterine artery ascends as far as the fundus, supplying many branches to the anterior and posterior surfaces of the uterus. It continues laterally, and divides into branches that supply the ovary and the fallopian tubes, forming a rich cruciate anastomosis with the ovarian arteries. The extensive anastomotic connections between the paired uterine and ovarian arteries ensure adequate blood supply. Any one of these vessels can support a normal pregnancy. Additional collateral supply is available from the aorta through the middle sacral artery, the ilio-lumbar arteries, and the inferior mesenteric artery, as well as from the deep and common femoral arteries through the pudendal, vaginal, and obturator arteries.

Venous drainage follows the arterial supply, except that the left ovarian vein drains to the left renal vein instead of into the vena cava.

NATURAL HISTORY

Preinvasive Disease

Most cervical carcinomas originate in the transformation zone. In this area, the endocervical cells are replaced by squamous metaplasia. Over 90% of cervical carcinomas are associated with human papillomavirus infection, which may result in dysplasia, squamous carcinoma in situ, and adenocarcinoma in situ. Chronic infection with a high-risk type of human papillomavirus, together with other poorly understood factors, results in squamous carcinoma in situ and adenocarcinoma in situ (1). These lesions represent precursor lesions for invasive squamous and adenocarcinomas. High-risk HPV types may cause severe squamous dysplasia or squamous carcinoma in situ without progression from mild squamous dysplasia. In one study, high-grade dysplasia occurred at a median time of 26 months after HPV detection. There was little progression from low-grade to high-grade dysplasia (9). Only about 15% of low-grade dysplasias will progress within 2 years, but about one-third of high-grade dysplasias will progress within 10 years if not treated (10, 11). High-grade dysplasia is detected up to 10 years before invasive carcinoma develops (1). Low-grade dysplasia and genital warts have a peak incidence in the 20s; high-grade dysplasia peaks in the mid-30s; and invasive cervical carcinoma is most often seen after age 40 (1,12).

Patterns of Spread

The malignant cells can break through the basement membrane to invade the cervical stroma. The lesion may be ulcerated, exophytic, or infiltrative, and may spread to adjacent vaginal fornices or to the paracervical and parametrial tissues; or, if untreated, to the bladder, the rectum, or both. Carcinoma of the uterine cervix has been found to extend into the lower uterine segment or endometrial cavity in 10% to 30% of patients (13).

Regional lymphatic or hematogenous spread may occur. Dissemination usually follows an orderly sequence, but occasionally a small carcinoma may metastasize to the pelvic lymph nodes, invade the bladder or the rectum, or produce distant metastasis. Carcinoma of the cervix may spread to the paracervical and parametrial lymphatics, metastasizing to the obturator lymph nodes, the hypogastric lymph nodes, and to other external iliac nodes. There may be tumor metastases to the common iliac or paraaortic lymph nodes (14, 15). Involvement of periaortic nodes without involvement of pelvic nodes is unusual. The incidence of metastasis to pelvic and paraaortic lymph nodes is listed in Table 22.1.

TABLE 22.1. *Rates of lymph node metastasis in patients with carcinoma of the cervix*

References	Primary Treatment	FIGO Stage IB			IIA			IIB			III		
		Patients	Pelvic Nodes (%)	PA Nodes (%)	Patients	Pelvic Nodes (%)	PA Nodes (%)	Patients	Pelvic Nodes (%)	PA Nodes (%)	Patients	Pelvic Nodes (%)	PA Nodes (%)
Girardi et al.[16]	RH	163	31		8	0	4	249	45				
Averette et al.[17]	RH	866	14	5	95	21							
Kamura et al.[18]	RH	211	12		48	17		86	34				
Alvarez et al.[19]	RH	401	12	1									
Ayhan et al.[20]	RH	207	21	6	38	57	(0/6)	25	40	(4/8)			
Delgado et al.[21]	RH	645	16										
Lee et al.[22]	RH	596	13		250	27		108	35				
Fuller et al.[23]	RH	285	15		133	22							
Barber[24]	RH/EX	273	14					283*	28		67	42	
Burghardi et al.[25]	RH	122	31		8	25		195	44				
Creasman et al.[26]	RH	258	14		10	10							
Boyce et al.[27]	RH	138	14										
Piver and Chung[28]	RH	73	27										
Boronow[29]	RH		26										
Sudarsanam et al.[30]	RH/RT	135		7	21		14	22	18	18	19		19
Stehman et al.[31]	RT	8	75	50				321		15	188	23†	37
LaPolla et al.[32]	RT	158		5	8	38	0	39	33	17	38	55	25
Berman et al.[33]	RT	22	27	23	25		12	240		19	180		17
Ballon et al.[34]	RT	143		6	16	38	19	32	16	33	24	38	30
Lagasse et al.[34a]	RT	16		25	22		18	58		7	61		33
Buchsbaum[35]	RT	21	38	0	4		0	15			104		33
Wharton et al.[36]	RT							67*	35	18	291		33
Nelson et al.[37]	RT				16		13	47		15	39		38
Guthrie et al.[38]	RT										37		35

PA, paraaortic; RH, radical hysterectomy, EX, exenteration; RT, radiation therapy.

* Stages IIA and IIB combined.

† Patients with positive paraaortics excluded.

From Eifel PJ, Berek JS, and Thigpen JT. Gynecologic cancers. In: DeVita VT Jr, Hellman S, Rosenberg SA, eds. *Cancer – Principles and practice of oncology,* Vol. 1, 5th ed. Philadelphia: Lippincott-Raven, 1997:1436.

In addition to the pelvic nodes, there are lymph nodes distributed throughout the parametrium. Girardi and associates (16) studied 359 specimens from radical hysterectomies: 132 clinical stage IB, eight stage IIA, and 219 stage IIB. Parametrial lymph nodes were identified in 280 patients (78%), with 63 (22.5%) of these patients having involvement of lymph nodes by malignancy. The incidence of positive nodes was 11.4% in stage IB and 21.5% in stage IIB. Involved lymph nodes were found in the medial parametrium (44.4%), in the lateral parametrium (38%), or in both areas (17.5%). There was a close correlation between involvement of the parametrial lymph nodes and the iliac lymph nodes. Of the patients with negative parametrial nodes, only 26% had positive iliac lymph nodes, however 81% of patients with positive parametrial lymph nodes also had metastatic involvement of the pelvic nodes. Hematogenous dissemination through the venous plexus and the paracervical veins occurs less frequently, but is seen in more advanced stages. Covens and co-workers analyzed the parametria of 842 patients subjected to radical hysterectomy (39). Though 33 patients had some lateral involvement, 25 of these had involvement of the parametria itself and eight had parametrial nodal involvement. No patient had both. There was a high correlation with tumor size and depth of invasion. These authors questioned the need to fully excise the parametrium for patients with limited disease.

The most common distant metastatic sites are the lungs, mediastinal and supraclavicular lymph nodes, bones, and liver (40).

When recurrence occurs after therapy, the majority of patients will be symptomatic, though asymptomatic recurrences may be found in the pelvis with periodic surveillance (41). The median interval to recurrence is 17 months, though a small percentage of recurrences may be detected after five years (42).

CLINICAL PRESENTATION AND DIAGNOSTIC EVALUATION

Preclinical Invasive Disease

Screening and Cytology

Detection of dysplasia and carcinoma *in situ* on Pap smears has led to a marked decrease in the incidence of and mortality from invasive cervical carcinoma in developed nations. Recommendations of the American Cancer Society are that asymptomatic and low-risk women age 20 and older, and sexually active women under the age of 20 have annual Pap smears for 2 consecutive years, and then every 3 years until age 65 (43).

The Bethesda System, created in 1988 in order to standardize terminology for reporting Pap smear results in a way that would provide clear implications for clinical management (44), accommodates the fact that changes due to HPV infection cannot be reliably separated from mild squamous dysplasia, and that moderate and severe squamous dysplasia cannot be consistently differentiated. Two categories of dysplasia are now used: the term *low grade squamous intraepithelial lesion* (LSIL) encompasses both HPV changes and mild squamous dysplasia, while *high grade squamous intraepithelial lesion* (HSIL) includes moderate and marked dysplasia, as well as squamous carcinoma *in situ*. The term *atypical squamous cells of undetermined significance* has been used to designate cells that have characteristics between those of reactive cells and dysplasia. Specimen adequacy is also addressed in the Bethesda System. This system was modified in 1991 (45), and again in 2001 (46). The categories LSIL and HSIL have been retained. However, because 10% to 20% of women with atypical squamous cells on Pap smear have underlying moderate or severe squamous dysplasia, and because 1 in 1000 may have invasive cancer (47), the 2001 classification altered terminology for Pap smears with these findings. In the 2001 Bethesda System, atypical squamous cells are classified as ''of undetermined significance (ASC-US)'' or ''cannot exclude HSIL (ASC-H).'' About 5% to 10% of atypical squamous-cell cases fall into the category of ''ASC-H'' (48–50). Abnormal glandular cells are classified as ''atypical endocervical, endometrial, or glandular cells''(46).

Colposcopy and Biopsy

Colposcopy evaluates the exocervix and a portion of the endocervix adjacent to the transition of the squamous and columnar epithelium. Colposcopy-directed biopsy and endocervical curettings provide a firm diagnosis in most patients. For some patients, colposcopy is not sufficient. Colposcopy must be considered inadequate if the transformation zone is not fully visualized, if a visible lesion extends into the endocervical canal, if the endocervical curettings reveal dysplastic fragments, or if there is discordance of more than one grade among the diagnostic evaluations. In such cases, conization biopsy should be performed. A more complete discussion of pre-invasive disease can be found in Chapter 19.

Conization Biopsy

Conization must be performed if no gross lesion of the cervix is observed and an endocervical tumor is suspected, colposcopy is inadequate, or a diagnosis of microinvasive carcinoma is made upon biopsy. Conization biopsy may also be therapeutic for a large number of patients.

Loop Excision

Loop diathermy excision is an acceptable alternative to cold knife conization. The technique allows conization to be done in an office setting. Randomized trials have shown the technique to be just as effective, quicker, and more reliable than laser excision (51,52).

Clinical Disease

Symptoms and Complaints

Often, the first symptomatic manifestation of cervical cancer is abnormal vaginal bleeding. Serosanguineous or yellowish vaginal discharge, at times foul-smelling, may also be noticed, particularly in patients with advanced necrotic lesions. If chronic bleeding occurs, the patient may suffer anemia, weight loss, fatigue, or other constitutional symptoms.

In patients who complain of pain in the lumbosacral or gluteal area, the possibility of iliac or paraaortic lymph node involvement with extension into the lumbosacral nerve roots or hydronephrosis should be considered. Urinary and rectal symptoms (e.g., hematuria, rectal bleeding) may suggest invasion of the bladder or rectum.

Physical Findings

The most common physical finding is a visible lesion on the cervix. Some lesions can be hidden from view in the endocervical canal, but appreciated on bimanual examination. The widest diameter of the lesion, and whether or not there is a free space between the tumor and the pelvic wall, should be assessed. Parametrial and uterosacral involvement can be clinically evaluated only by rectal examination. Node-bearing regions (groin, supraclavicular fossa) should be evaluated.

Diagnostic Biopsy

Any suspicious lesion of the cervix should be biopsied to an adequate depth, preferably at the margin, to confirm the diagnosis of invasive carcinoma. Specimens should be obtained from any suspicious area in all four quadrants of the cervix, and from suspicious areas in the vagina.

Staging

Clinical Staging Procedures

Assessment for clinical staging is best made by pelvic and rectal examination. Because of the advantage of having several examiners and the benefit of muscular relaxation, pelvic examination under anesthesia is recommended. Radiation and gynecologic oncologists should jointly evaluate patients who may be candidates for radiation therapy. Cystoscopy or rectosigmoidoscopy may be considered for patients with stage IVA disease, or for those with a history of urinary or lower gastrointestinal tract disturbances.

Laboratory Studies

Patients should have complete peripheral blood evaluation (hemogram, white blood cell count, differential, and platelet count), complete chemistry profile (with particular attention to blood urea nitrogen, creatinine, uric acid, and liver functions), and urinalysis.

Radiographic Studies

Chest radiographs and evaluation of ureteral integrity should be obtained in all patients. Computed tomography (CT) and magnetic resonance imaging (MRI) are extensively employed (53).

Heller and co-workers (54) reported a prospective evaluation of 320 patients with stage IIB, III, or IVA carcinoma of the cervix entered into a Gynecologic Oncology Group (GOG) protocol upon whom preoperative CT scan, lymphangiogram, and ultrasound of the aortic area were performed. Para-aortic node dissection was performed in patients with negative staging studies. The lymphangiogram, CT scan, and ultrasound had false-negative frequencies for pelvic lymph node evaluation of 14.2%, 25%, and 30%, respectively. The sensitivity was 79% for lymphangiogram, 34% for CT scan, and 19% for ultrasound. The specificity ratings of these tests were 73%, 96%, and 99%, respectively. Whether the limitations of these staging studies remain in light of significant improvements in imaging technology is not clear.

Computed tomography is used frequently as a single study. If performed with intravenous contrast, CT can substitute for intravenous pyelogram. Camilien (55) reported 61 patients with carcinoma of the uterine cervix who had both preoperative CT scans and exploratory laparotomy. The radiographic and surgical-pathologic findings were correlated, showing that 75% of the enlarged pelvic lymph nodes detected on CT scan contained metastases. Ninety-seven percent of the patients with negative nodes upon CT scan were pathologically negative (97% specificity). However, histologically positive pelvic nodes were often missed on CT scan (25% sensitivity). The CT scan has been found to be more valuable in the evaluation of the paraaortic lymph nodes.

Ohara and colleagues evaluated the prognostic significance of CT-based nodal assessment using strict measurement guidelines (56). Nodal status was assessed as "negative" if <5 mm, "possibly positive" if 5–10 mm, or "probably positive" if >10 mm. Significant differences were found between "negative" and "probably positive" status in all endpoints. "Negative" nodal status and "possibly positive" status was generally not prognostic, although there were significant differences in distant metastasis-free rate between "negative," "possibly positive," and "probably positive" (96.4%, 59.3%, and 35.1%, respectively). The authors concluded that radiographic staging and evaluation of nodal assessment are valuable, particularly when strict cutoff measurements are used.

MRI has been used for assessment of extracervical extension. Parametrial tumor can be identified on T2-weighted images from the low-intensity cervix and uterine ligaments.

MRI may be useful to define the volume treated, particularly if lateral fields are used (57,58). Abnormal or suspicious lymph node findings on CT or MRI should be confirmed with CT-guided thin-needle aspiration biopsies.

Positron emission tomography (PET) is increasingly utilized to evaluate patients with cervical carcinoma. Singh et al. performed pre-treatment PET scans in 47 stage IIIB patients (59). Without pathologic confirmation, the authors used the PET data to classify patients into 4 groups based on nodal status: no evidence; pelvis only; pelvic and paraaortic; and pelvis, paraaortic, and supraclavicular metastases. The 3-year estimates of cause-specific survival were 73%, 58%, 29%, and 0%, respectively, for these 4 groups. Although CT scans were also done in these patients, the authors did not report the findings relative to PET scan findings, making it difficult to know the value of PET scanning beyond that of more conventional imaging.

Lin et al. reported the results of PET scans in 50 patients with cervical cancers whose CT scans did not show evidence of paraaortic metastasis (60). Retroperitoneal lymph node dissections were carried out in all patients, and 14 patients were found to have adenopathy. There were 2 false-negative and 2 false-positive results in the 50 patients. The authors calculated that PET scanning had a sensitivity of 85.7%, a specificity of 94.4%, and an accuracy of 92% in their hands.

Park et al. obtained PET scans in 27 patients prior to surgical lymph node staging (61). Eight lymph node areas were specifically defined and correlated with both surgical specimen and PET findings. Although specificity was reasonably high, the sensitivity, particularly for metastases <1 cm, was limited.

FIGO and American Joint Committee Commission on Cancer (AJCC) Staging

The staging system widely used for cervical cancer is determined by FIGO, in collaboration with the World Health Organization and the International Union Against Cancer, and was last revised in 1995 (62). The 1985 FIGO revision (63) categorized minimal microscopic stromal invasion as stage IA_1, and invasion of 5 mm or less in depth or 7 mm or less in horizontal spread as stage IA_2. Kolstad (64) reviewed the results of therapy in 643 patients with early invasive carcinoma, reclassified as stage IA_1 or IA_2, confirming the validity of the staging modification. Similar conclusions were reached by Tsukamoto and co-workers (65). As revised in 1995, stage IA includes microscopic disease, and any clinically apparent case will be classified as stage IB. Stage IA is further divided into IA_1 (invasion up to 3 mm deep and 7 mm wide) and IA_2 (invasion between 3 and 5 mm deep and 7 mm wide). Stage IB is divided into IB_1 (lesions no greater than 4 cm in diameter) and IB_2 (lesions greater than 4 cm in diameter) (62).

A parallel TNM staging system has been proposed by the AJCC. The current criteria for the various stages are defined in Table 22.2 (66). All histologic types are included. When there is disagreement regarding the staging, the less advanced stage should be used. Most U.S. gynecologic and radiation oncologists report results using the FIGO classification.

The FIGO staging system is based on clinical evaluation (inspection, palpation, colposcopy); roentgenographic examination of the chest, kidneys, and skeleton; and endocervical curettage and biopsies. Lymphangiograms, arteriograms, CT findings, MRI, laparoscopy or laparotomy findings, and radiographically-directed biopsies are not to be used for clinical staging. Suspected invasion of the bladder or the rectum should be confirmed by biopsy. Bullous edema of the bladder and swelling of the mucosa of the rectum are not accepted as definitive criteria for staging.

For a lesion to be classified as stage IIIB, the tumor should definitely extend to the lateral pelvic wall, although fixation is not required. Patients with hydronephrosis or nonfunction of the kidney ascribed to extension of the tumor are classified as stage IIIB, regardless of the pelvic findings.

Surgical Staging Procedures

Van Nagell and co-workers (67) were among the first to quantitate the discrepancies between clinical, surgical, and pathologic findings. The GOG prospectively evaluated 290 patients with carcinoma of the cervix. Para-aortic node metastases were found in 19 of 58 patients (32.8%) with clinical stage IIB disease, and in 19 of 61 (31.1%) with stage IIIB disease (15).

A number of studies have compared the significance of para-aortic nodal metastases to other clinical and surgical findings with regard to progression-free survival and overall survival (31,68,69). In a multivariate analysis of 626 patients treated on GOG randomized studies, the relative risk associated with positive para-aortic nodes was 11.0 for modeling of time to recurrence and 6.2 for modeling of survival time. In addition to the significant increase in risk of relapse, patients with para-aortic nodal metastasis are more likely to have extrapelvic failure (33). It has not been demonstrated that surgical staging or metastatic periaortic node irradiation increases the probability of survival in these patients (32, 70).

Goff and associates evaluated the impact of surgical staging in 86 of 98 patients who were treated between 1993 and 1997 (71). They confirmed previous studies' conclusions that surgical staging was more sensitive than CT, and that patients with macroscopic nodal involvement fared poorly. They believed that concurrent chemoradiation improved outcomes. Their study design precluded a conclusion that surgical staging itself would improve survival overall. The value of debulking of nodes was addressed by Kupets and co-workers (72). In their model, the incremental overall benefit, by stage, was quite small.

TABLE 22.2. *Definition of TNM*

The definitions of the T categories correspond to the stages accepted by the Federation Internationale de Gynécologie et d'Obstetrique (FIGO). Both systems are included for comparison.

Primary tumor (T)

TNM categories	FIGO stages	Description
TX		Primary tumor cannot be assessed
T0		No evidence of primary tumor
Tis	0	Carcinoma *in situ*
T1	1	Cervical carcinoma confined to uterus (extension to corpus should be disregarded)
*T1a	IA	Invasive carcinoma diagnosed only by microscopy. Stromal invasion with a maximum depth of 5.0 mm measured from the base of the epithelium and a horizontal spread of 7.0 mm or less. Vascular space involvement, venous or lymphatic, does not affect classification
T1a1	IA1	Measured stromal invasion 3.0 mm or less in depth and 7.0 mm or less in horizontal spread
T1a2	IA2	Measured stromal invasion more than 3.0 mm and not more than 5.0 mm with a horizontal spread 7.0 mm or less
T1b	IB	Clinically visible lesion confined to the cervix or microscopic lesion greater than T1a/IA2
T1b1	IB1	Clinically visible lesion 4.0 cm or less in greatest dimension
T1b2	IB2	Clinically visible lesion more than 4.0 cm in greatest dimension
T2	II	Cervical carcinoma invades beyond uterus but not to pelvic wall or to lower third of vagina
T2a	IIA	Tumor without parametrial invasion
T2b	IIB	Tumor with parametrial invasion
T3	III	Tumor extends to pelvic wall and/or involves lower third of vagina, and/or causes hydronephrosis or nonfunctioning kidney
T3a	IIIA	Tumor involves lower third of vagina, no extension to pelvic wall
T3b	IIIB	Tumor extends to pelvic wall and/or causes hydronephrosis or nonfunctioning kidney
T4	IVA	Tumor invades mucosa of bladder or rectum, and/or extends beyond true pelvis (bullous edema is not sufficient to classify a tumor as T4)

Regional Lymph Nodes (N)

NX		Regional lymph nodes cannot be assessed
N0		No regional lymph node metastasis
N1		Regional lymph node metastasis

Distant Metastasis (M)

MX		Distant metastasis cannot be assessed
M0		No distant metastasis
M1	IVB	Distant metastasis

* All macroscopically visible lesions—even with superficial invasion—are T1b/IB.

American Joint Committee on Cancer (AJCC). Cervix Uteri. In: Greene FL, Page DL, Fleming ID, et al., eds. *AJCC Cancer Staging Manual*, 6th ed. New York: Springer, 2002:260.

PATHOLOGY

Squamous-Cell Carcinoma

Squamous carcinoma of the cervix includes both microinvasive squamous carcinoma and more deeply invasive carcinoma. Variants of invasive squamous carcinoma, which may be associated with differences in biologic behavior, include verrucous carcinoma, papillary squamous and transitional carcinoma, warty carcinoma, and lymphoepithelioma-like carcinoma.

Preinvasive Disease

Squamous carcinoma *in situ* is a precursor lesion of invasive squamous carcinoma. Squamous carcinoma *in situ* is characterized by full-thickness atypia of the cervical epithelium. Endocervical glands may also be involved. The normal maturation of squamous epithelium is absent. The epithelium is replaced by atypical cells that often have enlarged, oval nuclei, and increased nuclear to cytoplasmic ratios. Mitotic figures are present. There is no breach of the underlying basement membrane (Fig. 22.1).

Microinvasive Carcinoma

The Society of Gynecologic Oncologists (SGO) and FIGO have defined microinvasive carcinoma of the cervix differently. The SGO definition includes tumors that invade less than 3 mm below the base of the epithelium and have no lymphovascular space invasion. The FIGO definition does

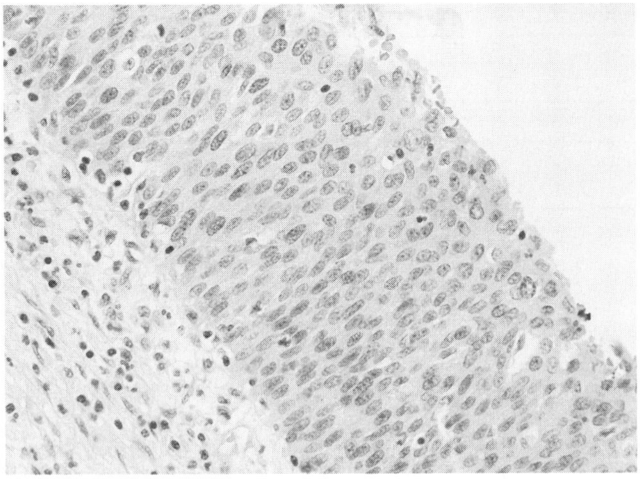

FIG. 22.1. Squamous-cell carcinoma *in situ*. The epithelium displays full thickness atypia. Cells have enlarged, hyperchromatic nuclei, and there is no evidence of maturation.

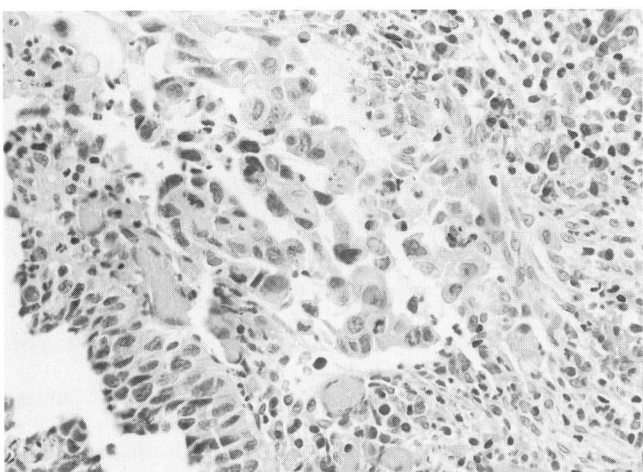

FIG. 22.2. Microinvasive squamous-cell carcinoma. There is an area of squamous carcinoma *in situ* (lower left). A nest of invasive carcinoma cells (center) has broken through the basement membrane. The invasive cells are larger, with more abundant cytoplasm and larger, more pleomorphic nuclei. A desmoplastic stroma response is present (right).

not include evaluation of lymphovascular space invasion. It divides microinvasive carcinoma into stage $1A_1$ (depth of invasion less than 3 mm, and horizontal dimension less than 7 mm) and stage $1A_2$ (depth of invasion more than 3 mm but less than 5 mm, and horizontal dimension less than 7 mm).

Microinvasive squamous carcinoma is associated with squamous intraepithelial neoplasia, and may arise from either the surface epithelium or from endocervical glands involved by dysplasia. It is characterized by small nests of cells that have escaped the basement membrane of the surface or glandular epithelium. Microinvasive carcinoma often displays cells that are larger, with more abundant eosinophilic cytoplasm than cells in the adjacent dysplasia (Fig. 22.2). A desmoplastic stromal reaction is usually present. The nests of microinvasive tumor are irregular and haphazardly arranged. These features are useful in distinguishing microinvasion from rounded, well-circumscribed endocervical glands involved by squamous dysplasia.

Depth of invasion should be measured from the basement membrane of the site of origin. If the tumor arises from surface epithelium, depth is the distance from the basement membrane of the surface epithelium to the deepest nest of invasive neoplasm. If the tumor arises from an endocervical gland, depth is measured from the basement membrane of the gland. If the site of origin is not clear, depth is measured from the basement membrane of the surface epithelium.

Nests of superficial invasion seen in small biopsies should be reported as such, with dimensions of the tumor. A diagnosis of microinvasive squamous carcinoma of the cervix requires a LEEP or conization biopsy that encompasses the entire lesion and has negative margins.

Invasive Squamous-Cell Carcinoma

Invasive cervical carcinoma arises from high-grade dysplasia, which may be detected up to 10 years before invasive

carcinoma develops (1). Untreated squamous carcinoma *in situ* results in invasive carcinoma in about 34% of cases over a period of 10 years (73). Invasive carcinoma occurs most often after the age of 40 years (12), although it may be seen in young women. It is associated with human papillomavirus infection; a recent study estimated a 99.7% incidence of HPV in cervical carcinomas (74). Risk factors for development of cervical squamous carcinoma are the same as those for sexually transmitted diseases, including lower socioeconomic groups, heterosexual activity beginning early in life, many pregnancies, and multiple sexual partners (75).

Most invasive squamous carcinomas of the uterine cervix arise at the transformation zone. They may extend into the ectocervix or endocervix. These tumors may consist of firm, indurated masses, or they may be ulcerated or polypoid. Microscopic examination reveals irregular, haphazardly infiltrating nests of cells with eosinophilic cytoplasm and enlarged, atypical, hyperchromatic nuclei (Fig. 22.3).

Mitoses may be numerous, and atypical forms may be present. There is typically a desmoplastic stromal response around the nests of invasive neoplasm. Lymphatic and vascular space invasion may be present, especially in more deeply invasive tumors. Invasive squamous carcinomas are classified as keratinizing or nonkeratinizing, although this classification has no prognostic significance. Keratinizing squamous carcinomas display at least some keratin pearl formation. Nonkeratinizing squamous carcinomas are composed of irregular nests of cells that may display abundant eosinophilic cytoplasm and intercellular bridges but do not contain keratin pearls. Some squamous carcinomas are composed of smaller cells without evidence of neuroendocrine differentiation; these neoplasms should be classified as nonkeratinizing squamous carcinomas.

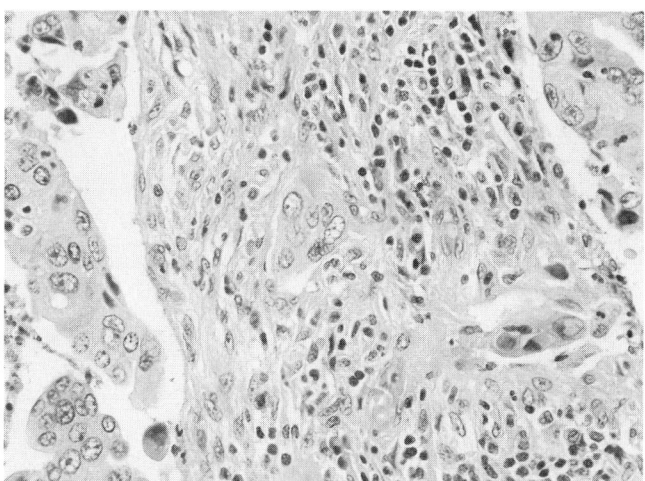

FIG. 22.3. Invasive squamous-cell carcinoma. Small, irregular nests of cells with markedly atypical nuclei are present. They are surrounded by desmoplastic stroma containing inflammatory cells.

Invasive squamous carcinomas are also graded (76–78), although treatment protocols do not depend on grade, and the histologic grade may not correlate with prognosis. Grade 1 (well-differentiated) tumors are not very common in the cervix. They display keratin pearls and large numbers of keratinized cells. Nuclei display only mild to moderate atypia, and mitoses are typically not numerous. Grade 2 (moderately differentiated) tumors represent the majority of invasive squamous carcinomas of the uterine cervix, and are usually nonkeratinizing squamous carcinomas with nuclear pleomorphism, numerous mitoses, and an infiltrative pattern. Grade 3 (poorly differentiated) tumors either have smaller cells without neuroendocrine differentiation, or are pleomorphic with anaplastic nuclei and sometimes a tendency to form spindle cells that must be distinguished from sarcoma by positive cytokeratin stains.

Variants of Squamous-Cell Carcinoma

Verrucous Carcinoma

Verrucous carcinoma occurs rarely in the uterine cervix (79–81). Examination of the cervix reveals a papillary excrescence that may resemble condyloma acuminatum. In fact, lesions termed ''giant condyloma of Buschke and Lowenstein'' in the past probably represent verrucous carcinomas. Microscopic examination displays papillary fronds of squamous epithelium not containing connective tissue cores. The fronds are often pointed and have a ''church spire'' appearance. Underlying connective tissue displays bulbous nests of squamous epithelium that invade the stroma with a pushing margin but display little cytologic atypia. Any lesion displaying significantly atypical nuclei does not represent verrucous carcinoma. The distinction between verrucous

carcinoma and regular squamous carcinoma is important because verrucous carcinoma invades locally but does not metastasize. In order to diagnose verrucous carcinoma, it is necessary to see the invasive portion of the neoplasm. Superficial biopsies are usually not diagnostic.

Papillary Squamous and Transitional Carcinoma

Some cervical neoplasms are characterized by papillary superficial architecture with substantial nuclear atypia not seen in verrucous carcinomas (82–85). The most common presenting symptoms are vaginal bleeding and abnormal Pap smears. Papillary, polypoid, or granular lesions are often evident upon examination of the cervix.

These tumors may have thin or thick papillae that contain a connective tissue core (Fig. 22.4). The papillary processes may be covered by highly atypical epithelium displaying keratinization, or the epithelium may consist of multiple layers of cells with oval, hyperchromatic nuclei that do not show keratinization, and resemble transitional cell epithelium. Nuclear grooves may be present. Some tumors display epithelium with mixed features. Immunohistochemical studies have shown that most of these tumors are cytokeratin 7–positive and cytokeratin 20–negative; these results are consistent with squamous differentiation (84). Human papillomavirus type 16 has been identified in these neoplasms (82).

Many papillary squamous and transitional carcinomas are associated with an underlying invasive carcinoma. The invasive neoplasm is often typical squamous carcinoma, but some cases of invasive transitional carcinoma have been described. Superficial biopsies display only the papillary portion of the neoplasm. LEEP or conization biopsy should be performed to evaluate the possibility of underlying invasive carcinoma.

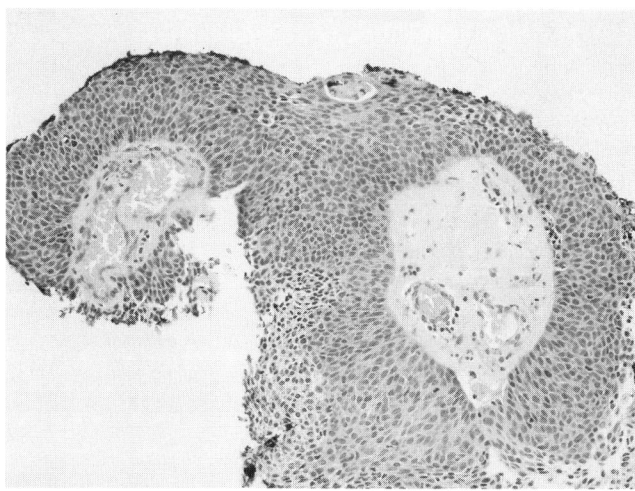

FIG. 22.4. Papillary squamous-cell carcinoma. Papillary fronds of tumor contain connective tissue cores, and are covered with multiple layers of atypical epithelial cells.

These neoplasms appear to behave in the same manner as similarly staged routine squamous carcinoma of the cervix, although they may be associated with late recurrences or metastases. They must be distinguished from verrucous carcinomas, which display little atypia and have a much more indolent clinical course.

Warty Carcinoma

Warty carcinoma of the cervix is a rare papillary neoplasm that displays marked condylomatous change, but has features typical of routine invasive squamous carcinoma at its deep margin (86,87). These tumors are associated with human papillomavirus (88), and may behave less aggressively than the usual type of invasive squamous carcinoma.

Lymphoepithelioma-like Carcinoma

Lymphoepithelioma-like carcinoma, more commonly seen in the nasopharynx, also occurs in the uterine cervix. Some patients may present with abnormal bleeding and have cervical masses, whereas others may have abnormal Pap smears and no visible cervical lesions (89). Lymphoepithelioma-like carcinoma of the cervix is seen most often in Asian women, and it has been associated with Epstein-Barr virus infection in those patients (90). In contrast, studies from Europe have not demonstrated Epstein-Barr virus DNA (91, 92), but some have suggested a role for human papillomavirus in the etiology of this neoplasm (92,93).

Microscopically, this tumor is characterized by nests of cells with lightly eosinophilic cytoplasm and large vesicular nuclei with prominent eosinophilic nucleoli. Cell borders are indistinct, giving the tumor cell nests a syncytial appearance. Aggregates of tumor cells are surrounded by a prominent inflammatory infiltrate that includes lymphocytes, plasma cells, and varying numbers of eosinophils. This neoplasm can be distinguished from glassy cell carcinoma (which is also accompanied by prominent inflammation) by the lack of prominent cell borders and granular eosinophilic cytoplasm in lymphoepithelioma-like carcinoma. A recent study demonstrated the predominant T-cell nature of the lymphocytic infiltrate in lymphoepithelioma-like carcinoma of the uterine cervix; most of the T cells were suppressor/cytotoxic CD8 cells (91).

Adenocarcinoma

While the incidence of squamous carcinoma of the cervix has decreased in the past decades owing to cytologic screening, the number of cases of cervical adenocarcinoma has increased (94–97). A 29% increase in the incidence between the 1970s and the 1990s has been reported (98). Adenocarcinoma of various types accounts for 20% to 25% of cervical carcinomas (95).

Adenocarcinoma *in situ* is a precursor of invasive adeno-

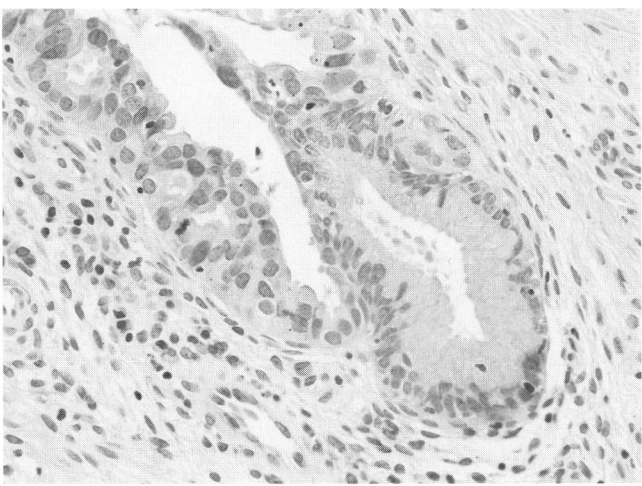

FIG. 22.5. Adenocarcinoma *in situ*. Part of this endocervical gland is normal (upper left corner). The remainder of the gland has been replaced by stratified cells with atypical, large nuclei and mitotic figures.

carcinoma. It is found adjacent to many invasive adenocarcinomas, often accompanied by squamous dysplasia. Both adenocarcinoma *in situ* and invasive adenocarcinoma of the cervix are associated with human papillomavirus (usually type 18, but sometimes type 16).

Adenocarcinoma *in situ* is characterized by preservation of the overall endocervical gland architecture. However, endocervical glands and surface epithelium are replaced to varying degrees by cells displaying atypia, including nuclear enlargement and stratification, nuclear hyperchromasia, and mitotic figures (Fig. 22.5). Most adenocarcinomas *in situ* occur near the transformation zone, and skip lesions are unusual (96).

Early Invasive Adenocarcinoma

Early invasive adenocarcinoma of the uterine cervix displays an alteration from the normal endocervical gland architecture. This abnormality may take the form of solid or cribriform nests of cells, architecturally irregular or incomplete glands lined by malignant cells, or small buds of highly atypical cells arising from glands involved by adenocarcinoma *in situ*. A desmoplastic stroma may be present.

Technically, the definitions of microinvasive carcinoma, according to both SGO and FIGO, apply to all types of carcinoma. Application of this term to glandular lesions of the cervix has not been generally accepted. Some gynecologic pathologists believe that these lesions should be classified as early invasive adenocarcinoma, with a best possible measurement of the depth of invasion (94,96), because an increased incidence of metastatic disease correlates with increasing depth of invasive disease. One author has suggested that depth of invasion should be measured from the luminal surface to the deepest invasive tumor nest so that, as in malignant melanomas, tumor thickness rather than depth of invasion is measured (96).

Mucinous Adenocarcinoma

There are several variants of mucinous adenocarcinoma of the cervix, including endocervical, intestinal, signet-ring cell, minimal deviation, and villoglandular variants.

Mucinous Adenocarcinoma, Endocervical Variant

The endocervical variant of mucinous adenocarcinoma is the most common type of cervical adenocarcinoma. It is composed of irregular, haphazardly arranged tubuloracemose glands lined by cells resembling those seen in normal endocervical glands, although they may sometimes have limited amounts of cytoplasmic mucin. Nuclei are basally located, stratified, and atypical (Fig. 22.6). Mitoses are present. Grade 1 (well-differentiated) tumors have uniform nuclei with minimal stratification and few mitotic figures. Grade 2 (moderately differentiated) adenocarcinomas have more marked cytologic atypia with frequent mitoses. They may also have solid areas accounting for less than half of the neoplasm. Grade 3 (poorly differentiated) adenocarcinomas contain more prominent solid areas, pleomorphic nuclei, and many mitoses. Desmoplastic stromal response is variable in this type of cervical adenocarcinoma.

Mucinous Adenocarcinoma, Intestinal-type, Signet-ring and Colloid Variants

Rare endocervical adenocarcinomas have glands containing goblet cells; these tumors display intestinal differentiation (99). Signet-ring cell carcinomas and colloid carcinomas

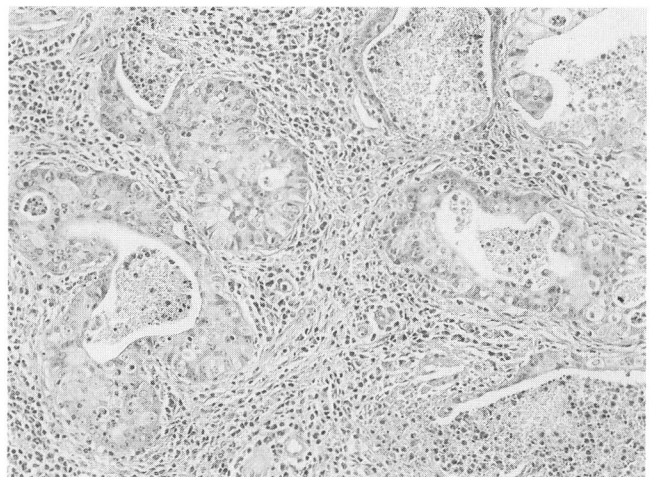

FIG. 22.6. Invasive adenocarcinoma. There is a haphazard invasion of the cervix by irregular glands lined by multiple layers of atypical cells.

are extremely rare (100,101), and must be distinguished from metastatic tumors from the gastrointestinal tract.

Mucinous Adenocarcinoma, Minimal Deviation Variant (Adenoma Malignum)

The term *adenoma malignum* was originally proposed by McKelvey and Goodlin (102) to describe a form of cervical adenocarcinoma that is so well-differentiated that it may be difficult to recognize as a malignant lesion. The term *minimal deviation adenocarcinoma* (103) is a more appropriate designation for this lesion. There is also a tendency for benign lesions of the uterine cervix to be overdiagnosed as minimal deviation adenocarcinoma (104), further emphasizing the difficulty of diagnosing this neoplasm.

This tumor is uncommon, and represents only about 1.3% of cervical adenocarcinomas (105,106). Patients range in age from 25 to 72 years (107). They may present with abnormal bleeding or a mucoid discharge. The cervix may appear normal, or it may display a firm area or a mass. The neoplasm is very difficult to diagnose on small biopsies because the infiltrative gland pattern cannot be appreciated. Conization specimens are more conducive to accurate diagnosis in this lesion, but some cases have been diagnosed only after hysterectomy.

Gross examination of hysterectomy specimens displays firm, tan-yellow neoplasms. Most cases contain mucinous glands, but some display endometrioid glands (108). Microscopically, glands infiltrate the cervical stroma in a haphazard manner; they do not conform to the normal endocervical gland pattern. They may display budding contours, and they typically have angular, sharply pointed outlines, in contrast to the rounded contours of benign endocervical glands. The glands of minimal deviation adenocarcinoma appear deceptively benign on low power. Lack of substantial cytologic atypia is a prerequisite for this diagnosis. However, high-power examination reveals at least some areas with mild to moderate atypia, in which some nuclear enlargement, stratification, and rare mitotic figures may be identified (Fig. 22.7). The infiltrating glands may be devoid of any surrounding desmoplastic reaction. Some authors (104,107) have described the utility of positive cytoplasmic staining for carcinoembryonic antigen (CEA) in these neoplasms after the possibility of squamous metaplasia has been excluded.

Minimal deviation adenocarcinoma may occur as a sporadic neoplasm, although patients with Peutz-Jeghers syndrome are at risk of developing this cervical tumor (107), along with ovarian mucinous neoplasms.

Mucinous Adenocarcinoma, Well-differentiated Villoglandular Variant

Well-differentiated villoglandular adenocarcinoma is a type of low-grade adenocarcinoma that displays similarities to villous adenomas of the intestine (109). Patients may pre-

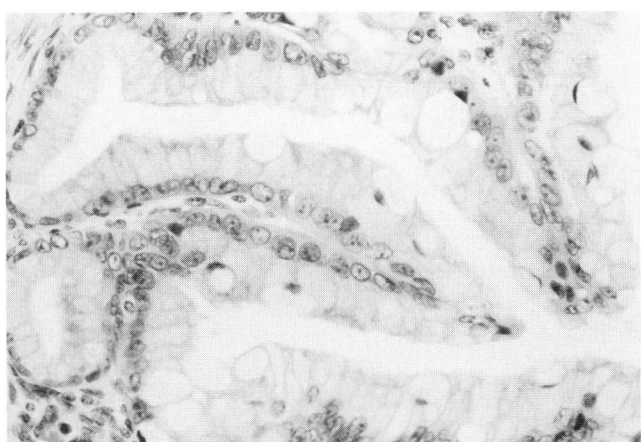

FIG. 22.7. Minimal deviation adenocarcinoma. This gland has some very bland cytologic features (left side), but enlarged, atypical nuclei are evident in other areas.

sent with polypoid or papillary endocervical masses upon pelvic examination, abnormal bleeding, or abnormal Pap smears. The age range has been 23 to 57 years, with most cases occurring in patients younger than 40 years of age (110–112).

Microscopic examination of these neoplasms reveals villous, papillary structures that may be either long and slender, or short and broad. These processes contain a connective tissue core that often displays inflammatory cells. The covering epithelium is a single layer of stratified cells with endocervical, endometrial, or intestinal differentiation. Nuclei display only mild to moderate atypia, and mitotic figures are infrequent (Fig. 22.8). Only tumors with low-grade cytologic atypia should receive this diagnosis, since other endocervical carcinomas may have papillary features (9). Invasive adeno-

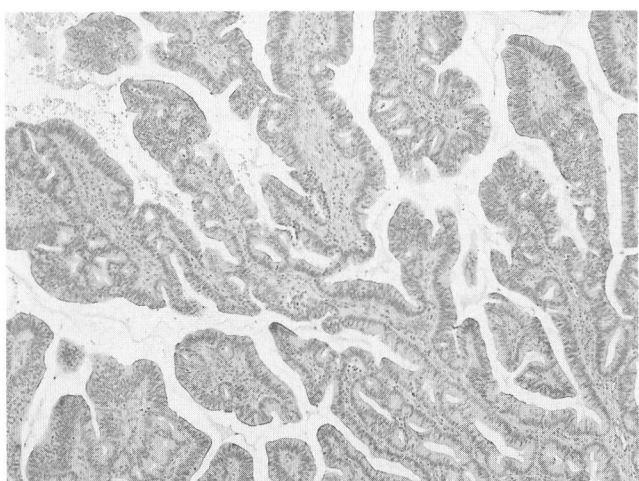

FIG. 22.8. Well-differentiated villoglandular adenocarcinoma. Long, slender villous processes are covered with epithelium displaying mild atypia. Nuclei are crowded, but they retain an oval shape and are uniform in size.

carcinoma may be seen deep to the papillary areas, and is characterized by branching glands lined by atypical cells and surrounded by desmoplastic stroma. These neoplasms do not display the marked nuclear atypia and epithelial tufting seen in the much more aggressive papillary serous carcinoma of the cervix. They may be associated with typical adenocarcinoma *in situ* of the cervix.

Some authors have found an association between well-differentiated villoglandular adenocarcinoma of the cervix and oral contraceptive use (111). More recently, these tumors have been shown to contain high-risk types of human papillomavirus (types 16 and 18) (112). Neither oncogene amplification nor tumor suppressor gene loss was identified (112).

Well-differentiated villoglandular carcinoma has not metastasized unless it was associated with more aggressive types of carcinoma. A few cases have recurred (112). Some cases have been successfully treated by conization if the tumor is completely excised and the patient wishes to retain fertility. Generally, this diagnosis should only be suggested on the basis of small biopsy specimens; definitive diagnosis should be made only in tumors seen on conization or hysterectomy specimens. Diagnosis of this type of neoplasm on the basis of only a small biopsy specimen could result in undertreatment of a potentially more aggressive neoplasm (95).

Endometrioid Adenocarcinoma

Endometrioid carcinomas of the uterine cervix are rare, and have probably been overdiagnosed (77); these tumors make up about 7% of all cervical adenocarcinomas (95,113). These neoplasms display histologic features identical to endometrial carcinoma. Therefore, the possibility of a primary endometrial adenocarcinoma with endocervical extension or drop metastasis must be excluded before the diagnosis of a primary endocervical endometrioid adenocarcinoma is established. A rare case has arisen from endocervical endometriosis (114).

Other Adenocarcinomas

Clear-Cell Adenocarcinoma

Clear-cell carcinoma of the cervix has been associated with intrauterine diethylstilbestrol (DES) exposure; however, it also occurs in the absence of DES exposure. Patients usually have a cervical mass. Microscopically, the tumor has three patterns that may occur individually, or as an admixture (115). The solid pattern of tumor displays sheets of cells containing abundant glycogen-rich clear cytoplasm, atypical nuclei, and mitoses. The tubulocystic pattern contains tubules and cystic spaces lined by oxyphilic, hobnail, or clear cells. The papillary pattern is the least common variant and often coexists with solid or tubulocystic areas.

Serous Adenocarcinoma

Papillary serous carcinoma of the uterine cervix (116,117) has a bimodal age distribution, occurring in patients younger than 40 years and patients older than 65 years. This age distribution has also been seen in well-differentiated villo-glandular carcinoma, but differs from the typical mid-life age of patients with cervical adenocarcinomas in general.

Gross examination may reveal a nodular mass, an indurated cervix, or no visible abnormality. Microscopically, these tumors are identical to serous tumors of the ovary, endometrium, and primary peritoneal serous carcinomas. Considering the rarity with which this type of neoplasm is seen in the cervix, the diagnosis of primary serous carcinoma of the uterine cervix should be made only after excluding metastasis or extension of disease from another site, especially the endometrium.

Histologic examination of serous carcinoma of the uterine cervix reveals fibrous papillae lined by atypical epithelial cells; secondary papillae and tufts of neoplastic epithelial cells are often present (Fig. 22.9). Glandular structures have irregular luminal borders due to tufting of tumor cells. Nuclei usually show high-grade atypia, and numerous mitoses are present.

These are aggressive tumors (117,118) that may metastasize to pelvic, periaortic, and inguinal lymph nodes. Larger tumors (>2 cm diameter) and tumors invading more than 10 mm are associated with a worse prognosis.

Mesonephric Adenocarcinoma

Remnants of the mesonephric ducts persist and can be seen in the lateral aspects of the cervix. They are often not identified because uteri are traditionally bivalved along their lateral aspects, and most microscopic sections are taken from

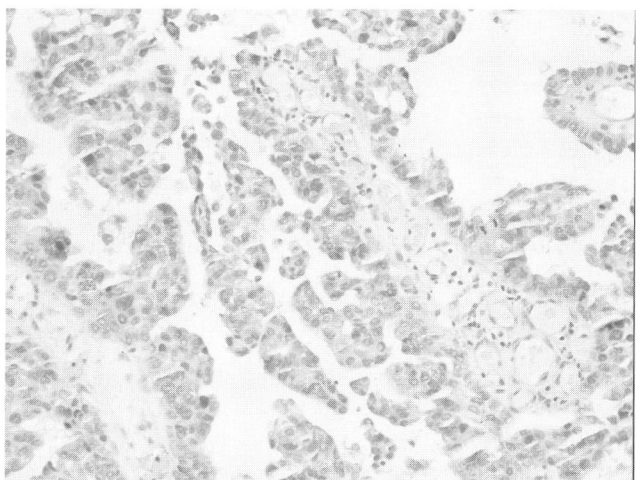

FIG. 22.9. Papillary serous adenocarcinoma. The papillary structures have a connective tissue core. There is marked tufting and stratification, and the nuclei are markedly atypical.

the anterior and posterior portions of the cervix. Mesonephric duct remnants are seen as lobules of small, round, glandular structures lined by flattened cuboidal epithelium and containing intraluminal PAS-positive material. The cells of mesonephric duct remnants do not contain intracytoplasmic mucin, unlike the cells lining endocervical glands. Mesonephric duct hyperplasia may occur in the cervix. Mesonephric adenocarcinomas are thought to arise from mesonephric duct remnants. Only about two dozen cases have been documented (119–121). Early reports of lesions termed mesonephric carcinoma are now known to represent clear cell carcinoma, with no relationship to the mesonephric duct remnants.

Patients have ranged in age from 52 to 55 years (106). Some patients have not had grossly apparent lesions, but most present with abnormal bleeding and have visible cervical masses. These neoplasms occur deep in the lateral cervical wall. Microscopically, most mesonephric carcinomas are adenocarcinomas (119,121), although some with a concomitant spindle cell component have been termed "malignant mesonephric mixed tumors" (120). Mesonephric carcinomas display a variety of histologic appearances, including ductal, tubular, retiform, solid, and sex cord–like patterns (120). Mesonephric hyperplasia may be associated with the carcinoma (119). Like mesonephric remnants, mesonephric carcinoma tumor cells contain no intracytoplasmic mucin; however glandular structures may display luminal PAS-positive material.

Microcystic Endocervical Adenocarcinomas

This type of endocervical adenocarcinoma was recently described (122). Eight cases have been seen; most patients presented with either abnormal Pap smears or vaginal bleeding. Abnormalities of the endocervix were visible in 3 patients. These tumors are characterized by numerous cystically dilated glands simulating the appearance of a benign lesion at low power. However, higher power examination reveals areas of significant cytologic atypia and mitotic activity. Areas of more typical mucinous or intestinal endocervical adenocarcinoma may also be present. These lesions may be deeply invasive. Only three patients have had significant follow-up data. One patient died after a debulking procedure for a pelvic recurrence two years after her initial diagnosis, and two other patients are alive without evidence of tumor at 1 and 6.5 years after diagnosis.

Other Epithelial Tumors

Adenosquamous Carcinoma

Adenosquamous carcinoma is a tumor composed of admixed malignant glandular and squamous elements. This term should not be used for poorly differentiated squamous carcinomas, in which mucicarmine stains show scattered mucin vacuoles. Likewise, it is different from collision tumors, which display adjacent adenocarcinoma and squamous carcinoma.

Glassy Cell Carcinoma

Glassy cell carcinoma is a form of poorly differentiated adenosquamous carcinoma that displays cells with eosinophilic cytoplasm, well-defined cell borders, prominent nucleoli, and a prominent infiltrate of eosinophils and plasma cells. This is a very rare tumor. Occasionally, this morphology may be seen in recurrences of adenocarcinomas or adenosquamous carcinomas that have been treated with radiation therapy (RT) (95).

Adenoid Cystic Carcinoma

Adenoid cystic carcinoma of the cervix is a rare but aggressive malignant neoplasm. The largest study of these tumors reported 14 cases (123). These lesions are typically seen in elderly patients, many of whom present with postmenopausal bleeding. Examination of the cervix typically shows a lesion.

Microscopic examination of these tumors reveals a cribriform gland pattern. The glands may contain hyaline or mucinous material. Nuclei are larger and more pleomorphic than those seen in adenoid basal epithelioma, and numerous mitoses as well as areas of necrosis are present in adenoid cystic carcinoma. Electron microscopy has shown basement membrane–like material around the nests of tumor cells as well as in some gland lumina (123). The tumor cells stain with cytokeratin. In contrast to adenoid cystic carcinoma of the salivary glands, this neoplasm in the cervix has not displayed unequivocal evidence of myoepithelial cells, either by immunohistochemical staining for S100 protein or by electron microscopy.

Adenoid cystic carcinoma of the cervix often recurs, and may metastasize. In the largest series reported, the only patients who were free of tumor at last followup had stage IB tumor. No patient with higher stage disease was alive and well (123).

Adenoid Basal Epithelioma (Carcinoma)

Adenoid basal epithelioma is a rare cervical neoplasm. It was originally called adenoid basal carcinoma. However, given its indolent clinical course, the term adenoid basal epithelioma is more appropriate.

The age of patients with adenoid basal epithelioma ranges from 30 to 91 years (106,124). This neoplasm is often seen in postmenopausal women who are asymptomatic, with normal-appearing cervices (123). These lesions are usually incidental findings in specimens obtained for the purpose of evaluating squamous intraepithelial neoplasia. A neoplastic squamous component is often an associated feature (106).

Microscopically, adenoid basal epithelioma is characterized by nests of cells that have a basaloid appearance, and may display peripheral palisading. Some gland lumina are present in the basaloid cell nests, although the number of glands is variable. Squamous metaplasia may also be seen. Mitotic figures are typically rare.

Adenoid basal epithelioma, in the absence of a coexisting invasive carcinoma, is a benign lesion with no reported cases of metastatic behavior (106). It must be distinguished from adenoid cystic carcinoma, which is an aggressive malignant neoplasm.

Neuroendocrine Tumors

A recent workshop sponsored by the College of American Pathologists and The National Cancer Institute (125) proposed standard terminology for neuroendocrine tumors of the uterine cervix. The previous lack of uniform nomenclature and diagnostic criteria for these neoplasms made it difficult to study their incidence and biologic behavior. Immunohistochemical or electron microscopic evidence of neuroendocrine differentiation is necessary for diagnosis of all neuroendocrine tumors except small-cell carcinoma. Chromogranin or synaptophysin stains are recommended for documentation of neuroendocrine differentiation. Chromogranin works best when cells contain numerous neuroendocrine granules; synaptophysin stains cells with fewer granules. Neuron-specific enolase is nonspecific by itself, but may be useful in conjunction with one of the other stains. Many cases of small-cell carcinoma will also stain for these markers. Neuroendocrine granules can also be seen by electron microscopy if fresh tumor tissue is available.

Carcinoid Tumors

Typical Carcinoid Tumors

Typical carcinoids of the cervix are rare neoplasms. This diagnosis should be made with caution, because most cervical neuroendocrine tumors are aggressive neoplasms. They display organoid architecture without nuclear atypia, mitotic figures, or necrosis. Immunohistochemical stains for chromogranin and synaptophysin demonstrate neuroendocrine differentiation. There are not enough documented cases of this neoplasm to permit assessment of biologic behavior.

Atypical Carcinoid Tumors

Atypical carcinoid tumors also display organoid nests of cells, but the cells display nuclear atypia and a mitotic rate of 5–10 MF/10 HPF. Necrosis may be present. These tumors are also rare, precluding evaluation of biologic behavior. However, they may metastasize. Immunohistochemical evidence of neuroendocrine differentiation is required for diagnosis (126).

Large-Cell Neuroendocrine Carcinoma

Large-cell neuroendocrine carcinomas (Fig. 22.10) display organoid nests of cells with peripheral palisading of nuclei, prominent nucleoli, variable amounts of necrosis, eosinophilic cytoplasmic granules and numerous mitotic figures (> 10 MF/10 HPF). Vascular/lymphatic space involvement is often seen, and many are associated with co-existing adenocarcinoma *in situ* or adenocarcinoma of the cervix (127). These tumors are highly aggressive neoplasms (127). Evidence of neuroendocrine differentiation is necessary for diagnosis and is most easily obtained with immunohistochemical stains for chromogranin and synaptophysin.

Small-Cell Carcinoma

Most neuroendocrine tumors seen in the uterine cervix represent small-cell carcinomas. Small-cell carcinoma is characterized by cells with scant cytoplasm, inconspicuous nuclei with finely stippled chromatin, nuclear molding, extensive necrosis, crush artifact, and numerous mitotic figures (Fig. 22.11). Single-cell infiltration of the stroma is common. Vascular/lymphatic space invasion is often seen (128,129). These tumors have morphology identical to that seen in small-cell carcinoma of the lung. They are aneuploid tumors (130) that show a strong association with type 18 HPV (126, 131) Immunohistochemical stains for neuroendocrine markers such as chromogranin and synaptophysin may be helpful in the diagnosis (132).

Mixed Epithelial and Mesenchymal Tumors

Mullerian adenosarcomas occur in the cervix (133,134). Patients range in age from 13 to 67 years, with a mean age of

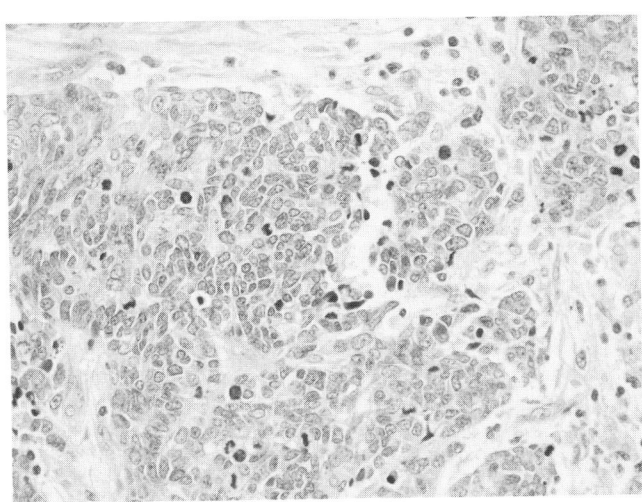

FIG. 22.11. Small-cell neuroendocrine carcinoma. This tumor displays cells that are smaller than those of squamous carcinoma. Nuclei are large and atypical with molding of adjacent nuclei. There is a very high mitotic rate.

37 years. They may present with abnormal bleeding. These neoplasms consist of polypoid or papillary masses. Microscopically, they display benign glands and sarcomatous stroma with a periglandular cuff of condensed stroma. The sarcomatous component contains variable numbers of mitotic figures and some cases display heterologous elements including cartilage and striated muscle. These tumors generally have a favorable prognosis, but deep invasion and sarcomatous overgrowth are adverse prognostic factors (133, 134).

Malignant mixed müllerian tumors may involve the cervix, although only about 30 cases have been reported (135). Patients have ranged in age from 23 to 87 years; the mean age is 65 years. Patients have presented with abnormal bleeding or an abnormal Pap smear, and all have had cervical masses (116). Various types of carcinoma can be seen in these tumors, including squamous carcinoma, basaloid carcinoma, adenocarcinoma, or adenoid cystic carcinoma (135, 136). The sarcomatous component may be homologous or heterologous. Some have suggested that malignant mixed müllerian tumors arising in the cervix have a better prognosis than those arising in the uterine corpus (135).

Other Malignant Tumors

Various sarcomas have been reported in the uterine cervix, although they are uncommon. They include leiomyosarcoma and endometrial stromal sarcoma. Primary cervical malignant melanoma is rare (137). Eleven cases of granulocytic sarcoma involving the uterine cervix were reported in 1997. Some represented the initial disease presentation, and others were identified during the course of acute myeloid leukemia (138). Primary extranodal lymphoma (139) and primitive neuroectodermal tumors (140,141) have been reported in the

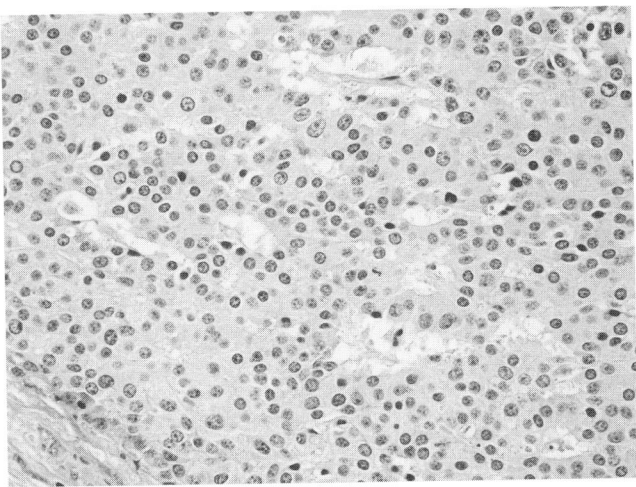

FIG. 22.10. Large-cell neuroendocrine carcinoma. This tumor displays organoid architecture. The tumor cells are much larger than those seen in small-cell carcinoma. They have abundant eosinophilic cytoplasm, and there are numerous mitotic figures. Areas of necrosis were present elsewhere in the tumor.

cervix. Primary germ-cell tumors of the cervix have also been described (99).

Secondary tumors of the cervix include those invading from contiguous organs and metastases from other sites (99). The former include tumors arising in the uterine corpus, urinary bladder, or rectum. Metastases can originate from many sites, including the ovary, uterus, and more distant primary tumors.

PROGNOSTIC FACTORS

Age, Race, and Socioeconomic Status

In older reports, carcinoma of the cervix has the same prognosis in younger and older patients (142,143). Others have observed decreased survival in women younger than 35 or 40 years, who have a greater frequency of poorly differentiated tumors (31,144). Two European studies have shown improved outcome for younger patients (145,146). This contradiction may be explained by Rutledge et al (147), who showed an interaction between age and stage in the relative hazard plots for 250 patients less than 35 years of age and those for matched controls.

Several investigators have observed a correlation between race or socioeconomic characteristics of patients and incidence of cervical cancer and outcome of therapy (148,149). African-American patients tend to have more exposure to risk factors, have more advanced disease at diagnosis, and are less likely to undergo curative therapy.

General Health

Jenkin and Stryker (150) observed a higher incidence of pelvic recurrences and complications in patients with hypertension. Kapp and others (151) found that neutrophil count, uterine position, and history of diabetes also contributed to poorer outcome. Patients who are HIV positive and who have either carcinoma *in situ* or invasive cervical cancer appear to be at very high risk (152–154).

Hypoxia and Anemia

The idea that decreased serum hemoglobin concentration worsens outcomes in patients with cervical cancer treated with RT has been around for decades. Possibly, this concept can be traced to a study done at the Norwegian Radium Hospital, in which 2 separate eras of treatment were compared. During the World War II years (1940 to 1945), anemic patients were unlikely to be transfused, in contrast with patients treated in a later era (1956 to 1958) (155). Patients with stages II and III disease treated in the later period had better outcomes when adjusted for stage. The authors recognized that there were potential confounding variables, such as tumor size, treatment improvements, etc. A subsequent randomized trial of transfusion by Bush et al. seemed to

support this conclusion (156). Recently, the results of the trial by Bush have been reconsidered, and a number of weaknesses and study biases were disclosed. In fact, using the modern statistical concept of intention-to-treat analysis, there is no overall difference in death from disease related to blood transfusion (157).

Fyles' et al. published an excellent review of the basic, translational, and clinical data regarding anemia and its potential impact on radiosensitivity and radiocurability (157). Clearly, the interactions are much more complex than previously believed. For example, in the presence of anemia, adaptive mechanisms come into play that shift the oxyhemoglobin dissociation curve to the right, providing a compensatory increase in oxygen released into the tissues. There is also an increase in tissue perfusion and oxygenation as hemoglobin decreases due to reduced blood viscosity. However, these effects are potentially less effective in patients with diabetes, smokers, or patients who are vasoconstricting in the presence of marginal cardiac output.

Furthermore, Fyles' work shows that the relationship between pre-treatment hemoglobin levels and direct measurements of oxygen tension in cervical cancers is tenuous (Fig. 22.12). Interestingly, there was a positive correlation between hemoglobin and tumor oxygenation in nonsmokers, but the correlation was negative in smokers. Dewhirst has also pointed out the complicated and unpredictable nature of the relationship between serum hemoglobin and tumor oxygen status (158).

Stehman et al. analyzed GOG patients with advanced disease, finding that nodal involvement and performance status were independent risk factors for survival and relapse, while hemoglobin was not (31). Nodal and distant metastases could be increased in anemic patients and patients with hy-

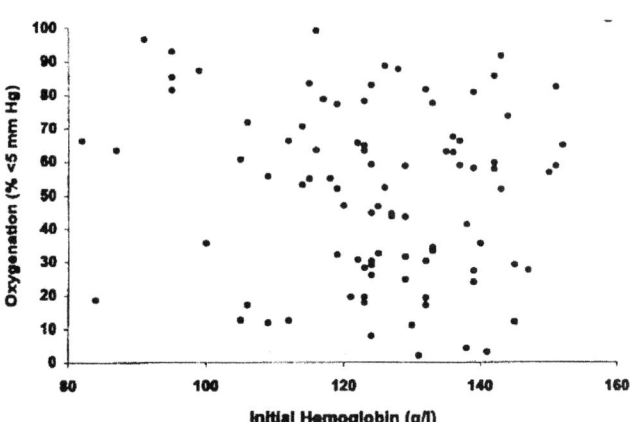

FIG. 22.12. The relationship between pretreatment hemoglobin level and the proportion of pO$_2$ values at <5 mm Hg (the hypoxic proportion, HP5). The graph shows HP5 (%) as a function of hemoglobin in 69 patients with cervical cancer. (From Fyles AW, Milosevic M, Pintilie M, et al. Anemia, hypoxia, and transfusion in patients with cervix cancer: a review. *Radiother Oncol* 2000;57:15.)

poxic tumors. Evidence for this also exists (159,160). Dehdashti et al. demonstrated the feasibility of using PET scanning to assess for tumor hypoxia, and also found that locoregional nodal metastases were increased in hypoxic tumors (161). Fyles et al. found a significant negative prognostic impact of tumor hypoxia only in node-negative patients. This was manifested by an increased risk of distant metastases rather than poorer pelvic tumor control (160).

A more important question therapeutically is whether correction of the anemia will improve oxygenation status and treatment outcomes. Human data from Sundfor show that only 50% of transfused patients will show an increase in tumor oxygenation (162). Similar data have been presented by Fyles et al. (157). Furthermore, the significant association between tumor hypoxia and tumor size suggests that improving oxygen delivery is unlikely to improve outcomes owing to factors unrelated to oxygenation, such as number of clonogens, suboptimal brachytherapy dose distributions, and greater risk of metastatic disease. Grogan et al. analyzed 475 patients treated with definitive RT $\pm$ chemotherapy at several institutions in Canada (163). It was found that presenting hemoglobin of <120 g/L vs. $\geq$12 g/L was significant prognostically, but only upon univariate analysis. In a multivariate analysis, only average weekly hemoglobin nadir was correlated with outcome. In 25 patients who had transfusion in order to raise hemoglobin levels, survival was similar to that in the 228 patients who remained at a level above 12 g/L without transfusion, and was significantly better than in the remaining patients, whose hemoglobin either remained low or fell during treatment.

It is tempting for clinicians to believe that anemia is related to inferior outcomes, since this is a situation that is potentially remediable. Whether correcting the anemia will impact tumor oxygenation and improve outcomes is less clear. Santin et al. have shown detrimental effects of blood transfusion on immune function in patients undergoing RT for cervical cancer (164). Additional clinical data raise the possibility that transfusion itself can lead to inferior outcomes, at least in patients who undergo surgery as primary therapy (165). Given the conflicting nature of the data, additional clinical research is necessary.

Tumor Size/Volume

Gauthier and associates (166) described a correlation between metastatic lymph nodes and tumors with deep stromal invasion. Furthermore, such patients had a lower 2-year relapse-free survival and a greater incidence of recurrence than patients with smaller tumors. Likewise, Inoue (167) observed a close correlation between the incidence of parametrial extension and pelvic nodal metastases according to the depth of stromal invasion in stages IB through IIB carcinoma of the cervix. Survival rates were significantly reduced when tumors invaded deeper than 2 cm (91.6% to 73.8%, p <0.001) and 3 cm (89.6% to 58.3%, p <0.001).

Delgado and coworkers (177) described 3-year disease-free survival rates of 94.8%, 88.1%, and 67.6%, respectively, for occult, $\geq$3 cm, and >3 cm stage I squamous cell carcinomas of the cervix treated by radical operation. Survival strongly correlated with depth of tumor invasion of the stroma: 86% to 94% for less than 10 mm, 71% to 75% for 11 to 20 mm, and 60% for 21 mm or greater. In patients without parametrial involvement, the survival rate was 84.9%, but it was 69.6% for those with parametrial tumor extension.

Several investigators have described a greater incidence of lymphatic and distant metastases in patients with bulky stages IB and IIA tumors treated by radical hysterectomy (28,167,168) This correlated with decreased 5-year actuarial survival. Volume of disease is more difficult to assess clinically in locally advanced disease (stages IIB and above). Yet, in patients with stage IIB disease, Kovalic and associates (169) observed no difference in 10-year disease-free survival between those with unilateral (61%) or bilateral (64%) parametrial extension. The collective GOG review indicates that tumor diameter is a more powerful prognosticator than bilaterality (31).

Van Nagell and colleagues (170) found that the recurrence rate after radical hysterectomy or irradiation for stage IB disease was 5% for tumors less than 2 cm in diameter treated with either modality, and they recommended radical surgery for these patients. However, in lesions 2 to 5 cm in diameter, the failure rate was 24% with surgery, but only 11% with irradiation.

In a retrospective analysis of 1178 patients, Perez and associates (171) reported pelvic failure rates of 6% (small post-conization lesions), 7.7% (<3 cm), 16% (>3 cm) in stage IB patients, and 10%, 12%, and 23% to 28% in stage IIA, respectively (Fig. 22.13). Stage IIB bulky primary tumors showed an 11% increase in the pelvic failure rate. Stage IIB pelvic failures were more frequent when disease extended into the lateral parametrium (25%), compared with that extending into the medial parametrium only (17%) (p = 0.01). Bilateral parametrial disease increased the pelvic failure rate in stage IIIB (48% versus 28%, p >0.01), but not in stage IIB disease (21%) (p = 0.83). Five-year disease-free survival for patients with IB tumors larger than 3 cm was 67%, versus 90% for those with tumors smaller than 3 cm (p = 0.01). In stage IIA, the rates were 70% and 40%, respectively. Stages IIB and IIIB central bulky disease (>5 cm in diameter) had decreased disease-free survival. Patients with stage IIB with lateral-half parametrial involvement had lower 5-year disease-free survival (58%) than those with medial involvement (70%) (p = 0.004).

Eifel and coworkers (172), in a review of 1526 patients with stage IB squamous-cell carcinoma of the uterine cervix treated with RT alone, also noted a strong correlation between central and pelvic tumor control, disease-specific survival, and tumor size. Pelvic tumor control was 97% with tumors less than 5 cm, and 84% with tumors 5 to 7.9 cm.

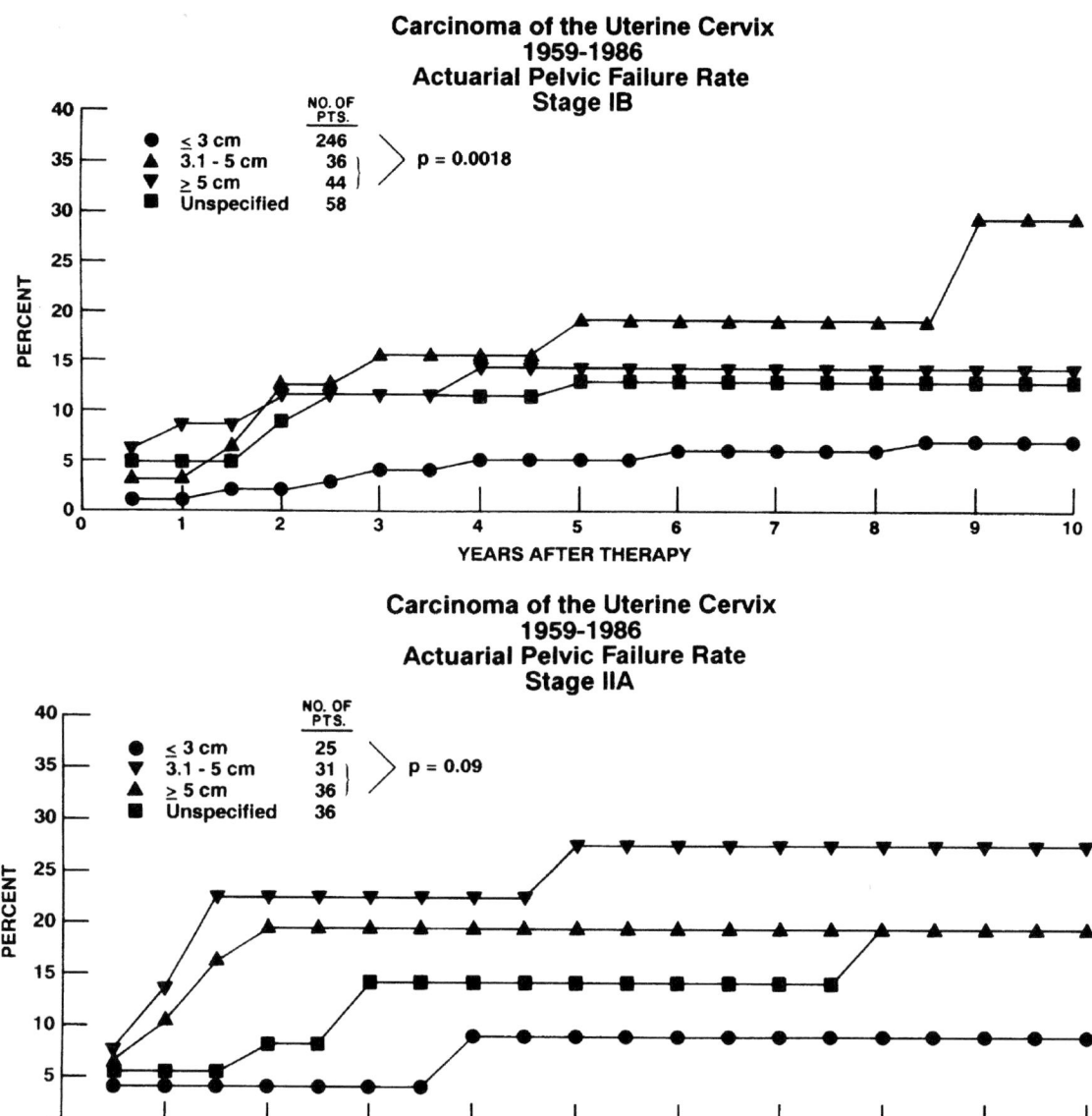

FIG. 22.13. Carcinoma of the uterine cervix (1959—1986): actuarial pelvic failure rate. **A:** Stage IB. **B:** Stage IIA. (From Stehman FB, Perez CA, Kurman RJ, et al. Uterine cervix. In: Hoskins WJ, Perez CA, Young RC, et al., eds. *Principles and Practice of Radiation Oncology*, 3rd ed. Philadelphia: Lippincott-Raven, 2000:890.)

In a multivariate analysis of prognostic factors related to nodal or distant metastases in 128 patients, Pitson and colleagues found that tumor size and tumor hypoxia were both independently predictive, whereas stage and hemoglobin concentration were not (173).

Tumor Stage

Fyles and associates (174), in 965 patients with invasive carcinoma of the cervix, identified FIGO stage as the most significant prognostic factor, followed by dose of irradiation to point A, and overall time of RT. When the analysis was limited to patients treated with doses of 75 Gy or more, irradiation dose was no longer a significant factor. The 10-year survival rate was 62% in 743 patients receiving doses of 85 Gy or higher to point A, in contrast to 53% for 222 patients receiving lower doses.

Stehman, reporting for the GOG on 626 patients treated on Phase III trials (31), confirmed the prognostic significance of tumor burden, whether measured by FIGO stage, centimeter size, or bilateral disease. All of these patients had been surgically staged. Para-aortic node metastases conferred a much greater risk than any of the measures of volume of tumor, however. This serves to emphasize the fact that FIGO staging does not take into account important prognostic information, such as nodal status. While some clinicians would place patients with known para-aortic nodal disease in the stage IV category, others would choose to stage according to approved clinical staging procedures, mainly pelvic examination. Furthermore, stage is only indirectly related to tumor volume, since there can be significant variability in this important prognostic factor within a given stage, resulting in substantial overlap within stage groupings.

Nodal Status

Lymph node involvement is, in most studies, the most significant negative prognostic factor. Reports emphasize higher 5-year survival rates (90% or higher) among surgically treated patients with no evidence of metastasis in the regional nodes, compared to patients with positive pelvic (50% to 60%) or para-aortic nodes (20% to 45%) (175,176). Delgado and co-workers (177) reported a 3-year disease-free survival of 85.6% for 545 patients with negative pelvic lymph nodes, compared with 74.4% for patients with one or more positive nodes. Decreasing 5-year survival rates have been associated with increasing numbers of positive pelvic nodes: 62% for one node, 36% for two, 20% for three or four, and no survivors for five or more (175).

Tinga et al. reported the survival rate to be 87% in 19 patients with a single node involved vs. 53% in 15 patients with multiple nodal involvement (p <0.02) (176). Extranodal infiltration was also an adverse prognostic factor.

Alvarez et al. conducted a retrospective study of 185 surgically treated patients with stages IB-IIA cervical cancer, 103 of whom received adjuvant pelvic RT (178). In multivariate analysis, only patient age, tumor size, and number of nodal metastases were significant factors in relation to overall survival and recurrence rate. The location of the nodal metastases and unilateral vs. bilateral metastases were not found to be significant factors in this analysis, although numbers were very small. Based on these data, the authors concluded that patients with primary tumor size <1 cm and no more than 2 pelvic lymph nodes were at a sufficiently low risk of recurrence following radical hysterectomy and pelvic lymphadenectomy, and that adjuvant RT is probably unnecessary.

Lymphovascular Space Invasion

Lymphovascular space invasion (LVSI) proved to be a significant prognostic factor in a surgical-pathologic study of 542 patients completed by the GOG (177). Disease-free survivals were 77% and 89%, respectively, in patients with and without LVSI. Furthermore, LVSI was shown to correlate strongly with pelvic adenopathy. Roman et al. have shown that quantitative assessment of the degree of LVSI

is possible, and this also correlates with risk of pelvic lymph node involvement by metastatic tumor (179).

Biomarkers

Multiple biomarkers with potential prognostic value have been evaluated in cervical cancer, often with conflicting results and conclusions (180). For example, measures of tumor proliferation parameters (e.g., potential doubling time, S phase fraction, labeling indices), apoptosis, and other cellular characteristics often correlate with clinical outcomes (181–183). What is less clear is how to use this information in a way that improves therapy in the individual patient.

Gaffney et al. performed immunohistochemical staining for epidermal growth factor receptor (EGFR), vascular endothelial growth factor (VEGF), topoisomerase-II alpha (TOPO-II), and cyclooxygenase-2 (COX-2) on specimens from 55 patients, and evaluated potential correlations between expression and outcome (184). On multivariate analysis, increased staining for VEGF and COX-2 correlated with an increased risk of death. Although the limitations of such analyses and the conflicting results in the literature are well recognized, such translational research has the potential to suggest additional therapeutic avenues for exploration.

Histopathologic Features

Microinvasive Squamous Carcinoma

In microinvasive squamous-cell carcinoma, factors that have been reported to increase an individual's risk for nodal metastases, recurrence, and death are: (1) depth of stromal invasion; (2) presence of lymphovascular space involvement; (3) tumor volume; and (4) status of the resection margin.

The lack of a uniform definition and methodology for measuring the depth of invasion together with variation in length of follow-up and treatment methods make interpretation of the published data difficult. Nonetheless, there is a consensus that depth of stromal invasion is the major factor in determining the outcome of patients with microinvasive carcinoma. The development of recurrent disease or death in patients with tumors invading less than 1 mm is extremely rare. In long-term follow-up studies involving 403 women, no patient with less than 1 mm of stromal invasion treated with a cone biopsy or simple hysterectomy died of her tumor (64,185). Recurrent disease occurs in approximately 1% of patients with tumors invading less than 3 mm, whereas recurrence occurs in approximately 5% of patients when there is 3.1 to 5 mm of invasion (186–190).

Confluence of neoplastic epithelium is not associated with pelvic metastases, vaginal recurrence, or cancer death. Lymph vascular space involvement is reported to occur in 0% to 8% of tumors invading less than 1 mm, and in 9% to

29% of tumors invading 1 to 3 mm. The clinical significance, however, of lymphovascular space involvement is controversial. Some studies have reported no direct relationship between the presence of lymphovascular involvement and lymph node metastases, whereas others have found it to be an adverse prognostic factor (185,189,190).

Although some authors have reported no pelvic node metastases in patients with tumors measuring up to 420 mm, this method of measuring volume is cumbersome and time-consuming (191). Other investigators have used lateral extent of spread as a surrogate for measuring tumor volume. This has been correlated with the frequency of residual neoplasia in postcone hysterectomy specimens (190).

The status of the cone margin is probably the most valuable single parameter in deciding the therapeutic approach to patients with early invasive squamous carcinoma. In most studies, women with cone margins positive for either squamous intraepithelial lesion or invasive disease are much more likely to have residual invasive disease in the hysterectomy specimen than are women with negative margins.

Histopathology

It is not clear whether there is a difference in survival between invasive squamous and invasive adenocarcinoma of the cervix. One study reported lower survival for stage II adenocarcinoma, but not for other stages (98), whereas other studies have not confirmed any survival difference for these two types of tumors (192–194).

A recent study of 505 patients with non–squamous-cell carcinoma of the cervix examined histologic features for prognostic significance (195). Stage was a strong prognostic factor; five-year survival for patients with FIGO stage I disease was 76%, compared with less than 50% for higher stage disease. No patients with tumor thickness less than 5 mm and horizontal tumor dimension less than 7 mm had lymph node metastases. In patients with FIGO stage I non–squamous carcinoma of the cervix, the presence of lymph node metastases, vascular invasion, and extension to the uterine corpus are independent negative prognostic factors (195). In comparison with tumor limited to the cervix, tumor extension to the uterine corpus was correlated with twice the risk of dying of tumor. The grade and specific type of adenocarcinoma were not of prognostic significance in this study, although well-differentiated villoglandular adenocarcinoma and minimal deviation adenocarcinoma were not evaluated. There is no prognostic significance in the distinction between mucinous and endometrioid adenocarcinoma of the cervix.

The presence of small-cell neuroendocrine carcinoma in any amount, even when associated with other types of neoplasm, is an independent prognostic factor associated with aggressive tumor behavior.

Human Papillomavirus

Human papillomavirus is strongly associated with cervical cancer. The association is independent of other risk factors (1). Types 6 and 11 cause condylomata acuminata (Fig. 22.14). Some HPVs are associated with both high-grade cervical dysplasia and invasive carcinoma of the cervix. These "high-risk" HPV types include HPV 16, 18, 31, 33, 35, 39, 45, 52, 54, 56, 58, 59, 66 and 68 (1,79,196). HPV types 16 and 18 account for over 70% of cervical cancers. A large study completed in 1999 found an incidence of HPV in cervical cancers of 99.7% (74).

HPV invades the basal cells of the cervical epithelium, usually at the transformation zone. High-risk viral types usually integrate their DNA into the host genome. HPV viral oncogenes E6 and E7 inhibit the action of tumor suppressor genes p53 and the retinoblastoma gene. This activity prevents repair of DNA damage and programmed cell death, enabling proliferation of damaged cells and resultant tumorigenesis.

HPV cannot be cultured by conventional techniques. Molecular methods are necessary for detection. There is one FDA-approved commercial system available; it detects high-

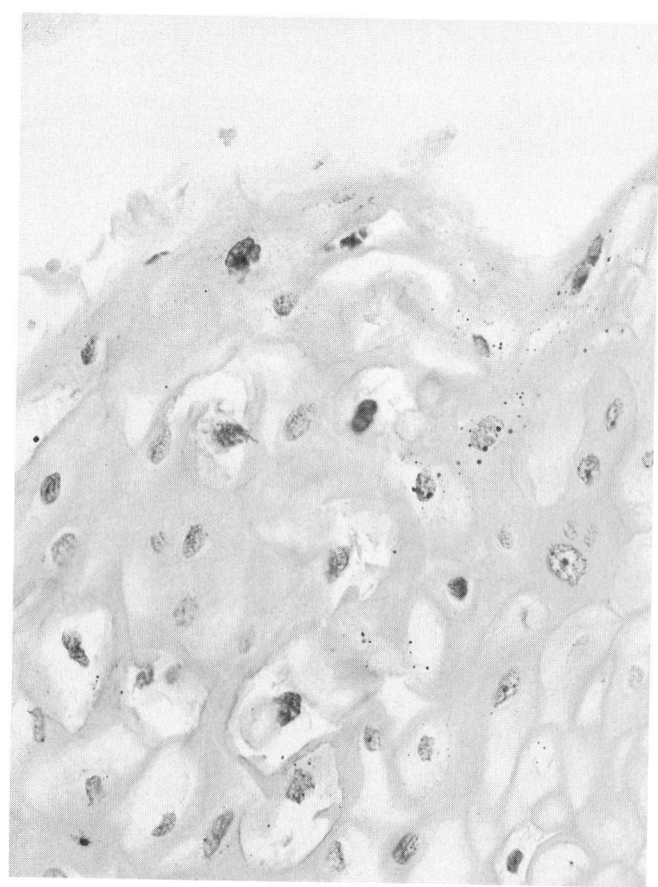

FIG. 22.14. Human papillomavirus changes. This squamous epithelium displays cells with large halos surrounding atypical nuclei (so-called koilocytotic atypia).

risk HPV types using a nucleic acid amplification technique. It is more sensitive, but less specific, than Pap smears for detection of high-grade dysplasia.

The presence of HPV type 18 appears to correlate with a poor prognosis in squamous carcinoma of the cervix (87). In one study, 45% of tumors associated with HPV type 18 recurred, in contrast to 16% of tumors associated with HPV type 16 (197). Other authors have also shown an increased risk of recurrence in HPV type 18 related tumors (198,199).

Cellular Oncogenes

Over-expression of ras genes is seen in many cervical carcinomas (99,200), and over-expression of the ras gene product p21 is associated with poor prognosis and an increased frequency of lymph node metastases (201,202). Alteration in the c-myc oncogene also occurs in some cervical carcinomas, and is associated with higher stage tumors and poor prognosis (99). After adjusting for age and stage, some authors found a correlation between amplification of *c-myc, c-erbB2,* and *H-ras* codons 12, 13, and 61 with the development of recurrent cervical cancer (203).

GENERAL MANAGEMENT

Carcinoma *In Situ*

Christopherson and co-workers (204) described 124 patients with carcinoma *in situ* (CIS) diagnosed by various forms of biopsy, 117 of whom showed the same lesion on conization. Fourteen patients also had microinvasive carcinoma; three had normal specimens and four showed residual dysplasia.

Patients with CIS are often treated with a total hysterectomy (205). When a patient wishes to have more children, CIS may be treated conservatively with a therapeutic conization (206,207), laser ablation (208), or cryotherapy (209). These various techniques have comparable efficacy. However, the loop excision is quicker and more reliable than laser excision (51,52).

Since patients with CIS have virtually no risk of pelvic adenopathy, it is also appropriate to treat with only intracavitary RT. Tumor control rates of 100% have been reported (205,210,211). Grigsby and Perez successfully treated 21 such patients with a single intracavitary implant, delivering a mean point A dose of 46.12 Gy; no treatment sequelae were observed (210). Others might choose to use 2 separate implants and slightly higher point A doses.

Stage IA

The concept of "microinvasion" (equating to FIGO stage IA) should define tumors that penetrate the basement membrane but have little or no risk of nodal involvement or dissemination. In 1994, the Montreal FIGO Congress defined stage IA_1 as stromal invasion ≤ 3 mm in depth and having horizontal extension no greater than 7 mm. Stage IA_2 was defined as having stromal invasion > 3 mm, but ≤ 5 mm, with horizontal extension ≤ 7 mm. Many clinicians also support the concept that tumors in this category should not exhibit lymphatic or vascular space involvement. All macroscopically visible lesions are considered stage IB tumors. Though there may be anecdotal reports of patients with superficial invasion and positive nodes, patients with ≤ 3 mm of invasion will have nodal involvement in no more than 0% to 4% of cases (189,212).

Use of a strict definition allows an appropriately conservative therapeutic approach. Published series indicate that patients with lesions up to 3 mm in depth may be safely treated with conization or loop excision (213–216). Total hysterectomy is the more commonly accepted therapy. Abdominal, vaginal, and laparoscopic procedures produce excellent results (190).

Microinvasive adenocarcinoma presents a special problem, since there are so few data about the disease and the role of limited therapy. Schorge and co-investigators treated five women with adenocarcinoma, invasive less than 3 mm and no wider than 7 mm, with cold-knife conization (217). All patients were between 26 and 33 years of age. No patient had capillary lymphatic space invasion. There were no recurrences with follow-up of 6 to 20 months.

Greer and associates (218) described histologically positive margins in 66% (33 of 50) of patients with stage IA_2 carcinoma of the cervix on whom a conization was performed. Residual invasive disease at the time of subsequent radical hysterectomy was found in 24% (4 of 17) of patients with negative margins. Two of the 50 patients (2%) had positive pelvic lymph nodes. Takeshima et al. performed lymphadenectomies on 29 patients with stage IA_2 tumors, finding positive nodes in only 1 (3.4%) (212).

Stage IA_2 carcinoma of the cervix is usually treated with a total or modified radical hysterectomy with or without pelvic lymphadenectomy in medically operable patients (186,219).

Patients with microinvasive cervical carcinoma can be treated with intracavitary brachytherapy alone (65 to 75 Gy to point A in one or two insertions) with excellent results. Hamberger reported no regional failure in 41 patients treated with only intracavitary therapy, and morbidity was minimal (220). Grigsby and Perez included 34 stage IA patients in their series, 13 of whom received only intracavitary RT; the remaining 21 also had external RT (210). Only 1 stage IA patient (who received both external RT and brachytherapy) suffered a recurrence. A complication rate of 5.9% was reported in this group, all complications occurring in patients receiving pelvic RT.

Fertility-Sparing Surgery/Radical Trachelectomy

Since 1998 there have been six publications in the English literature, each reporting different single-institution experi-

TABLE 22.3. *Pregnancies and outcomes following radical trachelectomy*

References	Years	Stages	No. of patients	Med. Age	Median follow-up	Recurrences	Deliveries
Burnett (221)	1995–2001	IA–IIA	21	30	32 mo	0	1
Covens (222)	1994–1998	IA–IB	32	31	23 mo	5%	37%
Dargent (225)	1987–1996	IA–IIB	47	not stated	52 mo	2	13
Roy (223)	1991–1998	IA–IIA	30	32	25 mo	one	4
Shepard (226)	1994–1998	Ibi	10	32	not stated	0	3
Schlaerth (224)	1995–1999	I	10		48 mo	0	2
Total			150			5	35

ences with radical vaginal trachelectomy and laparoscopic lymphadenectomy (221–226). Patients were carefully selected for younger age, lower body mass index, smaller tumors (<2 cm), negative nodes, and negative margins. The rate of recurrence appears to be acceptably low with more than two years of follow-up, but the number of patients so treated is still small. Even when the total results are pooled, the upper bound of the confidence interval is too high to make comparative conclusions. There is a risk of a type II error in such an interpretation. In some cases in which a cerclage stitch was used at the completion of the procedure, successful subsequent pregnancies have been reported (Table 22.3). This would appear to be a promising technique, offering selected patients the opportunity for fertility preservation that would not be possible following radical hysterectomy or radiation therapy. The technique has not been widely taught, so it is not widely available. On a positive note, these early reports reflect the learning curve of the reporting institutions, and it is reasonable to assume that results will improve with increased experience.

Stages IB and IIA

Both definitive irradiation and radical operation are accepted treatments for stages IB and IIA carcinoma of the cervix. The preference of one over the other depends on the institution, the oncologists involved, the general condition of the patient, and tumor characteristics. Though generally accomplished via the abdominal route, radical hysterectomy can be performed laparoscopically (227). Surgery has often been preferred in young women because of the desire to preserve ovarian function (228). However, according to some reports, ovarian function preservation has been observed in only 50% to 60% of surgically treated patients not receiving irradiation (229,230). In a report from Anderson and colleagues (229), only four of 24 (17%) patients with ovarian transposition who received postoperative pelvic irradiation had continued ovarian function. In a survey of 124 patients who had undergone radical hysterectomy and lymphadenectomy with ovarian transposition, 68 respondents were premenopausal at time of surgery. Six of 30 women (20%) with ovarian preservation experienced early hormonal failure (five had one ovary, and one patient had both preserved); two other women (6.5%) subsequently re-

quired oophorectomy for benign conditions (231). Follow-up on 102 patients up to 87 months who underwent ovarian transposition was reported by Buckers et al (232). Ovarian function was retained by patients who did not undergo radiation therapy. However, only 41% of patients who received postoperative radiation therapy retained ovarian function for a mean of 43 months. The mean age of menopause for these patients was 36.6 years.

According to some gynecologists, treatment with radical pelvic surgery may alter sexual function to a lesser degree than radiation therapy (233,234). Combined modalities appear to have a more pronounced effect than either radiation or operation alone (235). Radical operation will shorten the functional length of the vagina, but pliability and transudative lubrication are usually preserved. Radiation therapy can reduce length, caliber, and lubrication of the vagina; however, these symptoms can be alleviated in some patients with hormonal replacement and vaginal dilatation. The evidence to differentiate between surgery and radiation based on sexual function is poor. Bergmark and collegues were unable to demonstrate any treatment effect in 256 cervical cancer survivors who responded to a standardized questionnaire (236). The postmenopausal patient who is not sexually active may have complete obliteration of the vagina, precluding follow-up examination.

Results of therapy comparing modalities should include all patients evaluated for each therapeutic modality. This applies particularly to surgical series. Findings revealed at operation may change the treatment plan, excluding some high-risk patients. This is exemplified by a report by Delgado and associates (21) for the GOG. Member institutions entered 1125 patients prior to operation. There were 80 ineligible patients after strict pathology review. An additional 129 patients were explored, but the hysterectomy was abandoned because of intraoperative complications in 49 patients, or because of extent of disease beyond the uterus in 80. Failure to account for these patients in other series overestimates the efficacy of the operative procedure.

Whitney examined these GOG patients in depth and found that those 8.7% of patients who had hysterectomy abandoned had a median recurrence-free survival of 19 months compared to 84 months for the cohort who had completed radical hysterectomy (237). Brewster and co-workers examined the same question using SEER data (238). They found a survival advantage for the surgical intent-to-treat group when the tumor was 4 cm or less in size. However there was no treatment effect when the tumor was >4 cm.

In order to better understand about nodal status intraoperatively, Levenback and associates studied the usefulness of lymphatic mapping to identify positive sentinel nodes at laparotomy (239). A sentinel node was successfully identified in 33 of 39 patients preoperatively, and in all 39 at the time of operation. In four patients, radical hysterectomy was abandoned. There was one patient with a false-negative sentinel node.

There are few comparisons of radical operation and radical irradiation, and it is probable that the two modalities are comparable with respect to survival (240,241). Differences in outcomes are more likely related to patient prognostic variables and statistical adjustments of data than to true differences between the modalities. Newton (240) and Roddick and Greenlaw (241) reported comparable survival and pelvic recurrence rates in patients with stages IB and IIA carcinoma treated with radical hysterectomy or irradiation alone. Morley and Seski (242) described their 31-year experience with 446 patients with stage IB carcinoma of the cervix alternatively assigned to radiation therapy or operation (excluding patients under 35 years of age). The uncorrected and corrected survivals were nearly identical.

A randomized study in Italy (243) showed no significant difference in outcome when patients were treated with irradiation alone, or radical hysterectomy followed by radiotherapy based on pathologic findings. Other series of radical hysterectomy or definitive irradiation for patients with stage IB disease have confirmed cure rates in the range of 85% (244,245).

In an analysis of 98 patients with stages IB-IIB bulky endocervical carcinoma (≥6 cm) treated with irradiation alone (40 Gy to the whole pelvis, followed by two or more intracavitary insertions), Eifel et al. (246) noted that in 25 patients receiving less than 6000 mgh brachytherapy, the 5-year pelvic recurrence rate was 33%, in comparison with 16% for those receiving higher doses ($p = 0.03$). The 5-year actuarial survival rates were 44% and 60%, respectively ($p = 0.14$).

Radical operation has a less than 1% risk of operative mortality; yet, this exceeds the risk of direct mortality from irradiation (244, 247). Patients who are at increased risk of operative mortality because of medical status should receive radiation therapy rather than operation.

Radical hysterectomy can be accomplished via the laparoscopic route (248). Spirtos and associates operated on 78 consecutive patients with stages IA$_2$ and IB cervical cancer, completing the operation laparoscopically in 73. With at least three years of follow-up, there were four documented recurrences.

For most patients, the choice of treatment is made on the basis of comparative morbidity rather than risk of mortality. Younger patients may opt for an attempt at ovarian preservation rather than hormonal replacement. Adverse effects of operation tend to occur during or shortly following therapy. In addition to the risks of anesthesia and operation, radical hysterectomy carries a risk of injury to the urinary tract. Ureteral injury and ureterovaginal or vesicovaginal fistula have been reported to follow as many as 5% to 7% of radical hysterectomies (242). More recent studies have shown that a rate of 1% to 2% can be expected with current techniques (244). These fistulas may close spontaneously with urinary drainage, but some will require reoperation and repair. Urinary diversion or nephrectomy is rarely required. A number of patients will have persistent voiding dysfunction after radical hysterectomy. The degree of dysfunction relates to the extent of the procedure and the degree of denervation of the detrusor muscle (249).

In contrast, some adverse effects of radiation therapy may not occur until many years after treatment (250). Bowel fistulae are more common than urinary fistulae when irradiation is used. Fistulae following irradiation rarely close spontaneously, and frequently require diversion of the fecal stream. Although intestinal fistulae are uncommon, a sizable number of patients will have lesser disturbances of intestinal function. These patients usually respond to dietary restriction or antispasmodic therapy. Van Nagell and colleagues (251–253) identified several factors that predispose radiation therapy patients to intestinal injury, including young age, thin body habitus, smoking, diabetes, hypertension or other vascular disease, and pelvic inflammatory disease.

Node-positive Early-Stage (Operable) Cervical Carcinoma

Approximately 15% of patients with surgically amenable cervical carcinomas (FIGO stages I-IIA) will have positive pelvic nodes. Of these, a percentage less than 50% will have grossly positive nodes recognized intraoperatively. When this occurs, the dilemma becomes whether to proceed with the radical hysterectomy, or to abandon the surgery and opt for curative-intent RT. Whitney and Stehman reviewed the GOG #49 database, and found that, in 98 of 1127 patients with clinical stage IB tumors, the surgeon abandoned the operation. Sixty-eight of these were patients with squamous carcinomas whose surgery was abandoned not owing to medical reasons but rather to tumor extension beyond the uterus, forming the basis of their report (237). Of these, 17 (1.5% of the total group, 25% of the study group) patients had grossly positive pelvic lymph nodes, 12 (1.1% of the total group, 17.6% of the study group) of whom had this finding as the only manifestation of extrauterine disease. Most patients received curative-intent RT when feasible. Patients with positive pelvic nodes did poorly, with 8 of 12 failing, including 3 with distant disease. The median recurrence-free interval was only 10 months, and the median survival was 17 months. The main conclusion from this study was that it is invalid to directly compare results of surgical treatment with results from RT, since surgical series typically exclude the patients with a poor prognosis in whom the operation is abandoned, while these patients would be included in the RT series.

Bremer et al. reported considerably better outcomes in a series of 26 patients in whom the operation was aborted after the intraoperative finding of positive pelvic nodes. Five-year survival was 61% in this patient group (254). Morbidity was limited.

Probably the best data regarding whether to complete the hysterectomy come from Potter et al., who did a matched pair analysis of 30 patients with positive pelvic nodes. Patients undergoing hysterectomy also received pelvic RT (255). There was no survival or local control advantage conferred by completing the radical hysterectomy; however, local control data suggested a trend favoring definitive RT.

In patients with positive pelvic nodes, the use of concurrent chemotherapy would be advised based on the possibility of distant spread and the need to optimize pelvic control. Randomized data support the addition of chemotherapy to postoperative RT in these patients (256) (Fig. 22.15). Based on available data, it is difficult to conclude that completing the hysterectomy adds anything to the outcome. Possible disadvantages include delaying the initiation of RT, adding surgical morbidity, and utilizing two treatment modalities when one (RT) would likely suffice. Furthermore, leaving the uterus in place provides an appropriate conduit for intracavitary RT and probably lessens the risk of complications.

Recent data suggest an advantage for surgically resecting grossly positive lymph nodes prior to RT (257–259), although others have questioned the benefit in the vast majority of patients (72). Clinicians who believe that completing

the radical hysterectomy improves outcome, even with positive nodes, will point to data suggesting that patients who undergo radical hysterectomy, as a group, have a better outcome than the patients in whom the procedure is aborted (237,254). Others will point out that the groups are not prognostically similar and suggest that a reasonable approach is to have the surgeon resect or debulk grossly positive nodes and surgically stage the paraaortics but abort the radical hysterectomy. RT with chemotherapy would then become the primary therapy.

Stage IIIA Carcinoma of the Cervix

Cervical carcinomas extending to the lower third of the vagina without pelvic sidewall extension or hydronephrosis are uncommon, representing less than 2% of patients with cervical cancer. As a result, these patients are often not reported separately, although management presents a significant challenge to the radiation oncologist. In general, these patients have a better prognosis than stage IIIB patients, especially when there is limited parametrial extension, and the vaginal involvement is continuous with the cervix (260).

Cardinale et al. (261) reported 17 patients, 12 (71%) of whom obtained local control with RT. Five-year disease-free survival was 58%. Kavadi and Eifel (260) found a similar local control rate of 72% in 44 patients, but 5- and 10-year actuarial survival rates were 37% and 34%, respectively, reflecting the impact of distant failure seen in 13 patients. In this series, patients with no parametrial extension and direct extension from the cervix (as opposed to "skip" lesions in the lower vagina) had a 5-year survival of 73%.

The inguinal lymph node areas must be assessed clinically and radiographically. When this assessment is negative, RT is given to the inguinofemoral nodes prophylactically, typically necessitating an anteroposterior/posteroanterior (AP-PA) approach. When the lymph node assessment suggests gross disease, it might be appropriate to confirm this with needle biopsy or consider the role of inguinal lymph node dissection following RT. Alternatively, RT doses can be escalated to reflect the presence of gross tumor.

Treating the inguinal nodes adequately while limiting the dose to the underlying femoral heads is a significant challenge. An important first step is understanding the location of the inguinal nodes. This is best accomplished by measuring the depth of the femoral vessels by a cross-sectional imaging technique. As Koh et al. have shown, the depth of these nodes averages 6 cm, and can vary substantially and be beyond the range of typical electron energies (262). Dittmer and Randall have reported a simple photon-only technique that provides good coverage of inguinal nodes at depth, minimizes "hot" and "cold" spots, and respects the tolerance of the femoral heads in most cases (263) (Fig. 22.16). More difficult is the challenge of delivering tumoricidal doses of radiation to the entire vagina while respecting tolerances of the normal tissues, in particular the rectum.

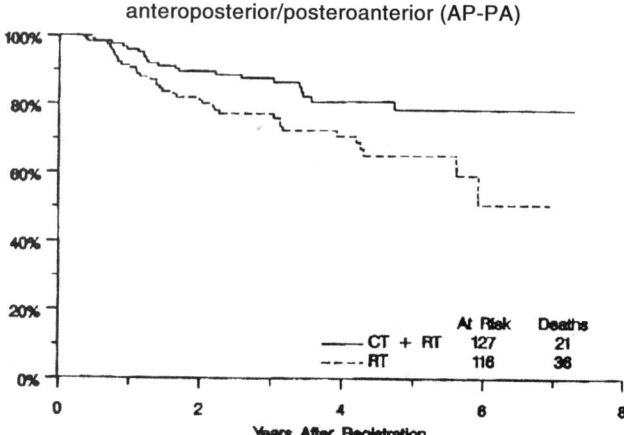

FIG. 22.15. Overall survival for 127 patients randomized to receive CT + RT and for 116 patients randomized to receive RT alone after radical surgery. (From Peters WA III, Liu PY, Rolland JB, et al. Concurrent chemotherapy and pelvic radiation therapy compared with pelvic radiation therapy alone as adjuvant therapy after radical surgery in high-risk early-stage cancer of the cervix. *J Clin Oncol* 2000;18:1609.)

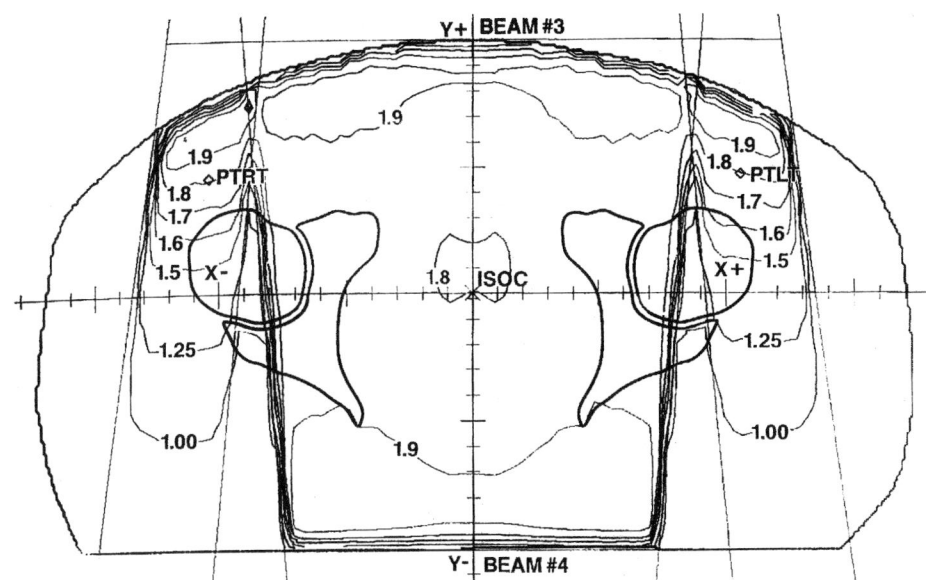

FIG. 22.16. Isodoses calculated for composite plan including posterior, anterior, and two anterior inguinal boost fields. A dose of 1.8 Gy is delivered at isocenter (ISOC), and to points PTRT (calculation point on the right) and PTLT (calculation point on the left), which are the estimated locations of the right and left inguinal nodes. Note reduced dose delivered to femoral head. (From Dittmer PH, Randall ME. A technique for inguinal node boost using photon fields defined by asymmetric collimator jaws. *Radiother Oncol* 2001;59:63.)

Given that virtually the entire length of rectum will be treated with an intracavitary approach, which encompasses the entire vagina, the tolerance will be lessened, and the risk of complications will increase. In addition, because of the typical "slope," or decrease, in patient thickness in the superior-inferior direction, there will be a dose gradient that can result in "hot" spots of 120% to 125%. This is potentially remediable with intensity-modulation techniques, although another approach is simply to measure the dose gradient and take it into account by raising the lower border accordingly, and/or taking the gradient into account during the brachytherapy portion of the treatment.

A general approach is to give external beam RT to the pelvis and entire vagina of approximately 40 to 44 Gy over 5 weeks (delivering 50 Gy to the inguinal areas at depth), and follow this with 1 or 2 intracavitary implants. An intrauterine tandem combined with Delclos rings permits delivery of a controlled, measurable dose to the vagina. One should aim for a total dose of approximately 65 Gy to the entire vagina, combining the external and intracavitary doses. One can consider a second implant that does not treat the entire vagina, typically with a Fletcher-Suit applicator, particularly when there is parametrial extension. Ideally, one will deliver 80 to 85 Gy to point A in this fashion, but if the maximum rectal dose is limited to 60 to 65 Gy some compromise in point-A dose may be required.

It is probably appropriate to administer cisplatin-based chemotherapy with the external RT, based on randomized studies that included these patients, with the hope of improving survival (264–266). However, concurrent chemotherapy will likely increase acute toxicities, particularly given the increased volume encompassed by the RT port, the use of the AP-PA technique, and the sensitivity of the vulva, generally, to RT. Furthermore, the randomized studies included very few stage IIIA patients, so dogmatism is to be avoided.

There is not a single "right" way to treat these patients. Considerable individualization of therapy is required, preferably directed by an experienced gynecologic radiation oncologist.

Stages IIB, IIIB, and IVA

Most patients with stages IIB and III tumors are best treated with concurrent chemoradiation, or in some cases, with irradiation alone. Patients with stage IVA disease (bladder or rectal invasion) can be treated either with irradiation or with pelvic exenteration. Unless a fistula is already present, exenteration is usually not necessary. Small fistulae will sometimes close during fractionated radiation therapy. Million and colleagues (267) saw 128 patients with bladder invasion, and selected 53 for definitive treatment. Five patients were treated with anterior exenteration alone, six with this operation combined with irradiation, and 42 with irradiation alone. Urinary diversion was done before treatment in nine patients because of vesicovaginal fistula and/or obstructive ureteropathy. Sixteen of the 53 patients (30%) survived 5 years. Only two vesicovaginal fistulas developed during treatment among the remaining patients. No patient experienced a new fistula after therapy.

Kramer and colleagues (268) reported that 9 of 48 patients (18%) with stage IVA disease survived 5 years after irradiation alone.

Special Considerations

Adenocarcinoma of the Cervix

Adenocarcinomas of the cervix can exist in the form of *in situ* or microinvasive disease, with clinical characteristics similar to equivalent stages of squamous carcinoma, except that it is more difficult to diagnose adenocarcinoma *in situ* (AIS) on screening cytology (269,270). This is possibly because these lesions typically arise in the transformation zone, where it is more difficult to obtain cells using traditional sampling methods. Similarities between AIS and microinvasive adenocarcinoma and their squamous counterparts include a significant amount of time before progression to invasive disease (in the case of AIS) (271), and the appropriateness of more conservative therapies than radical hysterectomy (in the case of microinvasive disease) (269). However, with regard to this latter point, it has been pointed out by Hirai et al. that it can be difficult to preoperatively evaluate the amount of tumor spread in cervical adenocarcinomas (272).

There have been several reports of similar survival rates for comparable stages of adenocarcinoma and squamous cell carcinoma. Look et al, for the GOG, found no additional risk associated with adenocarcinoma compared to squamous carcinoma among stage IB patients (273). When other risk factors are considered, including clinical stage, volume of disease, dose of irradiation, and presence of lymph node metastasis, no difference in tumor control or survival has been observed in adenocarcinomas when compared with epidermoid carcinoma (31,274–278). In contrast, data are conflicting regarding the prognosis of more advanced adenocarcinomas of the cervix compared to squamous carcinomas. Grigsby and colleagues (274) observed comparable 5-year disease-free survival rates (all stages combined) for 925 patients with squamous carcinoma and for 79 patients with adenocarcinoma treated with irradiation alone. The size of the primary lesion and dose of irradiation were significant variables for recurrence in the pelvis. Significant factors for distant metastatic disease were size of the primary lesion and metastatic lymph nodes at the time of diagnosis.

Similar observations were reported by Eifel and colleagues (279) for 334 patients with adenocarcinoma of the cervix. The 5-year relapse-free survival and locoregional control rates were 88% and 94%, respectively, for 91 patients with normal-sized cervix; 64% and 82%, respectively, for 102 patients with lesions 3 to 5.9 cm in diameter; but only 45% and 81%, respectively, for 22 patients with tumors greater than 6 cm in diameter. The incidence of distant metastases increased with the stage and size of the tumor.

Berek and colleagues (276) observed comparable 5-year survival rates in patients with stage I adenocarcinoma treated with irradiation alone or combined with surgery (81.5%); however, in stage II disease, the 5-year survival rate with irradiation alone was 39.7% (18 patients) and 68.2% (14 patients) with combined therapy. Moberg and colleagues (280) observed better survival in 251 patients with stages IB and IIA disease treated with combination irradiation and surgery than in those treated with radiation therapy alone. There was no difference in 5-year survival rates between patients with adenocarcinoma and those with other cervical malignant tumors. In contrast, Hopkins and associates (277)

reported better results with combination therapy compared with irradiation alone, although the differences were not statistically significant. In a Patient Care Evaluation study of 11,157 patients under the auspices of the American College of Surgeons, a multivariate analysis of patients with stage IB disease revealed that tumor size, nodal spread, and treatment other than surgery alone were independent prognostic factors. However, histologic type (adenocarcinoma, adenosquamous carcinoma, and squamous carcinoma) did not have a significant effect on survival.

Davidson et al. treated 1505 and 95 patients with squamous and adenocarcinomas, respectively, with radical RT (281). The actuarial 5-year survival for all stages was 54.6% for squamous carcinomas and 54% for adenocarcinomas. There were no significant differences when analyzed by stage.

However, Kleine et al. performed a matched-pair analysis of squamous carcinomas (268 patients) and adenocarcinomas (144 patients) of the cervix, finding significantly lower 5- and 10-year survivals in stages I-II adenocarcinomas (282). The authors pointed out that stages III and IV patients had roughly equivalent survival rates, irrespective of histology, arguing against a difference in radiosensitivity. Rather, the authors felt that the difference was most likely related to more frequent subclinical metastases in the adenocarcinoma group. Similar data were published by Randall et al. (283). The preponderance of the evidence supports the position that there are no clinically significant differences between squamous carcinomas and adenocarcinomas, irrespective of stage, that treatment decisions should be largely unaffected by histology, and that, when outcomes are controlled for important prognostic factors, definitive treatment is likely to produce equivalent results in both.

Small Cell Carcinoma of the Cervix

Reagan et al. divided squamous carcinomas of the cervix into three categories: keratinizing squamous cell carcinoma, large cell non-keratinizing squamous cell carcinoma, and small cell carcinoma (284). Later, it became apparent that the "small cell carcinoma" group consisted of a heterogeneous group of tumors, many displaying neuroendocrine differentiation. Tumors in this category have been designated carcinoids, neuroendocrine carcinomas, oat cell carcinomas, small cell carcinomas, and undifferentiated carcinomas. A recent study group advocated a nomenclature similar to that used for neuroendocrine tumors of the lung. Accordingly, neuroendocrine tumors are subdivided into typical carcinoid, atypical carcinoid, large cell neuroendocrine carcinoma, and small cell carcinoma (SCC) (285). The term "small cell" should be limited to those rare tumors with counterparts in the lung and other anatomic locations noted for a high proliferation rate and marked propensity to regional lymph node and distant metastases (126,129). These tumors account for less than 3% of cervical neoplasms.

Small-cell carcinomas are often not confined to the cervix and surrounding tissues at diagnosis. Therefore, work-up may include bone marrow aspiration and other tests to detect the metastatic spread characteristic of this histology. Lymph node involvement is also present in over 50%, and vascular invasion is frequently present.

Van Nagell et al. published a series of 41 patients with small-cell carcinomas, none of whom had chemotherapy (286). Seventy percent had stage I or II disease. Twenty-eight patients were treated with RT, and 13 with radical hysterectomy. Local failure was considerably less common in the stages I-II patients treated with RT than surgery (6% vs. 31%), and recurrence at any site was more common in the surgically treated patients (54%), compared with the RT patients (31%). This is understandable in view of the highly radiosensitive nature of these lesions. Although this series and other data (283) show that some patients with early stage disease will not have metastatic disease at presentation and are potentially curable with local therapies, the frequency of systemic disease and failure patterns cause many oncologists to utilize combination chemotherapy as part of standard therapy in all stages of disease.

Hoskins et al. utilized 4 cycles of etoposide (40 mg/m^2) and cisplatin (25 mg/m^2) for 5 days during weeks 1, 3, 5, and 7 (287). RT commenced on the second cycle. Prophylactic cranial RT was also given following this treatment, in the absence of progression. Of 11 patients treated in this fashion, at least 5 were stages IIIB-IV. Overall and failure-free survivals were 28% at 3 years. There was substantial hematologic and gastrointestinal toxicity, and 2 treatment-related deaths.

The same irradiation techniques as outlined for other histologic varieties of cervical carcinoma should be used in combination with the multiagent chemotherapy.

Carcinoma of the Cervical Stump

Historically, in patients who have undergone subtotal or supracervical hysterectomy, carcinoma of the cervical stump made up nearly 4% of cases treated with RT. Although the incidence has greatly declined, these increasingly rare patients remain at risk of developing cervical carcinoma. The natural history and patterns of spread of these cancers are similar to those of the cervix in the intact uterus. The diagnostic workup, clinical staging, and basic principles of therapy are the same. However, there are potentially important differences in treatment.

Radical operation for stage I cervical stump carcinomas (trachelectomy) is made more difficult by the previous procedure. Creadick (288) reported results in 83 patients, 25 of whom had radical trachelectomy and pelvic lymphadenectomy. The survival rate was 85.7% in squamous-cell carcinoma and 50% in adenocarcinoma (patients with stages I and II disease). Barillot et al. prospectively accrued 213 cases of cervical stump carcinoma; 77% received primary RT, 15%

received brachytherapy and surgery, and 8% received surgery alone for *in situ* carcinoma and subsets of stages IA, IB, and IIA disease (289). Stage for stage, local control and survival were equivalent among the surgically treated and the RT treated patients. However, lethal complications were much more likely in the surgically treated patients. Patients receiving RT including brachytherapy had significantly better results than those having only external RT. Severe complications with RT were similar to those observed among patients with intact uteri. Other investigators, however, have reported increased complication rates among patients with cervical stump cancers treated with RT versus patients treated with intact uteri (290,291).

It is thought that the higher complication rate relates to the lack of adequate uterine cavity length to accommodate a tandem containing two or three sources. However, some patients with a history of supracervical hysterectomy retain enough uterus to insert 2 standard cesium-137 sources. As many sources as technically feasible should be inserted in the remaining cervical canal without protruding active source length through the cervical os. Comparably higher activity sources should be used in the tandem, allowing a greater contribution from these sources to the point A dose and a correspondingly lower vaginal mucosal dose.

In early stage tumors, it is critical to maximize the brachytherapy portion of the treatment, because this allows higher doses to be delivered to the tumor while limiting dose to normal structures. Early mid-line shields (e.g., at 20 to 30 Gy) are desirable. Limiting the total external beam dose to 40 Gy, optimizing the intracavitary RT with proper packing and distribution of activity, and respecting the tolerances of the rectum and bladder will keep complication rates reasonably low. Limiting the maximum rectal dose to 65 or 66 Gy and the bladder dose to around 80 Gy is desirable, even if the point A dose is somewhat compromised (<80 Gy).

More advanced stages should be treated with 40 Gy to the pelvis, combined with the maximum intracavitary doses permitted within tolerance. Platinum-based chemotherapy will be indicated in most cases. Limited sidewall boosts may be necessary, depending on the dose to the sidewalls from the brachytherapy and the radiographic evaluation of the nodes. When there is no opportunity to insert any sources in the cervical canal, the whole pelvis dose should be increased to 45 Gy, and the primary tumor boosted to around 60 to 65 Gy with shrinking fields. Alternatively, interstitial therapy can be considered following the initial external RT. Total dose (external and brachytherapy) to the upper vaginal mucosa should not exceed 150 Gy.

The 5-year survival for carcinoma of the cervical stump treated with irradiation is similar to that reported for patients with carcinoma of the intact uterus (289–293). In the Barillot series of 213 patients, 5-year local control rates by stage were 100% in IA, 85% in IB, 82% in IIA, 71% in IIB, 45% in IIIA, 54% in IIIB, and 30% in IV. Corrected 5-year survival rates were 82%, 78%, 73%, 69%, 38% and 0% in stages IB, IIA, IIB, IIIA, IIIB, and IV, respectively (289). In 253 patients reported by Miller, median survival times were 203, 140, and 32 months for stages I, II, and III, respectively (290). In the series of 70 patients reported by Kovalic and colleagues (169), the 10-year disease-free survival rates were 100% for stage IA, 79% for stage IB, 66% for stage IIB, and 39% for stage IIIB disease. Pelvic failure rates were 10% in stage IB (2 of 19), 9% in stage II (2 of 12), and 50% in stage IIIB (3 of 6).

SURGICAL TECHNIQUES

Hysterectomy

There are several variations of hysterectomy used in the management of carcinoma of the uterine cervix (Table 22.4) (249). The description of the five classes of hysterectomy by Piver and associates (249) has found general acceptance.

Class I, or Total (Extrafascial) Abdominal Hysterectomy

Total abdominal hysterectomy consists of removal of the cervix, adjacent tissues, and a small cuff of the upper vagina in a plane outside the pubocervical fascia. There is minimal disturbance of the trigone of the bladder and the ureters. This procedure is preferred to the intrafascial hysterectomy, which does not ensure complete removal of all cervical tissue. This procedure is similar to the procedure commonly performed for benign indications.

Total hysterectomy may be performed for patients with preinvasive or microinvasive disease if childbearing has been completed. Though the procedure is indicated for invasive malignancy of the uterine corpus, it has little role in the therapy of invasive cervical cancer (293–295).

Class II, or Modified Radical (Extended) Hysterectomy

Modified radical hysterectomy removes the cervix and upper vagina, including paracervical tissues. The ureters are dissected in the paracervical tunnel to the point of entry into the bladder. Because the ureters are unsheathed and retracted laterally, parametrial and paracervical tissue can be safely removed medial to the ureter. This operation may be performed with or without pelvic lymphadenectomy.

As gynecologic oncologists select smaller tumors for operative therapy, it is reasonable to tailor the procedure to fit the patient and her disease. The class II hysterectomy is less morbid than the class III, and appears to be well suited for patients with 3 to 5 mm of invasion and small lesions that do not distort anatomy (296). In many institutions, the class II and class III procedures are blended into a continuum of radicality.

Class III, or Radical Abdominal Hysterectomy with Bilateral Pelvic Lymphadenectomy

Radical abdominal hysterectomy consists of a resection of the parametrial tissues to the pelvic wall, with complete dissection of the ureters from their beds and mobilization of the bladder and the rectum to allow for more extensive removal of tissues. Resection of at least 2 to 3 cm of vaginal cuff is done. A bilateral pelvic lymphadenectomy is usually carried out. The operative approach requires an understanding of the pelvic spaces, and is best characterized as a successful dissection of the ureters (297).

This operation is usually referred to as the Wertheim procedure or Meigs' procedure. Wertheim performed radical operations for cervical cancer starting in 1898 and published multiple reports between 1900 and 1910. Considering the lack of blood transfusion and antibiotics at the turn of the century, his accomplishments are formidable (298).

TABLE 22.4. *Types of abdominal hysterectomy*

Type of surgery	Intrafascial	Extrafascial type I	Modified radical type II	Radical type III
Cervical fascia	Partially removed	Completely removed	Completely removed	Completely removed
Vaginal cuff removal	None	Small rim removed	Proximal 1–2 cm removed	Upper one-third to one-half removed
Bladder	Partially mobilized	Partially mobilized	Partially mobilized	Mobilized
Rectum	Not mobilized	R.V. septum partially mobilized	R.V. septum part	Mobilized
Ureters	Not mobilized	Not mobilized	Unrooted in ureteral tunnel	Completely dissected to bladder entry
Cardinal ligaments	Resected medial to ureters	Resected medial to ureters	Resected at level of ureter	Resected at pelvic sidewall
Uterosacral ligaments	Resected at level of cervix	Resected at level of cervix	Partially resected	Resected at post-pelvic insertion
Uterus	Removed	Removed	Removed	Removed
Cervix	Partially removed	Completely removed	Completely removed	Completely removed

Type IV, extended radical hysterectomy (partial removal of bladder or ureter), in addition to type III.
From Stehman FB, Perez CA, Kurman RJ, et al. Uterine cervix. In Hoskins WJ, Perez CA, Young RC, eds. *Principles and Practice of Gynecologic Oncology*, 3rd ed. Philadelphia: Lippincott Williams & Wilkins, 2000:864.

There is as much controversy about whether or not to do the procedure as how to perform it. Most surgeons prefer to operate on young, healthy, slender, non-smokers with small tumors. Some intercurrent diseases, such as diabetes mellitus, pelvic inflammatory disease, hypertension, collagen disease, or adnexal masses, are considered contraindications to irradiation, and conversely, indications for radical hysterectomy (252,253).

The procedure can be done with the patient in the supine or lithotomy position through a vertical or transverse incision. The pelvic node dissection may be done before or after the hysterectomy. If the finding of nodal involvement would defer the operator from completion of the procedure, then the node dissection should be done first. Many gynecologic oncologists employ bladder drainage, even though the degree of dissection and devascularization is less than in the past (299). Elegant illustrations of the procedure are found in texts and atlases (300,301).

Class IV, or Extended Radical Hysterectomy

Extended radical hysterectomy is rarely performed. Patients with tumors that encroach upon the distal ureter or parametrium are best treated with irradiation. This operation differs from a class III operation in that the superior vesical artery is sacrificed, and more vaginal cuff is removed.

Class V Hysterectomy

Class V hysterectomy differs from the class IV procedure in that an involved portion of the distal ureter or bladder is excised.

Pre-treatment Nodal Staging

Pre-treatment nodal staging operations have been performed to evaluate the presence of metastases to the paraaortic or pelvic nodes. There has been no direct impact on survival to date. An extraperitoneal approach to lymph node dissection (33) has largely replaced transperitoneal staging as first practiced (36). Berman and colleagues (33) described a curvilinear left-flank incision similar to that used for renal transplantation.

Patients who have had pretreatment nodal staging followed by paraaortic irradiation encounter major complications more often (11.5%) after transperitoneal lymphadenectomy, compared with 3.9% after the extraperitoneal lymphadenectomy group ($p = 0.03$) (302). The identification of metastatic involvement of the para-aortic nodes usually modifies therapy, but pelvic node involvement may not (302). There may be some theoretical advantage to debulking large pelvic nodes, but data are lacking (72).

Paraaortic nodal sampling can be accomplished by minimally invasive surgery (laparoscopy) with shorter recovery time (303). The yield appears to be adequate, and no false negatives were encountered in Fowler and associates' experience (304).

Pelvic Exenteration

This procedure consists of *en bloc* removal of the pelvic viscera for centrally recurrent carcinoma of the cervix, and may be used in a very few selected patients with stage IVA disease. This operation encompasses a radical hysterectomy, pelvic lymph node dissection, and removal of the bladder (anterior exenteration) or rectum (posterior exenteration) or both (total exenteration). The ileum, transverse colon, or sigmoid has been the usual means of achieving urinary diversion (305,306). Use of continent diversion, anterior exenteration, and low-rectal anastomosis has reduced the overall morbidity for these patients (307,308). Before proceeding with exenteration, proof that there is no fixation to the pelvic wall and no extension of disease beyond the pelvis is mandatory. Metastases outside the pelvis, including those to para-aortic lymph nodes or any viscera, are contraindications to the procedure. Bilateral ureteral obstruction by tumor is also a relative contraindication (309,310).

Pelvic exenteration was formerly used in stage IVA carcinoma of the cervix with extension to the bladder (309,311). Pelvic exenteration was applied as primary therapy by Deckers and associates (311) for 65 patients with carcinoma of the cervix. An actuarial 5-year survival rate of 18.5% was achieved. The technique and indications have evolved over time. There have been improvements in operative mortality, and 5-year survival rates are associated with better techniques and patient selection (Table 22.5).

However, exenteration is rarely necessary because of modern radiation therapy. Million and co-workers (267) reported 18 of 53 selected patients (34%) with bladder involvement who survived without disease and with only 2 fistulae after definitive irradiation. These results were comparable to those obtained with exenteration. Upadhyay and associates (312) observed 43% local tumor control and 18% 5-year survival among 44 patients with stage IVA carcinoma of the cervix treated with definitive radiation therapy.

Preoperative evaluation and patient selection criteria for pelvic exenteration were described by Creasman and Rutledge (313) and by Rutledge et al. (314). Patients with weight loss, hydronephrosis, leg edema, and hip pain rarely benefit from the procedure and should be excluded from consideration. At examination under anesthesia, pelvic fixation of tumor correlates well with poor survival. If exploration reveals intra-abdominal metastases, positive nodes, ascites or positive washings, serosal breakthrough in the cul-de-sac of Douglas, or small-bowel adhesions to tumor, the procedure should be abandoned. Recent improvements in preoperative imaging with CT or MRI have reduced the number of patients undergoing exploration.

The operation carries a high morbidity, and this procedure cannot be compared with radical resections for bladder can-

TABLE 22.5. *Results after pelvic exenteration*

Author	No. of patients	(%) Operative	5-year survival rate (%)
Bricker et al. (1960)[311a]	150	10	25
Symmonds et al. (1975)[311b]	198	8.1	33
Rutledge et al. (1977)[314]	296	13.5	33.8
Morley et al. (1989)	100	2	61
Lawhead et al. (1989)[311c]	65	9.2	23

From Stehman FB, Perez CA, Kurman RJ, et al. Uterine cervix. In Hoskins WJ, Perez CA, Young RC, eds. *Principles and Practice of Gynecologic Oncology*, 3rd ed. Philadelphia: Lippincott Williams & Wilkins, 2000:865.

cer or rectal cancer, in which most patients have not been radiated. Patients who weigh over 200 pounds or who have received 60 Gy of pelvic radiation therapy are at substantial risk for major complications (313). Enteric complications, such as fistula or obstruction, are the most serious complications specifically associated with this procedure. Orr and associates (315) reported that 15% of their patients developed gastrointestinal-tract fistula. Intestinal anastomoses in irradiated intestine indicate significant risk. In the experience of Lichtinger and others (316), 22.5% of patients developed gastrointestinal fistulas, with a mortality rate of 53.3%. These investigators observed that small-bowel fistulas occurred most often at irradiated small-bowel anastomoses. Their recommendation is to perform enterocolostomy rather than entero-enterostomy if a small intestinal segment is to be used for urinary diversion.

The fate of patients who have recurrent cervical cancer and are explored but not resected is dismal. Hardman and Daly (317) observed three survivors among 45 patients on whom the procedure was abandoned. Stanhope and Symmonds (318) reported 59 patients who underwent exenterations that were retrospectively considered palliative, most commonly because of positive nodes. The 5-year survival rate was 23% among the patients with positive nodes after irradiation.

RADIATION THERAPY TECHNIQUES

The two main modalities of irradiation are external photon, or electron beam and brachytherapy. External photon irradiation is used to treat the whole pelvis and the parametria, including the common iliac and paraaortic lymph nodes, while the central disease (cervix, vagina, and medial parametria) is primarily irradiated with intracavitary sources.

External Irradiation

External pelvic irradiation is delivered before intracavitary insertions in patients with (1) bulky cervical lesions, to improve the geometry of the intracavitary application; (2) exophytic, easily bleeding tumors; (3) tumors with necrosis or infection; and (4) parametrial involvement.

Volume Treated

In the treatment of invasive carcinoma of the uterine cervix, it is imperative to deliver adequate doses of irradiation to the pelvic lymph nodes, depending on the stage of the primary tumor. Greer and associates (319) reported on intraoperative retroperitoneal measurements carried out in 100 patients at the time of radical surgery. Both common iliac bifurcations were cephalad to the level of the lumbosacral prominence in 87% of patients. Therefore, the superior border of the pelvic portal should be at the L4–5 interspace to include the external iliac and hypogastric lymph nodes. This margin should generally be extended to the L3–4 or even the L2–3 interspace if common iliac nodal coverage is indicated. The width of the pelvis at the level of the obturator fossae averaged 12.3 cm, and the distance between the femoral arteries at the level of the inguinal rings averaged 14.6 cm. Posterior extension of the cardinal ligaments in their attachment to the pelvic wall was consistently posterior to the rectum and extended to the sacral hollow. The uterosacral ligaments also extended posteriorly to the sacrum. These anatomic landmarks must be kept in mind in the correct design of lateral pelvic portals. The upper margins of the portals in patients with small stage IB tumors can be placed at the L5-S1 interspace, and for more advanced stages, at the L4–5, L3–4, or even L2–3 interspace (Fig. 22.17A and B). A 2-cm margin lateral to the bony pelvis is adequate. If there is no vaginal extension, the lower margin of the portal is at the mid-portion to inferior border of the obturator foramen. When there is vaginal involvement, the field should extend distally beyond the tumor a minimum of 4 cm, although some contend that the entire length of vagina should be treated down to the introitus. It is important to identify the distal extension of the tumor at the time of simulation by placing a radiopaque clip or bead on the vaginal wall, or by inserting a small rod with a radiopaque marker in the vagina. Often, vaginal extension will not be clearly defined by CT scan. In patients with involvement of the distal third of the vagina, portals should cover the inguinal lymph nodes because of the increased probability of metastases. For stage IB disease, 15 × 15 cm portals at the surface (about 16.5 cm at isocenter) usually will be sufficient. For patients with

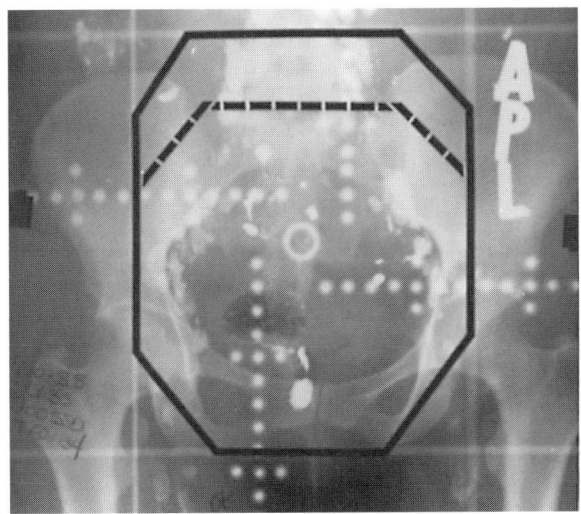
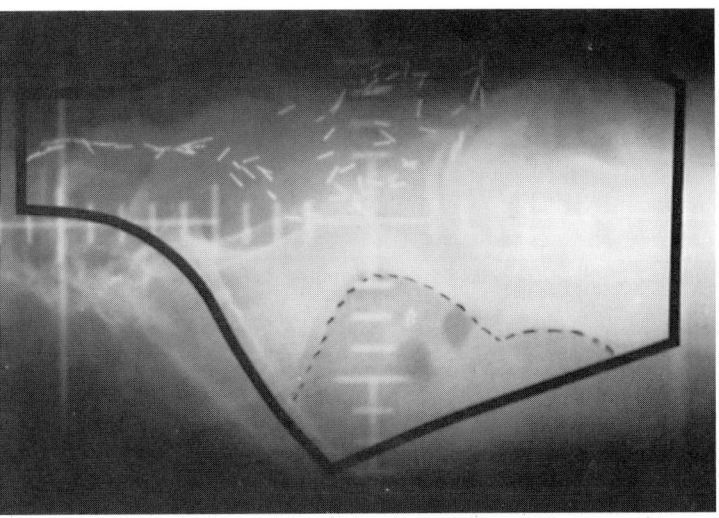

FIG. 22.17. A: Anteroposterior simulation film of the pelvis illustrating portals used for external irradiation. The 15 × 15 cm portals at SSD (source–skin distance) are used for stage IB (broken line), and 18 × 15 cm portals are used for more advanced disease (solid line). This allows better coverage of the common iliac lymph nodes. The distal margin is usually placed at the bottom of the obturator foramina. **B:** Lateral simulation film of the pelvis illustrating portals used for external irradiation. (From Stehman FB, Perez CA, Kurman RJ, et al. Uterine cervix. In Hoskins WJ, Perez CA, Young RC, et al., eds. *Principles and Practice of Radiation Oncology,* 3rd ed. Philadelphia: Lippincott-Raven, 2000:867.)

stage IIA, IIB, III, or IVA carcinoma, somewhat larger portals (18 × 15 cm at surface, 20.5 × 16.5 at isocenter) may be required to cover all of the common iliac nodes, in addition to the cephalad half of the vagina (320). Dittmer and Randall have published a convenient method of treating inguinal-femoral nodes using photons only while limiting the dose to femoral heads and avoiding some of the problems with junctioning fields, e.g., electrons (263) (Fig. 22.16).

The lateral portal anterior margin is placed anterior to the pubic symphysis to include the anterior extent of the external iliac nodes (321). A margin at the anterior edge of the symphysis pubis often will not suffice for adequate coverage of primary tumor as well (322,323) (Fig. 22–18A). The posterior margin usually covers at least 50% of the rectum in stage IB tumors, and will often extend to the sacral hollow in patients with more advanced tumors (Fig. 22.17B). Routinely placing the posterior border at the S2-S3 interspace frequently results in inadequate coverage of the planning target volume (322,323) (Fig. 22.18B). Kim et al., in a small retrospective series, documented higher local failure rates in patients with inadequate margins (322).

The use of lateral fields allows significant protection of small bowel. With a four-field technique, some radiation oncologists choose to weight the AP-PA beams in relation to the lateral fields, e.g., 60:40. While this increases small bowel dose slightly, it can avoid giving very high doses laterally, particularly in larger patients.

In the last decade, radiation oncologists have recognized the phenomenon of pelvic organ motion as a potential source of treatment error in prostate cancer and, more recently, cer-

vical cancer (324). This additional source of error and inadequate tumor coverage should be considered in planning external beam treatment. It is particularly important to recognize that this could be problematic in patients receiving treatment with intensity-modulated radiation therapy (IMRT) techniques.

Although common practice, the use of midline shields (MLS) during external beam RT for cervical cancer has not been well described, and there is no consensus regarding their use. There is variability in opinions and practice patterns regarding whether or not they should be used at all, patient selection, at what dose introduction is appropriate, "standard" versus "customized" blocks, the impact of intracavitary application geometry on the MLS's width and location, and how the use of an MLS affects the calculation of dose to point A. Radiation oncologists should recognize that the purpose of the MLS is to limit dose to the bladder and rectum in order to permit maximization of the intracavitary dose while still delivering sufficient doses to gross parametrial disease and microscopic or gross pelvic sidewall disease (nodal or tumor extension). Its use must be individualized, and experience helps avoid misuse. In very general terms, patients with earlier disease (stages I-IIA, or perhaps early IIB) benefit from earlier introduction of an MLS (20–30 Gy); patients with more advanced disease should not have an MLS placed before 40 Gy, and possibly not at all. It is crucial to perform pelvic examinations on a weekly basis in patients receiving primary RT for cervical cancer. An early favorable response might permit an earlier use of the MLS. Keeping in mind the purpose of the MLS, a fre-

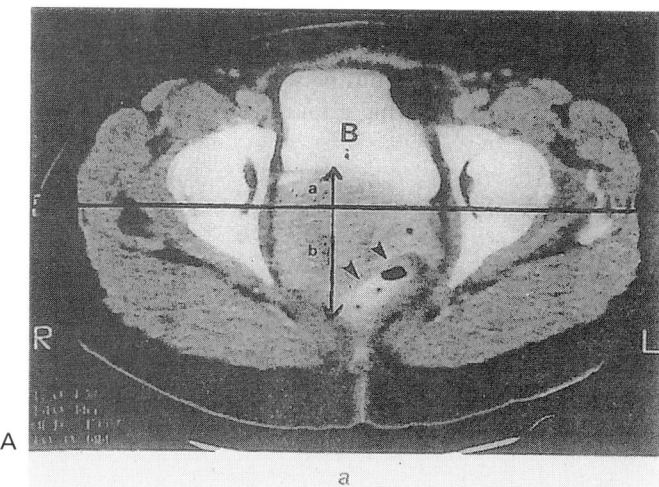

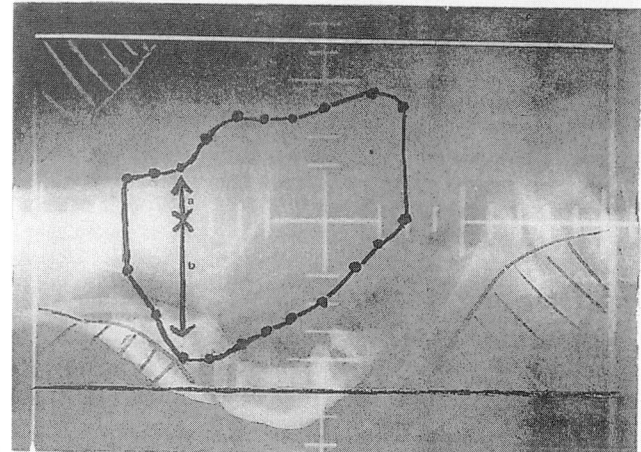

FIG. 22.18. A: Axial CT image at the level of the femoral head, showing cervical mass extension along the lateral aspect of the rectum *(arrow)*. Tumor extension anteriorly (a) and posteriorly (b) from the central axis. **B:** Conventional lateral pelvic portal showing inadequate margin at the rectal block in relation to the CT-defined tumor volume. (From: Kim RY, McGinnis LS, Spencer SA, et al. Conventional four-field pelvic radiotherapy technique without computed tomography—treatment planning in cancer of the cervix: potential geographic miss and its impact on pelvic control. *Int J Rad Oncol Biol Phys* 1995;31:111.)

quent practice is to use a standard-width shield (4 cm), and place it in midline position. This corresponds to the majority practice of academic centers (325). Generally, the pelvic dose delivered with the MLS is not added to the point A dose, but this dose is added to the nodal (sidewall, point B, point P) dose calculation. Unilateral sidewall boosts should be considered in patients who have only unilateral parametrial or sidewall involvement. Increasing parametrial doses correlate with risk of complications, particularly radiation proctitis (326) (Fig. 22.19).

In patients treated postoperatively, a sensible approach to limiting complications in selected patients was piloted by Kridelka et al. (327). Pelvic failure is by far the most frequent

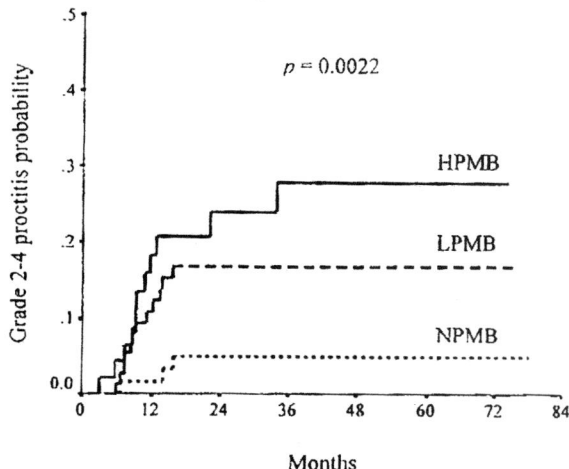

FIG. 22.19. Actuarial grades 2–4 proctitis probability among the three groups (HPMB = high parametrial boost; LPMB = low parametrial boost; NPMB = no parametrial boost). (From Huang EY, Lin H, Hsu HC, et al. High external parametrial dose can increase the probability of radiation proctitis in patients with uterine cervix cancer. *Gynecol Oncol* 2000;79:409.)

site of failure in early-stage cervical cancer patients, regardless of the initial treatment. However, in node-negative patients, the risk factors that indicate adjuvant RT following radical surgery are overwhelmingly related to a risk of failure in the central pelvis, including in the vaginal vault and paravaginal soft tissues. Given the well-known relationship between radiation volume and complication risk, Kridelka limited the adjuvant pelvic RT to fields smaller than "standard" (Fig. 22.20). In 25 patients with a risk of recurrence of at

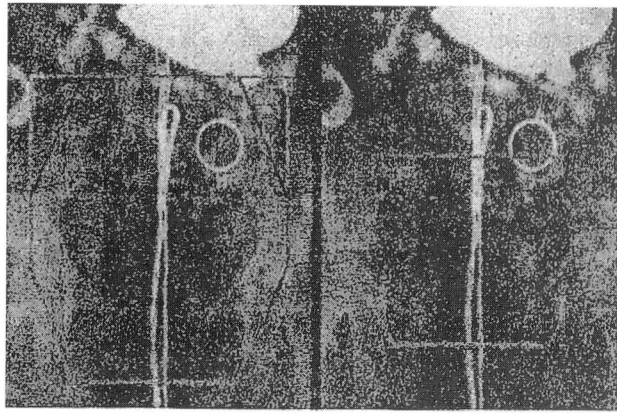

FIG. 22.20. Small bowel irradiation: standard field vs. small field. (From Kridelka FJ, Berg DO, Neuman M, et al. Adjuvant small field pelvic radiation for patients with high risk, stage IB lymph node negative cervix carcinoma after radical hysterectomy and pelvic lymph node dissection. *Cancer* 1999;86:2064.)

least 40%, as suggested by the GOG study (21), only 1 recurrence was noted, with a median follow-up of 32 months. As predicted, morbidity was very limited in quantity and grade. The authors compared disease-free survival curves of their experience and that of the observation arm in the GOG trial by Sedlis (328), finding small field pelvic RT to be significantly superior ($p = 0.005$).

A similar experience with small-field pelvic RT was reported recently by Ohara et al, in 42 patients with stages I-II node-negative squamous carcinoma of the cervix at significant risk of local recurrence (329). All patients so treated had deep cervical stromal invasion, parametrial extension, and/or positive or close (<5mm) surgical margins. Only 3 patients treated with small-field RT suffered recurrences, all in the pelvis. Serious toxicity was rare.

Technique of Extended Field Radiation Therapy

The reluctance among some radiation oncologists to utilize extended field radiation therapy (EFRT) either prophylactically or therapeutically in some cases relates to concern over increased acute and late toxicities rather than concern over efficacy or patient selection. This is largely because the PA chain is surrounded by organs of limited radiation tolerance, i.e. spinal cord, kidneys, small intestine. The use of opposed anterior and posterior fields is conceptually the easiest and cleanest from a dosimetric point of view, but delivers to a significant portion of the small bowel a radiation dose that will generally exceed tolerance if an appropriate dose for microscopic disease is delivered.

Various techniques have been utilized in an effort to deliver EFRT, all of which have both advantages and disadvantages. Carl et al. (330) advocate a biaxial four-segmental rotating technique that resulted in a very low risk of severe side effects. A more common approach is a four-field technique, which permits continuity with and use of a four-field approach in the pelvis, spares much of the small intestine, and shields the spinal cord and the vast majority of the kidneys from half of the beams. It is appropriate to perform an IVP or CT to accurately determine the kidneys' location. The dose to the kidneys can be kept within tolerance by preferentially weighting the anterior and posterior beams (e.g., 70:30 AP-PA to laterals). In most cases, this will be adequate to limit kidney doses within tolerance, even when delivering 40–45 Gy to the volume. Nevertheless, it is critical to know the kidney doses and the amount of the renal parenchyma receiving this dose when utilizing this technique. It is critical to perform off-axis dosimetry or CT planning and to approach each case individually.

Mutic et al. used positron-emission tomography (PET) data to assess for metastatic disease and to guide planning using IMRT techniques (331) (Fig. 22.21). In this fashion, it was feasible to escalate RT doses to 59.4 Gy while maintaining acceptable doses to surrounding tissues. However, in this approach, the clinical target volume received only .5

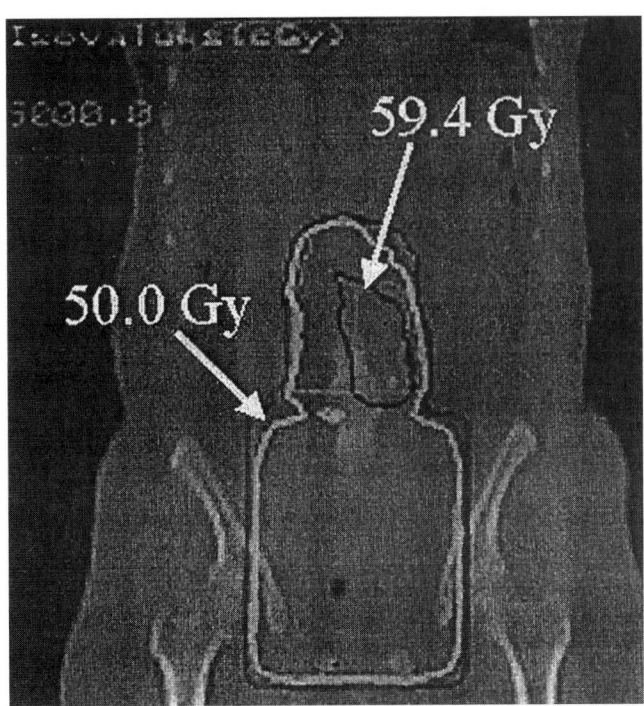

FIG. 22.21. Composite plan showing IMRT dose distribution for paraaortic region and whole pelvis dose. (From Mutic S, Malyapa RS, Grigsby PW, et al. PET-guided IMRT for cervical carcinoma w/ positive para-aortic lymph nodes—a dose-escalation treatment planning study. *Int J Radiat Oncol Biol Phys* 2003;55:34.)

Gy per fraction, and the radiobiologic implications of this are unclear. Furthermore, it remains to be seen if dose escalation for gross disease in the paraaortic chain can impact outcome.

Brachytherapy

Brachytherapy refers to the placement of radioactive sources at a short distance from the intended target. Because the anatomy of cervical cancer typically facilitates brachytherapy, and because brachytherapy permits very high doses to be safely delivered, it has long been a major factor in the ability of RT to cure cervical cancer. Several isotopes are available for cervical cancer brachytherapy, although at the present time ^{137}Cs is the most popular for low-dose-rate (LDR) brachytherapy. [192]Ir is frequently used for high-dose-rate (HDR) brachytherapy because of its high specific activity; it is also frequently used, in a lower activity, in removable LDR interstitial applications. Brachytherapy can be delivered with intracavitary techniques using applicators typically consisting of an intrauterine tandem and vaginal colpostats or, when necessary, vaginal cylinders. All state-of-the-art applicators are afterloading. Interstitial implants are typically done with permanent or removable isotopes, such as [198]Au and ^{192}Ir, respectively. Radiographs are always obtained using dummy sources, and the active sources can be afterloaded following review of films, if the position of the applicators is judged to be satisfactory.

Intracavitary Implants

Intracavitary brachytherapy is generally used in combination with external beam radiotherapy (EBRT), although it may be used alone in very early disease. LDR has been used since the early 1900s, but starting in the late 1950s, with the Cathetron Cobalt-60, HDR brachytherapy has become increasingly utilized.

Three brachytherapy systems were developed almost simultaneously: the Paris, Stockholm, and Manchester systems. They reached a surprising level of maturity and effectiveness by the late 1920s. The term "system" denotes a set of established rules, taking into account the source strength and the geometry, method, and duration of the application in order to obtain suitable dose distributions. In each of these systems, a brachytherapy insertion consisted of an intrauterine component (tandem) and a vaginal applicator. Treatment duration and loadings were developed empirically. Intracavitary treatment prescriptions were quantified in terms of milligram-hours; i.e., the product of the total mass of radium or radium equivalent (e.g., ^{137}Cs) contained in the sources, and the duration of the application in hours.

The classical Manchester system was the first system to use units of radiation exposure (roentgens) rather than mg-hrs to prescribe dose. The dose (in roentgens) was prescribed at specific points, termed A and B. Point A was originally defined as a point 2 cm lateral to the center of the uterine canal and 2 cm from the mucous membrane of the lateral fornix in the plane of the uterus. Point A was intended to represent the average dose to the "paracervical triangle." Point B was defined as 5 cm from the patient's midline at the same level as point A, and it was intended to quantify the dose received by the regional (obturator) lymph nodes. The various combinations of Manchester System ovoid dimensions and applicator loadings were designed to provide a reasonably constant point A dose rate of 50 to 55 cGy per hour. This approach heavily influenced intracavitary treatment practice patterns in the United States. The widely used Fletcher-Suit applicator system, Fletcher loadings, and the reference points A and B are all derived from this system.

A number of investigators have attempted to model the relationship between mg-hrs and point A dose by simple mathematical models. However, the approximate relationship of Point A cGy/mgh (0.80–0.85) applies only to the classical definition of point A, and for an implant of standard geometry. Many radiation oncologists have used revised definitions of point A that reference its location to the cervical os. This further obscures the relationship between point A dose and total mg-hrs prescription philosophies. In 91 Fletcher-Suit applications, using linear least-square regression, Potish and associates (332) observed a moderately

good correlation between mg-hrs and doses. However, the dose to point A was markedly affected by the positions of the colpostats and tandem, making it difficult to formulate a simple conversion factor between the two systems. Therefore computer-generated isodose curves provide the best means of determining the doses to point A, point B, bladder, and rectum (Fig. 22.22 A and B). ICRU Report No. 38 (333) defines the dose and volume specifications for reporting intracavitary therapy in gynecologic procedures. ICRU-38 recommended that reference points such as point A not be used, because "such points are located in a region where the dose gradient is high and any inaccuracy in the determination of the distance results in large uncertainties in the absorbed doses evaluated at those points." Instead, it introduced the concept of reference volume, i.e., the tissue volume encompassed by a reference isodose surface, recommending that the dimensions of the 60-Gy isodose surface be specified, including the contribution of the EBRT. They proposed that this pear-shaped reference volume be described in terms of its 3 dimensions: height (maximum dimension along the intrauterine sources), width (maximum dimension perpendicular to the intrauterine sources), and thickness (maximum dimension perpendicular to the intrauterine sources in the oblique sagittal plane), measured in the oblique, coronal, and sagittal planes containing the intracavitary sources. A number of weaknesses of the ICRU-38 recommendations have been pointed out, including the absence of rationale for the choice of 60 Gy. Widespread adoption is, therefore, lacking (334). However, the ICRU definitions of rectal and bladder points are frequently used.

If the vaginal vault is narrow, making it impossible to insert regular colpostats, miniovoids can be used (usually loaded with 10 mCi RaEq sources). When miniovoids cannot be inserted, an option is to use a protruding source in the vaginal vault, which is inserted in the afterloading tandem (usually 20 to 30 mCi RaEq) with an overlying plastic sleeve (Delclos ring). Afterloaded vaginal cylinders are used in conjunction with an intrauterine tandem to irradiate the vagina when the disease extends from the uterine cervix along the vaginal walls. Cylinders are available in various diameters (1–5 cm) and lengths to fit any vaginal width and length.

In general, the first intracavitary insertion is scheduled after 20–40 Gy of EBRT if patient and tumor geometry permit an adequate implant (typically early-stage patients, e.g., IB-early IIB). Otherwise, 30 to 45 Gy are delivered before the first application to decrease the size of the lesion and improve the relationship of the applicators to the cervix and vagina. The second application is performed 1 or 2 weeks later.

Intracavitary therapy, with its rapid dose fall-off with distance, yields a high dose to the uterus and paracervical tissues, but it is inadequate to treat the pelvic lymph nodes; external irradiation is necessary to supplement the dose. Therefore, the parametrial dose is primarily delivered with external irradiation. This combination technique affords a

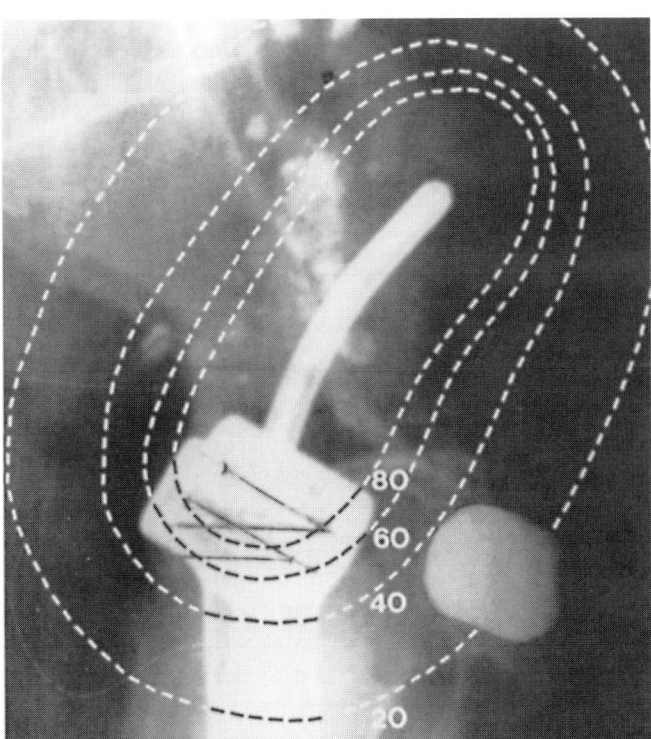

FIG. 22.22. (A) Anteroposterior and **(B)** lateral radiographs of standard intracavitary insertion with after-loading Fletcher-Suit tandem and ovoids. Slight deviation of the tandem to the left is apparent. However, there is good symmetry between the tandem and the ovoids. On the lateral projection, the tandem is crossing the ovoids near the center of the long axis. Radiopaque marker is present on the anterior lip of the cervix. A Foley balloon with Hypaque outlines the bladder neck. (From Stehman FB, Perez CA, Kurman RJ, et al. Uterine cervix. In Hoskins WJ, Perez CA, Young RC, et al., eds. *Principles and Practice of Radiation Oncology*, 3rd ed. Philadelphia: Lippincott-Raven, 2000:869.)

high central dose to the cervix, paracervical tissues, and parametria, as well as a moderate dose to the external iliac lymph nodes, without exceeding the bladder and rectal tolerance doses (Fig. 22.23).

Although the dose prescriptions for LDR brachytherapy are reasonably well established and practiced around the world, there remains some disagreement about whether the LDR intracavitary dose should be given in 1 or 2 implants (335–337). Rotman and Aziz have published a nice review of the literature regarding this controversy (338). Most radiation oncologists favor fractionating the intracavitary portion of the treatment (mostly 2 implants) because of theoretical and practical advantages that include: (1) tumor shrinkage between implants, allowing better dose coverage in the relevant isodose (higher dose to the tumor periphery); (2) repair of normal tissues between fractions, leading to fewer late effects; and (3) limiting the duration of bed rest and potential complications that can result. The clinical data tend to support the superiority of 2 implants over 1 implant, but this is not uniformly the case. There is a common, confounding variable, i.e., patients with more advanced disease are more likely to have only 1 implant because of the necessary reliance on external pelvic RT. Mitsuhashi et al. obtained im-pressive results in 293 patients with stages I-III squamous carcinoma of the cervix utilizing 3 LDR insertions (339). Treatment individualization, as usual, is to be recommended.

Dose Rate Considerations

The rate at which radiation is given is an important variable in the delivery of RT. Conventional EBRT typically uses dose rates of 100–300 cGy per minute but is fractionated. Brachytherapy dose rates can be much more variable, the exposure is often continuous, and dose gradients are infinitely greater than with external beam therapy.

The ICRU defines LDR as exposures between 40 and 200 cGy/hour, medium-dose-rate (MDR) as between 200 and 1200 cGy/hour, and HDR as >1200 cGy/hour (333). All agree that clinically significant differences exist between LDR, MDR, and HDR. In general, as the dose rate is lowered, the biologic effect of the radiation is decreased owing to the ability of tissues to repair sublethal radiation damage and to repopulate. While there is probably no inherent difference in these parameters between tumor and normal tissues, there is apparently a substantial difference when one considers acute responding (rapidly proliferating) vs. late respond-

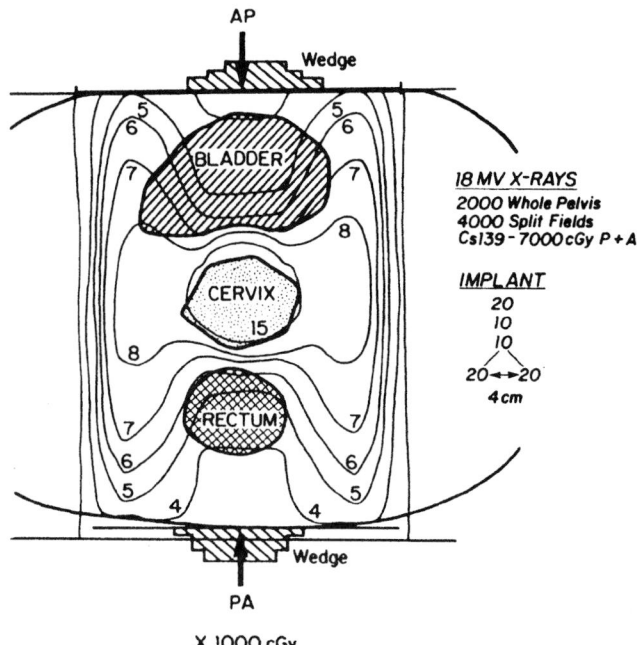

AP

Wedge

BLADDER

CERVIX

RECTUM?

Wedge

PA

18 MV X-RAYS
2000 Whole Pelvis
4000 Split Fields
Cs139 - 7000 cGy P + A

IMPLANT
20
10
10
20 ←→ 20
4 cm

X 1000 cGy

FIG. 22.23. Composite isodose curves through point A for patient with stage IIB carcinoma of the uterine cervix treated with external irradiation and two intracavitary insertions. Doses and source arrangement are shown. High doses can be delivered to the cervix and parametrial tissues with relative sparing of the bladder and rectum. (From Stehman FB, Perez CA, Kurman RJ, et al. Uterine cervix. In: Hoskins WJ, Perez CA, Young RC, et al., eds. *Principles and Practice of Radiation Oncology,* 3rd ed. Philadelphia: Lippincott-Raven, 2000: 870.)

ing (slowly proliferating) tissues. Late-responding tissues have a greater capability for repair than tumor or early-responding tissues, but this repair does not take place as fully with high dose rates (340). Therein lies the radiobiologic dilemma: higher dose rate or large doses per fraction cause relatively more severe late damage than tumor cell kill during HDR brachytherapy or external beam therapy.

Low Dose Rate

To a large degree, published data documenting the effectiveness of RT has been obtained with continuous LDR intracavitary techniques, which have been used for nearly a century. However, even within the dose-rate range considered LDR (0–200 cGy/hr), a strong dose-rate effect is likely. Lee et al. first pointed out the impact of increased dose rates on complications among patients treated for cervical cancer in 1976 (341). In comparing patients developing complications involving the bladder, rectum, and ureters, these authors found HDR rate to be a significantly better predictor of complications than either total dose or treatment time. Rodrigus et al. (342) reported a significant increase in late morbidity after increasing the intracavitary dose rate from the conven-

tional 0.54 Gy/hr to slightly greater than 1 Gy/hr, even though a 20% dose reduction was employed. Newman reported a series of 270 patients in whom an increase in grade 3 complications from 4% to 22% was observed after changing from a 75 cGy/hr dose rate to 150 cGy/hr, in spite of a 20% reduction in total dose (343). Lambin et al. confirmed this observation in a randomized trial between 2 dose rates in the LDR range (344). In a subsequent analysis of this randomized study, Haie-Meder et al. demonstrated that a true measure of complication rates must consider the prevalence of complications over time as well as the evolution of the complications, rather than relying on the analysis and grading of only the first complication reported (345).

Using a slightly higher dose rate (in the low MDR range), Patel et al. suggested, based on analysis of their clinical experience, that a dose reduction factor of approximately 30%, in comparison to a typical LDR range of 50–55 cGy/hr, would be required when using a dose rate of 220 cGy/hr at point A (346).

Pulsed LDR brachytherapy has also been investigated as a possible means of preserving the radiobiologic advantages of LDR while taking advantage of dose optimization offered by HDR technology. Swift et al. reported their experience in 65 patients, 42 of whom had cervical cancer (347). Median follow-up was only 15 months. In these patients with cervical cancer, 23 were alive without known disease at the time of the report. The 2-year actuarial survival rate was 65%, and the 2-year actuarial incidence of late complications was 14%. The authors concluded that pulsed LDR was feasible, and produced good local control rates. However, they recognized that significantly more experience and longer follow-up is required for pulsed LDR to be adequately evaluated.

High Dose Rate

The use of HDR techniques dates to the 1960s (348). The perceived advantages at that time included the elimination of radiation hazards (compared to those encountered in manually loaded LDR techniques) and improved patient convenience. It is clear that the radiobiology of changing dose rates was poorly understood at that time, and clinical data from these early years are lacking. Subsequently, additional benefits of HDR techniques have been suggested.

Orton and associates (349) suggested an LDR to HDR conversion factor of 0.54 to 0.6. Patel and colleagues (346) and Okawa and co-workers (350) calculated a similar dose rate correction factor of 0.58. In general, the α/β values are approximately 10 (Gy10) for tumor and early-responding tissues, and 3 to 5 (Gy3–5) for late-responding tissues.

To decrease the likelihood of increased late effects with HDR brachytherapy, it is necessary to use multiple HDR fractions and to decrease, as much as possible, the dose to late-responding tissues.

Conceptual Comparison of LDR and HDR

The use of HDR in the curative management of cervical cancer is becoming more and more accepted. However, controversy remains, because some question the accuracy of statements made regarding the advantages of HDR. For example, the virtual elimination of radiation exposure to personnel is a function of remote-afterloading technology, not of HDR. In addition, proponents suggest that outpatient HDR treatment improves patient convenience. Although most patients would prefer outpatient treatment, the multiple (5–12) insertions felt necessary to allow this technique to be practiced safely could limit patient convenience. Wright and colleagues (351) developed a questionnaire to elicit patient preference for LDR or HDR in cervical cancer. Subjects received descriptions of both treatment options and their probable outcomes. Preference was elicited for one LDR or three HDR fractions, and for two LDR or five HDR fractions, assuming both methods to be isoeffective. Strength of initial preference was measured by asking subjects how much of a change, in either the chances for cure or the chances for toxicity, would make them change preference. The questionnaire was completed by female staff at their center (n = 90), by a group of previously treated patients (n = 18), and by a group of newly diagnosed patients (n = 20). When both methods were assumed to be isoeffective, only 34% of the 38 patients preferred three fractions of HDR to one fraction of LDR. However, when HDR was assumed to be 2% more curative, or 6% less toxic, 50% said they would prefer HDR. Both preference and strength of preference for LDR were associated significantly with a greater traveling distance for treatments.

HDR has been suggested to have physical superiority over LDR techniques. For example, advocates suggest that it is possible to more vigorously pack or retract critical tissues away from the radioactive sources for the short time required to deliver an HDR treatment. Others would argue that this assertion is counter-intuitive, because a patient who is anesthetized for an LDR insertion should be better able to tolerate the kind of rectal and bladder retraction and packing that characterizes a well-done intracavitary insertion. Kim et al. found that adequacy of packing was better with general anesthesia (generally practiced for LDR insertions), compared with conscious sedation (often practiced for HDR insertions) (352). In addition, the same investigators directly compared vaginal packing between LDR and HDR implants, finding no consistent variation in packing adequacy (353). Also, proponents claim that limited applicator and source movement during HDR makes dose calculation more accurate. However, others argue that there is no evidence that the applicator positions are more stable during HDR insertions. Corn et al. (354) analyzed the positional stability of LDR Fletcher-Suit-Delclos applicators in 15 consecutive patients, finding a minimal amount of applicator shift and a median change in point A dose of only 1.4% over the course of the implants (median duration 56.5 hours). Finally, HDR users prefer the ability to "dose-optimize," meaning to specifically contour isodose shapes by varying dwell times and positions. Others would argue that modern LDR-based treatment of cervical carcinoma is somewhat individualized based on stage and anatomy, but is not based on the unrealistic expectation that the physician will be able to precisely determine, by physical or radiologic examination, the difference between normal and malignant tissue. It is unclear whether dose distributions can truly be optimized to conform precisely to the tumor volume.

The greatest concern regarding HDR is the potential for increasing complication rates in a patient population in which the majority will be cured. The literature reflects considerable inconsistency in terms of whether complication rates are increased with HDR over LDR. Possible reasons for this discrepancy are not known with certainty, but one possible explanation is the limited numbers of patients that have been treated and followed sufficiently to adequately assess late complications. This is particularly problematic when one considers the compelling clinical data from M. D. Anderson Cancer Center, demonstrating the continued risk of developing rectal and bladder complications as late as 20 to 25 years following RT (250). Other possible reasons include publication bias and patient selection factors. In a survey conducted by the American Brachytherapy Society (ABS) based on 1995 practice patterns, only 24% of responding institutions practiced HDR brachytherapy for cervical cancer, and only 16% of patients were treated in this fashion (355). It is possible that radiation oncologists are selecting some patients for HDR and others for LDR. If patients with anatomic limitations to good implant geometry are being selected for LDR, and patients with favorable geometry receive HDR implants, the advantage in therapeutic ratio from LDR will be obscured, resulting in misleading data.

Clinical Comparison of LDR and HDR

Many retrospective series of patients treated with HDR and LDR have been reported. The largest HDR series was that of Lorvidhaya et al., 1992 patients (356). Using a remote afterloading ^{60}Co system, the actuarial 5 year disease-free survival rate was 79.5%, 70.0%, 59.4%, 46.1%, 32.3%, 7.8%, and 23.1% in patients with stage IB, IIA, IIB, IIIA, IIIB, IVA, and IVB, respectively. Median follow-up was 96 months. Ferrigno and colleagues published separate reports of HDR (138 patients, stages II and III) and LDR (190 patients, stages I-III) treated patients at the same institution in Brazil (357,358). Median follow-up was 38 and 70 months in the HDR and LDR series, respectively. Although not randomized, actuarial 5-year overall survival rates in stage II were 61% in the HDR patients and 78% in the LDR patients. Stage III overall survival was 52% for HDR patients and 46% for LDR patients. These studies were strengthened by the use of actuarial methods for calculating complication rates. In the LDR series, 5-year actuarial rectal, small bowel, and urinary complication rates were 16.1%, 4.6%, and 7.6%, respectively (358). This compares with 16%, 11%, and 14% in the HDR series (357).

Petereit (359) reported the University of Wisconsin experience with 191 patients receiving LDR brachytherapy, and 173 receiving HDR brachytherapy with equivalent external beam irradiation techniques. For all stages combined, pelvic tumor control and survival were equivalent with the two treatment techniques. However, in the stage IIIB patients, pelvic control was only 44% at 3 years with HDR, vs. 75% with LDR ($p = 0.002$). This translated into a lower survival rate in stage IIIB patients (33% vs. 58%, $p = 0.004$).

Although no randomized trials in the United States have compared HDR and LDR brachytherapy for cervical cancer, there have been several performed elsewhere. Patel and associates (360) performed a randomized trial in India in 482 patients with previously untreated invasive squamous-cell carcinoma of the uterine cervix. Overall local tumor control with LDR was 79.7%, compared with 75.8% with HDR brachytherapy. The 5-year survival rates were comparable in all stages; however stage I patients had only a 75% 5-year survival. This study has been criticized for a number of reasons. Most problematic was the fact that patients were ''alternately'' randomized at the time of the implant, rather than at the start of treatment. Furthermore, implants were loaded only if the bladder and rectal doses were ≤60% of point A doses. Also, patients getting LDR brachytherapy received only 1 implant, and a treatment break of up to 4 weeks after external RT was given in some cases. Grade 3 and 4 complications were not significantly different between the two groups.

In a trial reported by Shigematsu and colleagues (361) in Japan, patients with stage IIB or III disease treated with HDR had both a higher 1-year local control rate (90% with HDR, and 77% with LDR) and rectal complication rate. The 5-year survival rate was 55% for both groups. This trial was not really randomized, since patients were assigned treatment based on registration number and bed availability (143 patients in HDR arm vs. 106 in LDR arm). Patients treated with LDR had widely varying time-dose parameters, in contrast to patients treated with HDR. Interestingly, subset analysis showed that stage IIB patients had better outcomes with LDR.

Teshima and associates (362) in Japan reported on a prospective randomized study of 430 patients with carcinoma of the uterine cervix treated with either LDR (171 patients) or HDR brachytherapy (259 patients), combined with external irradiation. Cause-specific survival and overall survival were comparable for each clinical stage with either modality, except for stage I overall survival. With HDR therapy, usually four fractions were delivered; and with LDR brachytherapy, two fractions. The incidence of pelvic failures was comparable in both groups. Grade 2 and 3 morbidity was

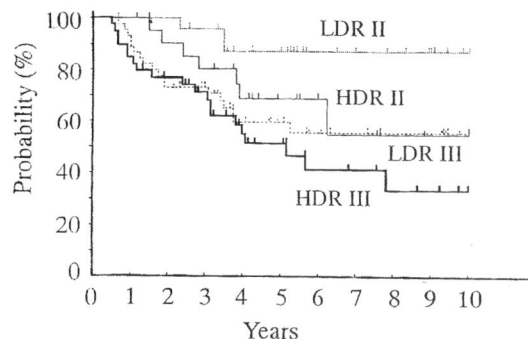

FIG. 22.24. The disease-specific survival rates of patients with carcinoma of the uterine cervix by stage and treatment group. HDR, high dose rate; LDR, low dose rate. (From Hareyama M, Sakata K, Oouchi A, et al. High-dose-rate vs. low-dose-rate intracavitary therapy for carcinoma of the uterine cervix. *Cancer* 2002;94:120.)

somewhat higher in the HDR group (about 10%), compared with the LDR group (4%) ($p = 0.002$).

More recently, Hareyama et al. published a randomized trial of 132 patients with stage II or IIIB disease (363). External RT doses were identical, and a conversion factor of 0.588 was used to convert LDR to HDR. The 5-year disease-specific survival rates were 69% and 51% with HDR in stages II and III, respectively. This compared with 87% and 60% with LDR (Fig. 22.24). Pelvic recurrence-free survivals with HDR were 89% and 73% for stages II and III, vs. 100% and 70%, respectively, in the LDR group (Fig. 22–25). Actuarial complication rates (≥ grade 3) at 5 years were 10% with HDR and 13% with LDR. These differences did not reach statistical significance, although stage II patients had a better survival than those treated with HDR.

Numerous studies, including Phase III randomized comparisons, have observed a deleterious effect of increasing dose rates on the incidence of radiation complications (344, 364–367). Fujikawa et al. reported a high incidence of severe

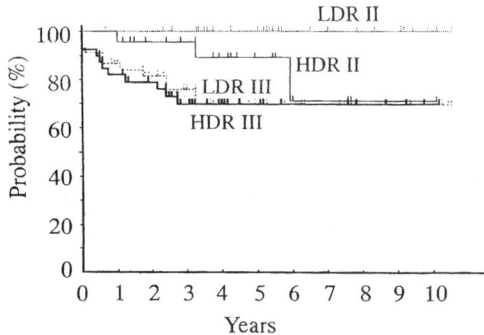

FIG. 22.25. The pelvic recurrence-free survival rates of patients with carcinoma of the uterine cervix by stage and treatment group. HDR, high dose rate; LDR, low dose rate. (From Hareyama M, Sakata K, Oouchi A, et al. High-dose-rate vs. low-dose-rate intracavitary therapy for carcinoma of the uterine cervix. *Cancer* 2002;94:120.)

urologic and gastrointestinal complications following radiation therapy with HDR brachytherapy in Japan, including a 2% risk of spontaneous rupture of the urinary bladder (368). These observations confirmed those of Ogina et al. (369) and Uno et al. (370). Wang et al. observed an increased risk of complications with HDR when compared to "existing results" of LDR techniques (371). Specifically, the 5-year actuarial rates were 38% for rectal injury and 9% for bladder complications. Other authors find serious complication rates to be comparable between LDR and HDR (360,372).

Dose and Fractionation in HDR Brachytherapy

The optimal time/dose/fractionation scheme and the technique for remote afterloading intracavitary HDR brachytherapy for cervical cancer have yet to be established. Data from Stanford University suggested that regimens using relatively few HDR treatments (as few as 1, mean 2.6 applications) give results as good as those using higher fraction numbers (373). Wayne State University uses a highly fractionated brachytherapy course with 8 to 12 HDR fractions (349), which was chosen to keep the rectal dose for each HDR fraction to between 2 and 2.5 Gy, in order to be consistent with doses considered tolerable for fractionated external beam irradiation.

Orton et al. have presented data detailing the large variability of HDR dose and fractionation schemes utilized in various institutions (349). Petereit and Pearcey (374) performed a literature review and analysis of published HDR dose and fractionation schedules, confirming the lack of consensus regarding dose prescription. The authors found that the HDR literature reported inadequate details of treatment and outcome, such as rectal and bladder doses and actuarial complication rates. Furthermore, no relationship was found between point A dose and either survival or pelvic control, nor was a relationship seen between dose and complication rate. It was concluded that the optimal fractionation schedule for HDR remains unknown, and that the quality of the current HDR literature is subject to considerable improvement. Petereit (374) used 45 Gy in 25 fractions external beam irradiation to the pelvis, combined with five HDR fractions (5.5 to 6 Gy per fraction), or four fractions of HDR brachy-

therapy (6.5 to 7 Gy in each fraction). The equivalent LDR brachytherapy at point A is 80 Gy, with 67 Gy delivered to the bladder or the rectum, assuming that these tissues receive 70% of the prescribed point A dose. For advanced stages, such as IIB or IIIB, the intracavitary dose may be increased to 7.5 Gy per fraction, to have an LDR equivalent dose of 85 to 90 Gy to point A. Based on his preliminary results and published reports in the literature, Petereit recommended the doses and fractionation schedules summarized in Table 22.6.

The current GOG cervical cancer protocols allow HDR brachytherapy. The recommended treatment schedule is 5 fractions of 6 Gy in addition to EBRT. However, as the GOG has moved toward international accrual, differences in practice patterns, particularly for HDR brachytherapy, are being acknowledged and discussed. For example, Toita et al. from Japan have reported good results in their patients using significantly lower HDR doses (375). Whether this observation can be explained by anatomic variation, different tumor biology, or other reasons is not clear at this time. Many more clinical data with close observation and extended follow-up are needed to establish optimum brachytherapy treatment schedules using nonstandard dose rates.

HDR Techniques

Dose specification reporting systems for HDR brachytherapy vary by institution. However, many combine the Tod and Meredith point A as a paracervical dose, with ICRU Report No. 38 reporting of bladder and rectal points (333). *In vivo* bladder and rectal dosimetry is performed during the HDR procedure by Roman and colleagues (376). Other centers obtain normal tissue doses from points located on dosimetry films. Clinical experience has demonstrated that some method of increasing the distance from the HDR sources to the rectal wall is mandatory to keep rectal doses and subsequent sequelae at acceptable levels. Various techniques, including rectal retractors, vaginal speculums, gauze packing, and intravaginal Foley catheter balloons, are used to achieve this goal.

Institutions that favor multiple (8–12) fractions of HDR brachytherapy often use an intrauterine stent so that applica-

TABLE 22.6. *Current HDR fractionation schedules used at University of Wisconsin for treating cervical cancer*

Stage	Whole pelvis	5 HDR fractions (LDR equivalent)	Point A Gy$_{10}$	LQED
I/II nonbulky	45 Gy	5.5 (35)	96	80
I/II bulky	45 Gy	6.0 (40)	102	85
IIIB	50.4 Gy	6.0 (40)	109	90

LQED, Linear quadratic effective dose for a 2-Gy fraction.
From Stehman FB, Perez CA, Kurman RJ, et al. Uterine cervix. In Hoskins WJ, Perez CA, Young RC, eds. *Principles and Practice of Gynecologic Oncology*, 3rd ed. Philadelphia: Lippincott Williams & Wilkins, 2000:902.

tors can be placed quickly, without cervical dilatation, using little or no sedation (377). Treatment planning is performed on the initial insertion, and is duplicated for all fractions by verifying the applicator position with fluoroscopy or radiographs.

Interstitial Implants

The use of brachytherapy is a significant factor in the successful management of patients with advanced cervical cancers. When intracavitary implants are impossible, options include EBRT alone, with a cone-down technique and interstitial brachytherapy.

Prempree (378) reported a 96% local tumor control rate and 61% 5-year disease-free survival rate in 23 patients with stage IIIB carcinoma of the cervix treated with a combination of external irradiation and intracavitary and interstitial implant to the parametrium. They described a 23% local failure rate and a 69% 5-year survival rate in 26 patients with similar stage carcinoma of the cervix treated in the same manner, but in whom the uterine cavity could not be probed or was absent. Overall, major complications were noted in 8% of 49 patients.

Aristizabal and associates (379) treated 21 patients with locally advanced invasive carcinoma of the uterine cervix with transperineal interstitial implants. With a mean follow-up of 26 months, local tumor control was noted in 18 patients (85%). Seven patients (33%) developed grade 2 or 3 complications, which included one vesicovaginal fistula, one rectovaginal fistula, and one patient with both fistulae. Three patients developed severe radiation proctitis or cystitis, or both (one each). The loading of the obturator needles or the use of the central cylinder sources probably contributed to the relatively high incidence of complications. The authors have discontinued the use of the obturator surface needles, except when there is gross residual tumor in the central area. In a later report, these authors observed a reduction in the incidence of serious radiation side effects from 33% to 6% (380). A higher risk of major complications with parametrial implants has been observed in other large series (381,382). In a group of patients treated in a GOG study (302) of surgical staging, the frequency of distal (pelvic) adverse effects was not related to the operative approach, but of 19 patients treated with interstitial implants, 5 (26.3%) had fistulae, compared with 6.4% of the 265 patients treated with conventional techniques.

In contrast, Nag et al. reported the use of interstitial brachytherapy to treat 31 patients with cervical cancer and 8 patients with vaginal cancer in whom intracavitary applications were said to be unfeasible (383). Reasons given for this included extensive parametrial involvement, extensive vaginal involvement, and poor vaginal anatomy. It appears that in most cases the decision to use interstitial therapy was made without first attempting intracavitary therapy, or because of an expectation that patients, particularly those with lateral parametrial extension, would have better outcomes with this technique. With a median follow-up of 36 months, there was a 51% local control rate and 34% actuarial 5-year survival rate in patients with cervical cancer. The complication rate was low, at 2.5%. This is potentially an underestimate, since the minimum follow-up was only 12 months.

The Martinez Universal Perineal Template (MUPIT) was designed as a multi-site applicator for treating various perineal and gynecologic malignancies. Homogeneity is emphasized, but dose rates are moderately high compared to the Syed-Neblett Interstitial Template (SNIT). Using the MUPIT, Martinez and co-workers (384) treated 37 patients with advanced or recurrent carcinoma of the cervix, and 26 with vaginal-urethral tumors. Doses of approximately 35 Gy were given, in addition to external irradiation (36 Gy to the whole pelvis and 14 Gy to pelvic side wall). They reported six local failures in the patients with cervical lesions, and five in the group with vaginal-urethral tumors. Gupta et al. updated this series, finding a grade 4 complication rate of 14%, which is substantial, especially considering the relatively low doses used (median 71 Gy) (385). Complications were more frequent in patients in whom the dose rate exceeded 70 cGy per hour.

Unlike intracavitary applications, vaginal packing cannot be used with interstitial templates. However, by paying close attention to concepts of preplanning, dose homogeneity, dose rate, and careful execution, complication rates can be lessened. Efforts to refine the transperineal implant procedure have largely focused on improved real-time imaging technologies (386,387). The use of endorectal magnetic resonance coils and transrectal ultrasound has been reported to facilitate needle placement by improving visualization of tumor and normal tissues in relation to needle position. In some cases, this is done in conjunction with open laparotomy or laparoscopy.

Patients are typically selected for interstitial therapy on the basis of practical difficulties that preclude intracavitary therapy; thus, they may not be comparable to patients treated in a more conventional manner. However, until further improvements and better data supporting the efficiency and safety of this technique are available, its use in locally advanced cervical cancer should be only in exceptional circumstances, and by experienced brachytherapists.

Doses of Irradiation

Invasive carcinoma of the cervix is treated with a combination of whole pelvis, intracavitary, and at times, interstitial therapy. Some institutions use lower doses of whole-pelvis external irradiation (10 Gy for stage IB and 20 Gy for stages IIA, IIB, and III), in addition to parametrial doses to complete therapy with an MLS. This brings total doses to 50 Gy in stage IB and IIA, or 60 Gy to the involved parametrial tissues for more advanced stages.

Other institutions prefer higher doses of whole pelvis external irradiation (usually 40 Gy), delivered by AP-PA or four-field box technique. This is usually combined with one or two LDR intracavitary insertions for approximately 4500 to 6000 mg-hrs (40 to 55 Gy to point A), depending on tumor stage (volume). Usual doses to point A from both the external irradiation to the whole pelvis and the LDR intracavitary brachytherapy range from 70 Gy for small (≤1 cm) stage IB tumors, to 90–95 Gy for stage IIB or IIIB tumors. In some patients, an additional parametrial dose (with midline 5 HVL rectangular block) is administered in patients with IIB, III, or IVA tumors (considering the dose delivered to the side wall by the brachytherapy). In patients with only unilateral parametrial involvement, consideration should be given to boosting only the involved side.

In the postoperative setting, patients generally should not receive more than 45 Gy to the whole pelvis. Doses up to 50.4 Gy are acceptable when treating smaller fields that exclude more small bowel. Brachytherapy or small-field external beam boosts can be given, within tolerance, to increase dose to the central pelvis. Additional means of limiting toxicity may include intensity-modulated RT techniques, radioprotectors, or other methods. The impact of concurrent chemotherapy on complication rates appears to be limited, but continued follow-up and research are needed.

Intraoperative Radiation Therapy

Intraoperative RT (IORT) refers to direct irradiation of a tumor bed, facilitated by direct visualization of the target volume and manual displacement and/or shielding of the surrounding normal tissues. Because of the necessarily invasive nature of the procedure, IORT is typically limited to single-fraction treatments, with dose depending on a number of factors, including amount and depth of residual disease, location, proximity to dose-limiting structures (small bowel, plexus, rectum, or bladder), and the prior RT dose.

Usually doses between 10 and 20 Gy are delivered using electron beam therapy of different energies (388). Crude rates of grade 3 or higher toxicity are around 35% in patients treated with IORT. Common toxicities include peripheral nerve injury, gastrointestinal damage (obstruction, perforation, and fistula formation), and ureteral stenosis.

Altered Fractionation

Conventional RT schedules typically employ fraction sizes of 180–200 cGy, given 5 days per week over a number of weeks. Altered fractionation refers to the use of nonstandard dose and fractionation schedules. Radiobiological research and modeling suggest that these different fractionation schedules could favorably impact control rates, complication rates, or both. Examples include hypofractionation (larger doses per fraction, lower total dose), hyperfractionation (smaller doses per fraction given more frequently,

e.g., 2 to 3 fractions per day, to a slightly higher total dose), accelerated fractionation (standard fraction sizes given more frequently, e.g., twice daily), and concomitant boost techniques (a larger volume is treated in standard fashion, while part of the volume, typically gross tumor, is treated with an additional smaller fraction on the same day, separated by 4 to 6 hours).

Wang (389) reported that hyperfractionation in the treatment of patients with pelvic tumors (1.5 Gy per fraction twice daily for 15 days to deliver 45 Gy to the primary tumor and pelvic lymph nodes in combination with brachytherapy) was well tolerated. Tumor control or survival was not reported. Komaki et al published an RTOG study of hyperfractionation in FIGO stages IB (bulky) to IVA cervical carcinoma (390). The whole pelvis received 24–48 Gy at 1.2 Gy per fraction. With 81 evaluable patients and a median 42-month follow-up, the study revealed no improvement in local control or late effects, compared with historic RTOG controls.

Varghese et al. reported a randomized trial of standard (50 Gy/25 fractions) vs. hyperfractionated RT (60 Gy at 1.2 Gy b.i.d.) in locally advanced cervical cancer (391). With very limited follow-up, the authors reported a significantly higher incidence of acute reactions and treatment breaks in the hyperfractionated arm. The GOG conducted two Phase I dose escalation studies using hyperfractionated pelvic RT in conjunction with chemotherapy (either hydroxyurea or 5FU + cisplatin) (392). RT doses were escalated from 48 Gy/40 fractions to 52.8 Gy/44 fractions to 57.6 Gy/48 fractions. Although the RT was reasonably tolerated, the incidence of late complications reached nearly 13% at the highest dose level.

Thomas et al. randomized 234 patients to a four-arm study: standard RT, standard RT with 5FU, partially hyperfractionated RT (5280 cGy in 33 fractions, b.i.d., RT on first 4 and last 4 days of RT), and partially hyperfractionated RT with 5FU (393). No significant difference was seen in survival or pelvic control.

Use of the concomitant boost technique in cervical cancer was reported by Kavanagh et al., who conducted a prospective trial in 22 patients (394). Pelvic RT of 45 Gy/25 fractions was given, and a concomitant boost of 14.4 Gy/9 fractions was given to gross tumor during weeks 3 to 5. Standard LDR brachytherapy was also given. Although the local control and survival rates were higher than a matched control group, the incidence of late bowel toxicity was sufficient to diminish enthusiasm for this approach until methods of lowering toxicity can be established.

Pallative or Emergent Irradiation

The radiation or gynecologic oncologist is often faced with treating a patient who requires palliation of pelvic pain, obstruction, or bleeding. If vaginal bleeding is the main concern, a single intracavitary implant with tandem and colpostats, about 50–55 Gy, to point A suffices. If the patients had prior RT, lower intracavitary doses should be prescribed (35–40 Gy) to point A. Alternatively, bleeding can be controlled by more conservative measures, such as vaginal packing, followed by the immediate institution of EBRT. In this circumstance, it can be appropriate to treat a slightly smaller pelvic volume and use doses per fraction slightly higher than standard, e.g., 250–300 cGy, allowing patients with localized disease to be approached with curative intent, without an excessive risk of complications.

Patients with stage IVB or incurable recurrent carcinoma often require palliation of pelvic pain or bleeding, and their general condition may not warrant a prolonged course of external irradiation. Short course, high-dose fractionation schedules with EBRT have been used, including 2 to 3 10-Gy fractions, with an interval of 4–6 weeks between courses, resulting in significant palliation in selected patients with advanced gynecologic malignancies. Although the response rate was 41% for patients completing the 3 courses, the actuarial incidence of grade 3–4 late gastrointestinal toxicity was unacceptable (45%) (395).

Spanos et al. reported on a Phase II study of daily multifraction split-course irradiation in patients with recurrent or metastatic pelvic malignancies (396). Irradiation consisted of 3.7 Gy per fraction given twice daily for two consecutive days, repeated at 3- to 6-week intervals for a total of 3 courses, to a total tumor dose of 44.4 Gy. Complete tumor response was noted in 15 patients (10.5%), and partial response in 32 (22.5%). In patients completing 3 courses of irradiation, the rate of complete or partial response was 45%. Twenty-seven patients survived longer than one year. The actuarial late complications rate was 5% at 12 months.

Subsequently, Spanos (397) reported for the Radiation Therapy Oncology Group on a Phase III study of accelerated split-course palliative irradiation in 284 patients. Patients received three courses of 14.8 Gy in four fractions over 2 days, with a rest of 2 to 4 weeks between courses, up to 44.4 Gy total dose. There were 136 patients randomized to rest periods of 2 or 4 weeks. There was a trend toward increased acute toxicity in patients with shorter rest periods (5 of 68, versus 0 of 68; $p = 0.07$). Late toxicity was not significantly different in the two groups, although length of follow-up was not sufficient to accurately assess it. Pelvic tumor response was comparable in both groups (34% versus 26%). More patients in the 2-week rest period group completed the three courses of therapy, but the most significant predictor for completion of therapy was Karnofsky Performance Status of 80 or higher. This schedule offers significant logistic benefits, and has been shown to result in good tumor regression and excellent palliation of symptoms.

CHEMOTHERAPY

Chemotherapy is increasingly utilized in the management of cervical cancer, both in primary management and for re-current and metastatic disease. Reviews have indicated that several chemotherapeutic agents from different classes are active in this disease (398,399). Conventional agents able to induce a response rate of at least 20% in measurable disease include cisplatin, ifosfamide, dibromodulcitol, porfiromycin, epirubicin, vindesine, chlorambucil, mitomycin C, and melphalan.

COMBINED MODALITIES

Invasive Carcinoma Treated with a Simple Hysterectomy

Given the frequency of simple hysterectomy or total abdominal hysterectomy (type I), it is not surprising that occasionally a patient is found to have an invasive cervical cancer unrecognized prior to surgery. Although this occurs uncommonly in an era of cytologic screening, it can occur in patients operated on for what is felt to be carcinoma *in situ*, ''microinvasive'' disease, or for ''benign'' indications.

If only microinvasive carcinoma is found, with no evidence of lymphatic-vascular space involvement, no additional therapy is necessary. However, in patients with more advanced disease, simple extrafascial abdominal hysterectomy is not curative, because the paravaginal/paracervical soft tissue, vaginal cuff, and pelvic lymph nodes are not removed.

It may be technically difficult to perform an adequate radical operation after previous simple hysterectomy, but this alternative deserves consideration for selected patients. Orr et al. advocated performing radical parametrectomy, upper vaginectomy, and pelvic lymphadenectomy in this settting. In 23 patients with negative margins after their initial surgery, completing the operation in this fashion found that 74% had no residual tumor, and none of the cancers recurred within 2 years. Of the 6 patients with residual, only 1 died of recurrent disease (400). Chapman et al. reported similar results in 18 patients with clear surgical margins and no apparent disease who underwent second operations. Three patients received RT for residual disease found during the reoperation (401). Both series reported acceptable acute and late morbidity with this approach.

Other authors have reported higher rates of failure and more significant complications. For example, in Kinney's series, reoperation documented residual disease in 4 of 27 patients, all of whom died of disease. Furthermore, there were 2 pelvic recurrences among the 23 patients in whom no additional tumor was found. In this series, the incidences of chronic lymphedema, urinary incontinence, and fistula formation diminished enthusiasm for reoperation (402).

Another approach favored by some is the use of adjuvant pelvic RT in patients with invasive disease of severity greater than microinvasive. Ampil and co-workers (403) described the results in 44 patients receiving postoperative irradiation after hysterectomy. Their results were similar, whether external irradiation was used alone or in combination with intracavitary therapy. They did not document an advantage in local control or 5-year survival rate with total external therapy doses greater than 40 Gy, compared with doses of less than 40 Gy ($p > 0.4$).

Andras and associates (404) treated 148 patients, and reported survival rates similar to those of the intact uterus when small volume disease is present in the surgical specimen. Patients with presumed microscopic residual disease did as well as patients treated initially in a stage-appropriate manner when postoperative irradiation was given.

Hopkins and colleagues (295), in a series of 92 patients treated with hysterectomy, noted a 5-year survival rate of 80% for squamous-cell carcinoma (64 patients) and 41% for adenocarcinoma (28 patients). Seven had parametrial involvement. Patients with squamous-cell carcinoma and less than 50% cervical invasion had a 96% survival rate, compared with 75% with more than 50% penetration. These authors reported 88% survival in patients receiving postoperative irradiation, compared with 69% in patients observed after surgery ($p = 0.10$). Significant complications related to irradiation occurred in 11 of 78 patients (14%), with a greater incidence noted in patients receiving over 80 Gy. The authors concluded that patients treated with standard hysterectomy and postoperative irradiation have a similar prognosis, but more complications than those treated initially with either radical surgery or irradiation.

Heller and associates (294) and Hopkins and colleagues (295) attempted to use retrospective FIGO staging to evaluate these patients. Patients with presumed IB disease had a 5-year survival rate of 78% with combined therapy. Those with presumed stage IIB disease had a 5-year survival rate of 67%. A significant difference in cumulative 5-year survival rate was observed between the patients with squamous-cell carcinoma (80%) and those with adenocarcinoma (41%, $p = 0.0001$). Others have not found such a difference based on histology (405).

Crane and Scheider published a retrospective series of 18 patients (405). In 4 patients, there remained gross residual, and 2 additional patients were left with microscopic residual at the resection margin (1 of these also had a positive lymph node), making this patient population relatively unfavorable compared to published experiences with reoperation. All patients were treated with adjuvant RT. Six had only external RT, and 12 had brachytherapy boosts to the vaginal cuff. One patient received chemo-radiation. With a median follow-up of 42 months, 5- and 10-year local control rates were 88%, and 5- and 10-year survival rates were 93%. Only 1 of 4 patients with gross residual relapsed, and 1 patient developed a significant late morbidity, a small bowel obstruction requiring surgery. Because patients with residual disease do poorly with this approach in comparison to RT, and patients with minimal, if any, disease do equally well with RT at a lower morbidity cost, these authors question the role of

reoperation. Therefore, they argue that adjuvant RT is the treatment of choice in these patients.

If the postoperative RT approach is chosen, postoperative irradiation should be administered immediately after recovery from operation, as prognosis is much worse if therapy is delayed (406,407). When there is gross tumor present in the vaginal vault, external irradiation to the whole pelvis (40–45 Gy) is required. In some cases, a small external beam boost might be advisable for an additional 10–15 Gy. An intracavitary insertion, as outlined previously, should be performed (35–60 Gy mucosal dose). If there is residual tumor, an interstitial implant, when feasible, should be carried out to increase the dose to this volume. The brachytherapist should note the possibility that small bowel is adherent to the vaginal cuff in the hysterectomized patient, representing a risk factor for complications with interstitial implants. Laparotomy or laparoscopy can be helpful in guiding the implant in these circumstances.

The potential contribution of concurrent platinum-based chemotherapy must be considered, particularly in view of the randomized study of patients treated after radical hysterectomy with high-risk features (256) (Fig. 22.15). Although not directly comparable, it is reasonable to extrapolate these results favoring concurrent chemotherapy to patients treated after simple hysterectomy for invasive disease, particularly in patients with gross residual, positive margins, positive nodes, lymphovascular space invasion, and, possibly, adenocarcinoma.

Adjuvant Hysterectomy after Radiation Therapy

Bulky endocervical tumors and the so-called barrel-shaped cervix have a higher incidence of central recurrence, pelvic and paraaortic lymph node metastasis, and distant dissemination (408). Early impetus for planned combined therapy for selected patients with cervical carcinoma was given by a series of articles from the M. D. Anderson Cancer Center (408–410). A greater incidence of failure was associated with lesions that expanded the isthmus of the cervix to 6 cm or greater. Patients who had planned extrafascial (type I) hysterectomy after RT had few central failures, but overall survival rates were only slightly affected. Jampolis and coworkers (408) examined factors associated with central failure. The limitation of brachytherapy doses with regard to the isthmus of the cervix and fundus and the ability of extrafascial hysterectomy to substitute for a second brachytherapy application appear to be supported by these reports.

Though some nonrandomized studies have shown a survival advantage for the patients who underwent adjuvant hysterectomy (172,411), other nonrandomized studies have shown no advantage for the combined modality approach (412,413). Perez et al. retrospectively compared RT alone (n = 892) with combined RT plus surgery (n = 306) (414). Patients treated with RT alone received combined external RT and brachytherapy dose of 70–85 Gy at point A for stages IB and IIA lesions, and 80–90 Gy for bulky tumors and IIB lesions. In patients receiving combined therapy, RT consisted of external and intracavitary RT of 60–70 Gy at point A. Cause-specific survivals (CSS) were equivalent with the two treatment approaches. Ten-year survival rate was 84% for IB patients, irrespective of treatment approach. For non-bulky stage IIA tumors treated with RT alone and with combined RT and surgery, the CSS was 66% and 71%, respectively. In the group with bulky stage IIA lesions, the CSS was 69% and 44% among patients treated with RT alone and with combined therapy, respectively ($p < 0.05$). Toxicities were comparable.

Thoms (415) and Eifel (246) and their associates at the M. D. Anderson Cancer Center carefully evaluated 1,526 patients, 371 of whom had lesions 6 cm or greater. They acknowledged numerous biases in treatment selection, but noted a statistically significantly higher survival rate at 10 years for patients treated with irradiation and surgery (64% vs. 45%). Tumor diameter was highly significant as a prognostic factor, and they concluded that only patients with lesions greater than 8 cm in diameter benefit from adjuvant hysterectomy.

Gallion and associates (411) reported on 75 patients with stage I disease that was greater than 5 cm in size, or barrel-shaped, or treated with either radiation therapy alone, or combined with extrafascial hysterectomy. Recurrent cancer was noted in 47% of patients treated with irradiation alone, compared with 16% of those treated with combined therapy ($p < 0.01$). The incidence of pelvic recurrence was reduced from 19% to 2%, and the incidence of extrapelvic recurrence from 16% to 7%. Einhorn and colleagues (416) found that as size of primary tumor increased, a progressively increasing

survival advantage was confirmed by combined therapy consisting of intracavitary irradiation followed by radical hysterectomy.

Perez and colleagues (414) found that tumors that do not regress promptly are more likely to recur. Morphologically persistent cancer in the surgical specimen at adjunctive hysterectomy was found to be a prognostically ominous sign by Russell and co-workers (417). Maruyama and associates (418) found an insignificant difference in tumor-free survival between patients with and without persistence at the time of hysterectomy.

The GOG performed a randomized trial in which 256 eligible patients with carcinomas of the cervix ≥4 cm were treated with either external beam and intracavitary irradiation, or with a slightly lower dose of intracavitary irradiation and the same external beam pelvic irradiation followed by an extrafascial hysterectomy (419). The survival rates were virtually identical in the irradiation alone and the combined irradiation and surgery groups (Fig. 22.26). The incidence of progression was somewhat higher in the irradiation alone group (46%), in comparison with the combined therapy group (37%) ($p = 0.07$). The reduction in the risk of progression or death for the combined treatment group was 23%, in comparison to the RT only group. In the irradiation alone group, the incidence of local recurrence at 5 years was 27%, and in the combined-therapy group it was 14% (Fig. 22.27). The distant metastasis rates were 16% and 20%, respectively. When analyzing the results of this study according to tumor size, the GOG study found that patients with tumor sizes of 4, 5, and 6 cm had an improved progression-free survival with combined therapy ($p = 0.06$), and a significant improvement in survival ($p = 0.007$) (419). Although ran-

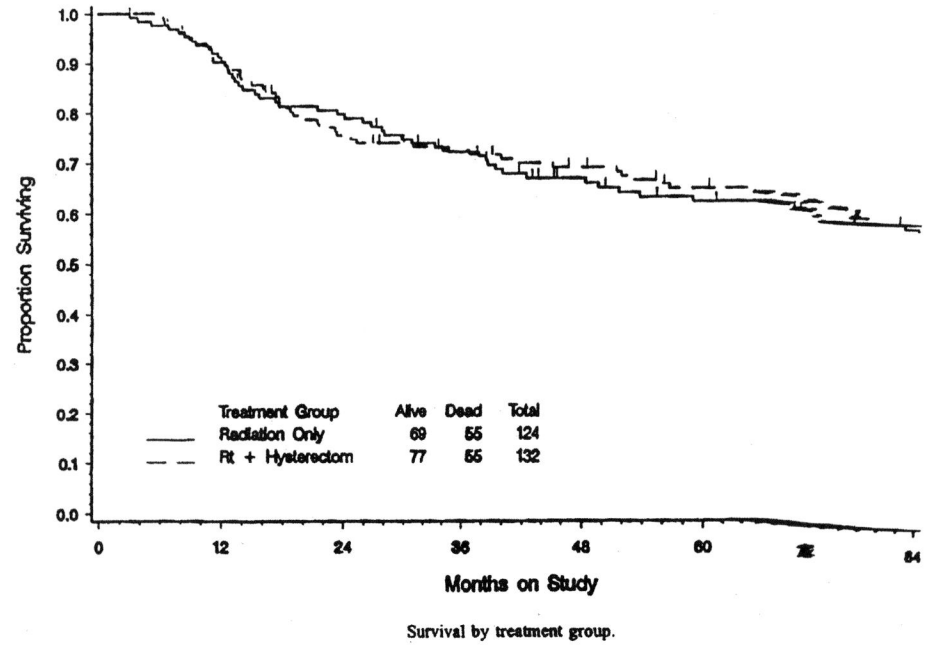

FIG. 22.26. Survival by treatment group for 2 treatment regimens: radiation only, and RT + hysterectomy. (From Keys HM, Bundy BN, Stehman FB, et al. Radiation therapy with and without extrafascial hysterectomy for bulky stage IB cervical carcinoma: a randomized trial of the Gynecologic Oncology Group. *Gynecol Oncol* 2003;89:348.)

Survival by treatment group.

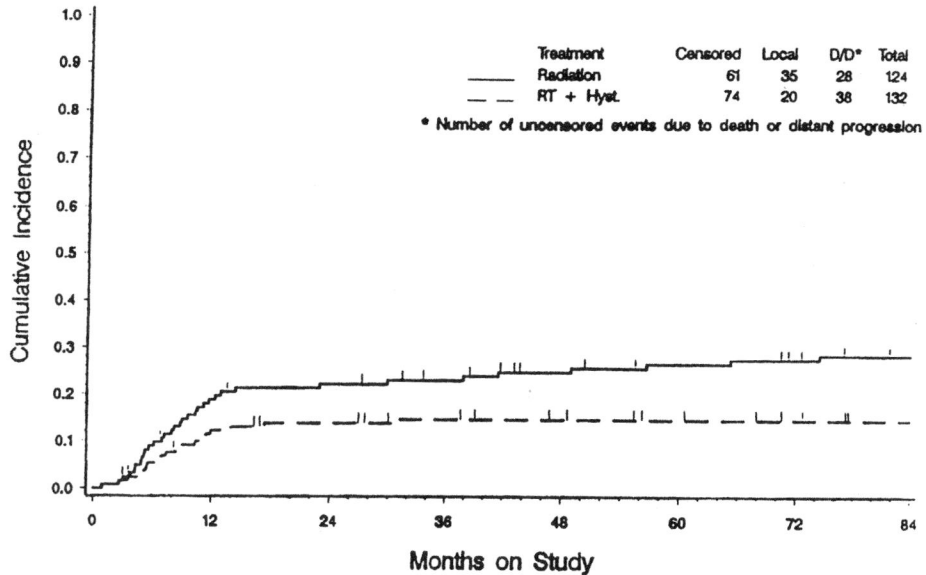

FIG. 22.27. Cumulative incidence of local relapse by treatment group (radiation and RT + hysterectomy). (From Keys HM, Bundy BN, Stehman FB, et al. Radiation therapy with and without extrafascial hysterectomy for bulky stage IB cervical carcinoma: a randomized trial of the Gynecologic Oncology Group. *Gynecol Oncol* 2003;89:349.)

domized, this study could be criticized for the relatively low point A doses given in the RT alone group (87% received 78 Gy or more), and the extended treatment times (49% completed RT within 60 days).

Interpretation of the literature regarding "bulky" stage IB cervical cancers can be difficult because of the variable definitions that have been used. Furthermore, selection bias is likely operative in retrospective series because unfavorable primary tumors that fail to adequately regress might be more likely to receive combined therapy. At the same time, patients with significant comorbid illness or other adverse factors (e.g., evidence of adenopathy) would be more likely to have RT alone. However, given the results of the GOG study, it appears that surgery does not contribute to increased survival compared to RT alone in patients with "bulky" stage IB disease. A favorable impact on the local recurrence rate is likely, and an improvement in survival for patients with tumors 4–6 cm in diameter is suggested.

Adjuvant Postoperative Pelvic RT

The most common failure pattern following radical surgery for cervical carcinoma is pelvic relapse. Factors predicting a higher failure rate include positive lymph nodes, a large primary tumor, involved surgical margins, lymphovascular space invasion, and depth of stromal invasion. The use of adjuvant RT has a long history in patients with risk factors for recurrence. The difficulty comes in defining a patient population at sufficient risk to warrant adjuvant RT, recognizing that many patients' tumors will not recur, even with no further therapy, and that patients with more advanced disease (especially involved lymph nodes) are at considerable risk of distant spread. More recently, the role of chemotherapy has become better established.

Conventional wisdom, retrospective data, and now pro-spective data suggest that adjuvant pelvic RT significantly improves pelvic control rates in patients with risk factors for recurrence who have completed radical surgery, which will likely translate to a survival benefit in an appropriately selected patient population.

Involved Pelvic Lymph Nodes

Metastatic disease in the pelvic lymph nodes is a poor prognostic sign. Pelvic nodal metastases may be associated with lesion size (28,177,178), deep stromal invasion (177, 178), and involvement of capillary or lymphatic vascular spaces (177). Postoperative pelvic radiation therapy has been advocated in the presence of these prognostic factors. No controlled studies show improved survival or pelvic control with postoperative pelvic RT in this circumstance.

Bianchi and colleagues observed a 65% 5-year survival rate in 60 patients who received external irradiation for pelvic node metastasis after radical hysterectomy (420). In contrast, in 15 patients who refused postoperative irradiation, only 3 survived 5 years (20%). The improvement in survival was particularly noticeable in the stage II patients. When pelvic irradiation was given after radical hysterectomy, the major complication rate was 21.1%, in comparison with 19.8% when hysterectomy was preceded by an intracavitary radium application, or 10.5% with surgery alone.

Kinney and colleagues (421) compared the results of therapy in 82 patients with stages IB and IIA carcinoma of the cervix found to have pelvic lymph node metastases at radical hysterectomy and bilateral lymphadenectomy without additional adjuvant therapy to a group of 103 similar patients who received 50 Gy to the pelvis postoperatively. From these 185 patients, 60 pairs matched for stage, tumor size, and number and location of positive nodes were analyzed. The 5-year survival rate was 72% for the surgery only group, and 64% for the group receiving adjuvant RT. The incidence of pelvic recurrences was 67% in the surgery only group, and 27% among patients receiving adjuvant irradiation. The lack of impact on overall survival is most likely related to the higher incidence of distant metastases in the irradiated patients.

Fuller and co-workers (422) treated 71 patients after radical hysterectomy who had positive pelvic lymph nodes with postoperative irradiation (40 Gy in 4 weeks). In 32 patients with one or two positive nodes, the 5-year survival rate in the irradiated group was slightly higher than in the non-irradiated group (about 60% and 40%, respectively). Lower survival was observed in seven patients with three or more involved nodes who received postoperative irradiation.

Stock et al. (423) analyzed the outcomes of 143 patients with stages I and II cervical carcinoma who underwent radical hysterectomy and lymph node dissection, and were found to have positive pelvic lymph nodes. Whole pelvic RT was administered in 108 patients, while 35 were observed. Patients receiving RT experienced significantly higher disease-free survival, overall survival, and pelvic control, compared to patients receiving no adjuvant therapy. Interestingly, relapse limited to the paraaortic chain occurred in 10%.

Soisson et al. analyzed 320 women who underwent radical surgery for stages IB and IIA cervical cancer (424). Postoperative RT was indicated and completed in 72 patients (22%). Nodal metatstases, tumor size >4 cm, histologic grade, race, and age >40 years were adverse prognostic factors for the entire group. Although it was recognized that the groups receiving and not receiving adjuvant RT were substantially different in risk profile, it was suggested that adjuvant RT did not improve survival in patients with unilateral nodal metastases or patients with large primary tumors with negative margins and no adenopathy. However, RT improved pelvic control, and GI and GU complications were not significantly different in the 2 groups. Systemic failure was the most common site of failure.

Hart et al. (425) reviewed 83 patients who received postoperative RT based on surgicopathologic risk factors. All patients received pelvic RT, followed by a brachytherapy boost using either LDR or HDR techniques. Five-year disease-free survivals were 89% and 72% for the LDR and HDR groups, respectively. Overall, pelvic control was 90%. Follow-up was much shorter for the HDR group as compared to the LDR group.

Fiorca et al. reviewed 50 patients who received RT following radical surgery (426). Most patients had multiple risk factors for recurrence, including lymph node metastases, large tumor, deep cervical stromal involvement, lower uterine segment involvement, and capillary-lymphatic space involvement. Actuarial survival and disease-free survival were 90% and 87%, respectively, at 70 months follow-up. The 10% risk of major GI complications was considered reasonable, in view of the potential benefit suggested.

An intergroup study was conducted by the Southwest On-cology Group (SWOG), GOG, and RTOG in women with FIGO stages IA$_2$, IB, or IIA carcinoma of the cervix found to have metastatic disease in the pelvic lymph nodes, positive parametrial involvement, or positive surgical margins at time of primary radical hysterectomy, and total pelvic lymphadenectomy with confirmed negative paraaortic lymph nodes (256). Eighty-five percent of patients accrued on this study were eligible based on pelvic node involvement. One hundred twenty-seven patients were randomized between pelvic external beam radiation therapy with 5-FU infusion and cisplatin, and 116 were treated with pelvic external beam irradiation alone. The median follow-up for survivors was 43 months. The 3-year survival on the adjuvant cisplatin/5-fluorouracil and irradiation arm was 87%, compared with 77% on the pelvic irradiation arm. The difference is statistically significant. Chemotherapy appeared to reduce both pelvic and extrapelvic recurrences. Acute toxicities were more common in the chemotherapy arm. Only 5% of patients accrued to this intergroup study had positive margins, probably because of the reluctance of clinicians to put these patients on a trial that did not allow brachytherapy boosts.

Close or Positive Margins

Estape et al. retrospectively analyzed 51 patients with close vaginal surgical margins following radical hysterectomy (defined as ≤ 5mm) (427). Twenty-three patients with negative nodes and close vaginal margins were studied. Although the 16 patients receiving RT had a preponderance of other risk factors, recurrence rates (12.5% vs 85.7%) and 5-year survival rates (81.3% vs 28.6%) significantly favored the group receiving adjuvant pelvic RT.

Kim and associates (428) described results on 38 patients receiving postoperative pelvic irradiation after radical hysterectomy for close surgical margins and/or metastatic pelvic lymph nodes. Patients with close surgical margins were treated with intracavitary vaginal ovoid insertions. Patients with positive margins fell into 2 groups: those with positive parametrial margins and those with involved vaginal margins. All 5 patients with involved parametrial margins treated with only cuff brachytherapy suffered local failures, compared with no pelvic failure in similarly treated patients with only vaginal margins positive for tumor. The authors recommended vaginal intracavitary irradiation alone only for those patients with carcinoma in situ (or, in our opinion, with minimally invasive carcinoma) at the vaginal margin of resection as the only risk factor. Figure 22.28 provides a possible explanation for this finding. In a postoperative RT series, Snijders-Keilholz et al. (429) reported that in only 1 of 17 patients with positive resection margins and in 2 of 6 with involved parametria did disease recur in the pelvis following adjuvant pelvic RT.

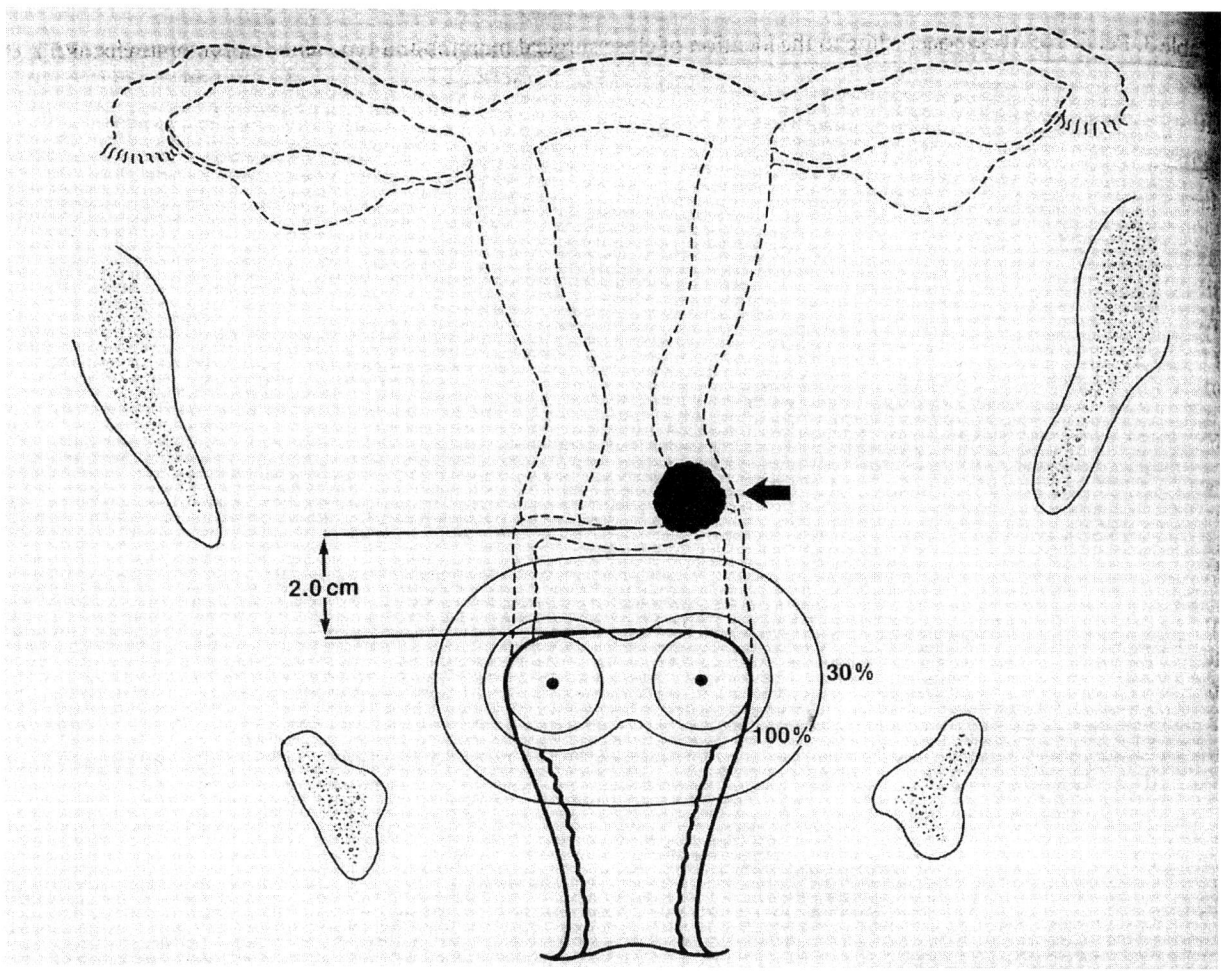

FIG. 22.28. Isodose line of vaginal ovoid irradiation in patient with radical hysterectomy. Note that shortened vagina is away from parametrial tissue (close paracervical margin, which is getting less than 30% of the tumor dose). (From Kim RY, Salter MM, Shingleton HM. Adjuvant postoperative radiation therapy following radical hysterectomy in stage IB carcinoma of the cervix: analysis of treatment failure. *Int J Radiat Oncol Biol Phys* 1988;14:445.)

Other Indications

Patients with negative nodes but other risk factors may benefit from adjuvant therapy (430). Large tumor size (>4 cm), deep cervical stromal invasion, or capillary-lymphatic space involvement without positive nodes is associated with increased tumor recurrence (177,178,424). In Alvarez's study (178), high-risk patients had a 13% survival, intermediate-risk patients had 56%-70% survival, and low-risk patients had 92% survival. It is possible that patients with multiple intermediate-risk factors may be at greater risk than patients with a single positive node (176).

Evidence to support adjuvant RT in high-risk, node-negative patients was presented by Snijders-Keilholz et al. (429). Ten patients had very significant risk profiles (capillary-lymphatic space invasion, tumor >4 cm, and high grade histology, or tumor size >4 cm and stromal invasion >15 mm). The authors reported no recurrences in this group, although the expected recurrence rate was 30–40% based on the GOG criteria (177).

Boronow reported a survival rate of 71.3% in patients with tumors greater than 6 cm who were treated initially with radical hysterectomy and postoperative RT and chemotherapy in all cases (431). Complications were reported to be minimal.

The GOG conducted a Phase III trial comparing radical hysterectomy alone with radical hysterectomy and postoperative pelvic RT in patients with node-negative stage IB cervical carcinomas, with prognostic features correlated with an intermediate risk of recurrence (approximately 30%) (328). Eligibility criteria for this study are given in Table 22.7. There were 277 patients randomized after radical hysterectomy: 137 to pelvic RT, and 140 to no further therapy. RT consisted of 46–50.4 Gy to a whole pelvic field. No brachytherapy was used. After a median follow-up of five years for living patients, recurrence was observed in 28% of

TABLE 22.7. *GOG 92 eligibility criteria*

CLS (*Capillary lymphatic space involvement*)	Stromal invasion	Tumor size
Positive	Deep 1/3	Any
Positive	Middle 1/3	≥2 cm
Positive	Superficial 1/3	≥5 cm
Negative	Deep or middle 1/3	≥4 cm

the patients in the control group, and in 15% of the radiated patients. There was a statistically significant reduction in the risk of recurrence (relative risk = 0.53, p = 0.008) in the irradiated group. Cox model analysis adjusting for risk factor combinations indicated that the risk of recurrence was decreased by 44% in the RT arm. A trend toward lower mortaliy with RT was observed, but had not reached statistical significance at the time of publication. Russell pointed out that more than 1 in 6 patients randomized to RT either refused treatment, or were substantially noncompliant, but were still analyzed in the RT arm, according to the intent-to-treat principle (432). While statistically appropriate, this methodology potentially underestimates therapeutic benefit. Severe or life-threatening adverse effects were observed in 7% of the radiated patients, versus 2.1% of the controls. Since many patients in this study had bulky tumors, typically indicating postoperative RT, a reasonable question posed by Russell is whether it is advisable to attempt radical surgery rather than primary RT in this patient population, since the complication rate will increase with the use of 2 treatment modalities rather than 1 (432).

Role of Chemotherapy

More than one-third of patients who suffer recurrences will develop extrapelvic disease (433,434). Early attempts to improve outcomes by using systemic therapies were generally unsuccessful. Curtin et al. (435) reported results from a Phase III randomized trial, comparing adjuvant sequential chemoradiation vs. RT alone following radical hysterectomy in high-risk stages IB-IIA cervical cancer. At a median follow-up of 36 months, there were no significant differences in recurrence rates or patterns of recurrences among the two treatment groups.

As mentioned, an intergroup study tested the addition of chemotherapy to pelvic RT in women with FIGO stages IA$_2$, IB, or IIA carcinoma of the cervix found to have metastatic disease in the pelvic lymph nodes, positive parametrial involvement, or positive surgical margins at time of primary radical hysterectomy (256). Patients randomized to pelvic EBRT with 5-FU infusion and cisplatin had a significantly improved 3-year survival rate of 87%, compared with 77% for women given only pelvic RT.

Strong consideration should be given to the use of concurrent chemotherapy with radiation therapy in women with stages I-IIA disease who have metastatic disease in the pelvic lymph nodes, positive parametrial disease, or positive surgical margins at the time of primary surgery.

Brachytherapy Alone

Kim and associates (428) recommended vaginal intracavitary irradiation alone only for those patients with carcinoma *in situ* (or, in our opinion, with minimally invasive carcinoma) at the vaginal margin of resection as the only risk factor.

Photopulos et al. reported 17 surgically treated node-negative patients with more than 50% cervical stromal invasion (436). Because of the perceived risk of local recurrence, vaginal cuff brachytherapy was given as the sole adjuvant treatment. With a mean follow-up of 39 months, no recurrence had been seen. Two patients with similar features who refused treatment suffered local recurrences. No morbidity was attributable to the brachytherapy.

Outpatient HDR brachytherapy is particularly suited for cervical cancer patients because it prevents the prolonged immobilization required for LDR brachytherapy. At Mallinckrodt Institute of Radiology, patients are treated with HDR brachytherapy with colpostats or a vaginal cylinder placed in the patient before each treatment with sedation and without anesthesia. An indwelling bladder catheter is used during the procedure, and gentle packing of the vagina with iodoform gauze helps to maintain the placement of the applicators. The position of the applicator(s) is verified with AP and lateral pelvic radiographs taken before the actual HDR treatment in each application. The usual dose per fraction prescribed at 0.5 cm depth is 6 to 7 Gy; three fractions are given 1 or 2 weeks apart.

Chemotherapy in Combinations for Localized Carcinoma of the Cervix

Concurrent Chemotherapy with Radiation Therapy

Although radiation therapy has maintained its place as the cornerstone of therapy for cervical cancer for nearly a century, local tumor control and cure rates are still considered inadequate, particularly in patients with larger lesions. Therefore, attempts have been made to improve the outcomes achievable to date. The most promising approach to date is concurrent chemotherapy and radiation.

The rationale for concomitant chemoradiation is twofold: (1) to increase the sensitivity of the tumor to the effects of the irradiation and (2) to eradicate microscopic systemic disease. A number of prospective trials have suggested that chemotherapy, particularly platinum-based, given concurrently with RT significantly improves outcomes, compared to RT alone.

Reports of concurrent chemotherapy with irradiation in

locally advanced disease have shown improved outcomes. These results have been confirmed in a number of randomized prospective trials: three by the GOG (265,266,437), one by the combined efforts of the GOG and the Southwest Oncology Group (SWOG) (256) and one by the RTOG (264). These five trials are all positive in favor of concurrent chemoradiation over radiation alone in most patients with stages IB-IVA disease (Table 22.8).

Whitney compared pelvic RT plus hydroxyurea versus 5-fluorouracil during pelvic irradiation in patients with inoperable stages IIB-IVA cervical cancer with negative paraaortic nodes (265). On both regimens, stage IIB patients received 40.8 Gy external beam therapy, followed by 40 Gy to point A, with 1 to 2 intracavitary implants. A parametrial boost to bring the dose to point B to 55 Gy was given if necessary. Patients with stages IIIB or IVA disease received 51 Gy EBRT, followed by 30 Gy to point A by 1–2 intracavitary implants, and a total of 60 Gy to point B with a parametrial boost if necessary. Patients assigned to hydroxyurea received 80 mg/kg twice weekly during EBRT. Those assigned to cisplatin plus 5-fluorouracil received cisplatin 50 mg/m^2 on days 1 and 29, and continuous infusion of 5-fluorouracil, 1000 mg/m^2/day on days 2–5 and days 30–33 of the EBRT. Of 368 patients, 177 were randomized to cisplatin plus 5-fluorouracil, and 191 to hydroxyurea. At a median of 8.7 years of follow-up for the survivors, the cisplatin/5-fluorouracil/radiation regimen demonstrated a superior progression-free survival ($p = 0.033$), with a 21% reduction in risk of progression or death (RR = 0.79). Survival was similarly superior for the cisplatin/5-fluorouracil/radiation regimen ($p = 0.018$), with a 26% reduction in risk of death (RR = 0.74).

The subsequent GOG study, #120, compared 3 different treatments: (1) RT plus weekly cisplatin vs. (2) RT plus cisplatin, 5-FU, and hydroxyurea vs. (3) RT plus hydroxyurea in patients with negative paraaortic nodes, and stages IIB, III, or IVA carcinoma of the cervix (the same population as that studied in GOG Protocol 85) (266). Radiation was given in all three arms in the same fashion as that described above for GOG Protocol 85. Patients assigned to hydroxyurea received 3 gm/m^2 twice weekly for six weeks during EBRT. Those assigned to cisplatin plus 5-fluorouracil plus hydroxyurea received cisplatin, 50 mg/m^2 on days 1 and 22, continuous infusion of 5-fluorouracil, 1000 mg/m^2/day days 2–5 and 23–26; and hydroxyurea 2 gm/m^2 twice weekly for six weeks during the EBRT. Those assigned to weekly cisplatin received cisplatin 40 mg/m^2 weekly for six weeks during the course of EBRT.

Of 526 patients, 173 were assigned randomly to cisplatin plus 5-FU plus hydroxyurea, 176 to weekly cisplatin, and 177 to hydroxyurea. At a median of 35 months of follow-up, both platinum-based regimens demonstrated a superior progression-free survival ($p < 0.001$), with a 43% reduction in risk of progression or death (RR = 0.57) for those treated with weekly cisplatin, and a 45% reduction (RR = 0.55) for those receiving the three-drug regimen. Survival was similarly superior for the weekly cisplatin regimen ($p = 0.004$), with a 39% reduction in risk of death (RR = 0.61), and, for the three-drug regimen, ($p = 0.002$) a 42% reduction in risk of death (RR = 0.58) (266). These results confirm the observations in GOG Protocol 85 for those patients with stages IIB-IVA disease.

The RTOG randomly selected patients with stages IB-IVA carcinoma of the cervix to radiation alone, or concurrently with cisplatin plus 5-FU (264). Unlike the GOG trials, not all patients had surgical staging of the paraaortic lymph nodes. On both arms of the study, patients received external beam radiation to the pelvis to a dose of 45 Gy. Those assigned to radiation alone also received 45 Gy to the paraaortic lymph nodes. Both arms received intracavitary radiation designed to deliver a total of 85 Gy to point A. Those assigned to receive cisplatin plus 5-FU received cisplatin 75

TABLE 22.8. *Chemoradiation in patients with cervical cancer: results of six randomized trials*

Trial Author	FIGO stage	Number of patients	Treatment regimen	Follow-up	Median 3-year survival (%)
Whitney et al (265)	IIB-IVA	177	EB + ICRT + PF	8.7 years	67
		191	EB + ICRT + HU		57
Morris et al (264)	IIB-IVA	195	EB + ICRT + PF	43 months	75
		193	EB + ICRT		63
Peters (256)	IA2-IIA	127	EB + PF	42 months	87
		116	EB		77
Rose (266)	IIB-IVA	176	EB + ICRT + P	35 months	65
		173	EB + ICRT + PFHU		65
		177	EB + ICRT + HU		47
Keys (437)	IB2 (> 4 cm)	183	EB + ICRT + P + S	36 months	83
		186	EB + ICRT + S		74
Pearcey (439)	IB (> 5 cm) – IVA	127	EB + ICRT + P	64 months	69
		126	EB + ICRT		66

EB = external beam, ICRT = intracavitary radiation therapy, P = cisplatin, F = 5-fluorouracil, HU = hydroxyurea, S = surgery.

mg/m^2 on day 1 every three weeks, followed by 5-FU 1000 mg/m^2/day for four days as a continuous intravenous infusion.

Of 388 patients, 193 were assigned randomly to radiation alone, and the other 195 to cisplatin plus 5-FU plus radiation. At a median of 43 months of follow-up, those receiving concurrent chemoradiation demonstrated a superior progression-free survival (p <0.001), with a 52% reduction in risk of progression or death (RR = 0.48). Survival was also superior for concurrent chemoradiation (p = 0.004), with a 41% reduction in risk of death (RR = 0.59). The rates of both locoregional and distant relapses were significantly reduced (RR = 0.47 and 0.39, respectively) by concurrent chemoradiation as compared to radiation alone. This study suggests that concurrent chemoradiation is the treatment of choice not only for stages IIB-IVA disease, as was suggested by the two GOG studies, but also for stages IB-IIA.

The GOG performed a randomized study of patients with stages IB-IIA carcinoma of the cervix. The treatment arms were radiation alone, or RT concurrently with weekly cisplatin, followed on both regimens by extrafascial hysterectomy (437). Patients on both regimens received EBRT to the pelvis to a dose of 45 Gy via a four-field box technique, followed by 30 Gy to point A by 1–2 intracavitary implants. The planned dose to point B was 55 Gy. Those randomized to weekly cisplatin received cisplatin 40 mg/m^2 weekly for six weeks during the EBRT. Both arms called for extrafascial hysterectomy after the completion of the radiation. Of 369 patients, 186 were assigned to radiation alone, and 183 to weekly cisplatin plus radiation. At a median of 36 months of follow-up, those receiving concurrent chemoradiation demonstrated a superior progression-free survival (p <0.001), with a 49% reduction in risk of progression or death (RR = 0.51). Survival was also superior for concurrent chemoradiation (p = 0.008), with a 46% reduction in risk of death (RR = 0.54).

An intergroup trial (SWOG, GOG, and RTOG) studied patients with stages IA$_2$, IB, and IIA with pelvic lymph node involvement, positive parametrial involvement, or positive surgical margins at the time of primary radical hysterectomy with pelvic lymphadenectomy and also negative common iliac and/or paraaortic lymph nodes (256). As previously discussed, eligible patients received radiation therapy with or without concurrent cisplatin plus 5-FU. Those getting concurrent chemoradiation received cisplatin 70 mg/m^2 day 1, plus 5-FU 1000 mg/m^2 daily for four days as a continuous infusion, repeated every three weeks for two cycles during the radiation. At a median 43 months follow-up, those receiving chemoradiation demonstrated a superior progression-free survival (p = 0.01). Survival was also superior for concurrent chemoradiation (p = 0.01), with a 51% reduction in risk of death (RR = 0.49). (Fig. 22.25) This study suggests that concurrent chemoradiation is the treatment of choice for selected postoperative patients with stages IA$_2$-IIA disease and the high-risk features noted above.

A study performed in Thailand and published by Lorvidhaya et al. assigned 926 patients randomly to 4 arms: standard RT alone, concurrent chemotherapy and RT, standard RT and adjuvant chemotherapy, and concurrent chemoradiation and adjuvant RT (438). The chemotherapy used was mitomycin-C (10 mg/m^2 IV on days 1 and 29) and 5-FU 200 mg/day orally for 3 courses of 4 weeks, with a 2-week rest every 6 weeks. With median follow-up of 89 months, the 5-year actuarial disease-free survival was highest in the concurrent chemoradiation arm, at 64.5%, and the loco-regional recurrence rate was lowest, at 14.3%. There was no significant difference in metastatic disease rates between the 4 arms; no significant increases in late effects were noted.

Not all controlled trials evaluating concurrent chemoradiation compared to RT alone are positive. Pearcy (439) reported the results of a National Cancer Institute of Canada trial, comparing pelvic RT with weekly cisplatin 40 mg/m^2/week for 6 cycles, vs. RT alone in 253 patients with stages IB-IVA squamous-cell carcinoma of the uterine cervix. Although there was a 13% improvement in relative risk of survival for the combination, this was not statistically significant (Table 22.8). In contrast to the GOG studies, surgical staging was not required, possibly diluting the benefit of combined therapy, since patients with paraaortic metastases would not have been curable with more localized RT. Furthermore, this trial lacked statistical power in the higher risk patients, as it was heavily weighted towards early stage patients, who have a lower risk of recurrence.

The clinical trials that have been performed to date have some flaws. For example, there are large discrepancies in outcomes from one trial to the next, even when the treatment is the same (hydroxyurea + RT arm in GOG trials #85 and #120). When RT alone has been given, it has been inadequate, compared with today's concept of acceptable RT in terms of overall treatment time and dose. Problems with patient selection and stratification have occurred (e.g., percent of patients with positive pelvic lymph nodes in RTOG 90–01). A significant percentage of patients drop out of protocol treatment (e.g., only 76% of patients completed chemotherapy per protocol in RTOG 90–01). Furthermore, Abu-Rustum has presented evidence that some patient populations, including the indigent, demonstrate a high drop-out rate with chemoradiation regimens because of acute toxicity and compliance difficulties, suggesting that the efficacy of chemoradiation regimens might not be equally realized in all patient populations (440). In an attempt to improve tolerance and full compliance with platinum-based chemoradiation, Higgins et al. utilized weekly carboplatin with RT in 31 evaluable patients (441). No treatment delays for neutropenia or gastrointestinal toxicity were seen, and a 90% objective response was reported.

	Treatment*	Control*	O–E	Variance
Platinum				
Wong (442a)	5/39	3/25	0·13	1·69
Whitney (265)	31/177	40/191	−3·15	14·34
Tseng (442b)	8/60	10/62	−0·85	3·87
Morris (264)	27/195	64/193	−18·73	17·46
Peters (256)	9/127	13/116	−2·50	5·01
Keys (437)	19/183	25/186	−2·82	9·71
Rose (266)	12/349	8/177	−1·27	4·30
Leborgne (442c)	8/75	13/78	−2·29	4·56
Subtotal	119/1205	176/1028	−31·49	60·95
Non-platinum				
Hernandez (442d)	3/37	0/18	0·98	0·64
Lorvidhaya (442e)	48/349	43/177	−12·37	16·83
Wong (442f)	6/110	10/110	−2·00	3·73
Roberts (442g)	7/78	15/82	−3·73	4·77
Subtotal	64/574	68/387	−17·11	25·97
Total	183/1779	244/1415	−48·60	86·91

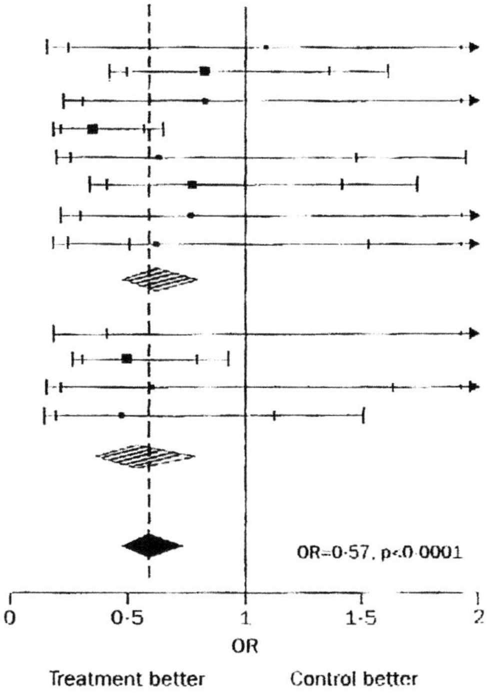

FIG. 22.29. Results for overall survival (O − E = observed minus expected; HR = hazard ratio. * indicates ratio of number of events/number of subjects entered, unpublished data). (From Green JA, Kirwan JM, Tierney JF, et al. Survival and recurrence after concomitant chemotherapy and radiotherapy for cancer of the uterine cervix: a systematic review and meta-analysis. *Lancet* 2001;358:781.)

Although some potentially valid criticisms of the studies supporting chemoradiation exist, the standard of care for stages IB$_2$-IVA disease is concurrent chemoradiation, based on the preponderance of evidence as described. A meta-analysis reported by Green et al. reviewed 19 published and 2 unpublished randomized studies of chemoradiation for cervical cancer (442). When combined, these studies included 4,580 randomized and 3,565 evaluable patients. A 12% absolute improvement in overall survival was noted (Fig. 22.29). Increased acute toxicity was confirmed, and the data were insufficient to evaluate the effect of chemotherapy on late toxicity. Additional work is ongoing to further refine the approach for maximum benefit.

Neoadjuvant Chemotherapy followed by Radiotherapy

Five randomized trials of neoadjuvant chemotherapy (NACT) followed by radiation versus radiation alone in patients with locally advanced cervical cancer (mainly stages III and IV) have been disappointing, in terms of both complete response rates and increase in survival that could be achieved with NACT (443–448). In fact, none of the five reported studies showed any survival benefit (Table 22.9). Pelvic failure was more common on the NACT arm in some of these trials, and a negative influence on survival was reported in two (446,448). In addition, treatment morbidity was sometimes severe (446). Explanation for these negative

TABLE 22.9. *Randomized trials of neoadjuvant chemotherapy followed by radiotherapy*

Author	Stage of disease	Number of patients	Chemotherapy (no. of cycles)	Local CRR CT + RT	Local CRR RT	Survival (FUP) CT + RT	Survival (FUP) RT
Souhami et al. (446)	IIIB	107	VBMP × 3	47	32	*23% (60)	*39% (60)
Tattersall et al. (447)	IIB–IVA	71	PVB × 3	65	73	141 wk‡	°169 wk‡
Chauvergne et al. (443)	IIB–III	151	VMCP × 2–4	77	75	42 mo‡	45 mo‡
Kumar et al (444, 445)	IIB–IVA	184	BIP × 2	63	69	38% (48)	36% (mo)
Tattersall et al (447)	IIB–IVA	260	EP × 3	43†	65†	62% (18)	

V = vincristine (in VBMP and VMCP), vinblastine (in PVB); B = bleomycin; P = cisplatin; I = ifosfamide; M = methotrexate, C = chlorambucil; E = epirubicin; Local CRR = Local complete response rate; FUP = Follow-up in months
* *p* = 0.02; † pelvic failures 29% vs 19% (*p*<0.003); ‡ median.

results cannot be given with certainty, but it has been suggested that chemotherapy could lead to an accelerated regrowth of surviving clones of cells, thus lessening the effect of subsequent radiotherapy (449). Another possibility is the development of cross-resistance between certain chemotherapeutic agents and radiation (450). Whatever the reason, NACT followed by radiotherapy for patients with locally advanced cervical cancer does not seem to be an option to follow any further.

Neoadjuvant Chemotherapy followed by Surgery

Numerous nonrandomized studies reported in the 1990s suggested that NACT followed by surgery might be an attractive approach to follow (451–460). Indeed, some but not all of the randomized trials show a trend in favor of this combined approach (461–465) (Table 22.10). Observations that have been made in the above-mentioned studies include the following: (1) cisplatin-based regimens are well tolerated, induce high response rates (particularly in earlier disease), and have little or no effect on surgical morbidity; (2) with NACT there is a reduced incidence of involved lymph nodes, capillary space involvement, deep invasion or undiagnosed parametrial disease; and (3) recurrence rates are reduced. Nevertheless, based on the available data, NACT remains investigational.

Adjuvant Chemotherapy

Several nonrandomized studies suggest a beneficial effect of adjuvant chemotherapy given after radical surgery in patients at high risk for recurrence (466–469). Two randomized trials with a very limited number of patients have tried to evaluate the effect of adjuvant chemotherapy in patients with high-risk cervical cancer after radical hysterectomy. The first study, with only 71 patients (all with lymph node metastases) compared postoperative radiation versus three cycles of postoperative chemotherapy (PVB; cisplatin, vinblastine, bleomycin) followed by radiation. In the second study 76 patients (with pelvic lymph node metastases and/or vascular invasion) randomly received adjuvant chemotherapy (carboplatin plus bleomycin) for six courses at 4-week intervals, standardized EBRT, or no further treatment. The results of both studies are inconclusive, but there were no apparent differences in the recurrence rates and patterns of recurrences or survival between those treated and those not treated with adjuvant chemotherapy.

TREATMENT OF RECURRENT CARCINOMA OF THE CERVIX

General Considerations

The main cause of death among women with cervical cancer is uncontrolled disease in the pelvis. Although this presents a difficult clinical problem, many patients with recurrent disease confined to the pelvis following definitive therapy, whether that therapy is surgery or RT, are potentially curable. Treatment selection and the likelihood of success are functions of the primary therapy, extent of disease at presentation, site of recurrence, local extent of the recur-

TABLE 22.10. *Randomized trials of neoadjuvant chemotherapy (NACT) followed by surgery*

Reference	FIGO stage	Number of patients per study arm[a]			Survival data
		NACT + S	NACT + RT	Control	
Sardi et al. (461)	All IB	102		103†	81% vs 66%, 8-yr FUP (p <0.05)
	IB 1	41		47†	82% vs 77%, 8-yr FUP (NS)
	IB2	61		56†	80% vs 61%, 9-yr FUP (p<0.01)
Sardi et al. (462)	IIIB	53	54	54‡	63% vs 53% vs 37%*, 4-yr FUP (p<0.05)
Benedetti-Panici et al. (463)	IB2-III	211		202‡	OS: 68.5% vs 60% (p=0.005) PFS: 52% vs 44% (p=0.02) (median FUP 27 months)
Sardi et al. (464)	IIB	76		75†	OS: 65% vs 41% (p<0.001) (median FUP 84 months)
Chang et al. (465)	B/IIA	68		52‡	OS: 79% vs 79% (NS) (median FUP 39 months)

* NACT + S versus NACT + RT, non-significant; NACT + S versus control, p = 0.005; NACT + RT versus control, p = 0.025
† Surgery ± radiation therapy
‡ Radiation therapy
RT = radiation therapy; S = surgery; NS = not significant; FUP = follow-up period; OS = overall survival; PFS = progression-free survival; NACT = cisplatin, vincristine, and bleomycin in references 461, 462, 464, and 465; NACT = platinum-based in reference 463

rence, disease-free interval, perfomance status, and co-morbidities.

When curative-intent salvage treatment is contemplated, the local recurrence should be biopsy-proven, and the patient should be evaluated for regional and distant metastasis by physical examination and imaging. A clinical diagnosis of pelvic sidewall involvement can almost always be made in the presence of a triad of sciatic pain, leg edema, and hydronephrosis. PET scanning is of potential benefit in the detection of recurrent cervical cancers following treatment, particularly in the subgroup of patients who have clinical findings suspicious for recurrence (470–472). However, biopsy confirmation of recurrence remains the gold standard for diagnosis, and will generally be required prior to embarking on salvage therapy.

Generally, patients with pelvic or regional recurrences after definitive surgery alone are managed with EBRT, often with brachytherapy. Concurrent cisplatin-based chemotherapy may also be recommended. Salvage options for patients with central recurrence after definitive or adjuvant RT are limited to radical, usually exenterative, surgery, and in selected patients, re-irradiation using interstitial radiation implants or highly conformal EBRT. Chemotherapy-responsive patients can obtain meaningful palliation in many cases.

Salvage Treatment after Definitive Radiation Therapy: Re-irradiation

Recurrent cervical carcinoma following definitive RT within previously irradiated areas presents a difficult management problem. Salvage surgery, usually exenterative in nature, can be offered to younger patients with limited, centrally recurrent lesions, if age and general condition permit. However, radical surgery following RT is accompanied by operative mortality in some, severe morbidity in many, and substantial loss of structure and function in all. Therefore, the applicability of salvage surgery is limited by physician and patient acceptance, as well as by clinical parameters. Even among patients meeting rigorous preoperative criteria, salvage surgery will be aborted in about one-fourth of patients (473).

Re-irradiation is typically better tolerated acutely, has little operative mortality, and often preserves structure and function of pelvic organs. When contemplating re-irradiation, it is important to analyze the techniques used in the initial treatment (beam energy, volume, doses delivered with external or intracavitary irradiation). The period of time between the two treatments must be taken into consideration, because it is postulated that some repair of the initial damage may take place in the interval.

Previously irradiated tissues do not have the same tolerance as newly irradiated tissues. Therefore, severe late effects have been frequently observed, particularly in older series that predominantly used external beam techniques in poorly selected patients. Thomas and colleagues (474) noted a median survival of only 7 months for 242 patients with recurrent carcinoma of the uterine cervix (all stages) who were primarily treated with irradiation. All but one patient, who was salvaged by a hysterectomy for a central failure, died within 24 months. Prasasvinichai and coworkers (475) reported a 17.6% 5-year survival rate for 51 patients with recurrent tumors limited to the pelvis, and Prempree and colleagues (476) treated eight patients, with three surviving tumor-free for more than 5 years.

However, positive results have been published. Sommers and colleagues (477) described the results of retreatment in 376 patients with recurrent carcinoma of the uterine cervix. Ninety-one patients received irradiation to control bleeding. Significant morbidity was observed in only four patients. The usual dose for paraaortic lymph node metastases was 45 to 50 Gy, given in 5 weeks. Other metastatic sites were treated with about 35 to 40 Gy in 3 to 4 weeks. The probability of 5-year survival after treatment for recurrence was 30% for patients treated with combined surgery and external irradiation, 12% for patients treated with surgery, and 4% for patients receiving external irradiation. Patients failing only in the pelvis who were re-irradiated with a secondary curative aim had a 40% (2 of 5 patients) 5-year survival rate. Although patients failing after initial treatment have a poor prognosis, it is possible to salvage some of those with limited pelvic, and particularly, central recurrences with additional aggressive therapy.

More recently, evidence has been presented to suggest that re-irradiation, particularly with interstitial or intracavitary techniques, can be curative in a significant percentage of patients with small-volume central recurrences, or new primaries, particularly when there has been a long disease-free interval since the earlier diagnosis and treatment. Puthawala and associates (478) used interstitial implants to treat recurrences in the pelvis after definitive radiation therapy. Seven of 10 patients exhibited tumor control. Palliation of symptoms was obtained in about 80% of the patients. The authors reported no postoperative mortality. Thirty percent of the patients experienced mild to moderate symptoms of proctitis and cystitis. Severe complications (i.e., soft tissue necrosis, and one instance each of rectovaginal fistula, vesicovaginal fistula, enterovaginal fistula, and rectal stricture) occurred in 15% of the patients.

Randall et al., in a series of 13 patients, observed a 69% complete response rate and a 46% NED (no evidence of disease) rate with a minimum 2-year follow-up, and median follow-up of 59 months (479). Interstitial re-irradiation (IRI) doses of 30–55 Gy were employed, with low-dose-rate permanent and temporary implants (Fig. 22.30 A and B). Patients with squamous histology did significantly better than patients with adenocarcinoma histology. Other predictors for improved outcomes included smaller tumor volumes, higher implant doses, and vaginal wall/suburethra vs. vaginal cuff location. Late morbidity was limited to 1 rectovaginal fistula in a patient who also had recurrent tumor. Suggested advan-

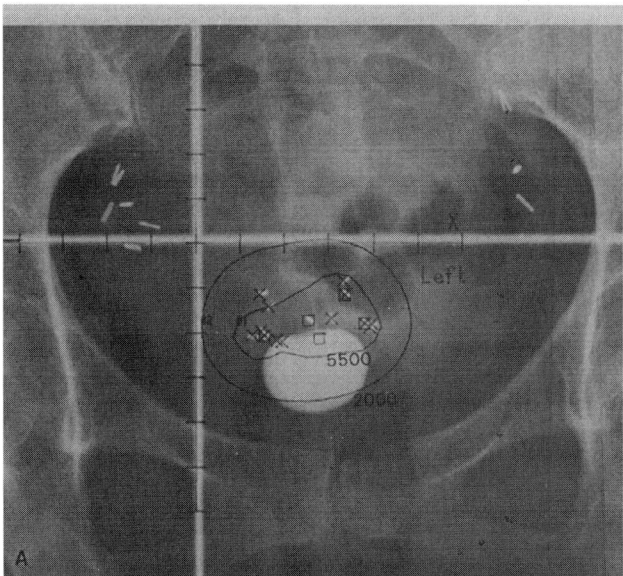

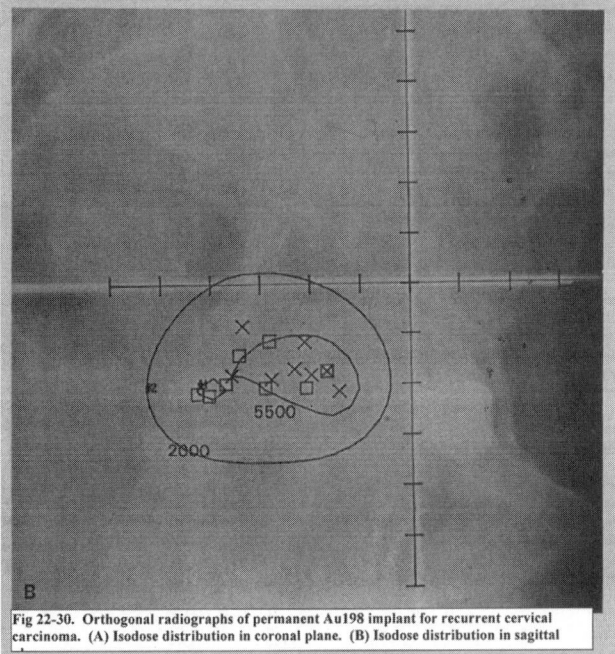

Fig 22-30. Orthogonal radiographs of permanent Au198 implant for recurrent cervical carcinoma. (A) Isodose distribution in coronal plane. (B) Isodose distribution in sagittal

FIG. 22.30. Orthogonal radiographs of permanent [198]Au implant for recurrent cervical carcinoma. **(A)** Isodose distribution in coronal plane. **(B)** Isodose distribution in sagittal plane. (From Randall ME, Evans L, Greven KM, et al. Interstitial re-irradiation for recurrent gynecological malignancies: results and analysis of prognostic factors. *Gynecol Oncol* 1993;48:29.)

tages and disadvantages of IRI and salvage surgery are shown in Table 22.11.

In a series of 73 patients with late recurrences of squamous carcinoma of the cervix in the vaginal canal following radiation therapy, Wang et al. (480) reported a 5-year survival rate of 40%. Sixty-one patients received only radiation therpay, mainly with fractionated brachytherapy techniques such as

TABLE 22.11. *Comparison of advantages and disadvantages of salvage surgery and interstitial re-irradiation*

Surgery
+ Ability to assess extent of disease and act accordingly
+ Applicable to large-volume recurrences
− Perioperative morbidity and mortality particularly RT
− Prolonged hospitalization
− High rate of reoperation
− Expense
− Applicable only to selected patients with good overall medical condition
− Detrimental to patient self-image
Re-irradiation
+ Little perioperative morbidity or mortality
− Little or no hospitalization for permanent implants unless laparotomy is required
+ Relatively inexpensive
+ Preserves structure and function in most patients
+ Applicable to patients who are medically compromised or aged
− Extent of disease difficult to assess in some cases
− Risk of late radiation injury
− Applicable only to small-volume recurrences

From: Randall ME, Evans L, Greven KM, et al. Interstitial reirradiation for recurrent gynecologic malignancies: Results and analysis of prognostic factors. *Gynecol Oncol* 1993;48:30.

vaginal molds. Doses of 20–40 Gy in 3 to 5 fractions over 3 to 5 weeks, using both LDR and HDR techniques, were typically employed, sometimes followed by more focused boosts. Favorable prognostic factors included proximal location in the vagina and tumor size <4 cm. Significant complications occurred in nearly 25%, including a 12% rate of fistula formation. Complications were more common among patients with distally located tumors.

Song et al. presented a series of 20 patients who underwent IRI for recurrent gynecologic malignancies of various sites. Thirteen patients underwent permanent [198]Au seed implants, and 7 had temporary ^{192}Ir implants. Overall, 80% of patients had a complete response, and 11 (55%) remained well with NED from 5 to 71 months after re-irradiation. No significant complications were noted (481).

Re-irradiation is probably underutilized in the management of locally recurrent cervical cancer. As chemotherapy does not have curative potential and many patients will not be candidates for exenterative surgery or will refuse such surgery, re-irradiation, in many cases, will be the only feasible curative-intent therapy. Patient selection and careful brachytherapy technique are crucial to successful re-irradiation.

Recurrence in the Paraaortic Chain

Post–radiation therapy recurrences confined to the paraaortic nodal region are reported. Most of these patients are treated palliatively with RT, or with systemic or investigational therapy. Grigsby et al. reported 20 patients with recurrent cervical cancer confined to the paraaortic region following definitive RT (482). The median time between the initial diagnosis and the recurrence was 12 months. Although all patients died within 2 years after recurrence, median survivals were longer in patients receiving >45 Gy. A disease-free interval of >24 months was also a positive prognostic factor. This observation was confirmed by the experience reported by Kim et al (483). These investigators treated 12 patients with isolated paraaortic failures following RT with concurrent chemotherapy (mostly paclitaxel) and hyperfractionated RT. In patients who relapsed within 24 months of their initial treatment, the median survival following attempted salvage was 13 months. In contrast, patients having a disease-free interval >24 months had a median survival of 45 months with this therapy.

Salvage Treatment after Definitive Radiation Therapy: Radical Surgery

Pelvic Exenteration

Surgery for recurrent gynecologic cancer was considered futile until the report by Brunschwig in 1948 (309). Better patient selection and continued improvements in anesthesia, operative technique, and postoperative care have improved survival and decreased morbidity. Surgical mortality from pelvic exenteration is typically 5% to 8%.

Preoperative determination of significant local extension, aortic or pelvic lymph nodes, intraperitoneal disease, or malignant ascites contraindicates laparotomy and pelvic exenteration. More recently, PET scanning has been advocated as a useful re-staging tool (484). Shingleton defined 3 risk groups based on time from initial therapy to recurrence, size of recurrent tumor, and preoperative pelvic sidewall fixation. Patients in the highest risk group were those with tumors >3 centimeters, sidewall fixation, and recurrence within 1 year of treatment. All patients in this group died of operative complications and/or persistent cancer within 18 months of exenteration (485).

Pelvic exenteration is accompanied by substantial functional and psychological changes. Of 40 patients reported by Ratcliff et al., 21 (52%) did not resume sexual activity, typically because of self-consciousness about the urostomy or colostomy, vaginal discharge, and vaginal dryness (486). Surgical techniques such as urinary diversion, pelvic reconstruction, and low rectal anastomoses have improved postoperative body image.

Vaginal and perineal reconstruction following radical pelvic surgery for recurrent gynecologic cancer is done to restore vulvovaginal function and to minimize postoperative complications by covering the pelvic defect with healthy, well-vascularized tissue. Techniques used for benign disease (e.g., skin grafts, cutaneous flaps) might not be useful in heavily irradiated patients, or for reconstruction following exenterative surgery. Flaps reported to be useful for tissue reconstruction in radical pelvic surgery include the gracilis myocutaneous, anterolateral thigh fasciocutaneous, bulbocavernosus myocutaneous, rectus abdominis musculoperitoneal (TRAMP) or myocutaneous (TRAM), rectus femoris myocutaneous, tensor fasciae latae myocutaneous, inferior gluteal, and omental J-flap. No method of pelvic reconstruction is superior to all others, or applicable in all cases.

Pelvic Reconstruction

The purposes of vaginal and perineal reconstruction following radical pelvic surgery for recurrent gynecologic cancer are to restore or create vulvovaginal function, and to minimize postoperative complications by transferring to the pelvic defect healthy tissue with good blood supply. Many techniques employed for benign disease such as congenital vaginal agenesis (skin grafts, cutaneous flaps, bowel flaps) are not applicable to heavily irradiated patients, or for reconstruction of extensive defects following exenterative surgery.

Urinary diversion is usually required when the urinary tract is involved with recurrent carcinoma, or when adequate surgical resection will compromise bladder or urethral integrity. Genitourinary tract reconstruction has improved survival and quality of life after radical pelvic surgery. Many technical innovations were developed in children with congenital defects, or in adults undergoing treatment for bladder carcinoma. While these same procedures are applicable to patients with gynecologic cancer, equivalent surgical morbidity and mortality should not be expected. Most women with recurrent vaginal or cervical cancer will have received prior radiation therapy, leading to sub-optimal healing, and potentially, postoperative complications. Tunneled ureterointestinal anastomosis, using irradiated ureter and irradiated intestine, may be applicable to the non-irradiated patient, but may lead to stricture and urinary obstruction in the patient with recurrent gynecologic malignancy.

No method of pelvic reconstruction is superior to all others, or applicable to all cases. An individualized approach to patient care is paramount in the selection of reconstructive procedures.

Radical Hysterectomy

In highly selected patients with small cervical recurrences (<2 cm) and negative pelvic nodes, radical hysterectomy may be considered as an alternative to pelvic exenteration (487). Rutledge reviewed 47 patients who underwent conservative surgery for cervical carcinoma recurrent after RT. There were 8 urinary tract fistulas and 7 enteric fistulas: all required operative diversion (488). In a review by Rubin et al., 5-year survival was 62% among 194 patients with recurrent cervical carcinoma treated with radical hysterectomy.

Two patients died of postoperative complications, and the fistula rate was 48%. This data suggested that patients with recurrent cervical cancer, initial FIGO stage IB or IIA with recurrent tumors ≤ 2 cm in diameter, could be considered for more conservative surgery, although the complication risk is high (489). Maneo et al. published a similar series of 34 patients (490). Median tumor size was 3.2 cm. After radical hysterectomy, 59% of patients suffered recurrence, and 44% suffered major complications. The authors felt that radical hysterectomy should be offered and performed only in selected patients with early stage tumors at diagnosis and small (<4 cm) recurrences.

Salvage Treatment after Previous Surgery—Definitive Radiation Therapy

Ciatto et. Al (491) classified recurrent cervical cancer according to its location and extent as follows: (a) central: confined to the vagina or paravaginal tissues, or both, not extending to the pelvic wall; (b) peripheral-limited: tumor limited to one parametrium with extension to the pelvic wall, with or without involvement of the vaginal wall and/or bone involvement; and (c) peripheral-massive: bilateral extension to the pelvic wall, with or without vaginal wall or bone involvement. Patients with central or limited peripheral recurrences are candidates for curative-intent RT. In these groups, survival rates of 30%–70% have been reported (492–495).

In RT-naïve patients, pelvic EBRT of 40–50 Gy to the primary tumor and regional lymphatics is indicated. Inguinofemoral lymph node regions should be included in patients with involvement of the distal third of the vagina. The entire vagina should be treated in most patients with vaginal recurrences following hysterectomy. A dose of 60–65 Gy with EBRT and/or endocavitary brachytherapy is desirable. The gross tumor volume should receive additional radiation; doses of 15 to 30 Gy are administered with single, double-plane, or volume implants. Exceeding total vaginal mucosal doses from the external brachytherapy doses of 140 Gy in the proximal vagina, or 95 Gy in the distal vagina increases the risk of injury (496).

Monk et al. (497) utilized EBRT followed by laparotomy and ''open'' interstitial implant for recurrent cancer in the upper vagina following hysterectomy. This approach provided the ability to accurately assess the extent of the disease and to separate bowel and bladder adhesions from the area of the implant, facilitated placement of the interstitial brachytherapy needles, and allowed the placement of an omental pedicle graft to separate the bladder and rectum from the implant volume. In 28 patients, local control was 71%, and the long-term complication rate was 11%. Long-term NED survival was 36%. Lesions <6 cm in patients with no previous RT had high control rates.

Jobsen and associates (498) described 16 complete responses in 18 patients (88%), with post-surgical locoregional recurrence treated with 50 to 60 Gy to the pelvis. Four of sixteen patients (31%) developed a second pelvic failure. The 5-year survival rate was 44%.

Ten percent of 114 patients with inoperable locoregional recurrence lived 15 months or longer, and 5% survived 5 years or more, as reported by Evans and colleagues (499). Satisfactory palliation was observed in a large proportion of the patients. Friedman and Péarlman (500) observed a 42% tumor-free survival rate in 38 patients. The worst results were noted in 11 patients with persistent or recurrent peripheral pelvic tumor, and in 6 patients with massive pelvic recurrences, in whom only palliation was achieved.

Krebs and associates (433) reported on 40 recurrences, 11 of which were limited to the central pelvis. The 5-year salvage rate for the patients with recurrence was 13%. Webb and Symmonds (501) analyzed 104 recurrences following initial surgical treatment, and found only a 5.7% 5-year survival rate after treatment for the recurrence.

Larson and associates (434) reported 27 recurrences in 249 patients treated with radical hysterectomy and pelvic lymphadenectomy for stage IB disease of the cervix (11%). Seventeen patients had tumor recurrence in the pelvis or vulva; the other 10 patients developed recurrences outside the pelvis. Eight of 15 patients (53%) treated with irradiation for isolated recurrence in the pelvis or vulva were tumor free between 10 and 126 months after treatment of the recurrence.

Nori and colleagues (502) reported on 75 patients with recurrent cervical cancer treated with external, intracavitary, or interstitial irradiation, and occasionally with surgery. Relief of symptoms was obtained in 70% of patients. Ten percent of patients survived 5 years. Early complications were observed in 10 patients, and late complications requiring surgical intervention occurred in 5 patients.

Ito et al. (495) reported on 90 patients with central recurrences from cervical cancer after surgery treated with HDR-ICB, with or without EBRT. The 10-year survival for the entire series was 52%. They found survival to be greatly influenced by tumor size (72%, 48%, and 0% 10-year survival respectively for small or no palpable tumor, medium [<3 cm], and large [≥3 cm]). In addition, patients who achieved a complete response after RT had a 10-year survival of 63%, vs. 10% for those with residual disease.

Ijaz et al (494) reported a 5-year survival of 39% in 43 patients with isolated locoregional recurrences treated with EBRT and selective brachytherapy. In 16 patients with limited recurrences to the vagina and paravaginal tissues, the 5-year survival was 69% after radical RT.

Salvage Treatment after Previous Surgery—Chemoradiation

Concurrent cisplatin-based chemotherapy with RT has proven beneficial in locally advanced cervical cancer (264–266,437). Retrospective and prospective Phase II studies using concurrent RT with 5-FU chemotherapy (474,480,

503) and paclitaxel (504) are encouraging. Although randomized studies are unlikely in this patient population, this combined modality approach may improve the locoregional control and survival in patients with isolated pelvic recurrences.

Salvage Treatment—Role of Intraoperative Radiation Therapy

Patients with microscopically positive or close margins have a poor prognosis after salvage surgery (485,505,506). Intraoperative RT has been used in this situation to potentially sterilize residual disease after tumor debulking. IORT allows direct visualization of the target volume, and displacement and/or shielding of the surrounding normal tissues. The IORT dose is generally limited because of prior RT, proximity of critical normal structures, and the single-fraction nature of the treatment.

IORT has been used for treatment of locally advanced and recurrent carcinoma of the cervix. Most of this experience is based on the treatment of isolated central and nodal recurrences, generally amenable to surgical excision. Limitations in evaluating IORT include small patient numbers, short follow-up, and widely varying patient selection criteria. Locoregional recurrence and distant metastasis rates after IORT vary between 20% and 60%, and 20% and 58%, respectively. The actuarial survival is poor, with 8%–25% 3- to 5-year survivals (507–509). Others have reported good survival and local control rates when IORT was given as part of initial therapy in patients with locally or regionally advanced cervical cancer undergoing complete surgical resection. However, the number of patients is too small to make any significant conclusions (388,510).

By analyzing prognostic factors, Abe and Shibamoto (511) suggested that patients most likely to benefit from IORT are those with central recurrences, particularly in non-irradiated patients, and in irradiated patients who have undergone gross total resection of all recurrent tumor.

The available data seem to indicate that IORT, although feasible, does not dramatically improve prognosis and is associated with significant incidence of long-term complications. Patients with limited central recurrences who are candidates for pelvic exenteration but are found to have unfavorable prognostic factors for local recurrence such as close positive margins, lymphovascular space involvement, or perineural invasion, may benefit from IORT or intraoperative interstitial brachytherapy (512). The role of concurrent and/or adjuvant chemotherapy in this setting needs to be defined.

Sidewall Implants

Combined operative and radiotherapeutic treatment (CORT) was described by Hockel et al (513,514) for the treatment of post-irradiation recurrences infiltrating the pelvic sidewall. The procedure involves surgical exploration and absence of intra-abdominal disease, involved contralateral pelvic nodes, retroperitoneal and bilateral inguinal lymphadenopathy. Grossly involved ipsilateral pelvic nodes and ipsilateral inguinal nodes that can be completely resected are not contraindications. Total gross resection of the tumor is performed, leaving only microscopic margins at the pelvic side wall. A single plane interstitial implant is performed, encompassing the entire area of potential microscopic residual disease with a 2-cm margin. In order to improve the therapeutic index, a pelvic wall "plasty" is done, in which un-irradiated, well-vascularized, autologous tissue is transposed to the pelvis to protect the hollow organs and reduce late effects. Reconstruction of pelvis is performed as in an exenteration. The tumor bed at risk is irradiated postoperatively on days 10 to 14 using a high-dose-rate technique. The total dose is based on the interval to recurrence (30 Gy if <4 weeks to 54 Gy if >6 months). In 48 patients treated with CORT, the severe complication rate was 33% at 5 years. The 5-year survival rate was 44%, and the absolute local control rate was 60% for the first 20 patients, and 85% for the last 28 treated patients.

Salvage Treatment–Role of Chemotherapy

Cisplatin, at present, is considered the single most active cytotoxic agent, and its preferred schedule of administration in metastatic or recurrent disease is 50–100 mg/m^2, given intravenously every three weeks (398). Overall, the duration of the objective responses to cisplatin in patients with metastatic or recurrent disease remains disappointing (4–6 months) and survival in such patients is only approximately seven months (399). There is a suggestion of a dose-response relationship because in one trial comparing 50 mg/m^2 and 100 mg/m^2, the overall response rate increased from 21% to 31% (515). However, there was only a minimal increase in the complete response rate (from 10% to 13%), and no improvement in response duration, progression-free interval, or survival. A small study performed at the Memorial Sloan Kettering Cancer Center applying 200 mg/m^2 of cisplatin (and sodium thiosulfate nephroprotection) suggested no further increase in response rate with these higher dosages, and toxicity was unacceptably high (516).

Response rates with combination chemotherapy have varied from 0 to nearly 100% in individual reports, reflecting sample size, differences in response assessment criteria, and patient characteristics. However, cumulative data indicated that a response rate of about 40% can be expected in well-selected patients (399,400). There is no indication from randomized trials that adding other active agents to cisplatin improves overall survival (517–521) (Table 22.12). Nevertheless, in most studies a higher response rate is obtained with the cisplatin-based combinations, and in the GOG study ifosfamide/cisplatin resulted in slightly better progression-free survival than cisplatin alone. However, in all studies

TABLE 22.12. *Randomized studies of cisplatin-based combinations vs. single-agent cisplatin in patients with cervical cancer*

Arms of studies and study drug	Number of patients	CR n (%)	PR n (%)	CR+PR n (%)	Median survival (months)	Reference
MMC/VCR/BLM/CDDP	54	4 (7)	8 (15)	12 (22)	6.9	
vs						
MMC/CDDP	51	2 (4)	11 (21)	13 (25)	7	[25]
vs						
CDDP	9	1 (11)	2 (22)	3 (33)	17	
DVA/BLM/MMC/CDDP	143	11 (8)	33 (23)	44 (31)†	10	
vs						[26]
CDDP	144	8 (6)	20 (14)	28 (19)†	9.4	
DBD/CDDP	153 (147)*	14 (9)	17 (12)	31 (21)	7.3	
vs						
IFOSF/CDDP	155 (151)*	19 (12.5)	28 (18.5)	47 (31)‡	8.3	[27]
vs						
CDDP	146 (140)*	9 (6.5)	16 (11.5)	25 (18)‡	8	
BLM/IFOSF/CDDP	50 (46)*	12 (26)	12 (26)	24 (52)**	8	
vs						[28]
CDDP	56 (51)*	5 (10)	10 (20)	15 (29)**	6	

MMC, mitomycin C; VCR, vincristine; BLM, bleomycin; CDDP, cisplatin (dose in all studies and in all arms 50 mg/m²); DVA, vindesine; DBD, dibromodulcitol; IFOSF, ifosfamide

* Number in parentheses indicates the number of patients evaluable for response.
† $p = 0.03$
‡ $p = 0.004$
** $p < 0.01$

these gains were achieved at the cost of considerable toxicity, which makes their value as palliative therapy questionable. An individual approach to these patients is warranted, whereby identification of a subset of patients who indeed might benefit from chemotherapy would be a major issue. Any decision for treatment of cervical cancer patients in the palliative setting should be assessed against the benefit of best supportive care, which may provide the best option for some of these patients.

RESULTS OF STANDARD THERAPY

In evaluating outcomes of treatment for carcinoma of the cervix, direct comparisons of various retrospective reports are potentially misleading. Zola and associates reviewed 152 papers published in the United States and Europe before or during 1980 on results of treatment of stages IA, IB, IIA, and IIB cervical carcinoma with surgery, irradiation, or combination therapy (522). Fifty-four percent of the papers reported observations on single series, without any comparison to historic controls or concurrently treated control patients. Identification of prognostic factors and information on imbalances of the distribution of patients between treatment groups were adequately presented in only 46% of the papers. Only 13% of the papers reported frequency and severity of sequelae of therapy. The authors concluded that the existing literature at that time was of limited help in deciding the best treatment for patients with cervical carcinoma. Fortunately, the modern area of prospective randomized studies and statistically appropriate analyses has helped in understanding the relative effectiveness of various therapies.

Stages I and IIA

Stage IA₁ carcinoma is usually treated with conization or hysterectomy. The control rate approaches 100% (64,190, 523,524). Stage IA₂ is usually treated with total or radical hysterectomy with or without pelvic lymphadenectomy in medically operable patients (186,219). In medically inoperable patients, stage IA carcinoma is effectively treated with intracavitary ¹³⁷Cs insertions only. In 34 patients treated at Washington University, 13 with intracavitary therapy only, no local or regional failures were noted; the 5-year disease-free survival rate (corrected for intercurrent disease) was 100% (210).

Webb and Symmonds (501) reported on 564 patients treated with radical hysterectomy and bilateral pelvic lymphadenectomy for stages IB and IIA, and occasionally stage IIB cervical carcinoma. Five-year survival was 88% for 205 patients with stage IB, 68% for 72 patients with stage IIA, and 44% for 21 patients with stage IIB. Kielbinska and co-workers (525), in a long-term follow-up of 792 women treated with irradiation and 789 women treated with hysterectomy and irradiation for stage I cervical carcinoma, found no difference in survival, incidence of recurrent carcinoma, or incidence of second primaries.

Piver and colleagues (249) treated 103 women with stage IB cervical carcinoma with either a radical hysterectomy and bilateral pelvic lymphadenectomy (limited to tumors 3 cm or less in greatest diameter), or irradiation (tumors larger than 3 cm or medically inoperable). The 5-year estimated disease-free survival rate was 92.3% for the surgical group, and 91.1% for the radiation therapy group. Similar overall

5-year survival rates were noted in the patients treated with surgery or irradiation. In the surgical group, 16.4% of the patients had lymph node metastases, and 7.3% developed a recurrence after therapy. In the irradiation group, patients with lesions larger than 1 cm in diameter had a 14.5% incidence of recurrence. The authors concluded that tumors less than 3 cm in diameter may be equally treated by radical hysterectomy and pelvic lymphadenectomy, or by radiation therapy alone.

Patterns of Care Study data reported by Komaki et al. found 5-year disease-free survival rates of 72%–77% for stage I patients (526). In these surveys, 5-year pelvic control rates were 88%–92% for stage I patients. For patients with stage II disease (IIA and IIB), 5-year disease-free survival and 5-year pelvic control rates were 50%–57% and 65%–76%, respectively. Barillot et al reported results of treatment with RT alone in 1,875 patients treated from 1970–1993 (527). The 5-year specific survival rates were 83.5% and 81% in stages IB and IIA, respectively.

With the demonstration of improved efficacy of chemoradiation compared to RT alone, modern outcomes would be expected to compare favorably to these older series. In the randomized GOG study of bulky IB cancers by Keys et al. (437), the estimated survival at 36 months was 83% in the chemoradiation arm (74% in the preoperative RT only arm). Patients also had hysterectomies following this treatment. Similarly, in high-risk stages I-IIA patients treated adjuvantly with chemoradiation following radical hysterectomy, the projected progression-free survival was 80% (63% in the postoperative RT alone arm).

Stages IIB, III, and IV

Most patients in the United States with stage IIB disease are treated with curative-intent chemoradiation. With RT alone, the 5-year survival rate has historically been 60% to 65%, and the pelvic failure rate 18% to 39% (528). In an analysis of the Patterns of Care Study, in which 157 patients had stage IIB disease, Coia and associates (529) reported better 4-year survival (67% and 54%) and in-field tumor control (78% and 68%) in patients with unilateral as opposed to bilateral parametrial involvement.

Komaki and associates (526), analyzing the Patterns of Care Study data, found 5-year disease-free survival rates of 18%–39% for stage III patients (mostly stage IIIB). The 5-year pelvic control rates were 37%–69% for this group of patients. Others have reported similar outcomes in stage IIIB carcinomas treated with RT alone (530,531).

Arthur and colleagues (532), studying 89 patients with stage IIIB carcinoma of the cervix treated with external irradiation and brachytherapy, observed a locoregional tumor control rate of 22.5%, and a disease-free survival rate of 15% in 16 patients treated with 78 Gy or lower to point A in comparison with 53% and 47%, respectively, in 24 patients receiving higher doses.

In patients with stage IVA disease, the 5-year survival rate ranges from 18% (251,296) to 34% (267). Pelvic failures range from 55% to 80% after definitive irradiation (268). Kramer and associates (268) described 48 patients with stage IVA carcinoma treated with definitive radiation therapy delivering 70 to 80 Gy or more to point A. Fifteen patients also received paraaortic irradiation (40 to 45 Gy). Nine patients survived without recurrence (5-year actuarial survival rate of 18%). Patients with minimal disease had a 5-year survival rate of 46%, in comparison with only 5% for those with extensive parametrial tumor. The major complication rate was 22%.

Chemoradiation should result in outcomes that compare favorably to these older series. Considering all eligible patients with stages IIB-IVA carcinomas enrolled in GOG #85, a 55% survival rate with platinum-based chemotherapy with RT was demonstrated after a median follow-up of 8.7 years (265). In this same group of patients, GOG #120 found a 66%–67% survival rate with platinum-based chemoradiation (266). Outcomes within each stage were not reported.

Impact of Prolongation of Treatment Time on Outcome

Owing to the radiobiologic phenomena of tumor cell repopulation and accelerated re-population, clinicians have long assumed that treatment prolongation, beyond some reasonable point, would likely have a deleterious effect on outcome in patients treated with RT. Several studies have supported this assumption by demonstrating lower pelvic tumor control and survival rates after definitive RT in invasive carcinoma of the uterine cervix when the overall treatment time is prolonged (533–537).

Fyles and associates (533) demonstrated the adverse effect of increased treatment duration on pelvic tumor control in 830 patients with cervical carcinoma treated with irradiation alone. Loss of tumor control approximated 1% per day of treatment prolongation beyond 30 days. Exclusion of patients who had delays due to causes beyond the control of the physician (e.g., complications, poor response, etc.) did not affect the conclusion. This effect was predominantly seen in stages III and IV.

Lanciano and colleagues (535), in an analysis of 837 patients from the Patterns of Care Study treated with irradiation for squamous-cell carcinoma of the uterine cervix, also reported a highly significant decrease in pelvic tumor control and survival with prolongation of treatment time. They described a 4-year actuarial infield recurrence increase from 6% to 20% when total treatment time increased from 6 weeks or less to 10 weeks ($p = 0.0001$). This translated into significantly decreased survival. In multivariate analysis, stage, age, and overall treatment time were the only independent factors associated with pelvic control. Similar to the Fyles study, the effect was most significant in the stage III patients.

Perez and colleagues (537), in 1,330 patients treated with

definitive RT, noted a strong correlation between overall treatment time and tumor stage (<7 weeks: 90% for stage IB; 87%, stage IIA; 77%, stage IIB; 67%, stage III; and 65%, stage IVA). Interruptions of therapy accounting for prolongation of treatment time occurred in 25% to 30% of patients, and occurred most frequently because of holidays and weekends and side effects of therapy. Overall treatment time had a major impact on pelvic tumor control in stages IB, IIA, and IIB. In stage IB, 10-year actuarial pelvic failure rates were 5% with overall treatment time of 7 weeks or less; 22% with 7.1 to 9 weeks; and 36% with more than 9 weeks ($p \leq 0.01$). For stage IIA disease, the corresponding values were 14%, 27%, and 36% ($p = 0.08$). In stage IIB disease, pelvic failure rates were 20%, 28%, and 34%, respectively ($p = 0.09$). However, in stage III, pelvic failure was not significantly affected by treatment time, in contrast to the reports by Fyles et al. and Lanciano et al. (533,535). There was also a strong correlation between overall treatment time and cause-specific survival in stages IB, IIA, and IIB. The 10-year cause-specific survival rates in stage IB were 86% with overall treatment time of 7 weeks or less; 78% for 7.1 to 9 weeks; and 55% for more than 9 weeks ($p \leq 0.01$). The corresponding rates in stage IIA were 73%, 41%, and 43%, respectively ($p \leq 0.01$). For patients with stage IIB disease, cause-specific survival rates were 72% for overall treatment time of 7 weeks or less; 60% for 7.1 to 9 weeks; and 65% for more than 9 weeks ($p = 0.01$). Patients with stage IIIB disease had 38% to 42% 10-year cause-specific survival for the various treatment times ($p = 0.51$).

Prolongation of time had a significant impact on pelvic tumor control and cause-specific survival regardless of tumor size, except for stage IB disease 3 cm or less (537). Regression analysis of pelvic tumor control confirmed previous reports (533) that prolongation of overall treatment time resulted in an increased failure rate of 0.59% per day in stages IB and IIA, and 0.86% per day in stage IIB. Performance of all intracavitary insertions within 4.5 weeks from initiation of irradiation yielded lower pelvic failure rates (8.8% versus 18% in stages IB and IIA 5 cm or smaller tumors, and 12.3% versus 35% in stage IIB tumors) ($p \leq 0.01$).

In the study by Petereit et al. (536), 209 patients were analyzed. The median treatment duration was 55 days. When analyzed according to patients who completed treatment in <55 days vs. ≥55 days, the shorter treatment duration was associated with significantly improved 5-year survival and pelvic tumor control rates for stages IB, IIA, and III, but not stage IIB. Late complications were not affected by treatment duration.

Girinsky and colleagues analyzed 386 patients with stages IIB and II carcinoma of the cervix, finding a significant decrease in local control rates with treatment times beyond 52 days. Multivariate analysis supported their conclusion that treatment prolongation is an independent risk factor for local failure (534).

Combining the published results, one can suggest that pelvic control will suffer at an approximate rate of 1% per day that treatment extends beyond 52–55 days. This impact will be potentially seen in all stages of localized disease, and survival will be negatively affected. Eifel and Thames have pointed out some of the difficulties in drawing conclusions from the data presented (538); nevertheless they support the recommendation to avoid prolonging treatment beyond 8–9 weeks. Erridge et al. have pointed out that there is probably a limit to the relationship between treatment time and outcome (539). In a cohort of patients, almost all of whom completed treatment within 7 weeks, no impact of overall treatment time was observed. However, grade 4 toxicities were more common among patients completing treatment on a compact schedule of 29–32 days.

Measurements of potential doubling time (T_{pot}) using halogenated pyrimidines in both head and neck and cervical cancers demonstrated median values of 5 days, which is significantly shorter than the volume doubling times described and consistent with accelerated proliferation (181). Tsang has presented evidence to support a similar phenomenon in cervical cancer, offering a scientific basis for limiting treatment duration with RT (181).

Results of Elective Paraaortic Lymph Node Irradiation

Occult involvement of the paraaortic lymph nodes is a potential cause of treatment failure in carcinoma of the cervix. In a prospective clinical-pathologic study performed by the GOG Heller et al. found that stages IIB, III, and IVA had documented paraaortic lymph node involvement in 21%, 31%, and 13%, respectively (54). Given the orderly lymphatic spread of cervical carcinoma to pelvic and paraaortic lymph nodes, and its frequency in defined patient groups, adjuvant or elective extended field radiation therapy (EFRT) is a logical treatment strategy that seeks to avoid the risks and treatment delays associated with surgical staging. Its use may be considered both in patients with early stage disease who have undergone appropriate surgical treatment and have risk factors arguing for adjuvant postoperative RT, and in patients for whom RT is the primary treatment.

Retrospective data suggest that EFRT can be delivered safely and with reasonable efficacy in high-risk patients (540,541). In a large retrospective series from Japan, Horii et al. reported on patients who received adjuvant (in some cases, therapeutic) EFRT based on multiple positive pelvic lymph nodes, and/or radiographic evidence of paraaortic lymph node enlargement (542). The investigators found a significant survival advantage for patients receiving EFRT, compared to similar patients who received only pelvic RT. This survival advantage was particularly noticeable among stage II patients. No serious complications were reported.

Interest in adjuvant EFRT increased following the publication of 2 randomized studies. The EORTC study reported by Haie et al (543) included 441 patients with stages I-III disease who did not have surgical staging, but were considered at high risk of undetected paraaortic lymph node involvement. In the study group, the paraaortic area received 40–50 Gy with EBRT. Significant findings included a higher rate of gastrointestinal toxicity, a significantly lower rate of paraaortic failures in the EFRT group, and a significantly lower rate of distant metastases in patients receiving EFRT and achieving pelvic control. There was no statistically significant difference between the two treatment arms with regard to local control, distant metastases, disease-free survival at 4 years, or survival. The incidence of small bowel injury was 0.9% in the pelvic RT, and 2.3% in the EFRT, groups. A severe complication rate of 9% was observed in patients receiving EFRT, compared with 4.8% in those treated to the pelvis only. Rotman published 10-year results from RTOG 79–20 (544). In this study, 367 patients (stage IIB or stages IB-IIA ≥4 cm) were randomized to pelvic RT vs. EFRT. Overall survival was 67% at 5 years, and 55% at 10 years for the patients receiving elective EFRT, compared with 55% and 44%, respectively, for those treated to the pelvis only ($p = 0.02$). However, this survival rate for patients in the control arm is disturbingly low, considering the patient population. Loco-regional failures were similar at 10 years for both arms (pelvic only, 35%; EFRT, 31%). When the first disease failure patterns were examined, more patients failed distally when treated only with pelvic RT compared to those receiving EFRT ($p = 0.053$). The EFRT arm was associated with more grade 4 and 5 complications, particularly in patients with prior abdominal surgery (11% versus 2%).

Results from RTOG 90–01 show that pelvic RT combined with platinum-based chemotherapy is superior to adjuvant EFRT in patients with locally advanced disease (264). Therefore, enthusiasm for EFRT has now understandably declined. What is uncertain is whether EFRT combined with chemotherapy offers opportunities for improved outcomes in patients at particularly high risk of metastatic paraaortic disease. Given the apparent ability of EFRT to impact failure rates in the paraaortic chain, the concept is reasonable. However, the attractiveness of the concept must be weighed against the possibility that patients with paraaortic metastases will also have hematogenous micrometastatic disease. Another issue is the ability of patients to tolerate combined chemotherapy and EFRT. Retrospective and prospective data suggest that there is substantial but manageable toxicity (545,546).

It is difficult to strongly recommend that any specific subset of patients should receive adjuvant EFRT. However, possible indications for its consideration include high pelvic lymph nodes involved, e.g., common iliac; gross nodal metastases in pelvis; bilateral positive pelvic lymph nodes; adenocarcinoma histology with any number of positive pelvic lymph nodes; and squamous-cell histology with ≥4 positive pelvic lymph nodes. In all cases, the radiation oncologist must determine that that patient is in reasonably good general health, with no, or limited, significant risk factors for RT injury. Furthermore, there should also be an assessment that there is a good chance of pelvic control (in patients receiving primary RT), since the absence of pelvic control will render paraaortic control meaningless. In this situation, the potential benefits of EFRT are considerably less, and the risk of complications is increased in patients who are less likely to benefit. This possibly excludes patients with bilateral stage IIIB disease.

Results of Therapeutic Paraaortic Lymph Node Irradiation

Data from the GOG suggests that patients with stages IB, II, III, and IVA cervical cancer will have spread to the paraaortic lymph nodes in 5%, 16%–21%, 25%–31%, and 13%, respectively (54,33). Tumor involvement in paraaortic lymph nodes is quite uncommon in the absence of pelvic lymph node metastasis (33). The degree to which RT demonstrates curative potential in this group of patients is quite variable, and is mostly related to selection factors in the patient population so treated.

Fifteen patients with involved paraaortic lymph nodes who received EFRT were reported by Brookland et al. (547). At a mean follow-up of 65 months, the 3-year actuarial NED survival was 50% among 12 patients with stages I-II tumors, whereas all 3 patients with stages III-IV tumors with paraaortic lymph node involvement died of disease, even with EFRT. Only 1 complication related to EFRT was observed.

Nori and colleagues reviewed 27 patients with documented paraaortic lymph node spread who underwent EFRT, including boosts to the delineated areas of involvement (502). Five-year survival was 29%. All survivors had squamous-cell carcinomas and stages I-II tumors. Patients with only microscopic involvement and macroscopic involvement had long-term survival rates of 60% and 23%, respectively. No long-term survivor suffered a late complication.

Lovecchio and associates (548) reported a 50% 5-year survival rate in 36 patients with stage IB and IIA cervical carcinoma who were identified at pre-therapy surgical staging laparotomy to have histologically confirmed paraaortic lymph node metastases. The patients were treated with radiation therapy, including 45 Gy to the paraaortic lymph nodes. Fourteen of 31 evaluable patients developed pelvic recurrence (12 of them combined with distant metastases). Unfortunately, the authors did not specify how many patients had paraaortic recurrences, although they reported four abdominal failures.

Forty-three patients comprised the series of patients with known paraaortic lymph node disease published by Vigliotti et al. (549). Nineteen patients had microscopic or small volume (<2 cm) paraaortic involvement; 14 had moderate tumor burdens of 2–5 cm; and 10 patients had massive paraaortic tumors >5 cm. All patients received EFRT of 39.6 to 60 Gy (median 50.4). At an impressive median follow-up of 13.5 years, 53% had developed distant metastases, and 28% remained continuously disease-free at the time of analysis or until intercurrent death. Survival rates at 5 years for patients with microscopic, small volume, moderate, and massive paraaortic tumor were 50%, 33%, 23%, and 0%, respectively. Patients with disease extending to the L1-L2 level were rarely salvaged. Complication rates were minimized in patients having extraperitoneal rather than transperitoneal dissections, as well as in patients with doses limited to 50 Gy. The investigators concluded that patients with paraaortic lymph node involvement most likely to benefit from EFRT are those patients with no more than a 2-cm tumor burden that does not extend above L3, in those whose pelvic tumor has a reasonable chance of pelvic control.

Kim and associates reviewed 43 patients with known paraaortic lymph node spread who received curative-intent RT following surgical staging and removal of gross paraaortic disease, in some cases (483). Pelvic tumor size (<6 cm vs. ≥6 cm) was a significant factor in survival. It was noted that patients with no residual paraaortic disease following surgery had significantly better outcomes than those patients with gross residual tumor, raising the question of whether surgical excision of bulky paraaortic lymph node disease is advisable in this situation. In contrast, Grigsby et al. did not find that tumor stage (reasonably correlated with pelvic tumor volume) was a significant factor in patients with paraaortic lymph node involvement (482). In a series of 43 patients the overall survival rate was 32% and the median survival was 2.2 years, although only 20 patients manifested recurrence. The predominant failure pattern was distant spread, suggesting that effective systemic therapy is warranted. Severe toxicity occurred in only 2 patients.

Based on a retrospective review of 35 patients treated for documented paraaortic lymph node spread, Stryker and Mortel suggested that EFRT can contribute to cure in approximately 30% of these patients (550). Again, patients with only microscopic involvement had considerably better outcomes than those with gross disease (42% vs. 26% 5-year survival). Grade 4 morbidity was seen in 8.6%, although in all cases the morbidity was related to the pelvic portion of the treatment rather than the EFRT.

Given the 50%-60% incidence of distant failure in this patient group, the role of chemotherapy is an appropriate question. Grigsby and associates (551) reported 47% survival and 49% locoregional failure at 2 years in 29 patients with stage I to IV carcinoma of the cervix, with biopsy-proven paraaortic lymph node metastases treated with hyperfractionated irradiation (48 Gy; 1.2 Gy twice daily), and a boost to reduced fields (total dose of 54 to 58 Gy), in addition to intracavitary irradiation in combination with cisplatin (75 mg/m² on days 1 and 22) and 5-FU (1000 mg/m²/24 hours for 4 days, beginning on days 1 and 22).

Varia et al. completed a Phase II study of EFRT plus chemotherapy (546). The protocol called for cisplatin to be given at 50 mg/m² on day 1, and 5-FU to be given at 1000 mg/m² over 96 hours during weeks 1 and 5. Eighty-six evaluable patients were accrued, 85 of whom completed EFRT; 90% completed chemotherapy. Grade 3–4 gastrointestinal and hematologic toxicities were seen in 19% and 15%, respectively. The actuarial risk of late morbidity was 14% at 4 years, primarily from rectal injury. Three-year overall survival and progression-free survival rates were 39% and 34%, respectively. Overall survival was 50% among stage I patients. Approximately 40% of patients had a distant failure as the first site of relapse.

Therapeutic EFRT in patients with paraaortic metastases appears to be efficacious, resulting in long-term survivals of 25%-50%. Definable sub-groups may have an even higher rate of long-term survival. EFRT can reliably control microscopic disease in the paraaortic chain; however, the curability of the individual patient is more a function of the ability to gain control of the pelvic disease and the likelihood that the patient will develop other metastatic disease.

In the era of combined chemotherapy and radiation therapy leading to improved local control and decreased systemic failure, the potential contribution of EFRT to improved outcome in patients with documented paraaortic lymph node metastases deserves additional consideration.

Chemotherapy can feasibly be added to EFRT in these patients, and it is reasonable to approach patients in this fashion unless co-morbid illnesses contraindicate systemic therapy. The optimum chemotherapy agents and schedule remain to be determined, although weekly cisplatin is a reasonable suggestion, based on current knowledge. The potential impact of concurrent chemotherapy on complication rates is unclear.

External Irradiation Alone

Rarely, brachytherapy procedures cannot be performed because of medical reasons or unusual anatomic configuration of the pelvis or the tumor (e.g., extensive lesion and inability to identify the cervical canal). These patients may be treated with higher doses of external irradiation alone, although the results are inferior to those obtained with combined external beam and intracavitary irradiation (390,529, 530,552).

Coia and co-workers (529), in an analysis of 565 patients with various stages of cervical carcinoma treated in the Patterns of Care Study, reported better survival (67%) and pelvic tumor control (78%) in patients undergoing brachytherapy treatment, compared with patients who had no intracavitary brachytherapy applications (36% 4-year survival, and 47% infield failure). In a later report from the Patterns of Care Study, Komaki and associates (526) reported improved outcomes for stage III patients, concurrent with the increased use of brachytherapy in the Patterns of Care Study surveys of 1973, 1978, and 1983.

Hanks and associates (552) and Montana and colleagues (530) reported a higher incidence of central-pelvic recurrences in patients with stage III cervical carcinoma treated with external beam alone than in patients receiving brachytherapy in addition to EBRT (Table 22.12). The incidence of major complications was similar in both groups of patients.

Castro and co-workers (553) reported on 118 patients with invasive cervical carcinoma treated with 50–60 Gy to the whole pelvis and boosts to residual tumor with reduced AP-PA portals to complete 70-Gy. With doses below 50 Gy, no pelvic tumor control was obtained in 32 patients, but disease control and survival were significantly enhanced with higher doses. Complications increased with higher doses; severe sigmoiditis was not noted in 32 patients treated with 50 Gy, but it was seen in 1 of 28 receiving 60 Gy and in 4 of 44 in the 70-Gy group.

Likewise, Akine and associates (554) treated 104 of 2,701 patients with carcinoma of the uterine cervix with external irradiation alone (AP-PA, or four-field box techniques) because of inability to perform intracavitary brachytherapy. The local tumor control rate was 27% for patients with stage II; 19% for stage III; and 15% for stage IVA disease. The 5-year survival rates were 36%, 17%, and 5%, respectively. Four patients had major complications (usually proctitis) that required surgical treatment, and one patient died of rectal bleeding.

COMPLICATIONS AND SEQUELAE OF SURGERY AND IRRADIATION

Surgery-Related Complications

Radical operation carries all of the complications associated with a major operation and general anesthesia. These include infection, pneumonitis, pulmonary embolus, myocardial infarction, cerebrovascular accident, hemorrhage, and death. The gynecologic oncologist's opportunity to choose between operation and radiation therapy has helped to maintain a low rate of operative complications. Decreasing morbidity and mortality can be attributed to improved anesthesia critical care, antibiotics, surgical technique and training, and similar advances. At many medical centers, the operative mortality of radical hysterectomy and pelvic lymphadenectomy is 2% or less (240,242–244,555).

Complications requiring readmission or reoperation are most often associated with the urinary tract. Fistula formation between the ureter or bladder and the vagina can occur in as many as 8.8% of patients (242–244,525). Fistulas are more commonly seen among those who have had prior irradiation. Without preoperative radiation therapy, the fistula rate is 2% to 4% (252). One-third to one-half of these fistulas can be expected to heal spontaneously with drainage. The remainder require repair, such as a ureteroneocystostomy. Rarely is nephrectomy or diversion indicated.

Bladder atony and delay in the removal of the urinary catheter are experienced by 4.2% of patients in collected series (252). The most commonly observed disability after radical hysterectomy is urinary dysfunction, resulting from partial denervation of the detrusor muscle (540). Patients may have various degrees of loss of bladder sensation, inability to initiate voiding, residual urine retention, and incontinence. The bladder may be contracted and spastic in the early postoperative period, but may become overdistended and hypotonic later. Appropriate therapy depends on a complete evaluation of detrusor function and may include anticholinergics, Δ-adrenergics, antibiotics, change in voiding habits, or intermittent self-catheterization.

Some loss of defecatory urge associated with chronic rectal dysfunction has been observed and characterized by Barnes and associates following radical hysterectomy (557). Manometric studies suggest a disruption of the spinal arcs controlling defecation.

Although these complications may be more amenable to correction than are the late effects after irradiation, comparative studies indicate that the frequency of long-term complications is not greatly different between operation and irradiation (240–242,558). Symmonds (558) observed that "it is unfortunate that there is no standard of measuring morbidity which provides a real appraisal of the patient's postoperative condition." Although ovarian and vaginal function may be preserved, we should not underestimate the disruptions caused by radical operation. Loss of reproductive function is taken for granted with either radical operation or radiation therapy. The emotional impact of hysterectomy may be negative, making the patient feed scarred or neutered. On the other hand, some patients will be relieved to have their cancer excised.

Radiation Therapy–Related Complications

Early effects of RT are usually manageable and resolve soon after treatment. Pedersen and associates reviewed 442 consecutive patients treated with combined external and intracavitary RT (559). Medication was required for early morbidity in 68% of patients.

Late sequelae are often permanent or require some intervention to improve. Commonly reported late sequelae of pelvic radiation therapy involve the recto-sigmoid, the small intestine, the genitourinary tract, the vagina, and other sites or organs, resulting, for example, in lymphedema, lumbosacral plexopathy, and pelvic insufficiency fractures. Rectosigmoid complications include chronic proctosigmoiditis, rectal stricture, and rectal ulcer. Complications involving the small intestine include obstruction and malabsorption syndrome. Genitourinary toxicity includes chronic cystitis, bladder contracture, urethral stricture, and incontinence. Late sequelae involving the vagina include vaginal stenosis/fibrosis, dyspareunia, vault necrosis, and rectovaginal or vesicovaginal fistulas.

There is approximately a 5% rate of major late sequelae in patients with stage I cervical carcinoma treated with radiation therapy, and approximately 10% in patients with stages II-IVA disease. Grade 2 complications are seen in 10%–15%

of patients with all stages treated with RT alone (560,561). However, the risk is related to a number of factors, mainly dose and volume treated.

Perez et al. reported a <2% risk of severe small bowel toxicity when the pelvic sidewall dose was <50 Gy, and a 5% incidence with doses >60 Gy (560). Similar findings were reported by Lanciano et al. (562). In a multivariate analysis, Perez et al. found only total doses to rectal and bladder points to significantly impact morbidity (561). A number of other authors have found a significant relationship between radiation dose and complications (531,563–566). Strockbine and colleagues (567), Hamberger and associates (220), Quilty (568), and Unal and coworkers (569) noted a greater incidence of pelvic complications in patients treated with higher doses to the whole pelvis (40 to 50 Gy). The authors found that the intracavitary radium dose did not correlate with severe complications. Similar observations were made by Stryker and associates (570) in 132 patients who had a 9% incidence of fistulas, and a 14% incidence of grade 2 and 3 complications after delivery of 50 Gy or higher to the whole pelvis (1.8 Gy daily dose) combined with intracavitary insertion. They recommended that the whole pelvis dose not exceed 40 to 45 Gy when doses of approximately 40 Gy are delivered to point A with intracavitary insertions.

It is accepted that there are other predisposing factors for injury, particularly to small bowel, including history of abdominopelvic surgery and pelvic inflammatory disease. In addition, Sherrah-Davies (571) reported higher morbidity when patients were treated with higher daily fractions of EBRT (40 Gy in 16 fractions over 3 weeks). The use of fraction sizes >2 Gy is generally not advisable. Patients with significant acute toxicity during RT may have an increased risk of late injury (572,573).

Injury to the gastrointestinal tract is the most frequent late complication of RT for cervical cancer. The rate of chronic bowel injury is 5%–15% in most series of patients treated with pelvic RT (560,572). These injuries may take years to manifest, but most series report a median latency period of 8–12 months (564). A report by Eifel and colleagues (172) on 1,784 patients with stage IB carcinoma of the cervix indicates that the greatest risk is in the first 3 years after therapy. The risk of rectal complications declined after the first 2 years of follow-up to 0.06% per year. Major complications include intestinal obstruction, fistula formation, severe bleeding, and intractable diarrhea. Fortunately, these sequelae are relatively infrequent. These injuries generally result from fibrosis and ischemia secondary to the effect of RT on the small blood vessels and connective tissue. Conservative management might include a low-residue diet, antidiarrheal medications, and steroid or sucralfate enemas. Some cases of partial small bowel obstruction can be managed by bowel rest, decompression, and diet modification. Obstruction refractory to conservative management may require surgery involving intestinal resection, and/or end-to-end anastomoses (573).

Chronic urinary symptoms (urgency, incontinence, and frequency) are frequently seen following RT. Parkin and associates (574) reported a 26% incidence of these symptoms in patients treated with irradiation alone for cervical carcinoma. The authors carried out urodynamic studies in 42 women, all of whom were free of disease 5 to 11 years after therapy. Cystometrograms and urethral profiles were performed and compared with 28 women having urodynamic evaluations before and after treatment. There was no difference in the mean maximum flow rate or mean residual urine value in the two groups. However, mean volume of full bladder sensation was significantly lower in the postirradiation group than in the pretreatment group, as was the mean maximum cystometric capacity. It should be noted that this same dysfunction is noted in about 10% of the general female population (575), and that it increases in older women (576).

Severe genitourinary toxicities secondary to RT include hemorrhagic cystitis and fistula. In large series, the rate at which these occur is 2%–3% (560,561,575) The latency period between RT and symptom onset is considerably longer than for gastrointestinal sequelae (559,560,562). Maier et al. reported the mean time to urinary fistula to be 2.7 years after RT, compared with ureteral stenosis, at 5.7 years (575). In the longitudinal study by Eifel et al. (172), the risk of major urinary tract complications for survivors continued at 0.3% per year beyond 20 years. At 20 years, the actuarial risk of major complications was 14.4%. Lajer et al. prospectively gathered data regarding urologic morbidity in 177 consecutive patients treated curatively with RT (576). The 5-year actuarial incidences of grades $1+2+3$, $2+3$, and 3 were 62%, 32%, and 5%, respectively. In the long-term recurrence-free survivors, there was some evidence of some reversibility of grades 1 and 2 morbidities.

The impact of concurrent chemotherapy on complication rates awaits additional patients, follow-up, and analysis. Souhami et al. observed an unexpectedly high rate of late gastrointestinal complications in patients treated with RT (with HDR brachytherapy) and concurrent cisplatin (577). Furthermore, the time course of these complications was compressed, with a median time to complication of 11 months following treatment completion. Sood et al. observed an increase in complication rate with chemotherapy, in comparison to patients who did not receive concurrent chemoradiation (578). The RT regimen included external RT and 2 fractions of HDR brachytherapy.

Vaginal function can be affected by both radical surgery and RT. Surgery will shorten the functional length of the vagina, but pliability and transudative lubrication are often preserved. Jensen et al. performed a longitudinal study of sexual function and vaginal changes after radiotherapy for cervical cancer (579). Over one-third reported lack of lubrication, 55% had some degree of dyspareunia, and 30% were dissatisfied with their sexual life. However, 63% of patients who were sexually active before treatment remained so following RT. Although some gynecologists feel that radical pelvic surgery may affect vaginal function to a lesser degree than radiation therapy (233,234), a large Swedish study questions this belief. Using a control group of untreated subjects and comparing them to patients treated with surgery, RT, or combination therapy for stages IB-IIA cervical cancer, the investigators found that the type of treatment had virtually no effect on the prevalence of vaginal changes and sexual distress (580). Radiation therapy can reduce length, caliber, and lubrication of the vagina; however, these symptoms can be alleviated in some patients with hormonal replacement and vaginal dilatation.

Although extremely rare, lumbosacral plexopathy has been occasionally reported in patients treated for pelvic tumors with doses of 60 to 67.5 Gy (581–583). At the Mallinckrodt Institute of Radiology, this syndrome has been observed in four patients with cervical carcinoma receiving external pelvic irradiation (60 Gy to the parametria) and brachytherapy. Characteristically, these patients have lower motor neuron weakness of the legs combined with loss of deep reflexes and muscular fasciculation. Although cystometrograms have demonstrated bladder atonicity in some cases, several authors have failed to observe bladder or rectal sphincter disturbances.

Ashenhurst and associates (581) noted that several patients previously reported as having radiation myelopathy of the dorsolumbar spine may indeed have suffered a lumbar and sacral nerve plexopathy instead of, or in addition to, the spinal cord injury (582). The differential diagnosis with recurrent tumors is sometimes difficult. In a comparison of 20 patients with lumbosacral plexopathy after irradiation, and 30 patients with plexus damage from pelvic malignancy, Thomas and associates (583) pointed out that indolent leg weakness occurred early in radiation-induced plexopathy (pain occurred initially in 10% of the patients, although ultimately it was present in 50%), whereas pain was most frequently associated with tumor plexopathy. Muscular weakness, numbness, and paresthesia are common in both groups. Computed tomography is extremely helpful in the detection of pelvic masses or bone destruction caused by tumor.

Insufficiency fracture occurs with normal stress in bone with diminished elastic flexibility, a condition that can exist in irradiated bones (584). The usual presenting symptom is moderate to severe pelvic pain. Although rare, they are reported in patients treated for gynecologic malignancies (585–587). Huh et al. reported that 8 out of 463 patients (1.7%) developed this complication (588). All patients were post-menopausal, and 7 of 8 were treated with curative intent. Differential diagnosis can include metastatic disease, tumor recurrence, second malignancy, and benign causes. Because symptoms can resolve with conservative management, proper diagnosis is important.

Although extremely rare, radiation myelitis can occur with extended field RT combined with chemotherapy. In a case reported by Bloss et al., this devastating complication

was seen with only 45 Gy in 30 fractions given to the paraaortic chain along with cisplatin (50 mg/m^2), and 5-FU continuous infusion at 300 mg/m^2 per day during RT (589). A latent period of 4 months was observed in this case. Fortunately, current chemoradiation regimens have not been associated with this complication.

Grigsby et al. published a detailed review of the late effects of cancer treatment on the female reproductive tract (590). A grading system based on the SOMA methodology was proposed (Symptoms, Objective, Management, and Analytic). Evaluation of this tool suggests that these scales are feasible to administer, and are valid in assessing the early subjective morbidity from radiation therapy (591).

Low-dose-rate (and pulsed LDR) implants require hospitalization and bed rest. At typical dose rates of 50–60 cGy per hour, implants typically last 2 or 3 days. During this time, there is the potential for acute problems related to or during the hospital stay. Wollschlaeger et al. reviewed 170 implants in 128 patients to determine the frequency and type of acute morbidity, finding that these developed during 42 implants (24.7%) (592). In 95% of cases, only minor problems such as uncomplicated fever and gastrointestinal distress occurred. In 2 cases (5%), persistent fever was considered an acute morbidity of moderate severity. No severe problems were encountered in this series. There were no identifiable prognostic features, including co-morbid illness, that were statistically correlated with these acute events. Jhingran and Eifel reviewed 7,662 implants in 4,043 patients, finding fatal or life-threatening complications to be exceptionally rare (593). Older series suggest slightly higher rates of acute morbidity (594,595).

Complications of Combined-Modality Therapies

Irradiation and Surgery

In some series, the complication rate tends to be higher with preoperative irradiation combined with surgery than with either modality alone, particularly because of injury to the ureter or the bladder (172,596). The dose of irradiation, technique, and type of surgical procedure performed are important in determining the morbidity of combined therapy. O'Quinn and co-workers (410) noted a decrease in severe complications of combined therapy, from 11.6% to 4%, when the two modalities were properly integrated. Excessive irradiation dose to the vaginal apex was associated with increased complications. These authors recommended use of meticulous, sharp dissection in performance of extrafascial hysterectomy. Jacobs and co-workers (597) noted a major complication rate of 5% in 102 patients with invasive cervical carcinoma treated with low dose preoperative irradiation and a radical hysterectomy with lymphadenectomy, or high dose preoperative irradiation and a conservative extrafascial hysterectomy.

A retrospective analysis of 306 patients with carcinoma of

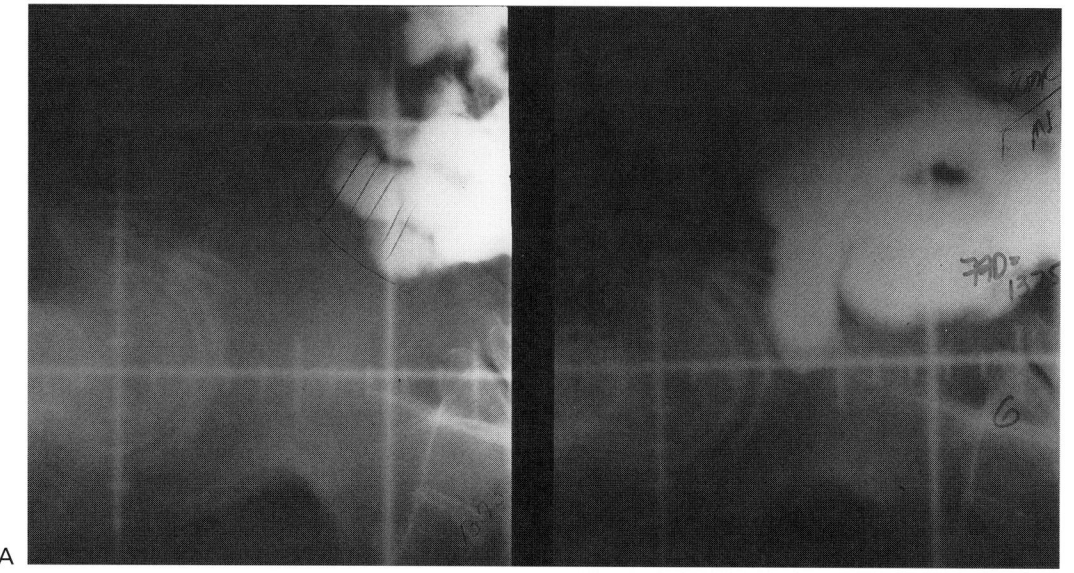

FIG. 22.31. Lateral radiographs, **(A)** with and **(B)** without bladder distention in a patient with contrast in small intestine.

the cervix receiving preoperative irradiation or postoperative irradiation showed morbidity in both groups comparable to that of irradiation alone (414). The most common moderate sequelae were cystitis, leg edema, and vault necrosis. The most common major sequelae were small-bowel obstruction/perforation (4.2%), ureteral stricture (2.6%), vesicovaginal fistula (1.6%), and rectovaginal fistula (1.3%). Eifel et al. found that the risk of rectovaginal fistula was doubled in patients who underwent extrafascial hysterectomy after RT, compared to those who had RT only (250).

The GOG performed a randomized trial in which 256 eligible patients with carcinomas of the cervix ≥4 cm were treated with either external beam and intracavitary irradiation, or with a slightly lower dose of intracavitary irradiation and the same external beam pelvic irradiation, followed by an extrafascial hysterectomy (419). In this series, the rates of grade 3 and 4 adverse effects were approximately 10% in both groups.

Surgery Followed by Irradiation

Radical operation commonly results in intestinal adhesions to denuded surfaces in the pelvis. When postoperative RT is recommended to selected patients, further complica-

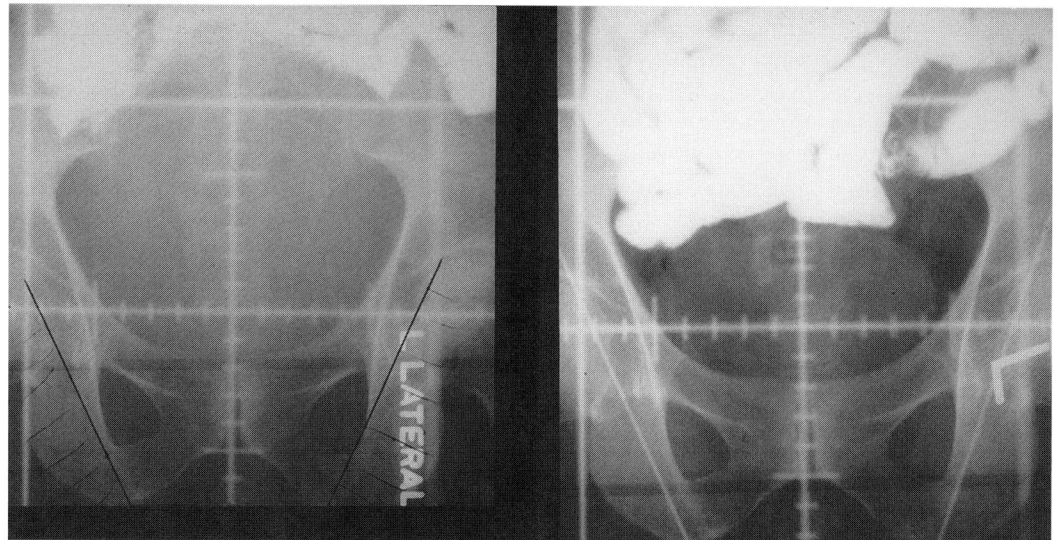

FIG. 22.32. Anteroposterior radiographs **(A)** with and **(B)** without bladder distention in a patient with contrast in small intestine.

tions of the additional therapy are expected. The Gynecologic Oncology Group demonstrated a significant increase in grades 2–4 late complications among patients undergoing pre-RT surgical staging, particularly with a transperitoneal approach compared with a retroperitoneal approach (302). Enteric complications, such as obstruction, fistula, or dysfunction were observed in 30% of patients so treated by Barter and associates (555) and in 24% of patients treated by Fiorica and colleagues (426). Other investigators, however, have reported no difference in the incidence of severe complications (424).

One complication that appears to be more common after combined treatment is lymphedema, which was observed in 23.4% of 402 patients treated by Martimbeau and others (598).

After pelvic irradiation or bilateral salpingo-oophorectomy with radical hysterectomy, vasomotor symptoms of menopause may occur. They can be treated with replacement hormones.

Decreased enteric morbidity has been observed by surgical modifications such as extraperitoneal lymphadenectomy to reduce intestinal adhesions to the posterior peritoneum (306,599,600) and by limiting radiation dose to the paraaortic nodes to 45 Gy (290,600). Methods to decrease the volume of small bowel irradiated will further lessen enteric morbidity. Figures 22.31 and 22.32 show the effect of treating patients in prone position with full bladder as a means of limiting the volume of small bowel irradiated.

REFERENCES

1. Garland SM. Human papillomavirus update with a particular focus on cervical disease. *Pathology* 2002;34:213–224.
2. Ferlay J, Bray F, Pisani P, et al. GLOBOCAN 2000: Cancer incidence, mortality and prevalence worldwide, Version 1.1, IARC Cancer Base No. 5, Lyon: IARC Press, 2001.
3. Franco EL, Duarte-Franco E, Ferenczy A. Cervical cancer: epidemiology, prevention and the role of human papillomavirus infection. *Can Med Assoc J* 2001;164:1017–1025.
4. Graham S, Priore R, Graham M, et al. Genital cancer in wives of penile cancer patients. *Cancer* 1979;44:1870–1874.
5. Schiffman MH, Brinton LA, Devesa SS, et al. Cervical cancer. In: Schottenfeld D, Fraumeni JF Jr, (ed). *Cancer epidemiology and prevention.* New York: Oxford University Press, 1996:1090–1116.
6. Winkelstein W. Smoking and cervical cancer: current status—a review. *Am J Epidemiol* 1990;131:945–957.
7. Jay N, Moscicki AB. Human papillomavirus infections in women with HIV disease: prevalence, risk and management. *AIDS Read* 2000;10:659–668.
8. Anson BJ, McVay CB. *Surgical anatomy.* 5th ed. Philadelphia: WB Saunders, 1971:800.
9. Woodman CBJ, Collins S, Winter R, et al. Natural history of cervical human papillomavirus infection in young women: a longitudinal cohort study. *Lancet* 2001;357:1831–1836.
10. Nasiell K, Roger V, Masiell M, et al. Behaviour of mild-cervical dysplasia during long-term follow-up. *Obstet Gynecol* 1986;67:665–669.
11. Holowaty P, Miller AB, Rohan T, et al. Natural history of dysplasia of the uterine cervix. *J Natl Cancer Inst* 1999;91:252–258.
12. Ho GY, Bierman R, Beardsley L, et al. Natural history of cervicovaginal papillomavirus infection in young women. *N Engl J Med* 1998;338:423–428.
13. Perez CA, Camel HM, Askin F, et al. Endometrial extension of carcinoma of the uterine cervix: a prognostic factor that may modify staging. *Cancer* 1981;48:170.
14. Henriksen E. The lymphatic spread of carcinoma of the cervix and of the body of the uterus: a study of 420 necropsies. *Am J Obstet Gynecol* 1949;58:924.
15. Lagasse LD, Creasman WT, Shingleton HM, et al. Results and complications of operative staging in cervical cancer: experience of the Gynecologic Oncology Group. *Gynecol Oncol* 1980;9:90.
16. Girardi F, Lichtenegger W, Tamussino K, Haas J. The importance of parametrial lymph nodes in the treatment of cervical cancer. *Gynecol Oncol* 1989;34:206.
17. Averette HE, Nguyen HN, Donato DM, et al. Radical hysterectomy for invasive cervical cancer: a 25-year prospective experience with the Miami technique. *Cancer* 1993;71:1422.
18. Kamura T, Tsukamoto N, Tsuruchi N, et al. Multivariate analysis of the histopathologic prognostic factors of cervical cancer in patients undergoing radical hysterectomy. *Cancer* 1992;69:181.
19. Alvarez HE, Potter ME, Soong SJ, et al. Rationale for using pathologic tumor dimensions and nodal status to subclassify surgically treated stage IB cervical cancer patients. *Gynecol Oncol* 1991;43:108.
20. Ayhan A, Tuncer ZS. Radical hysterectomy with lymphadenectomy for treatment of early stage cervical cancer: clinical experience of 278 cases. *J Surg Oncol* 1991;47:175.
21. Delgado G, Bundy BN, Fowler WC, et al. A prospective surgical pathological study of stage I squamous carcinoma of the cervix: a Gynecologic Oncology Group study. *Gynecol Oncol* 1989;35:314.
22. Lee YN, Wang KL, Lin MH, et al. Radical hysterectomy with pelvic lymph node dissection for treatment of cervical cancer: a clinical review of 954 cases. *Gynecol Oncol* 1989;32:135.
23. Fuller AF, Elliott N, Kosloff C, Hoskins WJ, Lewis JL. Determinants of increased risk for recurrence in patients undergoing radical hysterectomy for stage IB and IIA carcinoma of the cervix. *Gynecol Oncol* 1989;33:34.
24. Barber H. Cervical cancer: pelvic and para-aortic lymph node sampling and its consequences. *Baillieres Clin Obstet Gynaecol* 1988;2:769.
25. Burghardt E, Pickel H, Haas J, Lahousen M. Prognostic factors and operative treatment of stages IB to IIB cervical cancer. *Am J Obstet Gynecol* 1987;156:988.
26. Creasman WT, Soper JT, Clarke-Pearson D. Radical hysterectomy as therapy for early carcinoma of the cervix. *Am J Obstet Gynecol* 1986;155:964.
27. Boyce J, Fruchter R, Nicastri A, et al. Prognostic factors in stage I carcinoma of the cervix. *Gynecol Oncol* 1981;12:154.
28. Piver MS, Chung WS. Prognostic significance of cervical lesion size and pelvic node metastases in cervical carcinoma. *Obstet Gynecol* 1975;46:507.
29. Boronow RC. Stage I cervix cancer and pelvic node metastasis. *Am J Obstet Gynecol* 1977;127:135.
30. Sudarsanam A, Charyulu K, Belinson J, et al. Influence of exploratory celiotomy on the management of carcinoma of the cervix: a preliminary report. *Cancer* 1978;41:1049.
31. Stehman FB, Bundy BN, DiSaia PH, et al. Carcinoma of the cervix treated with irradiation therapy. I. A multi-variate analysis of prognostic variables in the Gynecologic Oncology Group. *Cancer* 1991;67:2776.
32. LaPolla JP, Schlaerth JB, Gaddis O, et al. The influence of surgical staging on evaluation and treatment of patients with cervical carcinoma. *Gynecol Oncol* 1986;24:194.
33. Berman ML, Keys H, Creasman W, et al. Survival and patterns of recurrence in cervical cancer metastatic to periaortic lymph nodes: a Gynecologic Oncology Group study. *Gynecol Oncol* 1984;19:8.
34. Ballon SC, Berman ML, Lagasse LD, et al. Survival after extraperitoneal pelvic and paraaortic lymphadenectomy and radiation therapy in cervical carcinoma. *Obstet Gynecol* 1981;57:90.
35. Buchsbaum H. Extrapelvic lymph node metastases in cervical carcinoma. *Am J Obstet Gynecol* 1979;133:814.
36. Wharton JT, Jones HW III, Day TG Jr, et al. Preirradiation celiotomy and extended field irradiation for invasive carcinoma of the cervix. *Obstet Gynecol* 1977;49:333.
37. Nelson JH, Boyce J, Macasaet M, et al. Incidence, significance, and

follow-up of para-aortic lymph node metastases in late invasive carcinoma of the cervix. *Am J Obstet Gynecol* 1977;128:336.

38. Guthrie RT, Buchsbaum HJ, White AJ, Latourette HB. Para-aortic lymph node irradiation in carcinoma of the uterine cervix. *Cancer* 1974;34:166.

39. Covens A, Rosen B, Murphy J, et al. How important is removal of the parametrium at surgery for carcinoma of the cervix? *Gynecol Oncol* 2002;84:145–149.

40. Carlson V, Delclos L, Fletcher GH. Distant metastases in squamous-cell carcinoma of the uterine cervix. *Radiology* 1967;88:961.

41. Bodurka-Bevers D, Morris M, Eifel PJ, et al. Post-therapy surveillance of women with cervical cancer—an outcomes analysis. *Gynecol Oncol* 2000;78:187–193.

42. Takehara K, Shigemasa K, Sawasaki T, et al. Recurrence of invasive cervical carcinoma more than 5 years after initial therapy. *Obstet Gynecol* 2001;98:680–684.

43. Smith RA, Cokkinides V, Eyre HJ. American Cancer Society guidelines for the early detection of cancer, 2003. *CA Cancer J Clin* 2003; 53:27–43.

44. National Cancer Institute Workshop. The 1988 Bethesda System for reporting cervical/vaginal cytologic diagnoses. *JAMA* 1989;262:931–934.

45. The 1991 Bethesda System for reporting cervical/vaginal cytologic diagnoses: report of the 1991 Bethesda Workshop. *JAMA* 1992;267:2892.

46. Solomon D, Davey D, Kurman R, et al. The 2001 Bethesda System: terminology for reporting results of cervical cytology (consensus statement). *JAMA* 2002;287:2114–2119.

47. Solomon D, Schiffman M, Tarone R for the ALTS Group. Comparison of three management strategies for patients with atypical squamous cells of undetermined significance: baseline results from a randomized trial. *J Natl Cancer Inst* 2001;93:293–299.

48. Sherman ME, Solomon D, Schiffman M for the ALTS Group. Qualification of ASCUS: a comparison of equivocal LSIL and equivocal HSIL cervical cytology in the ASCUS LSIL Triage Study. *Am J Clin Pathol* 2001;116:386–394.

49. Quddus MR, Sung CJ, Steinhoff MM, et al. Atypical squamous metaplastic cells: reproducibility, outcome and diagnostic features on ThinPrep Pap test. *Cancer* 2001;93:16–22.

50. Sherman ME, Tabbara SO, Scott DR, et al. "ASCUS, rule out HSIL": cytologic features, histologic correlates and human papillomavirus detection. *Mod Pathol* 1999;12:335–358.

51. Alvarez RD, Helm CW, Edwards RP, et al. Prospective randomized trial of LLETZ versus laser ablation in patients with cervical intraepithelial neoplasia. *Gynecol Oncol* 1994;52:175.

52. Mitchell MF, Tortolero-Luna G, Cook E, et al. A randomized clinical trial of cryotherapy, laser vaporization, and loop electrosurgical excision for treatment of squamous intraepithelial lesions of the cervix. *Obstet Gynecol* 1998;92:737.

53. Russell AH, Shingleton HM, Jones WB, et al. Diagnostic assessments in patients with invasive cancer of the cervix: A National Patterns of Care study of the American College of Surgeons. *Gynecol Oncol* 1996;63:159.

54. Heller PB, Malfetano JH, Bundy BN. Clinical pathologic study of stages IIB, III, and IVA carcinoma of the cervix: extended diagnostic evaluation for paraaortic node metastasis (a GOG study). *Gynecol Oncol* 1990;38:425.

55. Camilien L, Fordon D, Fruchter RG, et al. Predictive value of computerized tomography in the presurgical evaluation of primary carcinoma of the cervix. *Gynecol Oncol* 1988;30:209.

56. Ohara K, Tanaka YO, Tsunoda H, et al. Non-operative assessment of nodal status for locally advanced cervical squamous cell carcinoma treated by radiotherapy with regard to patterns of treatment failure. *Int J Radiat Oncol Biol Phys* 2003;55:354–361.

57. Mayr NA, Tali ET, Yuh WTC, et al. Cervical cancer: application of MR imaging in radiation therapy. *Radiology* 1993;189:601.

58. Russell AH, Walter JP, Anderson MW, et al. Sagittal magnetic resonance imaging in the design of lateral radiation treatment portals for patients with locally advanced squamous cancer of the cervix. *Int J Radiat Oncol Biol Phys* 1992;23:449.

59. Singh AK, Grigsby PW, Farroka D, et al. FDG-PET lymph node staging and and survival of patients with FIGO stage IIIb cervical carcinoma. *Int J Radiat Oncol Biol Phys* 2003;56:489–493.

60. Lin WC, Hung YC, Yeh LS, et al. Usefulness of 18F-fluorodeoxyglucose positron emission tomography to detect para-aortic lymph nodal metastasis in advanced cervical cancer with negative computed tomography findings. *Gynecol Oncol* 2003;89:73–76.

61. Park SY, Roh JW, Park YJ, et al. Positron emission tomography (PET) for evaluating para-aortic and pelvic lymph node metastasis in cervical cancer before surgical staging: A surgico-pathologic study. *Proc Am Soc Clin Oncol* 2003;22:456 (abstract).

62. Creasman WT. New gynecologic cancer staging. *Gynecol Oncol* 1995;58:157.

63. International Federation of Gynecologists and Obstetricians (FIGO). Changes in the definitions of clinical staging for the cervix and ovary. *Am J Obstet Gynecol* 1987;156:263.

64. Kolstad P. Follow-up study of 232 patients with stage IA1 and 411 patients with stage IA2 squamous cell carcinoma of the cervix (microinvasive carcinoma). *Gynecol Oncol* 1989;33:265.

65. Tsukamoto N, Kaku T, Matsukuma K, et al. The problem of stage IA (FIGO, 1985) carcinoma of the uterine cervix. *Gynecol Oncol* 1989;34:1.

66. American Joint Committee on Cancer (AJCC). Chapter 28: Cervix Uteri. In: Greene FL, Page DL, Fleming ID, et al., eds. *AJCC Cancer Staging Manual.* 6th ed. New York: Springer, 2002:260.

67. Van Nagell JR, Roddick JW, Lowin DM. The staging of cervical cancer: inevitable discrepancies between clinical staging and pathologic findings. *Am J Obstet Gynecol* 1971;110:973.

68. DiSaia PJ, Bundy BN, Curry SL, et al. Phase III study of the treatment of women with cervical cancer, stage IIB, IIIB, and IVA (confined to the pelvis and/or periaortic nodes) with radiotherapy alone versus radiotherapy plus immunotherapy with intravenous *Corynebacterium parvum*: A GOG study. *Gynecol Oncol* 1987;26:386.

69. Potish RA, Twiggs LB, Okagaki T, et al. Therapeutic implications of the natural history of advanced cervical cancer as defined by pretreatment surgical staging. *Cancer* 1985;56:956.

70. Rubin SC, Brookland R, Mikuta JJ, et al. Para-aortic nodal metastases in early cervical carcinoma: long-term survival following extended-field radiotherapy. *Gynecol Oncol* 1984;18:213.

71. Goff BA, Muntz HG, Paley PJ, et al. Impact of surgical staging in women with locally advanced cervical cancer. *Gynecol Oncol* 1999; 74:436–442.

72. Kupets R, Thomas GM, Covens A. Is there a role for pelvic lymph node debulking in advanced cervical cancer? *Gynecol Oncol* 2002; 87:163–170.

73. Spriggs AI, Boddington MM. Progression and regression of cervical lesions. Review of smears from women followed without initial biopsy or treatment. *J Clin Pathol* 1980;33:517–522.

74. Walboomers JMM, Jacobs MV, Manos MM, et al. Human papillomavirus is a necessary cause of invasive cervical cancer worldwide. *J Pathol* 1999;189:12–19.

75. Parazzini F, Franceschi S, La Vecchia C, et al. The epidemiology of female genital tract cancers. *Int J Gynecol Cancer* 1997;7:169–181.

76. Crissman JD, Makuch R, Budhraja ML. Histopathologic grading of squamous cell carcinoma of the uterine cervix. An evaluation of 70 stage Ib patients. *Cancer* 1985;55:1590–1661.

77. Kristensen GB, Abeler VM, Risberg B, et al. Tumor size, depth of invasion and grading of the invasive tumor front are the main prognostic factors in early squamous cell cervical carcinoma. *Gynecol Oncol* 1999;74:245–251.

78. Zaino RJ, Ward S, Delgado G, et al. Histopathologic predictors of the behavior of surgically treated stage IB squamous cell carcinoma of the cervix: A GOG Study. *Cancer* 1990; 69:1750–1758.

79. Faaborg LL, Smith ML, Newland JR. Case report: uterine cervical and vaginal verrucous squamous cell carcinoma. *Gynecol Oncol* 1979; 8:104–109.

80. Kashimura M, Tsukamoto N, Matsukuma K, et al. Verrucous carcinoma of the uterine cervix: report of a case with follow-up of 6½ years. *Gynecol Oncol* 1984;19:204–215.

81. Tiltman AJ, Atad J. Verrucous carcinoma of the cervix with endometrial involvement. *Int J Gynecol Pathol* 1982;1:221–226.

82. Randall ME, Andersen WA, Mills SE, et al. Papillary squamous cell carcinoma of the uterine cervix: a clinicopathologic study of nine cases. *Int J Gynecol Pathol* 1986;5:1–10.

83. Brinck U, Jakob C, Bau O, et al. Papillary squamous cell carcinoma

of the uterine cervix: report of three cases and a review of its classification. *Int J Gynecol Pathol* 2000;19:231–235.

84. Koenig C, Turnicky RP, Collins FK, et al. Papillary squamotransitional cell carcinoma of the cervix: a report of 32 cases. *Am J Surg Pathol* 1997;21:915–921.

85. Albores-Saavedra J, Young RH. Transitional cell neoplasms (carcinomas and inverted papillomas) of the uterine cervix. A report of five cases. *Am J Surg Pathol* 1995;19:1138–1145.

86. Kurman RJ, Norris HJ, Wilkinson E. Atlas of Tumor Pathology, Third Series, Fascicle 4. Tumors of the Cervix, Vagina and Vulva. Armed Forces Institute of Pathology, Washington, D.C., 1992.

87. Wright TC, Ferenczy A, Kurman RJ. Carcinoma and other tumors of the cervix. In Kurman RJ (ed). *Blaustein's pathology of the female genital tract.* 5th ed. New York: Springer Verlag, 2002:325–381.

88. Cho NH, Joo HJ, Ahn HJ, et al. Detection of human papillomavirus in warty carcinoma of the uterine cervix: comparison of immunohistochemistry, in situ hybridization and in situ polymerase chain reaction methods. *Pathol Res Pract* 1998;194:713–720.

89. Mills SE, Austin MB, Randall ME. Lymphoepithelioma-like carcinoma of the uterine cervix: a distinctive, undifferentiated carcinoma with inflammatory stroma. *Am J Surg Pathol* 1985;9:883–889.

90. Tseng CJ, Pao CC, Tseng LH, et al. Lymphoepithelioma-like carcinoma of the uterine cervix: association with Epstein-Barr virus and human papillomavirus. *Cancer* 2000;80:91–97.

91. Martorell MA, Julian JM, Calabuig C, et al. Lymphoepithelioma-like carcinoma of the uterine cervix. A clinicopathologic study of 4 cases not associated with Epstein-Barr virus, human papillomavirus, or simian virus 40. *Arch Pathol Lab Med* 2002;126:1501–1505.

92. Noel J, Lespagnard L, Fayt I, et al. Evidence of Human Papilloma virus infection but lack of Epstein-Barr virus in lymphoepithelioma-like carcinoma of uterine cervix: report of two cases and review of the literature. *Hum Pathol* 2001;32:135–138.

93. Saylam K, Anaf V, Fayt I, et al. Lymphoepithelioma-like carcinoma of the cervix with prominent eosinophilic infiltrate: an HPV associated case. *Acta Obstet Gynecol Scand* 2002;81:564–566.

94. Zaino RJ. Symposium Part I: Adenocarcinoma in situ, glandular dysplasia, and early invasive adenocarcinoma of the uterine cervix. *Int J Gynecol Pathol* 2002;21:314–326.

95. Young RH, Clement PB. Endocervical adenocarcinoma and its variants: their morphology and differential diagnosis. *Histopathology* 2002;41:185–207.

96. McCluggage WG. Endocervical glandular lesions: controversial aspects and ancillary techniques. *J Clin Pathol* 2003;56:164–173.

97. Hemminki K, Li X, Vaittinen P. Time trends in the incidence of cervical and other genital squamous cell carcinomas and adenocarcinomas in Sweden, 1958–1996. *Eur J Obstet Gynecol Reprod Biol* 2002;101:64–69.

98. Smith HO, Tiffany FF, Qualls CR, et al. The rising incidence of adenocarcinoma relative to squamous cell carcinoma of the uterine cervix in the United States: a 24-year population-based study. *Gynecol Oncol* 2000;78:97–105.

99. Fox H, Wells M, Harris M, et al. Enteric tumours of the lower female genital tract: a report of three cases. *Histopathology* 1988;12:167–176.

100. Haswani P, Arseneau J, Ferenczy A. Primary signet ring cell carcinoma of the uterine cervix: a clinicopathologic study of two cases with review of the literature. *Int J Gynecol Cancer* 1998;8:374–379.

101. Mayora M, Garcia-Valtuille A, Fernandez F et al. Adenocarcinoma of the uterine cervix with massive signet-ring cell differentiation. *Int J Surg Pathol* 1997;5:95–100.

102. McKelvey JL, Goodlin RR. Adenoma malignum of the cervix. *Cancer* 1963;16:549–557.

103. Silverberg SG, Hurt WG. Minimal deviation adenocarcinoma (''adenoma malignum'') of the cervix: a reappraisal. *Am J Obstet Gynecol* 1975;121:971–975.

104. Michael H, Grawe L, Kraus FT. Minimal deviation endocervical adenocarcinoma: clinical and histologic features, immunohistochemical staining for carcinoembryonic antigen, and differentiation from confusing benign lesions. *Int J Gynecol Pathol* 1984;3:261–276.

105. Kaminski PF, Morris HJ. Minimal deviation carcinoma (adenoma malignum) of the cervix. *Int J Gynecol Pathol* 1983;2:141–152.

106. Hart WR. Symposium Part II: Special Types of Adenocarcinoma of the Uterine Cervix. *Int J Gynecol Pathol* 2002;21:327–346.

107. Gilks CB, Young RH, Aguirre P, et al. Adenoma malignum (minimal deviation adenocarcinoma) of the uterine cervix: a clinicopathologic and immunohistochemical analysis of 26 cases. *Am J Surg Pathol* 1989;13:717–729.

108. Young RH, Scully RE. Minimal-deviation endometrioid adenocarcinoma of the uterine cervix. A report of five cases of a distinctive neoplasm that may be misinterpreted as benign. *Am J Surg Pathol* 1993;17:660–665.

109. Michael H, Sutton G, Hull MT, et al. Villous adenoma of the uterine cervix associated with invasive adenocarcinoma: a histologic, ultrastructural and immunohistochemical study. *Int J Gynecol Pathol* 1986; 5:163–169.

110. Young RH, Scully RE. Villoglandular papillary adenocarcinoma of the uterine cervix. A clinicopathologic analysis of 13 cases. *Cancer* 1989;63:1773–1779.

111. Jones MW, Silverberg SG, Kurman RJ. Well-differentiated villoglandular adenocarcinoma of the uterine cervix: a clinicopathological study of 24 cases. *Int J Gynecol Pathol* 1993;12:1–7.

112. Jones MW, Kounelis S, Papadaki H, et al. Well-differentiated villoglandular adenocarcinoma of the uterine cervix: oncogene/tumor suppressor gene alterations and human papillomavirus genotyping. *Int J Gynecol Pathol* 2000;19:110–117.

113. Schorge JO, Lee KR, Lee SJ, et al. Early cervical adenocarcinoma: selection criteria for radical surgery. *Obstet Gynecol* 1999;94: 386–390.

114. Chang SH, Maddox WA. Adenocarcinoma arising within cervical endometriosis and invading the adjacent vagina. *Am J Obstet Gynecol* 1971;110:1015–1017.

115. Blythe JG, Michael H, Hodel KA. Colposcopic and pathologic features in two cases of DES-related vaginal clear-cell adenocarcinoma. *J Reproduc Med* 1983;28:137–146.

116. Gilks CB, Clement PB. Papillary serous adenocarcinoma of the uterine cervix: a report of three cases. *Mod Pathol* 1992;5:426–431.

117. Zhou C, Gilks CB, Hayes M, et al. Papillary serous carcinoma of the uterine cervix; a clinicopathologic study of 17 cases. *Am J Surg Pathol* 1998;22:113–120.

118. Costa MJ, McIlnay KR, Trelford J. Cervical carcinoma with glandular differentiation: histological evaluation predicts disease recurrence in clinical stage I or II patients. *Hum Pathol* 1995;26:829–837.

119. Ferry JA, Scully RE. Mesonephric remnants, hyperplasia and neoplasia in the uterine cervix: a study of 49 cases. *Am J Surg Pathol* 1990; 14:1100–1111.

120. Clement PB, Young RH, Keh P, et al. Malignant mesonephric neoplasms of the uterine cervix: a report of eight cases, including four with a malignant spindle cell component. *Am J Surg Pathol* 1995;19; 1158–1171.

121. Silver SA, Devouassoux-Shisheboran J, Mezzetti TP, et al. Mesonephric adenocarcinomas of the uterine cervix: a study of 11 cases with immunohistochemical findings. *Am J Surg Pathol* 2001;25:379–387.

122. Tambouret R, Bell DA, Young RH. Microcystic endocervical adenocarcinomas: a report of eight cases. *Am J Surg Pathol* 2000;24: 369–374.

123. Ferry JA, Scully RE. ''Adenoid cystic'' carcinoma and adenoid basal carcinoma of the uterine cervix. *Am J Surg Pathol* 1988;12:134–144.

124. Brainard JA, Hart WR. Adenoid basal epitheliomas of the uterine cervix: a re-evaluation of distinctive cervical basaloid lesions currently classified as adenoid basal carcinoma and adenoid basal hyperplasia. *Am J Surg Pathol* 1998;22:965–975.

125. Albores-Saavedra J, Gersell D, Gilks B et al. Terminology of endocrine tumors of the uterine cervix. Results of a workshop sponsored by the College of American Pathologists and the National Cancer Institute. *Arch Pathol Lab Med* 1997;121:34–39.

126. Ambros RA, Park JS, Shah KV, et al. Evaluation of histologic, morphometric, and immunohistochemical criteria in the differential diagnosis of small cell carcinomas of the cervix with particular reference to human papillomavirus types 16 and 18. *Mod Pathol* 1991;4:586–593.

127. Gilks CB, Young RH, Gersell DJ, et al. Large cell carcinoma of the uterine cervix: a clinicopathologic study of 12 cases. *Am J Surg Pathol* 1997;21:905–914.

128. Abeler VM, Holm R, Nesland JM, et al. Small cell carcinoma of the cervix. A clinicopathologic study of 26 patients. *Cancer* 1994;73: 672–677.

129. Gersell DJ, Mazoujian G, Mutch DG, et al. Small-cell undifferentiated

carcinoma of the cervix. A clinicopathologic, ultrastructural, and immunocytochemical study of 15 cases. *Am J Surg Pathol* 1988;12:684–698.

130. Miller B, Dockter M, El Torky M, et al. Small cell carcinoma of the cervix: a clinical and flow-cytometric study. *Gynecol Oncol* 1991;42:27–33.

131. Stoler MH, Mills SE, Gersell DJ, et al. Small-cell neuroendocrine carcinoma of the cervix. A human papillomavirus type 18-associated cancer. *Am J Surg Pathol* 1991;15:28–32.

132. Conner MG, Richter H, Moran CA, et al. Small cell carcinoma of the cervix: a clinicopathologic and immunohistochemical study of 3 cases. *Ann Diagnostic Pathol* 2002;6:345–348.

133. Kerner H, Lichtig C. Mullerian adenosarcoma presenting as cervical polyps: a report of seven cases and review of the literature. *Obstet Gynecol* 1993;81:665–669.

134. Jones MW, Lefkowitz M. Adenosarcoma of the uterine cervix: a clinicopathological study of 12 cases. *Int J Gynecol Pathol* 1995;14:223–229.

135. Clement PB, Zubovits JT, Young RH, et al. Malignant mullerian mixed tumors of the uterine cervix: a report of nine cases of a neoplasm with morphology often different from its counterpart in the corpus. *Int J Gynecol Pathol* 1998;17:211–222.

136. Mathoulin-Portier MP, Penault-Llorca F, Labit-Bouvier C, et al. Malignant mullerian mixed tumor of the uterine cervix with adenoid cystic component. *Int J Gynecol Pathol* 1998;17:91–92.

137. Cantuaria G, Angioli R, Nahmias J, et al. Primary malignant melanoma of the uterine cervix: case report and review of the literature. *Gynecol Oncol* 1999;75:170–174.

138. Oliva E, Ferry JA, Young RH, et al. Granulocytic sarcoma of the female genital tract: a clinicopathologic study of 11 cases. *Am J Surg Pathol* 1997;21:1156–1165.

139. Muntz HG, Ferry JA, Flynn D, et al. Stage IE primary malignant lymphomas of the uterine cervix. *Cancer* 1991;68:2023–2032.

140. Tsao AS, Roth LM, Sandler A, et al. Cervical primitive neuroectodermal tumor. *Gynecol Oncol* 2001;83:138–142.

141. Malpica A, Moran CA. Primitive neuroectodermal tumor of the cervix: a clinicopathologic and immunohistochemical study of two cases. *Ann Diagn Pathol* 2002;6:281–287.

142. Berkowitz RS, Ehrmann RL, Lavizzo-Mourey R, et al. Invasive cervical carcinoma in young women. *Gynecol Oncol* 1979;8:311.

143. Kyriakos M, Kempson RL, Perez CA. Carcinoma of the cervix in young women. *Obstet Gynecol* 1971;38:930.

144. Dattoli MJ, Gretz HF III, Beller U, et al. Analysis of multiple prognostic factors in patients with stage IB cervical cancer: age as a major determinant. *Int J Radiat Oncol Biol Phys* 1989;17:41.

145. Meanwell CA, Kelly KA, Wilson S, et al. Young age as a prognostic factor in cervical cancer: analysis of population based on data from 10,022 cases. *Br Med J* 1988;296:386.

146. van der Graaf Y, Peer PGM, Zielhuis GA, et al. Cervical cancer survival in Nijmegan Region, The Netherlands 1970 to 1985. *Gynecol Oncol* 1988;30:51.

147. Rutledge FN, Mitchell MF, Munsell S, et al. Youth as a prognostic factor in carcinoma of the cervix: a matched analysis. *Gynecol Oncol* 1992;44:123.

148. Chen F, Trapido EJ, Davis K. Differences in stage at presentation of breast and gynecologic cancers among whites, blacks and Hispanics. *Cancer* 1994;73:2838.

149. Weiss LK, Kau TY, Sparks BT, et al. Trends in cervical cancer incidence among young black and white women in metropolitan Detroit. *Cancer* 1994;73:1849.

150. Jenkin RDT, Stryker JA. The influence of the blood pressure on survival in cancer of the cervix. *Br J Radiol* 1968;41:913.

151. Kapp DS, Fischer D, Gutierrez E, et al. Pretreatment prognostic factors in carcinoma of the uterine cervix: a multivariate analysis of the effects of age, stage, histology and blood counts on survival. *Int J Radiat Oncol Biol Phys* 1983;9:445.

152. Fruchter RG, Maiman M, Sillman FH, et al. Characteristics of cervical intraepithelial neoplasia in women infected with the human immunodeficiency virus. *Am J Obstet Gynecol* 1994;171:531.

153. Klevens RM, Fleming PL, Mays MA, Frey R. Characteristics of women with AIDS and invasive cervical cancer. *Obstet Gynecol* 1996;88:269.

154. Wright TC, Ellerbrock TV, Chiasson MA, et al. Cervical intraepithe-

155. Evans JC, Bergsio P. The influence of anemia on the results of radiotherapy in carcinoma of the cervix. *Radiol* 1965;84:709–717.

156. Bush RS, Jenkin RDT, Allt WEC, et al. Definitive evidence hypoxic cells influencing cure in cancer therapy. *Br J Cancer* 1987;37:302–306.

157. Fyles AW, Milosevic M, Pintilie M, et al. Anemia, hypoxia and transfusion in patients with cervix cancer: A review. *Radiother Oncol* 2000;57:13–19.

158. Dewhirst M. Concepts of oxygen transport at the microcirculatory level. *Semin Radiat Oncol* 1998;8:143–150.

159. Sundfor K, Lyng H, Rofstad E. Tumour hypoxia and vascular density as predictors of metastasis in squamous cell carcinoma of the uterine cervix. *Br J Cancer* 1998;76:822–827.

160. Fyles M, Milosevic M, Hedley D, et al. Tumor hypoxia has independent predictor impact only in patients with node-negative cervix cancer. *J Clin Oncol* 2002;20:680–687.

161. Dehdashti F, Grigsby PW, Mintun MA, et al. Assessing tumor hypoxia in cervical cancer by positron emission tomography with 60Co-STSM: Relationship to therapeutic response—A preliminary report. *Int J Radiat Oncol Biol Phys* 2003;55:1233–1238.

162. Sundfor K, Lyng H, Kongsgard U, et al. Polarographic measurements of pO2 in cervix carcinoma. *Gynecol Oncol* 1997;64:230–236.

163. Grogan M, Thomas GM, Melamed I, et al. The importance of hemoglobin levels during radiotherapy for carcinoma of the cervix. *Cancer* 1999;86:1528–1536.

164. Santin AD, Bellone S, Palmieri M, et al. Effect of blood transfusion during radiotherapy on the immune function of patients with cancer of the uterine cervix: Role of interleukin-10. *Int J Radiat Oncol Biol Phys* 2002;54:1345–1355.

165. Gemignani M, Zakashansky K, Venkatraman E, et al. Blood transfusion in radical hysterectomy and pelvic lymphadenectomy for invasive cervical cancer: Impact on recurrence and overall survival. *Proc Am Soc Clin Oncol* 2003;22:454 (abstract).

166. Gauthier P, Gore I, Shingleton H, et al. Identification of histopathologic risk groups in stage IB squamous cell carcinoma of the cervix. *Obstet Gynecol* 1985;66:569.

167. Inoue T. Prognostic significance of the depth of invasion relating to nodal metastases, parametrial extension and cell types. *Cancer* 1984;54:3035.

168. Van Nagell JR Jr, Donaldson ES, Wood EG, et al. The significance of vascular invasion and lymphocytic infiltration in invasive cervical cancer. *Cancer* 1978;41:228.

169. Kovalic JJ, Grigsby PW, Perez CA, Lockett MA. Cervical stump carcinoma. *Int J Radiat Oncol Biol Phys* 1991;20:933.

170. Van Nagell JR Jr, Rayburn W, Donaldson ES, et al. Therapeutic implications of patterns of recurrence in cancer of the uterine cervix. *Cancer* 1979;44:2534.

171. Perez CA, Grigsby PW, Nene SM, et al. Effect of tumor size on the prognosis of carcinoma of the uterine cervix treated with irradiation alone. *Cancer* 1992;69:2796.

172. Eifel PJ, Morris M, Wharton JT, et al. The influence of tumor size and morphology on the outcome of patients with FIGO stage IB squamous cell carcinoma of the uterine cervix. *Int J Radiat Oncol Biol Phys* 1994;29:9.

173. Pitson G, Fyles A, Milosevic M, et al. Tumor size and oxygenation are independent predictors of nodal disease in patients with cervix cancer. *Int J Radiat Oncol Biol Phys* 2001;51:699–703.

174. Fyles AW, Pintilie M, Kirkbride P, et al. Prognostic factors in patients with cervix cancer treated by radiation therapy: results of a multiple regression analysis. *Radiother Oncol* 1995;35:107.

175. Tanaka Y, Sawada S, Murata T. Relationship between lymph node metastases and prognosis in patients irradiated post-operatively for carcinoma of the uterine cervix. *Acta Radiol* 1984;23:455.

176. Tinga DJ, Timmer PR, Bouma J, et al. Prognostic significance of single versus multiple lymph node metastases in cervical carcinoma stage IB. *Gynecol Oncol* 1990;39:175.

177. Delgado G, Bundy B, Zaino R, et al. Prospective surgical-pathological study of disease-free interval in patients with stage IB squamous cell carcinoma of the cervix: A Gynecologic Oncology Group study. *Gynecol Oncol* 1990;38:352–357.

178. Alvarez RD, Soong SJ, Kinney WK, et al. Identification of prognostic factors and risk groups in patients found to have nodal metastasis at the time of radical hysterectomy for early stage squamous carcinoma of the cervix. *Gynecol Oncol* 1989;35:130.

179. Roman LD, Felix JC, Muderspach LI, et al. Influence of quantity of lymphovascular space invasion on the risk of nodal metastases in women with early stage squamous cancer of the cervix. *Gynecol Oncol* 1998;68:220–225.

180. Lee IJ, Park KR, Lee KK, et al. Prognostic value of vascular endothelial growth factor in stage IB carcinoma of the uterine cervix. *Int J Radiat Oncol Biol Phys* 2002;54:768–779.

181. Tsang RW, Fyles AW, Kirkbride P, et al. Proliferation measurements with flow cytometry Tpot in cancer of the uterine cervix: preliminary results. *Int J Radiat Oncol Biol Phys* 1995;32:1319–1329.

182. Tsang RW, Fyles AW, Li Y et al. Tumor proliferation and apoptosis in human cervix carcinoma I: Correlations between variables. *Radiother Oncol* 1999;50:85–92.

183. Tsang RW, Wong CS, Fyles AW, et al. Tumour proliferation and apoptosis in human uterine cervix carcinoma II: Correlations with clinical outcome. *Radiother Oncol* 1999;50:93–101.

184. Gaffney DK, Haslam D, Tsodikov A, et al. Epidemal growth factor receptor (EDFR) and vascular endothelial growth factore (VEGF) negatively affect overall survival in carcinoma of the cervix treated with radiotherapy. *Int J Radiat Oncol Biol Phys* 2003;56:922–928.

185. Burghardt E, Girardi F, Lahousen M, et al. Microinvasive carcinoma of the uterine cervix (International Federation of Gynecology and Obstetrics Stage IA). *Cancer* 1991;67:1037.

186. Buckley SL, Tritz DM, Van Le L, et al. Lymph node metastases and prognosis in patients with stage IA₂ cervical cancer. *Gynecol Oncol* 1996;63:4.

187. Copeland LJ, Silva EG, Gershenson DM, et al. Superficially invasive squamous cell carcinoma of the cervix. *Gynecol Oncol* 1992;45:307.

188. Sedlis A, Sall S, Tsukada Y, et al. Microinvasive carcinoma of the uterine cervix: a clinical-pathologic study. *Am J Obstet Gynecol* 1979;133:64.

189. Sevin BU, Nadji M, Averette HE, et al. Microinvasive carcinoma of the cervix. *Cancer* 1992;70:2121.

190. Van Nagell JR, Greenwell N, Powell DF, et al. Microinvasive carcinoma of the cervix. *Am J Obstet Gynecol* 1983;145:981.

191. Burghardt E, Holzer E. Diagnosis and treatment of microinvasive carcinoma of the cervix uteri. *Obstet Gynecol* 1977;49:641.

192. Anton-Culver H, Bloss JD, Bringman D et al. Comparison of adenocarcinoma and squamous carcinoma of the uterine cervix: a population based epidemiologic study. *Am J Obstet Gynecol* 1992;166:1507–1514.

193. Hale RJ, Wilcox FL, Buckley CH et al. Prognostic factors in uterine cervical carcinoma: a clinicopathological analysis. *Int J Gynecol Cancer* 2002;1:19–23.

194. Leminen A, Paavonen J, Forss M et al. Adenocarcinoma of the uterine cervix. *Cancer* 1990;65:53–59.

195. Alfsen CG, Kristensen GB, Skovlund E, et al. Histologic subtype has minor importance for overall survival in patients with adenocarcinoma of the uterine cervix. A population-based study of prognostic factors in 505 patients with nonsquamous cell carcinomas of the cervix. *Cancer* 2001;92:2471–2483.

196. International Agency for Research Cancer. Monographs on the Evaluation of the Carcinogenic Risks to Humans. Vol 64. Human papillomaviruses. Lyon: IARC, 1995.

197. Walker J, Bloss JD, Liao SY, et al. Human papillomavirus genotype as a prognostic indicator in carcinoma of the uterine cervix. *Obstet Gynecol* 1989;74:781–785.

198. Rose BR, Thompson CH, Simpson JM, et al. Human papillomavirus deoxyribonucleic acid as a prognostic indicator in early-stage cervical cancer: a possible role for type 18. *Am J Obstet Gynecol* 1995;173:1461–1468.

199. Burger RA, Monk BJ, Kurosake T, et al. Human papillomavirus type 18: association with poor prognosis in early stage cervical cancer. *J Natl Cancer Inst* 1996;88:1361–1368.

200. Skomedal H, Kristensen GB, Lie AD, et al. Aberrant expression of the cell cycle associated proteins TP53, MDM2, p21, p27, cdk4, cyclin D1, RB, and EGFR in cervical carcinomas. *Gynecol Oncol* 1999;73:223–228.

201. Hayashi Y, Hachisuga T, Iwasaka T, et al. Expression of ras oncogene product and EGF receptor in cervical squamous cell carcinomas and its relationship to lymph node involvement. *Gynecol Oncol* 1991;40:147–151.

202. Sagae S, Kuzumake N, Hisada T, et al. Ras oncogene expression and prognosis of invasive squamous cell carcinomas of the uterine cervix. *Cancer* 1989;63:1577–1582.

203. Soh LT, Heng D, Lee IW, et al. The relevance of oncogenes as prognostic markers in cervical cancer. *Int J Gynecol Cancer* 2002;12:465–474.

204. Christopherson WM, Parker JE. Relation of cervical cancer to early marriage and childbearing. *N Engl J Med* 1965;273:235.

205. Creasman WT, Rutledge FN. Carcinoma in situ of the cervix. *Obstet Gynecol* 1972;3:373.

206. Bjerre B, Eliasson G, Linell F, et al. Conization as only treatment of carcinoma in situ of the uterine cervix. *Am J Obstet Gynecol* 1976;125:143.

207. Burghardt E, Holzer E. Treatment of carcinoma in situ: evaluation of 1069 cases. *Obstet Gynecol* 1980;55:539.

208. Baggish MS. Management of cervical intraepithelial neoplasm by carbon dioxide laser. *Obstet Gynecol* 1982;60:378.

209. Bryson SCP, Lenehan P, Lickrish GM. The treatment of grade 3 cervical intraepithelial neoplasia with cryotherapy: an 11 year experience. *Am J Obstet Gynecol* 1985;151:201.

210. Grigsby PW, Perez CA. Radiotherapy alone for medically inoperable carcinoma of the cervix: stage IA and carcinoma in situ. *Int J Radiat Oncol Biol Phys* 1991;21:375.

211. Kolstad P, Klem V. Long-term follow-up of 1121 cases of carcinoma in situ. *Obstet Gynecol* 1976;48:125.

212. Takeshima N, Yanoh K, Tabata T, et al. Assessment of the revised International Federation of Gynecology and Obstetrics staging for early invasive squamous cervical cancer. *Gynecol Oncol* 1999;74:165–169.

213. Keighley E. Carcinoma of the cervix among prostitutes in a women's prison. *Br J Vener Dis* 1968;44:254.

214. Morris M, Mitchell MF, Silva EG, et al. Cervical conization as definitive therapy for early invasive squamous carcinoma of the cervix. *Gynecol Oncol* 1993;51:193.

215. Östör AG, Rome RM. Micro-invasive squamous cell carcinoma of the cervix: a clinico-pathologic study of 200 cases with long-term follow-up. *Int J Gynecol Cancer* 1994;4:257.

216. Kolstad P. Follow-up study of 232 patients with stage IA1 and 411 patients with stage IA2 squamous cell carcinoma of the cervix (microinvasive carcinoma). *Gynecol Oncol* 1989;33:265.

217. Schorge JO, Lee KR, Sheets EE. Prospective management of stage IA₁ cervical adenocarcinoma by conization alone to preserve fertility: A preliminary report. *Gynecol Oncol* 2000;78:217–220.

218. Greer BE, Figge DC, Tamimi HK, et al. Stage IA₂ squamous carcinoma of the cervix: difficult diagnosis and therapeutic dilemma. *Am J Obstet Gynecol* 1990;162:1406.

219. Creasman WT, Zaino R, Major FJ, et al. Early invasive carcinoma of the cervix (3 to 5 mm invasion): Risk factors and prognosis; A Gynecologic Oncology Group study. *Am J Obstet Gynecol* 1998:178;62.

220. Hamberger AD, Fletcher GH, Wharton JT. Results of treatment of early stage I carcinoma of the uterine cervix with intracavitary radium alone. *Cancer* 1978;41:980–985.

221. Burnett AF, Roman LD, O'Meara AT, et al. Radical vaginal trachelectomy and pelvic lymphadenectomy for preservation of fertility in early cervical carcinoma. *Gynecol Oncol* 2003;88:419–423.

222. Covens A, Shaw P, Murphy J, et al. Is radical trachelectomy a safe alternative to radical hysterectomy for patients with stage IA-B carcinoma of the cervix? *Cancer* 1999;86:2273–2279.

223. Roy M, Plante M. Pregnancies after radical vaginal trachelectomy for early-stage cervical cancer. *Am J Obstet Gynecol* 1998;179:1491–1496.

224. Schlaerth JB, Spirtos NM, Schlaerth AC. Radical trachelectomy and pelvic lymphadenectomy with uterine preservation in the treatment of cervical cancer. *Am J Obstet Gynecol* 2003;188:29–34.

225. Dargent D, Martin X, Sacchettoni A, et al. Laparoscopic vaginal radical trachelectomy. *Cancer* 2000;88:1877–1882.

226. Shepard JH, Crawford RAF, Oram D. Radical trachelectomy: a way to preserve fertility in the treatment of early cervical cancer. *Br J Obstet Gynaecol* 1998;105:912–916.

227. Spirtos NM, Schlaerth JB, Kimball RE, et al. Laparoscopic radical hysterectomy (type III) with aortic and pelvic lymphadenectomy. *Am J Obstet Gynecol* 1996;174:1763.

228. Webb GA. The role of ovarian conservation in the treatment of carcinoma of the cervix with radical surgery. *Am J Obstet Gynecol* 1975; 122:476.

229. Anderson B, LaPolla J, Turner D, et al. Ovarian transposition in cervical cancer. *Gynecol Oncol* 1993;49:206.

230. Feeney DD, Moore DH, Look KY, et al. The fate of the ovaries after radical hysterectomy and ovarian transposition. *Gynecol Oncol* 1995; 56:3.

231. Parker M, Bosscher J, Barnhill D, et al. Ovarian management during radical hysterectomy in the premenopausal patient. *Obstet Gynecol* 1993;82:187.

232. Buckers TE, Anderson B, Sorosky JI, et al. Ovarian function after surgical treatment for cervical cancer. *Gynecol Oncol* 2001;80:85–88.

233. Abitbol NM, Davenport JH. Sexual dysfunction after therapy for cervical carcinoma. *Am J Obstet Gynecol* 1974;119:181.

234. Siebel M, Freeman MG, Graves WL. Carcinoma of the cervix and sexual function. *Obstet Gynecol* 1979;55:484.

235. Flay LD, Matthews JHL. The effects of radiotherapy and surgery on the sexual function of women treated for cervical cancer. *Int J Radiat Oncol Biol Phys* 1995;31:399.

236. Bergmark K, Avall-Lundquist E, Dickman PW, et al. Vaginal changes and sexuality in women with a history of cervical cancer. *N Engl J Med* 1999;340:1383–1389.

237. Whitney C, Stehman FB. The abandoned radical hysterectomy: A Gynecologic Oncology Group study. *Gynecol Oncol* 2000;79: 350–356.

238. Brewster WR, Monk BM, Ziogas A,et al. Intent-to-treat analysis of Stage Ib and IIa cervical cancer in the United States: radiotherapy or surgery 1988–1995. *Obstet Gynecol* 2000;97:248–254.

239. Levenback C, Coleman RL, Burke TW, et al. Lymphatic mapping and sentinel node identification in patients with cervix cancer undergoing radical hysterectomy and pelvic lymphadenectomy. *J Clin Oncol* 2002;20:688–693.

240. Newton M. Radical hysterectomy or radiotherapy for stage I cervical cancer. *Am J Obstet Gynecol* 1975;123:535.

241. Roddick JW Jr, Greenlaw RH. Treatment of cervical cancer. *Am J Obstet Gynecol* 1971;119:754.

242. Morley GW, Seski JC. Radical pelvic surgery versus radiation therapy for stage I carcinoma of the cervix (exclusive of microinvasion). *Am J Obstet Gynecol* 1976;126:785.

243. Landoni F, Maneo A, Colombo A, et al. Randomised study of radical surgery versus radiotherapy for stage IB-IIA cervical cancer. *Lancet* 1997;350:535.

244. Artman LE, Hoskins WJ, Bibro MC, et al. Radical hysterectomy and pelvic lymphadenectomy for stage IB carcinoma of the cervix: twenty-one years' experience. *Gynecol Oncol* 1987;28:8.

245. Hoskins WJ, Ford JH Jr, Lutz MH, et al. Radical hysterectomy and pelvic lymphadenectomy for the management of early invasive cancer of the cervix. *Gynecol Oncol* 1976;4:278.

246. Eifel PJ, Thoms WW Jr, Smith TL, et al. The relationship between brachytherapy dose and outcome in patients with bulky endocervical tumors treated with radiation dose. *Int J Radiat Oncol Biol Phys* 1993; 28:113.

247. Benedet JL, Turko M, Boyes DA, et al. Radical hysterectomy in the treatment of cervical cancer. *Am J Obstet Gynecol* 1980;137:254.

248. Spirtos NM, Eisenkop SM, Schlaerth JB, et al. Laparoscopic radical hysterectomy (type III) with aortic and pelvic lymphadenectomy in patients with stage I cervical cancer: surgical morbidity and intermediate follow-Up. *Am J Obstet Gynecol* 2002;187:340–348.

249. Piver MS, Rutledge F, Smith JP. Five classes of extended hysterectomy for women with cervical cancer. *Obstet Gynecol* 1974;44:265.

250. Eifel PJ, Levenback C, Wharton JT, et al. Time course and incidence of late complications in patients treated with radiation therapy for FIGO stage IB carcinoma of the cervix. *Int J Radiat Oncol Biol Phys* 1995;32:1289.

251. Van Nagell JR, Maruyama Y, Parker JC, et al. Small bowel injury following radiation therapy for cervical cancer. *Am J Obstet Gynecol* 1974;118:163.

252. Van Nagell JR, Parker JC, Maruyama Y, et al. Bladder or rectal injury following radiation therapy for cervical cancer. *Am J Obstet Gynecol* 1974;119:727.

253. Van Nagell JR, Parker JC, Maruyama Y, et al. The effect of pelvic inflammatory disease on enteric complications following radiation therapy for cervical cancer. *Am J Obstet Gynecol* 1977;128:767.

254. Bremer GL, van der Putten HWHM, Dunselman GAJ, et al. Early stage cervical cancer: aborted versus completed radical hysterectomy. *Eur J Obstet Gynecol Repro Biol* 1992;47:147–151.

255. Potter ME, Alvarez RD, Shingleton HM, et al. Early invasive cervical cancer with pelvic lymph node involvement: to complete or not to complete radical hysterectomy? *Gynecol Oncol* 1990;37:78–81.

256. Peters WA III, Liu PY, Barrett RJ, et al. Concurrent chemotherapy and pelvic radiation therapy compared with pelvic radiation therapy alone as adjuvant therapy after radical surgery in high-risk early-stage cancer of the cervix. *J Clin Oncol* 2000;18:1606–1613.

257. Cosin JA, Fowler JM, Chen MD, et al. Pretreatment surgical staging of patients with cervical carcinoma; the case for lymph node debulking. *Cancer* 1998;82:2241–2248.

258. Hacker NF, Wain GV, Nicklin JL. Resection of bulky positive lymph nodes in patients with cervical carcinoma. *Int J Gynecol Cancer* 1995; 5(4):250–256.

259. Kinney WK, Hodge DO, Egorshin EV, et al. Surgical treatment of patients with stages IB and IIA carcinoma of the cervix and palpably positive pelvic lymph nodes. *Gynecol Oncol* 1995;57:145–149.

260. Kavadi VS, Eifel PJ. FIGO stage IIIA carcinoma of the uterine cervix. *Int J Radiat Oncol Biol Phys* 1992;24:211.

261. Cardinale J, Peschel RE, Gutierrez E, et al. Stage IIIA carcinoma of the uterine cervix. *Gynecol Oncol* 1986;23:199–204.

262. Koh WJ, Chiu M, Stelzer KJ, et al. Femoral vessel depth and the implications for groin node radiation. *Int J Radiat Oncol Biol Phys* 1993;27:969–974.

263. Dittmer PH, Randall ME. A technique for inguinal node boost using photon fields defined by asymmetric collimator jaws. *Radiotherapy Oncol* 2001;59:61–64.

264. Morris M, Eifel PJ, Lu J, et al. Pelvic radiation with concurrent chemotherapy compared with pelvic and para-aortic radiation for high-risk cervical cancer. *N Engl J Med* 1999;340(15):1137–1143.

265. Whitney CW, Sause W, Bundy B, et al. Randomized comparison of fluorouracil plus cisplatin versus hydroxyurea as an adjunct to radiation therapy in stage IIB-IVA carcinoma of the cervix with negative para-aortic lymph nodes: a Gynecologic Oncology Group study. *J Clin Oncol* 1999;17:1339.

266. Rose PG, Bundy BN, Watkins EB, et al. Concurrent cisplatin-based radiotherapy and chemotherapy for locally advanced cervical cancer. *N Engl J Med* 1999;340(15):1144–1153.

267. Million RR, Rutledge F, Fletcher GH. Stage IV carcinoma of the cervix with bladder invasion. *Am J Obstet Gynecol* 1972;113:239.

268. Kramer C, Peschel RE, Goldberg N, et al. Radiation treatment of FIGO stage IVA carcinoma of the cervix. *Gynecol Oncol* 1989;32: 323.

269. Schorge JO, Lee KR, Flynn CE, et al. Stage IA1 cervical adenocarcinoma; definition and treatment. *Obstet Gynecol* 1999;93:219–222.

270. Schoolland M, Segal A, Allpres S, et al. Adenocarcinoma *in situ* of the cervix. *Cancer* 2002;96:330–337.

271. Plaxe SC, Saltzstein SL. Estimation of the duration of the preclinical phase of cervical adenocarcinoma suggests that there is ample opportunity for screening. *Gynecol Oncol* 1999;75:55–61.

272. Hirai Y, Takeshima N, Tate S, et al. Early invasive cervical adenocarcinoma: its potential for nodal metastasis or recurrence. *BJOG: Internat J Obstet Gynecol* 2003;110:241–246.

273. Look KY, Brunetto VL, Clarke-Pearson DL, et al. An analysis of cell type in patients with surgically staged stage IB carcinoma of the cervix: A Gynecologic Oncology Group study. *Gynecol Oncol* 1996;63: 304.

274. Grigsby PW, Perez CA, Kuske RR, et al. Adenocarcinoma of the uterine-cervix: lack of evidence for a poor prognosis. *Radiother Oncol* 1988;12:289.

275. Randall ME, Constable WC, Hahn SS, et al. Results of radio-therapeutic management of carcinoma of the cervix with emphasis on the influence of histologic classification. *Cancer* 1988;62:48.

276. Berek JS, Castaldo TW, Hacker NF, et al. Adenocarcinoma of the uterine cervix. *Cancer* 1981;48:2734.

277. Hopkins MP, Schmid RW, Roberts JA, et al. Gland cell carcinoma (adenocarcinoma) of the cervix. *Obstet Gynecol* 1988;72:789.
278. Kilgore LC, Soong SJ, Gore H, et al. Analysis of prognostic features in adenocarcinoma of the cervix. *Gynecol Oncol* 1988;31:137.
279. Eifel PJ, Morris M, Oswald MJ, et al. Adenocarcinoma of the uterine cervix: prognosis and patterns of failure in 367 cases treated at the M.D. Anderson Cancer Center between 1965 and 1985. *Cancer* 1990; 65:2507.
280. Moberg PJ, Einhorn N, Silfversward C, et al. Adenocarcinoma of the uterine cervix. *Cancer* 1986;57:407.
281. Davidson SE, Symonds RP, Lamont D, et al. Does adenocarcinoma of uterine cervix have a worse prognosis than squamous carcinoma when treated by radiotherapy? *Gynecol Oncol* 1989;33:23–26.
282. Kleine W, Rau K, Schwoeorer D, Pfleiderer A. Prognosis of the adenocarcinoma of the cervix uteri: a comparative study. *Gynecol Oncol* 1989;35:145–149.
283. Randall ME, Kim JA, Mills SE, et al. Uncommon variants of cervical carcinoma treated with radical irradiation—A clinicopathologic study of 66 cases. *Cancer* 1986; 57:816–822.
284. Reagan JW, Hamonic MJ, Wentz WB. Analytical study of cells in cervical squamous cell cancer. *Lab Invest* 1957;6:241.
285. Albores-Saavedra J, Gersell D, Gilks CB, et al. Terminology of endocrine tumors of the uterine cervix: results of a workshop sponsored by the college of American Pathologists and the National Cancer Institute. *Arch Pathol Lab Med* 1997;121:34.
286. Van Nagell JR, Donaldson ES, Wood EG, et al. Small cell cancer of the uterine cervix. *Cancer* 1977;40:2243-2249.
287. Hoskins PJ, Wong F, Swenerton KD, et al. Small cell carcinoma of the cervix treated with concurrent radiotherapy, cisplatin, and etoposide. *Gynecol Oncol* 1995;56:218–225.
288. Creadick RN. Carcinoma of the cervical stump. *Am J Obstet Gynecol* 1958;75:565.
289. Barillot I, Horiot JC, Cuisenier J, et al. Carcinoma of the cervical stump: a review of 213 cases. *Eur J Cancer* 1993;29A:1231.
290. Miller BE, Copeland LJ, Hamberger AD, et al. Carcinoma of the cervical stump. *Gynecol Oncol* 1984;18:100.
291. Petersen LK, Mamsen A, Jakobsen A. Carcinoma of the cervical stump. *Gynecol Oncol* 1992;46:199–202.
292. Wimbush PR, Fletcher GH. Radiation therapy of carcinoma of the cervical stump. *Radiology* 1969;93:655.
293. Andras EJ, Fletcher GH, Rutledge F. Radiotherapy of carcinoma of the cervix following simple hysterectomy. *Am J Obstet Gynecol* 1973; 115:647.
294. Heller PB, Barnhill DR, Mayer AR, et al. Cervical carcinoma found incidentally in a uterus removed for benign indication. *Obstet Gynecol* 1986;67:187.
295. Hopkins MP, Peters WA, Anderson W, et al. Invasive cervical cancer treated initially by standard hysterectomy. *Gynecol Oncol* 1990; 36:7.
296. Photopulos GJ, Vander Zwagg R. Class II radical hysterectomy shows less morbidity and good treatment efficacy compared to class III. *Gynecol Oncol* 1991;40:21.
297. Knapp RC, Donahue VC, Friedman EA. Dissection of the paravesical and pararectal space in pelvic operations. *Surg Gynecol Obstet* 1973; 137:758.
298. Ballon SC. The Wertheim hysterectomy. *Surg Gynecol Obstet* 1976; 142:920.
299. Brunschwig A, Barber HRK. Surgical treatment of carcinoma of the cervix. *Obstet Gynecol* 1966;27:21.
300. Masterson BJ, ed. *Manual of Gynecologic Surgery.* 2nd ed. New York: Springer-Verlag, 1986.
301. Van Nagell JR Jr, DePriest PD, Higgins RV, et al. Surgical therapy for cervical cancer. In: Gershenson DM, DeCherney, Curry SL, eds. *Operative Gynecology.* Philadelphia: WB Saunders Co, 1993: 271.
302. Weiser EB, Bundy BN, Hoskins WJ, et al. Extraperitoneal versus transperitoneal selective paraaortic lymphadenectomy in the pretreatment surgical staging of advanced cervical carcinoma (a Gynecologic Oncology Group study). *Gynecol Oncol* 1989;33:283.
303. Querleu D. Laparoscopic paraaortic node sampling in gynecologic oncology: a preliminary experience. *Gynecol Oncol* 1993;49:24.
304. Fowler JM, Carter JR, Carlson JW, et al. Lymph node yield from laparoscopic lymphadenectomy in cervical cancer: a comparative study. *Gynecol Oncol* 1993;51:187.
305. Orr JW, Shingleton HM, Hatch KD, et al. Urinary diversion in patients undergoing pelvic exenteration. *Am J Obstet Gynecol* 1982;142:883.
306. Schlesinger RE, Berman ML, Ballon SC, et al. The choice of an intestinal segment for a urinary conduit. *Surg Gynecol Obstet* 1979; 148:45.
307. Hatch KD, Shingleton HM, Potter ME, et al. Lower rectal resection and anastomosis at the time of pelvic exenteration. *Gynecol Oncol* 1988;31:262.
308. Hatch KD, Shingleton HM, Soong SJ, et al. Anterior pelvic exenteration. *Gynecol Oncol* 1988;31:205.
309. Brunschwig A. Complete excision of the pelvic viscera for advanced carcinoma. *Cancer* 1948;1:177.
310. VanDyke AH, Van Nagell JR Jr. The prognostic significance of ureteral obstruction in patients with recurrent carcinoma of the cervix uteri. *Surg Gynecol Obstet* 1975;141:371.
311. Deckers PJ, Ketcham AS, Sugarbaker EV, et al. Pelvic exenteration for primary carcinoma of the uterine cervix. *Obstet Gynecol* 1971; 37:647.
311a. Bricker EM, Butcher HR Jr., et al. Surgical Treatment of advanced and recurrent cancer of the pelvic viscera: an evaluation of 10 years' experience. *Ann Surg* 1960;152:388.
311b. Symmonds RE, Pratt JH, Webb MJ. Exenterative operations: experience of 198 patients. *Am J Obstet Gynecol* 1975;121:907.
311c. Lawhead RA Jr, Clark DGC, Smith DH, et al. Pelvic exenteration for recurrent or persistent gynecologic malignancies: a 10-year review of the Memorial Sloan-Kettering Cancer Center experience (1972–1981). *Gynecol Oncol* 1989;33:279.
312. Upadhyay SK, Symonds RP, Haelterman M, et al. The treatment of stage IV carcinoma of cervix by radical dose radiotherapy. *Radiother Oncol* 1988;11:15.
313. Creasman WT, Rutledge FN. Preoperative evaluation of patients with recurrent carcinoma of the cervix. *Gynecol Oncol* 1972;1:111.
314. Rutledge FN, Smith JP, Wharton JT, et al. Pelvic exenteration: analysis of 296 patients. *Am J Obstet Gynecol* 1977;129:881–890.
315. Orr JW, Shingleton HM, Hatch KD, et al. Gastrointestinal complications associated with pelvic exenteration. *Am J Obstet Gynecol* 1983; 145:325.
316. Lichtinger M, Averette H, Girtanner R, et al. Small bowel complications after supravesicular urinary diversion in pelvic exenteration. *Gynecol Oncol* 1986;24:137.
317. Hardman A, Daly JW. Exploratory laparotomy in recurrent cervical cancer. *Obstet Gynecol* 1974;43:653.
318. Stanhope CR, Symmonds RE. Palliative exenteration: what, when, and why? *Am J Obstet Gynecol* 1985;152:12–16.
319. Greer BE, Koh WJ, Figge DC, et al. Gynecologic radiotherapy fields defined by intraoperative measurements. *Gynecol Oncol* 1990;38:421.
320. Greer BE, Koh WJ, Stelzer KJ, et al. Expanded pelvic radiotherapy fields for the treatment of locally-regionally advanced carcinoma of the cervix: outcome and complications. *Am J Obstet Gynecol* 1996; 174:1141.
321. Chun M, Timmerman R, Mayer R, et al. Radiation therapy of external iliac lymph nodes with lateral pelvic portals: identification of patients at risk for inadequate regional coverage. *Radiology* 1995;194:147.
322. Kim RY, McGinnis LS, Spencer SA, et al. Conventional four-field pelvic radiotherapy technique without computed tomography—treatment planning in cancer of the cervix: potential geographic miss and its impact on pelvic control. *Int J Radiat Oncol Biol Phys* 1994;31: 109–112.
323. Zunino S, Rosato O, Lucino S, et al. Anatomic study of the pelvis in carcinoma of the uterine cervix as related to the box technique. *Int J Radiat Oncol Biol Phys* 1999;44:53–59.
324. Kaatee RSJP, Olofsen MJJ, Verstraate MBJ, et al. Detection of organ movement in cervix cancer patients using a fluoroscopic electronic portal imaging device and radiopaque markers. *Int J Radiat Oncol Biol Phys* 2002;54:576–583.
325. Wolfson AH, Abdel-Wahab M, Markoe AM, et al. A quantitative assessment of standard vs. customized midline shield construction for invasive cervical carcinoma. *Int J Radiat Oncol Biol Phys* 1997;37: 237.
326. Huang EY, Lin H, Hsu HC, et al. High external parametrial dose can

increase the probability of radiation proctitis in patients with uterine cervix cancer. *Gynecol Oncol* 2000;79:406–410.

327. Kridelka FJ, Berg DO, Neuman M, et al. Adjuvant small field pelvic radiation for patients with high risk, stage IB lymph node negative cervix carcinoma after radical hysterectomy and pelvic lymph node dissection. *Cancer* 1999;86:2059–2065.

328. Sedlis A, Bundy BN, Rotman MZ, et al. A randomized trial of pelvic radiation therapy versus no further therapy in selected patients with stage IB carcinoma of the cervix after radical hysterectomy and pelvic lymphadenectomy: A Gynecologic Oncology Group study. *Gynecol Oncol* 1999;73:177–183.

329. Ohara K, Tsudoda H, Nishida M, et al. Use of small pelvic field instead of whole pelvic field in postoperative radiotherapy for node-negative, high-risk stages I and II cervical squamous cell carcinoma. *Int J Gynecol Cancer* 2003;13:170–176.

330. Carl U, Bahnsen J, Wiegel T. Radiation therapy of para-aortic lymph nodes in cancer of the uterine cervix. *Acta Oncologica* 1993;32:63–67.

331. Mutic S, Malyapa RS, Grigsby PW, et al. PET-guided IMRT for cervical carcinoma with positive para-aortic lymph nodes—a dose-escalation treatment planning study. *Int J Radiat Oncol Biol Phys* 2003;55:28–35.

332. Potish RA, Deibel FC Jr, Khan FM. The relationship between milli-gram-hours and dose to point A in carcinoma of the cervix. *Radiology* 1982;145:479.

333. International Commission of Radiation Units and Measurements. Dose and volume specification for reporting intracavitary therapy in gynecology. *ICRU Report 38.* Bethesda, Md., 1985.

334. Potter R, Limbergen EV, Gerstner N, et al. Survey of the use of the ICRU 38 in recording and reporting cervical cancer brachytherapy. *Radiother Oncol* 2001;58:11–18.

335. Marcial LV, Marcial VA, Krall JM, et al. Comparison of 1 vs 2 or more intracavitary brachytherapy applications in the management of carcinoma of the cervix, with irradiation alone. *Int J Radiat Oncol Biol Phys* 1991;20:81.

336. Rotmensch J, Connell PP, Yamada D, et al. One versus two intracavitary brachytherapy applications in early-stage cervical cancer patients undergoing definitive radiation therapy. *Gynecol Oncol* 2000;78:32–38.

337. Kraiphibul P, Srisupundit S, Pairachvet V, et al. Results of treatment in stage IIB squamous cell carcinoma of the uterine cervix: Comparison between two and one intracavitary insertion. *Gynecol Oncol* 1992;45:160–163.

338. Rotman M, Aziz H. Techniques in the radiation treatment of carcinoma of the uterine cervix. *Int J Radiation Oncol Biol Phys* 1991;20:173–175.

339. Mitsuhashi N, Takashashi M, Nozaki M, et al. Evaluation of external beam therapy and three brachytherapy fractions for carcinoma of the uterine cervix. *Int J Radiat Oncol Biol Phys* 1994;29:975–982.

340. Fowler JF. The linear quadratic formula and progress in fractionated radiotherapy: A review. *Br J Radiol* 1989;62:679.

341. Lee KH, Kagan AR, Nussbaum H, et al. Analysis of dose, dose-rate and treatment time in the production of injuries by radium treatment for cancer of the uterine cervix. *Brit J Radiol* 1976;49:430.

342. Rodrigus P, Winter KD, Venselaar JLM, et al. Evaluation of late morbidity in patients with carcinomas of the uterine cervix following a dose rate change. *Radiother Oncol* 1997;42:137.

343. Newman G. Increased morbidity following the introduction of remote afterloading, with increased dose rate, for cancer of the cervix. *Radiother Oncol* 1996;39:97–103.

344. Lambin P, Gerbaulet A, Kramar A, et al. Phase III trial comparing two low dose rates in brachytherapy of cervix carcinoma. Report at two years. *Int J Radiat Oncol Biol Phys* 1993;25:405–412.

345. Haie-Meder C, Kramar A, Lambin P, et al. Analysis of complications in a prospective randomized trial comparing two brachytherapy low dose rates in cervical carcinoma. *Int J Radiat Oncol Biol Phys* 1994;29:953–960.

346. Patel FD, Negi PS, Sharma SC, et al. Dose rate correction in medium dose rate brachytherapy for carcinoma of the cervix. *Radiother Oncol* 1998;49:317–323.

347. Swift PS, Purser P, Roberts LW, et al. Pulsed low dose rate brachytherapy for pelvic malignancies. *Int J Radiat Oncol Biol Phys* 1997;37:811.

348. Joslin CAF, O'Connell D, Howard N. The treatment of uterine carcinoma using the Cathetron. *Br J Radiol* 1967;40:895.

349. Orton CG, Seyedsadr M, Somany A. Comparison of high and low dose rate remote afterloading for cervix cancer and the importance of fractionation. *Int J Radiat Oncol Biol Phys* 1991;21:1425.

350. Okawa T, Sakata S, Kita-Okawa M, et al. Comparison of HDR versus LDR regimens for intracavitary brachytherapy of cervical cancer: Japanese experience. In Mould RF, ed. *International Brachytherapy.* Nucletron: Veenendaal, The Netherlands, 1992:13–17.

351. Wright J, Jones G, Whelan T, et al. Patient preference for high or low dose rate brachytherapy in carcinoma of the cervix. *Radiother Oncol* 1994;33:187.

352. Kim RY, Meyer JT, Plott WE, et al. Major geometric variation between multiple high-dose-rate applications of brachytherapy in cancer of the cervix: Frequency and types of variation. *Radiol* 1995;195:419–422.

353. Kim RY, Meyer JT, Spencer SA, et al. Major geometric variations between intracavitary applications in carcinoma of the cervix: High dose rate vs. low dose rate. *Int J Radiat Oncol Biol Phys* 1996;35:1035–1038.

354. Corn BW, Galvin JM, Soffen EM, et al. Positional stability of sources during low-dose-rate brachytherapy for cervial carcinoma. *Int J Radiat Oncol Biol Phys* 1993;26:513.

355. Nag S, Orton C, Young D, et al. The American Brachytherapy Society survey of brachytherapy practice for carcinoma of the cervix in the United States. *Gynecol Oncol* 1999;73:111–118.

356. Lorvidhaya V, Tonusin A, Changwiwit W, et al. High-dose-rate afterloading brachytherapy in carcinoma of the cervix: An experience of 1992 patients. *Int J Radiat Oncol Biol Phys* 2000;46:1185–1191.

357. Ferrigno R, Novaes PE, Pellizzon AC, et al. High-dose-rate brachytherapy in the treatment of uterine cervix cancer: Analysis of dose effectiveness and late complications. *Int J Radiat Oncol Biol Phys* 2001;50:1123–1135

358. Ferrigno R, Campos de Oliveira Faria SL, Weltman E, et al. Radiotherapy alone in the treatment of uterine cervix cancer with telecobalt and low-dose-rate brachytherapy: Retrospective analysis of results and variables. *Int J Radiat Oncol Biol Phys* 2003;55:695–706.

359. Petereit DG, Sarkaria JN, Potter DM, et al. High-dose-rate versus low-dose-rate brachytherapy in the treatment of cervical cancer: analysis of tumor recurrence—the University of Wisconsin experience. *Int J Radiat Oncol Biol Phys* 1999;45:1267–1274.

360. Patel FD, Sharma SC, Negi PS, et al. Low dose rate vs. high dose rate brachytherapy in the treatment of carcinoma of the uterine cervix: A clinical trial. *Int J Radiat Oncol Biol Phys* 1993;28:335.

361. Shigematsu Y, Nishiyama K, Masaki N, et al. Treatment of carcinoma of the uterine cervix by remotely controlled afterloading radiotherapy with high-dose-rate: a comparative study with a low-dose rate system. *Int J Radiat Oncol Biol Phys* 1983;9:351.

362. Teshima T, Inoue T, Ikeda H, et al. High-dose rate and low-dose rate intracavitary therapy for carcinoma of the uterine cervix. *Cancer* 1993;72:2409.

363. Hareyama M, Sakata KI, Oouchi A, et al. High-dose-rate versus low-dose-rate intracavitary therapy for carcinoma of the uterine cervix—a randomized trial. *Cancer* 2002;94:117–124.

364. Swamy K, Viswanathan N, Mohan DS, et al. Influence of brachytherapy dose rate on complications of carcinoma of the uterine cervix. *Endocuriether/Hypertherm Oncol* 1991;7:171.

365. Stout R, Hunter RD. Clinical trials of changing dose-rate in intracavitary low dose-rate therapy. In: Mould RF, ed. *Brachytherapy 2.* Leersum, The Netherlands: Nucletron International BV, 1989:219.

366. Symmonds RP, Jones RD, Laurie J, et al. The use of the cumulative radiation effect (CRE) formula to correct for the increased dose-rate when carcinoma cervix is treated with Selectron. In: Mould RF, ed. *Brachytherapy 2.* Leersum, The Netherlands: Nucletron International BV, 1989:49.

367. Van Lancker M, Storme G. Prediction of severe late complications in fractionated high dose-rate brachytherapy in gynecological applications. *Int J Radiat Oncol Biol Phys* 1990;20:1125.

368. Fujikawa K, Miyamoto T, Ihara Y, et al. High incidence of severe urologic complications following radiotherapy for cervical cancer in Japanese women. *Gynecol Oncol* 2001;80:21–23.

369. Ogino I, Kitamura T, Okamoto N, et al. Late rectal complication

following high dose rate intracavitary brachytherapy in cancer of the cervix. *Int J Radiat Oncol Biol Phys* 1995;31:725–734.

370. Uno T, Itami J, Aruga M, et al. High dose rate brachytherapy for carcinoma of the cervix: Risk factors for late rectal complications. *Int J Radiat Oncol Biol Phys* 1998;40:615–621.

371. Wang CJ, Leung SW, Chen HC, et al. High-dose-rate intracavitary brachytherapy (HDR-IC) in treatment of cervical carcinoma: 5-year results and implication of increased low-grade rectal complication on inititation of an HDR-IC fractionation scheme. *Int J Radiat Oncol Biol Phys* 1997;38:391–398.

372. Fu KK, Phillips TL. High-dose-rate versus low-dose-rate intracavitary brachytherapy for carcinoma of the cervix. *Int J Radiat Oncol Biol Phys* 1990;19:791.

373. Kapp K, Stuecklschweiger G, Kapp DS, et al. Low rate of significant morbidity following treatment of patients with inoperable carcinoma of the cervix with external beam radiation and high-dose rate brachytherapy. (abstract) *Int J Rad Oncol Biol Phys* 1995;32 (Suppl 1):227.

374. Petereit DG, Pearcey R. Literature analysis of high dose rate brachytherapy fractionation schedules in the treatment of cervical cancer: is there an optimal fractionation schedule? *Int J Radiation Oncol Biol Phys* 1999;43:359–366.

375. Toita T, Kakinohana Y, Ogawa K, et al. Combination external beam radiotherapy and high-dose-rate intracavitary brachytherapy for uterine cervical cancer: Analysis of dose and fractionation schedule. *Int J Radiat Oncol Biol Phys* 2003;56:1344–1353.

376. Roman TN, Souhami L, Freeman CR. High dose rate afterloading intracavitary therapy in carcinoma of the cervix. *Int J Radiat Oncol Biol Phys* 1991;20:921.

377. Ahmad K, Kim YH, Ezzell G, et al. Reproducibility of multifractionated outpatient high dose rate brachytherapy in carcinoma of the cervix using the Ahmad-Kim positioner. *Endocurie Hypertherm Oncol* 1992;8:171.

378. Prempree T. Parametrial implant in stage IIIB cancer of the cervix. III. A five-year study. *Cancer* 1983;52:748.

379. Aristizabal SA, Surwit EA, Hevezi JM, et al. Treatment of advanced cancer of the cervix with transperineal interstitial irradiation. *Int J Radiat Oncol Biol Phys* 1983;9:1013.

380. Aristizabal SA, Valencia A, Ocampo G, et al. Interstitial parametrial irradiation in cancer of the cervix stage IIB-IIIB: an analysis of pelvic control and complications. *Endocuriether Hypertherm Oncol* 1985;1:41.

381. Ampuero F, Doss LL, Khan M, et al. The Syed-Neblett interstitial template in locally advanced gynecological malignancies. *Int J Radiat Oncol Biol Phys* 1983;9:1897.

382. Gaddis O, Morrow CP, Klement V, et al. Treatment of cervical carcinoma employing a template for transperineal interstitial Ir 192 brachytherapy. *Int J Radiat Oncol Biol Phys* 1983;9:819.

383. Nag S, Martinez-Mongre R, Selman AE, et al. Interstitial brachytherapy in the management of primary carcinoma of the cervix and vagina. *Gynecol Oncol* 1998;70:27–32.

384. Martinez A, Edmundson GK, Cox RS, et al. Combination of external beam irradiation and multiple-site perineal applicator (MUPIT) for treatment of locally advanced or recurrent prostatic, anorectal, and gynecologic malignancies. *Int J Radiat Oncol Biol Phys* 1985;11:391.

385. Gupta AK, Vicina FA, Frasier AJ, et al. Iridium-192 transperineal interstitial brachytherapy for locally advanced or recurrent gynecological malignancies. *Int J Radiat Oncol Biol Phys* 1999;43:1055–1060.

386. Corn BW, Lanciano RM, Rosenblum N, et al. Improved treatment planning for the Syed-Neblett template using endorectal-coil magnetic resonance and intraoperative (laparotomy/laparoscopy) guidance: A new integrated technique for hysterectomized women with vaginal tumors. *Gynecol Oncol* 1995;56:255–261.

387. Stock RG, Chan K, Terk M, et al. A new technique for performing Syed-Neblett template interstitial implants for gynecologic malignancies using transrectal-ultrasound guidance. *Int J Radiat Oncol Biol Phys* 1997;37:819–825.

388. Haddock MG, Martinez-Monge R, Petersen IA, et al. Locally advanced primary and recurrent gynecologic malignancies. EBRT with or without IORT or HDR-IORT. In: Gunderson LL, Calvo F, Harrison LB, et al., eds. *Current Clinical Oncology: Intraoperative Irradiation: Techniques and Results.* New Totowa, NJ: Humana Press, 1999:397–419.

389. Wang CC. Altered fractionation radiation therapy for gynecologic cancers. *Cancer* 1987;60:2064.

390. Komaki R, Pajak TF, Marcial VA, et al. Twice-daily fractionation of external irradiation with brachytherapy in bulky carcinoma of the cervix. Phase I/II study of the Radiation Therapy Oncology Group 88–05. *Cancer* 1994;73:2619–2625.

391. Varghese C, Rangad F, Jose CC, et al. Hyperfractionation in advanced carcinoma of the uterine cervix: a preliminary report. *Int J Radiat Oncol Biol Phys* 1992;23:393–396.

392. Calkins AR, Harrison CR, Fowler WC, Jr., et al. Hyperfractionated radiation therapy plus chemotherapy in locally advanced cervical cancer: Results of two phase I dose-escalation Gynecologic Oncology Group trials. *Gynecol Oncol* 1999;75:349–355.

393. Thomas G, Dembo A, Ackerman I, et al. A randomized trial of standard versus partially hyperfractionated radiation with or without concurrent 5-fluorouracil in locally advanced cervical cancer. *Gynecol Oncol* 1998;69:137–145.

394. Kavanagh BD, Segreti EM, Koo D, et al. Long-term local control and survival after concomitant boost accelerated radiotherapy for locally advanced cervix cancer. *Am J Clin Oncol* 2001;24:113–119.

395. Spanos WJ, Wasserman T, Meoz R, et al. Palliation of advanced pelvic malignant disease with large fraction pelvic radiation and misonidazole: Final report of RTOG phase I/II study. *Int J Radiat Oncol Biol Phys* 1987;13:1479–1482.

396. Spanos WJ, Guse C, Perez CA, et al. Phase II study of multiple daily fractionations in the palliation of advanced pelvic malignancies. Preliminary report of the RTOG 85–02. *Int J Radiat Oncol Biol Phys* 1989;17:659–662.

397. Spanos WJ, Clery M, Perez CA, et al. Late effect of multiple daily fraction schedule for advanced pelvic malignancies (RTOG 8502). *Int J Radiat Oncol Biol Phys* 1994;29:961–967.

398. Thigpen JT, Vance R, Puneky L, Khansur T. Chemotherapy as a palliative treatment in carcinoma of the uterine cervix. *Semin Oncol* 1995;22 (Suppl. 3):16–24.

399. Vermorken JB. The role of chemotherapy in squamous cell carcinoma of the uterine cervix: a review. *Int J Gynecol Cancer* 1993;3:129–142.

400. Orr JW, Ball GC, Soong SJ, et al. Surgical treatment of women found to have invasive cervix cancer at the time of total hysterectomy. *Obstet Gynecol* 1986;68:353–356.

401. Chapman JA, Mannel RS, DiSaia PJ, et al. Surgical treatment of unexpected invasive cervical cancer found at total hysterectomy. *Obstet Gynecol* 1992;80:931–934.

402. Kinney WK, Egorshin EV, Ballard DJ, et al. Long-term survival and sequelae after surgical management of invasive cervical carcinoma diagnosed at the time of simple hysterectomy. *Gynecol Oncol* 1992;44:24–27.

403. Ampil F, Datta R, Datta S. Elective postoperative external radiotherapy after hysterectomy in early-stage carcinoma of the cervix: is additional vaginal cuff irradiation necessary? *Cancer* 1987;60:280.

404. Andras EJ, Fletcher GH, Rutledge F, et al. Radiotherapy of carcinoma of the cervix following simple hysterectomy. *Am J Obstet Gynecol* 1973;115:647.

405. Crane CH, Schneider BF. Occult carcinoma discovered after simple hysterectomy treated with postoperative radiotherapy. *Int J Radiat Oncol Biol Phys* 1999;43:1049–1053.

406. Durrance FY. Radiotherapy following simple hysterectomy in patients with stage I and II carcinoma of the cervix. *Am J Roentgenol Radium Ther Nuclear Med* 1968;102:165–169.

407. Davy M, Bentzen H, Jahren K. Simple hysterectomy in the presence of invasive cervical cancer. *Acta Obstet Gynecol Scand* 1977;56:105–108.

408. Jampolis S, Andras J, Fletcher GH. Analysis of sites and causes of failure of irradiation in invasive squamous cell carcinoma of the intact uterine cervix. *Radiology* 1975;115:681.

409. Fletcher GH. Cancer of the uterine cervix: Janeway Lecture. *Am J Roentgenol Radium Ther Nucl Med* 1971;111:225.

410. O'Quinn AG, Fletcher GH, Wharton JT. Guidelines for conservative hysterectomy after irradiation. *Gynecol Oncol* 1980;9:68.

411. Gallion HN, Van Nagell JR, Donaldson GS, et al. Combined radiation therapy and extrafascial hysterectomy in the treatment of stage IB barrel-shaped cervical cancer. *Cancer* 1985;56:262.

412. Gunderson LL, Weems WS, Hebertson RM, et al. Correlation of histopathology with clinical results following radiation therapy for carci-

noma of the cervix. *Am J Roentgenol Radium Ther Nucl Med* 1974; 120:74.

413. Kilgore LC, Soong SJ, Gore H, et al. Analysis of prognostic features in adenocarcinoma of the cervix. *Gynecol Oncol* 1988;31:137.

414. Perez CA, Grigsby PW, Camel HM, et al. Irradiation alone or combined with surgery in stage IB, IIA, and IIB carcinoma of uterine cervix: update of a nonrandomized comparison. *Int J Radiat Oncol Biol Phys* 1995;31:703..

415. Thoms WW, Eifel PJ, Smith TL, et al. Bulky endocervical carcinoma: a 23 year experience. *Int J Radiat Oncol Biol Phys* 1992;23:491.

416. Einhorn N, Patek E, Sjöberg B. Outcome of different treatment modifications in cervix carcinoma, stage IB and IIA: observation in a well-defined Swedish population. *Cancer* 1985;55:949.

417. Russell AH, Burt AR, Ek M, et al. Adjunctive hysterectomy following radiation therapy for bulky carcinoma of the uterine cervix: prognostic implication of tumor persistence. *Gynecol Oncol* 1987;28:220.

418. Maruyama Y, van Nagell JR, Yoneda J, et al. Dose-response and failure pattern for bulky or barrel-shaped stage IB cervical cancer treated by combined photon irradiation and extrafascial hysterectomy. *Cancer* 1989;63:70.

419. Keys HM, Bundy BN, Stehman FB, et al. Radiation therapy with and without extrafascial hysterectomy for bulky stage IB cervical carcinoma: A randomized trial of the Gynecologic Oncology Group. *Gynecol Oncol* 2003; 89:343–353.

420. Bianchi UA, Sartori E, Pecorelli S, et al. Treatment of primary invasive cervical cancer: considerations on 997 consecutive cases. *Eur J Gynecol* 1988;9:47.

421. Kinney WK, Alvarez RD, Reid GC, et al. Value of adjuvant whole-pelvis irradiation after Wertheim hysterectomy for early-stage squamous carcinoma of the cervix with pelvic nodal metastasis: a matched-control study. *Gynecol Oncol* 1989;34:258.

422. Fuller AF Jr, Elliott N, Kosloff C, et al. Lymph node metastases from carcinoma of the cervix, stages IB and IIA: implications for prognosis and treatment. *Gynecol Oncol* 1982;13:165.

423. Stock RG, Chen AS, Flickinger JC, et al. Node-positive cervical cancer: Impact of pelvic irradiation and patterns of failure. *Int J Radiat Onc Biol Phys* 1995;31:31.

424. Soisson AP, Soper JT, Clarke-Pearson DL, et al. Adjuvant radiotherapy following radical hysterectomy for patients with stage IB and IIA cervical cancer. *Gynecol Oncol* 1990;37:390–395.

425. Hart K, Han I, Deppe G, et al. Postoperative radiation for cervical cancer with pathologic risk factors. *Int J Radiat Oncol Biol Phys* 1997; 37:833.

426. Fiorca JV, Roberts WS, Greenberg H, et al. Morbidity and survival patterns in patients after radical hysterectomy and postoperative adjuvant pelvic radiotherapy. *Gynecol Oncol* 1990;36:343–347.

427. Estape RE, Angioli R, Madrigal M, et al. Close vaginal margins as a prognostic factor after radical hysterectomy. *Gynecol Oncol* 1998; 68:229.

428. Kim RY, Salter MM, Shingleton HM. Adjuvant postoperative radiation therapy following radical hysterectomy in stage IB carcinoma of the cervix: analysis of treatment failure. *Int J Radiat Oncol Biol Phys* 1988;14:445.

429. Snidjers-Keilholz A, Hellebrekers BWJ, Zwinderman AH, et al. Adjuvant radiotherapy following radical hysterectomy for patients with early-stage cervical carcinoma (1984–1996). *Radiother Oncol* 1999; 51:161–167.

430. Thomas GM, Dembo AJ. Is there a role for adjuvant pelvic radiotherapy after radical hysterectomy in early stage cervical cancer? *Int J Gynecol Cancer* 1991;1:1.

431. Boronow RC. The bulky 6-cm barrel-shaped lesion of the cervix: Primary surgery and postoperative chemoradiation. *Gynecol Oncol* 2000;78:313–317.

432. Russell AH. Truth or consequences. *Gynecol Oncol* 1999;73: 175–176.

433. Krebs HB, Helmkamp BF, Sevin BY, et al. Recurrent cancer of the cervix following radical hysterectomy and pelvic node dissection. *Obstet Gynecol* 1982;59:422.

434. Larson DM, Copeland LJ, Stringer CA, et al. Recurrent cervical carcinoma after radical hysterectomy. *Gynecol Oncol* 1988;30:381.

435. Curtin JP, Hoskins WJ, Venkatraman ES, et al. Adjuvant chemotherapy versus chemotherapy plus pelvic irradiation for high-risk cervical cancer patients after radical hysterectomy and pelvic lymphadenec-

tomy (RH-PLND): a randomized phase III trial. *Gyn Oncol* 1996;61: 3–10.

436. Photopulos GJ, Vander Swaag R, et al. Vaginal radiation brachytherapy to reduce central recurrence after radiacal hysterectomy for cervical carcinoma. *Gynecol Oncol* 1990;38:187–190.

437. Keys HM, Bundy BN, Stehman FB, et al. Cisplatin, radiation and adjuvant hysterectomy compared with radiation and adjuvant hysterectomy for bulky stage IB cervical carcinoma. *N Engl J Med* 1999; 340(15):1154–1161.

438. Lorvidhaya V, Chitapanarux I, Sangruchi S, et al. Concurrent mitomycin C, 5-fluorouracil, and radiotherapy in the treatment of locally advanced carcinoma of the cervix: A randomized trial. *Int J Radiat Oncol Biol Phys* 2003;55:1226–1232.

439. Pearcey R, Brundage M, Drouin P, et al. Phase III trial comparing radical radiotherapy with and without cisplatin chemotherapy in patients with advanced squamos cell cancer of the cervix. *J Clin Oncol* 2002;20:966–972.

440. Abu-Rustum NR, Lee S, Correa A, et al. Compliance with and acute hematologic toxic effects of chemoradiation in indigent women with cervical cancer. *Gynecol Oncol* 2001;81:88–91.

441. Higgins RV, Naumann WR, Hall JB, et al. Concurrent carboplatin with pelvic radiation therapy in the primary treatment of cervix cancer. *Gynecol Oncol* 2003;89:499–503.

442. Green JA, Kirwan JM, Tierney JF, et al. Survival and recurrence after concomitant chemotherapy and radiotherapy for cancer of the uterine cervix: a systematic review and meta-analysis. *Lancet* 2001;358: 781–786.

442a. Wong LC, Choo YC, Choy D, et al. Long-term follow up of potentiation of radiotherapy by cis-platinum in advanced cervical cancer. *Gynecol Oncol* 1989;35:159–163.

442b. Tseng CJ, Chang CT, Lai CH, et al. A randomized trial of concurrent chemoradiotherapy versus radiotherapy in advanced carcinoma of the uterine cervix. *Gynecol Oncol* 1997;66:52–58.

442c. Leborgne. Unpublished data.

442d. Hernandez JR, de la Huerta Sanchez R, Morales Canfield F, Fernandez Orozco A. Uterine cervix cancer. Clinical stage III. Combined radiotherapy and chemotherapy treatment. *Ginecol Obstet Mex* 1991; 59:238–242.

442e. Lorvidhaya V, Tonusin A, Sukthomya W, Changwiwit W, Nimmolrat A. Induction chemotherapy and irradiation in advanced carcinoma of the cervix. *Gan To Kagaku Ryoho* 1995;22:244–251.

442f. Wong LC, Ngan HYS, Cheung ANY, Cheng DKL, Ng TY, Choy DTK. Chemoradiation and adjuvant chemotherapy in cervical cancer. *J Clin Oncol* 1999;17:2055–2060.

442g. Roberts KB, Urdaneta N, Vera R, et al. Interim results of a randomized trial of mitomycin C as an adjunct to radical radiotherapy in the treatment of locally advanced squamous cell carcinoma of the cervix. *Int J Cancer* 2000;90:206–223.

443. Chauvergne J, Lhommé C, Rohart J, et al. Chimiothérapie néoadjuvante des cancers du col utérin aux stades IIb et III. Résultats éloignés d'un essai randomize pluricentrique portant sur 151 patients. *Bull Cancer (Paris)* 1993;80:1069–1079.

444. Kumar L, Kaushal R, Nandy M, et al. Chemotherapy followed by radiotherapy versus radiotherapy alone in locally advanced cervical cancer. A randomized study. *Gynecol Oncol* 1994;54:307–315.

445. Kumar L, Grover R, Pokharel YH, et al. Neoadjuvant chemotherapy in locally advanced cervical cancer: two randomized studies. *Aust NZ J Med* 1998;28:387–390.

446. Souhami L, Gil RA, Allan SE, et al. A randomized trial of chemotherapy followed by pelvic radiation therapy in stage IIIB carcinoma of the cervix. *J Clin Oncol* 1991;9:970-977.

447. Tattersall MHN, Ramirez C, Coppleson MA. A randomized trial comparing platinum-based chemotherapy followed by radiotherapy vs radiotherapy alone in patients with locally advanced cervical cancer. *Int J Gynecol Cancer* 1992;2:244–251.

448. Tattersall MHN, Lorvidhaya V, Vootiprux V, et al. Randomized trial of epirubicin and cisplatin chemotherapy followed by pelvic radiation in locally advanced cervical cancer. *J Clin Oncol* 1995;13:444–451.

449. Withers HR, Taylor JM, Maciejewski B. The hazard of accelerated tumor clonogen repopulation during radiotherapy. *Acta Oncol* 1988; 27:131–146.

450. Ozols RF, Masuda H, Hamilton TC. Keynote address: Mechanisms of

cross-resistance between radiation and antineoplastic drugs. *National Cancer Institute Monographs* 1988;6:159–165.

451. Benedetti-Panici P, Greggi S, Scambia G, et al. High-dose cisplatin and bleomycin neoadjuvant chemotherapy plus radical surgery in locally advanced cervical carcinoma: A preliminary report. *Gynecol Oncol* 1991;41:212–216.

452. Benedetti-Panici P, Scambia G, Baiocchi G, et al. Neoadjuvant chemotherapy and radical surgery in locally advanced cervical cancer. Prognostic factors for response and survival. *Cancer* 1991;67:372–379.

453. Dottino PR, Plaxe SC, Beddoe AM, et al. Induction chemotherapy followed by radical surgery in cervical cancer. *Gynecol Oncol* 1991;40:7–11.

454. Fontanelli R, Spatti G, Raspagliesi F, et al. A preoperative single course of high-dose cisplatin and bleomycin with glutathione protection in bulky stage IB/II carcinoma of the cervix. *Ann Oncol* 1992;3:117–121.

455. Eddy GL, Manetta A, Alvarez RD, et al. Neoadjuvant chemotherapy with vincristine and cisplatin followed by radical hysterectomy and pelvic lymphadenectomy for FIGO stage IB bulky cervical cancer: A Gynecologic Oncology Group pilot study. *Gynecol Oncol* 1995;57:412–416.

456. Zanetta G, Lissoni A, Pellegrino A, et al. Neoadjuvant chemotherapy with cisplatin, ifosfamide and paclitaxel for locally advanced squamous-cell cervical cancer. *Ann Oncol* 1998;9:977–980.

457. Sugiyama T, Nishida T, Muraoka Y, et al. Radical surgery after neoadjuvant intra-arterial chemotherapy in stage IIIb squamous cell carcinoma of the cervix. *Int Surg* 1999;84:67–73.

458. Marth C, Sundfor K, Kaern J, Tropé C. Long-term follow-up of neoadjuvant cisplatin and 5-fluorouracil chemotherapy in bulky squamous cell carcinoma of the cervix. *Acta Oncol* 1999;38:517–520.

459. Minagawa Y, Kigawa J, Irie T, et al. Radical surgery following neoadjuvant chemotherapy for patients with stage IIIB cervical cancer. *Ann Surg Oncol* 1998;5:539–543.

460. Meden H, Fattahi Meibodi A, Osmers R, et al. Wertheim's hysterectomy after neoadjuvant carboplatin-based chemotherapy in patients with cervical cancer stage IIB and IIIB. *Anticancer Res* 1998;18:4575–4579.

461. Sardi J, Giaroli A, Sananes C, et al. Long term follow-up of the first randomized trial using neoadjuvant chemotherapy in stage IB squamous carcinoma of the cervix: The final results. *Gynecol Oncol* 1997;67:61–69.

462. Sardi J, Giaroli A, Sananes C, et al. Randomized trial with neoadjuvant chemotherapy in stage IIIB squamous carcinoma cervix uteri: An unexpected therapeutic management. *Int J Gynecol Cancer* 1996;6:85–93.

463. Benedetti-Panici P, Landoni F, Greggi S, et al. Randomized trial of neoadjuvant chemotherapy (NACT) followed by radical surgery (RS) vs exclusive radiotherapy (RT) in locally advanced squamous cell cervical cancer (LASCCC). An Italian multicenter study. *Int J Gynecol Cancer* 1997;7(suppl 2):18 (abstract).

464. Sardi JE, Sananes CE, Giaroli AA, et al. Neoadjuvant chemotherapy in cervical carcinoma stage IIB: a randomized controlled trial. *Int J Gynecol Cancer* 1998;8:441–450.

465. Chang TC, Lai CH, Hong JH, et al. Randomized trial of neoadjuvant cisplatin, vincristine, bleomycin, and radical hysterectomy versus radiation therapy for bulky stage IB and IIA cervical cancer. *J Clin Oncol* 2000; 18:1740–1747.

466. Killackey MA, Boardman L, Carroll DS. Adjuvant chemotherapy and radiation in patients with poor prognostic stage Ib/IIa cervical cancer. *Gynecol Oncol* 1993;49:377–379.

467. Lai CH, Lin TS, Soong YK, et al. Adjuvant chemotherapy after radical hysterectomy for cervical carcinoma. *Gynecol Oncol* 1989;35:193–198.

468. Wertheim MS, Hakes TB, Daghestani AN, et al. A pilot study of adjuvant therapy in patients with cervical cancer at high risk of recurrence after radical hysterectomy and pelvic lymphadenectomy. *J Clin Oncol* 1985;3:912–916.

469. Sivanesaratnam V. Adjuvant chemotherapy in high-risk patients after Wertheim hysterectomy—10 year survivals. *Ann Acad Med Singapore* 1998;27:622–626.

470. Havrilesky LJ, Wong TZ, Secord AA, et al. The role of PET scanning

in the detection of recurrent cervical cancer. *Gynecol Oncol* 2003;90:186–190.

471. Grigsby PW, Siegel BA, Dehdashti F, et al. Post-therapy surveillance monitoring of cervical cancer by FDG-PET. *Int J Rad Oncol Biol Phys* 2003;55:907–913.

472. Ryu SY, Moon-Hong K, Suck-Chul C, et al. Detection of early recurrence with 18F-FDG PET in patients with cervical cancer. *Jour of Nuclear Med* 2003;44:347–352.

473. Miller B, Morris M, Rutledge F, et al. Aborted exenterative procedures in recurrent cervical cancer. *Gynecol Oncol* 1993;50:94–99.

474. Thomas GM, Dembo AJ, Black B, et al. Concurrent radiation and chemotherapy for carcinoma of the cervix recurrent after radical surgery. *Gynecol Oncol* 1987;27:254–263.

475. Prasavinichai S, Glassburn JR, Brady LW. Treatment of recurrent carcinoma of the cervix. *Int J Radiol Oncol Biol Phys* 1978;4:957.

476. Prempree T, Kwon T, Villa Santa U, et al. Management of late second or late recurrent squamous cell carcinoma of the cervix uteri after successful initial radiation treatment. *Int J Radiat Oncol Biol Phys* 1979;5:2053.

477. Sommers GM, Grigsby PW, Perez CA, et al. Outcome of recurrent cervical carcinoma following definitive irradiation. *Gynecol Oncol* 1989;35:150–155.

478. Puthawala AA, Syed AM, Fleming PA, et al. Re-irradiation with interstitial implant for recurrent pelvic malignancies. *Cancer* 1982;50:2810.

479. Randall ME, Evans L, Greven KM, et al. Interstitial re-irradiation for recurrent gynecological malignancies: Results and analysis of prognostic factors. *Gynecol Oncol* 1993;48:23–31.

480. Wang CJ, Lai CH, Huang HJ, et al. Recurrent cervical carcinoma after primary radical surgery. *Am J Obstet Gynecol* 1999;181:518–524.

481. Song G, Cardenes H, Randall ME. Interstitial reirradiation as salvage therapy for recurrent gynecologic malignancies. *Int J Gynecol Cancer* 2002;12:651–652 (abstract).

482. Grigsby PW, Vest ML, and Perez CA. Recurrent carcinoma of the cervix exclusively in the paraaortic nodes following radiation therapy. *Int J Radiat Oncol Biol Phys* 1994;28:451–455.

483. Kim JS, Kim SY, Kim KH, et al. Hyperfractionated radiotherapy with concurrent chemotherapy for para-aortic lymph node recurrence in carcinoma of the cervix. *Int J Radiat Oncol Biol Phys* 2003;55:1247–1253.

484. Sun SS, Chen TC, Yen RF, et al. Value of whole body 18F-fluoro-2-deoxyglucose positron emission tomography in the evaluation of recurrent cervical cancer. *Anticancer Res* 2001;21:2957–2961.

485. Shingleton HM, Soong SJ, Gelder MS, et al. Clinical and histopathologic factors predicting recurrence and survival after pelvic exenteration for cancer of the cervix. *Obstet Gynecol* 1989;73:1027–1034.

486. Ratliff CR, Gershenson DM, Morris M, et al. Sexual adjustment of patients undergoing gracilis myocutaneous flap vaginal reconstruction in conjunction with pelvic exenteration. *Cancer* 1996;78:2229–2235.

487. Coleman RL, Keeney ED, Freedman RS, et al. Radical hysterectomy for recurrent carcinoma of the uterine cervix after radiotherapy. *Gynecol Oncol* 1994;55:29–35.

488. Rutledge S, Carey MS, Prichard H, et al. Conservative surgery for recurrent or persistent carcinoma of the cervix following irradiation: is exenteration always necessary? *Gynecol Oncol* 1994;52:353–359.

489. Rubin SC, Hoskins WJ, Lewis JL. Radical hysterectomy for recurrent cervical cancer following radiation therapy. *Gynecol Oncol* 1987;27:316–322.

490. Maneo A, Landoni F, Cormio G, et al. Radical hysterectomy for recurrent or persistent cervical cancer following radiation therapy. *Int J Gynecol Cancer* 1999;9:295–301.

491. Ciatto S, Pirtoli L, Cionini L. Radiotherapy for postoperative failures of carcinoma of cervix uteri. *Surg Gynecol Obstet* 1980;151:621–624.

492. Lanciano R. Radiotherapy for the treatment of locally recurrent cervical cancer. *J Natl Cancer Inst Monogr* 1996;21:113–115.

493. Potter ME, Alvarez RD, Gay FL, et al. Optimal therapy for pelvic recurrence after radical hysterectomy for early-stage cervical cancer. *Gynecol Oncol* 1990;37:74–77.

494. Ijaz T, Eifel PJ, Burke T, et al. Radiation therapy of pelvic recurrence after radical hysterectomy for cervical carcinoma. *Gynecol Oncol* 1998;70:241–246.

495. Ito H, Shigematsu N, Kawada T, et al. Radiotherapy for centrally

recurrent cervical cancer of the vaginal stump following hysterectomy. *Gynecol Oncol* 1997;67:154–161.

496. Hintz BL, Kagan AR, Chan P, et al. Radiation tolerance of the vaginal mucosa. *Int J Radiat Oncol Biol Phys* 1980;6:711.

497. Monk BJ, Walker JL, Tewari KS, et al. Open interstitial brachytherapy for the treatment of local-regional recurrences of uterine corpus and cervix cancer after primary surgery. *Gynecol Oncol* 1994;52: 222–228.

498. Jobsen JJ, Lee JWH, Cleton FJ, et al. Treatment of loco-regional recurrence of carcinoma of the cervix by radiotherapy after primary surgery. *Gynecol Oncol* 1989;33:368.

499. Evans SR JR, Hilaris BS, Barber HRK. External vs. interstitial irradiation in unresectable recurrent cancer of the cervix. *Cancer* 1971;28: 1284.

500. Friedman M, Pearlman AW. Carcinoma of the cervix: radiation salvage of surgical failures. *Radiology* 1965;84:801.

501. Webb MJ, Symmonds RE. Site of recurrence of cervical cancer after radical hysterectomy. *Am J Obstet Gynecol* 1980;138:813.

502. Nori D, Valentine E, Hilaris BS. The role of paraaortic node irradiation in the treatment of cancer of the cervix. *Int J Radiat Oncol Biol Phys* 1985;11:1469–1473.

503. Maneo A, Landoni F, Cormio G, et al. Concurrent carboplatinum/ 5-fluorouracil and radiotherapy for recurrent cervical carcinoma. *Ann Oncol* 1999;10:803–807.

504. Cerrotta A, Gardan G, Cavina R, et al. Concurrent radiotherapy and weekly paclitaxel for locally advanced or recurrent squamous cell carcinoma of the uterine cervix. A pilot study with intensification of the dose. *Eur J Gynaecol Oncol* 2002;23:115–119.

505. Morley GW, Hopkins MP, Lindenauer SM, et al. Pelvic exenteration, University of Michigan: 100 patients at 5 years. *Obstet Gynecol* 1989; 74:934–943.

506. Averette HE, Lichtinger M, Sevin BU, et al. Pelvic exenteration: A 15-year experience in a general metropolitan hospital. *Am J Obstet Gynecol* 1984;150:179–184.

507. Mahe MA, Gerard JP, Dubois JB, et al. Intraoperative radiation therapy in recurrent carcinoma of the uterine cervix: Report of the French Intraoperative Group on 70 patients. *Int J Radiat Oncol Biol Phys* 1996;34:21–26.

508. Martinez-Monje R, Jurado M, Azinovic I, et al. Preoperative chemoradiation and adjuvant surgery in locally advanced or recurrent cervical carcinoma. *Rev Med Univ Navarra* 1997;41:19–26.

509. Garton GR, Gunderson LL, Webb MJ, et al. Intraoperative radiation therapy in gynecologic cancer: Update of the experience at a single institution. *Int J Radiat Oncol Biol Phys* 1997;37:839–843.

510. Martinez-Monje R, Jurado M, Aristu JJ, et al. Intraoperative electron beam radiotherapy during radical surgery for locally advanced and recurrent cervical cancer. *Gynecol Oncol* 2001;82:538–543.

511. Abe M, Shibamoto Y. The usefulness of intraoperative radiation therapy in the treatment of pelvic recurrence of cervical cancer. *Int J Radiat Oncol Biol Phys* 1996;34:513–514.

512. Beitler JJ, Anderson PS, Wadler S, et al. Pelvic exenteration for cervix cancer: Would additional intraoperative interstitial brachytherapy improve survival? *Int J Radiat Oncol Biol Phys* 1997;38:143–148.

513. Hockel M, Baussmann E, Mitze M, et al. Are pelvic side-wall recurrences of cervical cancer biologically different from central relapses? *Cancer* 1994;74:648–655.

514. Hockel M, Schlenger K, Hamm H, et al. Five-year experience with combined operative and radiotherapeutic treatment of recurrent gynecologic tumors infiltrating the pelvic wall. *Cancer* 1996;77: 1918–1933.

515. Bonomi P, Blessing JA, Stehman FB, et al. Randomized trial of three cisplatin dose schedules in squamous cell carcinoma of the cervix: A Gynecologic Oncology Group Study. *J Clin Oncol* 1985;3: 1079–1085.

516. Reichman B, Markman M, Hakes T, et al. Phase II trial of high-dose cisplatin with sodium thiosulfate nephroprotection in patients with advanced carcinoma of the uterine cervix previously untreated with chemotherapy. *Gynecol Oncol* 1991;43:159–163.

517. Alberts DS, Kronmal R, Baker LH, et al. Phase II randomized trial of cisplatin chemotherapy regimens in the treatment of recurrent or metastatic squamous cell cancer of the cervix: A Southwest Oncology Group Study. *J Clin Oncol* 1987;5:1791–1795

518. Vermorken JB, Zanetta G, De Oliveira CF, et al. Cisplatin-based com-bination chemotherapy (BEMP) versus single agent cisplatin (P) in disseminated squamous cell carcinoma of the uterine cervix (SCCUC): mature data of EORTC protocol 55863. *Ann Oncol* 1996; 7:67 (abstract)

519. Omura GA, Blessing JA, Vaccarello L, et al. Randomized trial of cisplatin versus cisplatin plus mitolactol (Dibromodulcitol) versus cisplatin plus ifosfamide in advanced squamous carcinoma of the cervix: A Gynecologic Oncology Group Study. *J Clin Oncol* 1997;15: 165–171.

520. Kumar L, Pokharel YH, Kumar S, et al. Single agent versus combination chemotherapy in recurrent cervical cancer. *J Obstet Gynaecol Res* 1998;24:401–409.

521. Moore DH, McQuellon RP, Blessing JA, et al. A randomized phase III study of cisplatin versus cisplatin plus paclitaxel in stage IVB, recurrent or persistent squamous cell carcinoma of the cervix: a Gynecologic Oncology Group study. Proceedings of ASCO 2001;20:201a (abst #801).

522. Zola P, Volpe T, Castelli G, et al. Is the published literature a reliable guide for deciding between alternative treatments for patients with early cervical cancer? *Int J Radiat Oncol Biol Phys* 1989;16:785–797.

523. Christopherson WM, Gray LA, Parker JE. Microinvasive carcinoma of the uterine cervix. *Cancer* 1976;38:629.

524. Tsukamoto N, Kaku T, Matsukuma K, et al. The problem of stage IA (FIGO, 1985) carcinoma of the uterine cervix. *Gynecol Oncol* 1989;34:1.

525. Kielbinska S, Ludwika T, Fraczek O. Studies of mortality and health status in women cured of cancer of the cervix uteri: comparison of long-term results of radiotherapy and combined surgery and radiotherapy. *Cancer* 1973;32:245.

526. Komaki R, Brickner TJ, Hanlon AL, et al. Long-term results of treatment of cervical carcinoma in the United States in 1973, 1978, and 1983: Patterns of Care study. *Int J Radiat Oncol Biol Phys* 1995;31: 973.

527. Barillot I, Horiot JC, Pigneux J, et al. Carcinoma of the intact uterine cervix treated with radiotherapy alone: A French cooperative study: Update and multivariate analysis of prognostic factors. *Int J Radiat Oncol Biol Phys* 1997;38:969–978.

528. Perez CA, Camel HM, Walz BJ, et al. Radiation therapy alone in the treatment of carcinoma of the uterine cervix: a 20 year experience. *Gynecol Oncol* 1986;23:127.

529. Coia L, Won M, Lanciano R, et al. The Patterns of Care Outcome Study for cancer of the uterine cervix: results of the 2nd National Practice Survey. *Cancer* 1990;66:2451.

530. Montana GS, Fowler WC, Varia MA, et al. Carcinoma of the cervix, stage III: results of radiation therapy. *Cancer* 1986;57:148.

531. Perez CA, Breaux S, Madoc-Jones H, et al. Radiation therapy alone in the treatment of carcinoma of uterine cervix. I. Analysis of tumor recurrence. *Cancer* 1983;51:1393.

532. Arthur D, Kaufman N, Schmidt-Ulrich R, et al. Heuristically derived tumor burden score as a prognostic factor for stage IIIB carcinoma of the cervix. *Int J Radiat Oncol Biol Phys* 1995;31:743.

533. Fyles A, Keane TJ, Barton M, Simm J. The effect of treatment duration in the local control of cervix cancer. *Radiother Oncol* 1992;25: 273–279

534. Girinsky T, Rey A, Roche B, et al. Overall treatment time in advanced cervical carcinomas: A critical parameter in treatment outcome. *Int J Radiat Oncol Biol Phys* 1994;27:1051–1056.

535. Lanciano, RM, Pajak TF, Martz K, et al. The influence of treatment time on outcome for squamous cell cancer of the uterine cervix treated with radiation: a Patterns of Care Study. *Int J Radiation Oncol Biol Phys* 1993;25:391.

536. Petereit DG, Sarkaria JN, Chappel R, et al. The adverse effect of treatment prolongation in cervical carcinoma. *Int J Radiat Oncol Biol Phys* 1995;32:1301–1307.

537. Perez CA, Grigsby PW, Castro-Vita H, et al. Carcinoma of the uterine cervix I. Impact of prolongation of treatment time and timing of brachytherapy on outcome of radiation therapy. *Int J Radiation Oncol Biol Phys* 1995;32:1275.

538. Eifel PJ, Thames HD. Has the influence of treatment duration on local control of carcinoma of the cervix been defined? *Int J Radiat Oncol Biol Phys* 1995;32:1527–1529.

539. Erridge SC, Kerr GR, Downing D, et al. The effect of overall treatment

time on the survival and toxicity of radical radiotherapy for cervical carcinoma. *Radiother Oncol* 2002;63:59–66.

540. Crawford JS, Harisiadis L, McGowan L, et al. Paraaortic lymph node irradiation in cervical carcinoma without prior lymphadenectomy. *Radiology* 1987;164:255–257.

541. Carl U, Bahnsen J, Wiegel T. Radiation therapy of para-aortic lymph nodes in cancer of the uterine cervix. *Acta Oncologica* 1993;32:63–67.

542. Horii T, Mitsumoto T, Noda K. Significance of para-aortic node irradiation in the treatment of cervical cancer. *Gynecol Oncol* 1988;31:371–383.

543. Haie C, Pejovic MH, Gerbaulet A, et al. Is prophylactic para-aortic irradiation worthwhile in the treatment of advanced cervical carcinoma? Results of a controlled clinical trial of the EORTC radiotherapy group. *Radiother Oncol* 1988;11:101–112.

544. Rotman M, Pajak TF, Choi K, et al. Prophylactic extended-field irradiation of para-aortic lymph nodes in stages IIB and bulky IB and IIA cervical carcinoma. *J Am Med Assoc* 1995;274:387.

545. Sood BM, Timmins PF, Gorla GR, et al. Concomitant cisplatin and extended field radiation therapy in patients with cervical and endometrial cancer. *Int J Gynecol Cancer* 2002;12:459–464.

546. Varia MA, Bundy BN, Deppe G, et al. Cervical carcinoma metastatic to para-aortic nodes: Extended field radiation therapy with concomitant 5-fluorouracil and cisplatin chemotherapy: A Gynecologic Oncology Group study. *Int J Rad Oncol Biol Phys* 1998;42:1015.

547. Brookland RK, Rubin S, Danoff BF. Extended field irradiation in the treatment of patients with cervical carcinoma involving biopsy proven para-aortic nodes. *Int J Radiat Oncol Biol Phys* 1984;10:1875–1879.

548. Lovecchio JL, Averette HE, Donato D, et al. 5-year survival of patients with periaortic nodal metastases in clinical stage IB and IIA cervical carcinoma. *Gynecol Oncol* 1989;34:43.

549. Vigliotti AP, Wen BC, Hussey DH, et al. Extended field irradiation for carcinoma of the uterine cervix with positive periaortic nodes. *Int J Radiat Oncol Biol Phys* 1992;23:501–509.

550. Stryker JA, Mortel R. Survival following extended field irradiation in carcinoma of cervix metastatic to para-aortic lymph nodes. *Gynecol Oncol* 2000;79:99–405.

551. Grigsby PW, Lu JD, Mutch DG, et al. Twice-daily fractionation of external irradiation with brachytherapy and chemotherapy in carcinoma of the cervix with positive para-aortic lymph nodes: Phase II study of the Radiation Therapy Oncology Group 92–10. *Int J Radiat Oncol Biol Phys* 1998;41:817.

552. Hanks GE, Herring DF, Kramer S. Patterns of Care Outcome Studies: results of the national practice in cancer of the cervix. *Cancer* 1983;51:959.

553. Castro JR, Issa P, Fletcher GH. Carcinoma of the cervix treated by external irradiation alone. *Radiology* 1970;95:163.

554. Akine Y, Hashida I, Kajiura Y, et al. Carcinoma of the uterine cervix treated with external irradiation alone. *Int J Radiat Oncol Biol Phys* 1986;12:1611.

555. Barter JF, Soong SJ, Shingleton HM, et al. Complications of combined radical hysterectomy-postoperative radiation therapy in women with early stage cervical cancer. *Gynecol Oncol* 1989;32:292.

556. Seski JC, Diokno AC. Bladder dysfunction after radical abdominal hysterectomy. *Am J Obstet Gynecol* 1977;128:643.

557. Barnes W, Waggoner S, Delgado G, et al. Manometric characterization of rectal dysfunction following radical hysterectomy. *Gynecol Oncol* 1991;42:116.

558. Symmonds RE. Morbidity and complications of radical hysterectomy with pelvic lymph node dissection. *Am J Obstet Gynecol* 1966;94:663.

559. Pedersen D, Bentzen SM, Overgaard J. Early and late radiotherapeutic morbidity in 442 consecutive patients with locally advanced carcinoma of the uterine cervix. *Int J Radiat Oncol Biol Phys* 1994;29:941.

560. Perez CA, Grigsby PW, Castro-Vita H, et al. Carcinoma of the uterine cervix. II. Lack of impact of prolongation of overall treatment time on morbidity of radiation therapy. *Int J Radiat Oncol Biol Phys* 1996;34:3–11.

561. Perez CA, Grigsby PW, Lockett MA, et al. Radiation therapy morbidity in carcinoma of the uterine cervix: dosimetric and clinical correlation. *Int J Radiation Oncol Biol Phys* 1999;44:855–866.

562. Lanciano RM, Martz K, Montana GS, et al. Influence of age, prior abdominal surgery, fraction size, and dose on complications after radiation therapy for squamous cell cancer of the uterine cervix: a pattern of care study. *Cancer* 1992;69:2124–2130.

563. Perez CA, Breaux S, Bedwinek JM, et al. Radiation therapy alone in treatment of the uterine cervix. II. Analysis of complications. *Cancer* 1984;54:235.

564. Kottmeier, HL. Complications following radiation therapy in carcinoma of the cervix and their treatment. *Am J Obstet Gynecol* 1964;88:854.

565. Pourquier H, Dubois JB, Deland R. Cancer of the uterine cervix: dosimetric guidelines for prevention of late rectal and rectosigmoid complications as a result of radiotherapeutic treatment. *Int J Radiat Oncol Biol Phys* 1982;8:1887.

566. Yudelev M, Kuten A, Tatcher M, et al. Correlations of dose and time-dose-fractionation factors (TDF) with treatment results and side effects in cancer of the uterine cervix. *Gynecol Oncol* 1986;23:310.

567. Strockbine MF, Hancock JE, Fletcher GH. Complications in 831 patients with squamous cell carcinoma of the intact uterine cervix treated with 3000 rads or more whole pelvis irradiation. *Am J Roentgenol Radium Ther Nucl Med* 1970;108:292.

568. Quilty PM. A report of late rectosigmoid morbidity in patients with advanced cancer of the cervix, treated with a 6 week pelvic brick technique. *Clin Radiol* 1988;39:297.

569. Unal A, Hamberger AD, Seski JC, et al. An analysis of the severe complications of irradiation of carcinoma of the uterine cervix: treatment with intracavitary radium and parametrial irradiation. *Int J Radiat Oncol Biol Phys* 1981;7:999.

570. Stryker JA, Bartholomew M, Velkley DE, et al. Bladder and rectal complications following radiotherapy for cervix cancer. *Gynecol Oncol* 1988;29:1.

571. Sherrah-Davies E. Morbidity following low dose rate Selectron therapy for cervical cancer. *Clin Radiol* 1985;36:131.

572. Jeremic B, Djuric LJ, Mijatovic LJ. Severe late intestinal complications afer abdominal or pelvic irradiation with high energy photon beams. *Clincial Oncol* 1991;3:100–104.

573. Marks GF, Mohiuddin M. The surgical management of the radiation-injured intestine. *Surgical Clinics of North America* 1983;63:81–96.

574. Parkin DE, Davis JA, Symonds RP. Urodynamic findings following radiotherapy for cervical carcinoma. *Br J Urol* 1988;61:213.

575. Maier U, Ehrenbock P, Hofbauer J. Late urological complication and malignancies after curative radiotherapy for gynaecological carcinomas: a retrospective analysis of 10,709 patients. *J Urol* 1997;158:814–817.

576. Lajer H, Thranov KR, Skovgaard LT, et al. Late urologic morbidity in 177 consecutive patients after radiotherapy for cervical carcinoma: A longitudinal study. *Int J Radiat Oncol Biol Phys* 2002;54:1356–1361.

577. Souhami L, Seymour R, Roman TN, et al. Weekly cisplatin plus external beam radiotherapy and high dose rate brachytherapy in patients with locally advanced carcinoma of the cervix. *Int J Radiat Oncol Biol Phys* 1993;27:871–878.

578. Sood BM, Gorla G, Garg M, et al. Two fractions of high-dose-rate brachytherapy in the management of cervix cancer: Clinical experience with and without chemotherapy. *Int J Radiat Oncol Biol Phys* 2002;53:702–706.

579. Jensen PT, Groenvold M, Klee MC, et al. Longitudinal study of sexual function and vaginal changes following radiotherapy for cervical cancer. *Int J Radiat Oncol Biol Phys* 2003;56:937–949.

580. Bergmark K, Avall-Lundqvist E, Dickman PW, et al. Vaginal changes and sexuality in women with a history of cervical cancer. *N Engl J Med* 1999;340:1383–1389.

581. Ashenhurst EM, Quartey GRC, Starreveld A. Lumbo-sacral radiculopathy induced by radiation. *Can J Neurol Sci* 1977;4:259.

582. Maier JG, Perry PH, Saylor W, et al. Radiation myelitis of the dorsolumbar spinal cord. *Radiology* 1969;93:153.

583. Thomas JE, Cascino TL, Earle JD. Differential diagnosis between radiation and tumor plexopathy of the pelvis. *Neurology* 1985;35:1.

584. Lundin B, Bjorkholm E, Jacobsson H. Insufficiency fractures of the sacrum after radiotherapy for gynaecological malignancy. *Acta Oncologica* 1990;29:211–215.

585. Konski A, Sowers M. Pelvic fractures following irradiation for endometrial carcinoma. *Int J Radiation Oncol Biol Phys* 1996;35:361–367.

586. Mumber MP, Greven KM, Haygood TM. Pelvic insufficiency frac-

tures associated with radiation atrophy: clinical recognition and diagnostic evaluation. *Skeletal Radiology* 1997;26:94–99.

587. Moreno A, Clemente J, Crespo C, et al. Pelvis insufficiency fractures in patients with pelvic irradiation. *Int J Radiation Oncol Biol Phys* 1999;44:61–66.

588. Huh SJ, Kim B, Kang MK, et al. Pelvic insufficiency fracture after pelvic irradiation in uterine cervix cancer. *Gynecol Oncol* 2002;86:264–268.

589. Bloss JD, DiSaia PJ, Mannel RS, et al. Radiation myelitis: A complication of concurrent cisplatin and 5-fluorouracil chemotherapy with extended field radiotherapy for carcinoma of the uterine cervix. *Gynecol Oncol* 1991;43:305–308.

590. Grigsby PW, Russell A, Bruner D, et al. Late injury of cancer therapy on the female reproductive tract. *Int J Radiation Oncol Biol Phys* 1995;31:1281–1299.

591. Routledge JA, Burns MP, Swindell R, et al. Evaluation of the LENT-SOMA scales for the prospective assessment of treatment morbidity in cervical carcinoma. *Int J Radiat Oncol Biol Phys* 2003;56:502–510.

592. Wollschlaeger K, Connell P, Waggoner S, et al. Acute problems during low-dose-rate intracavitary brachytherapy for cervical carcinoma. *Gynecol Oncol* 2000;76:67–72.

593. Jhingran A, Eifel PJ. Perioperative and postoperative complications of intracavitary radiation for FIGO stage I-III carcinoma of the cervix. *Int J Radiat Oncol Biol Phys* 2000;46:1177–1183.

594. Dusenbery KE, Carson LF, Potish RA. Perioperative morbidity and mortality of gynecologic brachytherapy. *Cancer* 1991;67:2786.

595. Lanciano R, Corn B, Martin E, et al. Perioperative morbidity of intracavitary gynecologic brachytherapy. *Int J Radiation Oncol Biol Phys* 1994;29:969–974.

596. Kjorstad KE, Martimbeau PW, Iversen T. Stage IB carcinoma of the cervix: the Norwegian Radium Hospital. Results and complications. III. Urinary and gastrointestinal complications. *Gynecol Oncol* 1983;15:42.

597. Jacobs AJ, Perez CA, Camel HM, et al. Complications in patients receiving both irradiation and radical hysterectomy for carcinoma of the uterine cervix. *Gynecol Oncol* 1985;22:273.

598. Martimbeau PW, Kjorstad KE, Kolstad P. Stage IB carcinoma of the cervix, the Norwegian Radium Hospital, 1968–1970: results of treatment and major complications. I. Lymphedema. *Am J Obstet Gynecol* 1978;131:389.

599. Bichel P, Jakobsen A. Histopathologic grading and prognosis of uterine cervical carcinoma. *Am J Clin Pathol* 1985;8:247.

600. Potish RA, Twiggs LB, Prem KA, et al. The impact of extraperitoneal surgical staging on morbidity and tumor recurrence following radiotherapy for cervical carcinoma. *Am J Clin Oncol* 1984;7:245.

CHAPTER 23

Corpus: Epithelial Tumors

Claes G Tropé, Kaled M. Alektiar, Paul J. Sabbatini, and Richard J. Zaino

The American Cancer Society estimated that there were 40,100 new cases of endometrial carcinoma in the United States in 2003 (1). Factors influencing its prominence are the declining incidence of cervical cancer, prolonged life expectancy, and earlier diagnosis. Currently, endometrial adenocarcinoma is the fourth most common cancer in females, ranking behind breast, bowel, and lung cancers. The roughly 6,800 deaths caused by endometrial carcinoma each year make it the seventh leading cause of death from malignancy in women. It is primarily a disease of the postmenopausal woman, although 25% of the cases occur in premenopausal patients, with 5% occurring in patients younger than 40 years of age (2,3).

In 75% of all cases, the tumor is confined to the uterine corpus at the time of diagnosis, and uncorrected survival rates of 75% or more are expected (4). In the past 50 years, the treatment of endometrial cancer has evolved from a regimen of preoperative intracavitary radium packing or external radiation therapy, followed in 6 weeks by hysterectomy, to a single application of intrauterine tandem and vaginal ovoids, followed immediately or in 6 weeks by hysterectomy, to a customized treatment program that uses hysterectomy and surgical staging as primary therapy and employs additional treatment depending on various risk factors. In 1988, this primary operative approach led the International Federation of Gynecology and Obstetrics (FIGO) to require surgical removal of the uterus to stage this disease (5).

In the past 30 years, a number of chemotherapeutic regimens have been tested as adjuvant treatment in the primary setting or for recurrent disease. Recently, the results of a randomized trial comparing whole abdominal radiotherapy versus chemotherapy as adjuvant treatment for FIGO stages III and IV disease were presented in abstract form and show an advantage for chemotherapy (6). This study has renewed interest in evaluating chemotherapy as an important part of adjuvant treatment, and current studies are considering whether it should be given either sequentially or concomitantly with radiation therapy. The administration of chemotherapeutic agents to patients with recurrent disease largely remains palliative, and novel approaches are under investigation (7).

The usual carcinoma of the endometrium is easily diagnosed, but the well-differentiated cancers may be difficult to separate from advanced atypical hyperplasia (3). In the past 10 years, helpful criteria have been adopted to permit differentiation of the two conditions into a benign lesion (atypical hyperplasia) and a neoplasm that is progressive (well-differentiated carcinoma).

ANATOMY

The uterus is situated in the pelvis between the bladder and the rectum. It is divided structurally and functionally into two parts—the body (corpus) and the cervix—that are separated by a slight narrowing of the uterus, known as the isthmus. This is the level of the internal os of the cervix. The cervix is divided into the supravaginal portion, which is closely approximated to the bladder, and the vaginal portion, which projects into the cavity of the vagina.

The principal ligaments of support for the uterus are the broad ligaments, the round ligaments, the uterosacral ligaments, and the cardinal ligaments. Blood is supplied to the uterus by the uterine artery, which is a branch of the hypogastric artery and which enters the wall of the uterus at the isthmus after it crosses over the ureter. It anastomoses with the ovarian artery in the ovarian ligament. The lymphatics

Claes G Tropé: Department of Gynecological Oncology, The Norwegian Radium Hospital, 0310 Oslo, Norway.

Kaled M. Alektiar: Department of Radiation Oncology, Memorial Sloan–Kettering Cancer Center, New York, New York 10021.

Paul J. Sabbatini: Department of Medicine, Memorial Sloan–Kettering Cancer Center, New York, New York 10021.

Richard J. Zaino: Department of Pathology, Penn State Milton S. Hershey Medical Center, Hershey, Pennsylvania 17033.

of the myometrium drain into the subserosal network of lymphatics, which coalesce into larger channels before leaving the uterus. Lymph flows from the fundus toward the adnexa and infundibulopelvic ligaments. The lymph flow from the lower and middle thirds of the uterus tends to spread in the base of the broad ligaments toward the lateral pelvic side wall (8). There are four drainage channels from the uterus: from the fundus, with the ovarian vessels; in the folds of the broad ligament; along the mesosalpinx and fallopian tubes; and along the round ligaments to the femoral lymph nodes.

EPIDEMIOLOGY AND RISK FACTORS

The clinical picture in endometrial carcinoma varies, including age at diagnosis, clinical course, histologic picture, ploidy, and hormone receptor status. This is likely to reflect a complex etiology involving both endogenous as well as exogenous factors (9,10). Most cases of endometrial carcinoma are thought to be sporadic; however, some cases clearly have a hereditary basis. Among women belonging to families with the autosomal dominant hereditary nonpolyposis colorectal cancer (HNPCC), the most common extracolonic cancer is endometrial carcinoma (11).

Environmental factors also appear to be important, and the increasing frequency of endometrial carcinoma has been attributed to an aging female population and to dietary and hormonal factors (12–16). Obesity and exogenous estrogen treatment for postmenopausal symptoms, especially when unopposed by cyclic progestagen, have been identified as risk factors for developing endometrial carcinoma (17–23). This is also the case for hormonal disturbances associated with diabetes mellitus, polycystic ovarian disease, and granulosa/theca cell tumors of the ovary (10,17,24–26). An inverse relation between parity and risk of endometrial carcinoma has been demonstrated in several epidemiologic studies (17,27,28), although, in some reports, the protective effect has been restricted to the first pregnancy (29,30). This increased risk among nulliparous women could be due to hormonal factors during pregnancy and lactation, representing a period with reduced exposure to unopposed estrogen (10,22,29). Shedding of malignant or premalignant cells at each delivery has been suggested as an alternative explanation (27,28) (Table 23.1).

Tamoxifen and Endometrial Cancer

Tamoxifen is a selective estrogen receptor modulator (SERM) with antiestrogenic properties in the breast and estrogenic effects in tissues such as bone and the cardiovascular system. It is an excellent breast cancer drug for all stages of the disease. Its SERM profile makes tamoxifen a valuable alternative to hormone replacement therapy, especially for women at high risk of breast cancer (31). Following the initial report by Killackey et al. (32) of endometrial cancer

TABLE 23.1. *Risks for endometrial carcinoma*

Characteristic	Increased risk
Obesity	
>30 lb	3
>50 lb	10
Nulliparous	2
Late menopause	2.4
"Bloody" menopause	4
Diabetes mellitus	2.8
Hypertension	1.5
Unopposed estrogen	9.5
Complex atypical hyperplasia	29

occurring in three breast cancer patients receiving antiestrogens, additional tamoxifen-associated uterine cancers have been reported (33–43). These reports illustrate the association between tamoxifen treatment for breast cancer and the development of endometrial cancer. The strongest data initially implicating tamoxifen use and the subsequent development of endometrial cancer were published in 1989 by Fornander et al. (36). The investigators reviewed the frequency of new primary cancers as recorded in the Swedish Cancer Registry for a group of 1,846 postmenopausal women with early breast cancer who were included in a randomized trial of adjuvant tamoxifen. They noted a 6.4-fold increase in the relative risk of endometrial cancer in 931 tamoxifen-treated patients compared to 915 patients in the control group. The dose of tamoxifen in this study was 40 mg/d, and the greatest cumulative risk of developing endometrial cancer was after 5 years of tamoxifen use.

Fisher et al. (35) published data regarding the association between tamoxifen use and the development of endometrial cancer when they reported the findings of the National Surgical Adjuvant Breast and Bowel Project (NSABP) B-14 trial. Data regarding the rates of endometrial and other cancers were analyzed on 2,843 patients with node-negative, ER-positive, invasive breast cancer randomly assigned to placebo or tamoxifen (20 mg/d) and on 1,220 tamoxifen-treated patients registered in NSABP B-14 subsequent to randomization. The average annual hazard rate for endometrial cancer in the placebo group was 0.2/1,000 and 1.6/1,000 for the randomized tamoxifen-treated group. The relative risk of an endometrial cancer occurring in the randomized, tamoxifen-treated group was 7.5. Similar results were seen in the 1,220 registered patients who received tamoxifen. The mean duration of tamoxifen therapy was 35 months, with 36% of the endometrial cancers developing within 2 years of therapy and six occurring less than 9 months after treatment was initiated, suggesting that some of the cancers may have been present prior to starting tamoxifen therapy.

Any conclusions drawn regarding the risks of tamoxifen treatment in inducing endometrial cancer must weigh the benefits of tamoxifen in reducing breast cancer recurrence and new contralateral breast cancers. In the B-14 trial, the cumulative rate/1,000 of breast cancer relapse was reduced from 227.8 in the placebo group to 123.5 in the randomized tamoxifen-treated group. In addition, the cumulative rate of contralateral breast cancer was reduced from 40.5 to 23.5, respectively, in the two groups. Taking into account the increased cumulative rate of endometrial cancer, there was a 38% reduction in the 5-year cumulative hazard rate in the tamoxifen-treated group. Thus, the benefit of tamoxifen therapy for breast cancer outweighs the potential increase in endometrial cancer being reported.

A report from the Yale Tumor Registry by Magriples et al. (39) suggested that uterine cancers occurring in breast cancer patients on tamoxifen may behave more aggressively and carry a worse prognosis. Other studies (34,35,43,44), however, have not been able to confirm these findings (Table 23.2). It would appear from the available literature that there is no difference in the stage, grade, or prognosis of endometrial cancers associated with tamoxifen use. Neven and Vergote (31) have reviewed the literature on the importance of tamoxifen's endometrial lesions and balance available evidence, and they give screening guidelines on how best to screen them. In a subset of tamoxifen users it seems advisable to assess the uterine cavity prior to intake with a yearly endometrial assessment as pointed out starting 3 years after initiation of treatment. In most cases, there is endometrial thickening on ultrasonographic assessment and additional tests such as hydrosonography or hysteroscopy are required to confirm an empty atrophic uterus, as remains the case in most asymptomatic women on tamoxifen.

Newer compounds, such as raloxifen, have a similar SERM profile to tamoxifen but are neutral on the uterus. This has recently been proven by 3 years of endometrial follow-up data. Long-term uterine safety should remain a point of priority for raloxifene if it is to compete with tamoxifen. Whether other SERMs in development are better, and which of them is better for the breast, is to be demonstrated in ongoing studies (31,45).

HYPERPLASIA

The current classification of endometrial hyperplasia accepted by both the International Society of Gynecologic Pathologists (ISGP) and the World Health Organization (WHO) is based on the schema of Kurman et al. (46), which divides hyperplasia on the basis of architectural features into simple or complex and on the basis of cytologic features into typical or atypical (Table 23.3). The resulting classification has four categories as follows: *simple hyperplasia* (SH), *complex hyperplasia* (CH), *simple atypical hyperplasia* (SAH), and *complex atypical hyperplasia* (CAH). Simple hyperplasia is defined as an increase in the number of endometrial glands, which may be dilated with little crowding or have an irregular outline and exhibit crowding. Complex hyperplasia is characterized by glands with irregular outlines, marked structural complexity, and back-to-back crowding. The designation atypical hyperplasia is used to denote a proliferation of glands exhibiting cytologic atypia, recognized as nuclear enlargement, the presence of nucleoli, or a change from an elongated to more ovoid or round nucleus. The chromatin may be either evenly or irregularly dispersed. The justification for this classification system rests on three retrospective studies which demonstrate a higher rate of progression of CAH to adenocarcinoma (46–48). It is sometimes difficult to apply this system that requires one to make a distinction between cytologically atypical nuclei and those without atypical nuclei since a spectrum of nuclear variability actually exists. As noted by Kendall et al. (49), the definitions of architectural complex-

TABLE 23.2. *Clinicopathologic data from series reporting on tamoxifen-associated uterine cancer*

	Magriples (39)	Barakat (34)	Fisher (35)	Fornander (44)	van Leeuwen (43)	Total (%)
No. patients	15	23	25	17	23	103
FIGO Stage						
I	7	15	21	14	17	74 (71.8)
II	0	2	1	2	3	8 (7.8)
III	2	5	1	0	0	8 (7.8)
IV	0	1	1	1	0	3 (2.9)
Unstaged	6	0	1	0	3	10 (9.7)
Histology						
Endometrioid	9	17	18	16	17	77 (74.8)
High-risk[a]	6	6	7	1	6	26 (25.2)
Grade (adenocarcinoma)						
Low (grade 1,2)	5	13	18	15	Not given	51 (72.9)[b]
High (grade 3)	10	4	5	0	Not given	19 (27.1)[b]
Deaths from uterine cancer	5 (33%)	5 (22%)	4 (16%)	3 (10%)	0 (0%)	17 (16.5)

[a] Includes papillary serous, clear cell, sarcoma.
[b] Grade only known for 70 patients.
Reprinted with permission from Barakat RR. The effect of tamoxifen on the endometrium. *Oncology* 1995;9:129.

TABLE 23.3. *Classification of endometrial hyperplasia*

Types of hyperplasia	Progressing to cancer (%)
Simple (cystic without atypia)	1
Complex (adenomatous without atypia)	3
Atypical	
Simple (cystic with atypia)	8
Complex (adenomatous with atypia)	29

ity and nuclear atypia potentially rest on a multitude of criteria, and some but not all criteria may be fully developed in any given case.

Three reports recently have addressed the reproducibility of diagnoses of hyperplasia (49–51). Intraobserver reproducibility was generally found to be moderate to good, whereas interobserver reproducibility was poor to moderate for various diagnostic categories. These studies probably overestimate the interobserver reproducibility since they used expert gynecologic pathologists and specified the classification to be used. In a currently active study by the Gynecologic Oncology Group (GOG), the ability to confirm a community-based diagnosis of atypical hyperplasia by means of an expert panel of pathologists is being evaluated. The current classification of hyperplasia relies on a combination of multiple architectural and cytologic criteria. It is hardly surprising that interobserver reproducibility is relatively low when multiple criteria are used to classify a lesion since each pathologist must assign a relative value or weight to each potentially conflicting criterion. Other factors contributing to low reproducibility include (a) the fragmentary nature of curettings, (b) the presence of borderline lesions, (c) uncertainty about the significance of focal hyperplasia, (d) the inadequacy of published descriptions and understanding of terms used to define architectural or cytologic atypia, and (e) the difficulty associated with the translation of verbal descriptions into light microscopic interobserver reproducibility for images.

Recently, Mutter et al. (52) have suggested that a new classification of endometrial precursor lesions based on a combination of molecular, morphometric, and morphologic data replace the current WHO system. They recommend that clonal, noninvasive lesions that lack the histologic features diagnostic of adenocarcinoma be classified as *endometrial intraepithelial neoplasia*, and that of the polyclonal lesions be grouped together simply as *hyperplasia*. The validity, applicability, and reproducibility of this proposal remain to be confirmed, but the need for a better concept and set of diagnostic terms is unquestionable.

The gross manifestations of endometrial hyperplasia are highly varied. The endometrium is often of diffusely increased thickness (5 to 10 mm or greater), vaguely nodular, tan, and soft without hemorrhage or necrosis.

However, hyperplasia may be focal or multifocal in a background of polyps or cycling endometrium, or even occasionally may be associated with a diffusely thin endometrial lining. Part of the variability may reflect a reduction in the endometrial thickness due to prior endometrial sampling. Coexistent adenocarcinoma is present in 1% to 40% of hysterectomies performed to treat hyperplasia, with the latter number reflecting the frequent co-occurrence of carcinoma with atypical complex hyperplasia.

Simple Hyperplasia

In simple hyperplasia, the endometrium is thicker than usual, with dilated glands that have outpouchings and invaginations, producing an irregular outline to the enlarged glands. The glands are crowded, the stroma is more densely cellular than usual, and some foam cells may exist within the stroma. Follow-up of patients with this condition reveals little or no progression to carcinoma.

Complex Hyperplasia

The endometrium is increased in thickness by back-to-back glands in cases of complex hyperplasia. Most glands have irregular outlines. There are papillary processes and intraluminal bridges. The two main features differentiating this from simple hyperplasia are the back-to-back glands and the intraluminal papillae. Epithelial pseudostratification is a frequent finding, producing an appearance of two to four cell layers. Mitotic activity is highly variable, but may range to up to ten mitotic figures per 10 high-power fields.

Atypical Hyperplasia

Atypical hyperplasia is characterized by cytologic atypia of the glands. The gland outlines may reflect simple or complex hyperplasia, although it is usually complex. The cells lining the glands are enlarged, show nuclear hyperchromatism and nuclear enlargement, and have an increased nucleus-cytoplasm ratio. Nuclei are irregular in size and shape and have a thickened nuclear membrane, prominent nucleoli, and a coarse chromatin texture. The nuclei may appear clear with scattered, coarse chromatin clumps.

Progression from Hyperplasia to Cancer

The natural history of endometrial hyperplasia is difficult to define for a variety of reasons, four of which follow: (a) pathologic criteria—criteria and terminology for the various forms of hyperplasia have changed repeatedly; (b) initial sampling—the method of initial diagnosis is often curettage, which removes part or all of the lesion to be studied; (c) coexisting lesions—other lesions such as adenocarcinoma may coexist at the time of diagnosis without our knowledge, since the curettage or biopsy samples only a minority of the endometrium; and (d) subsequent intervention—hormonal or surgical intervention usually interrupts observations of the natural history of the hyperplasia. Nevertheless, there are reasonably good data to support the following assertions: (a) endometrial hyperplasia is commonly a consequence of unopposed prolonged estrogen stimulation, (b) some hyperplasias may regress if the estrogenic stimulus is removed or in response to progestational or antiestrogenic treatment, (c) some hyperplasias coexist with, or progress to, invasive adenocarcinoma; and (d) the probability of progression to adenocarcinoma is related to the degree of architectural or cytologic atypia. Progression from hyperplasia to carcinoma occurs in only 1% of patients with simple hyperplasia and in 3% of patients with complex hyperplasia. Progression from atypical hyperplasia is much higher; 8% of patients with simple atypical hyperplasia and 29% of those with complex atypical hyperplasia develop carcinoma (46,53) (Table 23.3). Glandular complexity superimposed on atypia probably places the patient at greater risk than does cytologic atypia alone, but the point is unsettled.

CANCER PREVENTION AND SCREENING OF ENDOMETRIAL CANCER

Many endometrial cancers may be preventable, particularly those that are estrogen related. Prompt recognition of precursor lesions with institution of proper treatment is preventive. Because 95% of endometrial carcinomas occur in women 40 years old and older, and because endometrial hyperplasia, the precursor state, tends to be a premenopausal and perimenopausal condition, it is appropriate to evaluate individuals past their fourth decade of life if there is abnormal bleeding. Evaluation can be by endometrial biopsy or by dilatation and curettage (D&C) if the biopsy is unsuccessful or the results are unclear. Patients with complex and atypical hyperplasia may be treated by hysterectomy or by periodic use of progestins, depending on age and reproductive desires. Hysterectomy is the preferred treatment in the patient with complex atypical endometrial hyperplasia. This approach not only cures the usual presenting symptoms of abnormal bleeding, but also confers prophylaxis against the almost 30% risk of later developing endometrial carcinoma (46). Those treated with progestins should have a D&C performed before treatment to rule out the occasional occult carcinoma not detected by biopsy. A progestin should be administered at least 10 to 14 days each month, and endometrial biopsies should be performed at 3- to 4-month intervals to assess treatment results. Women with an intact uterus should never be prescribed estrogen-only preparations of hormone replacement therapy because this greatly increases their risk of endometrial cancer.

The addition of progestins to the regimens of patients treated with exogenous estrogen may prevent endometrial hyperplasia and subsequent cancer and may protect against the development of carcinoma (54,55). Several regimens exist, but the most important factor is administration of a progestin for at least 10 to 14 days each month.

Another preventive measure in the amenorrheic or hypermenorrheic perimenopausal patient with fluctuating levels of estrogen or in any patient with a suspected condition of unopposed endogenous estrogen production is periodic treatment with a progestin to create scheduled withdrawal bleeding and prevent hyperplasia. The ''progesterone challenge test'' as described by Gambrell et al. (56) may be helpful in defining this group of patients. This test involves challenging any nonpregnant amenorrheic patient with progesterone to see if withdrawal bleeding occurs (57). If bleeding does occur, endometrial sampling may be performed and a diagnosis established. Appropriate management can follow. Women with intact uteri who are taking tamoxifen for either treatment or prevention of breast cancer should be informed that endometrial cancer might be a possible consequence of this therapy; overweight/obese, nulliparous women with postmenopausal bleeding should be considered at high risk of endometrial cancer and should be investigated accordingly; and overweight/obese patients should be counseled that a healthy diet and regular exercise could reduce their risk of endometrial cancer (in addition to other known benefits) (31).

Considering the available knowledge about the disease and available tests, it seems unlikely that screening would be generally advised in the near future. This has also been the view in statements from official organizations like the International Union Against Cancer UICC (58) and the American Cancer Society (59). There are a few uncontrolled studies lending some support to the efficacy of screening programs (60,61). No randomized trials have been published. No health economic data have been presented in relation to the published reports. In spite of lacking evidence-based support, general screening is organized in high-risk women in Japan (60), and in some countries, women with a hereditary taint (HNPCC) are screened also regarding endometrial cancer. Screening of women on tamoxifen therapy with ultrasound or endometrial biopsies is not recommended (62). If new promising tests emerge, the procedure to evaluate them and then evaluate screening will take decades. It seems unlikely that mass screening aimed at endometrial cancer would be recommended during the first decades of the twenty-first century (63).

DIAGNOSTIC EVALUATION

Endometrial carcinoma occurs most often in the sixth and seventh decades of life, with an average age at onset of 60 years. Most patients are postmenopausal, and the remainder are usually in the climacteric, or so-called perimenopausal, years. It is estimated that 75% of the cases occur in patients

50 years old and older, and 95% occur in patients over 40 years of age (2). The disease, although reported in patients as young as age 16 years, is rare in patients younger than 30 years of age (2,3).

Symptoms of early endometrial carcinoma are few. However, 90% of patients have abnormal vaginal discharge; 80% of these show abnormal bleeding, usually postmenopausal, and 10% show leukorrhea. Other signs and symptoms of more advanced disease include pelvic pressure and other symptoms indicative of uterine enlargement or extrauterine tumor spread.

The standard method of assessing uterine bleeding and diagnosing endometrial carcinoma is the formal fractional D&C. Before dilating the cervix, the endocervix should be curetted. Careful sounding of the uterus is then accomplished; dilatation of the cervix is performed, followed by systematic curetting of the entire endometrial cavity. Cervical and endometrial specimens should be kept separate and forwarded for pathologic interpretation. Fractional D&C provides the maximum amount of tissue from the endometrial cavity and the opportunity for examination with the patient relaxed under anesthesia. Outpatient procedures, such as endometrial biopsy or aspiration curettage coupled with endocervical sampling, are definitive if positive for cancer (64,65). However, if sampling techniques fail to provide sufficient diagnostic information, the fractional D&C is mandatory (50).

Results of endometrial biopsies correlate well with endometrial curettings (66,67). However, the methods, individually or combined, may miss an existing endometrial carcinoma because the sampling is random and does not include the entire endometrium (68). If the endometrial sample is obtained by a biopsy or curettage, 15% to 25% of patients with the diagnosis of atypical hyperplasia may have a uterine carcinoma (69,70). Although a discrepancy of this extent may seem alarming, the carcinoma is invariably early stage and well managed by extrafascial hysterectomy (71). However, because of this discrepancy, patients with atypical hyperplasia treated by less than hysterectomy should be actively followed with endometrial sampling and D&C if results are unclear.

Pathologic Diagnosis

The International Society of Gynecologic Pathologists (ISGP) and the WHO last revised the classification of uterine tumors in 1992 (72), and the portion pertaining to carcinomas of the endometrium is presented in Table 23.4. This relatively simple classification scheme accommodates the vast majority of endometrial carcinomas and distinguishes among neoplasms of significantly different prognosis. Mixed carcinomas with two distinctive cell types are relatively common, and are defined as those carcinomas in which the secondary component constitutes at least 10% of the neoplasm.

TABLE 23.4. *Classification of endometrial carcinoma*

Endometrioid adenocarcinoma
    Papillary villoglandular
    Secretory
    Ciliated cell
    Adenocarcinoma with squamous differentiation
Mucinous carcinoma
Serous carcinoma
Clear-cell carcinoma
Squamous carcinoma
Undifferentiated carcinoma
Mixed types
Miscellaneous carcinomas
Metastatic carcinoma

In most endometrial samples, the distinction of adenocarcinoma from hyperplasia is straightforward. However, a small fraction of problematic cases with complex proliferations truly tax the abilities of experts as well as novices to classify them correctly. The diagnosis of a well-differentiated adenocarcinoma is made in the presence of any of the following criteria: (a) irregular infiltration of glands in an altered fibroblastic stroma, (b) a confluent glandular pattern that results in either a cribriform arrangement or confluent interconnected glands, or (c) extensive papillary growth of epithelium and stroma into glandular lumina (53).

Histologic Grade

The differentiation of a carcinoma is expressed as its grade. Grade 1 lesions (Fig. 23.1) are well differentiated

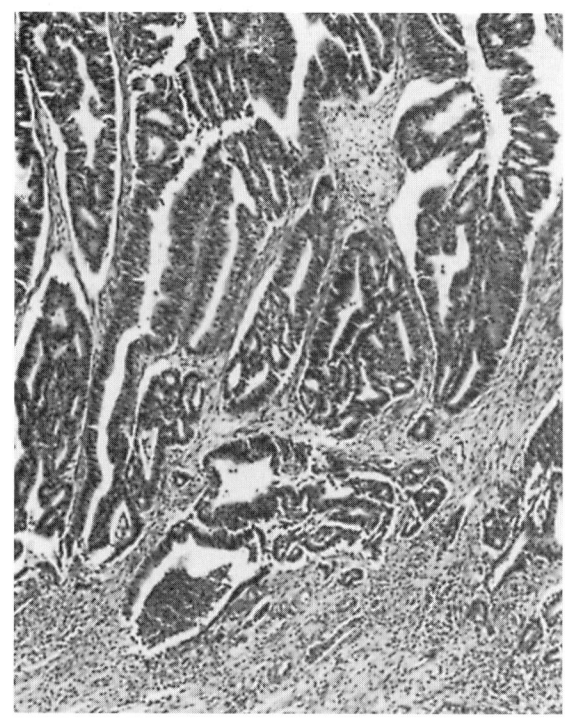

FIG. 23.1. Endometrioid carcinoma, grade 1.

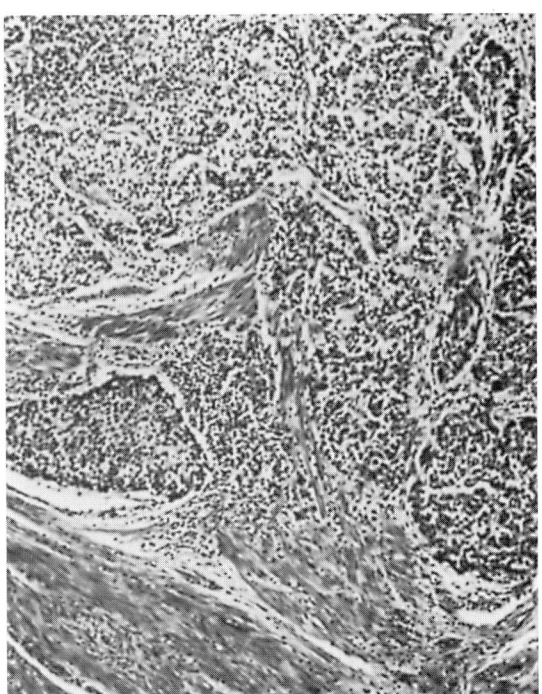

FIG. 23.2. Endometrial carcinoma, grade 3. Glands are not evident in most of the tumor.

and are generally associated with a good prognosis. Grade 2 tumors are moderately well differentiated and have an intermediate prognosis, and grade 3 (Fig. 23.2) reflects poorly differentiated lesions, which frequently have a poor prognosis. Both architectural criteria and nuclear grade are used in the FIGO and ISGP-WHO committee (73) classification of tumors and are easily applied to most cell types (Table 23.5). The architectural grade is determined as follows: grade 1: an adenocarcinoma in which less than 5% of the tumor growth is in solid sheets; grade 2: an adenocarcinoma in which 6% to 50% of the neoplasm is arranged in solid sheets of neoplastic cells; grade 3: an adenocarcinoma in which greater than 50% of the neoplastic cells are in solid masses. Regions of squamous differentiation are excluded from this assessment. The FIGO rules for grading state that notable nuclear atypia, inappropriate for architectural grade, raises the grade of a grade 1 or grade 2 tumor by 1. However, FIGO did not define notable nuclear atypia. Justification and clarification for this modification based on extreme nuclear pleomorphism were provided in a recent GOG study. For 715 women with nonserous endometrial carcinomas, three nuclear grades were defined as follows: grade 1: round to oval nuclei with even distribution of chromatin and inconspicuous nucleoli; grade 2: irregular, oval nuclei with chromatin clumping and moderate-size nucleoli; and grade 3: large, pleomorphic nuclei with coarse chromatin and large, irregular nucleoli. Patients with tumors of architectural grade

TABLE 23.5. *Corpus cancer surgical staging, FIGO 1988*

Stages/grades	Characteristics
IA G123	Tumor limited to endometrium
IB G123	Invasion to less than half of the myometrium
IC G123	Invasion to less than half of the myometrium
IIA G123	Endocervical glandular involvement only
IIB G123	Cervical stromal invasion
IIIA G123	Tumor invades serosa or adnexae or positive peritoneal cytology
IIIB G123	Vaginal metastases
IIIC G123	Metastases to pelvic or paraaortic lymph nodes
IVA G123	Tumor invades bladder and/or bowel mucosa
IVB	Distant metastases including intra-abdominal and/or inguinal lymph node

Histopathology, degree of differentiation
Cases should be grouped by the degree of differentiation of the adenocarcinoma:

G1	5% or less of a nonsquamous or nonmorular solid growth pattern
G2	6% to 50% of a nonsquamous or nonmorular solid growth pattern
G3	More than 50% of a nonsquamous or nonmorular solid growth pattern

Notes on pathologic grading
Notable nuclear atypia, inappropriate for the architectural grade, raises the grade of a grade 1 or grade 2 tumor by 1.
In serous adenocarcinomas, clear-cell adenocarcinomas, and squamous-cell carcinomas, nuclear grading takes precedence.
Adenocarcinomas with squamous differentiation are graded according to the nuclear grade of the glandular component.

Rules related to staging
Because corpus cancer is now surgically staged, procedures previously used for determination of stages are no longer applicable, such as the finding of fractional D&C to differentiate between stages I and II
It is appreciated that there may be a small number of patients with corpus cancer who will be treated primarily with radiation therapy. If that is the case, the clinical staging adopted by FIGO in 1971 would still apply, but designation of that staging system would be noted.
Ideally, width of the myometrium should be measured, along with the width of tumor invasion.

1 or 2, but with a majority of cells having nuclei of grade 3, had a significantly worse behavior, justifying an upgrading by one grade (74).

Taylor et al. (75) have recently proposed a two-tiered system for grading endometrial carcinoma based on a study of 85 patients with stages I and II endometrial cancer. They divided tumors at 10% intervals based on the percentage of solid tumor growth, and found that tumor recurrences were confined to the subset with greater than 20% solid tumor. They also found that this binary division yielded a higher degree of interobserver agreement than three architectural grades. Lax et al. (76) have presented preliminary data on a binary architectural grading system based on the presence of greater than 50% solid growth, a diffusely infiltrative growth pattern, and tumor cell necrosis. These methods will need to be replicated in a larger patient population before an assessment of their prognostic utility can be made.

Some cell types (i.e., serous, clear cell, ciliated, and undifferentiated) are not easily architecturally graded because their growth patterns are architecturally limited. In these, the nuclear grading is more universally applicable (77).

Cell Types

Endometrioid Adenocarcinoma

Endometrioid adenocarcinoma is the most common form of carcinoma of the endometrium, comprising 75% to 80% of the cases (78,79). It varies from well differentiated (Fig. 23.1) to undifferentiated (Fig. 23.2).

Characteristically, the glands of endometrioid adenocarcinoma are formed of tall columnar cells that share a common apical border, resulting in a smoothly delineated, round or oval luminal contour. With decreasing differentiation, there is a preponderance of solid growth rather than gland formation, and the cells lining glandular lumina become more numerous but not necessarily clearly stratified. Stromal invasion manifested by a desmoplastic host response or vascular invasion is often not evident in the biopsy or curettage specimen.

Villoglandular Carcinoma

There has been considerable confusion about the definition and significance of papillary carcinoma of the endometrium. A variety of cell types of endometrial adenocarcinoma with differing biologic behavior, including serous, clear-cell, mucinous, and villoglandular carcinoma may grow in a papillary fashion. Thus, the adjective *papillary* does not represent a cell type but rather an architectural pattern (78,80).

Villoglandular carcinoma is a relatively common subtype of endometrioid adenocarcinoma characterized by neoplastic columnar cells covering delicate fibrovascular cores. The apical cytoplasmic borders are straight, the nuclei are usually low grade, and the tumor cells architecturally resemble those of other endometrioid adenocarcinomas, with which they are often admixed. In the largest study to date, villoglandular carcinomas were better differentiated than endometrioid carcinomas, but the age at diagnosis, depth of myometrial invasion, nodal spread, and survival were similar to those of endometrioid carcinomas, justifying their classification as a subtype of endometrioid adenocarcinoma (81).

Secretory Carcinoma

Secretory carcinoma is a variant of endometrial carcinoma, but it is unusual and represents no more than 2% of the cases (82,83). It is identified by its well-differentiated glandular pattern, consisting of columnar epithelial cells containing intracytoplasmic vacuoles similar to secretory endometrium. It is usually grade 1 architecturally and by nuclear features. There is minimal cellular atypia, stratification, and pleomorphism. The intracellular secretions are not mucin but glycogen. The cellular features of secretory carcinoma differentiate it from clear-cell carcinoma, which is more papillary with more pleomorphic nuclei. By its lack of mucin, secretory carcinoma may be differentiated from mucinous carcinoma. Recognition of secretory carcinoma is important because it has a less virulent clinical course (83, 84), although the clinical profile of patients is similar to that of patients with adenocarcinoma. Confused identification may occur in patients who have been given progestogens before tissue sampling in what would have otherwise been an atypical hyperplasia or a well-differentiated endometrioid carcinoma. Atypical hyperplasia and endometrioid carcinoma may retain responsiveness to progestins and develop a secretory appearance. A good clinical history should be provided for the pathologist to avoid this confusion.

Ciliated Carcinoma

Ciliated carcinoma is rare. Grossly, it does not differ from ordinary endometrial carcinoma. Ciliated cells are more commonly identified in endometrial hyperplasia and in benign metaplasia (tubal metaplasia), but they may occur in endometrial carcinomas. Associated with prior exogenous estrogen use, this cell type is reported to have a good prognosis (85).

Adenocarcinoma with Squamous Differentiation

Foci of squamous differentiation are found in about 25% of endometrial adenocarcinomas (Fig. 23.3). Historically, the tumors were sometimes separated into adenoacanthoma or adenosquamous carcinoma based on whether the squamous component appeared histologically benign or malignant (86–90). However, in about 30% of cases, the squamous component is not clearly benign or malignant. In a GOG study of early-stage disease, it was noted that these tumors with squamous regions behave in a fashion similar to

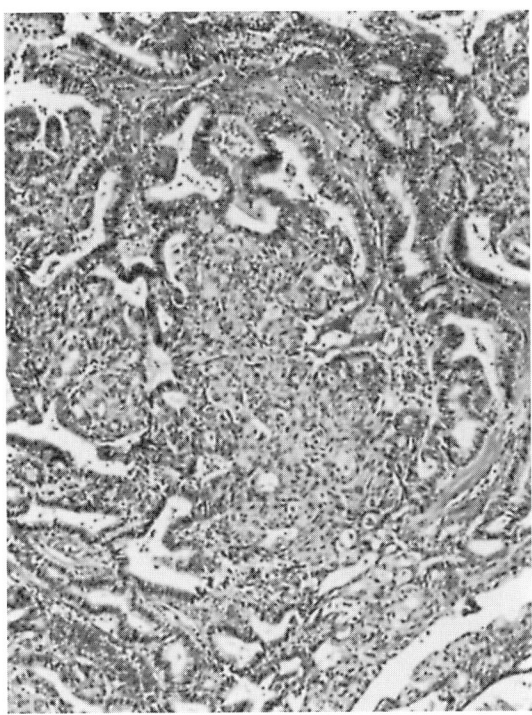

FIG. 23.3. Well-differentiated endometrioid carcinoma with bland squamous differentiation (adenoacanthoma).

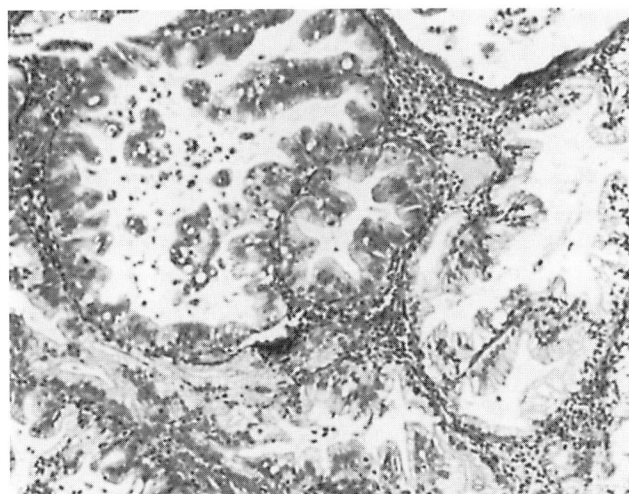

FIG. 23.4. Mucinous adenocarcinoma of the endometrium.

endometrioid carcinomas without squamous differentiation (91,a8). The squamous areas usually mirror the degree of differentiation, which, coupled with assessment of histologic grade and other conventional prognostic factors, is thus more useful for prognostication and determination of adjuvant therapy than the historic terms *adenoacanthoma* and *adeno-squamous carcinoma*, which are confusing and should be abandoned.

Mucinous Carcinoma

Mucinous adenocarcinoma is rare in the endometrium in contrast to its high frequency in the endocervix. It has been reported to represent between 1% and 9% of endometrial adenocarcinomas (92–94), but the former figure is probably more accurate. If present as the major cellular component of an endometrial carcinoma, this tumor resembles mucinous carcinoma seen in the ovary and endocervix. Two patterns occur: In one, the cells are columnar with basally oriented nuclei; in the other, the cells are more pseudostratified, as in an adenocarcinoma of the colon or mucinous carcinoma of the ovary (Fig. 23.4). The characteristic cellular pattern should represent over 50% of the entire tumor. Typically, there are papillary processes and cystically dilated glands lined by columnar or pseudostratified columnar epithelium. The cytoplasm is positive for carcinoembryonic antigen (CEA), mucicarmine, and periodic acid–Schiff stain (PAS), but it is diastase resistant (94). This tumor differs from clear-cell carcinoma and secretory endometrium by having more mucin and less glycogen. Ordinarily, atypia and mitotic figures are not prominent features. The glandular architecture is usually well maintained, and most are well differentiated (92). To establish the origin in the endometrium, exclusion of a primary endocervical tumor is required. If the endocervical sample demonstrates the same neoplasm, the site of origin must be carefully established because this cell type is common in the endocervix (95). Neither the pattern nor the type of mucin staining nor the presence of CEA can reliably distinguish mucinous adenocarcinoma of the endometrium from its more common counterpart in the endocervix (96, 97). Mucinous carcinoma of the endometrium has the same prognosis as common endometrial carcinoma (93).

Serous Carcinoma

Serous carcinoma of the endometrium closely resembles serous carcinoma of the ovary and fallopian tube because its papillary growth and cellular features are similar (Fig. 23.5). It is usually found in an advanced stage in older women (98). Fibrous papillary fronds are lined by epithelial cells, which are almost devoid of cytoplasm, but which manifest stratification, atypism, pleomorphism, mitotic figures, and bizarre forms. These fronds often detach or demonstrate a terminal growth of tiny papillary excrescences and individual cells, which detach easily. A second pattern of irregular gaping glands lined by cuboidal cells with scalloped, apical borders may be present, particularly in the deeper aspect of the tumor. Lymphatic invasion is commonplace in the myometrium. Distinction from clear-cell carcinoma may be difficult but can usually be accomplished on the basis of a greater degree of papillary processes, greater nuclear atypia, and less cytoplasm in papillary serous carcinoma. Psammoma bodies are frequently observed in serous carcinoma, but solid growth is more common in clear-cell carcinoma.

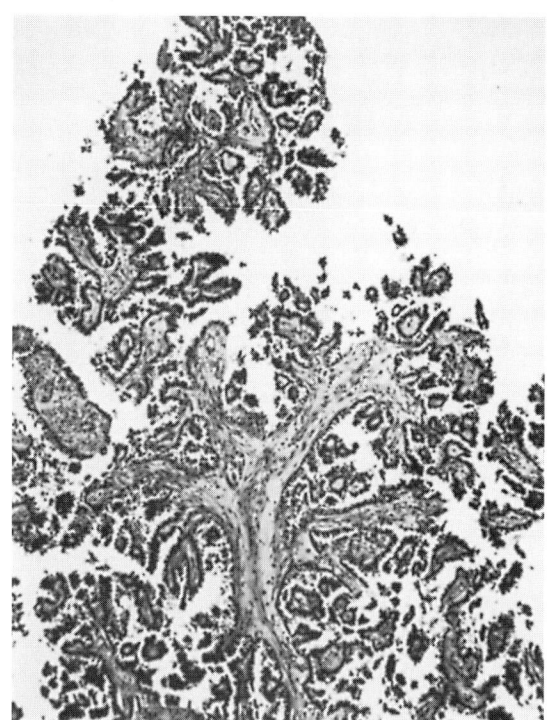

FIG. 23.5. Serous carcinoma of the endometrium. These tumors tend to occur in older women and behave aggressively.

Serous carcinoma represents approximately 10% of endometrial carcinomas, which is fortunate because it is an aggressive tumor. The tumors often deeply invade the myometrium, and unlike typical endometrioid adenocarcinoma, there is a propensity for peritoneal spread. Unfortunately, advanced-stage disease or recurrence is common even when serous carcinomas are apparently only minimally invasive or even confined to the endometrium in polyps (99,100). Since the metastatic disease is often identified only microscopically, about 60% of patients are upstaged following complete surgical staging (98,101,102). A recent report by Wheeler et al. (103) stressed the prognostic importance of meticulous surgicopathologic staging. They found that serous carcinoma truly confined to the uterus had an overall excellent prognosis, whereas patients with extrauterine disease, even if only microscopic in size, almost always suffered recurrence and death from tumor.

Endometrial intraepithelial carcinoma (EIC) has recently been recognized as a histologically distinctive lesion that is specifically associated with serous carcinoma of the endometrium (104–108). Serous carcinomas most often arise from a background of atrophy or polyps rather than hyperplasia (104,105,107), and they are not epidemiologically related to unopposed estrogen stimulation. EIC has been proposed to represent a form of intraepithelial tumor characteristic of serous carcinoma, and it is the likely precursor to invasive serous carcinoma. EIC is usually found in the endometrium harboring a serous carcinoma (105), but occasionally occurs

in the absence of any invasive carcinoma. In such cases, it may be associated with synchronous serous carcinoma in the peritoneum (106).

Clear-Cell Carcinoma

Clear-cell adenocarcinoma of the endometrium is generally recognized and defined on the basis of the distinctive clearing of the cytoplasm of neoplastic cells growing in any combination of solid, glandular, tubulocystic, or papillary configurations. About 4% of endometrial adenocarcinomas are of clear-cell type (109–116). In contrast with the diethylstilbestrol (DES)–related clear-cell carcinomas of the vagina and cervix, clear-cell carcinoma of the endometrium is almost exclusively a disease of menopausal women. The mean age at diagnosis is about 68 years, which is similar to that of serous adenocarcinoma and about 6 years older than that of typical endometrial adenocarcinoma (110,112,116). It is a biologically aggressive neoplasm, with a 5-year survival rate varying from only about 20% to 65% (110,112,114,116, 117).

The hallmark of clear-cell carcinoma is the presence of neoplastic cells with optically clear cytoplasm, reflecting an abundance of glycogen. Four basic architectural patterns of clear-cell adenocarcinoma exist, including solid, glandular, tubulocystic, and papillary, but most cases display an admixture of patterns. The solid pattern consists of masses of large neoplastic cells of polygonal shape with clear to faintly eosinophilic cytoplasm and distinct cell membranes. The glandular pattern is reminiscent of the tubular glands of endometrioid adenocarcinoma, whereas the tubulocystic pattern is formed of dilated spherical-appearing glands. The papillary pattern is architecturally identical to that of serous carcinoma, with generally short, branching fibrovascular cores, often hyalinized, covered by neoplastic cells. The latter three patterns often have lining cells with a hobnail appearance, resulting from the scalloped apex of individual neoplastic cells that project along the surface (Fig. 23.6).

Squamous Carcinoma

Although focal squamous differentiation is common in endometrial adenocarcinoma, pure squamous carcinoma of the endometrium is extremely rare, representing less than 1% of endometrial carcinoma, and with only about 60 reported cases (118–122). Most patients are postmenopausal, and the average age at diagnosis is about 65 years (118,120). Squamous carcinoma of the endometrium is established as primary in the endometrium after a cervical origin is ruled out. There must be no connection with or spread from benign or malignant cervical squamous epithelium. It is often associated with cervical stenosis, pyometra, and chronic inflammation. About 60% of the cases have been confined to the uterus, and the prognosis for these patients has been relatively good (118). In contrast, less than 15% of women with

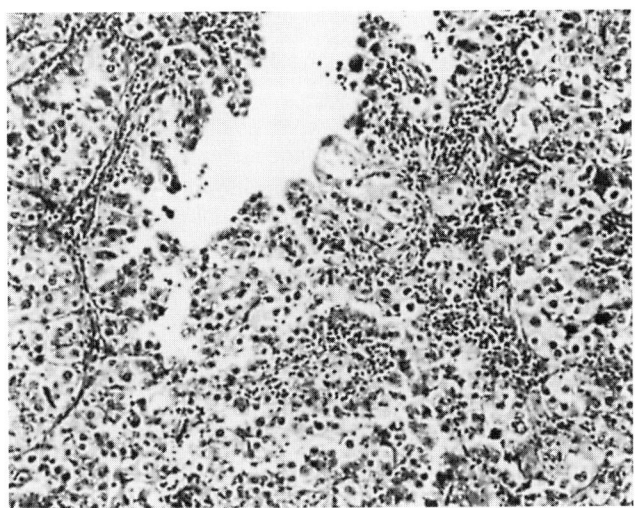

FIG. 23.6. Clear-cell carcinoma of the endometrium. This tumor occurs in older women and behaves aggressively.

advanced-stage disease have survived 2 years after diagnosis. Histologic grade does not appear to correlate with the probability of survival.

Undifferentiated Carcinoma

Undifferentiated carcinoma of the endometrium has no glandular, squamous, or sarcomatous differentiation in routinely stained sections. Most contain epithelial antigens detected by immunologic stains. Selected cases may contain argyrophilic cells or neurosecretory granules demonstrated by immunohistochemical stains or electron microscopy. Neurosecretory products are apparently not released into the patient's circulation or are not in an active form because no affected women have manifested symptoms. Neuroendocrine granules, therefore, have no clinical or prognostic significance (123,124).

A *glassy-cell carcinoma* has also been described, which comprises less than 1% of endometrial carcinomas. It is characterized by cytoplasm that has a ground-glass appearance, as in the cervix. Although few cases have been reported, like serous and clear-cell carcinomas, glassy-cell carcinoma appears to be aggressive (125,126).

Mixed Cell Type

If an endometrial carcinoma manifests two or more different cell types, each representing at least 10% or more of the tumor, the term *mixed cell type* is appropriate.

Metastatic Carcinoma to the Endometrium

Malignancies in other organs may metastasize to the endometrium. The most common extragenital sites are breast, stomach, colon, pancreas, and kidney, although any dissemi-

nated tumor could involve the endometrium. The ovaries are the most likely genital sources of metastasis. Metastatic carcinoma presents as abnormal vaginal bleeding, and the initial specimen for evaluation is usually a biopsy or curetting. Although the metastatic disease may appear as a large focus, individual and small groups of malignant cells may subtly intermingle with normal endometrium or myometrium. Lymphatics are usually involved. Special stains for mucin, CEA, or melanin may suggest that the cells are not of endometrial origin. In some instances, unusual cell types, such as signet-ring cells, may be present, suggesting a metastasis from the gastrointestinal tract. It is uncommon but not exceptional for the endometrial sample to be the first indication of an occult primary lesion (127,128).

Simultaneous Tumors

Cancers of an identical cell type may be discovered in the ovary and endometrium simultaneously (129). Usually, the primary site is assigned to the area having the largest tumor mass and most advanced stage. In certain situations, primary malignancies in the endometrium and ovary may coexist. This "field effect" of the "extended müllerian system" may occur in 15% to 20% of endometrioid carcinomas of the ovary (130,131). In a review of a GOG study of 74 patients with simultaneously detected endometrial and ovarian carcinoma with disease grossly limited to the pelvis, only 16% of women suffered a recurrence of disease, with a median follow-up of 80 months. This group of patients was atypical, with 86% having endometrioid histology in both sites. Recurrence was statistically related to the presence of microscopic metastases or high histologic grade (132).

Carcinomas of more advanced histologic grade and cell type are more difficult to assign to the field effect because of a higher probability of invasion and metastasis at the time of surgery (84). If the endometrial tumor is less than 5 cm in diameter, the ovarian lesion is unilateral, invasion is less than the middle third, vessels are not involved, and the endometrial carcinoma is well differentiated, metastasis to the ovary is unlikely (133).

PRETREATMENT AND STAGING STUDIES

After the diagnosis of endometrial carcinoma has been histologically confirmed, the patient should undergo a thorough evaluation. A complete physical examination can discover suspicious lymph nodes and areas of spread within the pelvis. These patients often have other medical problems that must be evaluated for their effect on treatment choices for the cancer. A chest radiograph is done to search for metastatic tumor and to help evaluate the cardiopulmonary status of the patient. In the past, a urinary imaging study, such as an intravenous pyelogram, was frequently ordered prior to surgery. The benefit of such a test in patients whose disease appears to be confined to the uterus is questionable. Cystoscopy and proctoscopy can be performed to determine whether the tumor has spread to the bladder or rectal mucosa in patients with locally advanced disease. Routine blood and urine studies should also be performed. Although a barium enema is not required as part of the evaluation for endometrial adenocarcinoma, patients who have intestinal symptoms may benefit from such a study or from a colonoscopy.

Diagnostic techniques, such as ultrasonography and magnetic resonance imaging (MRI), appear to be able to diagnose uterine invasion and lymph node involvement in a fairly accurate manner, with several reports indicating a 75% to 90% accuracy rate for determining muscle involvement (134–138). However, these techniques must be considered experimental until more data and information are available, particularly because they are costly and frequently require lengthy scan times. The only way to accurately diagnose the extent and depth of intrauterine invasion is by histologic examination of the hysterectomy specimen.

Serum levels of the antigenic determinant CA-125 are elevated in most patients with advanced or metastatic endometrial cancer (139). This observation was first reported by Niloff and others (140) in 1984. Values exceeding 35 U/mL were found in 14 (78%) of 18 patients with stage IV or recurrent disease, although none of 11 patients with stage I disease had elevations. Patsner and colleagues (141), in 1988, reported 81 patients with endometrial cancer that appeared to be confined to the uterus. At laparotomy, 20 (87%) of 23 of their patients with elevated CA-125 were found to have occult extrauterine disease. Conversely, only 1 of 58 patients with a normal value had occult extrauterine disease. In the largest study so far, Hsieh et al. (142) reviewed preoperative serum CA-125 levels, operative records, and pathologic reports in 141 patients diagnosed with endometrial carcinoma to find out if the preoperative level of CA-125 can provide additional information to determine the extent of lymphadenectomy required in the surgical staging and which cut-off is optimal in this respect. Of 141 patients, 124 were staged surgically and 24 (19%) were found to have lymph node metastasis. In the node-positive group, medium preoperative serum levels were 94 U/mL (range 17 to 363 U/mL). Mutivariate analysis showed lymph node metastasis had the most significant effect on the elevation of CA-125 levels (>40 U/mL). The sensitivity and specificity for screening lymph node metastasis were 78% and 84%, respectively. Hsieh et al.'s (142) data give evidence that preoperative CA-125 levels greater than 40 U/mL can be considered an indication for full pelvic and paraaortic lymphadenectomy in the surgical staging of endometrial carcinoma. These results are in accordance with others (143–147).

Rose and colleagues (148) found serial CA-125 measurements to be most useful in patients with high-risk disease whose initial stage was II, III, or IV, or whose tumor was grade 3 or of clear-cell or serous histology. Fifteen (94%) of 16 patients with recurrent disease had an elevated CA-125 level. If the initial value of CA-125 is elevated, serial

TABLE 23.6. *Corpus cancer clinical staging, FIGO 1971*

Stage	Characteristics
I	Carcinoma is confined to the corpus
IA	Length of the uterine cavity is 8 cm or less
IB	Length of the uterine cavity is more than 8 cm
Histologic subtypes of adenocarcinoma	
G1	Highly differentiated adenomatous carcinoma
G2	Differentiated adenomatous carcinoma with partly solid areas
G3	Predominantly solid or entirely undifferentiated carcinoma
II	Carcinoma involves the corpus and cervix
III	Carcinoma extends outside the uterus but not outside the true pelvis
IV	Carcinoma extends outside the true pelvis or involves the bladder or rectum

measurements may help indicate response to tumor therapy (see Chapter 7).

If the pretreatment studies are complete, the patient may be clinically staged if she is not a surgical staging candidate. The most universal clinical staging system is that proposed by the FIGO in 1971 (Table 23.6) (149). This clinical staging system is still applicable for cases that do not go to primary operative staging. Those that do undergo initial hysterectomy are staged by the 1988 FIGO system.

Two large prospective surgical staging trials conducted by the GOG were reported in 1984 and 1987 (150,151). These studies helped to define the prognostic factors of endometrial carcinoma and the current treatment approach for patients with this disease. In addition to evaluating the factors of age, race, and endocrine status, these studies confirmed that patient prognosis is directly related to the presence or absence of easily determinable uterine and extrauterine risk factors (Table 23.7) (77). The uterine factors are histologic cell type, tumor grade, depth of myometrial invasion, occult extension to the cervix, and vascular space invasion. The extrauterine prognostic factors are adnexal metastases, other extrauterine intraperitoneal spread, positive peritoneal cytology, pelvic lymph node metastases, and aortic lymph node involvement. Uterine size was previously believed to be a risk factor and was part of the older clinical staging system. However, recent information indicates that uterine size is not an independent risk factor but rather relates to cell type, grade, and myometrial invasion (151).

TABLE 23.7. *Risk factors in endometrial carcinoma*

Uterine factors	Extrauterine factors
Histologic type	Adnexal metastasis
Grade	Intraperitoneal spread
Myometrial invasion	Positive peritoneal cytology
Isthmus-cervix extension	Pelvic node metastasis
Vascular space invasion	Aortic node metastasis

Cell type and grade are factors that can be determined before hysterectomy, although grade, as determined by D&C, in some series has an overall 31% inaccuracy rate compared to grade in the hysterectomy specimen, and grade 3 tumors have a 50% inaccuracy rate (152). Recognition of all the other factors requires an exploratory laparotomy, peritoneal fluid sampling, and hysterectomy with careful pathologic interpretation of all removed tissue. This primary surgical approach led the FIGO, in 1988, to define endometrial cancer as a surgically staged disease, incorporating many of the prognostic factors into the staging process (Table 23.5) (5).

Surgical Staging

To stage appropriately by the FIGO criteria, the surgical procedure should minimally include an adequate abdominal incision (usually vertical), sampling of peritoneal fluid for cytologic evaluation (intraperitoneal cell washings), and abdominal and pelvic exploration with biopsy or excision of any extrauterine lesions suspicious for tumor. These procedures should be followed by total extrafascial hysterectomy and bilateral salpingo-oophorectomy. Any suspicious pelvic or paraaortic lymph nodes should be removed for pathologic evaluation. If certain high-risk factors are found, routine sampling is indicated if there are no suspicious retroperitoneal nodes.

All surgical specimens should be evaluated. Optimally, the unfixed uterus should be opened by the surgical pathologist, who can grossly estimate the depth of invasion, assess involvement of the cervix, and later sample the tumor for histologic assessment. There is no typical gross appearance of an endometrial carcinoma. Most are polypoid or ulcerative. Carcinoma usually differs in texture and color from the surrounding normal endometrium. The normal endometrium is irregular and tan, but a carcinoma is usually shaggy, white to gray-white, and focally hemorrhagic. If necrosis or papillary growth is a prominent feature, the tumor may be friable and may crumble with touch. Areas of myometrial invasion may be visible as gray-white to white, with yellow areas disclosing necrosis (Fig. 23.7). The texture may be soft, friable, or firm depending on the degree of necrosis.

Invasion of the myometrium may be more extensive microscopically than is evident visibly because of the characteristic infiltrative growth pattern of the tumor, although gross visual examination by the operating team of the cut uterine surface at the tumor site can accurately determine the depth of myometrial invasion in 91% of the patients (153). If the uterus is opened by the operating surgeon, care should be employed to avoid distortion of the anatomy. In a retrospective study by Goff and Riche (154), the gross estimation by pathologists of myometrial invasion in grades 2 and 3 tumors was poor. With invasion, the uterine cavity usually enlarges and the myometrium thickens, but a small uterus may have myometrial penetration to the serosa.

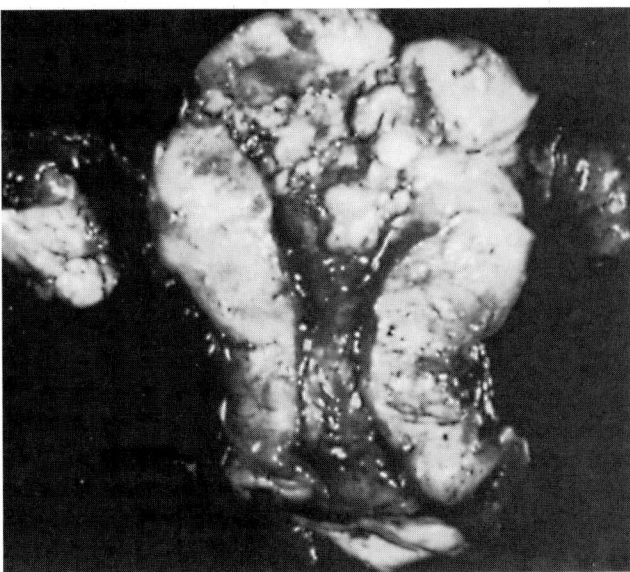

FIG. 23.7. Gross specimen of endometrial carcinoma. The carcinoma extends through the full thickness of the myometrium.

The endometrial carcinoma may be exophytic (papillary) or ulcerative. In general, carcinomas with a prominent papillary component tend to have a poor prognosis, probably due to the inclusion of serous and clear-cell types. Papillary endometrial adenocarcinoma is supported by fibrous stocks lined by well-differentiated cellular epithelium (102,155). The pathologic evaluation of specimens must determine cell type, histologic grade, depth of myometrial invasion, the presence of vascular invasion, and lymph node involvement. The evaluation must also include a thorough microscopic evaluation of the cervix for evidence of tumor extension. The pathology of lymphatic spread depends on the location of the tumor. The lower and middle portion of the uterus drains laterally to the parametrium and the paracervical and obturator lymph nodes. The upper corpus and fundus drain to the common iliac and paraaortic nodes, and a third pathway is along the round ligament to the inguinal nodes.

PATHOLOGIC FACTORS OF PROGNOSTIC SIGNIFICANCE

The importance of uterine risk factors is determined by how they affect the probability of pelvic and paraaortic lymph node involvement and subsequent survival. The importance of the extrauterine risk factors relates to positive retroperitoneal lymph nodes and survival.

FIGO Stage

The prognostic utility of surgicopathologic stage has been confirmed in multiple studies of large numbers of patients, using both univariate and multivariate analysis (74,109,150,

156–161). FIGO stage is often the single strongest predictor of outcome for women with endometrial adenocarcinoma in studies using multivariate analyses (109). Although the FIGO clinical staging system of 1971 was generally useful, retrospective comparison of the two methods demonstrated the clear superiority of surgicopathologic staging over clinical staging in predicting outcome.

Histologic Cell Types

The histologic classification of endometrial adenocarcinoma is important not only because it facilitates the recognition of lesions as carcinoma, but also because the cell type has consistently been recognized as being important in predicting the biologic behavior and probability of survival. Endometrioid adenocarcinoma accounts for the majority of tumors in the uterine corpus and fortunately usually has a relatively good prognosis. Consequently, the virulence of other cell types is usually related to endometrioid adenocarcinoma.

Adenocarcinoma with squamous differentiation is similar to typical endometrioid adenocarcinoma with respect to the distribution by age and frequency of nodal metastasis, and is associated with a slightly increased probability of survival. *Villoglandular carcinoma* has a biologic behavior similar to that of endoemetrioid adenocarcinoma (81,162). *Serous carcinoma* is often a lethal tumor, with overall survival rates varying from 40% to 60% at 5 years (80,101,112,163–167). *Clear-cell carcinoma* also has a highly aggressive behavior, with 5-year survival rates of 30% to 75% (110,111,116, 168–172).

Grade

The degree of histologic differentiation has long been considered to be one of the most sensitive indicators of tumor spread. The GOG and other studies have confirmed that as grade becomes less differentiated, there is a greater tendency for deep myometrial invasion and, subsequently, higher rates of pelvic and paraaortic lymph node involvement (Table 23.8) (151,173–175). In fact, 50% of grade 3 lesions have greater than one-half myometrial invasion, with pelvic and

paraaortic lymph node involvement approaching 30% and 20%, respectively. However, exceptions exist. Ten percent of grade 1 lesions have deep muscle invasion, and 7% of grade 3 lesions are limited to the endometrium. Although only 2.8% of all grade 1 lesions have spread to pelvic nodes and 1.7% to paraaortic nodes, 11% and 6%, respectively, are node positive if there is deep myometrial invasion (176).

Survival has also been consistently related to histologic grade, and in a GOG study of more than 600 women with clinical stage I or occult stage II endometrioid adenocarcinoma, the 5-year relative survival was as follows: grade 1 to 94%; grade 2 to 84%; grade 3 to 72% (151).

Myometrial Invasion

The depth of myometrial invasion should be recorded in all pathologic reports, preferably in both millimeters and in the percentage of total myometrial thickness. The optimal method for assessment of the depth of uterine invasion for prognostication remains unknown. The current FIGO staging of endometrial carcinoma subdivides stage I tumors as follows: IA, tumor limited to the endometrium; IB, invasion confined to the inner half of the myometrium; and IC, tumor invasion to the outer half of the myometrium.

Extension of tumor into adenomyosis is not regarded as invasion (177,178). The identification of residual endometrial stroma and a smooth regular outline to the area of question suggests adenomyosis. In true invasion, there is no stroma, there are irregular and ill-defined borders of invasion, and there may be a desmoplastic stroma around the malignant epithelium.

Deep myometrial invasion is one of the more important factors correlated with diminished proability of survival, and is associated with a higher probability of extrauterine tumor spread, treatment failure, and recurrence (150,179,180). In a GOG study of over 400 women with clinical stage I and occult stage II endometrioid adenocarcinoma, the 5-year relative survival was 94% when tumor was confined to the endometrium, 91% when tumor involved the inner third of the myometrium, 84% when the tumor extended into the middle third, and 59% when the tumor invaded into the outer third of the myometrium (161).

Although the depth of invasion is often inversely related

TABLE 23.8. *Histologic grade and depth of invasion*

Depth	Grade, no. of patients			Total (% of total)
	Grade 1 (%)	Grade 2 (%)	Grade 3 (%)	
Endometrium only	44 (24)	31 (11)	11 (7)	86 (14)
Superficial	96 (53)	131 (45)	54 (35)	281 (45)
Middle	22 (12)	69 (24)	24 (16)	115 (19)
Deep	18 (10)	57 (20)	64 (42)	139 (22)
Total	180 (100)	288 (100)	153 (100)	621 (100)

Reprinted from Creasman WT, Morrow CP, Bundy BN, et al. Surgical pathologic spread patterns of endometrial cancer (a Gynecologic Oncology Group study). *Cancer* 1987;60:2035.

to the degree of differentiation, myometrial invasion is an independent predictor of outcome for women with early-stage endometrial carcinoma (109,156,161,181–185). Regardless of grade, only 1% of patients with endometrial involvement have metastases to either the pelvic or paraaortic nodes, but the relative frequency of pelvic and paraaortic node involvement increases to 25% and 17%, respectively, for deep muscle invasion (151).

Isthmus-Cervix Extension

The location of tumor within the uterus has generally been considered to be important in the prediction of nodal spread. If only the fundus is involved, 8% of patients may have pelvic node metastases. This doubles to 16% if the isthmus-cervix (lower segment) is also involved. Only 4% of fundal lesions have metastases to paraaortic lymph nodes, and lower-segment lesions have a 14% risk of positive paraaortic nodes (151).

Vascular Space Invasion

Multiple studies have documented that lymphatic invasion is a strong predictor of tumor recurrence and death from tumor and is independent of depth of myometrial invasion or histologic differentiation (109,186–190). In one investigation of FIGO stage I endometrial adenocarcinoma, 9 of 15 patients with lymphatic invasion died of tumor, whereas none of the 78 without identified vascular invasion died of cancer (187). Zaino et al. (161) found that vascular invasion was a statistically significant indicator of death from tumor in early clinical stage but not early surgical stage endometrial adenocarcinoma. This suggests that lymphatic invasion helps to identify patients likely to have spread to lymph nodes or distant sites, but that its importance is diminished for those in whom thorough sampling of nodes has failed to identify metastasis. Capillary invasion is identified in 35% to 95% of serous carcinomas of the endometrium, where it has generally been associated with an elevated risk of tumor recurrence or death from disease (101,163,166).

Vascular space invasion or capillary-like space (CLS) involvement with tumor exists in approximately 15% of uteri containing adenocarcinoma (151,188,190). Pelvic lymph nodes are positive in 27% of cases, which is four times more often if malignant cells are found in the CLS than if absent. The relative risk of paraaortic node metastases is 19%, which is a sixfold increase over negative CLS involvement (151).

Adnexal Involvement

Six percent of clinical stage I and occult stage II patients have spread of tumor to the adnexa (151). Of these, 32% have pelvic node metastases compared with 8% pelvic node positivity if adnexal involvement is not present. Twenty per-

cent have positive paraaortic node metastases, which is four times greater than if adnexal metastases are not present.

Intraperitoneal Spread

Gross intraperitoneal spread without adnexal metastases correlates highly with involvement of pelvic and paraaortic lymph nodes. Fifty-one percent of patients with gross intraperitoneal spread have positive pelvic nodes, and only 7% without spread have positive pelvic nodes. The relative frequency of positive paraaortic nodes for patients with and without intraperitoneal spread is 23% and 4%, respectively (151).

Peritoneal Cytology

Twelve percent to 15% of patients who undergo surgical staging have positive peritoneal cytology. Of these, 25% have metastases to pelvic lymph nodes, and 19% have metastases to paraaortic lymph nodes. In addition, 35% of patients with extrauterine disease (adnexal, nodal, or intraperitoneal spread) have positive cytologic washings. However, 4% to 6% of patients with positive washings have no evidence of extrauterine disease (151,191). Published opinions are mixed about the significance of this finding (176,192–196). Several small series show no outcome differences (197–200). However, two large series show peritoneal cytology to be, by itself, a poor prognostic factor (201,202). Kadar and colleagues (203) found that positive peritoneal cytology had an adverse outcome on survival only if the endometrial cancer had spread to the adnexa, peritoneum, or lymph nodes, but not if disease was confined to the uterus, suggesting that not all cells that are found in the peritoneal cavity are capable of independent growth. Positive peritoneal cytology associated with extrauterine disease is a marker for aggressive disease and carries a worse prognosis.

Pelvic and Paraaortic Lymph Node Metastases

In the 1987 GOG (151) study of 621 clinical stage I and occult stage II patients, 70 (11%) had metastases to pelvic or paraaortic lymph nodes. Of this number, 22 patients had metastases to both the pelvic and paraaortic regions, and 12 had metastases to the paraaortic nodes only. The highest rate of paraaortic node metastases (32%) occurred if pelvic nodes were involved. The frequency of pelvic and paraaortic nodal metastases with respect to the other pathologic risk factors is shown in Table 23.9.

Ploidy

About two-thirds of endometrial adenocarcinomas are composed of diploid cells as measured by flow or static cytometry. Diploid tumors tend to be more frequently associated with less aggressive cell types, superficial invasion, and

TABLE 23.9. *Frequency of nodal metastasis among risk factors*

Risk factor	No. of patients	Pelvic no. (%)	Aortic no. (%)
Histology			
Endometrioid adenocarcinoma	599	56 (9)	30 (5)
Others	22	2 (9)	4 (18)
Grade			
1 Well	180	5 (3)	3 (2)
2 Moderate	288	25 (9)	14 (5)
3 Poor	153	28 (18)	17 (11)
Myometrial invasion			
Endometrial	87	1 (1)	1 (1)
Superficial	279	15 (5)	8 (3)
Middle	116	7 (6)	1 (1)
Deep	139	35 (25)	24 (17)
Site of tumor location			
Fundus	524	42 (8)	20 (4)
Isthmus-cervix	97	16 (16)	14 (14)
Capillary-like space involvement			
Negative	528	37 (7)	19 (9)
Positive	93	21 (27)	15 (19)
Other extrauterine metastasis			
Negative	586	40 (7)	26 (4)
Positive	35	18 (51)	8 (23)
Peritoneal cytology[a]			
Negative	537	38 (7)	20 (4)
Positive	75	19 (25)	14 (19)

[a] Nine patients did not have cytology reported.
Modified with permission from Creasman WT, Morrow CP, Bundy BN, et al. Surgical pathologic spread patterns of endometrial cancer (a Gynecologic Oncology Group study). *Cancer* 1987;60:2035.

better histologic differentiation (204–209). Survival has generally been higher for women with diploid tumors (204, 206,209), and the differences in progression-free survival among stage I patients have been as great as 94% for those with diploid tumors versus 64% for those with aneuploid cancers (204). In large studies employing multivariate analysis, ploidy has almost always remained a strong predictor of outcome (210–216). In a large study by Lundgren et al. (347 patients) (217), image cytometric DNA ploidy was the strongest predictor of outcome and was of value in predicting the risks for relapse.

Steroid Receptors

In most studies, the presence and quantity of steroid receptors have been positively correlated with histologic differentiation, FIGO stage, and survival (218–222). Various investigators have found, by univariate and multivariate analysis, that the presence of estrogen receptors (ERs) but not progesterone receptors (PRs), PR alone, or ER and PR were predictive of a low probability of recurrence or improved survival (220,223–227). Geisinger et al. (220) noted that both ER and PR were related not only to survival, but also to the clinical stage, histologic grade, and the absence of vascular invasion. Ehrlich et al. (223), in a study of 175 patients of all stages, reported that recurrence was related to the absence

of ERs or PRs, and that response to progestin therapy was more common in PR-positive tumors. Because of the diversity in published observations and high level of heterogeneity in the expression of steroid receptors within individual tumors, ERs and PRs are not routinely assessed as part of the primary assessment of the hysterectomy specimen in most institutions. In contrast, assessment of steroid receptors in metastases may be helpful in the decision about appropriate therapy for recurrent tumors.

Pathologic Models of Survival

Many patients with endometrial adenocarcinoma have a mixture of good and bad prognostic factors and do not fall into categories for which either the prognosis or need for adjuvant therapy is clear. When the data available from more than 1,000 women with clinical stages I and II endometrial adenocarcinoma entered on a GOG protocol were used, two models were created that can be applied to estimate the probability of survival after examining the factors described in the sections above (161). The first model is based on the clinical stage, whereas the second is restricted to those patients with surgical stage I or II disease. It should be emphasized that only 72% of clinical stage I or II endometrial adenocarcinomas were of surgical stage I or II.

For clinical stage I or II tumors, cell type, histologic grade,

TABLE 23.10. *Clinical stage I and II tumors: the proportional hazards modeling of relative survival time*

Variable	Regression coefficient	Relative risk	Significance test[a] (*p*-value)
Endometrioid			
Grade 1	0.00	1.0	
Grade 2	0.47	1.6	12.7 (.0004)
Grade 3	0.94	2.6	
Clear cell			10.5 (.001)
Grade 1	2.00	7.1	
Grade 2	1.33	3.8	2.7 (.1)
Grade 3	0.71	2.0	
Serous			6.7 (.01)
Grade 1	1.06	2.9	
Grade 2	1.47	4.4	2.7 (.1)
Grade 3	1.89	6.6	
Endometrioid with squamous differentiation			0.3 (.6)
Grade 1	0.25	0.8	
Grade 2	0.04	1.0	0.5 (.5)
Grade 3	0.17	1.2	
Villoglandular			2.2 (.1)
Grade 1	0.94	0.4	
Grade 2	0.28	1.3	3.2 (.08)
Grade 3	1.50	4.5	
Myometrial invasion			
Endometrium only	0.00	1.0	
Superficial	0.19	1.2	
Middle	0.46	1.6	23.9 (.0001)
Deep	1.08	3.0	
Positive washings	1.09	3.0	35.5 (.0001)
Age[b]	0.17		
Age squared[c]	0.000985		24.9 (.0001)
45 (arbitrary reference)	0.000	1.0	
55	0.715	2.0	
65	1.233	3.4	
75	1.554	4.7	
Vascular space involvement	0.41	1.5	4.6 (.03)

[a] Wald chi-square test; *p*-value for grading is for overall grade within cell type.
[b] Age as a linear variable, for each year >45 years of age.
[c] Patient's age squared, divided into four 10-year age groups.
From Zaino RJ, Kurman RJ, Diana KL, Morrow CP. Pathologic models to predict outcome for women with endometrial adenocarcinoma. *Cancer* 1996;77:1119.

depth of myometrial invasion, peritoneal cytology, vascular space invasion, and age are all statistically significant as independent risk factors in the multivariate proportional hazards model (Table 23.10). Each factor contributes to the probability of death and is associated with a specified relative risk of death from tumor. The product of the individual relative risks, or total relative risk, can then be used to estimate the probability of a patient dying from tumor by inspection of the predicted survival curves for various total relative risks (Fig. 23.8).

For surgical stage I or II tumors, the statistical significance of the cell type and grade is markedly reduced, whereas age and myometrial invasion persist as highly significant variables in the multivariate model (Table 23.11). One can infer from the differences between the two models that cell type and histologic grade are important in predicting the likelihood of extrauterine spread, but that if the tumor is confined to the uterus at the time of surgical exploration, then it is the depth of invasion that determines occult spread. Further, it should be noted that the survival for most women with early surgical stage disease is excellent (Fig. 23.9).

MOLECULAR ALTERATIONS IN THE PATHOGENESIS AND PROGRESSION OF ENDOMETRIAL ADENOCARCINOMA

Deletions or mutations of the *PTEN* gene, and microsatellite instability (MSI) due to hypermethylation of the promoter for the mismatch repair gene, *hMLH1*, are both relatively common and early events in the development of a significant proportion of endometrioid adenocarcinomas. In contrast, these molecular alterations do not appear to be critical in the pathogenesis of serous or clear-cell carcinoma. However, mutations in the *p53* gene are found with high

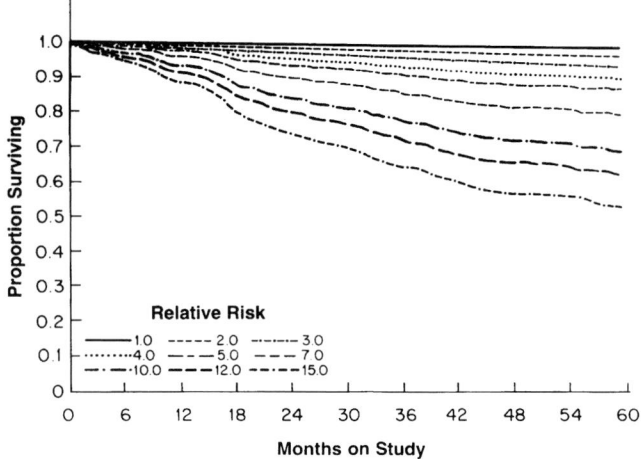

FIG. 23.8. Predicted survival time by initial tumor relative risk for clinical stages I and II patients. (Reprinted with permission from Zaino RJ, Kurman RJ, Diana KL, Morrow CP. Pathologic models to predict outcome for women with endometrial adenocarcinoma. *Cancer* 1996;77:1119.)

TABLE 23.11. *Surgical stages I and II tumors: the proportional hazards modeling of relative survival time*

Variable	Regression coefficient	Relative risk	Significance test[a] (*p*-value)
Endometrioid			
Grade 1	0.00	1.0	
Grade 2	0.28	1.3	2.7 (.1)
Grade 3	0.56	1.8	
Clear-cell			2.5 (.1)
Grade 1	1.62	5.1	
Grade 2	1.26	3.5	0.3 (.6)
Grade 3	0.91	2.5	
Serous			1.7 (.2)
Grade 1	0.80	2.2	
Grade 2	1.15	3.1	0.7 (.4)
Grade 3	1.49	4.4	
Endometrioid with squamous differentiation			0.1 (.7)
Grade 1	0.20	1.2	
Grade 2	0.01	1.0	0.3 (.6)
Grade 3	0.22	0.8	
Villoglandular			2.2 (.1)
Grade 1	4.91	0.01	
Grade 2	0.59	0.5	10.4 (.001)
Grade 3	3.73	41.9	
Myometrial invasion			
Endometrium only	0.00	1.0	
Superficial	0.39	0.5	
Middle	1.20	3.3	19.6 (.0002)
Deep	1.53	4.6	
Age[b]	0.17		
Age squared[c]	0.000837		20.7 (.0001)
45 (arbitrary reference)	0.00	1.0	
55	0.85	2.3	
65	1.52	4.6	
75	2.03	7.6	
Vascular space involvement	0.32	1.4	1.2 (.3)

[a] Wald chi-square test; *p*-value for grading is for overall grade within cell type.
[b] Age as a linear variable, for each year >45 years of age.
[c] Patient's age squared, divided into four 10-year age groups.
From Zaino RJ, Kurman RJ, Diana KL, Morrow CP. Pathologic models to predict outcome for women with endometrial adenocarcinoma. *Cancer* 1996;77:1120.

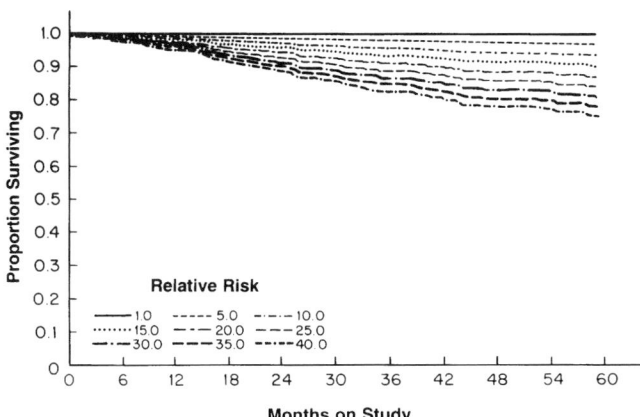

FIG. 23.9. Predicted survival time by initial tumor relative risk for surgical stages I and II patients. (Reprinted with permission from Zaino RJ, Kurman RJ, Diana KL, Morrow CP. Pathologic models to predict outcome for women with endometrial adenocarcinoma. *Cancer* 1996;77:1120.)

frequency not only in invasive serous carcinoma but also in endometrial intraepithelial carcinoma (108,228), the noninvasive precursor of serous carcinoma, suggesting that a different pathway is followed in the development of the second type of endometrial adenocarcinoma.

The function of the tumor-suppressor gene *PTEN* (MMAC1) includes inhibition of cell migration, spreading, and adhesion (229–232). The *PTEN* gene is located on chromosome 10q23 and about 40% of endometrial carcinomas display loss of heterozygosity of chromosome 10q23, which suggests the involvement of *PTEN* in this disease (233). *PTEN* mutations in 30% to 50% of endometrial carcinoma tumors make this the most frequent genetic alteration known in this disease (234–236). Risinger et al. (237) have in one study shown that inactivation of *PTEN* by mutation is associated with early disease in contrast to the study of Steck et al. (238) where *PTEN* gene alteration was linked to an advanced disease group.

MSI caused by shifts in allelic electrophenetric mobility results from replication error of repeated sequences. It was first described in HNPCC. One of the most common extracolonic tumors associated with this disease (11) is endometrial cancer, and MSI has been demonstrated in both hereditary and sporadic tumors. MSI in endometrial cancer has been reported to be between 9% and 43% (239–244). In 71% to 92% of sporadic endometrial carcinoma, MSI has been found to be associated with hypermethylation of the hMLH1 promoter region, whereas it seems to be less common in the promoter region of hMSH2 (245,246). It is likely that methylation of the promoter region is an important mechanism of *hMLH1* gene inactivation in endometrial carcinoma (247–251) and a precursor to MSI. Too few studies have been done to reach any conclusion regarding the importance of MSI as a prognostic factor in endometrial cancer.

p53 is a tumor-suppressor gene, the product of which is a protein involved in the regulation of the cell cycle at the G_1 checkpoint, permitting replication of cells that have acquired various mutations. Mutations of the *p53* gene often result in a protein with a longer half-life, which accumulates in the cell. Upregulation of wild-type (i.e., nonmutated) *p53* may occur after DNA damage and also results in overexpression that is detectable by immunohistochemistry. This appears to be an early event in the development of serous carcinoma, but it is a late event in endometrioid carcinomas for which it serves as an indicator of poor prognosis. In addition to the very frequent overexpression of p53 protein in serous carcinoma (252), it has also been related to a higher FIGO stage, clear-cell histology, higher histologic grade, and increased depth of myometrial invasion (114,210,253–266,a5). Lundgren et al. (217) studied *p53* in relation to clinicopathological variables in 376 consecutive patients with endometrial cancer stages I-IV. *p53* overexpression was found to be a strong significant factor with regard to relapse-free survival in univariate analysis, but it failed to retain its significance when submitted to multivariate analysis.

In contrast, *p53* mutations are not often found in low-grade endometrioid tumors (267). This suggests that different subgroups of endometrial cancers have different genetic pathways. Much more work is needed to understand the genetic mechanics at play and to translate this into use within the clinical and therapeutic field (268).

HER-2/*neu* is a proto-oncogene, the product of which is a transmembrane growth factor receptor, p185erb-2, which shares some homology with the epidermal growth factor receptor. It is normally expressed at low levels in the cycling endometrium. Gene amplification and/or overexpression occurs in about 20% to 40% of endometrial carcinomas, and has been associated with advanced stage (269,a3), decreased differentiation, aggressive cell types particularly including the clear-cell type (270,271,a7), and deep myometrial invasion (258). The significance of HER-2/*neu* amplification or overexpression as a predictor of survival is somewhat unclear, with no apparent association of overexpression to outcome being identified in several studies (213,261,270,272), but a statistically significant relationship in most others (210, 256,261,271,273–275) even after adjusting for other known risk factors (256,271,274). In addition to its potential utility as an indicator of poor prognosis, systemic therapy using antibodies directed against the HER-2/neu protein is currently being investigated for patients with tumors that express the protein at high levels.

Abnormal expression of the oncogenes *beta-* and *gamma-catenin* and *E-* and *P-cadherin* may play a critical role in the initiation and progression of endometrioid neoplasia (276,277). Moreno-Bueno et al. (277) have evaluated the immunoreactivity of *beta-* and *gamma-catenin* and *E-* and *P-cadherin* in 149 patients with premalignant and malignant endometrioid lesions to correlate their membranous expression with clinical pathologic data. Their data indicate that abnormal expression of catenin and cadherin was common in premalignant and malignant endometrial lesions. Nonendometrioid endometrial cancer showed a greater reduction in *E-cadherin* expression, upregulation of *P-cadherin*, and loss of heterozygosity at 16q21 than endometrial cancers. In contrast, nuclear accumulation of *beta-catenin* was frequently associated with a gene mutation characteristic of endometrioid lesions and may be an early event that is present in atypical endometrial hyperplasia. Reduced *E-cadherin* expression in endometrioid carcinomas is related to advanced stages, indicating a role for this molecule in tumor progression. Nuclear *beta-catenin* expression was found in 31.2% of endometrioid cancers and 3% of nonendometrioid cancers (*p* = .002) and was significantly associated with *beta-catenin* gene exon 3 mutations. *Beta-catenin* gene exon 3 mutations were associated with the endometrioid phenotype and were detected in 14 (15%) endometrioid cancers, but none of the nonendometrioid cancers (*p* = .02). *Gamma-catenin* nuclear expression was found in 10 endometrial cancer. It was not associated with the histologic type but was associated with more advanced stages (*p* = .04) (276).

The activation of *RAS* proto-oncogenes through either point mutations or gene amplification has been identified in various malignant tumors. Mutations in the K-*ras* oncogene have been reported in endometrioid cancer and also in endometrial hyperplasia, suggesting that K-*ras* activation may be an early event in the development of endometrioid malignancy (122). Mutations in codon 12 of K-*ras* occur in only about 10% to 15% of endometrial carcinomas, and their significance is unknown. In most studies, the presence of K-*ras* mutations has not been related to stage, grade, depth of invasion, or survival (278–281).

Further studies have identified mutations in several tumor-related genes such as *p16*, *hMLH1*, *hMSH2*, and *hMSH6* in endometrial cancer (282–284). Salvesen et al. (285) have shown that loss of nuclear p16 protein expression is not associated with promoter methylation but defines a subgroup of aggressive endometrial carcinoma with a poor prognosis and found to be a strong independent prognostic factor.

HISTORICAL TREATMENT

Of all the female pelvic malignancies, endometrial cancer seems to have more advocates for different treatment plans than any other. This is particularly true for tumors clinically confined to the uterine corpus, which represent 75% of all adenocarcinomas of this organ. The standard treatment for this disease has been and remains a total abdominal hysterectomy. However, through the years, preoperative and postoperative irradiation and, occasionally, chemotherapy and hormonal therapy have also been used.

The first significant report of employing irradiation in the management of patients with endometrial cancer was the publication of the "Stockholm Technique" by Heyman in

1935 (286). The use of intracavitary implants using Heyman's method became increasingly popular in the ensuing years. Subsequently, reports comparing results in patients treated with a single intrauterine tandem with those treated with multiple intrauterine capsules revealed a lower incidence of residual disease and an improved 5-year survival rate, favoring the patients treated with capsules (287–289). Lewis et al. (290), in cooperative studies in the late 1960s, showed that 25% of patients had deep myometrial invasion if treated initially by surgery, and only 8% had deep invasion if treated by preoperative irradiation. However, because pelvic and paraaortic node involvement seems to relate in part to depth of myometrial invasion, a significant predictor of spread of disease may be lost if preoperative irradiation is given and hysterectomy is delayed 4 to 6 weeks. In addition, some patients will not be adequately treated. Therefore, it appears that selective postoperative use is the most reasonable approach to irradiation as adjuvant treatment in the majority of patients.

Early uncontrolled trials suggested that progestin therapy after surgery or irradiation was associated with a decreased risk of recurrence in patients with disease confined to the uterus (291). However, large prospective randomized trials failed to show a survival advantage (199,292,293). Adjuvant cytotoxic chemotherapy versus no treatment has been studied in one large randomized trial, and no benefit was shown for patients treated with single-agent doxorubicin compared to an untreated control group (294). However, initial results of GOG study 122 comparing doxorubicin and cisplatin chemotherapy to whole abdominal radiotherapy as adjuvant treatment in patients with stage III or IV disease shows a benefit for patients receiving chemotherapy (6). The role of chemotherapy given either sequentially or concomitantly with more focused radiation approaches is under evaluation.

With improved preoperative and postoperative care, anesthesia administration, surgical techniques, and knowledge of tumor spread, the current treatment trend is to avoid preoperative irradiation or chemotherapy and to stage all patients surgically. Postoperative treatment whether chemotherapy or radiation therapy or both is reserved for those who are found to have poor prognostic factors after reviewing the surgicopathologic material (Table 23.12).

SURGICAL TECHNIQUE

After the diagnosis of endometrial carcinoma has been confirmed, the cell type and grade have been determined, and the appropriate studies to assess spread of disease have been performed, the patient is evaluated for suitability for major abdominal surgery. In a series of 595 consecutive patients, Marziale and colleagues (295) found an operability rate of 87%. Preparation for this surgery includes attention to any concurrent medical problems, such as hypertension and diabetes mellitus, which are frequent medical conditions

TABLE 23.12. *Contemporary treatment plan using surgical staging*

Treatment factors	Low risk	Intermediate risk	High risk
Stage	IA, G1,2	IA, G3 IB, IC (all grades) IIA, IIB (all grades) IIIA (+ cytology)	IIIA, IIIB, IIIC (all grades) IVA, IVB (all grades)
Postoperative treatment	None	Vaginal cuff irradiation Pelvic irradiation (questionable)	Vaginal cuff irradiation Pelvic irradiation Paraaortic irradiation (+ aortic nodes) Whole abdominal irradiation (intra-abdominal spread) or chemotherapy Clinical trials

G, grade.

of patients with endometrial cancer. Preoperative counseling includes obtaining permission to remove the uterus, tubes, and ovaries; permission for thorough intraabdominal exploration with biopsy and tumor removal as necessary; and permission to remove the pelvic and paraaortic lymph nodes.

The operative procedure is performed through an adequate abdominal incision that allows thorough intraabdominal exploration and retroperitoneal lymph node removal if necessary. On entry into the peritoneal cavity, fluid samples are obtained for subsequent cytologic determination. This is followed by thorough intraabdominal and pelvic exploration, with biopsy or excision of any lesion suspicious for tumor. The uterus should be particularly observed for tumor breakthrough of the serosal surface. The distal ends of the fallopian tubes are clipped or ligated to prevent possible tumor spill during uterine manipulation.

Total abdominal hysterectomy and bilateral salpingo-oophorectomy are the primary operative procedures for carcinoma of the endometrium. The plane of excision lies outside the pubocervical fascia and does not require unroofing of the ureters. The ovarian and fallopian tubes are removed en bloc with the uterus.

The advantage of the conservative approach is that surgery is usually straightforward, but the disadvantage is that it does not provide complete surgical staging. During recent years, this traditional model has been questioned for the following reasons: (a) there is a need for full surgical staging in order to ascribe the correct FIGO stage; (b) involved nodes are better removed than left undiscovered and then simply irradiated or indeed left unirradiated; (c) palpation of pelvic lymph nodes is not sufficiently accurate, with a sensitivity of 72% in a recent prospective study (296,297); and (d) a thorough lymphadenectomy that identifies no nodal metastases may be sufficient to avoid the need for adjuvant radiotherapy even with a high-risk tumor as assessed by the criteria previously outline (298,299).

For patients in whom paraaortic node sampling is indicated, sampling can be performed through a midline peritoneal incision over the common iliac arteries and aorta. Node sampling can also be performed on the right by mobilizing

the right colon medially and on the left by mobilizing the left colon medially. In each case, a sample of lymphatics and lymph nodes is resected along the upper common iliac vessels on either side and from the lower portion of the aorta and vena cava. On the left side, the lymph nodes and lymphatics are slightly posterior to the aorta, and on the right side, they lie primarily in the vena caval fat bed.

In some cases, pelvic lymph node sampling is indicated. This consists of a sample of lymph nodes taken from the distal common iliac and from the superior iliac artery and vein. A third sample of lymphatics is obtained from the group of nodes that lie along the obturator nerve. In a lymph node–sampling procedure, it is important to try to achieve an adequate sample of nodes from each anatomic site, but no attempt is made to perform a complete lymphadenectomy.

Some gynecologic oncologists advocate slicing open the uterus immediately following its removal in order to eyeball the degree of myometrial invasion or using microscopic frozen section (300) as a means of determining whether to proceed to lymphadenectomy (297). Doering and others (153) reported a 91% accuracy rate for 148 patients for determining the depth of myometrial invasion by gross visual examination of the cut uterine surface. A recent prospective study (297) indicates that visual inspection of <or> 50% correlated with microscopic assessment in 85% cases. However, the sensitivity of determining >50% was lower at 72%. If there is no gross residual intraperitoneal tumor, pelvic and paraaortic lymph nodes should be sampled for the following indications (Table 23.13): myometrial invasion, greater than one-half (outer half of myometrium); regardless of tumor grade, tumor presence in the isthmus-cervix; adnexal or other extrauterine metastases; the presence of serous, clear-

TABLE 23.13. *Indications for retroperitoneal node sampling*

Myometrial invasion more than 50%
Isthmus-cervix extension
Extrauterine spread
Serous, clear-cell, squamous, or undifferentiated cell types
Enlarged lymph nodes

cell, undifferentiated, or squamous types; and lymph nodes that are visibly or palpably enlarged. In a GOG study, 46% of the positive paraaortic lymph nodes were enlarged, and 98% of the cases with aortic node metastases came from patients with positive pelvic nodes, adnexal or intraabdominal metastases, or outer one-third myometrial invasion (185). These risk factors affected only 25% of the patients, yet they yielded most of the positive paraaortic node patients.

Lymph nodes need not be sampled for tumor limited to the endometrium, regardless of grade, because less than 1% of these patients have disease spread to pelvic or paraaortic lymph nodes (151,185,a4). A gray zone in deciding about lymph node sampling is represented by patients whose only risk factor is inner one-half myometrial invasion, particularly if the grade is 2 or 3. This group has 5% or less chance of node positivity (185). We favor node sampling in these instances if there seems to be any question about the degree of myometrial invasion. This includes invasion that approaches one-half of the myometrial thickness in patients who are medically fit to undergo the sampling procedures.

After these procedures, the patient is surgically staged according to the 1988 FIGO criteria (Table 23.5) (5). The overall surgical complication rate after this type of staging is approximately 20%. The serious complication rate is 6% (185).

Despite these above-mentioned rational points, there are still a large number of women treated worldwide who do not undergo a full surgical staging. The reasons for this are probably twofold (299):

1. There has never been a convincing evidence base to demonstrate the effectiveness of more extensive surgery in terms of improving survival. There have been no randomized trials of lymphadenectomy, and there are only retrospective data on which to rely. A case series that highlights the high cure rate with a standard lymphadenectomy is not useful in assessing the contribution of lymphadenectomy in terms of therapeutic effects. There is some value in terms of determining whether a negative lymphadenectomy can dispense with the need for adjuvant radiation. The only certain way to solve the therapeutic effect of lymphadenectomy will be by randomized trial and such a trial is currently ongoing in the United Kingdom coordinated by the Medical Research Council. In this trial, all women with stage I disease are randomized to have either "standard" total abdominal hysterectomy plus bilateral salpingo-oophorectomy or total abdominal hysterectomy plus salpingo-oophorectomy and lymphadenectomy. All surgery should be undertaken by gynecologists experienced in pelvic node dissection.

2. Many gynecologists are neither trained in the techniques of lymphadenectomy nor familiar with the concept of full surgical staging. Full staging and more complex surgery should be undertaken by specialized gynecologic oncologists.

An alternative method of surgically staging patients with clinical stage I endometrial cancer is gaining in popularity. This approach combines laparoscopically assisted vaginal hysterectomy with laparoscopic lymphadenectomy. Childers and colleagues (301,302) described their experience with this procedure in 59 patients with clinical stage I endometrial carcinoma. The laparoscopic procedure included a thorough inspection of the peritoneal cavity, obtaining intraperitoneal washings, and performing a laparoscopically assisted vaginal hysterectomy. Laparoscopic pelvic and aortic lymph node samplings were performed in all patients with grade 2 or 3 lesions, as well as in those patients with grade 1 lesions who were found to have greater than 50% myometrial invasion on frozen section. In two patients, laparoscopic lymphadenectomy was precluded by obesity. Six patients who were noted to have intraperitoneal disease at laparoscopy underwent exploratory laparotomy. Two additional patients required laparotomy for complications, including a transected ureter and a cystotomy. The mean hospital stay was 2.9 days.

Gemignani et al. (303) retrospectively compared the clinical outcomes and hospital charges for 69 women with early-stage endometrial cancer who underwent laparoscopically assisted vaginal hysterectomy compared to 251 who underwent an abdominal approach. Although the mean operating time was longer for the laparoscopic group, the overall complication rates, length of stay, and hospital charges were lower. Although follow-up was short, there was no significant difference in disease recurrence between the two groups.

Several other retrospective studies (242,303–307) have evaluated the validity of laparoscopic surgery in patients with endometrial cancer, but only in two of these studies have survival data been reported [Gemignani et al. (303) and Magrina et al. (305)]. In both studies, no differences in survival were found in laparoscopic vaginal surgery compared with laparotomy. The only prospective randomized trial published so far comparing laparoscopy-assisted vaginal versus abdominal surgery in patients with endometrial cancer is by Malur et al. (308). They randomized 70 patients with endometrial cancer FIGO stage I-III to laparoscopy-assisted simple or radical vaginal hysterectomy or simple or radical abdominal hysterectomy with or without lymph node resection. Thirty-seven patients were treated in the laparoscopic versus 33 patients in the laparotomy group. Lymph node resection was performed in 25 patients by laparoscopy and in 24 patients by laparotomy. Blood loss and transfusion rates were significantly lower in the laparoscopic group. The number of pelvic and paraaortic lymph nodes, duration of surgery, and incidence of postoperative complications were similar for both groups. No significant differences in disease recurrence rate and long-term survival were found between the laparoscopic and laparotomy groups (97.3% vs 93.3% and 83.9% vs 90.9%, respectively). No portal site metastases were noted. There was no difference in duration of surgery between the two groups. Malur et al. (308) explain this by an extensive exposure by laparoscopic surgery and laparoscopic lymphadenectomy in their team over the past 5 years which helped to save time. They also found a significantly shorter duration of hospital stay in the laparoscopic group, which also has been reported by others (242,304–306). Malur et al.'s (308) conclusion was that laparoscopic staging combined with laparoscopically assisted vaginal hysterectomy can be recommended for the treatment of women with endometrial cancer, offering a less invasive approach that is associated with less intraoperative and postoperative morbidity.

Although laparoscopically assisted surgical staging may provide an alternative approach to the management of endometrial cancer, its equivalence to the standard laparotomy approach remains unproven. The GOG is conducting a randomized trial of these two approaches to answer this question (GOG LAP-2).

Although results of long-term survival in laparoscopically treated endometrial cancer patients are still pending (309), some issues such as the risk of port site metastasis (310–312) and the higher incidence of positive peritoneal cytology (59) have been raised that weaken the enthusiasm for this technique. In this context, attempts to explore less invasive transabdominal incisions combining the specific advantages of each technique could represent a valid alternative to laparoscopy. For instance, a pilot study of minilaparotomy (length of incision from 4 to 10 cm) in patients with FIGO stage I–IV endometrial cancer has been studied by Fagotti et al. (309). Of 50 consecutive patients, 26 (52%) were considered eligible for minilaparotomy. All patients underwent total abdominal hysterectomy, bilateral salpingo-oophorectomy, and pelvic lymphadenectomy with and without omental and peritoneal biopsy. A mean number of 28 pelvic lymph nodes were removed. The complication rate was low. The mean hospital stay was 3.4 days. Intraoperative and postoperative parameters were compared to laparotomy controls and literature data on laparoscopy showing substantially comparable results. Fagotti et al. show that this technique offers the patients a cost-effective procedure that avoids many of the potential complications of standard therapy, prevents long hospital recovery periods, and accomplishes all of the important goals of standard recommendations.

Vaginal hysterectomy has often been cited as the simplest and least morbid approach to hysterectomy, with similar treatment outcomes in patients with clinical stage I endometrial cancer (313–316). It is often used as an alternative to an abdominal approach in obese and poor surgical–risk patients (317,318). Limitations include the lack of exploration of the intraperitoneal cavity, inability to procure cytologic washings, greater difficulty in performing an oophorectomy, and inability to perform lymph node sampling. Lymph node metastasis is related to such high-risk features as poor differentiation, unfavorable histologic subtypes, and deep myometrial invasion (302). Although it is true that risk of extrauterine disease can be estimated based on grade of tumor, accurate assessment requires surgical staging. Understaging in clinical stage I disease has been reported to occur in 19% to 22% of cases (319).

Adjuvant Treatment

A postoperative treatment plan should take into account the prognostic factors determined by the surgicopathologic staging. Patients can be classified to three categories: those who show a high rate of cure without postoperative therapy, those who yield a low rate of cure without postoperative therapy, and those who demonstrate a reduced rate of surgical cure but may or may not benefit from additional therapy.

The postoperative treatment plan should also consider the available postoperative treatment methods and their coincident morbidities. Chemotherapy as adjuvant treatment for patients with stages III and IV endometrial carcinoma has been recently supported as an alternative by data from the GOG study 122 and is discussed separately there in the section on adjuvant chemotherapy (6). The most pertinent question that is under active investigation is whether chemotherapy given sequentially or concomitantly with radiation therapy is superior to either modality alone.

ADJUVANT RADIATION THERAPY

Radiation therapy plays a significant role in the management of endometrial cancer. It is often used as an adjuvant treatment after surgery or as definitive treatment for patients who are medically inoperable or with local recurrence. In the past, most patients were treated with preoperative intracavitary brachytherapy with or without external beam radiotherapy followed by hysterectomy. This approach is not without its merit, especially in patients with gross cervical involvement. However, most patients nowadays undergo surgery first; then, depending on the prognostic features obtained from the pathology review, the need for radiotherapy is determined.

Early-Stage Disease

Most of the data on adjuvant radiation in endometrial cancer pertain to patients with early-stage (I-II) disease. The role of radiation in this group of patients, however, has been undergoing significant scrutiny is the last 5 years. Most of the debate focuses on the benefit of adjuvant radiation and to a lesser extent on the type of radiation that needs to be used.

Benefit of Adjuvant Radiation

Two recent prospective randomized trials compared surgery alone to surgery and postoperative external beam radiation. The first trial was conducted by the GOG (study 99) and presented only in abstract form where 390 patients with stage IB-IIB endometrial cancer who underwent total abdominal hysterectomy/bilateral salpingo-oophorectomy (TAH/BSO) and pelvic/paraaortic lymph node sampling were randomized to observation (n = 200) or postoperative pelvic radiation (n = 190) to a total dose of 50.4 Gy in 28 fractions (320). With a median follow-up of 56 months, the 3-year survival rate was 96% in the radiation arm compared with 89% in the observation arm (p = .09). The 2-year estimated progression-free survival rate was 96% versus 88% in favor of the irradiation arm (p = .004). Specifically, the rate of vaginal/pelvic recurrence was 9% in the surgery alone arm compared to 2% in the radiation arm. The second trial was the Postoperative Radiation in Endometrial Cancer (PORTEC) study where 714 patients with stage IB grade 2,3 and IC grade 1,2 were randomized after TAH/BSO and no lymph nodes sampling to observation (n = 360) or pelvic radiation (n = 354) to a total dose of 46 Gy in 23 fractions (321). With a median follow-up of 52 months, the 5-year vaginal/pelvic recurrence rate was 4% in the radiation arm compared to 14% in the observation arm (p <.001). The corresponding 5-year survival rates were 81% and 85%, respectively (p = .37).

Despite the fact that adjuvant radiation significantly improved locoregional control, most of the debate focuses on the lack of improvement in overall survival. Obviously the endpoint of overall survival is the gold standard for any randomized trial in cancer, but when dealing with early-stage endometrial cancer, the data should be interpreted with caution. First, because of relatively high incidence of other comorbidities such as hypertension, diabetes mellitus, and obesity as well as other cancers, the chance of dying from an intercurrent illness is as high if not higher than dying from endometrial cancer. In the RT arm of the PORTEC trial (322), the 8-year mortality rate from endometrial cancer was 9.6% compared to 14.4% from other causes and 5.3% from other cancers. In the no-RT group, the corresponding rates were 7.5%, 10.6%, and 5.3%. Similar data are emerging from GOG study 99. Thus, it is clear that the competing causes of death in this group of patients who have a low-mortality rate to start with make overall survival a very elusive endpoint to attain. Second, many of the patients who develop local recurrence after surgery alone are salvaged with subsequent radiation. Therefore, if we were to hypothesize that, in the surgery-alone group, salvage radiation was not offered to those who failed, then the overall survival might have been lower than that in the radiation therapy group. Third, even in patients who die from endometrial cancer, the most common cause is distant rather than local relapse. In the PORTEC trial, the 8-year mortality rate from local versus distant relapse was 1.1% and 7.9%, respectively, in the RT group and 2% and 5.2% in the surgery-alone group (322). It is unrealistic to expect a local treatment modality

such as radiation to alter this pattern of relapse. All these issues need to be considered when assessing the benefit of adjuvant radiation. Such debate is not new in the field of oncology, but it is important to note that other oncologists treating cancers of the breast or rectum, to name a few, when faced with similar results from prospective randomized trials, have recognized the importance of a multimodality approach.

Type of Radiation

There are two types of radiation (intravaginal brachytherapy or pelvic external beam radiation) that could be used either alone or in combination for early-stage endometrial cancer. Over the last three decades, the debate about the type of radiation to use has undergone a full circle. In the 1970s and mid 1980s, there was a shift from intravaginal brachytherapy alone to pelvic radiation plus intravaginal brachytherapy. Then in the late 1980s and early 1990s, there was a shift toward pelvic radiation alone. More recently, and with the increase in surgical lymph node staging, there has been a resurgence in the use of intravaginal brachytherapy alone.

Intravaginal Brachytherapy Alone or Combined with Pelvic Radiation. Aalders et al. (323) reported on 540 patients with stage IB-IC endometrial cancer who underwent TAH/BSO without lymph node sampling and postoperative intravaginal brachytherapy to 60 Gy to the vaginal mucosa. The patients then were randomized to observation (n = 277) or to supplemental pelvic radiation to 40 Gy (n = 263). A significant reduction in local recurrence rates was seen with the addition of pelvic radiation (1.9% vs 6.9%; p <.01). With regard to overall survival, there was no significant difference between the two arms of the study, but in the subset of patients with grade 3 disease and deep myometrial penetration, there was a survival advantage (cause-specific survival) of 18% versus 7% in favor of the pelvic radiation arm (323). The data from this trial somewhat contributed to the shift in treatment policies from intravaginal brachytherapy alone to external beam pelvic radiation.

Pelvic Radiation Alone or Combined with Intravaginal Brachytherapy. Greven et al. (324) reviewed the experience of two institutions in order to compare the outcome of the two approaches. In that study, there were 270 patients with stage I-II endometrial cancer: 173 were treated with postoperative pelvic radiation alone and 97 with a combination of intravaginal and pelvic radiation (324). The corresponding 5-year pelvic control and disease-free survival rates were 96% versus 93% (p = .32) and 88% versus 83% (p = .41). This study as well as others called into question whether the addition of vaginal radiation is needed (325,326). A number of other reports (327,328), however, suggest that vaginal vault radiation can be added to pelvic radiation with minimal morbidity and a very low rate of recurrences. Of interest, the two randomized trials (320,321) comparing surgery to adjuvant radiation both employed pelvic radiation alone with a local recurrence of only 2% to 4%.

Intravaginal Brachytherapy Alone. With the increase in surgical lymph node staging, the use of postoperative intravaginal brachytherapy alone regained its appeal, the rationale being that full surgical lymph node staging could potentially eliminate the need for pelvic radiation, whereas vaginal brachytherapy could still address the risk of vaginal cuff recurrence. Several reports in the past 5 years indeed showed a very low rate of recurrence either in the vagina or in the pelvis with such an approach (329–331).

From the above discussion, it is clear that the options available for patients with early-stage endometrioid endometrial cancer are numerous. Perhaps it is better to consider different options based on following factors. First, according to stage and grade; second, whether surgical lymph node staging was done; and third, based on the risk of nodal versus vaginal recurrence.

Stage IA Grade 1,2. The risk of pelvic lymph node positivity (151) is ≤3% and the 5-year progression-free survival rate in this group is of the order of 95% to 98%. It is unlikely that postoperative pelvic external beam radiation would add anything to the final outcome, and therefore radiation is not routinely recommended to this group of patients (327,332). The role of intravaginal radiation in these patients is also of questionable benefit because of an almost negligible risk of vaginal recurrence with surgery alone. Straughn et al. reported no vaginal recurrence in 103 patients with stage IA grade 1,2 treated with surgery alone (333).

Stage IA Grade 3. In GOG study 33, there were only eight patients with stage IA grade 3 disease, making it difficult to draw any meaningful conclusion (151). There were no relapses in the three patients receiving postoperative radiation as compared with one failure in the five patients who received no postoperative therapy. The risk of lymph node metastasis in this group of patients is negligible. Straughn et al. reported on eight patients with stage IA grade 3 disease treated with surgery alone, with two of patients developing isolated vaginal recurrence (333). Thus, these patients could be offered either intravaginal brachytherapy alone or observation.

Stage IB Grade 1,2. This group of patients constitutes the most common stage subgroup of all endometrial cancers. The outcome of patients who have lymph node dissection and no adjuvant radiation seems to be very good. Straughn et al. reported on 296 patients with IB grade 1,2 and found only nine (3%) vaginal recurrences and one (0.3%) pelvic recurrence (333). In comparison, data from Memorial Sloan–Kettering Cancer Center (MSKCC) on 233 patients with IB grade 1,2 showed a vaginal recurrence rate of only 1% and pelvic recurrence of 2% using postoperative intravaginal brachytherapy alone without routine surgical lymph node staging (334). Other investigators reported a vaginal recurrence rate of 0% to 1% and pelvic recurrence rate of 1% to 2% also using intravaginal brachytherapy (335–337).

Horowitz et al. reported on 62 patients who had surgical lymph node staging and received adjuvant intravaginal brachytherapy. There was one (1.6%) vaginal recurrence and no pelvic recurrence (329). Based on the data from the randomized trial by Aalders et al., it seems that pelvic radiation is not needed in this group of patients even without surgical lymph node staging. When the subset of patients with stage IB grade 1,2 was evaluated (n = 257), the rate of local recurrence either in the vagina or pelvis was 4% (5/126) in those treated with intravaginal brachytherapy alone compared to 2.3% (3/131) for those treated with brachytherapy and external radiation (323).

Thus, it seems reasonable to suggest that either observation or intravaginal brachytherapy (irrespective of surgical staging) is a reasonable option. But when deciding on whether adjuvant radiation is needed, it is important to address two issues. First, older patients tend to have higher rates of relapse. In the study by Straughn et al., eight of the ten vaginal/pelvic recurrences were in patients ≥60 years old (333). Second, often the indications for adjuvant radiation are rather arbitrarily based on the amount of myometrial invasion defined in thirds and on whether the tumor is grade 1 versus 2. Yet, the amount of myometrial invasion in this group of patients and whether an endometrial cancer is assigned as grade 1 as opposed to 2 in general does not appear to be a significant predictor of outcome (338,339).

Stage IB Grades 3-IC and 1,2,3. Up until the last 5 years, most of data in the literature on this group of patients were based on pelvic radiation either alone or in combination with intravaginal brachytherapy (326,327,340,341). But with the increase in surgical lymph node staging, a shift is occurring with regard to the role of radiation for stage IB grade 3 and even in stage IC disease. Therefore, the treatment decision is primarily based on whether the patient had surgical lymph node staging. The adequacy of the lymph node sampling/dissection should, at a minimum, meet the GOG guidelines of sampling the obturator, external iliacs, internal iliacs, common iliacs, and paraaortic lymph node stations.

Surgically Staged Patients. A recent multiinstitutional review of 220 patients with stage IC endometrial cancer by Straughn et al. compared adjuvant radiation to no radiation in patients with negative nodes on surgical staging (342). The investigators concluded that adjuvant radiation is not needed even though the 5-year disease-free survival was 74.5% for those treated with surgery alone compared to 92.5% for those treated with adjuvant radiation (*p* = .0134). It is unlikely that observation alone, even in those patients with full surgical staging, will be accepted by the radiation oncology community or even the patients when they see an 18% statistically significant difference in disease-free survival from a retrospective study in which most likely those patients with the worst prognostic features were the ones who received radiation.

A better alternative to observation in those patients who had surgical lymph node staging is intravaginal brachytherapy alone. Horowitz et al. reported on 81 patients with IB grade 3-IC who were treated with surgery including lymph node dissection followed by high-dose–rate intravaginal brachytherapy. Of the 81 patients, only 2 (2.4%) had vaginal recurrence and only 1 (1%) had pelvic recurrence (329). Chada et al. and Fanning reported on 38 and 39 patients, respectively, who were treated in a similar fashion. There was no vaginal or pelvic recurrence in either study (343, 344).

No Surgical Lymph Node Staging. In those patients with stage IB grade 3-IC without surgical lymph node staging, intravaginal brachytherapy alone does not seem to be adequate. In the Aalders et al. randomized trial, the rate of local recurrence in the subset of patients with IB grade 3 to IC was 9.3% (13/137) for those treated with brachytherapy alone compared to 1.3% (2/146) for those treated with brachytherapy and external radiation (323). This is not surprising since no lymph node sampling was done in that trial.

Whether intravaginal brachytherapy needs to be added to external beam therapy in this group of patients is debatable. Weiss et al. reported on 61 patients with stage IC endometrial cancer who were treated with postoperative pelvic radiation alone. With a median follow-up of 69.5 months, there was only one recurrence in the pelvis (1.6%). Their review of the published data from the literature on patients with stage IC showed a pelvic recurrence of 1.04% in 240 patients treated with pelvic radiation alone compared to 0.97% in 301 patients treated with pelvic and intravaginal radiation. Their conclusion was that pelvic radiation alone is sufficient, and effort should focus instead on trying to reduce the risk of distant relapse in this group of patients (345).

Stage II. It is important to recognize the distinction between gross and occult cervical involvement in endometrial cancer. Gross cervical involvement increases the risk of parametrial extension as well as spread to pelvic lymph nodes in a fashion similar to primary cervical cancer. Therefore, it should not be surprising that the treatment recommendations are similar. Patients with gross cervical involvement from endometrial cancer could undergo radical hysterectomy and pelvic lymph node dissection or preoperative radiation including pelvic radiation and intracavitary brachytherapy followed by simple hysterectomy. For occult cervical involvement, the treatment often consists of simple hysterectomy with or without lymph node surgical staging and adjuvant radiation. The type of radiation most often utilized is pelvic radiation and intravaginal brachytherapy. Pitson et al. reported on 120 patients treated with such a combination (346). The 5-year disease-free survival rate was 68% and the rate of pelvic relapse was 5.8% (7/120). There are also emerging data on the role of intravaginal brachytherapy alone in patients with occult cervical involvement who also had surgical lymph node staging. The rate of pelvic recurrence in four such series ranged from 0% to 6%, but the data need confirmation on a larger number of patients and longer follow-up (329,336,344,347).

Advanced-Stage Disease

This group of patients with advanced-stage disease is very heterogenous, with survival rates that range from about 10% for those with stage IVB to almost 95% for those with isolated positive pelvic washing.

Stage IIIA Disease (Positive Cytology)

In this subset of patients, the presence of other adverse features such as aggressive histologies or deep myometrial invasion should be determined first. If they are present, then the patients should be considered to be in a true advanced stage and be treated as such. On the other hand, if they are absent, then the true prognostic value of positive peritoneal cytology is still unclear (348). The literature regarding the benefits of treatment in this setting is mixed; even if treatment is beneficial, the appropriate modality still has to be defined. Based on the concept that the entire peritoneal cavity is at risk, intraperitoneal radioactive colloidal ^{32}P has been used by some with results that were better than in historic controls (349). Eltabbakh et al. reported on 27 patients with FIGO grade 1,2 and <50% myometrial invasion who were treated with intravaginal brachytherapy and megestrol acetate (Megace). None of the patients relapsed or died from their disease. Megace was given for 1 year, and at the end of therapy, 24 patients underwent second-look laparoscopy and peritoneal cytology. In 23 patients, the cytology was negative and the remaining patient, with persistent positive cytology, received an additional year of Megace after which cytology was confirmed to be negative (350). Unfortunately, there was no control group in this study to determine the true influence of Megace.

Stage IIIA Disease (Positive Adnexa or Serosa)

The outcome of patients with isolated adnexal involvement treated with pelvic radiation is reasonably good. Connell et al. reported on 12 patients treated with postoperative pelvic radiation with a 5-year disease-free survival of 70.9%. The weighted average of 5-year disease-free and overall survival rates from literature review in that study was 78.6% and 67.1%, respectively (351). Patients with isolated serosal involvement do worse than those with isolated adnexal involvement. Ashman et al. reported on 15 patients with isolated serosal involvement who were treated with pelvic radiation (352). The 5-year disease-free survival was only 41.5%.

Stage IIIB (Vaginal Involvement)

Vaginal involvement is a very uncommon presentation; these patients are usually not surgical candidates and are generally treated with definitive radiation including a combination of external beam and intracavitary/interstitial radiotherapy tailored to the extent of their disease (353).

Stage IIIC

If pelvic node involvement is the only major risk factor, treatment with postoperative pelvic radiotherapy can yield a 60% to 72% long-term survival rate in these patients (354–356). Patients with stage IIIC disease, by virtue of paraaortic node involvement, represent a particularly high-risk group. Following surgery, these patients are generally treated with extended field radiation to encompass the pelvis and the paraaortic regions. With this aggressive approach, several investigators have reported 30% to 40% survival rates in small patient populations (357–359).

The recognition that a significant number of patients with stage III disease fail in the abdomen (354,360) has prompted a number of investigators to evaluate whole abdominal radiotherapy in these patients (361,362). The GOG also did a pilot study (GOG study 94) on patients with maximally debulked stages III and IV disease using whole abdominal radiotherapy to a total dose of 30 Gy at 1.5 Gy per fraction followed by a pelvic boost for additional 19.8 Gy at 1.8 Gy per fraction. The 3-year disease-free and overall survival rates for the 77 patients with stage III-IV typical adenocarcinoma were 35% and 31%, respectively; for the 88 patients with stage III-IV papillary serous and clear-cell carcinoma, 3-year disease-free and overall survival rates were 31% and 33%, respectively (363). Using a different technique capable of delivering higher doses of radiation to the areas at risk for relapse in the abdomen, Stewart et al. reported 5-year disease-free and overall survival rates of 62% and 67%, respectively, in 62 patients with stage III endometrioid adenocarcinoma (364).

Stage IV

Stage IV disease usually has a dismal outcome, with survival rates in the range of 5% to 15%. Even in patients with tumor that can be thoroughly and optimally debulked, the results of whole abdominal radiation are still much inferior to those with stage III (362). In the above-mentioned GOG trial 94, there were 19 patients with stage IV endometrioid adenocarcinoma treated with whole abdomen radiation after maximal debulking. The 3-year disease-free and overall survival rates were far lower than were seen among stage III patients (G. P. Sutton, personal communication).

SPECIAL SITUATIONS

Medically Inoperable Stage I-II

Patients with medically inoperable uterine cancer are usually treated in a fashion similar to those with cervical cancer by using intracavitary applicators with or without pelvic ra-

diation. For patients with clinical stage I grade 1 or 2 and no evidence of myometrial invasion or lymph node metastasis on MRI, intracavitary brachytherapy alone is sufficient. Usually a Fletcher-Suit or Henschke applicator with one or two tandems (depending on uterus size) and ovoids is used to deliver 70 to 75 Gy to point A. The loading of the tandems is usually different than that in cervical cancer. This is done in order to provide wider coverage of the uterus laterally and superiorly. When pelvic radiation is added, the dose is usually 45 to 50 Gy supplemented with 30 to 35 Gy from intracavitary brachytherapy to bring the total dose to point A to 80 to 85 Gy. Rouanet et al. (365) treated 250 patients with endometrial cancer according to this approach, which yielded a 5-year disease-specific survival of 76.5%. An alternative brachytherapy approach would be to use the Hymen or Simon afterloading system that consists of multiple Teflon tubes that are inserted into the uterine cavity. With such a treatment approach, Grigsby et al. (366) reported that the 5-year progression-free survival rate of patients with clinical stage I disease treated with a combination of external and intracavitary radiotherapy was 94% for grade 1 disease, 92% for grade 2 disease, and 78% for grade 3 disease. More recently, high-dose–rate brachytherapy is also being employed (367,368).

SEROUS AND CLEAR-CELL HISTOLOGIES

Serous cancer and to a lesser extent clear-cell cancer tend to spread in a fashion similar to ovarian cancer with a high propensity for upper abdominal relapse. Therefore, whole abdomen radiation has been extensively studied in this group of patients (369). Lim et al. (270a) reported on 78 patients with stage I-IIIA papillary serous carcinoma: 58 were treated with whole abdomen radiation and 20 were not. The corresponding 5-year disease-specific survival rates were 74.9% and 41.3%, respectively ($p = .04$). In GOG study 94, the 3-year disease-free and overall survival for the 60 patients with stage III papillary serous or clear-cell carcinomas was 40.9% and 45.0%, respectively (363). The data on whole abdomen are somewhat encouraging, but the rate of relapse is still substantial, indicating the need for effective systemic therapy.

RADIATION THERAPY TECHNIQUES

Intravaginal Brachytherapy

The purpose of this treatment modality is to deliver the highest dose of radiation to the vaginal mucosa while limiting the dose to the surrounding normal structures such as the bladder, rectum, and small intestines. Intravaginal brachytherapy could be delivered with low-dose-rate ^{137}Cs sources, which requires admission to the hospital for a few days. The dose is usually 60 Gy prescribed to the vaginal mucosa or 30 to 35 Gy prescribed to 0.5 cm depth from the vaginal mucosa. The type of applicator used is generally the two ovoids from a Fletcher-Suit applicator, where only the vaginal cuff is irradiated. Alternatively, a cylinder could be used to treat one-half to two-thirds of the length of the vagina. Occasionally, the whole length of the vagina needs to be treated, especially in patients with grade 3 tumors, which have the tendency for relapse in the distal periurethral region. High-dose–rate brachytherapy using ^{192}Ir sources has been shown to be an attractive alternative to low-dose–rate brachytherapy. The treatment is given on an outpatient basis without the need for anesthesia and without the radiation exposure to medical personnel. At MSKCC, patients start their treatment 4 to 6 weeks postoperatively depending on the vaginal cuff healing. The treatment is given in three fractions of 7 Gy to a total dose of 21 Gy. The interval between each fraction is 1 to 2 weeks. The dose is prescribed to 0.5 cm depth from the mucosal surface. The treatment is usually delivered using a 3-cm diameter cylinder to treat one-half to two-thirds of the length of the vagina or the whole vagina in grade 3 tumors. Occasionally, the dose per fraction is lowered to 6 Gy instead of 7 Gy if the diameter of the cylinder is less than 3 cm. This is usually done to avoid a very high dose of radiation to the vaginal mucosa. The dose per fraction is also lowered to 4 to 5 Gy when pelvic radiation is added.

External Beam Radiation

Pelvic Radiation

Most patients are treated in the postoperative setting. At the time of simulation, the small bowel is opacified using oral contrast, a vaginal marker is used to define the vaginal cuff, and the rectum is opacified with barium or CT-compatible contrasts. Patients are usually placed in the prone position to displace the small intestines from the radiation field. The target volume consists of the pelvic lymph nodes, including obturator, external, internal, and lower common iliac groups, and the proximal two-thirds of the vagina. High-energy linear accelerators (15 MV) are preferred because of their sparing of the skin and subcutaneous tissue. The ideal beam arrangement with conventional radiation is the four-field pelvic-box technique to reduce the dose to the small intestines and to some extent the bladder and rectum. For the anteroposterior/posteroanterior (AP/PA) fields, the superior border is L5-S1, the inferior border is the bottom of the obturator foramina, and the lateral border is 2 cm beyond the widest point of the inlet of the true bony pelvis. For the lateral fields, the anterior border is in front of the pubis symphysis and the posterior border at least at S2–3. The superior and inferior borders are the same for the AP/PA fields. All fields are treated daily to a dose of 1.8 Gy. A total dose of 50.4 Gy is generally used when pelvic radiation is used alone or 45 Gy when combined with intravaginal brachytherapy.

Extended Field

This technique is mainly used for patients with documented positive paraaortic nodes. The preferred approach is the four-field box technique in order to lower the dose to the small intestines. However, attention should be paid to the dose that the kidneys might receive with the four-field arrangement. The lower border is the same as in pelvic radiation but the upper border is extended usually to the T11-T12 interspace. The typical dose is 45.0 Gy at 1.8 Gy or 1.5 Gy if patients develop acute gastrointestinal toxicity.

Whole Abdomen Radiation

The standard approach is AP/PA open fields with five HVL kidney blocks placed over the PA field only (if patient is lying supine) from the start of the treatment. The dose is usually 30.0 Gy at 1.5 Gy per fraction followed by 19.8 Gy boost to the pelvis at 1.8 Gy per fraction. The upper border is usually placed 1 cm above the diaphragm, and the lateral borders should extended beyond the peritoneal reflections. The lower border is usually at the bottom of the obturator foramen.

Complications of Radiation

Pelvic Radiation

In the PORTEC randomized trial (370), the overall (grades 1 to 4) rate of late complications was 26% in the RT group compared to 4% in the observation group ($p < .0001$). Most of the late complications in the RT group, however, were grades 1,2 (22%) and only 3% were grades 3,4. It is also important to note that many patients in this trial were treated with AP/PA fields in which the overall rate of complications was 30% compared to 21% for those treated with the four-field box ($p = .06$).

Whole Abdomen Radiation

The toxicity of whole abdomen radiation is more pronounced than that of pelvic radiation but not as high as expected. In GOG study 94, the rate of grade 4 gastrointestinal toxicity was seen in six patients (3.8%). Severe liver toxicity was seen in 3 of 158 evaluable patients (2%) with 2 of 3 recovering without sequelae. There were no grades 3,4 genitourinary toxicity (363).

Intravaginal Brachytherapy

The main advantage of intravaginal brachytherapy is its ability to deliver a relatively high dose of radiation to the vagina while limiting the dose to the surrounding normal structures such as the bowels and bladder. This advantage is manifested with the low rate of severe late toxicity seen with this treatment technique, ranging from 0% to 1% (329,

334,337). But such a very low rate of severe complications cannot be taken for granted because special attention needs to be paid to the depth of prescription, the dose per fraction, the length of vagina treated, and the diameter of the cylinder used (371).

ADJUVANT CHEMOTHERAPY

The role of adjuvant chemotherapy in the treatment of patients with endometrial cancer is evolving. Historically, adjuvant cytotoxic chemotherapy had only been studied in one large randomized trial (372). After surgical staging and TAH/BSO, the GOG treated 181 patients having poor prognostic factors with postoperative pelvic and paraaortic (if node positive) irradiation. In a random design, 92 patients were further treated with intravenous doxorubicin every 3 weeks to a total dose of 500 mg/m^2, and 89 patients received no further therapy (controls). At 5 years of observation, there was no difference in recurrence rates between the two groups.

Since extrapelvic failure is common in women with high-risk endometrial cancer, the impact of adjuvant radiation therapy on survival is limited. To address the issue of systemic failure, researchers at the M.D. Anderson Cancer Center re-treated 62 high-risk patients prospectively with adjuvant cisplatin (50 mg/m^2), doxorubicin (50 mg/m^2), and cyclophosphamide (500 mg/m^2), given every 4 weeks for six courses. Burke and colleagues (373) considered patients eligible for study if they had grade 2 disease with outer one-third or mid myometrial invasion, grade 3 tumor with any invasion, completely resected extrauterine disease, or high-risk histologies (clear-cell or papillary serous cancer). Actuarial 3-year survival was 82% for patients with disease confined to the uterus compared to 46% for those with extrauterine spread. Although adjuvant chemotherapy did not prevent distant failures in women with extrauterine disease, the survival rate for those with disease confined to the uterus was greater than expected.

The most significant development regarding the potential importance of chemotherapy comes with the initial reported results of GOG trial 122 in abstract form (6). This study randomized patients with surgical stage III or IV disease to whole abdominal irradiation versus doxorubicin and cisplatin chemotherapy. Pelvic and paraaortic lymph node sampling was optional if stage III or IV by other criteria. If paraaortic nodes were sampled and positive, negative scalene biopsy and chest CT were required. All patients underwent maximal debulking with no residual site >2 cm. Whole abdominal radiotherapy consisted of 30 Gy in 20 daily fractions of 150 cGy followed by a 15-Gy boost to the pelvis and to the paraaortic nodes if they were positive or not sampled. Chemotherapy consisted of doxorubicin 60 mg/m^2 and cisplatin 50 mg/m^2 every 21 days for eight courses. Doxorubicin was not given on cycle 8 to limit total anthracycline exposure to 420 mg/m^2. The primary endpoint was progression-free survival with overall survival and toxicity as secondary endpoints. Four hundred and twenty-two patients were randomized, with 396 patients analyzed. Patients were balanced with regard to stage, KPS, histology, and age. No other strata were included. Serous histology was present in approximately 20% in each arm. Therapy was completed in 84% (WART) versus 63% (chemotherapy). Toxicity was more prevalent in the chemotherapy arm with grades 3,4 toxicity: WBC 4% versus 62%, gastrointestinal 13% versus 20%, neurologic <1% versus 7%, and treatment-related deaths n = 4 versus 8. Progression-free and overall survival favored the chemotherapy-treated group: progression-free survival HR = 0.81 (CI 0.63 to 1.05) and overall survival HR 0.71 (CI 0.54 to 0.94) (6). Although these data establish a potential role for chemotherapy in the adjuvant treatment of patients with endometrial cancer, additional study is required to determine if an added benefit is present from combining chemotherapy with radiotherapy either sequentially or concomitantly. GOG study 184 is currently evaluating tumor volume–directed pelvic (with or without paraaortic) radiation followed by cisplatin and doxorubicin or by cisplatin, doxorubicin, and paclitaxel for patients with similar characteristics as in the above-mentioned GOG study 122; and pilot studies are determining tolerated doses and schedules for the concomitant use of platinum and taxane-based chemotherapy with both pelvic and whole abdominal radiotherapy.

Initial studies showing tumor response to alpha-hydroxyprogesterone stimulated the development of many clinical trials of progestins for this malignancy. Since that time, progestins have been used for treatment of all disease stages, and several reviews of progestin therapy for endometrial carcinoma have been published (374). Early uncontrolled trials suggested that progestin therapy after initial therapy with surgery or radiation was associated with a decreased risk of recurrence in patients with clinical stage I or II endometrial carcinoma (374). To evaluate these observations, several large randomized trials have been performed. An initial multiinstitutional trial by Lewis and colleagues (290) compared 500 mg of medroxyprogesterone acetate versus placebo given intramuscularly once weekly for 14 weeks and showed a 9% recurrence rate at 4 years for both groups.

MacDonald and colleagues (199) randomized 429 patients whose initial treatment consisted of surgery and radiation therapy followed by progestin treatment (i.e., hydroxyprogesterone caproate for 5 days followed by oral medroxyprogesterone acetate for 5 years) or observation. The projected overall 5-year survival rate was 76% for both treated and control patients even after adjustment for prognostic factors. A third trial by Vergote and colleagues (292), employing 1,084 patients with early endometrial cancer treated initially with surgery and radiation, compared 1 g of hydroxyprogesterone caproate (Delalutin), given intramuscularly twice weekly for 1 year, to observation. After a median follow-up period of 72 months, crude survival and relapse rates were not statistically different between the two groups. Although the median survival of the group of patients with cancer-related death was higher in the progestin group (30 months) compared with the control group (22 months; $p = .03$), death due to intercurrent nonmalignant disease was higher in the progestin group ($p = .04$). More recently, Minckwitz et al. randomized 388 largely stage I or II patients to medroxyprogesterone or tamoxifen or observation. No differences between progression-free or overall survival were seen among any of the three groups (293).

Kneale and colleagues (375) pointed out the difficulty of randomized trials of adjuvant therapy in patients with early-stage disease. They observed that these patients have an expected survival rate of 75%, and that approximately 40% of the deaths in these patients are unrelated to malignancy. The detection of a treatment-related benefit in survival of even 5% would require randomization of almost 2,000 patients, an enrollment goal not met in any of the published studies. Nontheless, from these data, adjuvant progestin therapy cannot be recommended as standard management.

Postoperative Estrogen

The postoperative use of supplemental estrogen as treatment for menopausal symptoms and prophylaxis against osteoporosis and heart disease appears to be safe, although only small numbers of patients have been evaluated. In retrospective reports by Creasman et al. (376), Lee et al. (377), and Baker (378), a total of 122 patients with stage I disease received postoperative estrogen. Of these, only one patient had a tumor recurrence. The patients in these reports were not randomized. However, it appears that survival is not decreased by the postoperative use of estrogen in patients with early-stage disease. The American College of Obstetricians and Gynecologists Committee Opinion (379) concluded that in women with a history of endometrial carcinoma, estrogens could be used for the same indications as for any other woman except that the selection of appropriate candidates should be based on prognostic indicators and the risk the patient is willing to assume. A randomized trial is being conducted by the GOG to prove conclusively the safety of estrogen replacement in this group of patients.

POSTOPERATIVE SURVEILLANCE

The frequency and extent of follow-up visits and surveillance tests for patients with a history of gynecologic cancer have traditionally been based on arbitrary guidelines that have been established and perpetuated at various institutions throughout the United States. The recent changes in medicine occurring throughout the country have led to a reevaluation of standard medical practices. With managed care contracts now being awarded to low-cost providers, there is an increased incentive to determine the most cost-effective manner of providing care. Endometrial cancer is the most common gynecologic malignancy in the United States. Since the majority of patients with endometrial cancer will do well, and there is no clear evidence that early detection of disease recurrence will improve outcome, it has become necessary to reevaluate the practice of routine intensive surveillance in women with a history of endometrial cancer. Whereas patients with medical complications, unexplained symptoms, or evidence of recurrent tumor require intense follow-up, guidelines will need to be set up for healthy, asymptomatic women who have been potentially cured and who continue to remain clinically free of disease.

One important consideration is that postoperative follow-up also allows for the incorporation of a health maintenance program, including evaluation of blood pressure, breast examination, and stool guaiac. One important issue that needs to be addressed is the psychologic support that routine follow-up visits provide for the cancer patient. The value of this support may be impossible to measure objectively. Although the cost savings due to less intensive surveillance will be substantial, physicians need to continue to provide emotional support and reassurance to their patients. Combining patient education with interval nursing phone contact and prompt evaluation of symptoms may help provide a more cost-effective method of practice, while continuing to provide the emotional support that cancer patients need and deserve.

In 1992, Barnhill and colleagues (380) reported on the clinical surveillance programs employed in the follow-up of gynecologic cancer patients as noted from the results of a survey of 94 members of the Society of Gynecologic Oncologists. For the asymptomatic patient with no clinical evidence of disease, the majority of respondents reported seeing patients in the clinic every 3 months for the first year following surgery, every 3 to 4 months the second year, every 6 months for the next 3 years, then annually thereafter. In the majority of cases, physical examination included the breasts, abdomen, lymph node regions, and pelvis. Aside from performing a pelvic examination, 84% reported doing a Papanicolaou (Pap) smear at each visit. In terms of surveillance studies, 72% obtained annual chest radiographs for the first 2 years after surgery, and this decreased to approximately 50% for the next 4 years. CT scans were obtained annually by approximately one-third of respondents for the first 2 years following surgery, a figure that steadily declined thereafter. Although these follow-up practices are used widely, there is no rationale for any particular surveillance protocol based on examination sensitivity, cost effectiveness, or survival benefit. Salvesen et al. (381) followed 249 women with diagnosed and treated endometrial carcinoma for a median period of 9 years (range 4 to 16) or until death to identify women with increased risk for recurrent disease. Forty-seven patients had recurrent disease, 32 within the first 2 years. Ten of the recurrences were diagnosed at routine follow-up, but only four were asymptomatic. In their follow-up program, one asymptomatic recurrence was detected for every

653 routine consultations. Low-risk groups with FIGO stage IA/IB, or patients below 60 years of age at primary operation, were identified in multivariate recurrence-free survival analysis. No asymptomatic recurrences were found in this group.

Several publications have attempted to address the issue of postsurgical surveillance in patients with endometrial cancer in an effort to devise a more efficient and cost-effective method of following these patients (285,382–384). Specific attention was paid to the value of history and physical examination, Pap smears, chest radiographs, and the CA-125 tumor marker in detecting recurrent disease. A great deal can be learned from these studies and applied to the development of future strategies for following these patients.

History and Physical Examination

Combining the data from the four studies (285,382–384), 188 patients (14%) developed disease recurrence, with 78 (42%) having no associated symptoms. Eighty-one percent of all recurrences were detected by either symptoms or physical findings. In patients who were asymptomatic at the time of recurrence, approximately 52% had disease detected by physical examination. Therefore, only 37 patients (48% of 78) had their recurrent disease detected by other diagnostic tests. In the symptomatic patients, the most frequent presenting complaint was pain, either abdominal or pelvic, followed by weight loss/lethargy and vaginal bleeding. Podczaski et al. (383) reported that only 2 of 23 symptomatic patients experienced abnormal bleeding, whereas 19 of 40 patients had vaginal bleeding in the series by Shumsky et al. (384). Clearly, patient education regarding the signs and symptoms of recurrent disease should be incorporated into a surveillance program. Physicians should act promptly to evaluate symptomatic patients with diagnostic tests targeted toward the symptoms.

Papanicolaou Smear

According to Barnhill et al. (380), 84% of asymptomatic patients being followed for a history of gynecologic cancer undergo Pap smears at each visit. Again, reviewing the findings of the four (285,382–384) published surveillance series, only 13 of the 188 patients (6.9%) with recurrent disease were found to have suspicious vaginal cytology; however, this was an isolated finding not associated with an abnormal physical examination or symptoms in only five (2.7%) of these patients. Obtaining Pap smears routinely at each follow-up visit does not appear to be beneficial.

Chest Radiographs

Surveillance chest radiographs are obtained by the majority of gynecologic oncologists during the first 2 years following surgery for early-stage endometrial cancer. Recurrent disease was detected by chest radiography in 27 of 188

(14.4%) of the patients reported in the pooled series. Although chest radiographs can document the presence of distant recurrences, their impact is limited by the poor outcome of patients with pulmonary metastases. Virtually all of these patients will succumb to their disease. The intent of routine surveillance is to detect the 10% to 15% of recurrences following primary treatment for endometrial cancer, with the hope that early initiation of therapy will improve the outcome. In view of the lack of effective systemic therapy for endometrial cancer and the poor prognosis of patients with pulmonary metastases, routine surveillance chest radiographs cannot be recommended.

CA-125

Elevated levels of the tumor-associated antigen CA-125 have been documented in patients with advanced/recurrent endometrial cancer, and are correlated with the clinical course of disease (148,a1). Rose at al. (148) noted that CA-125 levels were elevated in 19 of 33 (58%) patients with recurrent endometrial cancer. Reddoch et al. (285) detected recurrence by an elevated serum CA-125 level in 6 of 23 (26%) asymptomatic patients. None of the patients achieved long-term survival, probably reflecting the association between an elevated CA-125 level and widespread disease. In view of the short lead time between CA-125 elevation and diagnosis of recurrence, the value of surveillance CA-125 levels is limited and best reserved for patients with an elevated value at initial diagnosis.

Recommendations

Based on the knowledge that the majority of recurrences occur within the first 3 years after surgery, it is recommended that patients undergo semiannual pelvic examinations for 3 years, then annually thereafter. There is no evidence in the literature that routine chest radiographs improve survival, and these studies appear to indicate that routine Pap smears do not improve the outcome of patients with isolated vaginal recurrences. Based on these data, obtaining annual Pap smears appears to be reasonable. Whether this should be continued annually after 3 years is debatable, and one may consider discontinuing annual Pap smears after that time in favor of an every-3-year policy. Serial CA-125 determinations should be performed in patients with elevated levels at the time of diagnosis or with known extrauterine disease, but there is no evidence that such monitoring will improve patient outcome. Salvesen et al.'s (381) conclusion was that low-risk women should be considered for an alternative, less frequent follow-up. This would allow more detailed investigation of the high-risk women. Salvesen et al. (381) have suggested randomized studies comparing the actual number of consultations, and in particular, quality of life for women with and without routine follow-up visits (which are needed in order to impove our knowledge on this issue).

TREATMENT OF RECURRENT DISEASE

Patients with recurrent endometrial cancer must be fully evaluated for sites of recurrent disease. Depending on the site of the recurrence and prior therapy, patients may be treated for palliation or for cure. Treatment may consist of irradiation, surgery, endocrine therapy, or cytotoxic chemotherapy. These agents may be used singly or in combination. It is uncommon for patients with recurrent disease to be cured unless the recurrence is only in the vaginal cuff (central pelvis). Therefore, close follow-up after primary therapy with pelvic examinations and Pap smears cannot be overemphasized.

Radiation Therapy

Radiation Therapy for Local Recurrence

Radiation therapy can be curative in a select group of patients with small vaginal recurrences who have not received prior radiation. The 5-year local control rate ranges from 42% to 65% and the 5-year overall survival rate from 31% to 53% (385–387). Creutzberg et al. reported on survival after relapse from the PORTEC randomized trial (322). In patients who were initially randomized to surgery alone (n = 46/360), the 5-year survival after vaginal relapse was 65%. But before adopting salvage radiation as a treatment policy for all early-stage endometrial cancer, a few aspects of this trial need to be addressed. First, the 5-year survival rate from the PORTEC trial is much higher than what is reported in the literature. Most likely, the vaginal recurrences in this trial were detected very early, unlike patients in the community. The extent and size of local recurrence in endometrial cancer are very significant predictors of outcome (385). Second, this high rate of salvage pertains only to isolated vaginal recurrence. The rate of survival at 3 years for pelvic recurrence in the PORTEC trial was 0%. Third, although the trial does not mention any data on complications, it is not unrealistic to expect a higher complication rate than what is normally seen with adjuvant radiation. With salvage radiation, external beam RT and brachytherapy are often combined and the doses of radiation required are much higher than those used with adjuvant radiation. A recent study from M. D. Anderson Cancer Center by Jhingran et al. clearly highlights these issues (388). They reported on 91 patients who were treated with definitive radiation for isolated vaginal recurrence. The 5-year local control and overall survival rates were 75% and 43%, respectively. The median dose of radiation was 75 Gy, which often included external radiation and brachytherapy. The rate of grade 4 complications (requiring surgery) was 9%. Thus, when talking with a patient about adjuvant radiation versus radiation reserved for salvage, these issues need to be addressed and compared to the excellent local control and low morbidity obtained with adjuvant intravaginal brachytherapy.

Surgical Therapy

Isolated pelvic central recurrence after irradiation is rare. If it does occur, selected patients may benefit from pelvic exenterative surgery (294). There are no large published series, but some long-term survivors have been reported. Barakat et al. (389) reported the MSKCC experience with 44 patients who underwent pelvic exenteration for recurrent endometrial cancer between 1947 and 1994. Primary therapy usually consisted of TAH/BSO, with most receiving either preoperative or postoperative radiation therapy. Prior to exenteration, 10 of 44 (23%) patients had never received any form of radiation. The median interval between initial surgery and exenteration was 28 months (range 2 to 189 months). Exenteration was total in 23 patients (52%), anterior in 20 patients (46%), and limited to posterior in one patient. One vascular injury led to the only intraoperative death. Major postoperative complications occurred in 35 (80%) patients and included intestinal/urinary tract fistulas, pelvic abscess, septicemia, pulmonary embolism, and cerebrovascular accident. Median survival for the entire group of patients was 7.36 months, with nine (20%) patients achieving long-term survival (>5 years). Although only 20% of patients achieved long-term survival, this procedure remains the only potentially curative option for the few patients with central recurrence of endometrial cancer who have failed standard surgery and radiation therapy (389).

Endocrine Therapy

Hormonal agents have been found to be valuable, particularly in the patient with recurrent disease, and reviews of their use have been extensively published (390). Response rates to a variety of endocrine agents including progestins, antiestrogens, and aromatase inhibitors are presented in Table 23.14 (200,391–397).

The overall response to progestins is approximately 25%. However, some trials demonstrate lower response rates, usually in the range of 15% to 20%. These studies generally used more rigorous response criteria and had multiinstitutional participation. A higher dose of progestin does not appear to increase the response rate. In one randomized trial of 200 mg/d versus 1000 mg/d of medroxyprogesterone acetate (MPA), the overall response rate was actually 25% versus 15% favoring the low-dose arm (398,399). The time to treatment failure and median overall survival of the low- versus high-dose regimen, respectively, were 3.2 versus 2.5 months and 11.1 versus 7.0 months, all showing no advantage for an increased dose. Prognostic factors related to response were performance status, grade, and progesterone receptor level. The response rate was only 8% in poorly differentiated tumors. A Phase II trial of high-dose megestrol (800 mg orally daily) in 63 patients was associated with a response rate of 24% overall, which is similar to lower-dose regimens with doses of 40 mg po qid. As in the majority of studies with

TABLE 23.14. *Response to endocrine therapy*

Hormonal agent	References	Average dose	Approximate response rate (%)	Response range (%)
Hydroxyprogesterone caproate (Delalutin)	393,394	1–3 g IM q wk	29	9–34
Medroxyprogesterone acetate (Provera)	200	200–1000 mg IM q wk or po qd	22	14–53
Megestrol acetate (Megace)	394	40–800 mg po qd	20	11–56
Tamoxifen (Nolvadex)	396,397	20–40 mg po qd	10	0–53
Goserelin acetate	391	3.6 mg SC q month	11	NA
Anastrozole (SERM)	395	1 mg po q d	9	NA
Arzoxifene (SERM)	392	20 mg po q d	31	NA

NA, not applicable.

hormonal agents, response rates were statistically higher in patients with grade 1 or 2 lesions (37%) versus grade 3 lesions (8%); $p = .02$ (400). In addition to grade, a long disease-free interval (exceeding 2 or 3 years) and positive estrogen or progesterone receptor status have all been associated with an increased frequency of response (200,393, 398,400). Age, location of metastatic disease, number of metastatic sites, prior therapy, and weight have also been analyzed by several investigators, but they have not been convincingly linked with response.

Tamoxifen has been investigated in patients with recurrent disease in several studies (396,398,401). Results have varied, but in general, response rates have been modest in untreated patients. A recent GOG study evaluated 68 patients with advanced or recurrent disease receiving tamoxifen at 20 mg po bid and showed an overall response rate of 10% (90% CI 5.7 to 17.9%). The median progression-free interval was short at 1.9 months (90% CI 1.7 to 3.2 months) and the overall survival was 8.8 months (90% CI 7.0 to 10.1 months). One small randomized Phase II study comparing megestrol acetate to megestrol acetate with tamoxifen showed no advantage in response rate for the combination, with response rates of 20% versus 19%, respectively (402). The lack of synergistic response is supported by observations of endometrial carcinoma treated in a nude mouse model. Tumors treated with medroxyprogesterone or tamoxifen plus medroxyprogesterone were devoid of progesterone receptor during the growth inhibitory and regrowth phase of the tumor resulting from receptor downregulation (403). The possibility of alternating tamoxifen with megestrol acetate in order to exploit the recruitment of progesterone receptors by tamoxifen was also evaluated in GOG study 153 and is reported in abstract form. Fifty-six patients eligible for toxicity and response were given megestrol acetate at 160 mg/d for 3 weeks alternating with tamoxifen 40 md po q d for 3 weeks. An overall response rate of 26.5% (90% CI 17.3 to 38.4) with a 21.4% complete response rate was seen, with the duration of response exceeding 20 months in 8 of 15 responders. The response rate was 38% for patients with grade 1 disease and 22% for those with grade 3 disease. Although these Phase II results are intriguing, a randomized study

would be required to determine if alternating hormones is superior to single-hormone approaches (404). Positive receptor status has been associated with improved disease-free and overall survival rates (205,223,374). These data indicate that the receptor status provides important biologic information and that receptor-positive tumors tend to be better differentiated and slower growing than are their receptor-negative counterparts. Chemotherapy had no effect on hormone receptor capacity in a nude mouse model of xenografted endometrial cancer (405). Other factors, such as changes in vaginal cytology during treatment (406), and results in the subrenal capsule chemosensitivity assay (407) and in the nude mouse model (408), may help predict response to progestins.

Several studies have evaluated gonadotropin-releasing hormone analogs in patients with metastatic endometrial cancer. Gallagher and others (409) noted one complete and five partial responses to leuprolide or goserelin in 17 patients (35% response; 95% CI, 13% to 58%) with metastatic disease. Of note, the duration of remission ranged from 7 to 30 months, and 14 of the 17 patients had been previously treated with progestins. Another report described four responses in seven postmenopausal patients with endometrial cancer treated with goserelin (410). *In vitro* studies in human endometrial cancer cell lines have suggested that such growth inhibition may have been due to apoptosis (411). The GOG recently studied goserelin at 3.6 mg subcutaneously monthly in 40 patients with advanced or recurrent disease. Seventy-one percent of patients had received prior radiotherapy. There were two complete (5%) and three partial (7%) responses with an overall response rate of 11% (95% CI 4% to 27%). Goserelin is felt to have limited activity in this patient population, and no additional single-agent studies are planned (391).

Investigation is underway in patients with uterine cancer to evaluate the activity of SERMs. These agents have ER-antagonist activity in breast and uterine tissues and ER-agonist activity in bone. The first reported study to date is from the GOG and evaluated anastrozole at 1 mg po daily orally in 23 unselected patients (i.e., 9 patients had grade 2 tumors and 14 patients had grade 3 tumors) A partial response rate of 9% was seen (90% CI 3% to 23%). It is noted that the partial response rate of 9% in this study is similar to the 8% reported in grade 3 patients treated with standard progestins (395,400). A more recent study evaluated the investigational SERM arzoxifene in 37 patients. Twenty-six patients were ER positive and 22 were PR positive. A response rate of 31% (95% CI 25% to 51%) was seen in this selected patient population with a median duration of response of 13.9 months (392). Additional study of these agents in patients with well-differentiated tumors is warranted (412).

CYTOTOXIC CHEMOTHERAPY

Both single-agent and combination regimens are capable of inducing objective responses, yet the median time to treatment failure is on average 3 to 6 months and the overall survival of patients with metastatic endometrial cancer is generally less than 12 months. The role of chemotherapy in the recurrent disease setting remains palliative, and minimizing side effects is of equal importance when selecting a regimen. Responses to treatment are usually partial and have lasted an average of only 3 to 6 months. Also, the time to progression in most trials tends to be short, ranging from 4 to 6 months, with median survival averaging 7 to 10 months. Patients with complete response may have long progression-free intervals lasting 1 to 2 years, but such patients comprise only a minority of those treated. Particularly for patients with grade 1 histology, or small-volume asymptomatic metastatic disease, hormonal therapy may provide better initial palliation, reserving chemotherapy for rapidly progressive or symptomatic disease (413,414).

Single-Agent Trials

The wide variety of single agents that have been tested are presented in Table 23.15 (208,288,397,398,415–452). Despite the number of drugs evaluated, the most commonly used single agents today based on response rates of at least 20% include cisplatin, carboplatin, doxorubicin, epirubicin, ifosfamide, and paclitaxel, and recently topotecan has been added to this list.

The response rate to cisplatin dosages of 50 to 60 mg/m^2 given every 3 weeks was similar in patients with prior (25%) (425,447) and no prior chemotherapy (21%) (423,440,449). Carboplatin given in dosages of 300 to 400 mg/m^2 every 4 weeks has been associated with response rates of 29% (420, 426,433), which is similar to cisplatin. Doxorubicin in dosages of 55 to 60 mg/m^2 has been associated with an overall response rate of 26% (430,445,450) and epirubicin with a response rate of 26% (421). Liposomal doxorubicin was recently reported in a GOG study of 46 patients receiving 50 mg/m^2 every 4 weeks with an overall response rate of 9.5% (95% CI 2.7% to 26%). It is important to note that 32 patients had received prior doxorubicin therapy. Therefore, although liposomal doxorubicin appears to have limited activity in anthracycline-pretreated patients, an ongoing study is evaluating its efficacy in patients without prior chemotherapy treatment (79). Of the antimetabolites, 5-fluorouracil given in dosages of 15 mg/kg for 5 consecutive days and then every other day until dose-limiting toxicity has displayed a 21% response rate in 34 patients, whereas methotrexate (453) and mercaptopurine (424) have been inactive. Vincristine given in a weekly schedule was associated with a response rate of 18% in 33 untreated patients (419), but dose-limiting neurotoxicity was substantial. In a Phase II trial of paclitaxel conducted by the GOG (415), 28 patients with recurrent or advanced endometrial cancer received a dose of 250 mg/m^2 every 21 days. Patients who had received prior pelvic irradiation were treated at an initial dose of 200 mg/m^2. Complete responses were noted in four patients (14%) and partial responses in six (21%) for an overall response rate of 36%. A more contemporary GOG study evaluated paclitaxel at 200 mg/m^2 (175 mg/m^2 with prior radiotherapy) every 3 weeks in pretreated patients showing an overall response rate of 27.3% (95% CI 15% to 42.8%). The median duration of response was 4.2 months with an overall survival of 10.3 months (7). A similar study showed a response rate of 43% (95% CI 6% to 80%) in patients who had all previously been treated with platinum-based therapy (454).

Topotecan was evaluated in a Phase II trial of untreated advanced or recurrent endometrial cancer administered initially at 1.5 mg/m^2 every day for 5 days every 3 weeks. The trial was suspended for toxicity, but reopened and completed at 1 mg/m^2 q day for 5 days (or 0.8 mg/m^2/d for patients with prior radiotherapy). An overall response rate of 20% was seen with median duration of response of 8.0 months and overall survival of 6.5 months (455).

The frequent variability in response rate noted for the same agent is probably related to several factors, including prior treatment, performance status, extent of disease, and the response criteria used for evaluation. No current data suggest that dose-response relationships exist for single-agent therapy, and doses and schedules are generally adjusted to minimize toxicity for an individual patient.

Combination Therapy

The results of treatment with combination regimens are presented in Table 23.16 (425,445,456–472). The first combination to be explored was cyclophosphamide with doxorubicin in four trials in chemotherapy-naive patients (445,460, 465,469) using doxorubicin dosages of 40 to 50 mg/m^2 repeated every 3 to 4 weeks. The objective response rates for these trials were similar to single-agent doxorubicin and showed no advantage for the addition of cyclophosphamide. The GOG also compared doxorubicin alone with the same dose and schedule of doxorubicin plus cyclophosphamide (470). All patients had failed progestin therapy, had measurable lesions, and had no prior chemotherapy. The complete and partial response rates for patients receiving the doxorubicin (132 patients) and combination regimens (144 patients)

TABLE 23.15. *Single-agent trials*

Agent (ref.)	n	Prior treatment	No. of CR + PR	(%)	95% CI
Alkylating Agents					
Cyclophosphamide (500)	37	Some	4	11	3–25
Chlorambucil (500)	11	NS	0	0	0–28
Ifosfamide (416,444)	56	Some	4 + 4	14	6–26
Hexamethylmelamine (439,446)	54	Few	2 + 7	17	8–29
Cisplatin					
No prior Rx (425,447)	63	No	3 + 10	21	11–33
Prior chemo (423,440,449)	64	Yes	3 + 13	25	15–37
Carboplatin (420,426,433)	82	No	5 + 18	28	19–39
Anthracyclines/anthraquinones					
Doxorubicin (430,445,450)	161	No	18 + 24	26	19–34
Epirubicin (421)	27	No	2 + 5	26	11–46
Liposomal doxorubicin (79)	42	Yes	0 + 4	9.5	2.7–22.6
Pirarubicin (422)	28	7	2 + 0	7	1–30
Mitoxantrone (417,428,437)	46	32	0 + 2	4	1–15
Antimetabolites					
Fluorouracil (500)	34	NS	7	21	9–38
Methotrexate (453)	33	No	1 + 1	6	2–20
6-Mercaptopurine (424)	10	NS	0	0	0–31
Vincas/epipodophyllotoxins					
Vincristine (419,431)	38	5	1 + 5	16	6–31
Vinblastine (432,451)	48	Most	1 + 3	8	2–20
Etoposide (VP-16) (442)	29	Yes	0 + 1	3	1–29
Teniposide (VM-26) (436)	22	17	0 + 2	9	1–26
Investigational + other					
Aminothiodiazole (288)	21	12	0	0	0–16
Amonafide (434)	38	4	2 + 0	6	1–20
Amsacrine (AMSA) (418,427)	23	1	1 + 1	9	1–28
Cytembina (424)	30	Yes	10	33	17–53
Diaziquone (AZQ) (443)	26	20	1 + 1	8	1–25
Echinomycin (435)	21	Yes	1 + 0	5	1–23
Fludarabine (452)	19	Yes	0	0	0–18
Galactitol (443a)	17	Yes	0 + 1	6	1–27
Methyl-G (441)	21	11	3	14	3–36
Piperazinedione (448)	20	Most	0 + 1	5	1–25
Razoxane (ICRF-159) (429)	24	Yes	0	0	0–14
Semustine (MeCCNU) (438)	5	NS	0 + 2	40	5–85
Paclitaxel (7)	44	Yes	3 + 9	27.3	15–42.8
Topotecan (455)	42	No	3 + 5	20	

CR, complete response; NS, not stated; PR, partial response; 95% CI: The 95% confidence interval for complete and partial response.

were 22% and 30%, with a median progression-free interval of 3.2 and 3.9 months and a median survival of 6.9 and 7.3 months, respectively.

The addition of cyclophosphamide and doxorubicin to cisplatin (CAP) (425,459,462,463) and doxorubicin to cisplatin (AP) (457,466,468,472) has been associated with response rates ranging from 38% to 76%. The overlap of the 95% confidence intervals for CAP and AP regimens suggests no significant difference in response rates, thus allowing the AP regimen to become the "standard" to which more contemporary approaches are compared. Barrett and colleagues (457) studied a chronobiologically defined schedule of doxorubicin (60 mg/m^2 at 6:00 A.M.) and cisplatin (60 mg/m^2 at 6:00 P.M.) in an attempt to maximize the therapeutic index of the combination. The regimen in a Phase II trial produced

a 60% response rate, similar to other AP trials (466,468, 472), but the median survival of 14 months was somewhat longer than in other AP trials. Toxicity was substantial, with 43% of patients developing WBC counts of >1,000/mm^3. GOG 139 represented a randomized trial of standard versus circadian-timed cisplatin and doxorubicin, and preliminary analysis showed no difference in response rate (46% vs 49%) or progression-free (6.5 vs 5.9 months) or overall survival (11.2 vs 13.2 months) (473). The results of GOG 107 comparing doxorubicin (60 mg/m^2 every 3 weeks) with the same doxorubicin dose and cisplatin (50 mg/m^2 every 3 weeks) in 223 patients with advanced or recurrent endometrial cancer have shown a significantly higher response rate for the combination (45% vs 27%), but a progression-free and overall survival of 5.7 versus 3.8 months and 9.2 versus 9.0

TABLE 23.16. *Combination chemotherapy*

Reference	Drug	Dose (mg/m^2)	Schedule	Chemotherapy	n	CR + PR (%)	95% CI
Cyclophosphamide-doxorubicin-cisplatin (CAP)							
202	CYC	600	q 4 wk	No	19	27 (47)	2471
	DOX	50					
	CIS	60					
463	CYC	500	q 4 wk	No	18	55 (56)	3178
	DOX	50					
	CIS	50					
425	CYC	400	q 3 wk	No	16	05 (31)	1159
	DOX	40					
	CIS	40					
459	CYC	500	q 4 wk	No	87	1227 (45)	3456
	DOX	50					
	CIS	50					
462	CYC	500	q 3 wk	5	17	35 (47)	2372
	DOX	50					
	CIS	50					
Doxorubicin-cisplatin							
468	DOX	50	q 3 wk	No	9	12 (33)	770
	CIS	50					
472	DOX	50	q 4 wk	No	20	210 (60)	3681
	CIS	50					
466	DOX	60	q 4 wk	4/16	16	67 (81)	5496
	CIS	60					
457	DOX	60[a]	q 4 wk	No	30	612 (60)	4177
	CIS	60					
Cyclophosphamide-doxorubicin							
465	CYC	500	q 3 wk	No	11	32 (45)	1777
	DOX	37.5					
469	CYC	400500[AU:]	q 4 wk	No	26	08 (31)	1452
	DOX	4050					
445	CYC	500	q 3 wk	No	105	1519 (32)	2442
	DOX	50					
460	CYC	600	q 3 wk	No	13	15 (46)	1975
	DOX	50					
Other							
456	DOX	30	q 34 wk	No	42	310 (31)	1847
	CIS	50					
	VLB	5					
	VCR	1.5	q 3 wk	No	44	914 (52)	3768
	VM-26	100					
	CIS	60					
	CYC	500	q 3 wk	No	20	55 (50)	2773
	DOX	40					
	VCR	1.5					
	FU	500 (d2,3)					
464	MTX	30 (d1,15,22)	q 4 wk	No	25	15 (60)	3979
	VLB	3 (d2,15,22)					
	DOX	30 (d2)					
	CIS	70 (d2)					
Randomized trials-chemotherapy							
470	DOX		q 3 wk	No	90	(24)	1635
	vs						
	CYC			No	105	(32)	2442
	DOX						
471	DOX	60	q 3 wk	No	122	(27)	2744
	vs						
	DOX	60		No	101	(45)	5675
	CIS	50					
474	DOX	60	q 3 wk	No	157	40% (15% + n/a 35%)	
	CIS	50					
	VS						
	DOX	50			157	43% (17% + 26%)	
	PAC	150					

(continued)

TABLE 23.16. Continued

Reference	Drug	Dose (mg/m²)	Schedule	Chemotherapy	n	CR + PR (%)	95% CI
475	DOX	60			133	33% (7% + n/a 26%)	
	CIS	50					
	VS						
	DOX	45			133	57% (22% + 35%)	
	CIS	50					
	PAC	160					

CYC, cyclophosphamide; DOX, doxorubicin; CIS, cisplatin; CI, confidence interval; VLB, vinblastine; VCR, vincristine; VM-26, teniposide; FU, fluorouracil; MTX, methotrexate; PAC, paclitaxel.

[a] Circadian timed regimen doxorubicin at 0600 (6 A.M.) and cisplatin at 1800 (6 P.M.) hours.

months, respectively (472). Moderate to severe nausea and vomiting (16% vs 2%), platelet counts of 50,000 mm³ (14% vs 2%), and WBCs of 2,000 mm³ (61% vs 39%) were more common for the combination regimen. This study confirms a higher response rate with combination therapy, but the difference in progression-free survival is modest and likely not clinically meaningful; the overall survival is identical in the two groups.

Given the increased response rate of the doxorubicin combination, and the Phase II activity of single-agent paclitaxel, GOG trial 163 randomized patients with primary stage III and IV or recurrent endometrial cancer to doxorubicin and cisplatin or doxorubicin with 24-hour paclitaxel and granulocyte colony-stimulating factor (G-CSF). Preliminary results presented in abstract form only show response rates of 40% versus 44% with progression-free and overall survival of 7.2 versus 6.0 months and 12.4 versus 13,6 months, respectively, again showing no clinically meaningful survival differences between the two combinations (474).

The disadvantage of GOG trial 163 was the lack of platinum in the taxane-containing arm, which was subsequently studied in GOG 177 evaluating doxorubicin (60 mg/m² or 45 mg/m² in patients with prior radiotherapy) with cisplatin (50 mg/m²) as the standard arm versus paclitaxel (160 mg/m²) with doxorubicin (45 mg/m²) and cisplatin (50 mg/m²) and G-CSF as the investigational regimen. The primary objective was to determine if the addition of paclitaxel improved response rate and progression-free and overall survival, and a secondary objective explored the relationship between HER-2/neu overexpression and outcome with doxorubicin-based therapy. Two hundred and seventy-three patients were enrolled, and study was balanced for history of prior RT (50% vs 46%), serous carcinoma (15% vs 19%), stage, grade, and BSA. Grade III and IV platelet toxicity was higher in the three-drug arm (21% vs 2%), but other hematologic toxicity was ameliorated with G-CSF: ANC 36% versus 50% and neutropenic fever 3% versus 2%. Nonhematologic grade 3,4 toxicity was higher in the three-drug arm: gastrointestinal 59% versus 39% and metabolic 25% versus 13%. Response rates were better with the triplet: complete response 22% versus 7%, partial response 36% versus 27%, and overall RR 57% versus 34%. Median PFS was 8.3

months versus 5.3 months (p <.0005) and median overall survival was 15.3 months versus 12.1 months (p = .024). Responses were similar in serous (48%) versus nonserous histology (45%). Overall, TAP chemotherapy increased 12-month survival to 59% compared to 50% with AP with an HR of 0.75 (0.56 to 0.998). As the secondary objective, HER-2/neu testing was not done in approximately 12% of patients. Of those available, approximately 20% stained 3+, which was neither prognostic nor predictive of outcome in this patient population (475,476).

Although the TAP regimen produced an improvement in response rate and PFS, survival was minimally increased, and it is associated with greater toxicity. The combination of paclitaxel and carboplatin as a doublet has also been evaluated in a variety of Phase II trials with response rates in the 60% to 80% range (477,478). No direct Phase III comparisons between doxorubicin and platinum versus paclitaxel with platinum are available. A randomized Phase II study was recently presented in abstract form evaluating doxorubicin with cisplatin versus paclitaxel with carboplatin in 70 patients with advanced or recurrent endometrial cancer showing a response rate of 27.9% versus 35.3%, respectively, but a Phase III study would be required to comment on a progression-free or overall survival advantage (479).

The results of combining chemotherapy with progestin therapy are presented in Table 23.17 (370,458,461, 480–484). Complete and partial remission rates have ranged from 17% to 86%, although none is convincingly different than for chemotherapy alone. There are no data to suggest that endocrine therapy in conjunction with chemotherapy is superior to chemotherapy or endocrine therapy alone. Many of these trials have included small numbers of patients, and median survival rates have generally been less than 1 year. In most combined progestin-chemotherapy regimens, most patients had no prior progestin treatment, although in almost all of the chemotherapy trials most patients had prior progestins before entry.

Two other randomized trials compared different chemotherapy regimens with all patients receiving megestrol acetate (Megace) (461,482). Response rates for both these regimens were similar, with median survival times of approximately 7 and 10 months, respectively. In Horton's trial

TABLE 23.17. *Combination chemotherapy and progestin therapy*

Reference	Drug	Dose (mg/m²)	Schedule[a]	Chemotherapy	n	CR + PR (%)	95% CI
483	CYC	300	q 4 wk	No	15	54 (60)	3284
	DOX	30					
	CIS	50					
	MEG	120	Daily				
481	CYC	250–500	q 3 wk	No	15	41 (33)	1262
	DOX	30					
	CIS	50					
	MEG	80–160	Daily				
370	CYC	500	q 4 wk	No	15	8 (53)	2779
	DOX	50					
	CIS	50					
	MPA	300	Daily				
480	CYC	400	q 3 wk	No	29	85 (45)	2664
	FU	400					
	MEG	160	Daily				
458	CYC	400	d1,8 q 4 wk	No	7	06 (86)	4299
	DOX	30					
	FU	400					
	MPA	400 (IM)	TIW				
Randomized trials: chemotherapy plus endocrine therapy							
482	CYC	400	q 4 wk	No	56	411 (27)	1640
	DOX	40					
	MEG	80	TID				
	vs						
	CYC	250	q 4 wk		58	36 (16)	727
	DOX	30					
	FU	300	(d1-3)				
	MEG	80	TID				
461	L-PAM	7	4d q 4 wk	No	77	1217 (38)	2749
	FU	525[b]					
	MEG	180	q day 8 wk				
	vs						
	CYC	400	q 3 wk		78	1615 (36)	2951
	DOX	40					
	FU	400					
	MEG	180	q day 8 wk				

CYC, cyclophosphamide; DOX, doxorubicin; CI, confidence interval; CIS, cisplatin; MEG, megestrol acetate; MPA, medroxyprogesterone acetate; FU, fluorouracil; L-PAM, melphalan; TAM, tamoxifen; IM, intramuscular; alt q 3 wk, MPA and TAM alternate q 3 wk.

[a] For chemotherapy and progestin therapy, the progestin schedule is listed separately at the bottom of the column.
[b] Total dose.

(482), many patients had prior progestins, but this did not appear to affect the response to chemotherapy, and the response to prior progestin therapy was not related to treatment results. In the study by Cohen and others (461), response rate was also not related to prior progestin therapy, age, disease-free interval, metastatic site, or tumor grade.

FUTURE DIRECTIONS

Purdie and Green (485) recommend the following research agenda in epidemiology of endometrial cancer.

- To establish better biologic and epidemiologic data in order to disentangle the roles of age at first birth, age at last birth, number of births, and time since last birth in the development of endometrial cancer in relation to menopausal hormonal therapy.
- To determine the types of estrogens and progestogens, the appropriate doses, and the modes of administration that minimize cancer risk and maximize protection for osteoporosis and cardiovascular disease. Human studies need to be conducted into the mechanism of estrogen action in promoting proliferation of the endometrial stroma and its role in carcinogenesis. Examination of the role of genes that affect hormone metabolism and function, and whether mutations in these influence their endocrine effects.
- To establish more conclusively the independent and synergistic effects on weight, diet, exercise, alcohol consumption and smoking on occurrence of disease (485).

Ongoing clinical trials and future directions for the study of patients with endometrial cancer include refinement of diagnostic techniques, further clarification of treatment for patients with intermediate-risk factors, and definition of better treatment for those with advanced disease and recurrence.

Magnetic resonance imaging of the uterus requires more study. This may become an important aspect in determining who may benefit from extensive surgical staging or extension of irradiation treatment, particularly patients who are at increased surgical risk. The role of transvaginal color Doppler ultrasonography in the diagnosis and staging of endometrial carcinoma also requires further evaluation. Kurjak and colleagues (486) were able to detect 32 of 35 endometrial carcinomas by preoperative transvaginal color Doppler sonography. In addition, they were able to predict the extent of myometrial invasion in 18 of 19 cases.

The use of tumor markers, such as CA-125, warrants further study. They may aid in diagnosis and in monitoring therapeutic response. Much interest is being generated for the development of combinations of tumor markers to improve sensitivity and specificity. Lipid-associated sialic acid (LSA), CEA, CA-19-9, and CA-125 have been assayed in patients with endometrial cancer. LSA and CA-125 were significantly more sensitive than either CA-19-9 or CEA. The combined use of these and other tumor markers should be assessed in the hope of obtaining greater sensitivity. The clinical usefulness of combinations of tumor markers for endometrial cancer remains to be determined (139,142). Data from Hsieh et al. (142) provide evidence indicating that a preoperative CA-125 level greater than 40 U/mL can be considered a criterion for full pelvic lymphadenectomy in the surgical staging of endometrial cancer. However, prospective randomized studies are needed to establish the approximate cut-off value for serum CA-125 in this respect.

The judicious use of intravaginal brachytherapy in patients with adequate surgical lymph node staging should be an area of intense investigation, especially with regard to quality of life and sexual function. The therapeutic ratio of adjuvant external beam radiation is very likely to benefit from the advances in intensity modulated radiation therapy (IMRT) by providing the most conformal dose distribution to the tumor volume while sparing the surrounding normal structures. The high rate of relapse in locally advanced endometrial cancer treated with radiation indicates the need for systemic therapy. Adjuvant chemotherapy of high-risk localized endometrial cancer is a relatively unexplored area of clinical research. The current strategy is to define chemotherapy combinations with the highest response rates, and evaluate these in the adjuvant setting with comparison to the standard approach of radiation therapy. Concomitantly, GOG protocol 163 is randomizing patients between doxorubicin and cisplatin or paclitaxel and doxorubicin to determine the superior combination for additional evaluation.

The data from GOG study 122 showed promising results for combination chemotherapy in the adjuvant setting. But it is unlikely that chemotherapy alone is going to be sufficient, especially with more than 55% of patients still relapsing (388). Currently, GOG study 184 is evaluating pelvic with or without paraaortic radiation followed by either Adriamycin/cisplatin or Adriamycin/cisplatin/taxol in patients with stage III disease. Future studies should focus on trying to use concurrent rather than sequential radiation and chemotherapy to take advantage of the synergy of the two treatment modalities. Also needed is a prospective randomized trial of patients with clinical stage I disease and positive peritoneal cytology.

For recurrent disease, the GOG and other cooperative groups continue to study new agents in Phase II trials, a treatment strategy that is well founded considering present results. Furthermore, these patients should be considered for Phase I investigation with agents that offer theoretical promise.

The DNA content of tumor cells as a prognostic factor in patients with endometrial cancer requires investigation (214, 487–490). Preliminary studies suggest that application of DNA analysis correlates aneuploidy with advanced surgical stage, higher tumor grade, and poorer clinical outcome. The results of multivariate analyses would indicate that DNA ploidy is an independent prognostic factor in endometrial cancer. Application of this technique to low-stage endometrial cancers of high-grade or papillary serous type may be useful for selecting a subgroup of patients for adjuvant therapy. Although flow cytometric analyses may help identify a group of patients at increased risk for recurrence, the main challenge will be identifying what constitutes effective adjuvant therapy.

Further study of steroid-receptor levels may be helpful. In a subgroup of patients whose tumors are poor in both estrogen and progestin content, the survival is low, with 2- and 5-year survival rates of only 51% and 20.5%, respectively (491). Low hormone-receptor levels or lack of any detectable receptor may identify a group of patients who are at high risk of failure. With newer quantitative methods of immunohistochemical identification of the estrogen- and progestin-receptor protein, a precise relationship between the receptor status and outcome may be established, management may be directed, and survival may be predicted.

Several novel and strong prognostic markers in endometrial carcinoma have been identified. It is possible that the prognostic information derived from the tumor biomarkers also could reduce the need for extensive surgical staging. In order to answer this question, however, prospective studies relating the expression of tumor biomarkers in curettage material to the results from surgical staging as well as patient prognosis will be necessary.

The inhibition of angiogenesis is considered to be one of the most promising strategies that may lead to novel cancer therapies (492,493). The preliminary use of angiogenesis inhibitors (494–496) may further motivate the quantitation of intratumor microvessel density for decisions regarding therapeutic strategies as well as for prognostication.

Further studies of DNA repair genes, such as *hMLH1, hMSH2,* and *hMSH6* and the *PTEN* tumor-suppressor gene, seem particularly relevant in endometrial carcinoma. Little is known about the mechanisms involved in the inactivation of these genes as well as their prognostic significance in this disease. Hence, studies regarding protein expression and mechanisms for gene inactivation (promoter region methylation, mutation, and deletion) for the DNA repair genes and the *PTEN* tumor-suppressor gene are now in progress (381).

The ultimate goal is that the understanding of tumor biologic mechanisms involved in endometrial carcinoma should eventually lead to improved, individualized treatment. However, further identification of the underlying genetic defects in the tumors could allow development of more specifically targeted therapy. For other cancer types, identification of underlying genetic defects has been found to be related to treatment response (497) and contributed to the development of novel approaches in tumor treatment (498,499).

REFERENCES

1. Jemal A, Murray T, Samuels A, et al. Cancer statistics, 2003. *CA Cancer J Clin* 2003;53:5–26.
2. Gallup DG, Stock RJ. Adenocarcinoma of the endometrium in women 40 years of age or younger. *Obstet Gynecol* 1984;64:417.
3. Norris HJ, Tavassoli FA, Kurman RJ. Endometrial hyperplasia and carcinoma, diagnostic consideration. *Am J Surg Pathol* 1988;7:839.
4. International Federation of Gynecology and Obstetrics. Annual report on the results of treatment in gynecologic cancer. Stockholm: FIGO, 1985.
5. International Federation of Gynecology and Obstetrics. Corpus cancer staging. *Int J Gynaecol Obstet* 1989;28:190.
6. Randall ME, Brunetto G, et al. Whole abdominal radiotherapy versus combination doxorubicin-cisplatin chemotherapy in advanced endometrial carcinoma: a randomized phase III trial of the Gynecology Oncology Group. *Proc ASCO* 2003;22:3(abst).
7. Lincoln S, Blessing JA, Lee RB, Rocereto TF. Activity of paclitaxel as second-line chemotherapy in endometrial carcinoma: a Gynecologic Oncology Group study. *Gynecol Oncol* 2003;88:277–281.
8. Plentl AA, Friedman EA. *Lymphatic system of the female genitalia: the morphologic basis of oncologic diagnosis and therapy.* Philadelphia: WB Saunders, 1971:116.
9. Makar APH, Tropé CG. Endometrial and ovarian malignancies: epidemiology, etiology and prognostic factors. *Acta Obstet Gynecol Scand* 1992;71:331–336.
10. Rose PG. Endometrial carcinoma. *N Engl J Med* 1996;335:640–649.
11. Dunlop MG, Farrington SM, Carothers AD, et al. Cancer risk associated with germline DNA mismatch repair gene mutations. *Hum Mol Genet* 1977;6:105–110.
12. Beresford SAA, Weiss NS, Voigt LF, McKnight B. Risk of endometrial cancer in relation to use of oestrogen combined with cyclic progestagen therapy in postmenopausal women. *Lancet* 1997;349:458–461.
13. Goodman MT, Hankin JH, Wilkens LR, et al. Diet, body size, physical activity, and the risk of endometrial cancer. *Cancer Res* 1997;57:5077–5085.
14. Goodman MT, Wilkens LR, Hankin JH, et al. Associated of soy and fiber consumption with the risk of endometrial cancer. *Am J Epidemiol* 1997;146:294–306.
15. Potischman N, Hoover RN, Brinton LA, et al. Case-control study of endogenous steroid hormones and endometrial cancer. *J Natl Cancer Inst* 1996;88:1127–1135.
16. Weiderpass E, Baron JA, Adami HO, et al. Low potency oestrogen and risk of endometrial cancer: a case-control study. *Lancet* 1999;353:1824–1828.
17. De Ward F, De Ridder CM, Baanders-van Halewyn EA, Slotboom BJ. Endometrial cancer in a cohort screened for breast cancer. *Eur J Cancer Prev* 1996;5:99–104.
18. Grady D, Ernster VL. Hormone replacement therapy and endometrial cancer: are current regimens safe? *J Natl Cancer Inst* 1997;89:1088–1089.
19. Hulka BS, Kaukman DG, Fowler WC, et al. Predominance of early endometrial cancer after long-term estrogen use. *JAMA* 1980;244:2419–2422.
20. Key TJA, Pike MC. The dose-effect relationship between unopposed oestrogens and endometrial mitotic rate: its central role in explaining and predicting endometrial cancer risk. *Br J Cancer* 1988;57:205–212.
21. Pike MC, Peters RK, Cozen W, et al. Estrogen-progestin replacement therapy and endometrial cancer. *J Natl Cancer Inst* 1997;89:1110–1116.
22. Tretli S, Magnus K. Height and weight in relation to uterine corpus cancer morbidity and mortality: a follow up study of 570,000 women in Norway. *Int J Cancer* 1990;46:165–172.
23. Ziel HK. Estrogen's role in endometrial cancer. *Obstet Gynecol* 1982;60:509–515.
24. Dahgren E, Friberg LG, Johansson S, et al. Endometrial carcinoma; ovarian dysfunction—a risk factor in young women. *Eur J Obstet Gynecol Reprod Biol* 1991;41:143–150.
25. McDonald TW, Malkasian GD, Gaffey TA. Endometrial cancer associated with feminizing ovarian tumor and polycystic ovarian disease. *Obstet Gynecol* 1977;49:654–658.
26. Parazzini F, La Vecchia C, Negri E, et al. Diabetes and endometrial cancer: an Italian case-control study. *Int J Cancer* 1999;81:539–542.
27. Albrektsen G, Heuch I, Tretli G. Is the risk of cancer of the corpus uteri reduced by a recent pregnancy? A prospective study of 765,756 Norwegian women. *Int J Cancer* 1995;61:458–490.
28. Kvåle G, Heuch I, Ursin G. Reproductive factors and risk of cancer of the uterine corpus; a prospective study. *Cancer Res* 1988;48:6217–6221.
29. Franceschi S. Reproductive factors and cancer of the breast, ovary and endometrium. *Eur J Cancer Clin Oncol* 1989;25:1933–1943.
30. Parazzine F, La Vecchia C, Negri E, et al. Reproductive factors and risk of endometrial cancer. *Am J Obstet Gynecol* 1991;164:522–527.
31. Neven P, Vergote I. Tamoxifen, screening and new oestrogen receptor modulators. *Best Pract Res Clin Obstet Gynaecol* 2001;365–380.
32. Killackey MA, Hakes TB, Pierce VK. Endometrial adenocarcinoma in breast cancer patients receiving antiestrogens. *Cancer Treat Rep* 1985; 69:237.
33. Atlante G, Pozzi M, Vincenzoni C, Vacaturo G. Four case reports presenting new acquisitions on the association of breast and endometrial cancer. *Gynecol Oncol* 1990;37:378.
34. Barakat RR, Wong G, Curtin JP, et al. Tamoxifen use in breast cancer patients who subsequently develop corpus cancer is not associated with a higher incidence of adverse histologic features. *Gynecol Oncol* 1994;55:164.
35. Fisher B, Costantino JP, Redmond CK, et al. Endometrial cancer in tamoxifen-treated breast cancer patients: findings from the National Surgical Adjuvant Breast and Bowel Project (NSABP) B-14. *J Natl Cancer Inst* 1994;86:527.
36. Fornander T, Cedermark B, Mattsson A, et al. Adjuvant tamoxifen in early breast cancer: occurrence of new primary cancers. *Lancet* 1989;21:117.
37. Hardell L. Tamoxifen as risk factor for carcinoma of corpus uteri [Letter]. *Lancet* 1988;3:563.
39. Magriples U, Naftolin F, Schwartz PE, Carcangiu ML. High-grade endometrial carcinoma in tamoxifen-treated breast cancer patients. *J Clin Oncol* 1993;11:485.
40. Malfetano JH. Tamoxifen-associated endometrial carcinoma in postmenopausal breast cancer patients. *Gynecol Oncol* 1990;39:82.
41. Neven P, DeMuylder X, Van Belle Y, et al. Tamoxifen and the uterus and endometrium [Letter]. *Lancet* 1989;1:375.
42. Seoud MA-F, Johnson J, Weed JC. Gynecologic tumors in tamoxifen-treated women with breast cancer. *Obstet Gynecol* 1993;82:165.
43. van Leeuwen FE, Benraadt J, Coebergh JW, et al. Risk of endometrial cancer after tamoxifen treatment of breast cancer. *Lancet* 1994;343:448.
44. Fornander T, Hellstrom A-C, Moberger B. Descriptive clinicopatho-

logic study of 17 patients with endometrial cancer during or after adjuvant tamoxifen in early breast cancer. *J Natl Cancer Inst* 1993; 85:1850.

45. Cummings SR, Norton L, Eckert S, et al. Raloxifene reduces the risk of breast cancer and may decrease the risk of endometrial cancer in post menopausal women. Two year findings from the multiple outcomes of raloxifene evaluation (MORE) trial. *Proc Am Soc Clin Oncol* 1998;17:3(abst).

46. Kurman R, Kaminski P, Norris H. The behavior of endometrial hyperplasia. A long-term study of "untreated" hyperplasia in 170 patients. *Cancer* 1985;56:403–411.

47. Huang S, Amparo E, Fu Y. Endometrial hyperplasia: histologic classification and behavior. *Surg Pathol* 1988;1:215–225.

48. Hunter JE, Tritz DE, Howell MG, et al. The prognostic and therapeutic implications of cytologic atypia in patients with endometrial hyperplasia. *Gynecol Oncol* 1994;55:66–71.

48. Lahti E, Blanco G, Kauppila A, et al. Endometrial changes in postmenopausal breast cancer patients receiving tamoxifen. *Obstet Gynecol* 1993;81:660.

49. Kendall BS, Ronnett BM, Isacson C, et al. Reproducibility of the diagnosis of endometrial hyperplasia, atypical hyperplasia, and well-differentiated carcinoma. *Am J Surg Pathol* 1998;22(8):p1012–1019.

50. Bergeron C, Nogales F, Masseroli M, et al. A multicentric European study testing the reproducibility of the WHO classification of endometrial hyperplasia with a proposal of a simplified working classification for biopsy and curettage specimens. *Am J Surg Pathol* 1999;23: 1102–1108.

51. Skov BG, Broholm H, Engel U, et al. Comparison of the reproducibility of the WHO classifications of 1975 and 1994 of endometrial hyperplasia. *Int J Gynecol Pathol* 1997;16:33–37

52. Mutter GL. Endometrial intraepithelial neoplasia (EIN): will it bring order to chaos? The Endometrial Collaborative Group. *Gynecol Oncol* 2000;76:287–290.

53. Kurman R, Norris H. Evaluation of criteria for distinguishing atypical endometrial hyperplasia from well-differentiated carcinoma. *Cancer* 1982;49:2547–2559.

54. Gambrell RD Jr, Bagnell CA, Greenblatt RB. Role of estrogens and progesterone in the etiology and prevention of endometrial cancer: a review. *Am J Obstet Gynecol* 1983;146:696.

55. Persson I, Adami HO, Bergkvist L, et al. Risk of endometrial cancer after treatment with oestrogens alone or in conjunction with progestogens: results of a prospective study. *Br Med J* 1989;298:147.

56. Gambrell RD Jr, Massey FM, Castenada TA, et al. Use of the progesterone challenge test to reduce the risk of endometrial cancer. *Obstet Gynecol* 1980;55:732.

57. Gorodeski IG, Geier A, Lunenfeld B, Bahary CM. Progesterone challenge test in postmenopausal women with pathological endometrium. *Cancer Invest* 1988;6:481.

58. Miller AB, Chamberlain J, Day NE, et al. Report on a Workshop of the UICC Project on Evaluation of Screening for Cancer. *Int J Cancer* 1990;46:761–769.

59. Sonoda Y, Zerbe M, Smith A, et al. High incidence of positive peritoneal cytology in low-risk endometrial cancer treated by laparoscopically assisted hysterectomy. *Gynecol Oncol* 2001;80:378–382.

60. Nakagawa-Okamura C, Sato S, Tsuji I, et al. Effectiveness of mass screening for endometrial cancer. *Acta Cytol* 2002;46:277–283.

61. Vuento MH, Maatela JI, Tyrkko JE, et al. A longitudinal study of screening for endometrial cancer by endometrial biopsy in diabetic females. *Int J Gynecol Cancer* 1995;5:390–395.

62. Runowicz CD. Gynecologic suurveillance of women on tamoxifen: First do no harm. *J Clin Oncol* 2000;18:3457–3458.

63. Hogberg T. Screening in endometrial cancer. In: Luesley DM, Lawton F, Berchek A, eds. *Uterine cancer.* 2003.

64. Bamford DS, Hall EW, Newman MR. The Isaacs endometrial cell sampler: an evaluation in 100 patients. *Acta Cytol* 1984;28:101.

65. Walters D, Robinson D, Park RC, Patow WE. Diagnostic outpatient aspiration curettage. *Obstet Gynecol* 1975;46:160.

66. Grimes DA. Diagnostic office curettage; heresy no longer. *Contemp Obstet Gynecol* 1986;27:96.

67. Mattingly RF, Thompson JD. Dilatation of the cervix and curettage of the uterus. In: Mattingly RF, Thompson JD, eds. *Operative gynecology.* 6th ed. Philadelphia: JB Lippincott Co, 1985:495.

68. Fiorica JV, Hoffman MS, Roberts WS, et al. Detection of endometrial

carcinoma: clinical judgment versus histologic examination. *South Med J* 1990;83:759.

69. King A, Seraj IM, Wagner RJ. Stromal invasion in endometrial adenocarcinoma. *Am J Obstet Gynecol* 1984;149:10.

70. Tavassoli F, Kraus FT. Endometrial lesions in uteri resected for atypical endometrial hyperplasia. *Am J Clin Pathol* 1978;70:770.

71. Cowles TA, Magrina JF, Masterson BJ, Capen CV. Comparison of clinical and surgical staging in patients with endometrial carcinoma. *Obstet Gynecol* 1985;66:413.

72. Silverberg S, Kurman R. *Tumors of the uterine corpus and gestational trophoblastic disease.* Vol 3. Washington, DC: Armed Forces Institute of Pathology, 1992.

73. Zaino RJ, Silverberg SG, Norris HJ, et al. The prognostic value of nuclear versus architectural grading in endometrial adenocarcinoma: a Gynecologic Oncology Group study. *Int J Gynecol Pathol* 1994; 13:29.

74. Zaino RJ, Kurman RJ, Diana KL, Morrow CP. The utility of the revised International Federation of Gynecology and Obstetrics histologic grading of endometrial adenocarcinoma using a defined nuclear grading system. *Cancer* 1995;75:81.

75. Taylor R, Zeller J, Lieberman R, O'Connor D. An analysis of two versus three grades for endometrial carcinoma. *Gynecol Oncol* 1999; 74:3–6.

76. Lax S, Ronntet B, Pizer E, et al. A binary grading system for uterine endometrioid carcinoma is comparable to FIGO grading for predicting prognosis and has superior interobserver reproducibility. *Mod Pathol* 1999;12:118A.

77. Connelly PJ, Albershasky RC, Christopherson WW. Carcinoma of the endometrium. III. Analysis of 865 cases of adenocarcinoma and adenoacanthoma. *Obstet Gynecol* 1982;59:569.

78. Fanning J, Evans MC, Peters AJ, et al. Endometrial adenocarcinoma histologic subtypes: clinical and pathologic profile. *Gynecol Oncol* 1989;32:288.

79. Muggia FM, Blessing JA, et al. Phase II trial of the pegylated liposomal doxorubicin in previously treated metastatic endometrial cancer: a Gynecologic Oncology Group study. *J Clin Oncol* 2002;20: 2360–2364.

80. Sutton GP, Brill L, Michael H, et al. Malignant papillary lesions of the endometrium. *Gynecol Oncol* 1987;27:294.

81. Zaino FJ, Kurman RJ, Brunetto VL, et al. Villoglandular adenocarcinoma of the endometrium: a clinicopathologic study of 61 cases. *Am J Surg Pathol* 1998;22:1379.

82. Kusuyama J, Yoshida M, Imai H, et al. Secretory carcinoma of the endometrium. *Acta Cytol* 1989;33:127.

83. Toban H, Watkins GJ. Secretory adenocarcinoma of the endometrium. *Int J Gynecol Pathol* 1985;4:328.

84. Christopherson WM, Alberhasky RC, Connelly PF. Carcinoma of the endometrium: I. A clinicopathologic study of clear-cell carcinoma and secretory carcinoma. *Cancer* 1982;49:1511.

85. Hendrickson MR, Kempson RL. Ciliated carcinoma—a variant of endometrial adenocarcinoma. A report of 10 cases. *Int J Gynecol Pathol* 1983;2:1.

86. Alberhasky RC, Connelly PJ, Christopherson WM. Carcinoma of the endometrium. IV. Mixed adenosquamous carcinoma. A clinical-pathological study of 68 cases with long-term follow-up. *Am J Clin Pathol* 1982;77:655.

87. Julian CG, Daikoku NH, Gillespie A. Adenoepidermoid and adenosquamous carcinoma of the uterus. A clinicopathologic study of 118 cases. *Am J Obstet Gynecol* 1977;128:106.

88. Ng AB, Reagan JW, Storaasli JP, et al. Mixed adenosquamous carcinoma of the endometrium. *Am J Clin Pathol* 1973;59:765.

89. Salazar OM, DePapp EW, Bonfiglio T, et al. Adenosquamous carcinoma of the endometrium. An entity with an inherently poor prognosis? *Cancer* 1977;40:119.

90. Silverberg SG, Bolin MG, DeGiorgi LS. Adenoacanthoma and mixed adenosquamous carcinoma of the endometrium. A clinicopathologic study. *Cancer* 1972;30:1307.

91. Zaino RJ, Kurman RJ. Squamous differentiation in carcinoma of the endometrium. A critical appraisal of adenoacanthoma and adenosquamous carcinoma. *Semin Diagn Pathol* 1988;5:154.

92. Melhem MF, Tobon H. Mucinous adenocarcinoma of the endometrium: a clinicopathological review of 18 cases. *Int J Gynecol Pathol* 1987;6:347.

93. Ross J, Eifel P, Cox R, et al. Primary mucinous adenocarcinoma of the endometrium. *Am J Surg Pathol* 1983;7:715–729.

94. Tiltman A. Mucinous carcinoma of the endometrium. *Obstet Gynecol* 1980;55:244–247.

95. Maier RC, Norris HJ. Coexistence of cervical intraepithelial neoplasia with primary adenocarcinoma of the endocervix. *Obstet Gynecol* 1980;56:361.

96. Maes G, Fleuren GJ, Bara J, Nap M. The distribution of mucins, carcinoembryonic antigen, and mucus-associated antigens in endocervical and endometrial adenocarcinomas. *Int J Gynecol Pathol* 1988;7:112–122.

97. McCluggage WG, Roberts N, Bharucha H. Enteric differentiation in endometrial adenocarcinomas: a mucin histochemical study. *Int J Gynecol Pathol* 1995;14:250–254.

98. Wilson TO, Podratz KC, Gaffey TA, et al. Evaluation of unfavorable histologic subtypes in endometrial adenocarcinoma. *Am J Obstet Gynecol* 1990;162:418.

99. Lee K, Belinson J. Recurrence in noninvasive endometrial carcinoma. *Am J Surg Pathol* 1991;15:965–973.

100. Silva EG, Jenkins R. Serous carcinoma in endometrial polyps. *Mod Pathol* 1990;3:120–128.

101. Chambers JT, Merino M, Kohorn EI, et al. Uterine papillary serous carcinoma. *Obstet Gynecol* 1987;69:109–113.

102. Jeffrey JF, Krepart GV, Lotochi RJ. Papillary serous adenocarcinoma of the endometrium. *Obstet Gynecol* 1986;67:670.

103. Wheeler D, Bell K, Kurman R, Sherman M. Minimal uterine serous carcinoma: diagnostic and clinicopathologic correlation. *Am J Surg Pathol* 2000;24:797–806.

104. Ambros RA, Sherman ME, Zahn CM, et al. Endometrial intraepithelial carcinoma: a distinctive lesion specifically associated with tumors displaying serous differentiation. *Hum Pathol* 1995;26:1260–1267.

105. Sherman ME, Bitterman P, Rosenshein NB, et al. Uterine serous carcinoma. A morphologically diverse neoplasm with unifying clinicopathologic features. *Am J Surg Pathol* 1992;16:600–610.

106. Soslow R, Pirong E, Isacson C. Endometrial intraepitheial carcinoma with associated peritoneal carcinomatosis. *Am J Surg Pathol* 2000;24:726–732.

107. Spiegel G. Endometrial carcinoma in situ in postmenopausal women. *Am J Surg Pathol* 1995;19:417–431.

108. Zheng W, Khurana R, Farahmand S, et al. p53 Immunostaining as a significant adjunct diagnostic method for uterine serous carcinoma. *Am J Surg Pathol* 1998;22:1463–1473.

109. Abeler V, Kjørdstad K, Berle E. Carcinoma of the endometrium in Norway: a histopathological and prognostic survey of a total population. *Int J Gynecol Cancer* 1992;2:9–22.

110. Abeler VM, Kjorstad KE. Clear cell carcinoma of the endometrium: a histopathological and clinical study of 97 cases. *Gynecol Oncol* 1991;40:207–217.

111. Abeler VM, Vergote IB, Kjorstad KE, Trope CG. Clear cell carcinoma of the endometrium. Prognosis and metastatic pattern. *Cancer* 1996;78:1740–1747.

112. Christopherson W, Alberhasky R, Connelly P. Carcinoma of the endometrium II. Papillary adenocarcinoma: a clinicopathological study of 46 cases. *Am J Clin Pathol* 1982;77:534–540.

113. Kurman RJ, Scully RE. Clear cell carcinoma of the endometrium. An analysis of 21 cases. *Cancer* 1976;37:872.

114. Lax SF, Pizer ES, Ronnett BM, Kurman RJ. Clear cell carcinoma of the endometrium is characterized by a distinctive profile of p53, Ki-67, estrogen, and progesterone receptor expression. *Hum Pathol* 1998;29:551–558.

115. Miller B, Umpierre S, Tornos C, Burke T. Histologic characterization of uterine papillary serous adenocarcinoma. *Gynecol Oncol* 1995;56:425.

116. Webb GA, Lagios MD. Clear cell carcinoma of the endometrium. *Am J Obstet Gynecol* 1987;156:1486–1491.

117. Lackman FD, Craighead PS. Therapeutic dilemmas in the management of uterine papillary serous carcinoma. *Curr Treat Options Oncol* 2003;4:99–104.

118. Goodman A, Zukerberg LR, Rice LW, et al. Squamous cell carcinoma of the endometrium: a report of eight cases and a review of the literature. *Gynecol Oncol* 1996;61:54–60.

119. Melin JR, Wanner L, Schulz, DM, et al. Primary squamous cell carcinoma of the endometrium. *Obstet Gynecol* 1979;53:115.

120. Simon A, Kopolovic J, Beyth Y. Primary squamous cell carcinoma of the endometrium. *Gynecol Oncol* 1988;31:454–461.

121. Tagsjo EB, Rosenberg P, Simonsen E. Primary squamous cell carcinoma of the endometrium. Case report. *Eur J Gynaecol Oncol* 1993;14:308–310.

122. Yamashina M, Kobara TY. Primary squamous cell carcinoma with its spindle cell variant in the endometrium. A case report and review of literature. *Cancer* 1986;57:340–345.

123. Scully RE, Aguirre P, DeLellis RA. Argyrophilia, serotonin, and peptide hormones in the female genital tract and its tumor. *Int J Gynecol Pathol* 1984;3:51.

124. Ueda G, Yamasaki M, Inoue M, et al. A clinicopathologic study of endometrial carcinomas with argyrophil cells. *Gynecol Oncol* 1979;7:223.

125. Christopherson WM, Alberhasky PC, Connelly PJ. Glassy cell carcinoma of the endometrium. *Hum Pathol* 1982;13:418–421.

126. Hachisuga T, Sugimori H, Kaku T, et al. Glassy cell carcinoma of the endometrium. *Gynecol Oncol* 1990;36:134.

127. Kumar NB, Hart WR. Metastases to the uterine corpus from extravaginal cancers. A clinicopathologic study of 63 cases. *Cancer* 1982;50:2163.

128. Kumar NB, Schneider V. Metastases to the uterus from extrapelvic primary tumors. *Int J Gynecol Pathol* 1983;2:134.

129. Piura B, Glezerman M. Synchronous carcinomas of endometrium and ovary. *Gynecol Oncol* 1989;33:261.

130. Eifel P, Hendrickson M, Ross J, et al. Simultaneous presentation of carcinoma involving the ovary and uterine corpus. *Cancer* 1982;50:163.

131. Scully RE. *Tumors of the ovary and maldeveloped gonad.* AFIP Pamphlet No. 16. Washington, DC: Armed Forces Institute of Pathology, 1982:92.

132. Zaino RJ, Whitney C, Brady MF. Simultaneously detected endometrial and ovarian carcinomas: a clinicopathologic study of 74 cases. *Mod Pathol* 1998;11:118.

133. Ulbright T, Roth L. Metastatic and independent cancers of the endometrium and ovary. A clinicopathologic study of 34 cases. *Hum Pathol* 1985;16:28.

134. Chen SS, Rumancik WM, Spiegel G. Magnetic resonance imaging in Stage I endometrial carcinoma. *Obstet Gynecol* 1990;75:274.

135. Chun M, Ball HG, Doherty F, et al. Uterine thickness determination using real-time ultrasonography: a guide for intracavitary brachytherapy in the treatment of endometrial carcinoma. *Gynecol Oncol* 1990;36:176.

136. Fleischer AC, Kalemeris GC, Machin JE, et al. Sonographic depiction of normal and abnormal endometrium with histopathologic correlation. *J Ultrasound Med* 1986;5:445.

137. Gordon AN, Fleischer AC, Dudley BS, et al. Preoperative assessment of myometrial invasion of endometrial adenocarcinoma by sonography (US) and magnetic resonance imaging (MRI). *Gynecol Oncol* 1989;34:175.

138. Yazigi R, Cohen J, Munoz AK, Sandstad J. Magnetic resonance imaging determination of myometrial invasion in endometrial carcinoma. *Gynecol Oncol* 1989;34:94.

139. Olt G, Berchuck A, Bast RC Jr. The role of tumor markers in gynecologic oncology. *Obstet Gynecol Surv* 1990;45:570.

140. Niloff JM, Klug TL, Schaetzl E, et al. Elevation of serum CA 125 in carcinomas of the fallopian tube, endometrium, and endocervix. *Am J Obstet Gynecol* 1984;148:1057.

141. Patsner B, Mann WJ, Cohen H, et al. Predictive value of preoperative serum CA 125 levels in clinically localized and advanced endometrial carcinoma. *Am J Obstet Gynecol* 1988;158:399.

142. Hsieh CH, ChangChien CC, Lin H, et al. Can a preoperative CA 125 level be a criterion for full pelvic lymphadenectomy in surgical staging of endometrial cancer? *Gynecol Oncol* 2002;86:28–33.

143. Dotters DJ. Preoperative CA125 in endometrial cancer: is it useful? *Am J Obstet Gynecol* 2000;182:1328–1334.

144. Duk JM, Aalders JG, Fleuren GJ, de Bruijn HW. CA125: a useful marker in endometrial carcinoma. *Am J Obstet Gynecol* 1986;155:1097–1102.

145. Koper NP, Massuger LF, Thomas CM, et al. Serum CA 125 measurements to identify patients with endometrial cancer who require lymphadenectomy. *Anticancer Res* 1998;18:1897–1902.

146. Sood AK, Buller RE, Burger RA, et al. Value of preoperative CA125

level in the management of uterine cancer and prediction of clinical outcome. *Obstet Gynecol* 1997;90:441–447.

147. Soper JT, Berchuk A, Olt GJ, et al. Preoperative evaluation of serum CA125, TAG 72 and CA 15–3 in patients with endometrial carcinoma. *Am J Obstet Gynecol* 1990;163:1204–1209.

148. Rose PG, Sommers RM, Reale FR, et al. Serial serum CA-125 measurements for evaluation of recurrence in patients with endometrial carcinoma. *Obstet Gynecol* 1994;84:12.

149. International Federation of Gynecology and Obstetrics: classification and staging of malignant tumors in the female pelvis. *Int J Gynaecol Obstet* 1971;9:172.

150. Boronow R, Morrow C, Creasman W, et al. Surgical staging in endometrial cancer: clinical-pathologic findings of a prospective study. *Obstet Gynecol* 1984;63:825–832.

151. Creasman WT, Morrow CP, Bundy BN, et al. Surgical pathologic spread patterns of endometrial cancer (a Gynecologic Oncology Group study). *Cancer* 1987;60:2035.

152. Saint Cassia LJ, Weppelmann B, Shingleton H, et al. Management of early endometrial carcinoma. *Gynecol Oncol* 1989;35:362.

153. Doering DL, Barnhill DR, Weiser EB, et al. Intraoperative evaluation of depth of myometrial invasion in Stage I endometrial adenocarcinoma. *Obstet Gynecol* 1989;74:930.

154. Goff BA, Riche LW. Assessment of depth of myometrial invasion in endometrial adenocarcinoma. *Gynecol Oncol* 1990;38:46.

156. Creasman WT, Morrow CP, Bundy BN, et al. Surgical pathologic spread patterns of endometrial cancer. A Gynecologic Oncology Group Study. *Cancer* 1987;60[8 Suppl]:2035–2041.

157. Gal D, Recio FO, Zamurovic D. The new International Federation of Gynecology and Obstetrics surgical staging and survival rates in early endometrial carcinoma. *Cancer* 1992;69:200–202.

158. Homesly H, Zaino R. Endometrial cancer: prognostic factors. *Semin Oncol* 1994;21:71–8.

159. Kosary CL. FIGO stage, histology, histologic grade, age and race as prognostic factors in determining survival for cancers of the female gynecological system: an analysis of 1973–87 SEER cases of cancers of the endometrium, cervix, ovary, vulva, and vagina. *Semin Surg Oncol* 1994;10:31–46.

160. Wolfson A, Sightler S, Markoe A, et al. The prognostic significance of surgical staging for carcinoma of the endometrium. *Gynecol Oncol* 1992;45:142–146.

161. Zaino RJ, Kurman RJ, Diana KL, Morrow CP. Pathologic models to predict outcome for women with endometrial adenocarcinoma. *Cancer* 1996;77:1115.

162. Esteller M, Garcia A, Martinez-Palones JM, et al. Clinicopathologic features and genetic alterations in endometrioid carcinoma of the uterus with villoglandular differentiation. *Am J Clin Pathol* 1999;111:336–342.

163. Abeler VM, Kjorstad KE. Serous papillary carcinoma of the endometrium: a histopathological study of 22 cases. *Gynecol Oncol* 1990;39:266–271.

164. Carcangiu ML, Chambers JT. Uterine papillary serous carcinoma: a study on 108 cases with emphasis on the prognostic significance of associated endometrioid carcinoma, absence of invasion, and concomitant ovarian carcinoma. *Gynecol Oncol* 1992;47:298–305.

165. Chen J, Trost D, Wilkinson E. Endometrial papillary adenocarcinomas: two clinicopathologic types. *Int J Gynecol Pathol* 1985;4:279–288.

166. Hendrickson M, Martinez A, Ross J, et al. Uterine papillary serous carcinoma: a highly malignant form of endometrial adenocarcinoma. *Am J Surg Pathol* 1982;6:93–108.

167. Ward BG, Wright RG, Free K. Papillary carcinomas of the endometrium. *Gynecol Oncol* 1990;39:347–351.

168. Alektiar KM, McKee A, Lin O, et al. Is there a difference in outcome between stage I-II endometrial cancer of papillary serous/clear cell and endometrioid FIGO Grade 3 cancer? *Int J Radiat Oncol Biol Phys* 2002;54:79–85.

169. Aquino-Parsons C, Lim P, Wong F, Mildenberger M. Papillary serous and clear cell carcinoma limited to endometrial curettings in FIGO stage 1a and 1b endometrial adenocarcinoma: treatment implications. *Gynecol Oncol* 1998;71:83–86.

170. Carcangiu ML, Chambers JT. Early pathologic stage clear cell carcinoma and uterine papillary serous carcinoma of the endometrium:

comparison of clinicopathologic features and survival. *Int J Gynecol Pathol* 1995;14:30–38.

171. Kanbour-Shakir A, Tobon H. Primary clear cell carcinoma of the endometrium: a clinicopathologic study of 20 cases. *Int J Gynecol Pathol* 1991;10:67–78.

172. Malpica A, Tornos C, Burke TW, Silva EG. Low-stage clear-cell carcinoma of the endometrium. *Am J Surg Pathol* 1995;19:769–774.

173. Chambers SK, Kapp DS, Peschel RE, et al. Prognostic factors and sites of failure in FIGO stage I, grade 3 endometrial carcinoma. *Gynecol Oncol* 1987;27:180.

174. Sutton GP, Geiser HE, Stehman FB, et al. Features associated with survival and disease-free survival in early endometrial cancer. *Am J Obstet Gynecol* 1989;160:1385.

175. Wharton JT, Mikuta JJ, Mettlin C, et al. Risk factors and current management in carcinoma of the endometrium. *Surg Gynecol Obstet* 1986;162:515.

176. Yazigi R, Piver M, Blumenson I. Malignant peritoneal cytology as an indicator in Stage I endometrial cancer. *Obstet Gynecol* 1983;62:359–362.

177. Hall JB, Young RH, Nelson JH. The prognostic significance of adenomyosis in endometrial carcinoma. *Gynecol Oncol* 1984;17:32.

178. Hernandez E, Woodruff JD. Endometrial adenocarcinoma arising in adenomyosis. *Am J Obstet Gynecol* 1980;138:827.

179. Bucy GS, Mendenhall WM, Morgan LS, et al. Clinical Stage I and II endometrial carcinoma treated with surgery and/or radiation therapy: analysis of prognostic and treatment-related factors. *Gynecol Oncol* 1989;33:290.

180. Jones HW III. Treatment of adenocarcinoma of the endometrium. *Obstet Gynecol Surv* 1975;30:147.

181. Ambros R, Kurman R. Identification of patients with stage I uterine endometrioid adenocarcinoma at high risk of recurrence by DNA ploidy, myometrial invasion, and vascular invasion. *Gynecol Oncol* 1992;45:235–239.

182. Christopherson W, Connelly P, Alberhasky R. Carcinoma of the endometrium: V. An analysis of prognosticators in patients with favorable subtypes and stage I disease. *Cancer* 1983;51:1705–1709.

183. Eifel P, Ross J, Hendrickson M, et al. Adenocarcinoma of the endometrium: analysis of 256 cases with disease limited to the uterine corpus: treatment comparisons. *Cancer* 1983;52:1026–1031.

184. Lee KR, Vacek PM, Belinson JL. Traditional and nontraditional histopathologic predictors of recurrence in uterine endometrioid adenocarcinoma. *Gynecol Oncol* 1994;54:10–18.

185. Morrow CP, Bundy BN, Kumar RJ, et al. Relationship between surgical-pathological risk factors and outcome in clinical Stages I and II carcinoma of the endometrium. A Gynecologic Oncology Group study. *Gynecol Oncol* 1991;40:55.

186. Abeler VM, Kjorstad KE. Endometrial adenocarcinoma in Norway. A study of a total population. *Cancer* 1991;67:3093–3103.

187. Gal D, Recio FO, Zamurovic D, Tancer ML. Lymphovascular space involvement—a prognostic indicator in endometrial adenocarcinoma. *Gynecol Oncol* 1991;42:142–145.

188. Hanson M, van Nagell J, Powell D. The prognostic significance of lymph-vascular space invasion in Stage I endometrial cancer. *Cancer* 1985;55:1753–1757.

189. Inoue Y, Obata K, Abe K, et al. The prognostic significance of vascular invasion by endometrial carcinoma. *Cancer* 1996;78:1447–1451.

190. Sivridis E, Buckley CH, Fox H. The prognostic significance of lymphatic vascular space invasion in endometrial adenocarcinoma. *Br J Obstet Gynaecol* 1987;94:991.

191. Kennedy A, Peterson G, Becker S, et al. Experience with pelvic washings in stage I and II endometrial carcinoma. *Gynecol Oncol* 1987;28:50–60.

192. Creasman W, DiSaia P, Blessing J, et al. Prognostic significance of peritoneal cytology in patients with endometrial cancer and preliminary data concerning therapy with intraperitoneal radiopharmaceuticals. *Am J Obstet Gynecol* 1981;141:921–929.

193. Grimshaw R, Tupper W, Fraser R, et al. Prognostic value of peritoneal cytology in endometrial carcinoma. *Gynecol Oncol* 1990;36:97–100.

194. McLellan R, Dillon MB, Currie JL, Rosenshein NB. Peritoneal cytology in endometrial cancer: a review. *Obstet Gynecol Surv* 1989;44:711.

195. Sutton GP. The significance of positive peritoneal cytology in endometrial *cancer. Oncology* 1990;4:21.

196. Szpak C, Creasman W, Vollmer R, Johnston W. Prognostic value of cytologic examination of peritoneal washings in patients with endometrial carcinoma. *Acta Cytol* 1981;25:640–646.

197. Harouny V, Sutton G, Clark S, et al. The importance of peritoneal cytology in endometrial carcinoma. *Obstet Gynecol* 1988;72: 394–398.

198. Konski A, Poulter C, Keys H, et al. Absence of prognostic significance, peritoneal dissemination and treatment advantage in endometrial cancer patients with positive peritoneal cytology. *Int J Radiat Oncol Biol Phys* 1988;14:49.

199. Macdonald RR, Thorogood J, Mason MK. A randomized trial of progestogens in the primary treatment of endometrial carcinoma. *Br J Obstet Gynaecol* 1988;95:166.

200. Podratz KC, O'Brien PC, Malkasian GD Jr, et al. Effects of progestational agents in treatment of endometrial carcinoma. *Obstet Gynecol* 1985;66:106.

201. Creasman WT, Soper JT, McCarty KS Jr, et al. Influence of cytoplasmic steroid receptor content on prognosis of early stage endometrial carcinoma. *Am J Obstet Gynecol* 1985;151:922.

202. Turner D, Gershenson D, Atkinson N, et al. The prognostic significance of peritoneal cytology for stage I endometrial cancer. *Obstet Gynecol* 1989;74:775–780.

203. Kadar N, Homesley H, Malfetano J. Positive peritoneal cytology is an adverse risk factor in endometrial carcinoma only if there is other evidence of extrauterine disease. *Gynecol Oncol* 1992;46:145–149.

204. Britton L, Wilson T, Gaffey T, et al. Flow cytometric DNA analysis of stage I endometrial carcinoma. *Gynecol Oncol* 1989;34:317–322.

205. Geisinger K, Homesely H, Morgan T, et al. Endometrial adenocarcinoma. A multiparameter clinicopathologic analysis including the DNA profile and the sex steroid hormone receptors. *Cancer* 1986;58: 1518–1525.

206. Iversen O. Flow cytometric deoxyribonucleic acid index: a prognostic factor in endometrial carcinoma. *Am J Obstet Gynecol* 1986;155: 770–776.

207. Sorbe B, Risberg B, Frankendal B. DNA ploidy, morphometry, and nuclear grade as prognostic factors in endometrial carcinoma. *Gynecol Oncol* 1990;38:22–27.

208. Stendahl U, Strang P, Wagenius G, et al. Prognostic significance of proliferation in endometrial adenocarcinomas: a multivariate analysis of clinical and flow cytometric variables. *Int J Gynecol Pathol* 1991; 10:271–284.

209. van der Putten H, Baak J, Koenders T, et al. Prognostic value of quantitative pathologic features and DNA content in individual patients with stage I endometrial adenocarcinoma. *Cancer* 1989;63: 1378–1387.

210. Lukes AS, Kohler MF, Pieper CF, et al. Multivariable analysis of DNA ploidy, p53, and HER-2/neu as prognostic factors in endometrial cancer. *Cancer* 1994;73:2380–2385.

211. Nordstrom B, Strang P, Lindgren A, et al. Carcinoma of the endometrium: do the nuclear grade and DNA ploidy provide more prognostic information than do the FIGO and WHO classifications? *Int J Gynecol Pathol* 1996;15:191–201.

212. Pfisterer J, Kommoss F, Sauerbrei W, et al. Prognostic value of DNA ploidy and S-phase fraction in stage I endometrial carcinoma. *Gynecol Oncol* 1995;58:149–156.

213. Pisani AL, Barbuto DA, Chen D, et al. HER-2/neu, p53, and DNA analyses as prognosticators for survival in endometrial carcinoma. *Obstet Gynecol* 1995;85:729–734.

214. Susini T, Rapi S, Savino L, et al. Prognostic value of flow cytometric deoxyribonucleic acid index in endometrial carcinoma: comparison with other clinical-pathologic parameters. *Am J Obstet Gynecol* 1994; 170:527.

215. Trere D, Melchiorri C, Chieco P, et al. Interphase AgNOR quantity and DNA content in endometrial adenocarcinoma. *Gynecol Oncol* 1994;53:202–207.

216. Zaino RJ, Davis AT, Ohlsson-Wilhelm BM, Brunetto VL. DNA content is an independent prognostic indicator in endometrial adenocarcinoma. A Gynecologic Oncology Group study. *Int J Gynecol Pathol* 1998;17:312–319.

217. Lundberg C, Auer G, Frankendal B, et al. Nuclear DNA content, proliferative activity, and p53 expression related to clinical and histopathologic features in endometrial carcinoma. *Int J Gynecol Cancer* 2002;12:110–118.

218. Carcangiu M, Chambers J, Voynick I, et al. Immunohistochemical evaluation of estrogen and progesterone receptor content in 183 patients with endometrial carcinoma. Part II: Correlation between biochemical and immunohistochemical methods and survival. *Am J Clin Pathol* 1990;94:255–260.

219. Deligdisch L, Holinka C. Progesterone receptors in two groups of endometrial carcinoma. *Cancer* 1986;57:1385–1388.

220. Geisinger KR, Marshall RB, Kute TE, Homesley HD. Correlation of female sex steroid hormone receptors with histologic and ultrastructural differentiation in adenocarcinoma of the endometrium. *Cancer* 1986;58:1506-1517.

221. Kadar N, Malfetano J, Homesley H. Steroid receptor concentrations in endometrial carcinoma: effect on survival in surgically staged patients. *Gynecol Oncol* 1993;50:281–286.

222. McCarty K, Barton T, Fetter B, et al. Correlation of estrogen and progesterone receptors with histologic differentiation in endometrial adenocarcinoma. *Am J Pathol* 1979;96:171–184.

223. Ehrlich C, Young P, Stehman F, et al. Steroid receptors and clinical outcome in patients with adenocarcinoma of the endometrium. *Am J Obstet* 1988;158:796–807.

224. Fukuda K, Mori M, Uchiyama M, et al. Prognostic significance of progesterone receptor immunohistochemistry in endometrial carcinoma. *Gynecol Oncol* 1998;69:220–225.

225. Morris PC, Anderson JR, Anderson B, Buller RE. Steroid hormone receptor content and lymph node status in endometrial cancer. *Gynecol Oncol* 1995;56:406–411.

226. Nyholm HC, Christensen IJ, Nielsen AL. Progesterone receptor levels independently predict survival in endometrial adenocarcinoma. *Gynecol Oncol* 1995;59:347–351.

227. Tornos C, Silva EG, el-Naggar A, Burke TW. Aggressive stage I grade 1 endometrial carcinoma. *Cancer* 1992;70:790–798.

229. Lee JO, Yang H, Georgescu MM, et al. Crystal structure of the PTEN tumor suppressor: implications for its phosphoinositide phosphatase activity and membrane association. *Cell* 1999;99:323–334.

230. Li J, Yen C, Liaw D, et al. PTEN, a putative protein tyrosine phosphatase gene mutated in human brain, breast, and prostate cancer. *Science* 1997;275:1943–1947.

231. Maxwell GL, Risinger JI, Gumbs C, et al. Mutation of the PTEN tumor suppressor gene in endometrial hyperplasias. *Cancer Res* 1998; 58:2500.

232. Tamura M, Gu J, Matsumoto K, et al. Inhibition of cell migration, spreading, and focal adhesions by tumour suppressor PTEN. *Science* 1998;280:1614–1617.

233. Peiffer SL, Herzog TJ, Tribune DJ, et al. Allelic loss of sequences from the long arm of chromosome 10 and replication errors in endometrial cancers. *Cancer Res* 1995;55:1922–1926.

234. Kong D, Suzuki A, Zou TT, et al. PTEN1 is frequently mutated in primary endometrial carcinomas. *Nat Genet* 1997;17:143.

235. Risinger JI, Hayes AK, Berchech A, Barrett JC. PTEN/MMAC1 mutations in endometrial cancers. *Cancer Res* 1997;57:4736.

236. Tashiro H, Blazes MS, Wu R, et al. Mutations in PTEN are frequent in endometrial carcinoma but rare in other gynecological malignancies. *Cancer Res* 1997;57:3935–3940.

237. Risinger JI, Hayes K, Maxwell GL, et al. PTEN mutation in endometrial cancers is associated with favorable clinical and pathologic characteristics. *Clin Cancer Res* 1998;4:3005–3010.

238. Steck PA, Pershouse MA, Jasser SA, Y, et al. Identification of a candidate tumour suppressor gene, MMAC1, at chromosome $10_q23.3$ that is mutated in multiple advanced cancers. *Nat Genet* 1997;15: 356–362.

239. Caduff RF, Johnston CM, Svoboda-Newman SM, et al. Clinical and pathological significance of microsatellite instability in sporadic endometrial carcinoma. *Am J Pathol* 1996;148:1671–1678.

240. Duggan BD, Felix JC, Muderspach LI, et al. Microsatellite instability in sporadic endometrial carcinoma. *J Natl Cancer Inst* 1994;86: 1216–1221.

241. Helland A, Børresen-Dale AL, Peltomäki P, et al. Microsatellite instability in cervical endometrial carcinomas. *Int J Cancer* 1997;70: 499–501.

242. Martini M, Ciccarone M, Garganese G, et al. Possible involvement of hMLH1, p16(INK4a) and PTEN in the malignant transformation of endometriosis. *Int J Cancer* 2002;102:398–406.

243. Nagase S, Sato S, Tezuka F, et al. Deletion mapping on chromosome

10q25-q26 in human endometrial cander. *Br J Cancer* 1996;74: 1979–1983.

244. Risinger JI, Berchuck A, Kohler MF, et al. Genetic instability of microsatellite in endometrial carcinoma. *Cancer Res* 1993;53: 5100–5103.

245. Esteller M, Levine R, Baylin SB, et al. MLH1 promoter hypermethylation is associated with the microsatellite instability phenotype in sporadic carcinomas. *Oncogene* 1998;17:2413–2417.

246. Gurin CC, Federici MG, Kang L, Boyd J. Causes and consequences of microsatellite instability in endometrial carcinoma. *Cancer Res* 1999;59:462–466.

247. Baylin SB, Herman JG, Graff JR, et al. Alterations in DNA methylation: a fundamental aspect of neoplasia. *Adv Cancer Res* 1998;72: 141–196.

248. Herman JG, Latif F, Weng Y, et al. Silencing of the VHL tumor-suppressor gene by DNA methylation in real carcinoma. *Proc Natl Acad Sci U S A* 1994;91:9700–9704.

249. Jones PA, Laird PW. Cancer epigenetics comes of age. *Nat Genet* 1999;21:163–167.

250. Kowalski LD, Mutch DG, Herzog TJ, et al. Mutational analysis of MLH1 and MSH2 in 25 prospectively-acquired RER+ endometrial cancers. *Genes Chromosomes Cancer* 1997;18:219–227.

251. Merlo A, Herman JG, Mao L, et al. 5¹ CpG island methylation is associated with transcriptional silencing of the tumour suppressor p 16/CDKN2/MTS1 in human cancers. *Nat Med* 1995;1:686–692.

252. Tahiro H, Isacson C, Levine R, et al. p53 mutations are common in uterine serous carcinoma and occur as an early event in their pathogenesis. *Am J Pathol* 1997;150:177–185.

253. Ambros RA, Sheehan CE, Kallakury BV, et al. MDM2 and p53 protein expression in the histologic subtypes of endometrial carcinoma. *Mod Pathol* 1996;9:1165–1169.

254. Coppola D, Fu L, Nicosia SV, et al. Prognostic significance of p53, bcl-2, vimentin, and S100 protein-positive Langerhans cells in endometrial carcinoma. *Hum Pathol* 1998;29:455–462.

255. Geisler JP, Wiemann MC, Zhou Z, et al. p53 As a prognostic indicator in endometrial cancer. *Gynecol Oncol* 1996;61:245–248.

256. Hamel NW, Sebo TJ, Wilson TO, et al. Prognostic value of p53 and proliferating cell nuclear antigen expression in endometrial carcinoma. *Gynecol Oncol* 1996;62:192–198.

257. Jones MW, Kounelis S, Hsu C, et al. Prognostic value of p53 and K-ras-2 topographic genotyping in endometrial carcinoma: a clinicopathologic and molecular comparison. *Int J Gynecol Pathol* 1997;16: 354–360.

258. Khalifa MA, Mannel RS, Haraway SD, et al. Expression of EGFR, HER-2/neu, P53, and PCNA in endometrioid, serous papillary, and clear cell endometrial adenocarcinomas. *Gynecol Oncol* 1994;53: 84–92.

259. Kihana T, Hamada K, Inoue Y, et al. Mutation and allelic loss of the p53 gene in endometrial carcinoma. Incidence and outcome in 92 surgical patients. *Cancer* 1995;76:72–78.

260. Kohler MF, Carney P, Dodge R, et al. p53 Overexpression in advanced-stage endometrial adenocarcinoma. *Am J Obstet Gynecol* 1996;175:1246–1252.

261. Nielsen AL, Nyholm HC. p53 Protein and c-erbB-2 protein (p185) expression in endometrial adenocarcinoma of endometrioid type. an immunohistochemical examination on paraffin sections. *Am J Clin Pathol* 1994;102:76–79.

262. Nordstrom B, Strang P, Lindgren A, et al. Endometrial carcinoma: the prognostic impact of papillary serous carcinoma (UPSC) in relation to nuclear grade, DNA ploidy and p53 expression. *Anticancer Res* 1996; 16:899–904.

263. Risinger JI, Dent GA, Ignar-Trowbridge D, et al. p53 gene mutations in human endometrial carcinoma. *Mol Carcinog* 1992;5:250.

264. Tashiro H, Isacson C, Levine R, et al. p53 Gene mutations are common in uterine serous carcinoma and occur early in their pathogenesis. *Am J Pathol* 1997;150:177–185.

265. Taskin M, Lallas TA, Barber HR, Shevchuk MM. bcl-2 and p53 in endometrial adenocarcinoma. *Mod Pathol* 1997;10:728–734.

266. Yamauchi N, Sakamoto A, Uozaki H, et al. Immunohistochemical analysis of endometrial adenocarcinoma for bcl-2 and p53 in relation to expression of sex steroid receptor and proliferative activity [published erratum appears in *Int J Gynecol Pathol* 1996;15:369]. *Int J Gynecol Pathol* 1996;15:202–208.

267. Lax SF, Kendall B, Tashiro H, et al. The frequency of p53, K-ras mutation and microsatellite instability differs in uterine endometrioid and serous carcinoma. *Cancer* 2000;88:814–824.

268. Lalloo F, Evans G. Molecular genetics and endometrial cancer. *Best Pract Res Clin Gynaecol* 2001;15:355–363.

269. Berchuck A, Rodriguez G, Kinney R, et al. Overexpression of HER-2/neu in endometrial cancer is associated with advanced stage disease. *Am J Obstet Gynecol* 1991;164:15–21.

270. Reinartz JJ, George E, Lindgren BR, Niehans GA. Expression of p53, transforming growth factor alpha, epidermal growth factor receptor, and c-erbB-2 in endometrial carcinoma and correlation with survival and known predictors of survival. *Hum Pathol* 1994;25:1075–1083.

270a. Lim P, Al Kushi A, Gilks B, et al. Early stage uterine papillary serous carcinoma of the endometrium: effect of adjuvant whole abdominal radiotherapy and pathologic parameters on outcome. *Cancer* 2001; 91:752–757.

271. Rolitsky C, Theil K, McGaughy V, et al. HER-2/neu amplification and overexpression in endometrial carcinoma. *Int J Gynecol Pathol* 1999;18:138–143.

272. Backe J, Gassel AM, Krebs S, Muller T, Caffier H. Immunohistochemically detected HER-2/neu-expression and prognosis in endometrial carcinoma. *Arch Gynecol Obstet* 1997;259:189–195.

273. Hetzel D, Wilson T, Keeney G, et al. HER-2/neu expression: a major prognostic factor in endometrial cancer. *Gynecol Oncol* 1992;47: 179–85.

274. Nazeer T, Ballouk F, Malfetano JH, et al. Multivariate survival analysis of clinicopathologic features in surgical stage I endometrioid carcinoma including analysis of HER-2/neu expression. *Am J Obstet Gynecol* 1995;173:1829–1834.

275. Saffari B, Jones L, el-Naggar A, et al. Amplification and overexpression of HER-2/neu (c-erbB-2) in endometrial cancers: correlation with overall survival. *Cancer Res* 1995;55:5693–5698.

276. Moreno-Bueno G, Hardisson D, Sánchez C, et al. Abnormalities of the APC/β-catenin pathway in endometrial cancer. *Oncogene* 2002; 21:7981–7990.

277. Moreno-Bueno G, Hardisson D, Sarrió D, et al. Abnormalities of E- and P-cadherin and catenin (beta-, gamma-catenin, and p120ctn) expression in endometrial cancer and endometrial atypical hyperplasia. *J Pathol* 2003;199:471–478.

278. Caduff RF, Johnston CM, Frank TS. Mutations of the Ki-ras oncogene in carcinoma of the endometrium. *Am J Pathol* 1995;146:182–188.

279. Esteller M, Garcia A, Martinez-Palones JM, et al. The clinicopathological significance of K-RAS point mutation and gene amplification in endometrial cancer. *Eur J Cancer* 1997;33:1572–1577.

280. Ito K, Watanabe K, Nasim S, et al. K-ras point mutations in endometrial carcinoma: effect on outcome is dependent on age of patient. *Gynecol Oncol* 1996;63:238–246.

281. Semczuk A, Berbec H, Kostuch M, et al. K-ras gene point mutations in human endometrial carcinomas: correlation with clinicopathological features and patients' outcome. *J Cancer Res Clin Oncol* 1998;124: 695–700.

282. Katabuchi H, van Rees B, Lambers AR, et al. Mutations in DNA mismatch repair genes are not responsible for microsatellite instability in most sporadic endometrial carcinomas. *Cancer Res* 1995;55: 5556–5560.

283. Nakashima R, Fujita M, Enomoto T, et al. Alteration of p 16 and p 15 genes in human tumours. *Br J Cancer* 1999;80:458–467.

284. Winjen J, Leeuwen W, Vasen H, et al. Familial endometrial cancer in female carriers of MSH6 germline mutations. *Nat Genet* 1999;23: 142–144.

285. Salvesen HB, Das S, Akslen LA. Loss of nuclear p16 protein expression is not associated with promoter methylation but defines a subgroup of aggressive endometrial carcinomas with poor prognosis. *Clin Cancer Res* 2000;6:153–159.

286. Heyman J. The so-called Stockholm Method and the results of treatment of uterine cancer at the Radiumhemmet. *Acta Radiol* 1935;16: 129.

287. Arneson AN, Stanbro WW, Nolan JF. The use of multiple sources of radium within the uterus in the treatment of endometrial cancer. *Am J Obstet Gynecol* 1948;55:64.

288. Asbury RF, Blessing JA, McGuire WP, et al. Aminothiadiazole (NSC 4728) in patients with advanced carcinoma of the endometrium. A

Phase II study of the Gynecologic Oncology Group. *Am J Clin Oncol* 1990;13:39.

289. Nolan J, Arneson A. An instrument for inserting multiple capsules of radium within the uterus in the treatment of corpus cancers. *AJR Am J Roentgenol* 1943;49:504.

290. Lewis GC Jr, Slack NH, Mortel R, Bross ID. Adjuvant progestogen therapy in the primary definitive treatment of endometrial cancer. *Gynecol Oncol* 1974;2:368.

291. Kauppila A, Kujansuu E, Vihko R. Cytosol estrogen and progestin receptors in endometrial carcinoma of patients treated with surgery, radiotherapy, and progestin. Clinical correlates. *Cancer* 1982;50:2157.

292. Vergote I, Kjorstad K, Abeler V, Kolstad P. A randomized trial of adjuvant progestogen in early endometrial cancer. *Cancer* 1989;64:1011.

293. von Minckwitz G, Loibl S, Brunnert K, et al. Adjuvant endocrine treatment with medroxyprogesterone acetate or tamoxifen in stage I and II endometrial cancer—a multicentre, open, controlled, prospectively randomised trial. *Eur J Cancer* 2002;38:2265–2271.

294. Morley GW, Hopkins MP, Lindenauer SM, Roberts JA. Pelvic exenteration, University of Michigan: 100 patients at 5 years. *Obstet Gynecol* 1989;74:934.

295. Marziale P, Atlante G, Pozzi M, et al. 426 cases of Stage I endometrial carcinoma: a clinicopathological analysis. *Gynecol Oncol* 1989;32:278.

296. Arango HA, Hoffman Marit Scheistrøen, Roberts WS, et al. Accuracy of lymph node palpation to determine need for lymphadenectomy in gynecologic malignancies. *Obstet Gynecol* 2000;95:553–556.

297. Franchi M, Ghezzi F, Melpigano M, et al. Clinical value of intraoperative gross examination in endometrial cancer. *Gynecol Oncol* 2000;76:357–361.

298. COSA-NZ-UK. Endometrial Cancer Study Groups. Pelvic lymphadenectomy in high risk endometrial cancer. *Int J Gynaecol Cancer* 1996;6:102–107.

299. Kitchener HC. Surgery for endometrial cancer: what type and by whom. *Best Pract Res Clin Obstet Gynaecol* 2001;15:407–415.

300. Malviya VK, Deppe G, Malone JM Jr, et al. Reliability of frozen section examination in identifying poor prognostic indicators in Stage I endometrial adenocarcinoma. *Gynecol Oncol* 1989;34:299.

301. Childers JM, Brzechffa PR, Hatch KD, Surwit EA. Laparoscopically assisted surgical staging (LASS) of endometrial cancer. *Gynecol Oncol* 1993;51:33.

302. Childers JM, Surwit EA. Combined laparoscopic and vaginal surgery for the management of two cases of stage I endometrial cancer. *Gynecol Oncol* 1992;45:46–51.

303. Gemignani MI, Curtin JP, Zelmanovich J, et al. Laparoscopic-assisted vaginal hysterectomy for endometrial cancer: clinical outcomes and hospital charges. *Gynecol Oncol* 1999;73:5–11.

304. Boike G, Lurain J, Bruke J. A comparison of laparoscopic management of endometrial cancer with a traditional laparotomy. *Obstet Gynecol* 1994;52:105.

305. Magrina JF, Mutone NF, Weaver AL, et al. Laparoscopic lymphadenectomy and vaginal or laparoscopic hysterectomy with bilateral salpingo-oophorectomy for endometrial cancer. *Am J Obstet Gynecol* 1999;181:376–381.

306. Schribner DR, Mannel RS, Walker JL, Johnson GA. Cost analysis of laparoscopy versus laparotomy for early endometrial cancer. *Gynecol Oncol* 1999;75:460–463.

307. Spirtos NM, Schlaerth JB, Gross GM, et al. Cost and quality-of-life analyses of surgery for early endometrial cancer: laparotomy versus laparoscopy. *Am J Obstet Gynecol* 1996;174:1795–1799.

308. Malur S, Possover M, Wolfgang M, Schneider A. Laparoscopic-assisted vaginal versus abdominal surgery in patients with endometrial cancer: a prospective randomized trial. *Gynecol Oncol* 2001;80:239–244.

309. Fagotti A, Ferrandina G, Longo R, et al. Minilaparotomy in early stage endometrial cancer: an alternative to standard and laparoscopic treatment. *Gynecol Oncol* 2002;86:177–183.

310. Faught, W, Fung FK. Port site recurrence following laparoscopically managed early stage endometrial cancer. *Int J Gynecol Oncol* 1999;9:256–258.

311. Muntz HG, Goff BA, Madsen BL, You JL. Port-site recurrence after laparoscopic surgery for endometrial carcinoma. *Obstet Gynecol* 1999;93:807–809.

312. Wang PH, Yen MS, Yuan CC, et al. Port site metastasis after laparoscopic-assisted vaginal hysterectomy for endometrial cancer: possible mechanism and prevention. *Gynecol Oncol* 1997; 66:151–155.

313. Barakat RR, Park RC, Grigsby PW, et al. Corpus: epithelial tumors. In: Hoskins WJ, Perez CA, Young RC, eds. *Principles and practice of gynecologic oncology.* 2nd ed. Philadelphia: JB Lippincott Co, 1997:859–896.

314. Candiani GB, Belloni C, Maggi R, et al. Evaluation of different surgical approach in the treatment of endometrial cancer at FIGO stage I. *Gynecol Oncol* 1990;37:6.

315. Massi G, Savino L, Susini T. Vaginal hysterectomy versus abdominal hysterectomy for treatment of stage I endometrial adenocarcinoma. *Am J Obstet Gynecol* 1996;174:1320–1326.

316. Scarselli G, Savino L, Ceccherini R, et al. Role of vaginal surgery in the 1st stage endometrial cancer. Experience of the Florence School. *Eur J Gynaecol Oncol* 1992;13:15–19.

317. Bloss JD, Berman ML, Bloss LP, Buller RE. Use of vaginal hysterectomy for the management of stage I endometrial cancer in the medically compromised patient. *Gynecol Oncol* 1991;40:74–77.

318. Pitkin RM. Vaginal hysterectomy in obese women. *Obstet Gynecol* 1977;49:567–569.

319. Vardi JR, Tadros GH, Anselmo MT, Rafla SD. The value of exploratory laparotomy in patients with endometrial carcinoma according to the new International Federation of Gynecology and Obstetrics Staging. *Obstet Gynecol* 1992;80:204–208.

320. Roberts JA, Brunetto, Keyes HM, et al. A phase III randomized study of surgery vs. surgery plus adjunctive radiation therapy in intermediate-risk endometrial carcinoma (GOG 99) abstract 35. *Proc Soc Gynecol Oncol* 1998;70:

321. Creutzberg CL, van Putten WL, Koper PC, et al. Surgery and postoperative radiotherapy versus surgery alone for patients with stage-1 endometrial carcinoma: multicentre randomised trial. PORTEC Study Group. Post Operative Radiation Therapy in Endometrial Carcinoma. *Lancet* 2000;355:1404–1411.

322. Creutzberg CL, van Putten WL, Koper PC, et al. PORTEC Study Group. Survival after relapse in patients with endometrial cancer: results from a randomized trial. *Gynecol Oncol* 2003;89:201–209.

323. Aalders J, Abeler V, Kolstad P, et al: Postoperative external irradiation and prognostic parameters in stage I endometrial carcinoma: Clinical and histopathologic study of 540 patients. *Obstet Gynecol* 1980;56:419.

324. Greven KM, D'Agostino RB Jr, Lanciano RM, Corn BW. Is there a role for a brachytherapy vaginal cuff boost in the adjuvant management of patients with uterine-confined endometrial cancer? *Int J Radiat Oncol Biol Phys* 1998;42:101–104.

325. Randall ME, Wilder J, Greven K, et al. Role of intracavitary cuff boost after adjuvant external irradiation in early endometrial carcinoma. *Int J Radiat Oncol Biol Phys* 1990;19:49.

326. Rush S, Gal D, Potters L, et al. Pelvic control following external beam radiation for surgical stage I endometrial adenocarcinoma. *Int J Radiat Oncol Biol Phys* 1995;33:851–854.

327. Kucera H, Vaura N, Weghoupt K: Benefit of external irradiation in pathologic Stage I endometrial carcinoma: a prospective clinical trial of 605 patients who received postoperative vaginal irradiation and additional pelvic irradiation in the presence of unfavorable prognostic factors. *Gynecol Oncol* 1990;38:99.

328. Nori D, Merimsky O, Batata M, et al: Postoperative high dose-rate intravaginal brachytherapy combined with external irradiation for early stage endometrial cancer: A long-term followup. *Int J Radiat Oncol Biol Phys* 1994;30:831.

329. Horowitz NS, Peters WA 3rd, Smith MR, et al. Adjuvant high dose rate vaginal brachytherapy as treatment of stage I and II endometrial carcinoma. *Obstet Gynecol* 2002;99:235–240.

330. Mohan DS, Samuels MA, Selim MA, et al. Long-term outcomes of therapeutic pelvic lymphadenectomy for stage I endometrial adenocarcinoma. *Gynecol Oncol* 1998;70:165–171.

331. Orr JW Jr, Holimon JL, Orr PF. Stage I corpus cancer: is teletherapy necessary? *Am J Obstet Gynecol* 1997;176:777–788

332. Elliot P, Green D. The efficacy of postoperative vaginal irradiation in preventing vaginal recurrence in endometrial cancer. *Int J Gynecol Cancer* 1994;4:84.

333. Straughn JM Jr, Huh WK, Kelly FJ, et al. Conservative management of stage I endometrial carcinoma after surgical staging. *Gynecol Oncol* 2002;84:194–200.

334. Alektiar KM, McKee A, Venkatraman E, et al. Intravaginal high-dose-rate brachytherapy for Stage IB (FIGO Grade 1, 2) endometrial cancer. *Int J Radiat Oncol Biol Phys* 2002;53:707–713.

335. Anderson JM, Stea B, Hallum AV, et al. High-dose-rate postoperative vaginal cuff irradiation alone for stage IB and IC endometrial cancer. *Int J Radiat Oncol Biol Phys* 2000;46:417–425.

336. MacLeod C, Fowler A, Duval P, et al. High-dose-rate brachytherapy alone post-hysterectomy for endometrial cancer. *Int J Radiat Oncol Biol Phys* 1998;42:1033–1039.

337. Petereit DG, Tannehill SP, Grosen EA, et al. Outpatient vaginal cuff brachytherapy for endometrial cancer. *Int J Gynecol Cancer* 1999;9: 456–462.

338. Alektiar KM, McKee A, Lin O, et al. The significance of the amount of myometrial invasion in patients with Stage IB endometrial carcinoma. *Cancer* 2002;95:316–321.

339. Scholten AN, Creutzberg CL, Noordijk EM, Smit VT. Long-term outcome in endometrial carcinoma favors a two—instead of a three—tiered grading system. *Int J Radiat Oncol Biol Phys* 2002;52: 1067–1074.

340. Irwin C, Levin W, Fyles A, et al. The role of adjuvant radiotherapy in carcinoma of the endometrium—results in 550 patients with pathologic stage I disease. *Gynecol Oncol* 1998;70:247–254.

341. Piver M, Hempling R. A prospective trial of post-operative vaginal radium/cesium for grade 1–2 less than 50% myometrial invasion and pelvic radiation therapy for grade 3 or deep myometrial invasion in surgical stage I endometrial adenocarcinoma. *Cancer* 1990;66:133.

342. Straughn JM, Huh WK, Orr JW Jr, et al. Stage IC adenocarcinoma of the endometrium: survival comparisons of surgically staged patients with and without adjuvant radiation therapy. *Gynecol Oncol* 2003;89:295–300.

343. Chadha M, Nanavati PJ, Liu P, et al. Patterns of failure in endometrial carcinoma stage IB grade 3 and IC patients treated with postoperative vaginal vault brachytherapy. *Gynecol Oncol* 1999;75:103–107.

344. Fanning J. Long-term survival of intermediate risk endometrial cancer (stage IG3, IC, II) treated with full lymphadenectomy and brachytherapy without teletherapy. *Gynecol Oncol* 2001;82:371–374.

345. Weiss MF, Connell PP, Waggoner S, et al. External pelvic radiation therapy in stage IC endometrial carcinoma. *Obstet Gynecol* 1999;93: 599–602.

346. Pitson G, Colgan T, Levin W, et al. Stage II endometrial carcinoma: prognostic factors and risk classification in 170 patients. *Int J Radiat Oncol Biol Phys* 2002;53:862–867.

347. Ng TY, Nicklin JL, Perrin LC, et al. Postoperative vaginal vault brachytherapy for node-negative Stage II (occult) endometrial carcinoma. *Gynecol Oncol* 2001;81:193–195.

348. Milosevic MF, Dembo AJ, Thomas GM. The clinical significance of malignant peritoneal cytology in stage I endometrial carcinoma. *Int J Gynecol Cancer* 1992;2:225.

349. Soper JT, Creasman WT, Clarke-Pearson DL, et al. Intraperitoneal chromic phosphate ^{32}P suspension therapy of malignant peritoneal cytology in endometrial carcinoma. *Am J Obstet Gynecol* 1985;153: 191.

350. Eltabbakh GH, Piver MS, Hempling RE, Shin KH. Excellent long-term survival and absence of vaginal recurrences in 332 patients with low-risk stage I endometrial adenocarcinoma treated with hysterectomy and vaginal brachytherapy without formal staging lymph node sampling: report of a prospective trial. *Int J Radiat Oncol Biol Phys* 1997;38:373–380.

352. Ashman JB, Connell PP, Yamada D, et al. Outcome of endometrial carcinoma patients with involvement of the uterine serosa. *Gynecol Oncol* 2001;82:338–343.

353. Nicklin JL, Petersen RW. Stage 3B adenocarcinoma of the endometrium: a clinicopathologic study. *Gynecol Oncol* 2000;78:203–207.

354. Greven K, Corn B, Lanciano RM: Pathologic stage III endometrial carcinoma. *Cancer* 1993;71:3697.

355. Mariani A, Webb MJ, Keeney GL, et al. Stage IIIC endometrioid corpus cancer includes distinct subgroups. *Gynecol Oncol* 2002;87: 12–17.

356. Nelson G, Randall M, Sutton G, et al. FIGO stage IIIC endometrial carcinoma with metastases confined to pelvic lymph nodes: analysis of treatment outcomes, prognostic variables, and failure patterns following adjuvant radiation therapy. *Gynecol Oncol* 1999;75:211–214.

357. Corn BW, Lanciano RM, Greven KM, et al: Endometrial carcinoma with para-aortic lymphadenopathy: patterns of failure and opportunity for cure. *Int J Radiat Oncol Biol Phys* 1992;24:223.

358. Hicks ML, Piver S, Jeffrey LP, et al: Survival in patients with paraaortic lymph node metastases from endometrial adenocarcinoma clinically limited to the uterus. *Int J Radiat Oncol Biol Phys* 1993;26:607.

359. Rose PG, Cha SD, Tak WK, et al: Radiation therapy for surgically proven para-aortic node metastasis in endometrial carcinoma. *Int J Radiat Oncol Biol Phys* 1992;24:229.

360. Mariani A, Webb MJ, Keeney GL, et al. Endometrial cancer: predictors of peritoneal failure. *Gynecol Oncol* 2003;89:236–242.

361. Gibbons S, Martinez A, Schary M, et al: Adjuvant whole abdominopelvic irradiation for high-risk endometrial carcinoma. *Int J Radiat Oncol Biol Phys* 1991;21:1019.

362. Martinez A, Podratz K: Results of whole abdomino-pelvic radiation with nodal boost for patients with endometrial cancer at high risk of failure in the peritoneal cavity. *Hematol Oncol Clin North Am* 1988; 2:431.

363. Axelrod J, Bundy B, Roy T, et al. Advanced Endometrial Carcinoma (EC) treated with whole abdominal irradiation (WAI): A Gynecologic Oncology Group (GOG) Study. Presented at the Society of Gynecologic Oncologists' 26th Annual Meeting, 1995:136 (abst 99).

364. Stewart KD, Martinez AA, Weiner S, et al. Ten-year outcome including patterns of failure and toxicity for adjuvant whole abdominopelvic irradiation in high-risk and poor histologic feature patients with endometrial carcinoma. *Int J Radiat Oncol Biol Phys* 2002;54:527–535.

365. Rouanet P, Dubois JB, Gely S, Pourquier H. Exclusive radiation therapy in endometrial carcinoma. *Int J Radiat Oncol Biol Phys* 1993; 26:223–228.

366. Grigsby P, Kuske R, Perez CA, et al: Medically inoperable stage I adenocarcinoma of the endometrium treated with radiotherapy alone. *Int J Radiat Oncol Biol Phys* 1986;13:483.

367. Knocke TH, Kucera H, Weidinger B, et al. Primary treatment of endometrial carcinoma with high-dose-rate brachytherapy: results of 12 years of experience with 280 patients. *Int J Radiat Oncol Biol Phys* 15;37:359–365.

368. Nguyen TV, Petereit DG. High-dose-rate brachytherapy for medically inoperable stage I endometrial cancer. *Gynecol Oncol* 1998;71: 196–203.

369. Smith RS, Kapp DS, Chen Q, Teng NN. Treatment of high-risk uterine cancer with whole abdominopelvic radiation therapy. *Int J Radiat Oncol Biol Phys* 2000;48:767–778.

370. Creutzberg CL, van Putten WL, Koper PC, et al. PORTEC Study Group. The Postoperative Radiation Therapy in Endometrial Carcinoma. The morbidity of treatment for patients with Stage I endometrial cancer: results from a randomized trial. *Int J Radiat Oncol Biol Phys* 2001;51:1246–1255.

371. Sorbe BG, Smeds AC. Postoperative vaginal irradiation with high dose-rate afterloading technique in endometrial carcinoma Stage I. *Int J Radiat Oncol Biol Phys* 1990;18:305.

372. Morrow C, Bundy B, Homesley H, et al. Doxorubicin as an adjuvant following surgery and radiation therapy in patients with high-risk endometrial carcinoma, Stage I and occult Stage II: a Gynecologic Oncology Group study. *Gynecol Oncol* 1990;36:166.

373. Burke TW, Gershenson DM, Morris M, et al. Postoperative adjuvant cisplatin, doxorubicin, and cyclophosphamide (PAC) chemotherapy in women with high-risk endometrial carcinoma. *Gynecol Oncol* 1994; 55:47.

374. Kauppila A. Oestrogen and progestin receptors as prognostic indicators in endometrial cancer. A review of the literature. *Acta Oncol* 1989;28:561.

375. Kneale BL, Quinn MA, Rennie GC. A randomized trial of progestogens in the primary treatment of endometrial carcinoma. [Letter] *Br J Obstet Gynaecol* 1988;95:828.

376. Creasman WT, Henderson D, Hinshaw W, Clarke-Pearson DL. Estrogen replacement therapy in the patient treated for endometrial cancer. *Obstet Gynecol* 1986;67:326.

377. Lee RB, Burke TW, Park RC. Estrogen replacement therapy following treatment for Stage I endometrial carcinoma. *Gynecol Oncol* 1990; 36:189.

378. Baker D. Estrogen replacement therapy in patients with previous endometrial carcinoma. *Compr Ther* 1990;16:28.

379. ACOG Committee Opinion. Estrogen replacement therapy and endometrial cancer. August 1993; Number 126.

380. Barnhill D, O'Connor D, Farley J, et al. Clinical surveillance of gynecologic cancer patients. *Gynecol Oncol* 1992;46:275.

381. Salvesen HB. *Tumor biomarkers and prognostic factors in endometrial carcinoma.* Bergen, Norway: University of Bergen, 2000.

382. Berchuck A, Anspach C, Evans AC, et al. Postsurgical surveillance of patients with FIGO stage I/II endometrial adenocarcinoma. *Gynecol Oncol* 1995;59:20.

383. Podczaski E, Kamininski P, Gurski K, et al. Detection and patterns of treatment failure in 300 consecutive cases of early endometrial cancer after primary surgery. *Gynecol Oncol* 1992;47:323.

384. Shumsky AG, Stuart GE, Brasher PM, et al. An evaluation of routine follow-up of patients treated for endometrial carcinoma. *Gynecol Oncol* 1994;55:229.

385. Curran WJ, Whittington R, Peters AJ, et al: Vaginal recurrences of endometrial carcinoma: the prognostic value of staging by a primary vaginal carcinoma system. *Int J Radiat Oncol Biol Phys* 1988;15:803.

386. Sears J, Greven K: Prognostic factors and treatment outcome for patients with locally recurrent endometrial cancer. *Cancer* 1994;74:1303.

387. Wylie J, Irwin C, Pintilie M, et al. Results of radical radiotherapy for recurrent endometrial cancer. *Gynecol Oncol* 2000;77:66–72.

388. Jhingran A, Burke TW, Eifel PJ. Definitive radiotherapy for patients with isolated vaginal recurrence of endometrial carcinoma after hysterectomy. *Int J Radiat Oncol Biol Phys* 2003;56:1366–1372.

389. Barakat RR, Patel DA, Curtin JP, et al. Pelvic exenteration for recurrent endometrial adenocarcinoma. *Gynecol Oncol* 1996;250:163(abst).

390. Elit L, Hirte H. Current status and future innovations of hormonal agents, chemotherapy and investigational agents in endometrial cancer. *Curr Opin Obstet Gynecol* 2002;14:67–73.

391. Asbury RF, Brunetto VL, Lee RB, et al. Goserelin acetate as treatment for recurrent endometrial carcinoma: a Gynecologic Oncology Group study. *Am J Clin Oncol* 2002;25:557–560.

392. McMeekin DS, Gordon A, Fowler J, et al. A phase II trial of arzoxifene, a selective estrogen response modulator, in patients with recurrent or advanced endometrial cancer. *Gynecol Oncol* 2003;90:64–69.

393. Piver MS, Barlow JJ, Lurain JR, Blumenson LE. Medroxyprogesterone acetate (Depo-Provera) vs. hydroxyprogesterone caproate (Delalutin) in women with metastatic endometrial adenocarcinoma. *Cancer* 1980;45:268.

394. Quinn MA, Cauchi M, Fortune D. Endometrial carcinoma: steroid receptors and response to medroxyprogesterone acetate. *Gynecol Oncol* 1985;21:314.

395. Rose PG, Brunetto VL, et al. A phase II trial of anastrozole in advanced recurrent or persistent endometrial carcinoma: a Gynecologic Oncology Group study. *Gynecol Oncol* 2000;78(2):212–6.

396. Slavik M, Petty WM, Blessing JA, et al. Phase II clinical study of tamoxifen in advanced endometrial adenocarcinoma: a Gynecologic Oncology Group study. *Cancer Treat Rep* 1984;68:809.

397. Thigpen T, Brady MF, Homesley HD, et al. Tamoxifen in the treatment of advanced or recurrent endometrial carcinoma: a Gynecologic Oncology Group study. *J Clin Oncol* 2001;19:364–367.

398. Thigpen JT, Brady MF, Alvarez RD, et al. Oral medroxyprogesterone acetate in the treatment of advanced or recurrent endometrial carcinoma: a dose-response study by the Gynecologic Oncology Group. *J Clin Oncol* 1999;17:1736–1744.

399. Thigpen JT, Homesley HD. A randomized study of medroxyprogesterone acetate (MPA) 200mg versus 1000mg in the treatment of advanced, persistent or recurrent carcinoma of the endometrium. In: *Gynecologic Oncology Group Statistical Report*—February 1990: 177.

400. Lentz SS, Brady MF, Major FJ, et al. High-dose megestrol acetate in advanced or recurrent endometrial carcinoma: a Gynecologic Oncology Group Study. *J Clin Oncol* 1996;14:357–361.

401. Quinn MA, Campbell JJ, Murray R, Pepperell RJ. Tamoxifen and aminoglutethimide in the management of patients with advanced endometrial carcinoma not responsive to medroxyprogesterone. *Aust N Z J Obstet Gynaecol* 1981;21:226.

402. Pandya KJ, Yeap BY, Weiner LM, et al. Megestrol and tamoxifen in patients with advanced endometrial cancer: an Eastern Cooperative Oncology Group Study (E4882). *Am J Clin Oncol* 2001;24:43–46.

403. Satyaswaroop PG, Clarke CL, Zaino RJ, Mortel R. Apparent resistance in human endometrial carcinoma during combination treatment with tamoxifen and progestin may result from desensitization following downregulation of tumor progesterone receptor. *Cancer Lett* 1992; 62:107.

404. Fiorica J, Brunetto VL, et al. A Phase II study (GOG 153) of recurrent and advanced endometrial carcinoma treated with alternating courses of megestrol acetate and tamoxifen citrate. *Proc ASCO* 2000;22:1499(abst).

405. Vering A, Michel RT, Mitze M, et al. Influence of chemotherapy on hormone receptor concentration in a xenotransplanted endometrial cancer. *Eur J Obstet Gynecol Reprod Biol* 1992;45:131.

406. Bonte J, Decoster JM, Ide P. Vaginal cytologic evaluation as a practical link between hormone blood levels and tumor hormone dependency in exclusive medroxyprogesterone treatment of recurrent or metastatic endometrial adenocarcinoma. *Acta Cytol* 1977;21:218.

407. Stratton JA, Mannel RS, Rettenmaier MA, et al. Treatment of advanced and recurrent endometrial carcinoma: correlation of patient response to hormonal and cytotoxic chemotherapy and the response predicted by the subrenal capsule chemosensitivity assay. *Gynecol Oncol* 1989;32:55.

408. Zaino RJ, Satyaswaroop PG, Mortel R. Hormonal therapy of human endometrial adenocarcinoma in a nude mouse model. *Cancer Res* 1985;45:539.

409. Gallagher CJ, Oliver RT, Oram DH, et al. A new treatment for endometrial cancer with gonadotrophin releasing-hormone analogue. *Br J Obstet Gynaecol* 1991;98:1037.

410. De Vriese G, Bonte J. Possible role of goserelin, an LH-RH agonist in the treatment of gynaecological cancers. *Eur J Gynaecol Oncol* 1993;14:187.

411. Kleinman D, Douvdevani A, Schally AV, et al. Direct growth inhibition of human endometrial cancer cells by the gonadotropin-releasing hormone antagonist SB-75: role of apoptosis. *Am J Obstet Gynecol* 1994;170:96.

412. Chan S. A review of selective estrogen receptor modulators in the treatment of breast and endometrial cancer. *Semin Oncol* 2002;29[3 Suppl 11]:129–133.

413. Levine DA, Hoskins WJ. Update in the management of endometrial cancer. *Cancer J* 2002;8 [Suppl 1]:S31–S40.

414. Sonoda Y. Optimal therapy and management of endometrial cancer. *Expert Rev Anticancer Ther* 2003;3:37–47.

415. Ball H, Blessing JA, Lentz S, Mutch D. A phase II trial of Taxol in advanced and recurrent adenocarcinoma of the endometrium: a Gynecologic Oncology Group study. *Gynecol Oncol* 1996;62:278.

416. Barton C, Buxton EJ, Blachledge G, et al. A phase II study of ifosfamide in endometrial cancer. *Cancer Chemother Pharmacol* 1990;26 [Suppl]:S4.

417. Boadle DJ, Tattersall MH. Phase II study of mitoxantrone in advanced or metastatic endometrial carcinoma. *Aust N Z J Obstet Gynaecol* 1987;27:341.

418. Brenner DE, Garbino C, Kasdorf H, et al. A phase II trial of m-AMSA in the treatment of advanced gynecologic malignancies. *Am J Clin Oncol* 1982;5:291.

419. Broun GO, Blessing JA, Eddy GL, Adelson MD. A phase II trial of vincristine in advanced or recurrent endometrial carcinoma. A Gynecologic Oncology Group study. *Am J Clin Oncol* 1993;16:18.

420. Burke TW, Munkarah A, Kavanagh JJ, et al. Treatment of advanced or recurrent endometrial carcinoma with single-agent carboplatin. *Gynecol Oncol* 1993;51:397.

421. Calero F, Asins-Codoner E, Jimeno J, et al. Epirubicin in advanced endometrial adenocarcinoma: a phase II study of the Grupo Ginecologico Espanol para el Tratamiento Oncologico (GGETO). *Eur J Cancer* 1991;27:864.

422. Chauvergne J, Fumoleau P, Cappelaere P, et al. Phase II study of pirarubicin (THP) in patients with cervical, endometrial and ovarian cancer: study of the Clinical Screening Group of the European Organization for Research and Treatment of Cancer (EORTC). *Eur J Cancer* 1993;29A:350.

423. Deppe G, Cohen CJ, Bruckner HW. Treatment of advanced endometrial adenocarcinoma with cis-dichlorodiamine platinum (II) after intensive prior therapy. *Gynecol Oncol* 1980;10:51.

424. Dvorak O. Cytembena treatment of advanced gynecological carcinomas. *Neoplasm* 1971;18:461.

425. Edmonson JH, Krook JE, Hilton JF, et al. Randomized phase II studies of cisplatin and a combination of cyclophosphamide-doxorubicin-cisplatin (CAP) in patients with progestin-refractory advanced endometrial carcinoma. *Gynecol Oncol* 1987;28:20.

426. Green JB, Green S, Alberts DS, et al. Carboplatin therapy in advanced endometrial cancer. *Obstet Gynecol* 1990;75:696.

427. Hilgers RD, Legha SS, Johnston GA Jr, et al. m-AMSA and adenocarcinoma of the endometrium. A Southwest Oncology Group study. *Invest New Drugs* 1984;2:335.

428. Hilgers RD, Von Hoff DD, Stephens RL, et al. Mitoxantrone in adenocarcinoma of the endometrium: a Southwest Oncology Group study. *Cancer Treat Rep* 1985;69:1329.

429. Homesley HD, Blessing JA, Conroy J, et al. ICRF-159 (razoxane) in patients with advanced adenocarcinoma of the endometrium. A Gynecologic Oncology Group study. *Am J Clin Oncol* 1986;9:15.

430. Horton J, Begg CB, Arseneault J, et al. Comparison of Adriamycin with cyclophosphamide in patients with advanced endometrial cancer. *Cancer Treat Rep* 1978;62:159.

431. Jackson DV Jr, Jobson VW, Homesley HD, et al. Vincristine infusion in refractory gynecologic malignancies. *Gynecol Oncol* 1986;25:212.

432. Kavanagh JJ, Saul PB, Wharton JT, Rutledge FN. A trial of continuous-infusion vinblastine in refractory endometrial adenocarcinoma. *Gynecol Oncol* 1987;26:236.

433. Long HJ, Pfeifle DM, Wieand HS, et al. Phase II evaluation of carboplatin in advanced endometrial carcinoma. *J Natl Cancer Inst* 1988; 80:276.

434. Malviya VK, Liu PY, O'Toole R, et al. Phase II trial of amonafide in patients with advanced metastatic or recurrent endometrial adenocarcinoma. A Southwest Oncology Group study. *Am J Clin Oncol* 1994;17:37.

435. Muss HB, Blessing JA, DuBeshter B. Echinomycin in recurrent and metastatic endometrial carcinoma. A phase II trial of the Gynecologic Oncology Group. *Am J Clin Oncol* 1993;16:492.

436. Muss HB, Bundy BN, Adcock L. Teniposide (VM-26) in patients with advanced endometrial carcinoma. A phase II trial of the Gynecologic Oncology Group. *Am J Clin Oncol* 1991;14:36.

437. Muss HB, Bundy BN, DiSaia PJ, Ehrlich CE. Mitoxantrone for carcinoma of the endometrium: a phase II trial of the Gynecologic Oncology Group. *Cancer Treat Rep* 1987;71:217.

438. Omura GA, Shingleton HM, Creasman WT, et al. Chemotherapy of gynecologic cancer with nitrosoureas: a randomized trial of CCNU and methyl-CCNU in cancers of the cervix, corpus, vagina, and vulva. *Cancer Treat Rep* 1978;62:833.

439. Seski JC, Edwards CL, Copeland LJ, Gershenson DM. Hexamethylmelamine chemotherapy for disseminated endometrial cancer. *Obstet Gynecol* 1981;58:361.

440. Seski JC, Edwards CL, Herson J, Rutledge FN. Cisplatin chemotherapy for disseminated endometrial cancer. *Obstet Gynecol* 1982; 59:225.

441. Slayton R, Faraggi D. A phase II clinical trial of methyl-glyoxalbisguanylhydrazone (MGBG) in advanced endometrial cancer. *Proc Am Soc Clin Oncol* 1986;5:119(abst).

442. Slayton RE, Blessing JA, Delgado G. Phase II trial of etoposide in the management of advanced or recurrent endometrial carcinoma: a Gynecologic Oncology Group study. *Cancer Treat Rep* 1982;66:1669.

443. Slayton RE, Blessing JA, DiSaia PJ, Phillips G. A phase II clinical trial of diaziquone in the treatment of patients with recurrent endometrial carcinoma. A Gynecologic Oncology Group study. *Am J Clin Oncol* 1988;11:612.

444. Sutton GP, Blessing JA, Homesley HD, et al. Phase II study of ifosfamide and mesna in refractory adenocarcinoma of the endometrium. A Gynecologic Oncology Group study. *Cancer* 1994;73:1453.

445. Thigpen JT, Blessing J, DiSaia P, Ehrlich C. A randomized comparison of Adriamycin with or without cyclophosphamide in the treatment of advanced or recurrent endometrial cancer. *Proc Am Soc Clin Oncol* 1985;4:115(abst).

446. Thigpen JT, Blessing JA, Ball H, et al. Hexamethylmelamine as first-line therapy in the treatment of advanced or recurrent carcinoma of the endometrium: a phase II trial of the Gynecologic Oncology Group. *Gynecol Oncol* 1988;31:435.

447. Thigpen JT, Blessing JA, Homesley H, et al. Phase II trial of cisplatin as first-line chemotherapy in patients with advanced or recurrent endometrial carcinoma: a Gynecologic Oncology Group study. *Gynecol Oncol* 1989;33:68.

448. Thigpen JT, Blessing JA, Homesley HD, Petty W. Phase II trial of piperazinedione in the treatment of advanced or recurrent endometrial carcinoma. A Gynecologic Oncology Group study. *Am J Clin Oncol* 1986;9:21.

449. Thigpen JT, Blessing JA, Lagasse LD, et al. Phase II trial of cisplatin as second-line chemotherapy in patients with advanced or recurrent endometrial carcinoma. A Gynecologic Oncology Group study. *Am J Clin Oncol* 1984;7:253.

450. Thigpen JT, Buchsbaum HJ, Mangan C, Blessing JA. Phase II trial of Adriamycin in the treatment of advanced or recurrent endometrial carcinoma: a Gynecologic Oncology Group study. *Cancer Treat Rep* 1979;63:21.

451. Thigpen JT, Kronmal R, Vogel S, et al. A Phase II trial of vinblastine in patients with advanced or recurrent endometrial carcinoma. A Southwest Oncology Group study. *Am J Clin Oncol* 1987;10:429.

452. Von Hoff DD, Green S, Alberts DS, et al. Phase II study of fludarabine phosphate (NSC-312887) in patients with advanced endometrial cancer. A Southwest Oncology Group study. *Am J Clin Oncol* 1991;14: 193.

453. Muss HB, Blessing JA, Hatch KD, et al. Methotrexate in advanced endometrial carcinoma. A phase II trial of the Gynecologic Oncology Group. *Am J Clin Oncol* 1990;13:61.

454. Woo HL, Swenerton KD, Hoskins PJ. Taxol is active in platinum-resistant endometrial adenocarcinoma. *Am J Clin Oncol* 1996;19: 290–291.

455. Wadler S, Levy DE, Lincoln ST, et al. Topotecan is an active agent in the first-line treatment of metastatic or recurrent endometrial carcinoma: Eastern Cooperative Oncology Group Study E3E93. *J Clin Oncol* 2003;21(11):2110–4.

456. Alberts DS, Mason NL, O'Toole RV, et al. Doxorubicin-cisplatin-vinblastine combination chemotherapy of advanced endometrial carcinoma: a Southwest Oncology Group study. *Gynecol Oncol* 1987; 26:193.

457. Barrett RJ, Blessing JA, Homesley HD, et al. Circadian-timed combination doxorubicin-cisplatin chemotherapy for advanced endometrial carcinoma. A phase II study of the Gynecologic Oncology Group. *Am J Clin Oncol* 1993;16:494.

458. Bruckner HW, Deppe G. Combination chemotherapy of advanced endometrial adenocarcinoma with Adriamycin, cyclophosphamide, 5-fluorouracil, and medroxyprogesterone acetate. *Obstet Gynecol* 1977; 50:10s.

459. Burke TW, Stringer CA, Morris M, et al. Prospective treatment of advanced or recurrent endometrial carcinoma with cisplatin, doxorubicin, and cyclophosphamide. *Gynecol Oncol* 1991;40:264.

460. Campora E, Vidali A, Mammoliti S, et al. Treatment of advanced or recurrent adenocarcinoma of the endometrium with doxorubicin and cyclophosphamide. *Eur J Gynaecol Oncol* 1990;11:181.

461. Cohen CJ, Bruckner HW, Deppe G, et al. Multidrug treatment of advanced and recurrent endometrial carcinoma: a Gynecologic Oncology Group study. *Obstet Gynecol* 1984;63:719.

462. Dunton CJ, Pfeifer SM, Braitman LE, et al. Treatment of advanced and recurrent endometrial cancer with cisplatin, doxorubicin, and cyclophosphamide. *Gynecol Oncol* 1991;41:113.

463. Hancock KC, Freedman RS, Edwards CL, et al. Use of cisplatin, doxorubicin, and cyclophosphamide to treat advanced and recurrent adenocarcinoma of the endometrium. *Cancer Treat Rep* 1986;70:789.

464. Long HJ, Langdon RM, Wieand HS. Phase II trial of methotrexate, vinblastine, doxorubicin, and cisplatin (MVAC) in women with advanced endometrial cancer. *Proc Am Soc Clin Oncol* 1991;10: 184(abst).

465. Muggia FM, Chia G, Reed LJ, Romney SL. Doxorubicin-cyclophosphamide: effective chemotherapy for advanced endometrial adenocarcinoma. *Am J Obstet Gynecol* 1977;128:314.

466. Pasmantier MW, Coleman M, Silver RT, et al. Treatment of advanced endometrial carcinoma with doxorubicin and cisplatin: effects on both untreated and previously treated patients. *Cancer Treat Rep* 1985;69: 539.

467. Piver MS, Fanning J, Baker TR. Phase II trial of cisplatin, Adriamycin, and etoposide for metastatic endometrial adenocarcinoma. *Am J Clin Oncol* 1991;14:200.

468. Seltzer V, Vogl SE, Kaplan BH. Adriamycin and cis-diammine-dichloroplatinum in the treatment of metastatic endometrial adenocarcinoma. *Gynecol Oncol* 1984;19:308.

469. Seski JC, Edwards CL, Gershenson DM, Copeland LJ. Doxorubicin and cyclophosphamide chemotherapy for disseminated endometrial cancer. *Obstet Gynecol* 1981;58:88.

470. Thigpen JT, Blessing JA, DiSaia PJ, et al. A randomized comparison of doxorubicin alone versus doxorubicin plus cyclophosphamide in the management of advanced or recurrent endometrial carcinoma: a Gynecologic Oncology Group study. *J Clin Oncol* 1994;12:1408.

471. Thigpen T, Blessing J, Homesley H, et al. Phase III trial of doxorubicin +/- cisplatin in advanced or recurrent endometrial carcinoma: a Gynecologic Oncology Group (GOG) study. *Proc Am Soc Clin Oncol* 1993;12:261(abst).

472. Tropé C, Johnsson JE, Simonsen E, et al. Treatment of recurrent endometrial adenocarcinoma with a combination of doxorubicin and cisplatin. *Am J Obstet Gynecol* 1984;149:379.

473. Gallion H, Brunetto VL, et al. Standard timed doxorubicin plus cisplatin versus circadian timed doxorubicin plus cisplatin in patients with FIGO Stage III/IV or recurrent endometrial carcinoma. *Gynecol Oncol* 2002;84:487(abst 27).

474. Fleming G, Brunetto VL, et al. Randomized trial of doxorubicin plus cisplatin versus doxorubicin plus paclitaxel plus granulocyte colony stimulating factor in patients with advanced or recurrent endometrial cancer: a report on Gynecology Oncology Group Protocol. *Proc ASCO* 2000;19:1498(abst).

475. Fleming G, Brunetto VL, et al. Randomized trial of doxorubicin plus cisplatin versus doxorubicin plus cisplatin plus paclitaxel in patients with advanced or recurrent endometrial carcinoma: a Gynecologic Oncology Group Study. *Proc ASCO* 2002;21:807(abst).

476. Santin AD, Bellone S, Gokden M, et al. Overexpression of HER-2/neu in uterine serous papillary cancer. *Clin Cancer Res* 2002;8:1271–1279.

477. Hoskins PJ, Swenerton KD, Pike JA, et al. Paclitaxel and carboplatin, alone or with irradiation, in advanced or recurrent endometrial cancer: a phase II study. *J Clin Oncol* 2001;19(20):4048–4053.

478. Onishi Y, Nakamura T, et al. Evaluation of paclitaxel and carboplatin in patients with endometrial cancer. *Proc ASCO* 2003;22:1958(abst).

479. Weber B, Mayer F, et al. What is the best chemotherapy regimen in recurrent or advanced endometrial carcinoma? Preliminary results. *Proc ASCO* 2003;22:1819(abst).

480. Deppe G, Jacobs AJ, Bruckner H, Cohen CJ. Chemotherapy of advanced and recurrent endometrial carcinoma with cyclophosphamide, doxorubicin, 5-fluorouracil, and megestrol acetate. *Am J Obstet Gynecol* 1981;140:313.

481. Hoffman MS, Roberts WS, Cavanagh D, et al. Treatment of recurrent and metastatic endometrial cancer with cisplatin, doxorubicin, cyclophosphamide, and megestrol acetate. *Gynecol Oncol* 1989;35:75.

482. Horton J, Elson P, Gordon P, et al. Combination chemotherapy for advanced endometrial cancer. An evaluation of three regimens. *Cancer* 1982;49:2441.

483. Lovecchio JL, Averette HE, Lichtinger M, et al. Treatment of advanced or recurrent endometrial adenocarcinoma with cyclophosphamide, doxorubicin, cis-platinum, and megestrol acetate. *Obstet Gynecol* 1984;63:557.

484. Piver MS, Lele SB, Patsner B, Emrich LJ. Melphalan, 5-fluorouracil, and medroxyprogesterone aceatate in metastatic endometrial carcinoma. *Obstet Gynecol* 1986;67:261.

485. Purdie DM, Green AC. Epidemiology of endometrial cancer. *Best Pract Res Clin Obstet Gynaecol* 2001;15:341–354.

486. Kurjak A, Shalan H, Sosic A, et al. Endometrial carcinoma in postmenopausal women: evaluation by transvaginal color Doppler ultrasonography. *Am J Obstet Gynecol* 1993;169:1597.

487. Friberg L-G, Norén H, Delle U. Prognostic value of DNA ploidy and S-phase fraction in endometrial cancer Stage I and II: a prospective 5-year survival study. *Gynecol Oncol* 1994;53:64.

488. Ikeda M, Watanabe Y, Nanjoh T, Noda K. Evaluation of DNA ploidy in endometrial cancer. *Gynecol Oncol* 1993;50:25.

489. Newbury J, Schuerch C, Goodspeed N, et al. DNA content as a prognostic factor in endometrial carcinoma. *Obstet Gynecol* 1990;76:251.

490. Podratz KC, Wilson TO, Gaffey TA, et al. Deoxyribonucleic acid analysis facilitates the pretreatment identification of high-risk endometrial cancer patients. *Am J Obstet Gynecol* 1993;168:1206.

491. Chambers JT, MacLusky N, Eisenfield A, et al. Estrogen and progestin receptor levels as prognosticators for survival in endometrial cancer. *Gynecol Oncol* 1988;31:65.

492. Baillie CT, Winslet MC, Bradley NJ. Tumour vasculature—a potential therapeutic target. *Br J Cancer* 1995;72:257–267.

493. Hanahan D, Folkman J. Patterns and emerging mechanisms of the angiogenetic switch during tumorigenesis. *Cell* 1996;86:353–364.

494. Goldman CK, Kendall RL, Cabrera G, et al. Paracrine expression of a native soluble vascular endothelial growth factor receptor inhibits tumor growth, metastasis, and mortality rate. *Proc Natl Acad Sci U S A* 1998;95:8795–8800.

495. Maekawa R, Maki H, Yoshida H, et al. Correlation of antiangiogenic and antitumor efficacy of N-biphenyl sulfonyl-phenylalanine hydroxiamic acid (BPHA), an orally-active, selective matrix metalloproteinase inhibitor. *Cancer Res* 1999;59:1231–1235.

496. O'Reilly MS, Pirie-Shepherd S, Lane WS, Folkman J. Antiangiogenic activity of the cleaved conformation of the serpin antithrombin. *Science* 1999;285:1926–1928.

497. Aas T, Børresen AL, Geisler S, et al. Specific p53 mutations are associated with de novo resistance to doxorubicin in breast cancer patients. *Nat Med* 1996;2:811–814.

498. Bischoff JR, Kirn DH, Williams A, et al. An adenovirus mutant that replicates selectively in p-53-deficient human tumor cells. *Science* 1996;274:373–376.

499. Roth JA, Nguyen D, Lawrence DD, et al. Retrovirus-mediated wild-type p-53 gene transfer to tumors of patients with lung cancer. *Nat Med* 1996;2:985–991.

500. Carbone PP, Carter SK. Endometrial cancer: approach to development of effective chemotherapy. *Gynecol Oncol* 1974;2:348.

a1. Berchuck A, Soisson AP, Clarke-Pearson DL, et al. Immunohistochemical expression of Ca-125 in endometrial adenocarcinoma: correlation of antigen expression with metastatic potential. *Cancer Res* 1989;49:2091.

a3. Cianciulli AM, Guadagni F, Marzano R, et al. HER-2/neu oncogene amplification and chromosome 17 aneusomy in endometrial carcinoma: correlation with oncoprotein expression and conventional pathological parameters. *J Exp Clin Cancer Res* 2003;22:265–271.

a4. Kilgore LC, Partridge EE, Alvarez RD, et al. Adenocarcinoma of the endometrium: survival comparisons of patients with and without pelvic node sampling. *Gynecol Oncol* 1995;56:29–33.

a5. Kohlberger P, Gitsch G, Loesch A, et al. P53 protein overexpression in early stage endometrial cancer. *Gynecol Oncol* 1996;62:213.

a7. Tsuda H, Hirohashi S. Frequent occurrence of p53 gene mutations in uterine cancers at advanced clinical stage and with aggressive histological phenotypes. *Jpn J Cancer Res* 1991;83:1184.

a8. Zaino R, Kurman R, Herbold D, et al. The significance of squamous differentiation in endometrial carcinoma. *Cancer* 1991;68:2293–2302.

CHAPTER 24

Corpus: Mesenchymal Tumors

Gregory Sutton, John Kavanagh, Aaron Wolfson, and Carmen Tornos

Uterine sarcomas are rare malignancies that will account for as few as 6% of the estimated 40,100 cases of cancer of the uterine corpus in the United States in 2004 (1). Although the general prognosis of endometrial adenocarcinomas is excellent (a projected 6,800 disease-related deaths in 2004), uterine sarcomas are generally aggressive and overall mortality rates approached 90% in early reports (2). In a 1997 Norwegian survery, uterine sarcomas accounted for 26% of all deaths from uterine malignancies (3). Uterine sarcomas encompass a broad spectrum of neoplasms from pure smooth muscle tumors and endometrial stromal tumors (leiomyosarcomas and endometrial stromal sarcomas) to mixed epithelial/stromal tumors such as adenosarcoma and carcinosarcoma. Several classification systems exist (4), most based upon the original work of Ober (5); the World Health Organization histologic classification system of uterine sarcomas is summarized in Table 24.1.

EPIDEMIOLOGY AND RISK FACTORS

Leiomyosarcoma and Carcinosarcoma

The two major sarcomas, leiomyosarcoma and carcinosarcoma, are epidemiologically distinguishable in several ways including median age at diagnosis, racial distribution, appar-

ent relative incidence, method of diagnosis, and prior radiotherapy.

Median Age at Diagnosis

Figure 24.1 demonstrates mean ages at diagnosis for common uterine sarcomas and endometrial adenocarcinomas. Although impossible to subject to statistical scrutiny, patients with carcinosarcomas are on the average older [mean 65 (2), 67 (6) years] than those with endometrial adenocarcinomas [mean 59.1 years (7)], müllerian adenosarcomas [mean 57.4 (8), 58 (9) years], leiomyosarcomas [mean 53.5 (10), 55 (11), 56.2 (12) years], and endometrial stromal tumors [mean 41 (13), 46 (14), 48 (15) years]. Olah et al. (6) observed a bimodal age distribution in their review of 423 cases of uterine sarcoma; they attributed this to a premenopausal peak for patients with leiomyosarcoma and a postmenopausal peak for those with carcinosarcomas. Thus, many patients with carcinosarcomas are postmenopausal, whereas those with leiomyosarcomas may be premenopausal or perimenopausal at the time of diagnosis. In a review of 208 patients with leiomyosarcomas from the Mayo Clinic (11), only 41% were postmenopausal. Figures 24.2 and 24.3 demonstrate that the incidence of carcinosarcoma rises exponentially with age, especially for nonwhites, beginning at 50 to 54 years, whereas leiomyosarcoma plateaus in middle age regardless of race.

Racial Distribution

Zelmanowicz et al. (16) are the most recent investigators to note that women with carcinosarcomas are more likely to be of African-American descent (among 453 patients and controls, 28% versus 4%, $p = .001$) than those with endometrial adenocarcinomas. In the reviews of Mortel et al. and

Gregory Sutton: Division of Gynecologic Oncology, Obstetrics and Gynecology, St. Vincent Hospitals and Health Services, Indianapolis, Indiana 46260.

John Kavanagh: Department of Gynecologic Medical Oncology, M. D. Anderson Cancer Center, Houston, Texas 77030.

Aaron Wolfson: Department of Radiation Oncology, University of Miami, School of Medicine, Miami, Florida 33136.

Carmen Tornos: Department of Pathology, Memorial Sloan–Kettering Cancer Center, New York, New York 10021.

TABLE 24.1. *World Health Organization classification system of uterine sarcomas*

Mesenchymal tumors
Endometrial stromal and related tumors
  Endometrial stromal sarcoma, low grade
  Endometrial stromal nodule
  Undifferentiated endometrial sarcoma
Smooth muscle tumors
  Leiomyosarcoma
    Epithelioid variant
    Myxoid variant
  Smooth muscle tumor of uncertain malignant potential
  Leiomyoma, not otherwise specified
    Histologic variants
      Mitotically active variant
      Cellular variant
      Hemorrhagic cellular variant
      Epithelioid variant
      Myxoid
      Atypical variant
      Lipoleiomyoma variant
    Growth pattern variants
      Diffuse leiomyomatosis
      Dissecting leiomyoma
      Intravenous leiomyomatosis
      Metastasizing leiomyoma
Miscellaneous mesenchymal tumors
  Mixed endometrial stromal and smooth muscle tumor
  Perivascular epithelioid cell tumor
  Adenomatoid tumor
  Other malignant mesenchymal tumors
  Other benign mesenchymal tumors
Mixed epithelial and mesenchymal tumors
  Carcinosarcoma (malignant müllerian mixed tumor, metaplastic carcinoma)
  Adenosarcoma
  Carcinofibroma
  Adenofibroma
  Adenomyoma
    Atypical polypoid variant

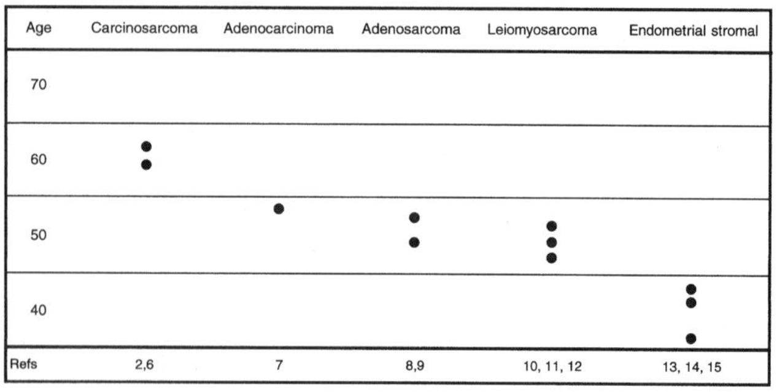

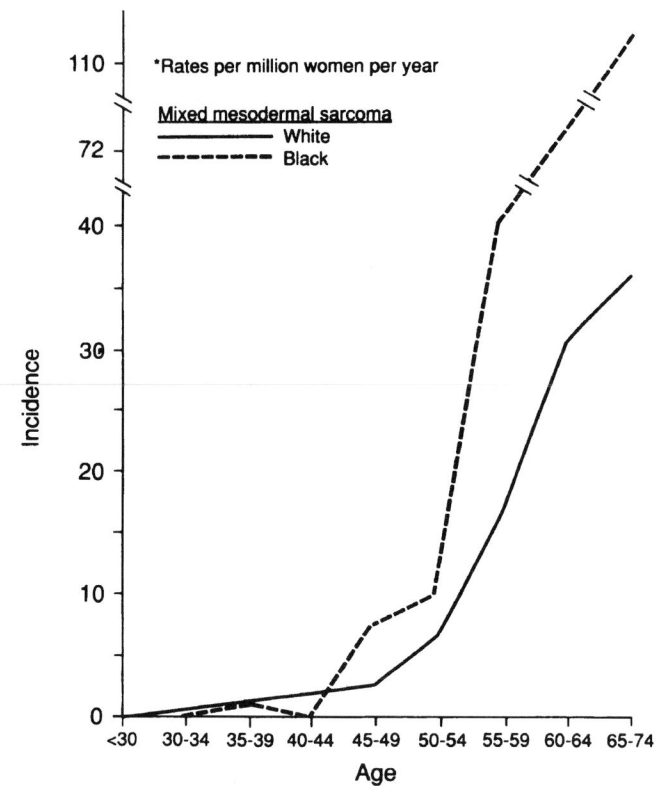

FIG. 24.2. Age distribution of patients with carcinosarcomas.

Age	Carcinosarcoma	Adenocarcinoma	Adenosarcoma	Leiomyosarcoma	Endometrial stromal
70					
60	• •				
50		•	• •	• •	
40					• • •
Refs	2,6	7	8,9	10, 11, 12	13, 14, 15

FIG. 24.1. Age at diagnosis of common uterine sarcomas.

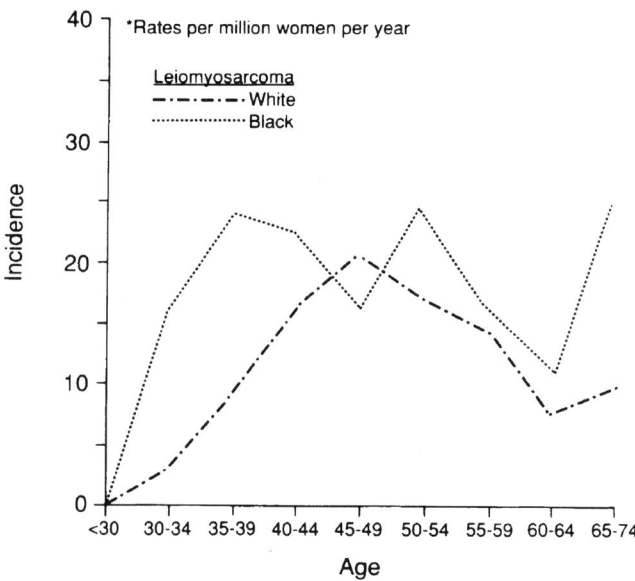

FIG. 24.3. Age distribution of patients with leiomyosarcomas.

Norris et al. (17,18), 33% and 24% of patients with carcinosarcomas were nonwhite, respectively. In contrast, a clinicopathologic review of patients with leiomyosarcoma by Silverberg et al. (12) found " . . . no racial predilection for this tumor."

Relative Incidence

Carcinosarcomas and leiomyosarcomas constitute about 4% and 1.5% of all uterine malignancies in clinical series, respectively (6). Echt et al. (19) reviewed 66 patients treated over 21 years at the University of Southern California and found carcinosarcoma in 48%, leiomyosarcoma in 36%, and endometrial stromal sarcoma in 15%. Because the risk profile of carcinosarcomas so closely parallels that of endometrial adenocarcinomas with regard to obesity, diabetes, anovulation, and low parity, Silverberg et al. (20) have suggested that they be regarded as "metaplastic" endometrial carcinomas instead of true sarcomas. Many other pathologists agree with this notion; malignant mixed mesodermal tumors are discussed with endometrial adenocarcinomas instead of with other malignant stromal tumors (21).

In series of uterine sarcomas referred for histopathologic diagnosis, leiomyosarcomas are seen more commonly than carcinosarcomas. The differentiation between benign, malignant, and uncertain malignant potential smooth muscle tumors is more subtle than the definitive determination of a high-grade carcinosarcoma.

Prior Radiotherapy

Although as many as a third of patients with carcinosarcomas in some series have a history of antecedent pelvic radiotherapy, this is rarely, if ever, an etiologic factor in patients with leiomyosarcoma of the uterus. Christopherson et al. (22) described two cases among 33 patients with uterine leiomyosarcoma who had a history of radiotherapy, which is one of the only citations in the literature for leiomyosarcomas. In the series of carcinosarcomas reported by Norris et al. (18), nine of 31 patients (29%) had received pelvic radiotherapy from 7 to 26 years prior to diagnosis. Among 1,208 uterine malignancies in the report by Meredith et al. (23), 30 occurred in patients exposed to pelvic radiotherapy. Only 8 of these 30 patients had been irradiated for a gynecologic malignancy, with the others being treated for uterine bleeding, polyps, or fibroids. Of irradiated patients, five (17%) developed carcinosarcomas, for a crude association of 11%. The risk of endometrial adenocarcinoma arising after radiation was 2%. It has been suggested that postirradiation carcinosarcomas occur at a younger average age than those arising *de novo* (24); latency is generally shorter in the older population, however (23). These tumors also tend to present at an advanced stage; this may reflect the fact that radiotherapy for either cervical cancer or benign uterine conditions is associated with a significant cervical stenosis, which prevents the cardinal symptom of carcinosarcomas, uterine bleeding.

Müllerian Adenosarcoma

Clinically, these neoplasms occur in women aged 14 to 89 years (median 58 years) (57), with no racial predilection or noteworthy reproductive characteristics. The most common symptoms were bleeding, pelvic pain, prolapse, and vaginal discharge. On clinical examination, about 40% of patients had tissue protruding from the cervical os (25). In the second series of Clement and Scully, five patients had a history of radiation therapy 8 to 30 years before diagnosis. Of note is the report in 1996 of Clement et al. (9) of six patients who developed müllerian adenosarcomas of the uterine corpus after taking tamoxifen for periods of 6 months to 4 years. An additional such case was reported by Bocklage et al. (26).

CLINICAL PRESENTATION

Vaginal bleeding is the most common presenting symptom in women with uterine sarcomas in general (27,28) and is nearly universal in those with carcinosarcomas (29), but may occur in as few as 40% of those with leiomyosarcomas. A typical presentation of carcinosarcoma is vaginal bleeding associated with a protuberant, fleshy mass from the cervix. Uterine enlargement is common with carcinosarcomas. These neoplasms arise in the endometrial lining but often grow in an exophytic pattern within the endometrial cavity (Fig. 24.3). Bleeding and uterine cramping are common as the uterus attempts to expel the globular mass.

Uterine enlargement and a presumptive diagnosis of uterine leiomyomas are nearly universal findings in patients with leiomyosarcoma (Fig. 24.4A and B). The incidence of leiomyosarcoma in all patients with clinical myomas is less than 1% but increases with age to slightly over 1% in the sixth decade of life (30). Whereas the diagnosis of carcinosarcoma is confirmed, or at least suggested, at the time of endometrial biopsy or curettage, leiomyosarcoma is rarely diagnosed before hysterectomy (11) unless the process is widespread.

DIAGNOSIS AND WORKUP

Berchuck et al. reported that in 14 patients with leiomyosarcomas undergoing dilatation and curettage, a prehysterectomy diagnosis was made in only 8 (31). Although the diagnosis of carcinosarcoma may be missed because endometrial biopsy or curettage does not adequately sample both the epithelial and stromal components of the tumor, appropriate preoperative referral is made because of the presence of a

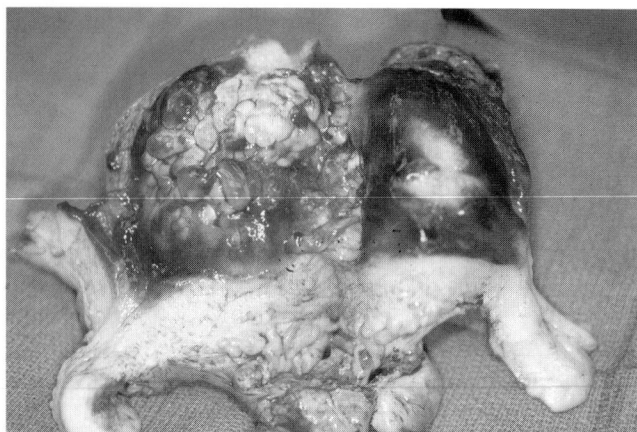

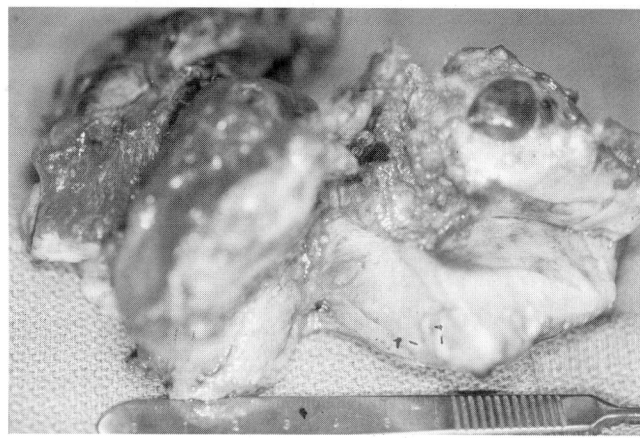

FIG. 24.4. A & B: Uterine leiomyosarcoma resulting in painful pelvic mass; diagnosis made on frozen section evaluation. Note uninvolved endometrium. (Courtesy St. Vincent Women's Hospital.)

malignancy, and staging is accomplished at the time of hysterectomy. Conversely, most leiomyosarcomas are diagnosed after hysterectomy at the time of histologic review of the surgical specimen. Referral and disposition decisions are therefore made *a posteriori*. More often than not, staging is omitted from the initial procedure. This dichotomy in the presentation of the two main uterine sarcomas was highlighted in a staging study published by the Gynecologic Oncology Group (GOG) (32). Far fewer patients with leiomyosarcomas were referred for enrollment in the study than those with the diagnosis of carcinosarcoma (301 carcinosarcomas, 59 leiomyosarcomas, and 93 endometrial stromal tumors and adenosarcomas). Restaging after primary surgery may have been an obstacle to entry of patients with leiomyosarcoma. In fact, the investigators who performed this study, Major et al. (32), deigned that "In light of the small number of leiomyosarcoma cases with positive lymph nodes, re-exploration [*solely for staging*] is not recommended in patients with leiomyosarcomas."

Patients with uterine carcinosarcomas, unless presenting with clinical metastases, should be managed in referral cen-

ters where appropriate surgical staging can be performed. Although vaginal sonography and magnetic resonance imaging may reveal myometrial involvement, the frequency of occult nodal and peritoneal metastases makes appropriate surgical evaluation paramount. Yamada et al. (33) underscored this fact in their staging study of 62 patients, 38 (61%) of whom had surgically detected extrauterine metastases.

Since the most common sites of metastases for uterine sarcomas other than leiomyosarcoma are pelvic and paraaortic lymph nodes, studies such as computed tomography of the abdomen and pelvis are probably not justified in patients with clinical stages I and II disease; on the other hand, if an extensive uterine mass is present, these evaluations may suggest a palliative rather than curative approach to the patient. Radionuclide bone scans and imaging of the brain are of little value in the absence of pulmonary metastases. Preoperative radiographs are helpful in excluding pulmonary metastases and are often medically indicated in patients of advanced age. The utility of chest tomography in uterine sarcomas has not been formally addressed but should be considered in patients with high-grade lesions, especially if palliation rather than curative therapy seems appropriate based upon advanced age and/or poor performance status.

Porter et al. (34) reviewed 600 patients with nonthoracic T2 soft-tissue sarcomas and concluded that routine chest CT identified metastases in 19.2% of patients but at a cost of $27,594 per patient with metastases. If scanning was limited to patients with high-grade histologies only, the cost per patient with metastases was reduced to $418 per patient with metastases. Since no specific data are in place for uterine sarcomas, CT scanning seems to be indicated in the triage of patients with high-grade sarcomas to differentiate between those with surgically resectable, and thus curable, lesions and those with more extensive pelvic lesions in whom the focus is control of symptoms.

STAGING AND NODAL INVOLVEMENT

By convention, the 1988 International Federation of Obstetrics and Gynecology (FIGO) staging criteria for endometrial cancer (see Table 23.5) are used to assign stages in cases of uterine sarcomas.

Whereas carcinosarcomas, like endometrial adenocarcinomas, commonly metastasize to pelvic or paraaortic lymph nodes, leiomyosarcomas rarely metastasize to nodal sites. In the review of 203 stages I and II carcinosarcomas surgically staged as part of a GOG study reported by Silverberg et al. (20), 34 cases (16.7%) were associated with nodal metastases. Nearly all had lymphatic or vascular involvement in the myometrium; lymphatic involvement was a much better predictor of nodal metastases than tumor grade or mitotic index. Doss et al. (2) confirmed that pelvic lymph nodes were the most common site of metastasis in carcinosarcomas, and others have confirmed a rate of nodal spread in clinically localized disease between 13.2% and 31.0% (33, 35).

Multiple nodal metastases were noted in 66% of patients with any nodal spread in Chen's report (36), and Norris et al. (18) described lymph node metastases in 90% of fatal cases.

In contrast, Major et al. (32) reported that only 3.5% of patients with clinically localized leiomyosarcomas had lymph node metastases identified at the time of surgical staging. In the recent Mayo Clinic series (11), 4 of 36 (11%) patients had nodal spread, but only 1 of these (2.6%) had isolated nodal metastases. Data from three series (28,30,37) indicate that lymph nodes were histologically positive only if clinically enlarged or associated with obvious intraabdominal spread. Thus, the need for lymph node dissection in patients with leiomyosarcomas remains unsubstantiated.

Among patients with müllerian adenosarcomas who underwent surgical staging including lymph node sampling (38), 20% were found to have spread outside the uterus to involve lymph nodes, vagina, parametrium, ovary, and malignant peritoneal washings.

PATHOLOGY

Malignant mesenchymal tumors can be classified in two groups: pure sarcomas and sarcomas associated with an epithelial component. Among the pure sarcomas, the most common is leiomyosarcoma, followed by endometrial stromal sarcomas, and rarely others including rhabdomyosarcoma, liposarcoma, angiosarcoma, chondrosarcoma, osteosarcoma, and alveolar soft part sarcoma. Sarcomas mixed with an epithelial component include carcinosarcomas (also called malignant mixed müllerian tumors), when the epithelial component is malignant, and adenosarcomas, when the epithelial component is benign.

Leiomyosarcoma and Smooth Muscle Tumors

Leiomyosarcomas are malignant smooth muscle tumors that usually arise *de novo* (unrelated to leiomyomas). Unlike leiomyomas, they are rare and they are not hormonally driven. Grossly, they are solitary poorly circumscribed masses that have a soft and fleshy consistency. The cut surface is variegated with gray areas intermixed with yellow areas of necrosis and sometimes hemorrhagic areas. The epicenter of the tumor is the myometrium. Most leiomyosarcomas are intramural, and occasionally they can extend into the cervix or beyond the uterus.

Microscopically, most leiomyosarcomas are overtly malignant and have hypercellularity, coagulative tumor cell necrosis, abundant mitoses [more than 10/10 high-power fields (HPFs)], atypical mitoses, marked cytologic atypia, and in-

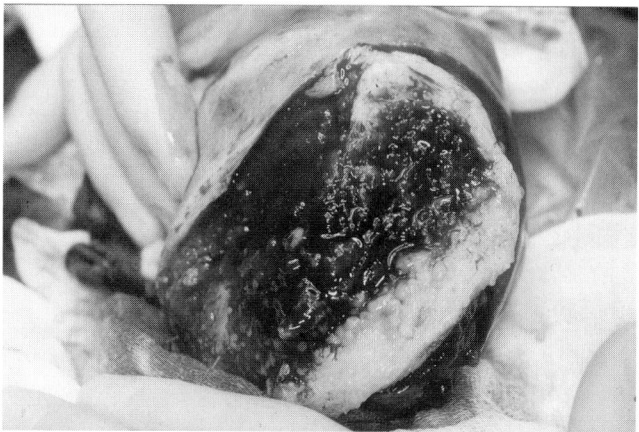

FIG. 24.5. Low-grade but extensive endometrial stromal sarcoma. (Courtesy St. Vincent Women's Hospital).

filtrative borders (Fig. 24.5). Some cases lack some of these features, and occasionally the differential diagnosis between a benign and a malignant lesion can be controversial. The three most important criteria are coagulative tumor cell necrosis, number of mitoses, and significant cytologic atypia (39). Coagulative tumor cell necrosis has an abrupt transition from viable to necrotic tissue (in contrast with hyaline necrosis that can be seen in leiomyomas and has an area of hyalinized tissue between the necrotic and the viable tumor). Some smooth muscle tumors have some worrisome features but not enough to render an unequivocal diagnosis of sarcoma. These tumors are either atypical leiomyomas, smooth muscle tumors with low malignant potential (low probability of an unfavorable outcome), or smooth muscle tumors of uncertain malignant potential (STUMP) (insufficient tumors have been studied to predict their behavior). Table 24.2 summarizes the current way of classifying uterine smooth muscle tumors based on their histologic characteristics. This classification is mostly based on a large retrospective study from Stanford University published in 1994 (39). In addition, two previous studies had already shown the benign behavior of most tumors with up to 15 mitoses per 10 HPF that clinically and pathologically appear to be leiomyomas (40,41). This group of tumors is currently classified as mitotically active leiomyomas. Leiomyomas are more likely to have a high mitotic count if they are excised during the secretory phase of the menstrual cycle, during pregnancy, or while patients are receiving exogenous progesterone therapy.

There are some tumors that are not represented in Table 24.2; for example, tumors without coagulative tumor cell necrosis, with focal or multifocal atypia, and more than 20 mitoses per 10 HPF. These tumors are very rare, and none has been reported in any of the published series. They should probably be considered of uncertain malignant potential. In addition, one sometimes encounters tumors that lack some of the three major criteria (mitoses, atypia, necrosis) but have other worrisome criteria such as infiltrative borders, vascular

TABLE 24.2. *Patterns of failure for patients with surgically staged uterine sarcomas managed by surgery with or without external beam pelvic irradiation (± vaginal brachytherapy ± chemotherapy)*

Reference	Stage	Vagina	Pelvis	Extrapelvis	Abdomen	Distant	Adjuvant treatment
92	I, II	Not Stated	14/112	Not Stated	Not Stated	Not Stated	Yes[a]
92	I, II	Not Stated	24/112	Not Stated	Not Stated	Not Stated	No[a]
97	I, II, III, IV	Not Stated	17/59	Not Stated	17/59	15/59	Mainly No[b]
117	I, II, III, IV	2/31	5/31	20/31	Not Stated	Not Stated	Yes[b]
117	I, II, III, IV	6/33	6/33	17/33	Not Stated	Not Stated	No[b]
114	I, II, III, IV	4/36	10/36	Not Stated	19/36	18/36	Mainly Yes[b]
Subtotals		12/100 (12.0%)	76/383 (19.8%)	37/64 (57.8%)	36/95 (37.9%)	33/95 (34.7%)	
Totals		–	88/383 (19.8%)	106/159 (66.7%)	–	–	

[a] Randomized.
[b] Nonrandomized.

invasion, or atypical mitotic figures. Classification of such cases is always problematic, and in most cases the tumors are best classified as tumors of uncertain malignant potential. These unusual cases should probably be reviewed by a gynecologic pathologist to offer a second opinion (Fig. 24.6).

Smooth muscle tumors with either myxoid or epithelioid features behave differently from typical spindled smooth muscle tumors, and they are classified using different histologic criteria. Epithelioid tumors have cells that are round instead of spindle shaped and have round nuclei. The term *epithelioid* is used because these tumors mimic epithelial lesions (carcinomas), and they can be positive for cytokeratin-like carcinomas. Malignant epithelioid smooth muscle tumors (epithelioid leiomyosarcomas) have significant cytologic atypia, at least three mitoses per 10 HPF, and usually coagulative tumor cell necrosis (42) (Fig. 24.7). At least one previous study suggests that epithelioid tumors may be overall more aggressive than the spindle cell ones with a higher tendency to metastasize (43).

Myxoid smooth muscle tumors of the uterus are rare. Histologically, they are deceiving because they usually lack cytologic atypia and necrosis, and their mitotic rate is low. The diagnosis of malignancy is based on the presence of infiltration of the myometrium and/or vascular invasion (44) (Fig. 24.8).

Carcinosarcomas

Uterine carcinosarcomas, also called malignant mixed müllerian tumors, are lesions that contain both carcinomatous and sarcomatous elements (Fig. 24.9). Recent studies suggest that both components derive from a single stem cell and that the lesion is monoclonal in origin based on molecular, immunohistochemical, tissue culture, and ultrastructural data (45,46).

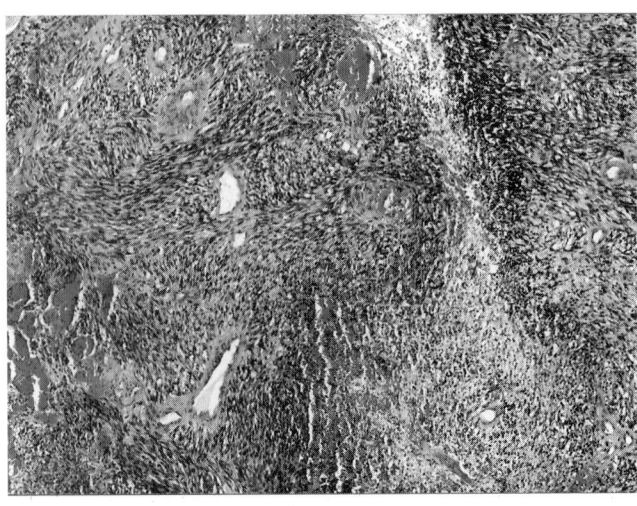

FIG. 24.6. Endometrial stromal nodule resected widely after treatment with tamoxifen (86). (Courtesy St. Vincent Women's Hospital.)

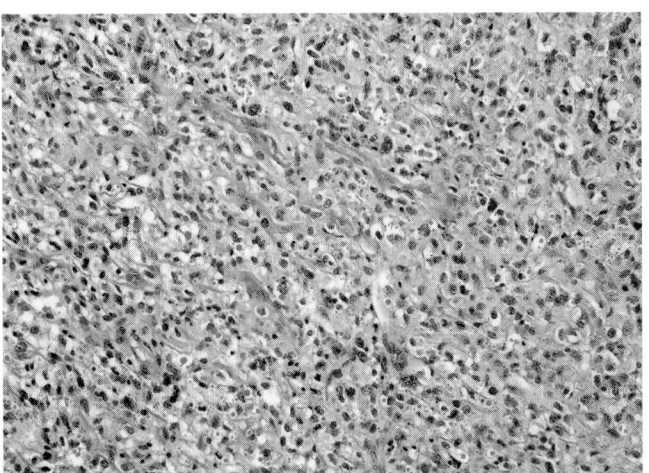

FIG. 24.7. Leiomyosarcoma with geographical distribution of necrotic and viable tumor.

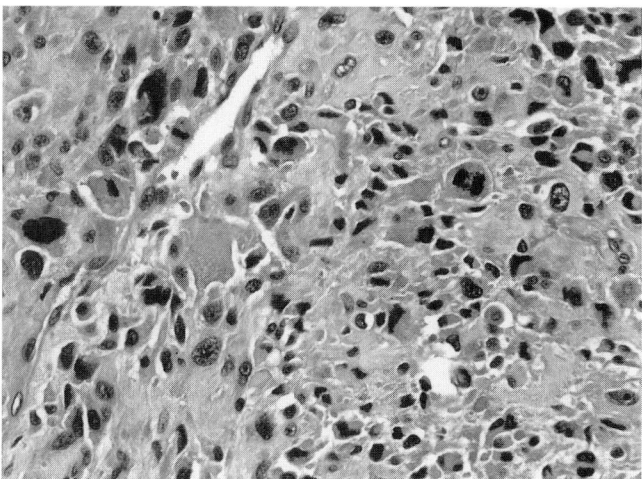

FIG. 24.8. Smooth muscle tumor of uncertain malignant potential with diffuse cytologic atypia, six mitoses per 10 HPF, focal infiltrative borders, but absence of necrosis.

Most carcinosarcomas are polypoid tumors that fill the endometrial cavity and may protrude through the cervical os. The tumors are soft and fleshy with areas of necrosis and hemorrhage. It is not uncommon to see obvious myometrial invasion on gross examination, and some cases extend into the cervix. The size of the tumor is variable. Some cases are small (<2 cm) and can be entirely removed by a curettage, whereas others can measure up to 20 cm.

Microscopically, the tumors have a typical biphasic pattern with a carcinomatous and a sarcomatous component. The carcinomatous component is usually a high-grade adenocarcinoma that can be endometrioid, serous, or clear cell. Occasionally, the carcinoma is squamous or undifferentiated. The sarcomatous component may be homologous or heterologous. Homologous sarcoma is present in 53% of

cases, usually a high-grade spindle or myxoid type resembling leiomyosarcoma, fibrosarcoma, malignant fibrous histiocytoma, or undifferentiated sarcoma. Heretologous sarcoma is seen in 47% of cases and contains rhabdomyosarcoma, chondrosarcoma, osteosarcoma, or liposarcoma in decreasing frequency. Most cases have myometrial invasion (78%). In 40% there is invasion of less than half of the myometrial wall, and in 38% there is deep myometrial invasion into or through the outer half of the myometrium (20). Lymphovascular invasion is present in 50%. The carcinoma is usually the component invading the myometrium and lymphovascular spaces.

Most studies suggest that the behavior of carcinosarcomas reflects the carcinomatous component. Tumors typically metastasize through lymphatic channels and spread in a way similar to endometrial carcinomas. Most metastases and recurrences are composed of pure carcinoma (75% of cases) (20,45,47). Cases in which the carcinomatous component is either serous or clear-cell carcinoma have a worse prognosis than cases with endometrioid carcinoma, at least in the largest reported series with detailed pathologic review (20). The type (homologous or heterologous), grade, and percentage of the sarcoma do not seem to affect prognosis (20,48,49).

Müllerian carcinosarcomas can occur in extrauterine sites. Most cases have occurred in the peritoneum (50–52) or retroperitoneum (53). Some cases have been seen in patients previously irradiated to that extrauterine site, and some cases may have arisen in areas of endometriosis.

Endometrial Stromal Neoplasms

Endometrial stromal lesions by definition are composed of cells identical to those found in the stromal componant of proliferative endometrium. They are usually subclassified in accordance with the seminal work of Norris and Taylor (54) into two broad groups of tumors based upon "pushing" or infiltrating, angioinvasive margins as stromal nodules or stromal sarcomas. Stromal sarcomas have been further subdivided into low-grade stromal sarcomas (also previously referred to as endometrial stromal myosis) or undifferentiated endometrial sarcomas based upon mitotic indices (less than 10 and 10 or more mitoses/10 HPFs, respectively). Several sources (13,14) suggest that undifferentiated endometrial sarcomas may actually be monophasic carcinosarcomas since they occur at older ages, often contain pleomorphic and anaplastic cells, are uniformly aggressive, and are often fatal.

Stromal Nodule

Stromal nodules are by far the least common of the pure endometrial stromal neoplasms (Fig. 24.10). Chang et al. (13) observed that many small benign stromal nodules of millimeter size were observed in hysterectomy specimens and were of only incidental interest. Conversely, stromal

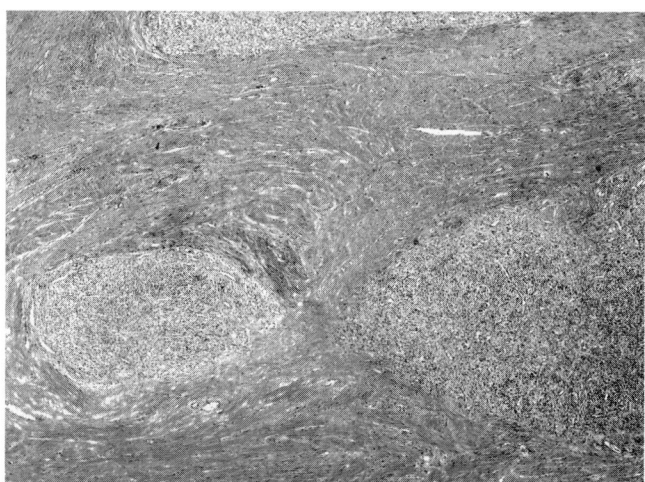

FIG. 24.9. Endometrial stromal nodule with numerous thick collagen bands.

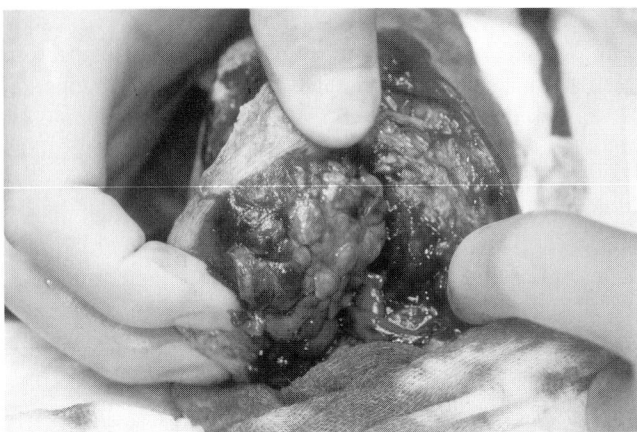

FIG. 24.10. Low-grade but extensive endometrial stromal sarcoma. (Courtesy St. Vincent Women's Hospital.)

nodules may become quite large and cause bleeding or uterine enlargement, which are the two most common symptoms associated with stromal tumors. In the review of 50 stromal nodules by Dionigi et al. (15), size ranged from 1.2 to 22 cm with an average of 7.1 cm.

On cut section, endometrial stromal nodules are fleshy and often tan-yellow. Microscopically, they are composed of uniform bland small cells resembling normal endometrial stromal cells with fusiform nuclei and scant cytoplasm and of abundant arterioles reminiscent of the spiral arterioles of the normal endometrium. The mitotic rate is low, with most tumors having less than 5 mitoses per 10 HPFs. Most endometrial stromal nodules are cellular, and some have variable amounts of intercellular collagen sometimes forming dense collagen bands or nodules (Fig. 24.11). Another common finding is the presence of clusters of foamy histiocytes within the tumor. The borders between the tumor and the adjacent

myometrium are microscopically well defined (pushing border). Occasionally, they may have more irregular borders with minimal areas of tumor extending into adjacent myometrium, usually within 3 mm of the main tumor mass (13–15). Endometrial stromal nodules lack associated lymphovascular invasion. Other changes that can be seen in endometrial stromal nodules include smooth muscle metaplasia, cystic degeneration, sex-cord–like areas, and necrosis.

Endometrial stromal nodules are commonly confused with cellular leiomyomas. Since both tumors are benign, the misdiagnosis of one for the other is probably of no clinical consequence if the tumor is found in a hysterectomy specimen. If the tumor is found in a curettage specimen, it is impossible for the pathologist to tell apart a stromal nodule versus a stromal sarcoma. If the tumor is misdiagnosed as a cellular leiomyoma in a curettage, the consequences may be more dramatic. There are some histologic features that favor a leiomyoma: blood vessels with thick muscular walls, cleft-like spaces, and merging with the adjacent myometrium. In addition, a battery of immunohistochemical stains can be of use. CD10 is usually positive in endometrial stromal cells, and desmin and h-caldesmon are usually positive in smooth muscle tumors (14)

Stromal Sarcoma

Endometrial stromal sarcomas can be low grade or high grade. The low-grade tumors have uniformly bland cells reminiscent of benign endometrial stromal cells. On gross examination, some show a single visible mass, and others have multiple masses or diffuse myometrial infiltration by worm-like masses. Microscopically, low-grade endometrial stromal sarcoma is similar to endometrial stromal nodule, and the differential diagnosis is based on the presence of unequivocal myometrial invasion and/or lymphovascular invasion (Fig. 24.12). Some endometrial stromal sarcomas

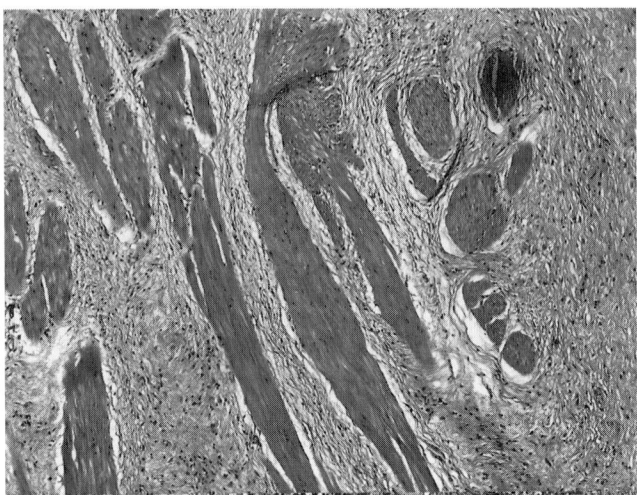

FIG. 24.11. Epithelioid leiomyosarcoma with "epithelioid cells" with round nuceli and round plump eosinophilic cytoplasm, marked cytologic atypia, and numerous mitoses.

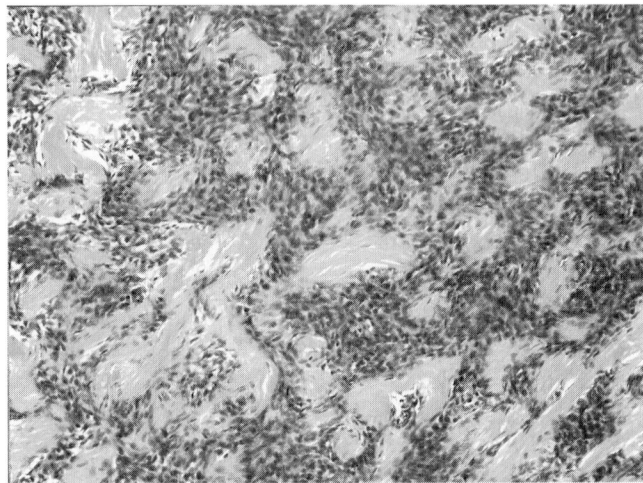

FIG. 24.12. Myxoid leiomyosarcoma with diffuse infiltration of myometrial smooth muscle.

have unusual histologic features that may render their diagnosis more difficult. These features include myxoid changes, fibroblastic and/or smooth muscle differentiation, epithelioid changes, and extensive endometrioid glandular differentiation (55–58).

Low-grade endometrial stromal sarcomas can occur in extrauterine sites including ovary, fallopian tube, cervix, vagina, vulva, pelvic cavity, abdominal cavity, retroperitoneum, and placenta (59–63). In some cases, the lesions have been associated with endometriosis. Histologically, they are similar to uterine endometrial stromal sarcomas, and a uterine tumor needs to be excluded before accepting the lesion as a primary extrauterine endometrial stromal sarcoma. The relapse rate for extrauterine endometrial stromal sarcoma is 62%, which is similar to high-stage low-grade uterine endometrial stromal sarcoma. Mitosis and atypia do not correlate with prognosis.

High-grade endometrial stromal sarcoma has marked cytologic atypia to the extent that the tumor can hardly be recognized as being of endometrial stromal origin. Morphologically, these high-grade lesions resemble undifferentiated mesenchymal tumors and behave as high-grade sarcomas (55). It may be advisable to refer to them as "high-grade sarcomas" or "poorly differentiated uterine sarcoma" (55) rather than as "endometrial stromal sarcoma," which, to some clinicians, conveys the idea of an indolent low-grade tumor. These tumors are usually seen in patients older than 50 years and have a recurrence rate of over 85%.

Most endometrial stromal tumors have cytogenetic abnormalities involving rearrangements of chromosomes 6, 7, and 17. The most characteristic translocation of these tumors, t(7;17) (p15;q21), generates a fusion of the *JAZF1* and *JJAZ1* genes. This fusion appears to be rarer among the high-grade lesions. The presence of this chromosomal abnormality may be of use in the diagnosis of difficult cases or recurrent tumors (64,65)

Uterine Tumor Resembling Ovarian Sex-Cord Tumor

In 1976, Clement and Scully (66) coined the description uterine tumors resembling ovarian sex-cord tumors (UTROSCTs) to describe a variant of endometrial stromal sarcomas in which benign glands and epithelioid cells are found. There is evidence that tumors predominantly containing epithelioid elements may behave more aggressively than other endometrial stromal sarcomas.

Müllerian Adenosarcoma

Clement and Scully (8) described müllerian adenosarcomas in 1974 and updated their experience with 100 cases in 1990 (25). These are mixed müllerian tumors that occupy a position midway between benign adenofibromas and carcinosarcomas. Histologically, they are composed of malignant stromal and benign epithelial components. They are dis-

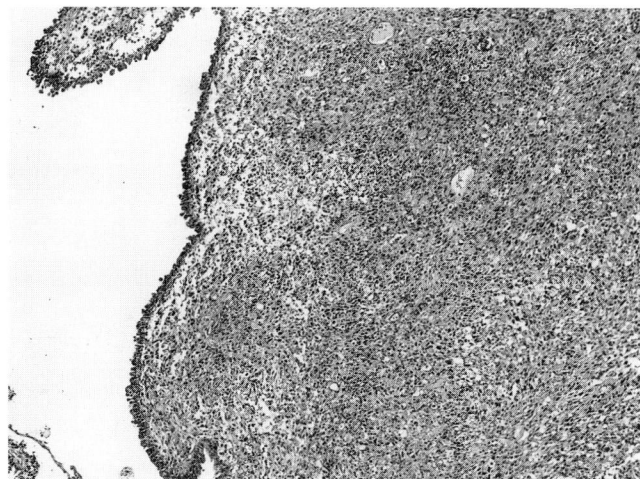

FIG. 24.13. Müllerian adenosarcoma with a polypoid leaf-like pattern of growth.

tinctly rare in that fewer than 200 cases had been reported as of 1990.

Most adenosarcomas arise in the endometrium and rarely in the endocervix, lower uterine segment, and myometrium (25). Grossly, the majority are solitary polypoid masses with a spongy appearance secondary to the presence of small cysts. Occasional cases appear as multiple polyps or masses and can be multicentric. Their size is variable, being from 1 to 17 cm (mean 5 cm) (Fig. 24.13).

Microscopically, the tumors have a benign epithelial component usually covering the surface of the polyps and in the form of benign glands uniformly distributed throughout the tumor. The mesenchymal component is usually a low-grade sarcoma that resembles endometrial stroma. The presence of hypercellular stroma around the glands is common, and some tumors have a leaf-like papillary growth pattern (Fig. 24.14). Sometimes the diagnosis of adenosarcoma can be

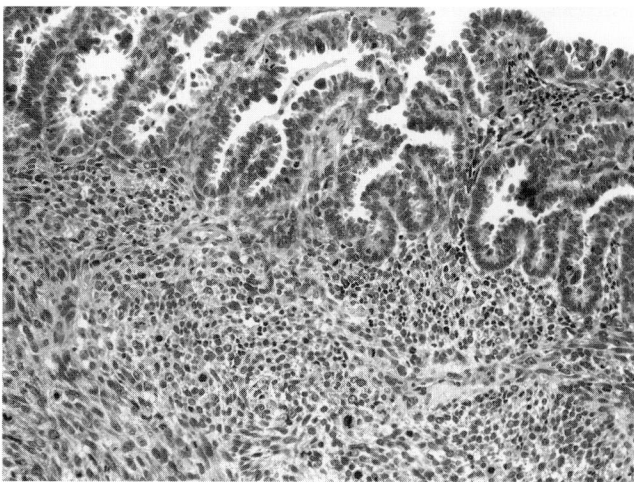

FIG. 24.14. Multiple nodules of endometrial stromal sarcoma infiltrating myometrium.

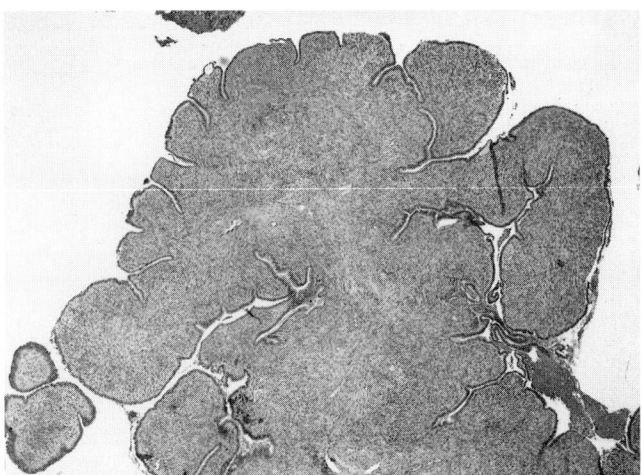

FIG. 24.15. Carcinosarcoma with serous carcinoma (**top**) and high-grade sarcoma (**bottom**).

difficult owing to the very low-grade nature of the sarcoma. Minimal criteria were described by Clement and Scully in a review of 100 cases of adenosarcoma published in 1990 (25). They include at least one of the following: two or more stromal mitoses per 10 HPF, marked stromal hypercellularity, and significant stromal cell atypia (67). Even with these criteria, some cases are deceivingly bland, and several cases have been seen in which the diagnosis was only possible after multiple ''recurrences'' of uterine polyps were reviewed. A minority of cases have ''sarcomatous overgrowth,'' when more than 25% of the tumor is composed of pure sarcoma. In these cases, the sarcoma is typically high grade (68) (Fig. 24.15).

Müllerian adenosarcomas have been described in extrauterine sites including the ovary and areas of endometriosis in the vagina (69,70), gastrointestinal tract (71), urinary bladder (72), pouch of Douglas (73), peritoneum (74), and liver (75).

PROGNOSTIC FACTORS

Stage at presentation is clearly an overriding prognosticator in all uterine sarcomas. Patients with extrauterine disease have a poor outlook regardless of adjuvant therapy, as do those with large tumors, uterine serosal spread, and lesions that are composed predominantly of an epithelial as opposed to stromal component. Fifty to 75% of patients with stage I or II carcinosarcomas survive their disease (33,76), whereas few with stages III and IV disease are cured (29). For leiomyosarcomas, the statistics are similar. There were no 2-year survivors among patients with extrauterine spread of uterine leiomyosarcomas in the studies of Hannigan (77) or Berchuck (31).

Major et al. reported that adnexal spread, lymph node metastases, tumor size, lymphatic and vascular space involvement, histologic grade, cell type, age, peritoneal cytol-

ogy, and depth of myometrial invasion affected progression-free survival on univariate analysis. On multivariate analysis of prognostic features, adnexal spread, nodal metastases, heterologous cell type, and grade were significant (32).

Leiomyosarcomas

Tumor stage is the best prognostic factor in leimyosarcomas (11,78–81). In addition, there are pathologic features that have been implicated as independent prognostic factors including mitotic count (48,78,79), vascular invasion (79–81), and grade (11,81). Mitotic count has been detected to be a strong independent prognostic parameter in several large studies with 126, 71, and 78 cases, respectively (48, 78,79). In one of these studies, mitotic count was an independent prognostic indicator in stage I tumors only (79). In these studies, there are statistically significant differences in survival in patients with less than 10 mitoses/10 HPF versus those with more than 10 mitoses/10 HPF (48,78,79). The presence of vascular space invasion has been associated with a worse prognosis in three recent studies with 71, 14, and 21 cases, respectively (79–81). In two of these studies, multivariate analysis showed that vascular space involvement had an impact on overall survival (79,80). In another study, univariate analysis showed that the absence of vascular invasion was associated with longer survival (81). The influence of tumor grading on prognosis has been addressed in two recent studies with 78 and 208 cases, respectively (11,48). In one study, grade had no impact on prognosis (48), and in the other one, multivariate analysis showed that high grade was associated with a significantly worse disease-specific survival (11). The grading system used in these two studies was different. In one study, the grading system included cytologic atypia, mitotic count, and tumor necrosis, which is the same three-tier system currently used to grade soft tissue sarcomas. In this study, grading proved not to be a prognostic factor for survival or relapse in either univariate or multivariate analysis (48). In the second study, the grading system was based solely on cytologic features without taking into account mitotic count or necrosis. In this study, tumors were graded as high grade or low grade. In both univariate and multivariate analyses, grade proved significantly to influence disease-specific mortality (11). The use of different grading systems may explain the different results of both studies. However, more studies are needed to establish the utility of either grading system in classifying uterine leiomyosarcomas.

There were 59 leiomyosarcomas in the GOG staging study reported by Major et al. (32). Nodal metastases, adnexal spread, and malignant peritoneal cytology occurred in 3.5, 3.5, and 5.3%, respectively. For 3 years, progression-free survival was 31% and multivariate analysis yielded only mitotic count as signicant in progression-free survival. At 3 years, zero, 61%, and 79% of women with 0 to 9, 10 to 20, or greater than 20 mitoses/10 HPFs, respectively, suffered relapses. Fewer mitoses/10 HPFs were also associated with longer survival in this study.

In the Mayo Clinic review, stage, grade, and oophorectomy influenced survival in patients with leiomyosarcoma in a Cox proportional hazards model (11).

Carcinosarcomas

Stage is the most important prognostic indicator in carcinosarcoma (48,50–52,56,80). Besides the histologic type of the carcinoma, other histopathologic features that have been implicated as prognostic factors in more than one study include depth of myometrial invasion (15,33,49,80,82) and lymphovascular invasion (15,33,80).

Silverberg's (20) review of carcinosarcomas in the GOG study demonstrated that features of the stromal component of these lesions had little bearing on the presence of metastases; however, high-risk epithelial constituents such as clear-cell and papillary serous malignancies influenced the frequency of metastases and, conversely, overall outcome. Other adverse prognostic indicators included deep myometrial invasion, lymphatic or vascular space involvement, or uterine isthmus or cervical spread. In this study, there was no difference in prognosis when purely homologous carcinosarcomas were compared with those containing heterologous elements.

Stromal Neoplasms

The most important prognostic indicator in low-grade endometrial stromal sarcoma is stage (13). However, even patients with stage I disease have a recurrence rate of 36%. It is impossible to predict histologically which patients will recur since most have no cytologic atypia and rare mitotic figures. When comparing stage I patients with more or less than 10 mitoses/10 HPF, the mitotic rate does not predict recurrences. In patients with high-stage disease (stages II, III, IV), a mitotic index of more than 10 mitoses/10 HPF correlates with a worse prognosis. High-stage tumors have a higher incidence of lymphovascular invasion compared to low-stage tumors (13); however, lymphovascular invasion is not an independent prognostic indicator (13,83).

Müllerian Adenosarcoma

Histopathologic factors that affect prognosis in müllerian adenosarcoma are myometrial invasion (25) and sarcomatous overgrowth (68,84,85). The recurrence rate is 12.7% for patients without myometrial invasion or stromal overgrowth, 46% for those with only myometrial invasion, and 70% in cases with stromal overgrowth (68). Patients with adenosarcoma with stromal overgrowth have a poor prognosis similar to that of carcinosarcoma (85). Also suggesting poor outcome were lymphatic or vascular space involvement

and rhabdomyosarcomatous differentiation. Any extrauterine spread was associated with a poor prognosis as was myometrial invasion.

GENERAL MANAGEMENT

Surgery

Women with the diagnosis of endometrial stromal nodule should have dilatation and curettage to ascertain the extent of the lesion; hysterectomy is the preferred means of therapy, but local excision has been performed successfully in young women who wish to maintain the potential for pregnancy. Before conservative surgery is undertaken, ultrasound or magnetic resonance imaging should be employed to define the limits of the lesion. Staging surgery is unnecessary for these tumors. Conservative management of endometrial stromal nodule with tamoxifen and local excision has been reported (86).

Endometrial stromal sarcomas and carcinosarcomas should be staged in the same careful fashion as are endometrial adenocarcinomas. Adnexal structures should be removed as well as lymph nodes in the distribution of the pelvic, common iliac, and aortic vessels. Peritoneal washings should be obtained because they are of prognostic value in carcinosarcomas (87). Omentectomy is a recognized part of staging such high-risk endometrial lesions as papillary serous and clear-cell cancers; it should be similarly recommended for these sarcomas.

Surgical staging of leiomyosarcomas is controversial. As noted previously, these malignancies are often diagnosed postoperatively. Since the risk of metastases to lymph nodes is small, reexploration for staging only is probably unnecessary.

In the rare instance when a young woman undergoes a myomectomy for leiomyomas and is found to have a low-grade leiomyosarcoma or smooth muscle tumor of "uncertain malignant potential," it may be possible to avoid hysterectomy. Conservative therapy must be undertaken only under ideal conditions, and the patient must understand the uncertainty of outcome. Careful follow-up with magnetic resonance imaging is essential. Although O'Connor and Norris (88) reported favorable outcomes in 13 of 14 patients treated with myomectomy alone in "mitotically active" leiomyomas, Berchuck et al. (31) identified two patients undergoing myomectomy who had residual leiomyosarcoma in the uterus at hysterectomy.

Recurrent leiomyosarcomas are often amenable to local resection of metastases.

Gardner and Daly (89) reported favorable results in patients with resected pulmonary metastases and determined that disease-free interval of over 12 months, radiographic doubling time of over 20 days, and number of metastases of four or less were favorable prognostic factors. Ueda et al. (90) found that grade of primary sarcoma was an important prognostic determinant. In a Memorial Sloan–Kettering review of 41 patients who had surgical resection of recurrent uterine leiomyosarcomas, 2-year survival was 71.2%, with time to first recurrence ≥12 months. Complete surgical resection was an important prognostic indicator (91).

Adjuvant Radiation Therapy

Since the primary management of patients with uterine sarcomas is surgical, radiation therapy is used adjuvantly in this group of patients. No prospectively randomized trial has shown a survival benefit for postoperative radiation therapy for patients with uterine sarcomas. A major impediment to any clinical trial involving these uncommon tumors is that it would require at least a decade to accrue sufficient patients for statistical validity.

The GOG has an open Phase III trial (protocol 150) for patients with all surgical stages of carcinosarcomas of the uterus (without extraabdominal spread) who have undergone optimal surgical debulking. Patients are randomized to receive adjuvant radiotherapy or combination chemotherapy. This study was designed to accrue 200 patients and is now projected to complete accrual by 2005.

The European Organization for Research and Treatment of Cancer (EORTC) completed a Phase III trial (protocol 55874) for surgical stage I and II patients with uterine sarcomas (103 leiomyosarcomas, 91 carcinosarcomas, and 28 endometrial stromal sarcomas) (92). This study closed in 2001. Although patterns of failure have not yet been reported, there were 12.5% (14 of 112) relapses in the adjuvantly treated cohort (pelvic external beam irradiation) versus 21.4% (24 of 112) recurrences in the observed group (p = .004). This study did not demonstrate a survival benefit for postoperative radiotherapy. The impact on pelvic control was only seen in patients with carcinosarcomas.

The following section will present a review of the patterns of failure from selected studies that incorporated surgical staging and attempted to investigate (prospectively or retrospectively) whether or not adjuvant radiotherapy had an impact upon the overall first site of failure. Techniques and complications of adjunctive radiation therapy will not be discussed here as they are dealt with in Chapter 23.

The literature is replete with reports in which administration of postoperative radiotherapy was left to the discretion of the treating physician (19,27,32,49,76,82,93–126). In addition, many of these studies involved only clinical rather than surgical staging. Most reports evaluated patients with several different cell types, whereas others focused on a specific histological entity (e.g., leiomyosarcoma).

The first group of reports (92,97,114,117) include studies that surgically staged patients with all types of uterine sarcomas. Almost all series were retrospective series, and most contained patients with stages I through IV disease. Thus, it is not surprising that there were more extrapelvic [66.7% (106 failures in 159 patients)] than pelvic failures [19.8% (88 failures in 383 patients)]. Also, many of these studies did not separate extrapelvic relapses into abdominal and distant locations of tumor recurrence. The combined pelvic and extrapelvic failure rates from the studies that predominantly did not use postoperative radiotherapy (92,97,117) were approximately 26% (53 pelvic failures in 204 patients) and 53.3% (49 extrapelvic failures in 92 patients) versus 19.6% (35 pelvic failures in 179 patients) and 85.1% (57 extrapelvic failures in 67 patients), respectively, for those receiving adjuvant (mainly pelvic external beam) radiotherapy (92,114, 117).

From this limited information, one cannot determine the impact of adjuvant radiation therapy on patterns of failure. Two autopsy series of uterine sarcomas (115,127) found the majority of recurrences were in the abdominal cavity. There was no appreciable difference in the sites of relapse among the three main histologic types of uterine sarcomas. Thus, one key factor in determining the potential role of adjuvant radiotherapy is differentiating between the risks of abdominal and distant (extraabdominal) failures.

Carcinosarcoma

The next set of reports (32,49,76,95,108,118,120,128) focused specifically on patients with uterine carcinosarcomas, also termed "metaplastic carcinoma" (20). Again there were limited data distinguishing between abdominal and extraabdominal recurrences. Three of these series (95,198,118) consisted exclusively of patients with surgical stage I and II patients, and the remainder included patients with all stages of disease. In these series, the pelvic/extrapelvic failure rates of 22.7% (135 pelvic failures in 594 patients) and 37.8% (262 extrapelvic failures in 694 patients) can be broken down further by no adjuvant (32,76,95,108,118) versus postoperative radiotherapy (32,49,76,93,108,118,120); namely 27.7% (80 pelvic failures in 289 patients) and 31.8% (92 extrapelvic failures in 289 patients) versus 18.0% (55 pelvic failures in 305 patients) and 55.7% (170 extrapelvic failures in 305 patients), respectively. There is a downward trend in pelvic relapses but an increase in failures in the abdomen and beyond.

For surgical stage I and II disease, the published recurrence rates range from 40% to 60% (113). The pelvic and extrapelvic recurrence rates of 39.2 % (20 pelvic failures in 51 patients) and 37.3% (19 extrapelvic failures in 51 patients), respectively, without subsequent radiation therapy (95,108,118) may be contrasted to 10% (4 pelvic failures in 40 patients) and 27.5% (11 extrapelvic failures in 40 patients) with the addition of pelvic radiotherapy (108,118).

From the previously cited GOG experience (32), only 19% (28/147) of patients with uterine carcinosarcoma of all stages relapsed outside the abdomen as the sole site of recurrent disease. This suggested that postoperative whole abdominal irradiation might impact on patterns of failure in this subset of uterine sarcomas. As noted earlier, a Phase III trial (GOG protocol 150) is nearing completion and will address this issue.

In one prospective pilot study of patients with clinical stage I or II uterine carcinosarcomas, 38 patients were scheduled to receive adjuvant platinum-containing chemotherapy followed by tailored radiotherapy (pelvic external beam and/or intracavitary vaginal brachytherapy) and then additional chemotherapy (35). Although only 21 of 38 (58%) patients ultimately received both modalities, the overall survival rate was 28 of 38 (74%). Those completing combined modality therapy had an overall survival of 20 of 21 (95%). Although the patterns of failure in this cohort were not delineated, this report suggests further exploration of adjuvant combined-modality therapy for patients with uterine carcinosarcomas.

Leiomyosarcoma

The third collection of restrospecitve studies (32,78,99) includes patients with uterine leiomyosarcomas. Only one (99) evaluated patients with surgical stages I and II tumors, whereas the others included patients with all stages of disease. The overall pelvic and extrapelvic relapse rates from this group were 16.6% (30 pelvic failures in 181 patients) and 42.0 % (76 extrapelvic failures in 181 patients), respectively. Once more there is minimal information separating upper abdominal and extraabdominal recurrences. The pelvic and extrapelvic recurrence percentages were 18.5% (22 pelvic failures in 119 patients) and 41.2% (49 extrapelvic failures in 119 patients), respectively, for the nonirradiated cohort and 12.9% (8 pelvic failures in 62 patients) and 43.5% (27 extrapelvic failures in 62 patients), respectively, for the irradiated cohort. This retrospective comparison does not suggest an effect of postoperative radiotherapy on recurrence rates for patients with uterine leiomyosarcoma. However, two of these series (32,78) combined to yield an 11.1% (4 pelvic failures in 36 patients) pelvic relapse rate with radiation versus 61.1% (22 pelvic failures in 36 patients) without adjuvant radiation therapy. The major obstacle with leiomyosarcoma is that the majority of patients have distant extraabdominal metastases, especially in the lung, despite having local (pelvic) control (32,78). This suggests that effective adjuvant systemic therapy must be added to at least pelvic irradiation in order to significantly impact the outcome of these patients.

Stromal Sarcoma

The final group of restrospective series (82,100,129) concentrates on patients with surgically staged endometrial stromal sarcomas. This category of uterine sarcomas can be subdivided (50) by the mitotic index into a low-grade category (also known as endolymphatic stromal myosis) associated with less than 10 mitotic figures/10 HPF or a true endometrial stromal sarcoma. The pelvic and extrapelvic rates of relapse from these reports are 42.2% (49 pelvic failures in

116 patients) and 33.3% (38 extrapelvic failures in 114 patients), respectively. Yet, only one (100) of the listed studies evaluates failure pattern as a function of mitotic index. This series reports no abdominal or distant recurrences (independent of the administration of adjuvant irradiation) among all stages of endolymphatic stromal myosis. However, there was a 33.3% (six failures in 18 patients) recurrence rate in the pelvis, and the majority did not receive radiation therapy. This suggests a possible role for pelvic external beam irradiation .

Pelvic, abdominal, and distant relapse rates for patients with high-grade endometrial stromal sarcomas are 34.8% (11 failures in 32 patients), 34.8% (11 failures in 32 patients), and 40.6% (13 failures in 32 patients), respectively. Further studies are indicated to determine if whole abdominal radiotherapy, combined pelvic irradiation and chemotherapy, or whole abdominal radiotherapy and chemotherapy would be the optimal choice of adjuvant therapy in these patients.

Systemic Therapy

Uterine sarcomas, although far less common than endometrial carcinomas, exhibit two features that increase the need for systemic therapy: a recurrence rate of at least 50%, even in stage I disease, and a high propensity for distant failure. Unfortunately, the comparatively low incidence of the disease has restricted the ability to perform meaningful randomized controlled trials to determine optimal systemic therapy. Despite this, cooperative group studies have provided data for the rational selection of systemic chemotherapy.

Crucial to the understanding of the use of chemotherapy in uterine sarcomas is the observation that these neoplasms are a heterogeneous mixture of various histologies, the majority of which are malignant mixed müllerian tumors (carcinosarcomas), which were previously known as the mixed mesodermal sarcomas, leiomyosarcomas, and endometrial stromal sarcomas. The first two of these, the malignant mixed müllerian tumors and the leiomyosarcomas, constitute 90% of cases entered into clinical trials. These two histologic subtypes are usually the only uterine sarcomas with sufficient numbers to permit meaningful Phase III studies; however, as these two histologic subtypes appear to respond differently to chemotherapy, they should be studied in separate patient populations.

Chemotherapy: Limited Disease

Uterine sarcoma has a high rate of distant metastases even in the absence of intraperitoneal or lymph node metastases. It has been concluded that this is due to the high rate of hematogenous and lymphatic dissemination (115). Even for surgical stage I disease, the recurrence is as high as 53% (32). To date, the largest randomized trial of adjuvant chemotherapy in patients with uterine sarcoma that has been performed did not segregate the different histologic subtypes. Although the recurrence rate and median survival of patients treated with doxorubicin compared to the control arm with no therapy were 39% versus 51% and 73 months versus 55 months, respectively, this GOG trial concluded that there was no significant difference (111). As with advanced disease, the later trials began to segregate the histologic subtypes. A nonrandomized study using adjuvant combination chemotherapy of etoposide, cisplatin, and doxorubicin demonstrated a 2-year survival of 92% of 23 patients with surgical stage I and stage II uterine carcinosarcomas. The fact that seven patients also received radiation therapy makes the result controversial (130). A more recent pilot study concluded that a multimodality treatment consisting of chemotherapy with epirubicin and cisplatin as well as radiation resulted in a 74% overall survival at a median follow-up of 55 months in 38 patients with surgical stages I and II carcinosarcomas (35). The investigators concluded that multimodality treatment might serve as the best treatment arm in future randomized trials.

To date, there has been no prospective study on patients with uterine leiomyosarcomas. Two factors continue to limit the study of adjuvant therapy in patients with uterine sarcomas: the relatively low frequency of the disease, which makes it difficult to complete randomized trials in a reasonable period of time, and the lack of highly active agents.

Chemotherapy: Advanced or Recurrent Disease

Leiomyosarcomas

Numerous single agents have been and continue to be tested in patients with leiomyosarcomas (Table 24.3). Unfortunately, the results have been unimpressive. In 1983, the GOG demonstrated seven responses among 28 patients (25%) treated with doxorubicin every 3 weeks as a single agent (131). To date, this has been considered to be the most active single agent. The GOG demonstrated ifosfamide to have moderate activity, with six partial responses among 35 patients (17%) (132,133), whereas limited activity was seen with single-agent paclitaxel, which was associated with a 9% overall response in 33 patients (134). Intravenous single-agent etoposide was shown to have overall response of 11%

in 28 patients (135), whereas prolonged oral etoposide had an overall response of 6.9% among 29 patients (136). Single-agent cisplatin also had a poor overall response of 3% to 5% in Phase II trials (137,138). A newer antifolate compound, trimetrexate, was used in a small study reported in 2002. It was associated with an overall response of 4.3% in 28 patients who had received prior treatment (139). Mitoxantrone (140), diaziquone (141), amonafide (142), aminothiadiazole (142), piperazinedione (143), and topotecan (140) were found to be inactive as single agents.

As in carcinosarcomas, combination chemotherapy in Phase II studies has been shown to have greater response rates. In 1983, the GOG demonstrated that the combination of doxorubicin and dacarbazine had an overall response rate of 30% (18%). Two years later, the same group demonstrated a 13% response rate using the combination of doxorubicin and cyclophosphamide (144). Both of these trials were too small to make any significant conclusion. However, as mentioned, the trials did serve the purpose of allowing researchers to observe that leiomyosarcomas had a different chemotherapeutic response profile compared to carcinosarcoma, resulting in the separation of the two different histologic entities in subsequent trials.

In 1996, the same group demonstrated an 18% overall response with a combination of dacarbazine, etoposide, and hydroxyurea (145). In the same year, using a combination of ifosfamide and doxorubicin, the GOG demonstrated an overall response of 30.3% in patients with advanced leiomyosarcoma with no history of prior treatment (146). The most recent effort from the GOG concluded that the use of combination of mitomycin, doxorubicin, and cisplatin produced an overall response rate of 23% in 35 patients albeit in exchange for significant pulmonary toxicity (147). The effort in leiomyosarcomas continues to focus on the identification of active drugs in Phase II trials. In conclusion, there is currently no evidence to support the use of combination chemotherapy in advanced or recurrent uterine leiomyosarcomas.

Carcinosarcomas

Several drugs have been studied in this group of tumors as single agents (Table 24.4). However, three drugs have

TABLE 24.3. *Single-agent activity in leiomyosarcoma of the uterus*

Drugs	N	Prior Rx	Schedule	Overall response (ref.)
Doxorubicin	28 (131)	No	60 mg/m² q 21 days	25%
Ifosfamide	35 (132,133)	No	1.5 g/m² + mesna 0.3 g/m² for 5 days q 28 days	17%
Cisplatin	33 (154)	No	50 mg/m² q 21 days	3%
	19 (138)	Yes	50 mg/m² q 21 days	5%
Etoposide	28 (135)	Yes	100 mg/m² for 3 days q 28 days	11%
	29 (136)	Yes	50 mg/m²/d orally for 21/28 days	6.9%
Paclitaxel	33 (134)	Yes	175 mg/m² q 21 days	9%
Trimetrexate	28 (139)	Yes	5 mg/m²/d orally for 5/14 days	4.3%

TABLE 24.4. *Single-agent activity in leiomyosarcoma of the uterus*

Drugs	N Overall response (ref.)	Prior Rx	Schedule
Doxorubicin	28 (131) 25%	No	60 mg/m² q 21 days
Ifosfamide	35 (132,133) 17%	No	1.5 g/m² + mesna 0.3 g/m² for 5 days q 28 days
Cisplatin	33 (154) 3%	No	50 mg/m² q 21 days
	19 (138) 5%	Yes	50 mg/m² q 21 days
Etoposide	28 (135) 11%	Yes	100 mg/m² for 3 days q 28 days
	29 (136) 6.9%	Yes	50 mg/m²/d orally for 21/28 days
Paclitaxel	33 (134) 9%	Yes	175 mg/m² q 21 days
Trimetrexate	28 (139) 4.3%	Yes	5 mg/m²/d orally for 5/14 days

demonstrated clear-cut activity: ifosfamide, cisplatin, and paclitaxel (131,137,138,148–154). Of the three drugs given as a single agent, ifosfamide is the most active single agent studied to date. In a 5-day schedule, ifosfamide produced five complete and four partial responses (overall response of 32%) among 28 patients with no prior chemotherapy (153).

In patients with prior chemotherapy, cisplatin produced an 18% response in 28 patients (137). A repeat trial in patients with no prior chemotherapy documented essentially the same response rate of 19% among a larger group of patients (138). Both trials used cisplatin at 50 mg/m² every 3 weeks. Investigators at M.D. Anderson Cancer Center employed a higher dose ranging from 75 mg/m² to 100 mg/m² every 3 weeks. Only 12 patients with measurable disease were entered into the trial, but one complete and four partial responses were observed (42%) (155). The lack of randomization and the small number of cases in this trial prohibit conclusions about the merits of the higher dose. Paclitaxel as a single agent has been observed to be associated with a response rate of 21.2% in a group of 33 patients with uterine sarcoma who have had prior chemotherapy (148).

Doxorubicin, generally regarded as the most active agent in soft tissue sarcomas, unfortunately demonstrated little activity in two trials of patients with carcinosarcomas. The first, conducted as one arm of a randomized trial, produced only four responses among 41 patients with a dose of 60 mg/m² every 3 weeks (131). The second, with a range of doses from 50 to 90 mg/m² every 3 weeks, resulted in no response among the nine patients with measurable disease (149). Demonstrating negligible activity in Phase II studies were etoposide (152), mitoxantrone (150), piperazinedione (143), diaziquone (151), and aminothiadiazole (142).

In the history of chemotherapy development, combination therapy has been considered to have the potential of producing a greater response. However, not all combination regimens have impacted survival. This is clearly seen in the treatment of uterine carcinosarcomas.

There have been numerous reports of combination chemotherapy for uterine sarcoma (Table 24.5). A combination of cyclophosphamide, vincristine, doxorubicin, and dacarbazine (DTIC) had a reported 23% (156) overall response rate. A combination of etoposide, hydroxyurea, and dacarbazine resulted in a response of 15% in 32 patients (157). More recently, EORTC reported a trial based on 48 patients with unresectable or recurrent carcinosarcoma who were treated with a combination of cisplatin, doxorubicin, and ifosfamide. The overall response rate was an impressive 56%. Unfortunately, this regimen was also associated with a high incidence of nephrotoxicity and hematologic toxicities. The group concluded that the next randomized Phase III trial based on this three-drug combination might answer the question of survival impact (158). Indeed, evaluation of the true value of combination chemotherapy requires randomized Phase III trials.

The first randomized study in 1983 by the GOG combined carcinosarcomas with other sarcomas, resulting in patient numbers being too small for subset analysis (131). Nonetheless, combining doxorubicin and DTIC resulted in an overall response of 23% and a trend toward greater response as compared to single-agent doxorubicin (10%). A significant improvement in the progression-free and overall survival also could not be demonstrated, but two conclusions could be drawn from this trial. The first was the fact that a greater response to chemotherapy was significantly associated with an increase in the overall survival and the disease-free survival. The second observation was that carcinosarcomas had a different response profile compared to leiomyosarcomas. Two years later, the GOG compared cyclophosphamide plus doxorubicin to single-agent doxorubicin. A response of 25% was seen in carcinosarcomas, but again, the numbers were too small to show any significant benefit compared to single-agent doxorubicin. The trial was also closed early because of failure to reach statistical significance (144).

TABLE 24.5. *Trials of chemotherapy in sarcomas of the uterus*

Histology	N	Intent	Drugs (ref.)	Results	p-value
Randomized trials					
OR					
Mixed müllerian tumors	72	P	Doxorubicin vs doxorubicin + DTIC (131)	10% (4/41) vs 23% (7/31)	Numbers too small to make subset analysis
Leiomyosarcoma	48			25% (7/28) vs 30% (6/20)	
Other sarcomas	26			18% (2/11) vs 20% (3/15)	
OR					
Mixed müllerian tumors	20	P	Doxorubicin vs doxorubicin + cyclophosphamide (144)	25%	Numbers too small to make subset analysis
Leiomyosarcoma	23			13%	
Other sarcomas	9			22%	
OR					
Mixed müllerian tumors	194	P	Ifosfamide vs ifosfamide + cisplatin (159)	36% (37/102) vs 54%(50/92)	p = .03
MPFS				4 months vs 6 months MOS	p = 0.02
				7.6 months vs 9.4 months	p = .07
MOS					
All histologic subtypes	156	A	Doxorubicin vs no chemotherapy (111)	73 months vs 55 months	No
Nonrandomized trials					
Mixed müllerian tumors	41	P	Doxorubicin + cisplatin + ifosfamide (158)	56%	NA
Mixed müllerian tumors	26	P	Cyclophosphamide + vincristine + doxorubicin + DTIC (156)	23%	NA
Mixed müllerian tumors	32	P	Etoposide + hydroxyurea + DTIC (157)	15%	NA
Mixed müllerian tumors	23	A	Etoposide + cisplatin + doxorubicin (130)	92% 2-year overall survival	NA
Mixed müllerian tumors	38	A	Epirubicin + cisplatin (35)	74%	
				Alive at median follow-up 55 months	NA
Leiomyosarcoma	33	P	Doxorubicin + ifosfamide (146)	30.3%	NA
Leiomyosarcoma	39	P	Hydroxyurea + DTIC + etoposide (145)	18.4%	NA
Leiomyosarcoma	23	P	Mitomycin + doxorubicin + cisplatin (157)	23%	NA

OR, overall response; A, adjuvant; P, palliative; MPFS, median progression-free survival; MOS, median overall survival; DTIC, dacarbazine (dimethyltriazenyl imidazole carboxamide).

With the recognition of the difference in response to therapy between carcinosarcomas and leiomyosarcomas, randomized trials began to regard each of the two major histologic subtypes as separate patient populations. Unfortunately, this increased the time necessary to complete clinical trials. Despite that, a large randomized trial was performed and reported in 2000. The GOG compared the addition of cisplatin to ifosfamide in 194 eligible patients and found that this improved the overall response rate from 36% to 54% and prolonged the median progression-free interval by an absolute 2 months. However, this advantage was not associated with a significant overall survival gain (159).

In conclusion, there is currently no evidence to support the use of combination chemotherapy in advanced or recurrent uterine carcinosarcomas.

Chemotherapy: Stromal Sarcoma

Patients with endometrial stromal sarcomas are often not classified separately in Phase II studies of uterine sarcomas, making it difficult to identify specific activity of various agents. The GOG reported on 21 patients treated with ifosfamide in a Phase II study; the overall response was 33.3% (160). However, interest in endometrial stromal sarcomas continues owing to the difference in the prognosis of patients with low-grade disease versus those with high-grade disease.

Hormonal Therapy

Although the role of hormonal therapy is clear in breast and endometrial cancers, few uterine sarcomas contain sufficient estrogen- or progesterone-receptor protein to influence therapy, the only exception being low-grade endometrial stromal sarcomas or stromal nodules. It has been found that a large proportion of uterine sarcomas possessed estrogen and progesterone receptors, but the median concentrations were substantially lower than those observed in breast or endometrial cancers (161). Uniquely, low-grade endometrial stromal sarcomas are hormonally responsive in roughly two-thirds of cases.

Lantta et al. (162) published two cases of extensive intra-peritoneal low-grade endometrial stromal sarcoma associated with high concentrations of progesterone receptor in complete remission with hormonal therapy. Three patients reported by Baker et al. (163) had partial responses or stabilization of disease on oral megestrol acetate; all had progesterone-receptor concentrations exceeding 674 fmol/mg. Piver et al. (164), in a collaborative survey of endolymphatic stromal myosis, recorded complete or partial responses to hormonal therapy in 6 of 13 patients (46%) treated with progestational agents. Scribner and Walker (165) reported a patient with an extensive endometrial stromal sarcoma of the uterus whose tumor was reduced to resectable size by the administration of leuprolide acetate and megestrol acetate. Endometrial stromal sarcomas of a lower grade have also been reported to express srp27, an estrogen-induced 24-kDK protein (166). Medroxyprogesterone acetate has induced major responses to pulmonary metastatic lesions from endometrial stromal sarcoma (32,167,168).

Hormonal therapy has not been extensively evaluated in mesenchymal uterine tumors. Estrogen and progesterone receptors were found in 55.5% and 55.8%, respectively, of samples from patients with various types of uterine sarcomas. Receptor levels were not influenced by stage, grade, or mitotic count; however, endometrial stromal sarcomas had higher receptor levels (161). There are anecdotal reports of responses to hormonal therapy in adenosarcomas and low-grade leiomyosarcomas but the area has not been well studied (169).

Systemic Therapy Summary

The current role of chemotherapy in the management of uterine sarcomas involves the use of single agents in the treatment of patients with advanced or recurrent disease, with an emphasis on palliative intent. In carcinosarcomas, the drug of choice is ifosfamide. For leiomyosarcomas, the only conclusively active drug has been doxorubicin. Hormonal therapy, particularly progestational agents, has a role in the treatment of advanced or recurrent endometrial stromal sarcomas. The use of other hormonal agents in the treatment of other histologic subtypes has not been studied. Efforts to identify additional active agents continue.

RESULTS OF THERAPY

Leiomyosarcoma

Reported progression-free survival at 3 years in the Major et al. (32) was 31% in patients with leiomyosarcoma. In the study of 423 uterine sarcomas of Olah et al. (6), overall 5-year survival was 31%; 42% patients with endometrial stromal sarcoma, 34% of those with leiomyosarcoma, and 33% with carcinosarcomas were alive at the end of the study period with median survival times of 30, 17, and 13 months, respectively. These researchers also found that stage, degree of differentiation, age, and histologic type were the four common factors influencing survival in a multiple regression analysis.

Carcinosarcoma and Adenosarcoma

Major et al. (32) reported a recurrence rate of 53% for 301 clinical stage I and II carcinosarcomas. This includes 61 patients (20%) who were "upstaged" based upon surgical findings. Median survival in patients with clinically recurrent or advanced-stage carcinosarcomas ranged from 4 to 13 months (2,8,76,77) despite therapy.

Kaku et al. (38), in a review of GOG materials, indicated that müllerian adenosarcomas usually were locally invasive; 30% of the 31 cases in their review suffered recurrences. Among the 100 patients of Clement and Scully (25), 26.1% developed recurrent disease. Generally, müllerian adenosarcomas are regarded as being locally invasive and are managed in some cases with local excision. However, sarcomatous overgrowth has been described in up as many as 57% of cases (38,68) and is associated with a fulminant clinical course and death.

Endometrial Stromal Sarcoma

Virtually no endometrial stromal nodule will recur after hysterectomy. In the series of Donigi et al. (15), there were no reported relapses in patients followed for a median of 43.5 months and a maximum of 214 months.

It may be difficult to determine the prognosis of endometrial stromal sarcoma in a given patient. Although mitotic count may be important, Chang et al. (12) suggested that stage (stage I versus stages II-IV) was more important in determining survival. Their series was largely referral material, and few patients had undergone complete surgical staging. Perhaps as a result, 36% of their stage I patients experienced relapse and 23% of these died of the disease. Remarkably, median time to relapse in patients with stage I tumors was 69 months. Patients with stage I endometrial stromal sarcomas most commonly experienced recurrences in the pelvis or abdomen, strongly suggesting a role for complete surgical staging and, perhaps, adjuvant radiotherapy in patients with extrauterine disease. Eight of 73 patients (11%) with stage I disease either presented with or developed pulmonary metastases. The median time to pulmonary relapse was 116 months!

Young et al. (170) and Berchuck et al. (129) have suggested that patients with ovarian preservation at the time of hysterectomy for endometrial stromal sarcoma were more likely to develop recurrences. Although this was not the case in the report of Chang et al. (13) (seven cases with no recurrences after hysterectomy), bilateral salpingo-oophorectomy would seem to be prudent given the potential for low-grade endometrial stromal sarcomas to express estrogen receptors and respond to hormonal therapy.

In the large series of Chang et al. (13), mitotic count successfully predicted outcome in patients with stage II-IV endometrial stromal sarcoma. Utilizing the 10 mitoses/10 HPF criteria, 8 of 13 (62%) patients with high-grade stromal sarcomas experienced disease recurrence compared with 35 of 77 (45%) of those with low-grade tumors.

Patterns of Failure

Although Echt et al. (19) reported no difference in recurrence patterns between patients with carcinosarcoma and leiomyosarcoma, others have reported a propensity for carcinosarcoma to relapse in the abdomen or pelvis and leiomyosarcomas to metastasize to the lung (171). In the follow-up of the GOG staging study reported by Major et al. (32), 28 of 301 patients with carcinosarcomas developed lung metastases (9.3%) versus 24 of 59 (40.7%) of those with leiomyosarcomas. Recurrences with a pelvic component were 63 (20.9%) and 8 (13.6%), respectively, for the two tumor types. The decision to use postoperative irradiation in this study was made by the treating physicians.

In patients whose tumors were initially confined to the uterus, there were purely distant recurrences in only 4 of 51 (7.8%) patients with carcinosarcomas reported by Nielsen et al. (128) and Shaw et al. (172) but 22 of 35 (62.9%) in the patients with leiomyosarcoma reported by Punnonen et al. (173) and Yu et al. (67). In a 10-year review of uterine leiomyosarcomas at Massachusetts General Hospital, Dinh et al. (174) reported that 20 of 27 patients either presented with or developed pulmonary metastases.

Sensitivity to Cisplatin Chemotherapy

When the GOG separated uterine sarcomas of different histologies in Phase II trials of cytotoxic agents, a major difference between carcinosarcomas and leiomyosarcomas was identified. Cisplatin has definite activity in treatment of refractory carcinosarcomas, but has limited effectiveness in leiomyosarcomas of the uterus. Thigpen et al. (138) reported a 19% response rate in chemotherapy-naive patients with carcinosarcomas given a dose of 50 mg/m^2 cisplatin intravenously every 3 weeks; cisplatin administration was associated with a response rate of 18% in patients with doxorubicin-refractory carcinosarcomas but only 5.3% of patients with similarly treated leiomyosarcomas (137). Of 33 chemotherapy-naive patients with recurrent or metastatic leiomyosarcoma, only one partial response (3%) was observed with cisplatin administration in the GOG study (138).

CLINICAL TRIALS

The GOG has played a leading role in developing new drugs for advanced and metastatic leiomyosarcomas and uterine carcinosarcomas through a series of Phase II studies in both previously treated and chemotherapy-naive patients.

It will be important to include available biologic and immunologic agents in this series of studies. The GOG has also completed one Phase III study of ifosfamide with or without cisplatin in patients with advanced or metastatic carcinosarcomas and is currently evaluating ifosfamide with or without paclitaxel in the same population. An existing Phase III study also evaluates whole abdomen radiotherapy versus combination chemotherapy (cisplatin plus ifosfamide) as adjuvant treatment in patients with essentially resected disease of all stages.

MOLECULAR BIOLOGY, GENETICS, FUTURE DIRECTIONS, AND CONCLUSIONS

There has been a slow evolution in the understanding of the basic science of sarcomas. The majority are felt to be sporadic with no specific etiology and most have complex karyotypes (175). However, in an increasing number of sarcomas, specific chromosomal translocations resulting in fusion genes that are constitutive and involve activation of transcription factors have been identified. Clear-cell sarcomas, myxoid liposarcomas, alveolar rhabdomyosarcomas, and alveolar soft-part sarcomas all have been associated with translocation-induced fusion genes that result in activated transcription factors and uncontrolled growth (175). Perhaps the most striking recent advance was the identification of c-*kit* tyrosine kinase activation in gastrointestinal stromal tumors (GISTs), which are histologically indistinguishable from leiomyosarcomas of the small bowel. The specific inhibitor of c-*kit*, imatinib mesylate, or STI-571 may produce long-term responses in patients with metastatic GISTs. Wang et al (176) recently reported that c-*kit* immunoreactivity was present in 12 of 16 uterine leiomyosarcomas evaluated. Whether this finding will translate into a role for imatinib in these malignancies remains to be seen.

In leiomyosarcomas, other avenues may be explored. Human immunodeficiency virus–immunocompromised pediatric patients are unusually susceptible to leiomyosarcomas. The causative agent in these tumors appears to be the Epstein-Barr virus (177). Similar smooth muscle tumors associated with the Epstein-Barr virus have been described in a few adult organ transplant recipients (178). Although evidence of this virus is lacking in immunocompetent adults with leiomyosarcomas (179), a common intermediary factor may exist which is as yet unrecognized.

Calponin, a tumor-suppressor gene, may be inactivated, suppressed, or poorly expressed in leiomyosarcomas (180). The role of *calponin* inhibition in the genesis of leiomyosarcomas and the possibility of restoring calponin activity as a therapeutic approach deserve evaluation.

Trials of adjuvant chemotherapy are appropriate in early stage, resected leiomyosarcomas. Recurrence rates after surgery alone are unacceptably high; the risk of mortality associated with recurrent leiomyosarcoma easily offsets any morbidity derived from adjuvant chemotherapy in this population of relatively young patients.

A variety of potential markers are overexpressed in uterine carcinosarcomas and include p53, mdm-2 (181), platelet-derived growth factor receptor-β, c-abl (182), HER-2/neu (183,184), vascular endothelial growth factor (185), and IGF-II and IGF-IR (186). None is associated with prognostic implications (187); the evolving concept of carcinosarcomas as metaplastic endometrial carcinomas may result in elucidation of new means of prevention and therapy. Combination or sequential radiation and chemotherapy has a great deal of appeal (31).

Endometrial stromal sarcomas have been associated with the translocation t(7;17) (p15–21;q12–21) in over a third of cases (188); this information, in addition to the established hormone responsiveness of low-grade stromal sarcomas, may provide a basis for therapeutic strategies in the future.

A basic understanding of uterine sarcomas and their differences is paramount to the understanding of surgical and adjuvant therapy as well as palliative treatment in patients with these rare neoplasms; this knowledge is critical in the practice of gynecologic oncology.

REFERENCES

1. Jemal A, Taylor M, Samuels A, et al. Cancer statistics, 2003. *CA Cancer J Clin* 2003;53:5–26.
2. Doss LL, Llorens AS, Henriquez EM. Carcinosarcoma of the uterus: a 40-year experience from the state of Missouri. *Gynecol Oncol* 1984;18:43–53.
3. Nordal RR, Thoresen SO. Uterine sarcomas in Norway 1956–1992: incidence, survival, and mortality. *Eur J Cancer* 1997;33:907–911.
4. Scully RE, Bonfiglio TA, Kurman RJ, et al. *World Health Organization international classification of tumour; histological typing of female genital tract tumors.* 2nd ed. Berlin: Springer, 1994.
5. Ober WB. Uterine sarcomas: histogenesis and taxonomy. *Ann N Y Acad Sci* 1959;75:689–703.
6. Olah KS, Dunn JA, Gee H. Leiomyosarcomas have a poorer prognosis than mixed mesodermal tumours when adjusting for known prognostic factors: the result of a retrospective study of 423 cases of uterine sarcoma. *Br J Obstet Gynaecol* 1992;99:590–594.
7. Ronnett BM, Zaino RJ, Ellenson LH, et al. Endometrial cancer. In: Kurman RJ, ed. *Blaustein's Pathology of the Female Genital Tract.* 5th ed. New York: Springer, 2002:501–560.
8. Clement PB, Scully. Mullerian adenosarcoma of the uterus: a clinicopathologic analysis of ten cases of distinctive type of mullerian mixed tumor. *Cancer* 1974;34:1138–1149.
9. Clement PB, Oliva E, Young RH. Mullerian adenosarcoma of the uterine corpus associated with tamoxifen therapy: a report of six cases and review of tamoxifen-associated endometrial lesions. *Int J Gynecol Pathol* 1996;15:222–229.
10. Bartsich EG, Bowe ET, Moore JG. Leiomyosarcoma of the uterus. *Obstet Gynecol* 1968;32:101–106.
11. Giuntoli RL, Metzinger DS, DiMarco CS, et al. Retrospective review of 208 patients with leiomyosarcoma of the uterus: prognostic indicators, surgical management, and adjuvant therapy. *Gynecol Oncol* 2003;89:460–469.
12. Silverberg SG. Leiomyosarcoma of the uterus; a clinicopathologic study. *Obstet Gynecol* 1971;28:613–628.
13. Chang KL, Crabtree GS, Kim Lim-Tan S, et al. Primary uterine endometrial stromal neoplasms. A clinicopathologic study of 117 cases. *Am J Surg Pathol* 1990;14:415–438.
14. Evans HL. Endometrial stromal sarcoma and poorly differentiated endometrial sarcoma. *Cancer* 1982;50:2170-2182.
15. Dionigi A, Oliva E, Clement PB, et al. Endometrial stromal nodules and endometrial stromal tumors with limited infiltration: a clinicopathologic study of 50 cases. *Am J Surg Pathol* 2002;26:567–581.
16. Zelmanowicz A, Hildesheim A, Sherman MA, et al. Evidence for a common etiology for endometrial carcinomas and malignant mixed mullerian tumors. *Gynecol Oncol* 1998;69:253–257.
17. Mortel R, Nedwich A, Lewis GC, et al. Malignant mixed mullerian tumors of the uterine corpus. *Obstet Gynecol* 1970;35:469–480.
18. Norris HJ, Roth E, Taylor HB. Mesenchymal tumors of the uterus. *Obstet Gynecol* 1966;28:57–63.
19. Echt G, Jepson J, Steel J, et al. Treatment of uterine sarcomas. *Cancer* 1990;66:35–39.
20. Silverberg SG, Major FJ, Blessing JA, et al. Carcinosarcoma (malignant mixed mesodermal tumor) of the uterus. A Gynecologic Oncology Group pathologic study of 203 cases. *Int J Gynecol Pathol* 1990;9:1–19.
21. Kurman RJ, ed. *Blaustein's Pathology of the Female Genital Tract.* 5th ed. New York: Springer, 2001.
22. Christopherson WM, Williamson EO, Gray LA. Leiomyosarcoma of the uterus. *Cancer* 1972;29:1512–1517.
23. Meredith RJ, Eisert DR, Kaka Z, et al. An excess of uterine sarcomas after pelvic irradiation. *Cancer* 1986;58:2003–2007.
24. Varela-Duran J. Nochomovitz LE, Prem KA, et al. Post irradiation mixed Mullerian tumors of the uterus. *Cancer* 1980;45:1625–1631.
25. Clement PB, Scully RE. Mullerian adenosarcoma of the uterus: A clinicopathologic analysis of 100 cases with a review of the literature. *Hum Pathol* 1990;21:363–381.
26. Bocklage T, Lee KR, Belinson JL Uterine mullerian adenosarcoma following adenomyoma in a woman on tamoxifen therapy. *Gynecol Oncol* 1993;44:104–109.
27. Larson B, Silfversward C, Nilsson B, et al. Mixed mullerian tumors of the uterus—prognostic factors: a clinical and histopathologic study of 147 casess. *Radiother Oncol* 1990:123–132.
28. Goff BA, Rice LW, Fleischhacker D, et al. Uterine leiomyosarcoma and endometrial stromal sarcoma: lymph node metastases and sites of recurrence. *Gynecol Oncol* 1993;50:105–109.
29. Iwasa Y, Haga H, Konishi I, et al. Prognostic factors in uterine carcinosarcoma: a clinicopathologic study of 25 patients. *Cancer* 1998;82:512–519.
30. Leibsohn S, d'Ablain G, Mischell DR, et al. Leiomyosarcoma in a series of hysterectomies performed for presumed uterine leiomyomas. *Am J Obstet Gynecol* 1990;162:968–974.
31. Berchuck A, Rubin SC, Hoskins WJ, et al. Treatment of uterine leiomyosarcoma. *Obstet Gynecol* 1988;71:845–854.
32. Major FJ, Blessing JA, Silverberg SG, et al. Prognostic factors in early-stage uterine sarcoma. *Cancer* 1993;71:1702–1709.
33. Yamada DS, Burger RA, Brewster WR, et al. Pathologic variables and survival for patients with surgically evaluated carcinosarcoma of the uterus. *Cancer* 2000;88:2782–2786.
34. Porter GA, Cantor SB, Ahmad SA, et al. Cost-effectiveness of staging computed tomography of the chest in patients with T2 soft tissue sarcomas. *Cancer* 2002;94:197–204.
35. Manolitsas T, Wain GV, Williams KE, et al. Multimodality therapy for patients with clinical stage I and II malignant mixed mullerian tumors of the uterus. *Cancer* 2001;91:1437–1443.
36. Chen SS. Propensity of retroperitoneal lymph node metastases in stage I sarcoma of the uterus. *Gynecol Oncol* 1989;32:215–219.
37. Gard GB, Mulvany NJ, Quinn MA. Management of uterine leiomyosarcoma in Australia. *Aust N Z J Obstet Gyneaecol* 1999;39:93–98.
38. Kaku T, Silverberg SG, Major FJ, et al. Adenosarcoma of the uterus: a Gynecologic Oncology Group clinicopathologic study of 31 cases. *Int J Gynecol Pathol* 1992;11:75–88.
39. Bell SW, Kempson RL, Hendrickson MR. Problematic uterine smooth muscle neoplasms. A clinicopathologic study of 213 cases. *Am J Surg Pathol* 1994;18:535–558.
40. Perrone T, Dehner LP. Prognostically favorable "mitotically active" smooth muscle tumors of the uterus. A clinicopathologic study of ten cases. *Am J Surg Pathol* 1988;12:1–8.
41. O'Connor DM, Norris HJ. Mitotically active leiomyoma of the uterus. *Hum Pathol* 1990;21:223–227.
42. Prayson RA, Goldblum JR, Hart WR. Epithelioid smooth muscle tumors of the uterus. A clinicopathologic study of 18 patients. *Am J Surg Pathol* 1997;21:383–391.
43. Jones MW, Norris HJ. Clinicopathologic study of 28 uterine leyomiosarcomas with metastases. *Int J Gynecol Pathol* 1995;14:243–249.
44. Kugami S, Kashimura M, Toki N, Katuhata Y. Myxoid leiomyosar-

coma of the uterus with subsequent pregnancy and delivery. *Gynecol Oncol* 2002;85:538–542.

45. McCluggage WG. Malignant biphasic uterine tumors: carcinosarcomas or metaplastic carcinomas? *J Clin Pathol* 2002;55:321–325.

46. Torenbeek R, Hermsen MA, Meijer GA, et al. Analysis by comparative genomic hybridization of epithelial and spindle cell components in sarcomatoid carcinoma and carcinosarcoma: histogenetic aspects. *J Pathol* 1999;189:338–343.

47. Bitterman P, Byungkyu C, Kurman RJ. The significance of epithelial differentiation in mixed mesodermal tumors of the uterus. A clinicopathologic and immunohistochemical study. *Am J Surg Pathol* 1990; 14:317–328.

48. Pautier P, Genestie C, Rey A, et al Analysis of clinicopathologic prognostic factors for 157 uterine sarcomas and evaluation of a grading score validated for soft tissue sarcoma. *Cancer* 2000;88: 1425–1431.

49. Inthasorn P, Carter J, Valmadre S, et al Analysis of clinicopathologic factors in malignant mixed mullerian tumors of the uterine corpus. *Int J Gynecol Cancer* 2002;12;348–353.

50. Garamvoelgyi E, Guillou L, Gebhard S, et al. Primary malignant mixed mullerian tumor of the female peritoneum. A clinical, pathologic and immunohistochemical study of three cases and review of the literature. *Cancer* 1994;74:854–863.

51. Rose PG, Rodriguez M, Abdul-Karim FW. Malignant mixed mullerian tumor of the female peritoneum: Treatment and outcome of three cases. *Gyneol Oncol* 1997;65:523–525.

52. Sumathi VP, Murnaghan M, Dobbs SP, et al. Extragenital mullerian carcinosarcoma arising from the peritoneum: report of two cases. *Int J Gynecol Cancer* 2002;12:764–767.

53. Shintaku M, Matsumoto T. Primary mullerian carcinosarcoma of the retroperitoneum: report of a case. *Int J Gynecol Pathol* 2001;20: 191–195.

54. Norris HJ, Taylor HB. Mesenchymal tumors of the uterus. I. A clinical and pathological study of 53 endometrial stromal tumors. *Cancer* 1966;19:755–766.

55. Oliva E, Young RH, Clement PB, Scully RE. Myxoid and fibrous endometrial stromal tumors of the uterus: a report of 10 cases. *Int J Gynecol Pathol* 1999;18:310–319.

56. Yilmaz A, Rush DS, Soslow RA. Endometrial stromal sarcomas with unusual histologic features: a report of 24 primary and metastatic tumors emphasizing fibroblastic and smooth muscle differentiation. *Am J Surg Pathol* 2002;26:1142–1150.

57. Oliva E, Clement PB, Young RH. Epithelioid endometrial and endometrioid stromal tumors: a report of four cases emphasizing their distinction from epithelioid smooth muscle tumors and other oxyphilic uterine and extrauterine tumors. *Int J Gynecol Pathol* 2002;21:48–55.

58. Clement PB, Scully RE. Endometrial stromal sarcomas of the uterus with extensive endometrioid glandular differentiation: a report of three cases that caused problems in differential diagnosis. *Int J Gynecol Pathol* 1992;11:163–173.

59. Chang KL, Crabtree GS, Soo Kim LT, et al Primary extrauterine endometrial stromal neoplasms: a clinicopathologic study of 20 cases and a review of the literature. *Int J Gynecol Oncol* 1993;12:282–296.

60. Irvin W, Pelkey T, Rice L, et al. Endometrial stromal sarcoma of the vulva arising in extraovarian endometriosis: a case report and literature review. *Gynecol Oncol* 1998;71:313–316.

61. Katsanis WA, O'Connor DM, Gibb RK, et al. Endometrial stromal sarcoma involving the placenta. *Ann Diagn Pathol* 1998;2:301–305.

62. Kondi-Paphitis A, Smyrniotis B, Liapis A, et al. Stromal sarcoma arising in endometriosis. A clinicopathologic and immunohistochemical study of 4 cases. *Eur J Gynaecol Oncol* 1998;19:588–590.

63. Boardman CH, Jefferies JA. Low grade endometrial stromal sarcoma of the ectocervix after therapy for breast cancer. *Gynecol Oncol* 2000; 79:120–123.

64. Koontz JI, Soreng AL, Nucci M, et al. Frequent fusion of the JAZF1 and JJAZ1 genes in endometrial stromal tumors. *Proc Natl Acad Sci U S A* 2001;98:6348–6353.

65. Micci F, Walter CU, Teixeira MR, et al. Cytogenetic and molecular genetic analyses of endometrial stromal sarcoma: nonrandom involvement of chromosome arms 6p and 7p and confirmation of JAZF1/JJAZ1 gene fusion in t(7;17). *Cancer Genet Cytogenet* 2003;144: 119–124.

66. Clement PB, Scully RE. Uterine tumors resembling ovarian sex-cord tumors. A clinicopathologic analysis of fourteen cases. *Am J Clin Pathol* 1976;66:512–525.

67. Yu KJ, Ho DM, Ng HT, et al. Leiomyosarcoma of the uterus: a review of 14 cases. *Chin Med J (Taipei)* 1989;44:109–115.

68. Clement PB. Mullerian adenosarcoma of the uterus with sarcomatous overgrowth. A clinicopathologic analysis of 10 cases. *Am J Surg Pathol* 1989;13:28–38.

69. Anderson J, Behbakht K, De Geest K, et al Adenosarcoma in a patient with vaginal endometriosis. *Obstet Gynecol* 2001;98:964–966.

70. Liu L, Davidsomn S, Singh M. Mullerian adenosarcoma of vagina arising in persistent endometriosis: report of a case and review of the literature. *Gynecol Oncol* 2003; 90:486–490.

71. Yantiss RK, Clement PB, Young RH. Neoplastic and pre-neoplastic changes in gastrointestinal endometriosis: a study of 17 cases. *Am J Surg Pathol* 2000;24:513–524.

72. Vara AR, Ruzis EP, Moussabeck O, et al. Endometrioid adenosarcoma of the bladder arising from endometriosis. *J Urol* 1990;143:813–815.

73. Murugasu A, Miller J, Proietto A, et al. Extragenital mullerian adenosarcoma with sarcomatous overgrowth arising in an endometriotic cyst in the pouch of Douglas. *Int J Gynecol Pathol* 2003;13:371–375.

74. Dincer AD, Timmins P, Pietrocola D, et al. Primary peritoneal adenosarcoma with sarcomatous overgrowth associated with endometriosis. *Int J Gynecol Pathol* 2002;21:65–68.

75. N'Senda P, Wendum D, Balladur P, et al. Adenosarcoma arising in hepatic endometriosis. *Eur Radiol* 2000;10:1287–1289.

76. Gerszten K, Faul C, Kounelis S, et al. The impact of aduvant radiotherapy on carcinosarcoma of the uterus. *Gynecol Oncol* 1998;68:8–13.

77. Hannigan EV, Gomez IG. Uterine leiomyosarcomas: a review of prognostic clinical and pathologic factors. *Am J Obstet Gynecol* 1979;134: 557–562.

78. Gadducci A, Landoni F, Sartori E, et al. Uterine leiomyosarcoma: Analysis of treatment failures and survival. *Gynecol Oncol* 1996;62: 25–32.

79. Mayerhofer K, Obermair A, Windbichler G, et al. Leiomyosarcoma of the uterus: a clinicopathologic multicenter study of 71 cases. *Gynecol Oncol* 1999;74:196–201.

80. Rovirosa A, Ascaso C, Ordi J, et al. Is vascular and lymphatic space invasion a main prognostic factor in uterine neoplasms with a sarcomatous component? A retrospective study of prognostic factors of 60 patients stratified by stages. *Int J Radiat Oncol Biol Phys* 2002;52: 1320–1329.

81. Bodner K, Bodner-Adler B, Kimberger O, et al. Evaluating prognostic parameters in women with uterine leiomyosarcoma. A clinicopathologic study. *J Reprod Med* 2003;48:95–100.

82. Bodner-Adler B, Bodner K, Obermair A, et al. Prognostic parameters in carcinosarcoma of the uterus: a clinicopathologic study. *Anticancer Res* 2001;21:3069–3074.

83. Nordal RR, Kristensen GB, Karen J, et al The prognostic significance of surgery, tumor size, malignancy grade, menopausal status, and DNA ploidy in endometrial stromal sarcoma. *Gynecol Oncol* 1996; 62:254–259.

84. Verschraegen CF, Vasuratna A, Edwards C, et al. Clinicopathologic analysis of mullerian adenosarcoma: the MD Anderson Cancer Center experience. *Oncol Rep* 1998;5:939–944.

85. Krivak TC, Seidman JD, McBroom JW, et al. Uterine adenosarcoma with sarcomatous overgrowth versus uterine carcinosarcoma: a comparison of treatment and survival. *Gynecol Oncol* 2001;83:89–94.

86. Schilder JM, Hurd WW, Roth LM, Sutton GP. Hormonal treatment of an endometrial stromal nodule followed by local excision. *Obstet Gynecol* 1999;93:805–807.

87. Szpak C

88. O'Connor DM, Norris HJ. Mitotically-active leiomyomas of the uterus. *Hum Pathol* 1990;21:223–229.

89. Gardner TE, Daly JM. Diagnosis and management of distant recurrence in soft-tissue sarcomas. *Semin Oncol* 20;5:456–461.

90. Ueda T, Uchida A, Kodama K, et al. Aggressive pulmonary metastasectomy for soft tissue sarcomas. *Cancer* 1993;72:1919–1925.

91. Leitao MM, Brennan MF, Hensley M, et al. Surgical resection of pulmonary and extrapulmonary recurrences of uterine leiomyosarcoma. *Gynecol Oncol* 2002;87:287–294.

92. Reed NS, Mangioni C, Malmstrom H, et al. First results of a randomized trial comparing radiotherapy versus observation postoperatively in patients with uterine sarcomas. an EORTC-GCG Study. *Int J Gynecol Cancer* 2003; 13[Suppl 1]:4.

93. Nielsen SN, Podratz KC, Scheithauer BW, O'Brien PC. Clinicalpathologic analysis of uterine malignant mixed mullerian tumors. *Gynecol Oncol* 1988;34:372–378.

94. Chauveinc L, Deniaud E, Plancher X, et al. Uterine sarcomas: the Curie Institut experience. Prognostic factors and adjuvant treatments. *Gynecol Oncol* 1999:72:232–237.

95. Chi DS, Mychalczak B, Saigo PE, et al. The role of whole-pelvic irradiation in the treatment of early-stage uterine carcinosarcoma. *Gynecol Oncol* 1997;65:493–498.

96. Coquard R, Romestaing P, Ardiet J-M, et al. Uterine sarcomas managed by surgery followed by radiation therapy. Clinical outcome, prognostic factors and role of radiation therapy. *Bull Cancer* 1997; 84:625–629.

97. El Husseiny G, Al Bareedy N, Mourad WA, et al. Prognostic factors and treatment modalities in uterine sarcoma. *Am J Clin Oncol* 2002; 25:256–260.

98. Ferrer F, Sabater S, et al. Impact of radiotherapy on local control and survival in uterine sarcomas: a retrospective study from the Grup Oncologic Catala-Occita. *Int J Radiat Oncol Biol Phys* 1999;44: 47–52.

99. Gadducci A, Fabrini MG, Bonuccelli A, et al. Analysis of treatment failures in patients with early-stage uterine leiomyosarcoma. *Anticancer Res* 1995;15:485–488.

100. Gadducci A, Sartori E, Landoni F, et al. Endometrial stromal sarcoma: analysis of treatment failure and survival. *Gynecol Oncol* 1996;63: 247–253.

101. Hoffman W, Schmandt S, Kortmann RD, et al. Radiotherapy in the treatment of uterine sarcomas. *Gynecol Obstet Invest* 1996;42:49–75.

102. Hornback NB, Omura G, Major FJ. Observations on the use of adjuvant radiation therapy in patients with stage I and II uterine sarcoma. *Int J Radiat Oncol Biol Phys* 1986;12:2127–2130.

103. Huang K-T, Chen C-A, Tseng G-C, et al. Endometrial stromal sarcoma: report of twenty cases. *Acta Obstet Gynecol Scand* 1996;75: 551–555.

104. Ishiko O, Wakasa K-I, Honda K-I, et al. Excellent results of postoperative radiotherapy for endometrial stromal sarcoma of low-grade malignancy. *Gynecol Obstet Invest* 2000;49:214–216.

105. Knocke TH, Kucera H, Dorfler D, et al. Results of postoperative radiotherapy in the treatment of sarcoma of the corpus uteri. *Cancer* 1998;83:1972–1979.

106. Knocke TH, Weitmann HD, Kucera H, et al. Results of primary and adjuvant radiotherapy in the treatment of mixed Mullerian tumors of the corpus uteri. *Gynecol Oncol* 1999;73:389–395.

107. Lotocki R, Rosenshein NB, Grumbine F, et al. Mixed Mullerian tumors of the uterus: clinical and pathologic correlations. *Int J Gynaecol Obstet* 1982;20:237–243.

108. Molpus KL, Redlin-Frazier S, Reed G, et al. Postoperative pelvic irradiation in early stage uterine mixed Mullerian tumors. *Eur J Gynaecol Oncol* 1998;19:541–546.

109. Moskovic E, MacSweeney E, Law M, et al. Survival, patterns of spread and prognostic factors in uterine sarcoma: a study of 76 patients. *Br J Radiol* 1992;66:1009–1015.

110. Olah KS, Gee H, Blunt S, et al. Retrospective analysis of 318 cases of uterine sarcoma. *Eur J Cancer* 1991;27:1095–1099.

111. Omura GA, Blessing JA, Major F, et al. A randomized clinical trial of adjuvant adriamycin in uterine sarcomas: a Gynecologic Oncology Group study. *J Clin Oncol* 1985;3:1240–1245.

112. Peters WA, Kumar NB, Fleming WP, et al. Prognostic features of sarcomas and mixed tumors of the endometrium. *Obstet Gynecol* 1984;63:550–556.

113. Perez CA, Askin F, Baglan RJ, et al. Effects of irradiation on mixed Mullerian tumors of the uterus. *Cancer* 1979;43:1274–1284.

114. Piura B, Rabinovich A, Yanai-Inbar I, et al. Uterine sarcoma in the south of Israel: study of 36 cases. *J Surg Oncol* 1997; 64:55–62.

115. Rose PG, Piver MS, Tsukada Y, et al. Patterns of metastasis in uterine sarcoma: An autopsy study. *Cancer* 1989;63:935–938.

116. Salazar OM, Bonfiglio TA, Patten SF, et al. Uterine sarcomas: natural history, treatment and prognosis. *Cancer* 1978;42:1152–1160.

117. Salazar OM, Bonfiglio TA, Patten SF, et al. Uterine sarcomas: analysis of failures with special emphasis on the use of adjuvant radiation therapy. *Cancer* 1978;42:1161–1170.

118. Sartori E, Bazzurini L, Gadducci A, et al. Carcinosarcoma of the uterus: a clinicopathological multicenter CTF Study. *Gynecol Oncol* 1997;67:70–75.

119. Soumarova R, Horova H, Seneklova Z, et al. Treatment of uterine sarcoma: a survey of 49 patients. *Arch Gynecol Obstet* 2002;266: 92–95.

120. Spanos WJ, Peters LJ, Oswald MJ. Patterns of recurrence in malignant mixed Mullerian tumors of the uterus. *Cancer* 1986;57:155–159.

121. Spanos WJ, Wharton JT, Gomez L, et al. Malignant mixed Mullerian tumors of the uterus. *Cancer* 1984;53:311–316.

122. Tinkler SD, Cowie VJ. Uterine sarcomas: a review of the Edinburgh experience from 1974 to 1992. *Br J Radiol* 1993;66:998–1001.

123. Vaccarello L, Curtin JP. Presentation and management of carcinosarcoma of the uterus. *Oncology* 1992;6:45–59.

124. Weitmann HD, Knocke TH, Kucera H, et al. Radiation therapy in the treatment of endometrial stromal sarcoma. *Int J Radiat Oncol Biol Phys* 2001;49:739–748.

125. Weitmann HD, Kucera H, Knocke T-H, et al. Surgery and adjuvant radiation therapy of endometrial stromal sarcoma. *Wien Klin Wochenschr* 2002;114:44–49.

126. Wheelock JB, Krebs H-B, Schneider V, et al. Uterine sarcoma: Analysis of prognostic variables in 71 cases. *Am J Obstet Gynecol* 1985; 151:1016–1022.

127. Fleming WP, Peters WA, Kum NB, et al. Autopsy findings in patients with uterine sarcoma. *Gynecol Oncol* 1984;9:168–172.

128. Nielsen SN, Podratz KC, Scheithauer BW, O'Brien PC. Clinical-pathologic analysis of uterine malignant mixed mullerian tumors. *Gynecol Oncol* 1988;34:372–378.

129. Berchuck A, Rubin SC, Hoskins WJ, et al. Treatment of endometrial stromal tumors. *Gynecol Oncol* 1990;36:60–65.

130. Resnik E, Chambers SK, Carcangiu ML, et al. A Phase II study of etoposide, cisplatin, and doxorubicin chemotherapy in mixed mullerian tumors (MMT) of the uterus. *Gynecol Oncol* 1995;56:370–375.

131. Omura GA, Major FJ, Blessing JA, et al. A randomized study of adriamycin with and without dimethyl triazenoimidazole carboxamide in advanced uterine sarcomas. *Cancer* 1983;52:626–632.

132. Sutton GP, Blessing JA, Barrett RJ, McGehee R. Phase II trial of ifosfamide and mesna in leiomyosarcoma of the uterus: a Gynecologic Oncology Group study. *Am J Obstet Gynecol* 1992;166:556–559.

133. Sutton G, Blessing JA, McGuire W, et al. Phase II trial of ifosfamide and mesna in leiomyosarcomas of the uterus. *Gynecol Oncol* 1990; 36:295.

134. Sutton G, Blessing JA, Ball H. Phase II trial of paclitaxel in leiomyosarcoma of the uterus: a gynecologic oncology group study. *Gynecol Oncol* 1999;74:346–349.

135. Slayton RE, Blessing JA, Angel C, Berman M. Phase II trial of etoposide in the management of advanced and recurrent leiomyosarcoma of the uterus: a Gynecologic Oncology Group Study. *Cancer Treat Rep* 1987;71:1303–1304.

136. Rose PG, Blessing JA, Soper JT, Barter JF. Prolonged oral etoposide in recurrent or advanced leiomyosarcoma of the uterus: a Gynecologic Oncology Group study. *Gynecol Oncol* 1998;70:267–271.

137. Thigpen JT, Blessing JA, Wilbanks GD. Cisplatin as second-line chemotherapy in the treatment of advanced or recurrent leiomyosarcomas of the uterus: a phase II trial of the Gynecologic Oncology Group. *Am J Clin Oncol* 1986;9:18–20.

138. Thigpen JT, Blessing JA, Beecham J, et al. Phase II trial of cisplatin as first-line chemotherapy in patients with advanced or recurrent uterine sarcomas: a Gynecologic Group Study. *J Clin Oncol* 1991;9: 1962–1966.

139. Smith HO, Blessing JA, Vaccarello L. Trimetrexate in the treatment of recurrent or advanced leiomyosarcoma of the uterus: a phase II study of the Gynecologic Oncology Group. *Gynecol Oncol* 2002;84: 140–144.

140. Miller DS, Blessing JA, Kilgore LC, et al. Phase II trial of topotecan in patients with advanced, persistent, or recurrent uterine leiomyosarcomas: a Gynecologic Oncology Group Study. *Am J Clin Oncol* 2000; 23:355–357.

141. Slayton RE, Blessing JA, Look K, Anderson B. A phase II clinical trial of diaziquone (AZQ) in the treatment of patients with recurrent leiomyosarcoma of the uterus. A Gynecologic Oncology Group study. *Invest New Drugs* 1991;9:207–208.

142. Asbury R, Blessing JA, Smith DM, Carson LF. Aminothiadiazole in the treatment of advanced leiomyosarcoma of the uterine corpus. A Gynecologic Oncology Group study. *Am J Clin Oncol* 1995;18: 397–399.

143. Thigpen JT, Blessing JA, Homesley HD, et al. Phase II trial of piperazinedione in patients with advanced or recurrent uterine sarcoma. A Gynecologic Oncology Group study. *Am J Clin Oncol* 1985;8: 350–352.

144. Muss HB, Bundy B, DiSaia PJ, et al. Treatment of recurrent or advanced uterine sarcoma. A randomized trial of doxorubicin versus doxorubicin and cyclophosphamide (a phase III trial of the Gynecologic Oncology Group). *Cancer* 1985;15:1648–1653.

145. Currie J, Blessing JA, Muss HB, et al. Combination chemotherapy with hydroxyurea, dacarbazine (DTIC), and etoposide in the treatment of uterine leiomyosarcoma: a Gynecologic Oncology Group study. *Gynecol Oncol* 1996;61:27–30.

146. Sutton G, Blessing JA, Malfetano JH. Ifosfamide and doxorubicin in the treatment of advanced leiomyosarcomas of the uterus: a Gynecologic Oncology Group study. *Gynecol Oncol* 1996;62:226–229.

147. Edmonson JH, Blessing JA, Cosin JA, et al. Phase II study of mitomycin, doxorubicin, and cisplatin in the treatment of advanced uterine leiomyosarcoma: a Gynecologic Oncology Group study. *Gynecol Oncol* 2002;85:507–510.

148. Curtin JP, Blessing JA, Soper JT, DeGeest K. Paclitaxel in the treatment of carcinosarcoma of the uterus: a Gynecologic Oncology Group study. *Gynecol Oncol* 2001;83:268–270.

149. Gershenson DM, Kavanagh JJ, Copeland LJ, et al. High-dose doxorubicin infusion therapy for disseminated mixed mesodermal sarcoma of the uterus. *Cancer* 1987;59:1264–1267.

150. Muss HB, Bundy BN, Adcock L, Beecham J. Mitoxantrone in the treatment of advanced uterine sarcoma. A phase II trial of the Gynecologic Oncology Group. *Am J Clin Oncol* 1990; 13:32–34.

151. Slayton RE, Blessing JA, Clarke-Pearson D. A phase II trial of diaziquone (AZQ) in mixed mesodermal sarcomas of the uterus. A Gynecologic Oncology Group study. *Invest New Drugs* 1991;9:93–94.

152. Slayton RE, Blessing JA, DiSaia PJ, Christopherson WA. Phase II trial of etoposide in the management of advanced or recurrent mixed mesodermal sarcomas of the uterus: a Gynecologic Oncology Group Study. *Cancer Treat Rep* 1987;71:661–662.

153. Sutton GP, Blessing JA, Rosenshein N, et al. Phase II trial of ifosfamide and mesna in mixed mesodermal tumors of the uterus (a Gynecologic Oncology Group study). *Am J Obstet Gynecol* 1989;161:309–312.

154. Thigpen JT, Blessing JA, Orr JW Jr, DiSaia PJ. Phase II trial of cisplatin in the treatment of patients with advanced or recurrent mixed mesodermal sarcomas of the uterus: a Gynecologic Oncology Group study. *Cancer Treat Rep* 1986;70:271–274.

155. Gershenson DM, Kavanagh JJ, Copeland LJ, et al. Cisplatin therapy for disseminated mixed mesodermal sarcoma of the uterus. *J Clin Oncol* 1987;5:618–621.

156. Piver MS, DeEulis TG, Lele SB, Barlow JJ. Cyclophosphamide, vincristine, adriamycin, and dimethyl-triazeno imidazole carboxamide (CYVADIC) for sarcomas of the female genital tract. *Gynecol Oncol* 1982;14:319–323.

157. Currie JL, Blessing JA, McGehee R, et al. Phase II trial of hydroxyurea, dacarbazine (DTIC), and etoposide (VP-16) in mixed mesodermal tumors of the uterus: a Gynecologic Oncology Group study. *Gynecol Oncol* 1996;61:94–96.

158. van Rijswijk RE, Vermorken JB, Reed N, et al. Cisplatin, doxorubicin and ifosfamide in carcinosarcoma of the female genital tract. A phase II study of the European Organization for Research and Treatment of Cancer Gynaecological Cancer Group (EORTC 55923). *Eur J Cancer* 2002;39:481–487.

159. Sutton G, Brunetto VL, Kilgore L, et al. A phase III trial of ifosfamide with or without cisplatin in carcinosarcoma of the uterus. A GOG study. *Gynecol Oncol* 2000;79:147–153.

160. Sutton G, Blessing JA, Park R, et al. Ifosfamide treatment of recurrent or metastatic endometrial stromal sarcomas previously unexposed to chemotherapy: a study of the Gynecologic Oncology Group. *Obstet Gynecol* 1996;87:747–750.

161. Sutton GP, Stehman FB, Michael H, et al. Estrogen and progesterone receptors in uterine sarcomas. *Obstet Gynecol* 1986;68:709–714.

162. Lantta M, Kahanpaa K, Karkkainen J, et al. Estradiol and progesterone receptors in two cases of endometrial stromal sarcoma. *Gynecol Oncol* 1984;18:233–239.

163. Baker TR, Piver MS, Lele SB, Tsukada Y. Stage I uterine adenosarcoma: a report of six cases. *J Surg Oncol* 1988;37:128–132.

164. Piver MS, Rutledge FN, Copeland L, et al. Uterine endolymphatic stromal myosis. *Obstet Gynecol* 1984;63:725–745.

165. Scribner DR Jr, Walker JL. Low-grade endometrial stromal sarcoma: preoperative treatment with Depo-Lupron and Megace. *Gynecol Oncol* 1998;71:458–460.

166. Navarro D, Cabrera JJ, Leon L, et al. Endometrial stromal sarcoma expression of estrogen receptors, progesterone receptors and estrogen-induced srp27 (24K) suggests hormone responsiveness. *J Steroid Biochem Mol Biol* 1992;41:589–596.

167. Mansi JL, Ramachandra S, Wiltshaw E, Fisher C. Endometrial stromal sarcomas. *Gynecol Oncol* 1990;36:113–118.

168. O'Brien AA, O'Briain DS, Daly PA. Aggressive endometrial stromal sarcoma responding to medroxyprogesterone following failure of tamoxifen and combination chemotherapy. Case report. *Br J Obstet Gynaecol* 1985;92:862–866.

169. Krumholz BA, Lobovsky FY, Halitsky V. Endolymphatic stromal myosis with pulmonary metastases. Remission with progestin therapy: report of a case. *J Reprod Med* 1973;10:85–89.

170. Young RH, Prat J, Scully RE. Endometrioid stromal sarcomas of the ovary: a clinicopathologic analysis of 23 cases. *Cancer* 1984;1153:1143–1155.

171. Hornback N, Omura GA, Major FJ. Observations on the use of adjuvant radiation therapy in patients with stage I and II uterine sarcoma. *Int J Radiat Oncol Biol Phys* 1986;12:2127–2130.

172. Shaw RW, Lynch PF, Wade-Evans T. Mullerian mixed tumour of the uterine corpus: a clinical histopathological review of 28 patients. *Br J Obstet Gynaecol* 1983;90:562–570.

173. Punnonen R, Lauslahti K, et al. Uterine sarcomas. *Ann Chir Gynaecol* 1985;74[Supp]:11–15.

174. Dinh TA, Oliva EA, Fuller AF, et al. The treatment of gynecologic leiomyosarcoma. Results from a 10-year experience (1990–1999) at the Massachusetts General Hospital. *Gynecol Oncol* 2004;92:684–692.

175. Helman LJ, Meltzer P. Mechanisms of sarcoma development. *Nat Rev Cancer* 2003;3:685–694.

176. Wang L, Felix JC, Lee JL, et al. The proto-oncogene c-*kit* is expressed in leiomyosarcomas of the uterus. *Gynecol Oncol* 2003;90:402–406.

177. Rogatsch H, Bonatti H, Menet A, et al. Epstein-Barr virus–associated multicentric leiomyosarcoma in an adult patient after heart transplantation: case report and review of the literature. *Am J Surg Pathol* 2000;24:614–621.

178. Boman F, Gultekin H, Dickman PS. Latent Epstein-Barr virus infection demonstrated in low-grade leiomyosarcomas of adults with acquired immunodeficiency syndrome, but not in adjacent Kaposi's lesion or smooth muscle tumors in immunocompetent patients. *Arch Pathol Lab Med* 1997;121:834–838.

179. Hill MA, Araya JC, Eckert MW, et al. Tumor specific Epstein-Barr infection is not associated with leiomyosarcomas in human immunodeficiency virus negative individuals. *Cancer* 1997;80:204–210.

180. Horiuchi A, Nikaido T, Taniguchi S, Fujii S. Possible role of calponin h1 as a tumor suppressor in human uterine leiomyosarcoma. *J Natl Cancer Inst* 1999;91:790–796.

181. Seki A, Kodama J, Miyagi Y, et al. Amplification of the mdm-2 gene and p53 abnormalities in uterine sarcomas. *Int J Cancer* 1997;26:33–37.

182. Ramondetta LM, Burke TW, Jhingran A, et al. A Phase II trial of cisplatin ifosfamide and mesna in patients with advanced or recurrent malignant mixed mullerian tumors with evaluation of potential molecular targets. *Gynecol Oncol* 2003;90:529–536.

183. Nasu K, Kawano Y, Hirota Y. Immunohistochemical study of c-*erb*B-2 expression in MMMT of the female genital tract. *Int J Obstet Gynecol* 1996;22:347–351.

184. Costa MJ, Walls J. Epidermal growth factor receptor and c-*erb*B-2 oncoprotein expression in female genital tract carcinosarcomas (malignant mixed mullerian tumors). *Cancer* 1996;77:533–542.

185. Emoto M, Iwasaki H, Ishiguro M, et al. Angiogenesis in carcinosarcomas of the uterus: differences in the microvessel density and expression of vascular endothelial growth factor between the epithelial and mesenchymal elements. *Hum Pathol* 1999;30:1232–1241.

186. Roy RN, Gerulath AH, Cecutti A, Bhavnani BR. Loss of IGF-II imprinting in endometrial tumors: overexpression in carcinosarcoma. *Cancer Lett* 2000;153:67–73.

187. Iwasa Y, Haga H, Konishi I, Kobashi Y. Prognostic factors in uterine carcinosarcoma. *Cancer* 1998;82:512–519.

188. Hibshoosh H, Lattes R. Immunohistochemical and molecular genetic approaches to soft tissue tumor diagnosis: a primer. *Semin Oncol* 1997;24:515–525.

CHAPTER 25

Epithelial Ovarian Cancer

Robert F. Ozols, Stephen C. Rubin, Gillian M. Thomas, and Stanley J. Robboy

Epithelial ovarian carcinoma is the leading cause of death from gynecologic cancer in the United States. In 2003, there will be an estimated 24,400 new cases in the United States (4% of all cancer diagnoses), and approximately 14,300 women will die of this disease this year (1,2). Ovarian cancer is the fourth most frequent cause of cancer death in women and accounts for 5% of all cancer deaths. The death rate from ovarian cancer exceeds that of cervical and endometrial carcinomas combined. It has been estimated that, in the United States, 1 woman in 70 will develop ovarian cancer in her lifetime, and 1 woman in 100 will die of this disease.

EPIDEMIOLOGY

Incidence and Mortality

The age-specific incidence of ovarian cancer increases with age and peaks in the eighth decade. The incidence rates by age, depicted in Figure 25.1, are based upon cancer registry data collected by the Surveillance, Epidemiology, and End Results Program (SEER) of the National Cancer Institute (NCI) (3). Epithelial ovarian cancer is infrequent in women below the age of 40 years, after which the rate increases with age from 15 per 100,000 in the 40- to 44-year age group to a peak rate of 57 per 100,000 in the 70- to 74-year age group. The median age of diagnosis is 63 years, and 48% of patients are 65 years or older (3).

In African-American women, the average incidence is 10

per 100,000 compared to an average incidence of 13 to 15 in white women. The average incidence in African-American women has decreased 0.5% among women under 50 years old and increased 0.4% among older women. Overall, African-American women have a lower lifetime risk (1.05%) compared to white women (1.82%). In some databases, higher death rates were observed in African-American women (4), and it appears that minorities in general received less guideline therapy as defined by the National Institutes of Health Consensus Development Conference on Ovarian Cancer (5). The most recent American Cancer Society data, however, show both a similar stage distribution at diagnosis and 5-year survival for African-American women compared to white women with ovarian cancer (1).

In the last three decades, the overall incidence of ovarian cancer has been relatively unchanged, with a declining incidence for younger women but an increasing incidence for older women (6). During this same time period, some studies have found an increasing ovarian cancer mortality rate in older women (greater than 65 years) and a decreasing mortality in younger women (7). Increased oral contraceptive use may account for the decreasing incidence and mortality rates among younger women in the United States. Factors associated with the increasing mortality in older women remain to be defined. Younger women have earlier stage at diagnosis, and some studies have found that less aggressive treatment is frequently administered to elderly patients (4).

Overall, there has been little change in ovarian cancer mortality in the last quarter century, and the number of recorded deaths from ovarian cancer in the United States has been relatively stable in the last 8 years (1). There exist marked differences in survival rates for patients with epithelial ovarian cancer depending upon their age and stage of their disease. Five-year survival for women under 65 years of age is 65.8% compared to 32.9% for women 65 years and over (2). Women with advanced-stage epithelial ovarian

Robert F. Ozols: Division of Medical Science, Fox Chase Cancer Center, Philadelphia, Pennsylvania 19111.

Stephen C. Rubin: Department of Obstetrics and Gynecology, University of Pennsylvania Medical Center, Philadelphia, Pennsylvania 19104.

Gillian M. Thomas: Toronto, Ontario, Canada M5R 1V1.

Stanley J. Robboy: Department of Pathology, Duke University Medical Center, Durham, North Carolina 27710.

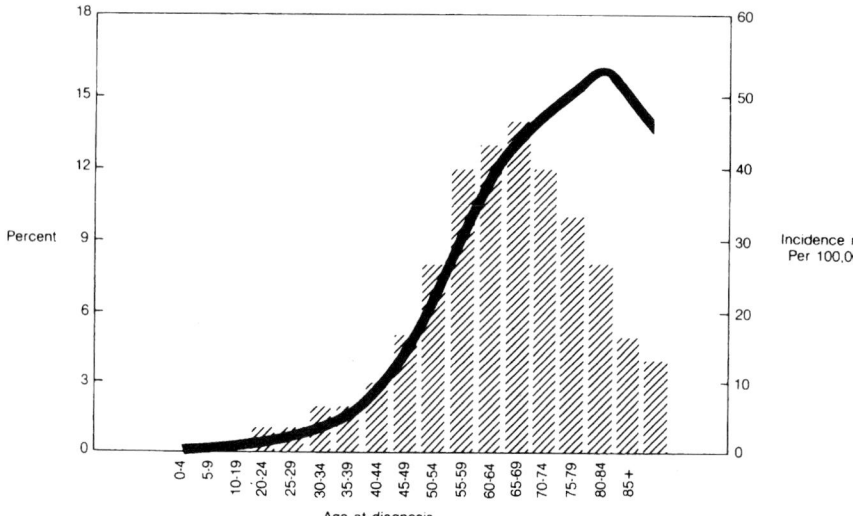

FIG. 25.1. Incidence rates by age for ovarian cancer. (Reprinted from Yancik R, Ries LG, Yates JW. Ovarian cancer in the elderly: an analysis of surveillance. *Am J Obstet Gynecol* 1986;154:639. Copyright 2004, with permission from Elsevier.)

cancer under the age of 45 years have a 45% survival rate compared to 13% for women 65 to 74 years of age.

Although overall survival has been relatively unchanged, there was a statistically significant improvement in 5-year survival rates from 1992 to 1998. Compared to the early 1970s when 5-year survival rates were 36%, by 1998, the 5-year survival rate had increased to 53% (1). As previously noted, in contrast to many other tumors, the stage-specific 5-year survival rates for white and African-American women are similar: localized disease, 95% versus 91%; regional disease, 81% for both; and advanced disease, 31% versus 28%, respectively (1).

Etiology

The molecular events leading to the development of epithelial ovarian cancer are unknown. Epidemiologic studies, however, have identified endocrine, environmental, and genetic factors as being important in the carcinogenesis of ovarian cancer. Epidemiologically established risk factors include nulliparity, family history, early menarche and late menopause, white race, increasing age, and residence in North America and Northern Europe (8).

Reproductive Factors

The majority of epidemiologic studies have demonstrated that parity is an important risk factor for ovarian cancer. Women who were ever pregnant have a 30% to 60% less risk of ovarian cancer than nulliparous women (8,9). Multiple pregnancies exert an increasingly protective effect. Compared to a relative risk of 1.0 for nulliparous women, one to two pregnancies result in a relative risk of 0.49 to 0.97. For women with greater than three pregnancies, the relative risk is further decreased to 0.35 to 0.76 (8). An associated

factor that also reduces the risk is a history of breast-feeding, although no consistent relationship has been established between breast-feeding duration and decreased risk. Epidemiologic data have also suggested a connection between risk for epithelial ovarian cancer and poorly understood ovulation abnormalities that reduce the likelihood of conception (10).

A case-cohort study examined the influence of ovulation-inducing drugs (clomiphene) on the risk for ovarian tumors in infertile women (11). The use of clomiphene for more than 12 ovulatory cycles was associated with a two- to threefold elevated risk. Most of the tumors were tumors of low malignant potential (LMP), previously referred to as borderline tumors of the ovary, in the infertile women on prolonged clomiphene. In a pooled analysis, ovarian cancer risk was increased among women who had used fertility drugs (odds ratio of 4.0 and 2.8 among women with LMP tumors and invasive cancer, respectively) (12).

Case-control studies have also consistently demonstrated that users of oral contraceptives have 30% to 60% less chance of developing ovarian cancer than do women without such contraceptive use (13–15). The relationship between the use of combined oral contraceptives and the risk of epithelial ovarian cancer has been investigated by the World Health Organization (WHO) in 368 women with ovarian cancer compared to 2,397 matched controls (14). The relative risk for women who had ever used oral contraceptives was 0.75. The risk further decreased with increasing time since cessation of use and, in contrast to other studies (15), the risk decreased with longer duration of use. The decreased risk was substantially greater in nulliparous women compared to parous women (0.16 vs 0.85, respectively). Oral contraceptives are estimated to have prevented over 1,700 cases of ovarian cancer per year in the United States (15).

The increased risk of ovarian cancer in women with a prior history of breast cancer as well as the two- to fourfold increased risk of breast cancer in women with a history of ovarian cancer provide further evidence of the importance of altered hormonal environment in the etiology of ovarian cancer (9,16). Although early individual epidemiologic studies did not establish a clear association between ovarian cancer risk and the use of hormone replacement therapy (17), a later meta-analysis of 21 studies showed the existence of a small increase in overall risk [relative risk (RR) 1.15, confidence interval (CI) 1.05 to 1.27] (18).

Several recent studies have established an association between hormone replacement therapy and risk of ovarian cancer. In the Cancer Prevention Study II, mortality from ovarian cancer was doubled in postmenopausal women who had used estrogens for 10 or more years (19). A cohort study in the United States confirmed an association with estrogen alone [odds ratio (OR) 1.6, 95% CI 1.2 to 2.0] but no association with combined hormones (20). A Swedish case-control study reported an increased risk associated with the use of unopposed estrogens (OR 1.43, 95% CI 1.02 to 2.0) and sequential preparations of estrogen and progestins (OR 1.54, 95% CI 1.15 to 2.05) but not with the use of continuous progestin regimens (21). Most recently, the results of The Women's Health Initiative Randomized Trial provided additional support regarding the effects of estrogen plus progestin on risk of ovarian cancer (22). Almost 17,000 postmenopausal women were randomized to placebo or one tablet per day of 0.625 mg of unconjugated estrogen plus 2.5 mg of medroxyprogesterone acetate. The trial was stopped early because of an increased risk of breast cancer. In addition, the hazard ratio for invasive ovarian cancer in women assigned to the estrogen plus progestin compared to placebo was 1.58; 95% CI 0.77 to 3.24. The low rates of ovarian cancer in the population, and the small number of cases (20 in the hormone arm and 12 in the placebo arm) limit the precision of the risk estimates, but the results are nevertheless worrisome. Although confirmation in another trial is awaited, these results do support the revised guidelines for the use of continuous combined estrogen plus progestin therapy (23).

The protective effects of parity, multiple births, history of breast-feeding, and oral contraceptive use supports the "incessant ovulation" hypothesis for the etiology of ovarian cancer (24,25). According to this hypothesis, ovarian cancer develops from an aberrant repair process of the surface epithelium, which is ruptured and repaired during each ovulatory cycle. The probability that ovarian cancer will develop is, therefore, a function of the total number of ovulatory cycles, together with a genetic predisposition and other, as yet undefined environmental factors. Consequently, the risk of ovarian cancer would be expected to fall as the number of ovulatory cycles is lowered. Alternatively, excessive gonadotropin secretion [follicle-stimulating hormone (FSH) or luteinizing hormone ([LH)] has been theorized to play a role in ovarian oncogenesis (26). Under excessive gonadotropin

stimulation and resulting estrogenic stimulation, the surface epithelium is entrapped in inclusion cysts and undergoes proliferation and malignant transformation. The protective effects of oral contraceptives and pregnancy on ovarian cancer risk are consistent with both hypotheses as oral contraceptives suppress ovulation and lower gonadotropin levels. Similarly, pregnancies decrease the number of ovulations and, during pregnancy, gonadotropin levels are decreased. However, not all epidemiologic data, including the results of recent studies of hormone replacement therapy and risk of ovarian cancer, fully support these hypotheses (27).

Another hypothesis has suggested a role for androgens and progestins in ovarian cancer development (16). Ovaries contain androgen receptors, the ovary is androgenic postmenopausally, and elevated androgen levels have been associated with an increased risk of ovarian cancer. Progestins may, on the other hand, be protective. Progestin levels are increased during pregnancy, progesterone receptors are present on ovarian epithelial cells, and progestin-only oral contraceptives that do not totally suppress ovulation have a protective effect similar to that observed with contraceptive preparations with a greater suppressive effect on ovulation (28).

Cramer (29) has recently hypothesized that ovarian cancer risk is associated with "stromal hyperactivity." He theorizes that granulosa and thecal cells remain in the ovarian stroma after ovulation and control steroid production. By reducing ovulatory cycles, the number of residual follicles in the stroma with functioning granulosa-thecal cells would also be decreased.

Another hypothesis for ovarian cancer development has been based on the association of endometriosis and pelvic inflammatory disease with increased risk of ovarian cancer. The inflammation hypothesis states that any inflammatory agent or condition increases the risk of ovarian cancer, and is also supported by epidemiologic data that the use of antiinflammatory agents, including aspirin and nonsteroidal antiinflammatory drugs, protects against ovarian cancer development (30).

Smith and Xu (31) have provided an alternative hypothesis based on their observation that loss of basement membrane is an early event leading to morphologic transformation of ovarian surface epithelium (32). In preovulatory stimulation of the ovarian surface epithelium by gonadotropins, the basement membrane of the ovarian surface is similarly degraded. Loss of basement membrane is mediated through prostaglandins produced by gonadotropin-induced COX-2. This observation provides a mechanism for the possible ovarian cancer preventive effect of COX-2 inhibitors.

None of these hypotheses for ovarian cancer development has accounted for all epidemiologic and experimental associations. It is apparent that ovarian cancer development is a complex process with the surface epithelial cells subject to numerous factors that may stimulate transformation, including hormones, stromal production of steroids, inflammatory cells, and other environmental factors.

Genetic Factors

Family history is an important factor in assigning an individual woman's probability for developing ovarian cancer. It is clinically useful to separate the genetic risk for ovarian cancer into familial ovarian cancer and hereditary ovarian cancer. Compared to the lifetime risk of 1.82% for the general population, a woman with a single family member affected by ovarian cancer has a 4% to 5% risk (33–35). In cases in which two relatives have ovarian cancer, a woman's risk increases to 7%. Women with hereditary ovarian cancer syndromes, defined as women with at least two first-degree relatives with ovarian cancer, may have a lifetime probability as high as 25% to 50% of developing ovarian cancer (8). Of note, only 7% of all ovarian cancer patients will report a first-degree relative with ovarian cancer (35). Although there has been an increased awareness of familial and hereditary ovarian cancer, leading to the establishment of ovarian cancer registries, such as the one at Roswell Park Memorial Institute (36) in Buffalo, New York, the precise incidence of familial ovarian cancer remains to be prospectively determined. Although hereditary ovarian cancer is uncommon, compared with the vastly more common sporadic form, these ovarian cancer kindreds are the focus of intense research efforts in that at least three genes that carry a genetic predisposition to ovarian cancer have already been identified (Table 25.1) (37–39).

Probably 10% of all epithelial ovarian carcinomas result from a hereditary predisposition. The molecular genetics of ovarian cancer are detailed in Chapter 2. Two distinct clinical syndromes associated with hereditary ovarian cancer are currently known (37–39) The most common of these is termed hereditary breast-ovarian cancer (HBOC). This syndrome accounts for 85% to 90% of all hereditary cancer cases currently identified. The vast majority of these cases are associated with mutations of the BRCA1 locus. BRCA1 consists of 22 coding exons and encodes for a protein of 1863 amino acids. BRCA1 is a tumor-suppressor gene that acts as a negative regulator of tumor growth. Inheritance of a cancer-predisposing mutant allele of BRCA1 is followed by loss of inactivation of the wild-type allele, which results in nonregulation of cell growth and progression toward malignancy. BRCA1 functions as a transcription factor and is important to the proper conduct of meiosis and regulation of the cell cycle. It is involved in the repair of damaged DNA and maintenance of genomic stability. Mutations of BRCA1 occur throughout the gene, and 80% of these mutations are loss of function and nonsense or frameshift alterations. Genetic epidemiologic studies have identified that specific mutations exist in certain populations and ethnic groups (37–39). The 185delAG and 5382insC mutations are present in 1% and 0.1% of the Ashkenazi Jews (European Jews, historically Yiddish speaking, who settled in central and northern Europe). In contrast to the association with hereditary ovarian cancer, somatic mutations of BRCA1 occurring in sporadic ovarian cancer are rare.

A second breast-ovarian cancer susceptibility gene, BRCA2, is localized to 13q12 (40). Tissue expression of BRCA2 resembles that of BRCA1 and the genes also share structural and functional similarities. There appears to be a regulated coordination of gene expression during cell cycle progression and both genes are involved in cell differentiation. Numerous mutations of BRCA2 have also been identified; the 6174delt mutation has been found in 1.4% of Ashkenazi Jews (37). It has been estimated that the probability of carrying a pathogenic BRCA1/2 mutation is approximately 40% among Ashkenazi Jewish patients with ovarian or peritoneal cancer (38). Similar to BRCA1, somatic mutations of the BRCA2 locus are rare in sporadic ovarian cancer (39).

Initial studies from families with evidence of linkage to BRCA1 suggested that a lifetime risk of ovarian cancer might be as high as 63% in women carrying BRCA1 mutations. Larger studies now show that the lifetime risk of ovarian cancer is 28% to 44% among women with BRCA1 mutations and 27% among those with BRCA2 mutations (41). Furthermore, in larger population studies on the Ashkenazi Jewish women who were unselected for family cancer history, the

TABLE 25.1. *Genes associated with hereditary ovarian cancer syndromes*

Gene	Syndrome	Location	Germline mutations/ ovarian tumors examined	%
BRCA1	Breast and ovarian cancer	17q21	23/565	4.1
BRCA2	Breast and ovarian cancer	13q12	6/180	3.3
Mismatch Repair	Hereditary nonpolyposis colorectal cancer		3/104	2.9
hMSH2		2p16		
hMLSH1		3p21		
pPMS2		7p22		
			Total	10.3

Reprinted with permission from Boyd J. Molecular genetics of hereditary ovarian cancer. *Oncology* 1998;12:399–406.

lifetime ovarian cancer risk is 16% for carriers of any of the three founder mutations described for *BRCA1* and *BRCA2* (42).

Based on family pedigrees revealing multiple cases of ovarian cancer without any apparent increase in breast cancer, a site-specific form of ovarian cancer had been theorized in addition to the well-established HBOC (43). Linkage studies, however, have not identified any locus other than *BRCA1*, which suggests that site-specific manifestation is not a distinct hereditary syndrome but rather represents a variant manifestation of HBOC in which early-onset breast cancer is infrequent (37).

In the second well-described hereditary syndrome, epithelial ovarian cancer is a component of the hereditary nonpolyposis colorectal syndrome (HNPCC) (44). It is also an autosomal dominant genetic syndrome, which was known previously as Lynch syndrome II (45). A predisposition to site-specific colorectal cancer exists with predilection for the proximal colon, early age of onset of excessive synchronous and metachronous colorectal cancers, and an increased predisposition for several other tumors including endometrial, ovarian, and stomach tumors. Mutations in DNA mismatch repair genes predispose to HNPCC. Ovarian cancer occurs in approximately 5% to 10% of HNPCC patients with one of the three described germline mutations (Table 25.1). A marked excess of carcinomas of the endometrium and ovary is particularly associated with mutations in *hMSH2*.

There appear to be distinct clinical and pathologic features of ovarian cancer with germline mutations of *BRCA1* compared to sporadic ovarian cancer. Among 53 patients with germline mutations of *BRCA1*, the average age of diagnosis was 48 years, and the vast majority of cancers were serous adenocarcinomas (46). Cancers associated with *BRCA1* mutations had a significantly more favorable course, with an actuarial median survival of 77 months in 43 patients with advanced disease compared to 29 months with matched controls (Fig. 25.2). These results have been confirmed in some, but not all, retrospective studies (47). The Gynecologic Oncology Group (GOG) is performing a prospective study of the clinical course of ovarian cancer patients with *BRCA1* mutations compared to the more common sporadic form of the disease.

The appropriate management of women with a hereditary ovarian cancer risk remains to be defined. Surveillance and screening, particularly with transvaginal sonography, are frequently employed, but there is no evidence that these measures result in risk reduction. The National Institutes of Health Consensus Development Panel recommended that prophylactic oophorectomy should be considered in women with hereditary ovarian cancer syndromes at age 35 years or after childbearing is completed (5). However, as will be discussed below, there is an increased risk for peritoneal carcinomatosis in women with hereditary ovarian cancer, which persists following prophylactic oophorectomy.

Oral contraceptive use may reduce the risk of ovarian

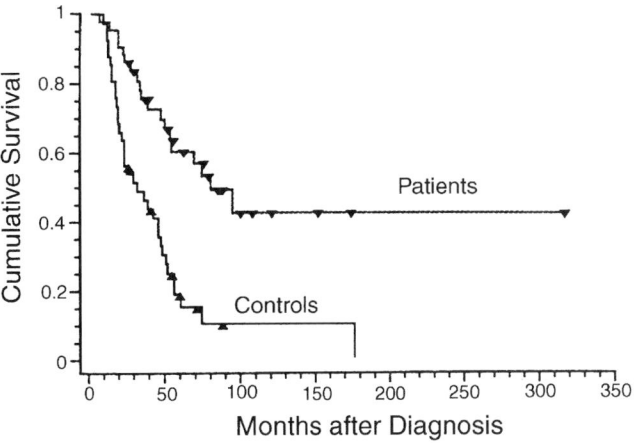

FIG. 25.2. Actuarial survival among 43 patients with advanced ovarian cancer and *BRCA1* mutations compared to matched controls without known mutations. (Reprinted with permission from Rubin SC, Benjamin I, Behbakht K, Takahashi H, et al. Clinical and pathological features of ovarian cancer in women with germ-line mutations of BRCA1. *N Engl J Med* 1996;335:1413. Copyright © 2004 Massachusetts Medical Society. All rights reserved.)

cancer in women with mutations in the *BRCA1* or *BRCA2* gene. In a case-control retrospective study (48), the risk ratio for ovarian cancer associated with the use of oral contraceptives was compared in 207 women with hereditary ovarian cancer against 161 of their sisters as controls. All 207 patients carried mutations in *BRCA1* or *BRCA2*, whereas the women of the control group were enrolled regardless of whether they had either mutation. The use of oral contraceptives for 6 or more years was associated with a 60% reduction in risk. The protective effect of oral contraceptive use was evident after adjusting for parity, tubal ligation, and ages at delivery of first and last child. In addition, increased parity also was protective against ovarian cancer to the same degree as in the general population. Although the data from this retrospective study suggest that oral contraceptive use should be considered in the prevention of cancer for women with *BRCA1* or *BRCA2* mutations, they are insufficient for specific recommendations with regard to age at which treatment should begin or to which specific formulation of oral contraceptives should be used.

Patient education and counseling by trained geneticists are essential components of any risk-assessment program (49). Studies are in progress to determine how best to integrate genetic testing into clinical practice, including selection of appropriate genetic tests, risk reduction using conventional screening techniques, role of prophylactic oophorectomy and chemoprevention, and behavioral studies in high-risk women.

Tumor-Suppressor Genes

While 10% of ovarian cancer is purported to develop on a hereditary basis, this figure may, in fact, be significantly underestimated (37,38). Other genetic mutations probably exist that confer a predisposition with low penetrance in a mendelian recessive fashion. In addition, there may be interactions with other susceptibility loci that are yet undefined. Both sporadic and hereditary ovarian cancer exhibit multiple genetic alterations implicating both tumor-suppressor genes and oncogenes. However, it remains uncertain which alterations are necessary for initiation or promotion of tumorigenesis and which result from genomic instability inherent in advanced tumors. Molecular probes have recognized restriction of fragment-linked polymorphisms or confirmed loss of genetic material in numerous chromosomes, suggesting the involvement of multiple tumor-suppressor genes in tumor development and progression. Loss of heterozygosity is common in ovarian cancer of specific loci chromosomes 3p, 6q, 11p, 13q, 17p, and 17q (37,38). These loci and others represent potential sites for other putative cancer-causing genes. Prowse et al. (38) have recently summarized the role of tumor-suppressor genes in ovarian cancer.

Mutations of the *p53* gene, which codes for a tumor-suppressor protein that likely acts as a transcription factor regulating gene expression, are the most frequently reported genetic alternations in ovarian cancer (50,51). Such mutations are associated with immunohistochemically detectable elevated levels of mutant protein and occur most frequently in serous tumors. The prognostic significance of *p53* expression in ovarian cancer has not been fully determined. In 284 patients with epithelial ovarian cancer, p53 immunoreactivity was detected in 177 (62%) (50). In a univariate analysis, but not in a multivariate analysis, *p53* expression was associated with decreased survival. In a subset of patients with early-stage disease, *p53* expression approached statistical significance as an independent prognostic factor. A recent GOG study in 125 patients with advanced-stage ovarian cancer confirmed that alterations in *p53* were a common event. It was reported that a mutation in *p53*, but not overexpression of *p53*, was associated with a short-term survival benefit. The initial risk reductions disappeared with longer follow-up (52). Expression of *p53* has not been reported in LMP tumors of the ovary and appears to be associated with an increasing histologic grade (53). Additional studies are required to define the role of *p53* and response to chemotherapy and survival.

Alternative molecular techniques have also helped to identify putative tumor-suppressor genes potentially involved in ovarian oncogenesis. Using differential RNA display to probe gene expression differences between normal rat ovarian surface epithelial cells and transformed cells, a gene, *LOT1*, was identified that showed lost or decreased expression in five of eight transformed rat surface epithelial cell lines (54). Overexpression of *LOT1* in an ovarian cancer line suppressed growth.

Using similar differential display techniques, *NOEY2* is another gene that was found to be expressed in normal surface epithelial cells but not in ovarian cancer cell lines (55).

Transformation of *NOEY2* into ovarian cancer cell lines resulted in suppression of growth. Both genes may exert their effect on tumorigenesis by perturbing signal transduction pathways.

An RNA fingerprinting strategy and Northern blot analysis identified that the gene *DAB2* was differentially expressed in epithelial ovarian cancer cells compared to normal human ovarian surface epithelial (HOSE) cells (56). *DAB2*, the expression of which closely correlates with morphologic transformation of the ovarian surface epithelial cells, may be a critical determinant of epithelial organization. Loss of *DAB2* is an early event in ovarian carcinogenesis, promoting epithelial cell transformation and disorganized growth (32).

Oncogenes

Abnormalities of dominant oncogenes are frequently found in ovarian cancer with at least 25 alterations in cellular oncogenes having been reported to date (38). Altered c-*myc*, H-*ras*, and Ki-*ras* are the most frequent findings (38,57). The protein product of *ras*, p21, is expressed in 44% and overexpressed in 18% of invasive epithelial tumors, with Ki-*ras* amplification being observed in 8%. However, mutational activation is uncommon (4%) in invasive tumors, whereas *ras* mutations are more common in LMP tumors (58). This difference suggests that *ras* mutations have little significance in invasive tumors, but are involved in the development of LMP tumors (58). There is no evidence that levels of p21 correlate with clinical outcome in advanced ovarian cancer (59).

Overexpressed c-*myc* in one study was relatively frequent (30%) but is without an established prognostic influence (38). Expression of growth-factor receptors is more common and may be associated with prognosis. Epidermal growth-factor receptor is expressed in one-half of ovarian tumors, and increased expression has been associated with a decrease in disease-free survival. The related growth-factor receptor *ERB*B2 was initially reported to be amplified and/or overexpressed in up to 32% of ovarian cancers (60), but in a GOG screening of over 800 patients with recurrent ovarian cancer, only 11.4% of the patients showed overexpression (61).

In addition to alterations in cell surface growth-factor receptors, downstream signal transduction pathways appear to be abnormally functioning or dysregulated in ovarian cancer (38,57). Besides *ras*, *AKT2* and *PIK3CA* are oncogenes involved in the pathogenesis of ovarian cancer whose protein products act within signal transduction pathways. AKT2 is a serine-3 threonine protein kinase that was found amplified in both primary human ovarian cancers and in ovarian cancer cell lines (62). Amplified *AKT2* gene was observed in 12% of ovarian carcinomas but not in benign or LMP ovarian tumors (63). Overexpressed *AKT2* was observed in an additional 3 of 25 of ovarian carcinomas negative for *AKT2* amplification. *AKT2* is rapidly activated by several mitogenic growth factors, such as epidermal growth factor (EGF) and

PI3-kinase (PIK3CA). PIK3CA has also been shown to have increased copy number in ovarian cancer (64). A tumor suppressor, PTEN, acts by opposing the action of PI3-kinase by dephosphorylating the signaling lipid phosphatidylinositol. PTEN is downregulated in some ovarian tumors and there is an inverse correlation between PTEN expression and AKT2 expression (65). This important pathway of cell signaling appears to be frequently disrupted in ovarian tumors by alterations in PTEN, PIK3CA, and/or AKT2. Although the exact mechanisms of how alterations in this EGF receptor (EGFR) signaling pathway contribute to ovarian cancer etiology and progression remain poorly defined, the identification of the involved oncogenes and suppressor genes may well provide new targets for prevention and treatment. The current status of oncogenes and tumor-suppressor genes in the etiology and progression of ovarian cancer is summarized in Chapter 5.

Ovarian tumors, a few of which are epithelial, occur with other genetic disorders. Peutz-Jeghers syndrome (i.e., mucocutaneous pigmentation and intestinal polyps) is associated with an increased risk for a distinctive tumor of sex-cord stromal origin (i.e., sex-cord tumor with annular tubules) and, very rarely, with mucinous tumors. Patients with mixed gonadal dysgenesis (46XY genotype or mosaic) can develop gonadoblastomas. Women with multiple nevoid basal-cell carcinomas are at increased risk for the development of ovarian fibromas.

Environmental Factors

Epithelial ovarian carcinoma has its highest incidence in industrialized Western countries. In Japan, however, the incidence is low. The risk in Japanese immigrants to the United States and to their offspring increases but does not reach the levels observed in the white population. Whereas some studies have associated a diet high in meat and animal fat, characteristic of industrialized nations (9), others, such as a case-control study in Utah between 1984 and 1987, failed to demonstrate that calories, fat, protein, fiber, or vitamins A and C appreciably altered the risk (66). Some reports suggest that obesity is associated with a slight increase in the relative risk.

Cramer et al. (67) evaluated the relationship between dietary factors and genetically determined levels of red blood cell galactose-1-phosphate uridyl transferase with the risk of developing ovarian cancer. This study was based on the hypothesis that ovarian cancer is a consequence of hypergonadotropic hypogonadism (high secretions of gonadotropins due to ovarian failure or absent feedback control of the pituitary) and to the experimental observation that dietary galactose consumption and decreased levels of transferase are associated with hypergonadotropic hypogonadism. In this case-control study, the mean transferase activity in patients with ovarian cancer was significantly lower than in controls. Furthermore, when the ratio of lactose consumption (often in the form of yogurt) to transferase (L/T) was calculated, patients with ovarian cancer had a mean L/T ratio of 1.17 compared to 0.98 for controls, with a highly significant trend toward increasing ovarian cancer risk with increasing L/T ratio.

Other dietary risk factors have also been investigated (8, 9). Coffee and tobacco usage has not been associated with ovarian cancer, although there appears to be a slight increased risk with alcohol consumption.

Earlier epidemiologic studies suggested a protective effect for mumps on the subsequent development of ovarian cancer. However, this may not be an independent risk factor, as women from large families are more likely to be exposed to mumps as children and, in turn, have large families themselves (8,9).

Although epidemiologic studies suggest environmental causes, definite associations with industrial exposure to carcinogens or to diagnostic and therapeutic radiation have not been established (8,9). There have been conflicting reports regarding the association of the use of talcum powder (which in the past had been shown to contain asbestos) and the development of ovarian cancer (68). Exposure to asbestos and talc particulates (primarily in the form of dusting powders) could lead to passage of such materials through the vaginal reproductive tract to the ovaries (69).

Prevention of Ovarian Cancer

The retrospective epidemiologic data describing a decreased incidence of ovarian cancer associated with oral contraceptive pills have led to the recommendation that they should be considered as primary prevention in women at an increased risk. As previously discussed, women with hereditary ovarian cancer due to *BRCA1* or *BRCA2* mutations have a marked reduction in risk with prolonged use of oral contraceptives (48). Further support for their use in risk reduction has been generated from the Cancer and Steroid Hormone (CASH) study and SEER data (13–15). The effect of oral contraceptive use on the incidence of epithelial ovarian cancer was determined in four groups of women: positive family history (not selected by genetic testing), negative family history, parous, and nulliparous (70). Five years of oral contraceptive use reduced the risk in nulliparous women to the same level as that for parous women who were nonusers. Furthermore, 10 years of use by women with a positive family history reduced their level of risk below that for women who were nonusers and without a family history of ovarian cancer. The exact mechanism of risk reduction by oral contraceptives remains to be defined. Although decreased ovulation may be a major mechanism, the progestational components of oral contraceptives may exert independent protective effects, including inducing apoptosis on surface epithelial cells (71).

A recent study also suggested that fenretinide, a synthetic retinoid, may also protect women against ovarian cancer

(72). This drug was administered to breast cancer patients at high risk for a new primary tumor or a contralateral tumor based on *in vivo* studies showing a protective effort against carcinogen-induced mammary carcinomas in rats. In a randomized trial, six patients in the control group of 1,427 women developed ovarian cancer, whereas no patient receiving fenretinide developed ovarian cancer. Although preliminary, these results demonstrate the potential feasibility of chemoprevention of ovarian cancer in high-risk groups. A placebo-controlled prospective randomized trial of fenretinide is in progress in high-risk women who have elected to undergo a prophylactic oophorectomy (73). A previous study has identified the existence of putative histopathologic biomarkers in ovaries from women with a hereditary risk for ovarian cancer (74). The purpose of this trial is to determine whether fenretinide can reduce the incidence or severity of this potential premalignant phenotype.

The Nurses' Health Study of 121,700 nurses was used to determine the effect of tubal ligation and hysterectomy on the subsequent risk of ovarian cancer (75). There was a strong inverse association between tubal ligation and ovarian cancer (RR 0.33). There was a weaker protective effect of hysterectomy (RR 0.67). The mechanism for the protective effects is unclear. Tubal ligation may affect circulating hormone levels by interfering with ovarian circulation.

Prophylactic oophorectomy has been recommended by some investigators for selected women in families with hereditary or familial ovarian cancer (5). However, a prophylactic oophorectomy will not be protective in all high-risk patients from such ovarian cancer families. In a retrospective study, 16 families were identified in which at least two first-degree relatives had documented ovarian cancer (76). Twenty-eight women in these families underwent prophylactic oophorectomy and were followed from 1 to 20 years.

Over time, three of these women developed disseminated intraabdominal carcinomatosis indistinguishable histopathologically from ovarian carcinoma. The time to the development of the intraabdominal malignancy ranged from 9 months to 11 years after the prophylactic oophorectomy. The most likely explanation for the failure of prophylactic oophorectomy is that tissues at risk may include the broader second müllerian system (tumors arising directly from the peritoneal mesothelium), which is the same tissue from which the ovaries are derived embryologically. The occurrence of *BRCA1* germline mutations in patients with primary peritoneal carcinoma has also been documented (77). Consequently, removal of the ovaries eliminates only one potential site for malignant transformation in patients with familial ovarian cancer.

A multicenter international study has been initiated to examine the effectiveness of prophylactic oophorectomy in inherited breast/ovarian cancer families (78). In 346 first-degree relatives who did not undergo oophorectomy, after 1,600 person-years of follow-up, eight ovarian cancers developed compared to two peritoneal carcinomatosis cases in 44 oophorectomized women with 460 person-years of follow-up. The results of this study support a protective effect of oophorectomy in high-risk women. This study also confirms the excess risk of peritoneal carcinomatosis in oophorectomized women with hereditary ovarian cancer.

Two additional studies have recently described the effects of prophylactic oophorectomy on carriers of *BRCA1* or *BRCA2* mutations. Rebbeck et al. (79) reported on 551 women with germline *BRCA1* or *BRCA2* mutations who were identified from high-risk registries and studied for the occurrence of ovarian and breast cancer. The incidence of ovarian cancer was examined in 259 women who underwent prophylactic oophorectomy and in 292 matched controls

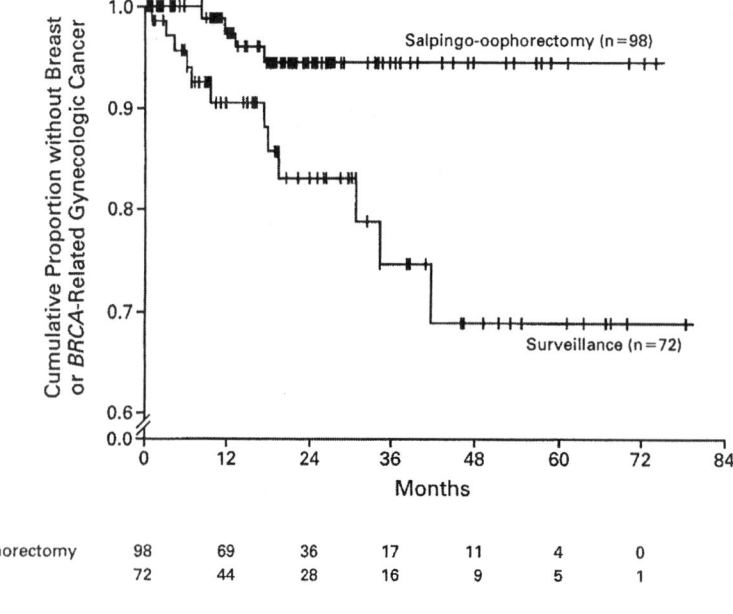

No. at Risk							
Salpingo-oophorectomy	98	69	36	17	11	4	0
Surveillance	72	44	28	16	9	5	1

FIG. 25.3. Kaplan-Meier estimates of the time to breast cancer or BRCA-related gynecologic cancer among women who underwent salpingo-oophorectomy and women who elected a surveillance policy (*p* = .006). (Reprinted with permission from Kauff ND, Satagopan JM, Robson MR, et al. Risk-reducing salpingo-oophorectomy in women with a *BRCA1* or *BRCA2* mutation. *N Engl J Med* 2002;346: 1609–1615. Copyright © 2004 Massachusetts Medical Society. All rights reserved.)

who had not undergone surgery. In six women who underwent prophylactic oophorectomy, previously unsuspected stage I ovarian cancer was found. Two women (0.8%) developed papillary serous peritoneal carcinoma 3.8 and 8.6 years after bilateral prophylactic oophorectomy. In the control population, 58 women (19.9%) developed ovarian cancer after a mean follow-up of 8.8 years. Prophylactic oophorectomy significantly reduced the risk of epithelial ovarian cancer (hazard ratio 0.04, 95% CI 0.01 to 0.16).

Kauff et al. (80) reported on a prospective follow-up study of 170 high-risk women, only some of whom chose to undergo either prophylaxis. As shown in Figure 25.3, there is a marked increase in the cumulative proportion without breast- or *BRCA*-related gynecologic cancer in women who underwent salpingo-oophorectomy compared to those on the surveillance regimen. During a mean follow-up of 2 years, breast cancer was diagnosed in 3 of the 98 women who chose surgery, and peritoneal cancer was diagnosed in one woman in this group. Among the 72 women who chose surveillance, breast cancer was diagnosed in eight, ovarian cancer in four, and peritoneal cancer in one. These studies provided further evidence that salpingo-oophorectomy in carriers of *BRCA1* mutations reduces the risk of both epithelial ovarian cancer and breast cancer.

Current screening techniques (as will be discussed) utilizing serum CA-125 levels, pelvic ultrasound, and frequent pelvic examinations are not likely to have the necessary sensitivity or the specificity markedly to increase the number of patients diagnosed with ovarian cancer at an earlier stage. Currently, the optimal management for women in the high-risk familial ovarian cancer syndromes with *BRCA1/2* mutations is a prophylactic oophorectomy. However, women should be counseled that they may be at risk for the development of intraabdominal carcinomatosis even when histologically normal ovaries are removed.

PATHOLOGY

Ovarian tumors, although inappropriately often considered as a single entity, consist of many types, each with subtypes. The classification in Table 25.2, presented in detail for the common epithelial tumors, has been developed and continuously updated under the auspices of WHO, the International Federation of Gynecology and Obstetrics (FIGO), the International Society of Gynecologic Pathologists, and the Society of Gynecologic Oncologists (SGO) (81).

The common epithelial tumors are by far the most frequently encountered forms of ovarian tumors, accounting

TABLE 25.2. *Histologic classification of common epithelial tumors of the ovary*

Serous tumors	Endometrioid tumors (continued)
Benign	Malignant
Cystadenoma and papillary cystadenoma	Adenocarcinoma
Surface papilloma	Adenoacanthoma
Adenofibroma and cystadenofibroma	Adenosquamous carcinoma
Tumor of low malignant potential	Malignant adenofibroma with a malignant
Cystadenoma and papillary cystadenoma	stromal component
Surface papilloma	Adenosarcoma
Adenofibroma and cystadenofibroma	Endometrial stromal sarcoma
Malignant	Carcinosarcoma, homologous and
Adenocarcinoma	heterologous
Surface papillary adenocarcinoma	Undifferentiated sarcoma
Malignant adenofibroma and	Clear-cell tumors
cystadenofibroma	Benign
Mucinous tumors	Tumor of low malignant potential
Benign	Malignant
Cystadenoma	Adenocarcinoma
Adenofibroma and cystadenofibroma	Transitional-cell tumors
Tumor of low malignant potential	Brenner's tumor
Intestinal type	Proliferating Brenner's tumor
Endocervical-like	Malignant Brenner's tumor
Malignant	Transitional cell carcinoma (non-Brenner type)
Adenocarcinoma	Squamous-cell carcinoma
Malignant adenofibroma	Mixed epithelial tumors (specify types)
Mural nodule arising in mucinous cystic	Benign
tumor	Tumor of low malignant potential
Endometrioid tumors	Malignant
Benign	Undifferentiated carcinoma
Adenoma and cystadenoma	
Adenofibroma and cystadenofibroma	
Tumor of low malignant potential	

Modified with permission from Tavassoli FA and Devilee P. *Tumours of the breast and female genital organs. World Health Organization Classification of Tumors.* Lyon, France: IARC Press, 2003.

for three-fifths of all ovarian neoplasms and nine-tenths of all ovarian cancers (Table 25.3). The single most common malignancy, the serous adenocarcinoma, occurs in approximately 1% of women.

General Features

It is generally accepted that most neoplasms of "common epithelial origin" arise from the surface epithelium (or serosa) of the ovary (82). During embryonic life, the coelomic cavity forms and is lined by a mesothelial lining of mesodermal origin, part of which becomes specialized to form the serosal epithelium covering the gonadal ridge. By a process of invagination, this same mesothelial lining gives rise to the müllerian ducts, from which arise the fallopian tubes, uterus, and wall of the vagina. On occasion, routine examination of the epithelium that covers the seemingly normal-appearing ovary discloses early, *de novo* microscopic forms of epithelial cancer.(83)

As the ovary develops, the surface epithelium extends into

TABLE 25.3. *Comparison of ovarian cancers[a]*

Cancer type	Mean age (yr) (%)	Frequency All tumors[b] (%)	Frequency Malignant and LMP (%)	Diameter (cm)	Bilaterality[c] (%)
Common epithelial		59			
Serous		46			
Benign	45	49		9	17
LMP	48	15	14	9	34
Malignant	56	36	32	9	73
Mucinous		36			
Benign	44	81			2
LMP	49	14	10	15	6
Malignant	52	5	3	18	47
Endometrioid		8			
Benign	40	4		10	
LMP	48	19	3		7
Malignant	57	77	13	11	33
Clear cell		3			
Benign	45				
LMP	45				
Malignant	53	3	6	12	13
Brenner's		2			
Benign	52	98			
LMP		1			
Malignant		1			
Squamous	56	<1			
Mixed		3	2		
Undifferentiated	62	2	3	10	53
Small cell	28				
Germ cell		27	6		
Sex cord stromal		10	4		
Steroid cell					
Metastatic		1	3		75
		100			

LMP, low malignant potential.

[a] Reprinted with permission from Robboy SJ, Duggan M, Kurman RT. The female reproductive system. In: Rubin E, Farber J, eds. *Pathology.* 2nd ed. Philadelphia: JB Lippincott, 1988; and based primarily on cases (referrals excluded) treated at King George V Memorial Hospital, Sydney (Russell P, Farnsworth A. Surgical pathology of the ovaries. 2nd ed. New York: Churchill Livingstone, 1997), and secondarily on the geographically based Cancer and Steroid Hormone Study, CDC (Dr. Robboy, unpublished). Data about age and bilaterality come additionally from large series of individual tumor types. Serous tumors for 46% of all common epithelial tumors, and benign serous tumors for 49% of all serous tumors.

[b] Indented figures sum to 100% and are subsets of the next higher order. For example, common epithelial tumors account for 59% of all ovarian tumors, serous tumors for 46% of all common epithelial tumors, and benign serous tumors for 49% of all serous tumors.

[c] Bilaterality is for all tumors regardless of stage. In general, bilaterality for stage 1 common epithelial tumors (confined to ovaries) is one-half that with stage 3 (peritoneal) spread. The greater bilaterality associated with higher stage reflects metastatic spread by implantation rather than independent primary tumor formation in both ovaries.

the ovarian stroma to form inclusion glands and cysts. The epithelium, in becoming neoplastic, exhibits a variety of müllerian-type cells, which are in order of decreasing frequency: (a) serous (resembling the fallopian tube); (b) mucinous (resembling the endocervix); (c) endometrioid (resembling endometrium); and (d) clear-cell (glycogen-rich cells resembling endometrial glands in pregnancy). The ovarian surface epithelium, within its repertoire of metaplasia, may also exhibit urothelial differentiation, that is, transitional cells (resembling Walthard's rests and bladder).

Specimen Examination

Although thorough sampling of an ovarian tumor for microscopic analysis is an often-stated requirement for optimal pathologic examination, thoroughness cannot be equated with a formula for a specified number of slides taken randomly, which often provides little additional information (84). Instead, careful gross examination and judicious sampling are key (85). For example, adhesions on the surface of an ovary, although usually inflammatory in origin, are sometimes an indication that a tumor has penetrated the capsule. As a routine, it is helpful if the surgeon marks the adhesions with a stitch. Tissue sections should be taken perpendicularly through the adhesion and the capsule.

The ovarian tumor specimen should be serially sectioned ("bread-loafed") at close intervals and each piece carefully examined for differences in texture. Serous tumors tend to show greater uniformity than mucinous tumors, which are notorious for great variation, with only a small percentage of slides disclosing features diagnostic of cancer. Mucinous adenocarcinomas are commonly composed almost exclusively of cysts typical of adenoma or LMP tumors, whereas only a few areas are solid and show the diagnostic features

of carcinoma. Solid areas preferentially should be submitted for microscopic examination. Benign serous tumors tend to be unilocular. Serous LMP tumors tend to have clusters of numerous papillae that are larger and more edematous than those of adenocarcinomas, which are solid or relatively fine. Blocks taken from the base of papillary processes are particularly helpful to avoid overlooking occult areas of poorly differentiated carcinoma. As transition forms between benign and malignant epithelia are well documented (86), careful gross examination of the specimen is mandatory to help identify both the regions of LMP tumor and the frankly invasive carcinoma.

General Features Based on Degree of Malignancy

Benign Tumors

Common epithelial tumors that are benign are almost always serous or mucinous, and generally arise in women between the ages of 20 and 60 years (87). The tumors are frequently large, often 15 cm in greatest dimension, and sometimes exceed 30 cm. Benign serous tumors are more commonly bilateral (one-sixth of cases) than the other types of benign epithelial tumors. Benign epithelial tumors are typically cystic; hence the term *cystadenoma* (e.g., serous or mucinous cystadenoma) (Fig. 25.4). Microscopically, a single layer of tall, columnar epithelium lines the cysts. Papillae, if present, consist of a fibrovascular core covered by a single layer of mature, tall, columnar epithelium identical to that of the cyst lining. A prominent fibrous component can be present, giving a grossly solid or papillary appearance to surface areas of the tumor, in which case the term *cystadenofibroma* or *adenofibroma* can be used. These variants are identical in behavior to cystadenomas.

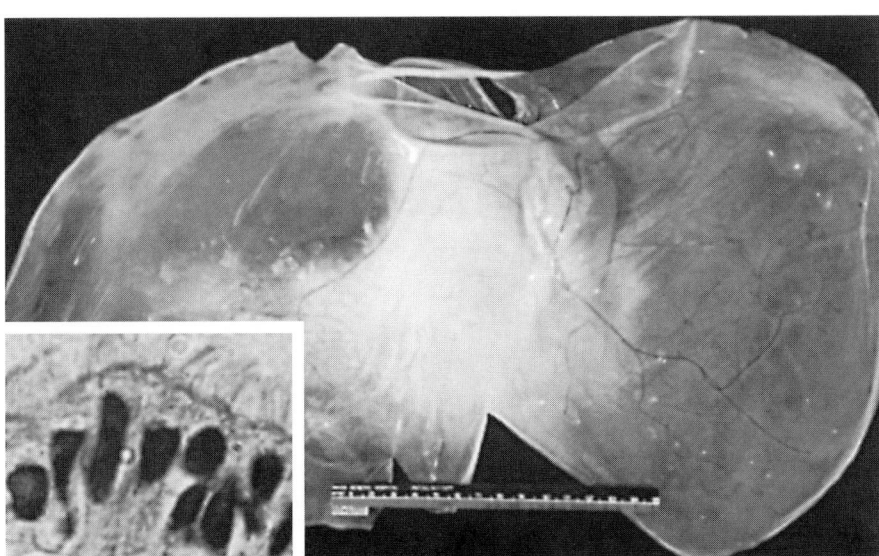

FIG. 25.4. Serous cystadenoma of ovary. The gross specimen is a unilocular cyst in which the wall is paper thin and the fluid filling the cyst is clear. (**Insert**) The epithelium lining the cyst wall is one layer thick and composed of ciliated, tall columnar cells resembling serous cells (H&E ×1250). (From Robboy SJ, Merino M, Kurman RT. The female reproductive system. In: Rubin E, Gorstein F, eds. *Pathology*. 4th ed. Philadelphia: JB Lippincott, 2004.)

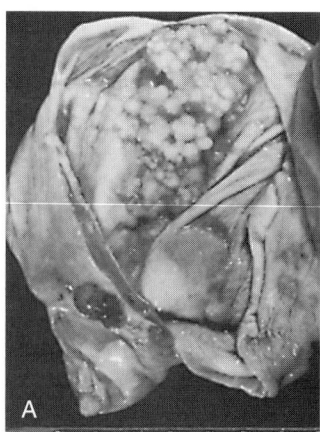
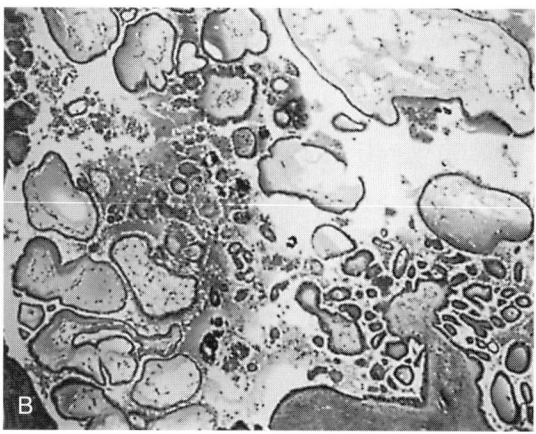

FIG. 25.5. Serous cystadenoma of low malignant potential. **A:** The tumor, which arises from the wall of a unilocular cyst, is a 6- × 3-cm mass with the appearance of a firm bunch of grapes. **B:** The grape-like structures are fibrovascular stalks lined by a mantle of serous cells one to several layers thick. Some cells are ciliated or display cytologic atypia. Mitoses are infrequent. (H&E ×64). (From Robboy SJ, Merino M, Kurman RT. The female reproductive system. In: Rubin E, Gorstein F, eds. *Pathology.* 4th ed. Philadelphia: JB Lippincott, 2004.)

Tumors of Low Malignant Potential

Patients with LMP tumors are in general older than patients with benign neoplasms and younger than ones with frank malignancies (Table 25.2). These tumors generally are associated with an excellent prognosis despite peculiar histologic features suggestive of cancer (88–96). Nearly all series report 5-year survival rates of 100% when the tumor is stage I or IIA. Even when the tumor involves the pelvis or abdomen, about 80% of patients will be alive after 5 years. Some fatalities are related to therapy rather than the tumor itself. Much effort has been focused during this past decade toward identifying those features associated with a poor prognosis, even to the point where all future cases might be classified as benign or malignant, removing the utility altogether of the LMP category (97).

The histologic features used to diagnose LMP tumors include (a) architectural complexity of glandular structures; (b) epithelial papillae (especially in serous tumors), with detached atypical cell clusters as single or small groups of cells; (c) cellular stratification (especially in mucinous tumors); (d) increased mitotic activity; and (e) nuclear atypia (increased nuclear:cytoplasmic ratios, hyperchromatism, and prominent nucleoli) (Fig. 25.5). Not infrequently, the differentiation between LMP tumor and frank malignancy must be made on the architectural basis of invasion (pushing borders vs destructive invasion, respectively) rather than on a cytologic basis of the cells themselves.

In recent years, as noted, the designation of "borderline tumors" has been generally replaced by "tumors of low malignant potential" (LMP). Another designation is "atypical proliferating tumor" (87), which reflects that stage I tumors are virtually always benign. Other terminologies used for LMP tumors as a generic group have subdivisions with "epithelial atypia" and "intraepithelial carcinoma"(98). At this time, there is no evidence that indicates these terms offer any advantage over the current system.

Microinvasion is a special category. Such tumors resemble typical LMP tumors except that foci of invasive carci-

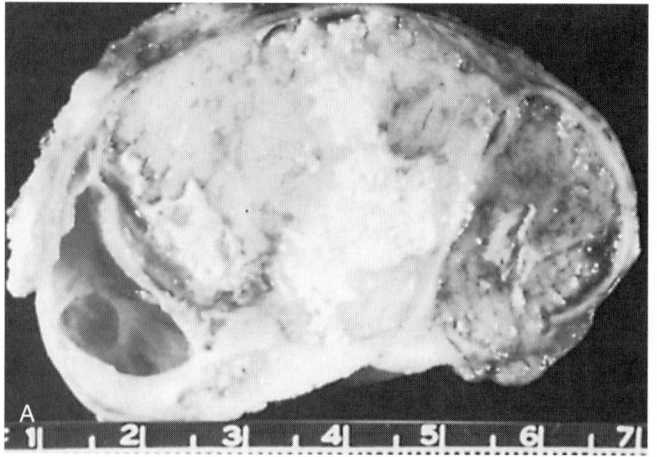
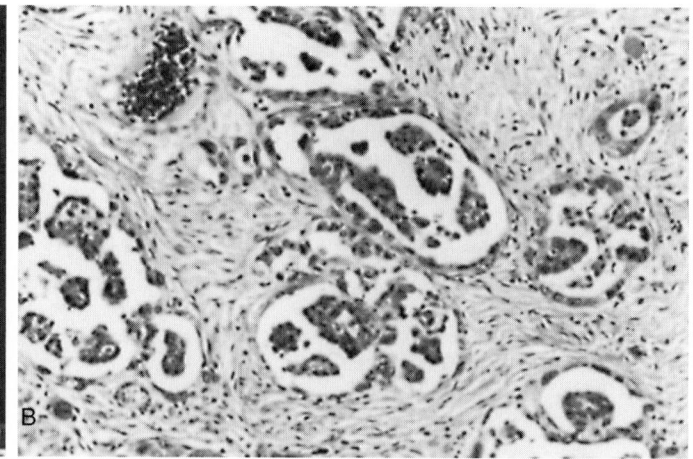

FIG. 25.6. Serous adenocarcinoma. **A:** The ovarian malignancy is solid with interspersed broad regions of necrosis. **B:** Numerous papillations of tumor cells destructively permeate the stroma. (From Robboy SJ, Merino M, Kurman RT. The female reproductive system. In: Rubin E, Gorstein F, eds. *Pathology.* 4th ed. Philadelphia: JB Lippincott, 2004.)

noma up to 3 mm in size are present in the stroma. Such foci consist predominantly of single cells or clusters of cells, sometimes with a cribriform pattern. A desmoplastic reaction to the tumor is often seen. Microinvasion does not seem to adversely alter the excellent prognosis of LMP tumors of the ovary (99).

Malignant Tumors (Invasive Carcinomas)

Histologically, malignant epithelial tumors are uncommon in women under the age of 35 years. Malignant ovarian tumors often present as solid masses, usually with areas of necrosis and hemorrhage (Fig. 25.6). By the time a carcinoma reaches a size of 10 to 15 cm, it has often already spread beyond the ovary and seeded the peritoneum.

Destructive growth, an important feature of malignancy, helps to distinguish frank malignancies from LMP tumors. Infiltrative destructive growth is best demonstrated by individual or small clusters of cells growing in a disorganized pattern with angulated, sharp borders that dissect into stromal planes and are usually associated with desmoplasia.

Although the histologic differentiation between a pushing border (characteristic of LMP tumors) and destructive invasion is usually readily apparent, clues in difficult cases include (a) altered tumor/stromal interface from a broad, uniform front to a focally irregular or ragged border; (b) change in the normal or edematous stroma to one that is desmoplastic; and (c) a chronic inflammatory cell infiltrate. The distinction between a pushing border and destructive infiltrative growth is important since it is often the only feature differentiating an adenocarcinoma from an LMP tumor.

SEROUS TUMORS

Serous tumors account for nearly half (46%) of all common epithelial tumors. About one-third are malignant, one of six are LMP tumors, and half are benign. The mean age for patients with cancer is 56 years. Patients with benign and LMP tumors are generally younger, with mean ages at diagnosis of 45 and 48 years, respectively. Approximately one of six serous adenomas is bilateral. Serous LMP tumors are bilateral in one-third of cases. In many cases, this represents implantation rather than a second independent primary lesion. Serous adenocarcinomas that are stage I are bilateral in one-third of cases. Those of higher stage are bilateral in two-thirds of cases. On a molecular basis, LMP and high-grade carcinomas differ, suggesting discordant pathogenic mechanisms (99).

Gross Appearance

Serous cystadenomas, defined as serous cysts larger than 1 cm in diameter, range typically from several centimeters to very large. The neoplasm is commonly unilocular and often has an extremely attenuated, translucent wall (Fig. 25.7). Sometimes adenomas exhibit slightly raised papillary excrescences, which typically are localized to a few areas of the wall.

Serous adenofibromas, required as being minimally 1 cm in diameter, are firm and white owing to the large stromal component. They generally have multiple small cysts and are found in about one-fifth of benign serous tumors.

Serous LMP tumors, including the variant micropapillary LMP tumors, are similar in most respects to their benign

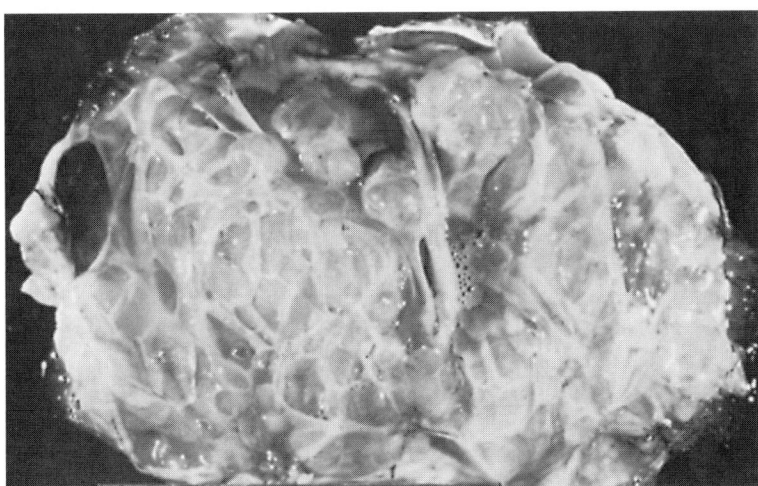
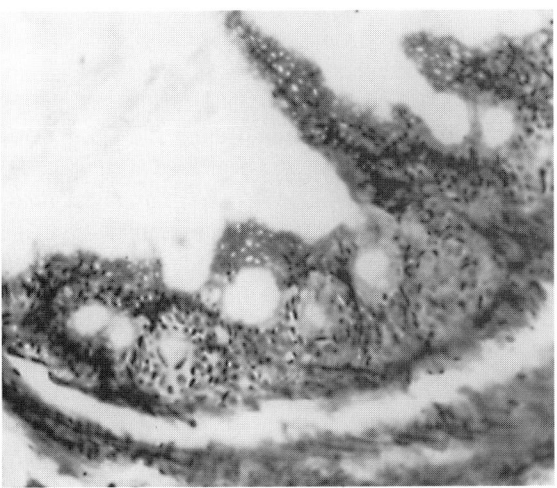

A   B

FIG. 25.7. Mucinous cystadenoma of low malignant potential. **A:** Tumors that are adenomas or "of low malignant potential" are typically multilocular, being composed of hundreds of locules up to several centimeters in diameter and filled with a thick, tenacious fluid. None of the locules is solid. The gross photograph is of a cystadenoma. **B:** Tumors of low malignant potential exhibit epithelial stratification up to several layers thick. The locule may appear as a garland composed of folds simulating a cribriform pattern. (From Robboy SJ, Merino M, Kurman RT. The female reproductive system. In: Rubin E, Gorstein F, eds. *Pathology.* 4th ed. Philadelphia: JB Lippincott, 2004.)

counterparts. The distinction on gross examination is that the papillations are usually pronounced. Polypoid structures resembling grapes 1 to 10 mm in greatest dimension are frequently seen (Fig. 25.5). Their surfaces frequently are covered by relatively fine papillae. Necrosis is absent. Serous LMP tumors often secrete a fluid that has a higher mucin content than benign adenomas. This should not be mistaken on gross examination for a mucinous neoplasm.

Serous adenocarcinomas have the most variegated appearance. They range in size from small (2 to 3 cm) to quite large. The tumors, similar to many other forms of ovarian malignancies of common epithelial origin, are usually relatively solid with areas of hemorrhage and necrosis (Fig. 25.6). Cysts and foci of papillarity are commonly present.

Microscopic Appearance

The epithelium that characterizes serous tumors resembles the lining of the normal fallopian tube. If well differentiated, the cells may display cilia as is seen in the normal tubal epithelium. If less well differentiated, they have only eosinophilic cytoplasm. The nucleus is relatively large. Mucin, if demonstrable, is confined to the apical border of the cell.

Serous adenomas are typically lined by epithelium that is extremely well differentiated. Psammoma bodies are usually few or absent. If present in moderate to large numbers, the diagnosis of serous adenoma of LMP must be strongly entertained. Papillae, if present, are few in number and are composed of loose stromal to fibromatous cores and lined by epithelial cells that are typically flattened to slightly cuboidal serous cells.

Serous LMP tumors are characterized microscopically by bulbous but sometimes fine to coarse papillary fronds, in which atypical, stratified neoplastic cells cover a thick core of fibrovascular stroma. Commonly, a small to moderate proportion of the papillae exhibit clusters of cells that appear as solid cellular buds that, because of tangential sectioning, appear to be detached from the epithelial lining. The degree of nuclear atypia as well as the number of figures is variable. Ciliated cells are common, as are psammoma bodies. The diagnosis of an LMP tumor requires that no area contain frank stromal invasion. The presence of small foci of microinvasive tumor does not alter the patient's otherwise excellent prognosis (98).

"Micropapillary carcinoma" is a variant of an LMP serous tumor that has been newly described and disputed (100–103). This tumor has been described to act in a slightly more aggressive and clinically malignant fashion than the usually indolent and clinically benign, more common, form of LMP tumor even when it has spread throughout the peritoneal cavity. The fibrovascular fronds of the typical LMP serous tumors display a mantle of epithelial cells on the surface that appear focally as a multilayered shell with irregular zones of filiform micropapillarity. In this form, the micropapillarity is diffuse and uniformly covers all of the fibro-

vascular cores. Although the investigators who first described this lesion suggested it should be classified as an adenocarcinoma, subsequent studies have shown that unless associated with invasive implants, it behaves as ordinary boderline tumors, suggesting that it should remain in the category of LMP tumors (125–131) Within the original description of micropapillarity was a second form of abnormality, that is, foci with a cribriform pattern, but most pathologists already interpret this as being an early form of grade 1 invasive cancer.

Destructive invasion in an LMP tumor, if greater than 3 mm, indicates the presence of a serous carcinoma. When papillae invade into the stroma, the stromal margins may appear to be retracted and display relatively pointed contours in relief. Solid clusters of cells may exhibit a cribriform pattern (intraglandular bridging) indicative of autonomous growth and, hence, adenocarcinoma. Usually, invasion is accompanied by a fibrous stromal reaction called desmoplasia.

During recent years, patients with LMP tumors of the ovary have been carefully staged and peritoneal biopsies obtained both at primary surgery and at second-look laparotomies. This has led to a better understanding of the types of serous lesions that can arise *de novo* in the peritoneum. The peritoneum, like the ovarian surface epithelium, is of mesothelial origin and, therefore, subject to the same disease processes. The implication of this hypothesis is that tumors arising in the peritoneum may be multicentric and independent of ovarian tumors, as they represent a "secondary müllerian system"(111).

In reality, LMP tumors that are found in the peritoneum, including the broad ligament (112), are similar to those arising in the ovary and the question of primary or metastatic (or implants) must be discerned. Like the borderline lesion arising in the ovary, the features characterizing the serous LMP tumor primary in the peritoneum are papillary processes, small clusters of cells, cell stratification, detached cellular clusters, nuclear atypia, and mitotic activity. Many LMP tumors in the peritoneum associated with a serous ovarian tumor of LMP malignancy are most likely metastases to the peritoneum (113).

In evaluating peritoneal biopsies, tumors must be distinguished from reactive peritoneal hyperplasia and benign epithelial inclusions. Reactive mesothelial proliferations commonly simulate serous differentiation. A particularly difficult differential diagnosis about which there is still considerable debate is the lesion in which only a few glands are found in the peritoneal biopsy, the epithelium is extremely well differentiated, and psammoma bodies are conspicuous. Some proponents consider these as being benign serous growths that are reactive and nonneoplastic, whereas others have shown that many may be LMP tumors (114). The term *endosalpingiosis* or *atypical endosalpingiosis* is often used to describe this lesion, but this name is probably inappropriate since the roots of the words themselves refer to a lesion that is benign, "-osis," and arising from epithelium related to the fallopian tube, "-salping-." If the neoplasms present in the peritoneal cavity are to be considered as LMP or malignant serous neoplasms, then the reactive forms should also probably be considered as serous, and given a name such as "serous metaplasia" or "serous adenoma" so as to achieve continuity of nomenclature.

Late recurrences (16 years mean duration) have been reported in some patients with stage IA or IB LMP serous tumors and, of these, about two-thirds have succumbed to the disease (115). These patients initially had "endosalpingiosis" found in the peritoneum, suggesting that what was considered to be endosalpingiosis might initially have been implanted tumor from ovarian LMP tumors (113,114).

Müllerian inclusion cysts are another finding to be considered when dealing with LMP serous tumors. These occur in the form of individual round to oval glands with an obvious lumen and are frequently found in both the omentum and lymph nodes. A peripheral basement membrane is present and cilia may be prominent. The epithelium is usually only one cell layer thick, and stratification, if present, is minimal. The nuclei are basally situated, mitotic activity is absent, and there is no nuclear atypia. Their resemblance to fallopian tube epithelium has led to the use of the terms *endosalpingiosis* if the lesion is in the peritoneal cavity and *müllerian inclusion cyst* if in a lymph node. These names should probably also be changed to "serous inclusion cyst" to reflect the nature of the tissue present. Although most reports have labeled these as benign, inclusion cysts may, in fact, be metastases even though their presence seems to have no impact on prognosis (114). Many cases are associated with LMP serous tumors of the ovary.

In addition to the above lesions, LMP serous tumors of the ovary can give rise to forms of more obvious metastases/implants to the peritoneum. They are (a) noninvasive with or without reactive desmoplasia or (b) invasive. The definition of noninvasive "implants" is controversial (94), as is the relation of this entity to long-term prognosis (115). Tumors with noninvasive implants progress slowly, if at all, and are associated with very low death rates. Noninvasive implants are superficially located on peritoneal structures and lack irregular infiltrative margins. The epithelium of noninvasive implants exhibits clusters of slightly atypical serous cells often admixed with variable numbers of psammoma bodies. They often have papillae filling smoothly contoured cystic invaginations lying on the peritoneal surface or between folds in the omentum.

The presence of desmoplasia, per se, is not considered to be a sign of invasive malignancy. A desmoplastic response to tumor, if present in the form of sharply circumscribed plaques, may represent implants that have plastered onto the peritoneal surface or even extended into septa between the lobules of omentum (116). The implants are not considered to be invasive until they are solid or invade irregularly as jagged, disordered nests of tumor cells. In some cases, this distinction can be very difficult if not impossible. The distinction is important, however, as the prognosis with invasive implants is significantly worse.

Some LMP tumors of the ovary may show signs of invasion, but only in the peritoneal implants (94). Although classified as "LMP" because of the microscopic findings in the ovarian primary (116), tumors with "invasive implants" are reported to act in a clinically aggressive manner and have been associated with a worse prognosis. Microscopically, invasive implants disclose an irregular, aggressive-appearing infiltration into the underlying tissue. The tumor glands show extensive intraglandular bridging or irregularly shaped solid nests of cells resembling tumors of low-grade serous adenocarcinoma. Severe cytologic atypia is present in most cases.

Of clinical significance is that invasive peritoneal lesions, although still called "LMP" by some, may be aggressive. We prefer to refer to these lesions as adenocarcinoma arising in an LMP tumor. In addition to invasiveness, three other features of implants regarded as LMP are associated with adverse outcomes. They include severe cytologic atypia, increased mitotic activity, and residual tumor in the peritoneum postoperatively.

Serous adenocarcinomas usually display obvious invasion. The tumor may appear as large sheets of cells growing autonomously without stromal support or as broad to fine clusters of cells related to papillae that irregularly dissect through the stroma.

Serous tumors are usually graded to reflect both architectural and cytoplasmic features of differentiation. Tumors of progressively higher grade generally have prognoses that are correspondingly worse. Grades 1 to 3 refer, respectively, to tumors that are histologically well differentiated, moderately differentiated, and poorly differentiated. Grade 1 tumors have fine, well-developed papillae nearly throughout. Grade 2 tumors disclose areas where sheets of tissue may form and disclose greater cellular atypicality and mitoses. Grade 3 tumors exhibit large sheets of undifferentiated cells. The mitotic rate and number of atypical mitoses increase progressively in the various grades (89).

High correlation has been observed between the stage and tumor grade (117). Nearly 90% of tumors that extend to the pelvic peritoneum, omentum, or beyond (stages IIB to IV) are grades 2 and 3. In contrast, 72% of tumors confined to the ovaries or the surfaces of the reproductive organs (stages I to IIA) are grade 1. Both stage and grade correlate highly with prognosis. Using extended forms of histopathologic grading based on multiple easily quantified microscopic parameters, several scoring indices have been developed that more precisely group patients, which have prognostic implications for lymph node metastases, recurrence, and survival (118–121) Better interobserver agreement also has been reported (120).

A positive correlation has also been reported between the presence of psammoma bodies and differentiation of tumor.

Psammoma bodies are common, and even sometimes extensive, in grade 1 tumors (58%), rarer in grade 2 tumors (12%), and uncommon in grade 3 tumors (5%). For reasons that are unclear, their presence also carries a significantly better prognosis for survival; patients with extensive psammoma bodies and high-stage tumors (stages II to IV) have 5-year survival rates that are approximately 20% higher than patients without this finding.

The serous psammocarcinoma is a rare variant of serous adenocarcinoma that is characterized by massive psammoma body formation. It is categorized as a carcinoma since it often displays destructive invasion or vascular invasion on microscopic examination; in half the cases, the extraovarian tumor also invades in peritoneal sites. Despite these features, the cytologic attributes are more in keeping with a low-grade neoplasm.

Similar to LMP tumors, a serous adenocarcinoma can arise as a primary tumor from the peritoneum. Its histologic features and biologic behavior resemble its ovarian counterparts (122). Ultrastructural features in the peritoneal tumor resemble some features of mesothelioma, suggesting that the serous carcinomas may arise from mesothelial cells modified by various müllerian influences. Serous tumors arising on the surface of the ovary, but not involving the ovarian parenchyma per se, are similar in most respects to tumors that arise in the ovary. They share identical microscopic features. Serous tumors arising on the surface, however, are nearly always more widespread at the time of diagnosis and, hence, have a more guarded prognosis.

MUCINOUS TUMORS

Mucinous tumors account for one-third (36%) of all common epithelial tumors. The great majority are benign (81%). About one-sixth are LMP, and only 5% are malignant. The mean age for patients with mucinous adenocarcinoma is 52 years, which, like serous adenocarcinoma, is substantially greater than the mean age of patients with benign and LMP tumors (44 and 49 years, respectively).

Patients with mucinous adenocarcinoma of the cervix sometimes develop an independent mucinous adenocarcinoma of the ovary. The coexistence of these two tumors is reported in particular with the Peutz-Jeghers syndrome. Pseudomyxoma peritonei is a rare condition characterized by copious mucin and clusters of well-differentiated mucinous cells that are scattered throughout the abdominal cavity. Although once believed to arise from LMP mucinous tumors of the ovary, current evidence indicates, in most cases, that the tumor arises in the appendix and is metastatic to the ovary (123). Finally, stromal luteinization in mucinous tumors can give rise to signs of virilism, or occasionally, hyperestrinism.

Gross Appearance

Mucinous tumors can grow to extremely large sizes, being among the largest of any recorded tumor in the body. Sizes exceeding 40 kg and 30 cm in greatest diameter are not uncommon. Tumors that are benign are rarely bilateral (2%), and those that are LMP are only slightly more commonly bilateral (6%). Malignant tumors, especially those of higher stage, are commonly bilateral (46%). Whether benign, LMP, or sometimes frankly malignant, the tumors are usually multilocular, with cyst size varying from area to area, but rarely exceeding 3 cm. A thick, tenacious fluid often fills the cysts.

Mucinous tumors, not uncommonly, have one or several regions that differ significantly from the rest of the specimen. It is of critical import that solid areas and areas with hemorrhage or necrosis be examined with exacting care. Firm areas among otherwise typical mucinous cysts are often cancerous. Anaplastic carcinoma, sarcoma, sarcoma-like proliferations, and benign mesenchymal growths are rare types of tumor that may appear as a solid nodule from one to many centimeters in size in the wall of mucinous tumors (124). When examining a mucinous tumor, all cysts should be opened since an occasional one will disclose hair, indicating the presence of and origin in a teratoma. Solid areas may disclose tissues such as carcinoid, also indicating that the neoplasm is a teratoma, but with a mucinous overgrowth. Finally, some conditions, such as pseudomyxoma peritonei, may occasionally be found with what appears grossly and microscopically to be an LMP mucinous tumor, but is cytokeratin 7 negative and cytokeratin 20 positive, indicative that the cancer is, in fact, metastatic, usually from the appendix (123,125,126). Finally, some occult tumors of the appendix and pancreas may metastasize to the ovary and resemble primary LMP mucinous tumors, for which reason routine immunohistochemical studies are recommended on all such mucinous tumors. The finding of positive reaction for cytokeratin 20 and a lack of reaction for cytokeratin 7 needs to be strongly evaluated for the possibility that the tumor originated outside the ovary (127). The distinction between primary and metastatic tumor to the ovary is discussed in more detail in another paper (128).

Microscopic Appearance

Mucinous cystadenomas are lined by cells that generally resemble the typical mucinous cell lining the normal endocervix. Only occasionally do they resemble the cells lining the normal colon. The mucinous cell has a foamy pale texture and amphophilic color.

Mucinous tumors of LMP disclose a wide spectrum of atypia. Like benign tumors, mucinous LMP tumors fall into two microscopic types: endocervical and intestinal, with the latter showing one or more cell types. Unlike benign tumors, the intestinal type of mucinous epithelium is found in five of six LMP tumors (90,129,130). Nearly half of the cases exhibit argyrophilic cells and sometimes even Paneth cells. The lining cells are usually one to three cell layers thick, the nuclear atypia is mild to moderate, and mitotic figures may be few, but sometimes are numerous (Fig. 25.7). To be classified as an LMP tumor, the epithelium lining the papillae should generally not exceed three cell layers in thickness and lack the following: a marked overgrowth of atypical cells; solid, cellular masses devoid of connective tissue support; severely anaplastic nuclear features; and destructive stromal invasion.

Mucinous adenocarcinomas are usually diagnosed by traditional morphologic criteria. The tumors present as sheets of cells, often in a cribriform pattern, or as tumor cells dissecting into the stroma. As mucinous tumors become less well differentiated, the cells often lose their intracytoplasmic mucinous component, and, therefore, may be difficult, if not impossible, to distinguish from serous and, especially, endometrioid carcinomas. If squamous differentiation or endometriosis is present, the tumor is more likely to be endometrioid. The overall better rates of survival of patients with mucinous compared to endometrioid and serous adenocarcinomas reflect that relatively few poorly differentiated tumors of advanced stage can be recognized as mucinous; those so identified have 5-year survival rates near 0%. Stromal invasion (greater than microinvasion), high nuclear grade, and capsular rupture are adverse prognostic features in stage I tumors (131).

Not all mucinous adenocarcinomas exhibit a cribriform pattern. A form described three decades ago appears to be microscopically like mucinous LMP tumors, but is four or more cell layers thick. Recent studies with long-term follow-up indicate that, in the absence of stromal invasion, such tumors are all clinically benign (131,132).

Unlike serous and endometrioid tumors, the cytologic characteristics of well-differentiated mucinous cancers may resemble those of benign or LMP tumors, and thus the distinction sometimes lies in the architectural pattern or the presence of invasion. Thus, the most difficult differential diagnosis of mucinous adenocarcinoma is LMP mucinous tumor. Studies with image analysis indicate that adverse morphologic features include (a) large-volume percentage of epithelium; (b) larger nuclei, especially those with an enlarged short axis; and (c) numerous mitoses.

ENDOMETRIOID TUMORS

Endometrioid tumors account for a relatively small proportion (8%) of the common epithelial tumors. Most endometrioid tumors are malignant. Up to a fifth of these tumors are of LMP. The mean age of patients with cancer is 57 years, which is substantially higher than that associated with benign and LMP tumors (40 and 48 years, respectively). Approximately 10% of cases, with reports of up to 40% (133), are associated with endometriosis, implying that, in at least some cases, this tumor arises as neoplastic transformation of the endometriosis (134). Over 10% of endometrioid tumors of the ovary are also associated with endometrial tumors of an identical histologic variant, each appearing as if it were primary in its respective organ (135). The similar

histology and subtype and high survival rate of these patients (80% at 10 years) suggest that the majority, if not most, are synchronous primaries rather than metastases (136). Many of these patients have coexisting endometriosis in addition (136,137).

Gross Appearance

Benign endometrioid tumors are rare and cannot be diagnosed as endometrioid on gross examination. They generally arise on an adenofibromatous background in which the firm, yellow-white stroma contains multiple cysts filled with clear or sometimes dark brown or chocolate-colored fluid. Endometrioid tumors generally resemble serous tumors in most respects.

LMP tumors range in size from small to large. They average 10 cm in diameter and are predominantly solid (93). Necrosis is rare. The cysts vary from small to about 9 cm in size and are filled with fluid that may be serous, mucinous, or hemorrhagic. Criteria for distinguishing these from adenocarcinoma are not well defined as this is a rare entity.

Endometrioid adenocarcinomas, like serous carcinomas, vary in size with an average of 10 cm. The tumors are often fleshy in character. Wide zones of necrosis are common, especially if the tumor is large or poorly differentiated. Endometrioid tumors are more cystic than serous tumors and surface papillations are relatively infrequent.

Microscopic Appearance

Adenoma

Benign endometrioid tumors are classified as such only when the predominant cell type resembles the lining of the endometrium as it occurs in the normal state, polyps, hyperplasia, or cancer. Endometriosis can be suspected if the tumor exhibits endometrial stroma or evidence of recurrent hemorrhage. Endometrioid adenofibromas may show squamous metaplasia.

LMP Endometrioid Tumors

Two variants of LMP tumors are recognized: the more common, which arises in adenofibromas, and the less common, which arises as a papilla. About 15% of the patients have associated endometriosis. Epithelial stratification above 5 mm helps separate benign and proliferative adenofibromas from LMP tumors (93).

An occasional LMP tumor may show microscopic foci of invasion. The few recorded cases have behaved in a clinically benign fashion, suggesting that, as with serous tumors, tiny microscopic foci of invasive mucinous tumor should have little influence on later clinical behavior.

Endometrioid adenocarcinomas resemble adenocarcino-

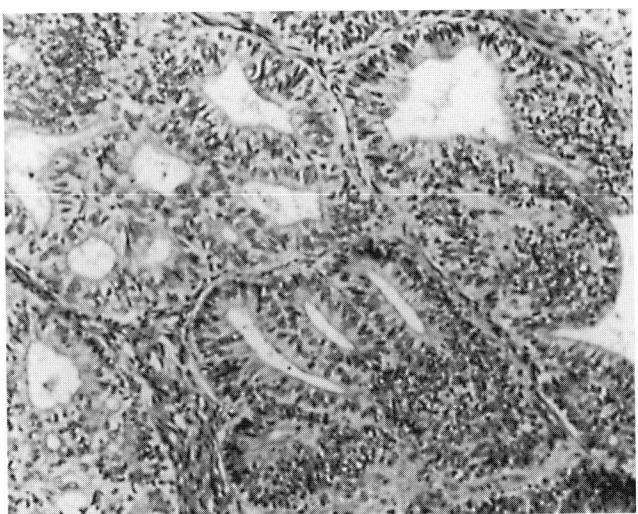

FIG. 25.8. Endometrioid adenocarcinoma. The tumor microscopically resembles adenocarcinoma of the endometrium. The glands are ovoid to circular and display greater regularity than serous carcinoma. Papillations, if present, tend to be blunter than the more jagged, sharply pointed papillations of serous adenocarcinoma (H&E ×135).

mas of the endometrium (Fig. 25.8). Like endometrial tumors, they can vary from well-differentiated (grade 1) to poorly differentiated (grade 3) and may show focal to extensive areas of well-differentiated squamous cells (endometrioid adenocarcinoma with squamous metaplasia, also known as adenoacanthoma) to poorly differentiated squamous cells (also known as adenosquamous carcinoma). Its lower frequency of occurrence than serous carcinoma reflects to a large degree that poorly differentiated endometrioid tumors cannot be distinguished with ease from poorly differentiated serous tumors, and thus such cases tend to be recorded as being serous. Endometrioid tumors are, therefore, proportionally more common if well differentiated, which may also account for the overall better prognosis of endometrioid compared to serous tumors. When controlled for stage, the survival rate for endometrioid tumors is similar to that of serous adenocarcinoma in some studies (138) but better in others (139).

Occasionally, the tumor may show extensive subnuclear vacuolization (so-called secretory pattern) or extensive ciliation (ciliated-cell adenocarcinoma) (140), which is a sign of a high degree of differentiation. Another unusual pattern is oxyphilic cell differentiation (141). Tumors with numerous small cavities may simulate the Call-Exner bodies of granulosa-cell tumors. However, an endometrioid tumor forms glands where a distinct rim of apical cytoplasm lines the lumen. In contrast, the cavities in granulosa-cell tumor are most likely degenerative, and the surface of the inner lining exhibits haphazardly arranged, irregular nuclei. The center of a classic Call-Exner body may also contain periodic acid–Schiff (PAS)–positive eosinophilic material. Numer-

ous tubules in a tumor sometimes resemble those of colonic cancers metastatic to the ovary. They may also resemble the seminiferous tubules found in Sertoli-Leydig tumors (142). Immunohistochemical approaches have been proven to be useful to separate the epithelial from sex-cord stromal tumors, with the former being cytokeratin 7 and BER-EP4 reactive and cytokeratin 20 and inhibin unreactive (143,144).

The category of "endometrioid tumor," regardless of which organ of the female genital tract is considered, encompasses a subclass of tumors that contains a stromal component. Endometrioid stromal sarcomas are tumors in which the neoplasm is composed exclusively of malignant endometrial-type stroma. The müllerian adenosarcoma displays a malignant stromal component and an epithelial component that is benign, but neoplastic nonetheless. As expected, spontaneous tumor rupture, high grade, or the presence of a high-grade sarcomatous component is associated with a poor prognosis (145). The carcinosarcoma, which has a poor prognosis when greater than stage I (146), is composed of stroma and epithelium where both are malignant. This latter category now encompasses the malignant mesodermal mixed tumor, which is a carcinosarcoma with heterologous elements, such as fat, cartilage, bone, and skeletal muscle (147). The gross and microscopic features of these tumors resemble closely similar tumors in the endometrium.

Most synchronous tumors of the ovary and endometrium are of the same histologic type. Endometrioid tumor with squamous metaplasia (adenoacanthoma) is the most common pattern.

Clear-Cell Tumors

Clear-cell tumors are uncommon (3% of all common epithelial tumors). The few that are benign or of LMP are adenofibromas. The mean age for patients with clear-cell adenocarcinoma is 53 years (148), which is similar to the other categories of cancers of common epithelial origin. About half of cases are associated with endometriosis (149).

Gross Appearance

Clear-cell tumors resemble endometrioid tumors on gross examination and cannot be distinguished with any reliability from serous tumors. Sometimes clear-cell tumors, when arising within an endometriotic cyst, may appear as a pedunculated polyp. Clear-cell adenocarcinoma is bilateral in under one-sixth of cases (13%) and, as such, has the lowest frequency of bilaterality of any of the more common forms of epithelial tumors (serous, mucinous, endometrioid, and clear-cell).

Microscopic Appearance

Clear-Cell LMP Tumors. The ability to distinguish the rare clear-cell LMP tumor from the frankly malignant tumor is often difficult since the latter, especially when small, may appear to be deceptively benign (87). A tumor is considered to be malignant when (a) the glands and islands of epithelial cells manifest high-grade cytologic characteristics of malignancy; and (b) invasion is present as evidenced by a desmoplastic or myxoid response of the stroma to the cells or a haphazard extension of cells into the stroma.

Clear-cell adenocarcinoma of the ovary is morphologically similar to the clear-cell adenocarcinoma that occurs sporadically in the endometrium of older women and in the vagina and cervix of young women who were exposed prenatally to diethylstilbestrol (DES) (Fig. 25.9) (150). Clear and ''hobnail'' cells are its hallmark. The clear appearance of the cytoplasm results from glycogen that has leached as the tissue specimen is prepared for microscopic examination. The hobnail cells are bulbous nuclei that protrude into the lumen well beyond the apparent cytoplasmic limits of the cell. The clear cells usually appear as sheets of cells that have the appearance of a solid growth, but may also line tubules. The hobnail cells, and sometimes flat cells, are encountered more commonly in the pattern of growth showing tubules and cysts.

The clear-cell adenocarcinoma may show any of several uncommon patterns. Oxyphilic clear-cell adenocarcinoma refers to a pattern in which the cytoplasm is abundantly eosinophilic, a variant often mistaken for a steroid cell tumor. The clear-cell tumor may also resemble the endodermal sinus tumor. Historically, the two tumors were considered as being the same until it was recognized that clear-cell tumors are müllerian in origin and endodermal sinus tumors

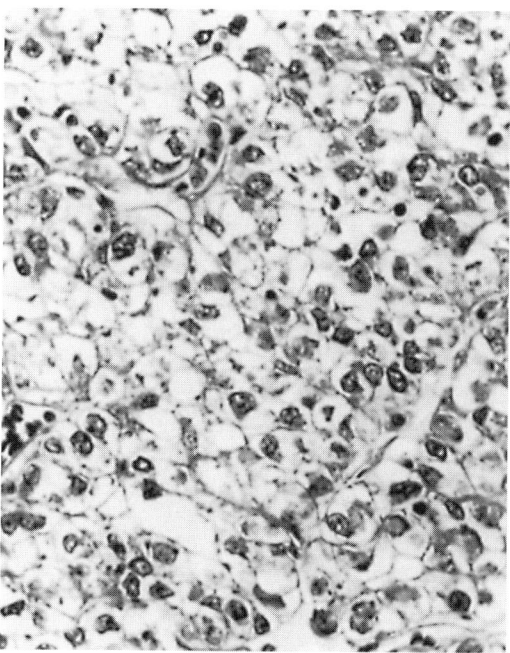

FIG. 25.9. Clear-cell adenocarcinoma. The sheets of tumor cells have clear cytoplasm (H&E ×350).

are of germ-cell origin. Dysgerminoma may also resemble a clear-cell adenocarcinoma, but has characteristic fibrous trabeculae that are permeated with lymphocytes. Finally, what may appear to be clear-cell adenocarcinoma of the the ovary may be clear-cell carcinoma metastatic from the kidney (151).

Uncertainty exists whether ovarian clear-cell adenocarcinoma is more aggressive than the other common epithelial malignancies (152). In some studies specifically addressing correlates of survival, advancing stage, and increased mitotic rate (>six mitoses/10 HPF or high MIB1 activity) were adverse prognostic indicators (153,154). Other investigators (155) emphasize young age, stage, or vascular invasion as being poor prognostic factors and the presence of a predominantly (>75%) papillary or tubulocystic morphology as a favorable prognostic factor. Overall, the 5-year survival for stage I tumors is 60% and 12% for all other stages. Many of the differences found in analyses appear to reflect the relative compositions of stage and grade and whether the more poorly differentiated tumors are correctly categorized by their true cell type.

Transitional-Cell Tumors

Brenner's Tumor

Brenner's tumor, a tumor of urothelial differentiation, is the rarest (2%) of the common epithelial tumors. It is believed to arise from the pelvic mesothelium through transitional-cell metaplasia, much in the same manner as Walthard's rests arise. Most of these tumors are small, benign, and discovered incidentally. Few benign tumors are large enough to cause symptoms (Fig. 25.10). Rarely are these LMP tumors or frankly malignant. Malignant tumors are of two types. Malignant Brenner's tumor, which is exceedingly rare, consists of a poorly differentiated transitional-cell–type epithelium in which definitive foci of benign Brenner's tumor are present. The transitional-cell carcinoma, which in some cases may be a malignant Brenner's tumor in which foci of benign Brenner's tumor cannot be found, is an entity that has been separated from the categories of malignant Brenner's tumor and undifferentiated carcinoma. This was done because of the opinion, now questionable(156), that the transitional-cell carcinoma is more amenable to combination chemotherapy than other common epithelial tumors that have spread beyond the ovary. There is also the opinion that the two are different as the Brenner's tumor has an immunophenotype-like urothelium, whereas the transitional-cell tumor more closely resembles poorly differentiated serous adenocarcinoma (157).

Gross Appearance. Benign Brenner's tumors are typically small, solid, and well circumscribed. The one-third that exceed 5 cm in diameter present like any other large ovarian tumor, for example, with nonspecific signs of a space-occupying mass. Some reach 15 kg and 30 cm in greatest dimension. Many Brenner's tumors are detected as small

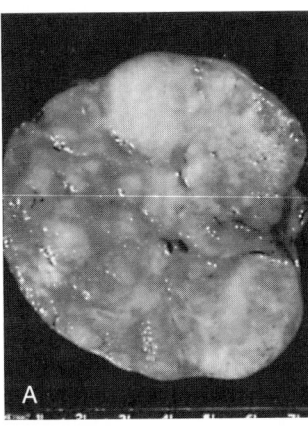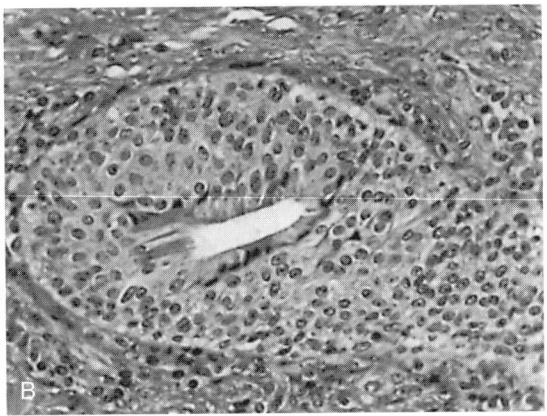

FIG. 25.10. Brenner's tumor. **A:** The tumor, which is solid, is characterized grossly by its extreme hardness and lack of necrosis and hemorrhage. The parenchyma is mottled brown to white. **B:** Embedded within the dense fibrous tissue are nests of transitional epithelium resembling transitional epithelium of the urinary tract. The most superficial layer of cells frequently exhibits mucinous differentiation (H&E ×315). (From Robboy SJ, Merino M, Kurman RT. The female reproductive system. In: Rubin E, Gorstein F, eds. *Pathology.* 4th ed. Philadelphia: JB Lippincott, 2004.)

nodules in the walls of mucinous tumors regardless of whether the mucinous tumor is of germ-cell origin or of common epithelial origin. About 7% are bilateral. Borderline Brenner's tumors usually occur as large cysts. Malignant Brenner's tumors tend to be substantially more solid, but sometimes contain cysts.

Microscopic Appearance. Brenner's tumors, unlike other common epithelial tumors, have two components. One is epithelial cords, which are composed of ovoid to polyhedral cells with large, longitudinally grooved nuclei (coffee bean shaped). The cellular arrangement often resembles a transitional-cell epithelium (urothelium-like) with a superficialmost layer of cells displaying copious, mucin-rich cytoplasm. The second component is a dense, fibrous stroma in which are found the nests of transitional cells. The stroma is typically prominent and at times so massive as to nearly obscure the epithelial component. Minute foci of stromal calcification are found in over half the tumors.

In contrast to benign Brenner's tumor, which usually presents no difficulty in diagnosis, the distinction between LMP and malignant Brenner's tumor may be difficult. LMP Brenner's tumors exhibit papillae lined by a proliferating transitional epithelium typical of that found in bladder tumors. Occasionally, the apicalmost layer of cells has mucin-rich cytoplasm. Malignant Brenner's tumors have transitional epithelium that may be high grade or focally resemble squamous-cell carcinoma. Both LMP and malignant Brenner's tumors have foci of a clearly identifiable benign Brenner's component. Studies of DNA content have shown that benign and nonaggressive lesions are diploid, whereas clinically aggressive lesions are aneuploid.

Transitional-Cell Carcinoma

Transitional-cell carcinoma is a second form of ovarian cancer with urothelial differentiation. Unlike malignant Brenner's tumor, which by definition arises from demonstrable preexisting benign or proliferative Brenner's tumor, the transitional-cell carcinoma lacks such a demonstrable component.

The transitional-cell carcinoma is considered to be a separate variant of ovarian cancer based on both clinical and histologic grounds. Patients with transitional-cell carcinoma present with tumors in higher stages than do patients with malignant Brenner's tumors. Transitional-cell carcinoma is also more aggressive, as many more women with low-stage tumors develop recurrences. Tumors progress much less often in patients with malignant Brenner's tumors (26%) even if the tumor is cytologically atypical and demonstrates stromal invasion. Distinguishing the transitional-cell carcinoma from other epithelial tumors, especially serous carcinoma, is important. Transitional-cell carcinoma, even at high stage, is reported to respond well to chemotherapy, although this has now been contested, whereas undifferentiated carcinomas and poorly differentiated serous carcinomas do not.

In addition to clinical differences, there are differences in microscopic and immunohistochemical findings. Distinct areas of stromal calcification are present in a majority of both benign and malignant Brenner's tumors but absent in transitional-cell carcinoma of the ovary. Transitional-cell tumors of the ovary, although appearing as urothelial-like, show immunoreactivity differences from true urothelium. The tumor of ovarian origin is immunoreactive with cytokeratin 7, whereas the bladder tumors show no such reactivity (158). In our experience, tumors that are typical transitional-cell carcinoma in the ovary usually have metastases indistinguishable from serous adenocarcinoma.

Squamous-Cell Carcinoma

Squamous-cell carcinoma is the newest category of surface epithelial-stromal tumors recognized by the WHO classification scheme for ovarian tumors. As for most epithelial tumors, the average age at diagnosis is 56 years, and most of the tumors are stage II or III. The stage of the tumor and its grade correlate best with overall survival (159). This category is exceedingly rare.

Mixed Carcinoma

Approximately 3% of all ovarian tumors of common epithelial origin are mixed—when more than 10% of the neoplasm exhibits a second cell type. Mixtures of histologically benign types or of LMP have no adverse effects on prognosis beyond that on each component alone (160). One common specific malignant combination is mixed clear-cell and endometrioid carcinoma, both being related to endometriosis. Serous and endometroid carcinomas are also commonly encountered. Occasionally, these patterns can be difficult to distinguish from metastases (161).

Undifferentiated Carcinoma

Undifferentiated carcinoma refers to epithelial tumors that are so poorly differentiated as to preclude further classification into any of the types described above. Tumors may be considered to be undifferentiated even in the presence of small foci of glands or pools of mucin since these findings, if present in small quantities, are not specific for any single tumor type.

Small-cell carcinoma is a subgroup of undifferentiated tumor. This tumor, which is of at least two types, the hypercalcemic and pulmonary types, is enigmatic in both its histogenesis and classification (162). The hypercalcemic tumor typically occurs in young women (mean age 24 years) (163). Two-thirds have systemic hypercalcemia, which is commonly reversed after the tumor has been excised (164). This variety of small-cell carcinoma is virtually always unilateral, but has spread beyond the ovary in half of patients by the time of diagnosis. Diffuse sheets of small, closely packed cells punctuated by variable numbers of follicle-like spaces characterize its histology. The individual cells have scant cytoplasm and a single nucleus. Mitotic activity is typically brisk. Although the DNA content is nearly always diploid, over 60% of patients with stage IA tumor die of the disease or have recurrences. Features in stage IA tumors associated with a more favorable outcome are age <30 years, normal preoperative serum calcium, and small tumor size. A large-cell variant of the small-cell type has also been described (165).

The second form of small-cell carcinoma resembles small-cell ("oat-cell") carcinoma of the lung (166). The tumor occurs in older women (mean 59 years), and half of the tumors are bilateral. Neuron-specific enolase and synaptophysin (typically reported as being more sensitive than chromogranin) reactivity is common, whereas chromogranin reactivity is occasionally found. The majority of tumors are aneuploid. The mean survival to death is 8 months.

A third and rare form of undifferentiated carcinoma is the neuroendocrine tumor of the non–small-cell type (167). Microscopically, the neuroendocrine component immunoreactive for chromogranin is in sheets, usually as closely packed islands, cords, or trabeculae of epithelial cells with little intervening stroma. The prognosis is poor (168,169).

NATURAL HISTORY AND PATTERNS OF SPREAD

Epithelial ovarian cancers are thought to arise from embryologic derivatives of the ovarian surface epithelium. For the early part of their natural history, most remain confined as cystic growths within epithelial inclusion cysts in the substance of the ovary itself. Over time, the tumor penetrates through the surface of the ovarian capsule, allowing malignant cells to exfoliate into the peritoneal cavity. There the cells follow the normal circulation of peritoneal fluid up the right paracolic gutter and to the undersurface of the right hemidiaphragm, where they may implant and grow as surface nodules. The omentum is also a frequent site of involvement, and, indeed, all intraperitoneal surfaces are at risk. Such exfoliation and implantation are one of two primary modes of spread of ovarian cancer. The other is via the retroperitoneal lymphatics that drain the ovary. These follow the ovarian blood supply in the infundibulopelvic ligament to terminate in lymph nodes lying along the aorta and vena cava up to the level of the renal vessels. Lymph channels also pass laterally through the broad ligament and parametrial channels to terminate in the pelvic sidewall lymphatics, including the external iliac, obturator, and hypogastric chains (170). Spread may also occur along the course of the round ligament, resulting in involvement of the inguinal lymphatics. Lymph node metastases are correlated with the stage of disease, and retroperitoneal node involvement has been found in the majority of advanced ovarian cancer cases (171, 172).

The initial spread of ovarian cancer, by both the intraperitoneal and lymphatic routes, is clinically occult. A significant proportion of women with ovarian cancer that grossly appears to be confined to one or both ovaries have widespread disease. The extent of their disease can be detected only by histologic examination of visually normal tissues sampled during careful surgical staging (173,174). It has been estimated that approximately 10% of patients with apparently localized ovarian cancer that appears to be confined to the ovaries will have metastases to the aortic nodes (174). Many patients with apparently localized disease will also have occult disease in peritoneal washings or in biopsies of the diaphragm and omentum (Table 25.4).

TABLE 25.4. *Subclinical metastases in apparent early ovarian cancer*

Site	No. of patients with involvement	Total patients	% involved
Diaphragm	17	223	7.6
Omentum	21	294	7.1
Cytology	13	69	18.8
Peritoneal	6	61	9.8
Pelvic nodes	18	202	8.9
Aortic nodes	35	285	12.3

Modified with permission from Moore DH. Primary surgical management of early epithelial ovarian carcinoma. In: Rubin SC, Sutton GP, eds. *Ovarian cancer.* New York: McGraw-Hill, 1993.

DIAGNOSIS AND CLINICAL EVALUATION

Approximately 75% to 85% of patients with epithelial ovarian cancer are diagnosed at the time when their disease has spread throughout the peritoneal cavity. The most common presenting symptom is that of abdominal discomfort or pain, followed closely by abdominal distention due to the presence of malignant ascites or large intraabdominal masses. Gastrointestinal symptoms are also relatively frequent, and the symptoms of nausea, dyspepsia, early satiety, constipation, and/or obstipation are common but, unfortunately, nonspecific. Occasionally, patients will experience urinary frequency or dysuria and/or vaginal bleeding. This latter symptom, due to ovarian cancer, occurs more frequently in premenopausal patients.

The diagnosis of early-stage ovarian cancer (when the tumor is still confined to the pelvis) usually occurs by palpation of an asymptomatic adnexal mass during a routine pelvic examination. However, the vast majority of palpable adnexal masses are not malignant and, in premenopausal women, ovarian cancer represents less than 5% of adnexal neoplasms. In these women, the ovarian enlargement is usually due to either follicular or corpus luteum cysts. The vast majority of these functional cysts will regress in one to three menstrual cycles and, consequently, the initial approach to management for a palpable adnexal mass less than 8 cm in size in a premenopausal woman is to repeat the pelvic examination and imaging studies in 1 to 2 months.

In contrast, an adnexal mass in a premenarchal or postmenopausal woman, particularly when complex, has a higher likelihood of being a malignant tumor, and surgical exploration is usually indicated.

Abdominal ultrasonography is frequently used to aid in the evaluation of adnexal pelvic masses. Features that are more frequently associated with malignancy include irregular borders, multiple echogenic patterns due to the presence of solid elements with prominent papillary projections, dense multiple irregular septa, and bilateral tumors. Ultrasonography is also useful to demonstrate the presence of ascites, as well as involvement of adjacent organs. Other radiographic techniques, including computed tomography (CT) scans and magnetic resonance imaging (MRI), are not routinely necessary for preoperative evaluation of ovarian cancer but may provide useful information. The CT scan may provide additional evidence of the exact size of liver and pulmonary nodules, as well as abdominal and pelvic masses, which can be used to monitor the response of therapy. Lymphangiography has an accuracy of approximately 90% in detecting paraaortic lymph node involvement. Owing to poor patient acceptance and the high degree of expertise required of the radiologists interpreting the studies, lymphangiograms are not routinely performed, and CT scans are currently used to evaluate paraaortic and pelvic adenopathy.

Positron emission tomography (PET) utilizes a differential in metabolic activity between benign and malignant cells using the radiopharmaceutical 2-[^{18}F]fluoro-2-deoxy-D-glucose (^{18}FDG). PET imaging has not yet been shown to be useful in the differential diagnosis of ovarian cancer, but some studies suggest that PET/CT imaging may have a role in detecting residual or recurrent disease (175).

The use of other radiographic studies is dependent upon the results of the initial physical examination and the presence of patient symptoms. Brain scans and bone scans are unnecessary unless suggested by the patient's symptoms; metastases to these sites are extremely uncommon, particularly at the time of diagnosis. Barium studies of the gastrointestinal tract are not routinely indicated in premenopausal women unless there is occult blood in the rectum or symptoms to suggest intestinal obstruction. In postmenopausal women, in whom there is a higher likelihood that colorectal carcinoma is producing symptoms similar to those which can be observed with ovarian cancer, barium enema and proctoscopy may be useful in the differential diagnosis. Because of the association of ovarian cancer with breast cancer and because metastatic breast cancer can produce intraabdominal carcinomatosis as well, mammography is often performed to exclude the presence of primary breast cancer. A Papanicolaou (Pap) smear should be obtained, although ovarian cancer cells are unlikely to exfoliate through the uterus to the cervix, and their presence is associated with advanced stage.

The preoperative evaluation of patients with suspected ovarian carcinoma should include a a determination of the serum CA-125 level. CA-125 has proven to be the most useful, currently available marker for epithelial ovarian cancer, primarily because of its utility in monitoring the results of therapy (176). CA-125 determinants are glycoproteins, with molecular weights from 220 to >1,000 kD (177). OC-125 is a murine monoclonal antibody that recognizes the antigenic determinants of CA-125. A double-determinant immunoradiometric assay has been developed against these CA-125 determinants. It has been demonstrated that <1% of normal nonpregnant women have serum CA-125 levels >35 U/mL. In contrast, 80% to 85% of patients with epithelial ovarian cancer have elevated serum levels (178). The serous histologic subset of epithelial ovarian cancer has the highest incidence of elevated CA-125 levels (>85%), whereas mucinous tumors are associated with a low incidence of abnormally elevated serum CA-125 levels.

In postmenopausal women with asymptomatic pelvic masses, an elevated serum CA-125 (>65 U/mL) had a sensitivity of 97% and a specificity of 78% for ovarian cancer (179). In contrast, in premenopausal women, there is a higher prevalence of nonmalignant conditions that can produce elevated serum CA-125 levels (e.g., pregnancy, endometriosis, uterine fibroids, and pelvic inflammatory disease). In postmenopausal women with an adnexal mass, an elevated CA-125 level indicates the need for prompt surgical exploration, whereas in premenopausal women, additional noninvasive studies as described above are indicated.

SCREENING

No reliable procedures are currently available for the early detection of ovarian cancer (5). Available potential screening techniques have included pelvic examination (ovarian palpation), ultrasound examinations, CA-125 and other tumor markers, and combined modality approaches. Criteria have been established for a useful screening test(s) (180). Besides being accurate, a screening test should be inexpensive, safe, simple, and tolerable. Successful screening should result in a decrease in site-specific morbidity and mortality from a disease. The usefulness of a test can be assessed by measures of sensitivity, specificity, and positive predictive value. The sensitivity refers to the probability of a positive test when the disease is present, whereas the specificity represents the probability that the test will be negative in the absence of the disease and is a measure of the false-positive rate. The positive predictive value represents the number of diagnostic procedures (i.e., laparotomies) performed in women who do not have the disease for each woman who has ovarian cancer. Mathematically: sensitivity = true positives/(true positives false negatives); specificity = true negatives/(true negatives false positives); positive predictive value = true positives/ (true positives false positives).

What constitutes an acceptable positive predictive value for ovarian cancer has not been agreed upon, although some investigators feel that 10% is the minimum level (181). The positive predictive value varies with the incidence of the disease and, consequently, will be markedly affected by the population screened (Fig. 25.11). Assuming 100% sensitivity, a test will have to have a specificity of 99.6% and 90.0% for screening all women over 45 years in age and

BRCA1 mutant gene carriers, respectively, to achieve an arbitrary 10% positive predictive value.

Pelvic Examinations

The detection of an asymptomatic pelvic mass on routine physical examination may identify an ovarian carcinoma before abdominal dissemination, but there are no data on the frequency with which ovarian cancer is detected in asymptomatic women on the basis of an annual pelvic examination. Furthermore, there is no evidence that ovarian cancer detected in asymptomatic women on the basis of an abnormal pelvic examination alters morbidity or mortality. Thus, although frequent pelvic examination continues to be a common recommendation for women past the age of 40 years, its benefit as a screening procedure for ovarian cancer has not been established.

Ultrasonography

Transabdominal ultrasonography is a screening procedure that is easy to perform, has a good patient acceptability, and is essentially free of complications. However, ultrasonography is not sufficiently specific for use as a routine screening procedure. In a prospective study of 5,479 self-referred asymptomatic women undergoing annual transabdominal ultrasonography at King's College Hospital in London (182), five patients with primary ovarian cancer (three with LMP tumors) were identified from a total of 15,977 scans, of which 338 (2.3%) were initially abnormal. Of note, 326 laparotomies were performed to diagnose these five cases. An additional four patients were found to have metastatic ovarian cancer. Although the apparent detection rate was 100%, the false-positive rate was 2.3%, and the specificity was 97.7%. The odds that an abnormal transabdominal ultrasound indicated the presence of primary ovarian cancer were 1 in 67.

Transvaginal sonography has been proposed as a more specific alternative to abdominal sonography as a screening test (183–185) because of increased resolution capable of detecting minimal morphologic changes in the ovary. Transvaginal ultrasonography also does not require any patient preparation. At the University of Kentucky, 3,220 asymptomatic postmenopausal women were so screened (184,185). Surgery was performed in 44 women with ovarian abnormalities, with the following findings: two stage I ovarian cancers (one granulosa-cell and one epithelial carcinoma); one stage IIIB ovarian cancer; and 41 benign pathologies, including 21 serous cystadenomas. Thus, the sensitivity was 100%, specificity 98.7%, and positive predictive value 6.7% (i.e., 15 laparotomies were needed to find one ovarian cancer). These investigators have proposed that removal of cystadenomas may also decrease the risk of ovarian cancer since, based upon their histologic review, they feel that such tumors may be precursors of invasive epithelial cancers.

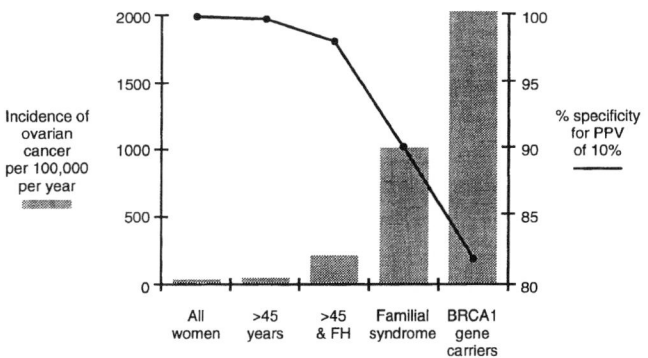

FIG. 25.11. The incidence of ovarian cancer in various population groups with different risks for ovarian cancer and the specificity required of screening tests to achieve a positive predictive value of 10%. (Reprinted from Jacobs I. Genetic, biochemical, and multimodal approaches to screening for ovarian cancer. *Gynecol Oncol* 1994;55:S22–S27. Copyright 2004, with permission from Elsevier.)

Transvaginal ultrasonography has been combined with Doppler flow studies (186,187) in an effort further to improve the accuracy of sonography and reduce the unacceptably high rate of false-positive results that currently have been reported with ultrasonography alone. Such a procedure detects intraovarian vascular changes, which principally are neovascularization and changes in impedance of blood flow that may help discriminate benign from malignant tumors. Initial results have demonstrated that morphologically normal ovaries show no neovascularization. Similarly, benign masses lacked neovascularization and had a pulsatility index markedly different from invasive ovarian cancers (even early-stage disease), which had clear evidence of neovascularization and marked differences in pulsatility index. Unfortunately, a recent study (187) reported that Doppler technology did not improve diagnostic accuracy when the transvaginal sonogram assessed both tumor volume and wall structure [morphology index (MI)]. Four hundred forty-two ovarian tumors were assigned a score of 0 to 10 based on increasing volume and morphologic complexity. Doppler flow studies were performed on 371 of these tumors. Only one malignancy was found in 315 tumors with an MI less than 5, whereas there were 52 malignancies in 127 tumors with an MI ≥5. The positive predictive value was 0.409. The addition of Doppler flow indices to MI did not improve the accuracy of predicting malignancy.

CA-125 Levels

The finding that approximately one-half of women with stage I and stage II ovarian cancer have serum CA-125 levels >65 U/mL has suggested that serum CA-125 levels are sufficiently sensitive to identify patients with early-stage disease (176). In a group of 915 Roman Catholic nuns, when the upper limit of normal for CA-125 was raised to 65 U/mL, only 0.5% of women past the age of 50 years had elevated tests (188). As previously noted, false-positive test results have been reported in a number of nonmalignant gynecologic conditions, such as peritonitis, pancreatitis, renal failure, and alcoholic hepatitis. Owing to the high false-positive rate relative to the low incidence of epithelial ovarian cancer, a single CA-125 assay is not useful in detecting early-stage disease. In a large study from Sweden, serum CA-125 levels were measured annually in 5,550 women over the age of 40 years (189). In women who had CA-125 levels >30 U/mL, surveillance was undertaken with sequential CA-125 levels every 3 months, and pelvic examinations and transabdominal ultrasounds were performed every 6 months. If the CA-125 doubled or was >95 U/mL at the time of screening, or if an adnexal mass was detected by either ultrasound or pelvic examination, the patients underwent a laparotomy. One hundred seventy-five women were found to have elevated CA-125 levels, and six ovarian cancers were detected clinically or sonographically (two stage IA, two stage IIB, and two stage III). Three women with normal CA-125 levels

developed ovarian cancer. For women less than 50 years old, a CA-125 value >35 U/mL had a specificity of 97% compared to 99% for women more than 50 years of age. Specificity was increased to 99.8% for both groups if the serum CA-125 level was set at 95 U/mL.

Multimodal Screening

The NCI-sponsored Prostate, Lung, Colorectal and Ovarian (PLCO) Cancer Screening Trial enrolled over 74,000 women from 1993 through 2000 at ten screening sites throughout the United States (190). Women were randomly assigned to either the intervention arm, which included baseline measurements of CA-125 levels and transvaginal ultrasonography followed by annual CA-125 readings for 5 years and TVUs for 3 years, or an observation arm. Participants will be followed for a minimum of 13 years. Initial results are expected in 2004 or 2005.

It is hoped that sequential measurements of CA-125 levels over a period of time can lead to substantial improvement of screening programs (191). The risk of ovarian cancer algorithm (ROCA) calculates the risk of ovarian cancer for an individual comparing each individual serial CA-125 level to the pattern in known cases of ovarian cancer and controls. The result is presented as the individual's estimated risk of having ovarian cancer during the year following the test. Currently, ROCA is being evaluated in a large United Kingdom screening trial as well as in a small pilot study of 2,400 high-risk women in the United States.

A large English study examined the sequential continuation of serum CA-125 and ultrasonography in screening 22,000 volunteers without a family history of ovarian cancer (192). If the serum CA-125 level ≥30 U/mL in the initial determination, women underwent abdominal ultrasonography followed by a laparotomy for an ovarian abnormality. Forty-one women had a positive screen, and 11 had ovarian cancer: two stage IA, one stage IB, one stage IIA, and seven stage III or IV. Eight of the 21,959 women who had a negative screen developed ovarian cancer. In this study, the positive predictive value was 26.8% for ovarian cancer of all stages but decreased to 9.8% for early-stage (III) disease. The specificity was 99.9%, with a sensitivity of 78.6% at 1 year and 57.9% at 2 years.

Based on these results, the same group of investigators performed a pilot randomized trial of screening in 22,000 postmenopausal women aged 45 years or older (193). Women randomized to screening underwent three annual screens that involved measurement of serum CA-125 levels, pelvic ultrasonography if the CA-125 was elevated, and referral to a gynecologist if there was an increased ovarian volume on sonography. In the screened group, there were 468 women with elevated CA-125 levels, 29 were referred for a gynecologic opinion, and cancer was detected in 6 of these women with 23 false-positive screening results. The positive predictive value was 21%. During the 7-year follow-up of this study, an additional 10 women were identified with ovarian cancer in the screened group and 20 in the control group. The median survival for women with cancer in the screened group was 73 months and in the control group was 42 months (p = .0112). However, the number of deaths from cancer did not significantly differ between the two groups. These results demonstrate that a multimodality approach to screening is feasible. Based on these results, a large-scale screening trial has begun, termed the United Kingdom Collaborative Trial of Ovarian Cancer Screening (UKCTOCS) (27). This is a randomized trial with a control group undergoing no screening, a multimodal group undergoing annual screening with serum CA-125 as the primary test and ultrasound as a secondary test, and an ultrasound-only group undergoing annual screening with an ultrasound as the primary test and repeat ultrasound in 6 to 8 weeks as a secondary test. An estimated 200,000 women are expected to enroll up until 2010, and ovarian cancer mortality will be assessed 7 years later.

These preliminary studies using serum CA-125 levels, pelvic examinations, and ultrasonography have demonstrated that ovarian cancer can be detected in asymptomatic women. However, these procedures are associated with a significant false-positive rate such that an unacceptably large number of negative laparotomies would result if each "positive" screening test resulted in surgical exploration aimed at diagnosing early ovarian cancer. Since a surgical procedure is required to diagnose ovarian cancer, there is a defined morbidity and mortality associated with screening. When the positive predicted value is below 10%, more harm (complications of unnecessary laparotomy) than good (diagnosing early-stage ovarian cancer) may come to a screened population. Furthermore, in a recent review of uncontrolled trials of ovarian cancer screening (194) in 36,208 women, 29 cases of ovarian cancer were identified, but only 12 (41%) were stage I. Survival is unlikely to be significantly affected by an earlier diagnosis of advanced-stage disease. Until the completion of the large randomized trials described above, the recommendations of the NIH Consensus Conference against routine screening of the general population remain in effect (5).

Even in women with a positive family history of ovarian cancer, there is no evidence that screening can affect mortality from this disease. In 1,502 asymptomatic women who were screened by transvaginal ultrasonography and who had at least one close relative with ovarian cancer, seven ovarian cancers (three of LMP) were found (195). In high-risk women who have two first-degree relatives with ovarian cancer or who are carriers of the *BRCA1* or *BRCA2* gene, the ability of screening tests to detect earlier-stage ovarian cancer has also not been established. Yet, it seems prudent to couple pelvic and ultrasound examinations with serum CA-125 determinations on a regular basis and also to consider a prophylactic oophorectomy after completion of childbearing.

Genomic and Proteomic Screening

While large-scale prospective randomized trials of currently available screening technologies, such as serum CA-125 levels and TVU, are in progress, additional studies are exploring potential novel markers identified using genomic and proteomic technologies. Following the identification of OC-125 as an antigen for screening, other ovarian cancer–associated antigens were identifed and corresponding antibody assays evaluated in pilot screening programs. NB/70K, OVX-1, and levels of macrophage colony-stimulating factor (M-CSF) were evaluated individually and, in some cases, as panels (196–198). Whereas initial studies reported encouraging sensitivity, specificity was not substantially improved. Similarly, lysophosphatidic acid (LPA) was reported in preliminary studies to be a predictive biomarker for ovarian cancer (199), but it has not been proven to be superior to CA-125 either singly or in combination.

Genomic, transcriptional profiling, and proteomic technologies are being used to identify novel cancer-specific screening markers (200). These markers may complement those found previously by antibody-based or candidate gene approaches. Mok et al. (201) used transcriptional profiling of ovarian cancer cell lines to identify potential candidate markers, including prostasin. At least 14 other candidate tumor markers have also been found through transcriptional profiling or other technologies, including serial analysis of gene expression, subtractive hybridization, and differential display (200). These novel markers may be used alone or in combination with other markers, such as mesothelin and NES-1, which were identified by monoclonal antibody and candidate gene approaches (27,200).

It has been suggested that early in the course of cancer development, low molecular serum proteins may be altered that reflect the pathologic changes occurring in the organs. Petricoin et al. (202) reported on a bioinformatics tool to identify proteomic patterns in serum with a potential for distinguishing neoplastic from nonneoplastic disease within the ovary. Proteomic spectra were generated by mass spectroscopy (surface-enhanced laser desorption and ionization). Spectra derived from serum from 50 unaffected women and 50 patients with ovarian cancer were analyzed by an iterative searching algorithm that identified a proteomic pattern capable of discriminating cancer from noncancer. This pattern correctly identified 50 ovarian cancer cases in a masked set, including all 18 stage I cases. Of the 66 cases of nonmalignancies, 63 were recognized as benign. Preliminary results yielded a sensitivity of 100% and a specificity of 95%. The specificity of 95% will still lead to too many false-positive laparotomies if applied to the general population (203). The technology is currently being refined in order to increase the specificity.

SURGICAL STAGING

Our understanding of the early natural history and patterns of spread of epithelial ovarian cancer forms the basis for a rational system for staging the disease and for the surgical management of apparent early ovarian cancer. The widely used FIGO staging system, revised in 1985, is presented in Table 25.5 (204).

The stage, defined as the extent of disease at the time of diagnosis, can be determined only following exploratory

TABLE 25.5. *Carcinoma of the ovary: FIGO nomenclature (Rio de Janeiro, 1998)*

Stage I	Growth limited to the ovaries.
IA	Growth limited to one ovary; no ascites present containing malignant cells. No tumor on the external surface; capsule intact.
IB	Growth limited to both ovaries; no ascites present containing malignant cells. No tumor on the external surfaces; capsules intact.
IC[a]	Tumor either stage IA or IB, but with tumor on surface of one or both ovaries, or with capsule rupture, or with ascites present containing malignant cells, or with positive peritoneal washings.
Stage II	Growth involving one or both ovaries with pelvic extension.
IA	Extension and/or metastases to the uterus and/or tubes.
IIB	Extension to other pelvic tissues.
IIC[a]	Tumor either Stage IIA or IIB, but with tumor on surface of one or both ovaries; or with capsule(s) rupture; or with ascites present containing malignant cells or with positive peritoneal washings.
Stage III	Tumor involving one or both ovaries with histologically confirmed peritoneal implants outside the pelvis and/or positive retroperitoneal or inguinal nodes. Superficial liver metastases equals stage III. Tumor is limited to the true pelvis, but with histologically proven malignant extension to small bowel or omentum.
IIIA	Tumor grossly limited to the true pelvis, with negative nodes, but with histologically confirmed microscopic seeding of abdominal peritoneal surfaces, or histologically proven extension to small bowel or mesentery.
IIIB	Tumor of one or both ovaries with histologically confirmed implants, peritoneal metastasis of abdominal peritoneal surfaces, not exceeding 2 cm in diameter; nodes are negative.
IIIC	Peritoneal metastasis beyond the pelvis >2 cm in diameter and/or positive retroperitoneal or inguinal nodes.
Stage IV	Growth involving one or both ovaries with distant metastases. If pleural effusion is present, there must be positive cytology to allot a case to stage IV. Parenchymal liver metastasis equals stage IV.

[a] In order to evaluate the impact on prognosis of the different criteria for allotting cases to stage IC or IIC, it would be of value to know if rupture of the capsule was spontaneous or caused by the surgeon, and if the source of malignant cells detected was peritoneal washings or ascites.

laparotomy and thorough evaluation of all areas at risk. Operations on women with a pelvic or adnexal mass that may represent ovarian cancer should be carried out through a vertical abdominal incision to allow access to the upper abdomen, which is difficult to visualize through a low transverse incision. On entering the abdomen, aspiration of ascites or peritoneal lavage should be performed to obtain specimens for cytologic examination. Separate specimens should be submitted from the pelvis, right and left paracolic gutters, and the undersurfaces of the right and left hemidiaphragms. An encapsulated adnexal mass should be removed intact, if possible, since rupture and spillage of malignant cells within the peritoneal cavity will increase the patient's stage and may adversely affect her prognosis. Adhesions should be noted and marked since they may represent occult areas of microscopic disease. If frozen section indicates the presence of ovarian cancer, a complete abdominal exploration should be carried out, including evaluation of all intestinal surfaces. Any suspicious areas should be biopsied. Omentectomy and random peritoneal biopsies should be performed. Aortic lymph node sampling (Fig. 25.12) should also be performed. Several reports (171,172,205) have demonstrated that the pelvic lymph nodes are involved by ovarian cancer at the same frequency as are paraaortic nodes and suggest the need for routine pelvic node sampling as well. The technique for surgical staging of apparent early ovarian cancer is summarized in Table 25.6.

Standardized protocols are used to record the specific details of operative and pathologic findings that have prognostic and therapeutic bearing on treatment and natural history (206). When a rigorous staging laparotomy is performed, a substantial number of patients initially felt to have localized disease will be upstaged. Young et al. (207) reported on ovarian cancer patients believed to have stage I or II disease following initial surgery who underwent repeat staging procedures. Almost a third (31%) of these women were upstaged following the second procedure (Table 25.7), and 77% of the upstaged patients actually had stage III disease. Before referral, only 25% of patients had an initial surgical incision that was adequate for proper staging. Similarly, McGowan et al. (208) examined the completeness of surgical staging in 291 women with ovarian cancer and concluded that 46% had been inadequately evaluated. When staging was performed by gynecologic oncologists, 97% of patients were properly staged as compared to 52% and 35% of cases operated on by obstetricians/gynecologists and general surgeons, respectively. These observations underscore the critical importance of having an experienced physician involved in the surgical staging of all patients with ovarian cancer.

The importance of meticulous staging cannot be overemphasized, since postoperative therapy is based upon anatomic stage, as well as other factors, discussed in the section on therapy below. In the past, inadequate surgery often led to understaging and subsequent inadequate postoperative therapy in a significant proportion of ovarian cancer patients.

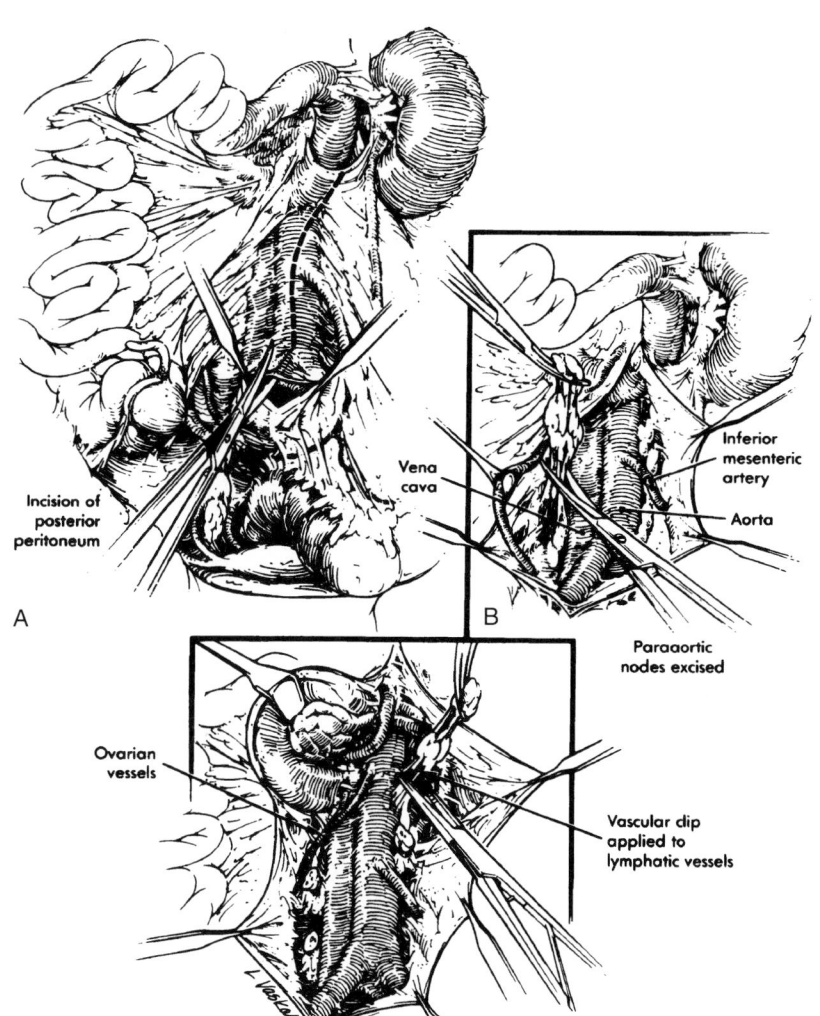

Incision of
posterior
peritoneum

Vena
cava

A

B

Inferior
mesenteric
artery

Aorta

Paraaortic
nodes excised

Ovarian
vessels

Vascular clip
applied to
lymphatic vessels

C

FIG. 25.12. Paraaortic node dissection for staging of apparent early ovarian cancer. The posterior parietal peritoneum overlying the aorta is incised **(A)**, and the nodal tissue stripped from the vena cava **(B)** and the aorta **(C)** to the level of the left renal hilus. (Reprinted from Rubin SC, Benjamin I. Surgery for ovarian cancer. In: Nicols DH, Clarke-Pearson DL, eds. *Gynecologic and obstetric surgery.* 2nd ed. St. Louis: Mosby, 2000. Copyright 2004, with permission from Elsevier.)

For example, patients were frequently treated with pelvic irradiation at a time when they already had distant, undetected metastases outside the radiation ports. A report from the NCI's SEER database indicated that only about 10% of American women with apparent early-stage ovarian cancer received appropriate surgical staging and recommended postoperative therapy (209).

Although ovarian cancer is surgically staged primarily on the basis of the anatomic sites of disease documented at laparotomy, stage IV disease may be documented by cytologically positive pleural fluid or fine-needle aspiration of supraclavicular adenopathy. The majority of patients will have advanced-stage disease (FIGO stages III to IV) after careful staging. The stage distribution of over 8,000 patients

TABLE 25.6. *Surgical staging of apparent early ovarian cancer*

Vertical incision
Multiple cytologic washings
Intact tumor removal
Complete abdominal exploration
Removal of remaining ovaries, uterus, tubes[a]
Omentectomy
Lymph node sampling
Random peritoneal biopsies, including diaphragm

[a] May be preserved in selected patients.

TABLE 25.7. *Results of repeat staging in apparent stages I and II ovarian cancer*

Initial stage	No. of patients	% upstaged
IA	37	16
IB	10	30
IC	2	0
IIA	4	100
IIB	38	39
IIC	9	33
Total	100	31

Reprinted with permission from Young RC, Decker DG, Wharton JT, et al. Staging laparotomy in early ovarian cancer. *JAMA* 1983;250:3072–3076.

TABLE 25.8. *Distribution by stage of ovarian cancer patients*

Stage	No. of patients	%
I	2,549	23
II	1,409	13
III	5,170	47
IV	1,784	16
Total	10,912	100

Reprinted from Pettersson F. International Federation of Gynecology and Obstetrics Report. Stockholm: FIGO, 1991:248.

depicted in Table 25.8 may still overestimate the percentage of patients with early-stage disease since not all patients in this series underwent a comprehensive laparotomy (210).

PROGNOSTIC FACTORS

Surgery accurately stages a patient and allows the evaluation of a series of clinicopathologic variables that are often used to select postoperative therapy. These prognostic factors are discussed below.

Tumor Stage

The 5-year survival of patients with epithelial ovarian cancer is directly correlated with the tumor stage. However, there have been major differences in survival reported for patients with the same FIGO stage, reflecting the inadequacy of early staging procedures that led to the frequent understaging of patients. Whereas early studies reported 5-year survivals for patients with stage I disease of approximately 60% to 80%, current studies utilizing a comprehensive staging laparotomy demonstrate that some subsets of patients with stage I disease have a 90% 5-year survival (209). Similarly, initial studies of patients with stage II disease reported the range of 5-year survivals from 0% to 40%. However, stage II disease frequently is upstaged to stage III disease, particularly when patients present with large-volume disease in the pelvis. The small number of patients who are found to have stage II disease following completion of a comprehensive laparotomy have a 5-year survival rate of approximately 80%. Patients with stage III disease have 5-year survival of approximately 15% to 20%, whereas patients with stage IV disease have less than a 5% 5-year survival (210).

Volume of Residual Disease

The volume of residual disease following cytoreductive surgery is directly correlated with survival (211–221) (Table 25.9). Patients who have been optimally cytoreduced have a 22-month improvement in median survival compared to those patients undergoing less than optimum resection. In these retrospective analyses of the importance of residual

TABLE 25.9. *Effect of the amount of residual tumor following primary cytoreduction on survival of patients with advanced ovarian cancer treated with chemotherapy*

Study (ref.)	Year	Survival (months)	
		Optimal[a]	Suboptimal[a]
Hacker et al. (211)	1983	18	6
Vogl et al. (212)	1983	40+	16
Delgado et al. (213)'	1984	45	16
Pohl et al. (214)	1984	45	16
Conte et al. (215)	1985	25+	14
Posada et al. (216)	1985	30+	18
Louie et al. (218)	1986	24	15
Redman et al. (219)	1986	37	26
Neijt et al. (220)	1987	40	21
Hainsworth et al. (221)	1988	72	13
Piver et al. (222)	1988	48	21
Sutton et al. (217)	1989	45	23
Mean		39	17

[a] Original investigator's definition.

volume upon survival, the size of the largest residual mass, and not the total number of lesions, has been believed to be the primary factor correlating with prognosis. Yet, the number of residual masses may be an important prognostic factor as well (222,223). Patients who have only a single residual mass following cytoreductive surgery have a significantly greater chance of achieving a surgically confirmed complete remission compared with those patients with multiple small nodules even though each nodule is less than 2 cm in size. Prospective confirmation of the importance of debulking surgery in the survival of patients with advanced disease, however, is lacking. It has been suggested that patients who present with small-volume disease that is optimally cytoreduced following hysterectomy with bilateral salpingo-oophorectomy and omentectomy have disease that is biologically less aggressive than do patients who are anatomically cytoreduced to the same amount of residual disease but require a maximal tumor reduction with removal of bulky disease throughout the peritoneal cavity. For example, in a study from Roswell Park Cancer Institute, it was demonstrated that cytoreductive surgery was successful in debulking 87% of patients with stages III and IV disease to less than 2-cm residual tumor masses (224). The percentage of patients in this study who were optimally cytoreduced was markedly higher than the 17% to 40% successful debulking rate reported in many other series (Table 25.9).

However, only 30% of patients in this study achieved a complete remission with chemotherapy even though only 13% of the patients had any residual mass greater than 2 cm after debulking surgery. Furthermore, progression-free survival was only 29% at 3 years. These results suggest that, in addition to the volume of disease, other unknown biologic factors influence survival in patients with advanced disease. A prospective randomized trial to assess the impact of cytoreductive surgery upon survival, however, is difficult to perform. The changes in the FIGO staging system may help retrospectively to answer the question of the importance of the volume of disease at the time of diagnosis upon survival. Stage III disease is now subdivided into three groups, based upon the volume of disease, before any attempt at surgical debulking (Table 25.5). This will permit a comparison of survival for patients who have small-volume disease prior to cytoreductive surgery (IIIA and IIIB) with that of patients who present with bulky disease (IIIC) and who are subsequently cytoreduced.

Histologic Subtype and Grade

In general, the histologic type has less prognostic significance than the other clinical factors, such as stage, volume of disease, and histologic grade. In some series, patients with mucinous adenocarcinomas have an overall better survival in comparison to endometrioid or serous adenocarcinomas. These findings reflect the rarity with which high-grade mucinous adenocarcinoma of the ovary is diagnosed. Few poorly differentiated tumors of advanced stage can clearly be identified as mucinous adenocarcinomas; patients with those tumors so identified have a 5-year survival rate near 0%. Endometrioid carcinoma also has been suggested to have a better prognosis than serous adenocarcinoma, as well as presenting with a lower histologic grade and clinical stage. Again, poorly differentiated endometrioid carcinoma cannot be differentiated with ease from poorly differentiated serous tumors and is generally classified as serous. Well-differentiated endometrioid carcinomas are, therefore, proportionally more common, which may account for the overall better prognosis for endometrioid than for serous tumors. Some analyses have suggested that ovarian clear-cell adenocarcinoma may be more aggressive than the other common epithelial malignancies on a stage-for-stage basis (225). In a literature review of nearly 400 cases of clear-cell tumor, the 5-year survival for stage I tumors is 60% and 12% for all other stages. However, similarly analyzed data for these other forms have not shown great differences and, in fact, indicate higher degrees of uniformity when stratified by stage and cell type (210).

The histologic grade of the tumor is a particularly important prognostic factor in patients with early-stage disease. As will be discussed, stage I patients with well- or moderately well-differentiated tumors have a greater than 90% 5-year survival when treated with surgery alone (226). In contrast, patients with stage I disease with poorly differentiated or clear-cell tumors have a significantly worse survival, and postoperative therapy is indicated. In advanced-stage pa-

tients treated with cisplatin-based chemotherapy, most studies have failed to demonstrate a significant correlation between histologic grade and survival (210). This may reflect variable degrees of intraobservational and interobservational variation in grading of ovarian tumors (227,228). In addition, different grading systems have been used at different institutions, leading to interinstitutional variability as well.

Surgical Prognostic Factors

Controversy remains about the prognostic importance of other surgical observations (229–233). Tumor size, bilaterality, and ascites without cytologically positive cells are not considered to be of prognostic significance in patients with early-stage disease. However, tumor spillage, capsular penetration, and cytologically malignant ascites (FIGO stage IC) are generally believed to be associated with a worse prognosis. As will be discussed below in the section on therapy for localized disease, a large multivariate analysis has been performed on clinical and pathologic variables that has identified surgical factors that are associated with an adverse effect on prognosis.

CA-125 Levels

The prognostic significance of preoperative and postoperative CA-125 levels has been established (234,235). Serum levels of CA-125 generally reflect volume of disease. Whereas prechemotherapy CA-125 levels have been shown on univariate analysis to be of prognostic significance, on multivariate analysis, they are usually not an independent prognostic factor owing to their association with volume of disease (235). In addition, high CA-125 levels may predict for unresectability and an inferior survival. Postoperative CA-125 levels appear to have greater prognostic significance. In a multivariate analysis, postoperative CA-125 levels were of independent prognostic significance in patients with or without residual disease (236).

Controversy also remains regarding the prognostic accuracy of the rate of decline of serum CA-125 levels and the absolute levels after one to three cycles of chemotherapy. In one study, a level greater than 100 U/mL after the third cycle of treatment was associated with a median survival of 7 months compared to a 50% 5-year survival for patients with a CA-125 level of 10 U/mL or less (237). In another study, there was a marked difference in prognosis for patients who had a greater than sevenfold decrease in CA-125 levels 1 month after chemotherapy compared to those with a lesser reduction (235). In a multicenter study from England, the predictive value of CA-125 levels after the third cycle of chemotherapy was confirmed (237). However, the false-positive rate for accurately predicting progression was 19%. The investigators in this study concluded that, although CA-125 levels are useful for predicting group outcomes, they do not have the predictive power to guide treatment decisions in individual patients. Consequently, although CA-125 levels are frequently drawn before each course of therapy, if the patient shows clinical improvement, treatment should be continued despite the level of CA-125 (234). If there is no change clinically, and if the CA-125 level markedly increases, changing treatment is a consideration. However, if there is no clinical change but the CA-125 is dropping or is not changing, treatment with the same regimen should continue.

Criteria have been proposed to define response to treatment based on serum CA-125 levels (237–239). Patient response and CA-125 levels in 277 patients were used to develop criteria for a serologic response that was then tested prospectively in 458 patients. Similar correlations between standard and CA-125 response criteria were also observed in patients treated with paclitaxel-based chemotherapy. Two definitions were proposed for CA-125 response: A 50% response occurred if, after two samples, there was a 50% decrease in serum CA-125 levels; a 75% response occurred if there was a serial decrease of serum CA-125 over three samples of greater than 75%. The CA-125 response rate was 66% compared with a GOG-defined response rate of 62%. The investigators suggested that the 50%/75% CA-125 definitions can be accepted as measurements of response and can be used in addition to or in place of standard criteria used by cooperative groups for patients receiving initial chemotherapy. In addition, CA-125 response definitions may be useful for regulatory authorities, such as the Food and Drug Administration (FDA), for the assessment of activity of new agents. The CA-125 response definitions have been studied in over 19 clinical trials with 14 different drugs in Phase II trials. The CA-125 response rate was 18% (CI 1.01–1.3) higher than the clinical response rate, such that if in a clinical trial the response rate using standard criteria was 20%, it would be 23.6% according to CA-125 criteria.

An elevated CA-125 has also been increasingly used as an indicator of progression following completion of chemotherapy. Clinical trials groups have established criteria for progression of disease based on elevations of CA-125 levels or the observance of physical or radiographic evidence of disease. The use of serum CA-125 levels to initiate second-line therapy will be discussed subsequently.

Investigational Prognostic Factors

More quantitative approaches to identify biologic factors associated with clinical prognostic significance are under investigation, which may decrease the subjectivity frequently associated with histologic prognostic factors.

Ploidy Analysis

The role of ploidy analysis for predicting the behavior of epithelial ovarian tumors remains controversial, with conflicting data in many studies (240–244). Although stage and extent of residual tumor after debulking surgery remain the most important clinical prognostic factors, ploidy analysis appears to be an independent prognostic factor and itself may offer additional insights. DNA content is aneuploid more commonly in higher than in lower-stage tumors (stages III to IV are 50% to 80% aneuploid; stages I to II are 10% to 80%) and, according to many studies, correlates with degree of differentiation (grade). Ploidy levels generally do not correlate with histologic type (240).

An important question the study of Gajewski et al. (240) addresses is whether DNA ploidy analysis has prognostic value in early-stage disease and whether this technique might help identify those patients at significantly higher risk of recurrence and who might benefit from adjuvant therapy. At 10 years' follow-up, the survival was 100% for the nine patients with diploid tumors and 58% for those with aneuploidy. Results related to second-look operations are also of interest; 94% of positive operations were aneuploid in contrast to only 47% where the operation was negative (53% diploid). Of even more importance, there were no recurrences (0%) with diploid tumors, but 43% for aneuploid tumors when the second-look operation was negative. Even if the tumors are in advanced stage (stages III to IV), ploidy analysis appears to offer new information about degrees of aggressiveness, with 5-year survival being about 45% for diploid tumors and 20% for aneuploid neoplasms.

Few data are available about the DNA content of serous LMP tumors and, like the carcinomas, many of the data are conflicting. Generally, most stage I and stage III tumors are DNA diploid. Some studies have suggested that DNA aneuploidy is associated with an adverse clinical outcome. Small numbers of mucinous LMP tumors have been examined, with nearly all being DNA diploid. Between two studies with matched controls, one reported a strong relation of DNA aneuploidy with an adverse outcome (241), whereas the other did not (244).

Genetic and Biologic Factors

The genetics of ovarian cancer and associated clinical implications are described in Chapter 5 and summarized earlier in this chapter. As previously noted, genetic alterations are common in epithelial ovarian cancers, and they have led to numerous reports on the prognostic impact of molecular markers. These molecular markers frequently can be categorized as abnormalities in oncogene products (HER-2/neu, p20), suppressor gene products (p53, p16, pRB), and measures of drug sensitivity (PgP, LRP, MRP, GST, BAX) (245, 246). In addition, there have been a series of reports regarding markers of proliferation (DNA index, S-Phase fraction, KI-67 index, proliferating cell nuclear antigen), DNA repair (leukocyte platinum, DNA excision repair, helicase complexes), serum cytokine levels (CSF-1, interleukin-6), and factors associated with tumor invasion and metastases

(NM23). Despite the large number of reports describing putative prognostic factors, they are not currently used in the routine selection of treatment for patients with either early-stage or advanced-stage disease. The prognostic information from many of these reports is limited because of the lack of substantial size and because of the fact that most studies do not compare putative markers with other experimental markers reported in the literature. Finally, many of the reports are contradictory with regard to conclusions regarding prognostic importance, for example, four of seven reports on *p53*, four of eight evaluating HER-2/neu, and three of four reports on EGFR found these molecular markers to be independent prognostic factors (246). However, whereas some reports measured more than one marker, none measured all three molecular markers.

Similarly, factors associated with drug resistance have also not been shown to be routinely useful in the management of patients with advanced ovarian cancer (247,248). Differing mechanisms of resistance to natural products and alkylating agents have been identified in ovarian cancer cell lines. Amplifications and expression of the multidrug resistance gene (*MDR*) and enzymes associated with glutathione metabolism and DNA repair are associated with resistance and natural products (e.g., paclitaxel, doxorubicin, vinblastine) and alkylating agents and platinum compounds, respectively. Increased levels of p-glycoprotein were detected in the minority of ovarian cancer samples from patients treated with doxorubicin. Utilizing more sensitive polymerase chain reaction (PCR) methods, expression of *MDR1* was detected in 65% of specimens from untreated patients (249). However, the expression of *MDR1* has not been shown to be of prognostic value (250). Similarly, although glutathione-S-transferase was found to be abundant by immunostaining in 89% of untreated ovarian cancers, no relationship could be demonstrated with survival and response to chemotherapy. Increased DNA repair is associated with cisplatin resistance, and tumors from clinically resistant ovarian cancer patients have been shown to have higher levels of expression of the DNA repair enzyme ERCC-1 (251). Retrospective studies have suggested that the extent of platinum-DNA adduct formation in DNA from white blood cells is related to the likelihood of response to patients treated with either cisplatin or carboplatin (252). A large prospective study is in progress using specimens obtained from patients entered on a GOG clinical trial of paclitaxel/carboplatin versus paclitaxel/cisplatin.

Genomics

As previously described, the use of genomic translational profiling and proteomic technologies to investigate DNA, RNA, and protein levels in tumors and biologic fluids may identify novel and more effective cancer-specific screening markers than currently available. Furthermore, such technology is also being used to identify genes involved in ovarian carcinogenesis as well as genes associated with response to therapy and prognosis. Ono et al. (253) analyzed gene expression profiles in nine ovarian tumors using a DNA marker consisting of 9,121 genes. In comparison to normal ovarian tissues, they identified 55 genes that were commonly upregulated and 48 genes that were downregulated in the cancer specimens. Hough et al. (254) used serial analysis of gene expression (SAG) to generate global gene expression profiles for various ovarian cell lines and tissues, including primary cancers, ovarian surface epithelial cells, and cells from cystadenomas. These profiles were used to compare overall patterns of gene expression and to identify differentially expressed genes. These investigators identified a number of genes highly differentially expressed between nontransformed ovarian epithelial and ovarian carcinomas. Some of the genes identified were known to be overexpressed in ovarian cancer, but the additional genes represent novel candidates. Ismail et al. (255) used C and DNA representational difference analyses to compare expressed genes in primary cultures of normal human ovarian surface epithelial (HOSE) and ovarian tumor–derived epithelial cells. Their results revealed 44 HOSE-specific and 16 tumor cell–specific genes that exhibited at least 2.5-fold difference in expression.

Suzuki et al. (256) used comparative genomic hybridization (CGH), a genomewide approach, for identification of genome aberrations in ovarian cancer that are associated with clinical endpoints. They demonstrated that loss of chromosome 16q24 and a total number of independent genome copy number aberrations greater than 7 are associated with reduced survival duration. Regions that frequently are abnormal and associated with altered survival duration are consequently strong candidates for high-resolution analysis and gene discovery and may ultimately be useful markers for prediction of clinical outcome. Aberrant DNA methylation is a frequent epigenetic event in ovarian cancer and represents an additional source of potential molecular markers. Wei et al. (257) investigated CpG island hypermethylation across stages III and IV ovarian tumors. Hierarchical clustering revealed two tumor groups with distinctly different methylation profiles. The duration of progression-free survival after chemotherapy was significantly shorter for patients whose tumors contained high levels of concurrent methylation compared to patients whose tumors had lower tumor methylation levels. These data suggest that CpG island methylation is associated with early disease recurrence after chemotherapy. The differential methylation hybridization assay they developed also identified a group of CpG island loci that are potentially useful as epigenetic markers for predicting treatment outcome in ovarian cancer patients. Additional large-scale studies are in progress to correlate the gene expression profiles in patients with advanced ovarian cancer and survival. Such analyses may identify patients with advanced-stage disease in whom standard therapy is likely to be ineffective and who may be candidates for experimental

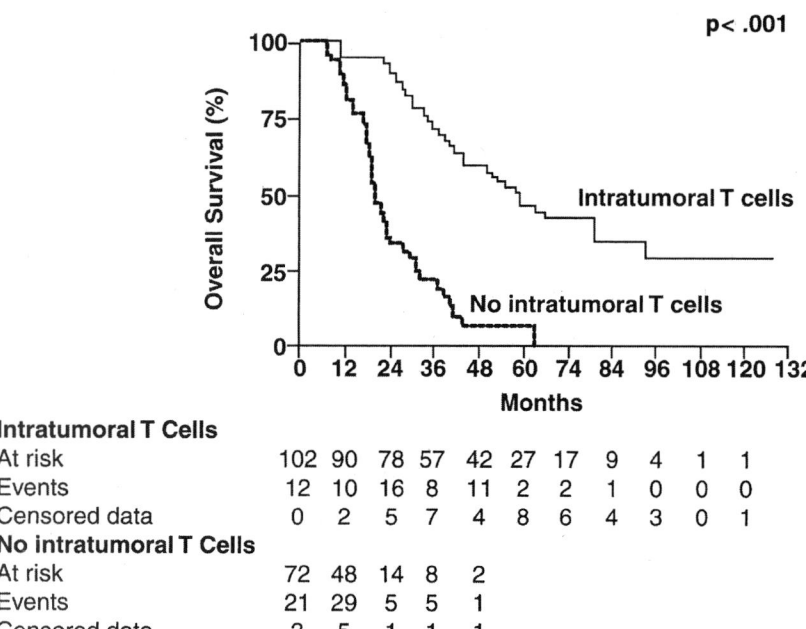

Intratumoral T Cells											
At risk	102	90	78	57	42	27	17	9	4	1	1
Events	12	10	16	8	11	2	2	1	0	0	0
Censored data	0	2	5	7	4	8	6	4	3	0	1
No intratumoral T Cells											
At risk	72	48	14	8	2						
Events	21	29	5	5	1						
Censored data	3	5	1	1	1						

FIG. 25.13. Kaplan-Meier curve for duration of survival according to presence or absence of intratumoral T cells in 173 patients with stage III or IV epithelial ovarian cancer. (Reprinted with permission by Zhang L, Conejo-Garcia JR, Katsaros D, et al. Intratumoral T cells, recurrence, and survival in epithelial ovarian cancer. *N Engl J Med* 2003;348: 203–213. Copyright © 2004 Massachusetts Medical Society. All rights reserved.)

treatments. Differential gene expression profiles will also be essential in the identification of novel molecular targets.

In addition to novel genetic markers, immunologic studies have also identified an association with clinical outcome and the presence of intratumoral T cells (258). CD3$^+$ tumor-infiltrating T cells were detected within tumor-cell islets in 102 of 186 tumors (54.8%). The 5-year survival rate was 38% for patients whose tumors contained T cells compared to 4.5% for patients without tumor-infiltrating T cells (Fig. 25.13).

TREATMENT CONSIDERATIONS

The selection of therapy for patients with epithelial ovarian tumors is based upon anatomic stage and the previously described clinicopathologic features. Therapeutic options may include cytoreductive surgery, chemotherapy, radiation therapy, or a combination of these modalities. However, most patients with advanced ovarian cancer are not cured with these treatments. Clinical trials are evaluating new treatment approaches in virtually all stages of ovarian cancer in an effort to define more effective treatments, and patients should be encouraged to participate in these studies.

Limited-Stage Epithelial Ovarian Cancer

Although only 10% to 15% of all patients with epithelial ovarian cancer after a comprehensive laparotomy are diagnosed with early-stage disease, approximately one-third of all cured patients are derived from stages I and II, highlighting its importance. An in-depth understanding of the management of early-stage disease has been hampered by several

interrelated factors. First, patients with early-stage disease have a much better prognosis than do patients with advanced disease. The relative infrequency of early-stage disease makes Phase III randomized trials (e.g., small numbers of patients and a low event rate) difficult to do.

Second, until recently, the FIGO staging classification for early-stage disease has been descriptive rather than prognostic. It had recognized nine subcategories of stage I. Subclasses A (unilateral), B (bilateral), and C (capsular penetration, tumor spillage, or positive peritoneal cytology) had each been further subdivided, according to differentiation, into three grades. However, the prognostic significance of this categorization has not been established. Two large studies failed to show that bilaterality, rupture, or capsular penetration had any influence on outcome (259). Data on the prognostic significance of positive peritoneal cytology in ovarian cancer are also scarce and inadequate. In an effort to address the limitations of previous retrospective analyses using sample sizes too small for independent prognostic variables to be detectable with sufficient power, a large retrospective study using an international database was used to identify the most important prognostic variables in patients with stage I disease (260). Over 1,500 patients with invasive epithelial ovarian cancer, FIGO stage I, were included in data extracted for univariate and multivariate analysis of disease-free survival in relation to various clinical and pathologic variables. This multivariate analysis identified degree of differentiation as the most powerful prognostic indicator of disease-free survival: moderately versus well differentiated (hazard ratio 3.13: 95% CI 1.68 to 5.85); poorly versus well differentiated (8.89: 95% CI 4.96 to 5.49); followed by rupture before surgery (2.65: 95% CI 1.53 to 4.56); rupture during surgery (1.65: 95% CI 1.07 to 2.51); FIGO stage IB versus IA (1.70: 95% CI 1.01 to 2.85); and age per year (1.02: 95% CI 1.0 to 1.03). None of the following was of prognostic value when the effects of these additional factors were accounted for: histologic type, dense adhesions, extracapsular growth, ascites, FIGO stage (1988), and site of the tumor. It should be pointed out that ascites was not an independent prognostic indicator. However, ascites was defined as in the FIGO 1973 classification (i.e., ascites in the opinion of the surgeon was pathologic or clearly exceeded normal amounts, or malignant cells were detected on peritoneal cytology). The FIGO1988 classification required information on the cytology of the peritoneal fluid. The new classification did not seem to be superior in this retrospective analysis to the 1973 FIGO classification. In this retrospective study, new prognostic factors, such as tumor-suppressor genes, oncogenes, molecular markers of angiogenesis, metastases, morphometric variables, proliferation markers, serum CA-125 concentrations, and DNA ploidy were not examined. Nevertheless, this study clearly demonstrated that the degree of differentiation is the most important independent prognostic factor and should be used in clinical decison making and in the FIGO classification of stage I ovarian cancer. Furthermore, cyst rupture before or during surgery decreases the disease-free survival independently and should be avoided whenever possible.

Third, most early studies of limited-stage patients in the past have not utilized comprehensive staging laparotomy, as outlined in the previous section. Consequently, survival data from studies performed before 1980 are difficult to compare to recent trials because now many patients with apparent early-stage disease have been upstaged on the basis of a meticulous staging laparotomy.

Furthermore, although the recent literature has emphasized the importance of thorough intraoperative exploration (staging) in patients with disease apparently localized to the ovaries, scant recognition has been made of the semantic difficulty presented by the concept of "extension to other pelvic (equals stage II disease) or abdominal (equals stage III disease) organs." No problem exists when the surgeon encounters discrete implants separate from the primary tumor or when solid tumor is found growing into adjacent structures. However, more often, apparently benign adherence of a cyst to adjacent structures, in the absence of metastatic implants or obvious direct tumor extension, is found. There is a considerable body of evidence suggesting that such "benign" adherence, when it is dense, is associated with a relapse risk equivalent to stage II, and that these patients should be considered not as having stage I but rather stage II disease (259). Adherence is considered to be dense when so described by the surgeon, when sharp dissection was required to mobilize the tumor, when a raw area was left in the place of adherence, or when cyst rupture resulted from dissecting the adhesions free. It is a common practice to advance the stage of nonmetastatic but densely adherent tumors to stage II, and this was done in the recent multicenter stages I and II study (261). However, as noted, the recent large retrospective international study failed to identify dense adhesions as an independent prognostic factor (260), and adhesions are not used by the GOG to "upgrade" apparent stage I patients without histologic confirmation of disease.

The optimal surgical procedure for all epithelial ovarian carcinomas is removal of the uterus along with both fallopian tubes and ovaries. In the younger patient who wishes to retain her childbearing potential and who appears to have a curable cancer (i.e., a localized tumor with favorable histology), it may be appropriate to preserve the uterus and other ovary if a wedge biopsy of this ovary confirms the absence of disease. However, there is a risk that such a procedure may have a higher recurrence rate, and completion of the more standard operation is indicated following childbearing.

External Beam Radiation

Clinical trials have evaluated the postoperative impact of both radiation therapy and chemotherapy upon the survival of patients with limited-stage disease. There have been two randomized studies of external beam pelvic radiation therapy in patients with stage I tumors, neither of which would be considered adequate by today's standards. In the GOG study (262), stage I patients were randomized postoperatively among observation, pelvic radiation therapy, and melphalan. Unfortunately, the elimination of almost half the entered patients from the analysis, as well as the absence of a requirement for complete surgical staging, makes it difficult to draw conclusions from this study. The Princess Margaret Hospital study (231) randomized stage IA patients between postoperative pelvic radiation therapy and observation but did not require comprehensive staging. Both studies failed to demonstrate superiority for any form of therapy. Although pelvic radiation produced a reduction in the rate of pelvic relapses, distant relapses occurred throughout the peritoneal cavity, leading to the same overall relapse rate.

Abdominopelvic radiation therapy has not been the subject of a Phase III trial in patients with stage I disease but has been retrospectively compared to pelvic radiation therapy or no treatment (263). No benefit was found in grade 1 patients, where the risk of relapse was under 5% overall. In grades 2 and 3, a statistically nonsignificant reduction in relapse risk was observed. In patients whose tumors were densely adherent, a significant reduction in relapse was associated with the use of abdominopelvic radiation therapy.

Intraperitoneal Radiocolloid Therapy

Since transcoelomic spread is the main route of dissemination of ovarian cancer, the intraperitoneal instillation of radiocolloids, which deliver high doses of radiation to the peritoneal surfaces, would seem intuitively attractive, particularly for patients with apparently localized disease who may be harboring distant, unsuspected metastases. Colloids labeled with radioactive isotopes of phosphorus (^{32}P) or gold (^{198}Au) have been administered intraperitoneally. Unlike ^{32}P, a pure beta emitter (short penetration electrons), ^{198}Au also emits gamma rays, and because these are a greater radiation hazard to patient contacts, it is no longer available in North America for this use. There have been no randomized trials of either ^{32}P or ^{198}Au against a no-treatment control arm in patients with early-stage disease.

Despite its simplicity and appeal, therapeutic use has not been widely accepted for radiocolloid therapy. Experimental data show that radiation dose distribution of the peritoneal surface is quite variable and unpredictable. The average energy of the electrons released by ^{32}P is 0.6 MeV, which means that penetration of useful doses of radiation does not occur beyond 2- to 3-mm depth. Thus, the dose to lymph nodes and the retroperitoneum is usually negligible, and the dose to residual nodules greater than 2 mm thick is also negligible. A multivariate analysis (retrospective) of the Norwegian Radium Hospital data showed a nonsignificant excess of relapses in patients who received ^{32}P or ^{198}Au compared to pelvic radiation therapy or to no adjuvant treatment in stages I and II (265). When given together with pelvic radiation therapy, unacceptably high bowel toxicity is encountered. Thus, the therapeutic value of ^{32}P, even in early-stage ovarian cancer, has not been established. Where the intent is to provide adequate radiation therapy to the entire peritoneal cavity, it may be better delivered with external beam radiation; the delivery of radiation is uniform, predictable, and adequately irradiates the entire abdominal contents.

Chemotherapy in Localized Disease

The role of chemotherapy in the adjuvant setting in patients with stages I and II disease has been studied in both randomized and nonrandomized trials. The first study of the GOG compared melphalan to observation (262). Outcome and conclusions were weakened by the exclusion of nearly half of the randomized patients from the analysis, but a nonsignificant advantage for the melphalan-treated patients was reported.

There have been two studies of adjuvant therapy by the GOG in early-stage epithelial ovarian cancer in which patients were treated on the basis of clinicopathologic characteristics following a comprehensive staging laparotomy (226). Table 25.10 lists the criteria used to separate early-stage patients into favorable and unfavorable prognostic groups. Patients in the favorable prognosis category were randomly assigned to receive no further therapy or oral intermittent melphalan (0.2 mg/kg daily for 5 days), with repeat cycles every 4 to 6 weeks, for a total of 12 courses or 18 months of therapy, whichever came first. After a comprehensive staging laparotomy and pathology review, 81 patients

TABLE 25.10. *Favorable vs unfavorable early-stage ovarian cancer*

Favorable	Unfavorable
Stage IA or IB disease	Stage IA or IB with poorly differentiated tumors
Well- or moderately well-differentiated tumors	Tumor on external surface
	Ruptured capsule
	Ascites or positive peritoneal washing
	All stage II

were available for analysis (38 patients who received no adjuvant therapy and 43 patients who received intermittent oral melphalan). With a median follow-up of greater than 6 years, there have been only six deaths in this group of patients: four in the observation group and two patients who received intermittent melphalan. Five of the deaths were directly related to ovarian cancer, and one patient died of aplastic anemia. The 5-year disease-free and overall survival rates for untreated patients were 91% and 94%, respectively. The disease-free survival and the overall survival rates were 98% for those patients who received melphalan.

This important study has identified a group of patients with early-stage ovarian cancer (stage IA1 or IB1 tumors with well-differentiated or moderately well-differentiated histologic features) who do not require adjuvant therapy. The overall 5-year survival is greater than 90%, and these patients can be spared the toxicity of chemotherapy. In particular, melphalan chemotherapy is associated with a known risk of myeloproliferative disorders, including acute leukemia, and although such complications are uncommon, decreasing the risk of such a catastrophic illness is a substantial benefit.

Randomized Trials of ^{32}P Versus Chemotherapy

Table 25.11 summarizes the results of randomized trials of ^{32}P versus chemotherapy in early-stage ovarian cancer. In the GOG study (227), patients with limited-stage disease but unfavorable prognostic features were randomized to receive melphalan (in the same dose and schedule as described for patients with favorable prognostic features) or intraperitoneal ^{32}P (15 mCi of chromic phosphate). A total of 141 patients were evaluated (73 randomized to ^{32}P and 68 to melphalan). Eighty-nine patients in this group had stage II disease (with the majority having stage IIB disease), the remainder had stage I disease, with the unfavorable prognostic criteria previously defined. With a follow-up exceeding 5 years, the 5-year disease-free survival rate was 80% in patients treated with either ^{32}P or melphalan. Similarly, the 5-year survival rates were 78% for ^{32}P and 81% for melphalan. The relapse rate was 19%, with 81% of the recur-

TABLE 25.11. *Randomized trials of ^{32}P vs chemotherapy in early-stage disease*

Series (ref.)	No. of patients	Study design	5-year disease-free survival (%)
GOG protocol 7602 (226)	141	^{32}P vs melphalan	80 vs 80
Norwegian Radium Hospital (265)	347	^{32}P vs cisplatin	81 vs 75; p = NS
NCIC (264)	257	Pelvic RT followed by: ^{32}P vs melphalan vs API	66 vs 61 vs 62; p = NS
GICOG (266)	161	^{32}P vs cisplatin	65 vs 85
GOG protocol 95 (267)	207	^{32}P vs cisplatin plus cyclophosphamide	66 vs 77 (Recurrence rates 31% lower with chemotherapy)

GOG, Gynecologic Oncology Group; NCIC, National Cancer Institute of Canada; GICOG, Gruppo Interregionale Collaborativo in Ginecologia; API, abdominopelvic irradiation; NS, not significant.

rences seen in the first 2 years of follow-up. However, 5 of the 27 recurrences were observed after 2 years (ranging from 30 to 84 months). The impact of treatment upon survival in this group of patients cannot be established, since an untreated observation group was not included. It is possible that neither treatment markedly affected survival and that the overall 5-year survival rate of 80% (which is much higher than previously reported for patients with stage II disease) represents the natural history for comprehensively staged patients with these unfavorable prognostic features.

The National Cancer Institute of Canada (NCIC) Clinical Trials Group (264) treated 257 patients with high-risk early-stage ovarian cancer, as well as with completely resected stage IIB or stage III disease, with pelvic radiation followed by randomization to either melphalan (8 mg/m² 4 days every 4 weeks for 18 cycles) or intraperitoneal ^{32}P (1,020 mCi) or to total abdominal radiation therapy (22.5 Gy in 20 fractions). Surgical staging was incomplete in this study, but all patients had an abdominal hysterectomy. With a median follow-up of 8 years, there was no difference in actuarial 5-year survival rates. The ^{32}P arm of the study was associated with a high incidence of delayed bowel complications and was closed prematurely.

The Norwegian Radium Hospital performed a large randomized trial in 347 completely resected stages I, II, and III ovarian cancer patients who received either cisplatin (50 mg/m² for six courses) or intraperitoneal ^{32}P (710 mCi) (265). Patients who were found to have extensive adhesions at surgery received ???abdominal/pelvic irradiation instead of ^{32}P. Surgical staging was extensive in this trial and included hysterectomy, bilateral salpingo-oophorectomy, omentectomy, evaluation of ascitic fluid, and examination of pelvic and retroperitoneal lymph nodes. There was no significant difference in the 5-year actuarial disease-free survival rates for patients treated with either cisplatin or ^{32}P. However, there was significant toxicity associated with the intraperitoneal instillation of ^{32}P, with a 5% rate of surgically treated small-bowel obstructions. Based on the excessive toxicity associated with ^{32}P, the Norwegian Radium Hospital group did not recommend further evaluation of ^{32}P for subsequent adjuvant studies.

A similar study was performed in a multicenter group in Italy (266) in which stage IC ovarian cancer patients received either cisplatin (50 mg/m² every 28 days for six cycles) or ^{32}P (12 mCi). Complete surgical staging was required. Disease-free survival was prolonged in the cisplatin group; however, there was no difference in 5-year survival (cisplatin 81% vs ^{32}P 78%).

The GOG has completed a trial of ^{32}P versus three cycles of cisplatin plus cyclophosphamide in patients with unfavorable early-stage disease (267). A total of 251 evaluable patients were randomized to receive either 15 mCi intraperitoneal ^{32}P or the combination of cyclophosphamide (1 g/m²) and cisplatin (100 mg/m²) for three cycles. The percentage of patients recurrence free at 10 years is 72% for chemotherapy and 65% for ^{32}P. After adjusting for stage and histologic grade, the estimated recurrence rate is 29% lower for chemotherapy compared to intraperitoneal ^{32}P. The death rate was 17% lower for patients treated with chemotherapy. The recurrence rate was 1.62 times greater for stage II than stage I (p = .05). The probability of surviving 10 years for stage I patients was 70% compared to 62% for stage II patients. Eight patients randomized to ^{32}P were not able to receive treatments and three patients had bowel perforation during catheter insertion. However, bone marrow suppression was more common with chemotherapy. It was concluded that the better progression-free interval for chemotherapy and the problems with adequate distribution and bowel toxicity associated with intraperitoneal ^{32}P make chemotherapy the standard for patients with early high risk for ovarian cancer who receive adjuvant therapy.

Chemotherapy Versus Observation

Recent clinical trials have attempted to determine whether any form of adjuvant treatment is superior to a policy of no immediate treatment for patients with early-stage ovarian cancer with poor prognostic features. A randomized trial with a no-treatment arm was conducted by the Italian Interregional Cooperative Group of Gynecologic Oncology (266). In this study, patients with stage IA or IB, grade 2 or 3 tumors were randomized to receive cisplatin (50 mg/m² every 28 days for six cycles) or to no immediate treatment. With a median follow-up time of 76 months, cisplatin reduced the relapse rate by 65%. The 5-year disease-free survival was 65% in the control arm and 83% in the chemotherapy arm. However, there was no difference in overall survival: 88% for cisplatin and 82% for patients randomized to no initial treatment. The lack of a survival advantage in the treated arm reflects the efficacy of cisplatin administered at the time of recurrence.

The results of two large prospective randomized trials that compared no immediate chemotherapy versus chemotherapy for patients with early-stage ovarian cancer were recently reported. In addition, a combined analysis of the two trials was also performed. The International Collaborative Ovarian Neoplasm 1 (ICON1) (268) and the Adjuvant Chemotherapy in Ovarian Neoplasm (ACTION) (269) trials each had almost 500 patients who underwent similar randomization procedures to either platinum-based adjuvant chemotherapy immediately following surgery or to no adjuvant chemotherapy until clinical progression indicated the necessity for treatment. In both trials, there was flexibility about the specific chemotherapeutic regimen used but both required a platinum-based drug to be included. There were marked differences in patient inclusion criteria for these two trials. The ICON1 trial required that the patient have histologically confirmed ovarian cancer of epithelial origin and that the clinician was uncertain as to whether to offer immediate adjuvant chemotherapy (268). It was required that all visible tumor be removed and thorough surgical staging was recommended with total hysterectomy and bilateral salpingo-oophorectomy, where appropriate, and omentectomy. The ACTION trial, on the other hand, required surgical staging

and patients were eligible with stages IA and IB, grades 2 and 3; all stages IC and II; and all stages I and IIA with clear-cell epithelial cancer of the ovary (269). In cases of stage IA cancer, unilateral salpingo-oophorectomy followed by surgical staging was permitted. Surgical staging had to consist of at least careful inspection and palpation of all peritoneal surfaces with biopsies of any suspect lesions. A more comprehensive staging laparotomy was strongly advised, which included omentectomy, peritoneal washings, blind biopsies from the perineum, pericolic gutters, and the right hemidiaphragm as well as iliac and paraaortic lymph node sampling. Staging was considered to be optimum if all these requirements were met. Three other less comprehensive staging categories were defined: modified, minimal, and adequate.

Despite these differences in trial design and patient eligibility, the analysis of the combined results showed better overall survival for patients in the adjuvant chemotherapy arm than for patients with no immediate chemotherapy (270). The difference in overall survival was 8% in favor of chemotherapy (82% vs 74%, $p = .008$) (Fig. 25.14). Similarly, recurrence-free survival was also better for patients in the adjuvant chemotherapy arm than for patients in the no–immediate treatment arm (76% vs 65%, $p = .001$). In a separate study, the survival of stage I patients who relapsed after a policy of observation only was similar to that of stage III patients and ''salvage'' was possible in only 20% (271).

Despite the improvement in survival observed in the combined analysis, the question of whether they represent ''definitive proof'' of the benefit of platinum-based adjuvant chemotherapy for all patients with early-stage ovarian cancer has been questioned (272). The ICON1 trial, with its broad

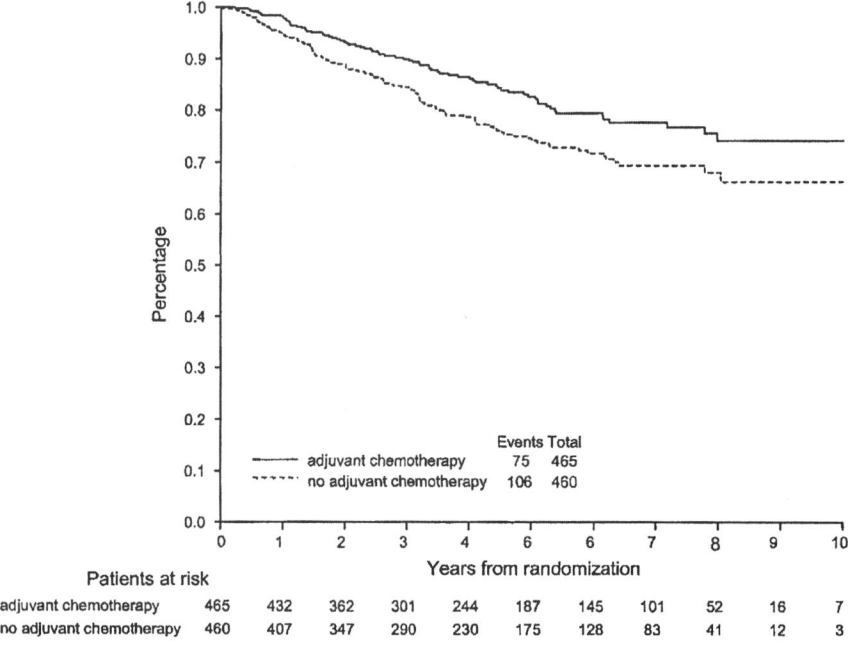

FIG. 25.14. Kaplan-Meier curves for overall survival in early state ovarian cancer patients treated with adjuvant chemotherapy (*solid line*) and no adjuvant chemotherapy (*dotted line*). Five-year survival rate was 74% for women without adjuvant chemotherapy and 82% for the adjuvant chemotherapy group. (Reprinted with permission from International Collaborative Ovarian Neoplasm 1 (ICON1) and European Organization for Research and Treatment of Cancer Collaborator–Adjuvant Chemotherapy in Ovarian Neoplasm (EORTC-ACTION). International collaborative ovarian neoplasm trial 1 and adjuvant chemotherapy in ovarian neoplasm trial: Two parallel randomized phase III trials of adjuvant chemotherapy in patients with early-stage ovarian carcinoma. *J Natl Cancer Inst* 2003;95:105–112.)

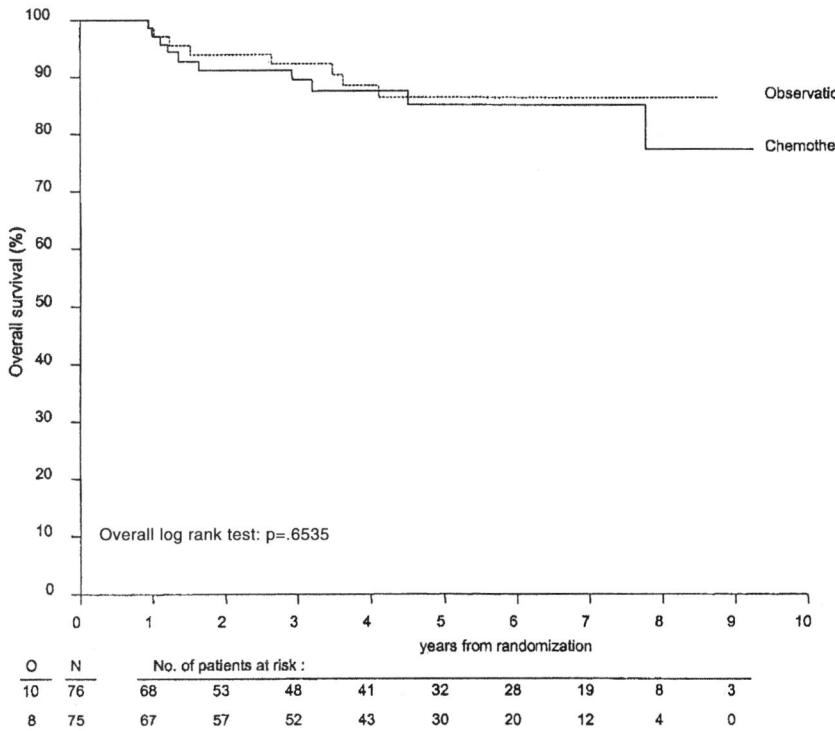

FIG. 25.15. Kaplan-Meier curves for overall survival for patients optimally staged who received immediate adjuvant chemotherapy (N = 76) (*solid line*) compared to optimally staged patients in the observation arm. (Reprinted with permission from Trimbos JB, Vergote I, Bolis G, et al. Impact of adjuvant chemotherapy and surgical staging in early-stage ovarian carcinoma: European Organization for Research and Treatment of Cancer—adjuvant chemotherapy in ovarian neoplasm trial. *J Natl Cancer Inst* 2003;95:113–125.)

entry criteria, included patients who would not have been eligible for other such trials, that is, patients with well-differentiated tumors and patients who may have had occult stage III disease since a comprehensive laparotomy was not mandatory. It should also be pointed out that in the ACTION trial, where comprehensive surgical staging was required, only one-third of the patients had optimal surgical staging retrospectively. In this retrospective subset analysis, there was no improvement in either overall survival or relapse-free survival in patients who had optimal surgical staging (Fig. 25.15). These results suggest that platinum-based adjuvant chemotherapy is primarily of benefit to patients who were incompletely staged. Patients with high-risk, early-stage, epithelial ovarian cancer who are either incompletely staged or in whom staging data are incomplete or unavailable should receive platinum-based chemotherapy because their survival will be compromised if chemotherapy is delayed until time of clinical progression. It is planned that the next European Organization for Research and Treatment of Cancer (EORTC) trial will attempt prospectively to confirm the subset findings from the current trial that adjuvant chemotherapy in early-stage ovarian cancer is not effective after optimal surgical staging. Possible protocol design will randomly assign nonoptimally staged patients to restaging (i.e., to make sure the patient is optimally staged) followed by observation or immediate adjuvant chemotherapy without staging. It is also clear from these large randomized trials that only a minority of patients with early-stage cancer benefit from chemotherapy. In the combined analysis, 18% of patients were not cured by adjuvant chemotherapy. Molecu-

lar markers, including gene expression profiles, are needed to better differentiate good and poor prognosis early-stage patients and to better identify patients who are candidates for immediate adjuvant therapy. In addition, it is also evident that better adjuvant therapies are needed to improve survival in that subset of early-stage ovarian cancer patients who, despite the minimal disease and optimal therapy, still are not cured.

The preliminary results of the most recent GOG randomized trial in early-stage ovarian cancer have recently been presented (273). Following a comprehensive staging laparotomy as previously defined by the GOG, patients were randomized to either three or six cycles of paclitaxel (175 mg/m^2 infused over 3 hours) followed by carboplatin (dosed to an AUC of 7.5 infused over 30 minutes). Cycles were repeated every 21 days. Four hundred fifty-seven patients were accrued to this protocol and 321 patients (70%) met all eligibility criteria. However, 20% of the patients were deemed to be ineligible owing to incomplete surgical staging. With a median surveillance of 4.5 years, 75% (241 patients) are alive without recurrence. In the standard three-cycle arm, the estimated probability of cancer recurrence within 5 years was 27% compared to 19% in the six-cycle arm. The risk of recurrence was 32% lower than for patients treated with six cycles of chemotherapy (relative hazard 0.672; 95% CI 0.416 to 1.08). If the treatment comparison includes patients considered to be ineligible due to incomplete surgical staging, then the recurrence rate was 24% less with six cycles of chemotherapy (relative hazard 0.762; 95% CI 0.499 to 1.16). There was more toxicity, particularly anemia, granulocytopenia, and neurotoxicity, for the six cycles of treatment. The investigators concluded that the addition of three more cycles of carboplatin and paclitaxel over the standard three cycles did not significantly alter the rate of recurrence. The current GOG trial continues to utilize three cycles of chemotherapy with paclitaxel and carboplatin as the control arm. In an experimental arm, patients also receive three cycles of the same chemotherapy but, in addition, they are treated with 26 weekly paclitaxel administrations to determine if maintenance therapy is effective.

The following treatment approaches are recommended for patients with early-stage invasive epithelial ovarian cancer. For patients with early-stage epithelial ovarian cancer with favorable prognostic criteria (Table 25.10.), no postoperative treatment is indicated. Since patients with early-stage tumors with any of the poor prognostic features in Table 25.10 have a relapse risk of at least 20%, postoperative treatment is justified. The primary treatment option for this group of patients is carboplatin plus paclitaxel chemotherapy. Total abdominal and pelvic radiation remains an option, although the vast majority of patients, at least in the United States, are treated with chemotherapy. ^{32}P has been shown to be less effective than chemotherapy and is no longer recommended. There is no evidence that a second-look operation after completion of any adjuvant therapy improves outcome in patients with early-stage disease and it is not routinely recommended.

MANAGEMENT OF LMP TUMORS

Early-Stage Disease

Surgery is the cornerstone of treatment for early-stage ovarian tumors of LMP; most patients have not received postoperative adjuvant therapy, and 5-year survivals have ranged from 90% to 100%. It is important to note that the same principles of surgical staging detailed earlier in this chapter with regard to invasive cancers apply equally to tumors of LMP. Since many women with LMP tumors are in the childbearing years, the efficacy and safety of conservative surgery have been important. There is no evidence that a conservative surgical approach has an adverse effect on survival in patients with stage I tumors of LMP (274,275). Even though patients treated with a unilateral oophorectomy have a higher recurrence rate than patients treated with a total hysterectomy and bilateral oophorectomy, effective surgery for recurrent disease leads to equivalent survival. Whether even more conservative surgery (e.g., cystectomy) has an adverse impact on survival remains a subject of debate. Although cystectomy may increase the recurrence rate, it may not have an adverse effect on survival. However, in order to avoid recurrences and still maintain fertility, there appears to be little, if any, disadvantage to performing a unilateral oophorectomy. In patients who present with stage II LMP tumors, a total abdominal hysterectomy and bilateral salpingo-oophorectomy with appropriate staging of the peritoneal cavity is recommended.

There are numerous small clinical trials in the literature in which patients with stage I LMP tumors of the ovary have been treated with adjuvant therapy, including single-agent and combination chemotherapy, pelvic or abdominopelvic radiation, and intraperitoneal radioactive colloids. In a collective review of patients treated with any of these modalities, only three patients died of persistent disease (275). The overall percentage of untoward events (death, recurrence of disease, or persistence of disease) was 11.2%. In contrast, in 450 patients with stage I disease who did not receive any form of adjuvant therapy, there were only two deaths from LMP tumors, with a 4.4% rate of untoward events. There has been only one prospective randomized trial of adjuvant therapy in stage I LMP tumors (276). Following surgery, which included at a minimum a total abdominal hysterectomy and bilateral salpingo-oophorectomy, 55 patients with LMP tumors were randomized to either no further treatment, pelvic radiation, or oral intermittent melphalan. Since there was only one patient who had a recurrence, the conclusion from this study and the collected literature series is that adjuvant therapy for stage I tumors of LMP is not necessary.

Data are extremely limited on the use of adjuvant therapy in patients with stage II LMP tumors. There is no evidence that adjuvant therapy with either radiation or chemotherapy can decrease the recurrence rate or prolong survival in this group of patients (275).

The results of the large GOG trials in early-stage ovarian cancer have direct relevance to the necessity for adjuvant therapy in patients with LMP tumors (226). Eligibility criteria for entry into study included a demonstration of invasive epithelial ovarian carcinoma. However, after central review, it was established that 51 patients had LMP tumors: 27 patients in the trial of favorable-prognosis early-stage ovarian cancer (12 randomized to melphalan and 15 to observation), and 24 patients in the trial for patients with unfavorable-prognosis early-stage ovarian cancer (10 randomized to receive melphalan and 14 to receive intraperitoneal ^{32}P). Only 4% (2 of 51 patients) with LMP tumors who entered into these two randomized trials have died. Furthermore, it is not clear that either death was actually caused by persistent tumor growth. These studies provide additional evidence that patients with early-stage ovarian cancer with LMP tumors do not benefit from adjuvant therapy.

Stages III and IV

Approximately 20% of patients with ovarian tumors of LMP will present with stage III or IV disease at the time of diagnosis. According to our current understanding of the disease process, the primary surgical management of these patients should be identical to that used in patients with invasive ovarian cancers. The benefit of postsurgical therapy in this group of patients has not been well established. In a collective series of 139 patients (275) with stage III LMP tumors, 52% received adjuvant therapy, including single-agent alkylating drugs and various combination therapy regimens. An additional 23% of the patients were treated with either external beam irradiation or intraperitoneal administration of radioactive colloids, and 15% of the patients received combined-modality treatment. Only 10% of the patients received no postsurgical treatment. The percentage of deaths or recurrences was higher in the untreated group (50%) compared to those receiving postoperative chemotherapy (42%). However, such a retrospective comparison cannot be used to make a strong case for the efficacy of adjuvant therapy in advanced LMP tumors.

There have been several reports of findings at second-look surgery in patients with LMP ovarian tumors following therapy. In 15 patients with stage III LMP tumors treated with cisplatin-based chemotherapy in a GOG study, 6 were found to have no disease at second look (277). Similarly, Gershenson and Silva (278) surgically determined the response to chemotherapy in 20 patients with metastatic serous ovarian tumors of low malignant potential who had macroscopic residual disease after initial surgery. The overall response rate was 80% (40% complete remission and 40% partial).

Even without an established benefit from postoperative therapy, 5-year survivals for patients with advanced-stage LMP ovarian tumors have ranged from 64% to 96% (276). However, there is a steady decline in survival after 5 years, with an overall mortality rate of 25% to 30% (275). The indolent clinical course suggests that LMP ovarian tumors have a low growth fraction, which likely also accounts for their lack of responsiveness to chemotherapy.

There is, however, a subset of patients who have an aggressive clinical course in whom chemotherapy has been used because of rapid disease recurrence after surgery. Kaern et al. (241) have used cellular DNA content to identify patients with LMP tumors of the ovary who have an unfavorable prognosis and who may benefit from chemotherapy. In this study from Norway, 12% to 14% of all ovarian tumors were of the LMP type. Patients over the age of 60 years with advanced LMP diploid mucinous or serous tumors had a 15-year survival of 75% compared to a 20% survival if the LMP tumors were aneuploid (Fig. 25.16). Other investigators have confirmed the prognostic significance of aneuploidy in LMP tumors of the ovary (279,280). A prospective demonstration that patients with aneuploid ovarian tumor of LMP benefit from combination chemotherapy, however, has not been reported.

The management of LMP tumors with "invasive implants" remains an area of controversy (281). Seidman and Kurman (282) have suggested that some advanced-stage LMP tumors should be classified as "micropapillary serous carcinomas" since they are frequently associated with invasive implants and a high risk for relapse. In a collected series, invasive implants were associated with a fourfold increase

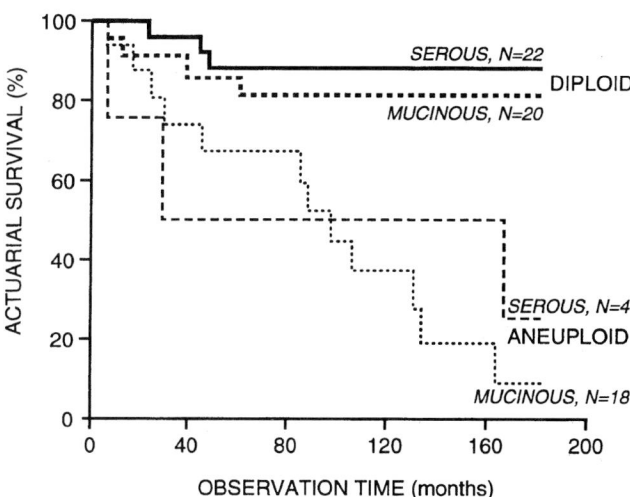

FIG. 25.16. Survival of patients with aneuploid and diploid low malignant potential tumors of the ovary. (Reprinted from Kaern J, Trope C, Kjorstad KE, et al. Cellular DNA content as a new prognostic tool in patients with low malignant potential tumors of the ovary. *Gynecol Oncol* 1990;38:452–457. Copyright 2004, with permission from Elsevier.)

in relapse rate and a sixfold increase in death rate compared to noninvasive peritoneal implants. Although invasive implants appear to confer an adverse prognosis, it has not been established that postoperative chemotherapy is effective in either decreasing the relapse rate or improving survival.

The GOG performed a study to define the natural history of LMP tumors and to determine the efficacy of therapy with melphalan and cisplatin (274). After a comprehensive laparotomy, patients with no gross residual disease were followed without treatment until the time of clinical progression. Patients with residual disease after their initial laparotomy were carefully followed with CT scans and ultrasound studies. Patients underwent a second-look laparotomy if they did not have disease progression after 1 year. Patients who demonstrated disease progression, either documented clinically or at second look, were treated initially with melphalan. Patients who progressed on melphalan were subsequently treated with cisplatin therapy. Patients with clinically evident residual disease after initial surgery immediately received postoperative oral intermittent melphalan followed by cisplatin at the time of progression. The systematic follow-up and treatment of patients with LMP ovarian tumors in this GOG study will provide prospective information about the natural history of this disease and about the efficacy of intervention with chemotherapeutic agents.

Advanced Epithelial Ovarian Cancer

Cytoreductive Surgery

Despite decades of effort aimed at improving methods of early detection and diagnosis, the majority of cases of cancer of the ovary are not diagnosed until the disease has spread beyond the ovary (Table 25.8). Often, patients with advanced disease will present with an abdomen distended with ascites and obviously bulky tumor masses in the pelvis and upper abdomen. For most human solid tumors, aggressive surgical resection is justified only if all known tumor can be removed, rendering the operation potentially curative. For epithelial cancer of the ovary, however, there is substantial theoretical and clinical support for the concept that debulking, or cytoreduction, of large tumor masses can be beneficial to the patient even in the absence of complete tumor removal. Griffiths (283) has reviewed the theoretical basis for cytoreductive surgery. Removal of bulky tumor masses in a patient with advanced ovarian cancer may improve the patient's comfort, reduce the adverse metabolic consequences of the tumor, and enhance the patient's ability to maintain her nutritional status. Such effects are likely to increase her ability to tolerate the intensive chemotherapy that is required. Perhaps, more importantly, removal of large tumor masses may enhance the response of the remaining tumor to chemotherapy. Large tumor masses with a relatively poor blood supply may provide a pharmacologic sanctuary where viable tumor cells can escape exposure to adequate concentrations of cytotoxic drugs. Additionally, such poorly vascularized masses may have a low growth fraction [i.e., a larger proportion of cells in the nonproliferating (G_0) phase of the cell cycle] when they are relatively insensitive to the effects of cytotoxic drugs (see Chapter 15).

According to the mathematical model of Goldie and Coldman (284), chemotherapy resistance develops, in part, as the result of random spontaneous mutations that occur at a rate related to the growth rate and number of tumor cells present. It is, therefore, possible that surgical cytoreduction may also decrease the development of chemoresistant clones of tumor cells. Also, it has been suggested that removal of tumor bulk enhances immune function, although strong confirmatory experimental evidence is lacking.

In 1968, Munnell (285), who introduced a concept of the "maximum surgical effort" for ovarian cancer, reported an improved survival in patients who had a "definitive operation" compared to "partial removal" or "biopsy only." In 1969, Delclos and Quinlan (286) reported 25% versus 9% survival in stage III ovarian cancer patients when disease was cytoreduced surgically to "nonpalpable" versus "palpable." Griffiths (283) was the first to accurately quantify residual disease following primary surgery and to correlate this with survival in a group of 102 patients receiving chemotherapy (single-agent melphalan) for stage II or III ovarian cancer. Using a multiple linear regression model, he found that survival duration was significantly related to residual tumor size, and he reported a median survival of 39 months for patients with no residual tumor compared to 12.7 months for patients with residual tumor >1.45 cm in maximum diameter. He also noted an important limitation of cytoreductive surgery: Extensive resection of tumor bulk with failure

to remove all masses >1.5 cm in diameter did not influence survival.

In 1978, Young et al. (287) reported the first randomized trial of multiagent nonplatinum chemotherapy versus single-agent alkylating therapy of advanced ovarian cancer, showing that patients reduced to "optimal disease" were more likely to achieve a complete clinical response, as well as a pathologic complete response. Other investigators utilizing platinum-based regimens have also supported the role of primary cytoreductive surgery. Omura et al. (288), reporting a GOG study comparing two cisplatin-based regimens, found a statistically significant difference in progression-free interval, survival, and proportion of patients achieving negative second-look laparotomy in those with no gross residual disease compared to those with gross residual ≤1 cm. In clinical trials in which the percentage of patients who were optimally cytoreduced was reported (Table 25.12), the median survival for optimally cytoreduced patients was 39 months as compared to 17 months for those not optimally cytoreduced. In addition, Fuks et al. (297) and Dembo (298) have reported beneficial effects of primary cytoreduction when radiation is used following surgery, as well.

More recently, several investigators have published results supporting the role of primary cytoreduction. Hoskins et al. (299), analyzing GOG data, reported on the effect of residual disease size on survival after primary cytoreductive surgery. The patient population studied was relatively homogeneous because it included only patients with suboptimal residual disease according to the GOG definition (>1 cm). This removes an important source of bias present in most prior studies since patients found to have only small-volume disease (or debulked to very small-volume disease) are excluded. Among their study group of 294 patients, they noted a statistically significant improvement in survival in patients who had 1- to 2-cm residual disease as compared to those with >2-cm residual disease ($p < .01$). These data, when

TABLE 25.12. *Success in achieving optimal[a] primary cytoreduction in stages III and IV epithelial ovarian cancer*

Study (ref.)	Year	Total patients	% optimal cytoreduction
Young et al. (287)	1978	80	24
Smith et al. (289)	1979	792	24
Delgado et al. (213)	1984	75	17
Neijt et al. (290)	1984	186	41
Wharton et al. (291)	1984	395	39
Redman et al. (219)	1986	86	40
Heintz et al. (292)	1986	70	70
Neijt et al. (293)	1987	191	49
Pive et al. (222)	1988	40	87
Potter et al. (294)	1991	185	64
Eisenkop et al. (295)	1992	126	82
Baker et al. (296)	1994	136	83
Total mean		2,362	51.6

[a] Original investigator's definition.

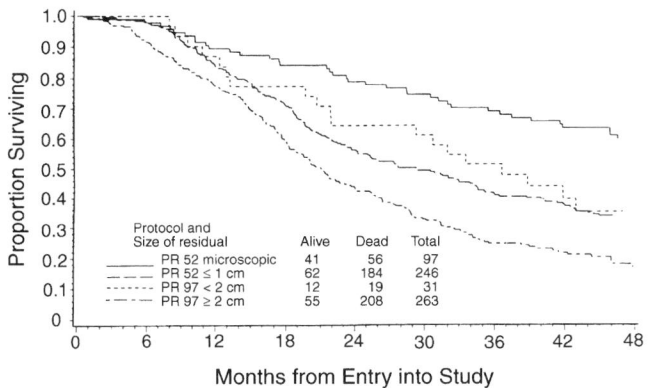

FIG. 25.17. Survival time by initial abdominal tumor description (except omentum). (Reprinted from Hoskins WJ, McGuire WP, Brady MR, et al. The effect of diameter of largest residual disease on survival after primary cytoreductive surgery in patients with suboptimal residual epithelial ovarian carcinoma. *Am J Obstet Gynecol* 1994:170:974–979. Copyright 2004, with permission from Elsevier.)

combined with data from GOG protocol 52, in which patients with stage III or IV disease had optimal (<1 cm) residual disease, provide a striking example of the prognostic importance of the extent of residual disease (Fig. 25.17) (299). Eisenkop et al. (300), in a small study, found a survival benefit to the complete elimination of all visual peritoneal implants using such modalities as CO_2 laser, argon-beam coagulator, and the cavitron ultrasonic surgical aspirator. Retrospective reports confirm that aggressive primary (and secondary) cytoreductive operations are associated with minimal morbidity and mortality when performed by experienced surgeons (301). The National Institutes of Health Consensus Development Conference on Ovarian Cancer held in April of 1994 concluded that "aggressive attempts at cytoreductive surgery as the primary management of ovarian cancer will improve the patient's opportunity for long-term survival." (Final Statement, NIH Consensus Development Conference on Ovarian Cancer, Bethesda, 1994) (5).

Stage IV ovarian cancer patients present special considerations with regard to cytoreduction. Most of the studies supporting cytoreductive surgery have included both stage III and stage IV patients but have not analyzed them separately. Four recent retrospective studies that have examined the prognostic significance of optimal debulking in stage IV ovarian cancer have all shown a statistically significant improvement in survival in patients with small-volume residual tumor (Table 25.13) (302–305). Based on these data, it seems reasonable to attempt cytoreduction in medically fit patients with stage IV disease if optimal residual disease is achievable.

The actual percentage of patients with advanced ovarian cancer who can successfully be cytoreduced remains to be established. The percentage of patients optimally cytoreduced has ranged from 87% to 17% in different studies in the literature, with a mean of 35% (Table 25.12). This wide range is due to several factors in addition to the skill and experience of the surgeon. There has not been universal agreement as to the size of residual masses that place the patient in the "optimal" category. Furthermore, the patient populations may not be comparable with regard to volume of disease at surgery or are not controlled for surgery prior to referral to the investigator.

Since many patients cannot be successfully cytoreduced at initial surgery, the benefit of a brief induction course of chemotherapy prior to debulking surgery has been explored. Two to three cycles of chemotherapy substantially increase the percentage of patients who will be successfully cytoreduced. Two studies (306,307) provided retrospective comparisons of advanced-stage patients treated with neoadjuvant chemotherapy compared to patients treated with surgery followed by chemotherapy. Both studies demonstrated the feasibility of neoadjuvant chemotherapy and the results have led to an ongoing EORTC randomized trial of neoadjuvant chemotherapy versus surgical debulking followed by chemotherapy in selected patients with advanced disease.

Ng et al (308) reported on a series of 38 patients with advanced ovarian cancer managed by a program of "chemosurgical debulking" as part of a clinical trial at Memorial Sloan–Kettering Cancer Center. Thirty-eight patients with bulky (5 to 25 cm) ovarian cancer underwent primary surgery followed by two courses of high-dose intravenous cisplatin and cyclophosphamide. The patients were then explored for repeat debulking prior to the administration of intraperitoneal chemotherapy. At the conclusion of the second debulking procedure, 30 (79%) of this poor-prognosis group had been cytoreduced to <1-cm disease. Following

TABLE 25.13. *Effect of debulking on survival in stage IV ovarian cancer*

Study (ref.)	Year	Surgical result	No. of patients	Optimal (%)	Median survival (months)	p
Curtin et al. (303)	1997	Optimal (<2 cm)	41	45	40	.01
		Suboptimal	51		18	
Liu et al. (304)	1997	Optimal (<2 cm)	14	30	37	.02
		Suboptimal	33		17	
Munkarah et al. (305)	1997	Optimal (<2 cm)	31	34	25	.02
		Suboptimal	61		15	
Bristow et al. (302)	1998	Optimal (1 cm)	25	30	38	.0004
		Suboptimal	59		10	

intraperitoneal chemotherapy, 47% of the patients achieved a surgically confirmed complete remission (309).

There is conflicting evidence from two large prospective randomized trials whether interval debulking can improve survival in certain patients with advanced ovarian cancer (310,311). In a multicenter trial conducted by the EORTC (310), patients with suboptimal (>1-cm) disease remaining after primary cytoreduction were treated with three cycles of cyclophosphamide and cisplatin. Those without progression were randomized to interval debulking surgery and additional chemotherapy versus additional chemotherapy alone. With approximately 150 patients randomized to each arm, patients undergoing the interval debulking showed a statistically significant improvement in both progression-free interval and median survival (Fig. 25.18). The interval surgery was generally well tolerated.

More recently, the GOG has reported the results of proto-col 152, a prospective randomized trial of interval secondary cytoreduction in patients with advanced ovarian cancer with suboptimal residual disease (311). Five hundred fifty patients were enrolled in this study within 6 weeks of initial surgery. After three cycles of paclitaxel and cisplatin, patients without evidence of tumor progression were randomized to receive either secondary cytoreduction and three additional cycles of chemotherapy or chemotherapy alone. At the time of the report, median progression-free survival and overall survival for the interval cytoreduction group were 10.5 months and 33.9 months, respectively, compared to 10.7 months and 33.7 months for the chemotherapy-alone group. The overall survival for the two groups is shown in Figure 25.18.

Several possibilities have been advanced to explain the difference in outcome between the GOG and European studies, both large prospective randomized trials. Probably most

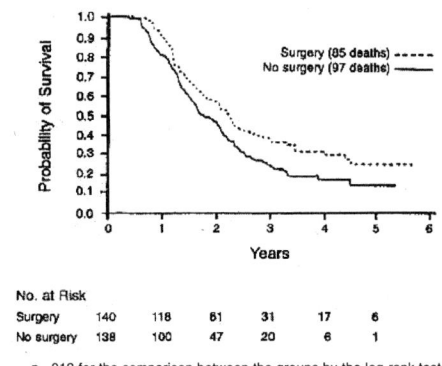

A   p=.012 for the comparison between the groups by the log-rank test

Overall Survival
by Treatment Group

Treatment	Alive	Dead	Total
Debulking surgery	65	151	216
No Debulking	63	145	208

Months from Randomization

B

FIG. 25.18. A: Survival of patients with advanced ovarian cancer who underwent internal debulking surgery compared to treatment with chemotherapy only (EORTC study). (From van der Berg MEL, van Lent M, Byuse M, et al. The effect of debulking surgery after induction chemotherapy on the prognosis in advanced epithelial ovarian cancer. *N Engl J Med* 1995;332:629–634. Copyright © 2004 Massachusetts Medical Society. All rights reserved.) B: Survival of patients with advanced ovarian cancer who underwent internal debulking surgery compared to treatment with chemotherapy only. (GOG study) (Reprinted with permission from Rubin, Sutton GP, eds. Ovarian Cancer, New York: McGraw Hill, 1993.)

important of these is the difference in the training and experience of the surgeons involved. In the GOG trials, both the initial and interval cytoreductive operations were performed almost exclusively by trained gynecologic oncologists, whereas in the EORTC trial the initial surgery was most often done by general gynecologists. As a result, residual disease following primary surgery measured <5 cm in about two-thirds of the GOG patients as compared to one-third of the patients in the EORTC trial. Following chemotherapy, residual disease >1 cm was found in 56% of the GOG patients versus 65% of the European patients. This resulted in a higher likelihood of successful cytoreduction in the EORTC trial, with conversion from suboptimal to optimal residual tumor in 45% of patients as compared to 36% in the GOG trial.

Additionally, the chemotherapeutic regimen used in the GOG trial, paclitaxel and platinum, may have reduced the benefit of interval cytoreduction relative to the EORTC trial, which used a platinum and cyclophosphamide combination. Differences in outcome may also be related to differing post-treatment surveillance, and to the availability of more effective second-line therapies since the EORTC trial completed accrual in May of 1993.

The available evidence from the prospective trials of interval cytoreduction suggests that although this technique should not be a routine management strategy, certain selected patients may benefit depending on the aggressiveness of the initial cytoreductive surgery, the geographic distribution and size of the remaining disease, and the response to the initial several cycles of chemotherapy.

Postoperative Chemotherapy

Surgery is rarely, if ever, curative for patients with advanced ovarian cancer, even in patients without gross residual disease after successful cytoreduction. Ovarian cancer is a highly chemosensitive tumor, and chemotherapeutic agents from a wide variety of different classes have shown activity. Clinical trials during the past three decades have explored single-agent therapy and combination chemotherapy as well as comparisons of individual drugs to combination regimens. The platinum compounds remain the most active agents in ovarian cancer and are the cornerstone of combination drug regimens. In the past decade, a series of novel compounds have been identified to be clinically active in recurrent ovarian cancer. Paclitaxel, the prototypic drug of a new class of agents termed *taxanes*, was the first of these agents to be included as part of initial chemotherapeutic regimens for patients with advanced disease. Currently, the standard of care, as will be discussed below, for most patients with ovarian cancer consists of the combination of paclitaxel and carboplatin.

Platinum Compounds

The demonstration that cisplatin was active in previously treated patients with advanced ovarian cancer led to a series of prospective randomized clinical trials in which the role of cisplatin in the combination chemotherapy of previously untreated patients was evaluated. The GOG performed the largest comparative trial of a platinum-containing regimen versus a non–platinum-containing regimen (312). In this study, 227 patients with advanced ovarian cancer were randomized to receive treatment with either the combination of Adriamycin (doxorubicin) plus cyclophosphamide versus the CAP regimen (cisplatin, Adriamycin, and cyclophosphamide). A total of 120 patients receiving the cyclophosphamide plus Adriamycin regimen had measurable residual ovarian cancer following surgery compared to 107 patients treated with CAP regimen. The complete response rate for CAP chemotherapy was 51% compared to 26% for the two-drug regimen ($p < .001$). Similarly, the CAP regimen was superior with regard to response duration (median 14.6 vs 8.8 months), progression-free interval (13.1 vs 7.7 months), and overall survival (15.7 vs 9.7 months). This study, together with a trial from the Netherlands Cancer Institute comparing a cisplatin-containing regimen (CHAP-5) to the hexamethylmelamine, cyclophosphamide, methotrexate, and 5-fluorouracil (Hexa-CAF) combination (290), as well as the Mayo Clinic trial (313) of cyclophosphamide plus cisplatin versus cyclophosphamide, established the basis for the routine use of cisplatin in combination chemotherapy for previously untreated patients with advanced cancer.

Carboplatin is a second-generation platinum coordination compound that, in Phase I trials, was less nephrotoxic, neurotoxic, and emetogenic than was cisplatin (314–316). The absence of nephrotoxicity permits the administration of carboplatin in an outpatient setting without the necessity for forced hydration. Carboplatin has a dose-limiting toxicity of myelosuppression, which has primarily manifested as thrombocytopenia. The effects of myelosuppression may be decreased by autologous bone marrow transplantation, cytokines, or peripheral stem-cell transfusions that have facilitated the dose-intensity studies described in the section on experimental therapy below.

Carboplatin is rapidly excreted in the kidney following intravenous administration. Consequently, the area under the concentration-time curve (AUC) will be greater in patients who have a decrease in glomerular filtration rate (GFR). Carboplatin hematologic toxicity correlates with the AUC. Retrospective studies have also suggested that there is a relationship to tumor response and AUC, with a response plateau being reached at an AUC of 6 to 7 (317). Calvert (318) has developed a formula to individualize dose based upon a desired AUC and the patient's GFR: dose (mg) = AUC $\times$ GFR + 25. In the Calvert formula, the GFR was estimated by renal clearance of EDTA (CrEDTA). However, creatinine clearance can be used to substitute for GFR and can either be measured or estimated from the patient's age and serum creatinine.

At least 12 randomized trials have been performed comparing single-agent carboplatin with cisplatin or in combination regimens in patients with advanced disease (319). Ten of these trials showed equivalent efficacy. Two meta-analyses have been performed comparing cisplatin and carboplatin in randomized trials totaling approximately 2,200 patients with 1,750 deaths (320,321). As seen in Figure 25.19, the hazard ratio is essentially at unity in comparing cisplatin and carboplatin. Furthermore, the long-term follow-up of the first randomized study of cisplatin versus carboplatin in untreated patients with advanced ovarian cancer has demonstrated no significant differences in survival (5-year survivals of 15% vs 19%, respectively, for cisplatin and carboplatin) with a minimum follow-up of 8 years (322). With a minimum follow-up duration of 8 years, there were no statistically significant differences in survival, that is, 5-year survival rates of 15% and 19% for cisplatin and carboplatin, respectively.

Three prospective randomized trials have compared carboplatin-containing nontaxane combination regimens to cisplatin-containing combination regimens. In North America, the combination of carboplatin plus cyclophosphamide has been compared to the standard cisplatin plus cyclophosphamide regimen in previously untreated patients with suboptimal disease in studies performed by the Southwest Oncology Group (SWOG) (323) and by the NCIC (324). There have been no reported survival differences for patients treated with carboplatin or cisplatin in these combinations. European investigators reported long-term follow-up on a comparison of a cisplatin combination versus a carboplatin regimen in which there may be differences in survival. This study compared the CHAP-5 regimen to the CHAC (cyclophosphamide, hexylmethylmalamine, methotrexate, and carboplatin) regimen in which carboplatin replaced cisplatin in 341 patients with advanced disease (325). The complete remission rate for the CHAP-5 regimen was 32% versus 27% for patients treated with the carboplatin-containing combination. In patients with no or <1 cm residual disease, there was a trend toward improvement in survival for patients randomized to the cisplatin combination. In patients with bulky disease, there were no survival differences.

Long-term follow-up from single-institution trials is also informative because it often reflects the results of a uniform approach to therapy. Sutton et al. (217) reported on 56 patients who received chemotherapy with the CAP regimen and who were followed for a minimum of 10 years. In this study, 91% of the patients had either suboptimal stage III

(No. events/no. entered)

	Carboplatin	Cisplatin	O-E	Variance
Single Agent				
Royal Marsden 2	58/67	57/64	-0.02	28.62
Adams	37/45	33/43	0.68	17.41
GICOG	72/88	73/85	0.24	36.16
Subtotal	167/200	163/192	0.90	82.18
Combination				
MOCG	23/27	23/29	-0.78	11.31
EORTC	126/169	120/170	4.24	61.32
MAYO	42/50	43/54	4.51	20.78
GONO	65/83	67/82	-2.67	32.90
NCICCTG	189/224	188/223	-2.76	94.08
SWOG	156/171	149/171	4.65	75.89
GOCA	44/87	41/86	2.26	21.18
Athens	62/73	64/76	-0.12	30.92
Japan	5/29	5/23	-1.16	2.32
Subtotal	712/913	700/914	8.18	350.70
Total	879/1113	863/1106	9.08	423.88

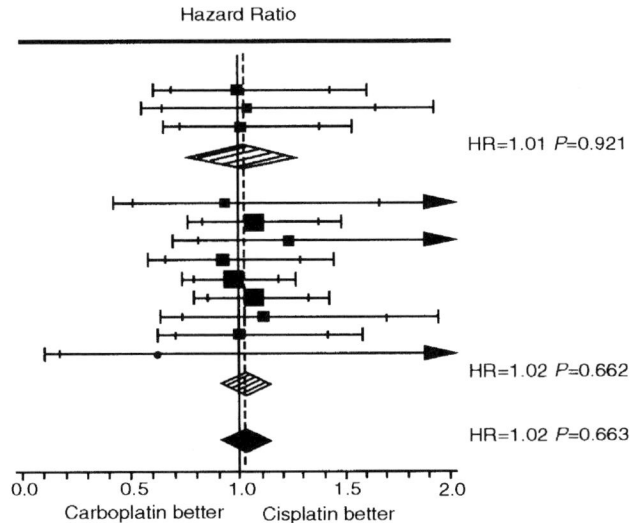

HR=1.01 P=0.921

HR=1.02 P=0.662

HR=1.02 P=0.663

Carboplatin better — Cisplatin better

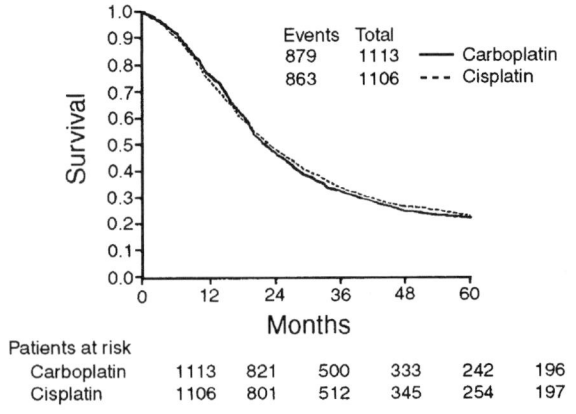

	Events	Total	
	879	1113	— Carboplatin
	863	1106	--- Cisplatin

Patients at risk

	0	12	24	36	48	60
Carboplatin	1113	821	500	333	242	196
Cisplatin	1106	801	512	345	254	197

FIG. 25.19. Hazard ratio (HR) plot for cisplatin vs carboplatin from randomized clinical trials of single-agent comparisons or combinations that include cisplatin or carboplatin. The overall HR is 1.02 (95% CI 0.93–1.12). (Reprinted with permission from Aabo K, Adams P, Adnitt P, et al. Chemotherapy in advanced ovarian cancer: four systematic meta-analyses of individual patient data from 37 randomized trials. *Br J Cancer* 1998;78:1479–1487.)

or stage IV disease, with the majority of patients having high-grade lesions. Eight patients (14%) had a negative second-look laparotomy, and three were alive without evidence of disease from 133 to 144 months after diagnosis. Five patients who did achieve a surgically confirmed complete remission died of disease 2 to 123 months after a negative second-look laparotomy. This study demonstrated that late recurrences can occur after a negative second-look laparotomy, and that more than 5 years of survival data are necessary to evaluate the overall effect of chemotherapy upon survival.

The long-term survival data from the Netherlands in almost 400 patients confirmed the superiority of CHAP-5 to Hexa-CAF. For Hexa-CAF, 5-year and 10-year survivals were 18% and 9%, compared to 32% and 21%, respectively, for patients treated with CHAP-5 (290). Hexa-CAF–treated patients received platinum at the time of recurrence. Such a sequential use of cisplatin was inferior to immediate platinum-based chemotherapy. In a study from the NCI (218), survival data were reported on 62 consecutive patients with advanced ovarian cancer who received chemotherapy with the Chex-UP regimen [cyclophosphamide, hexamethylmelamine, 5-fluorouracil (5-FU), and cisplatin]. The overall response to chemotherapy was 69%, with 19% of patients achieving a surgically confirmed complete remission. Seven of the 12 patients have had disease recurrence, with median duration of remission following a negative second-look laparotomy of 53 months. However, the median duration of survival for patients achieving a surgically confirmed complete remission will exceed 7.5 years. Overall, 9 of the 62 patients (15%) were alive more than 4 years after treatment. In this group of surviving patients, there were no patients who had stage IV disease. Six of the patients had residual bulky disease after the initial laparotomy and, nevertheless, had prolonged survival. This study confirmed the importance of a surgically confirmed complete remission. Patients who did not achieve a pathologically confirmed complete remission had a median disease-free survival of only 8.5 months compared to 53 months for those with a surgically documented complete remission. In this study, late recurrences (53 and 55 months) were also observed after a pathologic complete remission.

The impact of specific chemotherapeutic regimens on long-term survival of patients with advanced ovarian cancer has been an area of controversy. Two meta-analyses comparing survival in patients treated with platinum-based combination chemotherapeutic regimens versus non–platinum-based combination chemotherapy have addressed this issue (320,321). Four survival comparisons were made from 53 trials with over 8,000 patients:

1. Single nonplatinum agents versus nonplatinum combinations (e.g., melphalan vs Hexa-CAF)
2. Single nonplatinum agents versus a platinum combination (e.g., chlorambucil vs CAP)

3. The addition of platinum to a combination regimen (e.g., AC [Adriamycin & cyclophosphamide] vs CAP).
4. Single-agent platinum versus a platinum combination (e.g., platinum vs PC [cisplatin, cyclophosphamide]).

Overall, there was no difference in survival for patients treated with a single nonplatinum compound compared to combinations that did not include a platinum drug. For patients who received platinum as part of the initial drug regimen, there was statistically significant improvement in survival ($p = .02$) with a 12% reduction in risk of death (hazard ratio of 0.88) (320). This, in turn, translates into a 5% improvement in survival at both 2 and 5 years (Fig. 25.20). It can be concluded that cisplatin-based chemotherapy has produced a substantial clinical improvement (increased response rate, increased duration of response, and increased time to progression). However, the overall effect upon survival has been modest. A relatively small increased risk of secondary leukemia has been identified in ovarian cancer patients treated with platinum-based chemotherapy (326). However, the clinical benefit of platinum treatment outweighs the leukemia risk.

Doxorubicin (Adriamycin) and Platinum Combinations

The role of additional agents, in particular doxorubicin, when used in combination with cisplatin, has also been investigated in several large, well-controlled clinical trials. The GOG compared cisplatin plus cyclophosphamide (CP) versus the PAC combination in 349 patients with advanced disease (288). The pathologically confirmed complete remission (PCR) rates were similar (30% vs 33%) for the two

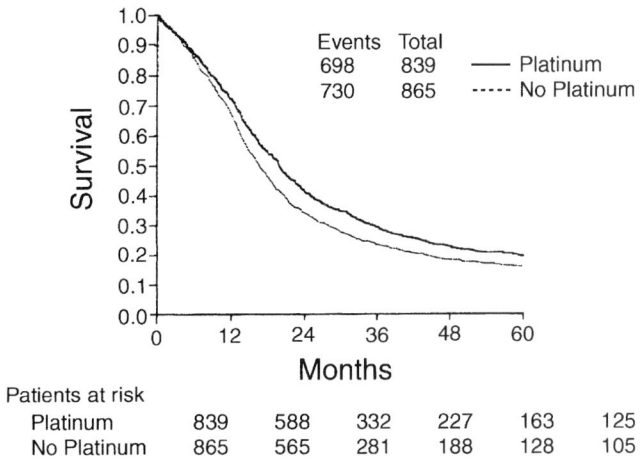

FIG. 25.20. Survival of patients treated with a platinum regimen or a nonplatinum regimen as initial therapy for advanced ovarian cancer. Meta-analysis shows a 5% reduction in mortality with cisplatin at both 5 and 10 years. (Reprinted with permission from Aabo K, Adams P, Adnitt P, et al Chemotherapy in advanced ovarian cancer: four systematic meta-analyses of individual patient data from 37 randomized trials. *Br J Cancer* 1998;78:1479–1487.)

treatment regimens. There was also no significant difference in progression-free interval (median 22.7 vs 24.6 months) or in overall survival (median 31.2 vs 38.9 months). The better general survival in this group of patients reflects the eligibility criteria, which included patients with stage III ovarian cancer having <1-cm residual lesions. Similarly, the Netherlands Cancer Institute comparison of CP versus CHAP-5 failed to demonstrate an advantage for the four-drug regimen (293). However, after 7 years of follow-up, a large Italian clinical trial comparing PAC versus CP has demonstrated a significantly higher PCR rate (62% vs 40%) and a 10-month increase in median survival for patients treated with the doxorubicin-containing regimen (327).

Meta-analyses pooling the data from these two trials, as well as those from two additional randomized studies of doxorubicin versus nondoxorubicin regimens, demonstrated a survival benefit between 5% and 7% from years 2 to 6 for the doxorubicin-treated patients (328,329). However, the interpretation of clinical trials comparing cisplatin plus CP to the PAC regimen has been limited by differences in toxicity and in dose intensity. Equitoxic regimens have not been routinely compared and, in most studies, doxorubicin was merely added to platinum plus CP administered at their standard doses. This has usually led to an increased dose intensity for the PAC regimen. Only the GOG study was performed with regimens that produced comparable hematologic toxicity, which was achieved by increasing the CP dose to 1,000 mg/m^2 in the two-drug regimen and lowering it to 500 mg/m^2 in the three-drug regimen (288).

Whereas the meta-analyses suggested a clinical benefit for doxorubicin, a large randomized trial (330) failed to confirm any survival disadvantage for the PAC regimen compared to single-agent carboplatin (Fig. 25.21). In this interna-

tional study, 1,526 patients were randomized to either carboplatin at an AUC of 5 or to the standard PAC regimen: cisplatin (50 mg/m^2), doxorubicin (50 mg/m^2), and cyclophosphamide (500 mg/m^2). Based on the absence of any survival advantage in this trial, it is unlikely that doxorubicin will be further studied in clinical trials in patients with previously untreated advanced ovarian cancer.

Paclitaxel

Paclitaxel was reported to have significant activity in advanced ovarian carcinoma in 1989 (331). A series of Phase I and Phase II trials (332–336) exploring the activity of paclitaxel as a single agent or in combination with platinum compounds was followed by prospective randomized trials comparing cisplatin plus paclitaxel versus standard therapy of cisplatin plus cyclophosphamide (Table 25.14) (337,338). Based on the superiority of the paclitaxel regimen, most investigators now consider the combination of paclitaxel plus a platinum compound to be the preferred regimen for previously untreated patients with advanced ovarian cancer (363).

Paclitaxel is the prototypic drug of a new class of agents termed *taxanes* that exert their cytotoxic effects by a unique mechanism of action. Paclitaxel was initially isolated in a crude extract from the bark of the Pacific yew, *Taxus brevifolia*. The structure of paclitaxel is shown in Figure 25.22. The cytotoxicity of paclitaxel is due to its unique effects on microtubules. In addition to their primary function in the formation of the mitotic spindle apparatus, microtubules also play a role in maintenance of cellular shape and motility and in the mediation of signals between surface receptors and the nucleus (339). Microtubules are polymers of tubulin and microtubule-associated proteins (MAPs). There is a dynamic equilibrium with tubulin heterodimers that are composed of alpha and beta protein subunits that exist as isotypes consisting of slightly different amino acid sequences. Paclitaxel binds to microtubules and shifts the equilibrium toward microtubule assembly. This is in contrast to other clinically useful antimicrotubule agents that lead to disassembly of microtubules. Paclitaxel binds preferentially to the β-subunit, leading to stable polymerized microtubules that inhibit the dynamic reorganization of the microtubule network. Morphologic effects of paclitaxel and microtubules include formation of microtubule bundles and abnormal mitotic asters. Paclitaxel arrests cells in G$_2$/M. Although the cytotoxic effect is felt to be primarily related to the disruption of mitoses, some antitumor effects of taxanes are not dependent on antimitotic activity (340). Paclitaxel has antiangiogenic properties, modifies the motility of ovarian cancer cells *in vivo*, and induces apoptosis by modulating genes involved in apoptotic regulation.

There appear to be multiple mechanisms of resistance associated with taxanes. The taxanes are good substrates for the 170-kD Pgp efflux pump encoded by the *mdr1* gene, and

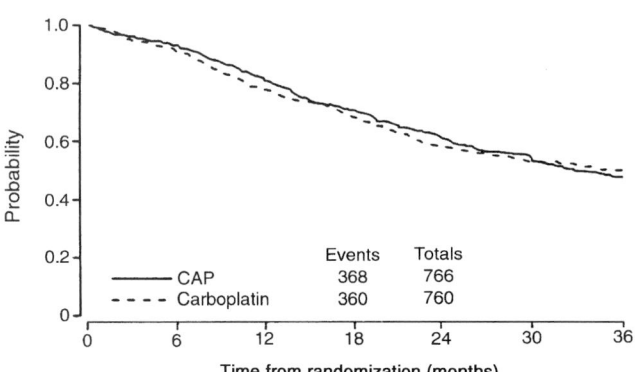

FIG. 25.21. Kaplan-Meier survival plot for patients randomized to CAP (766 patients) or to single-agent carboplatin (760 patients). (From ICON Collaborators. ICON2: randomized trial of single-agent carboplatin against three drug combination of CAP (cyclophosphamide, doxorubicin, and cisplatin) in women with ovarian cancer. *Lancet* 1998;352:1571–1576. Reprinted with permission from Elsevier.)

TABLE 25.14. *Paclitaxel/cisplatin vs cyclophosphamide in advanced ovarian cancer*

Patient characteristics	GOG 111[a]		OV10[b]	
	Stage III/IV with suboptimal disease		Stage IIBIV	
Regimens				
Paclitaxel	135 mg/m² 24-hr IV		175 mg/m² 3-hr IV	
Cisplatin	75 mg/m²		75 mg/m²	
Cyclophosphamide	750 mg/m²		750 mg/m²	
	q 3 wk 6 cycles		q 3 wk d9 cycles	
Response by treatment arm	Paclitaxel/ cisplatin	Cyclophosphamide/ cisplatin	Paclitaxel/ cisplatin	Cyclophosphamide/ cisplatin
Complete response (%)	51	31	41	27
Overall response (%)	73	60	59	45
Progression-free survival (mo)	18	13	15.5	11.5
Overall survival (mo)	38	24	35.6	25.8

[a] From McGuire WP, Hoskins WJ, Brady MF, et al. Cyclophosphamide and cisplatin compared with paclitaxel and cisplatin in patients with stage III and stage IV ovarian cancer. *N Engl J Med* 1996;334:1–6.
[b] Piccart MJ, Bertelsen K, James K, et al. Randomized Intergroup Trial of cisplatin-paclitaxel versus cisplatin-cyclophosphamide in women with advanced epithelial ovarian cancer: three-year results. *J Natl Cancer Inst* 2000;92:699–708.

resistance to paclitaxel has been associated with increased expression of this gene. In addition, alterations in the interaction of taxanes with microtubules have also been reported in resistant cells (340). Mutations of specific tubulin isotype genes may also confer resistance to taxanes.

Taxanes in Recurrent Disease

The initial Phase I trials of paclitaxel were associated with significant hypersensitivity reactions that were successfully

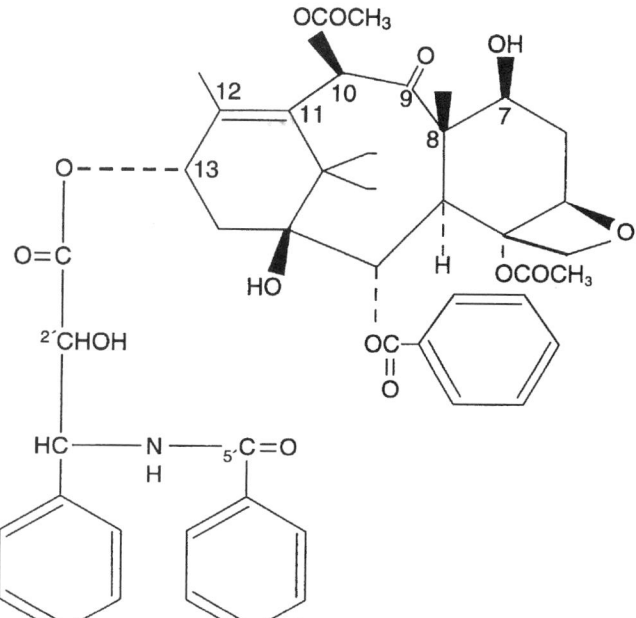

FIG. 25.22. Structure of paclitaxel. (Reprinted with permission from Rowinsky EK, Donehower RC. Drug therapy. *N Engl J Med* 1995;13:1004. Copyright © 2004 Massachusetts Medical Society. All rights reserved.)

overcome using a 24-hour infusion schedule together with premedication consisting of steroids, cimetidine, and diphenhydramine. The Phase II trials in previously treated ovarian cancer patients demonstrate an overall response rate of approximately 30% to 40% (335,336). Of particular importance was the observation that paclitaxel was active as a single agent in platinum-resistant patients, defined as patients having disease progression while on cisplatin or having a duration or remission lasting less than 6 months. In the GOG trial, in 43 patients with recurrent, persistent, or progressive ovarian cancer during or after a platinum-based chemotherapy, the overall response rate to single-agent paclitaxel was 37%, including a clinical complete remission rate of 18% (335). The median progression-free interval was 4.2 months, and median survival was 16 months. In this study, there were 27 platinum-resistant patients in whom paclitaxel had an overall response rate of 33%. Major toxicities associated with paclitaxel included alopecia, myelosuppression (which was manifested primarily as neutropenia with little effect upon platelets), myalgias, and peripheral neuropathy. In these early trials, paclitaxel was administered at a dose range from 110 to 175 mg/m².

Docetaxel, a semisynthetic taxane derived from the European yew, *T. baccata*, is an analog of paclitaxel that appears to have similar activity in recurrent ovarian cancer but has a different spectrum of toxicity (341). The primary toxicity of docetaxel is myelosuppression, although peripheral edema and weight gain are common. This latter toxicity can be managed by steroids and diuretics.

Paclitaxel/Cisplatin Combinations as Primary Therapy

Based on the activity of paclitaxel in refractory patients with ovarian cancer, Phase I studies were initiated in combination with cisplatin. Based on sequencing studies (334), a subsequent GOG prospective randomized trial (GOG protocol 111) compared paclitaxel at a dose of 135 mg/m^2 in a 24-hour infusion in combination with cisplatin at a dose of 75 mg/m^2 versus the standard therapy consisting of cyclophosphamide at 750 mg/m^2 and cisplatin at 75 mg/m^2 (337). Only patients with suboptimal stage III disease or stage IV disease were entered in this trial. A second-look laparotomy was to assess pathologic response in patients who achieved a clinical complete remission. Among 216 women with clinically measurable disease, the paclitaxel combination resulted in a significantly higher complete response rate than cyclophosphamide/cisplatin (51% vs 31%, $p = .01$), a higher overall response rate (73% vs 60%, $p = .01$), and a statistically significant improvement in progression-free survival (18 months vs 13 months, $p < .001$). Most importantly, median survival was also improved in the paclitaxel-treated patients (38 months vs 24 months, $p < .001$). Follow-up on this study now exceeds 60 months, and there is a 20% reduction of risk progression and a 34% reduction in risk of death in patients randomized to cisplatin/paclitaxel (Fig. 25.23).

A subsequent European and Canadian trial (338) (OV10) provided collaborative results to the GOG protocol (Table 25.14). This study differed from the GOG study in that the paclitaxel was administered at 175 mg/m^2 over a 3-hour infusion and the paclitaxel was available as salvage therapy for patients on the cisplatin/cyclophosphamide arm who failed treatment. The selection of a 3-hour paclitaxel infusion regimen was based on a prior European-Canadian trial (342) in which previously treated patients with advanced ovarian cancer were randomized in a 2 × 2 bifactorial design to receive either paclitaxel by a 24- or 3-hour infusion and two different doses of paclitaxel, 175 or 135 mg/m^2. All patients received standard premedications. This study demonstrated that a 3-hour infusion of paclitaxel could be safely administered and was associated with significantly less neutropenia. In addition, there was a slight increase in time to progression for patients who received the higher dose and, consequently, a 3-hour infusion at 175 mg/m^2 became the accepted paclitaxel dose and schedule for patients with recurrent ovarian cancer. While the therapeutic results of OV10 were essentially identical to those reported by GOG protocol 111, there was a significant difference in toxicity. Eighteen percent of the patients on the paclitaxel arm experienced grade 3 neurotoxicities compared to only 1% on the cyclophosphamide arm. This increased neurotoxicity was due to the shorter duration of infusion of paclitaxel in the European study compared to the 24-hour infusion in the GOG trial.

The subsequent GOG trial in patients with suboptimal stages III and IV ovarian cancer compared cisplatin (100 mg/m^2) or a 24-hour infusion of paclitaxel (200 mg/m^2) to the combination of paclitaxel (135 mg/m^2) plus cisplatin (75 mg/m^2) (343). Six hundred fourteen eligible patients were treated with the monotherapy or the combination. Single-agent therapies were discontinued more frequently [cisplatin because of toxicity or patient refusal (17%) and paclitaxel

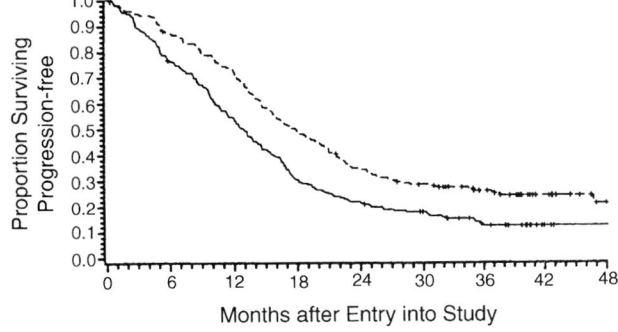

	No. Progression-free	No. with Treatment Failure	Total	Median Progression-free Survival (mo)
Treatment				
—— Cisplatin + cyclophosphamide	28	174	202	13
- - - Cisplatin + paclitaxel	45	139	184	18

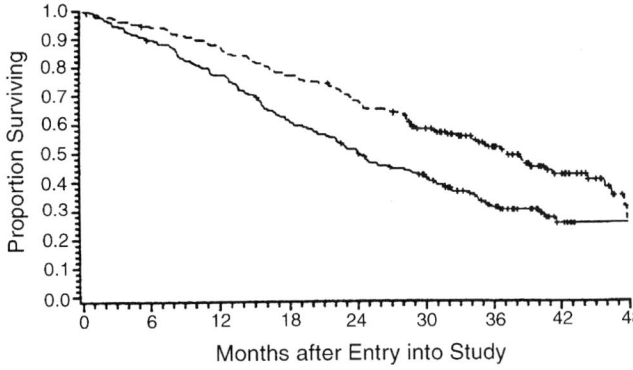

	No. Alive	No. Dead	Total	Median Survival (mo)
Treatment				
—— Cisplatin + cyclophosphamide	65	137	202	24
- - - Cisplatin + paclitaxel	86	98	184	38

FIG. 25.23. Progression-free survival and survival of previously untreated patients with suboptimal stage III and stage IV ovarian cancer randomized to cisplatin + cyclophosphamide or cisplatin + paclitaxel. (Reprinted with permission from McGuire WP, Hoskins WJ, Brady MR, et al. Cyclophosphamide and cisplatin compared with paclitaxel and cisplatin in patients with stage III and stage IV ovarian cancer. *N Engl J Med* 1996;334:1–6. Copyright © 2004 Massachusetts Medical Society. All rights reserved.)

because of progression (20%)] compared to combination chemotherapy in which 7% of patients discontinued because of toxicity and 6% because of disease progression. Neutropenia, fever, and alopecia were more severe with paclitaxel-containing treatments, whereas cisplatin-containing regimens resulted in more anemia, thrombocytopenia, neurotoxicity, nephrotoxicity, and gastrointestinal toxicity. The overall response rate to paclitaxel was significantly lower compared with the cisplatin regimens (42% vs 67%, $p < .01$). The relative hazard of first progression or death was significantly greater among those randomized to paclitaxel when compared with cisplatin treatment. The hazard ratio did not differ significantly between the two cisplatin treatments. Median durations of survival were 30.2, 25.9, and 26.3 months for those patients randomized to cisplatin, paclitaxel, and the combination regimen, respectively. The differences in overall death rates were not statistically significant. Patients randomized to single-agent therapy frequently crossed over to the alternative drug, at times even before clinical progression. Since overall survival was similar in three arms and the combination therapy had a better toxicity profile, the combination of cisplatin and paclitaxel remained the preferred initial treatment.

Paclitaxel/Carboplatin Combinations as Primary Therapy

Despite the results of meta-analyses that demonstrated no significant difference in efficacy of carboplatin versus cisplatin in ovarian cancer patients, there was concern that carboplatin may not be as effective in patients with optimal stage III ovarian cancer (344). This was based on the retrospective subset analysis of the randomized comparison of Chex-UP versus CHAP-5 in which, as previously described, there was a trend toward improved survival in patients with <1-cm residual disease who were randomized to the cisplatin combination. As a result, three large randomized Phase III trials have been performed comparing paclitaxel/carboplatin versus paclitaxel/cisplatin in the United States and Europe. In these trials, paclitaxel was administered at a 3-hour infusion and carboplatin was administered at an AUC of 5.0 to 7.5. Bookman et al. (345) demonstrated that paclitaxel and carboplatin could be administered at full therapeutic doses when AUC dosing was used for carboplatin and if paclitaxel was administered in a 3-hour infusion. This outpatient regimen was associated with modest nonhematologic toxicity, and despite the use of both drugs at full therapeutic doses with manageable hematologic toxicity, <2% of cycles were associated with grade 4 thrombocytopenia or febrile neutropenia. The importance of AUC dosing for carboplatin is shown in Figure 25.24, which compares carboplatin AUC dosing and body-surface area. The median dose of carboplatin at an AUC of 7.5 was 471 mg/m². This combination was shown to be highly active in the Phase II trial, with an overall response rate of 75% and a 67% clinical complete response rate. A European study confirmed the activity of this combination in a similar Phase II study.

On the basis of the results of the GOG pilot (345), protocol 158 was designed as a noninferiority study to compare the efficacy and toxicity of carboplatin plus paclitaxel with cisplatin plus paclitaxel for patients with small-volume, stage III disease (346). Seven hundred ninety-two eligible patients were enrolled in the study, and prognostic factors were similar in the treatment groups. Gastrointestinal, renal, and metabolic toxicity and grade 4 leukopenia were significantly more frequent in patients receiving the cisplatin regimen. Grade 2 or greater thrombocytopenia was more frequent in

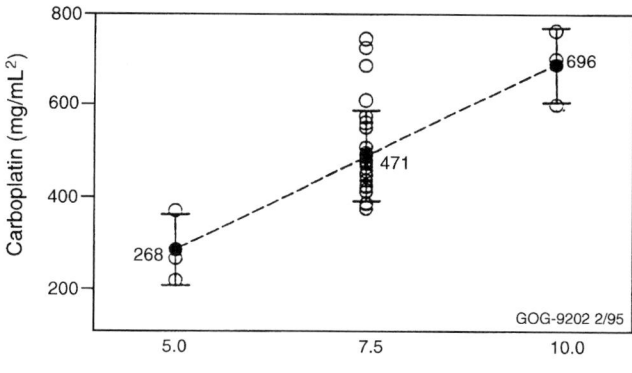

FIG. 25.24. Comparison of carboplatin dosage by AUC and body surface. The Calvert formula was used to calculate the dose at an AUC between 5 and 10. An AUC dose of 7.5 could be combined with paclitaxel at 175 mg/m² with acceptable toxicity. (Reprinted with permission from Bookman MA, McGuire WP, Kilpatrick D, et al. Carboplatin and paclitaxel in ovarian carcinoma: a phase I study of the Gynecologic Oncology Group. *J Clin Oncol* 1996;14:1895. Reprinted with permission from the American Society of Clinical Oncology.)

patients receiving the paclitaxel combination. Neurologic toxicity was similar in both treatment groups. Median progression-free survival and overall survival were 19.4 and 48.7 months, respectively, for patients receiving the cisplatin regimen compared with 20.7 and 57.4 months, respectively, for patients receiving the carboplatin treatment. The relative risk of progression for the carboplatin plus paclitaxel-treated patients was 0.88 (95% CI 0.75.0 to 1.03) and the RR of death was 0.84 (95% CI 0.70 to 1.02) (Fig. 25.25). It was concluded that the carboplatin plus paclitaxel arm resulted in less toxicity, was easier to administer, and was not inferior when compared with cisplatin plus paclitaxel.

A smaller trial from the Netherlands and Denmark randomized 190 women with stages IIB to IV ovarian cancer to receive paclitaxel at a dose of 175 mg/m² in a 3-hour infusion combined with either carboplatin dosed to an AUC of 5 or cisplatin at a dose of 75 mg/m² (347). This trial was not sufficiently powered to evaluate any differences in progression-free interval or survival. Virtually identical results to the GOG 158 study were reported from the Arbeitsgemeinschaft Gynaekologische Onkologie (AGO) Ovarian Cancer Study Group, who also performed a randomized clinical trial of cisplatin plus paclitaxel versus carboplatin plus paclitaxel as first-line treatment for patients with stages IIB to IV ovarian cancer (348). Quality of life was evaluated using the EORTC quality of life questionnaire. The proportion of patients without progression at 2 years was not statistically significantly different between the two treatments. Median progression-free survival in the carboplatin arm was 17.2 months and in the cisplatin arm was 19.1 months. These differences were not statistically significantly different. Similarly, there was no significant difference for median overall

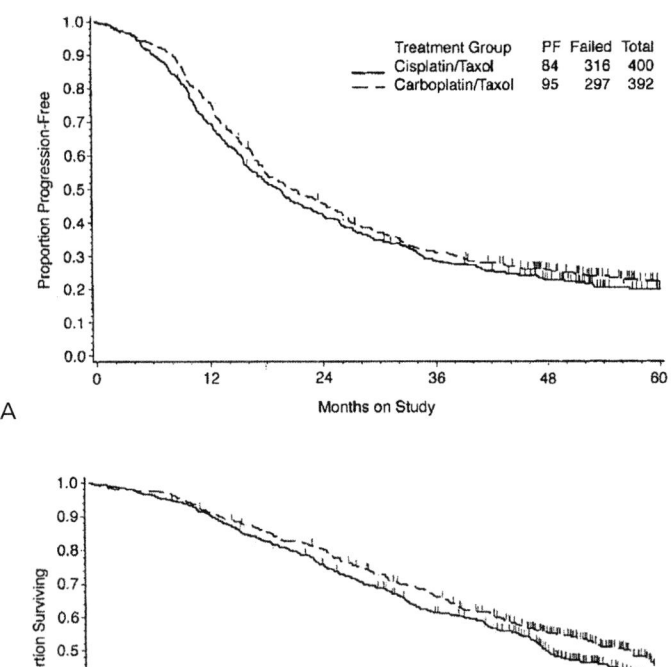

A

B

FIG. 25.25. A and **B**: Progression-free survival and overall survival for optimal stage III ovarian cancer patients randomized to cisplatin plus paclitaxel or carboplatin plus paclitaxel. (From Ozols RF, Bundy BN, Greer BE, et al. Phase III trial of carboplatin and paclitaxel compared with cisplatin and paclitaxel in patients with optimally resected stage III ovarian cancer: a Gynecologic Oncology Group Study. *J Clin Oncol* 2003;21:3194–3200. Reprinted with permission from the American Society of Clinical Oncology.)

survival (43.3 months for patients receiving the carboplatin arm vs 44.1 months for the cisplatin-treated patients). The carboplatin regimen was associated with a higher frequency of hematologic toxicity but lower frequency of gastrointestinal and neurologic toxicity than the platinum-treated group of patients. Mean and global quality of life scores at the end of treatment were statistically significantly better in the carboplatin-treated patients compared to the cisplatin-treated group. Based on these randomized trials that demonstrated no lack of efficacy but a decrease in toxicity, carboplatin plus paclitaxel is now considered the preferred combination regimen for patients with advanced ovarian cancer.

The ICON investigators performed a prospective randomized trial of paclitaxel plus carboplatin versus standard chemotherapy with either single-agent carboplatin or the three-drug combination of cyclophosphamide, doxorubicin,

and cisplatin (CAP) in women with stages I to IV ovarian cancer (349). There was a median follow-up of 51 months with 1,265 deaths. Survival curves show no difference in overall survival between paclitaxel plus carboplatin and control (hazard ratio 0.98, 95% CI 0.87 to 1.10, $p = .74$) (Fig. 25.26). Median survivals were essentially identical: 36.1 months on paclitaxel plus carboplatin and 35.4 months on control therapy. Similarly, median progression-free survival was 17.3 months on paclitaxel plus carboplatin and 16.1 months on the control treatment. The combination caused more alopecia, fever, and neuropathy than the carboplatin alone and more sensory neuropathy than the three-drug combination. These investigators concluded that single-agent carboplatin and CAP were as effective as paclitaxel plus carboplatin as first-line treatment for women requiring ovarian cancer treatment. The more favorable toxicity profile of single-agent carboplatin suggested that this drug may be a reasonable option as first-line chemotherapy for ovarian cancer. These results appear to be in contradiction with the results from the GOG protocol 111 and the OV10 trial that demonstrated that paclitaxel plus cisplatin was superior to cisplatin plus cyclophosphamide in terms of progression-free survival and overall survival. The reason for these discordant results remains controversial (350). The GOG continues to use paclitaxel plus carboplatin as the standard therapy for patients with advanced ovarian cancer, and all prospective randomized trials in previously untreated pa-

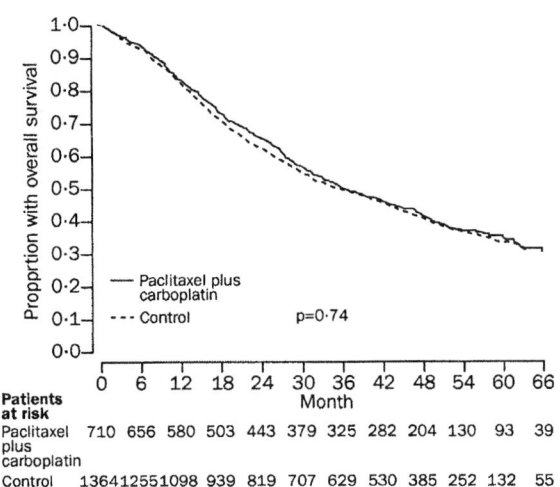

FIG. 25.26. Survival for 2074 ovarian cancer patients randomized to treatment with paclitaxel plus carboplatin or to a control of either single agent carboplatin or the three-drug PAC combination (cisplatin, doxorubicin, and cyclophosphamide). (From the International Collaborative Ovarian Neoplasm (ICON) Group. Paclitaxel plus carboplatin versus standard chemotherapy with either single-agent carboplatin or cyclophosphamide, doxorubicin, and cisplatin in women with ovarian cancer: the ICON3 randomised trial. *Lancet* 2002; 360:505–515. Reprinted with permission from Elsevier.)

tients with advanced ovarian cancer continue to use paclitaxel plus carboplatin as the control regimen.

Dose and Dose Intensity of Platinum and Paclitaxel

Despite the fact that platinum compounds have been clinically used in the treatment of ovarian cancer for almost two decades, questions still remain regarding the role of dose and dose intensity for these agents. A retrospective study of 33 published trials in ovarian cancer provided early evidence for the importance of cisplatin dose intensity expressed as milligrams per square meter per week (351). Doses of cisplatin beyond 100 mg/m^2 have been associated with unacceptable toxicity, primarily neurotoxicity. This has limited an in-depth prospective evaluation of the importance of clinical dose intensity. However, randomized trials have compared different platinum-dose intensities over a limited clinically relevant range (352–357). There was no advantage for higher dose intensity in the majority of these studies. The GOG trial was the largest, and 458 patients with bulky stages III and IV disease were randomized to receive either eight cycles of cisplatin (50 mg/m^2) plus cyclophosphamide (500 mg/m^2) every 3 weeks or four cycles of cisplatin (100 mg/m^2) plus cyclophosphamide (1,000 mg/m^2) every 3 weeks (355). The actual received dose intensity for the low-dose regimen was 0.95, and for the high-dose regimen, 1.90. There was no significant difference in overall response rate or survival in patients who received the regimen with the twofold increase in dose intensity. However, as expected, the high-dose regimen was associated with significantly more myelosuppression. Similarly, the large Italian trial also failed to demonstrate any improvement for patients who received a double-dose intensity of cisplatin. In the Gruppo Interegionale Coopartivo Oncologico Ginecologia (GICOG), 306 patients were randomized to either six cycles of cisplatin (356) (75 mg/m^2) every 3 weeks or nine cycles of cisplatin (84) (50 mg/m^2) every week. In these trials, the only variable was the dose intensity of cisplatin, with each regimen delivering the same total dose of drugs. Two other large randomized trials increased both the total dose and the dose intensity of cisplatin in the experimental arm. In the Gruppo Oncologico Nord-Ovest (GONO) trial (352), 145 patients with bulky disease were randomized to receive cisplatin at either 50 or 100 mg/m^2 every 4 weeks for six cycles with all patients receiving cyclophosphamide (600 mg/m^2) plus epirubicin (60 mg/m^2). There were no differences in response rate, progression-free survival, or overall survival. In contrast, the Scottish trial (354) randomized 159 patients with stages IC to IV disease to either high-dose (50 mg/m^2) or low-dose (100 mg/m^2) cisplatin every 3 weeks for six cycles with all patients receiving cyclophosphamide (750 mg/m^2) with each cisplatin administration. When the results were initially reported with a median follow-up of 127 weeks, the trial showed a highly significant difference in progression-free survival and overall survival in favor of the high-dose arm,

and the accrual ceased with a total of 191 patients being randomized. After a median follow-up of 4 years and 9 months, 159 patients with advanced ovarian cancer were dead. The overall survival for the high-dose and low-dose patients was 32.4% and 26.6%, respectively. With longer follow-up, there was a marked reduction in the overall benefit. However, toxicity, particularly neurotoxicity, was still evident in the fourth year in patients treated with a high-dose regimen, and the investigators recommended that the dose of cisplatin not be increased beyond 75 mg/m^2, representing a possible balance between efficacy and toxicity (357).

In two other trials, patients were randomized to different doses of carboplatin using AUC dosing. Gore et al. (358) reported on a trial by the London Gynecologic Oncology Group in which 227 patients with advanced ovarian cancer were randomized to carboplatin at an AUC of 6 for six courses or an AUC of 12 for four courses. Owing to the unacceptable toxicity of high-dose carboplatin, the received percentage total dose increase was only 20%. However, there was no difference in progression-free or overall survival between the two treatment arms. The overall survival rate at 5 years was 31% and 34%, respectively, for patients treated at an AUC of 6 or 12. Danish investigators randomized patients with advanced-stage ovarian cancer to receive carboplatin at an AUC of 4 or 8, with all patients receiving 500 mg/m^2 of cyclophosphamide with each cycle (359). There was no difference in the surgically confirmed complete remission rate (32% vs 30%), and, similarly, there was no significant difference in overall survival. These studies are consistent with retrospective studies correlating response with AUC, and indicate that there appears to be a plateau in response at an AUC of 4 to 6 (317).

Single-institution trials initially suggested that there was a steep dose-response relationship with paclitaxel dose in previously treated patients with advanced ovarian cancer. High-dose paclitaxel (250 mg/m^2) in an NCI study (360) resulted in a 48% to 50% response rate, which appeared to be superior to previous studies in which paclitaxel was used at a dose of 135 to 175 mg/m^2 with a resulting response rate of approximately 30%. However, in the European-Canadian trial in previously treated patients who were randomized in a bifactorial design to receive either 175 or 135 mg/m^2 of paclitaxel over either 24 or 3 hours, the response was only slightly higher (not statistically different) at 175 mg/m^2 (20%) compared to 135 mg/m^2 (15%) (342). Progression-free survival was, however, significantly longer in the high-dose group (19 vs 14 weeks) and response rates were similar in the 24- and 3-hour groups (19% vs 16%). Based on modest dose effect with longer time to progression, the dose of 175 mg/m^2 in a 3-hour infusion became the standard schedule for treatment of patients with recurrent disease. GOG investigators performed a randomized trial of a 24-hour infusion of paclitaxel at different doses in previously treated patients with advanced disease (361). For 271 patients with measurable disease, high-dose paclitaxel [250 mg/m^2 plus granulocyte colony-stimulating factor (G-CSF)] gave a higher response rate (36% vs 27%) than that for patients treated with 175 mg/m^2. However, progression-free survival and overall survival were similar. The median duration of overall survival was 13.1 months and 12.3 months for paclitaxel 175 and 250 mg/m^2, respectively. Despite cytokine support, high-dose paclitaxel is associated with increased platelet toxicity, anemia, neurotoxicity, and gastrointestinal toxicity. These prospective randomized trials suggest that there is, at best, a modest dose-response effect for paclitaxel in previously treated patients. A subsequent prospective randomized trial in previously untreated advanced ovarian cancer patients compared two different doses of paxlitaxel (175 vs 225 mg/m^2), with all patients receiving carboplatin at an AUC of 5. No improvement in survival was reported for the higher dose paxlitaxel regimen (362).

Fennelly et al. (363) performed a Phase I and pharmacologic study of paclitaxel administered weekly in patients with relapsed ovarian cancer. Maximum tolerated dose was 80 mg/m^2 in this heavily pretreated group of patients. Partial responses were observed in 30% of assessable patients including patients with progressive disease on a standard 3-week paclitaxel schedule. The weekly paclitaxel was associated with less toxicity, particularly alopecia. Subsequent Phase II trials have evaluated higher doses of weekly paxlitaxel (80 mg/m^2) and reported response rates of 32% to 47% in platinum-refractory patients (364,365).

Treatment of Patients Following Induction Chemotherapy

The optimum management of patients with advanced ovarian cancer following an induction course of chemotherapy remains to be determined and is an area of active clinical investigation. Approximately two-thirds of patients with advanced ovarian cancer will achieve a clinical complete remission following chemotherapy, that is, no evidence of disease on physical examination or in radiographic studies, together with a serum CA-125 level in the normal range. However, only one-third of all patients with advanced ovarian cancer will be disease free at a second-look laparotomy following cisplatin-based chemotherapy. As previously described, the most important prognostic factor that influences the likelihood of achieving a surgically confirmed complete remission is the volume of disease at the time chemotherapy was initiated. Patients who have suboptimal disease have a four- to fivefold decreased likelihood of achieving a complete remission as compared to those patients who were optimally cytoreduced. In addition, patients with large-volume disease who do achieve a complete remission have a higher likelihood of a subsequent relapse than do patients with small-volume disease. At least 50% of all patients who do achieve a surgically confirmed complete remission will ultimately experience recurrence (366–368). In the GOG study (369) of intraperitoneal radioactive phosphorus versus ob-

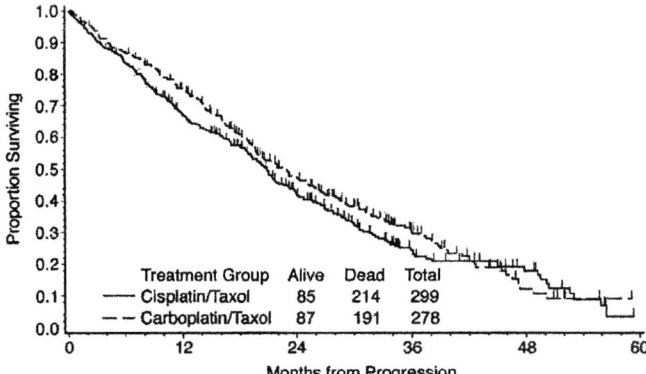

FIG. 25.27. Survival from time of recurrence for optimal stage III patients who were treated on GOG protocol 158 with either cisplatin/Taxol or carboplatin/Taxol. (From Ozols RF, Bundy BN, Greer BE, et al. Phase III trial of carboplatin and paclitaxel compared with cisplatin and paclitaxel in patients with optimally resected stage III ovarian cancer: a Gynecologic Oncology Group study. *J Clin Oncol* 2003;21:3194–3200. Reprinted with permission from the American Society of Clinical Oncology.)

servation, 64% of patients who achieved a surgically confirmed complete remission relapsed (median follow-up 63 months).

The survival of patients who recur after a complete remission is poor. Although some patients will benefit from second-line therapy, <10% will achieve a clinical complete remission, and the median survival is less than 1 year. Figure 25.27 depicts survival of optimal stage III patients who were treated with either six cycles of carboplatin plus paclitaxel or cisplatin plus paclitaxel (346). Median survival after progression is less than 2 years, and there is no evidence for curative potential after relapse, although the prolonged median survival suggests that treatment after progression may extend survival.

Maintenance Therapy and Consolidation

As previously noted, most patients with advanced ovarian cancer achieve a clinical complete remission after cytoreductive surgery and combination chemotherapy. However, the majority of these patients experience disease recurrence. Consequently, an effective consolidation of maintenance therapy that would prevent recurrences after clinical complete remission could have a potentially greater impact on survival in patients with advanced ovarian cancer. Consolidation therapy and maintence therapy have been studied in a series of clinical trials after induction chemotherapy. Consolidation therapies are focused on short-term treatments that have included high-dose chemotherapy with stem-cell transplant, whole abdominal radiation therapy, or intraperitoneal administration of ^{32}P or antibodies conjugated with a variety of radioisotopes. The results of the GOG trial comparing intraperitoneal radioactive phosphorus (^{32}P) versus observation after negative second-look laparotomy for advanced-stage ovarian cancer have recently been reported (369). Two hundred two eligible patients were randomly selected to receive either 15 mCi IP ^{32}P (n = 104) or no further therapy (n = 98). There was no difference in tumor recurrence rate (65%) in the IP ^{32}P group and in the observation arm (64%). There was also no statistically significant difference in overall survival (p = .19); relative risk of death 0.85, 90% CI 0.62 to 1.16. Despite a complete pathologic remission following second-look laparotomy after initial surgery and chemotherapy with a platinum-based regimen, 61% of stage III ovarian cancer patients had tumor recurrence within 5 years of a negative second-look laparotomy. The results of the randomized trial from the Swedish-Norwegian Ovarian Cancer Study Group (370) consolidation treatment with radiotherapy are discussed below. Currently, no form of consolidation radiation has been shown statistically to improve overall survival, and the toxicities of whole abdominal radiation limit potential future studies.

Curie et al. (371) conducted a prospective randomized trial of high-dose chemotherapy and peripheral blood stem-cell support as consolidation in patients with responsive, low-burden, advanced ovarian cancer. One hundred ten patients were randomized to receive high-dose therapy with carboplatin and cyclophosphamide or three cycles of conventional dose maintenance therapy. There was an 11-month improvement in median disease-free survival for patients receiving the high-dose chemotherapy. A multivariate analysis identified a selective population of young women with chemosensitive advanced disease and small residual disease at second-look surgery in whom high-dose consolidation chemotherapy resulted in a significantly improved disease-free survival compared to conventional dose maintenance. This and other trials have failed to demonstrate any improvement in overall survival for high-dose chemotherapy with stem-cell support.

Maintenance therapies have focused on prolonged administration of single-agent chemotherapy (372–375), extended cycles of induction chemotherapy (376–378), intraperitoneal chemotherapy (379), hormonal therapy, immunotherapy, including interferon (380), vaccines targeting CA-125 (381), radioimmunoconjugates (382,383), and matrix metalloproteinase inhibitors (384). No randomized control trial of maintenance therapy has been shown to extend survival in patients with advanced ovarian cancer (although some studies are still in progress).

Several studies have further explored the use of maintenance intravenous chemotherapy in patients achieving a clinical complete remission. A SWOG/GOG study demonstrated that 12 cycles of intravenous paclitaxel (175 mg/m^2) administered every 28 days to women in clinical complete remission following induction chemotherapy with a platinum plus paclitaxel–based regimen resulted in a 7-month improvement in median progression-free survival compared with those who received three cycles of paclitaxel (372). This

trial was discontinued at a time when there was a statistically significant improvement in time to progression but no difference in overall survival between the treatment arms (Fig. 25.28). A survival comparison will not be possible since patients assigned to three cycles of therapy were permitted the option of receiving an additional nine cycles of treatment when the study was closed, and with the early closure, insufficient patients were randomized ever to detect a survival difference. Maintenance therapy for 12 months was also associated with significantly more toxicity compared to treatment with three cycles of treatment. Additional trials of maintenance paclitaxel are also in progress in Europe.

The preliminary results of European trials of maintenance topotecan have recently been reported.(374,375). Over 1,300 patients with advanced ovarian cancer who responded to intial chemotherapy were randomized to observation or four cycles of monthly topotecan. No significant difference in progression-free survival or overall survival was observed for patients receiving topotecan. A previous European study had also demonstrated that maintenace therapy with epirubicin (387) did not improve survival in patients who achieved a clinical complete remission following platinum-based induction chemotherapy. At this point, no consolidation or maintenance therapy can be routinely recommended for patients achieving a clinical complete remission following induction therapy. It is possible that gene expression arrays may identify subsets of patients with advanced ovarian cancer in whom chemotherapy or molecular-targeted therapies may prove to be an effective maintenance strategy. Such trials should also incorporate formal quality of life assessments, with both progression-free survival and overall survival being primary endpoints (385,386).

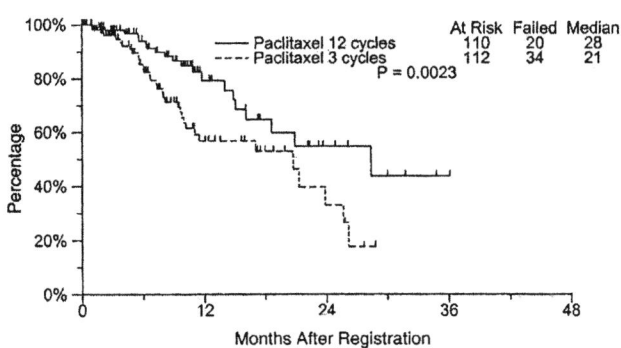

FIG. 25.28. Progression-free survival of patients treated with either 3 monthly cycles or 12 monthly cycles of paclitaxel as maintenance therapy of advanced stage ovarian cancer patients who were in a clinical complete remission after platinum/paclitaxel-based chemotherapy. (From Markman M, Liu PY, Wilczynski S, et al. Phase III randomized trial of 12 versus 3 months of maintenance paclitaxel in patients with advanced ovarian cancer after complete response to platinum and paclitaxel-based chemotherapy: a Southwest Oncology Group and Gynecologic Oncology Group Trial. *J Clin Oncol* 2003; 21:2460–2465. Reprinted with permission from the American Society of Clinical Oncology.)

FOLLOW-UP OF PATIENTS IN REMISSION

Most patients with ovarian cancer who enter a clinical complete remission have been followed with a combination of pelvic examinations, computerized abdominal tomograms, and monitoring of serum CA-125 levels. A rising serum CA-125 level can indicate tumor progression many months prior to clinical evidence of recurrence. The appropriate management of an asymptomatic patient following induction chemotherapy who has a rising CA-125 level without other evidence of disease remains undetermined. Although it is theoretically advantageous to reinstitute chemotherapy at the time of lowest tumor burden, there is no evidence that initiating chemotherapy for a rising CA-125 level will improve survival. A rising CA-125 in a patient with a clinical complete remission accurately predicts for recurrence in over 95% of patients (388). The median lead time before other manifestations of disease progression in the literature has been 35 months (389). However, a significant proportion of patients (approximately 30%) may have lead times of greater than 6 months. A prospective randomized trial is in progress to determine whether early institution of second-line treatment at the time the patient has a rising CA-125 produces an improvement in disease-free and overall survival, as well as an enhancement in quality of life, compared to treatment at the time of a symptomatic recurrence or at the time the patient develops measurable disease radiologically or on physical examination. Since the primary goal in recurrent disease is palliation, some investigators recommend tamoxifen for use in asymptomatic women with a rising CA-125 level in the absence of detectable disease (390). Frequent measurements of serum CA-125 levels in women who are asymptomatic and in a clinical complete remission are a source of patient anxiety since the prognostic significance of disease recurrence is well known. Similarly, frequent CT scans of the pelvis and abdomen have also not been shown to be a cost-effective measure in decreasing symptoms or in improving survival. Similarly, there currently is no established role for the use of indium 111 satumomab pendetide in the monitoring of patients who achieve a clinical complete remission or who have elevated CA-125 levels without other evidence of disease. Immunoscintigraphy with this indium-labeled monoclonal antibody can detect recurrences of ovarian cancer but has a 17% false-positive rate (391).

In premenopausal women with ovarian cancer, the initial staging and cytoreductive laparotomy results in a surgical castration. Consequently, these women frequently experience hot flashes, and those who do achieve long-term survival are at increased risk for osteoporosis and heart disease. Since some ovarian cancer cells have estrogen and progesterone receptors, there has been concern regarding the use of hormone replacement therapy in this patient population. A retrospective study from the United Kingdom failed to demonstrate that hormone replacement therapy had a detrimental effect on the prognosis of patients with ovarian cancer who are under 50 years of age at the time of diagnosis (392). In the absence of a prospective, randomized, controlled clinical trial, hormone replacement therapy can be administered to premenopausal women with ovarian cancer following surgery and chemotherapy if they have severe vasomotor symptoms, although, as previously discussed, recent data have identified an association of ovarian cancer risk and exogenous hormone administration. If hormonal therapy is administered, it may be prudent to limit the duration as much as possible.

SECOND-LOOK PROCEDURES

Laparotomy and Laparoscopy

Patients with advanced ovarian cancer have frequently undergone abdominal explorations after induction chemotherapy. However, although surgery is necessary to assess the response to therapy accurately and is often required for management of intestinal obstruction, there is no evidence that any type of surgical procedure after initial chemotherapy prolongs overall survival. The term *second-look laparotomy* has been incorrectly used to refer to several distinctly different types of surgery. These include secondary operations to resect known residual or recurrent disease and secondary operations performed for relief of cancer-related symptoms, such as intestinal obstruction. In current usage, the term should be reserved for a systematic surgical exploration in asymptomatic patients who have completed a planned course of chemotherapy for ovarian cancer. Following initial cytoreductive surgery, many patients with ovarian cancer will have no measurable disease at the time they begin chemotherapy and will remain free of detectable tumor during their entire chemotherapeutic treatment. In that circumstance, objective assessment of response to treatment by repeat laparotomy can define the response to treatment.

In 1966, during an era when single-agent alkylating therapy for advanced ovarian cancer was standard, Rutledge and Burns (393) reported on 288 patients treated with melphalan and asked the question: Should laparotomy be used more often when a patient has an unusually good response to determine whether the drug should be discontinued? In their report, 28 patients underwent surgery for this reason; 12 had no tumor detected. The investigators felt that ''good response to the drugs is the reason for laparotomy,'' but pointed out that patients with a negative reexploration may relapse, as did two in their series (395). Interest in second-look laparotomy as a means of determining when chemotherapy could be discontinued was stimulated during the 1970s, when reports began to appear linking the long-term use of alkylating agents to the development of acute leukemia (394,395).

With the introduction of platinum-based chemotherapy in the mid to late 1970s and the use of aggressive primary debulking, up to 50% of patients treated with chemotherapy for advanced cancer had no clinically detectable tumor at the completion of their chemotherapy. Since it was known that many of these women harbored occult residual cancer, a number of investigators tested noninvasive methods of detecting such disease. Imaging techniques such as CT, sonography, and MRI are generally unable to detect intraperitoneal tumor masses smaller than 1 to 2 cm and, in fact, may miss much larger masses (396). Some investigators (397) have suggested that the cytologic analysis of peritoneal fluid obtained by culdocentesis may be a means of assessing response in women under treatment for ovarian cancer. The accuracy of this technique in detecting residual disease is quite low, however. In a recent study of 96 women reexplored for ovarian cancer who had multiple cytologic washings taken at the time of laparotomy, only 34% of patients with biopsy-proven gross intraperitoneal disease had positive washings (398). In patients with only microscopic disease, 28% had positive washings.

Several groups have used laparoscopy as an alternative to second-look laparotomy. In 1981, Berek et al. (399) reported 119 consecutive laparoscopic examinations performed in 57 patients. Fourteen percent of their patients had major complications requiring laparotomy, most of which involved bowel perforation. At the NCI, laparoscopy was routinely used to assess response to chemotherapy (400). In their series, no patient required a surgical exploration because of a laparoscopy complication. In 66 restaging laparoscopies, residual tumor was found in 33 (50%) and provided the only evidence for disease in 24 cases (36%). These latter patients were spared an unnecessary second-look laparotomy. However, if the laparoscopy was negative, residual disease was documented in 55% of patients at laparotomy.

More recently, the group from the Memorial Sloan–Kettering Cancer Center has reported their experience with the use of laparoscopy for second-look evaluation in 150 patients with advanced ovarian cancer following chemotherapy (401). The majority of patients (87%) had stage III or IV disease at initial surgery; the remainder were stage II or unstaged. Eighty-two patients (54%) had optimal cytoreduction at the time of their initial surgery. All patients had completed primary chemotherapy and were clinically disease free based on imaging studies and CA-125 levels at the time of second look. Sixty-nine patients (46%) were found to have pathologically negative second looks; thus, the rate of positive second-look evaluations was 54%. The rate of conversion to laparotomy was 18 of 150 (12%). In three cases, this was secondary to bowel injury; one patient sustained a bladder injury; the remainder of conversions to laparotomy were for secondary cytoreduction. There was only one case in which the patient was found to have extensive adhesions and laparoscopy was abandoned. The overall rate of major complications was 2.7%. Although long-term follow-up is not available, the rate of negative evaluations and the rate of recurrences in patients with negative second looks appear

to be equivalent to those described in studies of second-look assessment by laparotomy.

Serum tumor markers, in particular CA-125, have been proven to be clinically useful in monitoring the course of ovarian cancer, and this has led to studies assessing their accuracy in patients with clinical complete remissions in an effort to obviate the need for surgical reassessment in ovarian cancer patients. Although an elevated CA-125 level is highly accurate as an indicator of persistent disease, numerous studies have shown that, even with a normal serum CA-125 level, a significant number of patients in clinical complete remission will have residual disease at laparotomy. Rubin et al. (402) measured CA-125 levels at the time of secondary surgery in 96 ovarian cancer patients, all of whom had had documentation of an elevated CA-125 level at the time when the tumor was first diagnosed and were, therefore, "marker-positive." Persistent disease was found in 62% of patients who had a normal CA-125 level at the time of surgery. These findings have been confirmed in other studies (403). Consequently, if the primary purpose of the second-look laparotomy is to determine whether the patient has residual ovarian cancer, an elevated CA-125 level makes such a procedure unnecessary.

A second-look laparotomy itself is intended as a thorough reexploration of the peritoneal cavity and selected retroperitoneal structures. Immediately prior to surgery, a pelvic examination under anesthesia is performed. Cystoscopy and proctoscopy may be useful in symptomatic patients or in those with prior tumor involvement of the bladder or lower gastrointestinal tract.

The abdomen should be entered through a generous vertical excision, extending from the pubic symphysis to well above the umbilicus. If obvious tumor is found, frozen-section confirmation should be obtained. The goal of the operation becomes removal of as much tumor as possible. If no obvious tumor is found, the surgeon must undertake a meticulous, systematic search for areas of occult tumor. Saline washings are obtained from multiple sites within the peritoneal cavity, usually including the pelvis, both paracolic gutters, and the undersurfaces of both hemidiaphragms. All adhesions should be lysed and portions submitted for histologic analysis since adhesions often form at the site of tumor nodules. The upper abdomen should be explored carefully, with any suspicious areas biopsied. The residual omentum should be palpated, as should the aortic lymph nodes. The intestines must be carefully examined. A thorough exploration of the pelvic cavity is performed. Throughout this evaluation, particular attention should be paid to areas where residual disease was left at the initial operation. If suspicious areas are identified, frozen-section confirmation should be obtained and areas of tumor resected as completely as possible.

If no tumor is identified, a series of biopsies is performed from areas that may harbor occult disease. The stumps of the infundibulopelvic ligaments, which carry the ovarian blood and lymphatic supplies, should be identified in the

TABLE 25.15. *Findings at second-look laparotomy from 71 combined series*

Finding	Number	%
No tumor found	2,417	47
Tumor found	2,773	53
Total	5,190	100

Modified with permission from Barter JF, Barnes WA. Second-look laparotomy. In: Rubin SC, Sutton GP, eds. *Ovarian cancer*. New York: McGraw-Hill, 1993:269–300.

TABLE 25.17. *Findings at second-look laparotomy by extent of residual disease following primary cytoreduction*

Residual	No. negative	Total patients	% negative
None	331	460	72
Optimal[a]	330	655	50
Suboptimal[a]	158	682	23

[a] Original investigator's definition.

Modified with permission from Barter JF, Barnes WA. Second-look laparotomy. In: Rubin SC, Sutton GP, eds. *Ovarian cancer*. New York: McGraw-Hill, 1993:269–300.

retroperitoneum and biopsied. Other surgical pedicles in the pelvis should be examined and biopsied if suspicious. If the uterus was not removed at the initial operation, hysterectomy should be performed. Peritoneal biopsies should be taken from multiple sites within the abdominal cavity, including the pelvis, paracolic gutters, and both hemidiaphragms. Some have suggested the use of a laparoscope or sterile proctoscope to facilitate inspection of the diaphragms. Any remaining areas of omentum should be removed. Many surgeons remove the appendix if present. Paraaortic and pelvic lymph nodes should be thoroughly sampled. A second-look operation at which no tumor is identified will take several hours and will produce 20 to 30 individual biopsy specimens.

Over the last 10 years, there have been many published series on second-look laparotomy. Table 25.15 summarizes several reports in which about 55% of the patients with no clinical evidence of disease were found to have cancer present at reexploration (404). These findings are a clear indication of our current inability to identify persistent cancer by noninvasive means.

Several clinical and histologic factors have been shown to relate to the likelihood of tumor being found at the time of second-look laparotomy. The most important factors are stage and the volume of tumor remaining following initial cytoreductive surgery. As shown in Table 25.16, patients with stages III and IV disease had a substantially lower proportion of negative second-look operations than did those with stages I and II, 33% versus 70% to 80%, respectively.

The amount of residual disease remaining following the initial operation for ovarian cancer is also a major determinant of the likelihood of disease being found at the time

of second-look laparotomy. Table 25.17 summarizes pooled data on 2,616 patients, providing information on the relationship of the extent of residual disease following primary surgery to findings at second look. Patients with suboptimal residual disease after primary surgery had only a 23% likelihood of a negative second look as compared to 50% for those with optimum residual and 72% in those with no known residual tumor. Many series have included stage I patients in their analysis of the effect of residual disease on findings at second-look laparotomy. As all stage I patients would be included in the no-residual disease group, this would account, in part, for the improved prognosis of this group. Even considering this bias, there seems to be a strong correlation between extent of residual disease and the likelihood of finding disease at reexploration.

The histologic grade of the tumor, as distinct from the cell type, has been shown to be a significant prognostic factor, although it has been suggested that, in advanced-stage patients treated with platinum-containing chemotherapy, grade may be of less importance. Numerous series have correlated the surgical findings at a reexploration with tumor grade (Table 25.18). Earlier series demonstrated a stronger relationship between grade and second-look findings, perhaps because more of the patients in these series were treated with chemotherapeutic regimens that did not contain platinum. Overall, women with poorly differentiated tumors seem to have a somewhat lower chance of having a negative second-look laparotomy, although it should be remembered that these data are not controlled for other important prognostic variables, including stage and the amount of residual tumor.

Second-look laparotomy is a highly invasive diagnostic procedure that results in significant expense, discomfort, and

TABLE 25.16. *Findings at second-look laparotomy related to stage of disease from 31 combined series*

Stage	No. negative	Total patients	% negative
I	268	331	81
II	190	276	69
III	441	1,120	39
IV	59	177	33

Modified with permission from Barter JF, Barnes WA. Second-look laparotomy. In: Rubin SC, Sutton GP, eds. *Ovarian cancer*. New York: McGraw-Hill, 1993:269–300.

TABLE 25.18. *Findings at second-look laparotomy related to histologic grade*

Grade	No. negative	Total patients	% negative
1	163	283	58
2	167	389	43
3	259	619	42

Modified with permission from Barter JF, Barnes WA. Second-look laparotomy. In: Rubin SC, Sutton GP, eds. *Ovarian cancer*. New York: McGraw-Hill, 1993:269–300.

time in the hospital for the patient; however, it is associated with little serious medical morbidity. Although many reports on second-look surgery have not discussed complications, among seven major series published since 1980 that specifically report complications, no deaths were seen in 682 operations (229). The most common complications were infections of the surgical wound (6.3%), the urinary tract (5.6%), and the lungs (2.8%).

Our understanding of the prognostic significance of the findings at second-look laparotomy has evolved significantly in recent years. The finding of large-volume residual tumor carries a grave prognosis. In some series, when survival is reported separately for patients with gross tumor, approximately 80% died within 3 years of second-look laparotomy. Patients who have only microscopic disease detected at second look fare considerably better. Copeland et al. (405) reported on 50 patients with microscopic disease followed for a median of 40 months from second look. Survival rates were 96% and 71% at 2 and 5 years, respectively.

Because even the most carefully performed second-look operation may miss microscopic areas of tumor and because ovarian cancer may occasionally spread beyond the areas assessed at surgery, a negative second-look operation is not synonymous with cure of cancer. Papers reporting the incidence of recurrence following negative second-look laparotomy have often included patients treated with different chemotherapeutic regimens for variable durations and followed for relatively short periods of time. This has made the true incidence of and the risk factors for recurrence following negative second-look laparotomy difficult to determine. In a prior review that included 12 reports published from 1980 to 1986, it was calculated that the overall recurrence rate was 18%, including 10.9% in stages I and II and 26% for patients with stage III or IV disease (229). In 1988, Rubin et al. (406) reported a 50% risk of recurrence following a negative second-look laparotomy in patients treated with platinum-based chemotherapy. A multivariate analysis demonstrated that stage, histologic grade, and extent of residual disease remaining after primary cytoreduction were significant predictors of recurrence following a negative second look. Patients who do recur have a poor prognosis, and few, if any, can be cured by currently available salvage therapies. As will be discussed, patients who have a prolonged disease-free interval (>12 months) have a 30% to 50% likelihood of responding to second-line therapy. Some patients will have a prolonged secondary response, although only a few patients will have a response to second-line therapy that lasts longer than 12 months.

There is presently no evidence that any type of additional therapy can improve survival in patients who do achieve a surgically confirmed complete remission (see section on Maintenance Therapy and Consolidation above). There is also no evidence that second-look laparotomy per se is a therapeutic procedure (366). Although there are no prospective trials in which patients in a clinical complete remission

have been randomized either to a second-look operation or to medical follow-up, retrospective studies comparing the survival of patients who underwent a second-look laparotomy versus patients in whom a second-look was not performed have failed to show any difference in survival. Consequently, it has been proposed that a second-look laparotomy no longer be considered a routine procedure in patients who achieve a complete remission.

An alternative to second-look laparotomy is second-look laparoscopy. A second-look laparoscopy is usually performed as a same-day procedure with patients being discharged home the day of surgery or 1 day postoperatively. It remains the most accurate test to determine disease status and allows for insertion of intraperitoneal catheters if intraperitoneal chemotherapy is considered. With modern laparoscopic techniques, a second-look laparoscopy provides excellent visualization and access to the peritoneal and extraperitoneal spaces where ovarian cancer may be detected. The laparoscopic approach is associated with less operating time, fewer complications, less blood loss, fewer or less costly hospital charges, and shorter hospitalization than laparotomy. The majority of cases can be completed by the laparoscopic approach, with approximately 10% to 15% of cases requiring conversion to laparotomy to complete the procedure satisfactorily. If a second-look operation is planned, the laparoscopic approach should be considered as the initial step as it may provide all the necessary information and avoid the potential morbidity and hospitalization associated with the open approach.

Recent data from GOG protocol 158, comparing carboplatin and paclitaxel versus cisplatin and paclitaxel in optimal residual stage III ovarian cancer patients, have a bearing on the issue of second-look laparotomy (346). Although not randomly allocated to a second look, almost 400 patients (50%) in this study elected the procedure. Approximately half of the patients had no evidence of disease at second-look laparotomy. Patients with residual disease at the second look underwent a variety of treatments with the majority of patients receiving more systemic chemotherapy with paclitaxel and carboplatin. There was no difference in progression-free or overall survival between the patients electing second-look laparotomy and those declining the procedure and treated only at the time of clinical progression. The group with the pathologically documented complete remission had better overall survival than the group with residual disease at the second look. Consequently, the potential value of a second-look surgery to identify patients who could potentially benefit from treatment of residual disease was not substantiated in this study. Given the fact that many of these patients who had optimal residual disease following their initial surgery had no disease or only small-volume disease found at the second look, relatively few, if any, would be expected to benefit from secondary cytoreduction during the operation. The usefulness of a second-look laparotomy to assess the results of therapy accurately in the setting of a clinical trial is unequivocal. However, in a nonclinical trial situation, there appears to be little justification for a second-look laparotomy merely to obtain prognostic information. If, on the other hand, therapeutic decisions will be based upon findings at second look, such a procedure may be justified. However, the patient must be aware that there is no evidence that any form of subsequent therapy has been shown to significantly prolong survival. These observations are consistent with the recommendations from the NIH Consensus Conference (Final Statement, NIH Consensus Development Conference on Ovarian Cancer, Bethesda, 1994) (5).

Secondary Cytoreductive Surgery

The benefit of secondary cytoreductive operations in ovarian cancer, at the time of second-look laparotomy or otherwise, has not been clearly demonstrated. Since about one-half of patients who do undergo second-look laparotomy will have disease found, and in about 80% of these patients macroscopic disease will be present, approximately 40% of all patients having second-look laparotomy are candidates for secondary cytoreduction. Technically, secondary cytoreduction can be accomplished, with reported success rates ranging from 24% to 84% (408–411). There is less information available, however, on the effect of secondary cytoreduction on survival. Chambers et al. (412) concluded that residual tumor size following secondary cytoreduction did not influence survival after comparing 23 patients with microscopic residual disease and 6 with macroscopic disease. Luesley et al. (409) found no survival benefit in patients cytoreduced to microscopic disease compared to patients with residual macroscopic disease or small-volume gross residual disease. On the other hand, Podratz et al. (413) reported an actuarial 4-year survival rate of 55% in patients with microscopic residual disease compared to 19% for those with macroscopic disease. In a series reported by Hoskins et al. (410), patients cytoreduced to microscopic residual disease at the time of the second look had a 5-year survival of 51%. This was similar to the survival of patients found to have only microscopic disease at the second look, and was significantly better than the survival in patients left with gross disease. Lippman et al. (414) examined the effect of extensive tumor resection at second-look laparotomy on survival for patients with >2 cm gross residual disease. Patients undergoing optimum resection (<2 cm residual tumor) had a significantly better survival than those undergoing suboptimal resection, suggesting that there is a survival benefit associated with optimal cytoreduction at second-look laparotomy.

Segna et al. (411) reported on 100 patients with advanced ovarian cancer initially treated with cisplatin-based therapy who were explored at the time of recurrence. Sixty-one percent of patients were left with optimal (<2 cm) disease after secondary cytoreduction. These patients had a significant improvement in their median survival compared with pa-

tients with suboptimal residual disease (27 vs 9 months, $p = .0001$). It appears that, in patients whose tumors remain sensitive to chemotherapy, cytoreduction to small-volume disease prior to secondary chemotherapy can be of benefit. However, there has been no prospective comparative trial assessing the survival impact of secondary cytoreductive surgery in this setting.

PALLIATIVE SURGERY

For the majority of women with ovarian cancer, the disease eventually progresses within the abdominal cavity. Such tumor growth often produces compromise of the intestinal lumen, leading to intestinal obstruction that requires hospitalization for intravenous hydration and decompression of the intestinal tract. Since these patients generally have no impairment of other vital organ systems, they are often completely alert and in little or no pain. If conservative measures fail to result in relief of the obstruction, the patient and her physician must then confront a difficult decision: prolonged in-hospital (or at-home) intravenous hydration and gastric decompression, or an attempt at surgical relief of the obstruction. In making this decision, one must consider a number of factors, including the patient's overall physical condition, the current status of her cancer and future therapeutic options, the site of the intestinal obstruction, and the extent of her prior therapy, including prior surgical procedures, intraperitoneal chemotherapy, and radiation therapy. A number of investigators have attempted to identify clinical factors that would allow selection of patients unlikely to benefit from surgery for intestinal obstruction so that these women might be saved exploration. Krebs and Goplerud (415) identified a series of variables, including advanced age, poor nutritional status, the presence of palpable tumor masses, the presence of ascites, and a history of previous radiation therapy to the pelvis or whole abdomen, that were associated with a poor outcome. Other studies (414) have reported that the serum albumin level, nutritional status, and the amount of residual ovarian cancer at the completion of bowel obstruction surgery were significantly associated with postoperative survival. On the other hand, in one study (416), no clinical features could be identified that would predict operability or survival following surgery. These differences may be accounted for, in part, by variation in patient selection and preoperative and postoperative care.

The site of intestinal obstruction in ovarian cancer patients is most commonly the small intestine. If the patient is felt to be an operative candidate, consideration should be given to the use of preoperative total parenteral nutrition to improve the patient's nutritional status and decrease the risk of perioperative complications related to malnutrition. Total parenteral nutrition is generally not indicated in patients in whom no surgery is planned. In a series of 54 operations performed for intestinal obstruction in ovarian cancer patients, Rubin et al. (417) reported that the site of obstruction was in the small intestine in 44%, the large intestine in 33%, and involved both small and large intestines in the remaining 22% of cases. A definitive surgical procedure for relief of obstruction was performed in 79% of the patients in this series; the remaining patients were explored and judged to be inoperable. Among the patients undergoing a definitive procedure, about 80% were discharged from the hospital with restoration of intestinal function sufficient to allow a regular or low-residue diet. The mean postsurgical survival among these patients was 6.8 months. In a more recent report from the Memorial Sloan–Kettering Cancer Center (418), the investigators retrospectively reviewed all patients undergoing surgery for intestinal obstruction due to recurrent ovarian cancer from 1994 to 1999. During the study period, 68 operations were performed on 64 patients. The mean time from original diagnosis of ovarian cancer to obstruction was 2.8 years. Surgical correction (intestinal surgery performed for relief of obstruction) was attained in 57 of 68 (84%) cases. Successful palliation (the ability to tolerate a regular or low-residue diet at least 60 days postoperatively) was achieved in 71% of cases in which surgical correction was possible. The rate of major surgical morbidity was 22%. There was one death from pulmonary embolus and one from peritonitis. Two other deaths occurred because of progression of disease, for an overall perioperative mortality rate of 6%. Postoperative chemotherapy was administered in 45 of 57 (79%) cases in which surgical correction was possible. The median survival of the entire cohort was 8 months. If surgery resulted in successful palliation, median survival was 11.6 versus 3.9 months for all other patients. Although survival is relatively brief, by restoring intestinal function, at least temporarily, these patients can leave the hospital and enjoy an improved quality of life for their remaining months. In the absence of criteria that clearly predict operability, survival, and quality of life following surgery for intestinal obstruction in ovarian cancer patients, an active surgical approach should remain a management option. For patients who are deemed to be unsuitable for surgical exploration or found to be inoperable at exploration, gastrostomy, which can usually be accomplished percutaneously, offers a more comfortable alternative to prolonged nasogastric drainage (418).

MANAGEMENT OF ASCITES

Ascites is a common finding at the time of initial presentation in patients with advanced ovarian cancer. Generally, ascites does not produce any significant discomfort or respiratory embarrassment. Although the fluid may reaccumulate in the days following initial surgery, once chemotherapy is begun, it usually resolves quickly. In the occasional patient in whom massive ascites causes respiratory compromise, either before or after surgery, paracentesis may be performed safely for temporary relief prior to the initiation of chemotherapy. Cruikshank and Buchsbaum (419), using hemo-

dynamic monitoring, showed that large quantities of ascites can be rapidly removed from ovarian cancer patients without untoward effects. This also appears to have little significant effect on serum proteins. The failure of ascites to resolve after the initiation of chemotherapy or its reappearance later in the course of treatment is an indication of lack of response to treatment and a grave prognostic sign.

Although the majority of patients with advanced ovarian cancer will eventually experience progression of disease, most do not develop clinically significant ascites. For those who do, therapeutic options are limited. Instillation of bleomycin into the peritoneal cavity as a nonspecific sclerotic agent has been reported but has been minimally effective in ovarian cancer (420,421). Experience with implanted peritoneovenous shunts has been poor, with a significant rate of blockage and the risk of embolization and implantation of tumor cells (422). In the absence of effective therapy for the patient's underlying cancer, it is usually not possible to control ascites other than on a temporary basis.

RADIATION THERAPY

The use of radiation therapy in the management of ovarian cancer continues to be controversial despite data supporting its use. Controversy arises as a result of several factors, including the early use of inappropriate techniques and doses of radiation and the selection of inappropriate patients for such therapy.

In the past decade, refinements in our knowledge of the possible benefits of radiation therapy in ovarian cancer have been achieved. The extensive analysis of the prognostic factors predicting for long-term survival after radiation therapy has allowed better definition of the subgroups of patients in whom it is appropriate to use radiation as the first-line postoperative modality of treatment with curative intent.

Pivotal to the use of curative radiation in ovarian cancer is a recognition that ovarian cancer has a dominant route of dissemination throughout the peritoneal cavity, and that tumor remains confined to the abdominal cavity for extended periods of time. In fact, at first relapse, regardless of therapy, tumor is confined to the abdominal cavity in the vast majority of patients. Thus, for radiation to be of curative benefit, techniques that encompass the whole peritoneal cavity, rather than just the pelvis or lower abdomen alone, are likely to be most beneficial. Several studies have compared treatment using abdominopelvic radiation therapy with pelvic radiation therapy alone or combined with single-agent alkylating chemotherapy (423,424). These studies demonstrate a superior outcome using abdominopelvic radiation therapy for patients with minimal residual disease after primary surgery.

The dose of radiation that can be delivered safely to the upper abdomen is considerably lower than that which would be considered optimal and sufficient for the successful treatment of solid tumors. The efficacy of radiation in eradicating

TABLE 25.19. *Whole abdomen radiation in patients with residual disease*

Study endpoint (ref.)	Volume of residual disease prior to radiation	
	<2 cm	>2 cm
Percent 10-yr RFR (424)	38%	6%
Percent 15-yr FFR (425)	50%	14%
Percent 10-yr RFS (426)	62%	0%
Percent 10-yr survival (427)	42%	10%
Surviving fraction at 6 yrs (428)	0.41	
Percent 9-yr RFR (429)	62%	8%

RFR, relapse-free rate; FFR, failure-free rate; RFS, relapse-free survival.

residual tumors is dependent on the number of clonogenic cells present. Thus, the limitations imposed by the tolerance of the normal tissues in the abdomen, particularly the gastrointestinal tract, imply that whole abdominal irradiation would produce a modest improvement in tumor control in the upper abdomen, but this benefit would be seen only in patients with small numbers of residual clonogenic cells or microscopic disease residuum in the upper abdomen. Clinical trials have supported that conclusion. There is little or no curative potential for abdominal irradiation in patients with bulky disease in the upper abdomen (Table 25.19).

Choice of Radiation Technique

Several techniques for delivering radiation to the entire peritoneal cavity have been developed. The two most commonly used are the moving-strip technique, in which a small part of the abdomen is irradiated daily sequentially, and the open-field technique, in which the whole volume is treated daily. The moving-strip technique was initiated in an era when radiation therapy equipment could not adequately encompass the large volumes required in one portal. It was justified because a biologically higher dose could be delivered sequentially to the smaller volumes than could be delivered simultaneously to the whole volume in the open-field technique. The duration of the entire treatment course, however, using the moving-strip technique was approximately twice that of the open-field technique. Theoretically, the prolonged treatment course might allow accelerated proliferation of tumor (430) and possible reseeding of tumor metastases from the untreated area of the peritoneum back to the previously treated area. Given the movement of the abdominal contents from day to day, there is also some uncertainty about the dose received by mobile organs. These two techniques have been compared with the commonly used radiation doses and fractionation schemes (431,432). In both studies, the difference in 5-year survival between the two treatment approaches was less than 1%. The analysis of the Princess Margaret Hospital study shows the two techniques

to be comparable in all patient subgroups regardless of stage, histology, grade, or tumor residuum. Furthermore, there were no differences in acute toxicity between the two treatment techniques. Although late complications were infrequent with either method, they were less commonly encountered with the open-field technique. The open-field technique (Fig. 25.29) has become the standard in most centers because of shorter duration of treatment, technical simplicity, and reduced long-term toxicity. Variations in the open-field technique include adding a T-shaped boost portal to the paraaortic nodes and medial domes of the diaphragm and treating the upper and lower abdomen through separate portals. Figure 25.29 and Table 25.20 depict the recommended treatment volume and technical principles of whole abdominopelvic radiation therapy.

Although the technique of radiation is likely to continue to be that of the open field, recent radiobiologic information suggests theoretical strategies to change radiation fractionation schemes to increase the biologically effective dose delivered without increasing radiation toxicity. The effect of a simple dose escalation using the same 1-Gy dose per frac-

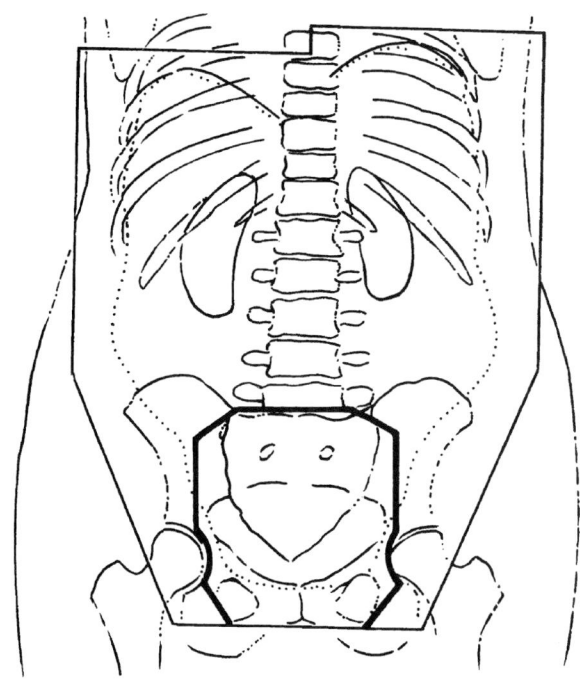

FIG. 25.29. Treatment volume for abdominopelvic radiotherapy in patients with ovarian cancer. The entire peritoneal cavity must be encompassed. Liver shielding is not used. The kidneys are shielded to keep the renal core at 18–20 Gy. The true pelvis is given a boost dose in 0.18- to 0.22-Gy fractions to a total dose of 45–50 Gy. Parallel opposing portals are used with beam energy sufficient to ensure dosage variation of <5%. (From Dembo AJ. Adominopelvic radiotherapy in ovarian cancer: a 10-year experience. *CANCER* 1985;55: 2285–2290. Copyright © 2004 American Cancer Society. Reprinted by permission of Wiley-Liss Inc., a subsidiary of John Wiley & Sons, Inc.)

TABLE 25.20. *Technical principles of curative radiotherapy*

1. The entire peritoneal cavity must be encompassed.
2. The moving-strip and open-field techniques are equally effective, but the latter is preferred.
3. No liver shielding is used. This limits the upper abdominal dose to 2,500–2,800 cGy in 100- to 120-cGy daily fractions.
4. Partial kidney shielding is used to keep the renal dose at 1,800–2,000 cGy.
5. The true pelvis is given a boost dose in 180–220 cGy.
6. Use parallel-opposing portals, with beam energy sufficient to ensure a dosage variation no greater than 5%.

Reprinted with permission from Dembo AJ. Epithelial ovarian cancer: the role of radiotherapy. *Int J Radiat Oncol Biol Phys* 1992;22:838–845.

tion of abdominal irradiation was examined in a randomized trial (432). Escalation to a total abdominal dose of 27.5 Gy in 27 fractions did not result in improved disease or overall survival nor was toxicity increased. Possible changes in radiation fractionation schemes include delivering two to three fractions per day of fraction size less than 1 Gy. Using such a scheme, Morgan et al. (433), with an open-field technique, were able to deliver 30.6 Gy in 0.8-Gy fractions twice daily with a pelvic boost of 1,519.2 Gy to the pelvis; treatment was well tolerated and did not appear to result in any increased late toxicity. Changed fractionation schemes, with or without accompanying sensitizing ''chemotherapy,'' warrant exploration to determine whether they will be of increased curative benefit in patients with optimal disease or whether they will even be useful treatment for some patients with suboptimal disease.

Curative Radiation Therapy

The results presented in Table 25.19 provide evidence that radiation therapy is primarily effective in patients who have no macroscopic residual disease after primary surgery. However, the overall results do not indicate how many additional patients were cured by irradiation since some are cured by surgery alone. Thus, the curative potential for irradiation is best assessed by determining the outcome of treatment in patients with known macroscopic residual disease after their initial laparotomy. Since 95% of recurrences develop within 5 years of treatment, 8- and 10-year relapse-free and survival rates provide a more accurate estimate of the actual cure rate associated with any treatment. Table 25.19 summarizes the long-term survival or relapse-free rates in six published studies of whole abdomen radiation therapy for patients with advanced ovarian cancer (424–429). All patients had known macroscopic residual disease when treated with irradiation. The cure rates were determined by the stage at presentation and by the volume of residual disease. For those studies with more than 10-year follow-up, the outcomes were similar. Between 38% and 62% of patients with small residual lesions (<2 cm) were cured after whole abdomen and pelvic

irradiation. There was a higher cure rate for patients with stage II disease in whom the pelvis was treated to a higher dose than was the upper abdomen. For patients with larger residual lesions (>2 cm), the probability of cure was only 0% to 14%. Although these studies provide strong evidence that whole abdomen irradiation is able to cure patients with small-volume residual ovarian cancer, certain questions have been raised about interpretation of the results. These studies were performed before the period when aggressive cytoreductive surgery and comprehensive exploration of abdominal contents were accepted as the standard operative procedures for patients with ovarian cancer. Thus, in general, the presence and volume of residual disease may have been understated. Contrarily, if patients were determined as having only small-volume residual disease and had not had aggressive cytoreduction, their disease may have been inherently more favorable than that described now after aggressive cytoreduction.

These data, however, showing similar long-term, failure-free survival rates in patients with known small residual amounts of disease postoperatively, are strong evidence that radiation therapy is curative in selected patients with ovarian cancer.

Toxicity of Abdominopelvic Radiation Therapy

Abdominopelvic irradiation is associated with both acute and chronic side effects; the acute effects of irradiation usually resolve within 2 to 3 weeks after completion of treatment. The common effects reported by most patients include fatigue, which increases during the course of irradiation. Gastrointestinal toxicity is common, with some degree of nausea or anorexia experienced by most patients. The former symptom is well relieved by the new antinauseants, such as ondansetron. About 75% of patients do develop diarrhea, with or without some abdominal cramping. Hematologic toxicity is usually acceptable. If the patient has received no prior antineoplastic therapy with systemic agents, interruption of the course of radiation therapy is very rarely required for thrombocytopenia (<50,000 platelets/ mm^2) or neutropenia (<1,000/mm^2).

The late effects of radiation include asymptomatic basal pneumonitis or fibrosis detectable in 15% to 20% of patients on radiographic films. This results from the necessity of including 1 to 2 cm of lung field in the radiation portal in order to adequately encompass the leaves of the diaphragms. With upper abdominal doses of 0.220.25 Gy in 22 to 25 fractions, about 50% of patients will develop transient elevations of alkaline phosphatase from hepatic irradiation a few months after radiation therapy. Fewer than 1% of patients develop jaundice or ascites (424).

Late gastrointestinal toxicity is the complication concerning most investigators. The frequency and severity are dependent on the total dose of radiation, the dose per fraction, and the extent and number of previous operations. There

Stage	Residuum	Grade 1	Grade 2	Grade 3
I	0	96 ± 2% (n=80)	78 ± 5 (71)	62 ± 8 (39)
II	0	91 ± 4 (45)	73 ± 7 (46)	52 ± 7 (47)
II	<2 cm	No Relapses (5)	78 ± 14 (9)	21 ± 11 (14)
III	0	63 ± 14 (15)	26 ± 14 (12)	29 ± 11 (20)
III	<2 cm	88 ± 12 (8)	45 ± 11 (20)	39 ± 10 (27)

FIG. 25.30. Percent 5-year relapse-free rates ± standard deviation in groups according to stage, residuum, and grade. The numbers in parentheses indicate the number of patients in each cell. Low-risk patients are shown by the hatched lines; intermediate risk by the unshaded boxes enclosed in bold lines; high-risk by shaded boxes. (Fourteen patients without specific grade assignments were excluded.) (Reprinted with permission from Carey M, Dembo AJ, Fyles AW, et al. Testing the validity of a prognostic classification in patients with surgically optimal ovarian carcinoma: a 15-year review. *Int J Gynecol Cancer* 1993;3:24–35.)

appears to be an increased risk of late complications if lymph node sampling was performed as part of the initial operation. If the technical principles of whole abdominal radiation therapy, as depicted in Table 25.20, are followed, the risk of serious bowel complications may be minimized. Generally, about 10% to 15% of patients may report some diarrhea or persistent bloating related to particular dietary intolerance, but frank malabsorption is extremely rare. Obstruction requiring surgical correction is much more uncommon than most appreciate. In four studies with almost 1,100 patients in total, 5.6% (range 1.4% to 14%) of the patients required bowel surgery for late treatment-associated complications of radiation. In these collected series, less than 0.5% (four patients) died as a result of radiation-induced bowel damage.

Selecting Patients for Abdominopelvic Radiation Therapy

Abdominopelvic radiation therapy has been used during the past 15 years in all stages and extents of ovarian cancer (263,423,424). From these randomized and nonrandomized studies, considerable data have defined the patient and tumor factors that will predict a favorable outcome after the use of abdominopelvic radiation therapy. Besides the general medical condition of the patients and their suitability for such therapy, the tumor factors that determine suitability include the extent of disease at presentation, the amounts and sites of residual disease in the pelvis and abdomen, and the histopathological findings (grade and type) of the tumor (424).

A multivariate analysis of pathologic prognostic factors was performed for an initial cohort of patients treated between 1971 and 1978 (434). A second cohort of patients treated between 1979 and 1985 was examined to test the validity and reproducibility of the original prognostic classification. The derived prognostic classification shown in Figures 25.30 and 25.31 has been used to select treatment by classifying patients with ovarian cancer into low-, intermediate-, or high-risk categories. The low-risk group is composed of patients with stage I ovarian cancer, who by multifactorial analysis of prognosis within stage I have been determined to have such a good survival (96% ± 2%) that no postoperative therapy is warranted. These patients at low risk for recurrence after surgery alone are those with stage I, grade 1 disease, without evidence of dense adherence or ascites. The remainder of patients with stage I disease, that is, those with grade 2 or 3, or with dense adherence or ascites, have a significant risk of relapse and fall into the intermediate-risk

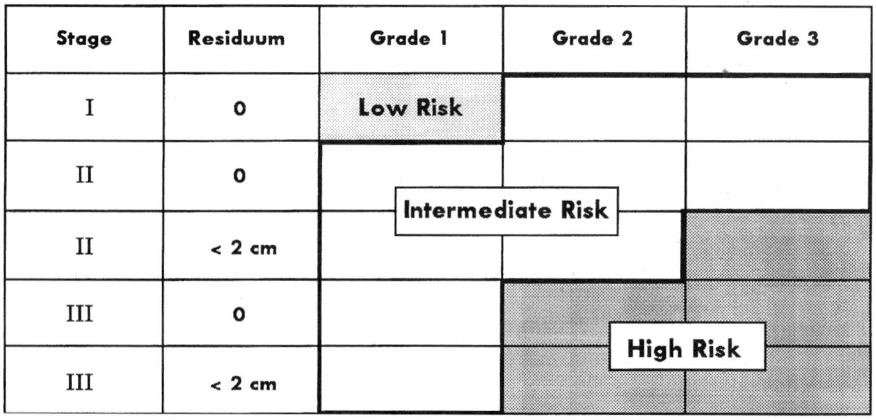

Stage	Residuum	Grade 1	Grade 2	Grade 3
I	0	Low Risk		
II	0		Intermediate Risk	
II	< 2 cm			
III	0			High Risk
III	< 2 cm			

FIG. 25.31. Prognostic subgroupings according to stage, residuum, and grade in patients with stages I to III disease and small or no tumor residuum. Abdominopelvic radiation therapy is recommended as the sole postoperative treatment in the intermediate-risk patient group. (Reprinted from Dembo AJ. Epithelial ovarian cancer: the role of radiotherapy. *Int J Radiat Oncol Biol Phys* 1992;22:835–845. Copyright 2004, with permission from Elsevier.)

group. Currently, the randomized studies in the management of stage I disease have failed to show a significant advantage for treatment (231,262,428,435). Although a curative benefit for abdominopelvic radiation therapy has not been established in stage I disease, except for those with dense adherence, it has been established as curative therapy for a large proportion of patients with stage II disease whose residuum is less than 2 cm. Thus, it seems appropriate at this time to consider that abdominopelvic radiation therapy and platinum-based chemotherapy are both rational options for management of the high-risk patient with stage I disease, that is, those with grade 2 or 3 tumors, with large-volume ascites and/or positive peritoneal cytologic findings, and those with dense adherence.

In selecting patients with stages II and III disease for whom abdominopelvic radiation therapy is appropriate, the amount and site of residual disease and the tumor grade are strong determinants of success of outcome. Given the restrictions imposed on the dose deliverable to the upper abdomen and pelvis, abdominopelvic irradiation should be used only in patients with no macroscopic disease in the upper abdomen and with small macroscopic (0 to 2 cm) residual disease in the pelvis. Figures 25.30 and 25.31 show the data and classification of patients into the three definable and separate risk groups on the basis of the stage of disease, the amount of residual disease postoperatively, and the tumor grade. This classification of patients into risk groups has been validated by other investigators (426–429,436, 437). The patients in the intermediate-risk category constitute about 33% of the total patient population with ovarian cancer. It is in this intermediate-risk group that abdominopelvic radiation therapy is the most appropriate as the sole postoperative treatment method. This group comprises mainly patients with stages I and II disease, including those with dense adherence. Those with stage III disease are suitable for this treatment alone if their macroscopic residual tumor is less than 2 cm, is located in the pelvis, and is grade 1. Using abdominopelvic radiation therapy, more than 67% of intermediate-risk patients were alive and disease-free 10 years after treatment with minimal late morbidity (264).

Five- and 10-year survivals for 46 patients in the intermediate-risk group were 60% and 54%, respectively. An abdominal dose of ≥36 Gy significantly reduced abdominal recurrence from 49% to 18%, $p = .006$, and was associated with longer survival independent of stage, grade, and amount of residual disease. Although this study suggests a dose-control relationship, a higher rate of small bowel obstruction was observed. Total abdominal dose of >30 Gy and a pelvic dose >50 Gy were associated with 40% small bowel obstruction, whereas with lower doses only 4% had small bowel obstruction. Patients shown as being high risk in Figure 25.31 have an approximately 20% 10-year failure-free rate when treated with abdominopelvic radiation therapy alone (437). Recognition of this poor outcome has led us to examine, in a nonrandomized study, the use of six cycles of cisplatin-based combination chemotherapy followed by abdominopelvic radiation therapy (437). In these high-risk, optimally cytoreduced patients, the sequential therapy appeared to improve their median survival time and relapse-free rate significantly compared to those achieved by radiation therapy alone.

These sequential studies, with confirmation by others, reveal that abdominopelvic radiation therapy provides a significant curative benefit to patients defined as intermediate risk by our prognostic classification system. Radiation therapy is, therefore, considered to be a rational choice of therapy for a large proportion of patients with optimally cytoreduced ovarian cancer.

Radiation Therapy versus Chemotherapy

The relative effectiveness of abdominopelvic radiation therapy and combination platinum-based chemotherapy in patients with small or no macroscopic residual ovarian cancer has often been debated. A literature review does not resolve which of these two treatments is preferred. Most of the series in the literature with whole abdominal radiation therapy are older and have not utilized rigorous staging or aggressive cytoreductive surgery, as has been the case for the more recent chemotherapy studies. The extent of disease in the radiation studies might be underestimated, and the results of this form of treatment may be actually better than reported. On the other hand, in the older series, patients who had small macroscopic residual disease after surgery (which did not require extensive cytoreduction) may have a more favorable prognosis than do patients treated by chemotherapy who had minimum macroscopic disease after more aggressive debulking surgery. In addition, new diagnostic techniques and more accurate staging procedures have changed the stage distribution of ovarian cancer, further complicating retrospective comparisons. The recognition that cisplatin alone or in combination produces response rates of approximately 60% to 80% in patients with advanced disease leads to initial optimism that overall cure rates in ovarian cancer would be substantially improved. More recently, long-term survival rates or progression-free rates have been reported for the use of cisplatin-based chemotherapy in advanced disease. Unfortunately, no group has been able to successfully complete a randomized comparison of the effectiveness of abdominopelvic radiation therapy with cisplatin-based combination chemotherapy. Although a number of cooperative groups have attempted to perform comparative trials, they have been unsuccessful in answering this question. The two treatment methods are so different that it is likely that investigator bias and difficulty entering patients in the trials severely limited patient accrual and were the probable causes that resulted in premature closure of the studies. With all of the theoretical and possible limitations on comparing treatment results of the use of one modality versus the other in nonrandomized trials, an examination of long-term disease-free survivals in various independent studies using platinum-based chemotherapy or radiation therapy is illuminating. Overall, the survival rates reported for whole abdominopelvic radiation therapy in stage III optimal disease are approximately 30% to 35% (424,438). In GOG protocol 158 (346), almost 800 optimal stage III patients were treated with platinum-based chemotherapy with a median progression-free survival of less than 2 years and a disease-free survival at 4 years of 25% to 30% (Fig. 25.25). It would be expected that 10% to 15% more of these patients would relapse when the duration of follow-up is extended beyond 4 years. Thus, it would appear in comparing separate trials, with all of the inherent limitations of that process (but acknowledging that there are no better available pertinent data), that the long-term survival results for whole abdominal radiation therapy and chemotherapy are very similar. It is clear that radiation therapy is an effective agent for the management of ovarian cancer, and if it is to be used as primary postoperative therapy, the criteria for selecting patients and technical recommendations for therapy must be strictly adhered to.

The similarity of the long-term survivals for patients treated with platinum-containing chemotherapy or radiation therapy should stimulate a reinterest in the use of radiation therapy in ovarian cancer. Although many investigators were quick to discard radiation therapy from the armamentarium for management of ovarian cancer when cisplatin was believed to be a promising agent for improved cure rates, it is now apparent that that decision may have been ill conceived. No other single agent with the level of activity that radiation has in ovarian cancer has been discarded from the treatment armamentarium for any solid tumor, including ovarian cancer. It would now appear to be appropriate to investigate further the role of radiation therapy, either as a sole agent or as part of a multimodality armamentarium, in the primary management of ovarian cancer. With the demonstration that paclitaxel is a highly active cytotoxic agent in ovarian cancer and that interaction may occur between this agent and radiation, it would seem appropriate to explore their concurrent use in ovarian cancer.

None of these studies is definitive, and none addresses the question of how abdominopelvic radiation therapy compares to treatment with cisplatin or paclitaxel-based combination chemotherapy. Although a number of cooperative groups have attempted to perform a comparative randomized clinical trial, they have been unsuccessful in answering this question. The two treatment methods are so different that investigator bias severely limited patient accrual and led to closure of the studies. If radiation therapy is to be used, the apparent criteria for selecting patients and technical recommendations in Table 25.20 and in Figure 25.29 must be strictly adhered to.

Radiation Therapy After Chemotherapy in Advanced Disease

Fuks and colleagues (297) were among the first to propose the use of sequential cisplatin-based chemotherapy and secondary cytoreductive surgery, followed by whole abdomen radiation therapy, in patients with advanced disease. Since that time, numerous reports of sequential multimodality therapy have appeared. A recent review of the role of salvage or consolidative radiation therapy (438) examined the published results. This article reported on a total number of 713 patients in 28 literature series, yet it was impossible to reach definitive conclusions about the value of sequential therapy since most studies reported were single-arm trials without appropriate controls. Overall, the balance of evidence was against a significant curative benefit for radiation therapy as salvage or consolidation treatment, at least in the situations in which it had been used. However, it is important to consider the possible causes of failure to show a benefit for radiation in order to guide the design of future studies that should rigorously examine the role of salvage radiation therapy in advanced disease. The review of studies in the literature confirmed that, in many situations, patient selection was inappropriate in that it was based on large-volume residual disease following chemotherapy. Where studies reported the amount of residual disease in patients so treated, survival was clearly dependent on the tumor residuum prior to radiation therapy. The survival of those with macroscopic disease postchemotherapy and cytoreductive surgery was only 17% and is probably no different from that achieved with primary surgery and chemotherapy (Tables 25.21 and 25.22). It suggests that salvage radiation therapy is inappropriate for most patients with any disease residuum after chemotherapy that is more than microscopic in volume. Survivals after multimodality therapy were better for those with microscopic or <5 mm residual disease and for those with

TABLE 25.21. *Survival results reporting benefit for sequential therapy in patients with zero or microscopic residual disease prior to radiation therapy*

	No. of surviving/no. at risk	
Study (ref.)	Zero residuum	Microscopic or <5 mm
Chiara et al. (440)	6/9	5/11
Greiner et al. (441)	14/15	5/9[a]
Reddy et al. (441a)		4/5
Kuten et al. (441b)	5/5	12/18
Solomon et al. (441c)		4/12
Kong et al. (445)		3/5
Rosen et al. (441d)	4/4	3/4
Haie et al. (441e)	14/23	
Kersh et al. (441f)	1/4	10/15
Goldhirsch et al. (441g)	19/24	
Menczer et al. (441h)	9/10[b]	
Morgan et al. (433)		8/8[a]

[a] <1 cm residuum.
[b] Result interpreted as negative by investigators.
Reprinted with permission from Thomas GM. Is there a role for consolidation or salvage radiotherapy after chemotherapy in advanced epithelial ovarian cancer? *Gynecol Oncol* 1993;51:97–103.

TABLE 25.22. *Survival by tumor residuum prior to radiation therapy*

No residuum	Microscopic or <5 mm	Microscopic
76% (86/113)	49% (77/158)	17% (34/202)

Note: Survival following sequential surgery, chemotherapy, and whole-abdominopelvic radiation therapy appears dependent on tumor residuum prior to radiation. Data extracted from 28 literature series containing 713 patients, of which 473 had sufficient information to estimate residuum.

Reprinted with permission from Thomas GM. Is there a role for consolidation or salvage radiotherapy after chemotherapy in advanced epithelial ovarian cancer? *Gynecol Oncol* 1993;51:97–103.

no residual disease. They were 49% (77 of 158) and 76%, respectively. It is unclear whether the better survivals of those with no microscopic residual disease are attributable to the abdominal radiation therapy employed or rather to the inherently better prognostic features of these tumors. The observed outcomes are compatible with the variability of already known prognostic factors in ovarian cancer, such as age, grade, and previous response to chemotherapy, and, therefore, do not unequivocally establish a treatment effect for radiation therapy. The better results, however, for those with microscopic or no residual disease suggest that at least some possible benefit may accrue to these patients and helps direct the future selection of patients in whom such therapy should be explored in a controlled fashion.

Whereas most reported series had insufficient patients to do meaningful analyses of possible prognostic and treatment factors determining the observed outcome, the data of Schray et al. (450) are valuable because of the method of analysis and presentation. These investigators performed a multivariate analysis of factors significant for disease-free survival and established significance for the grade of tumor (70% survival for grades 1 and 2 vs 10% for grades 3 and 4); the initial residuum prior to chemotherapy (50% survival for <2 cm vs 14% for >2 cm); and patient age (54% for <50 years vs 20% for >50 years). They also looked at the amount of residual disease at the time of radiation therapy. Where the disease was microscopic, three of five patients remained disease-free following radiation therapy. Where macroscopic disease was debulked to microscopic prior to consolidative radiation therapy, only five of 21 patients remained disease-free. Importantly, they also analyzed the outcome according to the number of the favorable factors present, that is, the pre–chemotherapy residuum, the pre–radiation therapy residuum, and the grade of the tumor. If no favorable factors were present, 0% (0 of 17) remained disease-free; with one factor present, 29% (4 of 14); two factors present, 53% (8 of 15); and three factors present, 67% (4 of 6) remained disease-free.

Appropriate selection of patients for studies of salvage radiation therapy should be guided by this type of informa-

tion. Selection should also be guided by extrapolation from the pertinent situations in which radiation therapy used as the sole postoperative therapy has been shown to be of curative benefit. Radiation therapy is appropriate only as the sole postoperative therapy for patients with no macroscopic disease in the upper abdomen and small or no macroscopic residual disease in the pelvis (298,434,435). Since radiation is not beneficial as curative therapy in groups with larger volumes of residual disease, it is unlikely (because of many biologic factors that may be operative, including accelerated clonogen proliferation) that salvage radiation therapy would be of curative benefit in similar patients who have already received extensive surgery (including secondary debulking and chemotherapy to which resistance may have already been demonstrated).

In an effort to deliver an increased biologically effective whole abdominal radiation dose and to decrease toxicity, hyperfractionation techniques are being investigated. The delivery of two to three small radiation fractions per day to a similar or greater cumulative dose during the same period as achieved by conventional daily fractionation may take advantage of differences in cell kinetics between tumor cells and normal cells, improving the therapeutic ratio primarily by decreasing toxicity. One of the theoretical explanations for the lack of efficacy of consolidative radiation therapy is the existence of true cross resistance between cisplatin chemotherapy and irradiation. Human ovarian cancer cell lines with acquired resistance to cisplatin develop relative radiation resistance *in vitro* (451). It is also possible that any therapy that leads to rapid cytoreduction (chemotherapy or irradiation) may lead to an accelerated proliferation of remaining clonogenic tumor cells. Withers et al. (430) performed a detailed analysis of the relationships between irradiation with fractionation schemes of different durations and therapeutic benefit for patients with head and neck cancer. They demonstrated that accelerated proliferation did occur during a course of fractionated radiation treatment and that the magnitude of radiation dose required to overcome the accelerated proliferation was on the order of 0.6 Gy per day. Consequently, accelerated tumor proliferation may account for treatment failure after a previous course of cytoreductive therapy, and this principle applies equally to cytoreduction by radiation therapy or by chemotherapy. Thus, a strategy of using hyperfractionated and accelerated irradiation may be a useful one to overcome these biologic limitations.

Morgan and co-workers (433) used hyperfractionation to treat 15 stage III patients with known residual disease after induction therapy with cisplatin-based regimens. Using an open-field technique, they were able to deliver 30.6 Gy in 0.8-Gy fractions twice daily with a pelvic boost of 1,519.2 Gy to gross disease in the pelvis. Limiting the kidney and liver doses to 20.0 and 30.4 Gy, respectively, all patients completed the planned treatment course, and only two patients required a treatment break for thrombocytopenia. No episodes of small-bowel obstruction occurred. Kong and colleagues (444) treated patients with sequential chemotherapy, second-look surgery, and whole abdomen radiation therapy. In that study, a total dose of 30 Gy was delivered to the abdomen in 1-Gy fractions twice daily, and only one patient developed bowel obstruction.

Although overall there does not appear to be a curative benefit in the situations in which consolidative therapy has been employed, it is probable that treatment strategies employing sequential multimodality therapy will be beneficial in a small, select group of patients. Clearly, patient selection should be based on identification of those most likely to fail following chemotherapy and those most likely to benefit from salvage radiation therapy. Two studies give some degree of optimism that subsets of patients may be aided by this sequential multimodality therapy. In a report from Toronto (452), consolidation abdominopelvic radiation therapy following six cycles of cisplatin-based combination chemotherapy in the high-risk, optimally cytoreduced patients was performed. Forty-four of 51 eligible patients seen between 1981 and 1985 with optimally cytoreduced stage II or III disease were entered into this nonrandomized study. Their survival was compared to that of 48 eligible historical control patients matched for age, stage, and residual disease treated with radiation therapy alone between 1978 and 1981. The median follow-up time was 6.6 years. The combined therapy led to an extension of the median survival from 2.4 to 5.7 years, and 42.6% of patients receiving combined therapy were free of relapse at 5 years compared to 21.6% ($p = .03$) in the historical control group treated with abdominopelvic irradiation alone. Since the control group received radiation therapy alone, it cannot be certain that the entire benefit that was observed was attributable to the combined sequential therapy, that is, whether the consolidation/radiation therapy provided improvement over that achievable in a comparable group treated with chemotherapy alone. There is evidence, however, that the radiation therapy did appear to be additive.

The Swedish Norwegian Ovarian Cancer Study Group (370) recently reported the long-term results of their multicenter study, which closed in April 1993. One hundred seventy-two patients of an initial total of 741 were randomized after four courses of cisplatin/doxorubicin chemotherapy followed by second-look surgery to receive consolidation therapy. Patients were stratified according to the amount of residual disease at second-look surgery. Stratum one consisted of 98 patients with microscopic or no macroscopic residual disease. These patients were randomized to receive one of three possible treatments: whole abdominal therapy, continued chemotherapy with cisplatin/doxorubicin to ten courses in total, or observation only. Although the patient groups are relatively small, follow-up is substantial, and a significant improvement in survival was observed for those receiving whole abdominal radiation therapy. In the subgroup with complete surgical and pathologic remission, progression-free survival was significantly better ($p = .032$) in the radiotherapy group (56% at 5 years) than in the chemotherapy group (36% at 5 years) and the untreated control group (35% at 5 years). Overall survival was also improved in patients receiving radiotherapy ($p = .08$) (Fig. 25.32). In the subgroup with microscopic residuum, no benefit was observed. Late grade 3 bowel complications occurred in 10%.

Many studies of abdominopelvic radiation therapy after chemotherapy have reported a higher complication rate than for radiation therapy alone (438,453). Several explanations may account for the increased complications associated with radiation therapy in this situation: (a) high radiation doses, that is, pelvic dose above 0.45 Gy or abdominal dose above 0.220.25 Gy; and (b) multiple or at least second-look laparotomies before whole abdominal irradiation.(446). Because the benefit of using abdominopelvic radiation therapy after chemotherapy is equivocal and confined probably to a small subset of patients, the risk of complications is a major con-

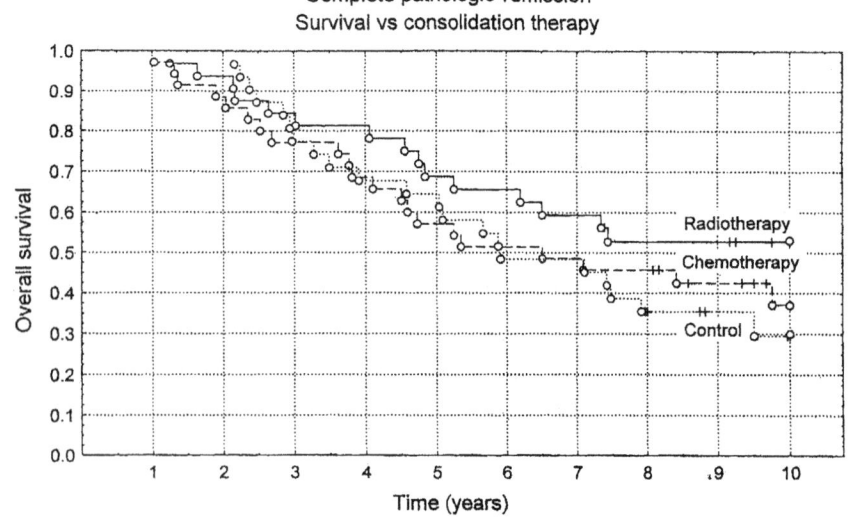

Complete pathologic remission
Survival vs consolidation therapy

FIG. 25.32. Overall survival versus type of consolidation treatment in patients with a surgically confirmed complete remission after induction chemotherapy. Radiotherapy-treated patients had borderline improved survival, ($p = .084$). (Reprinted with permission by B. Sorbe on Behalf of the Swedish-Norweigian Ovarian Cancer Study Group. Consolidation treatment of advanced (FIGO stage III) ovarian carcinoma in complete surgical remission after induction chemotherapy: A randomized, controlled, clinical trial comparing whole abdominal radiotherapy, chemotherapy, and no further treatment. *Int J Gynecol Cancer* 2003;13: 278–286.)

sideration. This risk can be minimized by restricting the radiation dose in patients who have had second-look operations.

To date, no studies have been reported examining either the toxicity or efficacy of salvage or consolidative whole abdominopelvic irradiation after paclitaxel-based chemotherapy.

In summary, it would seem that radiation therapy as consolidative treatment should be confined to those patients who have negative or microscopic disease at second-look laparotomy, whose prechemotherapy bulk is minimally larger than those with optimal disease, whose chemotherapy is restricted to six courses of therapy with effective agents that provide the least toxicity to the bone marrow, and whose radiation therapy is delivered with a dose and technique providing acceptable complication rates or one that explores the possible theoretical benefits of hyperfractionated irradiation to somewhat higher than conventional accepted doses (454).

PALLIATION

Recurrent or persistent ovarian cancer after first-line chemotherapy is incurable. Patients are often symptomatic, with generalized or localized abdominal symptoms from intraperitoneal disease. Usually, second-, third-, or fourth-line chemotherapy is used in attempts to prolong life and palliate symptoms. Few specific data are available to evaluate the quality of life achieved or degree of symptom palliation. As will be subsequently reviewed, reported response rates for chemotherapy range between 10% and 43% and are associated with various toxicities. Radiation therapy as a palliative modality in ovarian cancer is often neglected, but may be very useful if the sole or dominant symptomatic problem for the patient is localized to a site and volume that may be safely encompassed in a radiation field. For example, a fixed pelvic mass eroding the vaginal mucosa causing bleeding, pain, or bowel or bladder dysfunction may occur without obvious disseminated symptomatic peritoneal disease. Tumor regression or symptomatic relief can often be obtained in these situations from local irradiation. Similarly, radiation may be employed to treat localized masses elsewhere in the abdomen, such as the retroperitoneal nodes. Palliative irradiation may also be useful for extraabdominal disease, particularly supraclavicular or inguinal node masses and bony or brain metastases. Radiation therapy may be beneficial for the acute relief of painful hepatomegaly due to capsular distention.

Limited data are available from the literature concerning the palliative efficacy of radiation therapy in these settings (455–458) Using large single-fraction irradiation, one to three fractions of 10 Gy, investigators at the M.D. Anderson Cancer Center (449) reported overall response rates of 55% and 71% among ovarian cancer patients palliated for pain and bleeding, respectively. However, 6 of 42 patients so treated did develop severe bowel radiation injury that may

be attributable to the large fractions employed. Another report of palliative radiation therapy used after initial management with cisplatin-containing regimens documented that radiation therapy produced a mean symptom-free interval of 8.5 months in a group of patients with a median survival of 19.5 months (457). A study from Fox Chase Cancer Center (455) reported the use of fractionated palliative irradiation in 33 patients with symptomatic ovarian cancer in 47 irradiated sites. For the entire group, complete palliative response was seen in 51% of patients, and overall palliative responses occurred in 79%. The median duration of palliation was 4 months, which reflected palliation until death in 90% of cases. Vaginal or rectal bleeding was controlled in 90% and 85%, respectively, and pain relief occurred in 83%. A range of radiation doses was employed, but it is unclear whether patients with better performance status received the higher doses. Palliation was improved in those with higher Karnofsky performance status and in those who received biologically effective doses (BED) of at least 44 Gy (e.g., 35 Gy in 14 fractions). In a recently reported study from the Memorial Sloan–Kettering Cancer Center, variable doses of palliative irradiation were given to a group of 33 patients with platinum-refractory disease who had not previously received paclitaxel. Complete subjective or objective responses were observed in 70% (458). Firm recommendations on the optimal dose for palliation cannot be made; none of the papers provides sufficient detail to do a multivariate analysis of factors predictive of the observed palliative response. Also, the palliative dose fractionation schemes employed do not allow the construction of a dose-response curve. However, it is clear that durable palliation may be achieved with local radiation therapy for ovarian cancer recurring after cisplatin-based chemotherapy, particularly in patients with good performance status.

INTRAPERITONEAL ^{32}P IN PATIENTS WITH ADVANCED OVARIAN CANCER

Intraperitoneal ^{32}P has been used in patients with advanced epithelial ovarian cancer, primarily in two clinical situations: (a) in an attempt to decrease the recurrence rate in patients who achieve a surgically confirmed complete remission following induction chemotherapy; and (b) in patients who have microscopic or minimal residual disease documented at second look. In a small pilot study with an historical comparison to a no-treatment control group, there was a suggestion that ^{32}P treatment was associated with a lower recurrence rate in patients who achieved a complete remission (459). As previously described (369) (see section on Maintenance Therapy and Consolidation above), intraperitoneal ^{32}P in a randomized comparison against observation did not decrease the risk of relapse or improve survival in patients with a surgically confirmed complete remission (Fig. 25.33).

In patients with residual disease at second-look laparot-

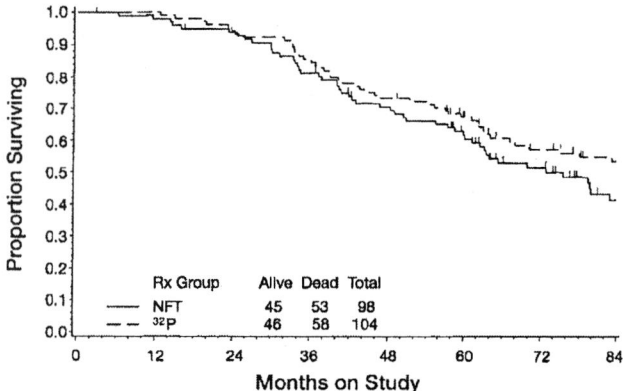

FIG. 25.33. Overall survival for patients in a surgically confirmed complete remission who received no further therapy (NFT) or ^{32}P chronic phosphate suspension. Overall survival is not significantly different. (From Varia MA, Stehman FB, Bundy BN, et al. Intraperitoneal radioactive phosphorus (^{32}P) versus observation after negative second-look laparotomy for stage III ovarian carcinoma: a randomized trial of the Gynecologic Oncology Group. *J Clin Oncol* 2003;21:2849–2855. Reprinted with permission from the American Society of Clinical Oncology.)

omy, there have been conflicting reports about the efficacy of intraperitoneal ^{32}P (459). There are no randomized trials demonstrating that intraperitoneal ^{32}P is curative in patients who have residual disease. In addition, adequate distribution throughout the peritoneal cavity may also be a problem secondary to adhesions in patients who have undergone prior surgical staging and debulking. Prospective evaluation of intraperitoneal ^{32}P versus other forms of therapy in patients with known residual disease after induction chemotherapy awaits completion of the trial of intraperitoneal therapy versus observation in patients with a negative second-look laparotomy. If intraperitoneal ^{32}P cannot prevent or delay the recurrence rate in an optimum situation of microscopic disease, it is unlikely that this modality of therapy will be beneficial in patients who have larger amounts of residual disease.

INTRAPERITONEAL CHEMOTHERAPY

The ability of intraperitoneal chemotherapy to control the accumulation of malignant ascites has been known since the 1950s. However, the modern era of intraperitoneal chemotherapy began in 1978, when the intent switched from palliation to a treatment modality administered with curative intent. The new approach was based on pharmacologic modeling studies of the physiologic and anatomic characteristics of the peritoneal cavity and the chemical properties of antineoplastic drugs. These characteristics suggested that the intraperitoneal administration of anticancer agents in a large volume to peritoneal tumors would lead to a pharmacologic advantage compared to intravenous therapy (460).

Following the demonstration that such large-volume intermittent dialysis was feasible via a semipermanent Tenckhoff catheter (461), numerous pharmacologic Phase I trials were performed using virtually all the drugs active against human ovarian cancer (461,462).

These studies have demonstrated that intraperitoneal therapy is technically feasible in the majority of patients. However, in a significant number (20% to 30%), uniform distribution of drug-containing dialysate (as measured by CT scans) throughout the peritoneal cavity is not possible, primarily due to adhesions (463). The complication rate and patient acceptance have improved with the development of a totally implantable peritoneal access device (portacath) (464). The portacath system allows the peritoneal cavity to be accessed by inserting a needle through the skin and stopper into a port. Catheter blockage, which occurs in approximately 8% of patients, is usually due to the formation of a fibrous reaction around the outside of the catheter (465). Infectious complications, occasionally manifested as peritonitis, occur in approximately 8% of patients (466).

The intraperitoneal administration of most drugs with established activity via the intravenous route has produced a marked pharmacologic advantage in ovarian cancer patients. Paclitaxel has recently been added to the list of active agents that can be safely administered infrequently while producing a pharmacologic advantage. The pharmacologic advantage, defined as the ratio of peak peritoneal concentration to peak plasma concentration or as the ratio of the AUC of the peritoneal cavity to the plasma AUC, has ranged from 7 for methotrexate to over 1,000 for mitoxantrone and paclitaxel (Table 25.23) (466).

The pharmacology and efficacy of cisplatin and cisplatin combinations have been extensively studied in patients with

TABLE 25.23. *Pharmacologic advantage for intraperitoneal chemotherapy*

Drug	Ratio of drug level in peritoneal cavity to plasma concentration[a]	
	Peak	AUC
Cisplatin	20	12
Carboplatin		18
Melphalan	93	65
Adriamycin	474	
Mitomycin	71	
Mitoxantrone		1,400
5-fluorouracil	298	367
Methotrexate	92	100
Paclitaxel[b]		1,000

AUC, area under the curve.
[a] From Markman M. Intraperitoneal chemotherapy. *Semin Oncol* 1991;18:248.
[b] From Markman M, Rowinsky E, Hakes T, et al. Phase I trial of intraperitoneal taxol: a Gynecologic Oncology Group study. *J Clin Oncol* 1992;10:1485–1491.

residual or recurrent ovarian cancer. Cisplatin has been of particular interest owing to its high intrinsic activity against ovarian cancer and because cytotoxic plasma levels can be achieved after intraperitoneal administration. Under these circumstances, the outer rim of a peritoneal tumor should be exposed to high levels of drug by direct diffusion from the peritoneal surface, whereas cytotoxic concentrations would theoretically be achieved in the inner core owing to drug delivery via the microcirculation (466). Approximately one-third of patients with residual ovarian cancer have been documented at third-look laparotomy to have had a complete response to the intraperitoneal administration of cisplatin (466–468). The intraperitoneal administration of combinations of agents, particularly cisplatin and VP16, has led to somewhat higher response rates (469,470), although prospective evidence of the superiority of intraperitoneal combination chemotherapy is lacking.

In these studies, responses have been primarily limited to patients with small-volume disease. Furthermore, responses have been observed to intraperitoneal cisplatin, primarily in patients with a prior response to intravenous cisplatin. This is the same group of patients, discussed in the section on second-line therapy, who also have the greatest benefit from retreatment with systemic therapy. This raises the possibility that the primary benefit of intraperitoneal therapy results from its systemic effects. These studies suggest that, once acquired resistance to cisplatin develops, the pharmacologic advantage achieved by the intraperitoneal route is insufficient to increase cytotoxicity substantially. Although the simultaneous administration of IV sodium thiosulfate as a systemic neutralizing agent permits even greater doses of cisplatin to be administered intraperitoneally (468), it has not been shown to lead to a higher response rate. Although Phase II trials have produced substantial responses to intraperitoneal chemotherapy, there has been no prospective randomized trial comparing this form of treatment to systemic therapy in patients with small-volume residual disease after a standard course of intravenous induction therapy.

Sequential intravenous and intraperitoneal chemotherapy has been administered in clinical trials in untreated patients with ovarian cancer. Markman (471) reported a high complete remission rate (47%) for a treatment approach that included debulking surgery, high-dose intravenous cisplatin, and secondary cytoreduction followed by intraperitoneal cisplatin. Barakat et al. (472) reported results of a Phase II trial of intraperitoneal cisplatin and etoposide as consolidation therapy in patients with stages II to IV ovarian cancer who had achieved a surgically confirmed complete remission to induction therapy. Survival was compared to a cohort of patients undergoing observation only. Median disease-free survival has not been reached for patients undergoing consolidation and was 28.5 months for the controls. The results of long-term follow-up for intraperitoneal chemotherapy at the Memorial Sloan–Kettering Cancer Center have recently been updated by Barakat et al. (379). Median survival was reported for patients based on amount of residual disease at the time intraperitoneal therapy was initiated: no residual (8.7 years), microscopic (4.8 years), <1 cm (3.3 years), and >1 cm (1.2 years).

Randomized Comparisons of Intraperitoneal versus Intravenous Chemotherapy

Howell et al. (473) reported a 74% 4-year survival for patients with small-volume residual disease who were treated with cisplatin or cisplatin combined with other agents. Since patients had small-volume disease, it cannot be concluded, however, that patients in this study survived because of the intraperitoneal therapy or because they had a favorable natural history. Subsequently, an intergroup study compared intraperitoneal and intravenous cisplatin in patients with small-volume disease (474). Eligible patients for this trial had no tumor masses >2 cm residual following initial surgery. Patients were randomized to six courses of intraperitoneal cisplatin (100 mg/m^2) or to intravenous cisplatin at the same dose. All patients received 600 mg/m^2 of cyclophosphamide intravenously. Of the 539 eligible patients, 385 had <0.5-cm residual disease after surgery. Median follow-up was almost 4 years. The median survival of patients receiving the intraperitoneal chemotherapy was 49 months and was significantly longer than the median survival of 41 months for the patients who received both drugs intravenously. In addition, there was less clinical hearing loss and neutropenia in patients treated with intraperitoneal platinum.

A follow-up GOG trial of sequential intravenous and intraperitoneal chemotherapy has been completed in patients with optimal stage III disease (475). In this study, the control arm consisted of intravenous cisplatin plus paclitaxel. The experimental arm consisted of two cycles of carboplatin dosed to an AUC of 9 followed by six cycles of intraperitoneal cisplatin and intravenous paclitaxel. A total of 462 patients with small-volume stage III ovarian cancer were evaluable. Neutropenia, thrombocytopenia, and gastrointestinal and metabolic toxicities were greater in the experimental arm, and 18% of patients received less than two courses of IP therapy and discontinued because of toxicity. Progression-free survival was superior for patients randomized to the experimental arm (28 months vs 22 months, $p = .01$). There was a borderline improvement in overall survival associated with the intraperitoneal regimen (median 63 months vs 52 months, $p = .05$). Because the improvement in overall survival was of borderline statistical significance and the toxicity was greater with the experimental arm, it was not recommended for routine use.

A subsequent Phase II trial by the GOG of intraperitoneal paclitaxel demonstrated a high degree of activity in patients with small-volume disease (476). Of 28 assessable patients with previously treated ovarian cancer who had microscopic disease at the start of intraperitoneal paclitaxel (60 mg/m^2

weekly for 16 weeks), 17 patients (61%) achieved a surgically defined complete response. In contrast, only 1 of 31 patients (3%) with any microscopic disease achieved a complete remission.

Based on the demonstration of high degree of activity in this Phase II trial, and results of the previously mentioned two randomized trials, the GOG performed a third randomized trial of intraperitoneal therapy versus intravenous therapy (GOG protocol 172) (477). In this study, patients with optimal stage III disease were randomized to receive intravenous paclitaxel (135 mg/m^2 in a 24-hour infusion) together with cisplatin (75 mg/m^2) or to the experimental combination consisting of intravenous paclitaxel (135 mg/m^2 over 24 hours on day 1) followed by 100 mg of cisplatin intraperitoneally on day 2 and paclitaxel at 60 mg/m^2 intraperitoneally on day 8, with cycles administered every 21 days. The preliminary results of this trial have been reported (470). Nineteen percent of patients treated with the intraperitoneal regimen could not complete therapy owing to toxicity. In the intraperitoneal arm, there was significantly more grades 3 and 4 toxicity, including leukopenia (31% vs 14%), thrombocytopenia (12% vs 4%), gastrointestinal toxicity (46% vs 24%), neurologic toxicity (19% vs 9%), infection (16% vs 5%), and pain (11% vs 1%). The relative risk of recurrence was 0.73 for patients receiving the intraperitoneal chemotherapy and immature survival data are trending toward the experimental arm. At this point, the GOG is not performing any randomized trials of intraperitoneal chemotherapy owing to the excessive toxicity of intraperitoneal therapy and the absence of clearly defined improvement in survival. Phase I studies of intraperitoneal carboplatin and paclitaxel are planned since this combination may have less toxicity (478–480).

The results of an EORTC trial of intraperitoneal cisplatin versus no further treatment in ovarian cancer patients with a pathologically complete remission after platinum-based intravenous chemotherapy have been reported (479). With a median follow-up of 8 years, there was no statistically significant difference in the hazard ratios for progression-free survival and overall survival: 0.89 (CI 0.59 to 1.33) and 0.82 (CI 0.52 to 1.29), respectively.

The reasons for the pharmacologic advantage associated with intraperitoneal administration of platinum-based chemotherapy having a limited effect on survival of patients with small-volume ovarian cancer are not clear. It is possible that the retroperitoneal nodes involved with tumor are sanctuary sites. In addition, although a pharmacologic advantage clearly exists with regard to the ratio of drug levels in the peritoneal cavity versus the systemic circulation, it has not been established that substantially more drug is actually delivered to intraperitoneal tumor nodules. In a rat model, the depth of penetration of cisplatin was only 1 to 2 mm into intraperitoneal tumors following intraperitoneal therapy, and the actual platinum concentration in the periphery of these tumors was only two to three times greater than that achieved

with intravenous administration (481). It is also possible that current studies have overestimated the frequency of uniform drug distribution throughout the peritoneal cavity, and that adhesions may produce pharmacologic sanctuaries.

As previously noted, approximately 30% to 50% of patients who achieve a surgically confirmed complete remission ultimately suffer a relapse. This high relapse rate suggests that many negative second-look laparotomies are false negatives, and that patients have microscopic residual disease that is undetected at surgery. It is in this situation that intraperitoneal chemotherapy may be beneficial since the problem of poor penetration into macroscopic tumor nodules will be avoided. Results are not available from a European study in which patients who achieved a complete remission were randomized to receive intraperitoneal therapy or observation.

Surgical Considerations for Intraperitoneal Chemotherapy

The three common methods of obtaining access to the peritoneal cavity are single-use percutaneous catheters, semipermanent percutaneous catheters, and implanted subcutaneous port and catheter systems. Reported complications for all catheters include intestinal injury, catheter blockage, and infections involving the peritoneal cavity or the abdominal wall (482,483). The implanted subcutaneous port and catheter systems have the advantages of a lower risk of infection and better patient acceptance. In the largest series reported to date, Davidson et al. (484) analyzed data on 249 catheters placed in 227 patients. No injuries occurred at the time of catheter placement. Significant complications occurred in 17.6% of patients, including catheter blockage (8.8%) and infection (8.8%). In eight patients, late erosion of the catheter into the intestinal lumen was noted. Recommendations from this study concluded that catheters should not be placed at the time of colon surgery because of a possible increase in the risk of infection, and that intraperitoneal chemotherapy should not be administered until 7 to 14 days following catheter placement to allow time for wound healing. Strict aseptic technique should be used when catheters are accessed. The implanted subcutaneous port and catheter systems have an acceptable level of morbidity for delivery of intraperitoneal therapy. The major technical impediment to successful intraperitoneal therapy is the formation of adhesions within the peritoneal cavity, which leads to catheter blockage and poor distribution of drugs instilled into the cavity. Recent experience suggests that catheters designed for intravenous use may be used for intraperitoneal chemotherapy. The smaller diameter of the IV catheter, together with the absence of side holes, may produce fewer intraperitoneal adhesions as compared to the catheters designed for IP use (480).

SECOND-LINE CHEMOTHERAPY

Patients who do not respond to their initial chemotherapeutic regimen or who relapse after achieving a prior response overall have a relatively poor prognosis and neither group has a substantial cure rate. However, the response rates and duration of clinically significant remissions to second-line therapy are markedly different in these two groups of patients. In patients who achieve a complete remission to initial therapy with a platinum-based regimen and have a disease-free interval greater than 6 months, treatment with carboplatin at the time of initial recurrence produces an approximately 30% response rate (315,485). Similarly, these patients can often be effectively retreated with cisplatin (486–488). However, carboplatin has a better toxicity profile in this setting since many of the patients will have residual neuropathy from prior cisplatin. For patients who experienced severe myelosuppression with their first courses of carboplatin, retreatment with carboplatin may produce unacceptably severe hematologic toxicity and, in that situation, cisplatin may be a better alternative for salvage therapy. As will be described, some recent trials suggest that carboplatin combinations may be more effective than single-agent platinum compounds in these platinum-sensitive patients.

Most patients with advanced disease are now being treated with a combination of paclitaxel plus a platinum compound as their initial chemotherapeutic regimen. The likelihood of achieving a secondary response to paclitaxel is similar to that for the platinum compounds, that is, the longer the initial disease-free interval, the more probable that paclitaxel retreatment will be effective (489). As discussed previously, novel schedules of paclitaxel, including a 96-hour infusion and weekly administration, have been studied. Whereas a 96-hour schedule appears to be inactive in ovarian cancer (490), a weekly schedule has produced a 32% to 47% response rate in patients refractory to the conventional 3-week schedule (364,365).

Those patients who do not respond to platinum- or paclitaxel-based induction chemotherapy have a lower response rate to second-line treatment, and these patients should be encouraged to enter experimental clinical trials (489,491). There is almost complete cross-resistance between carboplatin and cisplatin and, consequently, outside of a clinical trial situation, therapy should be with nonplatinum compounds.

It has recently been identified that in addition to the disease-free interval, the probability of response to chemotherapy following platinum-based treatment for ovarian cancer is related to other clinical factors as well. Eisenhauer et al. (492) reported on a multivariate analysis of 704 patients who received prior treatment with platinum-based chemotherapy. Eleven factors were examined in a univariate analysis and only three factors remained significant as independent predictors of response: serous histology, number of disease sites, and tumor size. In their analysis, time from last treatment, when evaluated as a continuous variable, was not found in the final model and was highly correlated with tumor size.

A series of new agents have been shown to have activity in the second-line treatment of patients with recurrent ovarian cancer including topotecan (493,494), oral VP16 (495), gemcitabine (496,497), vinorelbine (498), docetaxel (341,499, 500), and liposomal doxorubicin (501,502).

Topotecan is a second-generation semisynthetic camptothecin analog which inhibits topoisomerase I, an intranuclear enzyme that relieves torsion in DNA induced by replication. Myelosuppression was the dose-limiting toxicity in Phase I trials and activity was noted at a dose of 1.5 mg/m^2 daily $\times$ 5 schedule. In Phase II studies in patients who progressed after one or more platinum-based regimens, topotecan produced a response rate ranging from 14% to 25% on various schedules (493,494). In a Phase III randomized study, patients who were treated with topotecan after platinum-based therapy without prior paclitaxel had a response rate of 20.5%, compared with 13.2% in patients who received paclitaxel (503). The GOG subsequently evaluated topotecan in platinum-sensitive patients (504). The overall response rate was 33% in 46 patients, including two complete responses. Median progression-free interval was 9.6 months. Grade 4 neutropenia occurred in 45 patients, and 21 patients received G-CSF. Bookman et al. (493) reported on 139 patients with previously treated ovarian cancer in whom 81% had resistance to platinum. The overall response rate was 13.7%, with a 12.4% response rate in platinum-resistant patients and 19.2% response rate observed in platinum-sensitive patients. The median duration of response and time to progression were 18.1 and 12.1 weeks, respectively. The median survival was 47 weeks. Grade 4 neutropenia was the primary toxicity and occurred in 82% of the patients. Owing to the substantial myelosuppression of a daily $\times$ 5 schedule, alternative treatment schedules with topotecan are being studied, including a weekly schedule that appears to be active and associated with less toxicity (505). Additional trials are in progress to confirm the activity and toxicity as well as to determine the optimal dosing of a weekly schedule.

Whereas intravenous etoposide has been shown to have little, if any, clinical activity in patients with recurrent ovarian cancer, prolonged oral etoposide was shown to be an active second-line therapy for platinum-resistant and platinum-sensitive ovarian cancer patients. In a Phase II GOG trial, 97 patients were assessable for toxicity and 82 for response (495). Among 41 platinum-resistant patients, a 27% response rate, including a 7.3% clinical complete response rate, was observed. Median response duration was 4.3 months and the median progression-free interval was 5.7 months. Median survival time in these poor-prognosis platinum-resistant patients was 10.8 months. In platinum-sensitive patients, there was a 34% response rate, including a 15% clinical complete response rate. Median response ratio in this more favorable group of patients was 7.5 months and median survival time was 16.5+ months. Grade 3 or 4 hematologic toxicity was common (grade 3 or 4 leukopenia occurred in 41% of patients). The dose of 50 mg/m² per day for 21 days every 28 days was well tolerated for nonhematologic side effects.

Gemcitabine is a novel pyrimidine analog with broad activity in solid tumors, including lung cancer, pancreatic cancer, and breast cancer. Lund et al.(496) reported on a Phase II study in previously treated ovarian cancer patients and reported a 19% response rate in 42 patients. The median response duration was 8.5 months. Seven of the eight responders were resistant to first-line platinum-containing combination chemotherapy. Leukocytopenia and thrombocytopenia were the primary toxicities and were managed by dose reductions. Gemcitabine was also shown to have activity in patients resistant to both platinum and paclitaxel, with a partial response rate of 13% (497).

Liposomal doxorubicin (501,502), a preparation of doxorubicin and a liposome that contains surface-grafted segments of the hydrophilic polymer methoxypolyethylene glycol, was shown in a Phase II study to produce a response rate of 26%. The median progression-free survival was 5.7 months, with a median overall survival of 11 months. Grades 3 and 4 nonhematologic skin and mucosal toxicities (either hand-foot syndrome or stomatitis) were common.

A large randomized trial (474 patients) compared the efficacy and safety of liposomal doxorubicin and topotecan in patients with platinum-sensitive and platinum-resistant ovarian cancer (506). The overall progression-free survival was similar between the two arms, as were the overall response rates for liposomal doxorubicin and topotecan (19.7% vs 17.0%, $p = .39$). Median overall survival times were also similar: 60 versus 56.7 weeks, respectively. In a retrospective analysis in platinum-sensitive patients, there was a statistically significant benefit to overall survival for liposomal doxorubicin (108 vs 71 weeks). Both doxorubicin and topotecan had lower response rates in platinum-resistant patients compared to platinum-sensitive patients (12.3% vs 28.4%) for liposomal doxorubicin, and 6.5% vs 28.8% for topotecan in platinum-sensitive and platinum-resistant patients, respectively. Severe hematologic toxicity is more common with topotecan, whereas liposomal doxorubin resulted in more palmar-plantar erythrodysesthesia (PPE). Both topotecan and liposomal doxorubin were administered at FDA-approved doses (1.5 mg/m² per day for 5 consecutive days vs 50 mg/m² every 4 weeks, respectively). However, in clinical practice, these doses have been found to be excessively toxic and patients are usually treated with 1.0 to 1.25 mg/m² days 1 through 5 with topotecan and 40 mg/m² every 4 weeks for liposomal doxorubicin.

In addition to these agents, drugs such as hexamethylmelamine and ifosfamide also have activity in recurrent ovarian cancer. Similar to drugs such as topotecan and liposomal doxorubicin, these agents also have low response rates in platinum-resistant patients compared to platinum-sensitive patients (489).

Combination chemotherapeutic regimens have also been used as second-line treatment for patients with ovarian cancer. Rose et al. (507) reported on the activity of second-line therapy with paclitaxel and carboplatin in patients who had received prior treatment with paclitaxel and platinum. Patients had received a prior clinical complete remission that lasted for greater than 6 months with initial therapy with paclitaxel and a platinum compound. In this highly favorable group of patients, second-line therapy with paclitaxel plus carboplatin produced a 70% clinical complete remission rate, with an additional 20% achieving a partial response. The majority of patients developed recurrence after secondary therapy at a median interval of 9 months. In a retrospective study from the Memorial Sloan–Kettering Cancer Center, platinum-sensitive patients treated with the same combination of paclitaxel and carboplatin had a higher than expected complete response rate (42%) (508). Similarly, a combination of gemcitabine and carboplatin also produced a high response rate (62.5%) in platinum-sensitive patients (509).

The heterogeneous nature of ovarian cancer and the large number of prognostic factors that influence response to therapy necessitate the prospective randomized trials to eliminate bias in selection factors even in patients with recurrent ovarian cancer. Recently, a randomized trial comparing paclitaxel plus platinum with conventional platinum-based therapy in patients with platinum-sensitive recurrent ovarian cancer was reported (510). Eight hundred patients with platinum-sensitive ovarian cancer relapsing after 6 months were enrolled in an international trial conducted in five countries. Patients were randomly assigned to paclitaxel plus platinum (80% of patients receiving paclitaxel plus carboplatin) or conventional platinum-based chemotherapy (71% of patients receiving carboplatin alone). With a median follow-up of 42 months, survival curves (Fig. 25.34) show a difference in favor of paclitaxel plus platinum (hazard ratio 0.82, 95% CI 0.69 to 0.97, $p = .02$), corresponding to an absolute difference in 2-year survival of 7% between the paclitaxel/platinum combination and conventional treatment groups (57% vs 50%, 95% CI for difference of 1% to 12%). Similarly, there was a 5-month improvement in median survival (29 months vs 24 months) for patients treated with the paclitaxel/platinum combination. The progression-free survival curves also showed a difference in favor of paclitaxel plus platinum (hazard ratio 0.76, 95% CI 0.66 to 0.89, $p = .0004$), corresponding to an absolute difference in a 1-year progression-free survival of 10% (50% vs 40%) and in median progression-free survival of 3 months. This was the first reported randomized trial in patients with platinum-sensitive recurrent ovarian cancer that demonstrated a beneficial effect for paclitaxel in combination with platinum chemotherapy on survival and progression-free survival. The AGO has also performed a prospective randomized trial in a similar group of patients who were randomized to single-agent car-

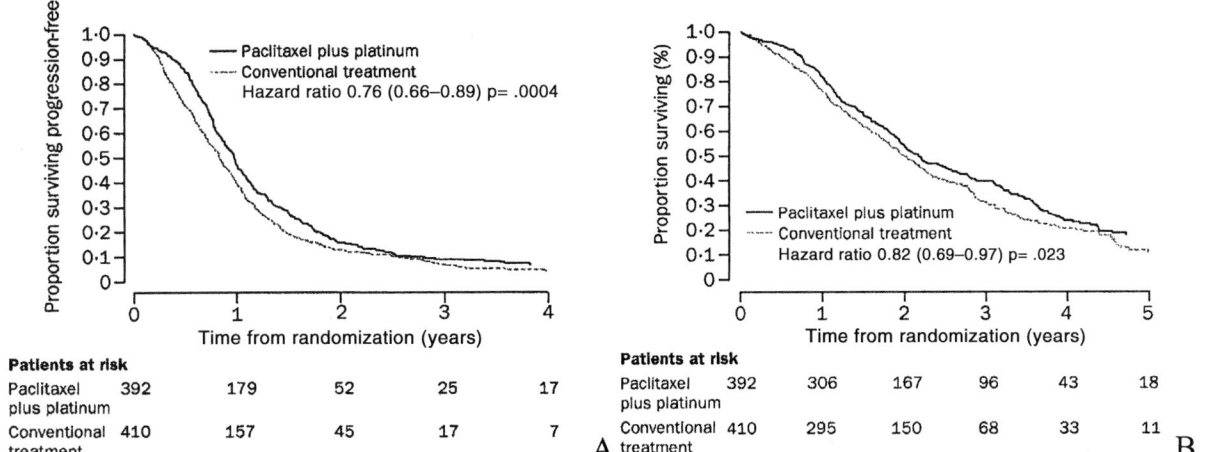

FIG. 25.34. **A** and **B**: Progression-free and overall survival for paclitaxel plus platinum or conventional treatment in advanced ovarian cancer patients who relapsed more than 6 months after initial chemotherapy. (From The ICON and AGO Collaborators. Paclitaxel plus platinum-based chemotherapy versus conventional platinum-based chemotherapy in women with relapsed ovarian cancer: the ICON4/AGO-OVAR-2.2 trial. *Lancet* 2003;361:2099–2106. Reprinted with permission from Elsevier.)

boplatin or the combination of carboplatin plus gemcitabine based on their Phase II results with the two-drug combination (509). These two trials are not definitive in addressing the issue of whether combination chemotherapy is superior compared to the use of the same drugs in sequence in patients with platinum-sensitive ovarian cancer. In the United States, the GOG is developing a multiarm randomized trial in platinum-sensitive patients that may resolve issues about which combination is superior and whether these combinations are superior to single agents used in sequence.

HORMONAL THERAPY

A wide variety of hormonal therapies have been used in patients with ovarian cancer (511,512). Progestational agents have been used primarily on the basis of a possible similarity in biologic behavior between endometrioid ovarian cancer and endometrial cancer. Clinical interest in hormonal therapy for ovarian cancer has been further stimulated by the finding that human ovarian tumors frequently have estrogen and androgen receptors. Clinical trials of various hormonal manipulations, in addition to progestational agents, have been reported, including antiandrogens (513), gonadotropin-releasing hormone analogs (leuprolide acetate) (514), and antiestrogens (515,516). Overall, the response rate to progestational agents and antiestrogens has been only 15% and 4% to 5%, respectively. Similar response rates have been reported for leuprolide acetate (17%) and cyproterone acetate (7%) (513,514). In the GOG study, there was a 13% complete response rate to tamoxifen at a dose of 20 mg PO b.i.d., which is twice the common dose for breast cancer (515,516). Eight of the nine patients achieving a complete remission had elevated levels of estrogen receptor.

A large clinical trial evaluated chemohormonal therapy in patients with previously untreated advanced disease (517). One hundred patients were treated with a combination of cisplatin plus doxorubicin, with half of the patients randomized to receive concomitant tamoxifen. However, there was no difference in overall or progression-free survival between these two patient groups.

Taken as a group, hormonal therapies produce an approximate 10% response rate in previously treated patients. A correlation may exist between the presence of hormone receptors and a response to therapy. Even though hormonal therapy does have a low response rate, it remains a viable therapeutic option in patients who have failed cytotoxic chemotherapy or who cannot tolerate its toxic effects.

EXPERIMENTAL THERAPY

Clinical research in the treatment of ovarian cancer is focused upon four major objectives:

1. Improving the complete remission rate with chemotherapy and cytoreductive surgery
2. Preventing or delaying recurrences after achievement of a complete remission (discussed previously)
3. Understanding the mechanisms of antineoplastic drug resistance and developing pharmacologic techniques capable of reversing or preventing drug resistance
4. Developing effective molecular-targeted and immunotherapy approaches

NEW DRUGS AND COMBINATIONS

As discussed previously, platinum and paclitaxel have resulted in a significant improvement in the treatment of patients with advanced ovarian cancer. However, numerous questions still remain regarding the optimum use of these agents, including dose, duration of administration, and combination with other active agents. Whether paclitaxel was the optimum taxane to use in combination with carboplatin was evaluated in a large prospective randomized trial in Europe (518). Over 800 patients with advanced disease were randomized to treatment with carboplatin (AUC = 6) plus paclitaxel (175 mg/m²) or to carboplatin (AUC = 6) plus docetaxel (75 mg/m²). Previous Phase II trials had demonstrated that docetaxel produced a response rate comparable to paclitaxel in platinum-resistant patients (20% to 35%). The randomized study in untreated patients was designed as a superiority trial; however, the preliminary results have failed to show an improvement in either progression-free survival or overall survival. The paclitaxel patients experienced more neurotoxicity, whereas docetaxel led to more myelosuppression, allergic reactions, and diarrhea. These investigators have chosen docetaxel plus carboplatin as the control arm of future randomized trials, whereas all other randomized trials of new therapies continue to use carboplatin plus paclitaxel as the standard regimen.

Based on the activity of the newer agents as second-line treatments in paclitaxel- and platinum-resistant patients, Phase I and Phase II trials has been performed with either three-drug combinations or novel doublets. Subsequently, a series of prospective randomized trials has been initiated comparing experimental triplets and doublets to standard therapy with carboplatin plus paclitaxel (Table 25.24 and Fig. 25.35).

A three-drug triplet in which gemcitabine is combined with carboplatin and paclitaxel was first developed by Hansen et al. (519). It was shown that gemcitabine (800 mg/m² on day 1 and day 8) could be combined with full-dose carboplatin (AUC = 5) and paclitaxel (175 mg/m²) in a 3-hour infusion. This three-drug combination resulted in a response rate of 100% in previously untreated patients with advanced ovarian cancer. Look et al. (520) piloted a similar triplet in the GOG. Owing to the unacceptably incidence of complicated neutropenia and grade 4 thrombocytopenia, the starting doses of carboplatin were selected to be an AUC of 5 on day 1 and paclitaxel 135 mg/m² on day 1, and gemcitabine 800 mg/m² on day 1 and day 8. The majority of patients received eight complete cycles without dose modification, excessive delay, or support with hematologic growth factors.

European investigators added epirubicin to paclitaxel and

TABLE 25.24. *Prospective randomized trials of new combination chemotherapeutic regimens*

Triplets
  Paclitaxel + carboplatin + epirubicin
  Paclitaxel + carboplatin + gemcitabine
  Paclitaxel + carboplatin + topotecan
  GOG 182/ICON 5
Doublets
  Docetaxel + carboplatin
  Gemcitabine + carboplatin
  Topotecan + cisplatin
  GOG 182/ICON 5
Other
  Paclitaxel + carboplatin plus interferon-γ

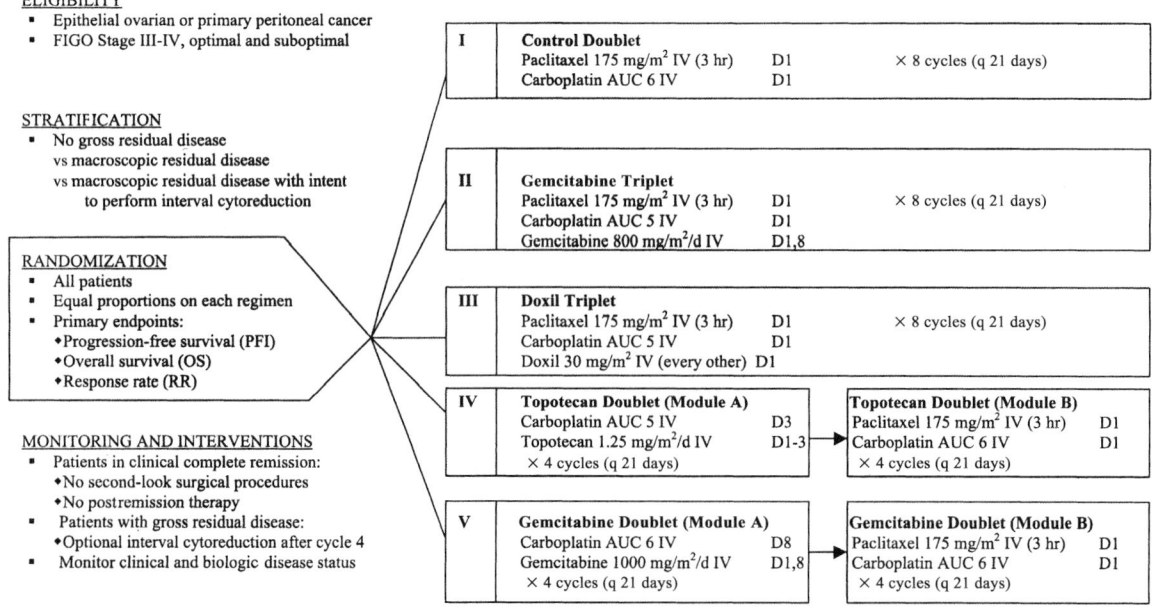

FIG. 25.35. Schema for GOG 182: a phase III randomized trial of paclitaxel and carboplatin versus triplet or sequential doublet combinations in patients with epithelial ovarian or primary peritoneal carcinoma.

carboplatin in Phase I and Phase II studies (521). The maximum tolerated dose of epirubicin was 60 mg/m^2 combined with a 3-hour infusion of paclitaxel 175 mg/m^2 and carboplatin dosed to an AUC of 5. The preliminary results of randomized trials comparing paclitaxel plus carboplatin versus the three-drug combination incorporating epirubicin have recently been reported (522,523). Initial results suggest that there may be improvement in progression-free survival for patients receiving the three-drug combination, although there are no data available currently on overall survival. The three-drug combination was associated with more myelosuppression compared to standard therapy with paclitaxel plus carboplatin. Rose et al. (524) conducted a Phase I evaluation of liposomal doxorubicin in combination with carboplatin plus paclitaxel. Owing to dose-limiting hematologic toxicity, the recommended doses for the triplet combination necessitated decreasing the dose to 30 mg/m^2 and administering it only every other cycle in combination with carboplatin and paclitaxel. Rose et al. (525) also completed a Phase I study of oral etoposide with carboplatin (AUC = 5) and paclitaxel (175 mg/m^2) that established a recommended etoposide dose of 50 mg/m^2 per day × 10 days. In this study, 3 of 52 patients, however, developed acute myelogenous leukemia that occurred between 16 and 35 months after completion of therapy. Further development of this combination is unlikely owing to the unacceptably high risk of secondary leukemia in newly diagnosed patients receiving front-line therapy.

A three-drug combination of paclitaxel, cisplatin, and topotecan also produced a high response rate (60% clinical complete response and 27% partial response) in previously untreated patients in a Phase I pharmacologic study (526). Neutropenia was the dose-limiting toxicity of this combination and required significant dose reductions in paclitaxel (110 mg/m^2 on day 1) and cisplatin (75 mg/m^2 on day 2) followed by topotecan (dosed to 0.3 mg/m^2 per day for days 2 through 6). In addition, G-CSF support was also necessary. Excessive toxicity and the requirement for growth-factor support make this combination problematic, although a randomized comparison of paclitaxel plus carboplatin versus a three-drug combination of topotecan, paclitaxel, and carboplatin is in progress in Italy (527). Phase II studies of sequential couplets of cisplatin/topotecan followed by paclitaxel and platinum have been developed with less toxicity. Hoskins et al. (528) reported on 44 patients who were treated with cisplatin 50 mg/m^2 on day 1 and topotecan 0.75 mg/m^2 on days 1 through 5 administered at 21-day intervals for four cycles. Patients were then treated with paclitaxel 135 mg/m^2 over 24 hours on day 1 and cisplatin 75 mg/m^2 on day 2 at 21-day intervals for an additional four cycles. The overall response rate was 78%. In addition, 77% of patients with elevated CA-125 levels at baseline had normalization of CA-125 levels at the end of therapy. Myelotoxicity was the major toxicity but it was of a short duration. Since paclitaxel plus carboplatin has replaced paclitaxel plus cisplatin as the standard therapy, the investigators have developed a new regimen in which the paclitaxel/cisplatin couplet is replaced by a couplet of paclitaxel (175 mg/m^2) plus carboplatin (AUC = 5). Consequently, in an international study of the EORTC and the NCIC Clinical Trials Group, the experimental arm consists of four cycles of cisplatin plus topotecan followed by four cycles of carboplatin plus paclitaxel. The control arm is eight cycles of carboplatin plus paclitaxel.

Several studies have demonstrated that gemcitabine can be combined with cisplatin or carboplatin (509,529). Based on high levels of activity in recurrent ovarian cancer as well as in pilot studies in previously untreated patients with advanced ovarian cancer, an industry-sponsored (Eli Lilly) trial is currently in progress in which previously untreated patients with advanced ovarian cancer are randomized to treatment with carboplatin plus paclitaxel or gemcitabine plus carboplatin.

As will be discussed subsequently, immunologic therapies are also under evaluation in ovarian cancer. A prospective randomized trial comparing carboplatin plus paclitaxel to the two-drug combination with interferon-γ is also currently in progress in the United States. This study is based upon a smaller randomized trial in Europe in which previously untreated patients with advanced ovarian cancer were treated with cisplatin plus cyclophosphamide or cisplatin plus cyclophosphamide plus interferon-γ (530). The interferon-treated patients had improvement in time to progression and in overall survival.

No evidence currently exists to indicate whether optimal combinations should utilize sequential single agents, doublets, or triplets (531). The triplet combinations have increased bone marrow toxicity, and individual drug doses are lower than comparable single agents or doublets, creating the possibility that tumor efficacy may be compromised. However, combinations that include some of the newer agents that inhibit DNA repair, including topotecan and gemcitabine, may enhance the effects of platinum and, consequently, to achieve optimum therapeutic benefit may not require the higher doses as used when the drugs are administered as single agents. The use of sequential doublets appears to permit higher doses of individual drugs, and it is also possible that sequential utilitzation of more than one regimen with a different mechanism of action may prevent the emergence of drug-resistant tumors. GOG protocol 182/ICON5 (Fig. 25.35) was designed so that each of the experimental regimens should be given for at least four cycles to provide an opportunity to observe treatment-related benefit from the new agent, and that each arm should also contain at least four cycles of carboplatin and paclitaxel to maintain benefit from this standard regimen (531). The experimental triplets with gemcitabine and liposomal doxorubicin each contained eight cycles, although the liposomal doxorubicin, as noted, can only be administered every other cycle based on toxicity data obtained in a GOG pilot study. A sequential doublet uses topotecan (daily × 3) with carboplatin administered on day 3 based on pilot studies by the GOG of different sequences of these two agents. A sequential doublet with gemcitabine also utilizes the "reverse" sequence (carboplatin on day 8) for four cycles followed by four cycles of carboplatin and paclitaxel. The control arm consists of carboplatin (AUC = 6) together with paclitaxel (175 mg/m^2) in a 3-hour infusion. All five regimens are administered for a total of eight cycles. Until the completion of these randomized Phase III trials, carboplatin plus paclitaxel remains the primary standard of care for previously untreated patients with advanced ovarian cancer.

DOSE INTENSIFICATION AND HIGH-DOSE CHEMOTHERAPY WITH STEM-CELL SUPPORT

An alternative approach to the development of new drugs and drug regimens has been to intensify the dose of standard chemotherapy combinations. As previously noted, a doubling of the dose intensity of platinum compounds has not been associated with any improvement in survival in prospective randomized trials in previously untreated patients with bulky ovarian cancer. Subsequent studies attempted to determine whether survival could be improved if the dose intensity was increased five- to tenfold. Many of these studies focused on increasing the dose intensity of carboplatin and decreasing its dose-limiting toxicity of myelosuppression, especially thrombocytopenia. The clinically available cytokines do not permit a more than two- to threefold increase in dose intensity, which may not be clinically meaningful.

Shpall et al. (532) summarized the results of early Phase I and Phase II trials of high-dose chemotherapy with hematologic support in ovarian cancer patients. More than ten individual Phase I and Phase II trials have been reported, although the number of patients in these trials is small. More than 200 women with advanced-stage ovarian cancer, however, have now received high-dose chemotherapy in these clinical studies. The overall response rate was approximately 70% to 80%, which is higher than that reported for other second-line therapies. However, the median duration of response in these studies was less than 9 months. Subsequently, high-dose chemotherapy was focused on patients with small-volume disease and drug-sensitive tumors.

Stiff et al. (533) reported on their experience in 100 patients who had received high-dose chemotherapy with autologous transplantation for persistent or relapsed ovarian cancer. The majority of patients were treated with a high-dose regimen consisting of carboplatin, mitoxantrone, and cyclophosphamide, although 25 patients were treated with a combination of high-dose melphalan and mitoxantrone with or without paclitaxel. Univariate and multivariate analyses were performed to identify factors associated with prolonged survival following high-dose chemotherapy with a transplant. Tumor bulk and cisplatin sensitivity were identified as the best predictors for progression-free survival. The median progression-free and overall survival for 20 patients

with platinum-sensitive disease with <1 cm of volume was 19 and 30 months, respectively. These investigators concluded that patients with platinum-resistant and bulky disease should not be transplanted owing to their poor survival following high-dose chemotherapy.

A similar retrospective study on high-dose chemotherapy with bone-marrow transplant was reported by the European Group for Blood and Marrow Transplant (EBMT) (534). This registry included results on 254 patients who had received a transplant in different disease categories, that is, patients in first or second remission with or with no residual disease or microscopic/macroscopic residual after standard-dose treatment. The median survival following transplantation in patients in a complete remission was 33 months, which was significantly better than the 14 months in the other disease categories. Deaths related to the procedure occurred in 4.7%. Based on these results, a Phase III trial of high-dose therapy in selected stages III and IV patients is in progress by the EBMT.

A limiting factor of autologous bone-marrow transplantation has been the inability to administer more than one to two cycles of high-dose therapy. Peripheral blood progenitor cell transplants have been shown to be feasible and effective in reversing drug-induced bone-marrow suppression. These cells can be harvested on an outpatient basis and permit administration of multiple cycles of high-dose chemotherapy. Peripheral blood stem-cell transplantation and its potential role in gynecologic malignancies have recently been reviewed by Cooper (535) and Lewis et al. (536). The largest single trial has been reported by investigators at the Memorial Sloan–Kettering Cancer Center (537). In their initial study, cyclophosphamide (3 g/m^2) was administered every 2 weeks for three cycles followed by four carboplatin treatments. Multiple leukaphereses were performed following each dose of cyclophosphamide to harvest peripheral blood stem cells, which were reinfused following high-dose carboplatin. Carboplatin doses could be escalated to 800 to 1200 mg/m^2 with an intertreatment interval of approximately 2 weeks. These investigators subsequently added paclitaxel to this regimen. In their pilot study, a total of 13 patients were evaluable for response. The overall response rate was 100%, with 92% of the patients achieving microscopic residual disease with a complete response rate of 38%.

Based upon these results, pilot studies of multiple cycles of high-dose carboplatin and paclitaxel followed by reinfusion of peripheral stem cells were conducted in previously untreated patients by investigators from the Memorial Sloan–Kettering Cancer Center (538) and Fox Chase Cancer Center (539). Both studies demonstrated a high degree of activity (34% surgically confirmed complete response and 67% clinical complete response, respectively).

Consequently, a multiinstitutional GOG trial of high-dose therapy in optimal stage III disease was performed (540). In this trial, peripheral blood stem cells were collected by leukaphoresis after mobilization with cyclophosphamide (3 gm/m^2), paclitaxel (300 mg/m^2), and G-CSF. Patients subsequently received three cycles of carboplatin (AUC = 15), paclitaxel (250 mg/m^2), and peripheral blood stem cells followed by G-CSF. Patients then received one cycle of high-dose melphalan (140 mg/m^2) and hematologic support. Nine patients ended the trial and received all planned cycles of chemotherapy. However, of the eight patients who consented to surgical reassessment upon completing therapy, only one patient had a pathologically confirmed complete response. The estimated probability of pathologic complete response was 12.5% (95% CI 0.3 to 52.7%). Hematologic toxicity was severe but manageable. Nevertheless, 25% of cycles resulted in hospital admission for neutropenic fever and other complications of treatment. The low pathologic complete response rate did not justify the toxicity. It should be noted that the standard six cycles of carboplatin plus cyclophosphamide in the same group of patients in GOG protocol 158 produced a negative second-look rate in approximately 50% of the patients (346). Consequently, this pilot study did not support further evaluation of high-dose chemotherapy with stem-cell support in previously untreated patients with advanced ovarian cancer. No such trials are in progress in the United States. No prospective trial of high-dose therapy with peripheral stem-cell transplantation has established clinical benefit in any patient population either previously treated or untreated.

REVERSAL OF DRUG RESISTANCE

Acquired drug resistance is a major factor that limits the effectiveness of chemotherapy in patients with advanced ovarian cancer. Patients with recurrent disease after an initial response to chemotherapy rarely, if ever, are cured with chemotherapy (Fig. 25.27). In part, this is related to the broad cross resistance that develops toward antineoplastic agents from different pharmacologic classes. An additional 20% to 25% of patients have intrinsically drug-resistant tumors at the time of diagnosis and never respond to any chemotherapeutic regimen. It remains to be established whether the mechanisms responsible for acquired drug resistance are the same as those present in intrinsically drug-resistant patients.

The biochemical and molecular mechanisms associated with primary drug resistance and cross resistance in ovarian cancer have been extensively studied. Resistance to bifunctional alkylating agents and to platinum complexes is multifactorial and includes:

1. Alterations in drug accumulation
2. Increased inactivation by detoxification enzymes, such as glutathione-S-transferases (GST)
3. Direct binding to nonprotein thiols, such as glutathione (GSH), or to protein thiols, e.g., metallothionein
4. Increased removal of lethal DNA adducts by activated DNA repair enzymes

The observation that drug-resistant human ovarian cancer cell lines have higher levels of cellular GSH and that lowering GSH levels increases the potential for the cytotoxicity of alkylating agents and platinum complexes is of possible clinical relevance since inhibition of GSH biosynthesis is pharmacologically feasible. Buthionine sulfoximine (BSO) irreversibly inhibits the enzyme gamma-glutamyl-cysteine synthetase and produces a 90% reduction in GSH levels in cell lines and in animals. Furthermore, in a nude mouse model system in which the animals die of intraabdominal carcinomatosis following intraperitoneal transplantation of human ovarian cancer cells, BSO significantly increased the cytotoxicity of melphalan. A Phase I trial of BSO plus melphalan demonstrated that BSO can be safely administered to patients at doses that produce an 80% reduction in GSH levels in circulating lymphocytes in the majority of drug-resistant patients (541). Further evaluation of this strategy has been limited by limited availability of BSO and the toxicity of treatment. However, the GSH pathway continues to be a target for novel therapeutic approaches, including the evaluation of novel alkylating agents that are activated by GST π, which is elevated in drug-resistant tumors (542,543).

The findings that alkylating-agent and platinum resistance is associated with increased DNA repair capacity (544) are of clinical interest, since inhibition of DNA repair enzymes may be possible. Experimentally, inhibition of DNA repair enzymes has been shown to also restore sensitivity to platinum compounds in drug-resistant tumors. Aphidicolin, an inhibitor of DNA polymerase alpha, was effective in restoring sensitivity to cisplatin in human ovarian cancer cells *in vitro* (545). Clinical trials have demonstrated that the drug is essentially nontoxic and that the necessary plasma levels may be achievable. However, clinical evaluation of cisplatin plus aphidicolin was not performed owing to drug availability. However, gemcitabine also inhibits DNA repair pathways, and this may account, in part, for the high response rate (43%) reported for the combination of gemcitabine plus cisplatin in platinum-resistant ovarian cancer patients (including responses in four of six patients who were resistant to gemcitabine as a single agent) (546). The GOG is performing a confirmatory study of this combination in platinum-resistant patients.

A decrease in the net accumulation of structurally unrelated antineoplastic drugs is a major mechanism for pleiotropic (multidrug) resistance frequently associated with the use of natural products such as Adriamycin, vincristine, and VP16 (547). This type of resistance is due to increased expression/amplification of the *MDR1* gene, which codes for a protein that acts as an efflux pump. The binding of antineoplastic drug to this efflux pump can be inhibited by drugs such as verapamil, which restores drug sensitivity by increasing intracellular drug levels. Drug-sensitive human ovarian cancer cell lines exposed to Adriamycin *in vitro* develop this form of multidrug resistance. However, it does not appear that increased expression of *MDR* is a clinically relevant mechanism of drug resistance in most patients currently treated with combination chemotherapy. Increased *MDR1* expression has been observed in 20% to 30% of tumors from resistant ovarian cancer patients following therapy with a drug regimen that included a natural product, usually doxorubicin. Increased expression of *MDR1* has not been observed in tumors from patients treated with alkylating agents plus cisplatin (548). Since doxorubicin is not commonly used in most induction regimens, clinical trials of agents that modulate *MDR1* resistance are not likely to be relevant for most patients with ovarian cancer. However, resistance to the natural product paclitaxel is associated with *MDR1* expression, and *MDR1*-modulating agents will be studied in paclitaxel-resistant patients.

In addition to the 170-kD multidrug-resistant *MDR1* gene, overexpression of proteins, particularly the 190-kD MDR-associated protein (MRP), has also been associated with the multidrug resistance phenotype in preclinical cancer models. A series of novel agents capable of reversing multidrug-resistant phenotype has undergone Phase I and Phase II evaluation in ovarian cancer patients. Based on the activity and toxicity of the cyclosporin analog PSC-833 (549), a prospective randomized Phase III was performed in which patients received paclitaxel and carboplatin with or without this *MDR*-modulating agent. The preliminary results of this trial have failed to show any clinical benefit for PSC-833. Biricodar, a novel agent that reverses multidrug resistance conferred by overexpression of both *MDR1* and MRP in preclinical models, has undergone a Phase I study in combination with paclitaxel in drug-resistant patients (550). The acceptable toxicity profile of biricodar supports its further evaluation in patients with *de novo* or acquired resistance to paclitaxel caused by overexpression of *MDR1* and/or MRP.

BIOLOGIC AND MOLECULAR-TARGETED THERAPY OF OVARIAN CANCER

The immunobiology and principles of immunotherapy and molecular-targeted therapy for gynecologic malignancies have recently been reviewed (551,552). Ovarian cancer has long been a target of immunotherapeutic approaches. Initially, nonspecific immunostimulants were extensively studied in patients with ovarian cancer. However, randomized trials of melphalan, with or without *Corynebacterium parvum*, or combination chemotherapy with or without BCG [bacille Calmette-Guérin (vaccine)] failed to demonstrate any improvement in survival when administered either subcutaneously or intravenously. More recently, as previously described, a randomized trial demonstrated improvement in survival for patients treated with systemic interferon-γ together with a chemotherapeutic regimen consisting of cyclophosphamide plus cisplatin compared to treatment with chemotherapy alone (530).

A Phase I/II trial with adoptive immunotherapy in patients with ovarian cancer has also been reported (553). Patients in this study received intraperitoneal interleukin-2 (IL-2) together with lymphokine-activated killer (LAK) cells. Although evidence for clinical activity was found, the peritoneal toxicity of this approach was substantial, and further trials to evaluate the effectiveness of adoptive immunotherapy await the circumvention of the peritoneal fibrosis associated with this form of treatment. Intraperitoneal IL-2 alone is associated with less toxicity and has been associated with long-term survival in a select group of recurrent ovarian cancer patients (554). Among 34 patients with small-volume recurrent disease, there were seven surgically confirmed complete responses and two partial responses. Of particular interest was the observation that six patients were alive and disease-free for more than 5 years. As with other noncontrolled studies in this group of patients with small-volume residual disease, randomized comparisons are required to confirm any potential therapeutic advantage. As previously described in the section on Prognostic Factors above, the presence of intratumoral T cells independently correlated with delayed recurrence or delayed death (258), and in a multivariate analysis was also associated with increased expression of interferon-γ, IL-2, and lymphocyte-attracting chemokines within the tumor. Furthermore, the absence of intratumoral T cells was associated with increased levels of vascular endothelial growth factor. These data suggest that vascular endothelial growth factor may affect the behavior of ovarian cancer cells, not only by promoting angiogenesis, but by also reducing the number of T cells (552). In addition, chemokines have been shown to induce T-cell–mediated rejection of tumors in experimental models and, likewise, interferon-γ and Il-2 may have antitumor effects as well. These studies provide additional support for further trials of T-cell therapy in patients with ovarian cancer (552). Earlier strategies, as noted, used peripheral blood lymphocytes, tumor-associated lymphocytes, or tumor-infiltrating lymphocytes that were expanded and activated *ex vivo*.

Recent advances in immunobiology have indicated that T-cell costimulation is essential for proper T-cell activation and effective function and may partially explain the lack of efficacy of prior adoptive immunotherapy strategies (555). Coukos et al. (551) have summarized strategies to improve costimulatory signaling to T cells. Oligoclonal expansion of tumor-specific T cells may be possible with artificial antigen-presenting cells, tumor-cell–dendritic-cell hybrids, or tumor cells expanding costimulatory molecules in association with CD28 stimulation. Additional expansion and activation of T cells may be achieved through CD3 cross linking with CD28 costimulation. Such a "superactivated vector T-cell" population may be more effective for adoptive immunotherapy than using T cells obtained in the absence of costimulatory signals.

Monoclonal antibodies against surface markers of epithelial ovarian tumor cells or against the transferrin receptor have been used in early Phase I/II clinical trials. Murine monoclonal antibodies themselves are nontoxic unless linked to radioisotopes, such as ^{125}I or ^{131}I, or to toxins, such as recombinant ricin A chain or *Pseudomonas* endotoxin. Both immunotoxins and radioisotope conjugates have been associated with substantial toxicity in the early Phase I/II trials. Pancytopenia has been the dose-limiting toxicity associated with ^{131}I monoclonal antibodies, whereas immunotoxins have produced significant central nervous system and peripheral neurotoxicity.

Epenetos et al. (556), using a ^{131}I-labeled monoclonal antibody directed against placental alkaline phosphatase, reported prolonged survival in patients with small-volume residual disease who responded to the intraperitoneal administration of this radioconjugate. Other ^{131}I-labeled antibodies (e.g., OC125 against CA-125 and B72.3 against TAG72) have demonstrated localization in intraperitoneal ovarian tumors. The clinical utility of radioimmunoscintigraphy has not yet been established, but, as previously discussed in the section on Maintenance Therapy and Consolidation, radioimmunoconjugates (382,383) and antibodies against CA-125 (381,557) are currently being studied in patients who achieve a clinical complete remission following induction chemotherapy.

Overexpresssion of HER-2/*neu*, as previously described (60), may have prognostic implications in ovarian cancer. The GOG performed a Phase II trial of recombinant humanized anti–HER-2/*neu* in patients with recurrent ovarian cancer with overexpression of antigen as detected by immunohistochemistry (61). Only 11.4% of patients overexpressed HER-2/*neu*, and the objective response rate to the antibody was only 7%.

The tendency of ovarian cancer to remain confined to the peritoneal cavity makes it attractive to target cellular mechanisms associated with tumor-induced angiogenesis and invasion. Conventional therapy with cytoreductive surgery followed by paclitaxel/platinum–based chemotherapy produces a clinical complete remission rate in approximately 70% of patients with advanced disease. However, most of these patients have small-volume disease at the completion of therapy and remain at high risk for clinical relapse. It is in this clinical context that antiangiogenesis and antimetastasis drugs, such as angiostatin, endostatin, TNP-470, carboxyamidomidazole (CAI), and thalidomide, have the potential to prevent or delay recurrences (551,552). Clinical trials of CAI are planned by the GOG based upon demonstration that this agent inhibits metastases *in vivo* in a nude mouse model of ovarian cancer. As noted, however, the matrix metalloproteinase inhibitor BAY-129566 was not effective in delaying relapses in patients who achieved a clinical complete remission (384).

Tumor vaccines have also been extensively studied in ovarian cancer. Table 25.25. summarizes strategies for preparation of tumor vaccines as recently reviewed by Coukos et al. (551,552). In a Phase I trial using dinitrophenol (DNP)–modified autologous ovarian cancer tumor cells in stage III patients, some patients developed a measurable im-

TABLE 25.25. *Strategies for preparation of tumor vaccines*

Whole-cell vaccines
  Autologous or allogeneic tumor cells
  Tumor cells modified with physical or chemical agents
    Radiation
    Dinitrophenol
Tumor cells modified with biologic agents
  BCG
Autologous dendritic cells
  Dendritic cells with tumor cells modified by radiation or cell fragmentation
Antigen-based vaccines
  Tumor-specific antigens enriched by adjuvants
  Autologous dendritic cells incubated with antigens
DNA vaccines
  Recombinant virus carrying tumor-specific antigen cDNA

BCG, Bacille Calmette-Guérin (vaccine).
Adapted with permission from Coukos et al. Advances in biologic therapy. In: Ozols RF, ed. *American Cancer Society atlas of clinical oncology.* Hamilton, Ontario: BC Decker, 2003:194–212.

munoresponse, although no clinically meaningful responses were observed (558). Viruses are also being studied to determine whether they can make vaccines more immunogenic, and small trials in select ovarian cancer patients have reported some responses to such strategy, including the use of ultraviolet (UV)–radiated influenza A virus to produce an oncolysate vaccine prepared with established ovarian cancer cell lines (552). Dendritic-cell vaccines have also been developed owing to the recognition of their importance as antigen-presenting cells. Methodologies have been developed to generate clinically meaningful quantities of dendritic cells from peripheral blood precursors and such approaches will be tested in ovarian cancer and other tumors. Numerous tumor-associated antigens have also been identified in ovarian cancer which have been used to generate antibodies for vaccine trials (551,552).

Molecular-targeted therapies are also being evaluated in ovarian cancer patients. Inhibitors of tumor invasion, angiogenesis, and signal transduction pathways are at the forefront of molecular-targeted therapies in ovarian cancer and other solid tumors (559,560). Antibodies and small-molecule tyrosine kinase inhibitors have undergone early evaluation targeting the EGFR. The EGFR consists of an extracellular ligand-binding domain, a transmembrane region, and a cytoplasmic region containing a tyrosine kinase domain. The EGFR is expressed in many normal human tissues and overexpressed in many types of human cancer, including ovarian cancer. Binding of a stimulatory ligand to the extracellular domain of the EGFR [e.g., transforming growth factor-α (TGF-α)] and the epidermal growth factor (EGF) results in receptor dimerization, activation of the cytoplasmic tyrosine kinase, and the initiation of multiple intracellular signal transduction cascades. The net result is the stimulation of multiple bichemical pathways associated with the malignant phenotype, including increased cell proliferation, induction of angiogenesis, and inhibition of apoptosis (559,560). Phase II trials have been reported in preliminary form with OSI-6774 and ZD1839, potent, specific inhibitors of tyrosine kinase activity that compete with adenosine triphosphate for its binding site on the intracellular domain of the receptor. OSI-6774 (561) produced objective responses in some patients, whereas in the GOG trial of ZD1839, no objective responses were observed, but there may be prolongation of time to progression (562). The monoclonal antibody C225 blocks binding of EGF and TGF-α to EGFR and inhibits ligand-induced activation of its tyrosine kinase receptor. C225 is currently under investigation in Phase II studies as a single agent and in combination with paclitaxel plus carboplatin in previously untreated patients with advanced ovarian cancer. Other signal transduction inhibitors and molecular-targeted therapies currently under investigation are summarized in Table 25.26, which was adapted from a recent review by DiSaia and Bloss on new strategies for the treatment of ovarian cancer (560).

The genetic abnormalities associated with ovarian cancer development and progression have been previously summarized in this chapter and reviewed in detail in Chapter 5. Several strategies for gene therapy in ovarian cancer are under development based on specific molecular abnormalities and have been recently summarized (550,551,560,561). Numerous technical and biologic issues have limited the application of gene therapy to ovarian cancer and other solid tumors. For example, mutation of the *p53* tumor-suppressor gene is observed in more than half of ovarian cancer patients, and *p53* gene replacement therapy has been investigated. Replication-deficient adenovirus encoding human recombi-

nant wild-type *p53* [rAd/p53 (SCH58500)] was studied in a Phase I and Phase II trial in patients with recurrent ovarian cancer. Administration of this vector was well tolerated and led to a Phase III placebo-controlled trial. However, this trial was discontinued because no apparent benefit was seen in the patients who received the rAD/p53 (563).

One of the other technical limitations of gene therapy is the frequent inability to deliver a therapeutic or corrective gene into the cancer cells. Hortobagyi et al. (564) reported the results of a Phase I clinical trial of *E1A* gene transfer in ten women with metastatic ovarian cancer who expressed HER-2/*neu*. This trial was based on studies that had shown that the adenovirus type 5 *E1A* gene repressed HER-2/*neu* expression at the transcriptional level and was able to suppress tumor cell growth when transvected into human ovarian cancer cells that overexpressed HER-2/*neu*. *E1A*-bearing cationic liposomes were administered intraperitoneally on a weekly schedule. *E1A* gene expression was detected in tumor cells and was accompanied by downregulation in HER-2/*neu* expression, increased apoptosis, and reduced tumor-cell proliferation. Fever, nausea, vomiting, and discomfort at the injection site were observed, and Phase II trials are planned.

Herpes simplex–based vectors are a major category of gene therapy vectors. Transduction of "suicide vectors," such as herpes simplex virus (HSV) thymidine kinase (TK) gene into tumor cells, makes these cells sensitive for killing by the antiviral nucleoside ganciclovir (551,552,560). Neighboring cells that are not transduced have been shown to be killed ("bystander effect") when ganciclovir is administered to cells transduced by *HSVTK*. The mechanism of this effect has not been determined but may relate to the secondary effect of immune cells acting against the dying transduced cells. Clinical evaluation of the strategy, however, in ovarian cancer patients has been limited.

BRCA1 gene replacement therapy has also been studied in both Phase I and Phase II trials (565,566). Based on a Phase I clinical trial with the IP retroviral LXSN-*BRCA1sv* in which a minimal antibody response tumor reduction. was observed (557), a Phase II trial with intraperitoneal infusion of the vector in patients with less disease was initiated (558). This Phase II trial was terminated after six patients were treated. No responses were observed, and no disease stabilization was achieved. There was no vector stability, and rapid antibody production was noted. The reasons why more vector degradation was observed in the Phase II studies than in previous Phase I studies are uncertain, but may relate to differences in immune status between more heavily treated patients with extensive disease who were entered on Phase I studies compared to patients with small-volume disease who were entered on the Phase II trial. Effective gene therapy may require the development of less immunogenic vectors or coadministration of immunosuppressive agents with retroviral gene therapy.

Biotherapeutic approaches will likely increase in the com-

TABLE 25.26. *Molecular-targeted-based therapies for ovarian cancer*

Target	Agents
Signal transduction	ZD1839 (gefitinib);OSI-774 (erlotinib); C225 (cetuximab); CI-1040; STI-57I (imatinib mesylate); 2C4; trastuzamab; CCI-779
Farnesyltransferase inhibitors	BMS-214662 Manumycin
Antiangiogenesis	Thalidomide Bevacizumab LY317615
Antisense oligonucleotides	G3139 PKC-α ISIS 3521
Proteosomes	PS-341 (bortezomib)
Cyclooxygenase-2 (COX-2)	Celecoxib Rofecoxib
Apoptosis	Exisulind

Adapted with permission from DiSaia PJ, Bloss JD. Treatment of ovarian cancer: new strategies. *Gynecol Oncol* 2003;90:S24–S32.

ing decade as new molecular-targeted therapies are developed. Genetic profiling of a patient's tumor may be useful in selecting potential molecular-targeted therapies that are tailored to the aberrant expression of receptors and genes in a patient's tumor. In addition, how best to combine molecular-targeted therapies with traditional chemotherapy remains an area of active investigation. Furthermore, it is also possible that, in some situations, targeting a single component of a complex biological network may not produce a relevant degree of tumor growth inhibition, which may require the use of several different biologic-targeted therapies in combination. The stimulation of the antitumor immune mechanisms will be a continuing area of research. Enhancement of immune recognition and immune-mediated tumor destruction through therapeutic vaccines, adoptive immunotherapy, biologic response modifiers, and monoclonal antibodies will be tested in rationally designed prospective clinical trials.

REFERENCES

1. Jemal A, Murray T, Samuels A, et al. Cancer statistics, 2003. *CA Cancer J Clin* 2003;53:5–26.
2. Harlan LC, Clegg LX, Trimble EL. Trends in surgery and chemotherapy for women diagnosed with ovarian cancer in the United States. *J Clin Oncol* 2003;21:3488–3494.
3. Yancik R, Ries LG, Yates JW. Ovarian cancer in the elderly: an analysis of surveillance, epidemiology, and end results. *Am J Obstet Gynecol* 1986;154:639–647.
4. McGuire V, Jesser CA, Whittemore AS. Survival among U.S. women with invasive epithelial ovarian cancer. *Gynecol Oncol* 2002;84: 399–403.
5. National Institutes of Health Consensus Development Conference Statement. Ovarian cancer: screening, treatment, and follow-up. *Gynecol Oncol* 1994;55:S4.
6. Ries LAG, Kosary CL, Hankey BF, et al., eds. SEER cancer statistics review: 1973–1994, National Cancer Institute. Bethesda, MD: National Institutes for Health, 1997.
7. Oriel KA, Hartenbach EM, Remington PL. Trends in United States ovarian cancer mortality, 1979–1995. *Obstet Gynecol* 1999;93: 30–33.
8. Daly M, Obrams GI. Epidemiology and risk assessment for ovarian cancer. *Semin Oncol* 1998;25:255–264.
9. Greene MH, Clark JW, Blayney DW. The epidemiology of ovarian cancer. *Semin Oncol* 1984;11:209–226.
10. Whittemore AS, Wu ML, Paffenbarger RS, et al. Epithelial ovarian cancer and the ability to conceive. *Cancer Res* 1989;49:4047–4052.
11. Rossing MA, Daling JR, Weiss NS, et al. Ovarian tumors in a cohort of infertile women. *N Engl J Med* 1994;331:771–776.
12. Whittemore AS. The risk of ovarian cancer after treatment for infertility. *N Engl J Med* 1994;331:805–806.
13. Anonymous. The reduction in risk of ovarian cancer associated with oral-contraceptive use. The Cancer and Steroid Hormone Study of the Centers for Disease Control and the National Institute of Child Health and Human Development. *N Engl J Med* 1987;316:650–655.
14. Anonymous. Epithelial ovarian cancer and combined oral contraceptives. The WHO Collaborative Study of Neoplasia and Steroid Contraceptives. *Int J Epidemiol* 1989;18:538–545.
15. Cramer DW, Hutchison GB, Welch WR, et al. Factors affecting the association of oral contraceptives and ovarian cancer. *N Engl J Med* 1982;307:1047–1051.
16. Risch HA. Hormonal etiology of epithelial ovarian cancer, with a hypothesis concerning the role of androgens and progesterone. *J Natl Cancer Inst* 1998;90:1774–1786.
17. Daly MB. Epidemiology. In: Ozols RF, ed. *American Cancer Society atlas of clinical oncology.* Hamilton, Ontario: BC Decker, 2003: 39–48.
18. Garg PP, Kerlikowske K, Subak L, et al. Hormone replacement therapy and the risk of epithelial ovarian cancer: a meta analysis. *Obstet Gynecol* 1998;92:472–479.
19. Rodriguez C, Patel AV, Calle EE, et al. Estrogen replacement therapy and ovarian cancer mortality in a large prospective study of US women. *JAMA* 2001;285:1460–1465.
20. Lacey JV, Mink PJ, Lubin KH, et al. Menopausal hormone replacement therapy and risk of ovarian cancer. *JAMA* 2002;288:334–341.
21. Riman T, Dickman PW, Nilsson S, et al. Hormone replacement therapy and the risk of invasive epithelial ovarian cancer in Swedish women. *J Natl Cancer Inst* 2002;94:497–504.
22. Anderson GL, Judd HL, Kaunitz AM, et al. Effects of estrogen plus progestin on gynecologic cancers and associated diagnostic procedures. *JAMA* 2003;290:1739–1748.
23. US Preventive Services Task Force. Postmenopausal hormone replacement therapy for primary prevention of chronic conditions: recommendations and rationale. *Ann Intern Med* 2002;137:834–839.
24. Casagrande JT, Louie EW, Pike MC, et al. "Incessant ovulation" and ovarian cancer. *Lancet* 1979;2:170–173.
25. Fathalla, MF. Incessant ovulation—a factor in ovarian neoplasia. *Lancet* 1971;2:163.
26. Cramer DW, Welch WR. Determinants of ovarian cancer risk. II. Inferences regarding pathogenesis. *J Natl Cancer Inst* 1983;71: 717–721.
27. Modugno F. Ovarian Cancer and High-Risk Women Symposium Presenters. Ovarian cancer and high-risk women—implications for prevention, screening, and early detection. *Gynecol Oncol* 2003;91: 15–31.
28. Shildkraut JM, Calingaert B, Marchbanks PA, et al. Impact of progestin and estrogen potency in oral contraceptives on ovarian cancer risk. *J Natl Cancer Inst* 2002;94:32–38.
29. Cramer DW, Barbieria RL, Fraer AR, et al. Determinants of early follicular phase gonadotrophin and estradiol concentrations in women of late reproductive age. *Hum Reprod* 2002;17:221–227.
30. Ness RB, Cottreau C. Possible role of ovarian epithelial inflammation in ovarian cancer. *J Natl Cancer Inst* 1999;91:1459–1467.
31. Smith ER, Xu X-X. Etiology of epithelial ovarian cancer: a cellular mechanism for the role of gonadotropins. *Gynecol Oncol* 2003;91: 1–2.
32. Yang DH, Smith ER, Cohen C, et al. Molecular events associated with dysplastic morphologic transformation and initiation of ovarian tumorigenicity. *Cancer* 2002;94:2380–2392.
33. Kerlikowske K, Brown JS, Grady DG. Should women with familial ovarian cancer undergo prophylactic oophorectomy? *Obstet Gynecol* 1992;80:700–707.
34. Schildkraut JM, Thompson WD. Familial ovarian cancer: a population-based case-control study. *Am J Epidemiol* 1988;128:456–466.
35. Whittemore AS. Characteristics relating to ovarian cancer risk: implications for prevention and detection. *Gynecol Oncol* 1994;55: S15–S19.
36. Piver MS, Baker TR, Jishi MF, et al. Familial ovarian cancer. A report of 658 families from the Gilda Radner Familial Ovarian Cancer Registry 1981–1991. *Cancer* 1993;71:582–588.
37. Boyd J. Molecular genetics of hereditary ovarian cancer. *Oncology* 1998;12:399–406.
38. Prowse A, Frolov A, Godwin AK. Genetics. In: Ozols RF, ed. *American Cancer Society atlas of clinical oncology.* Hamilton, Ontario: BC Decker, 2003:49–82.
39. Lynch HT, Lynch JF, Casey MJ, et al. Genetics of gynecologic cancer. In: Hoskins WJ, Perez CA, Young RC, eds. *Principles and practice of gynecologic oncology.* 3rd ed. Philadelphia: Lippincott–Raven, 1997: 29–53.
40. Wooster R, Neuhausen Sl, Mangio J, et al. Localization of a breast cancer susceptibility gene, BRCA2, to chromosome 13q12–13. *Science* 1994;265:2088–2090.
41. Frank TS. Testing for hereditary risk of ovarian cancer. *Cancer Control* 1999;6:327–334.
42. Struewing JP, Hartge P, Wacholder S, et al. The risk of cancer associated with specific mutations of BRCA1 and BRCA2 among Ashkenazi Jews. *N Engl J Med* 1997;336:1401–1408.
43. Lynch HT, Bewtra C, Lynch JF. Familial ovarian cancer. Clinical nuances. *Am J Med* 1986;81:1073–1076.

44. Bewtra C, Watson P, Conway T, et al. Hereditary ovarian cancer: a clinicopathological study. *Int J Gynecol Pathol* 1992;11:180–187.
45. Lynch HT, Casey MJ, Lynch J, et al. Genetics and ovarian cancer. *Semin Oncol* 1998;25:265–280.
46. Rubin SC, Benjamin I, Behbakht K, et al. Clinical and pathological features of ovarian cancer in women with germ-line mutations of BRCA1. *N Engl J Med* 1996;335:1413–1416.
47. Boyd J, Rubin SC. Hereditary ovarian cancer: molecular genetics and clinical implications. *Gynecol Oncol* 1997;64:196–206.
48. Narod SA, Risch H, Moslehi R, et al. Oral contraceptives and the risk of hereditary ovarian cancer. Hereditary Ovarian Cancer Clinical Study Group. *N Engl J Med* 1998;339:424–428.
49. Daly, MB. Genetic counseling. In: Ozols RF, ed. *American Cancer Society atlas of clinical oncology*. Hamilton, Ontario: BC Decker, 2003:91–100.
50. Hartmann LC, Podratz KC, Keeney GL, et al. Prognostic significance of p53 immunostaining in epithelial ovarian cancer. *J Clin Oncol* 1994;12:64–69.
51. Kupryjanczyk J, Thor AD, Beauchamp R, et al. p53 gene mutations and protein accumulation in human ovarian cancer. *Proc Natl Acad Sci U S A* 1993;90:4961–4965.
52. Havrilesky L, Darcyk M, Hamdan H, et al. Prognostic significance of P53 mutation and P53 overexpression in advanced epithelial ovarian cancer: a Gynecologic Oncology Group study. *J Clin Oncol* 2003;21:3814–3825.
53. Berchuck A, Kohler MF, Hopkins MP, et al. Overexpression of p53 is not a feature of benign and early-stage borderline epithelial ovarian tumors. *Gynecol Oncol* 1994;52:232–236.
54. Abdollahi A, Roberts D, Godwin AK, et al. Identification of a zinc-finger gene at 6q25: a chromomsomal region implicated in development of many solid tumors. *Oncogene* 1997;14:1973–1979.
55. Yu, Y, Xu F, Peng H, et al. NOEY2 (ARHI), an imprinted putative tumor-suppressor gene in ovarian and breast carcinomas. *Proc Natl Acad Sci U S A* 1999;96:214–219.
56. Mok SC, Wong KK, Chan RK, et al. Molecular cloning of differentially expressed genes in human epithelial ovarian cancer. *Gynecol Oncol* 1994;52:247–252.
57. Auersperg N, Edelson MI, Mok SC, et al. The biology of ovarian cancer. *Semin Oncol* 1998;25:281–304.
58. Teneriello MG, Ebina M, Linnoila RL, et al. p53 and Ki-ras gene mutations in epithelial ovarian neoplasms. *Cancer Res* 1993;53:3103–3108.
59. Milner BJ, Allan LA, Eccles DM, et al. P53 mutation is a common genetic event in ovarian carcinomas. *Cancer Res* 1993;53:2128–2132.
60. Slamon DJ, Godolphin W, Jones LA, et al. Studies of the HER-2/neu proto-oncogene in human breast and ovarian cancer. *Science* 1989;244:707–712.
61. Bookman MA, Darcy KM, Clark-Pearson D, et al. Evaluation of monoclonal humanized anti-HER2 antibody, trastuzumab, in patients with recurrent or refractory ovarian or primary peritoneal carcinoma with overexpression of HER2: a Phase II Trial of the Gynecology Oncology Group. *J Clin Oncol* 2003;21:283–290.
62. Cheng JQ, Godwin AK, Bellacosa A, et al. AKT2, a putative oncogene encoding a member of a subfamily of protein-serine/threonine kinases, as amplfied in human ovarian carcinomas. *Proc Natl Acad Sci U S A* 1992;89:9267–9271.
63. Bellacosa A, de Feo D, Godwin AK, et al. Molecular alterations of the AKT2 oncogene in ovarian and breast carcinomas. *Int J Cancer* 1995;64:280–285.
64. Shayesteh L, Lu Y, Kuo WL, et al. PIK2CA is implicated as an oncogene in ovarian cancer. *Nat Genet* 1999;21:99–102.
65. Kurose K, Zhou XP, Araki T, et al. Frequent loss of PTEN expression is linked to elevated phosphorylated Akt levels, but not associated with p27 and cyclin D1 expression, in primary epithelial ovarian carcinomas. *Am J Pathol* 2001;158:2097–2106.
66. Slattery ML, Schuman KL, West DW, et al. Nutrient intake and ovarian cancer. *Am J Epidemiol* 1989;130:497–502.
67. Cramer DW, Harlow BL, Willett WC, et al. Galactose consumption and metabolism in relation to the risk of ovarian cancer. *Lancet* 1989;2:66–71.
68. Longo DL, Young RC. Cosmetic talc and ovarian cancer. *Lancet* 1979;2:1011–1012.
69. Cramer DW, Welch WR, Scully RE, et al. Ovarian cancer and talc. A case-control study. *Cancer* 1982;50:372–376.
70. Gross TP, Schlesselman JJ. The estimated effect of oral contraceptive use on the cumulative risk of epithelial ovarian cancer. *Obstet Gynecol* 1994;83:419–424.
71. Rodriguez GC, Walmer DK, Cline M, et al. Effect of progestin on the ovarian epithelium of macaques: cancer prevention through apoptosis? *J Soc Gynecol Invest* 1998;5:271–276.
72. DePalo, G, Veronesi U, Camerini T, et al. Can fenretinide protect women against ovarian cancer? *J Natl Cancer Inst* 1995;87:146–147.
73. Szarka CE, Hamilton TC, Klein-Szanto AJP, et al. Chemoprevention of ovarian cancer. In: Jacobs IJ, Shepherd JH, Oram DH, et al., eds. *Ovarian cancer*. Oxford, UK: Oxford University Press, 2002:153–160.
74. Salazar H, Godwin A, Daly MB, et al. Microscopic benign and invasive malignant neoplasms and a cancer-prone phenotype in prophylactic oophorectomies. *J Natl Cancer Inst* 1996;88:1810–1820.
75. Hankinson SE, Hunter DJ, Colditz GA, et al. Tubal ligation, hysterectomy, and risk of ovarian cancer. A prospective study. *JAMA* 1993;270:2813–2818.
76. Tobacman JK, Kase R, Greene MH, et al. Intra-abdominal carcinomatosis after prophylactic oophorectomy in ovarian-cancer-prone families. *Lancet* 1982;2:795–797.
77. Bandera CA, Muto MG, Schorge JO, et al. BRCA1 gene mutations in women with papillary serous carcinoma of the peritoneum. *Obstet Gynecol* 1998;92:596–600.
78. Struewing JP, Watson P, Easton DF, et al. Prophylactic oophorectomy in inherited breast/ovarian cancer families. *J Natl Cancer Inst Monogr* 1995;17:33–35.
79. Rebbeck TR, Lynch HT, Neuhausen SL, et al. Prophylactic oophorectomy in carriers of BRCA1 or BRCA2 mutations. *N Engl J Med* 2002;346:1616–1622.
80. Kauff ND, Satagopan JM, Robson ME, et al. Risk-reducing salpingo-oophorectomy in women with a BRCA1 or BRCA2 mutation. *N Engl J Med* 2002;346:1609–1615.
81. Robboy SJ, Anderson MC, Russell P. *Pathology of the female reproductive tract*. London: Churchill Livingstone, 2002.
82. Dietl J, Marzusch K. Ovarian surface epithelium and human ovarian cancer. *Gynecol Obstet Invest* 1993;35:129–135.
83. Friedman-Koss D, Crespo CJ, Bellantoni MF, et al. The relationship of race/ethnicity and social class to hormone replacement therapy: results from the Third National Health and Nutrition Examination Survey 1988–1994. *Menopause* 2002;9:264–272.
84. Raab SS, Robinson RA, Jensen CS, et al. Mucinous tumors of the ovary: interobserver diagnostic variability and utility of sectioning protocols. *Arch Pathol Lab Med* 1997;121:1192–1198.
85. Robboy SJ, Anderson MC, Russell P. Cutup. In: Robboy SJ, Anderson MC, Russell P, eds. *Pathology of the female reproductive tract*. London: Churchill Livingstone, 2002:861–875.
86. Puls LE, Powell DE, DePriest PD, et al. Transition from benign to malignant epithelium in mucinous and serous ovarian cystadenocarcinoma. *Gynecol Oncol* 1992;47:53–57.
87. Russell P, Farnsworth A. *Surgical pathology of the ovaries*. 2nd ed. New York: Churchill Livingstone, 1992:715.
88. Barnhill DR, Kurman RJ, Brady MF, et al. Preliminary analysis of the behavior of stage 1 ovarian serous tumors of low malignant potential: a Gynecologic Oncology Group study. *J Clin Oncol* 1995;13:2752–2756.
89. Buttini M, Nicklin JL, Crandon A. Low malignant potential ovarian tumours: A review of 175 consecutive cases. *Austral N Z J Obstet Gynaecol* 1997;37:100–103.
90. de Nictolis M, Montironi R, Tommasoni S, et al. Benign, borderline, and well-differentiated malignant intestinal mucinous tumors of the ovary—a clinicopathologic, histochemical, immunohistochemical, and nuclear quantitative study of 57 cases. *Int J Gynecol Pathol* 1994;13:10–21.
91. Kennedy AW, Hart WR. Ovarian papillary serous tumors of low malignant potential (serous borderline tumors). A long-term follow-up study, including patients with microinvasion, lymph node metastasis, and transformation to invasive serous carcinoma. *Cancer* 1996;78:278–286.
92. Kuoppala T, Heinola M, Aine R, et al. Serous and mucinous borderline

tumors of the ovary: a clinicopathologic and DNA-ploidy study of 102 cases. *Int J Gynecol Cancer* 1996;6:302–308.

93. Norris HJ. Proliferative endometrioid tumors and endometrioid tumors of low malignant potential of the ovary. *Int J Gynecol Pathol* 1993;12:134–140.

94. Silva EG, Kurman RJ, Russell P, et al. Symposium: ovarian tumors of borderline malignancy. *Int J Gynecol Pathol* 1996;15:281–302.

95. Sykes PH, Quinn MA, Rome RM. Ovarian tumors of low malignant potential: a retrospective study of 234 patients. *Int J Gynecol Cancer* 1997;7:218–226.

96. Tan LK, Flynn SD, Carcangiu ML. Ovarian serous borderline tumors with lymph node involvement—clinicopathologic and DNA content study of seven cases and review of the literature. *Am J Surg Pathol* 1994;18:904–912.

97. Seidman JD, Ronnett BM, Kurman RJ. Pathology of borderline (low malignant potential) ovarian tumours. *Best Pract Res Clin Obstet Gynaecol* 2002;16:499–A4.

98. Bell KA, Kurman RJ. A clinicopathologic analysis of atypical proliferative (borderline) tumors and well-differentiated endometrioid adenocarcinomas of the ovary. *Am J Surg Pathol* 2000;24:1465–1479.

99. Nayar R, Siriaunkgul S, Robbins KM, et al. Microinvasion in low malignant potential tumors of the ovary. *Hum Pathol* 1996;27: 521–527.

100. Singer G, Kurman RJ, Chang HW, et al. Diverse tumorigenic pathways in ovarian serous carcinoma. *Am J Pathol* 2002;160:1223–1228.

101. Burks RT, Sherman ME, Kurman RJ. Micropapillary serous carcinoma of the ovary: a distinctive low-grade carcinoma related to serous borderline tumors. *Am J Surg Pathol* 1996;20:1319–1330.

102. Seidman JD, Kurman RJ. Subclassification of serous borderline tumors of the ovary into benign and malignant types: a clinicopathologic study of 65 advanced stage cases. *Am J Surg Pathol* 1996;20: 1331–1345.

103. Kempson RL, Hendrickson MR. Ovarian serous borderline tumors: the citadel defended. *Hum Pathol* 2000;31:525–526.

104. Seidman JD, Kurman RJ. Ovarian serous borderline tumors: a critical review of the literature with emphasis on prognostic indicators. *Hum Pathol* 2000;31:539–557.

105. Eichhorn JH, Bell DA, Young RH, Scully RE. Ovarian serous borderline tumors with micropapillary and cribriform pattern: a study of 40 cases and comparison with 44 cases without these patterns. *Am J Surg Pathol* 1999;23:397–409.

106. Deavers MT, Gershenson DM, Tortolero-Luna G, et al. Micropapillary and cribriform patterns in ovarian serous tumors of low malignant potential. A study of 99 advanced stage cases. *Am J Surg Pathol* 2002; 26:1129–1141.

107. Gilks CB, Alkushi A, Yue JJW, et al. Advanced-stage serous borderline tumors of the ovary: a clinicopathological study of 49 cases. *Int J Gynecol Pathol* 2003;22:29–36.

108. Goldstein NS, Ceniza N. Ovarian micropapillary serous borderline tumors—clinicopathologic features and outcome of seven surgically staged patients. *Am J Clin Pathol* 2000;114:380–386.

109. Prat J. Serous tumors of the ovary (borderline tumors and carcinoma) with and without micropapillary features. *Int J Gynecol Pathol* 2003; 22:25–28.

110. Prat J, de Nictolis M. Serous borderline tumors of the ovary —a long-term follow-up study of 137 cases, including 18 with a micropapillary pattern and 20 with microinvasion. *Am J Surg Pathol* 2002;26: 1111–1128.

111. Smith Sehdev AE, Sehdev PS, Kurman RJ. Noninvasive and invasive micropapillary (low-grade) serous carcinoma of the ovary: a clinicopathologic analysis of 135 cases. *Am J Surg Pathol* 2003;27:725–736.

112. Lauchlan SC. The secondary mullerian system revisited. *Int J Gynecol Pathol* 1994;13:73–79.

113. Segal GH, Hart WR. Ovarian serous tumors of low malignant potential (serous borderline tumors). The relationship of exophytic surface tumor to peritoneal "implants." *Am J Surg Pathol* 1992;16:577–583.

114. Moore WF, Bentley RC, Berchuck A, et al. Some mullerian inclusion cysts in lymph nodes may sometimes be metastases from serous borderline tumors of the ovary. *Am J Surg Pathol* 2000;24:710–718.

115. Silva EG, Tornos C, Zhuang Z, et al. Tumor recurrence in stage I ovarian serous neoplasms of low malignant potential. *Int J Gynecol Pathol* 1998;17:1–6.

116. Gershenson DM, Silva EG, Tortolero-Luna G, et al. Serous borderline tumors of the ovary with noninvasive peritoneal implants. *Cancer* 1998;83:2157–2163.

117. Scully RE, Young RH, Clement RB. Tumors of the ovary, maldeveloped gonads, fallopian tube, and broad ligament. In: *Atlas of tumor pathology*. Vol 23, 3rd ed. Washington, DC: Armed Forces Institute of Pathology, 1998.

118. Russell P, Robboy SJ, Anderson MC. Ovarian tumors: classification and clinical perspective. In: Robboy SJ, Anderson MC, Russell P, eds. *Pathology of the female reproductive tract*. London: Churchill Livingstone, 2002.

119. Shimizu Y, Kamoi S, Amada S, et al. Toward the development of a universal grading system for ovarian epithelial carcinoma: testing of a proposed system in a series of 461 patients with uniform treatment and follow-up. *Cancer* 1998;82:893–901.

120. Shimizu Y, Kamoi S, Amada S, et al. Toward the development of a universal grading system for ovarian epithelial carcinoma. I. Prognostic significance of histopathologic features—problems involved in the architectural grading system. *Gynecol Oncol* 1998;70:2–12.

121. Ishioka S, Sagae S, Terasawa K, et al. Comparison of the usefulness between a new universal grading system for epithelial ovarian cancer and the FIGO grading system. *Gynecol Oncol* 2003;89:447–452.

122. Sato Y, Shimamoto T, Amada S, et al. Prognostic value of histologic grading of ovarian carcinomas. *Int J Gynecol Pathol* 2003;22:52–56.

123. Piura B, Meirovitz M, Bartfeld M, et al. Peritoneal papillary serous carcinoma: study of 15 cases and comparison with stage III-IV ovarian papillary serous carcinoma. *J Surg Oncol* 1998;68:173–178.

124. Ronnett BM, Kurman RJ, Zahn CM, et al. Pseudomyxoma peritonei in women: a clinicopathologic analysis of 30 cases with emphasis on site of origin, prognosis, and relationship to ovarian mucinous tumors of low malignant potential. *Hum Pathol* 1995;26:509–524.

125. Baergen RN, Rutgers JL. Mural nodules in common epithelial tumors of the ovary. *Int J Gynecol Pathol* 1994;13:62–72.

126. Moore WF, Bentley RC, Kim KR, et al. Goblet-cell mucinous epithelium lining the endometrium and endocervix: evidence of metastasis from an appendiceal primary tumor through the use of cytokeratin-7 and -20 immunostains. *Int J Gynecol Pathol* 1998;17:363–367.

127. Ronnett BM, Kurman RJ, Shmookler BM, et al. The morphologic spectrum of ovarian metastases of appendiceal adenocarcinomas: a clinicopathologic and immunohistochemical analysis of tumors often misinterpreted as primary ovarian tumors or metastatic tumors from other gastrointestinal sites. *Am J Surg Pathol* 1997;21:1144–1155.

128. Cathro HP, Stoler MH. Expression of cytokeratins 7 and 20 in ovarian neoplasia. *Am J Clin Pathol* 2002;117:944–951.

129. Lee KR, Young RH. The distinction between primary and metastatic mucinous carcinomas of the ovary: gross and histologic findings in 50 cases. *Am J Surg Pathol* 2003;27:281–292.

130. Guerrieri C, Hogberg T, Wingren S, et al. Mucinous borderline and malignant tumors of the ovary. A clinicopathologic and DNA ploidy study of 92 cases. *Cancer* 1994;74:2329–2340.

131. Kikkawa F, Kawai M, Tamakoshi K, et al. Mucinous carcinoma of the ovary. Clinicopathologic analysis. *Oncology* 1996;53:303–307.

132. Rodriguez IM, Prat J. Mucinous tumors of the ovary: a clinicopathologic analysis of 75 borderline tumors (of intestinal type) and carcinomas. *Am J Surg Pathol* 2002;26:139–152.

133. Nomura K, Aizawa S. Noninvasive, microinvasive, and invasive mucinous carcinomas of the ovary: a clinicopathologic analysis of 40 cases. *Cancer* 2000;89:1541–1546.

134. Takahashi K, Kurioka H, Irikoma M, et al. Benign or malignant ovarian neoplasms and ovarian endometriomas. *J Am Assoc Gynecol Laparosc* 2001;8:278–284.

135. Stern RC, Dash R, Bentley RC, et al. Malignancy in endometriosis: frequency and comparison of ovarian and extraovarian types. *Int J Gynecol Pathol* 2001;20:133–139.

136. Grosso G, Raspagliesi F, Baiocchi G, et al. Endometrioid carcinoma of the ovary: a retrospective analysis of 106 cases. *Tumori* 1998;84: 552–557.

137. Zaino R, Whitney C, Brady MF, et al. Simultaneously detected endometrial and ovarian carcinomas—a prospective clinicopathologic study of 74 cases: a Gynecologic Oncology Group study. *Gynecol Oncol* 2001;83:355–362.

138. McMeekin DS, Burger RA, Manetta A, et al. Endometrioid adenocarcinoma of the ovary and its relationship to endometriosis. *Gynecol Oncol* 1995;59:81–86.

139. Zwart J, Geisler JP, Geisler HE. Five-year survival in patients with endometrioid carcinoma of the ovary versus those with serous carcinoma. *Eur J Gynaecol Oncol* 1998;19:225–228.

140. Tornos C, Silva EG, Khorana SM, et al. High-stage endometrioid carcinoma of the ovary. Prognostic significance of pure versus mixed histologic types. *Am J Surg Pathol* 1994;18:687–693.

141. Eichhorn JH, Scully RE. Endometrioid ciliated-cell tumors of the ovary: a report of five cases. *Int J Gynecol Pathol* 1996;15:248–256.

142. Pitman MB, Young RH, Clement PB, et al. Endometrioid carcinoma of the ovary and endometrium, oxyphilic cell type: a report of nine cases. *Int J Gynecol Pathol* 1994;13:290–301.

143. Usadi RS, Bentley RC. Endometrioid carcinoma of the endometrium with sertoliform differentiation. *Int J Gynecol Pathol* 1995;14:360–364.

144. Guerrieri C, Franlund B, Malmstrom H, et al. Ovarian endometrioid carcinomas simulating sex cord stromal tumors: a study using inhibin and cytokeratin 7. *Int J Gynecol Pathol* 1998;17:266–271.

145. Hildebrandt RH, Rouse RV, Longacre TA. Value of inhibin in the identification of granulosa cell tumors of the ovary. *Hum Pathol* 1997;28:1387–1395.

146. Eichhorn JH, Young RH, Clement PB, et al. Mesodermal (mullerian) adenosarcoma of the ovary: a clinicopathologic analysis of 40 cases and a review of the literature. *Am J Surg Pathol* 2002;26:1243–1258.

147. Ariyoshi K, Kawauchi S, Kaku T, et al. Prognostic factors in ovarian carcinosarcoma: a clinicopathological and immunohistochemical analysis of 23 cases. *Histopathology* 2000;37:427–436.

148. Le T, Krepart GV, Lotocki RJ, et al. Malignant mixed mesodermal ovarian tumor treatment and prognosis: a 20-year experience. *Gynecol Oncol* 1997;65:237–240.

149. Behbakht K, Randall TC, Benjamin I, et al. Clinical characteristics of clear cell carcinoma of the ovary. *Gynecol Oncol* 1998;70:255–258.

150. Toki T, Fujii S, Silverberg SG. A clinicopathologic study on the association of endometriosis and carcinoma of the ovary using a scoring system. *Int J Gynecol Cancer* 1996;6:68–75.

151. Matias-Guiu X, Lerma E, Prat J. Clear cell tumors of the female genital tract. *Semin Diagn Pathol* 1997;14:233–239.

152. Young RH, Hart WR. Renal cell carcinoma metastatic to the ovary: a report of three cases emphasizing possible confusion with ovarian clear cell adenocarcinoma. *Int J Gynecol Pathol* 1992;11:96–104.

153. Tammela J, Geisler JP, Eskew PNJ, et al. Clear cell carcinoma of the ovary: poor prognosis compared to serous carcinoma. *Eur J Gynaecol Oncol* 1998;19:438–440.

154. Kennedy AW, Biscotti CV, Hart WR, et al. Histologic correlates of progression-free interval and survival in ovarian clear cell adenocarcinoma. *Gynecol Oncol* 1993;50:334–338.

155. Morimura Y, Hoshi K, Hang XL, et al. Evaluation with MIB1 antibody of proliferative activity in ovarian clear cell adenocarcinoma. *Int J Gynecol Pathol* 1996;15:315–319.

156. O'Brien ME, Schofield JB, Tan S, et al. Clear cell epithelial ovarian cancer (mesonephroid): bad prognosis only in early stages. *Gynecol Oncol* 1993;49:250–254.

157. Hollingsworth HC, Steinberg SM, Silverberg SG, et al. Advanced stage transitional cell carcinoma of the ovary. *Hum Pathol* 1996;27:1267–1272.

158. Riedel I, Czernobilsky B, Lifschitz-Mercer B, et al. Brenner tumors but not transitional cell carcinomas of the ovary show urothelial differentiation: immunohistochemical staining of urothelial markers, including cytokeratins and uroplakins. *Virchows Archiv* 2001;438:181–191.

159. Soslow RA, Rouse RV, Hendrickson MR, et al. Transitional cell neoplasms of the ovary and urinary bladder: a comparative immunohistochemical analysis. *Int J Gynecol Pathol* 1996;15:257–265.

160. Pins MR, Young RH, Daly WJ, et al. Primary squamous cell carcinoma of the ovary. Report of 37 cases. *Am J Surg Pathol* 1996;20:823–833.

161. Shappell HW, Riopel MA, Sehdev AES, et al. Diagnostic criteria and behavior of ovarian seromucinous (endocervical-type mucinous and mixed cell-type) tumors. *Am J Surg Pathol* 2002;26:1529–1541.

162. Che MX, Tornos C, Deavers MT, et al. Ovarian mixed-epithelial carcinomas with a microcystic pattern and signet-ring cells. *Int J Gynecol Pathol* 2001;20:323–328.

163. Dickersin GR, Scully RE. Ovarian small cell tumors: an electron microscopic review. *Ultrastruc Pathol* 1998;22:199–226.

164. Young RH, Oliva E, Scully RE. Small cell carcinoma of the ovary, hypercalcemic type. A clinicopathological analysis of 150 cases. *Am J Surg Pathol* 1994;18:1102–1116.

165. Matias-Guiu X, Prat J, Young RH, et al. Human parathyroid hormone-related protein in ovarian small cell carcinoma. An immunohistochemical study. *Cancer* 1994;73:1878–1881.

166. Ferlicot S, Bessoud B, Martin V, et al. Large cell variant of small cell carcinoma of the ovary, hypercalcemic type. *Ann Pathol* 1998;18:197–200.

167. Eichhorn JH, Young RH, Scully RE. Primary ovarian small cell carcinoma of pulmonary type. A clinicopathologic, immunohistologic, and flow cytometric analysis of 11 cases. *Am J Surg Pathol* 1992;16:926–938.

168. Eichhorn JH, Lawrence WD, Young RH, Scully RE. Ovarian neuroendocrine carcinomas of non-small-cell type associated with surface epithelial adenocarcinomas. A study of five cases and review of the literature. *Int J Gynecol Pathol* 1996;15:303–314.

169. Strobel SL, Graham R. Primary non-small cell neuroendocrine carcinoma of the ovary. *J Histotechnol* 2003;26:73–76.

170. Mangan CE, Rubin SC, Rabin DS, et al. Lymph node nomenclature in gynecologic oncology. *Gynecol Oncol* 1986;23:222–226.

171. Burghardt E, Pickel H, Lahousen M, et al. Pelvic lymphadenectomy in operative treatment of ovarian cancer. *Am J Obstet Gynecol* 1986;155:315–319.

172. Wu PC, Lang JH, Huang RL, et al. Lymph node metastasis and retroperitoneal lymphadenectomy in ovarian cancer. *Baillieres Clin Obstet Gynaecol* 1989;3:143–155

173. Knapp RC, Friedman EA. Aortic lymph node metastases in early ovarian cancer. *Am J Obstet Gynecol* 1974;119:1013–1017.

174. Piver MS, Barlow JJ, Lele SB. Incidence of subclinical metastasis in stage I and II ovarian carcinoma. *Obstet Gynecol* 1978;52:100–104.

175. Bristow RE, del Carmen MG, Pannu HK, et al. Clinically occult recurrent ovarian cancer: patient selection for secondary cytoreductive surgery using combined PET/CT. *Gynecol Oncol* 2003;90:519–528.

176. Olt GJ, Berchuck A, Bast RC. Gynecologic tumor markers. *Semin Surg Oncol* 1990;6:305–313.

177. Davis HM, Zurawski VR Jr, Bast RC, et al. Characterization of the CA-125 antigen associated with human epithelial ovarian carcinomas. *Cancer Res* 1986;46:6143–6148.

178. Niloff JM, Bast RC Jr, Schaetzl EM, et al. Predictive value of CA 125 antigen levels in second-look procedures for ovarian cancer. *Am J Obstet Gynecol* 1985;151:981–986.

179. Malkasian GD Jr, Knapp RC, Lavin PT, et al. Preoperative evaluation of serum CA125 levels in premenopausal and postmenopausal patients with pelvic masses: discrimination of benign from malignant disease. *Am J Obstet Gynecol* 1988;159:341–346.

180. Hulka BS. Cancer screening. Degrees of proof and practical application. *Cancer* 1988;62:1776–1780.

181. Jacobs I. Genetic, biochemical, and multimodal approaches to screening for ovarian cancer. *Gynecol Oncol* 1994;55:S22–S27.

182. Campbell S, Bhan V, Royston P, et al. Transabdominal ultrasound screening for early ovarian cancer. *BMJ* 1989;299:1363–1367.

183. DePriest PD, van Nagell JR, Jr, Gallion HH, et al. Ovarian cancer screening in asymptomatic postmenopausal women. *Gynecol Oncol* 1993;51:205–209.

184. van Nagell JR, DePriest PD, Puls LE, et al. Ovarian cancer screening in asymptomatic postmenopausal women by transvaginal sonography. *Cancer* 1991;68:458–462.

185. van Nagell JR Jr., Higgins RV, Donaldson ES, et al. Transvaginal sonography as a screening method for ovarian cancer. A report of the first 1000 cases screened. *Cancer* 1990;65:573–577.

186. Karlan BY, Platt LD. The current status of ultrasound and color Doppler imaging in screening for ovarian cancer. *Gynecol Oncol* 1994;55:S28–S33.

187. Ueland FR, DePriest PD, Pavlik EJ, et al. Preoperative differentiation of malignant from benign ovarian tumors: the efficacy of morphology indexing and Doppler flow sonography. *Gynecol Oncol* 2003;91:46–50.

188. Zurawski VR, Broderick SF, Pickens P, et al. Serum CA125 levels in a group of nonhospitalized women: relevance for the early detection of ovarian cancer. *Obstet Gynecol* 1987;69:606–611.

189. Einhorn N, Sjovall K, Knapp RC, et al. Prospective evaluation of

serum CA 125 levels for early detection of ovarian cancer. *Obstet Gynecol* 1992;80:14–18.

190. Prorok PC, Andriole GL, Bresalier RS, et al. Design of the Prostate, Lung, Colorectal and Ovarian (PLCO) Cancer Screening Trial. *Control Clin Trials* 2000;21:273S-309S.

191. Skates SJ, Xu F-J, Yu Y-H, et al. Toward an optimal algorithm for ovarian cancer screening with longitudinal tumor markers. *Cancer* 1995;76:2004–2010.

192. Jacobs I, Davies AP, Bridges J, et al. Prevalence screening for ovarian cancer in postmenopausal women by CA 125 measurement and ultrasonography. *BMJ* 1993;306:1030–1034.

193. Jacobs IJ, Skates SJ, MacDonald N, et al. Screening for ovarian cancer: a pilot randomised controlled trial. *Lancet* 1999;353:1207–1210.

194. Westhoff C. Current status of screening for ovarian cancer. *Gynecol Oncol* 1994;55:S34–S37.

195. Bourne TH, Campbell S, Reynolds K, et al. The potential role of serum CA 125 in an ultrasound-based screening program for familial ovarian cancer. *Gynecol Oncol* 1994;52:379–385.

196. Knauf S, Urbach GI. Identification, purification, and radioimmunoassay of NB/70K, a human ovarian tumor-associated antigen. *Cancer Res* 1981;41:1351–1357.

197. Ramakrishnan S, Xu FJ, Brandt SJ, et al. Elevated levels of macrophage colony stimulating factor (MCSI) in serum and ascites from patients with epithelial ovarian cancer. *Proc SGO* 1990;21:40.

198. Woolas RP, Xu FJ, Jacobs IJ, et al. Elevation of multiple serum markers in patients with stage I ovarian cancer. *J Natl Cancer Inst* 1993; 85:1748–1751.

199. Xu Y, Shen Z, Wiper DW, et al. Lysophosphatidic acid as a potential biomarker for ovarian and other gynecologic cancers. *JAMA* 1998; 280:719–723.

200. Mills GB, Bast Jr RC, Srivastava S. Future for ovarian cancer screening: novel markers from emerging technologies of transcriptional profiling and proteomics. *J Natl Cancer Inst* 2001;93:1437–1439.

201. Mok SC, Chao J, Skates S, et al. Prostasin, a potential serum marker for ovarian cancer: identification through microarray technology. *J Natl Cancer Inst* 2001;93:1458–1464.

202. Petricoin EF III, Ardekani AM, Hitt BA, et al. Use of proteomic patterns in serum to identify ovarian cancer. *Lancet* 2002;359: 572–577.

203. Daly MB, Ozols RF. The search for predictive patterns in ovarian cancer: proteomics meets bioinformatics. *Cancer Cell* 2002;1: 111–112.

204. Staging Announcement: FIGO Cancer Committee. *Gynecol Oncol* 1986;25:383.

205. Burghardt E, Pickel H, Holzer E, et al. The significance of lymphadenectomy in therapy of ovarian carcinoma. *Am J Obstet Gynecol* 1983; 146:111–112.

206. Robboy SJ, Duggan M, Kurman RT. The female reproductive system. In: Rubin E, Farber J, eds. *Pathology*. 2nd ed. Philadelphia: JB Lippincott, 1988.

207. Young RC, Decker DG, Wharton JT, et al. Staging laparotomy in early ovarian cancer. *JAMA* 1983;250:3072–3076.

208. McGowan L, Lesher LP, Norris HJ, et al. Misstaging of ovarian cancer. *Obstet Gynecol* 1985;65:568–572.

209. Munoz KA, Harlan LC, Trimble EL. Patterns of care for women with ovarian cancer in the United States. *J Clin Oncol* 1997;15:3408–3415.

210. Pettersson F. *Annual report on the results of treatment in gynecological cancer*. Vol. 20. International Federation of Gynecology and Obstetrics. Stockholm: Panorama Press AB, 1988:110.

211. Hacker NF, Berek JS, Lagasse LD, et al. Primary cytoreductive surgery for epithelial ovarian cancer. *Obstet Gynecol* 1983;61:413–420.

212. Vogl SE, Pagano M, Kaplan BH, et al. Cis-platin based combination chemotherapy for advanced ovarian cancer. High overall response rate with curative potential only in women with small tumor burdens. *Cancer* 1983;51:2024–2030.

213. Delgado G, Oram DH, Petrilli ES. Stage III epithelial ovarian cancer: the role of maximal surgical reduction. *Gynecol Oncol* 1984;18: 293–298.

214. Pohl R, Dallenbach-Hellweg G, Plugge T, et al. Prognostic parameters in patients with advanced ovarian malignant tumors. *Eur J Gynaecol Oncol* 1984;5:160–169.

215. Conte PF, Sertoli MR, Bruzzone M, et al. Cisplatin, methotrexate,

216. Posada JG, Jr, Marantz AB, Yeung KY, et al. The cyclophosphamide, hexamethylmelamine, 5-fluorouracil regimen in the treatment of advanced and recurrent ovarian cancer. *Gynecol Oncol* 1985;20:23–31.

217. Sutton GP, Stehman FB, Einhorn LH, et al. Ten-year follow-up of patients receiving cisplatin, doxorubicin, and cyclophosphamide chemotherapy for advanced epithelial ovarian carcinoma. *J Clin Oncol* 1989;7:223–229.

218. Louie KG, Ozols RF, Myers CE, et al. Long-term results of cisplatin-containing combination chemotherapy regimen for the treatment of advanced ovarian carcinoma. *J Clin Oncol* 1986;4:1579–1585.

219. Redman JR, Petroni GR, Saigo PE, et al. Prognostic factors in advanced ovarian carcinoma. *J Clin Oncol* 1986;4:515–523.

220. Neijt JP, ten Bokkel Huinink WW, van der Berg ME, et al. Long-term survival in ovarian cancer. Mature data from The Netherlands Joint Study Group for Ovarian Cancer. *Eur J Cancer* 1991;27: 1367–1372.

221. Hainsworth JD, Grosh WW, Burnett LS, et al. Advanced ovarian cancer: long-term results of treatment with intensive cisplatin-based chemotherapy of brief duration. *Ann Intern Med* 1988;108:165–170.

222. Piver MS, Lele SB, Marchetti DL, et al. Surgically documented response to intraperitoneal cisplatin, cytarabine, and bleomycin after intravenous cisplatin-based chemotherapy in advanced ovarian adenocarcinoma. *J Clin Oncol* 1988;6:1679–1684.

223. Heintz AP, van Oosterom AT, Trimbos JB, et al. The treatment of advanced ovarian carcinoma (1): clinical variables associated with prognosis. *Gynecol Oncol* 1988;30:347–358.

224. Piver MS, Lele SB, Marchetti DL, et al. The impact of aggressive debulking surgery and cisplatin-based chemotherapy on progression-free survival in stage III and IV ovarian carcinoma. *J Clin Oncol* 1988;6:983–989.

225. Vergote IB, Kaern J, Abeler VM, et al. Analysis of prognostic factors in stage I epithelial ovarian carcinoma: importance of degree of differentiation and deoxyribonucleic acid ploidy in predicting relapse. *Am J Obstet Gynecol* 1993;169:40–52.

226. Young RC, Walton LA, Ellenberg SS, et al. Adjuvant therapy in stage I and stage II epithelial ovarian cancer. Results of two prospective randomized trials. *N Engl J Med* 1990;322:1021–1027.

227. Baak JP, Langley FA, Talerman A, Delemarre JF. The prognostic variability of ovarian tumor grading by different pathologists. *Gynecol Oncol* 1987;27:166–172.

228. Cramer SF, Roth LM, Ulbright TM, et al. Evaluation of the reproducibility of the World Health Organization classification of common ovarian tumors with emphasis on methodology. *Arch Pathol Lab Med* 1987;111:819–829.

229. Rubin SC, Lewis JL, Jr. Second-look surgery in ovarian carcinoma. *Crit Rev Oncol Hematol* 1988;8:75–91.

230. Friedlander ML. Prognostic factors in ovarian cancer. *Semin Oncol* 1998;25:305–314.

231. Dembo AJ, Bush RS, Beale FA, et al. The Princess Margaret Hospital study of ovarian cancer: stage I, II and asymptomatic III presentations. *Cancer Treat Rep* 1979;63:249–254.

232. Sevelda P, Vavra N, Schemper M, Salzer H. Prognostic factors for survival in Stage I epithelial ovarian carcinoma. *Cancer* 1990;65: 2349–2352.

233. Webb M, Decker D, Mussey E, et al. Factors influencing survival in Stage I ovarian cancer. *Am J Obstet Gynecol* 1973;116:222–228.

234. Fayers PM, Rustin G, Wood R, et al. The prognostic value of serum CA 125 in patients with advanced ovarian carcinoma: an analysis of 573 patients by the Medical Research Council Working Party on Gynaecological Cancer. *Int J Gynecol Cancer* 1993;3:285–292.

235. Makar AP, Kristensen GB, Kaern J, et al. Prognostic value of pre- and postoperative serum CA 125 levels in ovarian cancer: new aspects and multivariate analysis. *Obstet Gynecol* 1992;79:1002–1010.

236. Mogensen O. Prognostic value of CA 125 in advanced ovarian cancer. *Gynecol Oncol* 1992;44:207–212.

237. Rustin GJ, Gennings JN, Nelstrop AE, et al. Use of CA-125 to predict survival of patients with ovarian carcinoma. North Thames Cooperative Group. *J Clin Oncol* 1989;7:1667–1671.

238. Rustin GJ, Nelstrop AE, Bentzen SM, et al. Use of tumour markers in monitoring the course of ovarian cancer. *Ann Oncol* 1999;10: S21–S27.

239. Rustin GJ, Nelstrop AE, McClean P, et al. Defining response of ovarian carcinoma to initial chemotherapy according to serum CA125. *J Clin Oncol* 1996;14:1545–1551.

240. Gajewski WH, Fuller AF Jr., Pastel-Ley C, et al. Prognostic significance of DNA content in epithelial ovarian cancer. *Gynecol Oncol* 1994;53:5–12.

241. Kaern J, Trope C, Kjorstad KE, et al. Cellular DNA content as a new prognostic tool in patients with borderline tumors of the ovary. *Gynecol Oncol* 1990;38:452–457.

242. Kaern J, Trope CG, Kristensen GB, et al. Evaluation of deoxyribonucleic acid ploidy and S-phase fraction as prognostic parameters in advanced epithelial ovarian carcinoma: a prospective study. *Am J Obstet Gynecol* 1994;170:479–487.

243. Trope C, Kaern J. DNA ploidy in epithelial ovarian cancer: a new independent prognostic factor? *Gynecol Oncol* 1994;53:1–4.

244. Harlow BL, Fuhr JE, McDonald TW, et al. Flow cytometry as a prognostic indicator in women with borderline epithelial ovarian tumors. *Gynecol Oncol* 1993;50:305–309.

245. Bookman MA, Ozols RF. Factoring outcomes in ovarian cancer. *J Clin Oncol* 1996;14:325–327.

246. Eisenhauer EA, Gore M, Neijt JP. Ovarian cancer: should we be managing patients with good and bad prognostic factors in the same manner? *Ann Oncol* 1999;10:S9–S15.

247. Izquierdo MA, van der Zee AG, Vermorken JB, et al. Drug resistance-associated marker Lrp for prediction of response to chemotherapy and prognoses in advanced ovarian carcinoma. *J Natl Cancer Inst* 1995;87:1230–1237.

248. van der Zee AG, Hollema H, Suurmeijer AJ, et al. Value of P-glycoprotein, glutathione S-transferase pi, c-erbB-2, and p53 as prognostic factors in ovarian carcinomas. *J Clin Oncol* 1995;13:70–78.

249. Fojo A, Hamilton TC, Young RC, et al. Multidrug resistance in ovarian cancer. *Cancer* 1987;60:2075–2080.

250. Holzmayer TA, Hilsenbeck S, von Hoff DD, et al. Clinical correlates of MDR1 (P-glycoprotein) gene expression in ovarian and small-cell lung carcinomas. *J Natl Cancer Inst* 1992;84:1486–1491.

251. Dabholkar M, Bostick-Bruton F, Weber C, et al. ERCC1 and ERCC2 expression in malignant tissues from ovarian cancer patients. *J Natl Cancer Inst* 1992;84:1512–1517.

252. Reed E, Ozols RF, Tarone R, et al. Platinum-DNA adducts in leukocyte DNA correlate with disease response in ovarian cancer patients receiving platinum-based chemotherapy. *Proc Natl Acad Sci U S A* 1987;84:5024–5028.

253. Ono K, Tanaka T, Tsunoda T, et al. Identification by cDNA microarray of genes involved in ovarian carcinogenesis. *Cancer Res* 2000;60:5007–5011.

254. Hough CD, Sherman-Baust CA, Pizer ES, et al. Large-scale serial analysis of gene expression reveals genes differentially expressed in ovarian cancer. *Cancer Res* 2000;60:6281–6287.

255. Ismail RS, Baldwin RL, Fang J et al. Differential gene expression between normal and tumor-derived ovarian epithelial cells. *Cancer Res* 2000;60:6744–6749.

256. Suzuki S, Moore DH 2nd, Ginzinger DG, et al. An approach to analysis of large-scale correlations between genome changes and clinical endpoints in ovarian cancer. *Cancer Res* 2000;60:5382–5385.

257. Wei SH, Chen CM, Strathdee G, et al. Methylation microarray analysis of late-stage ovarian carcinomas distinguishes progression-free survival in patients and identifies candidate epigenetic markers. *Clin Cancer Res* 2002;8:2246–2252.

258. Zhang L, Conejo-Garcia JR, Katsaros D, et al. Intratumoral T cells, recurrence, and survival in epithelial ovarian cancer. *N Engl J Med* 2003;348:203–213.

259. Dembo AJ, Davy M, Stenwig AE, et al. Prognostic factors in patients with stage I epithelial ovarian cancer. *Obstet Gynecol* 1990;75:263–273.

260. Vergote I, DeBrabanter J, Fyles A, et al. Prognostic importance of degree of differentiation and cyst rupture in stage I invasive epithelial ovarian carcinoma. *Lancet* 2001;357:176–182.

261. Zwart J, Geisler JP, Geisler HE. Five-year survival in patients with endometrioid carcinoma of the ovary versus those with serous carcinoma. *Eur J Gynaecol Oncol* 1998;19:225–228.

262. Hreshchyshyn MM, Park RC, Blessing JA. The role of adjuvant therapy in stage I ovarian cancer. *Am J Obstet Gyncol* 1980;138:139–145.

263. Bush RS, Allt WE, Beale FA. Treatment of epithelial carcinoma of the ovary: operation, irradiation and chemotherapy. *Am J Obstet Gynecol* 1977;127:692–704.

264. Klaassen D, Shelley W, Starreveld A, et al. Early stage ovarian cancer: a randomized clinical trial comparing whole abdominal radiotherapy, melphalan, and intraperitoneal chromic phosphate: a National Cancer Institute of Canada Clinical Trials Group report. *J Clin Oncol* 1988;6:1254–1263.

265. Vergote IB, Vergote-DeVos LN, Abeler VM, et al. Randomized trial comparing cisplatin with radioactive phosphorus or whole abdomen irradiation as adjuvant treatment of ovarian cancer. *Cancer* 1992;69:741–749.

266. Bolis G, Colombo N, Pecorelli S, et al. Adjuvant treatment for early epithelial ovarian cancer: results of two randomised clinical trials comparing cisplatin to no further treatment or chromic phosphate (32P). GICOG: Gruppo Interregionale Collaborativo in Ginecologia Oncologica. *Ann Oncol* 1995;6:887–893.

267. Young RC, Brady MF, Nieberg RK, et al. Adjuvant treatment for early ovarian cancer: a randomized phase III trial of intraperitoneal ^{32}P or intravenous cyclophosphamide and cisplatin—a Gynecologic Oncology Group Study. *J Clin Oncol* 2003;21:4350–4355.

268. Colombo N, Guthrie D, Chiari S, et al. International Collaborative Ovarian Neoplasm trial 1: a randomized trial of adjuvant chemotherapy in women with early-stage ovarian cancer. *J Natl Cancer Inst* 2003;95:125–132.

269. Trimbos JB, Vergote I, Bolis G, et al. Impact of adjuvant chemotherapy and surgical staging in early-stage ovarian carcinoma: European Organisation for Research and Treatment of Cancer-Adjuvant Chemotherapy in Ovarian Neoplasm Trial. *J Natl Cancer Inst* 2003;95:113–125.

270. Trimbos JB, Parmar M, Vergote I, et al. International Collaborative Ovarian Neoplasm trial 1 and Adjuvant ChemoTherapy in Ovarian Neoplasm trial: two parallel randomized phase III trials of adjuvant chemotherapy in patients with early-stage ovarian carcinoma. *J Natl Cancer Inst* 2003;95:105–112.

271. Kolomainen DF, A'Hern R, Coxon FY, et al. Can patients with relapsed, previously untreated, stage I epithelial ovarian cancer be successfully treated with salvage therapy? *J Clin Oncol* 2003;21:3113–3118.

272. Young RC. Early-stage ovarian cancer: to treat or not to treat. *J Natl Cancer Inst* 2003;95:94–95.

273. Bell J, Brady M, Lage J, et al. A randomized phase III trial of three versus six cycles of carboplatin and paclitaxel as adjuvant treatment in early stage ovarian epithelial carcinoma: a Gynecologic Oncology Group study. 34th Annual Meeting Society of Gynecologic Oncologists (abst 1).

274. Barnhill DR, Kurman RJ, Brady MF, et al. Preliminary analysis of the behavior of stage I ovarian serous tumors of low malignant potential: a Gynecologic Oncology Group study. *J Clin Oncol* 1995;13:2752–2756.

275. Chambers JT. Borderline ovarian tumors: a review of treatment. *Yale J Biol Med* 1989;62:351–365.

276. Creasman WT, Park R, Norris H, et al. Stage I borderline ovarian tumors. *Obstet Gynecol* 1982;59:93–96.

277. Sutton GP, Bundy BN, Omura GA, et al. Stage III ovarian tumors of low malignant potential treated with cisplatin combination therapy (a Gynecologic Oncology Group study). *Gynecol Oncol* 1991;41:230–233.

278. Gershenson DM, Silva EG. Serous ovarian tumors of low malignant potential with peritoneal implants. *Cancer* 1990;65:578–585.

279. Drescher CW, Flint A, Hopkins MP, et al. Prognostic significance of DNA content and nuclear morphology in borderline ovarian tumors. *Gynecol Oncol* 1993;48:242–246.

280. Padberg BC, Arps H, Franke U, et al. DNA cytophotometry and prognosis in ovarian tumors of borderline malignancy. A clinicomorphologic study of 80 cases. *Cancer* 1992;69:2510–2514.

281. Gershenson DM. Contemporary treatment of borderline ovarian tumors. *Cancer Invest* 1999;17:206–210.

282. Seidman JD, Kurman RJ. Subclassification of serous borderline tumors of the ovary into benign and malignant types. *Am J Surg Pathol* 1996;20:1331–1345.

283. Griffiths CT. Surgical resection of tumor bulk in the primary treatment of ovarian carcinoma. *Natl Cancer Inst Monogr* 1975;42:101–104.

284. Goldie JH, Coldman AJ. A mathematic model for relating the drug

sensitivity of tumors to their spontaneous mutation rate. *Cancer Treat Rep* 1979;63:1727–1733.

285. Munnell EW. The changing prognosis and treatment in cancer of the ovary. A report of 235 patients with primary ovarian carcinoma 1952–1961. *Am J Obstet Gynecol* 1968;100:790–805.

286. Delclos L, Quinlan EJ. Malignant tumors of the ovary managed with postoperative megavoltage irradiation. *Radiology* 1969;93:659–663.

287. Young RC, Chabner BA, Hubbard SP, et al. Advanced ovarian adenocarcinoma. A prospective clinical trial of melphalan (L-PAM) versus combination chemotherapy. *N Engl J Med* 1978;299:1261–1266.

288. Omura GA, Bundy BN, Berek JS, et al. Randomized trial of cyclophosphamide plus cisplatin with or without doxorubicin in ovarian carcinoma: a Gynecologic Oncology Group Study. *J Clin Oncol* 1989;7:457–465.

289. Smith JP, Day TG Jr. Review of ovarian cancer at the University of Texas Systems Cancer Center, M.D. Anderson Hospital and Tumor Institute. *Am J Obstet Gynecol* 1979;135:984–993.

290. Neijt JP, ten Bokkel Huinink WW, van der Burg ME, et al. Randomised trial comparing two combination chemotherapy regimens (Hexa-CAF vs CHAP-5) in advanced ovarian carcinoma. *Lancet* 1984;2:594–600.

291. Wharton JT, Edwards CL. Cytoreductive surgery for common epithelial tumors of the ovary. *Clin Obstet Gynaecol* 1983;10:235–244.

292. Heintz AP, Hacker NF, Berek JS, et al. Cytoreductive surgery in ovarian carcinoma: feasibility and morbidity. *Obstet Gynecol* 1986;67:783–788.

293. Neijt JP, ten Bokkel Huinink WW, van der Burg ME, et al. Randomized trial comparing two combination chemotherapy regimens (CHAP-5 vs CP) in advanced ovarian carcinoma. *J Clin Oncol* 1987;5:1157–1168.

294. Potter ME, Partridge EE, Shingleton HM, et al. Intraperitoneal chromic phosphate in ovarian cancer: risks and benefits. *Gynecol Oncol* 1989;32:314–318.

295. Eisenkop SM, Spirtos NM, Montag TW, et al. The impact of subspecialty training on the management of advanced ovarian cancer. *Gynecol Oncol* 1992;47:203–209.

296. Baker T, Piver MS, Hempling RE. Improved long-term survival by cytoreductive surgery to less than 1 cm, induction cisplatin and monthly cisplatin, Adriamycin, cyclophosphamide in advanced ovarian adenocarcinoma. *Proc Am Soc Clin Oncol* 1994;13:A861.

297. Fuks Z, Rizel S, Anteby SO, et al. Current concepts in cancer: ovary—treatment for stages III and IV. The multimodal approach to the treatment of stage III ovarian carcinoma. *Int J Radiat Oncol Biol Phys* 1982;8:903–908.

298. Dembo AJ. Radiotherapeutic management of ovarian cancer. *Semin Oncol* 1984;11:238–250.

299. Hoskins WJ, McGuire WP, Brady MF, et al. The effect of diameter of largest residual disease on survival after primary cytoreductive surgery in patients with suboptimal residual epithelial ovarian carcinoma. *Am J Obstet Gynecol* 1994;170:974–979.

300. Eisenkop SM, Nalick RH, Wang HJ, et al. Peritoneal implant elimination during cytoreductive surgery for ovarian cancer: impact on survival. *Gynecol Oncol* 1993;51:224–229.

301. Venesmaa P, Ylikorkala O. Morbidity and mortality associated with primary and repeat operations for ovarian cancer. *Obstet Gynecol* 1992;79:168–172.

302. Bristow RE, Montz FJ, Lagasse LD, et al. Survival impact of surgical cytoreduction in stage IV epithelial ovarian cancer. *Gynecol Oncol* 1999;72:278–287.

303. Curtin JP, Malik R, Venkatraman ES, et al. Stage IV ovarian cancer: impact of surgical debulking. *Gynecol Oncol* 1997;64:9–12.

304. Liu PC, Benjamin I, Morgan MA, et al. Effect of surgical debulking on survival in stage IV ovarian cancer. *Gynecol Oncol* 1997;64:4–8.

305. Munkarah AR, Hallum AV 3rd, Morris M, et al. Prognostic significance of residual disease in patients with stage IV epithelial ovarian cancer. *Gynecol Oncol* 1997;64:13–17.

306. Schwartz PE, Rutherford TJ, Chambers JT, et al. Neoadjuvant chemotherapy for advanced ovarian cancer: Long-term survival. *Gynecol Oncol* 1999;72:93–99.

307. Vergote I, De Wever I, Tjalma W, et al. Neoadjuvant chemotherapy or primary debulking surgery in advanced ovarian carcinoma: a retrospective analysis of 285 patients. *Gynecol Oncol* 1998;71:431–436.

308. Ng L, Rubin S, Hoskins W, et al. Aggressive chemosurgical debulking in patients with advanced ovarian cancer. *Gynecol Oncol* 1990;38:358–363.

309. Hakes T, Markman M, Reichman B, et al. Pilot trial of high intensity intravenous cyclophosphamide/cisplatin and intraperitoneal cisplatin for advanced ovarian cancer: a preliminary report. *Proc Am Soc Clin Oncol* 1989;8:152.

310. van der Burg ME, van Lent M, Buyse M, et al. The effect of debulking surgery after induction chemotherapy on the prognosis in advanced epithelial ovarian cancer. Gynecological Cancer Cooperative Group of the European Organization for Research and Treatment of Cancer. *N Engl J Med* 1995;332:629–634.

311. Rose PG, Nerenstone S, Brady M, et al. A phase III randomized study of interval secondary cytoreduction in patients with advanced stage ovarian carcinoma with suboptimal residual disease: a Gynecologic Oncology Group study. *Proc Am Soc Clin Oncol* 2002;21:201a(abst 802).

312. Omura G, Blessing JA, Ehrlich CE, et al. A randomized trial of cyclophosphamide and doxorubicin with or without cisplatin in advanced ovarian carcinoma. A Gynecologic Oncology Group Study. *Cancer* 1986;57:1725–1730.

313. Decker DG, Fleming TR, Malkasian GD Jr, et al. Cyclophosphamide plus cis-platinum in combination: treatment program for stage III or IV ovarian carcinoma. *Obstet Gynecol* 1982;60:481–487.

314. Calvert AH, Harland SJ, Newell DR, et al. Early clinical studies with cis-diammine-1,1-cyclobutane dicarboxylate platinum II. *Chemother Pharmacol* 1982;9:140–147.

315. Canetta R, Bragman K, Smaldone L, et al. Carboplatin: current status and future prospects. *Cancer Treat Rev* 1988;15:17–32.

316. Curt GA, Grygiel JJ, Corden BJ, et al. A phase I and pharmacokinetic study of diamminecyclobutane-dicarboxylateoplatinum (NSC 241240). *Cancer Res* 1983;43:4470–4473.

317. Jodrell DI, Egorin MJ, Canetta RM, et al. Relationships between carboplatin exposure and tumor response and toxicity in patients with ovarian cancer. *J Clin Oncol* 1992;10:520–528.

318. Calvert AH, Newell DR, Gumbrell LA, et al. Carboplatin dosage: prospective evaluation of a simple formula based on renal function. *J Clin Oncol* 1989;7:1748–1756.

319. Go RS, Adjei AA. Review of the comparative pharmacology and clinical activity of cisplatin and carboplatin. *J Clin Oncol* 1999;17:409–422.

320. Aabo K, Adams M, Adnitt P, et al. Chemotherapy in advanced ovarian cancer: four systematic meta-analyses of individual patient data from 37 randomized trials. Advanced Ovarian Cancer Trialists' Group. *Br J Cancer* 1998;78:1479–1487.

321. Stewart LA, Guthrie D, Parmar MK et al. Chemotherapy in advanced ovarian cancer. *BMJ* 1991;304:119.

322. Taylor AE, Wiltshaw E, Gore ME, et al. Long-term follow-up of the first randomized study of cisplatin versus carboplatin for advanced epithelial ovarian cancer. *J Clin Oncol* 1994;12:2066–2070.

323. Alberts DS, Green S, Hannigan EV, et al. Improved therapeutic index of carboplatin plus cyclophosphamide versus cisplatin plus cyclophosphamide: final report by the Southwest Oncology Group of a phase III randomized trial in stages III and IV ovarian cancer. *J Clin Oncol* 1992;10:706–717.

324. Swenerton K, Jeffrey J, Stuart G, et al. Cisplatin-cyclophosphamide versus carboplatin-cyclophosphamide in advanced ovarian cancer: a randomized phase III study of the National Cancer Institute of Canada Clinical Trials Group. *J Clin Oncol* 1992;10:718–726.

325. ten Bokkel Huinink WW, van der Burg ME, van Oosterom AT, et al. Carboplatin in combination therapy for ovarian cancer. *Cancer Treat Rev* 1988;15:9–15.

326. Travis LB, Holowaty EJ, Bergfeldt K, et al. Risk of leukemia after platinum-based chemotherapy for ovarian cancer. *N Engl J Med* 1999;340:351–357.

327. Bruzzone M, Repetto L, Chiara S, et al. A randomized trial comparing PC vs PAC chemotherapy in epithelial ovarian cancer: 7 years follow-up. *Proc Am Soc Clin Oncol* 1990;9:157a (abst610).

328. A'hern RP, Gore ME. Impact of doxorubicin on survival in advanced ovarian cancer. *J Clin Oncol* 1995;13:726–732.

329. Omura GA, Buyse M, Marsoni S, et al. Cyclophosphamide plus cisplatin versus cyclophosphamide, doxorubicin, and cisplatin chemo-

therapy of ovarian carcinoma: a meta-analysis. The Ovarian Cancer Meta-Analysis Project. *J Clin Oncol* 1991;9:1668–1674.

330. The ICON Collaborators. ICON2: randomized trial of single-agent carboplatin against three-drug combination of CAP (cyclophosphamide, doxorubicin, and cisplatin) in women with ovarian cancer. ICON Collaborators. International Collaborative Ovarian Neoplasm Study. *Lancet* 1998;352:1511–1576.

331. McGuire WP, Rowinsky EK. Old drugs revisited, new drugs and experimental approaches in ovarian cancer therapy. *Semin Oncol* 1991;18:255–269.

332. Einzig AI, Wiernik PH, Sasloff J, et al. Phase II study and long-term follow-up of patients treated with taxol for advanced ovarian adenocarcinoma. *J Clin Oncol* 1992;10:1748–1753.

333. Kohn EC, Sarosy G, Bicher A, et al. Dose-intense taxol: high response rate in patients with platinum-resistant recurrent ovarian cancer. *J Natl Cancer Inst* 1994;86:18–24.

334. Rowinsky EK, Gilbert MR, McGuire WP, et al. Sequences of taxol and cisplatin: a phase I and pharmacologic study. *J Clin Oncol* 1991; 9:1692–1703.

335. Thigpen JT, Blessing JA, Ball H, et al. Phase II trial of paclitaxel in patients with progressive ovarian carcinoma after platinum-based chemotherapy: a Gynecologic Oncology Group study. *J Clin Oncol* 1994;12:1748–1753.

336. Trimble EL, Adams JD, Vena D, et al. Paclitaxel for platinum-refractory ovarian cancer: results from the first 1,000 patients registered to National Cancer Institute Treatment Referral Center 9103. *J Clin Oncol* 1993;11:2405–2410.

337. McGuire WP, Hoskins WJ, Brady MF, et al. Cyclophosphamide and cisplatin compared with paclitaxel and cisplatin in patients with stage III and stage IV ovarian cancer. *N Engl J Med* 1996;334:1–6.

338. Piccart MJ, Bertelsen K, James K, et al. Randomized intergroup trial of cisplatin-paclitaxel versus cisplatin-cyclophosphamide in women with advanced epithelial ovarian cancer: three-year results. *J Natl Cancer Inst* 2000;92:699–708.

339. Rowinsky EK, Donehower RC. Paclitaxel (Taxol). *N Engl J Med* 1995;1004–1014.

340. Dumontet C, Sikic BI. Mechanisms of action of and resistance to antitubulin agents: microtubule dynamics, drug transport, and cell death. *J Clin Oncol* 1999;17:1061–1070.

341. Piccart MJ, Gore M, ten Bokkel Huinink W, et al. Docetaxel: an active new drug for treatment of advanced epithelial ovarian cancer. *J Natl Cancer Inst* 1995;87:676–681.

342. Eisenhauer EA, ten Bokkel Huinink WW, Swenerton KD, et al. European-Canadian randomized trial of paclitaxel in relapsed ovarian cancer: high-dose versus low-dose and long versus short infusion. *J Clin Oncol* 1994;12:2654–2666.

343. Muggia FM, Braly PS, Brady MF, et al. Phase III randomized study of cisplatin versus paclitaxel versus cisplatin and paclitaxel in patients with suboptimal stage III or IV ovarian cancer: a Gynecologic Oncology Group study. *J Clin Oncol* 2000;18:106–115.

344. Vermorken JB, ten Bokkel Huinink WW, Eisenhauer EA, et al. Advanced ovarian cancer. Carboplatin versus cisplatin. *Ann Oncol* 1993; 4:S41–S48.

345. Bookman MA, McGuire WP 3rd, Kilpatrick D, et al. Carboplatin and paclitaxel in ovarian carcinoma: a phase I study of the Gynecologic Oncology Group. *J Clin Oncol* 1996;14:1895–1902.

346. Ozols RF, Bundy BN, Greer BE, et al. Phase III trial of carboplatin and paclitaxel compared with cisplatin and paclitaxel in patients with optimally resected stage III ovarian cancer: a Gynecologic Oncology Group study. *J Clin Oncol* 2003;21:3194–3200.

347. Neijt JP, Engelholm SA, Tuxen MK, et al. Exploratory phase III study of paclitaxel and cisplatin versus paclitaxel and carboplatin in advanced ovarian cancer. *J Clin Oncol* 2000;18:3084–3092.

348. duBois A, Lück H-J, Meier W, et al. A randomized clinical trial of cisplatin/paclitaxel versus carboplatin/paclitaxel as first-line treatment of ovarian cancer. *J Natl Cancer Inst* 2003;95:1320–1330.

349. International Collaborative Ovarian Neoplasm Group. Paclitaxel plus carboplatin versus standard chemotherapy with either single-agent carboplatin or cyclophosphamide, doxorubicin, and cisplatin in women with ovarian cancer: the ICON3 randomised trial. *Lancet* 2002;360:505–515.

350. Sandercock J, Parmar MK, Torri V. First-line chemotherapy for ad-

351. Levin L, Hryniuk WM. Dose intensity analysis of chemotherapy regimens in ovarian carcinoma. *J Clin Oncol* 1987;5:756–767.

352. Conte PF, Bruzzone M, Carnino F, et al. High-dose versus low-dose cisplatin in combination with cyclophosphamide and epidoxorubicin in suboptimal ovarian cancer: a randomized study of the Gruppo Oncologico Nord-Ovest. *J Clin Oncol* 1996;14:351–356.

353. Dittrich C, Obermair A, Kurz C, et al. Prospective randomized trial of cisplatin/carboplatin versus conventional cisplatin/cyclophosphamide in epithelial ovarian cancer: first results of the impact of platinum dose-intensity on patient outcome. *Proc Am Soc Clin Oncol* 1996;15:279.

354. Kaye SB, Lewis CR, Paul J, et al. Randomised study of two doses of cisplatin with cyclophosphamide in epithelial ovarian cancer. *Lancet* 1992;340:329–333.

355. McGuire WP, Hoskins WJ, Brady MF, et al. Assessment of dose-intensive therapy in suboptimally debulked ovarian cancer: a Gynecologic Oncology Group study. *J Clin Oncol* 1995;13:1589–1599.

356. Colombo N, Pittelli M, Parma G, et al. Cisplatin dose-intensity in advanced ovarian cancer: a randomized study of conventional dose versus dose-intense cisplatin monochemotherapy. *Proc Am Soc Clin Oncol* 1993;12:255a(abst 806).

357. Kaye SB, Paul J, Cassidy J, et al. Mature results of a randomized trial of two doses of cisplatin for the treatment of ovarian cancer. Scottish Gynecology Cancer Trials Group. *J Clin Oncol* 1996;14:2113–2119.

358. Gore M, Mainwaring P, A'Hern R, et al. Randomized trial of dose-intensity with single agent carboplatin in patients with epithelial ovarian cancer. *J Clin Oncol* 1998;16:2426–2434.

359. Jakobsen A, Bertelsen K, Andersen JE, et al. Dose-effect study of carboplatin in ovarian cancer: a Danish Ovarian Cancer Group study. *J Clin Oncol* 1997;15:193–198.

360. Kohn EC, Sarosy G, Bicher A, et al. Dose-intense Taxol: high response rate in patients with platinum-resistant recurrent ovarian cancer. *J Natl Cancer Inst* 1994;86:18–24.

361. Omura GA, Brady MF, Look KY, et al. Phase III trial of paclitaxel at two dose levels, the higher dose accompanied by filgrastim at two dose levels in platinum-pretreated epithelial ovarian cancer: an intergroup study. *J Clin Oncol* 2003;21:2843–2848.

362. Scarfone G, Parazzini F, Sciatta C, et al. A multicenter randomized trial comparing two different doses of Taxol (T) plus a fixed dose of carboplatin (C) in advanced ovarian cancer (AOC). *Proc Am Soc Clin Oncol* 2001;20:205a(abst 816).

363. Fennelly D, Aghajanian C, Shapiro F, et al. Phase I and pharmacologic study of paclitaxel administered weekly in patients with relapsed ovarian cancer. *J Clin Oncol* 1997;15:187–192.

364. Kaern J, Tropé CG, Baekelandt M, et al. Phase II trial of weekly single agent paclitaxel (P) in platinum (PLAT) and paclitaxel refractory ovarian cancer (OC). *Proc Am Soc Clin Oncol* 2001;20:203a(abst 810).

365. Markman M, Baker ME, Hall JB, et al. Phase 2 trial of weekly single agent paclitaxel in platinum and paclitaxel-refractory ovarian cancer. *Proc Am Soc Clin Oncol* 2000;19:396a(abst 1567).

366. Ho AG, Beller U, Speyer JL, et al. A reassessment of the role of second-look laparotomy in advanced ovarian cancer. *J Clin Oncol* 1987;5:1316–1321.

367. Lund B, Williamson P. Prognostic factors for outcome of and survival after second-look laparotomy in patients with advanced ovarian carcinoma. *Obstet Gynecol* 1990;76:617–622.

368. Rubin SC, Hoskins WJ, Saigo PE, et al. Prognostic factors for recurrence following negative second-look laparotomy in ovarian cancer patients treated with platinum-based chemotherapy. *Gynecol Oncol* 1991;42:137–141.

369. Varia MA, Stehman FB, Bundy BN, et al. Intraperitoneal radioactive phosphorus (^{32}P) versus observation after negative second-look laparotomy for stage III ovarian carcinoma: a randomized trial of the Gynecologic Oncology Group. *J Clin Oncol* 2003;21:2849–2855.

370. Sorbe B on behalf of the Swedish-Norwegian Ovarian Cancer Study Group. Consolidation treatment of advanced (FIGO stage III) ovarian carcinoma in complete surgical remission after induction chemotherapy: a randomized, controlled, clinical trial comparing whole abdominal radiotherapy, chemotherapy, and no further treatment. *Int J Gynecol Cancer* 2003;13:278–286.

371. Cure H, Battista C, Guastalla J, et al. Phase III randomized trial of high-dose chemotherapy (HDC) and peripheral blood stem cell (PBSC) support as consolidation in patients (pts) with responsive low-burden advanced ovarian cancer (AOC): preliminary results of a GINECO/FNCLCC/SFGM-TC study. *Proc Am Soc Clin Oncol* 2001; 20:204a(abst 815).

372. Markman M, Liu PY, Wilczynski S, et al. Phase III randomized trial of 12 versus 3 months of maintenance paclitaxel in patients with advanced ovarian cancer after complete response to platinum and paclitaxel-based chemotherapy: a Southwest Oncology Group and Gynecologic Oncology Group trial. *J Clin Oncol* 2003;21:2460–2465.

373. Rothenberg ML, Liu PY, Wilczynski S, et al. Phase II trial of oral altretamine for consolidation of clinical complete remission in women with stage III epithelial ovarian cancer: a Southwest Oncology Group trial (SWOG-9326). *Gynecol Oncol* 2001;82:317–322.

374. Pfisterer J, Lortholary A, Kimmig R, et al. Paclitaxel/carboplatin (TC) vs. paclitaxel/carboplatin followed by topotecan (TC-Top) in first-line treatment of ovarian cancer FIGO stages IIb-IV. Interim results of a gynecologic cancer intergroup phase III trial of the AGO Ovarian Cancer Study Group and GINECO. *Proc Am Soc Clin Oncol* 2003; 22:446a(abst 1793).

375. Pignata S, Deplacido S, Scambia G, et al. Topotecan vs nihil after response to carboplatin and paclitaxel in advanced ovarian cancer. Early results of the MITO-1 (Multicenter Italian Trials in Ovarian Cancer) study. *Proc Am Soc Clin Oncol* 2003;22:446a(abst 1791).

376. Lambert HE, Rustin GJ, Gregoary WM, et al. A randomized trial of five versus eight courses of cisplatin or carboplatin in advanced epithelial ovarian carcinoma: a North Thames Ovary Group study. *Ann Oncol* 1997;8:827–833.

377. Hakes TB, Chalas E, Hoskins WJ, et al. Randomized prospective trial of 5 versus 10 cycles of cyclophosphamide, doxorubicin, and cisplatin in advanced ovarian carcinoma. *Gynecol Oncol* 1992;45:284.

378. Bertelsen K, Jakobsen A, Stroyer J, et al. A prospective randomized comparison of 6 and 12 cycles of cyclophosphamide, adriamycin, and cisplatin in advanced epithelial ovarian cancer: a Danish Ovarian Study Group trial (DACOVA). *Gynecol Oncol* 1993;49:30–36.

379. Barakat RR, Sabbatini P, Bhaskaran D, et al. Intraperitoneal chemotherapy for ovarian carcinoma: results of long-term follow-up. *J Clin Oncol* 2002;20:694–698.

380. Hall G, Coleman R, Stead M, et al. Maintenance treatment with interferon for advanced ovarian cancer. *Proc Am Soc Clin Oncol* 2000; 19:386a(abst 1529).

381. Berek J, Ehlen T, Gordon A, et al. Interim analysis of a double blind study of Ovarex® mAb B43.13 (OV) versus placebo (PBO) in patients with ovarian cancer. *Proc Am Soc Clin Oncol* 2001;20:210a(abst 837).

382. Epenetos AA, Verheijen R. Safety of radioimmunotherapy in international ovarian cancer study. *Proc Am Soc Clin Oncol* 2000;19: 387a(abst 1533).

383. Nicholson S, Bell S, McCormack M, et al. A randomised phase III trial of adjuvant intraperitoneal radioimmunotherapy in ovarian cancer. *Proc Am Soc Clin Oncol* 2000;19:383a (abst 1514).

384. Hirte HW, Vergote IB, Jeffrey JR, et al. An international multicentre phase III study of BAY 12–9566 (BAY) versus placebo in patients (pts) with advanced ovarian cancer (OVCA) responsive to primary surgery/paclitaxel + platinum containing chemotherapy (CT). *Proc Am Soc Clin Oncol* 2001;20:211a(abst 843).

385. Ozols RF. Maintenance therapy in advanced ovarian cancer: progression-free survival and clinical benefit. *J Clin Oncol* 2003;21: 2451–2453.

386. Thigpen T. Maybe more is better. *J Clin Oncol* 2003;21:2454–2456.

387. Scarfone G, Merisio C, Garavaglia E, et al. A phase III trial of consolidation versus NIHIL (NIL) for advanced epithelial ovarian cancer (AEOC) after complete remission (CR). *Proc Am Soc Clin Oncol* 2002;21:204a(abst 812).

388. Niloff JM, Knapp RC, Lavin PT, et al. The CA125 assay as a predictor of clinical recurrence in epithelial ovarian cancer. *Am J Obstet Gynecol* 1986;155:56–60.

389. Vergote IB, Bormer OP, Abeler VM. Evaluation of serum CA125 levels in the monitoring of ovarian cancer. *Am J Obstet Gynecol* 1987; 157:88–92.

390. van der Velden J, Gitsch G, Wain GV, et al. Tamoxifen in patients with advanced epithelial ovarian cancer. *Int J Gynecol Cancer* 1995; 5:301–305.

391. Surwit EA, Childers JM, Krag DN, et al. Clinical assessment of 111In-CYT-103 immunoscintigraphy in ovarian cancer. *Gynecol Oncol* 1993;48:285–284.

392. Eeles RA, Tan S, Wiltshaw E, et al. Hormone replacement therapy and survival after surgery for ovarian cancer. *BMJ* 1991;302:259–262.

393. Rutledge F, Burns BC. Chemotherapy for advanced ovarian cancer. *Am J Obstet Gynecol* 1966;96:761–772.

394. Kaldor JM, Day NE, Pettersson F, et al. Leukemia following chemotherapy for ovarian cancer. *N Engl J Med* 1990;322:1–6.

395. Reimer RR, Hoover R, Fraumeni JF Jr, et al. Acute leukemia after alkylating-agent therapy for ovarian cancer. *N Engl J Med* 1977;297: 177–181.

396. Lund B, Jacobsen K, Rasch L, et al. Correlation of abdominal ultrasound and computed tomography scans with second- or third-look laparotomy in patients with ovarian carcinoma. *Gynecol Oncol* 1990; 37:279–283.

397. McGowan L, Bunnag B. The evaluation of therapy for ovarian cancer. *Gynecol Oncol* 1976;4:375–383.

398. Rubin SC, Dulaney ED, Markman M, et al. Peritoneal cytology as an indicator of disease in patients with residual ovarian carcinoma. *Obstet Gynecol* 1988;71:851–853.

399. Berek JS, Griffiths CT, Leventhal JM. Laparoscopy for second look evaluation in ovarian cancer. *Obstet Gynecol* 1981;58:192–198.

400. Ozols RF, Fisher RI, Anderson T, et al. Peritoneoscopy in the management of ovarian cancer. *Am J Obstet Gynecol* 1981;140:611–619.

401. Husain A, Chi DS, Prasd M, et al. The role of laparoscopy in second-look evaluations for ovarian cancer. *Gynecol Oncol* 2001;80:44–47.

402. Rubin SC, Hoskins WJ, Hakes TB, et al. Serum CA-125 levels and surgical findings in patients undergoing secondary operations for epithelial ovarian cancer. *Am J Obstet Gynecol* 1989;160:667–671.

403. Berek JS, Knapp RC, Malkasian GD, et al. CA125 serum levels correlated with second-look operations among ovarian cancer patients. *Obstet Gynecol* 1986;67:685–689.

404. Barter JF, Barnes WA. Second-look laparotomy. In: Rubin SC, Sutton GP, eds. *Ovarian cancer*. New York: McGraw-Hill, 1993.

405. Copeland LJ, Gershenson DM, Wharton JT, et al. Microscopic disease at second-look laparotomy in advanced ovarian cancer. *Cancer* 1985; 55:472–478.

406. Rubin SC, Hoskins WJ, Hakes TB, et al. Recurrence after negative second-look laparotomy for ovarian cancer: analysis of risk factors. *Am J Obstet Gynecol* 1988;159:1094–1098.

407. Bookman MA, Greer BE, Ozols RF. Optimal therapy of advanced ovarian cancer: carboplatin and paclitaxel versus cisplatin and paclitaxel (GOG158) and an update on GOG0182-ICON5. *Int J Gynecol Cancer* 2003;13:1–7.

408. Berek JS, Hacker NF, Lagasse LD, et al. Survival of patients following secondary cytoreductive surgery in ovarian cancer. *Obstet Gynecol* 1983;61:189–193.

409. Luesley DM, Chan KK, Fielding JW, et al. Second-look laparotomy in the management of epithelial ovarian carcinoma: an evaluation of fifty cases. *Obstet Gynecol* 1984;64:421–426.

410. Hoskins WJ, Rubin SC, Dulaney E, et al. Influence of secondary cytoreduction at the time of second-look laparotomy on the survival of patients with epithelial ovarian carcinoma. *Gynecol Oncol* 1989; 34:365–371.

411. Segna RA, Dottino PR, Mandeli JP, et al. Secondary cytoreduction for ovarian cancer following cisplatin therapy. *J Clin Oncol* 1993;11: 434–439.

412. Chambers SK, Chambers JT, Kohorn EI, et al. Evaluation of the role of second-look surgery in ovarian cancer. *Obstet Gynecol* 1988;72: 404–408.

413. Podratz KC, Schray MF, Wieand HS, et al. Evaluation of treatment and survival after positive second-look laparotomy. *Gynecol Oncol* 1988;31:9–24.

414. Lippman SM, Alberts DS, Slymen DJ, et al. Second-look laparotomy in epithelial ovarian carcinoma. Prognostic factors associated with survival duration. *Cancer* 1988;61:2571–2577.

415. Krebs HB, Goplerud DR. Surgical management of bowel obstruction in advanced ovarian carcinoma. *Obstet Gynecol* 1983;61:327–330.

416. Clarke-Pearson D, DeLong ER, Chin N, et al. Intestinal obstruction in patients with ovarian cancer. Variables associated with surgical complications and survival. *Arch Surg* 1988;123:42–45.

417. Rubin SC, Hoskins WJ, Benjamin I, et al. Palliative surgery for intes-

tinal obstruction in advanced ovarian cancer. *Gynecol Oncol* 1989; 34:16–19.

418. Pothuri B, Vaidya A, Aghajanian C, et al. Palliative surgery for bowel obstruction in recurrent ovarian cancer: an updated series. *Gynecol Oncol* 2003;89:306–313.

419. Cruikshank DP, Buchsbaum HJ. Effects of rapid paracentesis. Cardovascular dynamics and body fluid composition. *JAMA* 1973;225: 1361–1362.

420. Ostrowski MJ, Halsall GM. Intracavitary bleomycin in the management of malignant effusions: a multicenter study. *Cancer Treat Rep* 1982;66:1903–1907.

421. Paladine W, Cunningham TJ, Sponzo R, et al. Intracavitary bleomycin in the management of malignant effusions. *Cancer* 1976;38: 1903–1908.

422. Souter RG, Wells C, Tarin D, et al. Surgical and pathologic complications associated with peritoneovenous shunts in management of malignant ascites. *Cancer* 1985;55:1973–1978.

423. Dembo AJ, Bush RS, Beale FA, et al. Ovarian carcinoma: improved survival following abdominopelvic irradiation in patients with a completed pelvic operation. *Am J Obstet Gynecol* 1979;134:793–800.

424. Dembo AJ. Abdominopelvic radiotherapy in ovarian cancer: a 10–year experience. *Cancer* 1985;55:2285–2290.

425. Martinez A, Schray MF, Howes AE, et al. Postoperative radiation therapy for epithelial ovarian cancer: the curative role based on a 24-year experience. *J Clin Oncol* 1985;3:901–911.

426. Fuller DB, Sause WT, Plenk HP, et al. Analysis of postoperative radiation therapy in stage I through III epithelial ovarian carcinoma. *J Clin Oncol* 1987;5:897–905.

427. Weiser EB, Burke TW, Heller PB, et al. Determinants of survival of patients with epithelial ovarian carcinoma following whole abdomen irradiation (WAR). *Gynecol Oncol* 1988;30:201–208.

428. Goldberg N, Peschel RE. Postoperative abdominopelvic radiation therapy for ovarian cancer. *Int J Radiat Oncol Biol Phys* 1988;14: 425–429.

429. Hruby G, Bull CA, Langlands AO, et al. WART revisited: the treatment of epithelial ovarian cancer by whole abdominal radiotherapy. *Australas Radiol* 1997;41:276–280.

430. Withers HR, Taylor JM, Maciejewski B. The hazard of accelerated tumor clonogen repopulation during radiotherapy. *Acta Oncol* 1988; 27:131–146.

431. Dembo AJ, Van Dyk J, Japp B, et al. Whole abdominal irradiation by a moving-strip technique for patients with ovarian cancer. *Int J Radiat Oncol Biol Phys* 1979;5:1933–1942.

432. Fyles AW, Thomas GM, Pintilie M, et al. A randomized study of two doses of abdominopelvic radiation therapy for patients with optimally debulked Stage I, II, and III ovarian cancer. *Int J Radiat Oncol Biol Phys* 1998;41:543–549.

433. Morgan L, Chafe W, Mendenhall W, et al. Hyperfractionation of whole-abdomen radiation therapy: salvage treatment of persistent ovarian carcinoma following chemotherapy. *Gynecol Oncol* 1988;31: 122–136.

434. Carey MS, Dembo AJ, Simm JE, et al. Testing the validity of a prognostic classification in patients with surgically optimal ovarian carcinoma: a 15-year review. *Int J Gynecol Cancer* 1993;3:24–35.

435. Dembo AJ, Bush RS, Brown TC. Clinico-pathological correlates in ovarian cancer. *Bull Cancer* 1982;69:292–297.

436. Dembo AJ, Bush RS. Current concepts in cancer: ovary—treatment of stages III and IV. Choice of postoperative therapy based on prognostic factors. *Int J Radiat Oncol Biol Phys* 1982;8:893–897.

437. Dembo AJ. Epithelial ovarian cancer: the role of radiotherapy. *Int J Radiat Oncol Biol Phys* 1992;22:835–845.

438. Thomas GM. Is there a role for consolidation or salvage radiotherapy after chemotherapy in advanced epithelial ovarian cancer? *Gynecol Oncol* 1993;51:97–103.

439. Chiara S, Orsatti M, Franzone P, et al. Abdominopelvic radiotherapy following surgery and chemotherapy in advanced ovarian cancer. *Clin Oncol* 1991;3:340–344.

440. Greiner R, Goldhirsch A, Davis BE, et al. Whole abdomen radiation in patients with advanced ovarian carcinoma after surgery, chemotherapy and second-look laparotomy. *J Cancer Res Clin Oncol* 1984;107: 94–98.

441. Reddy S, Hartsell W, Graham J, et al. Whole-abdomen radiation ther-

apy in ovarian carcinoma: its role as a salvage therapeutic modality. *Gynecol Oncol* 1989;35:307–313.

442. Kuten A, Stein M, Steiner M, et al. Whole abdominal irradiation following chemotherapy in advanced ovarian carcinoma. *Int J Radiat Oncol Biol Phys* 1988;14:273–279.

443. Solomon HJ, Atkinson KH, Coppleson JVM, et al. Ovarian carcinoma: abdominopelvic irradiation following re-exploration. *Gynecol Oncol* 1988;31:396–401.

444. Kong JS, Peters LJ, Wharton JT, et al. Hyperfractionated split-course whole abdominal radiotherapy for ovarian carcinoma: tolerance and toxicity. *Int J Radiat Oncol Biol Phys* 1988;14:737–743.

445. Rosen EM, Goldberg ID, Rose C, et al. Sequential multiagent chemotherapy and whole abdominal irradiation for stage III ovarian carcinoma. *Radiother Oncol* 1986;7:223–231.

446. Haie C, Pejovic-Lenfant MH, George M, et al. Whole abdominal irradiation following chemotherapy in patients with minimal residual disease after second look surgery in ovarian carcinoma. *Int J Radiat Oncol Biol Phys* 1989;17:15–19.

447. Kersh CR, Randall ME, Constable WC, et al. Whole abdominal radiotherapy following cytoreductive surgery and chemotherapy in ovarian carcinoma. *Gynecol Oncol* 1988;31:113–121.

448. Goldhirsch A, Greiner R, Dreher E, et al. Treatment of advanced ovarian cancer with surgery, chemotherapy, and consolidation of response by whole abdominal radiotherapy. *Cancer* 1988;62:40–47.

449. Menczer J, Modan M, Brenner J, et al. Abdominopelvic irradiation for stage II-IV ovarian carcinoma patients with limited or no residual disease at second-look laparotomy after completion of cisplatinum-based combination chemotherapy. *Gynecol Oncol* 1986;24:149–154.

450. Schray MF, Martinez A, Howes AE, et al. Advanced epithelial ovarian cancer: salvage whole abdominal irradiation for patients with recurrent or persistent disease after combination chemotherapy. *J Clin Oncol* 1988;6:1433–1439.

451. Louie KG, Behrens BC, Kinsella TJ, et al. Radiation survival parameters of antineoplastic drug-sensitive and resistant human ovarian cancer cell lines and their modification by buthionine sulfoximine. *Cancer Res* 1985;45:2110.

452. Ledermann JA, Dembo AJ, Sturgeon JF, et al. Outcome of patients with unfavorable optimally cytoreduced ovarian cancer treated with chemotherapy and whole abdominal radiation. *Gynecol Oncol* 1991; 41:30–35.

453. Whelan TJ, Dembo AJ, Bush RS, et al. Complications of whole abdominal and pelvic radiotherapy following chemotherapy for advanced ovarian cancer. *Int J Radiat Oncol Biol Phys* 1992;22: 853–858.

454. Randall ME, Barrett RJ, Spirtos NM, et al. Chemotherapy, early surgical reassessment, and hyperfractionated abdominal radiotherapy in stage III ovarian cancer: results of a Gynecologic Oncology Group study. *Int J Radiat Oncol Biol Phys* 1996;34:139–147.

455. Corn BW, Lanciano RM, Boente M, et al. Recurrent ovarian cancer. Effective radiotherapeutic palliation after chemotherapy failure. *Cancer* 1994;74:2979–2983.

456. Adelson MD, Wharton JT, Delclos L, et al. Palliative radiotherapy for ovarian cancer. *Int J Radiat Oncol Biol Phys* 1987;13:17–21.

457. May LF, Belinson JL, Roland TA. Palliative benefit of radiation therapy in advanced ovarian cancer. *Gynecol Oncol* 1990;37:408–411.

458. Gelblum D, Mychalczak B, Almadrones L, et al. Palliative benefit of external-beam radiation in the management of platinum refractory epithelial ovarian carcinoma. *Gynecol Oncol* 1998;69:36–41.

459. Varia M, Rosenman J, Venkatraman S, et al. Intraperitoneal chromic phosphate therapy after second-look laparotomy for ovarian cancer. *Cancer* 1988;61:919–927.

460. Dedrick RL, Meyers CE, Bungay PM, et al. Pharmacokinetic rationale for peritoneal drug administration in the treatment of ovarian cancer. *Cancer Treat Rep* 1978;62:1–11.

461. Myers C. The use of intraperitoneal chemotherapy in the treatment of ovarian cancer. *Semin Oncol* 1984;11:275–284.

462. McClay EF, Howell SB. A review: intraperitoneal cisplatin in the management of patients with ovarian cancer. *Gynecol Oncol* 1990; 36:1–6.

463. Piccart MJ, Speyer JL, Markman M, et al. Intraperitoneal chemotherapy: technical experience at five institutions. *Semin Oncol* 1985;12: 90–96.

464. Pfeifle CE, Howell SB, Markman M, et al. Totally implantable system for peritoneal access. *J Clin Oncol* 1984;2:1277–1280.

465. Rubin SC, Hoskins WJ, Markman M, et al. Long-term access to the peritoneal cavity in ovarian cancer patients. *Gynecol Oncol* 1989;33:46–48.

466. Markman M. Intraperitoneal therapy in ovarian cancer. *Semin Oncol* 1998;25:356.

467. Zimm S, Clearly SM, Lucas WE, et al. Phase I/pharmacokinetic intraperitoneal cisplatin and etoposide. *Cancer Res* 1986;47:1712.

468. Howell SB, Pfeifle CL, Wung WE, et al. Intraperitoneal cisplatin with systemic thiosulfate protection. *Ann Intern Med* 1982;97:845–851.

469. Reichman B, Markman M, Hakes T, et al. Intraperitoneal cisplatin and etoposide in the treatment of refractory/recurrent ovarian carcinoma. *J Clin Oncol* 1989;7:1327–1332.

470. Howell SB, Kirmani S, Lucas WE, et al. A phase II trial of intraperitoneal cisplatin and etoposide for primary treatment of ovarian epithelial cancer. *J Clin Oncol* 1990;8:137–145.

471. Markman M. Intraperitoneal chemotherapy. *Semin Oncol* 1991;18:248–254.

472. Barakat RR, Almadrones L, Venkatraman ES, et al. A phase II trial of intraperitoneal cisplatin and etoposide as consolidation therapy in patients with Stage II-IV epithelial ovarian cancer following negative surgical assessment. *Gynecol Oncol* 1998;69:17–22.

473. Howell SB, Zimm S, Markman M, et al. Long-term survival of advanced refractory ovarian carcinoma patients with small-volume disease treated with intraperitoneal chemotherapy. *J Clin Oncol* 1987;5:1607–1612.

474. Alberts DS, Liu PY, Hannigan EV, et al. Intraperitoneal cisplatin plus intravenous cyclophosphamide versus intravenous cisplatin plus intravenous cyclophosphamide for stage III ovarian cancer. *N Engl J Med* 1996;335:1950–1955.

475. Markman M, Bundy BN, Alberts DS, et al. Phase III trial of standard-dose intravenous cisplatin plus paclitaxel versus moderately high-dose carboplatin followed by intravenous paclitaxel and intraperitoneal cisplatin in small-volume stage III ovarian carcinoma: an intergroup study of the Gynecologic Oncology Group, Southwestern Oncology Group, and Eastern Cooperative Oncology Group. *J Clin Oncol* 2001;19:1001–1007.

476. Markman M, Brady MF, Spirtos NM, et al. Phase II trial of intraperitoneal paclitaxel in carcinoma of the ovary, tube, and peritoneum: a Gynecologic Oncology Group Study. *J Clin Oncol* 1998;16:2620–2624.

477. Armstrong DK, Bundy BN, Baergen R, et al. Randomized phase III study of intravenous (IV) paclitaxel and cisplatin versus IV paclitaxel, intraperitoneal (IP) cisplatin and IP paclitaxel in optimal stage III epithelial ovarian cancer (OC): a Gynecologic Oncology Group trial (GOG 172). *Proc Am Soc Clin Oncol* 2002;21:201a(abst 803).

478. Fujiwara K, Sakuragi N, Suzuki S, et al. First-line intraperitoneal carboplatin-based chemotherapy for 165 patients with epithelial ovarian carcinoma: results of long-term follow-up. *Gynecol Oncol* 2003;90:637–643.

479. Piccart MJ, Floquet A, Scarfone G, et al. Intraperitoneal cisplatin versus no further treatment: 8-year results of EORTC 55875, a randomized phase III study in ovarian cancer patients with a pathologically complete remission after platinum-based intravenous chemotherapy. *Int J Gynecol Cancer* 2003;13:196–203.

480. Alberts DS, Markman M, Armstrong D, et al. Intraperitoneal therapy for stage III ovarian cancer: a therapy whose time has come! *J Clin Oncol* 2002;20:3944–3946.

481. Los G, Mutsaers PHA, Lenglet WJM, et al. Platinum distribution in intraperitoneal tumors after intraperitoneal cisplatin treatment. *Cancer Chemother Pharmacol* 1990;25:389–394.

482. Jenkins J, Sugarbaker PH, Gianola FJ, et al. Technical considerations in the use of intraperitoneal chemotherapy administered by Tenckhoff catheter. *Surg Gynecol Obstet* 1982;154:858–862.

483. Braly P, Doroshow J, Hoff S. Technical aspects of intraperitoneal chemotherapy in abdominal carcinomatosis. *Gynecol Oncol* 1986;25:319–333.

484. Davidson SA, Rubin SC, Markman M, et al. Intraperitoneal chemotherapy: analysis of complications with an implanted subcutaneous port and catheter system. *Gynecol Oncol* 1991;41:101–106.

485. Ozols RF, Ostchega Y, Curt G, et al. High-dose carboplatin in refractory ovarian cancer patients. *J Clin Oncol* 1987;5:197–201.

486. Gershenson DM, Kavanagh JJ, Copeland LJ, et al. Retreatment of patients with recurrent epithelial ovarian cancer with cisplatin-based chemotherapy. *Obstet Gynecol* 1989;73:798–802.

487. Markman M, Rothman R, Hakes T, et al. Second-line platinum therapy in patients with ovarian cancer previously treated with cisplatin. *J Clin Oncol* 1991;9:389–393.

488. Ozols RF, Ostchega Y, Myers CE, et al. High-dose cisplatin in hypertonic saline in refractory ovarian cancer. *J Clin Oncol* 1985;3:1246–1250.

489. Ozols RF. Treatment of recurrent ovarian cancer: increasing options—''recurrent'' results. *J Clin Oncol* 1997;15:2177–2180.

490. Markman M, Rose PG, Jones E. Ninety-six-hour infusional paclitaxel as salvage therapy of ovarian cancer patients previously failing treatment with 3-hour or 24-hour paclitaxel infusion regimens. *J Clin Oncol* 1998;16(5):1849–1851.

491. Blackledge G, Lawton F, Redman C, et al. Response of patients in phase II studies of chemotherapy in ovarian cancer: implications for patient treatment and the design of phase II trials. *Br J Cancer* 1989;59:650–653.

492. Eisenhauer EA, Vermorken JB, van Glabbeke M. Predictors of response to subsequent chemotherapy in platinum pretreated ovarian cancer: a multivariate analysis of 704 patients. *Ann Oncol* 1997;8:963–968.

493. Bookman MA, Malmstrom H, Bolis G, et al. Topotecan for the treatment of advanced epithelial ovarian cancer: an open-label phase II study in patients treated after prior chemotherapy that contained cisplatin or carboplatin and paclitaxel. *J Clin Oncol* 1998;16:3345–3352.

494. Hoskins P, Eisenhauer E, Beare S, et al. Randomized phase II study of two schedules of topotecan in previously treated patients with ovarian cancer: a National Cancer Institute of Canada Clinical Trials Group study. *J Clin Oncol* 1998;16:2233–2237.

495. Rose PG, Blessing JA, Mayer AR, et al. Prolonged oral etoposide as second-line therapy for platinum-resistant and platinum-sensitive ovarian carcinoma: a Gynecologic Oncology Group study. *J Clin Oncol* 1998;16:405–410.

496. Lund B, Hansen OP, Theilade K, et al. Phase II study of gemcitabine (2′,2′-difluorodeoxycytidine) in previously treated ovarian cancer patients. *J Natl Cancer Inst* 1994;86:1530–1533.

497. Shapiro JD, Millward MJ, Rischin D, et al. Activity of gemcitabine in patients with advanced ovarian cancer: responses seen following platinum and paclitaxel. *Gynecol Oncol* 1996;63:89–93.

498. Bajetta E, DiLeo A, Biganzoli L, et al. Phase II study of vinorelbine in patients with pretreated advanced ovarian cancer: activity in platinum-resistant disease. *J Clin Oncol* 1996;14:2546–2551.

499. Kavanagh JJ, Kudelka AP, de Leon CG, et al. Phase II study of docetaxel in patients with epithelial ovarian carcinoma refractory to platinum. *Clin Cancer Res* 1996;2:837–842.

500. Vasey PA. Role of docetaxel in the treatment of newly diagnosed advanced ovarian cancer. *J Clin Oncol* 2003;21:S136–144.

501. Muggia FM, Hainsworth JD, Jeffers S, et al. Phase II study of liposomal doxorubicin in refractory ovarian cancer: antitumor activity and toxicity modification by liposomal encapsulation. *J Clin Oncol* 1997;15:987–993.

502. Gordon AN, Granai CO, Rose P, et al. Phase II study of liposomal doxorubicin in platinum- and paclitaxel-refractory epithelial ovarian cancer. *J Clin Oncol* 2000;18:3093–3100.

503. ten Bokkel Huinink W, Gore M, Carmichael J, et al. Topotecan versus paclitaxel for the treatment of recurrent epithelial ovarian cancer. *J Clin Oncol* 1997;15:2183–2193.

504. McGuire WP, Blessing JA, Bookman MA, et al. Topotecan has substantial antitumor activity as first-line salvage therapy in platinum-sensitive epithelial ovarian carcinoma: a Gynecologic Oncology Group Study. *J Clin Oncol* 2000;18:1062–1067.

505. Rowinsky EK. Weekly topotecan: an alternative to topotecan's standard daily x 5 schedule? *Oncologist* 2002;7:324–330.

506. Gordon AN, Fleagle JT, Guthrie D, et al. Recurrent epithelial ovarian carcinoma: a randomized phase III study of pegylated liposomal doxorubicin versus topotecan. *J Clin Oncol* 2001;19:3312–3322.

507. Rose PG, Fusco N, Fluellen L, et al. Second-line therapy with paclitaxel and carboplatin for recurrent disease following first-line therapy with paclitaxel and platinum in ovarian or peritoneal carcinoma. *J Clin Oncol* 1998;16:1494–1497.

508. Dizon DS, Hensley ML, Poynor EA, et al. Retrospective analysis of

carboplatin and paclitaxel as initial second-line therapy for recurrent epithelial ovarian carcinoma: application toward a dynamic disease state model of ovarian cancer. *J Clin Oncol* 2002;20:1238–1247.

509. duBois A, Lück HJ, Pfisterer J, et al. Second-line carboplatin and gemcitabine in platinum sensitive ovarian cancer—a dose-finding study by the Arbeitsgemeinschaft Gynäkologische Onkologie (AGO) Ovarian Cancer Study Group. *Ann Oncol* 2001;12:1115–1120.

510. The ICON and AGO Collaborators. Paclitaxel plus platinum-based chemotherapy versus conventional platinum-based chemotherapy in women with relapsed ovarian cancer: the ICON4/AGO-OVAR-2.2 trial. *Lancet* 2003;361:2099–2106.

511. McGuire WP, Rowinsky EK. Old drugs revisited, new drugs and experimental approaches in ovarian cancer therapy. *Semin Oncol* 1991;18:255.

512. Thigpen JT, Vance RB, Balducci L, et al. New drugs and experimental approaches in ovarian cancer treatment. *Semin Oncol* 1984;11:314–326.

513. Thompson P, Osborne R, Slevin M, et al. A phase II study of cyproterone acetate in advanced ovarian cancer. London Gynecology Oncology Group. *Proc Am Soc Clin Oncol* 1990;9:160.

514. Kavanagh JJ, Roberts W, Townsend P, et al. Leuprolide acetate in the treatment of refractory or persistent ovarian cancer. *J Clin Oncol* 1989;7:115–118.

515. Markman M, Iseminger KA, Hatch KD, et al. Tamoxifen in platinum-refractory ovarian cancer: a Gynecologic Oncology Group Ancillary Report. *Gynecol Oncol* 1996;62:4–6.

516. Hatch KD, Beecham JB, Blessing JA, et al. Responsiveness of patients with advanced ovarian carcinoma to tamoxifen. A Gynecologic Oncology Group study of second-line therapy in 105 patients. *Cancer* 1991;68:269–271.

517. Schwartz PE, Chambers JT, Kohorn EI, et al. Tamoxifen in combination with cytotoxic chemotherapy in advanced epithelial ovarian cancer. *Cancer* 1989;63:1074–1078.

518. Vasey PA, on behalf of the Scottish Gynaecological Cancer Trials Group. Survival and longer-term toxicity results of the SCOTROC study: docetaxel-carboplatin (DC) vs. paclitaxel-carboplatin (PC) in epithelial ovarian cancer (EOC). *Proc Am Soc Clin Oncol* 2002;21:202a(abst 804).

519. Hansen SW, Anderson H, Boman K, et al. Gemcitabine, carboplatin, and paclitaxel (GCP) as first-line treatment of ovarian cancer FIGO, stages IIB-IV. *Proc Am Soc Clin Oncol* 1999;18:357a(abst1379).

520. Look KY, Bookman MA, Brady M, et al. Update of the phase I feasibility trial of carboplatin, paclitaxel, and gemcitabine in patients with previously untreated epithelial ovarian or primary peritoneal cancer (EOC/PPC): A Gynecologic Oncology Group (GOG) study. *Proc Soc Gynecol Oncol* 2000;32:A154(abst).

521. duBois A, Lück HJ, Bauknecht T, et al. First-line chemotherapy with epirubicin, paclitaxel, and carboplatin for advanced ovarian cancer: a phase I/II study of the Arbeitsgemeinschaft Gynäkologische Onkologie Ovarian Cancer Study Group. *J Clin Oncol* 1999;17:46–51.

522. Kristensen G, Vergote I, Stuart G, et al. First line treatment of ovarian cancer FIGO stages IIb-IV with paclitaxel/epirubicin/carboplatin (TEC) vs. paclitaxel/carboplatin (TC). Interim results of an NSGO-EORTC-NCIC CTG Gynecological Cancer Intergroup phase III trial. *Proc Am Soc Clin Oncol* 2002;21:202a(abst 805).

523. du Bois A, Weber B, Pfisterer J, et al. Epirubicin/paclitaxel/carboplatin (TEC) vs. paclitaxel/carboplatin (TC) in first-line treatment of ovarian cancer FIGO Stages IIb-IV. Interim Results of an AGO-GINECO Intergroup Phase III Trial. *Proc Am Soc Clin Oncol* 2001;20:202a(abst 805).

524. Rose PG, Greer BE, Markman M, et al. A phase I study of paclitaxel, carboplatin, and liposomal doxorubicin in ovarian, peritoneal, and tubal carcinoma: a Gynecologic Oncology Group study. *Proc Am Soc Clin Oncol* 2000;19:387a(abst 1531).

525. Rose PG, Rodriguez M, Waggoner S, et al. Phase I study of paclitaxel, carboplatin, and increasing days of prolonged oral etoposide in ovarian, peritoneal, and tubal carcinoma: a Gynecologic Oncology Group study. *J Clin Oncol* 2000;18:2957–2962.

526. O'Reilly S, Fleming GF, Baker SD, et al. Phase I trial and pharmacologic trial of sequences of paclitaxel and topotecan in previously treated ovarian epithelial malignancies: a Gynecologic Oncology Group study. *J Clin Oncol* 1997;15:177–186.

527. Scarfone G, Bolis G, Parazzini F, et al. A multicenter, randomized,

528. Hoskins P, Eisenhauer E, Vergote I, et al. Phase II feasibility study of sequential couplets of cisplatin/topotecan followed by paclitaxel/cisplatin as primary treatment for advanced epithelial ovarian cancer: a National Cancer Institute of Canada Clinical Trials Group Study. *J Clin Oncol* 2000;18:4038–4044.

529. Bauknecht T, Hefti A, Morack G, et al. Gemcitabine combined with cisplatin as first-line treatment in patients 60 years or older with epithelial ovarian cancer: a phase II study. *Int J Gynecol Cancer* 2003;13:130–137.

530. Windbichler GH, Hausmaninger H, Stummvoll W, et al. Interferon-gamma in the first-line therapy of ovarian cancer: a randomized phase III trial. *Br J Cancer* 2000;82:1138–1144.

531. Bookman MA. Developmental chemotherapy. In: Ozols RF, ed. *American Cancer Society atlas of clinical oncology*. Hamilton, Ontario: BC Decker, 2003:168–193.

532. Shpall EJ, Jones RB, Bearman SI, et al. Future strategies for the treatment of advanced epithelial ovarian cancer using high-dose chemotherapy and autologous bone marrow support. *Gynecol Oncol* 1994;54:357–361.

533. Stiff PJ, Bayer R, Kerger C, et al. High-dose chemotherapy with autologous transplantation for persistent/relapsed ovarian cancer: a multivariate analysis of survival for 100 consecutively treated patients. *J Clin Oncol* 1997;15:1309–1317.

534. Ledermann JA, Herd R, Maraninchi D, et al. High dose chemotherapy in ovarian cancer: an analysis of the experience of the European Group for Blood and Marrow Transplant (EBMT) over 7 years. *Proc Am Soc Clin Oncol* 1999;18:360a.

535. Cooper DL. Peripheral blood stem cell transplantation. In: DeVita VT Jr, Hellman S, Rosenberg SA, eds. *Principles and practice of oncology*. Philadelphia: PPO Updates, 1994:1–12.

536. Lewis NL, Schilder RJ. High dose chemotherapy. In: Ozols RF, ed. *American Cancer Society atlas of clinical oncology*. Hamilton, Ontario: BC Decker, 2003:213–224.

537. Fennelly D, Schneider J, Spriggs D, et al. Dose escalation of paclitaxel with high-dose cyclophosphamide, with analysis of progenitor-cell mobilization and hematologic support of advanced ovarian cancer patients receiving rapidly sequenced high-dose carboplatin/cyclophosphamide courses. *J Clin Oncol* 1995;13:1160–1166.

538. Aghajanian C, Fennelly D, Shapiro F, et al. Phase II study of "dose-dense" high-dose chemotherapy treatment with peripheral-blood progenitor-cell support as primary treatment for patients with advanced ovarian cancer. *J Clin Oncol* 1998;16:1852–1860.

539. Schilder RJ, Gallo JM, Millenson MM, et al. Phase I trial of multiple cycles of high-dose carboplatin, paclitaxel, and topotecan with peripheral-blood stem-cell support as front-line therapy. *J Clin Oncol* 2001;19:1183–1194.

540. Schilder RJ, Brady MF, Spriggs D, et al. Pilot evaluation of high-dose carboplatin and paclitaxel followed by high-dose melphalan supported by peripheral blood stem cells in previously untreated advanced ovarian cancer: a Gynecologic Oncology Group study. *Gynecol Oncol* 2003;88:3–8.

541. O'Dwyer PJ, Hamilton TC, LaCreta FP, et al. Phase I trial of buthionine sulfoximine in combination with melphalan in patients with cancer. *J Clin Oncol* 1996;14:249–256.

542. Rosen LS, Brown J, Laxa B, et al. Phase I study of TLK286 (glutathione S-transferase P1–1 activated glutathione analogue) in advanced refractory solid malignancies. *Clin Cancer Res* 2003;9:1628–1638.

543. Kavanagh JJ, Kudelka AP, Garcia A, et al. Phase 2 study of TLK286 (GST P1–1 activated glutathione analog) administered weekly in patients with platinum refractory or resistant ≥ third-line advanced ovarian cancer. *Proc Am Soc Clin Oncol* 2003;22:452a(abst 1816).

544. Masuda H, Ozols RF, Lai GM, et al. Increased DNA repair as a mechanism of acquired resistance to cis-diamminedichloroplatinum (II) in human ovarian cancer cell lines. *Cancer Res* 1988;48:5713–5716.

545. Lai GM, Ozols RF, Smyth JF, et al. Enhanced DNA repair and resistance to cisplatin in human ovarian cancer. *Biochem Pharmacol* 1988;37:4597–4600.

546. Rose PG, Mossbruger K, Fusco N, et al. Gemcitabine reverses cis-

platin resistance: demonstration of activity in platinum- and multi-drug-resistant ovarian and peritoneal carcinoma. *Gynecol Oncol* 2003; 88:17–21.

547. Louie KG, Hamilton TC, Winker MA, et al. Augmentation of adriamycin accumulation and metabolism in adriamycin sensitive and resistant human ovarian cancer cell lines. *Biochem Pharmacol* 1986; 35:467–472.

548. Bourhis J, Goldstein LJ, Riou G, et al. Expression of a human multidrug resistance gene in ovarian carcinomas. *Cancer Res* 1989;49: 5062–5065.

549. Joly F, Joly F, Mangioni C, et al. A phase 3 study of PSC 833 in combination with paclitaxel and carboplatin (PC-PSC) versus paclitaxel and carboplatin (PC) alone in patients with stage IV or suboptimally debulked stage III epithelial ovarian cancer or primary cancer of the peritoneum. *Proc Am Soc Clin Oncol* 2002;21:202a(abst 806).

550. Rowinsky EK, Smith L, Wang YM, et al. Phase I and pharmacokinetic study of paclitaxel in combination with biricodar, a novel agent that reverses multidrug resistance conferred by overexpression of both MDR1 and MRP. *J Clin Oncol* 1998;16:2964–2976.

551. Coukos G, Rubin SC. Gene therapy for ovarian cancer. *Oncology* 2001;15:1197–1204, 1207.

552. Coukos G, Gray HJ, June CH. Advances in biologic therapy. In: Ozols RF, ed. *American Cancer Society atlas of clinical oncology.* Hamilton, Ontario: BC Decker, 2003:194–212.

553. Steis RG, Urba WJ, VanderMolen LA, et al. Intraperitoneal lymphokine-activated killer-cell and interleukin-2 therapy for malignancies limited to the peritoneal cavity. *J Clin Oncol* 1990;8:1618–1629.

554. Edwards RP, Lembersky BC, Kunschner AJ, et al. Intraperitoneal interleukin2 (IL2) produces durable responses for refractory ovarian cancer. *Proc Am Soc Clin Oncol* 1995;14:333.

555. Lamers CH, Boljuis RL, Warnaar SO, et al. Local but no systemic immunomodulation by intraperitoneal treatment of advanced ovarian cancer with autologous T lymphocytes re-targeted by a bi-specific monoclonal antibody. *Int J Cancer* 1997;73:211–219.

556. Epenetos AA, Munro AJ, Stewart S, et al. Antibody-guided irradiation of advanced ovarian cancer with intraperitoneally administered radiolabeled monoclonal antibodies. *J Clin Oncol* 1987;5:1890–1899.

557. Wagner U, Köhler S, Reinartz S, et al. Immunological consolidation of ovarian carcinoma recurrences with monoclonal anti-idiotype antibody ACA125: immune responses and survival in palliative treatment. *Clin Cancer Res* 2001;7:1154–1162.

558. Berd D, Kairys J, Dunton C, et al. Autologous, hapten-modified vaccine as a treatment for human cancers. *Semin Oncol* 1998;25:646–653.

559. Hanahan D, Weinberg RA. The hallmarks of cancer. *Cell* 2000;100: 57–70.

560. DiSaia PJ, Bloss JD. Treatment of ovarian cancer: new strategies. *Gynecol Oncol* 2003;90:S24–32.

561. Finkler N, Gordon A, Crozier M, et al. Phase 2 evaluation of OSI-774, a potent oral antagonist of the EGFR-TK in patients with advanced ovarian carcinoma. *Proc Am Soc Clin Oncol* 2001;20: 208a(abst 831).

562. Schilder RJ, Kohn E, Sill MW, et al. Phase II trial of gefitinib in patients with recurrent ovarian or primary peritoneal cancer: Gynecology Oncology Group 170C. *Proc Am Soc Clin Oncol* 2003;22; 451a(abst 1814).

563. Berek JS, Schultes BC, Nicodemis CF. Biologic and immunologic therapies for ovarian cancer. *J Clin Oncol* 2003;21:168–174.

564. Hortobagyi GN, Ueno NT, Xia W, et al. Cationic liposome-mediated E1A gene transfer to human breast and ovarian cancer cells and its biologic effects: a phase I clinical trial. *J Clin Oncol* 2001;19: 3422–3433.

565. Tait DL, Obermiller PS, Hatmaker AR, et al. Ovarian cancer BRCA1 gene therapy: Phase I and II trial differences in immune response and vector stability. *Clin Cancer Res* 1999;5:1708–1714.

566. Tait DL, Obermiller PS, Redlin-Frazier S, et al. A phase I trial of retroviral BRCA1sv gene therapy in ovarian cancer. *Clin Cancer Res* 1997;3:1959–1968.

CHAPTER 26

Ovarian Germ-Cell Tumors

Daniela E. Matei, Anthony H. Russell, Carolyn J. Horowitz,
David M. Gershenson, and Elvio Silva

Significant improvements in the management of ovarian germ-cell tumors have been achieved during the past two decades. The development of more effective chemotherapeutic regimens is clearly the leading cause for improved outcome for these patients. In addition, advancements in other disciplines led to the development of a more precise surgical staging system, improved radiographic imaging, more sophisticated pathology techniques, as well as improved supportive care and symptom control. A substantial majority of patients with ovarian germ-cell tumors are long-term survivors and suffer minimal morbidity from treatment. Fertility-sparing surgical procedures enable a large proportion of young women with ovarian germ-cell tumors to preserve their reproductive potential. These results illustrate the value of collaboration between different specialties (surgery, medical oncology, pathology, imaging).

PATHOLOGY

The World Health Organization (WHO) classification of germ-cell tumors of the ovary is presented in Table 26.1 (1). These tumors can be divided into three major categories: benign tumors, almost all of which are accounted for by dermoid cysts; malignant tumors arising from constituents of dermoid cysts; and primitive malignant germ-cell tumors, which recapitulate normal embryonic and extraembryonic cells and

D. E. Matei: Department of Hematology/Oncology, Indiana University, Indianapolis, Indiana 46202

A. H. Russell: Department of Radiation Oncology, Massachusetts General Hospital, Boston, Massachusetts

C. J. Horowitz: The Radiation Oncology Center, Willow Ridge Complex, Marlton, New Jersey

D. Gershenson: Department of Gynecologic Oncology, The University of Texas M. D. Anderson Cancer Center, Houston, Texas 77030

E. Silva: Department of Pathology, The University of Texas M. D. Anderson Cancer Center, Houston, Texas

structures. The most important of the third group of tumors are the dysgerminoma, the yolk-sac tumor, the immature teratoma, and the mixed primitive germ-cell tumor. Dermoid cysts, which account for one-quarter to one-third of all ovarian tumors, are most common in young women but are also encountered rarely in children and occasionally in elderly women. Malignant tumors arising from constituents of dermoid cysts account for 2% to 3% of ovarian cancers. These tumors are most commonly squamous carcinomas and follow an age-incidence curve similar to that of carcinomas derived from ovarian surface epithelium. Primitive germ-cell tumors account for 2% to 3% of all ovarian cancers and occur usually in young women. The peak age incidence for development of these tumors is the early twenties.

Dermoid Cysts

Dermoid cysts (mature cystic teratomas) are teratomatous cysts lined predominantly by epidermis with skin appendages. In 12% of cases, dermoid cysts occur bilaterally. The cyst lumen contains sebaceous material and hair. In two-thirds of cases, mature elements reflecting differentiation into tissues normally derived from all three embryonic germ layers (ectoderm, mesoderm, endoderm) are present. Any of these constituents has the potential for undergoing benign or malignant neoplastic transformation leading to formation of a tumor within a tumor. In patients older than 40 years, malignant transformation of dermoid cysts should be excluded. It is rare to note malignant lesions in dermoid cysts before this age. These malignant areas present as small nodules in the wall of the cyst, and can be recognized only after careful removal of the entire content of the cyst (2). The most common secondary tumor is squamous carcinoma (3, 4), which is found in about 1% of dermoid cysts, and appears grossly as an eccentric solid mass in the cyst wall or as a polypoid mass within the lumen. The natural history of squamous carcinoma arising in a dermoid cyst mimics squa-

TABLE 26.1. *World Health Organization classification of ovarian germ-cell tumors*

Dysgerminoma
  Variant: with syncytiotrophoblast cells
Yolk-sac tumor (endodermal sinus tumor)
  Variants: polyvesicular vitelline tumor
    Hepatoid
    Glandular
      Variant: "endometrioid"
Embryonal carcinoma
Polyembryoma
Choriocarcinoma
Teratomas
  Immature
  Mature
    Solid
    Cystic (dermoid cyst)
      With secondary tumor formation (specify type)
    Fetiform (homunculus)
  Monodermal and highly specialized
    Struma ovarii
      With thyroid tumor (specify type)
    Carcinoid
      Insular
      Trabecular
    Strumal carcinoid
    Mucinous carcinoid
    Neuroectodermal tumors
    Sebaceous tumors
    Others
  Mixed (specify types)
Mixed (specify types)

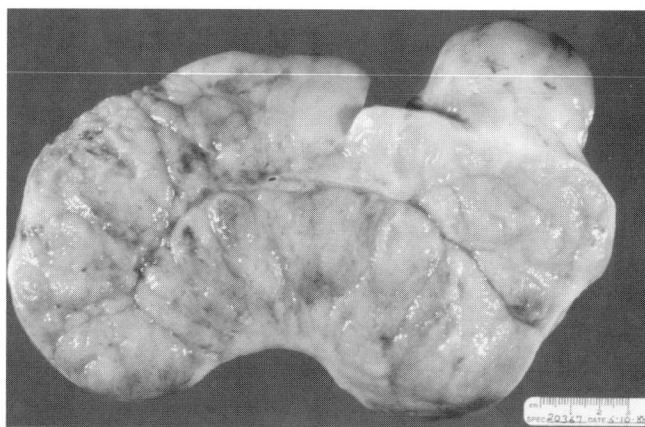

FIG. 26.1. Dysgerminoma—solid, lobulated, uniform clear surface cut.

mous carcinoma arising in other primary sites. Spread may be by direct extension or regional lymphatic metastases (paraaortic lymph nodes), and peritoneal dissemination may occur following cyst rupture (2,5). Curative management can be accomplished with aggressive local therapies (surgery, radiation, chemoradiation), even when cancer has extended beyond the ovary to involve regional structures, in a fashion analogous to the curative management of squamous cancer arising at other anatomic sites.

Other tumors arising in dermoid cysts include basal cell carcinomas, sebaceous tumors, malignant melanomas, adenocarcinomas, sarcomas, and neuroectodermal tumors. Endocrine-type tumors include struma ovarii and carcinoid tumors (6); such tumors are malignant in less than 5% of cases. The stroma is rarely functional, but carcinoid tumors can induce carcinoid syndrome in one-third of cases. The syndrome is almost always curable by removal of the tumor.

Dysgerminoma

Dysgerminoma accounts for about half of the primitive germ-cell tumors of the ovary, and is grossly bilateral in approximately 10% of cases (7,8). In addition, up to 10% of normal-appearing contralateral ovaries may contain elements of dysgerminoma on microscopic inspection. Typi-

cally, dysgerminoma appears as a solid, pink to cream-colored mass that is lobulated both on its external and on its cut surfaces (Fig. 26.1) (8). Microscopic examination reveals a monotonous proliferation of large, polyhedral clear cells rich in cytoplasmic glycogen with slightly flattened, round, uniform, central nuclei containing one or a few prominent nucleoli (Fig. 26.2). Tumor cells resemble closely the primordial germ cells of the embryo. A pure lymphocytic infiltrate of varying prominence is almost invariably present in the stroma. Occasionally noncaseating granulomas are encountered. About 5% of dysgerminomas contain syncytiotrophoblast cells as single or small groups of cells. Their presence may be associated with human chorionic gonadotropin (hCG) production; with estrogenic changes such as sexual precocity; and, less commonly, with androgenic manifestations. Recently, c-*kit* expression was recorded in dysgerminoma (9), and activating c-*kit* mutations (D816H missense mutations) were described in the phosphotransferase

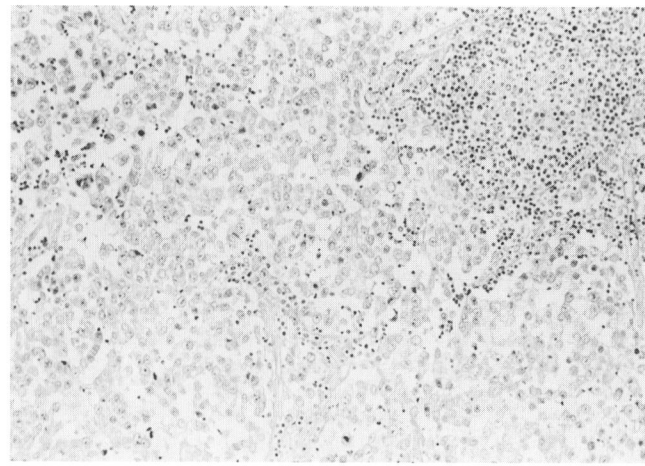

FIG. 26.2. Dysgerminoma—uniform cells with pale cytoplasm and nuclei, with prominent nucleolar groups of lymphocytes seen in the stroma.

domain of the receptor (10), suggesting that these tumors might be amenable to treatment with inhibitors of the c-*kit* receptor kinase, such as imatinib mesylate (Gleevec or STI571; Novartis, Basel).

Dysgerminoma can occur in dysgenetic ovaries (11,12); hence a normal female karyotype (or at least a normal phenotype) should be confirmed if the contralateral ovary will be preserved at surgery. Searching for residual, normal ovarian tissue in the sections of the removed ovary and inspection of the contralateral ovary are usually sufficient. However, if review of permanent sections reveals an association with gonadoblastoma or with a gonadal streak, which are common in 46,XY or in mosaic genotypes, search and removal of the contralateral gonad are required because of an increased risk for recurrence or for developing gonadoblastoma in the remaining ovary.

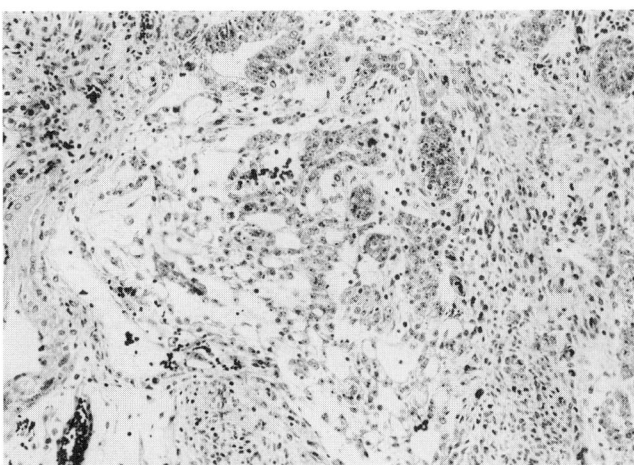

FIG. 26.4. Yolk sac tumor—extensive reticular pattern with focal glandular differentiation.

Yolk-Sac Tumors

Yolk-sac tumors (YSTs), or endodermal sinus tumors, are bilateral in less than 5% of cases and account for approximately 20% of primitive germ-cell tumors of the ovary. On gross examination, they typically form solid masses that are yellowish and more friable than dysgerminoma. YSTs are often focally necrotic and hemorrhagic, with cystic degeneration and rupture (Fig. 26.3). The most common microscopic pattern (reticular) reflects extraembryonic differentiation, with formation of a network of irregular, anastomosing spaces lined by primitive epithelial cells. In many cases, single papillae lined by tumor cells and containing a central vessel (Schiller-Duval bodyies) project into these spaces (endodermal sinus pattern) (Fig. 26.4). Occasionally, small vesicles resembling the yolk-sac vesicle of the normal embryo are present. When these structures predominate, the tumor is

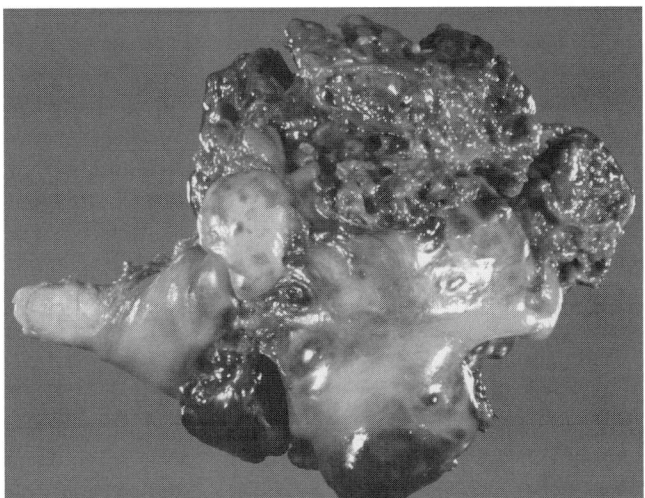

FIG. 26.3. Yolk sac tumor—solid and cystic areas with focal hemorrhage at the bottom.

designated a polyvesicular vitelline tumor. Like the normal yolk-sac vesicle, which divides into a vestigial primary yolk-sac vesicle and a secondary yolk-sac vesicle from where the gastrointestinal tract and its appendages develop, the neoplastic yolk sac rarely gives rise to tumors of embryonal type. These tumors recapitulate primitive gut (glandular yolk-sac tumor) and primitive liver (hepatoid yolk-sac tumor). Yolk-sac tumors commonly contain periodic acid–Schiff (PAS)–positive hyaline bodies and almost always contain cells that stain immunohistochemically for alpha fetoprotein (AFP).

Immature Teratomas

Immature teratomas account for approximately 20% of primitive germ-cell tumors and are usually unilateral. Bilateral tumors occur in less than 5% of cases, but benign neoplasms, usually dermoid cysts, can be found in the contralateral ovary in 10% of cases. Immature teratomas are predominantly solid, but may be cystic. The sectioned surface of an immature teratoma displays soft and solid areas, which correspond to its nervous system components, cartilage and bone; and cysts, which may be filled with serous or mucinous fluid or sebaceous material and hair (Fig. 26.5). Microscopic examination reveals a disorderly mixture of tissues derived from all three germ layers, with at least some of the components having an immature, embryonic appearance. The immature elements are almost always neuroectodermal. They consist mainly of primitive neuroectodermal tubules and sheets of small, round, malignant cells that may be associated with glia formation (Fig. 26.6).

Immature teratomas are graded from 1 to 3 based on the amount of immature neural tissue they contain, which is measured as the number of low-power microscopic fields containing neuroepithelium. The histologic grade correlates

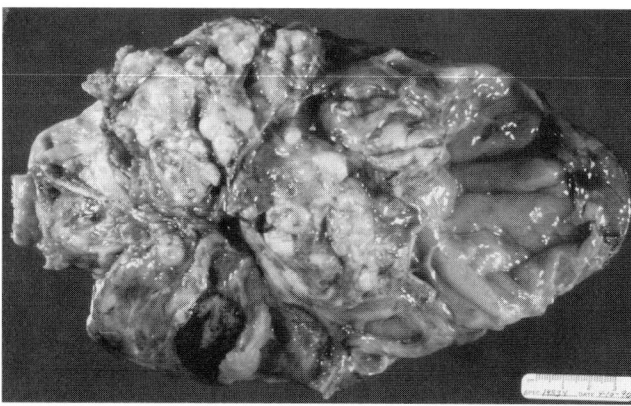

FIG. 26.5. Immature teratoma—multiple nodules of white hard tissue in the wall of a cyst.

closely with prognosis and is a determining factor for treatment in stage I tumors. For instance, in a series of 58 patients with stage I immature teratomas treated with surgery alone, survival was 81% for women with grade 1 tumors and 60% and 30% for patients with grade 2 and grade 3, respectively (13). Because of high interobserver variability noted in the distinction between grades 2 and 3, O'Conner and Norris have proposed changing the grading system to two grades (14): low grade, which includes the previous grade 1, and high grade, encompassing previous grades 2 and 3.

Immature teratomas and solid mature teratomas are occasionally associated with miliary peritoneal implants composed exclusively of mature glial tissue (gliomatosis peritonei, GP). The presence of gliomatosis has no impact on tumor stage or prognosis. Indeed, patients with diffuse peritoneal implants composed exclusively of mature glial tissue fare well (15,16). Sporadically, peritoneal implants grow slowly and require surgery for removal. Rarely, glial peritoneal implants undergo malignant transformation, which portends an ominous prognosis (17,18). The origin of peritoneal implants is unclear. To determine whether glial peritoneal

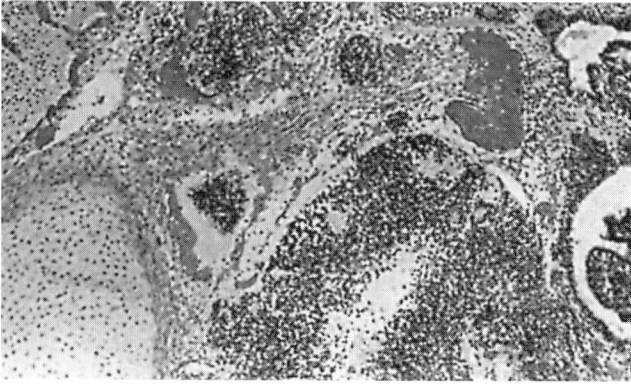

FIG. 26.6. Immature teratoma. A rounded nodule of small primitive neuroectodermal cells lies to the right of a nodule of fetal-appearing cartilage.

implants arise from elements of teratoma or whether they represent glial metaplasia of the pluripotent müllerian cells in the peritoneum, DNA analysis at microsatellite (MS) loci was performed for two cases (19). Whereas teratoma cells are homozygotic at the MS loci (maternal chromosomal copies), the glial implants contain cells with heterozygotic DNA content. This observation suggests that peritoneal glial implants in GP arise from müllerian stem cells, which contain dual (paternal and maternal) genetic material.

The *growing teratoma syndrome*, well recognized in testicular germ-cell tumors, has also been recorded in patients with ovarian immature teratomas (20). Enlarging tumor masses during chemotherapy for germ-cell tumors, associated with decreasing or normalized tumor markers, are highly suggestive of a growing teratoma (21). In these cases, even when the original tumor is immature, most of the tumor found in the metastases is mature teratomatous tissue. Treatment consists of surgical removal of the mass to prevent local mechanical complications (e.g., obstruction or compression of adjacent organs) or malignant transformation of the teratoma. If the resected tumor contains elements of viable neoplasm, additional chemotherapy should be given and be tailored on a case-by-case basis.

Embryonal Carcinomas and Choriocarcinomas

Embryonal carcinomas and choriocarcinomas of the ovary are extremely rare in pure form. Foci of choriocarcinoma or embryonal carcinoma are present in primitive germ-cell tumors of mixed histology. Embryonal carcinoma presents with a variety of patterns similar to those encountered in the testis, where the tumor is far more common. Choriocarcinoma is composed of nests of cytotrophoblast and intermediate trophoblast enveloped by syncytiotrophoblast. Both embryonal carcinoma and choriocarcinoma may produce hCG, and therefore could cause endocrine changes such as sexual precocity and irregular bleeding of endometrial origin.

Mixed Primitive Germ-Cell Tumors

Mixed primitive germ-cell tumors account for approximately 10% of primitive germ-cell tumors of the ovary. Bilateral ovarian involvement depends on the presence or absence of a dysgerminomatous component. If dysgerminomatous elements are present, the contralateral ovary is involved in 10% of cases. Mixture of dysgerminoma and yolk-sac tumor is the single most common combination encountered. The existence of this tumor category emphasizes to the pathologist the importance of extensive and judicious sampling of all primitive germ-cell tumors of the ovary since different components may require different therapy. According to some investigators, the prognosis of these tumors depends not only on the nature of their components but also on the proportion of specimen occupied by the most malignant element. However, with improvement in systemic chemotherapy in recent years, this distinction has become less important.

Poorly Differentiated Small-Cell Carcinoma

The poorly differentiated small-cell carcinoma of the ovary is a rare but distinct entity that deserves mention. It is classically associated with hypercalcemia (22) and may have germ-cell origin, as suggested by immunostaining for α_1-antitrypsin, the presence of PAS-positive intracellular globules, the presence of foci of intercellular basement membrane material, and focal laminin immunoreactivity (23). These tumors occur usually in young women and are invariably associated with dismal prognosis (24,25). Treatment with a germ-cell–type chemotherapeutic regimen is probably justified, although data are scant and inconclusive given the rarity of such tumors.

BIOLOGY OF OVARIAN GERM-CELL TUMORS

Biologically, ovarian germ-cell tumors, like testicular cancer, are derived from primordial germ cells, which undergo defective meiosis. Karyotypic abnormalities are common and include aneuploidy or chromosomal rearrangements. In contrast, benign teratomas have a normal karyoptype. One report notes chromosomal abnormalities in 7% of mature teratomas (26,27). Analysis of centromeric heteromorphisms suggests that 65% to 70% of benign teratomas result from a postmeiosis I type error (homozygotes), whereas the remaining 30% to 35% are caused by defective meiosis I, as demonstrated by heterozygosity of centromeric markers (26). Among malignant ovarian germ-cell tumors, aneuploidy and chromosomal translocations or truncations similar to those encountered in testicular carcinoma have been widely reported (28,29). The presence of an isochromosome 12p (i12p) has been noted in ovarian tumors (30), albeit less commonly than in testicular cancer. Other chromosomal aberrations such as loss or gain in chromosomes 1, 11, 12, 16, and X can be identified (31). The association between dysgerminoma and dysgenetic gonads (12) is well recognized and should be managed accordingly, as will be discussed.

CLINICAL FEATURES

Malignant germ-cell tumors of the ovary occur mainly in girls and young women. In the University of Texas M. D. Anderson Cancer Center (UTMDACC) series, the age of the patients ranged from 6 to 40 years, with a median age of 16 to 20 years depending upon histologic type (32).

Signs and symptoms in these patients were rather consistent. Abdominal pain associated with a palpable pelvic-abdominal mass was present in approximately 85% of patients (8,33). Approximately 10% of patients presented with acute abdominal pain, usually caused by rupture, hemorrhage, or torsion of these tumors. This finding may be somewhat more common in patients with endodermal sinus tumor or mixed germ-cell tumors and is frequently misdiagnosed as acute appendicitis. Less common signs and symptoms include abdominal distention (35%), fever (10%), and vaginal bleeding (10%). A few patients will exhibit isosexual precocity, presumably owing to hCG production by the tumor.

In a small percentage of cases, ovarian germ-cell tumors occur during pregnancy or in the immediate post partum period (8). For instance, in the series reported by Gordon et al., 20 of 158 patients with dysgerminoma were diagnosed during pregnancy or after delivery (11). Nondysgerminomatous ovarian tumors occur less frequently during pregnancy, but rare cases have been reported (34–37). Marked increase in AFP heralds the presence of a germ-cell tumor with yolk-sac component. By and large, patients with ovarian tumors diagnosed during pregnancy can be treated successfully without compromising the health of the fetus. Surgical resection of tumors and chemotherapy has been performed safely in the mid and third trimesters. However, rapid disease progression and pregnancy termination/miscarriage have been recorded, especially for nondysgerminomatous tumors (38).

Many germ-cell tumors possess the unique property of producing biologic markers that can be detected in serum. The development of specific and sensitive radioimmunoassay techniques to measure hCG and AFP led to dramatic improvement in the monitoring of patients with these tumors. Serial measurements of serum markers aid the diagnosis and, more importantly, are useful for monitoring response to treatment and detection of subclinical recurrences. Table 26.2 illustrates the typical findings in sera of patients with various tumor histologic types. Endodermal sinus tumor and choriocarcinoma are prototypes for AFP and respectively for hCG production. Embryonal carcinoma can secrete both hCG and AFP, but most commonly produces hCG. Mixed tumors may produce either, both, or none of the markers depending on the type and quantity of elements present. Dysgerminoma is commonly devoid of hormonal production, although a small percentage of tumors produce low levels of hCG if multinucleated syncytiotrophoblastic giant cells are present within the tumor tissue. The presence of an elevated level of AFP or high level of hCG (>100 U/mL) denotes the presence of tumor elements other than dysgerminoma. Therapy should be adjusted accordingly. Although immature teratomas are associated with negative markers, a few tumors can produce AFP.

TABLE 26.2. *Serum tumor markers in malignant germ-cell tumors of the ovary*

Histology	AFP	hCG
Dysgerminoma	−	±
Endodermal sinus tumor	+	−
Immature teratoma	±	−
Mixed germ-cell tumor	±	±
Choriocarcinoma	−	+
Embryonal carcinoma	±	+
Polyembryoma	±	+

A third tumor marker is lactic dehydrogenase (LDH). LDH is frequently elevated in patients with ovarian germ-cell tumors, particularly in dysgerminoma. Unfortunately, it is less specific than hCG or AFP, which limits its usefulness. The level of CA-125 is also elevated in some patients with ovarian germ-cell tumors, but this is also nonspecific (39).

SURGERY

Operative Findings

Malignant germ-cell tumors of the ovary tend to be quite large. In the UTMDACC series, these tumors ranged in size from 7 to 40 cm with a median size of 16 cm (33). Predominance of right-sided over left-sided involvement was noted. Bilaterality of tumor involvement (especially true stage IB disease) is exceedingly rare except in the case of dysgerminoma. Bilateral involvement occurs in 10% to 15% of dysgerminoma patients, although it has been reported to be lower in some series and higher in others (11,40–43). For nondysgerminomatous tumors, bilateral involvement almost always signifies advanced disease with metastatic spread to the contralateral ovary or a mixed germ-cell tumor with a prominent dysgerminomatous component.

Ascites may be noted in approximately 20% of cases. Rupture of tumors, either preoperatively or intraoperatively, can occur in approximately 20% of cases. Torsion of the ovarian pedicle was documented in 5% of patients in the UTMDACC series.

Benign cystic teratoma is associated with 5% to 10% of malignant germ-cell tumors. These coexistent teratomas may occur in the ipsilateral ovary, in the contralateral ovary, or bilaterally. Likewise, a preexisting gonadoblastoma may be noted in some patients (12). These patients generally have dysgenetic gonads associated with a 46,XY karyotype.

Malignant germ-cell tumors generally spread in one of two ways: along the peritoneal surface or through lymphatic dissemination. Although the relative frequency of these two principal mechanisms is difficult to discern, it is generally accepted that these neoplasms more commonly metastasize to lymph nodes than epithelial tumors. The high prevalence of inadequate staging procedures makes the true incidence of lymph node involvement uncertain. It is our impression that although still uncommon, malignant germ-cell tumors have a somewhat greater predilection than epithelial tumors to metastasize hematogenously to the parenchyma of liver or lung.

The stage distribution is also very different from that of epithelial tumors. In most large series, approximately 60% to 70% of tumors will be stage I (11). The next most common stage is III, accounting for 25% to 30% of tumors. Stages II and IV are relatively uncommon.

Extent of Primary Surgery

The initial treatment approach for a patient suspected of having a malignant ovarian germ-cell tumor is surgery, both for diagnosis and for therapy. After an adequate vertical midline incision, a thorough determination of disease extent by inspection and palpation should be made. If the disease is confined to one or both ovaries, it is imperative that proper staging biopsies be performed (see below).

The type of primary operative procedure depends upon the surgical findings. Because many of these patients are young women, for whom preservation of fertility is a priority, minimizing the surgical resection while ensuring removal of tumor bulk has to be balanced. As noted previously, bilateral ovarian involvement with tumor is exceedingly rare except for the case of pure dysgerminoma. Bilateral involvement may be found in cases of advanced disease (stages II to IV) in which there is metastasis from one ovary to the opposite gonad or in cases of mixed germ-cell tumors with a dysgerminomatous component. Therefore, fertility-sparing unilateral salpingo-oophorectomy with preservation of the contralateral ovary and of the uterus can be performed in most patients with malignant ovarian germ-cell tumors (44, 45). If the contralateral ovary appears to be grossly normal on careful inspection, it should be left undisturbed; however, in the case of pure dysgerminoma, biopsy may be considered because occult or microscopic tumor involvement occurs in a small percentage of patients. Unnecessary biopsy, however, may result in future infertility due to peritoneal adhesions or ovarian failure. If the contralateral ovary appears to be abnormally enlarged, a biopsy or ovarian cystectomy should be performed. If frozen examination reveals a dysgenetic gonad or if there are clinical indications suggesting a hermaphroditic phenotype, then bilateral salpingo-oophorectomy is indicated. However, it is difficult to establish this diagnosis on frozen section. Ideally, this determination should be made preoperatively (by determining a normal female karyotype). If benign cystic teratoma is found in the contralateral ovary (which occurs in approximately 5% to 10% of cases), then ovarian cystectomy with preservation of remaining normal ovarian tissue is recommended.

An important, albeit very rare, problem is bilateral gonadal involvement in a patient who desires to preserve fertility and who is a candidate for postoperative chemotherapy. There are no data regarding the ability of chemotherapy to eradicate a primary ovarian tumor. In testicular cancer, there are presumptive data suggesting that tumor may persist after chemotherapy in the gonad and that the testis may be a drug sanctuary. In exceptional situations, it may be reasonable to preserve an involved ovary in a patient who will be receiving chemotherapy. However, it is conceivable that ovarian preservation could increase the risk for recurrence in these selected cases. The decision to preserve an involved ovary is difficult and must be made carefully considering the individual patient's wishes.

The advent of in vitro fertilization technology should have an impact on operative management (46). Convention has dictated that if a bilateral salpingo-oophorectomy is necessary, a hysterectomy should also be performed. However, with current assisted reproduction technologies involving donor oocyte and hormonal support, a woman without ovaries could potentially sustain a normal intrauterine pregnancy. Similarly, if the uterus and one ovary are resected because of tumor involvement, current techniques provide the opportunity for oocyte retrieval from the remaining ovary, *in vitro* fertilization with sperm from her male partner, and embryo implantation into a surrogate's uterus. Therefore, traditional guidelines concerning fertility no longer apply for the surgical treatment of young patients with gynecologic tumors.

Surgical Staging

Surgical staging information is essential for determining extent of disease, for providing prognostic information, and for guiding postoperative management. A meticulous approach is important for every patient, but is of critical importance in those patients with early clinical disease in order to detect the presence of occult or microscopic metastases. Staging of ovarian germ-cell tumors follows the same principles applicable to epithelial ovarian tumors, as described by the International Federation of Gynecologists and Obstetricians (FIGO) (Table 26.3). Proper staging procedures consist of the following:

TABLE 26.3. *FIGO staging of ovarian germ-cell tumors*

Stage	Description
I	Tumor limited to ovaries.
IA	Tumor limited to one ovary, no ascites, intact capsule.
IB	Tumor limited to both ovaries, no ascites, intact capsule.
IC	Tumor either stage IA or IB, but with ascites present containing malignant cells or with ovarian capsule involvement or rupture or with positive peritoneal washings.
II	Tumor involving one or both ovaries with extension to the pelvis.
IIA	Extension to uterus or tubes.
IIB	Involvement of both ovaries with pelvic extension.
IIC	Tumor either stage IIA or IIB, but with ascites present containing malignant cells or with ovarian capsule involvement or rupture or with positive peritoneal washings.
III	Tumor involving one or both ovaries with tumor implants outside the pelvis or with positive retroperitoneal or inguinal lymph nodes. Superficial liver metastases qualify as stage III.
IIIA	Tumor limited to the pelvis with negative nodes but with microscopic seeding of the abdominal peritoneal surface.
IIIB	Negative nodes, tumor implants in the abdominal cavity <2 cm.
IIIC	Positive nodes or tumor implants in the abdominal cavity >2 cm.
IV	Distant metastases present.

1. Although a transverse incision is cosmetically superior, a vertical midline incision is usually necessary for adequate exposure, for appropriate staging biopsies, and for resection of large pelvic tumors or metastatic disease in the upper abdomen.

2. Ascites, if present, should be evacuated and submitted for cytologic analysis. If no peritoneal fluid is noted, cytologic washings of the pelvis and bilateral paracolic gutters should be performed prior to manipulation of the intraperitoneal contents.

3. The entire peritoneal cavity and its structures should be carefully inspected and palpated in a methodical manner. We generally prefer to start with the subphrenic spaces and move caudad toward the pelvis. The subdiaphragmatic areas, omentum, colon, all peritoneal surfaces, the entire retroperitoneum, and small intestinal serosa and mesentery should be checked. If any suspicious areas are noted, they should be submitted for biopsy or excised.

4. Next, the primary ovarian tumor and pelvis should be examined. Both ovaries should carefully be assessed for size, the presence of obvious tumor involvement, capsular rupture, external excrescences, or adherence to surrounding structures.

5. If disease seems to be limited, that is, confined to the ovary or localized to the pelvis, then random staging biopsies of structures at risk should be performed. These sites should include the omentum (with generous biopsies from multiple areas) and the peritoneal surfaces of the following sites: bilateral paracolic gutters, cul-de-sac, lateral pelvic walls, vesicouterine reflection, and subdiaphragmatic areas. Any adhesions should also be generously sampled.

6. The paraaortic and bilateral pelvic lymph node–bearing areas should be carefully palpated. Any suspicious nodes should be excised or sampled. There is no evidence that a complete paraaortic and/or pelvic lymphadenectomy is advantageous.

7. If obvious gross metastatic disease is present, it should be excised if feasible, or at least sampled to document disease extent. The concept of cytoreductive surgery and evidence to support it will be discussed below.

The gynecologic literature is replete with examples of inadequate surgical staging. The assumption that surgical staging in the 1990s is superior to that of several years ago may be erroneous. Most patients still undergo initial surgery in community hospitals and are inadequately staged. Upon referral of such a patient to a university or tertiary care center, the oncologist is faced with the dilemma of inadequate staging information. In such cases, postoperative studies including computed tomography of the abdomen and lymphangiography, if available, are recommended. If histopathologic and limited anatomic information from the first surgery clearly indicates the use of systemic chemotherapy, it is generally inadvisable to consider reexploration solely for the purpose of precise staging information. Reoperation to complete comprehensive staging may be appropriate under clinical circumstances in which careful surveillance observation after complete staging may be a sensible alternative to chemotherapy.

Cytoreductive Surgery

If widely spread tumor is encountered at initial surgery, it is recommended that the same principles concerning cytoreductive surgery applied in the surgical management of advanced epithelial ovarian cancer be followed. Specifically, as much tumor as technically feasible and safe should be resected. However, there is scant information in the literature on the subject of cytoreductive surgery of malignant germ-cell tumors because of their rarity.

Slayton et al., in a study of the Gynecologic Oncology Group (COG) (47), found that 15 of 54 (28%) patients with completely resected disease at primary surgery failed chemotherapy with a combination of vincristine, dactinomycin, and cyclophosphamide (VAC) as opposed to 15 of 22 (68%) patients with incompletely resected disease treated with the same regimen. Furthermore, a higher percentage of patients with bulky residual disease (82%) failed chemotherapy compared to those with minimal residual disease (55%). In a subsequent GOG study reported by Williams, in which patients received the combination regimen of cisplatin, vinblastine, and bleomycin (PVB), patients with tumors other than dysgerminoma who had clinically nonmeasurable disease after surgery had a greater likelihood of remaining progression-free than those with measurable disease (65% vs 34%) (48). In addition, patients who had been surgically debulked to optimal disease had an outcome intermediate between patients with suboptimal disease and those with optimal disease without debulking.

Even with epithelial tumors, the relative influence of tumor biology, surgical skill, and aggressiveness remains uncertain. Germ-cell tumors, especially dysgerminomas, are generally much more chemosensitive than epithelial ovarian tumors. Therefore, aggressive resection of metastatic disease in these cases, especially resection of bulky retroperitoneal nodes, is questionable. The surgeon must exercise thoughtful and mature intraoperative judgment when encountering such situations, carefully weighing the risks of cytoreductive maneuvers in the setting of chemosensitive tumors. There is no substitute for surgical experience and a clear understanding of the biologic behavior of these neoplasms. Even in the face of extensive metastatic disease, it is possible to perform a fertility-sparing procedure with preservation of a normal contralateral ovary.

The value of secondary cytoreductive surgery in the management of malignant ovarian germ-cell tumors is even less clear than that of primary cytoreductive surgery. Although secondary cytoreduction is of questionable benefit for patients with refractory epithelial ovarian cancer (49,50), germ-cell tumors are relatively more chemosensitive than

epithelial tumors and are more likely to respond to second-line therapy. Therefore, if a patient has an isolated focus of persistent tumor after first-line chemotherapy in an area such as the lung, liver, retroperitoneum, or brain, then surgical extirpation should be considered before changing chemotherapeutic regimens. Although this clinical situation is extremely rare, it has been observed in other chemosensitive tumors such as gestational trophoblastic disease and testicular cancer.

Unlike testicular cancer, the finding of a residual mass after completion of chemotherapy is much less common in patients with ovarian germ-cell tumors because these women are likely to have considerable tumor debulking at the time of the diagnostic surgical procedure, and thus they enter chemotherapy with significantly less tumor burden. At completion of chemotherapy, men with nonseminomatous tumors or seminoma may have persistent mature teratoma or desmoplastic fibrosis. In patients with bulky dysgerminoma, residual masses after chemotherapy are very likely to represent desmoplastic fibrosis. Although a number of patients with pure ovarian immature teratomas or mixed germ-cell tumors have persistent mature teratoma at the completion of chemotherapy, as documented by second-look laparotomy (51), the majority are left with multiple small peritoneal implants rather than with a true mass. However, it is now recognized that occasional patients who have received chemotherapy for immature teratoma or mixed germ-cell tumor containing teratoma will have bulky residual teratoma after chemotherapy. The natural history or biologic implications of this finding are not clear. In testicular cancer, patients with bulky residual teratoma may experience slow progression of the tumor or tumors (52). Furthermore, there is presumptive evidence that these patients may in time develop overtly malignant tumors within the persistent teratoma (53–56). There are anecdotal reports of progressive mature teratoma in ovarian germ-cell tumor patients after chemotherapy (20, 57,58). Considering this information, it seems appropriate to resect persistent masses in patients with negative markers after chemotherapy for germ-cell tumors containing immature teratoma. If viable neoplasm is found in the resected masses, additional chemotherapy should be considered depending on the clinical circumstances.

Second-Look Laparotomy

Since 1960, second-look laparotomy has been incorporated in the routine management of patients with epithelial ovarian cancer to assess disease status after a fixed interval of chemotherapy. It was only natural that such an approach would be extrapolated to the management of patients with malignant ovarian germ-cell tumors. In a review of the experience with second-look laparotomy at UTMDACC, findings were negative in 52 of 53 patients (59). The one patient with positive findings at second look laparotomy had an elevated AFP level prior to surgery, which accurately predicted residual disease. This patient received subsequent chemotherapy with PVB, entering prolonged remission. Of the patients with negative findings, one woman relapsed 9 months after the negative second-look surgery and subsequently died. Thirteen patients in this series had biopsy-proven evidence of residual mature teratoma (so-called "chemotherapeutic retroconversion") at second-look laparotomy; treatment was discontinued in all patients, and none developed recurrence. Thus, in this series, second-look surgery did not add prognostic information or alter the therapeutic management of patients. The role of second-look surgery is further obscured in the setting of advancement in imaging techniques [computed tomographic (CT) scanning, positron emission tomography (PET), magnetic resonance imaging (MRI)] and in an era in which tumor marker measurements are part of routine care of patients with germ-cell tumors.

The GOG experience with second-look laparotomy in ovarian germ-cell tumors has been reviewed (51). One hundred seventeen patients enrolled prospectively on one of three GOG protocols using brief cisplatin-based chemotherapy after initial surgical staging and cytoreduction (GOG protocols 45, 78, and 90) underwent second-look surgical procedures. Of these, 45 surgical procedures were performed in patients who received three courses of cisplatin, etoposide, and bleomycin (BEP) after complete tumor resection. In this subgroup, 38 patients had negative findings, two patients had immature teratoma, and five patients had mature teratoma. One of the patients with residual immature teratoma received further chemotherapy and one did not. Both of them and the rest of patients are disease free. One patient with negative second-look surgery findings subsequently relapsed and succumbed to disease. Hence, in the subgroup of patients with completely resected primary ovarian germ-cell tumors, the benefit of second-look surgery is nil. In contrast, 72 patients in this series treated with similar chemotherapy had advanced incompletely resected tumor before beginning adjuvant treatment. In this subgroup, 48 patients did not have teratomatous elements in their primary tumor. At second-look surgery, 45 patients had no residual tumor and three patients displayed persistent endodermal sinus tumor or embryonal carcinoma. All three of the latter patients died despite further treatment. Five patients with negative second laparotomies recurred, of which only one was salvaged with chemotherapy. Thus, the value of second-look surgery in patients with incompletely resected germ-cell tumors not containing teratoma is arguably minimal. However, in the subgroup of patients with incompletely resected tumors containing teratomatous elements (total of 24 patients), second-look surgery had an impact on subsequent management. Of these patients, 16 were found to have mature teratoma at second look, which was bulky or progressive in seven cases. Four additional patients were found to have residual immature teratoma. Fourteen of the total 16 patients with teratoma and 6 of the 7 women with bulky residual tumor remain disease free after surgical resection. Therefore, whereas sec-

TABLE 26.4. *Results of second-look surgery in patients enrolled on GOG protocols*

Primary surgery	Total no.	Positive second look: progression free/total no.	Negative second look: progression free/total no.
Completely resected tumor	45	7/7[a]	37/38
Incompletely resected tumor			
Teratoma present	24	16/20[b]	4/4
Teratoma absent	48	0/3[c]	41/45

[a] Five mature teratomas and two immature teratomas.
[b] Sixteen mature teratomas and four immature teratomas.
[c] Three embryonal carcinoma and yolk-sac tumors.
Reprinted with permission from Williams SD, Blessing JA, DiSaia PJ, et al. Second-look laparotomy in ovarian germ cell tumors: the Gynecologic Oncology Group experience. *Gynecol Oncol* 1994;52:287–291.

ond-look laparotomy is not necessary in patients with tumor completely resected primarily or in those patients with initially incompletely resected tumor not containing teratoma, clinical benefit can be derived in those patients with incompletely resected primary tumor that contains elements of teratoma (Table 26.4).

Advances in imaging technology, including the advent of PET scanning, may further obviate the need for surgical reexploration. Whereas PET scanning is sensitive for detecting active (malignant) tumor, its usefulness in evaluating residual mature teratoma is more limited (60–63). A positive PET scan in the setting of a residual mass after treatment is highly indicative of viable tumor, and when used in conjunction with traditional radiographic techniques (CT, MRI) and tumor marker determinations, can predict relapses with accuracy. A recent series demonstrates that in patients with residual masses after treatment for seminoma, a positive PET scan is strong evidence that the residual mass contains persistent tumor, whereas in the more common situation when the PET scan is negative, the residual mass is very unlikely to contain tumor. The specificity of the PET scan in this situation was 100%, the sensitivity was 80%, and the positive and negative predictive values were 100% and 95%, respectively (64).

CHEMOTHERAPY

Chemotherapy: From VAC to BEP

One of the great triumphs of cancer treatment in the 1970s and 1980s was the development of effective chemotherapy for testicular germ-cell tumors (65,66). The lessons learned from prospective, frequently randomized trials in testicular cancer have been applied to ovarian germ-cell tumors. Nowadays, the overwhelming majority of patients with ovarian germ-cell tumors survive their disease with the judicious use of surgery and cisplatin-based combination chemotherapy. There are many similarities and a few important differences between testicular cancer and ovarian germ-cell tumors.

Historically, the first regimens used successfully for women with ovarian germ-cell tumors were VAC or VAC-type regimens. Indeed, such treatment had curative potential. However, among patients with advanced disease, the number of long-term survivors after VAC therapy remained under 50%. For instance, in the series reported from the UTMDACC, although 86% of patients with stage I tumors were cured with VAC, the efficacy of the regimen was significantly less for patients with advanced disease (32). Only 57% of stage II patients and 50% of patients with stage III achieved long-term control. The two patients with stage IV tumors succumbed to their disease in this report. Similarly, in a study of the GOG, only 7 of 22 of patients with incompletely resected ovarian tumors achieved long-term disease control after treatment with VAC as compared to 39 of 54 patients with completely resected tumors (67). In this report, 11 of 15 patients with stage III and both patients with stage IV disease failed within 12 months of follow-up. These data suggest that VAC chemotherapy was insufficient for the treatment of advanced-stage and/or incompletely resected ovarian germ-cell tumors.

Because of the experience gained from the treatment of testicular germ-cell tumors demonstrating the superiority of cisplatin-based regimens, new platinum-based regimens were tested in patients with ovarian germ-cell tumors. Gershenson et al. reported efficacy of PVB in a small series of patients treated at the UTMDACC (68). Among 15 patients in this report, 7 patients received PVB in the adjuvant setting, and 9 patients received the combination at the time of recurrence. Six of seven patients treated with PVB up front are long-term survivors. Among them, three patients had optimally debulked stage III disease.

Subsequently, the PVB combination was evaluated prospectively in GOG protocol 45 (48). In this series, 47 of 89 patients with nondysgerminomatous ovarian tumors (53%) are continuously disease-free with a median follow-up of 52 months. The latest treatment failure occurred at 28 months. Eight other patients had durable remissions with second-line therapy and a few other patients had nonprogressive or slowly progressive immature teratoma. Thus, the 4-year overall survival was approximately 70%. Of note, 29% of patients enrolled in this trial had received prior radiation or chemotherapy, which might have affected negatively the overall outcome. As discussed previously, patients who were debulked to optimal disease fared better than those who were not. Histologic type and marker elevation before treatment were not associated with adverse outcome. However, even among patients with nonmeasurable (and presumably small volume) disease and without prior treatment, 8 of 30 patients treated with PVB ultimately failed.

In testicular cancer, subsequent experience documented that etoposide is at least equivalent to vinblastine and pro-

TABLE 26.5. *The BEP regimen*[a]

Cisplatin	20 mg/m² days 1–5
Etoposide (VP-16)	100 mg/m² days 1–5
Bleomycin	30 units IV weekly

[a] Three to four courses given at 21-day intervals.

duces improved survival in patients with high tumor volume (66). Furthermore, the use of etoposide in place of vinblastine led to reduced neurologic toxicity, abdominal pain, and constipation. The latter two adverse effects are particularly important for patients with ovarian tumors, as many will have had recent abdominal surgery. These observations led to the evaluation of the combination of cisplatin, etoposide and bleomycin (BEP) (Table 26.5) in patients with ovarian germ-cell tumors. In a series from the UTMDACC, long-term remissions have been recorded in 25 of 26 patients treated with BEP (69). The only patient who succumbed to disease had been noncompliant with treatment, monitoring, and follow-up. Four patients with measurable disease (radiographically or clinically) after surgery had complete remissions after treatment in this report. Hence, BEP chemotherapy was evaluated prospectively by the GOG in patients with ovarian germ-cell tumors (70). With this regimen, 91 of 93 enrolled patients remained free of disease at follow-up at the expense of tolerable and reversible toxicity, as will be described later. Based on these data, although BEP and VAC have not been compared head-to-head prospectively in patients with ovarian germ-cell tumors, BEP emerged as the preferred regimen.

The inclusion of cisplatin in the treatment of ovarian tumors resulted indisputably in an improvement in survival and disease control, as shown by the results of GOG studies, as well as by other clinical series reported from different groups (71–73).

Differences in Outcome for Patients with Completely Resected Tumors Versus Advanced-Stage Disease

It is clear that several prognostic factors impact significantly the outcome of patients with ovarian germ-cell tumors and that there are important differences between testicular and ovarian germ-cell neoplasms. For instance, surgery plays a central role in the management of ovarian tumors. In the hands of an experienced surgeon, the majority of women with ovarian tumors are debulked to minimal and often clinically undetectable disease before starting chemotherapy. Therefore, unlike patients with testicular cancer, most women who are candidates for chemotherapy have minimal or no residual disease. However, even in this circumstance, there seems to be little doubt that adjuvant therapy is appropriate in the majority of cases. The anticipated risk of relapse with surgery alone in the few patients studied is 75% to 80%. Patients with embryonal carcinoma, endoder-

TABLE 26.6. *Adjuvant chemotherapy*

Institution	Regimen	Progression free/total (%)
GOG (66)	BEP	89/93 (96)
Australia (51)	Multiple	9/10 (90)
Hospital 12 de Octubre (32)	PVB or BEP	9/9 (100)
M.D. Anderson (18)	PVB	4/4 (100)
Instituto Nazionale Tumori (3)	PVB	9/10 (90)
M.D. Anderson (19)	BEP	20/20 (100)

BEP, cisplatin, etoposide, bleomycin; PVB, cisplatin, vinblastine, bleomycin.

mal sinus tumors, and mixed tumors containing these elements are considered to be at very high risk of recurrence without postoperative therapy. This risk can be minimized by the use of adjuvant chemotherapy. In the GOG protocol 78, 50 of 51 patients with completely resected ovarian germ-cell tumors remained without evidence of disease when three cycles of BEP were given adjuvantly. Although BEP and VAC regimens have not been directly compared in a randomized trial, the superiority of BEP is thought to have been demonstrated. Other studies using cisplatin-based therapy have given similar results (Table 26.6). The recommended treatment for most patients (with the exception of patients with grade 1, stage IA immature teratoma) is adjuvant chemotherapy with three courses of BEP. In summary, virtually all patients with early-stage, completely resected disease will survive after careful surgical staging and cisplatin-based adjuvant chemotherapy.

More recently, clinical series and observations are beginning to suggest that surveillance with careful follow-up after surgery may be an acceptable alternative for carefully selected patients, as will be discussed below. Further studies are clearly needed in this area, and such a course of action should be taken only after very careful consideration given the fact that surgery followed by chemotherapy is curative for most patients.

In contrast, most clinical series have shown a worse clinical outcome for patients with metastatic disease or with incompletely resected tumors (Table 26.7). Current clinical trials in testicular germ-cell tumors separate patients with small tumor volume and a resultant excellent prognosis from

TABLE 26.7. *Chemotherapy of advanced disease*

Institution	Regimen	Progression free/total (%)
GOG (67)	PVB	47/89 (53)
Australia (51)	Multiple	42/46 (91)
Hospital 12 de Octubre (32)	PVB or BEP	15/19 (79)
M.D. Anderson (18)	PVB	7/11 (64)
Instituto Nazionale Tumori (13)	PVB	7/14 (50)
M.D. Anderson (19)	BEP	5/6 (83)

BEP, cisplatin, etoposide, bleomycin; PVB, cisplatin, vinblastine, bleomycin.

those with bulky tumor or liver or brain involvement (74). Patients in the former group will usually be complete responders to chemotherapy and long-term survivors, whereas only about 50% to 60% of the latter patients will survive. Hence, clinical trials for patients with good prognostic factors investigate shorter or less toxic chemotherapy aiming at minimizing toxicity (75) while preserving efficacy; whereas clinical trials for patients with advanced disease are evaluating more intensive chemotherapeutic regimens with the goal of improving the likelihood of cure (76,77). This is not the case for patients with incompletely resected or with advanced ovarian germ-cell tumors. Except for the subgroup of patients with dysgerminoma, there are no identifiable patients who have a sufficiently high cure rate to warrant less intensive therapy. Whether this is an inherent biologic difference between ovarian germ-cell tumors and testicular cancer or merely an underestimation of tumor volume because of intraperitoneal spread is not clear.

The role of high-dose chemotherapy with stem-cell rescue is being investigated for patients with intermediate or high-risk testicular cancer in an ongoing multiinstitutional clinical protocol (ECOG protocol 3894). Patients considered to have high risk for relapse are randomized to receive four cycles of BEP (control arm) versus two cycles of BEP followed by high-dose chemotherapy with autologous stem-cell rescue in the form of two (tandem) courses using carboplatinum, etoposide, and cyclophosphamide as a conditioning regimen (experimental arm). Because of the paucity of ovarian germ-cell tumors and because of the more aggressive initial surgical approach rendering the majority of patients nearly disease free, thus far it has not been possible to define a subgroup of patients who are at higher risk for recurrence. At present, the role of high-dose chemotherapy is not being evaluated as primary treatment for women with ovarian germ-cell tumors.

Management of Residual or Recurrent Disease

The large majority of patients with ovarian germ-cell tumors are cured with surgery and platinum-based chemotherapy. However, a small percentage of patients has persistent or progressive disease during treatment or that recurs after completion of treatment. Like in testicular cancer, these treatment failures are categorized as platinum-resistant (progression during or within 4 to 6 weeks of completing treatment) or platinum-sensitive (recurrence beyond 6 weeks from platinum-based therapy).

Most recurrences occur within 24 months from primary treatment. In a series from the UTMDACC, 42 treatment failures were identified among 160 patients with ovarian germ-cell tumors treated between 1970 and 1990 (78). Treatment failure in these patients was attributed to inadequate surgery in 14 patients, inadequate radiation in 5 patients, inadequate chemotherapy in 16 patients (underdosing and noncompliance), treatment-related toxicity in 1 patient, and unidentifiable causes in 6 patients. Of note is that a significant number of patients included in this series had received VAC-based chemotherapy, which may account for a higher than expected rate of recurrence (42 of 160 patients). Specifically, 17 of 26 patients treated up front with chemotherapy received VAC as primary treatment.

Given the high curability rate of ovarian germ-cell tumors with primary treatment, the management of recurrent disease represents a complex and often difficult issue, and should be preferably performed in a specialized center. Data to guide the management of patients with recurrent ovarian germ-cell tumors are scant, and by and large are derived or extrapolated from the clinical experience gained from treatment of testicular cancer patients. Approximately 30% of patients with recurrent platinum-sensitive testicular cancer can be salvaged with second-line chemotherapy (VeIP: vinblastine, ifosfamide, platinum) (76). In patients with recurrent or persistent testicular germ-cell tumors, there is now presumptive but strong evidence that high-dose therapy with carboplatin, etoposide with or without cyclophosphamide or ifosfamide, and stem-cell rescue is superior to standard-dose salvage therapy (79,80). Generally, one course of standard-dose therapy, usually cisplatin, vinblastine, and ifosfamide, is given. If an initial response is seen, then two subsequent courses of high-dose chemotherapy with stem-cell rescue are given (81). There is understandably scant experience with this approach in female germ-cell tumor patients, but presumably the concepts are similar.

The single most important prognostic factor in patients with testicular cancer is whether or not they are refractory to cisplatin. In patients who are truly cisplatin refractory, the likelihood of long-term survival and cure following high-dose therapy is less than 5% and high-dose therapy is of debatable appropriateness (82). On the other hand, the likelihood of cure with high-dose salvage therapy in patients who relapse from a complete remission after initial therapy is as high as 50%. A more recent report from Indiana University shows that with the use of tandem high-dose chemotherapeutic regimens and autologous stem-cell transplant in the setting of modern supportive care, as many as 42% of patients with platinum-refractory disease (defined as progression within 4 weeks from completing chemotherapy) can be failure-free survivors at 2 years (83). No disease-free survivors at 2 years among patients with absolute platinum-resistant disease (progression through platinum-based chemotherapy) were recorded in this report. Although this approach has not been and most probably will never be tested prospectively in women with recurrent platinum-sensitive ovarian germ-cell tumors because of the small numbers of patients, the concepts are very similar and support the use of high-dose therapy in this setting. Referral to a specialized center for management of recurrent disease is desirable. Patients with platinum-resistant disease cannot be cured. Active agents in this setting include ifosfamide, taxanes, and gemcitabine

(84–86); referral for treatment with investigational agents is appropriate.

Immediate Toxicity of Chemotherapy

Acute adverse effects of chemotherapy can be substantial, and affected patients should be treated by physicians experienced in their management. About 25% will have febrile neutropenic episodes during chemotherapy and will require hospitalization and broad-spectrum antibiotics (87). Cisplatin can be associated with nephrotoxicity. This adverse event can almost always be avoided by ensuring adequate hydration during and immediately after chemotherapy and avoidance of aminoglycoside antibiotics. Bleomycin can cause pulmonary fibrosis (87). Pulmonary function testing is frequently used to follow these patients. However, the value of carbon monoxide diffusion capacity to predict early lung disease has been challenged (88). The most effective method for monitoring germ-cell tumor patients is careful physical examination of the chest. Findings of early bleomycin lung disease are a lag or diminished expansion of one hemithorax or fine basilar rales that do not clear with cough. These findings can be very subtle, but if present mandate immediate discontinuation of bleomycin. It is important to note that randomized trials in good-prognosis testicular cancer have suggested that bleomycin is an important component of the treatment regimen, particularly if only three courses of therapy are given (89). Other randomized trials have shown that carboplatin is inferior to cisplatin and cannot be substituted for cisplatin without worsening therapeutic outcome (91,92).

Patients with advanced ovarian germ-cell tumors should receive three to four courses of treatment given in full dose and on schedule. There is presumptive evidence in testicular cancer that the timeliness of chemotherapy may be associated with outcome. Thus, treatment is given regardless of hematologic parameters on the scheduled day of treatment. The impact of the hematopoietic growth factors [granulocyte colony-stimulating factor (G-CSF), granulocyte-macrophage colony-stimulating growth factor (GM-CSF)] on the management of the myelosuppressive complications of this type of chemotherapy has not yet been precisely defined. As most patients will not develop neutropenic fever or infection, hematopoietic growth factors are not necessary for most patients (93). It is reasonable to use hematopoietic growth factors to avoid dose reductions for patients with previous episodes of neutropenic fever or in unusually ill patients (who are at a higher risk of myelosuppressive complications) or those who received prior radiotherapy. Modern antiemetic therapy (an example of which is shown in Table 26.8) has greatly lessened chemotherapy-induced emesis.

By following these guidelines and by providing supportive care as indicated, virtually all patients can be treated on schedule and in full or nearly full dose. Chemotherapy-re-

TABLE 26.8. *A typical antiemetic regimen*

Granisetron 1 mg IV 30 min prior to cisplatin daily for 5 days

or

Ondanesietron 0.15 mg/kg IV 30 min prior and 4 hours after cisplatin daily for 5 days

plus

Dexamethasone 20 mg IV 30 min prior to cisplatin on days 1 and 2

lated mortality should be less than 1%. Late effects of chemotherapy will be discussed subsequently.

IMMATURE TERATOMA

The situation of patients with immature teratoma (IT) is more complex. Immature teratomas are categorized as grade 1, 2, or 3 depending on the amount of immature neuroepithelium in the tumor [based on Thurlbeck and Scully's system, which was modified by Norris (13)]. Our current appreciation of recurrence risk in these patients is based on an early study by Norris (14). This report demonstrated that prognosis of patients with IT directly relates to tumor grade. Specifically, only 1 of 14 patients with grade 1 IT recurred, whereas 13 of 26 patients with grade 2 and 3 tumors recurred. This study set the current standard of care for women with stage I teratoma, which is surveillance for grade 1 immature teratoma and adjuvant chemotherapy with three courses of BEP for patients with grades 2 and 3 tumors. However, a significant limitation of the Norris report is the probable underestimation of tumor stage. Hence, in the modern era of complete surgical staging of ovarian neoplasms, it might be appropriate to reconsider the role of routine adjuvant therapy in these patients. Obviously, such an approach must be done with great caution, as surgery followed by adjuvant therapy will cure virtually all patients with localized high-grade teratoma. However, it is possible that the risk of relapse will be low in a defined population of well-staged patients, and that with careful follow-up, nearly all relapsing patients can be diagnosed with relatively small-volume tumor and cured with subsequent chemotherapy for metastatic disease. Although some issues are different in testicular cancer, a deferral of chemotherapy has been shown to be an appropriate therapeutic alternative in resected stage II tumors as well as for patients with clinical stage I disease. Surveillance for stage I ovarian IT is supported by experience from other groups.

First, an intergroup study of the Pediatric Oncology Group and the Children's Cancer Group reported that surveillance after complete surgical resection in 41 girls with ovarian immature teratoma was sufficient (94,95). Only one recurrence (which was salvaged with BEP) was noted during 24 months of follow-up. Of note is that in this series, 13 patients

had grades 2 and 3 IT and 10 patients had mixed tumors containing IT plus yolk-sac tumor.

Second, investigators at Mt. Vernon and Charing Cross Hospitals in England have observed 15 patients with stage IA tumors after initial surgical treatment (96). Of these, nine patients had grade 2 or 3 immature teratoma and six had elements of endodermal sinus tumor. There were three recurrences in this series: one of nine in the pure immature teratoma group and two of six in the mixed histology group. Two of these patients were salvaged with chemotherapy and one patient died of pulmonary embolus. Of note is that the patient who died became pregnant 4 months after diagnosis and could not be followed adequately owing to her pregnancy.

Third, investigators at the University of Milan reported the clinical outcome in a group of 32 patients with pure ovarian IT followed prospectively (97). In this group, nine patients had grades 2 and 3 stage IA immature teratomas and were treated with surgery and intensive surveillance. Only two recurrences were noted in this group. They consisted of one case of mature teratoma and one case of gliosis. The mature teratoma was resected and the patient with gliosis was followed without treatment. Both patients are alive and well and never received chemotherapy. Furthermore, among four patients with stage IC tumors treated with surgical resection and surveillance, there was one case of gliosis and one recurrence with mature tissue, which was resected (no chemotherapy). All patients are currently free of disease.

When considering these issues, it is important not to overstate the toxicities of adjuvant therapy. In earlier times, chemotherapy-induced emesis was a very significant problem. However, with modern antiemetics such as the 5HT3 antagonists, emesis is greatly reduced and, although sometimes unpleasant, rarely is a major complication of chemotherapy. Acute treatment-related mortality, particularly from bleomycin-related lung disease, is rare. In GOG protocol 78, there were no acute toxic deaths in 93 entered patients. Nonetheless, such chemotherapy is certainly unpleasant, produces universal alopecia, occasionally causes severe emesis, and has a remote risk of serious acute toxicity and drug-induced mortality. Considering this information, it may be appropriate to consider surveillance with careful follow-up in well-staged adult patients with ovarian stage IA immature teratoma. Although this concept is supported by evidence derived from the pediatric literature and by two small clinical series as discussed, this hypothesis has not been tested prospectively in the context of a clinical protocol and should therefore be approached with caution.

DYSGERMINOMA

Dysgerminoma is the female equivalent of seminoma. This disease differs from its nondysgerminomatous counterpart in several respects. First, it is more likely to be localized to the ovary at the time of diagnosis (stage I). Bilateral involvement is more common, as is its spread to retroperitoneal lymph nodes. While less relevant now than before the era of modern chemotherapy, dysgerminoma is very sensitive to radiation (7,11,42).

Observation for Stage I Tumors

As many as 75% to 80% of dysgerminoma patients used to be considered stage I at diagnosis (41,98). However, with more precise surgical staging, as done currently, the true figure is probably somewhat less. Still, as many as two-thirds of dysgerminoma patients are likely to be stage I at presentation. Traditionally, most of these women received postoperative radiotherapy. An alternative option for low-risk patients who desire to maintain fertility is postsurgical clinical surveillance given the fact that pelvic radiotherapy is associated with a high incidence of subsequent gonadal dysfunction and sterility (99). In a previous era, clinical observation was deemed to be appropriate for women with tumors <10 cm and without contralateral ovarian involvement, whereas adjuvant radiotherapy used to be recommended for tumors >10 cm (100). However, the size-based distinction was subsequently called into question (98,101). In a series reported by LaPolla, seven of nine patients with stage IA dysgerminoma followed without postoperative radiotherapy remained disease free (98). All but one had tumors >10 cm. In another report, among 14 patients with stage IA dysgerminoma treated with surveillance, 5 recurred. Of those, four patients were salvaged with radiation and one was salvaged with radiation followed by chemotherapy. All stage IA patients are alive and free of disease (7). Similarly, Gordon reported that the 5-year survival among 72 patients with stage IA pure dysgerminoma treated conservatively was 95% (11). The recurrence rate in this case series was 17%, with four deaths being attributable to disease (salvage chemotherapy was offered to only one patient).

Currently, many clinicians believe that well-staged IA dysgerminoma patients can be observed after unilateral salpingo-oophorectomy regardless of the size of the primary tumor if preservation of fertility is an issue. Careful follow-up is required because as many as 15% to 25% of patients will experience a recurrence. However, because of the tumor's chemosensitivity, virtually all dysgerminoma patients can be salvaged successfully at the time of recurrence if adequate follow-up and early detection have been accomplished (Table 26.9).

Radiation Therapy

In the past, many stage I patients and all patients with higher stage tumors received radiotherapy. De Palo and associates recommended radiation therapy for all stages I to III patients (41). Radiation therapy was delivered to the ipsilateral hemipelvis (with shielding of the contralateral ovary and the head of the femur) and to the paraaortic nodes. A single field incorporating these areas was used. In either case, the upper limit of the field was set at T10–T11. The lower limit of the spinal field was at L4–L5 level. The investigators recommended that all stage IB patients receive postoperative radiation therapy to the whole pelvis and paraaortic nodes. For stage III retroperitoneal disease (found at surgery), they offered curative radiation therapy set up in the same fashion as for stage I with the addition of a prophylactic field including the mediastinum and supraclavicular nodes. In the presence of peritoneal involvement, the whole abdomen and pelvis, mediastinum, and supraclavicular nodes were irradiated. They gave 30 Gy (7.5 to 9.0 Gy/week) as prophylactic irradiation. For curative irradiation, 35 to 40 Gy total dose was given and a boost (10 Gy) was delivered to involved nodes. When irradiating above the diaphragm, De Palo et al. gave 30 Gy 3 to 6 weeks after completion of irradiation below the diaphragm. When irradiating the entire abdominal cavity, the fields were similar to those used for epithelial tumors. They gave a total dose of 25 Gy (6.0 to 7.5 Gy/week). The kidneys were shielded. Similarly, Lawson and Adler reported giving 30 Gy (10 Gy/week) to pelvic and paraaortic fields (102). In their series, only two patients were treated to the whole abdomen, one with the moving strip technique and one with open fields. The patients treated with the moving strip technique received 22.5 Gy to the whole abdomen and 45.0 Gy to the pelvis.

Others reported similar treatment plans. Freed and associates gave external pelvic irradiation for disease limited to the pelvis (20 to 30 Gy in 2 to 3 weeks) (103). If the paraaortic nodes were positive histologically or by lymphangiogram, the fields were extended to cover this area. In this

TABLE 26.9. *Results of clinical surveillance after surgery in patients with stage IA dysgerminoma*

Institution (ref.)	Period	Progression free/ total no. (%)	Overall survival/ total no. (%)
AFIP (8)	1969	46/57 (80)	52/57 (91)
Hopkins (11)	1930–1981	58/72 (80)	67/72 (94)
Mayo Clinic (7)	1950–1984	9/14 (64)	14/14 (100)
Iowa Hospitals (98)	1935–1985	7/7 (100)	7/7 (100)
M. D. Anderson (100)	1976	5/5 (100)	5/5 (100)
Mt. Vernon Hospital (96)	1973–1995	6/9 (66)	9/9 (100)

case, prophylactic radiation therapy to the mediastinum and supraclavicular nodes (25 Gy in 2.5 to 3 weeks) was also given. If extranodal spread or intraabdominal disease was found, total abdominal therapy (25 to 30 Gy in 3 to 5 weeks) with a pelvic boost (15 to 20 Gy in 1.5 to 3 weeks) and paraaortic boost (15 Gy in 2 weeks) were recommended (100,103,104).

Historically, patients with testicular seminoma received prophylactic treatment to the mediastinum. However, over time, this line of reasoning has been challenged (105). Currently, most investigators consider this form of treatment to be obsolete because of the small number of patients who would derive a potential benefit, and because of the subsequent reduced tolerance for chemotherapy in this population. Furthermore, considering the recent developments in the field of chemotherapy, it is accepted that primary chemotherapy is equally or more effective than irradiation of extensive normal tissue volumes, and is substantially less likely to compromise salvage therapy when patients relapse after primary therapy. Given that most patients will be cured of their ovarian tumors, and that most patients are of relatively young age at diagnosis, some consideration should also be given to the delayed carcinogenic effects of intermediate-dose radiation in young women. Although this issue has not been specifically addressed in women with ovarian germ-cell tumors, it is logical to extrapolate from the experience of younger women who are frequently successfully treated with radiation for cancer of the uterine cervix, and in whom the risk of second malignancies (both within and remote from the primary radiation fields) may be elevated two or three decades following successful initial treatment (106).

Results of radiation therapy are reasonably good. De Palo et al. reported that all 13 stage I patients (12 stage IA and 1 with stage IB) were alive and free of disease with a median follow-up of 77 months (41). The 5-year relapse-free survival for the 12 stage III patients was 61.4% and the overall survival was 89.5%. Median follow-up was 67 months. Only one death was reported in this group. Earlier De Palo and associates (41) reported 100% overall 5-year survival and 90% recurrence-free 5 year survival in 31 stages IA, IB, and IC patients. At 4 years, the overall survival was 80% and the recurrence-free survival was 57% in stage III patients. Lawson and Adler reported that 10 of 14 stages I to III patients were alive with a median follow-up of 54 months (102). In this small series, there was no correlation between survival and either the initial stage of the disease or the size of the primary tumor found at laparotomy. Others have reported similar results with overall progression-free rates varying between 70% and 90% when radiotherapy followed surgical resection (42,43) (Table 26.10). However, despite the remarkable radiosensitivity of dysgerminoma, radiotherapy is rarely performed nowadays since chemotherapy is equally or more effective, is less toxic, and permits preservation of gonadal function.

TABLE 26.10. *Effects of radiotherapy in women with pure dysgerminoma*

Institution (ref.)	Period	Stage	Progression free/total no. (%)
AFIP (8)	1969	I–III	12/14 (85)
Mayo Clinic (7)	1950–1984	I–IV	16/20 (80)
M. D. Anderson (100)	1976	I–III	26/31 (84)
Florence (43)	1960–1983	IC–III	21/26 (80)
NCI Milan (41)	1970–1982	I–III	21/25 (84)
Iowa Hospitals (98)	1935–1985	I–III	12/13 (92)
Sweden (42)	1927–1984	I–IV	49/60 (83)
Egypt (139)	1978–1989	II–III	10/15 (66)
Prince of Wales Hospital (102)	1969–1983	II–III	10/14 (72)

Chemotherapy

There is an increasing amount of information available about chemotherapy for patients with advanced ovarian dysgerminoma. Dysgerminoma is very responsive to cisplatin-based chemotherapy, even more so than other types of tumors (69,107). Since 1984, patients with advanced dysgerminoma were eligible for GOG protocols. Patients received three to four courses of either PVB or BEP. In the most recent analysis, there were 20 patients evaluable (108). All had stage III or IV disease, and most of them had suboptimal (>2 cm) residual tumor. Eleven patients had clinically measurable tumor and ten responded completely. Fourteen patients underwent second-look laparotomy, and the results were negative in all cases, including the one patient who was only a partial clinical responder. Overall, 19 of the 20 women were disease-free with a follow-up of 9 to 66 months (26-month median). Nearly all patients with advanced dysgerminoma treated with chemotherapy will be durable complete responders. Considering that patients with stage III dysgerminoma would require extensive radiation and still carry a risk of failure, and that such patients probably fare worse with subsequent chemotherapy, it is clear that these patients should be treated primarily with chemotherapy.

As in other germ-cell tumors, these results may have implications for the management of patients with resected early-stage dysgerminoma. In most patients, preferred adjuvant therapy for patients who had conservative surgery and are desirous of maintaining fertility is BEP. This regimen will almost invariably prevent recurrence in tumors other than dysgerminoma and certainly will also do so in dysgerminoma. Furthermore, most patients will retain fertility. The effectiveness and tolerability of chemotherapy have made it the preferred adjuvant regimen even if fertility preservation is not an issue.

The implications of elevated hCG or AFP levels should be emphasized. These tumor markers are useful methods to follow the clinical course in patients with tumors other than dysgerminoma. As is the case in seminoma, AFP elevation denotes the presence of elements other than dysgerminoma and treatment should be tailored accordingly. However, an elevated hCG level can be occasionally seen in pure dysgerminoma. The finding of a high hCG should not alter therapy, but should prompt reexamination of the tumor specimen to determine whether syncytiotrophoblastic cells are present or if the tumor contains other neoplastic elements (mixed germ-cell tumor).

In summary, the majority of dysgerminoma patients have stage I disease at diagnosis. These patients can usually be treated with unilateral salpingo-oophorectomy, and if fertility is an issue, they can be observed carefully with regular pelvic examinations, abdominal CT, and tumor markers including LDH. Fifteen percent to 25% of patients treated with surveillance will experience a recurrence and will require chemotherapy at that time. In patients with more advanced but resected disease, risk of recurrence is significant enough to warrant adjuvant treatment. Alternatives are chemotherapy or radiation. For the majority of patients, chemotherapy is the clear choice because of ease of administration, predictable and minimal toxicity, and fertility-sparing properties. Chemotherapy is also recommended for patients with metastatic or incompletely resected tumor and for patients who recur after previous radiotherapy. Radiation might be considered as initial treatment in unusual circumstances, such as in older patients or in those with serious concomitant illness that would preclude the use of systemic chemotherapy.

LATE EFFECTS OF TREATMENT

As the prognosis of patients with malignant ovarian germ-cell tumors has dramatically improved with the evolution of modern combination chemotherapy, attention is focused on the late effects of therapy. There is a considerable body of literature on the late effects of treatment in testicular cancer patients, yet the information available for women with ovarian germ-cell tumors remains scant. However, many analogies can be drawn.

Sequelae of Surgery

Young patients with malignant ovarian germ-cell tumors undergo at least one, if not multiple, surgical procedures. Although there is no available information on the long-term effects of surgery on these patients, future infertility related to pelvic surgery with subsequent peritoneal and tubal adhesions is well described. Therefore, meticulous surgical technique and avoidance of unnecessary operative maneuvers (e.g., biopsy of a normal contralateral ovary) are required to prevent future complications (44,109,110). Another cause of infertility in this population is unnecessary bilateral salpingo-oophorectomy and hysterectomy. The M. D. Anderson series includes several patients who underwent surgical sterilization without good indication before referral to this center. It is expected that this phenomenon will be less frequent as information concerning the natural history of ovarian germ-cell tumors becomes more widely disseminated. In a series from Milan, among 55 patients treated with fertility-sparing surgery, without further chemotherapy, 12 of 12 patients who attempted conception became pregnant and 12 normal deliveries were recorded (111). Two additional pregnancies occurred in this group and resulted in termination, one of which was due to *in utero* detection of fetal malformation.

As with any group of patients with a history of pelvic surgery, patients with malignant ovarian germ-cell tumors may develop functional cysts in their residual ovary. Muram et al. reported their experience with 27 patients with ovarian germ-cell tumors who underwent unilateral salpingo-oophorectomy and were followed for 12 to 215 months after completion of therapy (112). Of the 18 patients who maintained ovarian function, 13 (72%) developed a functional ovarian cyst during the follow-up period. Trial of oral contraceptives and serial ovarian surveillance with sonography are helpful in distinguishing these functional cysts from tumor recurrence.

Sequelae of Radiation Therapy

There is limited information about the late effects of radiotherapy in dysgerminoma patients. In a review of the late effects of radiotherapy in patients receiving abdominal therapy for ovarian dysgerminoma at UTMDACC, a slight increase in dyspareunia and in the number of bowel movements was recorded (99). Somewhat surprisingly, none of 43 patients developed small bowel obstruction 3.3 to 34.6 years later (median follow-up 12.4 years). Furthermore, there were no other significant intestinal or bladder problems noted. No patients conceived after receiving radiotherapy, although three patients treated with fertility-sparing surgery spontaneously resumed menses. Although the late effects of radiotherapy in this population seem to be few with the notable exception of effects on gonadal function (113), such observations may soon be of only historical interest. As discussed earlier, there has been a strong trend away from radiotherapy and toward chemotherapy as the preferred postoperative therapy of dysgerminoma patients. Concern over the preservation of gonadal function has been the driving force behind this transition (40,114).

Sequelae of Chemotherapy

The evolutionary development and refinement of combination chemotherapy have resulted in the cure of a high percentage of patients with chemosensitive tumors, such as lymphomas, testicular cancer, gestational trophoblastic disease, and malignant ovarian germ-cell tumors. Within the last few years, several reports have described the long-term effects of chemotherapy on these patients. As expected, most reports refer to the more common lymphomas and testicular cancers.

A recently recognized effect of chemotherapy used in the treatment of germ-cell tumors is the risk of secondary malignancies. The epipodophyllotoxins teniposide and etoposide are associated with the development of acute myelogenous leukemia (AML) with certain morphologic and cytogenetic features (115–119). This treatment complication appears to be dose (115,116) and schedule dependent (118). Of 348 male germ-cell tumor patients receiving three to four courses of BEP as first-line therapy at Indiana University, two developed etoposide-related leukemia. None of 67 patients who received only three courses developed AML (115). Similarly, in the study reported by Pedersen-Bjergaard, 5 of 212 patients developed acute leukemia or myelodysplastic syndrome after etoposide therapy (116). However, all patients who developed AML received more than 2,000 mg/m² of etoposide. None of the 130 patients who received less than this dose developed AML. Morphologically, these leukemias are usually monocytic or myelomonocytic (M4 or M5). Characteristic chromosomal translocations (mostly involving the 11q23 region) are frequently, but not always, present. Leukemia after etoposide treatment occurs within 2 to 3 years compared to alkylating agent–induced AML, which has a longer latency period. Late occurrence of chronic myelogenous leukemia after treatment of testicular cancer has been reported (120). In the GOG protocol testing the efficacy of BEP in women with ovarian germ-cell tumors, one case of AML was recorded among 91 patients treated (70). An additional case of lymphoma was diagnosed during follow-up in this series, yet a correlation between chemotherapy and lymphoproliferative disorders has not been reported to date.

Considering these issues, most clinicians continue to believe that BEP is the chemotherapeutic regimen of choice. The incidence of second neoplasms is quite low, particularly in patients receiving low cumulative etoposide doses that should be required for all but a small minority of patients. In testicular cancer, etoposide is more effective than vinblastine and certainly is less toxic (66). Vinblastine-induced abdominal pain and ileus are quite troublesome for some patients, particularly for those who have had recent abdominal surgery, such as women with ovarian germ-cell tumors. The risk/benefit ratio continues to favor etoposide over vinblastine.

There also continues to be considerable focus on the long-term effects of chemotherapy on gonadal function. Studies of patients with a variety of cancers suggest that, although ovarian dysfunction or failure is a risk of chemotherapy, the majority of survivors can anticipate normal menstrual and reproductive function (121–123). Factors such as older age at initiation of therapy, greater cumulative drug dose (124), and longer duration of therapy (123) have an adverse effect on future gonadal function. Successful pregnancies after treatment with combination chemotherapy have been well documented in other types of malignancies, including Hodgkin's disease, non-Hodgkin's lymphomas, and leukemia.

There are similar reports in patients with malignant ovarian germ-cell tumors (111,125–128).

In a review of the UTMDACC series (125), 27 (68%) of 40 patients who had retained a normal contralateral ovary and uterus maintained regular menses consistently after completion of chemotherapy, and 33 (83%) were having regular menses at the time of follow-up. Of 16 patients who had attempted to become pregnant, 12 did so. One patient had an elective first-trimester abortion, and the other 11 patients bore 22 healthy infants over time, none of which had a major birth defect. In a series from Milan, among 169 patients with ovarian germ-cell tumors, 138 underwent fertility-sparing surgery, and of these, 81 underwent adjuvant chemotherapy (111). After treatment, all but one woman recovered menstrual function, and 55 conceptions were recorded. Forty normal full-term babies were delivered, and four cases of congenital malformations were reported (one in a patient who did not receive chemotherapy and three in women who had received chemotherapy; the difference was not statistically significant).

Although limited reports are available concerning other late effects of chemotherapy on patients with ovarian germ-cell tumors (129,130), there are several reports on this topic involving patients with testicular cancer (131–136). In male patients who received cisplatin-based combination regimens, principally PVB, late toxicities include high-tone hearing loss (131), neurotoxicity (131,134,136), Raynaud's phenomenon (132,136), ischemic heart disease (136,137), hypertension (136), renal dysfunction (136), and pulmonary toxicity (133,135). Fortunately, despite these observations, most patients have excellent overall health and functional status (135). Indeed, in a prospective study of immediate chemotherapy versus observation and chemotherapy at the time of relapse in patients with early-stage testicular cancer, the treated patients had only an increased incidence of paresthesias compared to the patients who were monitored without chemotherapy (138). Hypertension, cardiac disease, and stroke were rare and of similar incidence in chemotherapy-treated and chemotherapy-untreated patients at a median follow-up of 5.1 years. The late effects of treatment are more pronounced among children receiving treatment for germ-cell tumors (129). Specifically, neurotoxicity, growth abnormalities, pulmonary toxicity, and gastrointestinal toxicity have been reported in a higher proportion than in adult patients. The GOG recently completed an analysis evaluating the quality of life and psychosocial characteristics of survivors of ovarian germ-cell tumors compared to matched controls. In this analysis, the survivors appeared to be well adjusted, were able to develop strong relationships, and were free of significant depression. The impact on fertility was modest or none in those patients who underwent fertility-sparing surgeries. Overall, these women appeared to be free of any major physical illnesses at a median follow-up of 10 years (S. D. Williams, personal communication).

SUMMARY

Virtually all patients with early-stage, completely resected nondysgerminomatous tumors will survive after careful surgical staging and three courses of adjuvant BEP. Furthermore, 50% to 80% of patients with incompletely resected or advanced tumors will survive their disease as well. Current and future clinical trials should address the latter group of patients in an effort to improve therapeutic results. Acute toxicity of treatment is relatively modest. An important, but fortunately unusual, late complication of treatment is etoposide-induced leukemia. Patients receiving the usually administered cumulative dose of etoposide are at low risk for developing AML. Otherwise, late consequences of chemotherapy are limited. Efforts should concentrate on fertility preservation for patients who desire subsequent pregnancies.

The majority of dysgerminoma patients have stage I disease at diagnosis. These patients usually can be treated with unilateral salpingo-oophorectomy and careful postoperative observation without adjuvant treatment. Chemotherapy is offered at the time of recurrence. In patients with more advanced but resected disease, the risk of recurrence is significant enough to warrant up-front adjuvant treatment, which for most patients is chemotherapy because of its near universal effectiveness and limited impact on fertility. In patients with incompletely resected tumor or for patients who recur after previous radiation, chemotherapy similar to that given for tumors other than dysgerminoma is appropriate.

Surgery continues to have a pivotal role in the management of all patients with ovarian germ-cell tumors. Initial careful surgical staging is important for selection of appropriate subsequent therapy. The role of cytoreductive surgery is under study but the evidence supports its judicious use. However, an operation done strictly for debulking when the diagnosis is established does not seem warranted. Second-look laparotomy is not necessary in patients who have no residual tumor after their initial surgical procedure and who receive adjuvant chemotherapy. This procedure also does not seem to be warranted in patients with advanced tumors without elements of teratoma. However, patients with incompletely resected tumors containing teratomatous elements are likely to benefit from such surgery.

The judicious use of surgery followed by chemotherapy will cure the majority of patients with ovarian germ-cell tumors at the expense of minimal and predictable immediate and late toxicities. In most circumstances, fertility can be preserved.

REFERENCES

1. AT. Germ cell tumors of the ovary. In: Kurman RJ. (ed.). *Blaustein's pathology of the female tract*. New York: Springer-Verlag, 1987:268.
2. Pins MR, Young RH, Daly WJ, Scully RE Primary squamous cell carcinoma of the ovary. Report of 37 cases. *Am J Surg Pathol* 1996; 20:823–833.
3. Powell JL, Stinson JA, Connor BS, et al. Squamous cell carcinoma arising in a dermoid cyst of the ovary. *Gynecol Oncol* 2003;9: 526–528.
4. Mayer C, Miller DM, Ehlen TG. Peritoneal implantation of squamous cell carcinoma following rupture of a dermoid cyst during laparoscopic removal. *Gynecol Oncol* 2002;84:180–183.
5. Rose PG, Tak WK, Reale FR. Squamous cell carcinoma arising in a mature cystic teratoma with metastasis to the paraaortic nodes. *Gynecol Oncol* 1993;50:131–133.
6. Takemori M, Nishimura R, Sugimura K, et al. Ovarian strumal carcinoid with markedly high serum levels of tumor markers. *Gynecol Oncol* 1995;58:266–269.
7. Buskirk SJ, Schray MF, Podratz KC, et al. Ovarian dysgerminoma: a retrospective analysis of results of treatment, sites of treatment failure, and radiosensitivity. *Mayo Clin Proc* 1987;62:1149–1157.
8. Asadourian LA, Taylor HB. Dysgerminoma. An analysis of 105 cases. *Obstet Gynecol* 1969;33:370–379.
9. Malpica A, BR, Deavers MT, Kavangh J, Silva EG. Tyrosine kinases in ovarian dysgerminoma. *Mod Pathol* 2003;16:200A.
10. Tian Q, Frierson HF Jr, Krystal GW, Moskaluk CA. Activating c-kit gene mutations in human germ cell tumors. *Am J Pathol* 1999;154: 1643–1647.
11. Gordon A, Lipton D, Woodruff JD. Dysgerminoma: a review of 158 cases from the Emil Novak Ovarian Tumor Registry. *Obstet Gynecol* 1981;58:497–504.
12. Hart WR, BD. Germ cell neoplasms occurring in gonadoblastomas. *Cancer* 1979;43:669–678.
13. Norris HJ, Zirkin HJ, Benson WL. Immature (malignant) teratoma of the ovary: a clinical and pathologic study of 58 cases. *Cancer* 1976; 37:2359–2372.
14. O'Connor DM, Norris HJ. The influence of grade on the outcome of stage I ovarian immature (malignant) teratomas and the reproducibility of grading. *Int J Gynecol Pathol* 1994;13:283–289.
15. Nielsen SN, Scheithauer BW, Gaffey TA. Gliomatosis peritonei. *Cancer* 1985;56:2499–2503.
16. Truong LD, Jurco S 3rd, McGavran MH. Gliomatosis peritonei. Report of two cases and review of literature. *Am J Surg Pathol* 1982; 6:443–449.
17. Shefren G, Collin J, Soriero O. Gliomatosis peritonei with malignant transformation: a case report and review of the literature. *Am J Obstet Gynecol* 1991;164:1617–1620; Discussion 1620–1611.
18. Dadmanesh F, Miller DM, Swenerton KD, Clement PB. Gliomatosis peritonei with malignant transformation. *Mod Pathol* 1997;10: 597–601.
19. Ferguson AW, Katabuchi H, Ronnett BM, Cho KR. Glial implants in gliomatosis peritonei arise from normal tissue, not from the associated teratoma. *Am J Pathol* 2001;159:51–55.
20. Geisler JP, Goulet R, Foster RS, Sutton GP. Growing teratoma syndrome after chemotherapy for germ cell tumors of the ovary. *Obstet Gynecol* 1994;84:719–721.
21. Tonkin KS, Rustin GJ, Wignall B, et al. Successful treatment of patients in whom germ cell tumour masses enlarged on chemotherapy while their serum tumour markers decreased. *Eur J Cancer Clin Oncol* 1989;25:1739–1743.
22. Dickersin GR, Kline IW, Scully RE. Small cell carcinoma of the ovary with hypercalcemia: a report of eleven cases. *Cancer* 1982;49: 188–197.
23. Ulbright TM, Roth LM, Stehman FB, et al. Poorly differentiated (small cell) carcinoma of the ovary in young women: evidence supporting a germ cell origin. *Hum Pathol* 1987;18:175–184.
24. Seidman JD. Small cell carcinoma of the ovary of the hypercalcemic type: p53 protein accumulation and clinicopathologic features. *Gynecol Oncol* 1995;59:283–287.
25. Scully RE. Small cell carcinoma of hypercalcemic type. *Int J Gynecol Pathol* 1993;12:148–152.
26. Surti U, Hoffner L, Chakravarti A, Ferrell RE. Genetics and biology of human ovarian teratomas. I. Cytogenetic analysis and mechanism of origin. *Am J Hum Genet* 1990;47:635–643.
27. Deka R, Chakravarti A, Surti U, et al. Genetics and biology of human ovarian teratomas. II. Molecular analysis of origin of nondisjunction and gene-centromere mapping of chromosome I markers. *Am J Hum Genet* 1990;47:644–655.
28. Baker BA, Frickey L, Yu IT, et al. DNA content of ovarian immature

teratomas and malignant germ cell tumors. *Gynecol Oncol* 1998;71: 14–18.

29. Murty VV, Dmitrovsky E, Bosl GJ, Chaganti RS. Nonrandom chromosome abnormalities in testicular and ovarian germ cell tumor cell lines. *Cancer Genet Cytogenet* 1990;50:67–73.

30. Speleman F, De Potter C, Dal Cin P, et al. i(12p) in a malignant ovarian tumor. *Cancer Genet Cytogenet* 1990;45:49–53.

31. Shen DH, KU, Zhang Y, Cheung ANY. Cytogenetic study of malignant ovarian germ cell tumors by chromosome in situ hybridization. *Int J Gynecol Cancer* 1998;8:222–232.

32. Gershenson DM, Copeland LJ, Kavanagh JJ, et al. Treatment of malignant nondysgerminomatous germ cell tumors of the ovary with vincristine, dactinomycin, and cyclophosphamide. *Cancer* 1985;56: 2756–2761.

33. Gershenson DM, Del Junco G, Copeland LJ, Rutledge FN. Mixed germ cell tumors of the ovary. *Obstet Gynecol* 1984;64:200–206.

34. Christman JE, Teng NN, Lebovic GS, Sikic BI. Delivery of a normal infant following cisplatin, vinblastine, and bleomycin (PVB) chemotherapy for malignant teratoma of the ovary during pregnancy. *Gynecol Oncol* 1990;37:292–295.

35. Farahmand SM, Marchetti DL, Asirwatham JE, Dewey MR. Ovarian endodermal sinus tumor associated with pregnancy: review of the literature. *Gynecol Oncol* 1991;41:156–160.

36. Horbelt D, Delmore J, Meisel R, et al. Mixed germ cell malignancy of the ovary concurrent with pregnancy. *Obstet Gynecol* 1994;84: 662–664.

37. Rajendran S, Hollingworth J, Scudamore I. Endodermal sinus tumour of the ovary in pregnancy. *Eur J Gynaecol Oncol* 1999;20:272–274.

38. Bakri YN, Ezzat A, Akhtar, et al. Malignant germ cell tumors of the ovary. Pregnancy considerations. *Eur J Obstet Gynecol Reprod Biol* 2000;90:87–91.

39. Sekiya S, Seki K, Nagai Y. Rise of serum CA 125 in patients with pure ovarian yolk sac tumors. *Int J Gynaecol Obstet* 1997;58:323–324.

40. Ayhan A, Bildirici I, Gunalp S, Yuce K. Pure dysgerminoma of the ovary: a review of 45 well staged cases. *Eur J Gynaecol Oncol* 2000; 21:98–101.

41. De Palo G, Lattuada A, Kenda R, et al. Germ cell tumors of the ovary: the experience of the National Cancer Institute of Milan. I. Dysgerminoma. *Int J Radiat Oncol Biol Phys* 1987;13: 853–860.

42. Bjorkholm E, Lundell M, Gyftodimos A, Silfversward C. Dysgerminoma. The Radiumhemmet series 1927–1984. *Cancer* 1990;65: 38–44.

43. Santoni R, Cionini L, D'Elia F, et al. Dysgerminoma of the ovary: a report on 29 patients. *Clin Radiol* 1987;38:203–206.

44. Schwartz PE. Surgery of germ cell tumours of the ovary. *Forum (Genova)* 2000;10:355–365.

45. Peccatori F, Bonazzi C, Chiari S, et al. Surgical management of malignant ovarian germ-cell tumors: 10 years' experience of 129 patients. *Obstet Gynecol* 1995;86:367–372.

46. Saunders DM, Ferrier AJ, Ryan J. Fertility preservation in female oncology patients. *Int J Gynecol Cancer* 1996;6:161–167.

47. Slayton RE, Hreshchyshyn MM, Silverberg SC, et al. Treatment of malignant ovarian germ cell tumors: response to vincristine, dactinomycin, and cyclophosphamide (preliminary report). *Cancer* 1978;42: 390–398.

48. Williams SD, Blessing JA, Moore DH, et al. Cisplatin, vinblastine, and bleomycin in advanced and recurrent ovarian germ-cell tumors. A trial of the Gynecologic Oncology Group. *Ann Intern Med* 1989; 111:22–27.

49. Scarabell, C, Gallo A, Carbone A. Secondary cytoreductive surgery for patients with recurrent epithelial ovarian carcinoma. *Gynecol Oncol* 2001;83:504–512.

50. Parazzini F, Raspagliesi F, Guarnerio P, Bolis G. Role of secondary surgery in relapsed ovarian cancer. *Crit Rev Oncol Hematol* 2001;37: 121–125.

51. Williams SD, Blessing JA, DiSaia PJ, et al. Second-look laparotomy in ovarian germ cell tumors: the gynecologic oncology group experience. *Gynecol Oncol* 1994;52:287–291.

52. Andre F, Fizazi K, Culine S, et al. The growing teratoma syndrome: results of therapy and long-term follow-up of 33 patients. *Eur J Cancer* 2000;36:1389–1394.

53. Chen RJ, Huang PT, Lin MC, et al. Advanced stage squamous cell carcinoma arising from mature cystic teratoma of the ovary. *Acta Obstet Gynecol Scand* 2001;80:84–86.

54. Ronnett BM, Seidman JD. Mucinous tumors arising in ovarian mature cystic teratomas: relationship to the clinical syndrome of pseudomyxoma peritonei. *Am J Surg Pathol* 2003;27:650–657.

55. Vartanian RK, McRae B, Hessler RB. Sebaceous carcinoma arising in a mature cystic teratoma of the ovary. *Int J Gynecol Pathol* 2002; 21:418–421.

56. Shen DH, Khoo US, Xue WC, Cheung AN. Ovarian mature cystic teratoma with malignant transformation. An interphase cytogenetic study. *Int J Gynecol Pathol* 1998;17:351–357.

57. Itani Y, Kawa M, Toyoda S, et al. Growing teratoma syndrome after chemotherapy for a mixed germ cell tumor of the ovary. *J Obstet Gynaecol Res* 2002;28:166–171.

58. Kattan J, Droz JP, Culine S, et al. The growing teratoma syndrome: a woman with nonseminomatous germ cell tumor of the ovary. *Gynecol Oncol* 1993;9:395–399.

59. Gershenson D M, Copeland LJ, del Junco G, et al. Second-look laparotomy in the management of malignant germ cell tumors of the ovary. *Obstet Gynecol* 1986;67:789–793.

60. Albers P, Bender H, Yilmaz H, et al. Positron emission tomography in the clinical staging of patients with Stage I and II testicular germ cell tumors. *Urology* 1999;53:808–811.

61. Hain SF, O'Doherty MJ, Timothy AR, et al. Fluorodeoxyglucose positron emission tomography in the evaluation of germ cell tumours at relapse. *Br J Cancer* 2000;83:863–869.

62. Kollmannsberger C, Oechsle K, Dohmen BM, et al. Prospective comparison of [18F]fluorodeoxyglucose positron emission tomography with conventional assessment by computed tomography scans and serum tumor markers for the evaluation of residual masses in patients with nonseminomatous germ cell carcinoma. *Cancer* 2002;94: 2353–2362.

63. Sanchez D, Zudaire JJ, Fernandez JM, et al. 18F-fluoro-2-deoxyglucose-positron emission tomography in the evaluation of nonseminomatous germ cell tumours at relapse. *BJU Int* 2002;89:912–916.

64. De Santis M, Becherer A, Bokemeyer C, et al. FDG-PET as prognostic indicator for seminoma residuals: an update from the SEMPET study. *Proc ASCO* 2003;

65. Einhorn LH, Donohue J. Cis-diamminedichloroplatinum, vinblastine, and bleomycin combination chemotherapy in disseminated testicular cancer. *Ann Intern Med* 1977;87:293–298.

66. Williams SD, Birch R, Einhorn LH, et al. Treatment of disseminated germ-cell tumors with cisplatin, bleomycin, and either vinblastine or etoposide. *N Engl J Med* 1987;316:1435–1440.

67. Slayton RE, Park RC, Silverberg SG, et al. Vincristine, dactinomycin, and cyclophosphamide in the treatment of malignant germ cell tumors of the ovary. A Gynecologic Oncology Group Study (a final report). *Cancer* 1985;56:243–248.

68. Gershenson DM, Kavanagh JJ, Copeland LJ, et al. Treatment of malignant nondysgerminomatous germ cell tumors of the ovary with vinblastine, bleomycin, and cisplatin. *Cancer* 1986;57:1731–1737.

69. Gershenson DM, Morris M, Cangir A, et al. Treatment of malignant germ cell tumors of the ovary with bleomycin, etoposide, and cisplatin. *J Clin Oncol* 1990;8:715–720.

70. Williams S, Blessing JA, Liao SY, et al. Adjuvant therapy of ovarian germ cell tumors with cisplatin, etoposide, and bleomycin: a trial of the Gynecologic Oncology Group. *J Clin Oncol* 1994;12:701–706.

71. Culine S, Lhomme C, Kattan J, et al. Cisplatin-based chemotherapy in the management of germ cell tumors of the ovary: The Institut Gustave Roussy Experience. *Gynecol Oncol* 1997;64:160–165.

72. Segelov E, Campbell J, Ng M, et al. Cisplatin-based chemotherapy for ovarian germ cell malignancies: the Australian experience. *J Clin Oncol* 1994;12:378–384.

73. Dimopoulos MA, Papadopoulou M, Andreopoulou E, et al. Favorable outcome of ovarian germ cell malignancies treated with cisplatin or carboplatin-based chemotherapy: a Hellenic Cooperative Oncology Group study. *Gynecol Oncol* 1998;70:70–74.

74. Einhorn LH. Curing metastatic testicular cancer. *Proc Natl Acad Sci U S A* 2002;99:4592–4595.

75. Einhorn LH, Williams SD, Loehrer PJ, et al. Evaluation of optimal duration of chemotherapy in favorable-prognosis disseminated germ cell tumors: a Southeastern Cancer Study Group protocol. *J Clin Oncol* 1989;7:387–391.

76. Einhorn LH. Salvage therapy for germ cell tumors. *Semin Oncol* 1994; 21: 47–51.
77. Bokemeyer C, Kollmannsberger C, Meisner C, et al. First-line high-dose chemotherapy compared with standard-dose PEB/VIP chemotherapy in patients with advanced germ cell tumors: a multivariate and matched-pair analysis. *J Clin Oncol* 1999;17:3450–3456.
78. Messing MJ, Gershenson DM, Morris M, et al. Primary treatment failure in patients with malignant ovarian germ cell neoplasms. *Int J Gynecol Cancer* 1992;2:295–300.
79. Broun ER, Nichols CR, Turns M, et al. Early salvage therapy for germ cell cancer using high dose chemotherapy with autologous bone marrow support. *Cancer* 1994;73:1716–1720.
80. Broun ER, Nichols CR, Gize G, et al. Tandem high dose chemotherapy with autologous bone marrow transplantation for initial relapse of testicular germ cell cancer. *Cancer* 1997;79:605–1610.
81. Lotz JP, Andre T, Donsimoni R, et al. High dose chemotherapy with ifosfamide, carboplatin, and etoposide combined with autologous bone marrow transplantation for the treatment of poor-prognosis germ cell tumors and metastatic trophoblastic disease in adults. *Cancer* 1995;75:874–885.
82. Nichols CR, Tricot G, Williams SD, et al. Dose-intensive chemotherapy in refractory germ cell cancer—a phase I/II trial of high-dose carboplatin and etoposide with autologous bone marrow transplantation. *J Clin Oncol* 1989;7:932–939.
83. Vaena D, AR, Einhorn LH. Long term survival after high-dose salvage chemotherapy for germ cell malignancies with adverse prognostic variables. *Proc ASCO* 2003;(abst 1538).
84. Loehrer PJ Sr, Gonin R, Nichols CR, et al. Vinblastine plus ifosfamide plus cisplatin as initial salvage therapy in recurrent germ cell tumor. *J Clin Oncol* 1998;16:2500–2504.
85. Hinton S, Catalano P, Einhorn LH, et al. Phase II study of paclitaxel plus gemcitabine in refractory germ cell tumors (E9897): a trial of the Eastern Cooperative Oncology Group. *J Clin Oncol* 2002;20:1859–1863.
86. Nichols, CR, Roth BJ, Loehrer PJ, et al. Salvage chemotherapy for recurrent germ cell cancer. *Semin Oncol* 1994;21:102–108.
87. Mann JR, Raafat F, Robinson K, et al. The United Kingdom Children's Cancer Study Group's second germ cell tumor study: carboplatin, etoposide, and bleomycin are effective treatment for children with malignant extracranial germ cell tumors, with acceptable toxicity. *J Clin Oncol* 2000;18:3809–3818.
88. McKeage MJ, Evans BD, Atkinson C, et al. Carbon monoxide diffusing capacity is a poor predictor of clinically significant bleomycin lung. New Zealand Clinical Oncology Group. *J Clin Oncol* 1990;8:779–783.
89. Loehrer PJ Sr, Johnson D, Elson P, et al. Importance of bleomycin in favorable-prognosis disseminated germ cell tumors: an Eastern Cooperative Oncology Group trial. *J Clin Oncol* 1995;13:470–476.
90. de Wit R, Stoter G, Kaye SB, et al. Importance of bleomycin in combination chemotherapy for good-prognosis testicular nonseminoma: a randomized study of the European Organization for Research and Treatment of Cancer Genitourinary Tract Cancer Cooperative Group. *J Clin Oncol* 1997;15:1837–1843.
91. Bajorin DF, Sarosdy MF, Pfister DG, et al. Randomized trial of etoposide and cisplatin versus etoposide and carboplatin in patients with good-risk germ cell tumors: a multiinstitutional study. *J Clin Oncol* 1993;11:598–606.
92. Horwich A, Sleijfer DT, Fossa SD, et al. Randomized trial of bleomycin, etoposide, and cisplatin compared with bleomycin, etoposide, and carboplatin in good-prognosis metastatic nonseminomatous germ cell cancer: a Multiinstitutional Medical Research Council/European Organization for Research and Treatment of Cancer Trial. *J Clin Oncol* 1997;15:1844–1852.
93. American Society of Clinical Oncology. Recommendations for the use of hematopoietic colony-stimulating factors: evidence-based, clinical practice guidelines. *J Clin Oncol* 1994;12:2471–2508.
94. Cushing B, Giller R, Ablin A, et al. Surgical resection alone is effective treatment for ovarian immature teratoma in children and adolescents: a report of the Pediatric Oncology Group and the Children's Cancer Group. *Am J Obstet Gynecol* 1999;181:353–358.
95. Marina NM, Cushing B, Giller R, et al. Complete surgical excision is effective treatment for children with immature teratomas with or without malignant elements: a Pediatric Oncology Group/Children's Cancer Group Intergroup Study. *J Clin Oncol* 1999;17:2137–2143.
96. Dark GG, Bower M, Newlands ES, et al. Surveillance policy for stage I ovarian germ cell tumors. *J Clin Oncol* 1997;15:620–624.
97. Bonazzi C, Peccatori F, Colombo N, et al. Pure ovarian immature teratoma, a unique and curable disease: 10 years' experience of 32 prospectively treated patients. *Obstet Gynecol* 1994;84:598–604.
98. LaPolla JP, Benda J, Vigliotti AP, Anderson B. Dysgerminoma of the ovary. *Obstet Gynecol* 1987;69:859–864.
99. Mitchell MF, Gershenson DM, Soeters RP, et al. The long-term effects of radiation therapy on patients with ovarian dysgerminoma. *Cancer* 1991;67:1084–1090.
100. Krepart G, Smith JP, Rutledge F, Delclos L. The treatment for dysgerminoma of the ovary. *Cancer* 1978;41:986–990.
101. Thomas GM, Dembo AJ, Hacker NF, DePetrillo AD. Current therapy for dysgerminoma of the ovary. *Obstet Gynecol* 1987;70:268–275.
102. Lawson AP, Adler GF. Radiotherapy in the treatment of ovarian dysgerminomas. *Int J Radiat Oncol Biol Phys* 1988;14:431–434.
103. Freed JH, CJ, Pierce VK, et al Dysgerminoma of the ovary. *Cancer* 1979;43:798.
104. Marks RD, Underwood PB, Othersen HB, et al. Dysgerminoma—100% control with combined therapy in six consecutive patients with advanced disease. *Int J Radiat Oncol Biol Phys* 1978;4:453–456.
105. Thomas GM, Rider WD, Dembo AJ, et al. Seminoma of the testis: results of treatment and patterns of failure after radiation therapy. *Int J Radiat Oncol Biol Phys* 1982;8:165–174.
106. Boice JD Jr, Engholm G, Kleinerman RA, et al. Radiation dose and second cancer risk in patients treated for cancer of the cervix. *Radiat Res* 1988;116:3–55.
107. Culine S, Lhomme C, Kattan J, et al. Cisplatin-based chemotherapy in dysgerminoma of the ovary: thirteen-year experience at the Institut Gustave Roussy. *Gynecol Oncol* 1995;58:344–348.
108. Williams SD, Blessing JA, Hatch KD, Homesley HD. Chemotherapy of advanced dysgerminoma: trials of the Gynecologic Oncology Group. *J Clin Oncol* 1991;9:1950–1955.
109. Perrin LC, Low J, Nicklin JL, et al. Fertility and ovarian function after conservative surgery for germ cell tumours of the ovary. *Aust N Z J Obstet Gynaecol* 1999;39:243–245.
110. Kanazawa K, Suzuki T, Sakumoto K. Treatment of malignant ovarian germ cell tumors with preservation of fertility: reproductive performance after persistent remission. *Am J Clin Oncol* 2000;23:244–248.
111. Zanetta G, Bonazzi C, Cantu M, et al. Survival and reproductive function after treatment of malignant germ cell ovarian tumors. *J Clin Oncol* 2001;19:1015–1020.
112. Muram D, Gale CL, Thompson E. Functional ovarian cysts in patients cured of ovarian neoplasms. *Obstet Gynecol* 1990;75:680–683.
113. Howell, S, Shalet S. Gonadal damage from chemotherapy and radiotherapy. *Endocrinol Metab Clin North Am* 1998;27:927–943.
114. Casey AC, Bhodauria S, Shapter A, et al. Dysgerminoma: the role of conservative surgery. *Gynecol Oncol* 1996;63:352–357.
115. Nichols CR, Breeden ES, Loehrer PJ, et al. Secondary leukemia associated with a conventional dose of etoposide: review of serial germ cell tumor protocols. *J Natl Cancer Inst* 1993;85:36–40.
116. Pedersen-Bjergaard J, Daugaard G, Hansen SW, et al. Increased risk of myelodysplasia and leukaemia after etoposide, cisplatin, and bleomycin for germ-cell tumours. *Lancet* 1991;338:359–363.
117. Pui CH. Epipodophyllotoxin-related acute myeloid leukaemia. *Lancet* 1991;338:1468.
118. Pui CH, Ribeiro RC, Hancock ML, et al. Acute myeloid leukemia in children treated with epipodophyllotoxins for acute lymphoblastic leukemia. *N Engl J Med* 1991;325:1682–1687.
119. Ratain MJ, Kaminer LS, Bitran JD, et al. Acute nonlymphocytic leukemia following etoposide and cisplatin combination chemotherapy for advanced non–small-cell carcinoma of the lung. *Blood* 1987;70:1412–1417.
120. Pedersen-Bjergaard J, Brondum-Nielsen K, Karle H, Johansson B. Chemotherapy-related—late occurring—Philadelphia chromosome in AML, ALL and CML. Similar events related to treatment with DNA topoisomerase II inhibitors? *Leukemia* 1997;11:1571–1574.
121. Horning SJ, Hoppe RT, Kaplan HS, Rosenberg SA. Female reproduc-

tive potential after treatment for Hodgkin's disease. *N Engl J Med* 1981;304:1377–1382.

122. Byrne J, Mulvihill JJ, Myers MH, et al. Effects of treatment on fertility in long-term survivors of childhood or adolescent cancer. *N Engl J Med* 1987;317:1315–1321.

123. Siris ES, Leventhal BG, Vaitukaitis JL. Effects of childhood leukemia and chemotherapy on puberty and reproductive function in girls. *N Engl J Med* 1976;294:1143–1146.

124. Nicosia SV, Matus-Ridley M, Meadows AT. Gonadal effects of cancer therapy in girls. *Cancer* 1985;55:2364–2372.

125. Gershenson DM. Menstrual and reproductive function after treatment with combination chemotherapy for malignant ovarian germ cell tumors. *J Clin Oncol* 1988;6:270–275.

126. Brewer M, Gershenson DM, Herzog CE, et al. Outcome and reproductive function after chemotherapy for ovarian dysgerminoma. *J Clin Oncol* 1999;17:2670–2675.

127. Pektasides D, Rustin GJ, Newlands ES, et al. Fertility after chemotherapy for ovarian germ cell tumours. *Br J Obstet Gynaecol* 1987;94:477–479.

128. Rustin GJ, Pektasides D, Bagshawe KD, et al. Fertility after chemotherapy for male and female germ cell tumours. *Int J Androl* 1987;10:389–392.

129. Hale GA, Marina NM, Jones-Wallace D, et al. Late effects of treatment for germ cell tumors during childhood and adolescence. *J Pediatr Hematol Oncol* 1999;21:115–122.

130. Swenson MM, MacLeod JS, Williams SD, et al. Quality of life among ovarian germ cell cancer survivors: a narrative analysis. *Oncol Nurs Forum* 2003;30:380.

131. Hansen SW, Helweg-Larsen S, Trojaborg W. Long-term neurotoxicity in patients treated with cisplatin, vinblastine, and bleomycin for metastatic germ cell cancer. *J Clin Oncol* 1989;7:1457–1461.

132. Hansen SW, Olsen N. Raynaud's phenomenon in patients treated with cisplatin, vinblastine, and bleomycin for germ cell cancer: measurement of vasoconstrictor response to cold. *J Clin Oncol* 1989;7:940–942.

133. Hansen SW, Groth S, Sorensen PG, et al. Enhanced pulmonary toxicity in smokers with germ-cell cancer treated with cis-platinum, vinblastine and bleomycin: a long-term follow-up. *Eur J Cancer Clin Oncol* 1989;25:733–736.

134. Roth BJ, Greist A, Kubilis PS, et al. Cisplatin-based combination chemotherapy for disseminated germ cell tumors: long-term follow-up. *J Clin Oncol* 1988;6:1239–1247.

135. Boyer M, Raghavan D, Harris PJ, et al. Lack of late toxicity in patients treated with cisplatin-containing combination chemotherapy for metastatic testicular cancer. *J Clin Oncol* 1990;8:21–26.

136. Stoter G, Koopman A, Vendrik CP, et al. Ten-year survival and late sequelae in testicular cancer patients treated with cisplatin, vinblastine, and bleomycin. *J Clin Oncol* 1989;7:1099–1104.

137. Nichols CR, Roth BJ, Williams SD, et al. No evidence of acute cardiovascular complications of chemotherapy for testicular cancer: an analysis of the Testicular Cancer Intergroup Study. *J Clin Oncol* 1992;10:760–765.

138. Williams SD, Stablein DM, Einhorn L H, et al. Immediate adjuvant chemotherapy versus observation with treatment at relapse in pathological stage II testicular cancer. *N Engl J Med* 1987;317:1433–1438.

139. Zaghloul MS, Khattab TY. Dysgerminoma of the ovary: good prognosis even in advanced stages. *Int J Radiat Oncol Biol Phys* 1992;24:161–165.

CHAPTER 27

Ovarian Sex Cord–Stromal Tumors

David M. Gershenson, Lynn C. Hartmann, and Robert H. Young

The intraovarian matrix that supports the germ cells and is covered by the surface epithelium consists of cells originating from the sex cords and mesenchyme of the embryonic gonad. Granulosa cells and Sertoli cells, generally considered to be homologs, are derived from the sex cord cells, whereas the pluripotential mesenchymal cells are the precursors of the theca cells, Leydig cells, and fibroblasts. Neoplastic transformation of these cellular constituents, either singly or in various combinations collectively, results in neoplasms that are termed sex cord–stromal tumors (SCSTs). The classification of the sex cord–stromal tumors provides the template from which this chapter endeavors to stratify and define these tumor entities according to their morphologic characteristics (Table 27.1).

The SCSTs account for approximately 7% of all malignant ovarian neoplasms (1). Annually, 26,000 new cases of ovarian cancer are diagnosed in the United States, and therefore, an estimated 1,800 new cases of SCSTs will be detected annually. Although these tumors account for a decreasing proportion of all ovarian malignancies with advancing age, the annual age-related incidence continues to increase through the seventh decade of life (2). Overall, the majority of these tumors are of low malignant potential and associated with a favorable long-term prognosis. In addition, a significant proportion of SCSTs are diagnosed in patients prior to age 40 years and have the potential to produce a variety of steroid hormones. Hence, adequate knowledge of the natural history of each of these tumors is imperative to diagnose and individualize appropriately definitive surgical and adjuvant therapy.

D. M. Gershenson: Department of Gynecologic Oncology, The University of Texas M. D. Anderson Cancer Center, Houston, Texas 77030.

L. C. Hartmann: Department of Oncology, Mayo Clinic Cancer Center, Rochester, Minnesota 55905.

R. H. Young: Department of Pathology, Massachusetts General Hospital, Boston, Massachusetts 02114.

Sex cord–stromal tumors account for nearly 90% of all functioning ovarian neoplasms (3). With the exception of fibromas, the clinical presentation of patients with SCSTs is frequently governed by the clinical manifestations resulting from the endocrinologic abnormalities. Excessive estrogen production, whether from increased tumor synthesis or peripheral conversion of androgens, influences end-organ responses, which are usually age-dependent and can range from isosexual precocious puberty to menometrorrhagia to postmenopausal bleeding. In addition, the associated risks for endometrial cancer and possibly breast cancer must be

TABLE 27.1. *Classification of sex cord–stromal tumors*

Granulosa-stromal cell tumors
Granulosa-cell tumor
Adult type
Juvenile type
Tumors in the thecoma-fibroma group
Thecoma
Fibroma-fibrosarcoma
Sclerosing stromal tumor
Sertoli-stromal cell tumors
Sertoli-cell tumor
Leydig-cell tumor
Sertoli-Leydig cell tumor
Well-differentiated
Of intermediate differentiation
Poorly differentiated
With heterologous elements
Retiform
Mixed
Sex cord tumor with annular tubules
Unclassified
Gynandroblastoma
Steroid-cell tumors
Stromal luteoma
Leydig-cell tumor
Hilus-cell tumor
Leydig-cell tumor, nonhilar type
Steroid-cell tumor not otherwise specified

recognized (4–6). Conversely, the rapid onset of signs ranging from early defeminization to frank virilization heralds a hyperandrogenic state. Elevated circulating levels of testosterone and/or androstenedione provide strong evidence for the presence of a SCST. Although granulosa-cell, theca-cell, and Sertoli-cell tumors are generally considered to be estrogenic, and Sertoli-Leydig cell and steroid-cell tumors are predominantly androgenic, the functional endocrinologic capacities of these tumors are impossible to predict based on their morphologic features. It should also be noted that miscellaneous ovarian tumors, both primary and metastatic, that are not in the SCST family may be androgenic or estrogenic if their stroma is stimulated to undergo luteinization.

GRANULOSA-CELL TUMORS

Although granulosa-cell tumors (GCTs) of the ovary were initially described by Rokitansky in 1859 (7), the etiopathogenesis of these neoplasms remains ill defined. At least in part, this is a reflection of the low incidence of GCTs, and hence the limited number of cases witnessed at any single institution. Granulosa-cell tumors comprise only 5% of all ovarian malignancies and account for approximately 70% of malignant sex cord–stromal tumors (4–6,8–15). The annual incidence of GCTs in the United States and other developed countries varies from 0.4 to 1.7 cases per 100,000 women (5,6,14,16–18). Although GCTs have been diagnosed from infancy through the tenth decade of life, the peak incidence for these tumors occurs during the perimenopausal decade. The average age at the time of diagnosis in over 750 cases was 52 years (4–6, 9,11–14). Considering that GCTs occurring after the third decade of life appear to be histologically distinct in most instances from those occurring in children and younger adults, the clinical and pathologic characteristics for the juvenile and adult GCTs will be addressed separately.

Granulosa-Cell Tumors: Adult Type

Adult-type granulosa-cell tumors (AGCTs), as histologically described below, account for 95% of all GCTs. The majority of patients will present with one or a combination of the following clinical symptoms: abnormal vaginal bleeding, abdominal distention, and abdominal pain (5,6,11–14,19). The latter symptoms are most frequently attributable to the gross size of the tumor at the time of diagnosis, with the majority exceeding 10 cm in diameter and many exceeding 15 cm (5,12,14). In a recent series, 12% had ascites at diagnosis (19). Notwithstanding the accompanying discomfort from capsular distention, stretching of suspensory ligaments, and compression of adjacent structures, the etiology of acute severe pain is generally adnexal torsion, hemorrhage into the tumor, or rupture of a cystic component. However, in many series, menometrorrhagia, oligomenorrhea, or amenorrhea in premenopausal women or bleeding in postmeno-

pausal women is the most common reason for seeking medical assistance. These and other clinical manifestations such as breast tenderness, uterine myohypertrophy, and endometrial hyperplasia are consistent with the presence of an estrogen-secreting tumor.

The endocrine function of AGCTs, specifically the production of estrogens, has been repeatedly demonstrated by assessment of the end organ, the endometrium, and measurements of peripheral levels of estrogen before and after surgery. In a detailed retrospective analysis of endometrial specimens from patients (n = 69) with GCTs, Gusberg and Kardon (20) observed histologic features consistent with unopposed estrogen, including atypical adenomatous hyperplasia in 42% of the evaluated cohort, adenocarcinoma *in situ* (4) in 5%, and invasive adenocarcinoma in 22%. Similarly, Evans et al. (4) noted endometrial hyperplasia in 55% and adenocarcinoma in 13% of their GCT study population. Other investigators have corroborated the high prevalence of glandular hyperplasia and have reported adenocarcinoma frequencies ranging from 3% to 27% (5–6,9,11–14,21–22). Selective ovarian venous catheterizations during surgery have documented hormonal production, including the secretion of large quantities of estrogen from the ovary harboring the GCT. The return of serum estrogen to physiologic levels after definitive treatment has been witnessed repeatedly. Occasionally, patients with GCTs present with endometrial changes (decidual reaction of the stroma or secretory characteristics of the glands) consistent with tumor production of progesterone (23). Rarely, virilizing changes such as oligomenorrhea, hirsutism, and other masculinizing signs may accompany GCTs (24,25).

Pathology

AGCTs have an average diameter of approximately 12 cm, but a subset, 10% to 15% of the cases, are small and not appreciated on pelvic examination (26). Most characteristically, they are predominantly cystic with numerous locules filled with fluid or clotted blood and separated by solid tissue (Fig. 27.1), or they are solid with large areas of hemorrhage. The solid tissue may be gray-white or yellow and soft or firm. A rare tumor is cystic, usually thin walled, but occasionally thick walled, and multilocular or unilocular (24).

Microscopic examination reveals an almost exclusive population of granulosa cells or, more often, an additional component of theca cells, fibroblasts, or both. The granulosa cells grow in a wide variety of patterns. The better-differentiated tumors usually have microfollicular, macrofollicular, insular, or trabecular patterns. The microfollicular pattern is characterized by numerous small cavities (Call-Exner bodies) (Fig. 27.2) that may contain eosinophilic fluid, one or a few degenerating nuclei, hyalinized basement-membrane material, or rarely basophilic fluid. The microfollicles are typically separated by well-differentiated granulosa cells

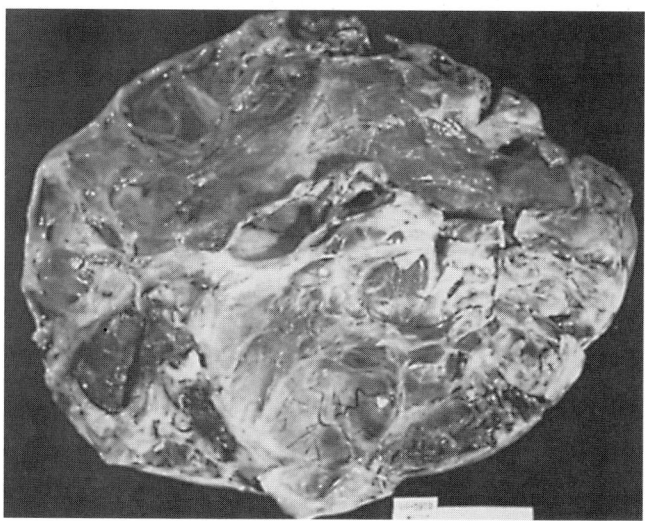

FIG. 27.1. Granulosa-cell tumor. The sectioned surface is composed predominantly of multiple cysts filled with blood. (Reprinted with permission from Case Records of the Massachusetts General Hospital, Case 89–1961. *N Engl J Med* 1961;265:1210.)

that contain scanty cytoplasm and pale, angular or oval, often grooved nuclei arranged haphazardly in relation to one another and to the follicles. The uncommon macrofollicular pattern is characterized by cysts lined by well-differentiated granulosa cells beneath which theca cells are present. The trabecular and insular forms of granulosa-cell tumors are characterized by bands and islands of granulosa cells separated by fibromatous or thecomatous stroma. The less well-differentiated forms of the adult granulosa-cell tumor typically have a water silk (moire silk), gyriform, or diffuse (sarcomatoid) pattern alone or in combination. The first two patterns are manifested by parallel undulating or zigzag rows

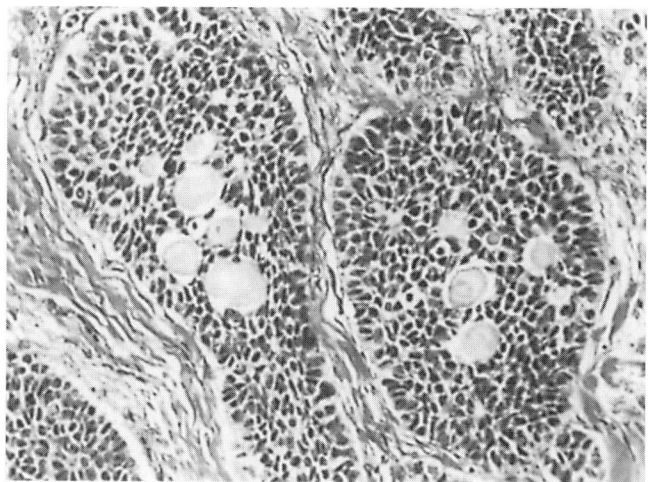

FIG. 27.2. Granulosa-cell tumor, adult type, microfollicular pattern. Several nests of granulosa-cells with small oval and angular nuclei enclose multiple Call-Exner bodies.

of granulosa cells, generally in single file, whereas the diffuse form is characterized by a monotonous, patternless cellular growth. In some adult granulosa-cell tumors, the neoplastic cells have moderate to abundant quantities of dense or vacuolated cytoplasms; the term *luteinized granulosa-cell tumor* is appropriate when such cells predominate (23). The cells in GCTs usually have round to oval, pale, and often grooved nuclei (Fig. 27.2), but rarely the cells are spindle-shaped, resembling a cellular fibroma or low-grade fibrosarcoma; mitotic figures may be numerous, but are rarely atypical. There is usually only mild nuclear atypia, but approximately 2% of tumors contain mononucleate and multinucleate cells with large, bizarre, hyperchromatic nuclei, the presence of which does not appear to worsen the prognosis (27).

Natural History

Adult granulosa-cell tumors are low-grade malignancies with a propensity to remain localized and demonstrate indolent growth. Ninety percent are stage I at diagnosis (22). The 10-year survival rate for stage I disease ranges from 86% to 96%; for more advanced disease at diagnosis, 26% to 49% (22). Bilaterality is infrequent (less than 10%) (19). For patients who recur, the median time to recurrence is 6 years. The median survival after recurrence is 5.6 years, consistent with indolent growth features (4,9). Tumor rupture occurred in 22% of a series of 97 cases (19). A unique feature of GCTs is the occurrence of recurrences at extended time intervals from primary therapy, suggesting the presence of persistent occult disease with a very indolent growth rate. Numerous investigators have witnessed recurrences more than a decade after primary treatment (28,29).

Prognostic Factors

The staging system for GCTs is the same as that used for epithelial ovarian cancer (International Federation of Gynecology and Obstetrics, FIGO). Whereas surgical stage has been recognized as the most important prognostic factor for GCTs, tumor size, rupture, histologic subtype, nuclear atypia, and mitotic activity have been correlated with survival with varying degrees of success (18,30,31). As noted above, GCTs are large and therefore prone to rupture. Rupture appears adversely to impact survival in stage I patients, justifying stratification as stage IC (9). However, the prognostic importance of positive cytology and surface involvement is less defined in stage I GCTs (18). Larger, well-characterized series are necessary to clarify these apparent discrepancies. Traditionally, tumor size was considered to be prognostically significant but appears to lose independent predictability when assessed according to stage (5,10,14,16). Both the increasing degree of nuclear atypia and the increasing mitotic frequency per 10 high-power fields (HPFs) have been correlated inversely with prognosis. Specimens from patients with more advanced disease were associated with a higher grade of atypia and/or more mitotic figures (5,9, 10,14). Of note is the observation that nuclear grade, despite its somewhat subjective assessment, has been reported to be a reliable prognostic indicator in stage I cases (9,14). The significance of histologic subtypes and ploidy status has been debated and appears to be of minimal value. Several investigative groups (4,5,8–10,14) have failed to confirm Kottmeier's (32) report of the prognostic importance of histologic patterns alone in GCTs. Similarly, the reported studies utilizing flow cytometric analysis of DNA content have been inconsistent. Klemi et al. (33) reported a significant survival advantage for patients with tumors demonstrating normal ploidy and/or an S-phase fraction of less than 6%. In contrast, other investigators have suggested that nondiploid GCTs are infrequently encountered (34,35). Chadha et al. (34) observed three of five aneuploid tumors from a sample population of 43 pathologically diagnosed GCTs to be vimentin negative but positive for cytokeratin and epithelial membrane antigen, and therefore cautioned that such highly aneuploid tumors may represent undifferentiated carcinomas. Indeed, it is clear that some series of GCTs in the literature are "contaminated" by the inclusion of undifferentiated carcinomas not otherwise specified or recently recognized entities, such as the large-cell carcinoma of hypercalcemic type. Series with unusually large numbers of late-stage or poor-prognosis cases should accordingly be evaluated cautiously.

Investigators have analyzed several potential molecular markers, including p53 status, telomerase, Ki-67, c-myc, and Her-2/neu in GCTs (36–40). To date, no molecular marker provides prognostic information for GCTs beyond what is known from stage and histopathologic parameters.

Ala-Fossi et al. stained 30 GCTs for the inhibin subunit. All 24 stages I and II tumors were positive, whereas 4 of 6 stages II to IV tumors were negative. Those that were negative were poorly differentiated and exhibited rapid disease progression. Stage was the sole independent prognostic factor (41).

Serum Markers

Recognizing that the majority of patients presenting with advanced GCTs will recur, the identification of a specific serum tumor marker(s) would facilitate early detection of recurrent disease and monitoring of treatment effectiveness (4,5,12,14). As noted above, serum estrogens are generally produced by GCTs and have been utilized as an indicator of disease status (42). Unfortunately, serum estradiol levels are occasionally not elevated, and more frequently are only marginally increased. Hence, they are not ideal for monitoring in a significant number of cases. Several proteins derived from granulosa cells, including inhibin, follicle-regulating protein, and müllerian-inhibiting substance, are readily assayable in serum and forwarded as useful diagnostic monitoring markers (43–51). In a prospective evaluation of 27 patients with GCTs, Jobling et al. (45) demonstrated that serum inhibin levels are typically elevated sevenfold above normal follicular phase levels prior to primary surgical management and can become elevated again several months prior to clinical detection of recurrent disease. In recent years, inhibin has become available as a marker that can be evaluated immunohistochemically to assist in the diagnosis of GCTs and, for that matter, other SCSTs (52).

Granulosa-Cell Tumors: Juvenile Type

Ovarian neoplasms are relatively rare in childhood and adolescence, and when encountered, the majority are of germ-cell origin, with only 5% to 7% being SCSTs. The latter, which consists predominantly of the granulosa-cell type in this age group, demonstrates a tumor biology that appears to be different from the typical granulosa-cell tumor (AGCT) considered above (53). Approximately 90% of the granulosa-cell tumors diagnosed in prepubertal girls and in most women less than 30 years of age will be of the juvenile type (JGCT). In a clinicopathologic analysis of 125 cases of JGCT, 44% of the tumors occurred prior to age 10 years and only 3% after the third decade of life (54). The majority of prepubertal patients present with clinical evidence of isosexual precocious pseudopuberty, which may include breast enlargement, development of pubic hair, increased vaginal secretions, advanced somatic development, and other secondary sex characteristics (54–58). Serum estradiol levels were reported as being elevated in 17 of 17 cases of JGCTs and pseudopuberty (56). In addition, elevated levels of serum progesterone (six of ten) and testosterone (six of eight) were likewise observed, as well as suppressed levels of luteinizing hormone and follicle-stimulating hormone. The occasional patient will harbor an androgen-secreting JGCT accompanied by virilization (54,56,57). Although the signs of either precocious pseudopuberty or virilization are dramatic, the most consistent clinical sign at presentation in patients with JGCTs is increasing abdominal girth. Young et al. (54) indicated that in only 2 of 113 nonpregnant patients with JGCTs was the treating physician unable to palpate a mass on abdominal, pelvic, and/or rectal examination. Abdominal pain, dysuria, and constipation may occur. Infrequently, a surgical emergency is encountered following spontaneous rupture or torsion of the enlarged ovary. Juvenile granulosa-cell tumors can occur in infants, in whom the prognosis appears to be more favorable than in older individuals (59).

The frequency of bilaterality for JGCTs is estimated to be 5%, similar to AGCTs (60). When stage was assigned based on surgical and histologic parameters, 88% were stage IA, 2% stage IB, 8% stage IC, and 3% stage II. As noted, extraovarian spread is infrequently encountered at exploration, whereas rupture of the tumor is noted in approximately 10% of cases. Ascites contributes to the abdominal distention in 10% to 36% of cases (54,56).

JGCTs have been reported in association with enchondromatosis alone (Ollier's disease) or concomitantly with hemangiomas (Maffucci's syndrome) (56,61–63). Individuals with these relatively uncommon mesodermal dysplasias generally present prior to puberty and frequently develop secondary neoplasms, most commonly sarcomas, after the second decade of life. Juvenile granulosa-cell tumors are the next most frequent tumor associated with these disorders and become evident during the first and second decades of life. These observations appear to imply more than coincidental occurrences and suggest a generalized mesodermal dysplasia, perhaps contributing to the pathogenesis of these neoplastic processes. In addition, congenital bilateral JGCTs of the ovary have been reported in leprechaunism, a disease characterized by insulin resistance resulting from an insulin-receptor defect (64).

Pathology

The appearances of JGCTs are similar to the adult form; a solid and cystic neoplasm, in which the cysts contain hemorrhagic fluid, is common (54,55,58). Uniformly solid and uniformly cystic neoplasms are also encountered; the latter may be multilocular or, in rare instances, unilocular. The solid component is typically yellow-tan or gray and occasionally exhibits extensive necrosis, hemorrhage, or both.

Microscopic examination typically reveals a predominantly solid cellular tumor with focal follicle formation, but occasionally, a uniformly solid or a uniformly follicular pattern is seen. In the solid areas, the neoplastic cells may be arranged diffusely or as multiple nodules of various sizes. The follicles typically vary in size and shape; Call-Exner bodies are rarely encountered, and the follicles rarely reach the large size of those in the macrofollicular AGCT. The follicular lumens in the juvenile tumor contain eosinophilic or basophilic fluid, which stains with mucicarmine in approximately two of three cases.

The two characteristic cytologic features of the neoplastic juvenile granulosa cells that distinguish them from those of the AGCT are their generally rounded, hyperchromatic nuclei, which almost always lack grooves, and their almost invariable moderate to abundant eosinophilic or vacuolated (luteinized) cytoplasm (Fig. 27.3). Nuclear atypia in JGCTs varies from minimal to marked; in approximately 13% of the cases, severe degrees are present. The mitotic rate also varies greatly but is generally higher than that seen in AGCTs, often being five or more per HPF (54,58).

Natural History

In the initial series by Young et al., 98% of 125 patients with JGCTs were less than 35 years of age, and 78% were 20 years or less (54). Notwithstanding the customary presenting complaint of increased abdominal girth and the clinical documentation of a large mass (64% >10 cm), 90% of the

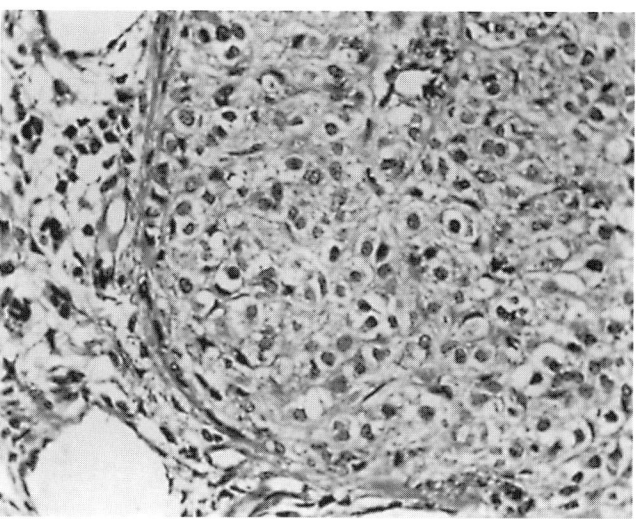

FIG. 27.3. Granulosa-cell tumor, juvenile type. A nodule of tumor is composed of large cells with abundant cytoplasm and slightly pleomorphic, hyperchromatic nuclei.

JGCTs analyzed by Young et al. (54) were stage IA or IB. The corresponding survival rate for these patients with an average follow-up of 3.5 years was 97%. Included were nine stage IA2 patients with rupture of the tumor, all of whom were alive and free of disease. Patients presenting with associated isosexual pseudoprecocious puberty may have a more favorable prognosis. Assessing 80 such cases accrued from 212 reported JGCTs, only two cancer-related deaths (2.5%) were observed. Presumably, the clinical manifestations lead to early medical intervention and reflect the excellent outcomes (54,56–58).

Although the early symptoms and presentation with localized disease are similar to AGCTs, several behavioral characteristics are notably different when comparing these histologic variants. Although the natural history of the adult form frequently includes a latency period with recurrences remote from initial diagnosis, the juvenile counterpart is characteristically aggressive in advanced stages and the time to relapse and death of limited duration. Thirteen cases of stage II, III, or IV disease were abstracted from three analyses with a combined sample size of 180 patients (54,56,57). Of these 13 cases, only three patients (23%) were alive when reported, and notably, the recurrences and deaths occurred within a relatively brief interval. In contrast to the AGCTs, no recurrence or death from JCGT was witnessed after 3 years in the three largest reports to date in the literature (54, 56,58).

Prognostic Factors

Young et al. (54) noted surgical stage to represent the most reliable prognostic indicator. Tumor size, mitotic activity, and nuclear atypia appeared to be significant when tumors were analyzed without regard to stage. However, these parameters lost discriminating value when applied to only stages IA1 and IB1 tumors. In that series, rupture did not correlate with outcome. Schneider et al. reported on a group of 54 sex cord–stromal tumors in children and adolescents from Germany (45 JGCTs and 9 others) (65). They addressed the outcome of patients with ''accidental'' stage IC disease, defined as violation of the tumor capsule during surgery, versus ''natural'' stage IC tumors, with preoperative rupture or malignant ascites. Among 12 pateints with accidental stage IC disease, there were no recurrences. In contrast, five of the nine patients with natural stage IC disease recurred ($p = .001$). Assessment of DNA content via flow cytometry in JGCTs demonstrated that nearly half of such tumors harbored nondiploid patterns (66,67). Jacoby et al. (66) were unable to correlate DNA ploidy or S-phase fraction (SPF) with either stage of disease or prognosis in patients with localized disease. In the series by Schneider et al., mitotic activity correlated with prognosis (65). There were no relapses in 35 patients whose tumors exhibited low or moderate mitotic activity. Among those with high mitotic activity (>19 mitoses/10 HPFs), approximately half recurred.

Although the information in the literature is limited, the various tumor markers as discussed above for AGCTs would appear to be applicable to JGCTs for the monitoring of advanced disease. Nishida et al. (67) have reported elevated preoperative serum estradiol and inhibin levels in a 3-year-old girl with isosexual pseudoprecocious puberty and JGCT. Surgical excision of the JGCT resulted in a return to undetectable estradiol and inhibin levels postoperatively.

TUMORS IN THE THECOMA-FIBROMA GROUP

Considering that the ovarian stromal cell is the precursor of both fibroblasts and theca cells, pure thecomas and pure fibromas appear to represent extremes in a continuum, with a significant percentage of the tumors having admixtures of lipid-laden, steroid-secreting cells and collagen-producing spindle cells. Nonetheless, the vast majority of tumors in the thecoma-fibroma group are readily subcategorized based on relatively distinct clinical and histologic characteristics. The major subcategories include thecoma, fibroma-fibrosarcoma, and the sclerosing stromal-cell tumor.

Thecoma

Theca-cell tumors (TCTs), or thecomas (Fig. 27.4), are composed of lipid-laden stromal cells, occasionally demonstrating luteinization, and are almost invariably clinically benign (4,68,69). Thecomas account for approximately 1% of ovarian neoplasms and occur at a more advanced age than other sex cord–stromal tumors. The majority of patients are in their sixth and seventh decades at the time of diagnosis (4,68). Combining two large series totaling over 140 patients, less than 10% presented prior to age 30 years. Notably, the luteinized tumors are an exception to this generaliza-

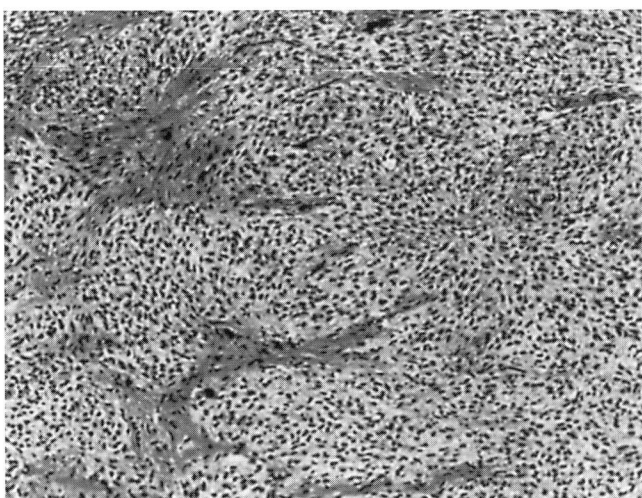

FIG. 27.4. Thecoma. The tumor is composed of a mass of clear, vacuolated cells with round to oval nuclei intersected by bands of fibromatous tissue. (Reprinted with permission from Morris JM, Scully RE. *Endocrine pathology of the ovary.* St. Louis: Mosby, 1958.)

tion, with 30% occurring in women before their fourth decade of life (70). Assessing a compendium of nearly 300 cases, bilaterality occurs with a frequency of approximately 2% and extraovarian spread occurs rarely if at all (4,68,69, 71).

The primary presenting signs and symptoms in patients with TCTs are abnormal genital bleeding and/or an abdominal/pelvic mass (68,69,71). The former urges initiation of medical intervention in the majority of postmenopausal patients, whereas an increasing abdominal girth or a palpable mass is more frequently the main presenting complaint of premenopausal patients. Lesion size has been reported to vary from <1 to 40 cm in diameter (68,69,71). Ascites is occasionally encountered.

Thecomas are considered to be among the most hormonally active of the sex cord–stromal tumors. The abnormal bleeding encountered in 60% of patients is presumably attributable to excess estrogen production (68,69). In the series reported by Evans et al. (4), endometrial hyperplasia was observed in 37% of the evaluable patients, and adenocarcinoma consistent with an unopposed estrogen effect was documented in an additional 27%. All the uterine cancers were well differentiated and minimally invasive, but two patients subsequently died of endometrial carcinoma. Other coexisting uterine pathologic findings potentially influenced by elevated circulating estrogen levels included leiomyomata, myohypertrophy, and endometrial polyps. Conversely, Zhang et al. (70) noted that nearly one-half of the evaluated luteinized thecomas were either nonfunctional or androgenic, resulting in a relatively significant frequency of masculinization.

An enigmatic tumor that has been considered to be a variant of luteinized thecoma has been associated with sclerosing peritonitis (72). These tumors are often bilateral and frequently have a brisk mitotic rate but have not been shown to have a metastatic potential. Sclerosing peritonitis has, however, been fatal owing to complications pursuant to it.

Fibroma-Fibrosarcoma

Fibromas represent the most commonly encountered sex cord–stromal tumor, accounting for approximately 4% of all ovarian neoplasms. These endocrine-inert tumors are seldom bilateral and vary in size from microscopic to extremely large masses. Although infrequently diagnosed prior to age 30 years, fibromas can occur at any age; the average age of diagnosis is the latter half of the fifth decade of life (73). These tumors become more edematous as their size increases, which frequently is accompanied by the escape of increasing quantities of fluid from the tumor surfaces. Ascites is detected in association with 10% to 15% of ovarian fibromas exceeding a diameter of 10 cm (74). Furthermore, 1% of patients develop a hydrothorax in addition to the hydroperitoneum, both resulting from excessive fluid loss from the ovarian fibroma (Meigs' syndrome) (75). Gorlin's syndrome represents an inherited predisposition to the development of ovarian fibromas along with several other abnormalities, the most frequent of which is the appearance of basal-cell nevi at an early age (76).

Although ovarian fibromas are generally considered to be benign lesions, approximately 10% will demonstrate increased cellularity and varying degrees of pleomorphism and mitotic activity. Fibromatous tumors characterized histologically by an increased cellular density and brisk mitotic activity are designated cellular fibromas and are considered to be tumors of low malignant potential, particularly if ruptured or associated with adhesions (77). In contrast, fibrosarcomas are highly malignant neoplasms. These tumors are distinguished by their greater cellular density and, most notably, moderate to marked pleomorphism (77).

Sclerosing Stromal-Cell Tumors

Sclerosing stromal-cell tumors (SSTs) were initially described by Chalvardjian and Scully (78) in 1973 as a distinct subgroup within the thecoma-fibroma family of ovarian tumors. Accounting for less than 5% of sex cord–stromal tumors, this relatively rare tumor characteristically differentiates itself histologically and clinically from both thecomas and fibromas (79,80). Histologically, the presence of pseudolobulation of cellular areas separated by edematous connective tissue, increased vascularity, and prominent areas of sclerosis are distinguishing features. Clinically, SSTs commonly become manifest during the second and third decades of life, with 80% being diagnosed prior to age 30 years, which is unique among ovarian stromal tumors (81). The signs and symptoms that most commonly necessitate medical evaluation include menstrual irregularities and/or

pelvic pain (82). Despite the relatively large tumor size, which ranges from clinically undetectable to 20 cm or more in greatest diameter, ascites is seldom encountered; this further contrasts SSTs from fibromas (82). In contrast to thecomas, SSTs were originally considered to be inactive endocrinologically (78). However, a limited number of cases have been subsequently reported in which steroidogenic activity has been clinically demonstrable (82–85). To date, all SSTs have been clinically benign, and with one exception (86), all have been unilateral. Although a recent report noted an elevated CA-125 level, which the investigators speculated was perhaps nonspecific (87), no specific tumor marker has been identified for SSTs to date.

Natural History

Thecomas, fibromas, and sclerosing stromal tumors are considered to be benign ovarian neoplasms, and any associated morbidity or mortality that would be encountered would be attributed to the treatment modalities or the sequelae of concurrent disease (4,68,71,73,88). Examples of the latter are deaths from endometrial carcinoma resulting from the unopposed estrogen produced by the thecomas (4). Although several cases of "malignant thecomas" have been reported, critical reappraisal of such tumors invariably results in histologic reassignment as sarcomas or diffuse granulosa-cell tumors (89). Furthermore, DNA ploidy assessment in both thecomas and fibromas not infrequently demonstrates aneuploid patterns that do not correlate with prognosis, rendering the significance of these observations questionable (90).

Prognostic Factors

The prognosis for patients diagnosed with cellular fibromas is generally considered to be quite favorable. Recurrences of these tumors of low malignant potential are generally correlated with adherent disease, rupture, or incomplete removal at the time of primary cytoreduction (77). Fibrosarcomas are associated with an extremely poor prognosis, but are fortunately rare.

SERTOLI-STROMAL CELL TUMORS

Neoplasms arising in the ovary exhibiting morphologic characteristics similar to those of the testes during various stages of gonadogenesis were recognized and elegantly described by Meyer (91,92). He reasoned that the origin of these tumors was the male blastema and coined the term *arrhenoblastoma*. Considering the functional nature of these male homologs and the varying degrees of associated defeminization and/or masculinization, the term *androblastoma* was also adopted. However, Morris and Scully (93), in 1958, contended that both designations implied masculinization, which is frequently absent, and furthermore facilitated the inclusion of a variety of unrelated androgen-producing ovarian tumors. Therefore, they recommended the adoption of the morphologic designation Sertoli-Leydig cell tumor (SLCT), which also allowed a consistent nomenclature for the general classification of sex cord–stromal tumors of the ovary. The SLCTs include tumors composed of Sertoli cells only, Leydig cells only, and a combination of Sertoli and Leydig cells.

Sertoli-Cell Tumors

Sertoli-cell tumors are rare, accounting for less than 5% of all SLCTs. In a review of the literature in 1984, Young and Scully (81) accepted only 23 reported cases based on histologic description. The average age at presentation was 27 years, but they noted this lesion can occur at any age. Evidence of estrogen production has been observed in approximately two-thirds of the reported cases. Consistent with excess estrogen production, isosexual precocious puberty has been witnessed during the first decade of life, menstrual disorders during the reproductive decades, and postmenopausal bleeding in the decades after the climacteric. Reflecting tumor size (average 9 cm), capsular distention and/or adnexal torsion, and abdominal distention and/or pain are frequent complaints. Pelvic examination generally confirms the presence of the tumor under these circumstances. The frequency with which excessive renin production has been associated with Sertoli cells appears to exceed mere chance (94–96). Evaluation of refractory hypertension and hypokalemia has rarely eventuated in the discovery of a Sertoli-cell tumor as the origin of the excess renin. An occasional Sertoli-cell tumor has arisen in a patient with the Peutz-Jeghers syndrome (PJS) (97).

Pathology

On gross examination, these rare tumors are typically solid, lobulated, and yellow (81,98). Microscopic examination typically shows hollow or solid tubules lined by cells that usually have relatively bland cytologic features, but rare tumors exhibit moderate to severe nuclear atypia. In most tumors, a tubular pattern predominates, but occasionally a diffuse pattern is conspicuous.

Prognosis

The great majority of these rare tumors have been unilateral stage I lesions. The greater majority of Sertoli-cell tumors are well differentiated, and only a single report in the literature described an anaplastic lesion that was rapidly fatal (81). Also, this case represents the sole published death associated with these tumors (81). Excision of the tumor results in prompt resolution of the hyperestrogenic state. (Leydig-cell tumors are discussed in the section on Steroid-Cell Tumors below.)

Sertoli-Leydig Cell Tumors

Sertoli-Leydig cell tumors (SLCTs) are extremely uncommon, accounting for less than 0.2% of all ovarian tumors. As implied by their designation, the tumors contain both Sertoli- and Leydig-cell elements. Many of the clinical characteristics are related to the degree of histologic differentiation and the presence of a retiform pattern and/or heterologous elements (described below). The average patient age at diagnosis is approximately 25 years, with the majority (70% to 75%) of the tumors becoming clinically manifest during the second and third decades of life. Less than 10% occur either prior to menarche or after the climacterium. Patients harboring well-differentiated tumors present at an average age of 35 years, or 10 years later than patients with intermediate or poorly differentiated lesions. Conversely, tumors with retiform patterns are generally detected 10 years earlier than the intermediate and poorly differentiated tumors (99–101). Based on the compiled data from three reported series totaling over 300 patients, the frequency of extraovarian spread of disease at the time of diagnosis is approximately 2% to 3%. In addition, the likelihood of encountering bilateral tumors is even less frequent (99–101).

The most frequent complaints at the time of presentation of these generally healthy adolescents and young adults are menstrual disorders, virilization, and nonspecific symptoms resulting from an abdominal mass. Nearly one-half of the patients experience sufficient abdominal pain or discomfort or note abdominal distention or palpate a mass on self-examination to prompt professional assessment. Whereas capsular distention and/or intralesional hemorrhage or necrosis of the tumor and/or adjacent visceral compression by the tumor account for the associated chronic or intermittent pain, acute abdominal pain necessitating emergency intervention invariably reflects vascular compromise from torsion. While lesion size varies according to histologic differentiation (approximately 5 cm for well-differentiated tumors to >15 cm for poorly differentiated tumors), abdominal, vaginal, and/or rectal examination readily identifies an adnexal mass in approximately 95% of symptomatic patients. The most common premonitory symptoms, namely, menstrual disorders and subtle androgenic manifestations, predate by several months, and less often, by years, the recognition of the overt clinical signs or symptoms. Irregular bleeding, oligomenorrhea, and postmenopausal bleeding, retrospectively, have been attributed to either excess androgens or estrogens. The etiology of the latter is presumably the peripheral conversion of androgens to estrogens or, rarely, from an estrogen-secreting SLCT. Frank virilization occurs in 35% of the patients with SLCTs, and another 10% to 15% have some clinical manifestations consistent with androgen excess. The most frequent androgenic symptom complex encountered includes amenorrhea, voice deepening, and hirsutism. In addition, breast atrophy, clitorimegaly, loss of female contour, and temporal hair recession, for example, are signs of masculinization witnessed in patients with SLCTs (99–101). The prevalence of androgenic manifestations appears to be independent of the degree of histologic differentiation but is observed less frequently in heterologous SLCTs and only occasionally in patients harboring retiform lesions (100, 102–105). Although the preoperative diagnosis of SLCT in the absence of androgenic excess may be impossible, this neoplastic entity should constitute the primary preoperative diagnosis in patients with androgenic manifestations presenting during the second through the fourth decades of life with a unilaterally palpable adnexal mass.

Uncommonly, estrogen manifestations are witnessed in the context of presumed end-organ estrogenic responses, including postmenopausal bleeding and endometrial polyp formation, hyperplasia, and adenocarcinoma. Cautious interpretation of such observations is required, realizing that peripheral conversion of androgens to estrogens may be as plausible as a primary estrogen-secreting SLCT. As expected from the clinical findings, most patients demonstrating signs of defeminization or virilization have elevated plasma testosterone levels (99–101). Whereas plasma androstenedione may occasionally be elevated, the urinary 17-ketosteroids, including dehydroepiandrosterone, are usually normal, with the occasional patient presenting with a slightly elevated level. An elevated testosterone/androstenedione ratio generally suggests the presence of an androgen-secreting ovarian tumor, most likely an SLCT. Recognizing that certain gonadotropin-releasing hormone (GnRH) agonists modulate androgen production by downregulating gonadotropin levels and through a direct effect on the ovary, Pascale et al.(106) demonstrated successful suppression of testosterone and androstenedione in five virilized women with the administration of GnRH agonists. Their data suggest that androgen-secreting tumors of the ovary appear to be less autonomous than such tumors originating in the adrenal gland. Surgical excision of the SLCTs results in a precipitous drop in androgen levels and, over time, partial to complete resolution of the clinical manifestations associated with androgen excess is observed.

The coexistence of other diseases with SLCTs has been chronicled. The frequency with which thyroid disease is observed in these patients appears to exceed mere chance. Furthermore, several cases of other mesenchymal tumors have occurred in patients with SLCTs, including sarcoma botryoides of the cervix as well as Ollier's disease (100,107). The latter is a rare disease, but it is associated with other sex cord–stromal tumors, specifically JGCTs, as noted above. Finally, a tendency toward familial occurrence appears to exist (100).

Pathology

Gross Features

Sertoli-Leydig cell tumors vary in size from small to huge masses, but most are between 5 and 15 cm in diameter. The

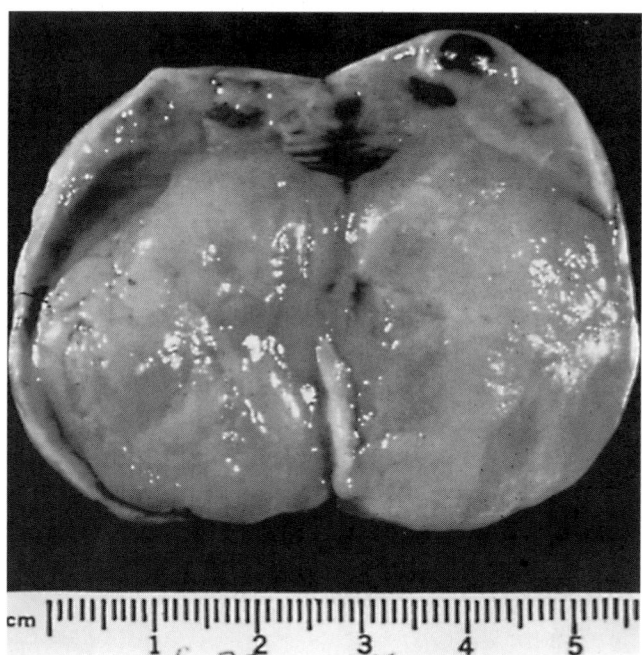

FIG. 27.5. Sertoli-Leydig cell tumor. The sectioned surface of the tumor is focally lobulated and was yellow in the fresh state.

majority are solid, often yellow, and lobulated (Fig. 27.5), but many are solid and cystic. Pure cystic tumors are exceptionally rare, in contrast to the situation with granulosa-cell tumors. Poorly differentiated tumors tend to be larger than those more differentiated, and contain areas of hemorrhage and necrosis more frequently (100). Tumors with heterologous or retiform components are more often cystic than other tumors in this category (102,103,105,108). The heterologous tumors occasionally simulate mucinous cystic tumors on gross examination, and retiform tumors may contain large edematous intracystic papillae, resembling serous papillary tumors, or may be soft and spongy with varying degrees of cystification (105).

Microscopic Features

Well-differentiated SLCTs are characterized by a predominantly tubular pattern (109). On low-power examination, a nodular architecture is often conspicuous, with fibrous bands intersecting lobules composed of small, round, hollow, or, less often, solid tubules lined by well-differentiated cells and separated by variable numbers of Leydig cells.

Sertoli-Leydig cell tumors of intermediate and poor differentiation form a continuum characterized by a variety of patterns and combinations of cell types (99–101). Some tumors exhibit intermediate differentiation in some areas and poor differentiation in others, and less commonly, tumors of intermediate differentiation contain well-differentiated foci. Both the Sertoli cells and the Leydig cells may exhibit varying degrees of immaturity. In tumors of intermediate differentiation, immature Sertoli cells have small, round, oval, or angular nuclei and generally scanty cytoplasm and are arranged typically in ill-defined masses, often creating a lobulated appearance on low power; solid and hollow tubules, nests, broad columns of Sertoli cells, and, most characteristically, thin cords resembling the sex cords of the embryonic testis are often present (Fig. 27.6). These structures are separated by stroma, which ranges from fibromatous to densely cellular to edematous, and typically contains clusters of well-differentiated Leydig cells (Fig. 27.6). Cysts containing eosinophilic secretion may be present and create a thyroid-like appearance, and follicle-like spaces are encountered rarely. The Sertoli-cell and Leydig-cell elements, singly or in combination, may contain varying and sometimes large amounts of lipid in the form of small or large droplets. When a significant amount of the stromal component is made up of immature, cellular mesenchymal tissue with high mitotic activity resembling a nonspecific sarcoma, the tumor is poorly differentiated.

Fifteen percent of SLCTs have a substantial retiform component, and are so designated because they are composed of a network of elongated tubules and cysts, both of which may contain papillae, resembling the rete testis (27). This pattern is usually accompanied by other patterns of SLCTs, but sometimes an entire tumor has a retiform pattern.

Heterologous elements occur in approximately 20% of Sertoli-cell tumors (106,110). In a series of these tumors, 18% contain glands and cysts lined by moderately to well-differentiated intestinal-type epithelium (106). Mesenchymal heterologous elements, encountered in 5% of Sertoli-cell tumors, include islands of cartilage arising on a sarcomatous background, areas of embryonal rhabdomyosarcoma, or both (110).

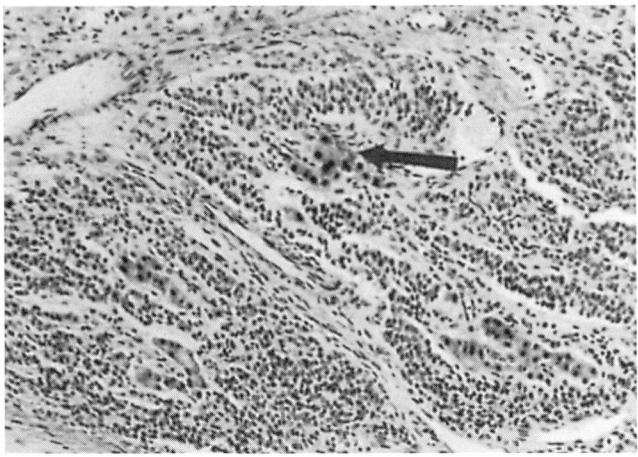

FIG. 27.6. Sertoli-Leydig cell tumor, intermediate differentiation. Nests of large Leydig cells (*arrow*) lie among bands of immature Sertoli cells. (Reprinted with permission from Morris JM, Scully RE. *Endocrine pathology of the ovary.* St. Louis: Mosby, 1958.)

Natural History

SLCTs display characteristics that differ markedly from their epithelial counterparts, notably in regard to their malignant potential. Despite an average size of approximately 16 cm, only 2% to 3% of SLCTs have demonstrable extraovarian spread at the time of detection. Furthermore, Young and Scully (54) identified only 29 clinically malignant cases in their series of 220 SLCTs having variable observation intervals, and they noted an 18% malignancy rate among 164 patients with adequate follow-up. At least in part, the more favorable prognosis reflects the abrupt onset of androgenic manifestations and the early detection of nonspecific symptoms, which promote prompt medical assessment. Nevertheless, the natural history of the malignant variant includes early recurrences, with approximately two-thirds becoming evident within 1 year of treatment and only 6% to 7% recurring after 5 years. The abdominal cavity (including the pelvis) and the retroperitoneal nodes are the most frequent sites for recurrences. In addition, the contralateral ovary, lungs, liver, and bone are other reported sites of recurrent metastatic disease. The collective salvage rates in patients with clinically malignant disease are low, with extrapolated estimates being less than 20%.

Prognostic Factors

Stage is the most important predictor of outcome in SLCTs. Fortunately, 97% of SLCTs are reportedly stage I at diagnosis, and less than 20% of these localized tumors become clinically malignant. The most cogent phenotypic prognostic determinant for stage I SLCTs is the degree of histologic differentiation (99–101). Approximately one-half of the reported SLCTs are of intermediate differentiation, 10% well differentiated, 20% heterologous, and the remainder poorly differentiated. No extraovarian spread or subsequent recurrences were encountered by Young and Scully (109) among 23 well-differentiated SLCTs. However, approximately 10% of intermediate and 60% of poorly differentiated tumors as well as 20% of heterologous tumors demonstrated clinically malignant behavior (100). The heterologous tumors contain either endodermal elements such as gastrointestinal epithelium and carcinoids or mesenchymal elements including skeletal muscles and/or cartilage. The endodermal elements are typically associated with intermediate-differentiated homologous elements and represent 75% of the heterologous SLCTs. Their corresponding prognosis parallels that of the intermediate-differentiated homologous tumors. In contrast, heterologous tumors containing mesenchymal elements account for 5% of all SLCTs and invariably coexist with a poorly differentiated homologous component. The clinically aggressive malignant behavior of poorly differentiated heterologous tumors is witnessed in the extremely low survival (100).

Retiform patterns, tumor size, mitotic activity, and tumor

rupture appear to increase in frequency as the degree of tumor differentiation decreases (99–101). Approximately 10% of neoplasms express histologic patterns resembling the rete testis. They are more commonly observed in younger patients (average age 15 years) and are generally larger, possibly secondary to the less frequent association of androgenic manifestations and hence a later clinical presentation (102–105). Sertoli-Leydig cell tumors harboring a retiform pattern are associated with a 20% malignancy rate, significantly higher than the 12% nonretiform SLCT rate. Young and Scully (105) noted 14 of 25 retiform cases were of intermediate differentiation, with 1 demonstrating poorly differentiated homologous histology and 10 exhibiting heterologous elements (3 intermediate and 7 poorly differentiated). Arguably, the less favorable prognosis reflects the frequency of associated heterologous and/or poorly differentiated homologous lesions. This concept is supported by the findings that the majority of the metastatic lesions do not contain retiform patterns (105). However, the adverse characteristics of the retiform component are witnessed when examining tumors of intermediate differentiation. Although only 4 of over 100 reported intermediate-differentiated SLCTs were clinically malignant, 3 of the 4 contained retiform patterns (100).

Tumor size, mitotic activity, and tumor rupture have been reported to influence prognosis (100,101). The size, mitotic index, and rupture frequency appear to increase as histologic dedifferentiation increases. Notwithstanding these associations, substratification of intermediate and poorly differentiated lesions according to these parameters identifies significant prognostic differences.

The frequency of androgen excess has been addressed above, with 50% or more of patients diagnosed with SLCTs either directly or indirectly displaying clinical manifestations of hyperandrogenism. Serum testosterone levels are invariably elevated when virilization is present, and selective venous catheterization has documented the ovary as the site of origin (111,112). In addition, immunostaining was positive for testosterone in eight SLCTs analyzed, including a limited number of tumors from patients without clinical signs or symptoms of androgen excess (2,113). The Leydig cells, as anticipated, were shown to be the cell of origin for the synthesis of testosterone. Following cytoreductive surgery, the serum testosterone levels are rapidly cleared from the circulation and have been reported on occasion to increase again as a function of the burden of recurrent metastatic disease.

Other unique secretory products, namely, inhibin and alpha fetoprotein (AFP), have been reported in a limited number of SLCTs and are proteins generally equated with granulosa-cell tumors (GCTs) and germ-cell tumors, respectively (103,105,112–114). In addition to GCTs, the Sertoli and Leydig cells have been shown to produce inhibin in testicular tissues, and presumably these same cell types are the site of origin in the SLCTs. Motoyama et al. (114) summarized the literature and reported the fourteenth case of an elevated serum AFP accompanying SLCTs. A clinically malignant course was appreciated in 43% of the described population, which had a mean age of 16 years. In addition, the majority (57%) was described as having a retiform component, a frequency substantially higher than the 10% usually seen in larger SLCT samples. Perhaps preferential AFP sampling accounts for a portion of this seemingly unusually high frequency in that, histologically, the retiform pattern may be confused with an endodermal sinus tumor, particularly in the absence of clinical androgenic manifestations. The Sertoli and Leydig cells appear to be the cells of origin for AFP within the tumor. Employing immunostaining, Gagnon et al. (113) confirmed that Leydig cells appear to be the predominant site for AFP synthesis, but Sertoli cells are also capable of producing this oncoprotein. Testing four retiform and four nonretiform SLCTs, they demonstrated a 50% positivity rate in both histologic subtypes. The precise frequency of both inhibin and AFP positivity and their correlation with disease activity await larger confirmatory assessments.

OVARIAN SEX CORD TUMOR WITH ANNULAR TUBULES

In 1970, Scully (60) described a limited series of unique ovarian tumors characterized by either simple or complex ring-shaped tubules and proposed the morphologic designation ovarian sex cord tumor with annular tubules (SCTATs). The distinctive cellular elements of these neoplasms were judged to be histologically representative of an intermediate between Sertoli-cell and granulosa-cell tumors. Shen et al. (115) reported that SCTATs accounted for 6% of the sex cord tumors treated at their institution. An association with PJS was likewise recognized, and in a subsequent report of 74 cases of SCTAT, Young et al. (116) noted approximately one in three SCTATs occurred in patients with PJS. Ovarian sex cord tumors with annular tubules occurring in association with PJS are typically small (many microscopic), multifocal, calcified, and bilateral. The average age of presentation is the early to mid portion of the fourth decade of life (116,117). The non-PJS tumors are considerably larger, seldom multifocal or calcified, and invariably unilateral. The average age of these patients is the mid to latter portion of the third decade of life.

Abnormal vaginal bleeding is the most common presenting complaint, including menstrual irregularities during the reproductive era and postmenopausal bleeding during the mature years. Menometrorrhagia followed by prolonged episodes of amenorrhea is commonly experienced in the non-PJS patients. Abdominal pain or discomfort is less frequently encountered but generally accompanies grossly involved adnexa or other incidental pelvic pathology. In addition, the signs and symptoms accompanying intussusception secondary to colonic polyp formation may be manifested in PJS-associated patients. The majority of PJS-associated SCTATs are not detectable via clinical examination and are appreciated unexpectedly during surgical or pathologic assessment. In contrast, the majority of non-PJS SCTATs are palpable on abdominal and/or vaginal examination. Although these tumors are seldom encountered during the first decade of life, isosexual precocity is invariably witnessed when SCTATs are diagnosed in affected children (116–119).

Considering the rarity of both PJS, an autosomal dominant disorder, and SCTAT, the frequency of concurrency of these two processes suggests a potential linkage in their pathogenesis. Approximately 36% of SCTATs are observed in patients with PJS. In addition, 15% of PJS-associated SCTATs also develop adenoma malignum of the cervix, a neoplasm that defies early diagnosis and is associated with a relatively high mortality (116,120–122). A recent report of 34 patients with PJS demonstrated a significantly elevated risk (relative risk = 20.3) of breast and gynecologic malignancies in women (123); one patient had a Sertoli-Leydig tumor and three had sex cord tumors with annular tubules. The PJS gene was mapped to chromosome 19p13.3 (124) and was later identified as a novel serine threonine kinase, STK11 (125). Because of the wide variety of malignancies occurring in individuals with PJS, STK11 is believed to function as a general tumor-suppressor gene.

Contingent on the patient's age, precocious puberty, menstrual irregularities, or postmenopausal bleeding are clinical manifestations of SCTATs, indirectly attesting to their endocrine activity (116–120,122,126,127). These signs of hyperestrogenism and the corresponding effects on the endometrium were readily recognized in the initial description of these unique tumors (53). Numerous reports have confirmed the presence of endometrial hyperplasia and/or polyp formation, particularly in PJS-associated SCTATs. Although similar signs in endometrial histology can be observed in non-PJS SCTATs, clinical histories of menorrhagia followed by episodes of amenorrhea are more frequently obtained (115–118,126,127). Endometrial sampling in a limited population of such patients has demonstrated a spectrum from atrophic glandular to secretory or decidualized endometrium suggestive of significant levels of progesterone production (115,117,127). Assessment of circulating steroid levels has confirmed the presence of excessive estrogen in essentially all SCTAT cases (115,126–128). However, normal progesterone levels have been observed in PJS-associated tumors, but elevated quantities of progesterone have been documented in non-PJS patients (115,126–128). Chen et al. (115) demonstrated elevated estrogen and progesterone levels (and normal testosterone levels) in two SCTAT patients without PJS having documented glandular atrophy and decidual stromal changes. Utilizing selective ovarian venous sampling, Crain (127) demonstrated a significant progesterone gradient between peripheral and ovarian venous serum in a non-PJS patient with pseudodecidual changes of the endometrium. Complete resolution of the manifestations attributed to these hormonal imbalances has been routinely witnessed with surgical extirpation of the ovarian neoplasm.

Pathology

Grossly, the PJS-associated tumors are solid and yellow. The non–PJS-associated neoplasms may be similar, but in some cases, they are solid and cystic or mostly cystic. This tumor is characterized microscopically by the presence of simple and complex annular tubules (Fig. 27.7). The simple tubules have the shape of a ring, with the nuclei oriented around the periphery and around a central hyalinized body composed of basement membrane material; an intervening anuclear cytoplasmic zone forms the major component of the ring. The more numerous complex tubules are rounded structures made up of intercommunicating rings revolving around multiple hyaline bodies. In patients with PJS, the tumors are typically multifocal and exhibit calcification.

Prognostic Factors

Notwithstanding their histologic similarities, the differences in the natural history and hence long-term prognosis for SCTATs associated with PJS and SCTATs independent of PJS are readily apparent. Those detected in women with PJS are benign. Important in the management of this entity, however, is the recognition that approximately 15% of these patients will harbor an adenoma malignum of the cervix (AMC). As a result of delayed declaration of symptoms, the diagnosis of AMC is frequently made following examination of the hysterectomy specimen. As evident in the recent review by Srivatsa et al. (122), the prognosis for PJS patients with SCTAT and AMC is ominous, reflecting high AMC recurrence rates and refractoriness to treatment.

Based on the compiled data from four reported series total-

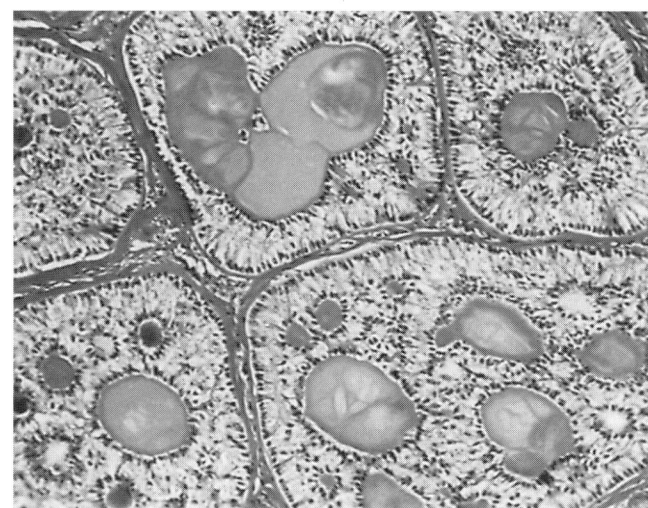

FIG. 27.7. Sex cord tumor with annular tubules. Numerous rounded tubules encircle multiple hyaline bodies.

ing 63 patients with SCTATs without clinically apparent PJS, the clinical malignancy rate approximated 20% (115–118). Primary extraovarian extension and/or the recurrence frequency has been correlated with the original tumor size and mitotic activity. The tumor characteristically has a relatively long doubling time, a propensity for lymphatic dissemination, and an aptness to remain lateralized. As the primary ovarian lesion is invariably unilateral, the lymphatic metastases are invariably ipsilateral, extending within the confines from the paraaortic region to the supraclavicular area. The nature of the retroperitoneal metastases generally facilitates surgical resection and repeat cytoreduction. The tumor's indolent growth pattern, coupled with the relative ease of resection, affords patients extended palliation.

Because SCTATs possess characteristics of both granulosa cells and Sertoli cells, tumor markers elicited by either or both cell types might find utility in the diagnosis and surveillance of these tumors as well. The observed increased serum estrogen levels and the corresponding clinical manifestations recognized with SCTATs suggest utility in monitoring hormone levels. Unfortunately, serum estradiol lacks adequate sensitivity, particularly when the residual tumor volume is limited. However, recent reports demonstrate the potential value and sensitivity of two unique secretory proteins as tumor markers for SCTATs. Gustafson et al. (128) illustrated the applicability of monitoring serum inhibin and müllerian-inhibiting substance (MIS) in the management of a patient with advanced, recurrent SCTAT. More recently, Puls et al. (129) likewise reported an excellent correlation between serum inhibin and MIS levels and the clinical status of a patient with SCTAT during chemotherapy administration. The ultimate utility of these tumor markers awaits accrual of sufficient numbers of patients with SCTATs to address adequately sensitivity and specificity issues.

SEX CORD–STROMAL TUMORS, UNCLASSIFIED

This ill-defined group of tumors, which accounts for less than 10% of those in the sex cord–stromal category, comprises those in which a predominant pattern of testicular or ovarian differentiation is not clearly recognizable. Talerman and his associates (130) have recently segregated from within this category a group of tumors for which they have proposed the designation ''diffuse nonlobular androblastoma.'' The six ovarian tumors they reported were mostly estrogenic and had a predominant diffuse proliferation of cells resembling theca cells, granulosa cells, or both, but five of the six cases also contained steroid-type cells and tubules typical of Sertoli-cell neoplasia.

Sex cord–stromal tumors may be particularly difficult to subclassify when they occur in pregnant patients because of alterations in their usual clinical and pathologic features (131). Their nature is rarely suggested clinically because during pregnancy estrogenic manifestations are not recognizable, and androgenic manifestations are rare. In one

study, 17% of 36 SCSTs that were removed during pregnancy were placed in the unclassified group, and many of those that were classified in the granulosa-cell or Sertoli-Leydig cell category had large areas with an indifferent appearance (131).

Gynandroblastoma

Gynandroblastoma is an extremely rare SCST if strict morphologic criteria are followed to establish the diagnosis. Microscopically, these tumors must demonstrate readily identifiable (at least 10%) granulosa cells and tubules of Sertoli cells. Not surprisingly, the corresponding stromal cells, namely, theca and/or Leydig cells, may also be present in varying degrees. Martin-Jimenez and colleagues (132) recently reviewed the world literature and were able to identify only 17 authenticated cases of gynandroblastoma. Patients presented at an average age of 29.5 years (range 16 to 65 years) with primary symptoms of menstrual disturbances consistent with the predominant functional status of the tumor. Commonly, a hyperandrogenic clinical profile is elicited, but signs and symptoms of excessive estrogens or no endocrine manifestations can be encountered. Amenorrhea, hirsutism, and clitorimegaly are frequently noted in association with elevated testosterone levels. Conversely, the common end-organ responses to hyperestrogenism include menometrorrhagia, postmenopausal bleeding, and endometrial hyperplasia. Although the unilateral masses are typically small, 75% are palpable prior to surgical exploration and are characterized by well-differentiated ovarian and testicular constituent elements. Regardless of the associated hormonal activity, gynandroblastomas are considered to be tumors of low malignant potential. To date, only a single case was reported to have been clinically malignant and resulted in death of the patient (133). Recently, a gynandroblastoma in pregnancy was reported (134).

Steroid-Cell Tumors

Steroid-cell tumors (SCTs) constitute only 0.1% of all ovarian neoplasms. The predominant components of these tumors are steroid hormone–secreting cells including lutein cells, Leydig cells, and adrenocortical cells. Until recently, the term *lipid-cell tumors* was applied to these neoplasms, but Hayes and Scully (135) noted that 25% of such designated tumors did not contain appreciable intracellular fat. Hence, the functional designation, steroid-cell tumors, was suggested and stratified into three subclasses: stromal luteoma, Leydig-cell tumor, and steroid-cell tumors not otherwise specified. The first two categories are essentially invariably benign, but some in the third group are malignant.

Stromal Luteoma

In 1964, Scully (136) described the stromal luteoma as a distinctive type of steroid-cell tumor. These relatively small

(<3 cm) tumors are localized within the parenchyma of the ovary and account for approximately 25% of SCTs. They are thought to arise from luteinized stromal cells or their precursors. Histologically, the adjacent ovarian matrix as well as the contralateral ovary demonstrate stromal hyperthecosis in the vast majority of cases. The distinction between nodular hyperthecosis and stromal luteomas has been arbitrarily based on size, with lesions <5 mm being referred to as nodular hyperthecosis. In contrast to stromal hyperthecosis, stromal luteomas are rarely bilateral.

The average age at which stromal luteomas are diagnosed is the latter half of the sixth decade of life, with 80% occurring after the climacterium (135). Considering the predominant functional profile is estrogenic, the result of either direct tumor secretion or peripheral conversion of androgens, it is not surprising that abnormal vaginal bleeding is the primary complaint. In a series of 25 cases reported by Hayes and Scully (135), information regarding the histologic architecture of the endometrium was known for 17 cases, which included 14 cases of hyperplasia and a single case of a well-differentiated adenocarcinoma of the endometrium. Conversely, 12% of the patients presented with clinical manifestations of hyperandrogenism. In their analysis, 20% of the tumors were functionally quiescent and were detected incidentally during histologic assessment of surgical specimens processed for a variety of other indications.

Prognostic Factors

Considering the small size and lack of atypical histology, the posttreatment course is benign. To date, we are unaware of a single adverse outcome. Any untoward sequelae related to the stromal luteoma would presumably reflect secondary events from prolonged excessive hormone secretions such as an endometrial carcinoma.

Leydig-Cell Tumors

Leydig-cell tumors account for only 15% to 20% of SCTs. Histologically, the cellular elements are indistinguishable from lutein cells or adrenocortical cells except for the presence of crystals of Reinke, a requirement based on either light or electron microscopy for definitive diagnosis. Roth and Sternberg (137) subdivided these tumors according to location and possibly the cell of origin; namely, Leydig-cell tumors of hilar type versus nonhilar type. Whereas the latter presumably arise from ovarian stromal cells and are extremely rare, the former tumors are located in the hilus of the ovary and encroach on or extend into the ovarian stroma in varying degrees. Other tumors containing features of Leydig-cell tumors (such as location in the ovarian hilus or adjacent to nonmedullated nerve fibers, location within a continuum of hilar-cell hyperplasia, fibrinoid vascular changes in the tumor, clustering of cells around vessels) but lacking crystals of Reinke are preferably categorized as steroid-cell

tumors not otherwise specified (138). By combining two reviews (138,139) that summarize the English-language literature prior to and after 1966, 38 Reinke-positive cases affording adequate abstraction were identified. These invariably unilateral tumors are typically small, ranging in size from 0.7 to 15 cm, with a mean of 2.7 cm, and are therefore frequently not detectable via clinical examination or pelvic imaging. Similar to stromal luteomas, the age of diagnosis is 58 years (range 37 to 86 years), with only a small percentage occurring prior to the climacterium. The initial clinical manifestations are usually consistent with a hyperandrogenic state. Overt signs of virilization are observed in greater than 80% of the patients. These include one or more of the following: hirsutism, acne, deepening of the voice, breast atrophy, clitorimegaly, and male-pattern baldness. In contrast to the frequently dramatic onset and progression of virilization witnessed with SLCTs, ovarian Leydig-cell tumors are generally characterized by a more indolent course. Paraskevas and Scully (138) reported an interval of 7 years between recognized onset of signs and symptoms of androgen excess and diagnosis. Analysis of serum androgens demonstrated testosterone to be consistently elevated while urinary 17-ketosteroids were normal or marginally increased. These observations suggest minimal production of androstenedione or dehydroepiandrosterone by these tumors.

Conversely, estrogenic manifestations are occasionally witnessed, such as irregular menses or postmenopausal bleeding (138,139). Pathologic assessment of the uterus may reveal endometrial hyperplasia, polyp formation, and/or carcinoma in the presence or absence of leiomyomata and/or myohypertrophy. Whether the hyperestrogenic features are a result of tumor secretion of estrogens or peripheral conversion of androgens to estrogens remains to be ascertained.

Prognostic Factors

In a review of the English literature through 1988, 38 Reinke-positive cases were accrued and only a single case of a clinically malignant lesion was identified (138,139). Based on tumor size (15 cm) alone, this sole example might be considered to be an outlier. Hence, similar to stromal luteomas, ovarian Leydig-cell tumors are essentially benign neoplasms with the primary postsurgical concerns consisting of regression of the androgen-induced alterations. Generally speaking, significant regression is witnessed, but significant residual sequelae are appreciated in approximately one-half of the patients.

Steroid-Cell Tumors Not Otherwise Specified

Neoplasms identified as steroid-cell tumors but lacking the specific characteristics of stromal luteomas or Leydig-cell tumors are collectively classified as steroid-cell tumors not otherwise specified (SCTNOS). These tumors constitute the majority of steroid-cell tumors and undoubtedly include both Leydig-cell tumors and stromal luteomas that fail to meet specific identification criteria already noted. Although serving as a catchment for an undefined percentage of steroid hormone–secreting tumors, as a group, the SCTNOS have nonetheless unique characteristics. The natural history and biology of these tumors are significantly different when compared to Leydig-cell tumors or stromal luteomas.

Although the average age at presentation of patients harboring SCTNOS is 43 years (10 to 15 years earlier than stromal luteomas and/or Leydig-cell tumors), these tumors have been diagnosed from early childhood to the ninth decade of life (140). In addition, these generally solid yellow tumors are larger than the other SCTs. The average size at diagnosis approximates 8.5 cm (range 1.2 to 45.0 cm). Furthermore, a higher frequency of bilaterality (5%) in advanced disease is encountered with these neoplasms. In their review of 63 collated cases, Hayes and Scully (140) reported that 81% of cases had localized disease (stage I), 6% had stage II disease, and 13% had stage III or IV disease. Curiously, they noted the average age (54 years) of patients with advanced disease was 10 years older than the group as a whole. At least in part, these findings reflect the absence of documented advanced malignancies during the first two decades of life.

Clinical signs and/or symptoms of androgen excess ranging from heterosexual precocity in prepubertal girls to amenorrhea, hirsutism, and/or virilization during the reproductive and/or postmenopausal ages prompt the majority of patients to seek medical advice (140,141). Not infrequently, the duration of these androgenic changes may have extended over many years (142). Additional concerns at presentation include increasing abdominal girth reflecting tumor size and, rarely, ascites, abdominal pain, cushingoid symptoms, and irregular uterine bleeding. The latter may represent clinical manifestations of estrogen excess (140,143), which has been suggested to occur at a frequency of 6% to 23%. Whether the source of estrogen is *de novo* synthesis by the tumor or from peripheral conversion of androgens remains to be determined. Isosexual precocious pseudopuberty has been detected in young girls harboring SCTNOS (140,144–145). An additional 10% to 15% of patients are asymptomatic, with tumors being detected incidentally during routine pelvic examination or at the time of hysterectomy or other surgical interventions.

The steroid hormone–secreting capacities of SCTNOS are more diverse than those of most sex cord–stromal tumors. Whereas approximately one in four patients do not demonstrate clinical manifestations of hormonal imbalances, the majority of patients with SCTNOS have evidence of androgen excess (10% to 15% estrogen excess) and a lesser percentage of cortisol excess. These excesses are demonstrable via assessment of end-organ responses and serum/plasma steroid levels. Whereas elevated plasma levels of corticosteroids are typically observed in conjunction with SCT-NOS, the number of overt presentations with Cushing's

syndrome is limited (144,146–148). However, 17% of the clinically malignant tumors reported by Hayes and Scully (140) were associated with Cushing's syndrome. The serum testosterone and androstenedione levels are invariably elevated, as are urinary 17-ketosteroids; presumably, the latter reflect the level of excess androstenedione production.

Pathology

Gross Features. The tumors are typically solid, well circumscribed, occasionally lobulated (Fig. 27.8), and average 8.4 cm in diameter (140). Approximately 5% are bilateral. They are typically yellow or orange but are occasionally red, dark brown, or black. Necrosis, hemorrhage, and cystic degeneration are occasionally observed.

Microscopic Features. On microscopic examination, the tumor cells are typically arranged diffusely but occasionally grow in nests, irregular clusters, thin cords, and columns. The polygonal to rounded tumor cells have distinct cell borders, central nuclei, and moderate to abundant amounts of cytoplasm that varies from eosinophilic and granular to vacuolated and spongy (Fig. 27.9). In approximately 60% of the cases, nuclear atypia is absent or minimal and mitotic activity is low (less than 2 MF/10 HPFs). In the remaining cases, grades 1 to 3 nuclear atypia (Fig. 27.3) is present, usually associated with an increase in mitotic activity (up to 15 MFs/10 HPFs).

Prognosis

In contrast to the benign natural history of both ovarian Leydig-cell tumors and stromal luteomas, SCTNOS are associated with a relatively high rate of clinical malignancy.

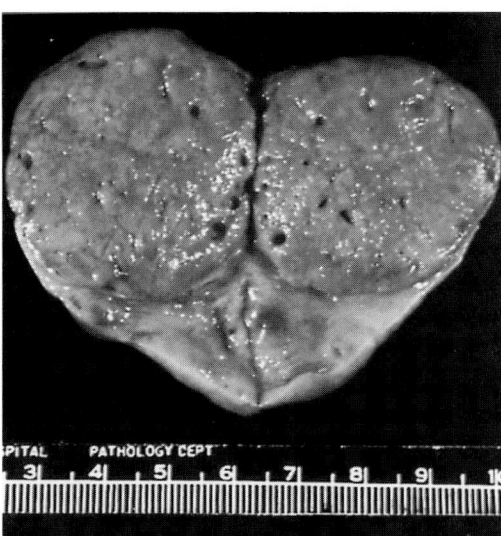

FIG. 27.8. Steroid-cell tumor, unclassified. The sectioned surface of the tumor is lobulated and was yellow-orange in the fresh state. This tumor was from a 9-year-old virilized girl.

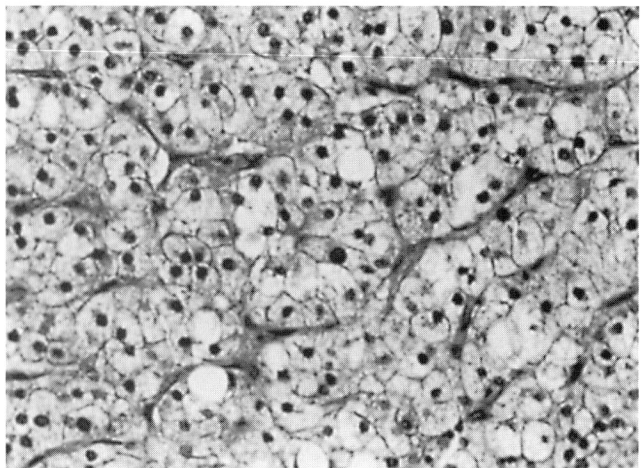

FIG. 27.9. Steroid-cell tumor. The tumor cells are large and rounded and laden with lipid vacuoles. (Reprinted with permission from Hayes MC, Scully RE. Ovarian steroid-cell tumors not otherwise specified [lipid cell tumors]: a clinico-pathologic analysis of 63 cases. *Am J Surg Pathol* 1987;11: 835.)

In the largest series in the literature, 43% of patients with follow-up of 3 or more years demonstrated extraovarian disease either at primary surgery or during subsequent follow-up (149). Unfortunately, to date, salvage therapy has been abysmal. Multiple factors appear to correlate with the frequency of disseminated disease including age, stage, tumor size, mitotic activity, tumor necrosis, hemorrhage, and symptoms of Cushing's syndrome. The average age of patients with clinical malignancies was 16 years older than patients without metastatic disease and having had 3 or more years of observation. No clinically malignant cases have been reported to date in patients less than 20 years of age. All malignant SCTNOS were reported to measure 7 cm or more in greatest diameter (140). In fact, 78% of all tumors 7 cm or larger were malignant, whereas only 21% of all benign tumors exceeded this dimension. The most cogent determinant correlating with malignant potential was mitotic activity, with 92% of malignant tumors displaying 2 or more mitotic figures per 10 HPFs. Similarly, in the presence of necrosis, 86% were malignant; if hemorrhage was present, 77% were malignant. In addition, three of four patients (17% of all malignant cases) with recognizable Cushing's syndrome harbored clinically malignant disease (140).

Although the majority of recurrences become clinically manifest within 3 years of diagnosis, Hayes and Scully (140) reported that 22% of recurrences occurred after 3 years and that, in fact, all of these cases occurred after 5 years; the longest interval witnessed was 19 years. Therefore, the duration of posttreatment surveillance should be adjusted accordingly. The only currently available utilizable markers for SCTNOS include the steroid hormones that were elevated prior to definitive treatment.

TREATMENT

The definitive management of sex cord–stromal tumors is dependent on one or more of the following therapeutic determinants: surgical stage, histologic subtype, patient's age and desire for procreation, and various prognostic factors. Surgery alone is sufficient for several SCSTs lacking malignant potential, whereas postoperative adjunctive therapy generally should be considered for patients with advanced disease and Sertoli-Leydig cell tumors with poor differentiation or heterologous elements (150).

Operative Management

Surgery remains the cornerstone of treatment for patients with SCSTs. Definitive therapy for SCSTs commences with an abdominal exploration through an adequate vertical midline incision. Following securing of peritoneal washings for cytologic assessment, inspection and palpation of the viscera are conducted to detect macroscopic disease. Fertility-sparing surgery with unilateral salpingo-oophorectomy seems to be appropriate management for patients with stage IA disease who are desirous of retaining their reproductive potential. For older patients or those with advanced-stage disease or bilateral ovarian involvement, abdominal hysterectomy and bilateral salpingo-oophorectomy is usually indicated. Frozen section examination of the ovarian tumor should be performed to confirm the diagnosis of a sex cord–stromal tumor. Resection of the ovarian tumor will constitute sufficient therapy for the essentially benign neoplasms, including thecomas, fibromas, gynandroblastomas, stromal luteomas, and Leydig-cell, sclerosing stromal, Sertoli-cell, and well-differentiated SLCTs. Furthermore, sex cord tumors with annular tubules associated with PJS are also considered to be benign and can be similarly managed, but it is imperative that the endocervix be evaluated and subsequently monitored for the potential development of an adenoma malignum of the cervix. Conversely, histologic confirmation of granulosa-cell tumors, intermediate or poorly differentiated Sertoli-Leydig cell tumors, sex cord–stromal tumors with annular tubules (independent of PJS), and steroid-cell tumors not otherwise specified will require definitive surgical staging. This includes multiple biopsies from high-yield sites, omentectomy, and pelvic and paraaortic lymph node sampling/dissection, although the benefit of comprehensive staging in those tumors has not been established.

Following careful surgical staging and in the absence of extraovarian disease, conservation of the uterus and contralateral ovary is reasonable in patients wishing preservation of fertility. However, when electing conservative, fertility-sparing treatment, a thorough curettage must be performed in all patients with estrogen-producing tumors whether they are considered to be benign or potentially malignant (4). If fertility is not an issue or if extraovarian spread of disease is documented, a hysterectomy and residual salpingo-oophorectomy should be performed. Although no scientific evidence exists pertaining to the efficacy of cytoreduction in SCSTs, based on the benefits observed with their epithelial counterparts, we endorse an aggressive maximum effort at primary surgery if metastatic disease is encountered. The value of secondary tumor reduction continues to be controversial but appears to be meritorious in the more indolent tumor types such as GCTs and SCTATs (those not associated with PJS). Repeat cytoreduction frequently affords these patients extended palliation. It is therefore mandatory that the surgeon have adequate familiarity with the natural history of the various SCSTs and the technical expertise to facilitate optimal surgical management.

POSTOPERATIVE MANAGEMENT AND MANAGEMENT OF RECURRENT DISEASE

Granulosa-Cell Tumors (Adult)

The vast majority of women with stage I disease have an excellent prognosis after surgery alone and do not require adjuvant therapy. For those with stage IC disease, consideration can be given to adjuvant therapy on an individualized basis. Most women presenting with stages II to IV disease would be advised to have postoperative therapy depending on their individual characteristics.

Whereas some investigators have reported improved outcomes in patients treated with adjuvant radiation therapy, other investigators have found no clear value to the use of adjuvant radiation therapy (4,6,12,151). Because of the rarity of granulosa cell tumor, it is difficult to conduct prospective trials in these patients. Two retrospective reports provide some data on the use of radiotherapy. Savage et al. reviewed the courses of 62 women treated for adult GCTs at the Royal Marsden Hospital from 1969 to 1995 (152). Thirty-eight (61%) had stage I disease. Eleven of the stage I patients had adjuvant pelvic radiation. The 10-year disease-free survival of these patients was 77% versus 78% for stage I patients treated with surgery alone. Unfortunately, neither complete surgical staging information nor the features that led to the selection of patients for adjuvant radiation were provided. For eight patients with inoperable disease (or residual disease postoperatively), radiation resulted in complete responses in four (50%) that lasted 16 months to 5 years.

Wolf et al. reported on 34 patients with GCTs treated with radiation at M.D. Anderson Cancer Center, 14 of whom had measurable disease (151). Six of the 14 (43%) had a clinical complete response. Three of the responders were alive without evidence of disease 10 to 21 years after radiation.

The Gynecologic Oncology Group (GOG) has reported the largest series of women with ovarian SCSTs treated with chemotherapy. They used four cycles of cisplatin, bleomycin, and etoposide (153). Eligible patients had incompletely resected stage II to IV or recurrent disease. Seventy-five patients entered but 18 were ineligible because of incorrect histology or disease status. Of the 57 eligible patients, 41 had recurrent disease and 16 primary disease. Thirty-nine had gross residual disease following surgery. Forty-eight had GCTs, seven had SLCTs, one a malignant thecoma, and one an unclassified SCST. This chemotherapy combination was considered to be active, with 11 of 16 primary-disease patients and 21 of 41 recurrent-disease patients remaining progression free at a median follow-up of 3 years. Recognizing the prolonged natural history of these tumors, longer follow-up of this cohort will be important. The regimen was fairly toxic, with two bleomycin-related fatalities among the first six patients treated with the initial bleomycin dose of 20 U/m^2 (maximum 30 U) weekly for 9 weeks. The bleomycin dose was then reduced (20 U/m^2 every 3 weeks × 4 cycles) with no mention of further toxicity. Grade 4 myelotoxicity occurred in 61% of the patients. The value of bleomycin in the treatment of this tumor type remains in question (154).

Gershenson et al. (155) also reported on the use of bleomycin, etoposide, and cisplatin in a group of nine women with poor-prognosis SCSTs of the ovary (seven had metastatic disease). The median progression-free survival was 14 months, with a median survival time of 28 months. These investigators, in the same publication, describe activity with paclitaxel in patients with granulosa-cell tumors who have failed platinum-based therapies. In an earlier series, Gershenson et al. (149) found that cisplatin, doxorubicin, and cyclophosphamide were shown to have activity in the treatment of metastatic ovarian stromal tumors, including two Sertoli-Leydig cell tumors. The overall response rate was 63% in this series.

The management of patients with recurrent disease must be individualized. Given the characteristic inolent growth pattern of GCTs, with long disease-free intervals, surgical resection of disease recurrence is often the initial step in the management of appropriate patients. Pecorelli et al. treated 38 patients with advanced (n = 7) or recurrent (n = 31) GCTs with cisplatin, vinblastine, and bleomycin (PVB) on a prospective trial through the EORTC (156). Of the seven women who presented with advanced disease (stages II to IV), one was alive and disease-free at 81 months. Five died between 4 and 12 months after the start of PVB, and another was alive with disease at two months. Among the 31 women with recurrent disease, 7 were alive without further evidence of disease from 24 to 81 months from the start of PVB. Consistent with the indolent course observed with GCTs in some women, another 11 women were alive with disease at a mean of 45 months from the start of PVB (median 39 months).

The wisdom of using a germ cell–like regimen for stromal tumors is questionable. Uygun et al. reported on a small series of 11 women with recurrent GCTs (157). Most had cyclophoshamide, Adriamycin (doxorubicin), and cisplatin (CAP) in the adjuvant setting. Four were treated with cyclophosphamide and cisplatin for recurrence and survived 35 to 73 months after recurrence. A case report of a dramatic response to paclitaxel in a patient with a GCT 2 years following cessation of platinum-based therapy has also been published (158). The GOG is currently conducting a phase II trial of paclitaxel in women with stromal tumors with measurable disease (GOG protocol 187)—either previously untreated or recurrent. At M. D. Anderson Cancer Center, taxane-based chemotherapy (usually the combination of paclitaxel and carboplatin) has been employed for patients with either newly diagnosed or recurrent sex cord–stromal tumors for the past few years. Preliminary analysis indicates that taxane-based chemotherapy appears to be promising, and the final analyses are in the process of being completed.

Considerable rationale exists for the utilization of hormone-based approaches in GCTs. A proportion of these tumors express steroid hormone receptors (159). Responses of GCTs, occasionally long-term, to medroxyprogesterone acetate and to GnRH antagonists have been reported (160–163). Fishman et al. (164) treated six patients with recurrent or persistent GCTs with monthly intramuscular injections of leuprolide acetate. Four patients had received prior cisplatinum-based chemotherapy. Five patients had evaluable disease: two had partial responses and three had stable disease. The leuprolide was well tolerated.

Granulosa-Cell Tumors (Juvenile)

Calaminus et al. (165) reported the outcome of 33 patients with JGCTs—24 treated with surgery alone and 9 with surgery and cisplatinum-based chemotherapy. There have been six relapses, with 60 months median follow-up: 2 of 20 stage IA, 2 of 8 stage IC, and 2 of 5 stages IIC to IIIC. Three patients with stage IIC to IIIC disease treated with adjuvant cisplatinum-based therapy remain disease free at 46 to 66 months after diagnosis. Furthermore, Powell and Otis (166) reported short-term disease control in two teenagers with stage III JGCTs following surgery and cisplatinum-based chemotherapy.

German investigators published their 15-year experience (1985 to 2000) with 54 sex cord–stromal tumors in children and adolescents (65). Forty-five were JGCTs. Twelve received adjuvant chemotherapy for stages IC to IIIC disease. Bleomycin, etoposide, and cisplatin (BEP), and cisplatin, etoposide, and ifosfamide (PEI) were the most commonly used regimens. Six patients remained in remission after adjuvant chemotherapy from 15 to 106 months later. A seventh developed a contralateral JGCT 10 years after her initial primary tumor. Five of the 12 have recurred, 3 of whom died 16 to 28 months from diagnosis.

Powell et al. have reported a patient with long-term disease-free survival following salvage chemotherapy for recurrent JGCT (167). The patient had presented with stage IIIC disease initially treated by resection of all gross disease followed by carboplatin and etoposide for six cycles. She recurred 13 months later with limited disease in the liver and a mass at the inferior aspect of the spleen. She underwent gross total resection followed by six cycles of bleomycin and paclitaxel. She was disease-free 44 months later, delivering a normal baby at cesarean section.

Sertoli-Leydig Cell Tumors

Therapy for those few individuals presenting with high-stage SLCTs, as well as for individuals with recurrent disease must be individualized. The effectiveness of radiation therapy is unknown (101). Reports exist of responses to vincristine, actinomycin D, and cyclophosphamide (VAC) and cisplatinum, doxorubicin, and cyclophosphamide (149,168). Schneider et al. reported three patients with SLCTs who were treated with platinum-based chemotherapy (65). One patient with stage IC disease with intermediate differentiation received two cycles of the combination of cisplatin and etoposide and was disease-free at 47 months. Two other patients, both of whom had stage IC poorly differentiated SLCTs, were dead of tumor at 7 and 19 months after receiving either BEP or PEI. Given the functional hormonal nature of many of these neoplasms, consideration could also be given to some form of hormonal manipulation, such as luteinizing hormone–releasing agonists or antagonists (169).

Sex Cord Tumor with Annular Tubules

Given the rarity of this tumor, the collective experience with systemic therapy for SCTATs is scant. Their endocrine activities suggest that the tumors may retain responsiveness to perturbation of gonadotropin levels. A recent case report documents a complete response to etoposide, bleomycin, and cisplatinum in a patient with recurrent SCTAT (129).

BIOLOGY

Epidemiology

The etiopathogenesis of ovarian cancer remains unknown. One frequently forwarded hypothesis contends that the exposure of the gonad to persistently high levels of pituitary gonadotropins facilitates malignant transformation (170). This hypothesis received support from epidemiologic work suggesting an increased risk of epithelial tumors, borderline and malignant, in women who had received fertility-promoting agents (171). In contrast, Unkila-Kallio et al. (172) questioned a possible link between fertility-promoting agents and GCTs based on a study using the nationwide Finnish Cancer Registry. They analyzed the occurrence of GCTs in Finland during the time period 1965 to 1994 against sales statistics for ovulation inducers. In fact, the incidence of GCTs declined by nearly 40% from 1965–1969 to 1985–1994, whereas the use of clomiphene citrate increased 13-fold and that of human menopausal gonadotropin increased

200-fold. Of interest, oral contraceptive use increased fivefold. To date, no inherited predisposition to GCTs has been identified (173). Moreover, major risk factors for GCTs have not been defined. Reproductive factors, including the use of fertility-promoting agents and oral contraceptives, do not correlate consistently with the development of disease.

The natural history of sex cord–stromal tumors is uniquely different from that of their epithelial counterparts and provides an intriguing tumor model. The vast majority of these neoplasms are characteristically of low malignant potential. They are typically unilateral and remain localized, retain hormone-secreting functions, and infrequently develop recurrences, many of which are delayed. In contrast, a small percentage of otherwise phenotypically similar tumors demonstrate a more virulent course and are generally refractory to therapy. The SCST subtypes display a bimodal age distribution, with notably JGCTs, SSCTs, SLCTs, and SCTATs occurring predominantly during the first three decades of life. Furthermore, the association of these tumors with several uncommon congenital disease entities, such as enchondromatosis, leprechaunism, and PJS, occurs at frequencies that exceed mere chance. Uniquely, several of these functioning neoplasms, including AGCTs, JGCTs, SLCTs, and SCTATs, overexpress growth-regulatory substances including inhibin, müllerian-inhibiting substance, and follicle-regulating protein. Given the limited number of ovarian SCSTs available for study, our current understanding of the mechanism of oncogenesis in these tumors is recognizably meager.

GENETICS, PHYSIOLOGY, AND MOLECULAR BIOLOGY

Conventional cytogenetic studies suggest that trisomy 12 may be a characteristic, nonrandom numerical chromosomal anomaly in select ovarian tumors. As a sole abnormality, trisomy 12 has most often been associated with sex cord–stromal tumors, including fibromas, fibrothecomas, thecomas, and GCTs (174–176). Fluorescent *in situ* hybridization (FISH) techniques, using probes for the alpha satellite region of chromosome 12, enable the study of paraffin-embedded tissue. This allows the analysis of larger numbers of cases while avoiding *in vitro* culture artifact. Utilizing this technique in the study of chromosome 12 in sex cord–stromal tumors, Persons et al. (177) confirmed the occurrence of trisomy 12 in 40% of 20 fibromas. However, the examination of 24 AGCTs showed no evidence of trisomy 12. Other investigators have demonstrated trisomy 12 in JGCTs (178,179). A gain of a whole chromosome may impart a proliferative advantage to a neoplastic clone by affecting the dosage of a gene or multiple genes located on that chromosome. A candidate gene on chromosome 12 is K-*ras*; however, Yang-Feng et al. (180) failed to demonstrate amplification of K-*ras* in ovarian tumors with trisomy 12.

Thus, further investigation is necessary to determine the possible pathologic role of trisomy 12 in sex cord–stromal tumors. Monosomy 22 and trisomy 14 have been reported in GCTs in case reports (181,182).

Our current knowledge regarding various autocrine and endocrine regulatory mechanisms influencing ovarian function, the overexpression of inhibin in several SCSTs, the alterations in ovarian steroidogenesis, and the changes in circulating gonadotropin levels in SCSTs provide several probable clues regarding the pathogenesis of these tumors. Investigations to date exploring the interactive regulatory mechanisms of inhibin, activin, follistatin, and follicle-stimulating hormone (FSH) have predominantly utilized GCTs. Follicle-stimulating hormone provides a fundamental regulatory role in the differentiation processes of granulosa cells during the early stages of follicle development. Specifically, FSH stimulates cell proliferation (mitosis), increases the availability of cell-surface prolactin and luteinizing hormone receptors, and induces aromatase activity, resulting in increased estradiol production. Other growth-regulatory factors such as insulin-like growth factor and epidermal growth factor modulate these actions, including the enhancement of the mitogenic effects of FSH. In addition, FSH secretion from the anterior pituitary is modulated in part by the serum levels of inhibin, activin, and estrogens and/or androgens.

Inhibin, a heterodimeric glycoprotein hormone composed of an alpha-subunit and one of two beta-subunits, is secreted by the granulosa cells of the ovary (183). Inhibin A consists of alpha and beta A; inhibin B, alpha and beta B. Petraglia et al. (184) studied the molecular form of inhibin in adult GCTs and epithelial ovarian cancers. Serum inhibin B was dramatically increased in eight of nine patients with GCTs. Inhibin A was slightly increased in all patients. Its major physiologic function is to inhibit the secretion of FSH by the anterior pituitary gland (185). Inhibin is expressed in excessive quantities by GCTs. Although it maintains its regulatory function pertaining to FSH suppression, it appears to be ineffective in controlling estrogen production and cell proliferation within the gonad. Robertson has recently reviewed the various serum-based assays for inhibin (186).

Activin, also a peptide hormone of ovarian granulosa-cell origin, is composed of two beta-subunits that are identical to those of inhibin. In contrast to inhibin, activin stimulates the secretion of FSH, induces the production of estradiol while having a negative impact on progesterone production, and serves as a promoter of differentiation of granulosa cells (187). Furthermore, follistatin, an additional peptide hormone, is functionally similar to inhibin (it suppresses secretion of FSH and estradiol production), but importantly is an activin-binding protein (185,187).

Biology-Genetics

Mayr et al. performed a comprehensive study of genetic aberrations in GCTs using a paraffin-embedded resource

(188). They studied 17 adult and 3 juvenile GCTs, combining comparative genomic hybridization (CGH); FISH using DNA-specific probes for chromosomes 12, 17, 22, and X; DNA cytometry and immunohistochemistry for inhibin, p53, and Ki-67. DNA cytometry showed 16 of the 20 tumors to be diploid (80%). However, by FISH, 6 of the 16 diploid tumors (37%) had chromosomal aberrations. Namely, FISH showed monosomy 22 in 8 of 18 cases (40%); trisomy 12 in 5 of 20 (25%); monosomy X in 2 of 20 (10%); and loss of chromosome 17 in a single case. The main CGH findings were gains of chromosomes 12 (six cases, 33%) and 14 (six cases, 33%) and losses of chromosomes 22 (seven cases, 35%) and X (one case, 5%), mainly comprising whole chromosomes or chromosomal arms. Immunohistochemistry revealed inhibin expression in 100% of tumors and p53 expression in 95% of tumors. All their patients had surgery at the University of Munich between 1985 and 2000. They had complete follow-up information for 15 of the 20 cases, with an average length of follow-up of 7.2 years. None of the immunohistochemical or genetic analyses provided statistically significant prognostic information.

The etiology of GCTs is poorly understood. P53 status has been assessed by several groups. Whereas one report found no mutations in p53 in GCTs (88), studies using immunohistochemistry to assess protein levels have produced variable results (39,189). The inhibin locus on 2q has also been studied. The frequency of loss of heterozygosity was low (1 of 17 tumors) in one study (188,189).

Given the centrality of FSH in the regulation of granulosa cells, different laboratories have studied the integrity of the FSH receptor in ovarian SCSTs. Kotlar et al. (190) detected a possible mutation (versus polymorphism) in the transmembrane domain of the receptor in a large proportion of a series of sex cord tumors. However, Fuller et al. (191) recognized that this alteration represents a polymorphism. To date, no activating mutations in the FSH receptor gene have been detected in GCTs (192).

Several laboratories have confirmed the presence of increased serum inhibin levels in patients with GCTs, which prior to surgical intervention are typically elevated several times above the normal premenopausal follicular-phase levels and may again become elevated months prior to clinical detection of recurrent disease (45,48,51,67,86). Lappohn et al. (48) and Healy et al. (86) have demonstrated a negative correlation between the serum concentrations of inhibin and FSH. These observations are consistent with the autonomous production of a biologically active form of inhibin by GCTs. A recent report by Sluijimer et al. (51), employing selective ovarian vein and tissue sampling, confirmed the bioactivity of GCT-secreted inhibin via measurement of FSH suppression in cultured rat pituitary cells. Furthermore, Gurusinghe et al. (193), utilizing immunohistochemical techniques, localized the site of excess inhibin-alpha and activins in the GCT to the granulosa cells. These data suggest that a structurally altered (nonfunctional) inhibin receptor might account for the uncontrolled proliferation of granulosa cells stimulated by other positive factors, including activin.

Considering that inhibin, a growth-suppressor protein, is secreted in excessive quantities by nearly all the potentially malignant SCSTs (including AGCTs, JGCTs, SLCTs, and SCTATs), the anticipated future investigative efforts will include the determination of the level of expression and functionality of inhibin, activin, and follistatin; the structural integrity of inhibin and activin receptors; and additional studies of relevant regulatory pathways.

REFERENCES

1. Koonings PP, Campbell K, Mishell DR Jr, et al. Relative frequency of primary ovarian neoplasms: a 10-year review. *Obstet Gynecol* 1989; 74:921–926.
2. Cramer DW, Devesa SS, Welch WR. Trends in the incidence of endometrioid and clear cell cancers of the ovary in the United States. *Am J Epidemiol* 1981;114:201–208.
3. Tavassoli FA. Ovarian tumors with functioning manifestations. *Endocrinol Pathol* 1994;5:137.
4. Evans AT, Gaffey TA, Malkasian GD Jr, et al. Clinicopathologic review of 118 granulosa and 82 theca cell tumors. *Obstet Gynecol* 1980;55:231–238.
5. Malmstrom H, Hogberg T, Risberg B, Simonsen E. Granulosa cell tumors of the ovary: prognostic factors and outcome. *Gynecol Oncol* 1994;52:50–55.
6. Ohel G, Kaneti H, Schenker JG. Granulosa cell tumors in Israel: a study of 172 cases. *Gynecol Oncol* 1983;15:278–286.
7. Rokitansky CV. Über abnormalities des corpus luteum. *Allg Wien Med Z* 1859;4:253.
8. Bjorkholm E. Granulosa cell tumors: a comparison of survival in patients and matched controls. *Am J Obstet Gynecol* 1980;138: 329–331.
9. Bjorkholm E, Silfversward C. Prognostic factors in granulosa-cell tumors. *Gynecol Oncol* 1981;11:261–274.
10. Fox H, Agrawal K, Langley FA. A clinicopathologic study of 92 cases of granulosa cell tumor of the ovary with special reference to the factors influencing prognosis. *Cancer* 1975;35:231–241.
11. Pankratz E, Boyes DA, White GW, et al. Granulosa cell tumors. A clinical review of 61 cases. *Obstet Gynecol* 1978;52:718–723.
12. Piura B, Nemet D, Yanai-Inbar I, et al. Granulosa cell tumor of the ovary: a study of 18 cases. *J Surg Oncol* 1994;55:71–77.
13. Schweppe KW, Beller FK. Clinical data of granulosa cell tumors. *J Cancer Res Clin Oncol* 1982;104:161–169.
14. Stenwig JT, Hazekamp JT, Beecham JB. Granulosa cell tumors of the ovary. A clinicopathological study of 118 cases with long-term follow-up. *Gynecol Oncol* 1979;7:136–152.
15. Young RH, Scully RE. Ovarian sex cord-stromal tumours: recent advances and current status. *Clin Obstet Gynaecol* 1984;11:93–134.
16. Bjorkholm E, Silfversward C. Granulosa- and theca-cell tumors. Incidence and occurrence of second primary tumors. *Acta Radiol Oncol* 1980;19:161–167.
17. Muir CS, Waterhouse JAH, Mack TM, et al. *Cancer incidence in five continents.* IARC Scientific Publications No. 88, Vol V. Lyon, France: International Agency for Research on Cancer, 1987.
18. Schumer ST, Cannistra SA. Granulosa cell tumor of the ovary. *J Clin Oncol* 2003;21:1180–1189.
19. Cronje HS, Niemand I, Bam RH, et al. Review of the granulosa-theca cell tumors from the Emil Novak Ovarian Tumor Registry. *Am J Obstet Gynecol* 1999;180:323–327.
20. Gusberg SB, Kardon P. Proliferative endometrial response to theca-granulosa cell tumors. *Am J Obstet Gynecol* 1971;111:633–643.
21. Stuart GC, Dawson LM. Update on granulosa cell tumours of the ovary. *Curr Opin Obstet Gynecol* 2003;15:33–37.
22. Chen VW, Ruiz B, Killeen J, et al. Pathology and classification of ovarian tumors. *Cancer* 2003;97[10 Suppl]:2631–2642.
23. Young RH, Oliva E, Scully RE. Luteinized adult granulosa cell tumors

of the ovary: a report of four cases. *Int J Gynecol Pathol* 1994;13: 302–310.

24. Nakashima N, Young RH, Scully RE. Androgenic granulosa cell tumors of the ovary. A clinicopathologic analysis of 17 cases and review of the literature. *Arch Pathol Lab Med* 1984;108:786–791.

25. Norris HJ, Taylor HB. Virilization associated with cystic granulosa tumors. *Obstet Gynecol* 1969;34:629–635.

26. Fathalla MF. The occurrence of granulosa and theca tumours in clinically normal ovaries. *J Obstet Gynaecol Br Commonw* 1967;74: 279–282.

27. Young RH, Scully RE. Ovarian sex cord-stromal tumors with bizarre nuclei: a clinicopathologic analysis of 17 cases. *Int J Gynecol Pathol* 1983;1:325–335.

28. Spencer HW, Mullings AM, Char G, et al. Granulosa-theca cell tumor of the ovaries. A late metastasizing tumour. *West Indian Med J* 1999: 48:33–35.

29. Dubuc-Lissoir J. Case report: Bone metastasis from a granulosa cell tumor of the ovary. *Gynecol Oncol* 2001;83:400–404.

30. Miller BE, Barron BA, Wan JY, et al. Prognostic factors in adult granulosa cell tumor of the ovary. *Cancer* 1997;79:1951–1955.

31. Fujimoto T, Sakuragi N, Okuyama K, et al. Histopathological prognostic factors of adult granulosa cell tumors of the ovary. *Acta Obstet Gynecol Scand* 2001;80:1069–1074.

32. Kottmeier HL. *Carcinoma of the female genitalia.* Baltimore: Williams & Wilkins, 1953.

33. Klemi PJ, Joensuu H, Salmi T. Prognostic value of flow cytometric DNA content analysis in granulosa cell tumor of the ovary. *Cancer* 1990;65:1189–1193.

34. Chadha S, Cornelisse CJ, Schaberg A. Flow cytometric DNA ploidy analysis of ovarian granulosa cell tumors. *Gynecol Oncol* 1990;36: 240–245.

35. Evans MP, Webb MJ, Gaffey TA, et al. DNA ploidy of ovarian granulosa cell tumors. Lack of correlation between DNA index or proliferative index and outcome in 40 patients. *Cancer* 1995;75:2295–2298.

36. Ala-Fossi SL, Maenpaa J, Aine R, et al. Prognostic significance of p53 expression in ovarian granulosa cell tumors. *Gynecol Oncol* 1997; 66:475–479.

37. Kappes S, Milde-Langosch K, Kressin P, et al. p53 mutations in ovarian tumors, detected by temperature-gradient gel electrophoresis, direct sequencing and immunohistochemistry. *Int J Cancer* 1995;64: 52–59.

38. King LA, Okagaki T, Gallup DG, et al. Mitotic count, nuclear atypia, and immunohistochemical determination of Ki-67, c-myc, p21-ras, c-erbB2, and p53 expression in granulosa cell tumors of the ovary: mitotic count and Ki-67 are indicators of poor prognosis. *Gynecol Oncol* 1996;61:227–232.

39. Liu FS, Ho ES, Lai CR, et al. Overexpression of p53 is not a feature of ovarian granulosa cell tumors. *Gynecol Oncol* 1996;61:50–53.

40. Dowdy SC, O'Kane DJ, Keeney GL, et al. Telomerase activity in sex cord-stromal tumors of the ovary. *Gynecol Oncol* 2001;82:257–260.

41. Ala-Fossi SL, Aine R, Punnonen R, et al. Is potential to produce inhibins related to prognosis in ovarian granulosa cell tumors? *Eur J Gynaecol Oncol* 2000;21:187–189.

42. Kaye SB, Davies E. Cyclophosphamide, Adriamycin, and cis-platinum for the treatment of advanced granulosa cell tumor, using serum estradiol as a tumor marker. *Gynecol Oncol* 1986;24:261–264.

43. Boggess JF, Soules MR, Goff BA, et al. Serum inhibin and disease status in women with ovarian granulosa cell tumors. *Gynecol Oncol* 1997;64:64–69.

44. Gustafson ML, Lee MM, Asmundson L, et al. Müllerian inhibiting substance in the diagnosis and management of intersex and gonadal abnormalities. *J Pediatr Surg* 1993;28:439–444.

45. Jobling T, Mamers P, Healy DL, et al. A prospective study of inhibin in granulosa cell tumors of the ovary. *Gynecol Oncol* 1994;55: 285–289.

46. Lane AH, Lee MM, Fuller AF Jr, et al. Diagnostic utility of Mullerian inhibiting substance determination in patients with primary and recurrent granulosa cell tumors. *Gynecol Oncol* 1999;73:51–55.

47. Lappohn RE, Burger HG, Bouma J, et al. Inhibin as a marker for granulosa cell tumor. *Acta Obstet Gynecol Scand Suppl* 1992;155: 61–65.

48. Lappohn RE, Burger HG, Bouma J, et al. Inhibin as a marker for granulosa-cell tumors. *N Engl J Med* 1989;321:790–793.

49. Rey RA, L'homme C, Marcillac I, et al. Antimullerian hormone as a serum marker of granulosa cell tumors of the ovary: comparative study with serum alpha-inhibin and estradiol. *Am J Obstet Gynecol* 1996;174:958–965.

50. Rodgers KE, Marks JF, Ellefson DD, et al. Follicle regulatory protein: a novel marker for granulosa cell cancer patients. *Gynecol Oncol* 1990;37:381–387.

51. Sluijmer AV, Heineman MJ, Evers JL, et al. Peripheral vein, ovarian vein and ovarian tissue levels of inhibin in a postmenopausal patient with a granulosa cell tumour. *Acta Endocrinol (Copenh)* 1993;129: 311–324.

52. McCluggage WG. Value of inhibin staining in gynecological pathology. *Int J Gynecol Pathol* 2001;20:79–85.

53. Scully RE. Stromal luteoma of the ovary: a distinctive type of lipoid-cell tumor. *Cancer* 1964;17:769.

54. Young RH, Dickersin GR, Scully RE. Juvenile granulosa cell tumor of the ovary. A clinicopathological analysis of 125 cases. *Am J Surg Pathol* 1984;8:575–596.

55. Lack EE, Perez-Atayde AR, Murthy AS, et al. Granulosa theca cell tumors in premenarchal girls: a clinical and pathologic study of ten cases. *Cancer* 1981;48:1846–1854.

56. Plantaz D, Flamant F, Vassal G, et al. Granulosa cell tumors of the ovary in children and adolescents. Multicenter retrospective study in 40 patients aged 7 months to 22 years. *Arch Fr Pediatr* 1992;49: 793–798.

57. Vassal G, Flamant F, Caillaud JM, et al. Juvenile granulosa cell tumor of the ovary in children: a clinical study of 15 cases. *J Clin Oncol* 1988;6:990–995.

58. Zaloudek C, Norris HJ. Granulosa tumors of the ovary in children: a clinical and pathologic study of 32 cases. *Am J Surg Pathol* 1982;6: 513–522.

59. Bouffet E, Basset T, Chetail N, et al. Juvenile granulosa cell tumor of the ovary in infants: a clinicopathologic study of three cases and review of the literature. *J Pediatr Surg* 1997;32:762–765.

60. Scully RE. Sex cord tumor with annular tubules: a distinctive ovarian tumor of the Peutz-Jeghers syndrome. *Cancer* 1970;25:1107–1121.

61. Asirvatham R, Rooney RJ, Watts HG. Ollier's disease with secondary chondrosarcoma associated with ovarian tumour. A case report. *Int Orthop* 1991;15:393–395.

62. Tamimi HK, Bolen JW. Enchondromatosis (Ollier's disease) and ovarian juvenile granulosa cell tumor. *Cancer* 1984;53:1605–1608.

63. Tanaka Y, Sasaki Y, Nishihira H, et al . Ovarian juvenile granulosa cell tumor associated with Maffucci's syndrome. *Am J Clin Pathol* 1992;97:523–527.

64. Brisigotti M, Fabbretti G, Pesce F, et al. Congenital bilateral juvenile granulosa cell tumor of the ovary in leprechaunism: a case report. *Pediatr Pathol* 1993;13:549–558.

65. Schneider DT, Calaminus G, Wessalowski R, et al. Ovarian sex cord-stromal tumors in children and adolescents. *J Clin Oncol* 2003;21: 2357–2363.

66. Jacoby AF, Young RH, Colvin RB, et al. DNA content in juvenile granulosa cell tumors of the ovary: a study of early- and advanced-stage disease. *Gynecol Oncol* 1992;46:97–103.

67. Swanson SA, Norris HJ, Kelsten ML, et al. DNA content of juvenile granulosa tumors determined by flow cytometry. *Int J Gynecol Pathol* 1990;9:101–109.

68. Bjorkholm E, Silfversward C. Theca-cell tumors. Clinical features and prognosis. *Acta Radiol Oncol* 1980;19:241–244.

69. Norris HJ, Taylor HB. Prognosis of granulosa-theca tumors of the ovary. *Cancer* 1968;21:255–260.

70. Zhang J, Young RH, Arseneau J, et al. Ovarian stromal tumors containing lutein or Leydig cells (luteinized thecomas and stromal Leydig cell tumors)—a clinicopathological analysis of fifty cases. *Int J Gynecol Pathol* 1982;1:270–285.

71. Barrenetxea G, Schneider J, Centeno MM, et al. Pure theca cell tumors. A clinicopathologic study of 29 cases. *Eur J Gynaecol Oncol* 1990;11:429–432.

72. Clement PB, Young RH, Hanna W, Scully RE. Sclerosing peritonitis associated with luteinized thecomas of the ovary. *Am J Surg Pathol* 1994;18:1–13.

73. Dockerty MB, Mason JC. Ovarian fibromas: clinical and pathologic study of 283 cases. *Am J Obstet Gynecol* 1944;47:741.

74. Samanth KK, Black WC. Benign ovarian stromal tumors associated with free peritoneal fluid. *Am J Obstet Gynecol* 1970;107:538–545.

75. Meigs JV. Fibroma of the ovary with ascites and hydrothorax: Meigs' syndrome. *Am J Obstet Gynecol* 1954;67:962.

76. Raggio M, Kaplan AL, Harberg JF. Recurrent ovarian fibromas with basal cell nevus syndrome (Gorlin syndrome). *Obstet Gynecol* 1983; 61[Suppl 3]:95S-96S.

77. Prat J, Scully RE. Cellular fibromas and fibrosarcomas of the ovary: a comparative clinicopathologic analysis of seventeen cases. *Cancer* 1981;47:2663–2670.

78. Chalvardjian A, Scully RE. Sclerosing stromal tumors of the ovary. *Cancer* 1973;31:664–670.

79. Gee DC, Russell P. Sclerosing stromal tumours of the ovary. *Histopathology* 1979;3:367–376.

80. Lam RM, Geittmann P. Sclerosing stromal tumor of the ovary. A light, electron microscopic and enzyme histochemical study. *Int J Gynecol Pathol* 1988;7:280–290.

81. Young RH, Scully RE. Ovarian Sertoli cell tumors: a report of 10 cases. *Int J Gynecol Pathol* 1984;2:349–363.

82. Suit PF, Hart WR. Sclerosing stromal tumor of the ovary. An ultrastructural study and review of the literature to evaluate hormonal function. *Cleve Clin J Med* 1988;55:189–194.

83. Cashell AW, Cohen ML. Masculinizing sclerosing stromal tumor of the ovary during pregnancy. *Gynecol Oncol* 1991;43:281–285.

84. Ismail SM, Walker SM. Bilateral virilizing sclerosing stromal tumours of the ovary in a pregnant woman with Gorlin's syndrome: implications for pathogenesis of ovarian stromal neoplasms. *Histopathology* 1990;17:159–163.

85. Katsube Y, Iwaoki Y, Silverberg SG, et al. Sclerosing stromal tumor of the ovary associated with endometrial adenocarcinoma: a case report. *Gynecol Oncol* 1988;29:392–398.

86. Healy DL, Burger HG, Mamers P, et al. Elevated serum inhibin concentrations in postmenopausal women with ovarian tumors. *N Engl J Med* 1993;329:1539–1542.

87. Van Winter JT, Podratz KC, Gaffey TA. Sclerosing stromal tumor of the ovary in a 13–year-old girl. *Adolesc Pediatr Gynecol* 1993;6:164.

88. Mancuso A, Grosso M, D'Anna R, et al. Anatomo-clinical considerations on the ovarian fibroma. *Clin Exp Obstet Gynecol* 1995;22:115–119.

89. Waxman M, Vuletin JC, Urcuyo R, et al. Ovarian low-grade stromal sarcoma with thecomatous features: a critical reappraisal of the so-called "malignant thecoma." *Cancer* 1979;44:2206–2217.

90. Lage JM, Weinberg DS, Huettner PC, et al. Flow cytometric analysis of nuclear DNA content in ovarian tumors. Association of ploidy with tumor type, histologic grade, and clinical stage. *Cancer* 1992;69:2668–2675.

91. Meyer R. Pathology of some special ovarian tumors and their relation to sex characteristics. *Am J Obstet Gynecol* 1931;22:697.

92. Novak E. Life and works of Robert Meyer. *Am J Obstet Gynecol* 1947;53:50.

93. Morris M, Scully RE. *Endocrine pathology of the ovary.* St. Louis: Mosby, 1958.

94. Aiba M, Hirayama A, Sukurada M, et al. Spironolactone body-like structure in renin-producing Sertoli-cell tumors of the ovary. *Surg Pathol* 1990;3:143.

95. Ehrlich EN, Dominguez OV, Samuels LT, et al. Aldosteronism and precocious puberty due to an ovarian androblastoma (Sertoli cell tumor). *J Clin Endocrinol Metab* 1963;23:358.

96. Korzets A, Nouriel H, Steiner Z, et al. Resistant hypertension associated with a renin-producing ovarian Sertoli cell tumor. *Am J Clin Pathol* 1986;85:242–247.

97. Ferry JA, Young RH, Engel G, et al. Oxyphilic sertoli cell tumor of the ovary: a report of three cases, two in patients with the Peutz-Jeghers syndrome. *Int J Gynecol Pathol* 1994;13:259–266.

98. Tavassoli FA, Norris HJ. Sertoli tumors of the ovary. A clinicopathologic study of 28 cases with ultrastructural observations. *Cancer* 1980;46:2281–2297.

99. Roth LM, Anderson MC, Govan AD, et al. Sertoli-Leydig cell tumors: a clinicopathologic study of 34 cases. *Cancer* 1981;48:187–197.

100. Young RH, Scully RE. Ovarian Sertoli-Leydig cell tumors with a retiform pattern: a problem in histopathologic diagnosis. A report of 25 cases. *Am J Surg Pathol* 1983;7:755.

101. Zaloudek C, Norris HJ. Sertoli-Leydig tumors of the ovary. A clinicopathologic study of 64 intermediate and poorly differentiated neoplasms. *Am J Surg Pathol* 1984;8:405–418.

102. Roth LM, Slayton RE, Brady LW, et al. Retiform differentiation in ovarian Sertoli-Leydig cell tumors. A clinicopathologic study of six cases from a Gynecologic Oncology Group study. *Cancer* 1985;55:1093–1098.

103. Talerman A. Ovarian Sertoli-Leydig cell tumor (androblastoma) with retiform pattern. A clinicopathologic study. *Cancer* 1987;60:3056–3964.

104. Young RH. Sertoli-Leydig cell tumors of the ovary: review with emphasis on historical aspects and unusual variants. *Int J Gynecol Pathol* 1993;12:141.

105. Young RH, Scully RE. Ovarian Sertoli-Leydig cell tumors. A clinicopathological analysis of 207 cases. *Am J Surg Pathol* 1985;9:543–569.

106. Pascale MM, Pugeat M, Roberts M, et al. Androgen suppressive effect of GnRH agonist in ovarian hyperthecosis and virilizing tumours. *Clin Endocrinol (Oxf)* 1994;41:571–576.

107. Weyl-Ben Arush M, Oslander L. Ollier's disease associated with ovarian Sertoli-Leydig cell tumor and breast adenoma. *Am J Pediatr Hematol Oncol* 1991;13:49–51.

108. Young RH, Prat J, Scully RE. Ovarian Sertoli-Leydig cell tumors with heterologous elements. I. Gastrointestinal epithelium and carcinoid: a clinicopathologic analysis of thirty-six cases. *Cancer* 1982;50:2448–2456.

109. Young RH, Scully RE. Well-differentiated ovarian Sertoli-Leydig cell tumors: a clinicopathological analysis of 23 cases. *Int J Gynecol Pathol* 1984;3:277–290.

110. Prat J, Young RH, Scully RE. Ovarian Sertoli-Leydig cell tumors with heterologous elements. II. Cartilage and skeletal muscle: a clinicopathologic analysis of twelve cases. *Cancer* 1982;50:2465–2475.

111. Cohen I, Shapira M, Cuperman S, et al. Direct in-vivo detection of atypical hormonal expression of a Sertoli-Leydig cell tumour following stimulation with human chorionic gonadotrophin. *Clin Endocrinol (Oxf)* 1993;39:491–495.

112. Ohashi M, Hasegawa Y, Haji M, et al. Production of immunoreactive inhibin by a virilizing ovarian tumour (Sertoli-Leydig tumour). *Clin Endocrinol (Oxf)* 1990;33:613–618.

113. Gagnon S, Tetu B, Silva EG, et al. Frequency of alpha-fetoprotein production by Sertoli-Leydig cell tumors of the ovary: an immunohistochemical study of eight cases. *Mod Pathol* 1989;2:63–67.

114. Motoyama I, Watanabe H, Gotoh A, et al. Ovarian Sertoli-Leydig cell tumor with elevated serum alpha-fetoprotein. *Cancer* 1989;63:2047–2053.

115. Shen K, Wu PC, Lang JH, et al. Ovarian sex cord tumor with annular tubules: a report of six cases. *Gynecol Oncol* 1993;48:180–184.

116. Young RH, Welch WR, Dickersin GR, et al. Ovarian sex cord tumor with annular tubules: review of 74 cases including 27 with Peutz-Jeghers syndrome and four with adenoma malignum of the cervix. *Cancer* 1982;50:1384–1402.

117. Hart WR, Kumar N, Crissman JD. Ovarian neoplasms resembling sex cord tumors with annular tubules. *Cancer* 1980;45:2352–2363.

118. Ahn GH, Chi JG, Lee SK. Ovarian sex cord tumor with annular tubules. *Cancer* 1986;57:1066–1073.

119. Solh HM, Azoury RS, Najjar SS. Peutz-Jeghers syndrome associated with precocious puberty. *J Pediatr* 1983;103:593–595.

120. Nomura K, Furusato M, Nikaido T, et al. Ovarian sex cord tumor with annular tubules. Report of a case. *Acta Pathol Jpn* 1991;41:701–706.

121. Podczaski E, Kaminski PF, Pees RC, et al. Peutz-Jeghers syndrome with ovarian sex cord tumor with annular tubules and cervical adenoma malignum. *Gynecol Oncol* 1991;42:74–78.

122. Srivatsa PJ, Keeney GL, Podratz KC. Disseminated cervical adenoma malignum and bilateral ovarian sex cord tumors with annular tubules associated with Peutz-Jeghers syndrome. *Gynecol Oncol* 1994;53:256–264.

123. Boardman LA, Thibodeau SN, Schaid DJ, et al. Increased risk for cancer in patients with the Peutz-Jeghers syndrome. *Ann Intern Med* 1998;128:896–899.

124. Hemminki A, Tomlinson I, Markie D, et al. Localization of a susceptibility locus for Peutz-Jeghers syndrome to 19p using comparative genomic hybridization and targeted linkage analysis. *Nat Genet* 1997;15:87–90.

125. Jenne DE, Reimann H, Nezu J, et al. Peutz-Jeghers syndrome is caused by mutations in a novel serine threonine kinase. *Nat Genet* 1998;18: 38–43.

126. Benagiano G, Bigotti G, Buzzi M, et al. Endocrine and morphological study of a case of ovarian sex-cord tumor with annular tubules in a woman with Peutz-Jeghers syndrome. *Int J Gynaecol Obstet* 1988; 26:441–452.

127. Crain JL. Ovarian sex cord tumor with annular tubules: steroid profile. *Obstet Gynecol* 1986;68[Suppl 3]:75S-79S.

128. Gustafson ML, Lee MM, Scully RE, et al. Müllerian inhibiting substance as a marker for ovarian sex-cord tumor. *N Engl J Med* 1992; 326:466–471.

129. Puls LE, Hamous J, Morrow MS, et al. Recurrent ovarian sex cord tumor with annular tubules: tumor marker and chemotherapy experience. *Gynecol Oncol* 1994;54:396–401.

130. Talerman A, Hughesdon PE, Anderson MC. Diffuse nonlobular ovarian androblastoma usually associated with feminization. *Int J Gynecol Pathol* 1982;1:155–171.

131. Young RH, Dudley AG, Scully RE. Granulosa cell, Sertoli-Leydig cell, and unclassified sex cord-stromal tumors associated with pregnancy: a clinicopathological analysis of thirty-six cases. *Gynecol Oncol* 1984;18:181–205.

132. Martin-Jimenez A, Condom-Munro E, Valls-Porcel M, et al. Gynandroblastoma of the ovary. Review of the literature. *J Gynecol Obstet Biol Reprod* 1994;23:391–394.

133. Novak ER. Gynandroblastoma of the ovary: review of 8 cases from the Ovarian Tumor Registry. *Obstet Gynecol* 1967;30:709–715.

134. Kalir T, Friedman F Jr. Gynandroblastoma in pregnancy: case report and review of literature. *Mt Sinai J Med* 1998;65:292–295.

135. Hayes MC, Scully RE. Stromal luteoma of the ovary: a clinicopathological analysis of 25 cases. *Int J Gynecol Pathol* 1987;6:313–321.

136. Scully RE, Young RH, Clement PB. *Tumors of the ovary, maldeveloped gonads, fallopian tube, and broad ligament.* Washington, DC: Armed Forces Institute of Pathology, 1998.

137. Roth LM, Sternberg WH. Ovarian stromal tumors containing Leydig cells. II. Pure Leydig cell tumor, non-hilar type. *Cancer* 1973;32: 952–960.

138. Paraskevas M, Scully RE. Hilus cell tumor of the ovary. A clinicopathological analysis of 12 Reinke crystal-positive and nine crystal-negative cases. *Int J Gynecol Pathol* 1989;8:299–310.

139. Dunnihoo DR, Grieme DL, Woolf RB. Hilar-cell tumors of the ovary. Report of 2 new cases and a review of the world literature. *Obstet Gynecol* 1966;27:703–713.

140. Hayes MC, Scully RE. Ovarian steroid cell tumors (not otherwise specified). A clinicopathological analysis of 63 cases. *Am J Surg Pathol* 1987;11:835–845.

141. Harris AC, Wakely PE Jr, Kaplowitz PB, et al. Steroid cell tumor of the ovary in a child. *Arch Pathol Lab Med* 1991;115:150–154.

142. Davidson BJ, Waisman J, Judd HL. Long-standing virilism in a woman with hyperplasia and neoplasia of ovarian lipidic cells. *Obstet Gynecol* 1981;58:753–759.

143. Taylor HB, Norris HJ. Lipid cell tumors of the ovary. *Cancer* 1967; 20:1953–1962.

144. Adeyemi SD, Grange AO, Giwa-Osagie OF, et al. Adrenal rest tumour of the ovary associated with isosexual precocious pseudopuberty and cushingoid features. *Eur J Pediatr* 1986;145:236–238.

145. Dengg K, Fink FM, Heitger A, et al. Precocious puberty due to a lipid-cell tumour of the ovary. *Eur J Pediatr* 1993;152:12–14.

146. Clement PB, Young RH, Scully RE. Clinical syndromes associated with tumors of the female genital tract. *Semin Diagn Pathol* 1991;8: 204–233.

147. Donovan JT, Otis CN, Powell JL, et al. Cushing's syndrome secondary to malignant lipoid cell tumor of the ovary. *Gynecol Oncol* 1993;50: 249–253.

148. Young RH, Scully RE. Ovarian steroid cell tumors associated with Cushing's syndrome: a report of three cases. *Int J Gynecol Pathol* 1987;6:40–48.

149. Gershenson DM, Copeland LJ, Kavanagh JJ, et al. Treatment of metastatic stromal tumors of the ovary with cisplatin, doxorubicin, and cyclophosphamide. *Obstet Gynecol* 1987;70:765–769.

150. Gershenson DM. Chemotherapy of ovarian germ cell tumors and sex cord stromal tumors. *Semin Surg Oncol* 1994;10:290–298.

151. Wolf JK, Mullen J, Eifel PJ, et al. Radiation treatment of advanced or recurrent granulosa cell tumor of the ovary. *Gynecol Oncol* 1999; 73:35–41.

152. Savage P, Constenla D, Fisher C, et al. Granulosa cell tumours of the ovary: demographics, survival and the management of advanced disease. *Clin Oncol* 1998;10:242–245.

153. Homesley HD, Bundy BN, Hurteau JA, et al. Bleomycin, etoposide, and cisplatin combination therapy of ovarian granulosa cell tumors and other stromal malignancies: a Gynecologic Oncology Group study. *Gynecol Oncol* 1999;72:131–137.

154. Colombo N, Parma G, Franchi D. An active chemotherapy regimen for advanced ovarian sex cord-stromal tumors. *Gynecol Oncol* 1999; 72:129–130.

155. Gershenson DM, Morris M, Burke TW, et al. Treatment of poor-prognosis sex cord-stromal tumors of the ovary with the combination of bleomycin, etoposide, and cisplatin. *Obstet Gynecol* 1996;87: 527–531.

156. Pecorelli S, Wagenaar HC, Vergote IB, et al. Cisplatin (P), vinblastine (V) and bleomycin (B) combination chemotherapy in recurrent or advanced granulosa (-theca) cell tumours of the ovary. An EORTC Gynaecological Cancer Cooperative Group Study. *Eur J Cancer* 1999; 35:1331–1337.

157. Uygun K, Aydiner A, Saip P, et al. Clinical parameters and treatment results in recurrent granulosa cell tumor of the ovary. *Gynecol Oncol* 2003;88:400–403.

158. Tresukosol D, Kudelka AP, Edwards CL, et al. Recurrent ovarian granulosa cell tumor: a case report of a dramatic response to Taxol. *Int J Gynecol Cancer* 1995;5:156–159.

159. Chadha S, Rao BR, Slotman BJ, et al. An immunohistochemical evaluation of androgen and progesterone receptors in ovarian tumors. *Hum Pathol* 1993;24:90–95.

160. Fishman A, Kudelka A, Edwards C, et al. GnRH agonist (Depot-Lupron) in the treatment of refractory or persistent ovarian granulosa cell tumor (GCT). *Proc Am Soc Clin Oncol* 1994;13:236(abst).

161. Isaacs R, Forgeson G, Allan S. Progestogens for granulosa cell tumours of the ovary [Letter]. *Br J Cancer* 1992;65:140.

162. Malik ST, Slevin ML. Medroxyprogesterone acetate (MPA) in advanced granulosa cell tumours of the ovary—a new therapeutic approach? *Br J Cancer* 1991;63:410–411.

163. Martikainen H, Penttinen J, Huhtaniemi I, et al. Gonadotropin-releasing hormone agonist analog therapy effective in ovarian granulosa cell malignancy. *Gynecol Oncol* 1989;35:406–508.

164. Fishman A, Kudelka AP, Tresukosol D, et al. Leuprolide acetate for treating refractory or persistent ovarian granulosa cell tumor. *J Reprod Med* 1996;41:393–396.

165. Calaminus G, Wessalowski R, Harms D, et al. Juvenile granulosa cell tumors of the ovary in children and adolescents: results from 33 patients registered in a prospective cooperative study. *Gynecol Oncol* 1997;65:447–452.

166. Powell JL, Otis CN. Management of advanced juvenile granulosa cell tumor of the ovary. *Gynecol Oncol* 1997;64:282–284.

167. Powell JL, Connor GP, Henderson GS. Management of recurrent juvenile granulosa cell tumor of the ovary. *Gynecol Oncol* 2001;81: 113–116.

168. Schwartz PE, Smith JP. Treatment of ovarian stromal tumors. *Am J Obstet Gynecol* 1976;125:402–411.

169. Emons G, Schally AV. The use of luteinizing hormone releasing hormone agonists and antagonists in gynaecological cancers. *Hum Reprod* 1994;9:1364–1379.

170. Whittemore AS, Harris R, Intyre J. Characteristics relating to ovarian cancer risk: collaborative analysis of 12 US case-control studies. IV. The pathogenesis of epithelial ovarian cancer. Collaborative Ovarian Cancer Group. *Am J Epidemiol* 1992;136:1212–1220.

171. Rossing MA, Daling JR, Weiss NS, et al. Ovarian tumors in a cohort of infertile women. *N Engl J Med* 1994;331:771–776.

172. Unkila-Kallio L, Leminen A, Tiitinen A, et al. Nationwide data on falling incidence of ovarian granulosa cell tumours concomitant with increasing use of ovulation inducers. *Hum Reprod* 1998;13: 2828–2830.

173. Werness BA, Ramus SJ, Whittemore AS, et al. Histopathology of familial ovarian tumors in women from families with and without germline BRCA1 mutations. *Hum Pathol* 2000;31:1420–1424.

174. Fletcher JA, Gibas Z, Donovan K, et al. Ovarian granulosa-stromal

cell tumors are characterized by trisomy 12. *Am J Pathol* 1991;138:515–520.

175. Halperin D, Visscher DW, Wallis T, et al. Evaluation of chromosome 12 copy number in ovarian granulosa cell tumors using interphase cytogenetics. *Int J Gynecol Pathol* 1995;14:319–323.

176. Pejovic T, Heim S, Alm P, et al. Isochromosome 1q as the sole karyotypic abnormality in a Sertoli cell tumor of the ovary. *Cancer Genet Cytogenet* 1993;65:79–80.

177. Persons DL, Hartmann LC, Herath JF, et al. Fluorescence in situ hybridization analysis of trisomy 12 in ovarian tumors. *Am J Clin Pathol* 1994;102:775–779.

178. Schofield DE, Fletcher JA. Trisomy 12 in pediatric granulosa-stromal cell tumors. Demonstration by a modified method of fluorescence in situ hybridization on paraffin-embedded material. *Am J Pathol* 1992;141:1265–1269.

179. Tanyi J, Rigo J Jr., Csapo Z, et al. Trisomy 12 in juvenile granulosa cell tumor of the ovary during pregnancy. *J Reprod Med* 1999;44:826–832.

180. Yang-Feng TL, Li SB, Leung WY, et al. Trisomy 12 and K-ras-2 amplification in human ovarian tumors. *Int J Cancer* 1991;48:678–681.

181. Lindgren V, Waggoner S, Rotmensch J. Monosomy 22 in two ovarian granulosa cell tumors. *Cancer Genet Cytogenet* 1996;89:93–97.

182. Van den Berghe I, Dal Cin P, De Groef K, et al. Monosomy 22 and trisomy 14 may be early events in the tumorigenesis of adult granulosa cell tumor. *Cancer Genet Cytogenet* 1999;112:46–48.

183. Burger HG. Inhibin. *Reprod Med Rev* 1992;1:1.

184. Petraglia F, Luisi S, Pautier P, et al. Inhibin B is the major form of inhibin/activin family secreted by granulosa cell tumors. *J Clin Endocrinol Metab* 1998;83:1029–1032.

185. Ying SY. Inhibins, activins, and follistatins: gonadal proteins modulating the secretion of follicle-stimulating hormone. *Endocr Rev* 1988;9:267–293.

186. Robertson DM, Stephenson T, Pruysers E, et al. Characterization of inhibin forms and their measurement by an inhibin alpha-subunit ELISA in serum from postmenopausal women with ovarian cancer. *J Clin Endocrinol Metab* 2002;87:816–824.

187. Hasegawa Y, Eto Y, Ibuki Y, et al. Activin as autocrine and paracrine factor in the ovary. *Horm Res* 1994;41[Suppl 1]:55–62.

188. Mayr D, Kaltz-Wittmer C, Arbogast S, et al. Characteristic pattern of genetic aberrations in ovarian granulosa cell tumors. *Mod Pathol* 2002;15:951–957.

189. Watson RH, Roy WJ Jr, Davis M, et al. Loss of heterozygosity at the alpha-inhibin locus on chromosome 2q is not a feature of human granulosa cell tumors. *Gynecol Oncol* 1997;65:387–390.

190. Kotlar TJ, Young RH, Albanese C, et al. A mutation in the follicle-stimulating hormone receptor occurs frequently in human ovarian sex cord tumors. *J Clin Endocrinol Metab* 1997;82:1020–1026.

191. Fuller PJ, Verity K, Shen Y, et al. No evidence of a role for mutations or polymorphisms of the follicle-stimulating hormone receptor in ovarian granulosa cell tumors. *J Clin Endocrinol Metab* 1998;83:274–279.

192. Hannon TS, King DW, Brinkman AD, et al. Premature thelarche and granulosa cell tumors: a search for FSH receptor and G5alpha activating mutations. *J Pediatr Endocrinol Metab* 2000;15:891–895.

193. Gurusinghe CJ, Healy DL, Jobling T, et al. Inhibin and activin are demonstrable by immunohistochemistry in ovarian tumor tissue. *Gynecol Oncol* 1995;57:27–32.

CHAPTER 28

Carcinoma of the Fallopian Tube

Maurie Markman, Richard J. Zaino, Peter A. Fleming, and Mary L. Gemignani

Primary carcinoma of the fallopian tube remains an enigma to the pathologist and oncologist. The pathologic criteria for distinguishing these tumors from those of the ovary are imprecise, and no method for early detection exists. However, their rarity, in a tissue that shares histology, embryology, and response to sex steroids with other organs of the genital tract, may ultimately provide clues to the pathogenesis of ovarian, tubal, and endometrial carcinomas.

The fallopian tube is the least common site of origin for malignant neoplasms of the female genital tract, although the epithelial surface area is much greater than that of the ovary, an organ that gives rise to carcinoma more than 20 times as frequently (1).

EMBRYOLOGY

The paramesonephric duct arises as a longitudinal invagination of the coelomic epithelium on the anterolateral surface of the urogenital ridge. The cranial portion of the duct opens into the coelomic cavity via a funnel-like structure, crosses the mesonephric duct in its horizontal intermediate portion, and then meets in its caudal vertical aspect with its contralateral partner. The first two parts form the fallopian tube, whereas the third portion rapidly fuses to form the uterine canal. The epithelium of the fallopian tube thus shares a common embryologic derivation with that of the endometrium and cervix and is not distant in origin from the coelomic epithelium of the gonadal ridge that covers the ovary. The stroma and muscular walls of the fallopian tube, uterine corpus, and cervix are all formed from the mesenchyme that surrounds the paramesonephric duct (2). In male embryos, the elaboration of müllerian-inhibiting substance by the testes results in regression of the paramesonephric ducts. The logic of treating women with tumors of paramesonephric origin with müllerian-inhibiting substance is thus appealing.

ANATOMY

The oviduct is a muscular tube that averages 12 cm in length. It has an external diameter that varies from 2.0 mm proximally to about 1.5 cm distally. It is situated in the edge of the mesosalpinx and extends from the superior, lateral angle of the uterus to the side of the pelvis. The lumen communicates proximally with the endometrial cavity, where it has a diameter of 1 to 2 mm, and distally with the peritoneal cavity, where the diameter is 2 to 4 mm. It is divided along its length into four portions: the pars interstitialis, that portion that transverses the myometrium; the isthmus, the narrow medial portion; the ampulla, the widest and longest section; and the infundibulum, the lateral, funnel-shaped portion that is terminally drawn into finger-like processes called fimbriae.

The fallopian tube has an external serosal layer, an internal mucosal layer, and an intermediate muscular layer. The serosa is covered by mesothelial cells that are continuous with the visceral peritoneum of the uterus. The muscle layer consists of an incomplete, and sometimes ill-defined, external longitudinal layer and a thicker, internal circular layer. When the tube is opened, multiple longitudinal folds of mucosa can be seen; in cross section, these folds appear as a maze of profusely branching papillae, or plicae. The complexity of the mucosal folds increases from the interstitial portion through the ampulla. The mucosa is formed of a lamina

M. Markman: Department of Hematology and Medical Oncology, The Cleveland Clinic Foundation, Cleveland, Ohio 44195

R. J. Zaino: Department of Pathology, Milton S. Hershey Medical Center, The Pennsylvania State University, Hershey, Pennsylvania 17033

P. A. Fleming: Department of Radiation Oncology, The Cleveland Clinic Foundation, Cleveland, Ohio 44195

M. L. Gemignani: Department of Obstetrics and Gynecology, Cornell University Medical College, Department of Surgery, Memorial Sloan–Kettering Cancer Center, New York, New York 10021

propria that is formed of a fibrovascular stroma, which focally may resemble the stroma of the endometrium, covered by a tall, simple columnar epithelium. This epithelium consists principally of ciliated cells (70%), which have motile function, and nonciliated cells (30%), which display secretory activity (3). Intercalary, or peg, cells represent exhausted secretory cells, and small lymphocytes are often also found between epithelial cells. Well-defined reserve cells are not convincingly identified at the light microscopic level.

Because the epithelium is the source for the majority of fallopian tube neoplasms, the ciliated and secretory cells are considered in more detail. Ciliogenesis occurs in the endometrium in response to estrogen stimulation, and ciliated cells are also most abundant in the fallopian tube at mid cycle, followed by deciliation during the secretory phase (4). Secretory cells also display maximal secretory activity at mid cycle, with exhaustion during the secretory phase (4). Pregnancy and prolonged progestin therapy cause secretory exhaustion and suppression, respectively. Atrophy of the epithelium typically occurs as a late postmenopausal effect and may be associated with fibrosis of the lamina propria and simplification of plicae. Many of the changes observed in the endometrial gland cells are thus replicated in the tubal epithelium, although to a much lesser degree.

EPIDEMIOLOGY AND PATHOGENESIS

Primary malignancy of the fallopian tube is a rare neoplasm; fewer than 2,000 cases have been reported in the literature, representing less than 1% of all gynecologic malignancies, with an average of 0.3% (5–9). The theoretical incidence is 3.0 to 3.6/1,000,000 women per year (10). There is a reported 14% higher incidence in whites than in blacks (10).

The age range for this tumor has been reported to be from 18 to 87 years, with most occurrences in the fifth and sixth decades of life. In a review of 393 patients, a mean age of 55.0 years was described (11), which is consistent with a mean age of 56.7 years in a meta-analysis of 577 patients (12). The clinical profile of these patients reveals a relatively low parity rate (13–18), with a mean parity of 1.0 to 1.7 (14,16,17a).

Although the pathogenesis of most fallopian-tube carcinomas remains unknown, during the past 5 years, evidence has emerged of a relationship between some cases of carcinoma of the fallopian tube and mutations in either the *BRCA1* or *BRCA2* gene. The data initially came from individual case reports (18a,19), followed by a very recent systematic epidemiologic analysis. Aziz and colleagues reviewed all of the pathologically confirmed cases of fallopian tube carcinoma identified from the Ontario Cancer Registry between 1990 and 1998, and found germline mutations in the *BRCA1* or *BRCA2* gene in 7 of 44 patients (16%) in whom blood samples were available for screening (20). Approached from a different perspective, thorough gross and microscopic exam-

ination of prophylactic oophorectomy specimens from women with either a family history or a known *BRCA1* or *BRCA2* mutation have revealed the presence of occult invasive or *in situ* carcinoma in the fallopian tube as often or even more often than in the ovary (19,21–24). In this setting, the tumors may be found anywhere throughout the entire length of the fallopian tube from the intrauterine portion to the fimbriated end. It appears that germline mutations in the *BRCA1* or *BRCA2* gene bear a relationship to carcinogenesis in the fallopian tube that is similar to that of development of carcinoma in the ovary or pelvic peritoneum. Other data relating specific mutations to fallopian tube cancer remain very incomplete. Comparative genomic hybridization performed on 12 fallopian tube carcinomas displayed a high level of genetic instability, most frequently with a DNA copy gain involving 3q, 1q, or 2q or a loss involving 16q or 22q (25). However, these mutations have not been associated with any known tumor-suppressor gene or oncogene.

CLINICAL PRESENTATION

Tumors of the fallopian tube cause early clinical signs and symptoms. Although the triad of pelvic pain, pelvic mass, and leukorrhea or vaginal bleeding, vaginal discharge, and lower abdominal pain have been described as pathognomonic of tubal carcinoma, the highest percentage of patients presenting with such a triad of symptoms has been only 11% (5). Another classic sign is hydrops tubae profluens, a sudden emptying of accumulated fluid in the distended fallopian tube that causes profuse, watery serosanguineous vaginal discharge associated with a decrease in pelvic mass size. Hydrops tubae profluens occurred in only 9% in a meta-analysis of 122 patients (17a).

The most common presenting sign of this tumor is metrorrhagia (11,12,14,16–18,26–29), followed by a colicky type of pain and vaginal discharge (11,18,27). The most common physical sign is a pelvic mass, occurring in 12% to 66% of patients (5,11,14,27).

DIAGNOSTIC WORKUP

Because of the rarity of primary malignancies of the fallopian tube and presenting signs that resemble those for salpingitis, ovarian abscess or tumor, pelvic inflammatory disease, and even ectopic pregnancy, it is difficult to diagnose most cases before surgical exploration (30). It has been reported in many series that the correct diagnosis was missed entirely in their working differential (8,15,16,31).

Some investigators have advocated the use of Papanicolaou (Pap) smears as a preoperative screening tool in patients with nonspecific symptoms, with positive results ranging from 0% to 60% (5,8,17,18,32). The use of endometrial sampling has produced equally unpromising results (18).

Many different modalities for detection of fallopian tube

cancers are under investigation, including nuclear-medicine imaging techniques with radioactive nucleotides, magnetic resonance imaging (MRI), ultrasound, and some tumor markers.

Hysteroscopy and Hysterosalpingography

Although hysteroscopy and hysterosalpingography can diagnose abnormal masses of the fallopian tube, they are nonspecific, and it is possible that their use may cause intraperitoneal tumor seeding in cases of malignancy when the ampulla is patent (33).

Ultrasonography

In combination with other screening techniques, ultrasonography, with a vaginal transducer (TVS), has added more accurate assessment of adnexal pathology than pelvic ultrasound alone (34,35).

The addition of color flow and Doppler waveform measurements has increased the sensitivity of TVS (36,37). In malignant masses, there is typically a decreased amount of muscle in the lining of the tumor vessels, which, combined with increased arteriovenous shunting within the tumor, increases flow and results in abnormal pulsatile and resistance indices compared with those of normal vessels (37). Color flow alone in imaging of postmenopausal adnexal masses has a reported specificity of only 65%; assuming that flow is visible (36). Kurjak et al. (36) found that the differences in vessel resistance indices between benign and malignant tumors gave a sensitivity of 96% and a specificity of 95% ($p < 0.001$).

The drawbacks to TVS with color flow Doppler lie with the experience of the operator, quality of instrumentation used, and the change in imaging characteristics of tumors dependent on stage (36).

Computed Tomography and Magnetic Resonance Imaging

Some investigators report that MRI is superior to ultrasound and computed tomography (CT) in that it can better differentiate the fallopian tube from other pelvic organs (38, 39). However, the separation of benign from malignant processes is difficult, and ultrasound has been concluded to be superior to MRI as a screening modality in the evaluation of adnexal tumors (39).

Nuclear Scan Imaging

Radioimaging with a combination of immunolymphoscintigraphy and immunoscintigraphy with ^{131}I-labeled F(ab')$_2$ fragments of monoclonal OC-125 antibodies improved detection of retroperitoneal lymph node metastases, with a sensitivity of 90% and a specificity of 83% (40). These findings were correlated with abnormally elevated levels of CA-125, indicating that individuals with high circulating levels of this tumor marker are at a higher risk of having metastatic disease.

Based on the higher glucose metabolism in malignant tumors, positron emission tomography (PET) is being used extensively in many patients. Whole-body fluorodeoxyglucose-PET (FDG-PET) scanning was demonstrated to detect sites of metastatic fallopian tube carcinoma in areas of skin nodules and bone discomfort (41). Newer techniques using PET and CT (PET/CT) imaging are promising in the evaluation of patients with recurrent fallopian tube carcinoma. PET/CT imaging was noted to have greater sensitivity over CT scan alone. Further study into this modality is warranted (42).

Tumor Markers

CA-125

Levels of CA-125 >65 U/mL have been defined as being probable for fallopian tube malignancies, with a specificity of 98% and a sensitivity of 75% (35). However, serum antigen levels are found to be elevated in both benign and malignant conditions such as endometriosis, pelvic inflammatory disease, and early pregnancy (43). Levels below the upper limit were noted in two patients who at second-look laparotomy had disease recurrence (44), as well as in one patient diagnosed with stage II disease who had a normal CA-125 level (45).

Reports suggest screening with this tumor marker would be more effective if used in combination with ultrasound (37,43). It has been suggested that elevated levels of CA-125 in supposed early-stage disease in conjunction with the use of CA-125 immunoscintigraphy may be predictive of metastatic disease (40,46).

As in ovarian carcinoma, CA-125 probably has a greater role as a marker of response to chemotherapy than in the initial diagnosis of fallopian tube carcinoma. In a group of 23 patients treated with platinum-based therapy with initially elevated CA-125, measurements obtained prior to each new cycle, and evaluation after the third and sixth cycles, all responding and progressing patients were correctly identified using standard response criteria (47). Two patients with stable disease were incorrectly classified as being CA-125 responders.

PATHOLOGY

The gross appearance of the fallopian tube affected by papillary carcinoma is typically described as enlarged, deformed, or fusiform, with agglutination of the fimbriae and,

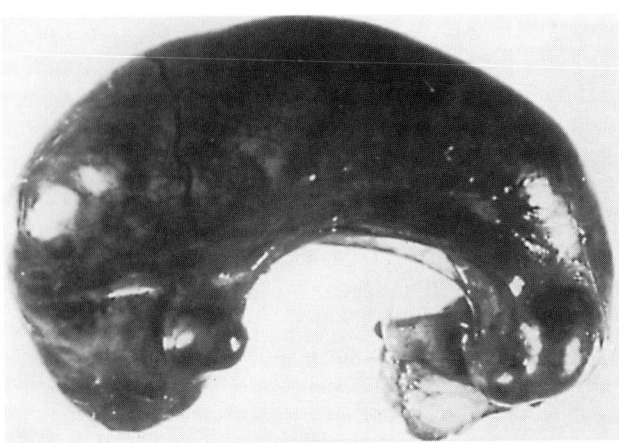

FIG. 28.1. Carcinoma of the fallopian tube. This gross photograph depicts the fusiform dilation of the tube with agglutination of the fimbria and distal obstruction. (Courtesy of Steven Silverberg, MD, Washington, DC.)

frequently, distal obstruction (Fig. 28.1) (48–51). When the tumor is confined to the mucosa, the tube is generally soft to palpation, and the initial impression of the surgeon is often hematosalpinx, pyosalpinx, or hydrosalpinx (48,52). Turbid fluid frequently fills the lumen, with a friable, exophytic, papillary, or nodular mass affixed to the mucosal surface. The most frequent site of origin is the ampulla, followed by the infundibulum (29,51,53).

In about 10% of cases in a recent large study, the tumor arose in the fimbriated end of the fallopian tube. All of these tumors were less than 3 cm in diameter (54,55).

Sometimes, multiple minute tumors stud the mucosal surface, or the entire lumen may be replaced by a necrotic mass. With more advanced disease, neoplastic cells penetrate the muscular wall and serosa of the tube, and extension to the ovary may result in a tubo-ovarian complex. In the latter situation, it is usually obvious that a malignant neoplasm has infiltrated the organs, but the distinction of tubal carcinoma from that of the ovary may not be possible, and reliance on arbitrary criteria usually results in the classification of the tumor as being ovarian in origin (see below).

Recently, a radically different presentation of fallopian tube carcinoma has been reported. Occult invasive or *in situ* carcinoma has been found to involve the fallopian tube in prophylactic salpino-oophorectomy specimens obtained from women with a strong family history of ovarian cancer or known *BRCA1* or *BRCA2* germline mutations (19,21–24, 56). Such tumors may not be visible macroscopically, and it is suggested that the entire fallopian tube as well as the ovary be serially sectioned and examined microscopically in this clinical setting.

The carcinoma affects the left and right tube with about equal frequency and displays bilateral involvement in about 5% to 30% of cases (11,15–17,28,52,57–63).

Historically, the tumors were classified microscopically

as papillary, alveolar, or medullary based on the formation of nests or diffuse masses. These terms are no longer familiar to many pathologists. The current World Health Organization (WHO) histologic classification of epithelial tumors of the fallopian tube is similar to that of other sites in the upper female genital tract and is divided into serous, mucinous, endometrioid, clear-cell, transitional, squamous, glassy-cell, and mixed carcinomas (55). This change in terminology reflects an increased recognition of both endometrioid and transitional-cell differentiation in carcinomas of the fallopian tube during the past 10 years.

Papillary serous adenocarcinoma is the most frequent primary malignant neoplasm of the fallopian tube, and was previously reported to represent about 90% of the 300 new cases annually occurring in the United States (1). In more recent studies, its frequency has been lower, reflecting the increasing recognition by pathologists that tumors of other cell types may legitimately arise in the fallopian tube (47, 64,65). In superficial lesions, the plicae, which are ordinarily covered by a simple columnar epithelium of ciliated and secretory cells, are replaced by multiple layers of columnar or cuboidal cells with pleomorphic and hyperchromatic nuclei (Figs. 28.2 and 28.3). The papillary configuration of the epithelium is usually preserved, but secretory activity and cilia are usually not preserved at the light microscopic level. Mitotic figures are frequent. Invasion of the muscular wall occurs early in the course of disease, and, as the tumor enlarges, necrosis becomes a common feature. It is critical for the pathologist to examine and liberally section the site of tumor carefully since the probability of survival is markedly different for women whose tumors are confined to the mucosa compared with those whose tumors either invade the muscular wall or extend to the serosa of the tube (63). Capillary or lymphatic vascular invasion is common even in early-stage disease, and has also been associated with a diminished probability of survival (28).

Endometroid carcinomas involving the fallopian tube are

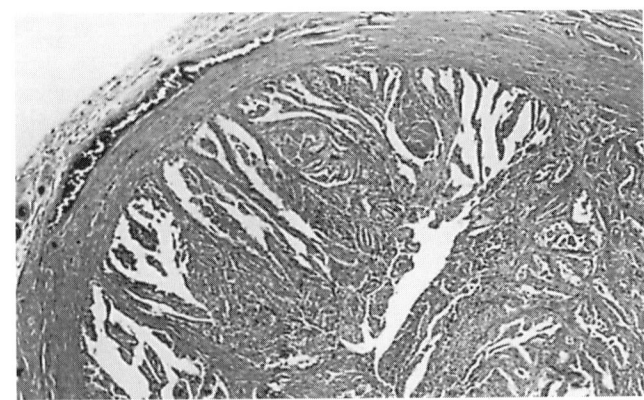

FIG. 28.2. Carcinoma of the fallopian tube. This low-magnification photomicrograph of a cross section of the tube displays extensive intraluminal papillary growth with preservation of the muscularis. (Original magnification ×25.)

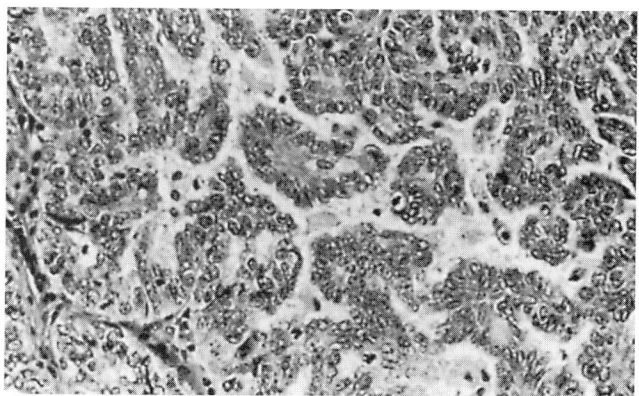

FIG. 28.3. Carcinoma of the fallopian tube. In this photomicrograph, fibrovascular papillae are covered by epithelial cells with atypical nuclei. (Original magnification ×100.)

more common than previously reported, and over 50 cases have been documented in the literature (55). They are formed of tubular glands, sometimes with foci of either benign- or malignant-appearing squamous differentiation (49,64, 66–72). In at least one case, the tumor arose in tubal endometriosis (67). The tumor usually resembles typical adenocarcinoma of the endometrium, but it may simulate female adnexal tumors of probable wolffian origin (55,73,74). It may be distinguished from the latter by the greater degree of cytologic atypia, mitotic activity, and at least focal endometrial-type gland formation (73,75). Many of the endometrioid carcinomas are either noninvasive or only superficially invasive, and appear to have a more favorable prognosis than serous carcinomas.

Transitional-cell carcinomas resemble tumors of urothelial type, with papillae formed of broad masses of cells covering a fibrovascular core (64,76–79). These papillae are distinguished from those of serous carcinomas by having a smooth surface rather than the scalloped surface of serous carcinoma and by the presence of longitudinal grooves in the nuclei of some cells. This was the predominant histologic pattern in 12 of 21 primary tubal carcinomas from Japan (79), but represented only about 10% of cases in a large series from the United States (64). The survival has been reported to be either better than or similar to that of serous carcinoma (55,79).

Too few cases of clear-cell, undifferentiated, or mixed types of carcinoma have been reported to characterize their behavior.

The histologic grade of fallopian tube carcinoma is usually simply designated as well, moderately, or poorly differentiated. In contrast to the depth of invasion, the degree of histologic differentiation has generally not been related to prognosis (15,16,28,29,50,53,80), although a few series have demonstrated a better probability of survival when the tumor was well differentiated (6,81). It is unclear whether this inability to prognosticate reflects the lack of biologic impor-

tance of histologic grade or simply the absence of reproducible criteria for grading.

Infiltrates of acute and chronic inflammatory cells are frequently identified in fallopian tubes with carcinoma. Whether their presence reflects an immune host response or the presence of secondary infection has not been established. No data relate the presence or density of the inflammatory infiltrate to prognosis.

The ultrastructural appearance of fallopian tube carcinoma resembles that of ovarian serous papillary carcinoma. Complex intercellular junctions provide evidence that the cells are epithelial, and membrane-bound granules indicate that limited secretory function is preserved. The neoplastic cells generally are devoid of cilia but display occasional microvilli along the apical surface (82,83).

No distinctive immunohistochemical markers of fallopian tube differentiation exist. Carcinoembryonic antigen is widely distributed in the lower intestinal tract during embryonic development and is present in mucinous neoplasms of the cervix and ovary, but it is absent from the postnatal normal or neoplastic fallopian tube. CA-125 can be detected immunohistochemically in both the benign and malignant fallopian tube (84,85); however, it is also found in endometrial and ovarian serous carcinomas, and thus cannot help the pathologist to discriminate whether a carcinoma has arisen in the fallopian tube or ovary. Determination of serum CA-125 levels also does not aid the early detection of fallopian tube carcinoma since elevated serum levels are usually associated with advanced primary carcinoma of the fallopian tube, uterus, or ovary (45,86–88). However, it helps monitor patients in whom the diagnosis has already been established since serum CA-125 is almost always a reliable indicator of recurrent carcinoma (44,45,85,88). Ca-1, an antibody directed against the Ca antigen, was initially thought to be largely confined to human cancer cells (89). However, subsequent work has indicated a broader specificity, and it is routinely detected in benign fallopian tube epithelium (89, 90).

ABH antigens are present on the mucosa of the normal and nonneoplastic fallopian tube but are diminished or lost in association with neoplastic transformation (91). It is not known whether precursor lesions might be identified by demonstrable loss of these blood group antigens. CA-19–9, a sialynated antigen of the Lewis blood group system, is present in the mucosa of the fallopian tube, as well as in the endocervix and endometrium. It has also been identified in the majority of adenocarcinomas arising in these organs, where the degree of expression, detected immunohistochemically, is inversely related to tumor differentiation (92).

The data are insufficient to offer conclusions about the frequency or significance of oncogene overexpression in fallopian tube carcinoma. In one study of HER-2/neu using a quantitative polymerase chain reaction assay, no tumors displayed amplification of the oncogene (93). The frequency of Her-2/*neu* overexpression has varied from 26% to 89% (94), whereas that of *p53* has ranged from 60% to 83% (25, 94). In contrast to ovarian carcinoma, their overexpression in fallopian tube carcinoma has not been associated with a worsened prognosis. Immunohistochemical overexpression of c-*myc* has also been reported in 61% of cases in one study (94). K-*RAS* point mutations in codon 12 have been reported to be present in seven of eight carcinomas of the fallopian tube (95).

Estrogen receptors have been identified in the nuclei of fallopian tube epithelium and in a minority of fallopian tube carcinomas (96); however, no data on the relationship between the presence of estrogen receptors and response to hormonal therapy for fallopian tube cancer exist.

RARE MALIGNANT NEOPLASMS OF THE FALLOPIAN TUBE

Most types of tumors found in the uterine corpus have also been reported to occur in the fallopian tube. About 50 cases of malignant mixed mesodermal tumors have been described (95,97–103). The average age at diagnosis is 58 years. The lesions grossly resemble those of fallopian tube carcinoma, with a dilated tube that contains an intraluminal papillary mass. However, in addition to a carcinoma arranged as glands or papillae, there is also a malignant stromal component. The tumors are further divided into homologous or heterologous types according to the absence or presence of differentiation of the stromal elements into cell types not normally found within the müllerian duct system, such as skeletal muscle or cartilage. The overall 5-year survival is about 15%, with a mean survival of about 17 months. The presence or absence of heterologous elements has not been related to outcome. A single positive observation is the markedly better probability of survival for women with tumors confined to the muscularis (102).

Three examples of primary squamous-cell carcinoma (104), immature teratoma (20), glassy-cell carcinoma (105), Wilms' tumor (65), and rare pure sarcomas, including leiomyosarcoma, angiosarcoma, malignant fibrous histiocytoma, stromal sarcoma, and fibrosarcoma, have been reported to occur in the fallopian tube (106–110). Other pure squamous carcinomas in the fallopian tube have been generally described as part of an extended *in situ* transformation that involves uterine cervix and corpus, frequently associated with cervical stenosis (see section Multifocal Carcinoma of the Müllerian System, Including the Fallopian Tubes below).

Serous, mucinous, and endometrioid tumors of low malignant potential occasionally occur in the fallopian tube (54, 111–113). Their biologic behavior appears to mimic that of low malignant tumors of the ovary.

About 100 cases of gestational choriocarcinoma arising in an ectopic tubal pregnancy have been reported (114). It displays pathologic and biologic characteristics identical to those of uterine choriocarcinoma (114,115). Nongestational choriocarcinoma of the fallopian tube has been reported in a prepubertal girl (59).

Papillary carcinoma of the tube typically occurs in menopausal women; however, in a handful of cases, it occurred in adolescent females or was discovered during pregnancy or at postpartum tubal ligation (105,116–118).

The precise, but awkward, appellation ''female adnexal tumors of probable wolffian origin'' has been given by Young and Scully to a rare neoplasm identified along the serosal surface of the distal portion of the fallopian tube or within the broad ligament or ovary (119). About 20 such tumors have been reported in women between 28 and 79 years of age. These tumors are typically unilateral, lobulated, grossly encapsulated, solid, or partially cystic masses that measure from 1 to 20 cm in diameter. A variety of microscopic patterns have been described, including cystic, closely packed tubules, sieve-like spaces, or diffuse proliferation. Usually, the cells have bland, oval nuclei and little mitotic activity. It is these cytologic features that help distinguish them from mesotheliomas or common epithelial malignancies. Intracytoplasmic mucin is absent. Although the majority of the tumors behave in a benign fashion, the presence of nuclear pleomorphism and, especially, increased mitotic activity (>10 mitoses/10 high-power fields) has been associated with more aggressive behavior.

PATTERNS OF SPREAD AND PROGNOSTIC FACTORS

The spread of fallopian tube carcinoma is relatively similar to that of the ovary, with frequent involvement of the peritoneum, omentum, bowel, and ovaries (18,29,120–123). In some series, half or more of all recurrences presented outside the peritoneal cavity; most often in the liver, lungs, and pleura, as well as in the vagina, kidney, brain, cervix, and skin (11,16,29). Although some investigators have reported that lymphatic spread is uncommon, this finding in part may have reflected a tendency not to perform lymph node dissections (63,123). The principal lymphatic drainage of the fallopian tube appears to be via the paraaortic lymph nodes (124). Pelvic or paraaortic lymph node involvement has been identified in 10% to 30% of patients at initial operation (124,125), in about one-third of women with recurrent disease (125), and in 75% (9 of 12) of patients at autopsy (125,126). As previously stated, the presence of capillary or lymphatic space involvement in early tubal carcinoma has been associated with diminished probability of survival at 5 years compared with patients in whom vascular invasion is not identified (29% vs 83%) (128).

Transcoelomic spread of tumor is an important mode of spread of fallopian tube carcinoma (15). Initially, exfoliation of neoplastic cells from the distal fimbriated end of the tube was suggested as the mechanism by which this occurred (123). However, it is difficult to reconcile this theory with the typical gross appearance of a dilated tube with a sealed distal tubal ostium (63). Further, Schiller and Silverberg (63), in a retrospective review of 76 published cases of fallopian tube carcinoma, documented the important relationship between the depth of invasion by tumor and survival. A crude 5-year survival of 91% was found for intramucosal lesions, 53% for tumors with mucosal wall invasion, and 25% or less for cases in which the tumors penetrated the tubal serosa. Using these data, they proposed a staging system for fallopian tube carcinoma based in part on the depth of invasion. Very similar 5-year survival rates by stage were recently reported in a study of 151 patients treated at the Norwegian Radium Hospital (47). In a univariate analysis of survival, the stage, presence of residual disease, ascites, depth of tubal invasion, a hydrosalpinx-like appearance, age, and vascular invasion, were all of statistical significance. However, several of these factors, such a depth of invasion and vascular space invasion, are interrelated. When subjected to a multivariate analysis, residual disease, stage, and a hydrosalpinx-like appearance retained strong statistical significance (47). In a subgroup analysis of 41 patients with stage I disease, depth of invasion and intraoperative tumor rupture were independent prognosticators. A study by Peters et al. (17) confirmed the importance of depth of invasion in predicting survival. Thus, the pathologist who examines a fallopian tube that contains carcinoma is recommended to provide information on the depth of invasion, the presence of lymphatic or capillary space involvement, and the degree of histologic differentiation.

DISTINCTION OF FALLOPIAN TUBE CARCINOMA FROM OVARIAN CARCINOMA

Because the gross and microscopic characteristics, as well as spread, of carcinoma of the fallopian tube closely resemble those of the ovary, it is sometimes difficult accurately to determine the site of origin of a tumor that forms a solid or cystic tubo-ovarian mass. In the past, some investigators have quite reasonably designated such tumors as tubo-ovarian carcinoma (49,81). Hu et al. (81), in 1950, proposed criteria for differentiating primary from metastatic carcinoma that involves the fallopian tube. These criteria, slightly modified, are outlined in Table 28.1 (123,126).

Many tumors of probable tubal origin fail to meet these stringent criteria. Because fallopian tube carcinomas are rel-

atively rare, it would seem logical to be restrictive in their definition. In this way, particular features about their pathogenesis, epidemiology, pathology, and clinical behavior would not be obscured by the inclusion of cases that might be of ovarian origin. The only fault with this approach is the possibility that the incidence of fallopian tube carcinoma will be underestimated.

HYPERPLASIA AND PREINVASIVE CARCINOMA OF THE FALLOPIAN TUBE

The sequence of histologic changes that precede the development of invasive adenocarcinoma of the fallopian tube has not been well described. Proliferation of the pseudostratified columnar cells in the absence of marked cytologic atypia or mitotic activity is referred to as epithelial hyperplasia (Fig. 28.4). The degree of proliferation varies and may result in a multilayered epithelium with focal tufting and, rarely, a cribriform pattern of cells. Tubal hyperplasia is more commonly observed as an incidental finding in patients with salpingitis (particularly tuberculous salpingitis), endogenous or exogenous estrogen stimulation, or serous ovarian tumors of low malignant potential (62,127). Moore and Enterline (128) prospectively sectioned entire oviducts from 124 nonselected hysterectomies and found hyperplasia in 19% of women, frequently as a focal lesion. The significance of hyperplasia is thus unknown, but the pathologist should be cautious not to overinterpret proliferative lesions as intraepithelial carcinoma.

Preinvasive carcinoma (dysplasia, carcinoma *in situ*) of the fallopian tube has been reported rarely (62,128,129). In contrast to hyperplasia, the diagnosis of carcinoma *in situ* requires the presence of marked cytologic atypia. The proliferation usually results in the formation of multilayered epithelium composed of cells with large, pleomorphic nu-

TABLE 28.1. *Criteria for pathologic diagnosis of primary fallopian tube carcinoma*

1. The main tumor is in the tube and arises from the endosalpinx.
2. The pattern histologically reproduces the epithelium of the mucosa and usually shows a papillary pattern.
3. If the wall is involved, the transition between benign and malignant tubal epithelium should be demonstrable.
4. The ovaries and endometrium are either normal or contain less tumor than the tubes.

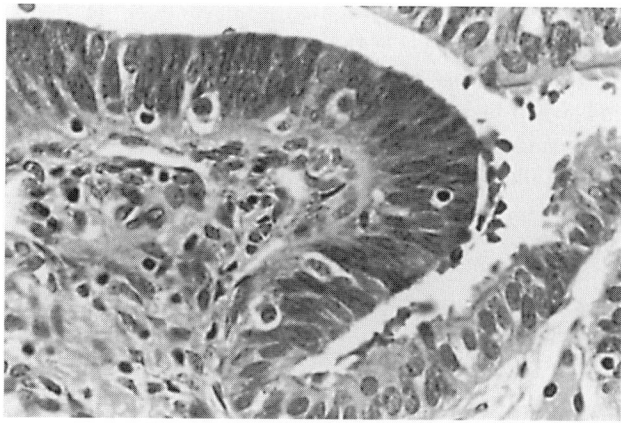

FIG. 28.4. Hyperplasia of the fallopian tube. Pseudostratification of cells and crowding of nuclei discovered as an incidental finding in a fallopian tube removed from a 49-year-old female with stress incontinence. (Original magnification ×100.)

clei, often prominent nucleoli, and interspersed mitotic activity. Whereas a papillary configuration is required by some investigators for the diagnosis of carcinoma *in situ*, the presence of a simple epithelium that displays severe cytologic atypia is considered by others to be sufficient for this diagnosis. The evidence that supports the designation of lesions as carcinoma *in situ* is their frequent occurrence in the transition between normal tubal epithelium and invasive carcinoma and their presence as part of multifocal *in situ* and early invasive neoplasia that involves the fallopian tube and ovary (62,129).

Chronic inflammation commonly coexists in fallopian tubes that contain carcinoma (5,63,124,126,130,131); this fact has resulted in speculation that acute and chronic salpingitis is a cause of fallopian tube cancer. However, it is more likely that inflammation is a response to the presence of the neoplasm coupled with obstruction of the fallopian tube rather than a carcinogenic factor. First, although acute salpingitis is usually a bilateral disease, the tube contralateral to the one that contains the carcinoma is frequently free of salpingitis. Second, fallopian tube carcinoma is a disease of postmenopausal women, a group with a low incidence of tubal infection. Nevertheless, in a pathologically based case-control study of the nonneoplastic contralateral tube from 14 women with fallopian tube carcinoma, changes significantly more common included luminal dilatation, plical atrophy, and chronic inflammation, which are all changes consistent with chronic, healed salpingitis (132).

In contrast to chronic salpingitis, the relationship between tuberculous salpingitis and carcinoma is more complex. More than two dozen cases of carcinoma arising in the tube affected by tuberculosis have been reported (133–135). Although some of the examples are well documented, with evidence of metastatic spread occasionally, there is some concern that not all of the cases truly represent coexisting invasive neoplasia. Hyperplasia of the mucosa is common in granulomatous salpingitis, and the proliferation of epithelium may be extreme, resulting in a cribriform pattern of epithelium associated with cytologic atypia (Fig. 28.5). In the absence of the granulomatous inflammation, this condition would be classified as dysplasia or carcinoma *in situ*. Designation of such lesions is problematic, however, since no data indicate their biologic potential in the presence or absence of inflammation. The diagnosis of invasive carcinoma should be made cautiously in the fallopian tube afflicted with tuberculosis and should be reserved for cases in which infiltration of the muscularis with a desmoplastic host response is obvious.

CYTOLOGY

Although exfoliative cervicovaginal cytology has been reported to be positive in as many as 40% to 60% of women with tubal carcinoma (28,123,136,137), in most series, abnormal Pap smears were distinctly uncommon (0% to 18%)

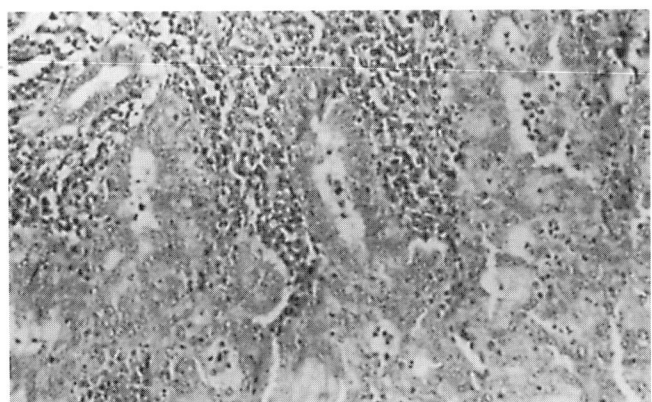

FIG. 28.5. Florid hyperplasia in a fallopian tube with chronic salpingitis. Marked proliferation of epithelial cells with focal cribriform growth pattern and moderate cytologic atypia accompanies dense inflammatory cell infiltrates. The lesion closely mimics carcinoma, but the pathologist should exercise great caution when granulomatous salpingitis or a tubo-ovarian complex is present. This 17-year-old woman was treated only with salpingectomy and remained free of disease after 7 years. (Original magnification ×64.)

(6,11,26,52,53,87,121,126,138). When present, the neoplastic cells are indistinguishable from those shed from endometrial adenocarcinoma, although several features may suggest that the tumor has arisen in the tube rather than the uterus. The malignant cells are scant in number and degenerate; malignant cells often present a spherical or papillary configuration; and the background is free of cellular debris (tumor diathesis) (139).

Because occult spread of tubal carcinoma outside the pelvis with serosal seeding occurs frequently, cytologic examination of peritoneal washings has been recommended (125). The presence of ascites or positive peritoneal cytology correlates well with an advanced stage of disease (27,139). A significantly worse prognosis has been reported for patients with exfoliated malignant cells in the peritoneum. In one study, the 5-year survival was 67% when the cytologic findings were negative but only 20% when malignant cells were present (128). Peritoneal fluid or washings should routinely be obtained at surgery for cytologic examination.

MULTIFOCAL CARCINOMA OF THE MÜLLERIAN SYSTEM, INCLUDING THE FALLOPIAN TUBE

Multifocal carcinomas that involve the fallopian tube can be divided into three patterns: synchronously detected multifocal neoplasia within the fallopian tubes; multifocal neoplasia that involves various genital organs, including the fallopian tube; and direct spread of carcinoma (frequently intraepithelial) along the mucosa of the cervix and endometrium to involve the fallopian tube.

About 20% of patients with fallopian tube carcinoma have

bilateral involvement. Although many specimens display a distinct site of mucosal tumor in each tube, it is unclear what percentage of patients reported to have bilateral disease actually have two, synchronously detected primary tubal neoplasms rather than metastasis from the contralateral tube (45). Unfortunately, most series do not include sufficient information to resolve this issue.

Multifocal carcinoma of the upper genital tract, including the fallopian tube, is relatively common (140–143). Sometimes, multiple papillary serous carcinomas are found in the ovary and on the serosa or in the lumen of the fallopian tube. These findings may reflect neoplastic transformation of the common embryologic field, which includes the coelomic epithelium that covers the ovary, fallopian tube, and other pelvic peritoneum (Fig. 28.6). At other times, endometrioid carcinomas are present in the endometrium, in the ovary, and in the mucosa of the tube. The frequent presence of endometriosis in these patients has led to the suggestion that it is the site of multifocal neoplastic transformation (142, 143). Multifocal neoplasia may be even more common than generally noted. In one series of 133 women with serous ovarian carcinoma, carcinoma *in situ* or early invasive carcinoma of the serially embedded fallopian tube was found in 4. The lesions were often focal, and none was grossly detected (129).

However, it is sometimes difficult to distinguish multiple primary neoplasms that arise in the fallopian tube and ovary or endometrium from endometrial or ovarian carcinoma metastatic to the tubal mucosa. For example, retrograde reflux of aggregates of neoplastic cells into the lumen of the fallopian tube may be observed in the hysterectomy specimen resected for endometrial adenocarcinoma (144). Occasionally, these refluxed tumor cells may implant and grow in the tubal mucosa since tumor types rarely observed primarily in the tube (such as clear-cell carcinoma or endometrioid carcinoma) coexist with endometrial carcinomas of these types. Direct spread of carcinoma *in situ* or invasive squamous carcinoma of the cervix along the mucosa of the endometrium and into the fallopian tubes has been occasionally reported (103,145–149). This extensive surface growth of malignant cells may reflect either horizontal spread with displacement of glandular epithelium by neoplasm or concurrent squamous metaplasia and neoplastic transformation in the cervix, endometrium, and fallopian tube (146). In view of the rarity of primary squamous carcinoma of the fallopian tube, the first hypothesis seems much more plausible.

CARCINOMA METASTATIC TO THE FALLOPIAN TUBE

The most common carcinoma that involves the fallopian tube is metastatic, generally from another site in the female genital tract. Carcinoma of the ovary is particularly likely to spread to the fallopian tube and may be found in up to half of patients with ovarian cancer (17,150a). Metastasis to the fallopian tube is reported to occur in 12% of patients with uterine corpus carcinoma and 4% of patients with cervical carcinomas (151,152). Although the tubal mucosa or muscular wall may be affected, primary involvement of the serosa is typical of ovarian carcinoma. Lymphatic or vascular space involvement is frequently identified in tumors metastatic from the uterus, and the entire wall of the fallopian tube may be permeated by tumor (151,152). Isolated examples of breast and bladder carcinoma metastatic to the fallopian tube have also been reported (153,154).

Endometrial stromal sarcomas, leiomyosarcomas, and malignant mixed mesodermal tumors that arise in the uterine corpus may invade directly into the adnexa and secondarily involve the fallopian tube. Lymphoma and leukemia also may spread to the fallopian tubes but usually do so as part of widespread organ involvement.

LESIONS THAT MIMIC PRIMARY CARCINOMA OF THE FALLOPIAN TUBE

The difficulty in distinguishing primary carcinoma of the fallopian tube from metastatic tumor has been addressed. In addition, several conditions, both neoplastic and nonneoplastic, may be confused with fallopian tube carcinoma (59, 155–158).

Salpingitis isthmica nodosa is the term given to a localized diverticulosis of the isthmic portion of the fallopian tube. The gross appearance, when visible, is of a firm, nodular expansion of the isthmus, with a diameter of less than 2 cm. Microscopically, a complex proliferation of branching glandular arrays is seen extending from the lumen to deep within the muscular wall (Fig. 28.7), often associated with hypertrophy of the muscularis. In spite of this architectural abnormality with pseudoinvasion, no cytologic atypia occurs, and the normal epithelial cell types of the fallopian tube mucosa may be readily identified.

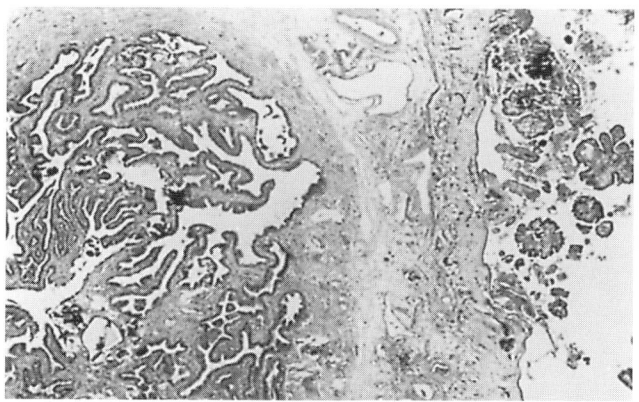

FIG. 28.6. Multifocal neoplasia involving the fallopian tube. Papillary carcinoma of low malignant potential is depicted on the serosa of the fallopian tube, whereas psammoma bodies are noted in the lumen. Histologically identical tumor was found in the ovaries. (Original magnification ×10.)

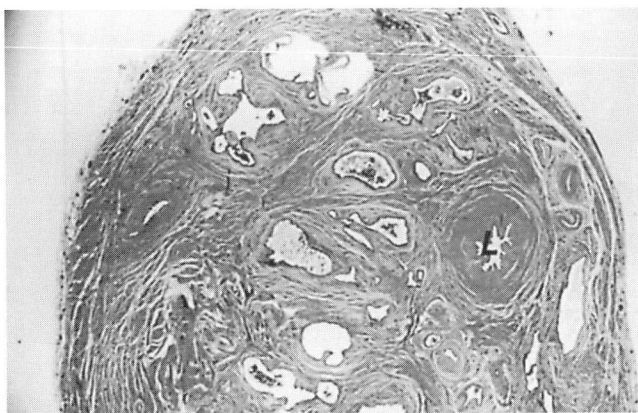

FIG. 28.7. Salpingitis isthmica nodosa. In this cross section of the fallopian tube, the luminal mucosa (L) appears unremarkable. However, the muscularis is thickened and nodular because of the proliferation of glands lined by a bland epithelium and surrounded by bundles of smooth muscle. (Original magnification ×4.)

Tuberculous salpingitis can closely mimic carcinoma both grossly and histologically (156,159). In the presence of granulomatous inflammation, the diagnosis of invasive carcinoma should be made only if one can identify tumor penetration into the muscularis associated with a host response. Two additional features provide some comfort to the pathologist who faces this diagnostic challenge. First, women with tubal carcinoma tend to be postmenopausal, whereas those having florid salpingitis are frequently young. Second, the nuclear atypia in carcinoma tends to be severe, whereas that of the reactive hyperplasia is mild or moderate with vesicular chromatin and small nucleoli.

Adenomatoid tumors represent benign mesotheliomas, which may occur along the serosa or deep muscularis of the fallopian tube (Fig. 28.8). They are usually small (1 to 2 cm

in diameter) nodular masses, formed of multiple, spherical, or slit-like channels lined by an attenuated layer of cells. The absence of cytologic atypia or significant mitotic activity permits the distinction from carcinoma. Immunohistochemical and ultrastructural studies provide convincing evidence of mesothelial cell differentiation for these lesions.

Metaplastic papillary tumor of the fallopian tube is a rare, incidental finding in pregnant or postpartum women. Focal, noncircumferential replacement of normal mucosa is accomplished by small papillae covered with large epithelial cells with abundant eosinophilic cytoplasm. Mitotic activity, severe cytologic atypia, and invasion are not seen. The behavior of these lesions is benign (92).

Cautery artifact in the fallopian tube results in elongation of epithelial cells with hyperchromasia of nuclei and smudging of chromatin (160). These changes resemble heat artifact in other epithelia and should not be confused with carcinoma.

STAGING

Because fallopian tube carcinoma has the propensity to spread intraabdominally, the most widely accepted staging system used in this malignancy is a modification of the International Federation of Gynecology and Obstetrics (FIGO) surgical staging of ovarian carcinoma, as first proposed by Dodson et al. (96). In 1992, FIGO formally established a staging classification for fallopian tube cancer (Table 28.2).

Scully and colleagues (55,64) have pointed out deficiencies in the current FIGO staging schema for fallopian tube carcinoma. The definition of stage 0 is inappropriate since *in situ* carcinoma is described as a tumor limited to the tubal mucosa—a structure that is composed of lamina propria as well as epithelium. Similarly, stage I tumors are described as tumors that extend into the submucosa—a structure that does not exist in the fallopian tube. Based on careful examination of the histology coupled with outcome in their large series of patients, Scully and colleagues have proposed a modification to the FIGO staging (Table 28.3). This modification corrects the nomenclature and emphasizes the prognostic impact of invasion into the muscular wall.

Unlike ovarian carcinoma, in which fully two-thirds of patients present with advanced-stage disease, the majority of patients with tubal cancer are diagnosed at an earlier stage. A review of eight series published over the past decade confirms the preponderance of early-stage disease in fallopian tube carcinoma (8,15,16,27–29,124). Of 558 patients, 33% were stage I, 33% were stage II, and 34% were stage III or IV.

GENERAL MANAGEMENT

Primary treatment of adenocarcinoma of the fallopian tube is surgical resection at the time of initial diagnosis. Extensive

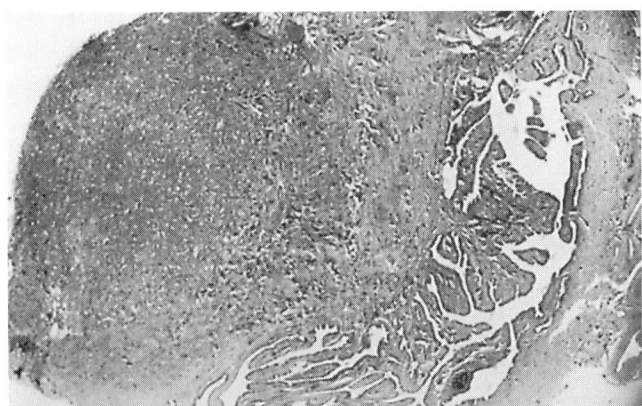

FIG. 28.8. Adenomatoid tumor. An eccentrically located subserosal mass is present in the fallopian tube. It can be distinguished from tubal carcinoma by its location and generally bland cytology. (Original magnification ×4.)

TABLE 28.2. *FIGO fallopian tube carcinoma staging*

Stage 0: Carcinoma *in situ* (limited to tubal mucosa).
Stage I: Growth limited to fallopian tubes.
Stage IA: Growth limited to one tube with extension into submucosa and/or muscularis but not penetrating serosal surface; no ascites.
Stage IB: Growth limited to both tubes with extension into submucosa and/or muscularis but not penetrating serosal surface; no ascites.
Stage IC: Tumor either stage IA or stage IB but with extension through or onto tubal serosa or with ascites containing malignant cells or with positive peritoneal washings.
Stage II: Growth involving one or both fallopian tubes with pelvic extension.
Stage IIA: Extension and/or metastasis to uterus and/or ovaries.
Stage IIB: Extension to other pelvic tissues.
Stage IIC: Tumor either stage IIA or IIB and with ascites containing malignant cells or with positive peritoneal washings.
Stage III: Tumor involving one or both fallopian tubes with peritoneal implants outside pelvis and/or positive retroperitoneal or inguinal nodes. Superficial liver metastasis equals stage III. Tumor appears limited to true pelvis but with histologically proved malignant extension to small bowel or omentum.
Stage IIIA: Tumor grossly limited to true pelvis with negative nodes but with histologically confirmed microscopic seeding of abdominal peritoneal surfaces.
Stage IIIB: Tumor involving one or both tubes with histologically confirmed implants of abdominal peritoneal surfaces, none exceeding 2 cm in diameter. Lymph nodes are negative.
Stage IIIC: Abdominal implants >2 cm in diameter and/or positive retroperitoneal or inguinal nodes.
Stage IV: Growth involving one or both fallopian tubes with distant metastases. If pleural effusion is present, cytologic fluid must be positive for malignant cells to be stage IV. Parenchymal liver metastasis equals stage IV.

Note: Staging for fallopian tube carcinoma is by the surgicopathologic system. Operative findings designating stage are determined before tumor debulking.

TABLE 28.3. *Modified FIGO staging for fallopian tube carcinoma[a]*

Stage 0: Carcinoma *in situ* (limited to tubal epithelium[b]).
Stage I: Growth limited to tube.
Stage IA: Growth limited to one tube without extension through or onto serosa, ascites containing malignant cells, or positive peritoneal washings.
Stage IA-0[c]: Growth limited to one tube with no extension into lamina propria.[b]
Stage IA-1[c]: Growth limited to one tube with extension into lamina propria[a] but no extension into muscularis.
Stage IA-2[c]: Growth limited to one tube with extension into muscularis.
Stage IB: Growth limited to both tubes without extension through or onto serosa, ascites containing malignant cells, or positive peritoneal washings.
Stage IB-0[c]: Growth limited to both tubes with no extension into lamina propria.[b]
Stage IB-1[c]: Growth limited to both tubes with extension into lamina propria,[b] but no extension into muscularis.
Stage IB-2[c]: Growth limited to both tubes with extension into muscularis.
Stage IC: Tumor either stage IA or IB but with extension through or onto tubal serosa or with ascites containing malignant cells or with positive peritoneal washings.
Stage I(F): Tumor limited to fimbriated end of tube(s) without invasion of tubal wall.
Stage II: Tumor involving one or both fallopian tubes with pelvic extension.
Stage IIA: Extension and/or metastasis to uterus and/or ovaries.
Stage IIB: Extension to other pelvic tissues.
Stage IIC: Tumor either stage IIA or IIB with ascites containing malignant cells or with positive peritoneal washings.
Stage III: Tumor involving one or both fallopian tubes with peritoneal implants outside pelvis, including superficial liver metastasis, and/or positive retroperitoneal or inguinal nodes. Tumor limited to pelvis except for histologically proven extension to small bowel or omentum.
Stage IIIA: Tumor grossly limited to pelvis with negative nodes but with histologically confirmed microscopic seeding of abdominal peritoneal surfaces.
Stage IIIB: Tumor involving one or both fallopian tubes with grossly visible, histologically confirmed implants of abdominal peritoneal surfaces, none >2 cm in diameter. Lymph nodes are negative.
Stage IIIC: Abdominal implants >2 cm in diameter and/or positive retroperitoneal or inguinal nodes.
Stage IV: Growth involving one or both fallopian tubes with distant metastases including parenchymal liver metastases. If pleural effusion is present, fluid must be positive cytologically for malignant cells.

[a]As suggested by Alvarado-Cabrero et al.
[b]Modification in terminology.
[c]Modifications to accommodate subsets of tumors that otherwise cannot be assigned a stage or to distinguish among subsets that may differ in their associated prognosis.

surgical resection and staging should be performed [total abdominal hysterectomy (TAH), omentectomy, and bilateral salpingectomy], as well as sampling of ascitic fluid or peritoneal washings and peritoneal sampling of diaphragm, bladder, and bowel. Recent reports advocate lymph node sampling, as nodal involvement may occur early in the course of disease spread. It may occur even earlier than the extent of pelvic spread may indicate (124,161). Numerous investigators have observed that the amount of residual tumor left behind at primary resection (>2 cm) has major prognostic implications (29). Some investigators have reported satisfactory results with conservative surgical treatment (unilateral salpingectomy only) in cases in which tumor has not invaded beyond the mucosa (162). Most patients, however, require some form of adjuvant treatment postoperatively to combat bulky residual disease or to treat assumed microscopic involvement. Hellstrom et al. (163), in a report of 128 patients

with fallopian tube carcinoma treated in Sweden, noted that 59 (46%) were treated with bilateral salpingo-oophorectomy (BSO), 47 (36%) with some form of hysterectomy and BSO, and the rest with incomplete surgery. The majority of the patients received adjuvant external or intracavitary irradiation, and 62 (48%) were treated with single or multiagent chemotherapy.

Most studies reporting results of adjuvant therapy are not based on prospective randomization of patients, and they use inconsistent staging schema and poorly reported or performed surgical staging.

Radiation therapy has been used as adjuvant therapy for fallopian tube carcinoma. It is difficult to evaluate its efficacy owing to variability in staging, surgical staging techniques, treatment volume, dose fractionation, and type of radiation used. All reported studies are retrospective and usually involve small numbers of patients treated over long periods (30).

SURGICAL MANAGEMENT

The surgical management of primary fallopian tube carcinoma closely parallels that of carcinoma of the ovary (164) (discussed in detail in Chapters 32, 33, and 34).

Fallopian tube carcinoma is rarely diagnosed preoperatively. The surgeon confronted with the diagnosis intraoperatively must therefore be prepared to perform the appropriate staging procedure. Improper staging procedures may erroneously lead to the downstaging of patients with more advanced disease. The importance of proper staging is highlighted by the tendency of fallopian tube carcinoma to metastasize to lymph nodes. Tamimi and Figge (124) reported a 53% incidence of lymph node metastases in 15 patients with tubal cancer. Five patients had disease in the paraaortic nodes, and, in two of these, this finding was the only evidence of metastases. Similarly, Schray et al. (161) noted a 35% incidence of nodal metastases in 34 patients. Five of nine patients with extrapelvic nodal metastases would otherwise have been classified as having stage I disease.

Patients with residual tumor mass of <1 cm after surgery enjoy a significantly higher survival rate than patients with larger residual tumor burdens; a situation identical to that observed in ovarian carcinoma (29). Surgical therapy for fallopian tube carcinoma should therefore follow similar guidelines as used in ovarian carcinoma.

The role of second-look laparotomy in the management of fallopian tube carcinoma is not clearly defined. The theoretical rationale for this procedure, based on experience with ovarian carcinoma, would be to determine the effectiveness of front-line therapy and provide information on disease status not reliably obtainable by noninvasive means (165). Approximately 86 cases of second-look procedures for tubal cancer have been reported in the medical literature (8,14, 28,29,107,138,139,167–170). Although 61% of these were negative, information regarding surgical stage before administration of chemotherapy or irradiation was not always available. Barakat et al. (107) reported the largest experience

to date regarding second-look laparotomy in tubal cancer; 21 of 35 platinum-treated patients had a negative second look. With a mean follow-up of 50 months, only four (19%) have had recurrence. This contrasts with advanced-stage ovarian carcinoma patients treated with platinum-based chemotherapy, among whom approximately 50% will experience recurrence after a negative second-look procedure, with a median interval of 14 months to recurrence (171). Based on their experience, the investigators recommend second-look laparotomy for patients with stages II to IV tubal cancer to assess tumor status more accurately, allowing for secondary cytoreduction and further treatment if necessary.

RISK-REDUCING SURGERY IN *BRCA* MUTATION CARRIERS

As previously noted, patients who harbor a mutation in the *BRCA* genes are also at increased risk for developing fallopian tube carcinoma (19,20,24). The incidence of occult gynecologic malignancies at the time of risk-reducing oophorectomy is estimated to be between 2% and 4% (21, 172–174). The incidental diagnosis of primary fallopian tube carcinoma has also been reported (56). The magnitude of the increased risk associated with fallopian tube cancer warrants removal of the entire tube at the time of risk-reducing oophorectomy. Variables such as genetic penetrance of the mutations and the risk of primary fallopian tube cancer have not been fully elucidated.

Some investigators have proposed performing a hysterectomy at the time of a risk-reducing oophorectomy to decrease the risk of subsequent fallopian tube carcinoma (23). It is known that a small amount of the interstitial portion of the fallopian tube will remain within the cornu of the uterus at the time of BSO. To date, there have been no reports of fallopian tube carcinoma arising subsequent to a risk-reducing BSO. Most fallopian tube cancers arise at the fimbria or in the isthmus portion of the fallopian tube and not within the interstitial portion where the mucosa is thinner and less complex (175). The scope of the surgical procedure would be significantly altered by adding a hysterectomy at the time of risk-reducing BSO. Thus, the additional risk associated with the surgical procedure may not be warranted in light of the limited data available of risk of subsequent fallopian tube carcinoma after risk-reducing BSO.

RADIATION THERAPY

Radiation therapy has long been used on an *ad hoc* basis as an adjunct therapy in the treatment of carcinoma of the fallopian tube following surgical resection of the primary tumor, with and without the addition of chemotherapy.

Irradiation techniques are similar to those used in treatment of ovarian carcinoma, including whole abdominal or pelvic external beam irradiation or intraperitoneal administration of radioactive colloids (^{32}P, ^{198}Au); better survival rates have been reported as compared with surgery alone (7, 29,121,162). There are too few data to support the use of radioactive colloids, and their use has no role in patients with bulky tumors (7,8,11).

The best results are achieved with a total dose of 50 Gy or greater to the pelvis in 5 to 6 weeks using megavoltage photon beams (5,14,16,46,176).

The following reports garnered from the literature, although all retrospective and nonrandomized, are instructional and may point to a rational basis of maneuvers.

Yoonessi (126) reported a retrospective study of 47 cases of primary fallopian tube adenocarcinoma seen before January 1975 at the University of Michigan Medical Center and the affiliated hospitals of the State University of New York at Buffalo and provided a literature survey. In stages I to IIB, 4 of 14 patients (29%) treated by surgery only and 5 of 14 patients (36%) treated with surgery and radiation therapy survived 5 years. Autopsy information was available in 12 of the 47 cases. Nine of these 12 patients (75%) had positive pelvic or aortic nodes; 6 (50%) had both pelvic- and paraaortic-positive nodes.

Roberts and Lifshitz (8) reported on a retrospective analysis of 28 cases of fallopian tube carcinoma. The survival data in this group of patients were combined with 74 cases published in the current literature to obtain a series of 102 evaluable cases. In all cases, either the tumor was completely resected or only minimal residual disease remained. At 5 years posttreatment, survival was 74.5% and 75.2% among stage I patients who underwent surgery only and surgery with pelvic irradiation, respectively; among stage II patients, the 5-year survival was 42.8% and 48.1%, respectively. The investigators concluded that there appeared to be no improvement in survival when pelvic irradiation was added to surgery.

Brown et al. (14) analyzed 21 patients. Postoperative irradiation was used in 14 patients. Either pelvic or whole abdominopelvic fields were treated using open-field techniques; one patient received pelvic and paraaortic irradiation. Five stage I patients received adjuvant postoperative irradiation, and three experienced long-term survival; in two of these patients, the uterus had been left for radium placement and the other received pelvic and paraaortic irradiation along with intravaginal radium. Nine patients had stage II disease. Three who underwent surgery and postoperative irradiation were disease free from 3 to 23 years later. Two of these three patients received abdominopelvic irradiation, and one received pelvic irradiation alone. Five patients had stage III disease, and one patient had stage IV disease. Postoperatively, three patients received abdominopelvic irradiation. The longest survivor had residual disease following surgery and remained alive and free of clinical disease for 11 years. The other two patients died within 1 year, although they had no clinical evidence of disease following surgery. Nine patients, five with stage IIB or III disease, were treated with

abdominopelvic or pelvic and paraaortic irradiation, and five of these remain free of disease.

Wong et al. (177) described their experience with primary carcinoma of the fallopian tube treated in Manchester, England, between 1966 and 1980. Ten patients received 30- to 45-Gy postoperative pelvic irradiation, resulting in five of ten patients surviving 2 years or more. Eight patients received no postoperative radiation therapy; six of eight patients survived at least 2 years.

Podratz et al. (29) reported on 47 patients with primary carcinoma of the fallopian tube treated at the Mayo Clinic. Three types of adjunctive radiation therapy were used: (a) intraperitoneal radioactive colloidal ^{32}P; (b) whole pelvic irradiation, with or without paraaortic inclusion; and (3) whole abdominopelvic irradiation. The total dose for whole pelvic irradiation (with or without paraaortic treatment) ranged from 35 to 55 Gy to the pelvis, with 9 of 16 patients receiving 50 Gy or more. Patients treated with whole abdominopelvic irradiation (with partial shielding of the liver and kidneys when necessary) received from 17 to 35 Gy, with additional doses to the pelvis and paraaortic regions in five of seven patients, resulting in a total pelvic dose of 38.0 to 52.2 Gy. The initial sites of treatment failure were known in 24 patients, with the abdominal cavity being identified as the site of failure in 21 patients (88%).

Tamimi and Figge (124) described results in 15 cases of primary adenocarcinoma of the fallopian tube. Information regarding lymph node metastases was obtained from pathologic material available at the time of initial diagnosis (five patients), recurrent disease (two patients), and at autopsy (one patient). Eight patients received radiation therapy as part of their treatment program following surgical treatment. Various radiation therapy regimens were used depending on the extent of the disease. The survival of the patients who received adjunctive chemotherapy, radiation therapy, or a combination was similar.

McMurray et al. (16) reported on 30 patients with adenocarcinoma of the fallopian tube treated with external irradiation (either ^{60}Co or betatron 22-MV x-rays) to the pelvis through anteroposterior-posteroanterior (AP-PA) parallel opposing fields. A midplane dose of between 36.0 and 50.4 Gy was delivered in 1.8- to 2.0-Gy daily doses with five fractions per week. Analysis of patterns of failure in stage I disease revealed one pelvic recurrence in six cases (17%) who did not receive pelvic irradiation, and in none of three patients who did receive pelvic irradiation; in stage II, one pelvic and one abdominal recurrence occurred in three patients (33%) who did not receive pelvic irradiation, and three pelvic and two abdominal recurrences occurred in eight patients who did receive pelvic irradiation (38%).

Higher pelvic recurrence rates in patients who have undergone complete tumor resection without postoperative pelvic irradiation have also been described by Denham and Maclennan (115) (i.e., 35% in stage I and 70% in stage II).

Muntz et al. reported on 19 patients with primary adenocarcinoma of the fallopian tube. Twelve patients received external radiation therapy (40- to 50-Gy midplane dose in 4 to 5 weeks to the pelvis or lower abdomen and pelvis). No patient received treatment to the upper abdomen, whole abdomen, or paraaortic chain. Two stage I patients, treated with pelvic irradiation, were both free of disease 5 and 20 years after diagnosis, respectively. Of three stage II patients who did not receive pelvic irradiation, one suffered a pelvic recurrence; of five patients treated with pelvic irradiation, none failed locally.

Ross (180) reviewed the records and pathologic materials of 40 patients with a primary malignancy of the fallopian tube. As of December 1988, 6 of 40 patients (15%) were disease free, with follow-up ranging from 22 to 141 months. Four early stage I or II tubal cancers were treated with adjuvant ^{32}P, with three of the patients having recurrences. Fifteen patients in this study underwent autopsy, with ten (67%) having paraaortic nodal metastases. Seven of these patients also had pelvic node metastases, but none had pelvic node metastasis without paraaortic node involvement.

Carlson et al. (97) reported, in 1993, on five new cases of malignant mixed müllerian tumor of the fallopian tube; four of five long-term survivors were disease free at 58 months (stage III, irradiation and chemotherapy), 75 months (stage II, irradiation and chemotherapy), 80 months (stage I, irradiation), and 205 months (stage II, irradiation and chemotherapy). Survivors were characterized by the absence of ascites and gross evidence of extension beyond the pelvis and tumor resectability. The irradiation was designed to deliver doses capable of eradicating microscopic residual foci to the original site of tumor and sites of possible occult metastases. Details of the irradiation techniques were not reported.

Other studies noted a 50% relapse rate when early-stage disease was treated with surgery alone or surgery and pelvic irradiation versus a greater than 50% 5-year survival rate when the abdomen and paraaortic areas were treated (14,29, 125).

Wolfson et al. (181) reported on 72 patients with carcinoma of the fallopian tube treated at six medical centers (24 stage I, 20 stage II, 24 stage III, and four stage IV). Adjuvant chemotherapy was administered to 54 patients and postoperative irradiation to 22 patients. Of these, 14 received whole pelvis external irradiation, five whole abdominal irradiation, two ^{32}P instillation, and one vaginal brachytherapy only. The 5-, 8-, and 15-year survival rates were 44%, 24%, and 19%, respectively, for patients treated with chemotherapy and 27%, 17%, and 14%, respectively, for those treated with irradiation. Significant prognostic factors included stage I versus more advanced stages and age at diagnosis (younger or older than 60 years). Patterns of failure included 2 vaginal, 5 pelvic, 24 abdominal, and 15 distant metastases. Abdominal failures were 21% in patients with stage I and 79% in patients with stages II, III, and IV disease. Patients experiencing abdominal relapse were more likely to die (32 of 72; 44%) than those without abdominal relapse (13 of 72; 18%) ($p = 0.001$).

In a study using the new FIGO staging system for fallopian tube carcinoma, researchers compared outcome for patients with carcinoma in situ versus stage I disease treated with either irradiation or cisplatin-based chemotherapy. Stage I patients treated with irradiation showed a significantly better prognosis than patients treated with chemotherapy ($p = 0.017$) (163). Some reports showed no benefit with irradiation using orthovoltage therapy, which is unable to deliver high doses to the deeper pelvic structures (182), or irradiating the pelvis only (8).

Klein et al. (183), in a retrospective analysis of 158 cases of fallopian tube cancer, reported on 95 cases of early disease, stage I (66 cases) and stage II (29 cases). All patients underwent a TAH/BSO, and 24 had undergone a radical pelvic/paraaortic lymphadenectomy. Of these latter patients, 30% were found to have positive nodes and were excluded from futher analysis (stage IIIC). The remaining 63 patients were distributed as either group 1 (32 patients) who received pelvic/paraaortic irradiation (45 to 52 Gy), with 11 cases also receiving whole abdominal irradiation (13 to 16 Gy), or group 2 (31 cases), who received six cycles of platinum chemotherapy. Group 1 patients experienced a median survival time of 57 months (95% CI 33 to 81), and group 2 had a median survival time of 73 months (95% CI 68 to 78) ($p = .476$). Patients who had undergone a pelvic/paraaortic lymphadenectomy experienced an 83% 5-year survival, with those patients whose surgical procedure was only a TAH/BSO having a 5-year survival of 58% ($p = .12$). In an update of this report (161), the investigators noted a 43-month median survial for patients who underwent a radical lymphadenectomy versus 21 months in individuals who did not have this procedure performed ($p = 0.095$).

Based on the above literature survey, the radiation therapy contribution to treatment of fallopian tube tumors may be summarized as follows:

1. In stage I and stage II carcinoma, failure to irradiate the pelvis, even in the absence of residual disease, results in a local recurrence rate of approximately 35% and 70%, respectively (15).
2. Pelvic irradiation for local tumor control is feasible; five stage II patients reported by Muntz et al. (137) had local control.
3. Despite locoregional control, intraperitoneal and extraperitoneal extrapelvic relapse is commonly observed. Indeed, in the series reported by McMurray et al. (16), almost half of the recurrences presented outside the peritoneal cavity, although usually in association with intraperitoneal metastases. The risk for paraaortic metastases has been identified by several investigators: 33% by Tamimi and Figge (124) and 67% by Ross (180).
4. Whole abdominal irradiation and intraperitoneal ^{32}P are controversial therapies. Whole abdominal irradiation has

been particularly well recorded in carcinoma of the ovary by Dembo (185) and Thomas and Dembo (2). The efficacy of whole abdominal irradiation in carcinoma of the fallopian tube is unknown, although institutional reports have documented anecdotal applications. The adequacy of doses in the range of 20 to 30 Gy by standard fractionation for sterilization of microscopic disease, as well as radiation toxicity, is to be determined. The instillation of ^{32}P has been used in carcinoma of the fallopian tube on an anecdotal basis with variable results; this modality would have little beneficial effect in the one-third of cases who have occult paraaortic metastases and would severely limit supplemental external irradiation. Satisfactory diffuse intraperitoneal distribution of isotope is also an important factor.

5. Based on the efficacy of radiation therapy in the case of occult microscopic disease, a rational approach to this rare disease for stages I to III (status postsurgical resection, no residual) might include external irradiation to pelvic and paraaortic nodes (i.e., 45 to 50.4 Gy, 1.8 Gy per fraction, five fractions per week, using megavoltage equipment) followed by chemotherapy (186).

CHEMOTHERAPY

The experience with chemotherapeutic agents for this malignancy is largely limited to case reports and small series; the overall experience closely parallels that of ovarian carcinoma.

One of the first reports of a response of fallopian tube adenocarcinoma to a chemotherapeutic agent was with the alkylating agent melphalan (Alkeran) (187). Single agents that have demonstrated activity in fallopian tube carcinoma include doxorubicin, cisplatin, and the alkylating agents melphalan, chlorambucil, cyclophosphamide, and thiotepa (126, 187). In general, responses in advanced disease to single agents have been short, although occasional long-term remissions (>2 years) have been reported (15).

The regimen of cyclophosphamide and doxorubicin has been reported to be active in several patients with advanced disease, with remissions lasting more than 2 years (136,169).

With the establishment of cisplatin as the most active drug in the treatment of advanced ovarian carcinoma, investigators have focused their attention on this drug in combination with cyclophosphamide or doxorubicin as therapy for fallopian tube carcinomas. More than 100 patients with adenocarcinoma of the fallopian tube have been reported to have been treated with a cisplatin-based combination regimen, with an overall response rate and survival that are similar to those observed in patients with advanced ovarian carcinoma (12,16,17,27,32,125,166,170,178,188–195). As paclitaxel has been documented to improve the effectiveness of cisplatin-based therapy of advanced ovarian cancer, it is reasonable to anticipate similar activity in fallopian tube carci-

nomas, although the experience with this combination in fallopian tube cancer remains limited (11,196,197). A recent report has documented the activity of topotecan in recurrent fallopian tube cancer (196).

Modest activity for combination chemotherapy with several agents, including cyclophosphamide, actinomycin, vincristine, doxorubicin, and dimethylthiazenoimidazole carboximide (DTIC), has been observed in the rare sarcomas of the fallopian tube (98,199,200).

As the normal fallopian tube responds in a cyclic fashion to hormonal influences, it is natural that progestational agents have been used in patients with fallopian tube carcinoma (27,32,187,201). Unfortunately, no convincing clinical data support the use of this class of agents in the management of this malignancy.

SUMMARY

Primary treatment of fallopian tube carcinoma is TAH and BSO. For early-stage tumors, less radical procedures may be considered depending on the age of the patient. Surgical therapy for fallopian tube carcinoma follows the guidelines for ovarian carcinoma. Second-look laparotomy is recommended for patients with stages II, III, and IV disease to determine tumor status and potential need for secondary cytoreduction and further chemotherapy.

Adjuvant therapy is recommended for all stages of carcinoma of the fallopian tube. In most circumstances, chemotherapy should be administered, although in rare circumstances radiation therapy may play a role.

REFERENCES

1. Berg JW, Lampe JG. High-risk factors in gynecologic cancer. *Cancer* 1981;48:429.
2. Thomas GM, Dembo AJ. Integrating radiation therapy into the management of ovarian cancer. *Cancer* 1993;71:1710.
3. Schulte BA, Rao KPP, Kreutner A, et al. Histochemical examination of glycoconjugates of epithelial cells in the human fallopian tube. *Lab Invest* 1985;52:207.
4. Donnez J, Casanas-Roux F, Caprasse J, et al. Cyclic changes in ciliation, cell height, and mitotic activity in human tubal epithelium during reproductive life. *Fertil Steril* 1985;43:554.
5. Hanton EM, Malkasian GD, Dahlin DC, Pratt JH. Primary carcinoma of the fallopian tube. *Am J Obstet Gynecol* 1966;94:832.
6. Momtazee S, Kempson RL. Primary adenocarcinoma of the fallopian tube. *Obstet Gynecol* 1968;32:649.
7. Phelps H, Chapman K. Role of radiation therapy in treatment of primary carcinoma of the uterine tube. *Obstet Gynecol* 1974;43:669.
8. Roberts JA, Lifshitz S. Primary adenocarcinoma of the fallopian tube. *Gynecol Oncol* 1982;13:301.
9. Rosen AC, Sevelda P, Klein M, et al. A comparative analysis of management and prognosis in stage I and II fallopian tube carcinoma and epithelial ovarian cancer. *Br J Cancer* 1994;69:577.
10. Rosenblatt KA, Weiss NS, Schwartz SM. Incidence of malignant fallopian tube tumors. *Gynecol Oncol* 1989;5:236.
11. Benedet JL, White GW, Fairey RN, Boyes DA. Adenocarcinoma of the fallopian tube: experience with 41 patients. *Obstet Gynecol* 1977;50:654.
12. Asmussen M, Kaern J, Kjoerstad K, et al. Primary adenocarcinoma

localized to the fallopian tubes: report on 33 cases. *Gynecol Oncol* 1988;30:183.

13. Boutselis JG, Thompson JN. Clinical aspects of primary carcinoma of the fallopian tube: a clinical study of 14 cases. *Am J Obstet Gynecol* 1971;111:98.

14. Brown MD, Kohorn EI, Kapp DS, et al. Fallopian tube carcinoma. *Int J Radiat Oncol Biol Phys* 1985;11:583.

15. Denham JW, Maclennan KA. The management of primary carcinoma of the fallopian tube: experience of 40 cases. *Cancer* 1984;53:166.

16. McMurray EH, Jacobs AJ, Perez CA, et al. Carcinoma of the fallopian tube: management and sites of failure. *Cancer* 1986;58:2070.

17. Nordin AJ. Primary carcinoma of the fallopian tube: a 20-year literature review. *Obstet Gynecol Surv* 1994;49:349.

17a. Peters WA, Andersen WA, Hopkins MP, et al. Prognostic features of carcinoma of the fallopian tube. *Obstet Gynecol* 1988;71:757.

18. Sedlis A. Carcinoma of the fallopian tube. *Surg Clin North Am* 1978; 58:121.

18a. Herbert-Blouin M, Koufogianis V, Gillett P, Foulkes W. Fallopian tube cancer in a BRCA1 mutation carrier: rapid development and failure of screening. *Am J Obstet Gynecol* 2002;186:53.

19. Rose PG, Shrigley R, Wiesner GL. Germline BRCA2 mutation in a patient with fallopian tube carcinoma: a case report. *Gynecol Oncol* 2000;77: 319.

20. Aziz S, Kuperstein G, Rosen B, et al. A genetic epidemiological study of carcinoma of the fallopian tube. *Gynecol Oncol* 2002;80:341.

21. Colgan TJ, Murphy J, Cole DE, et al. Occult carcinoma in prophylactic oophorectomy specimens: prevalence and association with BRCA germline mutation status. *Am J Surg Pathol* 2001;25:1283.

22. Hartley A, Rollason T, Spooner D. Clear cell carcinoma of the fimbria of the fallopian tube in a BRCA1 carrier undergoing prophylactic surgery. *Clin Oncol R Coll Radiol* 2000;12:58.

23. Paley PJ, Swisher EM, Garcia RL, et al. Occult cancer of the fallopian tube in BRCA1 germline mutation carriers at prophylactic oophorectomy: a case for recommending hysterectomy at surgical prophylaxis. *Gynecol Oncol* 2001;80:176.

24. Zweemer RP, Van Diest PJ, Verheijen RH, et al. Molecular evidence linking primary cancer of the fallopian tube to BRCA1 germline mutations. *Gynecol Oncol* 2000;76:45.

25. Heselmeyer K, Hellstrom A, Blegen H, et al. Primary carcinoma of the fallopian tube: comparative genomic hybridization reveals high genetic instability and a specific, recurring pattern of chromosomal aberrations. *Int J Gynecol Pathol* 1998;17:245.

26. Amendola BE, LaRouere J, Amendola MA, et al. Adenocarcinoma of the fallopian tube. *Surg Gynecol Obstet* 1983;157:223.

27. Eddy GL, Copeland LJ, Gershenson DM, et al. Fallopian tube carcinoma. *Obstet Gynecol* 1984;64:546.

28. Pfeiffer P, Mogensen H, Amtrup F, Honore E. Primary carcinoma of the fallopian tube: a retrospective study of patients reported to the Danish Cancer Registry in a 5-year period. *Acta Oncol* 1989;28:7.

29. Podratz KC, Podczaski ES, Gaffey TA, O'Brien PC, Schray MF, Malkasian GD Jr. Primary carcinoma of the fallopian tube. *Am J Obstet Gynecol* 1986;154:1319.

30. Ostapovicz DM, Brady LW. Fallopian tube. In: Perez CA, Brady LW, eds. *Principles and practice of radiation oncology.* 3rd ed. Philadelphia: Lippincott–Raven, 1998:1881.

31. Raghavan S, Chadaya R, Rani R, et al. A review of fallopian tube carcinoma over 20 years (1971–90) in Pondicherry. *Indian J Cancer* 1991;28:188.

32. Yoonessi M, Leberer JP, Crickard K. Primary fallopian tube carcinoma: treatment and spread pattern. *J Surg Oncol* 1988;38:97.

33. Hinton A, Bea C, Winfield AC, Entman SS. Carcinoma of the fallopian tube. *Urol Radiol* 1988;10:113.

34. Granberg S, Jansson I. Early detection of primary carcinoma of the fallopian tube by endovaginal ultrasound. *Acta Obstet Gynecol Scand* 1990;69:667.

35. Kol S, Gal D, Friedman M, Paldi E. Preoperative diagnosis of fallopian tube carcinoma by transvaginal sonography and CA-125. *Gynecol Oncol* 1990;37:129.

36. Kurjak A, Schulman H, Sosic A, Zalud I, Shalan H. Transvaginal ultrasound: color flow and Doppler wave form of the postmenopausal adnexal mass. *Obstet Gynecol* 1992;80:917.

37. Podobnik M, Singer Z, Ciglar S, Bulic M. Preoperative diagnosis of primary fallopian tube carcinoma by transvaginal ultrasound, cytological findings and CA-125. *Ultrasound Med Biol* 1993;19:587.

38. Kawakami S, Togashi K, Kimura I, et al. Primary malignant tumor of the fallopian tube: appearance at CT and MR imaging. *Radiology* 1993;186:503.

39. Thurnher S, Hodler J, Baer S, et al. Gadolinium-DOTA enhanced MR imaging of adnexal tumors. *J Comput Assist Tomogr* 1990;14:939.

40. Lehtovirta P, Kairemo KJ, Liewendahl K, Seppala M. Immunolymphoscintigraphy and immunoscintigraphy of ovarian and fallopian tube cancer using F(ab')2 fragments of monoclonal antibody OC 125. *Cancer Res* 1990;50[Suppl 3]:937s.

41. Karlan B, Hoh C, Tse N, et al. Whole body positron emission tomography with (fluorine-18)-2 deoxy-glucose can detect metastatic carcinoma of the fallopian tube. *Gynecol Oncol* 1993;49:383.

42. Makhija S. Howden N, Edwards R, et al. Positron emission tomography/computed tomography imaging for the detection of recurrent ovarian and fallopian tube carcinoma: a retrospective review. *Gynecol Oncol* 2002;85:53.

43. Davies AR, Fish A, Woolas R, Oram D. Raised serum CA-125 preceding the diagnosis of carcinoma of the fallopian tube: two case reports. *Br J Obstet Gynecol* 1991;98:602.

44. Tokunaga T, Miyazaki K, Matsuyama S, Okamura H. Serial measurement of CA 125 in patients with primary carcinoma of the fallopian tube. *Gynecol Oncol* 1990;36:335.

45. Lootsma-Miklosova E, Aalders JG, Willemse PHB, de Bruijn HW. Levels of CA 125 in patients with recurrent carcinoma of the fallopian tube: two case histories. *Eur J Obstet Gynecol Reprod Biol* 1987;24: 231.

46. Gadducci A, Madrigali A, Ciancia EM, et al. The clinical, serological, pathological and immunocytochemical features of a case of primary carcinoma of the fallopian tube. *Eur J Gynaecol Oncol* 1993;14:374.

47. Baekelandt M, Jorunn Nesbakken A, Kristensen G, et al. Carcinoma of the fallopian tube. *Cancer* 2000;89:2076.

48. Anbrokh YM. Macroscopic characteristics of cancer of the fallopian tube. *Neoplasma* 1970;17:557.

49. Green TH, Scully RE. Tumors of the fallopian tube. *Clin Obstet Gynecol* 1962;5:886.

50. Hee P, Pagel JD. Primary carcinoma of the fallopian tube. *Eur J Obstet Gynecol Reprod Biol* 1987;25:131.

51. Kneale BLG, Attwood HD. Primary carcinoma of the fallopian tube: report of 13 cases. *Am J Obstet Gynecol* 1966;94:840.

52. Meng ML, Gan-Gao, Scheng-Sun, et al. Diagnosis of primary adenocarcinoma of the fallopian tube. *J Cancer Res Clin Oncol* 1985;110: 136.

53. Semrad N, Watring W, Fu Y-S, et al. Fallopian tube adenocarcinoma: common extraperitoneal recurrence. *Gynecol Oncol* 1986;24:230.

54. Alvarado-Cabrero I, Navani SS, Young RH, Scully RE. Tumors of the fimbriated end of the fallopian tube: a clinicopathologic analysis of 20 cases, including 9 carcinomas. *Int J Gynecol Pathol* 1998;16: 189.

55. Scully R, Young R, Clement P. *Tumors of the ovary, maldeveloped gonads, fallopian tube, and broad ligament.* Vol 23. Washington, DC: Armed Forces Institute of Pathology, 1998.

56. Peyton-Jones B, Olaitan A, Murdoch JB. Incidental diagnosis of primary fallopian tube carcinoma during prophylactic salpingo-oophorectomy in BRCA2 mutation carrier. *BJOG* 2002;109:1413.

57. Dodson MG, Ford JH, Averette HE. Clinical aspects of fallopian tube carcinoma. *Obstet Gynecol* 1970;36:935.

58. Ingram FH, Hisley JC. Primary carcinoma of the fallopian tube. *South Med J* 1975;68:1153.

59. Janovski NA, Paramanandhan TL. Tumorous conditions of the fallopian tubes and ligaments of the female reproductive organs. In: Friedman E, ed. *Ovarian tumors: tumors and tumor-like conditions of the ovaries, fallopian tubes and ligaments of the uterus.* Vol 4. Philadelphia: WB Saunders, 1973;191.

60. Kinzel GE. Primary carcinoma of the fallopian tube. *Am J Obstet Gynecol* 1976;125:816.

61. Pauerstein CJ. Pathophysiology of the fallopian tube. *Clin Obstet Gynecol* 1974;17:89.

62. Pauerstein CJ, Woodruff JD. Cellular patterns in proliferative and anaplastic disease of the fallopian tube. *Am J Obstet Gynecol* 1966; 96:486.

63. Schiller HM, Silverberg SG. Staging and prognosis in primary carcinoma of the fallopian tube. *Cancer* 1971;28:389.

64. Alvarado-Cabrero I, Young RH, Vamvakas EC, Scully RE. Carcinoma of the fallopian tube: a clinicopathological study of 105 cases with observations on staging and prognostic factors. *Gynecol Oncol* 1999;72:367.

65. Bendit I, Johnston J, Valderrama E, et al. Molecular phenotype of a pediatric small round cell tumor. *Cancer* 1990;66:1534.

66. Czernobilsky B, Cornog JL. Squamous predominance in adeno-acanthoma of adnexa: report of a patient. *Obstet Gynecol* 1971;37:555.

67. Gaffney EF, Cornog J. Endometrioid carcinoma of the fallopian tube. *Obstet Gynecol* 1978;52:34s.

68. Imm FC. Primary adenosquamous carcinoma of the fallopian tube. *South Med J* 1980;73:678.

69. Moore DH, Woosley JT, Reddick RL, et al. Adenosquamous carcinoma of the fallopian tube: a clinicopathologic case report with verification of the diagnosis by immunohistochemical and ultrastructural studies. *Am J Obstet Gynecol* 1987;157:903.

70. Rorat E, Wallach RC. Endometrioid carcinoma of the fallopian tube: pathology and clinical outcome. *Int J Gynaecol Obstet* 1990;32:163.

71. Seraj IM, King A, Chase D. Malignant mixed müllerian tumor of the oviduct. *Gynecol Oncol* 1990;37:296.

72. Weiss PD, MacDougall MK, Reagan JW, Wentz WB. Primary adenosquamous carcinoma of the fallopian tube. *Obstet Gynecol* 1980;55:88s.

73. Daya D, Young RH, Scully RE. Endometroid carcinoma of the fallopian tube resembling an adnexal tumor of probable wolffian origin: a report of six cases. *Int J Gynecol Pathol* 1992;11:122.

74. Navani SS, Alvarado-Cabrero I, Young RH, Scully RE. Endometrioid carcinoma of the fallopian tube: a clinicopathologic analysis of 26 cases. *Gynecol Oncol* 1996;63:371.

75. Williamsom JM, Armour A. Microcystic endometrioid carcinoma of the fallopian tube simulating an adnexal tumour of probable wolffian origin. *Histopathology* 1993;23:578.

76. Chin H, Matsui H, Mitsuhashi A, et al. Primary transitional cell carcinoma of the fallopian tube: a case report and review of the literature. *Gynecol Oncol* 1998;71:469.

77. Federman Q, Toker C. Primary transitional cell tumor of the uterine adnexa. *Am J Obstet Gynecol* 1973;115:863.

78. Koshiyama M, Konishi I, Yoshida M, et al. Transitional cell carcinoma of the fallopian tumor: a light and electron microscopic study. *Int J Gynecol Pathol* 1994;13:175.

79. Uehira K, Hashimoto H, Tsuneyoshi M, Enjoji M. Transitional cell carcinoma pattern in primary carcinoma of the fallopian tube. *Cancer* 1993;72:2447.

80. Raju KS, Barker GH, Wiltshaw E. Primary carcinoma of the fallopian tube: report of 22 cases. *Br J Obstet Gynaecol* 1981;88:1124.

81. Hu CY, Taymor ML, Hertig AT. Primary carcinoma of the fallopian tube. *Am J Obstet Gynecol* 1950;59:58.

82. Johnson L, Diamond I, Jolly G. Ultrastructure of fallopian tube carcinoma. *Cancer* 1978;42:1291.

83. Rorat E, Fenoglio C. The ultrastructure of a poorly differentiated adenocarcinoma of the human tuba uterina. *Oncology* 1976;33:167.

84. Neunteufel W, Breitenecker G. Tissue expression of CA 125 in benign and malignant lesions of ovary and fallopian tube: a comparison with CA 19–9 and CEA. *Gynecol Oncol* 1989;32:297.

85. Puls LE, Davey DD, DePriest PD, et al. Immunohistochemical staining for CA-125 in fallopian tube carcinomas. *Gynecol Oncol* 1993;48:360.

86. Niloff JM, Klug TL, Schaetzl E, et al. Elevation of serum CA 125 in carcinomas of the fallopian tube, endometrium, and endocervix. *Am J Obstet Gynecol* 1984;148:1057.

87. Pinto MM, Bernstein LH, Brogan DA, Criscuolo E. Immunoradiometric assay of CA 125 in effusions: comparison with carcinoembryonic antigen. *Cancer* 1987;59:218.

88. Szymendera JJ. Clinical usefulness of three monoclonal antibody-defined tumor markers: CA 19–9, CA 50, and CA 125. *Tumour Biol* 1986;7:333.

89. McGee JO, Woods JC, Ashall F, et al. A new marker for human cancer cells. 2. Immunohistochemical detection of the Ca antigen in human tissues with the Ca1 antibody. *Lancet* 1982;2:7.

90. Woodhouse CS, Seiler C, Morgan AC. Immunohistochemical detection of the Ca antigen in normal and tumor tissues of humans by use of Ca1 monoclonal antibody. *J Natl Cancer Inst* 1985;74:383.

91. England D, Davidsohn I. Isoantigens A, B, and H in carcinoma of the fallopian tube. *Arch Pathol* 1973;96:350.

92. Scharl A, Crombach G, Vierbuchen M, et al. Antigen CA 19–9: presence in mucosa of nondiseased müllerian duct derivatives and marker for differentiation in their carcinomas. *Obstet Gynecol* 1991;77:580.

93. Stuhlinger M, Rosen AC, Dobianer K, et al. HER-2 oncogene is not amplified in primary carcinoma of the fallopian tube: Austrian Cooperative Study Group for Fallopian Tube Carcinoma. *Oncology* 1995;52:397.

94. Chung T, Cheung T, To K, Wong Y. Overexpression of p53 and HER-2/neu and c-myc in primary fallopian tube carcinoma. *Gynecol Obstet Invest* 2000;49:47.

95. Mizuuchi H, Mori Y, Sato K, et al. High incidence of point mutation in K-ras codon 12 in carcinoma of the fallopian tube. *Cancer* 1995;76:86.

96. Press MF, Holt JA, Herbst AL, Greene GL. Immunocytochemical identification of estrogen receptor in ovarian carcinomas: localization with monoclonal estrophilin antibodies compared with biochemical assays. *Lab Invest* 1985;53:349.

97. Carlson JA Jr, Ackerman BL, Wheeler JE. Malignant mixed müllerian tumor of the fallopian tube. *Cancer* 1993;71:187.

98. Hanjani P, Petersen RO, Bonnell SA. Malignant mixed müllerian tumor of the fallopian tube: report of a case and review of literature. *Gynecol Oncol* 1980;9:381.

99. Imachi M, Tsukamoto N, Shigematsu T, et al. Malignant mixed Müllerian tumor of the fallopian tube: report of two cases and review of literature. *Gynecol Oncol* 1992;47:114.

100. Kahanppa KV, Laine R, Saksela E. Malignant mixed müllerian tumor of the fallopian tube: report of a case with 5-year survival. *Gynecol Oncol* 1983;16:144.

101. Manes JL, Taylor HB. Carcinosarcoma and mixed mullerian tumors of the fallopian tube. *Cancer* 1976;38:1687.

102. Muntz HG, Rutgers JL, Tarraza HM, Fuller AF Jr. Carcinosarcomas and mixed müllerian tumors of the fallopian tube. *Gynecol Oncol* 1989;34:109.

103. Weber AM, Hewett WF, Gajewski WH, Curry SL. Malignant mixed müllerian tumors of the fallopian tube. *Gynecol Oncol* 1993;50:239.

104. Cheung AN, So KF, Ngan HY, Wong LC. Primary squamous cell carcinoma of fallopian tube. *Int J Gynecol Pathol* 1994;13:92.

105. Herbold DR, Axelrod JH, Bobowski SJ, Freel JH. Glassy cell carcinoma of the fallopian tube: a case report. *Int J Gynecol Pathol* 1988;7:384.

106. Abrams J, Kazal HL, Hobbs RE. Primary sarcoma of the fallopian tube: review of the literature and report of one case. *Am J Obstet Gynecol* 1958;75:180.

107. Barakat RR, Rubin SC, Saigo PE, et al. Second-look laparotomy in carcinoma of the fallopian tube. *Obstet Gynecol* 1993;82:748.

108. Chang KL, Crabtree GS, Lim-Tan SK, Kempson RL, Hendrickson MR. Primary extrauterine endometrial stromal neoplasms: a clinicopathologic study of 20 cases and a review of the literature. *Int J Gynecol Pathol* 1993;12:282.

109. Halligan AW, McGuinness EP. Malignant fibrous histiocytoma of the fallopian tube. *Br J Obstet Gynaecol* 1990;97:275.

110. Jacoby AF, Fuller AF Jr, Thor AD, Muntz HG. Primary leiomyosarcoma of the fallopian tube. *Gynecol Oncol* 1993;51:404.

111. Kayaalp E, Heller D, Majmudar B. Serous tumor of low malignant potential of the fallopian tube. *Int J Gynecol Pathol* 2000;19:398.

112. Seidman J. Mucinous lesions of the fallopian tube: a report of 7 cases. *Am J Surg Pathol* 1994;18:1205.

113. Zheng W, Wolf S, Kramer EE, et al. Borderline papillary serous tumour of the fallopian tube. *Am J Surg Pathol* 1996;20:30.

114. Ober WB, Maier RC. Gestational choriocarcinoma of the fallopian tube. *Diagn Gynecol Obstet* 1981;3:213.

115. Patton GW, Goldstein DP. Gestational choriocarcinoma of the tube and ovary. *Surg Gynecol Obstet* 1973;137:608.

116. Gatto V, Selim MA, Lankerani M. Primary carcinoma of the fallopian tube in an adolescent. *J Surg Oncol* 1986;33:212.

117. Schinfeld JS, Winston HG. Primary tubal carcinoma in pregnancy. *Am J Obstet Gynecol* 180;137:512.

118. Starr AJ, Ruffolo EH, Shenoy BV, Marston BR. Primary carcinoma

of the fallopian tube: a surprise finding in a postpartum tubal ligation. *Am J Obstet Gynecol* 1978;132:344.

119. Young RH, Scully SE. Ovarian tumors of probable wolffian origin: a report of 11 cases. *Am J Surg Pathol* 1983;7:125.

120. Gadducci A, Landoni F, Sartori E, et al. Analysis of treatment failures and survival of patients with fallopian tube carcinoma: a Cooperation Task Force (CTF) study. *Gynecol Oncol* 2001;81:150.

121. Henderson SR, Harper RC, Salazar OM, Rudolph JH. Primary carcinoma of the fallopian tube: difficulties in diagnosis and treatment. *Gynecol Oncol* 1977;5:168.

122. Hirai Y, Kaku S, Teshima H, et al. Clinical study of primary carcinoma of the fallopian tube: experience with 15 cases. *Gynecol Oncol* 1989; 34:20.

123. Sedlis A. Primary carcinoma of the fallopian tube. *Obstet Gynecol Surv* 1961;16:209.

124. Tamimi HK, Figge DC. Adenocarcinoma of the uterine tube: potential for lymph node metastases. *Am J Obstet Gynecol* 1981;141:132.

125. Maxson WZ, Stehman FB, Ulbright TM, et al. Primary carcinoma of the fallopian tube: evidence for activity of cisplatin combination therapy. *Gynecol Oncol* 1987;26:305.

126. Yoonessi M. Carcinoma of the fallopian tube. *Obstet Gynecol Surv* 1979;34:257.

127. Robey SS, Silva EG. Epithelial hyperplasia of the fallopian tube: its association with serous borderline tumors of the ovary. *Int J Gynecol Pathol* 1989;8:214.

128. Moore SW, Enterline HT. Significance of proliferative epithelial lesions of the uterine tube. *Obstet Gynecol* 1975;45:385.

129. Bannatyne P, Russel P. Early adenocarcinoma of the fallopian tube: a case for multifocal tumorigenesis. *Diagn Gynecol Obstet* 1981;3: 49.

130. Hershey DW, Fennell RH, Major FJ. Primary carcinoma of the fallopian tube. *Obstet Gynecol* 1981;57:367.

131. Yeung HHY, Bannatyne P, Russell P. Adenocarcinoma of the fallopian tubes: a clinicopathological study of eight cases. *Pathology* 1983; 15:279.

132. Demopoulos R, Aronov R, Mesia A. Clues to the pathogenesis of fallopian tube carcinoma: a morphological and immunohistochemical case control study. *Int J Gynecol Pathol* 2001;20:128.

133. Hameed K. Carcinoma arising in tuberculous fallopian tube. *Am J Obstet Gynecol* 1969;103:594.

134. Vinall PS, Buxton N, Cowen PN. Primary carcinoma of the fallopian tube associated with tuberculous salpingitis: a case report. *Br J Obstet Gynaecol* 1979;86:984.

135. Wiskind AK, Dudley AG, Majmudar B, Masterson KC. Primary fallopian tube carcinoma with coexistent tuberculous salpingitis: a case report. *J Med Assoc Ga* 1992;81:77.

136. Johnston GA. Primary malignancy of the fallopian tube: a clinical review of 13 cases. *J Surg Oncol* 1983;24:304.

137. Muntz HG, Tarraza HM, Granai CO, Fuller AF Jr. Primary adenocarcinoma of the fallopian tube. *Eur J Gynaecol Oncol* 1989;4:239.

138. Harrison CR, Averette HE, Jarrell MA, et al. Carcinoma of the fallopian tube: clinical management. *Gynecol Oncol* 1989;32:357.

139. Hirai Y, Chen J-T, Hamada T, et al. Clinical and cytologic aspects of primary fallopian tube carcinoma: a report of 10 cases. *Acta Cytol* 1987;31:834.

140. Jackson-York GL, Ramzy I. Synchronous papillary mucinous adenocarcinoma of the endocervix and fallopian tubes. *Int J Gynecol Pathol* 1992;11:63.

141. Qizilbash AH. Ovarian carcinoma identified by psammoma bodies in the cervicovaginal and endometrial smears. *Can Med Assoc J* 1974; 110:185.

142. Woodruff JD, Julian CG. Multiple malignancy in the upper genital canal. *Am J Obstet Gynecol* 1969;103:810.

143. Woodruff JD, Solomon D, Sullivant H. Multifocal disease in the upper genital canal. *Obstet Gynecol* 1985;65:695.

144. Creasman WT, Lukeman J. Role of the fallopian tube in dissemination of malignant cells in corpus cancer. *Cancer* 1972;29:456.

145. Hallgrimsson JT. Carcinoma in situ of the endocervix, corpus uteri and both oviducts. *Acta Obstet Gynecol Scand* 1967;46:268.

146. Kanbour AI, Stock RJ. Squamous cell carcinoma in situ of the endometrium and fallopian tube as superficial extension of invasive cervical carcinoma. *Cancer* 1978;42:570.

147. Mendez JA, Bedoya JM Jr, Matilla A, et al. Carcinoma in situ of the fallopian tube associated with cervical carcinoma. *Int J Gynaecol Obstet* 1976;14:353.

148. Punnonen R, Gronroos M, Vaajalahti P. Squamous cell carcinoma in situ from the uterine cervix to the distal end of the fallopian tube. *Acta Obstet Gynecol Scand* 1979;58:101.

149. Qizilbash AH, DePetrillo AD. Endometrial and tubal involvement by squamous carcinoma of the cervix. *Am J Clin Pathol* 1975;64:668.

150. McGarrity KA, Pettersson F, Ulfelder H, eds. *Annual report on the results of treatment of gynecologic cancer.* Vol 18. Stockholm: Radiumhemmet, 1982.

150a. Rauthe G, Vahrson HW, Burkhardt E. Primary cancer of the fallopian tube. Treatment and results of 37 cases. *Eur J Gynecol Oncol* 1998; 19:356.

151. Anbrokh GB, Anbrokh YM. Morphology of metastatic cancer of the fallopian tube in uterine cervix carcinoma. *Neoplasma* 1975;22:73.

152. Anbrokh GB, Anbrokh YM. Mechanism of development and morphology of secondary carcinomas of the oviducts in primary uterine corpus carcinoma. *Neoplasma* 1976;23:549.

153. Andriole GL, Garnick MB, Richie JP. Unusual behavior of low-grade, low-stage transitional cell carcinoma of bladder. *Urology* 1985;25: 524.

154. Case TC. Cancer of the breast with metastasis to the fallopian tube. *J Am Geriatr Soc* 1968;16:832.

155. Krebs H-B, Walsh J. An unusual case of ruptured tubo-ovarian abscess simulating ovarian carcinoma. *Diagn Gynecol Obstet* 1982;4:63.

156. Puflett D. Tuberculous salpingitis resembling adenocarcinoma. *Med J Aust* 1972;2:149.

157. Silverberg SG, Frable WJ. Prolapse of fallopian tube into vaginal vault after hysterectomy. *Arch Pathol* 1974;97:100.

158. Young RH, Clement PB. Pseudoneoplastic lesions of the lower female genital tract. *Pathol Ann* 1989;24:189.

159. Cheung A, Young R, Scully R. Pseudocarcinomatous hyperplasia of the fallopian tube associated with salpingitis: a report of 14 cases. *Am J Surg Pathol* 1994;18:1125.

160. Cornog JL, Currie JL, Rubin A. Heat artifact simulating adenocarcinoma of fallopian tube. *JAMA* 1970;214:1118.

161. Schray MF, Podratz KC, Malkasian GD. Fallopian tube cancer: the role of radiation therapy. *Radiother Oncol* 1987;10:267.

162. Saffos RO, Rhatagan RM, Scully RE. Metastatic papillary tumor of the fallopian tube: a distinctive lesion of pregnancy. *Am J Clin Pathol* 1980;74:232.

163. Klein M, Rosen A, Graf A, et al. Primary fallopian tube carcinoma: a retrospective survey of 51 cases. *Arch Gynecol Obstet* 1994;255: 141.

164. Hellström AC, Silfersvärd, Nilsson B, Pettersson F. Carcinoma of the fallopian tube: a clinical and histopathologic view. The Radiumhemmet series. *Int J Gynecol Cancer* 1994;4:395.

165. Kosary C, Trimble EL. Treatment and survival for women with fallopian tube carcinoma: a population-based study. *Gynecol Oncol* 2002; 86:190.

166. Rubin SC, Lewis JL. Second-look surgery in ovarian carcinoma. *Crit Rev Oncol Hematol* 1988;8:75.

167. Deppe G, Bruckner HW, Cohen CJ. Combination chemotherapy for advanced carcinoma of the fallopian tube. *Obstet Gynecol* 1980;56: 530.

168. Eddy GL, Copeland LJ, Gershenson DM. Second-look laparotomy in fallopian tube carcinoma. *Gynecol Oncol* 1984;19:182.

169. Guthrie D, Cohen S. Carcinoma of the fallopian tube treated with a combination of surgery and cytotoxic chemotherapy. *Br J Obstet Gynaecol* 1981;88:1051.

170. Jacobs AJ, McMurray EH, Parham J, et al. Treatment of carcinoma of the fallopian tube using cisplatin, doxorubicin, and cyclophosphamide. *Am J Clin Oncol* 1986;9:436.

171. Rubin SC, Hoskins WJ, Saigo PE, et al. Prognostic factors for recurrence following negative second-look laparotomy in ovarian cancer patients treated with platinum-based chemotherapy. *Gynecol Oncol* 1991;42:137.

172. Lu KH, Garber JE, Cramer DW, et al. Occult ovarian tumors in women with BRCA1 or BRCA2 mutations undergoing prophylactic oophorectomy. *J Clin Oncol* 2000;18:2728.

173. Rebbeck TR, Lynch HT, Neuhausen SL, et al. For the prevention and observation of surgical end points study group. Prophylactic oopho-

rectomy in carriers of BRCA1 or BRCA2 mutations. *N Engl J Med* 2002;346:1616.

174. Scheur L, Kauff N, Robson M, et al. Outcome of preventive surgery and screening for breast and ovarian cancer in BRCA mutation carriers. *J Clin Oncol* 2002;20:1260.

175. Wheeler JE. Diseases of the fallopian tube. In: Kurman RJ, ed. *Blaustein's pathology of the female genital tract.* New York: Springer-Verlag, 1994:529–532.

176. Fogh IB. Primary carcinoma of the fallopian tube. *Cancer* 1961;23:1332.

177. Wong WSF, Tindall NR, Wagstaff J, et al. Surgery and radiotherapy in the treatment of primary carcinoma of the fallopian tube: report of 18 cases. *Aust N Z J Obstet Gynaecol* 1985;25:211.

178. Cormio G, Maneo A, Gabriele A, et al. Treatment of fallopian tube carcinoma with cyclophosphamide, adriamycin, and cisplatin. *Am J Clin Oncol* 1997;20:143.

179. Baginski L, Yazigi R, Sandstad J. Immature (malignant) teratoma of the fallopian tube. *Am J Obstet Gynecol* 1989;160:671.

180. Ross WM. Primary carcinoma of the ovary: a review of 150 cases, with an appraisal of the fallopian tube as a pathway of spread. *Can Med Assoc J* 1966;94:1035.

181. Wolfson AH, Tralins KS, Greven KM, et al. Adenocarcinoma of the fallopian tube: results of a multi-institutional retrospective analysis of 72 patients. *Int J Radiat Oncol Biol Phys* 1998;40:71.

182. Singhal S, Sharma S, De S, et al. Role of radiotherapy in the management of primary carcinoma of the fallo pian tube. *Indian J Med Sci* 1991;45:58.

183. Thigpen JT, Blessing JA, Ball H, et al. Phase II trial of paclitaxel in patients with progressive ovarian carcinoma after platinum-based chemotherapy: a Gynecologic Oncology Group study. *J Clin Oncol* 1994;12:1748.

184. Klein M, Rosen A, Lahousen M, et al. The relevance of adjuvant therapy in primary carcinoma of the fallopian tube, stages I and II: irradiation vs. chemotherapy. *Int J Radiat Oncol Biol Phys* 2000;48:1427.

185. Dembo AJ. Epithelial ovarian cancer: the role of radiotherapy. *Int J Radiat Oncol Biol Phys* 1992;22:835.

186. Fletcher GH. Clinical dose-response curves of human malignant epithelial tumours. *Br J Radiol* 1973;46:1.

187. Boronow RC. Chemotherapy for disseminated tubal cancer. *Obstet Gynecol* 1973;42:62.

188. Barakat RR, Rubin SC, Saigo PE, et al. Cisplatin-based combination chemotherapy in carcinoma of the fallopian tube. *Gynecol Oncol* 1991;42:156.

189. Gurney H, Murphy D, Crouther D. The management of primary fallopian tube carcinoma. *Br J Obstet Gynaecol* 1990;97:822.

190. Morris M, Gershenson PM, Burke TW, et al. Treatment of fallopian tube carcinoma with cisplatin, doxorubicin, and cyclophosphamide. *Obstet Gynecol* 1990;76:1020.

191. Muntz HG, Tarraza HM, Goff BA, et al. Combination chemotherapy in advanced adenocarcinoma of the fallopian tube. *Gynecol Oncol* 1991;40:268.

192. Peters WA, Andersen WA, Hopkins MP. Results of chemotherapy in advanced carcinoma of the fallopian tube. *Cancer* 1989;63:836.

193. Wagenaar HC, Pecorelli S, Vergote I, et al. Phase II study of a combination of cyclophosphamide, adriamycin and cisplatin in advanced fallopian tube carcinoma. An EORTC gynecological cancer group study. European Organization for Research and Treatment of Cancer. *Eur J Gynaecol Oncol* 2001;22:187.

194. Wang PH, Yuan CC, Chao HT, et al. Prognosis of primary fallopian tube adenocarcinoma: report of 25 patients. *Eur J Gynaecol Oncol* 1998;19:571.

195. Young JA, Kossman CR, Green MR. Adenocarcinoma of the fallopian tube: report of a case with an unusual pattern of metastasis and response to combination chemotherapy. *Gynecol Oncol* 1984;17:238.

196. Gemignani ML, Hensley ML, Cohen R, Venkatraman E, et al. Paclitaxel-based chemotherapy in carcinoma of the fallopian tube. *Gynecol Oncol* 2001;80:16.

197. McGuire WP, Hoskins WJ, Brady MF, et al. Cyclophosphamide and cisplatin compared with paclitaxel and cisplatin in patients with Stage III and stage IV ovarian cancer. *N Engl J Med* 1996;334:1.

198. Dunton CJ, Neufeld J. Complete response to topotecan of recurrent fallopian tube carcinoma. *Gynecol Oncol* 2000;76:128.

199. Cass I, Resnik E, Chambers JT, et al. Combination chemotherapy with etoposide, cisplatin, and doxorubicin in mixed mullerian tumors of the adnexa. *Gynecol Oncol* 1996;61:309.

200. Piver MS, DeEulis TG, Lele SB, Barlow JJ. Cyclophosphamide, vincristine, Adriamycin and dimethyl-thiazeno imidazole carboxamide (CYVADIC) for sarcomas of the female genital tract. *Gynecol Oncol* 1982;14:319.

201. Smith JP. Chemotherapy in gynecologic cancer. *Clin Obstet Gynecol* 1975;18:109.

CHAPTER 29

Gestational Trophoblastic Diseases

Ross S. Berkowitz and Donald P. Goldstein

Gestational trophoblastic diseases (GTDs) comprise a group of interrelated diseases including complete and partial molar pregnancy, invasive mole, placental-site trophoblastic tumor, and choriocarcinoma that have varying propensities for local invasion and metastasis. Gestational trophoblastic tumors (GTTs) are one of the rare human malignancies that are highly curable with chemotherapy even with widespread metastases (1–4). Although GTTs most commonly follow a molar pregnancy, they may develop after any gestation. Important advances have been made in the diagnosis, treatment, and follow-up of patients with molar pregnancy and GTT. This chapter will review these advances and discuss basic principles in the management of patients with molar pregnancy and persistent GTTs.

EPIDEMIOLOGY

The reported incidence of GTDs varies dramatically in different regions of the world (5).The frequency of molar pregnancy in Asian countries is seven to ten times greater than the reported incidence in North America or Europe (6). Whereas hydatidiform mole occurs in Taiwan in 1 per 125 pregnancies, the incidence of molar gestation in the United States is about 1 per 1,500 live births. Variations in the incidence rates of molar pregnancy partly result from differences between reporting hospital-based versus population-based data.

R. S. Berkowitz: New England Trophoblastic Disease Center, Brigham and Women's Hospital and Dana Farber Cancer Institute, Division of Gynecologic Oncology, Gillette Center for Women's Cancers, Department of Obstetrics and Gynecology, Harvard Medical School, Boston, Massachusetts 02115

D. P. Goldstein: Trophoblastic Tumor Registry, Brigham and Women's Hospital and Dana Farber Cancer Institute, Division of Gynecologic Oncology, Gillette Center for Women's Cancers, Department of Obstetrics and Gynecology, Harvard Medical School, Boston, Massachusetts 02115

Jeffers et al. (7) reported a study from Ireland where all products of conception from first- and second-trimester abortions were referred for pathologic examination. The incidence of complete and partial mole was 1:1,945 and 1: 695 pregnancies, respectively.

The high incidence of molar pregnancy in some populations has been attributed to socioeconomic and nutritional factors. We have observed in a case-control study that the risk for complete molar pregnancy progressively increases with decreasing levels of consumption of dietary carotene (vitamin A precursor) and animal fat (8). Parazzini et al. (9) also reported from Italy that low carotene consumption was associated with an increased risk of GTD. Global regions with a high incidence of vitamin A deficiency correspond to areas with a high frequency of molar pregnancy. Vitamin A deficiency in the rhesus monkey produces degeneration of the seminiferous epithelium with production of primitive spermatogonia and spermatocytes (10). Dietary factors such as carotene may therefore partly explain the regional variations in the incidence of complete molar pregnancy.

The risk of having a complete molar pregnancy also increases with advanced maternal age (6). Women older than age 40 years have a five- to tenfold greater risk of having a complete molar gestation. Ova from older women may be more susceptible to abnormal fertilizations.

The risk for both complete and partial molar pregnancy is increased in women with a history of prior spontaneous abortion and infertility (11). Compared with women with no previous miscarriage, the risk for complete and partial mole was 3.1 and 1.9, respectively, among women with two or more prior miscarriages. Difficulty in conception or infertility problems was associated with an odds risk of 2.4 and 3.2, respectively, for complete and partial mole.

Certain epidemiologic features of complete and partial molar pregnancy differ markedly. Parazzini et al. (11) reported that the risk for partial mole was not associated with maternal age. Additionally, the risk for partial mole has been reported to be associated with the use of oral contraceptives and a history of irregular menstruation but not with dietary factors (12). Therefore, the risk for partial mole appears to be associated with reproductive history rather than dietary factors.

The risk for choriocarcinoma and GTT has been observed in a case-control study to be related to hormonal factors (13). Women with light menstrual flow and menarche after the age of 12 years were noted to be at increased risk for choriocarcinoma. Additionally, Palmer et al. (14) reported that the prior use of oral contraceptives was associated with an increased risk for choriocarcinoma.

IMMUNOBIOLOGY

The remarkable curability of GTTs may be partly attributable to a host immunologic response to paternal antigens expressed on trophoblastic cells (15). The prognosis of patients with gestational choriocarcinoma has been related to the intensity of lymphocytic and monocytic infiltration at the tumor-host interface (16). Because the lymphocytes and macrophages that infiltrate gestational choriocarcinoma are probably exposed to paternal antigens and oncoproteins, the immune cells may become activated. Immunologically active cells may promote the regression of GTTs through their release of cytokines. Cytokines have been reported to inhibit the proliferation of choriocarcinoma cells in vitro and to increase the HLA expression of choriocarcinoma cells in vitro, thereby increasing immunogenicity (17–19).

It has been theorized that the development and progression of persistent GTTs may be favored by histocompatibility between the patient and her partner. If the patient and her partner are histocompatible, the trophoblastic tumor that bears paternal antigens may not be immunogenic in the maternal host. The intensity of the host's immunologic response may depend upon the immunogenicity of the trophoblastic tumor. However, histocompatibility between the patient and her partner does not appear to be a prerequisite for the development or persistence of GTTs (20,21). The HLA system may, however, influence the clinical course of rapidly progressive and fatal GTT. Tomoda et al. (22) reported that drug-resistant choriocarcinoma was associated with increased histocompatibility between the patient and her partner. Similarly, Morgensen et al. (23) observed that histocompatibility between patients and partners was associated with a greater risk of metastatic GTT.

Because all chromosomes in a complete mole are paternal in origin, a complete molar pregnancy is a complete allograft and may stimulate a vigorous immunologic response by the maternal host. There is evidence for both a cellular and humoral immune response to complete molar pregnancy. As compared with normal placentas, molar implantation sites have a fivefold increased infiltration by helper T cells (24). Circulating immune complexes have also been measured in patients with complete mole and have been noted to increase as the patient entered gonadotropin remission (25).

Circulating immune complexes in patients with complete moles have been demonstrated to contain paternal HLA antigen (26). The maternal host with a complete mole is therefore sensitized to paternal HLA antigen. The distribution of HLA antigen in molar chorionic villi has been determined by immunofluorescence assays (27). HLA A, B, and C antigens were detected on the stromal cells of molar chorionic villi but not on the villous trophoblast. However, the molar villous fluid that bathes the stromal cells does not contain soluble HLA antigen (28). The maternal host may therefore be sensitized to paternal HLA antigen when the villous trophoblast layer is disrupted and HLA-positive villous stromal cells are released into the maternal circulation.

Molecular Pathogenesis

Several growth factors and oncogenes have been studied in molar tissues and choriocarcinoma (11). Increased expression of p53 and c-fms has been observed in complete mole and increased ras and c-myc RNA has been measured in choriocarcinoma (29–31).

We have investigated the expression of various growth factors and oncogenes in normal placenta, complete and partial mole, and choriocarcinoma (32,33). Complete mole and choriocarcinoma were characterized by overexpression of c-myc, c-erbB2, and bcl-2 and these oncoproteins may be important in the pathogenesis of GTD. Expression of c-fms protein did not differ between normal placenta and GTD. Complete mole and choriocarcinoma were also characterized by increased expression of p53, p21, Rb, and MdM2. The p53 gene was studied to detect any mutation in 22 complete moles and 11 choriocarcinomas that had increased expression of p53. Because only one nonsense mutation in p53 was detected by polymerase chain reaction analysis, it is likely that the overexpressed p53 protein was wild type. Although studies have identified increased expression of several growth factors in GTDs, the precise molecular pathogenesis has not been determined.

It was observed that the level of expression of epidermal growth-factor receptor (EGFR) in choriocarcinoma and the syncytiotrophoblast and cytotrophoblast of complete mole was significantly greater than the expression of EGFR in syncytiotrophoblast and cytotrophoblast of placenta and partial mole (34). This observation was consistent in both immunohistochemical and in situ hybridization studies. In complete mole, strong expression of EGFR and c-erbB3 in the extravillous trophoblasts was significantly associated with the development of postmolar tumor. The EGFR-related family of oncogenes may be important in the pathogenesis of gestational trophoblastic diseases.

Extracellular proteinases such as matrix metalloproteinases (MMPs) are thought to be important in modulating both cell-matrix interactions and the degradation of the basement membrane necessary for invasion and metastasis. Choriocarcinoma exhibits significantly stronger expression of

MMP-1 and MMP-2 and decreased expression of tissue inhibitor of MMP-1 (TIMP-1) than the syncytiotrophoblast of complete and partial mole and normal placenta (35). The increased expression of MMP-1 and MMP-2 and decreased expression of TIMP-1 in choriocarcinoma may contribute to the invasiveness of choriocarcinoma cells.

Certain genes are normally expressed on either the maternal or paternal allele, and this occurrence is described as parental imprinting. Modification of parental imprinting has been associated with tumor formation, and complete moles and choriocarcinomas have relaxation of parental imprinting (36). Relaxation in parental imprinting may be important in the pathogenesis of GTDs.

MOLAR PREGNANCY

Complete Versus Partial Molar Pregnancy

Pathologic and Chromosomal Features

Hydatidiform moles may be categorized as either complete or partial based upon gross morphology, histopathology, and karyotype (Table 29.1).

Complete hydatidiform moles have no identifiable embryonic or fetal tissues. The chorionic villi have generalized swelling and diffuse trophoblastic hyperplasia and the implantation-site trophoblast has diffuse, marked atypia (37, 38) (Fig. 29.1). Complete moles usually have a 46,XX karyotype, and the molar chromosomes are derived entirely from paternal origin (39). Most complete moles appear to arise from an anuclear empty ovum that has been fertilized by a haploid (23X) sperm, which then duplicates its own chromosomes (40). Whereas most complete moles have a 46,XX chromosomal pattern, approximately 10% of complete moles have a 46,XY karyotype (41). The 46,XY complete mole arises from fertilization of an anuclear empty ovum by two sperm. Whereas chromosomes in the complete mole are entirely of paternal origin, the mitochondrial DNA is of maternal origin (42).

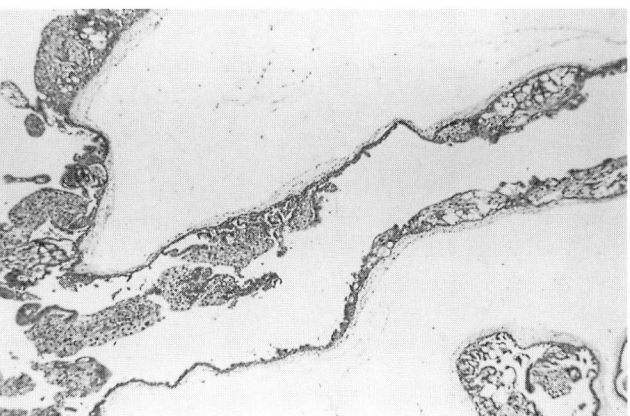

FIG. 29.1. Photomicrograph of a complete hydatidiform mole showing chorionic villi with generalized swelling and diffuse trophoblastic hyperplasia. (Magnification ×20.)

During the 1960s and 1970s, complete moles were primarily diagnosed in the second trimester. However, currently, most patients with complete moles are diagnosed in the first trimester both in the United States and abroad (43–45). The pathologic characteristics of a first-trimester complete mole are different than the classic features in the second trimester (44,46). Mosher et al. (46) compared pathologic findings of 23 current complete moles (1994 through 1997; mean gestational age, 8.5 weeks) with 20 historic complete moles (1969 through 1975; mean gestational age, 17 weeks). Histologically, current complete moles had a smaller mean maximal villous diameter (5.7 vs 8.2 mm), less circumferential trophoblastic hyperplasia (39% vs 75%), more primitive villous stroma (70% vs 10%), and less global necrosis (22% vs 54%). Current complete moles are often characterized by subtle morphologic alterations that may result in their misclassification as partial moles or nonmolar spontaneous abortions. Similarly, Keep et al. (47) described that early complete moles were characterized by focal trophoblastic hyperplasia, minimal villous cavitation, and a hypercellular primitive stroma.

Partial hydatidiform moles are characterized by the following pathologic features: (a) varying-sized chorionic villi with focal swelling and focal trophoblastic hyperplasia, (b) focal, mild atypia of implantation-site trophoblast, (c) marked villous scalloping and prominent stromal trophoblastic inclusions, and (d) identifiable fetal or embryonic tissues (48) (Fig. 29.2). Partial moles generally have a triploid karyotype, which results from the fertilization of an apparently normal ovum by two sperm (49). Lawler et al. (50) and Lage et al. (51) reported that 93% and 90%, respectively, of partial moles were triploid. When fetuses are identified with partial moles, they generally have stigmata of triploidy including growth retardation and multiple congenital anomalies. Genest et al. reviewed 19 putative nontriploid partial moles using standardized histologic diagnostic criteria and repeat flow cytometry and none of these cases on

TABLE 29.1. *Complete versus partial molar pregnancy: histopathologic and chromosomal features*

	Complete mole	Partial mole
Fetal or embryonic tissue	Absent	Present
Hydatidiform swelling of chorionic villi	Diffuse	Focal
Trophoblastic hyperplasia	Diffuse	Focal
Scalloping of chorionic villi	Absent	Present
Trophoblastic stromal inclusions	Absent	Present
Implantation-site trophoblast	Marked atypia	Mild atypia
Karyotype	46,XX (mainly); 46,XY	Triploid

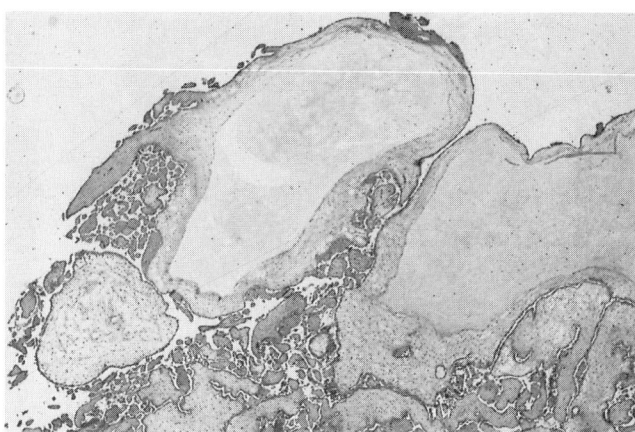

FIG. 29.2. Photomicrograph of a partial hydatidiform mole demonstrating varying-sized chorionic villi with focal swelling and focal trophoblastic hyperplasia. (Magnification ×50.)

reevaluation was convincingly a nontriploid partial mole (52). Nontriploid partial moles may not exist.

Complete Molar Pregnancy

Presenting Signs and Symptoms

The clinical presentation of a complete molar pregnancy has changed dramatically over the past two decades. Whereas complete mole was usually diagnosed in the second trimester in the 1960s and 1970s, the diagnosis of complete mole is now generally made in the first trimester (45). Earlier diagnosis is most likely attributable to the availability of accurate and sensitive tests for human chorionic gonadotropin (hCG) and the widespread use of ultrasound. The diagnosis of complete mole is now often made before the classic clinical signs and symptoms develop. Soto-Wright et al. (45) investigated the clinical presentation and outcome of patients with complete moles at the New England Trophoblastic Disease Center (NETDC) between 1988 and 1993 as compared with patients between 1965 and 1975.

Vaginal Bleeding

Vaginal bleeding is the most common presenting symptom in patients with complete moles; occurring in 89% to 97% of cases (53–55). Retained blood may undergo oxidation and prune juice–like fluid may leak from the endometrial cavity. Molar chorionic villi may separate from the decidua and disrupt vessels, leading to the distension of the endometrial cavity by large volumes of retained blood. Because bleeding used to be prolonged, occult, and considerable, 54% of our patients used to present with anemia (hemoglobin <10 g/100 mL). Vaginal bleeding continues to be the most common presenting symptom; occurring in 84% of our current patients (45). However, anemia was present in only 5% of our current patients with complete mole.

Theca Lutein Ovarian Cysts

The reported frequency of theca lutein ovarian cysts depends upon the method of diagnosis. Ultrasonography detected theca lutein ovarian cysts (>5 cm in diameter) in 23 (46%) of 50 patients with molar pregnancy (56). However, clinical examination detected theca lutein ovarian cysts in 26% of patients with molar pregnancy (57). Although theca lutein cysts are generally 6 to 12 cm in diameter, they may enlarge to more than 20 cm in size. They are usually multicystic and bilateral and contain serosanguineous or amber-colored fluid. Although theca lutein cysts are usually detected at the time of presentation, they may develop rapidly after molar evacuation.

Theca lutein cysts are detected exclusively in patients with very high serum hCG levels and result from hyperstimulation of the ovaries by high circulating levels of hCG (58). Other signs of ovarian hyperstimulation may infrequently develop, including ascites and pleural effusion. Theca lutein cysts generally resolve over an interval of 8 weeks (57).

Torsion or rupture of theca lutein ovarian cysts occurs infrequently. Kohorn (59) reported that 3 (2.3%) of 127 patients with molar pregnancy developed torsion of ovarian theca lutein cysts. Similarly, Montz et al. (57) noted that only 2 of 102 patients with theca lutein cysts developed torsion or rupture. If patients develop severe symptoms of pelvic or abdominal pressure or pain, theca lutein cysts may be decompressed by ultrasound-directed or laparoscopic aspiration (60). Ovarian rupture or torsion may also be managed by laparoscopy.

Excessive Uterine Size

Uterine size was excessively enlarged as compared with gestational age in about 38% to 51% of patients with complete moles (37,54,55). Both retained blood and chorionic tissues may expand the uterine cavity. Excessive uterine enlargement is commonly associated with markedly elevated hCG values from trophoblastic proliferation and overgrowth. Among current patients at the NETDC, excessive uterine size was diagnosed at presentation in only 28% of patients.

Hyperemesis Gravidarum

Hyperemesis requiring antiemetic therapy used to develop in 20% to 26% of patients with complete moles (37,59). Hyperemesis was associated with excessive uterine enlargement and high hCG values. High circulating levels of estrogen have been proposed as a cause of hyperemesis (61). Although hyperemesis used to be a common problem, only 8% of our current patients present with hyperemesis.

Preeclampsia

Preeclampsia used to be observed in 12% to 27% of patients with complete moles (54,62). Preeclampsia primarily developed in patients with excessive uterine size and high hCG levels. Eclamptic convulsions developed rarely. In contrast, between 1988 and 1993, only 1 of 74 patients with complete mole presented with preeclampsia at the NETDC.

Hyperthyroidism

Laboratory evidence of hyperthyroidism commonly used to be present in patients with complete moles. Galton et al. (63) reported that all 11 patients with complete mole had elevated thyroid function tests before molar evacuation. Hyperthyroidism occurred almost exclusively in patients with very high hCG values. There are conflicting data whether hCG is a thyroid stimulator in patients with molar pregnancy. Amir et al. (64) found no significant correlation between serum hCG levels and free T_4 and T_3 index values in 47 patients with complete mole. Similarly, Nagataki et al. (65) found no correlation between free T_4 and hCG in 10 patients. However, highly purified hCG may have intrinsic thyroid-stimulating activity, and some studies do report correlations between serum levels of hCG and total T_4 and T_3 (66).

Patients with poorly controlled or untreated hyperthyroidism may develop thyroid storm at the time of anesthesia induction and evacuation. Thyroid storm may be characterized by hyperthermia, delirium, coma, atrial fibrillation, and cardiovascular collapse. The diagnosis of thyroid storm must be made clinically so that treatment can be promptly instituted and not await the return of laboratory confirmation. Many of the cardiovascular and metabolic complications of thyroid storm may be prevented or reversed by the administration of beta-adrenergic blocking agents. A pulmonary artery catheter may be helpful to guide fluid replacement and to monitor cardiovascular status.

Between 1988 and 1993, none of our 74 patients with complete moles had clinical evidence of hyperthyroidism (45). However, during the past decade, one patient with a complete mole and a preevacuation hCG level of 1.4 million mIU/mL developed clinical and laboratory evidence of hyperthyroidism and required beta-adrenergic blockers to treat tachyarrhythmia.

Respiratory Insufficiency

Twiggs et al. (67) observed that 12 (27%) of 44 patients with a complete mole of at least 16-weeks size developed pulmonary complications. Respiratory insufficiency used to develop in 2% of our patients with complete moles (62). Pulmonary compromise was generally observed in patients with excessive uterine size and high hCG levels—the same group of patients who are at risk for preeclampsia and hyperthyroidism. During the past decade, none of our patients with complete moles developed respiratory failure.

Patients may present with anxiety, confusion, tachypnea, and tachycardia in the recovery room after molar evacuation.

Pulmonary insufficiency is multifactorial and results not only from embolization of molar tissue to the pulmonary vasculature, but also the cardiovascular complications of thyroid storm, preeclampsia, and massive fluid replacement. Chest radiography may show bilateral pulmonary infiltrates, and auscultation of the chest usually reveals diffuse rales. Arterial blood gases may indicate respiratory alkalosis and hypoxia. With appropriate cardiovascular and respiratory support, the signs and symptoms of respiratory distress usually resolve within 72 hours. However, it is vital to recognize that some patients may require mechanical ventilation to provide adequate oxygenation.

Partial Molar Pregnancy

Presenting Signs and Symptoms

Patients with partial molar pregnancy usually do not present with the classic clinical features that are characteristic of a complete mole. These patients generally present with the signs and symptoms of missed or incomplete abortion. Eighty-one patients were followed with partial moles at the NETDC between January 1979 and August 1984 (68). Excessive uterine size and preeclampsia were detected in only three and two patients, respectively. Szulman and Surti (48) and Czernobilsky et al. (69) reported that only 9 (11%) of 81 and 2 (8%) of 25 patients with partial moles had excessive uterine enlargement. Preeclampsia was reported in both studies in only 4% of patients. None of our patients had prominent theca lutein ovarian cysts, hyperthyroidism, or hyperemesis. The diagnosis of partial mole is usually made after histologic review of curettage specimens.

Ultrasonography and Diagnosis of Hydatidiform Mole

Ultrasonography is a sensitive and reliable technique for detecting complete molar pregnancy. Because of marked swelling of the chorionic villi, a complete mole produces a characteristic vesicular sonographic pattern. However, it may be difficult to distinguish an early complete mole from degenerating chorionic tissues, since small molar chorionic villi in the first trimester may be difficult to visualize on ultrasound. However, despite smaller chorionic villi, ultrasound is still able to detect most first-trimester complete moles (70). hCG measurement at the time of sonography may help in differentiating an early complete mole from a missed abortion (71).

Ultrasonography may also contribute to the diagnosis of partial molar pregnancy. Two sonographic findings are significantly associated with the diagnosis of partial mole: focal cystic changes in the placenta and a ratio of the transverse to anteroposterior dimension of the gestational sac >1.5 (72). Changes in the shape of the gestational sac may be part of the embryopathy of triploidy. When both findings were present, the positive predictive value for partial mole was 87%. On rare occasions, the sonogram will show the presence of a fetus with multiple congenital anomalies associated with a focally hydropic placenta. Naumoff et al. (73) also reported that partial moles may exhibit cystic spaces within the placenta with a growth-retarded fetus.

hCG Measurement and Diagnosis of Hydatidiform Mole

Patients with complete mole commonly have markedly elevated preevacuation hCG levels. Menczer et al. (74) reported that 30 (41%) of 74 patients with complete moles had preevacuation hCG values greater than 100,000 mIU/mL. Similarly, Genest et al. (75) noted that 46% of 153 patients with complete moles who were managed at the NETDC between 1980 and 1990 had preevacuation hCG levels above 100,000 mIU/mL. The measurement of markedly elevated hCG values is therefore suggestive of the diagnosis of complete mole.

Patients with partial mole less commonly present with markedly elevated hCG values. Czernobilsky et al. (69) reported that only 1 of 17 patients with partial moles presented with a urinary hCG value >300,000 mIU/mL. Likewise, we noted that only 2 of 30 patients with partial moles at the NETDC presented with hCG levels >100,000 mIU/mL (68).

Complete and partial moles also differ in their levels of free β- and α-subunits of hCG. Whereas complete moles have higher levels of percentage free β hCG, partial moles have higher levels of percentage free α hCG (76,77). The mean ratios of percentage free β hCG to free α hCG in complete and partial moles are 20.9 and 2.4, respectively.

Natural History of Molar Pregnancy and Prognostic Factors

Complete hydatidiform moles are well recognized to have a potential for developing uterine invasion or distant spread. Following molar evacuation, uterine invasion and metastasis occur in 15% and 4% of the patients, respectively (78). Although complete moles are now being diagnosed earlier in pregnancy, the incidence of postmolar tumors has not been affected (44,45).

Whereas the incidence of postmolar tumor is reported from 18% to 29% in the United States, the incidence of postmolar GTTs in Western Europe is reported from 8% to 10% of patients (2,54,59,79–83). Most centers in the United States define postmolar persistent GTTs by the presence of a reelevation or persistent plateau in hCG for at least 3 consecutive weeks. However, the definition of persistent disease does vary among American centers (84). The criteria for persistent GTTs in Western Europe are more stringent than American definitions. At the Charing Cross Hospital in London, the criteria for postmolar persistent tumors are: hCG

>20,000 IU/L more than 4 weeks after evacuation; progressively rising hCG levels, with a minimum of three rising values over 2 to 3 weeks; metastasis to the liver, kidney, brain, or gastrointestinal tract; metastasis to lung larger than 2 cm in diameter or three or more in number; or persistent hCG level 4 to 6 weeks after evacuation. The use of less stringent diagnostic criteria for postmolar tumors in the United States is partly motivated by the concern that some patients may be lost to follow-up. Among 333 recent patients with molar pregnancy at our center, 122 (37%) patients did not complete the entire hormonal follow-up and 13 (4%) patients were lost to follow-up without attaining even one undetectable hCG value (85). Furthermore, Massad et al. observed that among 40 indigent women with molar pregnancy, 33 (82%) did not fully comply with hCG follow-up and 5 (13%) were lost to follow-up before remission (86).

We reviewed 858 patients with complete moles to identify factors that predispose to postmolar tumors (53). At the time of presentation, 41% of the patients had the following signs of marked trophoblastic proliferation: hCG level >100,000 mIU/mL, uterine size greater than gestational age, and theca lutein cysts >6 cm in diameter. After evacuation, 31.0% of these patients developed uterine invasion and 8.8% developed metastases. The risk for persistent tumors is considerably less for patients who do not present with signs of marked trophoblastic growth. Following molar evacuation, only 3.4% of these patients developed invasion and 0.6% developed metastases. Similarly, Curry et al. (54) and Morrow (87) reported postmolar tumors in 57% and 55% of patients, respectively, with excessive uterine size and theca lutein ovarian cysts. Therefore, patients with complete moles and markedly elevated hCG levels and excessive uterine size are at increased risk of developing postmolar tumors, and are categorized as high risk.

An increased risk of postmolar GTTs has also been observed in women older than age 40 years. Tow (88) and Xia et al. (89) reported that 37% and 33%, respectively, of women more than 40 years old with complete molar pregnancy developed persistent tumors. In women over age 50 years, postmolar tumors were reported to have developed in 56% of patients (90). Complete moles in older women are more frequently aneuploid, and this may be related to their increased potential for local invasion and metastasis (91).

Patients with repetitive molar pregnancy are also at increased risk of developing persistent tumors in their later episodes of molar gestation. Between June 1965 and December 2001, we treated 34 patients with repeat molar gestations at the NETDC (92). Postmolar tumors developed following their first mole in 4 (20%) of 20 complete moles and in none of 14 partial moles. However, postmolar tumors developed following the second mole in 8 (44.4%) of 18 complete moles and 2 (12.5%) of 16 partial moles. Parazzini et al. (93) also reported a threefold increased risk of postmolar tumors in patients with repetitive molar disease.

The risk for persistent GTTs has been reported to be increased in complete moles with marked trophoblastic hyperplasia and atypia, high free β hCG levels, and heterozygous genotype. However, data concerning these three potential prognostic variables are inconsistent and conflicting (50,75, 76,94–98).

Sixteen (6.6%) of 240 patients who were followed for partial moles at the NETDC developed nonmetastatic persistent GTTs (99). Only one of these patients presented with the classic signs and symptoms of molar disease including excessive uterine enlargement, theca lutein ovarian cysts, and high hCG levels. Fifteen (94%) patients were thought to have a missed abortion before evacuation. Our patients with partial moles who developed persistent disease did not have clinical features that distinguished them from other patients with partial moles. Flow cytometric studies of partial moles that developed persistent tumors showed a triploid pattern in 11 (85%) of 13 cases with interpretable histograms (100).

The risk of developing persistent GTTs after partial moles has been reported from 0% to 11% (Table 29.2). Summarizing the data from nine centers, 39 (3.5%) of 1,125 patients with partial moles developed persistent GTTs and only 7 (18%) of these patients had metastases.

Multiple Conceptions with Molar Pregnancy and Coexisting Fetuses

Twin pregnancy consisting of a complete mole and a coexisting fetus has been estimated to occur in 1 per 22,000 to 100,000 pregnancies (101). We have reported our experience with eight cases of twin pregnancy with complete mole and a coexisting fetus and reviewed 14 additional published cases by other researchers (102). Furthermore, we described one case of a partial mole coexisting with a normal fetus

and placenta. As compared with singleton complete moles, twin pregnancies consisting of complete moles and coexisting fetuses have higher preevacuation hCG levels, have larger uteri, and are diagnosed later in pregnancy (103–105). Persistent GTT developed in 12 (55%) of 22 cases and 5 (22.7%) had metastatic tumor. Limited information is available to guide antenatal management of multiple gestations with complete moles and coexisting fetuses. These pregnancies are at risk for hemorrhage and preeclampsia. However, no patient died from obstetric or neoplastic complications, and five fetuses survived and no anomalies were detected. The increased availability of ovulation-induction drugs may result in more multiple gestations involving a molar pregnancy.

Surgical Evacuation

After diagnosing a molar pregnancy, the patient should be carefully evaluated to identify the potential presence of medical complications including preeclampsia, electrolyte imbalance, hyperthyroidism, and anemia that might complicate surgical evacuation. The patient is first stabilized and then a decision must be made concerning the most appropriate method of evacuation.

If the patient no longer desires to preserve fertility, hysterectomy may be performed and prominent theca lutein ovarian cysts may be aspirated at the time of surgery. Although hysterectomy eliminates the risks of local invasion, it does not prevent metastasis.

Suction curettage is the preferred method of evacuation regardless of uterine size in patients who desire to preserve fertility (106,107). As the cervix is being dilated, the surgeon may encounter brisk uterine bleeding due to the passage of retained blood. Shortly after commencing suction evacuation, uterine bleeding is generally well controlled and the uterus rapidly regresses in size. If the uterus is larger than 14-weeks size, one hand should be placed on top of the fundus and the uterus should be massaged to stimulate uterine contraction. When suction evacuation is thought to be complete, a sharp curettage should be performed to remove any residual chorionic tissue. Patients who are Rh negative should receive Rh immune globulin at the time of evacuation because Rh D factor is expressed on trophoblast.

Role of Prophylactic Chemotherapy

The use of prophylactic chemotherapy at the time of molar evacuation remains controversial (108). However, several investigators have reported that chemoprophylaxis reduces the risk of postmolar tumor (80,109).

Kim et al. (110) performed a randomized, prospective trial of chemoprophylaxis in patients with complete mole. Chemoprophylaxis significantly reduced the incidence of postmolar tumor from 47% to 14% in patients with high-risk complete moles. However, chemoprophylaxis did not

TABLE 29.2. *Persistent tumor after partial molar pregnancy*

Series (ref.)	No. of patients	No. of persistent tumors	No. of metastases
Czernobilsky et al. (69)	25	1	0
Goto et al. (243)	349	10	3
Lage et al. (100)	310	17	0
Lawler et al. (50)	51	0	0
Ohama et al. (244)	56	0	0
Stone and Bagshawe (245)	194	5	2
Szulman and Surti (246)	49	2	0
Vassilakos et al. (247)	56	0	0
Wong and Ma (248)	35	4	2
Total	1,125	39 (3.5%)	7 (0.6%)

significantly influence the occurrence of persistent tumors in patients with low-risk complete moles. Similarly, Limpongsanurak demonstrated in a double-blind randomized, controlled trial that actinomycin D reduced postmolar tumor in partients with high-risk complete moles from 50.0% to 13.8% (111).

We have also reported that prophylactic actinomycin D reduces the risk of persistent GTTs in patients with high-risk complete moles (78). Only 10 (11%) of 93 patients with high-risk complete moles developed postmolar tumor after prophylactic actinomycin D. Chemoprophylaxis failure more commonly occurred in patients with markedly elevated hCG values. Prophylactic chemotherapy may be of benefit in patients with high-risk complete moles, particularly when hormonal follow-up is unavailable or unreliable.

Hormonal Follow-Up

After molar evacuation, all patients must be followed with hCG measurements to assure remission. Patients are followed with weekly hCG values until they are normal for 3 weeks and then monthly values until they are normal for 6 months. After achieving nondetectable hCG levels, the risk of relapse appears to be very low (85).

Patients are encouraged to use effective contraception during the entire interval of follow-up. Intrauterine devices should not be inserted until the patient achieves normal hCG levels because of the risk of uterine perforation and infection if residual tumor is present. If the patient does not desire surgical sterilization, she is then confronted with the choice of using either hormonal contraceptives or barrier methods.

The incidence of postmolar tumor has been reported to be increased in patients who used oral contraceptives (112). However, data from the NETDC (113), the Gynecologic Oncology Group (114), and the Brewer Center (115) indicate that oral contraceptives do not increase the risk of postmolar trophoblastic disease. Ho Yuen and Burch (116) also reported that the use of oral contraceptives containing 50 μg or less of estrogen was not associated with an increased risk of postmolar tumor. They speculated that the conflicting data concerning the use of oral contraceptives and the risk of postmolar tumor may be explained by differences in the dosage of estrogen. We therefore believe that oral contraceptives may be safely prescribed after molar evacuation.

GESTATIONAL TROPHOBLASTIC TUMORS

Pathologic Considerations

After a molar pregnancy, persistent GTTs may have the histologic pattern of either molar tissue or choriocarcinoma. However, following a nonmolar gestation, persistent GTT may only have the histologic features of choriocarcinoma (117). Gestational choriocarcinoma does not contain chorionic villi but is composed of sheets of both anaplastic cyto- and syncytiotrophoblast.

Placental-site trophoblastic tumor (PSTT) is an uncommon variant of choriocarcinoma (118). This tumor is composed almost entirely of mononuclear intermediate trophoblast and does not contain chorionic villi. Because PSTTs secrete very small amounts of hCG, a large tumor burden may be present before hCG levels are detectable (119).

Natural History

Nonmetastatic Disease

Locally invasive GTTs develop in 15% of patients following evacuation of a complete mole and infrequently after other gestations (78). A trophoblastic tumor may perforate through the myometrium, producing intraperitoneal bleeding, or erode into uterine vessels, causing vaginal hemorrhage (Fig. 29.3). A bulky necrotic tumor may also serve as a nidus for infection.

Metastatic Disease

Metastatic GTTs occur in 4% of patients after evacuation of a complete mole and infrequently after other pregnancies

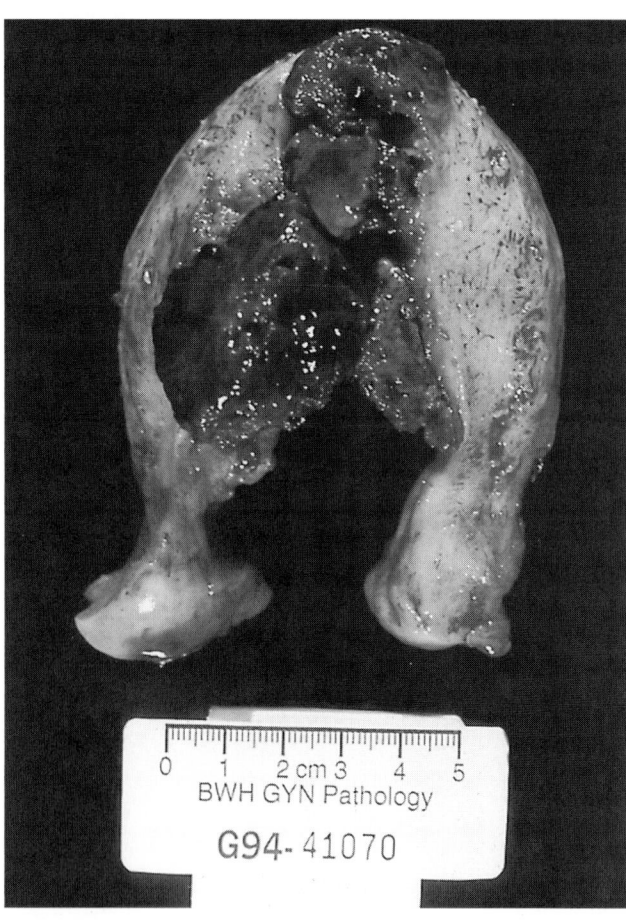

FIG. 29.3. Uterine choriocarcinoma invading and replacing fundal myometrium.

(78). A metastatic GTT is often associated with choriocarcinoma. Choriocarcinoma has a propensity for early vascular invasion with widespread dissemination. The most common metastatic sites are the lung (80%), vagina (30%), brain (10%), and liver (10%). Because trophoblastic tumors are perfused by fragile vessels, metastases are often hemorrhagic. Patients may present with signs and symptoms of bleeding from metastases such as hemoptysis or acute neurologic deficits. Cerebral and hepatic metastases are uncommon unless there is concurrent involvement of the lungs and/or vagina.

GTTs produce four principal radiologic patterns in the lung: (a) pleural effusion, (b) alveolar or snowstorm pattern, (c) discrete rounded densities, or (d) embolic pattern caused by pulmonary arterial occlusion (120–122). Patients may develop pulmonary hypertension in the absence of substantial parenchymal involvement. The extent of pulmonary involvement may differ greatly among centers owing to differences in the frequency of early detection. In Saudi Arabia, Bakri et al. (123) reported that >50% opacification of the lungs, pleural effusion, and more than 10 metastases were present in 33%, 48%, and 43% of patients, respectively, with pulmonary involvement. In contrast, in the United States, patients with pulmonary metastases generally have small nodules on chest radiography and infrequently present with prominent respiratory symptoms.

Patients with pulmonary metastases commonly have an asymptomatic lesion on chest radiography or may present with dyspnea, chest pain, cough, or hemoptysis. Trophoblastic emboli may cause pulmonary arterial occlusion and lead to right-heart strain and pulmonary hypertension (124). Gynecologic symptoms may be minimal or absent and the antecedent pregnancy may be remote in time. The patient may be thought to have a primary pulmonary disease because respiratory symptoms may be dramatic. Unfortunately, the diagnosis of GTT may only be considered and established after the performance of a thoracotomy. The diagnosis of GTT should be considered in any woman in the reproductive age group with unexplained systemic or pulmonary symptoms.

Early respiratory failure requiring mechanical ventilation may develop in patients with extensive pulmonary involvement. Kelly et al. (125) and Bakri et al. (123) reported 100% mortality in 11 and 8 patients, respectively, with early respiratory failure. However, Vaccarello et al. (126) reported one patient who was cured following mechanical ventilation for respiratory failure. Risk factors for early respiratory failure within 1 month of presentation include >50% lung opacification, dyspnea, anemia, cyanosis, and pulmonary hypertension. With chemotherapy, patients may develop bleeding into metastatic sites and potentially worsen pulmonary symptoms and radiologic findings. Importantly, Kelly et al. (125) noted that reducing the initial dose of chemotherapy did not protect against early respiratory failure and recommended administering intensive chemotherapy at the outset.

Vaginal lesions may present with irregular bleeding or purulent discharge and are most commonly located in the fornices or suburethrally. Vaginal metastases are highly vascular and may bleed vigorously if biopsied. Biopsy of vaginal metastases should be absolutely avoided; the desire to avoid hemorrhage should supersede the interest of obtaining an unequivocal pathologic diagnosis.

Most patients with cerebral metastases are symptomatic and present with vomiting, seizures, headache, hemiparesis, slurred speech, or visual disturbances (127,128). Neurologic symptoms usually result from increased intracranial pressure or intracerebral bleeding. Bakri et al. (129) and Athanassiou et al. (130) reported that 20 of 23 patients (87%) and 66 of 69 patients (96%), respectively, with brain involvement had neurologic complaints. Furthermore, Liu et al. (131) reported that all 34 patients with brain metastases presented with neurologic symptoms.

Patients with liver metastases less commonly present with symptoms that are related to hepatic involvement. Bakri et al. (132) noted that only 5 (26%) of 19 patients with liver metastases presented with jaundice, intraabdominal bleeding, or epigastric pain. Patients with liver metastases generally presented with symptoms related to pulmonary, vaginal, or cerebral involvement.

Staging System

The International Federation of Gynecology and Obstetrics (FIGO) reports data on GTTs using an anatomic staging system (Table 29.3). International staging enables a comparable reporting of data, which is critical to allow objective comparison of treatment results (133). Stage I includes all patients with persistently elevated hCG levels and tumor confined to the uterus. Stage II comprises all patients with tumor outside of the uterus but localized to the vagina and/or pelvis. Stage III includes all patients with pulmonary metastases with or without uterine, vaginal, or pelvic involvement. Stage IV patients have far-advanced disease with involvement of the brain, liver, kidneys, or gastrointestinal tract. Patients with Stage IV disease are most likely to be resistant to chemotherapy. Stage IV tumors generally have the histologic pattern of choriocarcinoma and commonly follow a nonmolar pregnancy, with protracted delays in diagnosis and large tumor burdens.

TABLE 29.3. *FIGO anatomic staging for gestational trophoblastic neoplasia*

Stage I	Disease confined to the uterus
Stage II	GTN extends outside of the uterus, but is limited to the genital structures (adnexa, vagina, broad ligament)
Stage III	GTN extends to the lungs, with or without known genital tract involvement
Stage IV	All other metastatic sites

GTN, gestational trophoblastic neoplasia.

It is also helpful to use prognostic variables to predict the likelihood of drug resistance and to assist in selecting appropriate chemotherapy. The current staging system combines both anatomic staging and a prognostic scoring system. The World Health Organization (WHO) has published a prognostic scoring system that reliably predicts the potential for chemotherapy resistance (Table 29.4). Bagshawe (1) first proposed, in 1976, a scoring system for risk factors in GTTs. When the prognostic score is 7 or greater, the patient is considered to be high-risk and requires intensive combination chemotherapy to achieve remission. In general, patients with stage I disease have a low-risk score and patients with stage IV disease have a high-risk score. Therefore, the distinction between low and high risk primarily applies to stages II and III GTTs.

The variables that are included in the prognostic score include tumor volume (hCG level, size of metastases, and number of metastases), site of involvement, prior chemotherapy exposure, and duration of disease. In 1965, Ross et al. (134) reported that patients with high hCG levels, prolonged delays in diagnosis, and brain or liver metastases were relatively resistant to single-agent chemotherapy. Hammond and colleagues (135) further observed in 1973 that patients with prior chemotherapy or an antecedent term pregnancy were also relatively unresponsive to single-agent chemotherapy. Several investigators have since strongly confirmed the importance and reliability of these prognostic factors (136–143).

Choriocarcinoma following term pregnancy has been noted to be a poor-prognosis factor and to have some distinctive clinical features (144–146). We reviewed the experience with postterm choriocarcinoma at the NETDC from 1964 to 1996 (147). Seven (16%) of 44 patients presented with clinical evidence of maternal-fetal bleeding, resulting in severe anemia and nonimmune hydrops or third-trimester bleeding. Although none of the infants had evidence of meta-static choriocarcinoma, rare cases of fetal involvement by choriocarcinoma have been reported and have generally resulted in fetal death. The time interval from delivery to diagnosis, sites of metastases, and pretreatment hCG level were all significant risk factors in predicting outcome. All 31 patients with a WHO score ≤8 survived, whereas 6 of 13 (46%) patients with a WHO score >8 died.

Diagnostic Evaluation

The optimal management of a GTT requires a thorough evaluation of the extent of the disease prior to treatment. All patients with persistent tumors should undergo a thorough assessment including a complete history and physical examination; hCG levels; hepatic, thyroid, and renal function tests; and chest radiograph. Asymptomatic patients with a normal pelvic examination and chest radiograph are very unlikely to have liver or brain metastases identified by further radiographic studies. However, patients with vaginal or lung metastases and/or choriocarcinoma should undergo computed tomographic (CT) scans or magnetic resonance imaging (MRI) scans of the head and abdomen to exclude brain and liver involvement.

Cerebral involvement may also be assessed in patients with metastatic GTTs and/or choriocarcinoma by measuring hCG levels in the cerebrospinal fluid (CSF). Bagshawe and Harland (148) reported that the plasma/CSF hCG ratio tends to be <60 in the presence of brain metastases. However, a single plasma/CSF hCG ratio may be misleading because very rapid changes in plasma hCG values may not be promptly reflected in the CSF (149). For example, Bakri et al. (150) observed that the serum/CSF hCG ratio was >60 in five of ten patients with cerebral involvement.

Pelvic ultrasonography may be useful to detect extensive uterine involvement by trophoblastic tumor and to identify

TABLE 29.4. *Modified WHO Prognostic Scoring System as adapted by FIGO*

Scores	0	1	2	4
Age	<40	≥40	–	–
Antecedent pregnancy	Mole	Abortion	Term	
Interval months from index pregnancy	<4	4–<7	7–<13	≥13
Pretreatment serum hCG (IU/L)	<10^3	10^3–<10^4	10^4–<10^5	≥10^5
Largest tumor size (including uterus)	–	3–<5cm	≥5cm –	
Site of metastases	Lung	Spleen, kidney	Gastrointestinal	Liver, brain
Number of metastases	–	1–4	5–8	>8
Previous failed chemotherapy	–	–	Single drug	2 or more drugs

Format for reporting to FIGO Annual Report: In order to stage and allot a risk factor score, a patient's diagnosis is allocated to a stage as represented by a roman numeral I, II, III, and IV. This is then separated by a colon from the sum of all the actual risk factor scores expressed in arabic numerals; e.g., stage 11:4, stage IV:9. This stage and score will be alloted for each patient.

TABLE 29.5. *Treatment protocol for stage 1 GTT (New England Trophoblastic Disease Center)*

Initial	Single-agent chemotheraphy or hysterectomy with adjunctive chemotherapy
Resistant	Combination chemoterapy
	Hysterectomy with adjunctive chemotherapy
	Local resection
	Pelvic infusion
Follow-up	
hCG	Weekly until normal 3
	Monthly until normal 12
Contraception	12 consecutive months of nomal hCG levels

hCG, human chorionic gonadotropin.

sites of resistant uterine disease (151). However, ultrasound should not be merely performed to document nonmetastatic disease (152). The sensitivity of ultrasonography may be further enhanced by the use of color flow Doppler as well as the vaginal probe (153–156). Ultrasonography may be helpful to select patients who will benefit from hysterectomy because it can accurately detect an extensive uterine trophoblastic tumor.

Management

Stage I

Tables 29.5 and 29.6 review the NETDC protocol for the management of stage I disease and the results of therapy. The selection of treatment is based mainly on the patient's desire to preserve fertility.

TABLE 29.6. *Stage I. Confined to uterine corpus (New England Trophoblastic Disease Center, July 1965 to May 2002)*

Remission therapy	No. of patients (%)	No. of remissions (%)
Initial	485 (91.9)	
Sequential MTX/Act-D		446 (92.0)
Hysterectomy		31 (6.4)
MAC		3 (0.6)
EMA		5 (1.0)
Resistant	43 (8.1)	
MAC		16 (37.2)
EMA		20 (46.5)
EITP		1 (2.3)
Hysterectomy		3 (7.0)
Local uterine resection		2 (4.7)
Pelvic infusion		1 (2.3)
Total	528	528 (100)

MTX, methotrexate; Act-D, actinomycin D; MAC, methotrexate, actinomycin D, cyclophosphamide; EMA, etoposide, methotrexate, actinomycin D; EITP, etoposide, ifosfamide, Taxol (paclitaxel), cisplatin.

If the patient no longer wishes to retain fertility, hysterectomy with adjuvant single-agent chemotherapy may be performed as primary treatment. Adjuvant chemotherapy is administered for three reasons: (a) to reduce the likelihood of disseminating viable tumor cells at surgery, (b) to maintain a cytotoxic level of chemotherapy in the bloodstream and tissues in case viable tumor cells are disseminated at surgery, and (c) to treat any occult metastases that may be already present at the time of surgery. Occult pulmonary metastases may be detected by CT scan in about 40% of patients with presumed nonmetastatic disease (157). Chemotherapy may be safely administered at the time of hysterectomy without increasing operative complications. Thirty-one patients were treated by primary hysterectomy and adjuvant chemotherapy at the NETDC and all achieved complete remission with no additional therapy.

Nonmetastatic PSTTs should be treated with hysterectomy because of their poor response to chemotherapy. Because PSTT is generally resistant to chemotherapy, there are few long-term survivors with metastases despite intensive multimodal therapy (158). Papadopoulos et al. (158) reviewed the clinical experience with 34 patients with PSTT at the Charing Cross Hospital. A long interval from the antecedent pregnancy to clinical presentation was the most important prognostic factor. Whereas all 27 patients survived when the interval from the antecedent pregnancy was less than 4 years, all 7 patients died when the time interval exceeded 4 years. Similarly, Lathrop et al. (119) reported in a review of 43 patients that all ten fatal cases of PSTT had a more than 2-year interval from antecedent pregnancy to diagnosis. However, whereas Lathrop et al. reported that the mitotic rate was prognostically important, Papadopoulos and colleagues observed that the mitotic rate of PSTT was not related to outcome.

Single-agent chemotherapy is the preferred treatment in patients with stage I disease who desire to retain fertility. Primary single-agent chemotherapy induced complete remission in 446 (92%) of 489 patients with stage I GTT. The remaining 43 resistant patients subsequently attained remission with either combination chemotherapy or surgical intervention. If the patient is resistant to chemotherapy and wants to preserve fertility, local uterine resection may be considered. When local resection is planned, ultrasound, MRI, and/or arteriogram may identify the site of resistant tumor. Two of our patients who underwent local uterine resection achieved remission, and one of these patients had a later term delivery by cesarean section.

Stages II and III

The NETDC protocol for the management of stages II and III disease and the results of treatment are outlined in Tables 29.7 to 29.9. Whereas low-risk patients are treated with primary single-agent chemotherapy, high-risk patients are managed with primary combination chemotherapy (159).

TABLE 29.7. *Treatment protocol for stages II and III GTTs (New England Trophoblastic Disease Center)*

Low risk[a]	
Initial	Single-agent chemotherapy
Resistant	Combination chemotherapy
High risk[a]	
Initial	Combination chemotherapy
Resistant	Second-line combination chemotherapy
Follow-up hCG	Weekly until normal 3
	Monthly until normal 12
Contraception	12 consecutive months of normal hCG levels

hCG, human chorionic gonadotropin.
[a]Local resection optional.

Between July 1965 and May 2002, 28 patients with stage II disease were treated at the NETDC and all achieved remission. Single-agent chemotherapy induced complete remission in 16 (80%) of 20 low-risk patients. In contrast, only two of eight high-risk patients achieved remission with single-agent treatment.

Single-agent chemotherapy is well recognized to be effective as primary treatment in low-risk metastatic GTTs (160). Summarizing the experience from four centers, single-agent chemotherapy induced complete remission in 128 (87.1%) of 147 patients with low-risk metastatic GTTs (139, 161–163). All patients who were resistant to single-agent chemotherapy later achieved remission with combination chemotherapy except two patients reported by Ayhan et al. (161).

Vaginal metastases may bleed profusely because they may

TABLE 29.8. *Stage II. Metastases to pelvis and vagina (New England Trophoblastic Disease Center, July 1965 to May 2002)*

Remission therapy	No. of patients	No. of remissions (%)
Low risk	20 (71.4%)	
Initial:		
Sequential MTX/Act-D		16 (80.0)
Resistant:		
MAC		2 (10.0)
EMACO		2 (10.0)
High risk	8 (28.6%)	
Initial:		
Sequential MTX/Act-D		2 (25.0)
MAC		4 (50.0)
Resistant:		
MAC		1 (12.5)
CHAMOCA		1 (12.5)
Total	28	28 (100)

MTX, methotrexate; Act-D, actinomycin-D; MAC, methotrexate, actinomycin D, cyclophosphamide; CHAMOCA, Bagshawe multiagent regimen; EMACO, etoposide, methotrexate, actinomycin D, cyclophosphamide, Oncovin (vincristine).

TABLE 29.9. *Stage III. Metastases to lung (New England Trophoblastic Disease Center, July 1965 to May 2002)*

Remission therapy	No. of patients	No. of remissions (%)
Low-risk	104 (68.0%)	
Initial:		
Sequential MTX/Act-D		85 (81.7)
Resistant:		
MAC		12 (11.5)
EMA		5 (4.8)
EMACO		2 (1.9)
High-risk	49 (32.0%)	
Initial:		
Sequential MTX/Act-D		13 (26.5)
MAC		14 (28.6)
EMACO		13 (26.5)
Resistant:		
MAC		2 (4.1)
CHAMOCA		1 (2.0)
5-FU-Adria		1 (2.0)
VPB		2 (4.1)
EMA		1 (2.0)
EMA-CE		1 (2.0)
Total	153	152 (99.3)

MTX, methotrexate; Act-D, actinomycin D; MAC, methotrexate, actinomycin D, cyclophosphamide; CHAMOCA, Bagshawe multiagent regimen; 5-FU-Adria, 5-fluorouracil, Adriamycin (doxorubicin); VPB, vinblastine, cisplatinum, bleomycin; EMA, etoposide, methotrexate, actinomycin D; EMACE, etoposide, methotrexate, actinomycin D, cisplatin, etoposide.

be highly vascular and friable. Bleeding may be controlled by packing the hemorrhagic lesion or performing wide local excision. Infrequently, angiographic embolization of the hypogastric arteries may be required to control hemorrhage from vaginal metastases. Yingna et al. reported that 18 (35.3%) of 51 patients with vaginal metastases presented with vaginal hemorrhage (164). Bleeding was controled by vaginal packing in 16 patients and angiographic embolization in 2 patients.

Between July 1965 and May 2002, 153 patients with stage III tumors were managed at the NETDC and 152 (99.3%) attained complete remission. Single-agent chemotherapy induced complete remission in 85 (81.7%) of 104 patients with low-risk disease and in 13 (26.5%) of 49 patients with high-risk disease. All patients who were resistant to single-agent treatment later achieved remission with combination chemotherapy.

Thoracotomy has a limited role in the management of stage III GTTs. Thoracotomy should be performed if the diagnosis is seriously in doubt. Furthermore, if a patient has a persistent viable pulmonary nodule despite intensive chemotherapy, pulmonary resection may be performed (165). However, an extensive metastatic survey should be obtained to exclude other sites of persistent tumor. It is important to emphasize that fibrotic nodules may persist indefinitely on the chest radiograph after complete gonadotropin remission is achieved. If a metastasis is persistent on radiography but is of questionable viability, a scan with radioisotope-labeled antibody to hCG or a positron emission tomography (PET) scan may be useful. A radioisotope hCG or PET scan may also be helpful in identifying occult sites of viable tumor (166,167). Tomoda et al. (168) reviewed their experience with pulmonary resection in 19 patients with chemotherapy-resistant GTTs. They proposed the following guidelines for successful resection: (a) good surgical candidate, (b) primary malignancy is controlled, (c) no evidence of other metastatic sites, (d) pulmonary metastasis is limited to one lung, and (e) hCG level is <1,000 mIU/mL. Complete remission was achieved in 14 of 15 patients who met all five criteria but in none of the 4 patients who had one or more unfavorable clinical features. Similarly, Jones et al. (169) reported that six (66.7%) of nine carefully selected patients with drug-resistant pulmonary GTTs attained complete remission following lung resection. Several investigators have reported that the achievement of nondetectable hCG levels within 1 to 2 weeks of resection of a solitary pulmonary nodule is highly predictive of a favorable outcome (170–173). Survival following salvage surgery is influenced by the number of preoperative chemotherapy regimens, number of disease sites, and the WHO score (174).

Hysterectomy may be required in patients with metastatic GTTs to control uterine hemorrhage or sepsis. Furthermore, in patients with bulky uterine tumor, hysterectomy may reduce the tumor burden and thereby limit the need for chemotherapy. Hammond et al. (175) reported that patients who underwent hysterectomy had a shorter duration of hospitalization and chemotherapy.

Stage IV

Tables 29.10 and 29.11 outline the NETDC protocol for the management of stage IV disease and the results of treatment. These patients are at high risk for developing rapidly progressive disease despite intensive therapy.

TABLE 29.10. *Treatment protocol for stage IV GTTs (New England Trophoblastic Disease Center)*

Initial
 Combination chemotherapy
  Brain: Whole head irradiation (30 Gy); craniotomy to manage complications
  Liver: Resection to manage complications
Resistant[a]
 Second-line combination chemotherapy
Follow-up
 hCG: Weekly until normal 3; monthly until normal 24
 Contraception: 24 consecutive months of normal hCG levels

hCG, human chorionic gonadotropin.
[a]Local resection optional.

TABLE 29.11. *Stage IV. Distant metastases (New England Trophoblastic Disease Center, July 1965 to May 2002)*

Remission therapy[a]	No. of remissions (%)	
<1975		
Initial: Sequential MTX/Act-D	5	6/20 (30)
Resistant: MAC	1	
>1975		
Initial: Sequential MTX/Act-D	2	15/19 (78.9)
Resistant:		
MAC	2	
HD MTX/Act-D	4	
MAC	1	
CHAMOCA	1	
VPB	1	
EMA	3	
EMACE	1	

HD, high dose; MTX, methotrexate; Act-D, actinomycin D; MAC, methotrexate, actinomycin D, cyclophosphamide; CHAMOCA, Bagshawe multiagent regimen; VPB, vinblastine, cisplatinum, bleomycin; EMA, etoposide, methotrexate, actinomycin D, EMACE, etoposide, methotrexate, actinomycin D, cisplatin, etoposide.
[a]Radiation therapy and surgery utilized when indicated.

All patients with stage IV disease should be treated with intensive combination chemotherapy and the selective use of radiation therapy and surgery (3,176). Before 1975, only 6 (30%) of 20 patients with stage IV disease attained complete remission. However, after 1975, 15 (78.9%) of 19 patients with stage IV tumors achieved remission. This dramatic improvement in survival resulted from the introduction of intensive multimodal therapy early in the course of treatment.

The management of hepatic metastases is particularly difficult and challenging. Hepatic resection may be required to control bleeding or to excise resistant tumor. Grumbine et al. (177) reported the use of selective occlusion of the hepatic arteries and concurrent combination chemotherapy in a patient with bleeding liver metastases who ultimately attained remission. Importantly, Wong et al. (178) noted that nine of ten patients with hepatic involvement achieved complete remission with primary intensive combination chemotherapy and without any hepatic irradiation. Bakri and colleagues (132) similarly reported that five of eight (62.5%) patients with liver metastases who were treated with combination chemotherapy alone attained complete remission.

If cerebral metastases are detected, whole brain irradiation is promptly instituted at the NETDC. The risk of spontaneous cerebral hemorrhage may be reduced by the concurrent use of chemotherapy and brain irradiation (179). Brain irradiation may be both hemostatic and tumoricidal. Yordan et al. (180) reported that deaths due to central nervous system involvement occurred in 11 (44%) of 25 patients treated with chemotherapy alone but in none of 18 patients treated with brain irradiation and chemotherapy.

However, Newlands et al. (181) have reported excellent remission rates in patients with cerebral metastases who were treated with chemotherapy alone. Thirty of 35 (86%) patients with cerebral lesions achieved sustained remission with intensive combination chemotherapy including high-dose intravenous and intrathecal methotrexate (MTX). None of their patients received external beam brain irradiation.

Craniotomy should be performed to manage life-threatening complications and thereby provide the opportunity for chemotherapy to induce complete remission. Craniotomy may be necessary to provide acute decompression or to control bleeding. Infrequently, cerebral metastases that are resistant to chemotherapy may be amenable to resection. Evans et al. (176) reported complete remission in three of four patients who underwent craniotomy to relieve intracranial pressure and in two of three patients undergoing craniotomy for resection of chemotherapy-resistant tumor. Athanassiou and colleagues (130) similarly reported that four of five patients undergoing craniotomy for acute intracranial complications were ultimately cured. Fortunately, most patients with cerebral metastases who achieve remission generally have no residual neurologic deficits (130).

Follow-Up

All patients with stages I, II, and III GTTs are followed with weekly hCG values until they are normal for 3 weeks and then monthly values until they are normal for 12 months. Patients are encouraged to use contraception during the entire interval of follow-up.

Patients with stage IV disease are followed with weekly hCG values until they are normal for 3 weeks and then monthly values until they are normal for 24 months. These patients require prolonged follow-up because they have an increased risk of late recurrence.

It is important for clinicians to recognize that hCG molecules in GTDs are more degraded or heterogeneous in serum than in normal pregnancy (182). Trophoblastic disease samples contain high proportions of free β hCG, nicked hCG, and β core fragment (183). When monitoring patients for GTD, it is therefore desirable to use an assay that detects not only intact hCG, but also all of its metabolites and fragments.

Many hCG assays have a degree of cross reactivity with luteinizing hormone. Following multiple courses of combination chemotherapy, ovarian steroidal function may be damaged, particularly in patients in their late 30s and 40s. When ovarian function is damaged, luteinizing hormone levels may rise, and owing to cross reactivity, the patient may be falsely thought to have persistent low levels of hCG. Patients who receive combination chemotherapy should therefore be placed on oral contraceptives to suppress luteinizing hormone levels and prevent problems with cross reactivity.

It is important to emphasize that some patients may have a false-positive elevation in serum hCG measurement owing to the presence of circulating heterophilic antibody (184). These patients with phantom hCG or phantom choriocarcinoma often have no clear antecedent pregnancy and no progressive rise in their hCG levels. The possibility of false-positive hCG measurement should be assessed by sending both serum and urine samples to a reference hCG laboratory. Patients with phantom hCG generally have no measurable hCG in a parallel urine sample.

Mutch and colleagues (185) reported recurrences after initial remission in 2% of patients with nonmetastatic GTTs, 4% of patients with good-prognosis metastatic GTTs, and 13% of patients with poor-prognosis disease. Relapses developed within 3 and 18 months in 50% and 85% of patients, respectively. Similarly, we observed relapse after initial remission in 2.9% of stage I, 8.3% of stage II, 4.2% of stage III, and 9.1% of stage IV patients (186). The mean time to recurrence from the last nondetectable hCG level was 6 months, and this did not differ among the four FIGO stages. All patients with stages I, II, and III GTTs who developed recurrence were subsequently cured, whereas both stage IV patients with recurrences died.

Chemotherapy

Single-Agent Chemotherapy

In 1956, Li et al. (187) reported the dramatic cure of metastatic choriocarcinoma in three women by using MTX. In 1961, Hertz and colleagues (188) reviewed the initial 5-year experience with chemotherapy in treating metastatic GTTs. Importantly, MTX alone induced complete remission in 28 (44%) of 63 patients with metastatic GTTs. After achieving impressive results in patients with metastatic disease, Hertz and coworkers (189) used MTX as the primary treatment of nonmetastatic GTTs. Complete remission was attained in all 16 women with nonmetastatic GTTs by administering MTX alone. Chemotherapy, therefore, obviated the need for hysterectomy and enabled patients to attain cure while retaining their fertility. Although MTX induced cure in many patients, it was still necessary to identify other active chemotherapeutic agents. Ross et al. (190) first used actinomycin D in 13 patients with MTX-resistant GTTs and 6 (46%) patients attained complete remission. Since the early 1960s, MTX and actinomycin D (Act-D) have remained the two central drugs in the treatment of patients with GTTs.

Single-agent chemotherapy with either Act-D or MTX has induced comparable and excellent remission rates in both nonmetastatic and metastatic GTTs (191). An optimal regimen should maximize the cure rate while minimizing toxicity. Many protocols have been evaluated for administering Act-D and MTX as single agents in nonmetastatic and low-risk metastatic GTTs (163,192–200). Several regimens of Act-D and MTX have induced complete remission in 70% to 100% of patients with nonmetastatic GTTs and in 50% to 70% of patients with low-risk metastatic disease. Fortunately, if a patient develops resistance to the initial single-agent chemotherapeutic treatment, it is still likely that the patient may achieve remission with an alternative single-agent.

Bagshawe and Wilde (201) first reported, in 1964, administering MTX with folinic acid (MTXFA) to reduce chemotherapeutic toxicity. MTXFA has remained the primary treatment of nonmetastatic and low-risk metastatic GTTs at the Charing Cross Hospital (192). Although MTXFA is highly effective, chemotherapy needed to be changed in 20% because of resistance and in 6% because of toxicity.

MTXFA has been the preferred single-agent regimen in the treatment of GTTs at the NETDC since 1974 (202–204). Between September 1974 and September 1984, 185 patients with GTTs were treated with primary MTXFA at the NETDC. Complete remission was induced with MTXFA in 162 (87.6%) patients, and 132 (81.5%) of these patients required only one course of MTXFA to achieve remission. MTXFA induced remission in 147 (90.2%) of 163 patients with stage I GTTs and in 15 (68.2%) of 22 patients with low-risk stages II and III GTTs. Among the 23 patients who were resistant to MTXFA, 14 (61%) achieved remission with Act-D and 9 attained remission with combination chemotherapy. Following MTXFA, thrombocytopenia, granulocytopenia, and hepatotoxicity occurred in only 11 (5.9%), 3 (1.6%), and 26 (14.1%) patients, respectively. No patient required platelet transfusions or developed sepsis due to myelosuppression and no patient developed alopecia. MTXFA only induces an excellent remission rate with minimal toxicity but also effectively limits chemotherapy exposure (205). The MTXFA regimen is administered over 8 days (MTX 1 mg/kg intramuscularly on days 1, 3, 5, and 7 and folinic acid 0.1 mg/kg intramuscularly or orally on days 2, 4, 6, and 8), and its effectiveness may be partly attributable to the prolonged exposure to MTX. When we administered MTX at a higher dosage (300 mg/m^2) over 12 hours and 30 minutes, the remission rate declined to 69% in patients with nonmetastatic disease (206).

Whereas MTX and Act-D are the two most commonly used single agents in the treatment of GTTs in the United States and in most of the world, 5-fluorouracil has been the preferred single-agent chemotherapy in China (207). Sung et al. reported that 5-fluorouracil induced complete remission in 93% of patients with stage I GTTs and in 86% of patients with stage II GTTs.

Combination Chemotherapy

Modified triple therapy with MTXFA, Act-D, and cyclophosphamide had been the preferred combination drug regimen at the NETDC (208). However, triple therapy is inadequate as an initial treatment in patients with metastatic disease and a high-risk score (score >7). Summarizing the experience from six centers, triple therapy induced complete remission in 47 (51%) of 92 patients with metastatic GTTs and a high-risk WHO score (score >7) (139,141,161,162, 209,210).

Etoposide (VP16) has been demonstrated to be a highly active antitumor agent in GTTs. Primary oral etoposide induced complete sustained remission in 56 (93.3%) of 60 patients with nonmetastatic or low-risk metastatic GTTs (211). Bagshawe (212) reported an 83% remission rate in patients with metastatic disease and a high-risk score using a combination regimen that included etoposide. This regimen (EMACO) includes etoposide, MTX, Act-D, cyclophosphamide, and Oncovin (vincristine) and is currently the preferred treatment for patients with metastatic GTTs and a high-risk score. Bolis et al. (213), Schink et al. (214), and Soper et al. (215) have similarly reported that EMACO induced complete remission in 13 (76.4%) of 17, in 5 (100%) of 5, and in 4 (67%) of 6 patients, respectively, with metastatic GTTs and a high-risk score. Furthermore, Bower et al. (216) and Kim et al.(217) reported that primary EMACO induced remission in 130 (86.1%) of 151 patients and in 87 (90.6%) of 96 patients, respectively, with high-risk metastatic GTTs (WHO score >7). Therefore, EMACO induces complete remission in 70% to 90% of patients with metastatic GTTs and a high-risk WHO score.

If patients experience resistance to EMACO, they may then successfully be treated with a modification of this regimen by substituting etoposide and cisplatin on day 8 (EMAEP) (216,218). Bower et al. (216) reported that EMAEP induced remission alone or in conjunction with surgery in 16 (76%) of 21 patients who were resistant to EMACO. When patients develop resistance to EMACO, surgical intervention may be necessary to remove sites of resistant tumor.

Unfortunately, the use of etoposide in GTTs has been reported to increase the risk of later secondary tumor including myeloid leukemia, melanoma, colon cancer, and breast cancer (219). The relative risk for leukemia, melanoma, colon cancer, and breast cancer was increased by 16.6, 3.4, 4.6, and 5.8, respectively. The increased risk for breast cancer did not become apparent until after 25 years. Among all patients who were treated with etoposide, 1.5% subsequently developed leukemia. Etoposide should therefore be used only in patients who require it to achieve remission; in particular, patients with metastatic GTTs and a high-risk score. When patients with nonmetastatic and low-risk metastatic GTTs experience resistance to MTX and Act-D, it is reasonable to consider administering triple therapy before treatment with regimens containing etoposide (220).

Second-line therapy with cisplatin, vinblastine, and bleomycin (PVB) may also be effective in patients with drug-resistant GTT. Gordon et al. (221), DuBeshter et al. (222), and Azab et al. (223) reported that PVB induced complete remission in 2 of 11 patients, 4 of 7 patients, and 5 of 8 patients, respectively, with drug-resistant GTTs.

The potential role of autologous bone marrow transplantation or stem-cell rescue in GTTs has yet to be defined. However, individual cases have been reported where high-dose chemotherapy with autologous bone marrow or stem-cell support has induced complete remission in patients with refractory GTTs (224,225).

Efforts continue to identify new agents that are effective in treating patients with GTTs. Although ifosfamide and paclitaxel (Taxol) are both active in treating GTTs, further studies must be performed to determine their potential role in either primary treatment or second-line therapy (226,227).

Patients who require combination chemotherapy must be treated intensively to attain remission. We administer combination chemotherapy as frequently as toxicity permits until the patient attains three consecutive normal hCG values. After the patient achieves normal hCG levels, three additional courses of chemotherapy are administered to reduce the risk of relapse.

SUBSEQUENT PREGNANCIES

Pregnancies After Hydatidiform Mole

Patients with complete molar pregnancies can anticipate normal reproduction in the future (92). Patients with complete moles who were treated at the NETDC had 1,278 later pregnancies between June 1965 and November 2001. These pregnancies resulted in 877 (68.6%) full-term live births, 95 (7.4%) premature deliveries, 11 (0.9%) ectopic pregnancies, and 7 (0.5%) stillbirths (Table 29.12). First-trimester spontaneous abortion occurred in 221 (17.3%) pregnancies, and major and minor congenital malformations were detected in only 40 (4.1%) infants. Primary cesarean section was performed in only 70 (18.8%) of 373 subsequent full-term and premature births between January 1979 and November 2001.

Limited information is available regarding the later pregnancy experience in patients with partial moles (Table 29.13). Between June 1965 and November 2001, patients with partial moles at the NETDC had 251 subsequent gestations that resulted in 189 (75.3%) term live births, 1 (0.4%) stillbirth, 1 (0.4%) ectopic pregnancy, and 4 (1.6%) premature deliveries. First-trimester spontaneous abortion occurred in 38 (15.1%) pregnancies, and major or minor congenital anomalies were detected in only 3 (1.5%) infants. The preliminary data concerning subsequent conceptions after partial moles are therefore reassuring.

When a patient has had a molar pregnancy, she is at increased risk of developing molar disease in later conceptions (228,229). Thirty-four (1:150) of our patients have had at least two molar gestations between June 1965 and November 2001 (92). Patients may have an initial complete or partial mole and then in a later pregnancy develop the other type of molar disease. Following two episodes of molar pregnancy, our 34 patients had 35 later conceptions, resulting in 20 (57.1%) full-term deliveries, 7 (20%) molar pregnancies (6 complete, 1 partial), 3 (8.6%) spontaneous abortions, 1 (2.9%) ectopic pregnancy, 1 intrauterine fetal death, and 3 (8.6%) therapeutic abortions. Bagshawe et al. (230) also reported that the risk of molar disease following two episodes of molar pregnancy was 15%. In six of our cases, the medical records clearly indicated that the patient had a different partner at the time of conception of different molar pregnancies (231). Patients with molar gestation appear to be at increased risk for later molar disease even with a different partner.

It therefore seems prudent to obtain an ultrasound in the first trimester of any subsequent pregnancy to confirm normal gestational development. An hCG measurement should also be obtained 6 weeks after the completion of any future pregnancy to exclude occult trophoblastic disease.

PREGNANCIES AFTER GTT

Patients with GTTs who are successfully treated with chemotherapy can also generally expect normal reproduction in

TABLE 29.13. *Subsequent pregnancies in patients with partial mole (New England Trophoblastic Disease Center, June 1, 1965 to November 20, 2001)*

Outcome	No. of patients	(%)	No./deliveries (%)
Term delivery	189	75.3	
Stillbirth	1	0.4	
Premature delivery	4	1.6	
Spontaneous abortion			
1st trimester	38	15.1	
2nd trimester	1	0.4	
Therapeutic abortion	11	4.4	
Ectopic pregnancy	1	0.4	
Repeat molar pregnancy	6	2.4	
Total pregnancies	251		
Congenital malformations (major and minor)			3/194 (1.5)
Primary cesarean section			29/194 (14.9)[a]

[a]January 1979 to November 2001.

TABLE 29.12. *Subsequent pregnancies in patients with complete mole (New England Trophoblastic Disease Center, June 1, 1965 to November 20, 2001)*

Outcome	No. of patients	(%)	No./deliveries (%)
Term delivery	877	68.6	
Stillbirth	7	0.5	
Premature delivery	95	7.4	
Spontaneous abortion			
1st trimester	221	17.3	
2nd trimester	8	0.6	
Therapeutic abortion	41	3.2	
Ectopic	11	0.9	
Repeat mole	18	1.4	
Total pregnancies	1,278		
Congenital malformations (major and minor)			40/979 (4.1)
Primary cesarean section			70/373 (18.8)[a]

[a]January 1979 to November 2001.

TABLE 29.14. *Subsequent pregnancies in patients with gestational trophoblastic tumors (New England Trophoblastic Disease Center, June 1, 1965 to November 30, 2001)*

Outcome	No. of patients	(%)	No./deliveries (%)
Term delivery	393	67.6	
Stillbirth	9	1.5	
Premature delivery	35	6.0	
Spontaneous abortion			
1st trimester	92	15.8	
2nd trimester	7	1.2	
Therapeutic abortion	28	4.8	
Ectopic pregnancy	7	1.2	
Repeat molar pregnancy	8	1.4	
Total pregnancies	581		
Congenital malformations (major and minor)			10/437 (2.3)
Primary cesarean section			68/335 (20.3)[a]

[a]January 1979 to November 2001.

the future (92). Patients with GTTs who were treated with chemotherapy at the NETDC had 581 pregnancies between June 1965 and November 2001. These later pregnancies resulted in 393 (67.6%) full-term live births, 35 (6.0%) premature deliveries, 7 (1.2%) ectopic pregnancies, and 9 (1.5%) stillbirths (Table 29.14). First-trimester spontaneous abortion occurred in 92 (15.8%) pregnancies and major and minor congenital anomalies were detected in only 10 (2.3%) infants. It is particularly reassuring that the frequency of congenital malformations is not increased because chemotherapy may be teratogenic and mutagenic. Primary cesarean section was performed in only 68 (20.3%) of 335 subsequent full-term and premature deliveries between January 1979 and November 2001. Later pregnancies have no increased risk for obstetric complications either prenatally or intrapartum.

Summarizing the experience from the NETDC with eight other centers, following chemotherapy for GTTs, data have been reported concerning the outcome of 2,657 later pregnancies (232–239). These subsequent pregnancies resulted in 2,038 (76.7%) live births, 71 (5.3%) premature deliveries, 34 (1.3%) stillbirths, and 378 (14.2%) spontaneous abortions. Although the frequency of stillbirth appears to be somewhat increased, congenital malformations were noted in only 37 infants (1.8%), which is consistent with the general population. Woolas et al. (239) noted that there was no difference in either the conception rate or pregnancy outcome between women treated with single-agent MTX and those receiving combination chemotherapy. Furthermore, only 7% of women who wished to become pregnant following chemotherapy for GTT failed to conceive (239).

PSYCHOSOCIAL CONSEQUENCES OF GTD

Women who develop GTDs may experience significant mood disturbance, marital and sexual problems, and con-

cerns over future fertility (240,241). Because GTD is a consequence of pregnancy, patients and their partners must confront the loss of a pregnancy at the same time they face concerns regarding malignancy. Patients may experience clinically significant levels of anxiety, fatigue, anger, confusion, sexual problems, and concern for future pregnancy that may last for protracted periods of time. Particularly, patients with metastatic disease and active disease are at risk for severe psychological reactions (240). Psychosocial assessments and interventions should be provided to patients with GTDs and their partners, and should be targeted particularly to patients in the metastatic and active disease groups. The psychologic and social stresses related to persistent GTTs may last for many years beyond achieving complete remission (242). Even 5 to 10 years after attaining complete remission, 51% of patients indicate that they would be somewhat likely to very likely to participate in a counseling program today to discuss psychosocial issues raised by having had GTT.

REFERENCES

1. Bagshawe KD. Risks and prognostic factors in trophoblastic neoplasia. *Cancer* 1976;38:1373.
2. Goldstein DP, Berkowitz RS. *Gestational trophoblastic neoplasms—clinical principles of diagnosis and management.* Philadelphia: WB Saunders, 1982:1.
3. Lurain JR. Advances in the management of high-risk gestational trophoblastic tumors. *J Reprod Med* 2002;47:451.
4. Martin BH, Kim JM. Changes in gestational trophoblastic tumors over four decades: a Korean experience. *J Reprod Med* 1998;43:60.
5. Palmer JR. Advances in the epidemiology of gestational trophoblastic disease. *J Reprod Med* 1994;39:155.
6. Bracken MB. Incidence and aetiology of hydatidiform mole: an epidemiologic review. *Br J Obstet Gynaecol* 1987;94:1123.
7. Jeffers MD, O'Dwyer P, Curran B, et al. Partial hydatidiform mole: a common but underdiagnosed condition. *Int J Gynecol Pathol* 1993; 12:315.
8. Berkowitz RS, Cramer DW, Bernstein MR, et al. Risk factors for complete molar pregnancy from a case-control study. *Am J Obstet Gynecol* 1985;152:1016.
8. Parazzini F, LaVecchia C, Mangili G, et al. Dietary factors and risk of trophoblastic disease. *Am J Obstet Gynecol* 1988;158:93.
10. O'Toole BA, Fradkin R, Warkany J. Vitamin A deficiency and reproduction in rhesus monkeys. *J Nutr* 1974;104:1513.
11. Fulop V, Mok SC, Gati I, Berkowitz RS. Recent advances in molecular biology of gestational trophoblastic diseases; a review. *J Reprod Med* 2002; 47:369–379.
11. Parazzini F, Mangili G, LaVecchia C, et al. Risk factors for gestational trophoblastic disease: a separate analysis of complete and partial hydatidiform moles. *Obstet Gynecol* 1991;78:1039.
12. Berkowitz RS, Bernstein MR, Harlow BL. Case-control study of risk factors for partial molar pregnancy. *Am J Obstet Gynecol* 1995;173: 788.
13. Buckley JD, Henderson BE, Morrow CP, et al. Case-control study of gestational choriocarcinoma. *Cancer Res* 1988;48:1004.
14. Palmer JR, Driscoll SG, Rosenberg L, et al. Oral contraceptive use and risk of gestational trophoblastic tumors. *J Natl Cancer Inst* 1999; 91:635.
15. Berkowitz RS, Goldstein DP, Anderson DJ. Recent advances in understanding the immunobiology of gestational trophoblastic disease—a review. *Trophoblast Res* 1987;2:123.
16. Ito H, Sekine T, Komuro N, et al. Histologic stromal reaction of the host with gestational choriocarcinoma and its relation to clinical stage, classification and prognosis. *Am J Obstet Gynecol* 1981;140:781.

17. Anderson DJ, Berkowitz RS. Gamma-interferon enhances expression of Class I MHC antigens in the weakly HLA-positive human choriocarcinoma cell line BeWo but does not induce MHC expression in the HLA-negative choriocarcinoma cell line Jar. J Immunol 1985; 135:2498.

18. Berkowitz RS, Hill JA, Kurtz CB, Anderson DJ. Effects of products of activated leukocytes (lymphokines and monokines) on the growth of malignant trophoblast cells in vitro. Am J Obstet Gynecol 1988; 158:199.

19. Steller MA, Mok S, Yeh J, et al. Effects of cytokines on epidermal growth receptor expression by malignant trophoblast cells in vitro. J Reprod Med 1994;39:209.

20. Berkowitz RS, Hornig-Rohan J, Martin-Alosco S, et al. HLA antigen frequency distribution in patients with gestational choriocarcinoma and their husbands. Placenta Suppl 1981;3:263.

21. Lawler SD, Klouda PT, Bagshawe KD. The HL-A system in trophoblastic neoplasia. Lancet 1971;2:834.

22. Tomoda Y, Fuma M, Saiki N, et al. Immunologic studies in patients with trophoblastic neoplasia. Am J Obstet Gynecol 1976;126:661.

23. Morgensen B, Kissmeyer-Nielsen F, Hauge M. Histocompatibility antigens on the HL-A locus in gestational choriocarcinoma. Transplant Proc 1969;1:76.

24. Berkowitz RS, Mostoufizadeh M, Kabawat SE, et al. Immunopathologic study of the implantation site in molar pregnancy. Am J Obstet Gynecol 1982;144:925.

25. Berkowitz RS, Lahey SJ, Rodrick ML, et al. Circulating immune complex levels in patients with molar pregnancy. Obstet Gynecol 1983;61:165.

26. Lahey SJ, Steele G Jr, Berkowitz RS, et al. Identification of material with paternal HLA antigen immunoreactivity from purported circulating immune complexes in patients with gestational trophoblastic neoplasia. J Natl Cancer Inst 1984;72:983.

27. Berkowitz RS, Anderson DJ, Hunter NJ, Goldstein DP. Distribution of major histocompatibility (HLA) antigens in chorionic villi of molar pregnancy. Am J Obstet Gynecol 1983;146:221.

28. Berkowitz RS, Hoch EJ, Goldstein DP, Anderson DJ. Histocompatibility antigens (HLA-A, B, C) are not detectable in molar villous fluid. Gynecol Oncol 1984;19:74.

29. Cheung ANY, Srivastava G, Chung LP, et al. Expression of the p53 gene in trophoblastic cells in hydatidiform moles and normal human placentas. J Reprod Med 1994;39:223.

30. Cheung ANY, Srivastava G, Pittaluga S, et al. Expression of c-myc and c-fms oncogenes in hydatidiform mole and normal human placenta. J Clin Pathol 1993;46:204.

31. Sarkar S, Kacinski BM, Kohorn EI, et al. Demonstration of myc and ras oncogene expression by hybridization in situ in hydatidiform mole and in the BeWo choriocarcinoma cell line. Am J Obstet Gynecol 1986;154:390.

32. Fulop V, Mok SC, Genest DR, et al. p53, p21, Rb, and MdM2 oncoproteins: expression in normal placenta, partial and complete mole and choriocarcinoma. J Reprod Med 1998;43:119.

33. Fulop V, Mok SC, Genest DR, et al. c-myc, c-erb B-2, c-fms, and bcl-2 oncoproteins—expression in normal placenta, partial and complete mole and choriocarcinoma. J Reprod Med 1998;43:101.

34. Tuncer ZS, Vegh GL, Fulop V, et al. Expression of epidermal growth factor receptor related family products in gestational trophoblastic diseases and normal placenta and its relationship with development of postmolar tumor. Gynecol Oncol 2000;77:389.

35. Vegh GL, Tuncer ZS, Fulop V, et al. Matrix metalloproteinases and their inhibitors in gestational trophoblastic diseases and normal placenta.Gynecol Oncol 1999;75:248.

36. Mutter GL, Stewart CL, Chaponot ML, et al. Oppositely imprinted genes H19 and insulin-like growth factor 2 are co-expressed in human androgenetic trophoblast. Am J Hum Genet 1993;53:1096.

37. Berkowitz RS, Goldstein DP, Bernstein MR. Evolving concepts of molar pregnancy. J Reprod Med 1991;36:40.

38. Montes M, Roberts D, Berkowitz RS, Genest DR. Prevalence and significance of implantation site trophoblast atypia in hydatidiform moles and in spontaneous abortions. Am J Clin Pathol 1996;105:411.

39. Kajii T, Ohama K. Androgenetic origin of hydatidiform mole. Nature 1977;268:633.

40. Yamashita K, Wake N, Araki T, et al. Human lymphocyte antigen expression in hydatidiform mole: androgenesis following fertilization by a haploid sperm. Am J Obstet Gynecol 1979;135:597.

41. Pattillo RA, Sasaki S, Katayama KP, et al. Genesis of 46, XY hydatidiform mole. Am J Obstet Gynecol 1981;141:104.

42. Azuma C, Saji F, Tokugawa Y. Application of gene amplification by polymerase chain reaction to genetic analysis of molar mitochondrial DNA: the detection of anuclear empty ovum as the cause of complete mole. Gynecol Oncol 1991;40:29.

43. Felemban AA, Bakri YN, Alkharif HA, et al. Complete molar pregnancy—clinical trends at King Fahad Hospital, Riyadh, Kingdom of Saudi Arabia. J Reprod Med 1998;43:11.

44. Paradinas FJ, Browne P, Fisher RA, et al. A clinical, histopathologic and flow cytometric study of 149 complete moles, 146 partial moles, 107 non-molar hydropic abortions. Histopathology 1996;28:101.

45. Soto-Wright V, Bernstein MR, Goldstein DP, Berkowitz R. The changing clinical presentation of complete molar pregnancy. Obstet Gynecol 1995;86:775.

46. Mosher R, Goldstein DP, Berkowitz RS, et al. Complete hydatidiform mole—comparison of clinicopathologic fea tures, current and past. J Reprod Med 1998;43:21.

47. Keep D, Zaragoza MV, Hasold T, et al. Very early complete hydatidiform mole. Hum Pathol 1996;27:708.

48. Szulman AE, Surti U. The syndromes of hydatidiform mole: II. Morphologic evolution of the complete and partial mole. Am J Obstet Gynecol 1978;132:20.

49. Szulman AE, Surti U. The syndromes of hydatidiform mole: I. Cytogenetic and morphologic correlations. Am J Obstet Gynecol 1978; 131:665.

50. Lawler SD, Fisher RA, Dent J. A prospective genetic study of complete and partial hydatidiform moles. Am J Obstet Gynecol 1991;164:1270.

51. Lage JM, Mark SD, Roberts D, et al. A flow cytometric study of 137 fresh hydropic placentas: correlation between types of hydatidiform moles and nuclear DNA ploidy. Obstet Gynecol 1992;79:403.

52. Genest DR, Ruiz RE, Weremowicz S, et al. Do nontriploid partial hudatidiform moles exist? A histologic and flow cytometric reevaluation of nontriploid specimens. J Reprod Med 2002; 47:363.

53. Berkowitz RS, Goldstein DP. Presentation and management of molar pregnancy. In: Hancock BW, Newlands ES, Berkowitz RS, eds. Gestational trophoblastic disease. London: Chapman and Hall, 1997:127.

54. Curry SL, Hammond CB, Tyrey L, et al. Hydatidiform mole: diagnosis, management and long-term follow up of 347 patients. Obstet Gynecol 1975;45:1.

55. Kohorn EI. Molar pregnancy: presentation and diagnosis. Clin Obstet Gynecol 1984;27:181.

56. Santos-Ramos R, Forney JP, Schwartz BE. Sonographic findings and clinical correlations in molar pregnancy. Obstet Gynecol 1980;56:186.

57. Montz FJ, Schlaerth JB, Morrow CP. The natural history of theca lutein cysts. Obstet Gynecol 1988;72:247.

58. Osathanondh R, Berkowitz RS, de Cholnoky C, et al. Hormonal measurements in patients with theca lutein cysts and gestational trophoblastic disease. J Reprod Med 1986;31:179.

59. Kohorn EI. Hydatidiform mole and gestational trophoblastic disease in southern Connecticut. Obstet Gynecol 1982;59:78.

60. Berkowitz RS, Goldstein DP, Bernstein MR. Laparoscopy in the management of gestational trophoblastic neoplasia. J Reprod Med 1980; 24:261.

61. Depue RH, Bernstein L, Ross RK, et al. Hyperemesis gravidarum in relation to estradiol levels, pregnancy outcome and other maternal factors: a seroepidemiologic study. Am J Obstet Gynecol 1987;156:1137.

62. Berkowitz RS, Goldstein DP. Pathogenesis of gestational trophoblastic neoplasms. Pathobiol Ann 1981;11:391.

63. Galton VA, Ingbar SH, Jimenez-Fonseca J, et al. Alterations in thyroid hormone economy in patients with hydatidiform mole. J Clin Invest 1971;50:1345.

64. Amir SM, Osathanondh R, Berkowitz RS, Goldstein DP. Human chorionic gonadotropin and thyroid function in patients with hydatidiform mole. Am J Obstet Gynecol 1984;150:723.

65. Nagataki S, Mizuno M, Sakamoto S, et al. Thyroid function in molar pregnancy. J Clin Endocrinol Metab 1977;44:254.

66. Nisula BC, Taliadouros GS. Thyroid function in gestational tropho-

blastic neoplasia: evidence that the thyrotropic activity of chorionic gonadotropin mediates the thyrotoxicosis of choriocarcinoma. *Am J Obstet Gynecol* 1980;138:77.

67. Twiggs LB, Morrow CP, Schlaerth JB. Acute pulmonary complications of molar pregnancy. *Am J Obstet Gynecol* 1979;135:189.

68. Berkowitz RS, Goldstein DP, Bernstein MR. Natural history of partial molar pregnancy. *Obstet Gynecol* 1986;66:677.

69. Czernobilsky B, Barash A, Lancet M. Partial mole: a clinicopathologic study of 25 cases. *Obstet Gynecol* 1982;59:75.

70. Benson CB, Genest DR, Bernstein MR, et al. Sonographic appearance of first trimester for complete hydatidiform moles. *J Ultrasound Obstet Gynecol* 2000; 16:188.

71. Romero R, Horgan JG, Kohorn EI, et al. New criteria for the diagnosis of gestational trophoblastic disease. *Obstet Gynecol* 1985;66:553.

72. Fine C, Bundy AL, Berkowitz RS. Sonographic diagnosis of partial hydatidiform mole. *Obstet Gynecol* 1989;73:414.

73. Naumoff P, Szulman AE, Weinstein B, et al. Ultrasonography of partial hydatidiform mole. *Radiology* 1981;140:467.

74. Menczer J, Modan M, Serr DM. Prospective follow-up of patients with hydatidiform mole. *Obstet Gynecol* 1980;55:346.

75. Genest D, Laborde O, Berkowitz RS, et al. A clinicopathologic study of 153 cases of complete hydatidiform mole (1980–1990): histologic grade lacks prognostic significance. *Obstet Gynecol* 1991;78:402.

76. Berkowitz RS, Ozturk M, Goldstein DP, et al. Human chorionic gonadotropin and free subunits' serum levels in patients with partial and complete hydatidiform moles. *Obstet Gynecol* 1989;74:212.

77. Ozturk M, Berkowitz RS, Goldstein DP, et al. Differential production of human chorionic gonadotropin and free subunits of gestational trophoblastic disease. *Am J Obstet Gynecol* 1988;158:193.

78. Berkowitz RS, Goldstein DP. Management of molar pregnancy and gestational trophoblastic tumors. In: Knapp RC, Berkowitz RS, eds. *Gynecologic oncology.* New York, McGraw-Hill, 1993:328.

79. Bagshawe KD. Trophoblastic neoplasia. In: Holland JF, Frei E III, Bast R Jr, et al., eds. *Cancer medicine.* 3rd ed. Baltimore: Williams & Wilkins, 1993:1691.

80. Fasoli M, Ratti E, Franceschi S, et al. Management of gestational trophoblastic disease: results of a cooperative study. *Obstet Gynecol* 1982;60:205.

81. Franke HR, Risse EKJ, Kenemans P, et al. Epidemiologic features of hydatidiform mole in the Netherlands. *Obstet Gynecol* 1983;62:613.

82. Lurain JR, Brewer JI, Torok EE, Halpern B. Natural history of hydatidiform mole after primary evacuation. *Am J Obstet Gynecol* 1983; 145:591.

83. Morrow CP, Kletzky OA, DiSaia PJ, et al. Clinical and laboratory correlates of molar pregnancy and trophoblastic disease. *Am J Obstet Gynecol* 1977;128:424.

84. Kohorn EI. Evaluation of the criteria used to make the diagnosis of non-metastatic gestational trophoblastic neoplasia. *Gynecol Oncol* 1993;48:139.

85. Feltmate CM, Batorfi J, Fulop V, et al. Human chorionic gonadotropin follow-up in patients with molar pregnancy: a time for reevaluation. *Obstet Gynecol* 2003;101:732.

86. Massad LS, Abu-Rustum NR, Lee SS, Renta V. Poor compliance with postmolar surveillance and treatment protocols by indigent women. *Obstet Gynecol* 2000;96:940.

87. Morrow CP. Postmolar trophoblastic disease: diagnosis, management and prognosis. *Clin Obstet Gynecol* 1984;27:211.

88. Tow WSH. The influence of the primary treatment of hydatidiform mole on its subsequent course. *J Obstet Gynaecol Br Commonw* 1966; 73:545.

89. Xia Z, Song H, Tang M. Risk of malignancy and prognosis using a provisional scoring system in hydatidiform mole. *Chin Med J* 1980; 93:605.

90. Tsukamoto N, Iwasaka T, Kashimura Y, et al. Gestational trophoblastic disease in women aged 50 or more. *Gynecol Oncol* 1985;20:53.

91. Tsuji K, Yagi S, Nakano RI. Increased risk of malignant transformation of hydatidiform moles in older gravidas: a cytogenetic study. *Obstet Gynecol* 1981;58:351.

92. Garner EIO, Lipson E, Bernstein MR, et al. Subsequent pregnancy experience in patients with molar pregnancy and gestational trophoblastic tumor. *J Reprod Med* 2002;47:380–386

93. Parazzini F, Mangili G, Belloni C, et al. The problem of identification of prognostic factors for persistent trophoblastic disease. *Gynecol Oncol* 1988;30:57.

94. Ayhan A, Tuncer ZS, Halilzade H, Kucukali T. Predictors of persistent disease in women with complete hydatidiform mole. *J Reprod Med* 1996;41:591.

95. Khazeli MB, Hedayat MM, Hatch KD, et al. Radioimmunoassay of free-beta subunit of human chorionic gonadotropin as a prognostic test for persistent trophoblastic disease in molar pregnancy. *Am J Obstet Gynecol* 1986;155:320.

96. Murad TM, Longley JV, Lurain JR, Brewer JI. Hydatidiform mole: clinicopathologic associations with the development of postevacuation trophoblastic disease. *Int J Gynecol Obstet* 1990;32:359.

97. Mutter G, Pomponio RJ, Berkowitz RS, Genest DR. Sex chromosome composition of complete hydatidiform moles: relationship to metastasis. *Am J Obstet Gynecol* 1993;168:1547.

98. Wake N, Fujino T, Hoshi S, et al. The propensity to malignancy of dispermic heterozygous moles. *Placenta* 1987;8:319.

99. Rice LW, Berkowitz RS, Lage JM, et al. Persistent gestational trophoblastic tumor after partial hydatidiform mole. *Gynecol Oncol* 1990; 36:358.

100. Lage JM, Berkowitz RS, Rice LW, et al. Flow cytometric analysis of DNA content in partial hydatidiform moles with persistent gestational trophoblastic tumors. *Obstet Gynecol* 1991;77:111.

101. Vejerslev LO. Clinical management and diagnostic possibilities in hydatidiform mole with coexistent fetus. *Obstet Gynecol Surv* 1991; 46:577.

102. Steller M, Genest DR, Bernstein MR, et al. Clinical features of multiple conception with partial or complete molar pregnancy and coexisting fetuses. *J Reprod Med* 1994;39:147.

103. Fishman DA, Padilla LA, Keh P, et al. Management of twin pregnancies consisting of a complete hydatidiform mole and normal fetus. *Obstet Gynecol* 1998;91:546.

104. Miller D, Jackson R, Ehlen T, McMurtrie E. Complete hydatidiform mole coexistent with a twin live fetus: clinical course of four cases with complete cytogenetic analysis. *Gynecol Oncol* 1993;50:119.

105. Steller M, Genest DR, Bernstein MR, et al. Natural history of twin pregnancy with complete hydatidiform mole and coexisting fetus. *Obstet Gynecol* 1994;83:35.

106. Berkowitz RS, Goldstein DP. Chorionic tumors. *N Engl J Med* 1996; 335:1740.

107. Hancock BW, Tidy JA. Current management of molar pregnancy. *J Reprod Med* 2002:47:347–354.

108. Goldstein DP, Berkowitz RS. Prophylactic chemotherapy of complete molar pregnancy. *Semin Oncol* 1995;22:157.

109. Kashimura Y, Kashimra M, Sugimori H, et al. Prophylactic chemotherapy for hydatidiform mole: five to 15 years follow-up. *Cancer* 1986;58:624.

110. Kim DS, Moon H, Kim KT, et al. Effects of prophylactic chemotherapy for persistent trophoblastic disease in patients with complete hydatidiform mole. *Obstet Gynecol* 1986;67:690.

111. Limpongsanurak S. Prophylactic actinomycin D for high-risk complete hydatidiform mole. *J Reprod Med* 2001;46:110.

112. Stone M, Dent J, Kardana A, Bagshawe KD. Relationship of oral contraception to development of trophoblastic tumour after evacuation of a hydatidiform mole. *Br J Obstet Gynaecol* 1976;83:913.

113. Berkowitz RS, Goldstein DP, Marean AR, Bernstein MR. Oral contraceptives and postmolar trophoblastic disease. *Obstet Gynecol* 1981; 58:474.

114. Curry SL, Schlaerth JB, Kohorn EI, et al. Hormonal contraception and trophoblastic sequelae after hydatidiform mole (a Gynecologic Oncology Group study). *Am J Obstet Gynecol* 1989;160:805.

115. Deicas RE, Miller DS, Rademaker AW, Lurain JR. The role of contraception in the development of postmolar gestational trophoblastic tumor. *Obstet Gynecol* 1991;78:221.

116. Ho Yuen B, Burch P. Relationship of oral contraceptives and the intrauterine contraceptive devices to the regression of concentrations of the beta subunit of human chorionic gonadotropin and invasive complications after molar pregnancy. *Am J Obstet Gynecol* 1983;145: 214.

117. Paradinas FJ, Fisher RA. Pathology and molecular genetics and trophoblastic disease. *Current Obstet Gynecol* 1995;5:6.

118. Feltmate CM, Genest DR, Wise L, et al. Placental site trophoblastic

tumor. a 17-year experience at the New England Trophoblastic Disease Center. *Gynecol Oncol* 2001;82:415.

119. Lathrop JC, Lauchlan S, Nayak R, Ambler M. Clinical characteristics of placental site trophoblastic tumor (PSTT). *Gynecol Oncol* 1988; 31:32.

120. Bagshawe KD, Garnett ES. Radiologic changes in the lungs of patients with trophoblastic tumours. *Br J Radiol* 1963;36:673.

121. Libshitz HI, Baber CE, Hammond CB. The pulmonary metastases of choriocarcinoma. *Obstet Gynecol* 1977;49:412.

122. Sung HC, Wu PC, Hu MH, Su HT. Roentgenologic manifestations of pulmonary metastases in choriocarcinoma and invasive mole. *Am J Obstet Gynecol* 1982;142:89.

123. Bakri YN, Berkowitz RS, Khan J, et al. Pulmonary metastases of gestational trophoblastic tumor: risk factors for early respiratory failure. *J Reprod Med* 1994;39:175.

124. Bagshawe KD, Noble MIM. Cardio-respiratory aspects of trophoblastic tumors. *Q J Med* 1966;137:39.

125. Kelly MP, Rustin GJS, Ivory C, Bagshawe KD. Respiratory failure due to choriocarcinoma: a study of 103 dyspneic patients. *Gynecol Oncol* 1990;38:149.

126. Vaccarello L, Apte SM, Diaz PT, et al. Respiratory failure from metastatic choriocarcinoma: a survivor of mechanical ventilation. *Gynecol Oncol* 1997;67:111.

127. Jones WB, Wagner-Reiss KM, Lewis JL Jr. Intracerebral choriocarcinoma. *Gynecol Oncol* 1990;38:234.

128. Sung H, Wu B. Brain metastasis in choriocarcinoma and malignant mole. *Chin Med J* 1979;92:164.

129. Bakri YN, Berkowitz RS, Goldstein DP, et al. Brain metastases of gestational trophoblastic tumor. *J Reprod Med* 1994;39:179.

130. Athanassiou A, Begent RHJ, Newlands ES, et al. Central nervous system metastases of choriocarcinoma: 23 years' experience at Charing Cross Hospital. *Cancer* 1983; 52:1728.

131. Liu TL, Deppe G, Chang QT, Tan TT. Cerebral metastatic choriocarcinoma in the People's Republic of China. *Gynecol Oncol* 1983;15:166.

132. Bakri YN, Subhi J, Amer M, et al. Liver metastases of gestational trophoblastic tumor. *Gynecol Oncol* 1993;48:110.

133. Kohorn EI. Negotiating a staging and risk factor scoring system for gestational trophoblastic neoplasia: a progress report. *J Reprod Med* 2002; 47:445.

134. Ross GT, Goldstein DP, Hertz R, et al. Sequential use of methotrexate and actinomycin D in the treatment of metastatic choriocarcinoma and related trophoblastic diseases in women. *Am J Obstet Gynecol* 1965;93:223.

135. Hammond CB, Borchert LG, Tyrey L, et al. Treatment of metastatic trophoblastic disease: good and poor prognosis. *Am J Obstet Gynecol* 1973;115:451.

136. Azab MB, Prejovic M-H, Theodore C, et al. Prognostic factors in gestational trophoblastic tumors. *Cancer* 1988;62:585.

137. Dijkema HE, Aalders JG, DeBruiju HWA, Laurini RN. Risk factors in gestational trophoblastic disease and consequences for primary treatment. *Eur J Obstet Gynecol Reprod Biol* 1986;22:145.

138. DuBeshter B. High-risk factors in metastatic gestational trophoblastic neoplasia. *J Reprod Med* 1991;36:9.

139. Dubuc-Lissoir L, Sweizig S, Schlaerth JB, Morrow CP. Metastatic gestational trophoblastic disease: a comparison of prognostic classification. *Gynecol Oncol* 1992;45:40.

140. Lurain JR, Casanova LA, Miller DS, Rademaker AW. Prognostic factors in gestational trophoblastic tumors: a proposed new scoring system based on multivariate analysis. *Am J Obstet Gynecol* 1991; 164:611.

141. Mortakis AE, Braga CA. Poor prognosis metastatic gestational trophoblastic disease: the prognostic significance of the scoring system in predicting chemotherapy failures. *Obstet Gynecol* 1990;76:272.

142. Ngan HYS, Lopes ADB, Lauder IJ, et al. An evaluation of the prognostic factors in metastatic gestational trophoblastic disease. *Int J Gynecol Cancer* 1994;4:36.

143. Soper JT, Clarke-Pearson DL, Hammond CB. Metastatic gestational trophoblastic disease: prognostic factors in previously untreated patients. *Obstet Gynecol* 1988;71:338.

144. Berkowitz RS, Goldstein DP, Bernstein MR. Choriocarcinoma following term gestation. *Gynecol Oncol* 1984;17:52.

145. Miller JM, Surwit EA, Hammond CB. Choriocarcinoma following term pregnancy. *Obstet Gynecol* 1979;53:207.

146. Olive DL, Lurain JR, Brewer JI. Choriocarcinoma associated with term gestation. *Am J Obstet Gynecol* 1984;148:711.

147. Rodabaugh KJ, Bernstein MR, Goldstein DP, Berkowitz RS. Natural history of postterm choriocarcinoma. *J Reprod Med* 1998;43:76.

148. Bagshawe KD, Harland S. Immunodiagnosis and monitoring of gonadotropin-producing metastases in the central nervous system. *Cancer* 1976;38:112.

149. Berkowitz RS, Osathanondh R, Goldstein DP, et al. Cerebrospinal fluid human chorionic gonadotropin levels in normal pregnancy and choriocarcinoma. *Surg Gynecol Obstet* 1981;153:687.

150. Bakri YN, Al-Hawashim N, Berkowitz RS. Cerebrospinal fluid/serum beta-subunit human chorionic gonadotropin ratio in patients with brain metastases of gestational trophoblastic tumor. *J Reprod Med* 2000; 45:94.

151. Berkowitz RS, Birnholz J, Goldstein DP, Bernstein MR. Pelvic ultrasonography and the management of gestational trophoblastic disease. *Gynecol Oncol* 1983;15:403.

152. Kohorn EI, McCarthy SM, Taylor KJW. Nonmetastatic gestational trophoblastic neoplasia: role of ultrasonography and magnetic resonance imaging. *J Reprod Med* 1998;43:14.

153. Dobkin GR, Berkowitz RS, Goldstein DP, et al. Duplex ultrasonography for persistent gestational trophoblastic tumor. *J Reprod Med* 1991; 36:14.

154. Hsieh FJ, Wu CC, Chen CA, et al. Correlation of uterine hemodynamics with chemotherapy response in gesta tional trophoblastic tumors. *Obstet Gynecol* 1994;83:1021.

155. Long MG, Boultbee JE, Langley R, et al. Preliminary Doppler studies on the uterine artery and myometrium in trophoblastic tumors requiring chemotherapy. *Br J Obstet Gynaecol* 1990;97:686.

156. Mangili G, Spagnolo D, Valsecchi L, Maggi R. Transvaginal ultrasound in persistent trophoblastic tumor. *Am J Obstet Gynecol* 1993; 169:1218.

157. Mutch DG, Soper JT, Baker ME, et al. Role of computed axial tomography of the chest in staging patients with nonmetastatic gestational trophoblastic disease. *Obstet Gynecol* 1986;68:348.

158. Papadopoulos AJ, Foskett M, Seckl MJ, et al. Twenty-five years clinical experience with placental site trophoblastic tumors. *J Reprod* 2002; 47:460.

159. Berkowitz RS, Goldstein DP. Gestational trophoblastic disease. *Cancer* 1995;76:2079.

160. Feldman S, Goldstein DP, Berkowitz RS. Low-risk metastatic gestational trophoblastic tumors. *Semin Oncol* 1995;22:166.

161. Ayhan A, Yapar EG, Deren O, Kisnisci H. Remission rates and significance of prognostic factors in gestational trophoblastic tumors. *J Reprod Med* 1992;37:461.

162. DuBeshter B, Berkowitz RS, Goldstein DP, et al. Metastatic gestational trophoblastic disease: experience at the New England Trophoblastic Disease Center, 1965–1985. *Obstet Gynecol* 1987;9:390.

163. Soper JT, Clarke-Pearson DL, Berchuck A, et al. Five day methotrexate for women with metastatic gestational trophoblastic disease. *Gynecol Oncol* 1994;54:76.

164. Yingna S, Yang X, Xiuyu Y, Hongzhao S. Clinical characteristics and treatment of gestational trophoblastic tumor with vaginal metastasis. *Gynecol Oncol* 2002;84:416.

165. Soper JT. Surgical therapy for gestational trophoblastic disease. *J Reprod Med* 1994;39:168.

166. Begent RH, Bagshawe KD, Green AJ. The clinical value of imaging with antibody to human chorionic gonadotropin in the detection of residual choriocarcinoma. *Br J Cancer* 1987;55:657.

168. Tomoda Y, Arii Y, Kaseki S, et al. Surgical indications for resection in pulmonary metastasis of choriocarcinoma. *Cancer* 1980;46:2723.

169. Jones WB, Romain K, Erlandson RA, et al. Thoracotomy in the management of gestational choriocarcinoma: a clinicopathologic study. *Cancer* 1993;72:2175.

170. Edwards JL, Makey AR, Bagshawe KD. The role of thoracotomy in the management of pulmonary metastases of gestational choriocarcinoma. *Clin Oncol* 1975;1:329.

171. Shirley RL, Goldstein DP, Collins JJ Jr. The role of thoracotomy in management of patients with chest metastases from gestational trophoblastic disease. *J Thorac Cardiovasc Surg* 1972;63:545.

172. Sink JD, Hammond CB, Young WG. Pulmonary resection in the man-

agement of metastases from choriocarcinoma. *J Thorac Cardiovasc Surg* 1981;81:830.

173. Wang Y, Song H, Xia Z. Drug resistant pulmonary choriocarcinoma metastasis treated by lobectomy. *Chin Med J* 1980; 93:758.

174. Lehman E, Gershenson DM, Burke TW, et al. Salvage surgery for chemorefractory gestational trophoblastic disease. *J Clin Oncol* 1994; 12:2737.

175. Hammond CB, Weed JC, Currie JL. The role of operation in the current therapy of gestational trophoblastic disease. *Am J Obstet Gynecol* 1980;136:844.

176. Evans AC Jr, Soper JT, Clarke-Pearson DL, et al. Gestational trophoblastic disease metastatic to the central nervous system. *Gynecol Oncol* 1995;59:226.

177. Grumbine FC, Rosenshein NB, Brereton HD, Kaufman SL. Management of liver metastases from gestational trophoblastic neoplasia. *Am J Obstet Gynecol* 1980;137:959.

178. Wong LC, Choo YC, Ma HK. Hepatic metastases in gestational trophoblastic disease. *Obstet Gynecol* 1986;67:107.

179. Brace KC. The role of irradiation in the treatment of metastatic trophoblastic disease. *Radiology* 1968;91:540.

180. Yordan EL Jr, Schlaerth J, Gaddis O, Morrow CP. Radiation therapy in the management of gestational choriocarcinoma metastatic to the central nervous system. *Obstet Gynecol* 1987;69:627.

181. Newlands ES, Holden L, Seckl MJ, et al. Management of brain metastases in patients with high-risk gestational trophoblastic tumor. *J Reprod Med* 2002;47:465.

182. Cole LA. hCG, its free subunits and its metabolites—roles in pregnancy and trophoblastic disease. *J Reprod Med* 1998;43:3.

183. Cole LA. New perspectives in measuring human chorionic gonadotropin levels for measuring and monitoring trophoblastic disease. *J Reprod Med* 1994;39:193.

184. Cole LA, Butler S. Detection of hCG in trophoblastic disease—the USA hCG Reference Service Experience. *J Reprod Med* 2002; 47: 433–444.

185. Mutch DG, Soper JT, Babcock CJ, et al. Recurrent gestational trophoblastic disease. Experience of the Southeastern Regional Trophoblastic Disease Center. *Cancer* 1990;66:978.

186. Goldstein DP, Zanten-Przybysz I, Bernstein MR, Berkowitz RS. Revised FIGO staging system for gestational trophoblastic tumors; recommendations regarding therapy. *J Reprod Med* 1998;43:37.

187. Li MC, Hertz R, Spencer DB. Effect of methotrexate therapy on choriocarcinoma and chorioadenoma. *Proc Soc Exp Biol Med* 1956; 93: 361.

188. Hertz R, Lewis JL Jr, Lipsett MB. Five year's experience with chemotherapy of metastatic choriocarcinoma and related trophoblastic tumors in women. *Am J Obstet Gynecol* 1961;82:631.

189. Hertz R, Ross GT, Lipsett MB. Primary chemotherapy of nonmetastatic trophoblastic disease in women. *Am J Obstet Gynecol* 1963; 86:808.

190. Ross GT, Stolbach LL, Hertz R. Actinomycin D in the treatment of methotrexate-resistant trophoblastic disease in women. *Cancer Res* 1962;22:1015.

191. Homesley HD. Single-agent therapy for nonmetastatic and low-risk gestational trophoblastic disease. *J Reprod Med* 1998;43:69.

192. Bagshawe KD, Dent J, Newlands ES, et al. The role of low-dose methotrexate and folinic acid in gestational trophoblastic tumours (GTT). *Br J Obstet Gynaecol* 1989;96:795.

193. DuBeshter B, Berkowitz RS, Goldstein DP, Bernstein MR. Management of low-risk metastatic gestational trophoblastic tumor. *J Reprod Med* 1991;36:36.

194. Homesley HD, Blessing JA, Schlaerth J, et al. Rapid escalation of weekly intramuscular methotrexate for nonmetastatic gestational trophoblastic disease: a Gynecologic Oncology Group study. *Gynecol Oncol* 1990;39:305.

195. Kohorn EI. Single-agent chemotherapy for nonmetastatic gestational trophoblastic neoplasia. *J Reprod Med* 1991;36:49.

196. Osathanondh R, Goldstein DP, Pastorfide GB. Actinomycin D as the primary agent for gestational trophoblastic disease. *Cancer* 1975;36: 863.

196. Rustin GJS, Newlands ES, Begent R, et al. Weekly alternating etoposide, methotrexate, actinomycin-D/vincristine and cyclophosphamide chemotherapy for treatment of CNS metastases of choriocarcinoma. *J Clin Oncol* 1989;7:900.

197. Petrilli ES, Twiggs LB, Blessing JA, et al. Single-dose actinomycin-D treatment for nonmetastatic gestational trophoblastic disease: a prospective phase II trial of the Gynecologic Oncology Group. *Cancer* 1987;60:2173.

198. Roberts JP, Lurain JR. Treatment of low risk metastatic gestational trophoblastic tumors with single agent chemotherapy. *Am J Obstet Gynecol* 1996;174:1917.

199. Rose PG, Piver MS. Alternating methotrexate and dactinomycin in nonmetastatic gestational trophoblastic disease. *J Surg Oncol* 1989; 41:148.

200. Wong LC, Choo YC, Ma HK. Methotrexate with citrovorum factor rescue in gestational trophoblastic disease. *Am J Obstet Gynecol 1985; 152:59.*201. Bagshawe KD, Wilde CE. Infusion therapy for pelvic trophoblastic tumors. *J Obstet Gynaecol Br Commonw* 1964;71:565.

202. Berkowitz RS, Goldstein DP. Methotrexate with citrovorum factor rescue and non-metastatic gestational trophoblastic neoplasms. *Obstet Gynecol* 1979;54:725.

203. Berkowitz RS, Goldstein DP, Bernstein MR. Methotrexate with citrovorum factor rescue as a primary therapy for gestational trophoblastic disease. *Cancer* 1982;50:2024.

204. Berkowitz RS, Goldstein DP, Bernstein MR. Ten years experience with methotrexate and folinic acid as primary therapy for gestational trophoblastic disease. *Gynecol Oncol* 1986;23:111.

205. Berkowitz RS, Goldstein DP, Jones MA, et al. Methotrexate with citrovorum factor rescue: reduced chemotherapy toxicity in the management of gestational trophoblastic neoplasms. *Cancer* 1980;45:423.

206. Garrett AP, Garner EIO, Goldstein DP, Berkowitz RS. Methotrexate infusion and folinic acid as primary therapy for nonmetastatic and low-risk metastatic gestational trophoblastic tumors—15 years of experience. *J Reprod Med* 2002;47:355–362.

207. Sung HC, Wu PC, Yang HY. Reevaluation of 5-fluorouracil as a single therapeutic agent for gestational trophoblastic neoplasms. *Am J Obstet Gynecol* 1984;150:69.

208. Berkowitz RS, Goldstein DP, Bernstein MR. Modified triple chemotherapy in the management of high-risk metastatic gestational trophoblastic tumors. *Gynecol Oncol* 1984;19:173.

209. Curry SL, Blessing JA, DiSaia PJ, et al. A prospective randomized comparison of methotrexate, dactinomycin and chlorambucil versus methotrexate, dactinomycin, cyclophosphamide, doxorubicin, melphalan, hydroxyurea, and vincristine in poor prognosis metastatic gestational trophoblastic disease: a Gynecologic Oncology Group study. *Obstet Gynecol* 1989;73:357.

210. Gordon AN, Gershenson DM, Copeland LJ, et al. High-risk metastatic gestational trophoblastic disease: further stratification into two clinical entities. *Gynecol Oncol* 1989;34:54.

211. Wong LC, Choo YC, Ma HK. Primary oral etoposide therapy in gestational trophoblastic disease, an update. *Cancer* 1986;58:14.

212. Bagshawe KD. Treatment of high-risk choriocarcinoma. *J Reprod Med* 1984;29:813.

213. Bolis G, Bonazzi C, Landoni F, et al. EMA/CO regimen in high-risk gestational trophoblastic tumor (GTT). *Gynecol Oncol* 1988;31:439.

214. Schink JC, Singh DK, Rademaker AW, et al. Etoposide, methotrexate, actinomycin D, cyclophosphamide and vincristine for the treatment of metastatic, high-risk gestational trophoblastic disease. *Obstet Gynecol* 1992;80:817.

215. Soper JT, Evans AC, Clarke-Pearson DL, et al. Alternating weekly chemotherapy with etoposide-methotrexate-dactinomycin/cyclophosphamide-vincristine for high-risk gestational trophoblastic disease. *Obstet Gynecol* 1994;83:113.

216. Bower M, Newlands ES, Holden L, et al. EMA/CO for high-risk gestational trophoblastic tumors: results from a cohort of 272 patients. *J Clin Oncol* 1997;15:2636.

217. Kim SJ, Bae SN, Kim JH, Kim CJ, Jung JK. Risk factors for the prediction of treatment failure in gestational trophoblastic tumors treated with EMA/CO regimen. *Gynecol Oncol* 1998;71:247.

218. Newlands ES, Bower M, Holden L, et al. Management of resistant gestational trophoblastic tumors. *J Reprod Med* 1998;43:111.

219. Rustin GJS, Newlands ES, Lutz JM, et al. Combination but not single-agent methotrexate chemotherapy for gestational trophoblastic tumors increases the incidence of second tumors. *J Clin Oncol* 1996;14:2769.

220. Soto-Wright V, Goldstein DP, Bernstein MR, Berkowitz RS. The management of gestational trophoblastic tumors with etoposide, methotrexate and actinomycin D. *Gynecol Oncol* 1997;64:156.

221. Gordon AN, Kavanaugh JJ, Gershenson DM, et al. Cisplatin, vinblastine, and bleomycin combination therapy in resistant gestational trophoblastic disease. *Cancer* 1986;58:1407.

222. DuBeshter B, Berkowitz RS, Goldstein DP, Bernstein MR. Vinblastine, cisplatin and bleomycin as salvage therapy for refractory high-risk metastatic gestational trophoblastic disease. *J Reprod Med* 1989; 34:189.

223. Azab M, Droz JP, Theodore C, et al. Cisplatin, vinblastine and bleomycin combination in the treatment of resistant high-risk gestational trophoblastic tumors. *Cancer* 1989;64:1829.

224. Giacalone PL, Benos P, Donnadio D, Laffargue F. High-dose chemotherapy with autologous bone marrow transplantation for refractory metastatic gestational trophoblastic disease. *Gynecol Oncol* 1995;58:383.

225. VanBesien K, Verschraegen C, Mehra R, et al. Complete remission of refractory gestational trophoblastic disease with brain metastases treated with multicycle ifosfamide, carboplatin, and etoposide (ICE) and stem all rescue. *Gynecol Oncol* 1997;65:366.

226. Jones WB, Schneider J, Shapiro F, Lewis JL Jr. Treatment of resistant gestational choriocarcinoma with Taxol: a report of two cases. *Gynecol Oncol* 1996;61:126.

227. Sutton GP, Soper JT, Blessing JA, et al. Ifosfamide alone and in combination in the treatment of refractory malignant gestational trophoblastic disease. *Am J Obstet Gynecol* 1992;167:489.

228. Lurain JR, Sand PK, Carson SA, Brewer JI. Pregnancy outcome subsequent to consecutive hydatidiform moles. *Am J Obstet Gynecol* 1982;142:1060.

229. Rice LW, Lage JM, Berkowitz RS, et al. Repetitive complete and partial hydatidiform mole. *Obstet Gynecol* 1989;74:217.

230. Bagshawe KD, Dent J, Webb J. Hydatidiform mole in England and Wales 1973–1983. *Lancet* 1986;2:673.

231. Tuncer ZS, Bernstein MR, Wang J, et al. Repetitive hydatidiform mole with different male partners. *Gynecol Oncol* 1999;75:224.

232. Ayhan A, Ergeneli MH, Yuce K, et al. Pregnancy after chemotherapy for gestational trophoblastic disease. *J Reprod Med* 1990;35:522.

233. Kim JH, Park DC, Bae SN, et al. Subsequent reproductive experience after treatment for gestational trophoblastic disease. *Gynecol Oncol* 1998;71:108–112.

234. Kjer JJ, Iversen T. Malignant trophoblastic tumors in Norway: fertility rate after chemotherapy. *Br J Obstet Gynecol* 1990; 97:623.

235. Kobayashi O, Matsui H, Takamizawa H. Analysis of pregnancy outcome after chemotherapy of trophoblastic disease. *Nippon Sanka Fujinka Gakkai Zasshi* 1986;38:181.

236. Ngan HYS, Wong LC, Ma HK. Reproductive performance of patients with gestational trophoblastic disease in Hong Kong. *Acta Obstet Gynecol Scand* 1988;67:11.

237. Song HZ, Wu PC, Wang Y, et al. Pregnancy outcome after successful chemotherapy for choriocarcinoma and invasive mole: long-term follow-up. *Am J Obstet Gynecol* 1988;158:538.

238. VanThiel DH, Ross GT, Lipsett MB. Pregnancies after chemotherapy of trophoblastic neoplasms. *Science* 1970;169:1326.

239. Woolas RP, Bower M, Newlands ES, et al. Influence of chemotherapy for gestational trophoblastic disease on subsequent pregnancy outcome. *Br J Obstet Gynaecol* 1998;105:1032.

240. Wenzel LB, Berkowitz RS, Robinson S, et al. The psychological, social, and sexual consequences of gestational trophoblastic disease. *Gynecol Oncol* 1992;46:74.

241. Wenzel LB, Berkowitz RS, Robinson S, et al. Psychological, social, and sexual effects of gestational trophoblastic disease on patients and partners. *J Reprod Med* 1994;39:163.

242. Wenzel L, Berkowitz RS, Newlands E, et al. Quality of life after gestational trophoblastic disease. *J Reprod Med* 2002; 47:387.

243. Goto S, Yamada A, Ishizuka T, Tomoda Y. Development of postmolar trophoblastic disease after partial molar pregnancy. *Gynecol Oncol* 1993;48:165.

244. Ohama K, Katsunori U, Okamoto E, et al. Cytogenetic and clinicopathologic studies of partial moles. *Obstet Gynecol* 1986;68:259.

245. Stone M, Bagshawe KD. Hydatidiform mole: two entities. *Lancet* 1976;1:535.

246. Szulman AE, Surti U. The clinicopathologic profile of the partial hydatidiform mole. *Obstet Gynecol* 1982;59:597.

247. Vassilakos P, Riotton G, Kajii T. Hydatidiform mole: two entities. *Am J Obstet Gynecol* 1977;127:167.

248. Wong LC, Ma HK. The syndrome of partial mole. *Arch Gynecol* 1984;234:161.

267. Zhuang H, Yamamoto AJ, Ghesani N, Alavi A. Detection of choriocarcinoma in the lung by FDG positron emission tomography. *Clin Nucl Med* 2001; 26:723.

CHAPTER 30

Breast Cancer

Beryl McCormick, Clifford Hudis, Mary Gemignani, D. David Dershaw,
Lee K. Tan, Carlos A. Perez, and Marie E. Taylor

HISTORY

Cancer of the breast existed in ancient times, and references to this disease can be found dating as far back as 3000 BC in an Egyptian papyrus (1). William Halsted, in the late nineteenth century, developed a radical operation that approached breast cancer as a disease that spread in an orderly fashion from the primary mass in the breast to the axillary lymph nodes, and beyond, to systemic or metastatic disease. In a report of his first 50 patients, published in 1884, he observed only three local failures (2). With additional patients and follow-up time, however, his patients' survival at 3 years from surgery was 42% (3). Yet, for the next 100 years, this operation or technical variations of it formed the cornerstone of the treatment of breast cancer. Additional local treatment, including postmastectomy chest-wall and nodal irradiation, had no significant impact on patient survival from breast cancer (4).

Studies of breast cancer in the last half of the twentieth century made observations inconsistent with Halsted's hypothesis, such as the 10% to 36% risk of recurrence seen after 20 years of follow-up among patients with node-negative disease (5–8). A similar challenge to the hypothesis arises from the observation that some patients, particularly those with multiple involved lymph nodes or with primary

B. McCormick: Department of Radiation Oncology, Memorial Sloan–Kettering Cancer Center, New York, New York 10021

C. Hudis: Department of Medicine, Memorial Sloan–Kettering Cancer Center, New York, New York 10021

D. D. Dershaw: Department of Radiology, Memorial Sloan–Kettering Cancer Center, New York, New York 10021

L. K. Tan: Department of Pathology, Memorial Sloan–Kettering Cancer Center, New York, New York 10021

C. A. Perez and M. E. Taylor: Department of Radiation Oncology, Mallinckrodt Institute of Radiology, Washington University School of Medicine, St. Louis, Missouri 63108

cancers larger than 5 cm, develop recurrence locally in the breast or chest wall despite macroscopic and microscopic clear margins of resections (9). Finally, there is difficulty explaining why some patients with no discernible primary disease in the breast, even at mastectomy, can present with metastatic breast cancer. Clearly, a more complex model than the one proposed by Halsted is required.

While the seeming randomness of metastatic spread has never been adequately explained, its cause, the successful establishment of viable micrometastases, has motivated the development of systemic adjuvant therapy. The simplest explanation for the development of metastases is that they are a consequence of three converging events: development of cells with metastatic growth potential, migration of these cells to distant sites, and the presence of a "fertile field" in which local conditions, including growth factors, are conducive to cancer cell viability. It remains impossible to identify patients in whom microscopic metastatic spread has occurred and those in whom it has not. The Fisherian hypothesis (or alternative hypothesis) addresses these issues by arguing that metastatic disease occurs so often and early in the course of breast cancer that the extent of local-regional treatment will have no impact on overall survival. From this follows the hypothesis, now clinically proven, that effective systemic therapy is necessary to gain significant improvements over those obtained through surgery alone (10).

In the 1970s, the first reports of true adjuvant systemic therapy trials appeared in the medical literature, starting with single-agent chemotherapy and compared with no chemotherapy, for patients with pathologic involvement of axillary lymph nodes at the time of mastectomy. One such trial, using melphalan, was reported by the National Surgical Adjuvant Breast and Bowel Project group (NSABP) (11). Fisher believed that most breast cancers had metastasized at the time of the patient's diagnosis, although neither available studies, nor the patient's extent-of-disease" workup, could demonstrate these occult metastases. Following this logic, the

NSABP group designed a series of innovative randomized trials to test this "Fisherian" approach to breast cancer (12). The B-06 trial randomized women to traditional mastectomy, or to a breast-conserving, "segmental" mastectomy with breast irradiation, or to breast-conservation surgery alone. All patients had an axillary lymph-node dissection, and those with nodal involvement also received systemic chemotherapy. Differences in local tumor control were observed favoring breast-conservation surgery plus irradiation over surgery alone, although no statistical differences in survival have been observed. Fortunately for women with breast cancer, all subsequent randomized studies comparing mastectomy to breast-conservation surgery plus irradiation demonstrated that survival is equivalent between the two different local procedures (13).

Progress in the use of systemic therapy as an adjuvant to local treatment for breast cancer continues, largely as the result of prospective randomized trials. The Milan Cancer Group published its results comparing multiagent cyclophosphamide, methotrexate, and fluorouracil (CMF) to observation after local surgery for those women with node-positive disease and continues to show a survival advantage in the chemotherapy arm 20 years from diagnosis (14). Newer regimens, now demonstrated to benefit both node-negative and node-positive breast cancer, will be discussed in more detail later in this chapter.

Yet sometimes patients with breast cancer and only local treatment are cured of their disease. Therefore, most recently, a view of early breast cancer that bridges the extremes of the Halsted and Fisher hypotheses has emerged. In this view, some but not all breast cancers are metastatic at diagnosis, but some are metastatic only in the regional area. These are called "oligometastases"(15), and the extent and efficacy of local treatments, coupled with systemic therapy, can make a difference in survival. The recent results reported for postmastectomy, postchemotherapy local-regional radiation treatments support this view, as they demonstrate both improved overall survival and local control for patients randomized to receive irradiation (16,17). Another provocative piece of data is provided by the preliminary results of several trials testing bisphosphonates as adjuvant therapy. In these trials, an expected reduction in bone metastases was associated with an unexpected reduction in other metastases (18, 19). Prevention of the first site of recurrent disease, be it chest wall or axilla or breast in the case of local therapy, or bone in the case of systemic therapy, may reduce the risk of subsequent metastases.

A discussion of the history of the treatment of breast cancer would not be complete without mention of the role of screening and prevention of this disease. Because of screening mammography projects in large populations, the median size of new breast cancers detected has decreased significantly, and the survival rates of women with this disease have improved (20).

Prevention of cancer has been a goal of the oncology community for many years. In 1998, results of the first large prevention trial for breast cancer by the NSABP were published, indicating that the risk of developing this disease (in women identified as having an increased risk and therefore qualifying for the study) could be reduced with the use of oral tamoxifen taken for 5 years (21).

Fisher et al. (22) reported on a risk-reduction study of 13,388 women at increased risk for breast cancer, age 60 years or older, or age 35 to 59 years (with a predicted breast cancer risk of at least 1.66%), or with a history of lobular carcinoma *in situ*. By random assignment, 6,707 women were given a placebo, and 6,681 received tamoxifen (20 mg/day) for 5 years. There was a decreased risk of invasive breast cancer of 49% in the women receiving tamoxifen and a reduction in incidence of noninvasive breast cancer of 50% (Fig. 30.1). This translated to an incidence of either type of breast cancer of approximately 10 cases per 1,000 at 48 months. The cumulative rate of invasive endometrial carcinoma was somewhat higher in the tamoxifen group (Fig. 30.2).

On the other hand, in a trial from the United Kingdom (23) in which 2,471 women 30 to 70 years of age with a family history of breast cancer were randomized to be treated with either tamoxifen (20 mg/day) or a placebo for as long as 8 years, the relative risk of breast cancer was 1.06 in each of the two groups; the trial showed that there was no difference in the incidence of breast cancer with administration of tamoxifen. A third trial was reported by Veronesi et al. (24) in which 5,408 women were randomized in 55 centers, half to be treated with tamoxifen (20 mg/day) for 5 years, the other half with a placebo. To be eligible, the patients needed to have had a hysterectomy. Women who took tamoxifen and hormone replacement therapy had a significantly lower incidence of breast cancer than those taking the

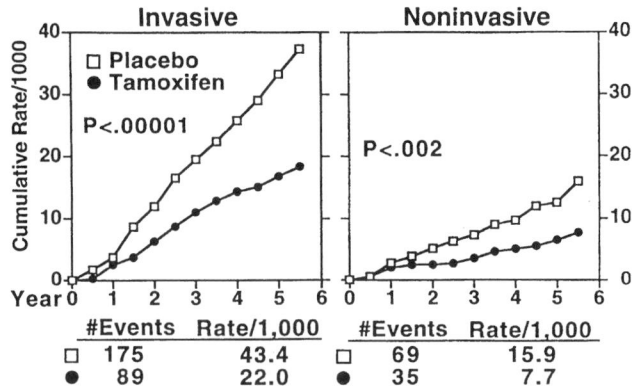

FIG. 30.1. Cumulative rates of invasive and noninvasive breast cancers occurring in participants receiving placebo or tamoxifen. The *p* values are two-sided. (Reprinted with permission of Oxford University Press, courtesy of Fisher B, for the National Surgical Adjuvant Breast and Bowel Project Investigators. *J Natl Cancer Inst* 1998;90:1371–1388.)

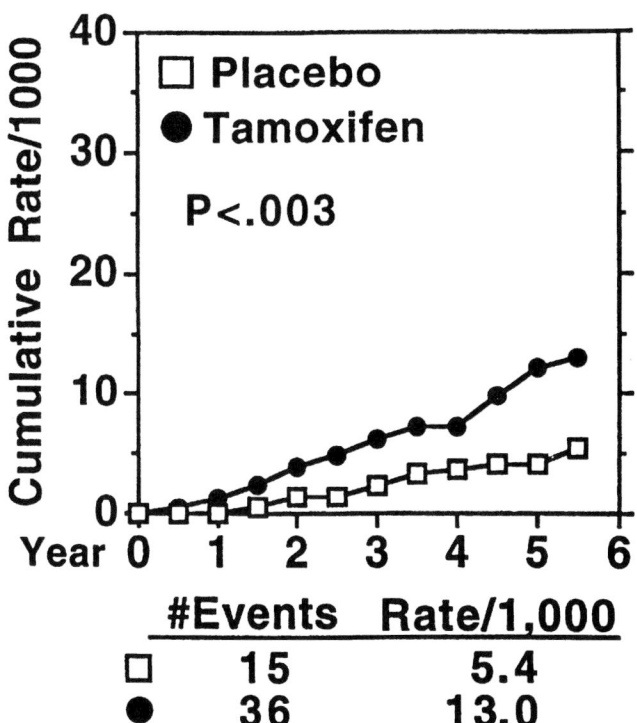

FIG. 30.2. Cumulative rates of invasive endometrial cancer occurring in participants receiving placebo or tamoxifen. The *p* value is two-sided. (Reprinted with permission of Oxford University Press, Courtesy of Fisher B, for the National Surgical Adjuvant Breast and Bowel Project Investigators. *J Natl Cancer Inst* 1998;90:1371–1388.)

placebo and hormonal replacement (one versus eight breast cancers). Women taking tamoxifen had significantly more vascular events and experienced more hypertriglyceridemia than women taking placebo.

The NSABP group is building on the data from their P-1 trial, despite differences with the United Kingdom study. The next trial is the P-2 or STAR (study of tamoxifen and raloxifene) trial, designed to address prevention. As in the P-1 trial, patients will be eligible if they meet the criteria for increased risk of developing breast cancer, as calculated by the Gail Model (25). The trial is designed to compare tamoxifen for 5 years to raloxifene for the same time period. Raloxifene is a selective estrogen-receptor modulator (SERM), originally tested for estrogen effects on bone metabolism, and now observed to decrease the risk of new breast cancers (26) (Fig. 30.3).

ANATOMY

The breast is made up of the mammary gland, fat, blood vessels, nerves, and lymphatics (Fig. 30.4) (27). The surface of the breast has deep attachments of fibrous septa, called *Cooper's ligaments*, which run between the superficial fascia (attached to the skin) and the deep fascia (covering the pectoralis major and other muscles of the chest wall) (28). The mammary gland lies over the pectoralis major muscle and extends from the second to the sixth rib on the vertical plane and from the sternum to the anterior or even midaxillary line on the horizontal plane (28). An additional layer of mammary tissue extends laterally into the axilla and, called the "tail," is sometimes quite prominent. The retromammary bursa lies between the deep layer of the superficial fascia and the deep fascia; it contains loose areolar tissue that allows for mobility over the chest wall. It is crossed by projections of the deep layer of the superficial fascia that join with the deep pectoral fascia to form the posterior suspensory ligaments of the breast. Deep projections of mammary parenchyma may extend between the muscle bundles of the pectoralis major muscle. The mamma consists of glandular tissue arranged in multiple lobes composed of lobules connected in ducts, areolar tissue, and blood vessels. The smallest lobules consist of clusters of rounded alveoli that open into the small branches of the lactiferous ducts; these unite and form larger ducts that eventually converge into single canals in the nip-

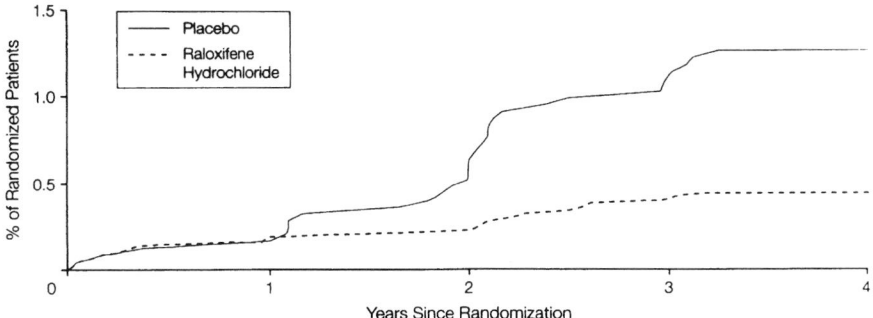

FIG. 30.3. Cumulative incidence of breast cancer among subjects in the placebo group and those in the combined raloxifene group and represented as a percentage of all patients randomized to either group. Statistical significance of the difference between the groups was tested by a log-rank test (p < 0.001). (Courtesy of Cummings SR, Eckert S, Krueger KA, et al. The effect of raloxifene on risk of breast cancer in postmenopausal women: results from the MORE randomized trial. *JAMA* 1999; 281:2192.)

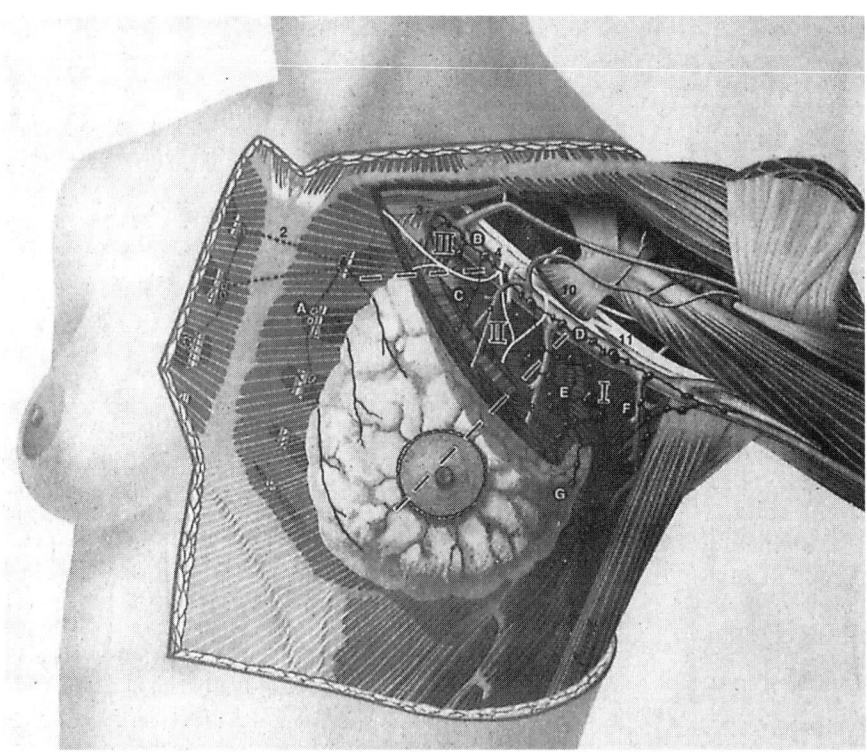

FIG. 30.4. Anatomy of the breast and lymphatic drainage. (Reprinted from Osborne MP. Breast development and anatomy. In: Harris JR, Hellman S, Henderson IC, Kinne DW, eds. *Breast diseases.* Philadelphia: JB Lippincott Co, 1987: 1–14.)

ple, corresponding to each lobe of the gland (15 to 20 galactophori).

A network of lymphatics is formed over the entire surface of the chest, neck, and abdomen and becomes dense under the areola. Mammary gland lymphatics begin in the interlobular or prelobular spaces, follow the ducts, and end in the subareolar network of lymphatics of the skin (28,29). The following lymphatic pathways originate mostly in the base of the breast: (a) the axillary or principal pathway, which passes from the upper and lower halves of the breast to the lateral chain of nodes situated between the second and third intercostal space; (b) the transpectoral pathway, which passes through the pectoralis major muscle to the supraclavicular lymph nodes; and (c) the internal mammary pathway, which passes through the midline, through the pectoralis major and intercostal muscles, usually close to the sternum,

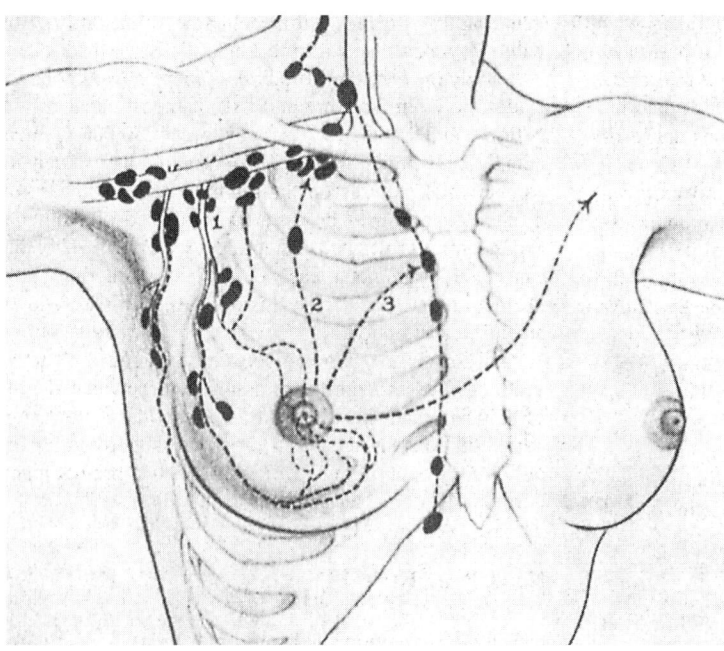

FIG. 30.5. Anatomy of the lymphatic routes of the breast. (Reprinted from del Regato JA, Spjut HJ, Harlan J, Cox J. *Ackerman and del Regato's cancer: diagnosis, treatment, and prognosis,* 6th ed. St. Louis: Mosby, 1985:853.)

to the nodes of the internal mammary chain. The main lymphatic channels of the breast are illustrated in Figure 30–5 (30).

EPIDEMIOLOGY

In the United States in 2003, approximately 211,300 new cases of breast cancer were diagnosed, and 39,800 women died of the disease (31). Breast and lung cancer are the foremost causes of cancer deaths in women. Breast cancer mortality has been stable for the last 50 years, although in recent years there has been a slight overall decline in contrast to pronounced peaks in incidence. Nearly all of the increase (83%) is accounted for by early diagnosis of *in situ* or invasive lesions less than 2 cm with screening mammography. Reduced mortality is a reflection of earlier diagnosis and more effective treatment, including adjuvant systemic therapy.

Although one of every ten women in the United States is projected to develop carcinoma of the breast, fortunately 80% to 92% of all breast masses are benign (32). Approximately 1% of breast cancers occur in men.

The risk factors for breast cancer in women are well documented: age over 50 years, personal or family history of breast cancer (e.g., mother, aunt), nulliparity, or birth of first child after age 30 (33). Madigan and colleagues (34) identified 193 women with breast cancer; the most important risk factors were age at the birth of first child and nulliparity, higher socioeconomic status, and family history. Several models now exist to estimate a woman's risk of breast cancer. The most widely distributed and used is the Gail Model (25).

Breast cancer is more frequent in Jewish women compared with non-Jewish women. Low incidence and mortality rates for female breast cancer are found in most Asian and African countries, intermediate rates in southern European and South American countries, and high rates in North America and northern European countries (35). Among the possible explanations for this variability are environmental factors, including diet.

Japanese women show lower rates of breast cancer than white women, a difference accounted for by an increased incidence of this cancer in postmenopausal white women. Postmenopausal breast cancer is also less common among Japanese who migrated to a Western country. After two or three generations, the incidence of female breast cancer among descendants of Japanese immigrants to Hawaii or to the mainland of the United States approaches that of white residents (35).

Newcomb and associates (36) noted that relative breast cancer risk among premenopausal women was reduced by a history of lactation (relative risk of 0.78) and by a cumulative lactation time exceeding 24 months.

Several large-scale studies have failed to demonstrate a correlation between the prolonged use of oral contraceptives and breast cancer (37–40). White and associates (41), in an analysis of 961 women born in 1944 or later who took oral contraceptives all of their reproductive life, reported no increase in breast cancer incidence. There was, however, a small increased risk, particularly for patients aged 35 or younger who used oral contraceptives for a long time, and for patients who used them in early reproductive life, or used high-progestin oral contraceptives for at least 1 year.

In 1995, Colditz and colleagues (42) noted that the combination of progestin and estrogen therapy in postmenopausal patients increased the risk of breast cancer (relative risk 1.41) compared with postmenopausal women who had never used hormones. Since then, a number of studies (43), including the Women's Health Initiative (WHI) randomized trial have established the link between combination estrogen plus progestin hormone replacement therapy and an increased risk of breast cancer. In the WHI study, this increase was observed in a relatively short period of time into the study (44). However, data on women taking unopposed estrogen replacement therapy only have not demonstrated a similar risk as those users of combination therapy (45).

Exposure to ionizing radiation during or after puberty increases the risk of developing carcinoma of the breast. Land and associates (46) reviewed reports on three populations of patients: one by Tokunaga and colleagues (47) on survivors of the atomic bombings in Hiroshima and Nagasaki; a report by Boice and Monson (48) on women in Massachusetts who had multiple fluoroscopic examinations of the chest for pulmonary tuberculosis; and a study by Shore and coworkers (49) of patients with postpartum mastitis exposed to multiple x-rays, in which nonexposed civilians were used as a control group. They concluded that the risk of irradiation-induced cancer of the breast increased approximately linearly with increasing doses and was heavily dependent on age at exposure. These observations were later confirmed by other investigators. In a study of 31,710 women who had tuberculosis and were examined with repeated fluoroscopic studies, a substantial proportion (26.4%) received doses to the breast of 10 cGy or more (50); the breast cancer risk was greatest among women who had radiation exposure between the ages of 10 and 14 (relative risk of 4.5 per cGy and an additive risk of 6.1 per 104 person-years per cGy), with substantially less excess risk with increasing age at first exposure.

In another study of 1,030 women with scoliosis who had multiple radiographic examinations over a period of 8.7 years, 11 cases of breast cancer were reported, compared with 6 expected (1.82 risk factor) (51); risk also increased with the number of x-ray examinations and estimated radiation doses to the breast (mean 0.13 Gy). Furthermore, in a cohort of 1,201 women who received x-ray treatment in infancy for enlarged thymus gland (estimated mean absorbed dose of radiation to the breast of 6.9 Gy), 22 breast cancers were diagnosed after an average of 36 years of follow-up, compared with 12 in 2,469 nonirradiated sisters (adjusted risk factor of 3.6) (52).

A high risk of solid tumors, especially breast cancer, has been described in women treated with radiation therapy for Hodgkin's disease at a young age. In a review of 1,380 women treated at 15 institutions before the age of 16 years, 17 women developed breast cancer: 7 after radiation therapy alone and 10 after irradiation and chemotherapy. Sixteen breast cancers appeared within or at the margin of the irradiation fields. The cumulative probability of breast cancer at 40 years of age was 35%. Women in this cohort of survivors had a risk of breast cancer 70 times higher than that of the general population (53).

Higher alcohol consumption has been correlated with increased risk of breast cancer (54). A study of 62,573 women from the Netherlands reported a relative risk for breast cancer of 1.3 in women who consumed up to 30 g of alcohol daily and 1.72 in those who consumed greater amounts (55). Longnecker and associates (56) also noted a 1.39 relative risk with about one drink daily, 1.69 with two, and 2.3 with three drinks daily.

High intake of total dietary fat has been implicated as a factor increasing the risk of breast cancer in animal studies (57) and in a meta-analysis of case-control studies (58). The meta-analysis was criticized for ignoring heterogeneities in the studies analyzed (59). Recently a report of 2,956 women diagnosed as having breast cancer was published comparing them with women obtaining 30.1% to 35% of their energy from fat and with women obtaining 20% or less of their energy from fat (60). The multivariate relative risk of breast cancer was 1.15, leading the authors to conclude that there was no evidence that lower fat intake or a specific major type of fat was associated with a decreased risk of breast cancer.

Analysis of 2,201 women between the ages of 30 and 62 years showed no significant association between degree of adiposity and the incidence of breast cancer, but suggested that increased central-to-peripheral body fat distribution may be a more specific marker than premalignant hormonal pattern predisposing to this disease (15).

In a review of 280,000 women, Byrne and associates (61) noted that women with 75% or greater breast density parenchymal patterns on the mammogram, as measured by the proportion of breast area composed of epithelial and stromal tissue, had a greater risk of breast cancer (fivefold). This parameter was independent of other prognostic factors, such as family history, age at the birth of first child, or level of alcohol consumption.

NATURAL HISTORY

The most common site of origin of breast cancer is the upper outer quadrant (38.5%), followed by the central area (29%), the upper inner quadrant (14.2%), the lower outer quadrant (8.8%), and the lower inner quadrant (5%). These rates correlate with the amount of breast tissue in the various quadrants. Cancer is somewhat more common in the left than in the right breast; it is unusual for cancer to appear in both breasts simultaneously (1% to 2%). Metachronous bilateral carcinoma of the breast has been observed in 5% to 8% of patients.

Using estimates of doubling time, it would take an average of approximately 5 years for a breast tumor to reach palpable size, and those lesions with slower doubling time would have an even longer latent period.

As the cancer grows, it travels along the ducts, eventually breaking through the basement membrane of the duct, invading adjacent lobules, ducts, fascial strands, and the mammary fat, spreading through the breast lymphatics and into the peripheral lymphatics. The tumor can grow through the wall of blood vessels, spread into the deep lymphatics of the dermis, and eventually produce edema of the skin (*peau d'orange*), which usually indicates that the superficial as well as the deep lymphatics are involved. Ulceration and infiltration of overlying skin, which may develop late in the course of the disease, are usually preceded by fixation and localized redness of the skin over the tumor (29) and are less frequently seen because of current emphasis on screening and early diagnosis.

A common route taken by breast carcinoma as it metastasizes is first through the axillary lymph nodes; the incidence of lymph-node metastasis increases with larger tumors. About 20% to 40% of newly diagnosed stage T1 and T2 breast cancers have pathologic evidence of axillary nodal metastases (62–64). Table 30.1 summarizes incidence of axillary metastases according to the size of the primary tumor.

Metastases to the internal mammary nodes are more frequent from medial and central lesions; these metastases

TABLE 30.1. *Incidence of metastatic axillary lymph nodes in carcinoma of breast correlated with primary tumor size*

Tumor size (cm)	Washington University[a]	Tinnemans et al (64)	Silverstein et al. (434)	Kambouris (62)
0.0–0.5	3/55 (5)	1/13 (7.7)	3/96 (3)	–
0.6–1.0	25/203 (12)	3/24 (12.5)	27/156 (17)	–
1.1–2.0	59/294 (20)	13/44 (29.5)	115/357 (32)	13/58 (22)
2.1–3.0	38/113 (34)	–	145/330 (44)[b]	15/25 (60)
3.1–4.0	9/31 (29)	–	–	1/7 (14)

Numbers in parentheses are percentages.
[a] Unpublished data.
[b] T2 tumors (2 to 5 cm).

TABLE 30.2. *Internal mammary (IM) node involvement related to location of primary tumor and axillary node involvement*

IM involvement	UIQ	LIQ	Central	UOQ	LOQ
Total	67/248 (27%)	20/61 (33%)	70/216 (32%)	54/382 (14%)	12/93 (13%)
Axilla not involved	20/143 (14%)	2/36 (6%)	5/76 (7%)	7/170 (4%)	2/40 (5%)
Axilla involved	47/105 (45%)	18/25 (72%)	65/140 (46%)	47/212 (22%)	10/53 (19%)

LIQ, lower inner quadrant; LOQ, lower outer quadrant; UIQ, upper inner quadrant; UOQ, upper outer quadrant.
From Handley RS. Carcinoma of the breast. *Ann R Coll Surg* 1975;57:59–66, with permission.

occur more frequently when there is axillary node involvement (Table 30.2) (65). The supraclavicular lymph nodes may be the target of metastatic deposits, usually after the high axillary or internal mammary lymph nodes have become involved with tumor.

Vascular invasion by tumor and hematogenous metastases to distant sites may be observed, even with small tumors. A highly significant correlation was found between tumor size and incidence of distant metastases (66). The distribution of tumor sizes and metastatic spread was log-normal, with a median diameter of 3.5 cm. The proportion of grade 1 tumors was higher in small tumors than in large ones, while the reverse was observed for grade 3 tumors; these data suggest that, during their growth, tumors progress toward higher grades (67).

A study by Hagemeister and colleagues (68) found more tumor involvement than had been clinically suspected in 166 patients who died of breast cancer and had autopsy; most of these patients had received treatment that included chemotherapy. There were 325 unsuspected metastases; areas of tumor involvement included the endocrine organs (40%), liver (30%), lungs (28%), cardiovascular system (21%), and genitourinary system (21%). Major causes of death were pulmonary insufficiency (26%), infection (24%), cardiac disease (15%), and hepatic insufficiency (14%). The most common cause of death was metastatic disease to various organs, accounting for 42% of all deaths; infection was the second most common cause of death.

A classic paper by Bloom and associates (69) outlined the natural history of breast cancer in 356 patients seen between 1805 and 1933 who were not treated by surgery or irradiation, 250 of whom had a pathologic diagnosis of cancer. There were no patients with stage I disease, 2.4% with stage II, 23% with stage III, and 74% with stage IV (Manchester System) (70). Survival in the untreated group was compared with that of a later group of patients treated with radical or modified radical mastectomy, with or without irradiation. They reported an overall 10-year survival of 34% in the treated patients and 3.6% in the untreated group; survival in both groups was dependent on the histologic grade of the tumor.

PATHOLOGY OF BREAST CANCER

The breast is a modified sweat gland that can be divided into two components: the large ducts and the terminal duct–lobular unit (TDLU). The large duct system of subsegmental, segmental, and lactiferous ducts converge and empty into the nipple. The TDLU is connected to the subsegmental ducts, represents the secretory unit of the gland, and is the site of origin of most pathologic entities of this organ, such as fibrocystic changes, ductal hyperplasia, and the majority of carcinomas including the ductal type (71,72).

Ductal Carcinoma *In Situ* (DCIS)

Ductal carcinoma *in situ* (DCIS) or intraductal carcinoma is a heterogeneous group of lesions, classified on the basis of their growth pattern as comedo and non-comedo types, with the latter encompassing the solid, cribriform, clinging/micropapillary, and papillary variants (73,74). Comedo-type DCIS is composed of a solid proliferation of large and pleomorphic epithelial cells within ducts, usually exhibiting numerous mitoses and central necrosis containing cellular debris (so-called "comedo-necrosis") (Fig. 30.6). The necrotic material often becomes calcified and these (coarse) calcifications have a distinctive mammographic appearance. Microinvasion is a feature more likely associated with comedo-type DCIS than other forms (Fig. 30.7) (75).

The solid, cribriform, papillary and micropapillary patterns of non-comedo DCIS are illustrated in Figs. 30.8 through 30.11. The micropapillary subtype differs from the papillary DCIS in that the papillary tufts lack fibrovascular

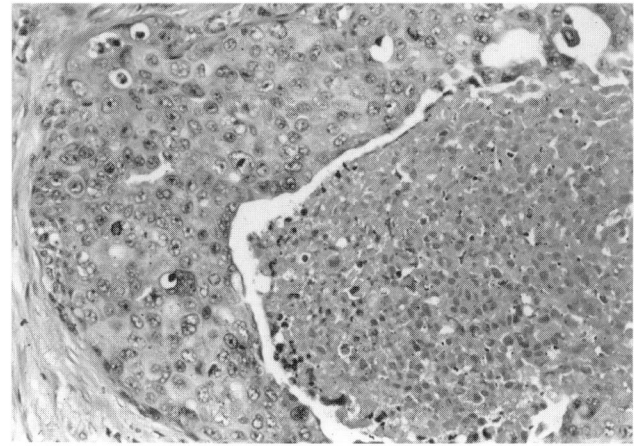

FIG. 30.6. Comedo-type/high-grade DCIS. The involved duct is distended by carcinoma cells growing in a solid pattern and exhibiting high nuclear grade, mitoses, and central necrosis.

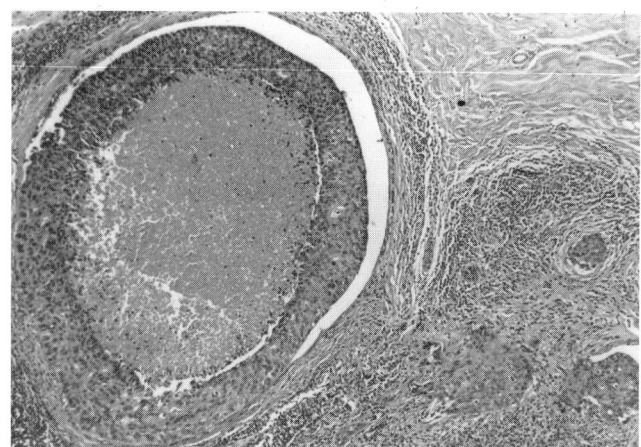

FIG. 30.7. Comedo-type/high-grade DCIS with microscopic clusters of microinvasion in the fibrotic and inflamed stroma.

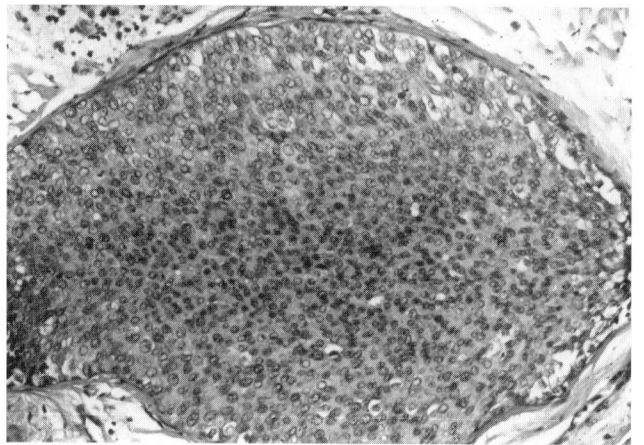

FIG. 30.8. Solid-type (noncomedo) DCIS with intermediate nuclear grade.

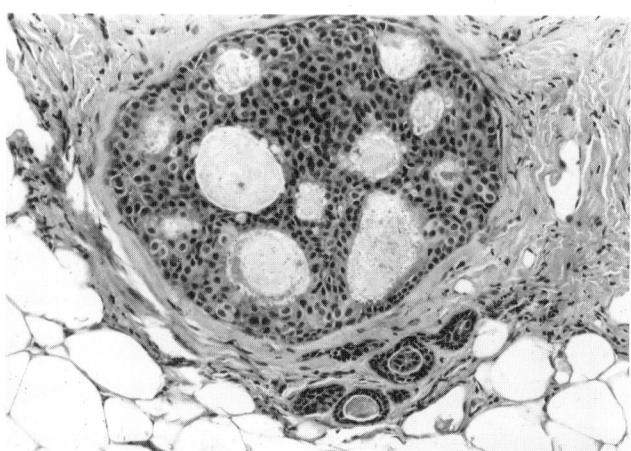

FIG. 30.9. Cribriform-type DCIS with low nuclear grade.

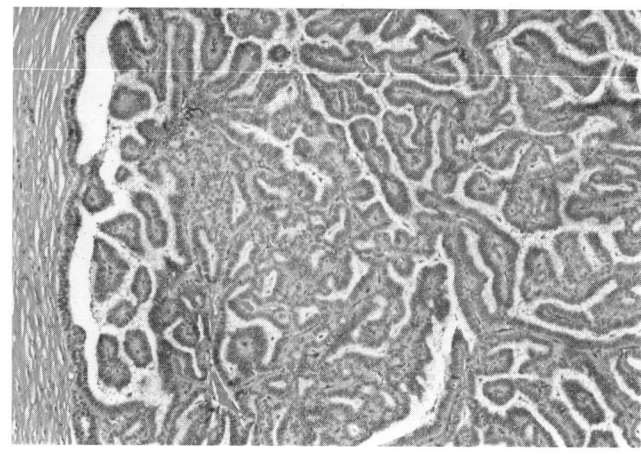

FIG. 30.10. Papillary-type DCIS with low nuclear grade.

cores. The "clinging" or "flat" type is usually associated with the micropapillary pattern and is believed to be a morphologic precursor of micropapillary DCIS. Microcalcifications may be associated with these non-comedo variants and may be detected by mammography. Their pattern of distribution, however, is less specific than that of the comedo DCIS and shows overlapping features with benign conditions.

Other, much less common "special" types include cystic hypersecretory, apocrine, clear-cell, signet ring–cell, and endocrine DCIS (76). The latter two types are often encountered in tumors with a papillary architecture (77–82). The classification of DCIS was not deemed to be clinically important and it served mainly to assist pathologists in making the diagnosis. There have been numerous attempts to identify predictors of successful breast-conservation therapy for DCIS, and the morphologic characteristics of these lesions have become important components in clinical decision-making. Even though several studies have demonstrated the association of comedo DCIS with higher recurrence rate re-

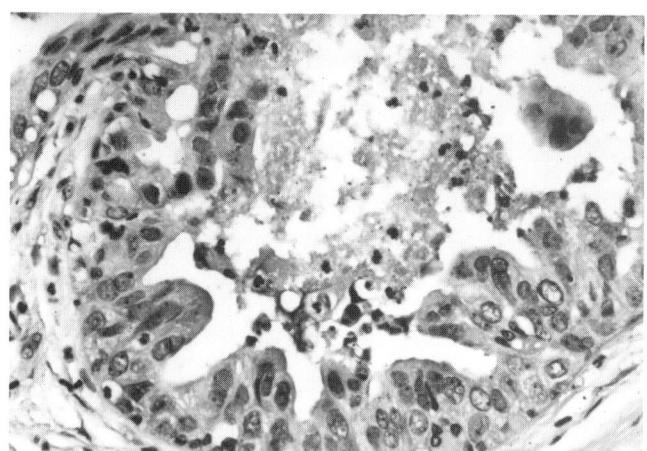

FIG. 30.11. DCIS with a micropapillary growth pattern, high nuclear grade, and focal necrosis.

TABLE 30.3. *Newly proposed classifications for DCIS according to Holland et al (90) and Silverstein et al (Van Nuys) (92)*

Designation by Holland et al/ Silverstein et al (Van Nuys)	Holland et al.	Silverstein et al (Van Nuys)
"Poorly differentiated"/high grade	Pleomorphic cells, frequent mitoses, minimal or no architectural differentiation, necrosis usually present, amorphous calcifications	High nuclear grade, any architectural pattern, necrosis may be present or absent
"Intermediately differentiated"/non–high grade with necrosis	Intermediate between the poorly and well-differentiated categories	Low to intermediate nuclear grade, any architectural pattern, substantial amounts of necrosis
"Well differentiated"/low grade	Monomorphic cells, few mitoses, pronounced architectural differentiation ("polarization"), necrosis uncommon, psammomatous calcifications	Low to intermediate nuclear grade without necrosis, any architectural pattern

gardless of treatment modality (75,83–87), the authors are not always in agreement with the dichotomous comedo-non-comedo definitions of DCIS: some require that the combination of a solid proliferation be present for the diagnosis of comedo DCIS, while others allow other architectural variants, such as cribriform and micropapillary, as long as the other two features of comedo DCIS (i.e., high nuclear grade and central necrosis) are identified. Conversely, not all solid DCIS lesions with central necrosis exhibit a high nuclear grade. In addition, a considerable number of DCIS cases show a mixed architectural pattern (88,89), making classification based on architecture a subjective exercise and comparison of outcome studies on long-term follow-up of DCIS difficult.

For these reasons, several alternative classification schemes of DCIS have been proposed (83,90–94), which take nuclear grade into account, and some also require evaluation of architectural patterns and/or the presence or absence of comedonecrosis. The DCIS classifications according to Holland et al (90) and Silverstein et al (Van Nuys classification) (92) are currently the most widely used in Europe and the United States, respectively. The differences between these two classification schemes are summarized in Table 30.3 (90,92), and examples of the three DCIS grades of the Van Nuys classification are illustrated in Figures 30.6 and 30.8 to 30.11.

Recent reports on the level of consistency among pathologists and on the prediction of recurrence using two or more of the new classifications have demonstrated a significant improvement over the conventional DCIS classification based on architecture, with the Van Nuys classification proving to be the easiest to implement (95–98). These observations indicate that nuclear grade and the presence or absence of comedonecrosis are two histologic features that are readily and reproducibly recognized by pathologists, although the nuclear grading of DCIS with apocrine cytology is still unsettled. Scott et al (94) recommend the recognition of the ''special'' types of DCIS as a separate group in order to better understand their natural history, while Holland et al (90) exclude them entirely and Silverstein et al (92) do not address the issue.

Other features that have been cited as significant for predicting outcome in patients with DCIS are surgical margin status and size of the lesion. Silverstein et al devised a prognostic index for DCIS by combining pathologic classification, tumor size, and margin width [the Van Nuys Prognostic Index (VNPI)] (Table 30.4) (99), a VNPI score of 3 being the most favorable and 9 the worst. With this method three distinct groups of DCIS can be stratified, each with a different probability for local recurrence after breast-conservation therapy. DCIS cases with VNPI scores of 3 or 4 are least likely to recur even if treated with excision only, those with VNPI scores of 8 or 9 are at high risk for local recurrence regardless of irradiation, and patients with intermediate scores of 5, 6 or 7 are shown to benefit the most from radiation therapy following breast-conserving surgery.

While the Van Nuys histologic classification of DCIS has been shown to produce the least interobserver variability and

TABLE 30.4. *The Van Nuys Prognostic Index (VNPI) scoring system*

Score	1	2	3
Pathologic classification	Non–high nuclear grade without necrosis	Non–high nuclear grade with necrosis	High nuclear grade with or without necrosis
Size of ductal carcinoma *in situ* (DCIS) (mm)	≤15	16–40	≥40
Closest margin width (mm)	≥10	1–9	<1

is easy to apply in clinical practice, the pathologic evaluation of lesion size and surgical margin are associated with several technical problems related to differences in processing techniques used in surgical pathology laboratories (100). To assess the extent of the lesion, Silverstein et al. (99) suggested to section each specimen serially at 2- or 3-mm intervals and to process the sections in sequence. However, this procedure has several disadvantages. First, tumor size measured in millimeters does not always reflect tumor volume, the latter being a much more accurate and meaningful evaluation of the extent of the DCIS. Second, if there is significant residual tumor present in the reexcision specimen, it is often impossible to determine the exact relationship between the first biopsy specimen and the reexcision material. Third, while serial sectioning at 2- or 3-mm intervals and submitting the entire specimen in sequence would be feasible in a low-volume surgical pathology laboratory, the process would add substantial costs and burden on the laboratory personnel in a high-volume laboratory.

The application of India ink and other dyes to assess surgical margins in pathologic specimens has been universally adopted. There is, however, disagreement over several aspects of margin assessment, including methods of margin sampling (perpendicular vs "orange-peel" technique, separate submission of margins by the surgeons) and the number of sections required (100).

It should be emphasized that DCIS represents a *spectrum* of ductal proliferations. At one end of the spectrum are the high-grade lesions in which microinvasive foci may be difficult to detect owing to periductal fibrosis and inflammation or may be missed because of inadequate sampling. The other end of the spectrum is represented by the low-grade DCIS that may be difficult to distinguish from atypical ductal hyperplasia (ADH) and may engender differing interpretations because of interobserver subjectivity compounded by the lack of consensus among pathologists with respect to the criteria used (101,102).

Paget disease of the nipple is a manifestation of ductal mammary carcinoma. It is almost invariably the result of intraepithelial spread from underlying (high-grade) intraductal carcinoma; in other words, the occurrence of DCIS in breast tissue of patients presenting with Paget disease is nearly 100%, and may or may not be associated with invasive carcinoma. A palpable mass is present in 50% to 60% of cases, and in these instances invasive ductal carcinoma is detected in more than 90% (103). In the absence of a palpable mass, invasive carcinoma occurs in less than 40% of cases. Histologically, Paget cells are large, pale-staining cells with prominent nucleoli and abundant cytoplasm occurring singly in the upper portions of the epidermis and forming groups in the basal layer.

Lobular Carcinoma *In Situ* (LCIS)

When Foote and Stewart described and introduced the term *lobular carcinoma in situ* (LCIS) more than 60 years ago, they already recognized three distinctive and important features of LCIS (104). The lesion is a microscopic finding and does not have any distinguishing gross pathologic features; it exhibits a multicentric distribution; and when invasive carcinoma develops following the diagnosis of LCIS, it can be of either the ductal or lobular type. We now also know that there are no specific mammographic features of LCIS (105). Microcalcifications were the most common indication for biopsy in those cases where LCIS was diagnosed, although the calcifications were rarely associated with the involved lobules and were seen in the adjacent ducts and lobules.

Microscopically, the lobules are typically distended by small, rather uniform, round cells with normochromic, round to oval nuclei and scant cytoplasm. Loss of cohesion and intracytoplasmic vacuoles containing mucin that sometimes are large enough to produce a signet ring–cell appearance are frequent findings. Often, the tumor cells extend into the neighboring (terminal) ducts by forming a continuous row beneath the nonneoplastic ductal epithelium, a process that is known as "pagetoid" spread of LCIS.

LCIS exhibiting the above-described cytologic features has been designated as "type A" or "classic." However, LCIS composed of larger cells with nucleoli has been encountered and has been referred to as "type B" LCIS (106). More recently, a "pleomorphic" type of LCIS composed of very large cells with peripherally located nuclei and occasional signet ring–cell features, has been described (107). The distinction between type B LCIS, so-called "pleomorphic" LCIS and DCIS may pose a diagnostic challenge even among experienced breast pathologists. Loss of expression of E-cadherin, a transmembrane glycoprotein that mediates cell-to-cell adhesion in epithelial tissues, has been shown to occur in most lobular-type carcinomas and is preserved in ductal-type lesions. For this reason, E-cadherin immunostaining is being used to classify ambiguous and difficult *in situ* lesions (108). It should be emphasized, however, that even though loss of E-cadherin expression has been shown in the so-called "pleomorphic" type of LCIS, its biologic behavior is not known at present time.

Invasive Carcinoma

For tumors to be classified as invasive, unequivocal stromal invasion must be identified; as with *in situ* carcinomas, the majority of invasive carcinomas can be divided into two major categories: *ductal* and *lobular* types.

Invasive Ductal Carcinoma

Invasive ductal carcinoma is morphologically diverse and its subclassification has incorporated various criteria, such as cell type (as in apocrine carcinoma), type of secretion (as in mucinous carcinoma), architectural patterns (as in papillary carcinoma or cribriform carcinoma), and pattern of spread (as in inflammatory carcinoma). Some of these subtypes are associated with a more indolent or more aggressive clinical behavior and are recognized as special types. The majority, however, which represent approximately 75% of invasive ductal carcinomas, have no specific features and are designated as not-otherwise-specified (NOS) type (109).

NOS invasive ductal carcinoma encompasses a multitude of tumors with various growth patterns (well-developed glands/tubules, solid nests, cords) and cytonuclear features. The most widely used microscopic grading of mammary ductal carcinomas is based on these two characteristics along with the evaluation of mitotic activity, also known as the Nottingham modification of the Bloom-Richardson system (110); the grade is obtained by adding up the scores for tubule formation, nuclear pleomorphism, and mitotic count, each of which is given 1, 2, or 3 points. This results in a total score of 3 to 9 points, which is translated into the final grade according to the following guidelines: 3 to 5 points = grade I (well differentiated), 6 to 7 points = grade II (moderately differentiated), and 8 to 9 points = grade III (poorly differentiated). The prognostic usefulness of this and related grading systems has been validated in a number of studies (111).

Special Types

Mucinous carcinoma, also known as mucoid or colloid carcinoma, usually occurs in postmenopausal women. Grossly, the tumor is well circumscribed, with a gelatinous cut surface. Microscopically, small clusters of tumor cells are seen to "float" in pools of mucin, producing a very distinct appearance (Fig. 30.12). It is important for prognostic reasons to restrict the diagnosis of mucinous carcinoma to those lesions exhibiting the characteristic feature throughout (so-called "pure" mucinous carcinoma), and to exclude those tumors showing areas of NOS-type invasive ductal carcinoma ("mixed" mucinous neoplasms) (6). The presence of signet ring cells in which the mucin is intracellular is uncommon in mucinous carcinoma, and tumors composed primarily of signet ring cells, so-called *signet ring–cell carcinoma* (see below), carries a much worse prognosis than mucinous carcinoma. In its pure or nearly pure form, mucinous carcinoma is associated with a very low incidence of nodal metastases (2% to 4%) (112) and has an excellent prognosis, particularly if the tumor measures less than 3 cm (6). Factors that have been associated with more aggressive behavior include large tumor size, increased tumor cellularity, and axillary lymph node metastases (112–114).

Tubular carcinoma is an invasive ductal carcinoma composed of very well-differentiated glands that can be difficult to distinguish from benign lesions such as radial scar or microglandular adenosis. Typically, the neoplastic tubules are angular with open lumina and are lined by a single layer of epithelial cells exhibiting apocrine-type "snouts" in their apical cytoplasm. These glands are distributed haphazardly in the cellular and often elastotic stroma (Fig. 30.13). In about two-thirds of the cases, a low-grade intraductal carcinoma is found admixed with and/or adjacent to the invasive component. Tubular carcinomas are usually small lesions, averaging about 1 cm in diameter (115–117). The increased detection of smaller tumors due to the widespread use of screening mammography has also increased the incidence of tubular carcinomas (118). Metastases to axillary lymph nodes occur in about 10% of the cases, with multifocal lesions having a higher rate of nodal metastases (116). The favorable prognosis of tubular carcinoma is limited to tumors composed of at least 75% well-differentiated tubular elements (114,119).

Medullary carcinoma usually affects patients under 50 years of age. Clinically, it is well circumscribed, may become large, and may mimic a benign tumor such as a fibroadenoma. Microscopically, the tumor cells grow in a solid pattern, are large, and are pleomorphic with prominent nucleoli

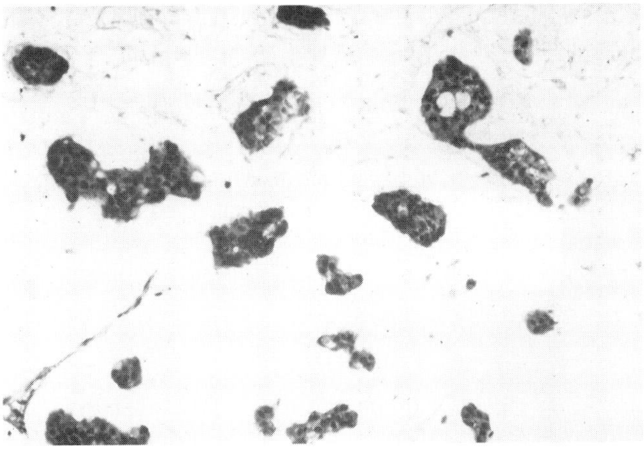

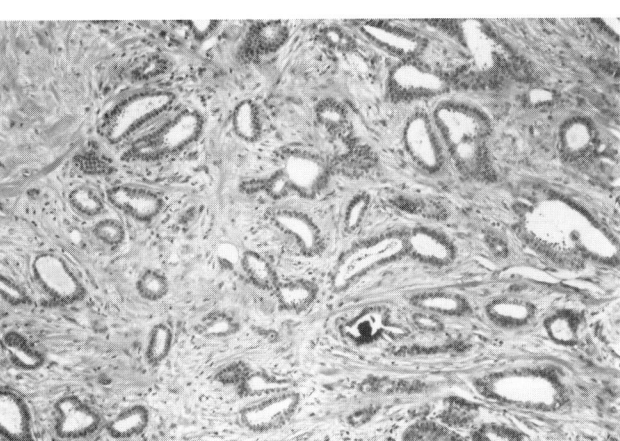

FIG. 30.12. Mucinous (colloid) carcinoma. Clusters of malignant cells in mucinous pools.

FIG. 30.13. Tubular carcinoma. Well-formed glands with open lumina infiltrating stroma.

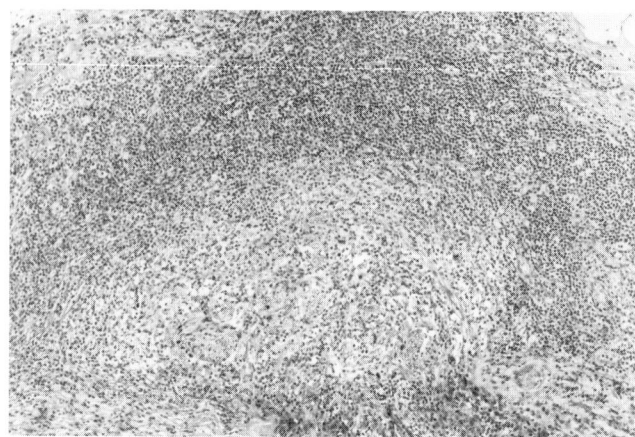

FIG. 30.14. Medullary carcinoma. The tumor cells (central lighter-staining area) show a syncytial growth pattern with pushing margins and are accompanied by a dense lymphoplasmacytic infiltrate (darker-staining zone around the tumor).

(Fig. 30.14). Mitoses are abundant, some of which are atypical. The cell borders are indistinct, giving the tumor a syncytial or sheet-like appearance. The tumor is accompanied by a dense lymphoplasmacytic reaction that is most conspicuous at its periphery, and while the tumor margins are circumscribed or "pushing," the inflammatory cells exhibit an infiltrative growth pattern into the surrounding tissue. Foci of solid high-grade intraductal carcinoma may be present adjacent to the main tumor mass. Tumor necrosis may be present and may lead to the formation of cystic areas within the tumor. Recent studies have shown a high prevalence of tumor histopathology reminiscent of medullary breast carcinoma in patients with *BRCA1* germline mutations (120,121).

Patients with medullary carcinoma tend to have a lower frequency of axillary lymph node metastases than patients with NOS-type invasive ductal carcinoma (122–124).

The prognosis of medullary carcinoma is better than for the ordinary or NOS-type invasive ductal carcinoma (122, 123) only if one adheres strictly to the following criteria in making the diagnosis: syncytial growth pattern, high nuclear grade, abundant mitoses, pushing tumor borders, and lymphoplasmacytic infiltrate. The term "atypical medullary carcinoma" or "invasive ductal carcinoma with medullary features" has been used to designate those tumors that show some but not all of the above histologic features. The disease-free survival of patients with these tumors is not statistically different from NOS invasive ductal carcinoma. It should be noted that even though the favorable prognosis of medullary carcinoma is commonly accepted, there is considerable difficulty in applying the diagnostic criteria and that this fact was never addressed in the published series reporting on the clinical outcome of medullary carcinomas (125, 126).

Invasive papillary carcinoma is a rare entity, and the great majority of them are *in situ* tumors. The invasive component

of a papillary carcinoma is in the majority of cases a microscopic lesion. It may show a papillary pattern or, more commonly, has the features of an ordinary invasive ductal carcinoma. Interestingly however, the *cytologic* features of the invasive carcinoma are similar to those of the *in situ* papillary component. Some papillary carcinoma exhibit a predominantly solid growth pattern, designated as *solid* papillary carcinoma. This subtype of papillary carcinoma occurs almost exclusively in women in their 70s, is often initially misdiagnosed as a benign papillary lesion (intraductal papilloma), and is frequently associated with neuroendocrine and mucinous differentiation (77,78). When invasion is present, the invasive carcinoma is usually of the mucinous type. As with the more conventional type of papillary carcinoma, the prognosis is excellent. The frequency of axillary lymph node metastases is low, a feature that is consistent with the sizes of the actual invasive component and the morphologically low-grade character of these carcinomas (127).

Metaplastic carcinoma is a nonspecific term for a ductal-type invasive carcinoma in which the predominant component of the tumor has an appearance other than an epithelial or glandular one. Two types of metaplastic carcinoma have been described: spindle cell (homologous) and sarcomatoid or pseudosarcomatous (heterologous). In the spindle-cell variant, foci of overt carcinomatous elements in the form of *in situ* and/or invasive ductal carcinoma are usually present. It is not uncommon to find transition areas in which the spindle cell and the carcinomatous components merge. The malignant spindle cells may be deceptively bland in appearance in some cases. Immunoreactivity for cytokeratin, a marker for epithelial differentiation, is often retained in the spindle-cell areas (128).

Sarcomatoid metaplastic carcinoma exhibits sarcoma-like components that may resemble osteosarcoma, chondrosarcoma, angiosarcoma, malignant fibrous histiocytoma, and fibrosarcoma. Immunohistochemically, the sarcomatoid elements have usually acquired a mesenchymal immunophenotype as evidenced by antibodies against vimentin, but occasionally still coexpress—albeit focally—epithelial markers.

The differential diagnosis of spindle-cell and sarcomatoid metaplastic carcinomas includes a malignant phyllodes tumor and a primary sarcoma of the breast, respectively. The prognosis of metaplastic carcinomas is difficult to ascertain because of their widely heterogeneous morphologic features. It appears though that metaplastic carcinoma behaves in a more aggressive fashion than an ordinary invasive ductal carcinoma (129). This is in part probably due to the poorly differentiated nature of these tumors, in particular the sarcomatoid type (130,131). Metastases tend to be hematogenous rather than to lymph nodes, reflecting the sarcomatous phenotype (129,131).

Secretory carcinoma, also known as *juvenile carcinoma,* is an exceedingly rare tumor affecting primarily, but not exclusively, children (132). Because of its relative circumscription, the clinical impression of secretory carcinoma is often that of a fibroadenoma. Typically, the microscopic growth pattern of the tumor is solid and focally papillary with a central area of hyalinization. The tumor cells have a vacuolated cytoplasm with low-grade nuclei, and form glandular lumina filled by an eosinophilic PAS-positive secretion, that is, they are immunoreactive with alpha-lactalbumin. The clinical behavior of secretory carcinoma is very indolent, and if axillary nodal metastases occur, they rarely involve more than three lymph nodes (133). The risk of recurrent or metastatic disease may be related to tumor size (larger than 2 cm) and presence of infiltrative tumor borders (134).

The term *inflammatory carcinoma* was originally used in a clinical setting in which patients presented with reddened and warm breasts simulating mastitis. Skin biopsies revealed extensive dermal lymphatic permeation by carcinoma in some cases. This led to the belief that the clinical appearance of an "inflammatory" breast is always associated with the pathologic finding of tumor emboli in the dermal lymphatics and vice versa. This assumption is not always true. Some patients may have extensive dermal lymphatic involvement by carcinoma without showing clinical features of inflammatory carcinoma. From a clinical standpoint, the presence of widespread (dermal) lymphatic permeation is an ominous sign irrespective of the physical findings (135). Although the clinical recognition of this entity by an experienced observer is quite reliable, it should be confirmed pathologically by a skin biopsy before deeming the tumor inoperable.

Other rare variants of invasive ductal-type carcinoma include adenoid cystic carcinoma and small-cell (oat-cell) carcinoma, which are morphologically similar to those encountered in the salivary gland and lung, respectively.

Invasive Lobular Carcinoma

The *classic type* of invasive lobular carcinoma is characterized by small, uniform tumor cells with scant cytoplasm and hyperchromatic nuclei growing in single file ("Indian file") and concentrically ("targetoid" pattern) around ducts and lobules (104,136,137). A desmoplastic stromal reaction is another typical feature of classic invasive lobular carcinoma. Over the last two decades the microscopic criteria of invasive lobular carcinoma have been expanded to include the so-called *variant forms*. Tumors with patterns of growth other than the classic linear formation, such as *solid, trabecular*, and *alveolar*, are considered variations of invasive lobular carcinoma as long as the relatively bland and uniform cytologic features of the tumor cells are maintained (138, 139). More recently, the concept has been expanded considerably by the inclusion of tumors with a *pleomorphic* cell population growing in single file (pleomorhic variant) (140–142). With the inclusion of the variant forms, invasive lobular carcinoma constitutes 10% to 14% of invasive breast carcinomas (139,143).

The prognosis of patients with invasive lobular carcinoma is not different from those with invasive NOS ductal carcinoma when stratified by stage (6,137). Although a few studies reported a slightly worse outcome for the variant forms, the difference is not statistically significant (137,143). A recent observation on the pleomorphic variant of invasive lobular carcinoma suggested a poorer prognosis when compared to the classic type (142); however, the number of cases is too small to draw a meaningful conclusion.

While the distinction between ductal and lobular types of invasive carcinoma has become more diluted owing to the widened morphologic criteria used, it is still a relevant one to make because of the higher incidence of bilaterality and multicentricity in the lobular-type group.

Special Variants

Tubulolobular carcinoma is morphologically a mixture of invasive lobular and tubular carcinomas, which merge with each other to form an invasive carcinoma that grows partially in single file but that also shows glandular elements seen in tubular carcinoma. Some authors have classified tubulolobular carcinoma as a variant of invasive lobular carcinoma, while others regard it as a variant of tubular carcinoma. Although the available data regarding the prognosis of tubulolobular carcinoma are limited, it appears that it is between that of pure tubular and that of invasive lobular carcinoma (116).

Signet ring–cell carcinoma is an invasive mammary carcinoma in which the predominant tumor cells show prominent intracytoplasmic mucin vacuoles, resulting in the typical signet ring appearance (144). The majority of this type of carcinoma show architectural and cytologic similarities to invasive lobular carcinoma and often coexist with it (the presence of signet ring cells is more commonly, but not exclusively, found in lobular carcinomas). Because of these reasons, signet ring–cell carcinoma is considered a variant of invasive lobular carcinoma. It is important to distinguish signet ring–cell carcinoma from mucinous (colloid) carcinoma because of the vastly different prognoses. Patients with a history of invasive lobular carcinoma who are then found to have carcinoma of the stomach with the clinical features of linitis plastica should be worked up for the possibility of metastatic lobular carcinoma. While strong positivity for estrogen receptors favors metastatic disease from the breast, some primary gastric adenocarcinomas have been found also to express estrogen receptor immunoreactivity. The recent differential staining for different cytokeratins has proved to be very helpful in such cases (145).

Other Unusual Malignant Primary Tumors

Cystosarcoma phyllodes, or phyllodes tumor, occurs in the same age group as breast carcinoma, with a median age of 45 years at presentation. These tumors may be encountered in younger patients but they are very uncommon (146). The histologic hallmarks of cystosarcoma phyllodes are stromal hypercellularity and the presence of benign glandular elements as an integral component of the tumor. These tumors have been classified as "benign," low-grade malignant and high-grade malignant, primarily based on the degree of cellularity, atypia, and mitotic activity of the stromal component. It must be noted that the distinction between a "benign" and low-grade malignant tumor is not always possible. The better-differentiated phyllodes tumors have a tendency for local recurrences if not completely excised, especially those with an infiltrative tumor margin. The cytologically high-grade malignant tumors typically show stromal overgrowth with sarcomatous features reminiscent of fibrosarcoma, malignant fibrous histiocytoma, or liposarcoma. Some tumors may exhibit heterologous stromal differentiation such as cartilage or bone. It is important to realize the potential of the high-grade lesions for distant metastases, which range from 3% to 12% in various studies. Axillary lymph node metastases are exceptional. The most common sites for distant metastases are lung and bone (147).

Angiosarcoma is the most common of the primary sarcomas occurring in the breast. The morphologic features of angiosarcoma are heterogeneous, ranging from lesions that are difficult to differentiate from benign vascular conditions to fully malignant tumors. Morphologically, the tumors are characterized by anastomosing vascular channels lined by atypical endothelial cells. The appearance may vary in the same tumor from that of a solid undifferentiated neoplasm to one that is quite bland cytologically. The latter may pose great difficulties in the assessment of surgical margins. The prognosis of angiosarcomas has been shown to correlate with the histologic differentiation (grade) of the neoplasms (148). The estimated 10-year disease-free survival is 15% for high-grade tumors, and 70% and 76% respectively for intermediate and low-grade neoplasms. Hematogenous metastases to bone, lung, liver, or contralateral breast and skin are more commonly found than is local recurrence.

PROGNOSTIC FACTORS

The prognostic factors influencing local relapse and survival can be divided into two groups, intrinsic or related to the characteristics of the tumor (e.g., histologic features, lymph node metastases), and extrinsic, including host factors, the type and adequacy of treatment, etc.

Intrinsic Prognostic Factors

The pathologic involvement of axillary lymph nodes is the single most important prognostic factor for breast cancer. The number of metastatic lymph nodes correlates extremely well with patient outcome, local and regional failure, development of distant metastases, and patient survival. Although prognostic categories of nodal involvement, such as one to three, four to nine, and ten or more positive nodes, have

been created for statistical analysis of patients, the number involved is in fact a continuing variable (149).

Haagensen (150) demonstrated a direct relationship between tumor involvement of axillary nodes and chest-wall recurrence, and an inverse correlation with survival in patients treated with radical or modified radical mastectomy. Fisher and associates (151) described diminishing survival after mastectomy with a greater number of metastatic axillary lymph nodes (152).

In addition, Valagussa and colleagues (153) noted that patients with involved internal mammary nodes had more recurrences than those without (27.9% 10-year relapse rate in patients with negative axillary nodes; 60% in patients with negative axillary nodes and involved internal mammary nodes) (154).

Tumor size is also an important prognostic factor, especially in patients who have uninvolved axillary lymph nodes. Patients with invasive cancers less than 1.0 cm in greatest diameter have an excellent prognosis if the lymph nodes are negative. Similarly, patients with certain "special" low-risk histologic subtypes of breast cancer up to 3.0 cm in diameter and with negative lymph nodes have a similarly favorable prognosis (6). For patients in the lymph-node–negative group with lesions larger than these, the likelihood of disease-free and overall survival decreases.

Another prognostic indicator for breast cancer outcome is the histologic grade of the tumor. Because of differences in grading systems used throughout the country and around the world, however, this factor is somewhat difficult to assess (155), as discussed in greater detail in the section on pathology.

Much has been written in recent years on the value of tumor markers for breast cancer. These intrinsic factors can be divided into two groups: those that are prognostic for the outcome of the patient, and those that predict a tumor response to a given therapeutic intervention. Controversy as to their usefulness resulted in several major organizations holding consensus meetings over the past 5 years. Table 30.5 summarizes the conclusions and recommendations of these meetings. Of note, both the ASCO guidelines and the St. Gallen's guidelines place value on only the estrogen- and progesterone-receptor status of the tumor. The ASCO guidelines place these markers in the "predictive" group, while the St. Gallen's guidelines place estrogen-receptor status in both the "prognostic" and "predictive" groups. Other markers, such as S phase and Ki-67, are noted only in the ACP guidelines, and there merit only the label "of possible value" (155). Although DNA flow cytometry provides important prognostic information, standardization of technique and histogram analysis, as well as quality control, need to be addressed before this technology can be used reliably on a wide scale (156). These markers are also discussed in the systemic therapy section of this chapter.

In the past several years' experience, c-*erb*B2 has proved to be a predictor of response to some chemotherapy agents.

TABLE 30.5. *Recommendations of four groups about what information might be used in prognostic/predictive assessment of breast-cancer patients*

Source	Prognostic factors	Predictive factors
NIH (1990)	Nodal status	Not addressed
	Tumor size	–
	ER, PgR	–
	Nuclear grade	–
	Histologic type	–
	Proliferation S phase	–
	Cathepsin D	–
St. Gallen's (1995)	Nodal status	Menopausal status
	Tumor size	ER
	Histologic grade	–
	Age	–
	ER	–
ACP (1995)	TNM	Not addressed
	Histologic type	–
	Histologic grade	–
	Of possible value	–
	Proliferation	–
	Mitotic count	–
	S phase	–
	Ki 67 MIB1	–
	*c-erb*B-2	–
	p53	–
	Angiogenesis	–
	Vascular invasion	–
ASCO (1996)	No laboratory-based measures	ER, PgR

ACP, American College of Pathology; ASCO, American Society of Clinical Oncology; NIH, National Institutes of Health.

From Ravdin PM. Prognostic factors in breast cancer. *American Society of Clinical Oncology educational book.* Denver, 1997:217, with permission.

This marker has demonstrated value in the treatment of node-positive patients with doxorubicin-based chemotherapy (157,158), and promises to predict response to trastuzimab (Herceptin) therapy as discussed later in this chapter.

In patients with gross multicentric disease or diffuse microcalcifications, it is difficult to perform breast-conservation surgery with satisfactory cosmetic results. Furthermore, these patients are at greater risk of breast relapse. In general, depending on the extent of the tumors, these patients are treated with a modified radical mastectomy.

Location of Primary Tumor

Fowble and coworkers (159) analyzed recurrence and survival in 886 patients with stages I and II breast cancer treated with breast-conservation therapy (median follow-up, 5 years). The patients were divided into four groups according to the primary tumor location: outer (495 patients), inner (202 patients), central (119 patients), and subareolar (70 patients). Subareolar tumors were defined as those immediately beneath the nipple-areolar complex or within 2 cm of the areolar margin. There were no significant differences in 5-year actuarial overall survival (91%, 86%, 92%, and 91%, respectively; $p = 0.34$), relapse-free survival (75%, 74%, 80%, and 79%, respectively; $p = 0.77$), or disease-free survival (82%, 78%, 87%, and 84%, respectively; $p = 0.29$) among the four groups.

In a review of 1,014 patients with early breast cancer treated with breast-conservation therapy, Haffty and associates (160) identified 98 patients who fulfilled the criteria of having a central/subareolar tumor. Ten of 98 patients had the nipple-areolar complex sacrificed at the time of surgery, while the remaining 88 patients had the entire area included in the boost cone-down field. The 10-year actuarial breast recurrence-free survival rate was 84%, distant disease-free survival was 88%, and overall survival was 79%, similar to patients with tumors in other locations. The nipple-areolar complex could be preserved in most patients, and there were no significant complications.

Histologic Features and Tumor Grade

Schnitt and associates (161) compared the results of tumor excision and irradiation in 49 patients with infiltrating lobular stages I and II carcinoma and 561 patients with similar stages of infiltrating ductal carcinoma. The 5-year actuarial risk of local recurrence was similar for both groups (12% versus 11%).

Weiss and colleagues (162) reported on 879 patients with stages I and II breast cancer treated with conservation surgery and irradiation. The patients were divided into seven groups based on histologic subtype: 368 patients with infiltrating and intraductal ductal carcinoma, 389 with pure infiltrating ductal carcinoma, 41 with infiltrating lobular carcinoma, 23 with combined infiltrating ductal and lobular carcinoma, 28 with medullary carcinoma, 12 with colloid carcinoma, and 18 with tubular carcinoma. There were no significant differences in 5-year actuarial overall survival, cause-specific survival, or relapse-free survival rates among the histologic categories. In addition, patterns of first local failure were not significantly different among the histologic groups.

Extensive Intraductal Carcinoma

According to the Harvard definition of extensive intraductal carcinoma (EIC), this condition exists when 25% or more of the primary tumor is intraductal carcinoma, and when intraductal carcinoma is seen outside (adjacent to) the infiltrating border (163,164). Ductal carcinoma *in situ* with microinvasion also fits this definition, which was first described as part of a research project to identify predictors for local failure after breast-conservation surgery and irradiation. Extensive intraductal carcinoma involving the primary tumor and adjacent tissues has been reported by some

TABLE 30.6. *Incidence of breast relapse correlated with extensive intraductal carcinoma (EIC) component in primary breast tumor or adjacent breast*

	Breast recurrence at 5 years	
Author	EIC present	EIC absent
Bartelink et al (171)	9% (79)	2% (208)
Boyages et al (172)	24% (166)	6% (418)
Eberlein et al (173)	27% (166)	7% (418)
Fisher et al (168)	11% (56)	9% (366)
Fowble et al (174)	22% (23)	4% (252)
Koper et al[a]	10% (283)	13% (283)
Kurtz et al (175)	18% (106)	8% (390)
MIR, Washington University[a]	10.7% (181)	4.2% (470)
Recht et al (176)	23% (143)	5% (302)
Schnitt et al (177)	15% (113)	1% (98)
Veronesi et al (178)		
Quadrantectomy	10% (22)	4% (338)
Tumorectomy	30% (38)	8% (307)
Zafrani et al (179)	11% (63)	6% (361)

Numbers in parentheses represent total number of patients in study.
MIR, Mallinckrodt Institute of Radiology.
[a] Unpublished data.

groups, particularly Harvard University (164,165) and Marseilles (166), to be associated with a higher incidence of breast recurrences. In contrast, Clarke and associates (167), Fisher and colleagues (168), and van Limbergen and co-workers (169) found no significant impact on local tumor control with extensive intraductal extension. This may be related to the pathologic criteria used in the definition of EIC, or to adequacy of tumor excision and doses of irradiation delivered to the boost volume. Vicini et al. (170) found that the predictive value of EIC disappeared when the surgeon took a larger volume of tissue from the breast, implying that the adequacy of the tumor excision explained in part the predictive value of EIC. Table 30.6 (168,171–179) summarizes reports of breast relapses in different series, correlated with presence of EIC.

Holland and coworkers (180) stated that an EIC component is associated with subsequent breast recurrence because of the presence of residual intraductal carcinoma in these patients. In a series of 214 women who underwent mastectomy, 71% of those with EIC had residual intraductal carcinoma after a wide excision biopsy, compared with 28% of those without that pathologic feature. In particular, 44% of the EIC-positive patients had prominent residual tumor in the mastectomy specimen, compared with 3% of those who were EIC-negative ($p < 0.00001$). Carefully assessed negative surgical margins and adequate irradiation should decrease or eliminate the significance of EIC for local failure.

BRCA *Genes*

BRCA1 is an important breast cancer–susceptibility locus identified in chromosome 17q21 via linkage analysis in fa-

milial breast and ovarian cancers. Of 97 patients studied (3 were males), 18 had familial breast cancer, 59 had sporadic unilateral breast cancer, and 20 had bilateral breast tumors and no family history of breast cancer. The high frequency of allelic imbalance (67%) was manifested at *BRCA1* in the 18 familial breast cancer patients. In the 20 patients with bilateral tumors, the corresponding percentage was considerably lower (181). A specific *BRCA1* mutation, 185delAG, was found to be associated with breast cancer (21%) in Jewish women younger than 40 years of age (182).

Eight breast cancer pedigrees with a high probability of containing individuals with the *BRCA1* gene mutation (odds 79.2% to 99.9%) were identified through genetic linkage analysis using probes located within q12–22 on the long arm of chromosome 17; 102 female relatives were successfully typed with one or both of adjacent markers, and 41 were probable non-*BRCA1* mutation carriers (183). Of the remaining 61 women classified as probable *BRCA1* carriers, breast cancer was diagnosed in 35; 13 of these had bilateral disease. Lifetime disease penetrance of the *BRCA1* gene was 88%, and this plateau was reached earlier (by age 65 years) than that estimated in segregation analysis. The survival curve of patients with breast cancer was less steep in *BRCA1* gene carriers than that in the general population; 5-, 10-, and 20-year survival rates not adjusted for noncancer deaths were 83%, 63%, and 41%, respectively. The 5-year survival rate was significantly higher in *BRCA1* carriers than that in an age-matched Scottish population ($p < 0.05$).

In another study, *BRCA1* was identified in 10% of 80 women diagnosed before the age of 35 who were not selected on the basis of family history (184). Easton and colleagues (185) estimated that more than half of women with *BRCA1* mutations develop breast cancer before the age of 50 and approximately 82% by age 70. One report suggested that women with breast cancer who harbor mutant *BRCA1* alleles may have a longer survival than unselected women with breast cancer (183).

Current techniques on isolation of *BRCA1* provide a unique opportunity to identify persons carrying this gene mutation, estimated to be 1 in 200 to 1 in 400 people in the United States. It is thought that the *BRCA1* gene accounts for 45% of familial breast cancers and perhaps 25% of breast cancer cases that occur before the age of 30.

Genetic studies in patients with breast cancer place a second susceptibility *BRCA2* locus in chromosome 13q12–13. As with *BRCA1*, *BRCA2* appears to confer high risk of early-onset breast cancer in women, as well as a substantially elevated risk of ovarian cancer (186). The risk of breast cancer in men carrying *BRCA2* mutations, although small, is probably greater than in men carrying *BRCA1* mutations. *BRCA2* is also associated with an increased risk of prostate, pancreatic, gall bladder and stomach cancers (186), and melanomas.

The identification of carriers of this gene will provide new opportunities for research in genetic and environmental etiology. Fundamental understanding of the function of *BRCA1* and *BRCA2* and ways to exploit that knowledge to diagnose, treat, and ultimately prevent breast cancer will be important subjects of prospective clinical trials (187) and bioethical discussions (and will have important implications in eligibility for healthcare coverage).

Extrinsic (Host) Prognostic Factors

Although the most important parameters for determining prognosis and patterns of failure in breast cancer are the intrinsic factors, some host factors are also highly relevant.

Age

The age of the patient at the time of diagnosis of the breast cancer has long been recognized to play a role in patient outcome. Several large population-based studies have demonstrated that all other factors being equal, patients between the younger age cutoff of 35 to 40 years and the older age cutoff of 75 to 80 years have the best prognosis for outcome of their disease. Women under the age of 40 or 35 years, or over the age of 75 or 80 years, have a poorer prognosis (188–191).

Young age is a risk factor for local breast recurrence after conservation surgery and irradiation, as well. Different investigators have used various age cutoffs such as 50, 40, 35, and 30 years. Vilcoq and colleagues (192) found a local-regional recurrence rate of 35% versus 4% in women younger than or older than 30 years, respectively. Kurtz and associates (193) reported a 19% incidence of local recurrence in 210 women younger than 40 years compared with 9% in 1,172 older women. This observation correlated with EIC, high tumor grade, and a major mononuclear cell reaction. The Harvard Joint Center's inferior results in younger women also correlated with the presence of EIC (194). These findings have also been reported by other authors (Fig. 30.15, Table 30.7) (167,169,178,193,196–203).

De la Rochefordiére and associates (204) noted that, in 1,703 premenopausal patients with stages I to III breast cancer, the youngest patients had significantly lower survival rates and higher local and distant relapse rates than the older patients. This was true for women treated with mastectomy, as well as after breast-conservation surgery and irradiation. The increases in local failure after mastectomy in the youngest patients were as striking as those in the conserved group. A log-linear function indicated a 4% decrease in recurrence for every year of age. These data strongly support the concept that younger patients have more aggressive cancer and may require different indicators for systemic treatment than older women with the same stage of disease.

Race

Black women are commonly diagnosed with more advanced stages of breast cancer than white women. In a re-

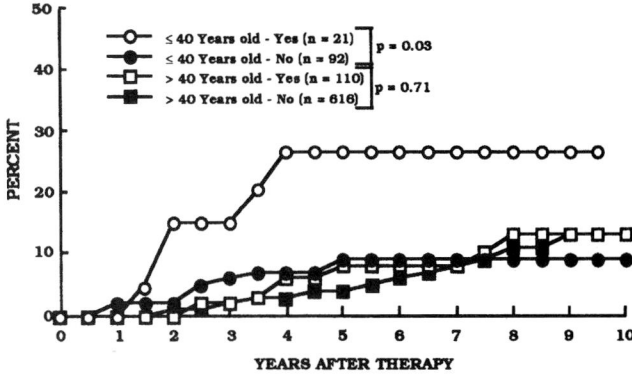

FIG. 30.15. Incidence of breast relapse correlated with extensive intraductal carcinoma (EIC) component and age for 839 patients treated at Mallinckrodt Institute of Radiology, Washington University. A higher breast relapse rate was seen in women younger than 40 years of age with EIC. (Reprinted with permission from Perez CA, Taylor ME. Breast: stage Tis, T1, and T2 tumors. In: Perez CA, Brady LW, eds. *Principles and practice of radiation oncology,* 3rd ed. Philadelphia: Lippincott–Raven,1998:1269.)

view of 10,502 women diagnosed with breast cancer (82% white and 18% African-American), Simon and Severson (205) observed that African-American women were more likely to present with regional or distant disease (45%) than white women (37%). White women had a better survival rate than African-American women during the first 4 years after diagnosis ($p < 0.0001$), but there were no significant differences in survival rates by race in women who lived longer than 4 years ($p = 0.64$). Furthermore, black women

TABLE 30.7. *Young age as risk factor for breast relapse in breast-conservation therapy*

	Breast recurrences		
Author	≤35 Years	≥35 Years	Follow-up (years)
Clarke and Martinez (197)	9% (32)	5% (424)	5 mean
Fowble et al (198)	24% (64)	13% (916)	8 actuarial
Haffty et al (199)	15% (34)	11% (349)	8.2 median
Halverson et al (200)	9% (37)	12% (474)	7 actuarial
Kurtz et al (193)	16% (91)	10% (1291)	11 mean
Matthews et al (201)	15% (72)	5% (306)	≥2
Nixon et al (202)	14% (107)	9% (1026)	8.3 median
Veronesi et al (178)	9% (95)	4% (1137)	6 median
Vicini et al (203)	21% (65)	9% (721)	5 actuarial
Vicini et al (203)	12% (44)	7% (554)	5 actuarial

Numbers in parentheses represent total number of patients in study.

are more likely than white women to report that they have not received a mammogram within 3 years prior to diagnosis. History of mammographic screening, however, accounted for less than 10% of the observed differences in stage at diagnosis (206).

In 887 black women and 265 white women with breast cancer analyzed by Ansell and associates (207), black women had lower 5-year breast cancer survival rates than white women (50.2% versus 60.2%; $p = 0.05$), and survival was lower when adjusted for stage and age. When adjusted for income in addition to stage and age, however, the effect of race on survival was reduced (from relative risk of 1.26 to 1.17).

Of note on this issue, among women who receive medical care through the Department of Defense and who should have uniform access to care, no difference in stage is demonstrated among white, African-American, and Hispanic women diagnosed with breast cancer (208, 209).

In 75 black and 615 white women with stages I and II breast cancer treated with breast-conservation therapy, cyclophosphamide, methotrexate, and 5-FU (CMF), with or without prednisone and tamoxifen, the 5-year actuarial local-only first failure rates were 5% for black women and 6% for white women ($p = 0.53$); regional-only failure rates were 9% for blacks and 1% for whites ($p = 0.002$), and regional recurrence as a component of first failure was 16% and 4%, respectively ($p = 0.001$) (210). Distant metastases as the only site of first failure were significantly greater in the black population (20% at 5 years versus 11% in white patients; $p = 0.01$). The 5-year overall survival rate for the black patients was 82% versus 91% for the white patients ($p = 0.01$).

Eley and associates (211) reported on a study of 612 black and 518 white women aged 20 to 79 years with primary invasive breast cancer. After controlling for geographic site and age, the risk of dying was 2.2 times greater for blacks than whites. Adjustment for stage reduced risk from 2.2 to 1.7; further adjustment for sociodemographic variables had no effect. They concluded that approximately 75% of the racial difference in survival was explained by the prognostic factors studied. Sociodemographic variables appeared to manifest largely in racial differences in stage at diagnosis.

Obesity

In a study of 923 women treated by mastectomy and axillary dissection, those who were obese (25% or more over optimal weight for height) at the time of primary breast cancer treatment were at significantly greater risk for recurrence (42%) compared with nonobese patients (32%) 10 years after diagnosis ($p < 0.01$) (212). On multivariate analysis, and after controlling for tumor size, number of positive axillary lymph nodes, age at diagnosis, and adjuvant chemotherapy, obesity remained a statistically significant prognostic factor, with a hazard ratio of 1.29. Recurrent disease developed in 32% of obese patients compared with 19% of nonobese women.

Pregnancy

Although in the past it was thought that pregnancy after the diagnosis of breast cancer was associated with a worse prognosis, recent evidence suggests the contrary (213). This subject will be discussed in detail later in this chapter.

CLINICAL PRESENTATION

The majority of patients with carcinoma *in situ*, T1, or T2 breast cancers present with a painless or slightly tender breast mass or have an abnormal screening mammogram. Patients with more advanced tumors may have breast tenderness, skin changes, bloody nipple discharge, or, occasionally, change in the shape and size of the breast. In the United States, patients rarely present with axillary lymphadenopathy or distant metastasis.

Mammography and Other Imaging Studies

An x-ray examination of the breast, a mammogram, can be performed as either a screening or diagnostic study, and can be done with film or digital recording. Although utilizing the same technology, these studies are designed to address differing clinical situations. It is important that the physician and the patient appreciate the different purpose of these two studies. Both digital and film mammography produce an image by passing an x-ray beam through the breast; the digital image is stored electronically and can be manipulated on a monitor while the film mammogram image is recorded on film. There is no demonstrated difference in the ability of film or digital mammography to screen for or characterize breast cancer. Additionally, imaging with sonography and magnetic resonance (MR) can be done to obtain additional information to that found by mammography.

Mammography practice in the United States is regulated by the Food and Drug Administration under the Mammography Quality Standards Act (MQSA) of 1992 (214). Federal regulation defines the training and experience needed by physicians, technologists, and medical physicists involved in mammography. A rigid quality-control program must be in place at each facility, monitoring x-ray equipment and film processors. Annual inspections of facilities are also performed. Practice outcome data must be obtained, as well as a record of follow-up on all women for whom biopsy has been recommended.

Mammographic Screening

The screening mammogram consists of two views of the breast, the top-to-bottom or craniocaudal (CC) view, and the angled side-to-side, or mediolateral oblique (MLO) view. In diagnostic mammography, additional views are commonly taken. Imaging the breast with these two views is designed to optimize the amount of breast tissue imaged on the mammogram and to maximize visualization of breast tissue in two different projections. This minimizes the possibility of acquiring a false impression that a lesion is present, due to overlying tissues, or of missing a cancer because the part of the breast containing it is not included on at least one of the two images. It also decreases the likelihood that a cancer will be obscured by overlying structures.

Screening mammography is used to evaluate the asymptomatic woman in order to discover early, nonpalpable breast cancer. Women who have any clinical suspicion of disease should not be studied with a screening mammogram. It is also an inappropriate examination for women who have breast implants or prior breast-conserving treatment for malignancy. Guidelines for screening mammography in the United States advise that a woman begin mammographic screening at age 40. The American College of Radiology and the American Cancer Society recommend that annual screening commence at this age, although some groups recommend biannual screening for women in their 40s.

With the agreement by the National Cancer Institute and general consesus that screening should begin at age 40 years, the controversy as to the usefulness of screening women in their 40s has largely ceased. This controversy had been based largely on the paucity, for many years, of statistically significant results from screening studies that would clearly indicate that there is a reduction in breast cancer mortality resulting from this intervention. Modern data, however, clearly refute this doubt as to the efficacy of screening these women. Results from the prospective randomized screening program in Gothenburg, Sweden, demonstrated a 44% breast-cancer mortality reduction for women in their 40s who were screened versus those who did not undergo screening (215). This reduction was statistically significant [95% confidence interval (CI), 0.32–0.98 relative risk of breast-cancer death in the screened group]. Results from the Malmo screening trial showed a 36% reduction in breast-cancer mortality (95% CI, 0.45–0.89 relative risk) for women in their 40s due to mammographic screening (216). These reductions were comparable to those for women 50 years old and older who underwent screening. Additionally, meta-analysis of all eight prospective randomized mammographic screening trials shows a statistically significant 29% reduction in breast-cancer mortality for screened women in their 40s (95% CI, 0.57–0.89 relative risk) (217). There are also data based on population-based screening in Sweden showing that the widespread use of this screening tool can produce mortality reduction in women 40 and older (218). Analysis of the cost of screening women with mammography beginning at age 40 has demonstrated that in the United States this intervention has a marginal cost per year of life saved at $16,100 to $18,800 (219). This is comparable to other mortality-reduction measures that are widely accepted (220).

Interestingly, an upper age limit for screening in the United States has never been established. A positive impact for mammographic screening up to age 80 has been demonstrated (221).

Diagnostic Mammography

Diagnostic mammography is performed to assess clinical signs or symptoms, to follow up women who have undergone breast conservation, and to image the augmented breast. Frequently, in all of these situations, more than the routine two screening views are required to fully evaluate the breast. For the augmented breast, at least four views are obtained, providing that the implant can tolerate displacement (222). In women who have undergone breast conservation, additional views are frequently necessary in order to adequately assess the tumorectomy site and to offset difficulties in positioning due to postirradiation fibrosis. All of these studies should be monitored by a radiologist while they are being done.

Mammography is sensitive for the detection of breast cancer, finding about 90% of cancer that can be found in a screening setting; however, it is not very specific. Of nonpalpable lesions that are found on mammography and are suspicious for carcinoma, only 20% to 40% will be found to be malignant at tissue sampling. In interpreting a mammogram, primary findings of tumor are those found within the primary cancer itself. These consist of the presence of a mass and/or calcifications. The pattern of masses formed by carcinomas is determined by the cellular proliferation of the tumor and the aggressiveness in invading surrounding tissue or inciting a scirrhous reaction in the surrounding breast. As breast masses are increasingly lobulated or spiculated, the likelihood that they are malignant increases (223) (Fig. 30.16). Spiculated masses can, however, be caused by nonmalignant entities such as scars, focal fibrosis, sclerosing adenosis, and radial scars. Also, masses that are either well defined and round or oval can be malignant, as in cases of intracystic papillary carcinomas or medullary and colloid cancers. In lesions that have some lobulation or spiculation of their contours, the possibility that they are malignant is great enough to warrant biopsy. In masses that are smooth, round or oval, the likelihood that they are malignant is less than 1%, and short-term mammographic follow-up after 6 months to ensure stability is appropriate (224).

As with masses, calcifications have a spectrum of mammographic patterns that vary according to the underlying histopathology (225). Large, coarse calcifications are invariably caused by tissue death, as in fat necrosis, and these are not a worrisome finding (Fig. 30.17). Round, punctate, and centrally lucent calcifications are also benign and should not lead to biopsy. Calcifications that are widely scattered throughout the breast with no clustering cannot be carcinoma either, since cancer is a focal, not diffuse, process. When calcifications are irregular, pleomorphic, and clus-

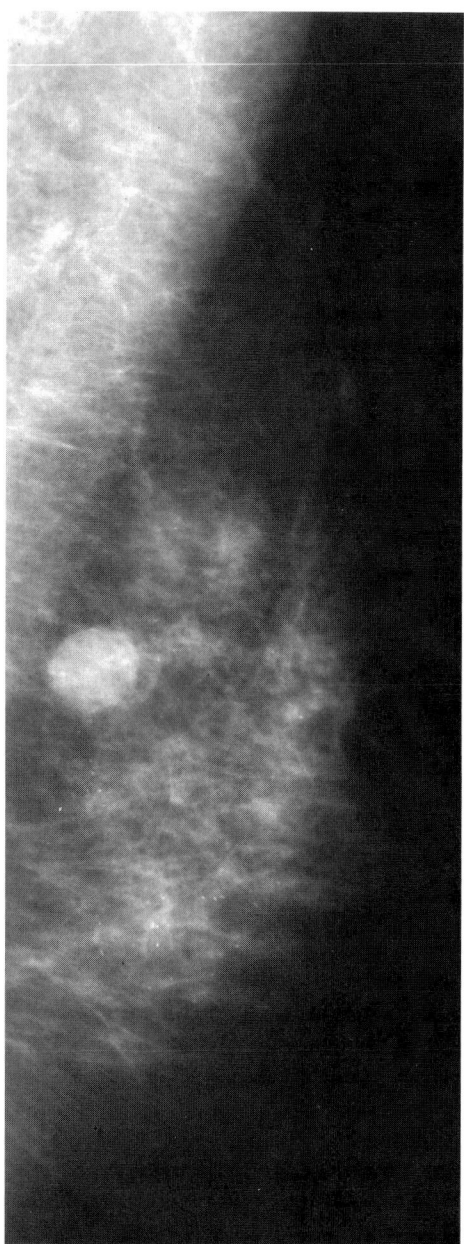

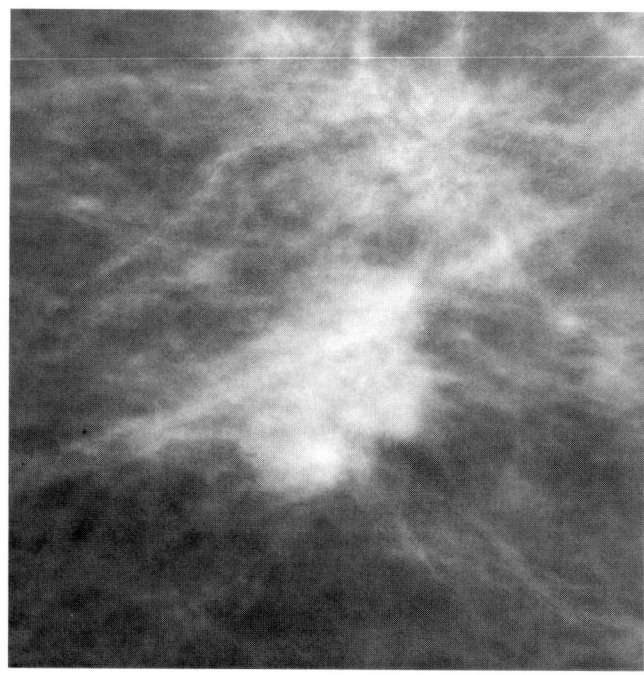

FIG. 30.16. A: Mammography demonstrates a well-defined, uncalcified, round mass in the upper breast. These characteristics are benign, reflecting the innocent nature of this cyst. **B:** This breast mass is irregular and spiculated. These characteristics reflect uncontrolled cellular proliferation and local invasion of this infiltrating ductal carcinoma.

tered, their pattern is nonspecific and will be due to cancer in about one-third of cases (226). Linear calcifications in the breast can be caused by the calcification of debris within the ducts. When the ducts are filled with carcinoma, their walls are irregular, and the pattern of these linear calcifications takes a similarly irregular form (Fig. 30.18). When ducts are free of cancer, their walls are smooth and parallel, and this becomes the pattern of these intraductal calcifications. Either of these types of intraductal, linear calcifications can also show branching patterns.

Secondary signs of carcinoma are findings beyond the primary tumor and can include architectural distortion, skin dimpling, nipple inversion, skin thickening, axillary adenopathy, and a prominent draining vein. When these signs are associated with mammographic or clinical patterns that suggest a possible breast cancer, they are supportive of that diagnosis. Their presence can also suggest more locally advanced tumor.

The American College of Radiology has produced a system for the standardization of mammography reporting. The Breast Imaging Reporting and Data System (BI-RADS) presents a uniform set of descriptors for mammographic findings (227). It also standardizes patient management recommendations based on the mammographic pattern (Table 30.8) (228). Inclusion of these management recommendations is required by the Food and Drug Administration in all mammogram reports. It is also required that mammography facilities notify all women of the results of their mammo-

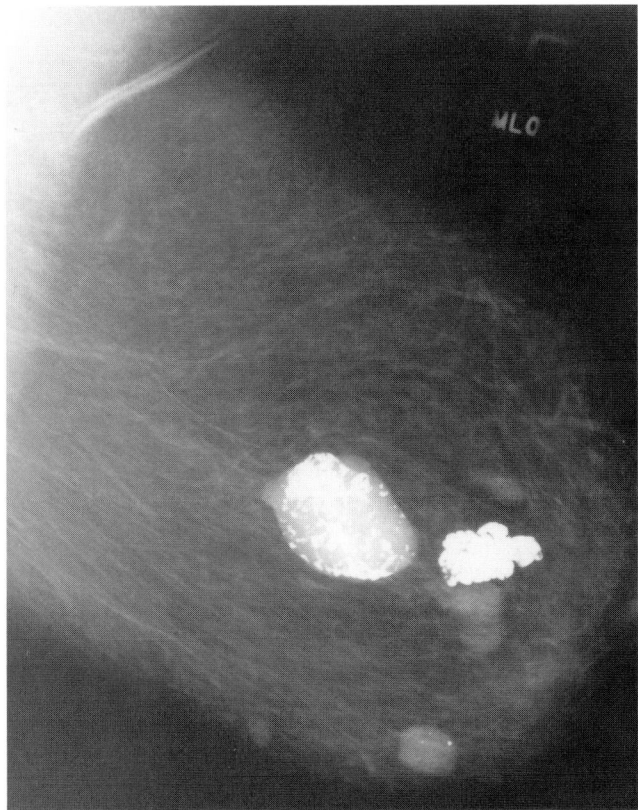

FIG. 30.17. Coarse calcifications are present in several well-defined masses. These are all fibroadenomas. The calcifications are dystrophic, caused by the calcification of dead tissue in these aging fibroadenomas.

gram in writing. This latter requirement does not, however, relieve a facility of the need to send a formal, medical report to the referring physician.

Screening for High-Risk Women and Non-mammographic Imaging Screening

For women at high risk for developing breast cancer at a young age, earlier mammographic screening is indicated. In its most recent breast cancer screening recommendations, the American Cancer Society recognized that these women may benefit from screening, although data to confirm this are not available (229). This group includes women with a personal history of breast cancer and a biopsy diagnosis of lobular carcinoma *in situ*. For these women, annual mammography commencing at the time of their diagnosis is indicated. For women who have been treated for Hodgkin's disease with mantle irradiation, irradiation-induced breast cancer can develop within 10 years of their treatment. Mammographic screening of these women is recommended commencing 8 years after their treatment (230).

For women with a strong family history, recommendations are based on the assumptions that these cancers fre-

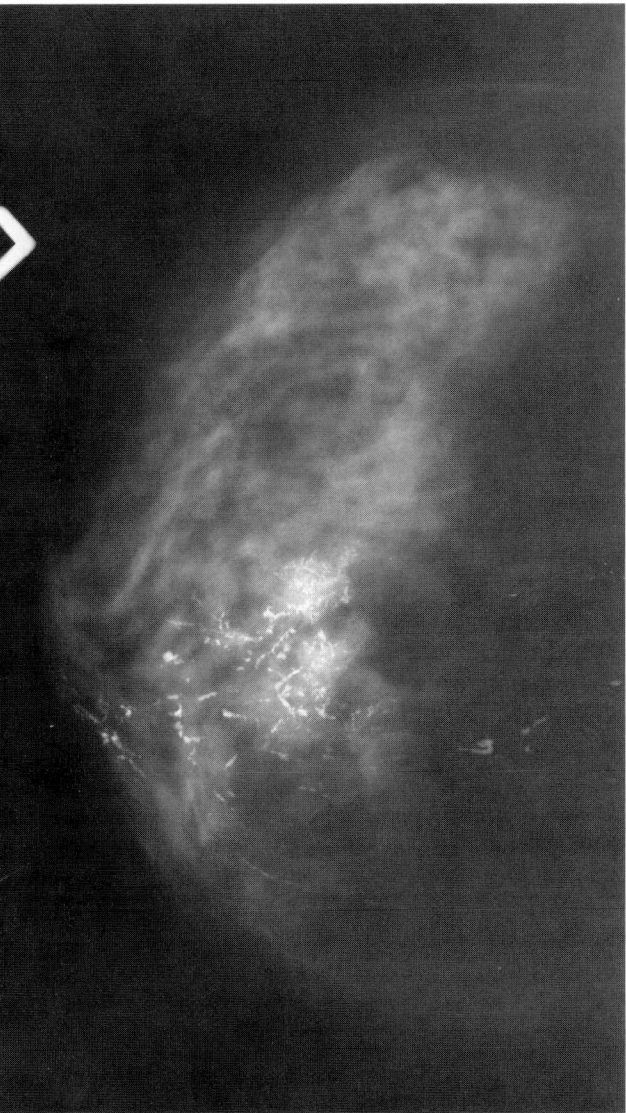

FIG. 30.18. This patient presented with possible Paget's disease of the nipple. Extensive, pleomorphic, fine calcifications are seen throughout much of the volume of the breast and are due to a large, infiltrating ductal carcinoma, which extends to the nipple and causes the finding of Paget's disease in this patient.

quently develop at an increasingly early age in succeeding generations and that mammography can diagnose breast cancers 2 to 4 years before they are clinically evident. Owing to the rarity of this disease in women under 25 years of age, however, as well as the difficulty in interpreting mammograms in many of these young women, and the sensitivity of the younger breast to radiation, screening mammography is not initiated before age 25 (231).

Experience with *BRCA*-positive women is very limited, and screening recommendations in this population are tentative. Mammographic screening should begin between 25 and 35 years of age. Determination of the age at which screening

TABLE 30.8. *The Breast Imaging Reporting and Data System (BI-RADS): patient management recommended by mammographic pattern*

Assessment categories
a. Assessment Is Incomplete:

Category 0
Need Additional Imaging Evaluation and/or Prior Mammograms For Comparison:
Finding for which additional imaging evaluation is needed. This is almost always used in a screening situation. Under certain circumstances this category may be used after a full mammographic work-up. A recommendation for additional imaging evaluation includes the use of spot compression, magnification, special mammographic views, ultrasound, and so forth.
Whenever possible, if the study is not negative and does not contain a typically benign finding, the current examination should be compared to previous studies. The radiologist should use judgement on vigorously to attempt obtaining previous studies. Category 0 should only be used for old film comparison when such comparison is **required** to make a final assesment.
b. Assessment Is Complete—**Final** Categories

Category 1
Negative:
There is nothing to comment on. The breasts are symmetric and no masses, architectural distortion, or suspicious calcifications are present.

Category 2
Benign Finding:
Like category 1, this is a "normal" assessment, but here, the interpreter chooses to describe a benign finding in the mammography report. Involuting, calcified fibroadenomas, multiple secretory calcifications, fat-containing lesions such as oil cysts, lipomas, galactoceles, and mixed-density hamartomas all have characteristically benign appearances and may be labeled with confidence. The interpreter may also choose to describe intramammary lymph nodes, vascular calcifications, implants, or architectural distortion clearly related to prior surgery while still concluding that there is no mammographic evidence of malignancy.
Note that both Category 1 and Category 2 assessments indicate that there is no mammographic evidence of malignancy. The difference is that Category 2 should be used when describing one or more specific benign mammographic findings in the report, whereas Category 1 should be used when no such findings are described.

Category 3
Probably Benign Finding(s)-Short-term Interval Follow-Up Suggested:
A finding placed in this category should have less than or equal to 2% risk of malignancy. It is not expected to change over the follow-up interval, but the radiologist would prefer to establish its stability.
There are several prospective clinical studies demonstrating the safety and efficacy of short-term follow-up for specific mammographic findings (1–5).
Three specific findings are described as being probably benign (the noncalcified circumscribed solid mass, the focal asymmetric density and the cluster of round [punctate] calcifications; the latter is anecdotally considered by some radiologists to be an absolutely benign feature). All the published studies emphasize the need to conduct a complete diagnostic imaging evaluation before making a probably benign (Category 3) assessment; hence it is inadvisable to render such as assessment in interpreting a screening examination. Also, all the published studies exclude palpable lesions, so the use of a probably benign assessment for a palpable lesion is not supported by scientific data. Finally, because evidence from all the published studies indicates the need for biopsy rather than continued follow-up when most probably benign finding increases in size or extent, it is inadvisable to render such an assessment when a finding that otherwise meets "probably benign" imaging criteria is either new or has increased in size or extent.
While the vast majority of findings in this category will be managed with an initial short-term follow-up (6 months) examination followed by additional examinations until longer-term (2 years or longer) stability is demonstrated, there may be occasions where biopsy is done (patient wishes or clinical concerns).

Category 4
Suspicious Abnormality – Biopsy Should Be Considered:
This category is reserved for findings that do not have the classic appearance of malignancy but have a wide range of probability of malignancy that is greater than those in Category 3. Thus, most reccommendations of breast interventional procedures will be placed within this category. By subdividing Category 4 into 4A, 4B, and 4C, it is encouraged that relevant probabilities for malignancy be indicated within this category so the patient and her physician can make an informed decision on the ultimate course of action.

Category 5
Highly Suggestive of Malignancy – Appropriate Action Should Be Taken:
These lesions have a high probability (=95%) of being cancer. This category contains lesions for which one-stage surgical treatment could be considered without preliminary biopsy, although current oncologic management may require percutaneous tissue sampling as, for example, when sentinel node imaging is included in surgical treatment or when neoadjuvant chemotherapy is administered at the outset.

Category 6
Known Biopsy Proven Malignancy – Appropriate Action Should Be Taken
This category is reserved for lesions identified on the imaging study with biopsy proof of malignancy prior to definitive therapy.

Reprinted with the permission of the American College of Radiology (ACR): ACR BI-RADS® – Mammography. 4th Edition. In: *ACR breast imaging reporting and data system, Breast Imaging Atlas.* Reston,VA, American College of Radiology, 2003. No other representation of this material is authorized without expressed, written permission from the American College of Radiology.

should begin can be calculated using the same formula as is used for those women with a strong family history (annual screening beginning 10 years earlier than the youngest first-degree relative presented with breast cancer, but not earlier than age 25).

The ability of non-mammographic imaging techniques to reduce breast cancer mortality has not been demonstrated. Multiple reports have shown that sonography and MRI are able to find breast cancers not seen on mammography. Many of these have been in breasts with known cancer or women with known cancer. There are no recommendations for the routine use of non-mammographic screening with an imaging modality for breast cancer. Studies are underway to assess the value of sonography and MR in screening, but outside of a study there is no indication for their use in this setting.

Breast Ultrasound

Sonography of the breast is an important adjunct to mammography in the diagnosis of breast disease (232). Its role was established based on its ability to differentiate a cyst from other masses in the breast. When the ultrasound criteria of a thin wall in a round or oval mass without internal echoes and with increased through-transmission are seen, a definitive diagnosis of a simple cyst can be made, and no further workup or biopsy is necessary (Fig. 30.19). Breast cysts, however, are often septated or contain internal echoes due to debris, and this can confound the diagnosis. Aspiration may be necessary for these lesions.

The sonographic diagnosis of solid masses is less reliable. Several criteria have been described that suggest the diagnosis of carcinoma (233). These include spiculation, angular

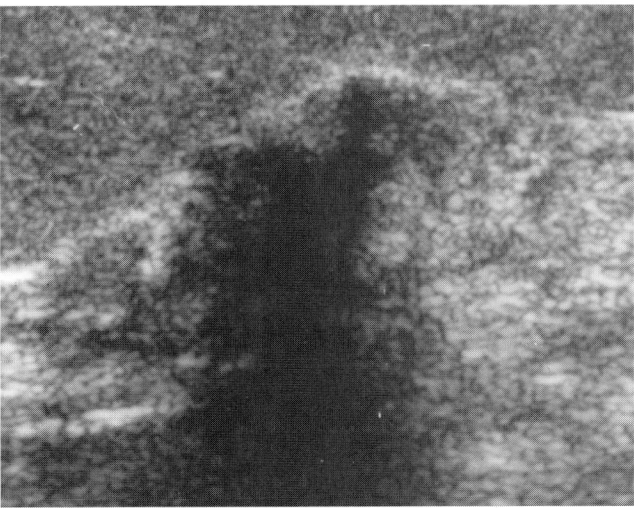

FIG. 30.20. The sonographic characteristics of this mass are that it is echo-dense, irregular, ill-defined, lobulated, and casts a shadow. These are all consistent with the diagnosis of infiltrating ductal carcinoma.

margins, marked hypoechogenicity, shadowing, the extension of the lesion into a duct, the presence of a branch pattern, and microlobulation. These are also often taller than they are wide (Fig. 30.20). Benign solid masses are most often characterized by the absence of the above findings, hyperechogenicity, minimal lobulation, ellipsoid shape, and a thin, echogenic pseudocapsule. Unfortunately, the sonographic pattern of a breast mass does not permit a definite diagnosis to be made (234). Therefore, tissue sampling of these lesions is often necessary.

Owing to the relative hypervascularity of breast cancer and the hypovascular nature of most benign lesions, sonographic interrogation using Doppler has been applied to breast masses to attempt to differentiate benign from malignant disease (235). This application has not found widespread acceptance, although it can augment information obtained from traditional gray-scale ultrasound.

In the workup of a young woman with a palpable mass, sonography is the first imaging study that is usually obtained. If it is possible to make a definitive diagnosis of a breast cyst, then no further workup is needed. If the mass is solid, mammography is useful to obtain additional information on the presence of calcifications within the lesion, or on the presence of other, nonpalpable disease within the breast.

Screening with sonography is not an accepted technique at this time. Because of the inability of sonography to image reliably microcalcifications commonly found with breast cancers, particularly with ductal carcinoma *in situ,* many cancers would be missed if screening were done with sonography. Sonography also has a very high false-positive rate, identifying many clinically unimportant lesions as requiring biopsy. Although published experience has demonstrated that some cancers that would otherwise go undetected can

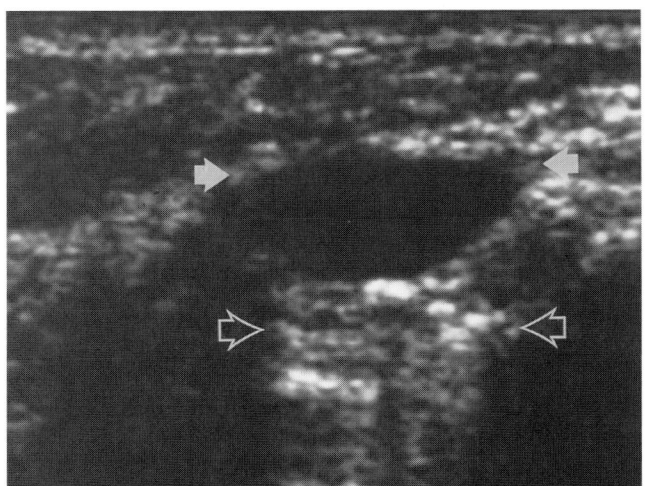

FIG. 30.19. Sonography was used to further assess this non-palpable mass that appeared on a mammogram. The mass (*solid arrows*) is oval, echo-free, and thin walled. There is enhancement of the sound beam beyond the lesion (*open arrows*). These characteristics are diagnostic of a simple cyst.

be found by sonography (236), the use of screening breast sonography is not presently accepted (232). It is, however, under investigation for select groups of women.

Sonography is also a useful tool in the evaluation of women with breast augmentation (237). In this setting it can be used to assess implant complications and palpable lesions. Sonographic criteria make it possible to differentiate silicone granulomas from other breast masses. Additionally, sonography is a valuable tool in guiding needle biopsy procedures.

Magnetic Resonance Imaging

Technical advances in the last decade have made magnetic resonance imaging (MRI) an increasingly utilized tool in the diagnosis and staging of breast cancer (238). Unlike mammography and sonography, however, MRI in this setting is considered minimally invasive because of the need to inject intravenous contrast material, which images tumor neovascularity. Owing to the ability of MRI to differentiate fat, silicone, and breast tissue, it is the best technique for the imaging diagnosis of implant complications and does not require an intravenous contrast agent (239). Although its ability to detect and stage ductal carcinoma in situ remains somewhat controversial, MRI appears to be reliable in imaging invasive cancer, often demonstrating the size and extent of the tumor within the breast with greater reliability than other imaging techniques (Fig. 30.21). It can therefore be a useful tool in assessing the extent of cancer in the breast in women with invasive carcinoma who are contemplating breast conservation (240). For the woman undergoing breast conservation in whom residual disease is suspected, MRI done after surgery can be useful in determining the adequacy of excision (241). Owing to the avascular pattern of scars and the hypervascular pattern of tumor recurrence, MRI can also be used to differentiate recurrent tumor from fat necrosis after breast conservation (242).

Some special applications of breast MRI include detection of the site of primary carcinoma in the breast in women with clinically evident axillary nodal metastases and no other evidence of breast tumor (243), assessment of possible axillary nodal metastases (244), and evaluation of response to nonsurgical treatment of women with locally advanced disease (245). Pitfalls in the interpretation of breast MRI have to do with false-positive examinations caused by enhancing normal glandular tissue in premenopausal women and focal benign lesions with an enhancement pattern similar to that of carcinoma. This pattern has been reported in hypercellular myxoid fibroadenomas, atypical hyperplasia, lobular carcinoma in situ, and other proliferative lesions of the breast (246). Increasingly, facilities have acquired the technology needed for MRI localization and MR-guided biopsy procedures. The absence of this technology has limited the clinical application of breast MR in the early twenty-first century, but this limitation appears increasingly not to be an issue.

Radiologic Workup of a Palpable Breast Mass

The imaging workup of the patient with a palpable breast mass depends on the communication of the presence of this mass to the radiologist, the age of the patient, the availability of prior studies for comparison, and the radiographic density of the breast. It is most important for the clinician to understand that the presence of a new, palpable breast mass without associated imaging findings does not indicate that the palpable lesion is not malignant. *A negative imaging workup does not negate the worrisome nature of a new palpable breast mass.* Additionally, young age does not negate the possibility of malignancy in a breast mass; it only makes it less likely than in the older patient. In women who have won litigation over the missed diagnosis of breast cancer, the most common presentation was a premenopausal patient (62% <50 years; 31% <40 years) complaining of a new, palpable mass that she has discovered (60%) (247).

The adequate workup of these patients requires communication of the presence of a palpable lesion to the radiologist examining the patient. Although the patient often communicates this information, the referring clinician should also convey it. It is of value to mark the site of the palpable mass on the skin of the breast to facilitate localization of the lesion so that the imaging assessment can be correctly directed to the site in question.

In some facilities the initial study in the workup of a palpable mass in all women 35 years old or younger is a sonogram;

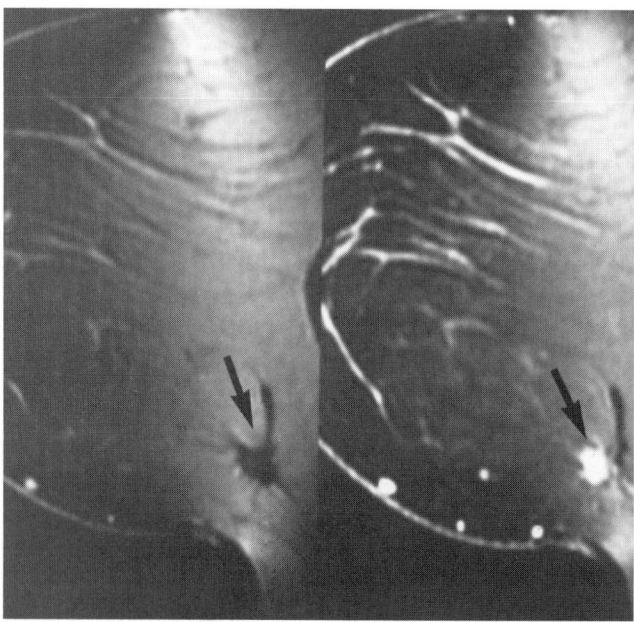

FIG. 30.21. A spiculated mass in the lower half of this breast (*arrows*) is imaged before and after intravenous contrast material (gadolinium) with magnetic resonance imaging. Enhancement of this breast carcinoma is due to tumor neovascularity. The configuration of the mass and its enhancement are virtually diagnostic for malignancy.

in other facilities this will be reserved for women 30 years old or younger. If this study demonstrates that a simple cyst is the reason for the mass, no further workup is necessary. If this is not found to be the case, mammography is performed (which might be diagnostic), or if there are other, non-palpable lesions present.

In the older woman, the workup begins with a two-view mammogram. In many facilities, a radiopaque marker will be placed over the palpable mass, documenting that the facility was aware of the presence of the lesion. Additional mammographic views may be done, including focal compression to displace surrounding tissue, magnification for better definition of the margins of a mass or the shape of associated calcifications, tangential views to displace the mass from obscuring dense breast tissue or augmentation prosthesis, and specialized views to image areas of the breast that are difficult to include on the routine two-view mammogram.

In the patient who has a noncalcified mass, additional information can often be obtained from sonography of the lesion. Even when a mass is palpable, however, sonography may not show a focal lesion in some cases, and this does not exclude the possibility of carcinoma (248). When calcifications are present within a mass, this excludes the diagnosis of a simple cyst, often making sonography unnecessary. Additionally, the pattern of calcifications often makes it possible to make a definitive diagnosis of degenerating fibroadenoma, or strongly suggests the possibility of malignancy. Spiculated masses are never due to a cyst, and sonography is not part of the workup of these lesions.

In those cases in which the imaging workup does not contribute to narrowing the differential diagnosis, the need for biopsy or clinical follow-up is based on the results of the physical examination and the patient history. In the case of women in whom a palpable lesion lies within a volume of breast tissue that is fatty on the mammogram, it is unlikely that the lesion is due to carcinoma (248).

DIAGNOSTIC WORKUP

Physical Examination and Findings

A complete clinical history and physical examination of the breast and axillary regions is of paramount importance in the evaluation of a patient suspected to have breast cancer. All examinations should begin with a thorough inspection of each breast, with special attention paid to any skin changes (such as discoloration, thickening, or dimpling), any changes in the nipple or areolar complex (including retraction, bleeding, discharge, or eczematous changes), and any readily evident abnormalities of symmetry of the breasts.

Changes in the skin may occur for multiple reasons. If a tumor is superficial, it will often cause a bulge of the overlying skin. It may also cause some retraction of skin owing to direct extension. Deeper tumors will on occasion also cause retraction of the skin by involvement of the fibrous septa of the breast (also known as Cooper's ligaments).

When present, edema of the breast is most often diffuse and known as *peau d'orange*. The most common cause of this physical finding is the presence of tumor within the dermal lymphatics causing obstruction of flow. It may, however, also be caused by bulky axillary adenopathy, or from prior surgery to the area. Therefore, it is not inevitably due to malignancy.

The supraclavicular, infraclavicular, and axillary lymph node basins must be palpated to determine whether there is clinically evident regional nodal disease. If axillary lymph nodes are palpable, it is important to classify the disease as N1 (mobile lymph nodes) or N2 (fixed or matted lymph nodes). Palpation of the breast should always be performed in both the sitting and the supine positions. Occasionally, tumors in close proximity to the chest wall may be difficult to palpate with the patient supine but will be readily apparent with the patient in a sitting position. Likewise, retroareolar tumors are sometimes best felt in a sitting position.

In addition to palpable, hard, and irregular masses, it is important to be cognizant of any asymmetric thickening of the breast. While this may simply be indicative of a normal distribution of breast tissue in the given patient, it may also be a carcinoma (249). It is important to note that the most common presentation of an infiltrating lobular carcinoma is not of a mass but a firm density (250).

Biopsy Methods in Cases of Palpable Disease

The evaluation of a dominant breast mass may consist of any of several techniques including fine-needle aspiration (FNA), core biopsy using a large-gauge needle, or open biopsy, whether it be excisional or incisional. Each method has its own advantages and disadvantages.

It is important to note that prior concerns about performing a first procedure in which the diagnosis of breast cancer is made and then following it with definitive therapy at a later time are unsubstantiated by current evidence. There is no adverse impact on either local control or long-term survival as the result of a two-stage procedure (251–253).

When a palpable mass is present, the most significant aspect of the evaluation is to determine whether it is cystic or solid. In order to make this determination, FNA provides a simple, quick, and relatively inexpensive means of determining whether a structure is fluid-filled or solid (254,255). It has the advantage of avoiding an unnecessary open biopsy in the case that a questionable palpable lesion is found to be a cyst. Two factors of paramount importance in evaluating the FNA should be considered. The first is the technical success rate of the person performing the FNA (255). If the performer of the procedure is uncomfortable with it, the likelihood that the findings will provide important information diminishes (256). Additionally, a benign finding should not dissuade a surgeon from an open biopsy if it is felt that a lesion is highly suspect for carcinoma. In those cases, as in cases in which a lesion is relatively small, there may be a sampling error that leads to inability to accurately diagnose a cancer (257). When FNA is positive for adenocarcinoma and a lesion is clinically suspicious, it may be extremely helpful to be aware of this in planning for a definitive surgical procedure. In an evaluation of 133 biopsy-proven carcinomas in which initial biopsy was performed using an FNA technique, the cytology was read as positive in 68%, suspicious in 17%, and benign in 6% (258). Additionally, this study showed that 9% of specimens were inadequate for evaluation.

In most instances, the likelihood of a false-positive result when a specimen is read by a skilled cytopathologist will vary between 0% and 0.5%, with the average rate being under 0.2% (256,259). An additional advantage of FNA is present when the technique is used for the evaluation of presumed recurrences in the site of scar tissue after breast-conservation therapy has been performed. In these cases, the accuracy of the aspiration is similar to that of a palpable lesion in a nonirradiated breast, and it avoids the significant wound-healing complications that may occur with open biopsy (260,261). One disadvantage of the FNA is the fact that it is usually not possible to distinguish between an *in situ* lesion and an invasive carcinoma using this technique. In these instances, it is extremely important to perform further biopsy to determine whether the mass is invasive prior to undertaking an evaluation of the axillary region.

Core Biopsy

Core biopsy remains an option for the surgeon but is currently performed in most instances by the radiologist for nonpalpable lesions. Indications for core biopsy in a patient with a palpable breast mass may include the ability to distinguish *in situ* from invasive disease more definitively than is possible with FNA. Additionally, this technique is often used in the patient in whom stage IV disease is present and definitive surgical therapy will therefore not be undertaken. In these cases, it allows one to obtain enough tissue to demonstrate certain histologic characteristics of the tumor and is most helpful in testing for estrogen and progesterone receptor status of a tumor.

In settings in which a skilled cytopathologist trained in breast pathology is not available, this procedure may provide material more easily evaluated by the pathologist than material from a fine-needle aspirate. Any concern about a lesion being suspicious for cancer should be addressed, even if core biopsy demonstrates the lesion to be histologically benign.

In the United States approximately one-fifth of the 600,000 breast biopsies done each year are for nonpalpable lesions. Using percutaneous needle biopsy procedures, the cost of these can be reduced by one-third to one-half (262). These biopsies can often be done more quickly than can open surgical techniques, they eliminate scarring, and they

provide a definitive diagnosis in 80% to 90% of cases, thereby eliminating the need for diagnostic surgery (263).

Imaging guidance for placement of the biopsy needle into the breast lesion can be done using either stereotactic or sonographic guidance. Less commonly, MRI guidance for these biopsies is now available. Stereotactic guidance is an x-ray imaging system, like mammography, that obtains angled views of the lesion so that the position of the lesion within the breast can be calculated by triangulation. Tissue acquisition can be done using FNA cytology, large-gauge gun-needle devices, directional vacuum-suction biopsy probes, or larger-gauge oscillating biopsy probes. Under sonographic guidance, positioning of the biopsy probe within the breast is usually done freehand; stereotactic positioning is automated.

Lesions should undergo biopsy only after there has been a complete imaging workup. This should not be replaced with tissue sampling. Clinical considerations that may preclude these procedures include inability of the patient to tolerate the biopsy procedure, and coagulopathy that might result in significant hemorrhaging during the biopsy. Small lesions without adjacent landmarks should not be biopsied unless a localizing clip can be put in place (264). If the lesion requires reexcision, localization of this site may not be possible, and the removal of a larger than usual volume of tissue may be required, resulting in cosmetic deformity (265).

Because calcifications are not reliably seen with sonography, calcifications are biopsied using stereotactic guidance (Fig. 30.22A and B). Sonographic guidance is desirable for biopsy of masses in patients with thin breasts that cannot accommodate the length of the biopsy probe when the breast is in compression for a stereotactic biopsy and in those who cannot tolerate positioning on a stereotactic device because of severe arthritis of the spine or shoulder. When a stereotactic prone table is used, masses in the axilla or near the chest wall may be difficult to image on some women; in these cases sonographic guidance should be used (266).

Major complications of these procedures are rare, reported in 0.2% of core biopsies (267), and these are equally divided between hemorrhage and infection. Minor complications occur in up to one-half of patients (268), and include ecchymosis, pain, and emotional stress.

Large-core needle biopsy of the breast can be performed with a variety of technologies. This biopsy technique was originally introduced using gun-needle devices that were first used in prostate biopsy. It has become generally accepted to use a needle gauge of at least 14 to ensure adequate sample size with minimization of biopsy artifact that can compromise the histologic analysis (269). After each core of tissue is obtained, the needle is removed from the breast and repositioned for consecutive cores to be obtained. Larger volumes of tissue can be excised using directional vacuum-suction technology (e.g., Mammotome). Although this technology is more expensive, the increased volume of tissue

FIG. 30.22. Stereotatic biopsy of breast calcifications. **A:** Mammography reveals a cluster of pleomorphic microcalcifications that could be due to carcinoma and require biopsy. **B:** Images obtained during the stereotactic biopsy show the calcifications at the leading edge of the biopsy needle (*arrow*). The needle will be fired into these to obtain the tissue sample. **C:** Specimen radiography of the tissue removed at core biopsy shows that calcifications are present in multiple specimens. Histologic diagnosis was apocrine metaplasia and cysts containing calcium. **D:** Because the calcifications were totally removed and there were no adjacent landmarks, a localizing clip (*arrow*) was placed in the breast at the end of the stereotactic biopsy. This makes it possible to easily localize the area if reexcision is necessary.

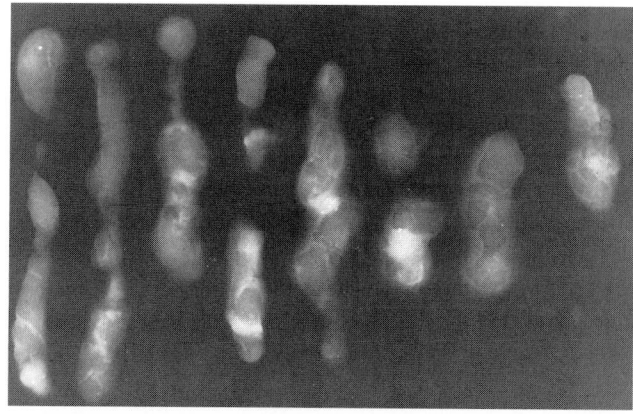

C

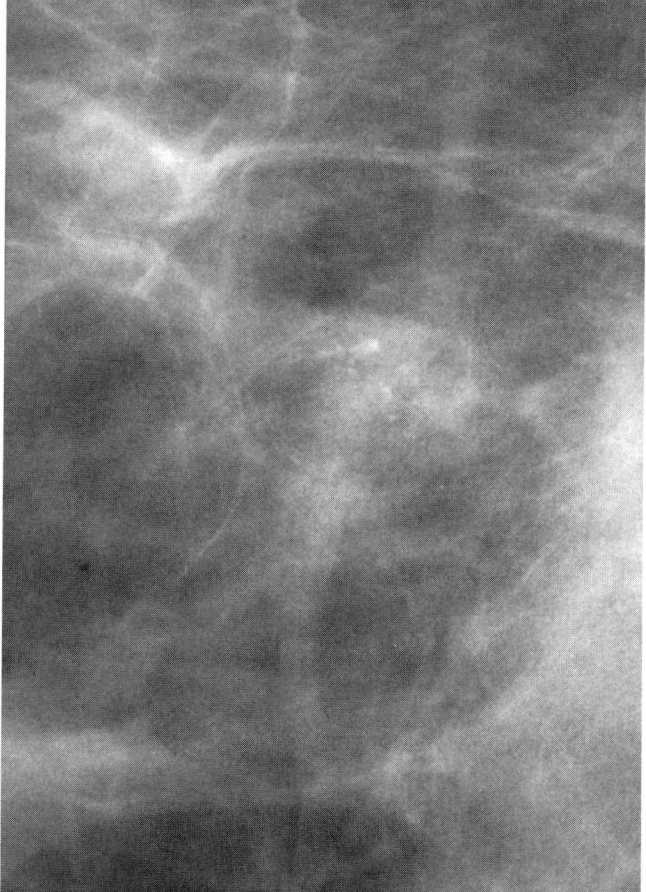

A

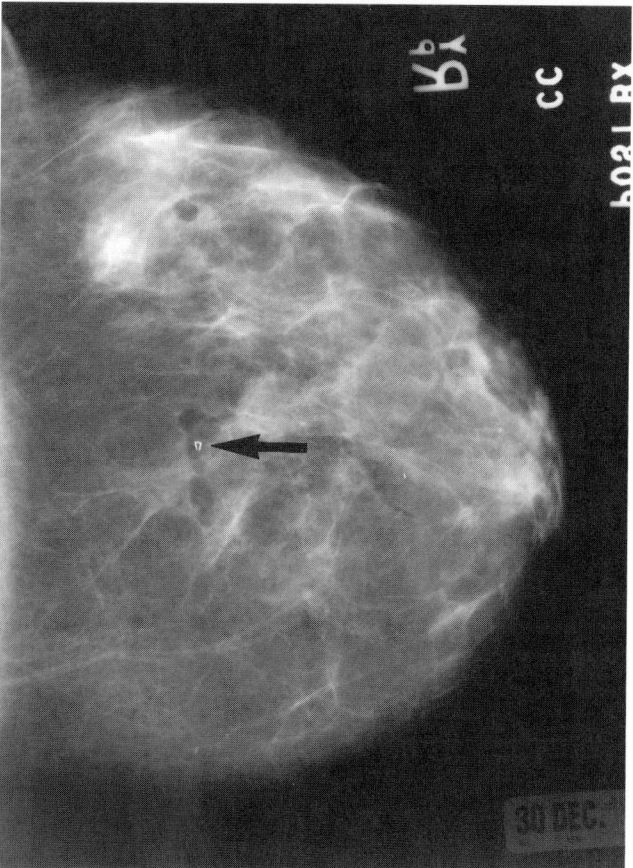

D

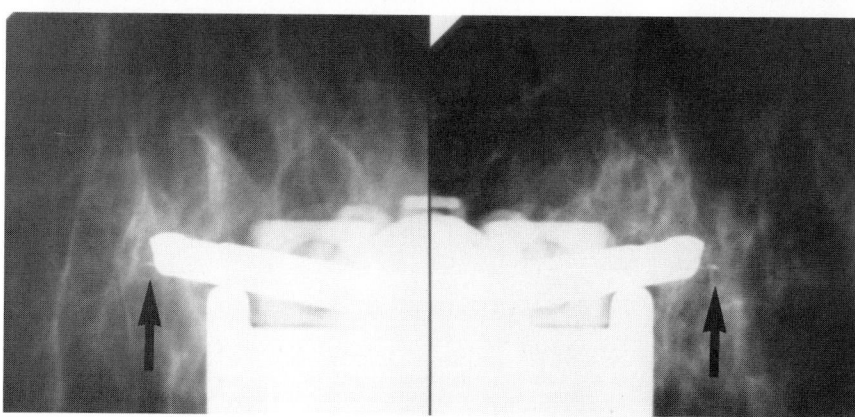

B

excised results in the more accurate diagnosis of some lesions, most importantly atypical ductal hyperplasia and ductal carcinoma *in situ* (270). When an 11-gauge vacuum-suction probe is used, a clip can be placed at the site of the lesion to mark its location (Fig. 30.22C and D). Localization for reexcision is therefore not compromised by total removal of these lesions.

Owing to the limited volume of tissue excised with needle biopsy procedures, some lesions will require surgical reexcision for a definitive diagnosis. Atypical ductal hyperplasia is routinely surgically excised, as coexistent carcinoma can be present. This has been found to be the case in up to 50% of women diagnosed with atypical ductal hyperplasia by 14-gauge core biopsy. Phyllodes tumors and some rare histopathologies require a larger volume of tissue for diagnosis than is usually obtained percutaneously. In some cases diagnosed as ductal carcinoma *in situ* at core biopsy, surgical excision will reveal areas of invasive cancer. This has been reported in 20% of cases diagnosed as ductal carcinoma *in situ* at 14-gauge core biopsy. In those lesions for which the histopathology is not concordant with the imaging pattern of the lesion, an assumption that the lesion was missed at the time of biopsy should be made, and rebiopsy of these lesions is indicated (268). There is controversy about the need for reexcision of some lesions including radial scar, papillary lesions, mucinous lesions, lobular carcinoma *in situ,* and atypical lobular hyperplasia. The management of these lesions will vary at different facilities.

Breast Biopsy with Preoperative Needle Localization

Of women who are sent to biopsy for nonpalpable lesions found on mammography or sonography, only about 20% to 40% will be found to have malignancy. The goals of preoperative wire localization are to ensure that the lesion in question is at least sampled at the time of surgical excision and to make it possible to achieve this with the removal of as little tissue as possible. These goals are most likely to be met when films are available for review by the radiologist before the needle localization is performed and when the radiologist and surgeon have agreed on the localization technique. Intraoperatively, specimen radiography should be available to monitor the success of the biopsy.

Failure to remove the lesion in question occurs in 1% to

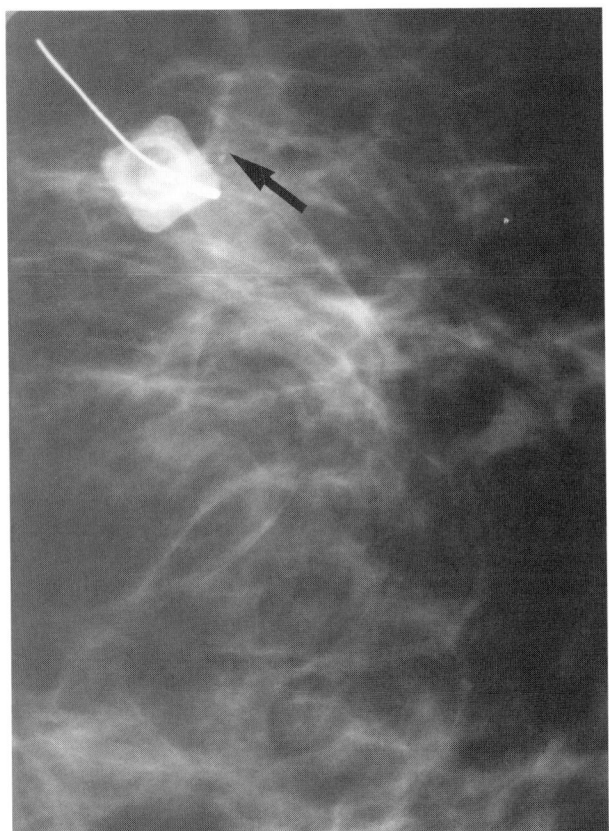
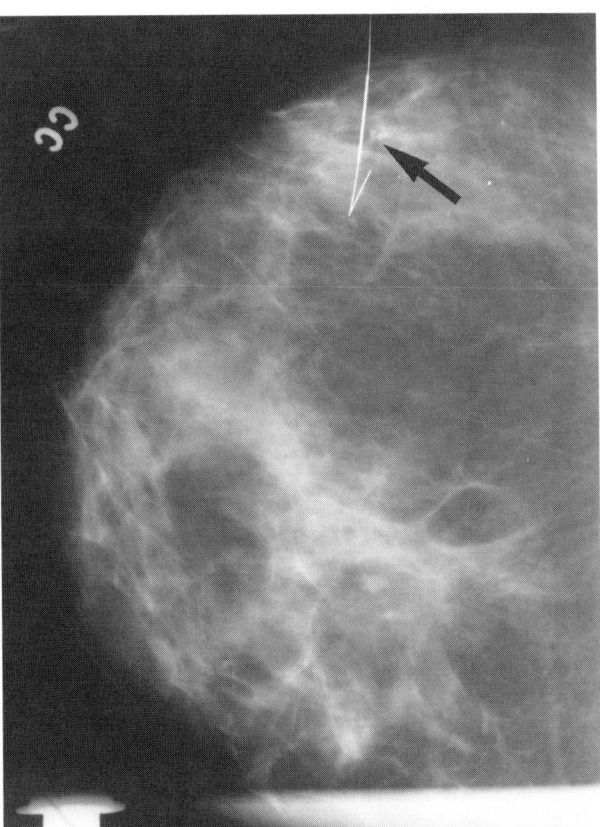

FIG. 30.23. Wire localization of nonpalpable breast calcifications. **A:** Needle containing a localizing wire has been positioned within a small cluster of microcalcifications. **B,C:** After accurate positioning of the needle, the needle is removed and the wire remains positioned in the breast, localizing the calcifications (*arrow*) on the craniocaudal (**B**) and mediolateral (**C**) views. Note the reinforced section of the wire near the end of the wire. (*Figure continues.*)

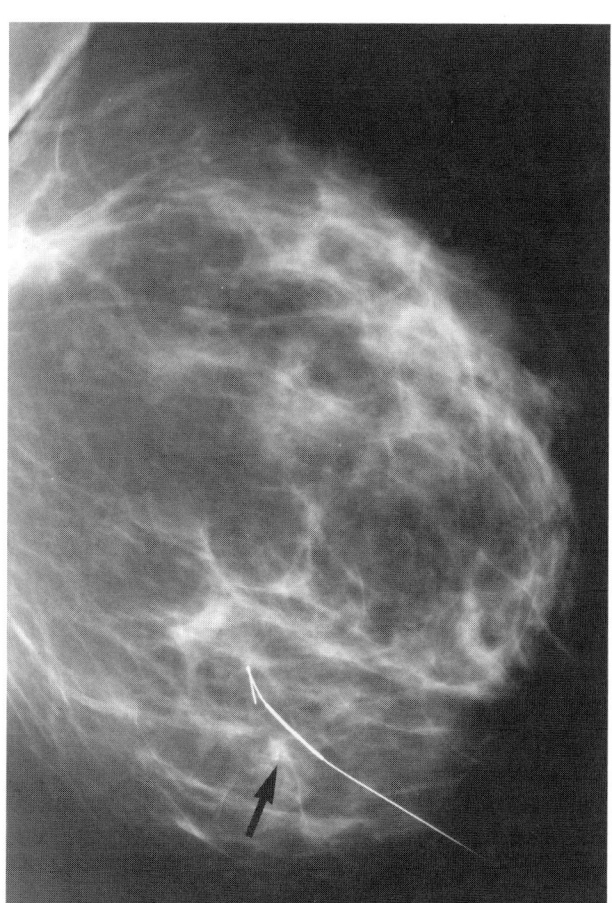

C

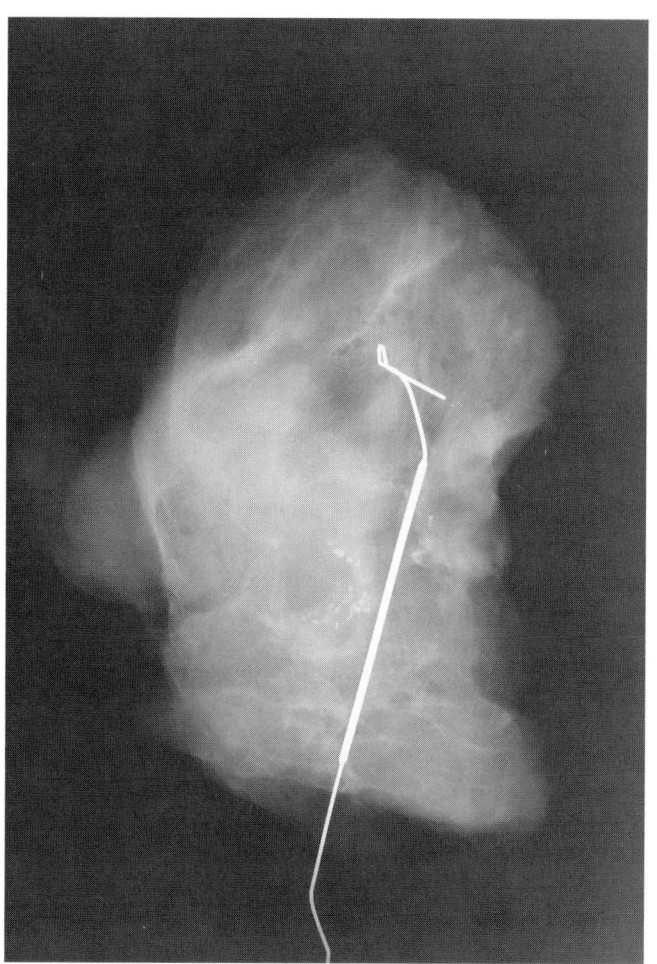

D

FIG. 30.23. Continued. **D:** Specimen radiograph of the removed tissue documents the presence of the worrisome calcifications within the specimen, surrounding the reinforced portion of the localizing wire. Histologic diagnosis was atypical ductal hyperplasia with calcifications.

8% of cases (271). Removal of more than one specimen may be necessary in 20% of cases.

Complications of the procedure are also rare. Fainting during the wire positioning is not uncommon, probably occurring in at least 1% of cases (272). This should not, however, result in cancellation of the procedure. Extreme pain and significant hemorrhaging during wire positioning are unusual occurrences. If the needle punctures the chest wall, pneumothorax can occur. Wires that are not adequately anchored to the skin can retract into the breast and become lost; they can then migrate within the breast and beyond. Transsection of the wire intraoperatively can result in the same occurrence.

Preoperative needle localization is easily performed and in most women is accomplished in about 30 minutes or less (Fig. 30.23). Preoperative sedation, if given, should not be administered until after the localization procedure. (Some facilities may give local anesthetic before the procedure, but this has been reported to be more painful than introduction of the wire into the breast) (273). The imaging studies on

which the procedure is to be based should have been reviewed. The patient is positioned for a mammogram, and the breast is compressed using a fenestrated compression paddle labeled with a grid. A single mammographic image is obtained, and location of the lesion to be localized is determined by its position on the grid coordinates. The skin over the lesion is cleansed, and a needle containing a wire is positioned at the appropriate depth within the breast corresponding to the previously identified grid coordinates. Two mammographic views are obtained. If necessary, the depth of the wire in the breast is adjusted. When appropriately positioned, the needle is withdrawn from the breast, and the localizing wire is left in place. A hook configuration at the wire tip stabilizes its position. The distal portion of the wire near the hook is thicker or "reinforced." This enables the surgeon to determine during dissection along the wire when the wire tip is being approached. After the wire has been positioned, a mammogram is obtained to demonstrate the relationship of the wire to the lesion; this is sent with the patient to surgery (274).

The wire tip or reinforced portion should be within 1 cm of the lesion to be excised. If a large volume of the breast is to be removed, such as in breast-conservation surgery for carcinoma, bracketing of the lesion can be accomplished by positioning more than one wire within the breast.

Lesions that are evident sonographically can be localized under sonographic guidance. Those seen only on one mammographic view can be localized using stereotaxis. In women who have augmentation prostheses in place, localization can usually be done without rupture of the prosthesis. However, it is wise to discuss this possibility with the patient and to note this discussion on the consent form.

Intraoperatively, for lesions seen mammographically, specimen radiography should be obtained. Specimen radiography can be performed using a mammography unit or an x-ray unit specifically designed for specimen radiography. This documents that the lesion in question has undergone biopsy and localizes its position within the removed tissue (Fig. 30.24). This enables the pathologist to direct histologic assessment to the appropriate site within the removed tissue. If the removed lesion is known to be malignant, specimen radiography is also useful in demonstrating extension of tumor to the margin of resection, indicating that further tissue should be removed.

Specimen radiography is reliable for the identification of calcification in the excised specimen. Most uncalcified masses can also be seen, although compression of the specimen may be needed. Areas of asymmetric density and architectural distortion are often difficult to identify on specimen radiography, which may be of little value when these lesions are excised.

Lesions seen only sonographically can have specimen sonography performed to document lesion removal and ascertain tumor transection. Lesions seen only on MR are identified by blood flow and therefore specimen imaging of these is not possible.

After histologic interpretation of the specimen has been performed, it is important that the imaging workup, localization films, and specimen radiographs be reviewed to ascertain that the suspicious lesion has been removed and diagnosed. If the lesion contains calcifications, the pathologist should note whether calcifications are seen and, if so, what histology is responsible for their formation. Failure to diagnose the lesion after its removal may require additional tissue sectioning. If calcifications are present within the lesion, radiography of the unsectioned tissue or the paraffin blocks can localize the area to be sectioned. If it is unclear whether the lesion has been excised or is still within the breast, repeat mammography may be necessary.

Open biopsy of physical abnormalities continues to be the gold standard for the evaluation of any suspected breast cancer. It provides information regarding the exact size and the histologic subtype of the tumor and makes it possible to assess the tumor margins and gives an indication of the presence of vascular and lymphatic invasion. Having this information may prove helpful in determining the appropriate definitive therapy for the patient.

It is also important to realize that open biopsy should be entertained in any patient in which a needle biopsy, whether it be an FNA or a core biopsy, demonstrates results discordant with the clinical or mammographic scenario. The concept of the "triple test" refers to the use of the clinical examination findings, the mammographic findings, and the results of an FNA to determine whether further investigation is warranted. When all three findings are consistent with a benign etiology of the mass, studies demonstrate a 99% predictive value for benign disease. If there is any discordance, however, open biopsy should be considered.

STAGING WORKUP

Once the diagnosis of breast cancer has been established, the patient requires a staging workup prior to any definitive treatment. For patients with only *in situ* lobular carcinoma, review of the mammograms and the pathology slides are sufficient, unless the patient opts for a total mastectomy. Laboratory studies, including a complete blood count and chemistry profile, would also be appropriate for this surgical procedure (275). For patients with ductal carcinoma *in situ*, review of the mammograms and pathology slides, paying particular attention to the status and width of the closest margin, is important (275). If breast conservation is selected by the patient, a postoperative mammogram demonstrating removal of any mammographic evidence of the disease is appropriate. If the patient chooses a total mastectomy, preoperative blood count and chemistry profile should be ordered as well.

For women with operable invasive breast cancer, the workup should include a blood count with platelets, liver

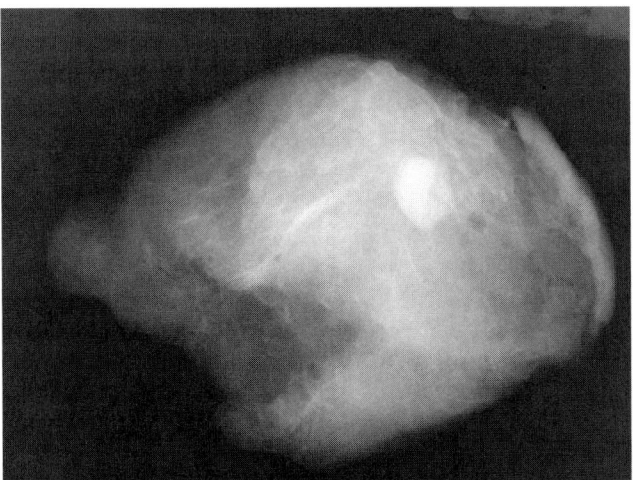

FIG. 30.24. Specimen radiograph of an excised mass documents the presence of a nonpalpable lesion within the specimen and not extending to the margins of resection. Histologic diagnosis was infiltrating ductal carcinoma.

function tests, a chest x-ray, bilateral mammograms with ultrasound as necessary, pathology review, and determination of intrinsic prognostic factors including estrogen and progesterone receptors and Her-2/*neu,* or ERB2, status. A bone scan and evaluation of the abdomen and pelvis by CT, ultrasound, or MRI are not likely to yield useful information in stage I disease, but are still part of the standard workup in many centers (275). For women with more advanced disease, these tests are important to rule out possible stage IV disease.

Staging Systems

The American Joint Committee on Cancer (AJCC) determines staging of breast cancer. The AJCC staging system is a clinical and pathologic staging system based on the tumor–node–metastasis (TNM) system. The new updated AJCC staging system (2002) incorporates sentinel node staging. It distinguishes micrometastasis from isolated tumor cells on the basis of size and histologic evidence of malignant activity. In the current AJCC staging system, supraclavicular lymph node metastasis is now classified as N3 disease, rather than M1 disease, as in the old system. Staging of the internal mammary nodes is also addressed (Table 30.9) (276).

MASTECTOMY IN THE TREATMENT OF BREAST CANCER

As early as the sixteenth century, rudimentary attempts to gain local control of breast cancer were made (277), and by the eighteenth century, the concept of an operative approach to breast cancer existed. It was at this time that Jean Louis Petit, the first director of the French Surgical Academy, advocated the removal of the breast, pectoral muscles, and axillary lymph nodes (278) for the treatment of breast cancer. While this should properly be considered the first radical mastectomy, it was not until the introduction of this procedure by Halsted in the late nineteenth century that the surgical community embraced it for the treatment of the majority of breast cancers (3,279). However, the concept of a less radical treatment for breast cancer quickly emerged, and as early as the 1920s, the need for a radical mastectomy was being questioned. While there were some early attempts at eradication of tumors by irradiation alone (280), the majority of early efforts to find an alternative were directed at reducing the extent of the surgical procedure. In 1948, Patey and Dyson (281) described what is now commonly referred to as the modified radical mastectomy, in which the breast tissue and the axillary contents are removed while a greater amount of overlying skin and the underlying pectoral muscles are preserved.

Several trials have now shown the modified radical mastectomy to be equivalent to treatment with a Halsted radical mastectomy with respect to local tumor recurrence and disease-free survival rates (282–284). In a randomized trial of

534 patients with stages I and II breast cancer, there was no difference in overall survival, disease-free survival, or local recurrence rates, regardless of the surgical procedure employed (284). A similar result was noted by Maddox et al. in 311 patients randomized to either procedure (283). By 1976, the American College of Surgeons survey found that modified radical mastectomy was the most commonly performed procedure for the treatment of early-stage breast cancer (285). Even today, with significant interest in breast-preservation procedures, it continues to be a widely used treatment option for early-stage breast cancer (286).

Concurrently a group of surgeons began to advocate more extensive surgical procedures, based on the concept of an orderly progression of disease and the belief that the internal mammary lymph nodes might also be involved in the progression; approximately 25% of the lymphatic drainage of the breast is directed toward the internal mammary lymph nodes (287), and these are not addressed by a standard radical mastectomy. The extended radical mastectomy was therefore developed to address these nodes and included either an en bloc or discontinuous dissection of the nodes in addition to a standard radical mastectomy.

The reported incidence of internal mammary node involvement varied in different series but averaged approximately 20% (288). Disease was most commonly seen with larger, inner-quadrant lesions. Additionally, the likelihood of involvement of the internal mammary nodes significantly correlated with involvement of the axillary lymph nodes. In one of the largest series of patients to undergo extended radical mastectomy, Urban and Marjani (289) at Memorial Sloan–Kettering Cancer Center found that internal mammary nodes were involved in only 7% of patients with negative axillary lymph nodes. Moreover, the incidence of clinical internal mammary lymph node recurrence in various studies was exceedingly low, ranging from 0% to 5% (290).

Two randomized, prospective trials directly compared radical mastectomy with extended radical mastectomy (291–293). Neither trial was able to show a survival advantage for patients undergoing internal mammary lymph-node dissection. To date, there is rarely an indication for the use of internal mammary lymph-node dissection.

BREAST-CONSERVATION THERAPY

Frances Williams (294) first reported the use of radiation as the sole therapeutic agent to successfully treat a group of patients at Boston City Hospital. At approximately the same time, Geoffrey Keynes (295) at St. Bartholomew's Hospital in London and Mustakallio in Finland (296) began to experiment with the use of radium implants or external radiation for breast cancer. Keynes treated 325 patients with local tumor removal. All patients had radium implantation at the site of the local excision as well as in the axilla. The 5-year survival ranged from 23.6% to 71%, dependent on the extent of disease at the time of initial presentation. These and other

TABLE 30.9. *American Joint Committee on Cancer staging for breast cancer*

DEFINITION OF TNM
Primary Tumor (T)
Definitions for classifying the primary tumor (T) are the same for clinical and for pathologic classification. If the measurement is made by physical examination, the examiner will use the major headings (T1, T2, or T3). If other measurements, such as mammographic or pathologic measurements, are used, the subsets of T1 can be used. Tumors should be measured to the nearest 0.1 cm increment.

TX	Primary tumor cannot be assessed
To	No evidence of primary tumor
Tis	Carcinoma *in situ*
Tis (DCIS)	Ductal carcinoma *in situ*
Tis (LCIS)	Lobular carcinoma *in situ*
Tis (Paget's)	Paget's disease of the nipple with no tumor

Note: Paget's disease associated with a tumor is classified according to the size of the tumor.

T1	Tumor 2 cm or less in greatest dimension
T1mic	Microinvasion 0.1 cm or less in greatest dimension
T1a	Tumor more than 0.1 cm but not more than 0.5 cm in greatest dimension
T1b	Tumor more than 0.5 cm but not more than 1 cm in greatest dimension
T1c	Tumor more than 1 cm but not more than 2 cm in greatest dimension
T2	Tumor more than 2 cm but not more than 5 cm in greatest dimension
T3	Tumor more than 5 cm in greatest dimension
T4	Tumor of any size with direct extension to (a) chest wall or (b) skin, only as described below
T4a	Extension to chest wall, not including pectoralis muscle
T4b	Edema (including peau d'orange) or ulceration of the skin of the breast, or satellite skin nodules confined to the same breast
T4c	Both T4a and T4b
T4d	Inflammatory carcinoma

REGIONAL LYMPH NODES (N)
Clinical

NX	Regional lymph nodes cannot be assessed (e.g., previously removed)
N0	No regional lymph node metastasis
N1	Metastasis to movable ipsilateral axillary lymph node(s)
N2	Metastasis in ipsilateral axillary lymph nodes fixed or matted, or in clinically apparent* ipsilateral internal mammary nodes in the *absence* of clinically evident axillary lymph node metastasis
N2a	Metastasis in ipsilateral axillary lymph nodes fixed to one another (matted) or to other structures
N2b	Metastasis only in clinically apparent* ipsilateral internal mammary nodes and in the *absence* of clinically evident axillary lymph node metastasis
N3	Metastasis in ipsilateral infraclavicular lymph node(s) with or without axillary lymph node involvement, or in clinically apparent* ipsilateral internal mammary lymph node(s) and in the *presence* of clinically evident axillary lymph node metastasis; or metastasis in ipsilateral supraclavicular lymph node(s) with or without axillary or internal mammary lymph node involvement
N3a	Metastasis in ipsilateral infraclavicular lymph node(s)
N3b	Metastasis in ipsilateral internal mammary lymph node(s) and axillary lymph node(s)
N3c	Metastasis in ipsilateral supraclavicular lymph node(s)

Clinically apparent is defined as detected by imaging studies (excluding lymphoscintigraphy) or by clinical examination or grossly visible pathologically.

Pathologic (pN)[a]

pNX	Regional lymph nodes cannot be assessed (e.g., previously removed, or not removed for pathologic study)
pN0	No regional lymph node metastasis histologically, no additional examination for isolated tumor cells (ITC)

Note: Isolated tumor cells (ITC) are defined as single tumor cells or small cell clusters not greater than 0.2 mm, usually detected only by immunohistochemical (IHC) or molecular methods but which may be verified on H&E stains. ITCs do not usually show evidence of malignant activity e.g., proliferation or stromal reaction.

pN0(i −)	No regional lymph node metastasis histologically, negative IHC
pN0(i +)	No regional lymph node metastasis histologically, positive IHC, no IHC cluster greater than 0.2 mm
pN0(mol −)	No regional lymph node metastasis histologically, negative molecular findings (RT-PCR)[b]
pN0(mol +)	No regional lymph node metastasis histologically, positive molecular findings (RT-PCR)[b]

[a]Classification is based on axillary lymph node dissection with or without sentinel lymph node dissection. Classification based solely on sentinel lymph node dissection without subsequent axillary lymph node dissection is designated (sn) for "sentinel node," e.g., pN0(i ++ (sn).
[b]RT-PCR: reverse transcriptase/polymerase chain reaction.

pN1	Metastasis in 1 to 3 axillary lymph nodes, and/or internal mammary nodes with microscopic disease detected by sentinel lymph node dissection but not clinically apparent**
pN1mi	Micrometastasis (greater than 0.2 mm, none greater than 2.0 mm)

(continued)

TABLE 30.9. *Continued*

pN1a	Micrometastasis in 1 to 3 axillary lymph nodes
pN1b	Metastasis in internal mammary nodes with microscopic disease detected by sentinel lymph node dissection but not clinically apparent**
pN1c	Metastasis in 1 to 3 axillary lymph nodes and in internal mammary lymph nodes with microscopic disease detected by sentinel lymph node dissection but not clinically apparent** (If associated with greater than 3 positive axillary lymph nodes, the internal mammary nodes are classified as pN3b to reflect increased tumor burden)
pN2	Metastasis in 4 to 9 axillary lymph nodes, or in clinically apparent* internal mammary lymph nodes in the *absence* of axillary lymph node metastasis
pN2a	Metastasis in 4 to 9 axillary lymph nodes (at least one tumor deposit greater than 2.0 mm)
pN2b	Metastasis in clinically apparent* internal mammary lymph nodes in the *absence* of axillary lymph node metastasis
pN3	Metastasis in 10 or more axillary lymph nodes, or in infraclavicular lymph nodes, or in clinically apparent* ipsilateral internal mammary lymph nodes in the *presence* of 1 or more positive axillary lymph nodes; or in more than 3 axillary lymph nodes with clinically negative microscopic metastasis in internal mammary lymph nodes; or in ipsilateral supraclavicular lymph nodes
pN3a	Metastasis in 10 or more axillary lymph nodes (at least one tumor deposit greater than 2.0 mm), or metastasis to the infraclavicular lymph nodes
pN3b	Metastasis in clinically apparent* ipsilateral internal mammary lymph nodes in the *presence* of 1 or more positive axillary lymph nodes; or in more than 3 axillary lymph nodes and in internal mammary lymph nodes with microscopic disease detected by sentinel lymph node dissection but not clinically apparent**
pN3c	Metastasis in ipsilateral supraclavicular lymph nodes

Clinically apparent is defined as detected by imaging studies (excluding lymphoscintigraphy) or by clinical examination.

***Not clinically apparent* is defined as not detected by imaging studies (excluding lymphoscintigraphy) or by clinical examination.

Distant Metastasis (M)

MX	Distant metastasis cannot be assessed
M0	No distant metastasis
M1	Distant metastasis

Used with the permission of The American Joint Committee on Cancer (AJCC), Chicago, Illinois. The original source for this material is the AJCC Cancer staging manual, 6th ed., 2002, published by Springer-Verlag, New York, www.springer-ny.com.

early reports regarding the long-term results of local surgery and irradiation in combination provided the impetus for later, randomized trials in the treatment of breast cancer.

Randomized Studies Comparing Breast-Conservation Therapy with Mastectomy

Since 1960, there have been seven randomized, prospective trials of breast-conservation therapy for invasive breast cancer. The earliest trial comparing breast conservation and radical mastectomy was conducted at Guy's Hospital in London (297). In this trial, 370 women with stages I and II breast cancer were randomized to either standard radical mastectomy or wide local excision and irradiation. The surgical excision was reported to encompass the tumor itself and approximately 3 cm of normal breast tissue. Whereas the patients undergoing a radical mastectomy had a standard dissection of the axilla, those patients who underwent a local excision did not have any surgical treatment for the axilla, even if there was clinical N1 disease. All patients in both groups were treated with what is now considered suboptimal radiation therapy of 35 to 38 Gy to the breast and 25 to 27 Gy to the axilla. In patients with clinical stage I disease, survival did not differ between the two groups. For patients

with stage II disease, however, survival was significantly lower in the group treated with local excision and irradiation. At 10 years of follow-up, local and regional recurrences were present in greater than 30% of patients with radiation, and with longer-term follow-up, the rate approached 50% (298).

Fortunately, multiple other randomized trials of breast-conservation therapy followed. From the National Tumor Institute of Milan in 1981, Veronesi (299) reported on 701 patients with tumors less than 2 cm and with clinically negative axillae who were randomized to be treated with either quadrantectomy and axillary dissection plus irradiation (50 Gy in 5 weeks to the breast and 10-Gy boost), or a standard Halsted radical mastectomy. Any woman found to have positive axillary lymph nodes on pathologic examination also received 12 cycles of adjuvant chemotherapy with Cytoxan, methotrexate, and 5-FU. Actuarial overall and disease-free survival rates were comparable in both groups; the crude incidence of local failure was 2.3% for patients who underwent radical mastectomy, and 8.8% for those with quadrantectomy and irradiation, at 20 years. Of note, a significant 66% of the failures in the breast-conserved group were outside of the index quadrant, representing true ipsilateral new breast cancers (300).

In the United States, the National Surgical Adjuvant

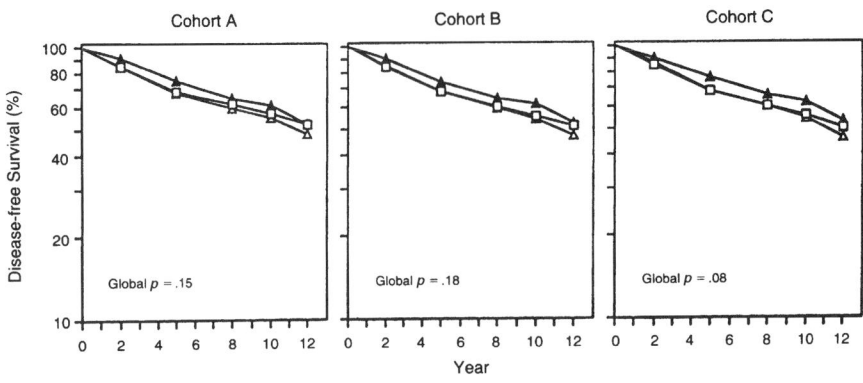

FIG. 30.25. Disease-free survival in three cohorts who were treated by total mastectomy, lumpectomy, or lumpectomy and breast irradiation. Cohort A represents patients analyzed according to randomized treatment assignment; Cohort B was analyzed according to analysis-per-protocol strategy (excluding 254 patients for various reasons); and Cohort C consisted of patients in Cohort B less all those enrolled by St. Luc's Hospital in Montreal. (Reprinted with permission from Fisher B, Anderson S, Redmond CK, et al. Reanalysis and results after 12 years of follow-up in a randomized clinical trial comparing total mastectomy with lumpectomy with or without irradiation in the treatment of breast cancer. *N Engl J Med* 1995;333:1456.)

Breast and Bowel Project (NSABP) performed a trial that not only compared modified radical mastectomy with segmental resection, axillary node dissection, and breast irradiation, but also included a third arm of patients who underwent segmental mastectomy without irradiation. The NSABP Protocol B-06 included 1,834 patients from multiple institutions with clinical stages I and II carcinoma less than 4 cm in size. The margins of the lumpectomy specimens were required to be grossly tumor-free; patients with margin involvement underwent total mastectomy. Irradiated patients received 50 Gy to the breast through tangential fields. Patients with positive axillary lymph nodes underwent adjuvant chemotherapy (301).

Fisher and colleagues updated the results of the NSABP Protocol B-06 in 2002; at 20 years (302) there is no significant difference in survival between patients treated with mastectomy or lumpectomy alone or in combination with irradiation (Fig. 30.25). The 20-year ipsilateral breast relapse rates were 39.2% for those with lumpectomy alone, and 14.3% in patients treated with lumpectomy and irradiation (Fig. 30.26).

The U.S. National Cancer Institute conducted a trial in which 237 patients with T1–2,N0,M0 disease were randomized to either modified radical mastectomy or breast-conservation therapy with lumpectomy and radiation therapy (45 to 50 Gy to breast plus boost) (303). After a median follow-up of 10 years, overall survival was 75% for the patients assigned to mastectomy and 77% for those treated with lumpectomy plus irradiation ($p = 0.89$). The rate of local-regional recurrence at 10 years was 10% after mastectomy and 5% after lumpectomy plus irradiation ($p = 0.17$) after patients with recurrences successfully treated with mastectomy were censored from the analysis.

Three other European randomized, prospective trials in-

clude the EORTC Breast Cancer Cooperative Group trial of 903 patients, 745 with stage II disease and the remainder with stage I, comparing modified radical mastectomy with breast-conservation surgery and radiation (304). Overall sur-

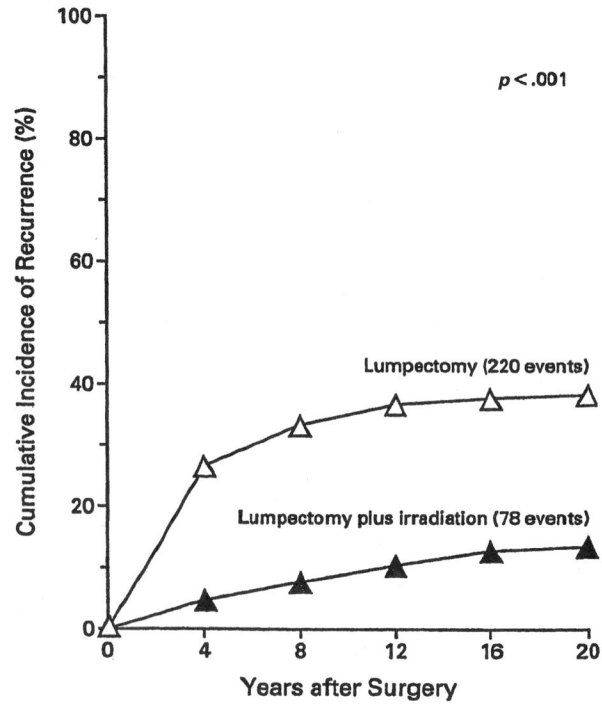

FIG. 30.26. Cumulative incidence of a first recurrence of cancer in the ipsilateral breast during 20 years of follow-up among 570 women treated with lumpectomy alone, and 567 treated with lumpectomy plus breast irradiation. The data are for women whose specimens had tumor-free margins. *N Engl J Med* 2002;347:1235.

vival and disease-free survival were comparable in both arms. The actuarial 8-year local tumor control rate was 91% in the mastectomy and 87% in the breast-conservation therapy groups (differences not statistically significant).

A Danish Cooperative Study randomized 905 women, of whom 859 patients were eventually evaluable (305). In high-risk patients (tumor >5 cm, invasion to skin and/or deep fascia, metastatic axillary lymph nodes) treated with breast-conservation therapy, the regional lymph nodes were also irradiated. Also, in high-risk patients treated with mastectomy, the same target volume was irradiated as in breast-conservation therapy, and all high-risk patients received adjuvant CMF. At 6 years the recurrence-free survival in 430 breast-conservation therapy patients was 70%, and in 429 patients in the mastectomy arm it was 66%. Overall survival rates were 79% and 82%, respectively. There were 12 breast relapses in the breast-conservation therapy patients (3%) and 19 chest-wall recurrences (4%) in the mastectomy group.

The Institut Gustave-Roussy also conducted a prospective randomized trial comparing mastectomy with local excision plus irradiation for women with cancers measuring 2 cm or less. Eighty-eight patients were treated with conservation surgery and irradiation, and 91 were treated with modified radical mastectomy without excision of the pectoral muscle (306,307). The 15-year disease-free survival rate was 55% for the tumorectomy group and 45% for the mastectomy group ($p = 0.23$). The 15-year local recurrence rate was 9% in the conservation surgery and irradiation group and 14% in the mastectomy group.

Nonrandomized Reports

Prior to the randomized, prospective trials detailed above, there were many nonrandomized trials of breast-conservation therapy. Additionally, many institutions continued to collect data on the outcomes experienced in the population of patients undergoing breast-conservation therapy in comparison with the outcomes of patients undergoing either radical or modified radical mastectomy.

Results described by multiple authors are summarized in Table 30.10 (167,169,171,195,196,308–326). Nonrandomized comparison of survival with radical mastectomy

TABLE 30.10. *Conservation surgery and irradiation in stages I and II breast cancer: results of selected nonrandomized studies*

Author	No. of patients	Stage	Irradiation dose (Gy) Breast	Irradiation dose (Gy) Boost	Local tumor control (%)	Excellent/good cosmesis (%)	10-year disease-free survival (%)
Amalric et al (308)	1,440	I, II	60	15–20	80	90	74
Barr et al (309a)	411	I, II, III	48.4	20	88	NS	NS
Bartelink et al (171)	585	T1,2	50	25	98	NS	T1 92[a], T2 85
Calle et al (309)	411	I, II	50	10	89	88	78
Clark et al (293)	1,504	T1,2NO	40/3 wk	5–15	86	NS	70
Clarke et al (167)	436	T1,2	45	15	90	NS	–
Delouche et al (195)	410	T1,T2	50–60	Yes	94 (T1), 86 (T2)	93	62.5
Dewar et al (310)	757	T0–2	45	15	92	–	68
Dubois et al (311)	231	I	45	10–15	91 (I)	90	I 84
	161	II	–	–	84 (II)	–	II 75
Fagundes et al (312)	425	T1, T2	50	10–15	92	77	74[b]
Fourquet et al (313)	518	T1,2	57–62	5–12	90	NS	NS
Fowble et al (314)	697	I, II	50	10–15	91	93	I 79, II 67
Gage et al (315)	1,870	I, II	45–50	10–20	87	NS	NS
Haffty et al (316, 317)	433	I, II	48	10–20	92	NS	81
	281	I	–	–	81	–	75
	–	II	<46	10–20	79	–	57
Kurtz et al (318)	1,593	I, II	50–60	20	89	–	86
Kuske et al (319)	417	I, II	50	10–20	91	81	I 80, II 52
Leborgne et al (320)	796	I, II	50	10–20	87	NS	82[c]
Montague (321)	134	I	50	15–20	94	–	78
	157	II	50	10–20	95	–	73
Osborne et al (322)	263	T1,2	45	10	85 (I), 81 (II)	–	54, 29
Plerquin et al (323)	245	I, II	50	10–20	90	82	75[c]
Recht et al (324)	366	I, II	50	10	96 (I), 90 (II)	–	–
Sarrazin et al (307)	179	T1, smT2	45	15	95	92	85[b]
Solin et al (325)	217	T1	45–50	10–15	95	90	T1 80[b]
	166	T2	45–50	10–15	92	90	T2 69[b]
van Limbergen et al (169)	235	T1,2(3)	40–65	8–20	90	–	T1 75.4, T2 61.9
Vicini et al (326)	1,396	I, II	50	10	92	87	NS
Vilcoq et al (196)	314	T1,2	50–55	10–20	90	–	84[b]
Washington University[d]	839	T1, T2	50	10–20	92	80	T1 82, T2 75

NS, Not stated.
[a] 6-year disease-free survival.
[b] 5-year disease-free survival.
[c] 15 years.
[d] Unpublished data.

TABLE 30.11. *Five-year survival correlated with treatment in stages I and II carcinoma of the breast: nonrandomized studies*

Author	Clinical stage	Conservation surgery and radiation therapy		Radical or modified mastectomy	
		No. of patients	5-year disease-free survival (%)	No. of patients	5-year disease-free survival (%)
Amalric et al (327)	I–II	1099	72	121	78
Janjan et al (328)	I–II	201	89	558	74
Montague (321)	I–II	134	85	224	88
	–	157	78	370	77
Peters (329)	I–II	203	86	609	82
Rissanen (330)	I–II	415	79	593	82

or breast-conservation therapy at various institutions in Europe and North America is detailed in Table 30.11 (321, 327–330).

Studies Comparing Lumpectomy Alone with Lumpectomy in Combination with Breast Irradiation

While randomized, prospective studies clearly showed that local excision followed by irradiation to the breast produces results comparable to those produced by modified radical mastectomy, the question of whether local excision alone might be an acceptable treatment alternative to modified radical mastectomy had not yet been answered. Several trials have now been performed, however, to address this question of the need for irradiation.

The Uppsala-Orebro Breast Cancer Study Group reported on a trial in which 184 women with stage I breast carcinoma were randomized to be treated with segmental resection, axillary dissection, and breast irradiation (54 Gy), while another 197 women were randomized to the same surgical procedures without irradiation (331). The actuarial local recurrence rates after median follow-up of 63 to 65 months were

2.3% in the irradiated group and 18.4% with surgery only. The 5-year disease-free survival rates were 91% and 87%, and the 5-year overall survival rates were 91% and 90%, respectively.

Clark and coworkers (293) reported on a randomized study of 421 patients with tumors 4 cm or less and negative nodes treated with wide-local excision and axillary dissection alone and 416 with the same surgery and breast irradiation (40 Gy in 3 weeks, 16 fractions; and 12.5-Gy boost in 5 fractions). With 7.6 years' median follow-up, breast recurrences occurred in 148 (35%) of the nonirradiated patients and in 147 (11%) of the irradiated patients (p <0.0001). Ninety-nine patients (24%) in the former and 87 (21%) in the latter group have died.

Results reported in several series are summarized in Table 30.12 (331–338).

Schnitt and coworkers (339) treated 90 patients with unicentric, 1 cm or less, ductal, mucinous, or tubular carcinoma with histologically negative lymph nodes by wide-local excision without breast irradiation. With a median follow-up of 55 months, 14 patients (16%) developed local recurrence. This finding prompted the observation that con-

TABLE 30.12. *Breast recurrence rate after tumor excision alone or combined with irradiation in stages I and II carcinoma of the breast*

Author	Tumor size (cm)	Surgery	Breast relapse	
			Tumor exclsion only	Tumor excision and irradiation
Cedermark et al (332)	≤2	Partial mastectomy	9/58 (15.5%)	6/204 (2.9%)
Clark et al (293)	≤5	Local excision	374 (29%)	1130 (14%)[a]
Clark et al (333)	–	–	421 (35%)	416 (11%)
Cooke et al (334)	–	Partial mastectomy	53 (21%)	44 (5%)
Fisher et al (335)[b]	≤4	– Axillary nodes	13/361 (37%)	45/377 (12%)
		+ Axillary nodes	9/211 (43%)	11/192 (6%)
Forrest et al (336)	–	Local excision, axillary dissection	72/294 (24.5%)	17/291 (5.8%)
Kantorowitz et al (337)	≤5	Local excision	22/77 (18.6%)	15/106 (14.2%)
		Quadrantectomy	4/18 (22.2%)	1/36 (2.8%)
Liijegren et al (Uppsala-Orebro Breast Study Group) (331)	≤2	Sector exclsion + axillary dissection	197 (18.4%)[c]	184 (2.3%)[c]
Whelan et al (338)	≤4	Lumpectomy + axillary dissection	396 (30%)[c]	403 (8%)[c]

[a] 10-year actuarial relapse.
[b] 8-year actuarial relapse.
[c] 5-year actuarial relapse.

servation surgery alone should rarely be considered as an alternative in standard treatment to limited surgery and breast irradiation or mastectomy for patients with small breast cancers.

In another trial, Veronesi and colleagues (340) in Milan randomly assigned 567 women with small breast cancer (<2.5 cm in diameter) to quadrantectomy followed by radiation therapy or to quadrantectomy alone. All patients underwent total axillary dissection. With median follow-up of 39 months (range 28 to 54 months), the incidence of local recurrence was 8.8% with quadrantectomy alone compared with 0.3% with breast irradiation ($p = 0.001$). The 5-year local failure rates for patients without EIC tumors were 28% with quadrantectomy alone and 9% with quadrantectomy and irradiation. Four-year overall survival was similar in the two treatment groups (approximately 76%).

The importance of irradiating the entire breast remains best documented in the NSABP B-06 trial, discussed in the prior section. In that trial, as in the Milan long-term results, it is important to keep in mind that with 20-year follow-up, new ipsilateral breast cancers develop, along with some late true local failures.

Selection Criteria for Breast-Conservation Therapy

It is important to be aware that, despite the fact that multiple randomized, prospective studies have demonstrated the equivalence of breast-conservation therapy and modified radical mastectomy, there will still be instances in which the best, or perhaps only, option will be to perform a mastectomy. Contraindications to breast conservation therapy exist because of the inability to radiate the breast or to remove all disease with an acceptable cosmetic result.

Patients who present in the first or second trimester of pregnancy are unable to receive radiation therapy owing to potential fetal harm. Thus, if a patient wishes to maintain her pregnancy, breast-conservation therapy may not be a treatment option.

When a patient presents with two or more macroscopic tumors of the breast in different quadrants, the cosmetic result from the surgery is less than optimal, and the local tumor control with irradiation decreases. Wilson and associates (341) from Yale studied the likelihood of recurrence in patients with multiple primary tumors treated with radiation therapy. They compared patients with multiple tumors treated with breast-conservation therapy to their population of patients with single tumors undergoing breast-conservation therapy. The risk of local recurrence at a median follow-up of 71 months was 23% (3/13) for the group with multiple tumors. The 5-year actuarial risk of local recurrence was 25% for this group, compared with 12% for single tumors. The survival rate in the population with multiple tumors was not significantly different from that of the entire population of patients undergoing local tumor resection followed by radiation therapy.

Patients who have undergone therapeutic irradiation to the breast region (often due to treatment for lymphoma at a younger age) are usually unable to have further irradiation to the region. Therefore, this group of patients should not be considered acceptable for treatment with breast-conservation therapy.

Finally, the presence of indeterminate or malignant-appearing calcifications throughout the breast suggests a diffuse disease process. In these instances, the breast cancer is best treated with mastectomy.

The relative contraindications to breast-conservation therapy exist because of the inability to eradicate all tumor cells and still achieve good cosmesis. Thus, patients with large tumors in a small breast may prefer a mastectomy with reconstruction. There are, however, some patients who would accept a significant degree of deformity in exchange for avoiding a modified radical mastectomy. Additionally, selected tumors in subareolar positions may often be treated with removal of the nipple-areolar complex, again affecting cosmesis. In many instances, this is preferable to a mastectomy for the patient.

There have been several anecdotal reports of severe fibrotic, postirradiation reactions in patients with active systemic lupus erythematosus and scleroderma (342,343). Because of this, many radiation oncologists are reluctant to treat such patients. Unfortunately, the true denominator of patients with connective-tissue disorders who have been treated with breast-conservation therapy is unknown.

An area of controversy regarding breast-conservation therapy has been the importance of negative margins of resection. Upon reexcision for positive margins at the time of initial excision of a tumor, 48% to 69% of patients will have residual tumor, and 8% will continue to have a positive margin (319,344,345). While some studies have shown the incidence of local recurrence to be equivalent regardless of whether a patient has negative or positive margins (346–348), others have shown a significant increase in local recurrence rates in patients with positive margins (24,175,254,281,349). These findings are summarized in Table 30.13. Based on the available data, it appears that margin status does have an impact on local recurrence rates. Re-excision is an appropriate next step for the surgeon and patient to take if the breast is large enough to technically allow it, but the patient must be aware that margin involvement is still possible after the additional surgery, and mastectomy may finally be necessary. Further, carefully assessed negative surgical margins and adequate irradiation may decrease or eliminate the significance of EIC for breast relapse, and today EIC per se is not considered a contraindication to breast-conservation therapy.

MANAGEMENT OF THE AXILLA

The inclusion of the axilla in the surgical management of the breast-cancer patient can be traced to the era of the Hal-

TABLE 30.13. *Breast recurrence correlated with microscopic margins of resection in breast-conservation therapy*

Author	Positive	Close	Negative	Unknown	Follow-up (years)
Abner et al (387)	13% (92)	4% (28)	2% (84)	–	6.2 median
Anscher et al (349a)	10% (32)	–	2% (132)	10% (98)	5 actuarial
Bartelink et al (171)	7% (32)	–	2% (242)	–	6 actuarial
Borger et al (349b)	16% (20)	–	2% (244)	6% (75)	5 actuarial
Clarke and Martinez (197)	9% (88)	–	4% (274)	–	5 mean
Fisher et al (349c)	–	–	12% (568)	–	10 actuarial
Ghossein et al (348)	10% (152)	–	12% (359)	–	7 median
Hartsell et al (349d)	11% (35)	–	2% (175)	3% (68)	3.4 median
Hunig et al (349e)	7% (15)	–	6% (90)	–	2.3 median
Pezner et al (349f)	–	–	2% (103)	11% (30)	5 actuarial
Ryoo et al (349g)	13% (23)	8% (87)	6% (283)	–	3.5 median
Schmidt-Ulrich et al (349h)	0% (46)	–	0% (61)	–	4.7 median
Slotman et al (349i)	10% (31)	8% (24)	3% (459)	–	5.7 median
Solin et al (349j)	2% (57)	11% (37)	7% (257)	9% (346)	5 actuarial
Washington University	7.5% (161)	–	6.7% (567)	8.1% (111)	5 actuarial
Zafrani et al (349k)	–	–	9%	–	10 actuarial

Numbers in parentheses represent total number of patients in study.

sted radical mastectomy. Over the years, as the theory of breast-cancer growth and dissemination has changed, the value of axillary lymph node dissection (ALND) has often been questioned. The potential benefits of such a dissection are important to analyze, however. First, knowledge regarding the status of the axillary nodes is extremely important in accurately staging a patient and evaluating risk of recurrence. Additionally, an appropriate axillary dissection serves to decrease the risk of a regional recurrence. Finally, adequate treatment of the axillary region may ultimately lead to a survival advantage (350).

Results obtained in clinical examination of the axillary nodes are notoriously inaccurate, with the sensitivity and specificity of a manual examination being only about 75% (351). Examination of the axilla with other radiologic procedures also appears to add little to the analysis of the status of the lymph nodes (352). Attempts to use multiple factors to demonstrate the probability of finding involved lymph nodes suffer from the fact that the accuracy is still not adequate (353). Arguments suggesting that axillary evaluation be abandoned in tumors of small size ignore the fact that there is no tumor size at which lymph-node involvement cannot be found (354). Multiple studies have shown that even in tumors less than 1 cm in size, lymph-node metastasis may be present in greater than 10% of patients (354–356). In a study of 81 patients with T1a and T1b breast cancers treated at Memorial Sloan–Kettering Cancer Center, the incidence of lymph-node metastasis was 10% in patients with T1a lesions and 15% in patients with T1b lesions (356). The authors were unable to identify any subgroup of low-risk patients in which axillary lymph-node dissection could be avoided. This correlates with data from the Surveillance, Epidemiology, and End Results Study in which almost 25,000 cases of breast cancer were evaluated (354). In this study, the incidence of lymph-node metastasis in patients with T1a tumors was 20.6%.

It is important to bear in mind that the extent of axillary dissection may be an important determinant not only of the risk of local recurrence but also of the ability to adequately stage the axilla. An axillary "sampling," in which lymph nodes are somewhat randomly removed from the axilla, has been shown to be less accurate in determining the extent of disease within the axilla than a standard axillary dissection (351,357,358). With axillary biopsy alone, Davies et al (351) demonstrated a 42% false-negative rate. Kissin's group (358) demonstrated an only slightly better rate of 24%. A mathematical model to assess the ability to accurately stage the axilla has shown that, in order to have 90% certainty that there is no nodal involvement in a T1 tumor, at least 10 lymph nodes should be removed (359). In order to avoid a high false-negative rate in patients under going an axillary dissection, various studies have shown that both level I and level II should be dissected (357,360). Danforth et al (357) found that, if level I and level II of the axilla are appropriately dissected, there is only a 3.1% chance of missing a positive lymph node present in level III. Rosen et al (360) and Boova et al (361) observed an even lower incidence of "skip" metastases (nodal disease that was present in level III and not in either of the first two levels).

The ability of a complete level I and level II axillary dissection to significantly diminish the likelihood of an axillary recurrence has been decisively demonstrated (362,363). When appropriately performed, the incidence should be less than 1% of cases. The effects of an axillary recurrence are not inconsequential, and this advantage of axillary dissection should therefore not be taken lightly. Perhaps less obvious is the effect that this recurrence might have on overall survival in the breast-cancer patient. The only trial that has directly addressed this is the NSABP B-04 trial (363,364). This trial randomized patients with clinically negative nodes to one of three groups—radical mastectomy, total mastectomy with regional nodal irradiation, or total mastectomy without nodal irradiation. Of patients undergoing radical mastectomy, the incidence of lymph-node metastasis was approximately 40%, and it was felt that the probability of this event would be similar in the other groups of patients. Thus, in theory 40% of patients undergoing mastectomy without regional nodal therapy should have recurrence in the axilla. In reality, only 65 of 365 patients (17.8%) did eventually develop a recurrence in the untreated axilla as the first site of disease. In all patients in this group, however, the survival was similar to that of patients in the other two groups, suggesting that axillary tumor control was not important in long-term survival.

Three other trials have now shown a survival disadvantage in patients who have not had adequate treatment of the axillary region. In the Southeast Scottish Study, 275 patients were randomized to receive either total mastectomy with irradiation or radical mastectomy (365), the rate of regional recurrence was significantly increased, and the survival rate decreased at 10 years in patients not undergoing an axillary dissection. In the study at the Institut Curie (359), 658 patients were randomized to lumpectomy and regional irradiation (including the breast and the axilla) or to lumpectomy, axillary dissection, and irradiation of the breast. The survival in the group of patients undergoing an axillary dissection was significantly higher than that in the group receiving axillary irradiation ($p = 0.014$) (359). It is important to note, however, that some patients in the group undergoing axillary dissection also underwent chemotherapy if lymph nodes were found to be involved.

A recent meta-analysis by Orr (350) attempted to correct for some of the biases of studies, such as NSABP B-04, in which partial-node dissection was performed in many patients randomized to no treatment. Orr analyzed six trials of clinical stage I breast cancer patients in which individuals were randomized either to axillary dissection or to observation only. Trials of radiation therapy to the axilla were not included. After a complicated correction for internal and external biases of each study, every study demonstrated a survival advantage for axillary node dissection.

If one concludes that axillary dissection is beneficial, it is important to balance its benefits with the complications of such a procedure. In following 106 patients after axillary dissection, Ivens et al (366) demonstrated that 15% of patients who underwent an axillary dissection complained of numbness, pain, and/or weakness that was significant enough to be noted on a daily basis, and at 2 years posttreatment, 14% of patients had a measurable arm lymphedema. Multiple other studies have indicated similar rates of lymphedema after axillary surgery (367,368). Thus, despite modern surgical techniques, the development of a major complication such as lymphedema continues to be significant.

Sentinel Lymph-Node Biopsy

The desire to prevent potential complications of axillary dissection in patients without axillary disease provided the impetus for the evaluation of sentinel lymph-node mapping and biopsy for breast cancer. The modern era of sentinel lymph-node biopsy was ushered in with its application to the treatment of malignant melanoma (369). The first reports of this technique in breast cancer were published in the early 1990s (370,371). Since that time, many groups have reported on their experience, including a multicenter study validating this technique's usefulness in the majority of instances (372–384). Varying techniques for identifying the sentinel lymph node, or nodes, as the case may be, have been reported. Some groups have used isotope localization only (373,374,378–380,382,383), others have used blue dye for localization only (375,377,378), and many use a combination of the two.

Ability to identify a sentinel lymph node ranged from 66% of cases to 100% of cases, with the majority of series demonstrating a node in approximately 90% of procedures, which is related to a learning curve for the technique. It is likely, however, that a certain rate of inability to identify an involved sentinel lymph node will always exist. In assessing the ability of each technique to identify the sentinel lymph node, it appears that isotope successfully localizes a lymph node more commonly than blue dye alone. The combination of the two techniques, however, has the greatest success rate (385). It appears that the majority of false-negative results (0% to 17%) occur in the initial cases that a surgeon performs (385). This is highlighted by the experience of Giuliano (377), who reported a 12% false-negative rate in his series of his first 174 patients but reported no false-negatives in the next 107 patients on whom he utilized the technique.

Further validation of the concept of a "true" sentinel node comes from the histopathologic analysis of negative sentinel lymph nodes and negative nonsentinel lymph nodes from a standard axillary dissection. Immunohistochemical (IHC) stains used in breast cancer are monoclonal antibodies against cytokeratins, AE1/AE3; CAM 5.2. Several studies have demonstrated an increase in the diagnostic yield of occult nodal metastases with the use of IHC analysis in patients thought to have negative nodes through standard histologic analysis using hematoxylin-eosin stains. Use of IHC stains can increase the yield of detection of tumor cells by 10% to 20% over standard histopathologic analysis. Metastases less than 2 mm in size are classified as micrometastases (386). The clinical significance of micrometastases is currently debated; however, the Ludwig study (387) has shown that patients with micrometastases have a worse 5-year survival than those with no metastases; namely, true node-negative patients. The impact on overall survival may be altered as adjuvant therapy is altered by enhanced histopathologic techniques and detection of metastatic disease. Sentinel lymph-node biopsy makes enhanced pathologic analysis logistically feasible and allows identification of a group of patients with increased risk of systematic relapse who might otherwise be unrecognized.

Turner and colleagues (388) performed immunohistochemical staining of all lymph nodes in a series of patients in whom the sentinel node and the axillary contents were negative by routine histopathologic sectioning. Of the 157 sentinel lymph nodes that were negative on routine sectioning, 10 (6%) demonstrated tumor with IHC methods. In contrast, of 1,087 nonsentinel lymph nodes, only 1 (0.1%) showed any evidence of metastatic cells with IHC staining. If the lymph node designated as a sentinel node were not actually that sentinel node, the rate of IHC-positive disease in the remaining lymph nodes should have been significantly higher.

Axillary sentinel lymph-node biopsy with lymphatic mapping should be a consideration in the management of any patient with invasive carcinoma. There are still certain cases, however, in which a standard axillary dissection may continue to be superior. In patients with suspicious palpable axillary disease, it is important to perform a complete dissection. Additionally, in a patient with a previous large biopsy cavity that is near the axilla, caution should be used in relying on the sentinel lymph-node biopsy because of the significant disruption of lymphatics that may have occurred from the prior excision. In general, larger tumors should not be considered absolute contraindications to the use of sentinel lymph-node biopsy. It is likely that the false-negative rate will remain constant at a level of 5% to 10%, and owing to the greater likelihood of axillary disease being present in patients with T2 and T3 tumors, the accuracy (true negatives plus true positives/total cases) may decrease slightly. Other situations in which axillary sentinel lymph-node biopsy may be difficult to use include those with true multifocal disease with gross invasive lesions in two separate quadrants of the breast, and those in which the true extent of disease is significantly greater than predicted by preoperative studies.

The issue of isolated micrometastatic disease in the SLN is an area of controversy. The question of whether everyone with a positive SLN needs a complete ALND is debated. The accuracy, value, and future of SLN biopsy currently is being evaluated in several prospective national trials. Among these trials is the American College of Surgeons Oncology Group (ACOSOG) Z0011 trial, which randomly assigns women with clinical T1 or T2,N0M0 breast cancer and a positive SLN to one of two treatment arms: ALND or no ALND. The primary endpoint is overall survival. Secondary endpoints are surgical morbidities and disease-free survival. If no difference is seen, patients can potentially be spared the morbidity of an ALND, even in the positive SLN setting. Until data are available, the standard of care for SLN-positive patients is ALND.

SURGICAL MANAGEMENT OF DUCTAL CARCINOMA *IN SITU*

The appropriate surgical management of the patient with ductal carcinoma *in situ* (DCIS) continues to evolve as increasing data regarding the disease become available. Historically, this carcinoma accounted for only 1% to 2% of all breast cancers (389,390), but with the increased use of screening mammography, by 2002 that proportion increased to 20% in the United States. Treatment options for this disease have changed in a similar fashion to those for invasive carcinomas.

Historically, DCIS was treated with a total mastectomy. In a small number of patients in which lesions were previously termed benign, but re-reviewed as DCIS, the likelihood of developing cancer after a biopsy only for DCIS ranged from 15% to 75% (29,391–396). On average, approximately one-third of patients whose DCIS was "untreated" developed an invasive breast cancer within a 10-year period (Table 30.14) (29,391–396).

In multiple series from various institutions, the risk of local recurrence after mastectomy approached zero. These results are summarized in Table 30.15 (63,79–81,392–395, 397–416).

Several factors have led to a shift away from the use of mastectomy for the treatment of DCIS. As breast-conservation therapy rapidly became the standard of care for patients with invasive breast cancer, it presented a troubling paradox that patients with early DCIS should be treated with mastectomy. Several pathologic features may influence management. In serial analysis of 82 mastectomy specimens (5-mm whole-organ sections), Holland and coworkers (417) found that DCIS involved one breast quadrant in 66%, extended over more than one quadrant in 23%, and was centrally located in 11%. The nipple or subareolar area was more frequently involved by comedo carcinoma (32 of 50, 64%) than by micropapillary and cribriform (11 of 32, 34%). In a review of 130 specimens, Bellamy and associates (85) commonly observed single-quadrant involvement with the comedo, solid, or cribriform subtypes of DCIS. In contrast, the micropapillary subtype of DCIS tended to have more diffuse involvement of the breast.

In 181 women, Silverstein and colleagues (418) noted that

TABLE 30.14. *Incidence of invasive breast carcinoma after a biopsy and excision only of ductal carcinoma* in situ

Author	Number of patients	Subsequent cancers[a]
Betsill et al (391)	10	7 (70%)
Farrow (392)	25	5 (20%)
Haagensen (29)	11	8 (73%)
Lagios et al (393)	20	3 (15%)
Lewis and Geshickter (394)	8	6 (75%)
Milils and Thynne (395)	8	2 (25%)
Page et al (396)	25	7 (28%)
Total	107	38 (35.5%)

[a] All developed within 10 years.

From Frykberg ER, Bland KI. Overview of the biology and management of ductal carcinoma in situ of the breast. *Cancer* 1994;74 [Suppl 1]:350–361, with permission.

TABLE 30.15. *Ductal carcinoma* in situ *of the breast: results after mastectomy*

Author	Number of patients	Local recurrences	Cancer deaths (DOD)	Follow-up (years)
Arnesson et al (397)	28	0%	0%	6.4
Ashikari et al (79)	111	2%	1%	1–10
Ashikari et al (398)	74	0%	0%	0 to 11
Brown et al (399)	40	0%	0%	5
Carter and Smith (400)	38	8%	8%	–
Ciatto et al (401)	210	1.4%	–	5.5
Cutuli et al (402)	34	3%	3%	6.8
Farrow (392)	200	4%	2%	5 to 20
Fentiman et al (403)	82	1%	1%	4.7 median
Fisher et al (404)	28	4%	3%	3.2 mean
Howard et al (405)	55[a]	3.6%	1.8%	1.5 to 12
Kinne et al (406)	80	1%	1%	11.5 median
Lagios et al (393)	53	6%	2%	–
Lewis and Geshickter (394)	36	0%	19%	2 to 36
Millis and Thynne (395)	20	0%	0%	<5 to >15
Ozzello (407)	22	5%	–	–
Petit et al (408)	127	7%	1.6%	7.6
Price et al (409)	25[b]	16%	NS	9 median
Rosner et al (410)	182	10%	2%	5
Schuh et al (411)	51	0%	2%	5.5 mean
Silverstein et al (63)	49	2%	0%	2.3 median
Silverstein et al (412)	98	1%	0%	4.9
Simpson et al (413)	34	0%	0%	17.7 mean
Sunshine et al (81)	70	4%	4%	>10
Temple et al (414)	116	0%	0%	7.5 mean
Von Rueden and Wilson (415)	47	2%	0%	–
Westbrook and Gallagher (80)	64	2%	0%	–
Wulsin and Schrelber (416)	12	0%	0%	NS

DOD, dead of disease; NS, Not specified.

[a] All nonlocal relapses were invasive, including axillary lymph nodes, contralateral breast, bone, etc.

[b] Including 19 total mastectomies and 6 subcutaneous mastectomies.

tumors larger than 2.5 cm in size had a greater tendency toward positive histologic margins on initial excision. Additionally, the presence of the comedo subtype of DCIS also increased the likelihood of positive margins. At reexcision, there was a significant incidence of residual intraductal breast carcinoma.

The size of a DCIS lesion may be related both to the ability to obtain free margins and to the risk of local recurrence after excision alone. In one study, lesions less than 15 mm in size had a local recurrence rate of 15%, whereas lesions measuring 16 to 25 mm had a local recurrence rate of 50% (419). These findings are similar to that of the NSABP B-17 trial; Fisher and colleagues (404) found that local failure occurred in 29% of patients with tumors less than 1 cm in size compared to 40% in larger lesions.

The importance of histologic features in the rate of local recurrence with excision alone has also been addressed in several studies. Controversy still exists as to their impact, however. In a study of 79 patients with mammographically detected DCIS, Lagios and Page (419) demonstrated that the risk of local recurrence was related to the nuclear grade of the DCIS. At a mean follow-up of 124 months, the risk of recurrence was 6%, 10%, and 33% for tumors with nuclear grades 1, 2, and 3, respectively. In contrast, the analysis by

Schwartz et al. (84) of 153 patients treated with local excision alone demonstrated no effect of nuclear grade.

While all of these data suggest that there are select instances in which excision alone may be effective therapy for DCIS, multiple studies confirm that the addition of radiation therapy decreases local relapse. Solin and coworkers (420) reported their findings of 261 breasts with DCIS in 259 women from nine institutions in Europe and the United States who had been treated with local excision and irradiation. The 10-year actuarial rate of local failure was 16% and that of distant metastases was 4% (Fig. 30.27) (420). Subsequently, the authors updated the results with 15-year follow-up rates (421): the cause-specific survival was 96%, breast relapse was 19%, and incidence of distant metastases was 3%. While the subtype involving comedo carcinoma plus nuclear grade 3 lesions had a greater incidence of local failures in the earlier years, at 10 years it was not different from other histologic subtypes (18% and 15%, respectively). Of 45 patients with local recurrence, 24 (53%) had invasive ductal carcinoma, and 21 (47%) had DCIS. Solin et al. (422) also described results of a patient subset of 110 women with unilateral, nonpalpable, mammographically detected DCIS of the breast who were treated with breast-conservation surgery and irradiation. With median follow-up of 9.3 years,

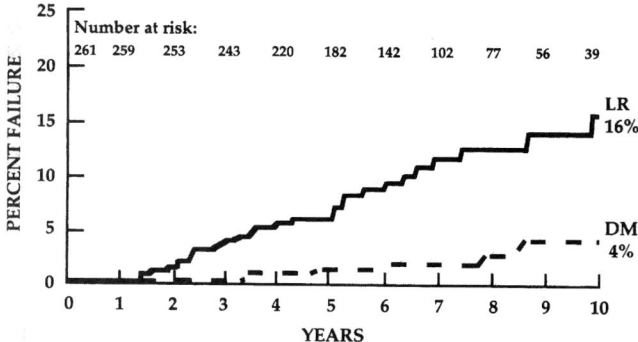

FIG. 30.27. Incidence of local-regional and distant metastases in patients with DCIS of the breast treated with breast-conservation therapy. LR, Local-regional; DM, distant metastases. (Reprinted with permission from Solin LJ, Recht A, Fourquet A, et al. Ten-year results of breast-conserving surgery and definitive irradiation for intraductal carcinoma [ductal carcinoma in situ] of the breast. *Cancer* 1991;68:2337.)

the local recurrence rates were 7% (3 of 42) in patients with negative final pathologic margins, 29% (5 of 17) in patients with positive or close final margins, and 14% (7 of 51) in patients whose final margins were unknown. Local recurrence developed in 14 of 56 (25%) of the women younger than 50 years of age but in only 1 of 54 (2%) of the older women; the median interval to local recurrence was 4.9 years in women younger than 50 and 8.7 years in the older group. There was no significant difference in 5-year local recurrence according to histologic subtype (8% for comedo and 2% for other). The 10-year actuarial cause-specific survival was 96%. A further subgroup of 21 patients was identified with characteristics (mammographic detection with microcalcifications alone, pathologically confirmed negative margins of excision, tumor size <2.5 cm) similar to those detailed by Lagios and colleagues (83), noted above for

treatment with local excision alone. With a median follow-up of 8.7 years, there were no local recurrences in the 21 patients in Solin's study with these characteristics treated with breast-conservation surgery and irradiation.

Two prospective randomized trials of excision alone versus excision and radiation therapy have been completed, and show similar results. The NSABP Protocol B-17 randomized 391 women to be treated with lumpectomy alone; 64 of the 391 (16.4%) developed ipsilateral breast cancer, compared with 28 of 399 (7%) randomized to be treated with lumpectomy and breast irradiation (423). The 5-year cumulative incidence of second cancers in the ipsilateral breast was reduced by irradiation from 10.4% to 7.5% for noninvasive cancer and from 10.5% to 2.9% for invasive lesions ($p = 0.055$ and $p < 0.001$, respectively) (423). In a 1999 update, with 8 year follow-up, the cumulative incidence of a second cancer of any kind in the lumpectomy only group increased to 31%, compared with 13% in the radiated group (log rank test PL 0.0001) (424).

The European Organization for Research and Treatment of Cancer (EORTC) designed a nearly identical Phase III trial for DCIS, comparing lumpectomy alone to lumpectomy plus irradiation. One thousand ten women were enrolled in the trial; with a median follow-up of 4.25 years, similar results were noted; local failure in the irradiated group was 8% compared to 16% with no radiation therapy (425).

The reported incidence of local recurrence after treatment of DCIS with conservation surgery and breast irradiation is higher but not significantly different from that seen after mastectomy (Table 30.16) (63,166,314,321,389,402,420, 423,426–433). More important, survival is comparable, and patients who have recurrences after lumpectomy and irradiation can be salvaged with mastectomy.

Routine node dissection has been eliminated for DCIS because so few patients have positive nodes. Silverstein and

TABLE 30.16. *Ductal carcinoma* in situ *of the breast: results of conservation surgery and irradiation*

Author	Number of patients	Local recurrence (%)	Cancer deaths	Median follow-up (years)
Baird et al (389)	8	25	–	3.2
Bornstein et al (426)	38	21	0	6.7
Cutull et al (402)	36	9	0	7
Fisher et al (423)	399	7.5	0	3.2[a]
Fowble et al (314)	46	4	0	2.9
Haffty et al (427)	60	9	0	3.6
Kurtz et al (166)	47	4	2	5
Kuske et al (428)	70	4	1	3.8
McCormick et al (429)	54	18	0	3
Montague (321)	34	3	0	5.5
Ray et al (430)	58	9	0	5
Silverstein et al (63)	103	10	1	5
Solin et al (420)	261	11	8	6.5
Stotter et al (431)	42	9	4	7.6
White et al (432)	52	6	2	5.6
Zafrani et al (433)	54	6	2	4.5

[a] Mean follow-up.

associates (434) analyzed axillary node positivity, disease-free survival, and breast-cancer–specific survival in six breast-cancer subgroups by T category. Nodal positivity for DCIS was 0% in 189 patients.

The NSABP recently reported on a trial, B-24, for DCIS in which all patients had breast-conservation surgery and irradiation and then were randomized to receive 5 years of tamoxifen or a placebo. Results of the irradiation-only arm matched the equivalent arm of the B-17 trial. Tamoxifen resulted in a significant further decrease in the risk of ipsilateral invasive breast cancer (44% reduction), but the decrease in ipsilateral noninvasive cancer did not reach significance. The anticipated impact of tamoxifen on the contralateral breast was observed (435). As well, the absolute risk reduction was small, tamoxifen side effects were observed, and the role of tamoxifen remains controversial.

PAGET'S DISEASE OF THE BREAST

This rare form of breast cancer makes up 1% to 4% of all breast tumors (436,437). Many of these patients have been treated with mastectomy, with favorable results (438, 439). A few reports have been published on conservation surgery and irradiation in treatment of this disease; Fourquet and colleagues (437) reported on 20 patients treated conservatively, with radiation therapy alone (17 patients), or with limited surgery and irradiation (three patients). Most patients received 50 to 55 Gy to the breast and axillary lymph nodes and 40 to 45 Gy to the internal mammary and supraclavicular lymph nodes. The 7-year actuarial disease-free survival rate for these patients was 81%, and the overall survival rate was 93%. Although Fourquet and associates (437) irradiated the axilla, at the present time this is not recommended owing to the low rate of incidence of axillary lymph nodes.

Pierce and colleagues (440) reported a review of 30 patients with Paget's disease treated at several institutions with breast-conservation therapy (50 Gy) with a boost (14 Gy). With a median follow-up of 62 months, three women developed a recurrence in the treated breast, and two additional patients failed in the breast as a component of first failure. The 8-year local-only failure rate was 16%; as a component of any failure, it was 23%. Four of five patients were salvaged by mastectomy. The 8-year disease-free survival rate was 95%.

ADENOCARCINOMA IN AXILLARY LYMPHADENOPATHY, NO DETECTABLE BREAST PRIMARY CANCER

Occasionally, the presence of a cancer of the breast is indicated only by an involved axillary lymph node (192). In addition to a careful physical examination involving the breast, bilateral mammograms, breast MRI, and chest x-rays should be obtained. An exhaustive radiographic workup, including CT scan of the chest, upper gastrointestinal studies,

TABLE 30.17. *Patients with isolated axillary adenopathy and histologically negative mastectomy specimens*

Source	No. of mastectomy specimens examined	No. (%) of negative specimens
Baron et al (441a)	35	11 (33)
Feuerman et al (441b)	10	3 (30)
Merson et al (442)	33	6 (18)
Owen et al (442a)	25	10 (40)
Westbrook and Gallager (442b)	12	3 (25)
Total	**115**	**33 (28.7)**

Modified from Vilcoq JR, Calle R, Fem F, et al. Conservative treatment of axillary adenopathy due to probable subclinical breast cancer. *Arch Surg* 1982; 117:1136–1138, with permission.

barium enema, and intravenous pyelogram, is not warranted (441). Often, after careful examination of mastectomy specimens, the primary tumor in the breast cannot be demonstrated (Table 30.17). These patients have a relatively good prognosis, with survival rates of 80% and 50% at 5 and 10 years.

An alternate local treatment for this group is irradiation of the breast and axillary dissection. Although a primary tumor is often not identified on mammograms, or more exhausting imaging with ultrasound or MRI (see imaging section), and boost doses cannot be delivered, the breast is treated with doses of 50 Gy. Campana et al (441) reported on 31 patients, some of whom were previously reported on by Vilcoq and colleagues (192). Initial treatment consisted of resection of the involved lymph nodes followed by irradiation in 14 patients, axillary dissection and radiation therapy in 8 patients, radiation therapy followed by axillary dissection in 6 patients, irradiation and modified radical mastectomy in 1 patient, and irradiation alone in 2 patients. All 31 patients received radiation therapy to the regional lymphatics (axillary, supraclavicular, and internal mammary chains) to doses of 60 Gy or higher; 10 patients received adjuvant chemotherapy. All 31 cases have been followed, with a median follow-up of 9 years. The overall 5- and 10-year survival rates were 76% and 71%, respectively. The risk of local-regional recurrence at 5 and 10 years was 14% and 25%, respectively, and the risk of developing distant metastases was 23.5% and 29%, respectively.

Merson and associates (442) analyzed 60 cases of axillary metastases. The number of pathologic metastatic nodes was 1 in 13 patients, 2 or 3 in 10 patients, and 4 or more in 23 patients; the number of metastatic nodes was not available in 14 cases. Extranodal invasion was seen in 92% of cases. Thirty-three patients underwent breast surgery at the time of histologic diagnosis of the axillary metastases; 6 patients were treated with radiation therapy to the breast, and 17 patients did not receive any immediate treatment to the breast (9 of these later developed a primary breast carcinoma).

Thirty-seven of 60 patients received adjuvant therapy (29 chemotherapy and 8 tamoxifen therapy). The 5- and 10-year survival rates were 77% and 58%, respectively. Survival was equivalent for patients treated with immediate surgery/ radiation therapy and for patients who were followed up without treatment to the breast. Adjuvant treatment did not improve prognosis.

Management of Lobular Carcinoma *In Situ*

For many years, management of lobular carcinoma *in situ* (LCIS) has consisted of biopsy of the involved and contralateral breasts (443). In 1974, Wheeler and associates (444) argued against mastectomy and proposed careful lifelong follow-up for patients with LCIS, an approach that is favored by most surgeons at the present time (445–447). Thus, LCIS is considered by most as a risk factor for developing a cancer, rather than a ''cancer'' itself.

The risk of breast cancer developing in these women averages about 0.7% per year, with a cumulative incidence of bilateral breast cancer of 4% to 26% (448). Two-thirds of the second breast cancers are metachronous. In the series from Haagensen and associates (449), of 211 untreated cases of LCIS with a mean follow-up of 14 years, an overall probability of developing invasive cancer in the ipsilateral breast was 10% and in the contralateral breast, 9%. In patients followed up for 16 to 25 years, the risk of invasive cancer increased to 22% in the ipsilateral breast compared with 15% in the contralateral breast. Haagensen recommended close follow-up for patients with LCIS owing to the equal risk of cancer in both breasts in these patients and the long interval in the development of invasive cancer.

Confirming these findings, Rosen and colleagues (450) reported on 84 patients with LCIS with an average follow-up of 24 years after biopsy only. The incidence of subsequent invasive carcinoma was 14% in the ipsilateral breast, 14% in the contralateral breast, and 8% for bilateral cancers. Overall, 36% of patients later developed invasive cancer.

In a review of 419 women, Lee and colleagues (448) found bilateral lobular breast cancer in 36 patients (8.6%) with a cumulative risk of 10% after 10 years. Prophylactic contralateral surgical procedures were performed on 105 women, leading to detection of 70 *in situ* and four invasive cancers. Patients undergoing contralateral prophylactic mastectomy had a better prognosis than those with unilateral tumors not treated prophylactically. There was no survival benefit, however, and the authors believe that contralateral prophylactic mastectomy should not be recommended.

Page and associates (451) noted that the incidence of invasive carcinoma after biopsy for LCIS at 15 years was 17%, and the recurrence rate was 8%. Partial mastectomy has been used in the treatment of these patients (445,452,453). Recurrences (either LCIS or infiltrating carcinoma) were observed in 1.5% to 21% of patients, and long-term mortality after mastectomy for recurrence ranged from 0% to 8.1%.

Singletary (454) described her experience with 45 women who had LCIS alone and 30 women who had LCIS associated with an ipsilateral stage I or stage II breast carcinoma but no abnormality in the opposite breast. There was a 1% incidence of synchronous and 5% incidence of metachronous nonlobular carcinoma *in situ* breast cancer in the contralateral breast. Another breast cancer developed in a different quadrant in 3 of 19 women (16%) with ipsilateral residual or intact breast tissue. The author endorsed the recommendation of lifelong, careful observation of patients with LCIS. Surveillance should consist of monthly self-examination, physical examination of the breast every 3 or 4 months, and annual mammogram.

Currently, there is no information regarding the use of breast irradiation in LCIS.

Management of Bilateral Carcinoma of the Breast

Among factors reported to be associated with increased risk of bilateral breast carcinoma are younger age (455–458), family history of breast cancer (455,457,459–461), lobular carcinoma (457,458,462), multicentric disease (460), histologic differentiation of the primary tumor, parity status (463), and positive PR assays (462).

Patients with bilateral carcinoma have been treated with total or modified radical mastectomy (406). Breast irradiation combined with tumor excision is an acceptable alternative therapy for appropriately selected women with bilateral carcinoma of the breast. Solin and associates (464) reported on 30 women receiving radiation therapy after breast-conservation surgery (11 with concurrent and 19 with bilateral carcinoma). Adjuvant chemotherapy was given to 10 patients. The 5-year disease-free survival rate after treatment of the first breast cancer was 79%, and the overall survival rate was 72%. In the 60 treated breasts, the 5-year actuarial local failure rate was 6%. In 25 treated breasts, with a minimum of 2 years of follow-up, 68% had excellent and 24% had good cosmetic results.

Ninety-five patients with bilateral carcinoma of the breast treated with mastectomy (60 patients), conservation of the breast (17 patients), or both (18 patients) were studied by Gustafsson and associates (465). Cumulative 5-year local tumor control rates were 94% for the 138 mastectomy patients and 90% for the 52 treated with breast-conservation therapy. The 5-year distant disease-free survival rate from treatment for the second carcinoma was 74%. Of the first carcinomas, 28% were stage I, compared with 43% of second carcinomas ($p < 0.05$). This percentage is most likely a reflection of the close follow-up after initial treatment. The interval between the diagnosis of the first and second carcinomas had a profound effect on outcome; the 5-year distant recurrence-free survival rate when second carcinomas were diagnosed within 5 years was 58%, compared with 95% for patients diagnosed more than 5 years after the first carcinoma.

De la Rouchefordière and coworkers (466) reported on 149 patients with simultaneous bilateral breast cancer (diagnosed within 6 months); of 298 tumors, 40% were T0 or T1, 45% were T2, and 15% were T3 or T4. The majority (83%) were clinically node-negative. Treatments were bilateral mastectomy in 43%, irradiation in 16%, and a combination of both in 41% of the patients. Fifty-one patients had bilateral breast-conservation therapy, and 24 were treated exclusively with irradiation. The 5-year disease-free survival rates were 70% to 86%, similar to those observed at their institution in patients with unilateral tumors.

Management of Cystosarcoma Phyllodes

These rare fibroepithelial tumors account for less than 0.5% of breast neoplasms in women (467). The diagnostic workup for this type of tumor is similar to that used for breast masses.

Treatment for cystosarcoma phyllodes is either mastectomy or generous wide-local excision, depending on the degree of malignancy or size of the lesion. Histologic grade appears to be the most important factor; only about 10% of benign tumors recur. Size of the tumor has not been shown to be a significant prognostic factor but may influence surgical margins. The presence of underlying or clearly malignant changes is, however, associated with a higher recurrence rate and distant metastases.

SYSTEMIC THERAPY

When it became clear that significant improvements in survival would require improved methods of delivering systemic therapy, effective drug therapy became the goal of investigators worldwide. As a result, there have been hundreds of clinical trials testing systemically administered drugs as an adjunct to local control obtained through surgery, with or without radiation therapy. These studies have supported the hypothesis that systemic therapy will improve distant disease-free and overall survival, although the impact to date has been far more modest than first anticipated.

Neoadjuvant Systemic Therapy

The early recognition that systemic therapy could alter the course of advanced breast cancer was followed by attempts to apply these treatments earlier in the disease process. In so doing, surgeons hoped first to provide the earliest possible systemic treatment in terms of time, and second, to shrink the primary disease so as to allow for less disfiguring surgery. Although the second goal has been achieved in certain patient subsets, the ideal integration of local surgery, radiation therapy, and systemic therapy remains controversial, and it seems likely that there will be no single answer, but rather differing solutions depending on the type of surgery, extent of disease, and specific systemic treatment options.

Preoperative, or neoadjuvant, chemotherapy is an attractive approach in several circumstances. The first is an unresectable tumor. In this case, if there is no evidence of systemic spread, the surgeon remains motivated to operate in the hopes of achieving cure, but the local extent of disease is such that a successful operation with clear margins is not possible. Specific examples include some patients with T3 lesions, almost all with T4, or N2, or N3 disease. A role for neoadjuvant treatment in patients with M1 disease manifested only by supraclavicular disease remains debatable (92). Certainly, in those patients with established stage IV disease, the goal of treatment is almost entirely to achieve local control, with little expectation that the early use of systemic therapy will result in a changed outcome compared with later use of the same agents.

Depending on the treatment selected, significant response to systemic chemotherapy in the breast is seen in 50% to 90% of all patients (92,468). This degree of response renders surgery an option in patients initially presenting with unresectable disease and also allows for downstaging of resectable tumors and, therefore, for less disfiguring surgery (468).

In addition to numerous Phase II and pilot trials, in a randomized, prospective trial (B-18) reported by the NSABP (469), 1,523 patients with initially operable breast cancer were randomly assigned to receive doxorubicin 60 mg/m^2 and cyclophosphamide 600 mg/m^2 ("AC") every 3 weeks for four cycles, either before or after standard surgery. Surgeons were asked to judge the appropriateness of limited excision and mastectomy for all patients at enrollment and were allowed to perform the optimal operation for each patient whether they were randomized to preoperative or postoperative chemotherapy. In the preoperative treatment group, limited tumor excisions were performed in 81% of cases, compared with 57% in the postoperative chemotherapy group. More striking results were seen among patients presenting with tumors of 5 cm or greater in size; a 175% increase in the use of lumpectomy was seen. In addition, a consistent reduction in the incidence and extent of positive ipsilateral axillary nodes was observed in all subgroups. This latter point is critical because it confounds the prognostic value of lymph node status and basing specific treatment options on the results. At the same time, there was no difference in disease-free or overall survival associated with preoperative versus postoperative chemotherapy. This suggests that "early" and "late" treatment, at least within the several-months interval tested in this trial, does not affect overall outcome. This is consistent with randomized data from other adjuvant trials that have also failed to show an advantage for early treatment (397). An example is a trial in which patients were randomly assigned to treatment with chemotherapy delivered on the day of surgery or to treatment delivered within a month or two of the operation (436). There was no advantage for immediate chemotherapy. Based on these results, it appears reasonable to consider preoperative chemotherapy for subgroups of patients who are expected to gain specific benefits. In addition to patients with unresectable disease, those who might refuse to undergo mastectomy but for whom a limited excision and radiation therapy would be acceptable might be most appropriate for this approach.

Given the effective downstaging seen with preoperative therapy, a patient with pathologic node-negative disease might have initially had positive nodes, or perhaps not. This introduces the problem of how to use nodal information when the surgery is performed after preoperative chemotherapy. NSABP B-27 addressed these issues; all patients receive preoperative AC, one-third of the patients receive no further chemotherapy, one-third receive docetaxel, 100 mg/m^2 intravenously for four courses preoperatively, and one-third undergo surgery and then receive the docetaxel. To date, the trial has shown an increase in response in the breast tumor when docetaxel precedes surgery compared to AC alone. Long-term outcomes data are awaited. The effect on primary tumor response of adding sequential Taxotere (docetaxel) to Adriamycin and cyclophosphamide was reported on preliminary results from NSABP Protocol B-27 (470). On the assumption that this trial is positive overall, the issue of which subsets are benefiting will remain. Moreover, if a large number of patients are treated who do not benefit, this will diminish the apparent impact of the taxane. On the other hand, even if the trial is positive, it may not allow for the optimal selection of patients for this more aggressive chemotherapy.

There are other reasons why treating all patients with neoadjuvant therapy may not be an optimal approach: most studies use anthracyclines, but many low-risk patients, for whom this more toxic drug does not offer proven advantage, may be overtreated. Such patients would be those with negative nodes, smaller tumors, and no amplification or overexpression of HER-2/*neu*; CMF might be just as effective and arguably less toxic for this group (471). Another possible difficulty concerns the method of diagnosis. Specific reasons for trying to avoid unnecessary use of anthracyclines include the increased risk of both acute toxicities, such as alopecia, neutropenia, and mucositis, and chronic or late toxicities, including cardiomyopathy and perhaps leukemia (472). In addition, there are some patients with negative nodes and small tumors for whom tamoxifen alone might be appropriate treatment (473). Finally, even though most patients have significant downstaging of their disease with neoadjuvant treatment, a small minority will have resistant disease and experience progression while undergoing treatment. At worst, this could result in some patients with marginally resectable breast cancer becoming unable to undergo successful mastectomy.

Because of the unpredictability of downstaging and all of the other reasons, clinicians treating patients outside of properly randomized clinical trials should continue to consider preoperative chemotherapy as most appropriate for patients with unresectable disease or for those for whom mas-

TABLE 30.18. *Current trials testing neoadjuvant therapy*

Design	Study
A→CMF versus AT→CMF versus AT→surgery →CMF, all receive Tam	INT-23/96, EU-97001
Preop AC versus preop AC → D versus preop and postop AC → D	NSABP-B-27
Preop versus postop FEC ×4	EORTC-10902
Preop versus postop (FLAC) with G-CSF	NCI-90-C-0044F
Neoadj FAC versus Neoadj CMF QOL	GOCS-08-BR-95-III

tectomy is not an acceptable option. If conservation surgery appears feasible at presentation, there is no clear advantage demonstrated for earlier systemic treatment (Table 30.18).

Prognostic Factors in Systemic Treatment of Breast Cancer

Risk assessment is key. Ideally, this effort could identify those patients with no risk of recurrence who could forego any systemic therapy and, at the same time, allow better treatment regimens for those at higher risk (474). An additional possibility is the identification of predictive factors. These are markers not associated with prognosis but that are useful in identifying patients more or less likely to respond to specific treatments (59). Host factors investigated for their role as prognostic features include age, concurrent illnesses, pregnancy, menstrual history, family history, and genetic phenotype (475). In general, these factors do not influence the course of established breast cancer but may, in some cases, speak to the etiology of the disease. For example, patients with breast cancer and a known mutation of *BRCA1* or *BRCA2* would seem to have an explanation for their disease (186,476–478). On the other hand, there is little evidence that patients with or without abnormal *BRCA1/2* have any differences in terms of prognosis or response to therapy (471,479–481). Age and pregnancy have been studied longer, although always in retrospective fashion. In general, youth is associated with worsened prognosis, but an important limitation on this interpretation is the frequent association of younger age with worsened pathologic findings such as less estrogen-receptor positivity, as will be discussed below (202). Pregnancy does not appear to have a consistent effect on prognosis (482).

Pregnancy may in some cases limit the diagnostic workup and the therapeutic interventions, however, leading in turn to less adequate care (483).

For many years, the single best risk factor has been the pathologic status of the ipsilateral axillary lymph nodes (7, 152). Until recently, evaluation of axillary nodes required a careful axillary dissection yielding at least nine or ten nodes for study (484,485). Recent evidence suggests that with proper training, *sentinel-node biopsy* may be sufficiently accurate to allow many patients with negative nodes to forgo axillary dissection (379), which will minimize the toxicity of the local surgical treatment for breast cancer without compromising our ability to assess risk.

Among patients with positive axillary nodes, there is a direct and almost linear correlation between the number of involved nodes on H&E sections and the risk of relapse (354,474,486,487). A newer wrinkle is the identification of microscopic spread in sentinel nodes negative on H&E sections (488). These studies include multiple thin sections through the sentinel nodes and the use of cytokeratin and other stains to identify malignant cells; polymerase chain-reaction studies are being used in some centers. In almost all studies, the finding of a positive node by any criteria leads to additional surgery as above. Emerging data, however, suggest that only rarely do patients with a sentinel node positive by special studies actually have any additional positive nodes by conventional testing (489). Hence, it is very possible that a new subset of node-negative patients with an intermediate prognosis between those with truly node-negative and node-positive disease may be identified, which may lead to further refinement in the staging system for breast cancer.

Tumor size is the second most important risk factor for recurrence and becomes the most important one in those patients with negative nodes (8); risk of relapse rises in direct proportion to the size of the invasive component. An important subset contains patients with invasive ductal or lobular carcinoma measuring up to 1 cm, who have only a 13% actuarial risk of relapse at 20 years. The impact of adjuvant therapy is sufficiently small that, historically, such patients have not been routinely treated. As well, caution in assessing size is warranted as the initial studies determining risk were based on macroscopic measurements made on gross specimens. Manipulation of tumor specimens to place them on glass slides may lead to erroneous measurements, particularly if the tumor has not been sectioned along its longest axis. In addition, the relative proportion of invasive and noninvasive components is important, as the preinvasive tumor (DCIS) should not contribute significant risk of relapse, as does the invasive component. For most invasive ductal or lobular carcinomas containing up to 25% intraductal component this is not a critical concern, but for the occasional smaller tumor with greater than 25% noninvasive component, risk assessment from size can be challenging. Histology is also an important consideration in assessing risk of relapse as it relates to tumor size (330,490,491). Invasive ductal and lobular carcinomas have a similar risk of relapse at similar sizes. Among patients with node-negative disease, however, those with special histologies such as pure tubular, mucinous (or colloid), papillary, or medullary carcinoma may have a better prognosis (491,492). In these subtypes, larger tumors of up to 2 or 3 cm appear to have the same excellent prognosis as is seen in invasive ductal or lobular

carcinomas measuring up to 1 cm. Of course, in the presence of positive nodes, the histologic subtype is less critical, although tumor size is still a significant contributor to risk (493). Perhaps the first successful prognostic factor beyond lymph node number and tumor size was estrogen-receptor (ER) assessment (494–498). When all else is equal, it is clear that tumors that express this hormone receptor or the progesterone receptor (PR) have a better outcome, with longer time to relapse and improved overall survival compared to those without (499,500). On the other hand, the differences are minimal, and the greatest utility of this assessment is to identify patients more or less likely to respond to tamoxifen (501). Note that tamoxifen is effective in patients with positive ER-PR assays and, specifically, that patients whose tumors are negative for the estrogen receptor but positive for the progesterone receptor should be offered tamoxifen (498).

There are a variety of other potential prognostic factors, including S-phase fraction, DNA ploidy, cathepsin-D levels determined by biochemical assay or immunohistochemistry, and HER-2/*neu* overexpression (502–507). For these and other markers, such as *p53* overexpression (a marker of mutated *p53* gene), retrospective analyses have suggested the possibility of an impact on prognosis. The tumor suppressor *p53* which, like HER-2/*neu*, is also located on chromosome 17 (17p), encodes for a 53-kD protein, and mutation can lead to accumulation of abnormal protein in the tumor tissue where it can be visualized by immunohistochemistry staining. Clinical correlation with immunohistochemical staining remains under investigation, however (508,509). Another limitation on the utility of these prognostic factors is that they often correlate with more easily measured variables, such as tumor size and degree of differentiation. An additional difficulty with this area of research is the general lack of standardization between and even within laboratories. A final obstacle to their routine use is the lack of a simple system for integrating the multiple, often conflicting, prognostic-factor data. As a result, some groups have gone so far as to develop computer models to integrate all of the available data for an individual patient to derive a specific prognosis. Whether this effort allows one to accurately identify patients who can forgo therapy (or vice versa) is not yet known (510,511). Because of their complexity and lack of reliability, these newer factors have not entered routine clinical practice, and the safest course in the clinic at present is to rely on established histopathologic measures alone in assessing prognosis (502).

A more recently explored factor that appears to be both prognostic and predictive is the HER-2/*neu* gene (512,513), an oncogene on chromosome 17. The HER-2/*neu* receptor is a member of a family of epidermal growth-factor receptors including HER-3/*neu*, HER-4/*neu*, and the epidermal growth-factor receptor, as well as others (514). The exact role of the HER-2/*neu* receptor in cell growth, viability, and death is not completely understood, but dimerization of

HER-2/*neu* with other members of the family appears to be critical. Hence, overexpression of the receptor, which presumably increases the chances for dimerization, could have profound biological impact (511); overexpression of the receptor, or amplification of the number of gene copies, is associated both in the laboratory and the clinic with poor prognosis of breast cancer (515,516). In general, those tumors with amplification and/or overexpression are more aggressive, respond better to anthracyclines, and can be effectively targeted for therapy by trastuzimab (Herceptin) (517).

Amplification and/or overexpression of the gene and protein, respectively, is seen in 25% to 50% of breast cancers, depending on the specific test utilized (512,518). Interobserver variability for specific tests, however, and the lack of agreed-upon standard methodology for testing remain major challenges to the widespread use of this test. Presently, the most widely available test for HER-2/*neu* overexpression is a polyclonal antibody stain that is sensitive but apparently less specific than the monoclonal antibody stain used in the development of therapy targeting this receptor. Hence, it is possible that the available laboratory tests will overstate the incidence of clinically significant HER-2/*neu* positivity and lead to apparent lesser activity for trastuzimab than is seen in more carefully selected patient populations.

For patients with node-negative disease, multivariate analysis of only a few of many studies and including a total of only 100 patients has found a weak correlation between HER-2/*neu* overexpression and prognosis, but this does not address its value as a predictive factor (516,519–524). On the other hand, HER-2/*neu* overexpression may predict relative sensitivity to doxorubicin, particularly at higher doses, although further studies are underway to confirm these findings (20,157). In advanced disease, tumors with HER-2/*neu* overexpression have in some series been found to be significantly more sensitive to taxanes when compared with tumors with low expression, but this is not a consistent finding (525).

Postsurgical Chemotherapy and Hormone Therapy

The effectiveness of systemic, as opposed to local, therapy for breast cancer was first established over 100 years ago with Beatson's publication of the results of oophorectomy for the treatment of breast cancer (526).

The efficacy of systemic therapy in metastatic breast cancer quickly ensured its use in the treatment of early-stage cancers. Obvious candidates for treatment were patients with locally advanced breast cancer; however, with the evolution in thinking concerning the natural history of the disease, the use of systemic therapy in the treatment of patients with no detectable disease was studied.

Oophorectomy, the first effective systemic therapy for stage IV breast cancer, was predicted to work against occult microscopic disease precisely because of its ability to counter demonstrable disease and was therefore the first therapeutic manipulation tested in the adjuvant setting. This is important because Skipper's argument for adjuvant treatment was based on assumptions drawn from a model of murine leukemia in which proportional cell-kill resulted from chemotherapy treatment (527). Even if correct (see below) this does not necessarily predict the efficacy of hormone therapy, which may exert its effect in alternative ways. The result of this situation is that the potential benefit for hormonal manipulations might be expected to be modest. In light of this, it is perhaps even more impressive that the series of studies undertaken in the 1940s and 1950s were positive and did succeed as the first proof of the principle that adjuvant therapy might be effective (528).

Treatment of Metastatic Breast Cancer

The treatment of metastatic breast cancer is largely driven by the need to palliate symptoms. In this setting, the job of clinicians is to balance the benefits and risks of treatment to help patients maintain the highest possible quality of life (529). The standard systemic treatment options for patients with breast cancer include hormone therapy, chemotherapy, and more recently, immunotherapy with a monoclonal antibody directed at the extracellular domain of HER-2/*neu*.

Most patients with metastatic breast cancer are treated with hormone therapy, when appropriate, and subsequently with chemotherapy, as hormone therapy is generally the least toxic approach and as hormone-responsive tumors can be somewhat more indolent in their natural history than receptor-negative tumors. Therapy generally consists of tamoxifen unless the patient has already received this drug, in which case an aromatase inhibitor, such as anastrozole or letrozole, is used (530–533). These agents offer an approximately 20% response, but a significant number of patients will experience disease stabilization and most patients can remain on these agents for prolonged periods of time. Third-line hormone therapy, while appropriate in selected patients with a series of prolonged responses to earlier hormonal treatments, is generally less effective, and when the time to treatment failure becomes short or visceral involvement becomes a greater issue, chemotherapy should be considered.

As previously discussed, the role of ovarian ablation as treatment for metastatic disease dates over a century (534). In premenopausal patients, this approach alone, or in combination with tamoxifen, is popular and effective. Whether it offers any advantage over tamoxifen alone is, however, not yet clear, although prospective studies continue to evaluate this possibility (535–538).

Upon the failure of hormone therapy, chemotherapy is the conventional next step. When the clinician has reason to doubt the potential benefits of hormone therapy (i.e., negative hormone-receptor assays, rapidly progressive visceral disease), chemotherapy may be used earlier. The use of chemotherapy in this setting is individualized, and the recent availability of newer active agents serves to further diversify treatment approach. Combination chemotherapy is most frequently used, although recent explorations of single agents in clinical trials have rekindled enthusiasm for this approach. Appropriate options include any of the standard doxorubicin-containing regimens (CAF, AC, single-agent), CMF regimens, and the taxanes (paclitaxel and docetaxel).

The role of combination therapy, while considered standard, is increasingly questioned. Combinations, as tested over the past few decades, offer increased tumor response, increased duration of response, and perhaps slight survival advantages. Recent studies with single agents have, however, challenged this view. Regimens such as CMF or CAF were developed without comparisons to sequential applications of the same agents. This reflected the bias of the era, that combinations had to be superior to single agents. The development of the taxanes and other new agents, some of which have overlapping toxicities with established drugs, have forced a re-examination of this concept using new combinations versus sequential applications of the same agents. A specific example is the combination of taxanes and anthracyclines, which, although initially appearing promising, was possibly associated with excess cardiac toxicity (539,540).

The Eastern Cooperative Oncology Group (ECOG) (541) performed a randomized trial of doxorubicin plus paclitaxel versus each of these agents given singly at their "optimal" dose levels. Single-agent doxorubicin was given at a dose of 60 mg/m^2, while paclitaxel was given as a 24-hour infusion at a dose of 175 mg/m^2; in each case, 3-week cycles were used. Even years after this study was designed, further explorations of doxorubicin and paclitaxel dosing have failed to identify more active dosing levels for these drugs. With regard to doxorubicin, an adjuvant trial, discussed below, in which patients were randomized to receive 60, 75, or 90 mg/m^2 of drug, failed to demonstrate benefit for the higher dose levels (542). For paclitaxel, a trial comparing 175, 210, or 250 mg/m^2 has not shown any significant differences in effectiveness, and a small advantage for 24-hour infusions, as compared with 3-hour ones, has been reported (543,544). Hence, the dose and schedule combinations tested remain appropriate.

The third arm of the ECOG trial tested concurrent administration of doxorubicin and paclitaxel, given at slightly lower doses of 50 mg/m^2 and 150 mg/m^2 for doxorubicin and paclitaxel, respectively, to avoid excess toxicity. For the patients on either of the single-dose arms, a critical and valuable component of the trial was the plan for crossover treatment with the opposite drug. Thus, patients treated with single-agent doxorubicin crossed over to paclitaxel at disease progression, and vice versa. Overall, 739 women with chemotherapy-naïve metastatic breast cancer were randomly assigned to one of three treatment arms, and the combination arm was associated with a higher response proportion than either single agent: 46% versus 33% or 34%. As is typical of multicenter Phase III trials, however, this result was far more modest than in the two similar European Phase II trials.

For patients on the single-agent arms, crossover from doxorubicin to paclitaxel (or vice versa) was associated with a 14% to 20% chance of secondary response, and the median time to overall treatment failure was actually longer for the sequential arms than for the combination, even though overall survival was not different. In this study, sequential single agents offered somewhat less toxicity, a longer overall treatment time, and no compromise in survival compared with combination therapy.

Another trial demonstrates the concept that an active single agent can be superior to an established combination; heavily pretreated patients were randomly assigned to single-agent therapy with docetaxel or to a standard combination of mitomycin C and vinblastine (MV) (545). Patients receiving docetaxel had an increased response proportion compared with MV and improved overall survival. One related trial from Europe compared a combination regimen followed by a second combination with a sequence of two single agents (546). As predicted by most prior trials, the response proportion was greater for the combination given initially as compared with the single agent. The overall survival, however, was equivalent on both arms, and the quality of life appeared to be significantly better with the single-agent arm.

In addition to studies of newer agents, a longstanding research effort has focused on the role of high-dose chemotherapy. The scientific basis for this hypothesis includes the expectation that, for some drugs, doses above certain levels will successfully overcome drug resistance, and this is supported by selected preclinical data (547,548); active drugs for which a steep dose-response relationship has been seen in the laboratory include most alkylating agents and anthracyclines. The clinical application of high-dose therapy is also based on laboratory studies suggesting that the use of high-dose alkylating agents following optional cytoreduction can eradicate viable tumor even when the same treatment is not curative if applied at an earlier stage, prior to an initial course of cytoreductive therapy (549). Initially referred to as "bone-marrow transplant," and more recently as "peripheral stem-cell transplant," high-dose chemotherapy usually involves the delivery of maximally tolerable doses of a combination of drugs supported by autologous stem cells. It was the development of reliable means of harvesting cells, initially from the marrow and later from the periphery, along with the discovery and development of hematopoietic growth factors, that made this field of treatment possible. Yet, the issue in high-dose therapy is not the supportive care but rather the anticancer effectiveness of the drugs. Hence, the origin of these cells, bone marrow or peripheral blood, is not particularly relevant in terms of eradicating breast cancer, although there may be differences in toxicity (550–553). Purging techniques are being developed to provide a purer infusion product, but again, the more basic issue is the effectiveness of the treatment *in vivo,* not the danger of infusing viable circulating cancer cells (554).

One of the first studies of autologous stem-cell–supported treatment was reported in 1966 with a small number of patients (555). Dozens of uncontrolled Phase II trials have since explored the feasibility of using cyclophosphamide, BCNU, cisplatin, etoposide, carboplatin, thiotepa, melphalan, mitoxantrone, and ifosfamide, along with other drugs, in various combinations at escalated doses and supported by various growth factors and harvested, autologous bone marrow or peripheral stem cells. In almost every case, feasibility for the tested regimen is suggested, and comparison with expected or historical outcomes is almost uniformly called "promising." This has led to widespread acceptance of high-dose chemotherapy as an appropriate option for patients with metastatic disease, even though Phase III trials have not been available for analysis (Table 30.19).

However, a prospective study in which patients with metastatic disease were treated with CAF and then randomized to receive high-dose therapy or CMF was most informative in that it demonstrated no differences in outcome (556).

Data on the impact of patient selection are provided by careful analyses of patients who did not undergo high-dose therapy. Investigators at M.D. Anderson Cancer Center re-evaluated over 1,500 patients treated on a series of 18 clinical trials of conventional-dose chemotherapy and identified a subset, about 40%, who would have been eligible for contemporaneous trials of high-dose therapy (198). Treatment with standard-dose doxorubicin-containing regimens yielded a complete response rate of 27% for high-dose chemotherapy candidates, versus 7% for noncandidates and a longer median time to progression and death. The promising results of nonrandomized trials of high-dose therapy could be partially explained by careful selection of patients with metastatic breast cancer.

The development and introduction of a recombinant humanized monoclonal antibody directed to the HER-2/neu protein (rhuMabHER2, trastuzimab: Herceptin) marks an exciting change in the approach to breast-cancer treatment. For the first time, a targeted treatment, in this case an immune therapy, can be effective (517,557). Moreover, ample laboratory evidence suggests at least additivity with chemotherapy for this and related epidermal growth-factor–receptor antibodies prompting the Phase III trial of AC or paclitaxel combined with trastuzimab reported in 1998 (518,558, 559). In the Phase III trial comparing chemotherapy (paclitaxel or AC depending on the patient's prior treatment history) to the same plus concurrent trastuzimab, there was a significant advantage for the latter arm. Unfortunately, in the case of doxorubicin, this was associated with a surprising risk of cardiac failure, and, while more active, it is probably not appropriate for most patients (560). On the other hand, the combination of paclitaxel and trastuzimab was associated with acceptable toxicity and is being studied in an upcoming generation of adjuvant-therapy trials.

Research to improve the palliative options for patients with metastases also continues; one development is the availability of bisphosphonates that act to decrease osteoclastic activity and lead to less bone loss. One of these agents, alendronate, is available for the treatment of osteoporosis, but two others, pamidronate and clodronate, are being studied and used to decrease the rate of progression of osteolytic bone metastases (561,562). Intriguingly, these relatively less toxic drugs may, by decreasing initial bone metastases, actually reduce visceral metastases "beyond" the bone. Adjuvant use of them could be reasonable and will be tested.

The Worldwide Overview of Adjuvant Therapy

Nonrandomized Phase II trials, although frequently performed to demonstrate the feasibility and potential activity of a regimen or approach, can almost never be used to identify appropriate standard treatments. Because the number of patients on such studies is usually small and there is no appropriate control group, placing the results of such studies in context is impossible. In addition, the heterogeneous natural history of breast cancer and the potential selection biases of even well-meaning investigators conspire to make interpretation very difficult. The randomized Phase III study must remain the gold standard for making treatment decisions. There have been, however, several hundred studies testing dozens of medical treatments with varying other treatments and modalities, with inconsistent follow-up. Overcoming this growing problem (the result of growing commitment, enthusiasm, and participation in randomized trials) requires a new approach to data analysis, and the meta-analysis performed by the Early Breast Cancer Trialists' Collaborative Group (EBCTCG) seeks to address this issue.

TABLE 30.19. *Trends in autotransplants for breast cancer reported to the ABMTR 1989–1995*

	1989–1990	1991–1992	1993–1994	1995
Average number of patients transplanted per year	310	920	1,400	1,700
Metastatic disease at transplant	88%	70%	64%	50%
100-day mortality	18%	8%	5%	5%

To clarify the real benefits of common therapies, the EBCTCG has performed four overviews of all available, randomized trials: the first was in 1985, the second was conducted in 1990, the third in 1995, and the fouth in 2000. Inclusion in the overviews required proper randomization in a given trial and at least 5 years of follow-up. Once the data were provided to the EBCTCG, trials testing similar interventions (i.e., tamoxifen) were grouped for analysis. For each study, the untreated control arm, if there was one, was used to define the risk of recurrence, or death, in the patient population, and a ratio of the risk in the treatment arm to the control arm was then calculated. The various calculations were combined, giving greater proportional weight to larger studies, and a ''bottom line'' was calculated for the treatment. The results were expressed in several ways, as will be discussed below.

Before considering the results of the overview, one should recognize both its strengths and weaknesses. First, as described, the overview is a process of homogenization wherein similar but not necessarily identical trials are grouped for analysis. For tamoxifen, 20 to 40 mg was the daily dose for a period of 2 to 5 years, making treatment heterogeneity less of a concern. Among the many combination chemotherapy regimens and trials, however, there is far greater variation in drugs, doses, durations of therapy, and schedules of administration, and the overall results are therefore less applicable to any specific regimen chosen for use by an individual practitioner. Second, there is a bias inherent in the overview process toward older trials, as at least 5 years of follow-up is required for inclusion; they are more likely to contain untreated control arms than newer trials. As a result, they often will demonstrate more striking differences in outcome than can be expected in comparisons of more or less effective treatments. Third, tempting as it is to compare the numbers generated when using one modality (e.g., tamoxifen) versus those from use of another (e.g., ovarian ablation or chemotherapy), such comparisons are indirect and, therefore, not necessarily based on the same patients or studies. Hence, they cannot be considered valid. Fourth, the overview is most powerful when examining very large, homogeneous groups. Thus, if one attempts to identify homogeneous subgroups, one loses statistical power. Finally, the overview results are reported in several ways, including relative or proportional odds reductions (which are constant) and absolute benefits (which vary in proportion to the underlying risk). It is critical to keep in mind the relationship between these two types of reported results. With a fixed benefit in proportional odds and a constant risk over time, the absolute benefits can be calculated to be larger among high-risk patients than lower-risk patients. If one focuses on the relative risk reductions, however, it would seem appropriate to treat every patient with early-stage disease. On the other hand, with a focus on the absolute benefits, one may miss the opportunity to offer significant improvements in outcome to lower-risk patients. Certainly, successful and appropriate application of these results to individual patients or groups of patients requires careful assessment of the underlying risk of recurrence.

Ovarian Ablation

Ovarian ablation can be achieved by surgery, radiation therapy, or medical therapy, all of which decrease estrogen production. Whether obtained by surgery or irradiation, ovarian ablation was assessed in the overview (563). As it is only the newer trials of temporary ablation that used GnRH analogues, there are not yet sufficently mature data or patient numbers to support conclusions from the overview. As menopausal status is often unknown for study patients, women up to 50 years of age at the time of randomization are considered premenopausal, and ovarian ablation is of value only for this group. Statistically significant benefits in rates of recurrence and survival are demonstrated, and the benefits are durable. Indirect comparisons suggest that the benefit of ovarian ablation is less in patients who also receive polychemotherapy treatment, but this comparison is further confounded by the greater likelihood that the patients with involved lymph nodes, and therefore worse prognoses, would have received chemotherapy in earlier trials. Conversely, most women with negative nodes did not receive chemotherapy. In comparing the relative risk reductions in patients in these two broad risk categories, a principle of the overview discussed above is again seen: the proportional benefits of treatment are the same, while the absolute benefits vary with the underlying risk. Hence, both groups benefit, but a larger absolute improvement is seen among those with involved nodes. As predicted from preclinical models and testing, ovarian ablation did not add a significant benefit in patients with ER-poor tumors, whereas an additive benefit was seen for those with ER-positive tumors even after accounting for the benefits of chemotherapy. Although one might hypothesize an impact on the incidence of contralateral new primary breast cancer, none was seen. Finally, as expected, postmenopausal women did not benefit from hormonal ablation, whether received on its own or in combination with chemotherapy.

Tamoxifen

The published report of the 1995 overview of tamoxifen included 87% of all patients randomized for treatment on any clinical trial to date. Overall, 55 trials and 37,000 women were included, drawn from a total of 63 properly randomized trials that enrolled in total more than 42,000 women. In general, this overview confirmed many of the previously known findings from single studies and validated and expanded on the results of the previous overview published in 1992 (564).

Treatment with tamoxifen is very effective in estrogen-receptor–positive or unknown patients and ineffective in those known to be ER-poor. Because of its limited impact in patients with ER-poor tumors, this subgroup was formally excluded from the analysis, leaving out about 30,000 evaluable patients. Included were about 18,000 with tumors overexpressing hormone receptors and an additional 12,000 for whom the receptor status was unknown (Table 30.20). A lack of hormone-receptor status to guide individual treatment decisions, while relatively common in previous decades, is a rare problem in current clinical practice. These patients are, however, included in the overview for tamoxifen because about two-thirds will, based on historical series, be hormonally responsive.

Tamoxifen significantly lowered the annual risks of breast cancer recurrence and death for all patients with receptor-positive disease regardless of level or risk. Again, patients with positive nodes gained more in absolute terms than those with negative nodes. Five years of therapy was significantly better than 1 or 2 years, and the beneficial effects were essentially consistent across all age groups. The possibility that longer durations might be even better, or possibly worse, as suggested by the second randomization of the NSAPB B-14 trial, could not be addressed, but future overviews may be able to assess more relevant data on this point (565).

At 10 years of follow-up after being treated with tamoxifen for 5 years, the proportional reductions in annual odds of recurrence and mortality were 47% and 26%, respectively. In women with node-negative breast cancer, the absolute risk of recurrence was reduced by 14.9% and mortality by 5.6%. Among patients with positive nodes, the respective numbers were 15.2% and 10.9%; these differences were highly statistically significant. Evaluation at 10 years showed that the beneficial effects exceeded the duration of the treatment but the benefits (with regard to recurrence) were greatest during the first 5 years. Over the first 10 years, mortality continuously decreased. In the overview, 20 mg

of tamoxifen daily appeared to be as effective as 30 to 40 mg; the effect of tamoxifen was independent of whether patients did or did not receive chemotherapy. In contrast to earlier reports, the 1995 overview clearly demonstrated benefit even for premenopausal patients, many of whom received chemotherapy. Because this seemed to represent a change from earlier results and interpretations, explanations for this apparent increase in effectiveness for tamoxifen have been sought. Possibilities include the exclusion of ER-poor patients from the analysis (as these would overly depress the apparent benefits in younger patients), the increased numbers of patients treated for 5 years, and perhaps the increased use of chemotherapy in those patients with resulting ovarian dysfunction. Certainly, if the tamoxifen effect is diminished by competition for the estrogen receptor by circulating estradiol, the frequent and modest ovarian dysfunction that results from chemotherapy might possibly increase the potential impact of tamoxifen even without overt menopause. Worth considering in this light are the several small, individual reports previously demonstrating reductions in mortality for younger women treated with tamoxifen, even absent chemotherapy or ovarian dysfunction (565,566).

The ideal duration of tamoxifen treatment remains indefinite; the overview showed that 5 years is superior to shorter treatment durations. In NSABP B-14 there is not only a lack of an additional benefit after 5 years but also a potentially detrimental effect (565). The emergence of tamoxifen-dependent cell lines, as can be obtained in the laboratory, may partially explain this effect. Certainly, in metastatic disease, the observation of a "tamoxifen-withdrawal response" suggests that this functional change in cellular responsiveness could be real. In addition, although only very few mature trials have examined durations beyond 5 years, some are positive in this direction (567). At present, and based on the

TABLE 30.20. *Tamoxifen in the overview*

| | | Annual risk reduction: recurrence (%) | | Annual risk reduction: mortality (%) | |
| | | Years of treatment | | Years of treatment | |
	Subgroup	2	5	2	5
All	All	25 ± 2	42 ± 3	15 ± 2	22 ± 4
Hormonal status	ER ÷	28 ± 3	50 ± 4	18 ± 4	28 ± 5
	ER unknown	28 ± 4	37 ± 8	15 ± 4	21 ± 9
	ER poor	13 ± 5	6 ± 11	7 ± 5	−3 ± 11
Lymph nodes	Positive	30 ± 3	43 ± 4	19 ± 3	28 ± 6
	Negative	28 ± 5	49 ± 4	11 ± 6	25 ± 5
Chemotherapy	C ÷ T versus C	22 ± 4	52 ± 8	16 ± 4	47 ± 9
Dose	20 mg	28 ± 3	45 ± 4	17 ± 4	21 ± 6
	30–40 mg	28 ± 4	49 ± 5	15 ± 4	32 ± 6
Age	<50	14 ± 5	45 ± 8	10 ± 6	32 ± 10
	50–59	32 ± 4	37 ± 6	19 ± 5	11 ± 8
	60–69	33 ± 4	54 ± 5	12 ± 5	33 ± 6
	≥70	42 ± 8	54 ± 13	36 ± 7	34 ± 13
	All ages	29 ± 3	47 ± 3	17 ± 3	26 ± 4
Number of trials	–	32	9	32	9
Number of patients	–	19,622	8,349	19,622	8,349

available data, discussed above, 5 years of adjuvant treatment with tamoxifen does seem to be a reasonable recommendation for women with hormone-receptor–positive or unknown breast cancers outside of clinical trials.

The possibility of using tamoxifen as a preventative agent must be addressed. This is further supported by the observation that women with a first diagnosis of invasive breast cancer have significantly increased risk for additional diagnoses (568). In particular, the most recent overview found a significant reduction in the incidence of contralateral breast cancer in studies in which tamoxifen was administered for longer than 1 year. Among the studies that included 5 years of treatment with tamoxifen, there was an almost 50% reduction in the annual risk of contralateral breast cancer, and this observation is directly comparable to the results of the NSABP Breast Cancer Prevention Trial (BCPT) (569). In the latter prospective study, tamoxifen was given, on a randomized basis, to women without known breast cancer but for whom a high risk was calculated using a risk-assessment model (21). As with the treatment effect discussed above, the protective effect was independent of age. Worth emphasizing is the fact that neither the hormone-receptor status nor other prognostic and predictive features of the primary cancer were associated with any impact on the preventative effect of tamoxifen. Unfortunately, the absolute impact of this protective effect is modest, such that perhaps 1 patient in 100 has a cancer prevented by treatment with tamoxifen. Moreover, at present, these results may confound our approach to patients with early-stage disease as we consider whether to treat only patients with tumors overexpressing hormone receptors and size exceeding 1 cm, or to perhaps treat all patients in order to reduce their risk of developing second primaries.

Many studies have shown an increase in the incidence of endometrial cancer associated with the use of tamoxifen, and this is confirmed in the overview (21,564). It is also possible that there is a trend toward a higher incidence of endometrial cancer in patients treated for 5 years compared with 1 or 2 years. In keeping with these results, in the P-1 trial, an annual incidence of endometrial cancer of 2.3 per 1,000 women was seen in the tamoxifen-treatment group compared to 0.9 per 1,000 in the placebo group. Although all of the cases of endometrial cancer on the study were early stage, and few of the excess cases were found in premenopausal women, these cancers can be lethal and are cause for concern. In contrast to earlier data, statistical evidence of more frequent gastrointestinal (stomach and colorectal) cancer was not confirmed by either the overview or the prevention trial (570).

Another important side effect of tamoxifen is a higher incidence of thromboembolic phenomena. Again, the NSABP prevention trial confirmed this toxicity with an annual rate of 0.69 per 1,000 treated women but a rate of only 0.23 in the placebo group.

A potential benefit of treatment with drugs exerting an estrogen-agonist effect is the prevention of osteoporosis. In the prevention trial, the incidence of fractures was reduced from an annual incidence of 5.28 per 1,000 women on the placebo arm to 4.29 on the treatment arm. The net effect of tamoxifen on bone density in young women is not completely clear, however. A relatively small European trial reported an increased loss of bone in premenopausal women treated with tamoxifen, at least in the first several years of therapy (571). It does appear that tamoxifen positively influences bone metabolism overall when given for more than a year or two, and certainly among menopausal women. Further study is needed, however, to address this issue in young patients.

The ideal timing of tamoxifen and chemotherapy is uncertain, and concurrent treatment raises the risk of thromboembolic events (572,573). Hence, tamoxifen should follow systemic chemotherapy outside of clinical trials.

The activity and toxicities of tamoxifen motivate the continued development of similar drugs. In general, drugs with mixed estrogen and antiestrogen effects can be called selective estrogen receptor modulators (SERMs), as their effect is dependent on the tissue under consideration; they are ''selective'' in their influence on the estrogen receptor. The ideal SERM is a drug with antiestrogenic activity on breast and uterine tissues, but estrogenic effects on the bone and cardiovascular system, among others. Multiple SERMs are in clinical development and offer the promise of an improved benefit-to-risk ratio in the future. To date, toremefene and raloxifene have been made available, although neither has yet been proven equivalent or better than tamoxifen as adjuvant breast cancer therapy (574–576); it is not possible to recommend any of these newer drugs in place of tamoxifen until randomized studies assure us of at least equivalent benefits.

Aromatase Inhibitors

Several selective inhibitors of aromatase, including anastrazole and letrozole (nonsteroidal) and exemestane (steroidal) are approved for the treatment of metastatic breast cancer in the United States (577). As a class, these agents are effective only in postmenopausal women because they cannot adequately suppress the robust ovarian aromatization. However in postmenopausal women they significantly reduce circulating functional estrogens and have been at least as active as tamoxifen in the first-line treatment setting with somewhat lesser toxicities. Based on this activity they have been tested in the adjuvant setting against tamoxifen.

The first trial, ATAC, compared anastrazole against tamoxifen and tamoxifen against a combination of anastrazole with tamoxifen in over 9,000 women (578). The latter comparison showed no significant differences but anastrazole alone was associated with a reduced event rate compared to tamoxifen. Over 93% of the women had known expression of hormone receptors and only a minority had received adjuvant chemotherapy. The toxicity profile for anastrazole was

TABLE 30.21. *Relative risk reductions for chemotherapy in the overview*

	Subgroup	Proportional risk reduction for recurrence (%)	Proportional risk reduction in mortality (%)
Age	All	23.8 ± 2.2	15.2 ± 2.4
	<40	37 ± 7	27 ± 8
	40–49	34 ± 5	27 ± 5
	50–59	22 ± 4	14 ± 4
	60–69	18 ± 4	8 ± 4
	70 and older	NR	NR
Chemotherapy regimen	CMF alone	24 ± 3	14 ± 4
	With additional drugs othe	20 ± 5	15 ± 5
	than CMF	25 ± 4	17 ± 4

CMF, cyclophosphamide, methotrexate, and 5-fluorouracil.

predictably different from tamoxifen and included less vaginal bleeding and uterine cancer but more musculoskeletal complaints and bone mineral density loss. Based on these data, anastrozole is approved for adjuvant use (579).

A second drug in this class, letrozole, was tested against placebo following the completion of 5 years of therapy with tamoxifen. This trial (MA17) led for the Breast Intergroup by the NCI of Canada, accrued over 5,000 patients and was recently reported earlier than anticipated because it demonstrated a statistically significant advantage for letrozole with a median follow-up of 2.4 years (580).

Taken together, these two large recent trials lead to several conclusions. First it is now clear that selective aromatase inhibitors are active in early stage breast cancer in postmenopausal women; and second, they clearly have different toxicity profiles as compared to tamoxifen. The optimal integration of these agents (How long should they be used? Should they be given instead of tamoxifen, following tamoxifen, or followed by tamoxifen?) remains uncertain. Based on the available evidence, anastrozole can be considered for use in place of 5 years of tamoxifen in postmenopausal women and letrozole can be considered for 5 years following completion of tamoxifen. Ongoing studies will provide additional information in the coming years.

Adjuvant Chemotherapy in the Overview

In the 1995 overview, 23,000 women drawn from 47 available randomized trials were included (581); the overview excluded the most recent trials because of their shorter follow-up. In women under the age of 50 years, the administration of multiple chemotherapy agents administered over several months or longer ("polychemotherapy") decreased the annual risk of relapse by 35% and mortality by 27%. With 10 years of follow-up, this translated into an absolute reduction in the risk of mortality of 7% in node-negative tumors and 11% in node-positive tumors. As is the case with tamoxifen, the relative risk reduction for both relapse rate and mortality was not significantly better for women with or without nodal involvement, but the absolute benefits were

higher in women with lymph node involvement. As discussed earlier, this is true because while the relative benefits are constant, patients with higher risk gain more in absolute terms than those with lower risk (Tables 30.21 and 30.22).

For women over the age of 50 years the benefits of chemotherapy were smaller but still significant; the annual risk reductions were 20% for recurrence and 11% for mortality. At 10 years of follow-up, this risk reduction translated into absolute gains of 2% and 3% in node-negative versus node-positive tumors, respectively.

A frequent concern is the duration of this effect. In view of this question, it is interesting to note that absolute reduction in mortality steadily increased during the first 10 years of follow-up and almost doubled between 5 and 10 years. Hence, a modest length of treatment (typically 6 months) in the first year leads to a significant and increasing benefit up to a decade later. At the moment, because of limited long-term follow-up, the degree of reduction in mortality beyond 10 years is not yet known. A slightly different pattern was seen with regard to relapse rate, which increased up to the fifth year but then remained stable in comparison to the control group.

An issue to consider in examining the results of the overview is the impact of treatment heterogeneity. Few of the chemotherapy trials, even those using cyclophoshamide, methotrexate, or 5-fluorouracil (CMF), actually delivered the same doses or schedules of drug. Hence, the chemotherapy regimens are more heterogeneous and the results less

TABLE 30.22. *Absolute risk reductions*

		Absolute risk reduction for recurrence (%)	Absolute risk reduction for mortality (%)
Node-negative	<50 years	10.4 ± 2.3	5.7 ± 2.1
	>50 years	15.7 ± 2.3	6.4 ± 2.3
Node-positive	<50 years	15.4 ± 2.4	12.4 ± 2.4
	>50 years	5.4 ± 1.3	2.3 ± 1.3
Anthracyclines versus CMF	–	3.2 ± 1.5	2.7 ± 1.4

CMF, cyclophosphamide, methotrexate, and 5-fluorouracil.

applicable to any particular version of CMF. Despite these limitations, when polychemotherapy was grouped into CMF alone, CMF with additional drugs, and other combinations of chemotherapy agents, the benefits of all three were highly significant but essentially the same. It remains possible, however, that a particularly effective version of CMF might exist but it would not be identified as such by the overview. Another possibility, however, that the inclusion of anthracyclines might improve outcomes, is addressable from the overview.

The ideal duration of chemotherapy is not defined. Indeed, there may not be one ideal duration; instead, it is possible that for individual regimens the ideal duration will be different, or even more challenging; perhaps the ideal duration varies with the patient and the pathology. The overview, however, confirms earlier findings that the use of CMF for more than 6 months is not beneficial (582).

Combination Chemohormonal Therapy

If both chemotherapy and hormone therapy are active, the possibilities that they may be additive or even conflicting must be considered. Consistently, several overviews have demonstrated additivity for these two modalities without evidence of significant negative interaction. In support of this conclusion, several recent large trials have extended this observation to postmenopausal women with positive nodes and in all age groups with negative nodes (583,584). Because the overview does not identify any patients with receptor-positive disease for whom tamoxifen and chemotherapy are not effective, including young women who are also treated with chemotherapy and older women already chosen for tamoxifen, it is reasonable to consider chemotherapy for postmenopausal patients treated with tamoxifen. Conversely, the addition of tamoxifen for younger women treated with chemotherapy is also reasonable.

Specific Chemotherapy Regimens

The most widely accepted standard treatment for breast cancer is probably the combination of cyclophosphamide, methotrexate, and 5-fluorouracil (CMF) regimens; these can be given in oral or intravenous forms and using a variety of schedules (every third or fourth week), doses, and durations. In general, CMF is a standard adjuvant therapy for low-risk patients, such as those with negative axillary nodes (14,585).

Given the high degree of activity seen for doxorubicin when given as a single agent, a variety of regimens incorporating it have been tested. The overview suggests that some of these non-CMF regimens, such as AC (doxorubicin and cyclophosphamide) and FAC (5-fluorouracil, doxorubicin, and cyclophosphamide) might even be more active than CMF. A subset analysis of 12 trials in which a CMF-type regimen was compared to a doxorubicin or epirubicin regimen (581) (Table 30.22) showed a small but statistically

significant advantage for anthracycline-containing regimens: the proportional risks for recurrence and mortality were reduced by 12% and 11%, respectively, and the absolute benefits were 3.2% and 2.7%, respectively.

A recent report of a randomized trial (Intergroup INT 0102) comparing CMF and CAF in high-risk node-negative patients with or without tamoxifen (586) enrolled 4,400 patients and stratified them into three risk groups: high (tumors of ≥2 cm or ER/PR-negative), low (<2 cm and ER/PR-positive), and uncertain (ER/PR-unknown). The high-risk patients were randomized to receive either CAF or CMF with or without tamoxifen for 5 years. The low-risk patients received no adjuvant therapy. The uncertain-risk patients were assigned to the high- or low-risk group based on the S-phase analysis of their tumors. Overall mortality was 8% with CAF and 9% with CMF, becoming 7% and 8%, respectively, when tamoxifen was added. The recurrence rate was 15% with CAF and 18% with CMF, and 13% and 15% with the addition of tamoxifen. Mortality and relapse rates were 4% and 11% in patients with small ER/PR-positive tumors. In this study of relatively low-risk node-negative patients, CAF may be marginally better, but more toxic, and this difference, while significant, is small.

Based on this possibility of superiority, as well as on the brevity and cost advantage of four cycles of AC as compared to six to eight cycles of CMF, many clinicians chose the former for many patients. It should be noted, however, that the toxicity profiles of the anthracycline-containing regimens differ from those of the CMF-type treatments (587). Specifically, alopecia and neutropenia are potentially greater with the anthracyclines, and the risk of cardiomyopathy is greater (588,589). As a result, one ongoing effort concerns the possibility of identifying patients whose tumors are more or less likely to benefit specifically from the use of anthracyclines. Presently, the most promising candidate in this regard is HER-2/*neu* status. In preclinical and more recent clinical testing, a trend is emerging for tumors that have amplified or overexpressed HER-2/*neu* to have increased responsiveness to doxorubicin while those lacking this trait do not. Hence, it may be possible in the future to offer anthracylines to patients with HER-2/*neu*–positive tumors and avoid these agents in those with HER-2/*neu*–normal expression (157, 513). At the same time, given the toxicities of anthracyclines, as well as this emerging evidence concerning the interaction between HER-2/*neu* overexpression, doxorubicin use, and doxorubicin dose, one can continue to recommend CMF, especially in low-risk patients with tumors not overexpressing HER-2/*neu*.

New Directions in Adjuvant Chemotherapy

Dose Escalation

Based on the promising laboratory data that suggest a steep dose-response relationship, particularly for alkylating agents, numerous pilot trials of very-high-dose, autologous stem cell–supported chemotherapy trials have been conducted, including many involving patients with high-risk early-stage disease. As a result, adjuvant therapy using high-dose chemotherapy was popularized and was often considered a standard treatment for high-risk breast cancer. High-dose adjuvant therapy followed by autologous bone-marrow transplant (ABMT) and/or peripheral stem-cell rescue (PSCR) was commonly used for women with more than 10 involved lymph nodes or with very large tumors. It has even been offered to women with much lower number of involved lymph nodes. Unfortunately, randomized studies now available do not support this approach.

Dose escalation has not emerged as an effective strategy even at lower dose levels. The NSABP B-22 trial was designed to test the value of intensifying the dose of cyclophosphamide (590). Postoperatively, patients with node-positive disease all received four cycles of doxorubicin, 60 mg/m^2, at 3-week intervals. They were, however, randomly assigned to concurrent treatment with four cycles of cyclophosphamide 600 mg/m^2, two cycles only with 1,200 mg/m^2, or four cycles at the higher dose. A subsequent trial from the NSABP (B-25) was similar in design but began at the higher dose of 1,200 mg/m^2 and doubled the dose intensity (2,400 mg/m$^2 \times$ 2) and the total dose (2,400 mg/m$^2 \times$ 4). Thus far, both of these trials fail to demonstrate significant advantages for any of the higher-dose arms. Moreover, a surprising incidence of myelodyscrasias and leukemia was identified on B-25, providing reason for caution (591). With regard to doxorubicin, a Cancer and Leukemia Group B trial (CALGB 9344) failed to show an advantage for doxorubicin dose escalation from 60 to 75 to 90 mg/m^2 given every third week for four cycles in combination with standard-dose (600 mg/m^2) cyclophosphamide (542). Given the emerging evidence concerning HER-2/*neu* status, it will be important to explore the HER-2/*neu* status of the patients on this trial.

Dose Density

Faced with the increasingly likely possibility that dose escalation for active drugs in breast cancer does not increase activity, alternative approaches are being developed. In addition, the models that first suggested value for adjuvant treatment also suggest that multiple cycles of treatment will be necessary for cure (592). Taken together, these two concepts lead to a treatment approach termed "dose density," in which treatment is intensified through the shortening of the intertreatment intervals. This method of dose intensification was first proposed by Norton and Simon (515), and has recently been the subject of clinical trials.

The first direct test of dose-dense therapy was the randomized trial from Milan of alternating versus sequential therapy using single-agent doxorubicin and CMF (593). Here, over 400 women with four or more involved axillary nodes received four cycles of doxorubicin and eight cycles of CMF.

TABLE 30.23. *Taxanes as (neo)-adjuvant Rx: randomized trials*

Study	Design	Result
9344	AC $\pm$ P	Positive
B28	AC $\pm$ P	Positive
Aberdeen	CAVp $\pm$ D	Positive
B27	AC $\pm$ D	Positive
BOIRG001	DAC versus FAC	Positive
MD Anderson	P→FAC versus FAC	Too Small ...? Positive
U.S. Oncology	DC versus AC	Positive? (early/small)

P, paclitaxel; D, docetaxel.

The less dose-dense arm utilized an alternating plan of two cycles of CMF followed by one cycle of doxorubicin, which can be represented as "CCACCACCACCA." The more dose-dense arm consisted of all four cycles of doxorubicin followed by all eight of CMF: "AAAACCCCCCCC." At 10 years of follow-up, the more dose-dense arm continues to demonstrate significant superiority. Based on this result, a pilot trial in which high-dose cyclophosphamide given at 2-week intervals replaced the CMF was performed with promising results (594). This led to the now completed SWOG-led randomized trial (SWOG 93–13) of concurrent versus sequential doxorubicin and cyclophosphamide (Table 30.23). Although not a positive trial, the confounding effects of differerent numbers of cycles and different dose sizes make interpretation difficult (595). A trial specifically designed to test the value of more frequent, alternate-week dosing is now completed and will be discussed below.

Taxanes

The most significant development in conventional chemotherapy in the past decade is the discovery of the efficacy, feasibility, and non–cross resistance of the taxanes, a new class of chemotherapeutic agents presently including docetaxel and paclitaxel, with other agents also being developed (596). Paclitaxel in particular has been extensively tested using a large variety of doses and schedules, but more recently dose-dense weekly applications of both taxanes are under development (597). Based on its promising activity, paclitaxel was added first to existing adjuvant regimens. The first use was as part of the sequential dose-dense regimen of doxorubicin and cyclophosphamide, and this trial, which also utilized escalated doses and increased frequency of treatment (every other week), yielded sufficiently promising results in high-risk patients to motivate a large Phase III study (598). The Intergroup, in a SWOG-led trial (SWOG 96–23), compared dose-dense sequential doxorubicin, paclitaxel, and cyclophosphamide versus concurrent AC followed by "conventional" high-dose autologous stem cell–supported consolidation in patients with four to nine involved axillary nodes. This study closed accrual early because of diminished interest, in the wake of the negative trials of high dose therapy as adjuvant therapy.

To determine the value of adding paclitaxel or docetaxel as adjuvant treatment, a variety of randomized trials are either underway or have been completed. The first completed trial is from the Cancer and Leukemia Group B (CALGB), which coordinated an intergroup trial designed to determine the impact of adding paclitaxel and also the value of escalating the dose of doxorubicin, as discussed above (599). A pilot trial had demonstrated the feasibility of utilizing AC followed by paclitaxel (600). A factorial design allowed the CALGB-led intergroup study to address two presumably unrelated questions. As discussed above, one randomization assigned patients to receive AC using 60 mg/m^2 versus 75 mg/m^2 versus 90 mg/m^2 of doxorubicin, and another assigned them to either receive four subsequent cycles of paclitaxel 175 mg/m^2 as 3-hour infusions or not (542). Over 3,000 patients were randomized in little more than 3 years, and at the final report, with a median follow-up of 69 months, the addition of paclitaxel was associated with a significant improvement in disease-free survival. The proportional reductions in risk of relapse and mortality were 17% and 18%, respectively. A recent report of NSABP B-28 testing virtually the same approach (AC with or without four doses of paclitaxel) (601) found the same disease-free survival benefit. In the same vein, a trial substituting 5-fluorouracil with docetaxel in the FAC regimen (hence, TAC vs FAC) was positive for the taxane (602).

The study of dose density, CALGB 9741, builds on these results; patients with node-positive breast cancer are treated with concurrent AC followed by paclitaxel (ACP) or sequential single agents (APC). On both arms, all patients receive four doses at standard dose levels for each of these three active drugs. To address the issue of dose density, patients are also randomly assigned to receive all of their chemotherapy at 2- or 3-week intervals, the former requiring granulocyte colony-stimulating factor (G-CSF). As with the earlier CALGB trial, this study utilizes a factorial design so as to allow for examination of two unrelated questions. At the first protocol-specified analysis, sequential and concurrent therapy (with AC together or sequentially) were equivalent but dose-dense therapy was superior in both disease-free and overall survival (603).

Additional information will be provided by many other related ongoing trials (Table 30.23) but it is already clear that taxanes are active in the adjuvant setting.

Radiation Therapy in Carcinoma of the Breast: Overview

In early-stage breast cancer, radiation therapy is usually given as one element of the primary local-regional treatment, in combination with a surgical procedure. After breast-conservation surgery, the entire breast is targeted for irradiation,

and depending on the extent of the axillary node dissection and the pathology of the nodes, the regional lymph nodes may also be included. Timing of irradiation will depend on the patient's need for systemic chemotherapy; in general, irradiation follows chemotherapy if the latter is prescribed.

For women who opt for mastectomy and who are at high risk for local failure, postoperative, post-chemotherapy irradiation to the chest wall and regional lymphatics is indicated. The definition of "high risk" has recently changed with the publication of two studies demonstrating that premenopausal patients with one to three involved axillary nodes benefit from this treatment in terms of both better local control and improved survival (16,17). Prior to these publications, "high risk" was defined as T3 lesions and the presence of four or more involved nodes. While these two studies from Overgaard in Denmark and Ragaz in Canada have been criticized for some evidence of less-than-optimal surgery, they focus attention on those patients who are at risk for local-regional failure not addressed by surgery and systemic treatment alone (604).

A recent retrospective study from the M.D. Anderson Cancer Center, which reviewed patterns of local failure in over 1,000 women treated with mastectomy and chemotherapy but not radiation, also suggests that the pathology findings of lymphovascular space involvement, gross multicentric disease, close or positive margins, or skin, nipple or pectoral fascia involvement, increases the risk of local-regional failure, and is reason to consider radiation post-mastectomy as well (605).

The other major role of irradiation in breast cancer is to palliate recurrent and metastatic disease. Irradiation is an effective treatment for metastatic lesions in the bone, brain, spinal cord, and other areas. It is also used to control local-regional disease in the chest wall and regional lymphatics.

Most irradiation treatments are given as a series of "external-beam" visits, where the patient comes daily for a fraction of the total dose prescribed. Linear accelerators most commonly produce these beams, although some cobalt units remain in use in North America. Treatment course times range from a few days, when rapid palliation is desired, to 6 to 7 weeks, in a primary situation, when the focus is on both cure and minimizing long-term side effects.

A second technique for delivering radiation is with the use of brachytherapy. For breast-cancer treatment, this may be done using a method in which a boost dose of additional radiation is delivered to the site of the primary cancer after irradiation of the entire breast has been completed. After-loading catheters can be placed intraoperatively in the biopsy cavity, and sources, usually ^{192}Ir, are temporarily loaded to deliver the desired dose. An alternate and more commonly used method of administering this boost involves the use of a more focused external-beam field of electrons. The rationale for primary treatment is discussed in the sections on surgery and chemotherapy, with information on prognostic factors in that section of this chapter.

Partial Breast Irradiation

Recently, several researchers have reported on their experience using both high dose–rate (HDR) and low dose–rate (LDR) brachytherapy as the sole radiation treatment of the intact breast (606–609). Since many breast recurrences after conservation surgery and whole breast radiation occur at or near the site of the index primary cancer, it is hypothesized that partial breast treatment may be as effective as whole breast treatment. Because a smaller volume of the breast is treated with this technique, the overall time course of these treatments has been shortened from the standard 6 weeks to 1 week, using a twice per day fractionation. Initial reports on both local control and cosmesis are encouraging, although few patients treated in this manner have been followed to the 5-year mark (610). Randomized studies comparing this to the standard 6 weeks of whole breast radiation are open for accrual (RTOG) (611,789 (new Vicini refs).

Intraoperative Radiation Therapy

Veronesi et al. developed an intraoperative radiation therapy (IORT) technique of a breast quadrant after the removal of the primary carcinoma using a mobile linear accelerator (linac) to deliver electron beams with energies from 3 to 9 MeV. Through a Perspex applicator, the radiation is delivered directly to the mammary gland and, to spare the skin from radiation, the skin margins are stretched out of the radiation field (Fig 30.28). To protect the thoracic wall, an aluminum-lead disc is placed between the gland and the pectoralis muscle. Different dose levels were tested from 10 to 21 Gy without important side effects. They estimated that a single fraction of 21 Gy is equivalent to 60 Gy delivered in 30 fractions at 2 Gy per fraction. The follow-up time of the 101 patients varied from 1 to 17 months (mean follow-up

time was 8 months); the IORT treatment was very well accepted by all patients. The authors believe that single-dose IORT after breast resection for small mammary carcinomas may be an excellent alternative to the traditional postoperative radiation therapy. However, a longer follow-up is needed for a better evaluation of the possible late side effects. At the Milan Cancer Center, a Phase III trial comparing IORT to whole breast radiation is ongoing (612).

Radiation Therapy Techniques for the Intact Breast

Following wide-local excision, segmental mastectomy, or quadrantectomy, the breast is irradiated with lateral and medial tangential portals. As noted above, consideration of regional lymphatic radiation depends primarily on the pathologic involvement of the excised axillary lymph nodes.

Treatment Volume

The entire breast, along with a small portion of underlying chest wall and lung, should be included in the irradiated volume. Radiopaque surgical clips placed at the margin of the tumor bed may assist in defining the target volume (613). The planning session is carried out in a special unit called the simulator, which is a diagnostic x-ray unit or CT scanner, with all the geometric characteristics of a high-energy treatment machine.

In order to prescribe a uniform dose to the entire breast, using a two-dimensional breast contour or three-dimensional data acquired with a CT simulator, a treatment plan using compensating wedges, filters, or with intensity modulation of the treatment beam is designed. The inhomogeneity throughout the entire treatment volume should be less than 10%. When treatment is delivered with a standard 6-MV photon beam to larger-sized patients, with tangential field separation of over 22 cm, there is still significant dose inhomogeneity in the breast, even with compensators (614). This problem can be minimized by using higher-energy photon beams with a ''spoiler'' to ensure adequate dose to the superficial breast tissue.

Other treatment positions than the standard supine position have been used to improve the dosimetry in patients with large, pendulous breasts. At the Institut Curie, these women are treated in the lateral decubitus position to flatten the breast contour (615). Irradiation in the prone position has been used at Memorial Sloan–Kettering Cancer Center (616), with reduction in the high-dose region of the irradiated breast, as well as reduction in volume of and dose to the underlying lung and heart, and reduction of scattered dose to the contralateral breast.

Doses and Beams

Tumor doses of 45 to 50 Gy are delivered to the entire breast in 5 to 6 weeks (1.8- to 2-Gy tumor-dose daily, five

Supine: Transverse Plane

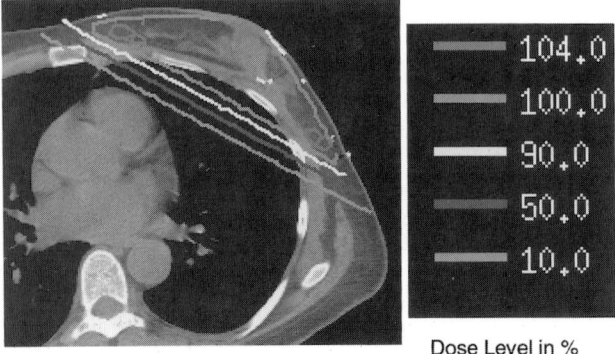

Dose Level in %

FIG. 30.28. Isodose curves for 6-MV x-rays, displayed in the transverse, sagittal and coronol planes, using IMRT planning. Prescription is to the 100% line. Prone position, compared with supine position, decreases lung dose.

weekly fractions). X-ray energies of 4 to 6 MV are preferred to treat the breast. Photon energies greater than 6 MV may underdose superficial tissues beneath the skin surface, but higher-energy photons may be helpful in large breasts in order to decrease the integral breast dose, as noted above.

"Boost" to Tumor Site

The so-called "boost" portion of the primary radiation treatment is a series of additional treatments directed only to the excisional biopsy site, since this region of the breast is most likely to harbor remaining tumor cells.

Fisher and colleagues (152) questioned the need for a "boost", and NSABP studies to date have not required a boost. A large randomized study from the EORTC group in Europe recently addressed this question. Over 5,500 women with stage I or II breast cancer were randomly assigned to whole breast treatment with or without a boost. At 5 years, the rate of local failure was 7.3% in the no-boost group, compared to 4.3% in the boost group. The largest benefit was seen in the youngest subset of women, those 40 years of age or younger. In that subset, the local failure rate was 19.5% without the boost, compared to 10.2% with the boost. In the oldest patient subset, the local failure rates were 4% without a boost compared to 2.5% with a boost. The authors concluded, after multivariate analysis, that "the absolute benefit of the additional dose justifies its use in patients 50 years old or younger" (617).

Margin width and post reexcision pathologic status of surgical margins must be considered in prescribing the boost dose as well. Boost doses range from 10 to 20 Gy.

Before the widespread availability of electron beam, interstitial brachytherapy, or a cone-down photon boost, was popular. Many institutions currently prefer electron-beam boost because of its relative ease in setup, the outpatient setting involved, its lower cost, the decreased time demanded of the physician, and its excellent results when compared with implants. Radiation oncologists who prefer the brachytherapy boost technique point to decreased skin dose and potential radiobiologic advantages when compared with electron-beam boost therapy.

Accurate target volume definition is critical with any boost technique. Methods vary from the simple and unsophisticated to such complex and expensive alternatives as ultrasound and CT definition of the target volume. The surgical clip method requires the cooperation of the surgical team; at the time of the wide excision, the surgeon places clips in the medial, lateral, superior, and inferior extents to the biopsy cavity, as well as a "deep" clip. During the simulation, these clips are localized with relation to the scar and setup marks and provide excellent guidance for the identification of the boost target volume.

Irradiation Dose to the Contralateral Breast

Fraass and colleagues (618) measured dose to the contralateral breast in 16 women treated to the intact breast with

TABLE 30.24. *Incidence of contralateral breast cancer in carcinoma of the breast treated with conservation surgery and irradiation or mastectomy*

Study	Conservation therapy	Mastectomy
Arrigada et al (436)	88 (14%)	91 (11%)
Broët et al (621)	1,819 (3.8%)	1,815 (3.9%)
Clark et al (293)	1,504 (3%)	–
Dewar et al (310)	757 (6%)[a]	–
Kurtz et al (674)	300 (6.5%)[b]	–
Washington University[f]	839 (6%)	–
Montague (321)	316 (1.9%)[c]	576 (5.2%)
Recht et al (324)	366 (9%)[d]	–
Rosen et al (754)	–	76 (10.7%) RT
		47 (9.4%) no RT
Sarrazin et al (622)	88 (9%)[c]	91 (9%)
Veronesi et al (623)	349 (5%)[e]	352 (5%)[f]

RT, radiation therapy.
[a] Actuarial relapse at 10 years.
[b] Actuarial risk at 20 years.
[c] Excludes simultaneous bilateral cancer.
[d] Actuarial risk at 5 years
[e] Actuarial risk at 12 years
[f] Unpublished data.

tangential fields and performed phantom measurements. For a typical treatment of 50 Gy, the contralateral breast received 0.5 Gy to 2 Gy. The volume of breast irradiated has minimal effect, but the use of portals for the regional lymph nodes increases dose to the contralateral breast. A careful dosimetric study demonstrated that most of the scatter dose received by the opposite breast originates in the collimator and accessories of the accelerator and can be significantly decreased by increasing the distance between the source and the patient's skin (619). The use of independent jaws combined with beam splitters following the contour of the chest wall of the patient can be very helpful in decreasing the dose to the contralateral breast. The use of dynamic wedges and of most forms of IMRT also significantly reduces the scatter to the contralateral breast (620). The clinical significance of this inadvertent radiation dose to the opposite breast is uncertain; various investigators have failed to show an increased risk of contralateral breast malignancy after treatment of the original breast by radiation therapy (Table 30.24) (321,436,621–623).

Irradiation of Regional Lymphatics

Supraclavicular Lymph Nodes

Irradiation of this area is prescribed if the patient has had a node dissection and more than three axillary lymph nodes are involved with carcinoma (275). If only the apex of the axilla is treated (after modified radical mastectomy or axillary dissection), the inferior border of the supraclavicular field is the first or second intercostal space. The medial border is 1 cm across the midline, extending upward, following

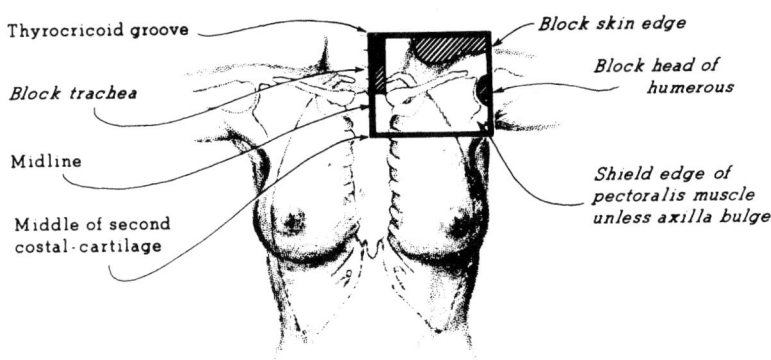

Thyrocricoid groove

Block trachea

Midline

Middle of second costal-cartilage

Block skin edge

Block head of humerous

Shield edge of pectoralis muscle unless axilla bulges

FIG. 30.29. Diagram illustrating the supraclavicular portal. When a 15-degree lateral angulation is used to avoid the spinal cord, the medial margin is 1 cm across the midline up to the sternal notch. The humeral head is at least partially blocked.

the medial border of the sternocleidomastoid muscle to the thyrocricoid groove. The lateral border may be at the level of the anterior axillary fold, although if the surgeon has left hemostasis clips in the axilla, these can guide the design of this field. The humeral head is blocked as much as possible without compromising coverage of the high axillary lymph nodes. This field is angled about 10 to 20 degrees laterally, to spare the spinal cord (Fig. 30.29). The total dose delivered to the supraclavicular field is 46 to 50 Gy, with consideration of a "boost" dose if biopsy-proven disease is identified in this region.

Axillary Lymph Nodes

When the axilla is treated, the supraclavicular field is extended to the second rib; the dose to the midplane of the axilla from the supraclavicular field is calculated at a point approximately 2 cm inferior to the midportion of the clavicle. The difference to this level is then made up by a supplemental dose delivered by a posterior axillary field to the complete dosage of 46 to 50 Gy.

Internal Mammary Lymph Nodes

The benefit of treatment to the internal mammary lymph nodes is an unresolved issue, since clinical failures at this site are very rare (624), and most patients at risk receive some form of adjuvant therapy. Treatment to the internal mammary nodes is not necessary in most patients; in patients with primary tumors in the medial quadrants, with tumors larger than 3 cm in diameter, or in those patients with multiple involved axillary nodes, or where involvement of these nodes is demonstrated by biopsy or imaging, every effort should be made to include them. This is technically demanding and can be accomplished by several techniques, including "wide tangent fields," a separate electron field, or a combination of both (625).

Irradiation Techniques after Mastectomy and for Local Chest-Wall Failure

Patients referred for adjuvant irradiation after mastectomy are at risk for both systemic and local-regional failure. The target volume required in this setting addresses the local-regional risk and includes the chest wall and regional lymphatics, with the same considerations for inclusion of the lower axilla and the internal mammary nodes as noted for treatment of the intact breast. Although the two studies from Canada and Denmark demonstrating the advantage of postmastectomy irradiation in node-positive, premenopausal women did include treatment of the internal mammary nodes, treatment to this area remains controversial (604).

Technique is determined by the patient's anatomy and whether or not a breast reconstruction has been done. For the patient with reconstruction, a three-field technique is used, as with the intact breast, with two tangent fields directed at the chest wall and reconstruction and a third, carefully matched field encompassing the supraclavicular nodal area and the apex of the axilla. Because the mastectomy scar and skin are considered at risk as sites of possible recurrence in this setting, the use of a bolus material is indicated to bring the surface dose up to the prescription dose. Photon beams are in the 4- to 6-MV range, and doses of 50 Gy over 5 weeks are appropriate, with a boost dose of 10 Gy to the mastectomy scar itself.

For women who have not had a breast reconstruction, this same three-field technique can be used. An alternate technique is the use of matching electron beams. For this, the patient is simulated and then CT scans throughout the target volume are obtained. This information is used to design custom electron-shaping cutouts and compensating bolus, to encompass, for example, the internal mammary and supraclavicular nodal areas with a beam energy that penetrates to a distance of 3.5 to 4.0 cm deep, and then matches with a custom cutout to cover the remainder of the chest-wall area, but with a lower electron energy based on the CT scan information. With this technique, little exit dose is received to underlying lung and heart; movement of the field junctions every other day is important to ensure a uniform dose in the match areas.

Recurrent disease in the chest wall or regional lymphatics is approached as potentially curative disease, provided that the recurrence is isolated. After surgical debulking, if technically feasible, irradiation design is again similar to the approach for the patient in the postmastectomy adjuvant irradiation setting, in terms of field design and dose. Any area where palpable disease is present is "boosted" to a dose higher than the 50 Gy appropriate for the entire local-regional area. The boost dose is individualized, depending on the volume of gross disease on physical and imaging evaluation.

Radiation for Distant Metastases

Radiation therapy for distant metastatic sites can often result in prompt relief of the patient's symptoms. Irradiation is most commonly used in breast-cancer management in this setting for disease in the bones, brain, and spinal cord, and to relieve pressure from metastatic disease in clinical situations such as superior vena cava syndrome or cranial nerve palsies. Treatment courses are often of shorter duration than curative courses, with a dose and fractionation scheme of 3 Gy per day for 10 days being most common in the United States.

FOLLOW-UP OF PATIENTS

After the acute phase of treatment for early-stage breast cancer, patients and physicians are motivated to pursue careful follow-up. Three obvious goals must be considered after treatment. One is the identification of new, curable disease; another is the early diagnosis of presymptomatic metastatic disease so as to facilitate preemptive palliation; and a third is to provide reassurance of good health.

Curable disease discovered during follow-up can include new primary ipsilateral or contralateral breast cancer, other primary malignancies, such as colorectal or cervical cancer, and other nonmalignant medical illnesses.

Patients with a personal history of one breast cancer are clearly at increased risk for the development of second primary breast cancers (568). Those undergoing breast conservation also have a risk of at least 5% of disease in the ipsilateral breast, even after optimal surgery and radiation therapy, that can represent recurrent, persistent, or new primary invasive cancer. Distinguishing between these possibilities is always challenging, and most patients in this category are treated for new primary disease if possible (626, 627). Women with *BRCA* mutations are at increased risk for breast-cancer–related events after breast conservation including increase in incidence of contralateral breast cancers (627). As is true in the case of any other defined high-risk group, screening should consist of regular history and physical examinations and screening mammography; however, the most appropriate interval for physical examination and mammography following treatment for breast cancer is not absolutely established. Retrospective studies have established the value of regular physical examinations combined with yearly mammographic screening. At minimum, patients who have completed treatment for one breast cancer should be followed at least as often as any other high-risk group. In keeping with the recommendations for screening in the

general population, patients with a history of breast cancer should be followed with at least a yearly history and physical examination and mammography. More frequent office visits may be justifiable, but the use of more frequent screening mammograms, although recommended by some clinicians, is not supported by prospective studies (628).

Although patients with a history of breast cancer may be at increased risk for other malignancies, there are no data supporting more intensive screening for them.

A particular concern in this regard among patients treated with tamoxifen as adjuvant therapy is surveillance for endometrial carcinoma (629) as patients on tamoxifen face an increased risk of uterine cancer (21,564).

Recent analysis from the NSABP data has noted a small number of uterine sarcomas among the number of patients taking tamoxifen with an intact uterus. These patients have already been included in the reported number of patients diagnosed with endometrial cancer.

In the NSABP trials (B-09, B-14, B-21, B-23, B-24, and P-1) a small number of uterine sarcomas were noted among 12 patients diagnosed with endometrial cancer. Nine of the 12 patients were diagnosed with a malignant mixed mesodermal tumor (MMMT) (carcinosarcoma). Overall, the rate of sarcoma in women taking tamoxifen was 0.17 per 1,000 women-years, which translates to less than one-tenth of 1%. AstraZeneca reviewed all available global data on tamoxifen through July 2001 for the occurrence of uterine malignancy. These data included worldwide literature reports and identified 942 uterine malignancies, of which 140 (15%) were uterine sarcomas. Seventy-three percent were the MMMT variant (630).

A new Food and Drug Administration warning on tamoxifen has been added to highlight the uterine cancer risk (both the endometrial and uterine sarcoma), and will also include the pulmonary embolism and stroke risks.

Annual pelvic examination should include an age-appropriate Papanicolaou smear if the woman has an intact uterus. The vast majority of women with tamoxifen-associated endometrial cancer present with vaginal spotting as an early symptom of their cancer. Therefore, prompt evaluation of vaginal spotting in the postmenopausal woman is essential.

At present, there is insufficient evidence to recommend the routine performance of uterine ultrasonography or endometrial biopsy for routine screening in asymptomatic women (631).

Concerns about a possible link between breast and ovary cancer, as demonstrated for some mutations of *BRCA1/2*, motivate the use of screening with serum CA-125 determinations and transvaginal ultrasound examinations. As in the general population, however, use of CA-125 marker as a screening test for ovarian cancer is not established, and investigating the false positives can be a difficult and fruitless pursuit, particularly since most elevations of CA-125 in patients with a personal history of breast cancer are due to metastatic breast cancer rather than ovarian disease.

Prophylactic Oophorectomy for Risk Reduction in *BRCA1/2* Carriers

It is known that women with *BRCA* mutations are at risk for developing breast and ovarian cancer. Although the risk of ovarian cancer is considerably lower than the risk of breast cancer in *BRCA* mutation carriers, the absence of reliable methods of early detection and the poor prognosis associated with advanced ovarian cancer have supported the recommendation of bilateral prophylactic oophorectomy after completion of childbearing in these women. The risk of primary peritoneal cancer (cancer of the lining of the peritoneal cavity) may still persist after bilateral salpingo-oophorectomy in this setting (632–634).

Breast cancer risk reduction in patients undergoing bilateral prophylactic oophorectomy has been reported. Retrospective reports indicate that in *BRCA1* mutation carriers a bilateral salpingo-oophorectomy may offer breast cancer risk reduction as well (635). Decreases in ovarian hormone exposure following surgical removal of the ovaries may alter breast cancer risk and may reach 50% risk reduction depending on the age of surgical menopause.

Two recent studies on bilateral salpingo-oophorectomy in carriers of *BRCA1* or *BRCA2* mutations reported the effectiveness of prophylactic oophorectomy in preventing ovarian cancer (636,637) The persistent risk of peritoneal tumors was approximately 1% in both studies after the risk reducing bilateral oophorectomy. The mean age of diagnosis of ovarian cancer was 50.8 years, which supports the recommendation for delaying oophorectomy until after the completion of childbearing. Risk reduction for breast cancer was from 25% to 50% in the patients undergoing bilateral salpingo-oophorectomy.

It is unlikely that a prospective randomized study on the use of bilateral salpingo-oophorectomy risk reduction will be performed. Discussion on the risk reduction offered by bilateral salpingo-oophorectomy is appropriate.

Follow-up after Treatment

A goal of follow-up is the detection of recurrent or metastatic disease. The purpose of this is to provide improved survival, delayed onset of symptoms, and possibly increased odds of cure, although curable metastatic disease is rare to nonexistent. The need to obtain accurate results for patients on clinical trials and a desire to reassure patients of their good health may also be motivating forces for clinicians. Tests include history and physical examination, serum liver-function assays, complete blood counts (CBC), serum-marker assays (CEA, CA-15–3, and possibly others), and a variety of radiographic studies. The use of nuclear bone scans, ultrasonography, CT, and MRI scans at regular intervals is particularly controversial in the absence of clinical signs or symptoms, as these are often expensive and can uncover nonmalignant abnormalities requiring invasive study for diagnosis.

Retrospective studies show that history and physical examinations detect 50% to 90% of all recurrences (638). Even among carefully followed patients, most recurrences are detected by investigation of a complaint or physical finding and not by any of the imaging studies. As a result, and based on historical standards, most investigators recommend 3- to 6-month intervals between physician visits for the first 1 to 5 years after diagnosis.

Many clinicians include a panel of blood and serum studies in their routine follow-up. In the case of the CBC, no data support its routine use, although it obviously can detect asymptomatic anemias and cytopenias that may be secondary to medical ailments or metastatic breast cancer. A remote possibility is the early detection of secondary leukemias, although these are unlikely to remain clinically silent for a significant period of time. Many investigators recommend at least a yearly CBC, but many others obtain this relatively inexpensive test far more often. Abnormal serum liver-function tests, including the alkaline phosphatase and SGOT, can be early indicators of liver or bone metastases and are widely included in most clinicians' follow-up schemas. For these two tests in particular, retrospective study has demonstrated both sensitivity and specificity of two serial elevations for recurrence (639).

In addition to liver-function testing, carcinoembryonic antigen (CEA) and the CA-15–3 (and analogues) are frequesntly used, with still others under development. The probability of establishing a diagnosis of metastatic breast cancer in patients with rising serial CEA determinations is between 15% and 68% (640). Unfortunately, with single determinations, false-positive rates range from 10% to 27%. In addition, the median lead time between detection of an elevated CEA and clinically detectable evidence of metastatic disease ranges from 5 to 7 months. In theory, palliation of an asymptomatic patient is not possible, although a delay in the onset of symptomatic disease may be (641).

The CA-15–3 and its analogues' assay for circulating levels of polymorphic epithelial mucin have been studied extensively and as with CEA; rising values over time accurately predict recurrent breast cancer with a median lead time of 9 months (642).

Chest radiography is often recommended on a yearly basis. Among smokers, it may be useful as a screening test for primary lung cancer, but in patients with a history of breast cancer it is typically used to screen for distant metastases (643). In a large retrospective study of high-risk patients with T3 or T4 tumors or positive nodes, patients underwent chest radiographs 6 months following diagnosis, 1 year following diagnosis, and yearly for 6 years (644). Presymptomatic disease, with a true positive rate of 1 of 76 examinations performed, was identified.

Because bone is a frequent site for recurrent breast cancer and may be the most frequent site of single metastases, the nuclear bone scan can be a sensitive means of detection. Treatment with radiation therapy including radiopharmaceuticals (^{89}Sr or ^{153}Sm) or orthopedic surgery may prevent pathologic fractures and subsequent pain, motivating many clinicians to advocate the routine use of nuclear bone scans in asymptomatic patients. One study demonstrated that the risk of conversion of bone scans from normal to abnormal after a diagnosis of stage I or II breast cancer was 7% and 45%, respectively; most conversions occurred in the first 24 months after diagnosis. Based on these data, some investigators recommend bone scans every 6 months for 2 years after diagnosis and to continue these examinations only in symptomatic patients (645). Evidence against routine use is provided by a retrospective review noting that the chance of finding metastatic disease on a bone scan was less than 1% if the patient was asymptomatic and had a normal chest radiograph, normal alkaline phosphatase level, and no other evidence of metastases (646). Some cooperative groups have recommended that this test not be performed on any asymptomatic patients beyond 3 years from diagnosis, and most modern trials do not require nuclear bone scans on a routine basis (647).

Considering the various methods for detecting recurrent stage IV breast cancer, Schapira and Urban (648) noted that patients themselves found 70.6% of all recurrent disease, physical examinations found 15.4%, nuclear bone scans detected 3.4%, chest radiographs, 2.7%, and serum blood tests, 5.9%. Mammography found an additional 2%, but this subset presumably does not represent metastatic disease. Similarly, Loprinzi (646) summarized the results of multiple reports of follow-up screening studies, finding that history and physical examinations detected 75% to 85% of all metastases, serum and liver-function tests found 1% to 12%, chest radiography, 0% to 5%, and nuclear bone scans, 0% to 8%. No data were available for markers such as CEA and CA-15–3.

In 1994, two randomized, prospective trials from Italy were reported in which ''intensive'' and ''nonintensive'' follow-up were compared. In the first trial, 1,243 patients under age 70 who were free of cancer were followed at 12 centers, and all patients had annual mammography and 3-month follow-up visits for 2 years and then 6-month follow-up visits thereafter. Patients were randomly assigned so that 621 underwent no other testing while 622 had chest radiographs and bone scans at 6-month intervals. There was slightly more distant disease noted in the intensive follow-up group as well as increased detection of isolated intrathoracic and bone involvement (18% versus 11.4%). Noteworthy, at 5 years of follow-up, there was no difference in the overall survival. Thus, early detection of metastasis did not change survival in this study (649).

A second but similar trial, the GIVIO study, followed 1,320 patients under age 70 at 26 treatment centers; 655 patients were randomly assigned to undergo yearly mammography as well as history and physical examination at 3-

month intervals for 2 years, and at 6-month intervals for 3 years. In the remaining group of 665 patients, chest radiographs were obtained every 6 months, along with yearly bone scans, liver sonograms, and laboratory testing, including serum liver-function tests. In addition to overall and disease-free survival, quality of life was also assessed using a panel of standard tools, but here there were no differences in any of these three endpoints (650).

BREAST CANCER PREVENTION

The ability to prevent breast cancer is a long-sought-after goal. An intriguing finding from the Early Breast Cancer Trialists' Collaborative Group was the observation of a 47% reduction in the annual odds of contralateral breast cancer among patients treated with tamoxifen (564). Similar preliminary observations in individual trials motivated the NSABP and NCI to launch the first prevention trial using this agent among over 13,000 research subjects identified as having a high risk for breast cancer, but no personal history except for lobular carcinoma *in situ* (21). There was almost a 50% reduction in breast cancer incidence in the tamoxifen group. The absolute benefits were modest, however, and the toxicities worrisome, making the routine use of tamoxifen as a preventative controversial in many quarters. At the same time, emerging evidence suggests the possibility that newer antiestrogens, such as raloxifene, may be effective and less toxic (651). As a result, the second large prevention trial, P-2, which plans for about 20,000 research subjects, also without a personal history of breast cancer except for lobular carcinoma *in situ,* is now open in North America. For patients with a personal history of breast cancer, the decision to use antiestrogens as a potential preventative agent, even if their primary tumor was receptor-negative, may be a difficult one to make and will be the subject of ongoing clinical research.

Prophylactic Breast Surgery

For patients at high risk for developing breast cancer, such as those with *BRCA1/2* mutations, the options of prophylactic mastectomy and/or oophorectomy should be discussed. Prophylactic, or risk-reducing, mastectomy may be performed in patients at increased risk of developing breast cancer. The two groups of patients that can consider this type of surgery are those with a known germline mutation in *BRCA1/2* or a strong family history of breast and/or ovarian cancer and patients with a personal history of unilateral breast cancer. The two types of prophylactic mastectomies commonly performed are the subcutaneous mastectomy and the total mastectomy. A subcutaneous mastectomy is usually performed through an inframammary incision and removes the entire breast tissue while leaving the overlying skin and nipple-areolar complex. A total mastectomy may be performed through an elliptical incision removing much of the skin and the entire nipple-areolar complex, but not the axillary lymph nodes. In both cases, a small amount of residual tissue is likely to be left behind in the skin, the inframammary fold, or in the axilla rendering the procedure less than 100% effective in preventing subsequent breast cancer.

Two large studies regarding the efficacy of prophylactic mastectomy have been reported in the past several years. The first by Hartmann et al. retrospectively reported on 214 patients deemed to be at high risk of breast cancer based upon family history alone (652); after a median follow-up of 14 years, 3 (1.4%) breast cancers were diagnosed. Compared to their sisters, of which 39% developed breast cancer, there was a reduction in incidence of approximately 90%. These authors subsequently genotyped 176 of these patients for *BRCA1/2* mutations and found 26 with germline mutations (653). None of these 26 patients developed breast cancer over a median follow-up of 13 years. Six incidental breast cancers were found at the time of prophylactic mastectomy. The second study was of 139 women with pathogenic *BRCA* mutations followed in a prospective manner (654). After a mean follow-up of only 3 years, no breast cancers developed in the prophylactic mastectomy group and eight cancers developed in the surveillance group. The 5-year incidence of breast cancer in the surveillance group was 17%. There were no incidental breast cancers noted at the time of prophylactic mastectomy in this study.

The largest study of women undergoing prophylactic contralateral mastectomy comes from the Mayo Clinic, in which 745 patients were followed for a median of 10 years after prophylactic contralateral mastectomy (655). Eight women developed a contralateral breast cancer for a risk reduction of approximately 95% based on expected rate of contralateral breast cancers in patients with a personal and family history of breast cancer. In a case-control study from City of Hope (656) 64 patients undergoing a prophylactic contralateral mastectomy were matched for multiple pathologic and clinical variables almost 3 to 1 with controls. In the prophylactic contralateral mastectomy group there were three incident breast cancers noted at the time of surgery, but no subsequent cancers in a mean follow-up of 6.8 years. In the control group there were 36 contralateral breast cancers identified subsequently. Despite a marked reduction in contralateral breast cancers for the patients undergoing a prophylactic contralateral mastectomy, there was not a statistically significant improvement in 15-year overall survival (64% vs 48%, $p = 0.26$); this was secondary to the development of metastatic disease. In this same study, there was an improvement in disease-free survival at 15 years even though overall survival was not statistically significant. From these studies it is clear that prophylactic contralateral mastectomy can dramatically reduce the risk of contralateral breast cancer in patients with unilateral disease. Whether or not this will have a significant effect for patients with early-stage disease will require further study.

In patients with *BRCA1/2* mutations, prophylactic bilateral salpingo-oophorectomy has the inherent benefit of risk reduction for ovarian cancer. Additionally, there is a breast cancer risk reduction of up to 50% in premenopausal patients. Whether the resulting reduction in the risk of breast cancer from this procedure is preferable to the risk-reducing bilateral mastectomy is likely to remain a personal decision for patients.

Radiographic Findings After Breast-Conservation Therapy

Dershaw (657) summarized the most frequent mammographic findings: parenchymal distortion and fibrosis at the tumor excision site (secondary to surgical scar and irradiation); skin thickening, seen in 90% of patients, which may be diffuse or more prominent at the surgical excision site; and calcifications, due to fat necrosis, that are coarse and round and have radiolucent centers. If these findings are stable, mammographic follow-up is sufficient; however, a change in number or characteristic pattern warrants a biopsy to rule out recurrent tumor.

Mammographic findings were correlated with clinical observations in several studies (658–660). These studies demonstrated that most changes were observed in the first 12 months after therapy, with stabilization achieved at 12 to 36 months after completion of therapy. Breast edema is mammographically present in virtually all patients at completion of therapy, with a steady decline in this observation over 36 months and approximate stabilization at 42 months (Fig. 30.30) (660).

Estrogen Replacement Therapy in Women with Breast Cancer

Traditionally, it was thought that estrogen replacement therapy was contraindicated in women who had a diagnosis of breast cancer. It is now, however, accepted that for healthy women approaching menopause, the short- and long-term benefits of estrogen replacement therapy may outweigh the risks (661).

In a control study of 3,130 women receiving hormonal replacement therapy compared with 3,698 controls, 36% of the former and 38% of the latter having received prior hormonal therapy (only 15% used combined estrogen and progestin regimens), Newcomb and associates (662) found no significant difference in risk of breast cancer. There was no significant increase in relative risk among women who had used hormone replacement therapy for at least 15 years compared with those who never used it. The relative risk (RR) was 1.11 for hormonal use for 15 years or longer and 1.05 in the control group.

Randomized trials have shown that such therapy improves common symptoms of menopause, including vasomotor disturbances and vaginal dryness (663). More recent studies have demonstrated improvement of quality of life with the

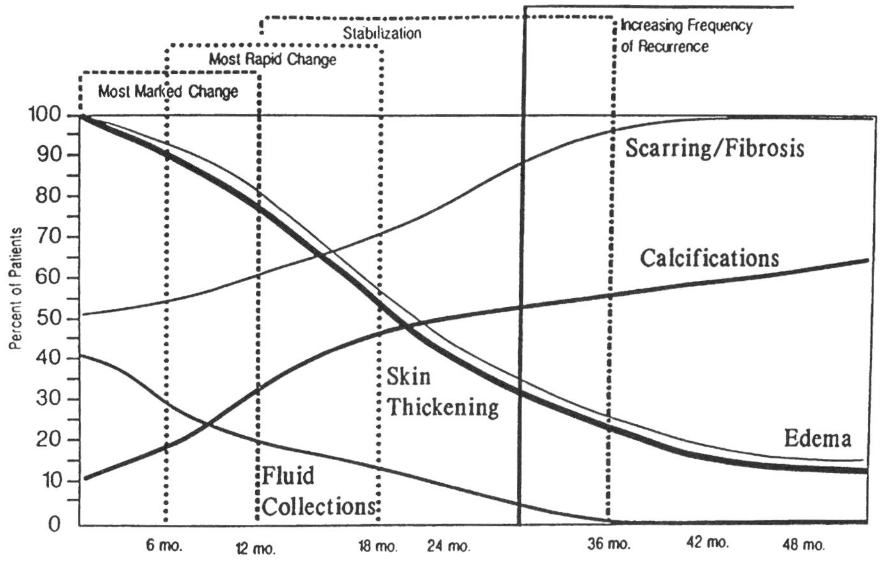

FIG. 30.30. Changing appearance of the conservatively treated breast. (Reprinted with permission from Mendelson EB. Evaluation of the postoperative breast. *Radiol Clin North Am* 1992;30:107.)

use of estrogen replacement therapy (664). Although it has been documented that the administration of unopposed estrogen to postmenopausal women is associated with an increased risk of developing endometrial cancer, this risk was thought avoidable with the addition of progesterone, until recently (665,666). Recent meta-analyses of studies of estrogen replacement therapy and hormone replacement therapy suggest that hormone users may have a slightly increased relative risk of developing breast cancer (1.3% at 15 years).

Recently, results from the Women's Health Initiative randomized controlled trial were reported. Between 1993 and 1998, 16,609 women with an intact uterus were randomized to receive combination HRT (0.625 mg/day conjugated equine estrogens and 2.5 mg/day medroxyprogesterone acetate) versus placebo. The planned duration of the trial was 8.5 years; however, the data and safety monitoring board of the committee recommended halting the trial because the incidence of invasive breast cancer after a mean of 5.2 years of follow-up had exceeded the stopping boundary that had been set at the initiation of the trial. The increased risk of breast cancer hazard ratio was 1.25 [95% confidence interval (CI), 1.00–1.59], for an individual woman a relatively small risk. There was also a reported increased risk of coronary heart disease (HR 1.29; 95% CI, 1.02–1.63), stroke (HR, 1.41;95% CI, 1.39–3.25). Beneficial effects included decreased risk in colorectal cancer (HR, 0.63; 95% CI, 0.43–0.92) and hip fracture (HR 0.66; 95% CI, 0.45–0.98). The data and safety monitoring board did not recommend stopping the estrogen-alone arm in women who had had a hysterectomy. Results of this part of the study are anticipated in 2005 (667).

The increased risk for breast cancer is apparent after 4 years of HRT use. The American College of Obstetricians and Gynecologists (ACOG) stresses the importance of addressing the reasons for initiating or continuing on HRT. It is no longer recommended to prevent heart disease in healthy women (primary prevention) or to protect women with preexisting heart disease (secondary prevention). In addition, it is no longer recommended solely for prevention of osteoporosis.

HRT is highly effective in treating vasomotor symptoms with limited effective alternative therapies. In this setting, short-term use (<5 years) can be considered, as data on short-term use does not show an increased association with breast cancer. However, in light of this study, and limited data on safety of hormone replacement therapy in patients with a history of breast cancer, alternatives to HRT in these breast cancer survivors should be considered.

Menstrual Period and Prognosis after Surgery

The issue of timing of surgery with respect to a particular phase of the menstrual cycle remains controversial. Several reports have noted improved survival among patients with positive axillary lymph nodes surgically treated in the later phase of the menstrual cycle, when progesterone levels are elevated. Biologic support for the influence of menstrual timing is provided by cyclical patterns of cell division and cell death observed in normal breast tissue, as well as by potential tumor-cell dissemination during surgery among patients with positive axillary nodes. Immune parameters, which also respond to cycling endogenous hormones, may influence the metastatic potential of circulating tumor cells (668).

In 96 premenopausal patients who underwent primary surgery for operable breast carcinoma, the 10-year disease-free and overall survival rates of patients whose initial surgery was 1 to 12 days after the starting date of the last menstrual period (follicular phase) were significantly poorer than the survival rates of those who underwent operation after more than 12 days from the last menstruation (luteal phase) (disease-free survival rate 40% versus 72%, $p = 0.002$; overall survival rate 40% versus 79%, $p = 0.001$) (669).

Senie and coworkers (670) noted in 283 premenopausal patients treated with mastectomy and axillary dissection that, when the tumor was excised during the follicular phase, a higher recurrence risk (43%) was observed compared with excision later in the menstrual cycle (29%) ($p = 0.02$).

Veronesi and associates (24) followed 1,175 premenopausal women treated for breast carcinoma (average 8 years). There were 192 unfavorable events among 525 patients operated on during the follicular phase (36.6%) and 192 in 650 patients operated on during the luteal phase (29.6%). The effect of phase was restricted to patients with positive axillary nodes. The 5-year relapse-free survival rates were 75.5% in 246 node-positive patients operated on during the luteal phase and 63.3% in 190 patients (both groups node-positive) who had surgery during the follicular phase.

On the other hand, Donegan and Shah (671) reviewed 97 women treated for operable stages of breast cancer; at operation, 55 were in the perimenstrual phase of the menstrual cycle (days 0 through 6 and days 21 through 36), and 42 were in the periovulatory phase (days 7 through 20). No relationship could be identified between the timing of surgical treatment and subsequent recurrences or survival. Lymph node status remains the most significant indicator for prognosis overall. Until additional data are available, there is no consensus as to the effect of menstrual cycle on prognosis, and currently no standard recommendations for when surgery should be insitituted.

Chronologic Rate and Location of Breast Relapses After Breast-Conservation Therapy

Most breast relapses (65% to 80%) after breast-conservation therapy within the initial 5 years after irradiation occur around the primary tumor site. Late breast recurrences occur into the second decade at a lower rate; the majority will not be in the immediate vicinity of the prior excision. They represent de novo breast cancers developing in other quadrants (672). Recht and associates (673), in an analysis of 607 patients with clinical stages I or II invasive carcinoma, described actuarial failure rates of 10% at 5 years and 16% at 10 years. The hazard rate in the first 5 years was approximately 2% per year until about 5 years after treatment and decreased to 0.5% per year after 8 years.

Kurtz and colleagues (318), in 1,593 patients with clinical stages I and II disease treated with conservation surgery and irradiation, noted a yearly actuarial risk of breast recurrence of 1.5% during both of the first two 5-year periods. After 10 years following therapy, the yearly risk decreased to 1.1%. During the first 10 years, about 80% of recurrences were located near the primary tumor. With increasing interval from primary treatment, only 45% of the breast recurrences were near the primary tumor. Kurtz and coworkers (674) also analyzed 300 patients who were disease-free 10 years after initial treatment: 16 patients (5.3%) developed recurrent carcinoma in the treated breast beyond the tenth year.

Fourquet and associates (313) reported on 518 patients treated with conservation surgery and irradiation (57 Gy to 65 Gy to the breast and 9-Gy to 12-Gy boost to tumor site). An increasing cumulative incidence of breast recurrences was noted with time, reaching over 20% at 20 to 25 years; 46% (26 of 56) of the recurrences were located in the same quadrant as the primary tumor.

Haffty and colleagues (675) described 82 breast relapses in 990 women treated with breast-conservation therapy, 47 of which were classified as true recurrences at the previously treated site and 33 as new primary tumors. True recurrences had a shorter median time to breast relapse (3.16 years) than new primary tumors (5.42 years). Both disease-free and overall survival rates were lower in patients with true breast recurrences (Fig. 30.31) (465). Residual disease occurred more frequently outside the recurrent tumor bed in patients with true recurrences compared with those with new primary lesions (48% versus 16%) ($p < 0.05$).

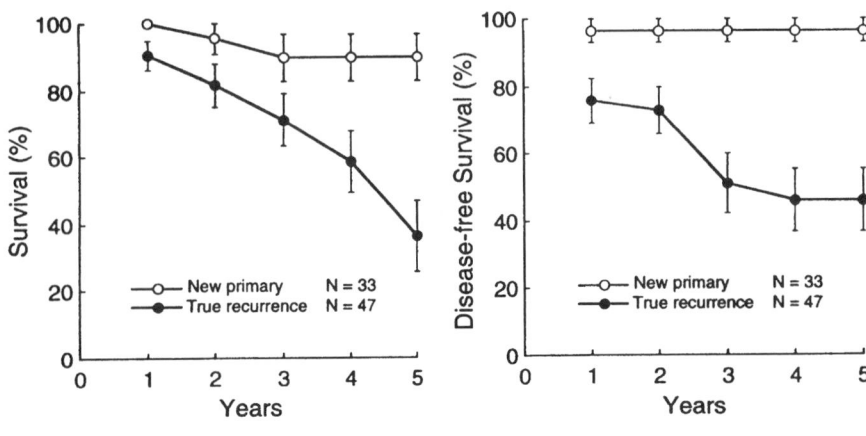

FIG. 30.31. Survival **(A)** and disease-free survival **(B)** after breast recurrence correlated with relapse classification. (Reprinted with permission from Haffty BG, Carter D, Flynn SD, et al. Local recurrence versus new primary: clinical analysis of 82 breast relapses and potential applications for genetic fingerprinting. *Int J Radiat Oncol Biol Phys* 1993;27:575.)

TABLE 30.25. *Incidence of regional node relapse after conservation surgery and radiation therapy for stages I and II breast cancer*

Author	Total no. patients	Follow-up	Regional node relapse (%)
Calle et al (309)	324	5 years minimum	2.1
Delouche et al (195)	410	11 years median	1.2
Fisher et al (301)	625	38.9 months mean	2.2
Fowble et al (676)	990	5 years actuarial	3
Halversion et al (624)	511	5 years actuarial	3
Leung et al (677)	493	10 years mean	1.2
Plerquin and Marin (678)	3,353	>5 years median	3
Recht et al (679)	1,624	–	2.3
Sarrazin et al (680)	592	78 months median	2
van Limbergen et al (169)	235	80 months median	3
Veronesl et al (681)	352	8 years median	2.3

From Fowble B, Solin LJ, Schultz, et al. Frequency, sites of relapse, and outcome of regional node failures following conservative surgery and radiation for early breast cancer. *Int J Radlat Oncol Biol Phys* 1989;17:703, with permission.

Failures in the regional lymph nodes are uncommon after breast-conservation treatment. Table 30.25 (169,195,301, 309,624,676–681) summarizes reports on the incidence of regional lymph-node relapse after conservation surgery and irradiation in stages I and II breast cancer.

Cosmesis

Host, surgical, radiotherapeutic, and chemotherapeutic factors may influence cosmetic outcome. Host factors include size and shape of the breast, age, race, compliance with care and hygiene, concurrent medical illnesses (such as hypertension, diabetes, and collagen vascular disease), and intrinsic sensitivity to irradiation (682). Surgical factors include the extent of surgical resection, reexcision, orientation and length of the scar, closure or not of the tylectomy cavity, separate or continuous axilla-tylectomy scars, extent of the axillary dissection, and whether or not an ellipse of skin over the tumor was removed. Radiation therapy factors include doses to the whole breast with tangential portals, beam energy, gradient of dose throughout the breast tissues (use of wedge or compensating filters), fractionation, overall duration of therapy including breaks, type and dose of boost, and volume treated (whether peripheral lymphatic irradiation is administered or not). Chemotherapy issues include cytotoxic agents used, timing and sequence relative to radiation therapy, and doses and combinations of drugs.

At Washington University, specific guidelines were established for each cosmetic endpoint for excellent, good, fair, and poor results. Questionnaires were completed by 458 patients and their radiation oncologists at regular 6-month intervals after treatment. Cosmetic outcome analysis of these patients was made for clinical and treatment-related factors (683). About 80% of patients had excellent/good cosmesis (Fig. 30.32). Clinical factors at presentation were analyzed by age, menopausal status, race, and tumor-related parameters of size, palpable status, and location (Table 30.26) (431). Patients older than 60 years had lower excellent cosmetic scores when compared with patients 60 years of age or younger. Tumor size significantly influenced cosmetic outcome, with 41% of patients with a tumor size of 2 cm

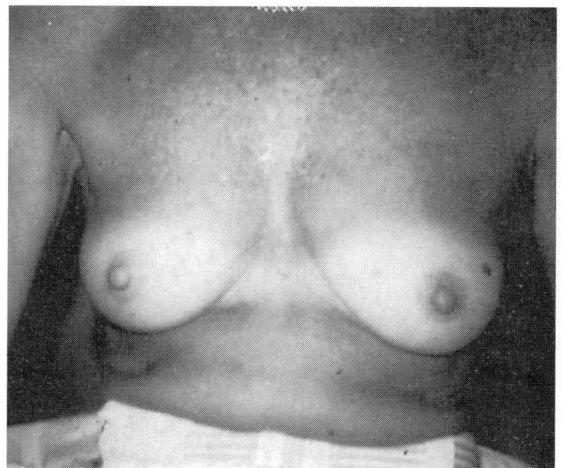
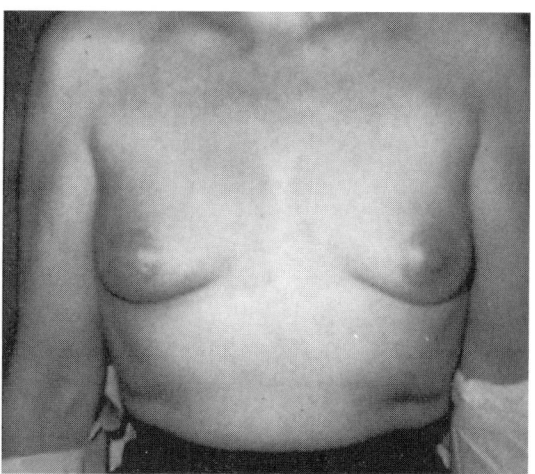

FIG. 30.32. A–B: Photographs of patients showing excellent cosmetic results obtained with conservation surgery and irradiation for patients with T1 and T2 carcinomas of the breast. *(Figure continues.)*

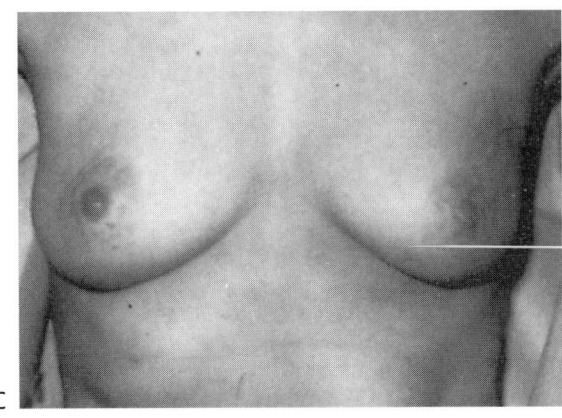
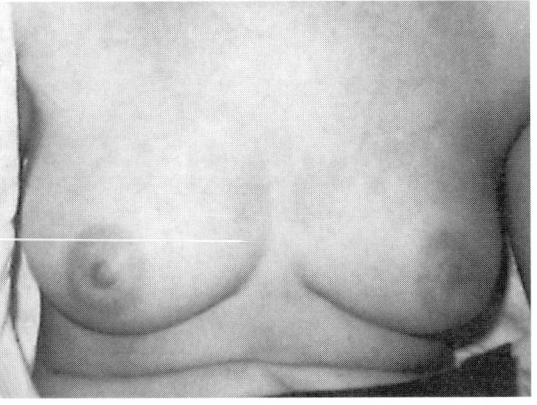

C

D

FIG. 30.32. Continued. **C–D:** The patient in **C** has minimal telangiectasis in the area with a boost (upper quadrant of left breast). (Reprinted with permission from Perez CA, Taylor ME. Breast: Stage Tis, T1, and T2 Tumors. In: Perez CA, Brady LW, eds. *Principles and practice of radiation oncology,* 3rd ed. Philadelphia: Lippincott–Raven,1998:1376.)

TABLE 30.26. *Cosmetic results correlated with patient and tumor characteristics*

	No. of patients	Cosmetic score			
		Excellent	Good	Fair	Poor
Age					
40 Years	75	31 (41%)	33 (44%)	3 (4%)	8 (11%)
41–60 Years	223	94 (42%)	92 (41%)	33 (15%)	4 (2%)
61–80 Years	150	45 (30%)	71 (47%)	28 (19%)	6 (4%)
>80 Years	10	3 (30%)	4 (40%)	3 (30%)	0
Menopausal status					
Premenopausal	141	63 (45%)	57 (40%)	11 (8%)	10 (7%)
Perimenopausal	31	15 (48%)	13 (42%)	3 (10%)	0
Postmenopausal	280	94 (34%)	126 (45%)	52 (18%)	8 (3%)
Race					
White	406	164 (40%)	171 (42%)	56 (14%)	15 (4%)
Black	50	9 (18%)	27 (54%)	11 (22%)	3 (6%)
Tumor size (mm)					
<10	140	63 (45%)	58 (41%)	16 (11%)	3 (2%)
11–20	202	76 (38%)	90 (45%)	29 (14%)	7 (3%)
21–50	107	32 (30%)	47 (44%)	20 (19%)	8 (7%)
Palpable mass					
Yes	236	86 (36%)	107 (45%)	33 (14%)	10 (4%)
No	124	52 (42%)	60 (48%)	9 (7%)	3 (2%)
Primary location in breast					
Upper outer and axillary tail	238	93 (39%)	101 (42%)	36 (15%)	8 (3%)
Upper inner	73	30 (41%)	33 (45%)	6 (8%)	4 (5%)
Lower outer	55	22 (40%)	24 (44%)	7 (13%)	2 (3%)
Lower inner	38	12 (32%)	18 (47%)	8 (21%)	0
Central	59	16 (30%)	23 (43%)	10 (19%)	4 (7%)

For excellent cosmetic score:
Age ≤40 to 60 years versus 61 to >80 years, $p = 0.001$.
Premenopausal and perimenopausal versus postmenopausal, $p = 0.02$.
White versus black, $p = 0.0034$.
Tumor size <10 to 20 mm versus 21 to 50 mm, $p = 0.05$.
Palpable mass versus no palpable mass, $p = 0.3976$.
Primary site of upper outer and axillary tail, upper inner, and lower outer versus lower inner and central, $p = 0.3407$.
From Taylor ME, Perez CA, Halverson KJ, et al. Factors influencing cosmetic results after conservation therapy for breast cancer. *Int J Radiat Oncol Biol Phys* 1995;31 : 753–764, with permission.

TABLE 30.27. *Cosmetic results correlated with breast surgical factors*

	No. of patients	Average volume of resection (cm³)	Cosmetic score			
			Excellent	Good	Fair	Poor
Type of breast surgery						
Excisional biopsy	127	40 ± 8.5	71 (56%)	46 (36%)	6 (5%)	4 (3%)
Wide excision	267	109 ± 8.9	93 (35%)	125 (47%)	39 (15%)	10 (4%)
Quadrantectomy	61	282 ± 50	8 (13%)	27 (44%)	22 (36%)	4 (7%)
Reexcision of primary site						
Yes	184	–	50 (27%)	85 (46%)	39 (21%)	10 (5%)
No	273	–	123 (45%)	114 (42%)	28 (10%)	8 (3%)
Scar orientation compliant with NSABP guidelines						
Yes	295	–	129 (44%)	126 (43%)	33 (11%)	7 (2%)
No	148	–	40 (27%)	66 (44%)	33 (22%)	9 (6%)

NSABP, National Surgical Adjuvant Breast Project.
For excellent cosmetic score:
  Excisional biopsy and wide excision surgery versus quadrantectomy, $p = 0.001$.
  Reexcision at primary site versus no re-excision, $p = 0.002$.
  Scar orientation compliant with NSABP guidelines versus noncompliance, $p = 0.0034$.
From Taylor ME, Perez CA, Halverson KJ, et al. Factors influencing cosmetic results after conservation therapy for breast cancer. *Int J Radiat Oncol Biol Phys* 1995;31:753–764, with permission.

or less having excellent cosmetic outcome compared with 30% for 2.1 to 5 cm ($p = 0.05$). Cosmetic outcome by race indicated 40% of whites had an excellent cosmetic rating compared with only 18% for African-Americans. Noteworthy, 30% of African-American patients received concurrent chemotherapy and/or hormonal therapy with irradiation compared with 23% of white patients. Of African-American patients, 14% were obese, 17% were hypertensive, 25% had both obesity and hypertension, and 4% had diabetes. Breast and axillary surgical factors affecting cosmesis are summarized in Table 30.27 (683).

In the Washington University survey, the type of breast surgery was important, with patients undergoing excisional biopsy having the highest rate of excellent cosmesis (56%) compared with wide excision (35%) and quadrantectomy (13%) ($p = 0.0001$). Scar-orientation compliance with NSABP guidelines was an important factor, with 44% of patients having excellent cosmetic ratings compared with 27% for patients with noncompliant scar orientations ($p = 0.0034$). Reexcision of the primary site also resulted in a lower rate of excellent cosmesis ($p = 0.0002$).

Radiation factors affecting cosmesis included treatment volume (tangential breast fields only versus three fields or more) ($p = 0.034$), whole-breast dose greater than 50 Gy ($p = 0.024$), total dose to the tumor site greater than 65 Gy ($p = 0.06$), and optimum dose distribution created with use of compensating filters (Table 30.28) (683).

Adjuvant chemotherapy may have a deleterious influence on excellent/good cosmetic results (Table 30.29) (683–687). In several studies, the main effect is a move from the "excellent" result category to the "good" result category. In par-

ticular, concomitant administration of chemotherapy and irradiation has a more pronounced effect on cosmesis.

Cosmetic Breast Surgery after Irradiation

It is estimated that 2 million women in the United States have received silicone-gel–filled implants for breast augmentation. Edelman and coworkers (688), in a review of case reports, found a lack of correlation between the incidence of breast cancer and silicone-gel implants. Incidence rates of breast cancer were similar to those expected in the general population.

Between 1980 and 1994, 680 patients with silicone-gel breast implants were identified in the Connecticut Tumor Registry, all with at least 1 year of follow-up. The control population consisted of 1,022 women who underwent tubal ligation between 1981 and 1985. There was no statistical difference in the breast-cancer rate within the two groups (0.59% in the implant group and 0.88% in the control group).

The Food and Drug Administration removed silicone-gel breast implants from the market, not because they were known to pose a risk, but because the manufacturers did not fulfill their legal responsibility to collect data on these questions (689). Saline-filled implants are available and should pose none of the potential problems ascribed to the silicone-gel implants.

A growing number of breast cancers occur in women with prior augmentation mammoplasty. The stage of breast cancer at diagnosis in women who have undergone augmentation mammoplasty has been examined, with conflicting results. In a retrospective review, Clark and associates (690) re-

TABLE 30.28. *Cosmetic results correlated with irradiation volumes, doses, and boost techniques*

	No. of patients	Median follow-up (months)	Cosmetic score			
			Excellent	Good	Fair	Poor
Type of radiation boost						
None	35	44	10 (29%)	13 (37%)	10 (28%)	2 (6%)
Electron	326	53	127 (39%)	147 (45%)	42 (13%)	10 (3%)
Implant	93	49	36 (39%)	40 (43%)	14 (15%)	3 (3%)
Daily fraction size without chemotherapy						
1.8 Gy	292	53	120 (41%)	126 (43%)	40 (14%)	6 (2%)
2.0 Gy	37	46	16 (43%)	14 (38%)	5 (14%)	2 (5%)
Daily fraction size with chemotherapy						
1.8 Gy	92	43	26 (28%)	47 (51%)	13 (14%)	6 (7%)
2.0 Gy	10	47	4 (40%)	2 (20%)	3 (30%)	1 (10%)
Treatment volume (field arrangements)						
Breast	302	48	125 (41%)	132 (44%)	39 (13%)	6 (2%)
Breast and supraclavicular nodes	29	67	6 (21%)	18 (62%)	4 (14%)	1 (3%)
Breast and supraclavicular and axillary nodes)	74	53	23 (31%)	31 (42%)	14 (19%)	6 (8%)
Breast and internal mammary nodes (± supraclavicular and axillary nodes)	53	67	19 (36%)	19 (36%)	10 (19%)	5 (9%)
Radiation dose to the breast (Gy)						
45–47	267	40	106 (40%)	123 (46%)	33 (12%)	5 (2%)
47.01–50	101	59	43 (43%)	37 (37%)	18 (18%)	3 (3%)
50.01–52	75	78	21 (28%)	34 (45%)	15 (20%)	5 (7%)
51.01–62	5	76	0	1 (20%)	1 (20%)	3 (60%)
Total Irradiation dose (breast and boost) (Gy)						
55–65	384	50	149 (39%)	170 (44%)	53 (14%)	12 (3%)
65.1+	74	58	24 (32%)	30 (41%)	14 (19%)	6 (8%)

For excellent cosmetic score:
  No boost versus electron or implant, $p = 0.30$.
  Daily fraction size of 1.8 versus 2 Gy without chemotherapy, $p = 0.9420$.
  Daily fraction size of 1.8 versus 2 Gy with chemotherapy, $p = 0.4748$.
  Breast versus breast and nodes, $p = 0.0340$.
  Radiation dose to breast of 45 to 50 Gy versus 50.01 to 62 Gy, $p = 0.0243$.
  For excellent versus good cosmetic score regardless of total radiation dose, $p = 0.06$.
From Taylor ME, Perez CA, Halverson KJ, et al. Factors influencing cosmetic results after conservation therapy for breast cancer. *Int J Radiat Oncol Biol Phys* 1995;31 : 753–764, with permission.

TABLE 30.29. *Impact of adjuvant chemotherapy on cosmesis in breast-conservation therapy*

Institution	Chemotherapy	Good-excellent cosmesis (%)	
		Radiation therapy without chemotherapy	Radiation therapy with chemotherapy
Harvard University (684)	CMF, A	92	67
Palo Alto (687)	CMF	88	73
NCI (685)	AC	80	70
University of Pennsylvania (686)	CMF ± P	89	81
Washington University (683)	CMF	81	78

A, Adriamycin; AC, Adriamycln, cyclophosphamide; CMF, cyclophosphamide, methotrexate, 5-FU; P, prednisone.

ported that 24% of 33 patients with augmented breasts and 42% of 1,735 patients with nonaugmented breasts had mammographically detected cancers (difference not significant). The incidence of DCIS in the two groups was similar (18% versus 15%). Sizes of the mammographically detected tumors in the two groups were comparable; however, palpable tumors in the augmented group were significantly smaller than those in the nonaugmented group. Axillary lymph-node involvement was detected in 19% of the augmented group and in 41% of the nonaugmented group. In the mammographically detected tumors, there was no significant difference in axillary lymph-node metastases between the patients with augmented breasts (13%) and those with nonaugmented breasts (15%).

There is debate regarding the use of breast implants in patients previously treated with breast irradiation. Evans and coworkers (691) reviewed the results in 39 irradiated breast implants and 338 nonirradiated implants in 297 patients. Several groups were identified, depending on the type of implant and the timing of the radiation therapy. After breast irradiation (average dose of 50 Gy) the implants were always placed submuscularly or beneath autogenous flaps. Significant capsular contracture or pain requiring implant removal occurred in 6 of 14 patients with implants in irradiated breasts. In comparison, 33 of 266 implants (12.4%) in nonirradiated breasts had similar complications. Ten of 25 implants placed beneath autogenous flaps in irradiated breasts had complications, in contrast to 6 of 72 implants placed beneath autogenous reconstructions without irradiation. Thus, irradiation had a significant negative impact on reconstructive outcome of the implants, and placing them under autogenous flaps did not have any protective effect. Contractures and complications were not affected by timing of irradiation, given either pre- or postoperatively, or by type of implant.

Breast-cancer patients with augmentations are currently being treated with conservation therapy, but no study has specifically investigated complications and cosmetic results of radiation therapy in this group of women.

In a report by Handel and colleagues (692), breast conservation was used in 17 augmented breast-cancer patients; 15 patients were available for follow-up. In 10 patients (67%), significant capsular contracture occurred in the irradiated breast an average of 12 weeks after completion of treatment. Four patients underwent revision surgery to correct symptoms arising from contracture. They concluded that irradiation of the breast for cancer in augmented women results in a high incidence of scar tissue contracture and poor cosmetic results.

In contrast, Guenther and coworkers (693) evaluated 20 women who developed breast cancer after augmentation mammoplasty (14 subcutaneous implants and 6 retromuscular implants). Patients were treated with wide-local tumor excision and levels I and II axillary lymph-node dissection. Irradiation was delivered to the breast (45 Gy to 50 Gy),

TABLE 30.30. *Survival following salvage surgery for isolated breast recurrence*

Author	No. patients	5-year survival rate (%)
Abner et al (387)	123	79
Amalric et al (308)	62	72
Calle et al (697)	19	74
Clark et al (243)	87	55
Dubois et al (311)	30	70
Fowble et al (698)	52	84
Haffty et al (316)	50	59
Keleti et al[a]	52	75
Kurtz et al (318)	159	69
Montague (301)	16	67
Osborne et al (699)	46	76
Recht et al (324)	65	63
Stotter et al (700)	49	63

[a] Unpublished data.

and a boost (14 Gy to 21 Gy) was given to the tumor excision site with either photons, electrons, or ^{192}Ir implant. With a median follow-up of 3.8 years (range, 6 months to 9.3 years), there were no local recurrences, although two patients developed distant metastases. Seventeen patients (85%) had good or excellent cosmetic results.

Management of Local Recurrences after Breast-Conservation Surgery

Most recurrences are invasive carcinoma, although *in situ* tumors are common. Approximately 40% have axillary lymph-node involvement; few demonstrate simultaneous distant metastasis. Mastectomy is the standard salvage procedure. Axillary lymph-node dissection, if not initially performed, may help guide adjuvant treatment as well as reduce the risk of a subsequent regional recurrence. Ipsilateral recurrence may be an independent prognostic factor for distant metastasis (694).

Unlike the prognosis for patients with local failures on the chest wall after radical mastectomy, the prognosis for patients whose failure occurs within the breast after conservation therapy is more favorable. As many as 80% of women who develop chest-wall recurrences after mastectomy will manifest distant metastases (695), whereas 40% or fewer of the women who develop isolated breast failure after conservation therapy develop distant disease (696).

Five-year survival is fairly comparable to that of women initially treated with mastectomy (Table 30.30) (297,308, 311,316,318,321,324,387,697–701).

SEQUELAE OF THERAPY

Conservation Surgery and Irradiation

The most frequent sequelae associated with conservation surgery plus irradiation are arm or breast edema, breast fibro-

TABLE 30.31. *Breast-conservation therapy, Washington University (1967–1991): incidence of treatment sequelae correlated with stage*

Sequelae	Stage T1			Stage T2		
	Grade 1	Grade 2	Grade 3	Grade 1	Grade 2	Grade 3
Breast fibrosis	16 (4%)	17 (5%)	4 (1%)	7 (5%)	8 (5%)	6 (4%)
Breast edema	20 (5%)	16 (4%)	2 (0.5%)	10 (7%)	3 (2%)	1 (0.7%)
Arm edema	19 (5%)	7 (2%)	3 (0.8%)	11 (8%)	3 (2%)	0
Soft tissue necrosis	3 (1%)	1 (0.3%)	1 (0.3%)	1 (0.7%)	2 (1%)	0
Rib or bone necrosis	1 (0.3%)	5 (1%)	–	0	1 (0.7%)	0
Pneumonitis	5 (1%)	4 (1%)	1 (0.3%)	2 (1%)	2 (1%)	0
Pericarditis	–	–	1 (0.3%)	–	–	–
Telangiectasia	9 (2%)	0	2 (0.5%)	3 (2%)	1 (0.7%)	3 (2%)
Fibrosis in other sites	–	–	–	4 (3%)	2 (1%)	1 (0.7%)

sis, painful mastitis or myositis, pneumonitis, and rib fracture. Apical pulmonary fibrosis is occasionally noted when the regional lymph nodes are irradiated.

Symptomatic pneumonitis is infrequent. This clinical syndrome is noted 1 to several months after irradiation (702). Patients present with dry cough (88%), shortness of breath (35%), or fever (53%), and on radiographic studies a pulmonary infiltrate is observed in the irradiated volume (703). The risk of developing radiation pneumonitis may be related to the volume of lung irradiated (702,704,705).

Lingos and colleagues (703) reported on radiation pneumonitis in a retrospective review of 1,624 patients treated with conservation surgery and irradiation. Overall, 1% of patients developed pneumonitis; no patient had late or persisting pulmonary symptoms. The incidence of radiation pneumonitis was correlated with the combined use of chemotherapy and a supraclavicular field ($p = 0.0001$); 14 of 17 patients who developed radiation pneumonitis had internal mammary lymph nodes treated. When patients treated with three-field technique received chemotherapy concurrently with irradiation, the incidence of radiation pneumonitis was 8.8% (8 of 92) compared with 1.3% (3 of 236) for those who received sequential chemotherapy and irradiation to the breast only and 0.5% (6 of 1,296) treated at the breast only with irradiation alone ($p = 0.002$). In this study, the volume of lung irradiated did not correlate with the risk of developing radiation pneumonitis.

Fuller and associates (706) evaluated irradiation doses given to the heart and coronary arteries during primary breast irradiation in 28 patients, 13 of whom were treated with breast-conservation surgery and megavoltage irradiation. Reconstruction of the anatomic position of the heart and irradiation doses received at each level were performed on CT scans obtained in the treatment position, including doses to each coronary artery. Extrapolated target doses were calculated using an α/β ratio of 4 Gy. The volume of heart irradiated to an extrapolated target dose of 5 Gy or more was significantly reduced in patients treated with megavoltage irradiation and breast-conservation therapy compared with the group previously treated with postmastectomy ortho-

voltage irradiation. For patients with left-sided tumors, this reduction was on the order of 42% ($p < 0.01$). The reduction in cardiac volume irradiated in patients with right-sided tumors was even greater. This study and the Oslo Report (707) describe an increased incidence of cardiac morbidity in patients treated postoperatively with tangential, internal mammary, and supraclavicular fields that include a large portion of the heart receiving high doses with ^{60}Co irradiation. With modern megavoltage irradiation, significantly smaller volumes of the left ventricle and coronary arteries are being treated, which results in a lower incidence of cardiac irradiation sequelae (708).

At Washington University, the most common grades 1 and 2 sequelae of conservation surgery and irradiation are breast and arm edema and breast fibrosis; the relative proportion of grade 3 sequelae is low (Table 30.31) (709). Likewise, McCormick and associates (710) showed that breast swelling was the most frequently noted symptom (31% of patients), followed by muscle pain (in motion), incision-site pain, and general breast discomfort (about 20%). Rib pain was noted by 13%. Forty-eight percent of patients reported more breast discomfort in the treated breast than in the untreated breast during sexual activity (64 sexually active patients).

The incidence of breast or arm edema after conservation therapy has varied, and it is related to performance and technique of axillary dissection (Table 30.32) (319,684,687,684,

TABLE 30.32. *Breast edema correlated with extent of axillary surgery in breast-conservation therapy*

	Dissection	
	Full	Limited
Beadle et al, 1983 (684)	44/109 (40%)	24/96 (25%)
Clarke et al, 1982 (711)	26/33 (79%)	5/43 (12%)
Kuske et al, 1990 (319)	7/46 (15%)	10/121 (8%)
Montague et al, 1983 (712)	9/9 (100%)	10/77 (13%)
Pezner et al, 1985 (713)	14/36 (39%)	2/11 (18%)
Ray and Fish, 1983 (687)	50/90 (56%)	6/40 (15%)

TABLE 30.33. *Arm and breast edema correlated with axillary dissection and lymph-node irradiation*

| Lymph node irradiation | Axillary dissection (n = 713) | | No axillary dissection (n = 126) | |
	Yes (n = 98)	No (n = 615)	Yes (n = 83)	No (n = 43)
Arm edema	22 (22%)	95 (15%)	0	1 (2%)
	p = 0.11			
Breast edema	15 (15%)	90 (15%)	5 (6%)	1 (2%)
	p = 0.98			
		p ≤0.01		

711–713), whether the axillary lymph nodes were irradiated, and doses of irradiation delivered.

At Washington University, arm and breast edema were observed in 15% to 22% of patients undergoing axillary dissection versus in 2% to 6% without this procedure; irradiation did not significantly increase these sequelae (Table 30.33).

On the other hand, Dewar and associates (714) reported a greater incidence of upper limb sequelae in patients undergoing axillary surgery and irradiation (33.7%) or irradiation alone (26%) than in patients treated with axillary dissection only (7.2%). The most frequent complications were edema, impaired shoulder mobility, pain on movement, sensory or motor deficit, and pectoral muscle fibrosis.

Brachial plexus dysfunction is a possible complication of regional nodal radiation therapy. Pierce and associates (715), in a review of 1,624 patients, encountered brachial plexus involvement in 1.8% of patients; other investigators have found the incidence to be less than 1% (174,195,716). Pierce and colleagues (715) found that the incidence of brachial plexopathy was significantly higher when the axillary dose was greater than 50 Gy (p = 0.004). However, dose alone did not determine whether a given patient would develop radiation damage; treatment technique (two versus three fields, p = 0.0009) and concomitant chemotherapy were also risk factors. Distinction between metastatic and radiation brachial plexopathy is very important but difficult to distinguish.

Gyenes and colleagues (717) reported on incidence of ischemic heart disease 15 to 20 years after adjuvant radiation therapy in 960 patients with breast cancer enrolled in the Stockholm Breast Cancer Trial. Of 37 long-term survivors, 20 received left-sided therapy, and 17 received right-sided therapy or no therapy. Radiation therapy consisted of ^{60}Co tangential fields for preoperative treatment and electron-beam portals, which included the internal mammary nodes, for postoperative therapy (45 Gy to 50 Gy). Evaluation consisted of electrocardiography, exercise stress tests with ^{99}Tc, myocardial perfusion scan, and careful history for cardiac risk factors. Results showed 5 of 20 patients (25%) treated with left-sided irradiation had ^{99}Tc defects compared with none of 17 control patients (p = 0.05). There was no left-ventricular dysfunction on echocardiogram. Conclusions were that left-chest irradiation may represent a risk factor

in the development of ischemic heart disease; however, left ventricular dysfunction was not related to previous irradiation.

Nixon and coworkers (718) reviewed 825 patients receiving irradiation to the left breast and 784 to the right breast as part of conservation therapy; median follow-up was 137 months. They found no significant difference in cardiac or breast-cancer mortality between the two groups.

Valagussa and associates (719) reported on cardiac effects after adjuvant chemotherapy and breast irradiation for operable breast cancer. They retrospectively evaluated 825 women in prospective trials with respect to irradiation, with or without administration of Adriamycin; 360 patients had breast-conservation therapy. With a median follow-up of 80 months, the overall incidence of congestive heart failure in all patients was 0.5%. Patients receiving Adriamycin chemotherapy without irradiation had a 0.8% incidence of congestive heart failure, and patients receiving both Adriamycin and left-breast irradiation had an incidence of 2.6%. Noted were two fatalities secondary to congestive heart failure in the latter group. Cardiac effects were believed to be greater in patients who were 55 years of age or older at the time of therapy, and risk factors for heart disease were important modifiers.

Pregnancy and Breast Cancer

Of all women who develop breast cancer, approximately 25% will do so in the premenopausal years, and many of these women may still wish to bear children. The incidence of breast cancer associated with pregnancy is estimated to be 1.5 to 2 in 10,000 pregnancies. Albrektsen and colleagues (720), in a study of 802,457 women from the Cancer Registry of Norway, observed a relative risk of breast cancer of 1.24% in the 3 to 4 years immediately after a pregnancy, followed by a decreased risk thereafter.

The most common presentation of a malignant tumor is a painless lump, usually discovered by the patient. According to Holmes (721), the two cardinal rules in evaluating breast problems in the pregnant patient are (1) ignore the pregnancy and evaluate the problem, and (2) keep the fetus out of evaluation procedures. The management of breast cancer in pregnancy should involve a team approach, including a breast surgeon, diagnostic radiologist, pathologist, obstetrician, breast counselor, medical oncologist, and radiation oncologist. Examining the breast in the pregnant patient is difficult because of engorgement and tenderness on palpation. Mammography is somewhat controversial, although the irradiation dose to the fetus is minimal (<0.50 mrem) (483). The increased density of the breast makes accurate interpretation difficult. Ultrasound and fine-needle aspiration (FNA) biopsy should be initially performed. After the diagnosis of cancer has been histologically confirmed, a thorough physical examination of the contralateral breast and all draining lymph node sites should be performed along with a search for distant metastases. Radiographic and scintigraphic imaging for staging should be minimized or deferred. A chest x-ray may be safely performed since the maximum dose to the fetus will be less than 50 mrad (722). Liberman and associates (483) reported on 85 women diagnosed with breast cancer associated with pregnancy; pretherapy mammogram was performed in 21. Findings were mass with calcification in nine (39%), uncalcified mass in four (17%), calcifications only in four (17%), and skin thickening in one. Twenty-two ductal carcinomas and one invasive lobular carcinoma were diagnosed. Mastectomy was performed in 19 (83%) and wide excision in four cases.

Several studies have reported that breast cancer associated with pregnancy has a worse prognosis, which may be related to delay in diagnosis (as pregnancy impedes early detection), and possibly to the biology of the tumor (482). A number of authors have commented on the unusually high percentage of pregnant patients who have lymph-node involvement compared with nonpregnant patients. Nugent and O'Connell (723) suggested that the poorer outcome relates to the young age of the patient and not necessarily to the pregnancy.

Treatment should not be altered or delayed (except irradiation or chemotherapy) because of pregnancy. Either a modified radical mastectomy or lumpectomy with axillary dissection is acceptable local treatment. Immediate breast reconstruction is not indicated. If the patient chooses breast-conservation therapy, irradiation should be deferred until the fetus is delivered, as 50 Gy to the breast even with external shielding will expose the fetus to 0.1 to 0.15 Gy when small and contained in the true pelvis. During later gestation, when the fetus is larger and high in the abdomen, some fetal areas may receive as much as 2 Gy (721). In another study performed with a phantom (film dosimetry), doses to the pelvis ranged from 4.3 Gy with 4-MV x-rays to 15.8 Gy with ^{60}Co (724). Although some question whether any dose of irradiation is safe for the fetus, Brent (724), in an extensive review of the literature, defined 0.05 Gy as a relatively safe upper limit of fetal exposure. Administration of chemotherapy in the first trimester is associated with a high risk of birth defects (17%, 24 of 139); this risk is less in the second and third trimesters (1.3%, 2 of 150) (probability of intrauterine growth retardation, prematurity, fetal malformation, or death) (725).

Some authors have suggested a therapeutic abortion based on a study by Adair (726), who reported in the early 1950s a better outcome in patients who terminated the pregnancy. Contrary to popular belief, however, pregnancy does not stimulate the growth of breast cancer (727). Thus, no justification exists for therapeutic abortion, which may be relevant only in the patient who has rapidly progressing disease, such as inflammatory breast cancer or metastatic disease.

With regard to pregnancy after breast cancer, Danforth (728) reviewed this issue with critical commentaries by Epstein and Henderson (729) and Wood (730). Nearly one-third of women of reproductive age who develop breast cancer will later have one or more pregnancies, and 70% of these will occur within 5 years of treatment. No data are available to suggest that subsequent pregnancy will hasten or induce breast-cancer recurrence. When matched by age and stage to nonpregnant patients, pregnant women with breast cancer do not have a worse outcome than patients with comparable stages (721).

Sutton and associates (731) reviewed 227 women 35 years of age or younger at diagnosis who became pregnant after treatment with CAF adjuvant chemotherapy. Twenty-five patients had 33 pregnancies. The median interval between completion of chemotherapy and pregnancy was 12 months (range, 0 to 87 months). Ten pregnancies were terminated, two had spontaneous abortion, two were still pregnant at the time of the report, and 19 produced normal full-term babies. The incidence of recurrences was 46% in patients without pregnancy compared with 28% in those who had subsequent pregnancies. Similarly, 38% of patients without subsequent pregnancy were deceased compared with 12% of patients who later became pregnant.

Zemlickis and associates (732) compared 118 women with breast cancer (119 pregnancies) with 269 nonpregnant controls. The distribution of breast-cancer stages among the 118 pregnant women was compared with that among 5,115 cases of breast cancer in nonpregnant women of reproductive age. Women having breast cancer in pregnancy were 2.5 times more likely to have metastatic disease (95% CI, 1.1–5.3) and had a significantly lower chance of having stage I disease ($p = 0.015$). Survival of pregnant women did not differ from that of the controls with similar stages.

On the other hand, on univariate analysis, a study of 1,885 patients with operable breast cancer (733) demonstrated better prognosis in patients who had never been pregnant compared with those who had (overall survival, 62% and 54%, respectively; $p = 0.01$; disease-free survival, 53% and 44%, respectively; $p = 0.005$) and in nulliparous compared with parous patients (overall survival, 62% and 53%, respectively; $p = 0.006$; disease-free survival, 52% and 44%, respectively; $p = 0.004$). Survival rates decreased with the number of pregnancies and deliveries. On multivariate analysis, parity remained an independent prognostic indicator in addition to classic highly significant prognostic factors (nodal involvement, tumor grade, and size).

A population-based matched survival study assessed the risk of death for breast cancer patients in relation to whether they delivered a live-born child subsequent to the cancer diagnosis (734). Among 2,548 women younger than 40 years old diagnosed with carcinoma of the breast, 91 experienced subsequent deliveries (10 months or longer after the diagnosis); 471 controls were matched for stage, age, and year of breast-cancer diagnosis. The controls had to survive at least the interval between the cancer diagnosis and the delivery of their matched counterparts. The controls had a 4.8-fold risk of death compared with those who delivered after the diagnosis of breast cancer. The authors' interpretation of this result is a "healthy mother effect" (only women who feel healthy give birth and those who are affected by the disease do not). Nevertheless, six of eight deaths among the 91 patients who did give birth were related to breast cancer.

Dow and coworkers (735) evaluated treatment outcome and quality of life in 23 patients with subsequent pregnancies in a group of 1,624 patients treated with breast-conservation surgery and irradiation. This group was compared with 23 patients without subsequent pregnancy, matched by age and stage at diagnosis and time to pregnancy without recurrence. There were 32 pregnancies and 30 live births; 6 of 23 (22%) women having children after breast-cancer therapy developed locally recurrent tumor compared with 29% in the case-matched group. One woman (4%) in the pregnancy group developed contralateral breast cancer compared with 11% in the case-matched group.

Although it has been recommended that a waiting period between treatment and pregnancy be observed, Epstein and Henderson (729) suggest that this is not necessary for low-risk patients. In patients receiving adjuvant chemotherapy, however, a minimum of 12 months between treatment and conception is advised. Lactation is contraindicated in patients receiving chemotherapy, as antineoplastic agents are excreted in the milk.

It is helpful to suggest that a waiting time (2 to 3 years) is needed for the patient to regain health before attempting the physical stress of pregnancy and that childbearing be deferred until after the period of greatest risk of recurrence of the tumor (728). The individual woman's prognosis, well-being, desire for children, support from spouse or significant other, and other sociodemographic factors must be carefully considered in this difficult decision-making process.

Lactation after Breast-Conservation Therapy

Successful breast-feeding from the untreated, as well as the treated breast, is possible after conservation surgery and irradiation. Higgins and Haffty (635) reviewed the records of 890 patients treated with radiation therapy for early-stage (stage I or II) breast cancer. Of 13 patients identified, 11 who subsequently experienced 13 pregnancies were interviewed. All patients reported little or no swelling of the treated breast during pregnancy. After delivery, lactation from the treated breast was present in four instances, absent in six, and pharmacologically suppressed in three. One patient successfully breast-fed from the treated breast for 4 months. In the majority of cases, breast-feeding from the untreated breast was successful. The interval from the time of treatment to the time of delivery did not appear to adversely affect lactation from the treated breast; one patient reported lactation from the treated breast 75 months after completion of treatment. The absence of lactation was associated with circumareolar incision in three patients (four pregnancies); thus lactation from the treated breast may be less likely to occur in the case of centrally located lesions.

Tralins (737) reported results of a survey describing 53 women who became pregnant after conservation therapy and breast irradiation. Eighteen exhibited some lactation, and 13 (24.5%) were able to feed from the involved breast. Pregnancy or lactation had no impact on prognosis; with 5.4 years' mean follow-up, tumor-free survival was 82%.

Psychoemotional Aspects of Breast-Cancer Therapy

Approximately 25% to 35% of patients diagnosed with breast cancer have significant levels of psychosocial distress, manifested by anxiety or depression, and some level of sexual dysfunction. These disruptive consequences of treatment remain bothersome for at least 2 years after initial therapy.

In a review of the literature studying psychosocial factors and their relation to breast cancer, Jensen (738) revealed major methodologic problems in evaluating data: small sample size, retrospective design, lack of cross-referencing for other important factors, cross-referencing studies instead of longitudinal studies, and insufficient statistical analysis. Regarding psychosocial factors, some of the most valid studies indicate that the risk of getting breast cancer may be connected with difficulties in expressing feelings, especially ones of aggression; coping strategy, amount of stress, and level of activity seem to be of possible influence on the prognosis. A possible connection between psyche and the immunologic system has been proposed, but there have been few data so far.

The specific types, magnitude, and duration of emotional dysfunction of women undergoing breast-conservation therapy compared with those treated with mastectomy are highly variable and require the attention and psychotherapeutic support of the treating physicians (739). Radical surgery produces more psychoemotional disruption in terms of feelings about the woman's body image, physical attractiveness, and sexuality, while lumpectomy and irradiation may interfere temporarily with the patient's lifestyle and cause worries about cancer and the perceived adverse effects of irradiation. At present, however, this assumption is not supported by research findings; the fear of recurrence has been reported to be similar in women undergoing either mastectomy or breast-conservation therapy (740).

A clinical decision analysis on the quality-adjusted life

expectancy of patients with breast cancer, comparing a group treated with mastectomy and one treated with breast-conservation therapy, showed that breast-conservation therapy yields better quality-adjusted life expectancy than mastectomy. There are, however, select subgroups of patients who should preferably undergo mastectomy (741).

In a comparison of psychologic effects on some patients randomized to NSABP Protocol B-06, Lasry and Margolese (742) noted that patients who underwent more radical surgery did not express less fear of cancer recurrence than those treated with lumpectomy. The expected trade-off between breast conservation and increased fear of cancer recurrence did not occur.

Body image, as a component of self-concept, was compared using mailed questionnaires in 257 patients treated with mastectomy, mastectomy with delayed reconstruction, mastectomy with immediate reconstruction, or conservation therapy (743). When analysis of covariance with age was used, body image in the conservation-therapy group was significantly more positive than in either the mastectomy group or the mastectomy and immediate reconstruction group. No differences in self-concept were evident among the four groups.

The advantage of breast-conservation therapy is psychologic, as preserving the configuration of the body maintains the sense of female identity and positive body image to a greater degree than is seen after mastectomy (744). Breast-conservation therapy does not, however, reduce the high frequency of anxiety phenomena, mental instability, and depression.

Psychosocial adjustment, body image, and sexual function were retrospectively assessed in 72 women who had partial mastectomy and in 147 women who had total mastectomy and immediate breast reconstruction (745). Questionnaires completed at a mean of 4 years after surgery (44% of questionnaires returned) showed that fewer than 20% of women reported good adjustment in the areas measured. Overall, 38% of women never or rarely worried about their tumor, 56% worried ''now and then'' to fairly frequently, and 6% worried almost continuously. There was no significant difference between the two groups with regard to body image, sexual attractiveness, or marital happiness. Of 184 women who answered the question, 109 (59%) felt cancer had brought them closer to their partner, 44 (24%) saw no significant impact, and 31 (17%) felt cancer had interfered with their relationships. With regard to frequency of sexual expression, desire for sex, or actual sexual activity, there was no significant difference between the two types of surgery groups. Pleasure with breast caressing had decreased since cancer treatment for 44% of women with partial mastectomy and for 83% of those with mastectomy and breast reconstruction. With regard to satisfaction with appearance of the breast, there was no significant difference between the surgical groups. Of 208 women who responded, 88% were moderately to extremely satisfied with their clothed appearance, and 59% were satisfied with their nude breast appearance.

Schain and colleagues (746) prospectively studied 142 women participating in clinical trials randomized to either mastectomy or lumpectomy and radiation therapy. Baseline assessments were made before randomization and at 6, 12, and 24 months after treatment. At 6 months, mastectomy patients reported significantly less control of events in their lives ($p = 0.003$) and more problems with sexual relations ($p = 0.021$) than did their conservatively treated counterparts. In addition, there were marked differences between mastectomy versus lumpectomy-irradiation patients in the degree of distress over body image ($p = 0.059$ at 24 months). This study concluded that breast-conservation therapy protects a woman's perception of her body but does not, over time, contribute to more positive sexual adjustment.

Levy and associates (747) reported on 129 stage I and stage II breast-cancer patients entered into a behavioral study. Approximately 70% of patients elected to have breast-conservation surgery (lumpectomy), with the remainder choosing mastectomy. Compared with mastectomy patients, breast-conservation patients were more functional 3 to 5 days after surgery, but they perceived themselves as having less energy and less emotional support, especially over the first 3 months of the recovery period.

With the increasing use of adjuvant chemotherapy in younger women with early-stage breast cancer, the long-term impact on quality of life, effects of premature menopause, and changes in perceived sexual attractiveness must be given a high priority in order for research to improve post-treatment adjustment and satisfaction in these patients (748,749). Women who received chemotherapy were more likely to worry about breast-cancer recurrence ($p = 0.001$), had sex less frequently ($p = 0.013$), tended to desire sex less frequently ($p = 0.032$), and had more vaginal dryness ($p < 0.001$) and dyspareunia ($p < 0.001$). Their ability to reach orgasm through intercourse tended to be reduced ($p = 0.043$), and their sexual satisfaction was significantly poorer ($p = 0.001$). The ability to have orgasm through noncoital caressing did not differ from that of other women. There was a significant correlation between the age of patient and the frequency of sexual desire and activity.

A study of 97 patients with stage I or II breast cancer who completed a set of questionnaires before initiating postoperative therapy demonstrated that 84% of the patients had difficulty communicating with the medical team (750). Most commonly reported problems were difficulty understanding physicians (49.5%), difficulty expressing feelings (46.3%), desire for more control over the medical team (45.3%), and difficulty asking questions of the physicians (42.6%). It is important for of physicians to foster interventions that enhance communications between patients with breast cancer and healthcare providers in order to improve each patient's psychologic adjustment to treatment and to decrease her distress.

Contralateral Breast Cancer

Administration of radiation therapy in the management of a first breast cancer is not a significant risk factor in the development of contralateral breast malignancy (462,751, 752). A report involving 27,175 women treated for breast cancer between 1960 and 1975 disclosed a relative risk of 1.2 to 1.4 of developing cancer in the contralateral breast in irradiated patients, in comparison with those who did not receive irradiation (753). The authors, however, concluded that the data did not indicate a pattern of relative risk consistent with an increased incidence of carcinoma of the breast in the opposite breast.

Rosen and coworkers (754) reported on 644 patients with T1 breast carcinoma treated primarily with mastectomy: 76 received adjuvant radiation therapy to the internal mammary and supraclavicular lymph nodes, 47 received irradiation to the regional nodes, and 5 patients had irradiation of the chest wall. Subsequent contralateral breast carcinoma was found in 10.9% of patients receiving adjuvant irradiation compared with 9.4% of those who did not receive postoperative irradiation.

Broët and colleagues (621), in an analysis of 4,748 women with invasive unilateral breast cancer, clinical stages I to III (3,768 were at risk at 5 years and 845 at 10 years), identified 282 metachronous contralateral breast cancers (median follow-up of 18 months). The cumulative rate was 4.1% at 5 years. Age less than 55 years at time of diagnosis of the first breast (RR, 1.4) and the presence of lobular invasive carcinoma (RR, 1.5) were associated with an increased risk of developing contralateral breast cancer. Adjuvant chemotherapy significantly decreased the risk (RR, 0.54). Of the total group of patients, 2,933 had breast-conservation treatment, and 1,815 had modified radical mastectomy (520). ^{60}Co breast irradiation was delivered to 1,819 patients as primary treatment. Mean dose to the breast was 57 Gy with surgery and 77.8 Gy without (reduced field after 57 Gy). The 5-year incidence of contralateral breast cancer was 3.9% without breast irradiation, 3.8% with total doses of 65 Gy or less to the tumor site, and 4.9% with higher doses (p = 0.42).

Singletary and associates (682) reported a 3.1% incidence of bilateral (synchronous or metachronous) breast cancer in 4,554 patients treated surgically for breast cancer. Fifty-five patients had a prior carcinoma of the breast, and 87 had a contralateral carcinoma of the breast detected within 4 months of enrollment. The frequency of metachronous breast cancer was relatively constant over time, with some clustering at years 1 to 4. The nodal status of the second breast cancer was related to the method of discovery rather than to the stage of the first carcinoma. Survival rates were similar for patients with metachronous or synchronous breast cancer. The contralateral cancers were more often found by mammography, were smaller, and were more frequently associated with negative axillary nodes than the first cancers.

Also, more contralateral breast cancers were diagnosed in the *in situ* stage.

Montague (321) reported six second-breast primary tumors in 316 patients (1.9% incidence) treated with conservation surgery and irradiation in contrast to 30 of 576 (5.2%) after radical or modified radical mastectomy alone.

Contralateral breast cancer developed during the second decade in 5 of 300 patients reported on by Kurtz and associates (674), with a cumulative risk of 6.5% at 20 years. Clark and colleagues (293) reported only a 3% incidence of contralateral breast primary tumors in 1,504 patients, and Recht and coworkers (324) noted a 9% incidence in 357 patients treated with conservation surgery and irradiation.

In an analysis of 6,406 women with stages 0 to III unilateral breast cancer, 319 patients (5%) developed a contralateral breast cancer (755). Median follow-up was 117 months from initial diagnosis and 52 months from detection of contralateral breast cancer. The proportion of early breast tumors (T1 or less) was significantly higher in the contralateral than in the first-treated breast (65% and 32%, respectively) (p <0.0001). The 5-year survival rate was 87%. Metachronous contralateral breast tumors did not have an adverse impact on overall survival of patients with breast cancer.

Table 30.24 (310,321,324,436,621–623,674,701,753). A summary of the reported incidence of contralateral cancer according to treatment modality is given in Table 30.24.

In a series by Nielsen and coworkers (460), 68% of 84 patients with a clinical diagnosis of invasive breast carcinoma had contralateral breast cancer on autopsy. Of the contralateral lesions, 49% were invasive and 51% were *in situ*. Ringberg and colleagues (756) reported a 40% incidence of unsuspected bilateral carcinoma and a 44% incidence in patients with initial *in situ* carcinoma in a group of 73 women with known unilateral breast carcinoma on whom contralateral subcutaneous mastectomy was performed as part of reconstructive surgery.

Boice and colleagues (757) evaluated the risk of second cancers associated with radiation therapy to the breast in 41,109 women registered with breast cancer in the Connecticut Tumor Registry between 1935 and 1982. They reviewed the records of 655 women in whom a second breast cancer developed 5 years or more after initial treatment and compared the radiation exposure with that of 1,189 matched controls who did not develop a second cancer. The average dose to the contralateral breast in women exposed to radiation was 2.82 Gy. The relative risk of developing a second breast cancer was 1.9 in the women who received radiation therapy; among patients who survived for 10 years or longer, the relative risk was 1.33. Women younger than 45 years of age had a 1.59 relative risk of developing a second breast cancer compared with 1.01 in older women.

On the other hand, Levitt and Mandell (758) estimated the dose delivered to the contralateral breast to be between 1 and 4 Gy. Assuming that 20,000 women undergo radiation therapy after conservation surgery and using data on the risk of developing breast cancer after various doses of ionizing radiation, they concluded that fewer than one additional case of breast cancer would occur after 10 years.

Storm and associates (759), in a case-controlled study of a registry-based cohort of breast-cancer patients in Denmark, also concluded that there was little, if any, risk of radiation-induced breast cancer associated with exposure of breast tissue to low-dose irradiation.

Incidence of Other Second Malignancy

Curtis and colleagues (760), in an analysis of the SEER Program data on 59,115 women with breast cancer diagnosed between 1973 and 1980, reported no cases of leukemia in a group of 1,988 women who received radiation therapy. In contrast, six cases of leukemia were observed (versus 1.58 expected) in 6,040 patients receiving chemotherapy in their first course of therapy. Five of six cases occurred in the third to seventh year after therapy. Parenthetically, the risk of developing leukemia in patients treated with surgery alone did not differ significantly from that of the general population. Curtis and associates (761) additionally reported the risk of leukemia after chemotherapy and radiation therapy for breast cancer based on a risk between leukemia and the amount of drug given in a cohort of 82,700 women diagnosed with breast cancer from 1973 to 1985 in the United States. Detailed information about therapy was obtained for 90 patients with leukemia and 260 matched controls. The dose of irradiation to the active marrow was estimated from individual radiation therapy records (mean dose, 7.5 Gy). The relative risk of acute nonlymphocytic leukemia was significantly increased after regional radiation therapy alone (RR, 2.4), alkylating agents alone (RR, 10.0), and combined irradiation and drug therapy (RR, 17.4). Dose-dependent risks were observed after radiation therapy and treatment with melphalan and cyclophosphamide; melphalan was 10 times more leukemogenic than cyclophosphamide (RR, 31.4 versus 3.1).

A rare complication after radical mastectomy is development of lymphangiosarcoma (762). It is associated with the development of lymphedema in the affected extremity and occurs in about 5 of 1,000 patients who have radical mastectomy and survive 5 years (763).

Souba and colleagues (764) described 10 patients with carcinoma of the breast in a group of 16 patients with radiation-induced chest-wall sarcomas. Of the 10, 6 tumors were malignant fibrohistiocytomas, 2 were osteosarcomas (1 of the rib and 1 of the sternum), 1 fibrosarcoma, and 1 supraclavicular mesenchymoma. The latency period between irradiation and the diagnosis of chest-wall sarcoma ranged from 5 to 28 years, with a mean of 13 years and a median of 10 years. Prognosis for these patients is extremely poor, with only one surviving past 2 years (died 48 months after treatment of sarcoma).

In a review of a Swedish regional healthcare cancer regis-
try, Karlsson and coworkers (765) noted 19 sarcomas in 13,490 women with previous breast-cancer diagnosis. The expected incidence for this tumor in that population was 8.7; thus, the relative risk of sarcoma in these patients with breast cancer was 2.2. There were six cases of angiosarcoma in the arm associated with lymphedema; all patients had received radiation therapy 7 to 14 years prior to detection of the sarcoma. In seven other cases, the sarcoma appeared in the vicinity of the treated breast cancer; six patients had received radiation therapy to the breast. The authors noted that the risk of soft-tissue sarcoma in patients treated with breast cancer is very low and pointed out that the integral dose delivered with modern breast-conservation therapy techniques is significantly lower than that given to the patients in this study.

Angiosarcomas arising in the field of radiation therapy are rare. Fineberg and Rosen (627) studied three patients with cutaneous angiosarcoma and four patients with atypical vascular lesions. All had breast-conservation surgery and axillary lymph-node dissection, and six patients received conventional high-energy postoperative doses of external-beam irradiation to the breast. Angiosarcoma was diagnosed 3.5, 3.7, and 5.25 years after radiation therapy. The three angiosarcomas were multifocal or diffuse and high grade, with solid cellular foci located mainly in the dermis. Two angiosarcoma patients underwent mastectomy; one died 10 months after diagnosis with recurrent local angiosarcoma, and the other was alive without angiosarcoma 2 months after diagnosis. Unlike other radiation-induced sarcomas, cutaneous angiosarcoma often occurs within a short time after irradiation. It is important to distinguish atypical vascular lesions from angiosarcoma, but currently there is no evidence that they represent a precursor to radiation-induced angiosarcoma.

Thirty-six cases of angiosarcoma after irradiation had been reported in the literature. Edeiken and coworkers (766) presented two additional patients treated with breast-conservation treatment who developed angiosarcoma in the field of prior irradiation. Seven cases of angiosarcoma after radiation therapy for breast-conserving treatment of breast carcinoma had been reported; the average time interval between the administration of radiation therapy and development of angiosarcoma was 8.6 years.

In a review of the literature, Wijnmaalen and colleagues (767) noted 13 cases of postirradiation angiosarcoma of the breast. They reported three additional cases from their experience of treating patients with breast-conservation surgery and irradiation. The mean interval between treatment of primary breast cancer and the development of angiosarcoma in these 16 patients was 76 months. The clinical aspect was typical, with multiple bluish or purple nodules of the skin, purple discoloration, and erythematous maculas or areas, sometimes combined with ulceration, edema, or a palpable mass. Mammography does not necessarily raise suspicion, and the interpretation of FNA or biopsy may be difficult. A mastectomy was performed in all patients. Follow-up data are available for 12 patients; 2 patients died of extensive local recurrences and 1 of distant metastases. In a series of 3,295 patients treated with conservation surgery and irradiation for breast cancer, Zucali and associates (768) observed three cases of soft-tissue sarcoma in the irradiated breasts. These authors believe that the risk of a second primary tumor in the irradiated breast is too low to justify modification of current policies of conservative therapy of breast cancer.

The number of patients with long-term follow-up after breast-conservation therapy is growing fast. Therefore, special attention should be paid to uncommon skin changes of the treated breast, since clinical suspicion is the main clue to the diagnosis of postirradiation angiosarcoma. The primary therapy is simple mastectomy if wide tumor-free margins can be achieved. At this time, there is no clear indication for standard adjuvant chemotherapy or irradiation.

REFERENCES

1. Breasted JH (trans). *The Edwin Smith surgical papyrus.* Vols 1 and 22. Chicago: University of Chicago Oriental Institute Publications, 1930.
2. Halsted WS. The results of operations for the cure of cancer of the breast performed at the Johns Hopkins Hospital from June 1889 to January 1894. *Johns Hopkins Hosp Rep* 1894;4:297.
3. Halsted WS. The results of radical operations for the cure of carcinoma of the breast. *Ann Surg* 1907;46:1.
4. Early Breast Cancer Trialists' Collaborative Group. Effects of radiotherapy and surgery in early breast cancer. *N Engl J Med* 1995;333:1444.
5. Quiet CA, Ferguson DJ, Weichselbaum RR, et al. Natural history of node-negative breast cancer: a study of 826 patients with long-term follow-up. *J Clin Oncol* 1995;13:1144.
6. Rosen PP, Groshen S, Kinne DW, et al. Factors influencing prognosis in node-negative breast carcinoma: analysis of 767 T1N0M0/T2N0M0 patients with long-term follow-up. *J Clin Oncol* 1993;11:2090.
7. Rosen PP, Groshen PR, Saigo PE, et al. A long-term follow-up study of survival in stage I (T1N0M0) and stage II (T1N1M0) breast carcinoma. *J Clin Oncol* 1989;7:355.
8. Rosen PP, Groshen S, Saigo P, et al. Pathological prognostic factors in stage I (T1N0M0) and stage II (T2N0M0) breast carcinoma: a study of 644 patients with median follow-up of 18 years. *J Clin Oncol* 1989;7:1239.
9. Union Internationale Contre le Cancer. *TNM atlas: illustrated guide to the classification of malignant tumours.* Berlin: Springer-Verlag, 1982.
10. Fisher B, Ravdin RD, Ausman RK, et al. Surgical adjuvant chemotherapy in cancer of the breast: results of a decade of cooperative investigation. *Ann Surg* 1968;168:337.
11. Fisher B, Carbone, P, Economou, SG, et al. L- Phenylalanine mustard (L-PAM) in the management of primary breast cancer: a report of early findings. *N Engl J Med* 1975;292:117.
12. Fisher B, Redmond, C, Fisher ER, et al. The contribution of recent NSABP clinical trials of primary breast cancer therapy to an understanding of tumor biology—an overview of findings. *Cancer* 1980;46:1009.
13. Morris A, Morris R, Wilson JF, et al. Breast-conserving therapy vs mastectomy in early-stage breast cancer: a meta-analysis of 10-year survival. *Cancer J Sci Am* 1997;3:6.
14. Bonadonna G, Valagussa P, Moliterni A, et al. Adjuvant cyclophosphamide, methotrexate, and fluorouracil (CMF) in node positive breast cancer: the results of 20 years of follow-up. *N Engl J Med* 1995;332:901.
15. Ballard-Barbash R, Schatzkin A, Carter CL, et al. Body fat distribution and breast cancer in the Framingham Study. *J Natl Cancer Inst* 1990;82:286.
16. Overgaard M, Hansen P, Overgaard J, et al. Postoperative radiotherapy in high-risk premenopausal women with breast cancer who receive adjuvant chemotherapy. *N Engl J Med* 1997;337:949.
17. Ragaz J, Jackson S, Le N, et al. Adjuvant radiotherapy and chemotherapy in node-positive premenopausal women with breast cancer. *N Engl J Med* 1997;337:956.
18. Diel I, Solomayer E, Costa S, et al. Reduction in new metastases in breast cancer with adjuvant clodronate treatment. *N Engl J Med* 1998;339:357.
19. Powles T, Paterson A, Nevantaus A, et al. Adjuvant clodronate reduces the incidence of bone metastases in patients with primary operable breast cancer. *Proc Am Soc Clin Oncol* 1998;17:468(abst).
20. Tabar L, Fagerberg G, Day NE, et al. Breast cancer treatment and natural history. *Lancet* 1992;339:412.
21. Fisher B, Costantino J, Wickerham D, et al. Tamoxifen for prevention of breast cancer: report of the National Surgical Adjuvant Breast and Bowel Project P-1 Study. *J Natl Cancer Inst* 1998;90:1371.
22. Fisher B, for the NSABP. Tamoxifen for prevention of breast cancer: Report of the NSABP P-1 study. *J Natl Cancer Inst* 1999;90:1371.
23. Powles T, Eeles R, Ashley S, et al. Interim analysis of the incidence of breast cancer in the Royal Marsden Hospital tamoxifen randomised chemoprevention trial. *Lancet* 1998;352:98.
24. Veronesi U, Luini A, Mariani L, et al. Effect of menstrual phase on surgical treatment of breast cancer. *Lancet* 1994;343:1545.
25. Gail MH, Brinton LA, Byar DP, et al. Projecting individualized probabilities of developing breast cancer for white females who are being examined annually. *J Natl Cancer Inst* 1989;81:1879.
26. Cummings SR, Eckert S, Krueger KA, et al. The effect of raloxifene on risk of breast cancer in postmenopausal women: results from the MORE randomized trial. *JAMA* 1999;281:2189.
27. Kinne DW, Kopans DB. Physical examination and mammography in the diagnosis of breast disease. In: Harris JR, Hellman S, Henderson IC, et al., eds. *Breast diseases.* Philadelphia: JB Lippincott, 1987:55.
28. del Regato JA, Spjut HJ, eds *Ackerman and del Regato's cancer: diagnosis, treatment, and prognosis.* 5th ed. St. Louis: Mosby, 1977:820.
29. Haagensen CD. *Diseases of the breast.* 2nd ed. Philadelphia: WB Saunders, 1971.
30. del Regato JA, Spjut HJ, eds. *Ackerman and del Regato's cancer: diagnosis, treatment and prognosis.* 6th ed. St. Louis: Mosby, 1985:853.
31. American Cancer Society. *Cancer facts and figures, 2003.* Atlanta: American Cancer Society, 2003.
32. Linsk JA, Franzen S. *Clinical aspiration cytology.* London: JB Lippincott, 1983:105.
33. Winchester DP, Bernstein JR, Paige ML, et al. *The early detection and diagnosis of breast cancer.* Atlanta: American Cancer Society, 1988:1.
34. Madigan MP, Ziegler RG, Benichou J, et al. Proportion of breast cancer cases in the United States explained by well-established risk factors. *J Natl Cancer Inst* 1987;87:1681.
35. Kelsey J. A review of the epidemiology of human breast cancer. *Epidemiol Rev* 1979;1:74.
36. Newcomb PA, Storer BE, Longnecker MP, et al. Lactation and a reduced risk of premenopausal breast cancer. *N Engl J Med* 1994;330:81.
37. Lippman ME, Allegra JC. Receptors in breast cancer. *N Engl J Med* 1978;299:930.
38. Rosner D, Lane WW. Oral contraceptive use has no adverse effect on prognosis of breast cancer. *Cancer* 1986;57:591.
39. Trapido EJ. A prospective cohort study of oral contraceptives and breast cancer. *J Natl Cancer Inst* 1981;67:1011.
40. Vessey M, Baron J, Doll R, et al. Oral contraceptives and breast cancer: final report of an epidemiologic study. *Br J Cancer* 1983;47:455.
41. White E, Malone KE, Weiss NS, et al. Breast cancer among young U.S. women in relation to oral contraceptive use. *J Natl Cancer Inst* 1994;86:505.
42. Colditz GA, Hankinson SE, Hunter DJ, et al. The use of estrogens

and progestins and the risk of breast cancer in postmenopausal women. *N Engl J Med* 1995;332:1589.

43. Collaborative Group on Hormonal Factors in Breast Cancer. Breast cancer and hormone replacement therapy: collaborative reanalysis of data from 51 epidemiological studies of 52,705 women with breast cancer and 108,411 women without breast cancer. *Lancet.* 1997;350: 1047–1059.

44. Chlebowski RT, Hendirx SL, Langer RD, et al. Influence of estrogen plus progestin on breast cancer and mammography in healthy postmenopausal women, The Women's Health Initiative Randomized Trial. *JAMA* 2003:289(24):.3243.

45. Li C, Malone K, Porter PL, el al; Relationship between long durations and different regimens of hormone therapy and risk of breast cancer. *JAMA* 2003:289(24):3254.

46. Land CE, Boice JD Jr, Shore RE, et al. Breast cancer risk from low-dose exposure to ionizing radiation. *J Natl Cancer Inst* 1980;65:353.

47. Tokunaga M, Norman JE Jr, Asano M, et al. Malignant breast tumors among atomic bomb survivors, Hiroshima and Nagasaki, 1950–1974. *J Natl Cancer Inst* 1979;62:1347.

48. Boice JD Jr, Monson RR. Breast cancer in women after repeated fluoroscopic examinations of the chest. *J Natl Cancer Inst* 1977;59: 823.

49. Shore RE, Hempelmann LH, Kowaluk E, et al. Breast neoplasms in women treated with x-rays for acute postpartum mastitis. *J Natl Cancer Inst* 1977;59:813.

50. Miller AB, Howe GR, Sherman GJ, et al. Mortality from breast cancer after irradiation during fluoroscopic examinations in patients being treated for tuberculosis. *N Engl J Med* 1989;321:1285.

51. Hoffman DA, Lonstein JE, Morin MM, et al. Breast cancer in women with scoliosis exposed to multiple diagnostic x-rays. *J Natl Cancer Inst* 1989;81:1307.

52. Hildreth NG, Shore RE, Dvoretsky PM. The risk of breast cancer after irradiation of the thymus in infancy. *N Engl J Med* 1989;321: 1281.

53. Bhatia S, Robison LL, Oberlin O, et al. Breast cancer and other second neoplasms after childhood Hodgkin's disease. *N Engl J Med* 1996; 334:745.

54. Willet WC, Stampfer MJ, Calditz GA, et al. Moderate alcohol consumption and risk of breast cancer. *N Engl J Med* 1987;315:1174.

55. van den Brandt PA, Goldbohm RA, et al. Alcohol and breast cancer: results from the Netherlands Cohort Study. *Am J Epidemiol* 1995; 141:907.

56. Longnecker MP, Newcomb PA, Mittendorf R, et al. Risk of breast cancer in relation to lifetime alcohol consumption. *J Natl Cancer Inst* 1995;87:923.

57. Prentice RL, Kakar F, Hursting S, et al. Aspects of rationale for the Women's Health Trial. *J Natl Cancer Inst* 1988;80:802.

58. Howe GR, Hirohata T, Hislop TG, et al. Dietary factors and risk of breast cancer: combined analysis of twelve case-control studies. *J Natl Cancer Inst* 1990;82:561.

59. Clark GM. Prognostic and predictive factors. In: JR Harris, Lippman ME, Morrow M, Hellman S, eds. *Diseases of the breast.* Philadelphia: Lippincott–Raven, 1996:461.

60. Holmes MD, Hunter DJ, Colditz GA, et al. Association of dietary intake of fat and fatty acids with risk of breast cancer. *JAMA* 1999; 281:914.

61. Byrne C, Schairer C, Wolfe J, et al. Mammographic features and breast cancer risk: effects with time, age, and menopause status. *J Natl Cancer Inst* 1995;87:1622.

62. Kambouris AA. Axillary node metastases in relation to size and location of breast cancers: analysis of 147 patients. *Am Surg* 1996;62: 519.

63. Silverstein MJ, Rosser RJ, Gierson ED, et al. Axillary lymph node dissection for intraductal breast carcinoma: is it indicated? *Cancer* 1987;59:1819.

64. Tinnemans JG, Wobbes T, Hollard R, et al. Treatment and survival of female patients with nonpalpable breast carcinoma. *Ann Surg* 1989; 209:249.

65. Handley RS. Carcinoma of the breast. *Ann R Coll Surg* 1975;57:59.

66. Koscielny S, Tubiana M, Le MG, et al. Breast cancer: relationship between the size of the primary tumour and the probability of metastatic dissemination. *Br J Cancer* 1984;49:709.

67. Tubiana M, Koscielny S. Natural history of human breast cancer: recent data and clinical implications. *Breast Cancer Res Treat* 1991; 18:125.

68. Hagemeister FB, Buzdar AU, Luna MA, et al. Causes of death in breast cancer: clinicopathologic study. *Cancer* 1980;46:161.

69. Bloom HJG, Richardson WW, Harries EJ. Natural history of untreated breast cancer (1805–1933). *BMJ* 1962;2:213.

70. Paterson R. *Treatment of malignant disease by radium and x-rays.* London: Arnold, 1948:309.

71. Wellings SR, Jensen HM, Marcum RG. An atlas of subgross pathology of the human breast with special reference to possible precancerous lesions. *J Natl Cancer Inst* 1975;55:231.

72. Faverly DR, Burgers L, Bult P, Holland R. Three-dimensional imaging of mammary ductal carcinoma in situ: clinical implications. *Semin Diagn Pathol* 1994;11:193.

73. Page DL, Rogers LW. Carcinoma in situ (CIS). In: Page D, Anderson TJ, eds. *Diagnostic histopathology of the breast.* New York: Churchill Livingstone, 1987:157.

74. Rosai J. Breast: In situ carcinoma. In: Rosai J, ed. *Ackerman's surgical pathology.* 8th ed. Vol 2. St. Louis: Mosby, 1996:1596.

75. Silverstein MJ, Waisman JR, Gamagami P, et al. Intraductal carcinoma of the breast (208 cases). Clinical factors influencing treatment choice. *Cancer* 1990;66:102.

76. Rosen PPR. Intraductal carcinoma. In: Rosen PP, ed. *Rosen's breast pathology.* Philadelphia: Lippincott–Raven, 1997: 227.

77. Maluf HM, Koerner FC. Solid papillary carcinoma of the breast. A form of intraductal carcinoma with endocrine differentiation frequently associated with mucinous carcinoma. *Am J Surg Pathol* 1995; 19:1237.

78. Tsang WYW, Chan JKC. Endocrine ductal carcinoma in situ (E-DCIS) of the breast. A form of low-grade DCIS with distinctive clinicopathologic and biologic characteristics. *Am J Surg Pathol* 1996; 20:921.

79. Ashikari R, Haydu SI, Robbins GF. Intraductal carcinoma of the breast (1960–1969). *Cancer* 1971;28:1182.

80. Westbrook KC, Gallagher HS. Intraductal carcinoma of the breast. A comparative study. *Am J Surg* 1975;130:667.

81. Sunshine JA, Moseley HS, Fletcher WS, et al. Breast carcinoma in situ: a retrospective review of 112 cases with a minimum of 10-years' follow-up. *Am J Surg* 1985;150:44.

82. Silverstein MJ, Barth A, Poller DN, et al. Ten-year results comparing mastectomy to excision and radiation therapy for ductal carcinoma in situ of the breast. *Eur J Cancer* 1995;31:1425.

83. Lagios MD, Margolin FR, Westdahl PR, et al. Mammographically detected duct carcinoma in situ. Frequency of local recurrence following tylectomy and prognostic effect of nuclear grade on local recurrence. *Cancer* 1989;63:618.

84. Schwartz GF, Finkel GC, Garcia JC, et al. Subclinical ductal carcinoma in situ of the breast. Treatment by local excision and surveillance alone. *Cancer* 1992;70:2468.

85. Bellamy CO, McDonald C, Salter DM, et al. Noninvasive ductal carcinoma of the breast: the relevance of histologic categorization. *Hum Pathol* 1993;24:16.

86. Solin LJ, Yeh I-T, Kurtz J, et al. Ductal carcinoma in situ (intraductal carcinoma) of the breast treated with breast-conserving surgery and definitive irradiation. Correlation of pathologic parameters with outcome of treatment. *Cancer* 1993;71:2532.

87. Fisher B, Dignam J, Wolmark N, et al. Lumpectomy and radiation therapy for the treatment of intraductal breast cancer: findings from the National Surgical Adjuvant Breast and Bowel Project B-17. *J Clin Oncol* 1998;16:441.

88. Patchefsky AS, Schwartz GF, Finkelstein SD, et al. Heterogeneity of intraductal carcinoma of the breast. *Cancer* 1989;63:731.

89. Lennington WJ, Jensen RA, Dalton LW, et al. Ductal carcinoma in situ of the breast. Heterogeneity of individual lesions. *Cancer* 1994; 73:118.

90. Holland R, Peterse JL, Millis RR, et al. Ductal carcinoma in situ: a proposal for a new classification. *Semin Diagn Pathol* 1994;11:167.

91. Poller DN, Silverstein MJ, Galea A, et al. Ductal carcinoma in situ of the breast: a proposal for a new simplified histological classification association between cellular proliferation and c-erbB2 protein expression. *Mod Pathol* 1994;7:257.

92. Silverstein MJ, Poller DN, Waisman JR, et al. Prognostic classification of breast ductal carcinoma in situ. *Lancet* 1995;345:1154.

93. Tavassoli FA. *Pathology of the breast.* Norwalk, CT: Appleton & Lange, 1992:238.

94. Scott MA, Lagios MD, Akelsson K, et al. Ductal carcinoma in situ of the breast: reproducibility of histological subtype analysis. *Hum Pathol* 1997;28:967.

95. Douglas-Jones AG, Gupta SK, Attanoos RL, et al. A critical appraisal of six modern classifications of ductal carcinoma in situ of the breast (DCIS): correlation with grade of associated invasive carcinoma. *Histopathology* 1996;29:397.

96. Bethwaite P, Smith N, Delahunt B, et al. Reproducibility of new classification schemes for the pathology of ductal carcinoma in situ of the breast. *J Clin Pathol* 1998;51:450.

97. Sloane JP, Amendoeira I, Apostolikas N, et al. Consistency achieved by 23 European pathologists in categorizing ductal carcinoma in situ using five classifications. European Commission Working Group on Breast Screening Pathology. *Hum Pathol* 1998;29:1056.

98. Badve S, A'Hern RP, Ward AM, et al. Prediction of local recurrence of ductal carcinoma in situ of the breast using five histological classifications: a comparative study with long follow-up. *Hum Pathol* 1998;29:915.

99. Silverstein MJ, Lagios MD, Craig PH, et al. A prognostic index for ductal carcinoma in situ of the breast. *Cancer* 1996;77:2267.

100. Consensus conference on the classification of ductal carcinoma in situ. The Consensus Conference Committee. *Cancer* 1997;80:1798.

101. Rosai J. Borderline epithelial lesions of the breast. *Am J Surg Pathol* 1991;15:209.

102. Schnitt SJ, Connolly JL, Tavassoli FA, et al. Interobserver reproducibility in the diagnosis of ductal proliferative breast lesions using standardized criteria. *Am J Surg Pathol* 1992;16:1133.

103. Chaudary MA, Millis RR, Lane EB, et al. Paget's disease of the nipple: a ten-year review including clinical, pathological and immunohistochemical findings. *Breast Cancer Res Treat* 1986;8:139.

104. Foote FW Jr, Stewart FW. Lobular carcinoma in situ: a rare form of mammary carcinoma. *Am J Pathol* 1941;17:491.

105. Pope TL, Fechner RE, Wilhelm MC, et al. Lobular carcinoma in situ of the breast: mammographic features. *Radiology* 1988;168:63.

106. Haagensen CD, Lane N, Lattes R. Neoplastic proliferation of the epithelium of the mammary lobules: adenosis, lobular neoplasia and small cell carcinoma. *Surg Clin North Am* 1972;52:497.

107. Frost AR, Tsangaris TN, Silverberg SG. Pleomorphic lobular carcinoma in situ. *Pathol Case Rev* 1996;1:27.

108. Jacobs, TW, Pliss N, Kouria G, Schnitt, SJ. Carcinomas in situ of the breast with indeterminate features: role of E-cadherin staining in categorization. *Am J Surg Pathol* 2001;25:229–236.

109. Berg JW, Hutter RV. Breast cancer. *Cancer* 1995;75:257.

110. Elston CW, Ellis IO. Pathological prognostic factors in breast cancer. I. The value of histological grades in breast cancer. Experience from a large study with long-term follow-up. *Histopathology* 1991;19:403.

111. Roberti NE. The role of histologic grading in the prognosis of patients with carcinoma of the breast: is this a neglected opportunity? *Cancer* 1997;80:1706.

112. Rasmussen BB, Rose C, Christensen IB. Prognostic factors in primary mucinous breast carcinoma. *Am J Clin Pathol* 1987;87:155.

113. Clayton F. Pure mucinous carcinomas of breast: morphologic features and prognostic correlates. *Hum Pathol* 1986;17:34–38.

114. Diab SG, Clark GM, Osborne CK, Libby A, Allred DC, Elledge RM. Tumor characteristics and clinical outcome of tubular and mucinous breast carcinomas. *J Clin Oncol* 1999;17:1442–1448.

115. McDivitt RW, Boyce W, Gersell D. Tubular carcinoma of the breast. Clinical and pathological observations concerning 135 cases. *Am J Surg Pathol* 1982;6:401.

116. Green I, McCormick B, Cranor M, et al. A comparative study of pure tubular and tubulolobular carcinoma of the breast. *Am J Surg Pathol* 1997;21:653.

117. Holland DW, Boucher LD, Mortimer JE. Tubular breast cancer experience at Washington University: a review of the literature. *Clin Breast Cancer* 2001;2:210–214.

118. Cody HS III. The impact of mammography in 1096 consecutive patients with breast cancer, 1979–1993. *Cancer* 1995;76:1579.

119. Winchester DJ, Sahin AA, Tucker SL, Singletary SE. Tubular carcinoma of the breast. Predicting axillary nodal metastases and recurrence. *Ann Surg* 1996;223:342–347.

120. Armes JE, Egan AJ, Southey MC, et al. The histologic phenotypes of breast carcinoma occurring before age 40 years in women with and without BRCA1 or BRCA2 germline mutations: a population-based study. *Cancer* 1998;83:2335–2345.

121. Eisinger F, Stoppa-Lyonnet D, Longy M, et al. Germ line mutation at BRCA1 affects the histoprognostic grade in hereditary breast cancer. *Cancer Res* 1996;56:471–474.

122. Ridolfi R, Rosen P, Port A, et al. Medullary carcinoma of the breast. A clinicopathologic study with 10 year follow-up. *Cancer* 1977;40:1365.

123. Wargotz ES, Silverberg SG. Medullary carcinoma of the breast. A clinicopathologic study with appraisal of current diagnostic criteria. *Hum Pathol* 1988;19:1340.

124. Fisher ER, Kenny JP, Sass R, et al. Medullary cancer of the breast revisited. *Breast Cancer Res Treat* 1990;16:215–229.

125. Gaffey MJ, Mills SE, Frierson HF, et al. Interobserver variability in histopathological diagnosis. *Mod Pathol* 1995;8:31–38.

126. Rigaud C, Theobald S, Noel P, et al. Medullary carcinoma of the breast. A multicenter study of its diagnostic consistency. *Arch Pathol Lab Med* 1993;117:1005–1008.

127. Lefkowitz M, Lefkowitz W, Wargotz ES. Intraductal (intracystic) papillary carcinoma of the breast and its variants: a clinicopathological study of 77 cases. *Hum Pathol* 1994;25:802.

128. Adem C, Reynolds C, Adlakha H, et al. Wide spectrum screening keratin as a marker of metaplastic spindle cell carcinoma of the breast: an immunohistochemical study of 24 patients. *Histopathology* 2002;40:556–562.

129. Rayson D, Adjei AA, Suman VJ, et al. Metaplastic breast cancer: prognosis and response to systemic therapy. *Ann Oncol* 1999;10:413–419.

130. Kaufman MW, Marti JR, Gallager HS, et al. Carcinoma of the breast with pseudosarcomatous metaplasia. *Cancer* 1984;53:1908.

131. Chieng C, Cranor M, Lesser ME, Rosen PP. Metaplastic carcinoma of the breast with osteocartilaginous heterologous elements. *Am J Surg Pathol* 1998;22:188.

132. Rosen PP, Cranor ML. Secretory carcinoma of the breast. *Arch Pathol Lab Med* 1991;115:141.

133. Krausz T, Jenkins D, Grontoft O, et al. Secretory carcinoma of the breast in adults; emphasis on late recurrence and metastasis. *Histopathology* 1989;14:25.

134. Richard G, Hawk JC 3rd, Baker AS Jr., Austin RM. Multicentric adult secretory breast carcinoma: DNA flow cytometric findings, prognostic features, and review of the world literature. *J Surg Oncol* 1990;44:238–244.

135. Fields JN, Kuske RR, Perez CA, et al. Prognostic factors in inflammatory breast cancer. Univariate and multivariate analysis. *Cancer* 1989;63:1225.

136. Foote FW Jr, Stewart FW. A histologic classification of carcinoma of the breast. *Surgery* 1946;19:74.

137. DiCostanzo D, Rosen PP, Gareen I, et al. Prognosis in infiltrating lobular carcinoma. An analysis of "classical" and variant tumors. *Am J Surg Pathol* 1990;14:12–23.

138. Fechner RE. Histologic variants of infiltrating lobular carcinoma of the breast. *Hum Pathol* 1975;6:373.

139. Martinez V, Azzopardi JG. Invasive lobular carcinoma of the breast. Incidence and variants. *Histopathology* 1979;3:467.

140. Eusebi V, Maghales F, Azzopardi JC. Pleomorphic lobular carcinoma of the breast: an aggressive tumor showing apocrine differentiation. *Hum Pathol* 1992;23:655.

141. Weidner N, Semple JP. Pleomorphic variant of invasive lobular carcinoma of the breast. *Hum Pathol* 1992;23:1167.

142. Bentz JS, Yassa N, Clayton F. Pleomorphic lobular carcinoma of the breast: clinicopathologic features of 12 cases. *Mod Pathol* 1998;11:814.

143. Dixon JM, Anderson TJ, Page DL, et al. Infiltrating lobular carcinoma of the breast. *Histopathology* 1982;6:149.

144. Frost AR, Terahata S, Yeh IT, et al. The significance of signet ring cells in infiltrating lobular carcinoma of the breast. *Arch Pathol Lab Med* 1995;119:64.

145. Wang NP, Zee S, Zarbo RJ, et al. Coordinate expression of cytokeratins 7 and 20 defines unique subsets of carcinomas. *Applied Immunohistochemistry* 1995;3:99–107.

146. Rajan PB, Cranor ML, Rosen PP. Cystosarcoma phyllodes in adoles-

cent girls and young women: a study of 45 patients. *Am J Surg Pathol* 1998;22:64.

147. Kessinger A, Foley JF, Lemon HM, et al. Metastatic cystosarcoma phyllodes: a case report and review of the literature. *J Surg Oncol* 1972;4:131.

148. Rosen PP, Kimmel M, Ernsberger D. Mammary angiosarcoma. The prognostic significance of tumor differentiation. *Cancer* 1988; 62: 2145.

149. Gamel JW, Meyer JS, Feuer E, et al. The impact of stage and histology on the long-term clinical course of 163,808 patients with breast carcinoma. *Cancer* 1996;77:459.

150. Haagensen CD. Treatment of curable carcinoma of the breast. *Int J Radiat Biol Phys* 1977;2:975.

151. Fisher B, Wolmark N, Bauer M, et al. The accuracy of clinical nodal staging and of limited axillary dissection as a determinant of histological nodal status in carcinoma of the breast. *Surg Gynecol Obstet* 1981;152:765.

152. Fisher B, Bauer M, Wickerham DL. Relation of number of positive axillary nodes to the prognosis of patients with primary breast cancer: a NSABP update. *Cancer* 1983;52:1551.

153. Valagussa P, Bonadonna G, Veronesi U. Patterns of relapse and survival following radical mastectomy: analysis of 716 consecutive patients. *Cancer* 1978;41:1170.

154. Donegan WL, Perez-Mesa CM, Watson FR. A biostatistical study of locally recurrent breast carcinoma. *Surg Gynecol Obstet* 1966; 122: 529.

155. Ravdin P. *Prognostic factors in breast cancer.* American Society of Clinical Oncology Educational Book. Denver: Karger 1997:217.

156. Osborne CK. Prognostic factors in breast cancer. *PPO Updates* 1990; 4:1.

157. Paik S, Bryant J, Park C, et al. erbB-2 and response to doxorubicin in patients with axillary lymph node-positive, hormone receptor-negative breast cancer. *J Natl Cancer Inst* 1998;30:1361.

158. Thor A, Berry D, Budman D, et al. erbB-2, p53, and efficacy of adjuvant therapy in lymph node-positive breast cancer. *J Natl Cancer Inst* 1998;90:1346.

159. Fowble B, Solin LJ, Schultz DJ, et al. Breast recurrence and survival related to primary tumor location in patients undergoing conservative surgery and radiation for early-stage breast cancer. *Int J Radiat Oncol Biol Phys* 1992;23:933.

160. Haffty BG, Wilson LD, Smith R, et al. Subareolar breast cancer: long-term results with conservative surgery and radiation therapy. *Int J Radiat Oncol Biol Phys* 1995;33:53.

161. Schnitt SJ, Connolly JL, Recht A, et al. Influence of infiltrating lobular histology on local tumor control in breast cancer patients treated with conservative surgery and radiotherapy. *Cancer* 1989;64:448.

162. Weiss MC, Fowble BL, Solin LJ, et al. Outcome of conservative therapy for invasive breast cancer by histologic subtype. *Int J Radiat Oncol Biol Phys* 1992;23:941.

163. Harris JR, Connolly JL, Schnitt SJ, et al. Clinical-pathologic study of early breast cancer treated by primary radiation therapy. *J Clin Oncol* 1983;1:184.

164. Harris JR, Connolly JL, Schnitt SJ, et al. The use of pathologic features in selecting the extent of surgical resection necessary for breast cancer patients treated by primary radiation therapy. *Ann Surg* 1985;201:164.

165. Schnitt SJ, Connolly JL, Recht A, et al. Breast relapse following primary radiation therapy for early breast cancer. II. Detection of pathologic features and prognostic significance. *Int J Radiat Oncol Biol Phys* 1985;11:1277.

166. Kurtz JM, Spitalier JM, Amalric R. Late breast recurrence after lumpectomy and irradiation. *Int J Radiat Oncol Biol Phys* 1983;9:1191.

167. Clarke DH, Le MG, Sarrazin D, et al. Analysis of local-regional relapses in patients with early breast cancers treated by excision and radiotherapy: experience of the Institut Gustave-Roussy. *Int J Radiat Oncol Biol Phys* 1985;11:137.

168. Fisher ER, Sass R, Fisher B, et al. Pathologic findings from the National Surgical Adjuvant Breast Project (Protocol 6). II. Relation of local breast recurrence to multicentricity. *Cancer* 1986;57:1717.

169. van Limbergen E, van den Bogaert W, van der Schueren E, et al. Tumor excision and radiotherapy as primary treatment of breast cancer: analysis of patient and treatment parameters and local control. *Radiother Oncol* 1987;8:1.

170. Vicini FA, Eberlein TJ, Connolly JL, et al. The optimal extent of resection for patients with stages I or II breast cancer treated with conservative sugery and radiotherapy. *Ann Surg* 1991;214:200.

171. Bartelink H, Borger JH, van Dogen JA, et al. The impact of tumor size and histology on local control after breast-conserving therapy. *Radiother Oncol* 1988;11:297.

172. Boyages J, Recht A, Connolly J, et al. Factors associated with local recurrence as a first site of failure following conservative treatment of early breast cancer. *Recent Results Cancer Res* 1989;115:92.

173. Eberlein TJ, Connolly JL, Schnitt SJ, et al. Predictors of local recurrence following conservative breast surgery and radiation therapy. *Arch Surg* 1990;125:771.

174. Fowble BL, Solin LJ, Schultz DJ, et al. Ten year results of conservative surgery and irradiation for stage I and II breast cancer. *Int J Radiat Oncol Biol Phys* 1991;21:269.

175. Kurtz JM, Jacquemier J, Amalric R, et al. Risk factors for breast recurrence in premenopausal and postmenopausal patients with ductal cancers treated by conservation therapy. *Cancer* 1990;65:1867.

176. Recht A, Danoff B, Solin LJ, et al. Intraductal carcinoma of the breast: results of treatment with excisional biopsy and irradiation. *J Clin Oncol* 1985;3:1339.

177. Schnitt SJ, Connolly JL, Harris JR, et al. Pathologic predictors of early local recurrence in stage I and II breast cancer treated by primary radiation therapy. *Cancer* 1984;53:1049.

178. Veronesi U, Salvador B, Luini A, et al. Conservative treatment of early breast cancer: long-term results of 1232 cases treated with quadrantectomy, axillary dissection and radiotherapy. *Ann Surg* 1990; 211:250.

179. Zafrani B, Fourquet A, Vilcoq JR, et al. Conservative management of intraductal breast carcinoma with tumorectomy and radiation therapy. *Cancer* 1986;57:1299.

180. Holland R, Connolly JL, Gelman R, et al. The presence of an extensive intraductal component following a limited excision correlates with prominent residual disease in the remainder of the breast. *J Clin Oncol* 1990;8:113.

181. Borg A, Zhang QX, Johannsson O, Olsson H. High frequency of allelic imbalance at the BRCA1 region on chromosome 17q in both familial and sporadic ductal breast carcinomas. *J Natl Cancer Inst* 1994;86:792.

182. FitzGerald MG, MacDonald DJ, Krainer M, et al. Germ-line *BRCA1* mutations in Jewish and non-Jewish women with early-onset breast cancer. *N Engl J Med* 1996;334:143.

183. Porter DE, Cohen BB, Wallace MR, et al. Breast cancer incidence, penetrance, and survival in probable carriers of BRCA1 gene mutation in families linked to BRCA1 on chromosome 17q12–21. *Br J Surg* 1994;81:1512.

184. Langston AA, Malone KE, Thompson JD, et al. *BRCA1* mutations in a population-based sample of young women with breast cancer. *N Engl J Med* 1996;334:137.

185. Easton DF, Bishop DT, Ford D, et al. Genetic lineage analysis in familial breast and ovarian cancer: results of 214 families. *Am J Hum Genet* 1993;52:678.

186. Cancer risks in BRCA2 mutation carriers. *J Natl Cancer Inst* 1999; 91(15):1310–1316.

187. Weber BL. Susceptibility genes for breast cancer [Editorial]. *N Engl J Med* 1994;331:1523.

188. Adami HO, Malker B, Meirik O, et al. Age as a prognostic factor in breast cancer. *Cancer* 1985;56:898.

189. Chung M, Chang HR, Bland KI, Wanebo HJ. Younger women with breast carcinoma have a poorer prognosis than older women. *Cancer* 1996;77:97.

190. Host H, Lund E. Age as a prognostic factor in breast cancer. *Cancer* 1986;57:2217.

191. Nemoto T, Vana J, Bedwani RN, et al. Management and survival of female breast cancer. *Cancer* 1980;45:2917.

192. Vilcoq JR, Calle R, Fem F, et al. Conservative treatment of axillary adenopathy due to probable subclinical breast cancer. *Arch Surg* 1982; 117:1136.

193. Kurtz JM, Spitalier JM, Amalric R, et al. Mammary recurrences in women younger than forty. *Int J Radiat Oncol Biol Phys* 1988;15: 271.

194. Recht A, Connolly JL, Schnitt SJ, et al. The effect of young age on tumor recurrence in the treated breast after conservative surgery and radiotherapy. *Int J Radiat Oncol Biol Phys* 1988;14:3.

195. Delouche G, Bachelot F, Premont M, et al. Conservation treatment of early breast cancer: long-term results and complications. *Int J Radiat Oncol Biol Phys* 1987;13:29.

196. Vilcoq JR, Calle R, Stacey P, et al. The outcome of treatment by tumorectomy and radiotherapy of patients with operable breast cancer. *Int J Radiat Oncol Biol Phys* 1981;8:1327.

197. Clarke DH, Martinez AA. Identification of patients who are at high risk for local regional breast cancer recurrence after conservative surgery and radiotherapy: a review article for surgeons, pathologists and radiation and medical oncologists. *J Clin Oncol* 1992;10:474.

198. Fowble BL, Schultz DJ, Overmoyer B, et al. The influence of young age on outcome in early stage breast cancer. *Int J Radiat Oncol Biol Phys* 1994;30:23.

199. Haffty BG, Fischer D, Rose M, et al. Prognostic factors for local recurrence in the conservatively treated breast cancer patients: a cautious interpretation of the data. *J Clin Oncol* 1991;9:997.

200. Halverson KJ, Perez CA, Taylor ME, et al. Age is a prognostic factor for breast and regional node recurrence following breast conserving surgery and irradiation in stage I and II breast cancer. *Int J Radiat Oncol Biol Phys* 1993;27:1045.

201. Matthews RH, McNeese M, Montague ED, et al. Prognostic implications of age in breast cancer patients treated with tumorectomy and irradiation or with mastectomy. *Int J Radiat Oncol Biol Phys* 1988; 14:659.

202. Nixon AJ, Neuberg D, Hayes DF, et al. Relationship of patient age to pathologic features of the tumor and prognosis for patients with stage I or II breast cancer. *J Clin Oncol* 1994;12:888.

203. Vicini FA, Recht A, Abner A, et al. The association between very young age and recurrence in the breast in patients treated with conservative surgery and radiation therapy. *Int J Radiat Oncol Biol Phys* 1990;19:132 (abstract)..

204. de la Rochefordière A, Asselain B, Campana F, et al. Age as a prognostic factor in premenopausal breast carcinoma. *Lancet* 1993;341: 1039.

205. Simon MS, Severson RK. Racial differences in survival of female breast cancer in the Detroit metropolitan area. *Cancer* 1996;77:308.

206. Jones BA, Kasl SV, Curnen MGM, et al. Can mammography screening explain the race difference in stage at diagnosis of breast cancer? *Cancer* 1995:75:2103.

207. Ansell D, Whitman S, Lipton R, et al. Race, income, and survival from breast cancer at two public hospitals. *Cancer* 1993;72:2974.

208. Zaloznik AJ. Breast cancer stage at diagnosis: Caucasians versus Afro-Americans. *Breast Cancer Res Treat* 1995;34:195.

209. Zaloznik AJ. Breast cancer stage at diagnosis: Caucasians versus Hispanics. *Breast Cancer Res Treat* 1997;42:121

210. Pierce L, Fowble B, Solin LJ, et al. Conservative surgery and radiation therapy in black women with early stage breast cancer: patterns of failure and analysis of outcome. *Cancer* 1992;69:2831.

211. Eley JW, Hill HA, Chen VW, et al. Racial differences in survival from breast cancer: results of the National Cancer Institute Black/White Cancer Survival Study. *JAMA* 1994;272:947.

212. Senie RT, Rosen PP, Rhodes P, et al. Obesity at diagnosis of breast carcinoma influences duration of disease-free survival. *Ann Intern Med* 1992;116:26.

213. Hornstein E, Skornick Y, Rozin R. The management of breast carcinoma in pregnancy and lactation. *J Surg Oncol* 1982;21:179.

214. Mammography Quality Standards Act of 1992. US Congress. Senate. 102nd sess, October 1, 1992. *S Rept* 102–448.

215. Bjurstam N, Bjorneld L, Duffy SW, et al. The Gothenburg breast cancer screening trial: preliminary results on breast cancer mortality for women aged 39–49. *Monogr Natl Cancer Inst* 1997;22:53.

216. Andersson I, Janzon L. Reduced breast cancer mortality in women under age 50: updated results from the Malmo mammographic screening program. *Monogr Natl Cancer Inst* 1997;22:63.

217. Hendrick RE, Smith RA, Rutledge JH III, Smart CR. Benefit of screening mammography in women aged 40–49; a new meta-analysis of randomized controlled trials. *Monogr Natl Cancer Inst* 1997;22: 87.

218. Duffy SW, Tabar L, Chen HH, et al. The impact of organized mammography service screening on breast carcinoma mortality in seven Swedish counties: a collaborative evaluation. *Cancer* 2002;95: 458–469.

219. Rosenquist CJ, Lindfors KK. Screening mammography beginning at age 40: a reappraisal of cost-effectiveness. *Cancer* 1998;82:2235.

220. Tengs TO, Adams ME, Pliskin JS, et al. Five-hundred life saving interventions and their cost-effectiveness. *Risk Anal* 1995;15:369.

221. Boer R, deKoning HJ, van Oortmarssen GJ, van der Maas PJ. In search of the best upper age limit for breast cancer screening. *Eur J Cancer* 1995;31:2040.

222. Eklund GW, Busby RC, Miller SH, Job TS. Improved imaging of the augmented breast. *AJR Am J Roentgenol* 1988;151:467.

223. Dershaw DD. Nonpalpable, needle-localized mammographic abnormalities: pathologic correlation in 219 patients. *Cancer Invest* 1986; 4:1.

224. Sickles EA. Periodic mammographic follow-up of probably benign lesions: results of 3,184 consecutive cases. *Radiology* 1991;179:463.

225. Shaw de Paredes E, Abbitt PL, Tabbarah S, Bickers MA, Smith DC. Mammographic and histologic correlations of microcalcifications. *Radiographics* 1990;10:577.

226. Liberman L, Abramson AF, Squires FB, et al. The Breast Imaging Reporting and Data System: positive predictive value of mammographic features and final assessment categories. *AJR Am J Roentgenol* 1998;171:35.

227. D'Orsi C. The American College of Radiology mammography lexicon: an initial attempt to standardize terminology. *AJR Am J Roentgenol* 1996;166:779.

228. American College of Radiology (ACR). Illustrated breast imaging reporting and data system (BI-RADS™), 3rd ed. Virginia: American College of Radiology, 1998.

229. Smith RA, Saslow D, Sawyer KA, et al. American Cancer Society guidelines for breast cancer screening: update 2003. *CA Cancer J Clin* 2003; 53:141–169.

230. Dershaw DD, Yahalom J, Petrek JA. Mammography of breast carcinoma developing in women treated for Hodgkin's disease. *Radiology* 1992;184:421

231. Dershaw DD. Indications for routine breast cancer screening of asymptomatic women less than 40 years old [letter]. *Am J Radiol* 1999;172:1136

232. Jackson VP. The role of US in breast imaging. *Radiology* 1990;177: 305.

233. Stanford JL, Weiss NS, Voigt LF, et al. Combined estrogen and progestin hormone replacement therapy in relation to risk of breast cancer in middle-aged women. *JAMA* 1995;274:137.

234. Skaane P, Engedal K. Analysis of sonographic features in the differentiation of fibroadenoma and invasive ductal carcinoma. *AJR Am J Roentgenol* 1998;170:109.

235. Kedar RP, Cosgrove DO, Bamber JC, Bell DS. Automated quantification of color Doppler signals: a preliminary study in breast tumors. *Radiology* 1995;197:39.

236. Kolb TM, Lichy J, Newhouse JH. Occult cancer in women with dense breasts: detection with screening US—diagnostic yield and tumor characteristics. *Radiology* 1998;207:191.

237. Harris KM, Gannott MA, Shestak KC, et al. Silicone implant rupture: detection with US. *Radiology* 1993;187:761.

238. Orel SG. High-resolution MR imaging for the detection, diagnosis, and staging of breast cancer. *Radiographics* 1998;18:903.

239. Gorczyca DP, DeBruhl ND, Ahn CY, et al. Silicone breast implant ruptures in an animal model: comparison of mammography, MR imaging, US and CT. *Radiology* 1994;190:227.

240. Orel SG, Schnall MD, Powell CM, et al. Staging of suspected breast cancer: effect of MR imaging and MR-guided biopsy. *Radiology* 1995; 196:115.

241. Orel SG, Reynolds C, Schnall MD, et al. Breast carcinoma: MR imaging before re-excisional biopsy. *Radiology* 1997;205:429.

242. Dao TH, Rahmouni A, Campana F, et al. Tumor recurrence versus fibrosis in the irradiated breast: differentiation with dynamic gadolinium-enhanced MR imaging. *Radiology* 1993;187:751.

243. Morris EA, Schwartz LH, Dershaw DD, et al. MR imaging of the breast in patients with occult primary breast carcinoma. *Radiology* 1997;205:437.

244. Mussurakis S, Buckley DL, Horsman A. Prediction of axillary lymph node status in invasive breast cancer with dynamic contrast-enhanced MR imaging. *Radiology* 1997;203:317.

245. Gilles R, Guinebretiere JM, Shapeero LG, et al. Assessment of breast

cancer recurrence with contrast-enhanced subtraction MR imaging: preliminary results in 26 patients. *Radiology* 1993;188:473.

246. Kaiser WA. False-positive results in dynamic MR mammography. *MRI Clin North Am* 1994;2:539.

247. Breast cancer study, June 1995. Physician Insurers Association of America. Washington, D.C.

248. Dershaw DD, Eddens G, Liberman L, et al. Sonographic and clinical findings in women with palpable breast disease and negative mammography. *Breast Dis* 1995;8:13.

249. Osuch JR, Bonham VL. The timely diagnosis of breast cancer. *Cancer* 1994;74:271.

250. Newstead GM, Bante PB, Toth HK. Invasive lobular and ductal carcinoma: mammographic findings and stage at diagnosis. *Radiology* 1992;184:632.

251. Abramson DJ. Delayed mastectomy after outpatient biopsy. *Am J Surg* 1976;132:596.

252. Bertario L, Reduzzi D, Piromalli D, et al. Outpatient biopsy of breast cancer: influence on survival. *Ann Surg* 1985;201:64.

253. Fisher ER, Sass R, Fisher B. Biologic considerations regarding the one- and two-step procedures in the management of patients with invasive carcinoma of the breast. *Surg Gynecol Obstet* 1985;161:245.

254. Donegan WL. Evaluation of a palpable breast mass. *N Engl J Med* 1992;327:937.

255. Ciatto S, Cariaggi P, Bulagresi P, et al. Fine needle aspiration cytology of the breast: review of 9533 consecutive cases. *Breast* 1993;2:87.

256. Lee KR, Foster RS Jr, Papillo JL. Fine needle aspirate of the breast: importance of the aspirator. *Acta Cytol* 1987;31:281.

257. Wollenberg NJ, Caya JB, Clowry LJ. Fine needle aspiration cytology of the breast: a review of 321 cases with statistical evaluation. *Acta Cytol* 1985;29:425.

258. Smith C, Butler J, Cobb C, State D. Fine needle aspiration cytology in the diagnosis of primary breast cancer. *Surgery* 1988;103:178.

259. Innes DJ Jr, Feldman PS. Comparison of diagnostic results obtained by fine needle aspiration cytology and Tru-cut or open biopsies. *Acta Cytol* 1983;27:350.

260. Malberger E, Edoute Y, Toledano O, et al. Fine-needle aspiration and cytologic findings of surgical scar lesions in women with breast cancer. *Cancer* 1992;69:148.

261. Pezner RD, Lorant JA, Terz J, et al. Wound-healing complications following biopsy of the irradiated breast. *Arch Surg* 1992;127:321.

262. Liberman L, Feng T, Dershaw DD, et al. US-guided core breast biopsy: use and cost-effectiveness. *Radiology* 1998;208:717.

263. Dershaw DD, Morris EA, Liberman L, et al. Non-diagnostic stereotaxic core breast biopsy: results of rebiopsy. *Radiology* 1996;198:323.

264. Shaw deParedes E. Patient selection and care for percutaneous breast biopsy. In: Dershaw DD, ed. *Interventional breast procedures.* New York: Churchill Livingstone, 1996:37.

265. Liberman L, Dershaw DD, Morris EA, et al. Clip placement after stereotactic vacuum-assisted breast biopsy. *Radiology* 1997;205:417.

266. Dershaw DD. Stereotaxic breast biopsy. *Semin Ultrasound CT MR* 1996;17:444.

267. Parker S, Burbank R, Jackman RJ, et al. Percutaneous large-core breast biopsy: a multi-institutional study. *Radiology* 1994;193:359.

268. Dershaw DD, Caravella BA, Liberman L, et al. Limitations and complications in the utilization of stereotaxic core breast biopsy. *Breast J* 1996;2:1.

269. Nath ME, Robinson TM, Tobon H, Chough DM, Sumkin JH. Automated large-core needle biopsy of surgically removed breast lesions: comparison of samples obtained with 14-, 16- and 18-gauge needles. *Radiology* 1995;205:203.

270. Burbank R. Stereotactic breast biopsy of atypical ductal hyperplasia and ductal carcinoma in situ lesions: improved accuracy with directional, vacuum-assisted biopsy. *Radiology* 1997;204:843.

271. Alexander HR, Candela FC, Dershaw DD, Kinne DW. Needle-localized mammographic lesions: results and evolving treatment strategy. *Arch Surg* 1990;125:1441.

272. Helvie MA, Ikeda DM, Adler DD. Localization and needle aspiration of breast lesions: complications in 370 cases. *AJR Am J Roentgenol* 1991;157:711.

273. Reynolds HE, Jackson VP, Musick BS. Preoperative needle localization in the breast: utility of local anesthesia. *Radiology* 1993;187:503.

274. Dershaw DD. Needle localization for breast biopsy. In: Dershaw DD, ed. *Interventional breast procedures.* New York: Churchill Livingstone, 1996:25.

275. Proceedings from the 14th Annual Conference of the National Comprehensive Cancer Network, February 26–March 2, 1999.

276. Green FL, Page DL, Fleming ID, et al., eds. *AJCC cancer staging manual,* 6th ed. New York, Springer-Verlag, 2002:209–220.

277. Degenshein GA, Ceccarelli F. The history of breast cancer surgery. Part I: Early beginnings to Halsted. *Breast* 1977;3:28.

278. Robbins G, ed. *Silvergirl's surgery: the breast.* Austin, TX: Silvergirl, Inc, 1984:31.

279. Virchow R (translated by Frank Chase). *Cellular pathology.* Philadelphia: JB Lippincott Co, 1863.

280. Keynes G. The radium treatment of carcinoma of the breast. *Br J Surg* 1931;19:425.

281. Patey DH, Dyson WH. The prognosis of carcinoma of the breast in relation to the type of operation performed. *Br J Cancer* 1948;2:7.

282. Delacrue NC, Anderson WD, Starr J. Modified radical mastectomy in the individualized treatment of breast carcinoma. *Surg Gynecol Obstet* 1969;129:79.

283. Maddox WA, Carpenter JT, Laws HL, et al. A randomized prospective trial of radical (Halsted) mastectomy versus modified radical mastectomy in 211 breast cancer patients. *Ann Surg* 1983;198:207.

284. Turner L, Swindell R, Bell WGT, et al. Radical versus modified radical mastectomy for breast cancer. *Ann R Coll Surg Engl* 1981;63:239.

285. Wilson RE, Donegan WL, Mettlin C, et al. The 1982 national survey of carcinoma of the breast in the United States by the American College of Surgeons. *Surg Gynecol Obstet* 1984;159:309.

286. Morrow M, White J, Moughan J, et al. Factors predicting the use of breast-conserving therapy in stage I and stage II breast carcinoma. *J Clin Oncol* 2001; 19(8):2254–2262.

287. Turner-Warnick RT. Lymphatics of the breast. *Br J Surg* 1959;46:524.

288. Lacour J, Bucalossi P, Caceres E, et al. Radical mastectomy versus radical mastectomy plus internal mammary dissection: five year results of an international cooperative study. *Cancer* 1976;37:206.

289. Urban JA, Marjani MA. Significance of internal mammary lymph node metastases in breast cancer. *Am J Roentgenol Radium Ther Nucl Med* 1971;3:130.

290. Fisher B, Slack NH, Cavanaugh PJ, et al. Post-operative radiotherapy in the treatment of breast cancer: results of the NSABP clinical trial. *Ann Surg* 1970;172:711.

291. Lacour J, Le M, Caceres E, et al. Radical mastectomy versus radical mastectomy plus internal mammary dissection: ten year results of an international cooperative trial in breast cancer. *Cancer* 1983;51:1941.

292. Meier P, Ferguson DJ, Karrison T. A controlled trial of extended radical versus radical mastectomy: ten year results. *Cancer* 1989; 63:188.

293. Clark RM, Wilkinson RH, Miceli PN, et al. Breast cancer: experiences with conservation therapy. *Am J Clin Oncol* 1987;10:461.

294. Williams FH. A further note on a new method of using roentgen rays: consideration of primary treatment of some early cases of breast cancer by these rays. *Boston Med Surg J* 1906;154:641.

295. Keynes G. Conservative treatment of cancer of the breast. *BMJ* 1937; 2:643.

296. Mustakallio S. Über die Möglichkeiten der Röntgentherapie bei der Behandlung des Brustkrebs. *Acta Radiol* 1945;26:503–511.

297. Atkins H, Hayward JL, Klugman DJ, et al. Treatment of early breast cancer: a report after 10 years of a clinical trial. *BMJ (Clin Res)* 1972; 2:423.

298. Hayward JL. The Guy's trial of treatments of ''early'' breast cancer. *World J Surg* 1977;1:314.

299. Veronesi U, Saccozzi R, del Vecchio M, et al. Comparing radical mastectomy with quadrantectomy, axillary dissection, and radiotherapy in patients with small cancers of the breast. *N Engl J Med* 1981; 305:6.

300. Veronesi U, Cascinelli N, Mariani L, et al. Twenty-year follow-up of a randomized study comparing breast-conserving surgery with radical mastectomy for early-stage breast cancer. *New Engl J Med* 2002; 347(16):1227–1232.

301. Fisher B, Bauer M, Margolese R, et al. Five-year results of a randomized clinical trial comparing total mastectomy and segmental mastectomy with or without radiation in the treatment of breast cancer. *N Engl J Med* 1985;312:665.

302. Fisher B, Anderson S, Redmond C, et al. Reanalysis and results after 12 years of follow-up in a randomized clinical trial comparing total mastectomy with lumpectomy with or without irradiation in the treatment of breast cancer. *N Engl J Med* 1995;333:1456.

303. Jacobson JA, Danforth DN, Cowan KH, et al. Ten-year results of a comparison of conservation with mastectomy in the treatment of stage I and II breast cancer. *N Engl J Med* 1995;332:907.

304. van Dongen JA. Randomized clinical trial to assess the value of breast conserving therapy in stage I and stage II breast cancer, EORTC 10801 Trial. *J Natl Cancer Inst Monogr* 1992;11:15.

305. Blichert-Toft M, Rose C, Andersen JA, et al. Danish randomized trial comparing breast conservation with mastectomy: six years of life-table analysis. *J Natl Cancer Inst Mongr* 1992;11:19.

306. Sarrazin D, Le M, Fontaine F, et al. Conservative treatment versus mastectomy in T1 or small T2 breast cancer: a randomized clinical trial. In: Harris JR, Hellman S, Silen W, eds. *Conservative management of breast cancer*. Philadelphia: JB Lippincott Co, 1983:101.

307. Sarrazin D, Le M, Rouesse J, et al. Conservative treatment versus mastectomy in breast cancer tumors with macroscopic diameter of 20 millimeters or less: the experience of the Institut Gustave-Roussy. *Cancer* 1984;53:1209.

308. Amalric R, Santamaria F, Robert F, et al. Conservation therapy of operable breast cancer: results of 5, 10 and 15 years in 2,216 consecutive cases. In: Harris HR, Hellman S, Silen W, eds. *Conservative management of breast cancer: new surgical and radiotherapeutic techniques*. Philadelphia: JB Lippincott Co, 1983:15.

309. Calle R, Vilcoq JR, Zafrani B, et al. Local control and survival of breast cancer treated by limited surgery followed by irradiation. *Int J Radiat Oncol Biol Phys* 1986;12:873.

309a. Barr LC, Brunt AM, Goodman, AG et al. Uncontrolled local recurrence after treatment of breast cancer with breast conservation. *Cancer* 1989;64:1203.

310. Dewar JA, Arriagada R, Benhamou S, et al. Local relapse and contralateral tumor rates in patients with breast cancer treated with conservative surgery and radiotherapy (Institut Gustave Roussy 1970–1982). IGR Breast Cancer Group. *Cancer* 1995;76:2260.

311. Dubois JB, Gary-Bobo J, Pourquier H, et al. Tumorectomy and radiotherapy in early breast cancer: a report on 392 patients. *Int J Radiat Oncol Biol Phys* 1988;15:1275.

312. Fagundes MA, Fagundes HM, Brito CS, et al. Breast-conserving surgery and definitive radiation: a comparison between quadrantectomy and local excision with special focus on local-regional control and cosmesis. *Int J Radiat Oncol Biol Phys* 1993;27:553.

313. Fourquet A, Campana F, Zafrani B, et al. Prognostic factors of breast recurrence in the conservative management of early breast cancer: a 25-year follow-up. *Int J Radiat Oncol Biol Phys* 1989;17:719.

314. Fowble BL, Solin SJ, Goodman RL. Results of conservative surgery and radiation for intraductal noninvasive breast cancer. *Am J Clin Oncol* 1987;10:110(abst).

315. Gage I, Recht A, Gelman R, et al. Long-term outcome following breast-conserving surgery and radiation therapy. *Int J Radiat Oncol Biol Phys* 1995;33:245.

316. Haffty BG, Fischer D, Beinfield M, et al. Prognosis following local recurrence in the conservatively treated breast cancer patient. *Int J Radiat Oncol Biol Phys* 1991;21:293.

317. Haffty BG, Goldberg NB, Fischer D, et al. Conservative surgery and radiation therapy in breast carcinoma: local recurrence and prognostic implications. *Int J Radiat Oncol Biol Phys* 1989;17:727.

318. Kurtz JM, Amalric R, Brandone H, et al. Local recurrence after breast-conserving surgery and radiotherapy: frequency, time course, and prognosis. *Cancer* 1989;63:1912.

319. Kuske R, Compaan P, Cross M, et al. Breast conservation therapy: 417 breast cancers with a minimum follow-up period of five years. *Int J Radiat Oncol Biol Phys* 1989;17:235.

320. Leborgne F, Leborgne JH, Ortega B, et al. Breast conservation treatment of early stage breast cancer: patterns of failure. *Int J Radiat Oncol Biol Phys* 1995;31:765.

321. Montague ED. Conservation surgery and radiation therapy in the treatment of operable breast cancer. *Cancer* 1984;53:700.

322. Osborne MP, Ormiston N, Harmer CL, et al. Breast conservation in the treatment of early breast cancer: a 20-year follow-up. *Cancer* 1984:53:349.

323. Pierquin B, Huart J, Raynal M, et al. Conservative treatment for breast cancer: long-term results (15 years). *Radiother Oncol* 1991;20:16.

324. Recht A, Silver B, Schnitt S, et al. Breast relapse following primary radiation therapy for early breast cancer. I. Classification, frequency and salvage. *Int J Radiat Oncol Biol Phys* 1985;11:1271.

325. Solin LJ, Fowble B, Martz KL, et al. Definitive irradiation for early stage breast cancer: the University of Pennsylvania experience. *Int J Radiat Oncol Biol Phys* 1988;14:235.

326. Vicini FA, Recht A, Abner A, et al. Recurrence in the breast following conservative surgery and radiation therapy for early-stage breast cancer. *NCI Monogr* 1992;11:33.

327. Amalric R, Santamaria F, Robert F, et al. Radiation therapy with or without primary limited surgery for operable breast cancer. *Cancer* 1982;49:30.

328. Janjan NA, Murray KJ, Walker A, et al. Prognosis for breast cancer surgery and radiation therapy compared with mastectomy alone: a retrospective analysis of 759 patients with stage I/II breast cancer. *Cancer* 1992;69:2842.

329. Peters MV. Wedge resection with or without radiation in early breast cancer. *Int J Radiat Oncol Biol Phys* 1977;2:1151.

330. Rissanen PM. A comparison of conservative and radical surgery combined with radiotherapy in the treatment of stage I carcinoma of the breast. *Br J Radiol* 1969;42:423.

331. Liljegren G, Holmberg L, Adami HO, et al. Sector resection with or without postoperative radiotherapy for stage I breast cancer: five-year results of a randomized trial. *J Natl Cancer Inst* 1994;86:717.

332. Cedermark B, Askergren J Alveryd A, et al. Breast-conserving treatment for breast cancer in Stockholm, Sweden, 1977 to 1981. *Cancer* 1984;53:1253.

333. Clark RM, Whelan T, Levine M, et al. Randomized clinical trial of breast irradiation following lumpectomy and axillary dissection for node-negative breast cancer: an update. *J Natl Cancer Inst* 1996;88:1659.

334. Cooke AL, Perera F, Fisher B, et al. Tamoxifen with and without radiation after partial mastectomy in patients with involved nodes. *Int J Radiat Oncol Biol Phys* 1995;31:777.

335. Fisher B, Redmond C, Poisson R, et al. Eight-year results of a randomized clinical trial comparing total mastectomy and lumpectomy with or without radiation in the treatment of breast cancer. *N Engl J Med* 1989;320:822.

336. Forrest AP, Stewart HJ, Everington D, et al. Randomised controlled trial of conservation therapy for breast cancer: 6-year analysis of the Scottish trial. *Lancet* 1996;348:708.

337. Kantorowitz DA, Poulter CA, Rubin P, et al. Treatment of breast cancer with segmental mastectomy alone or segmental mastectomy plus radiation. *Radiother Oncol* 1989;15:141.

338. Whelan T, Clark R, Roberts R, et al. Ipsilateral breast tumor recurrence postlumpectomy is predictive of subsequent mortality: results from a randomized trial. *Int J Radiat Oncol Biol Phys* 1994;30:11.

339. Schnitt SJ, Hayman J, Gelman R, et al. A prospective study of conservative surgery alone in the treatment of selected patients with stage I breast cancer. *Cancer* 1996;77:1094.

340. Veronesi U, Luini A, Del Vecchio M, et al. Radiotherapy after breast-preserving surgery in women with localized cancer of the breast. *N Engl J Med* 1993;328:1587.

341. Wilson LD, Beinfield M, McKhann CF, Haffty BG. Conservative surgery and radiation in the treatment of synchronous ipsilateral breast cancers. *Cancer* 1993;72:137.

342. Fleck R, McNeese MD, Ellerbroek NA, et al. Consequences of breast irradiation in patients with preexisting collagen vascular diseases. *Int J Radiat Oncol Biol Phys* 1989;17:829.

343. Robertson J, Clarke D, Pevzner M, et al. Breast conservation therapy: severe breast fibrosis after radiation therapy in patients with collagen vascular disease. *Cancer* 1991;68:502.

344. Gwin JL, Eisenberg BL, Hoffman JP, et al. Incidence of gross and microscopic carcinoma in specimens from patients with breast cancer after reexcision lumpectomy. *Ann Surg* 1993;218:729.

345. McCormick B, Kinne D, Petrek J, et al. Limited resection for breast cancer: a study of inked specimen margins before radiotherapy. *Int J Radiat Oncol Biol Phys* 1987;13:1667.

346. Fein DA, Fowble BL, Hanlon AL. The influence of pathologic margin status, adjuvant treatment and residual tumor within the re-excision

specimen on breast recurrence. *Int J Radiat Oncol Biol Phys* 1996; 36:275(abst).

347. Ghossein NA, Barba JP, Albert S, et al. Importance of adequate surgical excision prior to radiotherapy in the local control of patients treated conservatively for breast cancer. *Proc 17th Intl Cong Radiat Oncol* 1989;48(abst).

348. Ghossein NA, Vilcoq J, Stacey P, et al. Is it necessary to irradiate the breast after conservative surgery for local cancer? *Arch Surg* 1987; 122:913.

349. Mansfield CM, Komarnicky LT, Schwartz FG, et al. Ten year results in 1070 patients with stages I and II breast cancer treated by conservative surgery and radiation therapy. *Cancer* 1995;75:2328.

349a. Anscher MS, Jones P, Prosnitz LR, et al. Local failure and margin status in early-stage breast carcinoma treated with conservation surgery and radiation therapy. *Ann Surg* 1993;18:22.

349b. Borger J, Kemperman H, Hart A, et al. Risk factors in breast conservation therapy. *J Clin Oncol* 1994;12:653.

349c. Fisher B, Anderson S, Redmond C, et al. Reanalysis and results after 12 years of follow-up in a randomized clinical trial comparing total mastectomy with lumpectomy with or without irradiation in the treatment of breast cancer. *N Engl J Med* 1995;333:1456.

349d. Hartsell WF, Kelly CA, Greim KL, et al. Breast-conserving therapy: a boost dose of radiation therapy is not necessary when negative margins of excision are achieved. *Breast Cancer Res Treat* 1993;27: 190(abst).

349e. Hunig R, Walther E, Harder F, et al. The Basel Lumpectomy Protocol: 5 year experience with a prospective study for conservation treatment of breast cancer. In: Harris JR, Hellman S, Silen W, eds. *Conservation management of breast cancer*. Philadelphia: JB Lippincott Co, 1983;23.

349f. Pezner RD, Wagman LD, Ben-Ezra J, et al. Breast conservation therapy: local tumor control in patients with pathologically clear margins who receive 5000 cGy breast irradiation without local boost. *Breast Cancer Res Treat* 1994;32:261.

349g. Ryoo ME, Kagan AR, Wollin M, et al. Prognostic factors for recurrence and cosmesis in 393 patients after radiation therapy for early mammary carcinoma. *Radiology* 1989;172:555.

349h. Schmidt-Ullrich RK, Wazer DE, DiPetrillo T, et al. Breast conservation therapy for early stage breast carcinoma with outstanding 10-year locoregional control rates: a case for aggressive therapy to the tumor-bearing quadrant. *Int J Radiat Oncol Biol Phys* 1993;27:545.

349i. Slotman BJ, Meyer OWN, Njo KH, et al. Importance of timing of radiotherapy in breast conserving treatment for early stage breast cancer. *Radiother Oncol* 1994;30:206.

349j. Solin LJ, Fowble BL, Schultz DJ, et al. The significance of the pathology margins of the tumor excision on the outcome of patients treated with definitive irradiation for early stage breast cancer. *Int J Radiat Oncol Biol Phys* 1991;21:279.

349k. Zafrani B, Vielh P, Fourquet A, et al. Conservative treatment of early breast cancer: prognostic value of ductal in situ component and other pathologic variables on local control and survival: long-term results. *Eur J Cancer Clin Oncol* 1989;25:1645.

350. Orr RK. The impact of prophylactic axillary node dissection on breast cancer survival—a bayesian meta-analysis. *Ann Surg Oncol* 1999;6: 109.

351. Davies GC, Millis RR, Hayward JL. Assessment of the axillary lymph node status. *Ann Surg* 1990;192:148.

352. Bruneton JN, Caramella E, Hery M, et al. Axillary lymph node metastases in breast cancer. *Radiology* 1986;158:325.

353. Fourquet A, Zafrani B, Campana F, et al. Breast-conserving treatment of ductal carcinoma in situ. *Semin Radiat Oncol* 1992;2:116–124.

354. Carter C, Allen C, Henson D. Relation of tumor size, lymph node status, and survival in 24,740 breast cancer cases. *Cancer* 1989;63: 181.

355. McGee JM, Youmans R, Clingan F, et al. The value of axillary dissection in T1a breast cancer. *Am J Surg* 1996;172:501.

356. Rush Port E, Tan LK, Borgen PI, VanZee KJ. Incidence of axillary lymph node metastases in T1a and T1b breast carcinoma. *Ann Surg Oncol* 1998;5:23.

357. Danforth DN, Findlay PA, McDonald HD, et al. Complete axillary lymph node dissection for stage I-II carcinoma of the breast. *J Clin Oncol* 1986;4:655.

358. Kissin MW, Thompson EM, Price AB, et al. The inadequacy of axillary sampling in breast cancer. *Lancet* 1982;1:1210.

359. Cabanes PA, Salmon RJ, Vilcoq JR, et al. Value of axillary dissection in addition to lumpectomy and radiotherapy in early breast cancer. *Lancet* 1992;339:1245.

360. Rosen PP, Lesser ML, Kinne DW. Discontinuous or "skip" metastases in breast carcinoma. *Ann Surg* 1983;197:276.

361. Boova RS, Bonanne R, Rosato FE. Patterns of axillary nodal involvement in breast cancer. *Ann Surg* 1982;196:642.

362. Dewar J, Sarrazin D, Benhamou E, et al. Management of axilla in conservatively treated breast cancer. *Int J Radiat Oncol Biol Phys* 1987;13:475.

363. Fisher B, Redmond C, Fisher ER, et al. Ten year results of a randomized clinical trial comparing radical mastectomy and total mastectomy with or without radiation. *N Engl J Med* 1985;312:674.

364. Fisher B, Montague E. Comparison of radical mastectomy with alternative treatments for primary breast cancer. *Cancer* 1977;39:2829.

365. Langlands AO, Prescott RJ, Hamilton T. A clinical trial in the management of operable breast cancer. *Br J Surg* 1980;67:170.

366. Ivens D, Hoe AL, Podd TJ, et al. Assessment of morbidity from complete axillary dissection. *Br J Cancer* 1992;66:136.

367. Lin PP, Allison DC, Wainstock J, et al. Impact of axillary lymph node dissection on the therapy of breast cancer patients. *J Clin Oncol* 1993; 11:1536.

368. Werner RS, McCormick B, Petrek J, et al. Arm edema in conservatively managed breast cancer: obesity is a major predictive factor. *Radiology* 1991;180:177.

369. Morton DL, Wen DR, Wong JH, et al. Technical details of intraoperative lymphatic mapping for early stage melanoma. *Arch Surg* 1992; 127:392.

370. Giuliano AE, Kirgan DM, Guenther JM, et al. Lymphatic mapping and sentinel lymphadenectomy for breast cancer. *Ann Surg* 1994;220: 391.

371. Krag DN, Weaver DL, Alex JC, et al. Surgical resection and radiolocalization of the sentinel lymph node in breast cancer using a gamma probe. *Surg Oncol* 1993;2:335.

372. Albertini JJ, Lyman GH, Cox C, et al. Lymphatic mapping and sentinel node biopsy in the patient with breast cancer. *JAMA* 1996;276:1818.

373. Borgstein PJ, Meijer S, Pijpers R. Intradermal blue dye to identify sentinel lymph nodes in breast cancer. *Lancet* 1997;349:1668.

374. Borgstein PJ, Pijpers R, Comans EF, et al. Sentinel lymph node biopsy in breast cancer: guidelines and pitfalls of lymphoscintigraphy and gamma probe detection. *J Am Coll Surg* 1998;186:275.

375. Flett MM, Going JJ, Stanton PD, et al. Sentinel node localization in patients with breast cancer. *Br J Surg* 1998;85:991.

376. Galimberti V, Zurrida S, Zucali P, et al. Can sentinel node biopsy avoid axillary dissection in clinically node-negative breast cancer patients? *Breast J* 1998;7:8.

377. Giuliano AE, Jones RC, Brennan M, et al. Sentinel lymphadenectomy in breast cancer. *J Clin Oncol* 1997;15:2345.

378. Guenther JM, Krishnamoorthy M, Tan LR. Sentinel lymphadenectomy for breast cancer in a community managed care setting. *Cancer J Sci Am* 1997;3:336.

379. Krag D, Weaver D, Ashikaga T, et al. The sentinel node in breast cancer—a multicenter validation study. *N Engl J Med* 1998;339:941.

380. Krag DN, Ashikaga T, Harlow SP, et al. Development of sentinel node targeting technique in breast cancer patients. *Breast J* 1998;4: 67.

381. Offodile R, Hoh C, Barsky SH, et al. Minimally invasive breast cancer staging using lymphatic mapping with radiolabeled dextran. *Cancer* 1998;82:1704.

382. O'Hea BJ, Hill ADK, El-Shirbiny A, et al. Sentinel lymph node biopsy in breast cancer: initial experience at Memorial Sloan-Kettering Cancer Center. *J Am Coll Surg* 1998;186:423.

383. Pijpers R, Hoekstra OS, Collet GJ, et al. Impact of lymphoscintigraphy on sentinel node identification with technetium-99m-colloidal albumin in breast cancer. *J Nucl Med* 1997;38:366.

384. Roumen RMH, Valkenburg JGM, Geuskens LM. Lymphoscintigraphy and feasibility of sentinel node biopsy in 83 patients with primary breast cancer. *Eur J Surg Oncol* 1997;23:495.

385. Cody HS III. Sentinel lymph node mapping in breast cancer. *Oncology* 1999;13:25.

386. Abati AD, Kimmel M, Rosen PP. Apocrine mammary carcinoma: a clinicopathologic study of 72 patients. *Am J Clin Pathol* 1990;94:371.

387. Abner AL, Recht A, Eberlein T, et al. Prognosis following salvage mastectomy for recurrence in the breast after conservative surgery and radiation therapy for early-stage breast cancer. *J Clin Oncol* 1993; 11:44.

388. Turner RR, Ollila DW, Krasne DL, et al. Histologic validation of the sentinel lymph node hypothesis for breast carcinoma. *Ann Surg* 1997; 226:271.

389. Baird RM, Worth A, Hislop G. Recurrence after lumpectomy for comedo-type intraductal carcinoma of the breast. *Am J Surg* 1990; 159:479.

390. Smart CR, Myers MH, Gloeckler MA. Implications from SEER data on breast cancer management. *Cancer* 1978;41:787.

391. Betsill WL Jr, Rosen PP, Lieberman PH, et al. Intraductal carcinoma: long-term follow-up after treatment of biopsy alone. *JAMA* 1978;239: 1863.

392. Farrow JH. The James Ewing Lecture: current concepts in the detection and treatment of the earliest of the early breast cancers. *Cancer* 1970;25:468.

393. Lagios MD, Westdahl PR, Margolin FR, et al. Duct carcinoma in situ: relationship of extent of noninvasive disease to frequency of occult invasion, multicentricity, lymph node metastases and short-term treatment failures. *Cancer* 1982;50:1309.

394. Lewis D, Geshickter CF. Comedo carcinoma of the breast. *Arch Surg* 1938:36:225.

395. Millis RR, Thynne GSJ. In-situ intraductal carcinoma of the breast: a long term follow-up study. *Br J Surg* 1975;62:957.

396. Page DL, Dupont WD, Rogers LW, Landenberger M. Intraductal carcinoma of the breast: follow-up after biopsy only. *Cancer* 1982; 49:751.

397. Arnesson L-G, Smeds S, Fagerberg G, et al. Follow-up of two treatment modalities for ductal cancer in situ of the breast. *Br J Surg* 1989: 77:672.

398. Ashikari R, Huvos J, Snyder RE. Prospective study of non-infiltrating carcinoma of the breast. *Cancer* 1977;39:435.

399. Brown PW, Silverman J, Owens E, et al. Intraductal "noninfiltrating" carcinoma of the breast. *Arch Surg* 1976;111:1063.

400. Carter D, Smith RRL. Carcinoma in situ of the breast. *Cancer* 1977; 40:1189.

401. Ciatto S, Bonardi R, Cardona G. Intraductal breast carcinoma: review of a multicenter series of 350 cases. *Tumori* 1990;76:552.

402. Cutuli B, Teissler E, Piat JM, et al. Radical surgery and conservative treatment of ductal carcinoma in situ of the breast. *Eur J Cancer* 1992; 28:649.

403. Fentiman IS, Fagg M, Millis RR, et al. In situ ductal carcinoma of the breast: implications of disease pattern and treatment. *Eur J Surg Oncol* 1986;12:261.

404. Fisher ER, Sass R, Fisher B, et al. Pathologic findings from the National Surgical Adjuvant Breast Project (Protocol 6). I. Intraductal carcinoma (DCIS). *Cancer* 1986;57:197.

405. Howard PW, Locker AP, Dowle CS, et al. In situ carcinoma of the breast. *Eur J Surg Oncol* 1989;15:328.

406. Kinne DW, Petrek JA, Osborne MP, et al. Breast carcinoma in situ. *Arch Surg* 1989; 124:33.

407. Ozzello L. Intraepithelial carcinomas of the breast. In: Hollman KH, Verley JM, eds. *New frontiers in mammary pathology.* Vol 2. New York: Plenum Press, 1983:147.

408. Petit JY, Vilcoq JR, Contesso G, et al. Le traitement des cancers intracanalaires. In: Lansac J, Lefloch L, Bougnoux P, eds. *Depistage du cancer du sein et consequences therapeutiques.* Paris: Masson, 1989:115.

409. Price P, Sinnet HD, Gusterson B, et al. Duct carcinoma in situ: predictors of local recurrence and progression in patients treated by surgery alone. *Br J Cancer* 1990;61:869.

410. Rosner D, Bedwani RN, Vana J, et al. Noninvasive breast carcinoma: results of a national survey of the American College of Surgeons. *Ann Surg* 1980;192:139.

411. Schuh ME, Nemoto T, Penetrante RB, et al. Intraductal carcinoma: analysis of presentation, pathologic findings and outcome of disease. *Arch Surg* 1986;121:1303.

412. Silverstein MJ, Cohlan BF, Gierson ED, et al. Duct carcinoma in situ: 227 cases without microinvasion. *Eur J Cancer* 1992;28:630.

413. Simpson T, Thirlby RC, Dail DH. Surgical treatment of ductal carcinoma in situ of the breast. *Arch Surg* 1992;127:468.

414. Temple WJ, Jenkins M, Alexander F, et al. In situ breast cancer in Alberta 1951–1984. *Am J Clin Oncol* 1986;9:109(abst).

415. von Rueden DG, Wilson RE. Intraductal carcinoma of the breast. *Surg Gynecol Obstet* 1984;158:105.

416. Wulsin JH, Schreiber JT. Improved prognosis in certain patterns of carcinoma of the breast. *Arch Surg* 1962;85:111.

417. Holland R, Hendriks J, Verbeek A, et al. Extent, distribution, and mammographic/histological correlations of breast ductal carcinoma in situ. *Lancet* 1990;335:519.

418. Silverstein MJ, Gierson ED, Colburn WJ, et al. Can intraductal breast carcinoma be excised completely by local excision? *Cancer* 1994;73: 2985.

419. Lagios M, Page DL. Lagios experience. In: Silverstein MJ, Lagios MD, Poller DN, Recht A, eds. *Ductal carcinoma in situ of the breast.* Baltimore: Williams & Wilkins, 1997:361.

420. Solin LJ, Recht A, Fourquet A, et al. Ten-year results of breast-conserving surgery and definitive irradiation for intraductal carcinoma (ductal carcinoma in situ) of the breast. *Cancer* 1991;68:2337.

421. Solin LJ, Kurtz J, Fourquet A, et al. Fifteen-year results of breast-conserving surgery and definitive breast irradiation for the treatment of ductal carcinoma in situ of the breast. *J Clin Oncol* 1996;14:754.

422. Solin LJ, Fowble BL, Yen IT, et al. Microinvasive ductal carcinoma of the breast treated with breast-conserving surgery and definitive irradiation. *Int J Radiat Oncol Biol Phys* 1992;23:961.

423. Fisher B, Costantino J, Redmond C, et al. Lumpectomy compared with lumpectomy and radiation therapy for the treatment of intraductal breast cancer. *N Engl J Med* 1993;328:1581.

424. Fisher ER, Dignam J, Tan-Chiu E, et al. Pathologic findings from the National Surgical Adjuvant Breast Project (NSABP) eight-year update of Protocol B-17: intraductal carcinoma. *Cancer* 1999;86(3):429–438.

425. Julien JP, Bijker N, Fentiman IS, et al. Radiotherapy in breast-conserving treatment for ductal carcinoma in situ: first results of the EORTC randomized phase III trial 10853. *Lancet* 2000;355:528–533.

426. Bornstein BA, Peiro G, Connolly JL, et al. The influence of infiltrating lobular carcinoma on the outcome of patients treated with breast-conserving surgery and radiation therapy. *Int J Radiat Oncol Biol Phys* 1996;36:180(abst).

427. Haffty BG, Peschel RE, Papadopoulos D, et al. Radiation therapy for ductal carcinoma in situ of the breast. *Conn Med* 1990;54:483.

428. Kuske RR, Bean JM, Garcia D, et al. Breast conservation therapy for ductal carcinoma in situ. *Int J Radiat Oncol Biol Phys* 1993;26:391.

429. McCormick B, Rosen PP, Kinne D, et al. Duct carcinoma in situ of the breast: an analysis of local control after conservation surgery and radiotherapy. *Int J Radiat Oncol Biol Phys* 1991;21:289.

430. Ray GR, Adelson J, Hayhurst E, et al. Ductal carcinoma in situ of the breast: results of treatment by conservative surgery and definitive irradiation. *Int J Radiat Oncol Biol Phys* 1994;28:105.

431. Stotter AT, McNeese M, Oswald MJ, et al. The role of limited surgery with irradiation in primary treatment of ductal in situ breast cancer. *Int J Radiat Oncol Biol Phys* 1990;18:283.

432. White J, Levine A, Gustafson G, et al. Outcome and prognostic factors for local recurrence in mammographically detected ductal carcinoma in situ of the breast treated with conservative surgery and radiation therapy. *Int J Radiat Oncol Biol Phys* 1995;31:791.

433. Zafrani B, Fourquet A, Vilcoq JR, et al. Conservative management of intraductal breast carcinoma with tumorectomy and radiation therapy. *Int J Radiat Oncol Biol Phys* 1984;10:140(abst).

434. Silverstein MJ, Gierson ED, Waisman JR, et al. Axillary lymph node dissection for T1a breast carcinoma: is it indicated? *Cancer* 1994;73: 664.

435. Fisher B, Dignam J, Wolmark N, et al. Tamoxifen in treatment of intraductal breast cancer: NSABP B-24 randomised controlled trial. *Lancet* 1999;353:1993

436. Arriagada R, Le% MG, Rochard F, et al. Conservative treatment versus mastectomy in early breast cancer: patterns of failure with 15 years of follow-up data. *J Clin Oncol* 1996;14:1558.

437. Fourquet A, Campana F, Vielh P, et al. Paget's disease of the nipple without detectable breast tumor: conservative management with radiation therapy. *Int J Radiat Oncol Biol Phys* 1987;13:1463.

438. Maier WP, Rosemond GP, Harasym EL Jr, et al. Paget's disease in the female breast. *Surg Gynecol Obstet* 1969;128:1253.

439. Nance FC, DeLoach DH, Welsh RA, et al. Paget's disease of the breast. *Ann Surg* 1970;171:864.

440. Pierce L, McCormick B, Haffty B, et al. The use of radiotherapy in the conservative management of Paget's disease. *Int J Radiat Oncol Biol Phys* 1996;36:215(abst).

441. Campana F, Fourquet A, Ashby MA, et al. Presentation of axillary lymphadenopathy without detectable breast primary (T0N1b breast cancer): experience at Institut Curie. *Radiother Oncol* 1989;15:321.

441a. Baron PL, Moore MP, Kinne DW, et al. Occult breast cancer presenting with axillary metastases. *Arch Surg* 1990;125:210.

441b. Feuerman L, Attie JN, Rosenberg B. Carcinoma in axillary lymph nodes as an indicator of breast cancer. *Surg Gynecol Obstet* 1962; 114:5.

442. Merson M. Andreola S, Galimberti V, et al. Breast carcinoma presenting as axillary metastases without evidence of a primary tumor. *Cancer* 1992;70:504.

442a. Owen HW, Dockerty MB, Gray HK. Occult carcinoma of breast. *Surg Gynecol Obstet* 1954;98:302.

442b. Westbrook KC, Gallager HS. Breast carcinoma presenting as an axillary mass. *Am J Surg* 1971;122:607.

443. Smith BL, Bertagnolli M, Klein BB, et al. Evaluation of the contralateral breast: the role of biopsy at the time of primary breast cancer. *Ann Surg* 1992;216:17.

444. Wheeler JE, Enterline HT, Roseman JM, et al. Lobular carcinoma in situ of the breast: long-term follow-up. *Cancer* 1974;34:554.

445. Graham MD, Lakhani S, Gazet JC. Breast conserving surgery in the management of in situ breast carcinoma. *Eur J Surg Oncol* 1991;17:258.

446. Osborne MP, Hoda SA. Current management of lobular carcinoma in situ of the breast. *Oncology* 1994;8:45.

447. Walt AJ, Simon M, Swanson GM. The continuing dilemma of lobular carcinoma in situ. *Arch Surg* 1992;127:904.

448. Lee JSY, Grant CS, Donohue JH, et al. Arguments against routine contralateral mastectomy or undirected biopsy for invasive lobular breast cancer. *Surgery* 1995;118:640.

449. Haagensen CD, Lane N, Lattes R, et al. Lobular neoplasia (so-called lobular carcinoma in situ) of the breast. *Cancer* 1978;42:737.

450. Rosen PP, Kosloff C, Lieberman PH, et al. Lobular carcinoma in situ of the breast: detailed analysis of 99 patients with average follow-up of 24 years. *Am J Surg Pathol* 1978;2:225.

451. Page DL, Kidd TE Jr, Dupont WD, et al. Lobular neoplasia of the breast: higher risk for subsequent invasive cancer predicted by more extensive disease. *Hum Pathol* 1991;22:1232.

452. Bradley SJ, Weaver DW, Bouwman DL. Alternatives in the surgical management of in-situ breast cancer: a meta-analysis of outcome. *Am Surg* 1990;56:428.

453. Ringberg A, Andersson I, Aspergren K, et al. Breast carcinoma in situ in 167 women: incidence, mode of presentation, therapy and follow- up. *Eur J Surg Oncol* 1991;17:466.

454. Singletary SE. Lobular carcinoma in situ of the breast: a 31-year experience at the University of Texas M.D. Anderson Cancer Center. *Breast Dis* 1994;8:157.

455. Bodian C, Haagensen CD. Bilateral carcinoma of the breast. In: Haagensen CD, ed. *Diseases of the breast.* 3rd ed. Philadelphia: WB Saunders, 1986;440.

456. Chaudary MA, Millis RR, Hoskins EOL, et al. Bilateral primary breast cancer: a prospective study of disease incidence. *Br J Surg* 1984;71:711.

457. Hislop TG, Elwood JM, Coldman AJ, et al. Second primary cancers of the breast: incidence and risk factors. *Br J Cancer* 1984;49:79.

458. Lewis TR, Casey J, Buerk CA, et al. Incidence of lobular carcinoma in bilateral breast cancer. *Am J Surg* 1982;144:635.

459. Chaudary MA, Millis RR, Bulbrook RD, et al. Family history and bilateral primary breast cancer. *Breast Cancer Res Treat* 1985;5:201.

460. Nielsen M, Christensen L, Andersen J. Contralateral cancerous breast lesions in women with clinical invasive breast cancer. *Cancer* 1986; 57:897.

461. Sears HF, Janus C, McDermott A, et al. Bilateral breast carcinoma: prospective evaluation of factors assisting diagnosis. *J Surg Oncol* 1986;32:203.

462. Horn PL, Thompson WD. Risk of contralateral breast cancer: associations with histologic, clinical, and therapeutic factors. *Cancer* 1988; 62:412.

463. Michowitz M, Noy S, Lazebnik N, et al. Bilateral breast cancer. *J Surg Oncol* 1985;30:109.

464. Solin LJ, Fowble BL, Schultz DJ, et al. Bilateral breast carcinoma treated with definitive irradiation. *Int J Radiat Oncol Biol Phys* 1989; 17:263.

465. Gustafsson A, Tartter PI, Brower ST, et al. Prognosis of patients with bilateral carcinoma of the breast. *J Am Coll Surg* 1994;178:111.

466. de la Rochefordière A, Asselain B, Scholl S, et al. Simultaneous bilateral breast carcinomas: a retrospective review of 149 cases. *Int J Radiat Oncol Biol Phys* 1994;30:35.

467. Reinfuss M, Mitus J, Duda K, et al. The treatment and prognosis of patients with phyllodes tumor of the breast: an analysis of 170 cases. *Cancer* 1996;77:910.

468. Scholl SM, Fourquet A, Asselain B, et al. Neoadjuvant versus adjuvant chemotherapy in premenopausal patients with tumors considered too large for breast conserving surgery: preliminary results of a randomised trial. *Eur J Cancer* 1994;30A:645.

469. Fisher B, Brown A, Mamounas E, et al. Effect of preoperative chemotherapy on local-regional disease in women with operable breast cancer: findings from National Surgical Adjuvant Breast and Bowel Project B-18. *J Clin Oncol* 1997;15:2483.

470. NSABP. The effect on primary tumor response of adding sequential Taxotere to Adriamycin and cyclophosphamide: preliminary results from NSABP Protocol B-27. *Breast Cancer Treat Rep,* 2001: Abstract # 5.

471. Ravdin P, Chamness G. The c-erbB-2 proto-oncogene as a prognostic and predictive marker in breast cancer: a paradigm for the development of other macromolecular markers—a review. *Gene* 1995;159: 19.

472. Buzdar AU, Marcus C, Smith TL, et al. Early and delayed clinical cardiotoxicity of doxorubicin. *Cancer* 1985;55:2761.

473. Hudis C, Norton L. Adjuvant drug therapy for operable breast cancer. *Semin Oncol* 1996;23:475.

474. Campora E, Pronzato P, Amoroso D, et al. Prognostic factors in node positive primary breast cancer patients treated with adjuvant CMF. *Anticancer Res* 1992;12:1555.

475. Clark G, Sledge G, Osborne C. Survival from first recurrence: relative importance of prognostic factors in 1,015 breast cancer patients. *J Clin Oncol* 1987;5:5.

476. Marcus J, Watson P, Page D, et al. Hereditary breast cancer: pathobiology, prognosis, and BRCA1 and BRCA2 gene linkage. *Cancer* 1996; 77:697.

477. Offit K. BRCA1: a new marker in the management of patients with breast cancer? *Cancer* 1996;77:599.

478. Thompson M, Jensen R, Obermiller P, et al. Decreased expression of BRCA1 accelerates growth and is often present during sporadic breast cancer progression. *Nat Genet* 1995;9:444.

479. Collins F. BRCA1—lots of mutations, lots of dilemmas. *N Engl J Med* 1996;334:186.

480. Ford D, Easton D, Peto J. Estimates of the gene frequency of BRCA1 and its contribution to breast and ovarian cancer incidence. *Am J Hum Genet* 1995;57:1457.

481. Porter D, Cohen B, Wallace M, et al. Breast cancer incidence, penetrance and survival in probable carriers of BRCA1 gene mutation in families linked to BRCA1 on chromosome 17q12–21. *Br J Surg* 1994; 81:1512.

482. Petrek J. Breast cancer during pregnancy. *Cancer* 1994;74:518.

483. Liberman L, Giess CS, Dershaw DD, et al. Imaging of pregnancy-associated breast cancer. *Radiology* 1994;191:245.

484. Kiricuta CI, Tausch J. A mathematical model of axillary lymph node involvement based on 1446 complete dissections in patients with breast carcinoma. *Cancer* 1992;69:2496.

485. Wilking N, Rutqvist L, Carstensen J, et al. Prognostic significance of axillary nodal status in primary breast cancer in relation to the number of resected nodes. Stockholm Breast Cancer Study Group. *Acta Oncol* 1992;31:29.

486. Rakowsky E, Klein B, Kahan E, et al. Prognostic factors in node-positive operable breast cancer patients receiving adjuvant chemotherapy. *Breast Cancer Res Treat* 1992;21:121.

487. Recht A, Houlihan M. Axillary lymph nodes and breast cancer: a review. *Cancer* 1995;76:1491.

488. Cote RJ, et al Role of immunohistochemical detection of lymph-node

metastases in management of breast cancer. *Lancet*, 1999;354: 896–900.

489. Hill A, Tran K, Akhurst T, et al. Lessons learned from 500 cases of lymphatic mapping for breast cancer. *Ann Surg* 1999;229:528.

490. Fisher ER, Redmond C, Fisher B, et al. Prognostic factors in NSABP studies of women with node-negative breast cancer. *J Natl Cancer Inst* 1992;11:151.

491. Ridolfi RL, Rosen PP, Port A, et al. Medullary carcinoma of breast. *Cancer* 1977;40:1365.

492. Fisher E, Kenny J, Sass R, et al. Medullary cancer of the breast revisited. *Breast Cancer Res Treat* 1990;16:215.

493. Hellman S. Natural history of small breast cancers. *J Clin Oncol* 1994; 12:2229.

494. Brooks S, Saunders D, Singhakowinta A, et al. Relation of tumor content of estrogen and progesterone receptors with response of patients to endocrine therapy. *Cancer* 1980;46:2775.

495. Manni A, Arafah B, Pearson O. Estrogen and progesterone receptors in the prediction of response of breast cancer to endocrine therapy. *Cancer* 1980;46:2838.

496. Neville AM, Bettelheim R, Gelber RD, et al. Factors predicting treatment responsiveness and prognosis in node-negative breast cancer. *J Clin Oncol* 1992;10:696.

497. Osborne C, Yochmowitz M, Knight W, et al. The value of estrogen and progesterone receptors in the treatment of breast cancer. *Cancer* 1980;46:2884.

498. Ravdin P, Green S, Dorr T, et al. Prognostic significance of progesterone receptor levels in estrogen receptor-positive patients with metastatic breast cancer treated with tamoxifen: results of a prospective Southwest Oncology Group study. *J Clin Oncol* 1992; 10:1284.

499. Clark G, McGuire W, Hubay C, et al. Progesterone receptors as a prognostic factor in stage II breast cancer. *N Engl J Med* 1983;309: 1343.

500. Clark GM, McGuire WL. Steroid receptors and other prognostic factors in primary breast cancer. *Semin Oncol* 1988;15:20.

501. Rose C, Thorpe SM, Andersen KW, et al. Beneficial effect of adjuvant tamoxifen in primary breast cancer patients with estrogen receptor values. *Lancet* 1985;1:16.

502. American Society of Clinical Oncology. 1997 update of recommendations for the use of tumor markers in breast and colorectal cancer. Adopted on November 7, 1997 by the American Society of Clinical Oncology. *J Clin Oncol* 1998;16:793.

503. Clark GM, Mathieu M, Owens MA, et al. Prognostic significance of S-phase fraction in good-risk, node negative breast cancer patients. *J Clin Oncol* 1992;10:428.

504. Gnant MFX, Blijham GH, Reiner A, et al. Aneuploidy fraction but not DNA index is important for the prognosis of patients with stage I and II breast cancer: 10 year results. *Ann Oncol* 1993;4:643.

505. Isola J, Visakorpi T, Holli K, et al. Association of overexpression of tumor suppressor protein p53 with rapid cell proliferation and poor prognosis in node-negative breast cancer patients. *J Natl Cancer Inst* 1992;84:1109.

506. Isola J, Weitz S, Visakorpi T, et al. Cathepsin D expression detected by immunohistochemistry has independent prognostic value in axillary node-negative breast cancer. *J Clin Oncol* 1993;11:36.

507. Tandon AK, Clark G, Chamness GC, et al. Cathepsin D and prognosis in breast cancer. *N Engl J Med* 1990;322:297.

508. Clahsen P, van de Velde C, Duval C, et al. p53 protein accumulation and response to adjuvant chemotherapy in premenopausal women with node-negative early breast cancer. *J Clin Oncol* 1998;16:470.

509. Degeorges A, de Roquancourt A, Extra J, et al. Is p53 a protein that predicts the response to chemotherapy in node negative breast cancer? *Breast Cancer Res Treat* 1998;47:47.

510. McGuire WL, Clark GM. Prognostic factors and treatment decisions in axillary node-negative breast cancer, *N Engl J Med* 1992;326:1756.

511. Ravdin PM, Clark GM, Hilsenbeck SA, et al. A personal computer-based program for providing outcome estimates and cooperative group trial eligibility information for adjuvant therapy. *Proc Am Soc Clin Oncol* 1995;14:96(abst).

512. Rosen PP, Lesser ML, Arroyo CD, et al. Immunohistochemical detection of Her2/neu in patients with axillary lymph node-negative breast carcinoma. A study of epidemiologic risk factors, histologic features, and prognosis. *Cancer* 1995;75:1320.

513. Slamon DJ, Godolphin W, Jones LA, et al. Studies of the HER-2/neu proto-oncogene in human breast and ovarian cancer. *Science* 1989; 244:707.

514. Lippman ME. The development of biological therapies for breast cancer. *Science* 1993;259:631.

515. Prost S, Le M, Douc-Rasy S, et al. Association of c-erbB2-gene amplification with poor prognosis in non-inflammatory breast carcinomas but not in carcinomas of the inflammatory type. *Int J Cancer* 1994; 58:763.

516. Tanner B, Friedberg T, Mitze M, et al. C-erbB-2-oncogene expression in breast carcinoma: analysis by S1 nuclease protection assay and immunohistochemistry in relation to clinical parameters. *Gynecol Oncol* 1992;47:228.

517. Baselga J, Tripathy D, Mendelsohn J, et al. Phase II study of weekly intravenous recombinant humanized anti-p185HER2 monoclonal antibody in patients with HER2/neu-overexpressing metastatic breast cancer. *J Clin Oncol* 1996;14:737.

518. Slamon DJ, Leyland-Jones B. Shak S, et al. Use of chemotherapy plus a monoclonal antibody against HER2 for metastatic breast cancer that overexpresses HER2. *N Engl J Med* 2001;344(11):783–792.

519. Allred DC, Clark GM, Tandon AK, et al. HER-2/neu in node-negative breast cancer: prognostic significance of overexpression influenced by the presence of in situ carcinoma. *J Clin Oncol* 1992;10:599.

520. Bianchi S, Paglierani M, Zampi G, et al. Prognostic significance of c-erbB-2 expression in node negative breast cancer. *Br J Cancer* 1993; 67:625.

521. Gusterson B, Gelber R, Goldhirsch A, et al. Prognostic importance of c-erbB-2 expression in breast cancer. International (Ludwig) Breast Cancer Study Group. *J Clin Oncol* 1992;10:1049.

522. Kallioniemi O, Holli K, Visakorpi T, et al. Association of c-erbB-2 protein over-expression with high rate of cell proliferation, increased risk of visceral metastasis and poor long-term survival in breast cancer. *Int J Cancer* 1991;49:650.

523. McCann A, Dervan P, O'Regan M, et al. Prognostic significance of c-erbB-2 and estrogen receptor status in human breast cancer. *Cancer Res* 1991;51:3296.

524. Press MF, Bernstein L, Thomas PA, et al. HER-2/neu gene amplification characterized by fluorescence in situ hybridization: poor prognosis in node-negative breast carcinomas. *J Clin Oncol* 1997;15:2894.

525. Baselga J, Seidman A, Rosen P, et al. HER2 overexpression and paclitaxel sensitivity in breast cancer: therapeutic implications. *Oncology* 1997;11:43.

526. Beatson GT. On the treatment of inoperable carcinoma of the mamma: suggestions for a new method of treatment, with illustrative cases. *Lancet* 1986;2:104.

527. Skipper HE. Kinetics of mammary tumor cell growth and implications for therapy. *Cancer* 1971;28:1479.

528. Paterson R, Russell M. Clinical trials in malignant disease. Part II. Breast cancer: value of irradiation of the ovaries. *J Faculty Radiologists* 1959:10:130.

529. Seidman A. Chemotherapy for advanced breast cancer: a current perspective. *Semin Oncol* 1996;23:55.

530. Buzdar A, Jones S, Vogel C, et al. A phase III trial comparing anastrozole (1 and 10 milligrams), a potent and selective aromatase inhibitor, with megestrol acetate in postmenopausal women with advanced breast carcinoma. Arimidex Study Group. *Cancer* 1996;79:730.

531. Ingle J, Green S, Ahmann D, et al. Randomized trial of tamoxifen alone or combined with aminoglutethimide and hydrocortisone in women with metastatic breast cancer. *J Clin Oncol* 1986;4:958.

532. Muss H, Case L, Atkins J, et al. Tamoxifen versus high-dose oral medroxyprogesterone acetate as initial endocrine therapy of patients with metastatic breast cancer: a Piedmont Association Study. *J Clin Oncol* 1994;12:1630.

533. Nemoto T, Patel J, Rosner D, et al. Tamoxifen (Nolvadex) versus adrenalectomy in metastatic breast cancer. *Cancer* 1984;53:1333.

534. Beahrs OH, Henson DE, Hutter RWP, et al, eds. *Manual for Staging of cancer,* 4th ed. Philadelphia: JB Lippincott Co, 1992.

535. Ingle J, Krook J, Green S, et al. Randomized trial of bilateral oophorectomy versus tamoxifen in premenopausal women with metastatic breast cancer. *J Clin Oncol* 1986;4:178.

536. Lees A, Giuffre C, Burns P, et al. Oophorectomy versus radiation ablation of ovarian function in patients with metastatic carcinoma of the breast. *Surg Gynecol Obstet* 1980;151:721.

537. Pritchard K, et al. Randomized trial of cyclophosphamide, methotrex-

ate, and fluorouracil chemotherapy added to tamoxifen as adjuvant therapy in postmenopausal women with node-positive estrogen and/or progesterone receptor-positive breast cancer: a report of the National Cancer Institute of Canada Clinical Trials Group. Breast Cancer Site Group. *J Clin Oncol* 1997;15(6):2302–2311.

538. Sunderland MC, Osborne CK. Tamoxifen in premenopausal patients with metastatic breast cancer: a review. *J Clin Oncol* 1991;9:1283.

539. Dombernowsky P, Gehl J, Boesgaard M, et al. Treatment of metastatic breast cancer with paclitaxel and doxorubicin. *Semin Oncol* 1995;22:13.

540. Gianni L, Munzone E, Capri G, et al. Paclitaxel by 3-hour infusion in combination with bolus doxorubicin in women with untreated metastatic breast cancer: high antitumor efficacy and cardiac effects in a dose finding and sequence-finding study. *J Clin Oncol* 1995;13:2688.

541. Sledge GW, Neuberg D, Bernardo P, et al. Phase III trial of doxorubicin, paclitaxel, and the combination of doxorubicin and paclitaxel as front-line chemotherapy for metastatic breast cancer: an intergroup trial (E1193). *J Clin Oncol* 2003;21(4):588–592.

542. Henderson IC, Berry DA, Demetri GD, et al. Improved outcomes from adding sequential paclitaxel but not from escalating doxorubicin dose in an adjuvant chemotherapy regimen for patients with node-positive primary breast cancer. *J Clin Oncol* 2003;21:976–983.

543. Mamounas E, Brown A, Smith R, et al. Effect of Taxol duration of infusion in advanced breast cancer (abc): results from NSABP B-26 trial comparing 3- to 24-hr infusion of high-dose Taxol. *Proc Am Soc Clin Oncol* 1998;17:389(abst).

544. Winer E, Berry D, Duggan D, et al. Failure of higher dose paclitaxel to improve outcome in patients with metastatic breast cancer—results from CALGB 9342. *Proc Am Soc Clin Oncol* 1998;17:388(abst).

545. Nabholtz J, Thuerlimann B, Beswoda W, et al. Taxotere (t) improves survival over mitomycin c and vinblastine (mv) in patients (pts) with metastatic breast cancer (mbc) who have failed an anthracycline (ant) containing regimen: final results of a phase III randomized trial. *Proc Am Soc Clin Oncol* 1998;18:390(abst).

546. Joensuu H, Holli K, Heikkinen M, et al. Combination chemotherapy versus single-agent therapy as first- and second-line treatment in metastatic breast cancer: a prospective randomized trial. *J Clin Oncol* 1998;16:3720.

547. Frei I, E, Canellos G. Dose: a critical factor in cancer chemotherapy. *Am J Med* 1980;69:585.

548. Henderson IC, Hayes DF, Gelman R. Dose-response in the treatment of breast cancer: a critical review. *J Clin Oncol* 1988;6:1501.

549. Skipper HE. Laboratory models: the historical perspective. *Cancer Treat Rep* 1986;70:3.

550. Brockstein B, Ross A, Moss T, et al. Tumor cell contamination of bone marrow harvest products: clinical consequences in a cohort of advanced-stage breast cancer patients undergoing high-dose chemotherapy. *J Hematother* 1996;5:617.

551. Franklin W, Pflaumer S, Jones R, et al. The addition of stem cell factor (SCF) to filgrastim (r-metHuG-CSF) for mobilization of PBPC does not enhance mobilization of tumor cells into the peripheral blood of breast cancer patients. *Proc Am Soc Clin Oncol* 1997;16:A417(abst).

552. Franklin W, Shpall E, Archer P, et al. Immunocytochemical detection of breast cancer cells in marrow and peripheral blood of patients undergoing high dose chemotherapy with autologous stem cell support. *Breast Cancer Res Treat* 1996;41:1.

553. Weisdorf D, Miller J, Verfaillie C, et al. Cytokine-primed bone marrow stem cells vs. peripheral blood stem cells for autologous transplantation: a randomized comparison of GM-CSF vs. G-CSF. *Biol Blood Marrow Trans* 1997;3:217.

554. Bezwoda W. In vivo purging of peripheral stem cell products by high-dose CNVp: results from a randomized study comparing conventional dose chemotherapy (CNV) with double high-dose CNVp chemotherapy. *Proc Am Soc Clin Oncol* 1997;16:404(abst).

555. Redon H, Dupas M, Fasano J, et al. Intensive regional chemotherapy of certain cancers under protection of autologous bone marrow transfusion. *Presse Med* 1966;74:2619.

556. Stadtmauer, E, O'Neill A, Goldstein LJ, et al. Conventional dose chemotherapy compared to high-dose chemotherapy plus autologous hematopoietic stem-cell transplantation for metastatic breast cancer. Philadelphia Bone Marrow Transplant Group. *N Engl J Med* 2000;13:342(15):1069–1076.

557. Cobleigh M, Vogel C, Tripathy D, et al. Efficacy and safety of Herceptin™ (humanized anti-HER2 antibody) as a single agent in 222 women with HER2 overexpression who relapsed following chemotherapy for metastatic breast cancer. *Proc Am Soc Clin Oncol* 1998;17:376(abst).

558. Baselga J, Norton L, Albanell J, et al. Recombinant humanized anti-HER2 antibody (Herceptin™) enhances the antitumor activity of paclitaxel and doxorubicin against HER2/neu overexpressing human breast cancer xenografts. *Cancer Res* 1998;58:2825.

559. Baselga J, Norton L, Masui H, et al. Antitumor effects of doxorubicin in combination with anti-epidermal growth factor receptor monoclonal antibodies. *J Natl Cancer Inst* 1993;85:1327.

560. Hudis C, Seidman A, Paton V, et al. Characterization of cardiac dysfunction observed in the Herceptin™ (trastuzumab) clinical trials. *Breast Cancer Res Treat* 119:50:232.

561. Hortobagyi G, Theriault R, Porter L, et al. Efficacy of pamidronate in reducing skeletal complications in patients with breast cancer and lytic bone metastases. *N Engl J Med* 1996;335:1785.

562. Paterson A, McCloskey E, Ashley S, et al. Reduction of skeletal morbidity and prevention of bone metastases with oral clodronate in women with recurrent breast cancer in the absence of skeletal metastases (abst).

563. Early Breast Cancer Trialists' Collaborative Group. Ovarian ablation in early breast cancer: overview of the randomised trials. *Lancet* 1996;348:1189.

564. Early Breast Cancer Trialists' Collaborative Group. Tamoxifen for early breast cancer: an overview of the randomised trials. *Lancet* 1998;351:1451.

565. Fisher B, Dignam J, Bryant J, et al. The worth of five versus more than five years of tamoxifen therapy for breast cancer patients with negative lymph nodes and estrogen receptor-positive tumors. *J Natl Cancer Inst* 1996;88:1529.

566. Stewart HJ. The Scottish trial of adjuvant tamoxifen in node-negative breast cancer. *J Natl Cancer Inst Monogr* 1992;11:117.

567. Tormey D, Gray R, Falkson H, et al. Postchemotherapy adjuvant tamoxifen beyond five years in patients with lymph node-positive breast cancer. *J Natl Cancer Inst* 1996;88:1828.

568. Mamounas E, Bryant J, Fisher B, et al. Primary breast cancer (PBC) as a risk factor for subsequent contralateral breast cancer (CBC): NSABP experience from nine randomized adjuvant trials [Abstract 15]. 21st Annual San Antonio Breast Cancer Symposium, San Antonio, Texas, 1998.

569. Early Breast Cancer Trialists' Collaborative Group. Systemic treatment of early breast cancer by hormonal, cytotoxic, or immune therapy: 133 randomized clinical trials involving 31,000 recurrences and 24,000 deaths among 75,000 women. *Lancet* 1992;339:1,71.

570. Jordan V, Morrow M. Should clinicians be concerned about the carcinogenic potential of tamoxifen? *Eur J Cancer* 1994;30A:1714.

571. Powles T, Hickish T, Kanis J, et al. Tamoxifen preserves bone mineral density in postmenopausal women but causes loss of bone density in premenopausal women. *Proc Am Soc Clin Oncol* 1995;14:165(abst).

572. Pritchard K, Paterson AH, Paul NA, et al. Increased thromboembolic complications with concurrent tamoxifen and chemotherapy in a randomized trial of adjuvant therapy for women with breast cancer. *J Clin Oncol* 1996;14(10): 2731–2737. A recent SWOG study failed to demonstrate any advantage when tamoxifen was given concurrently with CAF as opposed to afterwards.

573. Pritchard KI, Thomson D, Myers RE, et al. Tamoxifen therapy in premenopausal patients with metastatic breast cancer. *Cancer Treat Rep* 1980;64:787.

574. Hard G, Iatropoulos M, Jordan K, et al. Major difference in the hepatocarcinogenicity and DNA adduct forming between toremifene and tamoxifen in female Crl:CD(BR) rats. *Cancer Res* 1993;53:4534.

575. Jordan V, Glusman J, Eckert S, et al. Incident primary breast cancers are reduced by raloxifene: integrated data from multicenter, double-blind, randomized trials in 12,000 postmenopausal women. *Proc Am Soc Clin Oncol* 1998;17:466(abst).

576. Jordan V. Designer estrogens. *Sci Am* 1998;279:60.

577. Dickler MN, Hudis CA: Aromatase inhibitors for treatment of breast cancer: from metastatic disease to prevention. *Prin Pract Oncol, Updates*, 2003;17(3):1–14.

578. The ATAC Group. Anastrozole alone or in combination with tamoxifen versus tamoxifen alone for adjuvant treatment of postmenopausal

women with early breast cancer: first results of the ATAC randomised trial. *Lancet* 2002;359:2131–2139.

579. Winer EP, Hudis C, Burstein HJ, et al. American Society of Clinical Oncology Technology Assessment Working Group update: use of aromatase inhibitors in the adjuvant setting. *J Clin Oncol* 2003;21:2597–2599.

580. Goss, PE, Ingle JN, Martino S, et al., A randomized trial of letrozole in postmenopausal women after five years of tamoxifen therapy for early-stage breast cancer. *N Engl J Med* 2003;349:1793–1802.

581. Early Breast Cancer Trialists' Collaborative Group. Polychemotherapy for early breast cancer: an overview of the randomised trials. *Lancet* 1998;352:930.

582. Tancini G, Bonadonna G, Valagussa P, et al. Adjuvant CMF in breast cancer: comparative 5-year results of 12 versus 6 cycles. *J Clin Oncol* 1983;1:2.

583. Albain K, Green S, Osborne K, et al. Tamoxifen versus cyclophosphamide, Adriamycin, and 5-FU plus either concurrent or sequential tamoxifen in postmenopausal, receptor (+) node (+) breast cancer: a Southwest Oncology Group phase III intergroup trial (SWOG-8814, INT-0100). *Proc Am Soc Clin Oncol* 1997;16:128a(abst).

584. Fisher B, Dignam J, DeCillis A, et al. The worth of chemotherapy and tamoxifen over tamoxifen alone in node-negative patients with estrogen-receptor positive invasive breast cancer: first results from the NSABP B-20. *Proc Am Soc Clin Oncol* 1997;16:1a(abst).

585. Engelsman E, Rubens RD, Klijn JGM, et al. Comparison of classical CMF with a three-weekly intravenous schedule in postmenopausal patients with advanced breast cancer: an EORTC study (Trial 10808). *Proc 4th Breast Cancer Working Conference*:1–5, 1987.

586. Hutchins L, Green S, Ravdin P, et al. CMF versus CAF with and without tamoxifen in high-risk node-negative breast cancer patients and a natural history follow-up study in low-risk node-negative patients: first results of intergroup trial Int 0102. *Proc Am Soc Clin Oncol* 1998;17:2(abst).

587. Fisher B, Redmond C, Wickerham DL, et al. Doxorubicin-containing regimens for the treatment of stage II breast cancer: the National Surgical Adjuvant Breast and Bowel Project experience. *J Clin Oncol* 1989;7:572.

588. Minow R, Benjamin R, Gottlieb J. Adriamycin (NSC 123127) cardiomyopathy. An overview with determination of risk factors. *Cancer Chemother Rep* 1975;6:190.

589. Von Hoff DD, Layard MW, Basa P, et al. Risk factors for doxorubicin-induced congestive heart failure. *Ann Intern Med* 1979;91:710.

590. Fisher B, Anderson S, Wickerham D, et al. Increased intensification and total dose of cyclophosphamide in a doxorubicin-cyclophosphamide regimen for the treatment of primary breast cancer: findings from National Surgical Adjuvant Breast and Bowel Project B-22. *J Clin Oncol* 1997;15:1858.

591. DeCillis A, Anderson S, Bryant J, et al. Acute myeloid leukemia (AML) and myelodysplastic syndrome (MDS) on NSABP B-25: an update. *Proc Am Soc Clin Oncol* 1997;16:130a(abst).

592. Skipper H, Schabel FJ, Wilcox W: Experimental evaluation of potential anticancer agents XIII: on the criteria and kinetics associated with ''curability'' of experimental leukemia. *Cancer Chemother Rep* 1964;35:1.

593. Bonadonna G, Zambette M, Valagussa P. Sequential or alternating doxorubicin and CMF regimens in breast cancer with more than three positive nodes. *JAMA* 1995;273:542.

594. Hudis C, Fornier M, Riccio L, et al. Five-year results of dose-intensive sequential adjuvant chemotherapy for women with high risk node-positive breast cancer: a phase II study. *J Clin Oncol* 1999;17:118.

595. Haskell, C, et al. Phase III comparison of adjuvant high-dose doxorubicin plus cyclophosphamide (AC) versus sequential doxorubicin followed by cyclophosphamide (A->C) in breast cancer patients with 0–3 positive nodes (intergroup 0137). *Proc Am Soc Clin Oncol* 2002;21:(abst 142).

596. D'Andrea G, Seidman A. Docetaxel and paclitaxel in breast cancer therapy: present status and future prospects. *Semin Oncol* 1997; 24:13–27.

597. Seidman A, Hudis C, Albanel J, et al. Dose-dense therapy with weekly 1-hour paclitaxel infusions in the treatment of metastatic breast cancer. *J Clin Oncol* 1998;16:3353.

598. Hudis C, Seidman A, Baselga J, et al. Sequential dose-dense doxoru-

bicin, paclitaxel, and cyclophosphamide for resectable high-risk breast cancer: feasibility and efficacy. *J Clin Oncol* 1999;17:93.

599. Henderson, IC, Berry DA, Demetri GD, et al. Improved outcomes from adding sequential paclitaxel but not from escalating doxorubicin dose in an adjuvant chemotherapy regimen for patients with node-positive primary breast cancer. *J Clin Oncol* 2003;21:976–983.

600. Demetri G, Berry D, Norton L, et al. Clinical outcomes of node-positive breast cancer patients treated with dose-intensified Adriamycin/cyclophosphamide followed by Taxol as adjuvant systemic chemotherapy (CALGB 9141). *Proc Am Soc Clin Oncol* 1997;16:143(abst).

601. Mamounas ED, Bryant J, Lembersky C, et al. Paclitaxel (T) following doxorubicin/cyclophosphamide (AC) as adjuvant chemotherapy for node-positive breast cancer: Results from NSABP B-28. *Proc Am Soc Clin Onc* 2003;4(abst 12).

602. Nabholtz JM, Pienkowski T, Mackey J, et al. Phase III trial comparing TAC (docetaxel, doxorubicin, cyclophosphamide) with FAC (5-fluorouracil, doxorubicin, cyclophosphamide) in the adjuvant treatment of node positive breast cancer (BC) patients: interim analysis of the BCIRG 001 study. *Proc Am Soc Clin Oncol* 2002;(abst 141).

603. Citron, ML, et al, Randomized Trial of Dose-Dense Versus Conventionally Scheduled and Sequential Versus Concurrent Combination Chemotherapy as Postoperative Adjuvant Treatment of Node-Positive Primary Breast Cancer: First Report of Intergroup Trial C9741/Cancer and Leukemia Group B Trial 9741. *J Clin Oncol* 2003;9:81.

604. Recht A, Bartleink H, Fourquet A, et al. Postmastectomy radiotherapy: questions for the twenty-first century. *J Clin Oncol* 1998;16:2886.

605. Katz A, Strom EA, Buchholz TA, et al. The Influence of Pathologic Tumor Characteristics on Locoregional Recurrence Rates Following Mastectomy. *Int J Radiation Oncology Biol Phys* 2001;50(3):735–742.

606. Vicini FA, Remouchamps V, Wallace M, et al. Ongoing clinical experience utilizing 3D conformal external beam radiotherapy to deliver partial-breast irradiation in patients with early-stage breast cancer treated with breast-conserving therapy. *Int J Radiat Oncol Biol Phys* 2003;57:1247–1253.

607. Vicini FA, Chen P, Fraile M, et al. Low-dose rate brachytherapy as the sole radiation modality in the management of patients with early-stage breast cancer treated with breast-conserving therapy: preliminary results of a pilot trial. *Int J Radiat Oncol Biol Phys* 1997;38(2):301–310.

608. Krishnan L, Jewell WR, Tawfik OW, et al. Breast conservation therapy with tumor bed irradiation alone in a selected group of patients with stage I breast cancer. *T Breast J* 2001;7(2):91–95.

609. Wazer DE, Berle L, Graham R, et al. Preliminary results of a phase I/II study of HDR brachytherapy alone for T1/T2 breast cancer. *Int J Radiat Oncology Biol Phys* 2002;53(4):889–897.

610. Veronesi U, Orecchia R, Luini A, et al. A preliminary report of intra-operative radiotherapy (IORT) in limited-stage breast cancers that are conservatively treated. *Eur J Cancer* 2001;37:2178–2183.

611. Vicini F, Arthur D, Polgar C, Kuske R. Defining the efficacy of accelerated partial breast irradiation: the importance of proper patient selection, optimal quality assurance, and common sense. *Int J Radiat Oncol Biol Phys* 2003;57:1210–1213.

612. Veronesi U, Orecchia R, Luini A, et al. A preliminary report of intra-operative radiotherapy (IORT) in limited-stage breast cancers that are conservatively treated. *Eur J Cancer* 2001;37:2178–2183.

613. Solin LJ, Danoff BF, Schwartz GF. A practical technique for the localization of the tumor volume in definitive irradiation of the breast. *Int J Radiat Oncol Biol Phys* 1985;11:1215.

614. Moody AM, Mayles WPM, Bliss JM, et al. The influence of breast size on late radiation effects and association with radiotherapy dose inhomogeneity. *Radiother Oncol* 1994;33:106.

615. Fourquet A, Campana F, Rosenwald J, et al. Breast irradiation in the lateral decubitus position technique of the Institut Curie. *Radiother Oncol* 1991;22:261.

616. Merchant TE, McCormick B. Prone position breast irradiation. *Int J Radiat Oncol Biol Phys* 1994;30:187.

617. Bartelink H, Horoit J, Poortmans P, et al. Recurrence rates after treatment of breast cancer with standard radiotherapy with or without addtional radiation. *New Engl J Med* 2001;345:1378–1387.

618. Fraass BA, Roberson PL, Lichter AS. Dose to the contralateral breast

due to primary breast irradiation. *Int J Radiat Oncol Biol Phys* 1985; 11:485.

619. Mueller-Runkel R, Kalokhe UP. Scatter dose from tangential breast irradiation to the uninvolved breast. *Radiology* 1990;175:873.

620. Chui CS, Hong L, Hunt M, McCormick B. A simplified intensity modulated radiation therapy technique for the breast. *Med Phys.* 2002; 29(4):522–529.

621. Broët P, de la Rochefordière A, Scholl SM, et al. Contralateral breast cancer: annual incidence and risk parameters. *J Clin Oncol* 1995;13: 1578.

622. Sarrazin D, Le MG, Arriagada R, et al. Ten-year results of a randomized trial comparing a conservative treatment to mastectomy in early breast cancer. *Radiother Oncol* 1989;14:177.

623. Veronesi U, Banfi A, Del Vecchio M, et al. Comparison of Halsted mastectomy with quadrantectomy, axillary dissection and radiotherapy in early breast cancer: long-term results. *Eur J Cancer Clin Oncol* 1986;22:1085.

624. Halverson KJ, Taylor ME, Perez CA, et al. Regional nodal management and patterns of failure following conservative surgery and radiation therapy for stage I and II breast cancer. *Int J Radiat Oncol Biol Phys* 1993;26:593.

625. Hunt MA, Shank B, McCormick B, et al. The use of lymphoscintigraphy in treatment planning of primary breast cancer. *Int J Radiat Oncol Biol Phys* 1989;17:597.

626. Bruce J, Carter DC, Fraser J. Patterns of recurrent disease in breast cancer. *Lancet* 1970;1:433.

627. Fineberg S, Rosen PP. Cutaneous angiosarcoma and atypical vascular lesions of the skin and breast after radiation therapy for breast carcinoma. *Am J Clin Pathol* 1994;102:757.

628. Kerlikowske K, Grady D, Rubin SM, et al. Efficacy of screening mammography. *JAMA* 1995;273:149–154.

629. Magriples U, Naftolin F, Schwartz PE, et al. High-grade endometrial carcinoma in tamoxifen-treated breast cancer patients. *J Clin Oncol* 1993;11:485.

630. Wickerham DL, Fisher B, Wolmark N, et al. Association of tamoxifen and uterine sarcoma. *J Clin Oncol* 2002;20(11):2758–2760.

631. Barakat, RR. The effect of tamoxifen on the endometrium. *Oncology* 1995;9:129.

632. Burke W, Daly M, Garber J, et al. Recommendations for follow-up of individuals with an inherited predisposition for cancer II. BRCA 1 and BRCA 2. Cancer Genetics Studies Consortium. *JAMA* 1997; 277:977–1003.

633. Piver MS, Jishi MF, Tsukada Y, Nava G. Primary peritoneal carcinoma after prophylactic oophorectomy in women with a family history of ovarian cancer. A report of the Gilda Radner Family Ovarian Cancer Registry. *Cancer* 1993;71:2751–2755.

634. Struewing JP, Watson P, Easton DF, et al. Prophylactic oophorectomy in inherited breast/ovarian cancer families. *J Natl Cancer Monogr* 1995;17:33–35.

635. Rebbeck TR, Levin AM, Eisen A, et al. Breast cancer risk after bilateral prophylactic oophorectomy in *BRCA1* mutation carriers. *J Natl Cancer Inst* 1999;91(17):1475–1479.

636. Rebbeck TR, Lynch HT, Neuhausen SL, et al. Prophylactic oophorectomy in carriers of *BRCA1* or *BRCA2* mutations. *N Engl J Med* 2002; 346(21):1616–1622.

637. Kauff NH, Satagopan JM, Robsin ME, et al. Risk-reducing salpingo-oophorectomy in women with a *BRCA1* or *BRCA2* mutation. *N Engl J Med* 2002;346(21):1609–1615.

638. Mansi JL, Earl HM, Powles TJ, et al. Tests for detecting recurrent disease in the follow-up of patients with breast cancer. *Breast Cancer Res Treat* 1988;11:249.

639. Hannisdal E, Gundersen S, Kvaloy S, et al. Follow-up of breast cancer patients stage I-II: a baseline strategy. *Eur J Cancer* 1993;29A:992.

640. Hayes DF, Kaplan WD. Evaluation of patients following primary therapy. In: Harris JR, Hellman S, Henderson IC, Kinne DW, eds. *Breast diseases.* 2nd ed. Philadelphia: JB Lippincott Co, 1991: 505–521.

641. Scanlon EF, Oviedo MA, Cunningham MP, et al. Preoperative and follow-up procedures on patients with breast cancer. *Cancer* 1980; 46:977.

642. Hayes DF, Zurawski VR, Kufe DW. Comparison of circulating CA15–3 and carinoembryonic antigen levels in patients with breast cancer. *J Clin Oncol* 1986;4:1542.

643. Ojeda MB, Alonso MC, Bastus R, et al. Follow-up of breast cancer stages I and II. An analysis of some common methods. *Eur J Cancer Clin Oncol* 1987;23:419.

644. Logager VB, Vestergaard A, Herrstedt J, et al. The limited value of routine chest x-ray in the follow-up of stage II breast cancer. *Eur J Cancer* 1990;26:553.

645. Feig SA. The role of new imaging modalities in staging and follow-up of breast cancer. *Semin Oncol* 1986;13:402.

646. Loprinzi CL. It is now the age to define the appropriate follow-up of primary breast cancer patients. *J Clin Oncol* 1994;12:881.

647. Wickerham L, Fisher B, Cronin W, et al. The efficacy of bone scanning in the follow-up of patients with operable breast cancer. *Breast Cancer Res Treat* 1984;4:303.

648. Schapira DV, Urban N. A minimalist policy for breast cancer surveillance. *JAMA* 1991;265:380.

649. Rosselli Del Turco MR, Palli D, Cariddi A, et al. Intensive diagnostic follow-up after treatment of primary breast cancer. *JAMA* 1994;271: 1593.

650. GIVIO Investigators. Impact of follow-up testing on survival and health-related quality of life in breast cancer patients. A multicenter randomized controlled trial. The GIVIO Investigators. *JAMA* 1994; 271:1587.

651. Cummings S, Norton L, Eckert S, et al. Raloxifene reduces the risk of breast cancer and may decrease the risk of endometrial cancer in post-menopausal women. Two-year findings from the multiple outcomes of raloxifene evaluation (MORE) trial. *Proc Am Soc Clin Oncol* 1998;17:3(abst).

652. Hartmann LC, Schaid DJ, Woods JE, et al. Efficacy of bilateral prophylactic mastectomy in women with a family history of breast cancer [see comments]. *N Engl J Med* 1999;340:77–84.

653. Hartmann LC, Sellers TA, Schaid DJ, et al. Efficacy of bilateral prophylactic mastectomy in BRCA1 and BRCA2 gene mutation carriers. *J Natl Cancer Inst* 2001;93:1633–1637.

654. Meijers-Heijboer H, van Geel B, van Putten WL, et al. Breast cancer after prophylactic bilateral mastectomy in women with a BRCA1 or BRCA2 mutation. *N Engl J Med* 2001;345:159–164.

655. McDonnell SK, Schaid DJ, Myers JL, et al. Efficacy of contralateral prophylactic mastectomy in women with a personal and family history of breast cancer. *J Clin Oncol* 2001;19:3938–3943.

656. Peralta EA, Ellenhorn JD, Wagman LD, et al. Contralateral prophylactic mastectomy improves the outcome of selected patients undergoing mastectomy for breast cancer. *Am J Surg* 2000;180:439–445.

657. Dershaw DD. Mammography in patients with breast cancer treated by breast conservation (lumpectomy with or without radiation). *AJR Am J Roentgenol* 1995;164:309.

658. Braw M, Erlandsson I, Ewers SB, et al. Mammographic follow-up after breast conserving surgery and postoperative radiotherapy without boost irradiation for mammary carcinoma. *Acta Radiol* 1991;32: 398.

659. Kuni CC, Weisensee AM, Lee CK. Mammographic changes following conservation surgery and radiation therapy for breast cancer. *Breast Dis* 1992;5:169.

660. Mendelson EB. Evaluation of the postoperative breast [Review]. *Radiol Clin North Am* 1992;30:107.

661. Pritchard KI, Sawka CA. Menopausal estrogen replacement therapy in women with breast cancer. *Cancer* 1995;75:1.

662. Newcomb PA, Longnecker MP, Storer BE, et al. Long-term hormone replacement therapy and risk of breast cancer in postmenopausal women. *Am J Epidemiol* 1995;142:788.

663. Coope J. Double-blind cross-over study of estrogen replacement therapy. In: Campbell S, ed. *Management of the menopause and the post-menopausal years.* Lancaster, England: MTP Press, 1976:159.

664. Daly E, Gray A, Barlow D, et al. Measuring the impact of menopausal symptoms in quality of life. *BMJ* 1993;307:836.

665. Henderson BE. The cancer question: an overview of recent epidemiologic and retrospective data. *Am J Obstet Gynecol* 1989;161:1859.

666. Voigt LF, Weiss NS, Chu J, et al. Progestagen supplementation of exogenous estrogens and risk of endometrial cancer. *Lancet* 1991; 338:274.

667. Rossouw JE, Anderson GL, Prentice RL, et al. Writing Group for the Women's Health Initiative Investigators. Risks and benefits of estrogen plus progestin in healthy postmenopausal women: principal

668. Senie RT, Rosen PP, Rhodes P, et al. Timing of breast cancer excision during the menstrual cycle influences duration of disease-free survival. *Ann Intern Med* 1991;115:337.

669. Saad Z, Bramwell V, Duff J, et al. Timing of surgery in relation to the menstrual cycle in premenopausal women with operable breast cancer. *Br J Surg* 1994;81:217.

670. Senie RT, Kinne DW. Menstrual timing of treatment for breast cancer. *J Natl Cancer Inst* 1994;16:85.

671. Donegan WL, Shah D. Prognosis of patients with breast cancer related to the timing of operation. *Arch Surg* 1993;128:309.

672. Lagios MD. Pathologic features related to local recurrence following lumpectomy and irradiation. *Semin Surg Oncol* 1992;8:122.

673. Recht A, Silen W, Schnitt SJ, et al. Time-course of local recurrence following conservative surgery and radiotherapy for early stage breast cancer. *Int J Radiat Oncol Biol Phys* 1988;15:255.

674. Kurtz JM, Amalric R, Delouche G, et al. The second ten years: long-term risks of breast conservation in early breast cancer. *Int J Radiat Oncol Biol Phys* 1987;13:1327.

675. Haffty BG, Carter D, Flynn SD, et al. Local recurrence versus new primary: clinical analysis of 82 breast relapses and potential applications for genetic fingerprinting. *Int J Radiat Oncol Biol Phys* 1993;27:575.

676. Fowble B, Solin LJ, Schultz DJ, et al. Frequency, sites of relapse, and outcome of regional node failures following conservative surgery and radiation for early breast cancer. *Int J Radiat Oncol Biol Phys* 1989;17:703.

677. Leung S, Otmezguine Y, Calitchi E, et al. Locoregional recurrences following radical external beam irradiation and interstitial implantation for operable breast cancer: a 23 year experience. *Radiother Oncol* 1986;5:1.

678. Pierquin B, Marin L. The past and future of conservative treatment of breast cancer. *Am J Clin Oncol* 1986;9:476.

679. Recht A, Pierce SM, Abner A, et al. Regional nodal failure after conservative surgery and radiotherapy for early-stage breast carcinoma. *J Clin Oncol* 1991;9:988.

680. Sarrazin D, Dewar JA, Arriagada R, et al. Conservative management of breast cancer. *Br J Surg* 1986;73:604.

681. Veronesi U, Zucali R, DelVecchio M. Conservative treatment of breast cancer with the QUART technique. *World J Surg* 1985;9:676.

682. Singletary SE, Taylor SH, Guinee VF. Occurrence and prognosis of contralateral carcinoma of the breast. *J Am Coll Surg* 1994;178:390.

683. Taylor ME, Perez CA, Halverson KJ, et al. Factors influencing cosmetic results after conservation therapy for breast cancer. *Int J Radiat Oncol Biol Phys* 1995;31:753.

684. Beadle GF, Come, S, Henerson C, et al. The effect of adjuvant chemotherapy on the cosmetic results after primary radiation treatment for early stage breast cancer. *Int J Radiat Oncol Biol Phys* 1984;10:2131.

685. Findlay P, Goodman R. Radiation therapy for treatment of intraductal carcinoma of the breast. *Am J Clin Oncol* 1983;6:281.

686. Hatschek T, Fagerberg G, Stal O, et al. Cytometric characterization and clinical course of breast cancer diagnosed in a population-based screening program. *Cancer* 1989;64:1074.

687. Ray GR, Fish VJ. Biopsy and definitive radiation therapy in stage I and II adenocarcinoma of the female breast: analysis of cosmesis and the role of electron beam supplementation. *Int J Radiat Oncol Biol Phys* 1983;9:813.

688. Edelman DA, Grant S, van Os WAA. Breast cancer risk among women using silicone gel breast implants. *Int J Fertil* 1995;40:274.

689. Kesler DA. The basis of the FDA's decision on breast implants. *N Engl J Med* 1992;326:1713.

690. Clark CP III, Peters GN, O'Brien KM. Cancer in the augmented breast. Diagnosis and prognosis. *Cancer* 1993;72:2170.

691. Evans GRD, Schusterman MA, Kroll SS, et al. Reconstruction and the radiated breast: is there a role for implants? *Plast Reconstr Surg* 1995;96:1111.

692. Handel N, Lewinsky B, Silverstein MJ, et al. Conservation therapy for breast cancer following augmentation mammoplasty. *Plast Reconstr Surg* 1991;87:873.

693. Guenther JM, Tokita KM, Giuliano AE. Breast-conserving surgery and radiation after augmentation mammoplasty. *Cancer* 1994;73:2613.

694. DiPaola RS, Orel SG, Fowble BL. Ipsilateral breast tumor recurrence following conservative surgery and radiation therapy. *Oncology* 1994:8:59.

695. Chu FC, Lin FJ, Kim JH, et al. Locally recurrent carcinoma of the breast. *Cancer* 1986;37:2677.

696. Kurtz JM, Amalric R, Brandone H, et al. Results of salvage surgery for mammary recurrence following breast-conserving therapy. *Ann Surg* 1988;207:347.

697. Calle R, Pilleron J, Schlienger P, et al. Conservative management of operable breast cancer: ten years' experience at the Foundation Curie. *Cancer* 1978;42:2045.

698. Fowble B, Solin LJ, Schultz DJ, et al. Breast recurrence following conservative surgery and radiation: patterns of failure, prognosis, and pathologic findings from the mastectomy specimens with implications for treatment. *Int J Radiat Oncol Biol Phys* 1990;19:833.

699. Osborne MP, Borgen PI, Wong GY, et al. Salvage mastectomy for local and regional recurrence after breast-conserving operation and radiation therapy. *Surg Gynecol Obstet* 1992;174:189.

700. Stotter A, Atkinson EN, Fairston BA, et al. Survival following local-regional recurrence after breast conservation therapy for cancer. *Ann Surg* 1990;212:166.

701. Barr LC,.Brunt AM, Goodman AG, et al. Uncontrolled local recurrence after treatment of breast cancer with breast conservation. *Cancer* 1989;64:1203.

702. Kaufman Z, Gunn W, Hartz AJ, et al. The pathophysiologic and roentgenologic effects of chest irradiation in breast carcinoma. *Int J Radiat Oncol Biol Phys* 1986;12:887.

703. Lingos TI, Recht A, Vinci F, et al. Radiation pneumonitis in breast cancer patients treated with conservative surgery and radiation therapy. *Int J Radiat Oncol Biol Phys* 1991;21:355.

704. Rothwell RI, Kelly SA, Joslin CAF. Radiation pneumonitis in patients treated for breast cancer. *Radiother Oncol* 1985;4:9.

705. Rotstein S, Lax I, Svane G. Influence of radiation therapy on the lung-tissue in breast cancer patients: CT-assessed density changes and associated symptoms. *Int J Radiat Oncol Biol Phys* 1990;18:173.

706. Fuller SA, Haybittle JL, Smith RE, et al. Cardiac doses in post-operative breast irradiation. *Radiother Oncol* 1992;25:19.

707. Host H, Brennhovd MD, Loeb M. Postoperative radiotherapy in breast cancer—long-term results from the Oslo study. *Int J Radiat Oncol Biol Phys* 1986;12:727.

708. Vallis KA, Pintilie M, Chong M, et al. Assesment of coronary heart disease morbidity and mortality after radiation for early breast cancer. *J Clin. Oncol* 2002;20(4):1036–1042.

709. Perez CA, Taylor ME, Halverson K, et al. Brachytherapy or electron beam boost in conservation therapy of carcinoma of the breast: a nonrandomized comparison. *Int J Radiat Oncol Biol Phys* 1996;34:995.

710. McCormick B, Yahalom J, Cox L, et al. The patient's perception of her breast following radiation and limited surgery. *Int J Radiat Oncol Biol Phys* 1989;17:1299.

711. Clarke D, Martinez A, Cox RS, et al. Breast edema following staging axillary node dissection in patients with breast carcinoma treated by radical radiotherapy. *Cancer* 1982;49:2295.

712. Montague ED, Pauleis DD, Schell SR, et al. Selection and follow-up of patients for conservation surgery and irradiation. *Front Radiat Ther Oncol* 1983;17:124.

713. Pezner RO, Patterson MP, Hill LR, et al. Breast edema in patients treated conservatively for stage I and II breast cancer. *Int J Radiat Oncol Biol Phys* 1985;11:1765.

714. Dewar JA, Sarrazin D, Benhamou E, et al. Management of the axilla in conservatively treated breast cancer: 592 patients treated at Institut Gustave-Roussy. *Int J Radiat Oncol Biol Phys* 1987;13:475.

715. Pierce SM, Recht A, Lingos TI, et al. Long-term radiation complications following conservative surgery (CS) and radiation therapy (RT) in patients with early stage breast cancer. *Int J Radiat Oncol Biol Phys* 1992;23:915.

716. Stotter AT, McNeese MD, Ames FC, et al. Predicting the rate and extent of locoregional failure after breast conservation therapy for early breast cancer. *Cancer* 1989;64:2217.

717. Gyenes G, Fornander T, Charlens P, et al. Morbidity of ischemic heart disease in early breast cancer 15–20 years after adjuvant radiotherapy. *Int J Radiat Oncol Biol Phys* 1994;28:1235.

718. Nixon AJ, Gelman R, Bornstein BA, et al. Non-breast cancer mortality

after conservative surgery and radiation therapy (RT) to the left breast. *Int J Radiat Oncol Biol Phys* 1996;36:181(abst).

719. Valagussa P, Zambetti M, Biasi S, et al. Cardiac effects following adjuvant chemotherapy and breast irradiation in operable breast cancer. *Ann Oncol* 1994;5:209.

720. Albrektsen G, Heuch I, Kvale G. The short-term and long-term effect of a pregnancy on breast cancer risk: a prospective study of 802,457 parous Norwegian women. *Br J Cancer* 1995;72:480.

721. Holmes FA. Breast cancer during pregnancy. *Cancer Bull* 1994;46:400.

722. Wagner LK, Lester RG, Saldana LR. The amount of radiation absorbed by the conceptus. In: *Exposure of the pregnant patient to diagnostic radiations: a guide to medical management.* Philadelphia: JB Lippincott Co, 1985:52.

723. Nugent P, O'Connell TX. Breast cancer and pregnancy. *Arch Surg* 1985;120:1221.

724. Brent RL. The effect of embryonic and fetal exposure to x-ray, microwaves, and ultrasound: counseling the pregnant and nonpregnant patient about these risks. *Semin Oncol* 1989;16:347.

725. Doll DC, Ringenberg S, Yarbro JW. Antineoplastic agents and pregnancy. *Semin Oncol* 1989;16:337.

726. Adair EA. Cancer of the breast. *Surg Clin North Am* 1953;33:313.

727. Isaacs JH. Cancer of the breast in pregnancy. *Surg Clin North Am* 1995;75:47.

728. Danforth DN Jr. How subsequent pregnancy affects outcome in women with a prior breast cancer. *Oncology* 1991;5:21.

729. Epstein RJ, Henderson IC. The Danforth article reviewed: the jury is in. *Oncology* 1991;5:30.

730. Wood WC. The Danforth article reviewed. *Oncology* 1991;5:35.

731. Sutton R, Buzdar AU, Hortobagyi GN. Pregnancy and offspring after adjuvant chemotherapy in breast cancer patients. *Cancer* 1990;65:847.

732. Zemlickis D, Lishner M, Degendorfer P, et al. Maternal and fetal outcome after breast cancer in pregnancy. *Am J Obstet Gynecol* 1992;166:781.

733. Korzeniowski S, Dyba T. Reproductive history and prognosis in patients with operable breast cancer. *Cancer* 1994;74:1591.

734. Sankila R, Heinavaara S, Hakulinen T. Survival of breast cancer patients after subsequent term pregnancy: "healthy mother effect." *Am J Obstet Gynecol* 1994;170:818.

735. Dow KH, Harris JR, Roy C. Pregnancy after breast-conserving surgery and radiation therapy for breast cancer. *Monogr Natl Cancer Inst* 1994;16:131.

736. Higgins S, Haffty BG. Pregnancy and lactation after breast-conserving therapy for early stage breast cancer. *Cancer* 1994;73:2175.

737. Tralins AH. Lactation after conservation breast surgery combined with radiation therapy. *Am J Clin Oncol* 1995;18:40.

738. Jensen AB. Psychosocial factors in breast cancer and their possible impact upon prognosis. *Cancer Treat Rev* 1991;18:191.

739. Schain WS. Psychosocial factors affecting treatment recommendations for primary breast cancer. NIH Consensus Development Conference, June 18–21, 1990:38–39.

740. Schain E, Edwards BK, Gorrell CR, et al. Psychosocial and physical outcomes of stage I primary breast cancer therapy: mastectomy vs excisional biopsy and irradiation. *Breast Cancer Res Treat* 1983;3:377.

741. Verhoef LCG, Stalpers LJA, Verbeek ALM, et al. Breast-conserving treatment or mastectomy in early breast cancer: a clinical decision analysis with special reference to the risk of local recurrence. *Eur J Cancer* 1991;27:1132.

742. Lasry JC, Margolese RG. Fear of recurrence, breast-conserving surgery, and the trade-off hypothesis. *Cancer* 1992;69:2111.

743. Mock V. Body image in women treated for breast cancer. *Nurs Res* 1993;42:153.

744. Blichert-Toft M. Breast-conserving therapy for mammary carcinoma: psychosocial aspects, indications and limitations. *Ann Med* 1992;24:445.

745. Schover LR, Yetman RJ, Tuason LJ, et al. Partial mastectomy and breast reconstruction: a comparison of their effects on psychosocial adjustment, body image, and sexuality. *Cancer* 1995;75:54.

746. Schain WS, D'Angelo TM, Dunn ME, et al. Mastectomy versus conservative surgery and radiation therapy: psychosocial consequences. *Cancer* 1994;73:1221.

747. Levy SM, Haynes LT, Herberman RB, et al. Mastectomy versus breast conservation surgery: mental health effects at long-term follow-up. *Health Psychol* 1992;11:349.

748. Glanz K, Lerman C. Psychosocial impact of breast cancer: a critical review. *Ann Behav Med* 1992;14:204.

749. Schover LR. Sexuality and body image in younger women with breast cancer. *J Natl Cancer Inst* 1994;16:177.

750. Langmuir VK, Poulter CA, Qazi R, et al. Breast cancer. In: Rubin P, ed. *Clinical oncology: a multidisciplinary approach for physicians and students.* 7th ed. Philadelphia: WB Saunders, 1993:193.

751. Basco VE, Coldman AJ, Elwood JM, et al. Radiation dose and second breast cancer. *Br J Cancer* 1985;52:319.

752. McCredie JA, Inch WR, Alderson M. Consecutive primary carcinomas of the breast. *Cancer* 1975;35:1472.

753. Hankey BF, Curtis RE, Naughton MD, et al. A retrospective cohort analysis of second breast cancer risk for primary breast cancer patients with an assessment of the effect of radiation therapy. *J Natl Cancer Inst* 1983;70:797.

754. Rosen PP, Groshen S, Kinne DW, et al. Contralateral breast carcinoma: an assessment of risk and prognosis in Stage I (T1N0M0) and Stage II (T1N1M0) patients with 20-year follow-up. *Surgery* 1989;106:904.

755. de la Rochefordière A, Mouret-Fourme E, Scholl S, et al. Role of metachronous contralateral breast carcinoma in the outcome of breast cancer. *Int J Radiat Oncol Biol Phys* 1995;32:212(abst).

756. Ringberg A, Palmer B, Linell F. The contralateral breast at reconstructive surgery after breast cancer operation: a histopathological study. *Breast Cancer Res Treat* 1982;2:151.

757. Boice JD Jr, Harvey EB, Blettner M, et al. Cancer in the contralateral breast after radiotherapy for breast cancer. *N Engl J Med* 1992;326:781.

758. Levitt SH, Mandell J. Benefits versus risks in conservation surgery with irradiation for breast cancer. *Am J Med* 1984;77:93.

759. Storm HH, Andersson M, Boice JD, et al. Adjuvant radiotherapy and risk of contralateral breast cancer. *J Natl Cancer Inst* 1992;84:1245.

760. Curtis RE, Hankey BF, Myers MH, et al. Risk of leukemia associated with the first course of cancer treatment: an analysis of the surveillance, epidemiology and end results section. *J Natl Cancer Inst* 1984;72:531.

761. Curtis RE, Boice JD, Stovall M, et al. Risk of leukemia after chemotherapy and radiation treatment for breast cancer. *N Engl J Med* 1992;326:1745.

762. Martin MB, Kon ND, Kawamoto EH, et al. Postmastectomy angiosarcoma. *Am Surg* 1984;50:541.

763. Durand JC, Poljicak M, Lefranc JP, et al. Wide excisaion of the tumor, axillary dissection, and postoperative radiotherapy as treatment of small breast cancers. *Cancer* 1984;53:2439.

764. Souba WW, McKenna RJ, Meis J, et al. Radiation induced sarcomas of the chest wall. *Cancer* 1986;57:610.

765. Karlsson P, Holmberg E, Johansson K-A, et al. Soft tissue sarcoma after treatment for breast cancer. *Radiother Oncol* 1996;38:25.

766. Edeiken S, Russo DP, Knecht J, et al. Angiosarcoma after tylectomy and radiation therapy for carcinoma of the breast. *Cancer* 1992;70:644.

767. Wijnmaalen A, van Ooijen B, van Geel BN, et al. Angiosarcoma of the breast following lumpectomy, axillary lymph node dissection, and radiotherapy for primary breast cancer: three case reports and a review of the literature. *Int J Radiat Oncol Biol Phys* 1993;26:135.

768. Zucali R, Merson M, Placucci M, et al. Soft tissue sarcoma of the breast after conservative surgery and irradiation for early mammary cancer. *Radiother Oncol* 1994;30:271.

Special Management Topics

CHAPTER 31

Management of Infections in Gynecologic Cancer Patients

Kent A. Sepkowitz, David L. Hemsell, and Donald Armstrong

Infection remains a major cause of morbidity and mortality in patients with gynecologic cancer. As always, the most common source of infection is the vaginal-cervical flora. In a healthy patient, this flora consists of a mixture of aerobes and anaerobes. The aerobes include gram-negative bacilli, such as *Escherichia coli*, *Klebsiella* species, and *Enterobacter* species, and gram-positive cocci, including streptococci and enterococci. The anaerobes include the *Bacteroides* and *Prevotella* species (e.g., *B. fragilis* and *P. bivius*), the *Clostridium* species, and anaerobic streptococci (Table 31.1) (1,2).

Gynecologic neoplasm, previous antibiotic use, and prior radiation therapy may alter the normal flora (3,4). Any of these organisms can become invasive and cause disease if the integrity of the protective integument of the vaginal wall or upper reproductive tract (uterus/fallopian tubes) is compromised.

The proximity of the gynecologic organs to the urinary system and the gastrointestinal tract, especially the colon, can predispose patients to infection even if the anatomic disruption appears to be minor. An indwelling intravenous, urinary, or other catheter can also allow easy access of bacteria or fungi into the bloodstream or favor formation of an abscess.

This chapter offers an overview of clinical situations commonly seen in gynecologic oncology and a more thorough account of each clinical disease category, such as wound infection or pneumonia. A patient with infection may have many predisposing factors, but it is still instructive to consider each factor separately.

APPROACH TO THE FEBRILE PATIENT

For the febrile gynecologic cancer patient, it is best first to consider the possible underlying mechanisms of disease (Table 31.2). Numerous factors can predispose a patient to infection, and awareness of specific risks of each clinical situation can often allow proper selection of empiric antibiotic therapy in advance of microbiologic culture results or radiographic studies.

Untreated Tumor

Unchecked growth of primary or metastatic tumor can result in infectious complications. Erosion of tumor through the vaginal wall or upper tract can allow vaginal flora to enter the peritoneum, leading to peritonitis or pelvic abscess.

Tumor can involve the bowel and cause obstruction or perforation of the bowel, resulting in peritonitis or abscess caused by bowel flora. Direct extension of tumor also can obstruct the urinary collecting system. This may result in urinary obstruction and infection, usually due to aerobic gram-negative rods.

Treatment for Tumor

Each therapeutic modality can predispose patients to a unique set of infections. The possible postoperative infectious complications of surgery include the routine postoperative sequence of "wind, wound, and water." Additional concerns in the patient with pelvic cancer are the problems of a nonsterile field, the proximity of the bowel to the involved area, the frequent need for prolonged Foley catheterization,

D. L. Hemsell: Division of Gynecology, Department of Obstetrics and Gynecology, University of Texas Southwestern Medical Center, Dallas, Texas 75235

D. Armstrong and K. A. Sepkowitz: Infectious Diseases Service, Memorial Sloan–Kettering Cancer Center, New York, New York 10021

TABLE 31.1. *Vaginal microflora in 209 women prior to elective hysterectomy for benign diagnoses*

Organisms recovered		Number
Aerobes		
Cocci		
	Enterococci faecalis	129
	Staphylococcus epidermidis	112
	Group B streptococci	54
	Streptococcus spp	36
	Staphylococcus aureus	30
Bacilli		
	Escherichia coli	145
	Klebsiella spp	27
	Proteus spp	26
	Enterobacter spp	15
	Other Enterobacteriaceae	19
	Subtotal	593
Anaerobes		
Cocci		
	Peptostreptococcus spp	249
Bacilli		
	Bacteroides spp	100
	Bacteroides fragilis group	93
	Fusobacterium spp	8
	Clostridium spp	5
	Subtotal	567

spp, species.
Modified with permission from Hemsell DL, Heard MC, Nobles BJ, et al. Alterations in lower tract flora after single-dose piperacillin and triple-dose cefoxitin at vaginal and abdominal hysterectomy. *Obstet Gynecol* 1988;72:875.

and surgery on an area already compromised by radiation therapy.

Chemotherapy can render an individual susceptible to infection by lowering the neutrophil count for days to weeks. Many patients develop bacteremia in this setting. Also, im-

TABLE 31.2. *Clinical situations that may predispose to infection*

Untreated tumor
Obstruction of gastrointestinal or urinary tract
  Erosion into bowel or vagina
Treatment of tumor
  Surgery
    Wound infection
    Intraabdominal infection
  Chemotherapy
    Neutropenia
    T-cell depression (e.g., corticosteroids)
  Radiation therapy
    Enteritis
    Urinary tract infection
    Poor wound healing
  Catheters
    Intravenous
    Intraperitoneal
    Foley and other urinary catheters
Specific cancers (e.g., vulvar)

munosuppressive agents such as corticosteroids can impair the immune response, predisposing the patient to certain infections. In addition, intraperitoneal and intravenous catheters that facilitate delivery of chemotherapy may predispose patients to infections (5,6). However, one study of 100 women with ovarian cancer found that early postoperative chemotherapy did not increase the risk of wound complications (7). The investigators recommended that concern for impaired wound healing should not result in a delay in postoperative chemotherapy.

Radiation therapy, including brachytherapy, predisposes patients to urinary tract infections, wound infections, and/or enteritis (8). Patients with specific cancers may be at higher risk for infection. Patients with vulvar carcinoma have up to a 2.5 times higher rate of admission for infection than did women with other types of pelvic cancer (9,10). The type of surgical therapy that was used in treatment and the older age of the patients (median 75 years) may have contributed to the increase.

Antibiotics

The continued development of new antibiotics has offered powerful therapies against a wide range of organisms. However, it is sometimes difficult to remember the differences in spectrum and toxic effects of each new antibiotic. In selecting antibiotics, the efficacy for the individual patient is of highest importance. However, with the worsening problem of bacterial resistance to antibiotics (11,12), attention to preserving overall bacterial susceptibility should also be kept in mind.

The following is an overview of selected antibiotics. Attention is given to their major uses and side effects (Tables 31.3 and 31.4). The reader should recognize that this is not a comprehensive list.

Penicillins

The penicillins belong to the group of beta-lactam antibiotics. Alteration of the original penicillin compound has yielded numerous semisynthetic compounds that have attained wide use in clinical practice.

Ampicillin was the first penicillin with activity against gram-negative bacilli. Its derivatives, including piperacillin, ticarcillin, mezlocillin, and azlocillin, have broad gram-negative activity, particularly against *Pseudomonas aeruginosa*. The addition of sulbactam to ampicillin (Unasyn), tazobactam to piperacillin (Zosyn), and clavulanic acid to ticarcillin (Timentin) and amoxicillin (Augmentin) further improved the spectrum of these antibiotics by reestablishing their activity to beta-lactamase–producing bacteria, including anaerobes.

Oxacillin and nafcillin have excellent activity against methicillin-sensitive *Staphylococcus aureus*.

TABLE 31.3. *Empiric therapy*

Infection	Treatment
Wound	No antibiotic treatment[a] (dressing changes q 6–8 h always necessary)
	Oxacillin or vancomycin[b]
	Ticarcillin/clavulanic acid
Abdomen[c]	Ampicillin/clindamycin or ampicillin/metronidazole/gentamicin
	Cefoxitin
	Levofloxacin, ciprofloxacin, or gatifloxacin and metronidazole
	Ceftriaxone/metronidazole
	Ticarcillin/clavulanic acid
	Imipenem or meropenem
Lung[c]	Penicillin
	Clindamycin
	Ceftriaxone
	Ticarcillin/clavulanic acid
	Imipenem
Urinary tract[c]	Cefazolin
	Trimethoprim-sulfamethoxazole
	Ciprofloxacin
	Vancomycin[d]
Intravenous catheter[c]	Oxacillin, cefazolin, or vancomycin[b]
	Ticarcillin/clavulanic acid
Unknown	Careful observation without treatment

[a]Antibiotics should be based on Gram's stain results and adjusted after the organism is isolated and the sensitivities are known.

[b]Oxacillin may be used if methicillin-resistant *Staphylococcus aureus* is not a problem at a given hospital. Otherwise, vancomycin must be used.

[c]An aminoglycoside (e.g., gentamicin, tobramycin, or amikacin according to hospital susceptibility patterns) should be added in patients with recent hospitalizations, recent past antibiotic use, or clinical instability.

[d]Vancomycin should be given if the patient is suspected of having an enterococcal infection.

Cephalosporins

Cephalosporins are also beta-lactam antibiotics. They are divided, somewhat arbitrarily, into "generations." In general, with each generation, gram-negative activity is enhanced and gram-positive activity is diminished. Some cephalosporins have excellent activity against anaerobes.

Cefazolin is a first-generation cephalosporin with excellent activity against many streptococcal species and methicillin-sensitive *S. aureus*. It is also active against some common gram-negative rods.

Cefoxitin and cefotetan are second-generation cephalosporins with good activity against anaerobes and gram-negative rods.

Ceftriaxone is a third-generation cephalosporin without anaerobic activity. It is more active against many gram-negative and gram-positive aerobes than is cefoxitin. Neither ceftriaxone nor cefoxitin is active against *P. aeruginosa*.

Ceftazidime is a third-generation cephalosporin with excellent activity against most gram-negative rods, including *P. aeruginosa*. It has unreliable activity against gram-positive cocci.

Cefepime is another expanded-spectrum cephalosporin with excellent activity against both gram-positive cocci and the Enterobacteriaceae.

Imipenem

Imipenem is a carbapenem. It has a very wide range of activity, including methicillin-sensitive *S. aureus*, *P. aeruginosa*, and anaerobes. Because of the possibility of encouraging resistance, many hospitals have limited the use of imipenem. Some patients who are allergic to penicillins or cephalosporins also are allergic to imipenem, but cross sensitivity is unpredictable. In general, imipenem is safe to administer to a patient with a beta-lactam allergy unless the allergic reaction included a blistering rash or bronchospasm.

Meropenem

Meropenem is the second Food and Drug Administration (FDA)–approved carbapenem. It does not require the addition of a dehydropeptidase-1 enzyme inhibitor, requires less frequent dosing, and may have less neurotoxicity. Efficacy was comparable with clindamycin/gentamicin in a multicenter study of 515 hospitalized women treated for acute pelvic infections (38).

Ertapenem

Ertapenem is the newest carbapenem and is administered once daily. Its spectrum is comparable to that of the others in the class, but without activity against *P. aeruginosa*, which is encountered almost exclusively in patients with neutropenia. It may be more useful for inpatient than outpatient management of women with pelvic infection (13).

Aztreonam

Aztreonam is a monobactam beta-lactam antibiotic with good activity against a wide range of gram-negative rods, including *P. aeruginosa* (14). It has no activity against gram-positive aerobes or against anaerobes. Patients with penicillin or cephalosporin allergies have a slightly increased risk of aztreonam allergy.

Sulfa Drugs

Trimethoprim-sulfamethoxazole remains useful for treating patients with simple urinary tract infections caused by many susceptible Enterobacteriaceae.

Quinolones

The first-generation quinolones, which include norfloxacin, levofloxacin, ciprofloxacin, and others, are most useful

TABLE 31.4. *Overview of some commonly used antibiotics*

Drug	Dose[a]	Activity[b]	Side effects[c]	Comment
Beta-lactam antibiotics				
Penicillin	2 million U q 4 h	*Clostridium* species	Seizures (all high-dose penicillins)	Anaphylaxis may occur with any penicillins
Ampicillin	12 g q 46 h	*E. coli* Enterococci (with an aminoglycoside)	Interstitial nephritis (all penicillins)	
Piperacillin[d]	3 g q 4 h	*P. aeruginosa* and other gram-negative rods Anaerobes		
Ticarcillin-clavulanic acid[e]	3.1 g q 4 h	*P. aeruginosa* and other gram-negative rods Anaerobes MSSA[f]		High obligate salt load (may be a problem with patients with congestive heart failure)
Oxacillin[g]	2 g q 4 h	MSSA[f]		
Cefazolin	12 g q 8 h	MSSA[f] Enteric gram-negative rod[h]		
Cefoxitin	12 g q 8 h	Enteric gram-negative rod[h] Anaerobes		
Ceftriaxone	1 g q 24 h	Enteric gram-negative rod	Cholecystitis	
Ceftazidime	12 g q 8 h	*P. aeruginosa* and other gram-negative rods		
Cefipime	12 g q 12 h	*P. aeruginosa* and other gram-negative rods		
Carbapenems and monobactams				
Imipenem	500,750 mg q 6 h	*P. aeruginosa* and other gram-negative rods MSSA[f] Anaerobes	Seizures, especially in patients with known CNS lesions	
Meropenem	5001,000 mg q 8 h	*P. aeruginosa* and other gram-negative rods MSSA[f] Anaerobes	Seizures, especially in patients with known CNS lesions	
Aztreonam	12 g q 8 h	*P. aeruginosa* and other gram-negative rods		Little cross allergy with penicillin-allergic patients
Ertapenem	1 g q 24 h	Gram negative rods EXCEPT *P. aeruginosa* Anaerobes MSSA		
Aminoglycosides				
Gentamicin[i]	45 mg/kg/d in 3 divided doses	Gram-negative rods, including *P. aeruginosa*	Ototoxicity and nephrotoxicity	Must monitor levels. q 24 h dosing if not neutropenic.
Amikacin	15 mg/kg/d in 2 or 3 divided doses	Gram-negative rods, including *P. aeruginosa*	Ototoxicity and nephrotoxicity	Must monitor levels. q 24 h dosing if not neutropenic.
Quinolones				
Ciprofloxacin	500–750 mg q 12 h PO or 400 mg IV q 12 h	*P. aeruginosa* and other gram-negative rods No anaerobic coverage; poor streptococcal and staphylococcal coverage		
Levofloxacin	500 mg PO/IV QD[11]	Similar to ciprofloxacin with enhanced streptococcal and staphylococcal coverage		

(continued)

TABLE 31.4. *Continued*

Drug	Dose[a]	Activity[b]	Side effects[c]	Comment
Gatifloxacin	400 mg PO/IV QD	Similar to levofloxacin but without *P. aeruginosa* coverage		
Cotrimoxazole	10 mg/kg/d in 4 divided doses	*E. coli*		
Clindamycin	300–900 q 8 h	Anaerobes MSSA[f]	Diarrhea, including *C. difficile* toxin-positive diarrhea	
Metronidazole	500 mg q 6–8 h	Anaerobes	Anorexia, antabuse-like reaction	
Vancomycin	1 g q 12 h	Gram-positive cocci, including MRSA[j]	Ototoxicity and nephrotoxicity (rare unless given with another ototoxic or nephrotoxic agent)	Must monitor levels Emergence of vancomycin resistance a significant concern.

[a]Doses must be adjusted for renal function, liver function, age, and weight.
[b]Only those organisms likely to be of concern in gynecologic oncology are included.
[c]All antibiotics may have unpredictable side effects, including fever, hepatitis, and rash. The side effects listed are those that the clinician should keep in mind when treating a patient with the given drug.
[d]Also includes ticarcillin, mezlocillin, and azlocillin.
[e]Piperacillin-tazobactam has a similar spectrum but is not adequate for pseudomonal infections. Ampicillin-sulbactam (Unasyn) has similar spectrum but is not active against *P. aeruginosa*.
[f]MSSA, *S. aureus* (methicillin-sensitive).
[g]Nafcillin has similar activity.
[h]Enterobacteriaceae and *Serratia*.
[i]Also includes tobramycin and netilmycin (12).
[j]MRSA, *S. aureus* (methicillin-resistant).
QD = daily

against aerobic gram-negative rods (15). Excellent oral absorption and once or twice a day dosing have made them an attractive alternative for many outpatient infections. The use of ciprofloxacin against gram-positive organisms, especially *S. pneumoniae* and *S. aureus*, is not recommended because resistant strains have already emerged. These quinolones have no activity against anaerobes and should not be used by themselves in outpatient therapy for a patient with intraabdominal infection.

Second-generation or extended-spectrum quinolones, such as gatifloxacin and moxifloxacin, have entered use in the United States. Although these agents have enhanced activity against many anaerobic bacteria, they should not be used to treat serious intraabdominal infection.

Metronidazole

Metronidazole retains excellent anaerobic activity. It is inactive against aerobes. It has been shown to promote the emergence of vancomycin-resistant enterococcus (VRE), presumably by altering the intestinal anaerobic flora (16). This, combined with its various side effects, most notably suppression of appetite, should be considered before routinely administering metronidazole to anyone with possible intraabdominal infection (17).

Macrolides and Lincomycins

The macrolides, erythromycin, clarithromycin (Biaxin), and azithromycin (Zithromax), have a limited role in management of infectious complications of the gynecologic cancer patient. Clindamycin, a lincomycin (named after Lincoln, Nebraska, where it was first identified in the soil), remains an excellent drug for patients with proven or presumed anaerobic infection, although increasing resistance among the *Bacteroides* species is occurring in many medical centers. Clindamycin also is active against methicillin-sensitive *S. aureus*. The production of *Clostridium difficile* diarrhea by clindamycin has resulted in appropriately cautious use (17).

Chloramphenicol

Concern about the development of aplastic anemia long ago sharply curtailed the use of chloramphenicol (17). Recent experience with this agent in the treatment of vancomycin-resistant *Enterococcus faecium*, however, has shown a surprisingly favorable toxicity profile (18). Because it remains a very active drug against most anaerobes, its use should be considered in patients with significant beta-lactam drug allergies or other contraindications to the other commonly used agents.

Vancomycin

Vancomycin is active against all gram-positive cocci and remains the drug of choice against methicillin-resistant *S. aureus*. Infection with *S. epidermidis* has become more common owing to increasing use of indwelling intravenous and intraperitoneal devices, and vancomycin still remains active against all strains. Concern about worsening vancomycin resistance, particularly of *E. faecium* isolates (19), has led to more restrictive use of this agent at many medical centers. In addition, the emergence of vancomycin-resistant *S. aureus* has emphasized the need to use this agent sparingly (12).

Aminoglycosides

The aminoglycosides, including gentamicin, tobramycin, and amikacin, are notorious for their ototoxicity and nephrotoxicity. Careful monitoring of blood levels can reduce, although not eliminate, these side effects. There appears to be no predictable difference in the degree of ototoxicity or renal toxicity among the aminoglycosides, which remain important in the management of cancer patients with fever and neutropenia (20). There are data in the treatment of women with acute pelvic infection confirming that single dosing (5 to 7 mg/kg/day) is as effective as and safer than more frequent dosing (21–23). It cannot be recommended in the treatment of neutropenic cancer patients.

PROPHYLAXIS IN GYNECOLOGIC CANCER SURGERY

Operative Site

Guidelines for the administration of antibiotics to uninfected patients undergoing pelvic surgical procedures were first proposed by Ledger and colleagues in 1975 (24). Prophylactic antibiotics are indicated for women undergoing pelvic surgery for malignancy. There have been very few studies evaluating this prophylaxis for women undergoing radical pelvic surgery for gynecologic malignancy, and the treatment in these studies has ranged from a single dose of doxycycline to 5 days of clindamycin and tobramycin.

Risk factors that have been associated with an increased incidence of infection in patients undergoing surgery for reproductive tract carcinoma include lower socioeconomic status, preoperative conization, failure to administer perioperative heparin, obesity, older patient age, a longer operative period, and a longer hospital stay before surgery (25). However, these risk factors were not uniform among investigators' evaluations.

Flora

The effects of lower reproductive tract flora in women with pelvic malignancy have been reported by Blythe (26),

Mead (27), Creasman et al. (28), and Hemsell et al. (29) among others. Blythe reported that the flora was similar to that of women without genital malignancy. Thadapalli et al. (30) reported that anaerobes were only rarely recovered from women with cervical cancer, and Mead (27) reported fewer gram-positive and gram-negative bacteria in women with pelvic cancer. Hemsell et al. (29) reported fewer gram-positive aerobic bacteria but more gram-negative anaerobes and *E. coli*. This variability, combined with the inconsistent evaluations of risk factors, implies that individual determination of the need for prophylaxis and the most effective agent is appropriate.

Clinical Investigation

The overall operative-site infection rate ranges from 6.7% to 44%. Retrospective data in these reports were contradictory. A decrease in significant operative-site infection was reported by Bell and Sevin (31) and by Mann and Orr (32). Gussman and colleagues reported a decreased incidence of pelvic infection with prophylaxis but not of overall operative-site infection (33).

Prospective data have not resolved this issue. Numbers of patients in comparative arms have been small, and the data may be, therefore, inadequate for detecting a statistically significant infection rate. No significant difference in overall operative-site infection was observed after perioperative prophylaxis by the research groups of Rosenshein (34) or Marsden (35), but significantly lower incidences of infection were reported by Sevin et al. (36) and Micha et al. (37). Sevin et al. (38) reported that a short course (three doses) of prophylaxis was as effective as a long course (12 doses) in preventing major infection after radical hysterectomy. If separate operative-site data from prospective studies are combined, the overall incidence of pelvic infection and wound infection was significantly reduced by the administration of prophylactic antimicrobials.

One patient population that has a significant surgical incision breakdown is that of women undergoing radical vulvectomy. Anecdotal experience indicates the principle pathogens to be *S. aureus* and *S. epidermidis*. The administration of broad-spectrum medications, such as piperacillin or mezlocillin, did not significantly reduce the incidence of postoperative wound infection; 8 of 12 women undergoing radical vulvectomy for vulvar carcinoma who were given single-dose piperacillin or mezlocillin developed postoperative infections (39). Drain sites fall into the same category. The foreign body undoubtedly contributes to the infections; local attention, rather than parenteral or oral antibiotics, is the appropriate preventive approach.

Agent Administration

Route of Administration

There are few prospective gynecologic oncology prophylaxis data comparing protection afforded by a particular regimen based on its route of administration. The protection afforded by 1 g cefazolin was identical whether it was given intramuscularly or intravenously to women undergoing elective abdominal hysterectomy for benign disease (40). However, there are potential disadvantages to intramuscular administration on the nursing unit, including pain, sterile abscess formation, and nerve irritation. Events may occur that delay or cancel the procedure, negating the need for the dose of antibiotic after it is given.

Intravenous administration of the antibiotic in the operating room avoids that problem. If given before anesthesia, the intravenous route also allows detection of an allergic reaction by the patient before the entire dose is administered. Intravenous administration produces higher serum and perhaps higher tissue concentrations of the agent than would be observed after intramuscular administration, but bacterial inoculation of the operative site with lower reproductive tract pathogens does not occur until vaginal entry, which is a late event in abdominal hysterectomy. Antibiotics have been administered to women undergoing hysterectomy for benign indications by suppository, by spray, and orally, with significant reduction in operative-site infection (41–43). There are no similar data for women undergoing hysterectomy for gynecologic cancer.

Timing of Drug Administration

The first dose of an antibiotic should be given intravenously in the operating room. Combination regimens and prolonged administration did not appear to offer superior infection prevention when compared with that provided by a single agent given once. If the interval between the first dose and opening the vagina exceeds 2.5 to 3 hours, a second intravenous dose should be given 15 to 30 minutes before the anticipated vaginal entry. This conclusion is based on data provided by Shapiro and others (44). This has not been clinically studied, but administration at longer fixed intervals has not enhanced protection at hysterectomy for benign indications.

Recommendations

Intravenous administration of 2 g cefazolin should be given in the operating room. Cefazolin provides activity against gram-negative and gram-positive aerobic and anaerobic bacteria; it is an uncommon therapeutic agent and is comparatively inexpensive—all beneficial attributes for a prophylactic antibiotic. A single dose of a prophylactic agent did not result in the selection of a resistant species, as did three doses of antibiotics at hysterectomy for benign disease (45). A 1-g dose may suffice, but 2 g was superior to 1 g for vaginal hysterectomy, and three 1-g doses over 16 hours were statistically inferior to a single 2-g dose for cesarean delivery (46,47). A single dose (1 g) of cefotetan was significantly ($p <.05$) superior to 1 g of cefazolin in

preventing operative-site infection after elective abdominal hysterectomy for benign diagnoses. Although the cost per vial was higher, there was an overall reduction in hospital costs owing to fewer infections and shorter hospital stays (48). Kobamatsu and co-investigators also found superior protection for women undergoing radical hysterectomy when using expanded-spectrum cephalosporins compared with first-generation agents (49). More prospective data are necessary for oncologic patients.

If the patient is allergic to cephalosporins or if she has a history of a type I immediate hypersensitivity reaction to a penicillin, and if she is not allergic to a tetracycline, the recommendation is 100 mg doxycycline orally at bedtime the night before surgery and again the day of surgery about 3 hours before departure for the operating room. This regimen has been evaluated prospectively in Parkland Memorial Hospital, but in a nonrandomized study using very few patients and no control regimen. If the woman is allergic to tetracycline, the recommendation is intravenous administration of 900 mg of clindamycin given preoperatively, as for cefazolin. The FDA recently approved an oral dose of trovafloxacin for hysterectomy and colorectal surgery prophylaxis. It may be particularly suited for the gynecologic cancer patient scheduled for pelvic surgery because of its spectrum of activity and half-life. It must not be administered with any antacids.

Bowel Preparation

Unobstructed Bowel

There are approximately 10^{11} bacteria in a gram of feces, making sepsis a major hazard if the colon is opened. It is desirable to reduce the patient's normal colonic microflora to diminish the postoperative infection rate in case it is necessary to perform colonic resection and reanastomosis. Preparation for colonoscopy is a regimen of clear liquids the day before surgery and 3 tbs of Fleet Phospho-Soda in one-half cup cool water at 4:00 and 6:00 PM the day before surgery. Patients should be cautioned to drink eight to ten 8–fl oz glasses of clear liquids the day before surgery. Additional clear fluid is acceptable. Some surgeons prefer to add a Fleet enema 2 hours before surgery. An alternative mechanical preparation is whole gut irrigation with chilled polyethylene glycol and electrolyte therapy or a similar lavage solution given orally at a rate of approximately 1 L/h until the rectal effluent is clear, but for not more than 4 hours.

In the antimicrobial approach, 1 g each of erythromycin and neomycin are given orally at 1:00, 2:00, and 11:00 PM the day before surgery. This regimen was initially proposed in 1971 by Nichols and Condon (50). An alternative is 1 g each of metronidazole and neomycin at 2:00 and at 11:00 PM the day before surgery. There should be no need to add further antimicrobial prophylaxis to 2 g of cefazolin or other agents. Because this may alter hydration status and serum electrolytes, many administer intravenous fluids to these patients.

Obstructed Bowel

There can be no mechanical prophylaxis for preoperative management of the obstructed bowel. Treatment principles include fluid and electrolyte therapy with mechanical decompression of the bowel from above and timed surgical intervention. Women with mechanical intestinal obstruction immediately after surgery may be able to be treated conservatively with decompression only. If necessary, surgery should be performed within 24 hours of the mechanical obstruction; these patients have the lowest mortality rate. A dose of intravenous antibiotic should be given in the operating room before the procedure, with a second dose given in the recovery room, and a third 8 hours later if it is necessary to enter the bowel lumen. The single-agent or combination regimen should provide broad coverage of both gram-positive and gram-negative aerobic and anaerobic bacterial species with a broader spectrum of antibacterial activity than with cefazolin. Evaluation has produced no evidence for a superior regimen. A single agent usually suffices unless the patient is septic, in which case triple antibiotics are appropriate because therapy, not prophylaxis, is necessary.

CLINICAL SYNDROMES

Peritonitis and Intraabdominal Abscess

Etiology

Infection in the patient with pelvic cancer most commonly involves the pelvis and abdomen. The potential causes of infection include complications of the primary tumor, surgery, and radiation therapy.

The tumor can compromise the integrity of the vaginal wall and allow seeding of endogenous vaginal flora into the pelvic and peritoneal cavities. Previous antibiotics, radiation therapy, and the tumor itself may alter the normal genital flora (3,4). The tumor can also erode into the bowel and allow entry of fecal material into the peritoneal cavity. Rare cases of several other syndromes arising from untreated pelvic tumor, including spontaneous clostridial gas gangrene and pneumoperitoneum, have been reported (51,52).

Peritonitis, with or without abscess formation, may occur postoperatively after hysterectomy or with bowel injury.

Radiation therapy to the pelvis can cause radiation enteritis, leading to a chronic diarrheal syndrome, which may develop years after radiation therapy is completed. These patients are also at higher risk for bowel adhesions and subsequent obstruction. There are conflicting reports about the effect of radiation on vaginal flora (3,4).

Signs and Symptoms

In the patient with pelvic cancer, peritonitis may develop at any time, including at initial diagnosis (e.g., tumor infiltra-

tion of bowel), immediately postoperatively, or days or weeks after surgery (e.g., tumor infiltration or radiation therapy). The signs are generally dramatic and familiar: abdominal pain, fever, and signs of peritoneal irritation. However, among postoperative patients or patients who have received radiation or corticosteroid therapy, the physical findings may resemble those of a routine postoperative patient, making the diagnosis more difficult. To assure proper diagnosis, frequent examinations and close observation are required.

Abscess formation can also occur in several settings. In some patients, a subclinical microperforation of bowel is successfully walled off by the body's immune system, forming a pericolic or intraperitoneal abscess. This has been shown to occur 7 to 10 days after microperforation (53). Fever or mechanical obstruction may be the only presenting signs. Subphrenic, psoas, or liver abscesses may present as a fever of unknown origin and may require a methodical, diligent evaluation for diagnosis.

A fistula, usually caused by tumor but also occurring postoperatively, may form between any two organ systems, including the bladder, vagina, bowel, or skin. Persistent suppuration despite therapy or the presence of a feculent discharge from skin, bladder, or vagina may suggest the development of a fistula.

Diagnosis

The diagnosis of peritonitis is usually made on clinical grounds. In patients who have clinical evidence of peritonitis but are unable to undergo surgery because of bulky tumor, multiple prior surgeries, or general debility, paracentesis with appropriate cultures may be useful in guiding antibiotic therapy.

Radiologic investigation is generally required to diagnose an abscess. Regular plain x-ray films of the abdomen are seldom revealing. A sonogram, computed tomographic (CT) scan, or magnetic resonance image (MRI) of the abdomen may show the collection. A gallium scan may also be helpful. In a particularly confusing case in which abnormalities of scans can represent an abscess, metastatic tumor, or postoperative changes, a labeled leukocyte scan may be required to diagnose the abscess with certainty.

The diagnosis of a fistula requires demonstration of abnormal drainage from one organ system to another. This can be shown by intravenous or intravesical injection of dye for fistulae arising from the bladder, oral or rectal instillation of dye for those arising from the gastrointestinal tract, or a fistulogram for a fistula involving the skin.

In all cases, laboratory abnormalities, including an elevated leukocyte count, an elevated erythrocyte sedimentation rate, and abnormal liver function tests may suggest the diagnosis and direct the workup.

The microbiologic diagnosis in each of these syndromes requires culture for aerobes and anaerobes. Blood cultures are only rarely positive. Some patients may have an unexplained bacteremia of enteric gram-negative rods or anaerobes. This is probably from a microperforation of the bowel. Any patient with pelvic tumor and enteric gram-negative rods or anaerobic bacteremia should be radiologically evaluated for evidence of perforation.

Therapy

Acute, generalized peritonitis where gastrointestinal perforation is suspected usually requires urgent surgery to irrigate the peritoneum and repair any perforation. Broad-spectrum antibiotic coverage with agents such as cefoxitin, ticarcillin–clavulanic acid, metronidazole, clindamycin with ampicillin, and an aminoglycoside such as gentamicin is generally effective for the polymicrobial infection (32). Addition of the aminoglycoside is particularly important for patients who have been recently or frequently hospitalized or who have had past courses of antibiotics. These situations predispose the patient to the development of resistant organisms.

Effective treatment of an abscess requires drainage. Percutaneous drainage is adequate in many cases, but laparotomy is occasionally required. Large or persistent abscesses may require placement of a suction drain. Patients with fistulae generally require resection of the involved tissue.

For intraabdominal infection, intravenous antibiotics directed at the recovered bacteria should continue for at least 5 to 7 days after drainage. Some patients who have been on antibiotics may have evidence of pus but no growth on cultures. In this situation, broad-spectrum antibiotics directed at enteric gram-negative rods and anaerobes should be administered. Laboratory parameters such as leukocyte counts should be followed to determine the exact duration.

Patients who are inoperable can be treated with chronic suppressive therapy, intravenously or orally. Oral agents such as amoxicillin–clavulanic acid (875 mg BID) or clindamycin (450 mg q 6 to 8 hours) may be effective. Ciprofloxacin and levofloxacin alone should not be used in this situation because they provide no anaerobic coverage.

Urinary Tract Infection

Etiology

Many clinical situations predispose a patient to urinary tract infection. Urinary tract infection continues to be the leading cause of infectious morbidity in this population. One study found that 54 (50%) of 109 patients with pelvic cancer admitted to the hospital because of infection had a urinary tract infection (54). *E. coli* was the most common organism isolated.

Another report found that the frequency of urinary tract infections is increased as much as threefold in patients undergoing pelvic irradiation (8).

Many patients who undergo pelvic surgery require pro-

longed bladder catheterization, usually with a Foley catheter. These patients may develop the well-recognized infectious complications of chronic bladder catheterization, the most common of which is recurrent infection. In addition, tumor can cause urinary obstruction and subsequent infection. The role of silver- or antibiotic-impregnated Foley catheters has not yet been defined.

Signs and Symptoms

Some patients with gynecologic malignancy and urinary tract infection have the familiar clinical picture of dysuria, fever, flank or suprapubic tenderness, elevated leukocyte count, and abnormal urinalysis. In many others, these signs and symptoms are obscured by the rest of the clinical picture. For instance, a postoperative patient may be expected to have abdominal tenderness, an elevated leukocyte count, and fever. The physician should consider the entire clinical setting before embarking on a course of therapy.

Diagnosis

Diagnosis is generally made on the basis of a urine culture, from a "clean catch" or through a catheter, but the initial urinalysis is extremely helpful. Pyuria is expected in any nongranulocytopenic patient with a urinary tract infection. Gram's stain of urinary sediment can direct antibiotic therapy in advance of the culture results.

A common problem confronting the physician is when patients, especially those with indwelling catheters or nephrostomy tubes, have positive urine cultures but do not appear to be ill. Differentiating colonization from invasive infection is never simple and requires clinical judgment. Any patient who is not granulocytopenic should also have pyuria along with positive urine cultures. The absence of pyuria in a patient with a positive urine culture suggests the likelihood of contamination/colonization. From a practical standpoint, in a clinically stable patient, it is reasonable to withhold antibiotics pending repeated urinalysis and urine culture. If an organism persists, therapy should be considered.

Therapy

Therapy should be based on the sensitivity pattern of the recovered organism. The choice of intravenous or oral therapy depends on how sick the patient is.

Optimal duration of therapy in a patient with a urethral stent or a permanent indwelling catheter is often difficult to determine. It is virtually impossible to eradicate an infection in the presence of a foreign body, and removal of the foreign object is the obvious therapy. However, removal is not always feasible. A patient with a urinary tract infection and a foreign body in the urinary collecting system should be considered for chronic suppressive therapy if she has recurrent infection. In general, among patients with gram-negative rods, chronic suppressive therapy may include ampicillin, trimethoprim-sulfamethoxazole, or ciprofloxacin. Patients with a chronic enterococcal infection may benefit from chronic suppressive therapy with amoxicilin–clavulanic acid (Augmentin) or amoxicillin alone.

In patients with pyuria and fever in whom a urinary tract infection is suspected, empiric antibiotic therapy should be given pending urine culture results. Gram's stain of urinary sediment may be helpful in directing treatment. However, for those cases in which Gram's stain is not helpful, broad-spectrum coverage should be given. For a patient who has had frequent or prolonged hospitalizations, effective coverage of potentially resistant gram-negative rods dictates that two drugs be given, preferably a beta-lactam and an aminoglycoside. Cefazolin (1 to 2 g IV, q 8 hours) and gentamicin (4 to 5 mg/kg/day IV in three divided doses) is a good empiric combination for many patients. For more debilitated patients or those with prolonged hospitalizations and frequent past courses of antibiotics, a third-generation cephalosporin, such as ceftazidime (1 to 2 g IV, q 8 hours), should be substituted for cefazolin. After culture results are known, antibiotics can be adjusted and the spectrum narrowed.

For any gynecologic cancer patient with an unexplained predisposition to recurrent urinary tract infection, a full investigation should be undertaken to exclude obstruction from tumor as the cause.

Wound Infections

There are important variables that influence the development of wound infection after surgery. These include hospital flora, patient flora, operative technique and variables, patient nutrition, and immunocompetency. Women being treated for reproductive tract cancer may be at risk because of specific problems with immunocompetency, possible prior chemotherapy or radiotherapy, poor nutritional status, hypoproteinemia, or low socioeconomic status. Additional risk factors for incisional infection include obesity and diabetes. Surgical variables include operative procedures in excess of 4 hours, breaks in surgical technique, excessive inoculum at the operative site, excessive cautery, passive drains, shaving of the area in which the incision is made immediately before surgery, and placement and types of sutures. Infections may range from a mild cellulitis to a devastating fasciitis or a deep infection with myonecrosis.

Cellulitis

Etiology

Cellulitis is a relatively frequent occurrence. The presence of a foreign body in a wound is an unavoidable risk factor in many cases, but this variable should be removed or reduced as much as possible. For example, suture material in the subcutaneous space should be kept to a minimum or not used. If suture is necessary, catgut, silk, and cotton may provoke inflammation, thereby increasing tissue ischemia. Absorbable sutures are much less reactogenic.

Devitalized tissue, especially fat, can also act as a foreign body. Excess cautery causes thermal injury; the charred tissue may act as a foreign body. The presence of significant amounts of devitalized tissue usually produces a wound defect. A mechanical wound retractor can cause fat necrosis, and there appears to be only minimal ability to resorb these areas during wound healing. These areas should be carefully identified and excised before closing the wound. If drains are used, they should be closed, and drains should be vacuumed. Drains should not exit through the wound but rather through an adjacent puncture site, and they should be removed as early as possible.

Staphylococcus aureus is recovered from 50% or more of wound infections. If the operative procedure involves transection of the vagina, the infections may harbor other species of normal flora of the lower reproductive tract, such as gram-positive and gram-negative anaerobes and Enterobacteriaceae.

Cellulitis of the leg occurs with increased frequency in patients after vulvectomy (55). The affected leg is not always edematous. Group B beta-hemolytic streptococci are frequently recovered. Prophylactic therapy with oral penicillin may reduce recurrences in some patients (55).

Signs and Symptoms

Cellulitis is almost uniformly associated with pain and erythema in the incisional margins, with an increase in local skin and tissue temperature, and many times with fever. Incisions are usually tender at examination. Incisional cellulitis may not become evident until the fourth postoperative day or later.

Diagnosis

The infected surgical incision should be explored. This can frequently be performed at the bedside. Opposing skin edges in such incisions are usually separated without difficulty and may expose underlying purulent material, seromas, hematomas, or any combination of these. The wound should be explored thoroughly, and, if the wound shows unusual features, aerobic and anaerobic cultures should be obtained. Foreign bodies such as sutures or drains should be removed, and obviously necrotic areas should be removed after the patient has been given parenteral pain medication. It is important to document deep fascial integrity. If this cannot be done at the bedside, it should be performed in the operating room.

Therapy

The wound should be packed open with fine-mesh gauze approximated to the incisional margins. Gauze is used to fill the intervening spaces after each dressing change. The dressing is changed two to four times daily, with chemical and mechanical débridement of necrotic areas. Commonly used solutions are hydrogen peroxide, acetic acid, and Dakin's solution (0.25% sodium hypochlorite). In general, these débriding solutions should be removed from the wound with sterile normal saline before packing because they may impede healing. Except in unusual instances, it is unnecessary to administer parenteral antimicrobials. These incisions may be left open to heal by secondary intent, or they may be closed before discharge from the hospital after the margins are completely granulated. The optimal time for secondary closure is about the fourth day after institution of wound therapy. Studies have shown that normal wound healing occurs as long as the hematocrit exceeds 17%, but that a lower level will impede healing (56).

Necrotizing Fasciitis

Necrotizing fasciitis is a potentially life-threatening infection of the soft tissues above deep fascia that can involve the abdominal wall or vulva with extension to the proximal thighs and buttocks. There are several descriptive names for this infection, such as beta-hemolytic streptococcal gangrene, hospital gangrene, gram-negative anaerobic cutaneous gangrene, nonclostridial gas gangrene, gangrenous erysipelas, or synergistic necrotizing cellulitis; but the name used by most is that coined by Wilson in 1952; that is, necrotizing fasciitis (57,58).

This significant infection has been reported in patients with endometrial cancer following irradiation and hysterectomy (54,59–61). It has also been found in endopelvic fascia, in a suprapubic catheter site during chemotherapy, in the vulva in diabetes, and after diagnostic laparoscopy (62–66).

Etiology

Bacteria recovered from necrotizing fasciitis infectious sites include anaerobes, particularly *Peptostreptococcus*, *Prevotella*, and *Bacteroides* species, as well as *E. faecalis*, *S. aureus*, and Enterobacteriaceae. These bacteria produce large quantities of proteolytic and other enzymes and toxins that allow rapid spread to contiguous tissues. Superficial vessels are occluded, depriving the affected areas of oxygen, other nutrients, and antibiotics. This deprivation interferes with bacterial eradication. Patients at particularly high risk of developing this infection include women older than 50 years of age and those with arteriosclerotic heart disease, diabetes, or other chronic diseases.

Signs and Symptoms

Early in the course of necrotizing fasciitis, the signs and symptoms are those of any wound cellulitis. Because there is no response to the usual methods of therapy, antibiotic therapy will frequently be initiated. The infection, however, seems to smolder initially, then rapidly progresses to involve the wound and to produce clinical sepsis. Mortality rates for this infection have been as high as 76%. The degree of disease evident on the skin is only a small fraction of the total amount of tissue that is involved because the skin is not the primary area of infection. Hallmarks of this infection include excessive pain, edema that is unusual for the apparently minimal degree of infection, and superficial tissue crepitance. The skin overlying the affected area becomes blue or brown as the disease progresses, and there may be formation of bullae. Edema progresses, and there may be seepage of grayish fluid from the skin, which slips over underlying tissue and does not bleed if cut. Lack of familiarity with this infection and failure to recognize its signs may delay diagnosis. Even when recognized and treated early, there is a high mortality rate.

Diagnosis

Diagnostic criteria as first outlined by Fisher and co-workers include (67):

1. Extensive necrosis of the superficial fascia with widespread undermining of surrounding tissue.
2. A moderate to severe systemic toxic reaction.
3. Absence of muscle involvement.
4. Failure to demonstrate *Clostridium* species in the wound or blood cultures.
5. Absence of major vascular occlusion.
6. Histologic demonstration of intense leukocytic infiltration, focal necrosis of the superficial fascia and surrounding tissues, and microvascular thrombosis characterize this infection.

Early diagnosis followed as soon as possible by appropriate treatment produces the highest cure rate. Radiologic evaluation, particularly with MRI, may confirm the diagnosis rapidly, and should be ordered whenever the disease is suspected. The average interval between diagnosis and initiation of treatment is approximately 5 days. If the interval is 4 days or less, survival rates are high, but an interval of 7 days or more is more likely to result in patient death because even intense antimicrobial therapy is rarely successful at this late stage.

Therapy

Although the administration of broad-spectrum antimicrobials is important, wide and often disfiguring surgical débridement is the treatment required for preservation of life. The excision must extend to areas that bleed. The areas of débridement should be treated as are areas of burns. Adjunctive therapy with whirlpool baths and perhaps hyperbaric oxygen may be of use.

Clostridial Myonecrosis

Clostridial myonecrosis (gas gangrene) was described by Altmeier and Furste (68). It is an infection that occurs in muscle and adjacent tissues beneath the deep fascia and is seen most commonly after trauma. However, it can be seen after intraabdominal surgery or surgery in an area that has been contaminated by feces. Mortality rates are about 25%, and poor-prognosis factors are leukopenia, advanced age, renal failure, and intravascular hemolysis.

Etiology

Clostridial myonecrosis is caused by *Clostridium perfringens* (80% to 95%), *C. novyi* (10% to 40%), or *C. septicum* (5% to 20%). It is usually seen in association with gastrointestinal mucosal ulceration or perforation because *Clostridium* species are normal inhabitants of the gastrointestinal tract. *C. perfringens* may be isolated from as many as 20% of the women with upper genital tract infections not involving sexually transmitted diseases (2). The mere presence of *C. perfringens* in a wound does not mean that the patient will develop gas gangrene; it develops in only 1% to 2% of wounds in which that species can be isolated.

Signs and Symptoms

Early signs and symptoms of clostridial myonecrosis are tense edema in tissue that is extremely tender and pain that rapidly intensifies. If an incision is open, it is not uncommon to see a swollen, herniated muscle. There is frequently a serosanguinous, dirty discharge that has many gram-positive or gram-variable rods but few leukocytes. There may also be gas bubbles, and the secretions have a particularly sweet, offensive odor. The surrounding tissue frequently has crepitus. The skin becomes red to green-purple and then turns yellow before becoming a characteristic bronze color. The usual incubation period is about 2 to 3 days, but it can be as short as 6 hours after the bacterial inoculation. With progression of the infection, the patient becomes obviously ill, pale, and sweaty, with increased pulse rate and decreased blood pressure. Temperature is usually elevated, but hypothermia may occur with shock.

Diagnosis

A positive wound culture may accompany the characteristic signs and symptoms of clostridial myonecrosis. X-ray films of the affected area frequently show gas deep in the tissues. Blood cultures grow clostridia in approximately 15% of the cases. It is common to find a decrease in hemoglobin and an increase in circulating leukocytes. Involved muscle is pale and edematous, with loss of elasticity, and it does not bleed or contract with stimulation. Histologic findings demonstrate coagulation necrosis of muscle fibers.

Therapy

Clostridial myonecrosis is another infection that requires prompt and extensive débridement in the operating room. Cultures must be performed, and because clostridia may develop plasmid-mediated antibiotic-resistance, repeated cultures with sensitivity testing may be required if a patient is slow to respond. In addition to wide débridement, the treatment of choice is penicillin G at a dose of 1 to 2 million units every 2 to 3 hours. Gram's stain also may indicate the presence of gram-negative bacteria, in which case coverage should be provided for those bacteria as well. Chloramphenicol is as effective against *Clostridium* species as it is against many gram-negative species. There has been little clinical experience with metronidazole, imipenem, or clindamycin, all of which have good *in vitro* activity against *C. perfringens*. An alternative is necessary in women who are truly allergic to penicillin. Other antibiotics with good *in vitro* activity include tetracycline, erythromycin, and rifampin. Hyperbaric oxygen may be adjunctive, but its efficacy has been debated.

Central Intravenous Catheter–Related Infections

Etiology

Indwelling central venous catheters (e.g., Broviac, Groshong, Hickman, Mediport) have greatly facilitated the administration of chemotherapeutic agents. However, catheter-related infections and thrombosis continue to be serious problems, causing considerable morbidity and occasional mortality (29,60). Patients often require prolonged and frequent hospitalizations for antibiotic therapy, and the catheter must be removed in about one-third of all catheters placed.

Infection can be introduced in two ways. The overlying skin or the catheter hub may be incompletely sterilized before use. Organisms that colonize the skin, such as *S. epidermidis*, *S. aureus*, *Bacillus* species, or diphtheroid species, may then enter the bloodstream and cause bacteremia. The water or solvent that contains the chemotherapeutic agent, heparin flush, or other infused agent may also be contaminated, resulting in introduction of bacteria into the bloodstream. Organisms that commonly inhabit water, such as *Stenotrophomonas maltophilia*, the *Acinetobacter* species, and the Enterobacteriaceae, should be anticipated in these circumstances.

Recent work has defined a pivotal role for the biofilm, the thin layer of slime that lines the inside of the catheter and/or hub (69). Most antibiotics appear to be unable to penetrate the area; furthermore, bacteria imbedded in the biofilm may slow the pace of their replication cycle, thereby thwarting the activity of those antibiotics that disrupt a certain point in replication.

Signs and Symptoms

Three general syndromes can suggest a catheter-related infection (70). First, the skin around the catheter entry site may become locally inflamed ("exit-site infection"). The patient may complain of pain and purulence and be febrile. Occasionally, the soft-tissue infection extends into the tunnel through which the catheter was burrowed. This infection ("tunnel infection") is more difficult to eradicate. Finally, bacteria introduced through the catheter ("luminal infection") may also cause a bacteremia without evidence of soft-tissue infection. The patient may complain of infusion-associated rigors and high fevers lasting an hour or more. In patients with two or more ports (i.e., on a Broviac catheter), infection may occur in one or both catheter ports.

Peripherally inserted central venous catheters (PICCs) are gaining popularity owing to their ease of insertion and removal. A recent study, however, has suggested that, among patients with various cancers, the complication rate of PICCs is identical to that of other central venous devices (71).

Diagnosis

The diagnosis of an exit-site or tunnel infection is made on clinical grounds. An inflamed, tender area along the tunnel or purulence at the exit site, with or without systemic complaints, should suggest infection. Gram's stain and culture of the site can reveal the infecting organism and allow prompt institution of antibiotic therapy.

Catheter-related, or luminal, bacteremias are diagnosed by blood culture. It is essential that, whenever possible, cultures be taken from peripheral and central sites. In persons with a catheter infection, after 24 hours of systemic therapy via a peripheral venous device, therapy can (and should) be delivered through the infected central catheter. When this is not possible, antibiotics may cautiously be directed through the central catheter at the start of therapy.

Therapy

Therapy should be guided by the Gram's stain and culture results. For patients with exit-site or tunnel infections and gram-positive cocci, vancomycin (1 g IV, q 12 hours) should be given pending sensitivity results. For patients with clinical tunnel infection only, empiric therapy with vancomycin (1 g IV, q 12 hours) should be given. For a patient with presumed catheter-related bacteremia, empiric therapy should be given pending culture results. A combination of antibiotics to cover gram-positive and gram-negative organisms, such as ticarcillin–clavulanic acid (3.1 g IV, q 4 hours), should be given with or without an aminoglycoside, such as gentamicin (3 to 5 mg/kg/day IV in three divided doses) or vancomycin (1 g IV, q 12 hours) with a fluoroquinolone such as ciprofloxacin (400 mg IV, q 12 hours). In patients with presumed catheter infection and chemotherapy-induced neutropenia, empiric therapy should include two agents for gram-negative rods, such as a third-generation cephalosporin and an aminoglycoside (72).

Treatment should continue for at least 7 days after cultures become negative. For patients with *P. aeruginosa*, consideration should be given for longer therapy. In patients with *S. aureus* alone, a possible source other than the catheter should be sought, including evidence of endocarditis, septic arthritis, or osteomyelitis. If an additional site of infection is identified, therapy for *S. aureus* may need to extend to 4 to 6 weeks. Patients who are clinically stable may receive much of their intravenous therapy as outpatients (72).

Intraperitoneal Catheter Infections

Etiology

Delivery of chemotherapeutic agents through an intraperitoneal catheter has enabled physicians to deliver high concentrations of drug locally while decreasing systemic side effects (73). However, intraperitoneal catheters can become infected at the exit site, along the catheter tunnel, or intraperitoneally. *S. epidermidis* is the most common organism found, followed by *S. aureus* and *Streptococcus* species. Gram-negative bacilli and anaerobes, presumably from the bowel, are also found. Patients who have been treated for bacterial peritonitis in the past may develop fungal peritonitis, particularly with *Candida albicans*.

Signs and Symptoms

With exit-site or tunnel infections, patients report discomfort at the site. Patients with peritonitis may complain of diffuse abdominal pain, with or without a change in bowel pattern. Fever may be absent in peritonitis, making the diagnosis more difficult because many patients with pelvic tumor have abdominal pain.

On examination, patients with exit-site or tunnel infections have redness and sometimes have discharge where the catheter has been inserted. Patients with peritonitis have tenderness and frequently have abdominal rebound.

Diagnosis

Diagnosis of exit-site and tunnel infections is made clinically, with support from a Gram's stain and culture of any discharge. Patients with suspected peritonitis should have withdrawal of peritoneal fluid for cell count and microbiologic evaluation. A rough guideline, derived from experience among patients receiving continuous ambulatory peritoneal dialysis, is that any leukocyte count in peritoneal fluid >100 cells/mm^3 suggests infection. Gram's stain and culture should reveal the specific organism.

Chemical peritonitis after instillation of chemotherapy can mimic infectious peritonitis. Differentiation of the two entities requires reliable microbiologic evaluation.

Therapy

Every attempt should be made to treat a patient without removing the central venous catheter, but in some circumstances, the catheter must be removed. In such instances, the catheter removal itself may be curative. If the catheter is removed, a 5- to 7-day course of intravenous antibiotics should be administered after removal. Every attempt should be made to delay insertion of the new catheter until blood cultures have become negative. If the infecting organism is *S. aureus* or *P. aeruginosa*, a longer course should be given.

For exit-site and tunnel infections, intravenous antibiotics are required, usually for 7 to 10 days, but longer for an extensive tunnel infection. Antibiotic choice should be dictated by the recovered organism.

For patients with peritonitis, intraperitoneal and systemic therapy is advised. Antibiotics directed at the recovered organism should be continued 10 days or longer, with serial peritoneal fluid cell counts guiding therapy. Specific doses of intraperitoneal antibiotics should be determined for each patient. The peritoneum provides a large absorptive surface, and antibiotics delivered intraperitoneally readily enter the intravascular space, sometimes causing additive toxic effects if intravenous antibiotics are being given as well.

Treatment of fungal peritonitis is a unique problem. Amphotericin B can cause adhesions if delivered intraperitoneally. Fluconazole, which can be administered orally or intravenously, was shown in one study of patients receiving continuous ambulatory peritoneal dialysis effectively to treat *C. albicans* peritonitis (50). Fluconazole may provide an alternative to amphotericin B among stable patients with fungal peritonitis.

Septic Pelvic Thrombophlebitis

Septic pelvic thrombophlebitis, also known as suppurative pelvic thrombophlebitis, is a disorder that has been diagnosed most frequently after antimicrobial therapy for pelvic infection after cesarean section or septic abortion, but it can be seen as a complication of infection after any type of pelvic surgery. The mortality rate observed in 1917 was 52% after surgical therapy (74). Fortunately, this complication of pelvic infection is now very rare. The use of antimicrobial prophylaxis and the enhanced antibacterial activity of current therapeutic regimens are presumed to be paramount in the disappearance of this potentially lethal infection.

Etiology

Septic pelvic thrombophlebitis is clot formation in the pelvic veins as a result of infection. It can be seen after hysterectomy, other pelvic operative procedures including brachytherapy, and in association with pelvic trauma or perirectal abscess. Classically, there is relative venous stasis before phlebitis that develops adjacent to pelvic infection. The intimal lining of the veins is invaded by bacteria, including Enterobacteriaceae, especially *E. coli*, aerobic and anaerobic streptococci, and *Bacteroides*. The veins involved may be the ovarian, hypogastric, or uterine, with essentially equal involvement in the right and left sides. If common iliac veins are involved, clot formation is more frequently seen on the left for unknown reasons. Infected clot may embolize to the lungs, kidneys, liver, brain, and spleen.

Signs and Symptoms

A clinical diagnosis may not be readily evident. Presentation is essentially that of a fever of unknown cause, and the physician must rule out infections such as pyelonephritis, pneumonia, and pelvic or abdominal abscess. The most frequent presentation currently seen is persistence of fever associated with tachycardia after clinical response to antimicrobial therapy for a pelvic infection. Physical examination is normal in most instances, but it may be possible to palpate tender cords in the vaginal fornices. In patients with bacteremia and septic emboli, chills are observed in as many as 67% of the patients, pyrexia may be elevated to 41°C, and the variations in temperature may be quite hectic. Dyspnea, tachypnea, pleuritic pain, cough, hemoptysis, restlessness, anxiety, and perhaps angina may all be seen with septic embolization.

Diagnosis

Compatible clinical presentation and CT or MRI scan are used for diagnosis (75). Criteria for diagnosis of venous thrombosis using CT studies include enlargement of the involved vein(s), sharply defined vessel walls enhanced by contrast media, and a low-density intraluminal mass (76). Diagnosis using MRI is based on intense intraluminal signals from clot in involved veins and a lack of signal with normal blood flow in uninvolved vessels; no contrast agent is needed. Blood culture should be performed if there is suspicion of septicemia. Tests for blood gases, a chest radiograph, and a ventilation-perfusion scan should be performed if there is suspicion of embolization. A gallium scintiscan may be necessary to identify very small septic embolic foci in the lungs.

Therapy

Early treatment of venous thrombosis was surgical (74). The first to advocate the use of anticoagulants in addition to antibiotics were Schulman and Zatuchni (77). There are cases in the literature in which patients with this diagnosis were successfully treated by antibiotics alone (78).

Heparin therapy regimens include 5,000 U subcutaneously every 4 hours or every 8 hours, 6,000 U IV every 6 hours, and continuous IV infusion after a bolus, with dose determined by clotting times two to three times the control values after steady state has been reached (4 to 8 hours). In the largest published study of heparin therapy, the mean time to become afebrile was 2.5 days, and the average duration of heparin therapy was 8 days (79,80). It was unnecessary to initiate warfarin sodium (Coumadin) therapy in patients without evidence of emboli. Thromboembolism during or after treatment with heparin was not reported. Antibiotic therapy must be continued. If there is significant improvement in the pulse rate and temperature pattern within 12 to 48 hours after addition of heparin, reassessment is mandatory. Treatment with low molecular weight heparin has not been studied or standardized for this condition (81).

Heparin therapy is not without complications. Between 2% and 5% of patients may have an allergic reaction; bleeding occurs in 7% to 10% of patients; and the most devastating effect is the development of the ''white clot syndrome'' (82). This occurs in <1% of patients, but it may be associated with major limb amputation in 20% of those suffering from it, and death has been reported for 50%. This phenomenon is a paradoxical arterial platelet aggregation associated with thrombocytopenia, and it should be suspected in patients with decreasing platelet counts or an increasing requirement of heparin to maintain adequate anticoagulation.

The only current indications for surgical intervention are embolization during heparin therapy or lack of response. The usual intervention is placement of a vena cava filter, which is a procedure usually performed by an interventional radiologist.

Osteomyelitis

Osteomyelitis of the pelvis can occur by direct extension in a patient with chronic pelvic infection. Severe pain, especially with ambulation, may suggest this diagnosis. Platelet count, leukocyte count, and erythrocyte sedimentation rate may be elevated. Bone scans can suggest the diagnosis, although the results may be misleading in patients with metastatic disease. An accurate diagnosis requires a bone biopsy and culture, with therapy being directed at the organism that is isolated. Therapy should continue for at least 6 weeks.

Neutropenia and Fever

Etiology

Chemotherapy very commonly induces prolonged neutropenia, placing patients at high risk for bacteremia (83). These patients have a particular risk for severe morbidity and mortality unless empiric intravenous antibiotic therapy is instituted at the first evidence of fever or clinical worsening.

Most commonly, the febrile neutropenic patient does not have an obvious source of fever. Even in those with bacteremia, the source is rarely clinically evident. Bacteria often enter the bloodstream through the gastrointestinal tract because of the small chemotherapy-induced ulcerations of the intestinal mucosa and the accompanying neutropenia and thrombocytopenia. Neutropenic patients may also develop a clinically diagnosed group of infections, including pneumonia and cellulitis. Neutropenic patients with these clinically diagnosed infections may progress very rapidly, may have exceedingly subtle clinical signs and symptoms, and always require early, aggressive therapy of their infections to achieve a response.

The remainder of this discussion considers only neutropenic patients without a clinically obvious source of fever.

Signs and Symptoms

Fever is often the only complaint of patients with neutropenia and bacteremia. Patients receiving chemotherapy should be instructed to take their own temperature at home twice a day (more frequently if a subjective feeling of fever develops) and to contact their treating physician for temperatures above 38.0°C or 100.4°F.

Diagnosis

Diagnosis is made by blood culture. Of all febrile, neutropenic patients from whom blood cultures are obtained, only 10% to 20% have an organism isolated (20). The others probably have enough organisms to cause fever and illness, but an insufficient load of organisms to be cultivated using current techniques.

A review of episodes of bacteremia from Memorial Sloan–Kettering Cancer Center revealed that the most common organisms isolated in the febrile, neutropenic host were E. coli (16%), Klebsiella species (15%), and Pseudomonas species (8%). Polymicrobic cultures, including E. coli, S. aureus, and Clostridium species, accounted for 21%, and S. aureus accounted for 6% (84). These results demonstrate the prevalence of enteric gram-negative rods as pathogens in the febrile, neutropenic cancer patient (Table 31.5). However, gram-positive coccal (particularly enterococci) and rod infections are also important in this group of patients. Many

TABLE 31.5. *Bacteria commonly recovered from neutropenic patients*

Gram-negative organisms
Echerichia coli
Klebsiella spp
Pseudomonas aeruginosa
Enterobacter spp
Gram-positive organisms
Staphylococcus aureus
Coagulase-negative *Staphylococcus* (*epidermidis* and *saprophyticus*)
Streptococcus pneumoniae
Group A beta-hemolytic streptococci
Viridans streptococci
Enterococcus faecalis
Corynebacterium spp

spp, species.
Modified with permission from Gordon AN, Martens M, LaPread Y, Faro S. Response of lower genital tract flora to external pelvic irradi ation. *Gynecol Oncol* 1989;35:233.

of these isolates are relatively resistant and require intravenous vancomycin (85).

Therapy

The Infectious Disease Society of America (IDSA) updates guidelines for management of the patient with fever and neutropenia. Full consideration of this complex topic is beyond the scope of this chapter (20). In general, however, a febrile, neutropenic patient should receive antibiotics with activity against *P. aeruginosa* pending results of blood cultures. Numerous regimens are effective, and their use should be determined according to sensitivity patterns for *P. aeruginosa* at a given hospital. In general, good results have been achieved with a beta-lactam antibiotic (e.g., semisynthetic penicillin such as ticarcillin–clavulanic acid or a third/fourth-generation cephalosporin such as ceftazidime or cefipime) or a carbapenem (imipenem or meropenem) with or without an aminoglycoside (Table 31.3).

Monitoring peak and trough levels of aminoglycosides is recommended to limit ototoxicity and nephrotoxicity. The choice of the specific aminoglycoside (e.g., gentamicin, tobramycin, amikacin) is dictated by the sensitivity patterns in a given hospital. Once-daily dosing of aminoglycosides is not recommended for the neutropenic patient but can be given in other settings.

The length of therapy for neutropenic patients is determined by many factors and must be individualized. Patients with prolonged neutropenia and fever should be followed by an infectious disease specialist.

Fungal Infections

Etiology

Patients with pelvic cancer may be at risk for the development of fungal infections, particularly those caused by *Candida* species, including *C. albicans*, *C. tropicalis*, *C. parapsilosis*, and *C. glabrata* (86). Infection may include fungemia, pelvic abscess, or infected urinary stents in a patient with extensive pelvic disease and urinary outflow obstruction.

Risk factors for the development of invasive candidiasis include prolonged courses (7 to 10 days) of intravenous broad-spectrum antibiotics; an intravenous catheter, particularly a central venous catheter; major abdominal surgery; prolonged neutrocytopenia, usually related to chemotherapy; and immunosuppressive therapy, especially with corticosteroids (87).

Signs and Symptoms

Patients with the appropriate risk factors who have unexplained fevers may be fungemic. Other than fevers, which can include rigors and hypotension and closely resemble bacteremia, there may be no other symptoms. Blood cultures are positive in only 50% of the patients with autopsy-proven disseminated candidiasis. Any blood culture positive for a yeast should be considered to be significant. A full evaluation for a hidden source should be completed, including a thorough reevaluation with history and physical examination, and appropriate laboratory tests that include repeat blood cultures. An ophthalmoscopic examination to exclude endophthalmitis should be performed since this complication may occur in up to 15% of patients with fungemia.

Much has been written suggesting that any patient with *Candida* species cultured from three sites (i.e., sputum, urine, wound) should be considered to have invasive disease and treated accordingly. Although somewhat helpful, antifungal therapy in all patients meeting this criterion should not be initiated until a full evaluation is performed. In many cases, no antifungal therapy will be required.

Candida species may cause urinary tract infection in a patient with such indwelling devices as a Foley catheter, internal stents, or percutaneous nephrostomies. Rarely a "fungus ball," consisting of a matted mass of yeast, may cause urinary obstruction.

Candida species almost never cause pneumonia except as a preterminal event in a critically ill intensive care unit patient. Thus, recovery of any yeast from a respiratory specimen should be considered to be most likely due to oral thrush contaminating the culture. In contrast, identification of a mold, such as *Aspergillus*, is an extremely serious finding that, thankfully, is quite unusual among gynecologic cancer patients.

Diagnosis

The diagnosis of a fungal infection is often quite difficult. The physician must differentiate between invasive disease, which must be treated, and colonization, which does not require therapy. The recovery of fungi from a urine, sputum, or wound culture does not necessarily mean that the fungus is pathogenic, and clinical judgment must be used to determine if a patient requires therapy. In general, cultures from sterile sites (e.g., blood, cerebrospinal fluid, pleural or peritoneal fluid) should be considered to represent invasive infection until a full evaluation is done. Also, fungi recovered from the initial specimen of drainage from an obstructed biliary or urinary tract should be considered to be pathogenic.

With most specimens however, the distinction between colonization and infection is not so simple. For urine, the presence or absence of pyuria is the simplest and most reliable means of differentiation: Those without pyuria are very likely only colonized and need no therapy. In such patients, a repeat urinalysis and culture may clarify the situation.

Therapy

Treatment options for fungal infections have expanded in recent years. Amphotericin B and associated amphotericin

B products (AmBisome and Ablecet) have the longest record for treatment of invasive fungal infections (86). The optimal duration of therapy for candidemia is not well defined and should be determined by individual responses. However, a 7- to 14-day course of therapy is probably adequate for most episodes (86).

In addition to amphotericin B products, both intravenous fluconazole therapy (400 mg daily) and caspofungin (70-mg load and then 50 daily IV) are very effective for nonneutropenic patients with fungemia (88,89). These agents offer comparable effectiveness but have fewer side effects than the amphotericin B products.

Patients who have *Candida* species consistently cultured from urine but no evidence of systemic fungal infection may benefit from bladder irrigation with amphotericin B. Given through a triple-lumen urinary catheter, daily infusion of 50 mg of amphotericin B in 1 L of fluid may eradicate the bladder colonization and prevent invasive fungal infection. Fluconazole is increasingly being given for this indication and appears to effective.

Pneumonia

Etiology

Postoperative pneumonia remains a common cause of fever in any surgical patient, including those with gynecologic cancer. Infection may occur from aspiration during intubation or extubation or from hypoaeration due to "splinting" in patients with severe postoperative pain. Postobstructive pneumonia may occur in patients with tumor metastatic to the lungs. In addition, pneumonia may occur in patients with chemotherapy-induced neutropenia (see above).

Signs and Symptoms

The familiar signs and symptoms of pneumonia are cough, fever, chest discomfort, and dyspnea and evidence of pulmonary consolidation on lung examination.

Diagnosis

The diagnosis is usually suggested by the clinical situation and by the findings on physical examination. These are further supported by chest radiographs and sputum examination and culture. Chest radiography may show consolidation. Gram-negative organisms predominate in the mouth flora of hospitalized patients, so an aspiration pneumonia occurring in a hospitalized patient is typically due to gram-negative rods. Although thought by many to be a substantial contributor, anaerobes seldom cause aspiration pneumonia in the hospital.

Therapy

Empiric, rather than pathogen-based, coverage of a postoperative patient with clinical pneumonia is usually necessary and varies according to the setting (90). For a patient who has been hospitalized less than 3 days and has had no other recent hospitalizations or recent courses of oral or intravenous antibiotics, single-drug therapy with levofloxacin or gatifloxacin is adequate (90). For the patient who has been hospitalized for a longer period or who has received recent antibiotics (increasing the likelihood of infection due to resistant organisms), *P. aeruginosa* should be covered by the addition of an aminoglycoside such as gentamicin (3 to 5 mg/kg/day in three divided doses), and a beta-lactam should be selected to cover the usual isolates in that hospital. Therapy should extend up to 10 days depending on clinical response. Various professional societies have codified recommendations for pneumonia management (91).

GASTROENTEROLOGIC SOURCES OF INFECTION

Diarrhea Associated with Antibiotics or Chemotherapy

Etiology

Diarrhea due to *C. difficile* can develop in patients who have received antibiotics or chemotherapy alone (92,93).

Signs and Symptoms

Antibiotic-associated diarrhea can occur at any time during an antibiotic course and for at least a month after discontinuation. Patients typically develop abdominal pain, fever, and frequent watery diarrhea; however, *C. difficile* colitis may sometimes cause abdominal pain and fever without diarrhea.

Diagnosis

Any patient with antibiotic- or chemotherapy-associated diarrhea should have a full evaluation of stool, including routine cultures and a test for evidence of *C. difficile* toxin (94). In patients with a highly suspicious clinical presentation but no evidence of *C. difficile* toxin in stool, sigmoidoscopy or colonoscopy may reveal the pathognomonic mucosal pseudomembranes. One study has suggested that evaluation of stool for *C. difficile* toxin is the only cost-effective test (92). A markedly elevated white blood cell count may also be a clue to diagnosis (95).

Therapy

Oral therapy with metronidazole (250 to 500 qid for 7 to 10 days) is adequate to treat most cases of antibiotic-associated diarrhea. Because of continued reports of vancomycin-resistant bacteria (96), the use of oral vancomycin is restricted in many hospitals. Oral vancomycin should be given only to patients with proven *C. difficile* diarrhea who have not responded to metronidazole. Some patients may require repeated or prolonged courses of metronidazole, particularly if their clinical course necessitates continuation of the provocative agent (i.e., continued antibiotics or chemotherapy). Antidiarrheal compounds such as Lomotil or Imodium should not be given routinely. If, however, diarrhea persists after appropriate tests and cultures, symptomatic therapy should be considered.

NONINFECTIOUS CAUSES OF FEVER

Not all patients with gynecologic malignancy and fever have an infection. Pulmonary embolus, drug-related fever, and tumor-related fever represent the main noninfectious sources of fever, but others, such as factitious fever and underlying collagen vascular disorder, must also be considered. The use of procalcitonin and neopterin levels may help distinguish between infected and noninfected patients (97).

Pulmonary embolus should be considered in a bed-bound or postoperative patient with any combination of fever, chest pain, dyspnea, or an abnormal chest radiograph. Patients with bulky pelvic tumors are also at risk. Diagnosis is notoriously difficult, although introduction of the "spiral chest CT" has sharply decreased the need for pulmonary angiograms. Therapy remains anticoagulation with heparin (usually low molecular weight) and then Coumadin. For patients who are unable to tolerate these drugs or who continue to have emboli despite therapy, an inferior vena cava umbrella may be required.

Any antibiotic may cause fever (98). Patients typically develop fever and a diffuse maculopapular rash after several days of therapy. Eosinophilia, although a helpful sign, is usually lacking. Mild elevations in liver function tests may be present. Atypical presentations of drug fever, including patients without rash or those who develop fever weeks into therapy or after completion of therapy, can also occur. The diagnosis is usually made by discontinuing the drug believed to be provocative and observing the patient. It is important to remember that some drug fevers may take as long as a week to resolve. Supportive measures, such as antipyretics and antipruritics, may decrease symptoms.

The diagnosis of tumor fever can be made only after systematic exclusion of all other potential causes of fever. Most patients with tumor fever have metastatic disease in the liver or lung. The fever may be as high as 40°C and accompanied by chills. The patient often feels relatively well if not febrile. Often, in a patient suspected of having tumor fever, a clinical trial of broad-spectrum antibiotics is given. If the fever does not abate and no other clear source is evident, the likelihood of tumor fever increases.

REFERENCES

1. Bartlett JG, et al. Quantitative bacteriology of the vaginal flora. *J Infect Dis* 1977;136(2):271–277.
2. Swenson RM, et al. Anaerobic bacterial infections of the female genital tract. *Obstet Gynecol* 1973;42:538–541.
3. Gilstrap LC 3rd, et al. Genital aerobic bacterial flora of women receiving radiotherapy for gynecologic malignancy. *Gynecol Oncol* 1986;23:35–39.
4. Gordon AN, et al. Response of lower genital tract flora to external pelvic irradiation. *Gynecol Oncol* 1989;35:233–235.
5. Gleeson NC, et al. Externalized Groshong catheters and Hickman ports for central venous access in gynecologic oncology patients. *Gynecol Oncol* 1993;51:372–376.
6. Nelson BE, et al. Experience with the intravenous totally implanted port in patients with gynecologic malignancies. *Gynecol Oncol* 1994;53:98–102.
7. Kolb BA, et al. Effects of early postoperative chemotherapy on wound healing. *Obstet Gynecol* 1992;79:988–992.
8. Widholm O, Mattsson T. Urinary tract infections in association with radium therapy for gynecological cancer. *Acta Obstet Gynecol Scand* 1972;51:247–250.
9. Brooker DC, et al. Infectious morbidity in gynecologic cancer. *Am J Obstet Gynecol* 1987;156:513–520.
10. Morgan LS, Daly JW, Monif GR. Infectious morbidity associated with pelvic exenteration. *Gynecol Oncol* 1980;10:318–328.
11. Neu HC. The crisis in antibiotic resistance. *Science* 1992;257:1064–1073.
12. Chang S, et al. Infection with vancomycin-resistant Staphylococcus aureus containing the vanA resistance gene. *N Engl J Med* 2003;348:1342–7.
13. Roy S, et al. Ertapenem once a day versus piperacillin-tazobactam every 6 hours for treatment of acute pelvic infections: a prospective, multicenter, randomized, double-blind study. *Infect Dis Obstet Gynecol* 2003;11:27–37.
14. Fishman A, et al. Aztreonam plus piperacillin—empiric treatment of neutropenic fever in gynecology-oncology patients receiving cisplatin-based chemotherapy. *Eur J Gynaecol Oncol* 1998;19:126–129.
15. King DE, Malone R, Lilley SH, New classification and update on the quinolone antibiotics. *Am Fam Physician* 2000;61:2741–2748.
16. Donskey CJ, et al. Effect of antibiotic therapy on the density of vancomycin-resistant enterococci in the stool of colonized patients. *N Engl J Med* 2000;343:1925–1932.
17. Kasten MJ, Clindamycin, metronidazole, and chloramphenicol. *Mayo Clin Proc* 1999; 74:825–833.
18. Lautenbach E, et al. The role of chloramphenicol in the treatment of bloodstream infection due to vancomycin-resistant Enterococcus. *Clin Infect Dis* 1998;27:1259–1265.
19. Frieden TR, et al. Emergence of vancomycin-resistant enterococci in New York City. *Lancet* 1993;342:76–79.
20. Hughes WT, et al. 1997 guidelines for the use of antimicrobial agents in neutropenic patients with unexplained fever. Infectious Diseases Society of America. *Clin Infect Dis* 1997;25:551–573.
21. Ali M, Goetz MB. A meta-analysis of the relative efficacy and toxicity of single daily dosing versus multiple daily dosing of aminoglycosides. *Clin Infect Dis* 1997;24:796–809.
22. Barza M, et al. Single or multiple daily doses of aminoglycosides: a meta-analysis. *BMJ* 1996;312:338–345.
23. Mitra AG, et al. A randomized, prospective study comparing once-daily gentamicin versus thrice-daily gentamicin in the treatment of puerperal infection. *Am J Obstet Gynecol* 1997; 177:786–792.
24. Ledger WJ, Gee C, Lewis WP. Guidelines for antibiotic prophylaxis in gynecology. *Am J Obstet Gynecol* 1975;121:1038–1045.
25. Velasco E, et al. Risk factors for infectious complications after abdominal surgery for malignant disease. *Am J Infect Control* 1996;24:1–6.
26. Blythe JG. Cervical bacterial flora in patients with gynecologic malignancies. *Am J Obstet Gynecol* 1978;131:438–445.
27. Mead PB. Cervical-vaginal flora of women with invasive cervical cancer. *Obstet Gynecol* 1978;52:601–604.
28. Creasman WT, et al. A trial of prophylactic cefamandole in extended gynecologic surgery. *Obstet Gynecol* 1982;59:309–314.
29. Hemsell DL, et al. Preventing major operative site infection after radical abdominal hysterectomy and pelvic lymphadenectomy. *Gynecol Oncol* 1989;35:55–60.
30. Thadepalli H, et al. Cyclic changes in cervical microflora and their effect on infections following hysterectomy. *Gynecol Obstet Invest* 1982;14:176–183.

31. Bell JG, SB. Prophylactic antibiotics in radical gynecology surgery. *Contemp Obstet Gynecol* 1985;26:57.

32. Mann WJ Jr, et al. Perioperative influences on infectious morbidity in radical hysterectomy. *Gynecol Oncol* 1981;11:207–212.

33. Gussman D, RJ, Carlson JA Jr. Prophylaxis for radical hysterectomy. *Infect Surg* 1987;6: 55.

34. Rosenshein NB, et al. A prospective randomized study of doxycycline as a prophylactic antibiotic in patients undergoing radical hysterectomy. *Gynecol Oncol* 1983;15:201–206.

35. Marsden DE, et al. Factors affecting the incidence of infectious morbidity after radical hysterectomy. *Am J Obstet Gynecol* 1985;152: 817–821.

36. Sevin BU, et al. Antibiotic prevention of infections complicating radical abdominal hysterectomy. *Obstet Gynecol* 1984;64:539–545.

37. Micha JP, et al. Prophylactic mezlocillin in radical hysterectomy. *Obstet Gynecol* 1987;69: 251–254.

38. Sevin BU, et al. Comparative efficacy of short-term versus long-term cefoxitin prophylaxis against postoperative infection after radical hysterectomy: a prospective study. *Obstet Gynecol* 1991:77:729–734.

39. van Lindert AC, et al. Single-dose prophylaxis with broad-spectrum penicillins (piperacillin and mezlocillin) in gynecologic oncological surgery, with observation on serum and tissue concentrations. *Eur J Obstet Gynecol Reprod Biol* 1990;36:137–145.

40. Hemsell DL, et al. Cefazolin for hysterectomy prophylaxis. *Obstet Gynecol* 1990;76: 603–606.

41. Smith CV, GD, Gibbs RL, et al. Oral doxycycline vs. parenteral cefazolin: prophylaxis for vaginal hysterectomy. *Infect Surg* 1989;99:64.

42. Turner, S., The effect of penicillin vaginal suppositories on morbidity in vaginal hysterectomy and on the vaginal flora. *Am J Obstet Gynecol* 1950;60:806.

43. Wright VC, Lanning MN, Natale R. Use of a topical antibiotic spray in vaginal surgery. *Can Med Assoc J* 1978;118:1395–1398.

44. Shapiro M, et al. Risk factors for infection at the operative site after abdominal or vaginal hysterectomy. *N Engl J Med* 1982;307: 1661–1666.

45. Hemsell DL, et al. Alterations in lower reproductive tract flora after single-dose piperacillin and triple-dose cefoxitin at vaginal and abdominal hysterectomy. *Obstet Gynecol* 1988;72:875–880.

46. Faro S, et al. Antibiotic prophylaxis: is there a difference? *Am J Obstet Gynecol* 1990; 162:900–907; Discussion 907–909.

47. Hemsell DL, et al. Single-dose cephalosporin for prevention of major pelvic infection after vaginal hysterectomy: cefazolin versus cefoxitin versus cefotaxime. *Am J Obstet Gynecol* 1987;156:1201–1205.

48. Hemsell DL, Johnson ER, Hemsell PG, et al. Cefazolin inferior to cefotetan for single-dose prophylaxis in women undergoing hysterectomy. *Clin Infect Dis* 1995;20:677.

49. Kobayamatsu Y, et al. Evaluation of the improvement of cephems on the prophylaxis of pelvic infection after radical hysterectomy. *Gynecol Obstet Invest* 1991;32:10102–6.

50. Nichols RL, Condon RE. Preoperative preparation of the colon. *Surg Gynecol Obstet* 1971;132:323–337.

51. Braverman J, et al. Spontaneous clostridia gas gangrene of uterus associated with endometrial malignancy. *Am J Obstet Gynecol* 1987;156: 1205–1207.

52. Douvier S, et al. Infectious pneumoperitoneum as an uncommon presentation of endometrial carcinoma: report of two cases. *Gynecol Oncol* 1989;33:392–394.

53. Weinstein WM, et al. Experimental intra-abdominal abscesses in rats: development of an experimental model. *Infect Immun* 1974;10: 1250–1255.

54. McNeeley SG Jr, et al. Infection on a gynecologic oncology service. *Gynecol Oncol* 1990; 37:183–187.

55. Bouma J, Dankert J. Recurrent acute leg cellulitis in patients after radical vulvectomy. *Gynecol Oncol* 1988;29:50–57.

56. Hunt TK, Rabkin J, von Smitten K. Effects of edema and anemia on wound healing and infection. *Curr Stud Hematol Blood Transfus* 1986; 53:101–113.

57. Bahary CM, Joel-Cohen SJ, Neri A. Necrotizing fasciitis. *Obstet Gynecol* 1977;50:633–637.

58. Wilson B. Necrotizing fascitits. *Am Surg* 1952;18:416.

59. Daly JW, King CR, Monif GR. Progressive necrotizing wound infections in postirradiated patients. *Obstet Gynecol* 1978;52[Suppl]:5S–8S.

60. Henderson W. Synergistic bacterial gangrene abdominal hysterectomy. *Obstet Gynecol* 1977:49:24S.

61. Husseinzadeh N, et al. Spontaneous occurrence of synergistic bacterial gangrene following external pelvic irradiation. *Obstet Gynecol* 1984; 63:859–862.

62. Bearman DM, Livengood CH 3rd, Addison WA. Necrotizing fasciitis arising from a suprapubic catheter site. A case report. *J Reprod Med* 1988;33:411–413.

63. Hoffman MS, Turnquist D. Necrotizing fasciitis of the vulva during chemotherapy. *Obstet Gynecol* 1989;74:483–484.

64. Roberts D. Necrotizing fasciitis of the vulva. *Am J Obstet Gynecol* 1987;157:568.

65. Pruyn SC. Acute necrotizing fasciitis of the endopelvic fascia. *Obstet Gynecol* 1978;52[Suppl]:25–45.

66. Sotrel G, Hirsch E, Edelin KC. Necrotizing fasciitis following diagnostic laparoscopy. *Obstet Gynecol* 1983;62[3 Suppl]:67s–69s.

67. Fisher JR, et al. Necrotizing fasciitis. Importance of roentgenographic studies for soft-tissue gas. *JAMA* 1979;241:803–806.

68. Altmeier WA. Gas gangrene. *Surg Gynecol Obstet* 1947;84:504.

69. Donlan RM, Costerton JW. Biofilms: survival mechanisms of clinically relevant microorganisms. *Clin Microbiol Rev* 2002;15:167–193.

70. Benezra D, et al. Prospective study of infections in indwelling central venous catheters using quantitative blood cultures. *Am J Med* 1988; 85:495–498.

71. Walshe LJ, et al. Complication rates among cancer patients with peripherally inserted central catheters. *J Clin Oncol* 2002;20:3276–3281.

72. O'Grady NP, et al. Guidelines for the prevention of intravascular catheter-related infections. *Infect Control Hosp Epidemiol* 2002;23: 759–769.

73. Sakuragi N, et al. Complications relating to intraperitoneal administration of cisplatin or carboplatin for ovarian carcinoma. *Gynecol Oncol* 2000;79:420–423.

74. Miller C. Ligation or excision of the pelvic veins in the treatment of puerperal pyaemia. *Surg Gynecol Obstet* 1917;25:431.

75. Twickler DM, et al. Imaging of puerperal septic thrombophlebitis: prospective comparison of MR imaging, CT, and sonography. *AJR Am J Roentgenol* 1997;169:1039–1043.

76. Zerhouni EA, Barth KH, Siegelman SS. Demonstration of venous thrombosis by computed tomography. *AJR Am J Roentgenol* 1980;134: 753–758.

77. Schulman H, ZG. Pelvic thrombophlebitis in the puerperal and postoperative gynecology patient. *Am J Obstet Gynecol* 1964;90:1293.

78. Brown CE, et al. Puerperal pelvic thrombophlebitis: impact on diagnosis and treatment using x-ray computed tomography and magnetic resonance imaging. *Obstet Gynecol* 1986;68:789–794.

79. Josey WE, Staggers SR Jr. Heparin therapy in septic pelvic thrombophlebitis: a study of 46 cases. *Am J Obstet Gynecol* 1974;120:228–233.

80. Brown CE, et al. Puerperal septic pelvic thrombophlebitis: incidence and response to heparin therapy. *Am J Obstet Gynecol* 1999;181: 143–148.

81. Lee AY, et al. Low-molecular-weight heparin versus a coumarin for the prevention of recurrent venous thromboembolism in patients with cancer. *N Engl J Med* 2003;349:146–153.

82. Stanton PE Jr, et al. White clot syndrome. *South Med J* 1988;81: 616–620.

83. Bodey GP, et al. Quantitative relationships between circulating leukocytes and infection in patients with acute leukemia. *Ann Intern Med* 1966;64:328–340.

84. Whimbey E, et al. Bacteremia and fungemia in patients with neoplastic disease. *Am J Med* 1987;82:723–730.

85. Shenep JL, et al. Vancomycin, ticarcillin, and amikacin compared with ticarcillin-clavulanate and amikacin in the empirical treatment of febrile, neutropenic children with cancer. *N Engl J Med* 1988;319: 1053–1058.

86. Rex JH, et al. Practice guidelines for the treatment of candidiasis. Infectious Diseases Society of America. *Clin Infect Dis* 2000;30:662–678.

87. Marsh PK, et al. Candida infections in surgical patients. *Ann Surg* 1983; 198:42–47.

88. Rex JH, et al. A randomized trial comparing fluconazole with amphotericin B for the treatment of candidemia in patients without neutropenia. Candidemia Study Group and the National Institute. *N Engl J Med* 1994;331:1325–1330.

89. Mora-Duarte J, et al. Comparison of caspofungin and amphotericin B for invasive candidiasis. *N Engl J Med* 2002;347:2020–2029.

90. Marik PE. Aspiration pneumonitis and aspiration pneumonia. *N Engl J Med* 2001;344: 665–671.

91. Bartlett JG, et al. Community-acquired pneumonia in adults: guidelines for management. The Infectious Diseases Society of America. *Clin Infect Dis* 1998;26:811–838.

92. Cirisano FD, et al. The etiology and management of diarrhea in the gynecologic oncology patient. *Gynecol Oncol* 1993;50:45–48.

93. Satin AJ, et al. Relapsing Clostridium difficile toxin-associated colitis in ovarian cancer patients treated with chemotherapy. *Obstet Gynecol* 1989;74:487–489.

94. Turgeon DK, et al. Six rapid tests for direct detection of Clostridium difficile and its toxins in fecal samples compared with the fibroblast cytotoxicity assay. *J Clin Microbiol* 2003; 41:667–670.

95. Wanahita A, Goldsmith EA, Musher DM. Conditions associated with leukocytosis in a tertiary care hospital, with particular attention to the role of infection caused by clostridium difficile. *Clin Infect Dis* 2002; 34:1585–1592.

96. Low DE, et al. Clinical prevalence, antimicrobial susceptibility, and geographic resistance patterns of enterococci: results from the SENTRY Antimicrobial Surveillance Program, 1997–1999. *Clin Infect Dis* 2001;32[Suppl 2]:S133–S145.

97. Ruokonen E, et al. Procalcitonin and neopterin as indicators of infection in critically ill patients. *Acta Anaesthesiol Scand* 2002;46:398–404.

98. Hirschmann J.V. Fever of unknown origin in adults. *Clin Infect Dis* 1997;24:291–300; Quiz 301–302.

CHAPTER 32

Management of Late Effects of Gynecologic Cancer Treatment

David G. Mutch, Perry W. Grigsby, Maurie Markman, and Stephen C. Rubin

The treatment of a serious illness such as cancer always involves the judicious search for a proper balance between efficacy and toxicity. Although we strive to maximize cure and minimize side effects, a certain acceptable level of treatment-related complications is unavoidable. This chapter reviews the management of the late complications of the major therapeutic modalities used in cancer treatment: chemotherapy, radiation therapy, and surgery. Although the distinction between the acute and late complications of therapy is arbitrary, we consider late toxic effects to be those that initially become clinically evident more than several months after the initiation of therapy.

CHEMOTHERAPY

Anemia, myelosuppression, and thrombocytopenia, which are among the most common acute complications of chemotherapy, may persist for months after the completion of treatment. In general, a delay in return of marrow function to normal does not imply that the patient will experience any long-term hematopoietic effects of treatment. However, if the patient requires future treatment with marrow-toxic drugs, it is likely that the marrow reserve will be limited.

Myelodysplastic Syndrome and Acute Nonlymphocytic Leukemia

Perhaps the most feared long-term complication of the administration of chemotherapeutic agents is the potential

D. G. Mutch: Division of Gynecologic Oncology, Washington University School of Medicine, St. Louis, Missouri 63110

P. W. Grigsby: Mallinckrodt Institute of Radiology, Washington University School of Medicine, St. Louis, Missouri 63110

M. Markman: Department of Hematology and Medical Oncology, The Cleveland Clinic Foundation, Cleveland, Ohio 44195

S. C. Rubin: Division of Gynecologic Oncology, University of Pennsylvania Medical Center, Philadelphia, Pennsylvania 19104

for the development of myelodysplasia and acute leukemia. Although first recognized more than a decade ago in patients with ovarian cancer treated with alkylating agents, it is now clearly documented that the *chronic* administration of this class of antineoplastic agents is associated with roughly a tenfold increased risk for the development of acute nonlymphocytic leukemia (1,2). Granulocytic leukemia is not a common disease; only approximately 12,000 cases are diagnosed in the United States each year. The peak incidence of secondary leukemia occurs 4 to 5 years after chemotherapy administration; an increased risk is noted for at least 8 years after the cessation of cytotoxic drug treatment.

Survival after the diagnosis of treatment-related acute nonlymphocytic leukemia is generally measured in months. Specific antileukemia therapy, although occasionally of clinical benefit, is usually unsuccessful in producing complete or long-lasting remission. In many patients with this clinical syndrome, it is most appropriate that the management plan involves supportive and comfort measures only (i.e., transfusions, antibiotic therapy, pain medications).

Current chemotherapy for gynecologic or other malignancies is quite different from the prolonged alkylating agent therapy reported to result in an unacceptably high incidence of acute leukemia. In ovarian cancer, studies have demonstrated that five or six treatment cycles or more prolonged treatment regimens produce equivalent therapeutic results (response rates and survival) (3,4). With fewer courses, both short-term (marrow suppression, emesis) and chronic side effects, including the risk of acute leukemia, should be reduced.

Because the majority of reports that estimated the risk of secondary leukemia after cytotoxic drug therapy in ovarian cancer were from the precisplatin chemotherapy era, an association between cisplatin and leukemia remains unsettled (5–10). One report has suggested the use of cisplatin in ovarian cancer may increase the risk for the development of acute leukemia by approximately fourfold (11). However, it is important to note that essentially all patients who received cisplatin in the prepaclitaxel era also received an alkylating agent (generally cyclophosphamide), a class of drugs known to be leukemogenic (2,12). Based on all available data, it is appropriate to state that even this small increase in the risk of developing acute leukemia is an acceptable price to pay for the substantial improvement in overall survival associated with the use of platinum agents in ovarian cancer.

In view of the documented risk of acute leukemia associated with the long-term use of alkylating agents in ovarian cancer and the known low response rate of the disease to this class of drugs (delivered at standard dose levels) in individuals who fail an initial cisplatin-based regimen (13), the administration of chronic oral alkylating agent therapy (chlorambucil, melphalan) as a second- or third-line treatment is strongly discouraged. Several studies have confirmed that the use of etoposide is strongly associated with the development of acute leukemia (14–17). This risk appears to be highly correlated with the total cumulative dose of the drug administered over time. Therefore, for diseases in which etoposide is an appropriate or required component of treatment (e.g., germ-cell tumors), management of the malignancy should include the use of optimal doses/schedules of the agent delivered for the minimal acceptable number of cycles.

Cardiac Toxicity

Doxorubicin, which has demonstrated activity in several gynecologic malignancies, is an important component of a number of commonly used treatment regimens (18). Its most serious potential side effect is cardiac toxicity (19). Whereas acute cardiac dysfunction (e.g., arrhythmias, pericarditis) may occasionally be observed, chronic heart failure is much more common. The incidence of subclinical and clinical congestive heart failure is directly related to the cumulative dose of doxorubicin administered (20). Cardiac abnormalities are rarely observed with a total doxorubicin dose <350 mg. With a cumulative dose of >550 mg/m^2, the incidence of cardiac dysfunction is 1% to 10%.

Risk factors for cardiac toxicity necessitating a lowering of the doxorubicin dose that can be safely administered include a history of significant hypertension or preexisting cardiac disease, prior cardiac or mediastinal irradiation, and age >70 years (19). Patients who have received cardiac irradiation are at a particularly high risk for developing cardiac complications even when the "safe" dose level of doxorubicin is reduced by 50% (250 mg/m^2) compared with those without such a history.

Doxorubicin-induced heart injury is unique, and specific histologic features are observed in tissue obtained through a cardiac biopsy during a right-heart catheterization (21). When morphologic abnormalities are graded, an objective scoring system appears to correlate well with the severity of the underlying pathologic process. However, although the results of a cardiac biopsy are predictive of future clinical symptoms, it is not a practical procedure to use in routine clinical practice.

Evaluation of serial ECG-gated blood-pool scans allows for a reasonably accurate assessment of the effect of doxorubicin on cardiac function (22,23). In most patients, a major drop in the cardiac ejection fraction is observed *before* the onset of clinical symptoms, allowing for discontinuation of the antineoplastic agent before more serious damage results.

Treatment of doxorubicin-induced heart failure focuses on improving myocardial contractility with afterload reduction and diuresis. Many patients improve symptomatically. Continued improvement in cardiac function has been noted more than a year after initial symptoms are observed.

Several methods have been used in standard clinical practice and experimentally to reduce the risk of the development of chronic cardiac dysfunction associated with doxorubicin, including administration by continuous infusion for several days (rather than by bolus instillation) (24) and the use of dexrazoxane, the first drug demonstrated to reduce anthracycline-induced cardiac injury (25). Neither technique appears to decrease the antineoplastic activity of doxorubicin compared with standard bolus administration.

The combination of doxorubicin and paclitaxel can result in an increased risk for cardiac toxicity compared with the use of doxorubicin alone (12). The appropriate sequencing of the drugs appears to reduce the risk of cardiac effects.

The combination of doxorubicin and herceptin (anti–HER-2/neu monoclonal antibody) also appears to potentiate the cardiac toxicity of doxorubicin and to a lesser extent that of paclitaxel (26). There is currently inadequate information available to recommend specific management strategies to reduce the risk of toxicity when either chemotherapeutic agent is combined with this novel monoclonal antibody.

Although paclitaxel itself has been considered to be an agent with potential cardiac toxicity, particularly in individuals with preexisting cardiac abnormalities, recent data have suggested most individuals can safely receive the drug without concern for the development of either acute (arrhythmias) or chronic (congestive heart failure) cardiac toxicities (27).

Pulmonary Toxicity

Bleomycin, an antitumor antibiotic, is a common component of the treatment regimen for patients with carcinoma of the cervix and malignant germ-cell tumors (18). The most serious toxic effect of bleomycin is subacute or chronic interstitial pneumonitis (28). This inflammatory process may progress to a fibrotic stage, with subsequent significant impairment of pulmonary function.

The most common early symptoms of bleomycin-induced pulmonary toxicity are cough and dyspnea. Bibasilar pulmonary infiltrates have been reported in as many as 5% of patients who receive total cumulative doses of bleomycin <450 mg. The incidence rises to 10% with higher cumulative doses. However, it should be noted that severe pulmonary toxicity has been observed at total bleomycin doses <100 mg.

In addition to the cumulative dose received, other risk factors for bleomycin-induced pulmonary dysfunction include preexisting emphysema, age >70 years, single doses >25 mg/m^2, and prior chest irradiation.

An interesting, potentially serious complication of bleomycin is the development of postoperative respiratory failure in patients previously treated with this agent (29). It has been postulated that bleomycin makes the lung more susceptible to oxygen toxicity. Lowering the inspired oxygen concentration during surgery to an F$_{IO_2}$ of 0.24 and avoiding fluid overload during surgery appear substantially to reduce the risk of postoperative respiratory insufficiency.

The pathogenesis of bleomycin-induced pulmonary dysfunction is not completely understood. The agent produces an inflammatory intraalveolar infiltrate with edema, followed by a proliferation of alveolar macrophages and subsequent interstitial fibrosis. In experimental systems, high concentrations achieved after bolus administration of bleomycin produced more pulmonary damage than either continuous infusion or delivery of low doses on a frequent dosing schedule. These data provide strong support for the clinical use of the agent either as a continuous intravenous infusion or on a low-dose weekly bolus schedule.

No specific treatment exists for bleomycin pulmonary toxicity except discontinuing the agent if pulmonary function tests, particularly the carbon monoxide–diffusing capacity, demonstrate a significant deterioration compared with baseline. Mild worsening in pulmonary function (10% to 15%) is common in patients treated with >240 mg of bleomycin. A more substantial worsening observed in pulmonary function tests should lead to the discontinuation of the antineoplastic drug. Steroid therapy may help reduce inflammation and improve symptoms, but it has little or no impact on established fibrotic lesions. Fortunately, most patients with subclinical disease or mild symptoms demonstrate improvement in symptoms, radiographic findings, and pulmonary function tests.

Mitomycin C, an antineoplastic agent used in patients with several gynecologic malignancies, can produce a syndrome similar to bleomycin-induced pulmonary insufficiency (17). Higher cumulative doses of the agent (20 mg/m^2) appear to increase the risk of mitomycin C–induced pulmonary dysfunction (30). Symptoms include cough and progressive dyspnea. Corticosteroids may be helpful, but patients can develop progressive pulmonary insufficiency. As many as 5% to 7% of patients treated with mitomycin C have been reported to have clinical or subclinical evidence of pulmonary toxicity (30).

Neurotoxicity

The dose-limiting side effect of cisplatin, one of the most important drugs in the management of gynecologic malignancies, is neurotoxicity (31–33). The neurologic effects of cisplatin include peripheral sensory neuropathy, ototoxicity, retinal toxicity, seizures, and autonomic dysfunction.

It is difficult to know the precise incidence of cisplatin-induced neurotoxicity because most early reports only occasionally noted this form of toxicity. In the past, the dose-limiting toxicity of cisplatin was acute renal dysfunction, and in most patients, it was not possible to administer high enough cumulative doses of cisplatin to observe nervous system toxicity (34). With the development of intensive hydration regimens, it has become possible significantly to increase the amount of cisplatin administered to individual patients.

Although cisplatin-induced neurotoxicity may occur after a single dose, most reports suggest that the incidence of this class of side effects increases with higher cumulative doses (31). A summary of the oncologic literature reveals that the incidence of cisplatin neurotoxicity is approximately 15% with a total cumulative dose <300 mg/m^2, but it rises to 85% with doses of >300 mg/m^2 (31).

The most common cisplatin-induced neurologic side effects result from toxicity to the peripheral sensory nerves. Patients complain of numbness, tingling, and paresthesia that involve the feet, legs, hands, and arms. Symptoms generally begin in the feet or hands and proceed proximally. Reflexes (ankle, knee) are lost, and vibratory sensation is greatly diminished. With continued treatment, patients may lose the ability to sense touch or pinprick. Ultimately, patients have difficulty walking and using their hands for fine motion (e.g., writing, picking up a fork).

Fortunately, recovery after cisplatin-induced peripheral neuropathy is common, although frequently not complete. Improvement in symptoms has been noted more than 2 years after the discontinuation of therapy, although most patients begin to note improvement within several months of stopping the antineoplastic drug.

Another important feature of cisplatin-induced neuropathy is that the initial symptoms may develop months after the last dose, and symptoms commonly worsen when the drug is stopped, only to improve several months later. This factor makes it difficult for the clinician to know whether a patient who experiences a mild neuropathy should continue to receive the agent because the ultimate severity of the current symptoms may not be known until after the next dose is scheduled to be given.

Cisplatin administration may also cause tinnitus and hearing loss in the high-frequency range (35). High-dose cisplatin regimens (100 mg/m^2 per dose) that achieve very high peak plasma levels appear to result in a greater incidence of ototoxicity than lower dose regimens (35,36). Paclitaxel (Taxol) can also produce a peripheral neuropathy, which is a dose-limiting toxicity of the agent (37). The neuropathy has been noted to worsen with higher cumulative dosing in some patients and to persist for considerable periods of time (>6 months) (37).

The combination of paclitaxel and cisplatin has been shown to have the potential to produce a higher incidence of peripheral neuropathy than either agent used alone. Of particular concern is the combination of cisplatin (75 mg/m^2) and 3-hour infusion of paclitaxel (175 mg/m^2), where several studies have demonstrated a 20% to 25% incidence of severe (grade 3) peripheral neuropathy (38,39).

Although less neurotoxic than cisplatin plus placitaxel, combination chemotherapy with carboplatin and paclitaxel, a commonly employed regimen in several gynecologic malignancies, also has the potential to produce distressing symptoms associated with the development of a peripheral neuropathy (40).

Renal Insufficiency

Cisplatin is the chemotherapeutic agent most commonly associated with renal compromise (34). Although the damage to the kidney is reversible in most patients, persistent abnormalities in renal function are common in patients who experience acute toxicity. In addition, severe irreversible renal toxicity secondary to cisplatin has been reported; fortunately, however, it is rare.

Cisplatin produces its nephrotoxic effects by damaging the renal tubules. Vigorous saline diuresis has been shown to prevent the development of major renal impairment in most patients who receive this agent, although significant decreases in creatinine clearance are common after standard cisplatin treatment programs for ovarian cancer (400 to 600 mg/m^2 cumulative dose).

In addition to abnormalities in renal function tests, hypomagnesemia secondary to renal magnesium wasting is common after cisplatin administration. Although this defect generally does not result in clinical symptoms of hypomagnesemia, renal magnesium wasting can be demonstrated in many patients more than a year after discontinuation of cisplatin.

Mitomycin may also be associated with renal damage and kidney failure of such severity that chronic dialysis is required (41).

Infertility and Mutagenic Potential

One of the greatest concerns of younger female patients who receive chemotherapy is its effect on fertility. The data that directly address the influence of antineoplastic agents on fertility are limited because accurate figures on the incidence of subsequent pregnancies are not available.

The development of amenorrhea during chemotherapy is influenced by patient age, as well as the specific drug used. Younger patients appear to be able to receive higher cumu-

lative doses of cytotoxic drugs than older women before amenorrhea occurs (42). Recent data reveal that the majority of young women treated with standard chemotherapy for gynecologic malignancies, including the intensive regimens employed in ovarian germ-cell tumors, have an excellent chance to maintain fertility (43–45).

One summary of the literature on the influence of chemotherapy on ovarian function concludes that, if a woman continues to menstruate after administration of cytotoxic antineoplastic therapy, no therapy-related impairment in her ability to become pregnant should exist (42). However, it remains uncertain whether such women will experience premature menopause; therefore, a woman must consider this factor in any decisions about family planning.

An additional important question about fertility is the risk of an increase in congenital abnormalities in the children of women treated with cytotoxic drug therapy. Again, although the available data in the medical literature that address this point are limited and conflicting, the consensus is that no significant increase of spontaneous abortions or fetal abnormalities in pregnancies occurs in this setting, and fetal development (including intellectual function) appears to be normal (46,47).

It is noteworthy that the administration of specific chemotherapeutic agents, most notably the antimetabolites (e.g., methotrexate), during early pregnancy is associated with the development of fetal abnormalities (46). In addition, followup of children exposed to antineoplastic agents *in utero* is of limited duration, and the ultimate impact of such therapy will be known only when long-term follow-up is available (47).

RADIATION THERAPY

Radiation therapy for gynecologic cancers has become increasingly refined and complex. Although multimodality treatment has improved disease outcome, it has also resulted in toxicities that clearly warrant further consideration and discussion (48,49). In the treatment of gynecologic malignancies, radiation therapy complications arise mainly from injuries to the bladder, ureter, rectosigmoid, and small bowel.

Early reactions develop gradually and may increase toward the end of the treatment. These reactions range from greater frequency and water content of stools to frank diarrhea associated with abdominal cramps. Acute reactions in the rectosigmoid may be manifested as increased mucus production or bloody stools. Urinary symptoms include frequency and dysuria. Hematuria during the acute phase is rare. Most of these early reactions, although common, are usually transient and easily managed by conservative measures. Delayed complications that involve the urinary and intestinal tracts generally occur 6 to 24 months after completion of radiation therapy.

Bladder complications, including hemorrhage or con-

TABLE 32.1. *Radiation Therapy Oncology Group morbidity grading system*

Grade	Morbidity
1	Minor symptoms requiring no treatment
2	Symptoms responding to simple outpatient management; lifestyle (performance status) not affected
3	Distressing symptoms altering patient's life style (performance status); hospitalization for diagnosis or minor surgical intervention (e.g., urethral dilatation) may be required
4	Major surgical intervention (e.g., laparotomy, colostomy, cystectomy) or prolonged hospitalization is required
5	Fatal complications

Reprinted with permission from Pilepich MV, Pajak T, George FW, et al. Preliminary report on phase III RTOG studies of extended-field irradiation in carcinoma of the prostate. *Am J Clin Oncol* 1983;6:485.

tracted bladder, usually occur later than those that involve the intestinal tract. Intestinal complications may include proctitis, sigmoiditis, bowel stricture, bowel obstruction, and fistulas. These sequelae may vary from mild symptoms with minimal mucosal changes or mucous discharge and bleeding to necrosis, ulceration or stenosis, perforation, and fistulas that require surgical intervention.

Until recently, the spectrum of radiation complications had not been accurately defined. In 1983, the Radiation Therapy Oncology Group published a meaningful grading system for radiation complications (Table 32.1) (50). This grading system is based on the effect of the treatment-related morbidity on the patient's performance status and the intervention required. More recently, the Gynecologic Oncology Group (GOG) has adopted a comprehensive common toxicity scale that is used at many centers in the United States [see www.gog.org and also the National Cancer Institute's (NCI) on-line publication www.rtog.org/members/toxicity/ctcmanual6–1-99.pdf]. Transient or mild treatment-related symptoms should not be classified as complications, but simply as anticipated treatment-related reactions. These symptoms are identified as complications only if they persist for more than 1 month after completion of therapy or if they progress to a higher grade at any time after therapy.

Many investigators have attempted to correlate early and late reactions. A significant correlation between excessive early reactions and eventual late damage to normal structures has never been shown (51–53).

Pathogenesis

The surface epithelium of the gastrointestinal tract has a rapid cell-replacement system to compensate for the natural exfoliation of the outermost layer of nonproliferative cells. The biologic effect of the most commonly used ionizing radiation produces damage to these cells. In general, the radiosensitivity of a particular tissue is related to the degree of mitotic activity of its cells (54). Gastrointestinal epithelial cells, with a rapid cycle time of 12 to 15 hours, are relatively sensitive to the biologic effects of radiation. The ensuing damage causes a depletion of the mucosal cells and a thinning of the mucosa. If the process progresses, it results in mucosal denudation. The acute inflammatory response and denudation of mucosa produce alterations that include malabsorption and fluid and electrolyte loss. The great proliferative and regenerative capacity of the stem cells generally allows total recovery of the mucosa from these early effects of irradiation.

The pathogenesis of late complications involves a different mechanism, which perhaps explains the lack of correlation between the severity of early and late complications. Late effects are the result of vascular endothelial damage. The gradual occlusion of blood vessels through capillary endarteritis and fibrosis in the submucosal tissues leads to narrowing of the vessels' lumina and tissue hypoxia. These changes may lead to ulceration, perforation, and fistula formation that can be precipitated or accelerated by infection or trauma.

Symptoms of radiation cystitis, which are similar to those of infectious irritation in the bladder, include urgency, frequency, dysuria, strangury, and hematuria. Perhaps the most incapacitating of these are bladder spasms, which can result in urinary retention and hemorrhage, and bladder contracture secondary to fibrosis.

Chronic changes in the urinary bladder may have a diffuse appearance and may be characterized by areas of extreme pallor that separate areas of intense erythema with petechiae. Occasionally, ulceration is present. Bladder capacity is often reduced (55). Histologic findings of radiation cystitis consist of mucosal atrophy interspersed with areas of hyperplasia, submucosal edema, and intimal proliferation of the submucosal vessels. An inflammatory infiltrate of the submucosa is characteristic, and, in severe injury, inflammatory infiltrates and fibrous scarring within the detrusor muscle are evident. Although rare, vesicovaginal, vesicoenteric, and vesicorectal fistulas are severe complications of radiation injury and occur as a result of higher doses. Such fistulas result from excessive destruction of the vasculature in the wall of the bladder and underlying tissues in patients treated with combination external beam and intracavitary irradiation (56–59). Fistulas generally develop from radiation ulcers that are punched out in appearance, with a clearly defined raised margin between the ulcer and adjacent mucosa. With progression of vascular damage, tissue breakdown and fistulization occur.

Biopsies of radiation ulcers should be avoided if the lesions have a typical appearance, location, and time interval after treatment because further injury can occur after repeated biopsies, which may precipitate fistula formation (60). If high radiation doses have been delivered to the anterior vaginal wall and bladder wall, as may occur in the treatment of cervical cancer, an equally high dose may also have been delivered to the posterior vaginal wall and anterior rectal wall. In some cases, vesicovaginal fistula and rectovaginal fistula can appear simultaneously (61). With advances in external therapy planning and computerized brachytherapy, the fistula rate may be as low as 2% (62).

Extravesical ureteral injury, which results in stricture and obstruction caused by radiation, is quite rare. Radiation strictures of the ureter are caused by a cicatricial contraction of the ureter wall that follows destruction of the ureteral mucosa. In two reviews published from the M. D. Anderson Cancer Center, covering two different time periods, 13 cases of late ureteral damage were reported in 1,800 cases of carcinoma of the cervix (0.7%) treated with irradiation alone (11, 20). In all cases, the strictures occurred at the ureterovesical junction that corresponded to the high-dose region with intracavitary irradiation. When definitive radiation therapy is combined with radical surgery, a higher incidence of ureteral damage may occur. Rotman and associates (63) reported a 60% incidence of prolonged unilateral or bilateral ureteral stricture in stage IIB cervical cancer in patients treated with irradiation and surgery. Periureteral fibrosis was considered to be a major factor in ureteral stricture. Twelve of 420 patients (2.8%) reported on by Muram and associates (64) developed this complication. Unilateral injury is a more common complication than bilateral injury (65,66).

The radiation tissue tolerance of the ureter is estimated at 75 to 80 Gy; a dose that exceeds the currently used doses of whole pelvis irradiation. In several large series, experience has shown that any ureteral abnormality or obstruction after radiation therapy must be regarded as active or recurrent disease until proven otherwise (67,68). The intramural ureter may be obstructed by entrapment within the fibrous scar of the bladder wall. Therefore, patients who exhibit severe chronic radiation cystitis are at high risk for associated ureterohydronephrosis.

Large bowel injury from radiation therapy becomes manifest within 2 years (median 6 to 18 months). Fistulas occur more frequently in the rectum than elsewhere in the gut and are confined almost exclusively to cases in which brachytherapy was used for gynecologic cancer. They occur along the anterior rectal wall posterior to the vaginal fornix.

Other chronic symptoms include strictures, tenesmus, bleeding, cramps, obstipation, diarrhea, and rectal urgency, which may require surgical intervention if severe enough. Radiographically, the most frequent appearance is a smooth, elongated narrowing. Alternatively, submucosal changes can give the appearance of a nodular or thumbprinting effect on the wall of the large bowel. Mesenteric shortening can produce retraction of the transverse colon.

Ulceration is frequent and sometimes simulates diverticulitis. Bleeding can occur from sites of ulceration and telangiectasis.

Mild cases of chronic irradiation injury to the large intestine can be managed by a low-residue diet and stool softeners (psyllium with loperamide or diphenoxylate with atropine). Fiber laxatives give a firmer consistency to the stool and soften it.

The extent of recommended surgical management for late bowel complications is controversial. Some favor an aggressive approach with lysis of all adhesions to free up the full length of the small bowel and resection of all severely involved segments. Others advocate a much more conservative approach of bypassing injured bowel by the simplest procedure available.

Vaginal stenosis and dyspareunia are distressing complications that may occur in patients who undergo primary radiation treatment for carcinoma of the cervix or combined surgery and irradiation for endometrial cancer. The degree of stenosis is a function of the total dose and length of vagina in the irradiation field. Jensen showed that many patients with advanced or recurrent cervical cancer have sexual dysfunction prior to radiation therapy (69). Symptoms may deteriorate following treatment. Estrogen therapy, when indicated, and vaginal dilators may help reduce the degree of functional disability (70,71). Femoral head fracture and necrosis, although a rare complication with megavoltage irradiation, can occur if the total dose to the femoral head exceeds 50 to 60 Gy (72). Other risk factors such as osteoporosis and trauma may also contribute to the development of this complication (39,73,74).

Predisposing Factors

The entire spectrum of predisposing factors for complications related to radiation therapy is not clearly understood. It is essential, however, to review some of the known predisposing factors to minimize the number of patients who will develop complications. These factors can be divided into three general categories: host, disease-related, and treatment-related. Host factors include inadequate oxygenation in the tissue that results from anemia, poor nutritional status, and metabolic or endocrine disorders that produce poor tissue oxygen perfusion, including hypertension and diabetes (74–78). The relationship between nutritional status and early and late bowel complications was studied by a group at the Institut Gustave- Roussy in Paris. It is essential that the patient's general nutritional condition be optimized before primary radiation therapy is delivered for a gynecologic malignancy (79). Preexisting pelvic pathology, such as colitis, diverticulitis, pelvic inflammatory disease, or previous abdominal or pelvic surgery, may significantly increase the chance of complications (63,80–83). Locally advanced cancer can directly or indirectly produce poor tissue oxygenation and can result in poor tissue tolerance to irradiation. Distorted pelvic anatomy from locally advanced cancer can also produce a suboptimal intracavitary dose distribution and can result in excessive irradiation of normal structures. Eifel reported an analysis of host factors including age, body mass index, race, tobacco smoking, diabetes, hypertension, and history of venereal disease in 3,489 patients with stage I or II squamous-cell carcinoma of the cervix (84). All but diabetes and hypertension had an impact on the incidence of late effects. Smoking was associated with high rates of bowel complications. Greater amount of smoking in terms of packs per day consumed also predicted a greater risk of late bowel injury. Obese women suffered greater bladder complications, whereas thin women had more bowel effects.

Treatment-related factors can also greatly contribute to the development of both early and late complications. External pelvic irradiation parameters include total dose, dose per fraction, beam energy, and number of treatment fields. Intracavitary irradiation factors include placement and type of applicator, dose rate, and total doses to the rectum, bladder, sigmoid, and small bowel (85).

Technical factors that affect normal tissue tolerance include total dose, dose per fraction, beam energy, treatment-field arrangement, and size of portals. Some reports in the literature have demonstrated a correlation between increased total external beam doses and higher complication rates (Table 32.2). Complication rates increase significantly when external beam doses >45 to 50 Gy, in addition to intracavitary/interstitial irradiation, are delivered to large pelvic fields without appropriate blocking of normal structures such as small bowel, rectum, and bladder (86–89). Logsdon analyzed a large group of patients with stage IIIB cervical cancer showed that external-beam doses >52 Gy had a > 50% major complications (90). Conversely, treatment strategies that limited external beam dose to <48 Gy and emphasized intracavitary brachytherapy had only 15% incidence of major complications. Shrinking-field techniques are highly recommended to minimize irradiation of large volumes in the pelvis, especially in patients with locally advanced disease (91,92). Parallel-opposed anterior and posterior portals with lower energy beams, such as cobalt 60 or 4- to 6-MV photons, deliver higher doses to superficially located normal tissue, such as small bowel and portions of bladder anteriorly and rectum and subcutaneous tissues posteriorly, compared with higher energy apparatuses (93,94). Four-field arrangement reduces the radiation dose to the normal tissues and at the same time facilitates appropriate shielding of these structures. The use of four fields instead of two and the need to treat all fields during each session have assumed greater importance recently based on the Patterns of Care Outcome Study and other reports (95–97).

Irradiation of the pelvis and paraaortic nodes by extended-field techniques increases the rate of complications. Some investigators suggest that doses >45 Gy in 5 weeks to the small bowel in the paraaortic fields are poorly tolerated, and if boost irradiation is considered beyond 44 Gy, it should be delivered with small portals (98–102). An increased rate of small bowel complications was observed in patients with cervical cancer who underwent surgical staging and received extended-field irradiation (98,102). Intestinal complications are less common with retroperitoneal surgical staging than with the transperitoneal approach. Early reports suggest that concurrent cisplatin with pelvic and paraaortic radiation can be achieved with acceptable acute and late toxicity (103). The Radiation Therapy Oncology Group studied twice-daily radiation fractionation (1.2 Gy BID to 48 Gy) to the pelvis and paraaortic nodal region in patients with paraaortic node–positive cervical cancers (104). Concurrent cisplatin and 5-flurouracil was administered. Toxicity was unacceptably high (17% late grade 4).

A number of reports in the literature indicate that total milligram-hours of the brachytherapy applications, a protruding vaginal source, deviated tandem, fixed tandem, and the use of a small intracavitary system (small ovoids) are factors related to high complication rates (65,87). Strockbine and colleagues (78) pointed out that protruding sources were used in 13 of 16 patients with rectal ulcers and 19 of 32

TABLE 32.2. *Incidence of grade 2 and 3 gastrointestinal complications (RTOG Scale) in relation to external pelvic irradiation dose*

Reference	No. of patients	Whole pelvic dose (Gy)	Complications (%)
Hamberger et al. (87)	192	40	3.1
	111	50	10
	15	60	20
Strockbine et al. (78)	11	30	0
	341	40	3
	85	50	8.5
	331	60	12
	63	70	26
			(all grades 3–5 complications)
Logsdon (90)	260	60	40
	301	70	17
	184	most > 52Gy	40
	162	most < 51Gy	17

Reprinted with permission from Logsdon, MD, Eifel, PJ. FIGO IIIB squamous cell carcinoma of the cervix: An analysis of prognostic factors emphasizing the balance between external beam and intracavitary radiation therapy. *Int J Radiat Oncol Biol Phys*, 1999;43(4):763–75.

patients with fistulas. Hamberger and associates (87) reported on 5 of 11 patients who developed rectal strictures when protruding sources or vaginal cylinders were used in addition to an external-beam dose of >50 Gy. A high-dose area can be formed at the ureterovesical junction by the acute angle formed between a laterally deviated tandem and the colpostat on the side of deviation. Sigmoid stenosis or fistula and ureteral strictures can occur because of deviated tandems. The introduction of afterloading techniques for intracavitary applications, together with computerized dosimetry and dose optimization, has greatly decreased the complications from brachytherapy.

The frequency of rectal and bladder complications is a function of the total dose received by these organs from both external beam and intracavitary irradiation, as well as the length or volume of these normal organs in the irradiation field (57,105). When the total maximum dose is >75 to 80 Gy to small volumes of the rectum or >80 Gy to the bladder, a significantly higher incidence of complications occurs (89, 106). If the ratio of bladder or rectum point dose to point A dose is less than 0.8, then complications are low (107).

Many women with early-stage IB cervical cancers are treated with a radical hysterectomy. Radiation therapy is indicated in an increasing proportion of these women who are found to have intermediate or high pathologic risk factors for tumor recurrence (108,109). Patients who require radiation therapy after a radical hysterectomy are known to have a greater risk for late toxicity (110). This crucial point is well illustrated in the prospective study reported by Landoni in which women with stages IB and IIA cervical cancer were randomized to definitive radiation therapy versus radical hysterectomy (110). Adjuvant radiation therapy was added to patients in the surgery arm for those with high-risk pathologic features. Although overall survival was equal in the two arms, long-term toxicity was experienced by 29% of patients in the surgery arm (nearly two-thirds required adjuvant radiation) versus 15% of patients treated with definitive radiation therapy. A follow-up study of surgical technique by the same group showed a similar incidence of late toxicity for patients treated with surgery and adjuvant radiotherapy (111).

The standard treatment for advanced cervical cancer is a combination of external beam and intracavitary irradiation and cisplatin-based chemotherapy (48,49). The long-term complication rate of this combined therapy is at present unknown (112).

Radiation Therapy Complications in the Treatment of Ovarian Cancer

Ovarian cancer is a disease that generally involves the entire peritoneal cavity; as such, the external irradiation fields that are used may be considerably larger than those used for other gynecologic malignancies. This practice increases the likelihood of acute toxicity, which usually consists of gastrointestinal symptoms and suppression of bone marrow activity. The incidence of diarrhea, vomiting, and weight loss during the course of treatment in a series of 167 patients who received high radiation doses (45 to 60 Gy) to the lower abdomen was 78% (113). In most patients, gastrointestinal symptoms subside within a few weeks after the completion of treatment. However, in 29% of patients in the cited report, diarrhea with or without gastrointestinal bleeding persisted over a period of a few months after treatment. In 24 of 167 patients (14%), severe bowel stenosis and bleeding developed, requiring surgical intervention (113). Fyles and colleagues prospectively collected toxicity data on 598 patients with ovarian cancer treated with abdominopelvic radiotherapy (114). Most patients had abdominal doses of 22.5 to 27.5 Gy with a pelvic dose of 45.0 Gy. Acute toxicity included severe nausea and vomiting in 6% and severe diarrhea in 6%. Treatment breaks were necessary in 10% of patients. Transient liver enzyme elevation was noted in 44% of patients, but only 2 patients had clinically apparent jaundice. Surgical intervention to relieve bowel obstruction was required in 2.7%, whereas six patients died from treatment complications.

Similar rates of acute and chronic radiation-induced enteritis have been reported by other investigators who used moving-strip techniques (115–117). Although the moving-strip technique was designed to decrease the morbidity of whole abdominal irradiation observed with the open-field technique, when the nominal standard dose (NSD) and the time-dose factor (TDF) values are compared, they show similar values. Because the NSD and TDF values provide an estimate of the normal tissue tolerances for a fractionated radiation therapy program, nearly identical values imply biologically equivalent programs (Table 32.3). Studies that compare the open-field and the moving-strip techniques have shown that the rates of acute morbidity and chronic complications are similar in patients treated with either technique (118–120).

Radiation-induced hepatitis and nephritis may occur with radiation doses that exceed 30 and 18 Gy, respectively. More recently, however, these symptoms have not commonly been observed because of careful application of appropriate protection to the liver and kidneys.

Late Complications of High-Dose–Rate Brachytherapy

Brachytherapy continues to play an important role in the treatment of cancers at several sites, including the cervix and endometrium. The physical advantages of brachytherapy result from superior localization of dose to the tumor volume. The two types of brachytherapy are intracavitary (using radioactive sources placed in body cavities in close proximity to the tumor volume) and interstitial (using radioactive seeds implanted into the tumor bed) (121).

Rapid developments have occurred in the brachytherapy technique with the introduction of remote afterloading. Ad-

TABLE 32.3. *Normal tissue tolerance to therapeutic irradiation*

Organ	TD 5/5 volume			TD 5/50 volume			Selected endpoints
	1/3	2/3	3/3	1/3	2/3	3/3	
Kidney	5,000	3,000[a]	2,300		4,000[a]	2,800	Clinical nephritis
Bladder	N/A	8,000	6,500	N/A	8,500	8,000	Symptomatic bladder contracture and volume loss
Bone: femoral head			5,200			6,500	Necrosis
Skin	10 cm²	30 cm²	100 cm²	10 cm²	30 cm²	100 cm²	Telangiectasia, necrosis, ulceration
			5,000			6,500	
	7,000	6,000	5,500			7,000	
Stomach	6,000	5,500	5,000	7,000	6,700	6,500	Ulceration/perforation
Small intestine	5,000		4,000a	6,000		5,500	Obstruction perforation/ fistula
Colon	5,500		4,500	6,500		5,500	Obstruction/perforation
Rectum	Volume 100 cm² No volume effect		6,000	Volume 100 cm² No volume effect		8,000	Severe proctitis/ necrosis/fis tula, stenosis
Liver	5,000	3,500	3,000	5,500	4,500	4,000	Liver failure
Bone marrow	4,000	1,000	400	4,500	1,000	650	
Spinal cord	5,000	5,000	4,700	7,000	7,000		

[a]<50% of volume does not make a significant change.

Reprinted with permission from Emami et al. Tolerance of normal tissue to therapeutic irradiation. *Int J Radiat Oncol Biol Phys* 1991;21:109.

vantages of remote afterloading systems, which allow the introduction of radioactive sources through nonradioactive applicators, include reduced radiation exposure to personnel, shorter treatment times, and better control of geometry (122). It was reported that better control rates are attained with afterloaded applicators than with nonafter loaded applicators (123).

Low-dose–rate (LDR) remote afterloading uses conventional treatment times. High-dose–rate (HDR) remote afterloaders permit shorter treatment times but require treatment fractionation and reduction in total dose to achieve results comparable with LDR brachytherapy (124). Although the application of remote afterloading did not become practical until the 1970s, it is now standard (125). With the introduction of remote afterloading, many centers have replaced LDR brachytherapy with HDR brachytherapy (122). Presently, a large number of HDR regimens exist. Most applicator types have been adapted for use with HDR machines (125).

The usual dose rate for HDR brachytherapy is 2 to 3 Gy/min, whereas traditional LDR brachytherapy is administered at a dose of 0.4 to 0.8 Gy/h (126–129). Evidence indicates that tumor control and treatment-related complications are roughly equivalent in both regimens (125,130–132). Some series have demonstrated a higher pelvic control rate with acceptable morbidity in patients treated with HDR therapy alone compared with a relatively high incidence of local recurrence in patients who receive <6,000 mgh (133).

However, the effectiveness of HDR brachytherapy is different for acutely responding and late-responding tissues (134). HDR brachytherapy may cause more damage to late-responding tissues, such as rectum and bladder, than does

LDR therapy. The majority of late complications of HDR brachytherapy in the treatment of cervical cancer involve the rectal and bladder mucosa and are a function of dose per fraction and total dose. Proctitis and cystitis are the most common late effects of HDR therapy. Orton and associates (135) reported significantly fewer late complications when the dose per fraction was <7 Gy, when compared with a dose >7 Gy. Swamy and colleagues (136) reported a significant influence of intracavitary dose rate on complications. The complication rate was 3% with 1.4 to 1.59 Gy/h, 14% with 1.6 to 1.89 Gy/h, and 27% with 1.9 to 2.2 Gy/h (136).

Endometrial Carcinoma

Although total abdominal hysterectomy and bilateral salpingo-oophorectomy are accepted as the primary standard for treatment of early-stage endometrial cancer, external beam irradiation is probably the only effective method of delivering a cancericidal dose to the pelvic lymphatics in high-risk patients (137,138). The rationale for the application of intracavitary brachytherapy administered either preoperatively or postoperatively is to reduce the frequency of vaginal tumor recurrence (134,139). For endometrial cancers, the highest risk of recurrence is in the vaginal vault (140). Adjuvant irradiation, regardless of technique, has been shown to reduce vaginal recurrences (141).

In recent years, gynecologic oncologists in the United States have become more likely to perform complete surgical staging on patients with clinical stage I endometrial cancer. The reporting of the GOG 99 trial (142) that randomized patients with intermediate-risk surgically staged endometrial cancer to observation versus adjuvant pelvic radiation has led to a decline in the recommendation of adjuvant pelvic radiation therapy by gynecologic oncologists in pathologic stage I intermediate-risk endometrial cancers (143). The abstract of GOG 99 reported improved pelvic control with radiation therapy but equivalent overall survival. The toxicity results of the Postoperative Radiation Therapy in Endometrial Cancer trial that randomized patients with clinical stage I disease to radiation or observation after hysterectomy without a lymph node dissection have contributed to this bias (144,145). This study reported a 26% incidence of grades 1 to 4 complications in patients receiving radiation therapy versus 4% in the group observed. Most complications were grade 1; only 3% of patients had late grades 3 to 4 gastrointestinal toxicity and no patient had late grades 3 to 4 genitourinary toxicity.

These findings with adjuvant external pelvic irradiation have led many physicians to favor adjuvant vaginal cuff brachytherapy alone; generally delivered via HDR vaginal cylinders. Horowitz reported no grades 3 to 4 complications in 164 patients with surgically staged IB and II endometrial cancer treated with this approach (146). Similarly, Alektiar had 1% grades 3 to 4 complications in 233 patients with pathologic IB grade 1 or 2 endometrial cancer (147). The majority of late complications resulting from HDR brachytherapy treatment of endometrial carcinoma involve the rectum, intestine, and bladder. Increased dose per fraction from 5 to 7 Gy to 7 to 10 Gy has resulted in an incremental increase in late complications with HDR vaginal radiation treatments. Complications of HDR vaginal brachytherapy are a function of dose per fraction and total radiation dose (external and intravaginal) and diameter of the vaginal cylinder (<2 cm cylinder results in higher complication rate). Another factor is length of the vagina irradiated (148). A series of 300 patients treated with external beam radiation and HDR brachytherapy for early-stage endometrial cancer revealed a posttreatment grade 1 to 2 complication rate of 9.5%, including cystitis (4.5%), vaginal stenosis (2.5%), proctitis (1.5%), vaginal necrosis (0.5%), and partial bowel obstruction (0.5%). Neither grade 3 to 4 complications nor additional late complications were observed (138).

Management of Complications

With modern treatment planning, both for external beam and intracavitary irradiation, the incidence and severity of radiation therapy complications can be reduced significantly. In the current era of combined-modality treatment, complications can also be minimized by judicious attention to the sequencing of chemotherapy and radiation treatments (120,149). The further development of intensity-modulated radiation therapy (IMRT) that uses beams of differential intensity of radiation to conform high-dose regions to target tissues and minimize exposure of normal tissue to ionizing radiation has the potential to further reduce late sequelae. An early report from the University of Chicago supports this

possibility in the setting of gynecologic malignancies (150). In this study, acute toxicity was both less frequent and less severe in patients treated with IMRT versus historic experience.

When radiation enteritis develops, it can be managed by an elemental diet that allows for total absorption in the proximal small intestine. Timely surgical intervention (discussed below) should be considered for symptoms of bleeding, pain, fistula formation, and obstruction (151–154). Although the occurrence of radiation enteritis is unusual with radiation-related fistulas, reports in the literature indicate that maintenance of electrolyte balance and nutrition by hyperalimentation may facilitate fistula closure (155).

Superimposed infections markedly worsen bladder symptoms and should always be considered if patients with radiation cystitis experience an acute exacerbation. Appropriate antibiotic therapy should be given if acute infection is documented. Anticholinergics may help increase bladder capacity and reduce bladder frequency. Instillation of 50 to 100 mL of a 10% solution of dimethyl sulfoxide has provided symptomatic relief in some patients (156). Irrigation of the bladder with corticosteroid solutions may also provide symptomatic relief.

For acute bleeding, diathermy cauterization via the cystoscope may be useful. Occasionally, intravesical instillation of 1% formalin may be of use in patients with severe chronic hematuria. A cystogram before instillation of formalin is important to rule out ureteral reflux or bladder leakage, as renal failure can result if formalin reaches the upper tracts, and significant perivesical fibrosis may occur with extravasation.

SURGERY

The complications of surgery per se occur almost exclusively in the perioperative period; therefore, a discussion of the role of surgery as it pertains to the late effects of therapy of gynecologic cancer is principally a discussion of the surgical management of irradiation injury to the intestinal and lower urinary tracts. The management of intraoperative and early postoperative complications, such as bleeding and surgical damage to the urinary and intestinal tracts, is covered only briefly in this chapter. Readers interested in detailed discussions of these topics are referred to excellent texts on the subject (157,158).

Intraoperative Urinary Tract Injuries

Intraoperative injury to the urinary tract is a relatively uncommon occurrence during surgery for gynecologic cancer. Recognized intraoperative injury to the ureter occurs in approximately 1% of nonirradiated patients undergoing radical hysterectomy for cervical cancer (159). This represents a significant improvement in the injury rate from series reported before 1980. Injuries can occur by a variety of mechanisms, but usually involve crushing or laceration of the ureter. Crushing injuries typically involve clamping and/ or ligation of the ureter. When identified intraoperatively, the clamp or ligature should be removed immediately and the ureter mobilized sufficiently from surrounding tissue so that it can be carefully inspected. Observation over a period of time may be necessary to assess the blood supply and extent of damage. Intravenous indigo carmine can be administered if there is concern about urinary leakage. If the ureter appears viable and there is no extravasation, the site of injury can be stented with a self-retaining stent (single or double pigtail) passed through either a ureterotomy or a cystotomy over a wire. The retroperitoneum near the site of injury should also be drained with a closed suction drain. Lesser degrees of injury such as those resulting from mass ligation of the ureter may not require stenting; simply removing the suture may suffice. Severe crushing injuries may require resection of the damaged segment of ureter and, depending on the site of the injury and the anatomy, either primary anastomosis or reimplantation into the bladder. Stenting should also be performed in these cases.

Ureteral lacerations that do not compromise the blood supply of the ureter can be closed primarily with absorbable suture over a stent. Larger injuries or complete transections will require primary repair or ureteroneocystostomy. Injuries below the pelvic brim can generally be managed by ureteroneocystostomy, with bladder mobilization and psoas muscle hitch if required. Those above the pelvic brim are often best managed by anastomosis, or intestinal interposition. Generally, a ureteroneocystostomy should be performed when possible, as the complication rate of this procedure is significantly lower than with other types of anastomosis. Permanent suture should never be used when suturing the uroendothelium.

Injuries above the pelvic brim can be managed with a variety of techniques, including transureteroureteral anastomosis, Boari flap, Demel technique, or intestinal interposition. Intestinal interposition uses a portion of the ilium as a ureteral extender and interposes a segment between distal ureter and bladder. The two flaps described must be raised carefully from medial to lateral, taking care to keep the superior vesicle artery intact. This will help keep the flap well vascularized. Transureteroureterostomy is potentially dangerous, because the function of both kidneys can be compromised if there is a technical problem with the anastomosis and, in the authors' opinion, should be avoided.

Intraoperative bladder injuries occur in approximately 1% to 2% of radical hysterectomy patients or other cases of radical surgery. They are generally easily repaired with a two-layer closure using absorbable suture, followed by bladder drainage for 5 to 14 days. Irradiated bladders generally should be drained longer than nonirradiated bladders.

Postoperative Urinary Tract Complications

With modern surgical techniques, the incidence of ureterovaginal fistula following radical hysterectomy has fallen to 1% to 2% from a rate of 10% to 20% several decades ago. Most become apparent from the fifth to the fourteenth day postoperatively. Placement of a vaginal tampon and instillation of intravesical methylene blue can allow discrimination of a bladder fistula from a ureteral fistula. Intravenous indigo carmine intravenous pyelography, cystoscopy, and retrograde pyelography may be useful to define the site of the problem. Initial therapy of ureterovaginal fistula is directed toward elimination of infection and maintenance of renal function. Retrograde stenting should be attempted, and, if successful, the stent should be left in place for several months. This will often allow spontaneous healing of the fistula. If a retrograde stent cannot be passed, percutaneous nephrostomy and antegrade stenting should be performed. If antegrade stenting cannot be accomplished, nephrostomy drainage should be established, and a decision made about the timing of surgical repair. If an active intraperitoneal urine leak is present, immediate repair is indicated. In the absence of this, many authorities prefer to wait 6 to 8 weeks before surgical repair, although there are also proponents of routine immediate repair.

Postoperative vesicovaginal fistulas are less common following radical hysterectomy and often heal spontaneously after prolonged bladder drainage. If surgical repair is necessary, most of these can be approached by the vaginal route. One of the most troubling complications after radical hysterectomy for cervical cancer is bladder dysfunction, a result of the necessary disruption of the nerve supply to the bladder that occurs during the radical pelvic dissection (55). Minor degrees of sensory and motor dysfunction, detectable by cystometrogram, are seen in essentially all patients, and approximately 2% to 3% of patients will have long-term clinically significant difficulties with bladder function that may require chronic intermittent self-catheterization.

Fistulas that occur after the patient has received a combination of radiation therapy and surgery are less likely to heal spontaneously and often require surgical intervention. Vesicovaginal fistulas resulting from radiation injury almost always require surgical correction. The repair can be achieved vaginally or abdominally. Vaginal repair often uses a portion of the bulbocavernosus muscle (Martius flap) (160, 161). Alternatively, abdominal repair may require using a flap of nonirradiated tissue such as the omentum between the bladder and vagina to improve the success of repair by including additional blood supply.

Urinary diversion is often required to divert the urinary stream in patients in whom it is felt a primary repair of the area cannot be achieved. The type of diversion can be continent or incontinent, depending on the clinical situation at the time that the repair is needed. Also, it will depend on the patient's willingness to care for an extraneous device. If the patient already has a colostomy, she may be more willing to care for such a device. Early complications of urinary diversion include urine leak and vascular complications. Urine leak that is clinically important is seen approximately

5% of the time (162,163). This may present as urine leaking from the perineum, incision, or stoma or through a cutaneous drain. Evidence of leakage may also manifest itself by fever with abscess formation, ileus, or decreased urine output with a contemporaneous rise in BUN or creatinine. Initial management should always be conservative. Percutaneous drains or nephrostomies can be placed by interventional radiology for drainage of the urine or abscess. The tracts will often close under appropriate conservative management. Surgical intervention should be avoided, as the operative mortality is exceedingly high. In the case of urinary diversion, one can occasionally consider an "undiversion." In this situation, the urinary conduit is attached to the dome of the bladder, reconnecting the urinary stream.

Penalever and colleagues (164) reported on the complications of continent urinary diversions. They observed a complication rate of 53% and a postoperative mortality of 9%. Early complications included stricture or obstruction, anastomotic leak, pyelonephritis, sepsis, and reservoir cutaneous fistula. Late complications included stricture or obstruction, incontinence, difficulty with catheterization, and urinary stones. All complications should be treated initially with drainage and nonoperative intervention until the complication is stabilized, then appropriate surgical management can be considered.

Intraoperative Intestinal Injuries

Intraoperative injury to the intestinal tract may occur from time to time in patients undergoing surgery for gynecologic cancers. Predisposing factors include prior extensive surgery, irradiation, inflammatory disease, and perhaps intraperitoneal chemotherapy. Intraoperative intestinal injuries generally lead to no serious sequelae, provided that the bowel has been adequately prepared and the injuries are recognized and repaired appropriately. The extent of the bowel preparation should be tailored to the surgical procedure being performed and the likelihood of intestinal injury. For high-risk patients or for those in whom intestinal resection is contemplated, a complete antibiotic and mechanical bowel preparation is indicated. (See the "Bowel Preparation" section of Chapter 11.) All bowel preparations can cause dehydration, and special attention should be given to the elderly patient to prevent dehydration with associated postoperative acute tubular necrosis; this may mean administering intravenous fluids during the bowel preparation.

Small injuries to the intestinal serosa usually do not require repair. Larger injuries or those occurring in irradiated bowel should be oversewn. Injuries that transgress both the serosa and the muscular layers of the bowel wall can be recognized by a bulging of the mucosa when gentle pressure is applied. These should be repaired, generally with a single layer of interrupted sutures. Injuries that enter the intestinal lumen must be dealt with according to their site and severity, as well as the condition of the intestine. Uncomplicated inju-

ries to the small intestine and to the well-prepared large intestine can usually be closed primarily. A common technique uses a first layer of continuous or interrupted absorbable suture, followed by an interrupted layer of permanent suture, such as 3–0 silk or Vicryl. In the presence of more extensive injury, vascular compromise, tumor, or obstruction, a more extensive procedure, such as resection and anastomosis, may be required. In the case of injury to the unprepared large bowel, diverting colostomy should be considered.

Postoperative Intestinal Complications

The spectrum of postoperative intestinal complications includes obstruction and leakage of intestinal contents. Postoperative mechanical obstruction generally results from adhesions forming in the early postoperative period. Initial management should be conservative, including gastric decompression and, possibly, intravenous nutritional support, as many postoperative obstructions will resolve spontaneously. Those that do not resolve with conservative management may require surgical correction (165).

Leakage of intestinal contents can be a devastating complication. It may occur at the site of intestinal injury or anastomosis or may develop spontaneously in unmanipulated bowel. Predisposing factors include the presence of tumor and distal obstruction. Prior radiation therapy not only increases the risk of intestinal complications, but also makes their management more difficult (discussed later in this chapter). Management must be individualized, but basic principles include cessation of oral intake, establishing a route of drainage for the leaking intestinal contents, and treatment of infection. Emergency operation and intestinal diversion may be required in the case of gross intraperitoneal leakage of intestinal contents. In less acute cases, such as enterocutaneous fistulas following surgery, supportive management with gastric suction, total parenteral nutrition, and the use of somatostatin may allow spontaneous healing.

The use of automatic-stapling devices to perform low-rectal anastomoses has greatly facilitated the avoidance of permanent colostomy in gynecologic cancer patients. The technical feasibility of the anastomosis, however, must be weighed against the risk of immediate and long-term complications. In patients at risk for poor healing of the anastomosis, a diverting colostomy should be considered. If a leak does occur postoperatively, simple diversion of the fecal stream usually prevents serious complications. The protective colostomy or ileostomy should be well out of the irradiated field if possible. A small proportion of patients undergoing low-rectal anastomosis with circular stapling devices will experience problems with long-term stenosis of the stapled anastomosis. It is important to use the largest staple cartridge that can be accommodated by the patient's intestinal lumen. Dilatation of the anastomosis under anesthesia may be effective in relieving symptomatic stenosis. Digital inspection of the anastomosis at regular office visits can help prevent progressive or recurrent stenosis. Very low anastomoses may also produce some degree of fecal urgency and incontinence, probably related to loss of the reservoir function of the rectal ampulla and denervation of the sphincter itself during the procedure. Radical pelvic resections as described above may also result in loss of bladder function and lead to atonic bladder; therefore, postvoid residuals should be checked during the postoperative period.

The reported frequency of anastomotic leaks varies significantly, depending on the type of anastomosis and site. The rate of clinical leak varies from 0% to 30%. This rate has been shown to be even higher when integrity of the anastomosis is investigated prospectively with water-soluble contrast material. Rectal anastomoses have a higher complication rate than all other anastomoses. The complication rate may also be related to the distance from the anal verge. Authors from the Mayo Clinic reported a 1% clinical leak rate in 402 patients undergoing hand-sewn colon anastomosis. Almost 6% (5 of 107) of the patients' colorectal anastomoses developed a leak (166,167). Pelvic abscess following an anastomosis may occur and is often heralded by high spiking fevers. The diagnosis is usually confirmed by CT scan and is usually best treated by percutaneous drainage under radiographic guidance (168).

A major long-term complication of colorectal anastomoses is stricture. This may occur in as many as 3% of very low anastomoses, particularly if the EEA stapler is used. The EEA stapler allows lower anastomoses than hand-sewn, but at a cost of increased risk of stricture, particularly if the area has been irradiated (167,169). It is unusual in anastomoses of the proximal rectum. The lower anastomoses, particularly those below the peritoneal reflection, can be dilated. Other more proximal strictures, including those of the small bowel, may require surgical correction (170).

Another common complication in gynecologic cancer patients is the small-bowel obstruction. Unfortunately, there is little information on management of this problem in our patients. Most of the management techniques are extrapolated from the general surgery literature. Small-bowel obstruction presents with dilated loops of small bowel, air fluid levels, and associated nausea and vomiting. If there is air in the rectum on abdominal x-ray, the diagnosis of obstruction secondary to ileus is made. This usually resolves with conservative management and nasogastric suction over 1 to 7 days. Any surgical procedure, whether peritoneal or extraperitoneal, may result in an ileus. Treatment for adynamic ileus is bowel rest with NG suction. Some have advocated agents to increase bowel motility, but this has not been shown to be effective in any peer-reviewed publications.

Mechanical small-bowel obstruction occurs in a significant portion of patients with gynecologic malignancies. The differential diagnosis is ileus, fecal impaction ischemia, and, of course, gastroenteritis. Treatment is immediate NG suction. This problem requires immediate medical attention, but

may no longer require immediate surgical attention. It is now generally accepted that a trial of conservative management is warranted in cases of small-bowel obstruction, provided that there is no evidence of ischemic bowel or evidence of strangulation. The majority of cases of partial small-bowel obstruction resolve with NG suction and electrolyte replacement, whereas fewer than 50% of cases of complete obstruction resolve with this treatment and ultimately require surgical intervention (171–173). The use of contrasted bowel studies is often helpful in distinguishing high-grade from low-grade obstruction and may be helpful in determining the site of obstruction. The type of contrast used is controversial. Barium often yields a better study, but can complicate subsequent operative procedures, as barium is quite caustic if spilled in the peritoneal cavity. Soluble contrast is safer, but often is diluted to such a degree that the study is not helpful (174). If one believes that there could be a large bowel obstruction, an enema with contrast should be performed before an upper GI study. If the obstruction is in the distal small bowel, evaluation by enema can also be helpful if the patient has an incompetent ileocecal valve.

The timing and advisability of surgery on a patient who has end-stage ovarian cancer is controversial and requires experience and associated judgment. If the physician feels that the patient's life expectancy is greater than 3 to 4 months and that the surgery is technically feasible, it is reasonable to proceed. Patients with disseminated carcinomatosis often have large segments of dysfunctional bowel, making resection necessary if the obstruction is to be relieved, and the risk of fistula is high. A gastrostomy tube and prolonged bowel rest should be used in this setting.

Large bowel obstructions often present with progressive symptoms of constipation and difficulty defecating. Once the obstruction is complete, surgical intervention is mandatory to avoid perforation at the cecum. The risk of cecal perforation increases when the cecum acutely dilates to more than 10 cm. Management is almost always a colostomy in the form of a loop or end, depending on the clinical situation (175).

Late medical complications of intestinal surgery include those that follow extensive resection of the ileum and right colon, which may produce chronic diarrhea from impaired absorption of water, fat, and bile salts, and problems related to poor absorption of nutrients, including the fat-soluble vitamins and vitamin B_{12}.

Postoperative Incisional Complications

Incisional complications after surgery include varying degrees of wound separation in the early postoperative period, as well as incisional hernias that become apparent in the later postoperative period. Superficial wound separations, involving only the skin and subcutaneous tissues, are generally minor problems. They may be managed by reclosure, if the tissues are in good condition, or allowed to heal by secondary intention. Wound separations involving the deep fascia are more serious. Fortunately, the use of single-layer bulk closure of the abdominal wall, a kind of "internal retention" suture, has made fascial dehiscence quite uncommon, even in high-risk patients. Fascial dehiscence must, of course, be repaired emergently.

Wound infection occurs in approximately 4% of patients undergoing a surgical procedure. Infection rate varies with the type of patient, her medical characteristics, and the type of wound. It is important to follow appropriate preoperative measures to minimize the wound infection rate (157).

Incisional hernia is a long-term complication that is also quite uncommon after single-layer bulk closure of the abdominal wall. However, the reported rate of hernias in the gynecologic oncology population is approximately 5% (176, 177). Incisional hernia occurs more often in patients who have factors that adversely affect healing, such as advanced malignancy, poor nutrition, and the use of radiation therapy and chemotherapy. It is also more common in patients who have had multiple prior operations and in those who have postoperative incisional complications, such as infection. The need for elective repair should be determined on an individual basis. Extensive hernias may require the use of a prosthetic material to bridge the fascial gap.

Surgical Management of Radiation Injury

The Patterns of Care Outcome Study of cervical cancer published in 1983 analyzed data on 706 patients treated with radiation therapy at 163 institutions across the United States (178). Major complications (those that required hospitalization) occurred in 86 patients (12%). Fewer than half of these complications required surgery for management.

Perez and associates (106), reporting on 811 patients with cervical cancer treated at the Mallinckrodt Institute of Radiology (St. Louis, Missouri), found that complications requiring surgery occurred in approximately 5% of patients. The most common intestinal complications included rectovaginal fistula, sigmoid stricture, small-bowel obstruction, and sigmoid perforation. The most common urinary-tract complications were bladder ulcer, vesicovaginal fistula, and ureteral stricture. In this report, irradiation dose and technique were the primary clinical features related to risk of complications. No relationship was demonstrated between complications and age or a history of previous pelvic disease. As mentioned previously, additional risk factors cited by other investigators include conditions that predispose to atherosclerosis, such as diabetes and hypertension (179). It is reasonable to estimate that approximately 5% to 7% of patients who undergo radiation therapy for cervical cancer will experience major treatment complications, including fistulas, that require surgery. The incidence of complications is significantly lower in women who receive irradiation for endometrial cancer, because of the lower central doses used. On the other hand, patients who undergo whole-abdominal irradiation as salvage treatment of ovarian cancer after chemotherapy failure have a risk of major complications reported in the range of 40% to 50% (180,181). Because of the high morbidity and low efficacy, this treatment has gained only limited acceptance.

Intestinal Tract

Radiation injury to the intestinal tract severe enough to require surgery generally becomes manifest in the first 2 years after treatment. In a series of 71 patients from the M.D. Anderson Cancer Center, who required surgery for radiation injury to the small intestine, Smith and coworkers (182) reported that 48% of the injuries developed within 1 year after completion of treatment and 74% developed within 2 years. Occasionally, however, complications may develop much later, perhaps as a result of the natural development of atherosclerosis that accompanies aging.

The most common sites of intestinal injury in patients who undergo pelvic irradiation are areas of the intestinal tract that typically lie in the pelvic field. The ileum is the most frequent site of injury, because of the greater radiosensitivity of the small intestine compared with the colon. In a series from the Mayo Clinic, Schmitt and Symmonds (183) reported that, among 93 patients who underwent surgery for radiation injury to the intestine, 78 (84%) had involvement of the ileum. The rectosigmoid colon and the cecum are also frequent sites of involvement.

The decision to operate on patients with radiation injury must never be made lightly. Surgery may be required in the management of radiation injury to the intestinal tract for palliation of severe symptoms that fail to respond to the previously outlined conservative management, as well as for relief of life-threatening complications, such as obstruction or perforation. In a review of all intestinal surgery performed during a 3-year interval on the Gynecology Service at Memorial Sloan–Kettering Cancer Center, Rubin and colleagues (184) reported that 79 (46%) of the 171 operations that involved intestinal surgery were performed in previously irradiated patients. The most common indications for these operations were intestinal obstruction (44%) and intestinal fistula or perforation (32%) that occurred in patients treated for cervical or corpus cancer.

Smith and DeCosse (15), in a review on radiation damage to the small intestine, emphasized three phases that can be applied to the management of radiation injury in all areas of the intestinal tract: stabilization, evaluation, and surgery. The patient's fluid, electrolyte, and nutritional status should be assessed and optimized before surgery; total parenteral nutrition is often required. Some investigators have suggested that the use of somatostatin to decrease gastrointestinal secretions may promote the healing of enteric fistulas (185). As mentioned previously, in contrast to fistulas in the nonirradiated intestine, those involving irradiated bowel only rarely heal with a program of intestinal rest and parenteral alimentation. In cases of bowel obstruction, intestinal intubation and decompression should be performed preoperatively. If infection is present, preoperative antibiotic therapy should be given.

Except in emergency situations, a careful evaluation of the entire intestinal tract should be made before any contemplated surgery. One should always bear in mind that recurrent cancer may, in part, be responsible for the intestinal problems; if cancer is present, the appropriate management may be altered. Radiographic studies of the large and small intestine should be performed. Cutaneous fistulas can be studied by injection of contrast medium, and stomas can be explored endoscopically. Evaluation of the ureters and bladder by intravenous pyelogram and cystoscopy may also provide useful information. As Marks and Mohiudden (186) pointed out, the extent of radiation injury may be greater than anticipated, and the patient must understand the possible need for intestinal or urinary diversion.

At operation, it is generally advisable to explore the entire abdominal cavity. Intestinal adhesions are frequently encountered, making exploration a difficult undertaking. Irradiated intestine must be handled with great care, and meticulous dissection must be used to lyse adhesions. Injuries to the intestinal wall that may be trivial in the nonirradiated patient may lead to fistulization of irradiated intestine. Frequently, in patients with gynecologic cancer, the surgeon encounters a matted mass of distal ileum densely fixed in the pelvis that is the site of obstruction or fistula. It is often not possible to release such a mass without damage to the involved intestine and risk of injury to adjacent structures, such as the urinary bladder and ureters, rectosigmoid colon, and major pelvic blood vessels. The decision whether to resect or bypass such an agglutinated mass of bowel may tax the judgment of even the most experienced surgeon. In general, such masses are best resected, particularly in the presence of intestinal necrosis, perforation, abscess formation, and fistulization, if resection can be accomplished without undue risk of gross contamination of the peritoneal cavity or damage to adjacent structures. Bypass procedures may be more likely to lead to the development of the blind-loop syndrome or to result in subsequent spontaneous perforation or fistulization of diseased defunctionalized intestine left *in situ*. In a series of 77 patients who underwent surgery for radiation injury to the small intestine, no difference in short-term complications was noted whether patients underwent resection or bypass, although it is likely that the two groups were not comparable in clinical features (182). The authors did believe that the long-term complications of fistula formation and continued small-bowel necrosis could be avoided by primary resection. In patients with peritonitis caused by perforation, Swan and coworkers (187) emphasized the option of ileostomy to avoid the risk of a failed intestinal anastomosis under these circumstances. In most cases, however, anastomosis can be performed. As pointed out by Hoskins and associates (188), anastomosis in the irradiated terminal ileum should be avoided by wide resection of the terminal ileum and ascending colon with ileocolonic anastomosis.

Decisions about bypass or resection of irradiated small intestine must also take into account the presence of enteric fistulas that are draining via the vagina, bladder, or skin. Smith and colleagues (189), reporting on 68 enteric fistulas managed on the Gynecology Service at Memorial Sloan–Kettering Cancer Center, emphasized that if fistulized loops cannot be resected, they should be totally excluded from the intestinal stream to minimize continued fistulous drainage. For example, in the common case of a terminal ileal fistula, this exclusion may be accomplished by dividing the ileum proximal to the fistula, performing an ileocolonic anastomosis, bringing out the ileal stump as a mucous fistula, and placing a staple line across the ascending colon to prevent reflux of intestinal contents through an incompetent ileocecal valve. The ultimate decisions as to the operative management of patients with irradiation injury to the small intestine must be in the hands of the operating surgeon. Under appropriate circumstances, satisfactory results may be obtained with either the resection or bypass procedure.

The surgical management of radiation injury to the large intestine presents a different set of considerations. Usually, the injury is to the rectosigmoid, where it may be manifested as proctitis, ulceration, stricture, perforation with abscess formation, or rectovaginal fistula (84). Lesser degrees of bleeding may be controllable by dietary modifications, hydrocortisone-containing enemas (Cortifoam, Proctofoam), or the use of the endoscopic YAG laser (190). Surgery is required for bleeding that fails to respond to conservative measures or is massive, recurrent, or associated with perforation. Colostomy alone, without resection of the involved intestinal segment, may be sufficient in some cases to control the bleeding, presumably by decreasing mechanical irritation and infection of the diseased area of the colon. In more severe cases, excision of the rectosigmoid is required, although this procedure may be technically difficult as a result of radiation fibrosis of the pelvic soft tissues. Under favorable circumstances, restoration of intestinal continuity by coloanal anastomosis may be feasible (191). The refinement of surgical stapling instruments over the last decade has extended the ability of the surgeon to perform such low anastomoses successfully.

Patients with rectal perforation and abscess formation may require urgent surgery after correction of fluid and electrolyte imbalance. The extent of the surgical procedure depends on the degree of radiation injury, the severity of the infection, and the general condition of the patient. Often, a diverting colostomy and drainage of the abscess control infection without the increased morbidity that may result from attempts at resection of the involved rectum. In chronic situations without active severe infection, resection and low anastomosis with a protective colostomy that can be closed several months after satisfactory healing has been demonstrated to be efficacious and may be considered.

Fistulization of the large intestine after pelvic radiation therapy usually occurs between the rectum and the vagina. Occasionally, the sigmoid colon or cecum may fistulize to the vagina, cervix, uterine fundus, or urinary bladder. Because these fistulas result from radiation necrosis of the intestinal wall, simple closure is doomed to failure. After a radiographic evaluation of the intestinal tract, generous biopsy specimens of the fistulous tract should be taken. If recurrent cancer is documented, a diverting colostomy is generally indicated for relief of symptoms, and attention should be given to further treatment of the cancer. If no evidence of recurrence is found, closure of the fistula can be attempted after fecal diversion. Successful fistula repair requires the delivery of a new vascular supply to the damaged area. Perhaps the simplest means of accomplishing this task is to develop the bulbocavernosus fat pad from the labium major for use as a vascular pedicle graft between the rectum and vagina, as described by Martius (192). Although short-term results appear satisfactory with this technique (193), late breakdown can occur (194). Graham (195) has described the use of the gracilis and rectus muscles in the closure of large rectovaginal fistulas after irradiation with good success. More recently, Bricker and Johnston (196) have described an innovative technique that uses a folded piece of normal colon as a patch over the fistula, with restoration of intestinal continuity above the level of the fistula (Fig. 32.1).

Urinary Tract

Serious urinary-tract complications after irradiation are somewhat less common than intestinal complications, presumably because of the greater resistance of the urinary tract to the damaging effects of ionizing radiation. Ureteral and bladder injuries that result from irradiation most often become manifest 1 to 3 years after therapy. In the series of Cushing and coworkers (95), 12.3 months was the mean interval for major radiation-related urinary-tract complications to develop in patients treated for carcinoma of the cervix. Ureteral injury occurred at a median time of 18 months in the report by Muram and coworkers (64), whereas the peak time of development of bladder injuries was 2 to 3 years in Kottmeier's (197) series. Occasionally, complications occur much later. Ureteral fistula as a complication of radiation therapy alone in the absence of surgery or recurrent cancer is extremely rare.

The incidence of ureteral stricture after pelvic radiation therapy has markedly diminished with the refinement of irradiation techniques in recent years. Everett (198), writing in 1939, noted a 15% incidence of severe ureteral obstruction in a small group of patients treated for carcinoma of the cervix. Kaplan (199) noted a 1% incidence of postirradiation ureteral obstruction in his patient population, but pointed out that this figure was probably an underestimate because patients were not routinely investigated. In the series of Un-

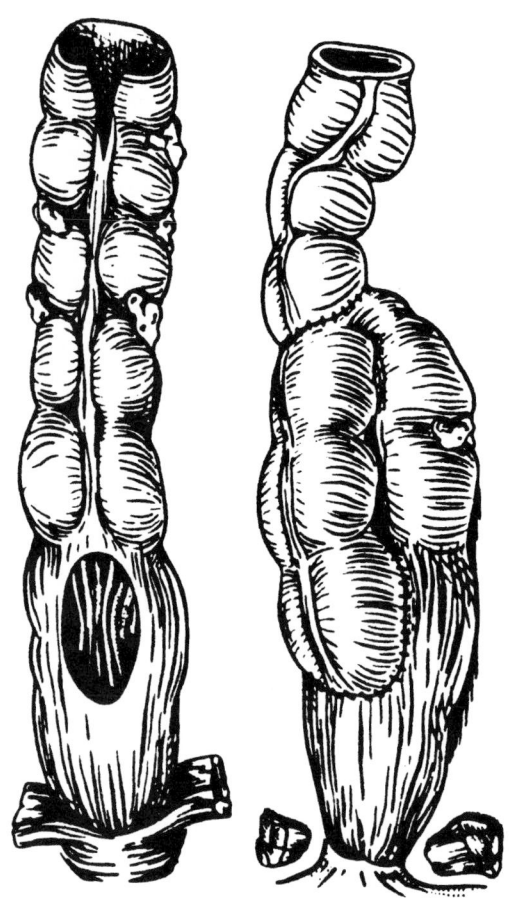

FIG. 3-1. Bricker's technique for repair of postirradiation rectovaginal fistula. The proximal end of the colon is anastomosed end-on to the fistula, or it can be increased by an antimesenteric slit to fit a larger fistulous defect. (Reprinted with permission from Bricker EM, Johnston WD. Repair of postirradiation rectovaginal fistula and stricture. *Surg Gynecol Obstet* 1979;148:499.)

derwood and colleagues (200), symptomatic ureteral stricture occurred in only 0.33% of 2393 patients who underwent radiation therapy for carcinoma of the cervix; however, pyelographic evidence of stricture was noted in 4% of 100 asymptomatic patients studied 5 or more years after treatment. Villasanta (66) has pointed out that ureteral stenosis generally occurs after cervicovaginal necrosis and parametritis and must be considered at least in part a complication of infection in irradiated patients. The most common site of ureteral stricture after pelvic irradiation appears to be 4 to 6 cm above the ureterovesical junction at the point at which the ureter passes through the parametrium (199), although obstruction may also occur at the ureterovesical junction (20) or may involve a long segment of ureter from the pelvic brim downward (201).

Because most patients who develop ureteral obstruction after irradiation for cancer of the cervix have recurrent cancer as the cause of obstruction, a thorough evaluation for recurrence must be undertaken before appropriate management can be determined. In addition to a complete physical examination and routine laboratory tests, patients should generally undergo an intravenous pyelogram. Creatinine clearance and isotope renography can be performed to determine precisely the degree of impairment of renal function. Computed tomography or magnetic resonance imaging of the abdomen and pelvis should be done to look for evidence of recurrent cancer, with needle biopsies of suspicious areas performed under radiologic guidance. All patients should undergo pelvic examination under anesthesia, with cystoscopy. Biopsies of the cervix, parametrium, and bladder may help detect recurrence. Antegrade or retrograde pyelography may be needed to determine the site of obstruction or the anatomy of the involved urinary tract. In some cases, exploratory laparotomy may be needed to document recurrent cancer; however, as Boronow (202) pointed out, given the lack of effective therapy for recurrent cervical cancer after radiation therapy, unless pelvic exenteration is contemplated, laparotomy for diagnosis of recurrence is seldom indicated. However, one must be wary of making a clinical diagnosis of recurrent cancer in the absence of histologic confirmation. In an autopsy series of 68 patients with fatal hydronephrosis and uremia, Kirchoff (203) found radiation fibrosis only as the cause of urinary obstruction in 18 patients.

Once recurrent cancer has been excluded, the site and length of the ureteral stricture have been determined, and differential renal function has been assessed, a plan of management may be developed. If infection is present in an obstructed renal unit, antibiotic treatment and decompression, usually by percutaneous nephrostomy, should be undertaken. In general, the goal of intervention is to eliminate infection and preserve renal function. A patient with a mild degree of hydronephrosis may be followed with serial evaluations. If significant impairment of renal function is present or develops under observation, intervention is indicated. Temporary relief of obstruction may be achieved by stenting of the ureter, either retrograde or antegrade, with an internal self-retaining stent. Although mechanical dilatation of radiation-related ureteral strictures has been attempted, it usually does not produce lasting relief of obstruction, probably owing to the intense degree of periureteral fibrosis present in these patients. Despite the common assumption that ureteral stricture resulting from irradiation should be a bilateral process, a summary of reports providing information on laterality of involvement shows that, in approximately 60% of patients, involvement was unilateral (Table 32.4). Temporization does have the advantage of allowing one to observe the patient for the development of stricture on the opposite side, because bilateral involvement may not always develop simultaneously.

If surgery is required, the specific operative intervention depends on the site and extent of the damage and the remaining renal function on the affected side. As reported by a number of authors, simple lysis of the ureter from its fibrotic bed in the retroperitoneum is rarely successful in eliminating

TABLE 32.4 *Laterality of irradiation-related ureteral obstruction*

| Reference | No. of obstructions | | |
	Unilateral	Bilateral	Total
Muram et al (64)	9	3	12
Kaplan (200)	10	1	11
Kirkinen et al. (209)	9	10 (7 simultaneous)	19
Underwood et al. (201)	3	5 (2 simultaneous)	8
Total	31 (62%)	19 (38%)	50

the obstruction (199,204). In general, it is necessary to resect the strictured segment of ureter and reconstruct the urinary tract using healthy tissue. Patients who have been heavily irradiated may have extensive fibrosis of the bladder, which makes direct reimplantation of the ureter difficult, particularly if a procedure such as bladder flap formation or psoas hitch is required to bridge the gap between the bladder and the ureter. In selected cases with minimal bladder fibrosis, satisfactory results may be obtained by ureteroneocystostomy, implanting the ureter into the lateral dome of the bladder, which usually has received a lesser dose of radiation. Often, the most prudent procedure is to interpose an isolated segment of intestine between the healthy ureter and the bladder (205,206). This bowel segment can also be used to increase bladder capacity if it has been significantly diminished as a result of irradiation. When considering how to reestablish intestinal continuity, one must remember that the ileum generally is heavily irradiated. Occasionally, a transureteroureterostomy above the irradiated field is appropriate, although one is naturally hesitant about the possibility of a complication that involves the opposite, relatively normal ureter. In extreme cases with bilateral ureteral injury or a bladder that can no longer function, urinary diversion may be required. This procedure is discussed fully in the section on pelvic exenteration, but may include continent urinary diversion, transverse or sigmoid colon conduit, or a Bricker-type conduit.

The bladder is subject to a spectrum of injuries from irradiation, which may produce sequelae including cystitis, hematuria, contracture, and, occasionally, severe necrosis and fistula formation. Bladder fistulas after irradiation for cancer of the cervix usually occur between the anterior vaginal wall and the posterior bladder wall because this area of the bladder receives the highest dose of radiation. In a series of 2,729 patients who underwent radiation therapy for cervical cancer at the M.D. Anderson Cancer Center, 34 patients (1.2%) experienced vesicovaginal fistula as a complication of irradiation in the absence of recurrent cancer (80). The incidence of fistula was related to the stage of the patient's cancer, with patients who had advanced-stage disease having a greater risk of this complication.

Conventional techniques of vesicovaginal fistula repair

that involve wide mobilization of the fistulous tract and a layered direct suture closure are usually not successful in the irradiated patient because of the fibrosis, poor tissue mobility, and compromised blood supply that follow irradiation (202). In the M.D. Anderson series, 20 patients underwent partial or complete colpocleisis for repair of radiation-induced vesicovaginal fistula (80). The authors were not enthusiastic about this technique, because several procedures were frequently required to achieve continence, coital function was often lost, and renal function was not improved and in many cases deteriorated. More often, once recurrent tumor has been ruled out and enough time has elapsed to allow for maturation of the fistula margins, closure may be attempted by a variety of techniques that involve the mobilization of well-vascularized tissue into the area. Boronow (202), who has contributed much to the subject, advises waiting 12 months between fistula formation and attempted closure. Gracilis muscle, omentum, and bulbocavernosus muscle have been used successfully (193,195,207,208).

Often, permanent urinary diversion is necessary. If one can subsequently repair the bladder, it is possible to attach the urinary conduit to the bladder dome in a procedure described by Boronow as the "undiversion."

In cases of bladder contracture that produces intolerable symptoms unresponsive to conservative measures, such as anticholinergic medications and bladder dilatation, augmentation cystoplasty may be indicated. Although some authors have suggested that bladder excision and replacement is preferable in radiation bladder disease (209), in the experience of others, augmentation generally suffices if the bladder mucosa is not grossly abnormal (210). Techniques of augmentation cystoplasty have been described using ileum, cecum, or colon (211). In general, a nonirradiated segment of intestine should be selected and detubularized to allow it to hold a larger volume and ensure better healing (212).

REFERENCES

1. Green MH, Boice JD, Greer BE, et al. Acute nonlymphocytic leukemia after therapy with alkylating agents for ovarian cancer: a study of five randomized clinical trials. *N Engl J Med* 1982;307:1416.
2. Kaldor JM, Day NE, Petterson F, et al. Leukemia following chemotherapy for ovarian cancer. *N Engl J Med* 1990;322:1.
3. Bertelsen K, Jakobsen A, Stroyer I, et al. A prospective randomized comparison of 6 and 12 cycles of cyclophosphamide, Adriamycin, and cisplatin in advanced epithelial ovarian cancer: a Danish Ovarian Study Group Trial (DACOVA). *Gynecol Oncol* 1993;49:30.
4. Hakes TB, Chalas E, Hoskins WJ, et al. Randomized prospective trial of 5 versus 10 cycles of cyclophosphamide, doxorubicin, and cisplatin in advanced ovarian carcinoma. *Gynecol Oncol* 1992;45:284.
5. Bassett WB, Weiss RB. Acute leukemia following cisplatin for bladder cancer. *J Clin Oncol* 1986;4:614.
6. Chambers SK, Chopyk RL, Chambers JT, et al. Development of leukemia after doxorubicin and cisplatin treatment for ovarian cancer. *Cancer* 1989;64:2459.
7. Ratain MJ, Kaminer KS, Bitran JD, et al. Acute nonlymphocytic leukemia following etoposide and cisplatin combination chemotherapy for advanced nonsmall-cell carcinoma of the lung. *Blood* 1987; 70:1412.
8. Reed E, Evans MK. Acute leukemia following cisplatin-based chemotherapy in a patient with ovarian cancer. *J Natl Cancer Inst* 1990; 82:431.
9. Travis LB, Curtis RE, Boice JD Jr, et al. Second malignant neoplasms among long-term survivors of ovarian cancer. *Cancer Res* 1996;56: 1564.
10. Winick NJ, McKenna RW, Shuster JJ, et al. Secondary acute myeloid leukemia in children with acute lymphoblastic leukemia treated with etoposide. *J Clin Oncol* 1993;11:209.
11. Slater JM, Fletcher GH. Ureteral strictures after radiation therapy for carcinoma of the uterine cervix. *Am J Roentgenol Radium Ther Nucl Med* 1971;111:269.
12. Gianni L, Munzone E. Capri G, et al. Paclitaxel by 3-hour infusion in combination with bolus doxorubicin in women with untreated metastatic breast cancer: high antitumor efficacy and cardiac effects in a dose-finding and sequence-finding study. *J Clin Oncol* 1995;13:2688.
13. Pater JL, Carmichael JA, Krepart GV, et al. Second-line chemotherapy of Stage III-IV ovarian carcinoma: a randomized comparison of melphalan to melphalan and hexamethylmelamine in patients with persistent disease after doxorubicin and cisplatin. *Cancer Treat Rep* 1987; 71:277.
14. Bajorin DF, Motzer RJ, Rodriguez E, et al. Acute non-lymphocytic leukemia in germ cell tumor patients treated with etoposide-containing chemotherapy. *J Natl Cancer Inst* 1993;85:60.
15. Smith DH, DeCosse JJ. Radiation damage to the small intestine. *World J Surg* 1986;10:189.
16. Stine KC, Saylors RL, Sawyer JR, Becton DL. Secondary acute myelogenous leukemia following safe exposure to etoposide. *J Clin Oncol* 1995;13:2688.
17. Verweij J, van der Burg MEL, Pinedo HM. Mitomycin C-induced hemolytic uremic syndrome: six case reports and review of the literature on renal, pulmonary and cardiac side effects of the drug. *Radiother Oncol* 1987;8:33.
18. Thigpen T, Vance R, Lambuth B, et al. Chemotherapy for advanced or recurrent gynecologic cancer. *Cancer* 1987;60:2104.
19. Von Hoff DD, Layard MW, Basa P, et al. Risk factors for doxorubicin-induced congestive heart failure. *Ann Intern Med* 1979;91:710.
20. Unal A, Hamberger AD, Seski JC, Fletcher GH. An analysis of the severe complications of irradiation of carcinoma of the uterine cervix: treatment with intracavitary radium and parametrial irradiation. *Int J Radiat Oncol Biol Phys* 1981;7:999.
21. Bristow MR, Mason JW, Billingham ME, et al. Doxorubicin cardiomyopathy: evaluation by phonocardiography, endomyocardial biopsy, and cardiac catheterization. *Ann Intern Med* 1978;88:168.
22. Alexander J, Dainiak N, Berger HJ, et al. Serial assessment of doxorubicin cardiotoxicity with quantitative radionuclide angiocardiography. *N Engl J Med* 1979;300:278.
23. Schwartz RG, McKenzie WB, Alexander J, et al. Congestive heart failure and left ventricular dysfunction complicating doxorubicin therapy: seven-year experience using serial radionuclide angiocardiography. *Am J Med* 1987;82:1109.
24. Legha SS, Benjamin RS, Mackay B, et al. Reduction of doxorubicin cardiotoxicity by prolonged continuous intravenous infusion. *Ann Intern Med* 1982;96:133.
25. Speyer JL, Green MD, Kramer E, et al. Protective effect of the bispiperazinedione, ICRF187, against doxorubicin-induced cardiac toxicity in women with advanced breast cancer. *N Engl J Med* 1988;319:745.
26. Slamon D, Leyland-Jones B, Shak S, et al. Addition of Herceptin (humanized anti-HER2 antibody) to first line chemotherapy for HER2 overexpressing metastatic breast cancer (HER2 + ?MBC) markedly increases anticancer activity: a randomized multinational controlled phase III trial. *Proc Am Soc Clin Oncol* 1998;17:98a.
27. Markman M. Kennedy A, Webster K, et al. Paclitaxel administration to gynecologic cancer patients with major cardiac risk factors. *J Clin Oncol* 1998;16:3483.
28. Blum RH, Carter SK, Agre K. A clinical review of bleomycin—a new antineoplastic agent. *Cancer* 1973;31:903.
29. Goldiner PL, Carlon GC, Critkovic E, et al. Factors influencing postoperative morbidity and mortality in patients treated with bleomycin. *BMJ* 1978;1:1664.
30. Verweij J, van Zanten T, Souren T, et al. Prospective study on the dose relationship of mitomycin C-induced interstitial pneumonitis. *Cancer* 1987;60:756.

31. Cersosima RJ. Cisplatin neurotoxicity. *Cancer Treat Rev* 1989;16: 195.

32. Hall DJ, Diasio R, Goplerud DR. Cisplatinum in gynecologic cancer. III. Toxicity. *Am J Obstet Gynecol* 1981;141:309.

33. Thompson SW, Davis LE, Kornfeld M, et al. Cisplatin neuropathy: clinical, electrophysiologic, morphologic, and toxicologic studies. *Cancer* 1984;54:1269.

34. Blachley JD, Hill JB. Renal and electrolyte disturbances associated with cisplatin. *Ann Intern Med* 1981;85:628.

35. Kopelman J, Budnick AS, Sessions RB, et al. Ototoxicity of high-dose cisplatin by bolus administration in patients with advanced cancers and normal hearing. *Laryngoscope* 1988;98:858.

36. Pollera CF, Marolla P, Nardi M, et al. Very high-dose cisplatin-induced ototoxicity: a preliminary report on early and long-term effects. *Cancer Chemother Pharmacol* 1988;21:61.

37. Donehower RC, Rowinsky EK, Grochow LB, et al. Phase I trial of Taxol in patients with advanced cancer. *Cancer Treat Rep* 1987;71: 1171.

38. Connelly E, Markman M, Kennedy A, et al. Paclitaxel delivered as a 3-hour infusion with cisplatin in patients with gynecologic cancers: unexpected incidence of neurotoxicity. *Gynecol Oncol* 1996;62:166.

39. Piccart MJ, Bertelsen K, James K, et al. Randomized intergroup rial of cisplatin-paclitaxel versus cisplatin-cyclophosphamide in women with advanced epithelial ovarian cancer: Three-year results. *J Natl Cancer Inst* 2000;92:669.

40. Neijt J, Engelholm S, Tuxen M, et al. Exploratory phase III study of paclitaxel and cisplatin versus paclitaxel and carboplatin in advanced ovarian cancer. *J Clin Oncol* 2000;18:3084.

41. Hamner RW, Verani R, Weinman EJ. Mitomycin-associated renal failure: case report and review. *Arch Intern Med* 1983;143:803.

42. Gradishar WJ, Schilsky RL. Ovarian function following radiation and chemotherapy for cancer. *Semin Oncol* 1989;16:425.

43. Tangir, J, Zelterman D, Wenging M, Schwartz P. Reproductive function after conservative surgery and chemotherapy for malignant germ cell tumors of the ovary. *Am College of Obstet Gynecol* 2003;101: 251

44. Bower M, Newlands E, Holden L, et. al. EMA/CO for high-risk gestational trophoblastic tumors: Results from a cohort of 272 patients. *J Clin Oncol* 1997;15:2636.

45. Brewer M, Gershenson D, Herzog C, et. al. Outcome and reproductive function after chemotherapy for ovarian dysgerminoma. *J Clin Oncol* 1999;17:2670.

46. Doll DC, Ringenberg QS, Yarbo JW. Antineoplastic agents and pregnancy. *Semin Oncol* 1989;16:337.

47. Garber JE. Long-term follow-up of children exposed in utero to antineoplastic agents. *Semin Oncol* 1989;16:427.

48. Keys HM, Bundy BN, Stehman FB, et al. Cisplatin, radiation and adjuvant hysterectomy compared with radiation and adjuvant hysterectomy for bulky Stage IB cervical carcinoma. *N Engl J Med* 1999; 340:1154.

49. Rose PG, Bundy BN, Watkins EB, et al. Concurrent cisplatin-based radiotherapy and chemotherapy for locally advanced cervical cancer. *N Engl J Med* 1999;340:114.

50. Pilepich MV, Pajak T, George FW, et al. Preliminary report on phase III RTOG studies of extended-field irradiation in carcinoma of the prostate. *Am J Clin Oncol* 1983;6:485.

51. Johnson R, D'Angio GJ, Tefft M, et al. Discussion: combined radiotherapy and chemotherapy. *Cancer* 1976;37:1214.

52. Kagan AR, DiSaia PJ, Wollin M, et al. The narrow vagina, the antecedent for irradiation injury. *Gynecol Oncol* 1976;4:291.

53. Kjorstad KE, Martimbeau PW, Iversen T. Stage IB carcinoma of the cervix. The Norwegian Radium Hospital: results and complications. III. Urinary and gastrointestinal complications. *Gynecol Oncol* 1983; 15:42.

54. Rubin P, Casarett GW. *Clinical radiation pathology*. Philadelphia: WB Saunders, 1968;1.

55. Farquarson DI, Shingleton HM, Soong SJ, et al. The adverse effects of cervical cancer treatment on bladder function. *Gynecol Oncol* 1987; 27:15.

56. Barber HRK. *Manual of gynecologic oncology*. Philadelphia: JB Lippincott Co, 1987:185.

57. Perez CA, Korba A, Purdy JA, et al. Dosimetric consideration in radiation therapy of carcinoma of the vagina. *Int J Radiat Oncol Biol Phys* 1976;1[Suppl]:67.

58. Phillips TL. The interaction of drug and radiation effects on normal tissue. *Int J Radiat Oncol Biol Phys* 1978;4:59.

59. Prempree T, Viravathona T, Slawson RG, et al. Radiation management of primary carcinoma of the vagina. *Int J Radiat Oncol Biol Phys* 1976;1[Suppl]:66.

60. Herbst AL. Cancer of the vagina. In: Gusberg SB, Frick HC, eds. *Corscaden's gynecologic cancer*. 5th ed. Baltimore: Williams & Wilkins, 1978:120.

61. Wharton JT, Smith JP, Delclos L, et al. Radiation therapy for cervical carcinoma. In: Buchsbaum HJ, Sciarra JJ, eds. *Gynecology and obstetrics*. Philadelphia: Harper & Row, 1983:1.

62. Maruyama Y, van Nagell JR. Radiation therapy in the treatment of cervical cancer. In: van Nagell JR, Barber HRK, eds. *Modern concepts of gynecologic oncology*. Bristol: Stonebridge Press, 1982:91.

63. Rotman M, John M, Roussis K, et al. The intracavitary applicator in relation to complications of pelvic radiation: the Ernst system. *Int J Radiat Oncol Biol Phys* 1978;4:951.

64. Muram B, Oxorn H, Currie RJ, et al. Postradiation ureteral obstruction: a reappraisal. *Am J Obstet Gynecol* 1981;139:289.

65. Aldridge CW, Mason JT. Ureteral obstruction in carcinoma of the cervix. *Am J Obstet Gynecol* 1980;60:1272.

66. Villasanta U. Complications of radiotherapy for carcinoma of the uterine cervix. *Am J Obstet Gynecol* 1972;114:717.

67. Bosch A, Frias Z, deValda G. Prognostic significance of ureteral obstruction in carcinoma of the cervix uteri. *Acta Radiol* 1973;47:56.

68. VanDyke AH, van Nagell JR. The prognostic significance of ureteral obstruction in patients with recurrent carcinoma of the cervix uteri. *Surg Gynecol Obstet* 1975;141:371.

69. Jensen, PT, et al., Longitudinal study of sexual function and vaginal changes after radiotherapy for cervical cancer. *Int J Radiat Oncol Biol Phys*, 2003;56:937.

70. Hartman P, Diddle AW. Vaginal stenosis following irradiation therapy for carcinoma of the cervix uteri. *Cancer* 1972;30:426.

71. Pitkin RM, Van Voorhis LW. Postirradiation vaginitis: an evaluation of prophylaxis with topical estrogen. *Radiology* 1971;99:417.

72. Grigsby PW, Roberts HL, Perez CA. Femoral neck fracture following groin irradiation. *Int J Radiat Oncol Biol Phys* 1995;32:63.

73. Delouche G, Burnet M, Guerin P, et al. Les lesions osseuses de la radiotherapie intensive des cancers gynecologiques: a propos de 20 cas releves au Centre Rene–Huguenin. *Ann Radiol (Paris)* 1970;13: 793.

74. Wollin M, Kagan AR. Optimization of the box technique to reduce femm dose in radiation therapy of the pelvis. *Int J Radiat Oncol Biol Phys* 1979;5:553.

75. Bourne RG, Kearsley JH, Grove WD, et al. The relationship between early and late gastrointestinal complications or radiation therapy for carcinoma of the cervix. *Int J Radiat Oncol Biol Phys* 1983;9:1445.

76. Fletcher GH. *Textbook of radiotherapy*. 3rd ed. Philadelphia: Lea & Febiger, 1980:720.

77. Roswit B, Malsky SJ, Reid CB. Radiation tolerance of the gastrointestinal tract. *Front Radiat Ther Oncol* 1972;6:160.

78. trockbine MF, Hancock JE, Fletcher GH. Complications in 831 patients with squamous cell carcinoma of the intact uterine cervix treated with 3000 rads or more whole pelvis irradiation. *Am J Roentgenol Radium Ther Nucl Med* 1970;108:293.

79. Donaldson S. Meeting of the Diet, Nutrition and Cancer Program Advisory Committee. *Cancer Lett* 1975;110:1.

80. Boronow RC, Rutledge F. Vesicovaginal fistula, radiation, and gynecologic cancer. *Am J Obstet Gynecol* 1971;111:85.

81. Choi K, Aziz H, Rotman M. Complications in the radiotherapeutic management of gynecological cancers. In: Nori D, Hilaris BS, eds. *Radiation therapy of gynecological cancer*. New York: Alan R. Liss, 1987:239.

82. Powell-Smith C. Factors influencing the incidence of radiation injury in cancer of the cervix. *Can Assoc Radiol J* 1967;16:132.

83. Yoonessi M, Romney S, Dayem H. Gastrointestinal tract complications following radiotherapy of uterine cervical cancer: past and present. *J Surg Oncol* 1981;18:135.

84. Eifel PJ, Jhringran A, Bodurka PC, et al. Correlation of smoking history and other patient characteristics with major complications of

pelvic radiation therapy for cervical cancer. *J Clin Oncol,* 2002;20: 3651.

85. Georgiou A, Grigsby PW, Perez CA. Radiation-induced lumbosacral plexopathy in gynecologic tumors: clinical findings and dosimetric analysis. *Int J Radiat Oncol Biol Phys* 1993;26:479.

86. Chadha M, Nori D, Hilaris BS, et al. Stage IIB carcinoma of the cervix managed with radiation therapy: an analysis of prognostic factors. *Endocurie Hypertherm Oncol* 1988;4:219.

87. Hamberger AD, Unal A, Gershenson DM. Analysis of the severe complications of irradiation of carcinoma of the cervix: whole pelvis irradiation and intracavitary radium. *Int J Radiat Oncol Biol Phys* 1983;9:367.

88. Nori D, Fuks Z. Radiation therapy in gynecologic cancer. *Curr Opin Oncol* 1989;1:97.

89. Pourquier H, Dubois JG, Delard R. Cancer of the uterine cervix: dosimetric guidelines for prevention of late rectal and rectosigmoid complications as a result of radiotherapeutic treatment. *Int J Radiat Oncol Biol Phys* 1982;8:1887.

90. Logsdon, MD, Eifel, PJ. FIGO IIIB squamous cell carcinoma of the cervix: An analysis of prognostic factors emphasizing the balance between external beam and intracavitary radiation therapy. *Int J Radiat Oncol Biol Phys*, 1999;43(4):763–75.

91. Cardiani P, Austoni E, Campiglio GL, et al. Repair of a recurrent urethrovaginal fistula with an island of bulbocavernous musculocutaneous flap. *Plastic Reconstr Surg* 1993;92:1393.

92. Cunningham DE, Stryker JA, Velkley DE, et al. Routine clinical estimation of rectal rectosigmoid and bladder doses from intracavitary brachytherapy in the cervix. *Int J Radiat Oncol Biol Phys* 1981;7: 653.

93. Alert J, Jimenez J, Beldarrain J, et al. Complications from irradiation of carcinoma of the uterine cervix. *Acta Radiol Oncol* 1980;19:13.

94. Allt, WEC. Supervoltage radiation treatment in advanced cancer of the uterine cervix: a preliminary report. *Can Med Assoc J* 1969;100: 792.

95. Cushing RM, Towell HM, Liegner LM. Major urological complications following radium and x-ray therapy for carcinoma of the cervix. *Am J Obstet Gynecol* 1968;101:750.

95a. Ellis F, Sorensen A, Lesorenier C. Radiation therapy schedules for opposing parallel fields and their biological effects. *Radiology* 1974; 111:701.

96. Stupar TA, Bahr GK, Elson HR, et al. Generation of iso-TDF maps: considerations for radiation therapy planning. *Radiology* 1978;126: 773.

97. Wilson CS, Hall EJ. On the advisability of treating all fields at each radiotherapy session. *Radiology* 1971;98:419.

98. Nori D, Valentine E, Hilaris BS. The role of paraaortic node irradiation in the treatment of cancer of the cervix. *Int J Radiat Oncol Biol Phys* 1985;11:1.

99. Piver MS, Barlow JJ, Krishnamsetty R. Five-year survival (with no evidence of disease) in patients with biopsy-confirmed aortic node metastasis from cervical carcinoma. *Am J Obstet Gynecol* 1981;139: 575.

100. Potish R, Adcock L, Jones T Jr, et al. The morbidity and utility of periaortic radiotherapy in cervical carcinoma. *Gynecol Oncol* 1983; 15:1.

101. Senoussi MAE, Fletcher GH, Borlase BC. Correlation of radiation and surgical parameters and complications in the extended field technique for carcinoma of the cervix. *Int J Radiat Oncol Biol Phys* 1979; 5:927.

102. Welander C, Pierce V, Nori D, et al. Pretreatment laparotomy in carcinoma of the cervix. *Gynecol Oncol* 1981;12:336.

103. Malfetano JH, Keys H, Cunningham MJ, et al. Extended field radiation and cisplatin for stage IIB and IIIB cervical carcinoma. *Gynecol Oncol,* 1997;67:203.

104. Grigsby PW, Keydow K, Mutch DG, et al. Long-term follow-up of RTOG 92–10: cervical cancer with positive para-aortic lymph nodes. *Int J Radiat Oncol Biol Phys,* 2001;51:982.

105. Perez CA, Camel HM, Kao MS, et al. Randomized study of preoperative radiation and surgery or irradiation alone in the treatment of Stage IB and IIA carcinoma of the uterine cervix: preliminary analysis of failures and complications. *Cancer* 1980;45:2759.

106. Perez CA, Breaux S, Bedwinek JM, et al. Radiation therapy alone

in the treatment of carcinoma of the uterine cervix. II. Analysis of complications. *Cancer* 1984;54:235.

107. Perez CA, Griguby BN, Lockett MA al. Radiation therapy morbidity in carcinoma of the uterine cervix: dosimetric and clinical correlation. *Int J Radiat Oncol Biol Phys* 1999; 44(4):855–66.

108. Sedlis A, Bundy BN, Rotman MZ, et al. A randomized trial of pelvic radiation therapy versus no further therapy in selected patients with stage IB carcinoma of the cervix after radical hysterectomy and pelvic lymphadenectomy: A Gynecologic Oncology Group Study. *Gynecol Oncol* 1999;73:177.

109. Peters WA 3rd, Liu PY, Barnett RJ, et al. Concurrent chemotherapy and pelvic radiation therapy compared with pelvic radiation therapy alone as adjuvant therapy after radical surgery in high-risk early-stage cancer of the cervix. *J Clin Oncol* 2000;18:1606.

110. Landoni F, Maneo A, Colombo A, et al. Randomised study of radical surgery versus radiotherapy for stage Ib-IIa cervical cancer. *Lance* 1997;350:535.

111. Landoni F, Maneo A, Colombo A, et al. Class II versus class III radical hysterectomy in stage IB-IIA cervical cancer: a prospective randomized study. *Gynecol Oncol* 2001;80:3.

112. Morris M, Eifel PJ, Lu J, et al. Pelvic radiation with concurrent chemotherapy compared with pelvic and para-aortic radiation for high-risk cervical cancer. *N Engl J Med* 1999;340:1137.

113. Fuks Z, Bagshaw MA. The rationale for curative radiotherapy for ovarian carcinoma. *Int J Radiat Oncol Biol Phys* 1975;1:21.

114. Fyles AW, Dembo AJ, Bush RS, et al. Analysis of complications in patients treated with abdomino-pelvic radiation therapy for ovarian carcinoma. *Int J Radiat Oncol Biol Phys* 1992;22:847.

115. Brady LW. Advances in the management of gynecological cancer in radiation therapy. *Cancer* 1975;36:661.

116. Dembo AJ, Bush RS, Beale FA. The Princess Margaret Study of ovarian cancer Stages I, II and asymptomatic III. *Cancer Treat Rep* 1979;63:249.

117. Wharton JT, Delclos L, Gallagher S. Radiation hepatitis induced by abdominal irradiation with the cobalt 60 moving strip technique. *Am J Roentgenol Radiat Ther Nucl Med* 1973;117:73.

118. Dembo AJ. Radiotherapeutic management of ovarian cancer. *Semin Oncol* 1984;11:238.

119. Dembo AJ. The sequential multiple modality treatment of ovarian cancer. *Radiat Oncol* 1985;3:187.

120. Fazekas JT, Maier JG. Irradiation of ovarian carcinoma: a prospective comparison of the open field and moving strip techniques. *Am J Roentgenol Radium Ther Nucl Med* 1974;120:118.

121. Nath R. New directions in radionuclide sources for brachytherapy. *Semin Radiat Oncol* 1993;3:278.

122. Deehan C, O'Donoghue JA. Biological equivalence of LDR and HDR brachytherapy. In: Mould RF, Batterman JJ, Martinez AA, Speiser BL, eds. *Brachytherapy from radium to optimization.* Leersum, The Netherlands: Nucletron, 1994:19.

123. Pettersson F. FIGO, annual report on the results of treatment in gynaecological cancer. Stockholm: International Federation of Gynecology and Obstetrics, Vol 20, 1988.

124. Hilaris B. Brachytherapy as we enter the year 2000. In: Nori D, ed. *The VIII brachytherapy update, 1988.* New York: Memorial Sloan-Kettering, 1988:137.

125. Crook J, Esche B. The uterine cervix. In: Cox J, ed. *Moss' radiation oncology: rationale, technique, results.* St. Louis: Mosby–Year Book, 1994:617.

126. Ahmad K, Young K, Orton C, et al. Fractionated high dose rate brachytherapy and concomitant teletherapy in the treatment of carcinoma of the cervix: technique and early results. *Endocurie Hypertherm Oncol* 1991;79:117.

127. Batterman JJ, Szabol BJ. Preliminary results of radiation therapy for carcinoma of the uterine cervix, using Selectron afterloading machine. In: Mould RF, ed. *Brachytherapy 2.* Proceedings of the 5th International Selectron Users' Meeting 1988. Leersum, The Netherlands: Nucletron, 1988:229.

128. Patel FD, Sharma SC, Negi PS, et al. Low dose rate vs. high dose rate brachytherapy in the treatment of carcinoma of the uterine cervix: a clinical trial. *Int J Radiat Oncol Biol Phys* 1994;28:335.

129. Teshima T, Inoue T, Ikeda H, et al. High dose rate and low dose rate intracavitary therapy for carcinoma of the uterine cervix: final results of Osaka University Hospital. *Cancer* 1993;72:2409.

130. Arai T, Takashi N, Shinroku M, et al. High dose rate remote afterloading intracavitary radiation therapy for cancer of the uterine cervix. *Cancer* 1992;69:175.

131. Iyer PS, Shanta A. Update of radionuclides used in endocurietherapy. *Endocurie Hypertherm Oncol* 1994;10:161.

132. Selke P, Roman TN, Souhami L, et al. Treatment results of high dose rate brachytherapy in patients with carcinoma of the cervix. *Int J Radiat Oncol Biol Phys* 1993;27:803.

133. Eifel P, Thoms W, Smith T, et al. The relationship between brachytherapy dose and outcome in patients with bulky endocervical tumors treated with radiation alone. *Int J Radiat Oncol Biol Phys* 1994;28:113.

134. Komaki R. The endometrium, the vagina, the vulva, and the female urethra. In: Cox JD, ed. *Moss' radiation oncology: rationale, technique, results.* St. Louis: Mosby–Year Book, 1994;683.

135. Orton CG, Seyesadr M, Somany A. Comparison of high and low dose rate afterloading for cervix cancer and the importance of fractionation. *Int J Radiat Oncol Biol Phys* 1991;21:1425.

136. Swamy K, Viswanathan N, Mohan D, Belliappa MS. Influence of brachytherapy dose rate on complications in the treatment of uterine cancer. *Endocurie Hypertherm Oncol* 1991;7:171.

137. Meerwaldt JH, Hoekstra CJM, Van Putten WLJ, et al. Endometrial adenocarcinoma: adjuvant radiotherapy tailored to prognostic factors. *Int J Radiat Oncol Biol Phys* 1990;18:299.

138. Nori D, Merimsky O, Batata M, Caputo T. Postoperative high dose-rate intravaginal brachytherapy combined with external irradiation for early stage endometrial cancer. *Int J Radiat Oncol Biol Phys* 1994;30:831.

139. Nori D. Principles of radiation therapy in the management of carcinoma of the endometrium. In: Nori D, Hilaris B, eds. *Radiation therapy of gynecological cancer.* New York: Allan R. Liss, 1987;115.

140. Maruyama Y, Ezzell G, Porter A. Afterloading high dose rate intracavitary vaginal cylinder. *Int J Radiat Oncol Biol Phys* 1994;30:473.

141. Sorbe B, Smeds AC. Postoperative vaginal irradiation with high dose rate afterloading technique in endometrial carcinoma stage I. *Int J Radiat Oncol Biol Phys* 1990;18:305.

142. Roberts JA, Brunetto VL, Keys HM, et al. A phase III randomized study of surgery vs. surgery plus adjunctive radiation therapy in intermediate risk endometrial adenocarcinoma. *Abstracts of the 29th Annual Meeting of the Society of Gynecologic Oncologists* 1998;30(70).

143. Naumann, R.W., R.V. Higgins, and J.B. Hall, The use of adjuvant radiation therapy by members of the Society of Gynecologic Oncologists. *Gynecol Oncol* 1999;75:4.

144. Creutzberg CL, van Putten WL, Koper PC, et al. Surgery and postoperative radiotherapy versus surgery alone for patients with stage-1 endometrial carcinoma: multicentre randomised trial. PORTEC Study Group. Post Operative Radiation Therapy in Endometrial Carcinoma. *Lancet* 2000;355(9213):1404–11.

145. Creutzberg CL, van Putten WL, Koper PC, et al. The morbidity of treatment for patients with Stage I endometrial cancer: results from a randomized trial. *Int J Radiat Oncol Biol Phys* 2001;51:1246.

146. Horowitz NS, Peters WA 3rd, Smith MR, et al. Adjuvant high dose rate vaginal brachytherapy as treatment of stage I and II endometrial carcinoma. *Obstet Gynecol* 2002;9:235.

147. Alektiar KM, McKee A, Venkatraman E, et al. Intravaginal high-dose-rate brachytherapy for Stage IB (FIGO Grade 1, 2) endometrial cancer. *Int J Radiat Oncol Biol Phys* 2002;53:707.

148. Nori D, Stitt PO. Role of high dose rate brachytherapy in carcinoma of the endometrium. In: Nag S, ed. *High dose rate brachytherapy.* Mt. Kisco, NY: Futura Publishing, 1994:385.

149. Conference on combined modality chemotherapy/radiotherapy. *Int J Radiat Oncol Biol Phys* 1978;5:1425.

150. Mundt AJ, Lujan AE, Rotmensch J, et al. Intensity-modulated whole pelvic radiotherapy in women with gynecologic malignancies. *Int J Radiat Oncol Biol Phys* 2002;52:1330.

151. Perkins DE, Spiut HJ. Intestinal stenosis following radiation therapy. *AJR Am J Roentgenol* 1962;88:953.

152. Reichelderfer M, Morrissey JF. Colonoscopy and radiation colitis. *Gastrointest Endosc* 1980;26:41.

153. Russell JC, Welch JP. Operative management of radiation injuries of the intestinal tract. *Am J Surg* 1979;137:433.

154. Smith RJ. Surgical management of radiation enteritis. *J Natl Med Assoc* 1979;71:441.

155. Macfayden BU, Dudrick SJ, Ruberg RL. Management of gastrointestinal fistulas with parenteral hyperalimentation. *Surgery* 1973;74:100.

156. Grigsby PW, Pilepich MV, Parsons CL, et al. Preliminary results of a phase I/II study of sodium pentosanpolysulfate in the treatment of chronic radiation-induced proctitis. *Am J Clin Oncol* 1990;13:28.

157. Morrow CP, Curtin JP, eds. *Gynecologic cancer surgery.* New York: Churchill Livingstone, 1996;141.

158. Orr JW, Shingleton HM. *Complications in gynecologic surgery.* Philadelphia: JB Lippincott Co, 1994.

159. Underwood PB, Wilson WC, Kreutner A, et al. Radical hysterectomy: a critical review of twenty-two years' experience. *Am J Obstet Gynecol* 1979;134:889.

160. Carmody E, Thurston W, Yueng E, Ho CH. Transrectal drainage of deep pelvic collections under fluoroscopic guidance. *Can Assoc Radiol J* 1993;44:429.

161. Hoskins WJ, Park RC, Long R, et al. Repair of urinary tract fistulas with bulbocavernous myocutaneous flaps. *Obstet Gynecol* 1984;63:588.

162. Hancock KC, Copeland LJ, Gershenson DM, et al. Urinary conduits in gynecologic oncology. *Obstet Gynecol* 1986;67:680.

163. Regan JB, Barrett DM. Stented versus non-stented ureteroileal anastomoses: is there a difference with regard to leak and stricture? *J Urol* 1985;134:1101.

164. Penalever MA, Angioli R, Mirhashimi R, Malik R. Management of early and late complications of ileocolonic continent urinary reservoir (Miami pouch). *Gynecol Oncol* 1998;69:185.

165. Montz FJ, Holschneider CH, Solh S, et al. Small bowel obstruction following radical hysterectomy: risk factors, incidence, and operative findings. *Gynecol Oncol* 1994;53:114.

166. Beard RW, Kelly KA. Randomized prospective evaluation of the EEA stapler for colorectal anastomosis. *Am J Surg* 1981;141:143.

167. Jex RK, Van Heersen JA, Wolf BG, et al. Gastrointestinal anastomoses: factors affecting early complications. *Ann Surg* 1987; 206:138.

168. Castro JR, Issa P, Fletcher GH. Carcinoma of the cervix treated by external irradiation alone. *Radiology* 1970;95:163.

169. Dziki AJ, Duncan JD, Harmon JW, et al. Advantages of hand-sewn over stapled anastomoses. *Dis Colon Rectum* 1991;34:44.

170. Max E, Sweeney WB, Bailey HR, et al. Results of 1,000 single layer continuous polyprolene intestinal anastomosis. *Am J Surg* 1991;162:461.

171. Brolin RE, Krasna MJ, Mast BA. Use of tubes and radiographs in the management of small bowel obstruction. *Ann Surg* 1987;206:126.

172. Snyder CL, Ferrel KL, Goodale RL, Leonard AS. Nonoperative management of small bowel obstruction with endoscopic long tube placement. *Ann Surg* 1990;56–587.

173. Sosa J, Gardner B. Management of patients diagnosed as acute intestinal obstruction secondary to adhesions. *Ann Surg* 1993;59:125.

174. Joyce WP, Delaney PV, Gorey TF, Fotzpatrick JM. The value of water soluble contrast radiology in the management of acute small bowel obstruction. *Ann R Coll Surg Engl* 1992;74:422.

175. Farmer KCR, Phillips RKS. True and false large bowel obstruction. *Baillieres Clin Gastroenterol* 1991;5:563.

176. Hoffman MS, Villa A, Roberts WS, et al. Mass closure of the abdominal wound with absorbable suture in surgery for gynecologic cancer. *J Reprod Med* 1991;36:356.

177. Shepard JH, Cavanaugh D, Riggs D, et al. Abdominal wound closure using a nonabsorbable single-layer technique. *Obstet Gynecol* 1983;61:248.

178. Hanks GE, Herring DF, Kramer S. Patterns of Care Outcome Studies: results of the national practice in cancer of the cervix. *Cancer* 1983;51:959.

179. van Nagell JR, Maruyuma Y, Parker JC, Dalton WL. Small bowel injury following radiation therapy for cervical cancer. *Am J Obstet Gynecol* 1974;118:163.

180. Kucera PR, Berman ML, Treadwell P, et al. Whole-abdominal radiotherapy for patients with minimal residual epithelial ovarian cancer. *Gynecol Oncol* 1990;36:338.

181. Linstadt DE, Stern JL, Quivey JM, et al. Salvage whole abdominal irradiation following chemotherapy failure in epithelial ovarian cancer. *Gynecol Oncol* 1990;36:327.

182. Smith ST, Seski JC, Copeland LJ, et al. Surgical management of irradiation-induced small bowel damage. *Obstet Gynecol* 1985;65:563.

183. Schmitt EH, Symmonds RE. Surgical treatment of radiation induced injuries of the intestine. *Surg Gynecol Obstet* 1981;153:896.

184. Rubin SC, Benjamin I, Hoskins WJ, et al. Intestinal surgery in gynecologic oncology. *Gynecol Oncol* 1989;34:30.

185. Curtin JP, Burt LL. Successful treatment of small intestinal fistula with somatostatin analog. *Gynecol Oncol* 1990;39:225.

186. Marks G, Mohiudden M. The surgical management of the radiation-injured intestine. *Surg Clin North Am* 1983;63:81.

187. Swan RW, Fowler WC Jr, Boronow RC. Surgical management of radiation injury to the small intestine. *Surg Gynecol Obstet* 1976; 142: 325.

188. Hoskins WJ, Burke TW, Weiser EB, et al. Right hemicolectomy and ileal resection with primary anastomosis for irradiation injury of the terminal ileum. *Gynecol Oncol* 1987;26:215.

189. Smith DH, Pierce VK, Lewis JL Jr. Enteric fistulas encountered on a gynecologic oncology service from 1969 through 1980. *Surg Gynecol Obstet* 1984;158:71.

190. Ahlquist DA, Gostout CJ, Viggiano TR, Pemberton JH. Laser therapy for severe radiation induced rectal bleeding. *Mayo Clin Proc* 1986; 61:927.

191. Schofield PF, Car ND, Holden D. The pathogenesis and treatment of radiation bowel disease. *J R Soc Med* 1986;79:30.

192. Martius H. Sphincter und Harnrohrenplastik aus dem M. bulbocavernosis. *Chirurgie* 1929;17:49.

193. Boronow RC. Repair of the radiation-induced vaginal fistula using the Martius technique. *World J Surg* 1986;10:237.

194. Aartsen EJ, Sindram IS. Repair of the radiation induced rectovaginal fistula without or with interposition of the bulbocavernosus muscle (Martius procedure). *Eur J Surg Oncol* 1988;14:171.

195. Graham JB. Vaginal fistulas following radiotherapy. *Surg Gynecol Obstet* 1965;120:1019.

196. Bricker EM, Johnston WD. Repair of postirradiation rectovaginal fistula and stricture. *Surg Gynecol Obstet* 1979;148:499.

197. Kottmeier HL. Complications following radiation therapy in carcinoma of the cervix and their treatment. *Am J Obstet Gynecol* 1964; 88:854.

198. Everett HS. The effect of carcinoma of the cervix uteri and its treatment upon the urinary tract. *Am J Obstet Gynecol* 1939;38:889.

199. Kaplan AL. Postradiation ureteral obstruction. *Obstet Gynecol Surv* 1977;32:1.

200. Underwood PB, Lutz MH, Smoak DL. Ureteral injury following irradiation therapy for carcinoma of the cervix. *Obstet Gynecol* 1977;49: 663.

201. Altvater G, Imholz G. Ureteral stenosis in carcinoma of the cervix uteri: prognostic significance and surgical treatment. *Geburtshilfe Frauenheilkd* 1960;20:1214.

202. Boronow RC. Urologic complications secondary to radiation alone or radiation and surgery. In: Delgado G, Smith JP, eds. *Management of complications in gynecologic oncology.* New York: John Wiley & Sons, 1982:163.

203. Kirchoff H. *Geburtshilfe Frauenheilkd* 1960;920:34.

204. Burns BC, Upton RT. Cancer of the uterus and ovary. Chicago: Year Book Medical Publishers, 1969.

205. Krupp P, Hoffman M, Roeling W. Terminal ileum as ureteral substitute. *Obstet Gynecol* 1970;35:416.

206. Perry CP, Massey FM, Moore TN, Erikson CA. Treatment of irradiation injury to the ureter by ileal substitution. *Obstet Gynecol* 1975; 46:517.

207. Bastiaanse M. Bastiaanse's method for surgical closure of very large radiation fistulae of the bladder and rectum. In: Youssef AF, ed. *Gynecologic oncology.* Springfield, IL: Charles C Thomas Publisher, 1960: 280.

208. Kirkinen P, Kauppila A, Kontturi M. Treatment of ureteral strictures after therapy for carcinoma of the uterus. *Surg Gynecol Obstet* 1980; 151:487.

209. Mundy AR. Cystoplasty. In: Mundy AR, ed. *Current operative surgery: urology.* Eastbourne, UK: Bailliere, 1986;140.

210. Barnard RJ, Lupton EW. Treatment of radiation urinary tract disease. In: Schofield PF, Lupton EW, eds. *The causation and clinical management of pelvic radiation disease.* London: Springer–Verlag, 1989: 123.

211. Goodwin WE. Experiences with intestine as a substitute for the urinary tract. In: King LR, Stone AR, Webster GD, eds. *Bladder reconstruction and continent urinary diversion.* Chicago: Year Book Medical Publishers, 1987:9.

212. Concepcion RS, Koch MO, McDougal S, Richards WO. Detubularized intestinal segments in urinary tract reconstruction: why do they work? *J Urol* 1988;139:310a.

CHAPTER 33

Management of Pain

Russell K. Portenoy, Annette Vielhaber, and Pauline Lesage

The heterogeneous patient population managed by gynecologic oncologists presents a broad range of problems in pain management. Acute pains are highly prevalent, including the rather straightforward incisional pain that follows surgical procedures. Chronic pain occurs in the context of numerous other physical and psychosocial symptoms, often in the population with advanced disease. The diversity of pain complaints and associated problems requires a systematic approach to assessment and analgesic therapy.

SCOPE OF THE PROBLEM

Pain is highly prevalent in the cancer population. Overall, 30% to 50% of patients undergoing active antineoplastic therapy and 75% to 90% of those with advanced disease experience chronic pain severe enough to warrant therapy (1–3). Although data specific to gynecologic tumors are meager, those extant suggest that the overall prevalence rates mirror these averages (1,4–6).

A 1994 survey of patients with ovarian cancer illustrates the prevalence and characteristics of chronic pain in this population (6). The sample included 111 inpatients and 40 outpatients. The median age was 55 years (range 23 to 86 years), and most patients (82%) had stage III or IV disease at presentation and active disease (69%) at the time of the survey. Forty-two percent (n = 63) reported "persistent or frequent pain" during the preceding 2 weeks. This pain had a median duration of 2 weeks (range <1 to 756 weeks) and was usually abdominal/pelvic (80%), frequent or almost constant (66%), and moderate to severe. Most patients reported that pain caused moderate or greater interference with various aspects of function, particularly activity (68%), mood (62%), work (62%), and overall enjoyment of life (61%). In a study of 97 outpatients with breast cancer (54% metastatic disease), 47% of patients experienced cancer-related pain substantially interfering with their mood, quality of life, and functional status (7). The most prevalent underlying pathology was postmastectomy syndrome (56%), followed by pain from bone metastasis (26%).

Although the prevalence of acute pain in patients with gynecologic cancers has not been determined, numerous surveys suggest that it too is extremely common. In general surgical populations, unrelieved postoperative pain has been reported in 25% to 70% of patients, and a survey of patients with chronic cancer pain observed that transient acute pains occurred in approximately two-thirds of the patients (8,9). As more cancer surgeries are performed in the ambulatory setting, the likelihood of inadequate management of postoperative pain may be increasing.

Patients with cancer, and particularly those with advanced disease, also experience numerous symptoms other than pain. In the aforementioned survey of patients with ovarian cancer, for example, the median number of symptoms per patient was nine (range 0 to 25) (Table 33.1)(6). In addition to pain, the most prevalent symptoms were fatigue ("lack of energy"), psychologic distress ("worrying," "feeling sad," and "feeling nervous"), and insomnia ("difficulty sleeping"). All of these symptoms had a prevalence of >50%. Compared to norms, approximately one-third of the patients in this survey recorded heightened psychologic distress. The most important predictor of heightened distress was progressive impairment in physical functioning.

Although the high prevalence of unrelieved pain in cancer populations, including those with gynecologic tumors, probably has many determinants, there is strong evidence that undertreatment is one of the most important (10,11). In routine practice settings, unrelieved cancer pain is far more

R. K. Portenoy: Department of Pain Medicine and Palliative Care, Beth Israel Medical Center, New York, New York 10003

A. Vielhaber: Department of Pain Medicine and Palliative Care, Beth Israel Medical Center, New York, New York 10003

P. Lesage: Department of Pain Medicine and Palliative Care, Beth Israel Medical Center, New York, New York 10003

TABLE 33.1. *Prevalence and characteristics of symptoms associated with ovarian cancer (n = 151)*

Symptom	Overall prevalence (%)	Intensity[a] (%)	Frequency[b] (%)	Distress[c] (%)
Worrying	71.7	55.4	33.5	25.0
Lack of energy	68.6	52.6	37.3	28.0
Feeling sad	63.8	46.4	22.8	22.2
Pain	61.8	50.4	32.9	24.1
Feeling nervous	61.5	39.9	25.0	19.6
Difficulty sleeping	57.3	44.0	30.7	20.7
Dry mouth	45.6	30.2	18.8	8.7
Feeling drowsy	45.3	32.7	15.9	9.3
Feeling irritable	45.9	33.8	12.2	10.8
Numbness/tingling in hands/feet	42.7	24.0	26.0	9.3
"I don't look like myself"	35.8	25.0		12.8
Nausea	35.6	18.8	9.4	8.1
Difficulty concentrating	34.7	16.0	7.3	11.3
Feeling bloated	34.7	26.0	17.3	8.7
Constipation	28.6	20.4		11.6
Lack of appetite	28.4	20.4	14.2	8.2
Change in the way food tastes	25.7	16.2		8.1
Hair loss	26.4	15.0		9.5
Cough	25.3	11.3	6.0	4.0
Itching	22.3	11.5	8.1	3.4
Diarrhea	20.8	10.1	6.0	4.0
Swelling of arms or legs	18.9	12.2		8.8
Shortness of breath	18.7	10.0	7.3	6.0
Weight loss	18.5	4.8		3.4
Problems with sexual interest or activity	17.6	14.9	10.9	6.8
Dizziness	16.2	5.4	2.7	2.7
Vomiting	13.3	8.7	3.3	6.0
Mouth sores	8.1	4.7	1.4	2.0
Nightmares	8.0	5.3	2.0	2.0
Problems with urination	7.3	5.3	4.0	3.3
Urinary accidents	7.4	4.1	0.7	1.4
Difficulty swallowing	5.4	3.4	2.7	2.0

[a]Percentage of sample describing the symptom as "moderate," "severe," or "very severe."
[b]Percentage of sample describing the frequency of the symptom as "frequently" or "almost constantly."
[c]Percentage of sample describing the distress associated with the symptom as "quite a bit" or "very much."
Reprinted with permission from Portenoy RK, Kornblith AB, Wong G, et al. Pain in ovarian cancer: prevalence, characteristics, and associated symptoms. *Cancer* 1994;74:907.

common than would be expected given the potential 70% to 90% success rate of simple pharmacologic approaches (12–15). For example, a survey of 1,308 outpatients with mixed tumor types revealed that 67% had pain during the previous week and that 42% of those with pain were not given adequate analgesic therapy (10). In a recent multinational survey of 1,095 patients with severe cancer pain requiring opioid medication, 66.7% of patients reported that the worst pain intensity during the day prior to the survey was 7 on a 10-point numeric scale (16,17).

Similarly, the potential for adequate analgesia in the setting of acute pain is much higher than the actual outcomes achieved in routine practice. In surveys of patient-controlled analgesia for postoperative pain, for example, almost all patients achieved analgesia (18). These success rates greatly exceed those reported in other studies of postoperative pain (8).

ASSESSMENT OF CANCER PAIN

The assessment of chronic pain in patients with gynecologic cancer requires an understanding of its phenomenology, pathophysiology, and syndromes. Optimally, this assessment must also consider the broad range of physical, psychologic, and social disturbances concurrently experienced by these patients. Patients with acute pain, particularly acute postoperative pain, pose less complex management problems, but could still potentially benefit from an ongoing comprehensive assessment.

Definition of Pain

According to the International Association for the Study of Pain, pain is "an unpleasant sensory and emotional experience associated with actual or potential tissue damage, or described in terms of such damage" (19). Reported pain may be perceived by the clinician to be greater than, or less than, the observable degree of tissue injury. In the cancer population, an organic process capable of explaining the pain can usually be identified, but this does not obviate the need for a careful assessment of other factors, including psychologic disturbances, that could be influencing the intensity of the pain or contributing to pain-related distress.

The definition of pain can be further clarified by the distinctions among nociception, pain, and suffering (Fig. 33.1) (20). Nociception is the activity produced in the afferent nervous system by potentially tissue-damaging stimuli. Clinically, nociception is inferred to exist whenever tissue damage is identified. Pain is the perception of nociception, and, like other perceptions, can be determined by more than the activity in the sensorineural apparatus alone. Although tissue damage related to the tumor or its treatment is common in those with cancer pain, a careful assessment is needed to infer the degree to which the pain report is consistent with the nociception presumed by the clinician on the basis of the physical findings. In all cases, factors other than nociception, including neuropathic processes that can sustain pain in the absence of ongoing tissue injury (see below) and psychologic disturbances, must be evaluated as other potential determinants of the pain. The failure to address these other factors while targeting therapy at the sources of nociception can lead to a poor outcome in which the focus of tissue damage is ameliorated but the pain continues.

Suffering, or "total pain," can be defined as a more global aversive experience determined by numerous perceptions, one of which may be pain (see below). Among the many other factors that may contribute to suffering are the perception of physical deterioration, the experience of symptoms other than pain, psychologic disturbances (e.g., depression or anxiety), disruption in the family, social isolation, and fear of death. Just as an inordinate focus on nociception, rather than pain, can lead to interventions that reduce tissue damage without alleviating symptoms, an emphasis on pain management alone in patients with profound suffering determined by other factors can fail to influence favorably the overall quality of life even if physical comfort is enhanced (21,22).

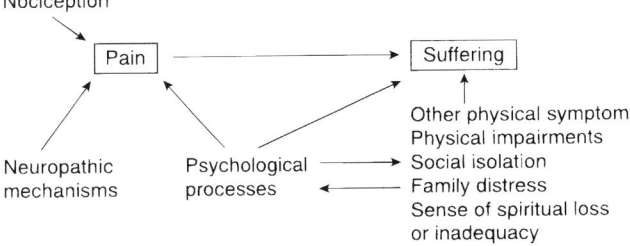

FIG. 33.1. Distinctions and interactions between nociception, pain, and suffering. (Reproduced with permission from Portenoy RK. Cancer pain: pathophysiology and syndromes. *Lancet* 1992;339:1026.)

Evaluation of the Pain Complaint

The comprehensive assessment of pain should include information about temporal characteristics (onset and duration), course (stable or changing since onset, relatively constant or widely fluctuating), severity (both average and worst), location, quality, and provocative and palliative factors. This evaluation is complemented by information about the patient's extent of disease, related medical and psychosocial conditions, and other issues.

Characteristics of Pain

Temporal

Acute pain usually has a well-defined onset and a readily identifiable cause (e.g., surgical incision). It may be associated with anxiety, overt pain behaviors (moaning or grimacing), and signs of sympathetic hyperactivity (including tachycardia, hypertension, and diaphoresis).

In contrast, chronic pain is characterized by an ill-defined onset and a prolonged, fluctuating course. Overt pain behaviors and sympathetic hyperactivity are typically absent, and vegetative signs, including lassitude, sleep disturbance, and anorexia, may be present. A clinical depression evolves in some patients. Most patients with chronic cancer pain also experience periodic flares of pain, or "breakthrough pain," an observation with important therapeutic implications (see below) (9).

Topographic

The distinctions among focal, multifocal, and generalized pains may influence both the assessment and treatment of the patient. Some therapies, such as nerve blocks and cordotomy, depend on the specific location and extent of the pain.

The distinction between focal and referred pain is similarly important. Focal pains are experienced superficial to the underlying nociceptive lesion, whereas referred pains are experienced at a site distant from the nociceptive lesion.

Pain may be referred from a lesion involving any of a large group of structures, including nerve, bone, muscle or other soft tissue, and viscera (23–25). Various subtypes can be distinguished: (a) pain referred anywhere along the course of an injured peripheral nerve (such as pain in the thigh or knee from a lumbar plexus lesion); (b) pain referred along a course of the nerve supplied by a damaged nerve root (known as radicular pain); (c) pain referred to the lower part of the body, usually the feet and legs, from a lesion involving the spinal cord (called funicular pain); and (d) pain referred to a site remote from the nociceptive lesion and outside the dermatome affected by the lesion (e.g., shoulder pain from diaphragmatic irritation).

Knowledge of pain referral patterns is needed in order to target appropriate assessment procedures. For example, a patient with recurrent cervical cancer who reports progressive pain in the inguinal region may require evaluation of numerous structures to identify the underlying nociceptive lesion, including the subjacent pelvic bones and hip joint, pelvic sidewall, paraspinal gutter at an upper lumbar spinal level, and intraspinal region at the upper lumbar level.

Etiologic

The etiology of acute pain is usually clear-cut. Further evaluation to determine the underlying lesion or pathophysiology of the pain is not indicated unless the course varies from the expected. In contrast, the etiology of chronic cancer-related pain may be more difficult to characterize. In most cases, pain is due to direct invasion of pain-sensitive structures by the neoplasm (21,26). The structures most often involved are bone and neural tissue, but pain can also occur when there is an obstruction of hollow viscus, distention of organ capsules, distortion or occlusion of blood vessels, and infiltration of soft tissues. The etiology of pain in less than a quarter of patients relates to an antineoplastic treatment, and less than 10% have pain unrelated to the neoplasm or its treatment (21,26,27).

These data suggest that a careful evaluation of cancer patients with pain is likely to identify an underlying nociceptive lesion, which will usually be neoplastic. A survey of patients referred to a pain service in a major cancer hospital noted that previously unsuspected lesions were identified in 63% of patients (28). This outcome altered the known extent of disease in virtually all patients, changed the prognosis for some, and provided an opportunity for a primary antineoplastic therapy in approximately 15%.

Pathophysiologic

Pain is labeled nociceptive if it is inferred that the sustaining mechanisms involve ongoing tissue injury. This injury can involve either somatic or visceral structures. The quality of somatic nociceptive pain is typically described as aching, stabbing, throbbing, or pressure-like. The quality of visceral nociceptive pain is largely determined by the structures involved. Obstruction of hollow viscus is usually associated with complaints of gnawing or crampy pain, whereas injury to organ capsules or mesentery is associated with an aching or stabbing discomfort.

Pain is labeled neuropathic if the evaluation suggests that it is sustained by abnormal somatosensory processing in the peripheral or the central nervous system (CNS). Neuropathic mechanisms are involved in approximately 40% of cancer pain syndromes and can be disease related (e.g., tumor invasion of nerve plexus) or treatment related (e.g., postmastectomy syndrome, chemotherapy-induced painful polyneuropathy) (17). Among those with metastatic disease, neuropathic pain usually results from neoplastic injury to

peripheral nerves (peripheral neuropathic pain). Other, less common, subtypes include (a) those in which the focus of activity is in the CNS (sometimes generically termed deafferentation pain); and (b) those in which the pain is believed to be maintained by efferent activity in the sympathetic nervous system (so-called sympathetically maintained pain) (29). Identification of a neuropathic mechanism is extremely important in clinical management because several specific therapies may be useful for these conditions (see below).

Neuropathic pain is diagnosed on the basis of the patient's verbal description of the pain and typically supported by evidence of nerve injury. Patients may use any of a variety of verbal descriptors but some, such as "burning," "shocklike," or "electrical," are particularly suggestive of neuropathic pain (30,31). Areas of abnormal sensations are often found on physical examination. These may include hypesthesia (a numbness or lessening of feeling), paresthesias (abnormal nonpainful sensations such as tingling, cold, or itching), hyperalgesia (increased perception of painful stimuli), hyperpathia (exaggerated pain response), and allodynia (pain

TABLE 33.2. *Cancer pain syndromes*

I.	Pain associated with direct tumor involvement
	A. Due to invasion of bone
	1. Base of skull
	2. Vertebral body
	3. Generalized bone pain
	B. Due to invasion of nerves
	1. Peripheral nerve syndromes
	2. Painful polyneuropathy
	3. Brachial, lumbar, sacral plexopathies
	4. Leptomeningeal metastases
	5. Epidural spinal cord compression
	C. Due to invasion of viscera
	D. Due to invasion of blood vessels
	E. Due to invasion of mucous membranes
II.	Pain associated with cancer therapy
	A. Postoperative pain syndromes
	1. Postthoracotomy syndrome
	2. Postmastectomy syndrome
	3. Postradical neck dissection
	4. Postamputation syndromes
	B. Postchemotherapy pain syndromes
	1. Painful polyneuropathy
	2. Aseptic necrosis of bone
	3. Steroid pseudorheumatism
	4. Mucositis
	C. Postirradiation pain syndromes
	1. Radiation fibrosis of brachial or lumbosacral plexus
	2. Radiation myelopathy
	3. Radiation-induced peripheral nerve tumors
	4. Mucositis
III.	Pain indirectly related or unrelated to cancer
	A. Myofascial pains
	B. Postherpetic neuralgia
	C. Chronic headache syndromes

induced by nonpainful stimuli such as a light touch or cool air) (32).

Psychologic factors may augment or alter the pain complaint, but are rarely the sole cause. If a credible pathophysiologic diagnosis is not apparent, it is best to label the pain idiopathic.

Pain Syndromes

Efforts to improve the assessment of cancer pain have been greatly encouraged by the description of numerous pain syndromes, each of which is defined by a cluster of symptoms and signs (Table 33.2)(21,26). Syndrome identification can help direct the diagnostic evaluation, clarify the prognosis, and target therapeutic interventions. Recognition of pain syndromes that occur commonly among patients with gynecologic cancers (Table 33.3) can also facilitate the assessment of these patients.

Comprehensive Assessment

A comprehensive assessment that incorporates this pain-related information can be used to elaborate a problem list that guides the priorities and direction of therapy (Table 33.4). In many situations, such as acute postoperative pain or chronic pain related to a well-characterized lesion (e.g., pathologic fracture), the assessment issues are simple and the problem list is brief and straightforward. Other patients, most often those with advanced disease, present a complex group of symptoms, medical disorders, and psychosocial disturbances. In these cases, a comprehensive assessment en-

TABLE 33.3. *Pain syndromes commonly encountered among patients with gynecologic cancer*

Acute pain syndromes
　At any stage of disease:
　　Postoperative pain
　　Mucositis
　In advanced stages of disease:
　　Recurrent bowel obstruction
　　Ureteral obstruction
　　Movement-related pain in brachial/lumbosacral
　　　plexopathy
　　Movement-related pain from bony lesions

Cancer-related chronic pain syndromes
　Brachial/lumbosacral plexopathy
　Chronic abdominal pain: bowel obstruction, ascites,
　　hepatomegaly
　Tenesmoid pain
　Bone pain from metastases

Treatment-related chronic pain syndromes
　Postmastectomy syndrome
　Radiation-induced plexopathy
　Chemotherapy-induced peripheral neuropathy (paclitaxel,
　　cisplatin)

TABLE 33.4. *Stepwise assessment of the patient with cancer pain*

Step 1: Data collection
　Pain-related history
　　Other relevant history
　　Disease related
　　Other symptoms
　　Psychiatric history
　　Social resources
　Available laboratory and imaging data
　　Radiographs and scans
　　Tumor markers
　　Hematologic parameters
　　Biochemical parameters
　　Pathology/histology
Step 2: Provisional assessment
　Provisional pain diagnosis
　　Syndrome identification
　　Inferred pathophysiology
　Global assessment
　Extent of disease
　Goals of care
　　Prolonging survival
　　Optimizing function
　　Optimizing comfort
　Concurrent concerns
　Other symptoms
　Untreated concurrent diseases
　Psychosocial needs
　Rehabilitative needs
　Financial needs
Step 3: Diagnostic investigations and other assessments
　Diagnostic investigations
　　Symptom specific
　　Extent of disease
　Other assessments
　　Psychological
　　Social
　　Financial
　　Functional
Step 4: Initial formulation and problem list
　Pain syndromes and pathophysiology
　Extent of disease
　Concurrent concerns
　Anticipated concerns
　Anticipated contingencies
Step 5: Patient review and formulation of prioritized problem lists
　Current problems
　Anticipated contingencies

Adapted with permission from Cherny NI, Portenoy RK. Cancer pain: principles of assessment and syndromes. In: Wall PD, Melzack R, eds. *Textbook of pain*. 3rd ed. Edinburgh: Churchill Livingstone, 1994:787.

courages efficient selection of an appropriate multimodal therapy.

Patients whose pain had been responsive to pain medication but experience an increase in pain intensity or a change in pain characteristics should be comprehensively reassessed as the initial step in management. The goal is to determine whether specific contributing factors can be identified. Relapse or disease progression, for example, may be amenable to primary therapeutic strategies, such as chemotherapy to address disease progression associated with loss of analgesic effectiveness. Other factors such as cord compression, systemic or local infection, and psychologic distress (e.g., depression) also may be treatable.

Management of Acute Pain

Although the treatment of patients with acute pain, particularly postoperative pain, is typically less challenging than the long-term management of chronic pain, the outcomes achieved in routine practice settings are often inadequate. In the surgical setting, studies have demonstrated that the failure to provide satisfactory analgesia may increase both psychologic and physiologic morbidity (33). In addition, there is evidence that early and adequate control of postoperative pain may decrease the likelihood of postsurgical chronic pain syndromes (34).

The need for a systematic assessment and expert management of postoperative pain is particularly important in the cancer population. Cancer patients may have concurrent medical problems, psychologic disturbances, and prior drug exposure that increase the heterogeneity of the population and diminish the likelihood that routine measures will provide adequate relief of pain.

"ROUTINE" APPROACH TO POSTOPERATIVE PAIN

Despite great variability in the pharmacokinetics and pharmacodynamics of single opioid doses (35), and the large proportion of patients who fail to attain adequate analgesia with routine postoperative care, many patients do respond adequately to an opioid, traditionally morphine or meperidine, administered "as needed" (8). In the cancer population, the starting dose must take into account the prior opioid exposure of the patient. A reasonable starting dose is the equivalent of 5% to 10% of the total opioid consumption during the previous 24 hours. If the drug or route of administration is changed, an equianalgesic dose table must be consulted to calculate the equivalent total daily dose of the new drug. Once a dose is selected, it can be initially administered every 2 to 3 hours as needed.

The proportion of cancer patients with postoperative pain who will be undertreated by an as-needed dosing schedule can be diminished if several factors are recognized. The variability in analgesic requirements may require changes in the starting dose, adjustment in the dosing interval during the immediate postoperative period, or both. Some patients require several dose adjustments. Similarly, variability in pain duration after any particular operation is great and the duration of opioid treatment must be flexible and be determined solely by patient response. Some patients have concerns about opioid-induced side effects and addiction, which may augment distress and diminish patient compliance with therapy unless strong reassurance is provided by the physician and other staff.

In some populations, the routine approach to postoperative pain management can be enhanced by the use of a nonopioid analgesic, specifically a nonsteroidal antiinflammatory drug (NSAID). In the United States, ketorolac has been approved for short-term parenteral use. In opioid-naïve patients, a standard dose of ketorolac can provide analgesia equivalent to a parenteral dose of morphine of 10 mg (36). The novel intravenous cyclooxygenase type 2 inhibitor parecoxib has been approved in Europe and is awaiting approval by the U.S. Food and Drug Administration (FDA). Intravenous parecoxib effectively decreased the PCA (patient-controlled analgesia) opioid requirement in patients undergoing major gynecologic surgical procedures (37). The addition of intravenous ketoprofen (not approved in the United States) to intravenous PCA with tramadol after major gynecologic cancer surgery also significantly reduced opioid consumption (38). At the present time in the United States, patients who are highly predisposed to opioid side effects or toxicity, such as those with severe preexisting lung disease, may benefit from a trial of ketorolac either in lieu of opioid therapy or in combination with an opioid. Ketorolac should not be used when NSAID treatment is contraindicated.

Patient-Controlled Analgesia

PCA has achieved great popularity in the management of postoperative pain (39–41) and is increasingly considered to be the standard treatment of pain after major surgery. Theoretically, the self-administration of small doses on a frequent basis allows the patient to tailor the dose to the pain and enhance a sense of personal control while achieving a more stable plasma drug concentration. Systematic reviews comparing PCA with conventional opioid analgesia provide some evidence that the use of PCA improves analgesia, decreases the risk of pulmonary complications, and increases patient satisfaction (42). However, not all studies of this modality have been positive. For example, a randomized controlled trial of 227 gynecologic cancer patients undergoing intraabdominal surgery found that patients who were switched from parenteral to oral morphine on the first postoperative day experienced the same degree of pain control as those who received parenteral morphine via PCA pump (43). The latter studies suggest that careful attention to dosing rather than the availability of a pump per se is the key factor in achieving adequate pain control.

Other Approaches to Acute Pain Management

Numerous alternative approaches to postoperative pain management have been explored. Some require the expertise of other specialists.

Oral Pretreatment

Pretreatment with sustained-release morphine reduces postoperative pain and analgesia requirements (44,45). This technique is seldom used but may be an option in patients whose postoperative pain management is expected to be problematic.

Intraspinal Analgesia

Experience in the use of epidural opioids or local anesthetics suggests that this approach is safe and offers a means to improve postoperative pain management and lower the risk of postoperative complications after major surgery (46, 47). Successful management requires careful attention to clinical monitoring during treatment. A randomized trial that compared optimized repetitive parenteral opioid dosing with epidural morphine in high-risk patients (morbidly obese patients undergoing gastroplasty) demonstrated improved relief of pain, mobilization, and respiratory recovery in those treated intraspinally (48). Epidural fentanyl resulted in significantly better pain control than PCA with morphine in patients who underwent thoracotomy (49). A study that evaluated 462 consecutive surgical cancer patients who underwent uncomplicated surgeries of the thorax or abdomen, or both, of more than 3 hours' duration showed that patients receiving epidural analgesia with 0.1% bupivacaine and 0.01% morphine sulfate experienced a faster recovery than those who received intravenous PCA (50). Pain control was satisfactory in both groups. A recent meta-analysis of patients who underwent abdominal surgical procedures concluded that postoperative analgesia with epidural local anesthetics reduced gastrointestinal paralysis compared with systemic or epidural opioids with comparable pain relief (51). In a small study of 18 patients, epidural analgesia compared with intravenous PCA offered improved pain control after mastectomy with immediate TRAM (transverse rectus abdominis muscle) flap reconstruction and resulted in a 25-hour reduction of time of hospitalization (52).

Although there is less clinical experience in the use of subarachnoid opioid administration for postoperative pain, the technique can provide excellent relief (53). For example, intrathecal morphine has been used successfully to manage pain following cesarean section (54), hysterectomy (55), and abdominal aortic surgery (56).

Regional Anesthetic Techniques

There are numerous regional anesthetic techniques that may be useful for the management of acute pain. The simplest is the application of aerosolized lidocaine at the surgical site, which has been shown substantially to reduce pain and opioid requirements during the first 24 hours after hysterectomy (57). Subcutaneous and topical local anesthesia after breast cancer surgery reduced pain and opioid consumption only slightly, but may be useful in patients with very high pain scores (58). Topical anesthetics that are longer acting are in development and may offer substantial benefits in the future.

Neural blockade capable of denervating the painful site is a potential approach in most cases. Catheters that deliver local anesthetic at a dose high enough to produce a sensory block can be placed in the epidural space or along peripheral nerves or plexus. Regional anesthesia can be used during an operation and then continued into the postoperative setting for pain control. In one study, for example, an intraoperative regional block with 1% ropivacaine in patients undergoing breast cancer surgery was combined with postoperative administration of oral mexiletine and significantly reduced the requirement for breakthrough pain medication (59).

Comprehensive Pain Service

The sophisticated use of regional anesthetic techniques usually requires the availability of pain specialists with expertise in the management of acute pain. Many hospitals have formed pain services, which are usually directed by anesthesiologists and provide expert assessment and comprehensive multimodality management of postoperative pain (60). Although this type of service has not been compared with an optimized standard approach by a well-educated medical staff, the care provided by these services clearly improves the outcome of routine pain management.

Other Approaches

Transcutaneous electrical nerve stimulation (TENS) has been suggested to be a useful modality for incisional pain after abdominal surgery (61,62). A meta-analysis demonstrated that TENS applied to the area surrounding the wound can significantly reduce analgesic consumption (63). Despite the evident simplicity and safety of the approach, there has been little application of its potential.

Cognitive approaches, including stress reduction, relaxation, hypnosis, and distraction techniques, have also reduced postoperative pain and analgesic requirements (64,65). These techniques are labor intensive and are almost never sufficient as the sole means of analgesia. Nonetheless, studies have established that higher levels of anxiety and depression can negatively influence postoperative pain and analgesic requirements (66) and efforts to reduce anxiety through preoperative education and postoperative psychologic interventions are likely to have salutary effects.

MANAGEMENT OF CHRONIC CANCER PAIN

The successful management of acute postoperative pain is an important concern of the gynecologic oncologist, and can usually be accomplished. The treatment of chronic pain is a far more challenging problem, particularly among those with advanced illness.

Cancer Pain, Symptom Distress, and Palliative Care

Most cancer patients who experience chronic pain also develop other physical and psychologic symptoms. Pain, fatigue, and psychologic distress are the most prevalent symptoms across populations (67,68). A broad assessment of symptom distress, followed by concurrent therapy of the most problematic symptoms other than pain, is a fundamental aspect of pain management.

Symptom distress, in turn, is only one aspect of the multifaceted problem of suffering, or "total pain" (21,69). The assessment of suffering requires an evaluation in multiple domains, including the physical, psychologic, social, and spiritual; this requires open and ongoing communication between the clinician and the patient.

The assessment and management of problems that relate to the broad constructs of suffering and quality of life are part of the therapeutic model of palliative care, which focuses on patients with progressive incurable illness and their families. This therapeutic approach aims to enhance the quality of life of the patient and family throughout the course of the disease. The effort to provide optimal palliative care should be considered to be one aspect of best practice for oncologists. Palliative care must intensify at the end of life, at which time the need for specialized care, such as that provided by hospice programs, may become evident.

General Principles of Pain Management

The development of a successful strategy for pain management must consider the etiology and pathophysiology of pain, the patient's medical status, and the goals of care. Although the main approach for the management of cancer pain is opioid-based pharmacotherapy, other interventions, including disease-oriented treatments (e.g., surgery, chemotherapy, or irradiation) or other analgesic techniques, may be appropriate in selected cases.

Role of Primary Therapies

Effective treatment of the pathology underlying the pain can be analgesic. Primary treatment includes antineoplastic therapies and interventions directed at other structural pathologies. For example, lysis of adhesions for bowel obstruction may also yield analgesia (60).

Although the palliative role of chemotherapy, especially its analgesic effects, has been poorly studied. Nonetheless, it is a common observation that patients who attain a partial or complete response also experience improved symptoms (70–72). In a study of patients with metastatic breast cancer,

palliative chemotherapy with doxorubicin with or without vinorelbine resulted in an improvement of pain in 60.4% of the 111 patients who suffered from pain at baseline; although patients with an objective tumor response were more likely to have an improvement in pain (84.9%), fully 61% of patients with stable disease also benefited (73). In a small study of patients with advanced ovarian cancer, palliative chemotherapy was associated with improvement in symptom control, emotional well-being, and global quality of life (74). In a study of patients with recurrent/advanced cervical cancer, 67% of patients experienced improvement of pain after alternating treatment with PBM (platinum, bleomycin, and methotrexate) and PFU [platinum and 5-fluorouracil (5-FU)] (75).

There is also evidence that radiation therapy can provide effective and durable palliation of pain and other symptoms in chemotherapy-refractory patients with ovarian cancer (74, 76,77) and cervical cancer (78,79). Radiation therapy can also provide analgesia to more than half the patients treated for bone metastases (51,78,80). Patients with widespread bone metastasis or bone pain refractory to local field radiotherapy may benefit from treatment with radiopharmaceuticals, such as strontium 89 (81,82). In addition, analgesia may be an expected result when irradiation is used to treat epidural disease, tumor ulceration, cerebral metastases, superior vena cava obstruction, and bronchial obstruction.

Unfortunately, many patients with chronic cancer pain have no option for primary antineoplastic therapy or did not achieve symptomatic relief from these interventions. The approach to these patients involves a diverse group of primary analgesic treatments (Table 33.5). Several concurrent interventions are often required to manage the pain.

The benefits of analgesic therapies must be balanced against the side effects they produce in a way that optimizes the outcome for the patient. Repeated assessments, performed as part of a broader approach to palliative care, are essential in this process and often lead to adjustments in the therapy (83–85).

TABLE 33.5. *Approaches used in the management of chronic cancer pain*

Primary therapies
Radiation therapy
Chemotherapy
Surgery
Antibiotics
Primary analgesic therapies
Pharmacologic approaches
Anesthetic approaches
Physiatric approaches
Neurostimulatory approaches
Psychological approaches
Complementary approaches

Therapeutic Approaches

Pharmacologic Management

Prospective trials indicate that more than 70% of patients can achieve adequate relief of cancer pain using a pharmacologic approach (2,3,13–15). Effective pain management requires expertise in the administration of three groups of analgesic medications: NSAIDs, opioid analgesics, and adjuvant analgesics. The term *adjuvant analgesic* is applied to a diverse group of drugs that have primary indications other than pain but can be effective analgesics in specific circumstances; for example, in the treatment of neuropathic pain.

A model approach to the selection of these drugs, known as the "analgesic ladder," has been developed by the World Health Organization (WHO) (Fig. 33.2)(3).

According to this approach, patients with mild to moderate cancer-related pain are first treated with acetaminophen (paracetamol) or a NSAID. This drug is combined with an adjuvant drug that can be selected either to provide additional analgesia (i.e., an adjuvant analgesic) or to treat a side effect of the analgesic or a coexisting symptom.

Patients who present with moderate to severe pain, or who do not achieve adequate relief after a trial of a NSAID, should be treated with an opioid conventionally used to treat pain of this intensity (previously designated a "weak" opioid), which is typically combined with a NSAID and may be administered with an adjuvant if there is an indication for one. Those who present with severe pain or who do not

achieve adequate relief following appropriate administration of drugs on the second rung of the "analgesic ladder" should receive an opioid conventionally used for severe pain (previously called a "strong" opioid), which may be combined with a NSAID or an adjuvant drug as indicated.

Nonsteroidal Antiinflammatory Drugs

The nonopioid analgesics, acetaminophen and the NSAIDs (Table 33.6), have a well-established role in the treatment of cancer pain (86–90). Based on clinical observations, NSAIDs appear to be especially useful in patients with bone pain or pain related to grossly inflammatory lesions and relatively less useful in patients with neuropathic pain (91). However, there is some evidence that NSAIDs may be useful in the management of all types of cancer pain regardless of the mechanism of pain involved (86,88,91). In addition, NSAIDs have an opioid-sparing effect that may be helpful to prevent the occurrence of dose-related side effects (92,93).

NSAIDS inhibit the enzyme cyclooxygenase (COX) to reduce production of prostaglandins, compounds that sensitize nociceptive primary afferent neurons, among other actions (94). A decline in peripheral and central prostaglandins presumably underlies the analgesic effects of the NSAIDs. There are two forms of COX, a constitutive form (COX-1) and an inducible form (COX-2). Compounds that inhibit COX-1 and COX-2 with similar potency (e.g., ibuprofen, naproxen, diclofenac) have a lower risk of inducing gastrointestinal adverse effects than compounds that are more selective for COX-1 (e.g., indomethacin) and a higher risk than those that are more selective for COX-2 (e.g., nabumetone); drugs that are highly selective for COX-2 inhibition, such as rofecoxib, celecoxib, and valdecoxib, are least likely to have these effects (88). There have been no comparative trials of selective COX-2 inhibitors and the nonselective NSAIDs in the cancer population.

NSAIDs should be administered with great caution to patients with a history of peptic ulcer disease or other significant risk factors for ulcer, such as advanced age and concurrent corticosteroid therapy (95). Antineoplastic therapy also may induce damage to upper gastrointestinal tract mucosa (96). For patients who are predisposed to ulcer disease or would have difficulty tolerating a gastrointestinal hemorrhage, the increased safety of the COX-2 selective drugs is likely to be an advantage. Coadministration of a proton pump inhibitor should also be considered as an approach to reduce the risk of gastrointestinal damage induced by NSAIDs (97–99) or antineoplastic therapy (94).

The potential for nephrotoxicity suggests that NSAIDs should also be used cautiously in patients with known renal insufficiency and those at high risk for renal impairment, including the elderly and patients receiving nephrotoxic chemotherapy. Selective COX-2 inhibitors and nonselective NSAIDs seem to be equally nephrotoxic and therefore

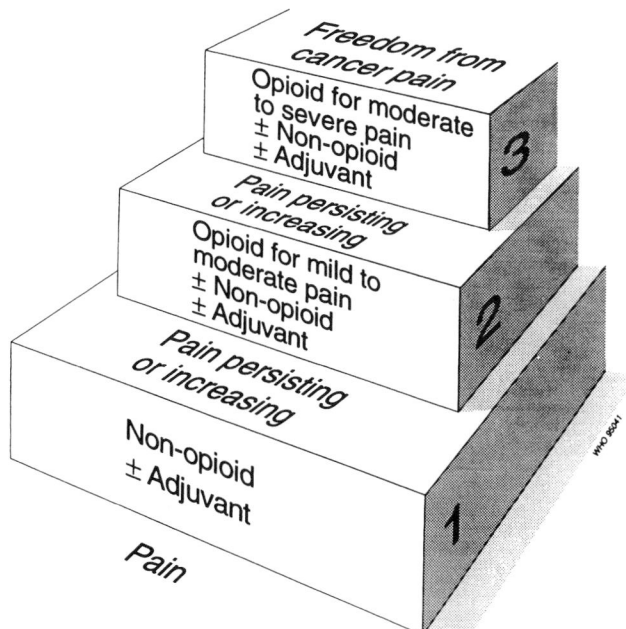

FIG. 33.2. The three-step "analgesic ladder" proposed by an expert committee of the Cancer Unit of the World Health Organization. (Reproduced with permission from the World Health Organization. *Cancer pain relief.* 2nd ed. Geneva: World Health Organization,1996.)

TABLE 33.6. *Nonsteroidal antiinflammatory drugs*

Class and generic name	Trade name	Approx. half-life (h)	Dosing schedule	Recommended starting dose[a]	Comment[b]
p-Aminophenol Derivatives					
Acetaminophen[c]	Tylenol, Datril, Panadol	3–4	q 4–6 h	650 mg q 4 h (5 doses daily)	Overdosage produces hepatic toxicity. Not anti-inflammatory and therefore not preferred as first-line analgesic or coanalgesic in patients with bone pain. Lack of GI or platelet toxicity, however, may be important in some cancer patients. At high doses, liver function tests should be monitored.
Naphthylalkanones					
Nabumetone	Relafen	22–30	q 24 h	500–1,000 mg q 12 h	Appears to have a relatively low risk of GI toxicity; once-daily dosing can be useful.
Salicylates					
Acetylsalicylic acid[c]	Aspirin	3–12[d]	q 4–6 h	650 mg q 4 h (5 doses daily)	Standard for comparison. May not be tolerated as well as some of the newer NSAIDs.
Diflunisal[c]	Dolobid, Dolobis	8–12	q 12 h	1000 × 1, then 500 q 12 h	Less GI toxicity than aspirin.
Choline magnesium trisalicylate[c]	Trilisate	8–12	q 12 h	500–1,000 mg q 12 h	Choline Mg trisalicylate and salsalate have minimal GI toxicity and no effect on platelet aggregation despite antiinflammatory effects. May therefore be particularly useful in some cancer patients.
Salsalate	Disalcid	8–12	q 12 h	500–1,000 mg q 12 h	
Proprionic acids					
Ibuprofen[c]	Motrin, Advil, Nuprin	3–4	q 4–8 h	400–600 mg q 8 h	Available over-thecounter.
Naproxen[c]	Naprosyn	13	q 12 h	250–500 mg q 12 h	Available as a suspension.
Naproxen sodium[c]	Aleve, Anaprox, Naprelan	13	q 12 h	275–550 mg q 12 h	
Fenoprofen	Nalfon, Fenopran, Progesic	2–3	q 6 h	200 mg q 6 h	
Ketoprofen	Orudis, Oruvail	2–3	q 6–8 h	25–50 mg q 8 h	
Flurbiprofen[c]	Ansaid	5–6	q 8–12 h	100 mg q 12 h	Experience too limited to evaluate higher doses, although it is likely that some patients would benefit.
Oxaprozin	Daypro	40	q 24 h	600 mg q 24 h	Once-daily dosing may be useful.
Acetic acids					
Indomethacin	Indocin, Indocid	4–5	q 8–12 h	25 mg q 8 h	Available in sustained-release and rectal formulations. Higher incidence of side effects, particularly GI and CNS, than proprionic acids.
Tolmetin	Tolectin	1	q 6–8 h	200 mg q 8 h	
Sulindac	Clinoril	14	q 12 h	150 mg q 12 h	Less renal toxicity than other NSAIDs.
Diclofenac	Voltaren	2	q 6–8 h	25 mg q 8 h	
Ketorolac[c]	Toradol	4–7	q 4–6 h	30–60 mg load then 15–30 mg q 6 h (parenteral); 10 mg q 6 h (oral)	Only parenteral formulation available. Approved for postoperative use. Experience too limited to evaluate higher doses.

(continued)

TABLE 33.6. *Continued*

Class and generic name	Trade name	Approx. half-life (h)	Dosing schedule	Recommended starting dose[a]	Comment[b]
Oxicams					
Piroxicam	Feldene	45	q 24 h	20 mg q 24 h	Administration of 40 mg for over 3 weeks is associated with a high incidence of peptic ulcer, particularly in the elderly.
Fenamates					
Mefenamic acid[c]	Ponstel, Ponstan	2	q 6 h	250 mg q 6 h	Not recommended for use longer than 1 week and therefore not indicated in cancer pain therapy.
Pyrazoles					
Phenylbutazone	Antadol, Butazoladin	50–100	q 68 h	100 mg q 8 h	Not a first-line drug owing to risk of serious bone marrow toxicity. Not preferred for cancer pain therapy.
COX-2 Inhibitors					
Celecoxib	Celebrex	11	q 12 h	100–200 mg q 12 h	Fewer GI side effects; no effect on platelet function
Rofecoxib	Vioxx	17	q 24 h	12.5–25.0 mg q 24 h	See celecoxib

CNS, central nervous system; GI, gastrointestinal.

[a]Starting dose should be one-half to two-thirds of the recommended dose for the elderly, those on multiple drugs, and those with renal insufficiency. Doses must be individualized. Low initial doses should be titrated upward if tolerated and clinical effect is inadequate. Doses can be incremented weekly. Studies of NSAIDs in the cancer population are meager; dosing guidelines are thus empiric.

[b]With all NSAIDs, stool guaiac and liver function tests, BUN, creatinine, and urinalysis should be monitored; frequency of monitoring should be increased for those on relatively high doses.

[c]Pain is approved indication.

[d]Half-life of aspirin increases with dose.

should be used with the same caution as nonselective NSAIDs (46). In these patients, acetaminophen is generally regarded as being safest, although some data suggest that this drug can also produce renal toxicity (100).

Other factors may also be important in the selection of an NSAID. First, there is substantial variability in the response of individual patients to different agents, and the response to an NSAID in the past should guide drug selection in the present. Second, it may be useful to consider the drug's duration of effect when selecting an NSAID. The need to improve treatment adherence or provide a simpler dosing regimen encourages the use of a drug that can be administered once daily (e.g., rofecoxib, nabumetone, oxaprozin, piroxicam, or sustained-release indomethacin) or twice daily (e.g., celecoxib, valdecoxib, diflunisal, naproxen, and many others), whereas the desire for as-needed dosing suggests the use of a short-duration drug (e.g., aspirin, acetaminophen, or ibuprofen). Finally, drug selection may be influenced by cost, which varies greatly among both drugs and pharmacies.

The most serious toxicities associated with the use of NSAIDs, bleeding peptic ulcer and renal failure, are dose related and often occult until severe morbidity occurs. Although patients with cancer pain are commonly treated with standard doses, it is reasonable to explore the dose range when patients respond and identify the minimal effective

dose for long-term therapy. Dose escalation in poor responders is limited by dose-related toxicities and a ceiling dose for analgesia above which additional dose increments fail to produce more relief. If an increase in dose maintains the therapy in the conventionally accepted safe range and provides more analgesia, it should be continued. The lack of additional pain relief following a dose increase, however, suggests that the ceiling has been reached, and the dose can then be lowered to the previously effective dose or the drug can be discontinued. All patients receiving an NSAID should be evaluated occasionally for occult fecal blood and the stability of renal function.

Opioid Analgesics

Expertise in the administration of opioid analgesics (Table 33.7) is the foundation of cancer pain management. The clinician should have knowledge of opioid pharmacology and a clear grasp of practical guidelines for dosing (101).

Opioid Classes. Based on receptor interactions, the opioid analgesics can be divided broadly into pure agonists and agonist-antagonists. The pure agonist drugs used in the management of chronic cancer pain are agonists at the μ receptor subtype. The agonist-antagonist drugs comprise a mixed agonist-antagonist subclass, which includes drugs that are

TABLE 33.7. *Opioid analgesics*

Drug	Dose (mg) equianalgesic to morphine 10 mg IM[a] PO	IM	Half-life (h)	Peak effect (h)	Duration (h)	Comment[c]
Morphine	20–30[b]	10	2–3	0.5–1.0	36	Standard for comparison.
Morphine CR	20–30	10	2–3	3–4	8–12	Various formulations are not bioequivalent.
Morphine SR	20–30	10	2–3	2–3	2–4	
Codeine	200	130	2–3	1.5–2.0	3–6	Combined with aspirin or acetaminophen. Usually for moderate pain. Also available without coanalgesic.
Hydromorphone	7.5	1.5	2–3	0.5–1.0	2–4	Potency may be greater; i.e., hydromorphone: morphine = 3:1 rather than 6.7:1 during prolonged use.
Oxycodone	20		2–3	1	3–4	Combined with aspirin or acetaminophen, for moderate pain; available orally without coanalgesic and useful for severe pain.
Oxycodone CR	20		2–3	2–3	8–12	
Oxymorphone	10 (rectal)	1	2–3	1.5–3.0	2–4	Available in rectal and injectable formulations.
Methadone	20	10	12–190	0.5–1.5	4–12	Although 1:1 ratio with morphine was in a single-dose study, there is a change with chronic dosing and large dose reduction (75%–90%) is needed when switching to methadone. Risk of delayed toxicity.
Levorphanol	4	2	12–15	0.5–1	4–6	Usage limited because only 2-mg tablets are available.
Fentanyl			7–12			Can be administered as a continuous IV infusion or SQ infusion; based on clinical experience, 100 μg/h is roughly equianalgesic to morphine 4 mg/h.
Fentanyl TTS			16–24		48–72	Based on clinical experience, 100 μg is roughly equianalgesic to morphine 4 mg/h. A ratio of oral morphine:transdermal fentanyl of 70:1 may also be used clinically.
Meperidine	300	75	2–3	0.5–1.0	3–4	Not preferred for cancer patients owing to potential toxicity.

[a]Dose that provides analgesia equivalent to 10 mg intramuscular morphine.
[b]Extensive survey data suggest that the relative potency of IM:PO morphine of 1:6 changes to 1:23 with chronic dosing.
[c]All opioids may produce various common side effects, (e.g., constipation, nausea, sedation). Respiratory depression is rare in cancer patients.

weak antagonists at the μ receptor and agonists at another receptor subtype, and a partial agonist subclass, which includes drugs that are partial agonists at the μ receptor (102). In the United States, the mixed agonist-antagonist drugs include pentazocine, nalbuphine, dezocine, and butorphanol and the partial agonists include buprenorphine.

All the agonist-antagonist drugs share properties that together suggest a limited role in the management of chronic cancer pain (102). These drugs have a ceiling dose for analgesia, and all have the potential to produce an abstinence syndrome in patients already physically dependent on an agonist drug. These characteristics indicate that the agonist-antagonist opioids can be used only in patients with no substantial prior opioid exposure and no need for relatively high

doses. Some of the mixed agonist-antagonists, particularly pentazocine, are also more likely to produce psychotomimetic effects than the pure agonist drugs. In patients with chronic pain, the lack of oral formulations for all but pentazocine also limits the utility of these drugs.

Agonist drugs (Table 33.7), the prototype of which is morphine, are preferred in the management of chronic cancer pain. To optimize the administration of these drugs, widely accepted dosing guidelines must be applied systematically.

"Weak" Versus "Strong" Opioids. Unlike the division of the opioids into agonist and agonist-antagonist classes, the distinction between "weak" opioids and "strong" opioids, which was originally incorporated into the WHO analgesic ladder approach, is more operational than pharmacologic (3).

The so-called weak opioids are now designated as those that are conventionally administered orally for moderate pain (second rung of the analgesic ladder), and the so-called strong opioids are those that are conventionally used to treat severe pain (third rung of the analgesic ladder). In the United States, the former group comprises codeine, hydrocodone, dihydrocodeine, oxycodone, propoxyphene, and occasionally meperidine. Tramadol, a unique centrally acting analgesic with a mechanism of action that is, in part, opioidergic, also is generally included with this group. The other opioids used for severe pain include morphine, hydromorphone, oxymorphone, levorphanol, fentanyl, and methadone.

Among those opioids conventionally used for moderate pain, codeine and propoxyphene are usually, but not always, combined with a coanalgesic (aspirin or acetaminophen); hydrocodone and dihydrocodeine are only available in combination products. Oxycodone, which is available both as a single entity and as a combination tablet combined with aspirin or acetaminophen, can be considered to be a drug for the second step of the ladder when used in combination with a coanalgesic and a drug for severe pain when used alone.

The designation of the drugs conventionally used to treat moderate pain as ''weak'' was a misnomer because none of these drugs is characterized by a ceiling effect that would limit its use. Rather, other considerations have led to the customary use of these opioids at doses limited to those capable of treating moderate pain in the relatively nontolerant patient. For example, the dose of any opioid combined in a single tablet with acetaminophen or aspirin can only be escalated until the dose of the nonopioid coanalgesic reaches a level associated with toxicity. As noted, hydrocodone and dihydrocodeine are available only in such combinations, and most of the other drugs in this group are typically administered in this form.

Propoxyphene and meperidine should not be used at higher doses because of the risk of enhanced toxicity due to accumulation of a metabolite. The metabolite of propoxyphene, norpropoxyphene, has not been a problem at the doses at which the parent compound is used clinically. However, the metabolite of meperidine, normeperidine, has been observed to produce clinically relevant side effects in the cancer population, including tremulousness, hyperreflexia, myoclonus, and even seizures (103). This risk suggests that meperidine should not be used in the management of cancer pain.

As suggested by the analgesic ladder, the simplest approach to the management of moderate pain in the cancer patient with limited or no prior exposure to opioids uses a combination product containing either aspirin or acetaminophen plus an opioid (codeine, oxycodone, hydrocodone, dihydrocodeine, or propoxyphene). The dose can be increased to maximally safe levels of the coanalgesic; for example, in products containing acetaminophen, this is usually 4 g per day. Although patients who do not benefit from this regimen are usually switched to an opioid, the fact that weak opioids have no ceiling effect provides additional flexibility.

Selection of an Opioid. The selection of an opioid for severe cancer pain is similarly empirical. Morphine often is considered to be the preferred first-line drug based on worldwide experience, ease of dosing, and the availability of numerous formulations, including extended-release forms with durations of effect of 12 hours (104) and 24 hours. Any of the other drugs may be better tolerated in the individual patient, and this variability suggests that therapeutic failure with one drug may be followed by remarkable success with another (105).

The predominant metabolic pathway for morphine is glucuronidation to morphine-3-glucuronide (M3G) and morphine-6-glucuronide (M6G) (106). The accumulation of morphine metabolites may be associated with side effects, such as myoclonus and chronic nausea (107–109). Probably as a consequence of first-pass glucuronidation through the liver, the ratios of M6G:morphine and M3G:morphine are higher with oral than parenteral administration (110,111). Liver dysfunction has a small effect on morphine kinetics (112), but renal insufficiency results in accumulation of M3G and M6G (113). For this reason, morphine should be administered cautiously to patients with renal insufficiency. The occurrence of morphine toxicity in these patients should be followed by a trial of an alternative opioid, such as hydromorphone or fentanyl.

The selection of an opioid for the treatment of severe cancer pain is also influenced by pharmacokinetic factors, the most salient of which is half-life. Because four to five half-lives are required to approach steady-state after dosing is initiated or changed, an opioid with a relatively long half-life requires a prolonged period to judge the full effect of a new dosing regimen. Although both levorphanol and methadone have half-lives longer than other opioids (Table 33.7), only methadone, which has a half-life that ranges between 12 and 190 hours, has been proven to be a problem in clinical practice. Substantial delayed toxicity has been observed many days after methadone treatment was begun or altered (114,115). Given the difficulties posed by the need for prolonged intensive monitoring with methadone, it is reasonable to view this drug as a second-line agent for patients predisposed to opioid side effects, including the elderly and those with major organ dysfunction, and those who are either noncompliant or difficult to evaluate.

The patient's previous favorable experience with opioid drugs should also be considered when choosing an opioid. The exception to this is meperidine, the toxic metabolite of which may accumulate with repeated dosing. A favorable experience with this drug during short-term administration should not be viewed as predictive of the response to chronic dosing.

Routes of Administration. The oral route is preferred in the management of chronic cancer pain owing to its safety, economy, and acceptability to patients. Alternative routes are often required, however, and the clinician must recognize their indications and be familiar with the accepted approaches. In a survey of patients with advanced cancer, more than half required two or more routes of administration prior to death and almost a quarter required three or more (116).

Transdermal Delivery. The transdermal route of administration is available for the highly lipophilic opioid fentanyl (117). This formulation, which offers a 48- to 72-hour dosing interval, has been quickly accepted into clinical practice. Comparative trials against controlled-release oral morphine suggest that this formulation is preferred by some patients and may be associated with relatively less constipation (118). The transdermal route may be very useful for the patient who is unable to swallow or absorb an orally administered opioid; this is particularly appropriate when the underlying pain syndrome is relatively stable. Pains that are rapidly fluctuating and require multiple supplemental doses may be more easily managed using an ambulatory infusion device with a PCA option. A trial of transdermal fentanyl also may be appropriate after other opioids have failed because of dose-limiting toxicity and after other therapies have become complicated by poor compliance with oral drug taking.

The pharmacokinetics of the transdermal system must be understood to optimize its use (117). The development of a subcutaneous depot under the patch results in a slow onset of effects following a dose change and a prolonged apparent elimination half-life (usually 24 hours) after the patch is removed. These characteristics relatively contraindicate the transdermal system in the management of acute pain or chronic pain that is rapidly increasing.

The limitations of transdermal fentanyl include the cost and the difficulties involved in delivering high doses. The potential advantages may also be lost if the patient requires frequent supplemental doses, which can only be administered via an alternative route, such as oral, rectal, or parenteral injection.

Continuous Infusion. Patients who are unable to swallow or absorb opioid drugs are candidates for long-term parenteral dosing. Repetitive intramuscular or subcutaneous injections are painful and should be rarely considered. Repetitive intravenous injections may be effective, but they usually require skilled nursing and may be associated with prominent "bolus" effects (toxicity at peak concentration, pain breakthrough at the trough, or both). Continuous intravenous infusion eliminates the fluctuations in plasma concentration and may be an effective means of providing sustained analgesia to these patients. Any opioid available in an injectable formulation can be used for continuous infusion.

The availability of continuous subcutaneous infusion using ambulatory infusion devices has markedly enhanced the clinical utility of infusion techniques (119,120). A diverse group of pumps that range considerably in features, complexity, and cost are now available, and the clinician often has the option of selecting a pump based on the needs

and resources of the patient. In most cities, skilled nursing organizations can assist in the management of therapy at home.

Improvements in pump technology provide the option for PCA in the home environment (120). For most patients, a continuous subcutaneous basal infusion is administered concurrent with an option for patient-controlled bolus injections to manage acute flares of pain. Drug concentration, dose, and lockout interval (minimum time between self-administered doses) are programmed into the pump by the clinician. Although there have been no controlled trials of this technique, patient acceptability has been high in clinical practice. In the future, these pumps may be supplanted, in part, by the advent of iontophoretic devices that can provide similar drug-delivery characteristics through the skin.

Intraspinal opioids. The discovery of opioid receptors in the spinal cord provided the foundation for the development of techniques to deliver opioid analgesics intraspinally (47, 121). Intraspinal administration can provide selective analgesia (i.e., without the sensory or motor blockade produced by local anesthetics) at doses lower than those required systemically. The strongest indication for a trial of intraspinal opioid administration is the occurrence of intolerable somnolence or confusion in patients who are not experiencing adequate analgesia during systemic opioid treatment of pain.

Many methods of intraspinal opioid administration are now in use (122). The most commonly used include a percutaneous epidural catheter, which is usually tunneled to the anterior abdominal wall and there connected to an ambulatory infusion pump; a totally implanted epidural catheter connected to a subcutaneous portal, which in turn is connected to an ambulatory pump; and an intrathecal catheter connected to a totally implanted continuous infusion device. The preferred drugs for chronic intraspinal infusion are morphine and hydromorphone, but many others are used empirically, and admixtures (e.g., opioid plus local anesthetic or clonidine, or both) are now commonplace.

Other routes of administration. The oral transmucosal formulation of fentanyl (OTFC) has been shown to be safe and efficacious when used as a "rescue" dose in cancer patients receiving a fixed-schedule opioid regimen for chronic cancer pain (101). In a double-blind, double-dummy, randomized, multiple crossover study of 134 adult cancer patients, OTFC was found to be more effective than immediate-release morphine sulfate in treating cancer-related breakthrough pain (123).

One study observed that absorption through the oral cavity actually can occur with any opioid, particularly those that are, like fentanyl, highly lipophilic (124). Any injectable formulation of an opioid could, therefore, be potentially used for sublingual administration. The inability to deliver high doses or prevent swallowing of the dose limits the suitability of this approach for most patients with cancer pain.

Rectal formulations of oxymorphone, hydromorphone, and morphine are available in the United States. The potency of opioids administered rectally is believed to approximate oral dosing (125). This route is generally used in the management of relatively nontolerant patients who develop a transient inability to use oral drugs.

Several other routes of administration are also feasible. Intranasal butorphanol is available, but this agonist-antagonist drug is rarely considered for cancer pain. Although buccal administration of morphine has been used occasionally, the limited transmucosal absorption of this compound (124) does not support wider use of this approach. Finally, intraventricular morphine has been used for cancer pain (126). The rationale for this approach is similar to that underlying the use of intraspinal opioids, and it usually has been considered for those patients with severe head or neck pain who develop intolerable CNS side effects from systemic administration of opioid drugs.

Guidelines for the Administration of Opioid Drugs. Dosing guidelines have been developed from extensive clinical experience and the known pharmacology of these agents.

Initial doses. A relatively opioid-naïve patient who has developed severe pain despite treatment using a combination drug that contains an opioid and a nonopioid should generally be switched to an opioid conventionally used on the third step of the analgesic ladder at a dose equivalent to 5 to 10 mg of intramuscular morphine or 15 to 30 mg of oral morphine every 4 hours. A table of equianalgesic doses (Table 33.7), derived from controlled studies of relative potency among opioid drugs, should be consulted in calculating the appropriate dose (127).

If a controlled-release opioid preparation is used, the total daily dose to initiate therapy is the same, but the dosing frequency is reduced. A recent study suggests that a simplified titration using sustained-release morphine once daily is equally effective as immediate-release morphine given every 4 hours, and patients report significantly less fatigue during the titration process (128).

As noted, knowledge of relative potency, as codified on the equianalgesic dose table (Table 33.7), guides the starting dose if an alternative to morphine is used or if the opioid drug or route of administration is changed during therapy. To switch to another opioid drug or route, the equianalgesic dose table is used to calculate a dose of the new drug that would be theoretically equianalgesic with the new drug or route. With few exceptions, the dosing regimen based on this calculated dose should be reduced by 25% to 50% to account for incomplete cross tolerance between drugs. A larger reduction, 75% to 90%, is prudent if the new drug is methadone (because of a unique pharmacology in this agent) or if the patient is significantly predisposed to opioid side effects. In contrast, no reduction in the equianalgesic dose is needed if the switch is to transdermal fentanyl (because a reduction is already built into the recommended equianalgesic ratios).

Dose titration. Following selection of a starting dose, dose adjustment is almost always required. Once a favorable balance between analgesia and side effects is obtained, this is usually maintained for a prolonged time unless there is progression in the pain-producing pathology. Although several large surveys have established that patients with stable disease usually demonstrate stable dosing patterns, most patients with cancer pain do not have stable disease (1,129). Recurrent pain or the new occurrence of side effects necessitates another period of dose titration. Inadequate adjustment of the dose is probably the most common reason for unsuccessful long-term management of cancer pain.

In all cases, the dose of an opioid should be increased until acceptable analgesia is produced or intolerable and unmanageable side effects supervene. Ceiling doses for the pure agonist opioids have not been identified clinically, and doses can, therefore, become extremely high as upward dose titration proceeds. Doses above the equivalent of 35,000 mg of morphine per day have been reported in rare patients (116). The absolute dose of the opioid is immaterial as long as the balance between analgesia and side effects remains acceptable for the patient.

Fixed versus as-needed dosing. For chronic pain, or frequently recurring pain, the best outcome for opioid usually is achieved if the drug is administered according to a fixed, around-the-clock schedule (130). In the relatively opioid-naïve patient, however, as-needed dosing may help define the opioid requirement in a manner that reduces the risk of side effects as the dose is increased.

Like the patient-controlled analgesia option described previously, the use of as-needed "rescue doses" may also provide a means of treating transitory pains (9). Clinical experience suggests that a short half-life drug should be used for these supplemental doses. With the exception of methadone, this can generally be the same drug administered on an around-the-clock basis. The rescue dose can be prescribed every 2 hours as needed at a dose equal to 5% to 15% of the total daily opioid consumption.

Tolerance, physical dependence, and addiction. The clinical implications of tolerance, physical dependence, and addiction are commonly misunderstood by patients and clinicians. These misapprehensions may lead to concern about adverse events and, possibly, undertreatment of pain.

Tolerance is a pharmacologic property of opioid drugs defined by the need for escalating doses in order to maintain effects (131–133). Patients may have other reasons for declining analgesic effects, however, among which are progressive nociception and increasing psychologic distress. Abundant survey data suggest that the most common reason for dose increase is worsening pain due to progression of a nociceptive lesion. Most patients with stable disease continue to require the same opioid dose for extremely long periods of time (129,134).

Fear of analgesic tolerance should never delay the implementation of opioid therapy. Furthermore, tolerance should not be invoked to explain the need for higher opioid doses unless a comprehensive reassessment has failed to identify an alternative explanation. If appropriately sought, a progressive or recurrent lesion is usually found (28).

Physical dependence is also a pharmacologic property of opioid drugs, which is defined by the occurrence of an abstinence syndrome following abrupt dose reduction or administration of an antagonist (131,133,135). Neither the dose nor the duration of dosing required to produce physical dependence is known, and it is prudent to assume that all patients who have received an opioid drug for more than a few days have the potential for withdrawal. This implies that dosing should not be discontinued suddenly and that antagonist drugs, including the agonist-antagonist opioids, should be avoided.

Patients who become physically dependent on opioids appear to develop increased sensitivity to the effects of antagonist drugs. Very small doses of naloxone may produce a severe abstinence syndrome. For this reason, the use of this drug should be limited to patients with symptomatic respiratory depression. When naloxone must be used in patients receiving chronic opioid therapy, only a dilute solution (e.g., 0.4 mg in 10 mL saline) should be administered and incremental doses should be given only until respiration improves. The goal of this intervention is improved respiration and not a return of consciousness, which may be associated with recurrent pain and withdrawal phenomena.

Both tolerance and physical dependence are distinct from addiction. Because the labels applied to patients can determine the attitudes and behaviors of caregivers, it is extremely important that appropriate terms are used to describe these phenomena. Patients who are perceived to have the capacity for withdrawal should be labeled physically dependent and not ''addicted.''

Addiction is a psychologic and behavioral syndrome characterized by loss of control over drug use, compulsive use, and continued use despite harm to the patient or others. Although abusable drugs, including opioids, can be shown to have reinforcing effects in animals, the capacity to produce addiction should not be considered an inherent property of the drug. Addiction presumably results from an interaction between the drug and a variety of factors that predispose the individual to compulsive use. These factors probably encompass genetic predispositions, situational aspects, and psychologic disturbances.

Cancer patients who engage in aberrant drug-taking behaviors, such as hoarding or selling, unsanctioned dose escalation, or manipulation of the medical system to obtain additional drugs, may or may not meet criteria for the diagnosis of addiction. If such aberrant behaviors are identified, measures should be taken to eliminate them while a detailed assessment is performed to clarify their meaning.

In some cases, aberrant drug-related behaviors appear to be driven by uncontrolled pain. This has been termed pseudoaddiction and is managed by improved efforts to provide pain relief. Occasionally, aberrant behaviors are related to a psychiatric disorder other than addiction or to the development of a mild encephalopathy, which leads to confusion about drug taking. The clinician must avoid the stigmatizing label of addiction for patients who have reasonable alternative explanations for aberrant behaviors, but be willing to render the diagnosis of addiction in those who actually have this disease. Consultation with an addiction medicine specialist may be useful in establishing the controls needed to stop inappropriate behavior and properly diagnose the condition.

The risk of true iatrogenic addiction is clearly relevant in judging the overall utility of opioid therapy for chronic cancer pain. There is substantial evidence that this risk is extremely low among those with no prior history of abuse or addiction (134,136–138). It is now widely accepted that fear of addiction should never be allowed to impede opioid therapy of severe cancer pain or the process of dose escalation required to optimize therapy. It is also clear that patients who have the disease of addiction and experience cancer pain must be treated aggressively for pain, and that successful outcomes in this group may require both skills in opioid pharmacotherapy and skills in addiction medicine approaches.

Management of Common Opioid Side Effects. Although there is no maximum dose or ceiling dose for the μ agonist opioids, the appearance of side effects imposes a practical limit on dose escalation. Given the importance of side effects in determining the response to an opioid, the successful management of common adverse side effects is a fundamental aspect of therapy (139). The most common side effects are related to gastrointestinal and neuropsychologic function (Table 33.8). The main strategies to address opioid-induced side effects are (a) effective symptomatic management, (b) opioid rotation or a switch in the route of administration, and (c) coadministration of a pharmacologic or nonpharmacologic treatment that reduces the opioid requirement (140–143).

Constipation is a highly prevalent side effect of opioid therapy. It may contribute to abdominal pain, distension, nausea, and worsening anorexia, and occasionally may progress to obstipation and bowel obstruction. The management of drug-induced constipation should begin with the elimination of nonessential constipatory drugs and, if possible, an increase in both fluid and fiber intake. Fiber should not be increased in those with likely partial bowel obstruction or marked debility because of the potential for worsening obstruction.

Laxative therapy should be considered whenever constipation cannot be controlled through nutritional measures. Routine laxative therapy should not be administered, however, if there is reason to believe that obstruction or impaction is present. These problems should be addressed before laxative therapy is initiated. Patients who are starting opioid therapy and have other predisposing factors for constipation should be considered for prophylactic laxative therapy.

There are numerous types of laxatives, including bulk-

TABLE 33.8. *Commonly used pharmacologic approaches in the management of opioid side effects*

Opioid side effect	Treatment

Constipation	Approaches for all patients:
	  Increase fluid intake and dietary fiber
	  Ensure comfort and convenience, etc.
	Discuss approaches with patient and select one or more:
	  Daily contact laxative plus stool softener (e.g., senna plus docusate)
	  Daily osmotic laxative or lavage agent
	  Intermittent use of laxative
	Consider alternative approaches in refractory cases:
	  Enema
	  Prokinetic agent (cisapride, metoclopramide)
	  Oral naloxone

Nausea	Several approaches:
	  If associated with vertigo or if markedly exacerbated by movement, antivertiginous drug (e.g., scopolamine, meclizine, dimenhydrinate)
	  If associated with early satiety, prokinetic agent (metoclopramide)
	  In other cases, dopamine antagonist drugs (e.g., prochlorperazine, chlorpromazine, haloperidol, metoclopramide)

Neuropsychologic	If analgesia is satisfactory, reduce opioid dose by 25% to 50% If analgesia is satisfactory and the toxicity involves confusion, consider a trial of a neuroleptic (e.g., haloperidol) If analgesia is satisfactory and the toxicity is somnolence, consider a trial of a psychostimulant (e.g., methylphenidate) Consider pharmacologic approaches to reduce the opioid requirement (addition of a coanalgesic or adjuvant) Consider trial of an alternative opioid If appropriate, consider nonpharmacologic analgesic approaches

forming agents, osmotic agents, lubricants, surfactants, contact cathartics, prokinetic drugs, agents for colonic lavage, and oral opioid antagonists. The conventional first-line approach is a combination of a stool softener and a cathartic agent. Most patients respond to this therapy. The recent advent of an oral lavage agent, propylethylene glycol, in a powered formulation offers another well-tolerated, and usually effective, approach. Osmotic agents, such as lactulose, are often tried in refractory cases.

Oral opioid antagonist therapy that can reverse opioid-induced constipation through local action on opioid receptors in the gut without causing systemic opioid withdrawal is available (144). At the present time, this treatment is implemented using oral naloxone, which is typically administered at a dose of 0.8 mg twice daily; the dose is doubled

every 2 to 3 days until favorable effects occur or side effects are experienced. The daily dose needed to reverse constipation is usually 12 to 18 mg/day. Trials of other quarternary opioid antagonists, such as methylnaltrexone (145–147), have been favorable and may expand the utility of this approach in the future.

Nausea or vomiting constitutes a problem for some 10% to 30% of cancer patients receiving opioid therapy (148). Potential contributing etiologies should be evaluated and the treatment adjusted accordingly. If the assessment suggests that factors other than opioids are contributing to the nausea, antiemetic therapy may be combined with specific interventions to reverse or minimize these factors.

Conventional antiemetic therapy can be administered on either an as-needed or fixed-schedule dosing regimen according to persistence of symptoms. There are many antiemetic drugs in diverse classes. The usual first-line drugs are the dopamine antagonists, including prochlorperazine, metoclopramide, and haloperidol.

Patients with refractory nausea may need other pharmacologic approaches. Although the antiemetic efficacy of corticosteroids is unexplained, these drugs are clearly beneficial for some patients. Others respond to a commercially available cannabinoid. Although ondansetron, granisetron, or dolasetron can be beneficial for patients with refractory symptoms, they are very costly and should be considered only after other therapies have failed. In difficult cases, combinations of drugs from unrelated classes often are tried. When behavioral factors appear to contribute, cognitive therapy has proven to be beneficial (149).

Data from prospective studies indicate that sedation or mental clouding occurs in 20% to 60% of patients starting oral opioid therapy for cancer pain (139). Significant impairment disappears in most patients with prolonged exposure to the drug. There is wide individual variation in response (150), however, and alterations in cognition, perception, or mood, as well as changes in the level of consciousness, can occur. When disturbances occur, their pattern and severity may be influenced by many factors, including the evolving medical condition and concurrent therapies. As a result, patients who develop neuropsychologic changes during opioid therapy require careful assessment and management.

If neuropsychologic side effects are mild, reassurance and education are usually sufficient interventions. When toxicity is severe or persistent enough to compromise the benefits of therapy, other interventions are needed. Treatment of potential etiologies other than the opioid (e.g., elimination of another nonessential drug or treatment of a metabolic disturbance), when feasible and indicated, is the first step in the management of neuropsychologic symptoms. If pain is well controlled, it is reasonable to try an opioid dose reduction of 25% to 50%.

Symptomatic therapies for opioid-induced sedation or mental clouding also should be considered (Table 33.8), but few have been well studied in clinical trials. Experience is greatest with psychostimulant therapy. For example, methylphenidate has been shown to decrease sedation in cancer patients taking opioids (151–154). The starting dose is 5 mg at breakfast and at lunchtime. Other psychostimulants that have been used empirically for this indication include dextroamphetamine, amphetamine, and modafinal.

Adjuvant Drugs

Most patients with cancer pain require multiple drugs for symptom management. Some of these adjuvant drugs are used to treat symptoms other than pain, particularly those that occur as side effects of the opioid (Table 33.8). Other drugs are used in an effort to provide additive analgesia. The latter drugs comprise the NSAIDs and the so-called adjuvant analgesics. Adjuvant analgesics may be defined as drugs that are commercially available for indications other than pain but may be analgesic in selected circumstances (155).

Many of the adjuvant analgesics may be considered for those with cancer pain (Table 33.9)(155). Treatment is generally considered after adequate titration of an opioid. They are particularly helpful in the treatment of pain syndromes that are often relatively less responsive to opioids, such as neuropathic pains. Although neuropathic pains, such as postmastectomy syndrome, painful polyneuropathy, and painful plexopathy (156–158), can respond well to an opioid regimen, they are relatively more likely to be poorly responsive and represent the most common target of the adjuvant analgesics.

Corticosteroids are among the adjuvant analgesics commonly used to treat neuropathic pain. These drugs also may improve anorexia, nausea, and fatigue, and are often used in open-ended therapy when cancer is relatively advanced.

Anticonvulsants, antidepressants, and oral local anesthetics have analgesic effects in neuropathic pain (155). Evidence for analgesic efficacy is best for the anticonvulsant gabapentin (159,160) and the tricyclic antidepressant amitriptyline (161–164). Gabapentin is often tried first, but is now considered to be only one of many potentially analgesic anticonvulsants. Others include the older drugs valproate, phenytoin, and clonazepam and the newer drugs lamotrigine, tiagabine, topiramate, oxcarbazepine, zonisamide, and levetiracetam.

The use of amitriptyline or one of the other analgesic tricyclic antidepressants often is limited by the high likelihood of side effects (163). Newer antidepressants, such as paroxetine, citalopram, and bupropion, also are analgesic and are better tolerated in the cancer population.

A trial with an oral local anesthetic usually is considered after antidepressant and anticonvulsant drugs have been tried (165). Intravenous or subcutaneous lidocaine may be useful in the treatment of severe, rapidly increasing neuropathic pain.

Other drugs also are used for neuropathic pain. There is extensive experience with the gamma-aminobutyric acid

TABLE 33.9. *Adjuvant analgesics*

Indication	Drugs
Neuropathic pain	Antidepressants
	Tricyclic antidepressants
	Amitriptyline
	Desipramine
	"Newer" antidepressants
	Fluoxetine
	Paroxetine
	Anticonvulsants
	Gabapentin
	Carbamazepine
	Phenytoin
	Valproate
	Clonazepam
	Lamotrigine
	Oral local anesthetics
	Mexiletine
	Tocainide
	Alpha$_2$-adrenergic agonists
	Clonidine
	Tizanidine
	NMDA receptor antagonists
	Ketamine
	Dextromethorphan
	Neuroleptics
	Pimozide
	Miscellaneous
	Baclofen
	Calcitonin
	Capsaicin
	Local anesthetics
	(e.g., lidocaine)
Bone pain	Bisphosphonates
	(e.g., pamidronate)
	Calcitonin
	Radiopharmaceuticals
	(e.g., strontium 89 and
	samarium 153)
Bowel obstruction	Scopolamine
	Glycopyrrolate
	Octreotide
Muscle spasms	Carisoprodol
	Methocarbamol
	Orphenadrine
	Baclofen
Multipurpose	Corticosteroids
	Dexamethasone
	Prednisone

(GABA) agonist baclofen and limited experience with the alpha$_2$-adrenergic drugs tizanidine and clonidine. Recently, interest has focused on the use of the n-methyl-d-aspartate inhibitors, three of which—dextromethorphan, amantadine, and ketamine—are commercially available in the United States. Small studies have suggested benefit from the addition of ketamine in cancer patients with difficult pain problems, including neuropathic pain (166–168). Ketamine can cause severe psychomimetic effects, however, such as nightmares and delirium, and the potential for this toxicity limits

its use in the routine clinical setting. There is some evidence that oral ketamine has a more favorable side effect profile than parenteral ketamine, with drowsiness being the most common problem (168).

The use of topical agents represent another adjuvant analgesic strategy. A lidocaine patch (Lidoderm) (169,170) is now available and has been shown to be effective in postherpetic neuralgia. In a recent study in cancer patients with surgical neuropathic pain (e.g., postmastectomy syndrome), topical capsaicin, a peptide that depletes substance P in small primary afferent neurons, was found to significantly decrease pain (171).

Opioid-refractory malignant bone pain is another syndrome for which adjuvant analgesics often are considered. The preferred drugs include bisphosphonates, radiopharmaceuticals, and calcitonin. There has been increasing evidence that the bisphosphonates improve overall morbidity associated with bone metastases, and a trial of one of these agents is typically considered first (172).

Adjuvant analgesics also are commonly employed in the setting of advanced bowel obstruction. Aggressive pharmacotherapy, particularly in those with advanced disease, may control symptoms and obviate the need for drainage procedures. Treatment usually involves the combination of anticholinergic drugs (e.g., scopolamine or glycopyrrolate), octreotide, corticosteroids, and opioids (173).

Alternative Approaches in Chronic Pain Management

Most patients with cancer pain can achieve adequate relief with pharmacologic approaches alone. It is important to recall, however, that a multimodality strategy is often needed to address the broader palliative care concerns of the patient and family, which derive from the complex interaction between pain and suffering (Fig. 33.1). The need for multiple treatments may relate to the persistence of pain despite optimal pharmacotherapy, or to the need to address multiple concurrent problems to achieve an outcome of pain therapy that is consistent with the larger goals of care and enhances overall quality of life.

When the focus is pain control, the potential alternative therapies include a large number of noninvasive and invasive approaches. Only a small minority of patients will require an invasive analgesic modality if the other therapies are optimally administered (10).

Anesthesiologic Approaches

Analgesic techniques traditionally considered to be within the purview of anesthesiologists play an important role in the management of chronic cancer pain. In addition to the use of intraspinal opioids, the many techniques of neural blockade represent extremely important therapeutic modalities.

Advances in the neuraxial infusion of opioids and other drugs (most often local anesthetics or clonidine) have largely supplanted the neurodestructive approaches that were employed in the past for pain syndromes refractory to systemic opioid therapy (see below). Neuraxial infusion is usually considered when intolerable side effects compromise systemic treatment with an opioid. In a recent controlled trial, continuous intrathecal infusion of morphine application via an implantable drug-delivery system yielded better pain control, less fatigue, and improved survival than comprehensive medical management alone (174).

Neural blockade comprises a diverse group of procedures that transiently or more permanently block sympathetic nerves, somatic nerves, or both (175,176). Somatic nerve blocks reduce afferent nociceptive input; sympathetic nerve blocks are used to block afferent input from viscera or occasionally to manage those cancer-related neuropathic pains that are presumed to be perpetuated at least in part by sympathetic efferent function.

Temporary nerve blocks with local anesthetic may be diagnostic, prognostic, or therapeutic. Diagnostic blocks elucidate the afferent pathways involved in the experience of pain. Prognostic blocks are implemented prior to a neurolytic procedure, and although extensive clinical experience indicates that a favorable response does not predict permanent relief following neurolysis, the failure to achieve pain relief with local anesthetic is commonly viewed as a contraindication to a destructive procedure. Repeated therapeutic blocks with local anesthetic are occasionally used in cancer patients who obtain substantial and fairly prolonged relief after such a temporary block.

Recently, local anesthetics have been used to provide more prolonged neural blockade through techniques of perineural or epidural infusion. Epidural local anesthetics, either alone or in combination with opioid drugs, can be used for prolonged periods to manage refractory pain (174,177).

Neural blockade with neurolytic solutions, usually alcohol or phenol, have been in use for many decades, and approaches have been developed to denervate virtually any area of the body (175,176). The short-term risks associated with the injection of these substances, such as damage to soft tissues and local hemorrhage or infection, combined with the long-term risks of neuritis and deafferentation pain, suggest that these techniques should generally be reserved for patients with refractory pain in the setting of advanced cancer. The advent of intraspinal opioids and continuous local anesthetic infusion has substantially reduced the proportion of patients for whom neurolytic techniques are appropriate.

The one generally accepted exception to the use of neurolysis as a last resort is celiac plexus blockade for the management of epigastric pain due to neoplastic invasion of the celiac axis. The response to neurolytic celiac plexus blockade in pain due to pancreatic cancer has been observed to be so satisfactory that earlier use is warranted whenever the typical pain syndrome occurs (178,179).

Trigger point injections may be considered within the purview of all practitioners. Myofascial pains are extremely common in patients with chronic cancer pain, and the use of local anesthetic injections into painful trigger points may be a useful adjunctive approach in these patients (180).

Intermittent nitrous oxide inhalation is an anesthetic technique that has been proven to be useful in the management of severe breakthrough pain in patients with advanced cancer (180). Although the availability of masks that reduce ambient leakage of the gas has increased the potential usefulness of this approach, it continues to be applied rarely.

Neurostimulatory Approaches

It has been appreciated for some time that stimulation of afferent neural pathways may result in analgesia. The best-known application of this principle is TENS. Other approaches include counterirritation (i.e., systematic rubbing of the painful part), percutaneous electrical nerve stimulation, dorsal column stimulation, deep brain stimulation, and acupuncture. Published experience in the use of these modalities for the management of cancer pain is meager. Surveys of the techniques that have been used most extensively in nonmalignant pain (TENS, acupuncture, and dorsal column stimulation) suggest that the majority of patients will achieve analgesia soon after the approach is implemented but only a few can obtain prolonged relief. A trial of TENS is usually considered in patients with neuropathic pain that has been proven to be difficult to manage with opioids.

A small series of patients successfully managed with deep brain stimulation suggests that some patients with cancer-related pain could potentially achieve long-term benefits from this modality (181). Nonetheless, because of the expertise required and the lack of confirmatory studies, it should only rarely be considered in this population.

Physiatric Approaches

The potential for analgesic effects from physiatric therapies, including the use of orthoses or prostheses, occupational therapy, and physical therapy, is not often recognized. For example, refractory movement-induced pains may be partially relieved by bracing the painful part, such as in patients with back pain due to metastatic lesions of the spine and those with arm pain related to a malignant brachial plexopathy.

The necessity for a well-fitting prosthesis in patients with traumatic or surgical limb amputation is well accepted. Patients with amputations for malignant disease who have persistent stump pain may benefit from intensive physical therapy using an appropriately designed prosthesis.

The rehabilitative consequences of physical therapy and occupational therapy are well known, and these approaches can yield salutary effects in patients forced to cope with repeated physical and psychologic losses. Equally important,

the techniques that are employed may have analgesic consequences, forestalling or reversing painful contractures or ankyloses in immobilized patients and providing an alternative approach to the management of painful trigger points.

Neurosurgical Approaches

Procedures designed to denervate the painful area surgically have been developed for every level of the nervous system from peripheral nerves to cortex (182). The most useful approach is cordotomy, which can be performed percutaneously in the awake patient and has been reported to provide more than 80% of patients with initial pain relief (16). Efficacy gradually declines over time, which suggests that the greatest utility of this technique is in the patient with relatively advanced disease. Potential adverse effects include ipsilateral leg paresis, ataxia, and bladder dysfunction. Post-cordotomy dysesthesia, a neuropathic pain that is often refractory to treatment, can appear many months after cordotomy and is an infrequent but potentially serious complication.

The use of other denervating procedures, such as neurectomy or rhizotomy, can be performed in patients with focal pain that can be effectively denervated by the sectioning of discrete nerves or roots. Like cordotomy, these procedures should only be considered for patients with a clear-cut nociceptive lesion underlying the pain.

Hypophysectomy, which can be performed surgically or chemically, has been reported to provide relief of pain in more than 60% of patients, with a median duration of approximately 3 months (179,183,184). The mechanism of action is not understood and the technique is now rarely considered. Similarly, neurosurgical procedures such as lobotomy or cingulotomy, which were advocated for refractory cases of cancer pain in the past, are now rarely performed.

Psychologic Approaches

Some patients or families who present with severe psychologic distress may benefit from a multidisciplinary approach in which psychologic interventions are emphasized within a program designed to palliate symptoms and provide family support. These goals may be accomplished in some cases through referral to a hospice or palliative care program. Occasionally, patients with psychiatric disorders are identified, indicating the need for further assessment and treatment by an appropriate specialist (185).

Specific cognitive and behavioral approaches have also been applied in the management of pain and related symptoms (186–190). Cognitive approaches include relaxation training, distraction techniques, hypnosis, and biofeedback, all of which may enhance a patient's sense of personal control and reduce pain. Although many of these approaches require experienced personnel to implement, several forms of relaxation training can be taught by the nonspecialist. Behavioral therapy, which has achieved wide acceptance in the management of nonmalignant pain, is occasionally considered in patients with limited disease whose level of functional impairment is perceived to be out of proportion to the effects of the neoplasm. Cognitive and behavioral psychologic approaches can focus the patient's attention on issues related to function and quality of life and reduce rumination about the disease.

Alternative or Complementary Medicine Approaches

Therapies that are typically considered to be complementary or alternative have had a growing role in pain management (191). These approaches often are very attractive to patients because they endorse a holistic strategy that is perceived as providing hope and self-control (192). Some interventions that are termed "complementary" are actually used routinely by specialists in pain medicine or palliative care. These include cognitive therapies (e.g., relaxation, meditation, and others), nutritional support, and acupuncture. Other interventions, such as homeopathy, naturopathy, and many others, are considered to be far outside the mainstream and are rarely suggested (193). Health-care professionals have the difficult task of expressing concerns about some of the latter therapies, although respecting patients' pursuit of complementary treatments that may be beneficial or, at least, offer no significant chance of harm.

CONCLUSION

Pain is highly prevalent among patients with gynecologic tumors. The clinicians involved in the care of these patients have a challenging task in being able to provide state of the art management approaches for both acute pain and chronic pain. Fortunately, the most effective strategy for both acute and chronic pain, namely, opioid-based pharmacotherapy, is clearly within the purview of all practitioners. The knowledge and skills necessary to optimize this therapy, and integrate it with the broader principles of palliative care, are fundamental to the practice of gynecologic oncology.

REFERENCES

1. Kanner RM. The scope of the problem. In: Portenoy RK, Kanner RM, eds. *Pain management: theory and practice*. Philadelphia: FA Davis Co, 1996:40.
2. Vainio A, Auvinen A. Prevalence of symptoms among patients with advanced cancer: an international collaborative study. *J Pain Symptom Manage* 1996;12:3.
3. World Health Organization. *Cancer pain relief*. 2nd ed. Geneva: World Health Organization, 1996.
4. Ferrell B, Smith S, Cullinane C, Melancon C. Symptom concerns of women with ovarian cancer. *J Pain Sympt Manage* 2003;25:528.
5. Olson SH, Mignone L, Nakrasieve C, Caputo TA, Barakat RR, Harlap S. Symptoms of ovarian cancer. *Obstet Gynecol* 2001;98:212.
6. Portenoy RK, Kornblith AB, Wong G, et al. Pain in ovarian cancer: prevalence, characteristics, and associated symptoms. *Cancer* 1994; 74:907.
7. Miaskowski C, Dibble SL. The problem of pain in outpatients with breast cancer. *Oncol Nurs Forum* 1995;22:791.
8. Edwards WT. Optimizing opioid treatment of postoperative pain. *J Pain Symptom Manage* 1990;5:S24.
9. Patt RB, Ellison N. Breakthrough pain. In: Aronoff GM, ed. *Evaluation and treatment of chronic pain*. 3rd ed. Baltimore: Williams & Wilkins, 1999:377.
10. Cleeland CS, Gonin R, Hatfield AK, et al. Pain and its treatment in outpatients with metastatic cancer. *N Engl J Med* 1994;330:592.
11. Von Roenn JH, Cleeland CS, Gonin R, et al. Physician attitudes and practice in cancer pain management. A survey from the Eastern Cooperative Oncology Group. *Arch Intern Med* 1993;119:121.
12. Moulin DE, Foley KM. Review of a hospital-based pain service. In: Foley KM, Bonica JJ, Ventafridda V, eds. *Advances in pain research and therapy*. Vol. 16. New York: Raven Press, 1990; 413.
13. Schug SA, Zech D, Dorr U. Cancer pain management according to WHO analgesic guidelines. *J Pain Symptom Manage* 1990;5:27.
14. Ventafridda V, Tamburini M, Caraceni A, et al. A validation study of the WHO method for cancer pain relief. *Cancer* 1987;59:850.
15. Walker VA, Hoskins PJ, Hanks GW, et al. Evaluation of WHO analgesic guidelines for cancer pain in a hospital-based palliative care unit. *J Pain Symptom Manage* 1988;3:145.
16. Arbit E. Anterolateral cordotomy. In: Arbit E, ed. *Management of cancer-related pain*. Mount Kisco, NY: Futura Publishing, 1993:321.
17. Caraceni A, Portenoy RK, a working group of the IASP task force on cancer pain. An international survey of cancer pain characteristics and syndromes. *Pain* 1999;82:263.
18. Lehman KA. Patient-controlled analgesia for post-operative pain. In: Max MM, Portenoy RK, Laska E, eds. *Design of analgesic clinical trials*. New York: Raven Press, 1991:481.
19. Merskey H, Bogduk N, eds. *Classification of chronic pain: descriptions of chronic pain syndromes and definitions of pain terms*. 2nd ed. Seattle: IASP Press, 1994.
20. Portenoy RK. Cancer pain: pathophysiology and syndromes. *Lancet* 1992;339:1026.
21. Cherny NI, Coyle N, Foley KM. Suffering in the advanced cancer patient: a definition and taxonomy. *J Palliat Care* 1994;10:57.
22. Portenoy RK. Pain and quality of life: theoretical aspects. In: Osoba D, ed. *Quality of life in cancer patients*. New York: CRC Press, 1991: 279.
23. Kellgren JG. On distribution of pain arising from deep somatic structures with charts of segmental pain areas. *Clin Sci* 1939;4:35.
24. Ness TJ, Gebhart GF. Visceral pain: a review of experimental studies. *Pain* 1990; 41:167.
25. Torebjork HE, Ochoa JL, Schady W. Referred pain from intraneural stimulation of muscle fascicles in the median nerve. *Pain* 1984;18: 145.
26. Foley KM. Pain syndromes in patients with cancer. In: Portenoy RK, Kanner RM, eds. *Pain management: theory and practice*. Philadelphia: FA Davis Co, 1996:191.
27. Twycross RG, Fairfield S. Pain in far-advanced cancer. *Pain* 1982; 14:303.
28. Gonzalez GR, Elliott KJ, Foley KM, Portenoy RK. The impact of a comprehensive evaluation in the management of cancer pain. *Pain* 1991;47:141.
29. Galer BS. Neuropathic pain of peripheral origin: advances in pharmacologic treatment. *Neurology* 1995;45:S17.
30. Boureau F, Doubrere JF, Luu M: Study of verbal description in neuropathic pain. *Pain* 1990;42:145.
31. Grond S, Radbruch L, Meuser T, et al. Assessment and treatment of neuropathic cancer pain following WHO guidelines. *Pain* 1999;79: 15.
32. Farrar JT, Portenoy RK: Neuropathic cancer pain: the role of adjuvant analgesics. *Oncology (Huntigt)* 2001;15:1435.
33. Cousins M. Acute and postoperative pain. In: Wall PD, Melzack R, eds. *Textbook of pain*. 4th ed. Edinburgh: Churchill Livingstone, 1999:
34. Carr DB, Goudas LC. Acute pain. *Lancet* 1999;353:2051.
35. Austin KL, Stapleton JV, Mather LE. Multiple intramuscular injections: a major source of variability in analgesic response to meperidine. *Pain* 1980;8:47.

36. Stouten EM, Armbruster S, Houmes RJ, et al. Comparison of ketorolac and morphine for postoperative pain after major surgery. *Acta Anaesth Scand* 1992;36:716.

37. Ng A, Smith G, Davidson AC. Analgesic effects of parecoxib following total abdominal hysterectomy. *Br J Anaesth* 2003;90:746.

38. Tuncer S, Pirbudak L, Balat O, Capar M. Adding ketoprofen to intravenous patient-controlled analgesia with tramadol after major gynecological cancer surgery: a double-blinded, randomized, placebo-controlled clinical trial. *Eur J Gynaecol Oncol* 2003;24:181.

39. Ferrante FM, Ostheimer GW, Covino BG, eds. *Patient-controlled analgesia.* Boston: Blackwell Science, 1990.

40. Joshi GP, White PF. Patient-controlled analgesia. In: Ashburn MA, Rice LJ, eds. *The management of pain.* Edinburgh: Churchill Livingstone, 1998:5778.

41. Sechzen PH. Patient-controlled analgesia: a retrospective. *Anesthesiology* 1990;72:735.

42. Ballantyne JC, Carr DB, Chalmers TC, et al. Postoperative patient-controlled analgesia: meta-analyses of initial randomized trials. *J Clin Anesth* 1993;5:182.

43. Pearl ML, McCauley DL, Thompson J, et al. A randomized controlled trial of early oral analgesia in gynecologic oncology patients undergoing intra-abdominal surgery. *Obstet Gynecol* 2002; 99:704.

44. Kay B, Healy TEJ. Premedication by controlled-release morphine. *Anaesthesia* 1984;39: 587.

45. Pinnock CA, Derbyshire DR, Elling AE, Smith G. Comparison of oral slow release morphine (MST) with intramuscular morphine for premedication. *Anaesthesia* 1985;40:1082.

46. Gambaro G, Perazella MA. Adverse renal effects of anti-inflammatory agents: evaluation of selective and nonselective cyclooxygenase inhibitors. *J Intern Med* 2003;253:643.

47. Benzon HT, Wong HY, Belavic AM Jr, et al. A randomized double-blind comparison of epidural fentanyl infusion versus patient-controlled analgesia with morphine for postthoracotomy pain. *Anesth Analg* 1993;76:316.

47. Grass JA. Epidural analgesia. In: Fleisher LA, Prough DS, Grass JA, eds. *Problems in anesthesia.* Vol 10. Philadelphia: Lippincott–Raven Publishers, 1998:45.

48. Rawal N, Sjostrand UH, Christoffersson E, et al. Comparison of intramuscular and epidural morphine for postoperative analgesia in the grossly obese: influence on postoperative ambulation and pulmonary function. *Anesth Analg* 1984;63:583.

50. De Leon-Casasola OA, Parker BM, Lema MJ, et al. Epidural analgesia versus intravenous patient-controlled analgesia. Differences in the postoperative course of cancer patients. *Reg Anesth* 1994;19:307.

51. Hoskins PJ, Paice P, Easton D, et al. A prospective randomized trial of 4 Gy or 8 Gy single doses in the treatment of metastatic bone pain. *Radiother Oncol* 1992;23:74.

52. Correll DJ, Viscusi ER, Grunwald Z, Moore JH Jr. Epidural analgesia compared with intravenous morphine patient-controlled analgesia: postoperative outcome measures after mastectomy with immediate TRAM flap breast reconstruction. *Reg Anesth Pain Med* 2001;26:444.

53. Gwirtz KH. Intrathecal analgesia. In: Fleisher LA, Prough DS, Grass JA, eds. *Problems in anesthesia.* Vol 10. Philadelphia: Lippincott–Raven Publishers, 1998:71.

54. Swart M, Sewell J, Thomas D. Intrathecal morphine for caesarean section: an assessment of pain relief, satisfaction and side-effects. *Anaesthesia* 1997;52:373.

55. Sarma VJ, Bostrom UV. Intrathecal morphine for the relief of post-hysterectomy pain—a double-blind, dose-response study. *Acta Anaesthesiol Scand* 1993;37:223.

56. Fleron MH, Weiskopf RB, Bertrand M, et al. A comparison of intrathecal opioid and intravenous analgesia for the incidence of cardiovascular, respiratory, and renal complications after abdominal aortic surgery. *Anesth Analg* 2003;97:2

58. Petterson N, Perbeck L, Hahn RG. Efficacy of subcutaneous and topical anesthesia for pain relief after resection of malignant breast tumours. *Eur J Surg* 2001;167:825.

59. Fassoulaki A, Sarantopoulos C, Melemeni A, Hogan Q. Regional block and mexiletine: the effect on pain after cancer breast surgery. *Reg Anesth Pain Med* 2001;26:223.

60. Ashburn MA. Anesthesia-based acute pain services: past, present and future. In: Fleisher LA, Prough DS, Grass JA, eds. *Problems in anesthesia.* Vol 10. Philadelphia: Lippincott–Raven Publishers, 1998:1.

61. Ali J, Yaffe CS, Serrette C. The effect of transcutaneous nerve stimulation on postoperative pain and pulmonary function. *Surgery* 1981;89: 507.

62. Cuschieri RJ, Morran CG, McArdle CS. Transcutaneous electrical stimulation for postoperative pain. *Ann R Coll Surg Engl* 1985;67: 127.

63. Bjordal JM, Johnson MI, Ljunggreen AE. Transcutaneous electrical nerve stimulation (TENS) can reduce postoperative analgesic consumption. A meta-analysis with assessment of optimal treatment parameters for postoperative pain. *Eur J Pain* 2003;7:181.

64. Good M, Anderson GC, Stanton-Hicks M, et al. Relaxation and music reduce pain after gynecologic surgery. *Pain Manag Nurs* 2002;3:61.

65. Weis OF, Sriwatanakul K, Weitraus M, Lasagna L. Reduction of anxiety and postoperative analgesic requirements by audiovisual instruction. *Lancet* 1983;1:43.

66. Ozalp G, Sarioglu R, Tuncel G, et al. Preoperative emotional states in patients with breast cancer and postoperative pain. *Acta Anaesthesiol Scand* 2003;47:26.

67. Curtis EB, Krech R, Walsh TD. Common symptoms in patients with advanced cancer. *J Palliat Care* 1991;7:25.

68. Portenoy RK, Thaler HT, Kornblith AB, et al. Symptom prevalence, characteristics and distress in a cancer population. *Qual Life Res* 1994; 3:183.

69. Cassell EJ. *The nature of suffering and the goals of medicine.* New York: Oxford University Press, 1991.

70. Ellison NM. Palliative chemotherapy. In: Berger A, Weissman D, Portenoy RK, eds. *Principles and practice of supportive oncology.* Philadelphia: Lippincott–Raven Publishers, 2002:667.

71. Hoy AM, Lucas CF. Radiotherapy, chemotherapy and hormone therapy: treatment for pain. In: Wall D, Melzack R, eds. *Textbook of pain.* 3rd ed. Edinburgh: Churchill Livingstone, 1994:1279.

72. MacDonald N, Osoba D. Principles governing the use of cancer chemotherapy in palliative medicine. In: Doyle D, Hanks GWC, MacDonald N, eds. *Oxford textbook of palliative medicine.* Oxford, UK: Oxford University Press, 1998:249.

73. Geels P, Eisenhauer E, Bezjak A, et al. Palliative effect of chemotherapy: objective tumor response is associated with symptom improvement in patients with metastatic breast cancer. *J Clin Oncol* 2000;18: 2395.

74. Doyle C, Crump M, Pintilie M, Oza AM. Does palliative chemotherapy palliate? Evaluation of expectations, outcomes, and costs in women receiving chemotherapy for advanced ovarian cancer. *J Clin Oncol* 2001;19:1266.

75. Chambers SK, Lamb L, Kohorn EI, et al. Chemotherapy of recurrent/advanced cervical cancer: results of the Yale University PBM-PFU protocol. *Gyncol Oncol* 1994;53:161.

76. Gelblum D, Mychalczak B, Almadrones L, et al. Palliative benefit of external-beam radiation in the management of platinum refractory epithelial ovarian carcinoma. *Gynecol Oncol* 1998;69:36.

77. Tinger A, Waldron T, Peluso N, et al. Effective palliative radiation therapy in advanced and recurrent ovarian carcinoma. *Int J Radiation Oncology Biol Phys* 2001;51:1256.

78. Ratanatharathorn V, Powers WE, Steverson N, et al. Bone metastasis from cervical cancer. *Cancer* 1994;73:2372.

79. Spanos WJ Jr, Pajak TJ, Emami B, et al. Radiation palliation of cervical cancer. *J Natl Cancer Inst Monogr* 1996;21:127

80. Pereira J. Management of bone pain. In: Portenoy RK, Bruera E, eds. *Topics in palliative care.* New York: Oxford University Press, 1998: 79.

81. Berna L, Carrio I, Alonso C, et al. Bone pain palliation with strontium-89 in breast cancer patients with bone metastases and refractory bone pain. *Eur J Nucl Med* 1995;22:1101.

82. Sciuto R, Festo A, Pasqualoni R, et al. Metastatic bone pain palliation with 89-Sr and 186-Re-HEDP in breast cancer patients. *Breast Cancer Res Treat* 2001;66:101.

83. Cherny NI, Portenoy RK. The management of cancer pain. *Cancer* 1993;72:3393.

84. Coyle N. A model of continuity of care for cancer patients with chronic pain. *Med Clin North Am* 1987;71:259.

85. Eisenberg E, Berkey CS, Carr DB, et al. Efficacy and safety of nonsteroidal antiinflammatory drugs for cancer pain: a meta-analysis. *J Clin Oncol* 1994; 12:2756.

85. Ventafridda V. Continuing care: a major issue in cancer pain management. *Pain* 1989;36:137.

86. Lomen PL, Samal BA, Lamborn KR, et al. Flurbiprofen for the treatment of bone pain in patients with metastatic breast cancer. *Am J Med* 1986;80:83.

88. Mercadante S. The use of anti-inflammatory drugs in cancer pain. *Cancer Treat Rev* 2001;27:51

89. Sunshine A, Olson NZ. Nonnarcotic analgesics. In: Wall PD, Melzack R, eds. *Textbook of pain.* 3rd ed. Edinburgh: Churchill Livingstone, 1994:923.

90. Wallenstein DJ, Portenoy RK. Nonopioid and adjuvant analgesics. In: Berger AM, Portenoy RK, Weissman DE, eds. *Principles and practice of palliative care and supportive oncology.* Philadelphia: Lippincott–Raven Publishers, 2002:84.

91. Mercadante S, Cassucio A, Agnello A, et al. Analgesic effects of nonsteroidal anti-inflammatory drugs in cancer pain due to somatic or visceral mechanisms. *J Pain Symptom Manage* 1999;17:351.

91. Rawlins MD. Non-opioid analgesics. In: Doyle D, Hanks GWC, MacDonald N, eds. *Oxford textbook of palliative medicine.* Oxford, UK: Oxford University Press, 1998:355.

92. Mercadante S, Sapio M, Caligara M, et al: Opioid-sparing effect of diclofenac in cancer pain. *J Pain Symptom Manage* 1997;14:15.

93. Mercadante S, Fulfaro F, Casuccio A. A randomised controlled study on the use of anti-inflammatory drugs in patients with cancer pain on morphine therapy: effects of dose-escalation and a pharmacoeconomic analysis. *Eur J Cancer* 2002;38:1358.

94. Vane JR, Bakhle YS, Botting RM. Cyclo-oxygenase 1 and 2. *Annu Rev Pharmacol Toxicol* 1998;38:97.

95. Hernandez-Diaz S, Rodriguez LA. Association between nonsteroidal anti-inflammatory drugs and upper gastrointestinal tract bleeding/perforation: an overview of epidemiologic studies published in the 1990s. *Arch Intern Med* 2000;160:2093.

96. Sartori S, Trevisani L, Nielsen I, et al. Randomized trial of omeprazole or ranitidine versus placebo in the prevention of chemotherapy-induced gastroduodenal injury. *J Clin Oncol* 2000;18:463.

97. Hawkey CJ, Karrasch JA, Szczepanski L, et al. Omeprazole compared with misoprostol for ulcers associated with nonsteroidal antiinflammatory drugs. Omeprazole versus Misoprostol for NSAID-Induced Ulcer Management (OMNIUM) study group. *N Engl J Med* 1998; 338:727.

98. Hawkey CJ: Progress in prophylaxis against nonsteroidal anti-inflammatory drug-associated ulcers and erosions. Omeprazole NSAID Steering Committee. *Am J Med* 1998; 104:67S; Discussion, 79S.

99. Yeomans ND, Tulassay Z, Juhasz L, et al. A comparison of omeprazole with ranitidine for ulcers associated with nonsteroidal antiinflammatory drugs. Acid Suppression Trial: Ranitidine versus Omeprazole for NSAID-associated Ulcer Treatment (ASTRONAUT) Study Group. *N Engl J Med* 1998;338:719.

100. McLaughlin JK, Lipwort L, Chow W-H, Blot WJ. Analgesic use and chronic renal failure: a critical review of the epidemiologic literature. *Kidney Int* 1998;54:679.

101. Portenoy RK, Lesage P. Management of cancer pain. *Lancet* 1999; 353: 1695.

102. Hoskins PJ, Hanks GW. Opioid agonist-antagonist drugs in acute and chronic pain states. *Drugs* 1991;41:326.

103. Kaiko RF, Foley KM, Grabinski PY, et al. Central nervous system excitatory effects of meperidine in cancer patients. *Ann Neurol* 1983; 13:180.

104. Portenoy RK, Maldonado M, Fitzmartin R, Kaiko R, Kanner R. Controlled-release morphine sulfate: analgesic efficacy and side effects of a 100 mg tablet in cancer pain patients. *Cancer* 1989;63:2284.

105. Galer BS, Coyle N, Pasternak GW, Portenoy RK. Individual variability in the response to different opioids: report of five cases. *Pain* 1992; 49:87.

106. Sjøgren P. Clinical implications of morphine metabolites. In: Portenoy RK, Bruera E, eds. *Topics in palliative care.* Vol 1. New York: Oxford University Press, 1997.

107. D'Honneur G, Gilton A, Sandouk P, et al. Plasma and cerebrospinal fluid concentration of morphine and morphine glucuronide after oral morphine. The influence of renal failure. *Anesthesiology* 1994;81:87.

107. Faura CC, Moore RA, Horga JF, et al. Morphine and morphine-6-glucuronide plasma concentrations and effect in cancer pain. *J Pain Symptom Manage* 1996;11:95.

108. Thogulava RK, Saxena A, Bhatnagar S, Barry A. Oral ketamine as an adjuvant to oral morphine for neuropathic pain in cancer patients. *J Pain Symptom Manage* 2002;23:60.

109. Tiseo PJ, Thaler HT, Lapin J, et al. Morphine 6-glucuronide concentrations and opioid-related side effects: a survey in cancer patients. *Pain* 1995;61:47.

110. Peterson GM, Randall CTC, Paterson J: Plasma levels of morphine and morphine glucuronides in the treatment of cancer pain: relationship to renal function and route of administration. *Eur J Clin Pharmacol* 1990;38:121.

111. Portenoy RK, Foley KM, Stulman J, et al. Plasma morphine and morphine-6-glucuronide during chronic morphine therapy for cancer pain: plasma profiles, steady-state concentrations and consequences of renal failure. *Pain* 1991; 47:13.

112. Sawe J: High-dose morphine and methadone in cancer patients: clinical pharmacokinetic consideration of oral treatment. *Clin Pharmacokinet* 1986;11:87.

113. Osborne RJ, Joel SP, Slevin ML: Morphine intoxication in renal failure: the role of morphine-6-glucuronide. *BMJ* 1986;292:1548.

114. Mercadante S. Morphine vs. methadone in the pain treatment of advanced-cancer patients followed-up at home. *J Clin Oncol* 1998;16: 3656.

115. Ripamonti C, Zecca E, Bruera E. An update on the clinical use of methadone for cancer pain. *Pain* 1997;70:109.

116. Coyle N, Adelhardt J, Foley KM, Portenoy RK. Character of terminal illness in the advanced cancer patient: pain and other symptoms in the last 4 weeks of life. *J Pain Symptom Manage* 1990;5:83.

117. Portenoy RK, Southam M, Gupta SK, et al. Transdermal fentanyl for cancer pain: repeated dose pharmacokinetics. *Anesthesiology* 1993; 28:36.

118. Ahmedzai S, Brooks D. Transdermal fentanyl versus sustained-release oral morphine in cancer pain: preference, efficacy and quality of life. *J Pain Symptom Manage* 1997;13:254.

119. Bruera E. Subcutaneous administration of opioids in the management of cancer pain. In: Foley KM, Bonica JJ, Ventafridda V, eds. *Advances in pain research and therapy.* Vol 16. New York: Raven Press, 1990: 203.

120. Swanson G, Smith J, Bulich R, et al. Patient-controlled analgesia for chronic cancer pain in the ambulatory setting: a report of 117 patients. *J Clin Oncol* 1989;7:1903.

121. Waldman SD, Leak DW, Kennedy LD, et al. Intraspinal opioid therapy. In: Patt RB, ed. *Cancer pain.* Philadelphia: JB Lippincott Co, 1993:285.

122. Waldman SD. Implantable drug delivery systems: practical considerations. *J Pain Symptom Manage* 1990;5:169.

123. Coluzzi PH, Schwartzberg L, Conroy JD Jr, et al. Breakthrough cancer pain: a randomized trial comparing oral transmucosal fentanyl citrate (OTFC) and morphine sulfate immediate release (MSIR). *Pain* 2001; 91:123.

124. Weinberg DS, Inturrisi CE, Reidenberg B, et al. Sublingual absorption of selected opioid analgesics. *Clin Pharmacol Ther* 1988;44:335.

125. Beaver WT, Feise GA. A comparison of the analgesic effect of oxymorphone by rectal suppository and intramuscular injection in patients with postoperative pain. *J Clin Pharmacol* 1977;17:276.

126. Cramond T, Stuart G. Intraventricular morphine for intractable pain of advanced cancer. *J Pain Symptom Manage* 1993;8:465.

127. Houde RW. Misinformation: side effects and drug interactions. In: Hill CS, Fields WS, eds. *Advances in pain research and therapy.* Vol 11. New York: Raven Press, 1989:145.

128. Klepstad P, Kaasa S, Jystad A, et al. Immediate- or sustained-release morphine for dose finding during start of morphine to cancer patients: a randomized, double-blind trial. *Pain* 2003,101:193.

129. Twycross RG. Clinical experience with diamorphine in advanced malignant disease. *Int J Clin Pharmacol Ther Toxicol* 1974;9:184.

130. Twycross RG, Lack SA. *Pain in advanced cancer.* London: Churchill Livingstone, 1994.

131. O'Brien CP. Drug addiction and drug abuse. In: Hardman JG, Limbind LE, Molinoff PB, Rudden RW, Gilman AG, eds. *The pharmacological basis of therapeutics.* 9th ed. New York: Macmillan, 1996:557.

132. Portenoy RK. Tolerance to opioid analgesics: clinical aspects. In: Hanks GW, ed. *Palliative medicine: problem areas in pain and symp-*

tom management. Plainview, NY: Cold Spring Harbor Laboratory Press, 1994:49.

133. Rinaldi RC, Steindler EM, Wilford BB, Goodwin D. Clarification and standardization of substance abuse terminology. *JAMA* 1988;259:555.

134. Kanner RM, Foley KM. Patterns of narcotic drug use in a cancer pain clinic. *Ann N Y Acad Sci* 1981;362:161.

135. Redmond DE, Krystal JH. Multiple mechanisms of withdrawal from opioid drugs. *Annu Rev Neurosci* 1984;7:443.

136. Perry S, Heidrich G. Management of pain during debridement: a survey of U.S. burn units. *Pain* 1982;13:267.

137. Portenoy RK. Opioid therapy for chronic non-malignant pain. A review of the critical issues. *J Pain Symptom Manage* 1996;11:203.

138. Porter J, Jick H. Addiction rare in patients treated with narcotics. *N Engl J Med* 1980;302:123.

139. Cherny N, Ripamonti C, Pereira J, et al. Strategies to manage the adverse effects of oral morphine: an evidence-based report. *J Clin Oncol* 2001;19:2542.

140. Drexel H, Dzien A, Spiegel RW, et al. Treatment of severe cancer pain by low-dose continuous subcutaneous morphine. *Pain* 1989;36:169.

141. McDonald P, Graham P, Clayton M, et al. Regular subcutaneous bolus morphine via an indwelling cannula for pain from advanced cancer. *Palliat Med* 1991;5:323.

142. Mercadante S, Portenoy RK. Opioid poorly-responsive cancer pain. Part 3. Clinical strategies to improve opioid responsiveness. *J Pain Symptom Manage* 2001;21:338.

143. Mercadante S, Casuccio A, Fulfaro F, et al. Switching from morphine to methadone to improve analgesia and tolerability in cancer patients: a prospective study. *J Clin Oncol* 2001;19:2898.

144. Culpepper-Morgan JA, Inturrisi CE, Portenoy RK, et al. Treatment of opioid-induced constipation with oral naloxone: a pilot study. *Clin Pharm* 1992;52:90.

145. Foss JF. A review of the potential role of methylnaltrexone in opioid bowel dysfunction. *Am J Surg* 2001,182:19S.

146. Kurz A, Sessler DI. Opioid-induced bowel dysfunction: pathophysiology and potential new therapies. *Drugs* 2003,63:649.

147. Thomas J, Portenoy RK, Moehl C, et al. A phase II randomized dose-finding trial of methylnaltrexone for the relief of opioid-induced constipation in hospice patients. *J Clin Oncol* 2003; 22: 729(abst 2933).

148. Campora E, Malini L, Pace M, et al. The incidence of narcotic-induced emesis. *J Pain Symptom Manage* 1991;6:428.

149. Burish TG, Tope DM. Psychological techniques for controlling the adverse side effects of cancer chemotherapy: findings from a decade of research. *J Pain Symptom Manage* 1992;7:287.

150. Zacny JP. A review of the effects of opioids on psychomotor and cognitive functioning in humans. *Exp Clin Psychopharmacol* 1995;3:432.

151. Bruera E, Miller MI, MacMillan D, Kuhen N. Neuropsychological effects of methylphenidate in patients reeiving a continuous infusion of narcotics for cancer pain. *Pain* 1992;48:163.

152. Bruera E, Driver L, Barnes E, et al. Patient controlled methylphenidate for cancer related fatigue: a preliminary report. *J Clin Oncol* 2003; 22:737(abst 2965).

153. Hanna AR, Sledge GW, Mayer ML, et al. Preliminary results of a phase II trial of methylphenidate in patients with breast carcinoma. *J Clin Oncol* 2003;22:727(abst 2922).

154. Wilwerding MB, Loprinzi CL, Maillard JA, et al. A randomized, crossover evaluation of methylphenidate in cancer pateints receiving strong opioids. *Support Care Cancer* 1995,3:135.

155. Portenoy RK. Adjuvant analgesics in pain management. In: Doyle D, Hanks GWC, MacDonald N, eds. *Oxford textbook of palliative medicine.* Oxford, UK: Oxford University Press, 1998:361.

156. Peltier AC, Russell JW. Recent advances in drug-induced neuropathies. *Curr Opin Neurol* 2002,15:633.

157. Sinclair R, Westlander G, Cassuto J, Hedner T. Postoperative pain relief by topical lidocaine in the surgical wound of hysterectomized patients. *Acta Anaesthesiol Scand* 1996;40:589.

158. Stevens PE, Dibble SL, Miaskowski CM. Prevalence, characteristics, and impact of postmastectomy pain syndrome: an investigation of women's experiences. *Pain* 1995;61:61.

159. Rowbotham M, Harden N, Stacey B, et al. Gabapentin for the treatment of postherpetic neuralgia: a randomized controlled trial. *JAMA* 1998;280.

160. Backonja M, Beydoun A, Edwards KR, et al. Gabapentin for the symptomatic treatment of painful neuropathy in patients with diabetes mellitus: a randomized controlled trial. *JAMA* 1998;280:1831.

161. Bosnjak S, Jelic S, Susnjar S, et al: Gabapentin for relief of neuropathic pain related to anticancer treatment: a preliminary study. *J Chemother* 2002;14:214.

162. Caraceni A, Zecca E, Martini C, et al. Gabapentin as an adjuvant to opioid analgesia for neuropathic cancer pain. *J Pain Symptom Manage* 1999;17:441.

163. Eija K, Tiina T, Neuvonen Pertti J: Amitriptyline effectively relieves neuropathic pain following treatment of breast cancer. *Pain* 1995;64:293.

164. Watson CPN: The treatment of neuropathic pain: antidepressants and opioids. *Clin J Pain* 2000;16:S49.

165. Sloan P, Basta M, Storey P, et al. Mexiletine as an adjuvant analgesic for the management of neuropathic cancer pain. *Anesth Analg* 1999;89: 760.

166. Mercadante S, Arcuri E, Tirelli W, et al. Analgesic effect of intravenous ketamine in cancer patients on morphine therapy: a randomized, controlled, double-blind, crossover, double-dose study. *J Pain Symptom Manage* 2000;20:246.

167. Ogawa S, Kanamura T, Noda K, et al. Intravenous microdrip infusion of ketamine in subanaesthetic doses for intractable terminal cancer pain. *Pain Clin* 1994;7:125.

169. Galer BS, Rowbotham MC, Perander J, et al. Topical lidocaine patch relieves postherpetic neuralgia more effectively than a vehicle topical patch: results of an enriched enrollment study. *Pain* 1999;80:533.

170. Gammaitoni AR, Davis MW. Pharmacokinetics and tolerability of lidocaine patch 5% with extended dosing. *Ann Pharmacother* 2002;36:236.

171. Ellison N, Loprinzi CL, Kugler J, et al. Phase III placebo-controlled trial of capsaicin cream in the management of surgical neuropathic pain in cancer patients. *J Clin Oncol* 1997;15:2974.

172. Bloomfield DJ. Should bisphosphonates be part of the standard therapy of patients with multiple myeloma or bone metastases from other cancers? An evidence-based review. *J Clin Oncol* 1998;16:1218.

173. Ripamonti C. Management of bowel obstruction in advanced cancer patients. *J Pain Symptom Manage* 1994;9:193.

174. Smith JT, Staats PS, Stearns LJ, et al. for the Implantable Drug Delivery Systems Study Group. Randomized clinical trial of an implantable drug delivery system compared with comprehensive medical management for refractory cancer pain: impact on pain, drug-related toxicity, and survival. *J Clin Oncol* 2002,19:4040.

175. Siddal PJ, Cousins MJ. Introduction to pain mechanisms. Implications for neural blockade. In: Cousins MJ, Bridenbaugh, PO, eds. *Neural blockade in clinical anesthesia and management of pain.* 3rd ed. Philadelphia: JB Lippincott Co, 1998:675.

176. Swarm RA, Cousins MJ. Anaesthetic techniques for pain control. In: Doyle D, Hanks GWC, MacDonald N, eds. *Oxford textbook of palliative medicine.* Oxford, UK: Oxford University Press, 1998:390.

177. Nitescu P, Appelgren L, Linder LE, et al. Epidural versus intrathecal morphine-bupivacaine: assessment of consecutive treatments in advanced cancer pain. *J Pain Symptom Manage* 1990;5:18.

178. Brown DL, Bielley CK, Quiel EC. Neurolytic celiac plexus block for pancreatic cancer pain. *Anesth Analg* 1987;66:869.

179. Patt RB, Cousins MJ. Techniques for neurolytic neural blockade. In: Cousins MJ, Bridenbaugh PO, eds. *Neural blockade in clinical anesthesia and management of pain.* Philadelphia: Lippincott–Raven Publishers, 1998:1035.

180. Fosburg MT, Crone RK. Nitrous oxide analgesia for refractory pain in the terminally ill. *JAMA* 1983;250:511.

181. Young RF, Brechner T. Electrical stimulation of the brain for relief of intractable pain due to cancer. *Cancer* 1986;57:1266.

182. Tasker RR. Surgical approaches to chronic pain. In: Portenoy RK, Kanner RM, eds. *Pain management: theory and practice.* Philadelphia: FA Davis Co, 1996:290.

183. Levin AB, Ramirez LL. Treatment of cancer pain with hypophysectomy: surgical and chemical. In: Benedetti C, Chapman CR, Moricca G, eds. *Advances in pain research and therapy.* Vol 7. New York: Raven Press, 1984:631.

184. Miles J. Pituitary destruction. In: Wall PD, Melzack R, eds. *Textbook of pain.* 3rd ed. Edinburgh: Churchill Livingstone, 1999:1159.

185. Massie MJ, Spiegel L, Lederberg MS, Holland JC. Psychiatric complications in cancer patients. *Textbook of clinical oncology.* 2nd ed. Atlanta: American Cancer Society, 1995:685.

186. Breitbart W, Passik SD, Payne D. Psychological and psychiatric interventions in pain control. In: Doyle D, Hanks GWC, MacDonald N, eds. *Oxford textbook of palliative medicine.* Oxford, UK: Oxford University Press, 1998:437.

187. Fleming U. Relaxation therapy for far-advanced cancer. *Practitioner* 1985;229:471.

188. Jacobsen PB, Hann DM. Cognitive-behavioral interventions. In: Holland JC, ed. *Psycho-oncology.* New York: Oxford University Press, 1998:717.

189. Meyer TJ, Mark MM. Effects of psychosocial interventions with adult cancer patients: a meta-analysis of randomized experiments. *Health Psychol* 1995;14:101.

190. Orne MT, Whitehouse WG. Nonpharmacologic approaches to pain relief: hypnosis, self-hypnosis, placebo effects. In: Aronoff GM, ed. *Evaluation and treatment of chronic pain.* 3rd ed. Baltimore: Williams & Wilkins, 1999:579.

191. Pan CX, Morrison S, Ness J, et al. Complementary and alternative medicine in the management of pain, dyspnea, and nausea and vomiting near the end of life: a systematic review. *J Pain Symptom Manage* 2000;20,374.

192. Wu W-H, Adewunni AA. Alternative medicine for chronic pain: a critical review. In: Aronoff GM, ed. *Evaluation and treatment of chronic pain.* 3rd ed. Baltimore: Williams & Wilkins, 1999:627.

193. Doan BD. Alternative and complementary therapies. In: Holland JC, ed. *Psycho-oncology.* New York: Oxford University Press, 1998: 817.

CHAPTER 34

Rehabilitation as an Integrative Model: Psychologic and Surgical Approaches

Paul Georg Knapstein, Sabine Hawighorst-Knapstein, Christian Stief, Michael Krychman, and Douglas A. Levine

Radical pelvic surgery for gynecologic cancers has advanced profoundly over the last two decades with the introduction of reconstruction procedures. The major objective for surgeon and patient alike is not only complete tumor resection, but also the production of an optimal anatomic, functional, and cosmetically pleasing result. Increasingly, greater emphasis has been placed on surgical procedures that restore or maintain approximately normal anatomy and function as it has been definitively shown that organ reconstruction reduces perioperative morbidity and has major impacts on the long-term postoperative quality of life of the patient. Gynecologic oncologists must not only be skilled technicians, competent in the various surgical techniques, they must also be true health-care providers, taking time to understand the patient's needs, expectations, and goals. Total patient care includes treatment of the disease as well as its consequences, both physical and psychosocial.

Psychologic rehabilitation as an integrative part of cancer therapy starts at the patient's first confrontation with the diagnosis of a primary or recurrent cancer. Modern treatment concepts offer increasingly more individualized multi-modality options. During a long process, the patient and her oncologist must cooperate intimately together, the latter acting as a professional counselor on somatic and psychosocial issues during the preoperative, perioperative, and long-term postoperative phase. Usually, the gynecologic surgeon

has neither the time nor the skills to provide extensive professional counseling. For example, it has been demonstrated that approximately 80% of cancer patients wish to have more time and opportunities to discuss their problems with their physician. On average, however, the time the patient was allowed to talk before being interrupted by the doctor was 18 seconds! Only 23% of the patients were able to finish their opening statements. Without interruption, the patients talked for no longer than 150 seconds. In other words, 2 minutes more of listening would enable the patient to express her major concerns (1,2). Therefore, the patient's medical staff team should include a gynecologist specialized in psychotherapy as well as a professional psychologist.

Sexual health programs are often multidisciplinary programs that consist of a comprehensive medical examination, sexual functioning assessment, and a psychiatric/ psychosexual evaluation by a certified sexual therapist. These clinics, when developed, offer a comprehensive approach to addressing the sexuality, intimacy, and fertility concerns of patients through the development of a dynamic team that can address the unique sexual problems of female cancer patients during and/or after cancer treatment. Patients may have access to a variety of specialists, including gynecologists, psychologists, psychiatrists, and pain-management clinicians, as well as others who have expertise in menopausal symptom management.

Sexual problems are common concerns for patients during the diagnosis, treatment, and recovery process of their cancer illness. As patients move from the acute crisis phase of illness, healthy sexual function may be viewed as an important step toward reestablishing a patient's sense of "normalcy" and well-being (3). Approximately one-half of women who survive breast or gynecologic cancers report severe, long-lasting sexual problems (4). Studies have shown that sexual dysfunction is highly prevalent in the cancer population at

P. G. Knapstein: Hospital University, Mainz, Germany (retired)

S. Hawighorst-Knapstein: Hospital University, Mainz, Germany

C. A. Stief: Department of Urology, Ludwigs-Maximilians-University, Munich, Germany

M. L. Krychman: Department of Surgery, Memorial Sloan-Kettering Cancer Center, New York, New York

D. A. Levine: Gynecology Service/Department of Surgery, Memorial Sloan-Kettering Cancer Center, New York, New York

large. Anderson reports that sexual functioning morbidity occurs in up to 90% of women with the most prevalent types of cancer (5). Others report posttreatment sexual dysfunction to range from 30% to 100% (4,6). Most commonly, people complain of low desire, hypoactive desire disorder, or dyspareunia, also know as painful intercourse.

New surgical procedures as well as innovative adjunctive therapies are enhancing and promoting a positive sense of self and enriching the survivor's quality of life (7). Sexual health is a key and critical component. Patient's expectations are now focused on survivorability with expectations, high functioning, and quality of life. Sexual health, intimacy, and a sense of human connectedness are paramount.

Several physiologic and psychologic factors may place patients at an increased risk for the development of sexual problems: advanced disease, radical surgery, pelvic radiation, menopausal symptoms, premorbid sexual dysfunction, and a negative self-concept/schema can influence sexual morbidity (8). Body image concerns present a psychologic barrier to intimacy and sexual desire. Partner conflicts and relationship miscommunications can be severe, debilitating, and painful.

A multidisciplinary approach is key to a successful program. Treatment plans are created and implemented by the sexual health-care professional team, which can include community gynecologists, gynecologic oncologists, and specialized sexual health programs if available. Therapeutic options may include hormonal manipulation, pain management, and skilled exercise as well as psychodynamic or cognitive behavioral therapy with a certified sex therapist. Educating patients concerning sexual myths and informing them on the possible effect that treatment may have on their sexual function as well as providing instructional guidance and support are integral parts of the psychologic evaluation and treatment. Compliance with preventative measures will be more likely if education and close follow-up are provided.

Sexual dysfunction is a common consequence of cancer treatment that may persist after treatment; unfortunately, however, sexual assessment and/or sexual counseling is not routinely provided in the oncology setting. Time constraints, personal physician embarrassment, lack of skills to deal with the sexually charged issues, or perhaps their own unresolved sexual dilemmas may factor into the decision of some health-care professionals not to address sexual health concerns with patients. Most patients will, however, welcome the opportunity to explore this essential aspect of their lives. To most, sexual contact and intimate contact are critical factors of humanness. A simple question to broach the topic can be, "Many patients who have experienced this type of cancer or therapy have had some issues with sexuality. Many are concerned about how their disease process or therapy may influence their sexual relationship. Do you have any of these or similar concerns?"

Even when sexual contact becomes secondary to a cancer diagnosis, physical expression of caring remains an important way of sharing intimacy. Sexuality is an important part of quality of life for cancer survivors.

INTEGRATIVE MODEL

Rehabilitation as an integrative model is a multidimensional process to restore and maintain the patient's functional and emotional well-being. George Engel, a psychoanalyst and internist, described the biopsychosocial model as an organizing principle and integrative concept for psychosocial education in medical settings (9). This model emphasizes the importance of understanding behavior in health and illness from a systems perspective, where multiple biologic, psychologic, and social systems interact and influence each other, and requires the physician to consider and integrate information from the patient at the interpersonal level.

The impact of reconstructive surgical procedures such as the creation of a neovagina and the helpfulness of newer techniques to create continent urine reservoirs or colostomies has been debated not only in terms of operative time, but also in terms of the patient's quality of life (10). Patients with central recurrences of cervical cancer or even with pelvic wall infiltration are candidates for pelvic exenteration, "if their psychologic and medical status will allow." The patient, however, is often unprepared for the complex situation she will have to face and may be hampered with unrealistic expectations. Thus, her psychologic status will reflect emotional discomfort owing to the life-threatening diagnosis of cancer and the radical treatment modality.

The psychologic and physical effects of organ loss owing to radical genital surgery are now widely accepted. Yet, only recently have the full impact and consequences of organ loss and reconstructive procedures become appreciated (11). According to the World Health Organization, health is defined as a "state of complete physical, mental and social well-being and not merely the absence of disease and infirmity" (12). In most clinical trials in oncology, physicians are asked to rate the performance status of their patients (13). During the 1980s, however, many studies documented low levels of interobserver reliability and low levels of agreement between ratings provided by clinicians versus those provided by patients themselves (14–16). Thus, only patient feedback can provide important insights into her physical and psychosocial problems before and after radical therapy. To evaluate these issues, the term *quality of life* has gained increasing attention. The goals of quality of life research include the evaluation of patient psychosocial and physical status before and after therapy, the comparative assessment of different treatment effects in terms of medical decision making, and the specification of potential improvements in patient care.

These days, there is general agreement that quality of life consists of the following dimensions: physical concerns (symptoms, pain); functional ability (daily activity); family well-being; emotional well-being; treatment satisfaction, including medical interaction; social and occupational functioning; and sexuality, including body image (17,18). The measurement of quality of life provides specific information about the interaction between the physical, psychologic, and social factors before and after surgery and will serve to improve the standards of patient-oriented research and patient care.

PREOPERATIVE PHYSICAL AND PSYCHOSOCIAL STATUS

For women with advanced or recurrent genital cancer, radical surgery may be the only chance for long-term survival, yet the 5-year survival rates even after this procedure are only 50%. Thus, quality of life after surgery is an important issue. To determine the patient's physical, psychologic, and social response to the genital cancer and its treatment, the pretreatment and posttreatment status must be compared. The physical functioning includes complaints such as having difficulty doing daily physical activities (e.g., walking, bending, or lifting, doing household chores, bathing, or preparing meals).

The pretreatment status of physical problems is related to the stage of the cancer. A patient with a primary diagnosis of genital cancer—leading to a standard Wertheim's procedure, for example—may have few or no physical problems. She may, however, be overwhelmed by the acute life-threatening situation and the surgical procedure. Unprepared for this situation, the patient will struggle through feelings of confusion, anxiety, anger, and depression. Patients with a persistent or recurrent cancerous disease, on the other hand, may have had time to develop a more adequate response (coping skills) to their physical and psychosocial problems. Although their physical status may be worse before surgery compared with the aforementioned patient group, there are no differences in preoperative anxiety among the various groups. Before surgery, many patients indicate that they do not have the energy they previously had. They fear that their disease and its treatment might interfere with their ability to work owing to their physical complaints such as fatigue and pain.

The patient's preoperative anxiety level is related to her physical complaints and represents an important predictive factor in her presurgical and postsurgical problems and in her global quality of life score after surgery (19). The global score for quality of life takes into account all dimensions of quality of life. Other factors, such as prior treatments or coexisting diseases, do not have a significant impact on quality of life before surgery. The psychosocial status includes psychologic problems such as feelings of anxiety, discomfort, or anger, medical interaction, sexuality, body image, and marital interaction. Highly anxious patients indicate difficulty sleeping and concentrating and feelings of upset or anger before surgery. However, the preoperative anxiety level is not related to the treatment modality. Patients who feel very anxious and uncomfortable before surgery indicate that medical interaction (e.g., waiting for the doctor, trying to understand the doctor's explanations and instructions) represents their greatest problem at that time.

The patient's preoperative anxiety level and coping skills will be an important determinant of her future well-being and quality of life after surgery as will the treatment modality itself. The patient's preoperative quality of life is affected by worries about whether the cancer is progressing, about not being able to care for herself and her family, about the physical changes in her body, and her concerns over her sexuality. A negative body image involves a lack of mental sensitivity in sexuality or a lack of positive statements about identification with and attractiveness of one's body, whereas feeling sexually attractive reflects a positive body image. According to Anderson et al. (20), there is a direct relationship between preoperative sexual self-schema/image and postoperative sexual functioning. A positive sexual self-image prior to an operative procedure can correlate with better adaptation in the postoperative, recovery phase. A patient's preoperative worries concerning her future sexuality, self-esteem, and partnership are important issues for discussion related to her postoperative quality of life. The patient and her partner—as well as the physician—often tend to neglect this important topic before surgery (21–23).

The treatment modality used will also influence the patient's body image and quality of life. With respect to partnership, patients diagnosed with an acute cancer and facing a radical hysterectomy, for example, seem to be more vulnerable in their psychosocial status compared with patients planned for a pelvic exenteration with recurrent cancer and longer persisting symptoms. This may be because the latter patient group has had an opportunity to adjust to their problems by improving their family support. Rarely is a long-persisting partnership disrupted because of the chronic disease. In other words, although patients in a stable partnership may struggle with the quality of their communication with a partner, those in a more problematic partnership may find their partnership disrupted under the especially acute burden of a cancer (24).

Many cancer centers now have specialized sexual health programs that specifically address patient concerns on how their cancer, surgical treatment, or adjuvant procedures (radiation, chemotherapy, or hormonal manipulation) may affect their sexual functioning. Most clinics consist of a multidisciplinary group of health-care providers that offer preoperative consultations. The teams often consist of a gynecologist who is well versed in sexuality as well as a trained therapist who can provide ongoing psychosexual or cognitive behavioral counseling.

These sexual rehabilitation clinics are an integral part of the comprehensive care for the cancer patient. They can also help to prevent and identify sexual problems occurring as a result of the cancer diagnosis or treatment. The programs can facilitate early interventions with therapeutic approaches to help lessen the severity of sexual dysfunction.

PREOPERATIVE COUNSELING

Interactions between patient, family, and staff around the time of diagnosis and before treatment have profound and long-term effects on quality of life. Not only do these interactions influence the patient's ability to come to terms with the diagnosis, but they also often set the tone for all future dealings with the medical community. The imperatives for the medical staff in this process are to provide both information and hope. These considerations require the care team to individualize their approach to each patient.

Counseling is a broad name for a wide variety of procedures for helping individuals adjust, such as giving advice, conducting therapeutic discussions, administering and interpreting tests, and providing vocational assistance. An emerging emphasis on preventive health, especially concerning healthy life styles for cancer patients (e.g., early detection, prevention through nutrition and daily activities), reveals effective counseling skills, based on patient satisfaction and time and financial issues.

Twenty percent of our communication is verbal and voluntary. The basic principles for an effective verbal counseling are effective listening, creating a caring and warm atmosphere with empathy and respect, and using open-ended questions to encourage the patient to describe her problems in her own words. Agreement between the patient and physician regarding the treatment plan and the exact role of the physician is an important aim to achieve. Highly anxious patients, in particular, indicate a desire for more communication and have greater dissatisfaction with the doctor-patient relationship (e.g., the doctor does not appear to listen, uses jargon, or talks down to the patient) than with technical competence (25,26). The traditional clinical method of short questions and answers tends to give the impression of a lack of feeling and therefore does not meet the patient's needs adequately, especially in cases of patients who are highly anxious before surgery (27). The majority of patients wish to be talked to as equals and do not want to be patronized (28,29).

Effective presurgical counseling for gynecologic cancer patients is based on three principles. First, it is important to obtain adequate information about the patient's problems, and her individual response to the current illness should be evaluated. The cancer patient is in a stressful situation before surgery. In the case of a newly diagnosed cancer, she may feel very upset and anxious, whereas in the case of persisting cancer, she may already have organized her support system in a more reliable way. A patient facing radical surgery will not only be shocked by the life-threatening diagnosis, but will also have to face the loss of her reproductive organs, such as her uterus, her ovaries, or even her vagina. In this situation, she will have to decide on the treatment modality and the surgical reconstructive procedure, taking into consideration possible associated complications, such as organ lesions, transfusions, pain management, and the impact her decision may have on her sexual functioning.

The woman's discomfort will also depend on her anxiety level: A very anxious woman will have more problems with the medical interaction than a woman who reacts with less anxiety. Questions regarding difficulties in sleeping, per-

forming daily functions, or concentrating may help determine the patient's state of underlying anxiety before surgery.

It may be helpful to start the medical interview with questions regarding the patient's familial situation, as this interest touches on the woman's worries directly and may therefore relieve her. Evaluation of the patient's support system is very important in creating a patient-doctor relationship based on mutual trust and also provides information about the patient's relationships within the family. Family structure can profoundly influence patient care and outcome. For example, family stability is associated with compliance with medical treatment. Social stress and lack of support are significant risk factors for most physical as well as mental illnesses (30, 31). A patient whose partner died 1 year ago, for example, may be more depressed and anxious compared with a patient whose spouse is present during the hospitalization and gives emotional support.

Evaluation of the patient's sexual relationship is an important preoperative requirement. The married, heterosexual woman may have different concerns than a single woman or a lesbian female. Wrongful assumptions that all women are involved in monogamous heterosexual relationships can lead to physician-patient conflict, distrust with the medical community, and hamper open, effective communication between the health-care professional and his or her patient.

The second principle is to help the patient understand the problems caused by the disease and to anticipate the treatment consequences to her postoperative daily life and individual situation. The treatment modality used will influence her quality of life profoundly. To create a neovagina may be essential for a patient's future body image and self-esteem whether or not she is living in a partnership (19,32). Ostomies for urine and/or feces and a colpectomy may reduce the patient's quality of life in the long run. Careful preoperative counseling on the patient's potential problems with her body image, sexuality, and partnership is necessary to facilitate her postoperative adjustment to the surgical treatment and may significantly impact the sexual problems that follow such surgical procedures. Statements before treatment, such as that the sexual relationship may be disturbed by a neovagina but will be better than without this procedure after colpectomy, may help the couple to talk about their intimate problems at that time. It may be difficult to raise this topic before surgery because the woman must face her life-threatening situation and may not be adequately adjusted to talk about her sexual problems. Referral to specialized sexual health programs within the cancer institutions may be appropriate. The patient's discomfort should be addressed, however, as this subject will influence her postoperative well-being profoundly.

The third principle of effective counseling is to devise a plan of action to resolve the aforementioned problems and those caused by the disease and its treatment. Interdisciplinary counseling, such as from other patients, support groups, or networks, may be helpful for giving advice on physical and psychosocial problems. The addition of social and psychologic services to help reduce financial, social, and emotional problems will improve the postoperative rehabilitation. The physician's task may also be to inform the patient about these possibilities and to give specific suggestions or referrals.

Paying closer attention to the setting (angle of facing, seating at eye level without barrier at the same level) as an integral part of nonverbal information also leads to a more effective rapport between physician and patient, especially in intimate situations such as medical interviews in gynecologic oncology. Sixty percent of all communication between individuals is nonverbal, generally involuntary, and cannot be hidden (33). Nonverbal communication includes kinesics (eye contact, attentive body posture), proxemics (spatial relationships), and paralanguage (voice tone, volume).

PREOPERATIVE PSYCHOSEXUAL COUNSELING

The loss of female genital organs because of a life-threatening disease and its treatment can affect the woman's self-esteem and body image. The illness may have already affected the patient's sexual life through pain, fatigue, and worry, and sexual dysfunction may have therefore occurred before surgery (34). Premature loss of ovarian function, vaginal dryness, and dyspareunia may be concerns.

Ostomies for urine and/or feces and a colpectomy can influence the patient's sexual life in the long-term. As stated previously, it is necessary to provide careful preoperative counseling to the patient regarding potential problems she may face with body image, sexuality, and partnership in order to facilitate her postoperative adjustment. Because the woman must initially face her life-threatening situation and therefore may not be psychologically prepared to discuss her sexual problems, it may be difficult to raise this topic in the presurgical setting. Nevertheless, it is extremely important to raise this subject, as it will influence her postoperative well-being profoundly.

A history of sexual problems should be obtained prior to surgery, and the patient should be encouraged to describe her problems in her own words. Several questions can be helpful to explore the patient's sexual situation before surgery. For example, one question can be, ''Has your illness interfered with your being a sexual partner?'' The second question may be, ''Has the disease altered your sexual life?'' A third should evaluate the patient's concerns regarding the impact the cancer may have on her sexual partnership.

A vaginal reconstructive procedure should be offered to every patient if her health status will allow it because this procedure will increase her self-esteem after organ loss and improve her body image even if intercourse will not be performed because of healing problems or marital problems. Physicians may be able to predict the patient's adjustment to the surgical procedures, and sexual problems may occur more often in patients without reconstructive procedures.

The evaluation of the physiologic-sexual response cycle according to Masters and Johnson may be an integrated part of a sexual-health intervention after nonreconstructive procedures and should be performed by a trained therapist. This detailed exploration of physiologic responses to sexual stimulation (excitement, plateau, orgasm, resolution) and sexual functioning can be an integral part of the preoperative health history before cancer surgery.

Sexual issues should be regarded as an important aspect of the patient's quality of life, and education about sexuality related to the surgical procedure should be mandatory.

POSTOPERATIVE PHYSICAL AND PSYCHOSOCIAL STATUS

Recent developments in surgical and medical care evoke questions regarding whether and how patient quality of life might be influenced, both physically and psychosocially. After surgery, the patient's quality of life is primarily affected by the surgical procedure. An evaluation of quality of life and body image demonstrates the benefits of newer techniques for organ reconstruction (10,19) (Figs. 34.1 and 34.2).

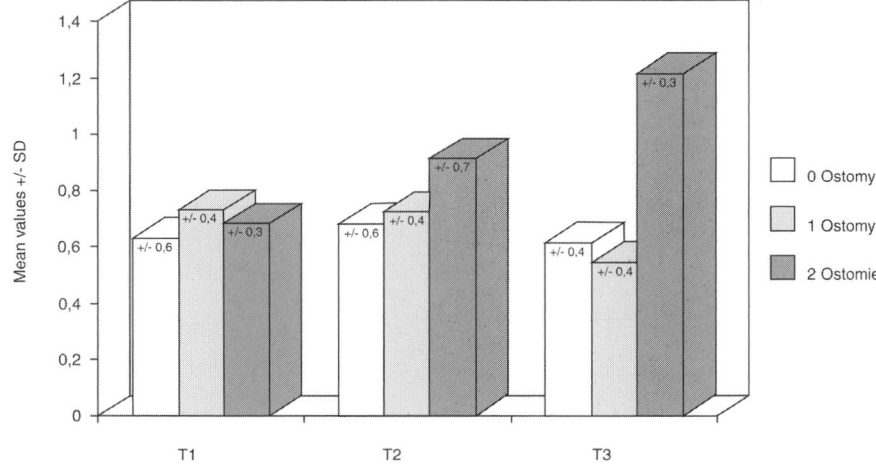

FIG. 34.1. Global score of quality of life including physical, psychologic, and social functioning: problems increase 1 year (T3) after surgery for women with to ostomies (no evidence of disease for all groups).

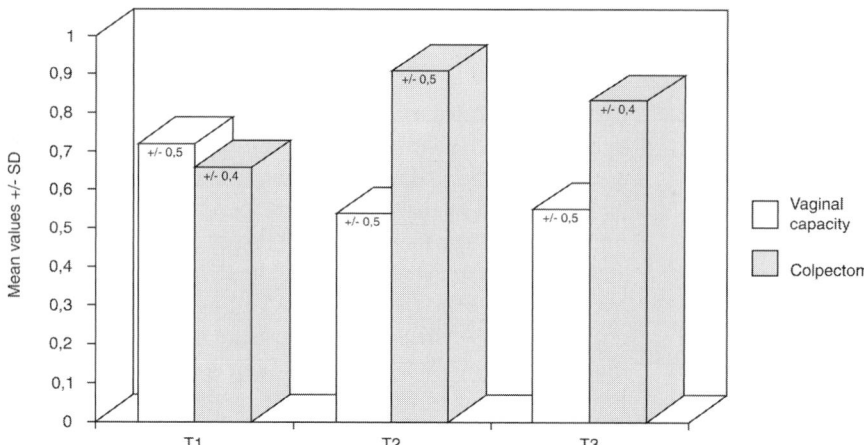

FIG. 34.2. Global score of quality of life including physical, phycologic, and social functioning: problems increase (T1, before; T2, 4; and T4, 12 months after surgery) for women with colpectomy (no evidence of disease for all groups).

Comparison of the postoperative physical and psychosocial problems among all groups, as defined by the different surgical techniques used in their treatment, reveals significant differences with regard to quality of life, body image, and sexuality for women with or without reconstructive procedures (21) (Figs. 34.3 and 34.4). Physical problems increase immediately after surgery and are dependent on the surgical technique used: Patients who have undergone a Wertheim's procedure suffer physical problems significantly more often after surgery compared with their preoperative status (35); patients with one or no ostomy indicate significantly fewer physical problems 1 year after surgery compared with those with two ostomies (19,36–38); and women with colpectomy report more physical problems compared with patients with a neovagina even 1 year postoperatively. Therefore, many women desire help for pain management and relief of physical problems following therapy.

With regard to psychosocial problems, women with two ostomies and/or colpectomy feel less attractive and self-confident compared with reconstruction-treated patients even if the latter group has no possibility of performing vaginal intercourse. The creation of a neovagina improves the quality of life and body image simply because the body seems to be "normal" (19,39).

After having overcome the acute situation of hospitalization and surgery, the patient's body image and self-confidence takes on greater importance, mainly for the woman herself, but also for her partner. For women with two ostomies and/or colpectomy, sexual and marital problems increase after surgery compared with reconstruction-treated women even until up to 1 year later. The physical and psychologic adjustment to visible ostomies represents an additional weight to the burden of the life-threatening disease. Women with reconstructive surgery such as neobladder, neovagina, and/or colon anastomosis indicate a significantly better outcome 1 year after surgery concerning sexual, marital, and psychosocial aspects of their quality of life and also in regard to body image. Thus, patients without reconstructive surgery after pelvic exenteration have the poorest outcome of all groups. This finding is not related to the stage of dis-

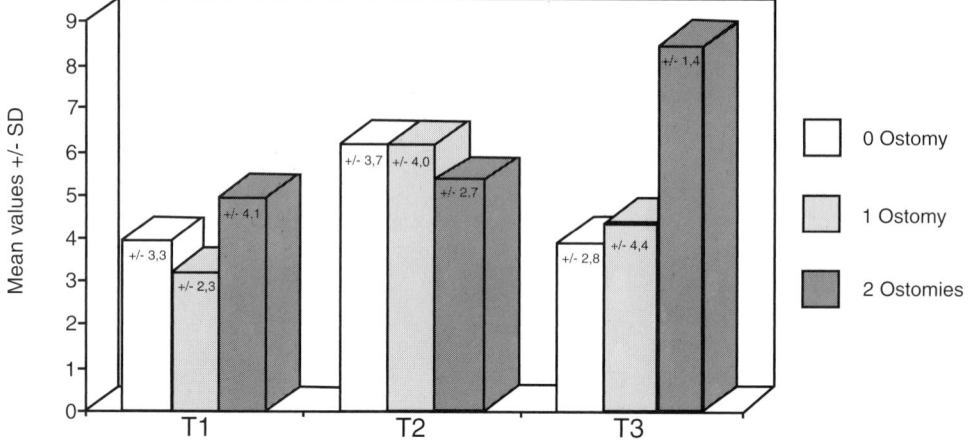

FIG. 34.3. Body image: uncertainty/discomfort increase 1 year (T3) after surgery for women with two ostomies (no evidence of disease for all groups).

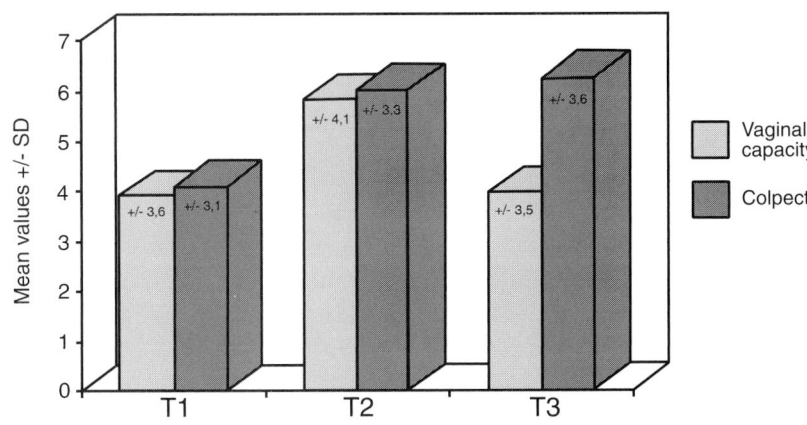

FIG. 34.4. Body image: uncertainty/discomfort increase 1 year (T3) after surgery for women with colpectomy (no evidence of disease for all groups).

ease before surgery. Nevertheless, it should be emphasized also that the overall quality of life of those surviving patients with one or two ostomies is quite acceptable. For many patients of all groups, worries about progression of tumor and not being able to care for themselves and their families remain the main problems postoperatively.

Women with a high anxiety level prior to surgery and who have two ostomies or one ostomy and/or a colpectomy as a surgical procedure also have the poorest outcome in terms of quality of life after surgery. Patients with reconstructive surgical procedures, on the other hand, tend to feel less anxious following therapy (40).

Another important aspect that has also been discussed in the literature is the role of partnership after recurrent cancer and mutilating surgery. Partnership or marital interaction is dependent on the time since initial diagnosis: The greater the time between the initial diagnosis and the onset of recurrence, the better the quality of marital interactions.

Thus, the different surgical techniques have significant impact on the patient's quality of life and body image and should be as radical as necessary and as reconstructive or organ-preserving as possible. Behavioral factors such as preoperative anxiety influence the postoperative health status, just as the treatment modality has an influence on emotional well-being. Therefore, in making decisions regarding medical therapy, the physician must understand that his or her decisions will significantly influence the patient's postoperative quality of life, and medical interactions should include the goal of decreasing patient anxiety (41).

POSTOPERATIVE COUNSELING

Each of the above-mentioned surgical procedures affects differently the patient's well-being. Medical counseling must therefore integrate the biologic and psychosocial factors of the individual patient. Owing to modern developments and an increasing number of treatment modalities, it is necessary to provide the patient with detailed and specific information regarding the physical and psychosocial long-term effects on the patient and her family members.

Even 1 year after surgery with no evidence of disease, cancer patients are aware that their life-threatening disease is their greatest concern. This concern, which includes worries about progression of the tumor and not being able to care for oneself and/or the family after surgery, is the main cause of anxiety for these patients. A high level of anxiety corresponds to a more problematic medical interaction. Integration of extended family members, spouses, partners, or social support networks may be helpful, however, as family structure also influences how patients cope with these worries: Family stability is associated not only with compliance with medical recommendations, but also with a better outcome concerning physical and psychiatric diseases (42).

Anxious patients who have undergone nonreconstructive procedures are in the most stressful situation and require very attentive counseling in the time of follow-up. It is necessary to provide patients with information about the problematic situation they may face owing to the possible impact of negative body image and problems concerning sexuality that occur after nonreconstructive surgery. This information should be integrated into patient-oriented counseling, with the aim of improving the patient's self-confidence through encouraging autonomy and avoidance of social isolation. Support groups and counseling networks are now easily accessible in cancer institutions via the internet. Many patients find posttreatment resource centers very helpful and informative.

Thus, the patient's somatic (side effects due to disease and treatment), physical (mobility), psychologic (anxiety), and social (family/personal interaction) interferences can be measured and should be the focus of clinical attention. In conclusion, we can summarize three phases of counseling:

1. The preoperative anxiety-level leads to increasing problems with medical interaction.
2. Physical problems are the patient's main concerns immediately following surgery.
3. Long-term effect problems with body image and sexuality are dominant and are often related to the surgical procedure; they may, however, be preexisting.

Prior to surgery, the main topic for the medical interview and counseling should be the patient's worries and concerns, as well as her family/social interaction, in an effort to reduce anxiety by allowing the patient to express her feelings and to incorporate her social support system. After surgery, the patient's physical problems and pain management should be the central point of the medical counseling. The patient's social functioning including sexuality, partnership, and body image issues should be integrated into the medical interview, both preoperatively when appropriate and in the postoperative period.

Women who had few or no problems before a surgical procedure, such as a Wertheim's procedure, and those who underwent nonreconstructive procedures, such as colpectomy and two ostomies, need special support and attention during their follow-up visits, as do patients who tend to be very upset, anxious, or angry.

Thus, many treatment and quality of life issues may be resolved for women with gynecologic cancer if the patient's medical and psychologic status will be considered in terms of an integrative model.

POSTOPERATIVE PSYCHOSEXUAL COUNSELING

This important quality of life issue is often overlooked after therapy, although sexuality and body image become increasingly important topics for the patients, especially those who have no evidence of disease and have undergone nonreconstructive procedures (19,34). Approximately 35% of patients with early cervical and about 80% of women with advanced genital cancer experience sexual problems (34). These problems do not necessarily damage marital stability, but do reduce the patient's self-esteem and body image, particularly in cases of nonreconstructive procedures. Sexuality should not be neglected by the doctor who carries out the follow-up check-up.

Sexual problems after therapy result mainly from the physical effects of the surgical procedure. Worries about progression of tumor and other psychologic worries may influence the patient's libido. The partner's attitude may also influence the patient's sexual behavior after surgery. Problems in marital interaction may result in sexual conflicts and further decrease the woman's self-esteem. Therefore, psychosexual counseling should also address the woman's partner and their concerns. It may be helpful to integrate the partner into the treatment decisions.

Besides counseling on how to use the neovagina, sexual counseling for women with urinary and bowel appliances is necessary. Women with continent neobladder reservoirs should catheterize before sexual activity and women with visible stomas may cover the pouches. Sexual arousal may stimulate bladder and bowel incontinence, which may be dietetic, and technical precautions should be taken before intercourse.

POSTOPERATIVE THERAPY

The therapeutic management for female sexual dysfunction after cancer therapy and treatment may consist of a complex approach. Treatment can include evaluation and treatment of previously neglected systemic illness(es) (uncontrolled hypertension, hypercholesterolemia and/or an underlying thyroid dysfunction), identification of medications that can affect the sexual response cycle and cause sexual dysfunction (e.g., antidepressants and antihypertensive medications), and behavioral modification (well-balanced nutrition, active exercise regimens, discontinuing tobacco use, and minimizing alcohol consumption). Specific, structured sexual tasks are often included in the management schema and include sensate focusing, guided imagery, relaxation techniques and the exploration of sexual fantasies, and enhancing alternate forms of sexual expression, such as mutual massage and manual, digital, or oral stimulation. Encouraging intercourse in alternative sexual positions such as side-to-side or female superior position may help limit deep pelvic thrusting, which can minimize vaginal discomfort during penetration.

Pain management can include guided imagery, meditation, deep muscle relaxation, and the active avoidance of lethargy. Pain management specialists can be consulted to adjust or reduce opioid regimens, add adjunctive analgesics, and modify dosing schedules to decrease fatigue and lethargy while maintaining adequate pain relief. When pain and fatigue are at a low level, sexual expression can be encouraged. Patient education regarding their genital anatomy and how the cancer diagnosis and therapeutic procedures have affected their sexual functioning is useful to debunk many long-standing sexual myths. Take-home items such as pamphlets, books, CD-ROMs, videos, and other visual aids can provide reinforcement and future reference. The American Cancer Society's booklet entitled *Cancer and Sexuality* is an excellent patient reference guide. It provides factual information and helpful suggestions to maintain and improve sexual functioning.

Certified sexual therapists trained to deal with cancer patients and associated body image issues, changes in intimacy, sexuality, self-esteem, and mood disturbances are helpful during the counseling process. Sexual health patients can be offered marital, individual, couples', and group therapy by a trained therapist who deals with both oncologic and sexually based issues. Pharmacologic intervention with hormonal manipulation may be a consideration if operative procedures have caused premature menopause resulting in vaginal atrophy and associated dyspareunia. The use of local vaginal estrogen tablets, rings, or creams, which are minimally absorbed, are becoming more widely accepted by patients and oncologists for the treatment of atrophic vaginitis. Local use of nonmedicated, nonhormonal vaginal moisturizers or vitamin E suppositories can provide alternative relief of the symptoms of vaginal dryness. These agents are recommended to be used two or three times weekly. In addition, patients are instructed to wear a light pad when using vitamin E suppositories because it may stain undergarments. The use of water-based vaginal lubricants with intercourse is also encouraged. However, lubricants and moisturizers that contain microbicides, perfumes, coloration, and flavors should be discouraged because these additives may be irritative to the vaginal mucosa.

Sexual devices can be used for patients who have undergone pelvic surgery or radiation therapy. Vaginal shortening, vaginal narrowing, and fibrotic scar tissue can often impede penetration, causing dyspareunia. Vaginal dilators with water-based lubricants can help lengthen and widen the vagina and loosen the scar tissue that contributes to pain and discomfort associated with vaginal intercourse. Ongoing supportive behavioral therapy is instrumental for continued compliance. Referral for a consultation by a subspecialist may be appropriate for certain clinical conditions. Consultants can include oncologists, social services providers, nutritionists, exercise therapists, and psychiatrists.

RECONSTRUCTIVE PELVIC SURGERY

Gynecologic oncologists commonly employ reconstructive techniques to repair tissue defects that are not amenable to primary closure to improve surgical and cosmetic outcomes. In this section, the techniques of pelvic reconstruction are described to provide an overview of select procedures so that the physician will have a working knowledge of these procedures and be able to provide appropriate counseling to patients. For additional surgical details, various well-written atlases are available (43–46).

Reconstruction of the Vulva

Owing to improved patient care and education as well as a greater understanding of the disease, large vulvar cancers that require an extended ''butterfly-type'' radical vulvectomy including en bloc groin resection have become rare. It has been demonstrated (see Chapter 29) that International Federation of Gynecology and Obstetrics (FIGO) stage I and certain stage II tumors can be safely removed with a combination of radical local excision and unilateral or bilateral lymph node dissection based upon depth of invasion. Currently, the use of sentinel lymph node mapping is under investigation as a possible alternative to formal groin dissection for selected patients. Known prognostic factors must be considered to individualize treatment for each patient.

Even after a radical local excision or simple vulvectomy, primary wound closure can often yield unsatisfactory cosmetic results or increase the risk of surgical complications. Pain, dyspareunia, and disturbances of micturition may occur. Therefore, a minor type of reconstruction is frequently required, as described below.

Newly diagnosed advanced vulvar tumors, FIGO stages III and IV, are initially treated by radiation and chemotherapy with better functional results and patient outcome than would otherwise be achieved with primary surgery. Since these tumors are often radioresponsive, a subsequent resection may be indicated. When performed, the procedure is usually more limited than would have been required at the outset and typically can preserve bowel and bladder functions.

The patient with recurrent disease is in a completely different situation with unique challenges, especially if she has received prior radiation therapy. The likelihood of cure is exceedingly low for recurrences that occur in the groin; yet local vulvar recurrences can occasionally be salvaged with radical surgery or combined modality treatment. Frequently, palliative surgery is required to alleviate intractable pain, body disfigurement, uncontrollable bleeding, or other constitutional symptoms. These operations invariably create sizable tissue defects that mandate reconstruction by either large transposition flaps or one of several available myocutaneous techniques.

Transposition Flaps

After radical or simple local excisions, small unilateral or bilateral defects of the vulva can be filled by using a simple transposition flap as described in Figure 34.5. The vulva can be easily reconstructed with a satisfactory cosmetic and functional result for defects up to an area of $60 \, \text{cm}^2$. A simple transposition flap is also useful for reconstruction after radiation therapy if the postirradiation sclerosis is not included in the perivulvar donor site. Other specific types of transposition flaps are described in Chapter 29 and illustrations with extensive detail can be found elsewhere (47).

The rhomboid transposition flap is frequently used to relieve tension on primary suture lines and prevent stenosis of the vaginal introitus. In several reported series, the morbidity has been acceptable with good functional results (48, 49). The V-Y advancement flap is also well suited for vulvar reconstruction where excessive tension would result from primary closure. The outcome of this type of flap has also been reassuring, and most morbidity can be managed conservatively (50,51). Larger defects of the vulva often involve the vagina and/or pelvic floor and are usually managed similarly to the vaginal/perineal defects created in conjunction with extended radical or exenterative surgery. Reconstruction of these defects is discussed in the vaginal reconstruction section below.

Defects of the Groin

Major tissue defects in the groin may develop in conjunction with a local recurrence of vulvar cancer in this region. Occasionally, a painful or disfiguring radiogenic scleroderma may require surgical intervention. After resection, these defects can often be repaired with a myocutaneous

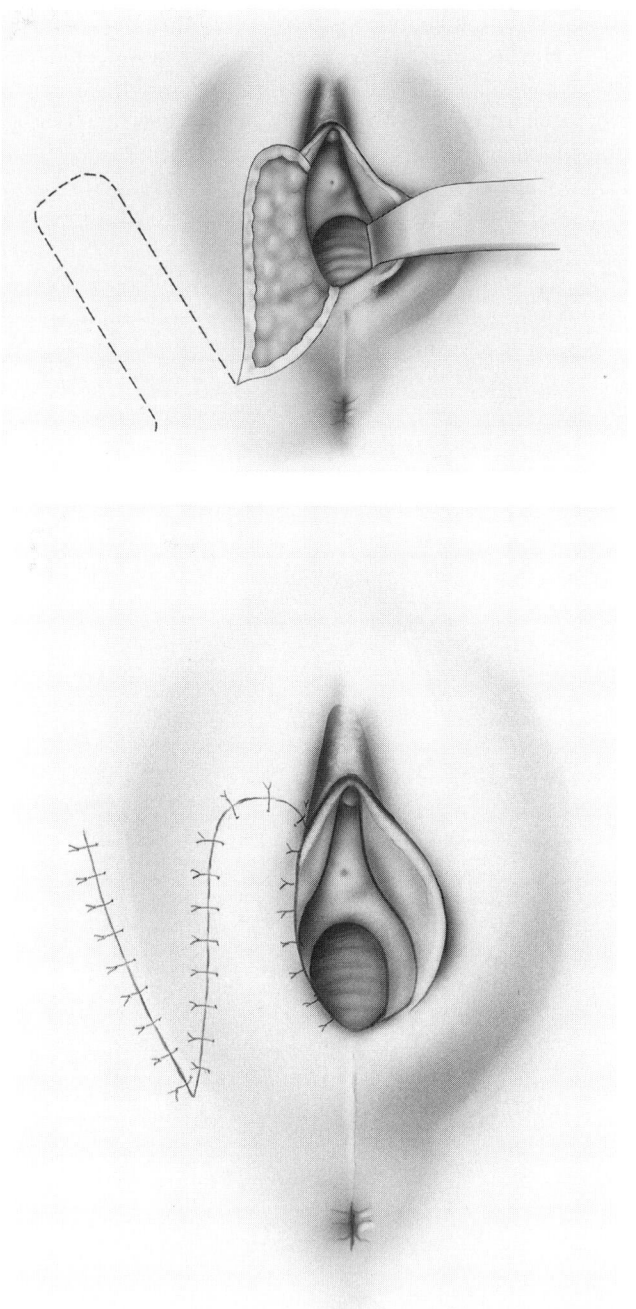

FIG. 34.5. Transposition skin flap for reconstruction of the partially or totally resected vulva. The size (up to 60 cm²) and shape of the perivulvar area to be used are outlined and then placed into the defect. When indicated, the technique can be used bilaterally.

tensor fascia lata flap. Excellent cosmetic results can be obtained with a flap area of up to 100 cm² or even greater in select cases. The resulting donor-site defect is quite acceptable. By modification of the design into an island flap, the arc of rotation can be extended to the periumbilical region where it can replace all layers of the abdominal wall as commonly occurs in association with bowel fistulas.

Perioperative Management

Optimal perioperative management is mandatory for good healing following reconstruction in the vulva, perineum, and vagina. Prior to a minor reconstruction, the rectum is cleansed using preoperative enemas to prevent contamination of the fresh wound with bowel flora. In addition, antibiotic prophylaxis is given prior to surgical incision. For major operations, a complete bowel preparation is initiated 2 days prior to the procedure. On day 1, the patient is instructed to drink only clear liquids. On the second day, a mechanical bowel preparation is begun and followed 6 to 10 hours later by one or more enemas until the stool is clear. Antibiotic prophylaxis is again given prior to surgical incision and may be continued postoperatively for up to 24 hours unless otherwise indicated. Artificial bowel paralysis is usually maintained by the opioid analgesia otherwise required for routine postoperative pain control. This beneficial side effect will usually suppress bowel activity for a period of 3 to 5 days and help prevent operative site infection.

The reconstructive procedures outlined and many others are currently employed in most major gynecologic centers. These techniques are safe when properly performed and are associated with a low risk of major morbidity. By individualizing treatment for each patient, choosing the best surgical options, observing intensive perioperative management, and employing proper technique, complications can be kept to a minimum. Each of the methods discussed is widely accepted and has been in use for many years.

Reconstruction of the Vagina

In recurrent disease of the cervix, uterus, or vagina, radical surgery may offer the only chance of cure or palliation of distressing symptoms. In these cases, the vagina often needs to be partially or completely removed. Many methods of partial or total vaginal reconstruction have been described. In this section, some of the more common techniques are described and illustrated.

Classification of Vaginal Defects

Until recently, there had been no uniform system to classify the type of vaginal defect introduced by radical cancer surgery. The utility of developing a reproducible classification system lies in the ability to apply particular reconstruction techniques to specific types of defects. A newly developed classification system attempts to create an algorithm for vaginal reconstruction (52). The vaginal defects are divided into partial (type I) defects and circumferential (type II) defects. Type I partial defects are subcategorized into those that involve the anterior or lateral wall of the vagina (type IA) and those that involve the posterior wall of the vagina (type IB). Type II circumferential defects are categorized into those that involve the upper one-third or two-thirds of the vagina (type IIA) and those that involve the entire vagina (type IIB). Although the defects created during radical pelvic surgery will vary widely, this classification system is categorized based upon the extent of resection and will be applicable to most oncologic resections.

Partial Vaginal Defects

Partial vaginal defects may occur during vaginal surgery, extended vulvar surgery, or radical exenterative procedures. Defects in the anterior and/or lateral vagina (type IA) can be repaired using a modified pudendal thigh fasciocutaneous flap. Originally described in the late 1980s for vaginal reconstruction and modified in the following decade, this flap has many advantages. It can be completed in a single stage, is reliable, is sensate, is technically simple, and has minimal donor site morbidity (53,54). Based on the terminal branches of the superficial perineal artery, the incision is carried from the skin to the level of the deep fascia, and the flap is then elevated over the proximal part of the adductor muscles. It is undermined in a parallel plane and tunneled medially beneath the labia. Although described here for partial vaginal defects, this flap can also be used to create a complete neovagina when performed bilaterally. Flap sizes of up to 16 × 6 cm have been reported. The pudendal thigh fasciocutaneous flap has generally been found to have low morbidity with wound dehiscence being described occasionally (55).

Posterior vaginal defects (type IB) can occur in conjunction with posterior exenteration, extended vulvar surgery, and vaginal surgery. When the defect is primarily in the lower posterior aspect of the vagina, a transposition flap or the pudendal thigh fasciocutaneous flap may be appropriate. More commonly, the defect involves the entire posterior wall of the vagina, in which case a rectus abdominis myocutaneous flap is more appropriate. To create a rectus abdominis myocutaneous flap, a vertical skin island is incised over the superior portion of the rectus abdominis muscle. The medial two-thirds of the muscle is dissected down to the anterior rectus sheath. The flap is transposed into position over the posterior aspect of the vagina and sutured into place (Fig. 34.6). This flap not only reconstructs the posterior wall of the vagina, but also provides sufficient bulk to fill in the dead space in the true pelvis often created during exenterative surgery.

Circumferential Vaginal Defects

Circumferential vaginal defects are frequently established during exenterative surgery. A supralevator exenteration will result in a defect that comprises the upper two-thirds of the vagina (type IIA). These defects can be reconstructed with a rolled rectus abdominis myocutaneous flap. Similar to the flap described for type IB defects in the previous section, the skin island is taken from the superior part of the muscle. To reconstruct the vaginal tube, a transverse skin island is used instead of a vertical skin island. Once harvested, the

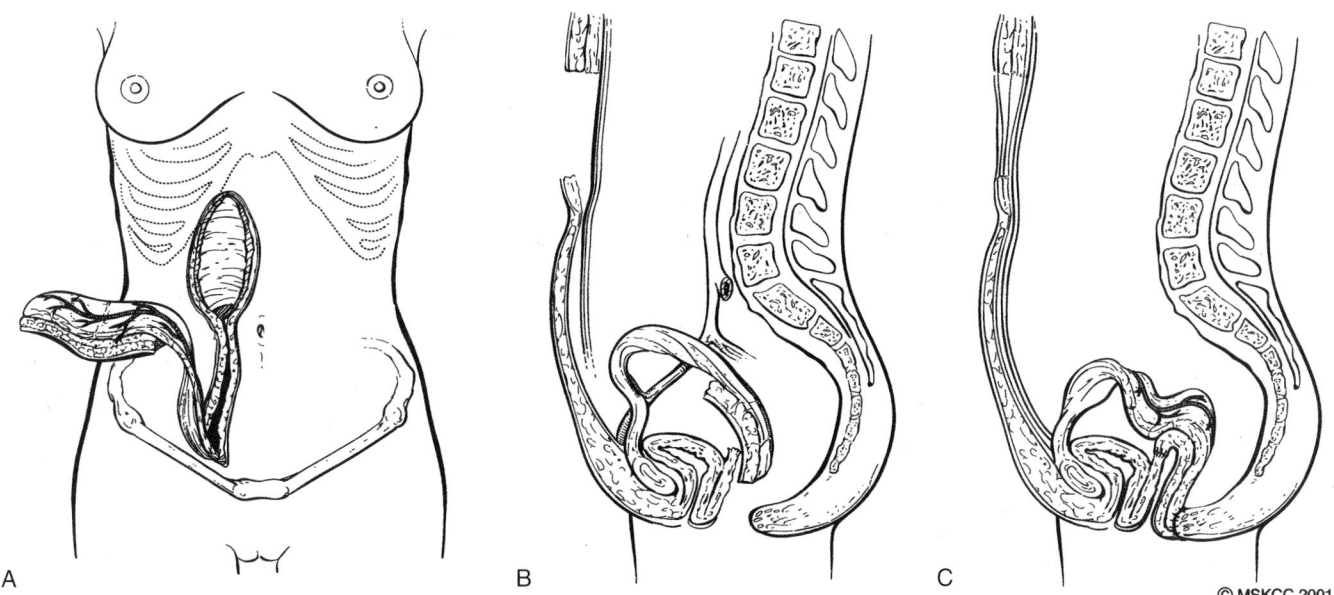

© MSKCC 2001

FIG. 34.6. A: The skin island and rectus muscle are dissected away from the anterior abdominal wall. Care is taken to preserve the inferior epigastric artery that runs longitudinally within the rectus abdominis muscle and serves as its blood supply. **B:** The flap is designed based on the size required to fill the defect and is placed into the pelvis. **C:** The completed flap is sutured to the remainder of the vagina and supports the posterior vaginal wall while filling in dead space within the pelvis. (© Memorial Sloan–Kettering Cancer Center.)

skin island is formed into a tube and the superior portion is used to close off the end that will ultimately become the vaginal apex. The flap is placed into the pelvis and the open end is sutured to the remaining vaginal tissue. Results have generally been acceptable with the rolled rectus abdominis myocutaneous flap, and the incidence of major and minor complications is approximately 10% to 20% (56–58). The reconstructed vagina is usually 6 to 8 cm in length and approximately 3 to 4 cm in width. If vaginal stenosis develops postoperatively, it can usually be relieved with vaginal dilators.

Vaginal defects that involve the entire vagina, as often occurs during a total infralevator pelvic exenteration, can be reconstructed using a bilateral gracilis myocutaneous flap. A skin incision is made over the proximal part of the gracilis muscle, which is supplied by the medial femoral circumflex artery. The flaps are undermined, taking care to preserve the vascular supply, and tunneled into the vaginal defect. They are sutured together and then rotated into position within the pelvis (Fig. 34.7). It is important to maintain the vascular supply of the muscle with the flap and leave the sensory innervation with the donor site. Alternatively, the tubed rectus abdominis myocutaneous flap described above can be used for complete vaginal defects.

The gracilis flap has been reported to have a higher complication rate in some series, and the donor site has an unpleasant appearance (58,59). However, the rectus abdominis flap is dependent on supply from the inferior epigastric artery, which is not always available and mandates that right lower quadrant stomas be placed through the oblique muscles rather than the rectus. Additionally, the rectus abdominis flap can interfere with abdominal closure. Both flaps provide sufficient bulk to fill the dead space within the true pelvis and have been employed successfully for years. In some patients, the gracilis flap donor site may be unavailable or suboptimal owing to lymphedema, thrombosis, radiogenic sclerosis, prior surgery, or other prior trauma.

Special Considerations

One of the most severe sequelae of high-dose radiation therapy to the pelvis or widely metastatic disease is the complete loss of vaginal function and fistulous tracts between the bladder and rectum. In this setting, organ reconstruction and fistula repair is usually not possible. In such cases, the best solution is likely to be a urinary diversion and end colostomy. In highly selected patients, an interval procedure can be performed where the urethra and posterior part of the bladder are resected, leaving the anterior part of the bladder to serve as a neovagina. Satisfactory results have been seen in a small number of patients treated to date.

The procedures described in this section are safe and yield good anatomic and functional outcomes. A minimal length of 4 to 6 cm for the reconstructed vagina is required for satisfactory sexual rehabilitation. The patient's personality and attitude that both she and her partner have regarding sexuality are as important as the purely anatomic result. Often, the neovagina is fully functional after surgical healing is complete, and for some patients, the use of vaginal dilators will be valuable. Although many patients will ultimately not end up having sexual intercourse for a variety of physical, oncologic, and psychologic reasons, it is important for the patient to know that she has this capacity. Body image and her overall quality of life may be profoundly affected by this knowledge.

Urologic Reconstruction

Surgical Strategy

Owing to the intimate anatomic relationship of the gynecologic, urologic, and intestinal organs within the true pelvis, advanced carcinomas of the corpus, cervix, or vagina often necessitate operating on several organs concurrently. Many advanced primary or recurrent carcinomas must be extirpated en bloc to avoid tumor spillage and improve patient outcome. When multiple organ resection is anticipated,

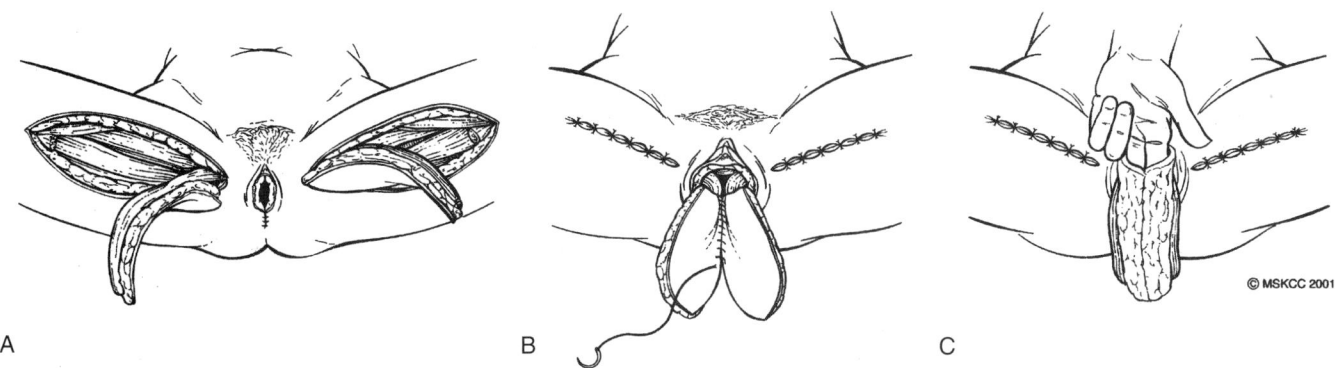

FIG. 34.7. A: Gracilis muscle is undermined taking care to preserve its vascular supply. **B:** The muscle is tunneled under the labia and sutured together. **C:** The completed flap is then rotated into the pelvis. (© Memorial Sloan–Kettering Cancer Center.)

careful preoperative planning can confirm that appropriate instrumentation and necessary personnel are available during the procedure. Unanticipated ureteral injuries must be expected, and the requisite instrumentation should either be in the operative suite or readily accessible.

In some centers, these combined procedures are performed solely by gynecologic oncologists operating as one or two teams and in other centers surgical colleagues are called upon to assist with urologic and colorectal reconstruction. The ablative phase of an exenteration procedure is typically performed by the gynecologic oncology team alone. Reconstruction of the urinary tract is then performed either by the same team, a second gynecologic oncology team, or a urologic team. Occasionally, an organ-preserving procedure (i.e., partial cystectomy, anterior sigmoid resection) may be appropriate. In these patients, however, the primary concern must be to obtain negative surgical margins and remove all viable tumor.

Preoperative Planning

When involvement of urologic or intestinal organs by an advanced gynecologic cancer is suspected based upon physical examination or radiographic studies, additional invasive diagnostic procedures are not usually required. However, if the discovery of metastatic disease would alter the surgical approach, a minimally invasive diagnostic procedures (i.e., laparoscopy or image-guided biopsy) may be warranted. The patient should be informed in detail of all preoperative findings and the possible intraoperative and postoperative sequelae, including the various options for anticipated reconstruction of the involved organs. A written informed consent should include the various surgical options discussed and the specific options preferred by the patient, their drawbacks and limitations, as well as potential operative complications.

If the bladder and/or rectum is involved and urinary or intestinal diversion is considered, patients should be seen preoperatively by an enterostomal therapist for consultation regarding the stoma position(s). The optimal stoma position will vary depending on the type of diversion and the patient's body habitus. Even in cases where careful preoperative planning has occurred, multiple stomal markings should be made since unanticipated intraoperative findings often necessitate

changing preoperative strategy. The surgeon further informs the patient on the principles of catheterization and assesses the physical and psychologic prerequisites for performing the necessary activities.

A complete mechanical bowel preparation (MBP) is often prescribed for all patients undergoing radical pelvic surgery to reduce the incidence of complications, such as fistula or infection. After a day of clear liquid diet, the patient completes a MBP followed by one or more enemas until the stool is clear. Oral antibiotics may also be prescribed for 24 hours prior to surgery. A significant body of literature has recently called into question the utility of preoperative MBP (60–62). Advocates cite the improved visualization and bowel handling after MBP as well as decreasing wound contamination by lowering the bacterial load. Opponents refer to the fact that most randomized trials to date have not shown a benefit to MBP. In addition, there is significant patient discomfort associated with MBP, and altering the normal microbiologic flora of the intestinal tract may be detrimental. Surgical site antibiotic prophylaxis is not controversial and is an important preoperative policy. Intravenous antibiotics should be administered prior to making the skin incision.

Ureteral Injuries

Ureteral injuries are not uncommon in gynecologic surgery and the likelihood of iatrogenic injury increases in proportion to the complexity of the operation. The key to proper management of ureteral injuries is to have a high index of suspicion so that when one does occur, it can be recognized and repaired intraoperatively. Injury to the ureters may occur by crushing, ischemia, ligation (partial or complete), transection (partial or complete), or segmental resection. The most common sites of injury during gynecologic oncology surgery are listed in Table 34.1. The appropriate repair depends upon the type and location of the injury. Minor crush injuries or suspected ischemia, which may occur from overzealous dissection, can be treated by stenting the ureter for 6 to 8 weeks. Partial transections or lacerations may be repaired primarily with a small-caliber suture over a ureteral stent. Prior to stent removal, an intravenous pyelogram or similar study should be obtained to ensure that the injury has been sufficiently repaired. If the defect is large or the ureter is

TABLE 34.1. *Sites of likely ureteral injury during gynecologic oncology surgery[a]*

Anatomic region	Ureter location	Procedure
Abdominal retroperitoneum	Lateral to aorta and vena cava	Aortic node dissection
Pelvic brim	Crossing over the external iliac vessels	Ligation of ovarian vessels
Pelvic retroperitoneum	In the obturator fossa	Pelvic node dissection
Cardinal ligaments	Beneath the uterine artery	Ligation of uterine artery
Vaginal apex	Near trigone at insertion into bladder	Transection of vagina and/or bladder mobilization

[a]The anatomic region, the location of the ureter within that region, and the procedure is commonly associated with injury in that location are indicated.

completely transected, a more extensive procedure is required.

For injuries occurring in the distal one-third of the ureter, direct reimplantation with or without a psoas hitch or Boari flap may be performed. If there is adequate ureteral length, the ureter can be directly reimplanted into the bladder through a submucosal tunnel. When a tension free anastomosis is not possible, the psoas hitch is the most reliable technique. It can be utilized for defects of up to approximately 7 cm (bifurcation of iliac vessels) from the bladder. After adequate mobilization of the bladder, a horizontal incision is made in the anterior bladder dome. The surgeon inserts two fingers and elevates the dorsolateral bladder above the iliac vessels. This region is fixed with traction sutures through the tendon of the psoas minor muscle, taking care not to pass the sutures deep enough to include the femoral nerve. The distal ureter then is implanted antirefluxively in this bladder "horn" using a submucosal tunnel (Fig. 34.8). The surgeon must pay careful attention to the ureter's deli-

cate blood supply to prevent ischemia while constructing a tension-free anastomosis.

If a psoas hitch will not result in a tension-free anastomosis, a pedicled flap of bladder wall (Boari flap) should be considered. This technique allows bridging of defects up to 12 cm and, in combination with the psoas hitch, even greater amounts of missing ureteral length may be replaced by a Boari flap. After full bladder mobilization, the bladder is filled to its utmost capacity and an ipsilateral-based flap is cut from the bladder wall. The distal ureter then is implanted antirefluxively through a submucosal tunnel after fixation of the flap to the psoas minor muscle (Fig. 34.9). For both techniques, a stent is placed in the reimplanted ureter and a suprapubic catheter is placed in the bladder.

For injuries to the upper ureter, the ureter may be directly reimplanted into the renal pelvis. When this is impossible or undesirable, an ileal interposition may be required to bridge the gap from the ureter to the bladder. Alternatively, a transureteroureterostomy can be established to implant the

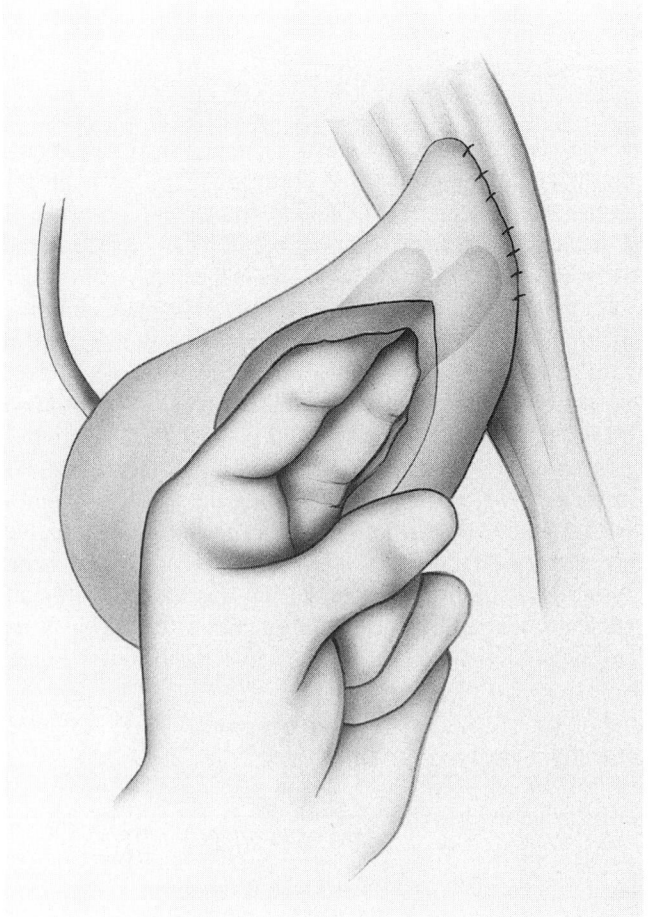

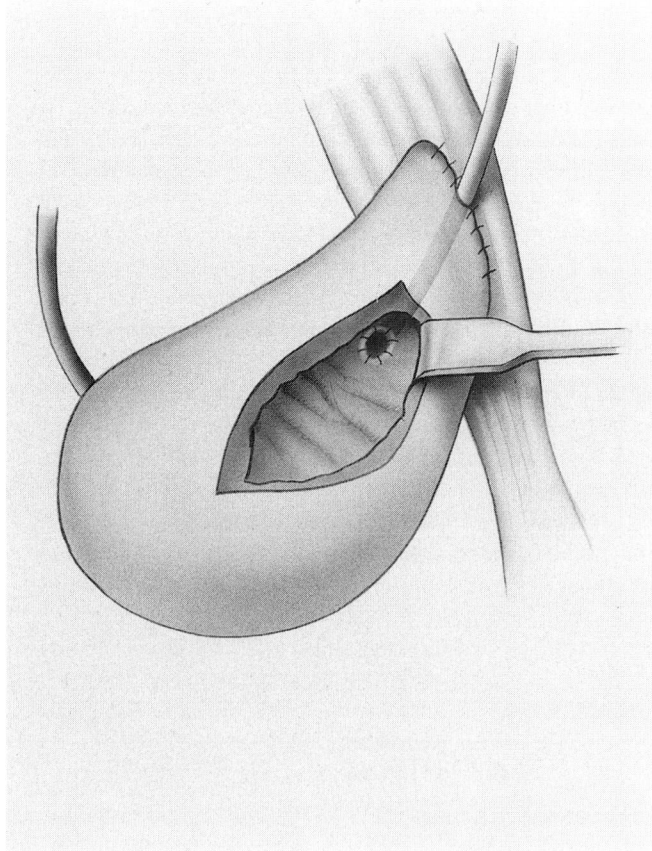

A

B

FIG. 34.8. A: After an oblique incision, two fingers are inserted into the bladder, pushing the bladder dome to the defect's ipsilateral psoas muscle. Here, the bladder is fixed by three to four interrupted sutures. **B:** The ureter is implanted antirefluxively through a submucosal tunnel in the dorsal aspect of the bladder wall.

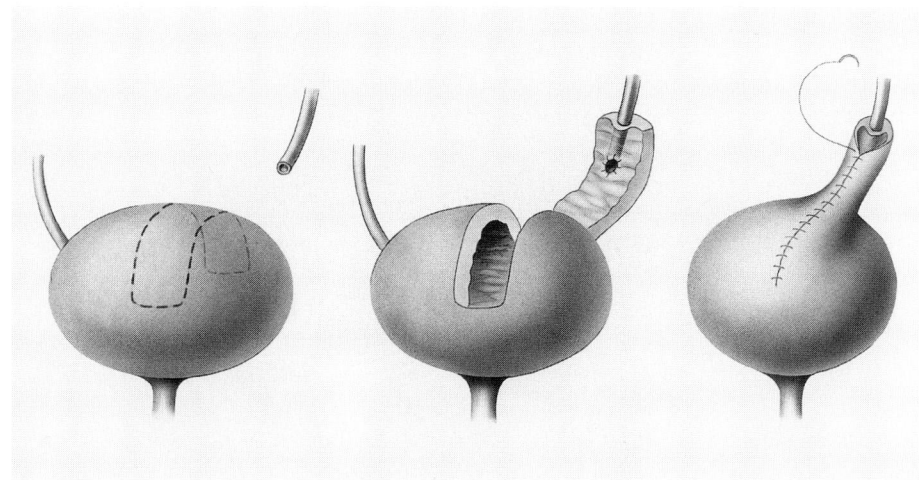

FIG. 34.9. For greater distal ureteral defects, a broad-based strip of bladder wall is dissected, then mobilized and fixed to the defect's ipsilateral psoas muscle. After antirefluxive implantation, the anterior bladder wall is closed by a running suture.

damaged ureter into the uninjured contralateral ureter and restore continuity to the upper collecting system. The decision to choose one procedure over another depends on the location of the injury, the length of ureter that needs to be replaced, and the experience of the operating surgeon.

Urinary Diversion

Whenever the lower urinary tract is scheduled for resection, urinary diversion and reconstruction will be required. Noncontinent diversion via an ileal conduit has been the most widely employed form of urinary diversion since the 1950s. In addition to the potential long-term complications of conduits, such as chronic infection, ureteroileal stenosis, and stone formation, some patients are unable to cope with an additional external appliance. In selected cases, various forms of continent urinary diversion can reduce the number of external appliances and lead to an improved quality of life.

Although the idea of a continent urinary reservoir is more attractive than a noncontinent type, the inherent disadvantages of such a complex surgical procedure must be carefully weighed against its assumed psychologic benefits. The creation of a continent diversion usually requires the use of more bowel and operating time than a simple ileal conduit and is associated with greater short- and long-term complications. In fact, some recent psychologic evaluations reveal no difference in satisfaction for patients with noncontinent diversions compared to patients with continent diversions (63,64). The indications for or against a specific diversion must be carefully considered for each individual patient.

Vascular supply is an important component of a successful urinary diversion. The blood supply of the ileum is derived from branches of the superior mesenteric artery. These branches form an intimate net of multiple arcades supplying the small bowel. In contrast, the colon is supplied by branches of both the superior and inferior mesenteric arteries. Here, the arterial blood supply does not form arcades within the mesentery but runs as isolated arteries through the mesentery, forming arcades only close to the large bowel itself. Therefore, much more attention must be paid to a sufficient blood supply when portions of large bowel are divided for bladder reconstruction as compared to use of the small bowel.

Noncontinent Urinary Diversion

Although there have been many advances in the use of continent reservoirs, the ileal conduit remains the standard for urinary diversion. The conduit requires relatively little operative time and a short bowel segment and is associated with low morbidity. It is especially useful in cases requiring additional time-consuming surgery or in patients with impaired renal function. The most common indication for urinary diversion in gynecologic oncology is total pelvic exenteration (TPE). Although many indications exist for TPE, most patients who are candidates for this procedure have recurrent cervical cancer and have previously received whole pelvic irradiation.

The creation of an ileal conduit begins by carefully mobilizing the ureters, taking care to avoid devascularizing them during the dissection. The ureters are usually transected at the pelvic brim so that a negative surgical margin is obtained and the portion of ureter to be used for the ileal anastomosis is not part of a prior radiation field. The left ureter is passed beneath the sigmoid mesentery toward the right. A refluxing ureteroileal anastomosis is created via the methods of Bricker or Wallace because of the low rates of stenosis associated with these procedures (65,66).

A 10- to 15-cm segment of distal ileum approximately 15 cm from ileocecal valve is isolated (Fig. 34.10A). A longer ileal segment may be isolated if the remaining ureters are particularly short or have limited mobility and there is concern that a tension-free anastomosis may not be possible. An ileoileostomy is performed to restore bowel continuity, and the butt-end of the isolated ileal segment is closed with

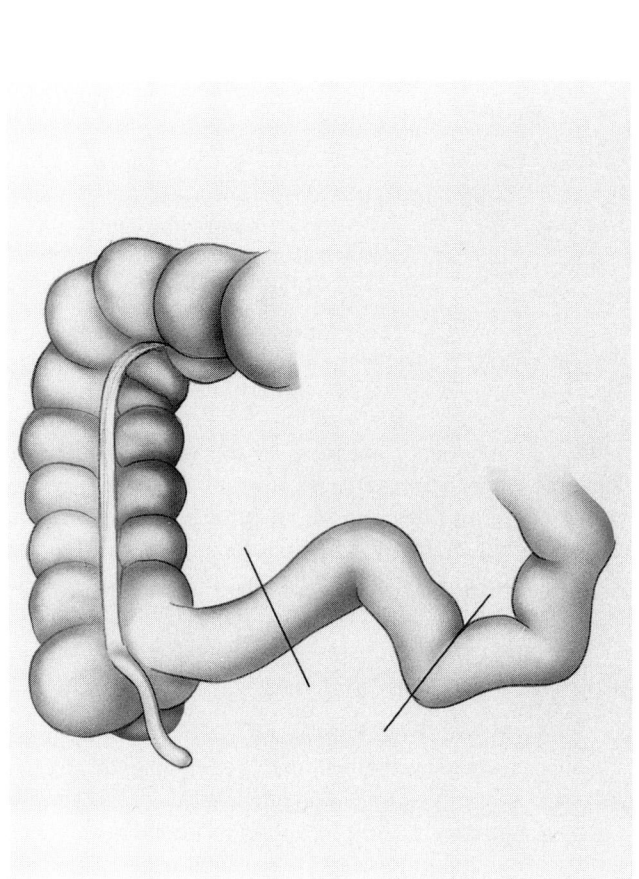

A

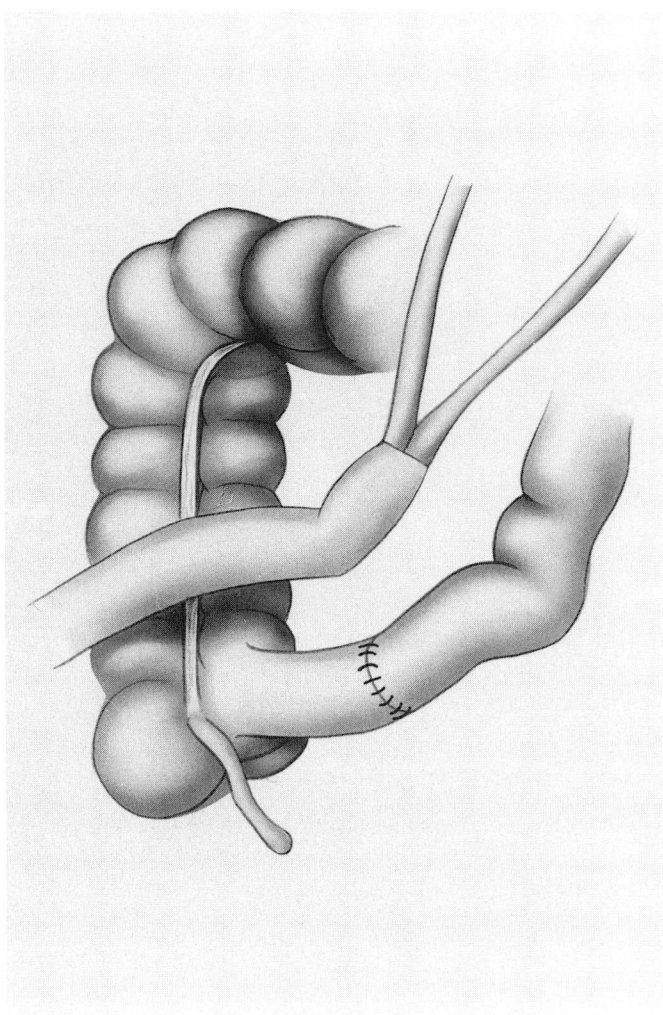

B

FIG. 34.10. A: A 10- to 15-cm segment of distal ileum is isolated approximately 15 cm from the ileocecal valve. **B:** An ileal conduit is constructed with refluxive ureteroileal anastomoses and continuity is restored to the ileum. The Wallace technique is shown.

a linear stapler or permanent silk suture. Single-J ureteral stents may be placed to bridge the ureteroileal anastomosis, although they are not required. A long fine-tipped clamp or Yankauer suction tip is passed through the isolated segment of ileum to the planned site of ureteroileal anastomosis. A small enterotomy is made sharply and stents, if used, are passed through the conduit. The ends of the ureters may be spatulated if they appear exceptionally narrow, although this too is usually not required. The ureteroileal anastomosis is performed near the butt-end of the ileal segment (Fig. 34.10B). The distal ileum is pulled through a separate incision in the abdominal wall and sutured in a rosebud fashion to ensure good stomal function.

A red rubber catheter is placed in the conduit for approximately 7 days to facilitate drainage during the early postoperative period. Radiographic imaging is not required, but may be obtained if there is concern for the continuity of the ure-

teroileal anastomosis. The patient is trained to care for the stoma as early as possible by an enterostomal therapist.

Specific Complications and Alternatives. Urinary leakage at the ureteroileal anastomosis is the most common early complication, especially in patients who have received previous pelvic radiation. The suspicion of a urinary leak should be raised when discharge from pelvic drains does not diminish or even increases throughout the early postoperative period. A conservative approach is justified for a small dehiscence at the anastomosis. Larger defects should undergo early formal revision. Late complications include ureteroileal stenosis, stomal stenosis, prolapse or retraction, urolithiasis, metabolic acidosis, and chronic pyelonephritis.

In patients with chronic small bowel disease, short small bowel, or heavily irradiated small bowel changes, a colon conduit is preferred. The colonic segment is chosen according to preoperative stomal considerations and intraoperative findings. Any segment of the colon (ascending, transverse, descending, or sigmoid) may be appropriate.

In addition to the continent urinary diversions discussed below, orthotopic bladder reconstruction is theoretically an option for gynecologic oncology patients undergoing exenterative surgery. In most situations, however, adequate urethral length would be available after completing an appropriate oncologic resection of recurrent disease. As well, many of the tissues required to create an orthotopic neobladder would have been previously irradiated, leading to a higher rate of complications. Finally, intermittent transurethral self-catheterization is often required during the postoperative period after creation of an orthotopic neobladder. Many patients have more difficulty self-catheterizing the urethra than managing an external stomal appliance or catheterizing a continent urinary diversion as described below.

Continent Urinary Diversions

Recent improvements in surgical techniques and perioperative care as well as presumed improvement in quality of life have paved the way for more frequent use of continent urinary diversions following radical pelvic surgery. The advent of intermittent catheterization has allowed some patients to receive a continent, catheterizable form of urinary reservoir. Several theoretical realizations have advanced our knowledge of continent reservoir function over the past few decades. An antimesenteric incision of the large bowel results in a detubularized plate that prevents synchronized peristalsis, resulting in a reduction of uninhibited contractions and consequently dramatically improving continence. The folding of this bowel plate increases the radius of the newly constructed reservoir, thereby creating a large-volume, low-pressure container sufficient for socially acceptable voiding patterns.

Owing to the location of recurrent disease and/or previous irradiation, most patients will not be able to use their natural urethral sphincter to control the outflow of urine, and a catheterizable reservoir offers an attractive therapeutic alternative. Usually, the efferent limb is connected to the umbilicus or right lower quadrant and the reservoir placed in the mid right abdomen. The reservoir is usually created from large bowel with or without an ileal patch to augment its size. Many continent catheterizable urinary diversions have been created by various investigators, each bearing a unique name. A comprehensive review is beyond the scope of this text and is available from other sources (67). In this section, one of the most common continent urinary diversions in gynecologic oncology, the Indiana pouch, is discussed and compared to a relatively new arrival onto the scene, the modified Penn pouch.

Indiana Pouch. The classic Indiana pouch, as originally described by Rowland in 1987, makes use of the ascending colon as the continent reservoir (68). The bowel is isolated from the distal ileum to the division of the right and middle colic arteries. It is opened along the anterior tenia coli to create a detubularized nonperistaltic pouch (Fig. 34.11A). An ileocolic anastomosis is then performed in the usual fashion to restore bowel continuity. Eight to 10 cm of terminal ileum is tapered to form the efferent catheterizable limb and the appendix, when present, is removed. The ileocecal valve is tapered with two rows of imbricating sutures over a 14 French red rubber catheter, which is brought out through the abdominal wall. The ureters are directly implanted into the distal part of the ascending colon prior to closing the reservoir in two layers (Fig. 34.11B, C). Submucosal tunneling of the ureters is not required and may increase the risk of anastomotic stenosis, offsetting any perceived benefit of preventing the reflux of urine into the upper collecting system. The anastomosis should be bridged by single-J ureteral stents that will remain *in situ* for less than 2 weeks.

Modifications of the technique have been described by various groups and provide useful alternatives. The University of Miami suggested including one-third to one-half of the transverse colon to increase the capacity of the reservoir (69). They also suggest using a purse-string suture to taper the distal ileum instead of two rows of imbricating sutures. Their modifications form the basis for the Miami pouch. The Florida pouch is similar to the Miami pouch except that two rows of imbricating sutures are placed opposite one another (70).

Ureteral stents remain *in situ* for 10 to 14 days and a Foley catheter remains in place for approximately 2 to 3 weeks to maintain decompression of the reservoir. A separate cecostomy tube or similar is placed into the reservoir in case the conduit should fail in the early postoperative period. Intermittent catheterization teaching is begun shortly before removing the Foley catheter and should be done in conjunction with an enterostomal therapist. Care is taken to ensure that the reservoir is completely emptied each time it is catheterized and irrigated intermittently to prevent mucus build-up. Initially after catheterization, residual urine volume is measured via the cecostomy tube, which usually confirms complete emptying of the reservoir.

Early complications include ureteral stricture, anastomotic leak, fistula, acute pyelonephritis, and difficult catheterization. Late complications include ureteral stricture, chronic pyelonephritis, pouchitis, incontinence, metabolic acidosis, difficult catheterization, stomal stenosis or retraction, parastomal hernia, and urolithiasis. Complications occur in approximately 50% of patients, and reoperation is necessary in approximately 15% of these patients (71–73).

Modified Penn Pouch. A modified Penn pouch, although more complex in design than the Indiana pouch, offers several theoretical advantages. In a similar manner to the continent, catheterizable urinary diversions described previously, the reservoir is fashioned from a detubularized segment of large bowel. However, the efferent limb is created from a

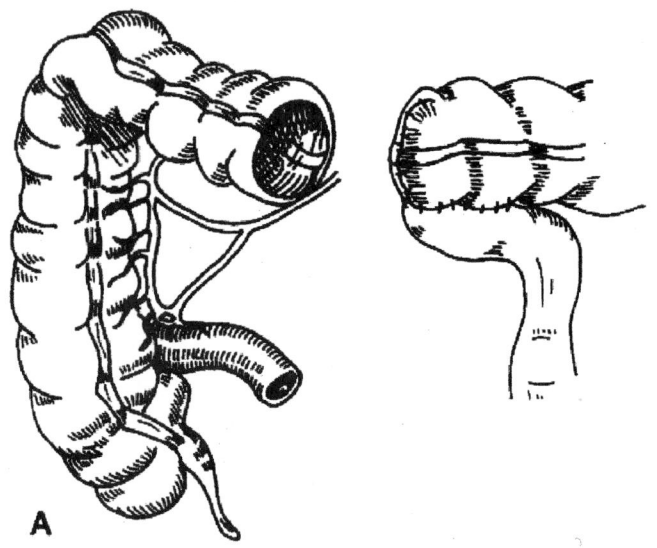

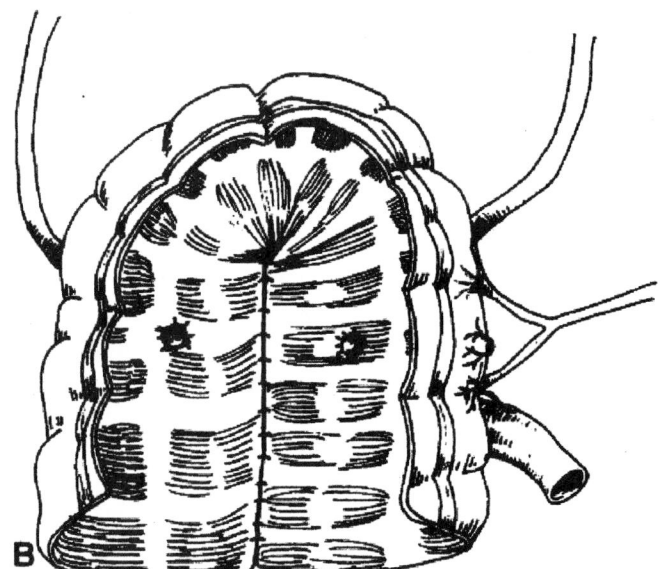

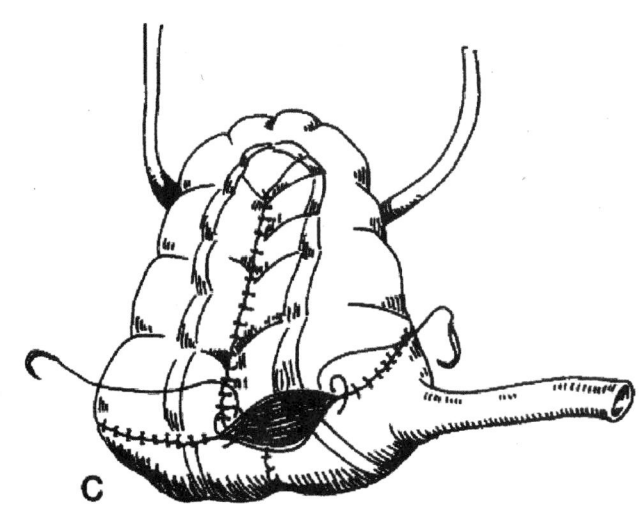

FIG. 34.11. A: The distal ileum, ascending colon, and a portion of the transverse colon are isolated. An ileocolic anastomosis is performed. **B:** The colon is detubularized and the appendix is removed, if present. The ureters are directly implanted into the dorsal aspect of the colon without tunneling. **C:** The colon is closed in two layers of running delayed absorbable suture. (Reprinted with permission from Walsh PC, Retik AB, Darracott E, Wein Vaughan Jr, eds. *Campbell's urology.* 8th ed. Philadelphia: WB Saunders, Fig 107–20.)

tunneled appendix using the Mitrofanoff principle to minimize stomal incontinence (74). As shown in Figure 34.12, the appendix is transfixed and buried in a submucosal tunnel that permits easy catheterization, a problem frequently encountered when the distal ileum is used as the catheterizable conduit. The ureters are implanted in the distal ileum that remains attached to the cecum through the native ileocecal valve. This design has two important benefits. The ileal segment can be lengthened to accommodate proximal nonirradiated ureteral segments. The ileocecal valve serves as an antireflux mechanism for the low-pressure high-capacity chamber, preventing a distended reservoir from overflowing into the upper collecting system.

If ureteral stents are placed intraoperatively, they are exteriorized through separate stab wounds since a 14 French red rubber catheter occupies the appendiceal limb. A cecostomy tube or similar is placed into the reservoir so that decompression is possible if the appendiceal limb functions improperly after catheter removal and serves as an alternative outlet while the patient is learning self-catheterization.

In several small series reported to date, the complications have been acceptable and the continence impressive (75). An alternative urinary diversion must be performed for patients who have undergone prior appendectomy or if the appendix is seriously damaged. Another consideration is that slightly more operative time is required to create a modified Penn pouch when compared to an Indiana-type pouch. Nonetheless, in gynecologic oncology patients undergoing radical pelvic surgery for recurrent cancer in the setting of heavy prior irradiation, this type of urinary diversion is likely to perform well with a low incidence of short- and long-term complications.

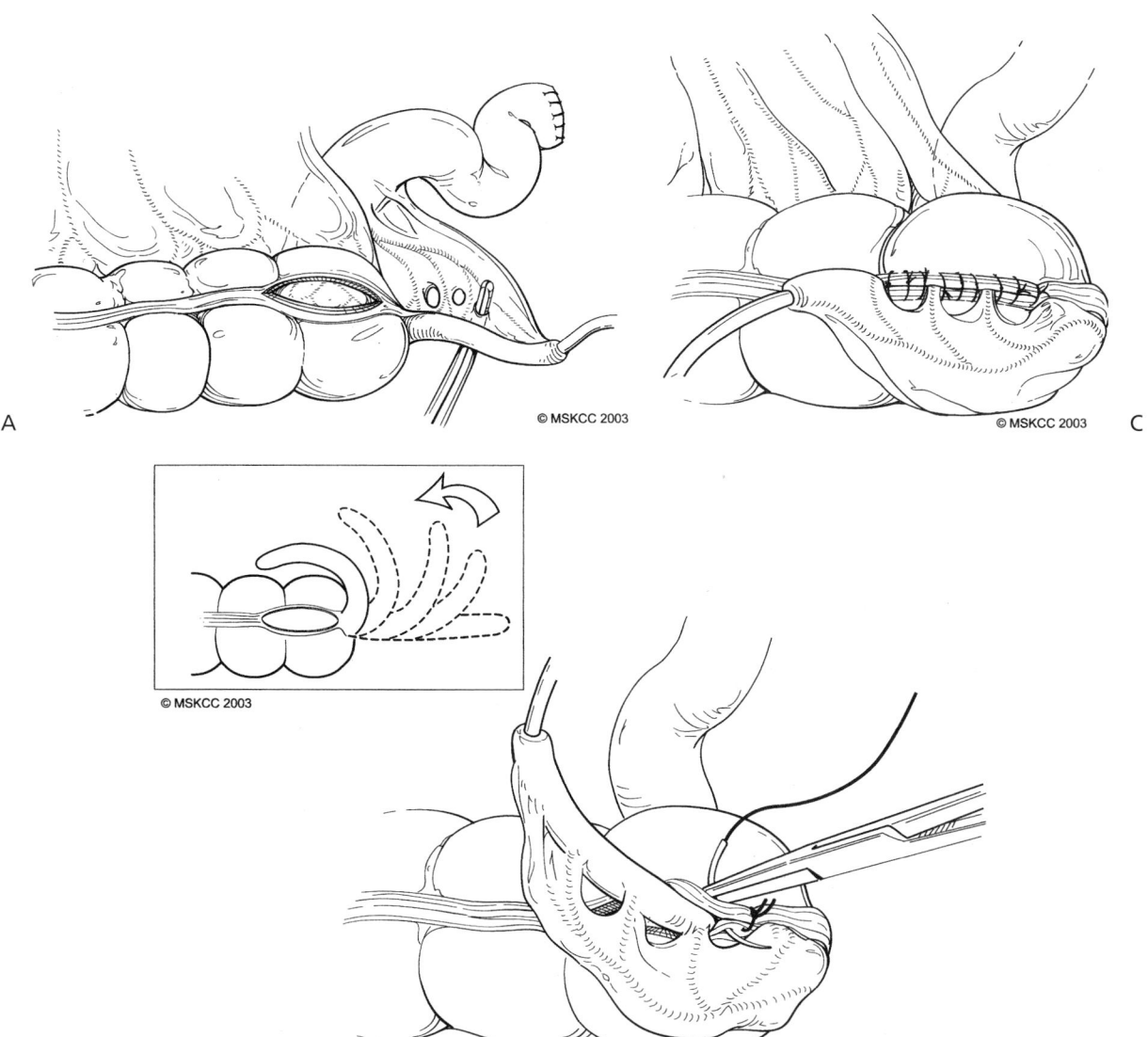

FIG. 34.12. A: A seromuscular incision along the anterior tenia coli is made for a distance of 4 to 5 cm and undermined. Three to four windows of Deaver are created in the mesoappendix. **B:** Permanent sutures from one edge of the seromuscular wall, through the windows of Deaver, and secured to the contralateral side. Starting at the first window, serial sutures are placed as the appendix is folded into the seromuscular chamber. **C:** When the tunneling is complete, approximately 2 cm of the appendix remains free for the formation of the cutaneous stoma. (© Memorial Sloan–Kettering Cancer Center.)

REFERENCES

1. Fallowfield L. Do psychological studies upset patients? In: Holland JC, ed. *Current concepts in psycho-oncology and AIDS: syllabus of the postgraduate course.* Memorial Sloan–Kettering Cancer Center, September 17–19, 1987, New York City. New York: Memorial Sloan–Kettering Cancer Center, 1987.
2. Mitchell GW, Glicksman AS. Cancer patients: knowledge and attitudes. *Cancer* 1977;40:61.
3. Schover, LR. *Sexuality and fertility after cancer.* New York: John Wiley & Sons, 1997.
4. Robinson JW. Sexuality and cancer. Breaking the silence. *Aust Fam Physician* 1998;27:45–47.
5. Andersen BL. How cancer affects sexual functioning. *Oncology (Huntingt)* 1990;4:81–88; Discussion 92–94.
6. Anderson BL., Woods XA, Copeland LJ. Sexual self schema and sexual morbidity among gynecological cancer survivors. *J Consult Clin Psychol* 1997;65:221–229.
7. van Tulder MW, Aaronson NK, Bruning PF. The quality of life of long-term survivors of Hodgkin's disease. *Ann Oncol* 1994;5:153–158.
8. Anderson BL. Surviving cancer: the importance of sexual self concept. *Med Pediatr Oncol* 1999;33:15–23.
9. Engel GL. The need for a new medical model: a challenge for biomedicine. *Science* 1977;196:129.
10. Cosin JA, Carter JR, Paley P, et al. A simplified method for detubularization in the construction of a continent ileocolic reservoir (Miami pouch). *Gynecol Oncol* 1997;64:436.
11. National Institutes of Health Consensus Development Conference statement on cervical cancer, April 13, 1996. *Gynecol Oncol* 1997;66:351.

12. *World Health Organization (WHO) Handbook for Reporting Results of Cancer Treatment,* Geneva, 1979.

13. Karnofsky DA, Burchenal JH. The clinical evaluation of chemotherapeutic agents in cancer. In: McCleod CM, ed. *Evaluation of chemotherapeutic agents.* New York: Columbia University Press, 1949: 191.

14. Schag CC, Heinrich RL, Ganz PA. Karnofsky performance status revisited: reliability, validity, and guidelines. *J Clin Oncol* 1984;2:187.

15. Selby PJ, Chapman JA, Etazadi-Amoli J, et al. The development of a method for assessing the quality of life of cancer patients. *Br J Cancer* 1984;50:13.

16. Slevin ML, Plant H, Lynch D, et al. Who should measure quality of life, the doctor or the patient? *Br J Cancer* 1988;57:109.

17. Aaronson NK, Bullinger M, Ahmedzai S. A modular approach to quality of life assessment in cancer clinical trials. *Recent Results Cancer Res* 1988;111:231–249.

18. Cella DF, Cherin EA. Quality of life during and after cancer treatment. *Compre Ther* 1988;14:69.

19. Hawighorst-Knapstein S, Schönefuß G, Hoffmann SO, Knapstein PG. Pelvic exenteration: effects of surgery on quality of life and body image—a prospective longitudinal study. *Gynecol Oncol* 1997;66:495.

20. Andersen BL, Woods XA, Copeland LJ. Sexual self-schema and sexual morbidity among gynecologic cancer survivors. *J Consult Clin Psychol* 1997;65:221–229.

21. Derogatis LR. Breast and gynecologic cancers. Their unique impact on body image and sexuality identity in women. *Front Radiat Ther Oncol* 1979;14:1–11.

22. Fisher S. *Body experience in fantasy and behavior.* New York: Appleton-Century-Crofts, 1970.

23. Weijmar Schultz WCM, Van De Weil HBM, Hahn DEE, Bouma J. Psychosexual functioning after treatment for gynecological cancer: an integrative model, review of determinant factors and clinical guidelines. *Int J Gynecol Cancer* 1992;2:281.

24. Hall JA, Roter DL, Rand CS. Communication of affect between patient and physician. *J Health Soc Behav* 1981;22:18.

25. Beckman HB, Frankel RM. The effect of physician behavior on the collection of data. *Ann Intern Med* 1984;101:692.

26. Comstock LM, Hooper EM, Goodwin JM, Goodwin JS. Physician behaviors that correlate with patient satisfaction. *J Med Educ* 1982;57: 105.

27. Buckman R. Communication in palliative care. In: Doyle D, Hanks GW, MacDonald N, eds. *Oxford textbook of palliative medicine.* Oxford, UK: Oxford University Press, 1992.

28. Baron RJ. An introduction to medical phenomenology: I can't hear you while I'm listening. *Ann Intern Med* 1985;103:606.

29. Weston WW, Brown JB. The importance of patients' belief. In: Stewart M, Roter D, eds. *Communicating with medical patients.* Newbury Park: Sage Publications, 1989:77–85.

30. Cohen F. Stress and bodily illness. *Psychiatr Clin North Am* 1981;4: 269.

31. Ruberman W, Weinblatt E, Goldberg JD, Chaudhary BS. Psychosocial influences on mortality after myocardial infarction. *N Engl J Med* 1984; 311:552.

32. Hawighorst-Knapstein S, Schönefuß G, Hoffmann SO, Knapstein PG. Pelvic exenteration: effects of surgery on quality of life and body image—a prospective longitudinal study. *Gynecol Oncol* 1997;66: 495.

33. Hall JA, Roter DL, Rand CS. Communication of affect between patient and physician. *J Health Soc Behav* 1981;22:18.

34. Andersen BL, Anderson B, de Prosse C. Controlled prospective longitudinal study of women with cancer: I. Sexual functioning outcomes. *J Consult Clin Psychol* 1989;57:683.

35. Hawighorst-Knapstein S. Pre- and postoperative counseling in gynecologic surgery. In: Neises M, Ditz S, eds. *Psychosomatische Grundversorgung in der Frauenheilkunde.* Stuttgart: Georg Thieme Verlag, 1999.

36. Baider L, Perez T, De-Nour AK. Gender and adjustment to chronic disease. A study of couples with colon cancer. *Gen Hosp Psychiatry* 1989;11:1.

37. MacDonald LD, Anderson HR. The health of rectal cancer patients in the community. *Eur J Surg Oncol* 1985;11:235.

38. Wirsching M, Druner HU, Herrmann G. Results of psychosocial adjustment to long-term colostomy. *Psychother Psychosom* 1975;26:245.

39. Andersen BL, Anderson B, de Prosse C. Controlled prospective longitudinal study of women with cancer: II. Psychological outcomes. *J Consult Clin Psychol* 1989;57:692.

40. Andersen BL, ed. *Women with cancer: Psychological perspectives.* New York: Springer-Verlag, 1986.

41. Elstein AS, Schulman LS, Sprafka SA. *Medical problem solving: an analysis of clinical reasoning.* Cambridge, MA: Harvard University Press, 1978.

42. Cohen-Cole SA. The biopsychosocial model in medical practice. In: Stoudemire A, ed. *Human behavior: an introduction for medical students.* Philadelphia: JB Lippincott Co, 1990.

43. Morrow CP, Curtin JP. *Gynecologic cancer surgery.* New York: Churchill Livingstone, 1996.

44. Levine DA, Barakat RR, Hoskins WJ. *Atlas of procedures in gynecologic oncology.* London: Martin Dunitz, 2003.

45. Knapstein PG, Friedberg V, Sevin BU. *Reconstructive surgery in gynecology.* New York: Thieme Medical Publishers, 1990:1–101.

46. McCraw JB, Arnold PG. *McGraw and Arnold's atlas of muscle and musculocutaneous flaps.* Norfolk, VA: Hampton Press, 1986: 265,357,389,423.

47. Mathes, S.J., Nahia, F. *Reconstructive surgery: principles, anatomy and technique.* Philadelphia: Elsevier Science, 1999.

48. Burke TW, Morris M, Levenback C, et al. Closure of complex vulvar defects using local rhomboid flaps. *Obstet Gynecol* 1994;84: 1043–1047.

49. Helm CW, Hatch KD, Partridge EE, Shingleton HM. The rhomboid transposition flap for repair of the perineal defect after radical vulvar surgery. *Gynecol Oncol* 1993;50:164–167.

50. Arkoulakis NS, Angel CL, DuBeshter B, Serletti JM. Reconstruction of an extensive vulvectomy defect using the gluteus maximus fasciocutaneous V-Y advancement flap. *Ann Plast Surg* 2002;49:50–54; Discussion, 54.

51. Tateo A, Tateo S, Bernasconi C, Zara C. Use of V-Y flap for vulvar reconstruction. *Gynecol Oncol* 1996;62:203–207.

52. Cordeiro PG, Pusic AL, Disa JJ. A classification system and reconstructive algorithm for acquired vaginal defects. *Plast Reconstr Surg* 2002;110:1058–1065.

53. Woods JE, Alter G, Meland B, Podratz K. Experience with vaginal reconstruction utilizing the modified Singapore flap. *Plast Reconstr Surg* 1992;90:270–274.

54. Wee JT, Joseph VT. A new technique of vaginal reconstruction using neurovascular pudendal-thigh flaps: a preliminary report. *Plast Reconstr Surg* 1989;83:701–709.

55. Monstrey S, Blondeel P, Van Landuyt K, et al. The versatility of the pudendal thigh fasciocutaneous flap used as an island flap. *Plast Reconstr Surg* 2001;107:719–725.

56. Smith HO, Genesen MC, Runowicz CD, Goldberg GL. The rectus abdominis myocutaneous flap: modifications, complications, and sexual function. *Cancer* 1998;83:510–520.

57. Tobin GR, Day TG. Vaginal and pelvic reconstruction with distally based rectus abdominis myocutaneous flaps. *Plast Reconstr Surg* 1988; 81:62–73.

58. Jurado M, Bazan A, Elejabeitia J, et al. Primary vaginal and pelvic floor reconstruction at the time of pelvic exenteration: a study of morbidity. *Gynecol Oncol* 2000;77:293–297.

59. Soper JT, Rodriguez G, Berchuck A, Clarke-Pearson DL. Long and short gracilis myocutaneous flaps for vulvovaginal reconstruction after radical pelvic surgery: comparison of flap-specific complications. *Gynecol Oncol* 1995;56:271–275.

60. Muzii L, Angioli R, Zullo MA, et al. Bowel preparation for gynecological surgery. *Crit Rev Oncol Hematol* 2003;48:311–315.

61. Guenaga KF, Matos D, Castro AA, et al. Mechanical bowel preparation for elective colorectal surgery. Cochrane Database Syst Rev. 2003; (2): CD001544. .

62. Zmora O, Mahajna A, Bar-Zakai B, et al. Colon and rectal surgery without mechanical bowel preparation: a randomized prospective trial. *Ann Surg* 2003;237:363–367.

63. Kitamura H, Miyao N, Yanase M, et al. Quality of life in patients having an ileal conduit, continent reservoir or orthotopic neobladder after cystectomy for bladder carcinoma. *Int J Urol* 1999;6:393–399.

64. Mansson A, Mansson W. When the bladder is gone: quality of life following different types of urinary diversion. *World J Urol* 1999;17: 211–218.

65. Bricker EM. Bladder substitution after pelvic evisceration. *Surg Clin North Am* 1950;30:1511–1521.

66. Wallace DM: Uretero-ileostomy. *Br J Urol* 1970;42:529–534.

67. Walsh PC, Retik AB, Darracott E, Wein Vaughan Jr, eds. *Campbell's urology*. 8th ed. Philadelphia: WB Saunders,

68. Rowland RG, Mitchell ME, Bihrle R, et al. Indiana continent urinary reservoir. *J Urol* 1987;137:1136–1139.

69. Bejany DE, Politano VA. Stapled and nonstapled tapered distal ileum for construction of a continent colonic urinary reservoir. *J Urol* 1988;140:491–494.

70. Lockhart JL. Remodeled right colon: an alternative urinary reservoir. *J Urol* 1987;138:730–734.

71. Penalver MA, Angioli R, Mirhashemi R, Malik R. Management of early and late complications of ileocolonic continent urinary reservoir (Miami pouch). *Gynecol Oncol* 1998;69:185–191.

72. Ramirez PT, Modesitt SC, Morris M, et al. Functional outcomes and complications of continent urinary diversions in patients with gynecologic malignancies. *Gynecol Oncol* 2002; 85:285–291.

73. Webster C, Bukkapatnam R, Seigne JD, et al. Continent colonic urinary reservoir (Florida pouch): long-term surgical complications (greater than 11 years). *J Urol* 2003;169:174–176.

74. Duckett JW, Snyder HM III. Use of the Mitrofanoff principle in urinary reconstruction. *Urol Clin North Am* 1986;13:271–274.

75. Bochner BH, McCreath WA, Aubey JJ, et al. Use of an ureteroileocecal appendicostomy urinary reservoir in patients with recurrent pelvic malignancies treated with radiation. *Gynecol Oncol* Forthcoming.

CHAPTER 35

Nutritional Support of Patients with Gynecologic Cancers

Moshe Shike and Mark Schattner

Cachexia and weight loss are common manifestations of cancer and exert major impacts on quality of life and survival. Malnutrition is a complex, multifactorial phenomenon that leads to progressive weight loss and deficiency of specific nutrients. Both the cancer and its various therapeutic modalities contribute to cachexia. Advances in understanding nutritional requirements and intermediary metabolism and major technologic progress in the ability to provide nutritional support have made it possible to feed almost any patient with cancer. Nevertheless, the indications for and the appropriate use of the various modalities of nutritional support are still evolving, and many questions remain unanswered.

Malnutrition in most patients with cancer is usually a manifestation of general calorie-protein deficits that result in progressive weight loss and weakness; however, it is important to recognize that, in some patients, specific nutrient deficiencies, such as magnesium deficiency or vitamin B_{12} deficiency, can be present even in the absence of weight loss and can contribute significantly to morbidity and even mortality.

Gynecologic malignancies and their multimodal therapies may be associated with severe malnutrition. Although some nutritional problems occur in patients with cervical and endometrial cancer, they are most commonly seen in those with ovarian cancer, particularly in advanced stages when intraabdominal metastasis severely impair gastrointestinal function. Because of the high incidence of malnutrition and its impact on the patient with cancer, nutritional assessment and appropriate therapy should be integral parts of the overall treatment plan.

NUTRITIONAL ASSESSMENT

Nutritional assessment in cancer patients is an ongoing process. It should be a part of the patient's initial evaluation and should be updated periodically. It is especially important to determine the nutritional state prior to therapeutic interventions as well as during and after an acute illness, with the goal of identifying those patients who could benefit from a specific form of nutritional support. The nutritional assessment method used must be simple, accurate, and inexpensive. Anthropometric parameters, serum protein measurements, and immunologic tests had classically formed the basis of the nutritional evaluation; however, they all have significant deficiencies.

Anthropometric and Biochemical Markers

Anthropometric measurements such as weight, skin fold thickness, mid arm muscle circumference, and creatinine/height index can all provide useful information but have major limitations. Change in weight is the single most useful measurement of the nutritional status when the change does not reflect changes in total body water. The often-present edema, effusions, ascites, or intravenous hydration limit the use of weight as a nutritional parameter. In addition, inaccuracies in scales and different clothing in hospitals and at home can often be sources of misleading information on changes in weight. Measurements of skin folds and mid arm muscle circumference (1) are useful tools in studies but have very limited use in clinical practice. A creatinine/height index derived by dividing the patient's 24-hour creatinine excretion by that of a healthy person of the same height offers a sensitive measure of early protein calorie malnutrition (2) but requires collection of a 24-hour urine specimen and is affected by alterations in renal function that may not be indicative of the nutritional state.

M. Shike: Cancer Prevention and Wellness Program, Memorial Sloan–Kettering Cancer Center, New York, New York 10021
M. Schattner: Department of Medicine, Memorial Sloan–Kettering Cancer Center, New York, New York 10021

Low levels of serum proteins such as albumin, prealbumin, transferrin, and retinol-binding protein were classically thought to represent malnutrition. However, in the malnourished sick patient, low levels of these proteins can be nonspecific. They are dependent on intact hepatic synthetic function as well as hydration status. At times, they can be low as a manifestation of severe illness (infection, metastatic cancer, multisystem organ failure) without being a reflection of the nutritional state. In addition, they can function as acute phase reactants and therefore be in the normal or elevated range in a clinically malnourished patient. The role of serum protein measurements in the nutritional assessment of an ill patient with cancer is therefore limited. Similar limitations apply to the role of immunologic parameters such as total lymphocyte count and delayed cutaneous hypersensitivity. In simple starvation, both of these measures may be decreased and can return to normal with initiation of nutritional support. However, in the cancer patient undergoing chemotherapy, surgery, or radiotherapy or in the midst of an acute illness, these parameters have little determinative value in the assessment of the nutritional state (3,4).

The above parameters have been combined to create numerous nutritional assessment indices. The most extensively studied is the Prognostic Nutritional Index (PNI) that factors measurements of serum albumin, serum transferrin, triceps skin fold, and delayed cutaneous hypersensitivity (5). Buzbey et al. prospectively studied the PNI in patients undergoing gastrointestinal surgery and found that it could accurately stratify patients into high, intermediate, or low risk of developing postoperative complications (6). It must be understood, however, that the index is only as good as the parameters from which it is calculated, and the same limitations outlined above are present in any of these indices.

Subjective Global Assessment

The clinical assessment of the nutritional status has always been used to some extent as part of the general medical history and physical examination. The validity of a formal clinical assessment of the nutritional status was demonstrated in a landmark study by Baker et al., who developed the Subjective Global Assessment (SGA) (7). The SGA is based on a complete history and physical examination with special emphasis on six areas: change in weight, dietary intake, gastrointestinal symptoms, functional capacity, physiologic stress, and physical signs of nutritional deficiencies. These data are used to place the patient into one of three groups. Group A (normal nutritional status) is made up of those patients without restriction of food intake or absorption, no change in functional status, and stable or increasing weight. Group B (mild malnutrition) consists of patients with evidence of decreased food intake and functional status but little or no change in body weight, whereas those with severe reduction in food intake, functional status, and loss of weight comprise group C (severe malnutrition).

The SGA has consistently been shown to be reproducible and reliable in identifying patients at risk for developing complications associated with malnutrition. In the initial study of 59 patients electively admitted to a general surgical ward, interobserver reproducibility in classification of the nutritional status was 81%, and in a later study of 202 patients, it was found to be 91% (7,8). Group assignment based on the SGA had prognostic significance on the ensuing clinical course. The initial study by Baker and colleagues showed a significant increase in incidence of infection, use of antibiotics, and length of hospitalization in group C when compared to group A (7). In the follow-up study of 202 patients undergoing gastrointestinal surgery, the rate of septic and nonseptic complications in group C was seven times greater than in group A (8). However, it must be recognized that although nutritional parameters are used to determine the SGA, the classification may still represent severity of illness rather than specific nutritionally related complications. Only a determination that the classification predicts which patients will respond favorably to nutritional support (with a decrease in complications) can validate the specificity of this technique. Nevertheless, the SGA provides a simple, reproducible, and accurate method to identify patients who are malnourished who could possibly benefit from nutritional support. Clinical assessments similar to the SGA have been shown to be superior to immunologic testing, plasma protein measurements, and bioelectrical impedance in providing a useful evaluation of nutritional status (7,9–12).

PREVALENCE OF MALNUTRITION

The prevalence of malnutrition depends on the tumor type and stage, the organs involved, and the anticancer therapy. Concurrent nonmalignant conditions such as diabetes and intestinal diseases can be important contributing factors.

The prevalence of weight loss during the 6 months preceding diagnosis of cancer was reported from a multicenter cooperative study of patients with 12 types of cancer (13). The lowest frequency (31% to 40%) and severity of weight loss were found in patients with breast cancer, hematologic cancers, and sarcomas. Intermediate frequency of weight loss was found in patients with colonic, prostatic, and lung cancer (54% to 64%). Patients with cancer of the pancreas and stomach had the highest frequency (over 80%) and severity of weight loss. Approximately 35% of the patients with lung cancer lost more than 5% of their body weight. This underscores the fact that even if the tumor does not involve the gastrointestinal tract directly, there can be significant weight loss because of systemic and metabolic derangements and loss of appetite. The study did not report on patients with gynecologic malignancies in whom weight loss can also be very frequent and severe. Other studies revealed that over 40% of patients receiving medical treatment for a variety of cancers were malnourished (14,15). Among surgical patients in a Veterans Administration hospital, 39% of those undergoing a major operation for cancer were malnourished, as judged by either a nutrition risk index or a combination of weight loss and low serum proteins (16). In a study from the Memorial Sloan–Kettering Cancer Center, the majority of patients with pancreatic cancer undergoing a curative resection were malnourished as determined by weight loss (17).

Data on the prevalence and impact of malnutrition in patients with gynecologic tumors are limited. The findings in these patients mirror the observations in patients with other cancers. A recent study of 67 consecutive patients hospitalized with gynecologic cancers at the University of Texas found that 54% of the women were malnourished as determined by the prognostic nutritional index (18). In 1983, Tunca (19) examined the nutritional state of gynecologic oncology patients at time of diagnosis using serum albumin, serum transferrin, immune response, and weight loss. Patients with advanced (stage III or IV) ovarian carcinoma had the highest incidence of severe malnutrition, whereas those with cancer of the cervix, endometrium, or vulva reported weight loss with no indication of malnutrition from serum markers or immune response testing. Twenty of the 21 patients with advanced ovarian carcinoma were anergic to recall antigens, and the mean levels of all serum markers examined were significantly lower than those found in patients with early (stage I or II) ovarian carcinoma or cancer of the cervix, vulva, or endometrium. Orr et al. (20,21) assessed the degree of protein-calorie malnutrition and evidence of vitamin deficiency in 78 patients with untreated cervical cancer. The incidence of protein-calorie malnutrition as assessed by anthropometrics, serum markers, and immune testing was directly related to tumor stage; 4% in stage I, 20% in stages II and III, and 60% in stage IV disease (20). Two-thirds of patients with untreated cervical cancer were found to have reduced blood levels of at least one vitamin. Mean serum levels of folate, beta-carotene, and vitamin C at the time of admission were all significantly below control values (21). Similar observations of significant protein-calorie malnutrition were seen in 25 patients with endometrial cancer (22).

At the Memorial Sloan–Kettering Cancer Center, 49 inpatients with gynecologic malignancies were referred to the clinical nutrition service over a 2-year period (1998 to 2000). This represented a diverse group of patients, with the vast majority being evaluated for support with parenteral nutrition and tended to represent the sickest population. Thirty-five of the patients had ovarian cancer, 6 had endometrial cancer, 7 had cervical cancer, and 1 patient had cancer of the vulva. Twenty patients had intestinal obstruction, 7 had enterocutaneous fistulae, 3 had intractable nausea and vomiting, 8 had prolonged ileus (>5 days), and the remainder had gastric outlet obstruction, mucositis, or dysphagia. The average weight loss in this group at the time of consultation was 8 kg, which represented a loss of 9.1% of the usual body weight. The weight loss in these patients was multifactorial in origin, secondary to the effects of the tumor and therapeu-

tic interventions on the gastrointestinal tract, decreased appetite, and possibly metabolic effects of the underlying malignancy. These patients representing the sickest of those with gynecologic malignancies demonstrate the association between the frequently seen complications (e.g., fistulae, intestinal obstruction, ileus) and significant weight loss.

SIGNIFICANCE OF MALNUTRITION

The impact of malnutrition on the cancer patient was demonstrated in a report by Warren in 1932 (23). Based on data from autopsies, the conclusion was that cachexia was the leading cause of death in a group of 400 patients with various cancers. More recent studies have confirmed the significant impact of malnutrition on the quality of life and prognosis of the cancer patient. In the aforementioned multicenter cooperative study of patients receiving chemotherapy (13), those who presented with weight loss at the time of diagnosis had decreased performance status and survival as compared with those without weight loss. In a study of patients with limited, inoperable lung cancer, weight loss was a major predictive factor for survival (14). The negative impact of malnutrition was also demonstrated in surgical patients with malignant and benign diseases. Malnourished patients undergoing a major operation were at greater risk for postoperative morbidity and mortality than were well-nourished patients (16,24).

The impact of malnutrition in patients with a primary gynecologic malignancy is striking. In 1988, while examining the role of total parenteral nutrition (TPN) in their patients, Terada and colleagues noted that those patients who developed major complications such as a fistula, wound infection, pneumonia, renal failure, respiratory failure, or died had significantly more weight loss and lower serum transferrin levels at the time of presentation (25). They concluded that these parameters might be of value in predicting clinical outcome in patients requiring nutritional support. Undernutrition also adversely affects surgical outcome in patients with primary gynecologic malignancies. Burnett et al. (26) reported that in 92 gynecologic oncology patients requiring colonic surgery, those who were classified as malnourished on the basis of serum markers were significantly more likely to develop major perioperative complications or die. Donato et al. (27) reported that of 104 patients with ovarian carcinoma undergoing intestinal surgery those considered to be malnourished on the basis of serum protein measurements and weight loss preoperatively had significantly more infectious complications, whereas other variables including preoperative bowel obstruction, extent of debulking, number of intestinal procedures, or hand versus stapled anastomosis failed to correlate with the rate of infectious complications (27). In 1993, Massad reported on 128 patients undergoing operations by the gynecologic oncology service at Barnes Hospital in St. Louis and showed that serum markers of malnutrition including decreased preoperative albumin and hemoglobin concentrations were strong indicators of increased length of hospitalization (28). Among women with gynecologic cancers who were hospitalized for any reason, malnutrition was associated with prolonged hospital stay (18).

ETIOLOGY OF MALNUTRITION

Cancer can induce a wide variety of derangements in the nutritional status ranging from generalized malnutrition with severe weight loss and muscle wasting to a single nutrient deficiency. The etiology of malnutrition in the cancer patient is multifactorial. Nutritionally relevant derangements can be induced by the tumor locally (i.e., gastrointestinal obstruction), by malabsorption, by humoral factors produced by the tumor itself, or by reaction of the immune system to the tumor. All modalities of cancer therapy—surgery, radiation, chemotherapy, immunotherapy, and palliative treatments—may be associated with side effects and complications that can impair the nutritional status.

The etiologic factors of malnutrition in the cancer patient whether caused by the tumor or antitumor therapies can be classified into three major categories: decreased food intake, malabsorption, and metabolic derangements that result in inefficient, wasteful metabolism.

Impaired Food Intake and Absorption

Both tumor and cancer treatment modalities can lead to decreased food intake through direct effects on the gastrointestinal tract or systemic effects leading to anorexia. Obstruction of the gastrointestinal tract can be caused by any gynecologic malignancy through external compression or, more rarely, by direct invasion. Although at times localized obstructions can be relieved surgically, the obstruction due to peritoneal carcinomatosis often seen in advanced ovarian cancer is particularly difficult to manage surgically. Often, draining gastrostomy with parenteral nutrition (when appropriate) is the only option for providing nutritional and symptomatic relief (29–31).

Tumors can induce anorexia without local involvement of the gastrointestinal tract. The pathophysiology of this phenomenon is not well understood. Norton et al. (32) utilized a model of surgically coupled tumor-bearing and normal rats with parabiotic cross circulation to show that tumor-induced anorexia is mediated by circulating substances. Tumor-induced impairment of smell and taste has been well described (24,33–36), but the mechanism has not been defined. There is growing evidence that cytokines play an important role in the pathogenesis of cancer cachexia. Bernstein et al. (37, 38) demonstrated in a rat model that infusion of tumor necrosis factor (TNF) mimics tumor-induced anorexia, and these effects are mediated via the area postrema and the caudal medial nucleus of the solitary tract in the central nervous system.

Therapies used for gynecologic malignancies often result in complications that impair nutrient intake and absorption. Surgical interventions can lead to fistulae, short bowel syndrome, infections, and ileus, all of which impair oral intake significantly. In a review of 12 years of colonic surgery in gynecologic oncology patients, the rate for major systemic complications (myocardial infarction, pulmonary embolism, renal failure, sepsis) was 13.7%, and the rate of major bowel complications (abscess, fistulae, hemorrhage, obstruction) was 12.1% (26). Adjuvant radiation and chemotherapy have been shown to increase the incidence of major complications after pelvic exenteration (39).

Radiotherapy can lead to various derangements in the structure and function of the gastrointestinal tract. Damage to the gastrointestinal tract following radiation to the abdomen and pelvis most commonly affects the small bowel, followed by the transverse colon, sigmoid, and rectum. Predisposing risk factors include pervious abdominal surgery, pelvic inflammatory disease, thin body habitus, hypertension, and diabetes mellitus (40). In general, a dose of 5,000 Gy is the threshold for significant injury. In the acute phase of radiation enteritis, virtually all patients experience anorexia, nausea, and vomiting that are thought to be mediated by effects of serotonin on the gut (41) and the central nervous system (42). This is followed 2 to 3 weeks later by diarrhea caused by direct injury to the intestinal mucosa resulting in diarrhea and mild to moderate malabsorption. Most patients will have complete resolution of these acute symptoms. However, a significant minority of patients who received radiotherapy will experience chronic dysfunction of the gastrointestinal tract (43). There is often a latent period of 1 to 2 years and possibly as long as 20 years before the symptoms of chronic radiation enteropathy surface (44,45). In a review of 102 patients with radiation enteritis after treatment for cervical or endometrial cancer, the median time to development of severe symptoms such as obstruction or perforation was 18 months (46).

Chronic radiation enteropathy is characterized pathologically by transmural injury leading to submucosal fibrosis, edema, lymphatic ectasia, and obliterative endarteritis, which can induce colicky abdominal pain, diarrhea, steatorrhea, ulceration, perforation, stricture, and fistula formation (40). Yeoh et al. (47) retrospectively studied the effects of pelvic irradiation given for the treatment of cervical cancer in 30 randomly selected women who had undergone radiotherapy 1 to 6 years earlier. Significant dysfunction of the gastrointestinal tract was detected. Nineteen of the patients had frequency of bowel movements, bile acid absorption, and vitamin B_{12} absorption outside of the control range. The investigators concluded that abnormal gastrointestinal function is essentially an inevitable long-term complication of pelvic irradiation (47). Husebye and colleagues (48) prospectively studied the gastrointestinal motility patterns in 41 patients with chronic abdominal complaints after radiotherapy for gynecologic cancer. Impaired fasting motility was found in 29% of patients, and motor response after a meal was attenuated in 24%.

Postparandial delay of the migrating motor complex was found to be an independent predictor of malnutrition as assessed by weight loss and serum albumin. Impaired motility of the small bowel, therefore, is a key factor in the symptoms experienced by patients with chronic radiation enteropathy (48). Chronic radiation enteritis predisposes to numerous secondary complications. Danielsson et al. (49) studied 20 patients with chronic or intermittent diarrhea occurring in women 2 or more years after receiving radiotherapy for gynecologic tumors. Bile acid malabsorption was detected in 65% of patients, whereas evidence of bacterial overgrowth on D-xylose or cholyl-glycine breath tests was found in 45%. Treatment with bile acid binders or antibiotics resulted in a significant decline in the number of daily bowel movements. The investigators concluded that treatment of these secondary complications of radiation-induced enteropathy can offer significant symptomatic relief. In 47 patients with gynecologic malignancies who had gastrointestinal complaints lasting more than 4 months after radiotherapy, Kwitko et al. (50) found 19 partial small bowel obstructions, 11 cases of malabsorption, and 5 fistulae. Improved fractionation of radiotherapy and protective shielding of the intestine where possible have reduced these complication rates (51). More recent studies of patients who received radiation therapy for uterine cancer found the prevalence of significant chronic radiation enteritis to be approximately 4% (52).

Chemotherapy is often associated with decreased food intake. Odynophagia, oral ulcers, and diarrhea are commonly seen during therapy with cytotoxic agents that affect the replicating cells of the intestinal mucosa such as 5-flourouracil, methotrexate, and bleomycin. The vinca alkaloids can cause ileus and constipation mediated by toxic effects on gastrointestinal neural pathways, whereas cisplatin and nitrosoureas are highly emetic (53,54). Significant nausea, vomiting, stomatitis, and diarrhea occur in 15% of patients receiving intravenous paclitaxel (Taxol) and 55% in those receiving the drug orally (55).

The psychologic impact of a malignancy and its associated therapies can also lead to decreased nutrient intake. Depression is a frequent cause of anorexia in this population, and learned food aversions are a common consequence of radiation or chemotherapy. As many as 56% of patients undergoing chemotherapy and 62% of those undergoing radiation therapy developed a learned food aversion in one study (56). This is characterized by a psychologic association between the consumption of a particular food and a temporally related unpleasant reaction to the therapy such as nausea and vomiting. This results in future avoidance of that particular food item. A recent Swedish study of patients with ovarian cancer showed that a multidisciplinary approach involving antiemetic drugs in conjunction with anxiolytics, training in relaxation techniques, nutritional advice, and continuity of nursing care resulted in significantly less cisplatin-induced emesis than antiemetics alone (57).

Metabolic Derangements

Even with normal nutrient intake, patients with cancer are at risk for malnutrition due to inefficient nutrient utilization and wasteful metabolic pathways. Compared to simple starvation, cancer cachexia is associated with altered metabolism of carbohydrates, fat, protein, vitamins, and minerals. Therefore, in order to optimize nutritional support in the cancer patient, it is imperative to consider metabolic derangements along with problems of ingestion, digestion, and absorption.

An increase in basal energy expenditure has been reported in many, but not all, studies of patients with malignancy (58–64). In patients with newly diagnosed small-cell lung cancer, Russell et al. (62) showed a mean increase of 37% in basal energy expenditure that fell substantially in those who responded to chemotherapy. Similar findings have been reported for gastric cancer (59) and sarcoma (65). Elevated basal energy expenditure will drop after tumor resection (66). There are limited data on the metabolic rate in patients with gynecologic cancers (64). Dickerson et al. (67) used indirect calorimetry to determine the resting energy expenditure in 31 patients with ovarian cancer and 30 patients with cervical cancer. Fifty-five percent of those with ovarian cancer were found to be hypermetabolic [basal energy expenditure (BEE) >110% predicted by the Harris-Benedict equation], whereas only 13% of patients with cervical cancer were hypermetabolic. These differences could not be explained by differences in the extent of disease, nutritional status, body temperature, or nutrient intake.

Abnormalities in carbohydrate metabolism in cancer patients include glucose intolerance and peripheral insulin resistance (68–71). These most often become apparent in the patient with advanced metastatic cancer found to have hyperglycemia that is refractory to high-dose insulin infusion (71, 72). In comparison, in simple starvation, patients are most often euglycemic or hypoglycemic. The hyperglycemia in cancer patients is exacerbated by increased hepatic gluconeogenesis. Shaw et al. (73) showed that this increase in glucose production is correlated with tumor burden and decreases after tumor resection. A number of energy-wasting metabolic cycles involving glucose have been identified. In the Cori cycle, glucose is converted to lactate by tumor cells and by the liver. This futile cycle results in a net loss of adenosine triphosphate (ATP) and may contribute to the loss of energy and weight experienced by the cancer patient (64, 74,75).

Lipid metabolism may also be abnormal in patients with a malignancy. There is often increased lipolysis with weight loss, and this leads to a decrease in fat mass that can be out of proportion to the loss of lean body mass (70,76). In addition, patients with cancer are often hyperlipidemic and this may be mediated by TNF-α (77). In contrast to normal homeostasis, cancer patients fail to suppress lipolysis with glucose infusion (73).

High total body protein turnover, with increased synthesis and catabolism, characterizes the alterations of protein metabolism seen in cancer patients (78,79). This results in depletion of muscle mass and loss of nitrogen and contrasts with the adaptive decrease in protein turnover seen in patients with uncomplicated starvation (80). TPN given to patients with cancer will result in gains of weight and body fat and net gains of total body nitrogen but no suppression of the high-protein flux (79,80).

Cytokines play an important role in inducing the metabolic derangements seen in the cancer patient (64). They mediate increased energy expenditure, whole body protein turnover, rise in serum triglyceride levels, and high glycerol turnover (23,81). TNF can be detected in the serum of cancer patients (82), and in animal models, it causes protein wasting, depletion of body fat, and anorexia (83,84). High serum levels of interleukin-1 and interleukin-6 are also present in patients with advanced cancer and cachexia. Interventions to downregulate these cytokines result in improved appetite, body weight, and quality of life (85).

The combined effects of these wasteful and inefficient alterations in metabolism make it difficult to restore nutritional status in the patient with cancer and cachexia despite the use of specialized nutritional support. This is in contrast with what is seen in patients with uncomplicated starvation who exhibit changes in metabolism that act to conserve energy and body tissues and in whom nutritional support is highly efficacious in reversing the effects of malnutrition.

NUTRITIONAL THERAPIES

There are four types of nutritional therapies: parenteral nutrition, enteral nutrition, oral dietary therapy, and drug therapy aimed at improving appetite and food intake. Depending on the patient's condition, nutritional support in the cancer patient has two distinct objectives: (a) provision of nutrition during anticancer therapies to counteract their nutritionally related side effects and improve outcome following these therapies; and (b) support in patients with long-term or permanent severe impairment of the gastrointestinal tract. In these patients, nutritional support may be required for indefinite periods of time. Results of numerous clinical trials support the use of nutritional support only in limited situations during anticancer therapies. In the group with prolonged gastrointestinal failure, nutritional support may be a lifesaving therapy because patients could die of starvation without TPN or enteral feeding.

Total Parenteral Nutrition

TPN is an effective method for delivery of nutrients directly into the blood, and thus overcomes the major causes of cancer cachexia, including decreased food intake and dysfunction of the gastrointestinal tract. Survival for more than 20 years in patients nourished exclusively by TPN clearly demonstrates the lifesaving role of this method of nutritional support. Initially, it seemed logical that TPN would be an effective adjuvant therapy for most cancer patients undergoing radiation therapy, surgery, or chemotherapy because of the accompanying cachexia and inability to eat adequately. Randomized studies, however, have shown that TPN only benefits a select subgroup of cancer patients during anticancer therapy.

Efficacy

In patients receiving chemotherapy with or without radiation therapy, TPN can lead to improvements of several nutritional parameters. Both body weight and body fat increase (80). Deficits of specific vitamins, minerals, and trace elements can be corrected and hydration status can be improved (80,86). TPN, however, does not alter many of the metabolic derangements encountered in the cancer patient. Increased glucose oxidation and turnover persist (73,87), as does muscle proteolysis (88,89) and increased lipolysis (90). Finally, TPN does not stop the overall losses of body nitrogen (91). The relevant issue for the clinician is the effect of TPN on the morbidity and mortality associated with cancer therapy and whether TPN can allow more intense therapy as was initially hoped. Numerous randomized trials have examined this issue. Studies of patients undergoing chemotherapy for carcinoma of the ovary (29), lung (92,93), colon (91), testes (94), lymphoma (95), and other tumors (96) have been conducted. However, the patients in these studies were largely unselected. Many were not malnourished and others had adequate oral intake with intact gastrointestinal function, thus making intravenous nutrition unnecessary and futile. Numerous meta-analyses concluded that nondiscriminatory use of TPN in patients undergoing chemotherapy offers no improvement in mortality, response to chemotherapy, or reduction in treatment-associated complications (97–99). This conclusion was echoed in a recent joint consensus statement from the National Institutes of Health, the American Society for Parenteral and Enteral Nutrition, and the American Society for Clinical Nutrition (100). The improvement in nutritional parameters afforded by TPN in patients receiving chemotherapy is not necessarily translated into improved clinical outcome. Thus, the routine use of TPN in these patients is not indicated. There are circumstances, however, in which nutritional support with parenteral nutrition should be considered. These include prevention of the effects of starvation in a patient unable to tolerate oral or enteral feedings for a prolonged period of time (usually more than 7 to 10 days), maximization of performance status in a malnourished patient prior to chemotherapy or surgery, and in patients undergoing bone marrow transplantation (101).

TPN may have a stimulatory effect on tumor cell cycle

kinetics (102). It has been suggested that this effect would induce improved tumor response to cell cycle–specific chemotherapy. Conclusive proof of such a response remains elusive.

A few randomized studies have examined the use of TPN in patients receiving radiotherapy to the abdomen and pelvis (103–106). Theses studies did not show any clear benefit from the routine administration of TPN.

The role of TPN in the perioperative period has been extensively studied (16,17,107–111). In an early study by Mueller et al. (111), 10 days of preoperative TPN was associated with nutritional improvement and significant reduction in major postoperative complications and mortality. These impressive results have not been confirmed in subsequent studies. At the Memorial Sloan–Kettering Cancer Center, a prospective study of 117 patients undergoing curative resection for pancreatic cancer randomized to receive TPN or intravenous fluids in the postoperative period showed no benefit from routine the use of postoperative TPN (17). The group receiving TPN had a significant increase in postoperative infectious complications. The largest prospective randomized trial investigating the role of TPN in the perioperative setting was the Veterans Administration Cooperative Study (16). In this study, 395 patients were randomized to receive 7 to 15 days of preoperative TPN and 3 days of postoperative TPN or oral feeding plus intravenous fluids. TPN did not improve morbidity or 90-day mortality. However, subgroup analysis showed that patients considered to be severely malnourished had fewer infectious complications if they received TPN. The investigators concluded that the routine administration of preoperative TPN should be limited to patients who are severely malnourished unless there are other specific indications.

Randomized studies specifically examining the role of perioperative TPN in patients with gynecologic malignancies are lacking. In a report by Terada (25), perioperative parenteral nutritional support was given to 84 of 99 patients. There were no major complications attributed to TPN, but 27% of the patients experienced minor complications: 11% due to central line placement or catheter sepsis, 2% due to fluid overload, and 13 % had metabolic complications. There was no report on overall perioperative morbidity or mortality in comparison to patients who did not receive perioperative TPN.

These data and others provide the basis for the recent joint consensus statement from the National Institutes of Health, the American Society for Parenteral and Enteral Nutrition, and the American Society for Clinical Nutrition regarding the use of perioperative TPN that states the following: (a) 7 to 10 days of preoperative TPN in a malnourished patient with gastrointestinal cancer results in a 10% reduction in postoperative complications; (b) routine use of postoperative TPN in malnourished surgical patients who did not receive preoperative TPN results in a 10% *increase* in complications; and (c) if by postoperative days 5 to 10, a patient is

TABLE 35.1. *Indications for TPN in hospitalized patients with gynecologic Cancers*

Perioperative
  7–10 days preoperatively in a malnourished patient (who cannot be fed enterally)
  Postoperative complications which prevent oral or enteral intake for more than 7–10 days
  Enterocutaneous fistula
  No indication for routine use
During radiation or chemotherapy
  Maximization of performance status prior to therapy in a malnourished patient who cannot be fed enterally
  Severe persistent (more than 7–10 days) mucositis, diarrhea, ileus, or emesis
  No indication for routine use
General
  After 7–10 days of inability to tolerate oral or enteral feeding due to any cause

unable to tolerate oral or enteral feedings, then TPN is indicated to prevent the adverse effects of starvation. This panel, however, cautions that in the majority of studies looking at perioperative TPN, the amount and type of parenteral nutrition given was not optimal, and often patients were given excess calories. Therefore, the results may differ with the provision of relatively hypocaloric formulas (100). It is reasonable to extend these recommendations to the gynecologic oncology patient undergoing surgery (Table 35.1).

Composition of TPN solution

Once the decision to proceed with parenteral nutritional support is made, access to a large-bore central vein should be obtained. This allows the use of calorically dense, hypertonic solutions that are often necessary in severely ill patients who may have restriction on the amount of intravenous fluids they can receive. When possible, this line should be used exclusively for TPN infusion and should be treated with strict aseptic technique. The composition of the TPN solution should be individualized based on the patient's condition and requirements, preferably by a dedicated nutritional support team (112). The solution must provide the protein and caloric needs, fluid, minerals, trace elements, and vitamins. Although indirect calorimetry and nitrogen balance can be used to determine energy and protein requirements, these measurements are too costly and cumbersome for routine use. There are numerous formulas, charts, and tables that can provide estimates of protein and caloric requirements. Estimates of nutritional requirements are based on weight and adjusted for the degree of physiologic stress encountered by the patient. Generally, patients require 30 Kcal/kg nonprotein calories, 1 g/kg amino acids, and about 2,000 mL of fluid. As illness severity increases, and organs' functions change, adjustments may be required. Thus, patients with kidney or liver failure require decreased amounts of amino acids, whereas those with heart failure require restriction of sodium and fluids. Nonprotein calories can be provided as dextrose or lipid and the relative amounts of these should also be individualized. Lipids provide 9.0 Kcal/g compared to 3.4 for dextrose. (In dextrose solutions, the glucose is present as glucosemonohydrate; hence a gram contains <4 Kcal.) Lipid calories are particularly useful in patients who have high caloric requirements but cannot tolerate a large fluid load. In addition, lipids are useful in patients with severe pulmonary or hepatic dysfunction as glucose metabolism produces more carbon dioxide, which can add to the burden of the ailing lung and can lead to fatty infiltration of the liver. Up to 60% of caloric requirements can be provided as lipid, but serum triglyceride levels must be monitored closely. Appropriate electrolyte content of TPN solutions is of critical importance. The amounts have to be tailored to the patients requirements and organ's function. Care must be taken to prevent potentially fatal hypokalemia or hypophosphatemia (particularly in the patient with severe weight loss) that can be precipitated by insulin-induced transport of the minerals to the intracellular space when inadequate amounts are given. Other electrolytic disorders such as cisplatin-induced hypomagnesemia and the syndrome of inappropriate secretion of antidiuretic hormone (SIADH) are common in the patient with gynecologic malignancy and must be addressed when ordering TPN. The TPN solution must also contain vitamins, minerals, and trace elements. Typically, these are available as standard commercial combination products. However, certain patients require specific modifications. For example, a patient with persistent diarrhea requires zinc supplementation in excess of the amounts present in standard trace element solutions.

Complications

Complications associated with TPN can be classified as catheter related, metabolic, or infectious. Catheter complications most often occur during placement of a central venous catheter and include pneumothorax, hemothorax, arterial injury, and hematoma. These can all be minimized when the procedure is performed by an experienced physician (113). Cobb et al. (114) reported a 3% incidence of pneumothorax, arrhythmia, thrombus, or bleeding during 523 intravenous catheter placements. A more recent study of subcutaneous peripheral infusion ports in women with gynecologic malignancies demonstrated a thrombosis rate of 26% during a mean follow up of 105 days. The investigators concluded that other types of vascular access devices may be preferable in this patient population (115).

Metabolic derangements are frequently encountered during support with TPN, and the prescribing physician must be well versed in the pathophysiology of these disorders. Hyperglycemia is the most common abnormality (113) and if not corrected can lead to an osmotic diuresis, dehydration, acidosis, and hyperosmolar coma. Patients receiving parenteral nutrition should have continuous monitoring for glycos-

uria, and if the dipstick is positive, the blood sugar concentration should be determined and sliding scale insulin coverage should be provided. One metabolic complication that deserves special mention is the "refeeding syndrome." In chronically ill patients with severe malnutrition, there is often a depletion of total body phosphorus and potassium. The phosphorus deficits may be masked by increased renal phosphorus absorption designed to maintain normal serum levels. When TPN is initiated, the infusion of a large glucose load with subsequent surge in insulin leads to increased cellular uptake of phosphorus and potassium that may induce severe life-threatening hypokalemia and hypophosphatemia (116,117). These disorders cause widespread tissue and organ dysfunction including muscle weakness, rhabdomyolysis, heart failure, cardiac arrhythmias, and repiratory failure and may result in death in extreme cases (117). Therefore, in patients with evidence of severe undernutrition, TPN should be initiated with small amounts of dextrose calories, supplemental phosphorus and potassium, and careful monitoring of serum phosphorus and electrolytes.

TPN has been associated with cholestatic liver disease as well as fatty infiltration of the liver and glycogen deposition. These abnormalities have been attributed to infusion of excessive glucose calories, imbalance of amino acids, and rarely fatty acid deficiency (118). Elevation of serum transaminases may occur, but it is generally mild (118,119). Severe liver dysfunction in adult TPN recipients is rare and requires a search for causes other than TPN.

Infections are particularly serious complications in patients with malignancy receiving TPN. In an evaluation of seven studies comparing TPN plus chemotherapy to chemotherapy alone, Koretz found four studies that showed an increase in infectious complications in patients receiving TPN1 (105). A meta-analysis by the American College of Nutrition showed a fourfold increase in infections when patients receiving chemotherapy were given TPN (97). In a prospective randomized study of TPN following pancreatic resection, recipients of TPN had significantly more infectious complications (17). Data from a VA randomized cooperative study showed that patients with mild to moderate malnutrition given perioperative TPN had increased rates of infections, whereas those with severe malnutrition developed significantly fewer infections when supported with TPN1 (16). Infectious complications are related to both central venous catheters and a variety of sites (wound infection, abscess, and pneumonia). Although there are now promising data to show that the use of catheters impregnated with antimicrobials may provide a significant reduction of catheter-related sepsis (120), it is not clear that the use of these catheters will eliminate the increase in infections in patients receiving TPN.

Home TPN

Long-term TPN in the home can be a lifesaving treatment in an appropriately selected group of patients. It is clear that cancer patients who have had severe gastrointestinal injury, such as massive intestinal resection or severe radiation enteritis, and in whom the cancer has been cured or is well controlled, can benefit from long-term TPN at home (121). Survival rates and TPN-related complications in such patients are comparable to those seen in patients with benign diseases (Crohn's disease, intestinal necrosis) who require home TPN. Among patients with widely metastatic disease and poor prognosis, home TPN offers very limited benefit (89). Only 15% of such patients survive longer than 1 year on home TPN (48). Recently developed techniques for placing feeding tubes make it possible to hydrate and feed patients enterally even in the presence of gastrointestinal obstruction (101), and thus obviate the need for home TPN in patients with upper gastrointestinal tract dysfunction. In terminally ill patients, TPN should be avoided. The concern that such patients should not be "starved to death" is not a justification for TPN. A recent noncontrolled study of terminally ill cancer patients hospitalized at a long-term care facility suggests that these patients did not experience hunger or thirst, and that in those who experienced such symptoms, small amounts of food alleviated the symptoms (122). In such patients, the utilization of TPN either in the home of at health-care facilities cannot be justified.

At the Memorial Sloan–Kettering Cancer Center, the clinical nutrition service prescribed home TPN for 20 patients with gynecologic malignancies (3 cervical, 15 ovarian, and 2 endometrial) from 1995 through 1998. This represented 9% of all cancer patients given this therapy. The indications for home TPN included bowel obstruction (ten patients), enterocutaneous fistula (seven patients), radiation enteritis (two patients), and short bowel syndrome (one patient). These patients were given home TPN because they had a good performance status or were considered to be candidates for further antitumor therapies. On average, they received home TPN for 163 days. Thirteen of the patients were able to resume oral or enteral feedings in amounts sufficient to sustain themselves after additional therapy and seven patients died while still dependent on TPN.

For patients with inoperable bowel obstruction due to metastatic ovarian cancer, predicting which patients will benefit from home TPN can be difficult (123). In a review of 9,897 days of home TPN administered to 75 patients with various cancers and intestinal obstruction, it was shown that a Karnofsky performance status >50 at the initiation of TPN could accurately predict which patients would have improved quality of life while on home TPN. The investigators concluded that home TPN should be avoided if the performance status is below this level (124). In addition, patients with a life expectancy of less than 2 to 3 months will not benefit from home TPN (89,124). In a study from Yale–New Haven Hospital of 17 patients with inoperable bowel obstruction due to malignancy, patients with ovarian cancer had the shortest survival (39 days) compared to patients with colonic cancer (90 days) and appendiceal cancer (184 days)

TABLE 35.2. *Indications for home total parenteral nutrition in patients with gynecologic cancers*

Severe chronic radiation enteropathy
Short bowel syndrome
Persistent enterocutaneous fistula
Selected patients with obstruction due to peritoneal carcinomatosis (Selection based on performance status and potential for further chemotherapy)

(125). Therefore, only a highly selected minority of patients with inoperable bowel obstruction can potentially benefit from home TPN. Currently, the best selection criteria for such patients are a fair or better performance status and the potential for further antitumor therapy (Table 35.2).

Enteral Nutrition

Enteral feeding delivers a liquid nutrient formula into the gastrointestinal tract through tubes placed into the stomach or small intestine. As in oral feeding, an adequately functioning small intestinal mucosa is required for absorption of nutrients. Enteral feeding can overcome many difficulties encountered in patients with a wide variety of gastrointestinal tract dysfunctions. A proximal gastrointestinal obstruction can be bypassed; tubes can be placed distal to obstructions as far as the jejunum and thus circumvent obstructing lesions of the oral cavity, esophagus, stomach, duodenum, or proximal jejunum (126,127). The liquid nutrient formula can be delivered as a slow, continuous infusion, thus maximizing absorption by a limited intestinal surface that can be overwhelmed by the higher volume delivered during oral feeding. Such an approach may be useful in patients with radiation enteritis, short bowel syndrome (with adequate remaining short bowel, usually 3 to 4 ft), or partial obstruction of the bowel.

Route of Administration and Nutrient Formula

Short-term (<2 weeks) access to the gastrointestinal tract can be obtained through nasogastric or nasoenteric tubes. Patients requiring longer nutritional support should have a gastrostomy or jejunostomy tube placed endoscopically, radiologically, or surgically. In comparison to nasal tubes, gastrostomy or jejumostomy tubes are wider (15 to 24 French) and therefore less likely to be obstructed by medications or nutrient solutions. In addition, they are fixed in the stomach or the upper intestine and do not migrate into the esophagus. Thus, the risk of aspiration is considerably decreased (126). These tubes are more comfortable and esthetically pleasing (128). These benefits were demonstrated in a recent randomized study of patients after an acute dysphagic stroke that showed patients fed with a gastrostomy tube had more optimal provision of nutrients, achieved a better nutritional state, and had less mortality than those fed with nasogastric tubes (129). Patients with gastrostomy tubes have been shown in prospective studies to receive over 90% of prescribed feedings compared to only 55% in patients fed through nasal tubes. These differences are largely attributed to nasogastric tube dislodgment (130). In a randomized study of 33 women with gynecologic malignancies, enteral feedings through a needle catheter jejunostomy maintained postoperative nutrition as measured by serum transferrin levels and was associated with few complications (131). The investigators concluded that women with gynecologic cancers should have a jejunostomy placed at the time of operation if it is anticipated that long-term nutritional support will be required.

Recently, the endoscopically placed percutaneous gastrostomy tube (PEG) has become the procedure of choice for placement of enteral feeding tubes because of its ease, safety, and the ability to perform it on an outpatient basis. Percutaneous jejunostomy (PEJ) tubes can also be placed endoscopically (127). PEJs allow for continued enteral feeding in patients with gastric resection, gastric outlet obstruction, or gastroparesis. Major complications (bleeding, peritonitis, abdominal wall abscess, colonic perforation, and aspiration) from PEG and PEJ placement are rare; occurring in 0% to 2.5% of patients, whereas minor complications (wound infection, tube migrations, or leak) are seen in 5% to 15% (65, 127,132,133). This favorably compares to the 2.5% to 16% complication rate and 1% to 6% mortality from a laparotomy required for surgical placement of feeding tubes (134–136).

More than 1,000 different enteral feeding formulas are currently commercially available (137). They are designed to provide either complete nutrition, single nutrients, or only fluids and electrolytes. Formulas differ in protein concentration, calories, osmolarity, and percentage of nonprotein calories delivered as carbohydrates or fats. Enteral feeding formulas that provide 1,500 to 2,000 Kcal/day normally contain all the necessary nutrients including proteins, vitamins, minerals, and trace elements. In addition, there are disease-specific formulations for patients with diabetes or hepatic, renal, or pulmonary dysfunction. The choice of formula should be individualized and often helps to minimize problems such as diarrhea, bloating, or hyperglycemia (126).

Enteral solutions may be administered by either bolus feedings or by continuous infusion (126,134,135). Bolus feeding is possible when the tip of the feeding tube is in an intact stomach. Up to 500 mL of a feeding formula can be infused over 10 to 15 minutes by a syringe or gravity into the stomach. The pyloric sphincter regulates flow into the duodenum. All bolus feedings should be done with the patient sitting upright to minimize the risk of aspiration. When the tip of the feeding tube is distal to the pylorus, continuous feeding must be employed to avoid abdominal distention and diarrhea. Rates as high as 150mL/h are generally well tolerated (126).

Efficacy

Data from randomized trials examining the efficacy of enteral nutrition given as an adjuvant therapy in patients receiving chemotherapy for a variety of cancers have failed to demonstrate a clear benefit in terms of survival or response to treatment (138–142). The validity of the conclusions of these studies, however, is limited by their small size and poor design. Similar difficulties plague the studies examining the role of standard enteral nutrition in the perioperative period (143–146). Although recent data examining early (postoperative day 1) enteral feeding in patients following resection of an upper gastrointestinal tract tumor showed improved protein metabolism, there is no evidence that this translates into improved clinical outcome (147). In a prospective randomized study of early enteral feeding in 195 patients after resection of upper gastrointestinal malignancy, there was no proven benefit. Complication rates, mortality, and length of hospital stay were not affected by early postoperative enteral feedings (148). Therefore, routine use of enteral nutritional support in patients receiving chemotherapy or undergoing operations for cancer cannot be justified. Accepted indications for enteral nutrition in cancer patients include (a) obstruction of the upper digestive tract in those who are not candidates for an operation, (b) the presence of chronic malnutrition due to inadequate oral intake, and (c) perioperative support of the malnourished patient (149).

Complications

Enteral nutrition is generally safe if careful attention is paid to the following: (a) choice of an appropriate formula, (b) infusion into an appropriate portion of the gastrointestinal tract, (c) use of the correct infusion method, and (d) an ongoing clinical and metabolic monitoring of the patient. The most serious complication of enteral feeding is aspiration, which occurs in 1% to 32% of patients (138,150,151). The risk is minimized by keeping patients upright during bolus feedings and using jejunal feedings if there is predisposition for aspiration, gastroparesis, or an impaired gag reflex. Diarrhea is reported in 5% to 30% of patients receiving enteral nutrition (152). Although the diarrhea may be related to underlying disorders of the gastrointestinal tract such as radiation enteritis or short bowel syndrome, a commonly overlooked cause is medications. Patients on enteral feeding often receive magnesium-containing antacids or antibiotics, both of which may induce diarrhea. Metabolic complications include dehydration, azotemia, hyperglycemia, and hyperkalemia. These are usually due to the patient's underlying disease and can be avoided with the choice of the proper formula and careful monitoring.

Home Enteral Nutrition

Home enteral nutrition (HEN) is increasingly being used to provide nutrients and fluids outside the hospital. Cancer is the most common indication for its use and accounts for 42% of all patients receiving HEN (121,126). It is a safe therapy in patients with cancer with only a 0.4% annual rate of complications requiring hospitalization (153). The overall 1-year survival for cancer patients on HEN is 30%; however, in patients with cancer of the head and neck who have been successfully treated, HEN has provided good nutrition for periods exceeding 7 years (65,126). Regular medical follow-up is essential to ensure appropriate functioning of the feeding tube and optimization of the nutritional regimen. This form of therapy is useful in patients with gynecologic malignancies with upper gastrointestinal tract obstructions that cannot be treated surgically.

Oral Dietary Therapy

Patients who are able to eat but have impairment of the gastrointestinal tract or have special metabolic requirements may benefit from a specialized oral dietary therapy (144). Often, this may obviate the need for more costly and complex interventions such as parenteral nutrition. In oral dietary therapy, the regular diet is modified based on the pathophysiologic changes induced by the underlying disorder with the goal of providing the most optimal nutrition possible (144). When the main problem is inadequate food consumption, various commercial oral supplements can be used, but usually for only short periods because they may become unpalatable after repeated ingestion. Some preparations provide complete nutrition, whereas others are intended to supplement deficits of specific nutrients. Problems common in patients with gynecologic malignancies such as partial small bowel obstruction, chronic radiation enteritis, and short bowel syndrome may all be amenable to dietary therapies. In partial small bowel obstruction or motility dysfunction, a diet comprising frequent, small, calorically dense meals with minimal amounts of fiber is indicated. Patients with radiation enteritis should receive a low-fat, low-fiber, and lactose-free diet. Dietary management of short bowel syndrome patients includes frequent small meals, limitation of fiber, lactose, and simple sugars, taking liquids separately from meals, and supplementation of calcium and zinc orally and magnesium and vitamin B_{12} parenterally.

Bye et al. (154) conducted a prospective, randomized trial of a low-fat, low-lactose diet in 143 women with gynecologic malignancies undergoing radiation therapy. The intervention group had significantly less diarrhea. Diarrhea in the control group correlated with increased fatigue and decreased physical function. The investigators concluded that diet intervention during radiotherapy reduced the severity of diarrhea, influenced patients' ability to cope with diarrhea, and gave them more control over their situation.

The successful implementation of prescribed diets depends to a large extent on a dietician converting the prescribed diet to a meal plan and working with the patient to implement it. In a prospective, randomized study of 57 patients undergoing chemotherapy for ovarian, breast, or lung cancer, those who received intensive dietary counseling had improved long-term food intake (155). Similar data have

been demonstrated in cancer patients undergoing radiotherapy (156) and in patients with acute leukemia undergoing induction chemotherapy (157).

Pharmacologic Agents

Agents that will reverse the wasting seen in advanced cancers have long been sought to complement or replace the provision of nutrients via the oral, enteral, or parenteral route. Hormones, appetite stimulants, and, most recently, cytokine antagonists have been examined. Studies of growth hormone (158,159), insulin-like growth factor I (IGF-I) alone (159), or IGF-I with insulin (160) in cancer-bearing rodent models showed significant attenuation of tumor-induced weight loss. In human clinical trials, these agents provided a modest gain in weight but no improvement in quality of life and no other benefits (161).

Appetite Stimulants

Anabolic steroids have no proven efficacy in treating cancer cachexia. In a murine model, administration of norandrolone propionate resulted in weight gain, but this was largely due to fluid retention (162). In human trials, steroids produced transient improvement of nutritional parameters and appetite, but continued use is associated with negative nitrogen balance, net calcium loss, glucose intolerance, and immunosuppression (161).

Megestrol acetate is a progestational agent that has been shown to improve appetite and ameliorate weight loss in numerous, but not all, studies of patients with cancer and cachexia (161). Doses in these studies ranged from 160 to 1,200 mg/day and maximal weight gain was generally seen within 8 weeks. However, the change in weight is largely due to increased adipose tissue and edema (163). Nevertheless, improvement in quality of life has consistently been demonstrated in several large prospective studies in patients with cancer cachexia treated with megestrol acetate (164,165). It is generally well tolerated but can exacerbate underlying diabetes mellitus and rarely lead to adrenal suppression. Dronabinol, a marijuana derivative, has shown some promise in small studies by improving appetite and causing weight gain; however, large randomized trials are lacking (161). The Food and Drug Administration (FDA) approval is currently limited to treatment of nausea and vomiting during chemotherapy and for cachexia in HIV-positive patients.

Cytokine Inhibitors

Inhibitors of cytokines involved in cancer cachexia and anorexia have the potential to be potent agents in the treatment of malnutrition in cancer. Monclonal antibodies against TNF lead to improved food intake and diminished loss of protein and fat in murine models of cancer cachexia (153). Similar data are available for anti–interleukin-6 (anti–IL-6)

TABLE 35.3. *Pharmacologic agents used for the treatment of cancer cachexia and anorexia*

Class of agent	Example	Efficacy	Adverse effects
Hormones	Insulin, IGF, GH	Attenuation of tumor-induced weight loss, *no* improvement in survival or quality of life demonstrated	Hypoglycemia; hypokalemia
Anabolic steroids	Oxandrolone, nandrolone	Transient improvement in appetite	Fluid retention; net loss of calcium and nitrogen; hyperglycemia; immunosuppression
Progestational agents	Megestrol acetate	Improved appetite, weight, and quality of life	Weight gain is mostly due to fluid retention and adipose tissue; may exacerbate diabetes mellitus; rare cases of adrenal insufficiency
Cannabinoids	Dorabinol	Improved appetite and weight gain in small studies	CNS effects (slurred speech, nausea, dizziness, sedation)
Cytokine inhibitors	Pentoxyfylline, thalidomide, suramin monoclonal antibodies to IL-1, IL-6, and TNF-α	Improved food intake and attenuation of protein loss in animal models	Clinical studies pending

(166,167) and anti–interferon-γ (anti–IFN-γ) (168). Suramin, a direct IL-6 receptor antagonist, decreased several key parameters of cachexia in tumor-bearing mice (169). A recent study form Japan of a novel inhibitor of IL-1 and TNF-α showed that direct injection of the drug into tumor did not alter tumor growth but did result in attenuation of loss of body weight and epididymal fat in tumor-bearing mice (170). Human studies utilizing the anticytokine approach are limited. Pentoxyfylline and thalidomide have been shown to inhibit TNF-α, but only thalidomide improved weight loss associated with AIDS and tuberculosis (171). Interestingly, recent data show that the clinical anticachexia effect of megestrol acetate are due, at least in part, to inhibition of cytokines (85) (Table 35.3).

ETHICAL CONSIDERATIONS

Prior to the advent of enteral and parenteral feedings, the inability to receive nutrients through oral intake inevitably led to wasting and death. Therefore, in the majority of patients, the natural history of cancer led to death because of dehydration and starvation (172). In patients with potentially curable or stable disease, nutritional support, when indicated, is an important and often critical part of the overall treatment plan. On the other hand, the role of nutritional support in the terminally ill is a subject filled with ethical and legal dilemmas. These problems come to light when the wishes of the patient or the patient's representative are not in agreement with the recommendations of the physicians. For example, a patient may wish to forego nutritional support despite recommendations that such a therapy should be given. Alternatively, patients or their representatives may want to initiate or continue TPN even after all anticancer therapies have failed and the patient is in a terminal state. Two general

principles apply: in the first case, autonomy and in the second, medical futility.

Autonomy is the right of competent patients to make decisions over their care and implies that the physician must solicit these decisions. It was not until the mid 1960s that autonomy began to supersede the Hippocratic tradition with its emphasis on the authoritarian role of the physician. This principle is clearly outlined in a report from the President's Commission for the study of Ethical Problems in Medicine and Biomedical and Behavioral Research that states:

> The voluntary choice of a competent and informed patient should determine whether or not life sustaining therapy will be undertaken, while healthcare institutions and professionals should try to enhance patients' abilities to make decisions on their own and to promote understanding of the available options (173).

With regard to most treatments (surgery, chemotherapy, radiation therapy), the patient's knowledge and experience may be very limited and thus the physician's recommendations may form the sole basis for the patient's decisions. This is not the case with nutrition. People understand the role of nutrition in sustaining life and it is often hard for a lay person to understand why parenteral nutrition may not be indicated or even harmful when the patient has no other source of nourishment. In such situations, it is the responsibility of the physician to explain thoroughly the reasons for withholding TPN.

The principle of medical futility often surfaces in discussion of nutritional support of the cancer patient, especially if the disease is advanced and unresponsive to therapy. There are four aspects to medical futility (174): (a) lack of physiologic rationale for the proposed therapy, (b) failure of the same therapy in a previous attempt, (c) all possible treatments for the underlying disease have failed, and (d) the therapy will not improve quality of life or achieve a goal of care (such as living to see a particular life event). In the case of parenteral (and rarely enteral) nutritional support of the cancer patients, aspects (c) and (d) may be specifically applicable.

It should be noted that these principles, autonomy and medical futility, should govern decisions for both initiation and withdrawal of an ongoing therapy. As stated in the report form the President's Commission,

> A justification that is adequate for not commencing a treatment is also sufficient for ceasing it. Moreover, establishing a higher requirement for cessation might unjustifiably discourage vigorous initial attempts to treat seriously ill patients that sometimes succeed (173).

Religious beliefs will often strongly influence decisions regarding nutritional support. Publicly stated opinions on the subject include (a) a statement form the Archbishop of Canterbury that removal from life support was permitted if it was better to allow the patient to die (175), (b) a report form the National Conference of United States Catholic Bishops that stated that Catholics are not required to use extraordinary means when recovery is hopeless and only the burden of care remains (176), and (c) a review of Orthodox Jewish rabbinical decisions that concluded "the imperative to preserve life, supersedes, with a few exceptions, quality of life considerations" (177).

For the gynecologic oncologist, management of the patient with an inoperable bowel obstruction due to peritoneal carcinomatosis is a difficult and recurrent problem. A recent review attempts to outline the role of parenteral nutrition in this population (123). TPN should be considered in only those patients with a good performance status, and careful attention must be paid to likely medical and symptomatic outcomes as well as ethical considerations. It is interesting to note the views of patients on various life-sustaining treatments. In a study from the University of Michigan, 90% of women undergoing treatment for a gynecologic cancer could envision a time when they would refuse ventilatory support, but only 37% could foresee a time when they would refuse artificial nutrition (178). It is important for the physician and other members of the health-care team to inform the patient and the family that in the terminally ill, provision of food and water by enteral or parenteral routes will not improve comfort (122,176) and, in fact, may add to discomfort (122, 179–181). At the Memorial Sloan–Kettering Cancer Center, TPN is used infrequently in patients with gynecologic cancer and bowel obstruction due to malignant carcinomatosis who do not receive any further anticancer therapy. TPN is used under these conditions only when it is judged that it will enhance the quality of life of a patient who is not at imminent risk of dying in spite of the widely metastatic disease. When considering the chance of improving the quality of life, the burden of TPN administration and monitoring, and the risk of complications have to be considered.

REFERENCES

1. Trosian M, Mullen JL. Nutritional assessment. In: Kaminski M, ed. *Hyperalimentation: a guide for clinicians.* New York: Marcel Dekker, 1985:47.
2. Nixon DW, Heymsfield SB, Cohen AE, et al. Protein-calorie undernutrition in hospitalized cancer patients. *Am J Med* 1980;69:491.
3. Dowd PS, Heatley RV. The influence of undernutrition on immunity. *Clin Sci Mol Med* 1984;66:241
4. Meakins JL, Christou NV, Shizgal HM, et al. Therapeutic approaches to anergy in surgical patients. *Ann Surg* 1979;190:286.
5. Mullen JL, Buzby GP, Waldman MT, et al. Prediction of operative morbidity and mortality by preoperative nutritional assessment. *Surg Forum* 1979;30:80.
6. Buzby GP, Mullen JF, Matthews DC, et al. Prognostic nutritional index in gastrointestinal surgery. *Am J Surg* 1980;139:160.
7. Baker JP, Detsky AS, Wesson DE, et al. Nutritional assessment: a comparison of clinical judgment and objective measurements. *N Engl J Med* 1982;306:969.
8. Detsky AS, Baker JP, O'Rourke K, et al. Predicting nutrition associated complications for patients undergoing gastrointestinal surgery. *JPEN J Parenter Enteral Nutr* 1987;11:440.
9. Detsky AS, Baker JP, Mendelson RA, et al. Evaluating the accuracy of nutritional assessment techniques applied to hospitalized patients: methodology and comparisons. *JPEN J Parenter Enteral Nutr* 1984; 8:153.
10. Crowe PJ, Snyman AM, Dent DM, Bunn AE. Assessing malnutrition in gastric carcinoma: bioelectrical impedance or clinical impression? *Aust N Z J Surg* 1992;62:390.
11. Ottow RT, Bruining HA, Jeekel J. Clinical judgement versus delayed hypersensitivity skin testing for the prediction of postoperative sepsis and mortality. *Surg Gynecol Obestet* 1984;159:475.
12. Pettigrew RA, Hill GL. Indicators of surgical risk and clinical judgement. *Br J Surg* 1986;73:47.
13. Dewys WD, Begg C, Lavin PT, et al. Prognostic effect of weight loss prior to chemotherapy in cancer patients. *Am J Med* 1980;69:491.
14. Lanzotti VJ, Thomas DR, Boyle LE. Survival with inoperable lung cancer. *Cancer* 1977;39:303.
15. Ollenschlager G, Viell B, Thomas W, et al. Tumor anorexia: causes, assessment, treatment. *Recent Results Cancer Res* 1991;121:249.
16. Veterans Affairs Total Parenteral Nutrition Cooperative Study Group, Perioperative total parenteral nutrition in surgical patients. *N Engl J Med* 1991;325:525.
17. Brennan MF, Pisters PWT, Posner M, et al. A prospective randomized trial of total parenteral nutrition after major pancreatic resection for malignanacy. *Ann Surg* 1994;220:436.
18. Santoso JT, Canada T, Latson B, et al. Prognostic nutritional index in relation to hospital stay with gynecologic cancer. *Obstet Gynecol* 2000;95:844.
19. Tunca JC. Nutritional evaluation of gynecologic cancer patients during initial diagnosis of their disease. *Am J Obstet Gynecol* 1983;147: 893.
20. Orr JW Jr, Wilson K, Bodiford C, et al. Nutritional status of patients with untreated cervical cancer. I. Biochemical and immunologic assessment. *Am J Obstet Gynecol* 1985;151:625.
21. Orr JW Jr, Wilson K, Bodiford C, et al. Nutritional status of patients with untreated cervical cancer. II. Vitamin assessment. *Am J Obstet Gynecol* 1985;151:632.
22. Orr JW Jr, Wilson K, Bodiford C, et al. Corpus and cervix cancer: a nutritional comparison. *Am J Obstet Gynecol* 1985;153:775.
23. Warren RS, Starnes HF, Gabrilove JL, et al. The acute metabolic effects of tumor necrosis factor administration. *Arch Surg* 1987;122: 1396.
24. Dempsey DT, Mullen JL, Buzby GP. The link between nutritional status and clinical outcome: can nutritional intervention modify it? *Am J Clin Nutr* 1985;47[Suppl 2]:352.
25. Terada KY, Christen C, Roberts JA. Parenteral nutrition in gynecology. *J Reprod Med* 1988;33:957.
26. Burnett AF, Potkul RK, Barter JF, et al. Colonic surgery in gynecologic oncology. Risk factor analysis. *J Reprod Med* 1993;38:137.
27. Donato D, Angelides A, Irani H, et al. Infectious complications after

gastrointestinal surgery in patients with ovarian carcinoma and malignant ascites. *Gynecol Oncol* 1992;44:40.

28. Massad LS, Vogler G, Herzog TJ, Mutch DG. Correlates of length of stay in gynecologic oncology patients undergoing inpatient surgery. *Gynecol Oncol* 1993;51:214.

29. Abu-Rustum NR, Barakat RR, Venkatraman E, Spriggs D. Chemotherapy and total parenteral nutrition for advanced ovarian cancer with bowel obstruction. *Gynecol Oncol* 1997;64:493.

30. Jong P, Sturgeon J, Jamieson CG. Benefit of palliative surgery for bowel obstruction in advanced ovarian cancer. *Can J Surg* 1995;38:454.

31. Zoetmulder FA, Helmerhorst TJ, Van Coevorden F, et al. Management of bowel obstruction in patients with advanced ovarian cancer. *Eur J Cancer* 1994;30A:1625.

32. Norton JA, Moley JF, Green MV, et al. Parabiotic transfer of cancer anorexia/cachexia in male rats. *Cancer Res* 1985;45:5547.

33. Carson JA, Gormican A. Taste acuity and food attitudes of selected patients with cancer. *J Am Diet Assoc* 1977;70:361

34. Dewys WD. Anorexia as a general effect of cancer. *Cancer* 1979;43:2013

35. Dewys WD, Walters K, Abnormalities of taste sensation in cancer patients. *Cancer* 1975;36:1988.

36. Trant AS, Serin J, Douglass HO. Is taste related to anorexia in cancer patients? *Am J Clin Nutr* 1982;36:45.

37. Bernstein IL. Neural mediation of food aversions and anorexia induced by tumor necrosis factor and tumors. *Neurosci Biobehav Rev* 1996;20:177.

38. Bernstein IL, Taylor EM, Bentson KL. TNF induced anorexia and learned food aversions are attenuated by area postrema lesions. *Am J Physiol* 1991;260:906.

39. Orr JW Jr, Shingleton HM, Hatch KD, et al. Gastrointestinal complications associated with pelvic exenteration. *Am J Obstet Gynecol* 1983;145:325.

40. Turtel PS, Shike M. Diseases of the small bowel. In: Shils ME, Olsen JA, Shike M, Ross AC, eds. *Modern nutrition in health and disease.* 9th ed. Philadelphia: Williams & Wilkins, 1999:1151.

41. Scarantino CW, Ornitz RD, Hoffman LG, Anderson RF Jr. On the mechanism of radiation-induced emesis: the role of serotonin. *Int J Radiat Oncol Biol Phys* 1994;30:825.

42. Bodis S, Alexander E 3rd, Kooy H, Loeffler JS. The prevention of radiosurgery-induced nausea and vomiting by ondansetron: evidence of a direct effect on the central nervous system chemoreceptor trigger zone. *Surg Neurol* 1994;42:249.

43. Sedgwick DM, Howard GC, Ferguson A. Pathogenesis of acute radiation injury to the rectum. A prospective study in patients. *Int J Colorect Dis* 1994;9:23.

44. Kinsella TJ, Bloomer WD. Tolerance of the intestine to radiation therapy. *Surg Gynecol Obestet* 1980;151:273.

45. Loiudice TA, Lang JA. Treatment of radiation enteritis: a comparison study. *Am J Gastroenterol* 1983;78:481.

46. Libotte F, Autier P, Delmelle M, et al. Survival of patients with radiation enteritis of the small and large intestine. *Acta Chir Belg* 1995;95:190.

47. Yeoh E, Horowitz M, Russo A, et al. A retrospective study of the effects of pelvic irradiation for carcinoma of the cervix on gastrointestinal function. *Int J Radiat Oncol Biol Phys* 1993;26:229.

48. Husebye E, Hauer-Jensen M, Kjorstad K, Skar V. Severe late radiation enteropathy is characterized by impaired motility of the proximal small intestine. *Dig Dis Sci* 1994; 39:2341.

49. Danielson A, Nhylin H, Persson H, et al. Chronic diarrhoea after radiotherapy for gynaecological cancer: occurrence and aetiology. *Gut* 1991;32:1180.

50. Kwitko AO, Pieterse AS, Hecker R, et al. Chronic radiation injury to the intestine: a clinico-pathological study. *Aust N Z J Med* 1982; 12:272.

51. Curran WJ. Radiation-induced toxicities: the role of radioprotectants. *Semin Radiat Oncol* 1998;4[Suppl 1]:2.

52. Kagei K, Tokuuye K, Okumura T, et al. Long-term results of proton beam therapy for carcinoma of the uterine cervix. *Int J Radiat Oncol Biol Phys* 2003;55:1265.

53. Bajorin D, Kelsen D. Toxicity of antineoplastic therapy. In: Turnbull ADM, ed. *Surgical emergencies in the cancer patient.* Chicago: Year Book Medical Publishers, 1987:14.

54. Mitchell EP, Schein PS. Gastrointestinal toxicity of chemotheraputic agents. *Semin Oncol* 1982;9:52.

55. Calbresi P, Chabner B. Chemotherapy of neoplastic diseases. In: Gilman AG, Rall TW, Nies AS, Taylor P, eds. *The pharmacologic basis of theraputics.* New York: Pergamon Press, 1990:1201.

56. Mattes RD, Curran WJ Jr, Alavi J, et al. Clinical implications of learned food aversions in patients with cancer treated with chemotherapy or radiation therapy. *Cancer* 1992;70:192.

57. Fletcher JC, Spencer EM. Incompetent patient on the slippery slope. *Lancet* 1995;345:271.

58. Arbiet JM, Lees DE, Corsey R, et al. Resting energy expenditure in controls and cancer patients with localized and diffuse disease. *Ann Surg* 1984;199:292.

59. Dempsey DT, Furer ID, Knox LS, et al. Energy expenditure in malnourished gastrointestinal cancer patients. *Cancer* 1984;53:1265.

60. Hansell DT, Davies JWL, Burns HJG. The relationship between resting energy expenditure and weight loss in benign and malignant disease. *Ann Surg* 1986;203:240.

61. Peacock JL, Inculet RI, Corsey R, et al. Resting energy expenditure and body cell mass alterations in sarcoma patients. *Surg Forum* 1986; 90:195.

62. Russel DM, Shike M, Marliss EB, et al. Effects of total parenteral nutrition and chemotherapy on the metabolic derangements in small cell lung cancer. *Cancer Res* 1984;44:1706.

63. Warnold I, Lundholm K, Schersten T. Energy balance and body composition in cancer patients. *Cancer Res* 1978;38:1801.

64. Gadducci A, Cosio S, Fanucchi, A, Genazzani AR. Malnutrition and cachexia in ovarian cancer patients: pathophysiology and management. *Anticancer Res.* 2001;21:2941.

65. Shike M, Berner YN, Gerdes H, et al. Percutaneous endoscopic gastrostomy and jejunostomy for long-term feeding in patients with cancer of the head and neck. *Otolaryngol Head Neck Surg* 1989;101: 549.

66. Lutetich JD, Mullen JL, Feurer ID, et al. Ablation of abnormal energy expenditure by curative tumor resection. *Arch Surg* 1990;125:337.

67. Dickerson RN, White KG, Curicllo PG, King SA. Resting Energy expenditure of patients with gynecologic malignancies. *J Am Coll Nutr* 1995;15:448.

68. Holroyde CP, Gabuzda TG, Putnam RC et al. Altered glucose metabolism in metastatic carcinoma. *Cancer Res* 1975;35:3710.

69. Holroyde CP, Skutches CL, Boden G, et al. Glucose metabolism in cachectic patients with colorectal cancer. *Cancer Res* 1984;44:5910.

70. Kern KA, Norton JA. Cancer cachexia. *JPEN J Parenter Enteral Nutr* 1988;12:286.

71. Lundhohm K, Holm G, Schersten T. Insulin resistance in patients with cancer. *Cancer Res* 1978;38:4665.

72. Cersosimo E, Pisters PW, Pesola G. et al. The effect of graded doses of insulin on peripheral glucose uptake and lactate release in cancer cachexia. *Surgery* 1991;109:459.

73. Shaw JH, Wolfe RR. Glucose and urea kinetics in patients with early and advance gastrointestinal cancer: the response to glucose infusion, parenteral feeding, and surgical resection. *Surgery* 1987;101:181.

74. Holroyde CP, Reichard GA. Carbohydrate metabolism in cancer cachexia. *Cancer Treat Rep* 1981;64:55.

75. Waterhouse C. Lactate metabolism in patients with cancer. *Cancer* 1974;33:66.

76. McAndrew PF. Fat metabolism and cancer. *Surg Clin North Am* 1986; 66:1003.

77. Beutler B, Cerami A. Cachectin and tumour necrosis factor as two sides of the same biological coin. *Nature* 1986;320:584.

78. Eden E, Ekman L, Bennegard K, et al. Whole body tyrosine flux in relation to energy expenditure in weight loosing cancer patients. *Metabolism* 1984;33:1020.

79. Norton JA, Stein TP, Brennan MF. Whole body protein synthesis and turnover in normal man and malnourished patients with and without known cancer. *Ann Surg* 1981;194:123.

80. Shike M, Russel DM, Detsky A, et al. Changes in body composition in patients with small cell lung cancer. The effect of total parenteral nutrition as an adjunct to chemotherapy. *Ann Intern Med* 1984;101: 303.

81. Warren RS, Donner DB, Starnes HF, et al. Modulation of endogenous hormone action by recombinant human tumor necrosis factor. *Proc Natl Acad Sci U S A* 1987;84:8619.

82. Balkwill F, Osborne R, Burke F, et al. Evidence for tumor necrosis factor/cachectin production in cancer. *Lancet* 1987;1:1229.

83. Fong Y, Mildawer LL, Merano M, et al. Cachectin/TNF or IL-1a induces cachexia with redistribution of body protein. *Am J Physiol* 1989;256:R659.

84. Tracey KJ, Wei H, Manoque KR, et al. Cachectin/TNF induces cachexia, anorexia and inflammation. *J Exp Med* 1987;7:1211.

85. Mantovami G, Maccio A, Lai P, et al. Cytokine activity in cancer-related anorexia/cachexia: role of megestrol acetate and medroxyprogesterone acetate. *Semin Oncol* 1998;6[2 Suppl]:45.

86. Lowry SF, Smith JC, Brennan MF. Zinc and copper replacement during total parenteral nutrition. *Am J Clin Nutr* 1981;34:1853.

87. Shaw JH, Humberstone DM, Wolfe RR. Energy and protein metabolism in sarcoma patients. *Ann Surg* 1988;207:283.

88. Jeevanandam M, Horowitz GS, Lowry SF, Brennan MF. Cancer cachexia and protein metabolism. *Lancet* 1984;1:1423.

89. Sharp JW, Roncagli T. Home parenteral nutrition in advanced cancer. *Cancer Pract* 1993;1:119.

90. Shaw JH, Wolfe RR. Fatty acid and glycerol kinetics in septic patients and in patients with gastrointestinal cancer. The response glucose infusion and parenteral feeding. *Ann Surg* 1987;205:368.

91. Nixon DW, Moffitt S, Lawson DH, et al. Total parenteral nutrition as an adjunct to chemotherapy of metastatic colorectal cancer. *Cancer Treat Rep* 1981;65[Suppl 5]:121.

92. Serrou B, Cupissol D, Plagne R, et al. Parenteral intravenous nutrition (PIVN) as an adjunct to chemotherapy in small cell anaplastic lung carcinoma. *Cancer Treat Rep* 1981;65[Suppl 5]:151.

93. Valdivieso M, Bodner GP, Benjamin RS, et al. Role of intravenous hyperalimentation as an adjunct to intensive chemotherapy for small cell bronchogenic carcinoma. *Cancer Treat Rep* 1981;65[Suppl 5]:154.

94. Samuels Ml, Selig DE, Ogden S, et al. IV hyperalimentation and chemotherapy for stage III testicular cancer: a randomized study. *Cancer Treat Rep* 1981;65:615.

95. Daly JM, Reynolds J, Thom A, et al. Immune and metabolic effects of arginine in the surgical patient. *Ann Surg* 1988;208:512.

96. Fletcher JP, Little JM. A comparison of parenteral nutrition and early postoperative enteral feeding on the nitrogen balance after major surgery. *Surgery* 1986;100:21.

97. American College of Physicians postition paper. Parenteral nutrition in patients receiving cancer chemotherapy. *Ann Intern Med* 1989;110:734.

98. Klein S, Simes J, Blackburn GL. Total parenteral nutrition and cancer clinical trials. *Cancer* 1986;58:1378.

99. McGeer AJ, Detsky AS, O'Rourke K. Parenteral nutrition in cancer patients undergoing chemotherapy: a meta-analysis. *Nutrition* 1990;6:233.

100. Klein S, Kinney J, Jeejeebhoy MB, et al. Nutrition support in clinical practice: Review of published data and recommendations for future research directions. *Am J Clin Nutr* 1997;66:683.

101. Weisdorf SA, Lysne J, Wind D, et al. Positive effects of prophylactic total parenteral nutrition on long term outcome of bone marrow transplantation. *Transplantation* 1987;43:833

102. Baron PL, Lawrence W, Chan WM, et al. Effects of parenteral nutrition on cell cycle kinetics of head and neck cancer. *Arch Surg* 1986;121:1282.

103. Ghavimi F, Shils ME, Scott BF, et al. Prospective study of nutritional support during pelvic irradiation: comparison of children requiring abdominal radiation and chemotherapy with and without total parenteral nutrition. *J Pediatr* 1982;4:530.

104. Kinsella TJ, Malcom A, Bothe A, et al. Prospective study of nutrition support during pelvic irradiation. *Int J Radiat Oncol Biol Phys* 1981;7:543.

105. Klein S, Koretz RL, Nutrition support in patients with cancer: what do the data really show? *Nutr Clin Pract* 1994;9:91.

106. Van Eys J, Copeland EM, Cangier A, et al. A clinical trial of hyperalimentation in children with metastatic malignancies. *Med Pediatr Oncol* 1980;8:63.

107. Detsky AS, Baker JP, O'Rourke K, Goel V. Perioperative parenteral nutrition: a metanalysis. *Ann Intern Med* 1989;107:195.

108. Fan ST, Lo M, Lai ECS, et al. Perioperative nutritional support in patients undergoing hepatectomy for hepatocellular carcinoma. *N Engl J Med* 1994;331:1547.

109. Hotler AR, Fischer JE. The effects of perioperative hyperalimentation on complications in patients with carcinoma and weight loss. *J Surg Res* 1977;23:31.

110. Hotler AR, Rosen HM, Fischer JE. The effects of hyperalimentation on major surgery in malignant disease: a prospective study. *Acta Chir Scand* 1976;86[Suppl]:466.

111. Mueller JM, Brenner U, Dienst C, et al. Perioperative parenteral feeding in patients gastrointestinal cancer. *Lancet* 1982;1:68.

112. Trager SM, Willimas GB, Milliren G, et al. Total parenteral nutrition by a nutrition support team: improved quality of care. *JPEN J Parenter Enteral Nutr* 1986;10:408.

113. Weisner RL, Bacon J, Butterworth LE. Central venous alimentation: a prospective study of the frequency of metabolic abnormalities among medical and surgical patients. *JPEN J Parenter Enteral Nutr* 1982;6:421.

114. Cobb DK, High KP, Sawyer RG, et al. A controlled trial of scheduled replacement of central venous and pulmonary artery catheters. *N Engl J Med* 1992;327:1062.

115. Cunningham MJ, Collins MB, Kredentser DC, Malfetano JH. Peripheral infusion ports for central venous access in patients with gynecologic malignancies. *Gynecol Oncol* 1996;60:397.

116. Solomon SM, Kirby DF. The refeeding syndrome: a review. *JPEN J Parenter Enteral Nutr* 1990;14:90.

117. Weisner RL, Krumdieck CL. Death resulting from overzelous total parenteral nutrition: the refeeding syndrome revisted. *Am J Clin Nutr* 1981;34:393.

118. Lowry SF, Brennan MF. Abnormal liver function during parenteral nutrition: relation to infusion excess. *J Surg Res* 1979;26:300.

119. Burt ME, Lowry SF, Gorschboth C, Brennan MF. Metabolic alterations in non-cachectic animal tumor systems. *Cancer* 1981;47:2138.

120. Darouiche RO, Issam IR, Heard SO, et al. A comparison of two antimicrobial-impregnated central venous catheters. *N Engl J Med* 1999;340:1.

121. Howard L, Ament M, Fleming R et al. Current use and clinical outcome of home parenteral and enteral nutrition therapies in the United States. *Gastroenterology* 1995;109:355.

122. McCann RM, Hall WJ, Groth-Junker A. Comfort care for terminally ill patients. *JAMA* 1994;272:1263.

123. Philip J, Depczynski B. The role of total parenteral nutrition for patients with irreversible bowel obstruction secondary to gynecological malignancy. *J Pain Symptom Manage* 1997;13:104.

124. Cozzaglio L, Balzola F, Cosentino F, et al. Outcome of cancer patients receiving home parenteral nutrition. Italian society of parenteral and enteral nutrition (S.I.N.P.E.) *JPEN J Parenter Enteral Nutr* 1997;21:339.

125. August DA, Thorn D, Fisher RL, Welchek CM. Home parenteral nutrition for patients with inoperable malignant bowel obstruction. *JPEN J Parenter Enteral Nutr* 1991;15:323.

126. Shike M. Enteral feeding. In: Shils ME, Olsen JA, Shike M, Ross AC, eds. *Modern nutrition in health and disease.* 9th ed. Philadelphia: Williams & Wilkins, 1999:1643.

127. Shike M, Latkany L. Direct percutaneous endoscopic jejunostomy. *Gastroenterol Clin North Am* 1998;8:569.

128. Daly JM. Malnutrition. In: Wilmore DW, Brennan MF, Harken AH, et al., eds. *Care of the surgical patient.* Section VII: *Special problems in perioperative care.* New York: Scientific American, 1994:1.

129. Norton B, Homer-Ward M, Donnelly MT, et al. A randomised prospective comparison of percutaneous endoscopic gastrostomy and nasogastric tube feeding after acute dysphagic stroke. *BMJ* 1996;312:13.

130. Di Lorenzo C, Lachman R, Hyman PE. Intravenous erythromycin for postpyloric intubation. *J Pediatr Gastroenterol Nutr* 1990;11:45.

131. Spirtos NM, Ballon SC. Needle catheter jejunostomy: a controlled, prospective, randomized trial in patients with gynecologic malignancy. *Am J Obstet Gynecol* 1988;158:1285.

132. Safadi BY, Marks JM, Ponsky JL. Percutaneous endoscopic gastrostomy. *Gastroenterol Clin North Am* 1998;8:551.

133. Ponsky JL, Gauderer MW, Stellato TA. Percutaneous endoscopic gastrostomy. Review of 150 cases. *Arch Surg* 1983;118:913.

134. Gallagher MW, Tyson KR, Ashcraft AW. Gastrostomy in pediatric patients: an analysis of complications and techniques. *Surgery* 1973;74:536.

135. Holder TM, Leape LL, Ashcraft KW. Gastrostomy: its use and dangers in pediatric patients. *N Engl J Med* 1972;286:1345.

136. Shellito PC, Malt RA. Tube gastrostomy. Techniques and complications. *Ann Surg* 1985;201:180.

137. Shils ME, Olsen JA, Shike M, Ross AC, eds. *Modern nutrition in health and disease.* 9th ed. Philadelphia: Williams & Wilkins, 1999: A-206.

138. Strong RM, Condon SC, Solinger MR, et al. Equal aspiration rates from postpylorus and intragastric-placed samll-bore nasoenteric feeding tubes: a randomized, prospective study. *JPEN J Parenter Enteral Nutr* 1992;16:59.

139. Evens WK, Nixon DW, Daly JM. A randomized study of oral nutritional support versus as lib nutritional intake during chemotherapy for advanced colorectal and non-small-cell lung cancer. *J Clin Oncol* 1987;5:113.

140. Elkort RJ, Baker FL, Vitale JJ, Cordano A. Long-term nutritional support as an adjunct to chemotherapy. *JPEN J Parenter Enteral Nutr* 1981;5:385.

141. Bozzetti F. Effects of artificial nutrition on the nutritional status of cancer patients. *JPEN J Parenter Enteral Nutr* 1989;4:406.

142. Bounous G, Gentile JM, Hugon J. Elemental diet in the management of the intestinal lesion produced by 5-fluorouracil in man. *Can J Surg* 1971;14:312

143. Smith RC, Hartemink RJ, Hollinshead JW, Gillett DJ. Fine bore jejunostomy feeding following major abdominal surgery: a controlled randomized clinical trial. *Br J Surg* 1985;72:458.

144. Shils ME, Shike M. Nutritional support of the cancer patient. In: Shils ME, Olsen JA, Shike M, Ross AC, eds. *Modern nutrition in health and disease.* 9th ed. Philadelphia: Williams & Wilkins, 1999:1297.

145. Ryan JA, Page CP, Babcock L. Early postoperative jejunal feeding of elemental diet in gastrointestinal surgery. *Am Surg* 1981;47:393.

146. Flynn MB, Leightty FF. Preoperative outpatient nutritional support of patients with squamous cancer of the upper aerodigestive tract. *Am J Surg* 1987;154:359.

147. Hochwald SN, Harrison LE, Heslin MJ, et al. Early postoperative enteral feeding improves whole body protein kinetics in upper gastrointestinal cancer patients. *Am J Surg* 1997;174:325.

148. Heslin MJ, Latkany L, Leung D, et al. A prospective, randomized trial of early enteral feeding after resection of upper gastrointestinal tract malignancy. *Ann Surg* 1997;226:577.

149. Kirby DF, Teran JC. Enteral feeding in critical care, gastrointestinal diseases, and cancer. *Gastroenterol Clin North Am* 1998;8:623.

150. Mullan H, Roubenhoff RA, Roubenhoff R. Risk of pulmonary aspiration among patients receiving enteral nutrition support. *JPEN J Parenter Enteral Nutr* 1992;16:160.

151. Montecalvo MA, Steger KA, Farber HW, et al. Nutritional outcome and pneumonia in critical care patients randomized to gasric versus jejunal tube feedings. The Critical Care Research Team. *Crit Care Med* 1992;20:1377.

152. Bliss DZ, Guenter PA, Settle RG. Defining and reporting diarrhea in tube-fed patients—what a mess! *Am J Clin Nutr* 1992;55:753.

153. Sherry BA, Gelin J, Fong Y, et al. Anticachectin/tumor necrosis factor-alpha antibodies attenuate development of cachexia in tumor models. *FASEB J* 1989;3:1956.

154. Bye A, Ose T, Jaasa S. Quality of life during pelvic radiotherapy. *Acta Obstet Gynecol Scand* 1995;74:147.

155. Ovensen L, Allingstrup L, Hannibal J, et al. Effects of dietary counseling on food intake, body weight, response rate, survival, and quality of life in cancer patients undergoing chemotherapy: a prospective, randomized study. *J Clin Oncol* 1993;11:2043.

156. Macia E, Moran J, Santos J, et al. Nutritional evaluation and dietetic care in cancer patients treated with radiotherapy: prospective study. *Nutrition* 1991;7:205.

157. Ollenschlager G, Thomas W, Konkol K, et al. Nutritional behaviour and quality of life during oncological polychemotherapy: results of a prospective study on the efficacy of oral nutrition therapy in patients with acute leukemia. *Eur J Clin Invest* 1992;22:546.

158. Bartlett DL, Stein TP, Torosian MH. Effect on growth hormone and protein intake on tumor growth and host cachexia. *Surgery* 1995;117: 260.

159. Ng EH, Rock CS, Lazarus DD, et al. Insulin-like growth factor preserves hast lean tissue mass in cancer cachexia. *Am J Physiol* 1992; 262:R426.

160. Tomas FM, Chandler CS, Coyle P, et al. Effects of insulin and insulin-like growth factors on protein and energy metabolism in tumour-bearing rats. *Biochem J* 1994;301:769.

161. Ottery FD, Walsh D, Strwford A. Pharmacologic management of anorexia/cachexia. *Semin Oncol* 1998;25[2 Suppl 6]:35.

162. Lyden E, Cvetkovska E, Westin T. Effects of nandrolone propionate on experimental tumor growth and cancer cachexia. *Metabolism* 1995; 44:445.

163. Strang P. The effect of megestrol acetate on anorexia, weight loss and cachexia in cancer and AIDS patients. *Anticancer Res* 1997;17: 657.

164. Beller E, Tattersall M, Lumley T, et al. Improved quality of life with megestrol acetate in patients with endocrine-insensitive advanced cancer; a randomised placebo-controlled trial. Australasian Megestrol Acetate Cooperative Study Group. *Ann Oncol* 1997;8:277.

165. Skarlos DV, Fountzilas G, Pavlidis N, et al. Megestrol acetate in cancer patients with anorexia and weight loss. A Hellenic Co-operative Oncology Group (HeCOG) study. *Acta Oncol* 1993;32:37.

166. Fujimoto-Ouchi K, Tamura S, Mori K, et al. Establishment and characterization of cachexia-inducing and non-inducing clones of murine colon 26 carcinoma. *Int J Cancer* 1995;61:522.

167. Gelin J, Moldawer LL, Lonnroth C, et al. Role of endogenous tumor necrosis factor alpha and interleukin 1 for experimental tumor growth and the development of cancer cachexia. *Cancer Res* 1991;51:415.

168. Matthys P, Dijkmans R, Proost P, et al. Severe cachexia in mice inoculated with interferon-gamma–roducing tumor cells. *Int J Cancer* 1991;49:77.

169. Strassmann G, Kambayashi T. Inhibition of experimental cancer cachexia by anti-cytokine and anti-cytokine receptor therapy. *Cytokines Mol Ther* 1995;1:107.

170. Yamamoto N, Kawamura I, Nishigaki F, et al. Effect of FR143430, a novel cytokine suppressive agent, on adenocarcinoma colon26-induced cachexia in mice. *Anticancer Res* 1998;18:139.

171. Haslett PA, Anticytokine approaches to the treatment of anorexia and cachexia. *Semin Oncol* 1998;2[Suppl 6]:53.

172. Warren S. The immediate causes of death in cancer. *Am J Med Sci* 1932;184:610.

173. President's Commission for the Study of Ethical Problems in Medicine and Behavior Research. Deciding to forego life sustaining treatment. A report on the ethical, medical, and legal issues in treatment decisions. Washington, DC: United State Government Printing Office, 1983;3,61.

174. Shils ME. Nutrition and medical ethics: the interplay of medical decisions, patients' rights, and the judicial system. In: Shils ME, Olsen JA, Shike M, Ross AC, eds. *Modern nutrition in health and disease.* 9th ed. Philadelphia: Williams & Wilkins, 1999:1689.

175. Coggan HD, Edwin Stevens Lecture. On dying and dying well. Moral and spiritual aspects. *Proc R Soc Med* 1977;70:75.

176. Position of the American Dietetic Association: legal and ethical issues in feeding permanently unconscious patients. *J Am Diet Assoc* 1995; 95:231.

177. Scostak RZ. Jewish ethical guidelines for resuscitation and artificial nutrition and hydration of the dying elderly. *J Med Ethics* 1994;20: 93.

178. Brown D, Roberts JA, Elkins TE, et al. Hard choices: the gynecologic cancer patient's end-of-life preferences. *Gynecol Oncol* 1994;55: 355.

179. Zerwekh JV. The dehydration question. *Nursing* 1983;13:47.

180. Schmitz P. The process of dying with and without feeding and fluids by tube. *Law Med Health Care* 1991;19:23.

181. Printz LA. Is withholding hydration a valid comfort measure in the terminally ill? *Geriatrics* 1988;43:84.

CHAPTER 36

Cancer in the Pregnant Patient

Ron E. Swensen, Barbara A. Goff, Wui-Jin Koh, Stephen H. Petersdorf, James G. Douglas, Elizabeth M. Swisher, and Benjamin E. Greer

Cancer is a crisis that is heightened when it is diagnosed during pregnancy. Such news is both devastating and unexpected to the gravid woman, occurring at a juncture in life that she has anticipated to bring only great joy. It is estimated that 1 of 1,000 to 1 of 1,500 live births is complicated by maternal malignancy (1,2). Although cancer is the second leading cause of death in women of reproductive age (3), it is fortunately rare as a cause of maternal mortality (4,5). As women continue to delay childbearing, the frequency of cancer during pregnancy will probably increase. Pregnancy will affect the choice and alter the utilization of standard treatment modalities, such as surgery, chemotherapy, and radiation.

Because cancer complicating pregnancy is both uncommon and unanticipated, its diagnosis may overwhelm the physician as well as the patient. Attention to the health of the mother in addition to the safety of the fetus often leads to therapeutic dilemmas. Appropriate treatment of an individual patient is determined not only by the strength of the indication for treatment, but also by ethical issues, cultural and religious attitudes, and, most importantly, the patient's desire to continue the pregnancy after being informed of potential risks and benefits of treatment. Optimal therapy for a woman with cancer complicating pregnancy thus requires an interdisciplinary approach that serves to educate the patient and her physicians about the benefits and potential risks of diagnostic procedures and treatment modalities in order to achieve the best possible outcome for both mother and fetus.

The decision to treat or delay treatment of a cancer is not difficult if, given current abortion laws, the pregnancy is unwanted and gestation is prior to 24 weeks, if the cancer is diagnosed after fetal maturity has been attained, or if the cancer is far advanced and a delay will not change the maternal prognosis. The difficult decision arises when the pregnancy is wanted and the fetus is not mature. Parents need to participate in the decision-making process and need adequate information on which to base their decision. Counseling should include the potential fetal effects of treatments such as chemotherapy and radiation.

When pregnancy is complicated by malignancy, timing of treatment becomes a crucial issue. One must weigh the benefit of delaying treatment toward achieving fetal maturity against the impact of delayed intervention on therapeutic success. Early delivery of the fetus warrants careful consideration. In the literature, arbitrary time limits of "fetal viability" have been used without inclusion of data regarding fetal mortality and morbidity. A review of 600 infants without congenital abnormalities from a neonatal intensive care unit (NICU) (6) demonstrated that the neonatal mortality decreased from 32.8% when the fetus was delivered at 26 to 27 weeks to 2.7% when allowed to mature to 34 to 35 weeks.

The principal risk to the premature infant is the development of respiratory distress syndrome (RDS) and the consequences related to the management of this condition. The risk of RDS decreased from 86.9% at 26 to 27 weeks to 12.7% at 34 to 35 weeks. Over that same interval, the rate of bronchopulmonary dysplasia (BPD) fell from 5.0% to 1.3%, and the rate of complicated intraventricular hemorrhage (IVH) fell from 32.7% to 1.3% (Table 36.1). In addi-

R. E. Swensen, B. A. Goff, E. M. Swisher: Division of Gynecologic Oncology, University of Washington School of Medicine, Seattle, Washington 98195

W.-J. Koh: Department of Radiation Oncology, University of Washington Medical Center, Seattle, Washington 98195

S. H. Petersdorf: Division of Medical Oncology, University of Washington Medical Center, Seattle, Washington 98195

J. G. Douglas: Departments of Radiation Oncology and Pediatrics, University of Washington Medical Center, Seattle, Washington 98195

B. E. Greer: Division of Gynecologic Oncology, University of Washington School of Medicine, Seattle, Washington 98195

TABLE 36.1. *Mortality, incidence of hyaline membrane (HMD), bronchopulmonary dysplasia (BPD), and complicated intraventricular hemorrhage (IVH) of 600 NICU infants by completed gestational weeks*

	Mortality (%)	HMD (%)	BPD (%)	IVH (%)
24–25 weeks, n = 30	66.7	93.3	50.0	36.7
26–27 weeks, n = 61	32.8	86.9	59.0	32.7
28–29 weeks, n = 67	20.9	71.6	34.3	34.2
30–31 weeks, n = 129	9.3	46.5	13.9	7.6
32–33 weeks, n = 163	1.2	33.7	2.4	1.8
34–35 weeks, n = 150	2.7	12.7	1.3	1.3

Reprinted with permission from Greer BE, Easterling TR, McLennan DA, et al. Fetal and maternal considerations in the management of stage I-B cervical cancer during pregnancy. *Gynecol Oncol* 1989;34:61–65.

tion to fetal age at delivery, birth weight for gestational age is also a predictor of fetal outcome (7).

The degree of morbidity attendant to RDS in prematurity is readily demonstrated by support requirements (Table 36.2). The mean length of mechanical ventilation and supplemental oxygen fell from 25.0 and 36.1 days, respectively, at 26 to 27 weeks to 0.7 and 1.3 days at 34 to 35 weeks. The total length of hospitalization, meanwhile, fell from 48.9 to 11.4 days during the same interval difference in gestational development (8). Survival of an infant born before 24 weeks is exceedingly rare.

These data indicate that for every additional 2 weeks of intrauterine life, there is significant decrease in morbidity and mortality for the premature infant. The low mortality and morbidity at 34 to 35 weeks is predominantly a reflection of lung maturity; specifically, the production of surfactant. Prospective studies have clearly demonstrated a decrease in the incidence of both RDS and mortality in premature infants treated with exogenous surfactant (9–12). This benefit is primarily seen in infants born at <28 weeks gestational age. The use of antenatal steroids alone has been shown to reduce

TABLE 36.2. *Ventilator dependent days, supplemental oxygen days, and total NICU days of 600 NICU infants by completed gestational weeks*

	Vent days	O₂ Days	NICU Days
24–25 weeks, n = 30	27.8	43.0	45.4
26–27 weeks, n = 61	25.0	36.1	48.9
28–29 weeks, n = 67	15.1	26.6	45.0
30–31 weeks, n = 12	4.5	9.7	25.9
32–33 weeks, n = 163	1.5	4.0	17.2
34–35 weeks, n = 150	0.7	1.3	11.4

NICU, neonatal intensive care unit.
Reprinted with permission from Greer BE, Easterling TR, McLennan DA, et al. Fetal and maternal considerations in the management of stage I-B cervical cancer during pregnancy. *Gynecol Oncol* 1989;34:61–65.

the overall incidence of RDS substantially (11), and when used in concert with surfactant, may potentiate the effect of surfactant. In addition, the use of surfactant may reduce the incidence of other neonatal complications, such as chronic pulmonary disease (13–15) and retinopathy of prematurity (ROP) (16–18), but it has not decreased the incidence of intracranial hemorrhage (ICH) and the ensuing developmental sequelae (15). If early delivery is elected, a skilled perinatology team should be assembled, and the appropriate predelivery assessment of lung maturity by amniotic fluid analysis should be performed.

The preceding data for premature infants are specific only to the neonatal period. Equally important are the long-term developmental sequelae of low birth weight infants. A 7-year longitudinal report of infants weighing <1,500 g at birth revealed deficits in IQ, visual-motor integration, and reading, with 54% of the low birth weight children requiring special education or resource help at 7 years of age (19). Complicated intraventricular hemorrhage is associated with major neurologic handicaps in childhood (20). Using comprehensive testing, only 26% of extremely low birth weight children were found to have optimal developmental abilities at preschool age (21).

The literature does not supply firm data to suggest that pregnancy itself precludes or potentiates the development of cancer. Thus, the most frequently diagnosed malignancies in pregnancy are those encountered in nonpregnant women of reproductive age, and include in decreasing order of prevalence: cancer of the cervix and breast, melanoma, Hodgkin's lymphoma, cancer of the ovary, colorectal cancer, and leukemia. Clear guidelines for the management of pregnant patients with cancer are difficult to establish; primarily because of the small number of reported cases of each of these malignancies occurring during pregnancy. The aim of the authors of this chapter is to review the current literature, and to render suggestions for workup and treatment of gynecologic cancers and the more common nongynecologic cancers when they occur in the pregnant patient. The fetal and maternal effects of radiation and chemotherapy also are presented.

RADIATION AND PREGNANCY

General Overview

The application of radiation during pregnancy, either for diagnostic or therapeutic reasons, raises difficult scientific, moral, and ethical issues. It is well recognized that ionizing radiation can substantially impact pregnancy outcome, but firm estimates of risks are difficult to determine since controlled clinical trials are obviously lacking. Much of the information that forms our current knowledge base regarding radiation and pregnancy outcome are extrapolated from animal experimental models or abstracted from human reports of cases and small series. Data from the large population-based experience of children exposed *in utero* among Japanese atomic bomb survivors have also contributed to our concern about the effects of radiation, but analysis is hampered by a lack of accurate dosimetry on which to base risk estimates, and confounding nonradiation variables related to the effects of war cannot be fully excluded.

Assessment of the actual risk of radiation exposure during pregnancy is further complicated by the variability in fetal susceptibility during different stages of *in utero* development, the difficulty of measuring *in vivo* dosimetry in individual patients, the dependence of age and scoring mechanisms (both physical and functional) in evaluating childhood effects, and the underlying rate of spontaneous congenital anomalies that exists in all animal species. Nevertheless, with an estimated 4,000 cases of concurrent pregnancy and maternal malignancy each year in the United States, clinical situations will arise when diagnostic and therapeutic irradiation is indicated (22).

The influence of radiation on pregnancy outcome may be divided into two distinct intervals of maternal exposure: (a) exposure in the prepregnant state, with consequences for subsequent fertility and genetic considerations in future pregnancies; and (b) exposure during pregnancy and impact on embryologic/fetal development (see Chapter 14).

Radiation and Effect on Future Pregnancies

The ovaries are among the most radiation-sensitive organs in the human body. Radiation-induced castration, with permanent amenorrhea and accompanying pronounced hormonal changes, essentially occurs in all women whose ovaries are exposed to more than 500 to 1,500 cGy. This effect is age-dependent, such that individuals over the age of 40 years may be rendered postmenopausal by much lower doses, whereas younger women, especially if prepubertal, are somewhat more resistant to the ovarian ablative effects of radiation (23). Many patients undergoing cancer therapy prior to pregnancy also receive chemotherapy in addition to radiation therapy, making the specific effects of each treatment modality on fertility and future induction of congenital abnormalities difficult to estimate.

Patients who require high-dose radiation therapy (4,000 to 4,500 cGy or more) to the whole pelvis, in addition to brachytherapy, as is often the case for gynecologic malignancies, should be counseled regarding the loss of reproductive capability. Not only is ovarian function typically lost, but radiation will also likely result in endometrial ablation, loss of uterine elasticity, and cervical and vaginal stenosis. Uterine structural effects from irradiation were first suggested by a study that reported fetal loss in 27 of 33 pregnancies in women who had previously been irradiated for menorrhagia. However, subsequent reports on survivors of the atomic bomb detonations in Hiroshima and Nagasaki did not corroborate these findings (24). In anecdotal cases, patients with early low vaginal cancers treated with brachytherapy alone have been reported to achieve pregnancy and

subsequently deliver vaginally (25). Additionally, the use of lateral and cephalad oophoropexy may conserve ovarian function in patients requiring pelvic radiation therapy, and, with increasing sophistication using *in vitro* fertilization techniques, preserve the option of future biologic offspring, albeit in surrogate mothers (26).

On the other hand, *in vivo* reproductive integrity may be preserved in patients who receive abdominal and limited pelvic radiation therapy. The largest experience comes from patients who have been treated for Hodgkin's disease. Aisner et al. (27) reviewed pregnancy outcomes in 43 women of childbearing age who were long-term survivors of Hodgkin's disease and had actively sought conception. The majority of patients had undergone staging laparotomy and midline oophoropexy. Sixteen patients were treated with radiation alone, all with some component of paraaortic or pelvic radiation therapy, four were treated with chemotherapy only, and 23 received combined-modality treatment consisting of both chemotherapy and radiation. The median age at treatment was 23 years. Of the 43 women desiring children, 35 (81%) subsequently became pregnant, delivering a total of 42 healthy children. Nine of the 43 patients had pelvic nodal radiation to a dose of 3,800 to 4,500 cGy, with central ovarian and uterine shielding, and 7 (78%) subsequently achieved pregnancy. In a review of the Stanford experience, Ortin et al. (28) obtained menstrual and pregnancy histories in 86 women who were treated for Hodgkin's disease before the age of 15 years. The majority of patients received radiation with or without chemotherapy. Overall, 75 patients (87%) maintained normal menstrual function. Of the 30 women who underwent pelvic nodal radiation (range 1,500 to 4,500 cGy; median 4,000 cGy), 19 (63%) retained normal menstrual function. With oophoropexy and proper shielding, the estimated average ovarian dose was 8% to 15% of the midplane pelvic tumor dose. The rate of ovarian failure was much higher among patients who received nitrogen mustard–based chemotherapy in addition to pelvic nodal radiation or in those who did not undergo oophoropexy. In contrast to this study, Byrne et al. (29) did not show any increased fertility deficit when alkylating agents were added to subdiaphragmatic radiation.

Green et al. (30) have recently reported pregnancy outcomes in female survivors of childhood cancer enrolled on national studies. Patients were eligible for evaluation if they were less than 21 years of age at the time of diagnosis, were >5 years from the time of diagnosis, and treated between 1970 and 1986. Four thousand and twenty-nine pregnancies were reported in 1,915 female cancer survivors. Pregnancy outcomes included 63% live births, 1% stillbirths, 15% miscarriages, 17% medical abortions, and 3% unknown or still in gestation at the time of the report. Compared to pregnancy outcomes of female siblings, survivors were less likely to have a live birth at a similar age and more likely to have a medical abortion. There were significantly more miscarriages reported by survivors of central nervous system tumors compared with female siblings ($p = .006$). Effects of both radiotherapy and chemotherapy were examined. The relative risk of miscarriage was increased among patients who received radiotherapy as part of their treatment and whose ovaries were in or near the radiation portal (30). Neither the rate of live births nor the rate of stillbirth were influenced by the various chemotherapeutic agents used in this cohort. Finally, the offspring of survivors were more likely to have birth weights <2,500 g than compared with the offspring of their siblings, and this was particularly true for those patients who received pelvic irradiation as part of treatment. Lower birth weights have also been described in women following total body irradiation as part of bone marrow transplantation (31).

Even if fertility is preserved, there is concern regarding induction of genetic abnormalities (germline mutations) by both radiation and chemotherapy. Such genetic effects could theoretically lead to malignancy or congenital abnormalities in future offspring even long after maternal cancer therapy is completed. Based on animal experiments and on observations of Japanese atomic bomb survivors, it is estimated that the dose of gonadal radiation required to produce an incidence of mutations equal to the baseline spontaneous rate in humans (mutation doubling dose) is approximately 100 to 150 cGy, with an approximate excess absolute risk of 100 incidents per 10,000 live-born children per 100-cGy exposure. For comparison, phantom measurements simulating standard mantle and paraaortic radiation for patients with Hodgkin's disease show an absorbed ovarian dose of about 80 cGy; suggesting that the genetic consequences of such radiation therapy to the individual, as well as society in general, is small (32,33). Mulvihill and Byrne (34) noted that in atomic bomb survivors and long-term cancer survivors, there was no significant increase in genetically linked disorders in future offspring as compared with matched control subjects or the general population, although a small adverse effect could not be definitively excluded. More recently, Boice et al. (32) have reported no increase in the incidence of genetic disorders in 4,214 children born to cancer survivors compared to sibling controls. The clinical experience of some investigators confirms a lack of detectable effect, especially genetically related, in future offspring of cancer treatment survivors (27,28). However, others have noted an increase in spontaneous abortions and low birth weight infants, particularly if conception occurred <1 year after cessation of radiation and/or chemotherapy (34,35). It may therefore be prudent to suggest delaying pregnancy for 6 to 12 months following completion of radiation in order to reduce the likelihood of an adverse fetal outcome (36,37).

Radiation During Pregnancy

The period of fetal development significantly influences the impact of *in utero* radiation exposure, affecting both radiosensitivity and the type of biologic effect observed.

Based primarily on animal data, and accounting for similar periods of organ development in humans, the gestational period *in utero* can be broadly divided into three intervals: preimplantation and early implantation, organogenesis, and fetal stage (22,38,39).

Preimplantation and Early Implantation

The period of preimplantation and early implantation, which corresponds roughly to the first 10 days postconception in humans, is the most sensitive stage to the *in utero* lethal effects of ionizing radiation. In mice, doses as low as 10 cGy have been shown to increase prenatal death and embryonic resorption, as expressed by decreased litter size. However, it has been noted in almost all animal experiments that survivors of *in utero* radiation exposure during this early stage of gestation develop no other congenital abnormalities (22,39). Although this all-or-nothing phenomenon has been widely accepted, several reports suggest that there may be an increased rate of malformations during the early preimplantation phase in certain strains of mice, a finding that as yet has not been substantiated in humans (40,41). A review of the human experience, based on Japanese atomic bomb survivors, as well as offspring of women exposed to therapeutic radiation while pregnant, support the animal-based observations (29,41). An explanation for this phenomenon lies in the fact that the embryo at this gestational stage consists of dividing, undifferentiated, totipotential cells. If a radiation exposure kills a sufficiently large fraction of the cells, the embryo becomes nonviable and is resorbed. On the other hand, if only a few cells are lost, the embryo can maintain viability, and a limited number of cell divisions will overcome the radiation-induced injury prior to cell differentiation and organogenesis (39,42).

Organogenesis

The period of organogenesis corresponds approximately to the interval from 10 days to 7 weeks postconception. However, in humans, major organogenesis does extend to 12 to 14 weeks, with substantial central nervous system (CNS) development continuing thereafter to term. Overall, the greatest incidence of gross structural malformations in animals irradiated *in utero* occurs during organogenesis. Intrauterine growth retardation is also frequently observed, although in experimental animals without other significant malformations, recovery to a normal adult weight may be achieved. Acute doses of 10 cGy or less in animals during this period result in a very low or undetectable (above the spontaneous baseline rate) incidence of congenital malformations or growth retardation, but a dose of 100 cGy will result in a near 100% incidence of gross morphologic anomalies observed at birth. In contrast to observations in animals, which demonstrate malformations of multiple organ systems, human exposure to radiation during this gestational period results primarily in intrauterine growth retardation and CNS-related abnormalities, specifically microcephaly, severe mental retardation, and eye anomalies. Visceral, limb, or other structural anomalies induced by radiation in humans are relatively infrequent. A dose threshold of perhaps 5 to 10 cGy has been suggested for observable growth retardation, microcephaly, and severe mental retardation based on data from Japanese atomic bomb survivors (22). Because CNS development in humans continues throughout gestation, the CNS effects of *in utero* radiation exposure extend beyond the interval encompassed by this period of primary organogenesis and have been observed with exposure up to 25 weeks postconception (22,43).

Fetal Stage

The fetal stage of gestational development extends approximately from the eighth week postconception to term, although in humans, there is considerable overlap with the interval of organogenesis, as discussed above. In experimental animals, radiation exposure during this period results in relatively few gross abnormalities, but can lead to permanent growth retardation presenting at birth and continuing to adulthood. Differential cognitive impairments also have been shown to occur in a mouse model during this period (44). In humans, as noted earlier, the CNS retains considerable sensitivity to the effects of radiation through approximately 25 weeks postconception, but at perhaps an increasing dose threshold, and with milder forms of microcephaly and mental deficiencies as compared with radiation exposure earlier in gestation (22,43). Growth retardation is also observed with doses >50 cGy (43). Substantially higher doses, on the order of several hundred centigrays, may lead to intrauterine death, manifesting as stillbirths.

Dose-Effect Considerations

The presence of a "threshold dose," the dose below which radiation would not be expected to affect the pregnancy adversely remains unresolved, and may be related to the specific fetal outcome measured (39,42). Several investigators have suggested that doses <10 cGy do not produce an observable effect on fetal development, as assessed by growth retardation, malformations, and mental deficiencies. At such low doses, the absolute risk to the fetus is minimal, and would be almost impossible to separate from the underlying spontaneous background congenital abnormality rate (38,39,45). Furthermore, the determination of a potential threshold dose may vary depending on the use of linear or exponential models of it from data obtained at higher doses. Fractionated exposure, as would be expected with therapeutic irradiation, would also reduce the likelihood of fetal damage as compared with a single acute exposure for a given

dose (22). On the other hand, radiation-related preimplantation loss of the embryo and induction of future cancer probably represent stochastic phenomena for which no threshold dose exists, and any dose of radiation may be capable of inducing genetic mutations that may not be expressed for years or even generations (42).

In addition to the general stage-specific effects of fetal radiation exposure, there is concern regarding the future induction of childhood cancer. The most compelling evidence in support of a causal link between antenatal radiation and childhood cancer comes from studies of twins at a time when radiographic pelvimetry of twin pregnancies was common practice (36,46). It has been estimated that *in utero* radiation of about 1 cGy approximately doubles the incidence of childhood malignancies during the first 10 years of life, with half of the induced cancers being leukemias. It should be emphasized that even with this relative risk of approximately 2, the absolute risk of cancer induction remains very low. Offspring of the Japanese atomic bomb survivors who were exposed during pregnancy do not show a similar excess of childhood cancers. However, continued follow-up indicates that there is an increase in cancer incidence in this population as it heads into its fifth decade of life (39,47).

It has been suggested that 10 cGy *in utero* exposure be used as a cutoff point beyond which a therapeutic abortion should be considered (39). Based on the preceding discussion, it would appear that a dose of 10 cGy might present an identifiable risk for adverse pregnancy outcome (other than possibly a very low incidence of induced childhood cancer) only for exposure during the early first trimester. In many cases, doses of up to 50 cGy during the first trimester are recorded before a substantial risk of malformation, growth retardation, and mental deficiency is recognized, with even higher doses being required to observe these effects following exposure in later pregnancy (22). The maximum permissible occupational radiation dose of 0.5 cGy throughout gestation is appropriately very conservative, but obviously not relevant in the context of maternal malignancy when diagnostic or therapeutic radiation is considered. Issues regarding radiation exposure of the pregnant patient, including the possibility of therapeutic abortion, will need careful consideration of all factors affecting the expectant mother and fetus.

Fetal Dose Estimates for Diagnostic and Therapeutic Radiation

Fetal exposure from diagnostic radiologic procedures and radiation therapy vary depending on equipment, technique, and the imaged or radiated site of interest. Table 36.3 provides fetal exposure estimates for various common diagnostic radiologic procedures in which ionizing radiation is used. The low doses, further minimized by appropriate technique and shielding, suggest that diagnostic radiation during pregnancy, judiciously applied, can be relatively safe.

TABLE 36.3. *Estimated fetal dose from common diagnostic radiologic exposures[a]*

Type of examination	Fetal dose range in cGY (rad)
Chest radiograph	0.00006
Abdomen-KUB flat plate	0.15–0.26
Lumbar spine	0.65
Pelvis	0.2–0.35
Hip	0.13–0.2
Intravenous pyelography	0.47–0.82
Upper GI series	0.17–0.48
Barium enema	0.82–1.14
Mammography	Essentially undetectable
CT head	0.007
CT upper abdomen	0.04[b]
CT pelvis	2.5
^{99m}Tc-MDP bone imaging	0.15[c]

KUB, kidneys, ureters, and bladder.
[a] Compiled from references 42, 275, and 276.
[b] For early pregnancy, with uterus confined to the pelvis.
[c] Based on an ovarian dose of 0.015 cGy per millicuries (mCi) of ^{99m}Tc-MDP, with a typical injected dose of 10 mCi. Bladder drainage should be used owing to high local dose from urinary excretion of the radiopharmaceutical.

Table 36.4 gives an overview of fetal dose estimates from maternal radiation therapy from information derived from clinical determinations and phantom measurements. Because the doses used in therapeutic radiation are orders of magnitude higher than those used in diagnostic procedures, the data in Table 36.4 reflect incidental fetal exposure from radiation therapy to sites distant from the pelvis or uterus. Obviously, the need for radiation therapy directed to the pelvis or abdomen during pregnancy will result in unacceptably high doses to the fetus, and should be completely avoided unless loss of pregnancy by spontaneous abortion or evacuation is expected.

There are three components to the ''scattered radiation'' that a fetus receives when maternal radiation therapy is used: (a) photon leakage through the treatment gantry head; (b) scattered radiation from the collimators and external beam modifiers, such as Cerrobend blocking; and (c) internal scatter within the patient. The first two components can be reduced by external shielding, whereas internal scatter cannot be modified for a given field setup. Although the relative contribution of each component to peripheral exposure outside the primary radiation field varies with field size, photon beam energy, and distance from the field edge, it has been suggested that, on average, leakage plus collimator scatter approximates the contribution of internal patient scatter, and the use of appropriate shielding may reduce exposure to critical sites outside the primary field of radiation by 50% or more (22,45,48). The use of high-energy photons also reduces fetal exposure as compared with cobalt 60 irradiation, although the production of photoneutrons with electron energies >10 MeV, coupled with the high radiobiologic effect

of neutrons, makes it prudent to treat pregnant patients with photons having a maximal energy of <10 MeV whenever feasible (22). Further reduction in scattered dose to the fetus can be achieved by judicious modification of standard radiation techniques, such as reducing field sizes or changing beam angles, or by the use of electrons when appropriate (22,49).

CHEMOTHERAPY IN PREGNANCY

In pregnant patients, the decision to initiate chemotherapy is often difficult given the potential mutagenicity of many of these agents while avoiding compromising the mothers' health (50,51). For patients with breast cancer, ovarian cancer, leukemia, and lymphomas, chemotherapy is usually a significant part of treatment (52). In many of these instances, chemotherapy may be given with relative safety. However, knowledge of the mechanism of action and possible side effects must be taken into consideration (53). Furthermore, many of the newer agents including chemotherapy such as the taxanes or monoclonal antibodies (rituximab, trastuzumab) have been only rarely given to pregnant patients despite their common use in breast cancer and lymphoma (54–57).

Numerous reports regarding the use of cancer chemotherapy in pregnancy have been published. The effects of chemotherapy on the fetus are influenced by several factors, including the timing of the exposure, duration and frequency of the exposure, and the ability of the drug to cross the placenta (58,59). Maternal factors that can alter fetal drug exposure include hypoproteinemia, which can increase free drug concentration, obesity, which can cause maternal sequestration of lipid-soluble drugs, and expanded plasma volume, which can reduce peak drug concentrations. Features of the chemotherapeutic agents favoring transplacental delivery include a preferential uptake of nonionized, slightly lipophilic molecules, low molecular weight (<1,000 D), and a low degree of protein binding (59,60). This is shared by most chemotherapeutic agents.

Chemotherapy typically affects rapidly dividing cells and is nonspecific in selecting cells to be killed (61). This property explains nonspecific side effects such as alopecia, mucositis, and myelosuppression. Chemotherapy will similarly affect the dividing cells of the fetus. The trimester of exposure is the most critical determinant for teratogenesis in pregnant patients. The first trimester is clearly the period when exposure of the fetus to antineoplastic agents is more likely to be associated with deleterious side effects, as this is the time when organogenesis occurs (62). During the first 2 weeks postconception, exposure to chemotherapy will produce either a spontaneous abortion or a normal fetus. During the remainder of the first trimester, administration of chemotherapy may result in congenital malformations and/or abortion. In a review by Doll et al. (60), 16% of pregnancies exposed in the first trimester to single-agent regimens and 17% exposed to combination chemotherapeutic regimens

TABLE 36.4. *Estimated fetal doses from extrapelvic and extraabdominal maternal radiotherapy*

Reference	Radiation site and details	Fetal gestational age	Fetal dose (cGy)

22	Distal tibia sarcoma—phantom measurements. 6-MV photons, 50-Gy prescribed tumor dose (no shielding)	25 weeks	Low fetus (at pubis): 1.5
			Mid fetus: 1.5
			Top of fetus: 1.2
			Top of fetus:
			  Unshielded: 3
			  External shields: 1.5

	Brain glioblastoma—phantom measurements. 6-MV photons, 60-Gy prescribed dose	13 weeks	Mid fetus:
			  Unshielded: 2.5
			  Shielded: 1.3
			Low fetus (at pubis):
			  Unshielded: 2.2
			  Shielded: 1.1
			Top of fetus:
			  Unshielded: 42
			  Shielded: 17

	Hodgkin's disease with mantle fields—phantom measurements. 6-MV photons, 38-Gy prescribed dose	34 weeks	Mid fetus:
			  Unshielded: 14
			  Shielded: 4
			Low fetus:
			  Unshielded: 6
			  Shielded: 2

206	Hodgkin's disease Mediastinum and neck—phantom measurements. 6-MV photons, 40-Gy prescribed tumor dose (with shielding)	5 fetuses, 18–31 weeks	Mid fetal level: 1.4–5.5 Upper fetal level: 8.2–20 Lower fetal level: 0.8–3 Mid fetal level: 10–13.6
	Cobalt 60, 40-Gy prescribed dose (with shielding)	4 fetuses, 16–26 weeks	Upper fetal level: 18.8–33.2
45	Brain gliomas—clinical and phantom measurements (no shielding)	Fetus #1, 26 weeks. 6-MV photons, 68 Gy to tumor	5.4–6.8
		Fetus #2, 27 weeks. 6-MV photons, 78 Gy to tumor	3.1
49	Hodgkin's disease: various supradiaphragmatic sites—clinical and phantom measurements. 16–30 Gy, various photon energies (no shielding)	7 fetuses, 12–32 weeks	2–50, measured as maximal fetal dose at top of uterine fundus

277	Breast cancer—phantom measurements. 6-MV photons, 50-Gy dose to breast	No fetus—doses specified to ovaries	Nonwedged fields:
			  Unshielded: 9
			  Shielded: 5
			With 30 wedges:
			  Unshielded: 18
			  Shielded: 8
			Measured doses much lower than estimated dose of 40 cGy extrapolated from published physics data sets.

were associated with congenital malformations. However, when the folate antagonists are excluded, the risk of fetal malformation in the first trimester is 6%. The background risk of major malformation for all births in the general population is 3%. In general, chemotherapy should be delayed whenever possible until after the first trimester. Therefore, the most difficult decisions usually occur in the first trimester when the option of therapeutic abortion versus the significant risks of teratogenicity from chemotherapy must be evaluated.

Antimetabolites, including the folic acid antagonists, are the agents most often associated with fetal abnormalities.

Methotrexate and aminopterin exposure during the first trimester may be associated with cranial dystocia, nasal and auditory canal abnormalities, micrognathia, and limb deformities (60,63). Other antimetabolites are less commonly associated with fetal abnormalities. Of 20 patients exposed to 6-mercaptopurine alone, there have been no documented abnormalities, although there has been an increased risk of spontaneous abortion. Cytosine arabinoside, alone or in combination, has been administered to at least 32 pregnant women with leukemia. Of six patients with documented first-trimester exposure, there were four normal children and two congenital malformations (64).

Other agents associated with an increased risk of fetal malformation when given in the first trimester are the alkylating agents, including busulfan, chlorambucil, cyclophosphamide, and nitrogen mustard (65). In a review of more than 70 women who received alkylating agents during pregnancy, the rate of fetal malformations was 14% in the first trimester but declined to 4% when given in the second and third trimesters.

Other agents that have been administered in the first trimester include the vinca alkaloids, vinblastine and vincristine (one malformation for 14 mothers exposed), and the antitumor antibiotics, such as the anthracyclines (60). The highly protein-bound nature of the vincas makes transplacental uptake inefficient. In addition, several studies have failed to demonstrate doxorubicin or its metabolites in significant amount in the amniotic fluid (66). In one series of 28 pregnant patients who received anthracyclines, including 3 women who were treated during the first trimester, there were no fetal malformations reported (67). This may be due the presence of MDR-1 p-glycoprotein in the gravid endometrium, which may provide a natural barrier to the fetus from the vinca alkaloids and anthracycline antibiotics (68). There are few data regarding the fetal risk of another group of natural chemotherapeutic agents, the epipodophylotoxins, VP-16 and VM-26. However, there may be a future risk to the mother who might receive these agents, as there is an increased risk of secondary acute myelogenous leukemia in patients who receive these drugs. The risk of developing leukemia appears to be related to the treatment schedule, cumulative dose, and additional agents. However, there have been no reports of pregnant women or newborns developing leukemia as a result of these agents (69).

Because organogenesis occurs during the first trimester, administration of chemotherapy in the second and third trimesters should not produce fetal malformations. However, antineoplastic agents given in the second and third trimesters are associated with low birth weight, intrauterine growth retardation, spontaneous abortion, and premature birth (51, 60). The prevalence of such abnormalities is not widely known owing to lack of data collection for all pregnant patients exposed to chemotherapy.

Agents commonly used in the practice of gynecologic oncology include paclitaxel (Taxol) and the platinum analogs cisplatin and carboplatin. Cisplatin distributes into most tissues and is teratogenic in several animal species. However, there is relatively little information regarding its use in human pregnancy. Several case reports have described administration of cisplatin in the second and third trimesters without adverse consequences. In the largest series reported, ten pregnant women were treated with cisplatin during the second and third trimesters (70). One-half of the infants demonstrated decreased fetal weight, one infant had persistent moderate bilateral hearing loss at birth, and there was also evidence of transient neonatal leukopenia. The risk associated with cisplatin administration in the first trimester is unknown, although neural development occurs during this period, and the teratogenic effects seen in animals typically affects neural development. Carboplatin also is embryotoxic during early pregnancy in rats (71). Limited case reports of carboplatin administration in the second and third trimester do not appear to carry substantial fetal risk; however, neonatal follow-up intervals are short (56,57,72).

The administration of chemotherapy near term may be particularly dangerous for several reasons. First, antineoplastic agents may not be excreted at term as there is no placental excretion and the neonatal liver and kidney may have a limited ability to metabolize agents such as the vinca alkaloids or cyclophosphamide. In addition, the mother may be neutropenic and thrombocytopenic if the chemotherapy is given within a few weeks prior to term. Therefore, the timing of exposure to antineoplastic agents near term must be closely coordinated with delivery of the fetus. It is reasonable either to plan delivery when the patient is not neutropenic or thrombocytopenic or one should avoid myelosuppressive chemotherapy for 3 weeks before the anticipated delivery date.

Administration of chemotherapy usually requires synchronous administration of supportive care medications such as antiemetics and growth factors. The experience with antiemetics is derived from experience with hyperemesis gravidarum. Although the phenothiazines appear to be safe in pregnancy, there are little data on the 5-HT3 receptor antagonists. In addition, there is no reliable information on the use of growth factors during pregnancy.

Because several chemotherapeutic agents, including hydroxyurea, cyclophosphamide, cisplatin, doxorubicin, and methotrexate, have been noted to be excreted in breast milk, breast-feeding is contraindicated for patients receiving chemotherapy (73).

Finally, there are few data about the delayed effects of *in utero* exposure to antineoplastic agents. Most of the data that do exist are from animal studies (74). Hypothetical long-term sequelae would include cardiotoxicity to those children exposed to anthracyclines *in utero*, decreased reproductive function, and impaired cognitive function because neuroblast development occurs in the second trimester, and impaired physical growth. However, the information documenting these concerns is anecdotal in nature owing to limited follow-up (75). The most extensive series is from Aviles, who reported on 84 children who received chemotherapy for hematologic malignancies *in utero* (76). These 84 children had normal birth weight and educational performance. With a median follow-up of more than 18 years, none of the children has had a malignancy and several have conceived children (77). The National Cancer Institute established a registry in 1985 to follow children who had *in utero* exposure to chemotherapy. Hopefully, this registry will provide more information on the long-term effects of chemotherapy *in utero*.

GYNECOLOGIC MALIGNANCIES AND PREGNANCY

Cervical Cancer in Pregnancy

Cervical carcinoma is the most frequently diagnosed malignancy in pregnancy, with roughly 1% of cervical cancers being diagnosed in gravid women. The reported incidence varies from 1.2 to 10.6 cases per 10,000 pregnancies among heterogeneous populations (78–80). Fortunately, with the improved screening programs in the United States, the incidence of invasive carcinoma in pregnancy is thought to have mirrored the decreased incidence seen in nonpregnant women (81). Pregnant women found to have cervical cancer were 3.1 times more likely than a nonpregnant matched historical cohort to be diagnosed with stage I disease (82).

Historically, there were concerns that pregnancy may have a deleterious effect on the natural history of cervical cancer. Two studies have confirmed that there is no difference in survival between women who are pregnant with cervical cancer and nonpregnant women when matched by age, stage, and year of diagnosis (81,82). Similarly, women who were pregnant at the time of diagnosis of clear-cell adenocarcinoma of the cervix and vagina had 5- and 10-year actuarial survival rates of 86% and 68%, respectively, and did not show any differences in survival or patterns of failure between pregnant and nonpregnant patients with this diagnosis (83).

Screening and Preinvasive Disease

For most women in developed countries, cervical cancer screening is routinely available, but the highest risk women are those least likely to receive appropriate screening services. Sampling of cervical cytology and cervical examination are routine components of early antenatal care. Physician contact during prenatal care provides caregivers a crucial window of opportunity to counsel patients who might not otherwise seek routine health care maintenance in the nongravid state regarding indications and benefits of annual cytologic screening and examination. As many as 5% of pregnant women exhibit cervical dysplasia (84).

Contrary to popular belief, screening of the cervix in preg-

nancy need not be vastly different from that practiced in the nongravid woman. As in the nonpregnant state, suspicious gross cervical lesions require biopsy with pregnancy notwithstanding. In a report reviewing the experience of a large urban county hospital, 67% (18 of 27) of pregnant women with cervical cancer were diagnosed in this manner (78). The normal-appearing cervix should be screened using conventional or liquid-based cervical cytology. The use of an endocervical brush and spatula to obtain a cytologic specimen, as compared with a cotton applicator and spatula, is safe in pregnancy and reduces the number of suboptimal smears (85,86). This is significant since the fraction of suboptimal smears in pregnant women is as high as 58% when using the conventional cotton swab versus 29% when using the cytobrush (87). In nonpregnant women, liquid-based cervical cytology is more sensitive and specific than conventional cytology for diagnosing cervical dysplasia and cervical cancer (88,89). However, this has not been confirmed in pregnant women. .

The Bethesda System is the standard classification system for reporting cervical cytology. Following an extensive period of international collaboration facilitated by internet discussion groups, this schema was updated at a consensus development conference held at the National Institutes of Health in April 2001. The consensus document and associated algorithms specifically address issues related to cervical cancer screening during pregnancy. As in nongravid patients, colposcopy with directed biopsies remains the principal procedure for the evaluation of abnormal cytology. Only endocervical curettage is deferred in pregnancy to prevent bleeding and premature rupture of membrances. Several well-done series have confirmed not only the safety and accuracy of colposcopy with directed biopsy in pregnancy, but also have provided a sound rationale for conservative management of biopsy-proven cervical dysplasia when invasive disease has been satisfactorily excluded (90–95). In one series of 6,286 patients evaluated for abnormal Papanicolaou (Pap) smears, 610 were pregnant at the time of evaluation. Colposcopy was performed in all cases (92). Of note, by the twentieth gestational week, all patients had undergone a ''satisfactory'' colposcopic evaluation. Colposcopically directed biopsy of any lesion seen was obtained without regard for perceived clinical severity. Histopathologic diagnoses of the biopsy specimens were concordant within one degree of severity with the colposcopic impression in 95% of cases, and no case of invasive cancer was missed. No major complication occurred, whereas minor delayed bleeding experienced in three patients was managed with only pressure to the bleeding site. Another series from Australia further supports these findings (93). Eight hundred and eleven women with abnormal cervical cytology were evaluated with colposcopy and biopsy of suspicious lesions. A punch biopsy was performed in 74% of patients undergoing colposcopy, and no complications were reported. Again, no cases of microinvasive or invasive carcinoma were missed. The histologically proven progression of intraepithelial dysplasia in pregnancy to a higher grade of dysplasia at postpartum evaluation was only 7%. No progression to microinvasive or invasive disease was seen. Highlighting the importance of colposcopy in pregnancy for evaluation of atypical cytology was a 14.5% discordancy between cytology revealing only atypia and colposcopically guided biopsy revealing cervical intraepithelial neoplasia grades 2 to 3 (32 of 331 patients). Unlike the nonpregnant state where an unsatisfactory colposcopy is an indication for a loop electrosurgical procedure (LEEP) or cone biopsy, pregnant women with unsatisfactory colposcopy should undergo repeat colposcopy in 6 to 12 weeks since the transformation zone tends to evert as pregnancy progresses. When cytologic lesions are followed by serial colposcopy during pregnancy, colposcopy should be repeated within 6 to 8 weeks after delivery and definitive treatment performed if indicated.

Atypical squamous cells of uncertain significance (ASC-US), the most common cytologic abnormality, should be evaluated during pregnancy in the same fashion as in the nonpregnant state. A variety of methods are acceptable including immediate colposcopy, colposcopy following a repeated abnormal cervical smear, or human papillomavirus testing followed by colposcopy when high-risk human papillomavirus types are detected.

Cervical smears that show atypical glandular cells (AGCs) are rare during pregnancy, and certain diagnostic pitfalls specifically associated with pregnancy must be considered in their interpretation. Decidual cells, endocervical gland hyperplasia, or glandular cells exhibiting an Arias-Stella reaction may appear very worrisome on cytologic interpretation, yet are benign changes related to pregnancy (96). It goes without saying that requisitions for cervical cytology in pregnant patients should identify the patient as being pregnant. Beyond this, both the pathologist and ordering physician should recognize the potential for false-positive interpretation of atypical-appearing glandular cells on cytology during pregnancy. In contrast to the nonpregnant state, AGCs identified during pregnancy may have a decreased likelihood of being associated with cervical adenocarcinoma or adenocarcinoma *in situ*. Kim et al. reported on 326 patients with AGCs (97). Altogether about 18% of women in their series were found to have squamous or glandular dysplasia or invasive adenocarinoma, whereas no malignancies were found in 22 pregnant members of this cohort and only 1 case of carcinoma *in situ* was identified. In most cases, colposcopy with biopsy (but without endocervical curettage) will resolve the issue. Because endocervical curettage and deep endocervical conization carry significant fetal risk, a review of the cytology with an expert cytopathologist to confirm the diagnosis is essential prior to considering these procedures.

Patients with low-grade or high-grade squamous intraepithelial lesions, LSILs or HSILs, respectively, as well as atypical squamous cells of uncertain significance—cannot rule out high-grade squamous intraepithelial lesion (ASC-H) should undergo colposcopy. The vast majority of low-grade and high-grade dysplastic lesions may be safely followed throughout gestation using serial colposcopy with biopsy (91,92,98). Given that the treatment of preinvasive lesions may be safely delayed until after delivery, the use of cryotherapy, LEEP, laser, or other ablative treatment is not routinely indicated during pregnancy.

Because the perinatal death rate following conization is 3% to 6% (99,100), the role of cervical conization has become narrowly limited in pregnancy, with traditional indications for diagnostic conization being altered. Conization during pregnancy is reserved for patients with persistent cytologic findings suggestive of invasive carcinoma that is unexplained by colposcopic findings, demonstration of minimal stromal invasion on biopsy, or any situation in which invasion cannot be ruled out satisfactorily by colposcopy and biopsy alone (91,101). Failure to visualize the entire transformation zone or inadequate colposcopic examination is not considered an indication for conization in the gravid patient (81,100). Because the squamocolumnar junction is typically everted during pregnancy, either a wedge biopsy or a shallow "coin biopsy," rather than the traditional cone biopsy, may be appropriate in those pregnant patients requiring further definition of the extent of disease. Such modified approaches may lessen the complications of conization, which typically include excessive hemorrhage and delayed cervical bleeding; noted in one series to be 8.9% and 3.7%, respectively (100). If necessary, conization of the cervix during pregnancy should be undertaken between 14 and 20 weeks or after fetal maturity.

Goldberg (102) introduced the concept of concurrent cerclage placement at the time of conization. McDonald cerclage placement was undertaken in 17 pregnant patients at 12 to 27 weeks' gestational age. A third of patients delivered prematurely; however, the earliest was at 35 weeks. No cases of hemorrhage, complications leading to hospital admission, or spontaneous abortion occurred. In comparison, Robinson (103) reported the Tulane experience with LEEP of the cervix in pregnancy. Twenty gravid women at 8 to 34 weeks' gestational age underwent loop excision, with two patients requiring blood transfusion and one instance of unexplained intrauterine fetal death 4 weeks following LEEP. Given no improvement in hemorrhagic complications and the issue of cautery artifact potentially obscuring margin and depth of invasion evaluation, we favor a modified cold knife approach to cervical conization when indicated.

To summarize, Figure 36.1 outlines a general algorithm for the evaluation of abnormal cervical cytology in pregnancy. By this algorithm, a pregnant patient with carcinoma *in situ* and microinvasive squamous carcinoma of 3 mm of invasion or less can deliver vaginally and be reevaluated and treated at 6 weeks postpartum. The management of invasive squamous cervical cancer will be discussed below. Invasive

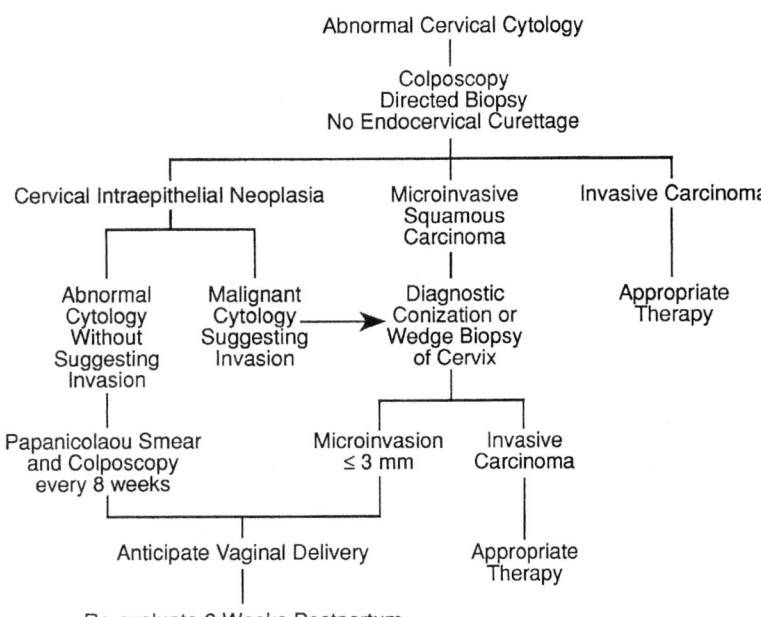

FIG. 36.1. Evaluation of patient with abnormal cytology during pregnancy. (Modified with permission from Hannigan EV. Cervical cancer in pregnancy. *Clin Obstet Gynecol* 1990;33:837.)

adenocarcinomas of the cervix should be treated as an invasive cancer regardless of the depth of invasion.

Invasive Cervical Carcinoma in Pregnancy

All patients with invasive cervical cancer in pregnancy should be counseled extensively regarding treatment options; ideally by the patient's physician together with input from gynecologic oncology, perinatologic, and neonatologic consultants. Recommendations for therapy are individualized in accordance with presenting stage, lesion size, and the patient's desire for the pregnancy, with the latter serving as the most important consideration. Fortunately, women with cervical cancer diagnosed during pregnancy are 3.1 times more likely than a nonpregnant matched historical cohort to be diagnosed with stage I disease (83). In the current literature, the majority of patients with cervical cancer during pregnancy are stage I, with 76% (85 of 112) being stage IB (6,78,81,104). Squamous-cell histology was demonstrated in 78% (88 of 112) of cases.

All series reporting outcome when treatment is intentionally delayed to optimize fetal maturity suggest no increased maternal risk in stage IA or IB disease; however, each of these retrospective reports comprises small, low-risk selected populations (Table 36.5). In sum total, experience in 91 patients with early cervical cancer and intentional treatment delays from 1 to 40 weeks revealed a recurrence rate of 4% (4 of 91). For example, Takushi et al. (105) reported on 12 early-stage patients who elected to delay treatment for 6 to 25 weeks. All remained disease free at >51 months of follow-up. Earlier studies by Sood (106), Duggan (78), Greer (6), and others have reported similar favorable outcomes. A truly informed patient, even with early-stage disease, has to

be willing to accept some undefined, but likely small, risk of progression before electing to delay treatment. On the other hand, as outlined above, delay of treatment to optimize fetal maturity provides a major, quantifiable benefit for the infant. Given this, planned treatment delay is generally acceptable for patients who are ≥20 weeks' gestational age at diagnosis with stage I disease and who desire to continue their pregnancy. However, as modern neonatal intensive care capabilities continue to decrease the threshold of fetal viability, these traditional guidelines of immediate termination of pregnancy prior to 20 weeks' gestation in the face of cervical cancer will likely also come to be influenced more readily in accordance with a patient's wishes to continue pregnancy.

For early-stage cervical cancer, radical surgery and radiation offer similar cure rates. Radical hysterectomy with bilateral retroperitoneal lymphadenectomy offers immediate

TABLE 36.5. *Planned delay in treatment of stage I cervical cancer in pregnant women*

Reference	n	Duration of delay (wks)	Recurrence
106	11	3–32	0
78	8	7–30	0
50	8	3–40	1
6	5	6–17	0
108	5	11–17	0
278	23	8–24	2
107	8	1–12	0
104	3	6–10	0
109	6	2–10	1
279	2	3	0
105	12	6–25	0
Total:	91	1–40	4(5%)

treatment for stages IA2 to IIA cervical cancer during pregnancy and has a demonstrated low associated morbidity, acceptable survival, and an opportunity for preservation of ovarian function (6,50,78,102,107–109). Furthermore, the gestational edema and more pronounced cleavage planes facilitate the dissection. At radical cesarean hysterectomy, a classic uterine incision is preferred. Bilateral oophoropexy is a reasonable consideration at the time of cesarean hysterectomy in the event that adjuvant radiation might be advisable postoperatively for patients with high-risk histopathologic features. In one series, 20 pregnant patients (95%) are alive and free of disease after radical hysterectomy with a mean follow-up of 40 months (104). In a subsequent study, Sood et al. (106) compared surgery for cervical cancer in pregnancy with outcomes in nonpregnant women in case-control fashion. Twenty-six patients underwent radical hysterectomy and four underwent extrafascial hysterectomy. A significantly higher blood loss was sustained in the pregnant as compared with the nonpregnant patients undergoing radical hysterectomy. However, this did not translate into a significant increase in blood transfusion, operative morbidity, or major complication rate. Survival was 97% in the pregnant patients and 90% in the controls at mean follow-up periods of 148 and 145 months, respectively. Thus, given the advantage of ovarian preservation and obviation of radiation-associated vaginal fibrosis, most young patients will benefit from radical surgery as opposed to radiation.

Pregnant patients with stage IIB, or more advanced, invasive cervical cancer, and patients either not medically fit or not interested in primary surgical treatment should undergo definitive radiation therapy together with adjuvant chemotherapy. Patients with advanced disease who elect delay in treatment should have documented fetal pulmonary maturity prior to classic cesarean section, and should start their radiation postoperatively following uterine involution. Pelvic and paraaortic lymph node dissection can be performed at the time of cesarean section to aid treatment planning; however, in interpreting the results of the lymphadenectomy, both the pathologist and gynecologic oncologist should be aware that decidual reaction may be present in normal lymph nodes in gravid women. These findings appear to be similar to metastatic squamous cells and must be correctly identified to allow appropriate assignment of prognosis and treatment (110).

Radiation planning for pregnant patients with cervical cancer requires careful adaptation in order to adjust for the anatomic distortion created by the gravid state. General guidelines for radiation therapy in cervical cancer are provided in Chapter 22. Traditional radiation therapy protocols and techniques may need to be modified in order to optimize individual patient treatment (111). Patients opting for primary radiation therapy with the intent of pregnancy termination should begin with external beam therapy with concurrent chemotherapy. It is common for the pregnancy to abort spontaneously when the woman is irradiated with >4,000 cGy of external beam radiation. In one series, however, 27% of 45 patients did not abort, and required subsequent surgical uterine evacuation (106).

For those patients electing treatment delay to allow fetal maturation, the mode of delivery remains controversial. It seems intuitively prudent to advise against attempts at vaginal delivery in patients with large and/or friable tumors given the risk of bleeding and potentially life-threatening hemorrhage that might force emergent hysterectomy under less than optimal circumstances. Patients with small-volume, early-stage tumors may be candidates for vaginal delivery. However, whether vaginal delivery promotes progression of disease is not yet clear. Two studies have demonstrated no difference in maternal survival on the basis of delivery route (81,82). However, a trend has been observed ($p = .08$) toward poorer survival in women delivering vaginally (112). Given this information, even in patients with small-volume disease, we favor cesarean delivery at the time of planned radical surgery and reserve vaginal delivery for those patients with preinvasive disease or stage IA1 invasive disease with planned postpartum fertility-sparing therapy.

There are 13 cases in the literature that describe implantation of malignancy at the episiotomy site (113). Ten of these recurrences were identified within 6 months of vaginal delivery. Six of the 11 women with follow-up data were free of disease after 10 months to >5 years following wide local excision and radiation therapy. Five of 11 women died of disease: 3 after radiation and/or chemotherapy and 2 after excision and radiation. All patients with invasive cervical cancer who deliver vaginally should have careful palpation of the episiotomy site or other repaired lacerations, particularly during the first 6 months following delivery. If recurrence is discovered at any of these sites, treatment should be excision followed by radiation therapy.

The survival of patients with stage I cervical cancer is excellent regardless of the time of diagnosis during pregnancy with reported survival rates of 85% to 95% (81,104). Overall survival for women who were pregnant and had invasive cervical cancer at all presenting stages is 80% (82).

Ovarian Neoplasms During Pregnancy

Adnexal masses are now detected in 1% to 2% of all pregnancies (114–117). In most cases, these are asymptomatic masses that are detected by routine obstetric ultrasound. In the majority of cases, the adnexal mass will be a small cyst (<5 cm) that resolves spontaneously and presents no risk to the pregnancy. The incidence of ovarian malignancy associated with pregnancy ranges from 1 in 8,000 to 1 in 20,000 deliveries (118,119). In the young patient, germ-cell malignancies are found most frequently. However, with increasing age, epithelial malignancies, especially those of low malignant potential, are more commonly encountered. The majority of adnexal masses that do not resolve spontaneously during pregnancy will be benign ovarian neoplasms.

However, even benign ovarian lesions can result in an adverse outcome of the pregnancy. Therefore, all adnexal masses in pregnancy need to be carefully evaluated and followed to determine the need for surgical intervention.

Management of the Adnexal Mass

The increasing use of prenatal ultrasound examinations is responsible for the increased detection of ovarian masses during pregnancy (114–117,120,121). Prior to the widespread use of ultrasound, most adnexal masses remained unrecognized until cesarean section or postpartum evaluation. Now, many asymptomatic masses are recognized as early as the first trimester. Recent studies suggest that finding an adnexal mass during pregnancy may not carry the same prognosis as it did in the preultrasound era (114).

The majority of adnexal masses found during pregnancy will be simple cysts <5 cm in diameter. In one recent study, 76% of masses were small, simple cysts and 24% were simple or complex, measuring >5 cm in diameter (114). Approximately 70% of adnexal masses will resolve by the early part of the second trimester. The histologic diagnosis and relative frequency of ovarian masses that persist into the second trimester are shown in Table 36.6, which contains data compiled from ten studies published from 1984 to 2003. Dermoid cysts are the most common ovarian neoplasm in pregnancy followed by serous cystadenomas. Overall, though, the most common masses detected in pregnancy are functional ovarian cysts; either follicular or corpus luteum cysts (120,121). These cysts are rarely >5 cm in diameter, although functional cysts as large as 10 cm have been reported. The vast majority of these cysts resolve as the pregnancy progresses and are undetectable by the fourteenth week of gestation. In a series of 90 pregnancies complicated by ovarian tumors reported by Struyk et al. (122), no functional cysts were noted in patients operated on during the eighteenth week of gestation.

Although most masses diagnosed during pregnancy are benign, there are still significant complications that may

arise and therefore result in the need for surgery. Torsion of an adnexal mass is probably more common in pregnancy, with a reported incidence of 5% to 15% (122–125). The majority of cases occur within the first 16 weeks, when the uterus is rising out of the pelvis, or during the puerperium, when the uterus is rapidly involuting. Other, less frequent complications can occur, including rupture of a cyst, hemorrhage into the mass, and infection. All of these complications are associated with an increased risk of spontaneous abortion or preterm labor, particularly when emergent abdominal surgery is performed in the third trimester (122–125).

Whereas there is a natural tendency to avoid any surgery during pregnancy, the likelihood that a pregnant woman with an adnexal mass will require surgery for the mass is not insignificant. For patients who present with symptoms consistent with torsion, rupture, or hemorrhage, emergent surgery will be necessary. In a series reported by Hess et al. (125), 15 of 54 pregnant women with an adnexal mass underwent an emergent exploratory laparotomy. There was also a high rate of complications in the 90 pregnancies with adnexal masses reported by Struyk et al. (122). Severe pain occurred in 26%, adnexal torsion in 12%, cyst rupture in 9%, and obstruction of labor in 17% of women. There were three cases of death in utero and seven cases of neonatal death, yielding an overall loss rate of 11%. Bromley et al. (115) reported on 125 women beyond 12 weeks' gestation with adnexal masses measuring ≥4 cm, 24 of whom underwent second-trimester laparotomy and 101 who were followed expectantly. For those followed expectantly, only one patient developed acute torsion at 39 weeks. There were no cases of premature labor, premature delivery, or other complications related to the mass.

For patients without acute symptoms, most investigators agree that the size and ultrasonographic characteristics of the ovarian mass will guide clinical management. Generally, simple cystic masses that are <6 cm in size do not require laparotomy during pregnancy as the risk of malignancy is under 1% (115,120). However, if the mass persists into the second trimester and is >8 cm, is rapidly growing, or is complex with an ultrasonographic appearance suspicious for malignancy, then surgery should be performed. Occasionally, magnetic resonace imaging (MRI) may help resolve whether a suspicious solid mass is adnexal in origin or is a uterine fibroid (126). In general, CA-125 levels are not useful because CA-125 can be elevated in pregnancy, especially in the first trimester (127). The ideal time to perform a laparotomy is at 16 to 18 weeks' gestation. Incidentally detected physiologic cysts will have resolved by this gestational age. Also, operations that might require removal of an ovary are preferably done in the second trimester because the placenta has completely replaced the hormonal function of the corpus luteum by 12 weeks of gestation. If an ovary with a corpus luteum must be sacrificed before 12 weeks of gestation, then progestational support for the pregnancy is recommended to avoid a first-trimester loss. If an adnexal mass is found in

TABLE 36.6. *Relative frequency of adnexal masses diagnosed during pregnancy[a]*

	n	%
Corpus luteum follicular cyst	131	17
Dermoid cyst	286	37
Cystadenoma	187	24
Paraovarian cyst	45	6
Endometrioma	38	5
Leiomyoma	24	3
Other	10	1
Malignancy	46	6

[a] Compiled from references 114, 115, 117, 121–123, 125, and 280–282.

the third trimester, surgery can probably be delayed until after vaginal delivery, or it can be performed at the time of cesarean section. Adnexal masses that persist following delivery should be removed or followed indefinitely by ultrasound with the expectation of prompt removal should features suggestive of malignancy be identified.

Patients who require surgery during the second trimester for an adnexal mass will usually need a vertical midline incision owing to the extrapelvic location of the adnexa (128). Attempts should be made to minimize manipulation of the gravid uterus. The contralateral ovary should be carefully inspected. If pathology is benign, a cystectomy should be attempted. Although the second trimester is the optimal time to perform a surgical intervention, there is still a risk of preterm labor and fetal loss. In a study by Platek et al. (85, 116), 19 patients underwent laparotomy. Complications within 12 hours of surgery included one spontaneous abortion and one patient with ruptured membranes. In a study by Bromley et al. (114,115), 24 women underwent a second-trimester laparotomy and there were no complications. Likewise, in a study by Bernhard et al. (62,114), 25 women had surgical removal of adnexal masses without complications. In a study by Kort et al. (120,129), there were two spontaneous abortions following adnexal surgery in 18 pregnant patients. In this study, prophylactic tocolytics were not shown to decrease the risk of preterm labor or preterm delivery in women who underwent nonobstetric surgery. However, in women who developed contractions in the third trimester, tocolytics did reduce the risk of preterm delivery.

Laparoscopic management of adnexal masses during pregnancy has been attempted by several investigators (130–132). Although laparoscopic management may be associated with a shorter period of bed rest, less postoperative pain, less analgesic requirements, and less use of tocolyics (132), there are potential hazards associated with the laparoscopy in the second trimester. At least two cases of fetal demise following laparoscopy have been reported (130,133). In one instance, a fetal demise occurred following an iatrogenic carbon dioxide pneumoamnion caused by unrecognized insertion of the Verres needle into the amniotic cavity. Patients in the second trimester who are subjected to laparoscopy should have the laparoscope inserted using the open technique. Additionally, the fetus may be at risk of acidosis due to maternal conversion of absorbed carbon dioxide gas into carbonic acid. For these reasons, laparoscopy for management of adnexal masses in pregnancy remains investigational at this time.

Management of Ovarian Cancer During Pregnancy

The most serious complication of a coexistent ovarian tumor and pregnancy is malignancy. Fortunately, the incidence of ovarian malignancy associated with pregnancy is low (118,119). For pregnant women with adnexal masses, the incidence of malignancy is approximately 6% (Table 36.6). However, the ultrasonographic appearance of the mass is an important consideration. In a study by Bromley et al. (115) of 131 adnexal masses diagnosed in the second trimester of pregnancy, only 1 was malignant (0.8%). The investigators noted that 14 of the masses were complex with features suspicious for malignancy. One of these masses did contain a malignancy and, therefore, the incidence of malignancy in this group was 7% (1 of 14). No mass with a benign appearance turned out to be malignant. In another series by Wheeler et al. (117), 34 patients were identified with complex ovarian masses that persisted into the second trimester. Three invasive malignancies and six tumors of low malignant potential were identified. In addition, these investigators found malignant tumors (invasive and low malignant potential) had a significantly lower pulsatility index than benign masses. However, there was considerable overlap of blood flow patterns between benign and malignant masses, which may limit the clinical usefulness of the pulsatility index. Interestingly, most ovarian malignancies are asymptomatic during pregnancy and are detected as an incidental finding at the time of routine ultrasound or cesarean section. Since the majority of these cancers are found fortuitously, most ovarian malignancies diagnosed during pregnancy are stage I (124).

The surgical management of ovarian cancer diagnosed during pregnancy should be the same as for a nonpregnant patient. Reliable frozen-section analysis of tumors is essential for appropriate intraoperative decisions. Because most tumors present as stage I, a unilateral oophorectomy or unilateral salpingo-oophorectomy with appropriate staging is the procedure of choice. Rarely will a hysterectomy be indicated. For more advanced stages, the extent of surgery, including cytoreduction, will depend on the stage of disease and fetal viability. Fortunately, this situation is rarely encountered in pregnancy (134,135).

The most common germ-cell malignancy associated with pregnancy is dysgerminoma; accounting for approximately 30% of ovarian malignancies in pregnancy (Table 36.7) (136). Dysgerminomas usually present as large solid masses.

TABLE 36.7. *Relative frequency of ovarian malignancies associated with pregnancy*

	n	%
Epithelial malignancies	24	35
Low malignant potential (*n* = 16)		
Adenocarcinoma (*n* = 8)		
Germ cell malignancies	23	33
Dysgerminoma (*n* = 19)		
Immature teratoma (*n* = 3)		
Endodermal sinus (*n* = 1)		
Gonadal stromal tumors	14	20
Feminizing (*n* = 11)		
Virilizing (*n* = 3)		
Sarcoma	2	3
Metastatic	6	9

Because they are heavy, they have a propensity for torsion as well as incarceration in the cul-de-sac. Dysgerminomas have a propensity for lymphatic spread; therefore, the optimal management for a dysgerminoma during pregnancy is a unilateral oophorectomy with ipsilateral pelvic and para-aortic lymph node dissection. The rate of bilaterality for dysgerminomas may be as high as 15%, although blind biopsy or wedge resection of a normal-appearing contralateral ovary is no longer recommended. For patients who are stage IA, no additional therapy is indicated and the pregnancy can continue. Recurrence rates for dysgerminoma confined to one ovary are approximately 10%. However, over 75% of recurrences can be cured with chemotherapy or radiation therapy (137). In patients with more advanced stages, adjuvant chemotherapy is indicated. Karlen et al. (138) reviewed 27 cases of dysgerminoma associated with pregnancy. Obstetric complications were common, including obstructed labor in 33% and fetal death in 24%. In this series, 30% of the 23 stage IA patients developed a recurrence. However, complete surgical staging, including pelvic and paraaortic lymph node dissection, was not performed in all patients assigned to stage IA.

For patients with other germ-cell tumors, a unilateral adnexectomy is the procedure of choice. Most of these patients will present with disease clinically confined to the ovary, and extended surgical staging has not been shown to improve survival. For patients with immature teratomas and endodermal sinus tumors, biopsies of the peritoneal surfaces and omentum should be submitted for histologic evaluation. The most frequent site of dissemination is the peritoneum, with the retroperitoneal lymph nodes being involved much less commonly (139). All patients with nondysgerminoma germ-cell tumors, except for immature teratoma stage IA grade 1, should receive adjuvant chemotherapy. The initiation of chemotherapy during pregnancy is controversial; however, for germ-cell tumors, which characteristically grow very rapidly, a delay could be deleterious. There are several published case reports of patients with germ-cell tumors receiving chemotherapy (bleomycin, etoposide, cisplatin and vinblastine, cisplatin, bleomycin) during the second and third trimesters. In each of these cases, there was successful outcome for both mother and infant (140–143).

Sex cord–stromal tumors are uncommon during pregnancy. In a series by Novak (136) of 100 ovarian tumors associated with pregnancy, there were 11 granulosa-cell tumors, 2 Sertoli-Leydig cell tumors, and 1 hilus-cell tumor. Young et al. (144) reported 36 sex cord–stromal tumors found during pregnancy. They found that these tumors were much less frequently associated with hormonal manifestations and more frequently complicated by rupture. Hemoperitoneum was present in 19% of patients and dystocia in 14%. Pathologically, the tumors differed from similar tumors in nonpregnant women by showing striking edema and prominent luteinization, whereas lacking recognizable differentiation in many areas. In all but one case, the patients were initially treated with conservative unilateral adnexal surgery. Two received chemotherapy and two radiation postoperatively. A total abdominal hysterectomy and bilateral salpingo-oophorectomy were performed in eight patients after delivery; no residual disease was found in any specimens. Follow-up was available for 30 patients and all were alive and well after a mean of 4.7 years.

Owing to the young age of most pregnant patients, ovarian tumors of low malignant potential are not uncommonly found. Studies show that, as in women who are not pregnant, the majority of these tumors will present as stage I and prognosis with unilateral salpingo-oophorectomy is excellent. Mooney et al. (145) observed more aggressive histology in women who were diagnosed with low malignant potential tumors during pregnancy. However, these features seem to regress with termination of the pregnancy and clinical outcomes were good.

Epithelial ovarian cancers discovered during pregnancy have a similar prognosis to those found in nonpregnant cases. Surgical staging should be performed in all apparent early-stage cases. However, whether to perform a total abdominal hysterectomy and salpingo-oophorectomy and a cytoreductive surgery for advanced-stage disease needs to be individualized, taking into consideration gestational age, fetal viability, and maternal wishes. With respect to chemotherapy, reports in the literature have indicated that most single- and multiagent regimens can be administered safely in the second and third trimesters without adverse fetal effects (52). Several case reports have been published documenting the treatment of advanced ovarian cancer in the second trimester with surgery followed by systemic chemotherapy with cyclophosphamide and cisplatin or carboplatin (72,146,147). In all of these cases, there were no adverse fetal or maternal effects. To date, there are only two reported cases where paclitaxel was used during pregnancy (56,57). In both cases, carboplatin and paclitaxel were administered during the second and third trimesters without apparent harm to the developing fetus. Each infant appeared to be normal over 15 months and 30 months of follow-up.

CA-125 levels during pregnancy may be unreliable. In a study by Kobayashi et al. (127), CA-125 was found to peak at 10 weeks' gestation and again at the time of delivery. During the second and third trimesters, serum levels were below 35 U/mL. CA-125 is very high in the amniotic fluid during the second trimester. These investigators conclude that elevated CA-125 levels in maternal sera are found at the time of chorionic invasion or placental separation. Although alpha fetoprotein (AFP) screening is used to detect neural tube defects, markedly elevated AFP levels are seen with endodermal sinus tumors. There are several case reports of asymptomatic pregnant women being diagnosed with yolk-sac tumors secondary to very high AFP levels detected in maternal serum (141). As for nonpregnant patients, lactate dehydogenase (LDH) can be assayed in pregnancy to follow the course of dysgerminoma. LDH levels do not change in pregnancy.

Other Gynecologic Cancers in Pregnancy

As the remaining gynecologic malignancies are uncommon in premenopausal women, their diagnosis during pregnancy is a rare event. Clear-cell carcinoma of the vagina was briefly discussed in the previous section on cervial cancer. Primary squamous-cell carcinoma of the vagina discovered during pregnancy is exceptionally rare. Leiomyosarcomas of the uterus and vulva have been reported (148,149), as has one case of mixed müllerian carcinoma of the endometrium (150).

Vulvar cancer is considered to be primarily a disease of the sixth or seventh decade. It is not surprising, therefore, that only 19 cases in pregnant women have been reported to date (151,152). Considering the paucity of reported cases, ample data upon which to formulate a management plan are unavailable. Meticulous attention to vulvar lesions with liberal use of punch biopsy will expedite diagnosis and treatment planning. Surgery has remained firmly established over the years as the primary mode of treatment for vulvar carcinoma. However, the past two decades have witnessed a shift in surgical philosophy from en bloc radical extirpation to limited radical dissection of the primary lesion with either separate or unilateral inguinal femoral lymphadenectomy (79,153,154). These modifications should be applied to the pregnant patient with invasive cancer of the vulva. Treatment should be delayed until the early second trimester. Of 19 reported cases, 9 women were surgically treated during pregnancy. None of these patients developed a recurrence. Five patients collectively identified among the reported series, in whom treatment was delayed until the postpartum period, developed recurrence and did not survive. Acknowledging limited data, we favor prompt treatment during pregnancy to secure a favorable outcome. After radical vulvectomy, women can successfully deliver vaginally provided that satisfactory vulvar healing has occurred without significant introital scarring. In small lesions with a low probability of lymph node metastasis, a two-stage approach can be considered in which the vulvar lesion is excised in a radial modified fashion during the pregnancy, delaying node dissection until after delivery, in order to limit groin wound morbidity during pregnancy.

Similarly, the association of pregnancy and endometrial cancer is rare. Although malignancy of the endometrium is the most common gynecologic cancer, only 10% of cases occur in women under the age of 40 years. Furthermore, it is well understood that endometrial carcinogenesis is commonly incited in an estrogen-dominated milieu, whereas pregnancy is characterized by elevated progesterone levels.

In a case report and review of the English literature, Vaccarello and colleagues (155) recently summarized 27 cases of endometrial carcinoma associated with pregnancy. In 12 of the cases, the diagnosis was made postpartum. Four of the 27 patients gave birth to live infants. Most of the cancers were focal, well differentiated, and minimally invasive. Thus, as predicted, the prognosis with surgical extirpation was excellent for the majority of patients.

Fertility Preservation in Women with Gynecologic Neoplasms

Most standard curative modalities for treatment of gynecologic cancer render the patient infertile. This fact must be considered by those women who are fertile at the time of diagnosis. Many of these women have completed their families and are unconcerned about treatment-induced infertility. However, for a subset of these young women, the prospect of losing their fertility during treatment for cervical cancer assumes paramount importance. Several investigators have attempted to modify treatment of these lesions to preserve the possibility of reproduction.

Cervical dysplasia may be treated in the outpatient clinic using cryotherapy, laser excision, or LEEP. All of these modalities appear to have minimal impact on the ability of a woman to become pregnant or to maintain the pregnancy successfully to term (156–158). In contrast, cold knife cone biopsy, which requires an outpatient surgical procedure, is associated with an increase in preterm delivery and low birth weight (159). The efficacy of treatment appears to be identical for each of these modalities (160). although the incidence of involved margins is slightly higher when LEEP is used versus cone biopsy (161). For these reasons, the indications for cone biopsy have progressively decreased; however, there remain clinical situations where a cone biopsy is the best diagnostic or therapeutic option.

Microinvasive squamous carcinoma of the cervix may be safely treated by cone biopsy or LEEP provided the cone margins and endocervical curettage are free of dysplasia or invasive malignancy, the depth of invasion is <3 mm, the lesion is <7 mm wide, and lymphovascular invasion is not present (162,163). In this setting, the probability of node metastasis is <2% and survival is excellent. Fertility rates following cone biopsy for microinvasive cervical carcinoma have been reported as 23% over 2 years of observation (164).

Fertility-preserving therapy of early stage IB1 cervical carcinoma has been attempted by a number of investigators. First performed in 1987, the Schauta radical vaginal hysterectomy was modified leaving the fundus in place but radically resecting the cervix and parametrial tissue (165). This radical vaginal trachelectomy was designed to treat locally invasive cervical carcinoma adequately, whereas leaving the uterine fundus intact for possible future fertility. The addition of a prophylactic cerclage at the initial procedure improved obstetric outcomes (165). Variations in this approach have been reported that include a radical abdominal trachelectomy (166). and various methods of lymph node dissection including groin incisions for retroperitoneal node dissection and, later, laparoscopic transperitoneal or retroperitoneal pelvic node dissection (167). In the selected populations where this approach has been used, there appears to be good control of the tumor. In summary, of the six major reported case series of 212 women with median follow-up intervals ranging between 23 and 52 months, only four recurrences have been noted (Table 36.8). Depending upon the series, 14% to 40% (average 27%) of patients receiving fertility-preserving surgery eventually attained pregnancy. Of those who became pregnant, 14% to 45% (average 28%) had a term delivery of a neonate following this procedure and an additional 10% to 33% (average 27%) had a preterm delivery.

Fertility-preserving surgery for ovarian neoplasms is appropriate for selected women with early-stage neoplasms of the ovary. Germ-cell ovarian neoplasms have a mean age of diagnosis during the late second or early third decade, an age when most women have not completed their families. Patients with clinically apparent stage IA germ-cell neoplasms who desire preservation of fertility may be treated effectively while leaving the uterus and opposite ovary in place as long as no gross disease is present in these organs. When an adequate staging procedure (including lymphadenectomy, omentectomy, and staging biopsies of peritoneal surfaces and suspicious lesions) proves the disease to be stage IA, dysgerminomas and grade 1 immature teratomas may be treated with surgery alone. Other germ-cell neoplasms are best treated following surgery with adjuvant bleomycin, etoposide, and cisplatin (BEP). Women receiving this regimen may suffer varying degrees of ovarian failure following chemotherapy but, perhaps owing to the young age of patients with germ-cell neoplasms, few suffer persistent premature ovarian failure. Gershenson et al. reported on 40 ovarian germ-cell patients successfully treated with conservative surgery and combination chemotherapy. In this report, 11 of 16 women seeking pregnancy delivered a total of 22 offspring, and only 1 patient was persistently infertile (168). Similar favorable results were reported by Low et al. (169). Among 73 women treated for ovarian germ-cell neoplasms, 61% experienced amenorrhea; however, all but

9% of these women returned to normal menstrual function after cessation of chemotherapy. There was only one case of infertility. Survival, even in advanced-stage cases, was excellent with 94% of patients being alive after a median of 53 months of follow-up. Although dysgerminomas are reported to have a 10% to 15% rate of bilateral involvement, most other germ-cell neoplasms only present with bilateral disease when generalized metastasis has occurred. For this reason, preservation of the opposite adnexa is safe and appropriate when fertility preservation is desired.

Early-stage epithelial tumors of the ovary may also be treated with conservative surgery under certain circumstances. Although the mean age of diagnosis is in the fifth decade, epithelial ovarian tumors of low malignant potential (LMP) are not uncommon in reproductive-age women. Women with early-stage LMP tumors of the ovary who seek to preserve fertility may safely preserve the uterus and contralateral ovary as long as no disease is present in these organs. Such procedures are associated with an increased frequency of recurrent LMP neoplasia but no increase in mortality (170,171).

Low-risk early-stage invasive epithelial ovarian cancer may also be safely treated with preservation of the uterus and contralateral ovary as long as disease does not involve these organs. A recent report by Schilder et al. retrospectively reviewed the combined experience of eight academic institutions (172). Fifty-two predominantly low-risk patients with stage I epithelial ovarian cancer were treated by unilateral salpingo-oopherectomy and adequate staging, occasionally followed by chemotherapy. They observed only five recurrences and two deaths during a median follow-up of 68 months, and 71% of those desiring pregnancy successfully bore offspring. These data demonstrate that women with low-risk early-stage epithelial ovarian cancer may be managed conservatively, thus preserving reproductive potential without compromising survival.

Endometrial cancer occurs very infrequently during the reproductive-age range. Occasionally, a woman will present with endometrial cancer and be very anxious to preserve fertility. This situation may arise as a consequence of chronic anovulation, a condition that predisposes to both infertility and endometrial hyperplasia. Several investigators have attempted treating these patients with progestins if thorough evaluation of the extent of the lesion using hysteroscopy, curettage, and imaging studies shows them to be at low risk of metastasis (173–175). In these reports, 42 women presented at young ages with grade 1, apparently localized endometrial cancer. After appropriate counseling, these women opted to receive hormonal treatment of endometrial cancer; in most cases with megestrol acetate. Twelve of the women did not respond to hormonal treatment and were treated surgically. Thirty of the women initially responded to treatment with progestins, but seven of them recurred, typically within several months of initiation of hormonal treatment. One of the women was found to have pelvic

TABLE 36.8. *Radical trachelectomy for fertility sparing treatment of early cervical cancer*[a]

	n	% preg
Total trachelectomies	212	
Recurrence	4	2
Number fertile	57	27
Total pregnancies	83	100
SAB/TAB	16	19
2nd trimester loss	13	16
Preterm	23	28
Term	23	28
Ongoing pregnancy	8	10

[a] Compiled from references 166, 168, and 283–286.

spread of her tumor, which was not controlled by further therapy. Although she had not yet expired of her disease, she remained alive with evidence of disease at the time of publication (174). Ten of the entire group of 42 women were successful in bearing children. An additional noteworthy case report highlights the inadequacy of progestin therapy followed by pregnancy reliably to eradicate endometrial carcinoma (176). A 28-year-old woman with a grade 1 endometrial carcinoma was given high-dose MPA for 1 year. Following multiple benign endometrial curettage specimens, she conceived following clomiphene citrate ovulation induction. During the postpartum interval, atypical cells were identified by hysteroscopy and endometrial curettage. A hysterectomy was performed where a small focus of noninvasive, grade 1 endometrioid adenocarcinoma was identified.

These extremely limited data are entirely inadequate to recommend progestin therapy alone for women with documented invasive endometrial cancer. Nevertheless, occasional patients will refuse definitive management because of their overwhelming desire to maintain their fertility potential. In the setting of a fully informed patient who clearly understands that she is assuming an additional, unquantified risk of progression and death, progestin therapy remains an experimental option for fertility-sparing treatment of endometrial cancer.

Gestational trophoblastic disease, by definition, occurs in women of reproductive age. Although treatment may rarely require hysterectomy, usually fertility may be safely preserved. Molar pregnancy may be treated with suction curettage, reserving single-agent chemotherapy if nonmetastatic or low-risk metastatic disease recurs. Pregnancy rates following this approach are about 68% with a 1% risk of subsequent molar pregnancy in later gestations (177). High-risk metastatic disease may require more aggressive chemotherapy typically using EMA/CO (etoposide, methotrexate, dactinomycin, vincristine, and cyclophosphamide) or MAC (methotrexate, dactinomycin, and cyclophosphamide or chlorambucil). Owing to the alkylating agents in these regimens, there tends to be more amenorrhea, especially for women who are nearing menopause. Nevertheless, 56% to 86% of women desiring future pregnancies were successful after receiving EMA/CO (178,179). Since pregnancy remains possible following treatment of gestational trophoblastic disease, and because beta human chorionic gonadotropin (HCG) is used as a sensitive tumor marker during follow-up, adequate contraception is critically important for these women during the initial follow-up interval.

NONGYNECOLOGIC MALIGNANCIES AND PREGNANCY

Breast Cancer

Reports of pregnancy-associated breast cancer have become more common in recent years as more women are delaying pregnancy until their 30s and 40s (180–185). Breast cancer is more common with increasing age, and so the delay in pregnancy likely accounts for increased risk of breast cancer. Furthermore, late first full-term delivery is a risk factor for breast cancer, placing these individuals at a greater risk of developing breast cancer during their late reproductive years. Breast cancer is among the most common malignancies associated with pregnancy, yet breast cancer during pregnancy is rare; occurring in approximately 3 of 10,000 pregnancies (183,186). Conversely, breast cancer during pregnancy accounts for 1% to 3% of all breast cancer cases.

Traditionally, breast cancer during pregnancy has been associated with a poor prognosis; however, more up-to-date data suggest that pregnant women, when matched for disease stage, have identical survival rates when compared with their nonpregnant cohorts (77,181). However, breast cancer in pregnant women is often diagnosed at a later stage than in nonpregnant women (77,187). In a series from the Memorial Sloan–Kettering Cancer Center, 56 pregnant patients with breast cancer were compared with 166 nonpregnant patients (188). Of the women with pregnancy-associated breast cancer, 61% had positive lymph nodes at diagnosis compared with 38% of their nonpregnant counterparts ($p <0.05$). For both groups with node-negative disease, the 5-year survival was 82%. Pregnant patients with positive nodes had a 47% 5-year survival versus 59% for their nonpregnant counterparts. Furthermore, only 31% of pregnant women had tumors <2 cm at surgery compared with 50% of nonpregnant patients. The Toronto group reviewed 102 women with pregnancy-associated breast cancer and 269 matched control subjects (77). Pregnancy-associated breast cancer in this study also included women diagnosed within the first year after delivery. The 5-year survival was identical for the pregnant population when compared with matched control subjects. Pregnant women were two and a half times more likely to present with metastatic disease and had a significantly lower chance of having stage I disease [45% vs 57.9% of control subjects ($p = .015$)]. While pregnancy-associated breast cancer may be diagnosed at a later stage, the prognostic factors including tumor size, nodal status, histologic grade, estrogen receptor status, and c-erbB-2 are similar to the prognostic factors seen in breast cancer in nonpregnant patients (189).

The normal physiologic changes in the pregnant breast may account for the delay in diagnosis. There is increasing firmness, nodularity, and hypertrophy that may make detection of a mass lesion more difficult. If either the physician or patient detects a mass, definitive evaluation must be pursued. Mammograms can be performed with limited risk of exposure to the fetus (Table 36.4). However, mammograms are less likely to provide useful information during pregnancy because of generalized radiographic density due to the hyperemia and increased water content of the breasts during pregnancy. Ultrasound may be helpful to differentiate a cyst from a solid mass and can be performed safely during pregnancy. Breast MRI may be performed safely, but experience with this modality in pregnancy and lactation is being accrued and may be subject to similar problems of detecting a mass in dense breast tissue (67). The detection of a mass mandates either a fine-needle aspiration or biopsy with ultrasound direction. Local anesthesia can be administered safely during all stages of pregnancy. A fine-needle aspirate requires an experienced cytopathologist, as the hyperproliferative state of mammary tissue may be difficult to distinguish from malignant tissue (190). As in nonpregnant women, infiltrating ductal carcinoma is the most common malignant histology. The spectra of malignant and nonmalignant conditions are similar in pregnant and nonpregnant women. In a series of 134 breast biopsies during pregnancy or lactation, 29 cases of cancer were diagnosed (1 per 4.6 biopsies) compared with 1 case per 5.4 biopsies in nonpregnant patients (191). The incidence of inflammatory breast cancer during pregnancy is approximately 3%, which is similar to the nonpregnant population. However, inflammatory breast cancer may be confused with mastitis. Therefore, several investigators have recommended that when an abscess due to mastitis in the pregnant patient is drained, a biopsy should be obtained (192).

The increased vascularity of the breast during pregnancy may increase the risk of bleeding, and biopsy of the lactating breast can lead to the development of a milk fistula and a higher risk of infection. However, these adverse effects can be minimized by careful techniques, including the use of core-needle rather than open biopsy, or successfully treated with antibiotics and temporary cessation of nursing. Although symptomatically bothersome, the possibility of developing such complications should not deter breast biopsy in the pregnant or lactating patient when a suspicious mass is identified given the more severe consequences of delayed diagnosis of malignancy (184).

The cancers discovered in pregnant women are often estrogen receptor (ER) negative and high grade, which is consistent with the age of the patient population. Where flow cytometry has been performed in pregnancy-related breast cancer, most tumors have a high S phase and are aneuploid. The value of hormone receptor status in pregnancy-related breast cancer is poorly defined. In a small series of ten patients, eight had ER-negative disease and two had low receptor-positive tumors (185). However, pregnancy may produce false-negative results, as increasing estrogen and progestin concentrations may downregulate ER levels. Furthermore, in pregnancy, all bound ERs may be occupied by endogenous hormone, so the results of the ligand-binding assay may be associated with a false-negative result. Immunocytochemical assays may avoid these problems; however, there are no accurate data regarding the assessment of hormone receptors by immunocytochemistry in pregnancy to verify this hypothesis (192).

Staging the pregnant patient with breast cancer is often limited to careful history, examination, blood tests, and ultrasound of the abdomen, as well as chest radiogrphy with abdominal shielding. Bone scans should be delayed until after delivery, whereas MRI may be useful to confirm bone, brain, and liver metastasis when suspected.

For pregnant women with early-stage disease, definitive surgery is the standard approach; typically consisting of a modified radical mastectomy. Because of concerns of fetal exposure to ionizing radiation, breast preservation with wide local tumor excision and node dissection followed by radiation therapy is usually not recommended for the first 6 months of pregnancy as primary management (192). In the last trimester, in suitable patients, a partial mastectomy (wide local incision) may be performed, and breast irradiation is then postponed until after delivery. Following mastectomy, patients with high-risk features, such as large primary tumor size, involved surgical margins, or multiple positive axillary nodes, require local adjuvant radiation. However, chest wall radiation therapy may be delayed for a few months, particularly if adjuvant chemotherapy is delivered during the interval between surgery and radiation therapy (193). Adjuvant therapy needs to be considered if the axillary nodes are positive or the cancer demonstrates adverse biologic characteristics, such as negative ER receptor status or high proliferation rate. For women who are within a few weeks of term, the chemotherapy can be delayed until after delivery. However, for most women in the second and third trimesters, adjuvant chemotherapy for node-positive disease continues to be considered the standard of care. The combination of doxorubicin (Adriamycin) and cyclophosphamide can be given relatively safely in the second and third trimesters. These drugs are standard agents for adjuvant therapy of breast cancer. Typically, four cycles of AC (Adriamycin and cyclophosphamide) can be started within 2 to 4 weeks of mastectomy (194). Methotrexate, an agent often used in the treatment of breast cancer, should be avoided whenever possible because of its teratogenic effects. Similarly, paclitaxel, which is often used for adjuvant therapy of breast cancer, should not be used given the lack of knowledge regarding its safety in pregnancy.

There are few data regarding the role of adjuvant hormonal therapy in the pregnant patient (186). A small series has not shown any benefit to oophorectomy in pregnant women with breast cancer (195). In laboratory animals, tamoxifen appears to cause defects in the müllerian system of the female offspring of exposed pregnant mice. Human data regarding the safety of hormonal therapy during pregnancy is limited to a small number of case reports. There is one case report of an infant exposed to tamoxifen who was born at 26 weeks and had Goldenhar's syndrome (microtia and hemifacial microsomia) (196). A second case report described ambiguous genitalia in an infant exposed to tamoxifen during the first and second trimesters (197). Owing to concerns about potential teratogenic effects, tamoxifen and aromatase inhibitors should be avoided during pregnancy (181).

For women with locally advanced or inflammatory breast cancer, the standard treatment is to administer neoadjuvant chemotherapy. In addition, for women with metastatic breast cancer, chemotherapy is the mainstay of treatment. In general, the pregnant patient with locally advanced, inflammatory, or metastatic breast cancer can be treated in a similar fashion. Management of such patients is often best approached in a multidisciplinary manner. For example, Berry et al. (198), from the M. D. Anderson Cancer Center, recently reported their approach to 24 patients who were diagnosed with breast cancer during pregnancy. These patients were managed with outpatient chemotherapy, surgery, or surgery plus radiation therapy as clinically indicated. Chemotherapy included 5-fluorouracil (5-FU), doxorubicin, and cyclophosphamide (198). The patients were managed in all trimesters of pregnancy and patients received a median of four cycles of combination chemotherapy. In these patients, there were no intrapartum complications attributable to therapy. The mean gestational age of delivery was 38 weeks and the Apgar scores, birth weights, and the immediate postpartum health were reported to be normal for all children (198). Although 5-FU was used in this study, most newer combinations use doxorubicin and cyclophosphamide without 5-FU.

The relatively positive outcome of the Berry study is in contrast to older series and suggests the need for a multidisciplinary approach to management (199). There have been relatively few reports regarding the outcome of pregnancies in women with breast cancer. In the review by the Toronto group, of 119 pregnancies occurring in conjunction with breast cancer, 22 were terminated by elective abortion and there were 12 miscarriages. Of the 85 deliveries, there were 83 live births and two stillbirths. There was a statistically lower mean birth weight for the babies born to women with breast cancer ($p = .002$) and a shorter mean gestational age ($p = .006$) (200).

Until 25 to 30 years ago, therapeutic abortion had been recommended to improve the outcome of pregnant women with breast cancer. However, recent studies have not demonstrated a benefit for therapeutic abortion. For example, in a series of 63 pregnant patients from the Mayo Clinic, 5-year survival was 59% in the women who carried to term and 43% in women who underwent therapeutic abortion (182). However, the group who had therapeutic abortions had higher stage disease. Similar studies do not suggest that therapeutic abortion alters the course of the disease (192).

Development of subsequent pregnancy after treatment for breast cancer does not confer a worse prognosis when compared with women who are treated for breast cancer and do not become pregnant. For example, Bunker and Peters (195) matched 96 patients who became pregnant after treatment for breast cancer with a similar cohort for age and stage who did not become pregnant. The patients who had subsequent pregnancies enjoyed better survival than control subjects, with a 72% 5-year survival for the patients who became pregnant versus 50% for the women who did not. Other investigators have confirmed the findings that subsequent pregnancy does not affect the outcome for women treated for breast cancer. In addition, the number of pregnancies and the interval between treatment and subsequent pregnancy or termination versus carrying the fetus to term does not affect the outcome (201). However, most investigators recommend delaying conception for 2 to 3 years after diagnosis because the greatest likelihood for recurrence is within the first 2 years, particularly in women with positive nodes. The concern is not that pregnancy would stimulate recurrence, but rather that the mother may not live long enough to raise the child. Therefore, the decision to become pregnant after the diagnosis of breast cancer must be individualized for each patient.

Hodgkin's Disease

The American Cancer Society estimates that there were 3,600 new cases of Hodgkin's disease affecting women in the United States in 2003, accounting for approximately 0.5% of all diagnosed female cancers (202). Because Hodgkin's disease presents at a median age of about 30 years, the disease and its treatment may have a significant impact both on concurrent and future pregnancies. It is estimated that Hodgkin's disease occurs in approximately 1 in every 6,000 pregnancies (203,204). In a large retrospective single-institutional review covering 35 years, 25 of 775 women (3.2%) treated for Hodgkin's disease were pregnant at diagnosis (111). Pregnancy itself does not appear to confer an adverse prognosis on the outcome of Hodgkin's disease (49, 204–206).

Hodgkin's disease most commonly presents with painless supradiaphragmatic lymphadenopathy either appreciated clinically in the cervical (neck nodes), supraclavicular, or axillary regions, or noted incidentally on chest radiography. In a large review, 92% of all patients presented with involvement of neck nodes and/or the mediastinum, with the axillary and lung hila being much less commonly affected. In this series of 719 patients, all of whom underwent staging laparotomy, Hodgkin's disease involving the spleen was noted in 27% of patients, with other abdominal sites (such as paraaortic nodes) being involved in 11% to 14% of cases. The presence of constitutional, so-called "B" symptoms, defined as the presence of fever above 38°C, night sweats, or unexplained weight loss of more than 10% in the 6 months preceding diagnosis, occurs in approximately 25% of patients and is associated with a higher stage of disease, affecting staging and treatment considerations (207).

The evaluation of Hodgkin's disease first requires an adequate nodal biopsy, with review by an experienced hematopathologist. Needle aspiration is inadequate to establish the diagnosis, and will not allow histopathologic subclassification. Hodgkin's disease is currently divided into four groups: lymphocyte predominant, nodular sclerosing, mixed cellularity, and lymphocyte depleted. This classification scheme has implications, albeit limited, for prognosis and treatment. Further workup includes a history with specific emphasis on the presence of B symptoms, drenching night sweats, fever above 38°C, and weight loss of 10% in 6 months, and a physical examination to assess all node-bearing regions of the body. In addition to routine blood counts, chemistry, and liver function tests, erythrocyte sedimentation rate and serum copper levels should be obtained, as the latter two may be useful as serologic markers for the disease in follow-up. However, pregnancy and the use of oral contraceptives will themselves cause significant elevations in serum copper levels. Currently recommended radiographic staging procedures include chest radiography and computed tomography (CT) scans of the chest, abdomen, and pelvis. The bipedal lymphangiogram is only performed in specific circumstances (208). To minimize diagnostic ionizing radiation exposure during pregnancy, ultrasound and MRI may be used in place of CT and bipedal lymphangiography, although these substitute tests have not been specifically compared with the standards in the staging of Hodgkin's disease. Positron emission tomography (PET) is frequently employed for staging in Hodgkin's disease but cannot be performed during pregnancy. A posterior iliac crest bone marrow biopsy is advised in patients with stages III and IV disease, particularly those with B symptoms, infradiaphragmatic disease, bony lesions, or an elevated serum alkaline phosphatase.

The staging laparotomy, which was widely used beginning in the late 1960s to provide information about the subdiaphragmatic patterns of spread in Hodgkin's disease, is currently rarely used. With the increased quality of diagnostic imaging, a better understanding of the clinical prognostic indicators that influence selection of therapy without laparotomy, and with effective multiagent chemotherapy, the role of this surgical procedure for staging has been virtually eliminated (209). Recent standard of practice has been to use abbreviated-course chemotherapy with involved-field radiation therapy. In particular, for this patient population, it has been shown that even among patients with clinical stage II disease, younger women (<27 years of age) with fewer than four sites of supradiaphragmatic involvement have a low risk of pathologic upstaging with laparotomy (143). Thus, for the woman who is pregnant with localized supradiaphragmatic Hodgkin's disease, it is certainly reasonable to consider omitting subdiaphragmatic staging and proceed with short-course chemotherapy and involved-field radiation therapy if appropriate shielding can be performed or, preferably, defer radiation until after term.

Current staging classification for Hodgkin's disease uses the Cotswold modification of the traditional Ann Arbor scheme and has been summarized elsewhere (208). Until recently, most patients with nonbulky stage I or IIA disease were treated with definitive radiation therapy. Standard techniques typically use initial "mantle" irradiation, covering the mediastinum, supraclavicular fossae, neck, and axilla to a dose of about 3,600 to 4,400 cGy, followed by matched paraaortic and splenic treatment 3 to 4 weeks after completion of the upper field. However, owing to concern about long-term sequelae associated with extensive radiotherapy, the current standard therapy is limited chemotherapy with four cycles of ABVD [Adriamycin (doxorubicin), bleomycin, vinblastine, and dacarbazine] followed by involved field radiotherapy. In pregnant patients who wish to retain the fetus, any subdiaphragmatic radiation should be deferred until after delivery. For patients with more advanced disease, multiagent chemotherapy, with or without consolidative radiation to sites of initial bulk disease, is the treatment of choice, with complete remission rates of 70% to 90% and overall cure rates of 65% to 75% when salvage regimens are included. The most common chemotherapy regimens in Hodgkin's disease have been MOPP (nitrogen mustard, vincristine, procarbazine, and prednisone) and ABVD or various similar combinations and hybrid schemes. However, the MOPP-based regimens have decreased in popularity with the recognition of the increased association of secondary malignancies and data suggesting that ABVD is associated with fewer long-term complications (210). The primary agents in ABVD include drugs that have been most widely used during pregnancy, with reportedly limited fetal effects (60).

There are several series that specifically describe patients who underwent treatment for Hodgkin's disease during pregnancy. Woo et al. (206) described 16 pregnant patients (estimated fetal gestational age of 6 to 32 weeks) presenting with clinically localized (two stage I and 14 stage II) supradiaphragmatic Hodgkin's disease who underwent definitive radiation therapy alone, typically using mantle fields. In 15 of the patients, subdiaphragmatic staging was completed after delivery, including lymphangiograms in ten and laparotomy in five. Eight patients received additional therapy after delivery consisting of further radiation and/or chemotherapy. Twelve of 16 patients have remained continuously disease free at follow-up times ranging from 1 to 31 years, and with successful salvage therapy in 2 of the 4 who relapsed, the 10-year actuarial determinate survival rate was 83%. All 16 patients delivered full-term normal babies without congenital anomalies, growth retardation, or subsequent childhood malignancies. In a survey of pregnancy and Hodgkin's disease, Lishner et al. (204) identified 22 women who underwent treatment while pregnant (16 radiation therapy, 1 chemotherapy, and 5 chemotherapy and radiation therapy) and compared them with matched control subjects. No intrauterine growth retardation or prematurity was noted, but treatment may have contributed to miscarriages, stillbirths (although not statistically significant), or a single case of congenital hydrocephalus in an infant treated with MOPP chemotherapy only during the first trimester. Other investigators have indicated that careful individualization of management of Hodgkin's disease during pregnancy, including close observation alone in selected cases, can result in successful outcomes for both mother and fetus (49,203).

Recent series by Anselmo et al. (205) have demonstrated that a prudent individualization of management may permit administration of chemotherapy and/or radiation therapy that will permit successful outcome for both the mother and fetus. In general, chemotherapy should be delayed until the second trimester of pregnancy. In this situation, standard chemotherapy with ABVD can be given. Adriamycin, bleomycin, and vinblastine are agents that can be given relatively safely in pregnancy. Alternatively, if chemotherapy needs to be administered near term to control disease and there is a desire to minimize exposure to the fetus, single-agent vinblastine may be administered to control the disease until delivery. However, for most women with Hodgkin's disease, individualization of therapy is appropriate. For women diagnosed in the first trimester, options include either therapeutic abortion or consideration of observation until the second trimester if therapy is not urgently needed (211). For women in the second and third trimesters, ABV can be given with relative safety, although there is some concern about dacarbazine. In general, radiation therapy should usually be withheld until after delivery.

Non-Hodgkin's Lymphoma

Although the incidence of non-Hodgkin's lymphoma (NHL) is higher in the overall population than Hodgkin's disease, NHL is less common than Hodgkin's disease during pregnancy; reflecting the fact that NHL most commonly presents after the reproductive years (212). The treatment of patients with NHL depends on the stage of the disease and histologic grade of the lymphoma. Most NHL patients present with disseminated disease. Staging studies should include careful history, physical examination, chest radiography with abdominal shielding, routine blood tests, and bilateral bone marrow biopsies. To limit ionizing radiation, MRI may be used in lieu of CT examination to stage pregnant patients with NHL.

The histologic subtype of NHL is the single most important determinant for treatment of the disease in both pregnant and nonpregnant patients. The low-grade lymphomas generally present with disseminated disease, but are indolent in nature, and so treatment can usually be delayed until after term. However, NHL in pregnancy is most commonly associated with more aggressive histologies (213). These intermediate- and high-grade lymphomas usually require treatment within several weeks of diagnosis. The published experience for treatment of NHL in pregnancy is not as extensive as that for Hodgkin's disease. In the largest published series, by Aviles et al. (214), 19 pregnant women with NHL were evaluated and treated over a 12-year period. Three mothers and their fetuses died during initial therapy owing to progressive lymphoma. Of the remaining 16 mothers, 6 women had high-grade lymphomas and 10 had intermediate-grade lymphomas. Eight patients received chemotherapy during the first trimester. All 16 mothers delivered live newborns, although six babies were small for gestational age at birth. There were no congenital malformations and none of the 16 children appeared to have had long-term effects. All patients received at least cyclophosphamide, vincristine, doxorubicin, and prednisone, and most were in remission at term. In a review by Ward of multiple case reports (212), similar favorable outcomes were reported for women with large-cell lymphoma treated in the second and third trimesters. The poor prognosis of pregnant patients with Burkitt's lymphoma is particularly notable; none of 18 reported pregnant patients with Burkitt's lymphoma survived, although the fetus survived in 4 patients to whom chemotherapy was given in the second and third trimesters.

Therefore, treatment guidelines for pregnant patients with indolent lymphoma include observation until after delivery when staging can be completed and appropriate therapy instituted. Radiation therapy to supradiaphragmatic sites with abdominal shielding can be performed for symptomatic stage I disease in the later stages of pregnancy. Alternatively, if chemotherapy is necessary, treatment with prednisone and either a vinca alkaloid or an anthracycline likely will control the disease until delivery of the child, after which standard therapy with alkylating agents can be administered. For patients with potentially curable intermediate- or high-grade lymphomas who present in the first trimester, a therapeutic abortion should be strongly considered, particularly for those women with unfavorable histologies, such as Burkitt's and lymphoblastic lymphoma, for whom aggressive combination chemotherapy and, occasionally, radiation therapy are required to offer the prospect of cure. For patients with intermediate-grade histologies presenting in the third trimester, an attempt to delay therapy until after delivery should be considered. For those patients presenting earlier in pregnancy or for those patients for whom treatment cannot be delayed, combination chemotherapy can be initiated relatively safely. The standard combination, CHOP [cyclophosphamide, doxorubicin (hydroxydaunomycin), vincristine (Oncovin), and prednisone] can be used for the patient with an intermediate-grade lymphoma who has stage III or IV disease presenting in the second or third trimester. These agents can be given relatively safely in pregnancy, but may be associated with the risk of intrauterine growth retardation. For patients with stage I or II intermediate-grade lymphomas, extremely successful outcomes can be achieved with an attenuated course of chemotherapy using three cycles of CHOP followed by involved-field radiation therapy (215). This approach should be pursued in the pregnant patient in the second and third trimester where the CHOP may be given and involved-field radiation therapy can be administered with appropriate shielding or deferred until after delivery.

Rituximab is a humanized anti-CD20 antibody frequently used in the management of B-cell lymphomas. As a humanized IgG molecule, it would be expected to cross the placenta. There has been one case report of this agent being used in combination with CHOP, which is a common regimen for most B-cell lymphomas starting at 21 weeks' gestation. A normal infant was delivered after three cycles and there was no evidence of B-cell depletion in the neonate (54). However, further investigation of this agent in pregnancy should be considered before confirming its safety.

Leukemia

Development of leukemia during pregnancy is a very uncommon event, occurring in approximately 1 per 75,000 pregnancies (216) This incidence is less than the 3.5 per 100,000 cases of leukemia for all inhabitants of the United States. The most likely explanation for this decreased incidence in pregnancy is that the reproductive years occur after the peak incidence of acute lymphoblastic leukemia (ALL) and before the peak age of patients with acute myelogenous leukemia (AML). The majority of pregnant women with acute leukemia develop AML. Chronic leukemia is less common in pregnant women, with the majority of patients developing chronic myelogenous leukemia (CML); chronic lymphocytic leukemia (CLL) is a disease of the elderly and is extremely rare in pregnant women.

The determination of appropriate therapy of acute leukemia in the pregnant patient requires knowledge of the overall prognosis for the mother, the trimester during which the leukemia is diagnosed, and the effect of the antileukemic agents on the fetus. For both AML and ALL, a complete remission rate of 65% to 75% can be achieved in previously untreated adults (158). The long-term disease-free survival, depending on prognostic features at diagnosis and subsequent postinduction treatment, can range from 25% to 50% for patients with either type of acute leukemia. There is no evidence that pregnancy alters the natural history or prognosis of acute leukemia *except when treatment is delayed.* Complete remission rates appear to be similar for pregnant and nonpregnant patients. In a series of 45 pregnant women with acute leukemias reported by Reynoso et al. (217), a complete remission rate of 72% for AML and 76% for ALL compare favorably with published results for nonpregnant patients.

Combination chemotherapy forms the basis of treatment for acute leukemia. The current chemotherapy used for treatment of acute leukemia, with the exception of methotrexate, is not typically associated with specific congenital abnormalities. However, the treatment of acute leukemia requires not only combination chemotherapy but intensive supportive care with antibiotics, antifungal agents, antiviral agents, antiemetics, and transfusions; all of which may affect the outcome of a pregnancy. For adults with ALL, standard agents used for induction include prednisone, vincristine, and daunorubicin. All of these agents have been given during the first trimester without evidence of a significant increase in the rate of congenital malformations, but there is a risk of prematurity, oligohydramnios, and fetal wastage (64,218,219).

For AML, standard induction therapy includes daunoru-

bicin and cytarabine. Delivery of this combination during the first trimester is associated with significant risk of teratogenesis; therefore, termination of the pregnancy in the first trimester should be strongly considered. In the largest reported series of 13 patients who were treated for acute leukemia in the first trimester, there was one spontaneous abortion, two elective abortions, eight premature births of whom two were stillbirths, and only two full-term pregnancies (64). The role of cytarabine in causing these malformations is unclear. Caligiuri and Mayer reported that of 30 women treated with cytarabine, 18 gave birth to normal offspring and 5 patients had elective termination (51). There have been reports of three additional successful pregnancies when chemotherapy was given in the first trimester (77,220). There have been 48 case reports of fetuses exposed to chemotherapy during the second and third trimesters (64, 77). Half of these births were premature, with three stillbirths and one case of spontaneous abortion. There has only been one congenital malformation (ocular) reported in association with chemotherapy exposure during the second or third trimester (217). This rate of malformation is similar to that of pregnant women in general without concurrent malignancy. There are relatively few data regarding the late effects of antileukemic chemotherapy on children exposed *in utero* (75). A summation of the literature describes the outcome in 28 children born to women receiving treatment for leukemia during pregnancy (64,217,221). Of these 28 children, 14 were exposed to therapy in the first trimester. Twenty-four of the 28 children are alive and well with follow-up extending to 17 years. The data from these series suggest that intrauterine exposure to antileukemic therapy does not produce identifiable late effects after birth.

Acute promyelocytic leukemia (APL) is a unique form of AML associated with a specific chromosomal abnormality (15,17) that produces a fusion protein, PML-RAR, affecting the retinoic acid receptor. APL is now treated with combination chemotherapy utilizing an anthracycline and cytarabine and all-*trans*-retinoic acid (ATRA). The risk of ATRA in pregnancy has not been described, but a similar agent, 13-*cis*-retinoic acid, causes a specific retinoic embryopathy when administered in the first trimester. There have been 11 cases of ATRA administered in pregnancy; most patients received this in the third trimester (222). No cases of embryopathy have been reported, but this agent should be used with caution in pregnancy.

The diagnosis and treatment of chronic leukemia is uncommon in pregnancy. If a pregnant patient is diagnosed with CLL, this disease usually has an indolent course and treatment can be delayed until after delivery. For patients who require therapy, the recommendations for indolent lymphoma apply to the management of these patients. Single-agent prednisone may be effective in controlling CLL until term. Alternatively, cyclophosphamide may be added in the second and third trimesters. Fludarabine has not been reported to have been administered during pregnancy. As mentioned previously, CML is the most common chronic leukemia diagnosed in pregnancy.

CML in the chronic phase is characterized by excessive production of mature myeloid elements; however, blast crisis that typically occurs 3 to 5 years after the initial diagnosis behaves like acute leukemia. Pregnancy does not adversely affect the course of CML, and therapy can usually be withheld until after delivery for those patients in chronic phase. For patients who require therapy because of leukocytosis, myelosuppressive therapy with hydroxyurea can be administered until definitive treatment is pursued, which should be delayed until delivery or termination of pregnancy (223). This is a low molecular weight antimetabolite that is likely to be teratogenic during the first trimester but that can be given during the subsequent stages of pregnancy (59). Standard therapy for CML has been allogeneic stem cell transplantation, but more recently, the tyrosine kinase inhibitor Imatinib is the standard therapy for CML. Tyrosine kinase inhibitors are presumably involved in fetal development, and so the use of Imatinib should be avoided until there are more data regarding its use in pregnancy (224). Leukopheresis is an option for women in the first trimester who are symptomatic owing to a high white blood cell count. Interferon-α has also been used in CML, but there are few data describing its use in pregnant patients; however, this agent is unlikely to cross the placenta given its high molecular weight.

For those women with hematologic malignancies who come to term, consideration should be given to collection of umbilical cord stem cells for potential use as a source of hematopoietic cells for transplantation should the mother relapse. A number of factors contribute to the suitability of cord blood as a potential source of stem cells, including HLA typing, number of cord blood cells obtained, and the size of the recipient. Nevertheless, collection of these cells can be performed safely and might permit additional avenues for treatment should the leukemia or lymphoma recur in the mother (225).

Malignant Melanoma

The incidence of melanoma has increased dramatically over the last 50 years (226,227). The median age of women diagnosed with malignant melanoma is 45 years. Studies have shown that of women who develop melanoma, 30% to 40% will be in their reproductive years, and approximately 8% of women are pregnant at the time of diagnosis (226, 228). The overall incidence of melanoma in pregnancy is estimated to be 0.14 to 2.8 cases per 1,000 births (228). Compared with men, women with melanoma have been found to have a more favorable prognosis (229–231).

In general, melanoma is not considered to be a hormone-dependent neoplasm. However, there are concerns that certain endocrine factors may influence the biologic behavior of melanoma. Nulliparous women may be at increased risk of developing melanoma compared with multiparous women

(232). In the first trimester of pregnancy, approximately 10% of women will experience signs of activation of nevi that typically disappear with birth. Increased pigmentation of the vulva, nipple, linea nigra, and preexisting nevi is a common characteristic of pregnancy. Pregnancy is associated with an increase in both adrenocorticotropic hormone (ACTH) and melanocyte-stimulating hormone (MSH), although a direct association between MSH and melanoma has not been found (233). Estrogen has been shown to increase melanocyte activity in animal studies, and there has been concern that hormonal changes in pregnancy could accelerate melanocyte growth (228). However, a recent case-control study found that pregnancy, oral contraceptive use, and estrogen replacement therapy were not associated with melanoma (234).

The majority of pregnant women with melanoma will have stage I disease (235,236). Studies have shown that there are no obvious differences in primary tumor location between pregnant and nonpregnant patients and that most lesions present on the extremities. Slingluff et al. (235) and MacKie et al.(237) have found that women diagnosed with melanomas in pregnancy have significantly thicker primary tumors, and Reintgen et al. (238) reported more unfavorable histopathologic features. Other investigators, however, have not confirmed these findings. The effect of pregnancy on survival of patients with melanoma has been controversial. Early reports, which were largely anecdotal and uncontrolled, gave the impression that melanoma arising in pregnancy was associated with a significant decrease in survival. More recent reports that have been controlled for prognostic variables have challenged such findings (226,228,235,236). In a case-control study by Travers et al. (239), melanomas diagnosed during pregnancy had significantly greater mean thickness, 2.28 versus 1.22 ($p = .007$). However, despite the increased thickness, pregnancy-associated melanomas had a slightly more favorable prognosis.

Analyses of survival data from multiple studies have shown no significant difference in overall survival rates of pregnant patients compared with nonpregnant patients after controlling for histopathologic parameters (227). Reintgen et al.(238) and Slingluff et al. (235) have found a significantly shorter disease-free interval for pregnant stage I patients. The shorter disease-free interval, however, did not affect overall patient survival. The incidence of nodal metastases was higher for pregnant women and time to nodal metastases was significantly shorter. These investigators suggest that pregnancy may be an indicator for elective node dissection because of the increased risk of nodal metastases. Currently, most patients with melanoma undergo sentinel node mapping and biopsy (227). If the sentinel node contains tumor, then a formal lymph node dissection is carried out. However, there are no reports of sentinel node mapping in pregnancy. Trapenznikov et al. (240) examined the effects of pregnancy termination on survival in women with melanoma. In their series, a significantly higher survival rate was observed in women who gave birth compared with those who underwent termination; the 5-year survival rates were 66.5% and 33.5%, respectively.

The only adjuvant therapy proven to improve survival in high-risk malignant melanoma patients has been high-dose interferon-α2b (227). The improvement in survival is only modest, and no reports of interferon use during pregnancy have been reported. The role of adjunctive radiation therapy in patients at high risk of locoregional relapse after primary resection (Clark's level IV or >4 mm thick lesion, positive regional lymphadenopathy) remains undefined. However, there is recent interest in the use of hypofractionated radiation (30 Gy in five fractions over 2.5 weeks), which in a large single-institution Phase II study has resulted in significant improvement in locoregional tumor control as compared with historical controls (227). The chemotherapeutic agent most commonly used to treat melanoma is dacarbazine, with response rates of approximately 20%. In some studies, the addition of tamoxifen to chemotherapy has improved results. Dipaola et al. (241) reported a case of a pregnant woman with rapidly progressive metastatic melanoma who was treated with tamoxifen and combination chemotherapy; the mother died of systemic disease, the baby was born alive and developed normally.

Melanoma is the most common cancer to metastasize to the placenta and fetus (242–245). In a report by Dildy et al. (246) of 53 cases of metastases to the placenta or fetus, 30% were due to melanomas. Of the 12 cases that involved metastasis to the fetus, 7 (58%) were due to melanoma. Spontaneous tumor regression has been described in infants born with transplacental metastasis (247). A more recent review by Alexander of placental metastasis demonstrated that melanoma accounted for 27 (31%) of 87 reported patients with placental disease. The fetus was affected in six of these patients and five of six infants died of melanoma. Thus, the placenta of woman with melanoma needs to be carefully examined by the pathologist.

Following a diagnosis of melanoma, women should be encouraged to delay pregnancy for 2 to 3 years since 80% to 90% of recurrences will develop within this time period (235,248). Several investigators have evaluated the outcome of patients who become pregnant following treatment of melanoma (226,237,238). Both disease-free interval and 10-year survival are similar between those with melanoma who become pregnant at a later date and those who did not, suggesting that subsequent pregnancy has no significant impact on long-term prognosis. In the past, oral contraceptives were not recommended for the patient who had recently been treated for melanoma. However, multiple studies have failed to demonstrate the presence of estrogen or progesterone receptors in benign and malignant melanocytic proliferative lesions (249).

Thyroid and Other Head and Neck Cancers

Malignancies of the thyroid are more common in women than in men, with an approximate ratio of 3:1. An estimated 13,500 new cases of female thyroid cancer were to have occurred in 1999 (5). Although the actual incidence of thyroid cancer in pregnancy is not known, approximately 50% of these malignancies occur in women between the ages of 15 and 44 years, substantially overlapping the childbearing years.

Most malignant tumors of the thyroid are of epithelial origin and are carcinomas. Papillary carcinoma represents the most common histologic type (75%) followed by follicular (15%), medullary (5%), and anaplastic (<5%) varieties. The diagnostic approach in a pregnant patient is similar to that for a nonpregnant patient with the exception that radioisotope scanning should be avoided. Fine-needle aspiration has emerged as the diagnostic test of choice. Thyroid suppression with exogenous thyroid hormone may be used for selected small nodules that have a benign appearance on aspiration and can safely be administered throughout pregnancy.

Surgical resection is the primary treatment for localized well-differentiated thyroid carcinomas, which include most cases of papillary and follicular cancers. In the pregnant patient, timing of surgery is an important decision (250). A retrospective analysis found equivalent thyroid cancer survival rates in pregnant women deferring surgery until the postpartum period compared with nonpregnant women who underwent immediate surgery, suggesting that surgery can be delayed until parturition without compromising long-term survival (251). The addition of thyroid hormone suppression or radioactive iodine (^{131}I) ablation after surgical resection decreases recurrence rates but has a limited impact on overall survival, which is in excess of 90% at 10 years for this favorable group.

For patients presenting with more extensive well-differentiated disease (either by direct invasion or metastases), surgery and the administration of ^{131}I may be necessary to provide optimal maternal treatment during pregnancy. Administration of ^{131}I during pregnancy carries the primary risk of causing fetal hypothyroidism, especially after the onset of the fetal thyroid iodine-concentrating ability at approximately 70 to 80 days of gestational age, whereas dose and effects on other tissues *in utero* are less clearly defined (252, 253). The precise risk of fetal hypothyroidism cannot be determined from the sporadic reports in the literature, but it would be prudent to counsel the mother on the potential sequelae of fetal hypothyroidism if treatment with ^{131}I is deemed necessary during pregnancy. It is imperative that the affected infant's thyroid status be determined shortly after birth so that replacement thyroid hormone can be initiated to avoid the potentially severe CNS sequelae. For patients who have previously received therapeutic ^{131}I for thyroid cancer, subsequent adverse pregnancy outcomes are very rare, although some have advocated delaying onset of pregnancy for a year following completion of ^{131}I administration (254,255).

Medullary thyroid carcinoma presents as two distinct clinical entities—a sporadic form and a familial version often in conjunction with other endocrine tumors as part of a multiple endocrine neoplasia syndrome. In either case, the treatment of choice is total thyroidectomy. In contrast to well-differentiated thyroid carcinoma, given the ineffectiveness of nonoperative ^{131}I salvage of recurrent or metastatic disease, surgery is more likely to be recommended shortly after diagnosis. Patients presenting with metastatic disease are not likely to respond significantly to any currently available chemotherapeutic regimens.

Patients presenting with anaplastic thyroid carcinoma have an extremely poor prognosis, with most patients dying within a year of diagnosis. Surgical resection is indicated for tumors that can technically be removed. However, most tumors are unresectable at presentation. Radiation therapy alone has not been shown to be an effective treatment. Recent attempts using combined chemotherapy and radiation therapy have shown some promise in prolonging survival, but long-term survival remains elusive (256).

Very rare instances of other head and neck epithelial cancers have been reported in conjunction with pregnancy (257, 258). The standard of treatment for most patients with head and neck cancer consists of surgery and/or radiation therapy depending on stage and site of presentation of the disease. Chemotherapy in combination with radiation has also been used with increasing success in advanced-stage disease (259). Dosimetric calculations for fetal exposure during head and neck radiation may be inferred from data in Hodgkin's disease and brain tumors (Table 36.4), and indicate that radiation therapy during pregnancy, if clinically indicated, results in acceptable doses to the fetus. In addition to the potential effects of fetal radiation exposure, one must also consider the consequences of decreased maternal nutritional intake as a result of acute mucositis commonly seen with head and neck radiation therapy.

Colorectal Cancer

Colorectal cancer is the third most common malignancy diagnosed in women, with an estimated 67,000 new cases (56,500 extrapelvic colon, 18,200 rectum) expected in 2003 (202). The age-specific incidence of the disease rises steadily with age through the eighth and ninth decades of life, with fewer than 10% occurring in patients younger than 40 years of age and approximately 2% under age 30 years (260). The incidence of early occurrence is increased in patients with high-risk conditions, such as familial adenomatous polyposis, Gardner's syndrome, inflammatory bowel disease, and a family history of hereditary nonpolyposis colorectal cancer. Colorectal cancer diagnosed during pregnancy is very rare, occurring in an estimated 0.001% to 0.002% of all pregnancies (261). A recent review indicated a total of about 300 reported cases of colorectal cancer in pregnant patients since the first described case in 1842 (262).

The presenting symptoms of colorectal cancer include rectal bleeding, alterations in bowel habits, pain, nausea, abdominal distension, and backache, symptoms that could be readily and erroneously associated with pregnancy itself, and therefore leading to delayed diagnosis (263). A high index of suspicion for patients with rectal bleeding and unexplained microcytic anemia should be maintained, especially in the high-risk-population subsets mentioned above. Given the concerns of radiation exposure associated with a barium enema, the primary means of diagnostic evaluation is with colonoscopy.

A survey and literature review of colorectal cancer in pregnancy (261) indicates that two-thirds or more of the malignancies arise in the rectum. This is in distinction to that of the general population, where two-thirds are found in the extrapelvic colon, with a progressive trend toward increasing numbers found proximally. Less than 30 total cases of colon cancer above the peritoneal reflection have been reported in association with pregnancy. When adjusted for stage and patient age, pregnancy itself appears to have no deleterious effect on colorectal cancer. However, patients diagnosed with the cancer during pregnancy generally present with a higher stage, which may reflect a delay in diagnosis or more aggressive tumor biology noted in younger patients with this malignancy.

The primary management of colorectal cancer is surgical resection. The predilection for a rectal site of origin during pregnancy may make surgical resection difficult in the presence of a gravid uterus, especially in the late second or third trimester. In such a situation, where fetal preservation is desired, a temporizing measure such as a diverting colostomy may be performed to address obstruction and bleeding, with a definitive procedure performed in conjunction with delivery immediately upon documentation of fetal pulmonary maturity. A cesarean section may be advisable secondary to the potential obstructive effects of a large rectal tumor.

Effective postsurgical adjuvant therapies have been identified in the management of patients with colorectal cancers. For patients with node-positive disease, chemotherapy with fluorouracil and levamisole or leukovorin has been shown significantly to reduce recurrence and improve overall survival (262,264,265). For rectal lesions, the use of fluorouracil-based chemotherapy in combination with pelvic radiation therapy significantly improves outcomes in patients with tumors that are node positive or have invaded into perirectal fat (266,267). These adjuvant treatments can be initiated in the immediate postpartum period.

Bone and Soft Tissue Sarcomas

Sarcomas of bone and soft tissues are rare; 4,800 new cases were expected to be diagnosed in women in 2003 (202). These tumors encompass a broad spectrum of histologic types, with diverse sites of origin and clinical characteristics. Within this group of mesenchymal tumors,

Ewing's sarcoma, rhabdomyosarcoma, and osteosarcoma are the most likely to occur prior to and during the childbearing years, with implications for coexisting or future pregnancies. The incidence of these tumors in pregnancy is undefined, with only anecdotal reports and a few small series being described in the literature (268–270).

Ewing's sarcoma occurs most frequently in the adolescent years. The most common sites of origin are the femur and the bones of the pelvis. Current treatment recommendations involve initial multiagent chemotherapy, such as with CAV [cyclophosphamide, doxorubicin (Adriamycin), and vincristine] followed by radiation therapy for local control. Surgery may be used in selected cases. Rhabdomyosarcoma, which is most common in early childhood, has a second peak of occurrence between 14 and 18 years of age. Common sites of presentation are the orbit, other head and neck sites, extremities, trunk, and genitourinary organs. General treatment approaches are similar to those for Ewing's sarcoma. Extremity and supradiaphragmatic lesions for both Ewing's sarcoma and rhabdomyosarcoma, with the exception of proximal femur tumors, may be irradiated, if indicated, with little risk to the fetus (Table 36.4). However, approximately 20% of these tumors arise in the pelvis, which may lead to delayed diagnosis and alteration of treatment algorithms during pregnancy (268).

The peak incidence of osteosarcoma occurs in the second and third decades of life. Most osteosarcomas arise from the long bones of the extremities, with about half presenting near the knee joint. Treatment for osteosarcoma involves neoadjuvant chemotherapy with agents such as doxorubicin, cisplatinum, methotrexate, and ifosfamide followed by surgical resection. Radiation therapy is usually considered only in unresectable lesions, which generally occur in the pelvis, or in cases where definitive surgical extirpation precludes limb-sparing considerations. Metastatic disease in the chest is not associated with the dismal prognosis of the past; patients with limited pulmonary metastases may be successfully salvaged with surgery and chemotherapy.

Other Tumors

Recent reports of rare tumors occurring during pregnancy include malignant brain glioma (45), liver carcinoma (271), renal-cell cancer (272), lung cancer (273), and pheochromocytoma (274). In addition to the principles of tumor management and maternal-fetal care that apply to most cases of cancers occurring during pregnancy, several unique considerations are presented by these specific malignancies. Primary hepatocellular carcinoma is associated with chronic hepatitis B infection, and is a very common cause of cancer death in certain areas of the world where endemic hepatitis exists. Abnormal serum alpha fetoprotein levels in hepatitis B–positive pregnant patients who are being screened for potential fetal neural tube defects should also alert the clinician to the possibility of a coexistent liver cancer (271). The

most common presenting symptoms of renal-cell cancer are hematuria and flank pain, which during pregnancy may be all too readily attributed to recurrent urinary tract infections. The use of abdominopelvic ultrasound to evaluate pregnant patients with recurrent or refractory urinary tract symptoms may lead to earlier diagnosis and treatment of a coexistent renal-cell cancer (272). As more women smoke at a younger age, the likelihood of encountering lung cancer during a pregnancy grows. Surgery is the preferred modality, but treatment planning is complicated by limitations on CT scanning; MRI would be a preferred option. Diagnosis may be delayed because of reluctance to obtain a chest radiograph in a pregnant patient with pulmonary symptoms. If chemotherapy is required, vinorelbine (a vinca alkaloid) and cisplatinum can be given with relative safety. Finally, even if not malignant, a pheochromocytoma secretes catecholamines that perturb the cardiovascular system, and intensive surveillance and medical management are required to achieve satisfactory maternal and fetal outcome (274).

CONCLUSIONS

The diagnosis of cancer during pregnancy often presents a management dilemma in that the lives of both the expectant mother and the fetus are directly affected simultaneously. Specific issues that are unique to this situation include decisions concerning termination of gestation, early delivery of the fetus, delay of maternal cancer therapy, and initiation of treatment during pregnancy. However, although therapeutically challenging, a diagnosis of cancer during pregnancy does not have to imply an adverse outcome for either the mother or the fetus. Treatment approaches have been discussed that allow preservation of pregnancy and yet provide sound maternal oncologic care. The management of cancer in pregnant patients is best achieved through close interaction between the patient, her family, and a multidisciplinary medical team that includes representatives from perinatology, neonatology, gynecologic oncology, medical oncology, radiation oncology, other surgical subspecialties and support services such as nursing and social work.

REFERENCES

1. Atrash HK, Koonin LM, Lawson HW, et al. Maternal mortality in the United States, 1979–1986. *Obstet Gynecol* 1990;76:1055–1060.
2. Donegan WL. Cancer and pregnancy. *CA Cancer J Clin* 1983;33:194–214.
3. From the Centers for Disease Control and Prevention. Maternal mortality—United States, 1982–1996. *JAMA* 1998;280:1042–1043.
4. Landis SH, Murray T, Bolden S, Wingo PA. Cancer statistics, 1998. *CA Cancer J Clin* 1998;48:6–29.
5. Landis SH, Murray T, Bolden S, Wingo PA. Cancer statistics, 1999. *CA Cancer J Clin* 1999;49:8–31, 1.
6. Greer BE, Easterling TR, McLennan DA, et al. Fetal and maternal considerations in the management of stage I-B cervical cancer during pregnancy. *Gynecol Oncol* 1989;34:61–65.
7. McIntire DD, Bloom SL, Casey BM, Leveno KJ. Birth weight in

relation to morbidity and mortality among newborn infants. *N Engl J Med* 1999;340:1234–1238.

8. Berman ML, DiSaia PJ. Pelvic malignancies, gestational trophoblastic neoplasia, and nonpelvic malignancies. In: Cresy RK, Resnick R, Eds. *Maternal-fetal medicine.* Philadelphia: WB Saunders, 1994;1112.

9. Bevilacqua G, Parmigiani S, Robertson B. Prophylaxis of respiratory distress syndrome by treatment with modified porcine surfactant at birth: a multicentre prospective randomized trial. *J Perinat Med* 1996; 24:609–620.

10. Corbet A, Long W, Schumacher R, et al. Double-blind developmental evaluation at 1-year corrected age of 597 premature infants with birth weights from 500 to 1350 grams enrolled in three placebo-controlled trials of prophylactic synthetic surfactant. American Exosurf Neonatal Study Group I. *J Pediatr* 1995;126:S5–S12.

11. Jobe AH, Mitchell BR, Gunkel JH. Beneficial effects of the combined use of prenatal corticosteroids and postnatal surfactant on preterm infants. *Am J Obstet Gynecol* 1993;168:508–513.

12. Kendig JW, Ryan RM, Sinkin RA, et al. Comparison of two strategies for surfactant prophylaxis in very premature infants: a multicenter randomized trial. *Pediatrics* 1998;101:1006–1012.

13. Gappa M, Berner MM, Hohenschild S, et al. Pulmonary function at school-age in surfactant-treated preterm infants. *Pediatr Pulmonol* 1999;27:191–198.

14. Pelkonen AS, Hakulinen AL, Turpeinen M, Hallman M. Effect of neonatal surfactant therapy on lung function at school age in children born very preterm. *Pediatr Pulmonol* 1998;25:182–190.

15. Sinkin RA, Kramer BM, Merzbach JL, et al. School-age follow-up of prophylactic versus rescue surfactant trial: pulmonary, neurodevelopmental, and educational outcomes. *Pediatrics* 1998;101:E11.

16. Bullard SR, Donahue SP, Feman SS, et al. The decreasing incidence and severity of retinopathy of prematurity. *J Aapos* 1999;3:46–52.

17. Kennedy J, Todd DA, Watts J, John E. Retinopathy of prematurity in infants less than 29 weeks' gestation: 3 1/2 years pre- and postsurfactant. *J Pediatr Ophthalmol Strabismus* 1997;34:289–292.

18. Termote J, Schalij-Delfos NE, Cats BP, et al. Less severe retinopathy of prematurity induced by surfactant replacement therapy. *Acta Paediatr* 1996;85:1491–1496.

19. Vohr BR, Garcia Coll CT. Neurodevelopmental and school performance of very low-birth-weight infants: a seven-year longitudinal study. *Pediatrics* 1985;76:345–350.

20. Papile LA, Munsick-Bruno G, Schaefer A. Relationship of cerebral intraventricular hemorrhage and early childhood neurologic handicaps. *J Pediatr* 1983;103:273–277.

21. Halsey CL, Collin MF, Anderson CL. Extremely low birth weight children and their peers: a comparison of preschool performance. *Pediatrics* 1993;91:807–811.

22. Stovall M, Blackwell CR, Cundiff J, et al. Fetal dose from radiotherapy with photon beams: report of AAPM Radiation Therapy Committee Task Group No. 36. *Med Phys* 1995;22:63–82.

23. Gradishar WJ, Schilsky RL. Ovarian function following radiation and chemotherapy for cancer. *Semin Oncol* 1989;16:425–436.

24. Otake M, Schull WJ, Neel JV. Congenital malformations, stillbirths, and early mortality among the children of atomic bomb survivors: a reanalysis. *Radiat Res* 1990;122:1–11.

25. Wharton JT, Rutledge FN, Gallager HS, Fletcher G. Treatment of clear cell adenocarcinoma in young females. *Obstet Gynecol* 1975; 45:365–368.

26. Chambers SK, Chambers JT, Kier R, Peschel RE. Sequelae of lateral ovarian transposition in irradiated cervical cancer patients. *Int J Radiat Oncol Biol Phys* 1991;20:1305–1308.

27. Aisner J, Wiernik PH, Pearl P. Pregnancy outcome in patients treated for Hodgkin's disease. *J Clin Oncol* 1993;11:507–512.

28. Ortin TT, Shostak CA, Donaldson SS. Gonadal status and reproductive function following treatment for Hodgkin's disease in childhood: the Stanford experience. *Int J Radiat Oncol Biol Phys* 1990;19: 873–880.

29. Byrne J, Mulvihill JJ, Myers MH, et al. Effects of treatment on fertility in long-term survivors of childhood or adolescent cancer. *N Engl J Med* 1987;317:1315–1321.

30. Green DM, Whitton JA, Stovall M, et al. Pregnancy outcome of female survivors of childhood cancer: a report from the Childhood Cancer Survivor Study. *Am J Obstet Gynecol* 2002;187:1070–1080.

31. Sanders JE, Hawley J, Levy W, et al. Pregnancies following high-dose cyclophosphamide with or without high-dose busulfan or total-body irradiation and bone marrow transplantation. *Blood* 1996;87: 3045–3052.

32. Boice JD Jr, Tawn EJ, Winther JF, et al. Genetic effects of radiotherapy for childhood cancer. *Health Phys* 2003;85:65–80.

33. Niroomand-Rad A, Cumberlin R. Measured dose to ovaries and testes from Hodgkin's fields and determination of genetically significant dose. *Int J Radiat Oncol Biol Phys* 1993;25:745–751.

34. Hawkins MM. Is there evidence of a therapy-related increase in germ cell mutation among childhood cancer survivors? *J Natl Cancer Inst* 1991;83:1643–1650.

35. Mulvihill JJ, McKeen EA, Rosner F, Zarrabi MH. Pregnancy outcome in cancer patients. Experience in a large cooperative group. *Cancer* 1987;60:1143–1150.

36. Hall EJ. Hereditary effects of radiation. In: Hall EJ, Ed. *Radiobiology for the radiologist.* Philadelphia: JB Lippincott Co, 1994;351.

37. Mulvihill JJ, Byrne J. Genetic counseling of the cancer survivor. *Semin Oncol Nurs* 1989;5:29–35.

38. Brent RL. The effect of embryonic and fetal exposure to x-ray, microwaves, and ultrasound: counseling the pregnant and nonpregnant patient about these risks. *Semin Oncol* 1989;16:347–368.

39. Hall EJ. Effects of radiation on the embryo and fetus. In: Hall EJ, ed. *Radiobiology for the radiologist.* Philadelphia: JB Lippincott Co, 1994;363.

40. Gu Y, Kai M, Kusama T. The embryonic and fetal effects in ICR mice irradiated in the various stages of the preimplantation period. *Radiat Res* 1997;147:735–740.

41. Pampfer S, Streffer C. Prenatal death and malformations after irradiation of mouse zygotes with neutrons or x-rays. *Teratology* 1988;37: 599–607.

42. Gaulden ME. Possible effects of diagnostic x-rays on the human embryo and fetus. *J Ark Med Soc* 1974;70:424–435.

43. Dekaban AS. Abnormalities in children exposed to x-radiation during various stages of gestation: tentative timetable of radiation injury to the human fetus. I. *J Nucl Med* 1968;9:471.

44. Sienkiewicz ZJ, Haylock RG, Saunders RD. Differential learning impairments produced by prenatal exposure to ionizing radiation in mice. *Int J Radiat Biol* 1999;75:121–127.

45. Sneed PK, Albright NW, Wara WM, et al. Fetal dose estimates for radiotherapy of brain tumors during pregnancy. *Int J Radiat Oncol Biol Phys* 1995;32:823–830.

46. Harvey EB, Boice JD Jr, Honeyman M, Flannery JT. Prenatal x-ray exposure and childhood cancer in twins. *N Engl J Med* 1985;312: 541–545.

47. Yoshimoto Y, Kato H, Schull WJ. Risk of cancer among children exposed in utero to A-bomb radiations, 1950–84. *Lancet* 1988;2: 665–669.

48. Fraass BA, van de Geijn J. Peripheral dose from megavolt beams. *Med Phys* 1983;10:809–818.

49. Nisce LZ, Tome MA, He S, et al. Management of coexisting Hodgkin's disease and pregnancy. *Am J Clin Oncol* 1986;9:146–151.

50. Sorosky JI, Sood AK, Buekers TE. The use of chemotherapeutic agents during pregnancy. *Obstet Gynecol Clin North Am* 1997;24: 591–599.

51. Sutcliffe SB. Treatment of neoplastic disease during pregnancy: maternal and fetal effects. *Clin Invest Med* 1985;8:333–338.

52. Doll DC, Ringenberg QS, Yarbro JW. Management of cancer during pregnancy. *Arch Intern Med* 1988;148:2058–2064.

53. Leslie KK. Chemotherapy and pregnancy. *Clin Obstet Gynecol* 2002; 45:153–164.

54. Herold M, Schnohr S, Bittrich H. Efficacy and safety of a combined rituximab chemotherapy during pregnancy. *J Clin Oncol* 2001;19: 3439.

55. De Santis M, Lucchese A, De Carolis S, et al. Metastatic breast cancer in pregnancy: first case of chemotherapy with docetaxel. *Eur J Cancer Care (Engl)* 2000;9:235–237.

56. Sood AK, Shahin MS, Sorosky JI. Paclitaxel and platinum chemotherapy for ovarian carcinoma during pregnancy. *Gynecol Oncol* 2001; 83:599–600.

57. Mendez LE, Mueller A, Salom E, Gonzalez-Quintero VH. Paclitaxel and carboplatin chemotherapy administered during pregnancy for advanced epithelial ovarian cancer. *Obstet Gynecol* 2003;102: 1200–1202.

58. Buekers TE, Lallas TA. Chemotherapy in pregnancy. *Obstet Gynecol Clin North Am* 1998;25:323–329.

59. Dipaola RS, Goodin S, Ratzell M, et al. Chemotherapy for metastatic melanoma during pregnancy. *Gynecol Oncol* 1997;66:526–530.

60. Doll DC, Ringenberg QS, Yarbro JW. Antineoplastic agents and pregnancy. *Semin Oncol* 1989;16:337–346.

61. Williams SF, Schilsky RL. Antineoplastic drugs administered during pregnancy. *Semin Oncol* 2000;27:618–622.

62. Beeley L. Adverse effects of drugs in the first trimester of pregnancy. *Clin Obstet Gynaecol* 1986;13:177–195.

63. Warkany J. Aminopterin and methotrexate: folic acid deficiency. *Teratology* 1978;17:353–357.

64. Caligiuri MA, Mayer RJ. Pregnancy and leukemia. *Semin Oncol* 1989; 16:388–396.

65. Glantz JC. Reproductive toxicology of alkylating agents. *Obstet Gynecol Surv* 1994;49:709–715.

66. Karp GI, von Oeyen P, Valone F, et al. Doxorubicin in pregnancy: possible transplacental passage. *Cancer Treat Rep* 1983;67:773–777.

67. Turchi JJ, Villasis C. Anthracyclines in the treatment of malignancy in pregnancy. *Cancer* 1988;61:435–440.

68. Arceci RJ, Baas F, Raponi R, et al. Multidrug resistance gene expression is controlled by steroid hormones in the secretory epithelium of the uterus. *Mol Reprod Dev* 1990;25:101–109.

69. Pui CH, Ribeiro RC, Hancock ML, et al. Acute myeloid leukemia in children treated with epipodophyllotoxins for acute lymphoblastic leukemia. *N Engl J Med* 1991;325:1682–1687.

70. Tomlinson MW, Treadwell MC, Deppe G. Platinum based chemotherapy to treat recurrent Sertoli-Leydig cell ovarian carcinoma during pregnancy. *Eur J Gynaecol Oncol* 1997;18:44–46.

71. Kai S, Kohmura H, Ishikawa K, et al. Teratogenic effects of carboplatin, an oncostatic drug, administered during the early organogenetic period in rats. *J Toxicol Sci* 1989;14:115–130.

72. Henderson CE, Elia G, Garfinkel D, et al. Platinum chemotherapy during pregnancy for serous cystadenocarcinoma of the ovary. *Gynecol Oncol* 1993;49:92–94.

73. Egan PC, Costanza ME, Dodion P, et al. Doxorubicin and cisplatin excretion into human milk. *Cancer Treat Rep* 1985;69:1387–1389.

74. Partridge AH, Garber JE. Long-term outcomes of children exposed to antineoplastic agents in utero. *Semin Oncol* 2000;27:712–726.

75. Garber JE. Long-term follow-up of children exposed in utero to antineoplastic agents. *Semin Oncol* 1989;16:437–444.

76. Aviles A, Neri N. Hematological malignancies and pregnancy: a final report of 84 children who received chemotherapy in utero. *Clin Lymphoma* 2001;2:173–177.

77. Zemlickis D, Lishner M, Degendorfer P, et al. Fetal outcome after in utero exposure to cancer chemotherapy. *Arch Intern Med* 1992;152:573–576.

78. Duggan B, Muderspach LI, Roman LD, et al. Cervical cancer in pregnancy: reporting on planned delay in therapy. *Obstet Gynecol* 1993;82:598–602.

79. Hacker NF, Leuchter RS, Berek JS, et al. Radical vulvectomy and bilateral inguinal lymphadenectomy through separate groin incisions. *Obstet Gynecol* 1981;58:574–579.

80. Manuel-Limson GA, Ladines-Llave CA, Sotto LS, Manalo AM. Cancer of the cervix in pregnancy: a 31-year experience at the Philippine General Hospital. *J Obstet Gynaecol Res* 1997;23:503–509.

81. Hopkins MP, Morley GW. The prognosis and management of cervical cancer associated with pregnancy. *Obstet Gynecol* 1992;80:9–13.

82. Zemlickis D, Lishner M, Degendorfer P, et al. Maternal and fetal outcome after invasive cervical cancer in pregnancy. *J Clin Oncol* 1991;9:1956–1961.

83. Senekjian EK, Hubby M, Bell DA, et al. Clear cell adenocarcinoma (CCA) of the vagina and cervix in association with pregnancy. *Gynecol Oncol* 1986;24:207–219.

84. Campion MJ, Sedlacek TV. Colposcopy in pregnancy. *Obstet Gynecol Clin North Am* 1993;20:153–163.

85. McCord ML, Stovall TG, Meric JL, et al. Cervical cytology: a randomized comparison of four sampling methods. *Am J Obstet Gynecol* 1992;166:1772–1777; Discussion 1777–1779.

86. Orr JW Jr, Barrett JM, Orr PF, et al. The efficacy and safety of the cytobrush during pregnancy. *Gynecol Oncol* 1992;44:260–262.

87. Rivlin ME, Woodliff JM, Bowlin RB, et al. Comparison of cytobrush and cotton swab for Papanicolaou smears in pregnancy. *J Reprod Med* 1993;38:147–150.

88. Abulafia O, Pezzullo JC, Sherer DM. Performance of ThinPrep liquidbased cervical cytology in comparison with conventionally prepared Papanicolaou smears: a quantitative survey. *Gynecol Oncol* 2003;90:137–144.

89. Bernstein SJ, Sanchez-Ramos L, Ndubisi B. Liquid-based cervical cytologic smear study and conventional Papanicolaou smears: a metaanalysis of prospective studies comparing cytologic diagnosis and sample adequacy. *Am J Obstet Gynecol* 2001;185:308–317.

90. Benedet JL, Boyes DA, Nichols TM, Millner A. Colposcopic evaluation of pregnant patients with abnormal cervical smears. *Br J Obstet Gynaecol* 1977;84:517–521.

91. DePetrillo AD, Townsend DE, Morrow CP, et al. Colposcopic evaluation of the abnormal Papanicolaou test in pregnancy. *Am J Obstet Gynecol* 1975;121:441–445.

92. Economos K, Perez Veridiano N, Delke I, et al. Abnormal cervical cytology in pregnancy: a 17-year experience. *Obstet Gynecol* 1993;81:915–918.

93. Woodrow N, Permezel M, Butterfield L, et al. Abnormal cervical cytology in pregnancy: experience of 811 cases. *Aust N Z J Obstet Gynaecol* 1998;38:161–165.

94. Yost NP, Santoso JT, McIntire DD, Iliya FA. Postpartum regression rates of antepartum cervical intraepithelial neoplasia II and III lesions. *Obstet Gynecol* 1999;93:359–362.

95. Palle C, Bangsboll S, Andreasson B. Cervical intraepithelial neoplasia in pregnancy. *Acta Obstet Gynecol Scand* 2000;79:306–310.

96. Michael CW, Esfahani FM. Pregnancy-related changes: a retrospective review of 278 cervical smears. *Diagn Cytopathol* 1997;17:99–107.

97. Kim TJ, Kim HS, Park CT, et al. Clinical evaluation of follow-up methods and results of atypical glandular cells of undetermined significance (AGUS) detected on cervicovaginal Pap smears. *Gynecol Oncol* 1999;73:292–298.

98. Ostergard DR, Nieberg RK. Evaluation of abnormal cervical cytology during pregnancy with colposcopy. *Am J Obstet Gynecol* 1979;134:756–758.

99. Averette HE, Nasser N, Yankow SL, Little WA. Cervical conization in pregnancy. Analysis of 180 operations. *Am J Obstet Gynecol* 1970;106:543–549.

100. Hannigan EV, Whitehouse HH 3rd, Atkinson WD, Becker SN. Cone biopsy during pregnancy. *Obstet Gynecol* 1982;60:450–455.

101. Choo YC, Chan OL, Hsu C, Ma HK. Colposcopy in microinvasive carcinoma of the cervix—an enigma of diagnosis. *Br J Obstet Gynaecol* 1984;91:1156–1160.

102. Goldberg GL, Altaras MM, Block B. Cone cerclage in pregnancy. *Obstet Gynecol* 1991;77:315–317.

103. Robinson WR, Webb S, Tirpack J, et al. Management of cervical intraepithelial neoplasia during pregnancy with LOOP excision. *Gynecol Oncol* 1997;64:153–155.

104. Monk BJ, Montz FJ. Invasive cervical cancer complicating intrauterine pregnancy: treatment with radical hysterectomy. *Obstet Gynecol* 1992;80:199–203.

105. Takushi M, Moromizato H, Sakumoto K, Kanazawa K. Management of invasive carcinoma of the uterine cervix associated with pregnancy: outcome of intentional delay in treatment. *Gynecol Oncol* 2002;87:185–189.

106. Sood AK, Sorosky JI, Krogman S, et al. Surgical management of cervical cancer complicating pregnancy: a case-control study. *Gynecol Oncol* 1996;63:294–298.

107. Lee RB, Neglia W, Park RC. Cervical carcinoma in pregnancy. *Obstet Gynecol* 1981;58:584–589.

108. Prem KA, Makowski EL, McKelvey JL. Carcinoma of the cervix associated with pregnancy. *Am J Obstet Gynecol* 1966;95:99–108.

109. van Vliet W, van Loon AJ, ten Hoor KA, Boonstra H. Cervical carcinoma during pregnancy: outcome of planned delay in treatment. *Eur J Obstet Gynecol Reprod Biol* 1998;79:153–157.

110. Cobb CJ. Ectopic decidua and metastatic squamous carcinoma: presentation in a single pelvic lymph node. *J Surg Oncol* 1988;38:126–129.

111. Russell AH. Contemporary radiation treatment planning for patients with cancer of the uterine cervix. *Semin Oncol* 1994;21:30–41.

112. Nevin J, Soeters R, Dehaeck K, et al. Cervical carcinoma associated with pregnancy. *Obstet Gynecol Surv* 1995;50:228–239.

113. Goldman NA, Goldberg GL. Late recurrence of squamous cell cervical cancer in an episiotomy site after vaginal delivery. *Obstet Gynecol* 2003;101:1127–1129.

114. Bernhard LM, Klebba PK, Gray DL, Mutch DG. Predictors of persistence of adnexal masses in pregnancy. *Obstet Gynecol* 1999;93: 585–589.

115. Bromley B, Benacerraf B. Adnexal masses during pregnancy: accuracy of sonographic diagnosis and outcome. *J Ultrasound Med* 1997; 16:447–52; quiz 453–454.

116. Platek DN, Henderson CE, Goldberg GL. The management of a persistent adnexal mass in pregnancy. *Am J Obstet Gynecol* 1995;173: 1236–1240.

117. Wheeler TC, Fleischer AC. Complex adnexal mass in pregnancy: predictive value of color Doppler sonography. *J Ultrasound Med* 1997;16:425–428.

118. Creasman WT, Rutledge F, Smith JP. Carcinoma of the ovary associated with pregnancy. *Obstet Gynecol* 1971;38:111–116.

119. Roberts JA. Management of gynecologic tumors during pregnancy. *Clin Perinatol* 1983;10:369–382.

120. Hogston P, Lilford RJ. Ultrasound study of ovarian cysts in pregnancy: prevalence and significance. *Br J Obstet Gynaecol* 1986;93:625–628.

121. Thornton JG, Wells M. Ovarian cysts in pregnancy: does ultrasound make traditional management inappropriate? *Obstet Gynecol* 1987; 69:717–721.

122. Struyk AP, Treffers PE. Ovarian tumors in pregnancy. *Acta Obstet Gynecol Scand* 1984;63:421–424.

123. Ballard CA. Ovarian tumors associated with pregnancy termination patients. *Am J Obstet Gynecol* 1984;149:384–387.

124. Beischer NA, Buttery BW, Fortune DW, Macafee CA. Growth and malignancy of ovarian tumours in pregnancy. *Aust N Z J Obstet Gynaecol* 1971;11:208–220.

125. Hess LW, Peaceman A, O'Brien WF, et al. Adnexal mass occurring with intrauterine pregnancy: report of fifty-four patients requiring laparotomy for definitive management. *Am J Obstet Gynecol* 1988;158: 1029–1034.

126. Sherer DM, Maitland CY, Levine NF, et al. Prenatal magnetic resonance imaging assisting in differentiating between large degenerating intramural leiomyoma and complex adnexal mass during pregnancy. *J Matern Fetal Med* 2000;9:186–189.

127. Kobayashi F, Sagawa N, Nakamura K, et al. Mechanism and clinical significance of elevated CA 125 levels in the sera of pregnant women. *Am J Obstet Gynecol* 1989;160:563–566.

128. Grendys EC Jr, Barnes WA. Ovarian cancer in pregnancy. *Surg Clin North Am* 1995;75:1–14.

129. Kort B, Katz VL, Watson WJ. The effect of nonobstetric operation during pregnancy. *Surg Gynecol Obstet* 1993;177:371–376.

130. Mathevet P, Nessah K, Dargent D, Mellier G. Laparoscopic management of adnexal masses in pregnancy: a case series. *Eur J Obstet Gynecol Reprod Biol* 2003;108:217–222.

131. Soriano D, Yefet Y, Seidman DS, et al. Laparoscopy versus laparotomy in the management of adnexal masses during pregnancy. *Fertil Steril* 1999;71:955–960.

132. Akira S, Yamanaka A, Ishihara T, et al. Gasless laparoscopic ovarian cystectomy during pregnancy: comparison with laparotomy. *Am J Obstet Gynecol* 1999;180:554–557.

133. Friedman JD, Ramsey PS, Ramin KD, Berry C. Pneumoamnion and pregnancy loss after second-trimester laparoscopic surgery. *Obstet Gynecol* 2002;99:512–513.

134. Dgani R, Shoham Z, Atar E, et al. Ovarian carcinoma during pregnancy: a study of 23 cases in Israel between the years 1960 and 1984. *Gynecol Oncol* 1989;33:326–331.

135. Moore JL Jr, Martin JN Jr. Cancer and pregnancy. *Obstet Gynecol Clin North Am* 1992;19:815–827.

136. Novak ER, Lambrou CD, Woodruff JD. Ovarian tumors in pregnancy. An ovarian tumor registry review. *Obstet Gynecol* 1975;46:401–406.

137. De Palo G, Pilotti S, Kenda R, et al. Natural history of dysgerminoma. *Am J Obstet Gynecol* 1982;143:799–807.

138. Karlen JR, Akbari A, Cook WA. Dysgerminoma associated with pregnancy. *Obstet Gynecol* 1979;53:330–335.

139. Gershenson DM, Del Junco G, Herson J, Rutledge FN. Endodermal sinus tumor of the ovary: the M. D. Anderson experience. *Obstet Gynecol* 1983;61:194–202.

140. Buller RE, Darrow V, Manetta A, et al. Conservative surgical management of dysgerminoma concomitant with pregnancy. *Obstet Gynecol* 1992;79:887–890.

141. Christman JE, Teng NN, Lebovic GS, Sikic BI. Delivery of a normal infant following cisplatin, vinblastine, and bleomycin (PVB) chemotherapy for malignant teratoma of the ovary during pregnancy. *Gynecol Oncol* 1990;37:292–295.

142. Horbelt D, Delmore J, Meisel R, et al. Mixed germ cell malignancy of the ovary concurrent with pregnancy. *Obstet Gynecol* 1994;84: 662–664.

143. Malone JM, Gershenson DM, Creasy RK, et al. Endodermal sinus tumor of the ovary associated with pregnancy. *Obstet Gynecol* 1986; 68:86S–89S.

144. Young RH, Dudley AG, Scully RE. Granulosa cell, Sertoli-Leydig cell, and unclassified sex cord-stromal tumors associated with pregnancy: a clinicopathological analysis of thirty-six cases. *Gynecol Oncol* 1984;18:181–205.

145. Mooney J, Silva E, Tornos C, Gershenson D. Unusual features of serous neoplasms of low malignant potential during pregnancy. *Gynecol Oncol* 1997;65:30–35.

146. King LA, Nevin PC, Williams PP, Carson LF. Treatment of advanced epithelial ovarian carcinoma in pregnancy with cisplatin-based chemotherapy. *Gynecol Oncol* 1991;41:78–80.

147. Malfetano JH, Goldkrand JW. Cis-platinum combination chemotherapy during pregnancy for advanced epithelial ovarian carcinoma. *Obstet Gynecol* 1990;75:545–547.

148. Kuller JA, Zucker PK, Peng TC. Vulvar leiomyosarcoma in pregnancy. *Am J Obstet Gynecol* 1990;162:164–166.

149. Lau TK, Wong WS. Uterine leiomyosarcoma associated with pregnancy: report of two cases. *Gynecol Oncol* 1994;53:245–247.

150. Scioscia AL, Merino MJ, Haas M, et al. Malignant mixed mullerian tumor of the uterus arising in association with a viable gestation. *Obstet Gynecol* 1988;71:1047–1050.

151. Del Priore G, Schink JC, Lurain JR. A two-step approach to the treatment of invasive vulvar cancer in pregnancy. *Int J Gynaecol Obstet* 1992;39:335–336.

152. Moore DH, Fowler WC Jr, Currie JL, Walton LA. Squamous cell carcinoma of the vulva in pregnancy. *Gynecol Oncol* 1991;41:74–77.

153. Burke TW, Stringer CA, Gershenson DM, et al. Radical wide excision and selective inguinal node dissection for squamous cell carcinoma of the vulva. *Gynecol Oncol* 1990;38:328–332.

154. DiSaia PJ, Creasman WT, Rich WM. An alternate approach to early cancer of the vulva. *Am J Obstet Gynecol* 1979;133:825–832.

155. Vaccarello L, Apte SM, Copeland LJ, et al. Endometrial carcinoma associated with pregnancy: a report of three cases and review of the literature. *Gynecol Oncol* 1999;74:118–122.

156. Ferenczy A, Choukroun D, Falcone T, Franco E. The effect of cervical loop electrosurgical excision on subsequent pregnancy outcome: North American experience. *Am J Obstet Gynecol* 1995;172: 1246–1250.

157. Weed JC Jr, Curry SL, Duncan ID, et al. Fertility after cryosurgery of the cervix. *Obstet Gynecol* 1978;52:245–246.

158. Spitzer M, Herman J, Krumholz BA, Lesser M. The fertility of women after cervical laser surgery. *Obstet Gynecol* 1995;86:504–508.

159. Kristensen J, Langhoff-Roos J, Wittrup M, Bock JE. Cervical conization and preterm delivery/low birth weight. A systematic review of the literature. *Acta Obstet Gynecol Scand* 1993;72:640–644.

159a. Gililland J, Weinstein L. The effects of cancer chemotherapeutic agents on the developing fetus. *Obstet Gynecol Surv* 1983;38:6–13.

160. Mathevet P, Chemali E, Roy M, Dargent D. Long-term outcome of a randomized study comparing three techniques of conization: cold knife, laser, and LEEP. *Eur J Obstet Gynecol Reprod Biol* 2003;106: 214–218.

161. Huang LW, Hwang JL. A comparison between loop electrosurgical excision procedure and cold knife conization for treatment of cervical dysplasia: residual disease in a subsequent hysterectomy specimen. *Gynecol Oncol* 1999;73:12–15.

162. Paraskevaidis E, Koliopoulos G, Lolis E, et al. Delivery outcomes following loop electrosurgical excision procedure for microinvasive (FIGO stage IA1) cervical cancer. *Gynecol Oncol* 2002;86:10–13.

163. Roman LD, Felix JC, Muderspach LI, et al. Risk of residual invasive

disease in women with microinvasive squamous cancer in a conization specimen. *Obstet Gynecol* 1997;90:759–764.

164. Morris M, Mitchell MF, Silva EG, et al. Cervical conization as definitive therapy for early invasive squamous carcinoma of the cervix. *Gynecol Oncol* 1993;51:193–196.

165. Dargent D, Martin X, Sacchetoni A, Mathevet P. Laparoscopic vaginal radical trachelectomy: a treatment to preserve the fertility of cervical carcinoma patients. *Cancer* 2000;88:1877–1882.

166. Rodriguez M, Guimares O, Rose PG. Radical abdominal trachelectomy and pelvic lymphadenectomy with uterine conservation and subsequent pregnancy in the treatment of early invasive cervical cancer. *Am J Obstet Gynecol* 2001;185:370–374.

167. Burnett AF, Roman LD, O'Meara AT, Morrow CP. Radical vaginal trachelectomy and pelvic lymphadenectomy for preservation of fertility in early cervical carcinoma. *Gynecol Oncol* 2003;88:419–423.

168. Gershenson DM. Menstrual and reproductive function after treatment with combination chemotherapy for malignant ovarian germ cell tumors. *J Clin Oncol* 1988;6:270–275.

169. Low JJ, Perrin LC, Crandon AJ, Hacker NF. Conservative surgery to preserve ovarian function in patients with malignant ovarian germ cell tumors. A review of 74 cases. *Cancer* 2000;89:391–398.

170. Morris RT, Gershenson DM, Silva EG, et al. Outcome and reproductive function after conservative surgery for borderline ovarian tumors. *Obstet Gynecol* 2000;95:541–547.

171. Morice P, Camatte S, El Hassan J, et al. Clinical outcomes and fertility after conservative treatment of ovarian borderline tumors. *Fertil Steril* 2001;75:92–96.

172. Schilder JM, Thompson AM, DePriest PD, et al. Outcome of reproductive age women with stage IA or IC invasive epithelial ovarian cancer treated with fertility-sparing therapy. *Gynecol Oncol* 2002;87:1–7.

173. Wang CB, Wang CJ, Huang HJ, et al. Fertility-preserving treatment in young patients with endometrial adenocarcinoma. *Cancer* 2002;94:2192–2198.

174. Kim YB, Holschneider CH, Ghosh K, et al. Progestin alone as primary treatment of endometrial carcinoma in premenopausal women. Report of seven cases and review of the literature. *Cancer* 1997;79:320–327.

175. Randall TC, Kurman RJ. Progestin treatment of atypical hyperplasia and well-differentiated carcinoma of the endometrium in women under age 40. *Obstet Gynecol* 1997;90:434–440.

176. Mitsushita J, Toki T, Kato K, et al. Endometrial carcinoma remaining after term pregnancy following conservative treatment with medroxyprogesterone acetate. *Gynecol Oncol* 2000;79:129–132.

177. Berkowitz RS, Tuncer ZS, Bernstein MR, Goldstein DP. Management of gestational trophoblastic diseases: subsequent pregnancy experience. *Semin Oncol* 2000;27:678–685.

178. Lok CA, van der Houwen C, ten Kate-Booij MJ, et al. Pregnancy after EMA/CO for gestational trophoblastic disease: a report from The Netherlands. *Bjog* 2003;110:560–566.

179. Bower M, Newlands ES, Holden L, et al. EMA/CO for high-risk gestational trophoblastic tumors: results from a cohort of 272 patients. *J Clin Oncol* 1997;15:2636–2643.

180. Barnavon Y, Wallack MK. Management of the pregnant patient with carcinoma of the breast. *Surg Gynecol Obstet* 1990;171:347–352.

181. Gwyn K, Theriault R. Breast cancer during pregnancy. *Oncology (Huntingt)* 2001;15:39–46; Discussion 46, 49–51.

182. King RM, Welch JS, Martin JK Jr, Coulam CB. Carcinoma of the breast associated with pregnancy. *Surg Gynecol Obstet* 1985;160:228–232.

183. Moore HC, Foster RS Jr. Breast cancer and pregnancy. *Semin Oncol* 2000;27:646–653.

184. Petrik JA. Breast cancer and pregnancy. In: Harris JR HS, Henderson IC, Kinne DW, eds. *Breast diseases*. Philadelphia: JB Lippencott Co, 1991;809.

185. Wallack MK, Wolf JA Jr, Bedwinek J, et al. Gestational carcinoma of the female breast. *Curr Probl Cancer* 1983;7:1–58.

186. Gallenberg MM, Loprinzi CL. Breast cancer and pregnancy. *Semin Oncol* 1989;16:369–376.

187. Max MH, Klamer TW. Pregnancy and breast cancer. *South Med J* 1983;76:1088–1090.

188. Petrek JA, Dukoff R, Rogatko A. Prognosis of pregnancy-associated breast cancer. *Cancer* 1991;67:869–872.

189. Reed W, Hannisdal E, Skovlund E, et al. Pregnancy and breast cancer: a population-based study. *Virchows Arch* 2003;443:44–50.

190. Finley JL, Silverman JF, Lannin DR. Fine-needle aspiration cytology of breast masses in pregnant and lactating women. *Diagn Cytopathol* 1989;5:255–259.

191. Byrd BF, Bayer DS, Roertson JC, et al. Treatment of breast tumors associated with pregnancy and lactation. *Am Surg* 1962;155:940.

192. Petrek JA. Breast cancer during pregnancy. *Cancer* 1994;74:518–527.

193. Buchholz TA, Austin-Seymour MM, Moe RE, et al. Effect of delay in radiation in the combined modality treatment of breast cancer. *Int J Radiat Oncol Biol Phys* 1993;26:23–35.

194. Stevenson J, Giantonio B, Boyd RL, Bruner JA. Adjuvant chemotherapy for breast cancer in pregnancy: can recommendations be made with confidence. *Semin Oncol* 1997;24:xxv–xxxvi; Discussion xxxvi, xxxix.

195. Bunker ML, Peters MV. Breast cancer associated with pregnancy or lactation. *Am J Obstet Gynecol* 1963;85:312–321.

196. Tewari K, Bonebrake RG, Asrat T, Shanberg AM. Ambiguous genitalia in infant exposed to tamoxifen in utero. *Lancet* 1997;350:183.

196a. Berry DL, Theriault RL, Holmes FA, et al. Management of breast cancer during pregnancy using a standardized protocol. *J Clin Oncol* 1999;17:855–861.

196b. Cullins S, Pridjian G, Sutherland C. Goldenhar's syndrome associated with tamoxifen given to the mother during gestation. *JAMA* 1994;271:1905–1906.

199. Keleher AJ, Theriault RL, Gwyn KM, et al. Multidisciplinary management of breast cancer concurrent with pregnancy. *J Am Coll Surg* 2002;194:54–64.

200. Zemlickis D, Lishner M, Degendorfer P, et al. Maternal and fetal outcome after breast cancer in pregnancy. *Am J Obstet Gynecol* 1992;166:781–787.

201. Danforth DN Jr. How subsequent pregnancy affects outcome in women with a prior breast cancer. *Oncology (Huntingt)* 1991;5:23–30; Discussion 30–31, 35.

202. Jemal A, Murray T, Samuels A, et al. Cancer statistics, 2003. *CA Cancer J Clin* 2003;53:5–26.

203. Jacobs C, Donaldson SS, Rosenberg SA, Kaplan HS. Management of the pregnant patient with Hodgkin's disease. *Ann Intern Med* 1981;95:669–675.

204. Lishner M, Zemlickis D, Degendorfer P, et al. Maternal and foetal outcome following Hodgkin's disease in pregnancy. *Br J Cancer* 1992;65:114–117.

205. Anselmo AP, Cavalieri E, Enrici RM, et al. Hodgkin's disease during pregnancy: diagnostic and therapeutic management. *Fetal Diagn Ther* 1999;14:102–105.

206. Woo SY, Fuller LM, Cundiff JH, et al. Radiotherapy during pregnancy for clinical stages IA-IIA Hodgkin's disease. *Int J Radiat Oncol Biol Phys* 1992;23:407–412.

207. Mauch PM, Kalish LA, Kadin M, et al. Patterns of presentation of Hodgkin disease. Implications for etiology and pathogenesis. *Cancer* 1993;71:2062–2071.

208. Urba WJ, Longo DL. Hodgkin's disease. *N Engl J Med* 1992;326:678–687.

209. Aisenberg AC. Problems in Hodgkin's disease management. *Blood* 1999;93:761–779.

210. Duggan DB, Petroni GR, Johnson JL, et al. Randomized comparison of ABVD and MOPP/ABV hybrid for the treatment of advanced Hodgkin's disease: report of an intergroup trial. *J Clin Oncol* 2003;21:607–614.

211. Pohlman B, Macklis RM. Lymphoma and pregnancy. *Semin Oncol* 2000;27:657–666.

212. Ward FT, Weiss RB. Lymphoma and pregnancy. *Semin Oncol* 1989;16:397–409.

213. Steiner-Salz D, Yahalom J, Samuelov A, Polliack A. Non-Hodgkin's lymphoma associated with pregnancy. A report of six cases, with a review of the literature. *Cancer* 1985;56:2087–2091.

214. Aviles A, Diaz-Maqueo JC, Torras V, et al. Non-Hodgkin's lymphomas and pregnancy: presentation of 16 cases. *Gynecol Oncol* 1990;37:335–337.

215. Miller TP, Dahlberg S, Cassady JR, et al. Chemotherapy alone compared with chemotherapy plus radiotherapy for localized intermediate- and high-grade non-Hodgkin's lymphoma. *N Engl J Med* 1998;339:21–26.

216. Feliu J, Juarez S, Ordonez A, et al. Acute leukemia and pregnancy. *Cancer* 1988;61:580–584.
217. Reynoso EE, Shepherd FA, Messner HA, et al. Acute leukemia during pregnancy: the Toronto Leukemia Study Group experience with long-term follow-up of children exposed in utero to chemotherapeutic agents. *J Clin Oncol* 1987;5:1098–1106.
218. Catanzarite VA, Ferguson JE 2nd. Acute leukemia and pregnancy: a review of management and outcome, 1972–1982. *Obstet Gynecol Surv* 1984;39:663–678.
219. Hansen WF, Fretz P, Hunter SK, Yankowitz J. Leukemia in pregnancy and fetal response to multiagent chemotherapy. *Obstet Gynecol* 2001; 97:809–812.
220. Zuazu J, Julia A, Sierra J, et al. Pregnancy outcome in hematologic malignancies. *Cancer* 1991;67:703–709.
221. Morishita S, Imai A, Kawabata I, Tamaya T. Acute myelogenous leukemia in pregnancy: fetal blood sampling and early effects of chemotherapy. *Int J Gynaecol Obstet* 1994;44:273–277.
222. Brell J, Kalaycio M. Leukemia in pregnancy. *Semin Oncol* 2000;27: 667–677.
223. Delmer A, Rio B, Bauduer F, et al. Pregnancy during myelosuppressive treatment for chronic myelogenous leukemia. *Br J Haematol* 1992;82:783–784.
224. Hensley ML, Ford JM. Imatinib treatment: Specific issues related to safety, fertility, and pregnancy. *Semin Hematol* 2003;40:21–25.
225. Fernandez MN, Millan I, Gluckman E. Cord-blood transplants. *N Engl J Med* 1999;340:1287–1288.
226. Kjems E, Krag C. Melanoma and pregnancy. A review. *Acta Oncol* 1993;32:371–378.
227. Lang PG Jr. Malignant melanoma. *Med Clin North Am* 1998;82: 1325–1358.
228. Wong DJ, Strassner HT. Melanoma in pregnancy. *Clin Obstet Gynecol* 1990;33:782–791.
229. Danforth DN Jr, Russell N, McBride CM. Hormonal status of patients with primary malignant melanoma: a review of 313 cases. *South Med J* 1982;75:661–664.
230. Rampen F. Malignant melanoma: sex differences in survival after evidence of distant metastasis. *Br J Cancer* 1980;42:52–57.
231. Shaw HM, Milton GW, Farago G, McCarthy WH. Endocrine influences on survival from malignant melanoma. *Cancer* 1978;42: 669–677.
232. Zanetti R, Franceschi S, Rosso S, et al. Cutaneous malignant melanoma in females: the role of hormonal and reproductive factors. *Int J Epidemiol* 1990;19:522–526.
233. Shiu MH, Schottenfeld D, Maclean B, Fortner JG. Adverse effect of pregnancy on melanoma: a reappraisal. *Cancer* 1976;37:181–187.
234. Smith MA, Fine JA, Barnhill RL, Berwick M. Hormonal and reproductive influences and risk of melanoma in women. *Int J Epidemiol* 1998;27:751–757.
235. Slingluff CL Jr, Reintgen DS, Vollmer RT, Seigler HF. Malignant melanoma arising during pregnancy. A study of 100 patients. *Ann Surg* 1990;211:552–557; Discussion 558–559.
236. Wong JH, Sterns EE, Kopald KH, et al. Prognostic significance of pregnancy in stage I melanoma. *Arch Surg* 1989;124:1227–30; discussion 1230–1231.
237. MacKie RM, Bufalino R, Morabito A, et al. Lack of effect of pregnancy on outcome of melanoma. For The World Health Organisation Melanoma Programme. *Lancet* 1991;337:653–655.
238. Reintgen DS, McCarty KS Jr, Vollmer R, et al. Malignant melanoma and pregnancy. *Cancer* 1985;55:1340–1344.
239. Travers RL, Sober AJ, Berwick M, et al. Increased thickness of pregnancy-associated melanoma. *Br J Dermatol* 1995;132:876–883.
240. Trapeznikov NN, Khasanov SR, Iavorskii VV. Melanoma of the skin and pregnancy. *Vopr Onkol* 1987;33:40–46.
241. Dipaola RS, Goodin S, Ratzell M, et al. Chemotherapy for metastatic melanoma during pregnancy. *Gynecol Oncol* 1997;66:526–530.
242. Ferreira CM, Maceira JM, Coelho JM. Melanoma and pregnancy with placental metastases. Report of a case. *Am J Dermatopathol* 1998; 20:403–407.
243. Baergen RN, Johnson D, Moore T, Benirschke K. Maternal melanoma metastatic to the placenta: a case report and review of the literature. *Arch Pathol Lab Med* 1997;121:508–511.
244. Marsh RD, Chu NM. Placental metastasis from primary ocular melanoma: a case report. *Am J Obstet Gynecol* 1996;174:1654–1655.
245. Alexander A, Samlowski WE, Grossman D, et al. Metastatic melanoma in pregnancy: risk of transplacental metastases in the infant. *J Clin Oncol* 2003;21:2179–2186.
246. Dildy GA 3rd, Moise KJ Jr, Carpenter RJ Jr, Klima T. Maternal malignancy metastatic to the products of conception: a review. *Obstet Gynecol Surv* 1989;44:535–540.
247. Rothman LA, Cohen CJ, Astarloa J. Placental and fetal involvement by maternal malignancy: a report of rectal carcinoma and review of the literature. *Am J Obstet Gynecol* 1973;116:1023–1034.
248. Schwartz JL, Mozurkewich EL, Johnson TM. Current management of patients with melanoma who are pregnant, want to get pregnant, or do not want to get pregnant. *Cancer* 2003;97:2130–2133.
249. Duncan LM, Travers RL, Koerner FC, et al. Estrogen and progesterone receptor analysis in pregnancy-associated melanoma: absence of immunohistochemically detectable hormone receptors. *Hum Pathol* 1994;25:36–41.
250. Vini L, Hyer S, Pratt B, Harmer C. Management of differentiated thyroid cancer diagnosed during pregnancy. *Eur J Endocrinol* 1999; 140:404–406.
251. Herzon FS, Morris DM, Segal MN, et al. Coexistent thyroid cancer and pregnancy. *Arch Otolaryngol Head Neck Surg* 1994;120: 1191–1193.
252. Arndt D, Mehnert WH, Franke WG, et al. Radioiodine therapy during an unknown remained pregnancy and radiation exposure of the fetus. A case report. *Strahlenther Onkol* 1994;170:408–414.
253. Shepard TH. Teratogenicity of therapeutic agents. In: Gluck L, ed. *Current problems in pediatrics*. Chicago: Year Book Medical Publishers, 1979.
254. Ayala C, Navarro E, Rodriguez JR, et al. Conception after iodine-131 therapy for differentiated thyroid cancer. *Thyroid* 1998;8:1009–1011.
255. Lin JD, Wang HS, Weng HF, Kao PF. Outcome of pregnancy after radioactive iodine treatment for well differentiated thyroid carcinomas. *J Endocrinol Invest* 1998;21:662–667.
256. Heron DE, Karimpour S, Grigsby PW. Anaplastic thyroid carcinoma: comparison of conventional radiotherapy and hyperfractionation chemoradiotherapy in two groups. *Am J Clin Oncol* 2002;25:442–446.
257. Matschke RG, Graber T, Panagiotopoulos A. A laryngeal cancer in pregnancy. *HNO* 1994;42:505–508.
258. Sevray B, Palaric JC, Cousin C, et al. Nasopharyngeal cancer and pregnancy. Review of the literature. Report of a case. *J Gynecol Obstet Biol Reprod (Paris)* 1991;20:431–435.
259. Brizel DM. Radiotherapy and concurrent chemotherapy for the treatment of locally advanced head and neck squamous cell carcinoma. *Semin Radiat Oncol* 1998;8:237–246.
260. Woods JB, Martin JN Jr, Ingram FH, et al. Pregnancy complicated by carcinoma of the colon above the rectum. *Am J Perinatol* 1992; 9:102–110.
261. Bernstein MA, Madoff RD, Caushaj PF. Colon and rectal cancer in pregnancy. *Dis Colon Rectum* 1993;36:172–178.
262. Cappell MS. Colon cancer during pregnancy. *Gastroenterol Clin North Am* 2003;32:341–383.
263. Skilling JS. Colorectal cancer complicating pregnancy. *Obstet Gynecol Clin North Am* 1998;25:417–421.
264. Laurie JA, Moertel CG, Fleming TR, et al. Surgical adjuvant therapy of large-bowel carcinoma: an evaluation of levamisole and the combination of levamisole and fluorouracil. The North Central Cancer Treatment Group and the Mayo Clinic. *J Clin Oncol* 1989;7: 1447–1456.
265. Moertel CG, Fleming TR, Macdonald JS, et al. Levamisole and fluorouracil for adjuvant therapy of resected colon carcinoma. *N Engl J Med* 1990;322:352–358.
266. Krook JE, Moertel CG, Gunderson LL, et al.. Effective surgical adjuvant therapy for high-risk rectal carcinoma. *N Engl J Med* 1991;324: 709–715.
267. Thomas PR, Lindblad AS. Adjuvant postoperative radiotherapy and chemotherapy in rectal carcinoma: a review of the Gastrointestinal Tumor Study Group experience. *Radiother Oncol* 1988;13:245–252.
268. Dhillon MS, Singh DP, Gill SS, et al. Primary bone malignancies in pregnancy. A report of four cases. *Orthop Rev* 1993;22:931–937.
269. Haerr RW, Pratt AT. Multiagent chemotherapy for sarcoma diagnosed during pregnancy. *Cancer* 1985;56:1028–1033.
270. Merimsky O, Le Cesne A. Soft tissue and bone sarcomas in association with pregnancy. *Acta Oncol* 1998;37:721–727.

271. To WK, Ghosh A. Primary liver carcinoma complicating pregnancy. *Aust N Z J Obstet Gynaecol* 1993;33:325–326.

272. Smith DP, Goldman SM, Beggs DS, Lanigan PJ. Renal cell carcinoma in pregnancy: report of three cases and review of the literature. *Obstet Gynecol* 1994;83:818–820.

273. Janne PA, Rodriguez-Thompson D, Metcalf DR, et al. Chemotherapy for a patient with advanced non–small-cell lung cancer during pregnancy: a case report and a review of chemotherapy treatment during pregnancy. *Oncology* 2001;61:175–183.

274. Sweeney WJ, Katz VL. Recurrent pheochromocytoma during pregnancy. *Obstet Gynecol* 1994;83:820–822.

275. Hall EJ. Diagnostic radiology and nuclear medicine: risk versus benefit. In: Hall EJ, ed. *Radiobiology for the radiologist.* Philadelphia: JB Lippincott Co, 1994;363.

276. Hart GC. Diagnostic medical exposures to ionizing radiation during pregnancy. *Nucl Med Commun* 1994;15:403–404.

277. Pennington EC, Staples J, Jani SK. A simple method for reducing ovarian dose during megavoltage irradiation of the breast. *Med Dosim* 1989;14:269–272.

278. Dudan R, Yon Y, Ford J, Averette H. Carcinoma of the cervix and pregnancy. *Gynecol Oncol* 1973;1:285.

279. Sood AK, Sorosky JI, Mayr N, et al. Radiotherapeutic management of cervical carcinoma that complicates pregnancy. *Cancer* 1997;80: 1073–1078.

280. Agarwal N, Parul, Kriplani A, et al. Management and outcome of pregnancies complicated with adnexal masses. *Arch Gynecol Obstet* 2003;267:148–152.

281. Sherard GB 3rd, Hodson CA, Williams HJ, et al. Adnexal masses and pregnancy: a 12-year experience. *Am J Obstet Gynecol* 2003;189: 358–362; Discussion 362–363.

282. Whitecar MP, Turner S, Higby MK. Adnexal masses in pregnancy: a review of 130 cases undergoing surgical management. *Am J Obstet Gynecol* 1999;181:19–24.

283. Roy M, Plante M. Pregnancies after radical vaginal trachelectomy for early-stage cervical cancer. *Am J Obstet Gynecol* 1998;179: 1491–1496.

284. Bernardini M, Barrett J, Seaward G, Covens A. Pregnancy outcomes in patients after radical trachelectomy. *Am J Obstet Gynecol* 2003; 189:1378–1382.

285. Shepherd JH, Mould T, Oram DH. Radical trachelectomy in early stage carcinoma of the cervix: outcome as judged by recurrence and fertility rates. *Br J Obstet Gynaecol* 2001;108:882–885.

286. Schlaerth JB, Spirtos NM, Schlaerth AC. Radical trachelectomy and pelvic lymphadenectomy with uterine preservation in the treatment of cervical cancer. *Am J Obstet Gynecol* 2003;188:29–34.

CHAPTER 37

AIDS and Women

Mary Jo Lechowicz and Otis W. Brawley

In 1981, an acquired immunodeficiency syndrome (AIDS) was described in a cohort of gay men presenting with Kaposi's sarcoma and *Pneumocystis carinii* pneumonia (PCP) (1–3). These reports would herald the beginning of an epidemic. Intravenous drug users (IVDUs) and recipients of human blood products were also subsequently found to be at high risk for contracting this disease at that time (4, 5). AIDS is due to an infection with a retrovirus now termed human immunodeficiency virus (HIV-1) (6–8).

It is estimated that there were 42 million people living with HIV infection or the condition known as AIDS at the beginning of 2003. An estimated 29.4 million (70%) live in Sub-Saharan Africa, 19.2 million (42%) of whom are women (9). The U.S. Centers of Disease Control and Prevention (CDC) estimates that 850,000 to 950,000 Americans are living with HIV infection, and 25% do not know that they are infected (10).

Treatment of HIV-1 is complex. This chapter is intended to give a clinical overview of the pertinent clinical topics seen in women infected with HIV-1.

EPIDEMIOLOGY

It is estimated that 40,000 new HIV infections occur each year in the United States. Seventy percent of these new cases are men and 30% are women. Of these newly infected people, half are younger than 25 years of age (11,12). Of the newly infected women in the United States, approximately 75% of women were infected through heterosexual sex and 25% through use of illegal intravenous drugs. Of the newly infected women, approximately 64% are African American, 18% are white, 18% are Hispanic, and a small percentage are members of other racial/ethnic groups (13).

The estimated number of AIDS cases reported through December 2002 in the United States was 886,575. Adult and adolescent AIDS cases totaled 877,275, with 159,271 cases in females. Through this same period, 9,300 AIDS cases were reported in children under age 13. The total number of deaths due to AIDS is 501,669, including 496,354 adults and adolescents, and 5,315 children under the age of 15 years. The estimated annual number of AIDS-related deaths in the United States fell approximately 14% from 1998 to 2002: 19,005 deaths in 1998 to 16,371 deaths in 2002. Of the estimated 16,731 AIDS-related deaths in 2002, approximately 51% were among African Americans, 28% among whites, 19% among Hispanics, and 1% among Asians/Pacific Islanders and American Indians/Alaskan Natives (4).

From 1985 to 2002, the proportion of adult/adolescent AIDS cases reported in American women increased from 7% to 26%. Over 70% of American women diagnosed with AIDS were between the ages of 20 and 44 years. During 2002, 158 pediatric AIDS cases were reported; 88% of these cases were in children with mothers with or at risk for HIV infection.

ETIOLOGY

Three years after the initial description of AIDS, the human T-lymphotropic virus-III /lymphadenopathy-associated virus (HTLV-III/LAV), now known as the human immunodeficiency virus type-1 (HIV-1), was identified as the causative agent of AIDS (14,15). HIV-1 is the most common cause of AIDS in the world (16). HIV-1 infection has been demonstrated to be a zoonotic infection that originated in chimpanzees. This lentivirus probably evolved from a simian immunodeficiency virus (SIV) crossing over to human beings in the early to mid twentieth century (17,18). A related retrovirus, human immunodeficiency virus-2 (HIV-2), may be an intermediate between HIV-1 and SIV. HIV-2 has 40% nucleotide similarity to HIV-1 and 75% nucleotide similarity to SIV (19–21).

M. J. Lechowicz: Department of Hematology and Oncology, Emory University, Atlanta, Georgia 30303

O. W. Brawley: Departments of Hematology and Oncology and Epidemiology, Emory University, Atlanta, Georgia 30303

HIV-2 was discovered in West Africa after the HIV-1/AIDS epidemic began (22,23). This virus has been isolated from patients with AIDS or AIDS-like diseases in western Africa who have no evidence of infection with HIV-1. HIV-2 seems to have been present in western Africa since at least 1966 (24,25). It also causes AIDS (26–31). AIDS in the HIV-2–infected patient presents with signs and symptoms similar to those associated with HIV-1 infection, but the time from infection with the HIV-2 virus and development of AIDS is longer than with HIV-1 (29–33). This chapter will concentrate on HIV-1 infection, which is the predominant infection in North America.

MOLECULAR BIOLOGY OF HIV-1

The development of drugs that have decreased HIV/AIDS mortality have stemmed from an increased understanding of the HIV-1 life cycle to prevent replication and production of infectious viral particles. Pharmaceutical developments hope to stop the virus from invading the healthy host cells before it even has a chance to replicate.

The molecular structure and life cycle of HIV facilitates understanding the diagnostic and therapeutic approaches to AIDS and the behavior and transmission of the HIV (34). In normal cellular function, deoxyribonucleic acid (DNA) is transcribed or copied to messenger ribonucleic acid (mRNA). Messenger RNA then acts as a template for protein synthesis in a process called translation. Retroviruses are a class of viruses that have ribonucleic acid (RNA) as their genetic material. They must convert this RNA to a DNA form in order to utilize the host cell machinery for reproduction (35). Reverse transcriptase (a specific DNA polymerase) is an enzyme that the virus brings with it into the cell. It transcribes viral RNA to a DNA form capable of encoding mRNA for subsequent gene expression using host cellular enzymes (36). An associated enzyme, integrase, is responsible for integration of the viral DNA into host cellular DNA. Reverse transcriptase and integrase are packaged within the viral core.

HIV-1 is 100 nm in diameter with a dense, cylindric nucleoid. The virus consists of a host-derived lipid envelope. A glycoprotein (gp), gp120, studs the outer lipid envelope. It is anchored to another glycoprotein, gp41, which transcends the lipid envelope. The gp120 of certain HIV strains has a high chemical affinity for the CD4 molecule (37–39). CD4 is found on the surface of T helper cells lymphocyte. A binding constant as high as 10^{-9} M has been measured between CD4 and gp120 in some strains of HIV-1 (40). Inside are two single plus sense strands of RNA, each consisting of 9,749 ribonucleotides (41). The RNA is contained within the cylindric nucleoid composed of core protein along with reverse trans-criptase and integrase.

In order for the HIV-1 to enter the cell, a fusion process takes place and the lipid bilayer of the virus is incorporated into the cell membrane as the viral core is internalized within the cell (42). This entire process lends itself to new types of antiviral drug class know as HIV entry inhibitors that are currently being investigated.

Once within the cell, the matrix protein and viral core layers are removed, exposing the viral RNA (as a ribonucleoprotein complex) to the cytoplasm. Viral reverse transcriptase then makes a single-strand DNA copy from one of the two plus strands of RNA, and a viral ribonuclease destroys the viral RNA as the reverse transcriptase makes yet a second copy of DNA using the first DNA as a template (43). The viral information, in DNA form, along with proteins and enzymes are transported to the nucleus. The viral enzyme integrase is responsible for inserting the viral DNA into the host DNA. The viral DNA may then remain latent, being duplicated along with the cell's own genes every time the cell divides. Both the viral reverse transcriptase and integrase are the targets of antiviral therapy, which is discussed below.

When activated, elements of the nucleotide sequences known as long terminal repeats (LTRs), located at each end of the viral DNA message, direct host cellular proteins to copy the integrated viral DNA into RNA. Some of this RNA serves as messenger RNA templates for structural proteins and enzymes, whereas additional RNA serves as genetic material for new virus. Viral replication is controlled by several of the viral genes interacting with the LTR and host cellular proteins. These viral genes act by promoting or repressing signals produced by the LTR (44,45).

When the cell is activated, transcribed HIV messenger RNA travels into the cytoplasm and is translated into viral structural proteins. The proteins that will make up the envelope of the virus are glycosolated in the cytoplasm and assembled to form the outer cell membrane. These glycoproteins are wrapped around the core in conjunction with the viral lipid bilayer as virus is extruded from the cell during the budding process. The final step for the HIV-1 virus to become infectious is cleavage of the gag polyproteins and enzymes by the virus-encoded protease. The drugs known as protease inhibitors function to block this maturation process.

HIV-1 GENOME

The HIV-1 genome contains the genes characteristic of all retroviruses: *gag, pol,* and *env* (46). These genes code structural proteins. The *gag* gene encodes the proteins in the core of the virion, whereas *pol* encodes four enzymes: reverse transcriptase (p50), integrase(p31), RNase H (p15), and protease (p10). The *gag* and *pol* products first appear as a *gag-pol* fusion protein. The *gag* gene product is the protein p55. p55 is ultimately cleaved by viral protease (4) during the process of viral maturation to form the viral proteins MA [matrix (p17)],CA [capsid (p24)], NC [nucleocapsid (p9)], and p6 (47). The *env* gene product is the polyprotein gp160, which is subsequently cleaved into the envelope glycoprotein gp120 and the transmembrane glycoprotein gp41 (48).

The HIV-1 genome then contains at least six other genes (*tat, rev, nef, vif, vpr,* and *vpu*). Three of these genes, *tat, rev,* and *nef,* have both positive and negative regulatory effects on the LTR region and HIV-1 replication. The *tat gene* is a transcriptional activator that is essential for HIV-1 replication (49). It acts principally to promote the elongation phase of HIV-1 transcription, so that full-length transcripts can be produced (50,51). The *rev* gene is a shuttle protein that binds to the *rev* response element (RRE) located on *env.* Transport of the viral transcripts to the cytoplasm depends on supply of *rev* (52).

HIV-1 contains an additional four genes, *nef, vif, vpr,* and *vpu,* that code for proteins that are important to the virulence of the virus and are less understood. The *nef* gene modifies the environment of the infected cell to optimize viral replication (53); and it reduces the expression of major histocompatibility complex (MHC) I determinants on the surface of the infected cell (54), which decreases the ability of CD8 cyctotoxic T cells from recognizing and killing infected cells. The absence of *nef* in infected monkeys and humans is associated with much slower clinical progression to AIDS (55,56).

It is known that *vpu* has two functions. One is the downmodulation of CD4 cells. This gene allows liberation of the viral envelope by triggering degradation of CD4 molecules complexed with *env* (57). The other role of *vpu* is enhancement of virion release. It has been shown that in the absence of *vpu,* large numbers of virions remain attached to the surface of infected cells (58). The *vpr* gene plays a role in the ability of HIV to infect nondividing cells by facilitating the nuclear localization of the preintegration complex (PIC) (59). As the name implies, the PIC is the complex of viral genetic material and proteins resulting from reverse transcription and has not been incorporated into the host cell genetic structure. The PIC includes double-stranded viral DNA, integrase, matrix, *vpr,* reverse transcriptase, and a high-mobility group DNA-binding cellular protein HMGI(Y) (60).

The *vif* gene plays an important, but not well-understood, role in the assembly of virions. HIV produced from heterokaryons in studies using permissive and nonpermissive cells showed nonpermissive cells' antiviral factor can be overcome by the expression of *vif* (61). The role of *vif* in nonpermissive cells implies that the *vif* protein is needed to overcome a negative factor for HIV infectivity and assembly.

TRANSMISSION OF HIV-1

In general, HIV-1 is transmitted through exposure and contact with infected bodily fluids. Those fluids most likely to be infected are blood, blood products, fluids contaminated with blood, and cerebrospinal fluid. HIV-1 has also been isolated from breast milk, cervical secretions, saliva, semen, tears, urine, and vaginal fluid (62). The virus is most efficiently transmitted through intimate sexual contact, transfusion of infected blood products, and the sharing of contaminated needles. HIV-1 may also be transmitted through exposure of open wounds or mucous membranes to blood or infected body fluid.

Sexual Transmission

Sexual transmission is the most common form of transmission of HIV-1. Many people who know they carry the infection do not change their sexual practices (63). One study found that 52% of sexually active HIV-positive men kept their serostatus secret from one or more sex partners (64).

Risk of HIV transmission can be decreased, but not eliminated, by limiting sexual partners and properly using latex condoms during genital-genital and anal-genital contact. Although HIV-1 transmission is reduced among couples properly using condoms, some studies indicate that as many as 17% of those regularly engaging in ''protected'' heterosexual intercourse with an infected individual may contract HIV-1 (65). Common misuse of condoms includes the use of substances that cause deterioration of latex such as petroleum jelly, vegetable shortenings, and oils as lubricants (66). Condoms made of animal intestine do not provide as much protection against HIV-1 transmission as do latex condoms (67,68). They have natural pores that are large enough to allow passage of the HIV.

Epidemiologic studies have demonstrated several factors that are associated with an increased risk of contracting HIV-1 through sexual contact. These include the number of sexual exposures, particularly the number of exposures to persons known to be infected with HIV-1, and the HIV-1 disease state of the source patient (69). There is evidence that patients with more advanced HIV-1 disease, as indicated by a low CD4 count, are more likely to transmit HIV-1 to their sexual partners when compared to patients with less advanced disease. Infectivity may be increased in a number of ways.

Primary infection may be associated with increased infectivity (70). Primary infection is the period of time between exposure to HIV and the appearance of antibodies. Plasma HIV RNA viral load levels and genital secretion HIV levels have been shown to be elevated, which may play a part in the increased level of infectivity at that time.

Concurrent sexually transmitted diseases also seem to increase viral infectivity. The presence of reproductive tract infections is strongly associated with susceptibility of HIV even after adjustment for sexual behavior (71). The prevalence of sexually transmitted diseases associated with ulcers (chancroid, syphilis, and herpes) is associated with increased risk of HIV infection (72,73). One study reported that men were more likely to seroconvert after sexual contact with women who had concurrent genital ulcer disease (74).

Sexual practices can alter infectivity of HIV. Sexual intercourse during a woman's menstrual period can increase a woman's risk of contracting HIV. Sexual practices that result in vaginal bleeding may also increase a woman's risk of developing HIV infection (75). Receptive anal intercourse, either male-male or male-female, is the sexual practice associated with the highest rate of HIV-1 transmission. Oral-genital contact (heterosexual and homosexual) has also been associated with HIV-1 transmission, although very infrequently (76–78).

The ''best therapy'' is prevention. Sexual abstinence or a mutually monogamous relationship between two uninfected people is the only sure way of preventing the sexual transmission of HIV-1.

Intravenous Drug Abuse

Another major risk factor for the transmission of HIV-1 is intravenous drug usage involving contaminated hypodermic needles. In 2001, the CDC data reported 39% of the cumulative AIDS cases in women were contracted through intravenous drug use. The risk of HIV-1 infection rises with the increasing frequency of injections and with the number of people who may have previously shared, borrowed or rented the needle (79). Both men and women frequently engage in prostitution in order to gain money to buy or in exchange for these drugs. Many people also become sexually uninhibited under the influence of ''crack'' cocaine or phencyclidine and engage in repetitive high-risk sexual behaviors.

Transmission of HIV-1 can be decreased in IVDUs with the use of clean needles. Cleaning used needles with bleach can also decrease the spread of the virus. Distribution of clean hypodermic needles is extremely controversial. Post-exposure prophylaxis has been used after the sharing of needles with an HIV-infected partner (80). When the source of exposure has a known high viral load or has previously been treated with a nucleoside reverse transcriptase inhibitor, it is recommended to use a protease inhibitor in the postexposure prophylaxis regimen (81).

Maternal-Fetal Transmission

In recent years, with the advent of early voluntary HIV screening in pregnant women and prophylaxis for fetal infection, the number of infant HIV cases has dropped dramatically. In 2000, only 174 pediatric AIDS cases were reported compared to almost 2,000 prior to antiviral prophylaxis guidelines in 1994. The possible mechanisms of viral infection may include absorption of the virus through the infant's digestive tract, maternal-fetal blood mixing during contractions, and cervical or vaginal exposure to the HIV-1. It is estimated that 70% of mother-child transmissions occur at delivery and about 30% of transmissions occur *in utero* (82). Infection increases with the presence of ruptured membranes and seems to be reduced with elective cesarean section (83).

In 1994, the results of the AIDS Clinical Trials Group

(ACTG) protocol 076 demonstrated a 67% reduction in perinatal HIV transmission in a double-blind, placebo-controlled trial of antepartum, intrapartum, and neonatal zidovudine (ZDV) (84). Afterward the United States Public Health Service (USPHS) published guidelines that all HIV-infected pregnant women and their babies be offered ZDV using the ACTG 076 regimen (85). In 1998, the guidelines were updated to include combination antiviral therapy for the pregnant woman if her health dictated it (86).

The Perinatal AIDS Collaborative Transmission Study looked at utilization and outcomes of the 1994 guidelines being prescribed in four U.S. cities from July 1, 1994 through June 30, 1998. A total of 1,025 children were born to 916 mothers. ZDV usage increased dramatically between 1994 and 1998. Completion of ZDV regimens increased from 41% to 70%. Women who used cocaine or heroine, had relatively high CD4 counts, or delivered preterm were less likely to receive the three-part ZDV regimen (87).

One factor that best predicts likelihood of infection of an infant is the viral load of the mother (88). Transmission is rare among women who are on effective antiretroviral therapies. There are also data to suggest that intrapartum and early neonatal prophylaxis without antepartum therapy can reduce the risk of maternal-child transmission (89).

There is ongoing controversy as to whether breast-feeding should be discouraged in all cases of HIV-1–infected mothers. HIV-1 has been isolated from the breast milk of HIV-1– infected mothers, and transmission of HIV-1 from mother to child by breast-feeding has been documented (90,91). Breast-feeding is thought to be responsible for approximately 300,000 HIV infections per year (92). Although formula feeding is advisable in countries where clean water and formula are available and affordable, the advantage of breast-feeding in preventing death from diarrheal disease may outweigh the risk of HIV transmission in some underdeveloped countries (93). The United Nations International Children's Emergency Fund (UNICEF) found increased use of breast-feeding could prevent 1.5 million child deaths per year (94,95). Presently, recommendations are for HIV-positive women to breast-feed for 6 months before introducing replacement feeding to optimize immunologic maternal protection and decrease gut damage from early introduction of replacement feeding. Studies are ongoing for the best recommendations on breast-feeding techniques as well as duration (96).

Maternofetal transmission of HIV can be decreased when women known to have HIV infection are treated. It has been suggested that one reason women refuse voluntary HIV testing is failure of their health-care provider to recommend it strongly (97).

A recent study showed that it is safe for a relatively healthy HIV-positive woman transiently to take ZDV monotherapy for prophylaxis of perinatal transmission of HIV (98). A European study looking at long-term effects of antiviral therapy *in utero* and in the early lives of children concluded that, with the exception of increased risk of premature delivery and reversible anemia, there was no adverse effect of antiviral therapy exposure in uninfected children born to HIV-infected women in the short or medium term (99). Table 37.1A shows some current guidelines for ZDV in pregnancy. Table 37.1B depicts the current data on antiretroviral therapy and carcinogenesis studies. We can aid in HIV prevention by recommending women that are high risk be tested for HIV, and if found to be positive, antiviral therapy should be strongly recommended.

Directives on how to counsel a woman about antiviral therapy in pregnancy is discussed in the Public Health Service Task Force Recommendations for Use of Antiretroviral Drugs in Pregnant HIV-1–Infected Women for Maternal Health and Interventions to Reduce Perinatal HIV-1 Transmission in the United States are regularly updated and available on the AIDS information website http://aidsinfo.nih.gov/guidelines/. Data regarding the effects on the fetus and newborn are in the updated results of the ACTG 076 trial. The concern for long-term effects and the risk of teratogenicity remain unknown and need to be discussed when counseling a woman about perinatal antiviral therapy.

Heath-Care Exposures

The majority of HIV-1–infected health-care personnel are members of high-risk groups, but by the end of 2001, there were 57 reported cases of HIV-1 seroconversions due to work-related exposure in the United States (100). There were an additional 138 infections among health-care personnel that were considered to be occupational HIV transmission. Injury with a needle contaminated from use in an HIV-1–infected patient is the most common ''work-related'' mode of transmission to health-care personnel. The estimated risk of transmitting the virus with a single percutaneous injury is 0.04% (101). Several large studies of health-care givers have been completed. One study involving 351 health-care professionals who had needle-stick or other sharp-object exposures

to the blood of HIV-1–infected patients reported that 3 persons with exposures (0.9%) seroconverted (102). A second study of 2,200 health-care workers injured in the same fashion reported that 16 contacts ultimately became seropositive (103).

Most cases of HIV-1 transmission to care givers have occurred through parenteral exposure to infected blood, although anecdotal reports of seroconversion following exposure to blood, urine, and other body fluids being splashed and contaminating cuts on hands, psoriatic rashes, and other abrasions exist (104). There is also evidence suggesting that the risk of occupational transmission is greater if the source patient has advanced disease (105). There is some evidence that the longer the exposure of the infected fluid to the wound the greater the risk of transmission. Immediate washing of the wound is indicated to dilute the inoculum. The CDC retrospectively found the risk of transmission of HIV to health-care workers was increased when the device causing the injury was inserted into an artery or vein, caused a deep injury, was visibly contaminated with blood, or the source patient died within 2 months of exposure (106).

Studies and reports of HIV-1 seroconversion due to occupational exposure illustrate the need for implementation of Universal Blood and Body Fluid Precautions. Even though the risk to hospital workers is small, blood and body fluid precautions should be practiced by all health-care givers on all patients (107,108). No patient, not even a patient who has recently tested negative for HIV-1, can be assumed to be free of infection with HIV-1 as a matter of general medical practice. The use of universal precautions will reduce the incidence of other diseases besides HIV-1 infection being transmitted from patients to health-care workers by blood and body fluids.

Currently, recommendations are for postexposure prophylaxis to be given to those believed to have been exposed to HIV infection. The CDC's retrospective case-control study of health-care personnel showed treatment with ZDV in the postexposure period was associated with an 81% reduction

TABLE 37.1A. *Zidovudine perinatal transmission prophylaxis regimen*

Antepartum	Initiation at 14–34 weeks gestation and continued throughout pregnancy of either Regimen A or B, as follows: **Regimen A.** Pediatric AIDS Clinical Trials Group protocol 076 regimen: ZDV 100 mg 5 times daily **Regimen B.** Acceptable alternative regimen: ZDV 200 mg 3 times daily or ZDV 300 mg 2 times daily
Intrapartum	During labor, ZDV 2 mg/kg of mother's body weight, intravenously for 1 hour, followed by a continuous infusion of 1 mg/kg of mother's body weight intravenously until delivery.
Postpartum	Oral administration of ZDV to the newborn infant (ZDV syrup, 2 mg/kg of infant's body weight every 6 hours) for the first 6 weeks of life, beginning at 8–12 hours after birth.

From Guidelines for the Use of Antiretroviral Agents in HIV-1 infected Adults and Adolescents., July 14, 2003. Department of Health and Human Services, Table 28 p.76.

TABLE 37.1B. *MMWR, November 22, 2002/S1 CRR18. U.S. Public Health Service 1–38 Task Force Recommendations for use of Antiretroviral Drugs in Pregnant HIV-1 Infected Women for Maternal Health and Intervention to Reduce Perinatal HIV Transmission in the United State.*

Antiretroviral drug	(FDA) pregnancy category[a]	Placental passage (newborn: mother drug ratio)	Long-term animal carcinogenicity studies	Animal teratogen studies
Nucleoside and nucleotide analogue reverse transcriptase inhibitors				
Zidovudine (Retrovir, AZT, ZDV)	C	Yes (human) (0.85)	Positive (rodent, noninvasive vaginal epithelial tumors)	Positive (rodent—near lethal dose)
Zalcitabine (HIVID, ddC)	C	Yes (rhesus monkey) (0.30–0.50)	Positive (rodent, thymic lymphomas)	Positive (rodent—hydrocephalus at high dose)
Didanosine (Videx, ddl)	B	Yes (human) (0.5)	Negative (no tumors, lifetime rodent study)	Negative
Stavudine (Zerit, d4T)	C	Yes (rhesus monkey) (0.76)	Not completed	Negative (but sternal bone calcium decreases in rodents)
Lamivudine (Epivir, 3TC)	C	Yes (human) (~1.0)	Negative (no tumors, lifetime rodent study)	Negative
Abacavir (Ziagen, ABC)	C	Yes (rats)	Not completed	Positive (rodent anasarca and skeletal malformations at 1,000 mg/kg (35× human exposure) during organogenesis; not seen in rabbits)
Tenofovir DF (Viread)	B	Yes (rat and monkey)	Not completed	Negative (osteomalacia when given to juvenile animals at high doses)
NonNucleoside reverse transcriptase inhibitors				
Nevirapine (Viramune)	C	Yes (human) (~1.0)	Not completed	Negative
Delavirdine (Rescriptor)	C	Unknown	Not completed	Positive (rodent—ventricular septal defect)
Efavirenz (Sustiva)	C	Yes (cynomologus monkey, rat, rabbit) (~1.0)	Not completed	Positive (cynomologus monkey—anencephaly, anophthalmia, microophthalmia)
Protease inhibitors				
Indinavir (Crixivan)	C	Minimal (human)	Not completed	Negative (but extra ribs in rodents)
Ritonavir (Norvir)	B	Minimal (human)	Positive (rodent, liver adenomas, and carcinomas in male mice)	Negative (but crypiorchidism in rodents)
Saquinavir (Forlovase – soft gel) (Invirase – hard gel)	B	Minimal (human)	Not completed	Negative
Nelfinavir (Viracept)	B	Minimal (human)	Not completed	Negative
Amprenavir (Agenerase)	C	Unknown	Not Completed	Negative (but deficient ossification and thymic elongation in rats and rabbits)
Lopinavir/Ritonavir (Kaletra)	C	Unknown	Not Completed	Negative (but delayed skeletal ossification and increase in skeletal variations in rats at maternally toxic doses)

[a] FDA pregnancy categories:

A, Adequate and well-controlled studies of pregnant women fail to demonstrate a risk to the fetus during the first trimester of pregnancy (and there is no evidence of risk during later trimesters); B, animal reproduction studies fail to demonstrate a risk to the fetus and adequate and well-controlled studies of pregnant women have not been conducted; C, safety in human pregnancy has not been determined, animal studies are either positive for fetal risk or have not been conducted, and the drug should not be used unless the potential benefit outweighs the potential risk to the fetus; D, positive evidence of human fetal risk based on adverse reaction data from investigational or marketing experiences, but the potential benefits from the use of the drug in pregnant women may be acceptable despite potential risks; X, studies in animals or reports of adverse reactions have indicated that the risk associated with the use of the drug for pregnant women clearly outweighs any possible benefit.

Prepared by L.M. Mofenson.

in the risk of HIV infection (109). It is important to remember that postexposure interventions do not protect completely. There have been reported cases of HIV infection in health-care personnel in the United States and elsewhere after having taken postexposure antiretroviral therapy. The most effective antiviral combination remains unknown.

It is important for an exposed health-care worker to be evaluated quickly in the event of an incident, have the patient and the health-care worker tested for HIV immediately, provide antiviral counseling, and begin prophylactic treatment as soon as possible.

Blood Transfusion

Prior to the development of a serologic test for HIV-1 infection in 1985, HIV-1 posed a significant threat to the safety of blood and blood products. Seventy percent of hemophiliacs in the United States are thought to be infected with HIV-1, and at least 12,000 individuals were infected from packed red blood cell and fresh frozen plasma transfusions before HIV-1 antibody testing became available.

Several public health measures have been instituted to make the blood supply safer. HIV-1 antibody testing became available in April 1985, and has decreased the risk of transfusion-acquired HIV-1 infection significantly (110). Additional analyses that are performed on donor blood include screening serum for elevated hepatic transaminases and testing for hepatitis B and C antigens. Testing of donor blood for HTLV-1 has recently been instituted, and testing for HIV-2 is being studied in the United States despite the low prevalence of HIV-2 in North America.

The older HIV tests were assays for antibodies to HIV. As such, there is a ''window period'' in which new infected persons will test negative until they have developed IgG antibodies. This window period is as long as 45 days (111). Newer enzyme immunosorbent tests are able to decrease the window period to an average of 25 days by testing for IgM and IgG (112). Some newer blood assays now look for the p24 antigen or involve nucleic acid amplification testing for HIV-1 and HIV-2. The evolution of technology over the past few years has brought down the estimated risk of transmission of HIV by screened blood from 1 in 450,000 to 1 in 660,000 blood donations in the United States (113).

Rigorous historical screening and questioning of donors for HIV-1 risk factors is also responsible for the increased safety of our blood supply. Voluntary donation and the confidential exclusion of patients with risk factors for these diseases are integral to safeguarding the blood supply available for transfusion. Many patients request direct donation from family members. This practice may circumvent these safeguards since individuals at high-risk for HIV-1 may feel obligated to donate and therefore this practice is not usually recommended.

DIAGNOSIS OF HIV-1 INFECTION

The development of a means of diagnosing HIV-1 infection in a patient prior to the patient developing AIDS is a major advancement in the fight against the epidemic. Routine screening is not generally recommended to date. However, if a patient's history or clinical information provides concern for significant risk to the patient, an HIV-1 test should be offered. It is imperative that patients receive counseling and information about both HIV-1 infection and testing prior to being evaluated and after the results of the test are known (114).

In March 1985, the U.S. Food and Drug Administration (FDA) licensed a commercially produced enzyme-linked immunoabsorbent assay (ELISA) to detect HIV-1 antibody in serum (115). The ELISA has become the most common method to screen for HIV-1 exposure and infection (116). Most laboratories use an ELISA or enzyme immunoassay (EIA) as an initial screening tool. The ELISA test is a general screening assay for antibody binding to HIV-1 (117,118). A test such as the HIV-1 ELISA, with a 99.8% specificity, will generate 20 false-positive test results in 10,000 tests. If the serum is positive in one of two additional tests, for a total of two of three tests, a confirmatory test, usually a Western blot, is performed.

The Western blot, also known as immunoblot enzyme linked immunoelectro transfer, is more time consuming but much more specific (119,120). The Western blot separates antigens by size and identifies antibodies to specific antigens of the virus (121). If antibodies exist for two of three of the p24, gp41, and gp120/160 proteins, the Western blot is considered to be positive. Samples positive on ELISA and confirmed with a positive Western blot should be considered to be positive. Samples positive by ELISA but negative by Western blot may generally be considered to be negative, but surveillance and testing of the patient over time is appropriate (122). If one has a high index of clinical suspicion, one should repeat the Western blot in 4 to 6 weeks for confirmation of a negative result.

The most common means of diagnosing HIV-1 infection remains serologic testing that demonstrates antibodies to HIV-1 using an ELISA test followed by a Western blot. Other tests that may be performed include HIV viral load and HIV-1 p24 antigen assays. The HIV-1 p24 antigen is, however, used for screening of donated blood. On average, it takes 6 days to detect p24 levels after HIV infection (123). The p24 antigen is helpful when one is concerned about early primary infection of HIV-1, but once antibodies begin to be produced, the levels of p24 antigen decrease (124,125).

Rapid Testing

New technology has allowed for development of more rapid testing of people to determine if they are HIV-1 positive. Perhaps a third of persons who are tested for HIV do not return for their HIV test results and counseling. Several rapid tests are now available and approved for use by the FDA. Because of the window period and the time required for the body to develop antibodies to the HIV-1 virus, a negative result from either of these two tests should prompt counseling for repeat testing in 8 to 10 weeks. These rapid HIV tests are believed to have comparable sensitivity and specificity to the enzyme immunosorbent assays (EIAs) regularly used in HIV-1 screening. Every reactive rapid test, however, must be confirmed with a supplemental test, that is, Western blot for diagnosis.

Neonatal Testing

The testing of neonates for HIV-1 infection is complex. A high percentage of neonates born to mothers infected with HIV-1 will have passively acquired anti–HIV-1 IgG, and thus will test positive by both ELISA and Western blot (126). Babies can maintain maternal IgG for up to 15 months. Some of these children, perhaps 50%, will not be infected with the virus, and over time, the maternal IgG will clear. With sequential testing, these children will have decreased titers and eventually test and remain antibody negative (127,128). A small number of HIV-1–infected babies do not form IgG for some time after birth and will test antibody negative after the clearing of maternal antibody, but these children will eventually seroconvert. Definitive diagnosis of HIV infection in early infancy requires nucleic acid amplification through polymerase chain reaction (PCR) or viral culture. HIV infection is diagnosed by two positive assays (PCR or viral culture) on two separate specimens. Infant HIV testing should be done as soon after birth as possible so appropriate treatment interventions can be implemented quickly (129).

CLINICAL STAGES OF HIV DISEASE

The clinical manifestations of HIV-1 disease vary greatly throughout the course of disease. HIV-1 infection can manifest with an acute viral infection syndrome followed by a prolonged asymptomatic period followed by advanced disease. HIV infection can be divided into four stages: primary HIV infection, clinically asymptomatic phase, symptomatic HIV infection, and progression from HIV to AIDS. A few patients may be long-term nonprogressors and never progress to advanced disease. However, most will continue through the phases of disease if untreated.

The acute HIV-1 infection syndrome, or primary HIV-1 infection, is a mononucleosis-like illness. Symptoms can include fevers, night sweats, malaise, fatigue, myalgias, arthralgias, headache, sore throat, diarrhea, generalized lymphadenopathy, macular erythematous eruption about the trunk, and thrombocytopenia (130). This illness may be mistaken for influenza, a "bad cold," or mononucleosis. Other neurologic sequelae have been noted such as meningitis, encephalitis, peripheral neuropathy, and myelopathy (131).

The symptoms of primary HIV-1 infection manifest 4 days to 4 weeks after exposure (132–134).

The syndrome is recognized or recalled by about 50% to 90% of patients (135,136). It may vary depending on the mode of transmission of HIV-1 to the patient. One observational study showed only 4.2% of IVDUs had symptomatic primary HIV-1 infection, whereas 47% of those who sexually acquired the infection were symptomatic (137). The difference may be related to the use of the medical care system, difference in patient recall, and the difference in familiarity with different clinicians with the presenting symptoms. Clinicians need to familiarize themselves with the symptoms and maintain a high index of suspicion for the disease.

There appears to be a prognostic significance in the presence and duration of primary HIV-1 infection. One large prospective study found 68% of symptomatic seroconverters had a significantly higher risk of developing AIDS at 56 months, whereas only 20% of asymptomatic patients had developed AIDS at 56 months. Also, another prospective study found an increased rate of progression to late-stage disease in symptomatic seroconverters with symptomatic primary infection greater than 14 days in length. Nearly 80% of those patients progressed to AIDS after 3 years compared with 10% for those with mild or no illness (138).

Primary HIV-1 infection is diagnosed by the presence of HIV-1 with the absence of HIV-1 antibodies. HIV-1 plasma viral load test can be measured if there is a high clinical suspicion for disease and ELISA or other antibody screening tests are negative.

After primary HIV-1 infection symptoms have resolved, there is a period of clinical latency. There is active HIV replication at this time. The length of asymptomatic HIV infection is variable. Although there are some patients who are long-term nonprogressors, many will go on to develop symptomatic HIV infection and AIDS without intervention. There is discussion in the literature as to the appropriate time to begin antiretroviral therapy during the asymptomatic HIV infection phase.

HIV-1–associated illnesses are a disease spectrum beginning with HIV-1 infection and continuing over time. The immune system becomes progressively more compromised and patients become prone to the development of infections and neoplasms that occur at significantly increased rates in immunocompromised patients. The CDC has defined AIDS as a clinical spectrum of diseases or syndromes that have been associated with infection with HIV-1. It is also important to remember that HIV-1–infected persons may also develop any illness that might occur in a non–HIV-1–infected person. These illnesses may present in unusual fashions, and are likely to be more severe in patients who are immunosuppressed because of infection with HIV-1.

A hallmark of HIV-1 infection, and a measure of disease progression, is the destruction and depletion of CD4-bearing T lymphocytes (139). Many of the immunologic abnormalities observed in AIDS can be explained by the ablation of the helper functions normally carried out or influenced by CD4-bearing T lymphocytes. This has led to the monitoring of CD4 cells as a marker of HIV-1 infection progression and immune status. Studies of natural killer (NK) T-cell targets, virally infected targets, and large granular lymphocytes that are active mediators of NK cell function also demonstrate impaired function with HIV-1 infection (140,141). Immunologic functions that may be affected include activation of macrophages; induction of specific B-cell function, induction of cytotoxic T cells and NK cells; suppressor T-cell activity; secretion of growth, differentiation or hematopoietic colony-stimulating factors; and secretion of factors that induce non–lymphoid cell function (142).

Polyclonal B-cell activation and hypergammaglobulinemia are common findings in patients infected with HIV-1 (143). The cause of this B-cell activation may be multifactorial. Infection with HIV-1 itself has been shown to induce polyclonal B-cell activation (144). Interleukin-6 (IL-6), a cytokine known to stimulate differentiation of B cells, found at circulating levels has been found to be increased in HIV-1–infected patients (145). In addition, patients infected with HIV-1 have increased numbers of circulating Epstein-Barr virus (EBV)–infected B cells (146). However, this increased immunoglobulin synthesis is nonspecific, and patients with HIV-1 infection actually have an impaired ability to produce specific antibodies in response to new antigenic stimulation (147,148).

A number of nonspecific symptoms can be seen as a patient's immune system becomes more impaired. Patients may also have oral thrush and oral hairy leukoplakia. Other conditions seen may include persistent diarrhea, unexplained fever, and weight loss. In addition, patients may develop HIV-1–associated encephalitis, neuropathy, myelopathy, and neuropsychiatric disorders (149). Dermatologic manifestations are quite common in HIV disease and include psoriasis, seborrheic dermatitis, molluscum contagiosum, tinea versicolor, tinea pedis, tinea capitis, alopecia, staphylococcal impetigo, and folliculitis. HIV-infected patients may also develop frequent and severe outbreaks of herpes simplex, reactivation of varicella zoster that can be multidermatomal, and severe outbreaks of condyloma acuminata that may disseminate.

Common findings in HIV-1–infected women are frequent or persistent vaginal candidiasis (150), persistent generalized lymphadenopathy, and leukopenia (151). Patients may have other external genital lesions including condylomata due to human papillomavirus (HPV) (152) and vulvar excoriations due to vulvovaginitis. Immunosuppressed women are prone to vaginal bacteriosis, trichomonias, and fungal vaginitis. There is also evidence that there is a greater incidence of severe pelvic inflammatory disease (PID) in HIV-infected women (153,154).

The CD4 lymphocyte count is a marker of immune deficiency. In the early epidemic, it was noted that patients with CD4 lymphocyte counts <200/mm³ developed an AIDS-defining illness at a rate of 30% per year (155,156). In 1993, the CDC definition of AIDS expanded to include patients with a CD4 count <200/mm³ or with an "AIDS-defining illness." AIDS-defining illnesses are opportunistic infections and cancers that are more prevalent in the immunosuppressed.

Patients with CD4 count <350/mm³ are at increased risk for herpes simplex virus, tuberculosis, oral or vaginal thrush, and herpes zoster ulcers. With a CD4 count <200/mm³, patients may present with *Pneumocystis carinii* pneumonia (PCP) and candidal esophagitis. Once a patient's CD4 count drops to <100/mm³, there is increased risk of cryptococcal meningitis, toxoplasmosis, encephalitis, and progressive multifocal leukoencephalopathy. Finally, once an HIV patient's CD4 count is <50/mm³, there is increased risk for *Mycobacterium avium* and cytomegalovirus infections.

HIV AND CANCER

As in patients with other immunodeficiencies, whether primary or iatrogenic, the HIV-1 infected are at increased risk for the development of cancer (157,158). The tumors originally associated with HIV-1 infection are Kaposi's sarcoma (KS) and non-Hodgkin's lymphoma (NHL). Epidemic KS was one of the earliest recognized manifestations of HIV-1 infection as well as one of the first AIDS-defining illnesses (159). NHL has been an AIDS-defining illness since 1985 (160). Invasive cervical cancer was added to the list of AIDS-defining illnesses in 1993 (161).

Kaposi's Sarcoma

KS rarely occurs in women. Nearly 30% of gay and bisexual AIDS patients have KS compared to less than 5% of all other AIDS patients (162). Initially, there was speculation of an infectious agent secondary to this observation. An unknown herpes virus was isolated from a KS lesion from an AIDS patient in the early 1990s (163). This virus was later to be known as the Kaposi's sarcoma herpes virus (KSHV), also known as human herpes virus 8 (HHV-8). Over 95% of KS lesions, no matter what their source, are found to be infected with KSHV (164).

HIV-1–associated KS is more fulminant than the classic form of the disease first described in 1872 by Moriz Kaposi (165,166). The predominant site of involvement with classic KS is the skin of the lower extremity. Although the most common initial presentation of epidemic KS is cutaneous disease, it can involve all organ systems, and the disease often follows a very fulminant course (167). Lesions typically can be found on the soles of the feet and in the head and neck area, particularly the oropharyngeal region (168). Visceral and lymphangitic obstruction may be seen late in the disease process. The gastrointestinal tract is the most common visceral site of KS. In excess of 50% of patients with HIV-1–related KS may have symptomatic bowel involvement resulting in enteropathy, pain, diarrhea, bleeding, and less frequently obstruction (169,170). Pulmonary involvement with KS should be considered in the differential diagnosis of patients with respiratory symptoms and known KS (171). Differentiation of pulmonary KS from an infectious process can be difficult. Because of the vascular nature of these tumors, the KS lesion may be the source of severe and even fatal hemorrhage, especially when there is involvement of the lung or gastrointestinal tract.

Since the use of highly active antiviral therapy (HAART) began the incidence of KS has decreased. KS lesions can regress because of HAART alone (172,173). Although HAART should be given patients with KS, some may need additional treatment. Those with gastrointestinal, pulmonary, and significant cutaneous disease will require local and systemic KS therapy. These can include local interventions such as focal radiation or intralesional or topical agents. For systemic disease, interferon-α and cytotoxic chemotherapy have been used. Liposomal doxorubicin and docetaxel are commonly used as single agents.

Non-Hodgkin's Lymphoma

In contrast to Kaposi's sarcoma, HIV-associated NHL does not appear to be limited to any particular risk group. There are currently no data to indicate that the overall development of HIV-1–associated lymphoma in women will be any different from that in men. The NHLs associated with HIV-1 disease usually are high-grade B-cell tumors. Histologies such as small noncleaved cell and large cell immunoblastic lymphomas are commonly seen in these patients and that are rare in the general population (174).

The most striking clinical findings of HIV-1–associated NHLs is their propensity to present with advanced-stage and extranodal sites of disease. In general, 11% of patients with HIV-1–associated NHLs have a primary CNS lymphoma, 17% will secondarily involve the CNS, 29% involve the bone marrow, 24% involve the liver parenchyma, and 22% involve the gastrointestinal tract, including several cases with rectal disease (175–181). Nearly every organ system has been reported as having been involved with AIDS-associated NHL. Patients with HIV-1–associated NHLs very frequently have constitutional or B symptoms (fever, night sweats, and weight loss). Overall 32% to 68% of patients in the initial reports had a previous defining illness prior to developing NHL (182,183).

The treatment of HIV-1–associated NHL has been disappointing. The prognostic factors related to a patient's underlying HIV-1 disease state appear also to be the most important prognostic factors for HIV-1–associated NHL (184–188). These tumors are much more difficult to treat when compared with the same tumors in the general population (189–191). Lymphomas in this population behave more aggressively, partially because these patients do not tolerate

chemotherapy well. More recently, with HAART and better supportive care, response rates to lymphoma treatment have improved. One report recently showed a complete remission in 74% of the 39 patients with B-cell lymphomas with a dose-adjusted chemotherapeutic regimen. In this group of patients, antiretroviral therapy was suspended while the patients received chemotherapy (192). This study questions the need for HAART during chemotherapy and if the interactions between HAART and chemotherapy may play in a role in response to treatment.

Other Lymphoma Types

Primary CNS lymphoma

Prior to the use of HAART, primary CNS lymphoma was found at autopsy in 10% of AIDS patients. AIDS patients had an incidence of primary CNS lymphoma (PCNSL) 3600-fold greater than in the general population (193). PCNSL is associated with EBV (194). Owing to HAART therapy, the incidence of primary CNS lymphoma in AIDS is falling (195).

Primary Effusion Lymphoma

Primary effusion lymphoma (PEL), also known as body cavity–based lymphoma, is a rare type of systemic lymphoma associated with AIDS. PEL is characterized by large anaplastic cells in a body cavity effusion; typically pleural effusion or ascites (196–198). These tumors are not unique to HIV patients and can be seen in other immunodeficiency states. The tumor cells frequently are found to have the genome of KSHV and EBV infection concurrently. As with PCNSL, there is a decreased incidence of PEL with the use of HAART.

Hodgkin's Lymphoma

There have now been multiple epidemiologic studies showing a greater than expected number of Hodgkin's lymphomas (HLs) in the HIV-positive population. HIV-related HL is generally more advanced at presentation and has a strong association with EBV (199). In the HAART era, HIV-related HL may be less clinically aggressive and with better survival than in the pre-HAART era (200,201).

Cervical Disease

Human papillomavirus (HPV) infection results in an increased incidence of malignancies in the setting of immunosuppression. HIV-1–induced immunosuppressed women are predisposed to cervical HPV infection and cervical dysplasia and neoplasia. It has even been suggested that the interaction between HIV and HPV may cause upregulation of latent oncogenic HPV (202–204).

In 1993, invasive cervical cancer was designated an AIDS-defining illness by the CDC (205). Cervical intrapithelial neoplasia (CIN) is diagnosed three times more often in HIV-infected women than in women who are HIV negative (206). The prevalence of cervical CIN in HIV-positive women ranges from 31% to 63% (207). The current opportunistic infection guidelines recommend HIV-1–infected women have a Papanicolaou (Pap) smear performed annually after two smears done at 6-month intervals are negative. More frequent Pap smears should be obtained if there is a previous abnormal Pap smear, or treatment of cervical dysplasia, or the woman has symptomatic HIV disease or a CD4 count $<200/mm^3$.

Anal Pap smears to assess for dysplasia and anal swabs to test for HPV may also be appropriate for patients who participate in receptive anal sexual activity. Although, it must be stressed that the screening value of these procedures is variable depending on the experience of the person performing the procedure and is still under investigation.

In HIV-positive patients, the prevalence and persistence of HPV infection increases with the lowering of the CD4 count and the elevation of the HIV RNA load (208). There has been speculation that the possibility of the reverse may also be true. HAART therapy is associated with varying levels of immune restoration. In a recent series looking at 168 HIV-infected women with CIN, HAART was found to have a significant level of increased regression of the patients (209). This is a promising study; however, further data would be required to change the intensive screening regimen recommended for HIV-positive women.

NON–AIDS-RELATED CANCER

Cancer is an increasing cause of death in the AIDS population (210). In addition to AIDS-defining cancers, recent linking between AIDS and cancer registries have shown a higher risk of AIDS patients developing non–AIDS-defining cancers. The HIV-infected population has a higher risk of HL, testicular seminoma, and lung, lip, and anal cancers (211–213).

Recent epidemiologic studies have found an increase in the incidence of lung cancer in HIV-positive patients (214, 215). Some postulate that the increased smoking rate in this population has not been adequately accounted for in assessment of risk. There are no data to suggest lung cancer should be treated differently in HIV-positive patients (216).

Although breast cancer is the most common carcinoma in women, the data do not support any increase in the incidence of breast cancer in the HIV-positive population (217). There is no evidence that breast cancer behaves differently in HIV-infected patients (218).

Australia has an excellent HIV Infection and Cancer Registry. The Australians attempted to divide cancer rates into the degree of immunosuppression based on date of HIV diagnosis. They showed a significant increase in cancer of the lip, anus, and connective tissue; Hodgkin's disease; myeloma; and leukemia. Interestingly, the Australian data did not show a significant increase in lung or testicular cancer. The other diagnoses seem to increase with increased levels of immune deficiency (219). An American study found an overall excess risk of many cancers in patients with AIDS, but a trend of worsening immunity could only be seen in KS and immunoblastic lymphomas (220).

Further studies will need to be done to assess the need for differences in treatment of patients with HIV and cancer. At present, there are no guidelines to suggest any variation for the treatment of a cancer patient with HIV infection. One may want to consider hematologic growth factors to decrease the possibility of complications related to chemotherapy and HAART.

TREATMENT OF THE HIV-1–INFECTED PATIENT

Treatment recommendations for the HIV-1–infected patient change frequently, and it takes dedication to keep current. In addition, it has been shown that a physician's experience is important in a patient's outcome. According to a 1998 survey, only 75% of patients who were starting antiretroviral therapy were assigned to the optimal regimens as defined by consensus guidelines (221,222).

Prophylactic Therapy

Treatment of the HIV-1–infected patient involves therapies aimed at HIV-1 itself as well as associated diseases. Patients who are extremely immunosuppressed benefit from measures to prevent opportunistic illness. Diseases that are strongly recommended for prophylactic therapy include PCP, mycobacterial tuberculosis, *Toxoplasma gondii* infection, varicella zoster virus infection, and *Mycobacterium avium* complex (MAC) infection. The CDC regularly provides guidelines for prophylactic treatment of patients with HIV-1 disease. Table 37.2 outlines some of the most recent guidelines for prophylactic therapies in adults and adolescents infected with HIV.

PCP is a common illness in HIV-1–infected patients. PCP prophylaxis should be administered to patients with HIV-1 infection who have had an episode of PCP or to patients with no previous history of PCP but <200 CD4 cells/mm^3 or CD4 cells $<14\%$ of the total lymphocyte count (223). Trimethoprim-sulfamethoxazole is currently the first choice for PCP prophylaxis. Dapsone, aerosolized pentamidine, and atovaquone are useful PCP prophylactic therapy alternatives, particularly for those who are allergic to sulfa-containing drugs. Trimethoprim-sulfamethoxazole or dapsone is also recommended for *T. gondii* prophylaxis in patients whose CD4 count is $<100/\mu L$.

Mycobacterial tuberculosis prophylaxis is based on the tuberculosis skin test results of the patient and those guide-

TABLE 37.2. *Prophylaxis to prevent first episode of opportunistic disease in adults and adolescents infected with HIV*

Pathogen	Preventive regimens		
	Indication	First choice	Alternatives
I. Strongly recommended as standard of care			
Pneumocystis carinii[a]	CD4+ count <200/μL or oropharyngeal candidiasis	Trimethoprim-sulfamethoxazole (TMP-SMZ), 1 DS po q.d. (AI) TMP-SMZ, 1 SS po q.d. (AI)	Dapsone, 50 mg po b.i.d. *or* 100 mg po q.d. (BI); dapsone, 50 mg po q.d. *plus* pyrimethamine, 50 mg po q.w. *plus* leucovorin 25 mg po q.w. (BI); dapsone 200 mg po plus pyrimethamine, 75 mg po plus leucovorin, 25 mg po q.w. (BI); aerosolized pentamidine, 300 mg q.m. via Respirgard II nebulizer (BI); atovaquone, 1500 mg po q.d. (BI); TMP-SMZ, 1 DS po t.i.w. (BI)
Mycobacterium tuberculosis Isoniazid sensitive[b]	TST reaction ≥5 mm or prior positive TST result without treatment or contact with case of active tuberculosis regardless of TST result (BIII)	Isoniazid, 300 mg po *plus* pyridoxine, 50 mg po q.d. × 9 mo (AII) or isoniazid, 900 mg po *plus* pyridoxine, 100 mg po b.i.w. × 9 mo (BII)	Rifampin, 600 mg po q.d. (BIII) × 4 mo or rifabuin 300 mg po q.d. (CIII) × 4 mo Pyrazinamide, 15–20 mg/kg po q.d. × 2 mo *plus* either rifampin, 600 mg po q.d. (BI) × 2 mo or rifabutin, 300 mg po q.d. (CIII) × 2 mo
Isoniazid resistant	Same as above; high probability of exposure to isoniazid-resistant tuberculosis	Rifampin 600 mg po (AIII) or rifabutin, 300 mg po (BIII) q.d. × 4 mo	Pyrazinamide 15–20 mg/kg po q.d. *plus* either rifampin, 600 mg po (BI) or rifabutin, 300 mg po (CIII) q.d. × 2 mo
Multidrug-(isoniazid and rifampin) resistant	Same as above; high probability of exposure to multidrug-resistant tuberculosis	Choice of drugs requires consultation with public health authorities. Depends on susceptibility of isolate from source patient	
Toxoplasma gondii[c]	IgG antibody to *Toxoplasma* and CD4+ count <100/μL	TMP-SMZ, 1 DS po q.d. (AII)	TMP-SMZ, 1 SS po q.d. (BIII): dapsone, 50 mg po q.d. *plus* pyrimethamine, 50 mg po q.w. *plus* leucovorin, 25 mg po q.w. (BI); dapsone, 200 mg po *plus* pyrimethamine, 75 mg po *plus* leucovorin, 25 mg po q w (BI); atovaquone, 1500 mg po q.d. with or without pyrimethamine, 25 mg po q.d. *plus* leucovorin, 10 mg po q.d. (CIII)
Mycobacterium avium complex[d]	CD4+ count <50/μL	Azithromycin, 1,200 mg po q.w., (AI) or clarithromycin,[d] 500 mg po b.i.d. (AI)*	Rifabutin, 300 mg po q.d. (BI); azithromycin, 1,200 mg po q.w. *plus* rifabutin, 300 mg po q.d. (CI)
Varicella zoster virus (VZV)	Significant exposure to chickenpox or shingles for patients who have no history of either condition or, if available, negative antibody to VZV	Varicella zoster immune globulin (VZIG), 5 vials (1.25 mL each) im, administered ≤96 h after exposure, ideally within 48 h (AIII)	
II. Generally Recommended			
Streptococcus pneumoniae[e]	CD4+ count ≥200/μL	23 valent polysaccharide vaccine, 0.5 mL im [BII]	None
Hepatitis B virus[f,g]	All susceptible (anti-HBc-negative) patients	Hepatitis B vaccine: 3 doses (BII)	None
Influenza virus[g,h]	All patients (annually, before influenza season)	Inactivated trivalent influenza virus vaccine: one annual dose (0.5 mL) im (BIII)	Oseltamivir, 75 mg po q.d. (influenza A or B) (CIII); rimantadine, 100 mg po b.i.d. (CIII), or amantadine, 100 mg po b.i.d. (CIII) (influenza A only)

(continued)

TABLE 37.2. *Continued*

Pathogen	Preventive regimens		
	Indication	First choice	Alternatives
Hepatitis A virus[f,g]	All susceptible (anti-HAV-negative) patients at increased risk for HAV infection (e.g., illicit drug users, men who have sex with men, hemophiliacs) or with chronic liver disease, including chronic hepatitis B or hepatitis C	Hepatitis A vaccine: 2 doses (BIII)	None

III. Evidence for Efficacy but Not Routinely Indicated

Pathogen	Indication	First choice	Alternatives
Bacteria	Neutropenia	Granulocyte colony-stimulating factor (G-CSF), 5–10 μg/kg sc q.d. × 2–4 w or granulocyte macrophage colony-stimulating factor (GM-CSF), 250 μg/m² sc iv × 2–4 w (CII)	None
Cryptococcus neoformans	CD4⁺ count <50/μL	Fluconazole, 100–200 mg po q.d. (CI)	Itraconazole capsule, 200 mg po q.d. (CIII)
Histoplasma capsulatum[i]	CD4⁺ count <100/μL, endemic geographic area	Itraconazole capsule, 200 mg po q.d. (CI)	None
Cytomegalovirus (CMV)[j]	CD4⁺ count <50/μL and CMV antibody positivity	Oral ganciclovir, 1 g po t.i.d. (CI)	None

NOTES: Information included in these guidelines might not represent Food and Drug Administration (FDA) approval or approved labeling for the particular products or indications in question. Specifically, the terms *safe* and *effective* might not be synonymous with the FDA-defined legal standards for product approval. The Respirgard II nebulizer is manufactured by Marquest, Englewood, CO. Letters and roman numerals in parentheses after regimens indicate the strength of the recommendation and the quality of evidence supporting it (see page 7). Anti-HBc, antibody to hepatitis B core antigen; b.i.w., twice a week; DS, double-strength tablet; HAART, highly active antiretroviral therapy; HAV, hepatitis A virus; HIV, human immunodeficiency virus; im, intramuscular; iv, intravenous; po, by mouth; q.d., daily; q.m., monthly; q.w., weekly; SS, single-strength tablet; t.i.w., three times a week; TMP-SMZ, trimethoprim-sulfamethoxazole; sc, subcutaneous; TST, tuberculin skin test.

[a] Prophylaxis should also be considered for persons with a CD4⁺ percentage of <14%, for persons with a history of an AIDS-defining illness, and possibly for those with CD4⁺ counts >200 but <250 cells/μL. TMP-SMZ also reduces the frequency of toxoplasmosis and some bacterial infections. Patients receiving dapsone should be tested for glucose-6-phosphate dehydrogenase deficiency. A dosage of 50 mg q.d. is probably less effective than 100 mg q.d. The efficacy of parenteral pentamidine (e.g., 4 mg/kg/month) is uncertain. Fansidar (sulfadoxine-pyrimethamine) is rarely used because of severe hypersensitivity reactions. Patients who are being administered therapy for toxoplasmosis with sulfadiazine-pyrimethamine are protected against *P. carinii* pneumonia and do not need additional prophylaxis against PCP.

[b] Directly observed therapy is recommended for isoniazid (e.g., 900 mg b.i.w.); isoniazid regimens should include pyridoxine to prevent peripheral neuropathy. If rifampin or rifabutin is administered concurrently with protease inhibitors or nonnucleoside reverse transcriptase inhibitors, careful consideration should be given to potential pharmacokinetic interactions (54). See discussion of rifamycin interactions in paragraph 11 in section on Tuberculosis. There have been reports of fatal and severe liver injury associated with the treatment of latent TB infection in HIV-uninfected persons treated with the 2-month regimen of daily rifampin and pyrazinamide; therefore it may be prudent to use regimens that do not contain pyrazinamide in HIV-infected persons whose completion of treatment can be assured (CDC. Update: Fatal and Severe Liver Injuries Associated with Rifampin and Pyrazinamide for Latent Tuberculosis Infection and Revisions in American Thoracic Society/CDC Recommendations, United States 2001 *MMWR* 50 (No. 34), Aug 31, 2001). Exposure to multidrug-resistant tuberculosis might require prophylaxis with two drugs; consult public health authorities. Possible regimens include pyrazinamide plus either ethambutol or a fluoroquinolone.

[c] Protection against toxoplasmosis is provided by TMP-SMZ, dapsone plus pyrimethamine, and possibly by atovaquone. Atovaquone may be used with or without pyrimethamine. Pyrimethamine alone probably provides little, if any, protection.

[d] See paragraph 9, in section on "Disseminated Infection with Mycobacterium avium complex" and references 53 and 54 for discussion of drug interactions.

*During pregnancy, azithromycin is preferred over clarithromycin because of the teratogenicity in animals of clarithromycin.

[e] Vaccination may be offered to persons who have a CD4⁺ T-lymphocyte count <200 cells/μL, although the efficacy is likely to be diminished. Revaccination 5 years after the first dose or sooner if the initial immunization was given when the CD4⁺ count was <200 cells/μL and the CD4⁺ count has increased to >200 cells/μL on HAART is considered optional. Some authorities are concerned that immunizations might stimulate the replication of HIV.

[f] Although data demonstrating clinical benefit of these vaccines in HIV-infected persons are not available, it is logical to assume that those patients who develop antibody responses will derive some protection. Some authorities are concerned that immunizations might stimulate HIV replication, although for influenza vaccination, a large observational study of HIV-infected persons in clinical care showed no adverse effect of this vaccine, including multiple doses, on patient survival (J. Ward, CDC, personal communication). Also, this concern may be less relevant in the setting of HAART. However, because of the theoretical concern that increases in HIV plasma RNA following vaccination during pregnancy might increase the risk of perinatal transmission of HIV, providers may wish to defer vaccination for such patients until after HAART is initiated.

[g] Hepatitis B vaccine has been recommended for all children and adolescents and for all adults with risk factors for hepatitis B virus (HBV). For persons requiring vaccination against both hepatitis A and hepatitis B, a combination vaccine is now available. For additional information regarding vaccination against hepatitis A and B, see CDC.

TABLE 37.3. *Antiretroviral drugs used against HIV-1*

Nucleoside/nucleotide reverse transcriptase inhibitors
    Abacavir
    Didanosine (DDI)
    Emtricitabine
    Lamivudine (3TC)
    Stavudine (D4T)
    Tenofovir
    Zalcitabine (DDC)
    Zidovudine (AZT)
Nonnucleoside reverse transcriptase inhibitors
    Delavirdine
    Efavirenz
    Vevirapine
Protease inhibitors
    Amprenavir
    Atazanavir
    Indinavir
    Loprinivir
    Nelfinavir
    Ritonavir
    Saquinavir
Fusion inhibitor
    Ebfuvirtide

lines are different for the HIV-positive patient. If an HIV-positive patient has a skin test that reacts >5 mm or the patient has a history of a positive skin test without treatment, prophylaxis is recommended. Also, if a patient has had contact with a patient with a case of active tuberculosis, regardless of the result of their skin test, prophylaxis is recommended. The specific drug regimen recommendations are based on sensitivity of tuberculosis to isoniazid and is also summarized in Table 37.2.

Other recommendations for prophylaxis are for varicella zoster virus and MAC. MAC prophylaxis is recommended for patients whose CD4 count is $<50/mm^3$. Azithromycin weekly or clarithromycin daily are the recommended first-line agents. Varicella zoster virus prophylaxis is recommended for patients who have a significant exposure to chickenpox or shingles and have no prior history of either disease (224).

Anti–HIV-1 Drugs

A number of anti-HIV drugs have been developed. Antiretroviral treatment has increased the lifespan and improved the quality of life of patients with HIV infection. A list of drugs currently available for the treatment of HIV-1 infection is given in Table 37.3. The guidelines for initiation of antiretroviral therapy are summarized in Table 37.4.

The goal of antiretroviral therapy until recently has been to decrease of the amount of HIV RNA and to improve immune function. It is currently believed the higher the level of HIV RNA, the faster the loss of CD4 cells and the shorter the duration from initial HIV infection to AIDS and death (225). Failure to decrease the HIV RNA level to below 50 copies per milliliter of plasma indicates inadequate suppression and risk of outgrowth of resistant virus (226).

The first class of drugs approved by the FDA for the treatment of HIV-1 were the nucleoside/nucleotide reverse transcriptase inhibitors (NRTIs). The NRTIs prevent the forma-

TABLE 37.4. *Guidelines for the Use of Antiretroviral Agents in HIV infected Adults and Adolescents, July 14, 2003. Table 6. The panel on Clinical Practices for the Treatment of HIV Infection. By HHS.*

Clinical category	CD4⁺ T-cell count	Plasma HIV RNA	Recommendation
Symptomatic (AIDS or severe symptoms)	Any value	Any value	Treat
Asymptomatic, AIDS	CD4⁺ T cells < 200/mm³	Any value	Treat
Asymptomatic	CD4⁺ T cells > 200/mm³ but < 350/mm³	Any value	Treatment should be offered, although controversial.ᵃ
Asymptomatic	CD4⁺ T cells > 350/mm³	> 55,000 (by RT-PCR or bDNA)ᵇ	Some experienced clinicians recommend initiating therapy, recognizing that the 3-year risk for untreated patients to develop AIDS is >30%; in the absence of increased levels of plasma HIV RNA, other clinicians recommend deferring therapy and monitoring the CD4⁺ T-cell count and level of plasma HIV RNA more frequently; clinical outcome data after initiating therapy are lacking.
Asymptomatic	CD4⁺ T cells > 350/mm³	< 55,000 (by RT-PCR or bDNA)	Many experienced clinicians recommend deferring therapy and monitoring the CD4⁺ T-cell count, recognizing that the 3-year risk for untreated patients to experience AIDS is <15%.

ᵃ Clinical benefit has been demonstrated in controlled trials only for patients with CD4⁺ T cells <200/mm³; however, the majority of clinicians would offer therapy at a CD4⁺ T-cell threshold <350/mm³. A recent evaluation of data from the Multicenter AIDS Cohort Study (MACS) of 231 persons with CD4⁺ T-cell counts >200 and <350.

tion of 3'-5' phosphodiester bonds between the DNA chain and the 5'-nucleoside triphosphates. They then act to terminate attachment and prevent ongoing viral DNA synthesis. Azidothymidine (AZT) and D4T are thymidine analogs. DDC and 3TC are cytidine analogs. DDI is an inosine analog and abacavir is a guanine analog. There is cross resistance between the nucleoside analogs. Drugs that are analogs to the same nucleoside are not to be used concurrently. Side effects of these drugs include lactic acidosis, pancreatitis, and neuropathy.

Delavirdine, nevirapine, and efavirenz are the nonnucleoside reverse transcriptase inhibitors (NNRTIs) currently in use. NNRTIs seem to be very effective in combination with NRTIs. There is a high degree of cross resistance in the NNRTI class. Protease inhibitors (PIs) are the most recent drugs used in HIV treatment. Indinavir, nelfinavir, saquinavir, and lopinavir/ritonavir are some of the drugs currently used. They inhibit the maturation of the HIV viral particles into virion. The viral particles are instead released and not able to infect the host cells.

There are continually updated guidelines developed by the Panel on Clinical Practices for Treatment of HIV convened by the Department of Health and Human Services for the most current data (http://www.cdc.gov/mmwr/preview/mmwrhtml/00054080.htm; last access 1/17/04). Two helpful websites are the AIDSinfo website, which is a service of the U.S. Department of Health and Human Services at http://aidsinfo.nih.gov/guidelines/ and the CDC division of HIV/AIDS prevention website at http://www.cdc.gov/hiv/treatment.htm. Combination antiretroviral therapy consisting of two nucleoside analog reverse transcriptase inhibitors and a protease inhibitor is the recommended standard treatment for HIV-1–infected adults (227).

A new class of drugs under investigation inhibit HIV entry into the cell. Future anti-HIV drug strategies include integrase inhibitors. These drugs interfere with HIV's ability to insert its gene into a cell's normal DNA.

HIV VACCINE

The development of a vaccine for primary prevention of HIV-1 disease is a priority. To date, there is not an available vaccine for prevention of HIV disease in humans. Various vaccines have been tested in monkeys and have kept viral loads undetectable, but they have not prevented HIV infection. Researchers are continuing to work to bring the HIV-1 vaccine to human subjects for testing.

CONCLUSIONS

Understanding of HIV-1 disease has greatly expanded over the last two decades. New classes of drugs are being introduced to block HIV from entering and damaging host immune cells. HIV-infected patients are living longer, and there is a great deal of interest in whether the HIV-1 disease,

the treatment for the disease, or the patient's immune system itself may play a role in secondary diseases as the patient ages. In the future, we will also need to have long-term data on the exposure to HAART in the fetus and newborn, not only related to HIV transmission. We are also beginning to learn about the differences between women's responses to standard HAART therapy and how it may differ from those of men.

What we do know is that the best treatment for HIV-1 infection is prevention. HIV-1 needs to be discussed with women so that they may take an active role in prevention from acquiring the disease.

REFERENCES

1. Gottlieb, MS, Schroff R, Schanker HM, et al. Pneumocystis carinii pneumonia and mucosal candidiasis in previously healthy homosexual men: evidence of a new acquired cellular immunodeficiency. *N Engl J Med* 305:1425, 1981.
2. Siegal FP, Lopes C, Hammer GS, et al. Severe acquired immunodeficiency in male homosexuals, manifested by chronic perianal ulcerative herpes simplex lesions. *N Engl J Med* 1981;305:1439.
3. Masur H, Michelis MA, Greene JB, et al. An outbreak of community-acquired Pneumocystis carinii pneumonia: initial manifestation of cellular immune dysfunction. *N Engl J Med* 1981;305:1439.
4. Peterman TA, Jaffe JW, Getchell FP, et al. Transfusion-associated acquired immunodeficiency syndrome in the United States. *JAMA* 1985;254:2913
5. Weiss SH, Goedert JJ, Sarngadharan MG, et al. Risk factors for HTLV-III infection among parenteral drug abusers (PDU). *Proc Am Soc Clin Oncol* 1986;5:3.
6. Barre-Sinoussi F, Chermann JC, Rey F, et al. Isolation of A T-lymphotropic retrovirus from a patient at risk for acquired immune deficiency syndrome (AIDS). *Science* 1983;220:868.
7. Gallo RC, Salahuddin SZ, Popovic M, et al. Frequent detection and isolation of cytopathic retroviruses (HTLV-III) from patients with AIDS and at risk for AIDS. *Science* 1984;224:500.
8. Gallo R, Wong-Staal F, Montagnier L, et al. HIV/HTLV nomenclature. *Nature* 1988;333:504.
9. WHO/UNAIDS AIDS Epidemic Update, 2002.
10. Fleming PL, Sweeney PA, Byers RH, et al. HIV Prevalence in the United States, 2000. 9th Conference on Retroviruses and Opportunistic Infections, Seattle, WA, Feb.24–28, 2002.
11. Centers for Disease Control and Prevention (CDC). HIV and AIDS—United States, 1981–2001. *MMWR Morb Mortal Wkly Rep* 2001;50:430–434.
12. Centers for Disease Control and Prevention HIV Prevention Strategic Plan through 2005. January 2001.
13. Center for Disease Control and Prevention. HIV/AIDS Surveillance Report 2002;14.
14. Francis DP, Curran JW, Essex M: Epidemic acquired immune deficiency syndrome (AIDS): Epidemiologic evidence for a transmitted agent. *J Natl Cancer Inst* 1983;71:1.
15. Essex M: Adult T-cell leukemia/lymphoma: Role of a human retrovirus of cats. *Adv Cancer Res* 1975;21:175.
16. Hahn BH, Shaw GM, De Cock KM, Sharp PM. AIDS as a zoonosis: scientific and public health implications. *Science* 2000;287:607–614.
17. Gao F, Bailes E, Robertson DL. Origin of HIV-1 in the chimpanzee Pan troglodytes *Nature* 1999;397:436–441.
18. Korber B. Theiler J, Wolinsky S. Limitations of a molecular clock applied to considerations of the origin of HIV-1. *Science* 1998;280:1868–1871.
19. Guyader M, Emerman M, Sonigo P, et al. Genome organization and transactivation of the human immunodeficiency virus type 2 *Nature* 1987;326:662–669.
20. Chakrabarti L, Guyader M, Alizon, et al. Sequence of simian immuno-

deficiency virus from macaque and its relationship to other human and simian retroviruses. *Nature* 1987;328:543–547.

21. Hirsch VM, Olmsted RA, Murphey-Corb M, et al. An African primate lentivirus (SIVsm) closely related to HIV-2. *Nature* 1989;339: 389–392.

22. Barin FS, M'Boup S, Denis F, et al. Serologic evidence for virus related to simian T-lymphotropic retrovirus III in residents of West Africa. *Lancet* 1985;2:1387.

23. Clavel F, Buetard D, Brun-Vezinet F, et al. Isolation of a new human retrovirus from West African Patients with AIDS. *Science* 1986;233: 343–346.

24. Bryceson A, Tomkins A, Ridley D, et al. HIV-2 associated AIDS in the 1970s [Letter]. *Lancet* 1988,2:221.

25. Kawamura M, Yamazaki S, Ishikawa K, et al. HIV-2 in West Africa in 1966 [Letter]. *Lancet* 1989,1:385

26. Clavel F, Mansinho K, Chamaret S, et al. Human immunodeficiency virus type 2 infection associated with AIDS in West Africa. *N Engl J Med* 1987;316:1180–1185.

27. Poulsen AG, Kvinesdal B, Aaby P, et al. Prevalence of and mortality from human immunodeficiency virus type 2 in Bissau, West Africa. *Lancet* 1989;1:827–831.

28. Brun-Vezinet F, Rey MA, Katlama C, et al. Lymphadenopathy-associated virus type 2 in AIDS and AIDS related complex. Clinical and virological features in four patients. *Lancet* 1987;1:128–132.

29. Le Guenno BM, Barabe P, Griffet PA, et al. HIV-2 and HIV-1 AIDS cases in Senegal:clinical patterns and immunological perturbations. *J Acquir Immune Defic Syndr* 1991;4:421–427.

30. Marlink RG, Ricard D, M'Boup S, et al. Clinical, hematologic, and immunologic cross-sectional evaluation of individuals exposed to human immunodeficiency virus type 2 (HIV-2). *AIDS Res Hum Retroviruses* 1988;4:137–148.

31. Norrgren H, Da Silva ZJ, Anderddon S, et al. Clinical features, immunological changes and mortality in a cohort of HIV-2 infected individuals in Bissau, Guinea-Bissau. *Scand J Infect Dis* 1998;30:323–329.

32. Marlink R, Kanki P, Thior I, et al. Reduced rate of disease development after HIV-2 infection as compared to HIV-1. *Science* 1994;265: 1587–1590.

33. Ancelle R, Bletry O, Baglin AC, et al. Long incubation period for HIV-2 infection. *Lancet* 1987;1:688–689.

34. Mitsuya H, Broder S: Strategies for antiviral therapy in AIDS. *Nature* 1987;325:773.

35. Haseltine WA, Wong-staal F. The molecular biology of the AIDS virus. *Sci Am* 1988;259:54.

36. Varmus H. Reverse transcription. *Sci Am* 1987;257:56–65.

37. Lasky LA, Nakamura G, Smith DH, et al. Delineation of a region of the human immunodeficiency virus type 1 gp120 glycoprotein critical for interaction with the CD4 receptor. *Cell* 1987;50:975.

38. McDougal JS, Kennedy MS, Sligh JM, et al. Binding of HTLV-III/LAV to T4+ T cells by a complex of the 110K viral protein and the T4 molecule. *Science* 1986;231:382.

39. McDougal JS, Mawle A, Cort SP, et al. Cellular tropism of the human retrovirus HTLV-III/LAV-I. Role of T cell activation and expression of the T4 antigen. *J Immunol* 1985;135:3151.

40. Deen KC, McDougal JS, Inacker R, et al. A soluble form of CD4 (T4) protein inhibits AIDS virus infection. *Nature* 1984;312:763.

41. Ratner L, Haseltine W, Patarca R, et al. Complete nucleotide sequence of the AIDS virus, HTLV-III. *Nature* 1985;212:277.

42. Dalgleish AG, Beverley PCL, Clapham PR. The CD4 (T4) antigen is an essential component of the receptor for the AIDS retrovirus. *Nature* 1984;312:763.

43. Centers for Disease Control, *MMWR Morb Mortal Wkly Rep Suppl*, Jan 1990.

44. Sodroski JG, Rosen CA, Haseltine WA. Trans-acting transcriptional activation of the long terminal repeat of human T-lymphotropic viruses in infected cells. *Science* 1984;225:381.

45. Sodroski JG, Patarca R, Rosen C, et al. Location of the trans-activating region on the genome of human T-cell lymphotropic virus type III. *Science* 1985;229:74.

46. Steffy K, Wong-Staal F. Genetic regulation of human immunodeficiency virus. *Microbiol Rev* 1991;55:193–205.

47. Gottlinger HG, Sodroski JG, Haseltine WA. Role of capsid precursor processing and myristoylation in morphogenesis and infectivity of human immunodeficiency type 1. *Proc Natl Acad Sci U S A* 1989; 86:5781–5785.

48. Haseltine W, Wong-Staal F. The molecular biology of the AIDS virus. *Sci Am* 1988;259:52.

49. Ruben S, Perkins A, Purcell R, et al. Structural and functional characterization of the human immunodeficiency virus tat protein. *J Virol* 1989;63:1–8.

50. Feinberg MB, Baltimore D, Frankel AD. The role of Tat in the human immunodeficiency virus life cycle indicated a primary effect on transcriptional elongation. *Proc Natl Acad Sci U S A* 1991;88:4045–4049.

51. Zhu Y, Pe'ery T, Ramanathan Y, et al. transcription elongation factor P-TEFb is required for HIV-1 tat transactivation in vitro. *Genes Dev* 1997;11:2622–2632.

52. Cullen BR. Retroviruses as model systems for the study of nuclear RNA export pathways. *Virology* 1998;249:203–210.

53. Doms RW, Trono D. The plasma membrane as a combat zone in the HIV battlefield. *Genes Dev* 2000;14:2677–2688.

54. Collins KL, Chen BK, Kalams SA, et al. Nef protein protects infected primary cells against killing by cytotoxic T lymphocytes. *Nature* 1998;391:397–401.

55. Kestler HW, Ringler DJ, Mori K, et al. Importance of nef gene for maintenance of high viral loads and for development of AIDS. *Cell* 1991;65:651–662.

56. Deacon NJ, Tsykin A, Soloman A, et al. Genomic structure of an attenuated quasi species of HIV-1 from a blood transfusion donor and recipient. *Science* 1995;270:988–991.

57. Willey RL, Maldarelli F, Martin MA, et al. Human immunodeficiency virus type 1 Vpu protein induces rapid degradation of CD4. *J Virol* 1992;66:7193–7200.

58. Klimkait T, Strebel K, Hoggan MA, et al. The human immunodeficiency virus type 1 specific protein vpu is required for efficient virus maturation and release. *J Virol* 1990;64:621–629.

59. Heinzinger NK, Bukinsky MI, Haggerty SA, et al. The Vpr protein of human immunodeficiency virus type 1 influences nuclear localization of viral nucleic acids in nondividing host cells. *Proc Natl Acad Sci U S A* 1994;91:7311–7315.

60. Miller MD, Farnet CM, Bushman FD. Human immunodeficiency virus type 1 preintegration complexes: studies of organization and composition. *J Virol* 1997;71:5382–5390.

61. Simon JH, Gaddis NC, Fouchier RA, Malim MH. Evidence for a newly discovered cellular anti-HIV-1 phenotype. *Nat Med* 1998;4: 1397–1400.

62. Friedland GH, Klein RS: Transmission of the human immunodeficiency virus. *N Engl J Med* 1987;317:1125.

63. Kilmarx PH, Hamers FF, Peterman TA. Living with HIV: experiences and perspectives of HIV-infected sexually transmitted disease clinic patients after posttest counseling. *Sex Transm Dis* 1998,25:28–37.

64. Marks G, Richarson JL, Maldonado N. Self-disclosure of HIV infection to sexual partners. *Am J Public Health* 1991;81:1321–1323.

65. April K, Schreiner W. The problem of the effectiveness of condoms against HIV infection. *Schweiz Med Wochenschr* 1990;30:120, 972–978.

66. Van de Perre P, Jacobs D, Sprecher-Goldberger S. The latex condom, an efficient barrier against sexual transmission of AIDS-related viruses. *AIDS* 1987;1:49.

67. Sprecher S, Soumenkoff G, Puissant F, Degueldre M. Vertical transmission of HIV in 15 week fetus [Letter]. *Lancet* 1986;2:288–289.

68. Jovaisas E, Koch MAS, Schafer A, et al. LAV/HTLV-III in 20-week fetus. *Lancet* 1985;2:1129.

69. Goedert JJ, Eyster ME, Biggar RG, Blattner WA. Heterosexual transmission of human immunodeficiency virus: association with severe depletion of T-helper lymphocytes in men with hemophilia. *AIDS Res Hum Retroviruses* 1987;3:355–361.

70. Jacquez JA, Koopman SJ, Simon CP, et al. Role of the primary infection in epidemics of HIV infection in gay cohorts. *J Acquir Immune Defic Syndr* 1994;7:1169–1184.

71. Wasserheit JN, Epidemiological synergy: interrelationships between human immunodeficiency virus infection and other sexually transmitted diseases. *Sex Transm Dis* 1992;19:61–77.

72. deVincenzi I. A longitudinal study of human immunodeficiency virus transmission by heterosexual partners. *N Engl J Med* 1994;331: 341–346.

73. Lazzarin A, Saracco A, Musicco M, et al. Man-to-woman sexual trans-

mission of human immunodeficiency virus: risk factors related to sexual behavior, man's infectiousness, and woman's susceptibility. *Arch Intern Med* 1991;151:2411–2416.

74. Cameron DW, Simonsen JN, D'Costa LJ, et al. Female to male transmission of human immunodeficiency virus type 1:risk factors for seroconversion on men. *Lancet* 1989;2:403–407.

75. Seidlin M, Vogler M, Lee E, et al. Heterosexual transmission of HIV in a cohort of couples in New York City. *AIDS* 1993;7:1247–1254.

76. Monzon OT, Capellan JMB. Female to female transmission of HIV [Letter]. *Lancet* 1987;2:40–41.

77. Marmar MM, Weiss LR, Lyden M, et al. Possible female-to-female transmission of human immunodeficiency virus. *Ann Intern Med* 1986;105:969.

78. Lyman D, Winkelstein W, Ascher M, Levy JA. Minimal risk of AIDS-associated retrovirus infection by oral genital contact [Letter]. *JAMA* 1986;255:1703.

79. Schoenbaum EE, Selwyn PA, Hartel D, et al. HIV seroconversion in intravenous drug abusers: Rate and risk factors. Presented at the II International Conference on AIDS, Wahington, DC, June 1987.

80. Katz MH, Gerberding JL. Postexposure treatment of people exposed to the human immunodeficiency virus through sexual contact or intravenous-drug use. *N Engl J Med* 1997;336:1097.

81. Katz MH, Gerberding JL. The care of persons with recent sexual exposure to HIV. *Ann Intern Med* 1998;128:306–312.

82. Minkoff H. Human immunodeficiency virus infection in pregnancy. *Obstet Gynecol* 2003:101;797–810.

83. Landesman S, Kalish L, Burns D, et al. The relationship of obstetric factors to the mother-to-child transmission of HIV-1. *N Engl J Med* 1996;334:1617–1623.

84. Connor EM, Sperling RS, Gelber R, et al. Reduction of materno-infant transmission of human immunodeficiency virus type 1 with zidovudine treatment. *N Engl J Med* 1994;331:1173–1180.

85. U.S. Center for Disease Control and Prevention. Recommendations of the Public Health Service Task Force on the use of zidovudine to reduce perinatal transmission of human immunodeficiency virus. *MMWR Morb Mortal Wkly Rep* 1994;43:1–21.

86. U.S. Center for Disease Control and Prevention. Public Health task Force recommendations for the use of antiretroviral drugs in pregnant women infected with HIV-1 for maternal health and for reducing perinatal HIV-1 transmission in the United States. *MMWR Morb Mortal Wkly Rep* 1998;47:1–31.

87. Orloff SL, Buterys M, Vink P, et al. Maternal characteristics associated with antenatal, intrapartum, and neonatal zidovudine use in four U.S. cities, 1994–1998. *J Acquir Immune Defic Syndr* 2001;28:65–72.

88. Garcia PM, Kalish LA, Pitt J, et al. Maternal levels of plasma human immunodeficiency virus type 1 RNA and the risk of perinatal transmission. *N Engl J Med* 1999;341:394–402.

89. Wade N, Birkhead GS, Warren BL, et al. Abbreviated regimens of zidovudine prophylaxis and perinatal transmission of human immunodeficiency virus. *N Engl J Med* 1998;339:1409–1414.

90. Hira SK, Mangrola UG, Mwale C, et al. Apparent vertical transmission of human immunodeficiency virus type 1 by breast-feeding in Zambia. *J Pediatr* 1990;117:421.

91. Thiry L, Sprecher-Goldberger S, Jonckeneer T, et al. Isolation of AIDS virus from cell-free breast milk of three healthy virus carriers. *Lancet* 1985;2:891.

92. UNAIDS. Report of the Global HIV/AIDS Epidemic: 2000. Geneva: INAIDS; UNAIDS/00.13E, 2000.

93. Pahwa S, Pahwa R, Saxinger C, et al. Influence of the human T-lymphotropic virus/lymphadenopathy-associated virus on functions of human lymphocytes: evidence for immunosuppressive effects and polyclonal B-cell activation by banded viral preparations. *Proc Natl Acad Sci U S A* 1985;82:8198–8202.

94. UNICEF. State of the World's Children: 1997. New York: UNICEF

95. Thapa S, Short RV, Potts M. Breast feeding, birth spacing and their effects on child survival. *Nature* 1988;335:679–682.

96. Ferrantelli F, Hofmann-Lehmann R, Rasmussen R, et al. Post-exposure prophylaxis with human monoclonal antibodies prevented SHIV89.6P infection or disease in neonate macaques. *AIDS* 2003;17:301–309.

97. Royce RA, Walter EB, Fernandez MI, et al. Barriers to universal prenatal HIV testing in four US locations in 1997. *Am J Public Health* 2001;91:727–733.

98. Bardeguez AD, Shapiro DE, Mofenson LM, et al. Effect of cessation of zidovudine prophylaxis to reduce vertical transmission on maternal HIV disease progression and survival. *J Acquir Immune Defic Syndr* 2003:32;170–181.

99. Hankin C, Thorne C, Peckham C, et al. Exposure to antiretroviral therapy in utero or early life: the health of uninfected children born to HIV-infected women. *J Acquir Immune Defic Syndr* 2003 32;4: 380–387.

100. Updated U.S. Public Health Service guidelines for the management of occupational exposures to HBV, HCV, and HIV and recommendations for postexposure prophylaxis. *MMWR Morb Mortal Wkly Rep* 2001;50:1–52.

101. Public Health Service Statement on Management of Occupational Exposure to Human Immunodeficiency Virus, Including Considerations Regarding Zidovudine Postexposure Use. *MMWR Morb Mortal Wkly Rep* 1990;39:1–14.

102. Curran JW, Jaffe HW, Hardy AM, et al. Epidemiology of HIV infection and AIDS in the United States. *Science* 1988;239:610.

103. Barnes DM: Health workers and AIDS: questions persist. *Science* 1988;241:161.

104. Centers for Disease Control: Update: Human immunodeficiency virus infection in health care workers exposed to blood of infected patients. *MMWR Morb Mortal Wkly Rep* 1987;36:285.

105. Bongaarts J, Reining P, Way P, Conant F. The relationship between male circumcision and HIV infection in African populations. *AIDS* 1989;3:373–377.

106. Cardo DM, Culver DH, Ciesielski CA, et al. A case-control study of HIV seroconversion in health care workers after percutaneous exposure. *N Engl J Med* 1997;337:1485–1490.

107. Recommendations for Prevention of HIV Transmission in Health-Care Settings, *MMWR Morb Mortal Wkly Rep* 1987;36S:4S–18S.

108. Centers for Disease Control: Acquired immune deficiency syndrome (AIDS): precautions for clinical and laboratory staffs. *MMWR Morb Mortal Wkly Rep* 1982:31:575.

109. Busch M, Lee LL, Satten GA, et al. Time course of detection of viral and serologic markers preceding human immunodeficiency virus type 1 seroconversion: implications for screening of blood and tissue donors. *Transfusion* 1995;35:91–97.

110. Selik RM, Ward JW, Buehler JW, et al. Demographic differences in cumulative incidence rates of transfusion-associated acquired immunodeficiency syndrome. *Am J Epidemiol* 1994;140:105–12.

111. Petersen LR, Satten GA, Dodd R, et al. Duration of time from the onset of human immunodeficiency virus type-1 infectiousness to development of detectable antibody. *Transfusion* 1994;34:283–289.

112. Busch MP, Lee LLJ, Satten GA, et al. Time course of detection of viral and serologic markers preceding human immunodeficiency virus type 1 seroconversion: implications for screening of blood and tissue donors. *Transfusion* 1995;35:91–97.

113. Lackritz EM, Satten GA, Aberle-Grasse J, et al. Estimated risk of transmission of the human immunodeficiency virus by screened blood in the United States. *N Engl J Med*.1995;333(26):1721–1725.

114. Benenson AS, Peddecord KM, Hofherr LK, et al. Reporting the results of human immunodeficiency virus testing. *JAMA*. 1990;262: 3435–3438.

115. Petricciani J. Licensed test for antibody to human T-lymphotropic virus type III: sensitivity and specificity. *Ann Intern Med* 1985;103: 726.

116. Marwick C. Blood banks give HTLV-III test positive appraisal at five months. *JAMA* 1985;254:1681.

117. Cockerill FR, Edson RS, Chase RC, et al. False positive antibodies to human immunodeficiency virus (HIV) detected by an enzyme-linked immunosorbent assay (ELISA) in patients at low risk for acquired immunodeficiency syndrome (AIDS). Presented at the 3rd International Conference on AIDS, Washington, DC, June 1–5, 1987: 34

118. Barin F, McLane MF, Allan JS, et al. Virus envelope protein of HTLV-III represents major target antigen for antibodies in AIDS patients. *Science* 1985;228:1094.

119. Towbin H, Staehelin T, Gordon J. Electrophoretic transfer of proteins from polyacrylamide gels to introcellulose sheets: procedures and some applications. *Proc Natl Acad Sci U S A* 1979;76:4350.

120. Tsang VCW, Peralta JM, Simons AR. Enzyme-linked immunoelectrotransfer blot techniques (EITB) for studying the specificities of anti-

gens and antibodies separated by gel electrophoresis. *Methods Enzymol* 1983;92:377.

121. Interpretation and use of the Western blot assay for serodiagnosis of human immunodeficiency virus type 1 infections. *MMWR Morb Mortal Wkly Rep* 1989;38:7:S1–S7.

122. Pahwa S, Kaplan M, Fikrig S. Spectrum of human T-Cell lymphotropic virus type III infection in children. Recognition of symptomatic, asymptomatic, and seronegative patients. *JAMA* 1986;255:2299.

123. Gallarda JL, Henrard DR, Liu D, et al. Early detection of antibody to human immunodeficiency virus type 1 by using an antigen conjugate immunoassay correlates with the presence of immunoglobulin M antibody. *J Clin Microbiol* 1992;30:2379–2384.

124. Zaaijer HL, von. Exel-Oehlers P, Kraaijeveld T, et al. Early detection of antibodies to HIV-1 by third-generation assays. *Lancet* 1992;340:770–772.

125. Henrard DR, Phillips J, Windsor I, et al. Detection of human immunodeficiency virus type 1 p24 antigen and plasma RNA: relevance to indeterminate serologic tests. *Transfusion* 1994;34:376–380.

126. Martin K, Katz BZ, Miller G. AIDS and antibodies to human immunodeficiency virus (HIV) in children and their families. *J Infect Dis* 1987;155:54.

127. Borkowsky W, Krasinski K, Paul D, et al. Human-immunodeficiency-virus infections in infants negative for anti-HIV by enzyme-linked immunoassay. *Lancet* 1987;1:1168.

128. Ragni MV, Urbach AH, Taylor S, et al. Isolation of human immunodeficiency virus and detection of HIV DNA sequences in the brain of an ELISA antibody-negative child with acquired immune deficiency syndrome and progressive encephalopathy. *J Pediatr* 1987;110:266.

129. Guidelines for the use of antiretroviral agents in pediatric HIV infection. HIV/AIDS Treatment Information Service (ATIS), November 26, 2003. [http://www.aidsinfo.nih.gov/guidelines/; last accessed 1/17/04]

130. Cooper DA, Gold J, MacLean P, et al. Acute AIDS retrovirus infection: definition of a clinical illness associated with seroconversion. *Lancet* 1985;1:537.

131. Tindall B, Cooper DA. Primary HIV Infection. Host responses and intervention strategies. *AIDS* 1991;5:1.

132. Cooper DA, Gold J, Maclean P, et al. Acute AIDS retrovirus infection. Definition of a clinical illness associated with seroconversion. *Lancet* 1985;2:537–540.

133. Schacker T, Collier AC, Hughes J, et al. Clinical and epidemiologic features of primary HIV infection. *Ann Intern Med* 1996;125:257–264.

134. Gaines H, von Sydow M, Pehrson PO, Lundbegh P. Clinical picture of primary HIV infection presenting as a glandular-fever-like illness. *BMJ* 1988;297:1363–8

135. Tindall B, Barker S, Donovan B, et al. Characterization of the acute clinical illness associated with human immunodeficiency virus infection. *Arch Intern Med* 1988;148:945–9

136. Pedersen C, Lindhardt BO, Jensen BL, et al. Clinical course of primary HIV infection: consequences for subsequent infection. *BMJ* 1989;299:154–7

137. Sinicco A, Fora R, Sciandra M, et al. Risk of developing AIDS after primary acute HIV-1 infection. *J AIDS* 1993;6:575–81

138. Pedersen C, Lindhardt BO, Jensen BL, et al. Clinical course of primary HIV infection: consequences for subsequent infection. *BMJ* 1989;299:154–157.

139. Ho DD, Pomerantz RJ, Kaplan JC. Pathogenesis of infection with human immunodeficiency virus. *N Engl J Med* 1987;317:278.

140. Rook AH, Masur H, Lane HC. Interleukin-2 enhances the depressed natural killer cell and cytomegalovirus specific cytotoxic activities of lymphocytes from patients with the acquired immunodeficiency syndrome. *J Clin Invest* 1983;72:398–403.

141. Cauda R, Tumbarello M, Ortona L. Inhibition of normal human natural killer cell activity by human immunodeficiency virus synthetic transmembrane peptides. *Cell Immunol* 1988;115:57–65.

142. Fisher AG, Ensoli B, Ivanoff L, et al. The sor gene of HIV-1 is required for efficient virus transmission in vitro. *Science* 1987;237:888.

143. Lane HC, Masur H, Edgar L, et al. Abnormalities of B-cell activation and immunoregulation in patients with the acquired immunodeficiency syndrome. *N.Engl J Med* 1983;309:453–458.

144. Yarchoan R, Guo H-G, Reitz M, et al. Alterations in cytotoxic and helper T cell function after infection of T cell clones with human T cell leukemia virus, type 1. *J Clin Invest* 1986;77:1466–1473.

145. Nakajima K, Martinez-Maza O, Hirano T, et al. Induction of IL-6 (B cell stimulatory factor 2/INF-B2) production by HIV. *J Immunol* 1989;142:531–536.

146. Birx DL, Redfield RR, Tosatao G. Defective regulation of Epstein-Barr virus infection in patients with acquired immunodeficiency syndrome (AIDS) or AIDS-related disorders. *N Engl J Med* 1986;314:874.

147. Simberkoff MS, El-Sadr W, Schiffman G. Streptococcus pneumonia infections and bacteremia in patients with AIDS. *Am Rev Respir Dis* 1984;130:1174–1176.

148. Shearer GM, Salahuddin SZ, Markham PH. Prospective study of cytotoxic T lymphocyte responses to influenza and antibodies to human T lymphotropic virus-III in homosexual men. *J Clin Invest* 1985;76:1699–1704.

149. Yarchoan R, Pluda JM. Clinical Aspects of infection with AIDS retrovirus: acute HIV infection, persistent generalized lymphadenopathy, and AIDS-Related Complex. In: DeVita JR, Hellman S, Rosenberg SA, eds. *AIDS, etiology, diagnosis, treatment, and prevention*. 2nd ed. Philadelphia: JB Lippincott Co, 1988:107–120.

150. Imam N, Carpenter CCJ, Mayer KH, et al. Hierarchical pattern of mucosa candida infection in HIV-seropositive women. *Am J Med* 1990;89:142.

151. State of Maryland, Communicable Disease Bulletin, May 1990

152. Vermund SH, Kelley KF, Klein RS, et al. High risk of human papillomavirus infection and cervical squamous intraepithelial lesions among women with symptomatic human immunodeficiency virus infection. *Am J Obstet Gynecol* 1991;165:392–400.

153. Hoegsberg B, Abulafia O, Sedlis A, et al. Sexually transmitted disease and human immunodeficiency virus infection among women with pelvic inflammatory disease. *Am J Obstet Gynecol* 1990;163:1135.

154. Safrin S, Dattel BJ, Haver L, et al. Seroprevalence and epidemiologic correlates of infection in women with pelvic inflammatory disease. *Obstet Gynecol* 1990;75:666.

155. Masur H, Ognibene FP, Yarchoan RY, et al. CD4 counts as predictors of opportunistic pneumonias in HIV infection. *Ann Intern Med* 1989;111:223.

156. Polk BF, Fox R, Brookmeyer R, et al. Predictors of AIDS developing in a cohort of seropositive homosexual men. *N Engl J Med* 1987;3116:61–66.

157. Penn I: The occurrence of malignant tumors in immunosuppressed states. *Prog. Allergy* 1986;37:259–300.

158. Kersey JH, Spector BD, Good RA. Primary immunodeficiency diseases and cancer. The immunodeficiency-cancer registry. *Int J Cancer* 1973;12:333–347.

159. Centers for Disease Control: Update on acquired immunodeficinecy syndrome (AIDS)-United States. *MMWR Morb Mortal Wkly Rep* 1982;31:507.

160. Centers for Disease Control. Revision of the case definition of acquired immunodeficiency syndrome for national reporting-United States. *MMWR Morb Mortal Wkly Rep* 1985;34:373–375.

161. CDC. 1993 classification system for HIV infection and expanded surveillance case definition for AIDS among adolescents and adults. Hyattsville, MD: U.S. Department of Health and Human Services. 1993; 1.

162. Selik RM, Starcher ET, Curran JW. Opportunistic diseases reported in AIDS patients: Frequencies, associations, and trends. *AIDS* 1987;1:175–182.

163. Chang Y, Cesarman E, Pessin MS, et al. Identification of herpesviruslike-DNA sequences in AIDS-associated Kaposi's sarcoma. *Science* 1994;266:1865–1869.

164. Antman K, Chang Y. Kaposi's sarcoma. *N Engl J Med* 2000;342:1027.

165. Mitsuyasu, RT, Taylor JMG, Glaspy J, et al. Heterogeneity of epidemic Kaposi's sarcoma: implications for therapy. *Cancer* 1986;57:1657–1661.

166. Kaposi, M.: Idiopathisches multiples Pigmentsarkom der Haut. *Arch Dermatol Syph* 1872;4:265–273.

167. Chachoua A, Krigel R, Lafleur F, et al. Prognostic factors and staging classification of patients with epidemic Kaposi's sarcoma. *J Clin Oncol* 1989;7:774–780.

168. Volberding PA. In: Ziegler JL, Dorfman RF, eds. *Kaposi's sarcoma:*

pathophysiology and clinical management. New York: Marcel Dekker, New York, 1988.

169. Heise W, Mostertz P, Skorde J, et al. Gastrointestinal Kaposi's sarcoma in AIDS—endoscopic findings. Vth International Conference on AIDS: The Scientific and Social Challenge, Montreal, June 4–9, 1989:349.

170. Krigel RL, Laubenstein LJ, Muggia FM. Kaposi's sarcoma: A new staging classification. *Cancer Treat Rep* 1983;67:531–533.

171. Gill PS, Akil B, Colletti P, et al. Pulmonary Kaposi's sarcoma: clinical findings and results of therapy. *Am J Med* 1989;87: 57–61.

172. Wit FW, Sol CJ, Renwick N, et al. Regression of AIDS-related kaposi's sarcoma associated with clearance of human herpesvirus-8 from peripheral blood mononuclear cells following the initiation of antiviral therapy. *AIDS* 1998,12:218–219.

173. Robles R, Lugo D, Gee L, et al. Effect of antiviral drugs used to treat cytomegalovirus end-organ-disease on subsequent course of previously diagnosed Kaposi's sarcoma in patients with AIDS. *J Acquir Immune Defic Syndr Hum Retrovirol* 1999;20:34–38.

174. Ziegler JL, Becksted JA, Volberding PA, et al. Non-Hodgkins's lymphoma in 90 homosexual men: relation to generalized lymphadenopathy and the acquired immunodeficiency syndrome. *N Engl J Med* 1984;311:565–570.

175. Bauer HM, Ting Yi, Greer CE, et al. Genital human papillomavirus infection in female university students as determined by a PCR-based method. *JAMA* 1991;265:472–477.

176. Kaplan LD, Abrams DI, Feigal E, et al. AIDS-associated non-Hodgkin's lymphoma in San Francisco. *JAMA* 1989;261:719.

177. Kalter SP, Riggs SA, Cabanillas F, et al. Aggressive non-Hodgkin's lymphomas in immunocompromised homosexual males. *Blood* 1985; 66:655.

178. Lowenthal DA, Strauss DJ, Campbell SW, et. al. AIDS-related lymphoid neoplasia: the Memorial Hospital experience. *Cancer* 1988; 61:2325–2337.

179. Bermudez MA, Grant K, Rodvien R, Mendes F. Non-Hodgkins lymphoma in a population; with or at risk for acquired immunodeficiency syndrome: indications for intensive chemotherapy. *Am J Med* 1989; 86:71.

180. Gill PS, Levine AM, Krailo M, et al. AIDS-related malignant lymphoma: Results of prospective treatment trials. *J Clin Oncol* 1987;5 1322.

181. Knowles DM, Chamulak GA, Subar M, et. al. Lymphoid neoplasia associated with the acquired immunodeficiency syndrome (AIDS): The New York University Medical Center experience with 105 patients (1981–1986). *Ann Intern Med* 1988;108:744–753.

182. Goedert JJ, Caussy D, Palefsky J, et al. Interaction of human immunodeficiency and papilloma viruses: association with anal epithelial abnormality in homosexual men. [Abstract] VIth International Conference on AIDS. Vol 3. San Francisco, June 20–24, 1990:326

183. Resnick RM, Cornelissen MTE, Wright DK, et al. Detection and typing of HPV in archival cervical cancer specimens using DNA amplification with consensus primers. *J Natl Cancer Inst* 1990;82: 1477–1484.

184. Lorintz AT, Schiffman MH, Jaffurs WJ, et al. Temporal association of human papillomavirus infection with cervical cytological abnormalities. *Am J Obstet Gynecol* 1990;162:645–651.

185. Marte C, Cohen M, Fruchter R, Kelly P. Pap test and STD finding in HIV + women at ambulatory care sites. VIth International Conference on AIDS. Vol 2. San Francisco, June 20–24, 1990:211(abst).

186. Tarricone NJ, Maiman M, Vieire J. Colposcopic evaluation of HIV seropositive women. VIth International Conference on AIDS. Vol 2. San Francisco, June 20–24, 1990(abst).

187. Vaccher E, Tirelli U, Spina M, et al. Age and serum lactate dehydrogenase level are independent prognostic factors in human immunodeficiency virus-related non-Hodgkin's lymphomas. *J Clin Oncol* 1996; 14:2217–2223.

188. Navarro JT, Ribera JM, Oriol A, et al. International Prognostic Index is the best prognostic factor for survival in patients with AIDS-related non-Hodgkin's lymphoma treated with CHOP: a multivariate study of 46 patients. *Haematologica* 1998;83:508–513.

189. Croxson T, Chabon AB, Rorat E et al. Intraepithelial carcinoma of the anus in homosexual men. *Dis Colon Rectum* 1987;27:325.

190. Feingold AR, Vermund S, Burk MD, et al. Cervical cytologic abnor-

malities and papillomavirus in women infected with human immunodeficiency virus. *J Acquir Immune Defic Syndr* 1990;3:896.

191. Vermund S, Kelley KF, Burk RD, et al. Risk of human papillomavirus (HPV) and cervical squamous intraepithelial lesion (SIL) highest among women with advanced HIV disease.VIth International Conference on AIDS. Vol 3. San Francisco, June 20–24, 1990:216(abst).

192. Little RF, Pittaluga S, Grant N, et al. Highly effective treatment of acquired immunodeficiency syndrome related lymphoma with dose-adjusted EPOCH: impact of antiretroviral therapy suspension and tumor biology. *Blood* 2003;101:4653.

193. Cote TR, Manns A, Hardy CR, et al. Epidemiology of brain lymphoma among people with and without acquired immune deficiency syndrome. AIDS/Cancer Study Group. *J Natl Cancer Inst* 1996;88: 675–679.

194. MacMahon EM, Glass JD, Hayward SD, et al. Epstein-Barr virus in AIDS-related primary central nervous system lymphoma. *Lancet* 1991;338:969–973.

195. Sparano JA, Anand K, Desai J, et al. Effect of highly active antiretroviral therapy on the incidence of HIV-associated malignancies at an urban medical center. *J Acquir Immune Defic Syndr* 1999;21[Suppl 1]:S18–S22.

196. Cesarman E, Chang Y, Moore PS, et al. Kaposi's sarcoma-associated herpesvirus-like DNA sequences in AIDS related body-cavity-based lymphomas. *N Engl J Med* 1995;332:1186–1191

197. Nador RG, Cesarman E, Chadburn A, et al. Primary effusion lymphoma: a distinct clinicopathologic entity associated with the Kaposi's sarcoma-associated herpes virus. *Blood* 1996;88:645.

198. Karcher DS, Alkan S. Human herpesvirus-8 associated body cavity-based lymphoma in human immunodeficiency virus-infected patients: a unique B-cell neoplasm. *Hum Pathol* 1997;28:801–808.

199. Vaccher E. Spina M. Tirelli U. Clinical aspects and management of Hodgkin's disease and other tumours in HIV infected individuals. *Eur J Cancer* 2001;37:1306–1315.

200. Mueller N, Grufferman S. The epidemiology of Hodgkin's disease. In: Mauch PM, Armitage JO, Diehl V, et al., eds. *Hodgkin's disease.* Philadelphia: Lippincott Williams & Wilkins, 1999:61–77

201. Glaser SL, Clarke CA, Gulley ML, et al. Population-based patterns of human immunodeficiency virus–related Hodgkin lymphoma in the Greater San Francisco Bay Area, 1988–1998. *Cancer.* 2003;98:300.

202. Schafer A, Friedmann W, Miekle M, et al. Increased frequency of cervical dysplasia-neoplasia in women infected with the human immunodeficiency virus is related to the degree of immunosuppression. *Am J Obstet Gynecol* 1991;164:593–599.

203. Maiman M, Fruchter RG, Clark M, et al. Cervical cancer as an AIDS-defining diagnosis. *Obstet Gynecol* 1997;89:76–80.

204. Minkoff HL, Eisenberger-Maitityahu D, Feldman J, et al. Prevalence and incidence of gynecologic disorders among women infected with human immunodeficiency virus. *Am J Obstet Gynecol* 1999;180: 824–836.

205. Centers for Disease Control and Prevention. 1993 classification system for HIV infection and expanded surveillance case definition for AIDS among adolescents and adults. Hyattsville, MD: U.S. Department of Health and Human Services, 1993;1

206. Chin KM, Sidhu JS, Janssen RS, et al. Invasive cervical cancer in human immunodeficiency virus–infected and uninfected hospital patients. *Obstet Gynecol* 1998;92:83–87.

207. Abercrombie PD, Korn AP. Lower genital tract neoplasia in women with HIV infection *Oncology* 1998;12:1735–1739.

208. Palefsky JM, Minkoff H, Kalish LA, et al. Cervicovaginal human papillomavirus infection in human immunodeficiency virus-1 (HIV)–positive and high risk HIV-negative women. *J Natl Cancer Inst* 1999;91:226–236.

209. Heard I, Tassie JM, Kazatchkine, et al. Highly active antiretroviral therapy enhances regression of cervical intraepithelial neoplasia in HIV-seropositive women. *AIDS* 2002;16:1799–1802.

210. Louis JK, Hsu LC, Osmond DH, et al. Trends in causes of death among patients with acquired immunodeficiency syndrome in the era of highly active antiretroviral therapy, San Francisco, 1994–1998. *J Infect Dis* 2002,186:1023–1027.

211. Franceschi S, Dal Maso L, La Vecchia C. Advances in the epidemiology of HIV-associated non-Hodgkin's lymphoma and other lymphoid neoplasms. *Int J Cancer* 1999;83:481–485.

212. Goedert JJ. The epidemiology of acquired immune deficiency syndrome malignancies. *Semin Oncol* 2000;27:390–401.

213. Lyter DW, Kingsley LA, Rinaldo CR, et al. Malignancies in the multicenter AIDS cohort (MACS) 1984–1994. *Proc Am Soc Clin Oncol* 1996;15:305.

214. Frisch M, Biggar R, Engels E, et al. Association of cancer with AIDS-related immunosuppression in adults. *JAMA* 2001;285:1736–1745.

215. Gallagher B, Zhengyan W, Schymaura M, et al. Cancer incidence in New York State aquired immunodeficiency syndrome patients. *Am J Epidemiol* 2001;154:544–556.

216. Bower MP, Powles T, Nelson M, et al. HIV-related lung cancer in the era of highly active antiretroviral therapy. *AIDS* 2003;17:371–375.

217. Grulich AE, Wan X, Law M, et al. Risk of cancer in people with AIDS. *AIDS* 1999;13:839–843.

218. Hurley J, Franco S, Gomez-Fernandez C. Breast cancer and human immunodeficiency virus: a report of 20 cases. *Clin Breast Cancer* 2001;3:215–220.

219. Grulich AE, Li Y, McDonald A, et al. Rates of non-AIDS-defining cancers in people with HIV infection before and after AIDS diagnosis. *AIDS* 2002;16:1155–1161.

220. Mbulaitey SM, Biggar RJ, Goedert JJ, et al. Immune deficiency and risk for malignancy among persons with AIDS. *J Acquir Immune Defic Syndr* 2003;32;527–533.

221. Bartlett JG. *Medical management of HIV infection.* Baltimore: Johns Hopkins University. Department of Infectious Diseases, 1998.

222. Volberding PA, Lagakos SW, Koch MA, et al. Zidovudine in asymptomatic human immunodeficiency virus infection: a controlled trial in persons with fewer than 500 CD4-positive cells per cubic millimeter. *N Engl J Med* 1990;322:941.

223. Centers for Disease Control: AIDS Weekly Surveillance Report. January 30, 1989.

224. USPHS/IDSA Guidelines for the Prevention of Opportunistic Infections in Persons Infected with HIV, November 28, 2001.

225. Mellors JW, Munoz A, Giorgi JV, et al. Plasma viral load and CD4 + lymphocytes as prognostic markers of HIV-1 infection. *Ann Intern Med* 1997;126:946–954.

226. Carpenter CCJ, Cooper DA, Fischl MA, et al. Antiretroviral therapy in adults: updated recommendations of the International AIDS Society—USA panel. *JAMA* 2000;283:381–390.

227. Centers for Disease Control and Prevention.. Guidelines for the use of antiretroviral agents in HIV-infected adults and adolescents. *MMWR Morb Mortal Wkly Rep* 2002;51:1–56.

CHAPTER 38

Quality of Life Issues in Gynecologic Cancer

Lari B. Wenzel and David Cella

In 2003, an estimated 83,700 new diagnoses of invasive gynecologic malignancies were predicted in the United States and 26,800 deaths were expected (1). Although survival varies by disease type and stage at diagnosis, it is estimated that approximately 666,000 women diagnosed with primary gynecologic cancer within the past 20 years are alive today (2). Therefore, as noted by Rowland and colleagues (3), cancer has become a curable disease for many, and a chronic disease for most.

Among the gynecologic cancers, survival gains are largely the result of advances in early detection and treatment (4). Treatment-related gains are often accompanied by a variety of side effects that diminish the patient's quality of life (QOL) during and after treatment. Standard cancer treatments, including surgery, chemotherapy, and radiation therapy, have the potential for reducing QOL, especially when they are not efficacious to the individual patient. In addition, the patient may experience disease-related symptoms that adversely affect QOL. Therefore, modern management of gynecologic cancer patients now includes consideration not only of the quantity of life, but also its quality. This chapter reviews the definition and measurement of QOL, and discusses quality of life issues relevant to the gynecologic malignancies (including site- and symptom-specific information).

QUALITY OF LIFE: DEFINITION AND MEASUREMENT

Defining Quality of Life

QOL assessment provides supplementary information about the impact of the disease and its treatment on cancer

L. B. Wenzel: Health Policy Research, University of California, Irvine, College of Medicine, Irvine, California 92697

D. Cella: Evanston Northwestern Healthcare, Institute for Health Research and Policy Studies, Evanston, Illinois 60201

patients. This information in turn aids physicians in selecting both antineoplastic and supportive-care therapy. Given the chronic and often incurable nature of many gynecologic malignancies, the toxicity and tolerability of a specific therapy can be as important as its efficacy, and all of these factors contribute to one's appraisal of health-related QOL. Quality of life evaluation allows us to confirm the assumption that the time added by therapy is of sufficient value to justify its cost, and to examine the value of therapies that do not add time to life, but appear to improve quality of life. The critical tradeoff is not always between toxicity and survival time; sometimes a treatment temporarily palliates tumor-induced symptoms without extending survival. Patients may find this desirable even in the face of competing toxicity. Only careful evaluation of patient-derived QOL can allow evaluation of tradeoffs between symptom relief and toxicity.

Since there is little consensus or understanding about how QOL considerations can be systematically used to make treatment decisions, it is essential that standardized definitions, approaches, and measures be advanced when examining and discussing treatment options. There is consensus that QOL is both subjective and multidimensional (5–9). An early working definition of QOL was developed that laid the groundwork for measurement: "Quality of life refers to patients' appraisal of and satisfaction with their current level of functioning as compared to what they perceive to be possible or ideal" (7). This definition was modified explicitly to incorporate the multidimensionality of QOL: "Health-related quality of life refers to the extent to which one's usual or expected physical, emotional and social well-being are affected by a medical condition or its treatment" (10). This definition provides minimum requirements for QOL measurement: the *patient's* perspective is obtained and areas of physical, mental, and social well-being are captured.

A review of available QOL questionnaires reveals over 30 different names for QOL dimensions (11). Careful review of the descriptions of these dimensions and available factor analytic studies suggest up to seven *distinct* dimensions: (a) physical concerns (symptoms, pain); (b) functional ability (activity); (c) social/family well-being; (d) emotional well-being; (e) treatment satisfaction (including financial concerns); (f) sexuality/intimacy (including body image); and (g) cognitive functioning. Two summary dimensions are also relevant but not always available with every QOL questionnaire: global evaluation of QOL (i.e., a single question rating the patient's global or overall perception of QOL or health status) and total score (i.e., the summation of dimension scores into an aggregate index of QOL) (11).

A typical approach combines a generic health status assessment such as the European Organization for Research and Treatment of Cancer QLQ-C30 (6), or the Functional Assessment of Cancer Therapy-General (FACT-G), with a more targeted set of questions specific to a given tumor type. The FACT-G (version 4), for example, includes a 27-item core questionnaire (FACT-G) that primarily evaluates the patient's physical, social/family, emotional, and functional well-being. In addition, several cancer-specific subscales can be useful in assessing QOL among gynecologic cancer patients (http://www.facit.org). The 13-item FACT-O is an ovarian cancer–specific subscale that assesses severity of problems that can be addressed through proper disease management (12–14). This subscale, as well as the FACT-Cx (cervix) (12), can be used alone or in combination with other scales and subscales of the FACT, such as the FACT/GOG-Ntx subscale (15), if neurotoxicity is of concern, or the Anemia subscale or Fatigue subscale if one is interested in these specific issues (16; http://www.facit.org). Each of these scales provides QOL information relevant to a specific condition for which intervention could be useful, thus potentially improving total patient care. Disease-specific and treatment-specific questions are usually of benefit when added to a general measure of QOL. Together they can provide comparability across different cancers and sensitivity to specific issues or symptoms relevant to a given malignancy or treatment.

QOL is indeed multidimensional, but it does not necessarily follow that reported QOL scores should always be reported by dimension. There are benefits to reporting QOL data in both disaggregated and aggregated forms. Disaggregated dimension scores give one a more detailed picture of the different areas of patient function and well-being, and are often preferred by the clinician. Aggregated scores and summary indices are critical, however, to enable decision makers more comfortably to adjust time for its quality. Treatment outcome evaluators, including health economists and health policy experts, prefer summary scores, although they lose some precision.

Approaches to Measuring Quality of Life

Over time, two approaches to measuring QOL have evolved: psychometric and utility. These approaches have evolved relatively independently of one another, largely be-

cause they were developed within different scientific disciplines. Psychometric approaches are derived from psychology, whereas utility approaches are derived from economics. Integrating these two approaches remains a critical challenge in QOL measurement.

Psychometric Approach

The psychometric approach includes generic health profile measurement and specific instruments intended to measure the multidimensional impact of a specific disease, treatment, or condition. This places heavy emphasis upon an individual's response and response variability across individuals. An important contribution of the psychometric approach is that it provides measurement of subjective or perceived well-being. Psychometric measures may or may not include a summary or total score. Only rarely have these summary scores been connected to patients' value for their current health status. This is problematic, because without a rating of patient preference, one cannot appropriately make a decision about the value of a given treatment to a given patient. For example, one of two patients with identical disease and treatment options may decline therapy, whereas the other will accept it enthusiastically. Because psychometric measures do not incorporate patient-specific weights for individual domains nor anchor states of health to a common standard, evaluating tradeoffs between quality and length of life, or between one dimension of QOL and another, is difficult. This presents a challenge in a clinical trial where the primary purpose for integrating QOL measurement is to incorporate data on the impact of treatment on both length and quality of life into conclusions about treatment effectiveness. The collection of patient preferences in clinical trials would allow the effect of treatment on quality-adjusted survival as well as on conventional outcome measures to be evaluated. Further, the addition of patient preference assessments to clinical trial outcome evaluation can make it possible to distinguish between patients who favor one treatment over another when both may have equivalent survival outcomes. A strategy for doing this has been described by Till and colleagues (17).

Utility Approach

The utility approach to health status measurement evolved from a tradition of cost-benefit analysis into cost-effectiveness approaches and, most recently, cost-utility approaches (18). The cost-utility approach extends the cost-effectiveness approach conceptually by evaluating the QOL benefit produced by the clinical effects of a treatment, thereby including the (presumed) patient's perspective. Cost-utility is a form of cost-effectiveness analysis that is often preferred by analysts who have reservations about valuing benefits in dollar terms. A utility is the numeric expression of the value an individual or society places on a particular health state, or a progression of health states over time. Utility assessment allows for QOL adjustments to a given set of treatment outcomes (typically, survival), whereas at the same time providing a generic outcome measure for cost comparisons and outcomes of different programs. The generic outcome, usually expressed as quality-adjusted-life-years (QALYs), is derived in each case by adjusting the length of time affected through the health outcome by the utility value, rated on a scale from 0 (death) to 1 (perfect health), of the resulting health status.

Two general cost-utility assessment methods are the standard gamble approach and the time tradeoff approach (19). In the standard gamble approach, people are asked to choose between their current state of health and a "gamble" in which they have various probabilities for death or perfect health (cure). The time tradeoff method is easier to perform and involves asking people how much time they would be willing to give up in order to live out their remaining life expectancy in perfect health. In practice, most cost-utility analyses employ expert estimates of utility weights, or in some cases, weights provided by healthy members of the general public. It is often assumed that these weights are reasonable approximations of patient preferences. However, it appears that utilities obtained from patients are generally higher than those provided by physicians, which are, in turn, higher than utilities for the same health states obtained from healthy individuals (20). There are practical impediments to collection of utilities directly from patients, including the complexity of the concepts involved and the requirement for an interviewer-administered questionnaire (often unfeasible in the cooperative group setting). In addition, utility assessments provide little information on important disease and treatment-specific problems, and are less sensitive than psychometric data to changes in physical health status over time (21–23).

QUALITY OF LIFE ISSUES IN GYNECOLOGIC CANCER

Although a number of factors may be responsible for both short and long-term QOL disruptions seen in gynecologic cancer patients, these disruptions are often articulated based on physical, functional, emotional, social, or sexual aspects of well-being. In general, these studies have described multiple challenges and quality of life disruptions (24–27). The literature suggests that the psychologic toll associated with a gynecologic cancer diagnosis can be severe as patients recognize the importance of both continued surveillance and possible recurrent cancer (27–31). Psychologic factors can include depression, sleeping difficulties, difficulty concentrating, and anxiety to a greater magnitude than many other cancer patient populations, and certainly greater than the general public (32–38), as well as changes in self-perception related to lost fertility or menopause and changes in the marital relationship (39–44).

Conceptual models in female survivorship have been de-veloped to predict risk for potential long-term psychologic maladaptation in cancer survivors (45–51). These historical models have been very instructive in conceptualizing general long-term gynecologic cancer survivorship experiences. For example, predisposing variables, such as age (52–53) and economic status, have been shown to interact with disease onset variables (i.e., disease stage, treatment toxicities, and physical performance) to determine a survivor's risk for psychologic vulnerability. In addition, premorbid psychologic well-being is widely considered to be an important determinant of well-being after treatment (27,54).

Cervical Cancer

After cancer treatment, it is common for cervical cancer patients to report fatigue, pain, bladder and bowel problems, and sexual dysfunction (36–38,52) with certain effects manifesting months after treatment completion (26,30–31, 55–56). Among cervical cancer survivors, a higher prevalence of psychologic concerns may occur in younger survivors (52) and Latina survivors (57–58), with the most common psychologic complaints being depressed mood and irritability. In a hallmark study of cervical cancer patients, contextual variables, general social support, and life stress were significant predictors of depression (59). Cancer-related variables, specifically physical symptoms associated with radiation, and practical barriers to receiving treatment, added significantly to the predictive model. It is important to note that Latina survivors also reported stress related to their socioeconomic and immigration status, and most wanted additional access to cancer-related support.

Long-term QOL can be affected in several ways in this vulnerable group. First, the anatomic changes resulting from the cancer or its treatment may permanently interfere with sexual function and reproductive ability and have a significant impact on self-image and social well-being (28,60). Many patients diagnosed with cervical cancer will be of childbearing age and may not have completed their anticipated family. Approximately one-third of patients report significant distress from treatment-related infertility (61).

We recently examined the reproductive concerns of long-term cervical cancer survivors (N = 51) compared to healthy controls (N = 50). As anticipated, cervical cancer survivors reported significantly more reproductive concerns ($p < 0.0001$). These concerns appeared to be related to sadness about their inability to bear children (31%), not being able to talk openly about their concerns (30%), frustration related to childbearing inability (25%), and mourning the loss of their ability to have children (25%). Among the cancer survivors, reproductive concerns were associated with greater gynecologic pain (.35, $p < 0.02$), younger age (.32, $p < 0.03$), worse general health (.29, $p < 0.04$), poorer physical well-being (.34, $p < 0.02$), poorer mental health (.36, $p < 0.009$), poorer psychologic well-being (.46, $p < 0.001$), less social support (.32, $p < 0.02$), and lower spiritual well-being scores

(.33, p <0.02). For healthy controls, reproductive concerns were associated with poorer mental health (.49, p <0.001), poorer social support (.54, p <0.0001), and lower spiritual well-being scores (.44, p <0.002). Other descriptive studies have documented mood disturbance, fear of recurrence, negative self-perception, concerns regarding infertility, relationship concerns, and sexual dysfunction beyond 5 years (39, 62).

The use of pelvic exenteration as a salvage therapy for recurrent cervical cancer can result in major alterations in body image and function. Depending upon the surgical techniques utilized, major changes in gastrointestinal and urinary tract function may result. Early studies suggested that patients receiving pelvic exenteration had satisfactory psychologic and emotional adjustment with ongoing psychotherapy (63–64). However, Anderson (65) and Fisher (66) found that pelvic exenteration patients experienced long-term distress and chronic sexual dysfunction including decreased sexual desire and frequency of sexual activity. Contemporary surgical techniques of continent urinary diversion and rectal reanastamosis have the potential to improve long-term QOL in this patient population. A report by Hawighorst surveyed 28 patients receiving pelvic exenteration preoperatively, 4 months, and 12 months after surgery using the Cancer-specific Rehabilitation and Treatment Planning questionnaire (CARES) (67,68). Patients with multiple ostomies reported lower QOL and poor body image compared to patients with no ostomy at 1 year after their surgery. Patients receiving vaginal reconstruction as part of their surgical procedure reported fewer QOL concerns and sexual problems. However, fear of recurrent disease remained a significant concern in all patients regardless of the surgical procedure performed. Patient selection and fitness for reconstructive surgery may bias subsequent QOL assessment. Ratliff et al. surveyed 95 patients who received gracilis myocutaneous vaginal reconstruction as part of their exenteration procedure (69). The attending physician determined that 70.4% of cases had a functional neovagina. Yet, 52% of patients reported not resuming sexual activity after surgery. Barriers to resuming sexual activity included altered body image related to urostomy or colostomy and vaginal dryness or discharge.

Ovarian Cancer

Ovarian cancer patients may experience QOL disruptions that include significant levels of distress, as well as impairment in physical, vocational, social, and sexual functioning (32,33,70). Issues of surgically induced menopause, loss of childbearing capacity, and impact of a major life-threatening illness figure prominently in the psychologic recuperation from ovarian cancer (71). Kornblith and colleagues (72) characterized the QOL of ovarian cancer patients over a 1-year period, in which they prospectively assessed the nature and extent of physical problems and psychologic distress, as well as determined medical and sociodemographic factors

predictive of distress. Since their sample included mainly patients with advanced disease, it is not surprising that many of the subjects (33%) presented with symptoms of anxiety and depression of moderate to severe intensity. Clinically significant depression and anxiety was also reported in 21% of 246 consecutive epithelial ovarian cancer patients (32). In this study, performance status was related to depression, anxiety, and QOL problems.

Importantly, in contrast to the one-third of ovarian cancer patients who experienced significant distress in the Kornblith study, there was also a resilient subset of patients (23%) who reported little distress. Resilience was also evident in long-term early-stage survivors (>5years), who reported few physical or psychosocial problems. Nevertheless, survivor-specific distress, such as fear of recurrence and future diagnostic tests, persisted (73). Other studies examining longer term (i.e., 2 to 9 years) survivorship sequelae have documented impairment in activity associated with peripheral neuropathy, a lack of energy, impaired hearing, and diminished sexuality (74–76). Overall, however, long-term survivors of ovarian cancer appear to experience a good QOL that includes satisfaction with life, supportive relationships, and aspects of existential well-being (e.g., hopefulness, high purpose in life, positive spiritual changes related to cancer) (73,76).

Future studies are needed in the study of recurrent ovarian cancer, where response rates are often limited, and the duration of responses generally brief. QOL will play an increasingly important role in future studies of promising agents for recurrent disease. Patients must play an integral and prominent role in the assessment of their own QOL (77). A number of studies have recognized discordance between the physician's and patient's perception of QOL (78). A study by Calhoun and colleagues surveyed a cohort of ovarian cancer patients and healthy gynecologic oncologists on issues of cisplatin-related toxicities (78). Using a modified time tradeoff methodology, ovarian cancer patients and physicians differed in their assessment of the impact of chemotherapy toxicities on QOL. Specifically, the treating physician's assessment of toxicity was less favorable then patients who had actually experienced complications related to cisplatin use. Prospective clinical trials will continue to teach the clinician the effects of interventions on QOL in gynecologic cancer patients.

Endometrial Cancer

Numerous posttreatment effects may be present in survivors of early endometrial cancer, and can include gastrointestinal, genitourinary, neurologic, vascular, and dermatologic effects; infections; vaginal stenosis; sexual dysfunction; menopausal symptoms; cardiovascular changes; and osteoporosis (79,80). Any of these complications have the potential to negatively disrupt QOL. Therefore, endometrial cancer survivors may experience QOL disruptions that include significant levels of distress, as well as impairment in physical, vocational, social, and sexual functioning (52). A 5-year follow-up of 75 endometrial cancer patients indicated that a sizable proportion (66%) of the women continued to experience emotional distress and impaired body image, which may have negatively impacted their social relationships (81). Related previous research suggests that half of the women who had received endometrial cancer treatment approximately 3 years earlier reported sexual functioning problems, where time since diagnosis was negatively associated with sexual functioning (82). Others have also associated sexual adaptation after endometrial cancer treatment with both positive and negative mediating variables (83,84).

Sexual Dysfunction

Alterations in sexuality and fertility are inherent in the diagnosis and treatment of gynecologic cancer, often resulting in varying degrees of sexual dysfunction (45,85–97). An estimated 50% of patients treated for gynecologic cancer may suffer from some type of sexual problem (96). Unfavorable changes in sexual desire or fulfillment have been attributed to radiation tissue changes, early menopause, vaginal shortening, and a change in one's body image (98). The psychosocial aspects of a cancer diagnosis may play an independent role in cancer-related sexual dysfunction.

Oophorectomy results in the loss of ovarian estrogen and testosterone production, both of which are needed to regulate female sexual function. Loss of estrogen can lead to hot flashes, vaginal mucosal dryness and atrophy, urinary incontinence, depression, and loss of libido, whereas loss of testosterone has been implicated in the loss of appetite, energy, memory, libido, orgasm, and genital sensation (99). Thus, premenopausal gynecologic cancer patients who undergo oophorectomy, like postmenopausal women, may experience a hormone-related decrease in vaginal lubrication and subsequent dyspareunia, decreases in desire, lack of arousal, and difficulty achieving orgasm (100). Orgasm is mediated by stimulation of the pudendal or pelvic nerve, and damage or destruction of these nerves during surgery can impair orgasmic ability. Further, chemotherapy or pelvic radiation therapy often affect ovarian function, resulting in decreases in sexual desire and orgasm (99). In addition, following pelvic radiation or intracavitary radiation, the vaginal tissue may become fibrous as the scarring process begins, with a resultant loss of the tissue's ability to stretch during intercourse (100). This, in turn, can further sexual dysfunction.

In addition, or as a consequence, a patient's self-esteem may be negatively impacted by untimely loss of reproductive function, disfiguring surgical treatment (e.g., radical vulvectomy), cosmetic issues (e.g., neovagina), and radiation- or chemotherapy-related alopecia. In turn, the loss of self-esteem can adversely affect sexual response, as well as the patient's intimate relationship with her sex partner. Women with a more negative sexual self-view show greater sexual morbidity following cancer than do women with a more positive self-view (97). Other psychologic factors that may interfere with sexual response are stress and depression (with or without anxiety), which can lead to decreased desire, arousal, and orgasm, as well as fatigue, which may leave the woman too exhausted to participate in sexual activity (99,100).

Early studies on hysterectomy and oophorectomy for benign disease suggested that approximately 40% of patients experience a decline of sexual function after surgery (101). However, Carlson reviewed eight studies on the effects of hysterectomy on sexual function and found that most patients receiving surgery for symptomatic, benign disease had improved QOL after their operation (102). In addition, sexual function was unchanged or improved in the majority of women. The diagnosis of gynecologic cancer appears to influence patients' sexuality beyond the physical changes associated with cancer and treatment. A study by Guidozzi et al. found that up to 80% of ovarian cancer patients experienced a decline in sexual frequency after their diagnosis, although there was no significant difference in sexual dysfunction in patients in clinical remission versus those with persistent or recurrent cancer (74). A separate study evaluated the physical and psychologic impact of gynecologic cancer in 96 newly diagnosed patients, and found a significant decrease in sexual activity and satisfaction (103). Bergmark and colleagues provided long-term follow-up information on vaginal function in patients treated for early-stage cervical cancer (60). Regular vaginal intercourse was reported among 68% of the 247 study participants. Cancer-related problems reported by patients included insufficient vaginal lubrication (26%), shortening of the vagina (26%), and insufficient vaginal elasticity (23%). Many cancer patients reported a reduction in sexual desire over the past 5 years, which was similar to a group of cancer free controls. However, cancer patients were more likely to find their reduced libido distressing.

Many pharmacologic and nonpharmacologic options are available for cancer patients experiencing female sexual dysfunction. If appropriate, hormone replacement therapy may be administered, although this is determined by the type and stage of the disease (99,100). Vaginal dryness may be ameliorated by use of lubricants, (e.g., water-soluble moisturizers, jellies, vitamin E oil or suppositories, estrogen cream, tablets, or rings). Vaginal stenosis commonly occurs as a result of radiation therapy but can usually be prevented by the use of a vaginal dilator or by having intercourse on a regular basis. Maintenance of vaginal patency is important not only to preserve sexual function, but also to permit adequate follow-up pelvic examinations. Patient education and counseling (preferably involving both partners) are very important components of managing sexual dysfunction in gynecologic cancer patients. Effective holistic care requires informing the patient about the basic concepts of female sexuality, patient history and physical examination techniques, the impact of her disease and its treatment on sexual function, and pharmacologic approaches to managing problems related to sexual function (104). Additionally, patients should be informed about nonpharmacologic treatments (including behavior modification) that are available for enhancing sexual function (e.g., changes in the environment, timing, methods of lovemaking, Kegel exercises).

Neurotoxicity

Neurotoxicity, particularly peripheral neuropathy, is an important side effect induced by chemotherapeutic agents commonly used in the gynecologic setting including the platinum compounds, taxanes, and vinca alkaloids (15). Depending on the agent used, peripheral neuropathy may primarily involve large-fiber sensory nerves, which control vibration and position sense, or both large- and small-fiber sensory nerves, the latter controlling touch, pain, and temperature sensations; however, motor nerves may also be affected (105).

Cisplatin, which affects the large sensory nerve fibers, initially causes sensations of burning, tingling, and numbness in the fingers and toes; impaired vibratory sense; and hypersensitivity to pain. The neuropathy may progress to diminished deep tendon reflexes with impairment of position sense, sensory ataxia, and neuropathic pain; however, motor function is preserved. Peripheral neuropathy usually develops when cumulative doses exceed 400 mg/m², and in patients given high doses (>500 mg/m²), symptoms may continue to worsen after cisplatin withdrawal (105,106). Cisplatin also commonly causes ototoxicity, with permanent high-tone hearing loss reported in up to 45% of patients receiving this agent (107). Carboplatin has activity similar to that of cisplatin, but is less neurotoxic. Peripheral neuropathy has been reported only rarely, and these cases occurred in patients who had previously received high-dose cisplatin therapy and had experienced mild neuropathy (106,108). Paclitaxel, which mainly affects the small sensory nerve fibers, is associated with an especially high incidence of neurotoxicity; that is, more than 50% of patients who receive doses exceeding 250 mg/m² develop significant neuropathy (15,106). Rapid-onset sensory neuropathy can occur, particularly with high-dose regimens, and, as indicated earlier, the use of this agent may be limited by cumulative peripheral neurotoxicity, which can severely impact the patient's QOL (109,110). Symptoms include a decrease in pain and temperature sensation (small fiber) as well as loss of vibration and position sense, deep tendon reflexes, muscle strength, and fine motor movement (large fiber). Peripheral neuropathy is increased when paclitaxel is given with cisplatin (111), given in doses >200 mg/m², or given to patients with preexisting conditions such as diabetes mellitus or alcoholism, or when high cumulative doses are administered. The symptoms often improve after discontinuation of treatment (106).

Fatigue

Fatigue is the most common symptom reported by cancer patients (112), having an estimated prevalence of about 78% (113–115). Like anemia, fatigue can profoundly affect QOL (116–120). Concomitant conditions that may contribute to fatigue include infection, dehydration, sleep disorders, pain, depression, and anxiety; however, anemia is often the major contributing factor (120).

In a presentation at the American Society of Clinical Oncology (2002), a significant correlation was reported to exist between greater decreases in hemoglobin levels and increases in fatigue interference with QOL ($r = -0.32$. $p = .05$) (121). In several earlier studies, relationships were demonstrated between hemoglobin levels and both fatigue and nonfatigue items on QOL scales (122,123). In a multicenter, randomized, double-blind, placebo-controlled study in which epoetin alfa, a recombinant human erythropoietin (rHuEPO), was administered to patients with anemia who were receiving nonplatinum chemotherapy, results of univariate analysis showed a strong and statistically significant (range $p = .0002$ to .0325) correlation between change in hemoglobin level and change in QOL for all primary variables evaluated: that is, FACT-G, FACT-An Fatigue subscale, the Cancer Linear Analog Scale (CLAS) items Energy Level, Ability to Do Daily Activities, and Overall QOL, and the Short Form 36 (SF-36) Physical Component Summary and Mental Component Summary (123). The clinical implications of fatigue for QOL in cancer patients have been examined in several surveys (113–115,124–126). Overall, these surveys demonstrated that fatigue is associated with significant physical, emotional, psychologic, social, and economic consequences.

Numerous placebo-controlled and open-label studies have shown that improvement in QOL can be achieved by correction of anemia with epoetin alfa (123,127–135). A retrospective analysis of the data for a subgroup of ovarian cancer patients from the once-weekly epoetin alfa study showed significant ($p < .017$) improvement in QOL measures (133). In all four studies [as well as in the retrospective subset analysis of gynecologic cancer patients (120)], the change in overall QOL correlated significantly with the change in hemoglobin level (range $p = .0002$ to $<.001$) (120,123, 127–129). These findings provided evidence that increasing hemoglobin levels by administration of epoetin alfa can significantly improve several aspects of QOL, including fatigue. Additional studies, including one that utilized minimally important difference (MID) analysis (136) and another that used a normative data comparison (134,137), confirmed the clinical relevance of the observed effects of epoetin alfa on QOL in the double-blind, placebo-controlled study, including those related to the FACT-An Fatigue and Anemia scales.

Long-term Issues in Gynecologic Cancer Survivorship

We recently examined long-term sequelae of gynecologic malignancies of women diagnosed 5 to 10 years earlier. To measure potential long-term emotional sequelae, we pooled ten items from the emotional well-being subscale of the Quality of Life-Cancer Survivorship (QOL-CS) measure (50). This survivor-specific distress subscale (Cronbach's alpha = .81) was significantly associated with age, with younger people being more distressed about their cancer (.43, p <0.002). In addition, more survivor-specific distress was associated with poorer quality of life (.77, p <0.0001), greater illness intrusiveness (.36, p <0.01), less social support (.32, p <0.02), and less confidence managing the illness (.34, p <0.02). There were trends of significant associations for depression (p = 0.06) and cancer-specific distress (p = 0.06). Such results suggest that there may be a subgroup of women who experience fears and concerns related to their disease that may be negatively influencing important aspects of their life despite the assurances that they are cured of their disease. This deserves careful consideration as we attempt to elucidate the strengths and vulnerabilities associated with being a long-term gynecologic cancer survivor.

Among the women of child-bearing age, approximately 60% of the participants indicated that that they would have attended a support group program during the initial treatment if it had been offered. In addition, approximately 55% expressed that they would likely participate in a counseling program today to discuss existing cancer-specific issues. Although these proportions are somewhat smaller for older survivors (ovarian and endometrial cancers), together these descriptive data suggest that aspects of long-term survivorship continue to be challenging and merit attention.

CONCLUSIONS AND FUTURE DIRECTIONS

The gynecologic cancer patient faces many challenges specific to the type of tumor and its treatment, as well as those common to the general oncologic population. Among the many challenges are treatment toxicities and side effects that can significantly diminish QOL, as well as the decreases in QOL intrinsic to the disease itself. Alleviation of these negative events can play a crucial role in enhancing or preserving the patient's QOL during and after treatment, enabling her to withstand and complete the most effective therapy. Caring for the patient, as well as her cancer, requires that measures to preserve or enhance the quality as well as the quantity of life are incorporated into the patient's treatment plan.

Gynecologic cancer can be particularly distressing for patients, both physically and emotionally, owing to the aggressiveness of the surgical and medical treatment administered, treatment-related side effects experienced, fears about disease recurrence or death, and changes in life style necessitated by the disease. Therefore, efforts must be made by the patients' health-care providers to furnish a comprehensive care program that will help the patients move through the trajectory from diagnosis to recovery or palliative care. Components of this program should include both patient and family education and psychosocial support. Psychosocial support can encompass a broad range of services such as emotional, nutritional, sexual, genetic, and financial counseling; steering patients and their families to institutional and community resources when possible; and providing referrals to organizations that offer general cancer information and support.

QOL research will continue to evolve and aid the therapeutic regimens in advancing the state of the science. The accrual of information over the past 5 years has demonstrated the importance of continuing examination and evaluation of QOL for those diseases in which clearly optimal treatments are not available or have significant potential for adverse sequelae. As a result, the opportunity to impact gynecologic cancer treatment positively will be maximized. QOL data may also be increasingly important in studies where problems such as sexual dysfunction, neurotoxicity, or fatigue may be considered to be severe and/or persistent. To that end, it is reasonable to begin systematically to introduce interventions aimed at preventing or diminishing the adverse effects of common treatments for gynecologic malignancies.

Finally, regarding decision analysis and support, it will be important to include QOL information in the discussion of disease management in patients with advanced, incurable disease. Today's local and systemic treatments for advanced cervical and ovarian cancer are controversial; for example, because they produce several complications and toxicities with marginal benefit. Therefore, it will be important to compare outcomes as a function of the treatment arm, and to determine the prognostic value of QOL data before and during therapy. Differentiation of likely responders from nonresponders as early as possible, using as much available data as possible is desirable, so that women can make informed decisions about continued treatment. A long-term goal should be to bring to the clinical setting information obtained from previous clinical trials and help women understand the likely negative and positive consequences of treatment options.

ACKNOWLEDGEMENTS

We acknowledge the support of the Office of Cancer Survivorship at the National Cancer Institute 1 R01 CA79039-01. We thank the Gynecologic Oncology Group and Rana Habbal, M.A., for their valuable contributions.

REFERENCES

1. American Cancer Society. Cancer facts and figures—2003. Atlanta: American Cancer Society, 2003.
2. SEER. Prevalence estimates applied to January 1998 U.S. population estimates from the Census Bureau. January 1998.
3. Rowland JH, Aziz NM, Tesauro G, Feuer EJ. The changing face of cancer survivorship. *Semin Oncol Nurs* 2001;17:236–240.
4. Armstrong DK. Relapsed ovarian cancer: challenges and management strategies for a chronic disease. *Oncologist* 2002; [Suppl 5]:20–28.

5. Aaronson NK: Quality of life: What is it? How should it be measured? *Oncology* 1988; 2:69–74.

6. Aaronson NK, Ahmedzai S, Bergman B, et al. The European Organization for the Research and Treatment of Cancer QLQ-C30: a quality of life instrument for use in international clinical trials in oncology. *J Natl Cancer Inst* 1993;85:365–376.

7. Cella DF, Cherin EA. Quality of life during and after cancer treatment. *Compr Ther* 1988;4:69–75.

8. Stewart AL, Ware JE, Brook RH. Advances in the measurement of functional status: construction of aggregate indexes. *Med Care* 1981; 19:473–488.

9. Schipper H, Clinch J, McMurray A, et al. Measuring the quality of life of cancer patients: the Functional Living Index-Cancer: development and validation. *J Clin Oncol* 1984; 2:472–483.

10. Cella DF. Measuring quality of life in palliative care. *Semin Oncol* 1995;22[2 Suppl 3]:73–81.

11. Kornblith AB, Holland JC. *Handbook of measures for psychological, social and physical function in cancer.* Vol 1: *Quality of life.* New York: Memorial Sloan–Kettering Cancer Center, 1994.

12. Cella DF, Tulsky DS, Gray G, et al. The functional assessment of cancer therapy (FACT) scale: development and validation of the general version. *J Clin Oncol* 1993;11:570–579.

13. Fish LS, Lewis BE. Quality of life issues in the management of ovarian cancer. *Semin Oncol* 1999;25[1 Suppl 1]:32–39.

14. Basen-Engquist K, Bodurka-Bevers D, Fitzgerald MA, et al. Reliability and validity of the Functional Assessment of Cancer Therapy-Ovarian. *J Clin Oncol* 2001;19:1809–1817.

15. Cella D, Peterman A, Hudgens S, et al. Measuring the side effects of taxane therapy in oncology. The Functional Assessment of Cancer Therapy-Taxane (FACT-Taxane). *Cancer* 2003; 98:822–831.

16. Yellen SB, Cella DF, Webster KA, et al. Measuring fatigue and other anemia-related symptoms with the Functional Assessment of Cancer Therapy (FACT) Measurement System. *J Pain Symptom Manage* 1997;13:63–74.

17. Till JE, Sutherland HJ, Meslin EM. Is there a role for preference assessments in research on quality of life in oncology? *Qual Life Res* 1992;1:31–40.

18. Drummond MF, Stoddart GL, Torrance GW. *Methods for economic evaluation of health care programmes.* Oxford, UK: Oxford University Press, 1987.

19. Torrance GW. Measurement of health state utilities for economic appraisal. *J Health Econ* 1986;5:1–30.

20. Boyd NF, Sutherland HJ, Heasman KZ, et al. Whose utilities for decision analysis? *Med Decis Making* 1990;10:58–67.

21. Tsevat J, Goldman L, Soukup JR, Lee TH. Stability of utilities in survivors of myocardial infarction. *Med Decis Making* 1990;10:323.

22. Canadian Erythropoietin Study Group. Association between recombinant human erythropoietin and quality of life and exercise capacity of patients receiving hemodialysis. *BMJ* 1990;300:573–578.

23. Tsevat J, Cook EF, Soukop JR, et al. Utilities of the seriously ill. *Clin Res* 1991; 39:589A(abst).

24. Andersen BL, Lutgendorf S. Quality of life as an outcome measure in gynecologic malignancies. *Curr Opin Obstet Gynecol* 2000;12: 21–26.

25. Schover LR. Quality counts: the value of women's perceived quality of life after cervical cancer. *Gynecol Oncol* 2000;76:3–4.

26. Klee M, Thranov I, Machin D. Life after radiotherapy: the psychological and social effects experienced by women treated for advanced stages of cervical cancer. *Gynecol Oncol* 2000;76:5–13.

27. Eisemann M, Lalos A. Psychosocial determinants of well-being in gynecologic cancer patients. *Cancer Nurs* 1999; 22(4):303–306.

28. McDonald TW, Neutens JJ, Fischer LM, Jessee D. Impact of cervical intraepithelial neoplasia diagnosis and treatment on self-esteem and body image. *Gynecol Oncol* 1989; 34:345–349.

29. Ferreira SE. Cervical intraepithelial neoplasia diagnosis: Emotional impact and nursing implications. *Clin Excel Nurse Pract* 1998;2: 218–224.

30. Andersen BL. Stress and quality of life following cervical cancer. *J Natl Cancer Inst Monogr* 1996;21:65–70.

31. Greimel ER, Freidl W. Functioning in daily living and psychological well-being of female cancer patients. *J Psychosom Obstet Gynaecol* 2000;21:25–30.

32. Boudurka-Beavers D, Basen-Engquist K, Carmack CL, et al. Depression, anxiety, and quality of life in patients with epithelial ovarian cancer. *Gynecol Oncol* 2000;78:302–308.

33. Hamilton AB. Psychological aspects of ovarian cancer. *Cancer Invest* 1999;17:335–341.

34. Fitch MI, Gray RE, Franssen E. Perspectives on living with ovarian cancer: older women's views. *Oncol Nurs Forum* 2001;28: 1433–1442.

35. Andersen BL, Anderson B, deProsse C. Controlled, prospective longitudinal study of women with cancer: II. Psychological outcomes. *J Consult Clin Psychol* 1989; 57:692–697.

36. Steginga SK, Dunn J. Women's experiences following treatment for gynecological cancer. *Oncol Nurs Forum* 1997;28:1403–1408.

37. Whelan TJ, Mohide EA, Willan AR, et al. The supportive care needs of newly diagnosed cancer patients attending a regional cancer center. *Cancer* 1997;80:1518–1524.

38. Lutgendorf SK, Anderson B, Rothrock N, et al. Quality of life and mood in women receiving extensive chemotherapy for gynecologic cancer. *Cancer* 2000;89:1402–1411.

39. Auchincloss SS. After treatment. Psychosocial issues in gynecologic cancer survivorship. *Cancer* 1995;76[10 Suppl]:2117–2124.

40. Wenzel LB. Psychosocial Consequences of gestational trophoblastic disease. In: Hancock B, Newlands E, Berkowitz R, eds. *Gestational trophoblastic disease.* 2nd ed. London: Chapman & Hall, 2002; 359–366.

41. Wenzel L. Psychosocial consequences of gestational trophoblastic disease. In: Hancock B, Newlands E, Berkowitz R, eds. *Gestational trophoblastic disease.* London: Chapman & Hall, 1997:233–239.

42. Wenzel LB, Berkowitz R, Newlands E, et al. Quality of life after gestational trophoblastic disease. *J Reprod Med* 2002;47:387–394.

43. Wenzel L, Berkowitz R, Robinson S, et al. The psychological, social and sexual effects of gestational trophoblastic disease on patients and their partners. *J Reprod Med* 1994; 39:163–167.

44. Wenzel L, Berkowitz R, Robinson S, et al. The psychological, social and sexual consequences of gestational trophoblastic disease. *Gynecol Oncol* 1992;46:74–81.

45. Andersen BL. Predicting sexual and psychologic morbidity and improving the quality of life for women with gynecologic cancer. *Cancer* 1993;71[4 Suppl]:1678–1690.

46. Wyatt GKH, Friedman LL. Development and testing of a quality of life model for long-term female cancer survivors. *Qual Life Res* 1996; 5:387–394.

47. Andersen B, Lutgendorf S. Quality of life in gynecologic cancer survivors. *CA Cancer J Clin* 1997;47:218–225.

48. Northouse L. A longitudinal study of the adjustment of patients and husbands to breast cancer. *Oncol Nurs Forum* 1989;16:511–516.

49. Ferrell B. Overview of breast cancer: Quality of life. *Oncol Patient Care* 1993;3:7–8.

50. Ferrell BR, Dow KH, Grant M. Measurement of the quality of life in cancer survivors. *Qual Life Res* 1995;4:523–531.

51. Ferrell BR, Dow KH, Leigh S, et al. Quality of life in long-term cancer survivors. *Oncol Nurs Forum* 1995;22:915–922.

52. Li C, Samsioe G, Iosif C. Quality of life in long-term survivors of cervical cancer. *Maturitas* 1999;32:95–102.

53. Wenzel LB, Fairclough DL, Brady MJ, et al. Age-related differences in the quality of life of breast carcinoma patients after treatment. *Cancer* 1999;86:1768–1774.

54. Shimozuma K, Ganz PA, Petersen L, Hirji K. Quality of life in the first year after breast cancer surgery: Rehabilitation needs and patterns of recovery. *Breast Cancer Res Treat* 1999;56:45–57.

55. Dow KH, Ferrell BR, Haberman MR, Eaton L. The meaning of quality of life in cancer survivorship. *Oncol Nurs Forum* 1999;26:519–528.

56. Andersen BL. Psychological interventions for cancer patients to enhance the quality of life. *J Consult Clin Psychol* 1992;60:552–568.

57. Spencer SM, Lehman JM, Wynings C, et al. Concerns about breast cancer and relations to psychosocial well-being in a multiethnic sample of early-stage patients. *Health Psychol* 1999;18:159–168.

58. Juarez G, Ferrell B, Borneman T. Perceptions of quality of life in Hispanic patients with cancer. *Cancer Pract* 1998;6:318–324.

59. Meyerowitz BE, Formenti SC, Ell KO, Leedham B. Depression among Latina cervical cancer patients. *J Social Clin Psychol* 2000; 19:352–371.

60. Bergmark K, Avall-Lundqvist E, Dickman PW, et al. Vaginal changes

and sexuality in women with a history of cervical cancer. *N Engl J Med* 1999;340:1383–1389.

61. Trapido EJ, Chen F, Davis K, et al. Cancer in south Florida Hispanic women. A 9-year assessment. *Arch Intern Med* 1994;154:1083–1088.

62. Corney RH, Crowther ME, Everett H, et al. Psychosexual dysfunction in women with gynaecological cancer following radical pelvic surgery. *Br J Obstet Gynaecol* 1993; 100:73–78.

63. RS Brown, B Haddox, A Psada, et al. Social and psychological adjustment following pelvic exenteration. *Am J Obstet Gynecol* 1972;114:162.

64. GM Dempsey, HJ Buchsbaum, J Morrison. Psychosocial adjustment to pelvic exenteration *Gynecol Oncol* 1975;3:325–334.

65. BL Andersen, NF Hacker. Psychosexual Adjustment following total pelvic exenteration. *Obstet Gynecol* 1983;61:331–338.

66. Fisher, SG. Psychosexual Adjustment following total pelvic exenteration. *Cancer Nurs* 1979; 2:219–225.

67. Hawighorst-Knapstein, Schonefub G, Hoffmann SO, Knapstein PG. Pelvic exteneration: effects of surgery on quality of life and body image—a prospective longitudinal study. *Gynecol Oncol* 1997;66:495–500.

68. Schag CA, Heinrich RL. Developing a comprehensive quality of life measurement tool: the Cancer Rehabilitation Evaluation System. *Oncology* 1990;4:135–138.

69. Ratliff CR, Gershenson DM, Morris M, et al. Sexual adjustments of patients undergoing gracilis myocutaneous flap vaginal reconstruction in conjunction with pelvic exenteration. *Cancer* 1996;78:2229–2235.

70. Cain MC, Wenzel LB, Monk BJ, Cella D. Palliative care and quality of life considerations in the management of ovarian cancer. In: Gershenson DM, McGuire WP, eds. *Ovarian cancer: controversies in management.* New York: Churchill Livingstone, 1998;281–307.

71. Auchincloss SS. Sexual issues in cancer patients: issues in evaluation and treatment. In: Holland JC, Rowland JC, eds. *Handbook of psychooncology.* New York: Oxford University Press, 1990:383–413.

72. Kornblith AB, Thaler HT, Wong G, et al. Quality of life of women with ovarian cancer. *Gynecol Oncol* 1995;59:231–242.

73. Wenzel LB, Donnelly JP, Fowler JM, et al. Resilience, reflection, and residual stress in ovarian cancer survivorship: a Gynecologic Oncology Group Study. *Psychooncology* 2002;11:142–154.

74. Guidozzi F. Living with ovarian cancer. *Gynecol Oncol* 1993;50:202–207.

75. Laurell G, Beskow C, Frankendal B, Borg E. Cisplatin administration to gynecologic cancer patients. Long-term effects on hearing. *Cancer* 1996;78:1798–1804.

76. Ersek M, Ferrell BR, Dow KH, Melancon CH. Quality of life in women with ovarian cancer. *West J Nurs Res* 1997;19:334–350.

77. Kahn SB, Houts PS, Harding SP. Quality of life and patients with cancer: a comparative study of patient versus physician perceptions and its implication for cancer education. *J Cancer Educ* 1992;7:241–249.

78. Calhoun E, Bennett C, Peeples P, et al. Perceptions of cisplatin-related toxicity among ovarian cancer patients and gynecologic oncologists. *Gynecol Oncol* 1998;71:369–375.

79. Potish RA, Dusenbery KE. Enterac mobidity of postoperative pelvic external beam and brachytherapy for uterine cancer. *Int J Radiat Oncol Biol Phys* 1990;18:1005–1010.

80. Stokes S, Bedwinek J, Breaux S, et al. Treatment of stage I adenocarcinoma of the endometrium by hysterectomy and irradiation: Analysis and complications. *Obstet Gynecol* 1985;65:86–92.

81. Neises M, Soedradjat F, Strittmatter HJ, et al. Quality of life of over 60-year-old patients with breast and uterine carcinoma, 5 years after primary operation. *Z Gerentol Geritr* 1996;29:136–142.

82. Cochran SD, Hacker NF, Wellisch D, Berek JS. Sexual functioning after treatment for endometrial cancer. *J Psycho Oncol* 1987; 5(2):47–61.

83. Lamb MA. Sexual adaptation of women treated for endometrial cancer. *Dis Abstr Int (B)* 1991;52:2994.

84. Bos-Branolte G, Rijshouwer YM, Zielstra EM, et al. Psychologic morbidity in survivors of gynecologic cancer. *Eur J Gynaecol Oncol* 1988;9:168–177.

85. Paavonen J. Sexual dysfunction associated with treatment of cervical cancer. *Sex Transm Infect* 1999;75:375–376.

86. Cull A, Cowie VJ, Farquharson DI, et al. Early stage cervical cancer:

psychosocial and sexual outcomes of treatment. *Br J Cancer* 1993;68:1216–1220.

87. Krumm S, Lamberti J. Changes in sexual behavior following radiation therapy for cervical cancer. *J Psychosom Obstet Gynaecol* 1993;14:51–63.

88. Schover LR, Fife M, Gershenson DM. Sexual dysfunction and treatment for early stage cervical cancer. *Cancer* 1989;63:204–212.

89. Andersen BL. Sexual functioning morbidity among cancer survivors. Current status and future research directions. *Cancer* 1985;55:1835–1842.

90. Lamb MA. Effects of cancer on the sexuality and fertility of women. *Semin Oncol Nurs* 1995;11:120–127.

91. Zacharias DR, Gilg CA, Foxall MJ. Quality of life and coping in patients with gynecologic cancer and their spouses. *Oncol Nurs Forum* 1994;21:1699–1706.

92. Andersen BL. Surviving cancer. *Cancer* 1994;74[4 Suppl]:1484–1495.

93. Andersen BL, Anderson B, deProsse C. Controlled prospective longitudinal study of women with cancer: I. Sexual functioning outcomes. *J Consult Clin Psychol* 1989; 57:683–691.

94. Andersen BL. How cancer affects sexual functioning. *Oncology (Huntingt)* 1990; 4:81–88; Discussion 92–84.

95. Andersen BL, van Der Does J. Surviving gynecologic cancer and coping with sexual morbidity: An international problem. *Int J Gynecol Cancer* 1994;4:225–240.

96. Andersen BL, Woods XA, Copeland LJ. Sexual self-schema and sexual morbidity among gynecologic cancer survivors. *J Consult Clin Psychol* 1997;65:221–229.

97. Andersen BL. Surviving cancer: the importance of sexual self-concept. *Med Pediatr Oncol* 1999;33:15–23.

98. Lamb MA. Psychosexual issues: the woman with gynecologic cancer. *Semin Oncol Nurs* 1990;6:237–243.

99. Brassil DF, Keller M. Female sexual dysfunction: definitions, causes, and treatment. *Urol Nurs* 2002;22:237–244.

100. Wilmoth MC. Sexual implications of gynecologic cancer treatments. *J Obstet Gynecol Neonatal Nurs* 2000;29:413–421.

101. Zussman L, Zussman, S, Sunley R, Bjornson E. Sexual response after hysterectomy-oophorectomy: recent studies and reconsideration of psychogenesis. *Am J Obstet Gynecol* 1981;140:725–729.

102. Carlson KJ. Outcomes of hysterectomy. *Clin Obstet Gynecol* 1997;40:939–946.

103. Harris R, Good RS, Pollack L. Sexual behavior of gynecologic cancer patients. *Arch Sex Behav* 1982;11:503–510.

104. Phillips NA. Female sexual dysfunction: evaluation and treatment [Review]. *Am Fam Physician* 2000;62:127–136, 141–142.

105. Sweeney CW. Understanding peripheral neuropathy in patients with cancer: background and patient assessment. *Clin J Oncol Nurs* 2002;6:163–166.

106. Plotkin SR, Wen PY. Neurologic complications of cancer therapy. *Neurol Clin North Am* 2003;21:279–318.

107. Adams M, Kerby IJ, Rocker I, et al. A comparison of the toxicity and efficacy of cisplatin and carboplatin in advanced cancer. The Swons Gynaecological Cancer Group. *Acta Oncol* 1989;28:57–60.

108. Heinzlef O, Lotz JP, Roullet E. Severe neuropathy after high dose carboplatin in three patients receiving multidrug chemotherapy. *J Neurol Neurosurg Psychiatry* 1998; 64:667–669.

109. Gordon AN, Stringer CA, Matthews CM, et al. Phase I dose escalation of paclitaxel in patients with advanced ovarian cancer receiving cisplatin: rapid development of neurotoxicity is dose-limiting. *J Clin Oncol* 1997;15:1965–1973.

110. Dunton CJ. Management of treatment-related toxicity in advanced ovarian cancer. *Oncologist* 2002;7[Suppl 5]:11–19.

111. McGuire WP, Hoskins WJ, Brady MF, et al. Cyclophosphamide and cisplatin compared with paclitaxel and cisplatin in patients with stage III and stage IV ovarian cancer. *N Engl J Med* 1996;334:1–6.

112. Portenoy RK, Kornblith AB, Wong G, et al. Pain in ovarian cancer patients. Prevalence, characteristics, and associated symptoms. *Cancer* 1994;74:907–915.

113. Vogelzang NJ, Breitbart W, Cella D, et al. The Fatigue Coalition. Patient, caregiver, and oncologist perceptions of cancer-related fatigue: results of a tripart assessment survey. *Semin Hematol* 1997; 34[Suppl 2]:4–12.

114. Curt G, Breitbart W, Cella D, et al. Impact of cancer-related fatigue on the lives of patients. *Proc Am Soc Clin Oncol* 1999;18:573a(abst).

115. Curt GA, Johnston PG. Cancer fatigue: the way forward. *Oncologist* 2003; 8[Suppl 1]:27–30.

116. Cella D. Factors influencing quality of life in cancer patients: anemia and fatigue. *Semin Oncol* 1998;25[Suppl 7]:43–46.

117. Groopman JE, Itri LM. Chemotherapy-induced anemia in adults: incidence and treatment [Review]. *J Natl Cancer Inst* 1999;91: 1616–1634.

118. Portenoy RK, Itri LM. Cancer-related fatigue: guidelines for evaluation and management. *Oncologist* 1999;4:1–10.

119. Sobrero A, Puglisi F, Guglielmi A, et al. Fatigue: a main component of anemia symptomatology. *Semin Oncol* 2001;28[Suppl 8]:15–18.

120. Campos S. The impact of anemia and its treatment on patients with gynecologic malignancies. *Semin Oncol* 2002;29[3 Suppl 8]:7–12.

121. Jacobsen PB, Thors CL, Cawley M, et al. Relation of decline in hemoglobin to cognitive functioning and fatigue during chemotherapy treatment. *Proc Am Soc Clin Oncol* 2002; 21:386a(abst 1542).

122. Cella D. The Functional Assessment of Cancer Therapy-Anemia (FACT-An) scale: a new tool for the assessment of outcomes in cancer anemia and fatigue. *Semin Hematol* 1997;34[3 Suppl 2]:13–19.

123. Littlewood TJ, Bajetta E, Nortier JWR, et al.; the Epoetin Alfa Study Group. Effects of epoetin alfa on hematologic parameters and quality of life in cancer patients receiving nonplatinum chemotherapy; results of a randomized, double-blind, placebo-controlled trial. *J Clin Oncol* 2001;19:2865–2874.

124. Curt GA. Impact of fatigue in quality of life in oncology patients. *Semin Hematol.* 2000; 37[Suppl 6]:14–17.

125. Curt GA. The impact of fatigue on patients with cancer: overview of FATIGUE 1 and 2. *Oncologist* 2000;5[Suppl 2]:9–12.

126. Curt GA, Breitbart W, Cella D, et al. Impact of cancer-related fatigue on the lives of patients: new findings from the Fatigue Coalition. *Oncologist* 2000;5:353–360.

127. Glaspy J, Bukowski R, Steinberg D, et al. Impact of therapy with epoetin alfa on clinical outcomes in patients with nonmyeloid malignancies during cancer chemotherapy in community oncology practice. *J Clin Oncol* 1997;15:1218–1234.

128. Demetri GD, Kris M, Wade J, et al. Quality-of-life benefit in chemotherapy patients treated with epoetin alfa is independent of disease response or tumor type: results from a prospective community oncology study. *J Clin Oncol* 1998;16:3412–3425.

129. Gabrilove JL, Cleeland CS, Livingston RB, et al. Clinical evaluation of once-weekly dosing of epoetin alfa in chemotherapy patients: improvements in hemoglobin and quality of life are similar to three-times-weekly dosing. *J Clin Oncol* 2001;19:2875–2882.

130. Crawford J, Cella D, Cleeland CS, et al. Relationship between changes in hemoglobin level and quality of life during chemotherapy in anemic cancer patients receiving epoetin alfa therapy. *Cancer* 2002;95: 888–895.

131. Fallowfield L, Gagnon D, Zagari M, et al. for the Epoetin Alfa Study Group. Multivariate regression analyses of data from a randomized, double-blind, placebo-controlled study confirm quality of life benefit of epoetin alfa in patients receiving non-platinum chemotherapy. *Br J Cancer* 2002;87:1341–1353.

132. Lahousen M, Andersson H, Antonopoulos M, Wilkinson PM. Epoetin alfa improves hematologic and quality of life (QOL) parameters in anemic ovarian cancer patients (pts) undergoing chemotherapy (CT). Proceedings of the 11th International Congress on Anti-Cancer Treatment 2002;170(abst).

133. Campos SM. Epoetin alfa 40,000 U once weekly significantly improves hemoglobin and quality of life in anemic patients with ovarian cancer. *Proc Am Soc Clin Oncol* 2003; 22:774(abst 3111).

134. Cella D. Control of cancer-related anemia with erythropoietic agents: a review of evidence for improved quality of life and clinical outcomes. *Ann Oncol* 2003;14:511–519.

135. Shasha D, George MJ, Harrison LB. Once-weekly dosing of epoetin alfa increases hemoglobin and improves quality of life in anemic cancer patients receiving radiotherapy and chemotherapy. *Cancer* 2003;

136. Patrick DL, Gagnon DD, Zagari MJ, et al. for the Epoetin Alfa Study Group. Assessing the clinical significance of health-related quality of life (HrQOL) improvements in anaemic cancer patients receiving epoetin alfa. *Eur J Cancer* 2003;39:335–345.

137. Cella D, Zagari MJ, Vandoros C, et al. Epoetin alfa treatment results in clinically significant improvements in quality of life in anemic cancer patients when referenced to the general population. *J Clin Oncol* 2003;21:366–373.

CHAPTER 39

End of Life Care

Joanna M. Cain, A. Peter M. Heintz, and Nikkie B. Swarte

End of life care is a very important part of palliative care. It requires total commitment of the entire health-care team. It not only includes medical interventions to relieve the suffering, but also psychosocial care. Communication skills are very important to assure effective end of life care. In this communication, the autonomy of the patient has to be respected. The caregivers have to realize that they have to respect the delicate balance between professional and personal involvement. Communication not only involves the patient, but also her relatives and friends. Psychologic and multiple physical symptoms need to be routinely assessed and addressed by physicians in the overall decision making concerning the end of life. Special attention should be paid to anxiety and depression. Although euthanasia is not universally available or approved by all societies, there are lessons to be learned for the terminal care of women from this experience.

GOALS OF CARE AT THE END OF LIFE

It is antithetical to most medical paradigms to imagine that our goal might be to make the exiting of life as important as the beginning of life. Yet, this is the goal of this chapter, and it is a medical goal more profound than merely relieving suffering. We fall far from this goal in most countries of the world, and particularly for dying women who seek to protect their families from anguish or financial harm by ignoring their needs or not asking for adequate pain control or support. Access to adequate pain control is only one small part—although a critical part—of this venture. The achievement of

end of life goals for a patient, the ability to passage from life with dignity, and the ability to create a positive meaning for those who remain as well as those who are leaving life—professional and family alike—all fall under the broad designation of goals of care at the end of life. In this chapter, attention will be paid to the psychologic and emotional care as well as the physical care that has to be given to patients in their last phase of life and to several aspects of the medical decisions concerning the end of life including euthanasia and physician-assisted suicide.

GOALS OF MEDICINE AND ETHICAL OBLIGATIONS OF PHYSICIANS: CARE AND CURE

Acknowledging or even identifying when women are "overmastered" by their disease is not accomplished easily. Is it the second or the sixth reemergence of their ovarian cancer? Is it different if you are 84 years old than if you are 33? Is it only when bowel obstruction or liver and renal failure impede further therapy or when a woman is relatively symptom free with progressive disease and further therapy will diminish her quality of life even though extending it? Furthermore, who should be the engineer of care and peaceful transitions? Should it be, and can it be, the same health professional that strenuously worked to cure the disease before this transition?

We live in a time when phenomenal abilities to prolong life exist, but the biggest challenge is identifying when the goals of medicine must shift from curing or controlling cancer to alleviating suffering and creating a peaceful transition to death. Seale has noted that "medical science has become so successful that what people fear most is not death itself but a slow death—locked behind hospital doors—that prolongs life and makes it a living hell" (1). As Callahan notes about the technology and advances that underpin health care now: "The most fundamental problem with technological medicine is two-fold: that it can give us a longer life and a

J. M. Cain: Department of Obstetrics and Gynecology, Oregon Health & Sciences University, Portland, Oregon 97239.

A. P. M. Heintz: Department of Gynecologic Oncology, University Medical Center Utrecht, Utrecht, the Netherlands.

N. B. Swarte: Department of Gynecologic Oncology, University Medical Center Utrecht, Utrecht, the Netherlands.

slower dying and that it can keep us alive when we might be better off dead'' (2). Our obligation to our patients requires us to identify when further curative therapy is more harmful than helpful in order to prevent suffering.

Two key issues define the time that goals of medicine shift from cure to comfort: One is the likelihood of success with continued efforts to cure disease and the second is the patient's goals and wishes regarding the side effects of treatments versus the potential benefit and impact on quality of life. The ideal role of the physician is to continue an ongoing conversation and relationship of truth telling and support in the physician-patient relationship. A conversation that reveals that there is no further therapy that is likely to cure or even control a cancer needs to take place as one that arises in a long line of conversations that have provided honest assessments of the medical status of disease along with exploring patient values and wishes and measuring them against the reality of the disease at the time. This conversation also must assure the patient that the presence and commitment of the physician to patient comfort care will be as aggressive as has been their commitment to a cure. There are, of course, some common glitches in this ideal description. First, the patient may—regardless of how carefully the physician has explored the issues—totally reject the idea that death is likely or even imminent. Second, the physician may not be able to provide ongoing care for multiple reasons including their own discomfort with terminal care. The physician still needs to make plans for maximal comfort and palliative care whether continuing with them or by referral regardless of the patient's rejection of the likelihood of death. Furthermore, resisting the urge to respond to the patient's denial by providing futile therapy is an ethical obligation as part of the axiom of nonmalificence—preventing greater harm than benefit from our interventions.

Telling the Truth and Nothing But the Truth?

In the recent past, telling the truth about cancer and impending death was ''not done.'' Patients were told that they had other conditions such as a severe infection, and that the doctor would do everything to save her and that she should not worry. Sometimes even the truth was only told to the family, which created a distance and a sense of distrust between the patient and her loved ones that was very painful for all involved. Even today in many countries, telling the truth is not common practice or is even considered to be cruel. In Western medicine, we acknowledge a patient's right to know everything about her illness and to make their own choice among treatment options. However, it is a mistake to translate this statement into ''patients must know everything about their illness and treatment options.'' It is more correct to say that patients have the right to know as much about their illness and treatment options as they want to know. If a patient asks a question, then an honest answer is expected. This does not mean that the patient wants a complete summary of all that medical knowledge has to offer or to be bludgeoned by the lack of any options. For example, information about complications and ways of dying that are very unlikely to occur will not contribute to her well-being. It is a responsibility of the physician to present the relevant data for the minute and consistently monitor what level of further information the patient is requesting. This requires a flexible state of mind because one patient may come in with data from the Internet and the other may be completely ignorant of the situation and prefer an ''ignorance is bliss'' approach to most things in her life. But for both patients, the same cautious approach to understanding where they are at the minute and presenting truthful information must be followed to help them to know what they need to know for their own

TABLE 39.1. *Key issues to address when the therapeutic focus shifts from cure to care*

Issue	Examples
Communication about terminal nature of cancer should occur in the course of ONGOING communication.	"We are not achieving the goals we set together with this chemotherapy." "The cancer is continuing to grow despite our efforts with this new agent."
Assess what the patient WANTS to know.	"I would not continue any further chemotherapy at this point, but feel we should focus on relieving your symptoms of . . . What do you think?" "Do you have questions about what we just discussed?"
Identify that, in fact, the patient's condition is terminal, and particularly if asked directly.	"Am I going to die of this?" "Yes, but our attention now needs to be focused on making whatever time you have as pain free and active as it possibly can be."
Identify the goals that the patient wants to achieve.	"Are there any special events or things that are on your agenda that we need to know about as we plan your treatment?"
Identify what resources the patient is planning to access (e.g., support systems as well as insurance coverage/hospice coverage).	"Have you talked to your . . . spouse /partner/children/ friends about your plans to be at home, and do they have ideas about how that will work?"
Make sure that the priority items for the patient are dealt with immediately.	"What is the number one issue for you right now?"

well-being as well as make decisions and conclude their private affairs (Table 39.1).

We also have to realize that having experienced the course of the disease, patients know very well that laboratory tests and imaging examinations can bring bad news. For this reason, whether or not they want to know the results and their meaning should be discussed with them before these tests are done. These tests should not be done if the answer is no, or if it is unclear how the results will change either the patient's thinking or the treatment planning options.

ROLE OF PATIENT IN DECISION MAKING

The most important way to understand each other is an honest and open communication. In daily practice, we have professional and personal relationships. In the end of life care, it is sometimes difficult to separate them because of the intimate and often personal contact that develops between the patient and the physician. The balance is critical. Sometimes a close personal relationship can be of benefit to both of them, but it also carries the risk of too much involvement and a too high emotional burden. This situation can hinder the fulfillment of the professional duties of the physician. The professional relationship between physician and patient is based on the trust the patient has in the physician. The patient believes and expects that the physician will do everything that is in her best interest, and that her autonomy is respected. The physician may expect respect and gratitude because of his or her help. An expectation of emotional mutuality on either side can lead to expectations that can undermine the professional role of the physician. If a physician finds himself or herself emotionally involved in ways that undermine decisions or influence care, then the physician should ask a colleague to take over and step back as they may not adequately assess the desires and needs of the patient.

Assuring that the patient's preferences about end of life care are documented is also a critical part of this transition from cure to care, and a responsibility of the care team. Although Do Not Resuscitate (DNR) policies and mechanisms vary state by state, this has become "part of the ritual of death" in our society and critical to assuring that a patient does not experience inappropriate interventions and suffering (3). It assures that the patient's values and wishes endure in a form that communicates their wishes to the multitude of health providers and care givers that they might potentially need to document this for.

A conversation about DNR policies also allows the health team to discuss legal mechanisms such as "living wills" or advance directives and durable power of attorney for health care that can assure that the patient's wishes are clearly stated and there is an individual identified who can speak for the patient's wishes if she cannot speak for herself. Most institutions will have experienced social workers or support staff that can assist patients with these instruments if desired.

ROLE OF FAMILY IN DECISION MAKING

Given the sequential and repetitive conversations described above, the inclusion of family and other support persons is almost universal and clearly preferable. For many patients, they are the ones with whom they have shared their lives and their dearest and deepest emotions. They are also the ones by whom the patient wants to be surrounded during the last phase of life. However, patients have the right to exclude or include whomever they wish in conversations, and occasionally medical events are so acute that they trigger discussions with family members without clarity about what the patient herself would have wished or without clarity about which family member truly speaks for the patient. Expert communication with the family then becomes the most critical means of assuring that the patient's best interests are served. Unfortunately, research suggests that communication is not as effective as it needs to be in these circumstances. Fifty-four percent of families did not understand basic information (diagnosis, prognosis, treatments) after physician-family meetings in an intensive care setting (4), a finding that could lead to the potential of conflict with families that could impede an appropriate transition to palliative care in any setting. Well-structured discussions that focus on the disease process, the goals of palliative therapy, and understanding the concerns of family members may help the family formulate decisions that support the dignity and choices that the patient herself would have chosen (5).

To prevent problems, it is wise to respect several rules:

- Always ask the patient if she has preferences in her contacts with friends and relatives. Often, she wants special persons to be more involved with than others.
- Ask the patient for one or two contact persons to organize the communication with family and friends. Communicate essential information always in the presence of them or of other relatives or friends chosen by the patient. In this way, the family and friends are well informed and they share the same information with the patient. They also can help the patient with the evaluation of the information afterward.
- Never talk about the patient "behind her back." If the physician does, and the patient finds out, the relationship of trust may be upset and take quite some time before it is restored. This also prevents the patient thinking that the family knows more than she does, which can also put pressure on the family relationships.
- In countries where health care can become a financial threat to the family, it is the responsibility of the physician that decision making concerning continuation of treatment or starting a treatment is based on the ethical principles of autonomy, beneficence, and nonmaleficence. It is not acceptable that this decision making is influenced by financial outside pressure.

At the end of life, we can expect emotional reactions by patients and their significant others, including family, to the inevitable life style changes and impending death. It is the task of the physician to try to understand the thoughts and behavior of the patient to death and dying as well as her worries and unfinished emotional and personal business. Information on the patient's values and beliefs should be sought; even information about very personal matters like relationships and sexuality might be needed for a proper assessment of her situation. Also, it is important to respect the balance, and the patient has to know that she has the choice to what extent she wants to participate in this assessment and what information she is comfortable to share both with the physician or care team and with her family and friends. In normal life, family and friends often meet the spiritual and emotional needs of a patient, and the role of the health team is to support these relationships.

An example regarding involvement of family at the end of life:

> Mrs. A was a 71-year-old woman who was admitted to the hospital for evaluation because of general malaise and pain. Three years earlier, she received radiotherapy for an IIb cervical cancer. She developed a severe radiation proctitis for which she was treated with a colostomy. More recently, a pelvic recurrence had been diagnosed. With general management and mild pain killers, her situation was effectively palliated and she took care of herself in her own apartment. On admission, she appeared to be in moderately good physical condition, but she did not want any active treatment and asked us to let her die. She had an incurable disease and life made no sense to her anymore. After a few days, it was noted that the woman seemed to be depressed, and although she had three adult children and five grandchildren, nobody came to visit her. We asked her if she wanted to talk about her family. Her first reaction was ''no,'' but the next day she started to talk spontaneously about her family. She and her husband had always been very busy running a clothing store. Her husband had died suddenly 8 years ago. After his funeral, there was a discussion between her and her children about the family relationships when they were young. The children told the mother that they had felt neglected because the store had always been first priority. The discussion had ended in a break up of the family relationship. The grandchildren were born after that quarrel, and she had never seen them. She had never admitted to herself how she missed them, but now, facing the end of life, she realized how wrong the situation was. She saw no way to restore the relationship. We asked her permission to contact the children, which she at first refused, but later said: ''Do whatever you need to do.'' After one telephone call with the eldest son, the children came to the hospital and had an emotional but very satisfying reunion with their mother. Later, the grandchildren came, and the general and mental condition of the patient improved. She did not talk about ''just let me go'' anymore and wanted optimal palliative treatment. In the circle of her family, the patient lived another 10 months and finally died peacefully in the presence of her children.

This example clearly demonstrates how personal information and family-based communication and intervention is sometimes needed to optimize palliative care, but also how such a situation should be approached with the wishes of the patient being the primary focus.

UNIQUE CIRCUMSTANCES FOR DECISION MAKING: PREGNANT PATIENTS

A rare, but particularly poignant, context of end of life decision making is that of the pregnant woman with terminal, metastatic cancer where survival even to the end of a normal pregnancy is unlikely. The choices for palliative therapy (e.g., pelvic radiation for control of local bleeding and pressure) may directly impact the likelihood of fetal survival and the possibility of delivery of the newborn—including prematurely with all the known consequences—with no living mother make the choices even more complex for the woman and for her family. Clearly, the primary objective is alleviation of symptoms for the woman, and choices to decrease the level of relief in order to facilitate fetal development should only be considered if strongly desired and pursued by the patient herself. There is no role for withholding appropriate and maximal pain and symptom management simply because the woman has a concurrent pregnancy (6). In addition, the premature timing of delivery of the child and the likelihood of maternal survival to the age of viability of the fetus have to be weighed against the supporting family's ability and choices about caring for a significantly premature child. Clearly, the role of the woman in fixing the parameters for balancing the fetal well-being against her own needs for alleviation of pain and suffering is central, and decisions that balance toward comfort rather than fetal outcomes must be equally supported by her health-care team.

SITE OF CARE

The site of end of life care is often restricted by insurance coverage, family or support person availability, and availability of hospice services and respite services. Despite a desire overall to die at home, many die in acute settings. Assuring that patients participate in the decision-making process even in the acute setting is important, but the physician's ability to predict the patient's preferred role is poor and patients need the opportunity to state how they would like decisions to be made (7). The availability of palliative-care teams in the acute setting can ameliorate this substantially and facilitate options that support both the patient and the care team. Although most individuals desire a chance to die at home, this falters in the face of an individual's concerns about the ability of their care givers to take the stress of their care, as well as the care givers themselves feeling inadequate to manage either the care expected or the actual death itself (8). Planning for this aspect of care early and engaging appropriate support services and counseling earlier may allow more individuals to access the comfort and familiarity of their home during the dying process. Facilitation of this by the oncologist is a gift not only to the patient, but also to her family and support network.

MAXIMIZING PALLIATION: MANAGING SYMPTOMS AT THE END OF LIFE

Pain Control Issues Unique to End of Life Care

Overall, the main approach to pain is to estimate the level of pain with different activities or circumstances, evaluate the source to focus the therapy, and aggressively to provide pain relief. The ability to assure that patient's dying process will be free of pain and still will be able to be with her family and friends mentally is possible with our present pain armamentarium, and if it is indeed intractable—then "there is a case for ensuring that a patient at least sleeps peacefully during the last few days or hours of life, if that is preferred" (9).

The mainstay of therapy at the end of life is usually opioid analgesics as patients have long passed just nonsteroidal antiinflammatory drugs and acetaminophen alone. However, the multiplicity of tumor-related and therapy-related pain syndromes that result in various neuropathies from invasion, radiation, or other therapy are real and often respond better to nerve-blocking therapies (10). Anticonvulsants are often cited as being useful for these in addition to opioids, but actual data are lacking (11). The most commonly used would be carbamazepine, which appears to have the same efficacy as gabapentin when used for neuropathic pain. Additionally, antidepressants (e.g., amitriptyline, desipramine) may be helpful as they may also treat underlying depression, have their own direct analgesic effect, and potentiate opioid analgesia (12). Often more appropriate is the use of sacral or regional nerve blocks or ablation of nerve roots. This regional approach is particularly helpful, along with such vehicles as indwelling epidural catheters, for pelvic-based pain.

The use of opioids focuses on full agonists, most commonly morphine, and noninvasive techniques are preferred. Oral dosing is always preferred, if possible, and usually a sustained-release "base" is established with every 8- to 12-hour dosing and breakthrough pain covered by an immediate-release form of morphine or with other agents. Sustained-release formulations are available for morphine, oxycodone, and hydromorphone. Rectal formulations also exist and are probably underutilized, although patients with prior radiation or painful lesions in the area may not be able to utilize this method. Although this may offer a means of avoiding expensive and cumbersome equipment for home use, the loss of a dose or variability in absorption limit this option (13). Also, buccal, sublingual, and liquid formulations of opioids and fentanyl can be used if oral methods are difficult because of swallowing difficulties or other concerns. The final option to avoid intravenous pain management is the transdermal fentanyl patch. This is particularly helpful, when stabilized dosing is reached, for individuals who require continuous baseline coverage but are unreliable about taking doses of pain medications. The downside is the long time to peak concentrations, which renders initial evaluation and titration of dosages difficult and requires significant use of short-term release opioids to cover (14).

The use of intravenous forms of opioids with patient controlled-analgesia pumps is well described in many publications. The use of a basal intravenous infusion with patient-controlled boluses is the preferred method. Subcutaneous infusion of opioids can also be used, with near equivalent efficacy, and it can be more easily managed in some home settings (15). For all methods, titration to comfort is the goal with management of secondary symptoms such as nausea or sleepiness as needed by the patient and within the context of her goals. The last few hours of life can be marked by both increased or decreased pain, and a strategy to address this needs to be in place as part of the pain-control program.

Nausea and Vomiting: Bowel Obstruction

The etiology of nausea and vomiting at the end of life can be related to medications but more often is related to malignant bowel obstruction. Ovarian and endometrial cancers have a higher likelihood of developing obstruction. It is critical to distinguish the obstructed bowel from constipation/obstipation for obvious reasons in terms of management. Since the majority of patients are already at risk for constipation from medications as well as low motility of the bowel, both peristalsis stimulants and fecal softeners are required for an adequate bowel program with rectal laxatives added as needed. Clearly, resolution of constipation and impaction will relieve nausea and vomiting from this source (16,17).

The consideration for surgery for bowel obstruction should be limited to those in whom their overall condition is otherwise good. Various studies have shown that advanced age, poor general health or nutritional status, diffuse peritoneal carcinomatosis, ascites, palpable masses, prior radiation, and multiple obstructed sites carry a higher mortality and morbidity with a gain of an average of 5.3 months for those who successfully negotiate the surgical intervention (18). In gynecologic oncology, carefully chosen individuals can achieve considerable relief (up to 75% success) with surgical intervention, and this can endure for months (19). The hallmarks of evaluation beyond overall status include imaging procedures (Gastrografin enemas, carefully chosen use of computed tomographic and limited upper gastrointestinal evaluations) that target the identification of multiple sites of obstruction. Failure to identify the presence of multiple sites of obstruction can lead to failure of the procedure and add to the pain and discomfort of the patient during the dying phase.

Symptom management is usually the path taken in the treatment of bowel obstruction. Nasogastric tubes provide quick relief, but are uncomfortable, and some reports suggest that they are ineffective in longer term management of symptoms (18). Gastrostomy tubes are generally more effective, but require surgical intervention or interventional radiology intervention that may not be desired by patients. Distal obstruction can sometimes be relieved through the use of stent placement (20,21) if that is available, and is worth consideration.

Additionally, there are pharmacologic options to consider, with haloperidol being a key choice for antiemetics in the setting of bowel obstruction (22). Additionally, hysocine hydrobromide and hysocine butyl bromide are helpful with patients experiencing colicky pain and nausea. Corticosteroids have been used to reduce inflammation, and potentially reduce the obstruction in some patients, and are worth a trial as part of conservative management. Dexamethasone in a dose of 4 to 8 mg per day for 3 to 5 days is generally used for this (23). Finally, somatostatin analogues such as octreotide can limit the secretions and motility and diminish the symptoms of bowel obstruction overall (24).

Nutritional Management: Hypoproteinemia

The value of end of life nutritional maintenance must be firmly set in the context of what the goal of the intervention is. Maintenance of nutrition as its own end goal is *not* a goal at the end of life, as it does not serve a goal of medicine and would be considered to be a futile intervention to which we are not ethically obligated. At times, however, management of nutrition as a trial to achieve another palliative or quality of life goal, for example, to relieve symptoms of hypoproteinemia and decrease peripheral edema that has not responded adequately to other interventions for comfort or to maximize stamina for a special event, with a limited time line for treatment may be an appropriate strategy. In this context, the nutritional support is to achieve greater palliation of symptoms or to reach a clearly defined goal of the patient, and both ends must have defined time lines set with patients ahead of time to assess the efficacy of this strategy in meeting these goals. In a sense, it allows patients to try to meet the energy needs for the energy expenditure they have set as a goal (e.g., attending a child's graduation or wedding) that they are otherwise unable to accomplish.

The options for nutrition are enteral if feasible and parenteral if not. Most patients at the end of life have tried increased oral feeding, but owing to low transit times with associated nausea and lack of appetite, have ceased trying to eat. If a time-limited option to increase appetite is desired, then corticosteroids such as dexamethasone can be considered, although their efficacy is limited. Additional appetite stimulants include progesterones such as Megace. Both can have a limited impact on oral intake. Diet supplements then form the basis for increasing nutritional input, including simple formulations such as instant breakfast or intact protein formulations with low lactose.

Other enteral feeding approaches generally focus on feeding tubes either placed under fluoroscopy via a nasogastric approach or surgically placed in the jejunum or the stomach. These use protein hydrolysates with timed feedings or continuous infusions. The discomfort of the nasogastric feeding tubes sometimes prevents this means of enteral feeding from being effective, but does allow for easy removal. J-tubes require surgical intervention in abdomens where landmarks are possibly obscured by tumor, and placement must be evaluated in light of the potential issues with the type of tumor and the likelihood of surgical difficulty. In patients with low motility and partial obstruction, the use of enteral feeding formulations may allow the patient to meet her goals without requiring the cumbersome and more difficult to adjust total parenteral nutrition (TPN).

TPN remains the final option for attempting to improve nutritional status transiently in end of life care. Undertaking TPN ties a patient to an intravenous line as well as incurring increased expense and potential for morbidity that could add to the burden of symptoms at the end of life. It is often more than a support person can take on at home, and may obligate the individual to undesired care settings. Furthermore, intavenous access with ports in the face of terminal disease and often-compromised immune surveillance can result in infections that diminish access not only for TPN, but also for needed pain control or other intravenous medications (25). This, therefore, must be understood in a framework that defines clear stopping parameters (failure to meet goals of symptom relief or improved stamina for an event) and a clear overall time line. In general, TPN is not of benefit in the end of life and terminal care setting.

Ascites Management

For women with ovarian cancer, ascites (and associated pleural effusions) create continual pressure, pain, and diminished pulmonary capacity that significantly impacts activities of daily life and their quality of life in the dying process. Management relies on elements of constriction of influx and increasing efflux. The pathophysiology of malignant ascites is not only obstructed efflux through lymphatics in the diaphragm (26), but also increased production of fluid. The fact that the protein content of the fluid is 85% of plasma levels versus 25% of plasma levels for transudates suggests that the vessel walls are compromised (26). The emerging culprit is vascular endothelial growth factor (VEGF) (27). This suggests that novel approaches to blocking the VEGF receptor might improve the options available for management of this problem.

The mainstay of ascites management remains paracentesis, and this has been improved through ultrasound guidance. The use of pleuracentesis kits and vacuum bottles allows this to to be done in outpatient settings or even at the bedside at home with ease, and many patients are managed simply with once or twice weekly removal of 1 to 4 L in an office setting, often without fluid replacement. Large volumes of fluid (10 L) can be removed (28), but this must be balanced with colloid infusions and risks further diminishing the intravascular albumin and protein concentrations (29), leading to worsening anasarca and associated symptoms.

Another common strategy in the management of ascites is the use of diuretics to diminish vascular volume and loss through the vascular tree. Spironolactone is the mainstay of managing ascites associated with cirrhosis and is worth considering for malignant ascites (30). Other diuretics can be considered as well, particularly furosemide, but their primary benefit may be the peripheral edema associated with hypoproteinemia. There have been no clear head-to-head studies of diuretics versus paracentesis and quality of life outcomes in these patients to guide therapy.

In the presence of a slow-growing malignancy, but a palliative stage of disease that requires frequent paracentesis, peritoneovenous shunts can be considered. Both Denver and Le Veen shunts have been used, with a complication rate of 25% being quoted in a review of multiple series by Helzberg (31). The general health status of the patient is the primary determinant of whether such an invasive approach is warranted, with a survival of at least 3 months being a rule of thumb (32). Concerns about potential tumor dissemination or emboli are less significant in applying this to end of life care (33).

Unique Aspects of Pulmonary Management

Among the most frightening symptoms for women and their families at the end of life are the symptoms of dyspnea and chest pain. Three etiologies stand out in metastatic gynecologic cancers: malignant pleural effusions, parenchymal metastases, and nodal/ mediastinal metastases with airway compromise. Although quite different in etiology, some basic principles form the basis of symptom management. These include the use of oxygen, relief of brochospasm, control of secretions, and measures to promote relaxation, which are helpful with all these etiologies.

Probably the most difficult issue to treat is pleural effusions, particularly as they compound the pulmonary constriction caused by ascites in ovarian cancer patients. Thoracentesis (with ultrasound guidance) gives immediate relief, but reaccumulations are common. Repeated thoracentesis may be a strategy appropriate to short-term management or if only needed every few weeks, with the 4% or greater risk of pneumothorax with each procedure as well as the concurrent discomfort (34). Alternatives are restricted to those who have recurrent symptomatic pleural fluid, where this is the primary source of symptomatology and the survival is expected to be more than a few weeks. The primary option for these patients is chemical pleuradesis, now virtually always done with talc by direct application with video-assisted thoracoscopic surgery (VATS) or through a chest tube (35,36) Success is quoted as being as high as 91%, but the setting of repeated prior thoracentesis often lends itself to scarring that can make the procedure less effective. Any suggestion of a trapped lung or an endobronchial obstruction further

diminishes success to the point that pleuradesis would not be a useful choice (37). Most individuals will have a fever and moderate to severe pain around the time of instillation, and complications include arrhythmias, pneumonitis, empyema, and respiratory failure. Such a procedure requires the patient to be in the hospital, occasionally in the intensive care unit for observation overnight if a VATS plus talc procedure is done, and creates costs and side effects that must be weighed carefully against the benefits. Clearly, pleuradesis should be restricted to individuals in whom this intervention has a significant chance of alleviating the primary symptoms to avoid exposing women unnecessarily to pain and side effects that further burden their dying phase of life.

Management of pulmonary metastases in the end of life setting, even if solitary, is focused on symptom relief. Many parenchymal lesions are asymptomatic, but pleural irritation can be problematic with coughing as well as hypoxemia. Lymphangitic carcinomatosis is less common in gynecologic malignancies than in others, such as breast or lung cancer, but dyspnea and hypoxemia with the thickened septa and interstitial edema are the primary symptoms to be managed. The dyspnea associated with lymphangitic spread is often symptomatically greater than the actual pulmonary disease present (38). Strategies to treat these symptoms are attention to environment, and diminishing walking or activity requires doing simple activities of daily living by changing the environment. The use of a fan for air circulation, nasal oxygen (with portable units), and trials of pursed lip breathing may all help. Certainly, consideration should be given to diuretic therapy if there is any component of fluid overload, and opiates, particularly morphine, are helpful. Morphine, often in use for pain control, also has a role in decreasing air hunger and dyspnea and should be tried in this setting if not already in use. Anxiolytics, although helpful for the anxiety component, often worsen symptoms by causing respiratory depression and should be used judiciously, if at all, for this component of symptom management.

Airway obstruction and cough have similar symptoms, and some of the therapy is similar. Cough may be due to multiple issues including conditions unrelated to malignancy such as asthma or sinusitis and from gastroesophageal reflux, which is more common with ascites. Therapies tailored specifically to these issues from the use of inhaled or intranasal steroids, antihistamines, and proton pump inhibitors for reflux are appropriate. Cough due to airway obstruction responds to narcotic suppression with morphine or codeine. Occasionally, steroid inhalers add additional relief from bronchial irritation induced by the metastatic disease. Even humidifiers may be helpful for some patients; particularly for coughs from irritated mucosal linings from prior mediastinal chest radiation. In some cases, radiation therapy targeted to specific areas of obstructing disease in the mediastinum, with an obviously longer survival estimate may be of value in managing symptoms. In sum, the therapies for pulmonary symptoms rely on local suppression of inflammation, suppression of cough and air hunger through opiates, and removal of fluid compression as needed.

Central Nervous System Involvement: Management of Seizures, Brain Metastases, Mental Status Changes

Mental status changes are present in the end of life population and management is often the key toward patients achieving their personal goals at the end of life, many of which center around being awake and conversant to bring closure with family and friends. Delirium is particularly distressing to family members who also are seeking closure with the dying patient. For both, the decline in function from a prior baseline heralds more losses to come and creates even greater anxiety. Etiologies can be metabolic abnormalities (sepsis, renal failure), innumerable drugs, and structural brain lesions with obvious differences in approach to treatment. There are clear predisposing factors including age, multisensory impairment, medical illness, depression, dehydration, and abnormal serum electrolyte levels are examples pertinent to the end stage of malignancies (39–41).

Understanding the nature of the delirium is important in addressing what may be more than one contributing factor. Assessing alertness, distractibility, the patient's ability to concentrate and talk easily, and simple cognitive disturbances of memory, reasoning, or perception all contribute to the delirium along with specific neurologic deficits or neuromuscular activity that can point to central nervous system metastases are all important. Laboratory and physical evaluation with infection, hypercalcemia, renal failure, hypoglycemia, hypomagnesemia, hypoxemia being key conditions to look for (42–44). Tuma and DeAngelis (45) noted that with appropriate workup, a significant number of patients can improve their symptoms (68%) even when terminal.

Obviously, addressing electrolytic abnormalities and treating infection have value when the goal is a clearer sensorium even if at the end of life. If opioid-induced delirium is the diagnosis, then rotation of types of opioids used or even a very low-level naloxone drip can be helpful in restoring function (46). If there are hallucinations and agitation, particularly in elderly dying patients, consideration of haloperidol or droperidol if more sedation is desired is appropriate (47,48). Given intravenously, haloperidol can be effective within 30 minutes and generally lasts for at least 4 hours. Given by mouth, the half-life of haloperidol is considerably longer, and could be used in mild delirium states. It is important to remember that these drugs have the potential of lowering the seizure threshold (49), as the more common electrolytic abnormalities associated with prior chemotherapy such as magnesium deficiency also may be present and compounds the risk. Finally, some patients may benefit from combining drugs and including a benzodiazepine. Some studies have noted that delirium in patients with advanced cancer more commonly requires more than one medication (50). The most commonly used are lorazepam (up to 2 mg) or midazolam, which is preferred if a subcutaneous route is to be used (51).

The other source of delirium or abnormalities in central nervous system function is brain metastasis. Initial therapy after diagnosis is the immediate use of corticosteroids to decrease local edema (52). This may, in fact, be all that is needed if the patient has a very short time to live as median survival with brain metastasis with steroids alone is about 2 months. However, if a patient is otherwise functional and treatment could improve their overall quality of life, then targeted radiation therapy should be considered. For this use, generally 300 Gy total dose given in 30-Gy fractions is administered (53). For care at the end of life, more aggressive resection and radiation is generally not appropriate.

Local Comfort Measures

Many of the measures for comfort at the end of life are related to common sense care that can escape notice but creates comfort for the dying woman (55). The environment itself gives comfort if familiar things are around, including sounds, smells, and pictures that hold meaning for the woman. The physician's role in assuring that the issues of access and fall prevention are addressed either by the physician or by a care team is important to the success of home care. Skin protection through rotation if the patient is bed bound and early identification and treatment of skin breakdown prevents unnecessary sources of pain and infection. Many patients derive great comfort from gentle massage and virtually all benefit from human touch and presence. Developing a plan for passive (or active) movement during the day alleviates pain and discomfort from decreased mobility. Eye care with artificial tears or even hydrogel eye patches may be needed. Perineal care and the use of catheters if needed to eliminate skin breakdown in the perineum are commonly used. While these are common sense, many families and patients need permission from their health-care team to make the environment home rather than a hospital at home. Yet, it is the breeze from the window, the smells of home, the sights of loved ones rocking in a chair beside them that bring the most comfort—and the physician must actively support choices that make this possible at the end of life.

Management of Fistulas in the Terminal Care Setting

The fistulas encountered at the end of life from both the urinary system and the gastrointestinal (GI) system are often the most difficult for family and care givers to deal with. The principles of management are relatively simple but difficult to achieve. The options are diversion, containment, and closure regardless of the site of the fistula.

Enterocutaneous fistulae can occur from every part of the

bowel, but those from the small bowel have high-frequency output and are highly irritating to the skin. Diversion is difficult in the setting of terminal cancer, primarily because the intraabdominal spread of disease is often the etiology of the fistula itself in association with prior therapies such as radiation. Occasionally, the options expand to surgical diversion (rather than resection with reanastamosis) if the terminal path does not include significant intraabdominal involvement solely to provide better control and better fit of pouches over the ostomy site than over a fistula site. As noted by Marsden et al., this does not remove the problem as there may still be a discharge from the site of tumor-related necrotic material that must be managed (55). If this is not possible, the only recourse—similar to bowel obstruction—is to attempt to diminish flow through the GI tract with somatostatin and then to minimize and manage skin irritation actively. Large bowel fistula, most commonly to the vagina, can be more easily diverted and this is the first choice if the patient is medically stable. Even a simple loop colostomy can provide relief from the volume of vaginal discharge. However, some discharge usually remains. The use of metronidazole for tumor necrosis and discharge in the vaginal area relieves some of the anaerobic odors, and sitz baths and douches as needed to control odor are also helpful.

Vesicovaginal and ureterovaginal fistulae are primarily handled by diversion if appropriate. The primary problem with diversion is the management of new percutaneous nephrostomies, and the additional factor that for some patients there may be a component of renal failure that there is no desire to reverse. Additionally, nephrostomies alone may not be adequate for resolution, and the use of ureteral occlusion with coils and sponge pledgets may also be helpful (56). Local measures, including scrupulous management of pelvic and perineal hygiene, the use of adult diapers, and the use of creams such as 1% silver sulfasalazine or skin barriers are primary measures. There are no vaginal means to control or contain the output that have so far been effective. Various measures such as the use of diaphragms glued to catheters or local tissue glues have generally been ineffective. There are reports of successful closure of fistulae with fibrin glue and bovine collagen (57), but not in the terminal setting.

Management of Bone Metastases

Bone metastases are rare in terminal gynecologic cancers, being primarily confined to unusually high-grade cell types such as glassy-cell, neuroendocrine tumors, small-cell, or clear-cell malignancies. When they occur, however, the pain associated with bone metastases can be the most excruciating of all the symptoms we deal with. If the metastases are limited in nature, radiation therapy on a palliative basis may supply additional pain relief with a success rate of 50% total pain relief and 80% to 90% of patients noting relief of pain (58). Relief of pain may be immediate or it may require

several months, and the use of antiinflammatory pain medications during treatment may aide in symptom relief until the effects of radiation become evident.

Key aspects of treatment include assuring that radiation fields encompass the entire area of bone involvement (59) and also the prevention of overlap with prior radiation fields. Multiple schemes have been used depending on the urgency and the overall expected survival time of the patient. However, longer radiation courses with higher doses do seem to have a slight advantage and should be considered in those patients with a longer life expectancy (60). Also, if there is a longer life expectancy, consideration should be given to prophylactic surgical fixation of weight-bearing bones with >50% cortical destruction or size >2.5 cm prior to radiation therapy (61,62).

Another option for consideration is the use of osteoblastaffinic agents such as strontium 89 or samarium 153 that deliver localized radiation to osteoblastic bony metastases. The primary problem in their use is the bone marrow suppression, which often limits their use in patients with ongoing residual suppression from their prior therapies. These agents are not appropriate for use in hypercalcemic patients, and the pain relief is slower in onset with duration of about 12 weeks. This option may require multiple doses to increase efficacy (63).

Regardless of the methods chosen, separate therapy for the bone metastases from that of pain medication can significantly improve palliation and pain control for the woman with bone metastases.

Psychologic Symptoms in Terminally Ill Cancer Patients

An important aspect of palliative care in terminally ill cancer patients is the recognition of psychologic symptoms. Depression and anxiety occur in a high percentage of cancer patients, particularly as disease advances and curative cancer treatment fails (64). Also, increasing physical disability has been found to be significantly correlated with an increased prevalence of depression and anxiety (65,66). The prevalence of depression in cancer patients has been the subject of numerous studies, and the reported rates have ranged from as high as 58.0% to as low as 4.5% depending on choices of study population and measurement instruments (67,68).

Anxiety in terminally ill cancer patients has received less attention than depression (69). Anxiety commonly increases as patients become aware of both the relative ineffectiveness of medical treatments in halting the progress of their disease and, consequently, their limited life expectancy (66). The awareness of the future death is likely to cause anxiety in terminally ill cancer patients. So far, little is known about depression and anxiety in terminally ill cancer patients in the last weeks before their death. Still, the treatment of these conditions has a place in the palliative care setting.

Recently, the prevalence of physical and psychologic

symptoms in terminally ill cancer patients with a life expectancy of less than 3 months was studied at the University Medical Center Utrecht, the Netherlands (70). The patients were from the departments of gynecology, internal medicine, lung diseases, hematology, and head and neck surgery. Depression and anxiety, depressive mood [Hospital Anxiety and Depression Scale (HADS)] and control of symptoms (Edmonton Symptom Assessment scale) were assessed in 80 patients with a life expectancy of less than 3 months. Fifty-six of the patients were women and the mean age was 61 years (range 32 to 84 years). The median period between the date the questionnaire was filled in and the date of dying was 1.3 months. There was a 14% prevalence of self-reported anxiety and 25% prevalence of self-reported depression. Anxiety and depression were primarily related to decreasing physical performance. Thirty-eight of the patients did not report anxiety or depression. The physical symptoms experienced by terminally ill cancer patients most related to anxiety and depression were shortness of breath, impaired well-being, pain, drowsiness, fatigue, and inactivity. The findings of a depression prevalence of 25% on the HADS coincides with the conclusion of Massie et al. (68) that among hospitalized cancer patients with significant levels of physical impairment, at least 25% suffer from clinical depression. An extensive review of Hotopf et al. showed that 29% of patients with advanced cancer scored ≥ 11 on the HADS depression subscale (71), which is also in agreement with our findings.

Breitbart suggests that the incidence of anxiety and depression in cancer patients increases with higher levels of disability, advanced illness, and pain (67). The closer the patient is to dying, the higher the score on depression and the lower the score on physical performance. In our study, anxiety and depression both increased with higher levels of pain.

Fishbain et al. also reviewed the relationship between the development of pain and the development of depression with similar linkages being found (72).

Although depression and anxiety are not routinely assessed in terminally ill patients prior to death, these data show that a relatively high percentage of terminally ill cancer patients suffer from psychologic distress a few weeks before death, which appears to be related to physical symptoms. This indicates that psychologic symptoms in terminally ill cancer patients need to be systematically assessed and considered by the physician in the overall decision making concerning the end of life. Treatment of anxiety and depression clearly also improves overall management of pain as well as making the process of closure more possible for dying women.

ROLE OF PHYSICIAN-ASSISTED SUICIDE AND EUTHANASIA ISSUES AND CONTEXT

The beginning and the end of life are probably the most emotional and impressive events a human can go through.

The newborn baby, as well as the patient who is dying, need all our attention and care. The very concept of palliative care is based on the basic commitment of the care giver to relieve all suffering. However, an important component of the suffering of cancer patients happens in their minds. Human beings have many emotional, spiritual, and social needs, and they can all contribute to the suffering of the patient. It is not always possible for any physician to meet all these needs. Even if everything possible has been done to relieve the symptoms of the patient including all the dimensions of suffering, physicians can find themselves at the limits of their professional abilities. The best the physician can do is to offer professional skills in combination with their own humanity. Sometimes, psychiatric or psychologic help is needed as well to deal with emotional levels of suffering. This balance between compassionate support and professional care can be difficult at the end of life for everyone involved, particularly physicians (73).

Sometimes, patients ask to end their life because of unbearable suffering. In most countries in the world, the law forbids assisted suicide or euthanasia. However, in the Netherlands, Belgium, and the United States (state of Oregon), access to euthanasia or assisted suicide is available for those experiencing unbearable suffering and is regulated. Decisions regarding assisted suicide are difficult for all concerned, and the concern that such access might diminish the attention paid to palliative care has been often expressed. However, data from Oregon (74) show that attention to and delivery of palliative care and home site of care and support at the end of life were both significantly improved by the presence of access to assisted suicide. Furthermore, this extended to development of a key hot-pink form that traveled with terminal patients from home to hospital settings, assuring that at all times the health-care team was aware of issues like DNR status and the patient's wishes about resuscitative care at the end of life (74).

Ethical Aspects

According to Krishna and Raffin, four principles—autonomy, beneficence, nonmaleficence, and justice—are necessary for a physician to make sound ethical decisions and should form the basis of decisions at the end of life, including decisions regarding assisted suicide (75):

Autonomy

The principle of autonomy supports the right for every patient who has a sound state of mind to self-determination over his or her own life. This translates into the right to choose among medically sound options (not just anything the patient desires for their care) or no care or intervention. How individuals—both patient and health-care professional—consider that these options can be interpreted differently depends on the religion and culture of the patient. Many religions consider life as a gift of God and nobody has the right to decide to end one's life, including the patient herself.

Beneficence

Beneficence is the core ethical principle of the Hippocratic oath. In today's language, the ethical principle of beneficence means that the primary responsibility of the physician is to achieve a goal of medicine (benefit the patient) through the proposed therapies. This principle obligates the physician to protect and promote the best medical interests of the patient. Among these are the following:

- The prevention of premature or unnecessary death
- The prevention, cure, or at least management of disease, injury, handicap, and unnecessary pain and suffering

Nonmaleficence

The physician should not do anything that can directly harm the patient. This principle is based on the Hippocratic principle whereby physicians were prohibited from administering drugs with the deliberate intention of causing a patient's death. It also is a constant reminder that unintended consequences occur from every beneficial intervention—some anticipated and some not. It is the role of the health professional to consider these harmful side effects, and not create greater harm than benefit in the course of care.

Justice

The fourth major ethical principle, justice, means that there must be a means of assuring that there is a just allocation and access to health care for all citizens (75,76). In considering the context of euthanasia and assisted suicide, it is helpful to recognize three different medical decisions concerning the end of life (MDEL) (77):

1. Nontreatment decisions.
2. Euthanasia and assisted suicide.
3. Alleviation of pain and other symptoms with medication that finally hastens the patient's death is also called "the principle of double effect."

These three MDEL all differ with respect to ethics and jurisprudence. The most important distinctions between them are the intention of the physician, the nature of the critical action, and the consent of the patient (78).

Nontreatment decisions and alleviation of pain and/or other symptoms with high dosages of opioids are medical decisions that belong to the domain of the physician. The decision is made in the best interest of the patient and the intention is to relieve the suffering even if that means shortening or not actively prolonging life. Like other medical

decisions at the end of life, the responsible physician makes these decisions in close cooperation with the team of care givers. The decision is then discussed with the patient and the family before it is executed.

Euthanasia and Assisted Suicide (EAS)

In the Netherlands, one of the very few countries in the world that has regulated euthanasia, this procedure is understood to mean "the intentional termination of the life of a patient at his or her request by a physician" (79,80). As a consequence of this definition, termination of life without the request of the patient (so-called "nonvoluntary" or "involuntary" euthanasia) as well as the so-called "principle of double effect" are not considered to fulfill the criteria of euthanasia (81).

Physician-assisted suicide is the provision by a physician of a means to a patient to end his or her life with the understanding that the person intends to use them to end his or her own life (78). The intention to end the patient's life makes this decision one that goes beyond the responsibility of the physician and raises questions about the fundamental principles on which the doctor/patient relationship is founded. Society as a whole is involved, and for this reason the policy concerning euthanasia and assisted suicide must be the result of in-depth discussions between all groups involved and finally needs judicial or legislative oversight and approval.

Those in favor of EAS argue that the principle of autonomy is the most important reason to agree to a voluntary request for EAS from a patient who has a sound mental state (78,82–86). Second, they claim that beneficence also supports euthanasia because sometimes continuation of life can cause more pain and suffering than death (78,87,88). Ending a human life in these exceptional circumstances is seen as a humane act or as a mercy killing.

Opponents of EAS, on the other hand, are of the opinion that a human life is always sacred and that ending it, even at the request of the patient, can never be approved (76). Rather than resorting to the option of euthanasia, physicians should be better trained in palliative therapies. So, they argue, beneficence alone cannot justify the legalizing of euthanasia (78). Ten Have and Welie have stressed that a physician will only agree to the request of a patient if he or she is confident that the patient is suffering intolerably and/or that the quality of life of the patient is very poor (80). According to them, it is impossible to make a decision about euthanasia based on both autonomy and beneficence as suggested by van Delden and co-workers (80,89). Others believe that the principle of beneficence is respected because the patient considers her suffering as unnecessary and every decision to prolong her life as disproportional suffering.

Modern medicine can prolong life far beyond the point where the patient would normally have died. By granting the request for euthanasia, it has been argued, the health team brings the patient back to the point that modern medicine has removed them from preventing harm (nonmaleficence) in the course of treatment. In this context, it must be clear that euthanasia and assisted suicide can only be allowed if the patient is able to make such a decision without any pressure (financial, social, emotional, medical) from outside. With that ideal in mind, EAS might only be considered in societies where equal health care without negative financial consequences for the family is available for all patients. As a consequence, EAS can only be practiced in a society that respects this equal allocation of care within the principle of justice.

How Can EAS Be Regulated?

The Netherlands was the first country in the world to regulate euthanasia. Until recently, the termination of the life of a severely suffering patient at his or her request remained a crime. Physician-assisted suicide and euthanasia were, theoretically, subject to criminal law. Legislation developed by Parliament concerned only the procedures for administering euthanasia without decriminalizing or legalizing it (79,80). Together with the Royal Dutch Society of Medicine, Parliament had developed precise criteria that needed to be fulfilled before EAS could be practiced. The Penal Code has recently been changed, and the present legislation decriminalizes euthanasia in situations where the specific criteria are met.

From November 1998, the notification procedure of euthanasia and assisted suicide has been in the hands of five regional committees (consisting of one physician, one lawyer, and one ethicist) who check the EAS procedure according to the precise criteria described below. This committee informs the public prosecutor within 6 weeks of the euthanasia or physician-assisted suicide. The aim of these committees is to increase reporting of euthanasia cases, to give feedback about the euthanasia process to the responsible physician, and to gain information about different aspects of euthanasia.

Reasons to Request Euthanasia

It is often suggested in the literature that a lack of adequate palliative care in the Netherlands may cause requests for euthanasia or physician-assisted suicide (79,90–92). In general, suffering by the dying patient goes far beyond physical pain that may be relieved but the suffering endures. Even relief of psychologic symptoms may not relieve the suffering endured by an individual at the end of life. Other factors (such as loss of mobility and activity) associated with increasing helplessness and dependence on others can cause distress. Another component of suffering is the loss of dignity. Although this is a very subjective component, it is considered by patients to be very important. That these are underlying causes for a request for euthanasia or physician-

assisted suicide is borne out by the results of the Dutch surveys. Van der Maas et al. found that patients requested euthanasia or physician-assisted suicide for the following reasons: loss of dignity (57% of cases), pain (46%), dying in an undignified way (46%), dependence on others (33%), or being tired of life (23%). In only 10 of the 187 cases was pain given as the single reason (81). These results correspond with those of a study by van der Wal et al., in which in only 5% of cases pain was found to be the most important reason for requesting euthanasia (93). Emanuel et al. concluded, after interviewing 155 oncologic patients, that patients experiencing pain are unlikely to desire euthanasia or physician-assisted suicide in contradistinction to patients suffering depression (94). It is possible that the oncologic patients in pain were worried that the palliative care and attempts to relieve pain would be reduced if euthanasia and physician-assisted suicide were legal (94).

At the University Medical Center Utrecht, we compared the records of 95 patients who died by euthanasia between 1992 and 1999 with 178 randomly selected control patients (2 per euthanasia case) who died of cancer in a natural way. The euthanasia group had more individuals who did not have a clear religion (79% vs 63%) and more gynecologic and head and neck cancers. The euthanasia patients had a better prognosis at the beginning of therapy and they had more surgeries. The control of pain was less optimal in patients who died of euthanasia (86% vs 99% at the day of dying). This might explain why the palliative care team was more often consulted for them. We know that pain plays an important role in 70% to 80% of all patients with terminal cancer. This group is consistent with the 10% of all terminally ill oncologic patients in whom it is not possible adequately to relieve all pain symptoms.

The most dominant physical complaints were gastrointestinal (64% in the euthanasia group and 71% in the control group), but these complaints were adequately treated in more than two-thirds of the patients. The diagnosis of depression was only made in one patient in the euthanasia group and in two in the control group, although all were examined for psychologic distress.

At the University Medical Center Utrecht, the reason to request euthanasia was primarily unbearable suffering and/or the hopelessness of their situation. It is noteworthy that in the control group, 52% of the patients were thought to have died as a consequence of their interventions for palliation (the principle of double effect). Both situations reflect a desire by patients to make autonomous decisions about the nature of the care they want to receive and the associated quality of life (95).

Guidelines for the Euthanasia Procedure

The discussion on euthanasia started in the Netherlands after the Postma case in February 1973, in which a family physician had administered a lethal injection of medicine to a terminally ill patient at her own explicit request. In the years after 1973, the discussion about euthanasia was concerned mainly with the acceptance of euthanasia and the development of appropriate criteria (96).

The courts drew up 25 specific criteria that had to be met if the physician were to avoid prosecution. These criteria reflected the discussions in Dutch society over 30 years. They can be summarized as follows:

- The patient must consider that his or her suffering is unbearable and hopeless. For this reason, it is important that the patient be well informed about his or her prognosis and the possibilities that palliative care has to offer.
- The wish to die must be well considered and persistent. This criterion includes the fact that the patient must be sound of mind, and the request for euthanasia must be done repeatedly.
- The request must be voluntary. This request has to be written down and signed by the patient. Furthermore, the wish to die may not be influenced by pressure from outside, from the relatives, or the medical personnel.
- The physician must consult at least one other physician. This consulted physician has to be independent and may not be involved in the treatment of the patient. He or she has to reconfirm the hopeless prognosis and the certainty of death.
- The request for euthanasia has to be discussed in a team of involved care givers: nurses, physicians, social workers, and preferably also the general practitioner. It is the task of this team to keep a close eye on the procedure and to determine whether all precise criteria have been precisely and carefully followed.
- The physician may not ascribe the death to natural causes and is obliged to keep proper records.

The relatives of the patients are always involved in the discussion after a request for euthanasia from a patient. However, the autonomy of the patient is considered as the most important factor, and the patient's request for euthanasia can still be approved even if the relatives disapprove. The above criteria for the practice of euthanasia have matured over 30 years of practice. The result is an open procedure that gives society much of the control. For the patient and the family, it is meant to guarantee a carefully considered procedure. It is important that the physician responsible for the patient meets these criteria.

Process of Euthanasia

Most terminal cancer patients fear the final phase of life. This fear will be discussed only when a relationship based on mutual trust exists between a patient and his or her physician; some patients may then express the wish for euthanasia. According to Hilhorst, this request for euthanasia can often be interpreted as an expression of the inner need to maintain a sense of intactness as an individual with personal control

over events. The simple fact that this possibility is not rejected outright gives a patient peace of mind and confidence (97). As van der Maas et al. reported, two-thirds of these requests never result in euthanasia because physicians can often offer alternatives (81).

On the basis of the Utrecht experience, the following factors can hinder adequate decision making with regard to euthanasia: (a) lack of information or conflicting information; (b) lack of knowledge of potential palliative terminal care; (c) difficulties coping with the concept of euthanasia; (d) frequent changes of personnel during days, nights, and weekends, leading to a lack of identification with the patient; and (e) ad hoc policy during evening and night shifts or during the weekends owing to the absence of attending physicians. To minimize the adverse influence of these five factors, the attending physician, as the one responsible for the interests of the patient, has to ensure an optimal exchange of information on the ward and within the team. Moreover, it is a strict rule that nobody is involved in the process of euthanasia against his or her own personal convictions. We consider this to be an important and precise criterion in the practice of euthanasia. Furthermore, it is very important that the moment of administration of the euthanaticum is planned carefully, so that the attending physician and nurse(s) can devote their attention entirely to the patient and his or her relatives (98–100).

Bereaved Family and Friends

Grief is a normal reaction to the death of a loved one and normally does not require any professional help. Sometimes grief is traumatic, which means that the grief symptoms take too long or too short, are not intense enough or too intense, or come too late. In the general population, 10% to 20% of bereaved people will suffer from traumatic grief. There are several risk factors for developing traumatic grief. The especially sudden loss of a partner or child are well-known risk factors. Unnatural death, such as suicide, also can cause severe grief reactions. Euthanasia is considered to be an unnatural death and, as such, it has been suggested that euthanasia may induce traumatic grief. However, the grief after suicide comes after an unexpected death, and frequently the relatives and friends did not have the opportunity to take leave of the person or achieve some closure with their own life issues. The grief after euthanasia or assisted suicide comes after a planned death and, in general, everybody had the opportunity to take leave of the dying person.

There were until recently no data in the literature about the mourning process of family and friends after euthanasia or assisted suicide in cancer patients. A recent cross-sectional study among family and friends of cancer patients who died by euthanasia and those of comparable cancer patients who died in a natural way has been published by the University Medical Center Utrecht (101). In this study, the bereaved family and friends of the euthanasia patients had less grief symptoms and posttraumatic stress reactions than the bereaved family and friends of the ones who died in a natural way. Adjustment for all other determinants for traumatic grief, including the duration of illness, did not influence the findings. The family and friends of the euthanasia group scored somewhat better on general well-being, whereas depressive symptoms were similar for both groups. A very important determinant of lower levels of grief symptoms was the possibility of saying goodbye and achieving closure. Another important factor is that the euthanasia process is executed without complications or unexpected situations. In our patients, the euthanasia processes went smoothly without unexpected situations. It is known from the study of Van der Boom that a complicated euthanasia process in AIDS patients was associated with complicated grief and added distress to the bereaved family and friends. This underlines strongly the importance of euthanasia being performed by experienced physicians who know what to do and how to do it.

The result of this study suggests that there is no reason to assume psychologic damage will occur to bereaved family and friends from the euthanasia experience. In fact, they experience a normal mourning process. The fact that the bereaved family and friends of the euthanasia patients experienced less grief symptoms can be explained by the fact that they had the opportunity to say goodbye while their loved ones were generally still fully aware. Besides, the bereaved family and friends of the euthanasia patients were better prepared for the way and day of the imminent death because they were able to talk openly with the patient and with the care team about death. These results underline how important this open communication and the possibility of saying goodbye are in terminal care in general. This is an important lesson for all health professionals regardless of their personal convictions about euthanasia. Assuring closure for the family with the patient is an important part of the terminal care for all patients.

Care for the Care Givers

Nothing is known about the effect euthanasia or assisted suicide has on the mental health of the involved physicians and nurses. Within palliative care in general and end of life care in particular, there is a tendency for patients and relatives to demand a more personal care and personal approach. Because of this contact-intensive nature of end of life care, it can be expected that physicians and nurses run a serious risk of depleting their emotional resources, especially when they cross the border between their professional and personal involvement. Finally, this can result in the burnout syndrome. Physicians and nurses should be aware of the risk factors in order to prevent this serious threat to their health. In oncology, and especially in end of life care, the stressors appear to be strongly related to the social and interpersonal aspects of the job, including the relationships with patients and co-workers on the team (102–105).

The fact that oncologists are regularly faced with their limited ability to alter the course of the illness is a major emotional discomfort. Another potential stressor is the concern about ethical issues and strong identification with the suffering of the patient. This can result in overcommitment and emotional exhaustion. Here we reach what can be called "the richness of oncology," which describes the situation that the patient has a strong, dependent relationship with the physician that is based on trust and belief in his or her abilities. The physician is seen as being competent and important. This can be very satisfying but it can also result in stress because of the heavy emotional burden and the emotional circumstances in which the relationship takes place and the pressure on the physician to avoid "failure."

To understand and prevent emotional exhaustion and burnout, physicians and nurses should be able to share their responses and feelings with others at work. This can be done by the organization of support groups at work where they can discuss what moved them and how they dealt with the situation (105–108). The participants get the opportunity to discuss the emotional aspects of the care of the terminal patient. On many occasions, this revisits conversations about life, death, and fertility with patients and their family. The team listens and discusses how these emotional events affected the person involved. Especially for younger and inexperienced personnel, this type of guidance by "peers" is very important. Young and inexperienced personnel always think that they are the first and only ones who ever experienced these emotions. As a result, they try to "reinvent the wheel," running the risk of an overly strong emotional involvement. The more experienced members of the team can provide perspective and insight into how to manage these difficult circumstances. For the more experienced members, the team meetings can work as control. Much experience can result in diminished emotional involvement and distancing the relationships to a routine. Comments, advice, and help of colleagues is one of the most important factors in staying mentally fit—again, a message for all health professionals, not just those involved in euthanasia.

CONCLUSIONS

End of life care is a very important part of palliative care. It requires total commitment of the entire health-care team. It includes medical interventions to relieve the suffering, but also psychosocial care. Communication skills are very important to assure effective end of life care. In this communication, the autonomy of the patient has to be respected. The care givers have to realize that they have to respect the delicate balance between professional and personal involvement. Communication not only involves the patient, but also her relatives and friends. It is important that this communication takes place in the presence of the patient as much as possible to avoid misunderstandings. Psychologic symptoms need to be routinely assessed and considered by physicians in the overall decision making concerning the end of life. Special attention should be paid to anxiety and depression.

End of life care in oncology does not mean that the physician has to postpone the inevitable as long as possible. In the course of adequate pain or symptom management, the side effects may shorten the time to death (principle of double effect), which is a well-recognized consequence of assuring maximal palliative care. This is a universally accepted consequence, and appropriate for end of life care. In the Netherlands and Belgium, euthanasia and physician-assisted suicide are accepted in end of life care, where the wish to die with dignity is the most important reported reason to request euthanasia.

Recent data have shown that euthanasia has no negative effect on the mourning process of family and friends; to the contrary, after euthanasia, we found less complicated grief in family and friends than after a natural death. This highlights the importance of paying attention to assuring that all patients and their families achieve closure and the ability to say goodbye when death is imminent. Unfortunately, little is known about the effect of euthanasia on physicians and nurses. However, we know that the intensive nature of palliative care in oncology is a risk factor for emotional exhaustion and burnout for all health providers. For this reason, good end of life care should not only include the patient and the family, but also the care givers.

REFERENCES

1. Seale C. *Constructing death*. Cambridge, UK: Cambridge University Press, 1998:31.
2. Callahan D. Living and dying with medical technology. *Crit Care Med.* 2003;31:S344–S346.
3. Burns JP, Edwards J, Johnson J, et al. Do-not-resuscitate order after 25 years. *Crit Care Med.* 2003;31:1543–1550.
4. Azoulay E, Chevret S, Leleu G, et al. Half the families of intensive care unit patients experience inadequate communication with physicians. *Crit Care Med* 2000;28:3044–3049.
5. Way J, Back AL, Curtis JR. Withdrawing life support and resolution of conflict with families. *BMJ* 2002;325:1342–1345.
6. Milliez J, Veronique C. Palliative care with pregnant women. *Best Pract Res Clin Obstet Gynecol.* 2001;15:323–331.
7. Heyland DK, Tranmer J, O'Callaghan CJ, Gafni A. The seriously ill hospitalized patient: preferred role in end of life decision making? *J Crit Care* 2003;18:3–10.
8. Evans N, Walsh H. The organization of death and dying in today's society. *Nurs Stand* 2002;16:33–38.
9. Lickiss JN, Hacker NF. Care of the patient close to death. *Best Pract Res Clin Obstet Gynecol* 2001;15:333–40.
10. Gordin V, Weaver MA, Hahn MB. Acute and chronic pain management in palliative care. *Best Pract Res Clin Obstet Gynecol* 2001;15: 203–234.
11. Wiffen P, Collins S, McQuay H, et al. Anticonvulsant drugs for acute and chronic pain. Cochrane Database of Systematic Reviews, 2002: Issue 4.
12. Hammond DL. Pharmacology of central pain-modulating networks (biogenic amines and non-opioid analgesics). *Adv Pain Res Ther* 1985;9:499–512.
13. Maloney CM, Kesner RK, Klein G, et al. The rectal administration of MS Contin: clinical implications of use in end stage cancer. *Am J Hospice Care* 1989;6:34–35.
14. Ashburn MA, Lipman AG. Management of pain in the cancer patients. *Anesth Analg* 1993;76;402–416.
15. Bruera E. Subcutaneous administration of opioids in the management of cancer pain. In: Foley K, Ventafridda V, eds. *Advances in pain research and therapy*. Vol. 16. New York: Raven Press, 1990: 203–218.
16. Sykes NP. Constipation management in palliative care. *Geriatr Med* 1997;27:55–57.
17. Agra Y, Sacristan A, Gonzalez M, et al. Efficacy of senna versus lactulose in terminal cancer patients treated with opioids. *J Pain and Symptom Manage* 1998;15:1–7.
18. Baines MJ. The pathophysiology and management of malignant intestinal obstruction. In: Doyle D, Hanks GWC, MacDonald N, eds. *Oxford textbook of palliative medicine*. Oxford, Uk: Oxford University Press. 1998:526–534.
19. Rubin SC, Hoskins WJ, Benjamin I, Lewis JL Jr. Palliative surgery for intestinal obstruction in advanced ovarian cancer. *Gynecol Oncol* 1989;34:16–19.
20. Diaz PL, Pinto PI, Fernandex LR, et al. Palliative treatment of malignant colorectal strictures with metallic stents. *Cardiovasc Intervent Radiol* 1999;22:29–36.
21. Tack J, Gevener AM, Rutgeerts P. Self-expandable metallic stents in the palliation of rectosigmoid carcinoma: a follow up study. *Gastrointest Endosc* 1998;48:267–271.
22. Baines MJ. Nausea, vomiting, and intestinal obstruction. In: Fallon M, O'Neill B, eds. *ABC of palliative care*. London: BMJ Books, 1998: 16–18.
23. Phillip J, Lickiss N, Grant PT, Hacker NF. Corticosteroids in the management of bowel obstruction in advanced ovarian cancer. *Gynecol Oncol* 1999;74:68–73.
24. Mangili G, Franchi M, Mariani A, et al. Octreotide in the management of bowel obstruction in terminal ovarian cancer. *Gynecol Oncol* 1996; 61:345–348.
25. Chang L, Tsai JS, Huang SJ, Shih CC. Evaluation of infectious complications of the implantable venous access system in a general oncologic population. *Am J Infect Control* 2003;31:34–9.
26. Nagy JA, Herzberg KT, Dvorak JM, Dvorak HF. Pathogenesis of malignant ascites formation: initiating events that lead to fluid accumulation. *Cancer Res* 1993;53:2631–2643.
27. Kraft A, Weindel K, Ochs A, et al. Vascular endothelial growth factor in the sera and effusions of patients with malignant and nonmalignant disease. *Cancer* 1999;85:178–187.
28. Arroyo V, Gines P, Planas R. Treatment of ascites in cirrhosis. Diuretics, peritoneovenous shunt, and large-volume paracentesis. *Gastroenterol Clin North Am* 1992;21:237–256
29. Gough IR, Balderson GA. Malignant ascites: a comparison of peritoneovenous shunting and nonoperative management. *Cancer* 1993;71: 2377–2382.
30. Greenway B, Johnson PJ, William R. Control of malignant ascites with spironolactone. *Br J Surg* 1982;69:441–442.
31. Helzberg JH, Greenberger NJ. Peritoneovenous shunts in malignant ascites. *Dig Dis Sci* 1985;30:1104–1107.
32. Souter RG, Tarin D, Kettlewell MG. Peritoneovenous shunts in the management of malignant ascites. *Br J Surg* 1983;70:478–481.
33. Fildes J, Narvaez GP, Baig KA, et al. Pulmonary tumor embolization after peritoneovenous shunting for malignant ascites. *Cancer* 1988; 61:1973–1976.
34. Bartter T, Mayo PD, Pratter MR, et al. Lower risk and higher yield for thoracentesis when performed by experienced operators. *Chest* 1993;103:1873–1876.
35. Light RW. Malignant pleural effusions. In: Light RW, ed. *Pleural diseases*. 3rd ed. Baltimore: Williams & Wilkins, 1995:90–116.
36. Kennedy L, Sahn SA. Talc pleuradesis for the treatment of pneumothrox and pleural effusion. *Chest* 1994;106:1215–1222.
37. Sahn SA. Malignancy metastatic to the pleura. *Clin Chest Med* 1998; 19:351–356.
38. Tucakovic M, Bascom R, Bascom PB. Pulmonary medicine and palliative care. *Best Pract Res Clin Obstet Gynecol* 2001;15:291–304.
39. Schor JD, Levkoff SE, Lipsitz LA, et al. Risk factors for delirium in hospitalized elderly. *JAMA* 1992;267:827–831.

40. Bruera E, Miller L, McCallion J, et al. Cognitive failure in patients with terminal cancer: a prospective study. *J Pain Symptom Manage* 1992;7:192–195.

41. Minagawa H, Yosuke U, Yamawaki S, Ishitani K. Psychiatric morbidity in terminally ill cancer patients: a prospective study. *Cancer* 1996; 78:1131–1137.

42. deStoutz ND, Tapper M, Faisinger RL. Reversible delirium in terminally ill patients. *J Pain Symptom Manage* 1995;10:249–253.

43. Seymour DG, Henschke PJ, Cape RDT, Campbell AJ. Acute confusional states and dementia in the elderly: the role of dehydration volume depletion, physical illness and age. *Age Ageing* 1980;9:137–146.

44. Bruera E. Severe organic brain syndrome. *J Palliat Care* 1991;7: 36–38.

45. Tuma R, DeAngelis L. Acute encephalopathy in patients with systemic cancer. *Ann Neurol* 1992;32:288.

46. Bruera E, Franco JJ, Maltoni M, et al. Changing pattern of agitated impaired mental status in patients with advanced cancer: association with cognitive monitoring, hydration and opioid rotation. *J Pain Symptom Manage* 1995;12:287–291.

47. Breitbart W, Marotta R, Platt MM, et al. A double blind trial of haloperidol, chlorpromazine, and lorazepan—the treatment of delirium in hospitalized AIDS patients. *Am J Psychiatry* 1996;153:231–237.

48. Resnick M, Burton B. Droperidol vs haloperidol in the initial management of acutely agitated patients. *J Clin Psychiatry* 1984;45:298–299.

49. Cold JA, Wells BG, Froemming JH. Seizure activity associated with antipsychotic therapy. *DICP* 1990;24:601–607.

50. Stiefel F, Fainsinger R, Bruera E. Acute confusional states in patients with advanced cancer. *J Pain Symptom Manage* 1992;7:94–98.

51. Bottomley D, Hanks G. Subcutaneous midazolam infusion in palliative care. *J Pain Symptom Manage* 1990;5:259–261.

52. Ruderman NB, Hall TC. Use of glucocorticoids in the palliative treatment of metastatic brain tumors. *Cancer* 1965;6:1–9.

53. Gaspar L, Scott C, Rotman M, et al. Recursive partitioning analysis (RPA) of prognostic factors in three radiation therapy oncology group (RTOG) brain metastases trials. *Int J Radiat Oncol Biol and Phys* 1997;37:745–751.

54. Cain JM. Practical aspects of hospice care at home. *Best Pract Res Clin Obstet Gynecol* 2001;15:305–311.

55. Marsden DE, Lickiss JN, Hacker NF. Gastrointestinal problems in patients with advanced gynecological malignancy. *Best Pract Res Clin Obstet Gynecol* 2001;15:253–263.

56. Farrell T, Wallace M, Hichs M. Long term results of transrenal occlusion with use of gianturco coils and gelatin sponge pledgets. *J Vasc and Interv Radiol* 1997;24:449–452.

57. Morita T, Akihiko. Successful endoscopic closure of radiation induced vesicovaginal fistula with fibrin glue and bovine collagen. *J Urol* 1999;162:1689–1690.

58. Carstens D. Palliative radiation therapy I female genital cancers. In: Vahrson HW, Brady LW, Heilmann HP, eds. *Radiation oncology of gynecological cancers*. New York: Springer, 1997:55–65.

59. Smith SC, Koh W. Palliative radiation therapy for gynecologic malignancies. *Best Pract Res Clin Obstet Gynecol* 2001;15:265–278.

60. Blitzer PH. Reanalysis of the RTOG study of the palliation of symptomatic osseous metastasis. *Cancer* 1985;55:1468–1472.

61. Fidler M. Incidence of fracture through metastasis in long bones. *Acta Orthop Scand* 1981;52:623–627.

62. Townsend PW, Smalley SR, Cozad SC, et al. Role of postoperative radiation therapy after stabilization of fractures caused by metastatic disease. *Int J Radiat Oncol Biol Phys* 1995;31:43–49.

63. McEwan AJ. Use of radionuclides for the palliation of bone metastases. *Semin Radiol Oncol* 2000;2:103–114.

64. Breitbart W. Identifying patients at risk for, and treatment of major psychiatric complications of cancer. *Support Care Cancer* 1995;3: 45–60.

65. Payne DK, Massie MJ. Anxiety in palliative care. In: Chochinov HM, Breitbart W, eds. *Handbook of psychiatry in palliative medicine*. Oxford, UK: University Press, 2000:63–74.

66. Williamson GM, Schulz R. Activity restriction mediates the association between pain and depressed affect: a study of younger and older adult cancer patients. *Psychol Aging* 1995;10:369–378.

67. Breitbart W, Bruera E, Chochinov HM, et al. Neuropsychiatric syndromes and psychological symptoms in patients with advanced cancer. *J Pain Symptom Manage* 1995;9:412–415.

68. Massie MJ, Holland JC. Depression and the cancer patient. *J Clin Psychiatry* 1990;51[Suppl]:12–17.

69. Shuster JL, Jones GR. Approach to the patient receiving palliative care. In: Stem TA, Herman JB, Slavin PL, eds. *The MGH guide to psychiatry in primary care*. New York: McGraw-Hill, 1998:147–165.

70. Swarte NB, van der Bom JG, van der Vaart CH, et al. Anxiety and depresssion in cancer patients prior to death. In: Swarte NB, ed. *Studies on euthanasia*. Academic Thesis, Utrecht University, 2003.

71. Hotopf M, Chidgey J, Addington-Hall J, et al. Depression in advanced disease: a systematic review Part I. Prevalence and case finding. *Palliat Med* 2002;16:81–97.

72. Fishbain DA, Cutler R, Rosomoff HL, Steele-Rosomoff R. Chronic pain associated depression: antecedent or consequence of chronic pain? A review. *Clin J Pain* 1997;13:116–137.

73. Randall F, Downie RS. *Palliative care ethics*. Oxford, UK: Oxford University Press, 1996.

74. Bascom PB, Tolle SW. Responding to requests for physician-assisted suicide: "These are uncharted waters for both of us . . .". *JAMA* 2002; 288(1):91–98.

75. Krishna G, Raffin TA. The dying thoracic patient. *Chest Surg Clin North Am* 1998;8:723–739.

76. Gordon M, Singer PA. Decisions and care at the end of life. *Lancet* 1995;346:163–166.

77. Van der Maas PJ, van der Wal G, Haverkate I, et al. Euthanasia, physician-assisted suicide, and other medical practices involving the end of life in The Netherlands, 1990–1995. *N Engl J Med* 1996;335: 1699–1705.

78. Emanuel EJ. Euthanasia. Historical, ethical and empiric perspectives. *Arch Intern Med* 1994;154:1890–1901.

79. Van den Akker B, Janssens RM, Ten Have HA. Euthanasia and international human rights law: prolegomena for an international debate. *Med Sci Law* 1997;37:289–295.

80. Ten Have HA, Welie JV. Euthanasia in The Netherlands. *Crit Care Clin* 1996;12:97–108.

81. van der Maas PJ, van Delden JJ, Pijnenborg L, Looman CW. Euthanasia and other medical decisions concerning the end of life. *Lancet* 1991;338:669–674.

82. Quill TE, Cassel CK, Meier DE. Care of the hopelessly ill. Proposed clinical criteria for physician-assisted suicide. *N Engl J Med.* 1992; 327:1380–1384.

83. Brock DW. Voluntary active euthanasia. Hastings Cent Rep Ref Type: Report, 10–22,1992.

84. Rachels J. *The end of life: euthanasia and morality.* New York: Oxford University Press; 1986.

85. Cassel CK, Meier DE. Morals and moralism in the debate over euthanasia and assisted suicide. *N Engl J Med* 1990;323:750–752.

86. Weir RF. The morality of physician-assisted suicide. *Law Med Health Care* 1992;20:116.

87. Angell M. Euthanasia. *New Engl J Med* 1988;319:1348–1350.

88. Brody H. Assisted death—a compassionate response to a medical failure. *N Engl J Med* 1992;327:1384–1388.

89. Delden JJM, Pijnenborg L and van der Maas PJ. The Remmelink study. Two years later. 23, 24–27. 1993. Hastings Cent Rep.

90. Block SD, Billings JA. Patient requests to hasten death. Evaluation and management in terminal care. *Arch Intern Med* 1994;154: 2039–2047.

91. Hendin H, Rutenfrans C, Zylicz Z. Physician-assisted suicide and euthanasia in The Netherlands. Lessons from the Dutch. *JAMA* 1997; 277:1720–1722.

92. Foley KM. Pain, physician-assisted suicide and euthanasia. *Pain Forum* 1995;4:163–178.

93. van der Wal G, Dillmann RJ. Euthanasia in The Netherlands. *BMJ* 1994;308:1346–1349.

94. Emanuel EJ, Fairclough DL, Daniels ER, Clarridge BR. Euthanasia and physician-assisted suicide: attitudes and experiences of oncology patients, oncologists and the public [Comments]. *Lancet* 1996;347: 1805–1810.

95. Swarte NB. *Psychosocial aspects of terminal cancer patients and their bereaved.* Academic Thesis, Utrecht University, 2003.

96. Legemaate J, Dillmann RJM. *Levensbeëindigend handelen door een arts: tussen norm en praktijk.* Stafleu Van Loghum, 1998.

97. Hilhorst HWA. Euthanasia in thinking and behaviour. In: Banck GA, et al., eds. *Gestalten van de dood [Statures of death]*. Baarn: Ambo, 1980:254–78.

98. Heintz AP. Euthanasia: can be part of good terminal care [Editorial]. *BMJ* 1994;308:1656.

99. Heintz AP. Euthanasia in gynaecological oncology [Editorial]. *Br J Obstet Gynaecol* 1992;99:941–943.

100. Heintz APM. Euthanasia: a personal experience in gynecologic oncology. *Int J Gynecol Cancer* 1995;5:71–75.

101. Swarte NB, van der Lee ML, van der Bom JG, et al. Effects of euthanasia on the bereaved family and friends: a cross sectional study.

102. Physician stress and burnout course. Texas Medical Association, 1999.

103. Penson RT, Dignan FC, Canellos GP, et al. Burnout: caring for the caregivers. *Oncologist* 2000;5:425–434.

104. Whippen D, Canellos GP. Burnout syndrome in the practice of oncology: results of a random survey of 1000 oncologists. *J Clin Oncol* 1991;9:1916–1920.

105. Halperin JD, Zabora JR, Brintzenhofe S. The emotional health of oncologists. *Oncol Issues* 1997;21:20–22.

106. Ramirez A, Graham J, Richards M, et al. Mental health of hospital consultants: the effects of stress and satisfaction at work. *Lancet* 1996; 347:724–728.

107. Ramirex A, Graham J, Richards M, et al. Burnout and psychiatric disorder among cancer clinicians. *Br J Cancer* 1995;71:1263–1269.

108. Creagan ET. Stress among medical oncologists: the phenomenon of burnout and a call to action. *Mayo Clin Proc* 1993;68:614–615.

APPENDIX

Source Information on International, National, and Grant-Making Organizations of Relevance to Gynecologic Oncology

Edward L. Trimble and Sergio Pecorelli

Gynecologic cancers affect women worldwide. The availability and reliability of cancer incidence data varies widely from country to country. The International Agency for Research on Cancer (1), a program of the United Nations, publishes a regular update on cancer incidence data (2).

In the United States, the National Cancer Institute (NCI), working with state and local cancer registries, tracks cancer incidence for 26% of the U.S. population through its Surveillance, Epidemiology, and End Results (SEER) (3) program. Both the NCI's SEER program and Centers for Disease Control (CDC) and Prevention's National Center for Health Statistics have made public-use electronic data files available via the Internet (4,5).

Breast cancer has been the most common cancer among women worldwide since 1975 followed by cervical cancer. In 2000, it has been estimated that 1,050,300 women were diagnosed with breast cancer and 470,000 women with cervical cancer (6). In the developed world, the incidence of cervical cancer has dropped dramatically over the last 50 years with the implementation of effective screening programs as well as the drop in parity. In developing countries, however, cervical cancer continues to be the second leading cause of cancer death.

For information on outcomes, we must rely on smaller in-depth studies, such as Surveillance, Epidemiology, and End Results (SEER) special studies, SEER-Medicare studies, regional surveys of care, and the grouped analyses of institutional outcomes in gynecologic cancer collated by the International Federation of Gynecology and Obstetrics (FIGO) (7).

Staging criteria for gynecologic cancers, excluding breast cancer, are established by FIGO (8). These criteria are updated periodically based on new data regarding prognosis for various subsets of patients. Staging for other malignancies, including breast cancer, is established by the American Joint Committee on Cancer and the International Union against Cancer (9,10).

In 2000, the European Commission Advisory Committee on Cancer Prevention issued a position paper on cancer screening, which included recommendations for cervical and breast cancer screening (11). Guidelines for cervical cancer screening in the developed world have been recently developed by the United States Preventive Services Task Force and the American Cancer Society (ACS) (12,13). The American Society of Colposcopy and Cervical Pathology (14) spearheaded the development of guidelines for the management of women with abnormal Papanicolaou (Pap) smears (15). The International Gynecologic Cancer Society (16) and FIGO have developed guidelines for the treatment of gynecologic malignancies. The International Atomic Energy Agency (17), a program of the United Nations, is working to develop guidelines for radiation therapy in the treatment of cervical cancer. In the United States, guidelines for treatment of gynecologic cancer have been published by the National Comprehensive Cancer Network (18), the Society of Gynecologic Oncologists (19), and the ACS. The NCI's Physician Data Query (PDQ) website maintains an evidence-based summary of published treatment reports for all stages of cancers (20). In addition, the Cochrane Collaboration Gynaecologic Group publishes meta-analyses of reported data in various gynecologic cancer settings (21).

E. L. Trimble: Department of Surgery, Cancer Therapy Evaluation Program, National Cancer Institute, Bethesda, Maryland 20892

S. Pecorelli: Department of Obstetrics and Gynecology, University of Brescia, Brescia, Italy

TABLE A.1. *Necessary elements for effective cervical cancer control programs*

1. Ongoing commitment of government and civil society to the goal of reducing the burden of cervical cancer.
2. Effective outreach to women at risk
3. Acceptable, inexpensive, sensitive, and specific screening modality
4. Immediate treatment of precancerous lesions
5. Timely referral of women with invasive cancers to treatment centers
6. Centers with expertise in the surgical management of cervical cancer
7. Centers with expertise in the management of cervical cancer with radiation and combined chemoradiation
8. Effective palliative care for women with advanced or recurrent cervical cancer

TABLE A.3. *Potential gaps in cancer care*

1. Patients with abnormal screening tests lost to follow-up or not referred for further evaluation
2. Incomplete evaluation of patients with abnormal screening tests or newly diagnosed cancer
3. Patients with newly diagnosed or recurrent cancer not referred to the appropriate cancer specialists
4. Cancer specialists with inadequate training for certain types and stages of cancer
5. Suboptimal coordination of multimodality care
6. Absent or inadequate health-care coverage for evaluation and treatment, HRQOL/survivorship issues, palliative and end of life care
7. Inadequate social and family support to ensure compliance with treatment recommendations
8. Lack of coordination between primary health care provider and cancer specialist of follow-up following treatment of cancer
9. Inadequate screening and intervention for HRQOL and survivorship issues
10. Inadequate palliative and end-of-life care

HRQOL, health-related quality of life.

The necessary elements for an effective cervical cancer control program are shown in Table A.1. In addition, the World Health Organization (WHO) has recently published a monograph on cancer prevention targeting the developing world (22).

Over the last 10 years, investigators have begun to study how best to maintain and enhance health-related quality of life (HRQOL) in patients with cancer. A partial list of validated HRQOL instruments that may be useful in gynecologic cancer studies is shown in Table A.2. The MAPI Research Institute also maintains a helpful database of HRQOL instruments and publications (23). A summary of some of the potential gaps in cancer care is shown in Table A.3.

In the United States, some of the larger databases that have been used for research into health-care delivery are listed in Table A.4. Potential funding sources for such research included both governmental and nongovernmental organizations (Table A.5).

SUPPORT FOR RESEARCH

Support for research may come from governments, nongovernmental organizations, such as foundations, professional societies, charities and advocacy groups, and from industry. The beginning investigator should explore all pos-

TABLE A.2. *Validated HRQOL instruments*

General
EORTC QLQ-C30-European Organization for Research and Treatment of Cancer Quality of Life Questionnaire
FACT-G-Functional Assessment of Cancer Therapy-General
Medical Outcomes Study 36-Item Short Form Health Survey (SF-36)
McGill Quality of Life Questionnaire
Quality of life index
Breast cancer
EORTC QLQ BR23- European Organization for Research and Treatment of Cancer Breast
Cancer-Specific Quality of Life Questionnaire
FACT-Breast
Gynecologic cancer
EORTC QLQ-OV 28- European Organization for Research and Treatment of Cancer Ovarian
Cancer-Specific Quality of Life Questionnaire
FACT-Ovarian Cancer
FACT-Cervical Cancer
FACT-Endometrial Cancer
Female sexuality
Groningen Sexual Arousability Score
McCoy Female Sexuality Questionnaire

HRQOL, health-related quality of life.

TABLE A.4. *Large United States databases for research into health-care delivery*

American College of Surgeons Commission on Cancer
National Cancer Data Base
    http://www.facs.org
Department of Health and Human Services (DHHS)
Center for Medicare and Medicaid Services
    http://www.cms.gov
    Medicare claims data
    Medicaid claims data
CDC National Breast and Cervical Cancer Early Detection Program (NBCCEDP)
    http://www.cdc.gov/nccdphp/bb_cancer/index.htm
Health Resources and Services Administration
    http://www..hrsa.gov/
National Center for Health Statistics
    http://www.cdc.gov/nchs/
    Behavior and Risk Factor Survey
    National Health and Nutrition Survey
    National Hospital Discharge Survey
    National Survey of Ambulatory Care
NCI Surveillance, Epidemiology, and End Results (SEER) Program
    http://www.seer.cancer.gov/

TABLE A.5. *Potential funding sources for research into health-care delivery*

Agency for Healthcare Research and Quality
   http://www.ahcpr.gov/
Center for Health Studies
   http://www.centerforhealthstudies.org
Center for Medicare and Medicaid Services
   http://www.cms.gov/
Health Canada
   http://www.hc-sc.gc.ca
Health Resources and Services Administration
   http://www.hrsa.gov/
Robert Wood Johnson Foundation
   http://www.rwjf.org

TABLE A.7. *Websites that offer advice on grantsmanship*

Albert Eisntein College of Medicine's "Faculty Grants Guide"
   http://www.aecomyu.edu/ogs/Guide/Guide.htm
NCI's Quick Guide for Grant Applications
   http://deainfo.nic.nih.gov/extra/extdocs/gntapp.htm
NIH Grants Review Criteria
   http://grants1.nih.gov/grants/peer/peer.htm
NIH Guide for Grants and Contracts
   http://grants1.nih.gov/grants/guide/index.html
Science Magazine's "Grants and Grant Writing"
   http://nextwave.sciencemag.org/cgi/content/full/1999/09/20/2

sible sources of support. Starter grants may be available at local hospitals and medical schools, whereas several professional societies and foundations have small grant programs for young investigators. Sources of larger grants include the National Institutes of Health (NIH) in the United States (24), Cancer Research U.K. in the United Kingdom (25), and the ACS. A list of private organizations that sponsor training and research grants applicable to gynecologic oncology is shown in Table A.6. Websites that offer advice on grantsmanship are shown in Table A.7. Biomedical grants from the NIH, NCI, CDC, Department of Defense (DOD), and the United Kingdom Medical Research Council are all coded uniformly using a Common Scientific Outline (CSO). In addition, the NCI, DOD, and the U.K. National Cancer Research Institute have developed an online database of current cancer research funded by the United States, United Kingdom, and private groups called the International Cancer Research Portfolio (26) and entered in an online database. Most biomedical grants from the U.S. federal government are summarized in a common database accessible via the Internet [Computer Retrieval of Information on Scientific Projects (CRISP) (27)].

TYPES OF INDIVIDUAL GRANTS

Grants can support additional training, specific research projects, and educational programs. Training can include

TABLE A.6. *Nonfederal sources of training and research support*

American Cancer Society
   http://www.cancer.org
American College of Obstetricians and Gynecologists
   http://www.acog.org
Avon Foundation
   http://www.avoncompany.com/women/avonfoundation/
Gynecologic and Obstetrical Society
   http://www.agosonline.org
Gynecologic Cancer Foundation
   http://www.wcn.org/gcf/
Robert Wood Johnson Foundation
   http://www.rwjf.org

both clinical and laboratory cancer research. In the United States, the largest single sponsor of grants is the NCI. A summary of NCI grant programs of interest to gynecologic oncology investigators is shown at the NCI website (http://ctep.cancer.gov/funding/surgon/awards/html#GYNECOLOGIC). NCI training grants are restricted to U.S. citizens, whereas NCI research grants are generally open to all investigators whether U.S. citizens or not.

SUPPORT FOR RESEARCH INFRASTRUCTURE

A number of major programs support the infrastructure for cancer research. In the United States, the NCI is the largest single sponsor of such programs. A list of the different grant mechanisms and programs supporting infrastructure for research is shown in Table A.8.

Outside the United States, support for cancer clinical trials infrastructure has been limited. Only a minority of the Clinical Trials Cooperative Groups that are members of the Gynecologic Cancer Intergroup, for example, receive substantial

TABLE A.8. *NIH and NCI programs supporting research infrastructure relevant to breast and gynecologic oncology*

Cancer Family Registries
   http://epi.grants.cancer.gov/CFR?
Clinical Trials Cooperative Groups
   http://www.nci.nih.gov/clinicaltrials/finding/cooperative-group-websites
Comprehensive Minority Biomedical Branch
   http://minorityopportunities.nci.nih.gov/index.html
Institutional Training Grants
   http://cancertraining.nci.nih.gov/
NCI Center for Bioinformation
   http://ncbi.cancer.gov/
NCI-designated Cancer Centers
   http://www3.cancer.gov/cancercenters/
National Center for Biotechnology Information
   http://ncbi.nlm.nih.gov
Specialized Programs of Research Excellence (SPORE)
   http://spores.nci.nih.gov/
Specimen and tumor banks
   http://www.cancerdiagnosis.nci.nih.gov/specimens/index.htm

TABLE A.9. *Clinical trials cooperative groups conducting research in breast and gynecologic cancer*

Breast cancer
   Eastern Cooperative Oncology Group (ECOG)
      http:ecog.dfci.harvard.edu
   European Organization for Research and Treatment of Cancer
      http://www.eortc.be/
   Cancer and Leukemia Group B (CALGB)
      http://www.calgb.org
   National Surgical Adjuvant Breast and Bowel Project (NSABP)
      http://www.nsabp.pitt.edu
   North Central Cancer Treatment Group (NCCTG)
      http://ncctg.mayo.edu
   Southwest Oncology Group (SWOG)
      http://www.swog.org
Breast and gynecologic cancer
   National Cancer Institute of Canada Clinical Trials Group
      (NCIC CTG)
      http://ctg.queensu.ca/
   Radiation Therapy Oncology Group (RTOG)
      http://www.rtog.org
Gynecologic cancer
   Arbeitgemeinschaft Gynaekologische Onkologie (AGO)
      http://www.ago-ovar.de
   Australia and New Zealand Gynecological Oncology Group
      (ANZGOG)
   European Organization for Research and Treatment of
      Cancer Gynecologic Cancer Cooperative Group
      (EORTC GCCG)
      http://www.eortc.be/home/GCG
   Grupo Espanol de Investigaction en Cancer de Ovario
      (GEICO)
   Group d'Investigateurs Nationaux pour l'Etude des
      Cancers Ovariens (GINECO)
      http://arcagy.nexenserves.com/tmro/index.htm
   Gynecologic Oncology Group (GOG)
      http://www.gog.org
   Japanese GOG (JGOG)
   Nordic Society of Gynecologic Oncology (NSGO)
      http://www.nsgo.org
   Scottish Gynaecologic Cancer Trials Group (SGCTG)
   United Kingdom Medical Research Council (MRC)
      http://www.mrc.ac.uk
Intergroup committees
   Breast Intergroup
   Gynecologic Cancer Intergroup
      http://ctep.cancer.gov/resources/gcig/index.html
   NIH intramural research

federal funding for their efforts (Table A.9). Of note, the All-Ireland Cancer Consortium and the British National Cancer Research Institute, both established since 2000, do support clinical trials networks in Ireland and the United Kingdom.

Clinical research is conducted at the NIH Clinical Center and the National Naval Medical Center. In general, only patients enrolled on research protocols may be treated at the NIH Clinical Center. Clinical areas of interest include chemotherapy for breast cancer, chemotherapy for advanced ovarian cancer, novel biologic approaches to cancer therapy, immunotherapy for cervical and ovarian cancer, and radiation for cervical cancer.

Young investigators may come to the NIH to work during high school and college, after college through medical school, and after residency. The programs through which investigators may work at the NIH may be reviewed at an NIH website (28). The Gynecologic Cancer Foundation (GCF) and the NCI have recently initiated a Scholar's Program to bring one or two young investigators to the NCI after fellowship training to help them start a research career. Additional information on training at the NCI in Bethesda is available at the NCI website (29).

Over the past 15 years, the fields of cancer research and

TABLE A.10. *Advocacy groups for cancer patients and families*

General
   American Cancer Society
      http://www.cancer.org
   Cancer BacUp
      http://www.cancerbacup.org.uk/
   CancerCare
      http://www.cancercare.org
   Gilda's Club
      http://www.glidasclub.org
   National Coalition of Cancer Survivors
      http://www.nccn.org
   The Wellness Community
      http://www.wellness-community.org
Gynecologic
   Donna (European breast cancer support)
      http://www.cancerworld.org/progetti/cancerworld/
      Europadonna/pagine/home/homefra meeudonna.html
   FORCE: Facing Our Risk of Cancer Empowered (for
      women at risk of breast and ovarian cancer)
      www.facingourrisk.org
   SHARE: Self-help for Women with Breast or Ovarian
   Cancer
      www.sharecancersupport.org
Breast
   Breast Cancer Action
      http://www.bcaction.org/
   National Breast Cancer Coalition
      http://www.natlbccc.org/bin/index.htm
   Susan G. Komen Breast Cancer Foundation
      http://www.komen.org/
   Y-Me
      http://www.y-me.org/
Ovarian
   CONVERSATIONS! The International Newsletter for
   Those Fighting Ovarian Cancer
      http://ovarian-news.com/
   National Ovarian Cancer Association
      http://www.ovariancanada.org
   National Ovarian Cancer Coalition
      http://www.ovarian.org
   Ovarian Cancer National Alliance
      http://ovariancancer.org/
Cervical
   Center for Cervical Health
      http://cervicalhealth.org
   National Cervical Cancer Coalition
      http://www.nccc-online.org

care have been strengthened by the development of many cancer advocacy groups. A variety of organizations, which have mobilized cancer survivors as well as relatives and friends of cancer patients, now play an active role in promoting cancer research, educating lay and medical audiences, and providing information to cancer patients and survivors. In the United States, organizations with a broad approach to cancer include the ACS, the National Coalition for Cancer Survivorship, and Cancer Care. In the United Kingdom, Cancer BacUp has a broad-based approach to cancer education. The Gynecologic Cancer Foundation, the ACS, and Cancer BacUp have extensive educational programs for women with breast and gynecologic cancer. Advocacy groups that focus on breast and gynecologic cancer may be found through various websites (Table A.10). Investigators should inform their cancer patients about resources available through these groups.

EDUCATIONAL MATERIALS

A variety of print and video materials as well as websites are now available for lay and patient audiences. The NIH, NCI, CDC, ACS, American College of Obstetricians and Gynecologists (ACOG), GCF, American College of Surgeons, and the American Society of Clinical Oncology (ASCO) have been particularly active in this regard. The National Library of Medicine's MEDLINE, which includes bibliographic databases both for the lay audience and for medical professionals, is also helpful (30). In addition, the

Cochrane Cancer Network maintains a database of all past and present controlled and randomized trials and systemic reviews (31). As mentioned above, the NCI also maintains the PDQ Cancer Information Summaries. Most PDQ screening, prevention, adult and pediatric treatment, genetics, complementary and alternative medicine, and supportive care summaries are available in patient versions. Additional educational material is also available from cancer advocacy and support groups. Information on available educational materials may be obtained from the various websites in Tables A.10 and A.11.

REFERENCES

1. IARC-http://www.iarc.fr/
2. Cancer Incidence in Five Continents-http://www.iarc.com.fr/ci5v8.htm
3. http:/www.seer.cancer.gov
4. (http://www.seer.cancer.gov/publicdata/).
5. http://www.cdc.gov/nchs
6. Parkin DM, Bray F, Ferlay J, et al. Estimating the world cancer burden: Globocan 2000. *Int J Cancer* 2001;94:153–156.
7. Pecorelli S, Benedet JL, Creasman WT, et al. FIGO Annual Report on the Results of Treatment in Gynaecologic Cancer: statement of results obtained in patients treated in 1990–1992, inclusive overall survival up to 1997. *J Epidemiol Biostat* 1998;3:1–168.
8. http://www.figo.org
9. http://www.cancerstaging.org/
10. http://www.uicc.org/
11. Patnick J. Review of recommendations on cervical cancer screening in the European Union. *Minerva Ginecol* 2003;55:293–295.
12. http://www.ahrq.gov/clnic/3rduspstf/cervcan.cervcanrr.htm
13. http://caonline.amcancersoc.org/cgi/content/short/52/6/342
14. http://www.asccp.org/
15. Wright TC Jr, Cosx JT, Massad LS, et al. 2001 Consensus Guidelines for the management of women with cervical cytological abnormalities. *JAMA* 2002;287:2120–2129.
16. http://www.igcs.org/
17. http://www.iaea.org.at/worldatom/
18. http://www.nccn.org/
19. http://www.sgo.org/
20. http://www.cancer.gov/ccancerinfo/pdq/
21. http://www.cochrane.org/cochrane/revabstr/GYNAECAAbstractIndex.htm
22. *Developing national cancer control programs.* Geneva: WHO, 2002.
23. http://www.mapi-research-inst.com
24. http://grants.nih.gov/grants/index.cfm
25. Cancer Research-UK-http://science.cancerresearchuk.org/fandm/?version=3
26. http://cancerportfolio.org
27. http://crisp.cit.nih.gov/
28. http://www.training.nih.gov/
29. http://cancer.gov/aboutnci/working/
30. http://www.nlm.nih.gov
31. Cochrane Cancer Network-http://canet.org/

TABLE A.11. *Information on available educational materials*

American Cancer Society
   http://www.cancer.org/docroot/LRN/LRN_0.asp?sitearea=
American College of Surgeons
   http://www.facs.org/public_info/ppserv.html
American Society of Clinical Oncology
   http://www.asco.org
Centers for Disease Control and Prevention
   http://www.cdc.gov/health/cancer.htm
National Cancer Institute
   http:www.nci.nih.gov/cancerinfo/
Women's Cancer Network (Gynecologic Cancer Foundation)
   http://www.wcn.org/

Subject Index

Page numbers followed by "f" denote figures and "t" denote tables

A

Abacavir, 1318t
ABC. *See* Abacavir
Abdomen
  infections of, 298
  surgical closure of, 322–323
Abdominopelvic radiation therapy, for
      ovarian cancer
  after chemotherapy, 960–961
  patient selection for, 956–957
  toxicity of, 955–956
ABH antigens, 1039
Abscess, intraabdominal, 298, 1180–1181
Absolute neutrophil count, 476
Absorbed dose, 402
ABX-EGF, 591
ACA-125, 136t, 147–148
Acantholytic squamous-cell carcinoma of
      vulva, 675–676
Acetaminophen
  cancer-related pain managed using,
      1223
  ovarian cancer prevention using, 192
  properties of, 1224t
Acetylsalicylic acid, 1224t
Acidosis
  metabolic, 292t, 293
  respiratory, 292t, 293
Acquired immunity, 124
Acquired immunodeficiency syndrome.
      See AIDS
ACT-D. *See* Dactinomycin
Actinomycin D. *See* Dactinomycin
Activating protein-1, 562–563
Activin, 163, 1029
Acute myelogenous leukemia, 1005, 1301
Acute nonlymphocytic leukemia, 523,
      1193–1194
Acute normovolemic hemodilution, 281
Acute pain
  definition of, 1217
  management of, 1220–1221
Acute promyelocytic leukemia, 1301
Acute quadriplegic myopathy syndrome,
      302
Acute renal failure, 275, 295
Acute respiratory distress syndrome, 287

Acute tubular necrosis, 295–296
Addiction, 1230
Adenocarcinoma
  breast cancer, 1119–1120
  cervical cancer. *See* Cervical cancer,
      adenocarcinoma
  clear-cell. *See* Clear-cell
      adenocarcinoma
  endometrioid
    of cervix, 754
    of vagina, 709
  mesonephric, 755
  microcystic endocervical, 755
  mucinous
    cervical cancer, 753–754
    endocervical variant, 753, 753f
    minimal deviation variant, 753, 754f
    vaginal cancer, 708–709
    well-differentiated villoglandular
        variant, 753–754, 754f
  papillary serous, 1038
  serous, 755, 755f
  skin appendage tumors, 678
Adenocarcinoma in situ
  cervical, 18–19, 647–648, 648f
  description of, 630
  incidence of, 18
Adenofibromas, serous, 907
Adenoid basal epithelioma, 756
Adenoid basal-cell carcinoma, 677
Adenoid cystic carcinoma, 756
Adenoma malignum, 235, 753, 1022
Adenomatoid tumors, 1044, 1044f
Adenosine triphosphate-binding cassette
      protein, 469
Adenosquamous carcinoma, 710,
      755–756
Adenoviruses, 61–62
Adnexal mass
  CA-125 for differential diagnosis of,
      159–160
  during pregnancy, 1290–1292
  ultrasound of, 250
Adnexectomy, 1293
Adoptive cellular therapy, 148
Adriamycin. *See* Doxorubicin
Adrucil. *See* 5-Fluorouracil

Adult-type granulosa-cell tumors
  characteristics of, 1012–1013, 1013f
  chemotherapy for, 1027–1028
  description of, 1012
  endocrine function of, 1012
  hormonal therapies for, 1028
  natural history of, 1013
  pathology of, 1012–1013, 1013f
  postoperative management of,
      1027–1028
  prognostic factors for, 1013–1014
  radiation therapy for, 1027
  recurrence of, 1027–1028
  serum markers, 1014
Advil. *See* Ibuprofen
Advocacy groups, 1364t
Afterloaded brachytherapy, 411, 413
Agenerase. *See* Amprenavir
AIDS. *See also* Human
        immunodeficiency virus
  carcinogenesis and, 62
  epidemiology of, 1313
  etiology of, 1313–1314
  history of, 1313
  prevalence of, 1313
Airway obstruction, 1349–1350
Airway pressure release ventilation, 286
AKT, 55, 77, 564, 593
AKT2, 77, 111t, 900
Albumin, 295t
Alcohol consumption
  ovarian cancer risks, 12
  uterine cancer risks, 7
Aleve. *See* Naproxen sodium
Alkalosis
  metabolic, 292t, 292–293
  respiratory, 292t, 293
Alkeran. *See* Melphalan
17-(Allylamino)-17-
        demethoxygeldanamycin, 597
Alopecia, 477, 520, 529
Alpha level, 213–214
Alpha particles, 379
Alpha-fetoprotein
  definition of, 162
  during pregnancy, 1293
  Sertoli-Leydig cell tumors and, 1021
  tumor production of, 162

1367